SCHRIER'S DISEASES OF THE KIDNEY

NINTH EDITION

SCHRIER'S DISEASES OF THE KIDNEY

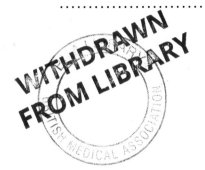

NINTH EDITION

VOLUME II

EDITED BY

THOMAS M. COFFMAN, MD
James R. Clapp Professor of Medicine
Chief, Division of Nephrology
Duke University and Durham VA Medical Centers
Durham, North Carolina
Program Director in Cardiovascular and Metabolic Disorders
Duke-NUS Graduate Medical School
Singapore

RONALD J. FALK, MD
Allen Brewster Distinguished Professor of Medicine
Director, UNC Kidney Center
Director, UNC Center for Transplant Care
Chief, Division of Nephrology and Hypertension
University of North Carolina
Chapel Hill, North Carolina

BRUCE A. MOLITORIS, MD
Professor of Medicine
Indiana University
Roudebush VA Medical Center
Indianapolis, Indiana

ERIC G. NEILSON, MD
Vice President for Medical Affairs
Lewis Landsberg Dean
Professor of Medicine and Cell and Molecular Biology
Feinberg School of Medicine
Northwestern University
Chicago, Illinois

ROBERT W. SCHRIER, MD, MACP, Honorary MRCP (UK)
Professor Emeritus
University of Colorado School of Medicine
Aurora, Colorado

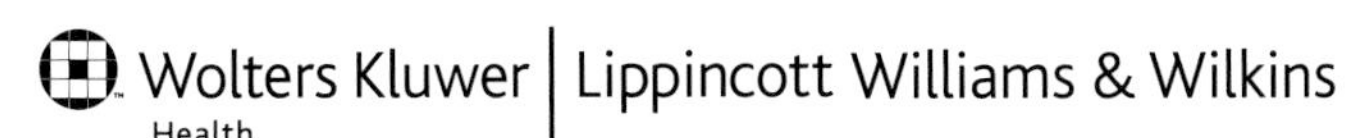

Philadelphia • Baltimore • New York • London
Buenos Aires • Hong Kong • Sydney • Tokyo

Acquisitions Editor: Julie Goolsby
Product Manager: Tom Gibbons
Vendor Manager: Alicia Jackson
Senior Manufacturing Manager: Benjamin Rivera
Marketing Manager: Kimberly Schonberger
Design Coordinator: Steve Druding
Production Service: Absolute Service, Inc.

Two Commerce Square
2001 Market Street
Philadelphia, PA 19103 USA
LWW.com

Printed in China

Library of Congress Cataloging-in-Publication Data
[978-1-4511-1075-3]
[1-4511-1075-8]
Schrier's diseases of the kidney. – 9th ed. / edited by Thomas M. Coffman
... [et al.].
p. ; cm.
Diseases of the kidney
Rev. ed. of: Diseases of the kidney & urinary tract. c2007.
Includes bibliographical references and index.
ISBN 978-1-4511-1075-3 (hardback : alk. paper) – ISBN 1-4511-1075-8
I. Coffman, Thomas M. II. Schrier, Robert W. III. Diseases of the kidney & urinary tract. IV. Title: Diseases of the kidney.
[DNLM: 1. Kidney Diseases. WJ 300]

616.6'1--dc23

2012024363

Care has been taken to confirm the accuracy of the information presented and to describe generally accepted practices. However, the authors, editors, and publisher are not responsible for errors or omissions or for any consequences from application of the information in this book and make no warranty, expressed or implied, with respect to the currency, completeness, or accuracy of the contents of the publication. Application of the information in a particular situation remains the professional responsibility of the practitioner.

The authors, editors, and publisher have exerted every effort to ensure that drug selection and dosage set forth in this text are in accordance with current recommendations and practice at the time of publication. However, in view of ongoing research, changes in government regulations, and the constant flow of information relating to drug therapy and drug reactions, the reader is urged to check the package insert for each drug for any change in indications and dosage and for added warnings and precautions. This is particularly important when the recommended agent is a new or infrequently employed drug.

Some drugs and medical devices presented in the publication have Food and Drug Administration (FDA) clearance for limited use in restricted research settings. It is the responsibility of the health care provider to ascertain the FDA status of each drug or device planned for use in their clinical practice.

To purchase additional copies of this book, call our customer service department at **(800) 638-3030** or fax orders to **(301) 223-2320.** International customers should call (301) 223-2300.

Visit Lippincott Williams & Wilkins on the Internet: at LWW.com. Lippincott Williams & Wilkins customer service representatives are available from 8:30 a.m. to 6:00 p.m., EST.

10 9 8 7 6 5 4 3 2 1

CCS0812

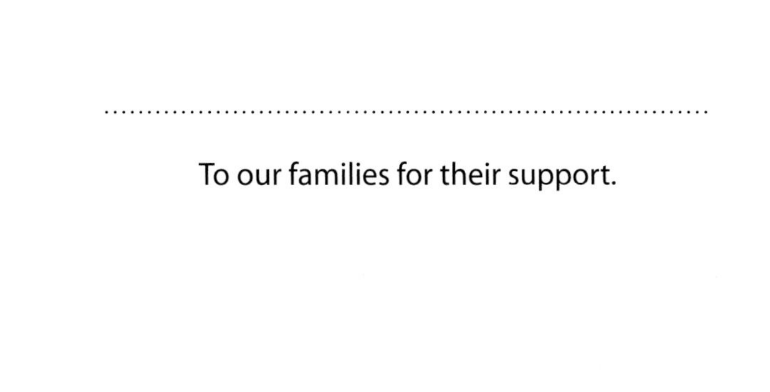

To our families for their support.

CONTENTS

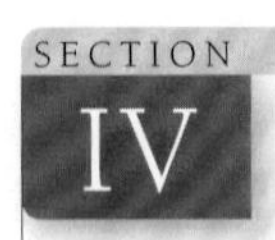

SECTION IV INFECTIONS OF THE URINARY TRACT AND THE KIDNEY 673

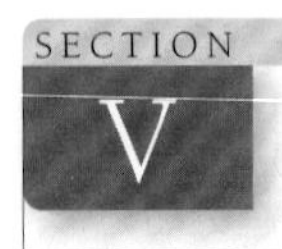

SECTION V ACUTE KIDNEY INJURY 785

*Deceased.

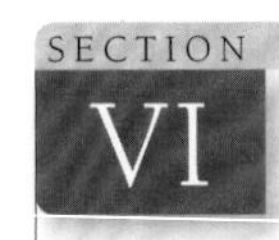

SECTION VI HYPERTENSION 1086

Volume II

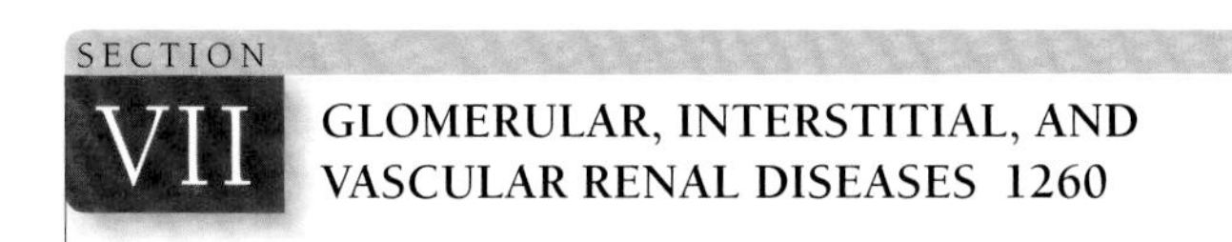

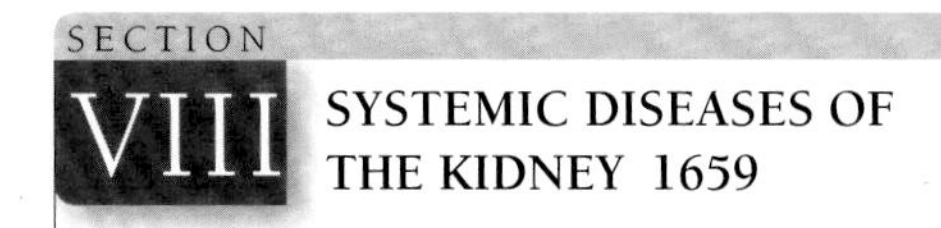

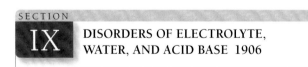

PREFACE

The recent advances in many aspects of kidney diseases have mandated a new edition of *Schrier's Diseases of the Kidney*. As in previous editions, a group of international experts was assembled to present this information in a comprehensive, authoritative, concise, and readily accessible fashion. The chapters have been extensively revised and updated.

Nephrology is a discipline that combines the basic and clinical sciences. Successful integration of this knowledge is the goal of this Ninth Edition. The 11 sections of the two-volume book are actually individual texts that can stand on their own.

The first section presents an overall view of the structural, physiologic, and biochemical aspects of the kidney. This section incorporates the latest developments in cellular and molecular biology, emphasizing the most current information and concepts on cell signaling, receptors, and ion channels. The subsequent 10 sections are disease oriented, with each section beginning with a pathophysiology chapter. The goal of *Schrier's Diseases of the Kidney* is to publish the most comprehensive material for practicing and academic physicians caring for patients with kidney disease and hypertension. The 11 sections of the book cover 86 chapters and are summarized as follows:

I **Structural and Functional Correlations in the Kidney** includes structural, hemodynamic, hormonal, ion transport, and metabolic functions in eight chapters.

II **Clinical Evaluation** is covered in five chapters on urinalysis, laboratory evaluation, urography, tomography, angiography, with indications and interpretations for renal biopsy.

III **Cystic and Tubular Disorders** in seven chapters covers genetic mechanisms, medullary cystic and sponge disorders, polycystic kidney disease, Alport syndrome, Fabry disease, and nail-patella syndrome, as well as isolated renal tubular disorders.

IV **Infections of the Urinary Tract and the Kidney** are contained in seven chapters, including host-defense mechanisms; urinary bacterial infections, including tuberculosis as well as fungal infections; renal abscesses; and cystitis.

V **Acute Kidney Injury** is described in 11 chapters, including the pathophysiology of renal cell ischemia and nephrotoxic injury, acute tubular necrosis, acute interstitial nephritis, and acute nephrotoxic renal disease.

VI **Hypertension** and its renal manifestations are covered in six chapters, which include pathophysiology, renal vascular, and endocrine-related hypertension as well as hypertension in pregnancy and in diabetes.

VII **Glomerular, Interstitial, and Vascular Renal Diseases** are discussed in 13 chapters, including collagen vascular diseases, chronic interstitial nephritis, primary glomerulonephritides, and vasculitides.

VIII **Systemic Diseases of the Kidney** are covered in eight chapters, including diabetes, hepatorenal syndrome, sickle cell disease, gout, myeloma/amyloidosis, and tropical diseases.

IX **Disorders of Electrolyte, Water, and Acid Base** are covered in nine chapters, including syndrome of inappropriate antidiuretic hormone secretion, central and nephrogenic diabetes insipidus, cardiac failure, cirrhosis, and the nephrotic syndrome.

X **Chronic Kidney Disease,** a section of six chapters, covers pathophysiology, anemia, osteodystrophy, the nervous system, cardiovascular complications, and metabolic and endocrine dysfunctions.

XI **Management of End-Stage Renal Disease** by transplantation, peritoneal dialysis and hemodialysis, including complications, outcomes, and ethical considerations, is discussed in six chapters.

As editors, we have substantial expertise in most of these areas of nephrology and are very pleased with the content of the Ninth Edition. Out of 86 chapters, 44 have new authors. We would like to thank our authoritative and remarkably talented contributing authors, whose dedication to nephrology is unmatched.

Thomas Coffman, MD
Ronald Falk, MD
Bruce Molitoris, MD
Eric Neilson, MD
Robert W. Schrier, MD

CONTRIBUTORS

William T. Abraham, MD, FACP, FACC, FAHA, FESC
Professor and Chair of Excellence in Cardiovascular Medicine
Ohio State University College of Medicine
Director, Division of Cardiovascular Medicine
Ohio State University Medical Center
Columbus, Ohio

Marcin Adamczak, MD, PhD
Assistant Professor
Department of Nephrology, Endocrinology and Metabolic Diseases
Medical University of Silesia
Katowice, Poland

Horacio J. Adrogué, MD
Professor of Medicine
Baylor College of Medicine
Chief of Nephrology
Methodist Hospital
Houston, Texas

Anupam Agarwal, MD
Professor of Medicine/Nephrology
Director, Division of Nephrology
University of Alabama at Birmingham
Birmingham, Alabama

Rajiv Agarwal, MD
Professor of Medicine
Indiana University School of Medicine
Indianapolis, Indiana

Rannar Airik, PhD
Postdoctoral Research Fellow in Pediatrics
University of Michigan
Ann Arbor, Michigan

Charles E. Alpers, MD
Professor of Pathology and Adjunct Professor of Medicine
University of Washington
Vice Chair, Department of Pathology
University of Washington Medical Center
Seattle, Washington

Sharon Anderson, MD
Professor of Medicine
Oregon Health and Science University
Chief, Division of Hospital and Specialty Medicine
Portland VA Medical Center
Portland, Oregon

William J. Arendshorst, PhD
Professor of Cell and Molecular Physiology
School of Medicine
University of North Carolina at Chapel Hill
UNC Kidney Center
Chapel Hill, North Carolina

Pierre Aucouturier, PhD, Professor
Director
Immune System and Conformation Diseases
UPMC/INSERM, UMRS 938
Director, Immunology Department
Groupe Hospitalier HUEP
Paris, France

Howard A. Austin III, MD
Adjunct Professor of Medicine
Uniformed Services University
Senior Clinical Investigator
National Institute of Diabetes and Digestive and Kidney Diseases
National Institutes of Health
Bethesda, Maryland

Kamal F. Badr, MD, ASCI, AAP
Professor of Medicine (Nephrology and Hypertension)
Associate Chair for Medical Education
American University of Beirut
Attending Physician (Nephrology and Hypertension)
American University of Beirut Hospital
Beirut, Lebanon

Kyongtae T. Bae, MD, PhD
Professor and Chairman of Radiology
University of Pittsburgh
University of Pittsburgh Medical Center
Pittsburgh, Pennsylvania

Sola Aoun Bahous, MD, PhD
Assistant Professor of Internal Medicine
Lebanese American University
Byblos, Lebanon
Assistant Professor of Internal Medicine
University Medical Center-Rizk Hospital
Beirut, Lebanon

James E. Balow, MD
Professor of Medicine
Uniformed Services University of the Health Sciences
Clinical Director, National Institute of Diabetes and Digestive and Kidney Diseases
Chief, Kidney Disease Section
National Institutes of Health
Bethesda, Maryland

Rashad S. Barsoum, MD, FRCP, FRCPE
Emeritus Professor of Internal Medicine
Cairo University
Chairman
The Cairo Kidney Center
Cairo, Egypt

George P. Bayliss, MD
Assistant Professor of Medicine
Warren Alpert Medical School of Brown University
Nephrologist, Division of Kidney Diseases and Hypertension
Rhode Island Hospital and The Miriam Hospital
Providence, Rhode Island

Anne M. Beck, MD
Professor of Pediatrics
Washington University
Pediatric Nephrologist
St. Louis Children's Hospital
St. Louis, Missouri

Laurence Beck, Jr., MD, PhD
Assistant Professor of Medicine
Boston University School of Medicine
Boston Medical Center
Boston, Massachusetts

Justin M. Belcher, MD
Clinical Research Fellow in Internal Medicine
Nephrology Section
Yale University
New Haven, Connecticut

William M. Bennett, MD
Professor of Medicine (Retired)
Oregon Health and Sciences University
Medical Director, Renal Transplant
Legacy Health System
Portland, Oregon

Daniel G. Bichet, MD
Professor of Medicine and Physiology
University of Montreal
Hôpital du Sacré-Couer de Montréal
Montreal, Canada

Scott D. Bieber, DO
Assistant Professor of Medicine
Nephrology Division
University of Washington
Seattle, Washington

Daniel J. Birmingham, PhD
Associate Professor of Internal Medicine
Division of Nephrology
Ohio State University
Columbus, Ohio

Annelie Brauner, MD, PhD
Professor of Microbiology, Tumor, and Cell Biology
Karolinska Institutet
Senior Consultant, Clinical Microbiology
Karolinska University Hospital
Stockholm, Sweden

Emmanuel L. Bravo, MD
Consultant
Department of Nephrology and Hypertension
Cleveland Clinic
Cleveland, Ohio

Frank Bridoux, MD
Professor of Nephrology
University of Poitiers
University Hospital Poitiers
Poitiers, France

Godela M. Brosnahan, MD
Associate Professor of Medicine
Division of Renal Diseases and Hypertension
University of Colorado Denver
Faculty
University of Colorado Hospital
Aurora, Colorado

Ruth Ellen Bulger, AM, PhD
Emeritus Professor of Anatomy, Physiology, and Genetics
Uniformed Services University of the Health Sciences
Bethesda, Maryland

Emmanuel A. Burdmann, MD, PhD
Associate Professor of Nephrology
University of São Paulo Medical School
São Paulo, Brazil

John M. Burkart, MD
Professor of Nephrology
Wake Forest Baptist Medical Center
Winston-Salem, North Carolina

Andrés Cárdenas, MD, MMSc, AGAF
Senior Specialist
GI Unit, Institute of Digestive Diseases and Metabolism
Hospital Clinic
Barcelona, Spain

Ivan P. Casserly, MB BCh
Assistant Professor of Cardiology
University of Colorado School of Medicine
Interventional Cardiologist, Cardiac and Vascular Center
University of Colorado Hospital
Aurora, Colorado

Neziha Celebi, MD
Resident in Pediatrics
PGY-1, Department of Pediatrics
Nassau University Medical Center
East Meadow, New York

Joumana T. Chaiban, MD
Medical Director
Joslin Diabetes Center at St. Vincent Charity Medical Center
Division Chief, Endocrinology and Metabolic Diseases
St. Vincent Charity Medical Center
Cleveland, Ohio

Laurence Chan, MD, PhD, FACP, RFCP, FHKCP (Hon)
Professor of Medicine
Division of Renal Diseases and Hypertension
University of Colorado Denver
Denver, Colorado
Director, Renal Transplant Fellowship Program and Transplant Nephrology Research
University of Colorado Hospital, Anschutz Medical Campus
Aurora, Colorado

Arlene B. Chapman, MD
Professor of Medicine
Assistant Fellowship Program Director
Renal Division
Emory University School of Medicine
Coprincipal Investigator, Atlanta Clinical and Translational Science Institute
Program Director, Clinical Interactions Network
Atlanta, Georgia

Ferdinand X. Choong, MD
Doctoral Student/Postgraduate Student
Department of Neuroscience
Karolinska Institutet
Stockholm, Sweden

Milan Chromek, MD, PhD
Researcher, Division of Pediatrics
Department of Clinical Science, Intervention and Technology
Karolinska Institutet
Pediatrician
Astrid Lindgren Children's Hospital
Karolinska University Hospital
Stockholm, Sweden

James E. Cooper, MD
Assistant Professor of Medicine
University of Colorado
Physician Affiliate
University of Colorado Hospital
Aurora, Colorado

William G. Couser, MD
Affiliate Professor of Medicine
University of Washington
Seattle, Washington

Byron P. Croker, MD, PhD
Professor of Pathology, Immunology and Laboratory Medicine
University of Florida
Chief, Department of Pathology and Laboratory Medicine Service
North Florida/South Georgia Veterans Health System
Gainesville, Florida

Brian S. Cummings, PhD
Associate Professor of Pharmaceutical and Biomedical Sciences
University of Georgia
Athens, Georgia

Marc E. De Broe, MD, PhD
Emeritus Professor of Medicine
University of Antwerp
Antwerp, Belgium

Jeroen K. J. Deegens, MD, PhD
Assistant Professor of Nephrology
Radboud University Nijmegen Medical Center
Nijmegen, The Netherlands

Louise M. Dembry, MD, MS, MBA
Professor of Medicine, Infectious Diseases and Epidemiology
Yale University School of Medicine
Hospital Epidemiologist and Codirector, Quality Improvement Support Services
Yale-New Haven Hospital
New Haven, Connecticut

Vimal K. Derebail, MD, MPH
Assistant Professor of Medicine
Division of Nephrology and Hypertension
University of North Carolina at Chapel Hill
Chapel Hill, North Carolina

Thomas D. DuBose, Jr., MD
Tinsley R. Harrison Professor and Chair of Internal Medicine
Wake Forest University School of Medicine
Wake Forest University Baptist Medical Center
Winston-Salem, North Carolina

Lance D. Dworkin, MD
Professor and Vice Chair of Medicine
Warren Alpert Medical School of Brown University
Director, Division of Kidney Disease and Hypertension
Rhode Island Hospital and The Miriam Hospital
Providence, Rhode Island

Jamie P. Dwyer, MD
Assistant Professor of Medicine
Division of Nephrology and Hypertension
Vanderbilt University School of Medicine
Nephrology Clinical Trials Center
Vanderbilt University Medical Center
Nashville, Tennessee

Allison A. Eddy, MD
Professor and Head, Pediatrics Department
University of British Columbia
Chief of Pediatrics
B.C. Children's Hospital
Vancouver, Canada

Charles L. Edelstein, MD, PhD, FAHA
Professor of Medicine
Division of Renal Diseases
University of Colorado Denver
University of Colorado Hospital
Aurora, Colorado

Garabed Eknoyan, MD
Professor of Medicine
Baylor College of Medicine
Houston, Texas

David H. Ellison, MD, FASN
Professor of Medicine
Oregon Health and Science University
Portland, Oregon

Ronald J. Falk, MD
Allen Brewster Distinguished Professor of Medicine
Director, UNC Kidney Center
Director, UNC Center for Transplant Care
Chief, Division of Nephrology and Hypertension
University of North Carolina
Chapel Hill, North Carolina

Tarek Fayad, MD
Assistant Professor of Internal Medicine
Cairo University
Consultant Nephrologist
Cairo University Hospitals and the Cairo Kidney Center
Cairo, Egypt

Andrew Fenves, MD
Clinical Professor of Medicine
UT Southwestern Medical School
Director, Nephrology Division
Baylor University Medical Center
Dallas, Texas

Gal Finer, MD, PhD
Assistant Professor
Northwestern University
Attending, Division of Pediatric Kidney Disease
Children's Memorial Hospital
Chicago, Illinois

Seth Furgeson, MD
Senior Instructor in Medicine
University of Colorado Denver
Physician
University of Colorado Hospital
Aurora, Colorado

Surafel F. Gebreselassie, MD
Associate Staff
Nephrology and Hypertension Department
Glickman Urological and Kidney Institute
Staff Physician
Cleveland Clinic
Cleveland, Ohio

Eric M. George, PhD
Instructor in Physiology and Biophysics
University of Mississippi Medical Center
Jackson, Mississippi

Gregory G. Germino, MD
Deputy Director
National Institute of Diabetes and Digestive and Kidney Disease
National Institutes of Health
Bethesda, Maryland
Adjunct Professor of Internal Medicine
Johns Hopkins University School of Medicine
Baltimore, Maryland

Pere Ginès, MD, PhD
Full Professor
University of Barcelona Medical School
Chairman, Liver Unit
Hospital Clinic
Barcelona, Spain

Amanda K. Goode, MA
Research Programs Development Manager
Department of Internal Medicine
Wake Forest School of Medicine
Winston-Salem, North Carolina

Elvira O. Gosmanova, MD, FASN
Assistant Professor of Medicine
Division of Nephrology
University of Tennessee Health Science Center
Staff Nephrologist
Methodist University Hospital
Memphis, Tennessee

Joey P. Granger, PhD
Professor of Physiology and Medicine
Director of Cardiovascular Renal Research Center
University of Mississippi Medical Center
Jackson, Mississippi

Martin Gregory, BM BCh, DPhil
Professor of Medicine
University of Utah Health Sciences Center
Clinical Chief, Nephrology Division
University of Utah Hospital
Salt Lake City, Utah

Rajan Gupta

Kenneth R. Hallows, MD, PhD, FASN
Associate Professor of Medicine and of Cell Biology
Renal-Electrolyte Division
University of Pittsburgh School of Medicine
Pittsburgh, Pennsylvania

Choli Hartono, MD
Assistant Professor of Clinical Medicine
Department of Transplantation Medicine and Extracorporeal Therapy
Division of Nephrology and Hypertension
Weill Cornell Medical College
New York Presbyterian Hospital
New York, New York

Erum Hartung, MD
Attending Physician
Department of Pediatrics
Children's Hospital of Philadelphia
Philadelphia, Pennsylvania

Imed Halal, MD
Postdoctoral Fellow in Medicine
University of Colorado Denver
Aurora, Colorado

Friedhelm Hildebrandt, MD
Professor of Pediatrics and of Human Genetics
University of Michigan
Ann Arbor, Michigan
Investigator
Howard Hughes Medical Institute
Chevy Chase, Maryland

Jonathan Himmelfarb, MD
Joseph W. Eschbach Endowed Chair in Kidney Research
Professor of Medicine
Director, Kidney Research Institute
University of Washington
Seattle, Washington

Michelle A. Hladunewich, MD, BSc, MSc, FRCP(C)
Assistant Professor of Medicine
University of Toronto
Director, Divisions of Nephrology and Obstetric Medicine
Sunnybrook Health Sciences Centre
Toronto, Canada

Ewout J. Hoorn, MD, PhD
Renal Fellow
Department of Internal Medicine-Nephrology
Erasmus Medical Center
Rotterdam, The Netherlands

Keith A. Hruska, MD
Professor of Pediatrics, Medicine, and Cell Biology/Physiology
Washington University School of Medicine
Director, Pediatric Nephrology
St. Louis Children's Hospital
St. Louis, Missouri

Lesley A. Inker, MD, MS
Associate Professor of Medicine
Tufts University
Attending, Department of Medicine
Tufts Medical Center
Boston, Massachusetts

J. Ashley Jefferson, MD, FRCP
Associate Professor of Nephrology
University of Washington
Seattle, Washington

J. Charles Jennette, MD
Brinkhouse Distinguished Professor and Chair
Department of Pathology and Laboratory Medicine
University of North Carolina at Chapel Hill
UNC Hospitals
Chapel Hill, North Carolina

Richard Johnson, MD
Professor of Medicine
Division of Nephrology
University of Colorado
Aurora, Colorado

Bruce A. Julian, MD
Professor of Medicine, Surgery, and Microbiology
University of Alabama at Birmingham
Attending Physician, Medicine and Surgery
University of Alabama Hospital
Birmingham, Alabama

Mehmet Kanbay, MD
Assistant Professor of Medicine
Division of Nephrology
Kayseri Training and Research Hospital
Kayseri, Turkey

Duk-Hee Kang, MD
Professor of Medicine
Division of Nephrology
Ewha Medical Research Center
Seoul, South Korea

Carol A. Kauffman, MD
Professor of Internal Medicine
University of Michigan
Chief, Infectious Diseases Section
Veterans Affairs Ann Arbor Healthcare System
Ann Arbor, Michigan

Maya Khairallah, MD
Assistant Professor of Medicine
Lebanese American University
Byblos, Lebanon

Edward D. Kim, MD
Professor of Surgery
Division of Urology
University of Tennessee Graduate School of Medicine
Knoxville, Tennessee

Radko Komers, MD, PhD
Assistant Professor of Medicine
Division of Nephrology and Hypertension
Oregon Health and Science University
Portland, Oregon

Jeffrey B. Kopp, MD
Adjunct Professor of Medicine
Uniformed Services University
Staff Clinician, Kidney Disease Section
NIH Clinical Center, National Institute of Diabetes and Digestive and Kidney Diseases
Bethesda, Maryland

Joel D. Kopple, MD
Professor of Medicine and Public Health
David Geffen School of Medicine at UCLA
Fielding UCLA School of Public Health Medicine
University of California, Los Angeles
Los Angeles, California
Division of Nephrology and Hypertension
Los Angeles Biomedical Research Institute at Harbor-UCLA Medical Center
Torrance, California

Sonal Krishnan, MD
Instructor in Radiology
University of Pittsburgh
University of Pittsburgh Medical Center
Pittsburgh, Pennsylvania

Wilhelm Kriz, MD
Professor Emeritus
Department of Anatomy and Cell Biology
University of Heidelberg
Heidelberg, Germany

Abhijit V. Kshirsagar, MD, MPH
Associate Professor of Medicine
Division of Nephrology and Hypertension
University of North Carolina
Chapel Hill, North Carolina

Warren Kupin, MD, FACP
Professor of Medicine
Division of Nephrology and Hypertension
University of Miami Miller School of Medicine
Associate Director, Transplant Nephrology
Jackson Memorial Hospital
Miami, Florida

Richard A. Lafayette, MD, FACP
Associate Professor of Nephrology
Stanford University
Director, Glomerular Disease Center
Stanford University Medical Center
Stanford, California

Craig B. Langman, MD
The Isaac A. Abt, MD, Professor of Kidney Diseases
Professor of Pediatrics
Feinberg School of Medicine, Northwestern University
Head, Kidney Diseases
Children's Memorial Hospital
Chicago, Illinois

Andrew S. Levey, MD
Dr. Gerald J. and Dorothy R. Friedman Professor of Medicine
Tufts University School of Medicine
Chief, William B. Schwartz Division of Nephrology
Tufts Medical Center
Boston, Massachusetts

Moshe Levi, MD
Professor and Vice Chair for Research
Departments of Medicine, Physiology, and Biophysics
University of Colorado
Denver, Colorado

Julia B. Lewis, MD
Professor of Medicine
Division of Nephrology
Vanderbilt University Medical Center
Nashville, Tennessee

Yeong-Hau Howard Lien, MD, PhD
Professor Emeritus of Medicine
University of Arizona
Nephrology Staff
University Medical Center
Tucson, Arizona

Stuart L. Linas, MD
Professor of Medicine
University of Colorado Denver
Aurora, Colorado
Chief, Division of Nephrology
Denver Health
Denver, Colorado

Valerie A. Luyckx, MB BCh
Associate Professor of Medicine
University of Alberta
Associate Professor, Division of Nephrology
University of Alberta Hospital
Edmonton, Canada

Etienne Macedo, MD, PhD
Associate Professor of Medicine
University of São Paulo
São Paulo, Brazil

Michael P. Madaio, MD
Professor and Chairman
Department of Medicine
Georgia Health Sciences University
Augusta, Georgia

Nicolaos E. Madias, MD
Maurice S. Segal, MD, Professor of Medicine
Tufts University School of Medicine
Chairman, Department of Medicine
St. Elizabeth's Medical Center
Boston, Massachusetts

Sreedhar A. Mandayam, MD
Associate Professor of Medicine
Division of Nephrology
Baylor College of Medicine
Houston, Texas

Julieanne G. McGregor, MD
Assistant Professor of Internal Medicine
University of North Carolina
Chapel Hill, North Carolina

Rajnish Mehrotra, MD
Professor of Medicine
David Geffen School of Medicine at UCLA
Los Angeles, California
Associate Chief, Division of Nephrology and Hypertension
Harbor-UCLA Medical Center
Torrance, California

Ravindra L. Mehta, MBBS, MD, DM, FACP, FRCP
Professor of Clinical Medicine
University of California San Diego
Vice Chair for Clinical Research
University of California San Diego Medical Center
San Diego, California

Keira Melican, PhD
Postdoctoral Fellow
Paris Cardiovascular Research Center
INSERM U970
Paris, France

Timothy W. Meyer, MD
Professor of Medicine
Stanford University
VA Palo Alto Health Care System
Palo Alto, California

Dennis J. Mikolich, MD*
Clinical Associate Professor of Medicine
Warren Alpert Medical School of Brown University
Chief, Division of Infectious Diseases
Veterans Affairs Medical Center
Providence, Rhode Island

William E. Mitch, MD
Gordon A. Cain Chair in Nephrology
Baylor College of Medicine
Houston, Texas

David B. Mount, MD, FRCPC
Assistant Professor of Medicine
Harvard Medical School
Physician, Renal Divisions
VA Boston Healthcare System
Brigham and Women's Hospital
Boston, Massachusetts

Thomas F. Mueller, MD
Associate Professor of Medicine
University of Alberta
University Hospital, Division of Nephrology
Edmonton, Canada

Laura L. Mulloy, DO
Professor of Medicine
Georgia Health Sciences University
Section Chief of Nephrology
Georgia Health Sciences Health System
Augusta, Georgia

Sean W. Murphy, MD, FRCPC
Associate Professor of Medicine
Memorial University of Newfoundland
Staff Nephrologist
Health Sciences Center
Newfoundland, Canada

Patrick H. Nachman, MD
Professor of Medicine
University of North Carolina
UNC Kidney Center
Chapel Hill, North Carolina

Tibor Nadasdy, MD
Professor of Pathology
Ohio State University
Director of Renal and Transplant Pathology
Wexner Medical Center at Ohio State University
Columbus, Ohio

Neha D. Nanda, MD
Assistant Professor of Medicine
Department of Internal Medicine, Section of Infectious Diseases
Yale University School of Medicine
New Haven, Connecticut

L. Gabriel Navar, PhD
Professor and Chair of Physiology
Tulane University
New Orleans, Louisiana

Lindsay E. Nicollé, MD, FRCPC
Professor of Medical Microbiology
University of Manitoba
Consultant, Infectious Diseases
Health Sciences Centre
Winnipeg, Canada

Yumi Noda, MD, PhD
Associate Professor of Nephrology and Chronic Kidney Disease
Tokyo Medical and Dental University
Tokyo, Japan

Charles R. Nolan, MD
Professor of Medicine and Surgery
University of Texas Health Sciences Center
Medical Director, Kidney Transplantation
University Hospital
San Antonio, Texas

Marina Noris, PhD
Head
Laboratory of Immunology and Genetics of Transplantation and Rare Diseases
Clinical Research Center for Rare Disease
"Aldo e Cele Daccò" Mario Negri Institute for Pharmacological Research
Bergamo, Italy

James E. Novak, MD, PhD
Assistant Professor of Medicine
Wayne State University
Associate Director, Nephrology Training Program
Medical Director, Home Dialysis
Henry Ford Health System
Detroit, Michigan

Jan Novak, PhD
Associate Professor of Microbiology
University of Alabama at Birmingham
Birmingham, Alabama

*Deceased

John W. O'Bell, MD
Assistant Professor of Medicine
Warren Alpert Medical School of Brown University
Nephrologist, Division of Kidney Disease and Hypertension
Rhode Island Hospital and The Miriam Hospital
Providence, Rhode Island

Ayodele Odutayo, BHSc, MD(C)
Medical Student
Department of Medicine
University of Toronto
Research Assistant, Nephrology Department
Sunnybrook Health Sciences Centre
Toronto, Canada

Ali J. Olyaei, PharmD
Professor of Nephrology and Hypertension
Oregon State University
Oregon Health and Science University Hospital
Portland, Oregon

William Charles O'Neill, MD
Professor of Medicine
Renal Division
Emory University School of Medicine
Atlanta, Georgia

Paul M. Palevsky, MD
Professor of Medicine
Renal-Electrolyte Division
University of Pittsburgh School of Medicine
Chief, Renal Section
VA Pittsburgh Healthcare System
Pittsburgh, Pennsylvania

Miguel F. Palma-Diaz, MD
Assistant Professor of Pathology and Laboratory Medicine
University of California, Los Angeles
Department of Pathology and Laboratory Medicine
David Geffen School of Medicine at UCLA
Los Angeles, California

Biff F. Palmer, MD
Professor of Internal Medicine
Division of Nephrology
University of Texas Southwestern Medical Center
Dallas, Texas

Patrick S. Parfrey, MD
University Research Professor in Medicine
Memorial University of Newfoundland
Staff Nephrologist
Eastern Health
Newfoundland, Canada

Chirag R. Parikh, MD, PhD
Associate Professor of Internal Medicine
Nephrology Section
Yale University
New Haven, Connecticut

Mark S. Pasternack, MD
Associate Professor of Pediatrics
Harvard Medical School
Chief, Pediatric Infectious Disease Unit
Physician, Infectious Disease Division
Massachusetts General Hospital
Boston, Massachusetts

Núria M. Pastor-Solar, MD
Assistant Professor of Medicine and of Cell Biology
Renal-Electrolyte Division
University of Pittsburgh School of Medicine
Pittsburgh, Pennsylvania

Mark A. Perazella, MD
Professor of Medicine
Section of Nephrology/Internal Medicine
Yale University School of Medicine
Director, Acute Dialysis Program
Yale-New Haven Hospital
New Haven, Connecticut

Alex Perino

Ryan B. Pickens, MD
PGY-5 Urology Resident
University of Tennessee Graduate School of Medicine
Knoxville, Tennessee

Kearkiat Praditpornsilpa, MD
Associate Professor of Medicine
Chulalongkorn University
King Chulalongkorn Memorial Hospital
Bangkok, Thailand

Darryl L. Quarles, MD
Professor and Chief
Division of Nephrology
University of Tennessee Health Science Center
Staff Nephrologist
Methodist University Hospital
Memphis, Tennessee

Muhammed A. Rafey, MD, MS, FASH
DNB Faculty
Consultant, Nephrology and Hypertension
Nephrology Department
Apollo Hospitals Hyderabad
Hyderabad, India

Rajeev Raghavan, MD
Assistant Professor of Medicine
Department of Nephrology
Baylor College of Medicine
Houston, Texas

Frederic Rahbari-Oskoui, MD, MS
Assistant Professor of Medicine
Department of Medicine-Renal Division
Emory University School of Medicine
Atlanta, Georgia

Asghar Rastegar, MD
Professor of Medicine
Nephrology Section
Yale University School of Medicine
Chief, Fitkin Firm
Yale-New Haven Hospital
New Haven, Connecticut

Berenice Y. Reed, PhD
Associate Professor of Medicine
University of Colorado Denver
Aurora, Colorado

W. Brian Reeves, MD
Professor of Medicine
Penn State University College of Medicine
Chief of Nephrology
Penn State Hershey Medical Center
Hershey, Pennsylvania

Giuseppe Remuzzi, MD
Director
Negri Bergamo Laboratories
Mario Negri Institute for Pharmacological Research
Director, Department of Immunology and Clinical Transplantation
Azienda Ospedaliera Ospedali Riunti di Bergamo
Bergamo, Italy

Agneta Richter-Dahlfors, PhD
Professor
Swedish Medical Nanoscience Center
Karolinska Institutet
Stockholm, Sweden

Professor Dr. Eberhard Ritz
Emeritus Professor of Nephrology
Ruperto Carola University
Heidelberg, Germany

Pierre Ronco, MD, PhD
Head
Inserm UMRS 702
UPMC University (Paris 6)
Chief, Nephrology and Dialysis
Tenon Hospital
Paris, France

Brad H. Rovin, MD
Professor of Medicine and Pathology
Nephrology Division
Ohio State University
Vice Chair for Research, Department of Internal Medicine
Ohio State University Hospitals
Columbus, Ohio

Robert H. Rubin, MD
Osborne Professor of Health Sciences and Technology
Professor of Medicine
Harvard Medical School
Director, Center for Experimental Pharmacology and Therapeutics
Massachusetts Institute of Technology
Associate Director, Division of Infectious Disease
Brigham and Women's Hospital
Boston, Massachusetts

Piero Ruggenenti, MD
Chief
Department of Renal Medicine
Mario Negri Institute for Pharmacological Research
Associate Professor of Immunology and Clinical Transplantation
Azienda Ospedaliera Ospedali Riuniti di Bergamo
Bergamo, Italy

David Salant, MD
Professor of Medicine
Boston University School of Medicine
Chief, Renal Section
Boston Medical Center
Boston, Massachusetts

Sei Sakaki, MD, PhD
Professor of Nephrology
Tokyo Medical and Dental University
Tokyo, Japan

Ramesh Saxena, MD
Professor of Internal Medicine
Nephrology Division
UT Southwestern Medical Center
Dallas, Texas

John A. Sayer, MD, PhD
Senior Clinical Lecturer in Nephrology
Institute of Genetic Medicine
Newcastle University
Consultant Nephrologist, Renal Services
Newcastle upon Tyne NHS Foundation Trust
Newcastle upon Tyne, United Kingdom

H. William Schnaper, MD
Professor and Vice Chair
Department of Pediatrics
Northwestern University Feinberg School of Medicine
Attending Physician, Division of Kidney Diseases
Ann and Robert H. Lurie Children's Hospital of Chicago
Chicago, Illinois

Rick G. Schnellmann, PhD
Distinguished University Professor and Chair
Department of Pharmaceutical and Biomedical Sciences
Medical University of South Carolina
Charleston, South Carolina

Robert W. Schrier, MD, MACP, Honorary MRCP (UK)
Professor Emeritus
Department of Medicine
University of Colorado School of Medicine
Aurora, Colorado

Fred G. Silva, MD
Nephropath, Inc.
Adjunct Clinical Professor of Pathology
University of Arkansas
Little Rock, Arkansas

Veronica Torres da Costa e Silva, MD
Assistant Professor of Nephrology
University of São Paulo
Assistant Physician
Hospital das Clinicas da FMUSP
São Paulo, Brazil

Visith Sitprija, MD, PhD
Emeritus Professor of Medicine
Chulalongkorn University
Director
Queen Saovabha Memorial Institute
Bangkok, Thailand

Eduardo Slatopolsky, MD
Joseph Friedman Professor of Renal Diseases in Medicine
Washington University School of Medicine
Physician
Barnes-Jewish Hospital
St. Louis, Missouri

Elsa Solà, MD
Liver Unit
University of Barcelona
Hospital Clinic
Barcelona, Spain

Stefan Somlo, MD
Professor of Medicine and Genetics
Chief, Section of Nephrology
Yale University
Attending Physician
Yale-New Haven Hospital
New Haven, Connecticut

Jessica L. Steffl, PharmD, BCPS
Lead Pharmacist
Department of Pharmacy Services
Oregon Health and Science University Hospital
Portland, Oregon

Terry B. Strom, MD
Professor of Medicine and Surgery
Harvard Medical School
Director, Immunology
Beth Israel Deaconess Medical Center
Boston, Massachusetts

Arohan R. Subramanya, MD
Assistant Professor of Medicine and of Cell Biology and Physiology
Renal-Electrolyte Division
University of Pittsburgh School of Medicine
Staff Physician, Renal Section
VA Pittsburgh Healthcare System
Pittsburgh, Pennsylvania

Manikkam Suthanthiran, MD
Stanton Griffis Distinguished Professor of Medicine
Weill Cornell Medical College
Chief, Department of Transplantation Medicine
New York Presbyterian Hospital
New York, New York

Andrew T. Taylor, MD
Professor of Radiology and Imaging Sciences
Director, Radioligand and Expert System Laboratory
Emory University School of Medicine
Atlanta, Georgia

Isaac Teitelbaum, MD
Professor of Medicine
University of Colorado School of Medicine
Medical Director, Acute and Home Dialysis Program
University of Colorado Hospital
Aurora, Colorado

Stephen C. Textor, MD
Professor of Medicine
Division of Nephrology and Hypertension
Mayo Clinic College of Medicine
Rochester, Minnesota

Ravi Thadhani, MD, MPH
Associate Professor of Medicine
Harvard Medical School
Director of Clinical Research in Nephrology
Masssachusetts General Hospital
Boston, Massachusetts

C. Craig Tisher, MD
Professor Emeritus of Medicine
University of Florida College of Medicine
Shands Hospitals and Clinics
Gainesville, Florida

Robert D. Toto, MD
Mary M. Conroy Professorship in Kidney Disease
Associate Dean, Translational Science
UT Southwestern Medical Center
Dallas, Texas

Ashish Upadhyay, MD
Assistant Professor of Medicine
Boston University School of Medicine
Attending Physician
Associate Director of Internal Medicine Residency Program
Boston Medical Center
Boston, Massachusetts

Peter N. Van Buren, MD
Division of Nephrology, Department of Internal Medicine
UT Southwestern Medical Center
Dallas, Texas

Nosratola D. Vaziri, MD, MACP
Professor of Medicine, Physiology and Biophysics
University of California, Irvine
University of California Irvine Medical Center
Orange, California

Joseph G. Verbalis, MD
Professor of Medicine
Georgetown University
Chief, Division of Endocrinology and Metabolism
Georgetown University Hospital
Washington, District of Columbia

Meryl Waldman, MD
Staff Physician and Clinical Investigator
National Institute of Diabetes and Digestive and Kidney Diseases
National Institutes of Health
Bethesda, Maryland

Terry Watnick, MD
Associate Professor of Medicine
Johns Hopkins School of Medicine
Baltimore, Maryland

I. David Weiner, MD
Professor of Medicine and Physiology and Functional Genomics
University of Florida College of Medicine
Staff Physician, Division of Nephrology, Hypertension and Transplantation
Shands Hospital at University of Florida
Chief, Nephrology and Hypertension Section
North Florida/South Georgia Veterans Health System
Gainesville, Florida

Astrid Weins, MD, PhD
Instructor in Pathology
Harvard University
Associate Pathologist
Brigham and Women's Hospital
Boston, Massachusetts

Steven D. Weisbord, MD, MSc
Assistant Professor of Medicine
Renal-Electrolyte Division
University of Pittsburgh School of Medicine
Staff Physician, Renal Section and Center for Health Equity Research and Promotion
VA Pittsburgh Healthcare System
Pittsburgh, Pennsylvania

Jack F. M. Wetzels, MD, PhD
Professor of Nephrology
Radboud University Nijmegen Medical Center
Nijmegen, The Netherlands

Andrzej Wiecek, MD, PhD, FRCP (Edin.)
Full Professor and Head
Department of Nephrology, Endocrinology and Metabolic Diseases
Medical University of Silesia
Katowice, Poland

Alexander C. Wiseman, MD
Associate Professor
Division of Renal Diseases and Hypertension
University of Colorado
Medical Director, Kidney and Pancreas Transplant Program
University of Colorado Hospital
Aurora, Colorado

Ikuyo Yamaguchi, MD, PhD
Assistant Professor of Pediatrics
University of Washington
Attending, Nephrology Department
Seattle Children's Hospital
Seattle, Washington

Jerry Yee, MD, FACP, FASN
Clinical Professor of Medicine
Wayne State University
Division Head, Nephrology and Hypertension
Henry Ford Health System
Detroit, Michigan

Luis Yu, MD
Associate Professor of Nephrology
University of São Paulo
Chief, AKI Group
Hospital das Clinicas da FMUSP
São Paulo, Brazil

Xueqing Yu, MD, PhD
Professor of Medicine
Sun Yat-Sen University
Director, Institute of Nephrology
First Affiliated Hospital, Sun Yat-Sen University
Guangzhou, China

Abolfazl Zarjou, MD
Postdoctoral Scholar
Department of Medicine/Nephrology
University of Alabama at Birmingham
Birmingham, Alabama

Xin J. Zhou, MD
Clinical Professor of Pathology
Texas A & M Health Science Center School of Medicine
Director, Renal Path Diagnostics, Pathologists BioMedical Laboratories
Baylor University Medical Center at Dallas
Dallas, Texas

Stephen H. Zinner, MD
Charles S. Davidson Professor of Medicine
Harvard Medical School
Boston, Massachusetts
Chair, Department of Medicine
Mount Auburn Hospital
Cambridge, Massachusetts

CHAPTER 45

Mechanisms of Immune Glomerular Injury

William G. Couser

INTRODUCTION

This chapter reviews the mechanisms of tissue injury that result in immune glomerular diseases, including glomerulonephritis and nephrotic syndrome (when presenting as a primary glomerular disease). The chapter is organized by individual diseases rather than by mechanisms to allow readers to appreciate more readily how the processes of tissue injury described here translate into the clinical disease entities encountered by clinicians and pathologists and covered in other chapters in this section. The mechanisms described derive from several decades of studies done at the molecular and cell culture levels in vitro as well as in an array of well-characterized animal models of glomerular diseases and in man. Cell cultures are not glomeruli or kidneys, and mice and rats are not humans, but years of experience have taught us that mechanisms defined in these experimental settings can be translated into an improved understanding of the very similar processes seen in human disease. For more information, the reader is referred to other reviews of the immune mechanisms that lead to glomerular disease.[1,2] A schematic overview of the major pathogenic sequences currently believed to be operative in human glomerulonephritis (GN), and their interactions, is presented in Figure 45.1.

BASIC IMMUNE MECHANISMS: AN OVERVIEW

The Innate Immune Response (Figure 45.1)

For many decades, studies of the pathogenesis of human GN have focused on the adaptive immune system involving antibodies and T cells. However, more recently, increased attention has been given to the more ancient and well-conserved elements of the innate immune response, which occurs immediately after an initiating event without the latent period involved in the processing of antigen, antigen presentation, and specific immune responses.[3] The innate immune system has two major arms: Toll-like receptors (TLRs) and complement, both of which may be involved in adaptive immunity as well.

TLRs are ancient and ubiquitous pattern recognition receptors present on all cell membranes and intracellularly between cytoplasm and endosomes.[3] Over 10 TLR isoforms have been characterized that recognize conserved molecular patterns like peptidoglycans, lipopolysaccharides, and bacterial and viral nucleic acids (pathogen-associated molecular patterns [PAMPs]). TLRs also respond to certain endogenous cell-derived patterns (danger-associated molecular patterns [DAMPs]). Another related cytoplasmic group of receptors called Nod-like receptors (NLR) has recently been described as well.[4] TLR ligation is central to activating the non–antigen-specific innate immune system in the immediate response to pathogens, but TLR activation is also required for adaptive, antigen-specific immune responses by facilitating conversion of dendritic cells to antigen-presenting cells.[3,4] TLRs activate multiple intracellular signaling pathways, primarily via nuclear factor kappa B (NF-κB), that lead to the local release of a variety of cytokines, chemokines, and other inflammatory mediators by all cells, including inflammatory cells like neutrophils and macrophages, as well as all three resident glomerular cells (Fig. 45.1).[3,4] Thus, TLRs and NLRs connect initiating pathogenic events like infection with a sequence of processes leading to immediate non–antigen-specific inflammation and tissue injury in GN that is associated with infections or autoimmunity or both (Fig. 45.1).

The Complement System (Figures 45.1 and 45.2)

The complement (C) system and its regulatory proteins are also ancient components of the innate immune system with multiple roles in human GN (Fig. 45.2).[5,6] C activation products are the principal mediators of antibody-induced GN. Nonimmunoglobulin zymogens, such as damaged cells and bacterial and viral proteins, can also activate C. C1q binding to immunoglobulins in the form of antigen–antibody complexes leads to classical pathway activation through C1, C4, and C2. Activation of the mannose-binding lectin (MBL) pathway is usually a consequence of microbial pathogens or galactosyl immunoglobulin G (IgG) binding to circulating MBL and proceeds through C4. The alternative C pathway (AP) is activated at low levels spontaneously, as well as by

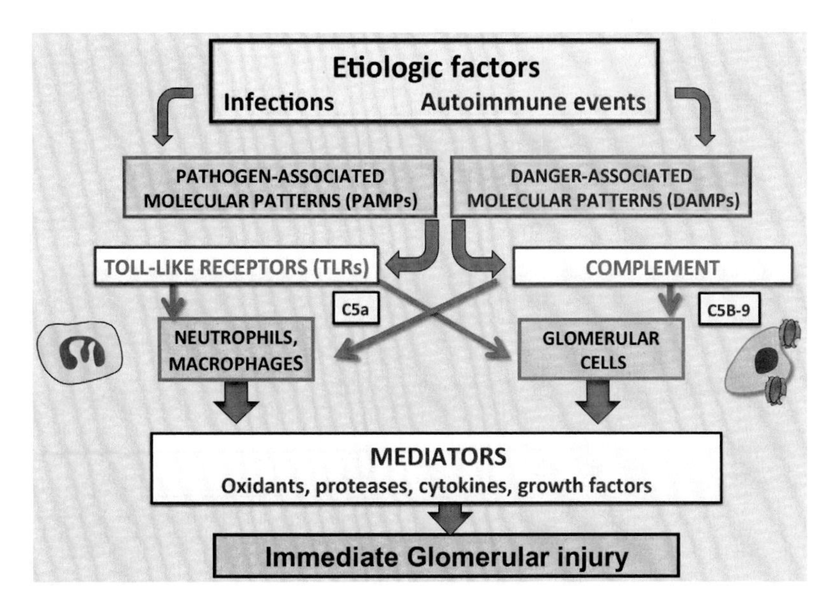

FIGURE 45.1 The innate immune system in glomerular disease. Etiologic factors, usually infections or autoimmune events, are presented to the immune system as pathogen-associated molecular patterns (PAMPs) or danger-associated molecular patterns (DAMPs). These interact with the two principal arms of the innate immune system, Toll-like receptors, and the complement system. Toll-like receptors are present on both circulating inflammatory cells like neutrophils and macrophages and on resident glomerular cells including endothelial and mesangial cells and podocytes. Toll-like receptor activation induces inflammation through release of multiple mediators including cytokines, growth factors, oxidants, proteases, eicosanoids, and others. Activation of complement also leads to the attraction of inflammatory cells through the generation of chemotactic factors such as C5a and to the conversion of resident glomerular cells to inflammatory cells following sublytic C5b-9 insertion into cell membranes. The mediators released by both infiltrating neutrophils and macrophages, and resident glomerular cells cause glomerular injury that leads to morphologic and functional changes in diseased glomeruli.

foreign surfaces such as some microbial products and damaged cells. AP activation begins at C3 without involving C1, C4, or C2. In individual complement-mediated diseases, several of these pathways may be involved.[5,6] Among the immunoglobulins, IgG subclasses IgG_1 and IgG_3 and IgM are classical C pathway activators, whereas IgG_2 and IgG_4 and normally glycosylated IgA activate C poorly.[7] However, C activation and its sequelae need not involve immunoglobulin deposits and may occur by other mechanisms even in the presence of immunoglobulin deposits. All C activation pathways lead to cleavage of C5 and release of chemotactic factors such as C5a that attract inflammatory cells (neutrophils, macrophages, platelets) when activation occurs within, or adjacent to, the circulatory compartment. Cleavage of C5 by C5 convertases also leads to the release of C5b and the addition of C6, C7, C8, and multiple C9 molecules to form the lipophilic terminal membrane attack complex (MAC or C5b-9) (Fig. 45.1).[8,9] Sublytic quantities of C5b-9 can insert into lipid bilayers of adjacent glomerular cell membranes and act in a fashion similar to receptor agonists. Sublytic C5b-9 initiates several signaling pathways and thus converts endothelial cells, mesangial cells, and podocytes to local inflammatory effector cells that can proliferate; release a variety of cytokines, growth factors, eicosanoids, oxidants, proteases, and other acute inflammatory mediators; as well as upregulate genes that encode matrix components and contribute to chronic overproduction of the extracellular matrix with scarring and sclerosis.[9] Immunoglobulin-induced C activation products like C5a can also activate TLRs, thus linking the innate and adaptive immune systems (Fig. 45.2).[10] C activation in vivo is tightly regulated by a number of circulating and cell-bound C regulatory proteins (CRPs) the functions of which, particularly those of CR1, factor H, membrane cofactor protein (MCP), and CD59, are also important in the development of several glomerular diseases (Fig. 45.2).[5,6]

The Adaptive Immune Response

Immunoglobulins

CD4 T-helper cells, activated by antigen-presenting dendritic cells and macrophages, stimulate B cells and plasma cells to make antibodies specific for nephritogenic antigens. Antigenic peptides capable of inducing GN may represent only a few amino acids of much larger proteins. Based on older studies of serum sickness in rabbits induced by single (acute) or repeated (chronic) injections of bovine serum albumin (BSA), glomerular immune deposits have long been attributed to the passive trapping of circulating, soluble antigen-IgG antibody complexes (ICs).[11,12] In acute serum sickness, a single exposure to BSA is followed by a latent period of 5 to 7 days and then the production of the IgG antibody. As antigen forms immune complexes and disappears from the circulation,

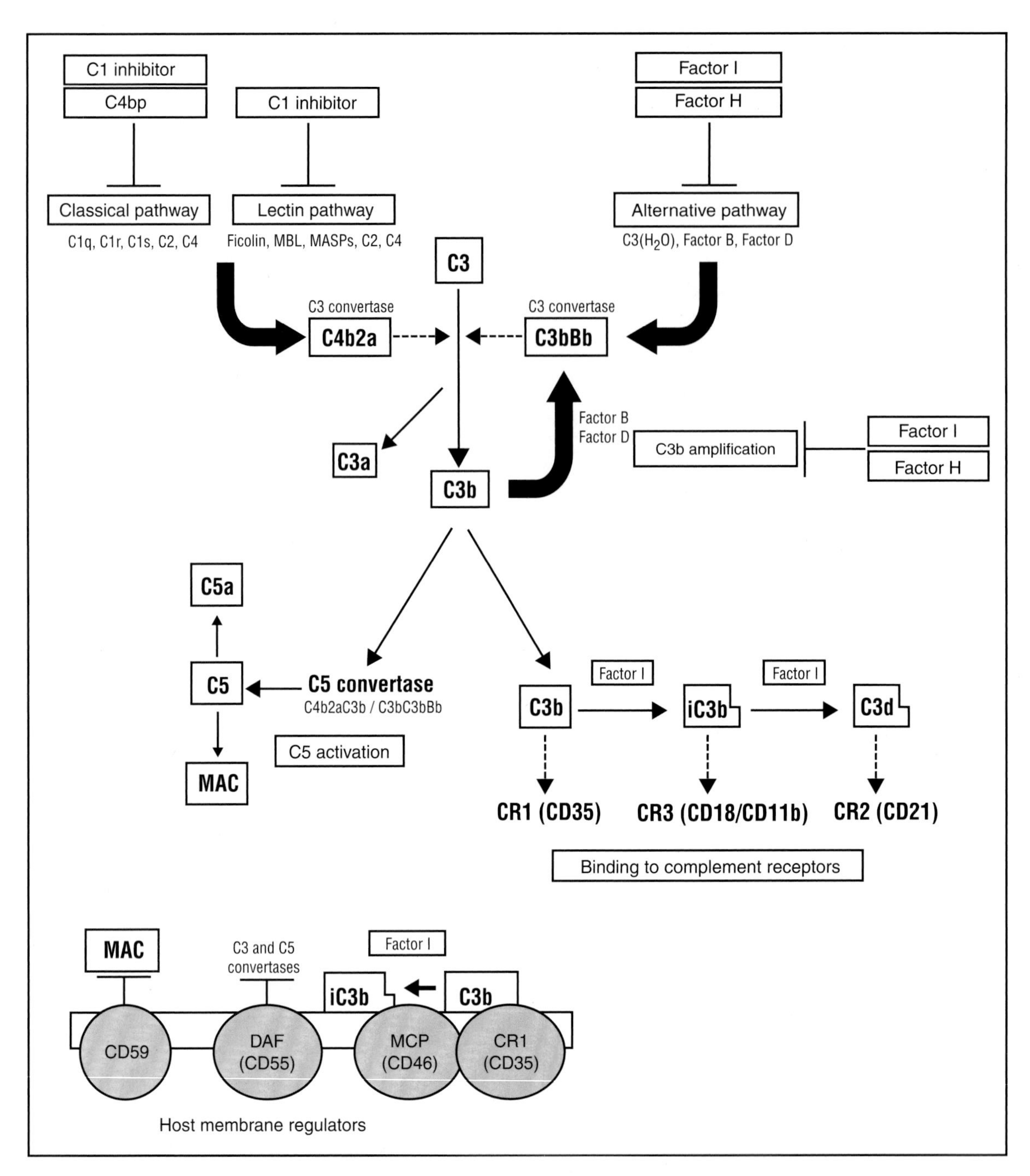

FIGURE 45.2 A schematic depiction of complement pathways and how they are activated as they relate to the pathogenesis of glomerulonephritis (GN). Activation via the classical, lectin, and alternative pathways leads to the formation of C3 convertases that cleave C3 to C3a and C3b. C3b can interact with complement receptors on cell surfaces such as CR1, CR2, and CR3 as well as contribute to the formation of C5 convertase. Cleavage of C5 results in the formation of the chemotactic factor C5a and C5b, which leads to the formation of the C5b-9 membrane attack complex (C5b-9) that is important in the mediation of several glomerular diseases. Factors H and I are circulating regulators of the alternative complement pathway, whereas CD59, decay accelerating factor (DAF), membrane cofactor protein (MCP), and complementary regulatory 1 (CR1) serve as membrane-bound regulators that protect cells from complement attack. *MBL*, mannose-binding lectin; *MASP*, MBL-associated serum protease; *MAC*, membrane attack complex (C5b-9) (Reproduced with permission from Pickering M, Cook HT. Complement and glomerular disease: new insights. *Curr Opin Nephrol Hypertens*. 2011;20(3):271–277.)

there is an initial phase of antigen excess leading to the formation of small, soluble immune complexes followed by equivalence with midrange size complexes that are believed to be trapped in tissues, and finally, to antibody excess with large complexes that are cleared through the mononuclear phagocyte system with eventual elimination of the antigen. Glomerular deposits of antigens and antibodies in acute serum sickness form primarily in the mesangium and in a subendothelial distribution. In chronic serum sickness, repeated antigen administration is provided to maintain slight antigen excess and is associated with more subepithelial deposits, again attributed to the passive glomerular trapping of small, preformed immune complexes that crossed the capillary wall to localize beneath podocytes.[12,13] Attribution of the tissue injury that occurs in serum sickness to the passive trapping of circulating complexes followed from observations that inflammation occurred only during the period that complexes could be detected in the circulation, corresponded with appearance of immune deposits in glomeruli and that both the antigen and antibody components of the immune complexes were constituents of the deposits.[13] However, later studies using passively administered preformed immune complexes did induce some glomerular deposits, but generally failed to replicate the tissue injury seen in either acute or chronic serum sickness.[14] Moreover, later measurements of circulating immune complex levels in human disease found little correlation between circulating complex levels, sizes, and disease activity. Other studies done in antiglomerular antibody (nephrotoxic nephritis [NTN]) models rather than in serum sickness demonstrated that antibody deposits activated C and other mediators that attracted circulating inflammatory cells—primarily neutrophils—which then caused tissue injury.[15] Some of these discrepancies were resolved in 1978 when it was shown that the classic subepithelial immune complex deposits in the Heymann models of membranous nephropathy (MN) in rats formed in situ and were unrelated to circulating immune complexes. Instead, they resulted from antibody binding to endogenous glomerular components localized on the podocyte (see Membranous Nephropathy, which follows).[14,16–18] Subsequent studies in both acute and chronic serum sickness using cationic BSA confirmed that deposits in these models involving exogenous antigens also formed locally and were unrelated to circulating immune complex levels or sizes.[19,20] This new paradigm allowed the mediation of immune complex nephritis to be studied directly rather than by being extrapolated from findings in models of anti-GBM disease.

The variables that determine biopsy findings and clinical consequences in immune complex GN include: (1) where deposits form in the glomerulus (ICs of the same composition that form in a subendothelial distribution lead to exudative inflammatory cell infiltrates, in the mesangium to mesangial cell [MC] proliferation and matrix expansion, and in a subepithelial distribution to a noninflammatory lesion with podocyte injury, foot process effacement, and heavy proteinuria)[18,21,22]; (2) the biologic properties of the antibody (or antigen) itself, especially the capacity to activate complement, the Fc receptor affinity, the ability to form lattices that are necessary for complement activation to occur, or cryoprecipitability[1,23]; (3) the mechanism of deposit formation (when ICs form in situ the process usually induces tissue injury at the site, whereas passive trapping of ICs formed in the circulation has not been shown to be nephritogenic)[1,14,18]; and (4) the quantity of immune deposits formed (the more deposits that form, the more severe the disease).

T Cells (Figure 45.3)

Although the existence of T cells sensitized to glomerular antigens was first demonstrated in glomerular basement membrane (GBM) disease over 40 years ago,[24] experimental verification of the pathogenicity of T cells was delayed by several factors. The rapid expansion of immunopathology using fluoresceinated antibodies to visualize and characterize antibody deposits in human renal biopsies, the lack of good T-cell markers in both rodent models and in humans, and the conviction that all forms of GN were antibody mediated resulted in little research in this area for 2 decades.[25] In 1984, the hypothesis that T cells could mediate GN independent of antibody was confirmed in ingenious experiments using bursectomized chickens that had no B cells, and later, in more conventional rodent models.[26] In addition to providing help for B cells,[28] antigen-specific CD4 T cells alone, sensitized to either self or nonself antigens that are localized in glomeruli, can induce antibody-independent tissue injury.[27,28] All subsets of T cells are now implicated in GN, including dendritic antigen-presenting cells (DC) and CD4 helper cells of the Th1, Th2, and T regulatory cell (Treg) lineages. The best-established mechanism of T-cell mediated glomerular injury involves the recruitment of macrophages, which then act as the inflammatory effector cells. However, interleukin 17 (IL-17) producing Th17 cells have attracted the most attention recently and now seem likely to account for much of the T cell-induced inflammation that occurs in GN.[29,30] Th17 cells are attracted by mechanisms involving chemokines and their receptors, and they release cytokines such as IL-9, IL-17, IL-21, IL-22, and tumor necrosis factor alpha (TNF-α),which induce other cells to produce additional proinflammatory chemokines that attract neutrophils and monocytes and also activate resident glomerular cells.[29,30] Th17 cells have now been demonstrated in renal biopsies in several forms of human GN.[31] The T-cell component of the adaptive immune response is regulated by CD4-derived Tregs (Fig. 45.3).[26]

DISEASES THAT USUALLY PRESENT AS GLOMERULONEPHRITIS

Postinfectious or Poststreptococcal Glomerulonephritis

The acute, diffuse exudative, and proliferative lesions of postinfectious or poststreptococcal glomerulonephritis (PSGN) were long regarded as the human equivalent of the acute

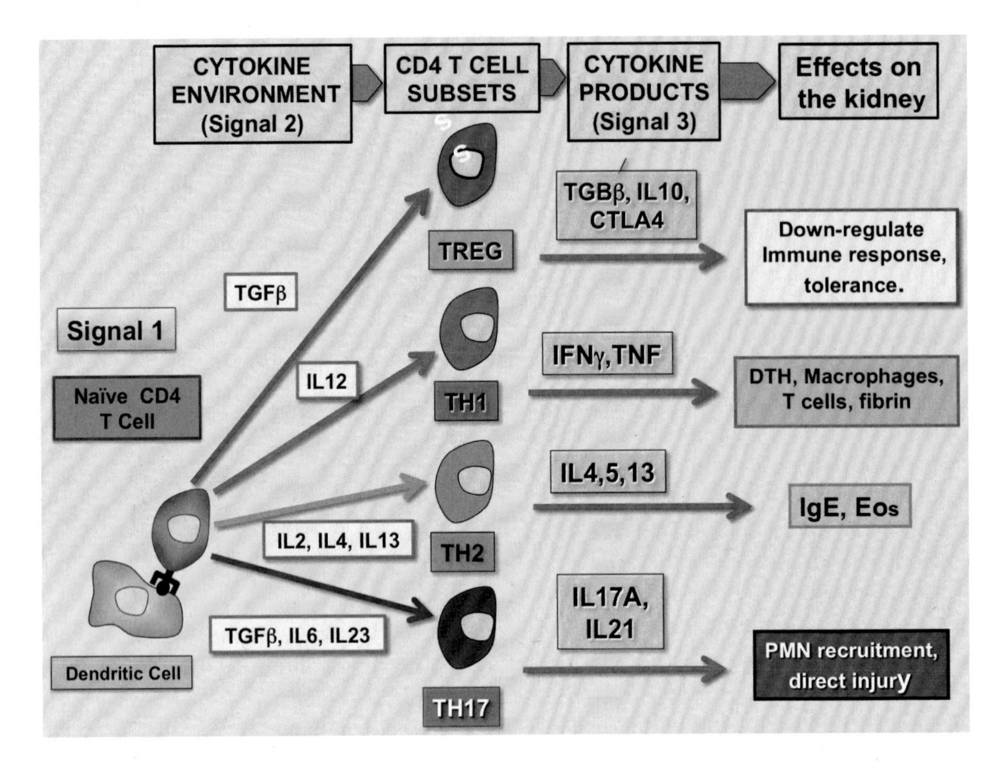

FIGURE 45.3 The T-cell component of the adaptive immune system in glomerulonephritis (GN). Antigen is presented to naïve CD4 T cells by dendritic cells (*Signal 1*). Depending on the predominant cytokine environment, T cells differentiate into CD4 T-cell subsets that play different roles in the pathogenesis of glomerular disease. In the presence of transforming growth factor beta (TGF-β), T regulatory cells (Tregs) develop that make TGF-β, interleukin 10 (IL-10), and cytotoxic T-lymphocyte antigen 4 (CTLA-4) that downregulate and control the immune response. IL-12 stimulates differentiation into Th1 cells that make interferon gamma (IFNγ) and TNF and produce traditional T-cell/macrophage-mediated delayed-type hypersensitivity (DTH) reactions. IL-2, IL-4, and IL-13 favor the development of Th2 cells that make IL-4, IL-5, and IL-13, and lead to allergic-type hypersensitivity reactions involving immunoglobulin E (IgE) and eosinophils (Eos). The CD4 T cells most implicated in the pathogenesis of GN are Th17 cells that differentiate in the presence of TGFβ, IL-6, and especially IL-17, and those that produce IL-17a and IL-21 that facilitate recruitment of other inflammatory cells such as neutrophils (PMNs) and also cause tissue injury directly.

"one shot" serum sickness model in rabbits, leading to a prolonged search for the "nephritogenic" streptococcal antigen that has extended over several decades. Although many candidate proteins have been proposed, most have failed to meet strict criteria for causality such as being demonstrable in deposits, particularly subepithelial "humps," inducing antibody that correlated with clinical disease, and inducing a similar disease in animal models.[32] However, streptococcal pyogenic exotoxin B (SpeB) meets most of these criteria. SpeB is a small (28 kDa), cationic (pK 9.3) cysteine protease with C activating and plasmin-binding properties and represents 90% of the secreted extracellular protein made in vivo by nephritogenic strains of group A streptococci.[32] Antibody to SpeB correlates with disease activity in PSGN and colocalizes with IgG and C3 in subepithelial "humps."[32,33] However, the intense exudative glomerular inflammatory response and subepithelial humps are not well explained by the analogy to acute serum sickness because intact circulating ICs do not form subepithelial IC deposits directly, and subepithelial IC deposits do not produce inflammation, presumably because complement activation products like C5a go directly into the urine and are not chemotactic for cells in the circulation.[14,18] Moreover, IgG is sometimes absent, or only a minor constituent of the deposits, whereas C3 deposition has been reported to both precede and exceed detectable IgG.[34,35] Several explanations for these apparent contradictions are plausible. They include observations that some subendothelial deposits are also present by electron microscopy (EM) in PSGN,[34,35] perhaps because the antibody to SpeB exhibits molecular mimicry with endothelial cell antigens, and antiendothelial antibody deposits are generally rapidly cleared.[36] In addition, SpeB alone is a zymogen that can activate C directly through the MBL pathway independent of IgG.[32] SpeB also exhibits plasmin-binding properties that can facilitate C activation and might cause proteolysis of GBM and facilitate the transit of dissociated subendothelial ICs to form subepithelial humps.[37] Finally, PSGN often exhibits autoimmune features including both IgM and IgG rheumatoid factors with cryoglobulin activity, antiendothelial antibodies, anti-DNA antibodies, and antineutrophil cytoplasmic antibodies (ANCA). Although the respective roles of these nonstreptococcal antibodies in mediating the disease, if any, remain undefined,

TABLE 45.1 The Most Common Complement Profiles and Autoimmune Features in Glomerulonephritis

Disease	Serum C Profile	Autoimmune Features	References
Poststreptococcal GN	AP, MBL; normal C1q, Low C3-C9	Anti-C1q, IgG AECA, anti-DNA, ANCA, PDI, cardiac myosin	37, 42, 45–48
IgA nephropathy	Normal, lectin pathway activation	Anti-glycan, mesangial cell	52, 53
Anti-GBM nephritis	Normal, CP	Anti-GBM, ANCA (20%)	88,107,108
ANCA-positive GN	Normal, AP	Anti-MPO, PR3, cPR3, NET, DNA, endothelial cell, LAMP2	110, 123, 137, 138,152
Lupus nephritis	CP, low C1q-C9	Anti-dsDNA, annexin, MPO, PR3, nucleosome, IgG, C1q, cardiolipin, MBL, NET	110, 123, 152
MPGN I	CP, low C1q-C9	Anti-C3 convertase (C3Nef),C4Nef, C1q IgM anti-IgG	
MCD/FGS	Normal	None	
Membranous nephropathy	Normal	Anti-PLA2R, DNA, NEP, aldose reductase, enolase SOD2	
Dense deposit disease	AP, normal C1q, low C3-C9	C3Nef, C4Nef, anti-CFH, factor B, C1q	
C3 nephropathy	AP, normal C1q, low C3-C9	C3Nef, anti-CFH	

Most forms of GN exhibit major features of autoimmunity. GN, glomerulonephritis; AP, alternative pathway; MBL, mannose-binding lectin; IgG, immunoglobulin G; AECA, anti-endothelial cell antibodies; ANCA, antineutrophil cytoplasmic antibody; PDI, protein disulfide isomerase; anti-MPO, antimyeloperoxidase; PR3, proteinase 3; cPR3, complementary proteinase 3; NET, neutrophil extracellular trap; NEP, LAMP2, lysosomal membrane protein 2; C3Nef, C3 nephritic factor; CP, cofactor protein; MPGN, membranoproliferative glomerulonephritis; MCD/FGS, minimal change disease/focal glomerulosclerosis; anti-PLA2R, anti-phospholipase A2 receptor; SOD2, superoxide dismutase 2; anti-CFH, anti-complement factor H. NEP, neutral endopeptidase.

these findings suggest an autoimmune component to postinfectious GN that is consistent with current thinking about most other immune glomerular diseases (Table 45.1).[38–40]

Other forms of postinfectious GN such as those associated with endocarditis, infected ventricular–atrial shunts, visceral abscesses, and *Staphylococcus aureus* infections with IgA deposits are clearly immunologically mediated, but the mechanisms involved in these diseases have been explored in much less detail.[41]

Immunoglobulin A Nephropathy

IgA nephropathy (IgAN) is the most common form of GN worldwide.[42] IgAN is characterized by a focal proliferation of mesangial cells and mesangial matrix expansion accompanying diffuse mesangial aggregates of IgA, and often IgG, C3, and C5b-9.[42–44] The disease is often associated with recurrent episodes of nephritis that immediately follow viral infections on mucosal surfaces of the upper respiratory or gastrointestinal tracts.[42–44] Although usually assumed to be mediated by a mesangial trapping of circulating ICs, no exogenous antigens have been consistently identified. Animal models of IgAN that closely mimic both the pathologic, immunopathologic, and the clinical features of IgAN have been challenging to produce, in part because of substantial differences between the rodent and human IgA immune systems. IgA in mesangial deposits, and in IC form in the circulation, is polymeric (mucosal) IgA_1 with a covalently linked secretory piece indicating a mucosal origin.[45,46] In IgAN, a population of these IgA_1 molecules exhibits deficient O-linked glycosylation at five sites in the hinge region of the molecule.[42–46] The failure to normally glycosylate IgA1 can be inherited and is commonly seen in family members without renal disease,[47] but the defect seems to occur epigenetically as well.[48] Although underglycosylated pIgA1 is produced by mucosal B cells and is usually assumed to originate from mucosal surfaces where it should not e-the bloodstream, it might also reach the circulation if abnormal trafficking of these cells to the bone marrow occurs.[49] Underglycosylated IgA_1 undergoes conformational change and exhibits altered biologic properties compared to normal IgA_1, including increased tendencies to self-aggregate, to activate C, and to bind to other molecules like fibronectin, IgG, and collagen IV.[45,46,50] In circulating macromolecular form, the underglycosylated IgA_1 aggregates lack the glycosylated sites necessary to interact with asialoglycoprotein and the CD 89 receptors in the liver and spleen, thus evading normal clearing mechanisms and facilitating mesangial localization.[45,46,51] It is not yet known if the "lanthanic" mesangial IgA deposits seen in 6% to 16% of normal donor kidneys without disease contain underglycosylated or normal IgA.[42]

Although IgG autoantibodies to MC antigens have been described in IgAN,[52] Suzuki et al.[53] were the first to report IgG antibodies directed to cryptic GalNac antigenic structures in the hinge region of aberrantly glycosylated IgA_1 molecules (antiglycan antibodies). IgG antiglycan antibodies appear to correlate with disease activity in a way that has not been demonstrated with serum levels of IgA, IgA immune complexes, or IgA-fibronectin aggregates.[53] Antiglycan antibodies form circulating ICs with underglycosylated IgA1 that can be passively trapped in the mesangium, although the mesangial trapping of ICs has not been demonstrated to be nephritogenic. Alternatively, IgG antiglycan antibodies could also lead to in situ IC formation with previously localized IgA aggregates. When IgG antibody does bind in situ to antigenic material in the mesangium[54] or on the MC membrane (the antithymocyte serum [ATS] model in rats),[56–59] the mesangial response to acute immune injury closely simulates the clinical and histopathologic features of human IgAN.[55,60]

In IgA nephropathy, MCs become activated through interactions between the IgA_1 deposits and IgA Fcα (CD89) receptors, TLRs (especially TLR4), and transferrin receptors (TfR, CD71).[61,62] Innate immunity and TLR activation by IgA aggregates, perhaps containing or accompanied by PAMPs, may account for the recurrent episodes of acute injury with hematuria, particularly those that immediately follow infections.[42,63] However, most experimental and clinical studies suggest a role for C in IgAN as well.[5,6,63,64] C5b-9 generated from C activation induced by the interaction of IgA_1 aggregates with MBL, or the in situ formation of ICs containing IgG antiglycan antibodies can induce MC transformation to a smooth muscle actin-expressing myofibroblastlike cells, upregulate genes for collagen I, and increase production of cytokines and growth factors such as IL-1, IL-6, TNF-α, platelet-derived growth factor (PDGF), transforming growth factor beta (TGF-β), epidermal growth factor (EGF), fibroblast growth factor (FGF), connective tissue growth factor (CTGF), and hepatocyte growth factor (HGF), all resulting in MC proliferation and matrix expansion.[5,6,8,9] Of these, the best-established mediators of the glomerular response to immune injury are PDGF, which is the principal growth factor involved in the proliferation of MC that follows immune injury and the CTGF/TGF-β pathway that induces overproduction of mesangial matrix.[65] The pattern of glomerular C deposition seen in active IgAN includes MBL, C4d, and C5b-9 (but not C1q) that colocalize with IgA_1 and suggest the activation of both MBL and AP.[66,67] Further evidence that C activation is important in IgAN includes observations that C deposits including MBL, C4d, and C5b-9 correlate with disease severity and prognosis.[66–68]

Rapidly Progressive, Crescentic Glomerulonephritis

Anti-Glomerular Basement Membrane Nephritis

Anti-GBM (aGBM) nephritis is characterized initially by an acute, focal necrotizing GN with crescents and linear deposition of IgG, usually with C3, on the GBM.[67] With pulmonary alveolar hemorrhage it becomes Goodpasture syndrome (GPS). The role of aGBM antibody deposition inducing C activation, chemotactic factor release, and neutrophil-mediated injury was defined in NTN models in the 1960s,[15] and the pathogenicity of human aGBM antibody was confirmed by the classic transfer studies of Lerner, Glassock, and Dixon[69] in 1967. Studies in mice deficient in C3 and C4 primarily implicate the classical C pathway,[56] which is activated by IgG1 and IgG3 aGBM that correlates with disease activity and recurrence in transplants.[57,58,67] Circulating and deposited aGBM antibodies are of the same specificity, indicating that available antigens to bind antibodies is limited, and they are primarily of the IgG1 and IgG3 subclasses.[58] Antibodies with apparently similar reactivity (but with lower titers, lower avidity, and primarily of the IgG2 and IgG4 subclasses) can be present in normal people.[59]

GBM antigens are also expressed in several extrarenal tissues, where they are sequestered by an endothelial cell layer impermeable to IgG.[70,71] The unique fenestrated endothelium in glomeruli allows for free access of IgG to GBM. The GBM antigen itself consists of two normally sequestered ("cryptic") epitopes, E_A and E_B, residing on the noncollagenous domain of both the a3 and a5 chains of the noncollagenous (NC)1 hexamer of type IV collagen and is synthesized in the glomerulus exclusively by podoctytes.[70,71] Antibody directed to the a5 chain is associated with worse renal outcomes.[71] Antibody deposition requires perturbation of the quaternary structure of the a3 45 NCI hexamer, possibly initiated by posttranslational modifications, proteolytic cleavage, or oxidant injury, which results in a conformational change in the a3 NCI and a5 NCI subunits ("autoimmune conformeropathy").[70,71] In animal models, the nephritogenic GBM antigen has been mapped to as few as three amino acid sequences in a core residue,[72] but both intermolecular and intramolecular epitope spreading occurs, suggesting immune reactivity may extend beyond the initial inducing autoantigen.[72] Pulmonary toxins such as infections, smoke, and volatile hydrocarbons may damage the endothelium and expose the antigen in alveolar capillaries, thus accounting for the pulmonary manifestations in GPS.[70,71] Whether such extrarenal events have any role in autoimmunization is not known.

T-cell reactivity to GBM antigens was first demonstrated 4 decades ago, and a pathogenic role for GBM antigen-specific "sensitized cells " was proposed,[24] but the hypothesis was given little credence at the time.[25] However, many subsequent studies have confirmed these original observations with newer technologies[73] and documented that nephritogenic GBM antigens can induce a T-cell mediated GN with crescents, proteinuria, and decreased renal function in the absence of aGBM antibody.[28,74,75] CD4 Th17 lymphocytes via the "IL-23/Th17 axis" have been shown to be central to the mediation of injury in aGBM models.[31,76] Another unique feature of the T-cell response to GBM is the appearance of long-lived Tregs and inversion of the T-cell effector/regulatory cell ratio later in the disease. This may account for why recurrences of anti-GBM disease are so infrequent compared to other autoimmune GNs where Treg activity is often impaired.[77]

The aGBM immune response in humans is strongly linked to human leukocyte antigen (HLA) DRB1 alleles 1501, 0701, and 0101with DRB 1501 conferring a relative risk of over 8, whereas 0701 and 0101 are protective.[78] This HLA linkage is the strongest yet identified in any autoimmune disease. Preceding infections or environmental toxins that might expose antigenic determinants in extrarenal tissue are possible triggering events. The disease can also be induced experimentally with a small nephritogenic T-cell epitope, pCol28-40 of Col4alpha3NC1, which exhibits molecular mimicry with PAMPs in some gram-negative bacteria, especially *Clostridia botulinum*.[79] Finally, glomerular-derived antigenic peptides that have been demonstrated in the urine can be taken up and degraded by tubular cells and then presented to interstitial dendritic cells, leading to induction of an immune response in regional lymph nodes.[80,81] The occurrence of ANCA antibodies and signs of vasculitis in up to 20% of aGBM patients and examples of aGBM disease occurring with MN, suggest that some of the proposed etiologic factors in ANCA-associated GN or MN could be operative in aGBM disease as well (Table 45.1).[82,83]

Antineutrophil Cytoplasmic Antibody-Associated Glomerulonephritis

Necrotizing crescentic GNs without immune deposits, later called "pauci-immune" GN, was first described in 1978,[84] and a decade later was linked to ANCA directed against myeloperoxidase (MPO) and proteinase 3 (PR3).[85] It is characterized by a focal necrotizing and crescentic GN with large "gaps" in the capillary wall associated with a smoldering, nephritic clinical course, usually in older individuals who may also exhibit extrarenal vasculitic disease.[84,85] The major entities associated with ANCA and GN are Wegener granulomatosis, Churg-Strauss syndrome, and microscopic polyangiitis (MPA), which may be renal limited.[86] Explorations of how anti-MPO and PR3 antibodies mediate GN without depositing in glomeruli have defined entirely new paradigms of immune glomerular injury.[87]

In vitro studies have shown that cytokines, released in response to infections, can "prime" neutrophils and up-regulate adhesion molecules on neutrophils and endothelial cells (L and E selectins, respectively) to facilitate localization in glomerular capillaries.[87,88] Cytokine-primed neutrophils redistribute MPO and PR3 contained in cytoplasmic primary granules to the cell surface by a mechanism involving CD177, thus permitting ANCA IgG to bind directly or through Fc or Fab′2 receptors.[89] ANCA binding induces a neutrophil respiratory burst with the release of cationic MPO and PR3 as well as other proteases and oxidants.[86–88,90] Neutrophil activation and neutrophil–platelet interactions also release neutrophil extracellular traps (NETs) containing entrapped MPO, PR3, and MPO DNA in a chromatin web that can mediate injury directly through TLRs as well as modulate the immune response.[91] In ANCA-GN, NETs are present in glomeruli and are colocalized with neutrophils and DCs, and anti-NET antibodies are present along with circulating MPO-DNA complexes (nucleosomes).[91] Activation of TLR2 and TLR9 exacerbate experimental crescentic GN.[92] Because of its highly cationic charge, MPO localizes readily in glomeruli by binding to endothelial cells on a charge basis, thus becoming a planted antigen that can form transient immune complexes in situ with the anti-MPO antibody or can interact with antigen-specific Th17 cells.[93] Finally, MPO can also cause glomerular injury directly through oxidative mechanisms involving the MPO-H2O2-halide system, resulting in halogenation of glomerular structures and severe glomerular injury.[93]

In 2002, Xaio et al.[94] provided the first compelling in vivo evidence for ANCA pathogenicity by transferring spleen cells and purified IgG from an MPO knockout mouse immunized with murine MPO to an immunologically compromised host to induce a T–cell-independent crescentic GN with proteinuria and reduced renal function. Other models have employed transfer of MPO+ bone marrow, adjuvants that enhance the immune response and increase cytokine levels, and mice with subclinical GN immunized to human MPO in which the crescentic GN that follows is mediated by the immune response to endogenous MPO.[87,95] Studies of the Xaio model have confirmed neutrophil dependence and, despite the absence of antibody deposits, a requirement for alternative C pathway activation involving C5a and C5a receptors.[87,96] Both alternate C pathway proteins and C5b-9 deposits have been demonstrated in glomeruli in the human disease.[96] A model of crescentic GN induced by transferring spleen cells from PR3 immunized nonobese diabetic (NOD) mice to immune deficient controls has also been described recently.[97]

Two other potentially nephritogenic ANCA antigens have also been identified. Lysosomal membrane protein 2 (LAMP2) exhibits molecular mimicry with the FimH group of adhesins on some gram-negative bacteria and is expressed on endothelial cells and neutrophils, and anti-LAMP antibodies have been correlated with disease activity and reported to induce a focal necrotizing and crescentic GN without immune deposits in animals.[98] However, these intriguing observations have not yet been confirmed. An antibody directed against complementary PR3 (cPR3)[99–101] encoded by the antisense strand of PR3 cDNA, has been detected in a minority (20%) of ANCA patients.[99] Anti-cPR3 IgG elicits an anti-idiotypic antibody response that is reactive with native (sense) PR3, suggesting a role for autoantigen complementarity in initiating the disease. Because amino acid sequences in cPR3 also have homologies with several infectious agents associated with PR3 disease including Ross River virus, *S. aureus*, and *Endamoeba histolytica*, this could represent another link to potentially etiologic infectious agents and the innate immune system.[100] Anti-cPR3 antibodies are also reactive, with plasminogen and might contribute to the delayed dissolution of clots in vitro potentially contributing to the prominent fibrin deposition seen in ANCA GN.[101]

Other groups have reasoned that the absence of antibody deposits in ANCA-positive GN, the limited correlation between ANCA levels and disease activity, and the absence of detectable ANCA in about 10% to 20% of patients with typical MPA[102] suggest a primary role for antibody-independent, T–cell-mediated immune mechanisms.[103,104] Consistent with this hypothesis is the persistent activation of T cells and the elevation of soluble T-cell products that correlate with disease activity,[105] the prominence of traditional Th1 delayed-type hypersensitivity markers like T cells, macrophages, fibrin, and occasional granulomas in ANCA-positive GN[104] and T-cell reactivity to ANCA antigens in some patients.[106–108] T cells alone, including Th17 cells, can induce focal necrotizing and crescentic GN when sensitized to a "planted" glomerular antigen (as might occur with "planted" cationic MPO).[27,109] A recent study using combinations of mice that were selectively deficient in T cells, B cells, or MPO demonstrated that active immunization with human MPO (in mice with subclinical glomerular injury) induced crescentic GN without immune deposits that required the presence of endogenous MPO and T-cell reactivity to MPO but did not require B cells or anti-MPO antibody.[95] Th17 cells and IL-17a, as well as TLRs 2 and 9, have recently been shown to be essential to the development of GN in a T–cell-dependent model.[92,109] Abnormalities in T-cell regulation and Tregs have also been described in ANCA disease with decreased Tregs associated with disease and increased levels with remission.[110]

Proposed etiologic agents in ANCA disease include environmental toxins such as silica, infectious agents including gram-positive (*S. aureus*) and gram-negative (FimH H adhesins) bacteria, viral infections, and several drugs.[86–88] There have also been significant but low level associations with potential susceptibility genes and their polymorphisms including ANCA antigens, HLA, immune response proteins, Fc receptors, cytokines, and others, but no high level associations have been described. The relatively frequent observation of ANCA antibodies in other autoimmune glomerular diseases including anti-GBM disease, systemic lupus erythematosus (SLE), and MN suggests that common etiologic and susceptibility factors may be present (Table 45.1).[82,111,112]

Lupus Nephritis

In lupus nephritis (LN), IgG, IgM, IgA, and C3 ("full house") deposits develop in the mesangium associated with mild disease (mesangial LN, class I to II) and extend along the subendothelial aspect of the capillary wall associated with increasing proliferative/inflammatory lesions in <50% (focal) or >50% (diffuse) proliferative LN, class III to IV. When deposits are primarily in a subepithelial distribution the lesion is membranous LN (class V), which usually presents with nephrotic syndrome and exhibits fewer tendencies to progression.[113] The autoimmune responses that underlie SLE have been extensively studied in mouse strains that develop the disease spontaneously and in humans, and are beyond the scope of this chapter.[114,115] The best-established functional immune abnormalities in SLE include a loss of tolerance to numerous self-antigens, B-cell hyperactivity with overproduction of autoantibodies, and defective T-cell regulation.[114]

IgG anti–double-stranded DNA antibodies (aDNA) in serum and in glomerular deposits are the most prominent serologic features of SLE.[114–116] The deposits are usually attributed to the passive trapping of DNA-aDNA ICs, although infusing aDNA or DNA-aDNA ICs has not achieved either significant glomerular localization or tissue injury in vivo.[14,115] Several other mechanisms by which anti-DNA antibodies might be nephritogenic have been proposed. Some monoclonal aDNA antibodies exhibit cross-reactivity with capillary wall antigens, especially laminin and actinin.[117] They may become internalized by cells within caveolae, achieve nuclear localization, and directly alter cell functions including apoptosis.[118] Antibody to MC annexin, which colocalizes with glomerular IgG and C3 deposits, and correlates with disease activity, has also been identified with mesangial deposits.[119] Most recent studies, however, suggest that deposited aDNA has reacted with extracellular DNA in the form of nucleosomes. Nucleosomes contain an anionic segment of DNA encircling a highly cationic histone core, giving the structure a net positive charge and thereby a high affinity for glomerular anionic sites along the endothelial surface of the capillary wall.[115,116] Defective apoptosis in SLE, perhaps related to an acquired defect in DNase I, leads to necrosis and the release of chromatin debris from apoptotic blebs, thus facilitating access of nucleosomes to antigen-presenting DCs as well as entry into the circulation.[114–116,120] Circulating nucleosomes are abundant in patients with lupus nephritis, antinucleosome antibodies correlate with disease, and both are present in membrane-associated electron dense deposits.[114–116] Although this could represent an epiphenomenon, nucleosomes are essential for aDNA antibody localization to occur in glomeruli.[115,116] Whether they localize initially as free antigenic material or are already in IC form is not known. Nucleosomes exhibit several other relevant biologic properties, including the ability to activate dendritic cells through binding to TLRs 2 and 9, and they likely directly activate resident glomerular cells through TLRs as well.[121,122] In that capacity, they may mimic infectious nonself structures to generate DAMPs that could lead to both a loss of tolerance and local inflammation through both the innate and adaptive immune systems.[122]

Other nonnucleosome autoantibodies have also been implicated in different aspects of the renal lesions in SLE, particularly lupus anticoagulant, anticardiolipin, antiphospholipid, and antibeta2 glycoprotein I antibodies in glomerular microthrombosis (Table 45.1).[123] Anti-C1q antibodies, mixed cryoglobulins containing rheumatoid factors, and others are also common (Table 45.1).[114,123,124] Recent studies in both experimental and human SLE have also implicated the Th2 immune response with B-cell differentiation, the activation of basophils, and the production of IgE anti-DNA antibodies that deposit in glomeruli.[125] B-cell activating factor (BAFF or Blys), a cytokine of the TNF ligand superfamily that activates B cells and modulates the immune response by inhibiting B-cell apoptosis, is increased in SLE, may contribute to autoantibody production, and is one of several potential new therapeutic targets.[126]

The subepithelial immune deposits in class V (membranous) LN[126] could form locally from dissociation of subendothelial ICs with transit across GBM to reform in a subepithelial location[37] or might represent reactivity of lupus autoantibodies to podocyte antigens analogous to the anti-PLA2R system identified in idiopathic MN and apparently operative in some patients with lupus MN (see the following).

C is believed to be a major mediator of tissue injury in LN through both intracapillary generation of neutrophil and macrophage chemotactic factors (classes 2 through 4) and the formation of C5b-9 (class V).[60,127] Disease severity is reduced in murine models that lack selected C proteins and increased with deficient regulatory proteins.[127,128] The observation that deficiencies of classical pathway proteins C1 > C4 > C2 are associated with an increased risk for SLE suggests protective roles for C as well.[5,6,127] For example, C1q is produced by dendritic cells and is involved in tolerance induction and clearance of both apoptotic cells and ICs.[5,6]

T cells exhibit several complex and abnormal phenotypes in SLE.[114,115] In active LN, activated T cells are expanded, provide excess help to B cells, localize in renal cell infiltrates, and produce IL-17, which correlates with disease activity, all implying CD4 and Th17 cell involvement.[114,115,129] Antigen-specific T-cell reactivity to nuclear antigens is well documented in LN,[129] and Th17 cells and IL-17 are increased in human and murine SLE and correlate with disease activity.[114,115,130] IL-17-producing T cells, either Th17 or $CD4^-$ $CD8^-$ (double negative) T cells, are present in nephritic kidneys and decreasing IL-17 production improves murine lupus nephritis.[115,130] In addition to increased CD4 activity in SLE, most studies also suggest an accompanying defect in Treg cell activity that would augment an autoimmune response.[114,115,131]

Epigenetic events, which might induce autoimmunity in SLE, include environmental exposures such as UV light and certain drugs and viral infections, especially Epstein-Barr virus (EBV).[114,116] Some of these are believed to interact with the immune system through inhibition of DNA methylation that can result in hypomethylated CD4 cells, the overproduction of IgG by B cells, and the overproduction of some cytokines.[132] Co-occurrences of LN with other GNs, including ANCA-positive GN,[111] IgA,[133] MN,[113] and even a minimal changelike podocytopathy,[135] are also sufficiently well established to suggest etiologic factors in common (Table 45.1).

Membranoproliferative Glomerulonephritis, Type I

Membranoproliferative glomerulonephritis, type 1 (MPGN I) has many similarities to a renal-limited LN clinically and pathologically, including the presence of frequent autoantibodies including rheumatoid factors, antinuclear, anticardiolipin, anti-C1q, anti-C3 convertase (C3 nephritic factor [C3Nef]), and antiendothelial antibodies (Table 45.1).[136–138] Hypocomplementemia with a classical pathway profile and increased disease susceptibility in the presence of C2 and C4 deficiency are also common to both entities.[5,6,127,133] The histologic features of capillary wall thickening, cellular proliferation, and infiltrating inflammatory cells associated with primarily mesangial and subendothelial deposits of IgG, IgM, and C3 are similar to LN and are also seen in a variety of chronic neoplasias (especially monoclonal gammopathies), infections, and other autoimmune processes.[136–138,139] However, in contrast to LN, MPGN I in adults is seen almost exclusively (>90%) in association with hepatitis C viral (HCV) infections, and the glomerular deposits have prominent features of cryoglobulins.[136,137,140,141]

The principal nephritogenic HCV antigen in MPGN I is believed to be a nonenveloped HCV E2 core protein, which can be demonstrated in circulating ICs and in glomerular deposits.[142,143] An IgG3 antibody bound to HCV E2 can interact with the globular domain of C1q, engage B cells through both B-cell receptors and TLR7, and elicit production of the monoclonal IgMκ antibody to polyclonal anti-HCV IgG (rheumatoid factor).[136–138,144] These soluble but cryoprecipitable aggregates of IgG, IgM, viral proteins/nucleic acids, and C1q make up the mesangial and subendothelial immune deposits characteristic of MPGN I. They cause local inflammation through direct interaction with TLRs 3, 7, and 9 on both infiltrating inflammatory cells and/or resident glomerular cells as well as by inducing more classical pathway C activation.[136–138,145–147] As in SLE, the subepithelial deposits often seen in MPGN I (and sometimes referred to type III MPGN) may represent subendothelial deposits that dissociate and reform, in situ, an antigen–antibody system involving a small cationic antigen or autoantibodies to as yet unidentified podocyte antigens.

As in SLE, C probably plays both nephritogenic and protective roles in MPGN I. C1q is important in mediating the initial interaction between IgM, IgG, HCV complexes, B cells, and TLRs,[136,144] and C activation by immune deposits through the classical pathway likely aggravates tissue injury,[5,6] although overexpression of a C regulatory protein, Crry, in a well-studied murine model did not significantly ameliorate the disease.[148]

The role of the CD4 effector and Tregs in MPGN I have not yet been well defined in either animal models or in humans.

DISEASES THAT USUALLY PRESENT WITH NEPHROTIC SYNDROME

The Minimal Change Disease/Idiopathic Focal Sclerosis Spectrum

There are many clinical and pathogenetic observations in minimal change disease (MCD) and idiopathic focal glomerulosclerosis (FGS), which suggest that they reflect differences in the glomerular response to similar mechanisms. Some patients with MCD are steroid resistant and develop FGS, whereas some with biopsy-documented FGS are steroid responsive and behave like MCD.[149–152] Both MCD and FGS can be triggered by multiple initiating events including infections, drugs, malignancies, and others.[149–152] Both are diseases of the podocyte and both have been associated with "permeability factors."[151–155] MCD and FGS can both recur immediately in transplants,[155,156] and can resolve when affected kidneys are placed in normal environments.[157,158] Differences between MCD and idiopathic FGS in morphologic phenotype and clinical expression could reflect (1) differences in either quantity or biologic activity of a similar primary mediator or group of mediators, or (2) genetic or epigenetic differences in the target podocyte leading to differences in response to, or recovery from, a common primary mediator. Many genes are now established that regulate podocyte responses related to the glomerular barrier function. An epigenetic factor that might also contribute to different phenotypes resulting from similar pathogenetic mechanisms is low birth weight, which is associated with lower nephron numbers, and increased vulnerability of individual nephrons to sclerosis. Alternatively, the response of normal podocytes to two different mediators has not been excluded.

Evidence continues to mount that both MCD and idiopathic FGS reflect the effect on podocytes of circulating, probably T–cell-derived, nonimmunoglobulin "permeability factors,"[151–155] a hypothesis first proposed by Shalhoub[153] in 1974. Studies by McCarthy and colleagues[155] over 15 years have demonstrated a factor in the serum of patients with recurrent FGS that can alter the albumin reflection coefficient of normal glomeruli in vitro, thus increasing glomerular permeability to albumin. In MCD, Koyama et al.[154] demonstrated that factor(s) secreted by T-cell hydridomas derived from patients with active MCD transferred a MCD-like lesion to normal rats. However, these observations were not followed up to identify the factor itself. Despite these in vitro and in vivo observations, identification of the responsible factor(s) has proven frustratingly difficult.[155] Many cytokines and other mediators, including hemopexin, soluble urokinase receptor (suPAR), TNF-α IL-13, angiopoietin-like 4, and cardiotropin-like cytokine 1 (CLC1), can be shown to be increased in MCD or FGS patients, and several also increase glomerular albumin permeability as measured using in vitro techniques.[151,155] suPAR has been implicated in altering podocyte β3 integrins leading to podocyte detachment and FGS,[159] and increased plasma levels of suPAR might contribute to proteinuria in both active and recurrent FGS through a similar integrin-related mechanism. Neutralization of CLC1 reduces permeability factor activity in FGS serum, as does galactose and normal serum and urine.[155]

Human studies document Th2 polarization and elevated levels of IL-13, a Th2 cytokine with podocyte receptors, in active MCD.[160] IL-13 alters podocyte function through CD-80, and overexpression of IL-13 induces albuminuria and foot process effacement.[161] Transferring CD34+ stem cells from patients with active MCD also transfers proteinuria and causes podocyte foot process effacement, although the responsible factor has not yet been established.[162] CD80 (B7.1) is a T-cell costimulatory molecule involved in antigen processing that is also expressed on podocytes. Podocyte CD80 activation through TLR4, independent of T cells, causes proteinuria and foot process effacement.[163] Recent studies by Garin et al.[164] have documented increased levels of CD80 expression in podocytes and CD80 protein in urine in active MCD (but not FGS), although measurement of urinary CD80 mRNA demonstrates higher levels in FGS than in MCD.[165] CD80 also functions as an inhibitory molecule in T cell–DC interaction and is downregulated by Treg-derived CTLA4, which is decreased in both serum and urine in active MCD.[164,166] Thus, an initiating event, or "first hit," such as an infectious process, might lead to the activation of podocyte CD80 via IL-13 or TLR4 leading to actin rearrangement and albuminuria with CD80 shedding in the urine.[166] The "second hit" would involve the defective CD80 regulation by either Tregs or podocyte-derived CTLA4.[166] Podocyte overexpression of angiopoeitinlike-4, which, like CD80, is increased in serum and podocytes in MCD patients, induces a steroid-sensitive MCD-like glomerular lesion with heavy proteinuria, suggesting a role for this molecule in the podocyte response in MCD/FGS as well.[167]

Membranous Nephropathy

Idiopathic MN is a noninflammatory glomerular lesion initially associated with essentially normal glomerular histology, accompanied by subepithelial deposits of IgG and C3 that are exclusively subepithelial in distribution and heavy proteinuria.[168] Active and passive Heymann nephritis (HN) are rat models described over 50 years ago that very closely mimic the human disease.[169] Although the subepithelial deposits in the Heymann models were initially attributed to the passive trapping of circulating ICs containing a tubular antigen, studies have since shown that IgG antibodies form subepithelial immune deposits in situ by binding to a podocyte protein complex now called megalin.[16,17,169] Unlike more inflammatory diseases in which the chemotactic factors generated by complement activation seem to play a primary role, proteinuria in experimental MN is complement dependent but mediated by sublytic C5b-9 attack on podocytes.[9,170] Sublytic C5b-9 activates several signaling pathways, alters the actin cytoskeleton, upregulates the expression of TGF-β and TGF-β receptors and matrix production leading to GBM thickening and "spike" formation, and increases the production of oxidants and proteases believed to damage underlying GBM leading to proteinuria.[9] C5b-9 also leads to podocyte DNA damage and impaired ability to complete the cell cycle, which may contribute to apoptosis, the shedding of podocytes in the urine, podocytopenia, and the development of glomerular sclerosis.[9,171]

Proof of principle that MN in humans can also result from an autoimmune mechanism analogous to the one defined in the Heymann models was first provided by Debiec et al.[172] who reported that alloimmunization of an infant to neutral endopeptidase (NEP) expressed on podocytes, resulting from a maternal NEP deficiency, leads to the transplacental transfer of anti-NEP IgG and typical MN in the newborn.[172] However, the anti-NEP mechanism is not operative in most cases of adult idiopathic MN. Recently, Beck et al. and Hofstra et al.,[173,174] using microdissection and proteomic technology, identified another antipodocyte autoantibody directed against the M-type phospholipase A2 receptor (PLA2R) in 70% to 80% of patients with idiopathic MN and showed that IgG anti-PLA2R is also present in the glomerular deposits and correlates with disease activity, response to therapy, and recurrence in transplants. Others have confirmed these findings.[175,176] Antibodies reactive with aldose reductase, enolase, and superoxide dismutase, as well as PLA2R, have also been eluted from MN glomeruli, but these may represent secondary phenomena related to oxidant stress rather than primary pathogenic mediators.[175] Idiopathic MN apparently induced by an exogenous antigen, analogous to the chronic serum sickness model in rabbits induced by cationic BSA, has recently been described.[177] Four children had idiopathic MN associated with cationic BSA, thought to derive from an exposure to cows' milk, with an antibody to it in the circulation and in the glomerular immune deposits. In this lesion, as well, subepithelial immune deposits appear to form locally independent of circulating immune complexes, and complement C3 and Cb-9 are present.[177]

Whether the role of C5b-9 in mediating proteinuria established in HN (and in the chronic BSA serum sickness models of MN as well)[178,179] mediates podocyte injury, and proteinuria in human MN is not established. C-independent mechanisms of proteinuria have also been well described with IgG antipodocyte antibodies in several models,[180] including HN,[181,182] although these models do not exhibit the prominent C3 and C5b-9 deposits seen in the C-dependent HN models and in humans. Despite the prominent C deposition in MN, deposited anti-PLA2R antibody is predominately of the poorly C-fixing IgG4 subclass, which induces poor C activation via the classical pathway. However, C activation might be induced by the lesser quantities of IgG1 and IgG3 usually present, as occurs with anti-NEP IgG.[172] However, in both human MN and HN, classical C-pathway components are often absent in glomerular deposits, suggesting that IgG4 might induce C activation via the MBL or alternative C pathways. In the rat, C-mediated injury also requires the inhibition of podocyte C-regulatory proteins.[9,183,184]

Once developed, the glomerular lesion in MN heals very slowly with proteinuria, often persistent for weeks or months after the immune response has abated and subepithelial deposits are no longer forming.[185] This likely explains why only 70% to 80% of patients with proteinuria and MN on biopsy have active disease as defined by elevated anti-PLA2R levels.[173,174] Glomerular deposition of C3c and urinary excretion of C5b-9 have both been established experimentally as valid biomarkers of ongoing immune deposit formation in MN,[185,186] but these should soon be supplanted by direct measurements of anti-PLA2R antibody.

Although a role for cytotoxic T cells has been proposed in C-independent models of HN,[187,188] T cells generally do not have access to podocytes or the subepithelial space and are rarely seen in most HN models or human MN.[183,189] No systematic studies of the role of T cells in human MN have been published.

No etiologic agents have been identified consistently in idiopathic MN. However, a genomewide association study has reported very strong associations with SNPs in genes that encode for HLA-DQA1 and PLA2R.[190] Whether these associations relate to rendering PLA2R antigenic or to altering its expression by podocytes is unclear. In secondary forms of MN, a number of potential etiologic agents have been identified, including hepatitis B virus (HBV) and HCV infections, several drugs, exposure to environmental toxins such as hydrocarbons, milk (in infants), formaldehyde, and solid organ tumors.[183,191] To date, these secondary forms of MN have only rarely been associated with anti-PLA2R, although up to 30% of patients with lupus MN had an anti-PLA2R antibody in one study.[191]

C3 Nephropathies

Dense Deposit Disease

Dense deposit disease (DDD) was formerly referred to as type II MPGN because a minority of cases resemble type I MPGN by light microscopy and have a similar nephritic/nephrotic clinical presentation.[192,193] However, DDD has little pathogenetic overlap with adult MPGN I and is probably better viewed as a C3 glomerulopathy, a form of GN characterized by deposits of C without immunoglobulins, usually associated with abnormalities in C regulation.[193–196] Thick linear deposits of C3, C5b-9, and other complement activation products without IgG characterize DDD along the contours of ribbon-like intramembranous electron-dense deposits within GBM and in the mesangium ("mesangial rings").[192,196] The C profile in serum and in glomerular deposits reflects alternative, or MBL, pathway activation.[5,6,192] Normally, the alternative pathway C3 convertase, C3bBb catalyzes spontaneous low levels of C3 activation (C3 "tick over"), but is tightly regulated by circulating factor H (CFH), which binds the active Bb site on the convertase to inactivate the enzyme.[5,6] Over 80% of DDD patients have an IgG autoantibody to the active site of the alternative pathway C3 convertase (C3 nephritic factor, C3Nef) that prevents normal CFH binding and, therefore, impairs regulation of the enzyme.[5,6,192,193,197] DDD can also be associated with congenital absence or the mutation of CFH, neutralization by an anti-CFH antibody or antibody to factor B.[197–200] Chronic unregulated C3 activation generates a variety of AP C activation products that accumulate, perhaps by charge interactions, along the inner GBM to form the classic dense deposits seen by EM.[200] In turn, this accumulation of proteins modifies the filtration barrier structure and integrity leading to proteinuria and nephrotic syndrome.

DDD is associated with other similar disorders of C regulation such as partial lipodystrophy, but no specific etiologic factors have been identified.

Isolated C3 Glomerulopathy

Glomerular deposits of C3 without immunoglobulin also characterize another glomerulopathy, sometimes termed isolated C3 deposition glomerulopathy, but the electron-dense deposits are seen primarily in mesangial and subendothelial sites rather than within GBM.[194,195] The lesion also may be associated with a spectrum of histologic abnormalities including MPGN I–like findings.[194,195, 200] The disorder(s) seems to affect younger patients who often have hematuria and proteinuria, but less commonly exhibit hypocomplementemia, nephrotic syndrome, or progression compared to DDD.[194,195] Evidence of disordered C regulation in the form of either mutated CRPs (H402 allele of factor H, factor I), anti-CFH, or antifactor B antibodies or C3Nef is also present in many of these patients.[194,195,196,198, 200] A familial form of isolated C3 glomerulopathy due to mutations in the CFHR5 gene has also been described in Greek Cypriots that is more likely to progress (30%) and is worse in men than women.[201] The composition of the deposits and the reason for their different distribution compared to DDD are not known.

CLOSING COMMENTS

Recent advances in the understanding the pathogenesis of immune glomerular diseases now link infectious processes, especially chronic viral ones, with autoimmunity and GN. Once viewed primarily as human equivalents of the antibody-mediated serum sickness (IC) or NTN (aGBM) models of GN in animals, most human GNs are now believed to be primarily autoimmune diseases involving both innate and acquired immune mechanisms, with distinction between the two becoming increasingly blurred. Moreover, T-cell as well as antibody-driven adaptive immune responses are considered of about equal importance (Fig. 45.1). Links to etiologic infectious agents more likely proceed through the recognition of PAMPs by TLRs and the triggering of autoimmune events than through direct effects of ICs containing exogenous antigens trapped from the circulation. However, progress in translating these scientific advances to better therapies has been slow, and in 2011, clinicians still rely almost entirely on corticosteroids and toxic and nonselective immunosuppressive agents for therapy, as described in the clinical chapters, which follow.

REFERENCES

1. Couser WG. Mediation of glomerulonephritis: basic and translational concepts. *J Am Soc Nephrol.* 2012;23(3):381–399.
2. Ponticelli C, Coppo R, Salvadori M. Glomerular diseases and transplantation: similarities in pathogenetic mechanisms and treatment options. *Nephrol Dial Transplant.* 2011;26(1):35–41.
3. Gluba A, Banach M, Hannam S, et al. The role of Toll-like receptors in renal diseases. *Nat Rev Nephrol.* 2010;6(4):224–235.
4. Gonçalves GM, Castoldi A, Braga TT, et al. New roles for innate immune response in acute and chronic kidney injuries. *Scand J Immunol.* 2011;73(5):428–435.
5. Pickering M, Cook HT. Complement and glomerular disease: new insights. *Curr Opin Nephrol Hypertens.* 2011;20(3):271–277.
6. Chen M, Daha MR, Kallenberg CGM. The complement system in systemic autoimmune disease. *J Autoimmun.* 2010;34(3):J276–J286.
7. Schroeder HW Jr, Cavacini L. Structure and function of immunoglobulins. *J Allergy Clin Immunol.* 2010;125(2 Suppl 2):S41–S52.
8. Couser WG, Baker PJ, Adler S. Complement and the direct mediation of immune glomerular injury: a new perspective. *Kidney Int.* 1985;28(6):879–890.
9. Cybulsky AV. Membranous nephropathy. *Contrib Nephrol.* 2011;169:107–125.
10. Stevens MG, Van Poucke M, Peelman LJ, et al. Anaphylatoxin C5a-induced toll-like receptor 4 signaling in bovine neutrophils. *J Dairy Sci.* 2011;94(1):152–164.
11. Dixon FJ, Feldman JD, Vazquez JJ. Experimental glomerulonephritis. The pathogenesis of a laboratory model resembling the spectrum of human glomerulonephritis. *J Exp Med.* 1961;113:899–920.
12. Wilson CB, Dixon FJ. Diagnosis of immunopathologic renal disease. *Kidney Int.* 1974;5(6):389–401.
13. Cochrane CG, Koffler D. Immune complex disease in experimental animals and man. *Adv Immunol.* 1973;16(0):185–264.
14. Couser WG, Salant DJ. In situ immune complex formation and glomerular injury. *Kidney Int.* 1980;17(1):1–13.
15. Cochrane CG, Unanue ER, Dixon F. A role of polymorphonuclear leukocytes and complement in nephrotoxic nephritis. *J Exp Med.* 1965;122:99–116.
16. Van Damme BJ, Fleuren GJ, Bakker WW, et al. Experimental glomerulonephritis in the rat induced by antibodies directed against tubular antigens. V. Fixed glomerular antigens in the pathogenesis of heterologous immune complex glomerulonephritis. *Lab Invest.* 1978;38(4):502–510.
17. Couser WG, Steinmuller DR, Stilmant MM, et al. Experimental glomerulonephritis in the isolated perfused rat kidney. *J Clin Invest.* 1978;62(6):1275–1288.
18. Couser WG. Mechanisms of glomerular injury in immune complex disease. (Nephrology Forum). *Kidney Int.* 1985;28(3):569–583.
19. Adler SG, Wang H, Ward HJ, et al. Electrical charge. Its role in the pathogenesis and prevention of experimental membranous nephropathy in the rabbit. *J Clin Invest.* 1983;71(3):487–499.
20. Ward HJ, Cohen AH, Border WA. In situ formation of subepithelial immune complexes in the rabbit glomerulus: requirement of a cationic antigen. *Nephron.* 1984;36(4):257–264.
21. Salant DJ, Adler S, Darby C, et al. Influence of antigen distribution on the mediation of immunological glomerular injury. *Kidney Int.* 1985;27:938–950.
22. Fries JW, Mendrick DL, Rennke HG. Determinants of immune complex-mediated glomerulonephritis. *Kidney Int.* 1988;34:333–345.

23. Wener MH, Mannik M. Mechanisms of immune deposit formation in renal glomeruli. *Springer Semin Immunopathol.* 1986;9(2–3):219–235.

24. Rocklin RE, Lewis EJ, David JR. In vitro evidence for cellular hypersensitivity to glomerular-basement-membrane antigens in human glomerulonephritis. 1970;283(10):497–501.

25. Dixon FJ. What are sensitized cells doing in glomerulonephritis? *N Engl J Med.* 1970;283(10):536–537.

26. Jiang H, Chess L. Regulation of immune responses by T cells. *N Engl J Med.* 2006;354:1166–1176.

27. Rennke HG, Klein PS, Sandstrom DJ, et al. Cell-mediated immune injury in the kidney: acute nephritis induced in the rat by azobenzenearsonate. *Kidney Int.* 1994;45(4):1044–1056.

28. Wu J, Hicks J, Borillo J, et al. CD4(+) T cells specific to a glomerular basement membrane antigen mediate glomerulonephritis. *J Clin Invest.* 2002;109(4):517–524.

29. Kim AH, Markiewicz MA, Shaw AS. New roles revealed for T cells and DCs in glomerulonephritis. *J Clin Invest.* 2009;119(5):1074–1076.

30. Kitching AR, Holdsworth SR. The emergence of Th17 cells as effectors of renal injury. *J Amer Soc Nephrol.* 2011;22(2):235–238.

31. Abdulahad WH, Stegeman CA, Kallenberg CG. Review article: The role of CD4(+) T cells in ANCA-associated systemic vasculitis. *Nephrology (Carlton).* 2009;14(1):26–32.

32. Rodríguez-Iturbe B, Batsford S. Pathogenesis of poststreptococcal glomerulonephritis a century after Clemens von Pirquet. *Kidney Int.* 2007;71(11):1094–1104.

33. Brodsky SV, Nadasdy T. Infection-related glomerulonephritis. *Contrib Nephrol.* 2011;169:153–160.

34. Edelstein CL, Bates WD. Subtypes of acute postinfectious glomerulonephritis: a clinic-pathological correlation. *Clin Nephrol.* 1992;38(6):311–317.

35. Sorger K, Gessler U, Hübner FK, et al. Subtypes of acute postinfectious glomerulonephritis. Synopsis of clinical and pathological features. *Clin Nephrol.* 1982;17(3):114–122.

36. Luo YH, Chuang WJ, Wu JJ, et al. Molecular mimicry between streptococcal pyrogenic exotoxin B and endothelial cells. *Lab Invest.* 2010;90(10):1492–1506.

37. Fujigaki Y, Batsford SR, Bitter-Suermann D, et al. Complement system promotes transfer of immune complex across glomerular filtration barrier. *Lab Invest.* 1995;72(1):25–33.

38. Sesso RC, Ramos OL, Pereira AB. Detection of IgG-rheumatoid factor in sera of patients with acute poststreptococcal glomerulonephritis and its relationship with circulating immune complexes. *Clin Nephrol.* 1986;26(2):55–60.

39. Vilches AR, Williams DG. Persistent anti-DNA antibodies and DNA-anti-DNA complexes in post-streptococcal glomerulonephritis. *Clin Nephrol.* 1984;22(2):97–110.

40. Ardiles LG, Valderrama G, Moya P, et al. Incidence and studies on antigenic specificities of antineutrophil-cytoplasmic autoantibodies (ANCA) in poststreptococcal glomerulonephritis. *Clin Nephrol.* 1997;47(1):1–5.

41. Satoskar AA, Nadasdy G, Plaza JA, et al. Staphylococcus infection-associated glomerulonephritis mimicking IgA nephropathy. *Clin J Am Soc Nephrol.* 2006;1(6):1179–1186.

42. Glassock RJ. The pathogenesis of IgA nephropathy. *Curr Opin Nephrol Hypertens.* 2011;20(2):153–160.

43. Tumlin JA, Madaio MP, Hennigar R. Idiopathic IgA nephropathy: pathogenesis, histopathology, and therapeutic options. *Clin J Am Soc Nephrol.* 2007;2(5):1054–1061.

44. Coppo R, Feehally J, Glassock R. IgA nephropathy at two score and one. *Kidney Int.* 2010;77(3):181–186.

45. Mestecky J, Tomana M, Crowley-Nowick PA, et al. Defective galactosylation and clearance of IgA1 molecules as a possible etiopathogenic factor in IgA nephropathy. *Contrib Nephrol.* 1993;104:172–182.

46. Novak J, Julian BA, Tomana M, et al. IgA glycosylation and IgA immune complexes in the pathogenesis of IgA nephropathy. *Semin Nephrol.* 2008;28(1):78–87.

47. Yu HH, Chu KH, Yang YH, et al. Genetics and immunopathogenesis of IgA nephropathy. *Clin Rev Allergy Immunol.* 2011;41(2):198–213.

48. Smith AC, de Wolff JF, Molyneux K, et al. O-glycosylation of serum IgD in IgA nephropathy. *J Am Soc Nephrol.* 2006;17(4):1192–1199.

49. Barratt J, Eitner F, Feehally J, et al. Immune complex formation in IgA nephropathy: a case of the 'right' antibodies in the 'wrong' place at the 'wrong' time? *Nephrol Dial Transplant.* 2009;24(12):3620–3623.

50. Kokubo T, Hiki Y, Iwase H, et al. Protective role of IgA1 glycans against IgA1 self-aggregation and adhesion to extracellular matrix proteins. *J Am Soc Nephrol.* 1998;9(11):2048–2054.

51. Novak J, Tomana M, Matousovic K, et al. IgA1-containing immune complexes in IgA nephropathy differentially affect proliferation of mesangial cells. *Kidney Int.* 2005;67(2):504–513.

52. Ballardie FW, Brenchley PE, Williams S, et al. Autoimmunity in IgA nephropathy. *Lancet.* 1988;2(8611):588–592.

53. Suzuki H, Fan R, Zhang Z, et al. Aberrantly glycosylated IgA1 in IgA nephropathy patients is recognized by IgG antibodies with restricted heterogeneity. *J Clin Invest.* 2009;119(6):1668–1677.

54. Mauer SM, Sutherland DE, Howard RJ, et al. The glomerular mesangium. 3. Acute immune mesangial injury: a new model of glomerulonephritis. *J Exp Med.* 1973;137(3):553–570.

55. Brandt J, Pippin J, Schulze M, et al. Role of the complement membrane attack complex (C5b-9) in mediating experimental mesangioproliferative glomerulonephritis. *Kidney Int.* 1996;49(2):335–343.

56. Sheerin NS, Springall T, Carroll MC, et al. Protection against anti-glomerular basement membrane (GBM)-mediated nephritis in C3- and C4-deficient mice. *Clin Exp Immunol.* 1997;110(3):403–409.

57. Zhao J, Yan Y, Cui Z, et al. The immunoglobulin G subclass distribution of anti-GBM autoantibodies against rHalpha3(IV)NC1 is associated with disease severity. *Hum Immunol.* 2009;70(6):425–429.

58. Yang R, Hellmark T, Zhao J, et al. Levels of epitope-specific autoantibodies correlate with renal damage in anti-GBM disease. *Nephrol Dial Transplant.* 2009;24(6):1838–1844.

59. Cui Z, Wang HY, Zhao MH. Natural auto antibodies against glomerular basement membrane exist in normal human sera. *Kidney Int.* 2006;69(5):894–899.

60. Moura IC, Benhamou M, Launay P, et al. The glomerular response to IgA deposition in IgA nephropathy. *Semin Nephrol.* 2008;28(1):88–95.

61. Monteiro RC. Role of IgA and IgA fc receptors in inflammation. *J Clin Immunol.* 2010;30(1):1–9.

62. Schlöndorff D, Banas B. The mesangial cell revisited: no cell is an island. *J Am Soc Nephrol.* 2009;20(6):1179–1187.

63. Coppo R, Amore A, Peruzzi L, et al. Innate immunity and IgA nephropathy. *J Nephrol.* 2010;23(6):626–632.

64. Oortwijn BD, Eijgenraam JW, Rastaldi MP, et al. The role of secretory IgA and complement in IgA nephropathy. *Semin Nephrol.* 2008;28(1):58–65.

65. Johnson RJ. Nephrology Forum: The glomerular response to injury. Progression or resolution? *Kidney Int.* 1994;45:1769–1782.

66. Stangou M, Alexopoulos E, Pantzaki A, et al. C5b-9 glomerular deposition and tubular alpha(3)beta(1)-integrin expression are implicated in the development of chronic lesions and predict renal function outcome in immunoglobulin A nephropathy. *Scand J Urol Nephrol.* 2008;42:373–380.

67. Salama AD, Levy JB, Lightstone L, et al. Goodpasture's disease. *Lancet.* 2001;358(9285):917–920.

68. Roos A, Rastaldi MP, Calvaresi N, et al. Glomerular activation of the lectin pathway of complement in IgA nephropathy is associated with more severe renal disease. *J Am Soc Nephrol.* 2006;17(6):1724–1734.

69. Lerner RA, Glassock RJ, Dixon FJ. The role of anti-glomerular basement membrane antibody in the pathogenesis of human glomerulonephritis. *J Exp Med.* 1967;126(6):989–1004.

70. Pedchenko V, Bondar O, Fogo AB, et al. Molecular architecture of the Goodpasture autoantigen in anti-GBM nephritis. *N Engl J Med.* 2010;363(4):343–354.

71. Pedchenko V, Vanacore R, Hudson B. Goodpasture's disease: molecular architecture of the autoantigen provides clues to etiology and pathogenesis. *Curr Opin Nephrol Hypertens.* 2011;20(3):290–296.

72. Bolton WK, Chen L, Hellmark T, et al. Molecular mapping of the Goodpasture's epitope for glomerulonephritis. *Trans Am Clin Climatol Assoc.* 2005;116:229–236.

73. Merkel F, Kalluri R, Marx M, et al. Autoreactive T-cells in Goodpasture's syndrome recognize the N-terminal NC1 domain on alpha 3 type IV collagen. *Kidney Int.* 1996;49(4):1127–1133.

74. Bolton WK, Chandra M, Tyson TM, et al. Transfer of experimental glomerulonephritis in chickens by mononuclear cells. *Kidney Int.* 1988;34(5):598–610.

75. Tipping PG, Holdsworth SR. T cells in crescentic glomerulonephritis. *J Am Soc Nephrol.* 2006;17:1253–1263.

76. Ooi JD, Phoon RK, Holdsworth SR, et al. IL23, not IL12, directs autoimmunity to the Goodpasture antigen. *J Am Soc Nephrol.* 2010;20(5):980–989.

77. Salama D, Chaudhry AN, Holthaus KA, et al. Regulation by CD25+ lymphocytes of autoantigen-specific T-cell responses in Goodpasture's (anti-GBM) disease. *Kidney Int.* 2003;64(5):1685–1694.

78. Phelps RG, Rees AJ. The HLA complex in Goodpasture's disease: a model for analyzing susceptibility to autoimmunity. *Kidney Int.* 1999;56(5):1638–1653.

79. Arends J, Wu J, Borillo J, et al. T cell epitope mimicry in antiglomerular basement membrane disease. *J Immunol.* 2006;176(2):1252–1258.

80. Macconi D, Chiabrando C, Schiarea S, et al. Proteasomal processing of albumin by renal dendritic cells generates antigenic peptides. *J Am Soc Nephrol.* 2009;20(1):123–130.

81. Sung SS, Bolton WK. T cells and dendritic cells in glomerular disease: The new glomerulotubular feedback loop. *Kidney Int.* 2010;77(5):393–399.

82. Lindic J, Vizjak A, Ferluga D, et al. Clinical outcome of patients with coexistent antineutrophil cytoplasmic antibodies and antibodies against glomerular basement membrane. *Ther Apher Dial.* 2009;13(4):278–281.

83. Hecht N, Omoloja A, Witte D, et al. Evolution of antiglomerular basement membrane glomerulonephritis into membranous glomerulonephritis. *Pediatr Nephrol.* 2008;23(3):477-480.

84. Stilmant MM, Bolton WK, Sturgill BC, et al. Crescentic glomerulonephritis without immune deposits: clinicopathologic features. *Kidney Int.* 1979;15(2):184–195.

85. Falk RJ, Jennette JC. Anti-neutrophil cytoplasmic autoantibodies with specificity for myeloperoxidase in patients with systemic vasculitis and idiopathic necrotizing and crescentic glomerulonephritis. *N Engl J Med.* 1988;318(25):1651–1657.

86. Falk RJ, Jennette JC. ANCA disease: where is this field heading? *J Am Soc Nephrol.* 2010;21(5):745–752.

87. Jennette JC, Xiao H, Falk R, et al. Experimental models of vasculitis and glomerulonephritis induced by antineutrophil cytoplasmic autoantibodies. *Contrib Nephrol.* 2011;169:211–220.

88. Flint J, Morgan MD, Savage COS. Pathogenesis of ANCA-associated vasculitis. *Rheum Ds Clin North Am.* 2010;36(3):463–477.

89. Jerke U, Rolle S, Dittmar G, et al. Complement receptor Mac-1 is an adaptor for NB1 (CD177)-mediated PR3-ANCA neutrophil activation. *J Biol Chem.* 2011;286(9):7070–7081.

90. Falk RJ, Terrell RS, Charles LA, et al. Anti-neutrophil cytoplasmic autoantibodies induce neutrophils to degranulate and produce oxygen radicals in vitro. *Proc Natl Acad Sci USA.* 1990;87(11):4115–4119.

91. Kessenbrock K, Krumbholz M, Schönermarck U, et al. Netting neutrophils in autoimmune small-vessel vasculitis. *Nat Med.*2009;15(6):623–625.

92. Summers SA, Steinmetz OM, Gan PY, et al. TLR2 induces Th17 myeloperoxidase autoimmunity, while TLR9 drives Th1 autoimmunity. *Arthritis Rheum.* 2011;63(4):1124–1135.

93. Johnson RJ, Lovett D, Lehrer RI, et al. Role of oxidants and proteases in glomerular injury. *Kidney Int.* 1994;45(2):352–359.

94. Xiao H, Heeringa P, Hu P, et al. Antineutrophil cytoplasmic autoantibodies specific for myeloperoxidase cause glomerulonephritis and vasculitis in mice. *J Clin Invest.* 2002;110(7):955–963.

95. Ruth AJ, Kitching AR, Kwan RY, et al. Anti-neutrophil cytoplasmic antibodies and effector CD4+ cells play nonredundant roles in anti-myeloperoxidase crescentic glomerulonephritis. *J Am Soc Nephrol.* 2006;17(7):1940–1949.

96. Xing GQ, Chen M, Liu G, et al. Complement activation is involved in renal damage in human antineutrophil cytoplasmic autoantibody associated pauci-immune vasculitis. *J Clin Immunol.* 2009;29(3):282–291.

97. Primo VC, Marusic S, Franklin CC, et al. Anti-PR3 immune responses induce segmental and necrotizing glomerulonephritis. *Clin Exp Immunol.* 2010;159(3):327–337.

98. Kain R, Exner M, Brandes R, et al. Molecular mimicry in pauci-immune focal necrotizing glomerulonephritis. *Nat Med.* 2008;14(10):1088–1096.

99. Pendergraft WF, Preston GA, Shah RR, et al. Autoimmunity is triggered by cPR-3(105-201), a protein complementary to human autoantigen proteinase-3. *Nat Med.* 2004;10:72–79.

100. Preston GA, Pendergraft WF III, Falk RJ. New insights that link microbes with the generation of neutrophil cytoplasmic autoantibodies: the theory of autoantigen complementarity. *Curr Opin Nephrol Hypertens.* 2005;14:217–222.

101. Bautz DJ, Preston GA, Lionaki S, et al. Antibodies with dual reactivity to plasminogen and complementary PR3 in PR3-ANCA vasculitis. *J Am Soc Nephrol.* 2008;19(12):2421–2429.

102. Chen M, Kallenberg CG, Zhao MH. ANCA-negative pauci-immune crescentic glomerulonephritis. *Nat Rev Nephrol.* 2009;5(6):313–318.

103. Tipping PG, Holdsworth SR. T cells in crescentic glomerulonephritis. *J Am Soc Nephrol.* 2006;17(5):1253–1263.

104. Cunningham MA, Huang XR, Dowling JP, et al. Prominence of cell-mediated immunity effectors in "pauci-immune" glomerulonephritis. *J Am Soc Nephrol.* 1999;10:499–506.

105. Nogueira E, Hamour S, Sawant D, et al. Serum IL-17 and IL-23 levels and autoantigen-specific Th17 cells are elevated in patients with ANCA associated vasculitis. *Nephrol Dial Transplant.* 2010;25(7):2209–2217.

106. King WJ, Brooks CJ, Holder R, et al. T lymphocyte responses to anti-neutrophil cytoplasmic autoantibody (ANCA) antigens are present in patients with ANCA-associated systemic vasculitis and persist during disease remission. *Clin Exp Immunol.* 1998;112(3):539–546.

107. Brouwer E, Stegeman CA, Huitema MG, et al. T cell reactivity to proteinase 3 and myeloperoxidase in patients with Wegener's granulomatosis (WG). *Clin Exp Immunol.* 1994; 98(3):448–453.

108. Yang J, Bautz DJ, Lionaki S, et al. ANCA patients have T cells responsive to complementary PR-3 antigen. *Kidney Int.* 2008;74(9):1159–1169.

109. Gan PY, Steinmetz OM, Tan DS, et al. Th17 cells promote autoimmune anti-myeloperoxidase glomerulonephritis. *J Am Soc Nephrol.* 2010;21(6):925–931.

110. Chavele KM, Shukla D, Keteepe-Arachi T, et al. Regulation of myeloperoxidase-specific T cell responses during disease remission in ant neutrophil cytoplasmic antibody-associated vasculitis: the role of Treg cells and tryptophan degradation. *Arthritis Rheum.* 2010 May;62(5):1539–1540.

111. Nasr SH, D'Agati VD, Park HR, et al. Necrotizing and crescentic lupus nephritis with antineutrophil cytoplasmic antibody seropositivity. *Clin J Am Soc Nephrol.* 2008;3(3):682–690.

112. Nasr SH, Said SM, Valeri AM, et al. Membranous glomerulonephritis with ANCA-associated necrotizing and crescentic glomerulonephritis. *Clin J Am Soc Nephrol.* 2009;4(2):299–308.

113. Markowitz GS, D'Agati VD. Classification of lupus nephritis. *Curr Opin Nephrol Hypertens.* 2009;18(3):220–225.

114. Rahman A, Isenberg DA. Systemic lupus erythematosus. *N Engl J Med.* 2008;358:929–939.

115. Crispín JC, Liossis SN, Kis-Toth K, et al. Pathogenesis of human systemic lupus erythematosus: recent advances. *Trends Mol Med.* 2010;16(2):47–57.

116. Mortensen ES, Rekvig OP. Nephritogenic potential of anti-DNA antibodies against necrotic nucleosomes. *J Am Soc Nephrol.* 2009;20(4):696–704.

117. Waldman M, Madaio MP. Pathogenic autoantibodies in lupus nephritis. *Lupus.* 2005;14(1):19–24.

118. Yanase K, Madaio MP. Nuclear localizing anti-DNA antibodies enter cells via caveoli and modulate expression of caveolin and p53. *J Autoimmun.* 2005;24(2):145–151.

119. Yung S, Cheung KF, Zhang Q, et al. Anti-dsDNA antibodies bind to mesangial annexin II in lupus nephritis. *J Am Soc Nephrol.* 2010;21(11):1912–1927.

120. Martinez-Valle F, Balada E, Ordi-Ros J, et al. DNase1 activity in systemic lupus erythematosus patients with and without nephropathy. *Rheumatol Int.* 2010;30(12):1601–1604.

121. Pawar RD, Patole PS, Ellwart A, et al. Ligands to nucleic acid-specific toll-like receptors and the onset of lupus nephritis. *J Am Soc Nephrol.* 2006;17(12): 3365–3373.

122. Smith KD. Lupus nephritis: Toll the trigger! *J Am Soc Nephrol.* 2006;17(12): 3273–3275.

123. Shen Y, Chen XW, Sun CY, et al. Association between anti-beta2 glycoprotein I antibodies and renal glomerular C4d deposition in lupus nephritis patients with glomerular microthrombosis: a prospective study of 155 cases. *Lupus.* 2010;19(10):1195–1203.

124. Pickering MC, Botto M. Are anti-C1q antibodies different from other SLE autoantibodies? *Nat Rev Rheumatol.* 2010;6(8):490–493.

125. Charles N, Hardwick D, Daugas E, et al. Basophils and the T helper 2 environment can promote the development of lupus nephritis. *Nat Med.* 2010;16(6):701–707.

126. Marston B, Looney RJ. Connective tissue diseases: Translating the effects of BAFF in SLE. *Nat Rev Rheumatol.* 2010;6(9):503–504.

127. Bao L, Quigg RJ. Complement in lupus nephritis: the good, the bad, and the unknown. *Semin Nephrol.* 2007;27(1):69–80.

128. Bao L, Haas M, Quigg RJ. Complement factor H deficiency accelerates development of lupus nephritis. *J Am Soc Nephrol.* 2011;22(2):285–295.

129. Lu L, Kaliyaperumal A, Boumpas DT, et al. Major peptide autoepitopes for nucleosome-specific T cells of human lupus. *J Clin Invest.* 1999;104(3):345–355.

130. Apostolidis SA, Crispín JC, Tsokos GC. IL-17-producing T cells in lupus nephritis. *Lupus.* 2011;20(2):120–124.

131. Valencia X, Yarboro C, Illei G, et al. Deficient CD4+CD25high T regulatory cell function in patients with active systemic lupus erythematosus. *J Immunol.* 2007;178(4):2579–2588.

132. Strickland FM, Richardson BC. Epigenetics in human autoimmunity. Epigenetics in autoimmunity—DNA methylation in systemic lupus erythematosus and beyond. *Autoimmunity.* 2008;41(4):278–286.

133. Coleman TH, Forristal J, Kosaka T, et al. Inherited complement component deficiencies in membranoproliferative glomerulonephritis. *Kidney Int.* 1983;24(5):681–690.

134. Vuong MT, Gunnarsson I, Lundberg S, et al. Genetic risk factors in lupus nephritis and IgA nephropathy—no support of an overlap. *PLoS One.* 2010;5(5):e10559.

135. Kraft SW, Schwartz MM, Korbet SM, et al. Glomerular podocytopathy in patients with systemic lupus erythematosus. *J Am Soc Nephrol.* 2005;16(1):175–179.

136. Alpers CA, Smith KD. Cryoglobulinemia and renal disease. *Curr Opin Nephrol Hypertens.* 2008;17(3):243–249.

137. Alchi B, Jayne D. Membranoproliferative glomerulonephritis. *Pediatr Nephrol.* 2010;25(8):1409–1418.

138. Vernon KA, Pickering MC, Cook HT. Experimental models of membranoproliferative glomerulonephritis, including dense deposit disease. *Contrib Nephrol*. 2011;169:198–210.
139. Sethi S, Zand L, Leung N, et al. Membranoproliferative glomerulonephritis secondary to monoclonal gammopathy. *Clin J Am Soc Nephrol*. 2010; 5(5):770–782.
140. Johnson RJ, Gretch DR, Yamabe H, et al. Membranoproliferative glomerulonephritis associated with hepatitis C virus infection. *N Engl J Med*. 1993;328(7):465–470.
141. Charles ED, Dustin EB. Hepatitis C virus-induced cryoglobulinemia. *Kidney Int*. 2009;76(8):818–824.
142. Sansonno D, Gesualdo L, Manno C, et al. Hepatitis C virus-related proteins in kidney tissue from hepatitis C virus-infected patients with cryoglobulinemic membranoproliferative glomerulonephritis. *Hepatology*. 1997;25(5):1237–1244.
143. Sansonno D, Lauletta G, Nisi L, et al. Non-enveloped HCV core protein as constitutive antigen of cold-precipitable immune complexes in type II mixed cryoglobulinaemia. *Clin Exp Immunol*. 2003;133(2):275–282.
144. Sansonno D, Tucci FA, Ghebrehiwet B, et al. Role of the receptor for the globular domain of C1q protein in the pathogenesis of hepatitis C virus-related cryoglobulin vascular damage. *J Immunol*. 2009;183(9):6013–6020.
145. Allam R, Anders HJ. The role of innate immunity in autoimmune tissue injury. *Curr Opin Rheumatol*. 2008;20(5):538–544.
146. Robson MG. Toll-like receptors and renal disease. *Nephron Exp Nephrol*. 2009;113(1):e1–e7.
147. Pawar RD, Patole PS, Zecher D, et al. Toll-like receptor-7 modulates immune complex glomerulonephritis. *J Am Soc Nephrol*. 2006;17(1):141–149.
148. Mühlfeld AS, Segerer S, Hudkins K, et al. Overexpression of complement inhibitor Crry does not prevent cryoglobulin-associated membranoproliferative glomerulonephritis. *Kidney Int*. 2004;65(4):1214–1223.
149. Cho MH, Hong EH, Lee TH, et al. Pathophysiology of minimal change nephrotic syndrome and focal segmental glomerulosclerosis. *Nephrology (Carlton)*. 2007;12 Suppl 3:S11–S14.
150. Waldman M, Crew RJ, Valeri A, et al. Adult minimal-change disease: clinical characteristics, treatment, and outcomes. *Clin J Amer Soc Nephrol*. 2007;2(3):445–453.
151. Ritz E, Amann K, Koleganova N, et al. Prenatal programming—effects on blood pressure and renal function. *Nat Rev Nephrol*. 2011 Mar;7(3):137–144.
152. Zhang SY, Audard V, Fan Q, et al. Immunopathogenesis of idiopathic nephrotic syndrome. *Contrib Nephrol*. 2011;169:94–106.
153. Shalhoub RJ. Pathogenesis of lipoid nephrosis: a disorder of T-cell function. *Lancet*. 1974;2(7880):556–560.
154. Koyama A, Fujisaki M, Kobayashi M, et al. A glomerular permeability factor produced by human T cell hybridomas. *Kidney Int*. 1991;40(3):453–460.
155. McCarthy ET, Sharma M, Savin VJ. Circulating permeability factors in idiopathic nephrotic syndrome and focal segmental glomerulosclerosis. *Clin J Am Soc Nephrol*. 2010;5(11):2115–2121.
156. Mauer SM, Hellerstein S, Cohn RA, et al. Recurrence of steroid-responsive nephrotic syndrome after renal transplantation. *J Pediatr*. 1979;95(2):261–264.
157. Ali AA, Wilson E, Moorhead JF, et al. Minimal-change glomerular nephritis. Normal kidneys in an abnormal environment? *Transplantation*. 1994; 58(7): 849–852.
158. Rea R, Smith C, Sandhu K, et al. Successful transplant of a kidney with focal segmental glomerulosclerosis. *Nephrol Dial Transplant*. 2001;16(2):416–417.
159. Wei C, Möller CC, Altintas MM, et al. Modification of kidney barrier function by the urokinase receptor. *Nat Med*. 2008;14(1):55–63.
160. Tain YL, Chen TY, Yang KD. Implications of serum TNF-beta and IL-13 in the treatment response of childhood nephrotic syndrome. *Cytokine*. 2003;21(3):155–159.
161. Lai KW, Wei CL, Tan LK, et al. Overexpression of interleukin-13 induces minimal-change-like nephropathy in rats. *J Am Soc Nephrol*. 2007;18(5): 1476–1485.
162. Sellier-Leclerc AL, Duval A, Riveron S, et al. A humanized mouse model of idiopathic nephrotic syndrome suggests a pathogenic role for immature cells. *J Am Soc Nephrol*. 2007;18(10):2732–2739.
163. Reiser J, von Gersdorff G, Loos M, et al. Induction of B7-1 in podocytes is associated with nephrotic syndrome. *J Clin Invest*. 2004;113(10):1390–1397.
164. Garin EH, Mu W, Arthur JM, et al. Urinary CD80 is elevated in minimal change disease but not in focal segmental glomerulosclerosis. *Kidney Int*. 2010;78(3):296–302.
165. Navarro-Muñoz M, Ibernon M, Pérez V, et al. Messenger RNA expression of B7-1 and NPHS1 in urinary sediment could be useful to differentiate between minimal-change disease and focal segmental glomerulosclerosis in adult patients. *Nephrol Dial Transplant*. 2011;26(12):3914–3923.
166. Shimada M, Araya C, Rivard C, et al. Minimal change disease: a “two-hit” podocyte immune disorder? *Pediatr Nephrol*. 2011;26(4):645–649.
167. Clement LC, Avila-Casado C, Macé C, et al. Podocyte-secreted angiopoietin-like-4 mediates proteinuria in glucocorticoid-sensitive nephrotic syndrome. *Nat Med*. 2011;17(1):117–122.
168. Fervenza FC, Sethi S, Specks U. Idiopathic membranous nephropathy: diagnosis and treatment. *Clin J Am Soc Nephrol*. 2008; 3(3):905–919.
169. Ronco P, Debiec H. Target antigens and nephritogenic antibodies in membranous nephropathy: of rats and men. *Semin Immunopathol*. 2007;29(4): 445–458.
170. Nangaku M, Couser WG. Mediators of renal injury in membranous nephropathy. *Arch Med Sci*. 2009;5(3A):S451–458.
171. Pippin JW, Durvasula R, Petermann A, et al. DNA damage is a novel response to sublytic complement C5b-9-induced injury in podocytes. *J Clin Invest*. 2003;111(6):877–885.
172. Debiec H, Guigonis V, Mougenot B, et al. Antenatal membranous glomerulonephritis due to anti-neutral endopeptidase antibodies. *N Engl J Med*. 2002;346(26):2053–2060.
173. Beck LH Jr, Bonegio RG, Lambeau G, et al. M-type phospholipase A2 receptor as target antigen in idiopathic membranous nephropathy. *N Engl J Med*. 2009;361(1):11–21.
174. Hofstra JM, Beck LH Jr, Beck DM, et al. Anti-phospholipase A_2 receptor antibodies correlate with clinical status in idiopathic membranous nephropathy. *Clin J Am Soc Nephrol*. 2011;6(6):1286–1291.
175. Prunotto M, Carnevali ML, Candiano G, et al. Autoimmunity in membranous nephropathy targets aldose reductase and SOD2. *J Am Soc Nephrol*. 2010;21(3):507–519.
176. Debiec H, Ronco P. PLA2R autoantibodies and PLA2R glomerular deposits in membranous nephropathy. *N Engl J Med*. 2011;364(7):689–690.
177. Debiec H, Lefeu, F, Kemper MJ, et al. Early-childhood membranous nephropathy due to cationic bovine serum albumin. *N Engl J Med*. 2011;364(22): 2101–2110.
178. Groggel GC, Adler S, Rennke HG, et al. Role of the terminal complement pathway in experimental membranous nephropathy in the rabbit. *J Clin Invest*. 1983;72(6):1948–1957.
179. Couser WG, Ochi RF, Baker PJ, et al. C6 depletion reduces proteinuria in experimental nephropathy induced by a nonglomerular antigen. *J Am Soc Nephrol*. 1991;2(4):894–901.
180. Salant DJ, Madaio MP, Adler S, et al. Altered glomerular permeability induced by F(ab')2 and Fab' antibodies to rat renal tubular epithelial antigen. *Kidney Int*. 1982;21(1):36–43.
181. Leenaerts PL, Hall BM, Van Damme BJ, et al. Active Heymann nephritis in complement component C6 deficient rats. *Kidney Int*. 1995;47(6):1604–1614.
182. Spicer ST, Tran GT, Killingsworth MC, et al. Induction of passive Heymann nephritis in complement component 6-deficient PVG rats. *J Immunol*. 2007;179(1):172–178.
183. Couser WG, Cattran D, Membranous nephropathy. In: Johnson RJ, Feehally J, Floege J, eds. *Comprehensive Clinical Nephrology*. 4th ed. London, England: Mosby International Publishers; 2010: 248–259.
184. Schiller B, He C, Salant DJ, et al. Inhibition of complement regulation is key to the pathogenesis of active Heymann nephritis. *J Exp Med*. 1998;188(7): 1353–1358.
185. Pruchno CJ, Burns MM, Schulze M, et al. Urinary excretion of the C5b-9 membrane attack complex of complement is a marker of immune disease activity in autologous immune complex nephritis. *Am J Pathol*. 1991;138(1):203–211.
186. Schulze M, Pruchno CJ, Burns M, et al. Glomerular C3c localization indicates ongoing immune deposit formation and complement activation in experimental glomerulonephritis. *Am J Pathol*. 1993;142(1):179–187.
187. Penny MJ, Boyd RA, Hall BM. Role of T cells in the mediation of Heymann nephritis. II. Identification of Th1 and cytotoxic cells in glomeruli. *Kidney Int*. 1997;51(4):1059–1068.
188. Penny MJ, Boyd RA, Hall BM. Permanent $CD8^{(+)}$ T cell depletion prevents proteinuria in active Heymann nephritis. *J Exp Med*. 1998;188(10):1775–1784.
189. Couser WG, Stilmant MM, Darby C. Autologous immune complex nephropathy. I. Sequential study of immune complex deposition, ultrastructural changes, proteinuria, and alterations in glomerular sialoprotein. *Lab Invest*. 1976;34(1):23–30.
190. Stanescu HC, Arcos-Burgos M, Medlar A, et al. Risk HLA-DQA1 and PLA(2)R1 alleles in idiopathic membranous nephropathy. *N Engl J Med*. 2011;364(7):616–626.
191. Qin W, Beck LH Jr, Zeng C, et al. Anti-phospholipase A2 receptor antibody in membranous nephropathy. *J Am Soc Nephrol*. 2011;22(6):1137–1143.
192. Alchi B, Jayne D. Membranoproliferative glomerulonephritis. *Pediatr Nephrol*. 2010;25(8):1409–1418.
193. Smith RJ, Harris CL, Pickering MC. Dense deposit disease. *Mol Immunol*. 2011;48(14):1604–1610.

194. Servais A, Frémeaux-Bacchi V, Lequintrec M, et al. Primary glomerulonephritis with isolated C3 deposits: a new entity which shares common genetic risk factors with haemolytic uraemic syndrome. *J Med Genet.* 2007;44(3):193–199.
195. Fakhouri F, Frémeaux-Bacchi V, Noël LH, et al. C3 glomerulopathy: a new classification. *Nat Rev Nephrol.* 2010;6(8):494–499.
196. Sethi S, Fervenza FC, Zhang Y, et al. Proliferative glomerulonephritis secondary to dysfunction of the alternative pathway of complement. *Clin J Am Soc Nephrol.* 2011;6(5):1009–1017.
197. Falk RJ, Sisson SP, Dalmasso AP, et al. Ultrastructural localization of the membrane attack complex of complement in human renal tissues. *Am J Kidney Dis.* 1987;9(2):121–128.
198. Noris M, Remuzzi G. Translational mini-review series on complement factor H: Therapies of renal diseases associated with complement factor H abnormalities: atypical haemolytic uraemic syndrome and membranoproliferative glomerulonephritis. *Clin Exp Immunol.* 2007;151(2):199–209.
199. Strobel S, Zimmering M, Papp K, et al. Anti-factor B autoantibody in dense deposit disease. *Mol Immunol.* 2010;47(7–8):1476–1483.
200. Sethi S, Gamez JD, Vrana JA, et al. Glomeruli of dense deposit disease contain components of the alternative and terminal complement pathway. *Kidney Int.* 2009;75(9):952–960.
201. Athanasiou Y, Voskarides K, Gale DP, et al. Familial C3 glomerulopathy associated with CFHR5 mutations: clinical characteristics of 91 patients in 16 pedigrees. *Clin J Am Soc Nephrol.* 2011 Jun;6(6):1436–1446.

CHAPTER 46

Acute Infectious Glomerulonephritis Including Poststreptococcal and Other Bacterial Infection–Related Glomerulonephritis

Laura L. Mulloy • Michael P. Madaio

Acute glomerulonephritis is characterized by the sudden appearance of hematuria, proteinuria, and red blood cell (RBC) casts. The differential diagnosis of this syndrome is listed in Table 46.1. The initial diagnostic approach includes clinical evaluation and serologic determinations, which can be classified as those diseases associated with a low versus a normal serum complement level. Histologic evaluation is very useful in confirming the diagnosis and defining the extent of inflammation and fibrosis. This chapter considers glomerulonephritis associated with bacterial infections. Glomerular diseases associated with other organisms are covered in subsequent chapters. Acute poststreptococcal glomerulonephritis (APSGN) is the prototype; however, the incidence has declined in industrialized countries over the last 50 years.[1] Furthermore, because other bacterial, viral, and parasitic organisms can be associated with acute glomerulonephritis, the term "acute postinfectious glomerulonephritis" (APIGN) is more appropriate.[2] The disease spectrum is also changing, involving more adults and fewer children.[3] The prevalence has also increased in diabetics, intravenous drug abusers, and alcoholics.[4]

The initial discussion focuses on APSGN, followed by consideration of other bacterial infections, with particular emphasis of APIGN associated with staphylococci. APSGN is distinguished from the other causes of acute glomerulonephritis by its characteristic serologic, histologic, and chronologic features. A link between streptococci and acute glomerulonephritis can be traced to epidemics of scarlet fever in the 18th century.[5] During the earlier part of the 20th century, it was recognized that infection with β-hemolytic streptococci could lead to glomerulonephritis.[5–8] Since this discovery, the clinical presentation and histologic features of the disease have been carefully documented, and considerable progress has been made in identifying the pathogenic mechanisms involved.

ACUTE POSTSTREPTOCOCCAL GLOMERULONEPHRITIS

Epidemiology and Incidence

APSGN is most prevalent in developing countries,[9] and it may occur sporadically or in epidemic form. Although the sporadic form is more common, analysis of epidemics has been particularly revealing.[10–25] It affects children more than adults, with peak age from 2 to 6 years (Table 46.2). Approximately 5% of cases are found among children younger than 2 years, with a slightly greater incidence (5%–10%) in adults older than 40. Spread between family members is common, and nephritogenic streptococci have been isolated from household pets.[26] Males have overt nephritis more commonly, and females tend to have more subclinical disease.[15,27] Cases of subclinical nephritis outnumber those of overt nephritis (4:1 to 10:1).[2,28] In temperate zones, APSGN occurs more commonly in winter months, and typically after pharyngitis; whereas in the tropics, skin infections during the summer are the initiating event.[29] Cyclical outbreaks of epidemic forms have been observed, although the reason for these cycles has not been fully explained.[21,30,31]

APSGN follows infection with only certain groups of streptococci, termed "nephritogenic." Group A streptococci are responsible for the majority of cases, and certain types predominate.[5,32,33] Nephritogenic group A streptococci have been characterized serologically by their cell wall proteins, M and T.[5,34–40] The risk of nephritis following infection with nephritogenic strains depends on the location of infection. For example, with type-49 streptococci, the risk of nephritis is five times greater with skin infections than with pharyngitis.

Nephritis following pyoderma with types 47, 55, 57, and 60 is also common.[5,15] The identification of nephritogenic strains suggests that there are factors unique to these

TABLE 46.1 **Major Causes of Acute Nephritis**

Low Serum Complement Level[a]	Normal Serum Complement Level
Systemic Diseases	**Systemic Diseases**
Systemic lupus erythematosus (focal ∼75%, diffuse ∼90%)[a]	Polyarteritis nodosa
	Wegener granulomatosis
Cryoglobulinemia (∼85%)	Hypersensitivity vasculitis
Subacute bacterial endocarditis (∼90%)	Henoch-Schönlein purpura
	Goodpasture syndrome
"Shunt" nephritis (∼90%)	Visceral abscess
Renal Diseases	**Renal Diseases**
Acute poststreptococcal glomerulonephritis (∼90%)	IgG-IgA nephropathy
	Idiopathic rapidly progressive glomerulonephritis
Membranoproliferative glomerulonephritis	Anti-glomerular basement membrane disease
Type I (∼50%–80%)[b]	Pauci-immune[c] (no immune deposits)
Type II (∼80%–90%)	Immune-deposit disease

Normal serum complement levels indicate that production of complement components is keeping up with consumption; it does not exclude participation of complement in the inflammatory process. Repeat measurements useful (2 to 3 × 1 week apart). Consistently normal serum levels are useful in narrowing the diagnostic possibilities.

[a]Percentages indicate the approximate frequencies of depressed C3 or hemolytic complement levels during the course of disease.

[b]Most common pathologic findings associated with hepatitis C infection.

[c]Pauci-immune indicates lack of significant glomerular deposition of immunoglobulin by direct immunofluorescence. Many patients have circulating ANCA.

Reprinted with permission from Madaio MP, Harrington JT. The diagnosis of glomerular diseases: acute glomerulonephritis and the nephrotic syndrome. *Arch Intern Med.* 2001;161.

strains that are pathogenically relevant (see later). However, host factors also play a role, as only approximately 10% of patients infected with nephritogenic strains develop overt disease. ASPGN has been reported following renal transplantation, although these patients are at no greater risk for the disease.[41]

Pathology (Table 46.3, Fig. 46.1)

Typically there is diffuse glomerulonephritis, with variable severity.[41,44,56,60–62] On light microscopy, there is cellular infiltration and glomerular cellular proliferation.[63] The predominant cell types depend on the timing of the biopsy. Within the first 2 weeks of disease, neutrophils, eosinophils, lymphocytes, and monocytes are present in the capillary lumen and in the mesangium, and endothelial and mesangial cell proliferation is prominent.[5,35,42] CD4 T cells usually exceed CD8 cells early on, whereas later CD8 cells predominate. Periglomerular accumulation of T cells may also be observed.[45] Occlusion of capillary lumen is not unusual, and mesangial expansion is typical.[44] Intracapillary fibrin thrombi and deposits and/or necrosis are observed in some cases. This pattern characterizes the so-called "exudative phase." During this period, intermittent thickening of capillary walls, corresponding to large subepithelial immune deposits, or "humps," are often observed (i.e., by trichrome staining). Focal capsular adhesions or segmental crescents are relatively common. Abundant crescent formation is unusual, but has been seen in more severe situations.[5,46] Over 4 to 6 weeks, polymorphonuclear neutrophils (PMNs) are no longer present, and hypercellularity with mononuclear cells (mesangial cells and/or infiltrating monocytes) predominates. During this latter phase, capillary lumens are usually patent. Glomerular hypercellularity usually slowly resolves, although mesangial hypercellularity may persist for months. Extraglomerular abnormalities are usually not as prominent

TABLE 46.2 **General Characteristics Of APSGN**

Age: Children > adults (5% < 2 years; 5% to 10% > 40 years)
Sex: Male > Female
Clinical manifestations: subclinical 4–10 × > overt nephritis
Site of infection: pharynx (temperate zones), skin (tropics)

TABLE 46.3 Pathology of APSGN

Light Microscopy

Diffuse proliferative glomerulonephritis

First 2 weeks (Exudative phase)
- Capillary lume: neutrophils, eosinophils, lymphocytes, monocytes
- Mesangial, endothelial cell, mesangial cell proliferation[5,35,42,43]
- Mesangial expansion typical; occasional occlusion of capillary lumen[44]
- CD4 T cells > CD8; occasional peri-glomerular[45]

Intracapillary fibrin thrombi and/or necrosis (less common)

Focal capsular adhesions or segmental crescents (relatively common; abundant crescents unusual[5,46,47])

Capillary wall thickening (second to subepithelial immune deposits, "humps")

Interstitial edema, ATN

Late phase (4 to 6 weeks)

Glomerular hypercellularity (second mesangial cells and monocytes) slowly resolves
- Interstitial infiltrates, and/or mild arteriolitis may be observed in either phase.[48] Severe vasculitis has been reported but is unusual.[49–51]

Immunofluorescence
- IgG, C3 diffuse granular/mesangial and capillary walls
- IgG disappears before C3
- IgM early, resolves slowly
- Properdin, (C5b-9) granular pattern, fibrin in severe cases
- Starry sky pattern of deposits associated with hypercellularity[52–55]
- Rope or garlandlike pattern: mesangial deposits with disease resolution[53–55]; persistent deposits associated with proteinuria and glomulerulosclerosis
- Significant IgA suggests IgAN or HSP
- Deposits in small vessels associated with vasculitis

Electron Microscopy
- Dome-shaped subepithelial electron-dense deposits resemble camel "humps"; (hallmark)[42]
- Most abundant in first month near slit pores[12,55–57] with proteinuria
- Remnant electron-lucent areas provide diagnostic clues[58]
- Subendothelial, mesangial, intramembranous deposits and smaller subepithelial deposits variably present and persist after resolution of subepithelial humps[58]
- Large subendothelial deposits associated with proteinuria and edema[59]
- Large intramembranous deposits associated with garlandlike pattern[55]
- GBM typically normal thickness[48]

ATN, acute tubular necrosis; GBM, glomerular basement membrane; HSP, Henoch-Schönlein purpura.

during either phase; however, interstitial edema, tubular necrosis, scattered mononuclear interstitial infiltrates, and/or mild arteriolitis have been observed.[48] Severe vasculitis has been reported but is unusual.[49–51]

By immunofluorescence microscopy, deposits of immunoglobulin G (IgG) and C3 are distributed in a diffuse granular pattern within the mesangium and capillary walls.[44,53–55,64] C3 is invariably present, whereas the quantity of IgG depends on the timing of the biopsy, and it is not uncommon to see only C3 deposits very early or late in disease. IgM can be present early in disease but may also be observed in smaller amounts later on. Significant amounts of IgA suggest an alternative diagnosis (e.g., IgA nephropathy or Henoch-Schönlein purpura). C1q and C4 are not usually detected; however, properdin and terminal complement components (C5b-9) are often present and in a granular pattern. Fibrin deposits can be detected in more severe cases. Different patterns of immune deposition have been observed, usually related to the timing of the renal biopsy. Early in the disease (the first few weeks), the fine granular appearance of immune deposits resemble a "starry-sky" appearance; this pattern is associated with glomerular hypercellularity.[53–55] With resolution of the disease (after 4–6 weeks), the immune deposits take on a more mesangial pattern, prior to

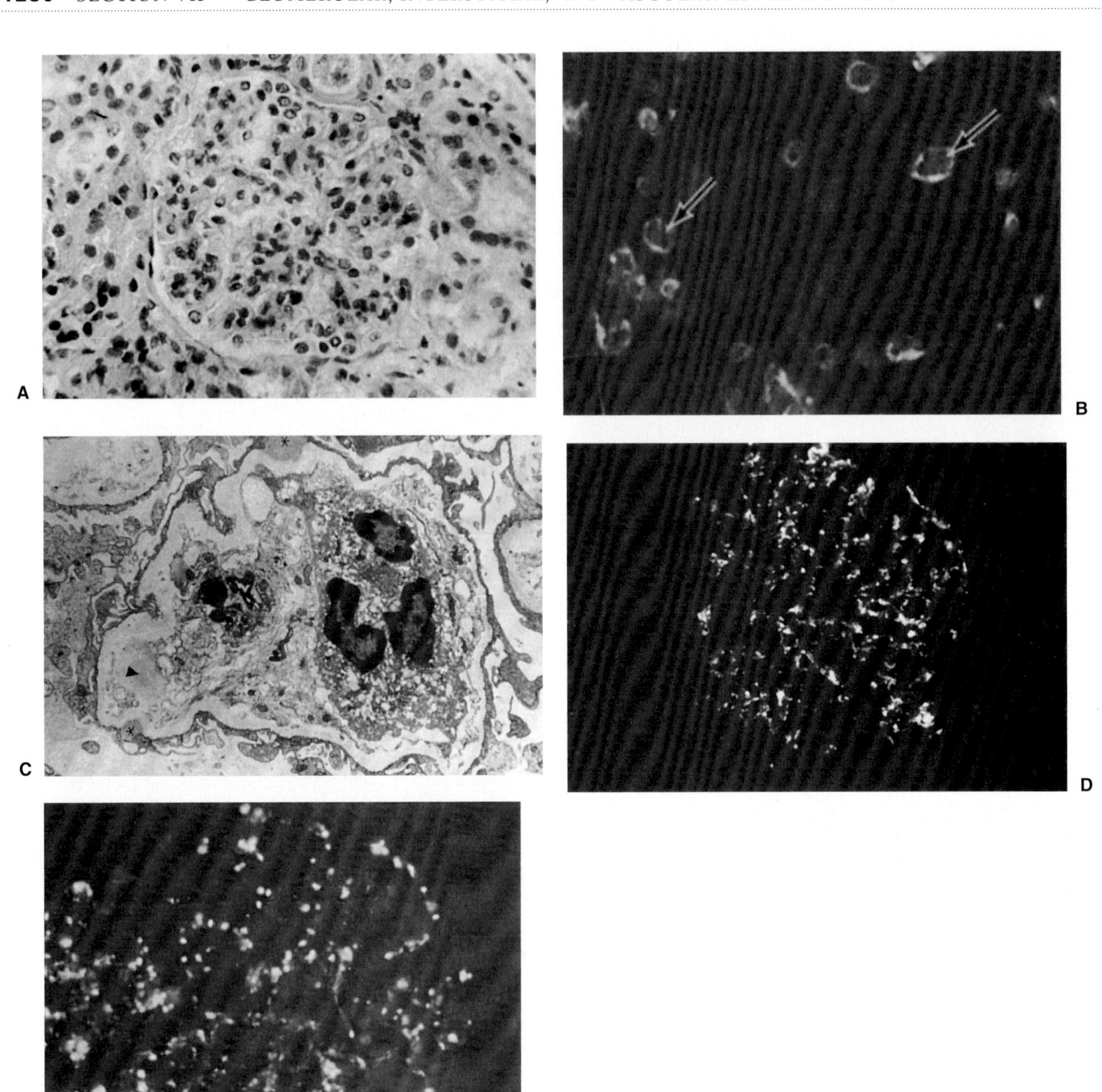

FIGURE 46.1 Pathology of poststreptococcal glomerulonephritis. **A:** Endocapillary proliferation with increased number of mesangial cells and glomerular infiltration with neutrophils (PMN). Biopsy specimen taken 10 days after the beginning of symptoms. (Hematoxylin & eosin ×500.) **B:** Intraglomerular cells reactive with OKM1 monoclonal antibody (*arrows*) in a biopsy specimen obtained 14 days after the initial symptoms. Monocytes and neutrophils are recognized by the antibody, and reactivity with antihuman lactoferrin (which identifies PMN) in serial sections was used to define glomerular monocyte infiltration. **C:** Glomerular capillary loop with PMNs in the lumen. Electron-dense deposits are present in subepithelial ("humps") (*) and subendothelial (<) locations. (×12,000). **D:** C3 deposits (+1) in the glomerular basement membranes and mesangium. (FITC-labeled antihuman ×500.) **E:** Glomerular deposition of the membrane attack complex of complement in a biopsy specimen obtained 16 days after onset identified with monoclonal poly-C9 antibody, which recognizes a neoantigen on C9. Pattern and localization of deposits is similar to the one found for C3 and C5. (**B** and **E** reproduced with permission from Parra G, Platt JL, Falk RJ, et al. Cell populations and membrane attack complex in glomeruli of patients with post streptococcal glomerulonephritis: identification using monoclonal antibodies by indirect immunofluorescence. *Clin Immunol Immunopathol.* 1984;33:324.)

disappearing. C3 may be present in the absence of detectable Ig, either very early in the disease (less than 2 weeks) or with disease resolution (i.e., with resolution of the IgG deposits). In about one fourth of cases, the deposits are large, and they aggregate in a rope or garlandlike pattern, and this pattern may be associated with persistent mesangial hypercellularity on light microscopy. When these type deposits are present, they may last for months and be associated with heavy proteinuria and development of glomerulosclerosis.[52–55] By contrast, transition to a mesangial pattern is usually associated with clinical and pathologic resolution. Immune deposits in small vessels may occur in the setting of vasculitis.

Dome-shaped subepithelial electron-dense Ig deposits, which resemble camel "humps," are the hallmark feature on electron microscopy.[42] These humps are most abundant within the first month, and frequently observed near epithelial slit pores.[12,55–57] They have been associated with heavy proteinuria, and resolve within 4 to 8 weeks. In later stages of the disease, they may be absent; however, remnant electron-lucent areas are occasionally observed and provide diagnostic clues.[58] Subendothelial, mesangial, and intramembranous deposits (along with smaller subepithelial deposits) are often present in variable amounts, and they usually persist after resolution of subepithelial humps.[58] Patients with large subendothelial deposits, without mesangial deposits, were found to have more proteinuria and edema.[59] Large intramembranous deposits are associated with the garlandlike pattern of immune deposits.[55] The basement membrane is usually of normal diameter, although thickening has occasionally been observed.[48] Cellular infiltration and proliferation relates to the timing of the biopsy, as described.

Pathophysiology

The association of APSGN with streptococcal infections from nephritogenic group A β-hemolytic streptococcus (GAS) implies that there are unique properties of these bacterial strains. Nevertheless, not all individuals infected with nephritogenic streptococci develop disease, suggesting that host factors are also important for disease expression. Four major mechanisms pertaining to the pathogenesis have been proposed, and they may be operative to varying degrees in individual patients. These mechanisms are summarized in Table 46.4.

Other factors may also contribute to disease susceptibility. Outbreaks among families during epidemics provide clues[27,61,83]; however, in contrast to rheumatic fever,[84] studies have thus far failed to support linkage. Nevertheless, bacterial systemic and host factors likely influence the specific characteristics and severity of disease,[45,55,85–87] and

TABLE 46.4 **Pathogenesis of APSGN**

1. **In situ immune complex formation.** Cell wall antigens (i.e., M proteins) from nephritogenic strains bind directly to glomeruli and activate the alternative complement pathway to initiate injury. Subsequently, antistreptococcal antibodies bind to glomerular-bound streptococcal antigens, leading to recruitment of polymorphonuclear leukocytes and mononuclear cells to amplify local inflammation via FcR engagement and classical complement activation. Candidate streptococcal antigens include: nephritis-associated plasmin receptor a glycolytic enzyme with glyceraldehyde-3–phosphate dehydrogenase (NAPIr-GAPDH) activity and streptococcal pyrogenic exotoxin B (SPE B) nephritis plasmin binding protein (NPBP), streptococcal pyrogenic exotoxin B precursor (SPE B), cationic proteinase produced by nephritogenic streptococci (related to an erythrogenic toxin),[65] heparin-inhabitable basement membrane binding protein,[66] streptococcal-derived kidney binding proteins,[67] and streptokinase.[43,67,68]
2. **Molecular Mimicry.** Antistreptococcal antibodies react with glomerular antigens,[36,69–71] including matrix and cell wall antigens.[36] Through either shared primary sequence homology or tertiary structure.[72–75]
3. **Altered IgG.** Streptococcal enzymes modify normal IgG; subsequently the altered IgG (a) elicits an immune response and (b) localizes in glomeruli (e.g., through charge-charge interactions).[76] Antibodies versus the deposited/altered IgG bind to the fixed or "planted" glomerular antigen to initiate inflammation.[77,78] In support of this mechanism: neuraminidase-producing streptococci desialate of IgG (making it more cationic),[79,80] elevated levels of serum rheumatoid factor, neuraminidase activity and free sialic acid are often present in patients with APSGN, and anti-Ig antibodies have been eluted from the kidney of a patient with this disease.[79,80] However, neuraminidase-producing streptococci are not unique to APSGN patients, and rheumatoid factor activity is present in many individuals with streptococcal infection who do not develop glomerulonephritis.
4. **Deposition of circulating streptococcal antigen-anti-streptococcal antibody immune complexes** (i.e., deposition based on affinity of exposed and complexed streptococcal protein fragments for glomeruli). Likely has a role in amplifying local inflammatory response, once disease is established.[81,82]

the relative role of host factors in glomerulonephritis is discussed in Chapter 48.

Clinical Manifestations (Table 46.5)

The symptoms of the disease are characteristic; however, most patients present with only a few features of the *acute nephritic syndrome*.[88] Typical presentations include edema, gross hematuria, and hypertension.[5,11,12,14,15,17,21,25,61,64,89] Anasarca is more common among children.[5] Occasionally, patients with gross hematuria will complain of dysuria. Hypertensive encephalopathy is unusual, but if untreated may be associated with seizures.[5,12] Encephalopathy may occur in the absence of significant hypertension due to cerebral vasculitis.[90] Some patients present with signs and symptoms of congestive heart failure; however, coexistence of rheumatic fever is rare.[15] Rapidly progressive glomerulonephritis with acute renal failure is unusual but well documented.[91] Hypertension and heart failure usually resolve after diuresis.

Children are more frequently affected than adults, although diagnosis may be delayed in the elderly.[5,15,21,27,31] During epidemics, most infected individuals develop only subclinical evidence of nephritis.[27,29,61,92] Nephrotic syndrome occurs in 5% to 10% of children and ~20% of adults,[5] and may occur either initially or later with improvement in glomerular filtration rate (GFR). Rapidly progressive glomerulonephritis occurs infrequently in children (~2%), and it is slightly more common in adults. In children, the clinical symptoms of acute glomerulonephritis usually resolve within 1 to 2 weeks; in adults, resolution may be more prolonged with a higher incidence of progressive renal disease.

The latent period between infection and nephritis depends on the site of infection: typically 1 to 3 weeks following pharyngitis, and 3 to 6 weeks after skin infection.[15] Shorter latent periods of days suggest an alternative diagnosis such as IgA nephropathy. The preceding infection may be accompanied by severe symptoms or be asymptomatic. In many cases, it is not possible to identify an antecedent infection. Regional lymphadenopathy may be present, even after other symptoms and signs of the primary infection have resolved. The acute nephritic syndrome usually lasts 4 to 7 days; however, it may be more prolonged in adults, especially in those with crescentic glomerulonephritis.[25] Coincident rheumatic fever or arthritis is unusual.[93,94] Recurrent episodes are uncommon, but repeated bouts of hematuria may occur during the initial episode. Although de novo disease involving transplanted kidneys is unusual, it may be associated with deterioration of graft function.[95] Extrarenal manifestations are uncommon but include arthritis and choroiditis.[96]

TABLE 46.5 Clinical and Laboratory Manifestations of APSGN[2,118]

Clinical	
Edema	85%
Gross hematuria	30%
Back pain	5%
Oliguria (transient)	50%
Hypertension	60%–80%
Nephrotic syndrome	5%
Laboratory	
Urinalysis: proteinuria, hematuria, casts	100%
Nephrotic range proteinuria	10%
Serum creatinine ≥2 mg/dL	25%
Streptococcal antibody profile (streptozyme)	
In patients with pharyngitis	>95%
In patients with skin infections	80%
False-positive rate	5%
Early abic Rx prevents antibody response	
C3, C4, and/or CH50 depressed	>90%
Hypergammaglobulinemia	90%
Cryoglobulinemia	75%
Rheumatoid factor	33%

Laboratory Findings (Table 46.5) and Diagnosis

Hematuria and proteinuria are invariably present, RBC casts and dysmorphic RBCs are common, and white blood cells often present. Proteinuria is characteristic, but nephrotic syndrome occurs in only 5% of patients at initial presentation.[60,97] Occasionally, there may be a transient increase in proteinuria to the nephrotic range with improvement in GFR, as the disease resolves.

At onset, the GFR is reduced and the serum creatinine is usually elevated, but may remain within the upper limits of the normal laboratory range; 25% of patients have a serum creatinine greater than 2 mg/dL.[2] Anemia may be present during the acute illness and early recovery period.[98] About 25% of patients will have a positive throat or skin culture,[99] although there is a greater yield of obtaining a positive skin culture in patients with impetigo.[100]

In the first 2 weeks of active nephritis C3 and CH50 levels are significantly depressed whereas C4 and C2 levels are usually normal or only mildly decreased—marked depression suggests another diagnosis.[5,88,101–103] Properdin levels are decreased in over 50% of patients, reflecting activation of the alternate complement pathway,[104] whereas increased plasma levels of C5b–9 reflect contribution of the membrane attack complex to pathogenesis.[105] Complement levels typically return to normal by 1 month, so they may be normal at initial presentation in some patients.[106] Persistent depression suggests another diagnosis.[101] C3 nephritic factor may be present in low amounts, but marked and/or persistent elevations are more typical of MPGN.[86]

Elevated titers of antibodies to extracellular products of streptococci, as measured in the streptozyme test, are positive in more than 95% of patients with pharyngitis and 80% of patients with skin infections.[5,15,40,107] This test measures five different streptococcal antibodies: antistreptolysin (ASO), antihyaluronidase (AHase), antistreptokinase (ASKase), antinicotinamide-adenine dinucleotidase (anti-NAD), and anti-DNAse B antibodies. The ASO, anti-DNAse B, anti-NAD, and AHase are more commonly positive after pharyngeal infections, whereas anti-DNAse B and AHase are more often positive following skin infections.[108–110] Overall, these tests are relatively specific for streptococcal infections, with a 5% false-positive rate. However, because the incidence of streptococcal infections in the general population is relatively high (especially in young children), they may be elevated in patients with unrelated streptococcal infection and glomerulonephritis. Antibody titers are elevated at 1 week, peak at 1 month, and fall toward their preinfection level after many months.[111,112] An increasing antibody titer is indicative of recent infection. Antibodies against M proteins are type-specific and confer strain-specific immunity.[39] They are detectable at 4 weeks following infection and persist for years; however, they are unrelated to the severity of disease. Early treatment with antibiotic therapy may prevent the antibody response to both extracellular products and M proteins but not nephritis; therefore, negative results in a patient who previously received antibiotics do not exclude the diagnosis.

Natural History and Prognosis

The overall prognosis is very good (<0.5% mortality; <5% end-stage renal disease [ESRD]).[13,16,18,19,21,23,24,60,113–116] Children have a better prognosis than adults whereas patients older than 40 years with rapidly progressing glomerulonephritis (RPGN) have a worse prognosis,[13,21,31,117] although RPGN associated with APSGN has a better prognosis than other forms of RPGN. Recovery after short-term dialysis dependence is not atypical, although renal function may not return to normal. Persistent urinary and histologic abnormalities are common in both adults and children and may last for years.[10,13,118] The persistence of proteinuria at 3 and 10 years is approximately 15% and 2%, respectively.[118] Patients with prolonged nephrotic syndrome or persistence of heavy proteinuria have a worse prognosis,[23,53–55,118] and persistent hypertension may contribute to progressive renal failure.[60,119]

Treatment and Prevention

Therapy is symptomatic with aims to control blood pressure and volume overload (e.g., with antihypertensives and overdiuretics). Dialysis may be necessary to treat hyperkalemia, volume overload, or uremia. Restriction of physical activity is appropriate during the first few days of the illness but is unnecessary once the patient feels well. The acute phase of the illness usually resolves within a week, and most patients undergo spontaneous diuresis after that interval.

Steroids, immunosuppressive agents, and/or plasmapheresis are generally not indicated. In adults with rapidly progressive renal failure with crescentic glomerulonephritis; however, treatment with a short course of intravenous pulse steroid therapy may be beneficial (500 mg to 1000 mg per 1.73 m^2 of intravenous methylprednisolone daily, for 3 days). More prolonged treatment with steroids or other immunosuppressive therapy is not recommended. Long-term antihypertensive therapy in patients with hypertension and chronic kidney disease is essential to limit progressive renal failure.

Specific therapy for streptococcal infections is important and includes treatment of the patient, family members, and close personal contacts.[120] Throat cultures should be performed on all these individuals and treatment with penicillin G (250 mg four times a day, for 7 to 10 days), or erythromycin (250 mg four times a day, for 7 to 10 days) in patients allergic to penicillin, is indicated to prevent both the development of nephritis in carriers and the spread of infection to others. Whether or not early treatment of infected patients prevents nephritis is not known. For patients with skin infections, attention to personal hygiene is also essential.

ACUTE POSTINFECTIOUS GLOMERULONEPHRITIS

Epidemiology and Changing Prognosis

As indicated, although the incidence of APSGN has declined over the over the past few decades, other infections (e.g., staphylococcal) have become more frequent causes of acute postinfectious glomerulonephritis.[4] For example, a retrospective review found *Staphylococcus* as the infectious agent in 60% of the cases of PIGN in adults in Taiwan. Of particular relevance, the patients were older (mean age 61 years) with male predominance, and there was an increased risk for developing chronic kidney disease.[121,122] A large review of APIGN in North America supported these observations, and almost 40% of the patients were immunocompromised with diabetes (~1/3), cancer, alcoholism, AIDS, and intravenous drug use as the most frequent associations.[2,123] The most common sites of primary infection were upper respiratory tract (24%), skin (17%), lung (17%), and heart (i.e., endocarditis, 12%).[4] Impaired overall health, immunity, poor hygiene, cutaneous ulcers, and poor dentition likely contribute to risk.[124,125] Alcoholism has been associated with a poor prognosis. APIGN may complicate diabetic glomerulosclerosis, because underlying staphylococcal infections are common in this group.[126,127] Complete remission rates are lower (25–50%) with an increased short-term mortality.[2,4,24,97,122,128,129]

Pathology

Although an array of lesions have been reported, three patterns dominate: diffuse endocapillary proliferation (70%–82%), focal proliferative, and exudative glomerulonephritis (8%–12%) or focal mesangial proliferative glomerulonephritis (<10%), whereas MPGN is observed in less than 10% of patients.[2–4] When APIGN and DGS coexist, mesangial and subendothelial deposits predominate with few small subepithelial deposits, IgA (vs. IgG) may predominate, and subepithelial humps are less frequently observed[4] or IF C3 deposits predominate with focal IgG deposition.[130]

Clinical Features

Most patients are male and elderly, with immunocompromised background. Classic features of AGN may not be present, and some present insidiously with the nephrotic syndrome. Overt history of infection is atypical.[2] Recurrent episodes are uncommon,[131] and PIGN is an uncommon etiology of de novo glomerulonephritis after renal transplantation.[132]

Therapy

Indications for immunosuppressive therapy over supportive care and antimicrobial therapy have included acute renal failure with/without crescents on renal biopsy. Corticosteroids have been most commonly used, although there is no clear evidence of benefit.[4] Treatment of the underlying conditions, strict control of blood pressure, and abstinence from alcohol may help overall outcome.

BACTERIAL ENDOCARDITIS

Epidemiology

Investigations to define the incidence of this complication have the typical limitations of retrospective studies and/or lacked histologic confirmation,[133,134] and effective antibiotic therapy may underestimate its frequency. Additionally, early and more effective therapies along with changes in the causative organisms have influenced the incidence of glomerulonephritis over recent years. Nevertheless, the incidence of glomerulonephritis associated with *Streptococcus viridans*–induced endocarditis has declined, and glomerulonephritis associated with acute bacterial endocarditis, particularly involving *Staphylococcus aureus,* has increased. Other organisms (e.g., *Bartonella henselae*, brucellosis, *Actinobacillus*) have also been linked.[133,134] The evolutionary trend with *S. viridans* and *S. aureus* is reviewed here.

In the preantibiotic era, glomerulonephritis was documented in a majority of patients dying from subacute bacterial endocarditis (SBE),[135–138] but with antibiotics, the prevalence decreased precipitously.[134–138] Early reports associated glomerulonephritis less frequently with acute bacterial endocarditis.[136] It was postulated that infection with less virulent organisms led to a more indolent and prolonged course, resulting in a greater antibody response that led to a higher incidence of immunologically mediated events.[119,134,139–141] More recent studies, however, suggest that either strain or host-dependent factors are operative.[134] Several factors contribute to this changing epidemiologic pattern, including use of prophylactic antibiotic regimens in patients with known valvular lesions, earlier recognition of bacteremia, and more effective antibiotics, among others.[138]

Coincident with this decline, there has been an increase in acute endocarditis in intravenous drug abusers. This is often due to *S. aureus* with infection of normal heart valves, and clinical evidence of glomerulonephritis has been found in 40% to 78% of patients with this condition.[134,142,143] Particularly noteworthy, the mean duration of clinical illness prior to the onset of glomerulonephritis is less than 10 days, and many patients are treated with antibiotics prior to overt disease.

Pathologic Features

Although, like ASPGN, many patterns have been reported, a few are more common. In general, the pathology can be divided into subacute and acute forms. Glomerular changes occurring with subacute endocarditis are usually less severe, with focal and segmental glomerulonephritis.[136,144] By contrast, patients with acute disease often have diffuse proliferative glomerulonephritis,[133] and crescents may be observed.[134,145] Rarely, features typical of membranoproliferative glomerulonephritis have been reported (e.g., double contours).[134,146,147] Edema and leukocyte infiltration are typical interstitial findings,[133,134,138,148] and they may be either immune-, infection-, or drug- (e.g., due to antibiotics) mediated.[133,149] Renal embolization has been reported in 30% to 60% of patients with fatal bacterial endocarditis and should be considered in the context of unexplained renal failure,[150] because peripheral manifestations of embolization are infrequent.[134] Mesangial and subendothelial capillary wall deposits of IgG, IgM, and complement (C3 > C1q) predominate,[133,148,151] with subendothelial and mesangial deposits.[148,151] Patients with acute *S. aureus* endocarditis often have subepithelial and intramembranous deposits.[151]

Clinical Features

The manifestations depend on the duration and severity of disease but are typical of acute glomerulonephritis,[152] hematuria is common,[134,148] and heavy proteinuria (nephrotic syndrome ~15%), hypertension, and renal dysfunction may develop, especially with delayed or ineffective therapy.[134,148,153–155] Gross hematuria should raise suspicion of either renal infarction or drug-induced interstitial nephritis[156]; pyuria is common (~2/3), and positive urine cultures are present in 15% to 30%.[157,158] Hypertension occurs infrequently (perhaps due to cardiac involvement),[134,159] and reduced GFR is variable, but may be a presenting symptom.[150]

Laboratory Findings (Table 46.6)

In general, laboratory findings do not correlate with disease activity. Primarily alternative pathway activation, particularly in patients with *S. aureus* endocarditis and glomerulonephritis, have been reported, suggesting that the bacterial wall antigens are capable of direct activation of either the alternative or mannose complement activation pathways, leading to nephritis prior to IgG deposition.[134,160] Normalization of complement levels usually occurs with bacteriologic cure and resolution of glomerulonephritis, whereas persistent hypocomplementemia suggests failure to control infection, which in turn may lead to progressive renal failure.[9]

Differential Diagnosis

In this setting, other considerations include renal emboli, drug-induced interstitial nephritis, and acute tubular necrosis and they are especially relevant in patients with deteriorating renal function.[9,47,169] Embolization of valvular vegetations to the kidney can result in infarction, producing the gross pathologic appearance of "flea-bitten" kidneys.[170] The clinical presentation is gross hematuria, sometimes associated with flank pain. Septic emboli may lead to renal abscesses, and endocarditis should always be considered in patients with multiple renal abscesses. The presence of heavy proteinuria, RBC casts, and dysmorphic RBCs suggests glomerulonephritis. Other considerations include drug-induced interstitial[134] and acute tubular necrosis and, occasionally, renal pathology is necessary to distinguish these entities.[62]

Treatment and Outcome

Eradication of infection with antibiotic and valve replacement (when appropriate) remain the mainstays of therapy.[9] The severity of the glomerulonephritis is related to the duration of infection prior to the initiation of antibiotic therapy.[134] Proteinuria and microscopic hematuria can persist for months after bacteriologic cure. The outcome of patients with severe renal dysfunction is variable, ranging from continued improvement over weeks to months in some, to persistent and progressive renal failure requiring dialysis in others, despite bacteriologic cure. Patients with a high proportion of glomerular crescents in renal biopsy specimens are more likely to have irreversible disease or progressive renal insufficiency.[9,134] With early and appropriate antibiotic therapy, mortality is less than 5%,[159] and GFR usually improves.[134] However, patients with advanced renal dysfunction at presentation may have further deterioration of the GFR, requiring dialysis. The mortality rate is high in this population, and this is most likely related to the combination of severe infection and renal failure.

The role of immunosuppressive therapy in patients with progressive renal failure, despite optimal antibiotic and surgical treatment, remains controversial. Anecdotal case reports suggested that plasmapheresis, corticosteroids, and cytotoxic agents, alone or in combination, may be useful in this situation.[145,163,171–175] However, in addition to the usual adverse effects of these agents, this therapy poses the risk of exacerbating the underlying infectious process. Therefore, these agents should only be considered under very specific circumstances, and there should be definitive clinical and laboratory evidence of bacteriologic cure. In one series, in 204 consecutive episodes of bacterial endocarditis, one third developed an elevated serum creatinine (≥2 mg/dL), and there was a fivefold increase in mortality in this subgroup.[176] Factors associated with an increased risk of acute renal failure included increased age, hypertension, thrombocytopenia, *S. aureus* infection, and prosthetic valve involvement.

TABLE 46.6 **Laboratory Findings of Glomerulonephritis Associated with Bacterial Endocarditis**

Rheumatoid factor: variable (10% to 70%)[161,162]
Circulating immune complexes (~90% nondiagnostic)[117,134,163–165]
Cryoglobulins (mixed >90%)[142,164]
ANCA + in patients with vasculitis[166–168]
Hypocomplementemia[134]
Depressed C3, C4[117,143,153,154,159,164]
Alternative pathway less commonly
Acute ~ 66%
Subacute 90%

Shunt Nephritis

Epidemiologic Patterns

Surgically implanted ventriculoatrial, ventriculojugular, and ventriculo-venal caval shunts have been commonly used to treat hydrocephalus.[169] Overall, infection occurs in 6% to 27% of patients with these ventriculovascular shunts,[169] with nephritis in 1% to 4% of those infected.[177] *Staphylococcus epidermidis* accounts for 75% of infections,[133,178] although other organisms have been isolated (e.g., *S. aureus*, diphtheroids, *Listeria monocytogenes*, *Peptococcus* species, *Serratia* species, *Bacillus subtilis*, *Corynebacterium bovis*, *Gemella morbillorum*, *Propionibacterium acnes*, fungi).[177,179–187] Ventriculoperitoneal devices are more resistant to colonization and infection, and associated glomerulonephritis is rare.[68,188] Most cases have been reported in children.[169,180,185] Recurrence of shunt nephritis in a transplanted kidney has not been reported.[47]

Clinical Manifestations

Symptoms may develop within weeks to years after the shunt placement. Fever is present in nearly all patients[169]; arthralgias, malaise, and weight loss suggest infection,[144,169] and purpura, lymphadenopathy, and hepatosplenomegaly is typical.[133,144] Hematuria (gross hematuria, ~50%), proteinuria (nephrotic syndrome, 28% to 43%), and renal failure (46% to 62%) are common at initial presentation.[133,169]

Laboratory Findings

C3 and C4 is low with active nephritis,[189] with normalization after treatment of the infection and resolution of glomerulonephritis. Persistently depressed levels suggest either inadequate therapy or another cause of glomerulonephritis.[190] Cryoglobulinemia may be present.[169,180,187,191] Blood cultures are often positive. However, sometimes the organisms are difficult to grow, with identification after culture of the removed shunt.

Pathologic Features

The typical lesions resemble MPGN type I[144,151,169] and, less commonly, diffuse proliferative changes similar to PIGN may be present.[192] Granular IgM (84%), IgG, (66%), and C3 (94%) deposits by IF and subendothelial and mesangial electron-dense deposits are typical.

Treatment and Outcome

Because antibiotic therapy alone is usually unsuccessful, treatment should include prompt removal of the infected shunt with external drainage and intravenous/intraventricular antibiotics.[193] Full recovery of renal function has been reported in two thirds of patients after eradication of infection,[178,181,189,194] whereas others observed either chronic kidney disease (CKD) or persistent urinary abnormalities.[133,169] Rarely, progression to ESRD has been reported.[169] Immunosuppressive therapy is not effective in these patients.[186]

Visceral Sepsis-Associated Glomerulonephritis

Epidemiology

Subacute or chronic infections including intrathoracic and intraabdominal abscesses, osteomyelitis, dental and maxillary sinus abscesses, septic abortions, and aortofemoral bypass graft infections have been associated with glomerulonephritis.[195–198] Glomerulonephritis has also been reported coincident with tuberculosis, pneumococcal pneumonia, *Campylobacter (Helicobacter) jejuni* enteritis, *Salmonella-Schistosoma mansoni* infections, and typhoid fever.[195–198]

Clinical Manifestations

Most patients have signs and symptoms associated with the underlying infection, typically with high fever and weight loss. The interval between the onset of infection and diagnosis of glomerulonephritis is variable (e.g., 2 weeks to 3 years).[195] Common manifestations include purpura, arthralgias (i.e., related to cryoglobulinemia),[195,199] hematuria, and proteinuria ± acute renal failure (with oliguria and hypertension).[195,199]

Laboratory Findings

Blood cultures are frequently negative, usually due to antecedent antibiotic administration. Mixed cryoglobulins are usually present at the time of diagnosis and disappear with eradication of infection.[195,199] The serum C3, C4, and CH50 levels are typically normal, unless there is an associated endovasculitis. C3 nephritic factor has occasionally been identified[144,200,201]; however, rheumatoid factor is usually absent.[200]

Pathologic Features

Proliferative glomerulonephritis is typical; however, a diverse group of lesions have been reported, including MPGN and[144,197,200] immune deposits consisting primarily of C3 (with/without IgG, IgM) in mesangial, subendothelial, or subepithelial locations. Subepithelial humps have been observed on occasion.[133]

Treatment and Outcome

Complete remission of glomerulonephritis is usually achievable with early and complete eradication of the underlying infection[196,197,200]; however, delayed and inadequate treatment may result in irreversible loss of renal function.[200]

Methicillin-Resistant *Staphylococcus*–Associated Glomerulonephritis

Methicillin-resistant *Staphylococcus* (MRSA)-associated glomerulonephritis differs from staphylococcal endocarditis-induced glomerulonephritis[202,203] in that serum complement levels are usually normal, there is polyclonal elevation of serum IgA and IgG levels, and IgA is often present within glomerular deposits with IgG and C3.[204,205] On average, glomerulonephritis occurs 5 to 6 weeks following the onset of MRSA infection and approximately 50% of infections are associated with pleural or abdominal abscesses. RPGN and/or the nephrotic syndrome is typical.[202] One third of patients have leukocytoclastic vasculitis and thrombocytosis occurs in three quarters. Renal pathology shows variable degrees of mesangial and/or endocapillary proliferation and crescents. IgA, IgG, and C3 deposit along with mesangial and capillary wall deposits on EM.

MRSA-associated glomerulonephritis often improves with effective eradication of infection[206]; however, some patients do not respond to antibiotic therapy and progress to ESRD.[207] Anecdotal experience with corticosteroids following apparent successful treatment of the underlying MRSA infection[206] led to relapse of the infection, with death from sepsis, raising concern over use prior to eradication.

Hemoperfusion with polymyxin B–immobilized fiber may be a useful therapy to reduce proteinuria in patients' refractory to antibiotic therapy.[208]

Reports of MRSA infections associated with renal amyloidosis, Henoch-Schönlein purpura, IgA nephropathy, and diabetic nephropathy underscore the importance of renal biopsy in distinguishing the underlying cause of disease,[209–211] and serum IgA subclass distribution may provide clues.[212] Overall, the incidence of MRSA-associated glomerulonephritis may be declining with better control of hospital-acquired MRSA infections.[205,213]

Syphilitic Glomerulopathy

Epidemiologic Patterns

The association between syphilis and renal disease has been known for more than a century.[214] Proteinuria is the most common manifestation. Nephrotic syndrome is more common with congenital syphilis (up to 8%) than in secondary forms (<1%).[209–212] Since the advent of mass screening and treatment campaigns, these forms of syphilis are now seen less commonly in developed countries. Primary syphilis is rarely a diagnostic dilemma, but secondary syphilis can be more difficult to diagnose, especially in homosexual males where no primary chancre develops.[215]

Pathology/Pathogenesis

The most common lesion resembles membranous nephropathy.[216] In some patients, mild mesangial and endothelial cell proliferation, associated with mesangial deposits of IgG and IgM, may be present.[144] Electron microscopy usually consists of variable thickening of the glomerular basement membrane (GBM) with subepithelial and occasional subendothelial dense deposits. Rarely, the histology resembles lesions associated with APSGN. Treponemes have been found in some cases within glomeruli, although other mechanisms may be operative.[217–219]

Clinical Manifestations

Affected children with congenital syphilis usually present at 1 to 4 months with edema and hypertension.[216,220,221] Rash and hepatosplenomegaly are common, and the typical radiologic findings associated with congenital syphilis are often present. Adults present with features of the nephrotic syndrome during active secondary syphilis.[216,220,221] Less commonly, AGN is the principal manifestation.[222]

Laboratory Findings

Positive results on serologic testing for syphilis in the appropriate clinical setting, in association with renal histologic findings, support the diagnosis. Serum complement levels (C3 and C4) are depressed in congenital syphilis, but normal in adults with secondary syphilis and nephropathy.[144]

Treatment

Penicillin is the treatment of choice.[144] For congenital syphilis, aqueous crystalline penicillin G, 50,000 units/kg/day, intravenously in divided doses for 10 days, or penicillin G procaine, 50,000 units/kg/day, intramuscularly for 10 days. For secondary syphilis, penicillin benzathine, 2.4 million units, intramuscularly (one dose), or penicillin G procaine, 600,000 units/day, intramuscularly for 8 days. Proteinuria subsides within 6 weeks of successful therapy in most patients. The prognosis is excellent with rapid recovery as the rule. CKD in treated patients has not been reported.[215]

REFERENCES

1. Tejani A, Ingulli E. Poststreptococcal glomerulonephritis. Current clinical and pathologic concepts. *Nephron.* 1990;55(1):1–5.
2. Montseny JJ, et al. The current spectrum of infectious glomerulonephritis. Experience with 76 patients and review of the literature. *Medicine (Baltimore).* 1995;74(2):63–73.
3. Wen YK, Chen ML. The significance of atypical morphology in the changes of spectrum of postinfectious glomerulonephritis. *Clin Nephrol.* 2010;73(3): 173–179.
4. Nasr SH, et al. Acute postinfectious glomerulonephritis in the modern era: experience with 86 adults and review of the literature. *Medicine (Baltimore).* 2008;87(1):21–32.
5. Rodriguez-Iturbe B. Acute poststreptoccal glomerulonephritis. In: Schrier R, ed. *Diseases of the Kidney*. Little Brown: Boston; 1993:1929–1947.
6. Rammelkamp CH. Acute hemmorhagic glomerulonephritis. In: McCarty M, ed. *Streptococcal Infections*. New York: Columbia University Press; 1954.
7. Rammelkamp CH, Weaver RS. Acute glomerulonephritis. The significance of variations in the incidence of disease. *J Clin Invest.* 1953;32:345.
8. Stetson CA, Rammelkamp CH, Krause RM. Epidemic acute nephritis: Studies on etiology, natural history and prevention. *Medicine.* 1955;34:431.
9. Neugarten J, Gallo GR, Baldwin DS. Glomerulonephritis in bacterial endocarditis. *Am J Kidney Dis.* 1984;3(5):371–379.
10. Berrios X, et al. Post-streptococcal acute glomerulonephritis in Chile—20 years of experience. *Pediatr Nephrol.* 2004;19(3):306–312.
11. Kaplan EL, et al. Epidemic acute glomerulonephritis associated with type 49 streptococcal pyoderma. I. Clinical and laboratory findings. *Am J Med.* 1970;48(1):9–27.
12. Lewy JE, et al. Clinico-pathologic correlations in acute poststreptococcal glomerulonephritis. A correlation between renal functions, morphologic damage and clinical course of 46 children with acute poststreptococcal glomerulonephritis. *Medicine (Baltimore).* 1971;50(6):453–501.
13. Lien JW, Mathew TH, Meadows R. Acute post-streptococcal glomerulonephritis in adults: a long-term study. *Q J Med.* 1979;48(189):99–111.
14. Morgan AG, et al. Proteinuria and glomerular disease in Jamaica. *Clin Nephrol.* 1984;21(4):205–209.
15. Nissenson AR, et al. Poststreptococcal acute glomerulonephritis: fact and controversy. *Ann Intern Med.* 1979;91(1):76–86.
16. Nissenson AR, et al. Continued absence of clinical renal disease seven to 12 years after poststreptococcal acute glomerulonephritis in Trinidad. *Am J Med.* 1979;67(2):255–262.
17. Poon-King, T, et al. Recurrent epidemic nephritis in South Trinidad. *N Engl J Med.* 1967;277(14):728–733.
18. Potter EV, et al. Clinical healing two to six years after poststreptococcal glomerulonephritis in Trinidad. *N Engl J Med.* 1978;298(14):767–772.
19. Potter EV, et al. Twelve to seventeen-year follow-up of patients with poststreptococcal acute glomerulonephritis in Trinidad. *N Engl J Med.* 1982; 307(12):725–729.
20. Richter ED. Epidemic nephritis. *N Engl J Med.* 1967;277:763–764.
21. Rodriguez-Iturbe B, Garcia R, Rubio L. Epidemic glomerulonephritis in Maracaibo. Evidence for progression to chronicity. *Clin Neph.* 1976;15:283–301.
22. Schacht RG, Gluck MC, Gallo GR. Progression to uremia after remission of acute postsrepococcal glomerulonephritis. *N Engl J Med.* 1976;295:977–981.
23. Sorger K, et al. Follow-up studies of three subtypes of acute postinfectious glomerulonephritis ascertained by renal biopsy. *Clin Nephrol.* 1987;27(3): 111–124.

24. Vogl W, et al. Long-term prognosis for endocapillary glomerulonephritis of poststreptococcal type in children and adults. *Nephron.* 1986;44(1):58–65.

25. Washio M, Oh Y, Okuda S. Clinicopathological study of poststreptococcal glomerulonephritis in the elderly. *Clin Neph.* 1994;41:265–270.

26. Svartman M, Potter EV, Finklea JF. Epidemic scabies and acute glomerulonephritis. *Lancet.* 1972;1(7744):249–251.

27. Rodriguez-Iturbe B, Rubio L, Garcia R. Attack rate of poststreptococcal nephritis in families. A prospective study. *Lancet.* 1981;1(8217):401–403.

28. Haas M. Incidental healed postinfectious glomerulonephritis: a study of 1012 renal biopsy specimens examined by electron microscopy. *Hum Pathol.* 2003;34(1):3–10.

29. Anthony BF, Kaplan EL, Wannamaker LW. Attack rates of actue nephritis after type 49 sterptococcal infection of the skin and respiratory tract. *J Clin Invest.* 1969;48:1697.

30. Muscatello DJ, et al. Acute poststreptococcal glomerulonephritis: public health implications of recent clusters in New South Wales and epidemiology of hospital admissions. *Epidemiol Infect.* 2001;126(3):365–372.

31. Rodriguez-Iturbe B. Epidemic poststreptococcal glomerulonephritis [clinical conference]. *Kidney Int.* 1984;25(1):129–136.

32. Barnham M, Thornton TJ, Lange K. Nephritis caused by Streptococcus zooepidemicus (Lancefield group C). *Lancet.* 1983;1(8331):945.

33. Pruksakorn S, et al. Epidemiological analysis of non-M-typeable group A Streptococcus isolates from a Thai population in northern Thailand. *J Clin Microbiol.* 2000;38(3):1250–1254.

34. Brandt ER, et al. Antibody levels to the class I and II epitopes of the M protein and myosin are related to group A streptococcal exposure in endemic populations. *Int Immunol.* 2001;13(10):1335–1343.

35. Brenner RM, Peterson J. Postinfectious glomerulonephritis. *Nephrology Rounds.* 2000;3:1–5.

36. Lange CF. Antigenicity of kidney glomeruli: evaluations by antistreptococcal cell membrane antisera. *Transplant Proc.* 1980;12(3 Suppl 1):82–87.

37. Nicholson ML, et al. Analysis of immunoreactivity to a Streptococcus equi subsp. zooepidemicus M-like protein to confirm an outbreak of poststreptococcal glomerulonephritis, and sequences of M-like proteins from isolates obtained from different host species. *J Clin Microbiol.* 2000;38(11): 4126–4130.

38. Ohkuni H, et al. Detection of nephritis strain-associated streptokinase by monoclonal antibodies. *J Med Microbiol.* 1991;35(1):60–63.

39. Stollerman GH. Streptococcal immunology: protection versus injury [editorial]. *Ann Intern Med.* 1978;88(3):422–423.

40. Stollerman GH, Lewis A, Schultz I. Relationship of immune response to group A streptococci to the course of acute and chronic recurrent rheumatic fever. *Am J Med.* 1956;20:163–169.

41. Sorof JM, et al. Acute post-streptococcal glomerulonephritis in a renal allograft. *Pediatr Nephrol.* 1995;9(3):317–319.

42. Kimmelstiel P. The hump-a lesion of acute glomerulonephritis. *Bull Pathol.* 1965;6:187.

43. Nordstrand A, Norgren M, Holm SE. An experimental model for acute post-streptococcal glomerulonephritis in mice. *Adv Exp Med Biol.* 1997;418: 809–811.

44. Feldman H, Mardiney MR, Shuler SE. Immunology and morphology of acute post-streptoccal glomerulonephritis. *J Clin Invest.* 1965;40:283–301.

45. Parra G, et al. Cell populations and membrane attack complex in glomeruli of patients with post-streptococcal glomerulonephritis: identification using monoclonal antibodies by indirect immunofluorescence. *Clin Immunol Immunopathol.* 1984;33(3):324–332.

46. Gruppe WE. Case records: 6–1975. *N Engl J Med.* 1975;292:307–312.

47. Haffner D, et al. The clinical spectrum of shunt nephritis. *Nephrol Dial Transplant.* 1997;12(6):1143–1148.

48. Earle DP, Jennings RB. Studies of poststreptococcal nephritis and other glomerular diseases. *Ann Intern Med.* 1959;51:851–860.

49. Bodaghi E, Kheradpir KM, Maddah M. Vasculitis in acute streptococcal glomerulonephritis. *Int J Pediatr Nephrol.* 1987;8(2):69–74.

50. Fordham CC III, et al. Polyarteritis and acute post-streptococcal glomerulonephritis. *Ann Intern Med.* 1964;61:89–97.

51. Ingelfinger JR, et al. Necrotizing arteritis in acute poststreptococcal glomerulonephritis: report of a recovered case. *J Pediatr.* 1977;91(2):228–232.

52. Freedman P, Peters JH, Kark RM. Localization of gamma-globulin in the diseased kidney. *Arch Intern Med.* 1960;105:524–535.

53. Sorger K. Postinfectious glomerulonephritis. Subtypes, clinico-pathological correlations, and follow-up studies. *Veroff Pathol.* 1986;125:1–105.

54. Sorger K, et al. The garland type of acute postinfectious glomerulonephritis: morphological characteristics and follow-up studies. *Clin Nephrol.* 1983;20(1):17–26.

55. Sorger K, et al. Subtypes of acute postinfectious glomerulonephritis. Synopsis of clinical and pathological features. *Clin Nephrol.* 1982;17(3): 114–128.

56. Fish AJ, et al. Epidemic acute glomerulonephritis associated with type 49 streptococcal pyoderma. II. Correlative study of light, immunofluorescent and electron microscopic findings. *Am J Med.* 1970;48(1):28–39.

57. Seegal BC, Andres JA, Hsu KC. Studies on the pathogenesis of acute and progressive glomerulonephritis in man by immunofluorescence and immunoferritin techniques. *Fed Proc.* 1965;24:100.

58. Tornroth T. The fate of subepithelial deposits in acute poststreptococcal glomerulonephritis. *Lab Invest.* 1976;35(5):461–474.

59. West CD, McAdams AJ. Glomerular deposits and hypoalbuminemia in acute post-streptococcal glomerulonephritis. *Pediatr Nephrol.* 1998;12(6): 471–474.

60. Baldwin DS, et al. The long-term course of poststreptococcal glomerulonephritis. *Ann Intern Med.* 1974;80(3):342–358.

61. Dodge WF, et al. Poststreptococcal glomerulonephritis. A prospective study in children. *N Engl J Med.* 1972;286(6):273–278.

62. Rose BD. *Pathophgysiology of Renal Disease*, 2nd ed. New York: McGraw-Hill; 1987:229.

63. Oda T, et al. Glomerular proliferating cell kinetics in acute post-streptococcal glomerulonephritis (APSGN). *J Pathol.* 1997;183(3):359–368.

64. Svartman M, et al. Epidemic scabies and acute glomerulonephritis in Trinidad. *Lancet.* 1972;1(7744):249–251.

65. Vogt A, et al. Cationic antigens in poststreptococcal glomerulonephritis. *Clin Nephrol.* 1983;20(6):271–279.

66. Bergey EJ, Stinson MW. Heparin-inhibitable basement membrane-binding protein of Streptococcus pyogenes. *Infect Immun.* 1988;56(7):1715–1721.

67. Glurich I, et al. Identification of Streptococcus pyogenes proteins that bind to rabbit kidney in vitro and in vivo. *Microb Pathog.* 1991;10(3):209–220.

68. Nordstrand A, et al. Streptokinase as a mediator of acute post-streptococcal glomerulonephritis in an experimental mouse model. *Infect Immun.* 1998;66(1): 315–321.

69. Becker C, Murphy G. The experimental induction of glomerulonephritis like that in man by infection with group A streptococci. *J Exp Med.* 1967;127: 1–38.

70. Markowitz AS, et al. Streptococcal related glomerulonephritis. II. Glomerulonephritis in rhesus monkeys immunologically induced both actively and passively with a soluble fraction from human glomeruli. *J Immunol.* 1967;98(1): 161–170.

71. Markowitz AS, et al. Streptococcal related glomerulonephritis. 3. Glomerulonephritis in rhesus monkeys immunologically induced both actively and passively with a soluble fraction from nephritogenic streptococcal protoplasmic membranes. *J Immunol.* 1971;107(2):504–511.

72. Fillit H, et al. Sera from patients with poststreptococcal glomerulonephritis contain antibodies to glomerular heparan sulfate proteoglycan. *J Exp Med.* 1985;161(2):277–289.

73. Kefalides NA, et al. Identification of antigenic epitopes in type IV collagen by use of synthetic peptides. *Kidney Int.*1993;43(1):94–100.

74. Kefalides NA, et al. Antibodies to basement membrane collagen and to laminin are present in sera from patients with poststreptococcal glomerulonephritis. *J Exp Med.* 1986;163(3):588–602.

75. Kraus W, Beachey EH. Renal autoimmune epitope of group A streptococci specified by M protein tetrapeptide Ile-Arg-Leu-Arg. *Proc Natl Acad Sci U S A.* 1988;85(12):4516–4520.

76. McIntosh LM, Kaufman DB, McIntosh JR. Glomerular lesions produced in rabbits by autologous serum and autologous IgG modified by treatment with a culture of hemolytic streptococcus. *J Med Microbiol.* 1972;(4):535.

77. Grubb A, et al. Isolation and some properties of an IgG Fc-binding protein from group A streptococci type 15. *Int Arch Allergy Appl Immunol.* 1982;67(4):369–376.

78. Kronvall G. A surface component in group A, C, and G streptococci with non-immune reactivity for immunoglobulin G. *J Immunol.* 1973;111(5):1401–1406.

79. Mosquera J, Katiyar V, Coello J. Neuraminidase production by streprococci from patients with glomerulonephritis. *J Infec Dis.* 1985;151:259–263.

80. Mosquera J, Rodriguez-Iturbe B. Extracellular neuraminidase production of stepococci associated with acute nephritis. *Clin Nephr.* 1984;21:21–28.

81. Treser G, et al. Antigenic streptococcal components in acute glomerulonephritis. *Science.* 1969;163(868):676–677.

82. Zack DJ, et al. Mechanisms of cellular penetration and nuclear localization of an anti- double strand DNA autoantibody. *J Immunol.* 1996;157(5): 2082–2088.

83. Wells WC. Observations on the dropsy which succeeds scarlet fever. *Trans Soc Imp Chir Knowledge.* 1812;3:167.

84. Layrisse Z, et al. Family studies of the HLA system in acute post-streptococcal glomerulonephritis. *Hum Immunol.* 1983;7(3):177–185.

85. Fillit HM, et al. Cellular reactivity to altered glomerular basement membrane in glomerulonephritis. *N Engl J Med.* 1978;298(16):861–868.

86. Rastaldi MP, et al. Adhesion molecules expression in noncrescentic acute post-streptococcal glomerulonephritis. *J Am Soc Nephrol.* 1996;7(11):2419–2427.

87. Reid HF, et al. Suppression of cellular reactivity to group A streptococcal antigens in patients with acute poststreptococcal glomerulonephritis. *J Infect Dis.* 1984;149(6):841–850.

88. Madaio MP, Harrington JT. Current concepts. The diagnosis of acute glomerulonephritis. *N Engl J Med.* 1983;309(21):1299–1302.

89. Jennings RB, Earle DP. Post-sreptococcal glomerulonephritis: histopathologic and early chronic late net phases. *J Clin Invest.* 1961;40:1525–1595.

90. Rovang RD, et al. Cerebral vasculitis associated with acute post-streptococcal glomerulonephritis. *Am J Nephrol.* 1997;17(1):89–92.

91. Couser WG, Johnson RJ, Alpers CE. Postinfectious glomerulonephritis. In: Neilson EG, Couser WG, eds. *Immunologic Renal Diseases.* Philadelphia: Lippincott Williams and Wilkins; 2001:899–930.

92. Sagel I, et al. Occurrence and nature of glomerular lesions after group A streptococci infections in children. *Ann Intern Med.* 1973;79(4):492–499.

93. Akasheh MS, et al. Rapidly progressive glomerulonephritis complicating acute rheumatic fever. *Postgrad Med J.* 1995;71(839):553–554.

94. Niewold TB, Ghosh AK. Post-streptococcal reactive arthritis and glomerulonephritis in an adult. *Clin Rheumatol.* 2003;22(4–5):350–352.

95. Moroni G, et al. Acute post-bacterial glomerulonephritis in renal transplant patients: description of three cases and review of the literature. *Am J Transplant.* 2004;4(1):132–136.

96. Besada E, Frauens BJ, Schatz S. Choroiditis, pigment epithelial detachment, and cystoid macular edema as complications of poststreptococcal syndrome. *Optom Vis Sci.* 2004;81(8):578–585.

97. Hinglais N, Garcia-Torres R, Kleinknecht D. Long-term prognosis in acute glomerulonephritis. The predictive value of early clinical and pathological features observed in 65 patients. *Am J Med.* 1974;56(1):52–60.

98. Becker A, et al. Anemia associated with acute post streptococcal glomerulonephritis. *Rev Med Chil.* 1994;122(11):1276–1282.

99. Blyth CC, Robertson PW, Rosenberg AR. Post-streptococcal glomerulonephritis in Sydney: a 16–year retrospective review. *J Paediatr Child Health.* 2007;43(6):446–450.

100. Sanjad S, et al. Acute glomerulonephritis in children: a review of 153 cases. *South Med J.* 1977;70(10):1202–1206.

101. Cameron JS, et al. Plasma C3 and C4 concentrations in management of glomerulonephritis. *Br Med J.* 1973;3(882):668–672.

102. Lewis EJ, Carpenter CB, Schur PH. Serum complement component levels in human glomerulonephritis. *Ann Intern Med.* 1971;75(4):555–560.

103. Sjoholm AG. Complement components and complement activation in acute poststreptococcal glomerulonephritis. *Int Arch Allergy Appl Immunol.* 1979;58(3):274–284.

104. McLean RH, Michael AF. Properdin anc C3 proactivator: alternate pathway components in human glomerulonephritis. *J Clin Invest.* 1973;52(3):634–644.

105. Matsell DG, et al. Plasma terminal complement complexes in acute poststreptococcal glomerulonephritis. *Am J Kidney Dis.* 1991;17(3):311–316.

106. Williams DG, et al. Studies of serum complement in the hypocomplementaemic nephritides. *Clin Exp Immunol.* 1974;18(3):391–405.

107. Zaum R, Vogt A, Rodriguez-Iturbe B. Analysis of the immune response to streoriciccal proteinase in poststrepococcal disease. Xth Lancefield International Symposium on Streoticiccal Diseases. Cologne, Germany; 1987:88.

108. Bisno AL, et al. Factors influencing serum antibody responses in streptococcal pyoderma. *J Lab Clin Med.* 1973;81(3):410–420.

109. Dillon HC Jr, Reeves MS. Streptococcal immune responses in nephritis after skin infections. *Am J Med.* 1974;56(3):333–346.

110. Wannamaker LW. Differences between streptococcal infections of the throat and of the skin (second of two parts). *N Engl J Med.* 1970;282(2):78–85.

111. Lyttle JD, Seegal D, Loeb E. The serum antistreptolysin titer in acute glomerulonephritis. *J Clin Invest.* 1938;17:632.

112. McCarty M. The antibody responce in streptococcal infections. In: McCarty M, ed. *Streptococcal Infections.* New York: Columbia University Press; 1954.

113. Drachman R, Aladjem M, Vardy PA. Natural history of an actue glomerulonephritis epidemic in childern. An 11 to 12 year follow up. *J Med Sci.* 1986;18:603.

114. Garcia R, Rubio L, Rodriguez-Iturbe B. Long-term prognosis of epidemic poststreptococcal glomerulonephritis in Maracaibo: follow-up studies 11–12 years after the acute episode. *Clin Nephrol.* 1981;15(6):291–298.

115. Kasahara T, et al. Prognosis of acute poststreptococcal glomerulonephritis (APSGN) is excellent in children, when adequately diagnosed. *Pediatr Int.* 2001:43(4):364–367.

116. Perlman LV, et al. Poststreptococcal glomerulonephritis. A ten-year follow-up of an epidemic. *JAMA.* 1965;194(1):63–70.

117. Kauffmann RH, et al. The clinical implications and the pathogenetic significance of circulating immune complexes in infective endocarditis. *Am J Med.* 1981;71(1):17–25.

118. Buzio C, et al. Significance of albuminuria in the follow-up of acute poststreptococcal glomerulonephritis. *Clin Nephrol.* 1994;41(5):259–264.

119. Baldwin DS. Chronic glomerulonephritis: nonimmunologic mechanisms of progressive glomerular damage. *Kidney Int.*1982;21(1):109–120.

120. Zoch-Zwierz W, et al. [The course of post-streptococcal glomerulonephritis depending on methods of treatment for the preceding respiratory tract infection]. *Wiad Lek.* 2001;54(1–2):56–63.

121. Wen YK. The spectrum of adult postinfectious glomerulonephritis in the new millennium. *Ren Fail.* 2009;31(8):676–682.

122. Wen YK. Clinicopathological study of infection-associated glomerulonephritis in adults. *Int Urol Nephrol.* 2010;42(2):477–485.

123. Keller CK, et al. Postinfectious glomerulonephritis—is there a link to alcoholism? *Q J Med.* 1994;87(2):97–102.

124. Gomez F, Ruiz P, Schreiber AD. Impaired function of macrophage Fc gamma receptors and bacterial infection in alcoholic cirrhosis. *N Engl J Med.* 1994;331(17):1122–1128.

125. Rimola A, et al. Reticuloendothelial system phagocytic activity in cirrhosis and its relation to bacterial infections and prognosis. *Hepatology.* 1984;4(1):53–58.

126. Nasr SH, et al. IgA-dominant acute poststaphylococcal glomerulonephritis complicating diabetic nephropathy. *Hum Pathol.* 2003;34(12):1235–1241.

127. Nasr SH, et al. Acute poststaphylococcal glomerulonephritis superimposed on diabetic glomerulosclerosis. *Kidney Int.* 2007;71(12):1317–1321.

128. Melby PC, et al. Poststreptococcal glomerulonephritis in the elderly. Report of a case and review of the literature. *Am J Nephrol.* 1987;7(3):235–240.

129. Moroni G, et al. Long-term prognosis of diffuse proliferative glomerulonephritis associated with infection in adults. *Nephrol Dial Transplant.* 2002;17(7):1204–1211.

130. D'Agati VD, Jeanette JC, Silva FG. *Atlas of Nontumor Pathology: Non-neoplastic Kidney Diseases.* Washington DC: American Registry of Pathology-Armed Forces Institute of Pathology; 2005:269–296.

131. Casquero A, et al. Recurrent acute postinfectious glomerulonephritis. *Clin Nephrol.* 2006;66(1):51–53.

132. Plumb TJ, et al. Postinfectious glomerulonephritis in renal allograft recipients. *Transplantation.* 2006;82(9):1224–1228.

133. Alder SG, Cohen AH. Glomerulonephriits with bactertial endocarditis. In: Schrier RW, Gottschalk CW, eds. *Diseases of the Kidney.* Boston: Little Brown; 1993.

134. Neugarten J, Baldwin DS. Glomerulonephritis in bacterial endocarditis. *Am J Med.* 1984;77(2):297–304.

135. Baehr G. Glomerular lesion of subacute bacterial endocarditis. *J Exp Med.* 1912;15:330.

136. Bell EJ. The glomerular lesion associated with endocarditis. *Am J Pathol.* 1932;8:639.

137. Keefer CS. Subacute bacterial endocarditis: Active cases without bacteremia. *Ann Intern Med.* 1937–1938;11:714.

138. Spain DM, King DW. The effect of penicillin on the renal lesion of subacute bacterial endocarditis. *Ann Intern Med.* 1952;36:1086–1095.

139. Glassock RJ. Secondary glomerular diseases. In: Brenner BM, Rector FC, eds. *The Kidney.* Little Brown: Boston; 1992:1493–1570.

140. Libman E. Characterization of various forms of glomerulonephritis. *JAMA.* 1923;80:813–818.

141. Pankey GA. Acute bacterial endocarditis at the University of Minnesota Hospitals, 1939–1959. *Am Heart J.* 1962;64:583–591.

142. Hurwitz D, Quismorio FP, Friou GJ. Cryoglobulinaemia in patients with infectious endocarditis. *Clin Exp Immunol.* 1975;19(1):131–141.

143. O'Connor DT, Weisman MH, Fierer J. Activation of the alternate complement pathway in Staph. aureus infective endocarditis and its relationship to thrombocytopenia, coagulation abnormalities, and acute glomerulonephritis. *Clin Exp Immunol.* 1978;34(2):179–187.

144. Madaio MP. Postinfectious glomerulonephritis. In: Jacobson HR, Striker GE, Klahr S, eds. *The Principles and Practice of Nephrology.* Mosby: St Louis; 1995:122–127.

145. Kannan S, Mattoo TK. Diffuse crescentic glomerulonephritis in bacterial endocarditis. *Pediatr Nephrol.* 2001;16(5):423–428.

146. Neufeld GK, et al. Infective endocarditis as a complication of heroin use. *South Med J.* 1976;69(9):1148–1151.

147. Spitzer RE, Stitzel AE, Urmson JR. Is glomerulonephritis after bacterial sepsis always benign? *Lancet.* 1978;1(8069):871.
148. Morel-Maroger L, et al. Kidney in subacute endocarditis. Pathological and immunofluorescence findings. *Arch Pathol.* 1972;94(3):205–213.
149. Colvin RB, Fang LST. Interstitial nephritis. In: Tisher CC, Brenner BM, eds. *Renal Pathology with Functional Correlation.* Lippincott: Philadelphia; 1989.
150. Lerner PI, Weinstein L. Infective endocarditis in the antibiotic era. *N Engl J Med.* 1966;274(7):388–393 concl.
151. Gutman RA, et al. The immune complex glomerulonephritis of bacterial endocarditis. *Medicine (Baltimore).* 1972;51(1):1–25.
152. Oda T, et al. Glomerular plasmin-like activity in relation to nephritis-associated plasmin receptor in acute poststreptococcal glomerulonephritis. *J Am Soc Nephrol.* 2005;16(1):247–254.
153. Boulton-Jones JM, et al. Renal lesions of subacute infective endocarditis. *Br Med J.* 1974;2(909):11–14.
154. Boyarsky S, Burnett JM, Barker WH. Renal failure in embolic glomerulonephritis as a complication of subacute bacterial endocarditis. *Bull Johns Hopkins Hosp.* 1949;84:207.
155. Williams RC Jr, Kunkel HG. Rheumatoid factor, complement, and conglutinin aberrations in patients with subacute bacterial endocarditis. *J Clin Invest.* 1962;41:666–675.
156. Glassock RJ. Clinical aspects of acute, rapidly progressive and chronic glomerulonephritis. In: Early LE, Gottschalk CW, eds. *Diseases of the Kidney.* Boston: Little Brown; 1979:691–763.
157. Lee BK, Crossley K, Gerding DN. The association between Staphylococcus aureus bacteremia and bacteriuria. *Am J Med.* 1978;65(2):303–306.
158. Musher DM, McKenzie SO. Infections due to Staphylococcus aureus. *Medicine (Baltimore).* 1977;56(5):383–409.
159. Gorlin R, Favour CB, Emery FJ. Long-term follow-up study of penicillin-treated subacute bacterial endocarditis. *N Engl J Med.* 1950;242(26):995–1001.
160. Pertschuk LP, et al. Glomerulonephritis due to Staphylococcus aureus antigen. *Am J Clin Pathol.* 1976;65(3):301–307.
161. Pelletier LL Jr, Petersdorf RG. Infective endocarditis: a review of 125 cases from the University of Washington Hospitals, 1963–72. *Medicine (Baltimore).* 1977;56(4):287–313.
162. Sheagren JN, et al. Rheumatoid factor in acute bacterial endocarditis. *Arthritis Rheum.* 1976;19(5):887–890.
163. Bayer AS, Theofilopoulos AN. Immunopathogenetic aspects of infective endocarditis. *Chest.* 1990;97(1):204–212.
164. Cabane J, et al. Fate of circulating immune complexes in infective endocarditis. *Am J Med.* 1979;66(2):277–282.
165. Hooper DC, et al. Circulating immune complexes in prosthetic valve endocarditis. *Arch Intern Med.* 1983;143(11):2081–2084.
166. Angangco R, Thiru S, Oliveira DB. Pauci-immune glomerulonephritis associated with bacterial infection. *Nephrol Dial Transplant.* 1993;8(8):754–756.
167. Soto A, et al. Endocarditis associated with ANCA. *Clin Exp Rheumatol.* 1994; 12(2):203–204.
168. Subra JF, et al. The presence of cytoplasmic antineutrophil cytoplasmic antibodies (C-ANCA) in the course of subacute bacterial endocarditis with glomerular involvement, coincidence or association? *Clin Nephrol.* 1998;49(1):15–18.
169. Arze RS, et al. Shunt nephritis: report of two cases and review of the literature. *Clin Nephrol.* 1983;19(1):48–53.
170. Horder TJ. Infective endocarditis with an analysis of 150 cases with special reference to the chronic form of the disease. *Q J Med.* 1909;2:289.
171. Daimon S, et al. Infective endocarditis-induced crescentic glomerulonephritis dramatically improved by plasmapheresis. *Am J Kidney Dis.* 1998;32(2):309–313.
172. Le Moing V, et al. Use of corticosteroids in glomerulonephritis related to infective endocarditis: three cases and review. *Clin Infect Dis.* 1999;28(5): 1057–1061.
173. McKenzie PE, et al. Plasmapheresis in glomerulonephritis. *Clin Nephrol.* 1979;12(3):97–108.
174. McKinsey DS, McMurray TI, Flynn JM. Immune complex glomerulonephritis associated with Staphylococcus aureus bacteremia: response to corticosteroid therapy. *Rev Infect Dis.* 1990;12(1):125–127.
175. Rovzar MA, et al. Immunosuppressive therapy and plasmapheresis in rapidly progressive glomerulonephritis associated with bacterial endocarditis. *Am J Kidney Dis.* 1986;7(5):428–433.
176. Conlon PJ, et al. Predictors of prognosis and risk of acute renal failure in bacterial endocarditis. *Clin Nephrol.* 1998;49(2):96–101.
177. Schoenbaum SC, Gardner P, Shillito J. Infections of cerebrospinal fluid shunts: epidemiology, clinical manifestations, and therapy. *J Infect Dis.* 1975;131(5):543–552.
178. Moncrieff MW, et al. Glomerulonephritis associated with Staphylococcus albus in a Spitz Holter valve. *Arch Dis Child.* 1973;48(1):69–72.
179. Balogun RA, et al. Shunt nephritis from Propionibacterium acnes in a solitary kidney. *Am J Kidney Dis.* 2001;38(4):E18.
180. Bolton WK, et al. Ventriculojugular shunt nephritis with Corynebacterium bovis. Successful therapy with antibiotics. *Am J Med.* 1975;59(3):417–423.
181. Caron C, et al. Shunt glomerulonephritis: clinical and histopathological manifestations. *Can Med Assoc J.* 1979;120(5):557–561.
182. Forrest JW Jr, et al. Immune complex glomerulonephritis associated with Klebsiella pneumoniae infection. *Clin Nephrol.* 1977;7(2):76–80.
183. Nagashima T, et al. Antineutrophil cytoplasmic autoantibody specific for proteinase 3 in a patient with shunt nephritis induced by Gemella morbillorum. *Am J Kidney Dis.* 2001;37(5):E38.
184. Peeters W, et al. Shunt nephritis. *Clin Nephrol.* 1978;9(3):122–125.
185. Pereria BJ, et al. Shunt nephritis associated with Staphylococcus aureus septicaemia. *J Assoc Phys Ind.* 1987;35:796.
186. Stickler GB, et al. Diffuse glomerulonephritis associated with infected ventriculoatrial shunt. *N Engl J Med.* 1968;279(20):1077–1082.
187. Strife CF, et al. Shunt nephritis: the nature of the serum cryoglobulins and their relation to the complement profile. *J Pediatr.* 1976;88(3):403–413.
188. Dobrin RS, et al. The role of complement, immunoglobulin and bacterial antigen in coagulase-negative staphylococcal shunt nephritis. *Am J Med.* 1975;59(5):660–673.
189. Levy M, Gubler MC, Habib R. Pathology and immunopathology of shunt nephritis in children: Report of 10 cases. in Proc 8th Int. Cong. Nephrol. Basel: Karger; 1981.
190. Wyatt RJ, Walsh JW, Holland NH. Shunt nephritis. Role of the complement system in its pathogenesis and management. *J Neurosurg.* 1981;55(1):99–107.
191. *Lancet.* 2001;358.
192. Toth T, Redl J, Beregi E. Shunt nephritis with crescent formation. *Int J Pediatr Nephrol.* 1987;8(4):231–234.
193. Bayston R, de Louvis J, Brown EM, et al. Treatment of infections associated with shunting for hydrocephalus. *Br J Hosp Med.* 1995;53:368–373.
194. Yeh BP, et al. Immune complex disease associated with an infected ventriculojugular shunt: a curable form of glomerulonephritis. *South Med J.* 1977; 70(9):1141–1143, 1146.
195. Beaufils M, et al. Acute renal failure of glomerular origin during visceral abscesses. *N Engl J Med.* 1976;295(4):185–189.
196. Boonshaft B, Maher JF, Schreiner GE. Nephrotic syndrome associated with osteomyelitis without secondary amyloidosis. *Arch Intern Med.* 1970;125(2): 322–327.
197. Boulton-Jones JM, Davidson AM. Persistent infection as a cause of renal disease in patients submitted to renal biopsy. A report from the glomerulonephritis registry of the United Kingdom MRC. *Q J Med.* 1986;58(58): 123–132.
198. Whitworth JA, et al. The significance of extracapillary proliferation. Clinicopathological review of 60 patients. *Nephron.* 1976;16(1):1–19.
199. Beaufils M. Glomerular disease complicating abdominal sepsis. *Kidney Int.*1981;19(4):609–618.
200. Beaufils M, et al. Glomerulonephritis in severe bacterial infections with and without endocarditis. *Adv Nephrol Necker Hosp.* 1977;7:217–234.
201. Madaio MP, Harrington JT. The diagnosis of glomerular diseases: acute glomerulonephritis and the nephrotic syndrome. *Arch Intern Med.* 2001;161(1):25–34.
202. Kobayashi M, Koyama A. Methicillin-resistant Staphylococcus aureus (MRSA) infection in glomerulonephritis—a novel hazard emerging on the horizon. *Nephrol Dial Transplant.* 1998;13(12):2999–3001.
203. Yoh K, et al. Cytokines and T-cell responses in superantigen-related glomerulonephritis following methicillin-resistant Staphylococcus aureus infection. *Nephrol Dial Transplant.* 2000;15(8):1170–1174.
204. Grcevska L, Polenakovic M. Garland pattern post-streptococcal glomerulonephritis (PSGN), clinical characteristics and follow-up [letter]. *Clin Nephrol.* 1996;46(6):413–414.
205. Koyama A, et al. Glomerulonephritis associated with MRSA infection: a possible role of bacterial superantigen. *Kidney Int.* 1995;47(1):207–216.
206. Nagaba Y, et al. Effective antibiotic treatment of methicillin-resistant Staphylococcus aureus-associated glomerulonephritis. *Nephron.* 2002;92(2): 297–303.
207. Yamashita Y, et al. Glomerulonephritis after methicillin-resistant Staphylococcus aureus infection resulting in end-stage renal failure. *Intern Med.* 2001;40(5):424–427.
208. Nakamura T, et al. Hemoperfusion with polymyxin B-immobilized fiber in septic patients with methicillin-resistant Staphylococcus aureus-associated glomerulonephritis. *Nephron Clin Pract.* 2003;94(2):c33–39.
209. Hirayama K, et al. Henoch-Schonlein purpura nephritis associated with methicillin-resistant Staphylococcus aureus infection. *Nephrol Dial Transplant.* 1998;13(10):2703–2704.

210. Pola E, et al. Onset of Berger disease after Staphylococcus aureus infection: septic arthritis after anterior cruciate ligament reconstruction. *Arthroscopy.* 2003;19(4):E29.
211. Yokota N, et al. Reversible nephrotic syndrome in a patient with amyloid A amyloidosis of the kidney following methicillin-resistant Staphylococcus aureus infection. *Nephron.* 2001;87(2):177–181.
212. Usui J, et al. Polyclonal activation of an IgA subclass against Staphylococcus aureus cell membrane antigen in post-methicillin-resistant S. Aureus infection glomerulonephritis. *Nephrol Dial Transplant.* 2006;(21):1448–1449.
213. Usui J, et al. Methicillin-resistant Staphylococcus-aureus-associated glomerulonephritis on the decline: decreased incidence since the 1990s. *Clin Exp Nephrol.* 2011;15(1):184–186.
214. Thompson IL. Syphilis of the kidney. *JAMA.* 1920;(75):17–20.
215. McPhee SJ. Secondary syphilis: uncommon manifestations of a common disease. *West J Med.* 1984;140(1):35–42.
216. Kleinknecht C, et al. Membranous glomerulonephritis with extrarenal disorders in children. *Medicine (Baltimore).* 1979;58(3):219–228.
217. Bhorade MS, et al. Nephropathy of secondary syphilis. A clinical and pathological spectrum. *JAMA.* 1971;216(7):1159–1166.
218. O'Regan S, et al. Treponemal antigens in congenital and acquired syphilitic nephritis: demonstration by immunofluorescence studies. *Ann Intern Med.* 1976;85(3):325–327.
219. Tourville DR, et al. Treponemal antigen in immunopathogenesis of syphilitic glomerulonephritis. Am *J Pathol.* 1976;82(3):479–492.
220. Choubrac P, et al. [Glomerulonephritis and secondary syphilis]. *Ann Med Interne (Paris).* 1977;128(5):483–486.
221. Pollner P. Nephrotic syndrome associated with congenital syphilis. *JAMA.* 1966;198(3):263–266.
222. Thomas EW, Schur M. Clinical nephropathies in early syphilis. *Arch Intern Med.* 1946;78:679–686.

CHAPTER

47 Viral Glomerulonephritis

Warren Kupin

Viral diseases represent a significant and often unrecognized cause of glomerular disease both in the United States and worldwide.[1,2] Viruses are associated with a variety of pathways leading to glomerular disease, which are not mutually exclusive or unique to a single virus species (Table 47.1). The main exception to this pattern is the singular association of type II cryoglobulinemia from IgMκ–IgG immune complexes with a hepatitis C infection, which does not occur with any other viral infection. Moreover, many viruses employ more than one pathway for mediating glomerular injury and can be associated with a diverse range of glomerular syndromes. The two primary pathways for viral-induced renal injury are the direct viral infection of renal tissue and the presence of viral-induced immune complex deposition in the kidney.

This chapter will detail the current understanding of the epidemiology, clinical presentation, diagnostic workup, pathogenicity, and therapeutic interventions for the spectrum of glomerular syndromes caused by different viral infections.

HEPATITIS C

Epidemiology

The hepatitis C virus (HCV) is the leading cause of cirrhosis and the need for liver transplantation in the United States.[3] HCV is an enveloped, spherical, positive-stranded RNA virus that belongs to the family Flaviviridae and has been assigned its own individual genus, Hepacivirus. This is the same viral family as yellow fever and dengue. Approximately 170 million people worldwide are chronic carriers of HCV, which represents 70% to 80% of all patients exposed to this virus as compared to a carrier rate of 15% for patients exposed to the hepatitis B virus (HBV).[4] According to the National Health and Nutrition Examination Survey (NHANES), there are 4.1 million people with HCV in the United States, accounting for 1.6% of the population.[5]

The most common methods for the acquisition of HCV are percutaneous exposure, especially from intravenous drug abuse (60%); nosocomial exposure due to failure to adhere to universal precautions; blood transfusions and blood products (prior to enzyme-linked immunosorbent assay [ELISA] screening); and the use of solvent detergents and interpersonal exposure (vertical transmission/sexual partners).[6] Once established in a carrier state, 30% of patients will eventually develop cirrhosis.

Differences in nucleotide sequences allow for the subclassification of HCV into six major genotypes (1 through 6) and further subgenotypes (1a and 1b, 2a and 2b, 3a and 3b, and 4a). These genotypes show significant geographic heterogeneity and differ not by virulence but by response to interferon (IFN) therapy.[7] The following data show the worldwide distribution of the different genotypes: Genotype 1 is present in 60% to 70% of HCV isolates in the United States; genotype 2 is found in the Caribbean and in Southeast Asia; genotype 3 is found in Asia; genotype 4 is noted in Africa and the Middle East; and genotypes 5 and 6 are found in both South Africa and Southeast Asia.[8]

The Pathophysiology of Infection

HCV is a hepatotropic virus that directly enters into hepatocytes through specific receptors: CD81, the Low density lipoprotein (LDL) receptor, the DC-SIGN, the L-SIGN, the human scavenger receptor SR-B1, and claudin-1.[9,10] Viral tropism exists for many other cell types, especially monocytes and B and T cells. After exposure to HCV, both humoral and cell-mediated immunity play a role in an effort to contain viral replication. IgG antibodies directed against both structural (envelope proteins E1 and E2) and nonstructural (NS3, NS4, NS5) proteins are almost universally present in HCV patients, but their presence does not correlate with viral clearance.[11] In fact, clearance of HCV can occur even in the absence of an antibody response.[12] The key element in achieving HCV control lies in the CD8 cytotoxic T-cell response in conjunction with natural killer (NK) cell proliferation. Production of IFN by these cells is downregulated in HCV carriers, thus allowing for viral replication, and this finding has led the way for the use of exogenous IFN as a therapeutic modality.[13]

The antibody response to HCV is measured through an ELISA, which does not distinguish between the individual targets of the IgG response. A recombinant immunoblot assay

TABLE 47.1 Mechanisms of Viral Mediated Glomerular Disease

Direct
Cytopathic effect on glomerular mesangial or epithelial cells
HIV
HIV-associated nephropathy
CMV
Glomerulitis/transplant glomerulopathy
Parvovirus
Collapsing FSGS
Cytopathic effect on glomerular endothelial cells
CMV
Thrombotic microangiopathy
HIV
Thrombotic microangiopathy
Parvovirus
Thrombotic microangiopathy
Hantavirus
Mesangial proliferative glomerulonephritis/nephrotic syndrome
Deposition of or in situ formation of immune complexes
Hepatitis C
Type I membranoproliferative glomerulonephritis
HIV
HIV immune complex disease of the kidney
Parvovirus
Acute proliferative glomerulonephritis
IgA nephropathy
Hepatitis B
Membranous glomerulopathy
Membranoproliferative glomerulonephritis
Polyarteritis nodosa
IgA nephropathy
Hepatitis A
Acute proliferative glomerulonephritis
IgA nephropathy
Indirect
Stimulation of host immune response – Cytokines/chemokines/growth factors
HIV
Hantavirus
Hepatitis B virus
Coxsackievirus B

CMV, cytomegalovirus; FSGS, focal segmental glomerulosclerosis.

(RIBA) can be used for confirmation, and this test can provide individual antibody specificities. There is no clinical relevance for measuring IgM antibodies to HCV because the detection of viremia is a more sensitive marker for acute and chronic infection. Following a positive ELISA/RIBA, the detection and quantification of HCV RNA is needed to determine the viral burden.[14] A reverse transcriptase polymerase chain reaction (RT-PCR) will provide not only a diagnostic value for HCV replication but also a means of following the response to therapy.

There are two special circumstances where the use of ELISA screening alone for HCV does not provide a high enough degree of specificity and must be complemented by a RT-PCR. These exceptions occur in patients unable to generate an antibody response to HCV and include HIV patients and patients with end-stage renal disease (ESRD). Approximately 5% to 10% of patients in these groups will have a negative ELISA but a positive RT-PCR. In both of these circumstances, reliance on ELISA screening is not enough to exclude active HCV infection.

Glomerular Syndromes

Extrahepatic disease is present in 30% to 40% of patients with chronic HCV infection and includes the following syndromes: mixed cryoglobulinemia with or without membranoproliferative glomerulonephritis type I (MPGN), autoimmune thyroiditis, porphyria cutanea tarda, Sjögren syndrome, pulmonary fibrosis, Mooren corneal ulcers, lichen planus, and diabetes mellitus.[15] In addition to MPGN type 1, HCV has been associated with a variety of other glomerular lesions, including membranous glomerulonephritis (GN), IgA nephropathy, postinfectious GN, focal and segmental GN, antineutrophil cytoplasmic antibodies (ANCA), positive vasculitis, and fibrillary glomerulonephritis (Table 47.2).[16]

TABLE 47.2 Glomerular Syndromes of Hepatitis B and Hepatitis C

Hepatitis B
Acute proliferative glomerulonephritis
Membranous nephropathy
Type I MPGN
FSGS
Polyarteritis nodosa
Hepatitis C
Type I MPGN
Membranous nephropathy
FSGS
IgA
Diabetic nephropathy

MPGN, membranoproliferative glomerulonephritis; FSGS, focal segmental glomerulosclerosis; IgA, immunoglobulin A.

In addition, a recent biopsy survey demonstrated the unexpected presence of diabetic nephropathy in 18% of HCV patients due to the high incidence of type II DM in HCV patients.[17]

Two important common findings are present among the diverse group of renal lesions seen with HCV: a lack of correlation with the degree of HCV liver disease and the ubiquitous presence of active HCV viremia.[18]

Membranoproliferative Glomerulonephritis Type I

MPGN type I comprises >85% of the glomerular lesions seen in HCV patients.[19] An essential characteristic of HCV-related MPGN in 80% of patients is the concomitant presence of cryoglobulinemia. In the Brouet classification, cryoglobulinemia is divided into three distinct types with the key differentiation among them being the nature of the protein that forms the cold dependent insoluble complex.[20] In each type of cryoglobulinemia, the primary protein is an immunoglobulin, usually an IgM antibody. In type 2 and Type 3 cryoglobulinemia, the IgM molecule targets the Fab or Fc portion of an IgG antibody. The difference between these two types lies in the character of the IgM antibody. In type 2 cryoglobulinemia, previously called mixed essential cryoglobulinemia, the IgM is a monoclonal IgMκ; whereas in type 3 cryoglobulinemia, the IgM is polyclonal. This IgM antibody for both types of cryoglobulinemia in HCV has rheumatoidlike activity. Unrecognized HCV is now considered to have been the cause of >90% of all previously described cases of mixed essential cryoglobulinemia.[21]

The IgG antibody that is the target of the IgM antibody in both type 2 and type 3 cryoglobulinemia has anti-HCV properties and is the antibody measured by the standard ELISA used for the diagnosis of HCV infection. These IgG antibodies target the HCV circulating RNA and the envelope proteins E1 and E2 and are complement fixing of the IgG1 and IgG3 subclasses. Consequently, the cryoglobulin immune deposit consists of IgMκ–IgG–E2/HCV RNA and is exceptionally large, resulting in deposition exclusively in the subendothelial space of the glomerular capillaries.[22]

On renal biopsy, instead of the typical subendothelial deposits seen in idiopathic MPGN type 1, HCV patients demonstrate extremely large pseudothrombi extending from the subendothelial space into the capillary lumen. On light microscopy these large, eosinophilic deposits can be easily confused with microthrombi such as those seen in a thrombotic microangiopathy, but on immunofluorescence and electron microscopy, their origin is clearly identified as being part of an immune deposit.

The typical Immunofluorescent pattern seen in the glomeruli of HCV patients is granular staining for IgM, IgG, C3, and C4. In addition, light chain staining reveals the predominant deposition of κ light chains in conjunction with IgM, indicating a clonal origin of this antibody.

Measurable cryoglobulinemia is present in approximately 50% of patients, regardless of the HCV genotype and geographic location. Typically, the cryocrit, a reflection of the quantity and potential pathogenicity of the cryoglobulins, is >2%. Importantly, despite the frequency of cryoglobulinemia, these immune complexes are clinically symptomatic in only 5% of patients.[23]

HCV-related cryoglobulinemia is rarely restricted to renal involvement alone and in >70% of cases, it is also associated with cutaneous, neurologic, and/or gastrointestinal disease.[24] The presence of multiorgan dysfunction and renal disease in a patient with long-standing HCV should raise the suspicion of cryoglobulinemia. Renal disease develops significantly more often with type II cryoglobulinemia as compared to type III cryoglobulinemia, possibly related to the solubility, charge, and size of the immune complexes.[25]

The clinical presentation seen with MPGN is typical of a patient with acute nephritis: new onset severe hypertension, acute kidney injury, active urinary sediment, and either nonnephrotic or nephrotic range proteinuria. Demographically, although more men than women are hepatitis C carriers (64% versus 36%), cryoglobulinemia tends to occur more frequently in women (56%).[26] This may have to do with the higher frequency of a TH2 response in women from a chronic antigenic stimuli like HCV, resulting in B-cell overactivity and consequent plasma cell antibody production.

There is an important time sequence leading to the development of MPGN from cryoglobulinemia in HCV patients. Initially, HCV patients demonstrate type III cryoglobulinemia as an early response to the HCV carrier state, and this phase occurs between 5 to 10 years after the acquisition of HCV. After 10 to 15 years in select patients, this type III cryoglobulinemia with a polyclonal IgM eventually transitions to a monoclonal IgM, changing it to a more virulent type II cryoglobulinemia.

Noncryoglobulinemic Membranoproliferative Glomerulonephritis

Not every case of type I MPGN secondary to HCV is related to the presence of cryoglobulinemia.[27] In 20% of MPGN cases in HCV patients, there is no evidence on renal biopsy of cryoglobulin deposition. These patients have the typical subendothelial immune deposits seen with type I MPGN, but their composition is distinct from the large eosinophilic pseudothrombi seen with cryoglobulinemia. HCV viral antigens, IgM and IgG, along with C3, are present by immunofluorescence.[28] In this circumstance, MPGN occurs in isolation from any systemic signs of vasculitis, and hypocomplementemia is not predictable as it is for cryoglobulinemia.

Laboratory Evaluation of Membranoproliferative Glomerulonephritis

Subclinical cases of MPGN have been reported from autopsy series of patients with HCV. A 5% incidence of HCV renal disease that was predominantly MPGN was noted, demonstrating the need for early detection. In addition, for patients undergoing liver transplantation who underwent routine renal biopsies, unsuspected MPGN was noted in 10% to 20% of samples in the presence of normal renal function.[29] This unsuspected frequency of MPGN in liver transplant recipients may explain the decline in renal function that occurs over time after transplantation, which previously may have been ascribed to calcineurin toxicity or pretransplant hepatorenal syndrome.

Clinically, the presence of HCV renal disease can be detected by the presence of albuminuria. In the NHANES study, the odds ratio for albuminuria was 1.84 in HCV-positive patients.[30] The urinalysis findings of patients with cryoglobulinemia are consistent with a nephritic syndrome, and both dipstick and microscopic analyses of urine samples are recommended at regular intervals in HCV patients.[31]

Prior to a renal biopsy, the presence of type II cryoglobulinemia can lend strong support for the presence of MPGN. Cryoglobulinemia is associated with activation of the classical pathway of complement, leading to systemic consumption of C3 and C4. It is rare to have clinically significant cryoglobulinemia in the absence of markedly depressed levels of both C3 and C4. In addition to directly measuring the cryoglobulin concentration, an indirect assessment of the presence of cryoglobulinemia is the presence of rheumatoid factor activity. The IgM monoclonal or polyclonal antibody directed against the HCV IgG antibody has crossover rheumatoid activity, which may provide an indirect quantitative reflection of the amount of cryoglobulins present. The assay for the measurement of cryoglobulin concentrations has been complicated with a high false-negative rate due to frequent improper collection and handling techniques, supporting the use of the rheumatoid factor in general clinical care.[32]

In patients with type II cryoglobulinemia, a serum protein and immune electrophoresis will show a gamma globulin spike of IgMκ. A free light assay will confirm the presence of abundant kappa light chain production with a kappa/lambda ratio >2.0. The selective presence of this unique type of monoclonal antibody is characteristic of the cryoglobulinemia of all genotypes of HCV.

Pathogenesis of Membranoproliferative Glomerulonephritis

The mechanisms responsible for the development of type I MPGN from HCV-induced type II cryoglobulinemia must take into consideration not only the link between the viral infection and cryoglobulin production, but also the pathway of injury caused by these immune complexes. Significant cryoglobulinemia is unique to HCV and is not typically seen with other forms of viral hepatitis. Consequently, the genesis of cryoglobulinemia is not related to the hepatotropic nature of this virus and must be a result of the unique lymphotropic properties of HCV.[33]

HCV has now been clearly shown to be B-cell lymphotropic with specific binding to the CD81 receptor, with additional receptors being identified as Toll-like receptors (TLR-3), scavenger receptors (SRB-1), and the LDL receptor.[34] The binding of HCV to B cells may result in both endocytic-mediated entry of the virus into the cell and also independently may directly stimulate the B cell. CD81 is a member of a signaling complex that involves CD19 and CD21 and lowers the threshold for cell activation and proliferation.[35] Clusters of B-cell aggregates have been identified on liver biopsies in patients with HCV cryoglobulinemia, confirming the separate proliferation of B cells distinct from the standard T-cell response seen in the liver from an HCV infection.[36]

CD5+ B cells appear to be a preferential cell type for HCV stimulation through CD81 and represent the primary cell phenotype seen in the peripheral blood and in liver tissues of patients with cryoglobulinemia.[37] CD5+ B cells are rare in adults and more common in fetal life, where they are responsible for innate immunity.[38] These cells have the propensity to produce IgM antibodies with a restricted set of immunoglobulin V genes, predominantly the VH/VL gene pair 51p1/kv325 with rheumatoidlike properties.[39] Once activated, CD5+ cells may produce interleukin (IL)-10 to catalyze further cell proliferation through an autocrine pathway. Patients with hepatitis B do not demonstrate this form of CD5+ clonal expansion because HBV is not lymphotropic.

In theory, the initial B-cell proliferation will lead to a generalized, broad-based antibody response that is associated with type III cryoglobulinemia. As discussed, this sequence of events occurs after 5 to 10 years of a chronic carrier state in up to 50% of patients. However, maturation of type III cryoglobulinemia into type II cryoglobulinemia requires the emergence of a B-cell clone. How a HCV infection results in clonal B-cell proliferation is still not definitely established, but the following two mechanisms have been suggested: chromosomal mutations and/or cytokine-mediated B-cell hyperplasia.

Initial studies suggested that B-cell clones in HCV type II cryoglobulinemia contained a chromosomal translocation identified as T(14;18).[40] This well-described mutation occurs in 80% of B-cell lymphomas and results in the translocation of the antiapoptotic gene BCL-2 from chromosome 18 to chromosome 14, leading to indefinite B-cell survival.[41] This acquired (somatic) genetic alteration would explain the B-cell clonality found in these patients, as well as the risk of B-cell lymphoma that is 35 times the rate in the general population. Recent work has cast doubt on this theory and has failed to confirm the widespread presence of this chromosomal aberration in HCV-related cryoglobulinemia.[42,43] Alternative hypermutations in antibody production from HCV CD81 binding independent of the T(14;18) translocation may still explain the generation of type II cryoglobulinemia.[44]

Alternatively, circulating IgG–HCV immune complexes may bind to a specific B-cell repertoire (RF+), stimulating the production of B-lymphocyte activating factor (BAFF), leading to further B-cell proliferation. However, the link to the production of a monoclonal IgM antibody from this B-cell proliferation still must be elucidated.

Once formed, the deposition of type II cryoglobulins in the kidneys occurs both in the subendothelial space and in the mesangium. HCV antigens have been colocalized to these regions, confirming their role in the formation of the immune complex.[45] The mesangial localization of the complexes results from binding to fibronectin with TLR-3 activation. The role of TLRs on mesangial cells is now recognized as an important mediator of renal injury from viral infections, particularly HCV immune complexes. The subsequent activation of IL-6, IL-1β, M-CSF, IL-8/CXCL8, RANTES/CCL5, MCP-1/CCL2, and ICAM-I all contribute to the cascade of intrarenal inflammation, leading to progressive loss of glomerular filtration rate (GFR).[46]

The Treatment of Membranoproliferative Glomerulonephritis

The identification of cryoglobulinemia as the primary cause of MPGN provides a key target for therapeutic intervention. Consequently, the removal of circulating cryoglobulins and the prevention of new immune complex production remain the goals of therapy. Ultimately, the prevention of further cryoglobulin production will rest on the control of HCV viremia, but achieving this endpoint is a slow and prolonged process. Current protocols on the use of pegylated or standard IFN mandate a 48-week period of therapy to achieve viral remission. Depending on the viral genotype, control of viral replication will be achieved in only 50% to 60% of patients.[47] This delay in controlling HCV and the unpredictable response and frequent intolerance to this therapy will not be able to attenuate the severity and permanency of glomerular injury.[48] Therefore, control of viremia must be complemented by efforts to reduce the inflammatory response to cryoglobulin deposition, to remove preformed immune complexes, and to directly target the B-cell clonal population.

The most extensive experience in the treatment of HCV-related MPGN comes from the previous studies in mixed essential cryoglobulinemia (MEC). Because it is now estimated that >90% of cases that were labeled as MEC were in fact related to HCV, data from those studies may be applicable in the current approach to therapy. The primary treatment consisted of high-dose corticosteroids, cyclophosphamide, and/or plasmapheresis with no antiviral therapy. Control of cryoglobulinemia and the normalization of serum complement occurred in only 25% and 30% of patients, respectively. Although none of the patients developed worsening liver disease, there were significant infectious complications, including pneumonia and sepsis.[49,50] Therefore, concerns over exacerbating the risk of HCV cirrhosis as a result of steroid and cytotoxic therapy do not appear to be major concerns as compared to their role in preventing life-threatening systemic vasculitic complications.

IFN alone for the treatment of MPGN can lead to a remission of MPGN in 40% to 50% of cases.[51] This is associated with a decrease in cryoglobulin levels and a normalization of serum complement.[52] Importantly, in patients that were able to achieve a viral response to IFN, a marked downregulation of CD81 was found on peripheral B cells, which increased during periods of relapse.[53] Control of MPGN is only achieved with a sustained viral remission, and relapses occurred with a breakthrough of HCV replication after IFN therapy was completed.

Rituximab, as a B-cell targeted therapy, has been successfully used in the treatment of non–viral-mediated cryoglobulinemia.[54] This experience has been applied to the treatment of HCV-related cryoglobulinemia and MPGN. In comparison to IFN therapy, patients treated with rituximab had a 25% higher rate of renal remission with an associated decrease in circulating cryoglobulinemia and normalization of serum complement levels. The HCV viral load increased with therapy but did not result in a clinical worsening of hepatic function. A review of the literature shows that the dose of rituximab used in most reported studies was 375 mg per square meter infused weekly for 4 consecutive weeks. Adjunctive steroids were always used in combination with rituximab. An overall response rate of clinical vasculitis was 80% to 93% with a relapse rate of 30% to 40% over 1 year of follow-up.[55]

As a consequence of the increased viral load seen with rituximab therapy, the next generation of trials have used a combination of IFN and rituximab. This combination resulted in a renal remission of >80% compared to <50% in patients receiving IFN only. Most importantly, there was a significant decrease in viral load in the combination arm similar to that in the IFN-only group.[56,57] Long-term safety of this combination over a 24-month period has been reported and also supports the option of retreatment with rituximab if a relapse occurs.[58]

The following treatment algorithm can be considered based on the published data and a consensus conference on the management of HCV cryoglobulinemia[59]:

1. For mild cases of cryoglobulinemia either isolated to the kidney without significant acute kidney injury (AKI) or with low-grade systemic involvement, IFN alone is a satisfactory option.
2. As the renal lesion intensifies or with more significant systemic organ involvement, rituximab can be added to IFN with term steroid therapy.
3. In life-threatening cases of necrotizing systemic vasculitis from cryoglobulinemia, plasmapheresis can be added in conjunction with rituximab, steroid therapy, and IFN.

Interferon Nephrotoxicity

Because IFN is now established to be the foundation for the treatment of HCV-related MPGN, attention must be placed on the potential nephrotoxicity of this therapy. As a consequence of the upregulation of cell-mediated and humoral-mediated immunity, IFN has been associated with de novo interstitial and glomerular syndromes as well as the exacerbation of underlying GN.[60] Most frequently, a combination of acute kidney injury with nephrotic syndrome has been reported with renal histology, demonstrating minimal change disease with or without an accompanying interstitial nephritis.[61,62] Acute kidney injury has been ascribed to coexisting acute tubular necrosis in most cases. Focal segmental glomerulosclerosis (FSGS) and MPGN have been described in IFN-treated patients, but they are rare manifestations that may or may not be related to the drug exposure.[63] In patients receiving IFN for hematologic malignancies, approximately 25% develop transient low-grade proteinuria and 10% experience acute kidney injury.[64] Recovery occurred after the discontinuation of therapy with remission of the nephrotic syndrome.

Differentiation between HCV-related MPGN and IFN nephrotoxicity can often be made by checking the HCV PCR and serum complement levels. In IFN-associated glomerulopathy characterized by minimal change disease and/or interstitial nephritis, both C3 and C4 will be normal and the viral load should reflect the control of viremia from the therapy. In HCV MPGN, the HCV PCR must reflect active viremia and the serum complement levels will be depressed due to the presence of cryoglobulinemia.

Hepatitis C Virus–Related Renal Disease after Transplantation

There are three scenarios where HCV may result in renal disease after organ transplantation: after kidney transplantation in a patient with known HCV, after combined liver/kidney transplantation in an HCV patient, and in the native kidneys after a liver transplant only in an HCV patient. The common link between each of these scenarios in the development of HCV-related renal disease is the presence of immunosuppression.

ESRD patients with HCV are considered viable kidney transplant candidates as long as there is no evidence of cirrhosis or active extrahepatic immune complex disease. The majority of these patients have ongoing low-level HCV viremia at the time of transplantation and may be at risk for posttransplant HCV-related renal disease. In the posttransplant period, type I MPGN due to cryoglobulinemia in the renal allograft remains the most frequently reported renal syndrome from HCV.[65] This may or may not represent recurrent renal disease because many HCV-positive patients on dialysis do not have prior native kidney biopsies to document their original cause of renal failure and may be first diagnosed with HCV at the time of the transplant workup or upon initiating dialysis therapy.

Cryoglobulinemia is detectable in up to 80% of HCV-positive renal transplant recipients, which represents a significantly higher incidence compared to the average of 40% to 50% in regular, nontransplant HCV patients.[66] The impact of posttransplant immunosuppression in promoting a greater degree of HCV viremia and altering the TH2/TH1 balance favoring the TH2 response may be responsible for this finding. Type III cryoglobulinemia was noted more frequently than type II cryoglobulinemia (78% versus 22%), supporting the low incidence of clinically significant cryoglobulinemic renal disease after transplantation.[67] MPGN may develop in 10% of patients with cryoglobulinemia posttransplant, which represents a higher incidence than in the general population (3%).[68]

Membranous nephropathy (MN) has also been reported posttransplant as a consequence of a preexisting HCV infection.[69] The presence of HCV was reported in 50% of cases of de novo postrenal transplant MN, and may be found more frequently in those patients treated with IFN prior to transplantation.[70] It is presumed that modulating the severity of the viremia before the exposure to immunosuppression may blunt the cryoglobulin production posttransplant, and only IgG–HCV immune complexes will be present, leading to a subepithelial localization and membranous disease.

In liver transplant recipients either with or without a simultaneous kidney transplant, the prevalence of posttransplant cryoglobulinemia is approximately 30%, with clinical renal disease being noted in 10% of cases.[71,72] This risk of cryoglobulinemic GN after liver transplantation is significantly higher than the 3% risk in patients with cryoglobulinemia in the general population.

The choice of treatment for posttransplant HCV-related MPGN is complicated by the risk of inducing acute antibody-mediated (humoral) rejection of the allograft by the use of IFN.[73] These antiviral agents also possess the capacity to increase human leukocyte antigen (HLA) class I and class II expression, leading to increased antigenicity of the allograft. They also increase the number of cytolytic immune effector cells and decrease T-suppressor cell function. The risk of rejection during and after a course of IFN in kidney transplantation has been reported to be between 50% and 100%.[74] In liver/kidney recipients, the use of IFN also may increase the risk of rejection of either or both organs.[75] Therefore, if left untreated, recurrent MPGN in a renal allograft is associated with eventual graft loss, and the treatment of MPGN with IFN may also lead to graft loss.

Ribavirin as a solitary therapy for HCV is not effective at reducing the progression to cirrhosis, but may have clinical use in posttransplant MPGN.[76] Anecdotal cases have shown a reduction in proteinuria and a stabilization of renal function with ribavirin alone and a relapse of renal disease with the cessation of treatment. This therapy was associated with a significant risk of anemia and is limited in its use based on the GFR. The presumed mechanism of action would be through a reduction of viral load with reduced immune complex generation.

Rituximab has been used in HCV patients posttransplant and has been associated with an improvement in renal function and a decrease in cryoglobulinemia.[77] However, in the absence of antiviral therapy, this agent leads to a significant increase in viral load and a potential worsening of the underlying liver function.[78]

The prevention of posttransplant HCV renal disease can be effectively achieved by reducing viremia prior to transplantation. The use of IFN therapy to induce a sustained viral remission prior to kidney transplantation significantly reduced the risk of posttransplant MPGN.[79] Currently, the guidelines for treatment of HCV prior to transplantation focus on reducing the risk of posttransplant cirrhosis but do not take into account the prevention of HCV-related renal disease in either liver or renal transplant recipients.

Hepatitis C Virus-Related Vasculitis

Chronic bacterial and viral infections have been associated with the development of antineutrophil cytoplasmic antibodies (ANCA) and antinuclear antibodies (ANA).[80–81] In HCV patients, a wide spectrum of autoantibodies have been reported in addition to ANCA and ANA, including antismooth muscle (ASM), antimitochondrial, antithyroid microsomal (ATM), antithyroglobulin (ATG), and anti–liver kidney microsomal (LKM1) autoantibodies. The titers of these autoantibodies are usually low and they are often transient in nature.[82] Of all cases of viral-related vasculitis, HCV was responsible for either C-ANCA or P-ANCA disease in 30% of patients. Both systemic and renal complications from small vessel vasculitis may be present, with renal disease characterized by hematuria and acute crescentic GN. This syndrome is distinguished from cryoglobulinemia-induced vasculitis by the absence of immune complexes and normal serum complement levels.

The presumed pathophysiology for the development of vasculitis in HCV is the chronic antigenic stimulation of B cells in HCV carriers. The expansion of CD5+ B-cell clones through stimulation of CD81 by HCV may increase the risk of autoimmunity, leading to ANCA generation. Limited experience is present, however, in the treatment of HCV-related vasculitis.

Focal Segmental Glomerulosclerosis and Immunoglobulin A Nephropathy

Case series have demonstrated an unexpected incidence of FSGS on the renal histology of HCV-infected patients.[83,84] In one case, the FSGS lesion appeared to resolve with IFN therapy and HCV was localized by in situ hybridization to renal tissue.[85]

IgA nephropathy has also been reported on pathology series in patients with HCV, especially in Asian and European case series.[86,87] These populations already have a high incidence of background IgA nephropathy, and it is not clear if this is a chance association between these two frequent diseases. Similar to the anecdotal FSGS case reported previously, IFN therapy has also resulted in the successful resolution of a case of IgA nephropathy in an HCV carrier.[88]

Diabetic Nephropathy

HCV patients have a significant risk for developing type II diabetes, with an odds ratio (OR) = 1.7.[89] This insulin-resistant state may be a consequence of postreceptor inhibition of insulin action by the HCV envelope proteins, especially E2.[90] Biopsy series of patients with HCV now demonstrate a frequency of diabetic nephropathy in 5% to 10% of cases with no coexisting evidence of MPGN or cryoglobulinemia.[91] Therefore, because diabetes is a direct result of HCV infection, diabetic nephropathy should be considered among the glomerular syndromes associated with HCV.

Kidney Disease: Improving Global Outcomes Guidelines for HCV Renal Disease

In 2003, a nonprofit foundation was formed to promote clinical guidelines based on the scientific review of the literature in the management of kidney disease. The Kidney Disease: Improving Global Outcomes (KDIGO) foundation has addressed the issue of HCV in chronic kidney disease (CKD), end stage renal disease (ESRD), and transplant recipients and published a set of guidelines on the diagnosis, evaluation, and management of this viral infection.[92] The following summary of the KDIGO recommendations is applicable to the area of HCV-related glomerular disease:

1. Testing is recommended annually for GFR, proteinuria, and hematuria in HCV patients to provide for the early detection of renal disease.
2. A kidney biopsy should be performed in cases suspected of HCV renal disease due to the diversity of renal syndromes that may occur.
3. Antiviral therapy with IFN and ribavirin (based on GFR) should be initiated in all cases of HCV renal disease and continued for 12 months.
4. Plasmapheresis, steroids, immunosuppressive agents, and antiviral therapy should be used for patients with active cryoglobulinemia.
   a. Immunosuppressive drug choices include rituximab or cyclophosphamide.
5. Ribavirin should be used with extreme caution in patients with Stages 3 through 5 CKD due to the risk of severe anemia.
6. Angiotensin converting enzyme inhibitors (ACEI)/angiotensin receptor blockers (ARB) therapy is recommended for patients with significant nephrotic syndrome as adjunctive therapy.

Key Points: Hepatitis C Virus and Glomerular Disease

1. HCV has unique B-cell tropism especially for CD5+ B cells, which is not a feature of other hepatidites.
2. The HCV virus not only enters the B cell, but can also directly stimulate B-cell proliferation and antibody production.
3. Approximately 50% of HCV patients develop cryoglobulinemia, but it is clinically symptomatic in only 3%, with a female predilection for disease.
4. Type III cryoglobulinemia is a precursor for the eventual transition to type II cryoglobulinemia, and is composed of an IgMκ monoclonal antibody with rheumatoid factor activity that is characteristic of HCV.
5. Type I MPGN is the most common glomerular lesion seen with HCV and results from type II cryoglobulinemia.

6. Controlling active HCV viremia is the therapeutic target for the treatment of HCV MPGN and systemic cryoglobulinemia, and this can best be achieved with IFN therapy.
7. Rituximab is considered the first adjunctive add-on therapy for more severe cases of renal and systemic disease, followed by plasmapheresis.
8. HCV renal disease may occur in the posttransplant period of either liver or kidney transplantation; however, IFN therapy is relatively contraindicated due to its association with a high risk of vascular rejection.
9. HCV may also be associated with ANCA-positive vasculitis due to the B-cell hyperplasia with diffuse autoantibody production.

HIV

Epidemiology

HIV infection has become a global pandemic, resulting in 35 million deaths since the initial description of AIDS in 1981. Currently, over 33 million people worldwide are carriers of the HIV virus with 65% of the cases residing in sub-Saharan Africa and 11% living in Asia, primarily in India.[93] Over 2.5 million new HIV cases are diagnosed each year. In the United States, 1.2 million people carry the HIV virus, with an annual incidence of >55,000 new cases reported each year.[94] Compared to the 330 million carriers of hepatitis B and the 170 million carriers of hepatitis C, HIV infection carries a significantly higher case fatality rate.

HIV genetically arose from the simian immunodeficiency virus and crossed over into a human pathogen from monkeys and chimpanzees in Cameroon and East Africa.[95] HIV is a lentivirus and consists of three main distinct groups: M, N, and O. The majority of infections seen worldwide belong to group M.[96] The M group is further categorized into 10 subtypes or clades (A through J), with subtype B being the most common species found in the United States and Europe.[97]

Demographically, the most common method of transmission of HIV worldwide is through heterosexual exposure, which explains the finding that 50% of HIV patients are women.[98] The vertical transmission of HIV occurs in one third of infected mothers and remains a major route of HIV acquisition in Africa. Parenteral transmission from intravenous drug abuse and homosexuality continue to be important ongoing sources of HIV infection.

In the United States, African American and Hispanic patients are overrepresented within the HIV population compared to their distribution in the general population.[99] Both of these ethnic groups each comprise 15% of the U.S. population, but account for 50% (African American patients) and 35% (Hispanic patients) of the HIV population.[100] This excess risk may be related to both socioeconomic as well as genetic susceptibility factors. Caucasian patients may carry a high rate of polymorphism for the primary HIV receptor: chemokine receptor 5 (CCXR5). Inheritance of these alleles either as a heterozygous or a homozygous expression for the altered receptor may prevent HIV cellular entry and provide a state of resistance to acquiring HIV disease after exposure. African American patients have a significantly lower rate of CCXR5 polymorphism and subsequently express the entire HIV receptor in its fully functional form.[101] In addition, genetic variation on chemokine receptor 2 and IL-2 expression may also play a pivotal role in the risk for acquiring HIV infection and in the development of systemic complications that may arise after a carrier state is established.

The Laboratory Diagnosis of HIV

HIV can be detected through both qualitative and quantitative assays. The serologic diagnosis of HIV is based on the detection of IgG antibodies targeting any of three specific HIV antigens: p24, gp120, and/or gp41. An ELISA is used as an initial screening test, and a positive result is confirmed through a Western blot, which yields a sensitivity and specificity of >99%.[102]

Quantification of the viral load is accomplished through measuring viral RNA by reverse transcription and subsequent PCR amplification. This test provides a reliable method to diagnose HIV infection and quantitatively follow therapeutic interventions.

Glomerular Syndromes and HIV

A variety of glomerular syndromes have been described as a direct consequence of HIV infection (Table 47.3).[103] In addition,

TABLE 47.3 Glomerular Syndromes in HIV Patients

Glomerular Syndromes in HIV Patients
HIV-associated nephropathy (HIVAN)
Collapsing variant of focal segmental glomerulosclerosis (FSGS)
HIV immune complex disease of the kidney (HIVICK)
Diffuse proliferative glomerulonephritis
IgA nephropathy
Proliferative glomerulonephritis (lupus-like variant)
Membranous glomerulonephritis
Mesangial proliferative glomerulonephritis
Thrombotic microangiopathy
Hepatitis-related glomerulonephritis (coinfection)
Hepatitis C
Type I membranoproliferative glomerulonephritis with cryoglobulinemia
Hepatitis B
Membranous glomerulonephritis
Membranoproliferative glomerulonephritis
"Classic" FSGS
Fibrillary glomerulonephritis
Postinfectious glomerulonephritis
Diabetic nephropathy
Amyloidosis

HIV patients are frequently coinfected with HCV (25% to 30%) and/or with HBV (2% to 9%), and these viral diseases may result in their own characteristic glomerular syndromes. Glomerular disease represents only a subset of all HIV-related renal diseases that otherwise involve a spectrum of acid base and electrolyte disorders, AKI, CKD, and highly active antiretroviral therapy (HAART)-related nephrotoxicity.

HIV-Associated Nephropathy

Epidemiology

The pathologic lesion of collapsing FSGS has been considered the hallmark of HIV renal disease and carries the designation HIV-associated nephropathy (HIVAN). This glomerular finding was originally described in AIDS patients in 1984 in New York and Miami.[104] Subsequently, HIVAN was documented to account for >90% of all glomerular disease found in HIV patients prior to the HAART era, which started in 1995. More recently, only 35% to 50% of renal biopsies in HIV patients demonstrate this classic lesion.[105]

HIVAN represents the third leading cause of ESRD in African American males ages 20 to 64 years old in the United States.[106] In the U.S. dialysis population, 1.6% of patients are HIV positive with HIVAN being responsible for approximately 50% of these cases of ESRD.[107] Looking at this data from the alternate perspective, non–HIVAN-related renal disease accounts for up to 50% of the cases of ESRD in HIV patients, and these etiologies may be related to HIV-associated immune complex disease of the kidneys (HIVICK), diabetes, hypertension, FSGS, HCV, and/or HAART therapy.

HIVAN is considered to be a consequence of uncontrolled viral replication, with the majority of patients having a CD4 count $<200/mm^3$ and having a markedly elevated viral load.[108] The presence of a low CD4 count with a low viral load confers a significantly greater risk for developing HIVAN (OR = 3.5) than the presence of a high viral load but with a CD4 count $>200\ mm^3$ (OR = 2.0). These data suggest that it is the biologic effect of the virus at the cellular level that is more important for the development of renal disease than simply the amount of circulating virus. The combined presence of both a low CD4 count and a high viral load resulted in the highest risk of HIVAN, with an OR of 6.1.

Conversely, the presence of a viral load <400 copies per milliliter is a strong negative predictor for the presence of HIVAN.[109] However, recent reports show that approximately 20% to 30% of HIV patients may have HIVAN in the absence of circulating viremia. In these patients, the detection of proviral DNA in peripheral blood mononuclear cells or renal tissue will demonstrate the HIV viral infection.[110]

Current estimates place a 2% to 10% lifetime risk of developing HIVAN in untreated HIV patients.[111] The most comprehensive data on the risk of HIVAN comes from sub-Saharan Africa, where a conservative estimate of 2.6 million cases of HIVAN may be present (10% of the total HIV population).[112] In the HAART naïve populations of Nigeria, Rwanda, and South Africa, the presence of proteinuria in the adult population with HIV ranged between 10% to 30%, with biopsy-proven HIVAN being present in 70% to 80% of these patients.[113]

HIVAN has a unique racial predisposition, with >95% of cases being diagnosed in Black patients. This overrepresentation of the Black race may be a consequence of multiple genetic risk factors influencing viral entry into cells and the host cytokine response. In addition to the polymorphism for the CCXR5 receptor, as previously discussed, the most recent genetic risk factor described for HIVAN deals with variants of the myosin heavy chain 9 (MHY9) protein. This IIa isoform is a nonmuscle-associated heavy chain that is present in the podocyte and is associated with actin and is coded for on chromosome 22.

Linkage disequilibrium studies have demonstrated 14 single nucleotide polymorphisms for this gene, which lead to a higher risk of ESRD and idiopathic FSGS but, in addition, resulted in a significant risk of HIVAN in Black patients.[114] The presence of these polymorphisms is rare in the Caucasian European population and may explain the marked susceptibility of Black patients to developing CKD and ESRD.[115]

More recent data suggest that the MHY9 polymorphisms may be a surrogate marker by linkage to inheritance of another gene disorder of the apolipoprotein 1 gene (APOL1).[116] This gene is also present on chromosome 22 and is highly associated with FSGS and ESRD in patients of African origin.[117] Variations in APOL1 (G1 and G2) confer resistance to trypanosome infections, which may explain the persistence of this recessively inherited gene in the African population.[118] The localization and role that APOL1 plays in podocyte function has not been defined and the expression of mRNA for APOL1 in the podocyte has only recently been demonstrated in the cell culture.[119]

Additional HIVAN susceptibility genes may be present, which interact with viral gene products to increase the risk of developing podocyte injury and renal disease.[120] In the mouse transgenic model for HIVAN (Tg26), three distinct gene loci have been identified, with one (HIVAN1) having a human counterpart on chromosome 3 and additional potential candidates for susceptibility genes being located on chromosomes 11,14, and 16.[121] The important contribution of a genetically susceptible host combined with virus-mediated gene products as a cause of HIVAN is becoming increasingly emphasized.

The method of acquisition of HIV has not been shown to be a risk factor for the development of HIVAN. Previous reports have linked intravenous heroin use with a risk of HIVAN based on the frequent finding of FSGS as part of the spectrum of heroin nephropathy.[122] However, the FSGS reported as part of heroin nephropathy differs from the collapsing variant of FSGS seen with HIVAN, and may have been related to adulterants of the heroin itself and therefore unrelated to undiagnosed HIV infections.[123]

HIVAN is not synonymous with heroin nephropathy and is a distinct disorder related directly to HIV, regardless of the method of exposure.

Clinical Diagnosis

There are six clinical clues that can be used to predict the diagnosis of HIVAN: (1) patient demographics, (2) the presence or absence of effective HAART therapy, (3) the degree of proteinuria, (4) the presence or absence of hypertension, (5) the radiologic appearance of the kidneys, and (6) the presence or absence of hematuria. Black race remains one of the most important discriminating features between HIVAN and HIVICK and non–HIV-related renal disease. HIVAN is distinctly unusual in non-Black patients (<10%), and this immediate demographic finding should lead to an alternative differential diagnosis other than HIVAN.[124]

Because HIVAN is a manifestation of uncontrolled HIV infection, the presence of a HAART-treated patient should raise suspicion that an alternative cause of renal injury is present. The measurement of the CD4 count and viral load, as discussed, will usually differentiate the risk of HIVAN from other causes of nephropathy.

As a consequence of the presence of collapsing FSGS, HIVAN should be suspected in any HIV patient with nephrotic-range proteinuria.[125] However, due to the presence of other glomerular diseases as a result of an HIV infection, the sensitivity and specificity of nephrotic-range proteinuria for HIVAN was 69% and 67%, respectively, with positive and negative predictive values of 52% and 80%. Although nephrotic range proteinuria is the most common presenting clinical finding for HIVAN, the diagnostic criteria for the presence of the nephrotic syndrome may not be fulfilled. HIVAN patients may have significant hypoalbuminemia but no evidence of edema on physical examination compared to the marked edema in classic FSGS patients. The etiology for this may be related to the production of high levels of nonspecific hypergammaglobulinemia, which may offset the loss of oncotic pressure in these patients, thus preventing edema formation.[126]

The predictive value of microalbuminuria in the early detection of HIVAN has not yet been defined. Overall, microalbuminuria has been detected in 11% of HAART-naïve HIV patients, with rates of 15% in Black patients and 7% in Caucasians.[127] In a longitudinal study, 15.7% of patients with microalbuminuria progressed to overt proteinuria, whereas 14% of patients without microalbuminuria developed microalbuminuria on follow-up.[128] Microalbuminuria was associated with lower CD4 counts and higher viral loads, suggesting that HIVAN and/or other tubulointerstitial injury may be a likely finding on renal biopsy. Renal biopsies in HIV patients with microalbuminuria have demonstrated unsuspected HIVAN lesions in >85% of patients.[129] Therefore, in addition to being a predictor of the development of CKD, increased cardiovascular morbidity, and mortality, microalbuminuria in HIV patients may be an early sign of HIVAN.

The Infectious Disease Society of America (IDSA) has now placed urinalysis screening as part of the workup in all HIV patients with a threshold of 1+ proteinuria requiring additional quantitation.[130] However, a screening urine dipstick target of this level has a sensitivity level of only 79% for significant proteinuria that may be clinically relevant as a sign of intrinsic disease.[131] Therefore, in light of the microalbuminuria data, a random urine microalbumin or albumin/creatinine ratio may be a more sensitive tool as compared to a urinalysis for the evaluation of renal disease in HIV patients.

Although classic FSGS patients universally have hypertension (HTN) associated with progressive CKD, only 12% to 20% of HIVAN patients will demonstrate HTN in the setting of collapsing FSGS. HIV-associated upregulation of cytokines leading to peripheral vasodilation and a possible renal tubular sodium natriuresis may counteract the development of HTN in patients with HIVAN.[132] The presence of significant HTN should lead to the consideration of an alternative differential diagnosis such as HIVICK, coexistent HBV or HCV renal disease, or HAART-related HTN.[133]

The presence of large size (>13 cm), highly echogenic kidneys on ultrasound have been widely promoted as markers for the presumptive diagnosis of HIVAN. However, on critical review, these findings do not have the predictive value to make them reliable clinical tools. HIVAN has been associated with large size kidneys due to the development of microtubular dilation.[134] This pathologic finding is not present in patients with HIVICK. However, only 12% to 28% of HIVAN patients have large kidney size by ultrasound with a sensitivity of 24% and a positive predictive value of only 44%.[135] In light of this data, the importance of kidney size has been overemphasized as an important feature of HIVAN.

The presence of increased renal echogenicity by ultrasound may be a better reflection of significant renal parenchymal disease. The level of echogenicity of the kidney is compared to the liver and can be graded qualitatively by categories of severity. When the degree of echogenicity is qualitatively defined (0 to 4+), then the predictive value at the extremes of the grades can have a sensitivity of 96% and a specificity of 51%.[136] Most radiology centers do not use a scale for determining the degree of echogenicity and, therefore, this finding is not a reliable clinical finding for HIVAN. Pelvicalyceal thickening has been reported as a highly specific finding in HIVAN, but this radiologic feature has not been further replicated in a large cohort.[137]

HIVAN should also be considered in patients with HIV that present with AKI. Overall, patients with HIV are more prone to AKI either from acute tubular necrosis (ATN) or nephrotoxic agents and experience a significantly higher mortality compared to AKI in the general community.[138] HIVAN was noted in the background of AKI in 20% of patients, indicating that this lesion should be considered a potential risk factor for AKI.[139] Any HIV patient with AKI should be evaluated for the presence of preexisting HIVAN.

The IDSA Guidelines also recommend estimating GFR in addition to a screening urinalysis for all HIV patients. HIVAN is often associated with a significant reduction in GFR, with the majority of patients having stage 3 CKD at the time of diagnosis.[140] The validity of using estimated GFR (eGFR) equations in HIV patients has not been established, although the Modification of Diet in Renal Disease (MDRD) formula appears to have superior accuracy compared to the Cockcroft and Gault equation in this population.[141] The new Chronic Kidney Disease Epidemiology Collaboration formula (CKD-EPI) formula has been compared to the MDRD equation and showed significantly closer correlation with isotopic measurements of GFR, especially at a GFR >60 mL per minute.[142]

Pathophysiology of HIV-Associated Nephropathy

HIVAN represents a unique constellation of four key pathologic findings in the renal biopsy: (1) collapsing FSGS, (2) microcystic dilation of the tubules, (3) interstitial nephritis, and (4) the presence of intracytoplasmic tubuloreticular bodies. By definition, the only specific requirement to fulfill the diagnosis of HIVAN is the presence of collapsing FSGS in the setting of an HIV infection with the remaining lesions being found in variable frequencies.

The glomerular lesion of collapsing FSGS seen in HIVAN is distinct from the immune complex proliferative GN of HIVICK and the classic perihilar and tip lesions seen with idiopathic FSGS. The hallmark of HIVAN is the proliferation and hypertrophy of the glomerular podocytes, leading not only to the physical involution of the glomerular tuft from the mass of overhanging cellular bulk, but also from the impaired synthesis of the normal glomerular basement membrane. The proper collagen composition of the basement membrane is dependent on podocyte function, and an increase in immature type IV collagen production was noted in HIVAN patients.[143] The decrease in GFR is subsequently related to the loss of ultrafiltration surface area as well as a loss of the ultrafiltration coefficient.

The cells that comprise the hyperplastic cap on top of the glomerular capillary tuft are not solely comprised of visceral epithelial cells but appear to also be of parietal cell origin based on the presence of specific parietal cell markers (CK8 and PAX2).[144] This finding of the coexistence of parietal and visceral epithelial cells in the collapsing lesion of FSGS is not unique to HIVAN and is also present in pamidronate-induced and idiopathic-collapsing FSGS.[145]

The current working hypothesis for the genesis of these hyperplastic cells is direct viral infection with the transcription of the viral genome leading to an uncoupling of cell differentiation.[146] HIVAN is categorized as a podocytopathy nicknamed the "dysregulated podocyte syndrome."[147] An HIV infection of renal cells is not restricted to only glomerular epithelial cells, but can also be found in tubular epithelial cells, collecting duct cells, and mesangial cells.[148] Indeed, renal tissue has been shown to be a potential reservoir for HIV even when there is no detectable viremia.[149]

The primary alteration of the podocyte by HIV is characterized by a physical change to a macrophage phenotype. The typical markers of a mature podocyte, including vimentin, synaptopodin, podocalyxin, and WT-1, are lost and the cell acquires new macrophage epitopes such as KP-1 and Ki-67.[150] In conjunction with the upregulation of these proliferation markers, there is a loss of p27 and p57, which usually downregulate the cell cycle. Podocytes normally do not replicate but, as a consequence of HIV infection, they now develop a dedifferentiated proliferative and hyperplastic capacity.[151]

A transgenic mouse model (Tg26) has demonstrated the importance of the cellular expression of the HIV genome as a cause of nephropathy.[152] These animals carry a noninfectious HIV construct in renal tissue, which leads to FSGS even when these kidneys are transplanted into normal littermates. In contrast, normal kidneys transplanted into the transgenic animals did not develop glomerular disease. These findings demonstrate the fact that circulating HIV virions are not important for the development of HIVAN, but rather, it is the presence of an intracellular HIV infection that dictates the expression of renal disease.[153]

The entry of HIV into renal cells must occur through a separate and distinct pathway compared to its ability to infect T lymphocytes. The CD4 receptor and the chemokine receptors (CCXR4 and CCXR5) have not been demonstrated in renal tissue. Possible methods for viral entry in the kidney include transcytosis, lipid rafts, microparticles, and C-type lectin receptors.[154–155]

Once viral entry is established, the 15 translation products from the nine genes of the HIV genome interplay to cause HIVAN.[156] Of these genes, at least three have been strongly implicated in directly causing the podocytopathy: Tat (transactivating protein), Nef (negative factor for viral replication), and Vpr (viral protein r). Both the Nef and Vpr genes independently and synergistically result in the development of podocyte dysregulation.[157] These gene products appear to exert their action by activating the Src kinase pathway with increased Stat3 and MAPK1.[158] In addition, Nef may cause proteinuria by interfering with the actin cytoskeleton of the podocyte by inducing a loss of stress fibers and increasing lamellipodia through the activation of Rac1 and the inhibition of RhoA.[159] The Tat protein complements these changes by causing increased glomerular permeability due to a marked reduction in nephrin expression.[160] Increased cytokine expression also plays a pivotal role in the development of HIVAN with increased vascular endothelial growth factor (VEGF) and nuclear factor kappa B (NF-κB) production by the podocyte.[161] These molecules promote further podocyte proliferation, leading to the collapsing lesion and increased cellular apoptosis both in the tubules and in the glomerulus.[162] Finally, newer pathophysiologic pathways have been identified, which include the mammalian target of rapamycin (mTOR) pathway and the notch signaling pathway, both of which are highly upregulated in HIVAN.[163,164] The complex interplay of all these pathways is still under investigation but remains a vital goal in order to better develop targeted therapy to interrupt the sequence of events that cause HIVAN.

The second major diagnostic feature of HIVAN after collapsing FSGS is the presence of microcystic dilation of the tubules, which can be found in 60% of cases.[165] By definition, these tubules are ectatic and assume a size three times larger than the diameter of a normal adjacent tubule. They result from the same altered rate of proliferation and apoptosis that occurs in the podocytes, and HIV gene expression can be isolated from the affected tubular cells. Multiple nephron segments are involved by the microcystic dilation, including the proximal and distal tubules and the collecting ducts.[166] Interestingly, as the tubular dilation increases and the epithelium becomes flattened, HIV gene expression ceases and the growth of the cysts becomes self-limiting.[167] This explains why the cysts never reach the size of those seen in autosomal dominant polycystic kidney disease and remain only microscopic and below the cortical surface. The mechanisms responsible for the loss of HIV gene transcription with cyst expansion have not been defined. The kidney size actually increases based on ultrasonography in 12% to 30% of patients due to the abundant tubular microcysts.

The third feature of HIVAN is the presence of an interstitial infiltrate consisting primarily of CD8+ T cells and plasma cells. The average CD4/CD8 ratio in the renal biopsy specimen is 0.35 and may reflect the systemic T-cell subset ratio. Often, the degree of interstitial inflammation may be out of proportion to the degree of glomerulosclerosis.[168] There is a marked upregulation of local α and γ IFN production, which further increases the antigenicity of the renal tubular cells by enhancing the expression of class II HLA antigens.[169] Additional inflammatory mediators are prominently activated within the interstitial infiltrate, especially NF-κB.[170] The presence of an interstitial infiltrate in the absence of collapsing FSGS in an HIV patient may occur in 20% of cases.[171] In these cases, the interstitial infiltrate usually represents an allergic drug reaction possibly to antibiotics, nonsteroidal anti-inflammatory drugs (NSAIDs), or HAART therapy.

The presence of tubuloreticular inclusion (TRI) bodies is the fourth most important feature of HIVAN and are present in >90% of cases. These lesions are found in glomerular and tubular endothelial cells as well as in infiltrating leukocytes.[172] TRI bodies are not pathognomonic of HIVAN because they may be seen in systemic lupus erythematosis (SLE). Morphologic analysis shows that these particles are approximately 20 to 25 nm tubule structures, are intracytoplasmic, and are located in the dilated cisternae of the endoplasmic reticulum and the perinuclear Golgi apparatus. TRI bodies are not viral particles but represent the effects of upregulation of IFN on the aggregation of acid glycoproteins. Therefore, an alternative name for the TRI bodies seen in HIVAN and SLE is interferon footprints.

Treatment of HIV-Associated Nephropathy

All treatment recommendations for HIVAN are based on individual center observational reports. In a Cochrane Database Review of HIVAN therapy, no randomized controlled trials were found in the literature and, therefore, the authors could not offer any proven guidelines for therapy.[173] The treatment strategies discussed in the following section are limited by the individual study designs, but they do offer a reasonable clinical scheme to follow based on the current scientific literature.

The strategy for the successful treatment of HIVAN is based on the basic premise that the glomerular disease results from active viral infection of renal tissue with the transcription of the HIV genome. Elimination of the viral load followed by efforts to reduce cytokine production, to decrease the interstitial infiltrate, and to reduce proteinuria comprise the goals of a coordinated therapeutic plan. Consequently, HAART therapy remains the a priori therapeutic intervention upon which all adjunctive treatments are then added.

HAART therapy can prevent the development of HIVAN in 60% of treated patients and, when initiated after the diagnosis of HIVAN, may reduce the rate of progression to ESRD by 38%.[174,175] In HIVAN patients who present with a decreased GFR, HAART therapy can result in an improvement in renal function.[176,177] Conversely, patients with HIVAN who stop HAART therapy experienced an accelerated decline of renal function.[178]

The benefit of HAART therapy on the real function in HIVAN can be correlated directly to the degree of viremia control.[179] The odds ratio in a multivariate analysis for an improvement of GFR with a decrease in viral load was 7.3. An average increase in GFR with HAART therapy was 10 mL per minute.[180]

The improvement in GFR with HAART therapy correlates with a reversal of the histologic lesions of HIVAN.[181] With control of HIV viremia, the podocyte phenotype can revert back to its normal nonproliferating state with a regression of the collapsing lesions. This is characterized by loss of the proliferative Ki67 markers and a reacquisition of synaptopodin, WT-1, and the other markers of a mature podocyte. In addition, the microcystic dilation of the tubules can regress with an improvement in the appearance of the interstitial space. The capacity for regression of HIVAN lesions likely is dependent on the degree of interstitial fibrosis and glomerulosclerosis that is present.

The role of HAART in the treatment of microalbuminuria in HIV patients is not established. Because the majority of HIV patients with microalbuminuria will have HIVAN on biopsy, this cohort appears to be an ideal target group for the early initiation of HAART. One study has demonstrated a decrease in microalbuminuria of 45% to 90% in more than 70% of treated patients.[182] Therefore, HAART has an antiproteinuric effect for patients with fully established nephrotic syndrome as well as in patients with microalbuminuria. The IDSA guidelines support the initiation of HAART therapy once the diagnosis of HIVAN is made.[183]

Corticosteroids have been successfully used in HIVAN as short-term therapy to improve renal function and to reduce proteinuria. Multiple retrospective case control and cohort studies using prednisone starting at 1 mg per kilogram per day tapered off over a 2 to 9 month period have supported the benefit of this therapy in HIVAN.[184–185] Steroid use was associated with an odds ratio for the development of ESRD of 0.20 to 0.29 (71% to 80% reduction in ESRD) and with a 40% improvement in GFR. Importantly, no significant increase in the rate of infectious complications was noted in the steroid-treated groups though a higher risk of avascular necrosis was noted.[186]

The mechanism of action of steroids may be primarily through the eradication of the inflammatory interstitial infiltrate and reducing local cytokine production.[187] Biopsy results before and after steroid therapy show a marked improvement in the interstitial nephritis without a major change in the glomerular lesion.[188] Steroids directly reduce NF-κB by increasing the natural inhibitor of this molecule I-κB and may attenuate the inflammatory cascade that results from HIV infection.[189]

The data appear to suggest that a short course of steroids carries an acceptable risk and is associated with an amelioration of proteinuria and an improvement in GFR. Theoretically, this therapy may be most effective when HIVAN is accompanied by a significant interstitial infiltrate, but can be tried on a short-term basis even in patients without interstitial nephritis as long as the degree of fibrosis is not pervasive.

Inhibition of the renin angiotensin system in nephrotic HIVAN patients has also been shown to be independently beneficial in lowering proteinuria and prolonging renal survival. The original study of ACEI in HIVAN was with the use of fosinopril in 44 HIVAN patients, showing three times an increase in renal survival with remission of the nephrotic syndrome in >70% of the treated patients.[190] Captopril similarly demonstrated four times an increase in renal survival in HIVAN and, in a multivariate analysis use of captopril or HAART therapy, were the only factors that influenced maintaining preservation of renal function.[191] ARB therapy with olmesartan was also associated with a protective effect on the development of HIVAN in the transgenic HIV mouse model, confirming the role of renin-angiotensin-aldosterone system (RAAS) inhibition in general as a beneficial focus of therapy in HIVAN.[192]

ACEI or ARB therapy may be beneficial through mechanisms beyond their effects on proteinuria and intraglomerular pressure. Angiotensin II is significantly upregulated in HIVAN and may directly and indirectly (through TGF-β) lead to podocyte injury and interstitial and glomerular fibrosis. Inhibition of angiotensin II with ARB therapy significantly ameliorated histologic podocyte damage in the transgenic mouse model for HIV.[193]

HIV Immune Complex Disease of the Kidneys

HIV immune complex disease of the kidneys (HIVICK) represents an emerging cause of glomerular disease in HIV patients and may be present in 30% to 45% of cases, making it the second most common glomerular disease after HIVAN.[194,195] This classification encompasses three major categories of glomerular disease: diffuse glomerulonephritis (DPGN, "lupus-like disease), MN, and IgA nephropathy.[196] The unifying feature of these three forms of HIVICK is the identification of mesangial and glomerular basement immune complexes associated with HIV antigens as an integral part of the complex.[197] HIV patients with coexisting hepatitis C or hepatitis B may develop renal lesions specific to those viral infections, and although immune complexes are present as the primary etiology of their glomerular injury, they do not involve HIV antigens. Therefore, these renal diseases will be discussed separately in the following text and are not considered part of HIVICK.

Pathophysiology of HIV Immune Complex Disease of the Kidneys

By definition, establishing the presence of immune complexes by immunofluorescence and/or by electron microscopy is a prerequisite for the diagnosis of HIVICK. These immune complexes may appear all by themselves in isolation or in the context of other features of HIV (TRI, microcystic tubular dilation, or interstitial nephritis) in 29% of cases. Therefore, the key distinguishing feature between HIVAN and HIVICK lies strictly in the glomerular pathology—either collapsing FSGS for HIVAN or immune complex–mediated GN in HIVICK.[198]

The development of HIVICK represents a unique variation of the immune response to HIV infection.[199] Hypergammaglobulinemia is a common finding in most HIV patients and indicates a generalized B-cell reaction to the HIV infection, often with low levels of ANCA, ANA, and other "autoimmune " markers being present. However, these are usually of low titer and are not associated with clinical disease. HIVICK is the end result of insoluble immune complexes formed, targeting an array of HIV antigens either in the peripheral circulation or in situ in the glomerular basement membrane. Specifically, in IgA nephropathy, an IgA-p24 immune complex has been identified, and in MPGN and membranous GN, both IgG–gp-120 and IgG-p24 complexes are present.[200]

HIV Immune Complex Disease of the Kidneys–Immunoglobulin A Nephropathy

IgA nephropathy is found in approximately 5% to 10% of renal biopsies in HIV patients, with an increased predominance in Caucasian and Asian populations.[201] Patients may present with nephrotic syndrome alone or with a combination of hematuria and nonnephrotic range proteinuria. It was initially suggested that IgA may occur by chance in any HIV population of Asian or Caucasian descent due to the high incidence of IgA in these general populations.[202] However, the finding of HIV p24 directly as part of the mesangial immune complexes bound to IgA confirms the role of HIV as an etiology for this glomerulopathy.

HIV Immune Complex Disease of the Kidneys–Lupus-like Glomerulonephritis

This form of diffuse and focal proliferative GN differs from other HIVICK lesions due to a marked predisposition in Black patients similar to HIVAN. The other HIVICK lesions have a significant predilection for patients that are Asian or Caucasian. This "lupus-like" glomerulonephritis lesion has a unique similarity to the DPGN seen in SLE, demonstrating both glomerular subendothelial ("wire loop"), mesangial, and subepithelial immune complexes associated with a "full house" staining on immunofluorescence of IgG, IgA, IgM, C1q, and C3.[203] An interstitial infiltrate may be present with predominant B cells as opposed to the T-cell infiltrate seen in HIVAN. A ubiquitous finding in the lesion is the presence of TRI, which is likely a result of heightened intrarenal IFN stimulation.

These histologic lesions closely resemble SLE nephritis with the caveat that the typical SLE autoimmune serology is negative and complement levels are not significantly depressed. Most of these patients have active HIV viremia and have had HIV for >10 years. The clinical presentation consists of hypertension, a decreased GFR with hematuria, and proteinuria consistent with a nephritic urinary sediment.[204] The patient course is one of rapid progression toward ESRD.

Treatment of HIV Immune Complex Disease of the Kidneys

Few studies address the treatment outcome of patients with HIVICK, although overall renal survival is more prolonged compared to untreated HIVAN.[205] HAART does not appear to have the same reproducible improvement benefit in HIVICK as it does for HIVAN, although anecdotal cases have shown some improvement in GFR.[206] In particular, the lupus-like proliferative glomerulonephritis variant of HIVICK progresses rapidly toward ESRD in <6 months with no response to corticosteroids and/or HAART. The lack of consistent benefit of HAART in HIVICK compared to HIVAN even though both are caused by active HIV infection can be explained by the method of renal injury. In HIVAN, the injury is related to alterations of the phenotype, which are clinically reversible. In HIVICK, there is extensive immune complex deposition that may not be remediable, leaving permanent scars and basement membrane damage. Controlling viremia in HIVICK does not affect the previously deposited immune complexes. The lupus-like variant would be particularly less likely to respond to HAART compared to IgA nephropathy and the membranous variants.

ACEI therapy has been used in HIVICK–IgA nephropathy with an improvement in proteinuria and a stabilization of GFR, but there are few reports of its use in other cases of HIVICK.[207] Consequently, establishing a firm diagnosis of HIVICK or HIVAN through a renal biopsy is essential in order to provide a more accurate prognosis for an individual patient.[208]

Coinfection of HIV and Hepatitis C Virus

Among all HIV carriers, coinfection with HCV is present in 25% to 30% of cases, whereas 8% to 10% of HCV patients are coinfected with HIV. This conservatively represents 250,000 patients in the United States and 10 million people worldwide who harbor both of these chronic viral infections. When both viral diseases are present together, the primary renal lesion often results from HCV and is a type I MPGN due to cryoglobulinemia. MPGN from HCV is present in 34% of cases, with HIVAN being present in only 9%.[209]

Nonspecific cryoglobulinemia can occur in low levels in up to 20% of HIV-only infected patients compared to an incidence of 50% in patients with HCV; however, they are rarely associated with renal disease.[210] The presence of HTN, systemic vasculitis, hematuria, and hypocomplementemia supports the diagnosis of MPGN in HCV/HIV coinfected patients compared to the lack of HTN and nephrotic sediment in HIVAN.[211]

Coinfection with HCV results in a more rapid rate of decline in GFR in HIV patients.[212] The presence of HCV coinfection with HIV also increased the risk of death sevenfold, and the presence of type I MPGN further resulted in an odds ratio for death of 6.0. Differentiation of HCV MPGN from HIV-associated nephropathy can be made clinically by the presence of hypertension, nephritic sediment, hypocomplementemia, and the presence of cryoglobulinemia, all of which are uncommon in HIV nephropathy (Table 47.4).[213]

Thrombotic Microangiopathy

Biopsy specimens from HIV patients prior to the HAART era in the 1980s frequently showed evidence of a thrombotic microangiopathy (TMA). The majority of these patients had advanced AIDS defined as a CD4 count <50/mm^3 and many had coexisting infections or malignancies.[214] Approximately 1.4% of pre-HAART HIV cases were complicated by TMA, with an autopsy incidence of 30% in AIDS patients. More recently, virtually no cases of TMA have been reported in the post-HAART era in patients under strict viral control.[215] The most likely causes of TMA in HAART-treated patients currently would be a consequence of a secondary malignancy, chemotherapy, or another infectious complication unrelated to the HIV virus.

With regard to the pathophysiology of this lesion in HIV patients, the HIV p24 antigen has been isolated directly from the endothelial cells in TMA cases, whereas the HIV gp120 antigen has been associated with the development of a procoagulant state.[216,217] In addition, HIV may induce endothelial injury through enhanced rates of endothelial cell apoptosis, acquired deficiency of von Willebrand factor cleaving protease, and by increased fibroblast growth factor activity.[218,219] Furthermore, TMA has also been reported to result not directly from HIV but from a coexisting active cytomegalovirus (CMV) infection as a secondary complication of immune dysregulation in these patients.[220]

The clinical presentation of TMA in the setting of HIV varies from the acute development of AKI to a more insidious onset of progressive CKD.[221] Histologic findings are typical of TMA in the general population, with glomerular thrombi and serologic evidence of hemolysis and platelet consumption. TMA may actually precede the clinical diagnosis of HIV and may be the first presenting complication of this viral infection.[222]

The treatment of active TMA in HIV patients has been attempted using combinations of plasmapheresis, corticosteroids, intravenous immunoglobulin (IVIG), plasma

TABLE 47.4 **Characteristic Features of HIV, HIVICK, HCV, and HBV**

	HIV	HIVICK	HCV	HBV
Racial predilection	Black	Caucasian	None	None
Gender	Male	1:1	Female	1:1
Renal histology	Collapsing FSGS Tubular microcysts Interstitial nephritis TRI	IgA, DPGN TRI Interstitial nephritis TRI	Type I MPGN IgMκ cryoglobulin Interstitial nephritis	MN MPGN IgA
Serum complement	Normal	Normal	Decreased C3, C4	Normal
Renal ultrasound	Increased echogenicity	Variable	Variable	Variable
HTN	Rare	Common	Marked elevation	Variable
Urinalysis	Nephrotic	Nephritic	Nephritic	Nephrotic
Mechanism	Direct viral infection	Immune complex (p24, gp120)	Immune complex (Cryoglobulinemia)	Immune complex (HBeAg)
Therapeutic options	HAART ACEI/ARB Steroids	HAART ACEI/ARB	Interferon Plasmapheresis Rituximab Steroids Cyclophosphamide	Antiviral IFN ACEI/ARB

HIVICK, HIV immune complex disease of the kidney; HCV, hepatitis C virus; HBV, hepatitis B virus; FSGS, focal segmental glomerulosclerosis; TRI, tubuloreticular inclusion; IgA, immunoglobulin A; DPGN, diffuse glomerulonephritis; MPGN, membranoproliferative glomerulonephritis; MN, membranous nephropathy; HTN, hypertension; HAART, highly active anti-retroviral therapy; ACEI/ARB, angiotensin converting enzyme inhibitors/angiotensin receptor blockers; IFN, Interferon.

infusions, and splenectomies.[223] However, these have been anecdotal case reports, and there is no consensus about the efficacy of these treatments in the setting of HIV. The successful prevention of TMA appears to be achieved primarily by control of viremia with HAART.[224]

Immunotactoid Glomerulonephritis

Only six cases have been reported in the literature of immunotactoid glomerulonephritis in patients with HIV.[225] Of these cases, 50% were associated with hepatitis C, and all cases presented with a combination of hematuria and proteinuria. A cause and effect relationship between HIV and immunotactoid disease has not been firmly established.

Diabetic Nephropathy

HIV patients may be at higher risk for diabetes as a result of coexistent HCV infection (OR = 3.7) or from the use of HAART therapy.[226] Diabetic nephropathy has now been noted on biopsy series in HIV patients at a frequency of 5% to 10%.[227] Therefore, although not directly related to the HIV virus, diabetic glomerulopathy needs to be considered in the differential diagnosis of the nephrotic syndrome, especially if the patient is on HAART therapy with well-controlled viremia, which significantly reduces the risk of HIVAN or HIVICK.

Key Points: HIV and Glomerular Disease

1. HIV glomerular disease may complicate 2% to 10% of patients with untreated HIV infection.
2. Although a variety of glomerular lesions may be present, the majority of cases are comprised of HIVAN, HIVICK, and glomerular disease from coinfection with HCV or HBV.
3. HIVAN represents a podocytopathy from direct HIV infection, resulting in reversion to a macrophage dedifferentiated phenotype.

4. The pathologic spectrum of HIVAN includes collapsing FSGS, microcystic dilation of the tubules, interstitial nephritis, and the presence of cytoplasmic tubuloreticular inclusions.
5. HIVAN responds to HAART therapy with reversal of the podocyte phenotype to normal and improvement of the interstitial lesions.
6. Steroid therapy may be beneficial in HIVAN patients with significant interstitial nephritis and acute kidney injury.
7. HIVICK is distinguished from HIVAN by the presence of glomerular basement membrane immune complexes composed of HIV antigens.
8. The pathologic spectrum of HIVICK primarily includes:IgA nephropathy, a lupus-like diffuse proliferative glomerulonephritis, and MN.
9. HIVICK does not predictably respond to HAART therapy.
10. TMA represents another variant of direct HIV infection of the kidney with significant endothelial injury.
11. Due to the heterogeneity of glomerular disease in HIV patients, a renal biopsy is necessary in most cases when a glomerular lesion is suspected in order to develop an effective prognostic and therapeutic plan.

HEPATITIS B

Epidemiology

Hepatitis B is a small partially double-stranded DNA virus of the Hepadnavirus family that is the leading cause of hepatocellular carcinoma, chronic hepatitis, and cirrhosis in the world.[228] Currently, it is estimated that more than one third of the world's population (2 billion people) have been exposed to HBV with the development of 400 million chronic carriers of hepatitis B antigens.[229] The prevalence of a chronic hepatitis B carrier state varies from 0.1% to 2.0% in low-prevalence areas (United States and Canada, Western Europe, Australia, and New Zealand), to 3% to 5% in intermediate-prevalence areas (Mediterranean countries, Japan, Central Asia, Middle East, and Latin and South America), to 10% to 20% in high-prevalence areas (southeast Asia, China, and sub-Saharan Africa). In the United States, it is estimated that there are 750,000 to 1 million HBV carriers.[230] The number of new cases in the United States has decreased over 80% in the past 20 years as a result of the implementation of routine hepatitis B vaccination, with 46,000 incident cases being reported in 2008.

The development of a carrier state after exposure to hepatitis B is related to the age of acquisition of the virus: 90% risk of a chronic carrier state after perinatal exposure, 10% to 20% risk after childhood exposure, and only a 5% risk after exposure as an adult. The risk of a carrier state is also directly related to the maturity of the immune system at the time of exposure, leading to the highest risk seen in infants from vertical or horizontal viral transmission as well as in immunocompromised individuals.[231]

Hepatitis B has been subdivided into eight genotypes (A through H), with genotype A being present primarily in North America, Europe, and Africa. Subgroup characterization may be important with regard to virulence and response to therapy, with genotype A demonstrating a higher response rate to IFN therapy than the other genotypes. In addition, genotypes A and D may be more frequently associated with certain types of hepatitis-related glomerular disease. Additional subdivisions of hepatitis B into serotypes based on surface epitopes (adr, adw, ayr, ayw) has not yet been linked to changes in clinical presentation.

Pathogenesis and Diagnosis of Acute Infection

The intact HBV molecule is called the Dane particle, which is a 42-nm structure consisting of an outer envelope and an inner core. The outer envelope contains lipids, proteins, and carbohydrates but importantly expresses the hepatitis B surface antigen (HBsAg). The inner core is composed of partially double-stranded circular, viral DNA polymerase, the hepatitis B core antigen:HBcAg, and the hepatitis B e antigen (HBeAg).[232]

Hepatitis B enters liver cells through endocytosis by way of specific receptors that have not been definitely identified but may be related to carboxypeptidase D. Although hepatitis B may be predominantly hepatotropic, a secondary reservoir for infection may also be present in lymphocytes. After entry into hepatocytes, the virus is not directly cytopathic, but hijacks the nuclear enzymes to replicate the viral DNA and produce additional virions. The primary injury to the liver is the indirect result of the immune response to the viral infection.

After exposure to hepatitis B, cell-mediated immunity is initially stimulated to control viral replication. The mobilization of cytotoxic lymphocytes is part of the adaptive immune response as opposed to the innate immune system. CD8+ T cells and NK cells are responsible for clearance of the virus through direct cell lysis and indirectly by the stimulation of antiviral cytokines such as IFN. CD4+ positive cells are subsequently recruited to develop an initial IgM neutralizing antibody response to HBcAg and eventually a long-term IgG–HBcAb and IgG– HBsAb. Importantly, IgM–HBcAb may persist for up to 2 years after the initial infection and, therefore, it is not always indicative of an acute infection.

IgG-HBsAb is usually representative of previous exposure and clearance of the virus; however, in chronic carriers, the presence of HBsAg may coexist with low nonneutralizing levels of HBsAb. In addition, in chronic HBsAg carriers, the presence of circulating HBeAg may also be present and represents a greater degree of infectivity and potential systemic complications (e.g., cirrhosis, renal disease).

Glomerular Syndromes

The association of renal syndromes with hepatitis B was initially reported in 1971 and, subsequently, a variety of renal lesions have been described as a consequence of either acute or chronic hepatitis B infection (Table 47.2).[233–234] Due to the heterogeneous nature of these lesions in natural history and in response to therapy, a renal biopsy is usually required, especially to classify the renal syndrome and to define the best treatment options. The most common renal syndromes from hepatitis B result from the chronic carrier state, but even in the acute phase of viral infection a transient glomerulonephritis may develop.

Acute Glomerulonephritis

A variety of extrahepatic autoimmune manifestations of hepatitis B may develop either during the acute phase of infection or in chronic carriers during episodes of acute viral exacerbation. During the initial immune response to hepatitis B exposure, 10% to 20% of patients may develop a systemic immune complex–mediated serum sickness reaction.[235] This syndrome is characterized by arthralgias, fever, rash, and an acute proliferative glomerulonephritis. The renal lesion rarely leads to permanent renal injury and recovers with the clearance of the HBsAg viremia. Renal biopsies in these patients demonstrated a pattern typical of postinfectious glomerulonephritis.[236] No long-term sequela result from this short-term self-limiting immune complex syndrome, and it is often clinically silent.

Membranous Nephropathy

The most common glomerular lesion seen in chronic hepatitis B carriers is MN and these cases may comprise 10% to 15% of all MN diagnoses in adults living in endemic areas for hepatitis B.[237] Although rare cases of membranous lesions have been reported within months of an acute hepatitis B exposure, the predominant pattern is the development of MN >2 years after the onset of a chronic carrier state. In terms of epidemiology, children develop MN more frequently than adults, and males predominate over females.

A genetic predisposition may be present with specific HLA loci (DRB1*1501) and infection with genotype A may be a risk factor for the development of MN.[238] There is no association of MN with the degree of hepatic enzyme elevation or liver histology, and the majority of patients have only mild serologic evidence of chronic hepatitis with no evidence of cirrhosis. This is in contrast to HIVAN and HIVICK, which usually develop only in the stages of advanced HIV infection, and with hepatitis C–related cryoglobulinemia and MPGN, which also develop very late in the course of active hepatic infection. In adults, there are two major types of MN lesions that have been identified isolated MN or MN with superimposed IgA staining.

Pathogenesis of Membranous Nephropathy

The histologic appearance of hepatitis B–related MN is indistinguishable from idiopathic MN with clearly defined subepithelial immune complex deposits. The source of these immune deposits, however, is distinct from the phospholipase A2 receptor that has now been shown to be the dominant antigen in idiopathic MN. The antigen for the immune deposits in hepatitis B MN may arise from three potential viral particles: HBsAg, HBcAg, or HBeAg. In addition, from a mechanistic standpoint, the deposit may form from either deposition of an IgG immune complex with one or more of the stated antigens or with the de novo formation of an immune complex after deposition of the circulating antigen in the basement membrane, first followed by deposition of the circulating antibody. The size and charge of the antigens are an important determinant of their pathogenicity and ability to traverse the glomerular basement membrane. HBeAg is the smallest of the three antigens at 17 kD with HBsAg measuring 35 to 50 kD and HBcAg at 22 kD.[239]

Indisputable evidence for the etiologic role of HBeAg in the formation of the subepithelial immune complexes comes from the use of monoclonal antibodies to localize these antigens in biopsy specimens. Approximately 90% of patients with chronic hepatitis B and biopsy proven MN have detectable HBeAg in the glomerulus, and >95% of these patients have measurable circulating HBeAg.[240]

Hepatitis B viral transcripts have been detected in >50% of renal biopsy specimens in MN, especially in proximal tubular epithelial cells and mesangial cells of both adults and children.[241] Southern blot and in situ hybridization studies of patients with MN demonstrate viral DNA in both nuclei and cytoplasm, suggesting that active viral replication may occur in renal tissue and their presence is not a matter of passive endocytosis from urine or blood.[242] Supporting the contributing role of cell injury from the presence of hepatitis B antigen deposition or expression is the finding that transgenic mice expressing HBsAg and HBcAg in renal tubular epithelial cells show the activation of both the complement and the coagulation cascade with the upregulation of acute phase reactants.[243] Sera of patients with hepatitis B increases the apoptotic cycle in proximal tubular cells via activation of the Fas gene expression.[244]

Mutational changes in the hepatitis B genome may alter its renal virulence, and specific genomic variations have been associated with MN in children.[245] Finally, the presence of podocytopenia in children with MN indicates a link between hepatitis B infection and podocyte injury, possibly through an increased apoptotic rate, thus further leading to proteinuria.[246]

All the aforementioned data support the primary role of viral antigenemia in MN, leading to immune complex formation with a potential role for renal tropism by hepatitis B, further enhancing the antigenicity of glomerular tissue.

Natural History and Treatment

Progression of hepatitis B–related MN toward ESRD occurs in approximately 25% to 35% of adults compared to a rate of <5% in children.[247] Spontaneous biopsy-proven histologic resolution of MN has been shown in children, which has been associated with systemic HBeAg clearance. These children may still remain HBsAg carriers, but the loss of the HBeAg with the emergence of HBeAb likely resulted in the cessation of immune complex formation followed by glomerular removal of preexisting subepithelial deposits. Therefore, the urgency to treat MN in children must be balanced not only by the potential side effects of the therapy, but also by the fact that the renal disease may remit spontaneously over time. This situation is not true in adults where the degree of nephrotic syndrome, hypertension, and loss of GFR tend to be more pronounced and unremitting.[248]

Because clearance of the virus is a prerequisite for ameliorating the renal lesion, therapy has consisted of antiviral therapy either in the form of subcutaneous IFN (standard or pegylated) or oral inhibitors of viral replication. The most common oral antiviral agents used are either nucleotide (tenofovir, adefovir) or nucleoside (lamivudine, entecavir, telbivudine) reverse transcriptase inhibitors.[249,250] In the treatment of hepatitis B MN, lamivudine (a cytidine analogue) has been the most commonly used agent.[251] Lamivudine therapy at 100 mg per day has been shown to reduce proteinuria, resulting in remission of the nephrotic syndrome, and is associated with a significant improvement in renal survival.[252] Approximately 75% to 85% of patients respond successfully to lamivudine, as demonstrated by a complete resolution of the HBeAg carrier state and the absence of hepatitis B viral replication. Renal remission often follows viral remission within 3 to 6 months.[253,254] Persistence of the nephrotic syndrome after 6 months of sustained viral remission is unusual and warrants additional investigation.

Long-term daily use of lamivudine may result in the viral acquisition of a drug resistance mutation at the YMDD locus. This amino acid sequence becomes altered to YIDD, leading to a threefold decrease in sensitivity of the viral transcriptase enzyme to inhibition from lamivudine. The resistant rate from this mutation is approximately 20% per year, requiring ongoing monitoring for breakthrough viral replication.[255]

Entecavir (a guanine analogue) has similarly been shown to effectively control viral replication and reduce proteinuria in hepatitis B–related MN and is associated with a significantly lower rate of viral drug resistant mutations (<0.2% per year) compared to lamivudine.[256] Therefore, this agent may evolve into the preferred choice of drugs for the treatment of hepatitis B–related MN.

IFN has also been successfully used to achieve viral clearance and a remission proteinuria at rates similar to those seen with lamivudine (50% to 90%). Intolerance to long-term subcutaneous IFN is present in 10% to 15% of patients and limits the use of IFN as a first-line therapy for MN. The efficacy, convenience, and tolerability of oral antiviral therapy provides a substantial advantage compared to IFN therapy.

Mycophenolate mofetil (MMF) has been used for hepatitis B MN with the expectation that it may provide similar efficacy as in idiopathic MN.[257] In vitro, MMF demonstrates viral inhibitory capacity for hepatitis B; however, in clinical practice MMF-treated patients showed a marked increase in hepatitis B viremia. Only partial remissions of proteinuria were noted and MMF was discontinued due to the risk of increased viral activity.

Corticosteroid therapy has been used in MN as sole therapy in the absence of concomitant antiviral treatment.[258] A clinical remission of the nephrotic syndrome has been reported in <10% of patients with clear evidence of an increase in viral load. In vitro and clinical data confirm the ability of corticosteroids to increase hepatitis B viral replication. Importantly, because corticosteroids may temporarily ameliorate the T-cell-mediated hepatic inflammation from hepatitis B, the withdrawal of steroids after the treatment of MN has been associated with significant rebound hepatitis.[259] As a consequence of the lack of efficacy of steroid therapy in hepatitis B MN and the risk of worsening viral load and liver function studies, steroid therapy is not a viable option in MN.

As a summary of all data reported at present, a meta-analysis of six clinical trials regarding the treatment of hepatitis B MN supports three major conclusions: (1) steroid therapy is ineffective in both adults and children with MN, (2) antiviral treatment results in a 90% remission rate in proteinuria, and (3) in contrast to earlier reports, spontaneous remission rates of proteinuria occur in 30% to 40% of both adults and children.[260]

Membranoproliferative Glomerulonephritis

Membranoproliferative glomerulonephritis (MPGN) represents the second most common renal glomerular syndrome in hepatitis B carriers after MN in both adults and children and is characterized by the typical lobular appearance of the glomerulus with splitting of the basement membrane and mesangial, subendothelial, and even subepithelial deposits.[261] Both type I and type III MPGN have been described in chronic hepatitis B carriers.[262] The clinical presentation is similar to patients with idiopathic MPGN and is characterized by the nephritic syndrome with or without nephrotic range proteinuria and decreased levels of serum complement (C3 and C4). An HLA association is present with an overrepresentation of DRB1*1502 in hepatitis B patients with MPGN. Care must be taken to exclude coinfection with hepatitis C as a cause of MPGN in hepatitis B carriers because up to 10% of patients worldwide carry both viral infections. The treatment of hepatitis C–related MPGN with cryoglobulinemia is completely distinct from the treatment of hepatitis B–related MPGN.

Pathogenesis of Membranoproliferative Glomerulonephritis

In contrast to the subepithelial localization of immune deposits in hepatitis B MN, patients with MPGN have predominant mesangial and subendothelial deposits. These immune complexes are composed of HBsAg and IgG, which, by nature, are significantly larger than HBeAg–IgG complexes, thus restricting their passage through the glomerular basement membrane. In rare cases, cryoglobulinemia has been present in hepatitis B patients, but the titers are often <3% and the renal histology has not been representative of classic cryoglobulin deposits. The presence of significant levels of cryoglobulins would be suggestive of a coinfection with hepatitis C.

Treatment of Membranoproliferative Glomerulonephritis

Because the pathogenesis of hepatitis B–related MPGN is related to viral antigenemia, the same treatment strategy should hold true for this disease as with MN. Steroids and immunosuppressive therapy have failed to produce any significant improvement in renal function in these patients. Successful clinical remission of MPGN has been achieved with lamivudine or IFN in rare individual cases.[263,264] Most patients achieve a viral remission but are left with nonnephrotic range proteinuria and CKD, consistent with the remnant scarring from extensive immune complex injury. Overall <50% of patients with MPGN will experience a significant improvement in renal function with IFN therapy.

Focal Segmental Glomerulosclerosis

The relationship between hepatitis B infection and the development of FSGS is circumstantial. Among seven well-reported cases in the literature, tissue immunohistochemistry demonstrated the presence of HBsAg and HBcAg in the glomerular basement membrane and mesangium in the absence of clearly defined immune complexes.[265] All patients responded to lamivudine therapy with a complete or partial resolution of proteinuria, but no follow-up biopsies were performed. Although the presence of viral antigens in the glomerulus may be a result of passive antigen trapping, the reported development of podocyte injury in hepatitis B patients may be the link between this viral infection and FSGS. At the present time, the management of hepatitis B carriers with FSGS remains viral control without a beneficial role for corticosteroids.

Immunoglobulin A Nephropathy

Most case series of renal biopsies in adults with chronic hepatitis B report a significant proportion of patients with IgA nephropathy, which may be more prevalent than MN or MPGN.[266] This preponderance of IgA nephropathy over MN is not seen in children with hepatitis B and is isolated to adults with HBV.[267] There are two potential explanations for this finding of IgA nephropathy exclusively in adult patients. One hypothesis argues that the geographic distribution of hepatitis B overlaps with the population at highest risk for IgA nephropathy.[268] Consequently, it would not be unexpected that IgA nephropathy would occur in patients who happen to have hepatitis B, but is unrelated by causality to the virus infection. The second explanation centers on IgA nephropathy as a direct syndrome related to hepatitis B.

In support of a direct cause and effect relationship of hepatitis B and IgA nephropathy is a detailed tissue analysis for hepatitis B antigens in a cohort of 50 patients with IgA nephropathy in the presence of a chronic hepatitis B carrier state (HBsAg positive but HBeAg negative). The presence of HBsAg and/or HBcAg was detected in both the mesangium and capillary loops in 82% of patients and in the tubular cytoplasm in 96% of biopsy samples.[269] Southern blot analysis and in situ hybridization studies demonstrated the integrated form of DNA for hepatitis B, suggestive of viral replication in renal tissue. The link between renal tissue expression of hepatitis B viral antigens and the presence of IgA immune complexes is not clear. Yet to be answered is why some patients develop a typical IgG response with immune complex formation, whereas others develop an IgA response, which could reflect individual genetic susceptibility and hepatitis B genotype variations.

There are no well-documented reports on the response of IgA nephropathy in patients with hepatitis B to either antiviral therapy or immunosuppressive agents. From the experience with MN, a reasonable approach would be the use of antiviral therapy to achieve control of viral replication.

Polyarteritis Nodosa

Hepatitis B is now considered by the American College of Rheumatology to be an important causative factor in the diagnosis of polyarteritis nodosa (PAN) and an essential part of the differential diagnosis. Prior to 1990, hepatitis B accounted for 40% to 50% of all cases of classic PAN with a progressive decline in the incidence to approximately 6% in 2000. This marked change in frequency is likely related to the widespread use of hepatitis B vaccinations, as well as a more successful control of chronic hepatitis B viremia with antiviral therapy.[270]

The largest review of hepatitis B–associated PAN has been published by the French Vasculitis Group and consists of 115 patients accumulated over a 20-year period.[271] From this predominantly European cohort, important demographic information has emerged regarding the clinical presentation of PAN in hepatitis B carriers. In only 30% of patients, hepatitis B was diagnosed prior to the onset of PAN, whereas in the remainder, the diagnosis of hepatitis B was made after the diagnosis of this systemic necrotizing medium and small vessel vasculitis. PAN appears to be a relatively early manifestation of chronic hepatitis B infection, often being diagnosed within a year of the initial diagnosis of an HBsAg carrier state. PAN tended to occur in the sixth decade and showed a strong male predominance (65%). Compared to classic PAN, hepatitis B–related PAN demonstrated more frequent gastrointestinal involvement, marked hypertension, and a higher risk of renal disease. Among the different hepatitis B genotypes, the risk of PAN is highest with genotype D in contrast to the risk of MN with genotype A. Similar to the risk for the development of MN, PAN was highly associated with a chronic carrier state that showed HBeAg persistence.[272]

In addition to the risk of PAN from being an HBeAg carrier, the use of a hepatitis B vaccination may also pose a risk for the development of PAN. Over 25 cases have been published in the literature, linking the acute development of PAN temporally to a recently administered hepatitis B vaccine.[273]

The Pathophysiology of Polyarteritis Nodosa

In hepatitis B carriers, the two most likely theories for the development of PAN include immune complex deposition in vascular epithelium or direct epithelial tissue infection with viral DNA.[274] The presence of hepatitis B immune complexes in PAN has been confirmed and forms the basis for the use of plasmapheresis in severe cases.[275] A different mechanism may exist for the pathogenesis of PAN in patients where vaccination may have caused the vasculitis. In these patients, stimulation of autoreactive T cells and antibody production may be the result of processes such as molecular mimicry and epitope spreading.[276,277] Exposure of genetically susceptible patients to hepatitis B antigens within the vaccine and the added adjuvant may produce cross-reactive lymphocytes that target self-antigens on the epithelium and endothelium.[278] ANCAs are routinely negative in hepatitis B–related PAN.

Therapy of Polyarteritis Nodosa

PAN is a fulminant, life-threatening systemic vasculitis that requires the urgent control of inflammation and the prevention of progressive organ damage from ischemia/infarction. Therefore, the use of antiviral therapy alone is usually not recommended due to the gradual and delayed clearance of viremia, which does not allow for the immediate control of the vasculitis. Concessions have to be made to use short-term steroid therapy with or without plasmapheresis in conjunction with antiviral therapy to effect a clinical remission. Cytotoxic therapy (i.e., cyclophosphamide) may markedly increase the risk of viremia and is not recommended as part of the adjuvant therapy in these patients.[279] A review of published reports on hepatitis B PAN has demonstrated the superiority of antiviral therapy (either lamivudine or IFN) over steroids in leading to a remission of systemic vasculitis (80% versus 50%) and reducing overall mortality (30% versus 46%).[3]

Remission and control of PAN has been achieved in 90% to 100% of patients that demonstrate systemic clearance of HBeAg, and relapses have been associated with a return to an HBeAg carrier state. Lamivudine, vidarabine, and IFN have been used in separate studies to successfully control HBeAg production in 60% to 66% of patients. Concomitant short-term steroids were used for a 2-week period and then were rapidly tapered off while plasmapheresis was started initially at 3 times a week and then gradually withdrawn based on the clinical response.

Preventive Strategy: Hepatitis B Vaccination

Ultimately, the most effective treatment of hepatitis B glomerular and vasculitic disease is the prevention of exposure and the acquisition of the virus. Worldwide institution of hepatitis B vaccination has had a significant impact on the development of hepatitis B–related renal disease. Mass vaccinations in China and in South Africa have reduced the incidence of hepatitis B carriage rate in the treated population by 95%, with a subsequent decrease in MN from hepatitis B by >95%.[280,281] Prior to 1983, Alaska had the highest incidence of hepatitis B–related vasculitis in the world. By 1989, hepatitis B vaccination campaigns resulted in the complete elimination of new cases of hepatitis B vasculitis.[282] Because the vaccination will not affect preexisting cases of hepatitis B in the population and the development of MN only occurs after years of a hepatitis B carrier state, the beneficial effect of vaccination on the incidence of MN will not be seen for up to 5 to 10 years after beginning a regionwide vaccination program.

Key Points: Hepatitis B and Glomerular Disease

1. Acute hepatitis B infection is associated with a self-limited immune complex–mediated acute proliferative GN.
2. Chronic hepatitis B carriers are at risk of three main immune complex–related glomerular diseases: MN secondary to HBeAg, MPGN secondary to HBsAg, or IgA nephropathy secondary to HBcAg and HBsAg.
3. PAN may develop in chronic hepatitis B from immune complex deposition in the vascular endothelium and is highly associated with HBeAg.
4. Antiviral therapy with lamivudine or IFN can successfully lead to a remission of MN and PAN.
5. Corticosteroids are not useful in the treatment of MN, MPGN, or IgA but may be used for short periods in severe PAN.
6. Advanced PAN can be treated with plasmapheresis in conjunction with antiviral therapy and a short course of corticosteroids.
7. The relationship of hepatitis B and FSGS has not been substantiated.

PARVOVIRUS

Epidemiology

Parvovirus B19 is a single-stranded DNA virus initially described in 1974 that has a worldwide distribution.[283] Three genotypes have been identified, with genotype 1 representing the majority of cases in North America and Europe. Clinical identification of specific genotypes is not clinically important due to the 90% sequence homology between them and the development of cross-reactive neutralizing antibodies that span across the genotypes.[284] Approximately 50% of children by age 15 test seropositive for antibodies against the viral capsid structural (VP1 and VP2) and nonstructural (NS1) proteins of parvovirus, indicating previous exposure, and by the sixth to seventh decade, 70% to 85% of the population demonstrates seropositivity.[285]

Acquisition of the virus occurs primarily through aerosolized droplet inhalation but may also result from vertical transmission, blood and plasma products (factor VIII and IX concentrates), or through organ transplantation (bone marrow and solid organ transplants). The majority of clinically symptomatic cases in children and young adults are the result of a primary parvovirus infection, whereas cases in the elderly usually represent reactivation of the disease due to an acquired impaired immune surveillance response.

There are two clinical presentations of parvovirus in the general immunocompetent population: erythema infectiosum (Fifth disease) and transient aplastic crises (TAC).[286] These are self-limited illnesses that typically last 4 to 8 days and resolve without long-term sequela. During the recovery phase of the illness, patients may develop a polyarthropathy syndrome as immune complexes form during the period of antibody excess with clearance of viremia. A third syndrome occurs in the immune-incompetent fetus even though the mother may have a normal immune response. Infection of the fetal liver and thymus can lead to fetal death from hydrops faetalis, particularly during the first 20 weeks of pregnancy. Finally, in immunocompromised patients (HIV, SLE, chemotherapy, organ transplant recipients), parvovirus B19 must be considered as an important cause of pure red cell aplasia (PRCA).[287]

Diagnosis

Parvovirus B19 infection can be diagnosed by a combination of quantitative PCR and ELISA antibody determination.[288] The presence of parvovirus B19 DNA in serum is indicative of ongoing or recent infection and the presence of an IgG or an IgM response can further define the time of onset of the disease.[289] In many cases, IgM may persist for up to 4 months after the initial infection and, therefore, it is not a sensitive marker for an active acute infection. The absence of IgM would be helpful in the presence of an IgG antibody as a potential indicator for chronic parvovirus infection. A blood PCR would still be needed to confirm active viremia.[290]

In immunocompromised patients, the lack of an adequate immune response relegates the diagnosis primarily to the PCR measurement. The presence of IgG or IgM may not be reliable in the setting of immunosuppression with impaired B-cell activity.[291]

Tissue PCR for parvovirus is a new technique that may supersede the use of blood PCR as a marker for active infection.[292] However, parvovirus DNA may persist in tissue for years after the initial infection even in asymptomatic patients, and the interpretation of this finding has not been defined for routine clinical use.

Glomerular Syndromes

Parvovirus B19 may result in two distinct forms of glomerular disease, corresponding to the time of either an acute or chronic viral infection.[293] In patients with acute parvovirus infection, a hypocomplementemic diffuse proliferative glomerulonephritis with mesangial and endocapillary immune complex deposition has been reported.[294–295] The usual age of onset is in the second and third decade before acquired natural immunity has developed, and a slight female predominance is present, as has been reported with other immune complex diseases such as cryoglobulinemia. The clinical presentation consists of acute kidney injury with both a nephritic and/or nephrotic syndrome.[296]

Immunohistochemistry has demonstrated the presence of parvovirus DNA and capsid antigens directly isolated from renal tissue with serologic evidence of an acute parvovirus infection confirmed by the presence of circulating IgM antibodies. The majority of these patients had a documented exposure to a parvovirus-infected individual and subsequently developed erythema infectiosum. In addition, most patients had clinical signs of systemic immune complex disease typical of a parvovirus infection: rash and/or symmetrical arthritis/arthralgias. Immunofluorescent studies showed a granular staining pattern for IgM/IgG and C3 in the peripheral capillary loops and the mesangium. Electron microscopy revealed the deposition of discrete subendothelial immune complexes with widening of the subendothelial space along with the mesangial deposits. Both C3 and C4 were transiently depleted in the serum and recovered to normal levels after resolution of the infection indicating activation of the classical complement pathway.[297]

Compared to the typical postinfectious glomerulonephritis seen with streptococcal infections, the renal lesions seen with acute parvovirus infection consist of subendothelial deposits instead of the typical subepithelial deposits, lack a significant exudative neutrophilic infiltrate and crescents, and are associated with only a mild decrease in GFR. Differentiation from SLE nephritis is essential and can be made by the absence of a "full house" Immunofluorescent staining on biopsy and the lack of serologic autoimmune titers.[298] Recovery has been predominantly spontaneous, but case reports of using short-term steroid therapy have been published with anecdotal improvement in renal function.

A high-risk group for parvovirus-related glomerulonephritis includes patients homozygous for sickle cell anemia.[299] Acute focal proliferative GN with or without crescents has been reported in this population coincident with active parvovirus infection. These lesions may resolve completely, but evolution to FSGS and chronic kidney disease has been documented.[300] The association of parvovirus with renal vasculitis from endothelial cell injury has been suggested as a cause of these lesions in sickle cell patients as well as the case reports showing an association of parvovirus with polyarteritis nodosa, Wegener granulomatosis, microscopic polyangiitis, and temporal arteritis.[301,302] These lesions clearly differ from the acute diffuse proliferative glomerulonephritis cases by the absence of immune complex deposition. The presence of parvovirus B19 in the vascular endothelium and failure to respond to the typical immunosuppressive therapy used for these lesions suggests a causal role of this virus in the pathogenesis of vasculitis.[303] The development and exacerbation of connective tissue disease by an active parvovirus infection has been described and may be related to the endothelial injury and production of vascular antigen-targeted autoantibodies.[304]

The parvovirus has also been linked to the development of both adult and childhood Henoch-Schönlein purpura. Analyses performed on skin biopsies and renal tissue has localized parvovirus DNA in the endothelium and glomeruli in conjunction with IgA deposits, suggesting that they are part of the immune complex formation.[305,306]

The association of parvovirus and collapsing FSGS has been an area of significant debate.[307] The original report by Tanawattanacharoen in 2000 showed the presence of parvovirus DNA in the parietal and visceral renal epithelial cells of 80% of patients with idiopathic FSGS and in 90% of patients with collapsing FSGS.[308] Among patients with minimal change disease and MN, there was also evidence of parvovirus DNA in 50% and 60% of samples, respectively. The lack of nucleic acid residues by in situ hybridization in any of the samples suggest that active viral replication was not currently present in those patients. Therefore, the role of parvovirus in the development of the glomerular lesions could not be substantiated and suggested that parvovirus may be an "innocent bystander" in renal tissue for many patients in the population.

A subsequent report linking parvovirus specifically with collapsing FSGS was published by Moudgil, confirming the tissue presence of parvovirus DNA in 78% of patients with collapsing FSGS but in only 15% of idiopathic FSGS and 26% of control kidney tissue samples.[309] Systemic parvovirus viremia was simultaneously noted in 87% of collapsing FSGS cases but only in $<10\%$ of the other renal diseases. This study appears to provide greater support for the relationship of parvovirus and collapsing FSGS. In contrast, in kidney transplant patients, no evidence for parvovirus was found in large series reviews of recurrent collapsing and idiopathic FSGS.[310]

Collapsing and noncollapsing FSGS have been reported in sickle cell patients with evidence of acute parvovirus infection. Nucleic acid detection of parvovirus in renal tissue was present in all three cases examined and all patients exhibited a rapid decline in renal function with no response to steroid therapy.[311]

Parvovirus can be a significant opportunistic pathogen after organ transplantation and is an important cause of posttransplant aplastic anemia.[312,313] Acute allograft dysfunction secondary to thrombotic microangiopathy has been associated with an active parvovirus infection in renal transplant patients.[314] Resolution of the renal lesions occurred concomitant with clearance of the viremia. No evidence of parvovirus DNA was noted in preimplantation biopsies of these patients and in control surveillance biopsies of well-functioning grafts. The etiology appears to be renal endothelial cell injury directly from parvovirus infection with no evidence of immune complex deposition. A combination of parvovirus infection coupled with calcineurin inhibitor therapy and ischemic–reperfusion injury to the grafts was felt to result in this thrombotic disorder.[315]

In contrast to CMV, which has been linked to the development of acute rejection, parvovirus does not appear to cause acute interstitial nephritis or rejection but has been demonstrated to be associated with chronic allograft injury.[316] The persistence of parvovirus DNA in renal tissue after transplantation on surveillance biopsies led to a higher risk for biopsy proven chronic allograft lesions:interstitial fibrosis, arteriolar hyalinosis, and glomerulosclerosis. Not every patient with intrarenal evidence of parvovirus infection had active viremia, although these patients still showed a higher risk of chronic injury.[317] This data suggests a potential role for tissue analysis for viral DNA as part of the routine histologic evaluation of renal transplant biopsy specimens.

Pathogenesis

Parvovirus B19 is a cytotoxic virus that targets the erythroid progenitor cells and CD36 positive erythroblasts.[318] The virus spares the erythroid stem cells because they lack the required receptor for viral entry:globoside (P blood group antigen).[319] Viral entry into the cell results in the initiation of the apoptotic cycle.[320] The P blood group antigen is also present on endothelial cells, which may be responsible for many of the systemic manifestations of the disease: myocarditis, synovitis, vasculitis, thrombotic microangiopathy, and glomerulonephritis. In addition to the P blood group, parvovirus uses the $\alpha5\beta1$ integrin for cellular entry and the nonstructural protein (NS3) may be an important mediator for the interruption of the cell cycle by stimulating DNA fragmentation.

Clearance of the virus results from the host IgG response to the viral capsid proteins, leading to antibody-dependent cell-mediated cytotoxicity but in addition host-cell-mediated immunity and cytokine response is also required for complete viral removal.[321,322] A neutralizing antibody against VP2 and VP1 is required for viral clearance and in patients with persistent parvovirus infection, patients often lack an adequate IgG response to VP1. Therefore, the presence of IgG antibodies to parvovirus B19 is not indicative of acquired resistance because the titer and specificity of these antibodies is not routinely measured.[323] Active viremia may still exist if the patient tests positive for parvovirus B19 IgG antibodies, and this infection should still be considered in the differential diagnosis until a confirmatory PCR study is obtained.

Treatment

The majority of patients with acute glomerulonephritis due to parvovirus have shown spontaneous resolution of the renal lesion with recovery and clearance of the infection. Anecdotal cases using steroids and cyclophosphamide for cases of crescentic GN have been published but lack control cohorts, and this therapy cannot be recommended. In immunocompromised patients, parvovirus B19 may require adjunctive therapy to achieve viral clearance. The two main forms of therapeutic intervention are a reduction of immunosuppression (in transplant recipients) and the use of IVIG.[324] A regimen of 400 mg per kilogram per day of IVIG for 5 to 10 days has been a recommended regimen, or a consolidated dose of 1 mg per kilogram per day over 2 days can be used.[325] Tacrolimus use may carry a higher risk for parvovirus replication and, therefore, conversion to a cyclosporine-based immunosuppression regimen may be beneficial in transplant recipients.

Key Points: Parvovirus and Glomerular Disease

1. Acute infection is associated with a self-limiting immune complex–mediated diffuse proliferative GN with hypocomplementemia.
2. Differentiation from postinfectious GN can be made by the presence of subendothelial immune complexes with parvovirus instead of the typical subepithelial location seen with other infections.
3. A high-risk group for renal disease are patients with sickle cell anemia and immunocompromised patients (i.e., transplant recipients).
4. IgA nephropathy/Henoch-Schönlein purpura/vasculitis may occur with acute parvovirus infection.
5. Thrombotic microangiopathy with AKI due to vascular endothelial injury from parvovirus has been reported in both the general population and in transplant recipients.
6. Chronic parvovirus infection has been associated with FSGS, particularly the collapsing variant with evidence of direct parvovirus infection of epithelial and mesangial cells.
7. Chronic allograft nephropathy, but not acute rejection, has been linked to persistent parvovirus infection after a kidney transplantation.
8. A blood or tissue PCR is more sensitive to active infection as compared to the IgG and IgM serologic response.
9. Treatment with IVIG and, when applicable in transplant patients, a reduction of immunosuppression may accelerate the clearance of the infection.

CYTOMEGALOVIRUS

Epidemiology

CMV is a double-stranded DNA virus that is a member of the herpes group virus family.[326] Specifically, of the eight defined herpes viruses, CMV is classified as human herpes virus-5 (HHV-5). CMV has a worldwide distribution affecting 60% to 80% of the adult population and is most well known for its ability to maintain a latent state. Acquisition of CMV occurs throughout early adolescence with 40% of children aged 10 to 12 years old demonstrating seropositivity, and this number increases progressively with age.[327] Both primary and secondary forms of CMV infection may occur in immunocompetent and immunocompromised patients, particularly HIV and organ transplant recipients.

CMV may cause a variety of extrarenal clinical syndromes: mononucleosis (21% of all cases), interstitial pneumonia, hepatitis, Guillain-Barré syndrome (polyradiculopathy), meningoencephalitis, myocarditis, thrombocytopenia with hemolytic anemia, skin rash, retinitis, and colitis.[328]

Glomerular Syndromes

CMV may result in three specific renal syndromes: glomerular disease, tubulointerstitial disease, and kidney transplant rejection with or without glomerular involvement.[329] Nephrotic syndrome due to MN with characteristic subepithelial immune deposits has been reported in infants and young children with a primary CMV syndrome.[330] The presence of CMV nucleic acids located directly in renal tissue was established by PCR performed on the biopsy specimen providing indirect evidence linking the viral disease with this immune complex nephropathy. Congenital CMV disease has been associated with a necrotizing and proliferative glomerulonephritis and CMV antigens have been detected in mesangial and glomerular endothelial cells.[331]

Reactivation of latent CMV may also be responsible for glomerular disease through direct and indirect mechanisms. A case of Henoch-Schönlein purpura with vasculitis was reported in a 13-year-old child and both PCR and in situ hybridization on renal tissue and blood vessels showed evidence of active CMV viral infection as a source of the immune complexes.[332] Adult IgA nephropathy has been associated with active CMV viremia, which resolved after viral therapy with ganciclovir. CMV antigenemia was detected in the mesangial cells of these patients by PCR. Overall, the association of CMV with IgA nephropathy is not fully established.[333]

In addition, CMV has been linked to the development of type II cryoglobulinemia with a secondary proliferative immune complex glomerulonephritis with systemic vasculitis as well as the development of type I MPGN in the native kidneys and posttransplant.[334–335] Collapsing FSGS has also been temporally related to an active CMV infection.[336] The sporadic nature of these reports similar to the reported association of IgA nephropathy with CMV fail to provide sufficient evidence for a significant causal association to be made of these glomerulopathies with CMV.

In renal transplant recipients, active CMV infection both primary and from reactivation has usually been associated with either asymptomatic tubular viral inclusions, acute graft rejection, and/or the development of chronic transplant glomerulopathy.[337] Intranuclear CMV inclusions in tubular and glomerular endothelial cells may be detected on biopsy specimens of renal allograft recipients in the absence of an interstitial infiltrate and typically are detected following a course of either induction therapy or treatment for rejection. The natural history of renal function in these patients is not clear and treatment has been variable, including a reduction in immunosuppression and antiviral therapy. It is felt that these inclusions represent sporadic CMV proliferation in the kidney from an overall state of increased immunosuppression.

More frequently, CMV tubular inclusions have been associated with a significant interstitial infiltrate of CD8+ T cells and mononuclear cells.[338] In these cases, it has been postulated that the host response to the CMV infection involves significant upregulation of γ-IFN increasing the antigenicity of the allograft through enhanced HLA expression.[339] This sequence of events leads to an acute interstitial nephritis from T-cell mediated rejection. The presence of acute renal injury and interstitial nephritis due to CMV has also been reported in bone marrow transplant recipients, indicating that in this circumstance it is the response to the CMV infection that leads primarily to the recruitment and migration of the interstitial cells.[340] In these patients, widespread renal tubular epithelial cell intranuclear inclusions of CMV were noted with a surrounding T-cell infiltrate in their native kidneys.

Less well established is the link between CMV and transplant glomerulopathy.[341] Although an initial report associated transplant glomerulopathy with CMV viremia in 1981, many subsequent studies have failed to confirm this association.[342] In this original report, a subset of five kidney transplant patients were noted to have absent tubulointerstitial infiltrates but an acute glomerular injury characterized by endothelial cell swelling and the deposition of a fibrillary-like material in the capillaries in the setting of active CMV viremia. Additional cases of acute CMV-related glomerular endothelial injury have been reported and substantiated on the basis of immunohistochemical localization of CMV in the glomerular capillaries.[343] The majority of patients reported with this lesion have improved with a reduction of immunosuppression and antiviral therapy.

CMV inclusions have been reported in glomerular endothelial cells but not glomerular epithelial cells.[344] Podocyte injury would appear to be through cytokine upregulation, but this pathway has not been explored in detail in transplant patients with CMV infection.[345] The term transplant glomerulopathy is typically used to denote the presence of a mesangiocapillary glomerular lesion with nephrotic syndrome in the setting of chronic allograft dysfunction. It is often associated with chronic humoral rejection. The cases of CMV-related glomerular disease in transplant patients is more typically representative of an acute glomerulitis.[346] Therefore, it would be more precise to label CMV as a cause of acute transplant glomerulitis and not an etiology of transplant glomerulopathy.[347]

In HIV patients and organ transplant recipients, CMV has been associated with thrombotic microangiopathy and renal injury.[348–349] CMV-infected renal endothelial cells were detected in 50% of patients with this syndrome and were absent in control patients. The link of CMV with thrombotic microangiopathy in organ transplant recipients is particularly important because this syndrome is most often associated with calcineurin inhibitor therapy and treated with a dose reduction or cessation of the agent. Failure to recognize the contributing effects of CMV may delay potential therapy and prolong the duration of infection. Finally, a single case of temporally associated CMV infection and immunotactoid glomerulopathy of the renal allograft was reported that resolved after treatment of the CMV viremia.[350]

Pathogenesis

CMV enters the cell through an endocytic pathway using a variety of preexisting receptors: PDGFRα, EGFR, $\alpha_2\beta_1$, $\alpha_6\beta_1$, $\alpha_v\beta_3$.[351] Direct cell invasion by CMV can occur in polymorphonuclear cells, T lymphocytes, salivary glands, epithelial cells, endothelial cells, neuronal cells, smooth muscle cells, and fibroblast monocytes and macrophages.[352] CMV is not an oncogenic virus and does not immortalize the cells like Epstein-Barr virus. CMV infection results in cell cycle arrest and diminished cell turnover.

CMV penetrates the nucleus of the cell and provides the genes for production of its own transcription factor, viral DNA polymerase. All renal cell lines in vitro have demonstrated CMV viral entry and early antigen production consistent with proliferation. CMV induces an upregulation of HLA class I and class II expression as a consequence of enhanced IFN and TNF-α expression.

Diagnosis

The most commonly used method for detecting active CMV infection is now the PCR assay. Previously, CMV required either viral culture through a "shell vial" technique using PMNs or detection of the CMV pp65 antigen in PMNs using a tagged monoclonal antibody.[353] The quantitative PCR assay appears to be the most sensitive and predictive assay of CMV disease. The exact cutoff level for viral copies that indicates significant infection has not been characterized and may vary based on the method used.[354,355]

The detection of patients with previous CMV exposure can be done by determining the presence or absence of CMV IgG antibodies using ELISA.[356] These nonneutralizing antibodies indicate prior exposure but do not guarantee viral control and active viremia can be present in spite of detectable circulating levels of CMV IgG antibodies. An IgM response to CMV does occur but may persist for months after the infection, limiting its use as a marker of acute infection. Histologic evidence of active CMV replication can be suggested by the presence of "owl-eye" intranuclear inclusion bodies, but these findings are infrequently seen. Tissue PCR for CMV is not standardized for routine use in making the diagnosis of CMV induced renal disease.

Treatment

CMV viremia may be treated with therapy, targeting the viral-induced DNA polymerase. These agents include ganciclovir, valganciclovir, foscarnet, and cidofovir. In addition, IVIG can be used to enhance viral clearance. Treatment of CMV has resulted in a remission of IgA nephropathy supporting a permissive role of this virus in the pathogenesis of the renal disease.[357] In transplant patients with CMV-associated tubulointerstitial or glomerular disease, a reduction of immunosuppression is a mandatory adjunctive intervention in addition to antiviral therapy.[358]

No clear recommendations can be made on the specific benefit of antiviral therapy on CMV renal disease.

Key Points: Cytomegalovirus and Glomerular Disease

1. A weak causal relationship has been reported between CMV and IgA nephropathy, immune complex–mediated glomerulonephritis, and cryoglobulinemic vasculitis.
2. In renal transplant patients, CMV leads primarily to renal tubular injury with a secondary inflammatory response and graft rejection.
3. In renal transplant recipients, CMV may also be associated with acute glomerular endothelial cell injury (transplant glomerulitis) with secondary podocyte dysfunction due to cytokine upregulation leading to AKI and possibly chronic allograft nephropathy.
4. Cases of thrombotic microangiopathy have been repeatedly linked to active CMV viremia in HIV patients and in solid organ transplant recipients and results from direct endothelial cell viral entry and subsequent injury.
5. Treatment of CMV with antiviral therapy has resulted in anecdotal improvement in the associated glomerular and vascular diseases.

HANTAVIRUS

Epidemiology and Diagnosis

Hantavirus is a single-stranded negative sense RNA virus, which belongs to the family Bunyaviridae and consists of 11 species which cause human infection. Rodents are the primary reservoir for this virus with the deer mouse (sin nombre hantavirus) being the major vector in the United States.[359] Hantavirus has a worldwide distribution with cases being reported in South America, Europe, Asia, Scandinavia, the Balkans, and Korea. Geographically, most North American cases occur in the western states such as New Mexico, California, Washington, and Texas. Few cases result directly from animal bites with the vast majority of exposure occurring from aerosolized virus from rodent urine, feces, or saliva.[360] Therefore, a high index of suspicion is required to diagnose this infection and should involve attention to high-risk exposure behaviors: travel to endemic areas, camping, farming, and animal exposure.

The virus uses surface glycoproteins to attach to integrins on vascular endothelial cells, platelets, and renal endothelial cells. A glycosylphosphatidylinositol (GPI)-anchored protein, decay accelerating factor, appear to be an essential component to allow virus entry from the apical portion of the cell.[361] The diagnosis of hantavirus infection is made by the ELISA detection of IgM and IgG antibodies. The ability to measure the hantavirus by PCR is available for most viral species and can provide a more rapid diagnosis compared to the delay in waiting for the change in IgM titers.[362]

Glomerular Syndromes

This virus is responsible for the development of two clinical syndromes: hemorrhagic fever and renal syndrome (HFRS) and hantavirus cardiopulmonary syndrome (HCPS). HFRS has been previously labeled as epidemic hemorrhagic fever, hemorrhagic nephritis, Songo fever, Korean hemorrhagic fever, and nephropathia epidemica.[363] Renal disease can occur in both syndromes but is most predominant in HFRS.

HFSR may affect >150,000 people annually worldwide. The clinical syndrome consists of high fever, systemic hemorrhage (DIC), circulatory collapse, and hypotension followed by oliguric AKI.[364] A diffuse capillary leak initiated by direct viral injury of endothelial cells has been implicated as the primary etiology for this syndrome. PCR studies have isolated hantavirus from renal vascular endothelial cells, especially in the outer medulla.[365]

Most importantly is the marked cytokine release that occurs in response to the endothelial cell injury that further promotes vascular permeability, vasodilation, and hypotension.[366] IFN-γ, TNF-α, IL-2, and IL-6 appear to be the primary mediators of vascular and renal injury from acute hantavirus infection. The magnitude of the cytokine response to hantavirus may be related to the viral species, but also may be genetically influenced.[367] The Asian and European strains of hantavirus are more virulent in the severity of HFSR compared to the sin nombre strain in North America.[368] Additional predictors of renal disease include the presence of hematuria, elevated white blood cell counts, and the presence of hepatic enzyme elevation.[369]

The renal lesion is more complex than simple ATN from hypoperfusion and is characterized by a prominent and pathognomonic interstitial infiltrate.[370] The interstitial nephritis is composed of CD8+ T cells and mononuclear cells associated with severe peritubular capillary congestion, interstitial hemorrhage, and edema.[371]

HFSR also involves glomerular injury in addition to the interstitial nephritis.[372] Most patients demonstrate a mesangial proliferative response without the presence of immune complexes and nonspecific localization of C3 and IgM. The majority of patients show a nephritic sediment with microhematuria and nonnephrotic range tubular proteinuria, but 25% may have fully established nephrotic syndrome.[373] In the absence of immune complexes, the proteinuria may be related to both direct viral mediated endothelial dysfunction and secondary podocyte dysfunction from the cytokine release. Rare cases of type I MPGN have also been reported with hantavirus infection that completely resolved with the resolution of the infection.[374]

There is no specific antiviral therapy for hantavirus, and HFRS is treated conservatively with supportive care. The need for temporary dialysis varies with the severity of illness and virus species. Between 5% to 40% of patients will require dialysis support during the period of oliguria, but most will recover renal function.[375] Mortality from HFRS differs based on the species of virus and can vary from 0.5% to 5% to 10%. Long-term renal outcomes appear to be consistent with most patients who experience dialysis requiring AKI of other causes with some patients developing HTN and CKD.[376] A single series with a 5-year follow-up found stage 3 CKD in 53% of patients that survived HCPS, which is likely the result of severe ATN.[377] However, in a separate cohort at a 10-year follow-up, the majority of patients recovered renal function back to their baseline levels.[378,379]

Key Points: Hantavirus and Glomerular Disease

1. Hantavirus is a rodent-borne viral illness with a worldwide distribution.
2. Kidney injury results from HFRS, which is associated with fever, capillary leak, hypotension, and oliguric AKI.
3. The pathogenesis of the disease is a result of diffuse endothelial injury from direct viral cellular entry with a secondary cytokine release syndrome.
4. Renal histology demonstrates a significant tubulointerstitial infiltrate of CT8+ T cells with hemorrhage and congestion.
5. Glomerular pathology consists of a mesangial proliferative lesion, with nephrotic syndrome being present in 25% of cases.
6. AKI requiring dialysis therapy may be present in up to 40% of patients with a mortality of 5% to 10%.
7. Treatment is supportive with the majority of survivors regaining renal function back to their baseline level.

HEPATITIS A

Glomerular Syndromes

Renal disease in hepatitis A occurs only in association with the acute period of active hepatitis because there is no chronic carrier state for this virus. IgA-associated acute GN has been reported with histologic evidence of mesangial and subendothelial deposits.[380] Resolution of the IgA nephropathy has occurred after recovery from hepatitis A.[381]

COXSACKIE B

The Coxsackie family of RNA viruses is part of the Enterovirus family and consists of two species: Coxsackievirus A (CVA) and Coxsackievirus B (CVB). These viruses have a worldwide distribution, are spread by the fecal–oral route, and are responsible for a flulike illness as well as aseptic meningitis, acute and chronic myocarditis, paralytic diseases, rhabdomyolysis, pleurodynia (Bornholm disease), and severe septic diseases in newborns. CVB has also been demonstrated to have a unique tropism for renal tissue and may be an unrecognized cause of glomerular disease.[382] In animal models, CVB gains entry into renal mesangial, tubular, and epithelial cells.[383] Cytopathic injury results in all cell types except mesangial cells, where a persistent state of infection may occur.

Acute glomerulonephritis with hematuria, proteinuria, and AKI has been reported in patients with CVB as well as in transplant recipients.[384,385] Biopsy and autopsy specimens have primarily shown a rapidly progressive GN with immune complex deposition, although renal vasculitis has also been reported.[386] In addition, both acute proliferative GN and IgA nephropathy can be induced in mice after inoculation with CVB.[387,388] In the mouse IgA model, mesangial infection with CVB resulted in a significant upregulation of γ-IFN and an exacerbation of the renal lesions.[389]

At present, the experimental animal models and clinical case reports provide strong support for the possibility that CVB may be a potential cause of acute GN in humans.

CONCLUSIONS

Viral diseases have now come to the forefront as unsuspected causes of glomerular diseases. The mechanisms of viral induced injury range from the direct viral infection of renal tissue to the development of immune complex deposition and the upregulation of intrarenal cytokines. This diversity represents a diagnostic challenge to the clinician and requires a systematic approach and an understanding of viral serologic testing, coupled with renal histology, and immunologic assays. Often, only a high index of suspicion will lead to the appropriate testing for specific viral infections based on the presentation and biopsy results.

Many answers are still required to further understand and define the pathways of HIV-related podocytopathy, the link between HCV and monoclonal IgM production, the relationship of many viruses to IgA nephropathy, and the mechanisms of HBV immune complex formation and injury. However, many successful therapeutic interventions have been developed for each viral-mediated renal injury based on the current understanding of the pathophysiology of the glomerular lesions, which truly supports the concept of "from bench to bedside."

REFERENCES

1. Lai AS, Lai KN. Viral nephropathy. *Nat Clin Pract Nephrol.* 2006 May;2(5):254–262.
2. di Belgiojoso GB, Ferrario F, Landriani N. Virus-related glomerular diseases: histological and clinical aspects. *J Nephrol.* 2002 Sep-Oct;15(5):469–479.
3. Kim WR, Terrault NA, Pedersen RA, et al. Trends in waiting list registration for liver transplantation for viral hepatitis in the United States. *Gastroenterology.* 2009 Nov;137(5):1680–1686.
4. Lavanchy D. Evolving epidemiology of hepatitis C virus. *Clin Microbiol Infect.* 2011 Feb;17(2):107–115.
5. Armstrong GL, Wasley A, Simard EP, et al. The prevalence of hepatitis C virus infection in the United States, 1999 through 2002. *Ann Intern Med.* 2006;144(10):705–714.
6. Soza A, Riquelme A, Arrese M. Routes of transmission of hepatitis C virus. *Ann Hepatol.* 2010;9 Suppl:33.
7. Simmonds P, Bukh J, Combet C, et al. Consensus proposals for a unified system of nomenclature of hepatitis C virus genotypes. *Hepatology.* 2005;42(4): 962–973.

8. Robertson B, Myers G, Howard C, et al. Classification, nomenclature, and database development for hepatitis C virus (HCV) and related viruses: proposals for standardization. International Committee on Virus Taxonomy. *Arch Virol.* 1998;143(12):2493–2503.
9. Sabahi A. Hepatitis C virus entry: the early steps in the viral replication cycle. *Virol J.* 2009 Jul 30;6:117.
10. Catanese MT, Ansuini H, Graziani R, et al. Role of scavenger receptor class B type I in hepatitis C virus entry: kinetics and molecular determinants. *J Virol.* 2010 Jan;84(1):34–43.
11. Netski DM, Mosbruger T, Depla E, et al. Humoral immune response in acute hepatitis C virus infection. *Clin Infect Dis.* 2005;41(5):667–675.
12. Logvinoff C, Major ME, Oldach D, et al. Neutralizing antibody response during acute and chronic hepatitis C virus infection. *Proc Natl Acad Sci USA.* 2004;101(27):10149–10154.
13. Cox AL, Mosbruger T, Lauer GM, et al. Comprehensive analyses of CD8+ T cell responses during longitudinal study of acute human hepatitis C. *Hepatology.* 2005;42(1):104–112.
14. Pawlotsky JM. Use and interpretation of hepatitis C virus diagnostic assays. *Clin Liver Dis.* 2003 Feb;7(1):127–137.
15. Zignego AL, Ferri C, Pileri SA, et al. Extrahepatic manifestations of hepatitis C virus infection: a general overview and guidelines for a clinical approach. *Dig Liver Dis.* 2007 Jan;39(1):2–17.
16. Hayat A, Mitwalli A. Hepatitis C and kidney disease. *Hepat Res Treat.* 2010;2010:534327.
17. Sumida K, Ubara Y, Hoshino J, et al. Hepatitis C virus-related kidney disease: various histological patterns. *Clin Nephrol.* 2010 Dec;74(6):446–456.
18. Meyers CM, Seeff LB, Stehman-Breen CO, et al. Hepatitis C and renal disease: an update. *Am J Kidney Dis.* 2003;42(4):631–657.
19. Kamar N, Izopet J, Alric L, et al. Hepatitis C virus-related kidney disease: an overview. *Clin Nephrol.* 2008 Mar;69(3):149–160.
20. Brouet JC. Cryoglobulinemias. *Presse Med.* 1983 Dec 24;12(47):2991–2996.
21. Ferri C. Mixed cryoglobulinemia. *Orphanet J Rare Dis.* 2008 Sep 16;3:25.
22. Charles ED, Dustin LB. Hepatitis C virus-induced cryoglobulinemia. *Kidney Int.* 2009 Oct;76(8):818–824.
23. Schott P, Hartmann H, Ramadori G. Hepatitis C virus-associated mixed cryoglobulinemia. Clinical manifestations, histopathological changes, mechanisms of cryoprecipitation and options of treatment. *Histol Histopathol.* 2001 Oct;16(4):1275–1285.
24. Ferri C, Zignego AL, Pileri SA. Cryoglobulins. *J Clin Pathol.* 2002 Jan;55(1): 4–13.
25. Cacoub P, Hausfater P, Musset L, et al. Mixed cryoglobulinemia in hepatitis C patients. *Ann Med Interne (Paris).* 2000 Feb;151(1):20–29.
26. Agnello V. Mixed cryoglobulinemia and other extrahepatic manifestations of HCV infection. In: Liang TJ, Hoofnagle JH, eds. *Hepatitis C.* San Diego, CA: Academic Press; 2000: 295–313.
27. Johnson RJ, Gretch DR, Yamabe H, et al. Membranoproliferative glomerulonephritis associated with hepatitis C virus infection. *N Engl J Med.* 1993;328(7): 465–470.
28. Meyers CM, Seeff LB, Stehman-Breen CO, et al. Hepatitis C and renal disease: an update. *Am J Kidney Dis.* 2003;42(4):631–657.
29. McGuire BM, Julian BA, Bynon JS Jr, et al. Brief communication: Glomerulonephritis in patients with hepatitis C cirrhosis undergoing liver transplantation. *Ann Intern Med.* 2006 May 16;144(10):735–741.
30. Tsui JI, Vittinghoff E, Shlipak MG, et al. Relationship between hepatitis C and chronic kidney disease: results from the Third National Health and Nutrition Examination Survey. *J Am Soc Nephrol.* 2006;17(4):1168–1174.
31. D'Amico G. Renal involvement in hepatitis C infection: cryoglobulinemic glomerulonephritis. *Kidney Int.* 1998;54(2):650–671.
32. Sargur R, White P, Egner W. Cryoglobulin evaluation: best practice? *Ann Clin Biochem.* 2010 Jan;47(Pt 1):8–16.
33. Zignego AL, Giannini C, Monti M, et al. Hepatitis C virus lymphotropism: lessons from a decade of studies. *Dig Liver Dis.* 2007; Sep;39 Suppl 1:S38–45.
34. Irshad M, Khushboo I, Singh S, et al. Hepatitis C virus (HCV): a review of immunological aspects. *Int Rev Immunol.* 2008;27(6):497–517.
35. Rosa D, Saletti G, De Gregorio E, et al. Activation of naïve B lymphocytes via CD81, a pathogenetic mechanism for hepatitis C virus-associated B lymphocyte disorders. *Proc Natl Acad Sci USA.* 2005 Dec 20;102(51):18544–18549.
36. Monteverde A, Ballarè M, Pileri S. Hepatic lymphoid aggregates in chronic hepatitis C and mixed cryoglobulinemia. *Springer Semin Immunopathol.* 1997;19(1):99–110.
37. Zuckerman E, Slobodin G, Kessel A. Peripheral B-cell CD5 expansion and CD81 overexpression and their association with disease severity and autoimmune markers in chronic hepatitis C virus infection. *Clin Exp Immunol.* 2002;128(2):353–358.
38. Pers JO, Jamin C, Predine-Hug F, et al. The role of CD5-expressing B cells in health and disease (review). *Int J Mol Med.* 1999 Mar;3(3):239–245.
39. Sasso EH. The rheumatoid factor response in the etiology of mixed cryoglobulins associated with hepatitis C virus infection. *Ann Med Interne (Paris).* 2000;151(1):30–40.
40. Zignego AL, Giannelli F, Marrocchi ME, et al. T(14;18) translocation in chronic hepatitis C virus infection. *Hepatology.* 2000 Feb;31(2):474–479.
41. Sasso EH, Martinez M, Yarfitz SL, et al. Frequent joining of Bcl-2 to a JH6 gene in hepatitis C virus-associated t(14;18). *J Immunol.* 2004 Sep 1;173(5): 3549–3556.
42. Abbas OM, Omar NA, Hassan ZK. T(14;18) is not associated with mixed cryoglobulinemia or with clonal B cell expansion in Egyptian patients with hepatitis C virus infection. *J Egypt Natl Canc Inst.* 2008 Jun;20(2):149–157.
43. Sansonno D, Tucci FA, De Re V, et al. HCV-associated B cell clonalities in the liver do not carry the t(14;18) chromosomal translocation. *Hepatology.* 2005 Nov;42(5):1019–1027.
44. Machida K, Cheng KT, Pavio N, et al. Hepatitis C virus E2-CD81 interaction induces hypermutation of the immunoglobulin gene in B cells. *J Virol.* 2005 Jul;79(13):8079–8089.
45. Cao Y, Zhang Y, Wang S, et al. Detection of the hepatitis C virus antigen in kidney tissue from infected patients with various glomerulonephritis. *Nephrol Dial Transplant.* 2009 Sep;24(9):2745–2751.
46. Wörnle M, Schmid H, Banas B, et al. Novel role of toll-like receptor 3 in hepatitis C-associated glomerulonephritis. *Am J Pathol.* 2006 Feb;168(2): 370–385.
47. Munir S, Saleem S, Idrees M, et al. Hepatitis C treatment: current and future perspectives. *Virol J.* 2010 Nov 1;7:296.
48. Garini G, Allegri L, Lannuzzella F, et al. HCV-related cryoglobulinemic glomerulonephritis: implications of antiviral and immunosuppressive therapies. *Acta Biomed.* 2007;78(1):51–59.
49. Beddhu S, Bastacky S, Johnson JP. The clinical and morphologic spectrum of renal cryoglobulinemia. *Medicine (Baltimore).* 2002 Sep;81(5):398–409.
50. D'Amico G. Renal involvement in hepatitis C infection: cryoglobulinemic glomerulonephritis. *Kidney Int.* 1998;54(2):650–671.
51. Saadoun D, Delluc A, Piette JC, et al. Treatment of hepatitis C-associated mixed cryoglobulinemia vasculitis. *Curr Opin Rheumatol.* 2008 Jan;20(1):23–28.
52. Alric L, Plaisier E, Thébault S, et al. Influence of antiviral therapy in hepatitis C virus-associated cryoglobulinemic MPGN. *Am J Kidney Dis.* 2004 Apr;43(4):617–623.
53. Kronenberger B, Herrmann E, Hofmann WP, et al. Dynamics of CD81 expression on lymphocyte subsets during interferon-alpha-based antiviral treatment of patients with chronic hepatitis C. *J Leukoc Biol.* 2006 Aug;80(2): 298–308.
54. Terrier B, Launay D, Kaplanski G, et al. Safety and efficacy of rituximab in nonviral cryoglobulinemia vasculitis: data from the French Autoimmunity and Rituximab registry. *Arthritis Care Res (Hoboken).* 2010 Dec;62(12):1787–1795.
55. Cacoub P, Delluc A, Saadoun D, et al. Anti-CD20 monoclonal antibody (rituximab) treatment for cryoglobulinemic vasculitis: where do we stand? *Ann Rheum Dis.* 2008 Mar;67(3):283–287.
56. Saadoun D, Resche Rigon M, Sene D, et al. Rituximab plus Peg-interferon-alpha/ribavirin compared with Peg-interferon-alpha/ribavirin in hepatitis C-related mixed cryoglobulinemia. *Blood.* 2010 Jul 22;116(3):326–334.
57. Saadoun D, Resche-Rigon M, Sene D, et al. Rituximab combined with Peg-interferon-ribavirin in refractory hepatitis C virus-associated cryoglobulinaemia vasculitis. *Ann Rheum Dis.* 2008 Oct;67(10):1431–1436.
58. Terrier B, Saadoun D, Sène D, et al. Efficacy and tolerability of rituximab with or without PEGylated interferon alfa-2b plus ribavirin in severe hepatitis C virus-related vasculitis: a long-term followup study of thirty-two patients. *Arthritis Rheum.* 2009 Aug;60(8):2531–2540.
59. Pietrogrande M, De Vita S, Zignego A, et al. Recommendations for the management of mixed cryoglobulinemia syndrome in hepatitis C virus-infected patients. *Autoimmun Rev.* 2011;10(8):444–454.
60. Ohta S, Yokoyama H, Wada T. Exacerbation of glomerulonephritis in subjects with chronic hepatitis C virus infection and interferon therapy. *Am J Kidney Dis.* 1999;33(6):1040–1048.
61. Willson RA. Nephrotoxicity of interferon alfa-ribavirin therapy for chronic hepatitis C. *J Clin Gastroenterol.* 2002 Jul;35(1):89–92.
62. Tovar JL, Buti M, Segarra A, et al. De novo nephrotic syndrome following pegylated interferon alfa 2b/ribavirin therapy for chronic hepatitis C infection. *Int Urol Nephrol.* 2008;40(2):539–541.
63. Coroneos E, Petrusevska G, Varghese F, et al. Focal segmental glomerulosclerosis with acute renal failure associated with alpha-interferon therapy. *Am J Kidney Dis.* 1996;28(6):888–892.
64. Izzedine H, Launay-Vacher V, Deray G. Antiviral drug-induced nephrotoxicity. *Am J Kidney Dis.* 2005 May;45(5):804–817.

65. Cruzado JM, Carrera M, Torras J, et al. Hepatitis C virus infection and de novo glomerular lesions in renal allografts. *Am J Transplantation.* 2001;1(2):171–178.

66. Faguer S, Kamar N, Boulestin A, et al. Prevalence of cryoglobulinemia and autoimmunity markers in renal-transplant patients. *Clin Nephrol.* 2008 Apr;69(4):239–243.

67. Sens YA, Malafronte P, Souza JF, et al. Cryoglobulinemia in kidney transplant recipients. *Transplant Proc.* 2005 Dec;37(10):4273–4275.

68. Hammoud H, Haem J, Laurent B, et al. Glomerular disease during HCV infection in renal transplantation. *Nephrol Dial Transplant.* 1996;11 Suppl 4:54–55.

69. Aline-Fardin A, Rifle G, Martin L, et al. Recurrent and de novo membranous glomerulopathy after kidney transplantation. *Transplant Proc.* 2009 Mar;41(2):669–671.

70. Morales JM, Pascual-Capdevila J, Campistol JM, et al. Membranous glomerulonephritis associated with hepatitis C virus infection in renal transplant patients. *Transplantation.* 1997;63(11):1634–1639.

71. Abrahamian GA, Cosimi AB, Farrell ML, et al. Prevalence of hepatitis C virus-associated mixed cryoglobulinemia after liver transplantation. *Liver Transpl.* 2000 Mar;6(2):185–190.

72. Duvoux C, Tran Ngoc A, Intrator L, et al. Hepatitis C virus (HCV)-related cryoglobulinemia after liver transplantation for HCV cirrhosis. *Transpl Int.* 2002 Jan;15(1):3–9.

73. Kamar N, Ribes D, Izopet J, et al. Treatment of hepatitis C virus (HCV) infection after renal transplantation: implications for HCV-positive dialysis patients awaiting a kidney transplant. *Transplantation.* 2006;82(7):853–856.

74. Morales JM. Hepatitis C virus infection and renal disease after renal transplantation. *Transplant Proc.* 2004 Apr;36(3):760–762.

75. Montalbano M, Pasulo L, Sonzogni A, et al. Treatment with pegylated interferon and ribavirin for hepatitis C virus-associated severe cryoglobulinemia in a liver/kidney transplant recipient. *J Clin Gastroenterol.* 2007 Feb;41(2):216–220.

76. Pham HP, Féray C, Samuel D, et al. Effects of ribavirin on hepatitis C-associated nephrotic syndrome in four liver transplant recipients. *Kidney Int.* 1998 Oct;54(4):1311–1319.

77. Basse G, Ribes D, Kamar N, et al. Rituximab therapy for de novo mixed cryoglobulinemia in renal transplant patients. *Transplantation.* 2005 Dec 15;80(11): 1560–1564.

78. Fabrizi F, Martin P, Elli A, et al. Hepatitis C virus infection and rituximab therapy after renal transplantation. *Int J Artif Organs.* 2007 May;30(5):445–449.

79. Cruzado JM, Casanovas-Taltavull T, Torras J, et al. Pretransplant interferon prevents hepatitis C virus-associated glomerulonephritis in renal allografts by HCV-RNA clearance. *Am J Transplant.* 2003;3:357.

80. Wu YY, Hsu TC, Chen TY. Proteinase 3 and dihydrolipoamide dehydrogenase (E3) are major autoantigens in hepatitis C virus (HCV) infection. *Clin Exp Immunol.* 2002;128(2):347–352.

81. Igaki N, Nakaji M, Moriguchi R, et al. [A case of hepatitis C virus-associated glomerulonephropathy presenting with MPO-ANCA-positive rapidly progressive glomerulonephritis]. *Nihon Jinzo Gakkai Shi.* 2000;42(4):353–358.

82. Bonaci-Nikolic B, Andrejevic S, Pavlovic M, et al. Prolonged infections associated with antineutrophil cytoplasmic antibodies specific to proteinase 3 and myeloperoxidase: diagnostic and therapeutic challenge. *Clin Rheumatol.* 2010 Aug;29(8):893–904.

83. Stehman-Breen C, Alpers CE, Fleet WP, et al. Focal segmental glomerular sclerosis among patients infected with hepatitis C virus. *Nephron.* 1999 Jan;81(1):37–40.

84. Kamar N, Izopet J, Alric L, et al. Hepatitis C virus-related kidney disease: an overview. *Clin Nephrol.* 2008 Mar;69(3):149–160.

85. Markowitz GS, Nasr SH, Stokes MB, et al. Treatment with IFN-α, -β, or -γ is associated with collapsing focal segmental glomerulosclerosis. *Clin J Am Soc Nephrol.* 2010 Apr;5(4):607–615.

86. Sumida K, Ubara Y, Hoshino J, et al. Hepatitis C virus-related kidney disease: various histological patterns. *Clin Nephrol.* 2010 Dec;74(6):446–456.

87. Gonzalo A, Navarro J, Bárcena R, et al. IgA nephropathy associated with hepatitis C virus infection. *Nephron.* 1995;69(3):354.

88. Ji F, Li Z, Ge H, et al. Successful interferon-α treatment in a patient with IgA nephropathy associated with hepatitis C virus infection. *Intern Med.* 2010;49(22):2531–2532.

89. White DL, Ratziu V, El-Serag HB. Hepatitis C infection and risk of diabetes: a systematic review and meta-analysis. *J Hepatol.* 2008;49(5):831–844.

90. Milner KL, van der Poorten D, Trenell M, et al. Chronic hepatitis C is associated with peripheral rather than hepatic insulin resistance. *Gastroenterology.* 2010;138(3):932–941.

91. Martin P, Fabrizi F. Hepatitis C virus and kidney disease. *J Hepatol.* 2008 Oct;49(4):613–624.

92. Kidney Disease: Improving Global Outcomes. KDIGO clinical practice guidelines for the prevention, diagnosis, evaluation, and treatment of hepatitis C in chronic kidney disease. *Kidney International.* 2008;73(Suppl 109):S1–S99.

93. Joint United Nations Programme on HIV/AIDS, World Health Organization. *UNAIDS: 2009 AIDS epidemic update. UNAIDS/09.36E/JC1700E.* Geneva, Switzerland: Authors; November 2009.

94. Centers for Disease Control and Prevention (CDC). Epidemiology of HIV/AIDS—United States, 1981–2005. *MMWR Morb Mortal Wkly Rep.* 2006;55(21): 589–592.

95. Heeney JL, Dalgleish AG, Weiss RA. Origins of HIV and the evolution of resistance to AIDS. *Science.* 2006;313(5786):462.

96. Archer J, Robertson DL. Understanding the diversification of HIV-1 groups M and O. *AIDS.* 2007;21(13):1693–1700.

97. Paraskevis D, Pybus O, Magiorkinis G, et al. Tracing the HIV-1 subtype B mobility in Europe: a phylogeographic approach. *Retrovirology.* 2009 May 20;6:49.

98. Beyrer C. HIV epidemiology update and transmission factors: risks and risk contexts–16th International AIDS Conference epidemiology plenary. *Clin Infect Dis.* 2007;44(7):981–987.

99. Hall HI, Song R, Rhodes P, et al. Estimation of HIV incidence in the United States. *JAMA.* 2008;300(5):520–559.

100. Centers for Disease Control and Prevention (CDC). HIV prevalence estimates—United States, 2006. *MMWR Morb Mortal Wkly Rep.* 2008;57(39):1073–1076.

101. Shrestha S, Strathdee SA, Galai N, et al. Behavioral risk exposure and host genetics of susceptibility to HIV-1 infection. *J Infect Dis.* 2006 Jan 1;193(1):16–26.

102. Daar ES, Pilcher CD, Hecht FM. Clinical presentation and diagnosis of primary HIV-1 infection. *Curr Opin HIV AIDS.* 2008;3(1):10–15.

103. Elewa U, Sandri AM, Rizza SA, et al. Treatment of HIV-associated nephropathies. *Nephron Clin Pract.* 2011 Feb 3;118(4):c346–c354.

104. Rao TK, Filippone EJ, Nicastri AD, et al. Associated focal and segmental glomerulosclerosis in the acquired immunodeficiency syndrome. *N Engl J Med.* 1984;310(11):669–673.

105. Wyatt CM, Morgello S, Katz-Malamed R, et al. The spectrum of kidney disease in patients with AIDS in the era of antiretroviral therapy. *Kidney International.* 2008;75(4):428–434.

106. Lu TC, Ross M. HIV-associated nephropathy: a brief review. *Mt Sinai J Med.* 2005;72(3):193–199.

107. Estrella ME, Fine DM, Gallant JE, et al. HIV Type 1 RNA level as a clinical indicator of renal pathology in HIV-infected patients. *Clin Infect Dis.* 2006;43(3): 1488–1495.

108. Winston JA, Klotman ME, Klotman PE. HIV-associated nephropathy is a late, not early, manifestation of HIV-1 infection. *Kidney International.* 1999;55(3): 1036–1040.

109. Estrella M, Fine DM, Gallant JE, et al. HIV type 1 RNA level as a clinical indicator of renal pathology in HIV-infected patients. *Clin Infect Dis.* 2006;43(3): 377–380.

110. Izzedine H, Acharya V, Wirden M, et al. Role of HIV-1 DNA levels as clinical marker of HIV-1-associated nephropathies. *Nephrol Dial Transplant.* 2011 Feb;26(2):580–583.

111. Ahuja TS, Borucki M, Funtanilla M, et al. Is the prevalence of HIV-associated nephropathy decreasing? *Am J Nephrol.* 1999;19(6):655–659.

112. Katz IJ, Gerntholtz T, Naicker S. Africa and nephrology: the forgotten continent. *Nephron Clin Pract.* 2010 Oct 15;117(4):c320–c327.

113. Fabian J, Naicker S. HIV and kidney disease in sub-Saharan Africa. *Nat Rev Nephrol.* 2009 Oct;5(10):591–598.

114. Kopp JB, Smith MW, Nelson GW, et al. MYH9 is a major-effect risk gene for focal segmental glomerulosclerosis. *Nat Genet.* 2008;40(10),1175–1184.

115. Kao WH, Klag MJ, Meoni LA, et al. MYH9 is associated with nondiabetic end-stage renal disease in African Americans. *Nat Genet.* 2008;40(10): 1185–1192.

116. Tzur S, Rosset S, Shemer R, et al. Missense mutations in the APOL1 gene are highly associated with end stage kidney disease risk previously attributed to the MYH9 gene. *Hum Genet.* 2010 Sep;128(3):345–350.

117. Genovese G, Friedman DJ, Ross MD, et al. Association of trypanolytic ApoL1 variants with kidney disease in African Americans. *Science.* 2010;329(5993): 841–845.

118. Genovese G, Tonna SJ, Knob AU, et al. A risk allele for focal segmental glomerulosclerosis in African Americans is located within a region containing ApoL1 and MYH9. *Kidney Int.* 2010;78(7):698–704.

119. Freedman BI, Kopp JB, Langefeld CD, et al. The apolipoprotein L1 (APOL1) gene and nondiabetic nephropathy in African Americans. *J Am Soc Nephrol.* 2010 Sep;21(9):1422–1426.

120. Quaggin SE. Genetic susceptibility to HIV-associated nephropathy. *J Clin Invest.* 2009 May;119(5):1085–1089.

121. Gharavi AG, Ahmad T, Wong RD, et al. Mapping a locus for susceptibility to HIV-1-associated nephropathy to mouse chromosome 3. *Proc Natl Acad Sci USA.* 2004 Feb 24;101(8):2488–2493.

122. Cunningham EE, Zielezny MA, Venuto RC. Heroin-associated nephropathy. A nationwide problem. *JAMA*. 1983;250(21):2935–2936.
123. Friedman EA, Tao TK. Disappearance of uremia due to heroin-associated nephropathy. *Am J Kidney Dis*. 1995;25(5):689–693.
124. Ross MJ, Klotman PE, Winston JA. HIV-associated nephropathy: Case study and review of the literature. *AIDS Patient Care STDS*. 2000;14(12):637–645.
125. Atta MG, Choi MJ, Longenecker JC, et al. Nephrotic range proteinuria and CD4 count as noninvasive indicators of HIV-associated nephropathy. *Am J Med*. 2005;118(11):1288.
126. Guardia JA, Ortiz-Butcher C, Bourgoignie JJ. Oncotic pressure and edema formation in hypoalbuminemic HIV-infected patients with proteinuria. *Am J Kidney Dis*. 1997 Dec;30(6):822–828.
127. Szczech LA, Grunfeld C, Scherzer R, et al., Microalbuminuria in HIV infection. *AIDS* 2007;21(8):1003–1009.
128. Szczech LA, Menezes P, Byrd Quinlivan E, et al. Microalbuminuria predicts overt proteinuria among patients with HIV infection. *HIV Med*. 2010 Aug;11(7):419–426.
129. Han TM, Naicker S, Ramdial PK, et al. A cross-sectional study of HIV-seropositive patients with varying degrees of proteinuria in South Africa. *Kidney Int*. 2006 Jun;69(12):2243–2250.
130. Gupta SK, Eustace JA, Winston JA, et al. Guidelines for the management of chronic kidney disease in HIV-infected patients: recommendations of the HIV Medicine Association of the Infectious Diseases Society of America. *Clin Infect Dis*. 2005;40(11):1559–1585.
131. Siedner MJ, Atta MG, Lucas GM, et al. Poor validity of urine dipstick as a screening tool for proteinuria in HIV-positive patients. *J Acquir Immune Defic Syndr*. 2008;47(2):261–263.
132. Herman ES, Klotman PE. HIV-associated nephropathy: epidemiology, pathogenesis, and treatment. *Semin Nephrol*. 2003;23(2):200–208.
133. Gazzaruso C, Bruno R, Garzaniti A, et al. Hypertension among HIV patients: prevalence and relationships to insulin resistance and metabolic syndrome. *J Hypertens*. 2003;21(7):1377–1382.
134. Di Fiori JL, Rodrigue D, Kaptein EM, et al. Diagnostic sonography of HIV-associated nephropathy: new observations and clinical correlation. *AJR Am J Roentgenol*. 1998;171(3): 713–716.
135. Symeonidou C, Standish R, Sahdev A, et al. Imaging and histopathologic features of HIV-related renal disease. *Radiographics*. 2008 Sep–Oct;28(5):1339–1354.
136. Atta MG, Longenecker JC, Fine DM, et al. Sonography as a predictor of human immunodeficiency virus-associated nephropathy. *J Ultrasound Med*. 2004;23(5):603–610.
137. Wachsberg RH, Obolevich AT, Lasker N. Pelvocalyceal thickening in HIV-associated nephropathy. *Abdom Imaging*. 1995 Jul–Aug;20(4):371–375.
138. Franceschini N, Napravnik S, Eron JJ Jr, et al. Incidence and etiology of acute renal failure among ambulatory HIV-infected patients. *Kidney Int*. 2005;67(4):1526–1531.
139. Naicker S, Aboud O, Gharbi MD. Epidemiology of acute kidney injury in Africa. *Semin Nephrol*. 2008;28(4):348–353.
140. Campbell LJ, Ibrahim F, Fisher M, et al., Spectrum of chronic kidney disease in HIV-infected patients. *HIV Med*. 2009;10(6):329–336.
141. Barraclough K, Er L, Ng F, et al. A comparison of the predictive performance of different methods of kidney function estimation in a well-characterized HIV-infected population. *Nephron Clin Pract*. 2009;111(1):c39–c48.
142. Bonjoch A, Bayés B, Riba J, et al. Validation of estimated renal function measurements compared with the isotopic glomerular filtration rate in an HIV-infected cohort. *Antiviral Res*. 2010 Dec;88(3):347–354.
143. Barisoni L, Kopp JB. Modulation of podocyte phenotype in collapsing glomerulopathies. *Microsc Res Tech*. 2002 May 15;57(4):254–262.
144. Dijkman HB, Weening JJ, Smeets B, et al. Proliferating cells in HIV and pamidronate-associated collapsing focal segmental glomerulosclerosis are parietal epithelial cells. *Kidney Int*. 2006 Jul;70(2):338–344.
145. Smeets B, Uhlig S, Fuss A, et al. Tracing the origin of glomerular extracapillary lesions from parietal epithelial cells. *J Am Soc Nephrol*. 2009 Dec;20(12): 2604–2615.
146. Kaufman L, Collins SE, Klotman PE. The pathogenesis of HIV-associated nephropathy. *Adv Chronic Kidney Dis*. 2010 Jan;17(1):36–43.
147. Barisoni L, Kriz W, Mundel P, et al. The dysregulated podocyte phenotype: a novel concept in the pathogenesis of collapsing idiopathic focal segmental glomerulosclerosis and HIV-associated nephropathy. *J Am Soc Nephrol*. 1999 Jan;10(1):51–61.
148. Bruggeman LA, Ross MD, Tanji N, et al. Renal epithelium is a previously unrecognised site of HIV-1 infection. *J Am Soc Nephrol*. 2000;11(11):2079–2087.
149. Winston JA, Bruggeman LA, Ross MD, et al. Nephropathy and establishment of a renal reservoir of HIV type 1 during primary infection. *N Engl J Med*. 2001;344(26):1979–1984.
150. Marshall CB, Shankland SJ. Cell cycle regulatory proteins in podocyte health and disease. *Nephron Exp Nephrol*. 2007;106(2):e51–59.
151. Papeta N, Sterken R, Kiryluk K, et al. The molecular pathogenesis of HIV-1 associated nephropathy: recent advances. *J Mol Med (Berl)*. 2011;89(5):429–436.
152. Rosenstiel P, Gharavi A, D'Agati V, et al. Transgenic and infectious animal models of HIV-associated nephropathy. *J Am Soc Nephrol*. 2009;20(11):2296–2304.
153. Bruggeman LA, Dikman S, Meng C, et al. Nephropathy in human immunodeficiency virus-1 transgenic mice is due to renal transgene expression. *J Clin Invest*. 1997;100(1):84–92.
154. Winston JA, Bruggeman LA, Ross MD, et al. Nephropathy and establishment of a renal reservoir of HIV type 1 during primary infection. *N Engl J Med*. 2001;344(26):1979–1984.
155. Mikulak J, Teichberg S, Faust T, et al. HIV-1 harboring renal tubular epithelial cell interaction with T cells results in T cell trans-infection. *Virology*. 2009 Mar 1;385(1):105–114.
156. Avila-Casado C, Fortoul TI, Chugh SS. HIV-associated nephropathy: experimental models. *Contrib Nephrol*. 2011;169:270–285.
157. Zuo Y, Matsusaka T, Zhong J, et al. HIV-1 genes vpr and nef synergistically damage podocytes, leading to glomerulosclerosis. *J Am Soc Nephrol*. 2006;17(10):2832–2843.
158. Lu TC, He JC, Klotman PE. Podocytes in HIV-associated nephropathy. *Nephron Clin Pract*. 2007;106(2):c67–71.
159. Lu TC, He JC, Wang ZH, et al. HIV-1 Nef disrupts the podocyte actin cytoskeleton by interacting with diaphanous interacting protein. *J Biol Chem*. 2008 Mar 28;283(13):8173–8182.
160. Doublier S, Zennaro C, Spatola T, et al. HIV-1 Tat reduces nephrin in human podocytes: a potential mechanism for enhanced glomerular permeability in HIV-associated nephropathy. *AIDS*. 2007 Feb 19;21(4):423–432.
161. Korgaonkar SN, Feng X, Ross MD, et al. HIV-1 upregulates VEGF in podocytes. *J Am Soc Nephrol*. 2008 May;19(5):877–883.
162. Ross MJ, Martinka S, D'Agati VD, et al. NF-kappaB regulates Fas-mediated apoptosis in HIV-associated nephropathy. *J Am Soc Nephrol*. 2005 Aug;16(8):2403–2411.
163. Sharma M, Callen S, Zhang D, et al. Activation of Notch signaling pathway in HIV-associated nephropathy. *AIDS*. 2010 Sep 10;24(14):2161–2170.
164. Kumar D, Konkimalla S, Yadav A, et al. HIV-associated nephropathy: role of mammalian target of rapamycin pathway. *Am J Pathol*. 2010 Aug;177(2):813–821.
165. D'Agati V, Suh JI, Carbone L, et al. Pathology of HIV-associated nephropathy: a detailed morphologic and comparative study. *Kidney Int*. 1989 Jun;35(6): 1358–1370.
166. Ross MJ, Bruggeman LA, Wilson PD, et al. Microcyst formation and HIV-1 gene expression occur in multiple nephron segments in HIV-associated nephropathy. *K Am Soc Nephrol*. 2001 Dec;12(12):2645–2651.
167. Ross MJ, Bruggeman LA, Wilson PD, et al. Microcyst formation and HIV-1 gene expression occur in multiple nephron segments in HIV-associated nephropathy. *J Am Soc Nephrol*. 2001 Dec;12(12):2645–2651.
168. Ross MJ, Fan C, Ross MD, et al. HIV-1 infection initiates an inflammatory cascade in human renal tubular epithelial cells. *J Acquir Immune Defic Syndr*. 2006;42(1):1–11.
169. Kimmel PL, Cohen DJ, Abraham AA, et al. Upregulation of MHC class II, interferon-alpha and interferon-gamma receptor protein expression in HIV associated nephropathy. *Nephrol Dial Transplant*. 2003;18(2):285–292.
170. Bruggeman LA, Adler SH, Klotman PE. Nuclear factor-kappa B binding to the HIV-1 LTR in kidney: implications for HIV-associated nephropathy. *Kidney Int*. 2001 Jun;59(6):2174–2181.
171. Parkhie SM, Fine DM, Lucas GM, et al. Characteristics of patients with HIV and biopsy-proven acute interstitial nephritis. *Clin J Am Soc Nephrol*. 2010 May;5(5):798–804.
172. Orenstein JM, Preble OT, Kind P, et al. The relationship of serum alpha-interferon and ultrastructural markers in HIV-seropositive individuals. *Ultrastruct Pathol*. 1987;11(5–6):673–679.
173. Yahaya I, Uthman AO, Uthman MM. Interventions for HIV-associated nephropathy. *Cochrane Database Syst Rev*. 2009 Oct 7;(4):CD007183.
174. Schwartz EJ, Szczech LA, Ross MJ, et al. Highly active antiretroviral therapy and the epidemic of HIV+ end-stage renal disease. *J Am Soc Nephrol*. 2005;16(8):2412–2420.
175. Lucas GM, Eustace JA, Sozio S, et al. Highly active antiretroviral therapy and the incidence of HIV-1-associated nephropathy: a 12-year cohort study. *AIDS*. 2004;18(3):541–546.
176. Kirchner JT. Resolution of renal failure after initiation of HAART: 3 cases and a discussion of the literature. *AIDS Read*. 2002 Mar;12(3): 103–105,110–112.
177. Atta MG, Gallant JE, Rahman MH, et al. Antiretroviral therapy in the treatment of HIV-associated nephropathy. *Nephrol Dial Transplant*. 2006;21(10): 2809–2813.

178. Scialla JJ, Atta MG, Fine DM. Relapse of HIV-associated nephropathy after discontinuing highly active antiretroviral therapy. *AIDS*. 2007;21(2):263–264.
179. Longenecker CT, Scherzer R, Bacchetti P, et al. HIV viremia and changes in kidney function. *AIDS*. 2009;23(9):1089–1096.
180. Kalayjian RC, Franceschini N, Gupta SK, et al. Suppression of HIV-1 replication by antiretroviral therapy improves renal function in persons with low CD4 cell counts and chronic kidney disease. *AIDS*. 2008;22(4):481–487.
181. Winston JA, Bruggeman LA, Ross MD, et al. Nephropathy and establishment of a renal reservoir of HIV type 1 during primary infection. *N Engl J Med*. 2001 Jun 28;344(26):1979–1984.
182. Gupta SK, Parker RA, Robbins GK, et al. The effects of highly active antiretroviral therapy on albuminuria in HIV-infected persons: results from a randomized trial. *Nephrol Dial Transplant*. 2005;20(10):2237–2242.
183. Hammer SM, Eron JJ Jr, Reiss P, et al. Antiretroviral treatment of adult HIV infection: 2008 recommendations of the International AIDS Society-USA panel. *JAMA*. 2008;300(5):555–570.
184. Eustace JA, Nuermberger E, Choi M, et al. Cohort study of the treatment of severe HIV-associated nephropathy with corticosteroids. *Kidney Int*. 2000;58(3):1253–1260..
185. Laradi A, Mallet A, Beaufils H, et al. HIV-associated nephropathy: outcome and prognosis factors. Groupe d' Etudes Nephrologiques d'Ile de France. *J Am Soc Nephrol*. 1998;9(12):2327–2335.
186. Miller KD, Masur H, Jones EC, et al. High prevalence of osteonecrosis of the femoral head in HIV-infected adults. *Ann Intern Med*. 2002;137(1): 17–25.
187. Briggs WA, Tanawattanacharoen S, Choi MJ, et al. Clinicopathologic correlates of prednisone treatment of human immunodeficiency virus-associated nephropathy. *Am J Kidney Dis*. 1996 Oct;28(4):618–621.
188. Briggs WA, Tanawattanacharoen S, Choi MJ, et al. Clinicopathologic correlates of prednisone treatment of human immunodeficiency virus-associated nephropathy. *Am J Kidney Dis*. 1996;28(4):618–621.
189. Ross MJ, Fan C, Ross MD, et al. HIV-1 infection initiates an inflammatory cascade in human renal tubular epithelial cells. *J Acquir Immune Defic Syndr*. 2006 May;42(1):1–11.
190. Wei A, Burns GC, Williams BA, et al. Long-term renal survival in HIV-associated nephropathy with angiotensin-converting enzyme inhibition. *Kidney International*. 2003;64(4):1462–1471.
191. Kimmel PL, Mishkin GJ, Umana WO. Captopril and renal survival in patients with human immunodeficiency virus nephropathy. *Am J Kidney Dis*. 1996;28(2):202–208.
192. Hiramatsu N, Hiromura K, Shigehara T, et al. Angiotensin II type 1 receptor blockade inhibits the development and progression of HIV-associated nephropathy in a mouse model. *J Am Soc Nephrol*. 2007 Feb;18(2):515–527.
193. Ideura H, Hiromura K, Hiramatsu N, et al. Angiotensin II provokes podocyte injury in murine model of HIV-associated nephropathy. *Am J Physiol Renal Physiol*. 2007 Oct;293(4):F1214–1221.
194. Fine DM, Perazella MA, Lucas GM, et al. Kidney biopsy in HIV: beyond HIV-associated nephropathy. *Am J Kidney Dis*. 2008 Mar;51(3):504–514.
195. Berliner AR, Fine DM, Lucas GM, et al. Observations on a cohort of HIV-infected patients undergoing native renal biopsy. *Am J Nephrol*. 2008;28(3): 478–486.
196. Cohen SD, Kimmel PL. Immune complex renal disease and human immunodeficiency virus infection. *Semin Nephrol*. 2008;28(6):535–544.
197. Gerntholtz TE, Goetsch SJ, Katz I. HIV-related nephropathy: a South African perspective. *Kidney International*. 2006;69(10):1885–1891.
198. Berggren R, Batuman V. HIV-associated renal disorders: recent insights into pathogenesis and treatment. *Curr HIV/AIDS Rep*. 2005 Aug;2(3):109–115.
199. Faulhaber JR, Nelson PJ. Virus-induced cellular immune mechanisms of injury to the kidney. *Clin J Am Soc Nephrol*. 2007 Jul;2 Suppl 1:S2–S5.
200. Kimmel PL, Phillips TM, Ferreira-Centeno A, et al. HIV-associated immune-mediated renal disease. *Kidney Int*. 1993;44(6):1327–1340.
201. Katz A, Bargman JM, Miller DC, et al. IgA nephritis in HIV-positive patients: a new HIV-associated nephropathy? *Clin Nephrol*. 1992;38(2):61–68.
202. Nebuloni M, Barbiano di Belgiojoso G, Genderini A, et al. Glomerular lesions in HIV-positive patients: a 20-year biopsy experience from Northern Italy. *Clin Nephrol*. 2009 Jul;72(1):38–45.
203. Haas M, Kaul S, Eustace JA. HIV-associated immune complex glomerulonephritis with "lupus-like" features: A clinicopathologic study of 14 cases. *Kidney Int*. 2005;67(4):1381–1390.
204. Tabechian D, Pattanaik D, Suresh U, et al. Lupus-like nephritis in an HIV-positive patient: report of a case and review of the literature. *Clin Nephrol*. 2003 Sep;60(3):187–194.
205. Cohen SD, Kimmel PL. Immune complex renal disease and human immunodeficiency virus infection. *Semin Nephrol*. 2008;28(6):535–544.
206. Szczech LA, Gupta SK, Habash R, et al. The clinical epidemiology and course of the spectrum of renal diseases associated with HIV infection. *Kidney Int*. 2004;66(3):1145–1152.
207. Górriz JL, Rovira E, Sancho A, et al. IgA nephropathy associated with human immunodeficiency virus infection: antiproteinuric effect of captopril. *Nephrol Dial Transplant*. 1997;12(12):2796–2797.
208. Dellow E, Unwin R, Miller R, et al. Protease inhibitor therapy for HIV infection: the effect on HIV-associated nephrotic syndrome. *Nephrol Dial Transplant*. 1999;14(3):744–747.
209. Izzedine H, Sene D, Cacoub P, et al. Kidney diseases in HIV/HCV-co-infected patients. *AIDS*. 2009 Jun 19;23(10):1219–1226.
210. Fabris P, Tositti G, Giordani MT, et al. Prevalence and clinical significance of circulating cryoglobulins in HIV-positive patients with and without co-infection with hepatitis C virus. *J Med Virol*. 2003;69(3):339–343.
211. Cheng JT, Anderson HL Jr, Markowitz GS, et al. Hepatitis C virus-associated glomerular disease in patients with human immunodeficiency virus coinfection. *J Am Soc Nephrol*. 1999 Jul;10(7):1566–1574.
212. Tsui J, Vittinghoff E, Anastos K, et al. Hepatitis C seropositivity and kidney function decline among women with HIV: data from the Women's Interagency HIV Study. *Am J Kidney Dis*. 2009;54(1):43–50.
213. Cheng JT, Anderson HL Jr, Markowitz GS, et al. Hepatitis C virus-associated glomerular disease in patients with human immunodeficiency virus coinfection. *J Am Soc Nephrol*. 1999 Jul;10(7):1566–1574.
214. Thompson CE, Damon LE, Ries CA, et al. Thrombotic microangiopathies in the 1980s: Clinical features, response to treatment, and the impact of the human immunodeficiency virus epidemic. *Blood*. 1992;80(8):1890–1895.
215. Gervasoni C, Ridolfo AL, Vaccarezza M, et al. Thrombotic microangiopathy in patients with acquired immunodeficiency syndrome before and during the era of introduction of highly active antiretroviral therapy. *Clin Infect Dis*. 2002;35(12):1534–1540.
216. Rivera H, Nikitakis NG, Castillo S, et al. Histopathological analysis and demonstration of EBV and HIV p-24 antigen but not CMV expression in labial minor salivary glands of HIV patients affected by diffuse infiltrative lymphocytosis syndrome. *J Oral Pathol Med*. 2003;32(7): 431–437.
217. Schecter AD, Berman AB, Yi L, et al. HIV envelope gp120 activates human arterial smooth muscle cells. *Proc Natl Acad Sci USA*. 2001;98(18):10142–10147.
218. Franchini M, Montagnana M, Targher G, et al. Reduced von Willebrand factor-cleaving protease levels in secondary thrombotic microangiopathies and other diseases. *Semin Thromb Hemost*. 2007;33(8):787–797.
219. Alpers CE. Light at the end of the TUNEL: HIV-associated thrombotic microangiopathy. *Kidney Int*. 2003;63(1):385–396.
220. Maslo C, Peraldi MN, Desenclos JC, et al. Thrombotic microangiopathy and cytomegalovirus disease in patients infected with human immunodeficiency virus. *Clin Infect Dis*. 1997;24(3):350–355.
221. Peraldi MN, Maslo C, Akposso K, et al. Acute renal failure in the course of HIV infection: A single-institution retrospective study of ninety-two patients and sixty renal biopsies. *Nephrol Dial Transplant*. 1999;14(6):1578–1585.
222. Sacristán Lista F, Saavedra Alonso AJ, Oliver Morales J, et al. Nephrotic syndrome due to thrombotic microangiopathy (TMA) as the first manifestation of human immunodeficiency virus infection: recovery before antiretroviral therapy without specific treatment against TMA. *Clin Nephrol*. 2001 May;55(5): 404–407.
223. Fine DM, Fogo AB, Alpers CE. Thrombotic microangiopathy and other glomerular disorders in the HIV-infected patient. *Semin Nephrol*. 2008 Nov;28(6): 545–555.
224. Becker S, Fusco G, Fusco J, et al. HIV-associated thrombotic microangiopathy in the era of highly active antiretroviral therapy: an observational study. *Clin Infect Dis*. 2004;39(Suppl 5):S267–S275.
225. Chen C, Jhaveri KD, Hartono C, et al. An uncommon glomerular disease in an HIV patient: value of renal biopsy and review of the literature. *Clin Nephrol*. 2011 Jan;75(1):80–88.
226. Tebas P. Insulin resistance and diabetes mellitus associated with antiretroviral use in HIV-infected patients: pathogenesis, prevention, and treatment options. *J Acquir Immune Defic Syndr*. 2008 Sep 1;49 Suppl 2:S86–S92.
227. Rachakonda AK, Kimmel PL. CKD in HIV-infected patients other than HIV-associated nephropathy. *Adv Chronic Kidney Dis*. 2010 Jan;17(1):83–93.
228. Hadziyannis SJ. Milestones and perspectives in viral hepatitis B. *Liver Int*. 2011 Jan;31 Suppl 1:129–134.
229. Lok AS, McMahon BJ. Chronic hepatitis B: update 2009. *Hepatology*. 2009;50(3):661–662.
230. Kim WR. Epidemiology of hepatitis B in the United States. *Hepatology*. 2009 May;49(5 Suppl):S28–34.
231. Heathcote EJ. Demography and presentation of chronic hepatitis B virus infection. *Am J Med*. 2008 Dec;121(12 Suppl):S3–11.

232. Chang KM. Hepatitis B immunology for clinicians. *Clin Liver Dis.* 2010 Aug;14(3):409–424.
233. Combes B, Stastny P, Shorey J, et al. Glomerulonephritis with deposition of Australia antigen antibody complexes in glomerular basement membrane. *Lancet.* 1971;2(7718):234–236.
234. Johnson RJ, Couser WG. Hepatitis B infection and renal disease: clinical, immunopathogenetic and therapeutic considerations. *Kidney Int.* 1990; 37(2):663.
235. Furuse A, Hattori S, Terashima T, et al. Circulating immune complex in glomerulopathy associated with hepatitis B virus infection. *Nephron.* 1982;31(3): 212–218.
236. Morzycka M, Slusarczyk J. Kidney glomerular pathology in various forms of acute and chronic hepatitis. *Arch Pathol Lab Med.* 1979 Jan;103(1):38–41.
237. Zeng CH, Chen HM, Wang RS, et al. Etiology and clinical characteristics of membranous nephropathy in Chinese patients. *Am J Kidney Dis.* 2008;52(4):691–698.
238. Park MH, Song EY, Ahn C, et al. Two subtypes of hepatitis B virus-associated glomerulonephritis are associated with different HLA-DR2 alleles in Koreans. *Tissue Antigens.* 2003 Dec;62(6):505–511.
239. Takekoshi Y, Tochimaru H, Nagata Y, et al. Immunopathogenetic mechanisms of hepatitis B virus-related glomerulopathy. *Kidney Int.* 1991 Dec;35: S34–39.
240. Lai KN, Ho RT, Tam JS, et al. Detection of hepatitis B virus DNA and RNA in kidneys of HBV-related glomerulonephritis. *Kidney Int.* 1996;50(6): 1965–1977.
241. He XY, Fang LJ, Zhang YE, et al. In situ hybridization of hepatitis B DNA in hepatitis B-associated glomerulonephritis. *Pediatr Nephrol.* 1998 Feb;12(2):117–120.
242. Lai KN, Ho RT, Tam JS, et al. Detection of hepatitis B virus DNA and RNA in kidneys of HBV related glomerulonephritis. *Kidney Int.* 1996;50(6): 1965–1977.
243. Ren J, Wang L, Chen Z, et al. Gene expression profile of transgenic mouse kidney reveals pathogenesis of hepatitis B virus associated nephropathy. *J Med Virol.* 2006 May;78(5):551–560.
244. Deng CL, Song XW, Liang HJ, et al. Chronic hepatitis B serum promotes apoptotic damage in human renal tubular cells. *World J Gastroenterol.* 2006 Mar 21;12(11):1752–1756.
245. Kim SE, Park YH, Chung WY. Study on hepatitis B virus pre-S/S gene mutations of renal tissues in children with hepatitis B virus-associated membranous nephropathy. *Pediatr Nephrol.* 2006 Aug;21(8):1097–1103.
246. Zhang Y, Zhou JH, Wang HT. Podocyte depletion in children with hepatitis B virus associated membranous nephropathy. *Zhonghua Er Ke Za Zhi.* 2007;45(5):344–348.
247. Gilbert RD, Wiggelinkhuizen J. The clinical course of hepatitis B virus-associated nephropathy. *Pediatr Nephrol.* 1994 Feb;8(1):11–14.
248. Lai KN, Li PK, Lui SF, et al. Membranous nephropathy related to hepatitis B virus in adults. *N Engl J Med.* 1991;324(21):1457–1463.
249. Tang S, Lai FM, Lui YH, et al. Lamivudine in hepatitis B-associated membranous nephropathy. *Kidney Int.* 2005;68(4):1750–1758.
250. Ikee R, Ishioka K, Oka M, et al. Hepatitis B virus-related membranous nephropathy treated with entecavir. *Nephrology (Carlton).* 2010 Mar;15(2):266.
251. Khedmat H, Taheri S. Hepatitis B virus-associated nephropathy: an International Data Analysis. *Iran J Kidney Dis.* 2010 Apr;4(2):101–105.
252. Mesquita M, Lasser L, Langlet P. Long-term (7-year) treatment with lamivudine monotherapy in HBV-associated glomerulonephritis. *Clin. Nephrol.* 2008;70(1):69–71.
253. Izzedine H, Massard J, Poynard T, et al. Lamivudine and HBV-associated nephropathy. *Nephrol Dial Transplant.* 2006;21(3):828–829.
254. Fabrizi F, Dixit V, Martin P. Meta-analysis: anti-viral therapy of hepatitis B virus-associated glomerulonephritis. *Aliment Pharmacol Ther.* 2006;24(5): 781–788.
255. Poordad F, Chee GM. Viral resistance in hepatitis B: prevalence and management. *Curr Gastroenterol Rep.* 2010 Feb;12(1):62–69.
256. Ikee R, Ishioka K, Oka M, et al. Hepatitis B virus-related membranous nephropathy treated with entecavir. *Nephrology (Carlton).* 2010 Mar;15(2):266.
257. Sayarlioglu H, Erkoc R, Dogan E, et al. Mycophenolate mofetil use in hepatitis B associated-membranous and membranoproliferative glomerulonephritis induces viral replication. *Ann Pharmacother.* 2005;39(3):573.
258. Lai KN, Tam JS, Lin HJ, et al. The therapeutic dilemma of usage of corticosteroid in patients with membranous nephropathy and persistent hepatitis B surface antigenaemia. *Nephron.* 1990;54(1):12–17.
259. Sheen IS, Liaw YF, Lin SM, et al. Severe clinical rebound upon withdrawal of corticosteroid before interferon therapy: incidence and risk factors. *J Gastroenterol Hepatol.* 1996;11(2):143–147.
260. Zhang Y, Zhou JH, Yin XL, et al. Treatment of hepatitis B virus-associated glomerulonephritis: a meta-analysis. *World J Gastroenterol.* 2010;16(6):770–777.
261. di Belgiojoso GB, Ferrario F, Landriani N. Virus-related glomerular diseases: histological and clinical aspects. *J Nephrol.* 2002 Sep–Oct;15(5):469–479.
262. Oner A, Tinaztepe K, Demircin G. Hepatitis-B-associated glomerulonephritis in children. *Turk J Pediatr.* 1997 Apr–Jun;39(2):239–246.
263. Wen YK, Chen ML. Remission of hepatitis B virus-associated membranoproliferative glomerulonephritis in a cirrhotic patient after lamivudine therapy. *Clin Nephrol.* 2006 Mar;65(3):211–215.
264. Abbas NA, Pitt MA, Green AT, et al. Successful treatment of hepatitis B virus (HBV)-associated membranoproliferative glomerulonephritis (MPGN) with alpha interferon. *Nephrol Dial Transplant.* 1999 May;14(5):1272–1275.
265. Khaira A, Upadhyay BK, Sharma A, et al. Hepatitis B virus associated focal and segmental glomerular sclerosis: report of two cases and review of literature. *Clin Exp Nephrol.* 2009 Aug;13(4):373–377.
266. Wang NS, Wu ZL, Zhang YE, et al. Existence and significance of hepatitis B virus DNA in kidneys of IgA nephropathy. *World J Gastroenterol.* 2005 Feb 7;11(5):712–716.
267. Ozdamar SO, Gucer S, Tinaztepe K. Hepatitis-B virus associated nephropathies: a clinicopathological study in 14 children. *Pediatr Nephrol.* 2003 Jan;18(1):23–28.
268. Panomsak S, Lewsuwan S, Eiam-Ong S, et al. Hepatitis-B virus-associated nephropathies in adults: a clinical study in Thailand. *J Med Assoc Thai.* 2006 Aug;89 Suppl 2:S151–156.
269. Wang NS, Wu ZL, Zhang YE, et al. Existence and significance of hepatitis B virus DNA in kidneys of IgA nephropathy. *World J Gastroenterol.* 2005 Feb 7;11(5):712–716.
270. Cacoub P, Terrier B. Hepatitis B-related autoimmune manifestations. *Rheum Dis Clin North Am.* 2009 Feb;35(1):125–137.
271. Guillevin L, Mahr A, Callard P, et al. Hepatitis B virus-associated polyarteritis nodosa: clinical characteristics, outcome, and impact of treatment in 115 patients. *Medicine (Baltimore).* 2005 Sep;84(5):313–322.
272. Cacoub P, Saadoun D, Bourlière M, et al. Hepatitis B virus genotypes and extrahepatic manifestations. *J Hepatol.* 2005;43:764–770.
273. de Carvalho JF, Pereira RM, Shoenfeld Y. Systemic polyarteritis nodosa following hepatitis B vaccination. *Eur J Intern Med.* 2008 Dec;19(8):575–578.
274. Mason A. Role of viral replication in extrahepatic syndromes related to hepatitis B virus infection. *Minerva Gastroenterol Dietol.* 2006 Mar;52(1):53–66.
275. Guillevin L, Ronco P, Verroust P. Circulating immune complexes in systemic necrotizing vasculitis of the polyarteritis nodosa group. Comparison of HBV-related polyarteritis nodosa and Churg-Strauss angiitis. *J Autoimmun.* 1990;3:789–792.
276. Chen RT, Pless R, Destefano F. Epidemiology of autoimmune reactions induced by vaccination. *J Autoimmun.* 2001;16:309–318.
277. Maya R, Gershwin ME, Shoenfeld Y. Hepatitis B virus (HBV) and autoimmune disease. *Clin Rev Allergy Immunol.* 2008 Feb;34(1):85–102.
278. Ram M, Shoenfeld Y. Hepatitis B: infection, vaccination and autoimmunity. *Isr Med Assoc J.* 2008;10(1):61–64.
279. Guillevin L, Mahr A, Cohen P, et al. Short-term corticosteroids then lamivudine and plasma exchanges to treat hepatitis B virus-related polyarteritis nodosa. *Arthritis Rheum.* 2004;51(3):482–487.
280. Xu H, Sun L, Zhou LJ, et al. The effect of hepatitis B vaccination on the incidence of childhood HBV-associated nephritis. *Pediatr Nephrol.* 2003 Dec;18(12):1216–1219.
281. Bhimma R, Coovadia HM, Adhikari M, et al. The impact of the hepatitis B virus vaccine on the incidence of hepatitis B virus-associated membranous nephropathy. *Arch Pediatr Adolesc Med.* 2003 Oct;157(10):1025–1030.
282. Sharlala H, Adebajo A. Virus-induced vasculitis. *Curr Rheumatol Rep.* 2008 Dec;10(6):449–452.
283. Cossart Y. Parvovirus B19 finds a disease. *Lancet.* 1981 Oct 31;2(8253): 988–989.
284. Servant-Delmas A, Lefrère JJ, Morinet F, et al. Advances in human B19 erythrovirus biology. *J Virol.* 2010 Oct;84(19):9658–9665.
285. Kishore J, Kapoor A. Erythrovirus B19 infection in humans. *Indian J Med Res.* 2000 Nov;112:149–164.
286. van Elsacker-Niele AM, Kroes AC. Human parvovirus B19: relevance in internal medicine. *Neth J Med.* 1999 Jun;54(6):221–230.
287. Florea AV, Ionescu DN, Melhem MF. Parvovirus B19 infection in the immunocompromised host. *Arch Pathol Lab Med.* 2007 May;131(5):799–804.
288. Doyle S. The detection of parvoviruses. *Methods Mol Biol.* 2011;665: 213–231.
289. Anderson LJ, Tsou C, Parker RA, et al. Detection of antibodies and antigens of human parvovirus B19 by enzyme-linked immunosorbent assay. *J Clin Microbiol.* 1986;24(4):522–526.

290. Koch WC, Adler SP. Detection of human parvovirus B19 DNA by using the polymerase chain reaction. *J Clin Microbiol.* 1990;28(1):65–69.
291. Zerbini M, Gallinella G, Cricca M, et al. Diagnostic procedures in B19 infection. *Pathol Biol (Paris).* 2002 Jun;50(5):332–338.
292. Daly P, Corcoran A, Mahon BP, et al. High-sensitivity PCR detection of parvovirus B19 in plasma. *J Clin Microbiol.* 2002 Jun;40(6):1958–1962.
293. Waldman M, Kopp JB. Parvovirus B19 and the kidney. *Clin J Am Soc Nephrol.* 2007 Jul;2 Suppl 1:S47–56.
294. Mori Y, Yamashita H, Umeda Y, et al. Association of parvovirus B19 infection with acute glomerulonephritis in healthy adults: case report and review of the literature. *Clin Nephrol.* 2002;57(1):69–73.
295. Podymow T, Muhtadie L. Pregnancy-associated parvovirus B19 infection causing postinfectious glomerulonephritis. *Hypertens Pregnancy.* 2010;29(4): 429–433.
296. Abeygunasekara SC, Peat D, Ross CN. Endocapillary glomerulonephritis secondary to human parvovirus B19 presenting with nephrotic syndrome: a report of two cases and a review of the literature. *Ren Fail.* 2010;32(7):880–883.
297. Takeda S, Takaeda C, Takazakura E, et al. Renal involvement induced by human parvovirus B19 infection. *Nephron.* 2001 Nov;89(3):280–285.
298. Ieiri N, Hotta O, Taguma Y. Characteristics of acute glomerulonephritis associated with human parvovirus B19 infection. *Clin Nephrol.* 2005 Oct;64(4): 249–257.
299. Tolaymat A, Al Mousily F, MacWilliam K, et al. Parvovirus glomerulonephritis in a patient with sickle cell disease. *Pediatr Nephrol.* 1999 May;13(4): 340–342.
300. Wierenga KJ, Pattison JR, Brink N, et al. Glomerulonephritis after human parvovirus infection in homozygous sickle-cell disease. *Lancet.* 1995 Aug 19;346(8973):475–476.
301. Li Loong TC, Coyle PV, Anderson MJ, et al. Human parvovirus associated vasculitis. *Postgrad Med J.* 1986;62(728):493–494.
302. Gabriel SE, Espy M, Erdman DD. The role of parvovirus B19 in the pathogenesis of giant cell arteritis: a preliminary evaluation. *Arthritis Rheum.* 1999;42(6):1255–1258.
303. Schwarz TF, Bruns R, Schröder C, et al. Human parvovirus B19 infection associated with vascular purpura and vasculitis. *Infection.* 1989;17(3):170–171.
304. Crowson AN, Magro CM, Dawood MR. A causal role for parvovirus B19 infection in adult dermatomyositis and other autoimmune syndromes. *J Cutan Pathol.* 2000;27(10):505–515.
305. Ferguson P, Saulsbury FT, Dowell SF, et al. Prevalence of human parvovirus B19 infection in children with Henoch-Schönlein purpura. *Arthritis Rheum.* 1996;39(5):880–881.
306. Cioc AM, Sedmak DD, Nuovo GJ, et al. Parvovirus B19 associated adult Henoch Schönlein purpura. *J Cutaneous Pathol.* 2002;29(10):602–607.
307. Swaminathan S, Lager DJ, Qian X, et al. Collapsing and non-collapsing focal segmental glomerulosclerosis in kidney transplants. *Nephrol Dial Transplant.* 2006;21(9):2607–2614.
308. Tanawattanacharoen S, Falk RJ, Jennette JC, et al. Parvovirus B19 DNA in kidney tissue of patients with focal segmental glomerulosclerosis. *Am J Kidney Dis.* 2000;35(6):1166–1174.
309. Moudgil A, Nast CC, Bagga A, et al. Association of parvovirus B19 infection with idiopathic collapsing glomerulopathy. *Kidney Int.* 2001;59(6): 2126–2133.
310. Schwimmer JA, Markowitz GS, Valeri A, et al. Collapsing glomerulopathy. *Semin Nephrol.* 2003 Mar;23(2):209–218.
311. Quek L, Sharpe C, Dutt N, et al. Acute human parvovirus B19 infection and nephrotic syndrome in patients with sickle cell disease. *Br J Haematol.* 2010 Apr;149(2):289–291.
312. Beckhoff A, Steffen I, Sandoz P, et al. Relapsing severe anaemia due to primary parvovirus B19 infection after renal transplantation: a case report and review of the literature. *Nephrol Dial Transplant.* 2007;22(12):3660–3663.
313. Ki CS, Kim IS, Kim JW, et al. Incidence and clinical significance of human parvovirus B19 infection in kidney transplant recipients. *Clin Transplant.* 2005;19(6):751–755.
314. Murer L, Zacchello G, Bianchi D, et al. Thrombotic microangiopathy associated with parvovirus B19 infection after renal transplantation. *J Am Soc Nephrol.* 2000;11(6):1132–1137.
315. Ardalan MR, Shoja MM, Tubbs RS, et al. Parvovirus B19 microepidemic in renal transplant recipients with thrombotic microangiopathy and allograft vasculitis. *Exp Clin Transplant.* 2008 Jun;6(2):137–143.
316. Barzon L, Murer L, Pacenti M, et al. Investigation of intrarenal viral infections in kidney transplant recipients unveils an association between parvovirus B19 and chronic allograft injury. *J Infect Dis.* 2009 Feb 1;199(3):372–380.
317. Helanterä I, Egli A, Koskinen P, et al. Viral impact on long-term kidney graft function. *Infect Dis Clin North Am.* 2010;24(2):339–371.
318. Servant-Delmas A, Lefrère JJ, Morinet F, et al. Advances in human B19 erythrovirus biology. *J Virol.* 2010 Oct;84(19):9658–9665.
319. Brown KE, Anderson SM, Young NS. Erythrocyte P antigen: cellular receptor for B19 parvovirus. *Science.* 1993 Oct 1;262(5130):114–117.
320. Wan Z, Zhi N, Wong S, et al. Human parvovirus B19 causes cell cycle arrest of human erythroid progenitors via deregulation of the E2F family of transcription factors. *J Clin Invest.* 2010 Oct 1;120(10):3530–3544.
321. Lindner J, Barabas S, Saar K, et al. CD4(1) T-cell responses against the VP1-unique region in individuals with recent and persistent parvovirus B19 infection. *J Vet Med B Infect Dis Vet Public Health.* 2005;52(7–8):356–361.
322. Norbeck O, Isa A, Pöhlmann C, et al. Sustained CD81 T-cell responses induced after acute parvovirus B19 infection in humans. *J Virol.* 2005;79(18): 12117–12121.
323. Corcoran A, Doyle S. Advances in the biology, diagnosis and host-pathogen interactions of parvovirus B19. *J Med Microbiol.* 2004 Jun;53(Pt 6):459–475.
324. Jordan SC, Toyoda M, Kahwaji J, et al. Clinical aspects of intravenous immunoglobulin use in solid organ transplant recipients. *Am J Transplant.* 2011 Feb;11(2):196–202.
325. Waldman M, Kopp JB. Parvovirus-B19-associated complications in renal transplant recipients. *Nat Clin Pract Nephrol.* 2007 Oct;3(10):540–550.
326. Gandhi MK, Khanna R. Human cytomegalovirus: clinical aspects, immune regulation, and emerging treatments. *Lancet Infect Dis.* 2004;4(12):725–738.
327. Cohen JI, Corey GR. Cytomegalovirus infection in the normal host. *Medicine (Baltimore).* 1985;64(2):100–114.
328. Gandhi MK, Khanna R. Human cytomegalovirus: clinical aspects, immune regulation, and emerging treatments. *Lancet Infect Dis.* 2004;4(12):725–738.
329. Battegay EJ, Mihatsch MJ, Mazzucchelli L, et al. Cytomegalovirus and kidney. *Clin Nephrol.* 1988 Nov;30(5):239–247.
330. Georgaki-Angelaki H, Lycopoulou L, Stergiou N, et al. Membranous nephritis associated with acquired cytomegalovirus infection in a 19-month-old baby. *Pediatr Nephrol.* 2009 Jan;24(1):203–206.
331. Beneck D, Greco MA, Feiner HD. Glomerulonephritis in congenital cytomegalic inclusion disease. *Hum Pathol.* 1986 Oct;17(10):1054–1059.
332. Murakami H, Takahashi S, Kawakubo Y, et al. Adolescent with Henoch-Schönlein purpura glomerulonephritis and intracranial hemorrhage possibly secondary to the reactivation of latent CMV. *Pediatr Int.* 2008 Feb;50(1): 112–115.
333. Park JS, Song JH, Yang WS, et al. Cytomegalovirus is not specifically associated with immunoglobulin A nephropathy. *J Am Soc Nephrol.* 1994 Feb;4(8):1623–1626.
334. Kramer J, Hennig H, Lensing C, et al. Multi-organ affecting CMV-associated cryoglobulinemic vasculitis. *Clin Nephrol.* 2006 Oct;66(4):284–290.
335. Lidar M, Lipschitz N, Langevitz P, et al. The infectious etiology of vasculitis. *Autoimmunity.* 2009 Aug;42(5):432–438.
336. Tomlinson L, Boriskin Y, McPhee I, et al. Acute cytomegalovirus infection complicated by collapsing glomerulopathy. *Nephrol Dial Transplant.* 2003 Jan;18(1):187–189.
337. Razonable RR, Eid AJ. Viral infections in transplant recipients. *Minerva Med.* 2009 Dec;100(6):479–501.
338. Toupance O, Bouedjoro-Camus MC, Carquin J, et al. Cytomegalovirus-related disease and risk of acute rejection in renal transplant recipients: A cohort study with case control analyses. *Transpl Int.* 2000;13(6):413–419.
339. Reischig T. Cytomegalovirus-associated renal allograft rejection: new challenges for antiviral preventive strategies. *Expert Rev Anti Infect Ther.* 2010 Aug;8(8):903–910.
340. van de Berg PJ, Heutinck KM, Raabe R, et al. Human cytomegalovirus induces systemic immune activation characterized by a type 1 cytokine signature. *J Infect Dis.* 2010 Sep 1;202(5):690–699.
341. Browne G, Whitworth C, Bellamy C, et al. Acute allograft glomerulopathy associated with CMV viraemia. *Nephrol Dial Transplant.* 2001 Apr;16(4): 861–862.
342. Richardson WP, Colvin RB, Cheeseman SH, et al. Glomerulopathy associated with cytomegalovirus viremia in renal allografts. *N Engl J Med.* 1981;305(2): 57–63.
343. Birk PE, Chavers BM. Does cytomegalovirus cause glomerular injury in renal allograft recipients? *J Am Soc Nephrol.* 1997 Nov;8(11):1801–1808.
344. Onuigbo M, Haririan A, Ramos E, et al. Cytomegalovirus-induced glomerular vasculopathy in renal allografts: A report of two cases. *Am J Transplant.* 2002;2(7):684–688.
345. Luo X, Rajagopal A, Ison M, et al. Two rare forms of renal allograft glomerulopathy during cytomegalovirus infection and treatment. *Am J Kidney Dis.* 2008 Jun;51(6):1047–1051.
346. Kashyap R, Shapiro R, Jordan M, et al. The clinical significance of cytomegaloviral inclusions in the allograft kidney. *Transplantation.* 1999;67(1):98–103.

347. Browne G, Whitworth C, Bellamy C, et al. Acute allograft glomerulopathy associated with CMV viraemia. *Nephrol Dial Transplant.* 2001;16(4):861–862.
348. Wei SH, Ho MC, Ni YH, et al. Cytomegalovirus-associated immune thrombocytopenic purpura after liver transplantation. *J Formos Med Assoc.* 2007 Apr;106(4):327–329.
349. Waiser J, Budde K, Rudolph B, et al. De novo hemolytic uremic syndrome postrenal transplant after cytomegalovirus infection. *Am J Kidney Dis.* 1999 Sep;34(3):556–559.
350. Rao KV, Hafner GP, Crary GS, et al. De novo immunotactoid glomerulopathy of the renal allograft: possible association with cytomegalovirus infection. *Am J Kidney Dis.* 1994;24(1):97–103.
351. Britt W. Virus entry into host, establishment of infection, spread in host, mechanisms of tissue damage. In: Arvin A, Campadelli-Fiume G, Mocarski E, eds. *Human Herpesviruses: Biology, Therapy, and Immunoprophylaxis.* Cambridge, United Kingdom: Cambridge University Press; 2007.
352. Sinzger C, Digel M, Jahn G. Cytomegalovirus cell tropism. *Curr Top Microbiol Immunol.* 2008;325:63–83.
353. Wreghitt TG, Teare EL, Sule O, et al. Cytomegalovirus infection in immunocompetent patients. *Clin Infect Dis.* 2003;37(12):1603–1606.
354. Boeckh M, Huang M, Ferrenberg J, et al. Optimization of quantitative detection of cytomegalovirus DNA in plasma by real-time PCR. *J Clin Microbiol.* 2004 Mar; 42(3):1142–1148.
355. Drew WL. Laboratory diagnosis of cytomegalovirus infection and disease in immunocompromised patients. *Curr Opin Infect Dis.* 2007 Aug; 20(4):408–411.
356. Mosca F, Pugni L. Cytomegalovirus infection: the state of the art. *J Chemother.* 2007 Oct;19 Suppl 2:46–48.
357. Ortmanns A, Ittel TH, Schnitzler N, et al. Remission of IgA nephropathy following treatment of cytomegalovirus infection with ganciclovir. *Clin Nephrol.*1998 Jun;49(6):379–384.
358. Kotton CN. Medscape. Management of cytomegalovirus infection in solid organ transplantation. *Nat Rev Nephrol.* 2010 Dec;6(12):711–721.
359. Schmaljohn CS, Hjelle B. Hantavirus: a global disease problem. *Emerg Infect Dis.* 1997;3(2):95–104.
360. Hjelle B, Jenison SA, Goade DE, et al. Hantaviruses: Clinical, microbiologic, and epidemiologic aspects. *Crit Rev Lab Sci.* 1995;32(5–6):469–508.
361. Krautkrämer E, Zeier M. Hantavirus causing hemorrhagic fever with renal syndrome enters from the apical surface and requires decay-accelerating factor (DAF/CD55). *J Virol.* 2008 May;82(9):4257–4264.
362. Heiske A, Anheier B, Pilaski J, et al. Polymerase chain reaction detection of Puumala virus RNA in formaldehyde-fixed biopsy material. *Kidney Int.* 1999 May;55(5):2062–2069.
363. Ferluga D, Vizjak A. Hantavirus nephropathy. *J Am Soc Nephrol.* 2008 Sep;19(9):1653–1658.
364. Peters CJ, Simpson GL, Levy H. Spectrum of hantavirus infection: hemorrhagic fever with renal syndrome and hantavirus pulmonary syndrome. *Annu Rev Med.* 1999;50:531–545.
365. Song JW, Song KJ, Baek LJ, et al. In vivo characterization of the integrin beta3 as a receptor for Hantaan virus cellular entry. *Exp Mol Med.* 2005 Apr 30; 37(2):121–127.
366. Markotić A. Immunopathogenesis of hemorrhagic fever with renal syndrome and hantavirus pulmonary syndrome. *Acta Med Croatica.* 2003;57(5):407–414.
367. Mustonen J, Partanen J, Kanerva M, et al. Genetic susceptibility to severe course of nephropathia epidemica caused by Puumala hantavirus. *Kidney Int.* 1996;49(1):217–221.
368. Clement J, Maes P, Van Ranst M. Acute kidney injury in emerging, nontropical infections. *Acta Clin Belg.* 2007 Nov–Dec;62(6):387–395.
369. Kim YK, Lee SC, Kim C, et al. Clinical and laboratory predictors of oliguric renal failure in haemorrhagic fever with renal syndrome caused by Hantaan virus. *J Infect.* 2007 Apr;54(4):381–386.
370. Muranyi W, Bahr U, Zeier M, et al. Hantavirus infection. *J Am Soc Nephrol.* 2005;16(12):3669–3679.
371. Settergren B. Clinical aspects of nephropathia epidemica (Puumala virus infection) in Europe: a review. *Scand J Infect Dis.* 2000;32(2):125–132.
372. Matthaeus T, Fries J, Weber M, et al. [Glomerular-type proteinuria in hantavirus nephritis]. *Med Klin (Munich).* 2004;99(5):223–227.
373. Ala-Houhala I, Koskinen M, Ahola T, et al. Increased glomerular permeability in patients with nephropathia epidemica caused by Puumala hantavirus. *Nephrol Dial Transplant.* 2002 Feb;17(2):246–252.
374. Mustonen J, Mäkelä S, Helin H, et al. Mesangiocapillary glomerulonephritis caused by Puumala hantavirus infection. *Nephron.* 2001 Dec;89(4):402–407.
375. Dara SI, Albright RC, Peters SG. Acute sin nombre hantavirus infection complicated by renal failure requiring hemodialysis. *Mayo Clin Proc.* 2005;80(5): 703–704.
376. Rippe B. Is there an increased long-term risk of hypertension and renal impairment after Puumala virus-induced nephropathy? *Kidney Int.* 2006 Jun;69(11):1930–1931.
377. Pergam SA, Schmidt DW, Nofchissey RA, et al. Potential renal sequelae in survivors of hantavirus cardiopulmonary syndrome. *Am J Trop Med Hyg.* 2009 Feb;80(2):279–285.
378. Braun N, Haap M, Overkamp D, et al. Characterization and outcome following Puumala virus infection: a retrospective analysis of 75 cases. *Nephrol Dial Transplant.* 2010 Sep;25(9):2997–3003.
379. Miettinen MH, Mäkelä SM, Ala-Houhala IO, et al. Ten-year prognosis of Puumala hantavirus-induced acute interstitial nephritis. *Kidney Int.* 2006 Jun;69(11):2043–2048.
380. Cheema SR, Arif F, Charney D, et al. IgA-dominant glomerulonephritis associated with hepatitis A. *Clin Nephrol.* 2004 Aug;62(2):138–143.
381. Han SH, Kang EW, Kie JH, et al. Spontaneous remission of IgA nephropathy associated with resolution of hepatitis A. *Am J Kidney Dis.* 2010 Dec;56(6): 1163–1167.
382. Pasch A, Frey FJ. Coxsackie B viruses and the kidney—a neglected topic. *Nephrol Dial Transplant.* 2006 May;21(5):1184–1187.
383. Conaldi PG, Biancone L, Bottelli A, et al. Distinct pathogenic effects of group B coxsackieviruses on human glomerular and tubular kidney cells. *J Virol.* 1997;71(12):9180–9187.
384. Aronson MD, Phillips CA. Coxsackievirus B5 infections in acute oliguric renal failure. *J Infect Dis.* 1975;132(3):303–306.
385. Page Y, Serrange C, Revillard JP, et al. [Letter: Coxsackie B virus infections in kidney transplantation]. *Nouv Presse Med.* 1976;5(25):1587–1588.
386. Aronson MD, Phillips CA. Coxsackievirus B5 infections in acute oliguric renal failure. *J Infect Dis.* 1975;132(3):303–306.
387. Isome M, Yoshida K, Suzuki S, et al. Experimental glomerulonephritis following successive inoculation of five different serotypes of group B coxsackieviruses in mice. *Nephron.* 1997;77(1):93–99.
388. Yoshida K, Suzuki J, Suzuki S, et al. Experimental IgA nephropathy induced by coxsackie B4 virus in mice. *Am J Nephrol.* 1997;17(1):81–88.
389. Kawasaki Y, Mitsuaki H, Isome M, et al. Renal effects of coxsackie B4 virus in hyper-IgA mice. *J Am Soc Nephrol.* 2006 Oct;17(10):2760–2769.

CHAPTER

48 Vasculitic Diseases of the Kidney

Julieanne G. McGregor • Patrick H. Nachman •
J. Charles Jennette • Ronald J. Falk

The field of vasculitis has been one of continuous advancements in knowledge for the past quarter of a century. Evolving understanding of the pathogenesis of these disorders, including the role of antineutrophil cytoplasmic antibodies (ANCA) and exogenous and host factors that prime an individual for onset of disease or relapse, have led to improved treatment strategies. This chapter reflects our current understanding of large-, medium-, and small-vessel vasculitis.

EPIDEMIOLOGY OF VASCULITIS

The incidence of vasculitis has been difficult to determine, largely because of an inconsistent classification strategy. The advent of the Chapel Hill Nomenclature System allowed for a more precise estimation of incidence and prevalence. The incidence of giant cell arteritis varies from 15 to 30 per million in individuals older than 50 years. There is an increased incidence with age and a female-to-male ratio of 2:1.[1] Giant cell arteritis is more common in Caucasians and is uncommon in African Americans. Takayasu arteritis has been described worldwide, but the disease is much more prevalent in Japan, where there are approximately 150 new cases per year. In Olmstead County, Minnesota, the incidence is 2.6 cases per mission per year.

The incidence of vasculitis associated with ANCA appears to be on the order of 10 to 20 cases per million.[1] In contrast, polyarteritis nodosa has become a rare disease. It is possible that the perceived increase in the incidence of microscopic polyangiitis (MPA) is a consequence of the development and widespread use of ANCA testing. Nonetheless, the incidence of MPA appears to have been more common in the 1990s than in the 1980s (19.8 versus 7 cases per million). Two interesting studies reported a much higher incidence of ANCA vasculitis. One study reported a much higher incidence in Alaskan Indians in which all cases were associated with hepatitis B.[2] The other report from Kuwait after the Gulf War found an increased incidence of 16 cases per million of polyarteritis nodosa and 24 cases per million of MPA.[3] The incidence of GPA was 0.7 per million per year from 1980 to 1986, increasing to 2.8 per million per year from 1987 to 1989. There was an increase in the annual prevalence from 28.8 per million in 1990 to 64.8 per million in 2005 in a primary care population.[4] In the 1990s the prevalence of granulomatosis with polyangiitis (GPA), formerly known as Wegener granulomatosis, was closer to 10.6 cases per million in the United Kingdom. The annual incidence of eosinophilic granulomatosis (EGPA) ranges between 0.5 and 6.8 cases per million.[5] The prevalence of polyarteritis nodosa (PAN), MPA, GPA, and EGPA in a large multiethnic suburb of Paris based on a three-source capture-recapture method during the calendar year 2000 was estimated per 1,000,000 adults to be 30 for PAN, 25 for MPA, 24 for GPA, and 11 for EGPA. The overall prevalence was 2.0 times higher for subjects of European ancestry than for non-Europeans (P = .01).[6]

DIAGNOSTIC CLASSIFICATION AND PATHOLOGY OF VASCULITIDES

ANCA vasculitis can affect any vessel in the body and thus can cause various clinical signs and symptoms. Most of these manifestations are indicative of vessel involvement in a particular organ rather than a specific pathologic category of disease. Therefore, ANCA vasculitis cannot be accurately diagnosed on the basis of clinical features alone. Serologic and other laboratory data can be very helpful in narrowing the differential diagnosis or providing additional support to a presumptive diagnosis, but data are rarely definitive. As with all tissues, vessels have a limited number of nonspecific patterns of response to injury. For example, many different inflammatory stimuli cause histologically indistinguishable acute and chronic inflammation with and without necrotizing or granulomatous features. To further complicate pathologic evaluation, vasculitic lesions evolve through various stages of active (Fig. 48.1) and sclerosing injury (Fig. 48.2). Specific categories of vasculitis have a particular predilection for involvement of certain types of vessels, although there is so much overlap that type of vessel involvement alone does not provide adequate categorization (Table 48.1, Fig. 48.3). Therefore, vasculitis cannot be diagnosed accurately on

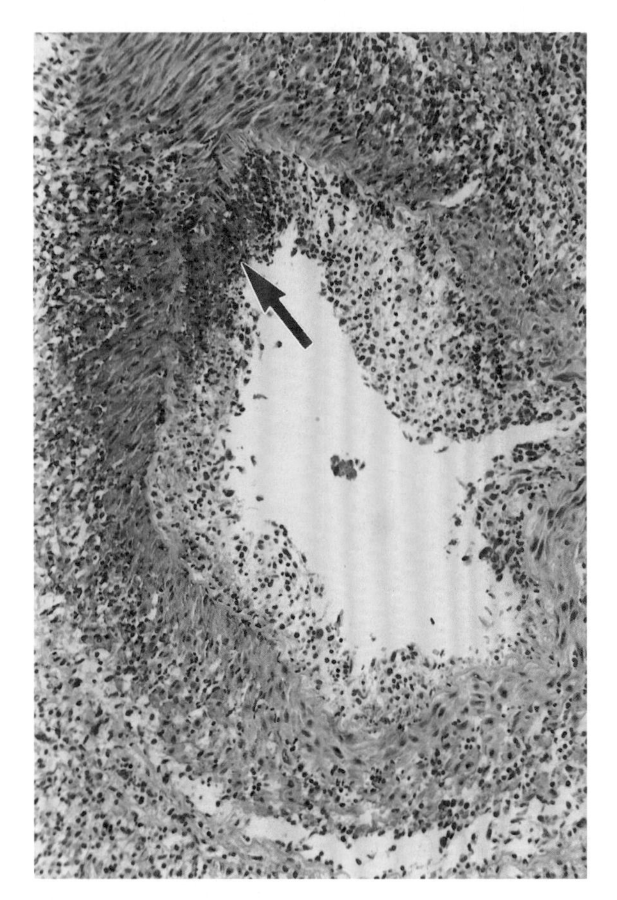

FIGURE 48.1 Acute necrotizing arteritis affecting a renal interlobar artery in a patient with Kawasaki disease. There is (*arrow*) transmural inflammation and necrosis. (Hematoxylin and eosin stain, magnification ×125.)

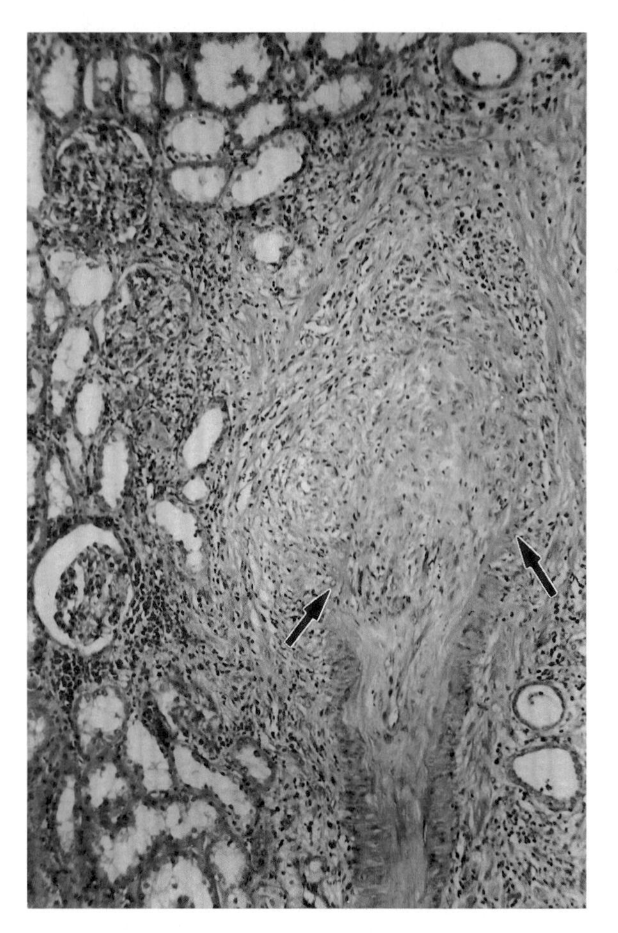

FIGURE 48.2 Chronic scarring in an arcuate artery from a patient with polyarteritis nodosa. The muscularis is completely destroyed (*arrows*), indicating that the sclerosis is secondary to a necrotizing arteritis rather than severe arteriosclerosis. (Hematoxylin and eosin stain, magnification ×75.)

the basis of pathologic features alone, especially if these are evaluated only by routine light microscopy. Recently, a pathologic classification system for ANCA vasculitis has been validated for prognostication of renal outcomes based on renal biopsy,[7] but the best approach to a specific diagnosis continues to be a combination of clinical, laboratory, and histologic data to identify distinctive clinicopathologic categories of vasculitis. Vasculitis categorization schemes will continue to be improved in the future; however, current systems provide valuable guidance for prognostication and for determining the most effective management strategy.

There are a number of approaches to the categorization of vasculitis. The system used in this chapter is a proposed modification of the Chapel Hill Nomenclature System, a system agreed upon by an international group of clinicians and pathologists with a special interest in vasculitis (Table 48.2).[8] There is a new nomenclature pending publication that recognizes a more specific categorization of vasculitides and abolishes eponyms.

Knowledge of the historical evolution of vasculitis categorization is helpful to understand the current diagnostic criteria for the classification of vasculitides. The following discussion of diagnostic classification includes a brief review of the historical events in the recognition of each category. The discussion is divided into sections discussing large-vessel vasculitis, medium-sized vessel vasculitis, and small-vessel vasculitis (Tables 48.1, Figs. 48.2 and 48.3). Large-vessel vasculitides were first recognized because of the reduced pulses and ischemic manifestations caused by chronic narrowing of major arteries. Medium-sized vessel vasculitides were first recognized because of the pseudoaneurysms caused by necrotizing lesions of medium-sized arteries, and small-vessel vasculitides were first recognized because of the glomerulonephritis and purpura caused by involvement of glomerular capillaries and dermal venules, respectively. Much of the discussion focuses on small-vessel vasculitides because these cause a higher frequency of renal disease.

TAKAYASU ARTERITIS AND GIANT CELL (TEMPORAL) ARTERITIS

Large-vessel vasculitis affects the aorta and its major branches, such as the arteries to the extremities and to the head and neck.[8] During the acute phase of disease, large-vessel vasculitis is characterized pathologically by inflammation that often

TABLE 48.1 **Major Diagnostic Categories of Vasculitis**

Large-vessel vasculitis (chronic granulomatous arteritis)
Giant cell arteritis
Takayasu arteritis
Medium-sized vessel vasculitis (necrotizing arteritis)
Polyarteritis nodosa
Kawasaki disease
Small-vessel vasculitis (necrotizing polyangiitis)
Pauci-immune small-vessel vasculitis (usually antineutrophil cytoplasmic antibody [ANCA] positive)
Microscopic polyangiitis
Granulomatosis with polyangiitis
Eosinophilic granulomatosis
Drug-induced ANCA vasculitis
Immune complex small-vessel vasculitis
Henoch-Schönlein purpura
Cryoglobulinemic vasculitis
Lupus vasculitis
Rheumatoid vasculitis
Goodpasture syndrome
Serum sickness vasculitis
Hypocomplementemic urticarial vasculitis
Drug-induced immune complex vasculitis
Infection-induced immune complex vasculitis
Behçet disease
Paraneoplastic small-vessel vasculitis
Lymphoproliferative neoplasm-induced vasculitis
Carcinoma-induced vasculitis
Myeloproliferative neoplasm-induced vasculitis
Inflammatory bowel disease vasculitis

contains giant cells in the inflammatory infiltrates during the active phase of disease. The chronic phase is characterized by extensive vascular sclerosis with little or no active inflammation. Inflammatory and sclerotic thickening of the aorta and the arteries causes narrowing of lumina, which in turn causes ischemia and the resultant clinical manifestations. Involvement of the renal artery may cause renovascular hypertension. The two major categories of large-vessel vasculitis are Takayasu arteritis and giant cell arteritis.

In 1856, William Savory described patients with diminished peripheral pulses who probably had Takayasu arteritis involving the major arteries to the extremities.[9] However, this category of vasculitis is named for Mikito Takayasu, a Japanese ophthalmologist who reported the ocular ischemic effects of this chronic granulomatous arteritis in 1908.[10] Takayasu arteritis, which also includes "aortic arch syndrome" and "pulseless disease," most often involves the aorta and its major branches, although the pulmonary arteries may be affected.[11] Takayasu arteritis is most common in Asia, although it occurs worldwide. It rarely occurs in patients older than 40 years and is usually diagnosed during the second decade of life. Clinically, it often presents with reduced pulses, vascular bruits, claudication, and renovascular hypertension.

Giant cell arteritis rarely occurs in patients younger than 50 years and is most common in patients of northern European ethnicity.[12] Like Takayasu arteritis, giant cell arteritis affects the aorta and its major branches; however, it has a much greater predilection for the extracranial branches of the carotid artery. Frequent clinical manifestations include headache, jaw claudication, blindness, deafness, tongue dysfunction, extremity claudication, and reduced peripheral pulses. Pathologic involvement of the renal artery is common in giant cell arteritis, but symptomatic renovascular hypertension is rare. This is in contradistinction to Takayasu arteritis, which often causes renovascular hypertension.

Giant cell arteritis has also been called "temporal arteritis," partly because one of the earliest descriptions of this type of vasculitis in 1890 by Hutchinson emphasized temporal artery involvement.[13] However, the term "giant cell arteritis" is more appropriate than "temporal arteritis" because (1) not all patients with giant cell arteritis have temporal artery involvement and (2) vasculitides other than giant cell arteritis can cause temporal artery inflammation, such as polyarteritis nodosa, granulomatosis with polyangiitis, and microscopic polyangiitis.[8] If a patient with clinical manifestations of temporal artery inflammation is found by temporal artery biopsy to have a necrotizing rather than a granulomatous arteritis, the differential diagnosis should include polyarteritis nodosa, MPA, GPA, and other forms of necrotizing vasculitis. The frequent association of polymyalgia rheumatica with giant cell arteritis is a useful diagnostic aid, although not all patients with giant cell arteritis have polymyalgia rheumatica and not all patients with polymyalgia rheumatica have giant cell arteritis.

Takayasu arteritis and giant cell arteritis cannot be accurately distinguished on the basis of pathologic evaluation of involved arteries. Polymyalgia rheumatica and involvement of branches of the carotid artery are more in favor of giant cell arteritis, and preferential involvement of the aorta and arteries to the extremities is slightly in favor of Takayasu arteritis. However, the best diagnostic discriminator is age. If a patient with clinical or pathologic features of chronic granulomatous arteritis is older than 50 years, a diagnosis of giant cell arteritis is warranted, whereas a diagnosis of Takayasu arteritis is warranted if the patient is younger than 50 years.[8] The presence of renovascular hypertension in a child or a young adult is suggestive of Takayasu arteritis. In a patient older than 50 years, renal artery involvement by a chronic sclerosing process is more likely secondary to atherosclerosis than to giant cell arteritis, and Takayasu arteritis is essentially ruled out by the age of the patient.

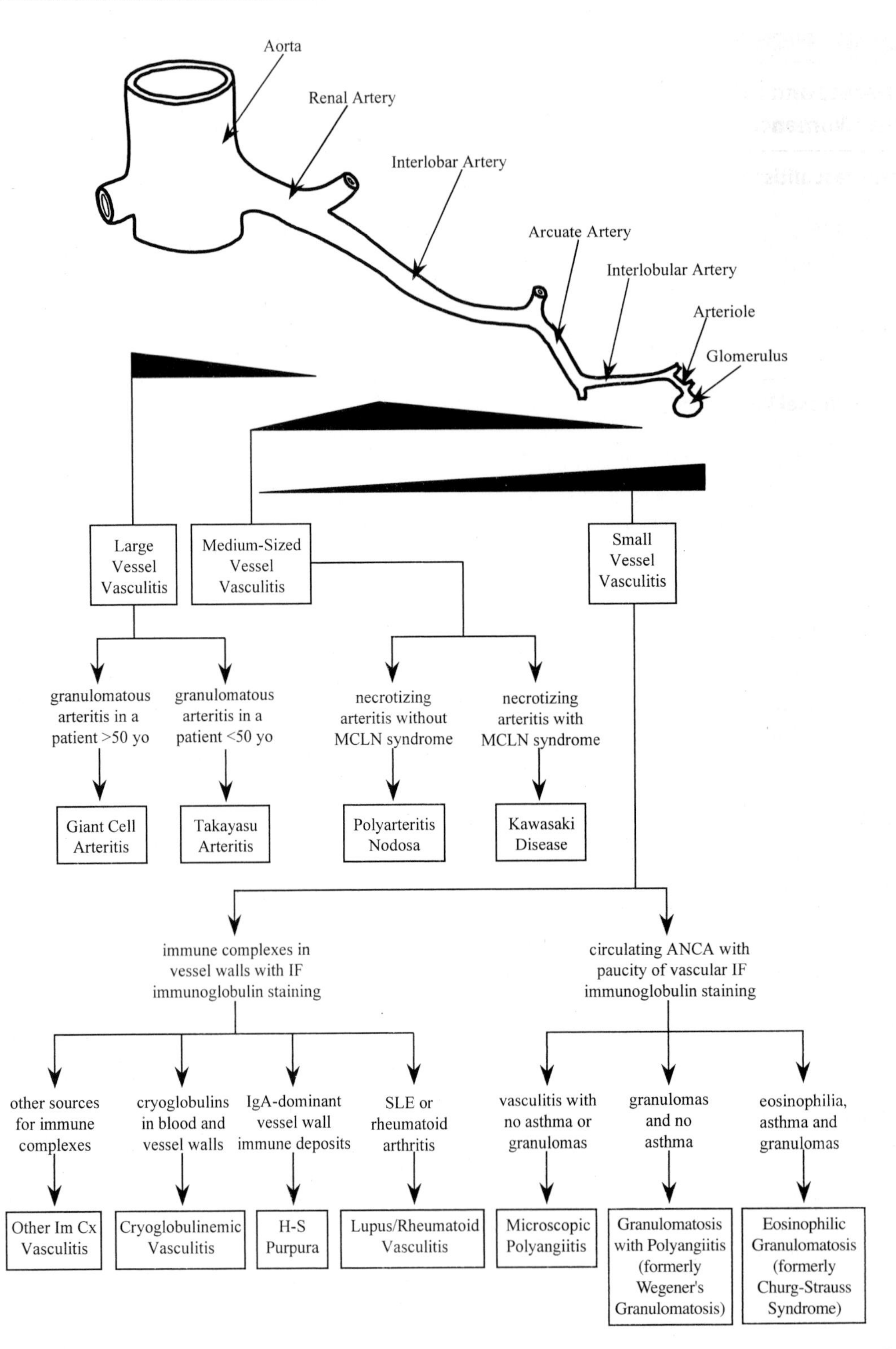

FIGURE 48.3 Predominant vascular involvement by large-vessel vasculitides, medium-sized vessel vasculitides, and small-vessel vasculitides as indicated by the positions and heights of the solid triangles. The algorithm suggests clinical and pathologic features that discriminate among different diagnostic categories of vasculitis. *yo*, years old; *MCLN*, mucocutaneous lymph node syndrome; *IF*, immunofluorescence microscopy; *ANCA*, antineutrophil cytoplasmic autoantibodies; *Im Cx*, immune complex; *SLE*, systemic lupus erythematosus; *H-S*, Henoch-Schönlein. (From Jennette JC, Falk RJ. Renal involvement in systemic vasculitis. In: Greenberg A, Cheung AK, Coffman TM, et al., eds. *National Kidney Foundation Nephrology Primer,* 2nd ed. San Diego, CA: Academic Press; 1998:200, with permission.)

TABLE 48.2 **Names and Definitions of Vasculitis Adopted by the Chapel Hill Consensus Conference on the Nomenclature of Systemic Vasculitis**

Large-vessel Vasculitis[a]	
Giant cell arteritis	Granulomatous arteritis of the aorta and its major branches, with a predilection for the extracranial branches of the carotid artery. Often involves the *temporal artery. Usually* occurs in patients older than 50 years and often is associated with *polymyalgia rheumatica.*
Takayasu arteritis	Granulomatous inflammation of the aorta and its major branches. Usually occurs in patients younger than 50 years.
Medium-sized Vessel Vasculitis[a]	
Polyarteritis nodosa	Necrotizing inflammation of medium-sized or small arteries without glomerulonephritis or vasculitis in arterioles, capillaries, or venules.
Kawasaki disease	Arteritis involving large, medium-sized, and small arteries, and associated with mucocutaneous lymph node syndrome. *Coronary arteries are often involved.* Aorta and veins may be involved. Usually occurs in children.
Small-vessel Vasculitis[a]	
Granulomatosis with polyangiitis[b] (formerly Wegener granulomatosis[c])	Granulomatous inflammation involving the respiratory tract, and necrotizing vasculitis affecting small-to medium-sized vessels, for example, capillaries, venules, arterioles, and arteries. Necrotizing glomerulonephritis is common.
Eosinophilic granulomatosis[c]	Eosinophil-rich and granulomatous inflammation involving respiratory tract and necrotizing vasculitis affecting small-to medium-sized vessels, and associated with asthma and blood eosinophilia.
Microscopic polyangiitis[c]	Necrotizing vasculitis with few or no immune deposits affecting small vessels, for example, capillaries, venules, or arterioles. Necrotizing arteritis involving small- and medium-sized arteries may be present. Necrotizing glomerulonephritis is very common. Pulmonary capillarities often occur.
Henoch-Schönlein purpura	Vasculitis with IgA-dominant immune deposits affecting small vessels, for example, capillaries, venules, or arterioles. Typically involves skin, gut, and glomeruli and is associated *with arthralgias or arthritis.*
Cryoglobulinemic vasculitis	Vasculitis with cryoglobulin immune deposits affecting small vessels, for example, capillaries, venules, or arterioles, and associated with cryoglobulins in serum. *Skin and glomeruli are often involved.*
Cutaneous leukocytoclastic angiitis	Isolated cutaneous leukocytoclastic angiitis without systemic vasculitis or glomerulonephritis.

[a]"Large artery" refers to the aorta and the largest branches directed toward major body regions (e.g., to the extremities and the head and neck); "medium-sized artery" refers to the main visceral arteries (e.g., renal, hepatic, coronary, and mesenteric arteries); and "small artery" refers to the distal arterial radicals that connect with arterioles. Note large and medium-sized vessel vasculitides do not involve vessels other than arteries.
[b]Modified nomenclature (Falk, Jennette JASN 2010).
[c]Strongly associated with ANCA.
From Jennette JC, Falk RJ, Andrassy K, et al. Nomenclature of systemic vasculitides. Proposal of an international consensus conference. *Arthritis Rheum.* 1994;37:187, with permission.

Aortitis is a common feature of Takayasu and giant cell arteritis but is also associated with other vasculitides such as syphilis, tuberculosis, mycosis, Behçet disease, and Kawasaki disease. The most commonly involved vessels are the subclavian arteries in more than 90% of patients. Diagnostic differentiation between Takayasu and giant cell arteritis is largely based on age, with patients younger than 40 years having Takayasu arteritis and those older than 50 having giant cell arteritis. Aortic aneurysm rupture represents a morbid complication of giant cell arteritis. Aortitis may result in ischemic symptoms or infarction of the area supplied by the involved vessel. Asymptomatic aortitis may be a more common phenomenon than previously thought.[14]

Clinical Presentation

According to the Giant Cell Arteritis Guideline Development Group[15] giant cell arteritis often presents with abrupt onset headache, which is classically temporal and unilateral but can be diffuse. Presenting complaints can also include scalp pain, jaw or tongue claudication, blurring of vision, diplopia or amaurosis fugax, fever, weight loss, fatigue, polymyalgic symptoms, or limb claudication. On physical exam, tender, thickened, or beaded temporal artery with diminished or absent pulse may be noted. Visual field defect, visual loss, or afferent papillary defect can be noted. Funduscopic exam classically reflects anterior ischemic optic neuritis with pale, swollen optic disc with hemorrhages. Central retinal artery occlusion, upper cranial nerve palsies, asymmetry of pulses and blood pressure, and bruits are also features of this disease.

Early presentation of Takayasu arteritis includes low-grade fever, malaise, night sweats, weight loss, arthralgia, and fatigue. Although clinical presentations vary significantly between patients, and Takayasu arteritis seems to be a relapsing and remitting syndrome, many patients have diminished or absent pulses, Reynaud phenomenon, vascular bruits, hypertension, mesenteric angina, retinopathy, aortic regurgitation, dizziness, seizures, or amaurosis fugax. Takayasu arteritis has been reported to accompany other autoimmune diseases including rheumatoid arthritis, ulcerative colitis, systemic lupus, Crohn disease, sarcoidosis, and amyloidosis.[16,17]

Laboratory Findings

Laboratory findings in large-vessel vasculitis include a mild anemia, elevated levels of C-reactive protein, elevated erythrocyte sedimentation rate, and a generalized elevation in γ-globulin levels. Takayasu arteritis patients may be p- or c-ANCA positive. Other serologic results, including tests for lupus and infections, are typically negative. Patients typically present with only mild hematuria and proteinuria, except in patients with concomitant amyloidosis. The most common presentation is associated with hypertension and renal insufficiency, whereas renal failure is uncommon.

Pathogenesis

The pathogenesis of giant cell and Takayasu arteritis is unknown. Current consensus is that large vessel vasculitis is likely autoimmune in origin. Chauhan et al. report that serum of patients with Takayasu arteritis contains antiaortic endothelial cell antibodies directed against 60 to 65 kDa heat-shock proteins.[18] Serum-containing antiaortic endothelial cell antibodies induced apoptosis of aortic endothelial cells. There is scant evidence for a direct link between antiaortic endothelial cell antibodies and the development of Takayasu arteritis, however.

There are several tantalizing clues that infectious agents may play a role in these diseases. In animals, there is evidence that gamma herpes virus 68 causes arteritis in mice lacking the interferon-γ receptor. In humans, an association exists between giant cell arteritis and parvovirus B19 infection.[19] However, a study using polymerase chain reaction (PCR) and immunohistochemistry techniques on 147 temporal artery biopsies found no evidence of parvovirus B19 DNA in the arteries of patients with giant cell arteritis.[20] A cyclic occurrence of disease, with a peak incidence occurring every 5 to 7 years, suggests an infectious cycle. Certain genetic factors are associated with the development of giant cell arteritis. This form of vasculitis is more common in individuals of Northern European descent living in Europe or the United States,[21] and there is clustering of cases among families.[22] The development of giant cell arteritis also correlates with the expression of HLA-DR4, which is also found in high frequency among patients with polymyalgia rheumatica.[23]

Giant cell arteritis may be a consequence of either or both the humeral and cellular immune responses. The clinical and experimental findings suggest that a cell-mediated process is most likely.[24] Most inflammatory cells that invade the vessel walls are CD4-positive T cells. Elevated levels of IL-6 correlate with the severity of the disease and decrease quite rapidly when glucocorticoids are administered.[25] Levels of several other cytokines and chemokines are similarly elevated. It is hypothesized that activated monocytes infiltrate the adventitia of large vessel walls via the vasa vasorum and become macrophages that then produce interferon-γ and recruit additional leukocytes, including macrophages. Unfortunately, the antigen responsible for these interactions has yet to be elucidated.

Renal Involvement

Renal involvement in Takayasu arteritis and giant cell arteritis is usually a consequence of inflammation and scarring of the aorta adjacent to the orifice of the renal artery, leading to stenosis of the renal artery and ischemic renal failure. One of the most common clinical presentations of this phenomenon is renovascular hypertension affecting more than 50% of patients with Takayasu arteritis. In Japan, Takayasu arteritis is an important cause of hypertension in adolescents.

Glomerular lesions and necrosis occurs in patients with large-vessel vasculitis, but this may be an overlap of a small-vessel vasculitis. Several cases of glomerulonephritis in the setting of Takayasu arteritis have been reported in the literature. The renal pathology in these cases varies from case to case, including focal segmental sclerosis, mesangial proliferation, membranoproliferative lesions, and crescentic lesions.

Treatment

The cornerstone of treatment of giant cell arteritis is based on the use of high-dose corticosteroids. Typically, prednisone is started at 1 to 1.5 mg/kg/day until the erythrocyte sedimentation rate is normal and the patient is asymptomatic. Initial treatment on an alternate-day basis is ineffective in the treatment of giant cell arteritis. When compared with patients receiving daily corticosteroids, only 30% (versus 85%) of patients treated with alternate-day dosing enter an early remission, and 75% (versus 15%) experience a flare of disease activity.[26] Intravenous pulses of methylprednisolone (1 g per day for 3 to 5 days) are recommended for patients with severe visual loss because this treatment seems to prevent additional visual loss or fellow-eye involvement after initiation of corticosteroids.[27] The initiation of corticosteroids within 2 weeks before a temporal artery biopsy does not change the characteristic pathologic findings.[28] A delay in treatment to obtain a temporal artery biopsy is therefore not warranted.

Once a clinical remission is attained, a slow taper of corticosteroids is undertaken by decreasing the dose by 10% every 2 weeks to a dose of 10 mg per day, then by 1 mg per day. Other similar tapering protocols have been suggested, but no critical assessment of these recommendations is available. Switching to an alternate-day regimen may be similarly efficacious and perhaps less toxic. Symptoms usually resolve within 2 to 3 days, and the erythrocyte sedimentation rate usually normalizes within 4 to 6 weeks. Most patients with giant cell arteritis require 2 years of corticosteroids, and a few remain on a low-dose regimen indefinitely. Patients who continue to require "maintenance" dosages of more than 15 mg per day may be considered "steroid resistant."

The high rate of complications attributable to the prolonged duration of corticosteroid therapy and the age distribution of patients with giant cell arteritis has led to an interest in identifying steroid-sparing alternative drugs. Dapsone, azathioprine, cyclosporine, antimalarials, cyclophosphamide, or gold have not been found to reduce corticosteroid toxicity and still maintain therapeutic effectiveness.[29] The reported beneficial effect on the rate of relapse of adding methotrexate to corticosteroids was not confirmed by a multicenter, placebo-controlled trial.[30] A retrospective study suggests that the concomitant use of low-dose aspirin decreases the rate of visual loss and cerebrovascular events in patients with giant cell arteritis.[31] Information on the use of tumor necrosis factor (TNF)-alpha-blocking agents in the treatment of giant cell arteritis is currently limited to very small case series.

The treatment of Takayasu arteritis is similarly based on high-dose corticosteroids. In a U.S. National Institutes of Health study, treatment was initiated at 1 mg per kg (up to 60 mg per day) for 1 to 3 months, followed by a slow taper to an alternate-day regimen over the following 4 to 8 weeks, and a subsequent slow taper over the following 6 to 12 months. This regimen is associated with a remission rate of 60% and an estimated median time to remission of 22 months.[32]

Unfortunately, relapses occur in as much as 45% of patients, leading to multiple or prolonged courses of corticosteroids. Up to 40% of patients require the addition of cytotoxic drugs such as cyclophosphamide or methotrexate. In an open-label study of 18 patients with persistent or refractory Takayasu arteritis despite treatment with corticosteroids alone, the use of methotrexate was associated with an 81% remission rate.[33] Fifty percent of patients achieved a corticosteroid-free remission on methotrexate, and half of these patients remained in remission after methotrexate was withdrawn. About 20% of patients did not attain remission despite corticosteroids and methotrexate. The successful use of infliximab has been reported in several case reports of patients with active Takayasu arteritis despite conventional therapy with corticosteroids and cyclophosphamide[34] or methotrexate.[35] The use of anti-TNF therapy was assessed in a pilot, open-label trial involving a total of 15 patients with active, relapsing Takayasu arteritis. Seven patients were initially treated with etanercept and eight with infliximab. The use of anti-TNF agents led to remission in 10 of the 15 patients that was sustained for 1 to 3.3 years without glucocorticoid therapy. Four patients achieved partial remission, with a >50% reduction in the glucocorticoid requirement. Two relapses occurred during periods when etanercept was interrupted, but remission was reestablished upon reinstitution of therapy.[36]

The optimal treatment of patients with Takayasu arteritis is further complicated by the results of biopsies of affected vessels obtained at the time of bypass surgery. These data revealed evidence of persistent vascular inflammation even in the absence of clinical signs or symptoms of active disease and in the setting of a normal erythrocyte sedimentation rate.[32,37] Surgical intervention is the definitive treatment of occlusive disease in patients with progressive Takayasu arteritis, especially in the absence of response to conventional therapy.

The diagnosis and treatment of hypertension represents a very important aspect of the care of patients with Takayasu arteritis because congestive heart failure, ischemic or hemorrhagic stroke, and renal failure account for most of the deaths from this disease.[38] The diagnosis of hypertension may be missed if it is based on measurement of blood pressure in the upper extremities alone, because of the high incidence of subclavian artery stenoses, which may be bilateral. In some cases, lesions in the thoracic or abdominal aorta or the iliac or femoral arteries may give misleading normal blood pressures in the lower extremities as well. It is thus recommended that arteriographic studies be performed with pressure transducers so that aortic pressures can be compared with extremity pressures, and to identify the extremity where blood pressure monitoring is most reliable and reflective of true blood pressure.[38]

MEDIUM-SIZED VESSEL VASCULITIS: POLYARTERITIS NODOSA AND KAWASAKI DISEASE

The medium-sized vessel vasculitides are necrotizing arteritides that have a predilection for arteries that lead to major viscera and their initial branches. In the kidneys, the major targets are the interlobar and arcuate arteries, with less frequent involvement of the main renal artery and interlobular arteries (Fig. 48.3). The two major categories of medium-sized vessel vasculitis are polyarteritis nodosa and Kawasaki disease. Pathologically, both are characterized in the acute phase by necrotizing arteritis with transmural inflammation that initially includes neutrophils and foci of fibrinoid necrosis (Fig. 48.1). The acute necrotizing inflammation often erodes completely through the artery wall and into the adjacent perivascular tissue, thereby forming a pseudoaneurysm (Fig. 48.4). Secondary complications of the arteritis include thrombosis, infarction, and hemorrhage. In only a few days, the lesions evolve from an acute neutrophil-rich inflammation to a "chronic" inflammation with predominantly mononuclear leukocytes. Sites of thrombosis and necrosis develop progressive scarring (Fig. 48.2). By definition, medium-sized vessel vasculitides do not cause glomerulonephritis, although they can cause hematuria, proteinuria (usually less than 2 g per 24 hours), and renal insufficiency as a result of renal infarction. Pseudoaneurysms near the renal surface may rupture and cause severe, even fatal, retroperitoneal and intraperitoneal hemorrhage.

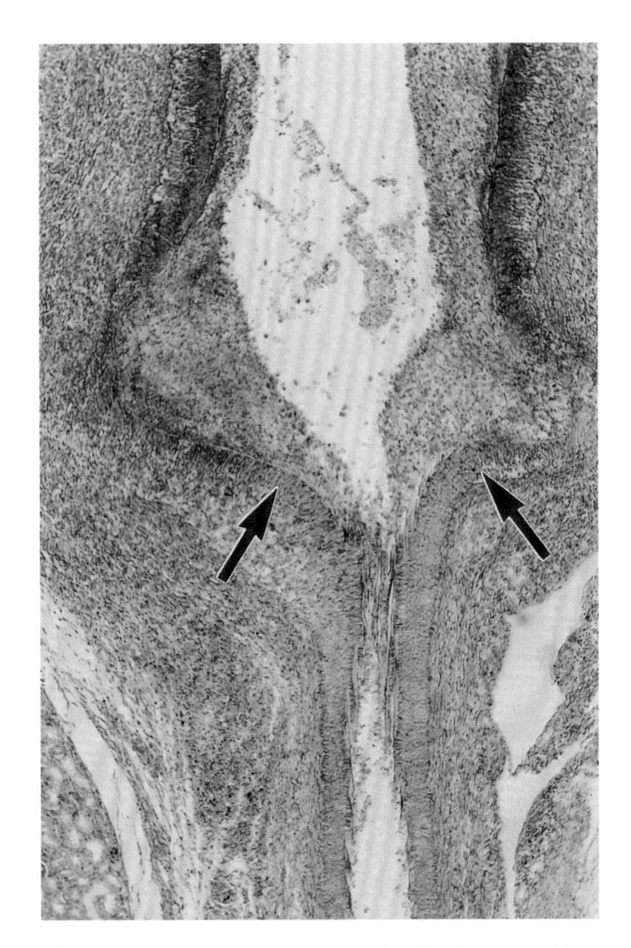

FIGURE 48.4 Acute necrotizing arteritis affecting a renal interlobar artery in a patient with Kawasaki disease. The necrotizing inflammation (*arrows*) has eroded into the perivascular tissue to produce a pseudoaneurysm. (Hematoxylin and eosin stain, magnification ×350.)

The meaning of the diagnostic term "polyarteritis nodosa" has evolved over the past century, and substantial confusion continues over how best to use it. The problem and the solution that we propose is best understood in historical context. Systemic necrotizing arteritis was first clearly described by Kussmaul and Maier in the mid-1800s.[39] They reported a patient with widespread visceral nodules caused by acute inflammation of arteries and called the process "periarteritis nodosa." Ferrari introduced the term "polyarteritis nodosa,"[40] which is more appropriate because the inflammation is transmural rather than perivascular. For approximately 50 years, essentially all patients with any pattern of necrotizing arteritis were included in the polyarteritis nodosa category. During the early to mid-1900s, astute investigators recognized that many patients with necrotizing arteritis had distinctive distributions of vascular inflammation or characteristic pathologic processes that warranted their separation from patients with arteritis alone. For example, Kawasaki disease, GPA, EGPA, and MPA were initially included in the category of polyarteritis nodosa but now are recognized as distinct entities.[8] The removal of these vasculitides from the polyarteritis nodosa category is justified not only on the basis of different patterns and distributions of vessel involvement, but also because they have different natural histories, prognoses, and treatment requirements.

The reduction of polyarteritis nodosa to a more homogeneous and clinically useful category of vasculitis began when Arnaout, among others, recognized that some patients with necrotizing arteritis had lesions that could be seen only by microscopic examination.[41] Circa 1950, Zeek et al.[42,43] and Godman and Churg[44] carried out careful evaluations of patients with arteritis and concluded that polyarteritis nodosa should be separated from the "microscopic" form of vasculitis that was characterized by involvement of not only small arteries but also venules and capillaries. As discussed later in the section on small-vessel vasculitis, Godman and Churg also concluded that polyarteritis nodosa was distinct not only from MPA but also from GPA and eosinophilic granulomatosis, and that MPA, GPA, and eosinophilic granulomatosis were related to one another.

The diagnostic approach that we advocate defines polyarteritis nodosa as necrotizing inflammation of medium-sized or small arteries without glomerulonephritis or vasculitis in arterioles, capillaries, or venules (Table 48.2).[8] This allows the separation of polyarteritis nodosa from other types of vasculitis, such as GPA, MPA, and eosinophilic granulomatosis, which have necrotizing arteritis as a component of a systemic polyangiitis that affects capillaries, venules, and arteries. By using this approach, the presence of glomerulonephritis rules out a diagnosis of polyarteritis nodosa and indicates the presence of some type of small-vessel vasculitis. Table 48.3 compares some of the features of polyarteritis nodosa and MPA. Note that glomerular capillaritis (glomerulonephritis) or pulmonary alveolar capillaritis with pulmonary hemorrhage rule out a diagnosis of polyarteritis nodosa and raise the possibility of MPA. Peripheral neuropathy is not a discriminator, because involvement of small epineural arteries in peripheral nerves may occur with polyarteritis nodosa or MPA. As discussed in more detail later, testing for ANCA is useful for distinguishing between polyarteritis nodosa and the ANCA-associated small-vessel vasculitides.[45–49] In a patient with necrotizing arteritis, a positive ANCA result decreases the likelihood of polyarteritis nodosa and increases the likelihood of MPA, GPA, or eosinophilic granulomatosis (i.e., increases the likelihood that the patient has or will develop necrotizing inflammation of vessels other than arteries, such as pulmonary alveolar capillaritis or glomerular capillaritis [glomerulonephritis]).

TABLE 48.3 **Clinical Differences Between Polyarteritis Nodosa and Microscopic Polyangiitis**

Clinical Feature	Polyarteritis Nodosa	Microscopic Polyangiitis
Rapidly progressive nephritis	No	Very common
Pulmonary hemorrhage	No	Yes
Peripheral neuropathy	Yes	Yes
Microaneurysms by angiography	Yes	Rare
Renovascular hypertension	Occasional	No
Positive hepatitis B serology	Uncommon	No
Positive antineutrophil cytoplasmic antibodies serology results	Rare	Frequent
Relapses	Rare	Frequent

From Guillevin L, Lhote F, Amouroux J, et al. Antineutrophil cytoplasmic antibodies, abnormal angiograms and pathological findings in polyarteritis nodosa and Eosinophilic granulomatosis: Indications for the classification of vasculitides of the polyarteritis nodosa group. *Br J Rheumatol.* 1996;35:958, with permission.

Necrotizing arteritis that is pathologically indistinguishable from the necrotizing arteritis of polyarteritis nodosa can occur in patients with Kawasaki disease (Figs. 48.1 and 48.3). Kawasaki disease is an acute self-limiting febrile illness, the second commonest vasculitis in childhood.[50] Kawasaki disease is characterized by the mucocutaneous lymph node syndrome, which includes nonsuppurative lymphadenopathy, polymorphous erythematous rash, erythema of the oropharyngeal mucosa, erythema of the palms and soles, conjunctivitis, indurative edema, and desquamation of the extremities. A major cause for morbidity and mortality in patients with Kawasaki disease is the development of a necrotizing arteritis. This arteritis has a predilection for coronary arteries but can occur anywhere, including the kidney (Figs. 48.1 and 48.3). Kawasaki disease is the most common cause of childhood-acquired heart disease.[50] Symptomatic renal involvement is rare in Kawasaki disease. Differentiation between the arteritis of Kawasaki disease and that of polyarteritis nodosa is very important because the treatment of Kawasaki disease differs from the treatment of polyarteritis nodosa (discussed in Treatment section).

The presence or absence of the mucocutaneous lymph node syndrome is an effective diagnostic discriminator between Kawasaki disease and polyarteritis nodosa.

Clinical Features

Patients with polyarteritis nodosa typically have constitutional symptoms, including fever and weight loss. The presence of mononeuritis multiplex, myalgias, and arthralgias, as well as skin lesions including nodules, ulcers, livedo reticularis, and digital ischemia in half of patients, characterize the disease. There is a spectrum of disease referred to as cutaneous polyarteritis nodosa associated with streptococcal infection.[50] Cutaneous polyarteritis nodosa has periodic exacerbations but is milder than classic polyarteritis nodosa. This presentation may be along the spectrum of systemic polyarteritis nodosa. Vasculitis of the coronary arteries may lead to cardiac symptoms. The renal disease seen in polyarteritis nodosa is primarily related to vasculitis of the renal arteries resulting in renovascular hypertension and/or renal parenchymal infarction. Patients with polyarteritis nodosa do not have evidence of small-vessel vasculitis, glomerulonephritis, or pulmonary capillaritis. In fact, the lung is rarely injured in polyarteritis nodosa, in contrast to the frequency of pulmonary disease in patients with GPA, MPA, or EGPA. Although not distinguishing features, gastrointestinal complaints and peripheral neuropathy are more common among patients with polyarteritis nodosa than patients with MPA. The skin lesions of polyarteritis nodosa closely mimic cholesterol emboli and calciphylaxis and therefore histopathologic confirmation of diagnosis is required. The prognosis of polyarteritis nodosa is really a reflection of the involvement of the kidneys, heart, central nervous system, or gastrointestinal tract.[51]

Tc-99m dimercaptosuccinic acid (DMSA) scanning of the kidneys can indirectly support the diagnosis of a medium-vessel vasculitis affecting the renal arteries by manifesting patchy areas of decreased isotope in the renal parenchyma.[52] Unquestionably, however, angiography of the renal, hepatic, and/or mesenteric vasculature via angiography is a superior approach for diagnosis of a medium vessel vasculitis. Demonstration of "aneurysms," narrowing of arteries, or pruning of the peripheral vascular tree suggest medium-vessel vasculitis. Large pseudoaneurysms, stenosis of the renal arteries or large branches, and resultant areas of ischemia or infarct within the kidney can be demonstrated by magnetic resonance angiography or computed tomography (CT) angiography.

Pathogenesis

The etiology of polyarteritis nodosa remains unclear, and most cases of polyarteritis nodosa are probably idiopathic. An association between polyarteritis nodosa and hepatitis B infection is evident by the fact that patients with hepatitis B antigenemia are at greater risk of developing polyarteritis nodosa. Hepatitis B virus has been implicated in up to one third of cases of polyarteritis nodosa.[54] A role for hepatitis B antigenemia in the pathogenesis of polyarteritis nodosa is further suggested by reports of vasculitis after hepatitis B vaccination.[55] Furthermore, treatment with antiviral agents and plasma exchange has led to resolution of the vasculitis in patients whose serology converts from being positive for the HBe or HBs antigens to the corresponding antibodies.[56,57]

Polyarteritis nodosa has been associated with a number of cancers, especially hairy cell leukemia.[58] Treatment of hairy cell leukemia with interferon-alpha (INF-α) may be associated with resolution of polyarteritis nodosa.[59] As opposed to patients with small-vessel vasculitis, patients with polyarteritis nodosa are ANCA-negative.[60]

Renal Manifestations

Both polyarteritis nodosa and Kawasaki disease are medium-sized vessel vasculitides that affect the kidney. These arteritides result in necrotizing lesions in the major renal arteries and aneurysm formation with thrombosis and renal infarction. The aneurysms are not true aneurysms but rather pseudoaneurysms. The arteritis of Kawasaki disease most commonly involves the coronary arteries, but in at least 25% of patients the lesions also involve the kidney. Tubulointerstitial nephritis is a not uncommon renal presentation in Kawasaki disease.[50] Renal manifestations of Kawasaki disease can lead to renal failure. Kawasaki disease is distinguished from polyarteritis nodosa by the pathognomonic sine qua non feature of mucocutaneous lymph node syndrome. Renal arterial involvement by polyarteritis nodosa, including interlobar and arcuate arteries, results in renal ischemia, infarction, and hemorrhage. One of the most painful and catastrophic consequences of this disease is rupture of an arterial pseudoaneurysm that causes retroperitoneal and sometimes intraperitoneal hemorrhage.

Treatment

The treatment of Kawasaki disease differs from the treatment of polyarteritis nodosa. Kawasaki disease usually is treated with aspirin and intravenous γ-globulin therapy,[53] whereas the treatment of polyarteritis nodosa classically has been based on the use of high-dose corticosteroids with the addition, in moderate to severe or organ-threatening cases, of cyclophosphamide. Unfortunately, most studies pertinent to the treatment of polyarteritis nodosa antedate the 1994 Chapel Hill consensus conference, which classified MPA among the small-vessel vasculitides separate from classic polyarteritis nodosa. Consequently, most of the older studies and reports include a substantial number of patients who would now be diagnosed with MPA and not classic polyarteritis nodosa. As a result of the consensus conference, the incidence of classic polyarteritis nodosa involving medium-sized vessels alone and without evidence for glomerulonephritis is very low and is not readily amenable to large-scale evaluation of various therapies. Fifty percent of classic polyarteritis nodosa is curable with 9 to 12 months of corticosteroid therapy alone.[61] The other 50% of polyarteritis nodosa will require cyclophosphamide therapy but once remission is obtained relapses are very uncommon.[62] The problem is compounded by the relatively recent recognition of the association of polyarteritis nodosa with hepatitis B virus (HBV) infection in a subset of patients with polyarteritis nodosa that varies from 10% to 50%, depending on the population studied.

In the absence of HBV infection, the mainstay of treatment of classic polyarteritis nodosa continues to rest on the use of high-dose corticosteroids. In patients without poor prognostic factors (no renal, cardiac, gastrointestinal, or central nervous system manifestations of disease), no survival difference was noted when treating polyarteritis nodosa with corticosteroids alone when compared to corticosteroids and cyclophosphamide.[63] Typically, prednisone is initiated at a dosage of 1 mg/kg/day for the first month. Over the course of the second month, the dosage is tapered to an alternate-day regimen so that the patient is receiving 1 mg per kg every other day by the end of the second month. It is subsequently tapered slowly by 5 mg per day weekly as tolerated. Should relapse occur after corticosteroid therapy, the addition of cyclophosphamide or azathioprine may be beneficial.[64] The addition of an alkylating agent such as cyclophosphamide in the treatment of polyarteritis nodosa is not as well established as in the treatment of MPA or GPA, although some studies report improved patient survival when these agents were added, especially in patients with poor prognostic factors.[64] In another study, the addition of cyclophosphamide to corticosteroids and plasma exchange led to decreased relapse in the cyclophosphamide-treated group, but no improvement in the 10-year survival rate.[65] In current practice, cyclophosphamide should be reserved for patients with severe or organ-threatening disease, with disease that fails to respond to treatment with corticosteroids alone, for patients who require unacceptably high doses of corticosteroids, or for patients who are intolerant to corticosteroid side effects. No randomized study exists to critically assess the value of a daily oral regimen of cyclophosphamide compared with pulse cyclophosphamide in the outcome of patients with classic polyarteritis nodosa; however, intravenous cyclophosphamide rather than an oral regimen is recommended, not to exceed 12 pulses.[64] In patients with poor prognostic factors, six intravenous pulse treatments with cyclophosphamide not followed by maintenance therapy were noted to have greater relapse rate than 12 intravenous infusions of cyclophosphamide. Although azathioprine has been used in the treatment of classic polyarteritis nodosa, this agent is better reserved for maintenance therapy or as a steroid-sparing agent. Current recommendations for patients with polyarteritis nodosa with poor prognostic factors are to obtain remission with pulse cyclophosphamide and then continue therapy with azathioprine for 12 to 18 total months of immunosuppression.[66] Plasma exchange does not seem to improve the outcome, decrease relapse, or improve long-term survival of patients with polyarteritis nodosa not associated with HBV.[67] The successful use of infliximab in PAN resistant to "conventional therapy" has been reported in a small number of cases.[68,69]

In the setting of HBV-associated polyarteritis nodosa, treatment with immunosuppression consisting of corticosteroids with or without cyclophosphamide is thought to be deleterious because it facilitates viral replication, delays the development of protective anti-HBV antibodies, and may lead to an aggravation of hepatic involvement.[70] For this reason, it has been advocated that only a short course of corticosteroids (1 mg/kg/day) be used for 1 week, followed by a rapid taper over the following week. The prompt institution of antiviral therapy may ameliorate the vascular inflammation. Treatment with plasma exchange has been advocated to clear circulating immune complexes thought to be important in the pathogenesis of this disease,[71] although no controlled trial has critically assessed the need for plasmapheresis. The antiviral agents used have included vidarabine, INF-α-2b, or more recently combination therapy of INF-α-2b in addition to lamivudine[72] or famciclovir.[57] No large-scale trials of antiviral therapy are available to critically assess the efficacy of these combinations in patients with HBV-related polyarteritis nodosa. Current work in the treatment of chronic HBV focuses on the use of INF-α-2b, modified purine analogs such as famciclovir, or L-stereoisomers of pyrimidine derivatives such as lamivudine.[73] In an uncontrolled study, the combination of a short course of corticosteroids followed by a 6-month course of lamivudine and scheduled plasma exchange (until hepatitis B antigen or anti-HBe antibody seroconversion) resulted in a clinical remission of the vasculitis.[74] In a recent retrospective analysis of 115 patients with HBV-associated polyarteritis nodosa (according to the Chapel Hill nomenclature) followed by the French Vasculitis Study Group between 1972 and 2002, the overall remission rate was 80.9% with a subsequent overall 9.7% relapse rate.[54] The rates of relapse or death were not significantly different among patients treated with antiviral agents (vidarabine, INF-α, or lamivudine) ($n = 80$) when compared to patients treated with corticosteroids alone, or with cyclophosphamide, or plasma exchanges ($n = 35$) (5% vs. 14.3% relapse; and 30% vs. 48.6% death, respectively). However, the use of antiviral agents has led to a significantly higher rate of seroconversions from HBeAg to anti-HBeAb (49.4% vs. 14.7%; $P < .001$). Such seroconversion was associated with a clinical remission and absence of relapse.

Outcome

Most studies examining patient outcome and predictors of patient survival in polyarteritis nodosa antedate the Chapel Hill consensus conference of 1994. These studies are based on cohorts of patients that include those with MPA, EGPA, and hepatitis B–associated classic polyarteritis nodosa. Earlier studies report a 5-year survival rate of approximately 55% in patients primarily treated with corticosteroids alone.[75] The addition of cyclophosphamide or immunosuppressive therapy to glucocorticoids seems to have improved the 5-year survival rate to about 80%. Patients with bowel infarction, serious gastrointestinal bleeding, or renal insufficiency had particularly poor prognosis. In a more recent prospective study including 342 patients, of whom 119 had classic polyarteritis nodosa without HBV (89 patients with HBV, 52 patients with MPA, 82 patients with EGPA),[51] proteinuria of 10 g per day, renal insufficiency, and gastrointestinal tract involvement were the major prognostic markers for a worse outcome.

SMALL VESSEL VASCULITIS

Microscopic Polyangiitis, Granulomatosis with Polyangiitis, and Eosinophilic Granulomatosis

Small-vessel vasculitides are characterized by necrotizing inflammation of multiple types of vessels. Arteries, veins, arterioles, venules, and capillaries may be affected; however, venules and capillaries are the most frequent targets. An understanding of the small-vessel vasculitides is important for nephrologists because these diseases often involve the kidneys and frequently cause glomerulonephritis. All of the small-vessel vasculitides listed in Table 48.1 can involve the kidneys. As mentioned in the discussion about the evolution of the definition of polyarteritis nodosa, small-vessel vasculitides with arterial involvement once were subsumed in the polyarteritis nodosa category. Zeek et al.[42,43] and Godman and Churg[44] were among the first to recognize that vasculitides that involve capillaries and venules in addition to arteries have clinical and pathologic features that are clearly distinct from those of polyarteritis nodosa.

The two major categories of small-vessel vasculitis include the "pauci-immune small vessel vasculitides" and the "immune complex–mediated small vessel vasculitides" (Table 48.1). Immune complex–mediated vasculitides, such as Henoch-Schönlein purpura (HSP), cryoglobulinemic vasculitis, lupus vasculitis, and antiglomerular basement membrane (anti-GBM) vasculitis, have extensive localization of immunoglobulin and complement in vessel walls as a consequence of deposition of circulating immune complexes or in situ immune-complex formation between circulating antibodies and planted or constitutive antigens. The pauci-immune small-vessel vasculitides have little or no vascular wall localization of immunoglobulins.[45] The pauci-immune small-vessel vasculitides often have necrotizing and crescentic glomerulonephritis as a component of the systemic necrotizing vasculitis. A pathologically identical pauci-immune necrotizing and crescentic glomerulonephritis also occurs as a renal-limited process, sometimes referred to as "idiopathic crescentic glomerulonephritis" or "renal vasculitis."[76] Pauci-immune crescentic glomerulonephritis, usually a component of systemic pauci-immune small-vessel vasculitis, is the most common type of crescentic glomerulonephritis (Table 48.4).

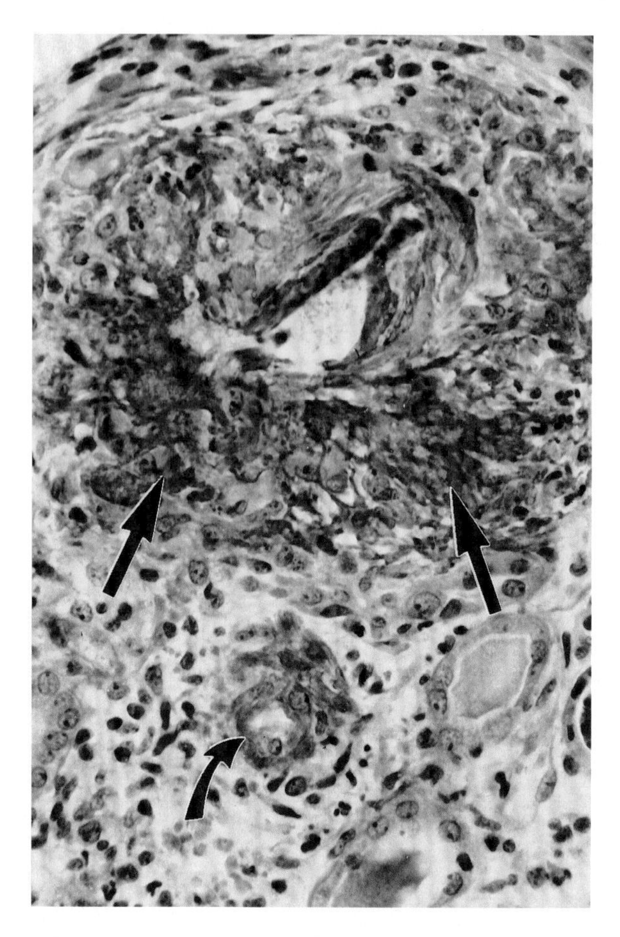

FIGURE 48.5 Necrotizing arteritis affecting an interlobular artery in a patient with microscopic polyangiitis. Note the extension of fibrinoid material into perivascular interstitium (*straight arrows*). Also note the necrotizing arteriolitis (*curved arrow*). (Masson trichrome, magnification ×350.)

TABLE 48.4 **Frequency of Immunopathologic Categories of Crescentic Glomerulonephritis in More Than 3,000 Consecutive Nontransplant Renal Biopsies Evaluated by Immunofluorescence Microscopy in the University of North Carolina Nephropathology Laboratory**

	Any Crescents (n = 540)	**>50% Crescents (n = 195)**	**Arteritis in Biopsy (n = 37)**
Immunohistology			
Pauci-immune (<2 positive immunoglobulin)	51% (277/540)	61% (118/195)[a]	84% (31/37)
Immune complex (≤2 positive immunoglobulin)	44% (238/540)	29% (56/195)	14% (5/37)[c]
Antiglomerular basement membrane	5% (25/540)[b]	11% (21/195)	3% (1/37)[d]

[a]Seventy of 77 patients tested for antineutrophilic cytoplasmic antibodies (ANCA) were positive (91%) (44 p-ANCA and 26 c-ANCA).
[b]Three of 19 patients tested for ANCA were positive (16%) (2 p-ANCA and 1 c-ANCA).
[c]Four patients had lupus and one poststreptococcal glomerulonephritis.
[d]This patient also had a p-ANCA (myeloperoxidase-ANCA).
From Jennette JC, Falk RJ. The pathology of vasculitis involving the kidney. *Am J Kidney Dis.* 1991;24:130, with permission.

The three major categories of systemic pauci-immune small-vessel vasculitis are microscopic polyangiitis (MPA), granulomatosis with polyangiitis (GPA) (formerly Wegener granulomatosis), and eosinophilic granulomatosis (EGPA).[44,77] Table 48.2 and Figure 48.3 provide an approach for differentiating these three vasculitides and for distinguishing them from other types of vasculitis. These three systemic vasculitic processes along with pauci-immune necrotizing and crescentic glomerulonephritis (renal-limited disease) can be broadly referred to as ANCA disease.

It is important to note that the eponym Wegener granulomatosis has been abandoned due to the history linking Friedrich Wegener to the Nazi party and his participation in Nazi war crimes. The disease process formerly referred to as Wegener granulomatosis is now known as granulomatosis with polyangiitis or GPA.[78–80]

MPA, GPA, and EGPA share a histologically identical necrotizing vasculitis that can affect arteries (Fig. 48.5), arterioles (Fig. 48.6), venules (Fig. 48.7), and capillaries, especially glomerular capillaries (Fig. 48.8). At all of these sites, the acute lesion is characterized by segmental necrosis with mural and perivascular fibrinoid material, sometimes accompanied by thrombosis in the vascular lumen. The initial inflammatory infiltrate has conspicuous neutrophils, often undergoing leukocytoclasia (Fig. 48.7), but this usually transforms into a predominantly mononuclear leukocyte infiltrate within a few days. The glomerular lesion of pauci-immune ANCA vasculitis begins with segmental fibrinoid necrosis (Fig. 48.8) that quickly leads to crescent formation (Fig. 48.9). At the time of renal biopsy, approximately 90% of patients with pauci-immune crescentic glomerulonephritis have some degree of glomerular necrosis and crescent formation, although this may involve fewer than 50% of glomeruli. Arteritis, arteriolitis, and medullary angiitis are seen in less than 20% of renal biopsy specimens. Medullary angiitis can be severe enough to cause focal papillary necrosis.

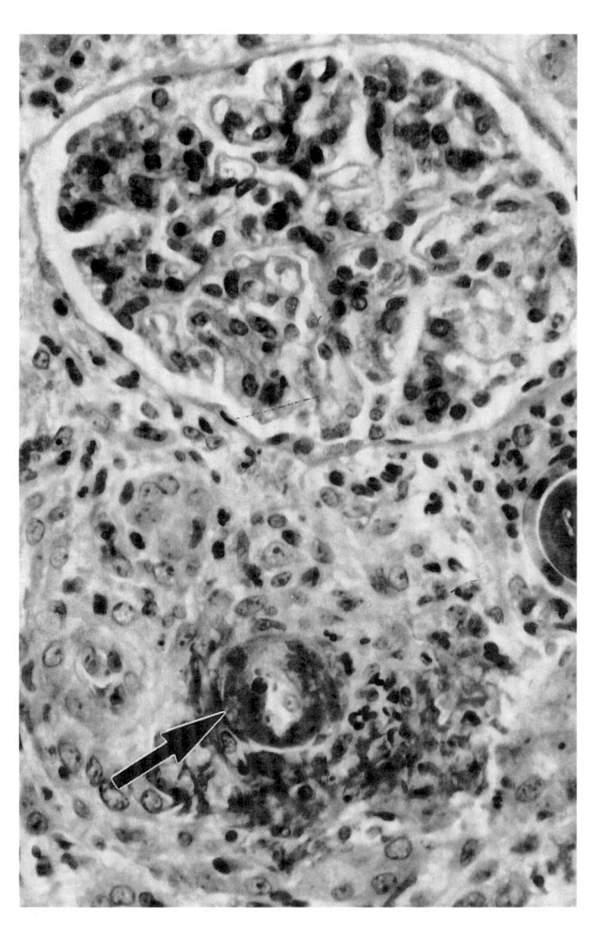

FIGURE 48.6 Necrotizing arteriolitis (*arrow*) affecting an arteriole in the renal cortex of a patient with microscopic polyangiitis. Note the fibrinoid material in the vessel wall and adjacent interstitium, and the focal perivascular leukocytoclasia. (Masson trichrome stain, magnification ×350.)

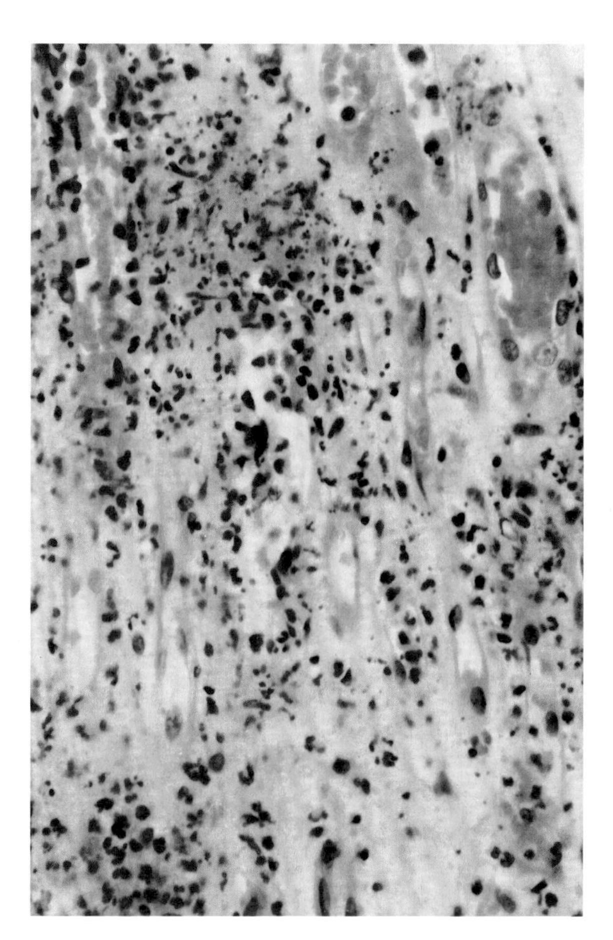

FIGURE 48.7 Leukocytoclastic medullary angiitis affecting the peritubular vasa recta in a patient with granulomatosis with polyangiitis. (Hematoxylin and eosin stain, magnification ×350.)

In addition to the renal vasculitic lesions illustrated in Figures 48.5 to 48.9, patients with all three systemic pauci-immune ANCA vasculitides share histologically identical inflammatory vascular lesions in other tissues, such as pulmonary hemorrhagic alveolar capillaritis, dermal

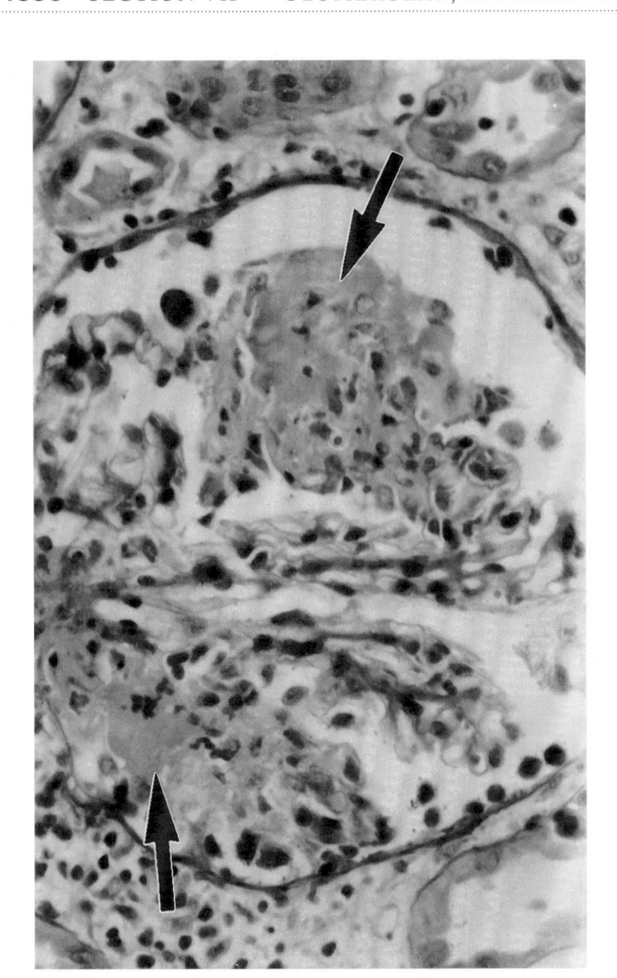

FIGURE 48.8 Segmental fibrinoid necrosis (*arrows*) in a glomerulus from a patient with microscopic polyangiitis. (Hematoxylin and eosin stain, magnification ×350.)

leukocytoclastic venulitis, and necrotizing inflammation of arteries in many tissues, including but not limited to peripheral nerves, skeletal muscle, gut, liver, pancreas, and skin. The diagnostic distinctions among the three diseases are not based on the pathologic or clinical features of vasculitis per se, but on the presence or absence of accompanying features, specifically granulomatous inflammation, asthma, and blood eosinophilia. As detailed in Table 48.2 and diagrammed in Figure 48.3, a diagnosis of MPA is warranted if a patient has systemic pauci-immune ANCA vasculitis with no evidence for necrotizing granulomatous inflammation or asthma. A diagnosis of GPA is warranted if a patient has systemic pauci-immune ANCA vasculitis with necrotizing granulomatous inflammation, usually in the upper or lower respiratory tract, and no asthma. A diagnosis of EGPA is warranted if a patient has systemic pauci-immune ANCA vasculitis with asthma and blood eosinophilia. Reaching these diagnostic conclusions does not necessarily require pathologic documentation of the lesions if reasonable clinical surrogates are identified. For example, in renal biopsy-proven pauci-immune necrotizing and crescentic glomerulonephritis, radiographic demonstration of cavitary lung nodules (in the absence of infection) or lytic bone lesions in the nasal septum are reasonable evidence for necrotizing granulomatous inflammation, warranting a diagnosis of GPA.

Serologic testing for ANCA is useful for making the diagnosis of pauci-immune ANCA vasculitis or renal-limited pauci-immune crescentic glomerulonephritis. As discussed in more detail in the "Laboratory Findings" section of this chapter, the major types of ANCA vasculitis are those that have specificity for proteinase 3 (PR3–ANCA) and for myeloperoxidase (MPO-ANCA).[46–49] In an indirect immunofluorescence microscopy assay, PR3–ANCA usually causes cytoplasmic staining of neutrophils (c-ANCA) and MPO-ANCA usually causes perinuclear staining (p-ANCA).

The clinical differential diagnosis of pauci-immune ANCA vasculitis also includes immune-complex ANCA vasculitis. Table 48.5 demonstrates significant overlap in organ system involvement among different types of pauci-immune ANCA vasculitis and immune-complex ANCA vasculitis. Upper or lower respiratory tract involvement has

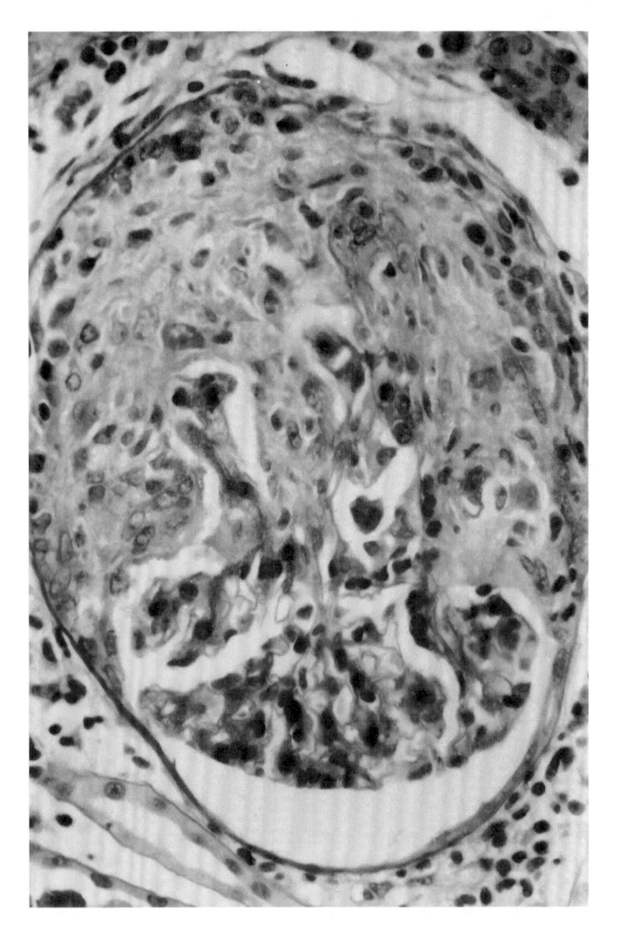

FIGURE 48.9 Cellular crescent in a glomerulus from a patient with microscopic polyangiitis. (Hematoxylin and eosin stain, magnification ×350.)

TABLE 48.5 **Comparison of Approximate Frequency of Manifestations of Microscopic Polyangiitis With Several Other Forms of Anca Vasculitis**

	Microscopic Polyangiitis	Granulomatosis with Polyangiitis	Eosinophilic granulomatosis	Henoch-Schönlein	Cryoglobulin Vasculitis
Cutaneous	40%	40%	60%	90%	90%
Renal	90%	80%	45%	50%	55%
Pulmonary	50%	90%	70%	<5%	<5%
Ear, nose, and throat	35%	90%	50%	<5%	<5%
Musculoskeletal	60%	60%	50%	75%	70%
Neurologic	30%	50%	70%	10%	40%
Gastrointestinal	50%	50%	50%	60%	30%

From Jennette JC, Falk RJ. Small vessel vasculitis. *N Engl J Med.* 1997;337:1512, with permission.

the greatest discriminatory value because respiratory tract involvement is common with pauci-immune ANCA vasculitis and rare with immune-complex ANCA vasculitis. Table 48.6 and Figure 48.3 detail a number of observations that can be used to conclusively differentiate among MPA, GPA, EGPA, cryoglobulinemic vasculitis, and HSP. Direct immunofluorescence microscopy of vessels in biopsy specimens, such as glomerular capillaries or dermal venules, is useful because this demonstrates immunoglobulin A (IgA)-dominant vascular immunoglobulin deposits in HSP, IgG, and IgM deposits in cryoglobulinemic vasculitis, and little or no immunoglobulin in pauci-immune small-vessel vasculitis.

TABLE 48.6 **Features That Allow Differentiation of Microscopic Polyangiitis from Several Other Forms of Anca Vasculitis**

	Henoch-Schönlein Purpura	Cryoglobulin Vasculitis	Microscopic Polyangiitis	Granulomatosis with Polyangiitis	Eosinophilic granulomatosis
Small-vessel vasculitis signs and symptoms[a]	+	+	+	+	+
IgA-dominant immune deposits	+	0	0	0	0
Cryoglobulins in blood and vessels	0	+	0	0	0
ANCA in blood	0	0	+	+	+
Necrotizing granulomas	0	0	0	+	+
Asthma and eosinophilia	0	0	0	0	+

[a]All of these small-vessel vasculitides can manifest any or all of the shared features of small-vessel vasculitides, such as purpura, nephritis, abdominal pain, peripheral neuropathy, myalgias, and arthralgias. Each is distinguished by the presence and just as importantly the absence of certain specific features.
From Jennette JC, Falk R. Small vessel vasculitis. *N Engl J Med.* 1997;337:1512, with permission.

Serologic testing also helps to focus the differential diagnosis, for example, testing for ANCA, anti-GBM, cryoglobulins, hepatitis C or B, antinuclear antibodies (ANA), and complement component levels.

In summary, the precise and accurate diagnosis of different categories of vasculitis, including ANCA vasculitis, requires the knowledgeable integration of clinical, laboratory, and pathologic data.

Demographics

ANCA vasculitis affects men and women equally. All ages are susceptible to disease, with a peak age of 74.[81] In the southeastern United States, approximately one third of all kidney biopsy patients are black. There appears to be a seasonal variation of the onset of disease, which most commonly occurs in the late fall and early spring.[82] It is possible that in northern latitudes, GPA predominates, whereas MPA is more common in southern climates.

Clinical Features

Renal Disease

The renal manifestations of ANCA vasculitis are several. Many, if not most, patients present with rapidly progressive glomerulonephritis with hematuria, proteinuria, and a rising serum creatinine over the course of days to weeks. This clinical presentation is associated with pathologic findings of glomerular necrosis and crescent formation. Invariably, interstitial inflammation results in interstitial fibrosis. At the other end of the spectrum are patients who present with much milder disease marked by isolated hematuria and low-grade proteinuria. On biopsy, these patients have focal areas of necrosis that result in areas of focal glomerulosclerosis. Persistent microscopic hematuria can be the harbinger of different renal outcomes. In some patients, persistent hematuria correlates with focal inflammation in the kidney that with additional inflammatory stimuli (e.g., infection and environmental exposure) transforms into an aggressive acute nephritis. The acute nephritic presentation is usually associated with renal insufficiency, hypertension, and biopsy findings of diffuse glomerular necrosis and crescent formation. In contrast, some patients with persistent microscopic hematuria without proteinuria have a clinically indolent disease that, in the absence of a renal biopsy, is ascribed to IgA nephropathy or thin basement membrane disease. Frequently, a renal biopsy is delayed until azotemia or significant proteinuria develops. By then, the biopsy reveals a picture of chronic glomerulonephritis with widespread glomerular sclerosis and only focal necrosis. Unfortunately in such cases, the persistent microscopic hematuria is a reflection of unrecognized, unchecked glomerular inflammation. The treatment of such patients must be evaluated on a case-by-case basis depending on the degree of scarring and renal insufficiency, as the risks of aggressive anti-inflammatory and immunosuppressive treatment may outweigh the potential benefits.

In the recently derived classification proposal for ANCA vasculitis, histopathologic renal disease was categorized based on percent of normal glomeruli, amount of cellular versus fibrous or sclerotic crescents, and degree of glomerulosclerosis.[7] Based on classifying the renal biopsy by these criteria, valuable information regarding renal outcome was validated. The information gained by this classification system may allow prediction of renal outcome based on biopsy and may eventually prove beneficial in making treatment decisions.

Proteinuria in ANCA vasculitis is usually due to glomerulosclerosis or severe necrotizing and crescentic glomerulonephritis. In most cases of acute nephritis or rapidly progressive glomerulonephritis, the amount of proteinuria is on the order of 500 to 3,000 mg per 24 hours. The mean 24-hour urine protein excretion of our patient population at presentation is only 800 mg per 24 hours. Certainly there are cases of nephrotic-range proteinuria typically associated with diffuse glomerulosclerosis.

Acute interstitial nephritis is an unusual expression of ANCA vasculitis. These patients generally present with pyuria and white blood cell casts without evidence of hematuria or proteinuria. In these cases, the glomeruli are completely spared, and inflamed vasa rectae are accountable for the clinical findings.

There are many examples of patients in whom ANCA vasculitis coexists with other forms of glomerular injury, the most common of these being anti-GBM disease. Typically patients with both ANCA and anti-GBM have vasculitis affecting vascular beds other than the kidney and the lung. Their clinical course is more consistent with an ANCA vasculitis than with anti-GBM disease. However, a retrospective analysis of patients with both ANCA vasculitis and anti-GBM suggests that these patients have more severe renal disease and a poorer prognosis than patients with ANCA alone,[83] although ANCA vasculitis patients have more frequent relapse. It is unclear whether patients with both antibodies and severe renal failure share the poor renal prognosis of dialysis-dependent patients with anti-GBM disease alone. Indeed, some patients may respond to treatment with a dialysis-free interval of months to years.

Similarly, there are patients with ANCA vasculitis and immune complex forms of glomerulonephritis (e.g., membranous glomerulopathy or IgA nephropathy). Typically, the renal biopsy reveals areas of crescent transformation or glomerular necrosis. The clinical finding of a sudden decrease in renal function and worsening of the hematuria herald this pathologic event. ANCA vasculitis may occur in patients with scleroderma, in whom the renal dysfunction is not attributable to a thrombotic microangiopathy, but to ANCA-induced necrosis and crescent formation.

As noted previously in this chapter, vessels larger than capillaries and venules are targets of inflammation. Small arteries, including the renal artery, can be injured. The most common clinical consequence of this process is renal infarction resulting in flank pain and renal insufficiency. Persistent disease of the renal artery causes stenosis and poststenotic dilation, with the clinical presentation of renovascular hypertension. Renal arteriography is necessary to delineate the degree of renal artery disease. Angioplasty or surgical correction of the stenotic vessel is frequently curative.

Skin Disease

Because the most commonly affected vessels of ANCA vasculitis are capillaries and postcapillary venules, the typical skin lesion is palpable purpura. Lesions tend to occur in "crops," primarily on the lower extremities. With time, the lesions flatten and either disappear or leave small hyperpigmented areas. In addition to this classic dermal presentation, there are several other cutaneous lesions, including petechiae, ecchymosis, ulceration, nodules, plaque-like lesions, livido reticularis, and urticaria. Several cases of urticarial vasculitis have been observed in the absence of hypocomplementemia and immune-complex deposition. In unusual circumstances, vasculitic lesions give rise to erythema nodosum or pyoderma gangrenosum–like lesions. Biopsy of the affected area reveals a leukocytoclastic angiitis. However, in the case of nodular lesions, a simple punch biopsy may not provide sufficiently deep material to sample an involved vessel of larger caliber. A deep "excisional" biopsy is necessary.

The differential diagnosis of renal dermal vasculitic syndromes is important. In addition to the ANCA vasculitides, systemic lupus erythematosus (SLE), cryoglobulinemia, and HSP cause cutaneous vasculitides and renal disease. Each of these conditions is associated with a different natural history and treatment approach. For instance, many patients with HSP require only supportive care. If the renal dermal vasculitic syndrome is a consequence of ANCA vasculitis or lupus, immunosuppressive therapy is warranted. In addition, cutaneous vasculitis is frequently the consequence of a drug reaction. There are numerous classes of drugs that cause leukocytoclastic lesions, the most common being propylthiouracil, minocycline, phenytoin, and penicillamine.

Pulmonary Disease

The pulmonary consequences of ANCA vasculitis are numerous and involve not only the lung parenchyma, but also the respiratory tract from the subglottis to the alveolar sacs. Several clinical presentations are common. Patients with MPA typically present with pulmonary infiltrates that are frequently initially ascribed to an infectious process. Generally, these patients describe hemoptysis, although many patients have no overt evidence of pulmonary bleeding. In some cases, the infiltrates wax and wane spontaneously. Infiltrates may coalesce, resulting in dyspnea and hypoxemia. The most alarming consequence of pulmonary capillaritis is the development of massive pulmonary hemorrhage. In our series, the occurrence of pulmonary hemorrhage was the most powerful predictor of death.[84] As discussed later, the prompt institution of plasmapheresis substantially decreased the mortality rate when compared with conventional immunosuppressive treatments.

Necrotizing granulomatous inflammation is a hallmark of GPA. Focal necrotizing lesions progress to confluent areas of necrosis that when surrounded by palisading histocytes, are called "geographic necrosis."[85] Nodular lesions are of varying size, from those that can only be seen by spiral CT to those that occupy a complete lobe of the lung. In general, the larger lesions tend to cavitate. The differential diagnosis must include aspergillus or tuberculous infection, as well as other opportunistic infections. Determining whether the nodular and cavitary lesions are due to granulomatous infection or are a consequence of an opportunistic infection can present a difficult diagnostic dilemma. These two processes may coexist at times.

Similarly, recurrent alveolar hemorrhage in immunosuppressed patients may be attributable to infection. Alveolar lavage is useful in determining if alveolar hemorrhage is due to an infectious cause rather than a consequence of ANCA vasculitis alone. Bronchioalveolar lavage should be performed carefully considering the possible deterioration in oxygenation immediately after the procedure. Careful attention to the protection of airway patency is mandatory. Transbronchial biopsy of the lung in patients with these diseases often results in nondiagnostic results. Open lung biopsy may be required for diagnosing the cause of pulmonary nodules, granulomas, or cavitary lesions. In addition to the characteristic pulmonary nodules of GPA, endobronchial lesions, similar to those found in the subglottic region and trachea, can cause airway obstruction and may result in areas of collapsed lung. The lesions are usually quite sensitive to systemic glucocorticosteroid treatment.

EGPA is characterized by the presence of asthma and eosinophilia in the circulation and within tissues. The pulmonary infiltrates tend to result in diffuse alveolar involvement but nodules and cavitations also occur. Eosinophilic pneumonia of other causes can be indistinguishable from the pulmonary presentation of EGPA. Therefore, it is important to verify that a small-vessel vasculitis exists before determining that the patient has EGPA.

Patients with subglottic masses or stenosis present with stridor or a sense of breathlessness. Results of flow–volume loop study results are abnormal. These lesions necessitate emergent attention to avoid life-threatening critical airway narrowing. Direct laryngoscopy with fiberoptic instrumentation allows visualization of the lesion. Glucocorticoid treatment is usually effective, but surgical intervention may be necessary. Areas of tracheal and bronchial granulomatous lesions can occur throughout the respiratory tree and result in bronchial obstruction.

The long-term consequences of intermittent pulmonary capillaritis result in pulmonary fibrosis. In some individuals, the diagnosis of idiopathic pulmonary fibrosis prompts consideration of ANCA vasculitis. Similarly, some patients with bronchiolitis obliterans with organizing pneumonia have had an underlying ANCA vasculitis.

Upper Respiratory Tract Disease

Vasculitis frequently affects the areas of the ear, nose, and throat. By far the most common localization occurs in the nose, especially in patients with GPA. Other areas of involvement include the nasopharynx, the paranasal sinuses, and within the larynx. With respect to the nose, persistent or repetitive episodes of rhinosinusitis are one of the first symptoms. Small ulcerations lead to a nasal discharge that becomes hemorrhagic. Once these lesions become inflamed, a thick purulent material oozes from bloody crusts covering much larger areas of ulceration and granulation tissue. Histologic evaluation of these tissues most commonly reveals nonspecific acute and chronic inflammation. With a good sample, one may find areas of fibrinoid necrosis or granulomatous inflammation. Focal areas of ischemia and infarction occur. Repetitive bouts of inflammation eventually lead to septal perforations, the loss of turbinates, and may result in a loss of support of the nasal bridge (saddle nose deformity of GPA). Even with treatment, the nasal mucosa becomes atrophic and crusty. The crusts cause epistaxis when patients sneeze or blow their nose. *Staphylococcus aureus* superinfections may be the root cause of these ulcerations and an important factor in their development. Topical treatment with antibacterial ointments or systemic treatment with antibiotics decreases nasal symptoms and limits the number of relapses.[86]

Sinusitis typically occurs with bloody nasal or postnasal discharge. Computed tomography may reveal bony erosions caused by granulomatous lesions typical of GPA. Necrotizing capillaritis associated with MPA or EGPA frequently causes necrotizing lesions in the sinuses as well but do not lead to bony erosions. Granulomatous inflammation that blocks the eustachian tubes leads to serous otitis media. Bacterial superinfections lead to infectious otitis media. Ventilating tubes placed in the tympanic membrane may lessen the problem. Facial nerve paralysis may occur as a result of entrapment of the nerve by granulomatous inflammation anywhere along the course of the nerve. Large granulomatous pseudotumors invade the orbit and may lead to loss of an eye.

Gastrointestinal Tract Disease

The gastrointestinal tract represents one of the least well-studied areas of involvement of ANCA vasculitis. In our experience, at least one third of patients with active necrotizing glomerulonephritis have abdominal complaints, either on presentation or at some point during the course of disease. One of the more common areas of vasculitic involvement is the gastric mucosa, causing nonhealing gastric or peptic ulcers. It is sometimes difficult to determine whether these ulcers are the consequence of vascular inflammation or glucocorticoid treatment. Endoscopic biopsy can provide a diagnosis, yet a presumptive diagnosis is made by a favorable response to glucocorticoid therapy. Similarly, pancreatitis, small bowel infarction, and ulcers throughout the gastrointestinal tract lead to abdominal pain. The most catastrophic of all abdominal vasculitic disease is transmural infarction of the bowel, leading to viscus perforation and polymicrobial sepsis. Prompt diagnosis and treatment is mandatory.

Autoimmune hepatitis and sclerosing cholangitis occur with p-ANCA that is not specific for MPO. The liver is usually not involved with necrotizing vasculitis.

Patients with ANCA vasculitis may have medium-sized artery involvement as well. Aneurysmal dilation and fibrinoid necrosis of mesenteric or renal arteries results in infarction of the affected organ. If a mesenteric artery is involved, infarctions cause substantial abdominal pain or an ischemic colitis. These patients require mesenteric arteriography to identify the areas of arterial involvement.

Neurologic Disease

Mononeuritis multiplex, or a pattern of multiple mononeuropathies, is caused by nerve impairment in anatomically separate regions. Most commonly, these areas of peripheral nerve ischemia are found in areas in the midthigh or mid upper arm, in watershed zones of poor vascular perfusion. Lesions of peripheral neuropathy occur abruptly and are very painful. The pain is described as a deep ache that is difficult to localize. Symptoms of the cutaneous distribution of the nerve occur several days after the onset of weakness and are described as a burning pain. Nerve biopsy should be performed in individuals with neuropathy as the major manifestation of vasculitis. A negative sural nerve biopsy result does not rule out the diagnosis. Repetitive biopsy of the nerve is almost useless. In a series of 200 patients with vasculitis and a neuropathy, only 27% had a vasculitis demonstrated in a muscular specimen only, 35% in a nerve only, and 27% in the nerve and the muscle.[87] Many patients develop distal peripheral sensory neuropathies. Whether these symptoms are a consequence of vasculitis, pharmaceutical treatment, or malnutrition is not clear.

The central nervous system is an uncommon locus for vasculitis disease. Vasculitis involving the central nervous system usually results in a headache,[88] without which the diagnosis is unlikely. Rarely, seizures are the presenting manifestation of central nervous system vasculitis. In GPA, meningeal disease can occur. Magnetic resonance imaging (MRI) with gadolinium infusion may reveal enhancing lesions in many separate foci. Most commonly, however, ANCA vasculitis affects vessels that are too small to produce a positive MRI scan. Cerebral angiography may reveal abnormalities in less than half of patients. If the patient has systemic hypertension, cerebrovascular disease from atherosclerosis, or renal insufficiency resulting in uremia, it may not be possible to ascertain the precise cause of central nervous system symptoms. Treatment with antihypertensive agents and dialysis can exclude or decrease the possibility that hypertension and uremia are the cause of the symptoms. Many patients with ANCA vasculitis are older adults, and vasculitis may be impossible to differentiate from atherosclerosis in that population.

Other Organ System Diseases

Any organ system or capillary bed may be inflamed by small vessel vasculitis, resulting in numerous other clinical manifestations. Ocular manifestations of disease include iritis, uveitis, and peripheral keratitis. These lesions result in a red eye and are observed using a slit lamp by a qualified ophthalmologist.

Polychondritis may also present as a feature of disease presentation in small vessel vasculitis or as a hallmark symptom of disease relapse. There are patients who have erythema and severe tenderness of the ears that precedes signs of vasculitis in other organ systems.

Cardiac vasculitic disease results in subendocardial ischemia. The lesions can be difficult to see by using coronary arteriogram. Whether patients have coronary vascular disease as a consequence of atherosclerotic disease or of vasculitis is difficult to determine. In our population, 5% of patients had myocardial infarction at the time of their generalized disease process. Pericarditis is much less common in patients with ANCA vasculitis than in those with lupus vasculitis. A pericardial friction rub should raise the specter of a separate disease process.

In more than 90% of our patients, constitutional features are hallmarks of disease. Fatigue represents a ubiquitous finding that persists even after all of the other specific manifestations of vasculitis appear to be in remission. In addition, fever, unexplained weight loss, myalgias, and arthralgias are common. Arthralgias are frequently migratory in which joint pain occurs in one joint, only to resolve and appear in another joint at another time. Frank arthritis with synovial thickening occurs in at least 10% of patients.

Thrombosis in ANCA Disease

About 10% of patients with ANCA vasculitis have venous thromboembolic events (VTE).[89] In a retrospective analysis of a large cohort of patients with systemic vasculitis (n = 1130), the frequency of thrombotic events was 8% among patients with ANCA vasculitis compared with 2.5% among patients with polyarteritis nodosa.[90] Sixty-eight percent of VTE occurred within 3 months before or 6 months after the diagnosis of systemic vasculitis or a relapse, corresponding to a rate of 7.26 per 100 person-year during these periods compared to 1.84 per 100 person-year during follow-up (and presumably diminished disease activity). The frequency of VTE did not differ significantly among patients with GPA, MPA, or EGPA or between those with PR3- versus MPO-ANCA.

Investigation continues regarding the etiology and mechanism underlying the increased propensity for thromboembolic events in ANCA vasculitis. Results of anticardiolipin antibodies, anti-beta2-glycoprotein antibodies, factor V Leiden, prothrombin gene mutation, and methylenetetrahydrofolate reductase gene mutation measurements do not adequately explain the increased propensity for VTE in ANCA vasculitis.[91] Other factors may contribute to the increased propensity for thrombotic events among ANCA vasculitis patients. One such factor could be the presence of antiplasminogen antibodies detected in a subset of patients with PR3-ANCA.[90] In these patients, plasminogen was identified as a target of antibodies directed against complementary PR3 (cPR3), a recombinant protein translated from the antisense strand of PR3 cDNA. Functionally, antiplasminogen antibodies delayed the conversion of plasminogen to plasmin and increased the dissolution time of fibrin clots.[90] Antiplasminogen antibodies were detected in 5 of 9 patients (56%) with PR3-ANCA and a thrombotic event, compared with 5 of 57 (9%) patients with idiopathic thrombosis (P = 0.002). In an independent United Kingdom and Dutch cohort of patients with ANCA vasculitis, 24% and 26% of patients respectively had antiplasminogen antibodies compared with <1% of controls.[92] Antiplasminogen antibodies were present in both PR3 and MPO positive patients. Investigators also identified antitissue plasminogen activator antibodies in 18% of patients. These antitissue plasminogen activator antibodies were more commonly found in the population with antiplasminogen antibodies. Serum containing antiplasminogen antibodies and antitissue plasminogen activator antibodies appeared to be associated with retarded fibrinolysis in vitro. Presence of these antibodies was also correlated to fibrinoid necrosis and cellular crescents on kidney biopsy and consequently more severely reduced renal function.[92]

LABORATORY FINDINGS

Abnormal laboratory findings in patients with ANCA vasculitis include normochromic and normocytic anemia, mild to marked leukocytosis, and mild thrombocytosis. Eosinophilia is uncommon in patients with GPA and MPA but is required for the diagnosis of EGPA. Several markers of inflammation such as the C-reactive protein and the erythrocyte sedimentation rate are elevated, especially at times of disease exacerbation. Rheumatoid factor levels are positive in some individuals.

In the differential diagnosis of ANCA vasculitis, a number of other vasculitic syndromes can be excluded by serologic tests. These include tests for lupus, including ANA, anti–double-stranded DNA (dsDNA) antibodies, serum complement levels, and cryoglobulins. Rarely, a patient may have an overlap syndrome of SLE and ANCA vasculitis, with positive ANA, anti-dsDNA, and usually anti-MPO antibodies. Unlike with polyarteritis nodosa, screening for infectious diseases usually yields negative results, including assays for hepatitis B and hepatitis C. Anti-GBM antibodies should be measured at least once in the differential diagnosis of crescentic glomerulonephritis. Tests for circulating immune complexes are not reliable.

The laboratory findings in patients with EGPA include eosinophilia in all patients. The degree of eosinophilia may reach 50% of the total leukocyte count. Elevated serum IgE levels and IgA containing immune complexes are found in some patients.[93]

ANCA Serologic Studies

Since Richard Davies reported eight patients with antibodies to neutrophils associated with necrotizing glomerulonephritis,[94] substantial advances have been made in the serologic analysis of ANCA. ANCA reacts not only to neutrophils, but also to monocytes. Effective ANCA testing must use both indirect immunofluorescent microscopy in conjunction with antigen-specific tests using highly purified MPO and PR3 antigens.[46–49] Indirect immunofluorescent microscopy has elucidated two different ANCA patterns. On ethanol-fixed human neutrophils, cytoplasmic ANCA (c-ANCA) result in diffuse immunofluorescent staining of the cytoplasm. In contrast, perinuclear ANCA (p-ANCA) stain the periphery of the nucleus using ethanol-fixed cells but have a cytoplasmic pattern when using formalin-fixed leukocytes. Most c-ANCA react with PR3, a serine proteinase found within the primary granule of neutrophils and monocytes. This serine proteinase has substantial homology with elastase and cathepsin G. Some c-ANCA (less than 10%) react with bacterial/permeability increasing protein. This pattern of reactivity is found mainly in patients with cystic fibrosis and inflammatory bowel disease.[95]

p-ANCA react with MPO in more than 90% of cases. MPO is a member of a multichain peroxidase family that also includes thyroperoxidase, eosinophil peroxidase, and lactoperoxidase. Many if not most of the p-ANCA found in diseases other than pauci-immune necrotizing glomerulonephritis and ANCA vasculitis do not react with MPO, such as in ulcerative colitis, primary sclerosing cholangitis, and Felty syndrome. The most confusing situation occurs in patients with lupus erythematosus. In these patients, p-ANCA are usually attributable to ANA, although in some rare cases, antilactoferrin and antielastase antibodies are found. Patients with lupus may have a false-positive anti-MPO test result by enzyme-linked immunosorbent assay (ELISA).[96]

The antigen specificity of circulating ANCA is not diagnostic for a particular clinicopathologic variant of ANCA vasculitis, although there are differences in the relative frequency of PR3-ANCA and MPO-ANCA in different types of pauci-immune small-vessel vasculitis (Table 48.7). For example, most patients with GPA have PR3-ANCA (c-ANCA), whereas most patients with renal-limited pauci-immune crescentic glomerulonephritis have MPO-ANCA (p-ANCA).

A positive ANCA result in a patient with strong clinical evidence for crescentic glomerulonephritis or another manifestation of ANCA vasculitis, such as purpura or pulmonary hemorrhage, has a high positive predictive value. A positive ANCA result in a patient with weak evidence for crescentic glomerulonephritis or ANCA vasculitis, such as isolated hematuria and proteinuria with normal renal function, has a much lower positive predictive value (Table 48.8). However, in a patient with weak clinical evidence for crescentic glomerulonephritis or ANCA vasculitis, a positive result increases the likelihood to a level that requires expeditious additional diagnostic evaluation, possibly including a renal biopsy, to confirm or refute the presence of a pauci-immune ANCA vasculitis or crescentic glomerulonephritis. It is important to note, however, that in serum from the Department of Defence Serum Repository on patients who developed GPA, with years of serum collected preceding disease manifestation, PR3 was noted to be significantly elevated up to 1.5 years prior to GPA diagnosis. Stable detectable PR3 is significantly associated with future incidence of GPA.[97] A negative ANCA result is more effective at ruling out pauci-immune crescentic glomerulonephritis in a patient with weak clinical evidence of ANCA vasculitis than in a patient with strong clinical evidence for small-vessel vasculitis (Table 48.8). Approximately

TABLE 48.7 **Approximate Frequency of Antineutrophil Cytoplasmic Antibodies (ANCAs) with Specificity for Proteinase 3 (PR3-ANCA, c-ANCA) or Myeloperoxidase (MPO-ANCA, p-ANCA) in Patients with Active Untreated Microscopic Polyangiitis, Granulomatosis with Polyangiitis, and Eosinophilic granulomatosis**

	Microscopic Polyangiitis	Granulomatosis with Polyangiitis	Eosinophilic granulomatosis	Renal-limited Vasculitis[a]
PR3-ANCA c-ANCA	40%	75%	10%	20%
MPO-ANCA p-ANCA	50%	20%	60%	70%
Negative ANCA	10%	5%	30%	10%

[a]Renal-limited vasculitis refers to pauci-immune necrotizing and crescentic glomerulonephritis with no apparent extrarenal vasculitis.

TABLE 48.8 **Predictive Value of Combined Indirect Fluorescent Antibody and Enzyme Immunoassay Antineutrophil Cytoplasmic Antibody Testing for Pauci-immune Crescentic Glomerulonephritis[a]**

Adult with	Prevalence Pretest Likelihood	Positive predictive Value Post-test Likelihood	Negative Predictive Value Post-test Unlikelihood
RPGN	47%	95%	85%
Hematuria, proteinuria (creatinine >3 mg/dL)	21%	84%	95%
Hematuria, proteinuria (creatinine 1.5–3 mg/dL)	7%	60%	99%
Hematuria, proteinuria (creatinine <1.5 mg/dL)	2%	29%	100%

[a]Data derived from an analysis of 2,315 patients, with ANCA assay sensitivity 81% and specificity 96%.
RPGN, rapidly progressing glomerulonephritis.
From Lim LC, Taylor JG III, Schmitz JL, et al. Diagnostic usefulness of antineutrophil cytoplasmic autoantibody serology. Comparative evaluation of commercial indirect fluorescent antibody (IFA) kits and enzyme immunoassay (EIA) kits. *Am J Clin Pathol.* 1999;111(3):363, with permission.

10% of individuals who present with pauci-immune necrotizing and crescentic vasculitis with or without systemic vasculitis will have negative serologies for ANCA. It is not clear how these individuals differ from those who present with ANCA-positive vasculitis. The clinical presentation of this group of ANCA-negative individuals is not distinct from ANCA-positive vasculitis and there is currently no difference in the approach of managing these two groups. Therefore, ANCA-negative individuals are broadly lumped into ANCA vasculitis until further study on this group mandates alterations on this course.

The ANCA result is typically negative in patients with polyarteritis nodosa, Takayasu arteritis, or giant cell arteritis. Some individuals have an overlapping disease with vasculitic involvement not only of large vessels, but also of small arteries. These patients have either PR3- or MPO-ANCA.

PATHOGENESIS

There has been an explosion of knowledge pertaining to the pathogenesis of ANCA vasculitis and pauci-immune necrotizing glomerulonephritis, but much still remains to be discovered. Although GPA, MPA, and EGPA share the hallmark of pauci-immune necrotizing ANCA vasculitis, each presents phenotypic differences. Further study into the causes of the granulomatous lesions of GPA or the stimulation of the eosinophilia and asthma in EGPA continue. Furthermore, the severity of disease varies from one patient to another. Investigations continue to evaluate the host factors that produce minimal disease in some patients and severe disease in others. Intriguing also is the observation that whereas vasculitis affects many capillary beds (e.g., kidney, skin, or lung) in some patients, it is limited to one organ in others. In many instances, the disease processes are focal. For example, only a segment of a capillary bed is affected, leaving an adjacent segment spared. This is exemplified by the observation that a segmental necrotizing lesion in a glomerulus may sit adjacent to an ostensibly normal glomerular segment.

Substantial in vitro and in vivo data suggest that ANCA play a pivotal role in the pathogenesis of pauci-immune vasculitis and glomerulonephritis.[45,89,98] ANCA are found in 85% to 90% of patients with pauci-immune glomerulonephritis and ANCA vasculitis. There is an absence of evidence for clearly delineated pathogenic mechanisms, such as immune-complex disease or direct antibody attack–mediated disease. ANCA titers tend to correlate with disease activity in some patients, although there is a paucity of evidence that ANCA titers can reliably predict disease severity or relapse. There is a clear description of transplacental transfer of MPO-ANCA from a mother with active MPA during pregnancy resulting in a pulmonary-renal vasculitic syndrome in the newborn infant.[99,100] In some human cases of a drug-induced ANCA vasculitis, cessation of the offending agent is associated with remission of small-vessel vasculitis and diminution of ANCA titers. In drug-induced ANCA vasculitis, there have been reports that the specificity is to human neutrophil elastase (HNE) ANCA. HNE belongs to the chymotrypsin family of serine proteases. HNE ANCA has been described in relation to cocaine-induced ANCA and ANCA related to antithyroid drugs.[101,102]

A number of laboratories have confirmed that ANCA induce neutrophil and monocyte activation using various methods. ANCA participate in the pathogenesis of vasculitis by interaction with MPO or PR3 that have translocated to the surface of the neutrophil or monocyte. Membrane-bound MPO/PR3 is expressed constitutively by neutrophils,[103] and this translocation is stimulated by low concentrations of TNFα and interleukin-γ and other cytokines.[104] Patients with ANCA vasculitis aberrantly express PR3 and MPO genes through epigenetic mechanisms, and this expression correlates with disease activity.[105–107] Interestingly, although the MPO and PR3 genes are on different chromosomes, message from both of these genes is coordinately increased, suggesting a similar, but unrecognized, transcription factor that may be regulating the production of many granular constituents.[106]

ANCA binding to MPO or PR3 induce premature respiratory burst in polymorphonuclear leukocytes and degranulation of primary and secondary granules[90,108–110] at the time of their margination and diapedesis. This process leads to the release of lytic enzymes and toxic oxygen metabolites at the site of the vessel wall, causing endothelial cell damage[111] and necrotizing inflammatory injury.

Neutrophils and monocytes are activated by two coordinated and separate signal transduction pathways. Previous controversy abounded as to whether ANCA activation of neutrophils and monocytes occurred by the Fc receptor alone or whether there was F(ab′)2 stimulation.[112] Human neutrophils constitutively express receptors for IgG, including FcRIIa and FcRIIIb. The former is a widely expressed receptor, whereas the latter is a low-affinity receptor with expression that is restricted to neutrophils and eosinophils.[113] Engagement of the Fc receptor results in a number of neutrophil-activation events, including respiratory burst, degranulation, phagocytosis, cytokine production, and upregulation of adhesion molecules.[111,112] Fc receptors are likewise engaged in the activation of neutrophils and monocytes by ANCA.[111,114] Polymorphisms of the Fc receptors could play an important role in the development of ANCA vasculitis. Whereas the FcRIIa single nucleotide polymorphisms appear unimportant,[115] evidence suggests that the FcRIIIb polymorphism may influence disease severity.[116] In addition to Fc receptor–induced activation, there are substantial data that the $F(ab')_2$ portion of the antibody molecule also plays a role in leukocyte activation. ANCA $F(ab')_2$ not only induce oxygen radical production,[112] but also induce the transcription of cytokine genes in normal human neutrophils and monocytes. Some genes are upregulated by both whole ANCA immunoglobulin and ANCA $F(ab')_2$, whereas other genes are upregulated by only one or the other.[116] It is most likely that $F(ab')_2$ portions of ANCA are capable of low-level neutrophil and monocyte activation.[112] The Fc portion of the molecule almost certainly causes leukocyte activation once the $F(ab')_2$ portion of the immunoglobulin has interacted with the antigen, either on the cell surface or in the microenvironment.[111] The signal transduction pathways of F(ab′)2 and Fc receptor activation have been nicely elucidated. Both of these possible activation pathways appear to activate a specific p21ras (Kristen-ras) through separate but coordinated pathways.[117] This important observation may provide a focus for a therapeutic target.

PR3 and MPO released from neutrophils and monocytes enter endothelial cells and cause cell damage. PR3 entry into the endothelial cells induces apoptosis via production of IL-8 and chemoattractant protein-1.[118–120] Likewise, MPO has been shown to be internalized into endothelial cells by an energy-dependent process,[121] and to transcytose intact endothelium to localize within the extracellular matrix. There, in the presence of the substrates H_2O_2 and NO_2^-, MPO catalyzes nitration of tyrosine residues on extracellular matrix proteins,[122] resulting in the fragmentation of extracellular matrix protein.[122,123] Evidence now supports endothelial cell injury by ANCA-activated neutrophils being mediated by serine proteases (PR3, elastase) instead of superoxide generation.[124]

There have been a number of in vitro models of ANCA neutrophil and endothelial cell interactions using flow models and intravital microscopy. With treatment using TNF, endothelial cells capture neutrophils from the circulation. With the addition of ANCA over these rolling neutrophils, a more substantial adhesion of leukocytes to endothelial cells and transmigration of leukocytes occur. This occurs through a conformational change on CD11b that reveals an activation epitope.[125]

The Role of T Cells

There is mounting evidence implicating T cells in the pathogenesis of ANCA vasculitis. It has long been known that there are circulating T cells in patients with ANCA vasculitis that have a Th1-type cytokine profile and are in a persistent state of activation. It has been difficult to demonstrate that circulating T cells derived from affected patients are activated by the ANCA target antigens. The predominance of IgG1 and IgG4 subclasses of ANCA denotes the effects of T-cell help and IL-4 on isotype switching.[126] Furthermore, in patients with ANCA glomerulonephritis, the concentrations of soluble IL-2 receptor, which is a marker of T-cell activation, neopterin, and soluble CD30 correlate well with disease activity.[127,128]

Memory T cell populations increase and naïve T cells are decreased.[129,130] T cells are found within granulomas and active vasculitic lesions in ANCA vasculitis.[131–133] Analysis of the profile of cytokine secretion by T cells derived from tissue with granulomatous inflammation (nasal mucosa or bronchiolar lavage fluid) as well as from peripheral blood T cells revealed a T-helper 1 (T_H1) pattern of cytokines.[134] This is corroborated by the finding that T cells from patients with GPA have a decreased expression of CD28 as compared to healthy controls.[135] CD28 costimulation promotes the production of T_H2 cytokines.[136] Conversely, a recent study looking at the cytokine profile of T cells from patients with ANCA vasculitis in complete remission and receiving *no* immunosuppressants revealed a T_H2 cytokine profile with elevated production of IL-6 and IL-10 and low production of interferon gamma (IFN-γ).[137] These differences in the detected cytokine profiles could be due to the state of disease activity. A subset of CD134+, GITR+ (glucocorticoid-induced

TNF-receptor-related protein) effecter memory T cells have been shown to be in greatly increased numbers in patients with GPA.[138] These cells were noted in active vasculitic lesions and are powerful immune cells that initiate and sustain immune responses.[139] Interestingly, effecter memory T cells have been noted in urine suggesting T cell migration to sites of active vasculitic lesions with disease activity.[140] T cells and monocytes are the predominant cell types in inflammatory vascular and perivascular lymphoid infiltrates in ANCA vasculitis.[133] Areas of lymphoid neogenesis or tertiary lymphoid organs are described in states of chronic inflammation[141] that resemble the structure of secondary lymphoid organs consisting of B cell follicles with a surrounding mantle zone of T cells and dendritic cells. T cells are activated via antigen presentation within these areas of lymphoid neogenesis. It is postulated that tissue-specific autoantigens are presented in these tertiary lymphoid organs[139,141] and due to lack of organized lymph flow and antigen-presenting cell trafficking (which are found in secondary lymphoid organs) antigens, antigen-presenting cells, and lymphocytes bathe in a persistent milieu of activation and autoimmunity. Granulomas are thought to be a form of these areas of lymphoid neogenesis or tertiary lymphoid organs.[132,142] PR3 within granulomas leads to TH1 activation via dendritic cells.[143,144] Speculation is that production of ANCA occurs in these areas of granulomas where affinity maturation of B cells is taking place.[139,142] Although granulomas are not commonly found in the kidney biopsies of patients with ANCA vasculitis, some form of lymphoid neogenesis has been noted.[138,145,146]

IL-17, produced by Th17 effecter T cells, stimulates activation and migration of neutrophils via secretion of TNF-α and IL-1β.[147] PR3 reactive Th17 cells have been shown to be expanded in patients in remission from GPA.[148,149] IL-17 is also produced via CD45RC T helper cells in ANCA vasculitis.[150] Migration of neutrophils via these factors may be an important factor in the pathogenesis of ANCA vasculitis.

Regulatory T cells that limit immune response may be dysfunctional in ANCA vasculitis.[151] Defects noted in regulatory T cells include failure to inhibit proliferation or cytokine production of effector T cells.[152,153] Dysfunctional regulatory T cells may be linked to effector memory T cell expansion and persistent T cell activation. One study has shown an increase in FoxP3+ regulatory T cells in patients in remission from ANCA vasculitis, although this finding was not noted by other investigators.[129,154]

In vitro analyses of peripheral blood T cell proliferation in response to MPO and PR3 yielded conflicting results. Studies have shown little or no difference in T-cell reactivity to PR3 between patients with ANCA vasculitis and controls.[155,156] In the largest study looking at T cell proliferative responses in 45 patients at various stages of disease (with and without treatment), PR3 responses were seen at all stages of disease activity, and to a lesser degree in healthy controls.[157] Interestingly, T cells from only two patients with PR3-ANCA, and none of the controls, proliferated in response to MPO.

Neutrophil Extracellular Traps

Recently, neutrophil extracellular traps (NETs) were reported to be present in kidney tissue affected by ANCA vasculitis.[158] Neutrophils release NETs, which are decondensed chromatin fibers containing PR3, MPO, elsastase, LL-37, and other cytoplasmic proteins. The function of NETs is entrapment and destruction of microbes.[159] With respect to autoimmunity, it is important to note that in ANCA vasculitis, LL-37 present in NETs can modify trapped DNA leading to activated dendritic cells and B cells via toll-like receptor sensing pathways.[160] Neutrophil release of NETs in ANCA vasculitis leads to IFN-α-stimulated plasmacytoid dendritic cells in the kidney.[158] It has been postulated that IFN-α may impair regulatory T cells thus promoting further inflammation.[161] Triggering of Toll-like receptors has also been postulated to lead to local B cell maturation and autoantibody production.[162]

Role of *Staphylococcus aureus* and Superantigens

Clinical studies reveal that 60% to 70% of patients with GPA have a chronic nasal carriage of *S. aureus*[86] that is associated with an eightfold increased rate of relapse.[163] Importantly, in a placebo-controlled randomized trial, patients with nasal carriage of *S. aureus* treated with trimethoprim-sulfamethoxazole had a significantly lower rate of relapse of the nasal or upper respiratory tract disease. *S. aureus* superantigens are most likely implicated in disease activity. For instance, patients with superantigen-positive *S. aureus* strains are more likely to have a relapse of disease than carriers of superantigen-negative strains.[164] The staphylococcal acid phosphatase appears to bind to the endothelium as a consequence of its cationic nature and is recognized by the sera of patients with GPA.[164] In addition, Brown-Norway rats immunized with staphylococcal acid phosphatase and then perfused with this same protein developed severe crescentic glomerulonephritis.[165]

Environmental Factors (Including Infections)

The first report of ANCA was an association in eight patients with necrotizing glomerulonephritis and arbovirus infection with the Ross River virus.[88] Several animal models suggest an association of arteritis and infection. For instance, parvovirus B19 is associated with a vasculopathy not only in humans, but also in the Aleutian mink.[166] These animals develop a chronic parvovirus illness that results in immune complex–mediated vasculitis. There are several animal models of infection-mediated vasculitis in which there may be direct invasion of the vascular wall.

Environmental factors, particularly exposure to silica dust and other silica-containing compounds, may increase the risk of developing a number of different autoimmune diseases including scleroderma, rheumatoid arthritis, systemic sclerosis, SLE, and vasculitis.[167] Early data were derived from studies that primarily evaluated cohorts of workers in occupations with high exposure to silica dust. This type of study is not ideal for assessing rare outcomes, such as autoimmune diseases. Case-control studies of specific autoimmune disorders have offered more insight into diseases potentially associated with silica dust exposure. Previous case-control studies have shown an association between ANCA vasculitides and exposure to silica dust or other silica-containing compounds[168,169] with odds ratios ranging from 4.4 to 14.0. More recently, a case-control study reported an association between primary systemic vasculitis and farming activities and exposure to occupational solvents, but the association with exposure to silica could not be ascertained.[170] In a study involving 129 patients with ANCA vasculitis with glomerulonephritis and 109 matched controls, only prolonged silica exposure (>23 years) was statistically significantly more common among patients than controls. There was no difference between the two groups in exposure to silica of shorter duration.[171] In contrast, exposure to silica dust was not associated with the development of lupus nephritis, in contrast to reports from occupational cohorts.[169,172,173]

Many drugs can induce vasculitis. In fact, 10% to 20% of cutaneous reactions to drug exposure are vasculitic in nature. A list of the most frequently implicated drugs includes anticonvulsants, antibiotics, penicillamine, hydralazine, nonsteroidal anti-inflammatory drugs, and propylthiouracil.[174] One of the drugs most commonly related to the development of anti-MPO–induced disease is propylthiouracil.[174] The story on cocaine is an interesting one. In 11 patients positive for MPO or PR3 ANCA with a history of cocaine use 5 patients were positive for both MPO and PR3, 8 had vasculitic rash, and 3 had renal disease involvement.[175] The hypothesis is that cocaine itself may not be the vasculitis promoting agent but in fact levamisole (an agent previously used for chemotherapy and for antihelminthic properties) that has recently been used for cutting cocaine may be associated with inducing ANCA vasculitis. This will need to be further investigated before definitive conclusions can be made.

Animal Models

There are now excellent animal models of ANCA vasculitis. The most direct evidence of the pathogenic role of anti-MPO antibodies stems from a model of transfer of either splenocytes or anti-MPO antibodies into Rag 2−/− mice.[176] In this model, MPO knockout mice (MPO−/−) were immunized with purified mouse MPO, and developed mouse anti-mouse-MPO antibodies. When splenocytes from these mice were transferred into Rag 2−/− mice, which lack functioning T and B cells, these animals developed a systemic necrotizing vasculitis and severe necrotizing and crescentic glomerulonephritis. When anti-MPO antibodies derived from immunized MPO knockout mice were transferred into Rag 2−/− mice, a pauci-immune necrotizing and crescentic glomerulonephritis was induced. This disease process occurred without antigen-driven T cells. Several follow-up studies have now been performed using this mouse model. In particular, the disease process was aggravated by the administration of lipopolysaccharide (LPS) into recipient mice by increasing the percentage of glomeruli involved with necrotizing and crescentic glomerulonephritis when anti-MPO antibodies were transferred into these mice.[177] The role of neutrophils in this response was highlighted by the abrogation of disease when the neutrophils of anti-MPO recipient mice were depleted by a selective antineutrophil monoclonal antibody (NIMP-R14).[178]

The pathogenic role of anti-MPO antibodies is also documented in a second animal model.[179] In this model, rats immunized with human MPO developed anti-rat-MPO antibodies. These animals then developed a necrotizing and crescentic glomerulonephritis, as well as pulmonary capillaritis. Microscopy of superior mesenteric vessels demonstrated that when a chemokine was applied to the vessel, the anti-MPO antibodies induced adherence and margination of leukocytes to the vessel wall. These two animal models document that anti-MPO antibodies are capable of causing a necrotizing and crescentic glomerulonephritis and a widespread systemic vasculitis, and also demonstrate that cytokines and chemokines exacerbate the injury in a manner that mimics the in vitro studies of ANCA-induced leukocyte activation.

A model of anti-PR3-induced vascular injury was developed in which a perivascular infiltrate was observed around cutaneous vessels in the setting of anti-PR3 antibodies and cytokine exposure.[89,180] Vasculitis and severe segmental and necrotizing glomerulonephritis was noted in nonobese diabetic mice with severe combined immunodeficiency given splenocytes from mice immunized with recombinant mouse PR3.[181] In summary, these animal studies document that both anti-MPO and proteinase-3 antibodies are capable of causing disease.

In immune-incompetent Rag′2 mice that developed ANCA vasculitis from the transfer of splenocytes of MPO knockout mice immunized with murine MPO, a previously unsuspected role of complement activation was demonstrated. Glomerulonephritis and vasculitis were completely blocked by complement depletion with cobra venom factor.[182] In this model, ANCA vasculitis failed to develop in mice deficient for complement factors C5 and B, whereas C4-deficient mice developed disease comparable with wild-type mice.[182] These results indicate that the alternative complement pathway (but not the classic or lectin pathways) is required for disease induction. Furthermore, the glomerulonephritis is completely abrogated or markedly ameliorated by treating the mice with a C5-inhibiting monoclonal antibody.[183] These results are corroborated by in vitro experiments that demonstrate that blockade of the C5a receptor on human neutrophils abrogated their stimulation.[184] In aggregate, results suggest an important role of complement activation in the pathogenesis of ANCA vasculitis; however, their relevance to disease in humans remains to be established.

The mannose receptor was highlighted by Chavele et al. as essential for producing crescentic glomerulonephritis in the mouse model of nephrotoxic nephritis.[185] The mannose receptor is a pattern recognition receptor present on alternatively activated macrophages (macrophages that appear to have a reparative function rather than a proinflammatory phenotype). In normal murine kidney, the mannose receptor is present primarily on mesangial cells. The mannose receptor is a lectin scavenger receptor with a role in clearance of endogenous material. This receptor binds to myeloperoxidase, collagen IV, and glycosylated immunoglobulins and has a role in Fc-mediated responses. Mannose receptor-deficient mice who displayed normal antibody and T cell function were protected from crescentic glomerulonephritis via mesangial cell apoptosis, diminishment of Fc-mediated responses, and generation of anti-inflammatory macrophages. The implications of these findings may eventually lead to targeted therapy that preserves adaptive immune responses.

Theories of Autoimmunity: Why Do Patients Make ANCA?

For all autoimmune diseases, the critical question is whether the most proximate cause is the formation of the autoantibody or the abnormal T cell clone. There have been a number of theories that may provide a basis for the alteration of self-antigens, the most plausible of which is known as the theory of molecular mimicry.[186] This theory suggests that there is an immune response directed against a microbial antigen that mimics the amino acid sequence or structure of a self-protein. To date, it has been difficult to demonstrate this theory in human autoimmune disease. A serendipitous finding in ANCA vasculitis has spawned a theory of autoantigen complementarity. Although the details of this theory and the proof that it may pertain to ANCA vasculitis is beyond the scope of this chapter, a brief description of this observation is germane for the understanding of ANCA vasculitis (Fig. 48.10).[187,188]

It has been known for decades that proteins transcribed and translated from the sense strand of DNA bind to proteins that are transcribed and translated from the antisense strand of DNA. Some patients with PR3 ANCA harbored antibodies to an antigen complementary to the middle portion of PR3. These anticomplementary PR3 antibodies formed an anti-idiotypic pair with PR3-ANCA. Moreover, cloned complementary PR3 proteins bind to PR3 and function as a serine proteinase inhibitor. What is the source of the complementary PR3 antigen? Preliminary data suggest that these proteins are found on a variety of microbes, some of which have been associated with ANCA vasculitis and also found in the genome of some patients with both PR3- and MPO-ANCA.[188] These studies need to be confirmed and expanded to understand what the source of the complementary PR3 antigen is in any given person, and just as importantly, whether these complementary proteins are capable of inducing disease. If these observations remain true, they may provide a promising avenue for the detection of the proximate cause of the autoimmune response in any given person.

There has been an alternate theory proposed for the genesis of pauci-immune necrotizing and crescentic glomerulonephritis based on the observation that some patients

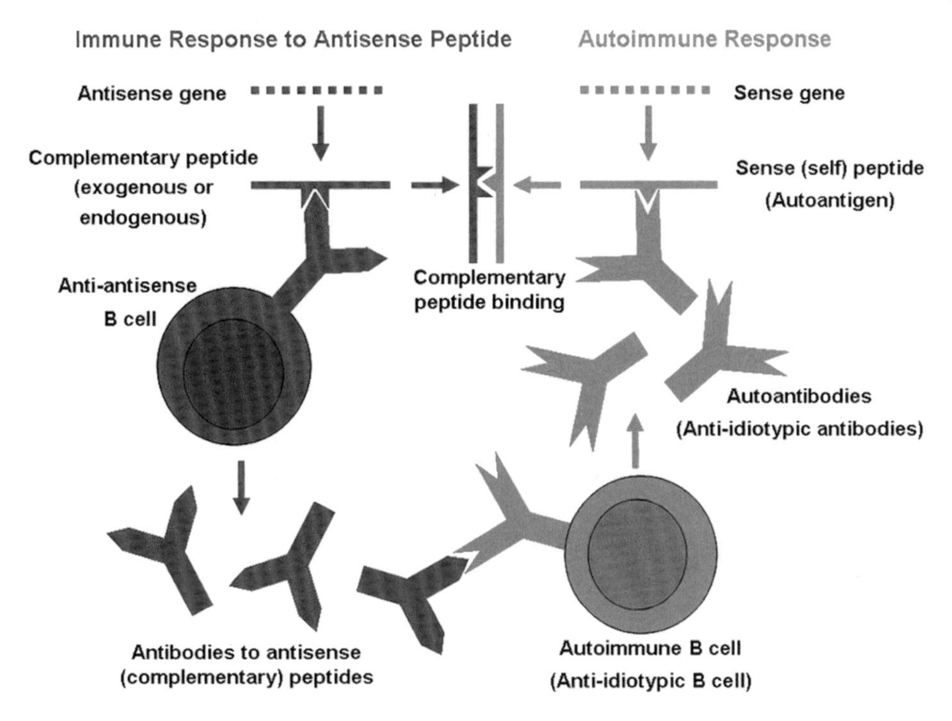

FIGURE 48.10 Schematic of a mechanism for the development of autoimmunity (theory of autoantigen complementarity) as a consequence of an immune response to a protein whose amino acid sequence is complementary to a self-protein.

with ANCA vasculitis have antibodies to another neutrophil protein, lysosome-associated membrane protein 2 (LAMP2). Kain et al. document that LAMP2 is capable of neutrophil activation and endothelial damage in vitro.[189] LAMP2 has homology to a protein expressed by fimbriated bacteria (FimH). Antibodies to either FimH peptides or LAMP2 peptides were shown to induce necrotizing and crescentic glomerulonephritis in rats. The theory proposed that anti-LAMP2 antibodies could therefore result from molecular mimicry as a result of infection with gram-negative organisms making FimH. From 680 ANCA patients between two academic centers, anti-LAMP-2 reactivity was present in 21% of ANCA sera and 16% of the control group with urinary tract infections. Titers of anti-myeloperoxidase and anti-proteinase 3 antibodies were 1,500-fold and 10,000-fold higher than anti-LAMP-2 titers, respectively. There was no correlation between anti-LAMP-2 antibodies and disease activity. Data do not support a mechanixtic relationship between anti-LAMP-2 antibodies and ANCA glomerulonephritis.[190,191]

Pathogenesis of Eosinophilic Granulomatosis

Eosinophilic granulomatosis is characterized by a necrotizing vasculitis involving primarily the small- and medium-size vessels, peripheral blood eosinophilia, allergic rhinitis, eosinophil-rich granulomatous inflammation presenting with pulmonary nodules, and upper airway and bronchial lesions leading to severe asthma. Forty percent of patients with EGPA are ANCA positive, usually directed against MPO.[192] ANCA-positive and -negative EGPA appear to differ to some extent with regard to the frequency and character of organ involvement. ANCA-positive patients are more likely to manifest signs of necrotizing glomerulonephritis, pulmonary hemorrhage, peripheral neuropathy, and purpura, whereas ANCA-negative patients are more likely to present cardiac involvement and pulmonary infiltrates.[62,192] Potential triggers of disease include desensitization treatment, inhaled antigens, free-base cocaine, and the use of leukotriene receptor antagonists (LTRA); however, only 23% of patients with EGPA report a potential triggering factor.[192] It is unclear whether the use of LTRAs stimulates a reduction in corticosteroid dose allowing for greater disease manifestation, whether they are prescribed to patients with severe asthma representing an early phase of the disease, or if LTRAs are causative of EGPA. Upon careful review of all cases of suspected drug-induced EGPA reported to the U.S. Food and Drug Administration (FDA) between 1996 and 2003 (n = 1274), the diagnosis could be confirmed in 181 cases, 90% of whom had a preceding exposure to LTRA.[193] A positive ANCA test was detected in 42% of the cases tested.

IL-5 and other Th2 cytokines seem to have a key role in the development of eosinophilia in EGPA[194] and patients with active EGPA appear to have elevated plasma levels of IL-5.[195] Peripheral blood mononuclear cell production of IL-5 may be increased in vitro in the setting of T cell activation.[194] IL5 induces terminal differentiation of committed eosinophil precursors,[196] prolongs their survival,[197] induces their degranulation and antibody-depended cytotoxicity,[198] and promotes their adhesion to endothelial cells and transmigration from the vasculature.[199]

T cells from patients with EGPA exhibit increased production of Th2 cytokines IL-4 and IL-13.[200] Migration of eosinophils to inflammatory sites appears to be mediated by Eotaxin-3.[201] Increased levels of Eotaxin-3 correlate to levels of disease activity and inflammation.[202]

Patients with EGPA have elevated production of the Th-1 cytokine IFNγ from peripheral T cell lines.[194] A recent study compared chronic eosinophilic pneumonia and asthma to EGPA and noted decreased CD4+ CD25+ T cells that produce IL-10 in active EGPA. These cells were noted to be increased in EGPA for patients in remission.[203] The relative importance of Th-1 and Th-2 responses may differ in patients with predominantly eosinophilic/allergic phenotype versus vasculitic/granulomatous manifestations of EGPA. Patients with active EGPA also exhibit decreased frequency of peripheral Treg cells,[204] and increased frequency of Th17 cells when compared to patients with asthma and chronic eosinophilic pneumonia.[203] Treg cells increase and Th17 cells decrease in EGPA remission.

TREATMENT

Induction

The treatment of ANCA vasculitis and glomerulonephritis rests primarily on the use of induction methylprednisolone, high-dose corticosteroids, cyclophosphamide, and most recently rituximab. As the serum creatinine concentration at the time of treatment is a significant determinant of long-term renal outcome, pulse methylprednisolone (7 mg/kg/day for 3 days) is used to curb the active inflammation as soon as possible. This is followed by instituting prednisone at a daily dosage of 1 mg/kg/day (not to exceed 80 mg per day for the first month of therapy). Corticosteroids are then tapered over the second month to an alternate-day dosing schedule and subsequently decreased every week by 10 to 20 mg per day until they are eventually discontinued by the end of the fourth to fifth month. In our population, patients maintained on corticosteroids beyond 6 months have no decrease in risk of relapse but do have a significantly greater risk of infections and a trend toward development of new onset diabetes mellitus. This is in contradistinction to meta-analysis data that noted a higher relapse rate in studies where corticosteroids were discontinued prior to 12 months of therapy.[205] This meta-analysis had significant heterogeneity among the studies included and duration of glucocorticoid dosing was not the primary treatment variable in any of the randomized controlled trials. Furthermore, this analysis was not based on patient-level data, and duration of glucocorticoid therapy was estimated from the described protocols. The rate of decrease in corticosteroid dosing should be tailored based on an assessment of each patient's disease activity.

The beneficial role of cyclophosphamide in the treatment of acute ANCA vasculitis is evidenced by the substantial improvement in the rate of remission (56% to 85%) and a threefold decrease in the risk of relapse associated with the use of this drug.[206] For many years cyclophosphamide has been administered as a daily oral regimen or as monthly intravenous pulses. When the intravenous route is used, it is usually started at a dose of 0.5 g per m^2 of body surface area, which is subsequently increased to a maximal dosage of 1 g per m^2. This dose is adjusted to maintain the 2-week leukocyte nadir at more than 3,000 per mm^3. When the daily oral regimen is used, cyclophosphamide is given at a daily dosage of 1.5 to 2 mg per kg.[206] To prevent severe leukopenia, careful attention to the leukocyte count must be maintained throughout this therapy. Cyclophosphamide was traditionally continued for a total of 6 to 12 months. Investigation into intravenous cyclophosphamide therapy has led the community away from using daily oral cyclophosphamide as first-line induction therapy. The intravenous regimen allows for a two to three times smaller total dose of cyclophosphamide than the oral regimen. A regimen of daily oral cyclophosphamide may be associated with a decreased risk of relapse.[207] However, in a meta-analysis of three randomized controlled trials comparing pulse versus oral continuous cyclophosphamide, pulse cyclophosphamide attained a statistically higher rate of remission, and lower rates of leukopenia and infections. Pulse cyclophosphamide was associated with a higher rate of relapse, which was not statistically significant.[208] The final outcomes of patients (death or end-stage kidney disease [ESKD]) were no different in the two groups despite the lower rate of relapse in the oral cyclophosphamide group.[208] The question of pulse versus oral cyclophosphamide was even more definitively addressed in a large, randomized controlled trial of pulse versus daily oral cyclophosphamide for induction of remission.[74] One-hundred and forty-nine patients with newly diagnosed ANCA vasculitis with renal involvement (creatinine < 500 μM per L) were randomized to receive either pulse cyclophosphamide, 15 mg per kg every 2 weeks for three infusions then an infusion every 3 weeks, or daily oral cyclophosphamide, 2 mg per kg per day. GPA, MPA, and renal-limited disease were evenly spread across the groups, as was serum positivity for PR3 versus MPO. Demographics, serum creatinine, and markers for disease severity were well matched between the groups. Primary outcome was time to remission. Change in renal function, adverse events, and cumulative dose of cyclophosphamide was also evaluated. Cyclophosphamide therapy was continued 3 months beyond the time of remission. All patients were then switched to azathioprine (2 mg/kg/day orally) until month 18, end of study follow-up. All patients received prednisolone starting at 1 mg per kg orally, tapered to 12.5 mg at the end of month 3 and to 5 mg at the end of the study (month 18). Median time to remission was 3 months for both groups. The two treatment groups did not differ in time to remission or proportion of patients who achieved remission at 9 months. No differences in renal function were noted between the two groups at any time point. Due to power constraints, the study could not detect a difference in relapse rates between the two groups. By 18 months, 13 patients in the pulse group and 6 in the daily oral group had a relapse (HR, 2.01 [CI, 0.77 to 5.30]). Absolute cumulative cyclophosphamide dose in the daily oral group was almost twice that in the pulse group with consequent statistically significant increased rate of leukopenia in the daily oral group. Serious infections did not differ between the two treatment groups. Overall, with the results of this randomized controlled trial confirming the similar rates and time to remission of the two cyclophosphamide regimens, and pulse cyclophosphamide being associated with about half of the cumulative dose of the medication and a significantly lower rate of leukopenia, the pulse regimen is considered first-line induction therapy for ANCA vasculitis. The trend toward a higher rate of relapse with pulse cyclophosphamide appears late (after 15 to 18 months) and is of unclear clinical significance on the long-term outcome of patients.

Strategy in the above study was to use cyclophosphamide three months after the documentation of remission followed by azathioprine for remission maintenance until 18 months (end of follow-up). In another report, cyclophosphamide was used for 3 months once remission was attained followed by azathioprine continued for 12 to 24 months.[209] This regimen offers the advantage of a limited use of cyclophosphamide and results in similar rates of remission and relapse as cyclophosphamide-only–based therapies.

In an uncontrolled study, 32 patients with 34 episodes of active ANCA vasculitis received induction treatment with oral MMF 1,000 mg twice daily for at least 12 months and oral prednisolone 1 mg per kg once daily for 6 weeks followed by a taper.[210] Complete remission was obtained in 78% of patients and partial remission in 19%. Relapse occurred in 52% of those who obtained complete remission and 100% after partial remission. The median relapse-free survival was 16 months and all but two patients were still on MMF at the time of relapse. Patients who had previously been treated successfully with cyclophosphamide responded better than those who had not, suggesting that MMF is unlikely to succeed in patients who are "resistant" to cyclophosphamide therapy.

In a controlled study of MMF plus corticosteroids compared to cyclophosphamide plus corticosteroids for induction therapy in ANCA vasculitis, 35 patients from Nanjing, China, were evaluated for remission at 6 months.[211] Follow-up beyond 6 months is not provided. The groups were well matched for demographic characteristics, activity score, duration and severity of kidney disease, and proteinuria. In the intention-to-treat analysis, assuming that those lost to follow-up did not respond, the remission rate at 6 months was 77.8% in the MMF group versus 47.1% in the cyclophosphamide group ($P = .09$ by Fisher's test). However, when patients lost to follow-up were excluded from the analysis, 61.5% of patients in the cyclophosphamide group had remission resulting in a difference of 16.3% between the groups ($P = .4$). The results of this study are limited by the small sample size and the very short duration of follow-up.

MMF was studied in 17 patients with MPO-positive pANCA MPA with active urine sediment or biopsy proven renal involvement and creatinine less than three with no life- or organ-threatening disease manifestations.[212] MMF 1,000 mg orally was given twice a day for 18 months in conjunction with corticosteroids (IV methylprednisolone 1 to 3 g followed by oral prednisone at 1 mg per kg per day tapered off by 6 months). Thirteen out of 17 patients reached the primary outcome of remission at 6 months with stable renal function. Of these, 12 patients remained in remission through month 18. Adverse events reported in this study were mild and treated by MMF titration in all but one patient who was deemed MMF intolerant.

Patients suffering primarily from mild ANCA vasculitis without renal involvement may benefit from the use of methotrexate in lieu of cyclophosphamide. In an uncontrolled study, methotrexate afforded rates of remission comparable to those published for cyclophosphamide.[213] An open-label study suggests that methotrexate could be used for maintenance therapy after the induction of remission with cyclophosphamide and corticosteroids,[214] but may be associated with a relatively high rate of relapse. In a randomized controlled trial of induction therapy among patients with "early" ANCA vasculitis comparing weekly methotrexate (15 mg per week escalating to a maximum of 20 to 25 mg per week by 12 weeks) to daily oral cyclophosphamide (2 mg/kg/day to a maximum of 150 mg per day), the rate of remission at 6 months was comparable among the two treatment groups (89.8% for methotrexate vs. 93.5% for cyclophosphamide, $P = .041$). However, the onset of remission in methotrexate-treated patients with relatively extensive disease or pulmonary involvement was delayed. Methotrexate was associated with a significantly higher rate of relapse than cyclophosphamide (69.5% vs. 46.5%), and 45% of relapses occurred while patients were receiving methotrexate.[215] Importantly, patients enrolled in this trial did not have organ- or life-threatening manifestations, or significant renal involvement. The dose of methotrexate must be reduced in patients whose creatinine clearance is less than 80 mL per min, and its use is contraindicated when creatinine clearances are less than 10 mL per min. Most experience of methotrexate in GPA has involved patients with no renal involvement or with glomerulonephritis and near-normal renal function.

Recent investigation into cyclophosphamide-sparing induction strategies for ANCA vasculitis has led to the possibility of using alternative induction therapy protocols including rituximab. Rituximab, a chimeric monoclonal antibody directed against the CD20 antigen, effectively depletes B lymphocytes, but not plasma cells. Two recent noninferiority randomized control trials evaluating rituximab and prednisone compared to cyclophosphamide with prednisone have been published.[216,217] **R**ituximab for **A**NCA-associated **V**asculitis (RAVE) is a placebo-controlled study of 197 patients with new-onset and relapsing ANCA vasculitis comparing oral cyclophosphamide and prednisone ($n = 99$) to four infusions of 375 mg per m^2 rituximab plus prednisone ($n = 98$).[216] There was no difference between the arms in complete remission (55% in cyclophosphamide arm, 64% in rituximab arm) off all therapy including prednisone at 6 months ($P = .21$). Adverse events and relapse within the first 6 months did not differ among patients with new onset disease. In patients presenting with relapse and randomized between the two arms, the rituximab protocol was significantly better. The RITUXVAS trial evaluated 44 patients with more severe disease.[217] This trial compared 6 to 10 infusions of cyclophosphamide followed by maintenance therapy with azathioprine to four infusions of 375 mg per m^2 rituximab in combination with two infusions of cyclophosphamide without maintenance therapy. Remission rates at 12 months of 76% in the rituximab group and 82% in the cyclophosphamide alone group were noted but adverse events were 45% and 36% in the rituximab and cyclophosphamide group respectively and 1-year mortality rate was 18% in both groups. In both RAVE and RITUXVAS, rituximab is noninferior to cyclophosphamide but enthusiasm is tempered by elevated adverse event rates that may signify no improvement in safety over cyclophosphamide. Analysis of long-term outcomes of these trials including sustained remission, rate of relapse, and safety data is anticipated, as rituximab has now received approval by the FDA.

Patients presenting with pulmonary hemorrhage also benefit from the institution of plasmapheresis in a regimen similar to that used for patients with Goodpasture disease. Although no controlled data are available, early and aggressive institution of plasmapheresis has in our experience substantially diminished the mortality rate associated with massive pulmonary hemorrhage.[218] Plasmapheresis is typically performed daily until the pulmonary hemorrhage ceases and then every other day for a total of 7 to 10 treatments. Plasma is replaced with a solution of 5% albumin, but two units of fresh-frozen plasma are administered at the end of the treatment to replace clotting factors and minimize the risk of persistent or renewed bleeding. In a randomized trial of plasma exchange versus methylprednisolone as additional therapy in patients with severe ANCA vasculitis (creatinine >500 μmol per L or dialysis dependent), the use of plasma exchange was associated with a significant improvement in the recovery of renal function and dialysis-free survival.[219] Meta-analyses of five studies confirmed the benefit of adjunct plasmapheresis noting a reduction in risk of requiring dialysis 12 months after therapy initiation.[220] Plasmapheresis is recommended as adjunct in ANCA vasculitis induction therapy for patients who present with life- or organ-threatening manifestations of vasculitis. On the basis of several relatively small studies, plasmapheresis does not seem to be of added benefit over the use of corticosteroids and cyclophosphamide in patients without pulmonary hemorrhage or severe renal involvement.[221,222] Further investigation into the effects of plasmapheresis in ANCA vasculitis is currently under way in a randomized control study.[223]

Treatment of Relapse

With the use of an alkylating agent, the rate of remission is on the order of 70% to 85%. Patients who require dialysis at the time of diagnosis have a decreased probability of recovering sufficient renal function to discontinue dialysis (about 50%). Patients that do recover sufficient renal function do so within the first 3 months of treatment. In a retrospective analysis of 523 patients with ANCA vasculitis followed over a median of 40 months, 136 patients reached ESKD.[224] Relapse rates of vasculitis were significantly lower on chronic dialysis (0.08 episodes per person-year) compared with the rate of the same patients before ESKD (0.20 episodes per person-year) or with patients with preserved renal function (0.16 episodes per person-year). Infections were almost twice as frequent among patients with ESKD on maintenance immunosuppressants and were an important cause of death. In the absence of active extrarenal vasculitis, immunosuppression may be stopped after 3 months if no signs of renal recovery have occurred as the risk/benefit ratio does not support the routine use of maintenance immunosuppression therapy in ANCA vasculitis patients on chronic dialysis.

Relapse in ANCA vasculitis occurs in about 45% of patients over a median of 44 months,[225] but relapse patterns are not uniform among patients. In our experience, 80% of relapses occur in the first 18 months after immunosuppressive therapy is discontinued. Others have not detected such a clustering of relapses in the early months after discontinuing therapy.[226] Recurrent disease may resemble clinically the initial presentation but is sometimes associated with new organ involvement.

The risk of relapse is not uniform among patients with ANCA vasculitis. Multivariate analysis of 258 patients with the disease who were treated and attained remission showed that presence of PR3-ANCA antibody and involvement of the lungs and upper respiratory tract were independent risk factors for relapse. Of the patients who presented none of these risk factors, 26% relapsed in a median of 62 months (median among those who relapsed was 20 months). In contrast, 47% of the patients who presented with a single risk factor experienced a risk for relapse (95% CI 1.1–3.9, $P = .038$). Of patients presenting with all three risk factors, 73% relapsed in a median of 17 months (median among those who relapsed was 15 months), corresponding to a 3.7-times increased risk of relapse (95% CI 1.4–9.7, $P = .007$) compared to those with no risk factors.[225] In a retrospective analysis of a separate large independent cohort of patients from the French Vasculitis Study Group, the presence of PR3-ANCA and lung involvement were found to be risk factors for relapse (hazard ratio 1.66 [95% CI 1.15–2.39] for PR3–ANCA and HR 1.56 [95% CI 1.11–2.20] for lung involvement).[227]

Recurrent glomerulonephritis is usually indicated by the recurrence or worsening of hematuria with an increase in serum creatinine. An increase in proteinuria alone or the gradual increase in serum creatinine without hematuria may be the result of progressive chronic scarring, rather than recurrent active inflammation. Repeated renal biopsy is sometimes indicated to best differentiate between recurrent disease and progressive scarring and to avoid unnecessary immunosuppression in the latter case.

Whether ANCA titers are predictive of a relapse is a matter of controversy. To determine the occurrence of a relapse, serial measurements of ANCA titers should be interpreted only in the context of the clinical history and physical and laboratory examination of the patient. Although ANCA titers correlate with disease activity when a group of patients are considered, the ANCA titer may not correlate in an individual patient. Some patients maintain a high titer level despite clinical remission, whereas others exhibit clinical evidence of active vasculitis in the absence of a rise in titer. ANCA titers are best used in serial measurements and interpreted in consideration with each patient's pattern.

Several studies have addressed whether ANCA could reliably predict the future occurrence of a relapse.[228] PR3-ANCA has been the focus of study in this regard with limited information pertaining to MPO-ANCA. One-hundred and fifty-six patients from Wegener granulomatosis etanercept (WEGET) study had serum collected every 3 months and the titers of antibodies to mature PR3 (PR3-ANCA) and to pro-PR3 were analyzed in relationship with disease activity and subsequent relapse.[229] In this study, there was only weak association between PR3-ANCA levels. The proportion of patients who had relapse within 1 year of an increase in PR3-ANCA levels was 40% for mature-PR3 and 43% for pro-PR3. These findings lack support for the use of PR3-ANCA levels in guiding immunosuppressive therapy.

Although a rise in ANCA titer may predict recurrent disease, the relapse may not occur for several months. In a study by Cohen Tervaert et al., one third of patients with a rise in titer did not experience clinical signs of relapse even after 18 months.[230] In this context, and considering the toxicities of immunosuppression, the prophylactic use of high-dose corticosteroids or cyclophosphamide to prevent relapse would needlessly expose many patients to their toxic side effects. If alternative, less toxic therapies are shown to be effective in the treatment of ANCA vasculitis, the risk–benefit ratio may make such a preemptive or prophylactic approach more appealing. To date, the evidence does not support the use of preemptive immunosuppressive therapy to prevent a relapse in patients with an increase in ANCA titer. Relapsing ANCA vasculitis responds to immunosuppression with corticosteroids and cytotoxic agents with a similar response rate as the initial disease. The decision regarding the repeated use of pulse methylprednisolone can be based on the total amount of corticosteroid that has been administered to the patient over the course of the disease, as well as the severity of the relapse. Patients with a history of relapsing disease pose a particular challenge because they are particularly subject to the cumulative toxic effects of cytotoxic agents and corticosteroids. Some may require the use of long-term "maintenance" immunosuppressive therapy with either low-dose prednisone or azathioprine. Although the use of trimethoprim-sulfamethoxazole or cotrimoxazole is beneficial in the prevention of relapses involving the nose and upper respiratory tract, no benefit is seen in disease affecting the kidneys or other organ systems.[231] The concomitant use of trimethoprim-sulfamethoxazole and methotrexate is contraindicated because it may result in severe bone marrow toxicity.

In an effort to limit the exposure to cytotoxic agents, a number of immunomodulatory drugs and antibodies are being evaluated for the treatment of patients with recurrent vasculitis. The various studies can conceptually be divided into two categories: studies aimed at treating patients who are resistant to conventional treatment with cyclophosphamide and corticosteroids, and studies aimed at the prevention of relapse. Table 48.9 summarizes various "novel" therapies that have been or are being evaluated. The efficacy of any such agents is currently not established, and they should not be considered as first-line therapies.

TABLE 48.9 **A Summary of Various "Novel" Therapies That Have Been or Are Being Evaluated in the Treatment of Anca Vasculitis and Glomerulonephritis**

Therapy	Possible Role	References
Plasmapheresis	Adjunctive therapy in patients with pulmonary hemorrhage or advanced renal disease	Gaskin, 2001[266]; Frasca, 1992, 1993[267,268]; Pusey, 199[145]; Zauner, 2002[269]; Klemmer, 2003[142]; Cole, 1992[144]; Jayne, 2007; Walters, 2010
Intravenous immunoglobulin	Adjunctive therapy in patients with persistent disease on standard therapy	Jayne et al.,[155] Martinez, 2008
Methotrexate	Alternative to cyclophosphamide in patients with "early disease" and without significant renal or pulmonary disease.	Sneller, 1995[148]; Langford, 2000[270]; DeGroot, 2005[150]
	Prevention of relapse?	Isaacs, 1996[161]; Booth, 2002[167]; Stegeman, 1997[271]
Azathioprine	Prevention of relapse?	Jayne, 2003[147]; Pagnoux, 2008; IMPROVE, 2010
Mycophenolate mofetil	Prevention of relapse?	Nowack, 1999[170]; Langford, 2004[272]; Stassen, 2007; Hu, 2008; Silva, 2010
Leflunomide	Prevention of relapse?	Metzler, 2004[273]
Rituximab	Adjunctive therapy for cyclophosphamide-resistant or relapsing patients?	Specks, 2001[274]; Keogh, 2005[156]; Eriksson, 2005[157]; Jones, 2009; Martinez, 2009
	Induction therapy	RAVE, RITUXVAS (Stone; Jones, 2010)
Infliximab	Adjunctive therapy for cyclophosphamide-resistant or relapsing patients?	Lamprecht, 2002[164]; Bartolucci, 2002[165]; Booth, 2004[166]; D'Haens, 1999[275]
Alemtuzumab	Adjunctive therapy for cyclophosphamide-resistant or relapsing patients?	Kirk, 2003[160]; Walsh, 2008
Etanercept	Shown NOT to be efficacious in the prevention of relapse	WGET[276]
Trimethoprim-sulfamethoxazole	Prevention of relapses that affect the upper respiratory tract	DeRemee, 1985[277]; Reinhold-Keller, 1996[278]; Stegeman, 1996[53]

Potential Adjunctive Treatment for Patients with Resistant Disease or Contraindications to Conventional Therapy

Several agents have been evaluated as adjunctive therapy for patients with resistant forms of ANCA vasculitis. Adjunctive therapy with intravenous immunoglobulin (IVIg) (single course of a total of 2 g per kg) was evaluated in a randomized controlled trial in patients with persistently active ANCA vasculitis despite conventional therapy. Patients treated with IVIg experienced a more rapid decline in disease activity (as measured by a 50% reduction in Birmingham Vasculitis Activity Score [BVAS]) and C-reactive protein at 1 and 3 months, but there was no significant difference between the two groups after 3 months with respect to disease activity or frequency of relapse.[232] The use of IVIg was also evaluated in a prospective, open-label study of 22 patients with relapsing ANCA vasculitis.[233] Patients received IVIg (0.5 g/kg/day for 4 days) administered monthly for 6 months as additional therapy to ongoing corticosteroids and/or immunosuppressants (cyclophosphamide, azathioprine, methotrexate, or MMF). Corticosteroid therapy could be continued or reintroduced with relapse; immunosuppressants could be maintained but could not be reintroduced. Serum creatinine >3.4 mg per dL or rapid rise in creatinine was reason for exclusion. One patient developed renal insufficiency after the first IVIg infusion. Ninety-five percent of patients achieved remission between months 1 and 5 but there was a 32% rate of relapse within 9 months. These results suggest that IVIg may induce remission in patients with relapsing ANCA vasculitis when added to baseline immunosuppression but should be avoided in patients with severe renal disease.

Evidence indicates that rituximab may have a role in the management of ANCA vasculitis that is resistant to or relapsing after standard therapy. As demonstrated in the RAVE trial, patients treated with rituximab for relapse had significantly improved outcome over patients treated with cyclophosphamide and corticosteroids.[216] Small, uncontrolled case series[156–158] used rituximab (375 mg per m^2 IV weekly × 4 or 500 mg IV weekly × 4 fixed doses) in conjunction with corticosteroids, resulting in remission in the majority of patients. In these reports rituximab was generally well tolerated. In contrast, in a fourth open label study of eight patients with severe, refractory GPA, the addition of rituximab (375 mg per m^2 every 4 weeks × 4 doses) to cyclophosphamide, mycophenolate mofetil, or methotrexate was associated with limited benefit.[234] Recent retrospective studies evaluating rituximab for refractory ANCA vasculitis report favorably for achievement of remission.[235]

Alemtuzumab (Campath-1H) is a humanized monoclonal IgG1 antibody directed against the CD52 antigen expressed on the surface of peripheral blood lymphocytes, monocytes, and macrophages.[236] Treatment with alemtuzumab results in complement-mediated lysis, antibody-dependent cellular cytotoxicity, and induction of apoptosis of target cells and results in depletion of T cells and B cells.[237] Alemtuzumab has been used to treat a select group of patients with refractory or relapsing autoimmune diseases, including 70 patients with ANCA vasculitis.[238] These patients received at least one course of 135 mg intravenous alemtuzumab over 5 days. Remission was achieved by 83% of surviving patients. Unfortunately, this treatment regimen was associated with high rates of serious infections and death (18% at 1 year) and a 43% rate of relapse. Recently, a cohort study on alemtuzumab in treatment of refractory or relapsing ANCA vasculitis showed high mortality with 31 deaths out of 71 patients.[239] In this study, 85% of patients entered remission but 72% of those patients had a relapse with a median time of 9.2 months. Mortality and infection risk limit the utility of this therapy.

Similarly, the chimeric monoclonal antibody directed against TNF-α[163] infliximab has been evaluated in four open-label uncontrolled trials of small numbers of patients.[240–243] In these studies, the treatment regimen included infliximab plus corticosteroids, and either cyclophosphamide or other immunosuppressive agents. In the largest of these trials, which included 32 patients with acute or resistant disease, infliximab was associated with a remission rate of 88% and a relapse rate of 20%.[166] These promising results are mitigated, however, by an elevated rate of serious infectious complications.

The immunosuppressant, 15-deoxyspergualin, used in Japan for the treatment of steroid-resistant renal transplant rejection, has also been evaluated for the treatment of refractory GPA.[244,245]

Maintenance Therapy

Azathioprine is the most well-validated maintenance therapy in ANCA vasculitis. In a controlled trial of 144 patients who achieved remission with daily oral cyclophosphamide and corticosteroids, a switch to azathioprine after 3 to 6 months was associated with equivalent relapse rates and long-term outcomes as 12 months of cyclophosphamide.[209]

Methotrexate offers no benefit over azathioprine in the prevention of relapse, and may be associated with a higher rate of serious adverse effects. Maintenance therapy with methotrexate compared to azathioprine in a randomized controlled fashion was evaluated after induction of remission with cyclophosphamide and corticosteroids.[246] The primary outcome measure was serious adverse events rather than the rate of relapse. One-hundred and twenty-six out of 180 treated patients attained remission and were randomized to azathioprine (2 mg/kg/day) or methotrexate (0.3 mg/kg/week initially and progressively increased to 25 mg per week) for 12 months followed by a tapered withdrawal over 3 months. Impaired renal function at randomization was not an exclusion criterion. The two groups were well matched for age, diagnosis, organ involvement, and serum creatinine. The azathioprine group included more patients with risk factors for relapse (PR3-ANCA and alveolar hemorrhage). There was no significant difference in the rate of relapse between the groups (36% and 33% respectively;

P = .71) with a mean randomization-to-relapse interval of 20.6 ± 13.9 months. Methotrexate was associated with a trend toward a higher rate of adverse events when compared to azathioprine (HR 1.65; 95% confidence interval 0.65 to 4.18; P = .29).

Methotrexate was compared to leflunomide for maintenance therapy in ANCA vasculitis in a controlled trial that was terminated early due to the rate of major relapses in the methotrexate limb.[247] Data does not support routine use of methotrexate for the prevention of relapse in ANCA vasculitis. Risk of serious adverse effects precludes the use of methotrexate in patients with decreased renal function.

In a large randomized control trial MMF was compared to AZA in 156 patients with ANCA vasculitis who attained remission with cyclophosphamide and corticosteroids.[248] Randomization was to MMF (2 g per day) versus azathioprine (2 mg/kg/day) and patients were followed for a median of 39 months. Relapses were more common in the MMF group compared to the azathioprine group (unadjusted HR for MMF 1.69, 95% CI 1.06–2.70; P = .03). Adverse events, disease activity score, glomerular filtration rate, and proteinuria did not differ between the groups.

Data is scarce on whether rituximab could be used for the prevention of relapses, but this remains an appealing concept.

Treatment of Eosinophilic Granulomatosis

Treatment of EGPA often parallels the approach to GPA and MPA. In a prospective, randomized open label trial of EGPA patients without renal impairment, cardiomyopathy, gastrointestinal tract, or central nervous system disease, patients entered remission with steroid treatment alone; however, relapse rate was 35%.[249] Attempts to sustain remission and avoid cyclophosphamide by use of azathioprine, MMF, or methotrexate for EGPA without poor prognostic factors have been reported.[249,250]

In five of seven patients with EGPA refractory to standard therapy given interferon-α with steroids went into remission although follow-up time was only 6 months.[250] There is case report evidence for use of the anti-IL-5 antibody mepolizumab and anti-IgE antibody omalizumab in refractory EGPA.[251,252] Interferon-α and mepolizumab have also been studied for maintenance treatment in EGPA.[252,253]

RENAL TRANSPLANTATION

Renal transplantation has been recognized as an option of renal replacement therapy in patients with GPA, MPA, or necrotizing crescentic glomerulonephritis. Although there is a risk of disease recurrence posttransplantation patient and graft outcomes in ANCA vasculitis are similar to those of renal transplant recipients with other causes of renal failure not including diabetes.[254] Successful renal transplantation in patients with ANCA vasculitis has been reported in patients who were in full remission and with negative ANCA test results, in patients with positive ANCA test results,[255,256] and even in patients with evidence of active vasculitis at the time of transplantation.[257] Recurrent vasculitis after transplantation has also been described as occurring as early as a few days posttransplantation and as late as several years posttransplantation. Just as with the initial ANCA vasculitis, reported recurrences after transplantation involve a spectrum of various organs and are not limited to the transplanted kidney.

Based on a pooled analysis,[258] ANCA vasculitis recurs in about 17% of all patients, with an average time from transplantation to relapse of 31 months. Case series report ANCA relapse rates after transplantation to range from 0.02 to 0.1 relapses per patient year.[257,259,260] The presence of ANCA at transplantation does not appear to increase the rate of relapse posttransplantation. Relapse rate was 9% (all extrarenal) at >1 year with no effect on graft function in a population where 80% were transplanted with induction therapy (66% using a depletion agent) and >80% maintenance therapy with tacrolimus or cyclosporine + MMF + prednisone.[261]

Patients with GPA had a relative risk of relapse of 2.75 when compared with patients with MPA or necrotizing crescentic glomerulonephritis alone. Conversely, ANCA pattern (c-ANCA or p-ANCA) or antigen specificity (PR3 or MPO) was not associated with differences in relapse rate posttransplantation.

A review of the reports of recurrent ANCA vasculitis posttransplantation reveal a good response to cyclophosphamide in the treatment of relapsing disease, although recurrent disease can lead to graft loss and even patient death.[262] Rituximab has been reported to be effective in treating posttransplant cyclophosphamide refractory recurrent ANCA disease.[263,264] In summary, renal transplantation is a beneficial option in the management of patients with ESKD associated with ANCA vasculitis. Although the presence of circulating ANCA is not a sufficient contraindication to transplantation, it is current practice not to perform transplantation in patients with active vasculitis, but to delay surgery until the disease is in remission. No data are currently available about the need to wait a certain period of time after remission is attained and before proceeding to transplantation.

BEHÇET DISEASE

Behçet disease is a systemic vasculitic syndrome classically characterized by a triad of recurrent oral ulcerations, genital ulcerations, and ocular lesions usually consisting of uveitis, iritis, or retinal vasculitis. Behçet disease can present with protean manifestations with multiple organ involvement, either concomitantly or consecutively. Other organ system involvement includes the skin, musculoskeletal system with arthralgias and myalgias, central nervous system, and lungs, and gastrointestinal, cardiac, and genitourinary systems. Vascular involvement may affect large blood vessels, capillaries, venules, and veins. The diagnosis of Behçet disease is based on an established set of criteria.[265] The criteria include the presence of oral ulcerations, and two or more of the following: recurrent genital ulcerations, eye lesions, skin lesions, and positive pathergy test results. The latter test represents a nonspecific skin hyperreactivity induced by intradermal needle prick.

Epidemiology

Although Behçet disease has been reported worldwide, the highest incidence of disease appears to be in Japan, the Middle East, and around the Mediterranean basin. The incidence ranges from 1 to 2 per 10,000 in Japan and Saudi Arabia to as low as 0.3 per 100,000 in Northern Europe. The peak age of onset is within the third decade, and there is a male preponderance in most published case series. Men are also reported to have more severe disease than women.

Pathogenesis

The etiology of Behçet disease remains unknown. Associations with infectious agents such as herpes simplex virus I, *Streptococcus sanguis,* parvovirus B19, and *Mycobacterium tuberculosis* have been hypothesized and evaluated to various degrees. However, no direct link has been convincingly established. Human leukocyte antigen (HLA) typing reveals a close association between Behçet disease and HLA-B51 (especially the allelic variants HLA-B*5101)[266] and HLA-B*5108 and HLA-B*57 among Caucasians.[267] Other studies point to an association with a microsatellite located between the HLA-B locus and the TNF gene rather than an association with the HLA-B*51 gene itself.[268] Therefore, the TNF promoter allele TNF-1031 was found to be independently associated with susceptibility to Behçet disease among Caucasians.[267] The presence of antibodies to a number of autoantigens such as alpha-tropomyosin[269] has been described. The role of such autoantibodies in the pathogenesis of the disease is unclear. Similarly, T cells are likely involved in the pathogenesis of Behçet disease as evidenced by an increase in $\gamma\delta$T cells,[270] a predominance of Th1 cell phenotype,[271] and autoreactive T cells.[272]

Renal Involvement

Renal involvement in Behçet disease appears to be more frequent than previously recognized. The spectrum of involvement ranges from subtle urinary abnormalities to end-stage renal disease and can conceptually be divided into five categories: (1) glomerulonephritis, (2) amyloidosis, (3) renal vascular involvement, (4) interstitial nephritis, and (5) other problems, such as complications of drug therapy or genitourinary system abnormalities.[273] The nephrotic syndrome and renal failure occurring in the setting of Behçet disease can be associated with the presence of AA amyloidosis more typically found in patients with long-standing disease.[274] Based on an extensive review of the published case reports (totaling 159 patients), amyloidosis was the most commonly reported lesion (43% of cases), whereas glomerulonephritis accounted for 32% of cases.[273] Although an early study reported the presence of hematuria, proteinuria, or both in about one third of patients,[275] a recent extensive retrospective review of more than 4,200 cases identified such urinary abnormalities in about 11% of patients tested and documented glomerulonephritis in only 7 (0.16%) patients.[276] The pathologic lesions associated with Behçet disease include focal and diffuse proliferative glomerulonephritis, membranoproliferative glomerulonephritis, focal segmental necrotizing glomerulonephritis with crescents, and minimal change disease. In Benekli's review, predominant IgA deposits are reported in 11 of 40 cases of glomerulonephritis associated with Behçet disease. The report of several cases of focal segmental necrotizing and crescentic glomerulonephritis[277] in the absence of immune complex deposition raises the question of an association with ANCA. The presence of such autoantibodies has been reported in rare cases,[278] but not in systematic screening of patients with Behçet disease.[279]

Treatment

A number of immunomodulatory and immunosuppressant agents are used in the treatment of Behçet disease. These include corticosteroids, calcineurin inhibitor, azathioprine, interferon-alpha, and rituximab.[280,281] More recently the use of agents that block the TNF pathway has also been reported.[282] Because of the rarity of glomerular involvement in Behçet disease, no definitive data for treatment are available. The use of corticosteroids has been reported with variable outcomes. In cases of Behçet disease with severe vasculitic disease or glomerulonephritis, the use of corticosteroids and immunosuppressive therapy with azathioprine or cyclophosphamide may be justified.

THERAPEUTIC CONSIDERATIONS COMMON TO ALL VASCULITIC SYNDROMES

As the mainstay of therapy of severe vasculitis remains based on corticosteroids and alkylating agents, it is associated with short- and long-term complications. The most prominent side effects of this form of therapy are infection, ovarian failure (especially with a prolonged course of cyclophosphamide), bone disease, and cataract formation. In addition, the prolonged use of cyclophosphamide is associated with a 15% risk of developing a transitional cell carcinoma of the bladder over the course of 5 to 10 years.[268] Whether the use of monthly pulse intravenous cyclophosphamide (which is associated with a smaller incidence cumulative dose and a lower incidence of hemorrhagic cystitis) can reduce the rate of bladder cancer is not yet ascertained.

The institution of attentive supportive care is crucial in minimizing the short- and long-term complications. Compulsive attention must be paid to the early detection and aggressive treatment of infections, because they remain an important cause of morbidity and death. Whenever possible, the use of trimethoprim-sulfamethoxazole for the prevention of *Pneumocystis carinii* pneumonia should be considered.

Whenever corticosteroids are used, measures must be taken to minimize the development of osteoporosis. Specific recommendations include calcium (1.2 g per day) and vitamin D supplementation and, in selected patients with established osteoporosis, calcitonin nasal spray or alendronate for patients in whom the drug is not contraindicated (e.g., azotemia or esophagitis). Rigorous control of blood pressure with sodium restriction and antihypertensive therapy is essential to minimize the additive effect of hypertension in loss of renal function after active nephritis. Current research directions include the preservation of gonadal function by hormonal manipulation during cytotoxic therapy. In a small study, the use of testosterone during cyclophosphamide treatment appeared to prevent azoospermia.[283] The gonadotropin-releasing hormone agonist leuprolide appears to be effective in the prevention of cyclophosphamide-induced ovarian failure based on a small prospective uncontrolled trial of patients with lupus nephritis.[284]

REFERENCES

1. Ntatsaki E, Watts RA, Scott DG. Epidemiology of ANCA-associated vasculitis. *Rheum Dis Clin North Am.* 2010;36:447–461.
2. McMahon BJ, Heyward WL, Templin DW, et al. Hepatitis B-associated polyarteritis nodosa in Alaskan Eskimos: clinical and epidemiologic features and long-term follow-up. *Hepatology.* 1989;9:97–101.
3. el Reshaid K, Kapoor MM, el Reshaid W, et al. The spectrum of renal disease associated with microscopic polyangiitis and classic polyarteritis nodosa in Kuwait. *Nephrol Dial Transplant.* 1997;12:1874–1882.
4. Watts RA, Al-Taiar A, Scott DG, et al. Prevalence and incidence of Wegener's granulomatosis in the UK general practice research database. *Arthritis Rheum.* 2009;61:1412–1416.
5. Pagnoux C, Guilpain P, Guillevin L. eosinophilic granulomatosis. *Curr Opin Rheumatol.* 2007;19:25–32.
6. Mahr A, Guillevin L, Poissonnet M, et al. Prevalences of polyarteritis nodosa, microscopic polyangiitis, Wegener's granulomatosis, and eosinophilic granulomatosis in a French urban multiethnic population in 2000: a capture-recapture estimate. *Arthritis Rheum.* 2004;51:92–99.
7. Berden AE, Ferrario F, Hagen EC, et al. Histopathologic classification of ANCA-associated glomerulonephritis. *J Am Soc Nephrol.* 2010;21:1628–1636.
8. Jennette JC, Falk RJ, Andrassy K, et al. Nomenclature of systemic vasculitides. Proposal of an international consensus conference. *Arthritis Rheum.* 1994; 37:187–192.
9. Savory WS. Case of a young woman in whom the main arteries of both upper extremities and of the left side of the neck were throughout completely obliterated. *Med Chir Trans Lond.* 1856;39:205–219.
10. Takayasu M. Case with unusual changes of the central vessels in the retina. *Acta Soc Opthamology.* 1908;12:554.
11. Arend WP, Michel BA, Bloch DA, et al. The American College of Rheumatology 1990 criteria for the classification of Takayasu arteritis. *Arthritis Rheum.* 1990;33:1129–1134.
12. Hunder GG, Bloch DA, Michel BA, et al. The American College of Rheumatology 1990 criteria for the classification of giant cell arteritis. *Arthritis Rheum.* 1990;33:1122–1128.
13. Hutchinson J. Diseases of the arteries. On a peculiar form of thrombotic arteries of the aged which is sometimes productive of gangrene. *Arch Surg.* 1890;1:323–329.
14. Rojo-Leyva F, Ratliff NB, Cosgrove DM III, et al. Study of 52 patients with idiopathic aortitis from a cohort of 1,204 surgical cases. *Arthritis Rheum.* 2000;43:901–907.
15. Dasgupta B. Concise guidance: diagnosis and management of giant cell arteritis. *Clin Med.* 2010;10:381–386.
16. Opastirakul S, Chartapisak W, Sirivanichai C. A girl with Takayasu arteritis associated with possible systemic lupus erythematosus. *Pediatr Nephrol.* 2004;19:463–466.
17. Hall S, Nelson AM. Takayasu's arteritis and juvenile rheumatoid arthritis. *J Rheumatol.* 1986;13:431–433.
18. Chauhan SK, Tripathy NK, Nityanand S. Antigenic targets and pathogenicity of anti-aortic endothelial cell antibodies in Takayasu arteritis. *Arthritis Rheum.* 2006;54:2326–2333.
19. Gabriel SE, Espy M, Erdman DD, et al. The role of parvovirus B19 in the pathogenesis of giant cell arteritis: a preliminary evaluation. *Arthritis Rheum.* 1999;42:1255–1258.
20. Rodriguez-Pla A, Bosch-Gil JA, Echevarria-Mayo JE, et al. No detection of parvovirus B19 or herpesvirus DNA in giant cell arteritis. *J Clin Virol.* 2004;31:11–15.
21. Salvarani C, Gabriel SE, O'Fallon WM, et al. The incidence of giant cell arteritis in Olmsted County, Minnesota: apparent fluctuations in a cyclic pattern [see comments]. *Ann Intern Med.*. 1995;123:192–194.
22. Mathewson JA, Hunder GG. Giant cell arteritis in two brothers. *J Rheumatol.* 1986;13:190–192.
23. Weyand CM, Hunder NN, Hicok KC, et al. HLA-DRB1 alleles in polymyalgia rheumatica, giant cell arteritis, and rheumatoid arthritis. *Arthritis Rheum.* 1994;37:514–520.
24. Weyand CM, Goronzy JJ. Giant cell arteritis as an antigen-driven disease. *Rheum Dis Clin North Am.* 1995;21:1027–1039.
25. Roche NE, Fulbright JW, Wagner AD, et al. Correlation of interleukin-6 production and disease activity in polymyalgia rheumatica and giant cell arteritis [see comments]. *Arthritis Rheum.* 1993;36:1286–1294.
26. Hunder GG, Sheps SG, Allen GL, et al. Daily and alternate-day corticosteroid regimens in treatment of giant cell arteritis: comparison in a prospective study. *Ann Intern Med.*. 1975;82:613–618.
27. Liu GT, Glaser JS, Schatz NJ, et al. Visual morbidity in giant cell arteritis. Clinical characteristics and prognosis for vision. *Ophthalmology.* 1994;101: 1779–1785.
28. Ray-Chaudhuri N, Kine DA, Tijani SO, et al. Effect of prior steroid treatment on temporal artery biopsy findings in giant cell arteritis. *Br J Ophthalmol.* 2002;86:530–532.
29. Nesher G, Sonnenblick M. Steroid-sparing medications in temporal arteritis—report of three cases and review of 174 reported patients. *Clin Rheumatol.* 1994;13:289–292.
30. Hoffman GS, Cid M, Hellmann DB, et al. A multicenter, placebo-controlled study of methotrexate (Mtx) in giant cell arteritis (GCA). [Abstract] *Arthritis Rheum* 2000;43:S115.
31. Nesher G, Berkun Y, Mates M, et al. Low-dose aspirin and prevention of cranial ischemic complications in giant cell arteritis. *Arthritis Rheum.* 2004;50:1332–1337.
32. Kerr GS, Hallahan CW, Giordano J, et al. Takayasu arteritis. *Ann Intern Med.* 1994;120:919–929.
33. Hoffman GS, Leavitt RY, Kerr GS, et al. Treatment of glucocorticoid-resistant or relapsing Takayasu arteritis with methotrexate. *Arthritis Rheum.* 1994;37:578–582.
34. Della RA, Tavoni A, Merlini G, et al. Two Takayasu arteritis patients successfully treated with infliximab: a potential disease-modifying agent? *Rheumatology (Oxford)*.. 2005;44:1074–1075.
35. Tanaka F, Kawakami A, Iwanaga N, et al. Infliximab is effective for Takayasu arteritis refractory to glucocorticoid and methotrexate. *Intern Med.* 2006;45: 313–316.
36. Hoffman GS, Merkel PA, Brasington RD, et al. Anti-tumor necrosis factor therapy in patients with difficult to treat Takayasu arteritis. *Arthritis Rheum.* 2004;50:2296–2304.
37. Kieffer E, Piquois A, Bertal A, et al. Reconstructive surgery of the renal arteries in Takayasu's disease. *Ann Vasc Surg.* 1990;4:156–165.
38. Hoffman GS. Treatment of resistant Takayasu's arteritis. *Rheum Dis Clin North Am.* 1995;21:73–80.
39. Kussmaul A, Maier R. Uber eine bisher nicht beschreibene eigenthumliche Arterienerkrankung (Periarteritis nodosa), die mit Morbus Brightii und rapid fortschreitender allgemeiner Muskellahmung einhergeht. *Dtsch Arch Klin Med.* 1866;1:484–518.
40. Ferrari E. Ueber Polyarteritis actua nodosa (sogenannte Periarteriitis nodosa), und ihre Beziehungen zur Polymyositis and Polyneuritis acuta. *Beitr Pathol Anat.* 1903;34:350–386.
41. Arnaout MA. A clinical and pathological study of periarteritis nodosa. A report of five cases, one histologically healed. *Am J Pathol.* 1930;6:426–429.
42. Zeek PM, Smith CC, Weeter JC. Studies on periarteritis nodosa. III. The differentiation between the vascular lesions of periarteritis nodosa and of hypersensitivity. *Am J Pathol.* 1948;24:889–917.
43. Zeek PM. Periarteritis nodosa: a critical review. *Am J Clin Pathol.* 1952; 22:777–790.

44. Godman GC, Churg J. Wegener's granulomatosis. Pathology and review of the literature. *Arch Pathol Lab Med.* 1954;58:533–553.

45. Jennette JC, Falk RJ. Small-vessel vasculitis [see comments]. *N Engl J Med.* 1997;337:1512–1523.

46. Guillevin L, Lhote F, Amouroux J, et al. Antineutrophil cytoplasmic antibodies, abnormal angiograms and pathological findings in polyarteritis nodosa and eosinophilic granulomatosis: indications for the classification of vasculitides of the polyarteritis nodosa group. *Br J Rheumatol.* 1996;35:958–964.

47. Kirkland GS, Savige J, Wilson D, et al. Classical polyarteritis nodosa and microscopic polyarteritis with medium vessel involvement—a comparison of the clinical and laboratory features. *Clin Nephrol.* 1997;47:176–180.

48. Jennette JC, Falk RJ. Anti-neutrophil cytoplasmic autoantibodies: Discovery, specificity, disease associations and pathogenic potential. *Adv Pathol Lab Med.* 1995;8:363–377.

49. Kallenberg CG, Brouwer E, Weening JJ, et al. Anti-neutrophil cytoplasmic antibodies: current diagnostic and pathophysiological potential. *Kidney Int.* 1994;46:1–15.

50. Dillon MJ, Eleftheriou D, Brogan PA. Medium-size-vessel vasculitis. *Pediatr Nephrol.* 2010;25:1641–1652.

51. Guillevin L, Lhote F, Gayraud M, et al. Prognostic factors in polyarteritis nodosa and eosinophilic granulomatosis. A prospective study in 342 patients. *Medicine (Baltimore).* 1996;75:17–28.

52. Basoglu T, Akpolat T, Canbaz F, et al. Tc-99m DMSA renal scan in polyarteritis nodosa with bilateral intraparenchymal renal artery aneurysms. *Clin Nucl Med.* 1999;24:201–202.

53. Newburger JW, Takahashi M, Burns JC, et al. The treatment of Kawasaki syndrome with intravenous gamma globulin. *N Engl J Med.* 1986;315:341–347.

54. Guillevin L, Mahr A, Callard P, et al. Hepatitis B virus-associated polyarteritis nodosa: clinical characteristics, outcome, and impact of treatment in 115 patients. *Medicine (Baltimore).* 2005;84:313–322.

55. De Keyser F, Naeyaert JM, Hindryckx P, et al. Immune-mediated pathology following hepatitis B vaccination. Two cases of polyarteritis nodosa and one case of pityriasis rosea-like drug eruption. *Clin Exp Rheumatol.* 2000;18:81–85.

56. Guillevin L, Lhote F, Sauvaget F, et al. Treatment of polyarteritis nodosa related to hepatitis B virus with interferon-alpha and plasma exchanges. *Ann Rheum Dis.* 1994;53:334–337.

57. Kruger M, Boker KH, Zeidler H, et al. Treatment of hepatitis B-related polyarteritis nodosa with famciclovir and interferon alfa-2b. *J Hepatol.* 1997;26: 935–939.

58. Hasler P, Kistler H, Gerber H. Vasculitides in hairy cell leukemia. *Semin Arthritis Rheum.* 1995;25:134–142.

59. Carpenter MT, West SG. Polyarteritis nodosa in hairy cell leukemia: treatment with interferon- alpha. *J Rheumatol.* 1994;21:1150–1152.

60. Agard C, Mouthon L, Mahr A, et al. Microscopic polyangiitis and polyarteritis nodosa: how and when do they start? *Arthritis Rheum.* 2003;49:709–715.

61. Guillevin L, Lhote F. Treatment of polyarteritis nodosa and microscopic polyangiitis. *Arthritis Rheum.* 1998;41:2100–2105.

62. Pagnoux C, Seror R, Henegar C, et al. Clinical features and outcomes in 348 patients with polyarteritis nodosa: a systematic retrospective study of patients diagnosed between 1963 and 2005 and entered into the French Vasculitis Study Group Database. *Arthritis Rheum.* 2010;62:616–626.

63. Gayraud M, Guillevin L, le Toumelin P, et al. Long-term followup of polyarteritis nodosa, microscopic polyangiitis, and eosinophilic granulomatosis: analysis of four prospective trials including 278 patients. *Arthritis Rheum.* 2001;44:666–675.

64. Guillevin L, Pagnoux C. Therapeutic strategies for systemic necrotizing vasculitides. *Allergol Int.* 2007;56:105–111.

65. Guillevin L, Jarrousse B, Lok C, et al. Longterm followup after treatment of polyarteritis nodosa and Churg-Strauss angiitis with comparison of steroids, plasma exchange and cyclophosphamide to steroids and plasma exchange. A prospective randomized trial of 71 patients. The Cooperative Study Group for Polyarteritis Nodosa [see comments]. *J Rheumatol.* 1991;18:567–574.

66. Guillevin L, Cohen P, Mahr A, et al. Treatment of polyarteritis nodosa and microscopic polyangiitis with poor prognosis factors: a prospective trial comparing glucocorticoids and six or twelve cyclophosphamide pulses in sixty-five patients. *Arthritis Rheum.* 2003;49:93–100.

67. Guillevin L, Lhote F, Cohen P, et al. Corticosteroids plus pulse cyclophosphamide and plasma exchanges versus corticosteroids plus pulse cyclophosphamide alone in the treatment of polyarteritis nodosa and eosinophilic granulomatosis patients with factors predicting poor prognosis. A prospective, randomized trial in sixty-two patients. *Arthritis Rheum.* 1995;38:1638–1645.

68. Al-Bishri J, le Riche N, Pope JE. Refractory polyarteritis nodosa successfully treated with infliximab. *J Rheumatol.* 2005;32:1371–1373.

69. Keystone EC. The utility of tumour necrosis factor blockade in orphan diseases. *Ann Rheum Dis.* 2004;63 Suppl 2:ii79–ii83.

70. Lam KC, Lai CL, Trepo C, et al. Deleterious effect of prednisolone in HBsAg-positive chronic active hepatitis. *N Engl J Med.* 1981;304:380–386.

71. Guillevin L, Lhote F, Jarrousse B, et al. Polyarteritis nodosa related to hepatitis B virus. A retrospective study of 66 patients. *Ann Med Interne (Paris).* 1992; 143 Suppl 1:63–74.

72. Wicki J, Olivieri J, Pizzolato G, et al. Successful treatment of polyarteritis nodosa related to hepatitis B virus with a combination of lamivudine and interferon alpha [letter]. *Rheumatology (Oxford).* 1999;38:183–185.

73. Torresi J, Locarnini S. Antiviral chemotherapy for the treatment of hepatitis B virus infections. *Gastroenterology.* 2000;118 (2 Suppl 1):83–103.

74. Guillevin L, Mahr A, Cohen P, et al. Short-term corticosteroids then lamivudine and plasma exchanges to treat hepatitis B virus-related polyarteritis nodosa. *Arthritis Rheum.* 2004;51:482–487.

75. Cohen RD, Conn DL, Ilstrup DM. Clinical features, prognosis, and response to treatment in polyarteritis. *Mayo Clin Proc.* 1980;55:146–155.

76. Cameron JS. Renal vasculitis: microscopic polyarteritis and Wegener's granuloma. *Contrib Nephrol.* 1991;94:38–46.

77. D'Amico G, Sinico RA, Ferrario F. Renal vasculitis. *Nephrol Dial Transplant.* 1996;11 Suppl 9:69–74.

78. Falk RJ, Gross WL, Guillevin L, et al. Granulomatosis with polyangiitis (Wegener's): an alternative name for Wegener's granulomatosis. *Arthritis Rheum.* 2011;63:863–864.

79. Falk RJ, Gross WL, Guillevin L, et al. Granulomatosis with polyangiitis (Wegener's): an alternative name for Wegener's granulomatosis. *Ann Rheum Dis.* 2011;70: 704.

80. Falk RJ, Gross WL, Guillevin L, et al. Granulomatosis with polyangiitis (Wegener's): an alternative name for Wegener's granulomatosis. *J Am Soc Nephrol.* 2011;22:587–588.

81. Watts RA, Scott DG. Epidemiology of the vasculitides. *Semin Respir Crit Care Med.* 2004;25:455–464.

82. Izzedine H, Rosenheim M, Launay-Vacher V, et al. Epidemiology of microscopic polyarteritis: a 16–year study. *Kidney Int.* 2004;65:741.

83. Levy JB, Hammad T, Coulthart A, et al. Clinical features and outcome of patients with both ANCA and anti-GBM antibodies. *Kidney Int.* 2004;66: 1535–1540.

84. Hogan SL, Nachman PH, Wilkman AS, et al. Prognostic markers in patients with antineutrophil cytoplasmic autoantibody-associated microscopic polyangiitis and glomerulonephritis. *J Am Soc Nephrol.* 1996;7:23–32.

85. Colby TV, Specks U. Wegener's granulomatosis in the 1990s—a pulmonary pathologist's perspective. *Monogr Pathol.* 1993;(36):195–218.

86. Stegeman CA, Tervaert JW, De Jong PE, et al. Trimethoprim-sulfamethoxazole (co-trimoxazole) for the prevention of relapses of Wegener's granulomatosis. Dutch Co-Trimoxazole Wegener Study Group. *N Engl J Med.* 1996;335:16–20.

87. Said G. Vasculitis neuropathies. In: Latov N, Wokke JHJ, Kelly JJ, eds. *Immunologic and Infectious Diseases of the Peripheral Nerves.* New York: Cambridge University Press; 1998:158–167.

88. Calabrese LH, Duna GF, Lie JT. Vasculitis in the central nervous system [see comments]. *Arthritis Rheum.* 1997;40:1189–1201.

89. Jennette JC, Xiao H, Falk RJ. Pathogenesis of vascular inflammation by anti-neutrophil cytoplasmic antibodies. *J Am Soc Nephrol.* 2006;17: 1235–1242.

90. Savage CO, Pottinger BE, Gaskin G, et al. Autoantibodies developing to myeloperoxidase and proteinase 3 in systemic vasculitis stimulate neutrophil cytotoxicity toward cultured endothelial cells. *Am J Pathol.* 1992;141:335–342.

91. Sebastian JK, Voetsch B, Stone JH, et al. The frequency of anticardiolipin antibodies and genetic mutations associated with hypercoagulability among patients with Wegener's granulomatosis with and without history of a thrombotic event. *J Rheumatol.* 2007;34:2446–2450.

92. Berden AE, Nolan SL, Morris HL, et al. Anti-plasminogen antibodies compromise fibrinolysis and associate with renal histology in ANCA-associated vasculitis. *J Am Soc Nephrol.* 2010;21:2169–2179.

93. Chumbley LC, Harrison EG Jr, DeRemee RA. Allergic granulomatosis and angiitis (eosinophilic granulomatosis). Report and analysis of 30 cases. *Mayo Clin Proc.* 1977;52:477–484.

94. Davies DJ, Moran JE, Niall JF, et al. Segmental necrotising glomerulonephritis with antineutrophil antibody: possible arbovirus aetiology? *Br Med J (Clin Res Ed).* 1982;285:606.

95. Cooper T, Savige J, Nassis L, et al. Clinical associations and characterisation of antineutrophil cytoplasmic antibodies directed against bactericidal/permeability-increasing protein and azurocidin. *Rheumatol Int.* 2000;19:129–136.

96. Jethwa HS, Nachman PH, Falk RJ, et al. False-positive myeloperoxidase binding activity due to DNA/anti-DNA antibody complexes: a source for analytical error in serologic evaluation of anti-neutrophil cytoplasmic autoantibodies. *Clin Exp Immunol.* 2000;121:544–550.

97. Owshalimpur D, Arbogast CB, Olson SW. Chronological serum antineutrophil cytoplasmic autoantibodies prior to the clinical presentation of Wegener's granulomatosis. [Abstract] *J Am Soc Nephrol.* 2006;20:408A.
98. Gomez-Puerta JA, Bosch X. Anti-neutrophil cytoplasmic antibody pathogenesis in small-vessel vasculitis: an update. *Am J Pathol.* 2009;175:1790–1798.
99. Bansal PJ, Tobin MC. Neonatal microscopic polyangiitis secondary to transfer of maternal myeloperoxidase-antineutrophil cytoplasmic antibody resulting in neonatal pulmonary hemorrhage and renal involvement. *Ann Allergy Asthma Immunol.* 2004;93:398–401.
100. Schlieben DJ, Korbet SM, Kimura RE, et al. Pulmonary-renal syndrome in a newborn with placental transmission of ANCAs. *Am J Kidney Dis.* 2005;45:758–761.
101. Wiesner O, Russell KA, Lee AS, et al. Antineutrophil cytoplasmic antibodies reacting with human neutrophil elastase as a diagnostic marker for cocaine-induced midline destructive lesions but not autoimmune vasculitis. *Arthritis Rheum.* 2004;50:2954–2965.
102. Slot MC, Links TP, Stegeman CA, et al. Occurrence of antineutrophil cytoplasmic antibodies and associated vasculitis in patients with hyperthyroidism treated with antithyroid drugs: A long-term followup study. *Arthritis Rheum.* 2005;53:108–113.
103. Van Rossum AP, Rarok AA, Huitema MG, et al. Constitutive membrane expression of proteinase 3 (PR3) and neutrophil activation by anti-PR3 antibodies. *J Leukoc Biol.* 2004;76:1162–1170.
104. Brouwer E, Huitema MG, Mulder AH, et al. Neutrophil activation in vitro and in vivo in Wegener's granulomatosis. *Kidney Int.* 1994;45:1120–1131.
105. Schreiber A, Otto B, Ju X, et al. Membrane proteinase 3 expression in patients with Wegener's granulomatosis and in human hematopoietic stem cell-derived neutrophils. *J Am Soc Nephrol.* 2005;16:2216–2224.
106. Yang JJ, Pendergraft WF, Alcorta DA, et al. Circumvention of normal constraints on granule protein gene expression in peripheral blood neutrophils and monocytes of patients with antineutrophil cytoplasmic autoantibody-associated glomerulonephritis. *J Am Soc Nephrol.* 2004;15:2103–2114.
107. Ciavatta DJ, Yang J, Preston GA, et al. Epigenetic basis for aberrant upregulation of autoantigen genes in humans with ANCA vasculitis. *J Clin Invest.* 2010;120:3209–3219.
108. Falk RJ, Terrell RS, Charles LA, et al. Anti-neutrophil cytoplasmic autoantibodies induce neutrophils to degranulate and produce oxygen radicals in vitro. *Proc Natl Acad Sci U S A.* 1990;87:4115–4119.
109. Cockwell P, Brooks CJ, Adu D, et al. Interleukin-8:A pathogenetic role in antineutrophil cytoplasmic autoantibody-associated glomerulonephritis [see comments]. *Kidney Int.* 1999;55:852–863.
110. Braun MG, Csernok E, Gross WL, et al. Proteinase 3, the target antigen of anticytoplasmic antibodies circulating in Wegener's granulomatosis. Immunolocalization in normal and pathologic tissues. *Am J Pathol.* 1991;139:831–838.
111. Porges AJ, Redecha PB, Kimberly WT, et al. Anti-neutrophil cytoplasmic antibodies engage and activate human neutrophils via Fc gamma RIIa. *J Immunol.* 1994;153:1271–1280.
112. Kettritz R, Jennette JC, Falk RJ. Crosslinking of ANCA-antigens stimulates superoxide release by human neutrophils. *J Am Soc Nephrol.* 1997;8:386–394.
113. Kimberly RP. Fcgamma receptors and neutrophil activation. *Clin Exp Immunol.* 2000;120 (Suppl 1):18–19.
114. Kocher M, Edberg JC, Fleit HB, et al. Antineutrophil cytoplasmic antibodies preferentially engage Fc gammaRIIIb on human neutrophils. *J Immunol.* 1998;161:6909–6914.
115. Tse WY, Abadeh S, McTiernan A, et al. No association between neutrophil FcgammaRIIa allelic polymorphism and anti-neutrophil cytoplasmic antibody (ANCA)-positive systemic vasculitis. *Clin Exp Immunol.* 1999;117:198–205.
116. Dijstelbloem HM, Scheepers RH, Oost WW, et al. Fcgamma receptor polymorphisms in Wegener's granulomatosis: risk factors for disease relapse. *Arthritis Rheum.* 1999;42:1823–1827.
117. Williams JM, Savage COS. Characterization of the regulation and functional consequences of p21ras activation in neutrophils by antineutrophil cytoplasm antibodies. *J Am Soc Nephrol.* 2005;16:90–96.
118. Taekema-Roelvink ME, van Kooten C, Heemskerk E, et al. Proteinase 3 interacts with a 111–kD membrane molecule of human umbilical vein endothelial cells. *J Am Soc Nephrol.* 2000;11:640–648.
119. Kurosawa S, Esmon CT, Stearns-Kurosawa DJ. The soluble endothelial protein C receptor binds to activated neutrophils: involvement of proteinase-3 and CD11b/CD18. *J Immunol.* 2000;165:4697–4703.
120. Taekema-Roelvink ME, van Kooten C, Janssens MC, et al. Effect of anti-neutrophil cytoplasmic antibodies on proteinase 3–induced apoptosis of human endothelial cells. *Scand J Immunol.* 1998;48:37–43.
121. Baldus S, Eiserich JP, Mani A, et al. Endothelial transcytosis of myeloperoxidase confers specificity to vascular ECM proteins as targets of tyrosine nitration. *J Clin Invest.* 2001;108:1759–1770.
122. Brennan ML, Wu W, Fu X, et al. A tale of two controversies: defining both the role of peroxidases in nitrotyrosine formation in vivo using eosinophil peroxidase and myeloperoxidase-deficient mice, and the nature of peroxidase-generated reactive nitrogen species. *J Biol Chem.* 2002;277:17415–17427.
123. Woods AA, Linton SM, Davies MJ. Detection of HOCl-mediated protein oxidation products in the extracellular matrix of human atherosclerotic plaques. *Biochem J.* 2003;370:729–735.
124. Lu X, Garfield A, Rainger GE, et al. Mediation of endothelial cell damage by serine proteases, but not superoxide, released from antineutrophil cytoplasmic antibody-stimulated neutrophils. *Arthritis Rheum.* 2006;54:1619–1628.
125. Calderwood JW, Williams JM, Morgan MD, et al. ANCA induces beta2 integrin and CXC chemokine-dependent neutrophil-endothelial cell interactions that mimic those of highly cytokine-activated endothelium. *J Leukoc Biol.* 2005;77:33–43.
126. Brouwer E, Tervaert JW, Horst G, et al. Predominance of IgG1 and IgG4 subclasses of anti-neutrophil cytoplasmic autoantibodies (ANCA) in patients with Wegener's granulomatosis and clinically related disorders. *Clin Exp Immunol.* 1991;83:379–386.
127. Schmitt WH, Heesen C, Csernok E, et al. Elevated serum levels of soluble interleukin-2 receptor in patients with Wegener's granulomatosis. Association with disease activity. *Arthritis Rheum.* 1992;35:1088–1096.
128. Stegeman CA, Tervaert JW, Huitema MG, et al. Serum markers of T cell activation in relapses of Wegener's granulomatosis. *Clin Exp Immunol.* 1993;91:415–420.
129. Marinaki S, Neumann I, Kalsch AI, et al. Abnormalities of CD4 T cell subpopulations in ANCA-associated vasculitis. *Clin Exp Immunol.* 2005;140:181–191.
130. Marinaki S, Kalsch AI, Grimminger P, et al. Persistent T-cell activation and clinical correlations in patients with ANCA-associated systemic vasculitis. *Nephrol Dial Transplant.* 2006;21:1825–1832.
131. Tipping PG, Holdsworth SR. T cells in crescentic glomerulonephritis. *J Am Soc Nephrol.* 2006;17:1253–1263.
132. Mueller A, Holl-Ulrich K, Lamprecht P, et al. Germinal centre-like structures in Wegener's granuloma: the morphological basis for autoimmunity? *Rheumatology (Oxford).* 2008;47:1111–1113.
133. Gephardt GN, Ahmad M, Tubbs RR. Pulmonary vasculitis (Wegener's granulomatosis). Immunohistochemical study of T and B cell markers. *Am J Med.* 1983;74:700–704.
134. Csernok E, Trabandt A, Muller A, et al. Cytokine profiles in Wegener's granulomatosis: predominance of type 1 (Th1) in the granulomatous inflammation. *Arthritis Rheum.* 1999;42:742–750.
135. Moosig F, Csernok E, Wang G, et al. Costimulatory molecules in Wegener's granulomatosis (WG): lack of expression of CD28 and preferential up-regulation of its ligands B7–1 (CD80) and B7–2 (CD86) on T cells. *Clin Exp Immunol.* 1998;114:113–118.
136. Rulifson IC, Sperling AI, Fields PE, et al. CD28 costimulation promotes the production of Th2 cytokines. *J Immunol.* 1997;158:658–665.
137. Popa ER, Franssen CF, Limburg PC, et al. In vitro cytokine production and proliferation of T cells from patients with anti-proteinase 3– and antimyeloperoxidase-associated vasculitis, in response to proteinase 3 and myeloperoxidase. *Arthritis Rheum.* 2002;46:1894–1904.
138. Wilde B, Dolff S, Cai X, et al. CD4+CD25+ T-cell populations expressing CD134 and GITR are associated with disease activity in patients with Wegener's granulomatosis. *Nephrol Dial Transplant.* 2009;24:161–171.
139. Wilde B, van PP, Witzke O, et al. New pathophysiological insights and treatment of ANCA-associated vasculitis. *Kidney Int.* 2011;79:599–612.
140. Abdulahad WH, Kallenberg CG, Limburg PC, et al. Urinary CD4+ effector memory T cells reflect renal disease activity in antineutrophil cytoplasmic antibody-associated vasculitis. *Arthritis Rheum.* 2009;60:2830–2838.
141. Aloisi F, Pujol-Borrell R. Lymphoid neogenesis in chronic inflammatory diseases. *Nat Rev Immunol.* 2006;6:205–217.
142. Voswinkel J, Mueller A, Kraemer JA, et al. B lymphocyte maturation in Wegener's granulomatosis: a comparative analysis of VH genes from endonasal lesions. *Ann Rheum Dis.* 2006;65:859–864.
143. Csernok E, Ai M, Gross WL, et al. Wegener's autoantigen induces maturation of dendritic cells and licences them for TH1 priming via the protease-activated receptor-2 pathway. *Blood.* 2006;107:4440–4448.
144. Capraru D, Muller A, Csernok E, et al. Expansion of circulating NKG2D+ effector memory T-cells and expression of NKG2D-ligand MIC in granulomatous lesions in Wegener's granulomatosis. *Clin Immunol.* 2008;127:144–150.
145. Segerer S, Heller F, Lindenmeyer MT, et al. Compartment specific expression of dendritic cell markers in human glomerulonephritis. *Kidney Int.* 2008;74:37–46.
146. Steinmetz OM, Velden J, Kneissler U, et al. Analysis and classification of B-cell infiltrates in lupus and ANCA-associated nephritis. *Kidney Int.* 2008;74:448–457.

147. Jovanovic DV, Di Battista JA, Martel-Pelletier J, et al. IL-17 stimulates the production and expression of proinflammatory cytokines, IL-beta and TNF-alpha, by human macrophages. *J Immunol.* 1998;160:3513–3521.
148. Abdulahad WH, Stegeman CA, Limburg PC, et al. Skewed distribution of Th17 lymphocytes in patients with Wegener's granulomatosis in remission. *Arthritis Rheum.* 2008;58:2196–2205.
149. Nogueira E, Hamour S, Sawant D, et al. Serum IL-17 and IL-23 levels and autoantigen-specific Th17 cells are elevated in patients with ANCA-associated vasculitis. *Nephrol Dial Transplant.* 2010;25(7):2209–2217.
150. Ordonez L, Bernard I, L'faqihi-Olive FE, et al. CD45RC isoform expression identifies functionally distinct T cell subsets differentially distributed between healthy individuals and AAV patients. *PLoS One.* 2009;4:e5287.
151. Brusko TM, Putnam AL, Bluestone JA. Human regulatory T cells: role in autoimmune disease and therapeutic opportunities. *Immunol Rev.* 2008;223:371–390.
152. Abdulahad WH, Stegeman CA, van der Geld YM, et al. Functional defect of circulating regulatory CD4+ T cells in patients with Wegener's granulomatosis in remission. *Arthritis Rheum.* 2007;56:2080–2091.
153. Morgan MD, Day CJ, Piper KP, et al. Patients with Wegener's granulomatosis demonstrate a relative deficiency and functional impairment of T-regulatory cells. *Immunology.* 2010;130:64–73.
154. Abdulahad WH, van der Geld YM, Stegeman CA, et al. Persistent expansion of CD4+ effector memory T cells in Wegener's granulomatosis. *Kidney Int.* 2006;70:938–947.
155. Brouwer E, Stegeman CA, Huitema MG, et al. T cell reactivity to proteinase 3 and myeloperoxidase in patients with Wegener's granulomatosis (WG). *Clin Exp Immunol.* 1994;98:448–453.
156. Mathieson PW, Oliveira DB. The role of cellular immunity in systemic vasculitis. *Clin Exp Immunol.* 1995;100:183–185.
157. King WJ, Brooks CJ, Holder R, et al. T lymphocyte responses to anti-neutrophil cytoplasmic autoantibody (ANCA) antigens are present in patients with ANCA-associated systemic vasculitis and persist during disease remission. *Clin Exp Immunol.* 1998;112:539–546.
158. Kessenbrock K, Krumbholz M, Schonermarck U, et al. Netting neutrophils in autoimmune small-vessel vasculitis. *Nat Med.* 2009;15:623–625.
159. Brinkmann V, Reichard U, Goosmann C, et al. Neutrophil extracellular traps kill bacteria. *Science.* 2004;303:1532–1535.
160. Leadbetter EA, Rifkin IR, Hohlbaum AM, et al. Chromatin-IgG complexes activate B cells by dual engagement of IgM and Toll-like receptors. *Nature.* 2002;416:603–607.
161. Yan B, Ye S, Chen G, et al. Dysfunctional CD4+,CD25+ regulatory T cells in untreated active systemic lupus erythematosus secondary to interferon-alpha-producing antigen-presenting cells. *Arthritis Rheum.* 2008;58:801–812.
162. Papayannopoulos V, Zychlinsky A. NETs: a new strategy for using old weapons. *Trends Immunol.* 2009;30:513–521.
163. Stegeman CA, Cohen Tervaert JW, Manson WL, et al. Chronic nasal carriage of *Staphylococcal aureus* in Wegener's granulomatosis identifies a subgroup of patients more prone to relapse. *Ann Intern Med.* 1994;120:12–17.
164. Popa ER, Stegeman CA, Bos NA, et al. Staphylococcal superantigens and T cell expansions in Wegener's granulomatosis. *Clin Exp Immunol.* 2003;132:496–504.
165. Brons RH, Klok PA, vanDijk NW, et al. Staphylococcal acid phosphatase induces a severe crescentic glomerulonephritis in immunized Brown-Norway rats: relevance for Wegener's granulomatosis? [Abstract] *Clin Exp Immunol.* 2000;120[Suppl 1]:44.
166. Dal Canto AJ, Virgin HW. Animal models of infection-mediated vasculitis. *Curr Opin Rheumatol.* 1999;11:17–23.
167. Parks CG, Cooper GS, Nylander-French LA, et al. Occupational exposure to crystalline silica and risk of systemic lupus erythematosus: a population-based, case-control study in the southeastern United States. *Arthritis Rheum.* 2002;46:1840–1850.
168. Nuyts GD, Van Vlem E, De Vos A, et al. Wegener granulomatosis is associated to exposure to silicon compounds: a case-control study [see comments] [published erratum appears in *Nephrol Dial Transplant.* 1995 Nov;10(11):2168]. *Nephrol Dial Transplant.* 1995;10:1162–1165.
169. Hogan SL, Satterly KK, Dooley MA, et al. Silica exposure in anti-neutrophil cytoplasmic autoantibody-associated glomerulonephritis and lupus nephritis. *J Am Soc Nephrol.* 2001;12:134–142.
170. Lane SE, Watts RA, Bentham G, et al. Are environmental factors important in primary systemic vasculitis?: A case-control study. *Arthritis Rheum.* 2003;48:814–823.
171. Hogan SL, Cooper GS, Nylander-French LA, et al. Duration of silican exposure and development of ANCA-associated small vessel vasculitis with glomerular involvement: a case-control study [Abstract]. *J Am Soc Nephrol.* 2004;15:16.
172. Sanchez-Roman J, Wichmann I, Salaberri J, et al. Multiple clinical and biological autoimmune manifestations in 50 workers after occupational exposure to silica [see comments]. *Ann Rheum Dis.* 1993;52:534–538.
173. Conrad K, Mehlhorn J, Luthke K, et al. Systemic lupus erythematosus after heavy exposure to quartz dust in uranium mines: clinical and serological characteristics. *Lupus.* 1996;5:62–69.
174. ten Holder S, Joy MS, Falk RJ. Drug-induced vasculitis: a review of cutaneous and systemic manifestations. [Abstract] *Clin Exp Immunol.* 2000;120 Suppl 1:60.
175. McGrath MM, Isakova T, Mottola AM, et al. Contaminated cocaine and drug-induced vasculitis. [Abstract] *J Am Soc Nephrol.* 2010;21:422A.
176. Xiao H, Heeringa P, Hu P, et al. Antineutrophil cytoplasmic autoantibodies specific for myeloperoxidase cause glomerulonephritis and vasculitis in mice. *J Clin Invest.* 2002;110:955–963.
177. Huugen D, Xiao H, van EA, et al. Aggravation of anti-myeloperoxidase antibody-induced glomerulonephritis by bacterial lipopolysaccharide: role of tumor necrosis factor-alpha. *Am J Pathol.* 2005;167:47–58.
178. Xiao H, Heeringa P, Liu Z, et al. The role of neutrophils in the induction of glomerulonephritis by anti-myeloperoxidase antibodies. *Am J Pathol.* 2005;167:39–45.
179. Little MA, Smyth CL, Yadav R, et al. Antineutrophil cytoplasm antibodies directed against myeloperoxidase augment leukocyte-microvascular interactions in vivo. *Blood.* 2005;106:2050–2058.
180. Pfister H, Ollert M, Froehlich LF, et al. Anti-neutrophil cytoplasmic autoantibodies (ANCA) against the murine homolog of proteinase 3 (Wegener's autoantigen) are pathogenic in vivo. *Blood.* 2004;104(5):1411–1418.
181. Primo VC, Marusic S, Franklin CC, et al. Anti-PR3 immune responses induce segmental and necrotizing glomerulonephritis. *Clin Exp Immunol.* 2010; 159:327–337.
182. Xiao H, Schreiber A, Heeringa P, et al. Alternative complement pathway in the pathogenesis of disease mediated by anti-neutrophil cytoplasmic autoantibodies. *Am J Pathol.* 2007;170:52–64.
183. Huugen D, van EA, Xiao H, et al. Inhibition of complement factor C5 protects against anti-myeloperoxidase antibody-mediated glomerulonephritis in mice. *Kidney Int.* 2007;71:646–654.
184. Schreiber A, Xiao H, Jennette JC, et al. C5a receptor mediates neutrophil activation and ANCA-induced glomerulonephritis. *J Am Soc Nephrol.* 2009; 20:289–298.
185. Chavele KM, Martinez-Pomares L, Domin J, et al. Mannose receptor interacts with Fc receptors and is critical for the development of crescentic glomerulonephritis in mice. *J Clin Invest.* 2010;120:1469–1478.
186. Oldstone MB. Molecular mimicry, microbial infection, and autoimmune disease: evolution of the concept. *Curr Top Microbiol Immunol.* 2005;296:1–17.
187. Pendergraft WF III, Pressler BM, Jennette JC, et al. Autoantigen complementarity: a new theory implicating complementary proteins as initiators of autoimmune disease. *J Mol Med.* 2005;83:12–25.
188. Pendergraft WF, Preston GA, Shah RR, et al. Autoimmunity is triggered by cPR-3(105–201), a protein complementary to human autoantigen proteinase-3. *Nat Med.* 2004;10:72–79.
189. Kain R, Exner M, Brandes R, et al. Molecular mimicry in pauci-immune focal necrotizing glomerulonephritis. *Nat Med.* 2008;14:1088–1096.
190. Cao Y, Schmitz JL, Yang J, et al. DRB1*15 Allele Is a Risk Factor for PR3–ANCA Disease in African Americans. *J Am Soc Nephrol.* 2011;22:1161–1167.
191. Roth AJ, Brown MC, Smith RN, et al. Anti-LAMP-2 antibodies are not prevalent in patients with antineutrophil cytoplasmic glomerulonephtritis. *J Am Soc Nephrol.* 2012;23(3):545–555.
192. Sable-Fourtassou R, Cohen P, Mahr A, et al. Antineutrophil cytoplasmic antibodies and the eosinophilic granulomatosis. *Ann Intern Med.* 2005;143:632–638.
193. Bibby S, Healy B, Steele R, et al. Association between leukotriene receptor antagonist therapy and eosinophilic granulomatosis: an analysis of the FDA AERS database. *Thorax.* 2010;65:132–138.
194. Hellmich B, Csernok E, Gross WL. Proinflammatory cytokines and autoimmunity in eosinophilic granulomatosis. *Ann N Y Acad Sci.* 2005;1051:121–131.
195. Schonermarck U, Csernok E, Trabandt A, et al. Circulating cytokines and soluble CD23, CD26 and CD30 in ANCA-associated vasculitides. *Clin Exp Rheumatol.* 2000;18:457–463.
196. Clutterbuck EJ, Hirst EM, Sanderson CJ. Human interleukin-5 (IL-5) regulates the production of eosinophils in human bone marrow cultures: comparison and interaction with IL-1, IL-3, IL-6, and GMCSF. *Blood.* 1989;73:1504–1512.
197. Yamaguchi Y, Suda T, Ohta S, et al. Analysis of the survival of mature human eosinophils: interleukin-5 prevents apoptosis in mature human eosinophils. *Blood.* 1991;78:2542–2547.
198. Fujisawa T, Abu-Ghazaleh R, Kita H, et al. Regulatory effect of cytokines on eosinophil degranulation. *J Immunol.* 1990;144:642–646.
199. Shahabuddin S, Ponath P, Schleimer RP. Migration of eosinophils across endothelial cell monolayers: interactions among IL-5, endothelial-activating cytokines, and C-C chemokines. *J Immunol.* 2000;164:3847–3854.
200. Kiene M, Csernok E, Muller A, et al. Elevated interleukin-4 and interleukin-13 production by T cell lines from patients with eosinophilic granulomatosis. *Arthritis Rheum.* 2001;44:469–473.

201. Zwerina J, Axmann R, Jatzwauk M, et al. Pathogenesis of eosinophilic granulomatosis: recent insights. *Autoimmunity.* 2009;42:376–379.
202. Polzer K, Karonitsch T, Neumann T, et al. Eotaxin-3 is involved in eosinophilic granulomatosis - a serum marker closely correlating with disease activity. *Rheumatology (Oxford).* 2008;47(6):804–808.
203. Saito H, Tsurikisawa N, Tsuburai T, et al. Cytokine production profile of CD4+ T cells from patients with active eosinophilic granulomatosis tends toward Th17. *Int Arch Allergy Immunol.* 2009;149 Suppl 1:61–65.
204. Tsurikisawa N, Saito H, Tsuburai T, et al. Differences in regulatory T cells between eosinophilic granulomatosis and chronic eosinophilic pneumonia with asthma. *J Allergy Clin Immunol.* 2008;122:610–616.
205. Walsh M, Merkel PA, Mahr A, et al. Effects of duration of glucocorticoid therapy on relapse rate in antineutrophil cytoplasmic antibody-associated vasculitis: A meta-analysis. *Arthritis Care Res (Hoboken).* 2010;62:1166–1173.
206. Nachman PH, Hogan SL, Jennette JC, et al. Treatment response and relapse in antineutrophil cytoplasmic autoantibody-associated microscopic polyangiitis and glomerulonephritis. *J Am Soc Nephrol.* 1996;7:33–39.
207. Guillevin L, Cordier JF, Lhote F, et al. A prospective, multicenter, randomized trial comparing steroids and pulse cyclophosphamide versus steroids and oral cyclophosphamide in the treatment of generalized Wegener's granulomatosis [see comments]. *Arthritis Rheum.* 1997;40:2187–2198.
208. de Groot K, Adu D, Savage CO. The value of pulse cyclophosphamide in ANCA-associated vasculitis: meta-analysis and critical review. *Nephrol Dial Transplant.* 2001;16:2018–2027.
209. Jayne D, Rasmussen N, Andrassy K, et al. A randomized trial of maintenance therapy for vasculitis associated with antineutrophil cytoplasmic autoantibodies. *N Engl J Med.* 2003;349:36–44.
210. Stassen PM, Cohen Tervaert JW, Stegeman CA. Induction of remission in active anti-neutrophil cytoplasmic antibody-associated vasculitis with mycophenolate mofetil in patients who cannot be treated with cyclophosphamide. *Ann Rheum Dis.* 2007;66:798–802.
211. Hu W, Liu C, Xie H, et al. Mycophenolate mofetil versus cyclophosphamide for inducing remission of ANCA vasculitis with moderate renal involvement. *Nephrol Dial Transplant.* 2008;23:1307–1312.
212. Silva F, Specks U, Kalra S, et al. Mycophenolate mofetil for induction and maintenance of remission in microscopic polyangiitis with mild to moderate renal involvement—a prospective, open-label pilot trial. *Clin J Am Soc Nephrol.* 2010;5:445–453.
213. Sneller MC, Hoffman GS, Talar-Williams C, et al. An analysis of forty-two Wegener's granulomatosis patients treated with methotrexate and prednisone. *Arthritis Rheum.* 1995;38:608–613.
214. Langford CA, Talar-Williams C, Barron KS, et al. Use of a cyclophosphamide-induction methotrexate-maintenance regimen for the treatment of Wegener's granulomatosis: extended follow-up and rate of relapse. *Am J Med.* 2003; 114:463–469.
215. de Groot K, Rasmussen N, Bacon PA, et al. Randomized trial of cyclophosphamide versus methotrexate for induction of remission in early systemic antineutrophil cytoplasmic antibody-associated vasculitis. *Arthritis Rheum.* 2005;52:2461–2469.
216. Stone JH, Merkel PA, Spiera R, et al. Rituximab versus cyclophosphamide for ANCA-associated vasculitis. *N Engl J Med.* 2010;363:221–232.
217. Jones RB, Tervaert JW, Hauser T, et al. Rituximab versus cyclophosphamide in ANCA-associated renal vasculitis. *N Engl J Med.* 2010;363:211–220.
218. Klemmer PJ, Chalermskulrat W, Reif MS, et al. Plasmapheresis therapy for diffuse alveolar hemorrhage in patients with small-vessel vasculitis. *Am J Kidney Dis.* 2003;42:1149–1153.
219. Jayne DR, Gaskin G, Rasmussen N, et al. Randomized trial of plasma exchange or high-dosage methylprednisolone as adjunctive therapy for severe renal vasculitis. *J Am Soc Nephrol.* 2007;18:2180–2188.
220. Walters GD, Willis NS, Craig JC. Interventions for renal vasculitis in adults. A systematic review. *BMC Nephrol.* 2010;11:12.
221. Cole E, Cattran D, Magil A, et al. A prospective randomized trial of plasma exchange as additive therapy in idiopathic crescentic glomerulonephritis. The Canadian Apheresis Study Group. *Am J Kidney Dis.* 1992;20:261–269.
222. Pusey CD, Rees AJ, Evans DJ, et al. Plasma exchange in focal necrotizing glomerulonephritis without anti-GBM antibodies. *Kidney Int.* 1991;40:757–763.
223. Jayne D, Merkel P, Walsh M. Plasma exchange and glucocorticoids for treatment of anti-neutrophil cycoplasm antibody (ANCA) vasculitis (PEXIVAS). http://clinicaltrials.gov/ct2/show/NCT00987389. 2011.
224. Lionaki S, Hogan SL, Jennette CE, et al. The clinical course of ANCA small-vessel vasculitis on chronic dialysis. *Kidney Int.* 2009;76:644–651.
225. Hogan SL, Falk RJ, Chin H, et al. Predictors of relapse and treatment resistance in antineutrophil cytoplasmic antibody-associated small-vessel vasculitis. *Ann Intern Med.* 2005;143:621–631.
226. Gordon M, Luqmani RA, Adu D, et al. Relapses in patients with a systemic vasculitis. *Q J Med.* 1993;86:779–789.
227. Pagnoux C, Hogan SL, Chin H, et al. Predictors of treatment resistance and relapse in antineutrophil cytoplasmic antibody-associated small-vessel vasculitis: Comparison of two independent cohorts. *Arthritis Rheum.* 2008;58:2908–2918.
228. Boomsma MM, Stegeman CA, van der Leij MJ, et al. Prediction of relapses in Wegener's granulomatosis by measurement of antineutrophil cytoplasmic antibody levels: a prospective study. *Arthritis Rheum.* 2000;43:2025–2033.
229. Finkielman JD, Merkel PA, Schroeder D, et al. Antiproteinase 3 antineutrophil cytoplasmic antibodies and disease activity in Wegener granulomatosis. *Ann Intern Med.* 2007;147:611–619.
230. Cohen Tervaert JW, Huitema MG, Hene RJ, et al. Prevention of relapses in Wegener's granulomatosis by treatment based on antineutrophil cytoplasmic antibody titre. *Lancet.* 1990;336:709–711.
231. Guillevin L, Cohen P, Gayraud M, et al. eosinophilic granulomatosis. Clinical study and long-term follow-up of 96 patients. *Medicine (Baltimore).* 1999;78:26–37.
232. Jayne DR, Chapel H, Adu D, et al. Intravenous immunoglobulin for ANCA-associated systemic vasculitis with persistent disease activity. *QJM.* 2000;93: 433–439.
233. Martinez V, Cohen P, Pagnoux C, et al. Intravenous immunoglobulins for relapses of systemic vasculitides associated with antineutrophil cytoplasmic autoantibodies: results of a multicenter, prospective, open-label study of twenty-two patients. *Arthritis Rheum.* 2008;58:308–317.
234. Aries PM, Hellmich B, Voswinkel J, et al. Lack of efficacy of rituximab in Wegener's granulomatosis with refractory granulomatous manifestations. *Ann Rheum Dis.* 2006;65:853–858.
235. Jones RB, Ferraro AJ, Chaudhry AN, et al. A multicenter survey of rituximab therapy for refractory antineutrophil cytoplasmic antibody-associated vasculitis. *Arthritis Rheum.* 2009;60:2156–2168.
236. Kirk AD, Hale DA, Mannon RB, et al. Results from a human renal allograft tolerance trial evaluating the humanized CD52–specific monoclonal antibody alemtuzumab (CAMPATH-1H). *Transplantation.* 2003;76:120–129.
237. Isaacs JD, Manna VK, Rapson N, et al. CAMPATH-1H in rheumatoid arthritis—an intravenous dose-ranging study. *Br J Rheumatol.* 1999;35:231–240.
238. Jayne DR. Campath-1H (anti-CD52) for refractory vasculitis: retrospective Cambridge experience 1989–1999. *Cleve Clin J Med.* 2002;69:Sii–s129.
239. Walsh M, Chaudhry A, Jayne D. Long-term follow-up of relapsing/refractory anti-neutrophil cytoplasm antibody associated vasculitis treated with the lymphocyte depleting antibody alemtuzumab (CAMPATH-1H). *Ann Rheum Dis.* 2008;67:1322–1327.
240. Lamprecht P, Voswinkel J, Lilienthal T, et al. Effectiveness of TNF-alpha blockade with infliximab in refractory Wegener's granulomatosis. *Rheumatology (Oxford).* 2002;41:1303–1307.
241. Bartolucci P, Ramanoelina J, Cohen P, et al. Efficacy of the anti-TNF-alpha antibody infliximab against refractory systemic vasculitides: an open pilot study on 10 patients. *Rheumatology (Oxford).* 2002;41:1126–1132.
242. Booth A, Harper L, Hammad T, et al. Prospective study of TNFalpha blockade with infliximab in anti-neutrophil cytoplasmic antibody-associated systemic vasculitis. *J Am Soc Nephrol.* 2004;15:717–721.
243. Booth AD, Jefferson HJ, Ayliffe W, et al. Safety and efficacy of TNFalpha blockade in relapsing vasculitis. *Ann Rheum Dis.* 2002;61:559.
244. Birck R, Warnatz K, Lorenz HM, et al. 15–Deoxyspergualin in patients with refractory ANCA-associated systemic vasculitis: a six-month open-label trial to evaluate safety and efficacy. *J Am Soc Nephrol.* 2003;14:440–447.
245. Flossmann O, Baslund B, Bruchfeld A, et al. Deoxyspergualin in relapsing and refractory Wegener's granulomatosis. *Ann Rheum Dis.* 2009;68:1125–1130.
246. Pagnoux C, Mahr A, Hamidou MA, et al. Azathioprine or methotrexate maintenance for ANCA-associated vasculitis. *N Engl J Med.* 2008;359:2790–2803.
247. Metzler C, Miehle N, Manger K, et al. Elevated relapse rate under oral methotrexate versus leflunomide for maintenance of remission in Wegener's granulomatosis. *Rheumatology (Oxford).* 2007;46:1087–1091.
248. Hiemstra TF, Walsh M, Mahr A, et al. Mycophenolate mofetil vs azathioprine for remission maintenance in antineutrophil cytoplasmic antibody-associated vasculitis: a randomized controlled trial. *JAMA.* 2010;304:2381–2388.
249. Ribi C, Cohen P, Pagnoux C, et al. Treatment of eosinophilic granulomatosis without poor-prognosis factors: a multicenter, prospective, randomized, open-label study of seventy-two patients. *Arthritis Rheum.* 2008;58:586–594.
250. Metzler C, Fink C, Lamprecht P, et al. Maintenance of remission with leflunomide in Wegener's granulomatosis. *Rheumatology (Oxford).* 2004;43:315–320.
251. Giavina-Bianchi P, Kalil J. Omalizumab administration in eosinophilic granulomatosis. *Eur J Intern Med.* 2009;20:e139.
252. Kahn JE, Grandpeix-Guyodo C, Marroun I, et al. Sustained response to mepolizumab in refractory eosinophilic granulomatosis. *J Allergy Clin Immunol.* 2010;125:267–270.

253. Metzler C, Csernok E, Gross WL, et al. Interferon-alpha for maintenance of remission in eosinophilic granulomatosis: a long-term observational study. *Clin Exp Rheumatol.* 2010;28:24–30.

254. Geetha D, Seo P, Specks U, et al. Successful induction of remission with rituximab for relapse of ANCA-associated vasculitis post-kidney transplant: report of two cases. *Am J Transplant* 2007;7:2821–2825.

255. Frasca GM, Neri L, Martello M, et al. Renal transplantation in patients with microscopic polyarteritis and antimyeloperoxidase antibodies: report of three cases. *Nephron.* 1996;72:82–85.

256. Rostaing L, Modesto A, Oksman F, et al. Outcome of patients with antineutrophil cytoplasmic autoantibody-associated vasculitis following cadaveric kidney transplantation. *Am J Kidney Dis.* 1997;29:96–102.

257. Schmitt WH, Haubitz M, Mistry N, et al. Renal transplantation in Wegener's granulomatosis [letter]. *Lancet.* 1993;342:860.

258. Nachman PH, Segelmark M, Westman K, et al. Recurrent ANCA-associated small vessel vasculitis after transplantation: A pooled analysis. *Kidney Int.* 1999;56:1544–1550.

259. Allen A, Pusey C, Gaskin G. Outcome of renal replacement therapy in antineutrophil cytoplasmic antibody-associated systemic vasculitis. *J Am Soc Nephrol.* 1998;9:1258–1263.

260. Elmedhem A, Adu D, Savage CO. Relapse rate and outcome of ANCA-associated small vessel vasculitis after transplantation. *Nephrol Dial Transplant.* 2003;18:1001–1004.

261. Gera M, Griffin MD, Specks U, et al. Recurrence of ANCA-associated vasculitis following renal transplantation in the modern era of immunosupression. *Kidney Int.* 2007;71:1296–1301.

262. Steinman TI, Jaffe BF, Monaco AP, et al. Recurrence of Wegener's granulomatosis after kidney transplantation. Successful re-induction of remission with cyclophosphamide. *Am J Med.* 1980;68:458–460.

263. Keogh KA, Ytterberg SR, Fervenza FC, et al. Rituximab for refractory Wegener's granulomatosis: report of a prospective, open-label pilot trial. *Am J Respir Crit Care Med.* 2006;173:180–187.

264. Stasi R, Stipa E, Poeta GD, et al. Long-term observation of patients with anti-neutrophil cytoplasmic antibody-associated vasculitis treated with rituximab. *Rheumatology (Oxford).* 2006;45:1432–1436.

265. : Criteria for diagnosis of Behcet's disease. International Study Group for Behcet's Disease. *Lancet.* 1990;335:1078–1080.

266. Koumantaki Y, Stavropoulos C, Spyropoulou M, et al. HLA-B*5101 in Greek patients with Behcet's disease. *Hum Immunol.* 1998;59:250–255.

267. Ahmad T, Wallace GR, James T, et al. Mapping the HLA association in Behcet's disease: a role for tumor necrosis factor polymorphisms? *Arthritis Rheum.* 2003;48:807–813.

268. Mizuki N, Ota M, Yabuki K, et al. Localization of the pathogenic gene of Behcet's disease by microsatellite analysis of three different populations. *Invest Ophthalmol Vis Sci.* 2000;41:3702–3708.

269. Mor F, Weinberger A, Cohen IR. Identification of alpha-tropomyosin as a target self-antigen in Behcet's syndrome. *Eur J Immunol.* 2002;32:356–365.

270. Freysdottir J, Lau S, Fortune F. Gammadelta T cells in Behcet's disease (BD) and recurrent aphthous stomatitis (RAS). *Clin Exp Immunol.* 1999; 118:451–457.

271. Frassanito MA, Dammacco R, Cafforio P, et al. Th1 polarization of the immune response in Behcet's disease: a putative pathogenetic role of interleukin-12. *Arthritis Rheum.* 1999;42:1967–1974.

272. de Smet MD, Dayan M. Prospective determination of T-cell responses to S-antigen in Behcet's disease patients and controls. *Invest Ophthalmol Vis Sci.* 2000;41:3480–3484.

273. Akpolat T, Akkoyunlu M, Akpolat I, et al. Renal Behcet's disease: a cumulative analysis. *Semin Arthritis Rheum.* 2002;31:317–337.

274. Akpolat I, Akpolat T, Danaci M, et al. Behcet's disease and amyloidosis. Review of the literature. *Scand J Rheumatol.* 1997;26:477–479.

275. Rosenthal T, Weiss P, Gafni J. Renal involvement in Behcet's syndrome. *Arch Intern Med.* 1978;138:1122–1124.

276. Altiparmak MR, Tanverdi M, Pamuk ON, et al. Glomerulonephritis in Behcet's disease: report of seven cases and review of the literature. *Clin Rheumatol.* 2002;21:14–18.

277. Herreman G, Beaufils H, Godeau P, et al. Behcet's syndrome and renal involvement: a histological and immunofluorescent study of eleven renal biopsies. *Am J Med Sci.* 1982;284:10–17.

278. Burrows NP, Zhao MH, Norris PG, et al. ANCA associated with Behcet's disease. *J R Soc Med.* 1996;89:47P-48P.

279. Ben Hmida M, Hachicha J, Kaddour N, et al. ANCA in Behcet's disease [letter]. *Nephrol Dial Transplant.* 1997;12:2465–2466.

280. Barnes CG. Treatment of Behcet's syndrome. *Rheumatology (Oxford).* 2006;45:245–247.

281. Davatchi F, Shahram F, Chams-Davatchi C, et al. Behcet's disease in Iran: analysis of 6500 cases. *Int J Rheum Dis.* 2010;13:367–373.

282. Melikoglu M, Fresko I, Mat C, et al. Short-term trial of etanercept in Behcet's disease: a double blind, placebo controlled study. *J Rheumatol.* 2005; 32:98–105.

283. Masala A, Faedda R, Alagna S, Set al. Use of testosterone to prevent cyclophosphamide-induced azoospermia. *Ann Intern Med.* 1997;126:292–295.

284. Dooley MA, Patterson CC, Hogan SL, et al. Preservation of ovarian function using depot leuprolide acetate during cyclophosphamide therapy for severe lupus nephritis. [Abstract] *Arthritis Rheum.* 2000;43:2858.

CHAPTER

49 Immunoglobulin A Nephropathy and Henoch-Schönlein Purpura

Jan Novak • Bruce A. Julian

Immunoglobulin A nephropathy (IgAN), the most common primary glomerulonephritis in the world,[1–3] is characterized by IgA-containing immune deposits in the glomerular mesangium. Berger and Hinglais described the disease in 1968 as a new entity based on the observation of "intercapillary deposits of IgA-IgG" using immunofluorescence examination of renal biopsy specimens from patients presenting with recurrent hematuria.[4] Subsequently, it was established that the IgA deposits are exclusively of the IgA1 subclass.[5] The same immunohistologic features are found in renal biopsy specimens from patients with Henoch-Schönlein purpura (HSP) and nephritis (HSPN) who have systemic findings of an IgA-associated vasculitis affecting the skin, gut, and joints.[6–9] On the other hand, biopsies of clinically normal skin of some patients with IgAN have deposits of IgA in the walls of dermal capillaries.[10] This finding, coupled with the shared biochemical abnormalities of circulating IgA1, has led to the postulate that the two diseases, IgAN and HSPN, represent the opposite ends of a spectrum of a disease process.[9,11]

IMMUNOGLOBULIN A NEPHROPATHY

Diagnosis

The histopathologic diagnosis of IgAN is usually clear and straightforward, with little need to consider a differential diagnosis. The key is the immunohistochemical identification of IgA deposition in the glomerular mesangium.

Immunofluorescence

A definitive diagnosis of IgAN can be made only by examination of renal cortical tissue with immunofluorescence microscopy or immunoperoxidase techniques. IgA is the dominant or codominant immunoreactant and is present predominantly in the mesangium, even in apparently normal or minimally affected glomeruli. Complement component C3 is usually found in the same distribution and is commonly accompanied by IgG, IgM, or both, although often with less intense fluorescence. Confocal microscopy has shown that when immune deposits show an outer layer of C3 rather than IgA, renal biopsy specimens exhibit more severe damage.[12] C1q and C4 are found rarely; if present in substantial quantities, the possibility of lupus nephritis should be entertained.[13]

Capillary loop fluorescence for IgA is observed most frequently in patients with clinically active disease. Such biopsy specimens may also show fibrinogen in the mesangium and capillary walls and IgM in areas of glomerular sclerosis. Walls of small and medium-sized blood vessels may contain abundant granular C3.

Light Microscopy

The light microscopic hallmark of IgAN is expansion of mesangial area with proliferation of mesangial cells and increased extracellular matrix. In patients with mild disease, these changes may be quite focal and segmental. Some glomerular tufts may appear to be normal. Capillary loops usually are patent, with normal configuration of capillary walls. However, in more florid disease, mesangial proliferative activity results in the matrix extending peripherally and circumferentially in the capillary walls, resulting in a double-contouring or "tram-tracking" effect, usually with lumen narrowing. In active disease, there may be tuft necrosis associated with an exudate of fibrin and infiltration of neutrophils, some of which may show karyorrhexis. This feature is often associated with crescents in Bowman's space.

In long-standing disease, areas of segmental tuft collapse and sclerosis, sometimes with overlying hyalinosis, are seen that usually are associated with broad synechiae. In progressive disease, the end result is glomerular obsolescence and sclerosis. All of these lesions may be found in one biopsy specimen. Focal segmental glomerulosclerosis may arise by several mechanisms, including postinflammatory scarring, compensatory hemodynamic changes after loss of nephrons, and primary damage to podocytes.[14–16]

Proportional to the degree of glomerular damage, there may be tubulointerstitial disease. When active glomerular disease is present, there often is interstitial edema associated with mild to moderate infiltrate of mononuclear cells and scattered neutrophils. Secondary tubular damage also may be evident. Interstitial scarring and tubular atrophy are features of advanced disease.[17] Hypertension-mediated damage may be seen patients with advanced disease. In an effort to standardize the description of the histologic features of the disease, an international consensus working group of nephrologists and nephropathologists has recently proposed a histologic classification scheme, the Oxford classification, based on light microscopic features.[18,19]

Electron Microscopy

Ultrastructural studies show varying degrees of expansion and proliferation of mesangial cells and extracellular matrix, and electron-dense deposits of differing sizes and amounts in the matrix. Deposits are particularly common in paramesangial areas. Corresponding to the segmental nature of the disease process, the distribution and amount of deposits may be quite patchy. Some mesangial sites may be distinctly free of deposits, yet others in the same glomerulus may be packed with them. These deposits are usually solid and homogeneous. Electron-dense deposits are occasionally found in the subepithelial and subendothelial areas of the glomerular basement membranes. Deposits in the latter location may be associated with focal necrotizing glomerular lesions on light microscopy.

Nephrotic syndrome with the pathologic features of minimal change disease has been noted in a few patients with IgAN.[20] In other patients, glomerular basement membranes are uniformly thin and this observation probably signifies the coexistence of two common conditions: IgAN and thin basement membrane nephropathy. However, one study of IgAN biopsies[21] described 40% with thin glomerular basement membranes, so perhaps mesangial IgA deposits interfere in some way with synthesis of normal glomerular basement membranes. The histologic features of IgAN are illustrated in Figure 49.1.

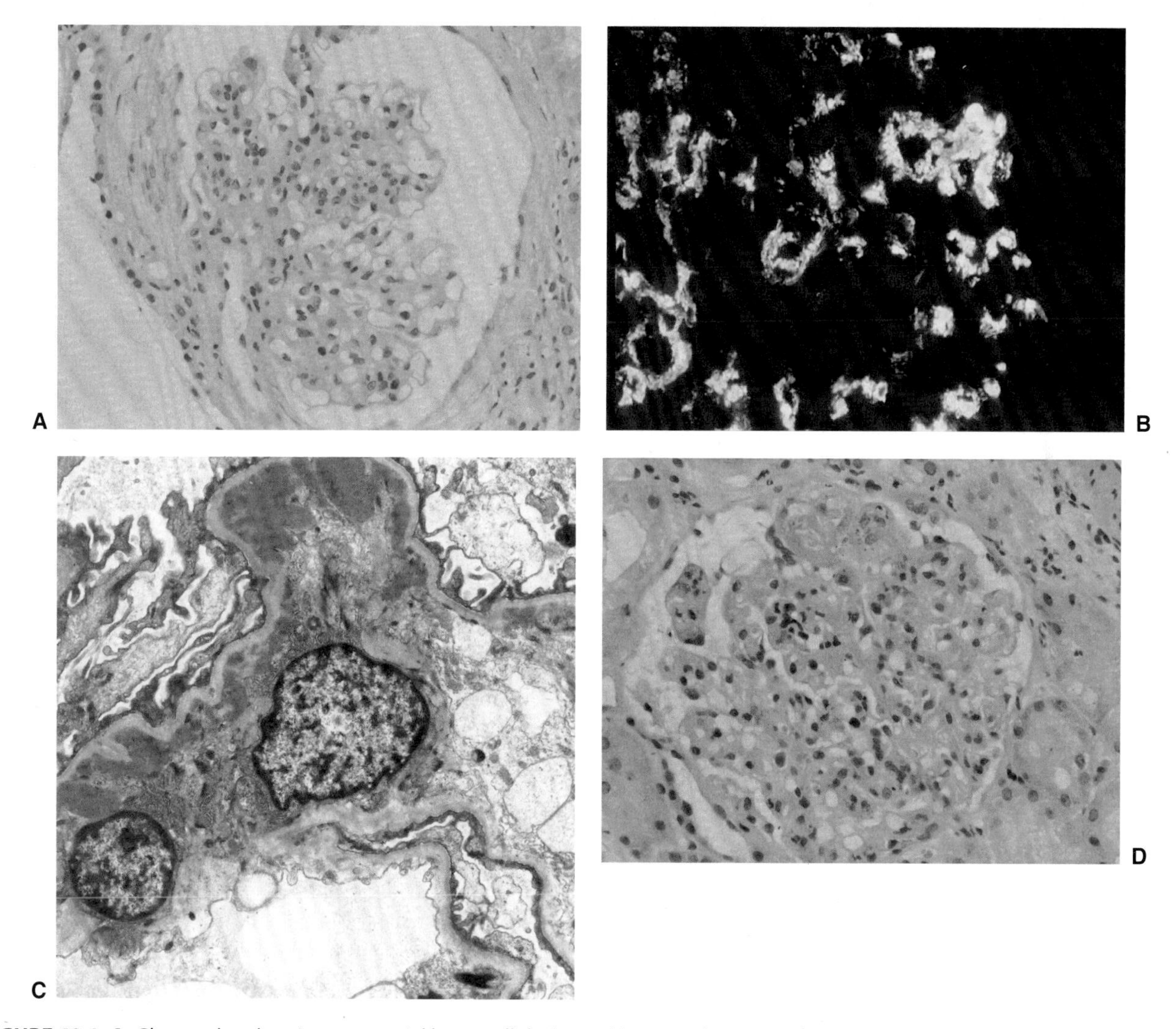

FIGURE 49.1 **A:** Glomerulus showing mesangial hypercellularity and increased mesangial matrix. (Hematoxylin and eosin stain, magnification, ×200.) **B:** Glomerulus, with brightly fluorescing mesangial deposits of IgA. (Fluorescinated antihuman IgA, magnification ×200.) **C:** Electron micrograph of glomerular mesangium showing multiple mesangial electron-dense deposits typical of IgA nephropathy. (Magnification ×3,000.) **D:** Glomerulus showing an acute lesion with segmental fibrinoid change and karyorhectic debris. (Hematoxylin and eosin, magnification ×200.) *(continued)*

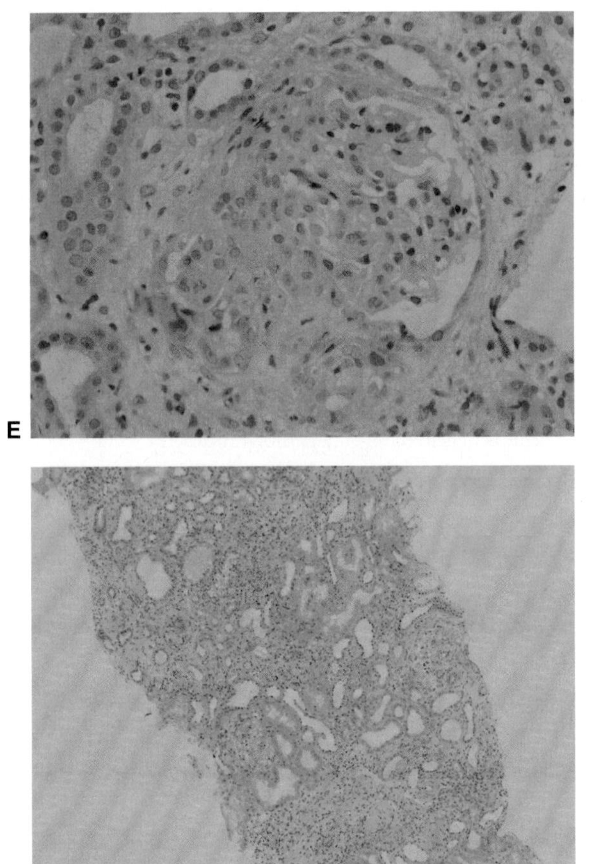

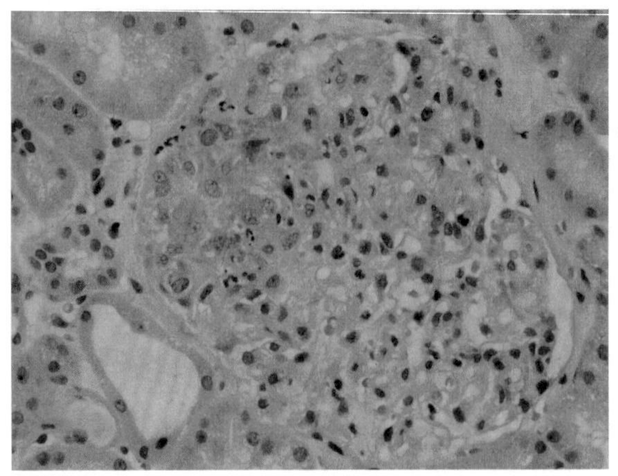

FIGURE 49.1 *(Continued)* **E:** Glomerulus showing an acute lesion with segmental crescent. (Hematoxylin and eosin, magnification ×200.) **F:** Sclerosing glomerulus with mesangial proliferation. (Hematoxylin and eosin, magnification ×200.) **G:** Low-power view of advanced IgAN, showing tubular dropout, interstitial fibrosis, and chronic inflammatory interstitial infiltrate. (Hematoxylin and eosin, magnification ×40.) (All photographs courtesy of Dr. James Nolan.)

Pathogenesis

Kidney as Innocent Bystander

IgAN recurs frequently in renal allografts.[22–26] Moreover, in isolated instances in which a kidney was transplanted from a donor with subclinical IgAN into a patient with non-IgA-nephropathy renal disease, the immune deposits cleared from the affected kidney within several weeks.[27] These clinical observations suggest that the cause of IgAN is extrarenal and there is considerable evidence indicating that the mesangial deposits originate from circulating IgA-containing immune complexes. It is well established that patients with IgAN frequently have elevated circulating levels of IgA and IgA-containing immune complexes.[28–30] Idiotypic determinants are shared between the circulating complexes and the mesangial deposits[31]; however, a disease-specific idiotype has not been identified.[32] Circulating immune complexes in patients with IgAN contain IgA1,[28,33,34] the only IgA subclass in the mesangial immunodeposits.

Analysis of the glycosylation of IgA1 in patients with IgAN has yielded novel insights into the mechanisms underlying immune complex formation and mesangial deposition.[30,34–40] Specifically, galactose deficiency in IgA1 *O*-glycans appears to be a key pathogenetic factor.[36] Circulating complexes in patients with IgAN contain IgA1 with galactose-deficient hinge-region *O*-linked glycans.[30,34,37,41] Notably, galactose-deficient IgA1 is the predominant glycosylation variant of IgA1 in the mesangial deposits, as determined by analyses of IgA1 eluted from glomeruli of nephrectomized kidneys or biopsy specimens from patients with IgAN.[42,43] A relationship between galactose deficiency and nephritis also has been underscored by two other observations: (1) galactose-deficient IgA1[44] and IgA-IgG circulating complexes[45] are found in sera of patients with HSPN but not in sera of patients with HSP and (2) patients with IgA1 myeloma have high circulating levels of IgA1, but only those with aberrantly glycosylated IgA1 develop immune-complex glomerulonephritis.[46,47]

Immunobiochemistry of IgA1: Galactose-deficient IgA1

IgA1 and IgA2 represent two structurally and functionally distinct subclasses of IgA in humans.[48] IgA1 contains a unique hinge-region segment between the first and second constant-region domains of the heavy chains (Fig. 49.2A), with a high content of proline, serine, and threonine, that is the site of attachment of *O*-glycans. Up to six of the nine possible sites are occupied in each hinge region. These IgA1 *O*-glycans consist of *N*-acetylgalactosamine with a β1,3-linked galactose that may be sialylated.[49–54] Sialic acid can be attached to *N*-acetylgalactosamine also

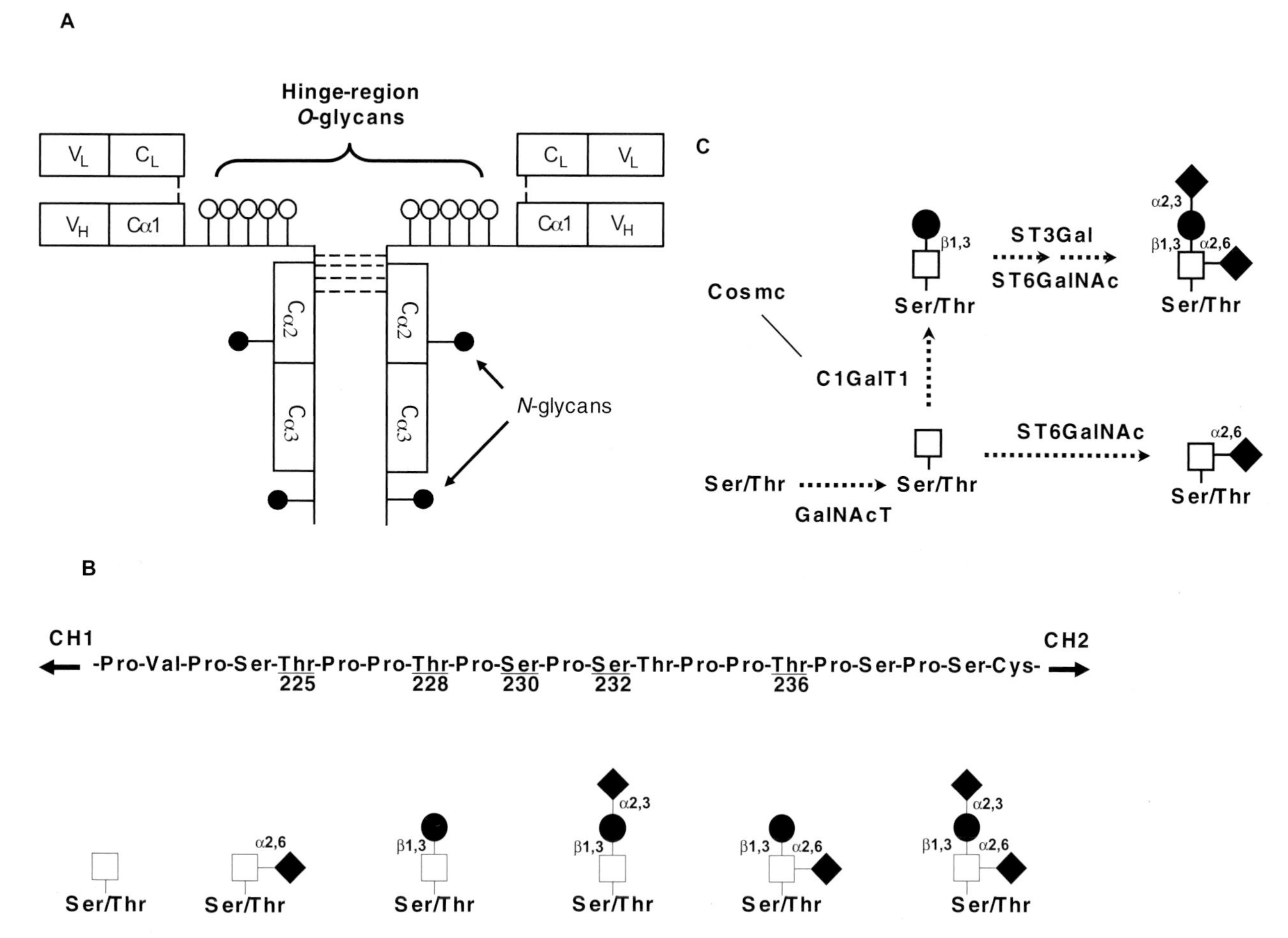

FIGURE 49.2 Structure and glycosylation of human IgA1. **A:** Monomer of IgA1 has two *N*-glycans and three to six *O*-glycans per heavy chain. **B:** Hinge-region amino acid sequence with common sites of *O*-glycan attachment and *O*-glycan variants of circulatory IgA1. The first two structures on the left side are galactose-deficient *O*-glycans. **C:** *O*-glycosylation of IgA1 is initiated by attachment of *N*-acetylgalactosamine to serine or threonine by UDP-*N*-acetylgalactosamine:polypeptide *N*-acetylgalactosaminyltransferases (GalNAc-Ts). The sites to be *O*-glycosylated and their order are determined by the specific set of GalNAc-Ts expressed in a particular cell type. *N*-acetylgalactosamine is then modified by addition of β1-3-linked galactose in a reaction catalyzed by UDP-galactose: *N*-acetylgalactosamine-α-Ser/Thr β,3-galactosyltransferase 1 (C1GalT1). Formation of active C1GalT1 depends on a specific chaperone, Cosmc. The *N*-acetylgalactosamine-galactose disaccharide can be further modified by attaching sialic acid to the galactose and/or *N*-acetylgalactosamine residues.

by an α2,6 linkage. The carbohydrate composition of the *O*-linked glycans in the hinge region of normal human serum IgA1 is variable (Fig. 49.2B). The prevailing glycans include galactose-*N*-acetylgalactosamine disaccharide and its mono- and di-sialylated forms.[30,51,54–58] Galactose-deficient variants with terminal *N*-acetylgalactosamine or sialylated *N*-acetylgalactosamine are rarely found in the *O*-glycans of normal serum IgA1.[51]

The first step in the *O*-glycosylation of the IgA1 hinge region, with selection of the sites to be modified and the control of the sequence in this process, is accomplished by one of the few enzymes of the UDP-*N*-acetylgalactosamine:polypeptide *N*-acetylgalactosaminyltransferase family. In the second step, *N*-acetylgalactosamine is then modified by addition of β1-3-linked galactose, as detailed in Figure 49.2C. Lastly, one or both sugars can be further modified by the addition of sialic acid.[59]

In patients with IgAN, the basis of the aberrant *O*-glycosylation of IgA1 has been determined by using immortalized IgA1-secreting cell lines generated from circulating mononuclear cells. The galactose deficiency develops due to changes in expression and activity of key enzymes involved in *O*-glycosylation in the IgA1-producing cells (Fig. 49.2C).[60] These changes in expression corresponded to decreased enzymatic activity of galactosyltransferase and elevated activity of sialyltransferase. Moreover, studies by other investigators identified mucosal, but not systemic, immune responses as the integral part of the aberrant *O*-glycosylation of IgA1.[61,62] However, mechanisms involved in these pathways and their regulation remain to be elucidated.

Aggregates of IgA1 and Immune Complexes with Antibody Specific for Galactose-deficient IgA1

Normal circulatory IgA has a relatively short half-life (~5 days) due to its rapid catabolism by hepatocytes.[63] Hepatocytes express the asialoglycoprotein receptor[52,64] that binds glycoproteins through terminal galactose or *N*-acetylgalactosamine residues.[52,64,65] Because the structural prerequisite for binding is a terminal galactose or *N*-acetylgalactosamine, the absence or enzymatic removal of the otherwise terminal sialic acid is essential for effective binding.

Galactose-deficient IgA1 is retained in the circulation for prolonged intervals.[66] Galactose deficiency in itself should not hinder disposal of IgA1 molecules because the asialoglycoprotein receptor recognizes terminal *N*-acetylgalactosamine as well as galactose.[65] However, if the *N*-acetylgalactosamine is linked to sialic acid or is occupied by an antibody, it cannot be recognized by the receptor.[41,67] Because galactose-deficient IgA1 is present primarily within immune complexes, it is plausible to speculate that this IgA1 does not effectively reach the hepatic asialoglycoprotein receptor. The larger size of the complexes, compared to that of uncomplexed IgA1, precludes binding to this receptor because the relatively small endothelial fenestrae block entry into the space of Disse. It is thus quite possible that immune complexes containing aberrantly glycosylated IgA1 are not efficiently cleared from the circulation and eventually deposit in the mesangium after passing through larger fenestrae in the glomerular capillaries.[69–72] In animals, high-molecular-mass immune complexes induce more severe glomerular lesions than do small complexes.[68]

Mesangial Deposition of IgA1 and Inducement of Mesangial Injury

Immune complexes containing aberrantly glycosylated IgA1 can activate human mesangial cells in vitro, resulting in a proliferative response and overproduction of extracellular matrix components and cytokines/chemokines.[37,41,73–75] Multiple studies have pointed to activation through an IgA-specific receptor(s) on mesangial cells. However, none of the known IgA receptors (CD89, asialoglycoprotein receptor, and polymeric immunoglobulin receptor) are expressed on human mesangial cells.[37,41,76] Among the candidate receptors that may mediate binding of IgA1 and IgA1 complexes are CD71 (transferrin receptor)[73,77,78] and the Fcα/μ receptor.[79] CD71 appears to be the major IgA1 receptor on proliferating human mesangial cells.[73,78,80] Notably, expression of CD71 is enhanced in the mesangia of IgAN patients and it colocalizes with IgA1 deposits.[81] Engagement of CD71 by IgA1 induces cellular proliferation and cytokine production (e.g., interleukin [IL]-6, tumor growth factor [TGF]-β).[80] This induction of cellular proliferation and cytokine production by IgA1 is inhibited completely by anti-CD71 antibody.[80] It is not clear, however, whether CD71 is the only receptor or if any other receptor(s) plays a role in the activation of mesangial cells.

Although the signaling pathways and detailed mechanisms of the activation of mesangial cells by IgA1-containing immune complexes remain to be elucidated, it is generally agreed that mesangial cells represent the primary target in IgAN. There are two hypotheses for mechanisms leading to activation of mesangial cells by IgA1 in IgAN (Fig. 49.3). Both theories propose multiple hits and involvement of aberrantly glycosylated IgA1 and antiglycan antibodies. The first assumes formation of immune complexes in the circulation and their subsequent mesangial deposition and activation of mesangial cells (Fig. 49.3, solid lines).[34,37,60,82] The other theory proposes that some of the aberrantly glycosylated IgA1 molecules are in the mesangium as lanthanic deposits, and later bound by newly generated antiglycan antibodies to form immune complexes in situ (Fig. 49.3, broken lines).[83]

Mesangial cells activated by immune complexes containing galactose-deficient IgA1 proliferate and overproduce extracellular matrix proteins, cytokines, and chemokines.[37,39,73,74,78,84–87] These processes, when unchecked for substantial periods of time, may lead to expansion of the glomerular mesangium and, ultimately, glomerular fibrosis with loss of glomerular filtration function. Furthermore, humoral factors (e.g., tumor necrosis factor [TNF]-α and TGF-β)[38,86,88,89] are released from mesangial cells activated by IgA1-containing immune complexes and alter podocyte gene expression and may thus increase glomerular permeability (Fig. 49.3). This mesangio-podocyte communication may be a mechanism to explain the occurrence of proteinuria and segmental glomerular sclerosis and tubulointerstitial injury in IgAN.[14,86] Moreover, pathogenicity of IgA1 immune complexes may be enhanced in the presence of systemic signs of oxidative stress, and it has been hypothesized that oxidative stress may affect expression and progression of the disease.[90]

Genetic Influences

Genetic factors are known to play an important role in susceptibility to IgAN, as indicated by worldwide reports of extended multiplex pedigrees.[91–98] Familial IgAN has offered a convenient tool for genetic studies and provided insight into the mechanism of inheritance. In some families, segregation of IgAN has been consistent with an autosomal-dominant transmission with incomplete penetrance. The incomplete penetrance, consistent with a complex-disease model, may reflect a requirement for additional genetic or environmental factors for clinical manifestation of the disease.

Gene mapping studies of diseases with complex determination are difficult and, thus far, no single mutation has been conclusively demonstrated to cause IgAN. Several genome-wide studies of familial IgAN have linked various loci with disease, including chromosomes 6q22-23 (named *IGAN1*), 4q26-31, 3p24-23, and 2q36.[95,99,100] In contrast to the linkage studies, association studies involve a collection of sporadic cases and a group of unrelated controls. These studies can be performed for specific preselected genes (candidate-gene association studies) or on a genome-wide

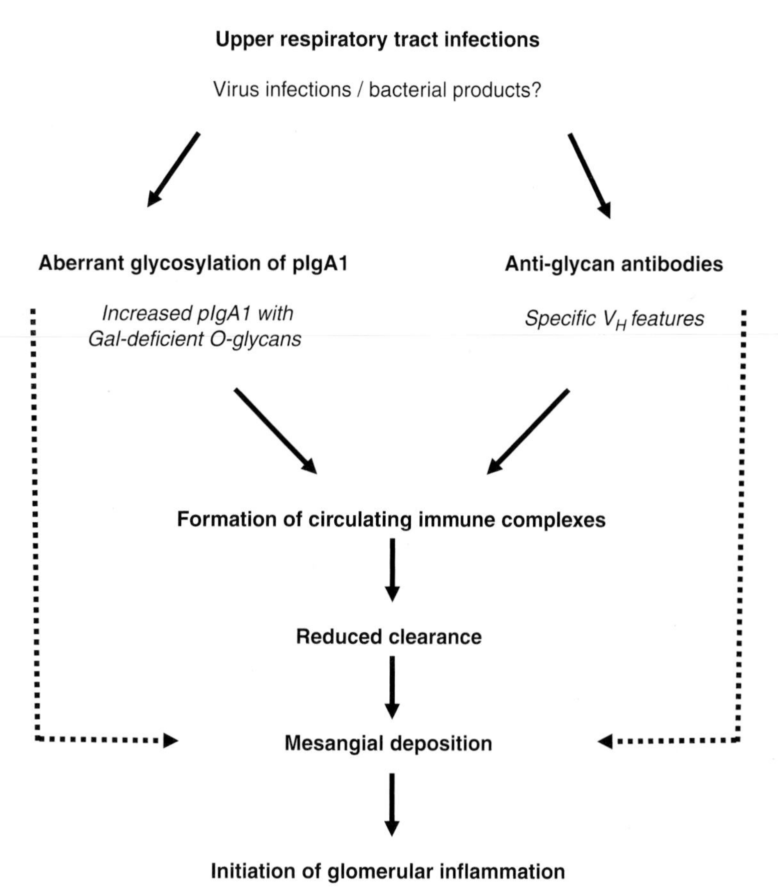

FIGURE 49.3 Mechanisms involved in IgAN pathogenesis. There are two hypotheses for mechanisms leading to the activation of mesangial cells by IgA1 in IgAN. Both theories propose multiple hits and involvement of aberrantly glycosylated IgA1 and antiglycan antibodies. The first assumes formation of immune complexes in the circulation and their subsequent mesangial deposition (*solid lines*).[34,82] Galactose-deficient IgA1 produced by a population of IgA1-secereting cells[60] is recognized by antiglycan antibodies with specific characteristics of variable region of the heavy chain[82] and, consequently, immune complexes are formed from autoantigen (galactose-deficient IgA1) and autoantibody (glycan-specific antibody). It further assumes that some of the circulating complexes are pathogenic—that is, able to deposit in the mesangium and activate the resident mesangial cells.[37] The other theory proposes that some of the aberrantly glycosylated IgA1 molecules are in the mesangium as lanthanic deposits, and later bound by newly generated antiglycan antibodies to form immune complexes in situ (*broken lines*).[83]

scale to provide an unbiased examination of the genome, with the ability to detect and correct for population stratification. Replication of findings in independent cohorts is necessary for validation of both approaches.[101]

A single, unreplicated genome-wide association study (GWAS) in a small European cohort (533 cases) has reported association of IgAN with a human leukocyte antigen (HLA) locus.[102] A recent replicated GWAS of a cohort of 3,144 IgAN cases of Chinese and European ancestry identified five loci.[103] These loci explained up to a tenfold variation in interindividual risk and cumulatively accounted for 4% to 7% of the disease variance and included three independent loci in the major histocompatibility complex, a common deletion of *CFHR1* and *CFHR3* at chromosome 1q32 (complement factor H-related genes) and chromosome 22q12. The risk allele frequencies also strongly paralleled the prevalence of IgAN in the different populations. Furthermore, many of the IgAN-protective alleles imparted increased risk for other autoimmune or infectious diseases, suggesting complex selective pressures on allele frequencies.[103] It is likely that studies with larger cohorts, and thus higher power, will define additional genetically influenced components in the pathogenesis of IgAN.

Recent studies of the glycosylation abnormalities of IgA1 offered prospects for a phenotypic biomarker for IgAN.[104–109] A new quantitative lectin-binding assay enabled investigation of the inheritance of galactose-deficient IgA1 in familial and sporadic forms of IgAN.[110] A high serum galactose-deficient IgA1 level was present in most index cases, as well as many of their first-degree relatives, whereas levels in spouses were indistinguishable from those in controls, eliminating an environmental effect. Segregation analysis of galactose-deficient IgA1 suggested inheritance of a major dominant gene with an additional polygenic component. The inheritance of galactose-deficient IgA1 has been confirmed in Chinese patients with familial and sporadic adult IgAN[39,111] and in pediatric patients with IgAN and HSPN.[94] Thus, aberrant IgA1 glycosylation is a common inherited defect that provides a unifying link in the pathogenesis of HSPN and familial and sporadic IgAN in many populations worldwide. GWAS studies using this new phenotype will likely provide information about the genetic and biochemical pathways leading to production of galactose-deficient IgA1 by IgA1-secreting cells.[60] Furthermore, elevated circulatory levels of galactose-deficient IgA1 are antecedent to disease. However, as most family members with elevated levels are asymptomatic, IgA1 glycosylation abnormalities are not sufficient to produce IgAN and additional cofactors, such as antiglycan antibodies,[82] are required to trigger formation of pathogenic immune complexes (Fig. 49.3).

Clinical Disease

Incidence and Prevalence

The reported incidence and prevalence of IgAN varies widely, and depends, to some degree, on variations in criteria for renal biopsy in different countries. Studies from Europe have estimated the incidence at 15 to 40 new cases per million population per year. The incidence is higher in Japan and Korea,[112,113] where screening for urinary abnormalities is routinely performed in school-aged children. Prevalence rates, expressed as a percentage of renal biopsy diagnoses, are reported to be 20% to 40% in Asia, Australia, Finland, and southern Europe. In the United States, the rate may be as low as 2% but in a large nephropathology referral practice IgAN accounted for 14% of nontransplant renal biopsies in adults aged 20 to 39 years.[114] Although local enthusiasm for detecting asymptomatic urinary abnormalities and then biopsying those individuals undoubtedly contributes greatly to these variations, there also appear to be important differences in susceptibility across different ethnic groups.[1–3,98] For example, IgAN is less common in central Africa and New Zealand Polynesians than in Caucasians of European origin. In African Americans, the prevalence is equal to that of European Americans in some regions of the United States.[115] Subclinical disease without urinary abnormalities is more common. In Japan, a study of renal allografts revealed mesangial IgA deposits in 16% of 510 kidneys at engraftment, of which 21% had mesangial proliferation.[116] In Singapore and Germany, IgA mesangial deposits were found in 2% and 4.8% of cases in two series of unselected autopsy examinations, respectively.[117,118]

Uncertainties about true incidence and different approaches to individuals with asymptomatic urinary abnormalities also affect estimations of prognosis. Patients with milder disease will exhibit a more benign clinical course and some will even enter clinical remission. However, most patients will have persistent urinary abnormalities (microscopic hematuria ± proteinuria), and 20% to 40% of untreated patients will progress to end-stage renal failure.[98,119] As a result, IgAN is a significant component in the national budgets for end-stage renal failure replacement therapy in many countries. For some patients, the interval to renal demise will be relatively short (months to several years) because of more aggressive disease and/or late presentation, whereas for others the interval may be decades.

Clinical Presentations

The variability of presentations and subsequent course is a feature of IgAN, and a list of the wide range of initial manifestations is shown in Table 49.1. There is an approximately 2–3:1 male preponderance.

TABLE 49.1 Patterns of Clinical Presentation of IgAN

Common
Synpharyngitic macroscopic hematuria ± loin pain
Microscopic hematuria, usually with proteinuria
Hypertension
Chronic renal failure
Henoch-Schönlein purpura
Uncommon
Malignant hypertension
Acute nephritic syndrome
Acute renal failure
Nephrotic syndrome

Macroscopic Hematuria. The most distinctive and, at least to the patient, dramatic presentation of IgAN is episodic macroscopic hematuria. This feature is the principal mode of presentation in children and young adults in the Western hemisphere.[120] There is a highly characteristic close temporal relationship between its onset and an upper respiratory tract infection, especially pharyngitis or tonsillitis, whereby visible hematuria occurs within 2 days of the sore throat. This timing led to the commonly used term "synpharyngitic hematuria," and differs from the 2- to 3-week gap between infection and macroscopic hematuria in postinfectious glomerulonephritis. Less frequently, macroscopic hematuria accompanies infections of other mucosal surfaces (e.g., gastroenteritis and urinary tract infections). This hematuria may be associated with systemic symptoms such as fever, malaise, fatigue, diffuse muscle aches, and abdominal or loin pain. It is usually short-lived, lasting less than a week, and its disappearance concurs with resolution of systemic symptoms. Occasionally there is associated transient acute renal impairment.

Differentiation from other causes of macroscopic hematuria (i.e., urinary tract infection or urolithiasis) is important because frequent and unnecessary radiographic and urologic investigations may ensue if the true cause is not recognized. Of utmost importance is the microscopic examination of the centrifuged urinary sediment, which displays dysmorphic red blood cells (altered in size and shape compared to normal red cells, indicating a glomerular origin[121]), plus granular and red-cell casts. Under these circumstances, renal biopsy is the appropriate first diagnostic procedure. Microscopic hematuria ± proteinuria usually persists between episodes of macroscopic hematuria. For reasons not yet clear, macroscopic hematuria due to IgAN rarely occurs after age 40, and such an event should raise suspicion for urinary tract malignancy or stones.

Asymptomatic Microscopic Hematuria and Proteinuria. At least one third of diagnoses of IgAN are made after investigating incidentally discovered microscopic hematuria, usually accompanied by proteinuria. This scenario can occur at any age, and is typical for older patients. Local attitudes to screening and evaluating asymptomatic urinary abnormalities dictate the frequency of such presentations. A common source of such referrals is medical examinations performed for work or insurance purposes.

Proteinuria and Nephrotic Syndrome. Proteinuria in the absence of hematuria is distinctly uncommon in IgAN. Nephrotic-range proteinuria is unusual, but can occur in the presence of either very active acute disease or advanced disease with considerable scarring. Occasionally, IgAN and minimal change disease occur together, and may simply be a chance association of two relatively common disorders. It is important to recognize this possibility because the nephrotic syndrome should be treated as for minimal change disease in isolation, with expectation of a similar response.[20]

Hypertension. IgAN is a major cause of hypertension in young adults. The widespread use of blood pressure screening programs may initially identify these patients. The dramatic presentation of malignant hypertension is also well recognized for IgAN, and renal biopsy findings often indicate severe and long-standing glomerular disease.

Acute Renal Failure. Acute renal failure is a rare presenting feature for IgAN. It may occur during episodes of macroscopic hematuria, possibly as a result of tubular obstruction/injury by red blood cells that resolves without specific therapy apart from occasional resort to temporary dialysis.[122] Alternatively, rapidly progressive renal dysfunction may be due to acute necrotizing, crescentic glomerular injury. It is important to document this severe manifestation of the disease by biopsy, as it is the strongest indication for aggressive therapy.

Chronic Kidney Disease. The proportion of patients with IgAN with chronic, established renal failure at presentation is uncertain because many who come to medical care late in their clinical course do not undergo the requisite renal biopsy. Undoubtedly some patients with end-stage renal failure with small kidneys had unrecognized IgAN for years. A reliable noninvasive marker for IgAN would clearly be helpful for the diagnosis of these patients. A presumptive, retrospective diagnosis can be made for renal transplant recipients for whom an allograft biopsy indicates IgAN.

Differential Diagnosis

Although clinical suspicion based on presenting features (e.g., synpharyngitic hematuria) will often lead to the correct diagnosis of IgAN, a renal biopsy is necessary for confirmation. No other investigation has been proven to reliably distinguish IgAN from other renal diseases. This fact is frustrating because it means that an invasive procedure is required for diagnosis, an approach often judged unnecessary in a person with isolated microscopic hematuria. Although microscopic hematuria and modest proteinuria are common in patients with membranoproliferative glomerulonephritis, Alport syndrome (hereditary nephritis), and thin basement membrane nephropathy, macroscopic hematuria is rare. Serum complement levels are typically reduced in patients with membranoproliferative glomerulonephritis. A family history of renal disease (without father-to-son transmission) often with concomitant hearing loss is typical of the X-linked form of Alport syndrome. Thin basement membrane nephropathy can be distinguished from IgAN only by renal biopsy with ultrastructural studies. Some persons undergoing renal biopsy for the evaluation of microscopic hematuria and modest proteinuria have no apparent immunohistologic abnormality.[123]

Disease Associations

The literature is replete with descriptions of associations of diseases with IgAN, although it is likely that many of these are chance occurrences.[124] Deposition of IgA in the mesangium is relatively common in severe liver disease due to alcoholic cirrhosis[125] and viral hepatitis.[126] Impaired clearance of IgA by the damaged hepatocytes is thought to contribute to this observation. IgAN has been associated with inflammatory bowel disease, more so ulcerative colitis than Crohn disease,[124] and with gluten sensitivity,[127] including celiac disease and dermatitis herpetiformis. Some investigators have postulated that intestinal inflammation leads to increased permeability of dietary antigens that induces synthesis of antigen-specific IgA antibodies to form immune complexes that later deposit in the mesangium.[128] Patients infected with human immunodeficiency virus (HIV) have increased circulating levels of immune complexes containing IgA and polymeric IgA1 rheumatoid factor. IgAN may be as frequent as 5% to 8% in these patients.[129,130] In this setting, IgA may bind to the viral capsid p24 protein to form immune complexes.

Clinical Course and Prognosis

IgAN is an important cause of end-stage renal disease in many countries, but predicting a patient's outcome at the time of diagnosis has been difficult. The clinical course is very clear at the time of diagnosis for those patients presenting with established renal impairment. An estimated glomerular filtration rate (eGFR[131]) <30 mL/min/1.73m^2 is generally deemed the "point of no return" whereby progression to end-stage renal failure is inevitable.[132] Patients with better eGFR at diagnosis usually follow one of four courses, although wide variations in screening and diagnosis approaches preclude a precise estimate of the frequency of each. The courses are: (1) clinical resolution of mild disease, (2) ongoing mild disease without progressive renal failure, (3) slowly progressive renal dysfunction, and (4) rapidly progressive renal failure.[98,119,133,134] Hypertension is a frequent association; it is invariable and often severe in patients with progressive disease. As discussed previously, many individuals with benign, asymptomatic disease with good prognosis likely never come to medical attention.

An important minority, perhaps 15% of those diagnosed, has mild disease at presentation (i.e., normal renal function, minimal proteinuria [<500 mg per day], and microscopic hematuria) and with time undergoes spontaneous resolution of all signs of renal disease. This course is more common in children than older patients. Mesangial IgA sometimes disappears.[135] About 50% of patients diagnosed with IgAN have persistent but benign disease. The typical pattern is ongoing low-grade microscopic hematuria, minimal or absent proteinuria, normal eGFR, and normotension or easily controlled hypertension. Such individuals should be monitored regularly, as significant changes in disease status may occur over years. Many of the remaining patients will have slowly progressive renal impairment, over years to decades, eventually leading to end-stage renal failure if lifespan permits. A more malignant shorter course is uncommon but well recognized. A rapidly progressive course is often foretold by focal necrotizing glomerular lesions in the diagnostic renal biopsy.

Clinical and histologic features can be used to generate meaningful prognostic information.[18,98,119,134,136] Poorly controlled hypertension, decrement in eGFR over a short interval, proteinuria >500 mg per day for more than 6 months, hyperuricemia, hyperlipidemia, and obesity are clinical risk factors for a poor prognosis.[137,138] Alternatively, eGFR at the time of biopsy is a relatively poor predictor for clinical course.[138] The Oxford classification found that, in biopsy specimens without crescents, four light-microscopy pathologic variables, mesangial hypercellularity, endocapillary hypercellularity, segmental glomerulosclerosis, and tubular atrophy/interstitial fibrosis, had independent value in predicting clinical outcome.[18,139] Furthermore, this value transcended age of the patient at biopsy and ancestry. If validated, this classification will better guide nephrologists in the care of individual patients.[18,139] The presence of cytotoxic T lymphocytes in the interstitium and within renal tubules was shown in a retrospective study to predict loss of renal clearance function in patients with normal or near-normal eGFR.[140] Also, increased urinary excretion of podocytes has been correlated with progressive glomerular scarring.[141] Glomerular crescents, even if relatively small, herald a poor clinical course[142] and the subset of patients with antineutrophil cytoplasmic autoantibodies (ANCA) exhibits particularly aggressive disease.[143] A calculated absolute renal risk for dialysis or death has been proposed, using hypertension, proteinuria ≥1 g per day, and severe histopathologic lesions at diagnosis.[144] Episodic macroscopic hematuria, initially deemed an unfavorable prognostic sign,[145] is now considered to indicate a benign prognosis, even after taking into account its higher frequency in children than adults. Individuals with continually normal blood pressure and proteinuria persistently <200 mg per day have a negligible risk of progression.[138] However, presentation with isolated microscopic hematuria may not be a reliable sign for a good long-term outcome.[146]

Disease Markers

Diagnosis of IgAN is based on evaluation of renal biopsy because of the absence of a valid alternative noninvasive test. As renal biopsy entails risk for serious complications, early detection of IgAN is frequently impossible and monitoring of the disease is compromised. Thus, a noninvasive diagnostic test will be very useful if it can detect subclinical IgAN, estimate the degree of activity, monitor the progression or abatement of renal injury, and assess response to treatment.

As the pathogenesis of IgAN is being uncovered and the roles of IgA1 and IgA1-containing immune complexes have been identified, serum levels of galactose-deficient IgA1 and antiglycan antibodies have been targeted as potential markers for diagnosis and disease progression.[39,60,82,105,111] Methodology includes lectin enzyme-linked immunosorbent assay (ELISA) for levels of galactose-deficient IgA1[60,105] or dot-blot test to semiquantitatively measure circulating IgG antibodies specific for galactose-deficient IgA1.[82] As these techniques are refined to improve sensitivity and specificity, they may become leading candidates to be developed into clinical assays.

Urine is another source of potential biomarkers, including galactose-deficient IgA1, immune complexes, or disease-specific peptides.[109,147–150] Several studies showed differential amounts of intact proteins and protein complexes in the urine of patients with IgAN, but no test has been developed into a clinically useful assay. More recently, it has been shown by modern proteomic/peptidomic techniques that urine includes many polypeptides and/or their proteolytic fragments that are disease-specific, including those specific for IgAN.[148,151–154] Thus, several approaches may be developed into clinically useful assays following the rules for clinical proteomics.[155,156]

Treatment

There is no known cure or disease-specific therapy for IgAN. Tactics to correct the glycosylation abnormality of IgA1 or to block the formation of nephritogenic IgA1-containing immune complexes remain at the conceptual stage and have yet to be tested in any disease model. Establishing efficacy of any treatment for IgAN is difficult because most patients have a benign course and the time course of progression is frequently slow, often measured in decades. As a result, the number of randomized controlled prospective clinical trials is quite limited and some trials have used reduction in proteinuria as a surrogate (proxy) endpoint, although the validity of this ploy has been questioned.[157] The therapeutic strategy for patients with glomerular renal diseases, including IgAN, is under review by a working group of the National Kidney Foundation in the United States, Kidney Disease: Improving

Global Outcomes (KDIGO), and its recommendations are slated to be published in 2012.

Preservation of Native Kidney Function

Current options mainly aim to control disease progression and, in general, do not differ significantly from recommended strategies for other progressive renal diseases. Patients with proteinuria <500 mg per day, normal blood pressure, normal eGFR, and little or no scarring on renal biopsy require regular observation and they should avoid use of tobacco,[158] maintain an appropriate weight, exercise regularly, and take aspirin 81 mg daily.

For children and adults at risk for progressive renal injury, additional therapy is indicated. There is an evidence-based consensus that the initial approach should be suppression of the renin-angiotensin-aldosterone system (RAAS[159–163]). This treatment is appropriate for control of hypertension and proteinuria. The target blood pressure for adults is <125/75 mm Hg. Proteinuria should be reduced to <500 mg per day. Angiotensin-converting enzyme (ACE) inhibitors and angiotensin receptor type 1 blockers (ARBs) act synergistically and this therapy delays loss of eGFR.[164] To attain these goals, additional measures may be necessary, such as restricting dietary sodium intake to <2.4 g per day and/or use of aldosterone antagonists or other diuretic agents. Importantly, patients with severe proteinuria (≥3 g per day) for whom treatment reaches and maintains excretion at ≤1 g per day have a clinical course similar to that for patients whose proteinuria was always <1 g per day.[137]

For patients with preserved renal function (e.g., eGFR >70 mL/min/1.73 m^2) who fail to reach the above treatment targets, immunosuppressive therapy has been recommended by some investigators based on a modest number of controlled prospective clinical trials.[165] Enthusiasm must be tempered by recalling that IgAN frequently recurs in renal allografts despite the use of corticosteroids, azathioprine, mycophenolate mofetil, cyclosporine, and tacrolimus in two- or three-drug combinations starting at the initial exposure of the kidney to a nephritogenic milieu. Glucocorticoids may be considered in a single-agent regimen using oral and parental therapy over a 6-month interval.[166] Clinical investigations under way in Germany will assess the efficacy of glucocorticoids added to suppression of RAAS.[167] Combining glucocorticoids with azathioprine was not helpful for adult patients at risk for progression and with eGFR >50 mL per min.[168] Cyclosphosphamide followed by azathioprine benefited patients with impaired renal function in a controlled prospective trial (serum creatinine >1.48 mg per dL [130 mmol per L] and higher by >15% in the prior year).[169] Patients with focal necrotizing glomerular lesions or cellular crescents frequently exhibit a rapid loss of eGFR and are often treated with cyclophosphamide, intravenous methylprednisolone, and oral prednisone (± plasmapheresis and ± antiplatelet agents), in a fashion similar to that for other forms of rapidly progressive, crescentic renal disease.[170,171] Unfortunately, high quality, randomized clinical trials have not been done, and there likely will be none in the near future. Small studies have shown an early response to treatment but a disappointing outcome for many patients over longer intervals. In weighing treatment with potent immunomodulating agents, it is important to respect the potentially serious toxicities and side effects. The occasional patient with nephrotic syndrome and histologic features of minimal change disease will respond well to standard glucocorticoid treatment for isolated minimal change disease.

Some investigators have advocated adjunctive therapy with omega-3 fatty acids (fish oil). Although the anti-inflammatory, antihypertensive, and antithrombotic effects may reduce proteinuria, its value for preserving renal clearance function is unproven.[172–174] Other agents have shown little benefit. Mycophenolate mofetil has been efficacious for patients with systemic lupus erythematosus, but treatment of patients with IgAN has shown mixed results.[175,176] Studies using a calcineurin inhibitor have been inconclusive.[160] Phenytoin, which reduces serum IgA levels, showed no usefulness.[177] There is also no advantage with methods to reduce antigen or antibody load, such as dietary gluten restriction or prophylactic antibiotics.

The dramatic presenting symptom of synpharyngitic hematuria has popularized tonsillectomy as a treatment option, particularly in Japan. Unfortunately, reports describing a clinical effectiveness for hematuria and proteinuria are limited to case series or nonrandomized trials, and patients were often concomitantly treated with immunosuppressive therapy.[178,179] There is little evidence that tonsillectomy ameliorates progression to end-stage renal failure.[180] Prospective randomized clinical trials are sorely needed before this surgical therapy can be recommended. Supportive therapy, including analgesia as required, is all that is required for acute episodes of macroscopic hematuria associated with biopsy-proven acute tubular injury not associated with crescentic glomerulonephritis.[181]

Transplantation

Kidney transplantation should be offered to all patients with IgAN without a contraindication, but it is not curative. The rate of recurrence (at least the appearance of IgA deposits) is at least 50% at 5 years after engraftment.[25,181] The risk of recurrence is higher if a prior allograft was lost to recurrent disease or the pretransplant course of disease was rapidly progressive and the biopsy showed crescentic glomerulonephritis.[182] The merit of three other factors to predict recurrence are more controversial: allografts from a genetically related donor, the lack of induction therapy with an anti-lymphocyte or antithymocyte agent, and presence of IgA deposits on biopsy at engraftment.[162]

Recurrent disease may be subclinical[25] and was often considered to be of little clinical significance,[183] but may have serious consequences.[184,185] Allograft loss due to recurrent IgAN is likely under-reported; unless immunofluorescence studies are routinely performed for transplant biopsy and nephrectomy specimens, losses may be erroneously attributed to chronic rejection or transplant glomerulopathy. High serum levels of aberrantly glycosylated IgA1 have not been associated with recurrent disease. Some genetic variants, including polymorphisms of TNF-α and interleukin-10, may be protective.[186] Despite these risks, the prognosis after transplantation for patients for IgAN is comparable with that for patients with other glomerulonephritis causes of end-stage renal failure.

Animal Models

The IgA1 isotype is present in only humans and hominoid primates. Consequently, progress in understanding the pathogenesis of IgAN has been hampered by the lack of animal models that recapitulate human disease. In spite of that, animal studies have identified multiple factors, including defective immunoregulation, mononuclear phagocyte function, and the role of antigen and complement, in the development of glomerular disease resembling human IgAN.

HIGA and ddY strains of mice develop IgAN-like deposits spontaneously with age.[187–192] ddY mice show mild proteinuria without hematuria and mesangioproliferative glomerulonephritis with glomerular IgA deposits, associated with increased serum IgA levels and some syntenic genetic loci.[191–193] These two models may offer opportunities to test some therapeutic approaches.[190,194] Another spontaneous model uses marmosets that exhibit wasting syndrome with glomerulonephritis and IgA deposits.[195]

Various genetic manipulations of mice induce renal pathology resembling IgAN.[196] A back-pack murine model used antigen-specific dimeric- and monomeric-IgA-producing hybridomas and the antigen to induce formation of immune complexes.[197] Only dimeric-IgA-containing complexes formed glomerular deposits. In other studies, assorted types of IgA-containing complexes have been used to generate passive models of IgAN that would be suitable for testing potential therapeutic strategies.[36,66,77,190,198–201]

HENOCH-SCHÖNLEIN PURPURA

HSP is a common vasculitis with IgA-dominant immune deposits affecting small vessels in skin, joints, and gut.[9,202–207] Historically, HSPN is a much older disease than IgAN, as it is a clinical syndrome readily recognized with its overt nonthrombocytopenic purpuric rash, arthritis, gut manifestations, and glomerulonephritis. Whereas Schönlein[6] in 1837 associated purpura and arthritis, and Henoch in 1874[7] recognized gastrointestinal and renal manifestations, the first clinical description of the disease was probably by Heberden in 1806.[208] Until the 1970s, most accounts of HSPN were descriptive, but the arrival of immunofluorescence technology allowed exploration of possible immunopathogenetic mechanisms. IgA immunofluorescence staining occurs in the glomerular mesangium and leukocytoclastic vasculitis lesions in the skin (especially purpuric lesions).[8]

Clinical Features

HSP most often manifests in the first decade of life (with male to female ratio of ~2 to 3:1) and has an increased prevalence in patients with familial Mediterranean fever. Susceptibility to disease or clinical features in some populations may be influenced by alleles at several genetic loci, including those for HLA, interleukin-8, and Toll-like receptors.[209–214] Most children exhibit a self-limited course with complete resolution, although a third of patients have a recurrence.[215] About 40% to 50% of patients with HSP develop glomerulonephritis, HSPN, and a nephritic or nephrotic syndrome and acute renal failure are more common manifestations than in IgAN. The renal disease is likely to be more severe in adults than in children[216]; skin involvement may include ulcers and renal disease more frequently progresses to end-stage renal disease.[203] As with IgAN patients, proteinuria carries significant weight in assessment of prognosis. Higher mean proteinuria over time[217] or proteinuria at 1 year after diagnosis[218] predicts a worse long-term outcome.

HSP commonly occurs soon after an upper respiratory tract infection. In one series, the prevalence of the major symptoms in children was purpura (100%), arthritis (82%), abdominal pain (63%), renal disease (40%), and gastrointestinal bleeding (33%).[33] The rash is distributed symmetrically, usually with greater involvement below the waist. Pain in multiple large joints (knees and ankles) without frank arthritis or permanent damage is typical, and abdominal pain may be disabling and accompanied by visibly bloody stools. Although these symptoms may cause much acute morbidity, recovery is usual. For those who develop renal involvement, it is generally apparent within 4 weeks of diagnosis.[219] As with IgAN, intermittent macroscopic hematuria or persisting microscopic hematuria are common.[11,203] Diagnosis of HSPN relies mostly on clinical signs and symptoms; because of risk of complications, only a few patients undergo renal biopsy to document the immunohistology.[220] Currently, no test predicts development of nephritis in HSP patients.

Renal Pathology

For those HSPN patients who undergo renal biopsy, the renal immunohistologic findings are indistinguishable from those of IgAN.[13,181,202,221] Clinical and laboratory evidence support a close relationship between IgAN and HSPN.[11,181,222] Proliferation of mesangial cells and expansion of extracellular matrix are found in patients with mild clinical disease, but progressive glomerular sclerosis and interstitial fibrosis lead to end-stage renal disease in 30% to 40% patients within 20 years after diagnosis.[202] HSPN recurs as IgA deposits in approximately 50% to 60% of renal allografts, usually without nonrenal manifestations.[23,24,223]

Pathogenesis

Aberrant glycosylation of IgA1 and IgA1-IgG circulating immune complexes of high molecular mass have been shown for patients with HSPN, similar to the findings for patients with

IgAN but not for patients with HSP without nephritis or with any other type of glomerulonephritis.[45,70,71,74,181,203,224,225] As in IgAN patients, high circulatory levels of galactose-deficient IgA1 in HSPN patients are inherited.[94] To date, no longitudinal study has examined whether this laboratory finding persists after resolution of clinical symptoms. HSPN patients, compared with HSP patients, have higher whole blood and urinary levels of leukotriene B_4 and lower levels of lipoxin A_4.[226] These findings may explain the prominent role of neutrophils in the vasculitis.

Treatment

To date, studies of children have failed to show that any therapy shortens duration of disease or prevents recurrence,[215] although a short course of glucocorticoids can reduce severity of abdominal pain or joint pain.[227] Anecdotal reports have described improvement after treatment with colchicine (as is used for familial Mediterranean fever) but this approach has not been systematically studied.[228] Glucocorticoids are not effective in preventing HSPN.[227,229–232] Despite the poor prognosis for HSPN in children, there is no firm evidence that treatment with glucocorticoids, azathioprine, cyclosphosphamide, cyclosporine, warfarin, dipyridamole, or mycophenolate mofetil, alone or in combination, confers benefit. Although randomized controlled trials have not been done, there is a general consensus that ACE inhibitors and ARBs should be used to treat hypertension and proteinuria in patients with HSPN.[233] Recent case reports indicated improvement in three children with refractory HSP treated with rituximab[234] and 14 children with HSPN treated with plasmapheresis alone[235] but neither approach has been rigorously tested. For adults, randomized trials to evaluate efficacy of any treatment are rare. One study found that adding cyclophosphamide to glucocorticoids for treatment of patients' severe HSP (most of whom had proteinuria ≥ 1 g/day and microscopic hematuria) was not advantageous.[236] As for patients with IgAN, renal transplantation is an excellent option for renal replacement therapy.[185]

REFERENCES

1. D'Amico G. The commonest glomerulonephritis in the world: IgA nephropathy. *Quart J Med.* 1987;64:709.
2. Levy M, Berger J. Worldwide perspective of IgA nephropathy. *Am J Kidney Dis.* 1988;12:340.
3. Julian BA, Waldo FB, Rifai A, et al. IgA nephropathy, the most common glomerulonephritis worldwide. A neglected disease in the United States? *Am J Med.* 1988;84:129.
4. Berger J, Hinglais N. Les dépôts intercapillaires d'IgA-IgG (Intercapillary deposits of IgA-IgG). *J Urol Nephrol.* 1968;74:694.
5. Conley ME, Cooper MD, Michael AF. Selective deposition of immunoglobulin A1 in immunoglobulin A nephropathy, anaphylactoid purpura nephritis, and systemic lupus erythematosus. *J Clin Invest.* 1980;66:1432.
6. Schönlein H. *Allgememe und Specielle Pathologe und Therapie*, 3rd ed, vol. 2. 1837.
7. Henoch E. Uber ein eigenthümliche Form von Purpura. *Berl Klin Wochenschr.* 1874;11:641.
8. Faille-Kuyber EH, Kater L, Kooiker CJ, et al. IgA-deposits in cutaneous blood-vessel walls and mesangium in Henoch-Schönlein syndrome. *Lancet.* 1973;1:892.
9. Davin JC. Henoch-Schönlein purpura nephritis: pathophysiology, treatment, and future strategy. *Clin J Am Soc Nephrol* 2011;6(3):679–689.
10. Faille-Kuyper EH, Kater L, Kuijten RH, et al. Occurrence of vascular IgA deposits in clinically normal skin of patients with renal disease. *Kidney Int.* 1976;9:424.
11. Davin JC, Ten Berge IJ, Weening JJ. What is the difference between IgA nephropathy and Henoch-Schönlein purpura nephritis? *Kidney Int.* 2001;59:823.
12. Muda AO, Feriozzi S, Rahimi S, et al. Spatial arrangement of IgA and C3 as a prognostic indicator of IgA nephropathy. *J Pathol.* 1995;177:201.
13. Jennette JC. The immunohistology of IgA nephropathy. *Am J Kidney Dis.* 1988;12:348.
14. Hill GS, Karoui KE, Karras A, et al. Focal segmental glomerulosclerosis plays a major role in the progression of IgA nephropathy. I. Immunohistochemical studies. *Kidney Int.* 2011;79:635.
15. El Karoui K, Hill GS, Karras A, et al. Focal segmental glomerulosclerosis plays a major role in the progression of IgA nephropathy. II. Light microscopic and clinical studies. *Kidney Int.* 2011;79:643.
16. Cook HT. Focal segmental glomerulosclerosis in IgA nephropathy: a result of primary podocyte injury? *Kidney Int.* 2011;79:581.
17. Haas M. Histologic subclassification of IgA nephropathy: A clinicopathologic study of 244 cases. *Am J Kidney Dis.* 1997;29:829.
18. Cattran DC, Coppo R, Cook HT, et al. The Oxford classification of IgA nephropathy: rationale, clinicopathological correlations, and classification. *Kidney Int.* 2009;76:534.
19. Roberts IS, Cook HT, Troyanov S, et al. The Oxford classification of IgA nephropathy: pathology definitions, correlations, and reproducibility. *Kidney Int.* 2009;76:546.
20. Mustonen J, Pasternack A, Rantala I. The nephrotic syndrome in IgA glomerulonephritis: response to corticosteroid therapy. *Clin Nephrol.* 1983;20:172.
21. Berthoux FC, Laurent B, Koller JM, et al. Primary IgA glomerulonephritis with thin glomerular basement membrane: a peculiar pathological marker versus thin membrane nephropathy association. *Contrib Nephrol.* 1995;111:1.
22. Coppo R, Amore A, Cirina P, et al. IgA serology in recurrent and non-recurrent IgA nephropathy after renal transplantation. *Nephrol Dial Transplant.* 1995;10:2310.
23. Odum J, Peh CA, Clarkson AR, et al. Recurrent mesangial IgA nephritis following renal transplantation. *Nephrol Dial Transplant.* 1994;9:309.
24. Coppo R, Amore A, Cirina P, et al. Characteristics of IgA and macromolecular IgA in sera from IgA nephropathy transplanted patients with and without IgAN recurrence. *Contrib Nephrol.* 1995;111:85.
25. Berger J. Recurrence of IgA nephropathy in renal allografts. *Am J Kidney Dis.* 1988;12:371.
26. Chandrakantan A, Ratanapanichkich P, Said M, et al. Recurrent IgA nephropathy after renal transplantation despite immunosuppressive regimens with mycophenolate mofetil. *Nephrol Dial Transplant.* 2005;20:1214.
27. Silva FG, Chander P, Pirani CL, et al. Disappearance of glomerular mesangial IgA deposits after renal allograft transplantation. *Transplantation.* 1982;33:241.
28. Czerkinsky C, Koopman WJ, Jackson S, et al. Circulating immune complexes and immunoglobulin A rheumatoid factor in patients with mesangial immunoglobulin A nephropathies. *J Clin Invest.* 1986;77:1931.
29. Coppo R, Basolo B, Piccoli G, et al. IgA1 and IgA2 immune complexes in primary IgA nephropathy and Henoch-Schönlein nephritis. *Clin Exp Immunol.* 1984;57:583.
30. Tomana M, Matousovic K, Julian BA, et al. Galactose-deficient IgA1 in sera of IgA nephropathy patients is present in complexes with IgG. *Kidney Int.* 1997;52:509.
31. Gonzales-Cabrero J, Egido J, Mampaso F, et al. Characterization of circulating idiotypes containing immune complexes and their presence in the glomerular mesangium in patients with IgA nephropathy. *Clin Exp Immunol.* 1989;76:204.
32. van den Wall Bake AWL, Bruijn JA, Accavitti MA, et al. Shared idiotypes in mesangial deposits in IgA nephropathy are not disease-specific. *Kidney Int.* 1993;44:65.
33. Coppo R, Basolo B, Martina G, et al. Circulating immune complexes containing IgA, IgG and IgM in patients with primary IgA nephropathy and with Henoch-Schönlein nephritis. Correlation with clinical and histologic signs of activity. *Clin Nephrol.* 1982;18:230.
34. Tomana M, Novak J, Julian BA, et al. Circulating immune complexes in IgA nephropathy consist of IgA1 with galactose-deficient hinge region and antiglycan antibodies. *J Clin Invest.* 1999;104:73.
35. Andre PM, Le Pogamp P, Chevet D. Impairment of jacalin binding to serum IgA in IgA nephropathy. *J Clin Lab Anal.* 1990;4:115.
36. Mestecky J, Tomana M, Crowley-Nowick PA, et al. Defective galactosylation and clearance of IgA1 molecules as a possible etiopathogenic factor in IgA nephropathy. *Contrib Nephrol.* 1993;104:172.

37. Novak J, Tomana M, Matousovic K, et al. IgA1-containing immune complexes in IgA nephropathy differentially affect proliferation of mesangial cells. *Kidney Int.* 2005;67:504.

38. Leung JC, Tang SC, Chan LY, et al. Synthesis of TNF-α by mesangial cells cultured with polymeric anionic IgA—role of MAPK and NF-κB. *Nephrol Dial Transplant.* 2008;23:72.

39. Tam KY, Leung JC, Chan LY, et al. Macromolecular IgA1 taken from patients with familial IgA nephropathy or their asymptomatic relatives have higher reactivity to mesangial cells *in vitro*. *Kidney Int.* 2009;75:1330.

40. Allen AC, Harper SJ, Feehally J. Galactosylation of *N*- and *O*-linked carbohydrate moieties of IgA1 and IgG in IgA nephropathy. *Clin Exp Immunol.* 1995;100:470.

41. Novak J, Vu HL, Novak L, et al. Interactions of human mesangial cells with IgA and IgA-containing circulating immune complexes. *Kidney Int.* 2002; 62:465.

42. Allen AC, Bailey EM, Brenchley PEC, et al. Mesangial IgA1 in IgA nephropathy exhibits aberrant *O*-glycosylation: Observations in three patients. *Kidney Int.* 2001;60:969.

43. Hiki Y, Odani H, Takahashi M, et al. Mass spectrometry proves under-*O*-glycosylation of glomerular IgA1 in IgA nephropathy. *Kidney Int.* 2001;59:1077.

44. Allen AC, Willis FR, Beattie TJ, et al. Abnormal IgA glycosylation in Henoch-Schönlein purpura restricted to patients with clinical nephritis. *Nephrol Dial Transplant.* 1998;13:930.

45. Levinsky RJ, Barratt TM. IgA immune complexes in Henoch-Schönlein purpura. *Lancet.* 1979;2:1100.

46. van der Helm-van Mil AHM, Smith AC, Pouria S, et al. Immunoglobulin A multiple myeloma presenting with Henoch-Schönlein purpura associated with reduced sialylation of IgA1. *Br J Haematol.* 2003;122:915.

47. Zickerman AM, Allen AC, Talwar V, et al. IgA myeloma presenting as Henoch-Schönlein purpura with nephritis. *Am J Kidney Dis.* 2000;36:E19.

48. Mestecky J, Moro I, Kerr MA, et al. Mucosal immunoglobulins. In: Mestecky J, Bienenstock J, Lamm ME, et al., eds. *Mucosal Immunology,* 3rd ed, vol. 1. Amsterdam: Elsevier Academic Press; 2005:153.

49. Baenziger J, Kornfeld S. Structure of the carbohydrate units of IgA1 immunoglobulin II. Structure of the *O*-glycosidically linked oligosaccharide units. *J Biol Chem.* 1974;249:7270.

50. Field MC, Dwek RA, Edge CJ, et al. *O*-linked oligosaccharides from human serum immunoglobulin A1. *Biochem Soc Trans.* 1989;17:1034.

51. Mattu TS, Pleass RJ, Willis AC, et al. The glycosylation and structure of human serum IgA1, Fab, and Fc regions and the role of *N*-glycosylation on Fcα receptor interactions. *J Biol Chem.* 1998;273:2260.

52. Tomana M, Kulhavy R, Mestecky J. Receptor-mediated binding and uptake of immunoglobulin A by human liver. *Gastroenterology.* 1988;94:887.

53. Tarelli E, Smith AC, Hendry BM, et al. Human serum IgA1 is substituted with up to six *O*-glycans as shown by matrix assisted laser desorption ionisation time-of-flight mass spectrometry. *Carbohydr Res.* 2004;339:2329.

54. Renfrow MB, Cooper HJ, Tomana M, et al. Determination of aberrant *O*-glycosylation in the IgA1 hinge region by electron capture dissociation Fourier transform-ion cyclotron resonance mass spectrometry. *J Biol Chem.* 2005; 280:19136.

55. Novak J, Tomana M, Kilian M, et al. Heterogeneity of *O*-glycosylation in the hinge region of human IgA1. *Mol Immunol.* 2000;37:1047.

56. Renfrow MB, MacKay CL, Chalmers MJ, et al. Analysis of *O*-glycan heterogeneity in IgA1 myeloma proteins by Fourier transform ion cyclotron resonance mass spectrometry: Implications for IgA nephropathy. *Anal Bioanal Chem.* 2007;389:1397.

57. Takahashi K, Wall SB, Suzuki H, et al. Clustered *O*-glycans of IgA1: Defining macro- and micro-heterogeneity by use of electron capture/transfer dissociation. *Mol Cell Proteomics.* 2010;9:2545.

58. Wada Y, Dell A, Haslam SM, et al. Comparison of methods for profiling *O*-glycosylation: Human Proteome Organisation Human Disease Glycomics/ Proteome Initiative multi-institutional study of IgA1. *Mol Cell Proteomics.* 2010;9:719.

59. Raska M, Moldoveanu Z, Suzuki H, et al. Identification and characterization of CMP-NeuAc:GalNAc-IgA1 α2,6-sialyltransferase in IgA1-producing cells. *J Mol Biol.* 2007;369:69.

60. Suzuki H, Moldoveanu Z, Hall S, et al. IgA1-secreting cell lines from patients with IgA nephropathy produce aberrantly glycosylated IgA1. *J Clin Invest.* 2008;118:629.

61. Bene MC, Faure GC. Mesangial IgA in IgA nephropathy arises from the mucosa. *Am J Kidney Dis.* 1988;12:406.

62. Smith AC, Molyneux K, Feehally J, et al. *O*-glycosylation of serum IgA1 antibodies against mucosal and systemic antigens in IgA nephropathy. *J Am Soc Nephrol.* 2006;17:3520.

63. Moldoveanu Z, Moro I, Radl J, et al. Site of catabolism of autologous and heterologous IgA in non-human primates. *Scand J Immunol.* 1990;32:577.

64. Stockert RJ, Kressner MS, Collins JD, et al. IgA interactions with the asialoglycoprotein receptor. *Proc Natl Acad Sci U S A.* 1982;79:6229.

65. Baenziger JU, Fiete D. Galactose and *N*-acetylgalactosamine-specific endocytosis of glycopeptides by isolated rat hepatocytes. *Cell.* 1980;22:611.

66. Mestecky J, Hashim OH, Tomana M. Alterations in the IgA carbohydrate chains influence the cellular distribution of IgA1. *Contrib Nephrol.* 1995;111:66.

67. Phillips JO, Komiyama K, Epps JM, et al. Role of hepatocytes in the uptake of IgA and IgA-containing immune complexes in mice. *Mol Immunol.* 1988;25:873.

68. Haakenstad AO, Mannik M. The biology of immune complexes. In: Talal N, ed. *Autoimmunity. Genetic, Immunologic, Virologic, and Clinical Aspects.* New York: Academic Press; 1977:277.

69. Novak J, Julian BA, Tomana M, et al. Progress in molecular and genetic studies of IgA nephropathy. *J Clin Immunol.* 2001;21:310.

70. Julian BA, Novak J. IgA nephropathy: an update. *Curr Opin Nephrol Hypertens.* 2004;13:171.

71. Couser WG. Glomerulonephritis. *Lancet.* 1999;353:1509.

72. Coppo R, Amore A. Aberrant glycosylation in IgA nephropathy (IgAN). *Kidney Int.* 2004;65:1544.

73. Moura IC, Arcos-Fajardo M, Sadaka C, et al. Glycosylation and size of IgA1 are essential for interaction with mesangial transferrin receptor in IgA nephropathy. *J Am Soc Nephrol.* 2004;15:622.

74. Novak J, Moldoveanu Z, Renfrow MB, et al. IgA nephropathy and Henoch-Schoenlein purpura nephritis: aberrant glycosylation of IgA1, formation of IgA1-containing immune complexes, and activation of mesangial cells. *Contrib Nephrol.* 2007;157:134.

75. Gomez-Guerrero C, Gonzalez E, Hernando P, et al. Interaction of mesangial cells with IgA and IgG immune complexes: a possible mechanism of glomerular injury in IgA nephropathy. *Contrib Nephrol.* 1993;104:127.

76. Leung JCK, Tsang AWL, Chan DTM, et al. Absence of CD89, polymeric immunoglobulin receptor, and asialoglycoprotein receptor on human mesangial cells. *J Am Soc Nephrol.* 2000;11:241.

77. Monteiro RC, Van De Winkel JG. IgA Fc Receptors. *Annu Rev Immunol.* 2003;21:177.

78. Moura IC, Centelles MN, Arcos-Fajardo M, et al. Identification of the transferrin receptor as a novel immunoglobulin (Ig)A1 receptor and its enhanced expression on mesangial cells in IgA nephropathy. *J Exp Med.* 2001;194:417.

79. McDonald KJ, Cameron AJM, Allen JM, et al. Expression of Fc α/μ receptor by human mesangial cells: a candidate receptor for immune complex deposition in IgA nephropathy. *Biochem Biophys Res Commun.* 2002;290:438.

80. Moura IC, Arcos-Fajardo M, Gdoura A, et al. Engagement of transferrin receptor by polymeric IgA1: evidence for a positive feedback loop involving increased receptor expression and mesangial cell proliferation in IgA nephropathy. *J Am Soc Nephrol.* 2005;16:2667.

81. Haddad E, Moura IC, Arcos-Fajardo M, et al. Enhanced expression of the CD71 mesangial IgA1 receptor in Berger disease and Henoch-Schönlein nephritis: Association between CD71 expression and IgA deposits. *J Am Soc Nephrol.* 2003;14:327.

82. Suzuki H, Fun R, Zhang Z, et al. Aberrantly glycosylated IgA1 in IgA nephropathy patients is recognized by IgG antibodies with restricted heterogeneity. *J Clin Invest.* 2009;119:1668.

83. Glassock RJ. The pathogenesis of IgA nephropathy. *Curr Opin Nephrol Hypertens.* 2011;20:153.

84. Chen A, Chen WP, Sheu LF, et al. Pathogenesis of IgA nephropathy: *in vitro* activation of human mesangial cells by IgA immune complex leads to cytokine secretion. *J Pathol.* 1994;173:119.

85. Gomez-Guerrero C, Lopez-Armada MJ, Gonzalez E, et al. Soluble IgA and IgG aggregates are catabolized by cultured rat mesangial cells and induce production of TNF-α and IL-6, and proliferation. *J Immunol.* 1994;153:5247.

86. Lai KN, Leung JC, Chan LY, et al. Activation of podocytes by mesangial-derived TNF-α: glomerulo-podocytic communication in IgA nephropathy. *Am J Physiol Renal Physiol.* 2008;294:F945.

87. Amore A, Cirina P, Conti G, et al. Glycosylation of circulating IgA in patients with IgA nephropathy modulates proliferation and apoptosis of mesangial cells. *J Am Soc Nephrol.* 2001;12:1862.

88. Lai KN, Leung JC, Chan LY, et al. Podocyte injury induced by mesangial-derived cytokines in IgA nephropathy. *Nephrol Dial Transplant.* 2009;24:62.

89. Coppo R, Fonsato V, Balegno S, et al. Aberrantly glycosylated IgA1 induces mesangial cells to produce platelet-activating factor that mediates nephrin loss in cultured podocytes. *Kidney Int.* 2010;77:417.

90. Camilla R, Suzuki H, Dapra V, et al. Oxidative stress and galactose-deficient IgA1 as markers of progression in IgA nephropathy. *Clin J Am Soc Nephrol* 2011;6:1903.

91. Julian BA, Quiggins PA, Thompson JS, et al. Familial IgA nephropathy. Evidence of an inherited mechanism of disease. *N Engl J Med.* 1985;312:202.
92. Beerman I, Novak J, Wyatt RJ, et al. Genetics of IgA nephropathy. *Nat Clin Pract Nephrol.* 2007;3:325.
93. Kiryluk K, Gharavi AG, Izzi C, et al. IgA nephropathy—the case for a genetic basis becomes stronger. *Nephrol Dial Transplant.* 2010;25:336.
94. Kiryluk K, Moldoveanu Z, Sanders JT, et al. Aberrant glycosylation of IgA1 is inherited in both pediatric IgA nephropathy and Henoch-Schönlein purpura nephritis. *Kidney Int.* 2011;80(1):79–87.
95. Gharavi AG, Yan Y, Scolari F, et al. IgA nephropathy, the most common cause of glomerulonephritis, is linked to 6q22-23. *Nat Genet.* 2000;26:354.
96. Gharavi AG, Scolari F, Lifton RP. Familial IgA nephropathy: Clinical features and genetic investigations. *Adv Nephrol Necker Hosp.* 2002;32:207.
97. Lavigne KA, Woodford SY, Barker CV, et al. Familial IgA nephropathy in southeastern Kentucky. *Clin Nephrol.* 2010;73:115.
98. Geddes CC, Rauta V, Gronhagen-Riska C, et al. A tricontinental view of IgA nephropathy. *Nephrol Dial Transplant.* 2003;18:1541.
99. Bisceglia L, Cerullo G, Forabosco P, et al. Genetic heterogeneity in Italian families with IgA nephropathy: suggestive linkage for two novel IgA nephropathy loci. *Am J Hum Genet.* 2006;79:1130.
100. Paterson AD, Liu XQ, Wang K, et al. Genome-wide linkage scan of a large family with IgA nephropathy localizes a novel susceptibility locus to chromosome 2q36. *J Am Soc Nephrol.* 2007;18:2408.
101. Manolio TA. Genomewide association studies and assessment of the risk of disease. *N Engl J Med.* 2010;363:166.
102. Feehally J, Farrall M, Boland A, et al. HLA has strongest association with IgA nephropathy in genome-wide analysis. *J Am Soc Nephrol.* 2010;21:1791.
103. Gharavi AG, Kiryluk K, Choi M, et al. Genome-wide association study identifies five susceptibility loci for IgA nephropathy, the most common form of glomerulonephritis. *Nat Genet.* 2011;43(4):321–327.
104. Lau KL, Wyatt RJ, Moldoveanu Z, et al. Serum levels of galactose-deficient IgA in children with IgA nephropathy and Henoch-Schoenlein purpura. *Ped Nephrol.* 2007;22:2067.
105. Moldoveanu Z, Wyatt RJ, Lee J, et al. Patients with IgA nephropathy have increased serum galactose-deficient IgA1 levels. *Kidney Int.* 2007;71:1148.
106. Mestecky J, Tomana M, Moldoveanu Z, et al. The role of aberrant glycosylation of IgA1 molecules in the pathogenesis of IgA nephropathy. *Kidney Blood Pres Res.* 2008;31:29.
107. Novak J, Julian BA, Tomana M, et al. IgA glycosylation and IgA immune complexes in the pathogenesis of IgA nephropathy. *Semin Nephrol.* 2008;28:78.
108. Novak J, Mestecky J. IgA Immune-complex. In: Lai KN, ed. *Recent Advances in IgA Nephropathy.* Hong Kong: Imperial College Press and the World Scientific Publisher; 2009:177.
109. Julian BA, Wyatt RJ, Matousovic K, et al. IgA nephropathy: a clinical overview. *Contrib Nephrol.* 2007;157:19.
110. Gharavi AG, Moldoveanu Z, Wyatt RJ, et al. Aberrant IgA1 glycosylation is inherited in familial and sporadic IgA nephropathy. *J Am Soc Nephrol.* 2008;19:1008.
111. Lin X, Ding J, Zhu L, et al. Aberrant galactosylation of IgA1 is involved in the genetic susceptibility of Chinese patients with IgA nephropathy. *Nephrol Dial Transplant.* 2009;24:3372.
112. Kitagawa T. Lessons learned from the Japanese nephritis screening study. *Pediatr Nephrol.* 1988;2:256.
113. Park YH, Choi JY, Chung HS, et al. Hematuria and proteinuria in a mass school urine screening test. *Pediatr Nephrol.* 2005;20:1126.
114. Nair R, Walker PD. Is IgA nephropathy the commonest primary glomerulopathy among young adults in the USA? *Kidney Int.* 2006;69:1455.
115. Wyatt RJ, Julian BA, Baehler RW, et al. Epidemiology of IgA nephropathy in central and eastern Kentucky for the period 1975 through 1994. *J Am Soc Nephrol.* 1998;9:853.
116. Suzuki K, Honda K, Tanabe K, et al. Incidence of latent mesangial IgA deposition in renal allograft donors in Japan. *Kidney Int.* 2003;63:2286.
117. Sinniah R. Occurence of mesangial IgA and IgM deposits in a control necropsy population. *J Clin Pathol.* 1983;36:276.
118. Waldherr R, Rambousek M, Duncker WD, et al. Frequency of mesangial IgA deposits in non-selected autopsy series. *Nephrol Dial Transplant.* 1989; 4:943.
119. D'Amico G. Natural history of idiopathic IgA nephropathy: role of clinical and histological prognostic factors. *Am J Kidney Dis.* 2000;36:227.
120. Haas M, Rahman MH, Cohn RA, et al. IgA nephropathy in children and adults: comparison of histologic features and clinical outcomes. *Nephrol Dial Transplant.* 2008;23:2537.
121. Kincaid-Smith P, Fairley K. The investigation of hematuria. *Semin Nephrol.* 2005;25:127.
122. Clarkson AR, Seymour AE, Thompson AJ, et al. IgA nephropathy: a syndrome of uniform morphology, diverse clinical features and uncertain prognosis. *Clin Nephrol.* 1977;8:459.
123. Tiebosch AT, Frederik PM, van Breda Vriesman PJ, et al. Thin-basement-membrane nephropathy in adults with persistent hematuria. *N Engl J Med.* 1989;320:14.
124. Pouria S, Barratt J. Secondary IgA nephropathy. *Semin Nephrol.* 2008;28:27.
125. Callard P, Feldmann G, Prandi D, et al. Immune complex type glomerulonephritis in cirrhosis of the liver. *Am J Pathol.* 1975;80:329.
126. McGuire BM, Julian BA, Bynon JS Jr, et al. Glomerulonephritis in patients with hepatitis C cirrhosis undergoing liver transplantation. *Ann Intern Med.* 2006;144:735.
127. Smerud HK, Fellstrom B, Hallgren R, et al. Gluten sensitivity in patients with IgA nephropathy. *Nephrol Dial Transplant.* 2009;24:2476.
128. de Moura CG, de Moura TG, de Souza SP, et al. Inflammatory bowel disease, ankylosing spondylitis, and IgA nephropathy. *J Clin Rheumatol.* 2006;12:106.
129. Gerntholtz TE, Goetsch SJ, Katz I. HIV-related nephropathy: a South African perspective. *Kidney Int.* 2006;69:1885.
130. Beaufils H, Jouanneau C, Katlama C, et al. HIV-associated IgA nephropathy—a post-mortem study. *Nephrol Dial Transplant.* 1995;10:35.
131. Levey AS, Bosch JP, Lewis JB, et al. A more accurate method to estimate glomerular filtration rate from serum creatinine: a new prediction equation. Modification of Diet in Renal Disease Study Group. *Ann Intern Med.* 1999;130:461.
132. Komatsu H, Fujimoto S, Sato Y, et al. "Point of no return (PNR)" in progressive IgA nephropathy: significance of blood pressure and proteinuria management up to PNR. *J Nephrol.* 2005;18:690.
133. Ibels LS, Gyory AZ, Caterson RJ, et al. Primary IgA nephropathy: Natural history and factors of importance in the progression of renal impairment. *Kidney Int.* 1997;61:S67.
134. Bartosik LP, Lajoie G, Sugar L, et al. Predicting progression in IgA nephropathy. *Am J Kidney Dis.* 2001;38:728.
135. Hotta O, Furuta T, Chiba S, et al. Regression of IgA nephropathy: a repeat biopsy study. *Am J Kidney Dis.* 2002;39:493.
136. Radford MG Jr, Donadio JV Jr, Bergstralh EJ, et al. Predicting renal outcome in IgA nephropathy. *J Am Soc Nephrol.* 1997;8:199.
137. Reich HN, Troyanov S, Scholey JW, et al. Remission of proteinuria improves prognosis in IgA nephropathy. *J Am Soc Nephrol.* 2007;18:3177.
138. Glassock RJ. IgA nephropathy: challenges and opportunities. *Cleve Clin J Med.* 2008;75:569.
139. Coppo R, Troyanov S, Camilla R, et al. The Oxford IgA nephropathy clinicopathological classification is valid for children as well as adults. *Kidney Int.* 2010;77:921.
140. van Es LA, de Heer E, Vleming LJ, et al. GMP-17-positive T-lymphocytes in renal tubules predict progression in early stages of IgA nephropathy. *Kidney Int.* 2008;73:1426.
141. Hara M, Yanagihara T, Kihara I. Cumulative excretion of urinary podocytes reflects disease progression in IgA nephropathy and Schönlein-Henoch purpura nephritis. *Clin J Am Soc Nephrol.* 2007;2:231.
142. Tumlin JA, Hennigar RA. Clinical presentation, natural history, and treatment of crescentic proliferative IgA nephropathy. *Semin Nephrol.* 2004;24:256.
143. Bantis C, Stangou M, Schlaugat C, et al. Is presence of ANCA in crescentic IgA nephropathy a coincidence or novel clinical entity? A case series. *Am J Kidney Dis.* 2010;55:259.
144. Berthoux F, Mohey H, Laurent B, et al. The absolute renal risk of dialysis/death in primary IgA nephropathy. *J Am Soc Nephrol.* 2011;22(4):752–761.
145. Bennett WM, Kincaid-Smith P. Macroscopic hematuria in mesangial IgA nephropathy: correlation with glomerular crescents and renal dysfunction. *Kidney Int.* 1983;23:393.
146. Szeto CC, Law MC, Wong TY, et al. Peritoneal transport status correlates with morbidity but not longitudinal change of nutritional status of continuous ambulatory peritoneal dialysis patients: a 2-year prospective study. *Am J Kidney Dis.* 2001;37:329.
147. Matousovic K, Novak J, Tomana M, et al. IgA1-containing immune complexes in the urine of IgA nephropathy patients. *Nephrol Dial Transplant.* 2006;21:2478.
148. Julian BA, Wittke S, Novak J, et al. Electrophoretic methods for analysis of urinary polypeptides in IgA-associated renal diseases. *Electrophoresis.* 2007; 28:4469.
149. Barratt J, Topham P. Urine proteomics: the present and future of measuring urinary protein components in disease. *CMAJ.* 2007;177:361.
150. Fliser D, Novak J, Thongboonkerd V, et al. Advances in urinary proteome analysis and biomarker discovery. *J Am Soc Nephrol.* 2007;18:1057.
151. Rossing K, Mischak H, Dakna M, et al. Urinary proteomics in diabetes and CKD. *J Am Soc Nephrol.* 2008;19:1283.

152. Julian BA, Suzuki H, Suzuki Y, et al. Sources of urinary proteins and their analysis by urinary proteomics for the detection of biomarkers of disease. *Proteomics Clin Appl.* 2009;3:1029.
153. Good DM, Zurbig P, Argiles A, et al. Naturally occurring human urinary peptides for use in diagnosis of chronic kidney disease. *Mol Cell Proteomics.* 2010;9:2424.
154. Haubitz M, Wittke S, Weissinger EM, et al. Urine protein patterns can serve as diagnostic tools in patients with IgA nephropathy. *Kidney Int.* 2005;67:2313.
155. Mischak H, Apweiler R, Banks RE, et al. Clinical proteomics: a need to define the field and to begin to set adequate standards. *Proteomics-Clin Appl.* 2007;1:148.
156. Mischak H, Allmaier G, Apweiler R, et al. Recommendations for biomarker identification and qualification in clinical proteomics. *Sci Transl Med.* 2010;2:46ps42.
157. Yusuf S, Teo KK, Pogue J, et al. Telmisartan, ramipril, or both in patients at high risk for vascular events. *N Engl J Med.* 2008;358:1547.
158. Yamamoto R, Nagasawa Y, Shoji T, et al. Cigarette smoking and progression of IgA nephropathy. *Am J Kidney Dis.* 2010;56:313.
159. Cheng J, Zhang W, Zhang XH, et al. ACEI/ARB therapy for IgA nephropathy: a meta analysis of randomised controlled trials. *Int J Clin Pract.* 2009;63:880.
160. Barratt J, Feehally J. Treatment of IgA nephropathy. *Kidney Int.* 2006; 69:1934.
161. Coppo R, Peruzzi L, Amore A, et al. IgACE: a placebo-controlled, randomized trial of angiotensin-converting enzyme inhibitors in children and young people with IgA nephropathy and moderate proteinuria. *J Am Soc Nephrol.* 2007;18:1880.
162. Coppo R, Feehally J, Glassock RJ. IgA nephropathy at two score and one. *Kidney Int.* 2010;77:181.
163. Hogg RJ. Immunoglobulin A nephropathy and related disorders. In Greenberg A, Cheung AK, Coffman TM, et al., eds. *Primer on Kidney Diseases*, 5th ed. Philadelphia: Saunders Elsevier; 2009:179.
164. Praga M, Gutierrez E, Gonzalez E, et al. Treatment of IgA nephropathy with ACE inhibitors: a randomized and controlled trial. *J Am Soc Nephrol.* 2003;14:1578.
165. Ballardie FW. Quantitative appraisal of treatment options for IgA nephropathy. *J Am Soc Nephrol.* 2007;18:2806.
166. Pozzi C, Andrulli S, Del Vecchio L, et al. Corticosteroid effectiveness in IgA nephropathy: long-term results of a randomized, controlled trial. *J Am Soc Nephrol.* 2004;15:157.
167. Eitner F, Ackermann D, Hilgers RD, et al. Supportive Versus Immunosuppressive Therapy of Progressive IgA nephropathy (STOP) IgAN trial: rationale and study protocol. *J Nephrol.* 2008;21:284.
168. Pozzi C, Andrulli S, Pani A, et al. Addition of azathioprine to corticosteroids does not benefit patients with IgA nephropathy. *J Am Soc Nephrol.* 2010;21:1783.
169. Ballardie FW, Roberts IS. Controlled prospective trial of prednisolone and cytotoxics in progressive IgA nephropathy. *J Am Soc Nephrol.* 2002;13:142.
170. Tumlin JA, Lohavichan V, Hennigar R. Crescentic, proliferative IgA nephropathy: clinical and histological response to methylprednisolone and intravenous cyclophosphamide. *Nephrol Dial Transplant.* 2003;18:1321.
171. Roccatello D, Ferro M, Cesano G, et al. Steroid and cyclophosphamide in IgA nephropathy. *Nephrol Dial Transplant.* 2000;15:833.
172. Miller ER III, Juraschek SP, Appel LJ, et al. The effect of n-3 long-chain polyunsaturated fatty acid supplementation on urine protein excretion and kidney function: meta-analysis of clinical trials. *Am J Clin Nutr.* 2009;89:1937.
173. Fassett RG, Gobe GC, Peake JM, et al. Omega-3 polyunsaturated fatty acids in the treatment of kidney disease. *Am J Kidney Dis.* 2010;56:728.
174. Hogg RJ. Idiopathic immunoglobulin A nephropathy in children and adolescents. *Pediatr Nephrol.* 2010;25:823.
175. Tan CH, Loh PT, Yang WS, et al. Mycophenolate mofetil in the treatment of IgA nephropathy: a systematic review. *Singapore Med J.* 2008;49:780.
176. Tang SC, Tang AW, Wong SS, et al. Long-term study of mycophenolate mofetil treatment in IgA nephropathy. *Kidney Int.* 2010;77:543.
177. Clarkson AR, Seymour AE, Woodroffe AJ, et al. Controlled trial of phenytoin therapy in IgA nephropathy. *Clin Nephrol.* 1980;13:215.
178. Miura N, Imai H, Kikuchi S, et al. Tonsillectomy and steroid pulse (TSP) therapy for patients with IgA nephropathy: a nationwide survey of TSP therapy in Japan and an analysis of the predictive factors for resistance to TSP therapy. *Clin Exp Nephrol.* 2009;13:460.
179. Wang Y, Chen J, Chen Y, et al. A meta-analysis of the clinical remission rate and long-term efficacy of tonsillectomy in patients with IgA nephropathy. *Nephrol Dial Transplant.* 2011;26(6):1923–1931.
180. Piccoli A, Codognotto M, Tabbi MG, et al. Influence of tonsillectomy on the progression of mesangioproliferative glomerulonephritis. *Nephrol Dial Transplant.* 2010;25:2583.
181. Barratt J, Feehally J. IgA nephropathy. *J Am Soc Nephrol.* 2005;16:2088.
182. Floege J, Burg M, Kliem V. Recurrent IgA nephropathy after kidney transplantation: not a benign condition. *Nephrol Dial Transplant.* 1998;13:1933.
183. Briganti EM, Russ GR, McNeil JJ, et al. Risk of renal allograft loss from recurrent glomerulonephritis. *N Engl J Med.* 2002;347:103.
184. Floege J. Recurrent IgA nephropathy after renal transplantation. *Semin Nephrol.* 2004;24:287.
185. Han SS, Sun HK, Lee JP, et al. Outcome of renal allograft in patients with Henoch-Schönlein nephritis: single-center experience and systematic review. *Transplantation.* 2010;89:721.
186. Coppo R, Amore A, Chiesa M, et al. Serological and genetic factors in early recurrence of IgA nephropathy after renal transplantation. *Clin Transplant.* 2007;21:728.
187. Imai H, Nakamoto Y, Asakura K, et al. Spontaneous glomerular IgA deposition in ddY mice: an animal model of IgA nephritis. *Kidney Int.* 1985; 27:756.
188. Miyawaki S, Muso E, Takeuchi E, et al. Selective breeding for high serum IgA levels from noninbred ddY mice: Isolation of a strain with an early onset of glomerular IgA deposition. *Nephron.* 1997;76:201.
189. Kamata T, Muso E, Yashiro M, et al. Up-regulation of glomerular extracellular matrix and transforming growth factor-β expression in RF/J mice. *Kidney Int.* 1999;55:864.
190. Tomino Y. Pathogenetic and therapeutic approaches to IgA nephropathy using a spontaneous animal model, the ddY mouse. *Clin Exp Nephrol.* 2011;15:1.
191. Nogaki F, Oida E, Kamata T, et al. Chromosomal mapping of hyperserum IgA and glomerular IgA deposition in a high IgA (HIGA) strain of DdY mice. *Kidney Int.* 2005;68:2517.
192. Suzuki H, Suzuki Y, Yamanaka T, et al. Genome-wide scan in a novel IgA nephropathy model identifies a susceptibility locus on murine chromosome 10, in a region syntenic to human IGAN1 on chromosome 6q22-23. *J Am Soc Nephrol.* 2005;16:1289.
193. Suzuki H, Suzuki Y, Aizawa M, et al. Th1 polarization in murine IgA nephropathy directed by bone marrow-derived cells. *Kidney Int.* 2007;72:319.
194. Hattori T, Sadakane C, Koseki J, et al. Saireito probably prevents mesangial cell proliferation in HIGA mice via PDGF-BB tyrosine kinase inhibition. *Clin Exp Nephrol.* 2007;11:275.
195. Schroeder C, Osman AA, Roggenbuck D, et al. IgA-gliadin antibodies, IgA-containing circulating immune complexes, and IgA glomerular deposits in wasting marmoset syndrome. *Nephrol Dial Transplant.* 1999;14:1875.
196. Nishie T, Miyaishi O, Azuma H, et al. Development of immunoglobulin A nephropathy-like disease in β1,4-galactosyltransferase-I-deficient mice. *Am J Pathol.* 2007;170:447.
197. Kennel-De March A, Prin-Mathieu C, Kohler CH, et al. Back-pack mice as a model of renal mesangial IgA dimers deposition. *Int J Immunopathol Pharmacol.* 2005;18:701.
198. Lamm ME, Emancipator SN, Robinson JK, et al. Microbial IgA protease removes IgA immune complexes from mouse glomeruli *in vivo*: potential therapy for IgA nephropathy. *Am J Pathol.* 2008;172:31.
199. Monteiro RC. Pathogenic role of IgA receptors in IgA nephropathy. *Contrib Nephrol.* 2007;157:64.
200. Launay P, Grossetete B, Arcos-Fajardo M, et al. Fcα receptor (CD89) mediates the development of immunoglobulin A (IgA) nephropathy (Berger's disease). Evidence for pathogenic soluble receptor-IgA complexes in patients and CD89 transgenic mice. *J Exp Med.* 2000;191:1999.
201. Emancipator SN. Prospects and perspectives on IgA nephropathy from animal models. *Contrib Nephrol.* 2011;169:126.
202. Emancipator SN. IgA nephropathy and Henoch-Schönlein syndrome. In Jennette JC, Olson JL, Schwartz MM, et al. eds. *Heptinstall's Pathology of the Kidney*. Philadelphia: Lippincott-Raven Publishers; 1998:479.
203. Fervenza FC. Henoch-Schönlein purpura nephritis. *Int J Dermatol.* 2003;42:170.
204. Davin JC, Weening JJ. Henoch-Schönlein purpura nephritis: an update. *Eur J Pediatr.* 2001;160:689.
205. Sanders JT, Wyatt RJ. IgA nephropathy and Henoch-Schönlein purpura nephritis. *Curr Opin Pediatr.* 2008;20:163.
206. Ozen S, Ruperto N, Dillon MJ, et al. EULAR/PReS endorsed consensus criteria for the classification of childhood vasculitides. *Ann Rheum Dis.* 2006; 65:936.
207. Ozen S, Pistorio A, Iusan SM, et al. EULAR/PRINTO/PRES criteria for Henoch-Schönlein purpura, childhood polyarteritis nodosa, childhood Wegener granulomatosis and childhood Takayasu arteritis: Ankara 2008. Part II: Final classification criteria. *Ann Rheum Dis.* 2010;69:798.
208. Heberden W. *Commentaries on the History and Cure of Diseases*. London; 1806:396.

209. Amoroso A, Berrino M, Canale L, et al. Immunogenetics of Henoch-Schoenlein disease. *Eur J Immunogenet.* 1997;24:323.
210. Amoli MM, Thomson W, Hajeer AH, et al. HLA-DRB1*01 association with Henoch-Schönlein purpura in patients from northwest Spain. *J Rheumatol.* 2001;28:1266.
211. Soylemezoglu O, Peru H, Gonen S, et al. HLA-DRB1 alleles and Henoch-Schönlein purpura: susceptibility and severity of disease. *J Rheumatol.* 2008;35:1165.
212. Peru H, Soylemezoglu O, Gonen S, et al. HLA class 1 associations in Henoch Schönlein purpura: increased and decreased frequencies. *Clin Rheumatol.* 2008;27:5.
213. Soylu A, Kizildag S, Kavukcu S, et al. TLR-2 Arg753Gln, TLR-4 Asp299Gly, and TLR-4 Thr399Ile polymorphisms in Henoch Schönlein purpura with and without renal involvement. *Rheumatol Int.* 2010;30:667.
214. Tabel Y, Mir S, Berdeli A. Interleukin 8 gene 2767 A/G polymorphism is associated with increased risk of nephritis in children with Henoch-Schönlein purpura. *Rheumatol Int.* 2011. Epub ahead of print.
215. Saulsbury FT. Henoch-Schönlein purpura. *Curr Opin Rheumatol.* 2010; 22:598.
216. Blanco R, Martinez-Taboada VM, Rodriguez-Valverde V, et al. Henoch-Schönlein purpura in adulthood and childhood: two different expressions of the same syndrome. *Arthritis Rheum.* 1997;40:859.
217. Coppo R, Andrulli S, Amore A, et al. Predictors of outcome in Henoch-Schönlein nephritis in children and adults. *Am J Kidney Dis.* 2006;47:993.
218. Edstrom Halling S, Soderberg MP, Berg UB. Predictors of outcome in Henoch-Schönlein nephritis. *Pediatr Nephrol.* 2010;25:1101.
219. Jauhola O, Ronkainen J, Koskimies O, et al. Renal manifestations of Henoch-Schönlein purpura in a 6-month prospective study of 223 children. *Arch Dis Child.* 2010;95:877.
220. Eiro M, Katoh T, Watanabe T. Risk factors for bleeding complications in percutaneous renal biopsy. *Clin Exp Nephrol.* 2005;9:40.
221. Emancipator SN, Mestecky J, Lamm ME. IgA nephropathy and related diseases. In: Ogra PL, Mestecky J, Lamm ME, et al., eds. *Mucosal Immunology.* San Diego: Academic Press; 1999:1365.
222. Meadow SR, Scott DG. Berger disease: Henoch-Schönlein syndrome without the rash. *J Pediat.* 1985;106:27.
223. Coppo R, Amore A, Roccatello D, et al. Complement receptor (CR1) and IgG or IgA on erythrocytes and in circulating immune complexes in patients with glomerulonephritis. *Nephrol Dial Transplant.* 1989;4:932.
224. Greer MR, Barratt J, Harper SJ, et al. The nucleotide sequence of the IgA1 hinge region in IgA nephropathy. *Nephrol Dial Transplant.* 1998;13:1980.
225. Lau KK, Suzuki H, Novak J, et al. Pathogenesis of Henoch-Schönlein purpura nephritis. *Ped Nephrol.* 2010:19.
226. Wu SH, Liao PY, Yin PL, et al. Inverse temporal changes of lipoxin A4 and leukotrienes in children with Henoch-Schönlein purpura. *Prostaglandins Leukot Essent Fatty Acids.* 2009;80:177.
227. Ronkainen J, Koskimies O, Ala-Houhala M, et al. Early prednisone therapy in Henoch-Schönlein purpura: a randomized, double-blind, placebo-controlled trial. *J Pediatr.* 2006;149:241.
228. Saulsbury FT. Successful treatment of prolonged Henoch-Schönlein purpura with colchicine. *Clin Pediatr (Phila).* 2009;48:866.
229. Huber AM, King J, McLaine P, et al. A randomized, placebo-controlled trial of prednisone in early Henoch Schönlein purpura [ISRCTN85109383]. *BMC Med.* 2004;2:7.
230. Chartapisak W, Opastiraku S, Willis NS, et al. Prevention and treatment of renal disease in Henoch-Schönlein purpura: a systematic review. *Arch Dis Child.* 2009;94:132.
231. Zaffanello M, Fanos V. Treatment-based literature of Henoch-Schönlein purpura nephritis in childhood. *Pediatr Nephrol.* 2009;24:1901.
232. Bogdanovic R. Henoch-Schönlein purpura nephritis in children: risk factors, prevention and treatment. *Acta Paediatr.* 2009;98:1882.
233. Ninchoji T, Kaito H, Nozu K, et al. Treatment strategies for Henoch-Schönlein purpura nephritis by histological and clinical severity. *Pediatr Nephrol.* 2011;26:563.
234. Donnithorne KJ, Atkinson TP, Hinze CH, et al. Rituximab therapy for severe refractory chronic Henoch-Schönlein purpura. *J Pediatr.* 2009;155:136.
235. Shenoy M, Bradbury MG, Lewis MA, et al. Outcome of Henoch-Schönlein purpura nephritis treated with long-term immunosuppression. *Pediatr Nephrol.* 2007;22:1717.
236. Pillebout E, Alberti C, Guillevin L, et al. Addition of cyclophosphamide to steroids provides no benefit compared with steroids alone in treating adult patients with severe Henoch Schönlein purpura. *Kidney Int.* 2010;78:495.

CHAPTER

50 Membranoproliferative Glomerulonephritis and Dense Deposit Disease

J. Ashley Jefferson • Miguel Palma-Diaz • Charles E. Alpers

Membranoproliferative glomerulonephritis (MPGN), sometimes referred to as mesangiocapillary glomerulonephritis, describes a pathologic pattern of injury characterized by thickening of peripheral capillary walls (membrano-), glomerular hypercellularity (-proliferative), with mesangial expansion leading to an accentuated lobular appearance of the glomerular tuft. Although there are idiopathic forms of this condition, the majority of cases of MPGN are associated with secondary causes—in particular, hepatitis C (Table 50.1). The various forms of MPGN have very different clinical courses and are described separately.

CLASSIFICATION

Prior classifications of MPGN have subdivided this entity into three different classes according to pathologic characteristics (Table 1). Type I is the most common and is an immune complex mediated disorder with primarily subendothelial and mesangial immune deposits leading to activation of the classical pathway of complement. Type III was described as having a similar histologic pattern, but with the additional finding of subepithelial immune deposits or a distinctive appearance of the capillary wall deposits identified by electron microscopy. It is increasingly recognized that cases previously considered as Type III MPGN do not represent a separate disorder, but rather are best considered a variant of Type I MPGN, or more commonly, a form of the recently described entity C3 glomerulopathy. Dense deposit disease (DDD; type II) results from dysregulation of the alternate pathway of complement, and it has become clear that only a minority of cases of DDD demonstrate an MPGN pattern on biopsy. In view of these points, we prefer to classify MPGN into primary and secondary causes (Table 50.2), and we follow an emerging consensus that DDD and C3 glomerulopathy are separate entities altogether.[1]

PRIMARY MEMBRANOPROLIFERATIVE GLOMERULONEPHRITIS

Epidemiology

Primary MPGN is a relatively rare form of glomerulonephritis in developed countries, where secondary forms of MPGN are much more common. The disease is usually found in children and young adults and, interestingly, the incidence appears to be decreasing worldwide.[2–5] This may be due to a true decrease in disease incidence, partly due to improved hygiene and environmental factors reducing the incidence of bacterial infections, but may also reflect the increased ability to detect secondary forms of MPGN (e.g., viral infections, monoclonal gammopathies). In developing countries, MPGN remains one of the most common forms of glomerulonephritis.[6–8] This classically has been considered secondary to the increased incidence of bacterial infections in these countries, but this has been questioned by Johnson et al., who found little evidence for active infection in cases of MPGN in Peru.[8] They have proposed that a shift in Th1/Th2 immune balance, induced by environmental and hygienic factors, may determine the incidence of a range of glomerular diseases worldwide.[9,10]

Primary MPGN is more common among whites than among black or Asian populations. A genetic susceptibility is supported by the finding of an extended HLA haplotype—HLA-B8, DR3, SCO1, GLO2—more frequently in patients with MPGN I and III (13%) than in the general Caucasian population (1%), although this haplotype is not specific for MPGN.[11] Familial forms of MPGN have been described, but these are rare.[12] Some of these may be secondary to mutations encoding complement proteins or their inhibitors (discussed below).

Pathogenesis

Primary MPGN is considered to be an adaptive immune response to a chronic antigenic stimulus leading either to the subendothelial and mesangial deposition of circulating immune complexes consisting of immunoglobulin G (IgG), C3, and antigen, or deposition of circulating antigens in the glomerular capillary walls (planted antigens) which then serve as a nidus for immune complex formation in situ. In secondary forms of MPGN a wide range of antigens (primarily infectious agents) have been implicated, but in primary MPGN the causative antigen remains unknown. The binding of the Fc portion of IgG or IgM in the immune complexes

TABLE 50.1 Former Classification of Membranoproliferative Glomerulonephritis

Classification	Pathologic Characteristics
Type I	Enlarged, lobulated glomerulus, mesangial hypercellularity Influx of mononuclear leukocytes Duplication of GBM with cellular interposition IgG, C1q, C3 deposition in mesangium and capillary wall Mesangial and subendothelial immune deposits
Type II (dense deposit disease)	Variable pattern on light microscopy C3 deposition in absence of IgG or C1q Ribbonlike dense deposits within GBM on electron microscopy
Type III	Histologic and immunofluorescence features similar to type I MPGN Additional subepithelial deposits with thickened irregular GBM

GBM, glomerular basement membranes; IgG, immunoglobulin G; MPGN, membranoproliferative glomerulonephritis.

TABLE 50.2 Current Classification of Membranoproliferative Glomerulonephritis

Classification	Associated Disorders
Primary MPGN	None
Secondary MPGN	
Infectious Disease	Viral: hepatitis C, hepatitis B, HIV Bacterial: shunt nephritis, visceral abscess, endocarditis Protozoan: quartan malaria, schistosomiasis, leprosy
Autoimmune Disease	Systemic lupus erythematosus, mixed cryoglobulinemia, scleroderma, Sjögren syndrome, hypocomplementemic urticarial vasculitis
Monoclonal Gammopathy	Monoclonal gammopathy of uncertain significance (MGUS), multiple myeloma, B cell lymphoma, chronic lymphocytic leukemia, Waldenström macroglobulinemia
Chronic Liver Disease	Chronic hepatitis, cirrhosis, α1-antitrypsin deficiency
Miscellaneous	Solid organ tumors; cystic fibrosis, sarcoidosis, sickle cell disease, hemolytic uremic syndrome, transplant glomerulopathy, drugs (heroin, α-interferon)
C3 Glomerulopathy	
Dense Deposit Disease (formerly type II MPGN)	Dysregulation of the alternate pathway of complement ■ C3 nephritic factor (partial lipodystrophy, retinal drusen) ■ Antifactor B autoantibody ■ Factor H dysfunction (inherited and acquired)
C3 Glomerulonephritis	Dysregulation of the alternate pathway of complement ■ C3 nephritic factor ■ Mutations in complement regulatory proteins (factor H, factor I, membrane cofactor protein)

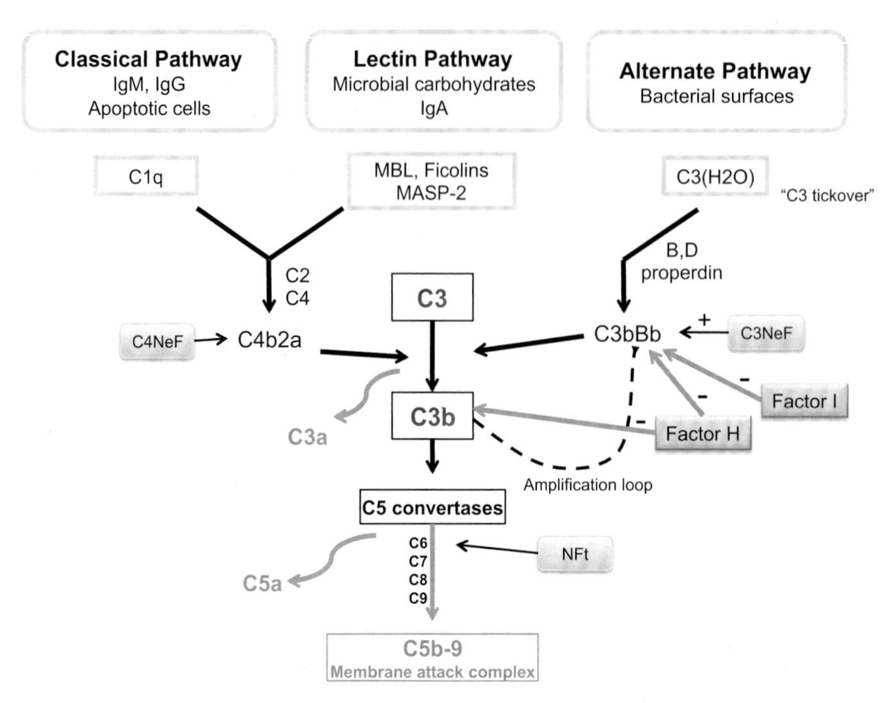

FIGURE 50.1 Complement pathways. Complement may be activated by one of three pathways. In MPGN type 1, the Fc portion of IgG or IgM in immune complexes binds C1q and activates the classical pathway, cleaving C3 to C3b. This process may be amplified by the alternate pathway (amplification loop). Cleavage fragment C3a acts as an anaphylatoxin, C3b binds to surfaces as an opsonin and further promotes the generation of the C5 convertases. These cleave C5 to form C5a (chemotactic factor), and lead to the formation of the membrane attack complex (C5b-9). In dense deposit disease, the usual low level activation (tickover) of the alternate pathway, which generates small amounts of C3 convertase (C3bBb), is dysregulated (either by C3 nephritic factor [C3NeF] or failure of factor H regulation) leading to a more profound activation of the alternate pathway and the generation of large amounts of C3b. Factor H is the major regulator of the alternate pathway. *MBL*, mannose binding lectin; *C4NeF*, C4 nephritic factor; *NFt*, nephritic factor of the terminal pathway; *C4b2a*, C3 convertase of classical pathway; *C3bBb*, C3 convertase of alternate pathway.

to C1q triggers activation of the complement via the classical pathway, but this initial activation may be amplified by the alternate pathway (amplification loop). The subsequent cleavage of C5 leads to the production of chemotactic factors (C5a), opsonins (C3b), and the membrane attack complex (C5b-9) (Fig. 50.1). In some cases, complement activation is enhanced by nephritic factors that stabilize either the classical pathway C3 convertase (C4 nephritic factor, C4NeF) or the alternate pathway C3 convertase (C3 nephritic factor, C3NeF) which may enhance the amplification loop.[13,14]

It is likely that the prominent monocyte influx that characterizes MPGN is the result of complex interactions including Fc portions of immunoglobulins within deposited immune complexes engaging Fc receptors on the surface of monocytes, as well as release of chemoattractant cytokines (e.g., colony stimulating factor 1 [CSF-1]) and other proinflammatory mediators by resident glomerular cells as a response to injury.[15,16] It is unknown whether the monocytes infiltrating human glomerulonephritis (GN) have a homogeneous phenotype, and are proinflammatory, or whether some or even a majority of these cells infiltrating at different time points of the disease course may be engaged in activities primarily directed to opsonization and phagocytosis of immune complexes, stabilization of disease, and repair of glomerular injury. Recent studies suggest systemic and local innate immune responses may also contribute to the pathogenesis of MPGN. For example, studies have demonstrated toll-like receptor 3 in human MPGN associated with viral infection,[17] and upregulated expression of toll-like receptor 4 on glomerular cells has been identified in an animal model of cryoglobulinemic MPGN,[18] but more specific immune mechanisms leading to glomerulonephritis have not been established.

Following an initial proliferative phase, a second reparative phase develops, which is characterized by the development of mesangial expansion and the formation of new basement membrane matrices resulting in double contours. These duplicated basement membrane matrices lead to the sequestering of immune complexes and entrapment of cells or cell processes between the matrices (cellular interposition) and presumably this sequestration reduces the stimulation for an acute inflammatory response by circulating leukocytes.

PATHOLOGY

The overall appearance of both primary and secondary types of MPGN often reveals enlarged glomeruli with accentuation of the normal lobular architecture (Fig. 50.2). Hypercellularity is mostly due to a combination of mesangial cell proliferation and infiltrating leukocytes. The mesangium is

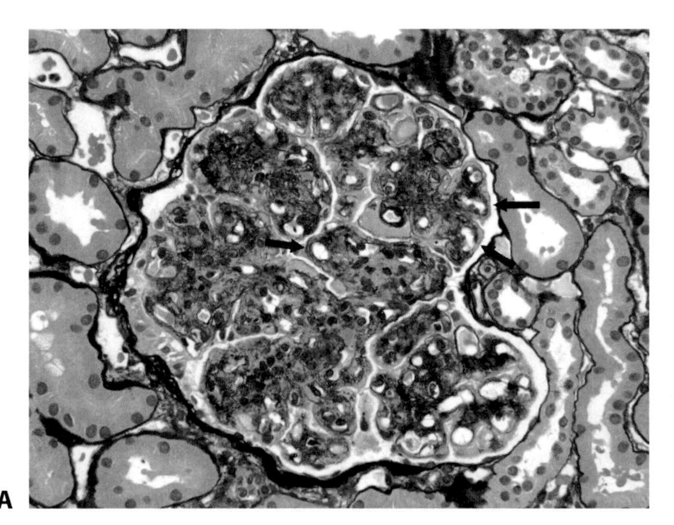
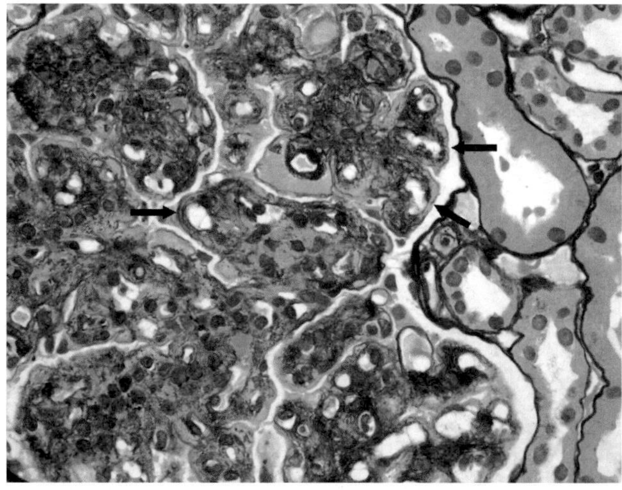

FIGURE 50.2 Membranoproliferative glomerulonephritis. **A:** Light microscopy showing prominent mesangial expansion due to increased cellularity and accumulation of extracellular eosinophilic material, diffuse thickening of glomerular basement membranes with segmental splitting (*arrows*), and influx of leukocytes (endocapillary proliferation). Jones' silver methenamine stain. **B:** Higher power view of this glomerulus shows the mesangial cell proliferation, the irregular thickening and focal splitting/duplication of basement membranes (*arrows*), and accumulation of acellular eosinophilic material, most likely deposits of immune complexes, in capillary walls and some mesangial regions. Jones' silver methenamine stain.

prominently expanded, both by increased matrix as well as increased cellularity, which may reduce the number of open capillary loops. PAS or methenamine silver stains of histologic sections may show a characteristic feature of duplication (sometimes referred to as splitting) of the glomerular basement membranes (GBM) due to the synthesis of new basement membrane material, with interposition of cells (mesangial, endothelial, or leukocyte) between the duplicated basement membrane matrices.

Immunofluorescence typically shows the presence of IgG and C3 in a peripheral capillary wall distribution (Fig. 50.3). C1q and C4 are also commonly present in keeping with activation by the classical pathway. IgM is not prominent in primary MPGN and, if present, may suggest the presence of a secondary form of MPGN (e.g., hepatitis C). Glomerulonephritis with an MPGN pattern but in which deposition of immune reactants is limited to C3 has traditionally been considered part of the spectrum of MPGN I or

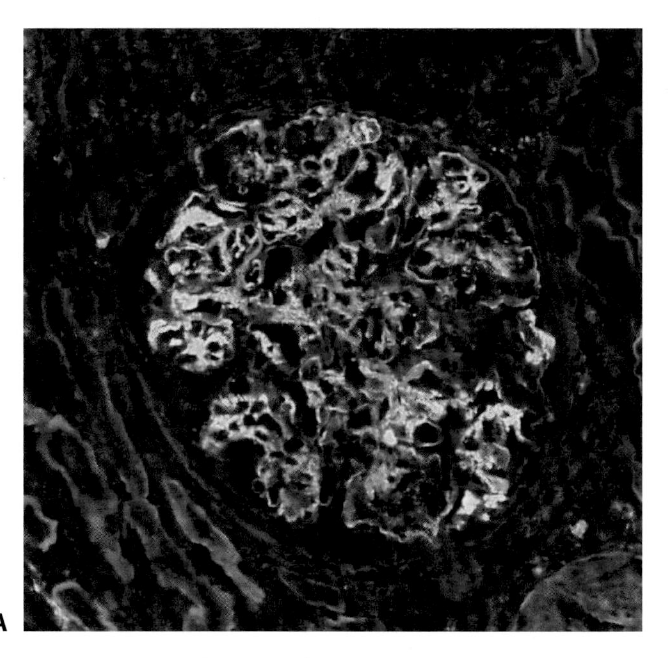
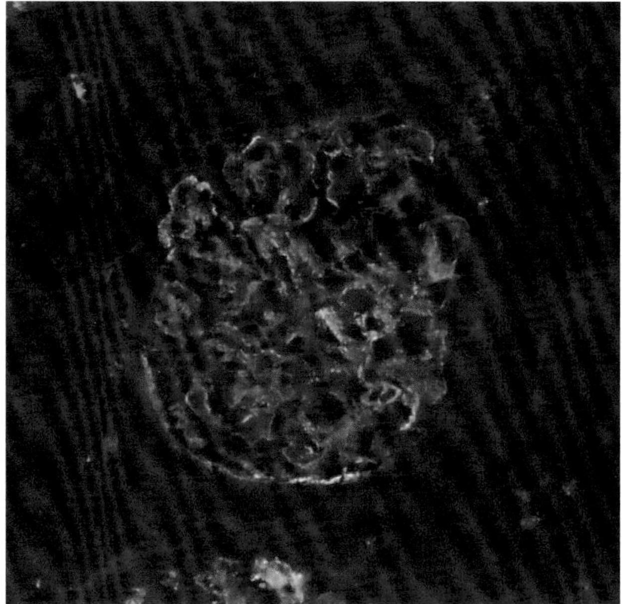

FIGURE 50.3 Membranoproliferative glomerulonephritis type I with characteristic deposition of **(A)** IgG and **(B)** C3 primarily involving peripheral capillary walls, with a granular pattern. Mesangial deposits are also present.

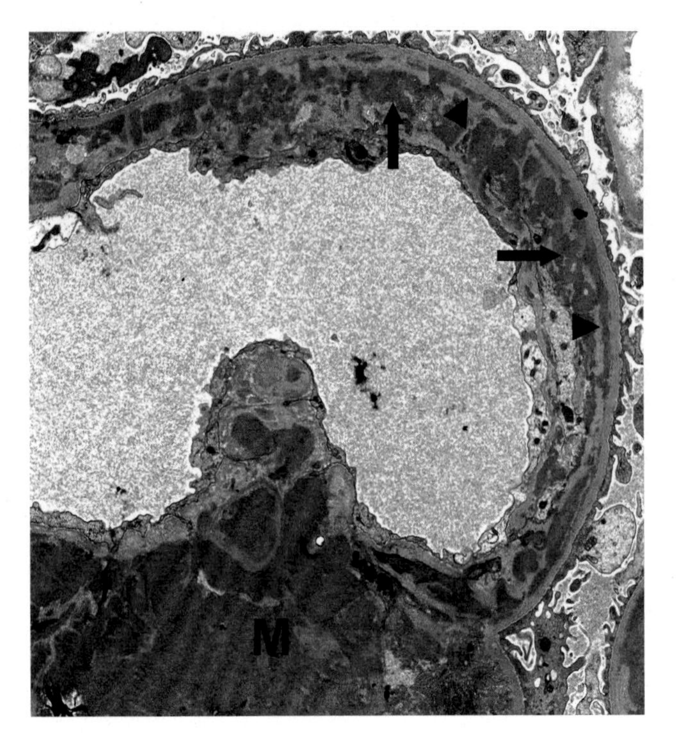

FIGURE 50.4 Membranoproliferative glomerulonephritis type I with characteristic discrete electron-dense immune complex deposits along the subendothelial aspect (*arrowheads*) of the original glomerular basement membrane and between duplicated basement membranes (*arrows*). Large, confluent electron-dense deposits are also identified within mesangial regions (*M*).

the former MPGN II. Recent data has suggested that many, if not all, of these cases can now be classified as DDD or manifestations of a distinct group of disorders tentatively termed C3 glomerulopathy (see later).[19]

On electron microscopy, subendothelial and mesangial deposits are typically present (Fig. 50.4). Subepithelial deposits may be present, but are usually scanty. Prominent subepithelial deposits are found in some patients, and some authors advocate a separate classification for this entity, MPGN type III, as described later.

It is usually impossible to differentiate secondary forms of MPGN from the primary disease, but suggestive features from common forms are described in Table 50.3. It should also be recognized that other clinical disorders may present with an MPGN pattern on renal biopsy. We have mentioned DDD, but other imitators may include thrombotic microangiopathy and other rare diseases (Table 50.4).

Clinical Features (Presentation and Clinical Manifestations)

Type 1 MPGN often presents in childhood or early teens with edema and nephrotic syndrome, and is often associated with hematuria and an active urine sediment (dysmorphic red cells and red cell casts). Constitutional symptoms including lassitude, fatigue, and weight loss may be present.

TABLE 50.3 Pathologic Features Suggestive of Underlying Secondary Disorders

Hepatitis C	Prominent IgM deposition Intracapillary eosinophilic globules (hyaline thrombi) Fibrillary or microtubular substructure to deposits (cryoglobulinemia)
Systemic lupus erythematosus	Hyaline thrombi or "wire loops" by histology C1q deposition and full house immunofluorescence Tubuloreticular structures
Monoclonal lympho-plasmacytic disorders	Heavy or light chain restriction of deposited immune reactants

TABLE 50.4 Disorders That Can Mimic MPGN on Renal Biopsy

Monoclonal lympho-plasmacytic disorders	Light chain deposition disease, immunotactoid glomerulonephritis, type 1 cryoglobulinemia; proliferative glomerulonephritis with monoclonal IgG deposits (PGNMID)
Thrombotic microangiopathy	See Chapter 55
Fibrillary glomerulonephritis and immunotactoid glomerulopathy	
Rare diseases	Collagen III glomerulopathy, fibronectin glomerulopathy, LCAT deficiency nephropathy
Transplant glomerulopathy	

LCAT, lecithin-cholesterol acyltransferase

A range of other modes of presentation may be found ranging from asymptomatic microhematuria or proteinuria on screening to an acute nephritic syndrome with gross hematuria, renal impairment, and hypertension. This is often initially diagnosed as a postinfectious glomerulonephritis, but the persistent hypocomplementemia and failure to resolve usually prompt a renal biopsy, if not already performed. In children the course is often slowly progressive, with 20% to 60% of treated patients progressing to end-stage renal disease (ESRD) over 10 to 15 years.[20–23] Risk factors for progression include the presence of nephrotic syndrome and a raised serum creatinine at presentation.

In adults, primary MPGN typically presents with an overlap between nephrotic and nephritic syndrome. Nephrotic range proteinuria is common, as are microhematuria, renal impairment, and hypertension, which may be prominent. The course is variable, but in the absence of a secondary cause, a progressive course is common.

Laboratory Findings

A major clinical clue to the diagnosis of MPGN is the presence of hypocomplementemia, due to activation of the classical pathway (Table 50.5). CH50, C3, and C4 are all depressed and may be persistent. C3 nephritic factor (C3NeF), an autoantibody stabilizing the C3 convertase of the alternate pathway, may occasionally be found (see dense deposit disease section).[13,14] C4 nephritic factor (C4NeF), an autoantibody stabilizing the classical pathway C3 convertase or a nephritic factor of the terminal pathway (Nft), have also been described,[24] occurring in ~20% of cases, either alone or with C3NeF.

TABLE 50.5 Causes of Hypocomplementemia in Kidney Disease[a]

Classical Pathway (↓C3, ↓C4)	Alternate Pathway (↓C3, ↔ C4)
Lupus nephritis	Postinfectious glomerulonephritis
Membranoproliferative glomerulonephritis (MPGN types I and III)	Dense deposit disease (C3 glomerulopathy)
Cryoglobulinemia (MPGN)	Hemolytic uremic syndrome
Endocarditis (MPGN)	
Shunt nephritis/abscess (MPGN)	

[a]Low C3 levels may also be seen in atheroembolism, liver disease, sepsis, and, rarely, heavy chain disease, rheumatoid vasculitis.

Treatment

The initial key to management is to rule out secondary causes with appropriate investigations. These may include screening for infections (e.g., hepatitis C, hepatitis B, endocarditis), autoimmune diseases (e.g., antinuclear antibody), monoclonal gammopathies (serum free light chains, serum protein electrophoresis), and complement disorders (e.g., nephritic factors).

Nonimmunosuppressive therapy is similar to that used in other forms of proteinuric kidney disease (see Chapter 75). Achieving excellent blood pressure control and renin angiotensin aldosterone system (RAAS) blockade with angiotensin-converting enzyme (ACE) inhibitors or angiotensin receptor blockers is the cornerstone of therapy. Supplemental therapies may include vitamin D supplementation, HMG-CoA synthetase inhibitors (statins), and aspirin. As with most glomerular disease there is an increased risk of cardiovascular disease.

Immunosuppressive Therapy

The role of immunosuppression is predicated on the accurate exclusion of secondary causes. The majority of evidence in children (mostly retrospective cohort studies) supports the use of an alternate day steroid regimen for prolonged periods of time. One report from the Cincinnati group, using prednisone 2 mg per kg alternate days for a minimum of 2 years, showed an 80% 10-year renal survival.[21] An early randomized controlled trial compared prolonged oral prednisone (40 mg per m^2) with placebo in 80 children with MPGN (a variety of subtypes), with a mean follow-up of 5.25 years.[25] Treatment failure was defined as an increase in serum creatinine >30% over baseline, or by 0.4 mg per dL, and was found in 33% of the prednisone group versus 58% of the placebo group. Adults with nephrotic syndrome or renal impairment are also typically treated with a 3- to 6-month course of steroids (prednisone 1 mg/kg/day). Notably, patients with subnephrotic proteinuria have a much better prognosis and may be treated more conservatively.[26]

The role of other immunosuppressive agents is less clear and, given the rarity of this condition, there is limited evidence to support their use. Two controlled prospective trials showed no benefit with dypiridamole[27] or combination cyclophosphamide, warfarin, and dypiridamole.[28] There are small series reporting beneficial results in steroid resistant disease with cyclosporine[29] or tacrolimus,[30] and with mycophenolate.[31] Rituximab may be considered, especially in the presence of a nephritic factor.[32]

Following kidney transplantation, idiopathic type 1 MPGN recurs in 20% to 30% of patients, and leads to graft loss in approximately 50% of these, although this historic data does not take into account the effect of separating cases of typical MPGN from those with C3 deposits only.[33]

MPGN TYPE III

MPGN Type III was originally described by Burkholder et al. in the 1970's as a separate entity with pathological features that overlap between membranous nephropathy and a proliferative glomerulonephritis.[34] It was characterized by the presence of epimembranous "spikes" of silver staining projections of matrix from the glomerular basement membranes, in addition to the usual features of MPGN, absent C1q and C4 deposition on immunofluorescence, and by the presence of prominent sub-epithelial immune deposits with thickening and irregularity of the GBM on electron microscopy (Figure 5). A second pattern of injury was described by the groups of Strife[35] and Anders[36], with histologic features of MPGN characterized ultrastructurally by permeation of an irregularly thickened glomerular basement membrane by electron dense deposits that are frequently poorly demarcated from the glomerular basement membrane, but are less electron dense than the deposits encountered in MPGN type I or dense deposit disease, and frequently contain areas of electron lucency. The clinical presentation of MPGN III is similar to MPGN type I, but patients tend to be older, with a more insidious presentation and hypertension is less common. Low C3 levels are typically found (~85%), but C4 is usually normal in keeping with activation of the alternate pathway.

It is now generally considered that MPGN III is not a separate class of MPGN, and modern classifications, as recently proposed by Sethi et al.[1], omit the use of this term (Figure 6). When immune complexes containing immunoglobulins are present, there is no compelling reason to consider MPGN III as a separate entity from MPGN I, as a distinct clinical course or outcome has not been defined, and pathologic features overlap with MPGN I. When only deposits of C3 are detected by immunofluorescence, a pattern present in most of the cases of Strife and Anders type, these cases fall into the broadly defined category of C3 glomerulopathy.

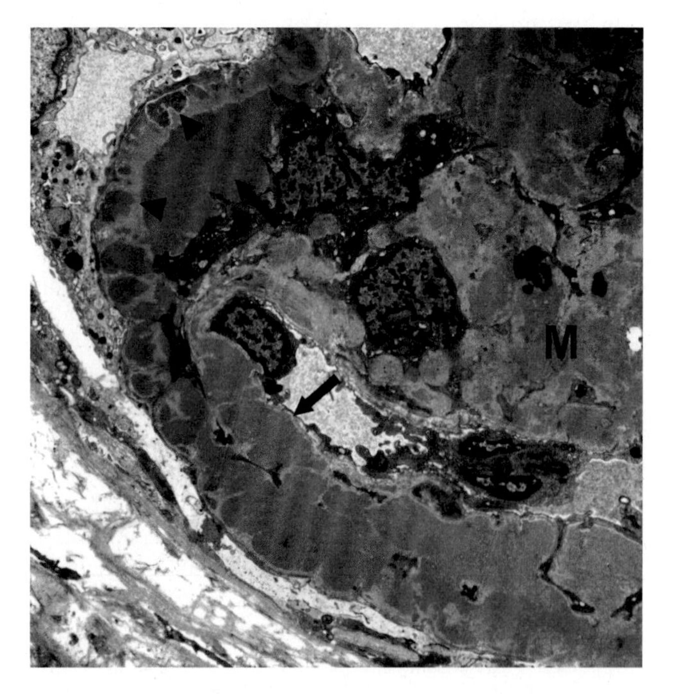

FIGURE 50.5 Membranoproliferative glomerulonephritis type III (Burkholder), now considered to be a variant of membranoproliferative glomerulonephritis, type I. There are thickened peripheral capillary walls showing massive electron dense deposits in subendothelial (*arrows*), intramembranous, and subepithelial locations (*arrowheads*). Similar deposits are also present in mesangial regions (*M*). There is extensive effacement of foot processes.

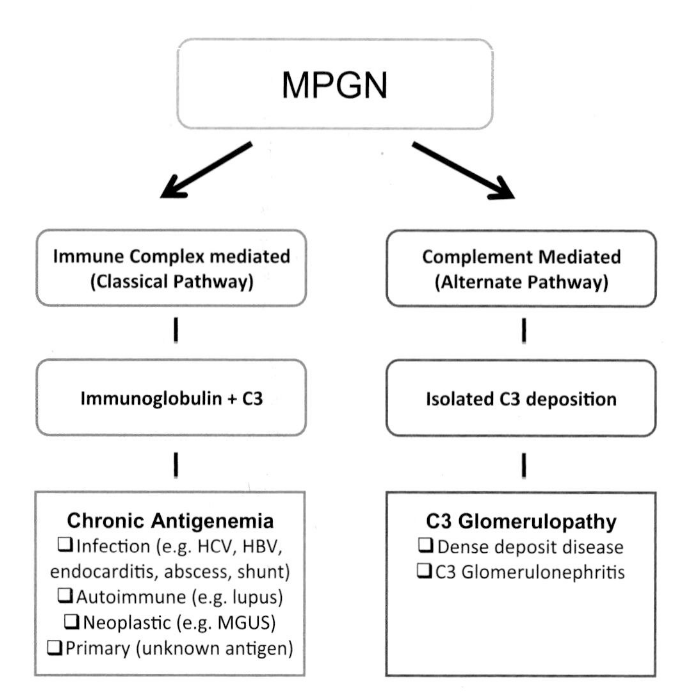

FIGURE 50.6 Pathophysiological classification of MPGN. MPGN may be subdivided into immune complex mediated and complement mediated pathways. Immune complexes derived from a chronic antigenic stimulus activate the classical pathway and are characterized by the glomerular deposition of both immunoglobulin and C3 seen by immunofluorescence microscopy. The finding of isolated C3 deposition by immunofluorescence, in the absence of immunoglobulin, suggests a form of C3 glomerulopathy due to dysregulated activation of the alternate pathway.

HEPATITIS C-ASSOCIATED MPGN

Hepatitis C virus (HCV) is a single-stranded RNA virus estimated to infect 170 million people worldwide. It is transmitted primarily by transfusion of blood products and intravenous drug use. Chronic infection occurs in 85% to 90% of exposed individuals and may progress to chronic active hepatitis, liver cirrhosis, and hepatocellular carcinoma. The association of HCV with cryoglobulinemic MPGN was first reported in 1993,[37] but a range of other renal diseases have also been reported with HCV infection (Table 50.6).

Cryoglobulinemic MPGN

Cryoglobulinemia refers to the presence of serum immunoglobulins that reversibly precipitate when cooled to 4°C,

TABLE 50.6 **Renal Manifestations of Hepatitis C Infection**

Renal Compartment	Mechanism	Clinical Disorder
Glomerular disease	Secondary to cryoglobulinemia	Membranoproliferative glomerulonephritis (type I and III) Immunotactoid glomerulopathy Fibrillary glomerulonephritis Crescentic necrotizing glomerulonephritis Amyloidosis
	Not associated with cryoglobulinemia	Membranoproliferative glomerulonephritis Mesangial-proliferative glomerulonephritis Membranous nephropathy Focal segmental glomerulosclerosis
Tubulointerstitial	Unknown	Hepatitis C-associated interstitial nephritis
Vascular	Secondary to cryoglobulinemia	Cryoglobulinemic vasculitis

and is classified according to the composition of the circulating cryoglobulins (Table 50.7). Type I cryoglobulins are composed of monoclonal immunoglobulins secondary to B cell disorders such as Waldenström macroglobulinemia or multiple myeloma. Type II and type III are mixed cryoglobulins consisting of polyclonal IgG complexed to another immunoglobulin which acts as an antiglobulin (anti-IgG rheumatoid factor [RF]). In type II this antiglobulin (usually IgM) is monoclonal, whereas in type III it is polyclonal. Evidence of HCV infection has been found in up to 95% of cases of type II cryoglobulinemia and 50% of type III cryoglobulinemia in some series.[38,39] The circulating cryoglobulins are typically composed of HCV antigen and anti-HCV antibody complexed to an IgM with rheumatoid factor activity. HCV RNA is found to be concentrated 10 to 100 times in the cryoprecipitate.[37,40]

The exact pathogenesis of the rheumatoid factor generation in HCV infected patients is still unknown, but may relate to B cell dysregulation following HCV infection. The E2 envelope protein of HCV has been shown to bind

TABLE 50.7 **Brouet Classification of Cryoglobulinemia[118]**

Type	Composition	Associated Disorders
I	Monoclonal IgG, IgM, or IgA	Monoclonal gammopathy of uncertain significance, multiple myeloma, B cell lymphoma, chronic lymphocytic leukemia, Waldenström macroglobulinemia
II	Polyclonal IgG with monoclonal IgM (positive rheumatoid factor)	Hepatitis C (~95% of cases); rarely hepatitis B, Epstein-Barr virus Lymphoproliferative disorders (especially B cell lymphoma) Essential mixed cryoglobulinemia Autoimmune disease (Sjögren syndrome, systemic lupus erythematosus)
III	Polyclonal IgG with polyclonal IgM	Infection: viral (hepatitis C [~50% of cases], hepatitis B, Epstein-Barr virus, HIV, cytomegalovirus); bacterial (endocarditis, poststreptococcal infection; leprosy); parasitic (schistosomiasis, toxoplasmosis, malaria) Autoimmune disease: systemic lupus erythematosus; rheumatoid arthritis Lymphoproliferative disorders Chronic liver disease Essential

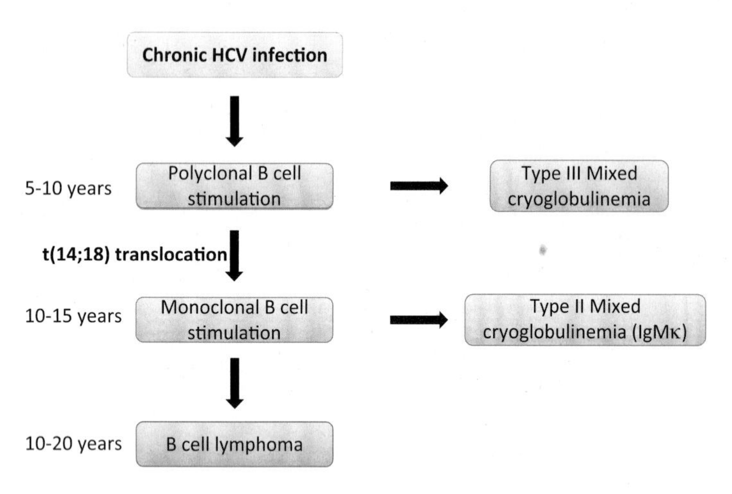

FIGURE 50.7 Hepatitis C-associated cryoglobulinemia. Binding of hepatitis C viral antigens to B cells leads to polyclonal proliferation and activation, with the development of a type II mixed cryoglobulinemia. Further clonal selection may generate a monoclonial type II mixed cryoglobulinemia, and long-term is a risk of developing B cell lymphoma. The figure depicts a postulated sequence but does not imply that a type III cryoglobulinemia always precedes type II cryoglobulinemia.

directly to B lymphocytes via CD-81 receptors leading to activation and proliferation.[41] A range of autoantibodies are commonly found with HCV infection with an increased incidence of autoimmune diseases such as thyroid disease, diabetes, and Sjögren syndrome. It is likely that earlier in the course of HCV infection, B cell stimulation produces polyclonal IgM leading to a type III cryoglobulinemia. Over time, a B cell clone emerges, due to the acquisition of somatic genetic alterations which enhance B cell survival, leading to a monoclonal IgM antiglobulin and type II cryoglobulinemia (Fig. 50.7). Notably, a t(14;18) translocation, which may lead to overexpression of the antiapoptotic gene *bcl-2*, has been described in 80% of patients with HCV and cryoglobulinemia, but is rare (<10%) in HCV patients without circulating cryoglobulins.[42]

The association of HCV with cryoglobulinemic MPGN is clear, although there remains debate over the role of HCV in noncryoglobulinemic MPGN.[43,44] Johnson et al. described 14 of 34 patients with MPGN and HCV infection that had no detectable cryoglobulins at presentation and, although many developed cryoglobulin positivity during follow-up, five remained persistently negative.[45] It is recognized that circulating cryoglobulins can be difficult to detect, and cryoglobulinemia may be missed. The clinical features and course appear to be identical to the cryoglobulinemic group.

Pathogenesis

Although there may be direct cytopathic effects of the virus on renal cells, the kidney disease is primarily felt to be a result of the host's adaptive immune response to viral infection. Circulating cryoglobulins may deposit in the glomerular capillaries and in the mesangial matrix, possibly due to the high affinity of the IgMκ constituent for fibronectin.[46] Viral RNA has been detected in glomerular tissue by in situ hybridization, and amplified from laser microdissected nephrons.[47] Some investigators[48,49] have been able to demonstrate the presence of HCV antigens in renal tissue using either immunohistochemistry or immunoelectron microscopy, but this has been difficult to replicate due in part to limitations of the detection methodology. The immune deposits likely consist of HCV antigen and anti-HCV antibody. Notably, in cryoglobulinemic MPGN, IgM is the predominant immunoglobulin, whereas in noncryoglobulinemic disease, IgG1 and IgG3 deposits are more commonly seen.[50] Cryoglobulinemia develops late in the course of HCV infection, often occurring years to decades after initial infection. The events that trigger the late development of cryoglobulinemia are unknown, as are the factors that cause only a small subset of HCV infected patients with evidence of cryoglobulinemia to develop MPGN or other HCV-associated glomerulopathies. Even the physiochemical properties that cause cryoglobulins to precipitate in the cold remain obscure.

Pathology

Histology reveals a pattern resembling type I MPGN; however, there are often more intense macrophage infiltrates and occasionally extensive hyaline thrombi (representing subendothelial and intraluminal cryoglobulinemic immune deposits) are found in glomerular capillary lumina (Fig. 50.8). A necrotizing vasculitis of small and medium vessels with glomerular crescents may occasionally be found. Immunofluorescence reveals C3 and IgG with predominant IgM deposition (Fig. 50.9). On electron microscopy the mesangial, subendothelial, and intraluminal deposits may have a distinct substructure, ranging from bundles of finely fibrillar tactoids similar in appearance to fibrin, to large microtubules similar to those encountered in immunotactoid glomerulopathy (Fig. 50.10). Demonstration of such features in a renal biopsy may suggest the diagnosis of otherwise clinically unsuspected cryoglobulinemia.

Clinical Presentation

Glomerulonephritis is typically a late complication of HCV, often occurring decades after the initial infection. The renal presentation usually includes microscopic hematuria, moderate to severe proteinuria, and mild renal impairment (chronic mixed nephritic/nephrotic picture). Hypertension is often prominent and difficult to control. Rarely, an acute oliguric presentation may occur. Extrarenal manifestations

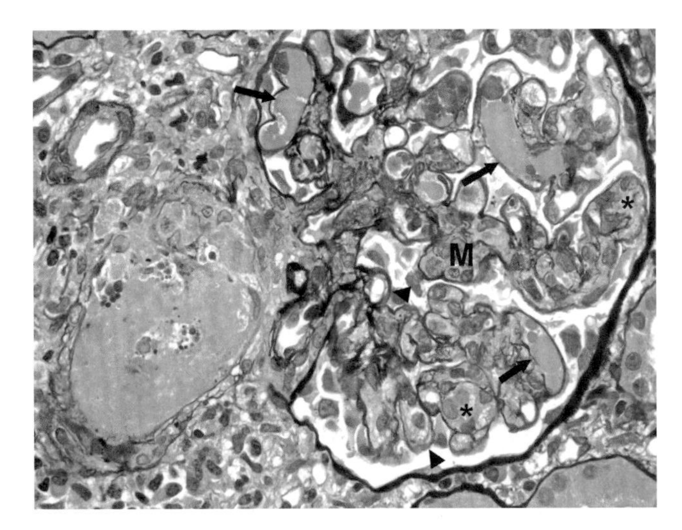

FIGURE 50.8 Cryoglobulinemic glomerulonephritis. Light microscopy showing accumulation of mononuclear leukocytes within capillary lumina and swelling of endothelial cells (endocapillary proliferation [*]), mesangial cell proliferation (*M*), and capillary wall abnormalities characterized by subendothelial accumulation of eosinophilic material and duplication of basement membrane matrices (*arrowheads*). Many capillaries are partially or completely occluded by globules of eosinophilic material, which are intracapillary aggregates of immune complexes in which cryoglobulins are a major component (*arrows*). The hilar arteriole is occluded by luminal accumulation of immune complexes similar to those present in glomerular capillaries. Jones' silver methenamine stain.

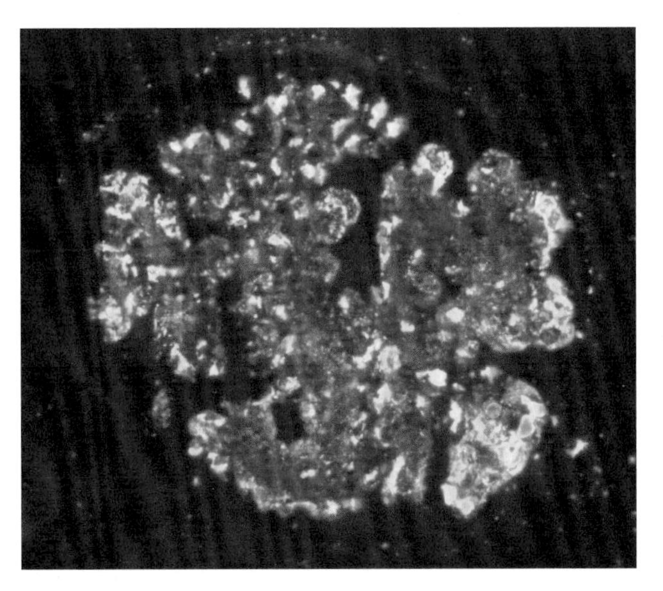

FIGURE 50.9 Cryoglobulinemic membranoproliferative glomerulonephritis with granular deposits of IgM along peripheral capillary walls. Note globular deposits of immune reactants (which also stain for IgG and C3 [not shown]) within capillary lumina that correspond to the intracapillary globules seen histologically in Figure 50.8.

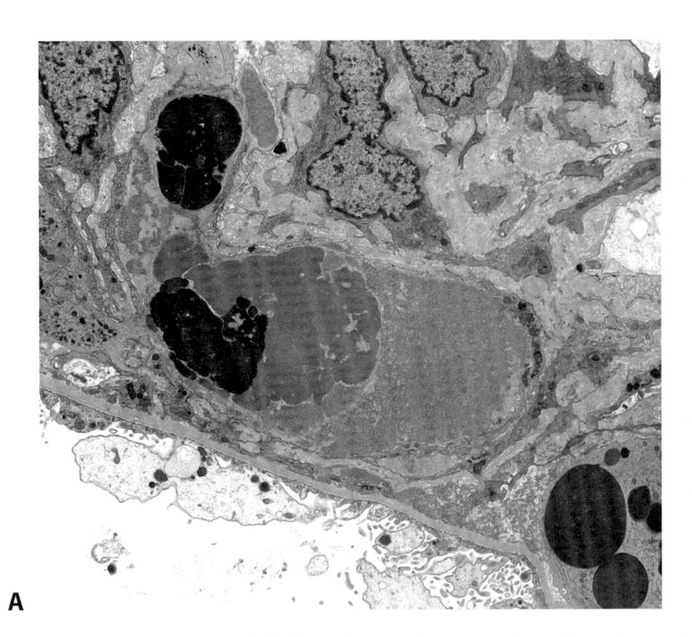

A

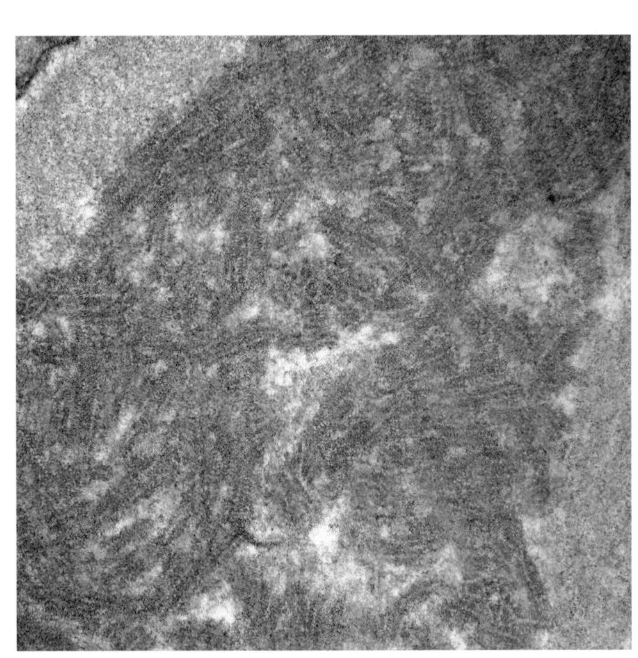

B

FIGURE 50.10 Cryoglobulinemic membranoproliferative glomerulonephritis. **A:** There are massive accumulations of electron dense deposits of immune complexes within some capillary loops, corresponding to the globules seen histologically in Figure 50.8 and the immune complexes identified in Figure 50.9. More discrete deposits are also present along the subendothelial aspect of the glomerular basement membrane. **B:** At higher magnification, the deposits reveal a microtubular substructure.

of the mixed cryoglobulinemia are often mild with palpable purpura, fatigue, and arthralgia, but more severe features of cryoglobulinemic vasculitis may develop including skin necrosis, peripheral neuropathy, central nervous system (CNS) vasculitis, or abdominal pain secondary to mesenteric vasculitis. Notably, the majority of HCV infected patients with cryoglobulinemia are asymptomatic, or have minimal nonspecific symptoms. In addition, clinically silent MPGN has been described in 27% of HCV infected patients who had normal urinalysis and renal function but underwent protocol renal biopsies at the time of liver transplantation.[51]

Investigations reveal hypocomplementemia with depression in CH50 (90%), C3 (50%), and often a marked decrease in C4 (75%). Circulating cryoglobulins can be detected (~75%), usually a type II mixed cryoglobulin in which the monoclonal rheumatoid factor is an IgMκ. Quantification of cryoglobulins (cryocrit) correlates poorly with organ involvement. Mild elevations of transaminases are commonly found (70%), and although patients may have no clinical evidence of liver disease, liver biopsy often reveals significant hepatic injury.[37] It should also be recognized that occasionally HCV antigens and antibody are bound up in the circulating cryoglobulins and false negative testing for HCV infection (anti-HCV IgG and HCV viremia by polymerase chain reaction) may occur. A high index of suspicion is required in this setting, and the diagnosis can be confirmed by polymerase chain reaction of the rewarmed cryoprecipitate.[52]

The clinical course of HCV-associated MPGN is usually indolent and, in general, the renal prognosis is good with only around 10% progressing to ESRD.[53,54] The extrarenal manifestations often follow a waxing and waning pattern, with long periods of quiescence. Mortality is much greater, however, secondary to a very high incidence of infection and cardiovascular disease. Indicators of a good outcome have not been clearly defined for this condition, but those with heavy proteinuria, renal dysfunction, high levels of viremia, and biopsy findings of marked monocyte infiltration or extensive glomerular deposits may be at greater risk of progression.

Treatment of HCV-MPGN

The primary treatment of HCV-MPGN is directed at eradication of the underlying hepatitis C, and thereby reducing the downstream B cell clonal expansion and generation of cryoglobulinemic antibodies. In cases with a more fulminant renal presentation, or with marked extrarenal manifestations of cryoglobulinemia, immunosuppression and/or plasmapheresis may be used prior to antiviral therapy (see Table 50.8).

Antiviral Therapy

Eradication of the virus by the host is limited as the virus has a high mutation rate with numerous subtypes allowing evasion from the immune system. Patients with mixed cryoglobulinemia and HCV viremia are candidates for antiviral therapy. A sustained viral response (SVR) is defined as clearance of HCV viremia during therapy that persists for 6 months post antiviral therapy. The most common antiviral therapy is currently a combination of ribavirin (a nucleoside antimetabolite) with pegylated interferon (PEG-IFN). HCV genotypes 1 and 4 are more resistant to therapy and require a longer duration of therapy (48 weeks) compared to genotypes 2 and 3 which are typically treated for 24 weeks. SVR occurs in only 30% to 50% of patients with genotype 1, compared to 65% to 90% with genotypes 2 or 3.[55] Factors predicting a poor response to treatment include a high viral load (>2 million copies per mL), viral genotype 1 or 4, liver cirrhosis, hepatic iron deposition in the liver, and longstanding infection.[56]

IFNα is often poorly tolerated secondary to adverse effects including flulike symptoms, weight loss, hypoalbuminemia,

TABLE 50.8 **Treatment of Hepatitis C-Associated Membranoproliferative Glomerulonephritis**

Clinical Presentation	Treatment
Nonnephrotic, normal renal function	Supportive therapy Consider antiviral therapy based on liver biopsy and/or renal course
Nephrotic or impaired renal function or extrarenal features of cryoglobulinemia	Pegylated interferon alfa-2a (180 μg weekly) + ribavirin (800–1200 mg/day) (+ telaprevir) Consider addition of rituximab (375 mg/m² weekly × 4)
Rapidly progressive glomerulonephritis (RPGN) or features of severe cryoglobulinemic vasculitis	Plasmapheresis (3 L ×3 per week for 2 to 3 weeks) IV methylprednisone 0.5 to 1 g × 3 days, oral prednisone 60 mg daily with slow taper over 2 to 3 months Rituximab or cyclophosphamide (2 mg/kg, adjusted for renal function) Antiviral therapy when cyclophosphamide discontinued and prednisone less than 20 mg/day

and anemia. It also has immuno-stimulatory effects which may induce autoimmune disorders such as thyroid or liver disease, or worsen the underlying glomerular disease in patients who do not achieve viral clearance.[57] Ribavirin is taken orally and is generally well tolerated, although the dose is often limited by the development of a reversible hemolytic anemia. As ribavirin is mainly eliminated through the kidneys, this adverse event is more common in kidney disease, and the drug must be used with caution when creatinine clearance is less than 50 mL per min.

Recent studies have demonstrated a dramatic increase in the SVR for genotype I patients using the NS3/4A protease inhibitors telaprevir[58,59] and boceprevir,[60,61] when added to standard anti-viral therapy of PEG-IFN and ribavirin.

Role of Immunosuppression and Plasmapheresis

Plasmapheresis (to remove circulating cryoglobulins) and immunosuppression (to decrease inflammation and reduce further cryoglobulin production) are reserved for those with a more aggressive renal or cryoglobulinemic disease during the acute phase. Typically this consists of intravenous methylprednisolone 0.5 to 1g for three days, followed by oral steroids (60 mg daily with slow taper over 2 to 3 months), plasmapheresis (3 L alternate × 3/week for 2 to 3 weeks) with warmed replacement fluid and cyclophosphamide 2 mg per kg for 2 to 4 months. This often controls the acute phase of the disease but is associated with a high relapse rate. Notably, although short courses of steroid do lead to increased HCV viremia, unlike chronic hepatitis B infection, a marked worsening of the underlying liver disease is uncommon.[62] Specific antiviral therapy is usually initiated as the immunosuppression is weaned (usually when the prednisone level is reduced to 20 mg per day or less).

Recent evidence suggests a very promising role for rituximab in HCV associated cryoglobulinemia. This monoclonal antibody targets B cells, which are chronically stimulated by HCV thus producing cryoglobulins and other autoantibodies. A small randomized controlled trial[63] and multiple small series have shown often dramatic responses in the clinical features of cryoglobulinemic vasculitis (purpura, arthralgias, peripheral neuropathy), which correlate with a decrease in serum cryoglobulins (RF) and rising serum C4 levels.[64–68] The exact role is still being clarified, however, as increased viremia,[69] and systemic drug reactions similar to serum sickness[70] have now been reported.

Cryoglobulinemic Glomerulonephritis (Not Associated with Hepatitis C)

It is important to recognize that cryoglobulinemic MPGN may occur in the absence of HCV infection.[62,71,72] In geographic regions where HCV infection is less prevalent—for example, Northern Europe—the majority of mixed cryoglobulinemia (MC) is the result of causes other than HCV infection.[73,74] Cryoglobulinemia is well described in patients with other infections, but the most common etiologies in several series are primary Sjögren syndrome and B cell lymphomas (Table 50.8). The term essential mixed cryoglobulinemia describes cases in which a secondary cause is not identified. Characteristic clinical features of MC include asthenia, arthralgia, purpura, and peripheral neuropathy. Notably, renal involvement typically occurs in the context of type II cryoglobulinemia.[72,73]

In one study from France, 20 patients with mixed cryoglobulinemia unrelated to HCV and MPGN were described.[72] Nine patients had primary Sjögren syndrome, one patient had a B cell lymphoma, and the remaining 10 patients were diagnosed with essential mixed cryoglobulinemia. The majority presented with nephrotic range proteinuria and microscopic hematuria, and investigations revealed a low or undetectable C4 with relatively normal C3 serum levels. All patients had type II cryoglobulins composed of polyclonal IgG and monoclonal IgMκ, similar to patients with HCV associated cryoglobulinemia. Renal biopsy showed MPGN with features of cryoglobulinemic glomerulonephritis including microtubular substructure of the deposits. Seven out of the 20 patients also had interstitial lymphocytic nodules, mostly composed of B cells. The patients were treated with a variety of therapies, including immunosuppression, and overall the renal outlook was favorable, but there was a 40% mortality from nonrenal causes. Notably, four out of 20 (20%) developed a B cell lymphoma during follow-up, and this group of patients requires close monitoring.

OTHER SECONDARY FORMS OF MPGN

MPGN Associated with Monoclonal Gammopathy

In a large biopsy series, a monoclonal gammopathy occurred in 22% of patients with a pathologic diagnosis of MPGN.[75] The majority (57%) of these were subsequently classified as a monoclonal gammopathy of uncertain significance (MGUS). Renal biopsy showed typical features of MPGN on light microscopy, with monoclonal deposition of IgG or IgM and either κ or λ light chain restriction. Clinical presentations were similar to other forms of MPGN, but the subsequent course was heavily determined by the etiology of the monoclonal protein (MGUS versus multiple myeloma). Notably, patients with an MGUS had a very high rate (66.7%) of recurrence post kidney transplantation, compared to MPGN patients without MGUS (30%).[76]

Notably, most forms of light and heavy chain deposition disease can present with patterns on light microscopy mimicking MPGN[77,78] (Table 50.4). A differential subgroup for this pattern of injury has been called proliferative glomerulonephritis with monoclonal IgG deposits (PGNMID).[79] This frequently presents with an MPGN pattern, with immunofluorescence demonstrating a single light and heavy chain subtype (most commonly IgG3κ).

MPGN Secondary to Chronic Infections

Although hepatitis C is the most common infectious cause of MPGN, many other chronic infections have been implicated (Table 50.1). Infective endocarditis,[80] shunt nephritis,[81] and chronic bacterial abscesses[82] are examples of chronic bacterial infections that are associated with MPGN. Persistent antigenemia resulting in the glomerular deposition of antigen-antibody immune complexes is the presumed pathogenesis.

Clinical features are variable, but hypocomplementemia is commonly seen, in keeping with activation of the classical pathway of complement (low C3, low C4). Treatment is directed at the underlying infectious etiology.

DENSE DEPOSIT DISEASE

The term DDD is derived from the finding of distinctive ribbonlike electron-dense deposits within the GBM that are revealed by electron microscopy. It was formerly considered a subtype of MPGN, and the clinical presentation is similar, but it is now clear that only a minority of cases of DDD present with an MPGN pattern on renal biopsy,[83] and DDD is now widely considered a separate glomerular disorder.

Epidemiology

DDD is primarily a disease that affects children and young adults, with a mean age of onset of 10–14 years.[84] It affects males and females equally, and may be more common in Caucasians. The finding of DDD in older patients suggests the presence of a monoclonal gammopathy, in which the MGUS protein may directly activate the alternate pathway of complement.[85] Familial DDD is rare, but a few cases have been reported, mostly secondary to inherited complement disorders.[86]

Pathogenesis

DDD is mediated by a persistent overactivation of the alternate pathway of complement. In health, the alternate pathway is in a state of balance. Spontaneous low level C3 activation due to a process called "tick-over" leads to the formation of the C3 convertase (C3Bb) (Fig. 50.1). This further cleaves C3 generating more C3Bb in a positive feedback process called the C3 amplification loop.[87] This process is controlled by a series of both fluid phase and surface bound proteins known as regulators of complement activation (RCA).[88] Factor H is the predominant RCA of the alternate pathway. It inhibits the C3 convertase of the alternate pathway (C3Bb) by cleaving Bb, and also serves as a cofactor for factor I which cleaves membrane bound C3b. Other RCA regulating the alternate pathway C3 convertase include factor I, MCP, DAF, CR1, and factor H related proteins. Enhanced progression through the complement pathway may occur due to increased early activation (e.g., by microbial pathogens in MPGN type I) or by failure of AP complement regulation due to mutations in, or antibodies to, the various RCA.

Animal models have helped to elucidate the role of factor H in DDD.[89,90] In a spontaneous porcine model of DDD, mutations in the factor H (CFH) gene led to structural changes which impaired protein secretion, leading to an absence of factor H in plasma.[91] Similarly, mice deficient in factor H develop a form of MPGN with subendothelial deposits, but without deposition of IgG.[92] Notably, double knockout mice (Cfh-/- Cfb -/-), deficient in both factor H and factor B, do not develop complement mediated renal disease confirming the need for alternate pathway activation.[92] Surprisingly, the Cfh-/- Cfi -/- double knockout mice did not show enhanced disease despite evidence of complement activation (low C3 and Cfb levels).[93] Indeed, they were protected from GBM abnormalities, suggesting that factor I is required for the generation of this model. It is suggested that it is the factor I dependent C3 fragment (iC3b) that targets the GBM as a component of the dense deposits, whereas excess plasma C3b may preferentially deposit in the mesangium.[94]

In human DDD, dysregulation of the AP leading to unregulated activation in the fluid phase may occur by several mechanisms.

C3 Nephritic Factor (C3NeF)

C3NeF is a heterogeneous group of antibodies which are found in about 80% of cases of DDD.[95,96] C3NeF binds to neoepitopes on Bb only when bound to C3b,[97] and stabilizes the nascent C3 convertase (C3Bb) making it resistant to inactivation by factor H, and other RCAs, thus amplifying the cleavage of C3. Notably, C3Nef may be found in some normal individuals, but is commonly seen in patients with partial lipodystrophy.[98] Adipsin, a surface protein on adipocytes, is identical to factor D of the alternate pathway and promotes complement activation on the adipocyte surface leading to cell lysis.[99] C3NeF has also been described in some patients with MPGN type 1, where it may amplify the classical pathway by enhancing the amplification loop of the alternate pathway. A nephritic factor of the classical pathway has also been described (C4NeF) which stabilizes the classical pathway C3 convertase (C4b2a) and may be found in 20% of cases of MPGN type 1.[100] A nephritic factor of the terminal pathway (NFt) is also described. This stabilizes the C5 convertase (C3bBbP).[101] Stabilization of the C3 convertase (C3Bb) has also been described in DDD due to autoantibodies to Factor B and C3b.[102,103]

Role of Factor H

Factor H is the most important regulator of complement activation (RCA) in the fluid phase. Impaired factor H function leads to uncontrolled activation of the complement pathway and has been associated with a number of renal diseases including DDD, atypical hemolytic syndrome, and C3 glomerulopathy.[19] Mutations in the CFH gene, both homozygous and heterozygous, have been associated with the development of DDD.[104–106] The majority of these mutations alter protein structure which impairs the secretion of factor H into the circulation.[107] Notably, even in cases of DDD secondary to C3NeF, a permissive genetic background is often found.[108] The His402 polymorphism in the CFH gene, which impairs the heparin and endothelial cell binding properties of factor H protein, has been described in 85% of patients with DDD.[109,110] This polymorphism is also common in age-related macular degeneration and retinal drusen, both conditions in

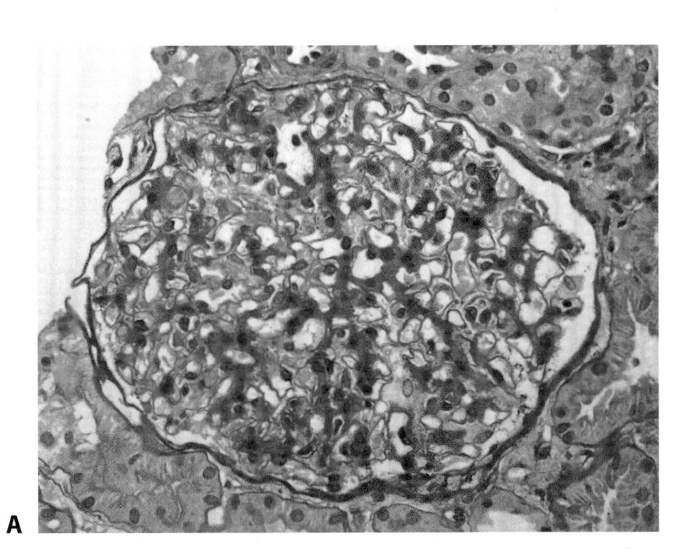

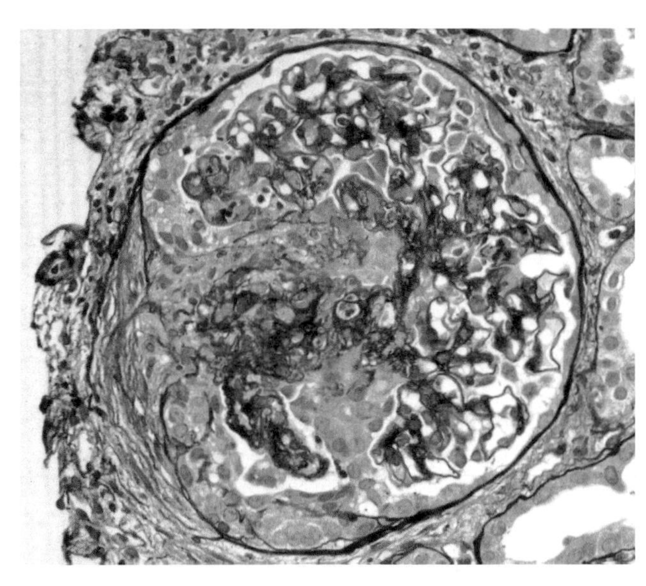

FIGURE 50.11 Dense deposit disease. **A:** Dense deposit disease can have histologic features indistinguishable from membranoproliferative glomerulonephritis type I, but many cases are characterized by a mesangial proliferative glomerulopathy, of varying severity, which in this case is only of minimal to mild severity. Periodic acid-Schiff stain. **B:** Dense deposit disease can also manifest as an acute crescentic injury with extracapillary proliferation of cells. Jones' silver methenamine stain.

which alternate pathway upregulation occurs.[111] Factor H mutations have also been described in atypical hemolytic uremic syndrome (aHUS), and it remains unclear why some patients develop aHUS versus DDD.[112,113] Interestingly, the mutations in aHUS typically map to the c-terminal end of the CFH gene, often do not reduce factor H levels, but inhibit the binding of factor H to membrane-bound C3b, whereas in DDD, the mutations are typically found in the n-terminal region with reduced circulating factor H levels.[106,114,115] Factor H activity may also be impaired by an autoantibody to factor H, which in some cases may be a monoclonal gammopathy.[85] Alternate pathway activation in DDD has also been described secondary to a mutation in the C3 gene, which produces a protein that upon cleaving to C3b, constructs a C3 convertase resistant to inactivation by fH.[116]

Pathology

Although initially described as a subtype of MPGN, it is now recognized that a variety of pathologic appearances by light microscopy may be encountered. In one study of 81 cases of DDD, the most common histologic pattern was a mesangial proliferative glomerulonephritis (43%), followed by MPGN (25%), crescentic glomerulonephritis (17%), acute proliferative and exudative glomerulonephritis (12%), and a few cases that could not be classified (3%).[83] Notably, subepithelial humps may be seen in some cases, and in others the mesangial proliferative pattern may be very mild and resemble minimal change disease by light microscopy (Fig. 50.11). The crescentic pattern usually occurs on a background of MPGN or mesangial proliferative disease (Fig. 50.11). Immunofluorescence shows intense C3 staining of the glomerular capillary walls and also the mesangium, but in the absence of immunoglobulin or C1q staining (Fig. 50.12). The morphologic hallmark of DDD is seen on electron microscopy which reveals dense, wavy, ribbonlike linear deposits within glomerular and tubular basement membranes (Fig. 50.13). Bowman's basement membrane may show similar deposits. The exact chemical composition of these dense deposits remains unclear, but they contain C3b and its breakdown products iC3b, C3dg, or C3c, and the terminal complement complex.[83,117]

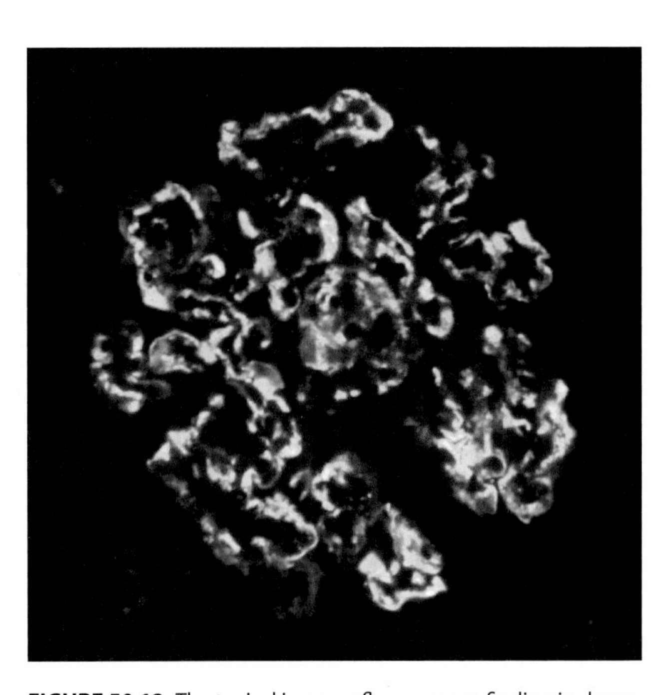

FIGURE 50.12 The typical immunofluorescence finding in dense deposit disease is strong, clumpy to confluent C3 deposition in mesangial regions and glomerular peripheral capillary walls.

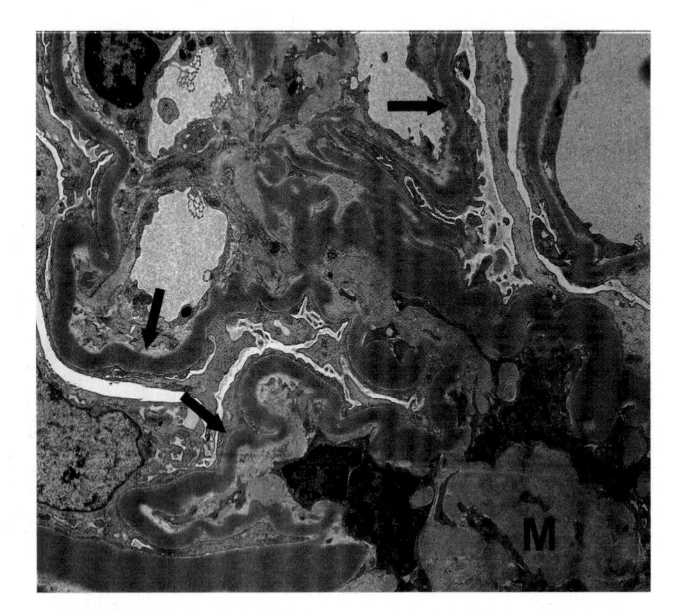

FIGURE 50.13 Pathognomonic of dense deposit disease is the presence of ribbonlike, confluent deposits with high electron density, extensively involving peripheral capillary walls (*arrows*) and mesangial regions (*M*) where such deposits may also be present in a more interrupted and less widespread distribution, and can involve other renal structures such as Bowman's capsules and tubular basement membranes.

Clinical Features

This is typically a disease of children who present with hematuria (may be macroscopic), proteinuria, and an acute nephritic or nephrotic syndrome, clinically indistinguishable from other forms of MPGN. Worsening proteinuria and hypertension predict a worse course. Laboratory testing reveals activation of the AP of complement with low C3 levels (805 to 100% children, 50% adults), normal C4 levels, and C3Nef (<80%). In some it may be associated with partial lipodystrophy or drusen in Bruch's membrane of the retina. An increased incidence of type I diabetes has been described.[118] The development of DDD in adults should prompt a search for a plasma cell dyscrasia.[119]

The long-term prognosis of DDD is often poor with ~50% of patients progressing to ESRD. Notably, neither the presence of C3NeF nor the serum C3 levels predict the clinical course.[120] Recurrent disease following kidney transplantation is common (affecting 50% to 100% of patients) and may occur as early as 12 days posttransplantation with 5-year graft loss around 50%.[121]

Treatment

The condition is diagnosed on biopsy, but a thorough investigation of the complement AP is required to determine the underlying disorder. This includes measures of complement activity (CH50, AP50), measurement of serum levels (C3, C4, factor H), mutation analysis of CFH, and testing for C3NeF. Further complement studies including factor B and factor I may be required.

The best treatment for this disease is unclear, and due to the rarity of the condition will not be guided by randomized controlled trials. The traditional therapy consists of high dose alternate day steroid therapy.[122] We advocate for additional treatment of DDD based on the individual pathogenesis.[123] In patients with C3NeF, one should consider the use of plasma exchange (to remove autoantibody) and therapy with mycophenolate or rituximab to try and eliminate autoantibody production. Plasmapheresis may also be considered in factor H deficiency to supply factor H with fresh frozen plasma. Recombinant active factor H may soon be available.[124] Eculizumab, a monoclonal antibody directed against complement C5 which inhibits the formation of the membrane attack complex, has been used successfully in the therapy of atypical hemolytic uremic syndrome,[125,126] and in a few cases of DDD.[127–129] In the future, the development of specific complement inhibitors may revolutionize the treatment of this condition.

C3 GLOMERULOPATHY

This term has been used to describe a range of disorders characterized by isolated deposition of C3, without the presence of immunoglobulin, due to uncontrolled activation of the alternate pathway of complement.[19] This group includes DDD, but also several other disorders with variable glomerular pathology. A consensus classification for these disorders does not yet exist, and the terms and groupings may change as better understanding of the genetic mutations and acquired abnormalities in the complement system is achieved.

C3 Glomerulonephritis

This subgroup has been defined by the presence of glomerular C3 deposition, in the absence of immunoglobulin, with electron-dense deposits, indistinguishable from immune complexes by electron microscopy, predominantly in a subendothelial and mesangial distribution, but also including subepithelial "hump-like" deposits.[115,130,131] It is synonymous with the prior description of MPGN type 1 with isolated C3 deposits but also includes cases formerly classified as MPGN III and cases of purely mesangial proliferative glomerulonephritis. There are many features analogous to DDD, but the characteristic intramembranous dense deposits of DDD are not seen. The majority of patients (75%) have an MPGN pattern on renal biopsy, whereas others had mesangial immune deposits, but without mesangial cell proliferation (Fig. 50.14). The clinical course is very variable (heterogeneous) with approximately 50% maintaining normal renal function, whereas 15% progressed to ESRD.

The absence of immunoglobulin and low serum levels of C3, but normal C4, are compatible with dysregulation of the alternate pathway of complement leading to isolated C3 deposition in the glomerulus. Both autoantibodies (C3NeF[~50%], anti-factor H[132]) and mutations in complement regulatory proteins (factor H, factor I, membrane cofactor protein) have been described in C3 glomerulonephritis.[19,90,95,115] However, the clinical experience with cases defined by this pathologic pattern is not yet sufficient to ascertain the proportion of such patients in which complement abnormalities can be identi-

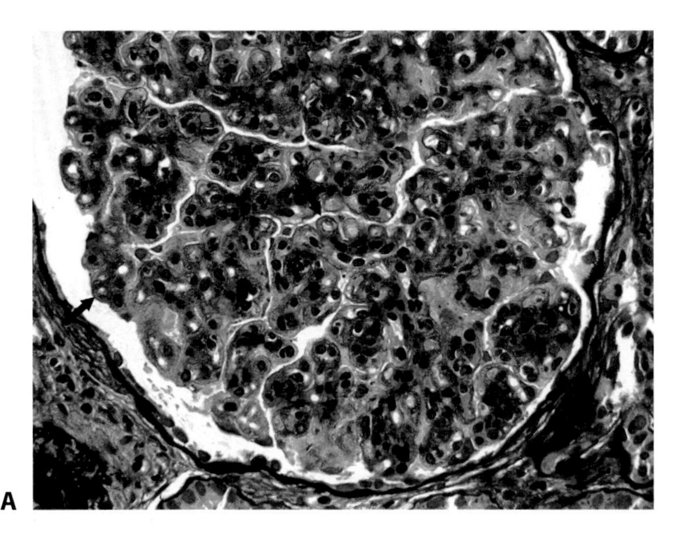

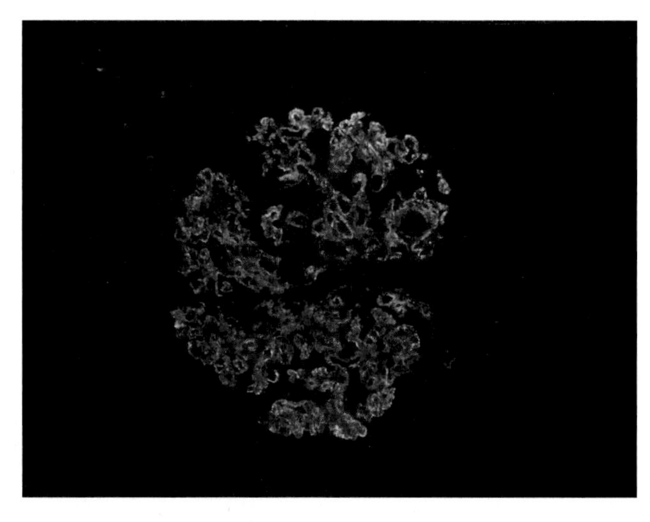

FIGURE 50.14 C3 glomerulonephritis. **A:** This case has a histologic appearance indistinguishable from membranoproliferative glomerulonephritis type I, with mesangial hypercellularity, leukocyte influx, and split/duplicated glomerular basement membranes (*arrows*). Jones' silver methenamine stain. **B:** Immunofluorescence microscopy demonstrates capillary wall and mesangial deposits of C3, but notably the absence of immunoglobulin heavy or light chains.

fied and implicated in causation, and the proportion of cases that may be due to other etiologies. C3GN has also been associated with a monoclonal gammopathy, which may present as a proliferative glomerulonephritis with isolated C3 deposits and large subepithelial humps that may be confused with a postinfectious glomerulonephritis.[133]

The identification of isolated glomerular C3 deposits should prompt an extensive evaluation of the complement system and the regulators of complement activation. Therapy for this condition is mostly supportive. With progressive disease, immunosuppression may be considered, but similar to DDD, the identification of specific complement abnormalities may result in focused treatments such as plasmapheresis, rituximab, or specific complement inhibitors (e.g., eculizumab).

Complement Factor H-related Protein 5 Nephropathy

There are five complement factor H-related proteins (CFHR1-5), encoded by genes within the RCA gene cluster on chromosome 1, which share some complement regulatory functions with factor H. In a Cypriot family, an inherited form of C3 glomerulopathy with autosomal dominant transmission has been described that was due to mutations in CFHR5.[134] Notably, the disease recurred posttransplant in one family member.[135] Isolated C3 deposition in the absence of immunoglobulin has also been described in familial MPGN3 linked to the same region.[136]

REFERENCES

1. Sethi, S. & Fervenza, F.C. Membranoproliferative glomerulonephritis—a new look at an old entity. *N Engl J Med.* 2012;366:1119–1131.

2. Progressively decreasing incidence of membranoproliferative glomerulonephritis in Spanish adult population. A multicentre study of 8,545 cases of primary glomerulonephritis. Study Group of the Spanish Society of Nephrology. *Nephron.* 1989;52:370–371.

3. Barbiano di Belgiojoso, G., et al. Is membranoproliferative glomerulonephritis really decreasing? A multicentre study of 1,548 cases of primary glomerulonephritis. *Nephron.* 1985;40:380–81.

4. Simon, P., et al. Epidemiology of primary glomerular diseases in a French region. Variations according to period and age. *Kidney Int.* 1994;46:1192–1198

5. Stratta, P., et al. Incidence of biopsy-proven primary glomerulonephritis in an Italian province. *Am J Kidney Dis.* 1996;27:631–639.

6. Asinobi, A.O., et al. The predominance of membranoproliferative glomerulonephritis in childhood nephrotic syndrome in Ibadan, Nigeria. *West Afr J Med.* 1999;18:203–206.

7. Chugh, K.S. & Sakhuja, V. Glomerular diseases in the tropics. *Am J Nephrol.* 1990;10:437–450.

8. Hurtado, A., et al. Distinct patterns of glomerular disease in Lima, Peru. *Clin Nephrol.* 2000;53:325–332.

9. Holdsworth, S.R., Kitching, A.R. & Tipping, P.G. Th1 and Th2 T helper cell subsets affect patterns of injury and outcomes in glomerulonephritis. *Kidney Int.* 1999;55:1198–1216.

10. Johnson, R.J., Hurtado, A., Merszei, J., Rodriguez-Iturbe, B. & Feng, L. Hypothesis: dysregulation of immunologic balance resulting from hygiene and socioeconomic factors may influence the epidemiology and cause of glomerulonephritis worldwide. *Am J Kidney Dis.* 2003;42:575–581.

11. Welch, T.R., Beischel, L., Balakrishnan, K., Quinlan, M. & West, C.D. Major-histocompatibility-complex extended haplotypes in membranoproliferative glomerulonephritis. *N Engl J Med.* 1986;314:1476–1481.

12. Bakkaloglu, A., Soylemezoglu, O., Tinaztepe, K., Saatci, U. & Soylemezoglu, F. Familial membranoproliferative glomerulonephritis. *Nephrol Dial Transplant.* 1995;10:21–24.

13. Ohi, H. & Yasugi, T. Occurrence of C3 nephritic factor and C4 nephritic factor in membranoproliferative glomerulonephritis (MPGN). *Clin Exp Immunol.* 1994;95:316–321.

14. Varade, W.S., Forristal, J. & West, C.D. Patterns of complement activation in idiopathic membranoproliferative glomerulonephritis, types I, II, and III. *Am J Kidney Dis.* 1990;16:196–206.

15. Guo, S., et al. Deletion of activating Fcgamma receptors does not confer protection in murine cryoglobulinemia-associated membranoproliferative glomerulonephritis. *Am J Pathol.* 2009;175:107–118.

16. Smith, K.D. & Alpers, C.E. Pathogenic mechanisms in membranoproliferative glomerulonephritis. *Curr Opin Nephrol Hypertens.* 2005;14:396–403.

17. Wornle, M., et al. Novel role of toll-like receptor 3 in hepatitis C-associated glomerulonephritis. *Am J Pathol.* 2006;168:370–385.

18. Banas, M.C., et al. TLR4 links podocytes with the innate immune system to mediate glomerular injury. *J Am Soc Nephrol.* 2008;19:704–713.

19. Fakhouri, F., Fremeaux-Bacchi, V., Noel, L.H., Cook, H.T. & Pickering, M.C. C3 glomerulopathy: a new classification. *Nat Rev Nephrol.* 2010;6:494–499.

20. Arslan, S., et al. Membranoproliferative glomerulonephritis in childhood: factors affecting prognosis. *Int Urol Nephrol.* 1997;29:711–716.

21. Braun, M.C., West, C.D. & Strife, C.F. Differences between membranoproliferative glomerulonephritis types I and III in long-term response to an alternate-day prednisone regimen. *Am J Kidney Dis.* 1999;34:1022–1032.

22. Garcia-de la Puente, S., Orozco-Loza, I.L., Zaltzman-Girshevich, S. & de Leon Bojorge, B. Prognostic factors in children with membranoproliferative glomerulonephritis type I. *Pediatr Nephrol.* 2008;23:929–935.

23. McEnery, P.T. Membranoproliferative glomerulonephritis: the Cincinnati experience—cumulative renal survival from 1957 to 1989. *J Pediatr.* 1990; 116:S109–114.

24. Clardy, C.W., Forristal, J., Strife, C.F. & West, C.D. A properdin dependent nephritic factor slowly activating C3, C5, and C9 in membranoproliferative glomerulonephritis, types I and III. *Clin Immunol Immunopathol.* 1989;50:333–347.

25. Tarshish, P., Bernstein, J., Tobin, J.N. & Edelmann, C.M., Jr. Treatment of mesangiocapillary glomerulonephritis with alternate-day prednisone—a report of the International Study of Kidney Disease in Children. *Pediatr Nephrol.* 1992;6:123–130.

26. Somers, M., et al. Non-nephrotic children with membranoproliferative glomerulonephritis: are steroids indicated? *Pediatr Nephrol.* 1995;9:140–144.

27. Donadio, J.V., Jr. & Offord, K.P. Reassessment of treatment results in membranoproliferative glomerulonephritis, with emphasis on life-table analysis. *Am J Kidney Dis.* 1989;14:445–451.

28. Cattran, D.C., et al. Results of a controlled drug trial in membranoproliferative glomerulonephritis. *Kidney Int.* 1985;27:436–441.

29. Bagheri, N., et al. Cyclosporine in the treatment of membranoproliferative glomerulonephritis. *Arch Iran Med.* 2008;11:26–29.

30. Haddad, M., Lau, K. & Butani, L. Remission of membranoproliferative glomerulonephritis type I with the use of tacrolimus. *Pediatr Nephrol.* 2007;22:1787–1791.

31. Jones, G., et al. Treatment of idiopathic membranoproliferative glomerulonephritis with mycophenolate mofetil and steroids. *Nephrol Dial Transplant.* 2004;19:3160–3164.

32. Dillon, J.J., et al. Rituximab therapy for Type I membranoproliferative glomerulonephritis. *Clin Nephrol.* 2012;77:290–295.

33. Briganti, E.M., Russ, G.R., McNeil, J.J., Atkins, R.C. & Chadban, S.J. Risk of renal allograft loss from recurrent glomerulonephritis. *N Engl J Med.* 2002;347:103–109.

34. Burkholder, P.M., Marchand, A. & Krueger, R.P. Mixed membranous and proliferative glomerulonephritis. A correlative light, immunofluorescence, and electron microscopic study. *Lab Invest.* 1970;23:459–479.

35. Strife, C.F., McEnery, P.T., McAdams, A.J. & West, C.D. Membranoproliferative glomerulonephritis with disruption of the glomerular basement membrane. *Clin Nephrol.* 1977;7:65–72.

36. Anders, D. & Thoenes, W. Basement membrane-changes in membranoproliferative glomerulonephritis: a light and electron microscopic study. *Virchows Arch A Pathol Anat Histol.* 1975;369:87–109.

37. Johnson, R.J., et al. Membranoproliferative glomerulonephritis associated with hepatitis C virus infection. *N Engl J Med.* 1993;328:465–470.

38. Agnello, V., Chung, R.T. & Kaplan, L.M. A role for hepatitis C virus infection in type II cryoglobulinemia. *N Engl J Med.* 1992;327:1490–1495.

39. Misiani, R., et al. Hepatitis C virus infection in patients with essential mixed cryoglobulinemia. *Ann Intern Med.* 1992;117:573–577.

40. Bichard, P., et al. High prevalence of hepatitis C virus RNA in the supernatant and the cryoprecipitate of patients with essential and secondary type II mixed cryoglobulinemia. *J Hepatol.* 1994;21:58–63.

41. Rosa, D., et al. Activation of naive B lymphocytes via CD81, a pathogenetic mechanism for hepatitis C virus-associated B lymphocyte disorders. *Proc Natl Acad Sci U S A.* 2005;102:18544–18549.

42. Zuckerman, E., et al. bcl-2 and immunoglobulin gene rearrangement in patients with hepatitis C virus infection. *Br J Haematol.* 2001;112:364–369.

43. D'Amico, G. Is type II mixed cryoglobulinaemia an essential part of hepatitis C virus (HCV)-associated glomerulonephritis? *Nephrol Dial Transplant.* 1995;10:1279–1282.

44. Garozzo, M., Finocchiaro, P., Martorano, C. & Zoccali, C. HCV and renal disease: not always associated with mixed cryoglobulinemia. *Clin Nephrol.* 2003; 60:361–363.

45. Johnson, R.J., et al. Hepatitis C virus-associated glomerulonephritis. Effect of alpha-interferon therapy. *Kidney Int.* 1994;46:1700–1704.

46. Fornasieri, A. & D'Amico, G. Type II mixed cryoglobulinaemia, hepatitis C virus infection, and glomerulonephritis. *Nephrol Dial Transplant.* 1996;11 Suppl 4:25–30.

47. Sansonno, D., et al. Hepatitis C virus RNA and core protein in kidney glomerular and tubular structures isolated with laser capture microdissection. *Clin Exp Immunol.* 2005;140:498–506.

48. Cao, Y., Zhang, Y., Wang, S. & Zou, W. Detection of the hepatitis C virus antigen in kidney tissue from infected patients with various glomerulonephritis. *Nephrol Dial Transplant.* 2009;24:2745–2751.

49. Sansonno, D., Gesualdo, L., Manno, C., Schena, F.P. & Dammacco, F. Hepatitis C virus-related proteins in kidney tissue from hepatitis C virus-infected patients with cryoglobulinemic membranoproliferative glomerulonephritis. *Hepatology.* 1997;25:1237–1244.

50. Barsoum, R.S. Hepatitis C virus: from entry to renal injury—facts and potentials. *Nephrol Dial Transplant.* 2007;22:1840–1848.

51. McGuire, B.M., et al. Brief communication: Glomerulonephritis in patients with hepatitis C cirrhosis undergoing liver transplantation. *Ann Intern Med.* 2006;144:735–741.

52. Van Thiel, D.H., et al. Cryoglobulinemia: a cause for false negative polymerase chain reaction results in patients with hepatitis C virus positive chronic liver disease. *J Hepatol.* 1995;22:464–467.

53. Roccatello, D., et al. Multicenter study on hepatitis C virus-related cryoglobulinemic glomerulonephritis. *Am J Kidney Dis.* 2007;49:69–82.

54. Tarantino, A., et al. Long-term predictors of survival in essential mixed cryoglobulinemic glomerulonephritis. *Kidney Int.* 1995;47:618–623.

55. Perico, N., Cattaneo, D., Bikbov, B. & Remuzzi, G. Hepatitis C infection and chronic renal diseases. *Clin J Am Soc Nephrol.* 2009;4:207–220.

56. Poynard, T., Yuen, M.F., Ratziu, V. & Lai, C.L. Viral hepatitis C. *Lancet.* 2003;362:2095–2100.

57. Ohta, S., et al. Exacerbation of glomerulonephritis in subjects with chronic hepatitis C virus infection after interferon therapy. *Am J Kidney Dis.* 1999;33:1040–1048.

58. Hezode, C., et al. Telaprevir and peginterferon with or without ribavirin for chronic HCV infection. *N Engl J Med.* 2009;360:1839–1850.

59. Jacobson, I.M., et al. Telaprevir for previously untreated chronic hepatitis C virus infection. *N Engl J Med.* 364:2405–2416.

60. Bacon, B.R., et al. Boceprevir for previously treated chronic HCV genotype 1 infection. *N Engl J Med.* 364:1207–1217.

61. Poordad, F., et al. Boceprevir for untreated chronic HCV genotype 1 infection. *N Engl J Med.* 364:1195–1206.

62. D'Amico, G. Renal involvement in hepatitis C infection: cryoglobulinemic glomerulonephritis. *Kidney Int.* 1998;54:650–671.

63. De Vita, S., et al. A randomized controlled trial of rituximab for the treatment of severe cryoglobulinemic vasculitis. *Arthritis Rheum.* 2012;64:843–853.

64. Dammacco, F., et al. Pegylated interferon-alpha, ribavirin, and rituximab combined therapy of hepatitis C virus-related mixed cryoglobulinemia: a long-term study. *Blood.* 2010;116:343–353.

65. Ferri, C., et al. Treatment with rituximab in patients with mixed cryoglobulinemia syndrome: results of multicenter cohort study and review of the literature. *Autoimmun Rev.* 2011;11:48–55.

66. Petrarca, A., et al. Safety and efficacy of rituximab in patients with hepatitis C virus-related mixed cryoglobulinemia and severe liver disease. *Blood.* 2010;116:335–342.

67. Saadoun, D., et al. Rituximab plus Peg-interferon-alpha/ribavirin compared with Peg-interferon-alpha/ribavirin in hepatitis C-related mixed cryoglobulinemia. *Blood.* 2010;116:326–334; quiz 504–325.

68. Terrier, B., et al. Efficacy and tolerability of rituximab with or without PEGylated interferon alfa-2b plus ribavirin in severe hepatitis C virus-related vasculitis: a long-term followup study of thirty-two patients. *Arthritis Rheum.* 2009;60:2531–2540.

69. Ennishi, D., et al. Monitoring serum hepatitis C virus (HCV) RNA in patients with HCV-infected CD20-positive B-cell lymphoma undergoing rituximab combination chemotherapy. *Am J Hematol.* 2008;83:59–62.

70. Sene, D., Ghillani-Dalbin, P., Amoura, Z., Musset, L. & Cacoub, P. Rituximab may form a complex with IgMkappa mixed cryoglobulin and induce severe systemic reactions in patients with hepatitis C virus-induced vasculitis. *Arthritis Rheum.* 2009;60:3848–3855.

71. Agnello, V. The etiology and pathophysiology of mixed cryoglobulinemia secondary to hepatitis C virus infection. *Springer Semin Immunopathol.* 1997;19:111–129.

72. Matignon, M., et al. Clinical and morphologic spectrum of renal involvement in patients with mixed cryoglobulinemia without evidence of hepatitis C virus infection. *Medicine (Baltimore).* 2009;88:341–348.

73. Saadoun, D., et al. Increased risks of lymphoma and death among patients with non-hepatitis C virus-related mixed cryoglobulinemia. *Arch Intern Med.* 2006;166:2101–2108.

74. Tervaert, J.W., Van Paassen, P. & Damoiseaux, J. Type II cryoglobulinemia is not associated with hepatitis C infection: the Dutch experience. *Ann N Y Acad Sci.* 2007;1107:251–258.

75. Sethi, S., et al. Membranoproliferative glomerulonephritis secondary to monoclonal gammopathy. *Clin J Am Soc Nephrol.* 2010;5:770–782.

76. Lorenz, E.C., et al. Recurrent membranoproliferative glomerulonephritis after kidney transplantation. *Kidney Int.* 2010;77:721–728.

77. Alpers, C.E. Glomerulopathies of dysproteinemias, abnormal immunoglobulin deposition, and lymphoproliferative disorders. *Curr Opin Nephrol Hypertens.* 1994;3:349–355.

78. Lin, J., et al. Renal monoclonal immunoglobulin deposition disease: the disease spectrum. *J Am Soc Nephrol.* 2001;12:1482–1492.

79. Nasr, S.H., et al. Proliferative glomerulonephritis with monoclonal IgG deposits. *J Am Soc Nephrol.* 2009;20:2055–2064.

80. Boseman, P., Lewin, M., Dillon, J. & Sethi, S. Marfan syndrome, MPGN, and bacterial endocarditis. *Am J Kidney Dis.* 2008;51:697–701.

81. Vella, J., et al. Glomerulonephritis after ventriculo-atrial shunt. *QJM.* 1995;88:911–918.

82. Elmaci, I., et al. Nocardial cerebral abscess associated with mycetoma, pneumonia, and membranoproliferative glomerulonephritis. *J Clin Microbiol.* 2007;45:2072–2074.

83. Walker, P.D., Ferrario, F., Joh, K. & Bonsib, S.M. Dense deposit disease is not a membranoproliferative glomerulonephritis. *Mod Pathol.* 2007;20: 605–616.

84. Lu, D.F., Moon, M., Lanning, L.D., McCarthy, A.M. & Smith, R.J. Clinical features and outcomes of 98 children and adults with dense deposit disease. *Pediatr Nephrol.* 2011;27:773–781.

85. Sethi, S., et al. Dense deposit disease associated with monoclonal gammopathy of undetermined significance. *Am J Kidney Dis.* 2010;56:977–982.

86. Meri, S., Koistinen, V., Miettinen, A., Tornroth, T. & Seppala, I.J. Activation of the alternative pathway of complement by monoclonal lambda light chains in membranoproliferative glomerulonephritis. *J Exp Med.* 1992;175:939–950.

87. Lachmann, P.J. The amplification loop of the complement pathways. *Adv Immunol.* 2009;104:115–149.

88. Zipfel, P.F. & Skerka, C. Complement regulators and inhibitory proteins. *Nat Rev Immunol.* 2009;9:729–740.

89. Licht, C. & Fremeaux-Bacchi, V. Hereditary and acquired complement dysregulation in membranoproliferative glomerulonephritis. *Thromb Haemost.* 2009;101:271–278.

90. Pickering, M. & Cook, H.T. Complement and glomerular disease: new insights. *Curr Opin Nephrol Hypertens.* 2011.

91. Hegasy, G.A., Manuelian, T., Hogasen, K., Jansen, J.H. & Zipfel, P.F. The molecular basis for hereditary porcine membranoproliferative glomerulonephritis type II: point mutations in the factor H coding sequence block protein secretion. *Am J Pathol.* 2002;161:2027–2034.

92. Pickering, M.C., et al. Uncontrolled C3 activation causes membranoproliferative glomerulonephritis in mice deficient in complement factor H. *Nat Genet.* 2002;31:424–428.

93. Rose, K.L., et al. Factor I is required for the development of membranoproliferative glomerulonephritis in factor H-deficient mice. *J Clin Invest.* 2008; 118:608–618.

94. Paixao-Cavalcante, D., Hanson, S., Botto, M., Cook, H.T. & Pickering, M.C. Factor H facilitates the clearance of GBM bound iC3b by controlling C3 activation in fluid phase. *Mol Immunol.* 2009;46:1942–1950.

95. Servais, A., et al. Acquired and genetic complement abnormalities play a critical role in dense deposit disease and other C3 glomerulopathies. *Kidney Int.* 2012.

96. Zhang, Y., et al. Causes of alternative pathway dysregulation in dense deposit disease. *Clin J Am Soc Nephrol.* 2012;7:265–274.

97. Daha, M.R., Austen, K.F. & Fearon, D.T. Heterogeneity, polypeptide chain composition and antigenic reactivity of C3 nephritic factor. *J Immunol.* 1978; 120:1389–1394.

98. Savage, D.B., et al. Complement abnormalities in acquired lipodystrophy revisited. *J Clin Endocrinol Metab.* 2009;94:10–16.

99. Choy, L.N., Rosen, B.S. & Spiegelman, B.M. Adipsin and an endogenous pathway of complement from adipose cells. *J Biol Chem.* 1992;267:12736–12741.

100. Halbwachs, L., Leveille, M., Lesavre, P., Wattel, S. & Leibowitch, J. Nephritic factor of the classical pathway of complement: immunoglobulin G autoantibody directed against the classical pathway C3 convetase enzyme. *J Clin Invest.* 1980;65:1249–1256.

101. West, C.D. & McAdams, A.J. Membranoproliferative glomerulonephritis type III: association of glomerular deposits with circulating nephritic factor-stabilized convertase. *Am J Kidney Dis.* 1998;32:56–63.

102. Chen, Q., et al. Combined C3b and factor B autoantibodies and MPGN type II. *N Engl J Med.* 2011;365:2340–2342.

103. Strobel, S., Zimmering, M., Papp, K., Prechl, J. & Jozsi, M. Anti-factor B autoantibody in dense deposit disease. *Mol Immunol.* 2010;47:1476–1483.

104. Levy, M., et al. H deficiency in two brothers with atypical dense intramembranous deposit disease. *Kidney Int.* 1986;30:949–956.

105. Licht, C., et al. Deletion of Lys224 in regulatory domain 4 of Factor H reveals a novel pathomechanism for dense deposit disease (MPGN II). *Kidney Int.* 2006;70:42–50.

106. Servais, A., et al. Heterogeneous pattern of renal disease associated with homozygous Factor H deficiency. *Hum Pathol.* 2011.

107. Dragon-Durey, M.A., et al. Heterozygous and homozygous factor h deficiencies associated with hemolytic uremic syndrome or membranoproliferative glomerulonephritis: report and genetic analysis of 16 cases. *J Am Soc Nephrol.* 2004;15:787–795.

108. Abrera-Abeleda, M.A., et al. Allelic variants of complement genes associated with dense deposit disease. *J Am Soc Nephrol.* 2011;22:1551–1559.

109. Abrera-Abeleda, M.A., et al. Variations in the complement regulatory genes factor H (CFH) and factor H related 5 (CFHR5) are associated with membranoproliferative glomerulonephritis type II (dense deposit disease). *J Med Genet.* 2006;43:582–589.

110. Lau, K.K., Smith, R.J., Kolbeck, P.C. & Butani, L. Dense deposit disease and the factor H H402 allele. *Clin Exp Nephrol.* 2008;12:228–232.

111. Bradley, D.T., Zipfel, P.F. & Hughes, A.E. Complement in age-related macular degeneration: a focus on function. *Eye (Lond).* 2010.

112. Noris, M., et al. Relative role of genetic complement abnormalities in sporadic and familial aHUS and their impact on clinical phenotype. *Clin J Am Soc Nephrol.* 5:1844–1859.

113. Noris, M. & Remuzzi, G. Atypical hemolytic-uremic syndrome. *N Engl J Med.* 2009;361:1676–1687.

114. Pechtl, I.C., Kavanagh, D., McIntosh, N., Harris, C.L. & Barlow, P.N. Disease-associated N-terminal complement factor H mutations perturb cofactor and decay-accelerating activities. *J Biol Chem.* 2011.

115. Servais, A., et al. Primary glomerulonephritis with isolated C3 deposits: a new entity which shares common genetic risk factors with haemolytic uraemic syndrome. *J Med Genet.* 2007;44:193–199.

116. Martinez-Barricarte, R., et al. Human C3 mutation reveals a mechanism of dense deposit disease pathogenesis and provides insights into complement activation and regulation. *J Clin Invest.* 2010;120:3702–3712.

117. Sethi, S., et al. Glomeruli of Dense Deposit Disease contain components of the alternative and terminal complement pathway. *Kidney Int.* 2009;75:952–960.

118. Lu, D.F., Moon, M., Lanning, L.D., McCarthy, A.M. & Smith, R.J. Clinical features and outcomes of 98 children and adults with dense deposit disease. *Pediatr Nephrol.* 2012;27:773–781.

119. Nasr, S.H., et al. Dense deposit disease: clinicopathologic study of 32 pediatric and adult patients. *Clin J Am Soc Nephrol.* 2009;4:22–32.

120. Appel, G.B., et al. Membranoproliferative glomerulonephritis type II (dense deposit disease): an update. *J Am Soc Nephrol.* 2005;16:1392–1403.

121. Braun, M.C., et al. Recurrence of membranoproliferative glomerulonephritis type II in renal allografts: The North American Pediatric Renal Transplant Cooperative Study experience. *J Am Soc Nephrol.* 2005;16:2225–2233.

122. McEnery, P.T. & McAdams, A.J. Regression of membranoproliferative glomerulonephritis type II (dense deposit disease): observations in six children. *Am J Kidney Dis.* 1988;12:138–146.

123. Smith, R.J., et al. New approaches to the treatment of dense deposit disease. *J Am Soc Nephrol.* 2007;18:2447–2456.

124. Schmidt, C.Q., Slingsby, F.C., Richards, A. & Barlow, P.N. Production of biologically active complement factor H in therapeutically useful quantities. *Protein Expr Purif.* 2011;76:254–263.

125. Kose, O., Zimmerhackl, L.B., Jungraithmayr, T., Mache, C. & Nurnberger, J. New treatment options for atypical hemolytic uremic syndrome with the complement inhibitor eculizumab. *Semin Thromb Hemost.* 36:669–672.

126. Lapeyraque, A.L., Fremeaux-Bacchi, V. & Robitaille, P. Efficacy of eculizumab in a patient with factor-H-associated atypical hemolytic uremic syndrome. *Pediatr Nephrol.* 26:621–624.

127. Bomback, A.S., et al. Eculizumab for Dense Deposit Disease and C3 Glomerulonephritis. *Clin J Am Soc Nephrol.* 2012.

128. Daina, E., Noris, M. & Remuzzi, G. Eculizumab in a patient with dense-deposit disease. *N Engl J Med.* 2012;366:1161–1163.

129. Vivarelli, M., Pasini, A. & Emma, F. Eculizumab for the treatment of dense-deposit disease. *N Engl J Med.* 2012;366:1163–1165.

130. Habbig, S., et al. C3 deposition glomerulopathy due to a functional factor H defect. *Kidney Int.* 2009;75:1230–1234.

131. Sethi, S., et al. Proliferative Glomerulonephritis Secondary to Dysfunction of the Alternative Pathway of Complement. *Clin J Am Soc Nephrol.* 2011.

132. Sethi, S., et al. Proliferative glomerulonephritis secondary to dysfunction of the alternative pathway of complement. *Clin J Am Soc Nephrol.* 2011;6:1009–1017.

133. Bridoux, F., et al. Glomerulonephritis with isolated C3 deposits and monoclonal gammopathy: a fortuitous association? *Clin J Am Soc Nephrol.* 2011; 6:2165–2174.

134. Gale, D.P., et al. Identification of a mutation in complement factor H-related protein 5 in patients of Cypriot origin with glomerulonephritis. *Lancet.* 2010;376:794–801.

135. Vernon, K.A., et al. Recurrence of complement factor H-related protein 5 nephropathy in a renal transplant. *Am J Transplant.* 2011;11:152–155.

136. Neary, J.J., et al. Linkage of a gene causing familial membranoproliferative glomerulonephritis type III to chromosome 1. *J Am Soc Nephrol.* 2002;13:2052–2057.

137. Brouet, J.C. Cryoglobulinemias. *Presse Med.* 1983;12:2991–2996.

CHAPTER 51

Membranous Nephropathy

Laurence Beck, Jr. • David Salant

Membranous nephropathy (MN) is one of the leading causes of primary nephrotic syndrome in adults. It is recognized by its characteristic subepithelial immune deposits as visualized by immunofluorescence and electron microscopy, in addition to the thickened glomerular basement membrane (GBM) that gives the disease its name. Primary MN is a glomerulus-specific autoimmune disease and accounts for about 75% to 80% of cases of MN. Recent work has found that most patients with primary MN have circulating autoantibodies to the phospholipase A_2 receptor (PLA_2R); the remainder can be considered idiopathic MN. Secondary MN accounts for the remaining 20% to 25% of cases. It may be a feature of systemic autoimmune disease, chronic infections, malignancy, or therapeutic drugs, and is rarely if ever associated with anti-PLA_2R antibodies. The course of primary MN is variable, and may be marked by spontaneous remissions and relapses. Although a proportion of those patients who fail to remit may have persistent proteinuria with maintained renal function, another 30% to 40% will progress to end-stage renal disease (ESRD). MN recurs in the kidney allograft in up to 40% of those cases that are transplanted. When treatment is deemed necessary, often for those with high levels of nephrotic-range proteinuria or worsening renal disease, immunosuppressive agents such as cyclophosphamide and cyclosporine have been shown to be effective. Several other agents have shown promise in small studies and may also turn out to be useful agents for the treatment of MN.

EPIDEMIOLOGY

Primary (or idiopathic) MN has been and remains the leading cause of adult nephrotic syndrome in many Caucasian-predominant populations, and is second only to focal and segmental glomerulosclerosis (FSGS) in others.[1–3] The estimated annual incidence of MN is 1 in 100,000.[4,5] Despite its relatively high incidence in Caucasian populations, it can be found worldwide in all racial groups. It is most common in the fourth through sixth decades, but can also occur in children or adolescents as well as the very elderly.[6,7] The primary form of MN is more common in males, with a male to female ratio of approximately 2:1. Secondary MN, related to autoimmune diseases, infections, malignancy, or drugs may also occur at any age, and is the form most often seen in children (especially hepatitis B-associated[8]). Malignancy-associated MN is more often a disease of older patients.

PRIMARY MEMBRANOUS NEPHROPATHY

As mentioned previously, primary MN is the most common form of this disease, representing 75% to 80% of all cases. It is a glomerulus-specific autoimmune disorder, characterized by the presence of subepithelial immune deposits containing IgG4 and associated in the majority of cases with circulating IgG4 autoantibodies to PLA_2R, a glycoprotein exposed on the podocyte surface (see Pathogenesis). The remainder of cases thought to be primary in nature may reflect a distinct disease with autoantibodies to another podocyte or glomerular protein, patients that remain proteinuric after the disappearance of anti-PLA_2R antibodies, or in fact cases of undiagnosed secondary disease. The primary form may recur after renal transplantation in up to 40% of cases.[9]

SECONDARY MEMBRANOUS NEPHROPATHY

Secondary cases of MN are suspected when the characteristic pathologic findings of MN are found in conjunction with another systemic condition or are associated with the use of a therapeutic agent or toxin. Due to a lack of available serologic markers (e.g., anti-PLA_2R autoantibodies) that could help to rule out primary disease, secondary cases were previously assumed to be present when MN was found in conjunction with one of the well- or lesser-known associations (Table 51.1).[10,11] There are many single case reports of MN occurring in conjunction with rare autoimmune diseases, infections, cancers, or therapeutic agents. It should be kept in mind that many of these may instead represent a coincidental finding of primary MN with these disorders, rather than a

TABLE 51.1 Causes of Membranous Nephropathy

Primary
- Anti-PLA_2R-associated
- Idiopathic

Secondary
- Autoimmune diseases
  - Systemic lupus erythematosus (class V lupus nephritis)
  - Other: rheumatoid arthritis, autoimmune thyroid disease, IgG4–related systemic disease
- Infection
  - Hepatitis B
  - Other chronic infections: hepatitis C, HIV, syphilis, schistosomiasis
- Alloimmunization
  - Fetomaternal alloimmunization
  - Graft-versus-host disease following hematopoietic stem cell transplantation
  - De novo membranous nephropathy in the renal allograft
- Drugs or toxins
  - Nonsteroidal anti-inflammatory drugs and Cox-2 inhibitors
  - Mercury-containing compounds
  - Other: gold salts, D-penicillamine, bucillamine
- Malignancy
  - Solid tumors (colon, stomach, lung, prostate)
  - Others: non-Hodgkin lymphoma, chronic lymphocytic leukemia, melanoma

disorder that is truly responsible for secondarily causing MN. Evidence for secondary MN comes in situations in which treatment of the underlying process (infection, autoimmune disease, malignancy) or removal of an offending drug is temporally associated with resolution of the nephrotic syndrome, but this still does not guarantee causation because primary MN undergoes spontaneous remission in one third of cases.

Despite these caveats, MN has been repeatedly found to be secondary to lupus and hepatitis B; in addition to being the most common secondary forms, the strength of the association is also the clearest. Malignancy-associated MN is another important secondary cause to be discussed later, but historically the association has been more controversial. In many cases, the pathologic lesion in secondary MN is similar to that of primary MN. However, there are often subtleties in terms of the location of the deposits, type of immunoglobulin deposited, or other additional features that are more supportive of a secondary cause.

Autoimmune Conditions

Various rheumatologic disorders have been described in association with MN (Table 51.1), of which systemic lupus erythematosus (SLE) is the most common. Ten to 20% of patients with lupus nephritis have an International Society of Nephrology/Renal Pathology Society Class V (membranous) lesion with predominantly subepithelial deposits (see Chapter 53). Clinically, the presentation is that of the nephrotic syndrome and is indistinguishable from idiopathic MN. The majority of these patients are young females, and the onset of the nephrotic syndrome may predate the development of other signs and symptoms of SLE. In a substantial proportion of these patients, the antinuclear antibody (ANA) titer may be low or undetectable, and the complement levels are usually normal. Therefore, there should be a high degree of suspicion for SLE in any young female with the nephrotic syndrome who is found to have MN by renal biopsy. With more established disease, ANA and anti–double-stranded DNA antibodies may be present, and complement levels may be slightly depressed. Several pathologic features on biopsy such as the presence of mesangial and/or subendothelial deposits, as well as the precise IgG subclass present in the deposits, may distinguish lupus-associated secondary MN from primary MN (see section on Pathology). Otherwise, the course of lupus-associated MN resembles that of the idiopathic form, with a good long-term prognosis for renal survival as compared to other forms of lupus nephritis.[12,13]

Rheumatoid arthritis is another autoimmune condition that has been historically linked to MN. However, this has usually, but not always, been in the setting of concurrent treatment of the arthritis with agents such as gold salts, D-penicillamine, or bucillamine (which are no longer commonly used), or nonsteroidal anti-inflammatory agents.[14] In these cases, proteinuria develops soon after exposure to the drug and resolves slowly over a period of months after the offending agent is withdrawn. The pathologic lesion is often identical to that of primary MN.

There are other autoimmune and systemic disorders that have been suggested to be rare secondary causes of MN, including autoimmune thyroid disease (Graves disease and Hashimoto thyroiditis),[10,15,16] IgG4–related systemic disease,[17,18] and sarcoidosis.[19,20] Whether or not these are truly causative etiologies or rather coincidental findings (that are likely to be reported in the literature due to this rare association of distinctive diseases) is not known at this point. As a case in point, a recent report described a patient with MN in which the diagnosis of sarcoidosis and the onset of proteinuria were temporally associated; however, the patient tested positive for anti-PLA_2R autoantibodies,[21] which suggests that the MN was in fact primary.

Infectious Diseases

Numerous infectious diseases have been associated with the development of MN (Table 51.1). In all cases, these represent chronic infections with longstanding and persistent antigenemia. The argument for an etiologic role of the infectious disease is strengthened when the nephrotic syndrome resolves with treatment of the infection, or when antigens produced by the microorganism are consistently found within the immune deposits.

The role of chronic infection with hepatitis B virus (HBV) is particularly strong and was first noted by Combes and colleagues in 1971.[22] HBV infection may account for 30% to 40% of cases of MN in Asia and is particularly prevalent in children in endemic areas, many of whom are asymptomatic carriers with no history of active hepatitis.[8,23–25] It is particularly noteworthy that the incidence of HBV-associated MN declined following the implementation of an active immunization program.[26] The serum transaminases tend to be normal or only mildly elevated, and the serology is positive for surface antigen, anti-core antibody, and usually e antigen. It appears that it is the e antigen and cationic anti-e antibody that are primarily deposited in the glomeruli.[8,25] HBV infection, along with membranous lupus nephritis, is the only other form of MN that may be associated with hypocomplementemia.[24] Although there may be spontaneous resolution of proteinuria in children, successful treatment of the underlying viral infection in adults with antiviral agents such as entecavir or lamivudine is typically necessary to achieve remission of the nephrotic syndrome.

MN has also been associated with many other chronic infectious diseases, although there is less evidence of causality, and MN is often not the predominant histologic lesion. For example, there are a number of case reports of MN in patients with chronic hepatitis C virus (HCV) infection,[27,28] but this agent is much more frequently associated with mixed cryoglobulinemia and the development of a membranoproliferative glomerulonephritis (MPGN) lesion. A membranous pattern has also been reported in patients infected with human immunodeficiency virus (HIV),[29–31] hepatosplenic schistosomiasis,[32] and congenital or acquired syphilis[33–35]; however, other forms of immune complex glomerulonephritis are more usual in these diseases. In several cases, microbial antigens such as those from treponemes in syphilis were found within the immune deposits.[36,37] As in lupus nephritis, the exact nature of the immune complex may determine whether it ultimately forms in a subepithelial versus a mesangial or subendothelial location.

Malignancy

The association of MN with cancer has long been a point of contention, in part due to the implications of screening for malignancy in a patient who has no other potential secondary causes for their MN. Proponents argue that screening a patient for malignancy may reveal an early occult tumor, whereas opponents argue that, because primary MN and malignancy are both diseases that occur with increased frequency in older individuals, the finding of both diseases in the same person is coincidental. The first report of a possible link between carcinoma and MN came in 1966[38] and this association has been reviewed virtually every decade since.[39–44] Although some may argue that detection bias can explain the association (i.e., patients who are found to have MN on biopsy are more likely to be screened for malignancy than their age-matched counterparts), a recent study that restricted the definition of malignancy-associated MN only to those in which the tumor was clinically evident before or at the time of the diagnosis of MN still found a higher than expected incidence of cancer compared to age- and gender-adjusted national cancer rates.[43] Thus, solid tumors, such as those of the gastrointestinal tract (colon and stomach), lung, and prostate, do appear to be detected in patients with MN at a greater frequency than would be expected for an age-matched national cohort. MN may also rarely occur secondary to non-Hodgkin lymphoma or chronic lymphocytic leukemia.[45] The association of MN and malignancy is strengthened by the temporal association, in several reports, of remission of the nephrotic syndrome following removal or treatment of the tumor. Some investigators have found evidence of tumor antigens such as CEA within the subepithelial immune deposits, and have been able to elute glomerular antibodies with reactivity to the tumor.[46,47]

Given evidence that seems to support both sides of the issue, it is likely that malignancy may be etiologically connected to MN in certain cases, but may only be coincidentally present with primary MN in other cases. This is reflected by a recent report that assayed 10 cases of malignancy-associated MN for the presence of anti-PLA_2R antibodies.[48] In 3 of 10 cases, there was evidence of circulating anti-PLA_2R antibodies and the predominant glomerular IgG subclass on examination of the biopsy material was IgG4, suggesting a coincidental occurrence of primary MN with a tumor. In the remaining seven cases, however, the patients were anti-PLA_2R negative, and the immune deposits were not positive for IgG4, suggesting a truly secondary cause of MN.[49] Future studies such as this may clarify the relationship between the two disease processes, and a positive test for autoantibodies may obviate the need for an extensive malignancy workup. For the time being, however, it is worth making sure that an elderly patient who is found to have MN on biopsy has had age- and gender-appropriate cancer screening, such as colonoscopy, prostate examination (and prostate-specific antigen testing), mammography, and chest imaging in patients with a history of past or current smoking.

Drugs and Toxins

Drug-associated MN can occur at any age and typically develops within 6 to 12 months of exposure to the offending agent, but the onset may be delayed for 3 to 4 years.[50] Historically, gold salts, D-penicillamine, and bucillamine used in the treatment of rheumatoid arthritis have been strongly linked to MN, although these agents are no longer in widespread use. The most common therapeutic agents currently implicated are the nonsteroidal anti-inflammatory drugs (NSAIDs), with mercury-containing compounds reflecting the most frequently encountered toxic exposure. The latter can be found as ingredients in certain skin-lightening agents, which have been linked to the development of MN in several reports.[51,52] Discontinuation of the drug leads to resolution of the proteinuria in virtually all cases.[50,53] However, studies with penicillamine, gold, and bucillamine indicate that protein excretion may continue to rise for several months after the cessation of therapy.[50] The mean time to resolution of the proteinuria is 9 to 12 months, although 2 to 3 years is required in some cases.

Although NSAID-induced nephrotic syndrome is more commonly associated with minimal change disease, it is evident that MN can also occur.[54,55] The association of NSAIDs with MN was illustrated in a study of 125 patients with a biopsy diagnosis of MN[55]; 23% reported regularly using NSAIDs and 13 of them were likely to have had NSAID-associated MN, as they demonstrated resolution of proteinuria within 1 to 36 weeks of discontinuing NSAIDs and had no recurrence of proteinuria at follow-up (5 months to 13 years). Many of the patients who developed MN had been treated with diclofenac, but probably any NSAID can be involved,[55] including cyclooxygenase-2 (Cox-2) inhibitors.[56]

Alloimmunity

MN may develop in situations when the immune system encounters non-self-antigens,[57] such as in renal transplantation or after allogeneic hematopoietic stem cell transplantation (HSCT). Although patients with a previous history of primary MN may develop recurrent disease in their allograft, more common is de novo MN, which may represent an alloimmune reaction to minor histocompatibility antigens on the allograft podocytes. The MN that occurs post-HSCT is likely to be a humoral manifestation of graft-versus-host disease, and is the most common cause of the nephrotic syndrome after HSCT.[58,59] It is of note that, like primary MN, these cases predominate in males, as opposed to the other causes of nephrotic syndrome after HSCT such as minimal change disease. A rare neonatal form of reversible MN due to fetomaternal alloimmunization has been described in babies born to mothers deficient in neutral endopeptidase (NEP), a protein expressed on podocytes (see Pathogenesis).[60,61]

Miscellaneous Conditions

Another form of pediatric MN was recently described in which circulating antibodies were found to be reactive with a cationic form of bovine serum albumin (BSA).[62] BSA, likely derived from cow's milk and absorbed as an undigested or partially digested protein, was detected in the glomerular immune deposits along with IgG. Moreover, specific anti-BSA antibodies could be eluted from the biopsy specimen in one case. MN has also been reported with diabetes, with or without associated diabetic nephropathy.[63] Although this may reflect a coincidental occurrence of MN with another common disease, there was evidence of porcine insulin within the immune deposits by immunostaining, and an improvement in proteinuria after switching from porcine to human insulin in a small case series.[64] There are also several reports of MN co-occurring with ANCA-positive crescentic glomerulonephritis. However, a recent report looking at the frequency of the two conditions in all renal biopsies performed at a single referral center concluded that the association was likely due to coincidence.[65]

PATHOLOGY

The name membranous nephropathy derives from the histopathologic appearance of the glomeruli of advanced cases of the disease in which expansion of the GBM is clearly visible on light microscopy and there is a paucity of inflammatory cells. Earlier in the course of the disease, however, the glomeruli may appear normal by light microscopy and further studies with immunofluorescence and electron microscopy are necessary for diagnosis. Conceptually, it is useful to think of the disease process as beginning with the formation or deposition of immune complexes beneath the podocyte, which then leads to podocyte injury and the deposition of new extracellular matrix between and around the immune deposits, culminating in a morphologically thickened GBM. Whereas several disparate conditions may underlie the development of MN and give rise to the formation of subepithelial immune deposits, as noted previously, the final pattern of injury is strikingly similar with some subtle differences discussed later. Although the histologic hallmarks of this disease—including GBM "spikes" visualized with the use of silver stains, and the fine granular deposition of IgG in a capillary loop pattern on immunofluorescence—were first described by Jones,[66] and Mellors and Ortega,[67] respectively, over 60 years ago, a definitive pathologic diagnosis depends on identifying the immune deposits with electron microscopy.

Light Microscopy

Light microscopy, with either hematoxylin and eosin (H&E) or periodic acid-Schiff (PAS) staining, reveals diffuse and generally uniform thickening of the GBM (Figs. 51.1 and 51.2). The heterogeneous character of the thickened GBM is best

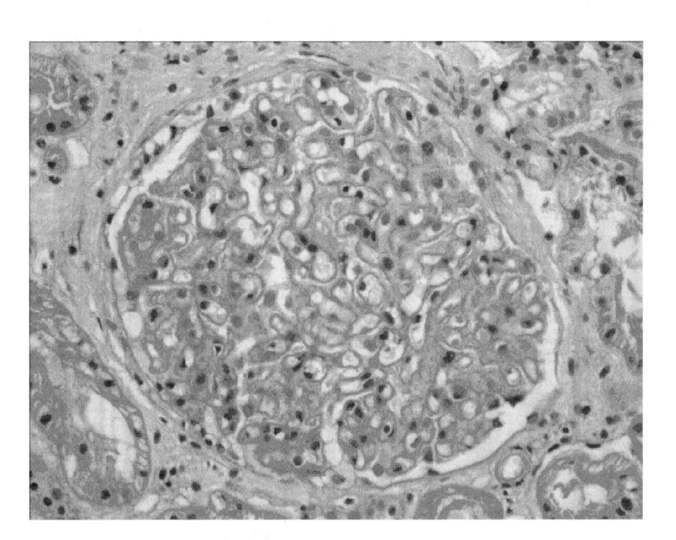

FIGURE 51.1 Hematoxylin and eosin stain (×250) of a glomerulus from a patient with idiopathic membranous nephropathy. There is diffuse thickening of the basement membrane without associated hypercellularity of the glomerular tuft. Inflammatory infiltrates are not seen and the capillary loops are widely patent. (Courtesy of Dr. Helen Cathro.)

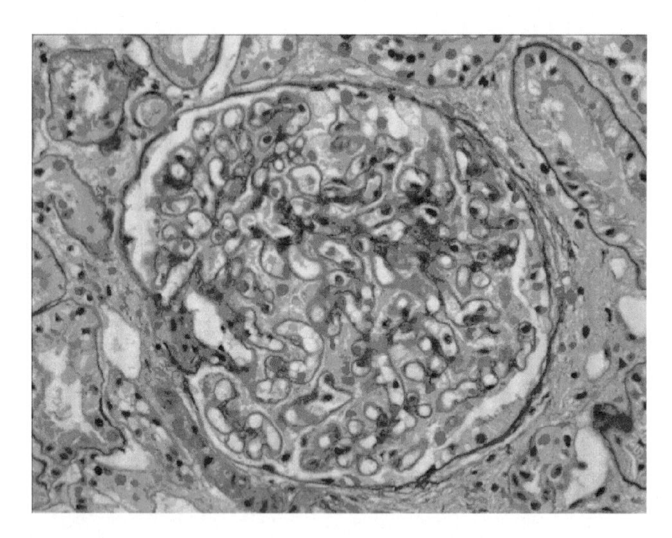

FIGURE 51.2 Periodic acid-Schiff stain of a glomerulus from a patient with idiopathic membranous nephropathy (×250). The basement membrane surrounding the capillary loops is diffusely thickened. (Courtesy of Dr. Helen Cathro.)

seen by silver methenamine (Jones' stain), which binds to basement membrane components but is not taken up by the immune deposits (Fig. 51.3). This staining, in appropriately advanced disease, reveals "spikes" of GBM present between deposits when the GBM is sectioned in cross-section, or "craters" or "pock-marks" caused by the nonsilver stained immune deposits when a tangential section of the GBM is encountered. These findings are pathognomonic for MN. The formation of immune deposits and the basement membrane response proceeds in stages according to the duration of disease (and repair). Ehrenreich and Churg (Table 51.2) classified this progression into four morphologic stages, which are more appropriate for describing the pathologic findings than correlating with clinical findings or prognosis.

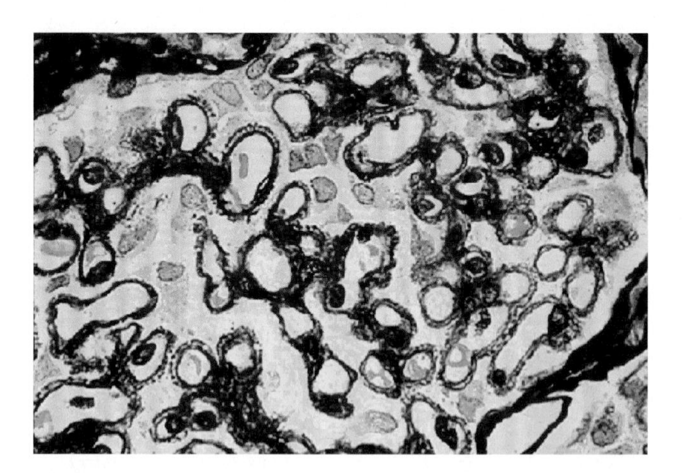

FIGURE 51.3 Jones silver stain (×250) of a glomerulus from a patient with idiopathic membranous nephropathy demonstrating "spikes" corresponding to newly synthesized basement membrane surrounding immune complexes. (Courtesy of Dr. Edward Klatt.)

TABLE 51.2 Pathologic Staging of Membranous Nephropathy

Stage	Electron Microscopy
I	Subepithelial electron-dense deposits
II	Subepithelial electron-dense deposits with intervening basement membrane ("spikes")
III	Incorporation of subepithelial electron-dense deposits into the basement membrane
IV	Reabsorption of deposits with loss of electron-dense deposits and development of lucent area in the basement membrane Remodeling of basement membrane and loss of electron-dense deposits

From Ehreneich T, Churg J. Pathology of membranous nephropathy. *Pathol Annu.* 1968;3:145.

Other compartments of the glomerulus usually appear normal. There is no evidence of mesangial cell proliferation or expansion except in the setting of SLE and other secondary forms. Importantly, there is typically no evidence of inflammatory cell infiltration (which argues against the continued use of the term "membranous glomerulonephritis"). Experimental studies suggested that this is on account of the subepithelial location of the immune deposits, which are separated from the capillary lumen and thereby unable to recruit inflammatory effector cells, as more readily occurs when immune deposits form in a mesangial or subendothelial location.[68]

With longer duration of disease and/or sustained heavy nephrotic proteinuria, tubulointerstitial damage can occur which is associated with decreased glomerular filtration rate (GFR) and a worsened renal prognosis. Similarly, lesions of secondary FSGS may also develop, also portending a worse prognosis and persistent proteinuria that is likely to be unresponsive to immunosuppression.

Immunofluorescence Microscopy

The finding of granular deposits of IgG in a capillary loop pattern on immunofluorescence is the sine qua non of both primary and secondary MN (Fig. 51.4). With the exception of class V lupus nephritis which may present with a "full house" pattern on immunofluorescence,[69] the deposits are predominantly IgG, with minimal staining for IgA and IgM, and tend to spare the mesangium. The complement component C3 is often seen, with the exception of very early disease. Although not typically performed, the characterization of IgG subclasses often helps to differentiate

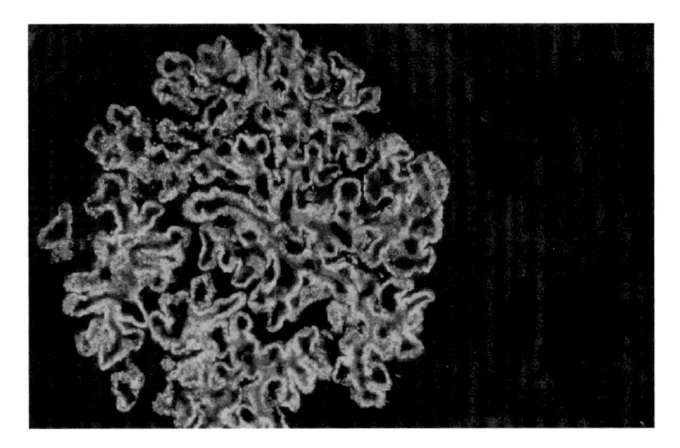

FIGURE 51.4 Immunofluorescence staining (anti-IgG) of a glomerulus from a patient with idiopathic membranous nephropathy (×250). Diffuse granular staining along the basement membrane is evident and corresponds to the deposition of immune complexes. Mesangial areas are free of immune deposits.

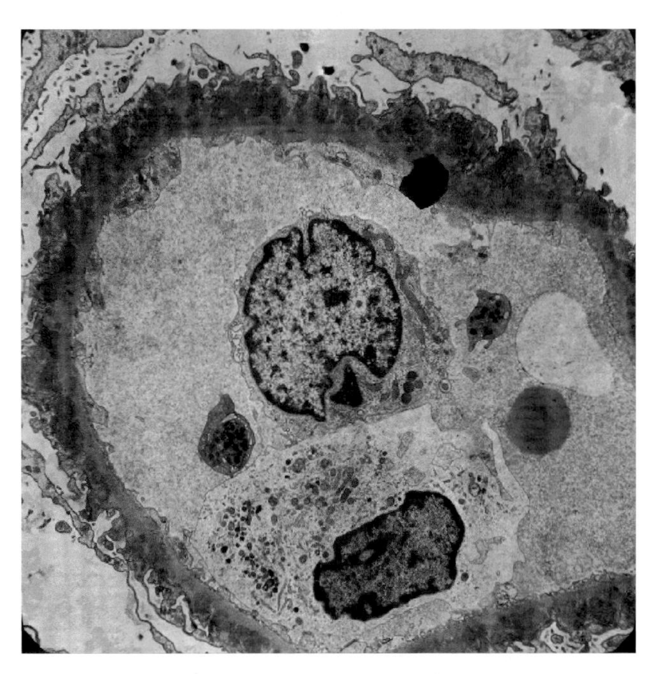

FIGURE 51.5 Electron micrograph of a glomerulus from a patient with idiopathic membranous nephropathy revealing characteristic electron-dense subepithelial deposits (×5,000). In this micrograph, basement membrane can be seen to encircle the deposits forming the spikes seen on Jones' silver staining (stages II and III). (Courtesy of Dr. Helen Cathro.)

primary from secondary disease, as the predominant IgG subclass in primary MN is IgG4. Secondary causes, in most cases, have a predominance of non-IgG4 subclasses, most notably in lupus-associated[69–71] and malignancy-associated MN.[49] The presence of C1q, an early component of the classical complement pathway, may also help distinguish between primary and secondary cases. Strong C1q staining is not typically found in primary MN (less than 20% of cases)[69,72] but is more common in lupus-associated MN.

Electron Microscopy

The hallmark of MN is the presence of subepithelial electron-dense deposits corresponding to the immune complexes (Fig. 51.5). Similar deposits are rare in the mesangium (but may be present in paramesangial areas) in primary MN, but are more common in secondary cases such as lupus- or NSAID-associated MN. These electron-dense deposits are typically homogeneous in nature, without visible substructure. Similar to other causes of the nephrotic syndrome, evidence of podocyte injury is present, with effacement (or "simplification") of the foot processes, microvillous changes, and the presence of protein reabsorption droplets within podocytes and proximal tubular cells. One additional finding on electron microscopy, the presence of tubuloreticular inclusions in the endothelial cells, may be strongly suggestive of lupus- or HIV-associated MN. However, these can be rarely found in primary disease as well.[73]

Variants

The presence of subepithelial electron-dense deposits in a segmental pattern (segmental MN) appears to be different than primary MN, with a childhood predominance and often an association with C1q deposition.[74] The finding of substructure in the deposits by electron microscopy is also atypical. A rare but distinctive form of MN characterized by "microspherules" within the deposits has been reported[75] and continues to be infrequently seen by pathologists. The nature of these particles and its association with other systemic diseases is unknown. Monoclonal immunoglobulin deposition disease usually gives rise to nodular glomerulosclerosis or a proliferative pattern of glomerular injury[76]; however, a histologic pattern mimicking MN through the presence of subepithelial deposits can also occur.[77–79] This form may be suggested by abnormal findings on serum or urine immunofixation electrophoresis, and is confirmed by demonstrating a kappa or lambda light chain restriction to the deposits on immunofluorescence.

PATHOGENESIS

Much of the proposed pathogenesis of MN has been elucidated from decades of study in the rat model of Heymann nephritis (HN).[80] In the past decade, a better understanding of the disease process in humans has been achieved due to the findings of autoantibodies to human podocyte proteins, especially the phospholipase A_2 receptor. Due to the historical importance of the Heymann nephritis model and the pathophysiologic lessons learned from it, we begin with a synopsis. Further information is available in several comprehensive reviews of the topic.[81–83]

In 1959, Walter Heymann published a description of the experimental rat model of immune deposition disease that morphologically and clinically mimics human MN and bears his name.[80] Rats actively or passively immunized against a proximal tubular brush border fraction (Fx1a) eventually develop nephrotic levels of proteinuria due to the subepithelial deposition of IgG-containing immune complexes.

Initial assumptions were that circulating immune complexes give rise to the glomerular subepithelial immune deposits. The size, charge, and affinity of the components of the immune complex were thought to determine their distribution into a subepithelial rather than subendothelial location. Using in vitro and ex vivo perfusion of isolated rat kidneys with anti-Fx1a antibodies, two independent research groups clearly demonstrated that the subepithelial deposits in HN form instead by the binding of immunoglobulin in situ to an antigen expressed on the basal surface of the podocyte foot processes.[84,85] The primary antigenic component of Fx1a was subsequently identified as the endocytic tubular brush border receptor megalin.[86–90] In rats, but not in humans, megalin is additionally present on the foot processes of the podocyte where it serves as the target for the circulating anti-Fx1a antibodies. These individual antibody-antigen interactions were shown to coalesce into small immune complexes through a process of "capping and shedding,"[91] and to ultimately aggregate in the GBM into the large electron-dense subepithelial deposits visible by electron microscopy.[92]

Further work in this experimental model unraveled the pathogenesis of the disease process.[81] Local complement activation by the immune complexes leads to the assembly of C5b-9, the membrane attack complex (MAC) that inserts into the plasma membrane of nearby podocyte foot processes. This instigates a series of maladaptive downstream signaling events leading to calcium influx, increased generation of arachidonic acid metabolites, and the production of reactive oxygen species. The resulting cytoskeletal changes lead to simplification or effacement of the foot processes, loss of slit diaphragms, and massive nonselective loss of protein into the urine. As a result of the signaling changes and loss of differentiated cell phenotype, the podocytes began to secrete and deposit extracellular matrix between and around the immune deposits, leading to an expansion of the GBM.[93] Despite the continued generation of C5b-9, the podocyte is not lethally injured as it is able to continually shed the MAC from its plasma membrane into the GBM and urine.

A similar process is presumed to take place in humans, and a role for complement activation in human MN is clear, because both C3 and C5b-9 have been shown to be present in the glomerular immune deposits[94] as well as in the urine.[95] However, the precise arm of the complement cascade responsible for these findings in MN is not clear. The absence of C1q[69,72] and the presence of IgG4 (IgG4 is generally considered to be unable to fix complement[96]) argue against a major role for the classical pathway, at least in primary MN. It is possible that the alternative or mannan-binding lectin pathways of complement activation may play a more important role in the cellular injury in primary MN, given the predominance of IgG4 in the deposits.

Because megalin, the target antigen in HN, is not expressed in the human glomerulus, it has long been hypothesized that an alternative protein expressed on the surface of the podocyte would serve as the target for antibody-mediated cytotoxicity in human disease. In a seminal case report,[60] Debiec and colleagues provided the first demonstration of such circulating antibodies reactive with an endogenous podocyte protein. A mother deficient in neutral endopeptidase (NEP), which is expressed by the podocyte, was immunized to this protein during a prior miscarriage. In a subsequent pregnancy, these anti-NEP alloantibodies crossed the placenta and into the fetal kidney, binding NEP at the surface of the fetal podocyte and causing the formation of subepithelial deposits. The infant was born with an antenatal form of MN, although the disease spontaneously resolved within several months after birth due to the eventual clearance of circulating maternal IgG. Several other cases of fetomaternal alloimmune MN in response to NEP have been described.[61] Importantly, infants were only proteinuric when mothers had both the complement-fixing IgG1 as well as the noncomplement-fixing IgG4 anti-NEP antibodies.

The next major advance in the field of primary MN came recently with the description of circulating autoantibodies to the M-type phospholipase A_2 receptor (PLA_2R) in the majority of patients with primary MN.[97] PLA_2R is a member of the mannose receptor family of transmembrane glycoproteins,[98,99] and is expressed by the human podocyte.[97] At least 70% of patients with primary MN have these autoantibodies when they are initially nephrotic. In contrast, such antibodies are absent in patients with secondary forms of MN, other glomerular diseases, and normal controls. Consistent with the known subclass distribution of IgG within the immune deposits of primary MN, the predominant circulating anti-PLA_2R subclass is IgG4, a marker of a type-2 helper T cell (Th2) response. These anti-PLA_2R autoantibodies have been found in patients with MN worldwide and of all major ethnicities. Antibodies from all anti-PLA_2R positive patients have exhibited reactivity only with the nonreduced protein, suggesting the presence of one or more conformation-dependent epitopes within the molecule, and likely in its N-terminal portion. IgG4 localizes with the PLA_2R antigen within the subepithelial immune deposits in primary (but not secondary) MN biopsy specimens,[97] which suggests that PLA_2R-anti-PLA_2R complexes are shed from the podocyte surface as noted earlier in the Heymann nephritis model. Furthermore, PLA_2R-reactive IgG can be specifically eluted from these biopsies.

A role for anti-PLA_2R autoantibodies in disease pathogenesis is suggested by observations that the presence of such antibodies is closely associated with clinical disease activity. Importantly, the anti-PLA_2R antibodies tend to disappear with a spontaneous- or treatment-induced remission and return with a relapse of the disease.[100] Further supportive of a pathogenic role is the repeated observation that changes in autoantibody precede corresponding changes in proteinuria by months. Indeed, biopsy studies have shown that residual evidence of the PLA_2R antigen may persist in deposits despite clearance from the circulation.[101] This lag time most likely represents the period of glomerular recovery, during which subepithelial deposits are slowly cleared, and podocyte cytoskeletal structure and the slit diaphragm apparatus returns to its baseline architecture. Final proof of pathogenicity awaits the creation of a suitable animal model.

The presence of anti-PLA_2R antibodies seems to largely be restricted to primary forms of MN; it is not found in lupus-, hepatitis-, or drug-associated MN, and is also not found in normal individuals or patients with other forms of glomerular disease.[48,97] Although not yet commercially available in the United States, it is anticipated that measurement of anti-PLA_2R antibodies may represent a powerful screening and monitoring tool, to be used adjunctively with renal biopsy and measurements of proteinuria.

Recent work has detailed the presence of antibodies against glomerular neoantigens, or podocyte proteins not expressed in the healthy state, but rather induced by disease. These include antibodies to aldose reductase and superoxide dismutase 2, which are normally intracellular proteins that appear to be expressed at the cell surface in MN.[102] The role of these antibodies in the initiation of disease activity is not clear; however, it is possible that they serve as progression factors that can lead to further immune complex formation and thus worsening of disease.

In all forms of MN, a complete clinical remission can occur with a reduction in proteinuria from nephrotic to completely normal levels. This is accompanied by the gradual disappearance of subepithelial and intramembranous deposits, reorganization of the podocyte foot processes, and reestablishment of slit diaphragms. Repeat biopsies performed in several patients who attained a complete remission after having been treated with the anti-B cell agent rituximab found a virtual disappearance of immunofluorescence staining for IgG4 (but not total IgG), a trend toward decreased C3 staining, as well as a complete or partial disappearance of the subepithelial deposits.[103] The structural changes that underlie a partial remission are less clear, but may reflect balanced rates of immune deposit formation and clearance, or incomplete restoration of the normal podocyte architecture due to the disordered GBM. Moderate proteinuria that persists despite the absence of immunologic activity may also be due to tubulointerstitial damage, nephron loss, and secondary FSGS. The transplantation of kidneys from rats with experimental HN into naïve rats revealed that, although a significant amelioration of proteinuria occurred in the absence of circulating antimegalin antibodies, the animals were left with permanent residual proteinuria due to persistent abnormalities of the glomerular capillary wall.[104]

The mechanisms for the formation of subepithelial deposits in secondary MN are not well understood, and may involve planted antigens or low-avidity circulating immune complexes rather than antibodies to native podocyte antigens. The presence of deoxyribonucleic acid (DNA)-histone complexes and the HBV e antigen have been variably demonstrated within the immune deposits of MN secondary to lupus or HBV infection, respectively.[8,105] Circulating immune complexes, which may have a net positive charge, eventually deposit on the outer aspect of the GBM, perhaps after dissociation and reassociation. Several isolated reports have detected various tumor antigens in the deposits in malignancy-associated MN, although it is unclear whether such antigens represent the initiators of disease or are only secondarily trapped within existing deposits. The molecular differences underlying the various locations in which immune complexes may deposit in lupus nephritis are not currently known. Similarly, the mechanisms whereby therapeutic drugs, toxins, or chronic infections lead to secondary MN have not yet been established.

The genetics of primary MN has highlighted both the major antigen PLA_2R and components of the antigen presentation system. Early studies documented an association with specific HLA molecules.[106,107] This was confirmed in a recent genome-wide association study (GWAS) that linked MN in a cohort of 585 European Caucasians with a single nucleotide polymorphism (SNP) in the HLA-DQA1 locus.[5] Remarkably, this study also showed an allelic association with *PLA2R1*, the gene that encodes PLA_2R. Surprisingly, no other loci were identified in this association study, although it is possible that studies in larger or ethnically different cohorts may identify further gene associations. Although this GWAS study was performed in an exclusively Caucasian population, two smaller studies in a Korean[108] and a Taiwanese[109] cohort have also defined SNPs within the *PLA2R1* coding region that are associated with primary MN. The implications of the studies in terms of the precise pathophysiology of the triggering events in primary MN are not yet known, nor are the implications for genetic testing.

Much work remains to be done to understand the early events that underlie the initiation of MN, although the finding of specific HLA molecules and a target antigen may stimulate further research in this vein. B cells are found within the renal interstitium in MN[110] and these or periglomerular or peritubular dendritic cells could serve as local antigen presenting cells.

CLINICAL FEATURES

The onset of clinical disease in MN is typically an insidious process, unlike the more explosive onset of the nephrotic syndrome as seen in minimal change disease or primary FSGS. The majority of patients present with weight gain, edema, proteinuria, and other signs of the nephrotic syndrome that have likely been developing over the course of months. Up to one third of cases may have hypertension at presentation as well. A smaller percentage of patients present with subnephrotic levels of proteinuria, perhaps detected by an abnormal urinalysis performed for an unrelated reason such as screening in pregnancy or for a life insurance examination. The proteinuria tends to be nonselective; that is, there is increased immunoglobulin as well as albumin excretion, as opposed to mainly albuminuria as seen in minimal change disease. Microscopic hematuria is present in up to 50% of cases despite the absence of frank glomerulonephritis, although red cell casts and macroscopic hematuria are typically not seen. Features of proximal tubular dysfunction such as glycosuria may be seen with especially heavy proteinuria. GFR is usually normal, unless the disease has been present but undetected for years. Other features of the nephrotic syndrome, including hypoalbuminemia, hyperlipidemia, low levels of 25-hydroxyvitamin D, and lipiduria are generally present.

Thromboembolic complications such as deep vein thrombosis, pulmonary embolism, and renal vein thrombosis can be the presenting feature in some patients with MN.[111] These complications are more common in MN than in other nephrotic conditions, even when adjusted for age and the degree of proteinuria, and MN is the most commonly associated condition in patients with renal vein thrombosis. Thromboembolic complications most frequently occur in patients with heavy, persistent proteinuria and serum albumin concentrations below 2 g per dL. Renal vein thrombosis may be asymptomatic and manifest for the first time with pulmonary embolism, or present with flank pain, hematuria, or deterioration in renal function.

LABORATORY FINDINGS

Laboratory findings in patients with MN reflect ongoing proteinuria and the nephrotic syndrome. Thus, hypoalbuminemia, hyperlipidemia, low levels of 25-hydroxyvitamin D and lipiduria (oval fat bodies, fatty casts) are common findings. The results of routine serologic studies, including complement levels, are all normal in primary MN. However, studies should be performed to exclude secondary causes of MN and include ANA, hepatitis B and C profiles, rapid plasmin reagin (RPR), as well as age-appropriate cancer screening. In addition, complement levels may be depressed in HBV- and lupus-associated secondary forms of MN. As in most cases of nephrotic syndrome, the erythrocyte sedimentation rate is typically elevated and is of no value in differentiating primary from secondary causes of MN. Currently, renal biopsy is the exclusive means for diagnosing MN and distinguishing primary disease from secondary etiologies. It is anticipated that circulating autoantibodies to PLA_2R may soon be used to support a diagnosis of primary MN. At this time, however, the test is only available in the research setting.

NATURAL HISTORY AND PROGNOSIS

Predicting the clinical course of an individual patient with MN at disease presentation is impossible given the variable and fluctuating disease course. It is a commonly taught dictum that one third of cases spontaneously remit, another third have persistent proteinuria that does not lead to a significant decline in renal function, and the final third progress inexorably to renal failure; however, these numbers vary considerably among different reports. Those patients that do undergo transplantation for ESRD have up to a 40% risk of recurrence of MN in the renal allograft.

The immunologic factors that trigger primary MN, impact its severity, or ultimately lead to its remission (and relapse) are not understood at this time. There have not been consistent links to any preceding infection; MN most often appears for no apparent reason in otherwise healthy middle-aged adults. Increased severity of proteinuria and longer duration of the nephrotic syndrome are clearly linked to poorer renal outcomes. The amount of time between a biopsy diagnosis of MN and the actual immunologic initiation of the disease (which is virtually never known) may determine in part the degree of proteinuria at presentation, as it may take many months before a patient develops peak proteinuria. In general, 75% of patients with primary MN are fully nephrotic at the time of biopsy diagnosis, whereas the remainder has nonnephrotic levels of proteinuria.[112] Patients who never develop nephrotic syndrome (approximately 40% of those who are nonnephrotic at presentation) have excellent prognosis, with a 10-year renal survival of nearly 100%. Nearly 70% of those who progress from nonnephrotic to nephrotic levels of proteinuria do so in the first year after diagnosis, and yet have a better renal prognosis than those who are nephrotic at presentation.[112]

Baseline demographic differences in natural history studies of MN appear to have blurred the overall prognostic picture, and are partially responsible for differences in opinion on whether or when to treat MN patients with immunosuppressive agents. A widely quoted single-center study involving 100 patients with untreated MN reported a 65% spontaneous remission rate and an 88% 5-year renal survival.[113] However, more than one third of the initial cohort in this study never had nephrotic range proteinuria, clearly biasing toward a more favorable prognostic picture. A more recent analysis that statistically corrected for the percentage of nonnephrotic patients has estimated that up to 50% of nephrotic patients with primary MN may reach ESRD over the course of 10 years.[114]

It is difficult to determine where an individual patient lies in the longitudinal spectrum of disease when relying only on proteinuria as a measure of clinical outcome. Either after a spontaneous remission or in response to treatment, the level of proteinuria may decline at a variable rate, and may or may not reach zero. Due to the severity and duration of structural changes in the glomerulus, or due to secondary changes such as tubulointerstitial damage and glomerular sclerosis, proteinuria may take months to years to normalize, or may remain persistently elevated, all in the absence of ongoing immunologic activity. A recent article by Polanco and colleagues shows that this decline in proteinuria can continue over years, even in those starting with very high levels of initial proteinuria.[115] Thus, a partial (incomplete) remission of proteinuria (typically, a greater than 50% decrease from baseline proteinuria to less than 3.5 g per day) does not provide an accurate account of the activity of the disease because several factors may cause a reduced but persistent level of proteinuria, including the hemodynamic changes induced by RAS and calcineurin inhibitors or immunologic remission with residual structural abnormalities.

Several prognostic factors have been identified that are associated with an unfavorable course. These include advanced age, male sex, reduced renal function at presentation, high levels of nephrotic-range proteinuria, urinary excretion of low molecular weight proteins such as β_2 microglobulin, hypertension, and tubulointerstitial fibrosis or glomerular sclerosis on renal biopsy. As has been shown in many renal diseases, the histologic presence of glomerular sclerosis, advanced vascular sclerosis, or tubulointerstitial disease generally portends an unfavorable renal prognosis.[116] However, these biopsy findings are also a function of age, the presence of concomitant hypertension, and were not independently predictive of poor prognosis when adjusted for creatinine clearance; nor did they predict severity of proteinuria, rate of progression, or response to treatment.[117] Thus, it appears that patients with these pathologic features merely have reduced renal reserve due to a later diagnosis, rather than an inherently more aggressive disease process. Although not commonly employed in treatment algorithms, this same study also showed that a higher degree of complement deposition was associated with a faster rate of disease progression.[117]

The factors that seem to be most important in predicting both a spontaneous remission and its durability are persistent, low grade (subnephrotic) proteinuria and female gender. Ethnicity may also be a factor, because a natural history study in 941 Japanese patients with MN showed excellent long-term outcomes.[118] Several groups have looked at the excretion of urinary proteins as predictors of prognosis in MN. Branten and colleagues found that the combination of high urinary β_2 microglobulin and high urinary IgG are excellent predictors of worsening renal function.[119]

As mentioned previously, this variable natural history of MN makes individual treatment decisions difficult, and interpretation of trials less than straightforward, as there is often no way to clearly differentiate a treatment response from a spontaneous remission, especially when it occurs very early after the start of treatment. Because only a subset of patients will progress to renal failure over an extended period of time, and due to the uncertainty of whether or not a spontaneous remission will occur, therapy with immunosuppressive agents must be tailored to those patients at greatest risk for a poor outcome. Cattran and colleagues have developed a predictive model using data from 184 patients with MN from the Metro Toronto Glomerulonephritis Registry.[120] Based on this model, it is generally acceptable to observe the patient (with the addition of conservative therapy) for 6 months to assess disease trajectory and to await a spontaneous remission, in the absence of rapidly worsening renal function or other life-threatening manifestations of the nephrotic syndrome such as pulmonary embolism. Those with normal renal function and lower amounts of proteinuria (<4 g per day) over 6 months constitute a group at low risk for developing progressive renal insufficiency from their disease. Intermediate levels of proteinuria (4 to 8 g per day) with stable renal function over 6 months represent an intermediate risk group. Those with persistent high grade nephrotic-range proteinuria (>8 g per day) over the course of 6 months, and/or reduced renal function at the outset or a progressive deterioration over 6 months, are at high risk (>75% likelihood) of having further renal deterioration.

A Dutch group follows a similar strategy, with a "wait-and-see" approach for those with nonnephrotic levels of proteinuria, and immediate immunosuppressive therapy for those with evidence of renal failure.[114] Patients with normal renal function are subjected to a risk assessment through the measurement of urinary markers such as β_2 microglobulin and IgG, which reflect both nonselective proteinuria at the level of the glomerulus as well as secondary tubular dysfunction. Those considered to be at high risk of progression to renal failure based on increased levels of excreted IgG and β_2 microglobulin are treated, whereas the rest are managed under a wait-and-see policy with reassessment at 1 year. Although this strategy is appealing in being able to immediately stratify those patients with normal renal function and nephrotic syndrome into those who should or should not be treated, these urinary indices have not been adopted widely.

The prognosis for renal survival that is associated with a response to treatment is in keeping with the tenet that sustained heavy proteinuria is detrimental to renal function. Patients achieving complete remission fare better than those who attain a partial remission, although both have improved renal survival over those who fail to remit at all.[121] Relapse occurs in nearly 25% of patients who achieve complete remission and nearly 50% of those with a partial remission, and renal survival is best in those that never relapse.[121]

Given that a high proportion of nephrotic patients may ultimately achieve remission spontaneously,[115] and that both spontaneous and treatment-induced remissions may take years to become fully apparent, the reader should interpret clinical therapeutic trials in MN cautiously; there are a large number of small trials with relatively short (1 to 2 years) follow-up, and only a few with long-term follow-up data.

THERAPY

It is important to differentiate primary from secondary causes of MN when establishing a treatment plan. Secondary forms of MN are best treated by focusing on the underlying disease process or therapeutic agent. Remission of proteinuria may gradually occur following successful treatment of underlying infection such as hepatitis B or syphilis, the withdrawal of an offending drug, or removal of an associated malignancy. The management of lupus-associated MN, often managed in conjunction with a rheumatologist, is similar to the approaches listed below for primary MN, using calcineurin inhibitors, cyclophosphamide, or mycophenolate.[122–127] The reader is also directed to excellent recent reviews on the therapy of primary MN for further details.[114,128]

The goals of therapy for patients with MN are the preservation of renal function, reduction of proteinuria, and minimization of complications from the nephrotic syndrome. These aims must be weighed against the risks associated with therapy, especially in light of the variable and unpredictable natural history of the disease itself. Although there have been a number of clinical trials in MN, small sample sizes due to the rarity of the disease as well as residual questions about the risk-benefit of each treatment option still preclude a consensus about first-line treatment in MN. Historically, the best evidence is for the use of alkylating agents or cyclosporine in conjunction with corticosteroids, but the toxicity of these agents and the emergence of newer agents with fewer side effects has maintained the controversy as to the optimal treatment regimen. Although the treatment of primary MN should largely be dictated by the nephrologist, there is certainly a role for a team care approach, including a pharmacist and dietician.

Conservative Therapy

All patients with MN should be started on angiotensin-converting enzyme (ACE) inhibitors or angiotensin II receptor blockers (ARBs) to reduce proteinuria. This recommendation comes in light of their effectiveness in most other proteinuric disease, although the data in MN does not support a major effect on disease outcome.[112,114,121] Diuretics and dietary salt restriction are necessary to treat the edema, due in part to sodium retention by the nephrotic kidney, and to enhance the antiproteinuric effect of inhibitors of the RAS. Additional antihypertensive agents should be added to achieve a target blood pressure goal of 125/75 mm Hg. Statins should be added and titrated to control hyperlipidemia.

Due to the high risk for thromboembolism in MN, prophylactic anticoagulation should be considered for those with serum albumin levels less than 2 g per dL, or even higher levels if the patient has an additional history of previous venous thromboembolism or has other risk factors, such as hereditary thrombophilia, malignancy, the use of oral contraceptives, or immobility. Anticoagulation is clearly indicated in those who present with or have a thromboembolic event in the course of their disease.

Other considerations for nonspecific treatment of the nephrotic state include supplementation with vitamin D, due to its loss with the vitamin D–binding protein in the urine, as well as careful surveillance for infectious disease, as the nephrotic syndrome is an acquired immunodeficiency state due to urinary losses of innate and adaptive immune factors.

Alkylating Agents: Cyclophosphamide and Chlorambucil

A meta-analysis of trials that investigated the use of corticosteroid monotherapy for the treatment of MN failed to show any evidence of efficacy.[129] Instead, typical immunosuppressive regimens for primary MN combine corticosteroids with alkylating agents for six to 12 months. Treatment with cyclophosphamide or chlorambucil in conjunction with corticosteroids is supported by several randomized controlled trials. Cumulative data suggests that 30% to 40% of those treated will achieve a complete remission from their disease. Another 30% to 50% will achieve a partial remission, with only 10% developing progressive renal disease. Relapse may occur in up to 30% of patients within 5 years of discontinuing the alkylating agent. However, these relapses can often be successfully treated with a repeat course of immunosuppressive therapy.

A series of reports from Italy provided convincing evidence for the efficacy of what has become known as the "Ponticelli regimen." This 6-month protocol alternates months of corticosteroid treatment with months of an alkylating agent.[130–132] Three daily 1-g doses of intravenous methylprednisolone are used to initiate the steroid months, followed by oral prednisone at 0.4 to 0.5 mg/kg/day for the remainder of the month. This regimen was originally alternated monthly with daily doses of oral chlorambucil (0.2 mg/kg/day), but a more recent study showed equivalent efficacy with fewer side effects with oral cyclophosphamide (2.5 mg/kg/day). The remission rate at 5 years was 73% for treated patients versus 40% for those who received only supportive therapy in the original study, in addition to better preservation of renal function. A subsequent report detailing 10 years of follow-up in this cohort demonstrated a 10-year dialysis-free survival of 92% (versus 60%) in the group treated with corticosteroids and chlorambucil.

Recently, Jha and colleagues provided confirmatory evidence from a 10-year follow-up of an Indian population with primary MN.[133] This open-label randomized controlled trial compared a 6-month treatment course consisting of alternating months of corticosteroids (as above) and oral cyclophosphamide (2 mg/kg/day) with supportive therapy alone. There were 34 remissions (15 complete) in the 51 treated patients who were followed for the full 10 years, versus only 16 remissions (5 complete) in the 46 patients treated with conservative therapy. Ten-year dialysis-free survival was higher in the treatment arm (89% versus 65%).

Despite the proven success of such cytotoxic therapy, concerns about adverse effects, such as infertility, hemorrhagic cystitis, and long-term bladder malignancy, limit its use, especially in lower risk patients in whom the risks of treatment may outweigh the benefits. Younger patients who desire to have children in the future should be encouraged to bank sperm or eggs prior to the initiation of therapy with alkylating agents, and all patients should be instructed to stop smoking tobacco to reduce the risk of bladder cancer.

The Calcineurin Inhibitors: Cyclosporine and Tacrolimus

Cyclosporine is an alternative, clinically validated immunosuppressive agent used in the treatment of MN.[134]

In 51 patients with steroid-resistant MN, treatment with cyclosporine plus corticosteroids for 6 months followed by a 4-week taper resulted in a 75% remission (complete and partial) rate, versus only 22% in the steroid-only control arm.[135] A frequently noted issue with the use of calcineurin inhibitors such as cyclosporine is the tendency for patients to relapse soon after discontinuation of therapy. Use of steroids in conjunction with cyclosporine appears to reduce relapse rates, as evidenced by a study investigating the use of cyclosporine, with or without steroids, over a 12-month treatment course. Although both groups achieved a remission rate of approximately 80% at 12 months, the relapse rate was lower in the group receiving the adjunctive corticosteroids.[136]

Longer courses of cyclosporine (1 to 2 years) with a slow taper may be necessary to avoid a high rate of relapse. Other investigators have demonstrated that tacrolimus induced a higher rate of remission than conservative treatment alone in heavily nephrotic patients.[137] However, nearly half of these patients had a nephrotic relapse within several months of tapering tacrolimus. Current trials are investigating the use of maintenance agents such as mycophenolate initiated during the taper of the calcineurin inhibitor, in an attempt to prevent these relapses. Thus far, a clinically validated combination has not been found.

The mechanism of cyclosporine in the reduction of proteinuria may be pleiotropic. There is a known effect on T cell activation as is seen in allograft immunosuppression, and there is also a vasoconstrictor effect that likely plays an additional role in the long-term nephrotoxicity of these agents. More recently, Faul and colleagues have provided intriguing evidence that cyclosporine may have direct effects on the podocyte, by inhibiting cathepsin L-mediated degradation of synaptopodin and maintaining the cytoskeleton in a more differentiated state that limits effacement and proteinuria.[138]

Adverse effects of the calcineurin inhibitors are well known, and may be dose limiting given the extended time periods that patients are required to remain on these agents in order to induce and maintain a clinical effect. Nephrotoxicity is of most concern, but other adverse effects include tremor, neuropathy, hypertension, gingival hyperplasia, and hyperglycemia (with tacrolimus).

Treatment of Advanced Disease

Patients sometimes present to medical attention after the disease has been present but undiagnosed for many months to years, and they may have developed significant renal dysfunction by that time. Several studies have shown that immunosuppressive therapy is still of use in selected patients, even in advanced renal disease. MN patients with heavy baseline proteinuria and progressive renal dysfunction who were randomized to cyclosporine had decreased proteinuria and slower progression of renal disease at 1 year, compared to those treated with supportive therapy alone.[139] Based on the toxicity of currently available therapies and this ability to successfully treat MN despite worsening renal function, Wetzels' group in the Netherlands has recommended a restrictive policy of treatment and has provided data that delaying treatment until there is evidence of renal disease progression does not alter long-term outcome.[140]

Alternative Agents

Due to the often severe adverse or nephrotoxic effects associated with the alkylating agents and calcineurin inhibitors, several newer and potentially less toxic agents are under evaluation for the treatment of MN. These studies tend to be of short duration and lack the benefit of long-term follow-up data.

Mycophenolate

Mycophenolate is another important immunosuppressive agent widely used in renal transplantation and lupus, but thus far has only been studied for the treatment of MN in the form of small trials of limited duration. The results have been varied. Initial studies[141,142] demonstrated that mycophenolate could reduce proteinuria in MN patients who had not responded to other conventional therapies. Although a recent randomized controlled trial demonstrated no effect of mycophenolate monotherapy in patients with normal renal function and nephrotic levels of proteinuria, compared to conservative antiproteinuric therapy alone,[143] its combination with corticosteroids may be more effective. Two randomized controlled trials[144,145] and one nonrandomized study that used a matched historically treated control group[146] all showed a composite remission rate of approximately 65% in response to 6 to 12 months of therapy with mycophenolate and steroids, compared to rates of 67% to 80% in the control groups treated with alkylating agents and steroids. The median lengths of follow-up ranged from 15 to 23 months. One study revealed a relapse rate of nearly 40% in the mycophenolate group.[146] Given these small studies with insufficient long-term follow-up, mycophenolate is not a first-line agent for the treatment of MN but may be considered, with adjunctive corticosteroids, if standard therapies are not effective or cannot be tolerated.

Rituximab

Rituximab is a B cell depleting humanized anti-CD20 antibody that has been widely used in the treatment of B cell lymphomas and a number of rheumatologic diseases. The rationale for its use in MN is plausible, given the role of humoral immunity and the presence of B cells within the kidney.[110] Although rituximab appears to induce remission with an initial efficacy that is similar to that provided by alkylating agents in combination with corticosteroids,[147] long-term data on dialysis-free survival have yet to be reported. In addition, there have not been consistent dosing protocols,[148–150] leaving the optimal treatment regimen still in question. A recent open-label trial that benefited from 24 months of follow-up involved the treatment of 20 high-risk MN patients with four weekly injections of 375 mg per m^2 body surface area.[151] Of the 18 patients who completed the 24 months (two were discontinued and switched to other agents due to a perceived lack of clinical benefit), there were 4 complete and 12 partial remissions. One other patient achieved a complete remission at 18 months, but had relapsed by the final time point. Patients who have not responded to other immunosuppressive therapies are not precluded from demonstrating a clinical response to rituximab.[152] Potential short-term adverse effects of rituximab seem limited to a mild infusion reaction, but longer term side effects such as the development of progressive multifocal leukoencephalopathy, as has been seen in patients with lupus treated with this agent, await longer term follow-up data.

Adrenocorticotrophic Hormone

Another intriguing agent that may have clinical utility in MN is adrenocorticotrophic hormone (ACTH). In an open-label study, Berg and colleagues treated 14 MN patients subcutaneously with a synthetic form of ACTH over an 8-week period, and achieved short-term results similar to those described previously.[153] Another small trial randomized 32 treatment-naïve patients with primary MN who had preserved renal function to either 1 year of ACTH therapy or 6 months of alternating therapy with alkylating agents and prednisone.[154] At 1 year, 87% in the ACTH group had achieved a complete or partial remission, versus 93% in the standard therapy group. Although not significant, there were twice as many complete remissions in the ACTH group. The synthetic formulation of ACTH used in these European studies differs from the form available in the United States, and there are no long-term follow-up studies that document the efficacy of this agent. Because exogenous corticosteroids given as monotherapy lack therapeutic effect in MN, the effects of synthetic ACTH are likely to extend beyond merely increased adrenal release of endogenous corticosteroids. The 13 N-terminal amino acids of ACTH comprise another small immunomodulatory hormone known as alpha-melanocyte stimulating hormone, and it is possible that some of the effect in MN may be due to these melanocortin peptides.

CONCLUSION

It is clear that a significant proportion of patients with MN will require treatment with immunosuppressive agents to cause remission of disease and to preserve their long-term renal function. A 6-month or longer period of conservative therapy with antiproteinuric therapy and diuretics is often warranted, in the absence of already-impaired or worsening renal function, to identify those who might spontaneously remit. Once the utility of anti-PLA_2R antibodies has been validated in larger studies, there might also be a role for the serologic monitoring of patients to assess immunologic disease activity. Clinically validated treatment protocols for MN include alkylating agents or cyclosporine, both in combination with corticosteroids, although newer agents such as rituximab or mycophenolate may also permanently join the armamentarium if the effects they have shown in small studies of limited duration hold up in the longer term.

REFERENCES

1. Braden GL, Mulhern JG, O'Shea MH, et al. Changing incidence of glomerular diseases in adults. *Am J Kidney Dis.* 2000;35:878–883.

2. Haas M, Meehan SM, Karrison TG, et al. Changing etiologies of unexplained adult nephrotic syndrome: a comparison of renal biopsy findings from 1976–1979 and 1995–1997. *Am J Kidney Dis.* 1997;30:621–631.

3. Korbet SM, Genchi RM, Borok RZ, et al. The racial prevalence of glomerular lesions in nephrotic adults. *Am J Kidney Dis.* 1996;27:647–651.

4. Leaf DE, Appel GB, Radhakrishnan J. Glomerular disease: why is there a dearth of high quality clinical trials? *Kidney Int.* 2010;78:337–342.

5. Stanescu HC, Arcos-Burgos M, Medlar A, et al. Risk HLA-DQA1 and PLA(2)R1 alleles in idiopathic membranous nephropathy. *N Engl J Med.* 2011; 364:616–626.

6. Chen A, Frank R, Vento S, et al. Idiopathic membranous nephropathy in pediatric patients: presentation, response to therapy, and long-term outcome. *BMC Nephrol.* 2007;8:11.

7. Moutzouris DA, Herlitz L, Appel GB, et al. Renal biopsy in the very elderly. *Clin J Am Soc Nephrol.* 2009;4:1073–1082.

8. Johnson RJ, Couser WG. Hepatitis B infection and renal disease: clinical, immunopathogenetic and therapeutic considerations. *Kidney Int.* 1990;37:663–676.

9. Dabade TS, Grande JP, Norby SM, et al. Recurrent idiopathic membranous nephropathy after kidney transplantation: a surveillance biopsy study. *Am J Transplant.* 2008;8:1318–1322.

10. Cahen R, Francois B, Trolliet P, et al. Aetiology of membranous glomerulonephritis: a prospective study of 82 adult patients. *Nephrol Dial Transplant.* 1989; 4:172–180.

11. Zeng CH, Chen HM, Wang RS, et al. Etiology and clinical characteristics of membranous nephropathy in Chinese patients. *Am J Kidney Dis.* 2008;52:691–698.

12. Bakir AA, Levy PS, Dunea G. The prognosis of lupus nephritis in African-Americans: a retrospective analysis. *Am J Kidney Dis.* 1994;24:159–171.

13. Kolasinski SL, Chung JB, Albert DA. What do we know about lupus membranous nephropathy? An analytic review. *Arthritis Rheum.* 2002;47:450–455.

14. Yoshida A, Morozumi K, Takeda A, et al. Membranous glomerulonephritis in patients with rheumatoid arthritis. *Clin Ther* 1994;16:1000–1006.

15. Ronco P, Debiec H. Pathophysiological lessons from rare associations of immunological disorders. *Pediatr Nephrol.* 2009;24:3–8.

16. Shima Y, Nakanishi K, Togawa H, et al. Membranous nephropathy associated with thyroid-peroxidase antigen. *Pediatr Nephrol.* 2009;24:605–608.

17. Saeki T, Imai N, Ito T, et al. Membranous nephropathy associated with IgG4–related systemic disease and without autoimmune pancreatitis. *Clin Nephrol.* 2009;71:173–178.

18. Watson SJ, Jenkins DA, Bellamy CO. Nephropathy in IgG4–related systemic disease. *Am J Surg Pathol.* 2006;30:1472–1477.

19. Dimitriades C, Shetty AK, Vehaskari M, et al. Membranous nephropathy associated with childhood sarcoidosis. *Pediatr Nephrol.* 1999;13:444–447.

20. Toda T, Kimoto S, Nishio Y, et al. Sarcoidosis with membranous nephropathy and granulomatous interstitial nephritis. *Intern Med.* 1999;38:882–886.

21. Knehtl M, Debiec H, Kamgang P, et al. A case of phospholipase A receptor-positive membranous nephropathy preceding sarcoid-associated granulomatous tubulointerstitial nephritis. *Am J Kidney Dis.* 2011;57:140–143.

22. Combes B, Shorey J, Barrera A, et al. Glomerulonephritis with deposition of Australian antigen-antibody complexes in glomerular basement membrane. *Lancet.* 1971;2:234–237.

23. Wrzolkowa T, Zurowska A, Uszycka-Karcz M, et al. Hepatitis B virus-associated glomerulonephritis: electron microscopic studies in 98 children. *Am J Kidney Dis.* 1991;18:306–312.

24. Yoshikawa N, Ito H, Yamada Y, et al. Membranous glomerulonephritis associated with hepatitis B antigen in children: a comparison with idiopathic membranous glomerulonephritis. *Clin Nephrol.* 1985;23:28–34.

25. Lai KN, Li PK, Lui SF, et al. Membranous nephropathy related to hepatitis B virus in adults. *N Engl J Med.* 1991;324:1457–1463.

26. Xu H, Sun L, Zhou LJ, et al. The effect of hepatitis B vaccination on the incidence of childhood HBV-associated nephritis. *Pediatr Nephrol.* 2003;18:1216–1219.

27. Hoch B, Juknevicius I, Liapis H. Glomerular injury associated with hepatitis C infection: a correlation with blood and tissue HCV-PCR. *Semin Diagn Pathol.* 2002;19:175–187.

28. Morales JM, Pascual-Capdevila J, Campistol JM, et al. Membranous glomerulonephritis associated with hepatitis C virus infection in renal transplant patients. *Transplantation.* 1997;63:1634–1639.

29. Cohen SD, Kimmel PL. Immune complex renal disease and human immunodeficiency virus infection. *Semin Nephrol.* 2008;28:535–544.

30. Haas M, Kaul S, Eustace JA. HIV-associated immune complex glomerulonephritis with "lupus-like" features: a clinicopathologic study of 14 cases. *Kidney Int.* 2005;67:1381–1390.

31. Nebuloni M, Barbiano di Belgiojoso G, Genderini A, et al. Glomerular lesions in HIV-positive patients: a 20-year biopsy experience from Northern Italy. *Clin Nephrol.* 2009;72:38–45.

32. Barsoum RS. Schistosomal glomerulopathies. *Kidney Int.* 1993;44:1–12.

33. Sanchez-Bayle M, Ecija JL, Estepa R, et al. Incidence of glomerulonephritis in congenital syphilis. *Clin Nephrol.* 1983;20:27–31.

34. Hunte W, al-Ghraoui F, Cohen RJ. Secondary syphilis and the nephrotic syndrome. *J Am Soc Nephrol.* 1993;3:1351–1355.

35. O'Regan S, Fong JS, de Chadarevian JP, et al. Treponemal antigens in congenital and acquired syphilitic nephritis: demonstration by immunofluorescence studies. *Ann Intern Med.* 1976;85:325–327.

36. Chen WP, Chiang H, Lin CY. Persistent histological and immunological abnormalities in congenital syphilitic glomerulonephritis after disappearance of proteinuria. *Child Nephrol Urol.* 1988;9:93–97.

37. Gamble CN, Reardan JB. Immunopathogenesis of syphilitic glomerulonephritis. Elution of antitreponemal antibody from glomerular immune-complex deposits. *N Engl J Med.* 1975;292:449–454.

38. Lee JC, Yamauchi H, Hopper J Jr. The association of cancer and the nephrotic syndrome. *Ann Intern Med.* 1966;64:41–51.

39. Alpers CE, Cotran RS. Neoplasia and glomerular injury. *Kidney Int.* 1986;30:465–473.

40. Beck LH Jr. Membranous nephropathy and malignancy. *Semin Nephrol.* 2010;30:635–644.

41. Bjorneklett R, Vikse BE, Svarstad E, et al. Long-term risk of cancer in membranous nephropathy patients. *Am J Kidney Dis.* 2007;50:396–403.

42. Burstein DM, Korbet SM, Schwartz MM. Membranous glomerulonephritis and malignancy. *Am J Kidney Dis.* 1993;22:5–10.

43. Lefaucheur C, Stengel B, Nochy D, et al. Membranous nephropathy and cancer: Epidemiologic evidence and determinants of high-risk cancer association. *Kidney Int.* 2006;70:1510–1517.

44. Row PG, Cameron JS, Turner DR, et al. Membranous nephropathy. Long-term follow-up and association with neoplasia. *Q J Med.* 1975;44:207–239.

45. Da'as N, Polliack A, Cohen Y, et al. Kidney involvement and renal manifestations in non-Hodgkin's lymphoma and lymphocytic leukemia: a retrospective study in 700 patients. *Eur J Haematol.* 2001;67:158–164.

46. Costanza ME, Pinn V, Schwartz RS, et al. Carcinoembryonic antigen-antibody complexes in a patient with colonic carcinoma and nephrotic syndrome. *N Engl J Med.* 1973;289:520–522.

47. Couser WG, Wagonfeld JB, Spargo BH, et al. Glomerular deposition of tumor antigen in membranous nephropathy associated with colonic carcinoma. *Am J Med.* 1974;57:962–970.

48. Qin W, Beck LH Jr, Zeng C, et al. Anti-phospholipase A2 receptor antibody in membranous nephropathy. *J Am Soc Nephrol.* 2011;22:1137–1143.

49. Ohtani H, Wakui H, Komatsuda A, et al. Distribution of glomerular IgG subclass deposits in malignancy-associated membranous nephropathy. *Nephrol Dial Transplant.* 2004;19:574–579.

50. Katz WA, Blodgett RC Jr, Pietrusko RG. Proteinuria in gold-treated rheumatoid arthritis. *Ann Intern Med.* 1984;101:176–179.

51. Chakera A, Lasserson D, Beck LH Jr, et al. Membranous nephropathy after use of UK-manufactured skin creams containing mercury. *QJM.* 2011;104:893–896.

52. Li SJ, Zhang SH, Chen HP, et al. Mercury-induced membranous nephropathy: clinical and pathological features. *Clin J Am Soc Nephrol.* 2010;5:439–444.

53. Hall CL, Jawad S, Harrison PR, et al. Natural course of penicillamine nephropathy: a long term study of 33 patients. *Br Med J (Clin Res Ed).* 1988;296:1083–1086.

54. Campistol JM, Galofre J, Botey A, et al. Reversible membranous nephritis associated with diclofenac. *Nephrol Dial Transplant.* 1989;4:393–395.

55. Radford MG Jr, Holley KE, Grande JP, et al. Reversible membranous nephropathy associated with the use of nonsteroidal anti-inflammatory drugs. *JAMA.* 1996;276:466–469.

56. Markowitz GS, Falkowitz DC, Isom R, et al. Membranous glomerulopathy and acute interstitial nephritis following treatment with celecoxib. *Clin Nephrol.* 2003;59:137–142.

57. Ronco P, Debiec H, Guigonis V. Mechanisms of disease: Alloimmunization in renal diseases. *Nat Clin Pract Nephrol.* 2006;2:388–397.

58. Brukamp K, Doyle AM, Bloom RD, et al. Nephrotic syndrome after hematopoietic cell transplantation: do glomerular lesions represent renal graft-versus-host disease? *Clin J Am Soc Nephrol.* 2006;1:685–694.

59. Terrier B, Delmas Y, Hummel A, et al. Post-allogeneic haematopoietic stem cell transplantation membranous nephropathy: clinical presentation, outcome and pathogenic aspects. *Nephrol Dial Transplant.* 2007;22:1369–1376.

60. Debiec H, Guigonis V, Mougenot B, et al. Antenatal membranous glomerulonephritis due to anti-neutral endopeptidase antibodies. *N Engl J Med.* 2002;346:2053–2060.

61. Debiec H, Nauta J, Coulet F, et al. Role of truncating mutations in MME gene in fetomaternal alloimmunisation and antenatal glomerulopathies. *Lancet.* 2004;364:1252–1259.

62. Debiec H, Lefeu F, Kemper MJ, et al. Early-childhood membranous nephropathy due to cationic bovine serum albumin. *N Engl J Med.* 2011;364:2101–2110.

63. Monga G, Mazzucco G, di Belgiojoso GB, et al. Pattern of double glomerulopathies: a clinicopathologic study of superimposed glomerulonephritis on diabetic glomerulosclerosis. *Mod Pathol.* 1989;2:407–414.

64. Furuta T, Seino J, Saito T, et al. Insulin deposits in membranous nephropathy associated with diabetes mellitus. *Clin Nephrol.* 1992;37:65–69.

65. Nasr SH, Said SM, Valeri AM, et al. Membranous glomerulonephritis with ANCA-associated necrotizing and crescentic glomerulonephritis. *Clin J Am Soc Nephrol.* 2009;4:299–308.

66. Jones DB. Nephrotic glomerulonephritis. *Am J Pathol.* 1957;33:313–329.

67. Mellors RC, Ortega LG. Analytical pathology. III. New observations on the pathogenesis of glomerulonephritis, lipid nephrosis, periarteritis nodosa, and secondary amyloidosis in man. *Am J Pathol.* 1956;32:455–499.

68. Salant DJ, Adler S, Darby C, et al. Influence of antigen distribution on the mediation of immunological glomerular injury. *Kidney Int.* 1985;27:938–950.

69. Haas M. IgG subclass deposits in glomeruli of lupus and nonlupus membranous nephropathies. *Am J Kidney Dis.* 1994;23:358–364.

70. Doi T, Mayumi M, Kanatsu K, et al. Distribution of IgG subclasses in membranous nephropathy. *Clin Exp Immunol.* 1984;58:57–62.

71. Kuroki A, Shibata T, Honda H, et al. Glomerular and serum IgG subclasses in diffuse proliferative lupus nephritis, membranous lupus nephritis, and idiopathic membranous nephropathy. *Intern Med.* 2002;41:936–942.

72. Moseley HL, Whaley K. Control of complement activation in membranous and membranoproliferative glomerulonephritis. *Kidney Int.* 1980;17:535–544.

73. Yang AH, Lin BS, Kuo KL, et al. The clinicopathological implications of endothelial tubuloreticular inclusions found in glomeruli having histopathology of idiopathic membranous nephropathy. *Nephrol Dial Transplant.* 2009;24(11):3419–3425.

74. Obana M, Nakanishi K, Sako M, et al. Segmental membranous glomerulonephritis in children: comparison with global membranous glomerulonephritis. *Clin J Am Soc Nephrol.* 2006;1:723–729.

75. Kowalewska J, Smith KD, Hudkins KL, et al. Membranous glomerulopathy with spherules: an uncommon variant with obscure pathogenesis. *Am J Kidney Dis.* 2006;47:983–992.

76. Salant DJ, Sanchorawala V, D'Agati VD. A case of atypical light chain deposition disease—diagnosis and treatment. *Clin J Am Soc Nephrol.* 2007;2:858–867.

77. de Seigneux S, Bindi P, Debiec H, et al. Immunoglobulin deposition disease with a membranous pattern and a circulating monoclonal immunoglobulin G with charge-dependent aggregation properties. *Am J Kidney Dis.* 2010;56:117–121.

78. Komatsuda A, Masai R, Ohtani H, et al. Monoclonal immunoglobulin deposition disease associated with membranous features. *Nephrol Dial Transplant.* 2008;23:3888–3894.

79. Nasr SH, Satoskar A, Markowitz GS, et al. Proliferative glomerulonephritis with monoclonal IgG deposits. *J Am Soc Nephrol.* 2009;20:2055–2064.

80. Heymann W, Hackel DB, Harwood S, et al. Production of nephrotic syndrome in rats by Freund's adjuvants and rat kidney suspensions. *Proc Soc Exp Biol Med.* 1959;100:660–664.

81. Cybulsky AV, Quigg RJ, Salant DJ. Experimental membranous nephropathy redux. *Am J Physiol Renal Physiol* 2005;289:F660–671.

82. Kerjaschki D, Neale TJ. Molecular mechanisms of glomerular injury in rat experimental membranous nephropathy (Heymann nephritis). *J Am Soc Nephrol.* 1996;7:2518–2526.

83. Nangaku M, Shankland SJ, Couser WG. Cellular response to injury in membranous nephropathy. *J Am Soc Nephrol.* 2005;16:1195–1204.

84. Couser WG, Steinmuller DR, Stilmant MM, et al. Experimental glomerulonephritis in the isolated perfused rat kidney. *J Clin Invest.* 1978;62:1275–1287.

85. Van Damme BJ, Fleuren GJ, Bakker WW, et al. Experimental glomerulonephritis in the rat induced by antibodies directed against tubular antigens. V. Fixed glomerular antigens in the pathogenesis of heterologous immune complex glomerulonephritis. *Lab Invest.* 1978;38:502–510.

86. Kerjaschki D, Farquhar MG. The pathogenic antigen of Heymann nephritis is a membrane glycoprotein of the renal proximal tubule brush border. *Proc Natl Acad Sci U S A.* 1982;79:5557–5561.
87. Kerjaschki D, Farquhar MG. Immunocytochemical localization of the Heymann nephritis antigen (GP330) in glomerular epithelial cells of normal Lewis rats. *J Exp Med.* 1983;157:667–686.
88. Makker SP, Singh AK. Characterization of the antigen (gp600) of Heymann nephritis. *Lab Invest.* 1984;50:287–293.
89. Raychowdhury R, Niles JL, McCluskey RT, et al. Autoimmune target in Heymann nephritis is a glycoprotein with homology to the LDL receptor. *Science.* 1989;244:1163–1165.
90. Saito A, Pietromonaco S, Loo AK, et al. Complete cloning and sequencing of rat gp330/"megalin," a distinctive member of the low density lipoprotein receptor gene family. *Proc Natl Acad Sci U S A.* 1994;91:9725–9729.
91. Camussi G, Noble B, Van Liew J, et al. Pathogenesis of passive Heymann glomerulonephritis: chlorpromazine inhibits antibody-mediated redistribution of cell surface antigens and prevents development of the disease. *J Immunol.* 1986;136:2127–2135.
92. Kerjaschki D, Miettinen A, Farquhar MG. Initial events in the formation of immune deposits in passive Heymann nephritis. *J Exp Med.* 1987;166:109–128.
93. Minto AW, Fogel MA, Natori Y, et al. Expression of type I collagen mRNA in glomeruli of rats with passive Heymann nephritis. *Kidney Int.* 1993;43:121–127.
94. Hinglais N, Kazatchkine MD, Bhakdi S, et al. Immunohistochemical study of the C5b-9 complex of complement in human kidneys. *Kidney Int.* 1986;30:399–410.
95. Brenchley PE, Coupes B, Short CD, et al. Urinary C3dg and C5b-9 indicate active immune disease in human membranous nephropathy. *Kidney Int.* 1992;41:933–937.
96. Aalberse RC, Stapel SO, Schuurman J, et al. Immunoglobulin G4: an odd antibody. *Clin Exp Allergy.* 2009;39:469–477.
97. Beck LH Jr, Bonegio RG, Lambeau G, et al. M-type phospholipase A2 receptor as target antigen in idiopathic membranous nephropathy. *N Engl J Med.* 2009;361:11–21.
98. Ancian P, Lambeau G, Mattei MG, et al. The human 180–kDa receptor for secretory phospholipases A2. Molecular cloning, identification of a secreted soluble form, expression, and chromosomal localization. *J Biol Chem.* 1995;270:8963–8970.
99. East L, Isacke CM. The mannose receptor family. *Biochim Biophys Acta.* 2002;1572:364–386.
100. Hofstra JM, Beck LH Jr, Beck DM, et al. Anti-phospholipase A2 receptor antibodies correlate with clinical status in idiopathic membranous nephropathy. *Clin J Am Soc Nephrol.* 2011;6(6):1286–1291.
101. Debiec H, Ronco P. PLA2R autoantibodies and PLA2R glomerular deposits in membranous nephropathy. *N Engl J Med.* 2011;364:689–690.
102. Prunotto M, Carnevali ML, Candiano G, et al. Autoimmunity in membranous nephropathy targets aldose reductase and SOD2. *J Am Soc Nephrol.* 2010;21: 507–519.
103. Ruggenenti P, Cravedi P, Sghirlanzoni MC, et al. Effects of rituximab on morphofunctional abnormalities of membranous glomerulopathy. *Clin J Am Soc Nephrol.* 2008;3:1652–1659.
104. Makker SP, Kanalas JJ. Course of transplanted Heymann nephritis kidney in normal host. Implications for mechanism of proteinuria in membranous glomerulonephropathy. *J Immunol.* 1989;142:3406–3410.
105. Kalaaji M, Fenton KA, Mortensen ES, et al. Glomerular apoptotic nucleosomes are central target structures for nephritogenic antibodies in human SLE nephritis. *Kidney Int.* 2007;71:664–672.
106. Chevrier D, Giral M, Perrichot R, et al. Idiopathic and secondary membranous nephropathy and polymorphism at TAP1 and HLA-DMA loci. *Tissue Antigens.* 1997;50:164–169.
107. Ogahara S, Naito S, Abe K, et al. Analysis of HLA class II genes in Japanese patients with idiopathic membranous glomerulonephritis. *Kidney Int.* 1992;41:175–182.
108. Kim S, Chin HJ, Na KY, et al. Single nucleotide polymorphisms in the phospholipase A(2) receptor gene are associated with genetic susceptibility to idiopathic membranous nephropathy. *Nephron Clin Pract.* 2010;117: c253–c258.
109. Liu YH, Chen CH, Chen SY, Lin YJ, et al. Association of phospholipase A2 receptor 1 polymorphisms with idiopathic membranous nephropathy in Chinese patients in Taiwan. *J Biomed Sci* 2010;17:81.
110. Cohen CD, Calvaresi N, Armelloni S, et al. CD20–positive infiltrates in human membranous glomerulonephritis. *J Nephrol.* 2005;18:328–333.
111. Glassock RJ. Prophylactic anticoagulation in nephrotic syndrome: a clinical conundrum. *J Am Soc Nephrol.* 2007;18:2221–2225.
112. Hladunewich MA, Troyanov S, Calafati J, et al. The natural history of the non-nephrotic membranous nephropathy patient. *Clin J Am Soc Nephrol.* 2009;4:1417–1422.
113. Schieppati A, Mosconi L, Perna A, et al. Prognosis of untreated patients with idiopathic membranous nephropathy. *N Engl J Med.* 1993;329:85–89.
114. du Buf-Vereijken PW, Branten AJ, Wetzels JF. Idiopathic membranous nephropathy: outline and rationale of a treatment strategy. *Am J Kidney Dis.* 2005;46: 1012–1029.
115. Polanco N, Gutierrez E, Covarsi A, et al. Spontaneous remission of nephrotic syndrome in idiopathic membranous nephropathy. *J Am Soc Nephrol.* 2010;21: 697–704.
116. Dumoulin A, Hill GS, Montseny JJ, et al. Clinical and morphological prognostic factors in membranous nephropathy: significance of focal segmental glomerulosclerosis. *Am J Kidney Dis.* 2003;41:38–48.
117. Troyanov S, Roasio L, Pandes M, et al. Renal pathology in idiopathic membranous nephropathy: a new perspective. *Kidney Int.* 2006;69:1641–1648.
118. Shiiki H, Saito T, Nishitani Y, et al. Prognosis and risk factors for idiopathic membranous nephropathy with nephrotic syndrome in Japan. *Kidney Int.* 2004;65: 1400–1407.
119. Branten AJ, du Buf-Vereijken PW, Klasen IS, et al. Urinary excretion of beta2–microglobulin and IgG predict prognosis in idiopathic membranous nephropathy: a validation study. *J Am Soc Nephrol.* 2005;16:169–174.
120. Cattran D. Management of membranous nephropathy: when and what for treatment. *J Am Soc Nephrol.* 2005;16:1188–1194.
121. Troyanov S, Wall CA, Miller JA, et al. Idiopathic membranous nephropathy: definition and relevance of a partial remission. *Kidney Int.* 2004;66: 1199–1205.
122. Austin HA III, Illei GG, Braun MJ, et al. Randomized, controlled trial of prednisone, cyclophosphamide, and cyclosporine in lupus membranous nephropathy. *J Am Soc Nephrol.* 2009;20:901–911.
123. Szeto CC, Kwan BC, Lai FM, et al. Tacrolimus for the treatment of systemic lupus erythematosus with pure class V nephritis. *Rheumatology (Oxford).* 2008;47: 1678–1681.
124. Tse KC, Lam MF, Tang SC, et al. A pilot study on tacrolimus treatment in membranous or quiescent lupus nephritis with proteinuria resistant to angiotensin inhibition or blockade. *Lupus.* 2007;16:46–51.
125. Radhakrishnan J, Moutzouris DA, Ginzler EM, et al. Mycophenolate mofetil and intravenous cyclophosphamide are similar as induction therapy for class V lupus nephritis. *Kidney Int.* 2010;77:152–160.
126. Waldman M, Austin HA III. Controversies in the treatment of idiopathic membranous nephropathy. *Nat Rev Nephrol.* 2009;5:469–479.
127. Beck LH Jr, Salant DJ. Treatment of membranous lupus nephritis: where are we now? *J Am Soc Nephrol.* 2009;20:690–691.
128. Fervenza FC, Sethi S, Specks U. Idiopathic membranous nephropathy: diagnosis and treatment. *Clin J Am Soc Nephrol.* 2008;3:905–919.
129. Hogan SL, Muller KE, Jennette JC, et al. A review of therapeutic studies of idiopathic membranous glomerulopathy. *Am J Kidney Dis.* 1995;25:862–875.
130. Ponticelli C, Zucchelli P, Passerini P, et al. A randomized trial of methylprednisolone and chlorambucil in idiopathic membranous nephropathy. *N Engl J Med.* 1989;320: 8–13.
131. Ponticelli C, Zucchelli P, Passerini P, et al. A 10–year follow-up of a randomized study with methylprednisolone and chlorambucil in membranous nephropathy. *Kidney Int.* 1995;48:1600–1604.
132. Ponticelli C, Altieri P, Scolari F, et al. A randomized study comparing methylprednisolone plus chlorambucil versus methylprednisolone plus cyclophosphamide in idiopathic membranous nephropathy. *J Am Soc Nephrol.* 1998;9:444–450.
133. Jha V, Ganguli A, Saha TK, et al. A randomized, controlled trial of steroids and cyclophosphamide in adults with nephrotic syndrome caused by idiopathic membranous nephropathy. *J Am Soc Nephrol.* 2007;18:1899–1904.
134. Cattran DC, Alexopoulos E, Heering P, et al. Cyclosporin in idiopathic glomerular disease associated with the nephrotic syndrome: Workshop recommendations. *Kidney Int.* 2007;72:1429–1447.
135. Cattran DC, Appel GB, Hebert LA, et al. Cyclosporine in patients with steroid-resistant membranous nephropathy: a randomized trial. *Kidney Int.* 2001;59:1484–1490.
136. Alexopoulos E, Papagianni A, Tsamelashvili M, et al. Induction and long-term treatment with cyclosporine in membranous nephropathy with the nephrotic syndrome. *Nephrol Dial Transplant.* 2006;21:3127–3132.
137. Praga M, Barrio V, Juarez GF, et al. Tacrolimus monotherapy in membranous nephropathy: a randomized controlled trial. *Kidney Int.* 2007;71:924–930.
138. Faul C, Donnelly M, Merscher-Gomez S, et al. The actin cytoskeleton of kidney podocytes is a direct target of the antiproteinuric effect of cyclosporine A. *Nat Med.* 2008;14:931–938.
139. Cattran DC, Greenwood C, Ritchie S, et al. A controlled trial of cyclosporine in patients with progressive membranous nephropathy. Canadian Glomerulonephritis Study Group. *Kidney Int.* 1995;47:1130–1135.

140. du Buf-Vereijken PW, Feith GW, Hollander D, et al. Restrictive use of immunosuppressive treatment in patients with idiopathic membranous nephropathy: high renal survival in a large patient cohort. *QJM.* 2004;97: 353–360.

141. Choi MJ, Eustace JA, Gimenez LF, et al. Mycophenolate mofetil treatment for primary glomerular diseases. *Kidney Int.* 2002;61:1098–1114.

142. Miller G, Zimmerman R III, Radhakrishnan J, et al. Use of mycophenolate mofetil in resistant membranous nephropathy. *Am J Kidney Dis.* 2000;36: 250–256.

143. Dussol B, Morange S, Burtey S, et al. Mycophenolate mofetil monotherapy in membranous nephropathy: a 1–year randomized controlled trial. *Am J Kidney Dis.* 2008;52:699–705.

144. Chan TM, Lin AW, Tang SC, et al. Prospective controlled study on mycophenolate mofetil and prednisolone in the treatment of membranous nephropathy with nephrotic syndrome. *Nephrology (Carlton).* 2007;12:576–581.

145. Senthil Nayagam L, Ganguli A, Rathi M, et al. Mycophenolate mofetil or standard therapy for membranous nephropathy and focal segmental glomerulosclerosis: a pilot study. *Nephrol Dial Transplant.* 2008;23:1926–1930.

146. Branten AJ, du Buf-Vereijken PW, Vervloet M, et al. Mycophenolate mofetil in idiopathic membranous nephropathy: a clinical trial with comparison to a historic control group treated with cyclophosphamide. *Am J Kidney Dis.* 2007;50:248–256.

147. Bomback AS, Derebail VK, McGregor JG, et al. Rituximab therapy for membranous nephropathy: a systematic review. *Clin J Am Soc Nephrol.* 2009;4:734–744.

148. Cravedi P, Ruggenenti P, Sghirlanzoni MC, et al. Titrating rituximab to circulating B cells to optimize lymphocytolytic therapy in idiopathic membranous nephropathy. *Clin J Am Soc Nephrol.* 2007;2:932–937.

149. Fervenza FC, Cosio FG, Erickson SB, et al. Rituximab treatment of idiopathic membranous nephropathy. *Kidney Int.* 2008;73:117–125.

150. Ruggenenti P, Chiurchiu C, Brusegan V, et al. Rituximab in idiopathic membranous nephropathy: a one-year prospective study. *J Am Soc Nephrol.* 2003;14:1851–1857.

151. Fervenza FC, Abraham RS, Erickson SB, et al. Rituximab therapy in idiopathic membranous nephropathy: a 2–year study. *Clin J Am Soc Nephrol.* 2010;5:2188–2198.

152. Cravedi P, Sghirlanzoni MC, Marasa M, et al. Efficacy and safety of rituximab second-line therapy for membranous nephropathy: a prospective, matched-cohort study. *Am J Nephrol.* 2011;33:461–468.

153. Berg AL, Nilsson-Ehle P, Arnadottir M. Beneficial effects of ACTH on the serum lipoprotein profile and glomerular function in patients with membranous nephropathy. *Kidney Int.* 1999;56:1534–1543.

154. Ponticelli C, Passerini P, Salvadori M, et al. A randomized pilot trial comparing methylprednisolone plus a cytotoxic agent versus synthetic adrenocorticotropic hormone in idiopathic membranous nephropathy. *Am J Kidney Dis.* 2006;47:233–240.

CHAPTER

52 Nephrotic Syndrome and the Podocytopathies: Minimal Change Nephropathy, Focal Segmental Glomerulosclerosis, and Collapsing Glomerulopathy

H. William Schnaper • Jeffrey B. Kopp

The term *nephrotic syndrome* refers to a classic tetrad of proteinuria, hypoproteinemia, edema, and hyperlipidemia. Although a relationship among these findings was recognized as early as the 15th century, the term *nephrosis* first achieved widespread acceptance in the early part of the 20th century, when Volhard and Fahr employed it as one of the major divisions of bilateral kidney disease.[1] Later developments, notably the advent of the percutaneous kidney biopsy, facilitated further delineation of the many forms of kidney disease that result in the nephrotic syndrome.[2,3] We have divided these diseases into three general categories, as shown in Table 52.1: (1) primary nephrotic syndrome, in which the process that initiates proteinuria is not immediately apparent from histopathologic evaluation; (2) inflammatory glomerular lesions; and (3) glomerulopathy secondary to other diseases that affect the kidney. Regardless of the underlying cause, all of these diseases share a common denominator in that each involves proteinuria of sufficient severity to produce hypoproteinemia. Typically, when the serum albumin concentration falls below a critical level of approximately 2 g per deciliter, the other clinical features of the nephrotic syndrome appear.

An analysis of the diseases underlying nephrosis is complicated because studies have used varied definitions; different methods of acquiring patient populations; and groupings that reflect clinical, functional, or histologic criteria. Clearly, the relative frequency of different causes of nephrosis varies with age and has changed over time. The data in Table 52.1 were developed more than 30 years ago and indicated that approximately 80% of children with renal disease had primary nephrotic syndrome, as opposed to only 25% of adults. Chronic glomerulonephritis was responsible for about half of the cases of nephrotic syndrome in adults but only 10% to 15% of childhood cases. These glomerulonephritides may result from a systemic disease, such as systemic lupus erythematosus, or they may be idiopathic, such as in membranous nephropathy. The remaining cases of nephrotic syndrome were associated with diseases such as diabetes mellitus and amyloidosis. They accounted for up to 20% of adult cases and only a very small percentage of childhood cases. This general pattern of causes for nephrotic syndrome is still observed in most industrial countries; additional causes are more likely to be seen in developing nations.[4–8]

This chapter focuses on the group of diseases subsumed under the category of *primary nephrotic syndrome*. We employ this term to describe the clinical picture of nephrotic syndrome that occurs in the absence of evidence for glomerulonephritis or systemic disease that would be sufficient to account for massive proteinuria. Primary nephrotic syndrome includes patients who have been described as having *minimal change nephropathy* (MCN), also called lipoid nephrosis, "nil" disease, idiopathic nephrotic syndrome of childhood, minimal change nephrotic syndrome (MCNS), or steroid-sensitive or steroid-responsive nephrotic syndrome. We have chosen to use MCN as the preferred term for this entity. Nephrosis is not always present in MCN, particularly in adult patients.[9,10] Although most pathologists require at least the presence of nephrotic-range proteinuria prior to treatment to make the diagnosis of MCN, occasionally, patients may lack edema, hypoalbuminemia, or hypercholesterolemia but have renal histology and ultrastructure that are otherwise typical. Furthermore, describing the lesion as a nephropathy offers a descriptor that is in parallel with the other forms of primary nephrotic syndrome, in that it is based on the defined histopathology rather than a potentially variable clinical picture. We will reserve the alternate term, MCNS, for the clinical presentation in which MCN has caused the nephrotic syndrome. Some patients with primary nephrotic syndrome have only a small amount of immunoglobulin M (IgM) deposited in the glomeruli, which usually is believed to be insignificant; some biopsy specimens reveal mild mesangial hypercellularity. These patients are considered to represent variants of MCN. A larger group of patients have significant extracellular matrix accumulation

TABLE 52.1 **Types of Kidney Disease Causing Nephrotic Syndrome in Pediatric and Adult Patients**

	Relative Incidence	
	Children	Adults
Primary nephrotic syndrome	79	24
Nephrotic syndrome associated with a glomerulopathy		
Chronic glomerulonephritis and systemic inflammatory disease	13	52
Secondary glomerulopathy	8	24

Data derived from: International Study of Kidney Disease in Children. A controlled therapeutic trial of cyclophosphamide plus prednisone vs. prednisone alone in children with focal segmental glomerulonephritis. *Pediatr Res.* 1980;14:1006; and Glassock RJ. The nephrotic syndrome. *Hosp Pract.* 1979;14:105.

or glomerular capillary collapse. These patients are defined as having *focal segmental glomerulosclerosis* (FSGS), also called focal sclerosis and hyalinosis, and *collapsing glomerulopathy*, respectively. A spectrum of pathologic findings may be observed. Moreover, some patients, regardless of the underlying pathology, respond to treatment with corticosteroids; others with an apparently identical histologic lesion are resistant to steroid therapy.

An examination of the incidence of these diseases illustrates both the age dependence of diagnoses and the changing nature of the underlying lesion. In a large series of renal biopsies of 1,000 consecutive patients who presented with the nephrotic syndrome to a referral center, the relative incidence of different causes of nephrosis changed over time, with significantly more FSGS and less MCN.[9] Although this study could reflect some degree of referral bias, it is likely that these numbers approximate the general distribution of histologic diagnoses in nephrotic patients. Of all children 0.5 to 19 years of age in the province of Ontario who were diagnosed as having nephrotic syndrome, the incidence of FSGS also increased over time.[11] The overall proportion of patients with primary nephrotic syndrome in children was greater than 90% compared with 50% in the adult study. The increasing incidence of FSGS (which more than doubled in both children and adults) is considered further in the section on *Focal Segmental Glomerulosclerosis, Collapsing Glomerulopathy, and Diffuse Mesangial Sclerosis*, later in this chapter.

In addition to the clinical observation that inflammation does not underlie the proteinuria of primary nephrotic syndrome, advances in our understanding of these disorders suggest that the origin of all these diseases resides in the specialized visceral epithelial cell of the glomerular filter, the podocyte. This cell contributes to the final barrier that determines the nature of the glomerular filtrate, and podocyte lesions appear to play a critical role in progressive forms of primary nephrotic syndrome. For this reason, an increasingly accepted term for the lesions causing primary nephrotic syndrome is the *podocytopathies*. In Table 52.2 taxonomy of the podocytopathies is shown grouped according to histologic characteristics.[12,13] An analysis of the pathology, physiology, and genetics of these diseases, and insight derived from examining acquired causes of each lesion, was used in this categorization. Patients who show few or no glomerular abnormalities by use of light microscopy include those with classical MCN and its histologic variants, and patients with Finnish-type congenital nephrotic syndrome. A second group has diffuse mesangial sclerosis and represents mostly young children with congenital forms of nephrosis, frequently resulting from a single gene mutation. The third category, FSGS, represents an entity the incidence of which is rising rapidly throughout the world. We have also chosen to define a fourth group: patients with collapsing glomerulopathy. Although this diagnosis previously has been thought to be a part of FSGS, the histologic appearance, the clinical course, and advances in our understanding of disease pathogenesis strongly suggest that it represents a distinct lesion. Further details regarding the definition of the categories in this table will be provided in this chapter.

It is important to note that the nephrotic syndrome has many physiologic consequences that are not limited to the classic tetrad of proteinuria, hypoalbuminemia, edema, and hyperlipidemia. These include abnormalities of electrolyte balance, coagulation, hormonal function, and immunity. This chapter reviews the mechanisms underlying these manifestations of nephrosis, our understanding of the pathogenesis of different forms of the podocytopathies, and the clinical features and management of patients with this entity.

PATHOPHYSIOLOGY OF THE NEPHROTIC SYNDROME

Virtually every abnormality observed in primary nephrotic syndrome can be traced directly or indirectly to the urinary loss of protein. Thus, the mechanisms responsible for this proteinuria have systemic consequences that are manifested in the clinical signs and symptoms of nephrosis.

TABLE 52.2 **Classification of Primary Podocytopathies**

Pathology	Genetic (Mendelian Inheritance)	Acquired	Medication Induced
Minimal change histology	■ Congenital NS, Finnish type *NPHS1* *NPHS1* + *NPHS2*	■ MCN ■ MCN variants Mesangial hypercellularity IgM nephropathy Glomerular tip lesion C1q nephropathy ■ MCN, association with Hodgkin disease, infection (see Table 52.4)	■ Nonsteroidal anti-inflammatory agents ■ Gold ■ Penicillamine ■ Lithium ■ Interferon-α and -β
Diffuse mesangial sclerosis (DMS) histology	■ Congenital presentation *LAMB2* (Pierson syndrome) ■ Childhood presentation *WT1* (Denys-Drash syndrome, isolated DMS)	■ Isolated DMS	
Focal segmental glomerulosclerosis (FSGS)	■ Congenital presentation *ITGB4* ■ Infancy/childhood presentation *NPHS2* *NPHS1* + *NPHS2* WT1 (Denys-Drash syndrome, Frasier syndrome) *PAX2* (renal-coloboma syndrome with oligomeganephronia) mtDNA (MELAS syndrome) *COQ2* *MYO1E* *PTPRO* ■ Adult presentation *INF2* *ACTN4* *CD2AP* *TRPC6* mtDNA (MELAS syndrome)	■ Primary FSGS Columbia classification 1. Not otherwise specified 2. Perihilar variant 3. Cellular variant 4. Tip lesion variant 5. Collapsing FSGS ■ C1q nephropathy ■ Adaptive FSGS Follows an adaptive response consisting of glomerular hyperperfusion and hypertrophy (a) Reduced nephron mass: renal dysplasia, oligomeganephronia, surgical renal mass reduction, reflux nephropathy, chronic interstitial nephritis (b) Initially normal nephron mass: obesity, increased muscle mass, sickle cell anemia, cyanotic congenital heart disease, hypertension*	■ Cyclosporine, tacrolimus ■ Interferon-α ■ Lithium ■ Pamidronate

(continued)

TABLE 52.2 **Classification of Primary Podocytopathies *(continued)***

Pathology	Genetic (Mendelian Inheritance)	Acquired	Medication Induced
Collapsing glomerulopathy	■ Action myoclonus-renal failure syndrome	■ Idiopathic collapsing glomerulopathy ■ C1q nephropathy ■ Collapsing glomerulopathy associated with infection HIV-1 Parvovirus B19 *Loa loa* filariasis Visceral leishmaniasis ■ Collapsing glomerulopathy, other associations Adult Still disease Allograft vascular diseases Multiple myeloma	■ Interferon-α ■ Pamidronate

A classification scheme for the MCN/FSGS/collapsing glomerulopathy spectrum is presented. The forms of FSGS that are assigned to the acquired and medication-induced categories may have genetic risk components that have not been well defined at present. The Columbia classification divides primary FSGS into five variants; in the present classification system the fifth variant, collapsing FSGS, has been termed idiopathic collapsing glomerulopathy. In recognition that there may be distinct forms of the glomerular tip lesion with divergent prognoses, this entity has been divided into two forms, glomerular tip lesion MCN variant and glomerular tip lesion FSGS variant (these forms may have distinct clinical outcomes but similar pathologic appearance). The diagnosis of adaptive FSGS requires the exclusion of specific glomerular disease, for example, immune-mediated glomerulonephritis and diabetic nephropathy (which may manifest focal and segmental scarring but are not considered FSGS). Possible associations of primary FSGS and collapsing glomerulopathy with other disease states have been treated somewhat conservatively, so that associations based on isolated case reports and controversial associations are excluded or designated with an asterisk. C1q nephropathy can present as MCN, FSGS, and collapsing glomerulopathy, as well as other forms of glomerulopathy. ACTN4, α-actinin-4; C1q, complement component 1q; CD2AP, CD2 associated protein; COQ2, coenzyme Q synthetase 2; IgM, immunoglobulin M; ITGB4, integrin β4; LAMB2, laminin β2; NPHS1, nephrin; NPHS2, podocin; MCN, minimal change nephropathy; MELAS, mitochondrial encephalopathy, lactic acidosis, and seizures; mtDNA, mitochondrial DNA; NS, nephrotic syndrome; TRPC6, transient receptor potential cation channel 6; WT1, Wilms tumor 1.

Mechanisms for Proteinuria

The renal factors contributing to albumin homeostasis include both glomerular filtration and tubular reabsorption. In its simplest form, the glomerulus functions as a means to promote fluid and solute flux from the blood vessel to the urinary space, from where most constituents of the filtrate are then reabsorbed. This model acquires significant complexity as solute particles approach the size limits that are characteristic of the glomerular filter. Furthermore, recent progress in understanding tubular handling of protein has demonstrated that the reabsorptive component also has a significant impact on albumin homeostasis.

Renal Handling of Macromolecules

The glomerular barrier to filtration consists of three layers: fenestrated endothelial cells, the trilaminar glomerular basement membrane (GBM), and the epithelial cell layer (Fig. 52.1). The epithelium does not constitute a continuous layer; rather, the interdigitating extensions from adjacent epithelial cells or podocytes are separated by spaces readily apparent on electron microscopy. The GBM has been considered a major barrier to filtration.[14] Experimental evidence supports a hypothetical construct in which the GBM is a thixotropic gel (one containing spicules that retard the passage of macromolecules through it).[15] Diffusion through this gel plays a significant role in restricting protein passage.[16] Thus, the filtration of protein is restricted in the same manner that regulates protein movement during gel electrophoresis, where small molecules most easily penetrate.[17] At the same time, other studies support a model in which macromolecules encounter a porous structure that limits the passage of larger molecules by steric hindrance.[18] Glomerular filtration is possible because a small portion of the urinary space separates the interdigitations of the podocytes. These spaces are partly occluded by the epithelial slit diaphragm (Fig. 52.1), which has pores[19,20] that likely constitute the limiting barrier structure, causing steric hindrance.[21] The barrier itself is composed primarily of nephrin, a cell–cell adhesion molecule that interdigitates between adjacent cell processes[22] and is supported by a slit-diaphragm complex that includes podocin, CD2-associated protein (CD2AP), FAT, Neph1, P-cadherin,

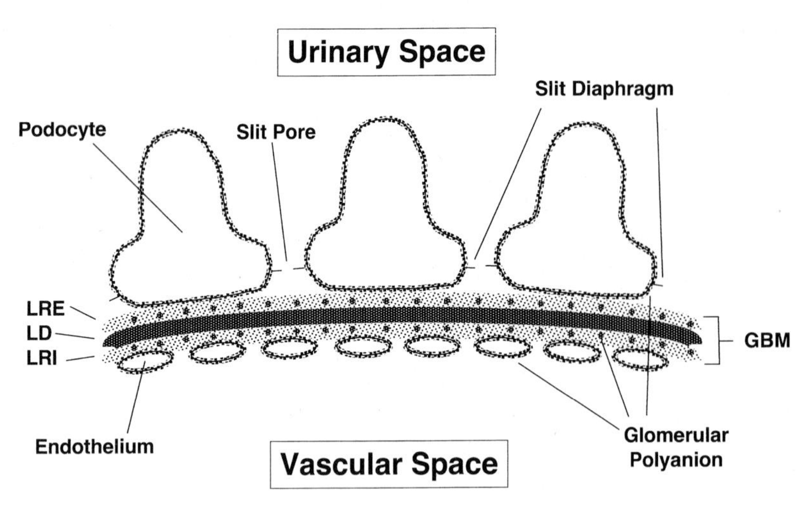

FIGURE 52.1 The glomerular filtration barrier. The distribution of glomerular polyanion in the glomerular basement membrane and on the endothelial and epithelial cell layers is shown. *LRE,* lamina rara externa; *LD,* lamina densa; *LRI,* lamina rara interna; *GBM,* glomerular basement membrane.

and vascular endothelial (VE)-cadherin.[23] The result is a latticework of proteins with openings of approximately 4 × 14 nm.[20,24] Therefore, both the GBM and the slit diaphragm contribute to steric influences on macromolecular filtration.

The porous component is demonstrated by permselectivity curves that plot the renal clearance of macromolecules, relative to the glomerular filtration rate (GFR), against the molecular radius, describing a sigmoid shape (Fig. 52.2) between approximately 2 and 5 nm (20 and 50 Å).[25] Therefore, some restriction in the filtration of dextrans occurs with molecules of about a 2-nm radius; restriction increases with increasing molecular size and approaches 100% for molecules of a radius of 5 nm.[26] In addition to size, the ability of macromolecules to cross the glomerular barrier is affected by molecular configuration, shape, deformability, and flexibility.[14] Permselectivity also is modified by glomerular hemodynamic factors, although the mechanisms for these effects remain a subject of some controversy.[17]

Initially, it was believed that macromolecule handling could be accounted for by an isoporous model for glomerular filtration, one in which the steric hindrance of the glomerular passage of macromolecules results from the presence of uniform pores in the barrier, each with a radius of approximately 5 nm. The size of these pores may be increased in models of increased permeability of the GBM.[27] However, it has become apparent that a heteroporous model may be more appropriate.[28] In this model, there are two pathways: one subject to classic steric hindrance, and a "shunt" pathway unaffected by size selectivity. As demonstrated by the clearance of very large dextrans, the glomerular filtration of macromolecules through this second pathway is enhanced in most forms of nephrosis and exacerbated by colloid volume expansion,[29] and is ameliorated in humans by antihypertensive therapy,[30] pressor doses of angiotensin II (in contrast to the effect in rats),[31] or indomethacin.[32] Therefore, there appears to be a hemodynamic component to the activation of this mechanism for proteinuria. The impact of this shunt is most noticeable for large molecules (greater than 6 nm); its effect on albumin clearance remains to be determined.

Steric hindrance is not sufficient to account for all aspects of permselectivity. Although proteins are handled in a manner similar to that for inert macromolecules,[14] protein clearances tend to be less than those of dextrans of comparable size.[14] Part of this difference is explained by the relatively rigid structure of the proteins. However, albumin, which has an effective molecular radius of 3.6 nm, is cleared by the normal kidney considerably less than are the equivalent-sized dextran molecules. Albumin carries a negative electrostatic charge, and its clearance is only slightly less than that of similarly sized dextran molecules carrying a negative charge.[33] This apparent charge selectivity has been attributed to negatively charged sialoglycoproteins in the glomerular filter,[34] which are present at regularly spaced intervals in the lamina rarae of the basement membrane,[35] at the endothelial fenestrae,[36] and lining the epithelial podocytes.[37] Collectively, these constitute the glomerular polyanions (Fig. 52.1). The presence of such negative-charge sites was proposed to be responsible for both the facilitated transport of polycations[38] and the restricted transport of polyanions[39] relative to that of neutral molecules of comparable size (Fig. 52.3). These effects are most apparent in the size range that is affected by some degree of steric hindrance.

Thus the determinants of glomerular permeability for a given particle are steric hindrance, glomerular hemodynamics, and electrostatic charge. The critical negative charges may not reside in the solid phase of the glomerular filter. The subpodocyte space creates a zone of delayed passage for larger macromolecules that cross the GBM.[40] Within this space, streaming potential establishes a flow-dependent charge gradient that is more negative on the urinary side of the GBM. A flow-dependent electrophoretic potential is accordingly established, driving negatively charged macromolecules back toward the vascular space.[41] The relative contribution of this gradient remains to be determined.

Tubular Handling of Protein

Renal protein metabolism also is affected significantly by tubular function. The glomerular filtrate normally contains a small amount of protein. A proximal tubular system has

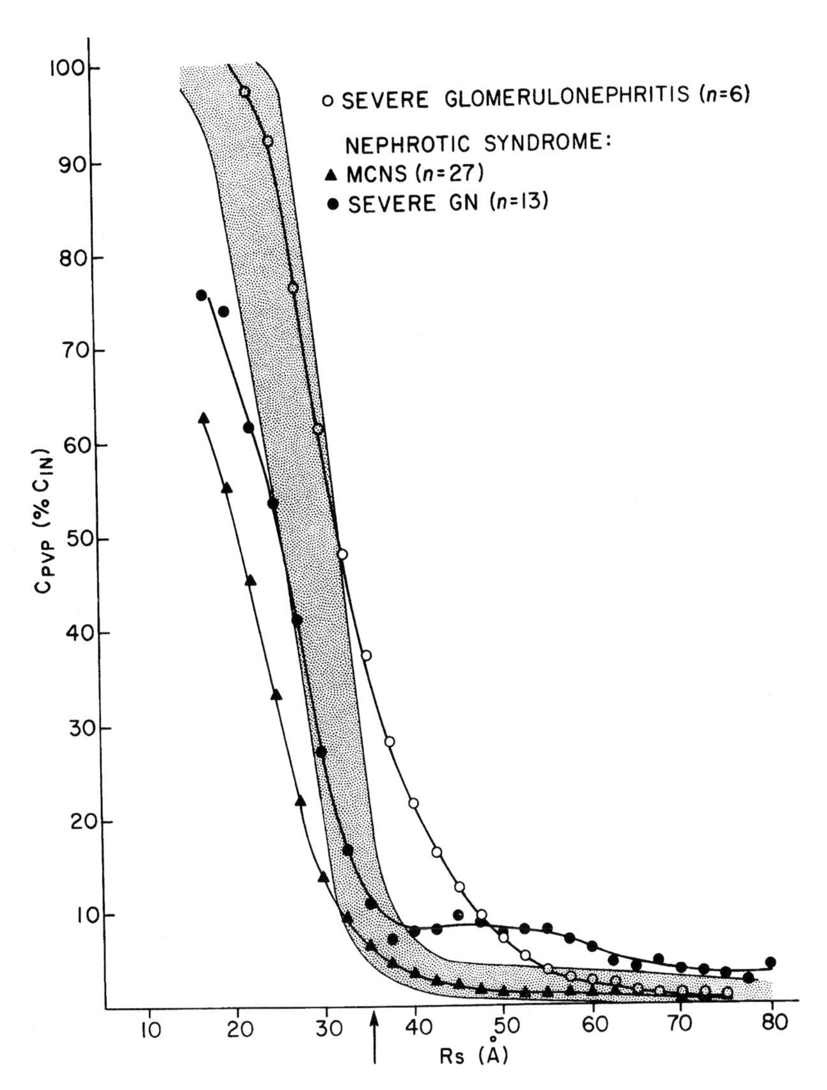

FIGURE 52.2 Permselectivity curves for patients with severe proliferative glomerulonephritis (GN) and for those with nephrotic syndrome secondary either to the minimal change nephropathy or to glomerulonephritis. Normal values are depicted by the *shaded area*. The *arrow* indicates the molecular size of albumin. The fractional clearance of larger macromolecules is increased in severe glomerulonephritis. In minimal change nephrotic syndrome (MCNS), the fractional clearance of smaller molecules is decreased. Patients with nephrotic syndrome secondary to glomerulonephritis show a hybrid curve. (Data modified from Robson AM, Cole BR. Pathologic and functional correlations in the glomerulopathies. In: Cummings NB, Michael AF, Wilson CB, eds. *Immune Mechanisms in Renal Disease*. New York: Plenum; 1982:109, with permission.)

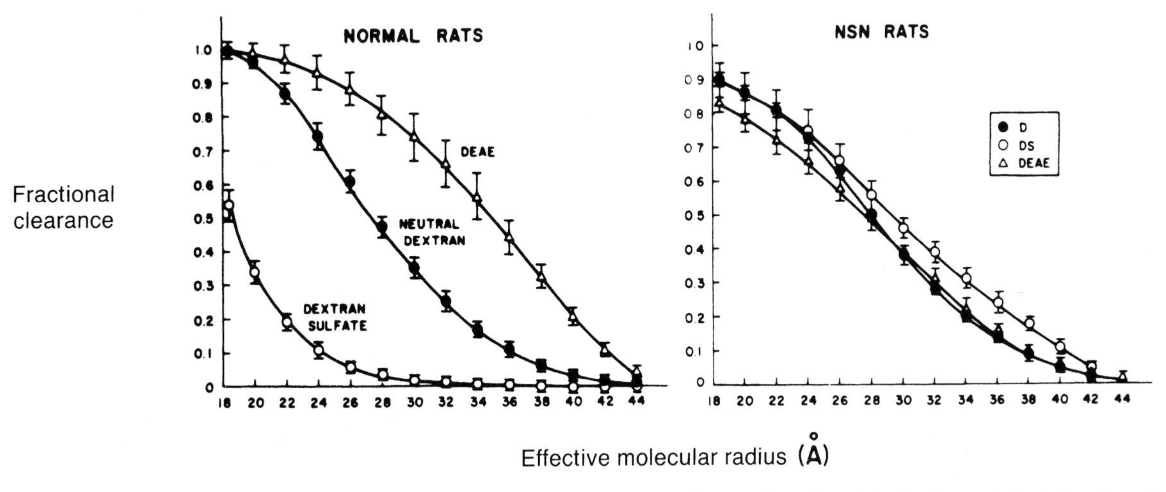

FIGURE 52.3 Clearance of neutral dextran (*D*), negatively charged dextran sulfate (*DS*), and positively charged diethylaminoethyl (*DEAE*) dextran of varying molecular size in normal rats and in those made albuminuric by treatment with nephrotoxic serum (NSN). In normal animals, the clearance of negatively charged dextrans is retarded, and that of cationic dextrans is enhanced, demonstrating charge selectivity by the glomerular filter. In NSN, charge discrimination is lost. (Reprinted from Bohrer MP, Baylis C, Humes HD, et al. Permselectivity of the glomerular capillary wall: facilitated filtration of circulating polycations. *J Clin Invest*. 1978;61:72; by copyright permission of the American Society for Clinical Investigation.)

sufficient capacity that, under physiologic conditions, little intact protein from the filtrate is present in the urine. For example, filtered albumin is subject to lysosomal degradation upon pinocytosis by the proximal tubular cell, with fragments appearing in both the plasma and the urine.[42] However, studies of rat kidneys, isolated but perfused in situ with radiolabeled albumin, indicate that some albumin is reabsorbed intact.[43] One mechanism of tubular protein reabsorption is demonstrated by its absence in Dent disease, a defect in chloride transport resulting from a mutation in the gene for a renal-specific, voltage-gated chloride channel, CLC-5, leading to hypercalciuric nephrolithiasis.[44] Proteinuria in this disease results from disruption of both receptor-mediated and fluid-phase endocytosis.[45] Patients with Dent disease have characteristic urinary losses of retinol-binding protein (RBP) and albumin.[46] The failure of protein reabsorption in this lesion has permitted an estimate that the glomerular filtrate contains 22 to 32 mg per liter of albumin, or roughly 3 to 6 g per day in the normal human adult, virtually all of which is reabsorbed under normal conditions. This represents greater than 4% of the total plasma albumin.[47]

This saturable mechanism for albumin reabsorption is mediated by three proteins that are associated with clathrin-coated pits in the proximal tubular cell.[48] Megalin is a 600-kDa, transmembrane protein and a member of the low-density lipoprotein-receptor family. It colocalizes in cultured opossum kidney (OK) cells with exogenous albumin and with cubilin, a 460-kDa protein that does not have a transmembrane domain. A third protein, amnionless, forms a complex with megalin and cubilin; the three proteins collaborate to reabsorb albumin.[49] Ligands for cubilin in the glomerular filtrate include not only albumin but also immunoglobulin light chain and apolipoprotein (apo)A-I. Megalin binds to the vitamin-binding proteins, RBP and vitamin D-binding protein, hormones, enzymes and β_2- and α_1- microglobulin, as well as albumin.[50,51] As will be discussed in the section to follow on Consequences of Proteinuria, the loss of many of these proteins has clinical significance in nephrotic syndrome. Another albumin "rescue" pathway that appears to facilitate reabsorption of intact albumin has been attributed to the FcRn immunoglobulin receptor.[52]

Altered Permselectivity in Nephrosis

Permselectivity patterns obtained in patients with MCNS[53,54] (Fig. 52.2) or animal models of selective albuminuria[39] (Fig. 52.3) show a relative decrease in macromolecular clearance even in the presence of marked proteinuria. In contrast, patients with glomerulonephritis show increased macromolecular clearances (Fig. 52.2), presumably due to structural damage to the GBM, which may be visible in renal biopsy material from patients in these disease states. This concept is supported by work in animals.[55] Thus the mechanisms for proteinuria in MCN and FSGS appear to be distinct from those in glomerulonephritis. In the former, proteinuria is relatively selective for albumin and occurs even though clearance of macromolecules comparable in size to albumin is decreased. In the latter, permselectivity of macromolecules that are 2.5 nm (25 Å) or larger is increased, resulting in poorly selective proteinuria. Patients with glomerulonephritis who have proteinuria that is sufficiently severe to cause the nephrotic syndrome may show a pattern of permselectivity (Fig. 52.2) that is a hybrid between those found in MCNS and those found in uncomplicated glomerulonephritis.[53] In these patients, as in MCNS, clearance of smaller molecules is relatively decreased. However, in contrast to the situation in MCNS, the relative clearance of larger molecules is increased. Similar hybrid curves have been described in diabetic glomerulosclerosis.[56]

Therefore, nephrotic proteinuria does not result from a simple defect in glomerular filter steric hindrance. Several theories have been advanced to account for albumin loss. A prominent one is a decrease in glomerular electrostatic charge selectivity. Renal biopsy material from patients with nephrotic syndrome shows decreased staining for glomerular polyanion.[57–60] Indeed, studies in MCNS patients suggested that albuminuria results from a reduction of fixed negative charge by approximately 50%.[61] Rats with nephrotic syndrome induced by puromycin amino nucleoside (PAN), which causes predominant albuminuria, show decreased staining by cationic dyes[62] and decreased sialic acid content.[63] Animals with PAN-induced nephrotic syndrome[64] as well as those with acute heterologous nephrotoxic serum nephritis[33] show increased clearance of negatively charged dextrans, with permselectivity curves approximating those of neutral dextrans. Further, the intravenous infusion of various polycations into animals results in a loss of staining for glomerular polyanion, increased porosity of the glomerular filter, and heavy proteinuria.[65–67] Unilateral renal artery infusion of the polycation protamine sulfate causes ipsilateral albuminuria and depletion of glomerular polyanion.[67] Finally, studies in patients suggest that the neutralization of vascular anionic charges may be systemic in nature[68,69] rather than confined to the kidney. This could result from effects of a protease present in the circulation such as hemopexin.[70,71] However, sieving curves generated in rats by glomerular localization of neutral or negatively charged polysaccharides were unable to demonstrate charge selectivity of the glomerular filter,[72] suggesting that technical factors or differences in the experimental approach could significantly affect the validity of experiments demonstrating charge selectivity. In these studies, bovine serum albumin (BSA) "uptake" was extremely high relative to other markers. A recent modification of the charge-selective model was proposed by Hausmann and colleagues.[41] In this flow-dependent model involving an electrochemical gradient across the filtration barrier, podocyte effacement disturbs flow, decreasing the negative charge in the urinary space. Consistent with this model, in PAN nephrosis increased albumin permeability occurs only in areas of podocyte dysfunction rather than diffusely, suggesting that the podocyte is more critical than the slit diaphragm in the pathogenesis of albuminuria.[73]

Another study found a role for negative charge in modulating renal protein handling in rats infused with neutral or anionic horseradish peroxidase. These results suggested that proteins may be more affected than polysaccharides by charge, but in this model charge selectivity was lost after inhibiting tubular protein uptake with lysine or ammonium chloride, suggesting the conclusion that charge selectivity does not reside in the glomerulus.[74] In mice, the plasma elimination rate of albumin (effective molecular radius of 36 Å) was comparable to that of much larger Ficoll molecules (≥ 65 Å). When the animals were treated with PAN, albumin clearance increased through an unknown renal mechanism.[75] Although charge selectivity could explain these findings, any mechanism that is involved could have affected either the glomerulus or the tubule. A study in analbuminemic rats treated with PAN showed no effect on renal size selectivity with treatment. There also was no change in the characteristics of urinary protein excretion.[76] Previously, it has been assumed that a greatly increased delivery of albumin to the proximal tubule saturated transport mechanisms or that the other proteins lost in the urine were bound to albumin, in either case causing loss of the nonalbumin proteins. However, the pattern of proteinuria observed in this study was similar to the findings in the CLC-5–null mouse, where low–molecular-weight proteinuria occurs, and suggests that at least some protein losses in nephrosis result from specific tubular mechanisms. These data support a significant role for the derangement of tubular protein handling in nephrotic syndrome.

Several investigators have suggested that impairment of the rescue pathway and other tubular, rather than glomerular, mechanisms are a significant cause of nephrotic proteinuria.[17,77] However, several lines of evidence suggest that this is not the case. Patients with Dent disease, and the CLC-5–null mouse, have "nephrotic-range" proteinuria but do not have nephrosis. The salvage of some of the 4% of the plasma albumin that is filtered per day[47] is likely to contribute positively to homeostasis, but a significant portion of albumin rescued by the tubule is degraded.[42] Assuming that half of the albumin is reclaimed intact, it is unlikely that losing 2% of plasma albumin per day will have a major effect on plasma albumin concentration. Finally, Deen and Lazzara[78] modeled the sieving coefficient for albumin. They performed a mass-transfer analysis to determine whether the sieving coefficient could be similar to, rather than greatly less than, that for neutral Ficoll of the same size. The higher value, which would have been required in the models supported by adherents of a causal role for tubular proteinuria, would generate tubular albumin concentrations located 1 mm distal to the glomerulus that are 20-fold higher than has been measured by rat micropuncture studies. The authors concluded that the glomerulus was the primary restricting site for albuminuria.[78] Although the possibility of charge selectivity was considered, it could not be tested by this analysis.

The alteration of podocyte architecture may account for the generally decreased fractional clearance of smaller macromolecules in nephrotic syndrome cited previously. It has been suggested that simplification of the foot process makes the glomerular pore less complex, thereby allowing for increased clearance of some long, narrow, rigid molecules. However, most plasma proteins are prolate ellipsoids (stubby cigar shaped) and show decreased clearance.[79] The effective pore radius was reported to be decreased in both MCNS and FSGS.[80] In this study, the ratio of total pore area to pore length was reduced by more than 50%. Further support for decreased pore area is found in studies indicating decreased filtration slit frequency (likely secondary to foot-process fusion)[81] or decreased pore number.[82] These findings would account for decreased macromolecular clearance but not enhanced albumin clearance.

An alternative to charge neutralization as an explanation of proteinuria is suggested by the data indicating that permselectivity patterns show enhanced clearance of larger neutral dextrans in FSGS.[82] Studies by Yoshioka and colleagues[83] suggest that there is enhanced clearance of albumin by less affected glomeruli, implicating hemodynamic factors related to hyperfiltration in remnant nephrons.[84] This could be accounted for by the heteroporous model in which a different class of pores greater than 60 Å in radius is increasingly used. This shunt pathway is active in angiotensin II–stimulated proteinuria[85] and Heymann nephritis.[86] Further, the hemodynamic implications of proposing a role for the shunt pathway are supported by the salient effect of angiotensin-converting enzyme (ACE) inhibition on glomerular size selectivity in disease.[87] However, because patients with MCN do not necessarily have increased use of the shunt pathway,[82] it is not clear that shunting represents a mechanism of proteinuria common to all causes of the nephrotic syndrome or is the major cause of nephrotic albuminuria.

A third hypothesis regarding the stimulus for proteinuria could account for changes in both charge and steric hindrance in the glomerular filtration barrier. Small anions such as Cl^- are freely filtered by the glomerulus, whereas negatively charged molecules such as albumin that are large enough to interact with the filtration barrier (but pass through) are affected by electrostatic hindrance. Modest increases in slit diaphragm pore size, perhaps mediated by alterations in cytoskeletal function,[88] may be sufficient to both decrease the steric hindrance of and reduce electrostatic interference with albumin transit, even before considering the amplifying effects of barrier charge neutralization or increased shunt pathway use.

Molecular Mechanisms of Podocyte Effacement

Given the importance of podocyte architecture in all of these models, the regulation of podocyte shape is an essential determinant of proteinuria. In podocyte effacement, the normally cortical distribution of the actin cytoskeleton, where structures extend from the periphery into the individual foot processes, is disrupted. Mundel and colleagues[89] have described a model system wherein the molecule B7-1 (also known as CD80), previously associated with lymphocyte costimulatory signals, is expressed in injured podocytes and binds to cytoskeletal structures, causing foot-process effacement.[89,90] It is expressed in the glomeruli of patients with MCN in relapse, but not in remission, and only marginally in patients with FSGS,[91] suggesting one mechanism by which podocyte architecture could be disrupted. In several mouse models of proteinuria, circulating levels of soluble urokinase receptor (suPAR) interfere with podocyte adhesive interactions through the adhesion molecules β3-integrin,[92] presumably disrupting podocyte architecture through this mechanism as well.

Consequences of Nephrotic Proteinuria

It is generally accepted that the central feature of the nephrotic syndrome, irrespective of its underlying renal cause, is hypoalbuminemia resulting from urinary loss. There is increased fractional catabolism of albumin in nephrotic syndrome,[93] mostly within the renal tubule after the increased filtration of plasma proteins.[94] Rates of hepatic synthesis of albumin are increased,[95] but this increase is inadequate to compensate for urinary losses.[96] Although gastrointestinal losses are possible through the transudation of albumin across the bowel wall in nephrosis, these are not likely to contribute significantly to decreased plasma albumin concentrations in the absence of significant bowel pathology.

Nonetheless, urinary losses cannot be considered an isolated phenomenon. It is apparent that a special relationship exists among protein synthetic capability, urinary loss of protein, and plasma protein concentrations. For example, patients undergoing chronic peritoneal dialysis lose "nephrotic range" amounts of protein, yet they usually have close to normal serum albumin concentrations.[97] In nephrosis, the rate of hepatic albumin synthesis is related to dietary protein intake. However, increasing protein intake leads to glomerular hyperfiltration[98,99] and enhanced loss of protein in the urine, resulting in lower serum albumin concentrations in patients on high protein diets.[100] The increase in dietary intake appears to stimulate selective hepatic expression of messenger ribonucleic acid (mRNA) for albumin, indicating that the stimulus is specific for albumin production and is not generalized to other proteins as well.[101] The dietary stimulus can be dissociated from potential effects of alterations in plasma oncotic pressure.[102] Although specific plasma amino acid content is unchanged, nitrogen balance is rendered more positive by ACE inhibition,[103] which decreases hyperfiltration and thus the amount of protein lost in the urine. Indeed, enalapril decreases $U_{Albumin}V$ (absolute albumin excretion) and fractional catabolism of albumin in normal or nephrotic rats on high protein diets.[104,105]

Edema Formation

One of the major consequences of hypoalbuminemia is edema formation. The major forces that maintain vascular volume are believed to be those described by Starling,[106] namely, the algebraic sum of hydrostatic and oncotic pressures acting at the level of the peripheral capillary beds (Fig. 52.4). Hydrostatic pressure is the dominant force at the arteriolar end of the capillary, where it is generated by

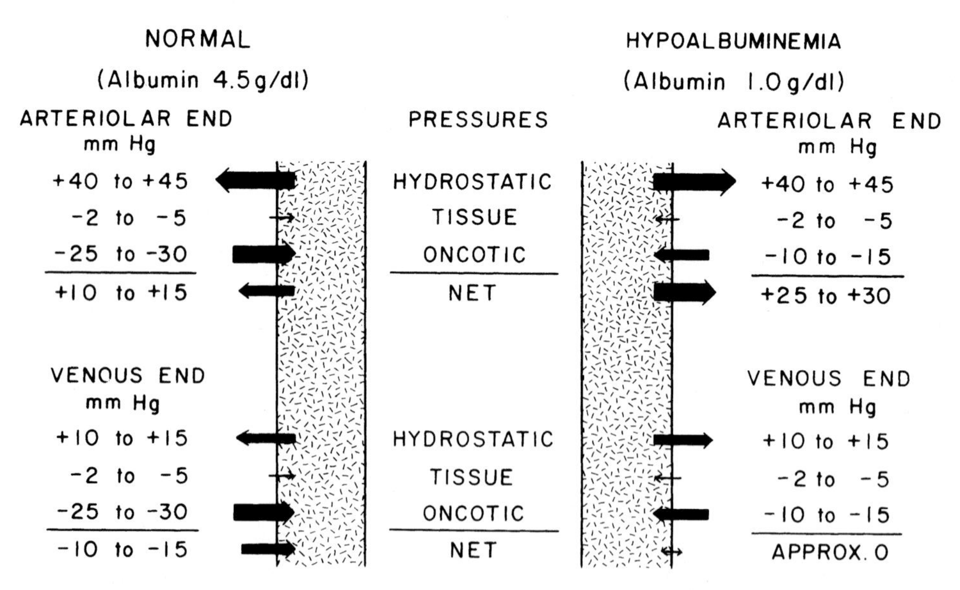

FIGURE 52.4 The forces that govern the movement of fluid across the peripheral capillary wall in healthy persons and in patients with primary nephrotic syndrome. The *shaded area* represents the lumina of the capillaries. The size and direction of the *arrows* are in proportion to the magnitude and direction of the force described by that arrow. In minimal change nephrotic syndrome, hypoalbuminemia causes a marked reduction in oncotic pressure. This increases the driving force for fluid out of the arteriolar end of the capillary and decreases the forces available for return of fluid at the venous end. The result is the development of increased amounts of fluid in the interstitial space and the beginning of edema formation. See text for more details. (From Robson AM. Edema and edema forming states. In: Klahr S, ed. *The Kidney and Body Fluids in Health and Disease*. New York: Plenum; 1984:119, with permission.)

arterial blood pressure. Pressure is lower in the capillaries (40 to 45 mm Hg) than in the arterial system, but it is markedly higher than tissue pressure, which ranges from 2 to 5 mm Hg. Hydrostatic pressure is opposed by plasma oncotic pressure (the osmotic pressure generated by colloidal solute), which is 25 to 30 mm Hg in healthy individuals. The resulting net force (10 to 15 mm Hg) drives an ultrafiltrate of blood from the capillaries into the interstitial fluid space. By the venous end of the capillary, hydrostatic pressure has been further dissipated (Fig. 52.4) and is exceeded by oncotic pressure, so that there is a net force for the return of fluid into the capillaries. In health, the loss of fluid at the arteriolar end of the capillaries slightly exceeds the amount resorbed at the venous end. The difference is returned to the circulation through the lymphatic system.[107]

Albumin, because of its abundance and its relatively small molecular size, is the plasma protein primarily responsible for the generation of oncotic pressure.[108] A decrease in plasma albumin concentration thus results in a decrease in oncotic pressure, so that the net driving force for loss of fluid at the arteriolar end of the capillary bed is increased and that for return of fluid at the venous end is reduced. Consequently, fluid accumulates in the interstitial space, initiating edema formation. This accumulation occurs first where tissue pressure is lowest, for example, in the eyelids or in the scrotum; it also appears in the most dependent parts of the body because venous hydrostatic pressure is highest at these sites and is transmitted to the venous end of the capillaries.

In this traditional model of nephrotic edema formation, often referred to as "underfilling,"[109] the translocation of fluid from the vascular to the interstitial fluid space as edema forms should decrease blood volume. The physiologic responses precipitated by such a reduction would then be important factors in producing the massive amounts of edema often seen in nephrotic syndrome. These changes include the release of antidiuretic hormone (ADH), the release of renin with increased production of angiotensin II, and decreases in renal blood flow and GFR.[110–112] All these changes favor renal retention and positive balances of both sodium and water unless intakes are decreased. Indeed, patients may exhibit increased thirst, which is probably stimulated both by angiotensin II[113] and by the decrease in blood volume monitored through baroreceptors and volume receptors. Retained sodium and water do not remain in the vascular space. Because of the hypoalbuminemia, they add to the edema.

In practice, the pathophysiology of edema formation in nephrotic syndrome is more complex than this traditional concept. Animal studies have documented that hypoproteinemia alone does not result in edema.[114] Humans with congenital analbuminemia do not develop nephrosis-like edema and have a normal plasma volume even in the virtual absence of serum albumin.[115] Furthermore, if the traditional theory is correct, patients in relapse of nephrotic syndrome should have decreased blood volumes and values should return to normal during remission from the disease. Although reduced values for blood volume have been reported,[116] normal or even increased levels have been documented too.[117,118] A survey of the literature[119] found that only 38% of patients with nephrosis had measurements indicating blood volumes reduced by 10% or more from normal, 48% had normal values, and 14% had increased values. In addition, patients with carefully documented MCNS studied during relapse and again during remission did not show a consistent increase in blood volumes with remission; indeed, in most, the values did not change.[119,120] Therefore, in contrast to the "underfilling" model, others have proposed an "overflow" hypothesis, in which the vascular tree is filled to excess, with increased hydrostatic pressure leading to fluid extravasation. Remarkably, nail bed micropuncture measurements in nephrotic patients did not support the notion that capillary overfilling occurs, but capillary leak appeared more important than underfilling in differentiating nephrotic from normal subjects.[121]

There are several possible explanations for these conflicting models, each of which appears valid in some cases. One is that the reported patients had varying underlying causes of their nephrotic syndrome, in some cases involving significantly decreased renal function. Nephrotic qsyndrome secondary to glomerulonephritis usually is associated with a normal or expanded blood volume.[122] A second potential confounding factor is that some patients were receiving treatment when studied. In addition to specific treatments, albumin infusion might enhance volume, and diuretic therapy may reduce both blood and interstitial fluid volume in nephrotic subjects.[123] A third issue is that measurements of blood volume are difficult to interpret because of methodologic problems. Labeled red cells may not circulate ideally in volume-depleted states, so that peripheral hematocrit may not reflect total body hematocrit; labeled albumin may have an increased volume of distribution in nephrotic syndrome, especially if vascular integrity to albumin is decreased.[124] Thus, both methods could be subject to errors.[122] Indeed, if the suggestion that nephrotic syndrome involves a generalized decrease of negative-charge sites[69] is correct, loss of such charge sites in capillary beds could cause increased losses of albumin into edema fluid.[125] This transfer not only would alter the apparent volume of distribution for albumin, but also might increase net extravascular oncotic pressure at the level of the capillaries. Support for this hypothesis is found in the observation that large changes in extracellular fluid volume cause little change in plasma volume in nephrotic patients.[126]

An attractive explanation for variations in reported blood volume is that the patients were studied in different phases of their disease process.[127] Blood volume could be reduced during the pathogenesis of the nephrotic state, particularly in MCNS, but return to normal as anasarca develops. The decrease in plasma volume after experimental depletion of serum proteins can be prevented by massive expansion of the extracellular fluid with saline solution.[128] Nephrotic subjects progress through a sodium-retaining phase but eventually enter into a new steady state in which they no longer accumulate edema and once again demonstrate the ability to excrete a sodium load.[111] With this new steady state, sodium and water retention may be so marked and edema accumulation may be so massive that tissue hydrostatic pressure is increased and blood volume is returned to normal. This may explain reports in which nephrotic subjects could be separated into those with high and those with low urine sodium concentrations.[120] The high-volume state, whether from massive fluid intake or decreased renal function, represents the overflow pathogenesis of nephrotic edema. It is likely that both underfilling and overflow occur, perhaps at different times in the same patient.

Hormonal Mechanisms

Regardless of whether underfilling or overflow is paramount, a third model suggests that hormonal mechanisms are of primary importance. Although we have emphasized a primary role for hypoalbuminemia in oliguria and sodium retention, patients with MCNS often undergo a marked, remission-induced diuresis beginning as soon as urinary albumin concentrations start to decrease and before the normalization of serum albumin. Initial studies of the pathophysiology of nephrosis suggested that fluid redistribution results in aldosterone-mediated sodium retention designed to replenish vascular volume.[129,130] Accordingly, aldosterone activity was thought to be more important in the genesis of fluid retention than either serum albumin or colloid osmotic pressure.[120] Consistent with this notion, patients with nephrotic syndrome show an increase in distal renal tubular sodium reabsorption.[111,131] Increased tubular sensitivity to aldosterone may further enhance edema formation.[132]

Renin–Angiotensin–Aldosterone System

Inconsistencies in reported plasma renin activity (PRA) results could be due to clinical factors similar to those that confound the interpretation of blood volume measurement. These include different stages of both disease process and sodium balance, as well as variations in therapeutic regimen. For example, immunofluorescence staining of renin-producing cells in renal biopsy material from nephrotic patients revealed increased numbers of these cells in hypoalbuminemic states. However, the increase correlated with a number of variables, most notably the presence of vascular disease.[133] In an attempt to standardize some of these variables, renin–sodium profiles were performed on patients with nephrotic syndrome. Two groups of patients were identified. In keeping with traditional concepts, the classic form was typically seen in patients with MCNS, in whom high levels of PRA and aldosterone activity were associated with vasoconstriction and hypoalbuminemia; values were further stimulated rather than suppressed by salt loading and decreased spontaneously before the occurrence of steroid-induced diuresis. In the hypervolemic, overfilling, form, seen typically with chronic glomerulonephritis and renal insufficiency, low renin activity was associated with sodium retention and increased normally with sodium depletion.[122] Other studies correlated PRA with plasma volume, serum albumin concentration,[134] or the state of sodium balance.[119] Natriuresis in MCNS was associated with an increase in PRA and presumably a decrease in plasma volume,[119] whereas that induced by water immersion, presumably mediated by an increase in blood volume, was associated with a measured decrease in PRA.[135] Therefore, PRA appears to correlate better with plasma volume than with the rate of urinary sodium excretion.

Difficulties in confirming a definitive role for the renin–angiotensin system in the genesis of nephrotic edema are similar to those in explaining edema formation in cirrhosis.[136] A multiplicity of interacting factors may be responsible in both of these disease states. Therefore, plasma renin levels could be controlled tightly by a variety of feedback mechanisms so that subtle changes, too small to be detected by current laboratory methods, are all that occur to maintain the altered homeostasis.

It was proposed that aldosterone could mediate sodium retention through its actions on the epithelial sodium channel, ENaC. In support of this hypothesis, ENaC shows increased apical targeting in nephrotic rats.[137] However, although adrenalectomy prevents this apical targeting, the adrenalectomized rats continue to show significant sodium retention and edema.[138] While these results do not rule out an alternative mechanism of aldosterone action, they implicate nonaldosterone mechanisms in nephrotic sodium retention.

Other Hormonal Regulators of Fluid and Electrolyte Balance

Other factors affecting volume status may include abnormal vascular tone,[139] altered levels of catecholamines,[140] and a variety of hormonal mechanisms.

Antidiuretic hormone secretion. 'Nephrotic patients with MCN may show decreased solute-free water excretion, although the capacity to generate solute-free water remains intact.[112] Increased ADH secretion may reflect a physiologic response to decreased intravascular volume.[116] In contrast, maximal urine osmolarity may be decreased in experimental rat nephrosis due to decreased renal tubular expression of aquaporin.[141,142]

Prostaglandin metabolism. Elevated levels of prostaglandin E_2 (PGE_2) were found in the serum of patients with nephrotic syndrome, the majority of whom had MCN.[143] The highest values were observed when the patients had clinically apparent edema. Urinary PGE_2 levels were increased in patients with idiopathic nephrotic syndrome who had a low urine sodium concentration as well as elevated plasma renin–aldosterone activity.[144] The observation that the administration of indomethacin to nephrotic patients results in an increase in body weight and a decrease in GFR suggests that prostaglandins may play a role in either the maintenance of GFR or amelioration of edema in nephrotic syndrome. Indomethacin also decreased proteinuria and PRA.[144] Response to indomethacin is dependent on concurrent sodium intake. When the agent was given to nephrotic patients on sodium-restricted diets, it resulted in a decrease in GFR. A similar drug regimen for patients with more liberal sodium intake did not affect renal hemodynamics.[145]

Atrial natriuretic peptide. Because atrial natriuretic peptide (ANP) causes renal vasodilation, an increase in GFR, and increased sodium excretion,[146] it has been suggested that abnormal metabolism of this hormone could mediate sodium retention in nephrosis. The acute increase of plasma volume following albumin infusion in nephrotic children is accompanied by a fivefold increase in ANP levels.[147] However, this may simply reflect a change from low plasma volume status before the infusion is begun in patients who likely have MCNS. Plasma concentrations of ANP were determined to be low in nephrotic patients compared to patients who had acute glomerulonephritis, and ANP levels correlated well with the degree of edema in nephritis but not in nephrosis.[148] Therefore, regulation of ANP appeared to be appropriate for presumed volume status. In rats with Adriamycin-induced nephrotic syndrome, changes in GFR after the infusion of ANP were similar to those in control animals, indicating that nephrosis does not alter glomerular filtration by changing ANP sensitivity.[149] In a similar model, no change was detected in ANP receptor density in nephrotic kidneys.[150] Nephrotic patients respond physiologically to ANP infusion,[151] although the mechanism by which this occurs may be different from that in normal subjects.[152] It has been proposed that ANP mediates the diuretic response to head-out immersion in nephrosis,[153] but the effect of ANP infusion, unlike that of immersion, is blocked by enalapril.[154]

Physical and Anatomic Factors Affecting Glomerular Filtration Rate

Taken together, these findings suggest that, although the secretion of ANP may in part mediate diuresis, physical factors are of greatest importance in the fluid retention of nephrosis, with abnormalities of ANP representing appropriate responses for the patient's physiology.[155] These physical factors may include a significant intrarenal component. Children with MCNS have decreases in both GFR and filtration fraction.[110,156,157] Decreased GFR could be due to a decrease in the ultrafiltration coefficient (K_f), causing a reduction in single-nephron GFR,[155] and has been suggested to result from effacement of the glomerular epithelial cell foot processes.[158] Alternatively, the decreased GFR could be a consequence of raised intratubular hydrostatic pressure in the proximal tubule secondary to the presence of filtered albumin, an increase in resistance to tubular flow,[159] or decreased proximal reabsorption of tubular fluid as a result of a reduction in peritubular capillary oncotic pressure.[155] There also may be a local role for the renin–angiotensin system, as saralasin infusion in experimental unilateral PAN-induced nephrotic syndrome resulted in an increase in single-nephron GFR in the experimental, but not in the control, kidney.[155] In another animal model of nephrotic syndrome, that of nephrotoxic serum nephritis, the K_f was reduced, but compensatory mechanisms maintained renal blood flow and whole-kidney and single-nephron GFR. These responses appeared to be intrarenal in origin and caused an increase in glomerular capillary pressure.[160]

Another factor affecting GFR is plasma albumin concentration. Hypoalbuminemia has been postulated to decrease glomerular plasma flow, thereby decreasing GFR. However, lower albumin also decreases plasma oncotic pressure, which should increase GFR. Löwenborg and Berg[161] report that GFR and filtration fraction vary directly with serum albumin but vary inversely with mean arterial blood pressure in children with MCNS. This finding supports a role for altered K_f in relapse, which is consistent with foot-process effacement. K_f is determined by the total filtration slit length, as shown by mathematical modeling of experimental data.[81] Some studies suggest that there is a weak correlation between the amount of proteinuria and the extent of foot-process effacement, but these studies included patients in relapse and in remission with MCN[162] and with multiple nephrotic diseases.[163] A study of 23 MCN patients in relapse showed no correlation between proteinuria and foot-process effacement ($r = 0.25$, $P = .25$).[164] The authors make the important point that assessment of the quantitative relationship between podocyte foot-process effacement and proteinuria should exclude patients in remission, as these patients have normal podocyte morphology (and therefore do not address the hypothesis that the degree of effacement correlates with proteinuria). Foot-process effacement reverses when patients undergo spontaneous or glucocorticoid-induced remission.

Other Physiologic Changes in Fluid and Electrolyte Metabolism

A curious phenomenon in primary nephrotic syndrome, perhaps related to decreased filtration fraction, is the occurrence of reversible or permanent renal failure unexplained by the underlying disease process. This has been reported in association with both MCN[165–167] and FSGS.[139] In some patients, renal failure was associated with the use of nonsteroidal anti-inflammatory drug (NSAID) therapy.[168,169] These episodes occur in the absence of renal vein thrombosis (vide infra) or other systemic symptoms. Because fractional excretion of sodium is low in these patients,[170] it is likely that the marked decrease in GFR occurs for hemodynamic reasons[171] rather than because of acute tubular necrosis or vasomotor nephropathy. In a study of 15 patients with MCNS and renal failure, GFR measured by inulin clearance was decreased out of proportion to clearance of para-aminohippurate (PAH), with filtration fraction reduced to between 3% and 9%.[172]

Improvement of renal function occurred in association with diuretic therapy either with or without albumin infusion. In patients who improved with pharmacologic diuresis, the serum creatinine level again rose on return to an edematous state. The authors postulate that glomerular hemodynamics were altered by the presence of intrarenal edema, which occurred concomitantly with peripheral edema.

Other circulatory abnormalities have been observed in patients with nephrotic syndrome. The occurrence of hypovolemic shock and hypotension has been related to a variety of medical procedures.[173] However, hypotension may occur spontaneously. These episodes usually are seen in patients during relapse who have an intercurrent illness causing fluid loss, such as emesis or diarrhea. The patients usually show marked responsiveness to small amounts of intravenous saline that are insufficient to replenish all fluid losses, suggesting a failure in maintenance of vascular tone. Recovery usually occurs if this complication is identified early and treated promptly. Sequelae may include acute tubular necrosis, renal vein thrombosis (RVT), or death.

Hyperlipidemia

Lipemic serum has long been recognized as a cardinal feature of the nephrotic syndrome.[174] Abnormalities in postprandial lipid metabolism were described more than 40 years ago.[175] Biochemical evaluation has shown that all lipid components of the plasma are increased, with cholesterol increasing more rapidly than phospholipid. Thus, as acute severity of the disease worsens, as measured by proteinuria, increased lipid levels[176] and the ratio of cholesterol to phospholipid increases.[177] Triglycerides are relatively normal at the initiation of relapse but increase as the disease continues[178]; lactescence occurs when the plasma triglyceride content exceeds 400 mg per deciliter. Hyperlipidemia may persist well into remission,[179] suggesting a residual effect of nephrosis on lipoprotein transport.[180]

Depending on the classification employed, the most common patterns of hyperlipoproteinemia seen in nephrosis are types II and IV[181] or types IIa, IIb, and V.[182] Low-density lipoproteins (LDLs) and very low-density lipoproteins (VLDLs) show the greatest increase in concentration. Values for high-density lipoprotein (HDL) cholesterol have been reported to be elevated,[183,184] normal,[185,186] or decreased.[178,187,188] This variation may relate to the age of the patients studied, the underlying cause of the nephrotic syndrome, the patient treatment, and whether renal insufficiency is present. Studies of lipoprotein cholesterol have produced conflicting results. The ratio of cholesterol to phospholipids or to triglycerides in various lipoproteins is altered, indicating abnormalities in quality as well as quantity of lipoproteins.

Several events may contribute to these abnormalities. Lipid metabolism is normally accomplished through a series of complex steps (Fig. 52.5). Through the action of 3-hydroxy-3-methylglutaryl coenzyme A (HMG CoA)

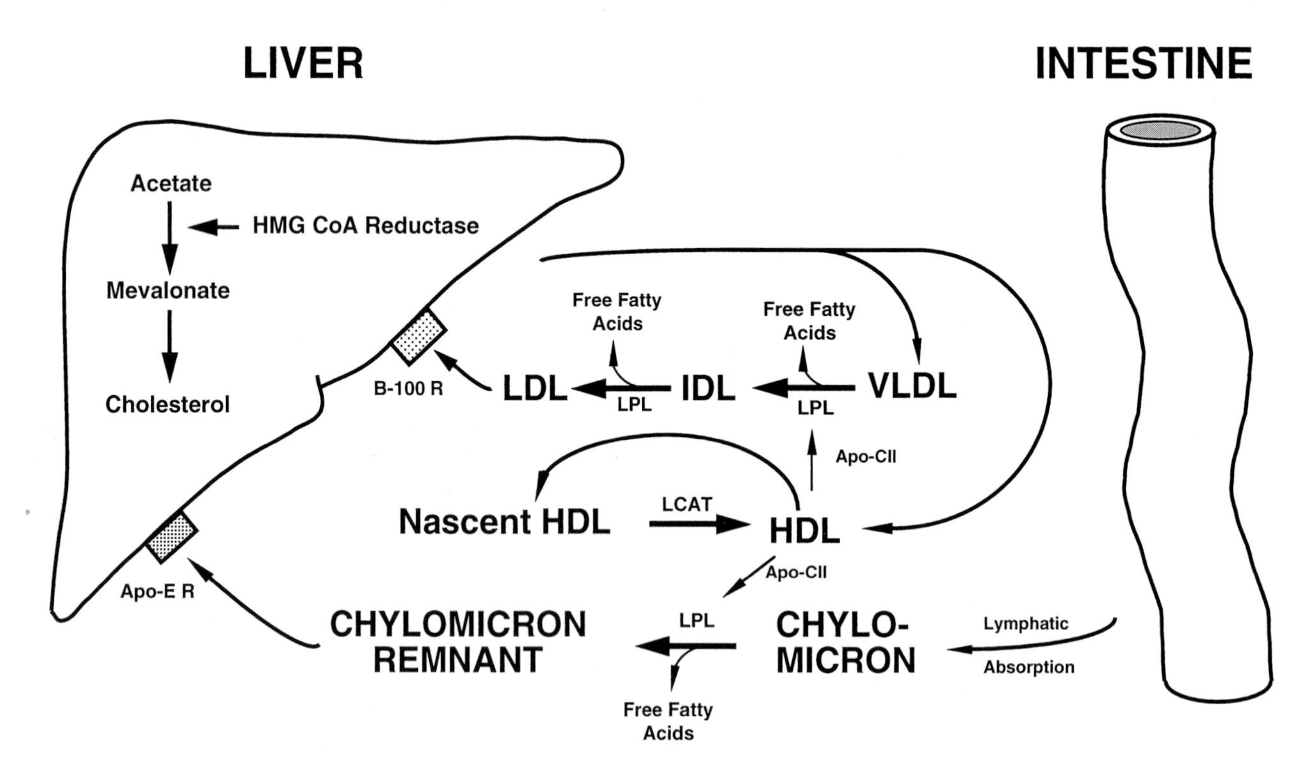

FIGURE 52.5 Normal pathways of lipid metabolism. *apo-CII*, apolipoprotein C-II; *Apo-E R*, chylomicron remnant (apo E) receptor; *B-100 R*, apolipoprotein B-100 (LDL) receptor; *HDL*, high-density lipoprotein; *IDL*, intermediate-density lipoprotein; *HMG CoA reductase*, 3-hydroxy-3-methylglutaryl coenzyme A reductase; *LCAT*, lecithin-cholesterol acyltransferase; *LDL*, low-density lipoprotein; *LPL*, lipoprotein lipase; *VLDL*, very-low-density lipoprotein. Figure composed with the assistance of Nader Rifai.

reductase, mevalonate is produced from acetate in the liver. This in turn is used to make cholesterol, which is incorporated into lipoproteins. The greater the triglyceride content of the lipoprotein, the less dense it is. Dietary fat absorbed from the intestine is formed into chylomicrons by being surrounded with a coat of apolipoprotein (apo) that is critical for transport of the hydrophobic lipid. The triglyceride content of the chylomicron is reduced in the periphery (mainly by the action of lipoprotein lipase [LPL]), and the resulting particle containing apo B-48 and apo E binds to the hepatocyte via a chylomicron remnant receptor. VLDL is synthesized in the liver and metabolized in the periphery through the action of LPL to intermediate-density lipoprotein (IDL), and then to LDL. LDL is bound to apo B-100, which is then taken up by the hepatocyte LDL receptor.[189,190] This brings additional cholesterol back to the liver, suppressing HMG CoA reductase activity and decreasing new cholesterol synthesis. The liver also produces HDL, which participates as a transport protein in the catabolism of lower density moieties, being regenerated by lecithin-cholesterol acyltransferase (LCAT). HDL also carries apo C-II, which activates LPL. Abnormalities at any step of metabolism from lipid uptake to the enterohepatic secretion of bile could result in the hyperlipidemia of nephrosis. Likely contributing factors include increased hepatic synthesis of lipoprotein, abnormal transport of lipid through the metabolic pathway, and abnormal catabolism secondary to decreased enzyme activity.

Lipoprotein Synthesis

It is clear that the hepatic synthesis of lipoproteins is increased in nephrotic patients.[177,191–194] The signal for this event appears to be related to hypoalbuminemia because the daily infusion of albumin into nephrotic patients, sufficient to raise serum levels, also decreases serum lipid, triglyceride, and cholesterol levels.[195] Increasing the plasma oncotic pressure in nephrotic patients or animals, by infusion of dextrans, decreases hepatic lipoprotein synthesis.[175,196] Additional laboratory studies suggest that the regulatory signal could be viscosity rather than oncotic pressure.[195,197,198] Cholesterol biosynthesis also has been investigated.[199,200] These studies show increased incorporation of ^{14}C from labeled mevalonate into cholesterol by the liver in experimental nephrosis. Although this result is consistent with the interpretation that rates of hepatic cholesterol synthesis are increased in nephrosis, artifactual changes due to the addition of exogenous substrate (mevalonate) could not be ruled out in these experiments.

Lipid Transport

Several aspects of lipid transport may be impaired in nephrosis. The major cholesterol-transporting protein associated with the LDLs in the plasma is apo B-100.[201] This also has been implicated as a significant apolipoprotein in atherogenesis. A recent study of nephrotic patients found that elevated serum concentrations of cholesterol, triglycerides, and phospholipids resulted mostly from changes in apo B-100–containing lipoproteins. The size of the apo B-100 pool in patients was two to three times that found in healthy subjects or in patients in remission. Fractional catabolism was decreased only slightly, suggesting that the major problem was overproduction rather than decreased breakdown.[180] Hepatic uptake of LDLs may be decreased[202] if the structural composition of LDLs in the circulating pool is abnormal, or if systemic neutralization of membrane negative charge leads to less efficient uptake of the largely cationic liposomes[203]; this would exacerbate hypercholesterolemia by decreasing negative feedback affecting hepatic synthesis. Alternatively, decreased hepatic uptake of LDLs could result from, rather than cause, hepatic overproduction of cholesterol.[201] Altered transport could also occur at the level of lipoprotein receptor expression, because the nephrotic liver shows increased endocytic HDL receptor mRNA and protein but decreased expression of scavenger receptor-BI expression. The latter may be regulated by a decrease in expression of PDZ-containing kidney protein-1, which protects SR-BI from degradation.[204]

Metabolism of Lipids

At least one report indicates that although LDL synthesis may be increased in nephrosis, VLDL catabolism is decreased.[194] Another study demonstrates that apolipoprotein E–rich IDL from nephrotic patients, but not from normal controls, inhibits sterol synthesis and cholesterol esterification.[205] This finding suggests that cellular apo E metabolism may be deranged in nephrosis. Consistent with this finding, genetic variations in the expression of *apo E* alleles may influence the degree of lipid abnormality in nephrotic patients.[206]

Interest regarding catabolism of lipids in nephrosis has focused on two enzymes: LPL, which facilitates the breakdown of ester bonds in glycerides, and LCAT, which catalyzes the reaction of lecithin and cholesterol to form lysolecithin and cholesterol ester.[207] In nephrotic children, elevated serum lipid levels correlate with decreased postheparin LPL activity.[208] In another study of nephrotic patients, most of whom had MCNS, hepatic LPL activity was normal, but serum and adipose tissue LPL activities were decreased in association with elevated plasma triglycerides.[184] Decreased hepatic[209] and adipose tissue[208] LPL activity in experimental rat models of nephrosis may contribute to altered lipoprotein levels in these animals. Such decreased activity may reflect decreased endothelial LPL expression.[210] LCAT activity also is decreased in experimental nephrosis,[211] with levels appearing to correlate with serum albumin concentration.[212]

Activity of these enzymes may be affected both directly and indirectly by urinary protein loss. Albumin binds to free fatty acids (FFAs); decreases in serum albumin concentration lead to FFA accumulation, thereby inhibiting LPL activity.[213] LPL activity also may be inhibited by cholesterol.[212] LCAT activity is inhibited by the accumulation of triglyceride and cholesterol esters,[214] suggesting that abnormal LCAT activity could be a result, rather than a cause, of nephrotic hyperlipidemia. However, lysolecithin, a reaction product that binds to albumin, inhibits LCAT activity in vitro; this feedback mechanism is blocked by the addition of physiologic levels of albumin.[214,215] Therefore, the urinary loss of albumin may lead to the inhibition of lipolytic enzyme function.

Albumin loss does not account entirely, however, for the elevated lipid levels. Although the infusion of albumin decreased serum lipid levels in an acute animal model of nephrotic syndrome, normalization occurred only after simultaneous infusion of heparin. This suggests the need for an additional factor that aids in clearing lipid from the plasma.[216] In further experiments with this model, nephrectomy resulted in greater improvement of the hyperlipidemia than did albumin infusions alone,[217] indicating that the factor may be lost in the urine. Further support for the loss of a specific regulatory molecule in the urine is provided by the observation that alteration of dietary protein intake markedly modulates the hepatic albumin synthetic rate but does not alter the hepatic synthesis of lipoproteins.[218] In this study, lipoprotein synthesis correlated directly with the urinary clearance of albumin, suggesting that albumin, or another substance lost in parallel with albumin, was needed to suppress lipoprotein synthesis. Experiments with analbuminemic rats indicate that albumin itself is not likely to be the critical molecule.[219] It has been suggested that the lost factor is LCAT.[177] HDL, which plays an essential role in catabolism of VLDL, also may be lost in the nephrotic urine.[220,221] Conversely, other studies indicate that HDL excretion is low,[196] especially in MCNS.[222] Apo C-II also may be lost in the urine.[201,223]

Clinical Significance

Regardless of the cause, the clinical significance of the lipid abnormalities in nephrosis must be considered. Hyperlipidemia has been associated with cardiovascular disease in otherwise healthy young adults, but studies evaluating such a correlation in nephrotic patients produced conflicting results. Premature coronary atherosclerosis[224] and a high incidence of myocardial infarction and other cardiovascular diseases[225,226] have been documented in nephrotic subjects, as well as a higher incidence of hypertension in nephrotic men than in control subjects.[227] Intimal-medial thickness ratios, as an index of atherosclerotic plaque formation, were increased as a function of the number of relapses that had occurred in children and young adults with steroid-sensitive nephrotic syndrome.[228] In addition, plasma levels of lipoprotein(a), a strong risk factor in cardiovascular disease, are increased.[229] Macrophage morphology and function are altered by the hyperlipidemia of nephrosis[230] and oxidized lipids are increased in the nephrotic syndrome,[231,232] potentially contributing to the development of atheromatous plaques. In contrast, other studies have not confirmed a predisposition to atherosclerosis in patients with nephrosis.[233,234] These discrepant results may reflect limitations of population base or selection bias.[184,222] In the studies that did not demonstrate an increased risk, it is unclear whether stratification of the patients into cohorts according to the degree of lipid abnormality would have shown an increased risk in patients with the highest consistent elevations in lipoprotein levels. Age, underlying diagnosis, disease course, and incidence of other complicating factors such as hypertension also may be important. Another significant consideration is the possible ameliorating effect of HDL on hyperlipidemia.[233–236] In several studies,[184,222] HDL levels were normal or increased in MCNS. This could have a protective effect and could decrease the likelihood of cardiovascular complications. A further study of larger groups of nephrotic patients would allow differentiation among patients with other cardiac risk factors in addition to the potential hazard of elevated serum lipid levels.

A second risk involves the role of lipids in causing or enhancing the progression of the renal disease itself.[237] Rats with PAN nephrosis fed high-cholesterol diets develop mesangial foam cells and mesangial proliferative changes.[238] The relationship of systemic hypertension and hyperlipidemia to atherosclerosis parallels the relationship of intraglomerular hypertension and high lipid levels to focal sclerosis.[238] Effective therapy of hyperlipidemia ameliorates single-nephron hyperfiltration[239] and retards progression of renal failure in obese Zucker rats[240] and in nephrotic rats with reduced renal mass.[241] In obese Zucker rats, a relative decrease in polyunsaturated fatty acids (PUFAs), rather than high cholesterol levels, may be the most important lipid-related factor in the progression of renal disease, because dietary supplementation with n-6 PUFA (sunflower oil) or n-3 PUFA (fish oil) slowed the progression of renal disease but only fish oil decreased serum cholesterol levels.[239]

In view of these considerations, and the fact that treatments for nephrosis such as steroids and diuretics may exacerbate hyperlipidemia, clinicians have invested increasing effort in controlling the lipid abnormalities of nephrosis.[242] Traditional dietary therapy is of marginal value, and may actually worsen the hyperlipidemia.[243] Cholestyramine may, by increasing the secretion of cholesterol into the bile, predispose one toward the development of cholesterol gallstones.[201] Nicotinic acid has significant side effects and has not been studied extensively. Probucol may cause concomitant loss of HDLs.[243] However, it has been shown experimentally to reverse lipid-mediated vasoconstriction[244] and to be effective in treating patients who were 5 to 20 years old.[245] Two other classes of drugs found to be effective in treating nephrotic hyperlipidemia are fibric acids and HMG CoA reductase inhibitors. Gemfibrozil, a fibric acid, caused a 51% reduction in serum triglyceride levels but only a 15% decrease in cholesterol when given at a dose of 600 mg twice a day to adult nephrotic patients; a 26% reduction in apo B was achieved.[246] Lovastatin, an inhibitor of HMG CoA reductase, caused a 27% to 29% reduction in total cholesterol, LDL cholesterol, and apo B at a dose of 20 mg twice daily in adult patients with nephrosis due to MCN or other diseases.[247] In patients with nephrotic-range proteinuria, doses up to 40 mg twice daily caused similar decreases regardless of whether the patients were on corticosteroid therapy. A slight increase was noted in serum HDL concentrations.[248] Kinetic studies showed that lovastatin enhances the catabolism of VLDL triglycerides and lowers LDL cholesterol by decreasing input rates for LDLs,[249] most likely through the inhibition of LDL–apo B synthesis from VLDL.[250] Atorvastatin also is effective in reducing nephrotic hyperlipidemia.[251] In children, HMG CoA reductase inhibitors may be effective, but some clinicians have urged caution regarding their use in the very young child, raising the possibility that inhibiting cholesterol synthesis might impair neural myelination. This potential concern needs to be weighed against the more immediate issues of cardiovascular complications and renal disease progression.

Disorders of Hemostasis

The association between nephrotic syndrome and intravascular coagulation has been known for more than a century, but it was not until 1948 that the concept of a thrombotic diathesis in nephrotic patients was proposed.[252] In a review of 3,377 children with nephrotic syndrome, the incidence of thromboembolic complications was 1.8%.[253] The prevalence of such complications in adult nephrotic subjects is much higher and averaged 26% in eight series of patients.[254] Thrombosis may occur at any stage during the course of the nephrotic syndrome, but it is most frequent in the early months.

Extent of Clinical Involvement

Deep vein thrombosis of the leg is the most common thrombotic complication in the nephrotic adult and was responsible for one third of the thromboembolic complications in the largest published series of nephrotic children.[253] Other reported sites of venous thromboses include the subclavian, axillary, external jugular, portal, splenic, hepatic, and mesenteric veins as well as the superficial cerebral cortical sinus, where thrombosis has been observed in both children and adults and may be fatal.[255,256] Arterial thrombosis occurs less frequently and is seen primarily in children. Thrombosis of the aorta and of the mesenteric, axillary, femoral, ophthalmic, carotid, cerebral, renal, pulmonary, and coronary arteries has been reported, as has intracardiac thrombosis.[255,256] The pulmonary[257] and femoral arteries are particularly susceptible, the former potentially resulting in infarction[258] and the latter usually as a complication of attempted blood sampling from the femoral vein. Although recanalization of the artery does occur, a relatively high proportion of patients with arterial thrombi die.[257]

The lesion that has attracted the most attention, however, is RVT. It is most often seen with membranous glomerulopathy[259] to the extent that at one time there was some controversy about whether RVT was the cause, rather than a complication, of the glomerular lesion. The reported frequency of RVT in patients with membranous disease has ranged from 4% to 51%, depending on the methods used to establish the diagnosis and to select the patient population for study.[260] The mean prevalence is 12%. There is a high incidence of RVT in mesangiocapillary glomerulonephritis and the nephritis of systemic lupus erythematosus, and RVT can complicate numerous other renal diseases.[255] It is relatively uncommon in nephrotic children except in those with congenital nephrotic syndrome of the Finnish type.[261]

The thrombosis may involve only the renal venous system or it may extend into the inferior vena cava. Therefore, it is not surprising that pulmonary emboli develop in about 40% of adult patients with RVT, although pulmonary emboli rarely occur in children. Death from pulmonary emboli is uncommon.[253,255]

The diagnosis of acute RVT is suggested by flank pain, costovertebral angle tenderness, gross hematuria, increased proteinuria, and acute reduction in renal function; intravenous pyelography may show ureteral notching or pelvicaliceal irregularities.[260] Ultrasonography may demonstrate only a large kidney or may visualize the thrombus if it extends into the renal vein or inferior vena cava. However, Doppler ultrasound analysis often shows decreased venous blood flow. A more chronic form of RVT may be asymptomatic and may be identifiable only by venography.[260,262] The mode of presentation of other thromboses depends on their site. Diagnosis can be difficult and the existence of arterial thrombosis may not be realized until autopsy. Ultrasonography and angiography are the preferred studies.

Regulators of Coagulation

The blood coagulation pathway represents a cascade of events that regulate the dynamic balance between the ability of the blood to remain fluid and its tendency to assume a gelled state in the presence of altered flow conditions or exposure to nonendothelial surfaces. Contributing to hemostatic balance are several opposing systems that contribute to a cascade through which a series of enzymes regulates fibrin polymerization (Fig. 52.6). Coagulation is initiated by the activation of prekallikrein to kallikrein (intrinsic pathway), or by exposure to nonendothelial tissues (extrinsic pathway). These pathways meet in the activation of factor IX, initiating a common pathway in which a central role is played by thrombin (factor IIa). This enzyme stimulates the activation of fibrinogen to fibrin and the aggregation of platelets. It also activates factors V, VIII, and XIII. Factor XIIIa triggers the cross-linking of fibrin monomer into a stable polymer. Two systems oppose clot formation and stability. Protein C is processed to activated protein C (aPC) by thrombin complexed with thrombomodulin. With free protein S as a cofactor, aPC inactivates factors Va and VIIIa. The other system that opposes coagulation is the fibrinolytic pathway, in which plasminogen activators convert plasminogen to plasmin, which degrades fibrin polymer. Several proteins inhibit these pathways: antithrombin III and α_2-macroglobulin inhibit

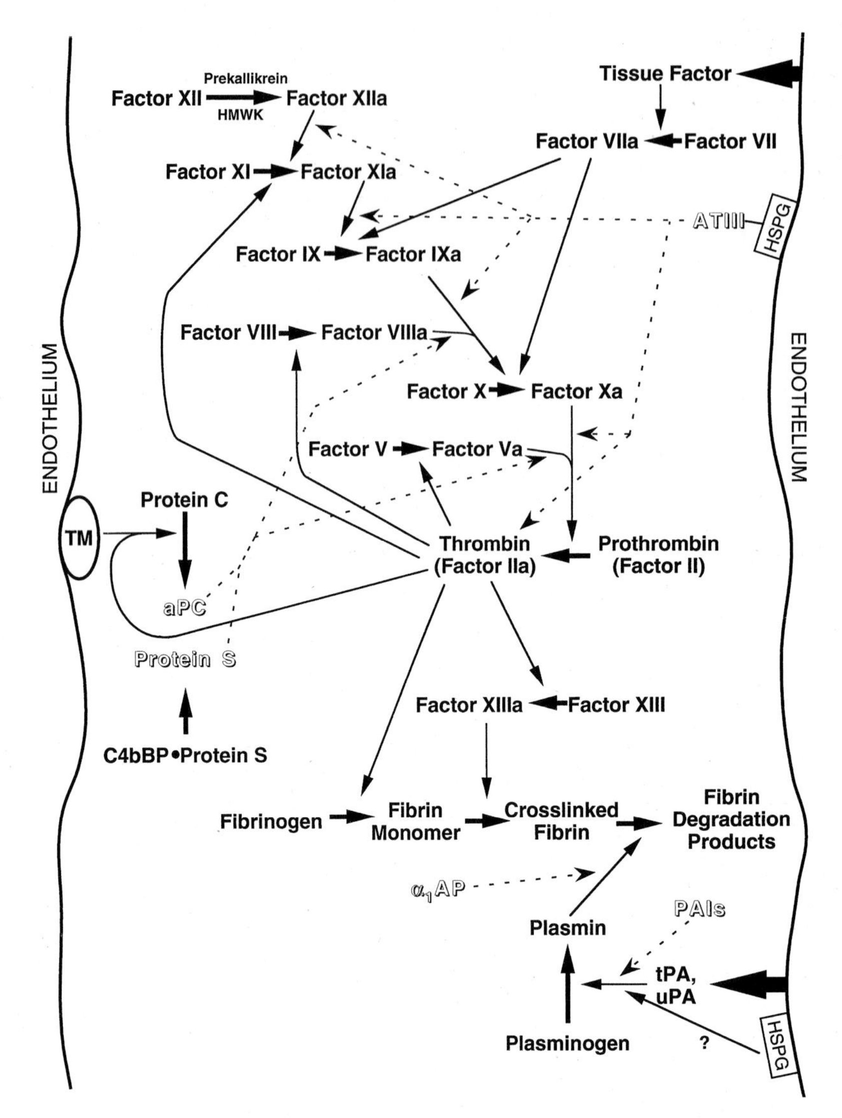

FIGURE 52.6 Interactions among circulating participants in the coagulation cascade. The intrinsic pathway begins in the upper left; the contact system of factor XII, prekallikrein, and high-molecular-weight kininogen (HMWK) that initiates the intrinsic cascade is shown in condensed form. The extrinsic pathway begins in the upper right. The action of factor VIIa on the activation of factor IX has blurred the distinction between these two limbs of the cascade. The common pathway begins with activation of factor X and results in thrombin activity and fibrin cross-linking. Coagulation is counteracted by the fibrinolytic pathway, including plasminogen activators and plasminogen/plasmin. In addition, there are several anticoagulant pathways, most notably inhibition of factors Va and VIIIa by the inhibitory cofactors protein S and activated protein C (aPC). Alpha-2-macroglobulin, which binds to and inhibits most of the enzymes in this system, is not shown here for the purpose of simplicity. The relationship between heparin sulfate proteoglycans (HSPGs) and plasminogen activator activity shown in the lower right should be regarded as hypothetical for human pathophysiology. *Thick solid lines with arrows* indicate reactions; *thin solid lines with triangular arrows* denote catalytic effects; *joining lines* show cofactors in catalysis. *Broken lines with fork-tailed arrows* represent inhibitory actions. PAI-1 and PAI-3 bind to aPC; this interaction may cause mutual inhibition of the action of these proteins. *α_1 AP,* α_1-antiplasmin; *ATIII,* antithrombin III; *C4bBP,* complement factor 4b-binding protein; *PAIs,* plasminogen activator inhibitors; *TM,* thrombomodulin; *tPA,* tissue-type plasminogen activator; *uPA,* urokinase plasminogen activator. (Figure composed with the assistance of G. A. Soff.)

thrombin; α_1-antiplasmin and α_2-macroglobulin inhibit plasmin; and the plasminogen activator inhibitors (PAIs) inhibit plasminogen activators and aPC. Activated protein C, in turn, opposes PAI effects. Many of the components of these pathways are altered in nephrosis. In addition, physical conditions of the nephrotic syndrome, such as venous stasis, hemoconcentration, increased blood viscosity, and possibly the administration of steroids, may also contribute to enhanced blood clotting. These nephrotic effects on coagulation pathways, which are listed in Table 52.3 and discussed in detail elsewhere,[255,262,263] are considered here briefly.

TABLE 52.3 Coagulation System Abnormalities in the Nephrotic Syndrome

Increased platelet aggregation
Thrombocytosis
β-Thromboglobulin
Platelet factor 4
Increased procoagulant activity
Physical factors
Hemoconcentration
Hyperviscosity
Increased factor production
Intrinsic pathway—factors VII and IX (variably)
Extrinsic pathway—factor VII (variably)
Common pathway
Fibrinogen
Factors V and VIII
Factors X and II (variably)
Urinary loss of anticoagulants
Antithrombin III
Free protein S
Increased inhibitors of anticoagulation
α_2-Macroglobulin
C4b-binding protein
Increased plasminogen

Platelet Aggregation

Platelets may play a role in the genesis of the coagulopathy of nephrotic syndrome. Thrombocytosis is commonly found, especially early in the disease course,[264] and platelets show markers of activation.[265] Platelet aggregability is increased and platelet degranulation has been described.[266] In addition, plasma levels of the platelet release substance β-thromboglobulin are increased.[264,267] Levels of platelet factor 4 are normal[268] or increased.[264] In contrast, platelet calcium ion release and ATP secretion have been found to be decreased in nephrosis.[269] The authors of that report suggest that platelets may become desensitized to platelet activating factor (PAF) because of exposure to consistently high ambient concentrations.

Platelet hyperaggregability correlates with the degree of proteinuria and with plasma cholesterol levels. It can be reversed by the addition of urine protein.[268] These findings suggest that the urinary loss of albumin[270] or of some factor that normally inhibits platelet aggregation is responsible for the changes seen in nephrotic syndrome. Alternatively, hyperlipidemia could result in the changes, because platelet aggregation is increased in patients with type II hyperlipoproteinemia to a degree that is comparable to that seen in nephrotic syndrome.[271] Altered platelet function could be a response to hypoalbuminemia, because the conversion of arachidonic acid into metabolites that aggregate platelets is known to be regulated by albumin.[272,273] Thus, platelets show greater production of thromboxane B_2 and malondialdehyde in nephrotic plasma than in normal plasma when challenged with arachidonic acid. The addition of albumin to the nephrotic plasma corrects this abnormality.[274] Finally, it is possible that alterations in platelet membranes could be responsible for increased platelet activity. Platelet membranes contain a sialoglycoprotein with a pK of 1.8 to 2.2.[275] This may be important in preventing spontaneous platelet aggregation or platelet interaction with the vessel wall.[276] Because systemic negative-charge sites may be reduced during relapses of nephrotic syndrome,[69] the same mechanism responsible for the reduction of negative-charge sites in the GBM could enhance platelet aggregation.

Coagulation Factors

Evidence that various functions of blood coagulation are activated in nephrosis is provided by increased concentration of the D-dimer of fibrinogen.[277] Elevated levels of this breakdown product of cross-linked fibrin indicate that both the coagulation and fibrinolytic pathways are concurrently activated. Plasma fibrinogen is consistently elevated in nephrotic syndrome due to increased hepatic synthesis. Chromatography demonstrates both increased polymerization and increased proteolytic derivatives of fibrinogen or fibrin. These changes reverse as patients with nephrotic syndrome enter remission.[278] This evidence for increased intravascular fibrin formation is supported by the finding of increased plasma levels of fibrinopeptide A, at least in FSGS.[278]

The concentration in nephrotic patients of coagulation factors that initiate fibrin formation likely reflects the balance between the increased hepatic synthesis of these proteins, triggered as part of a nonspecific response to hypoproteinemia, as described previously for lipoproteins, and urinary losses. Therefore, lower molecular-size proteins (approximately less than 70 kDa) may be lost in the urine, whereas higher molecular-size proteins (greater than 300 kDa) are likely to be increased in the plasma. For example, most studies agree that levels of factors V and VIII are increased in the plasma, whereas those of factors IX, XI, and XII are decreased[279] despite the possibility that production may still be increased. The magnitude of the increase in concentration of factors V and VIII, for example, correlates with the degree of reduction in serum albumin and the likely resulting increased hepatic synthesis of these factors, stimulated by hypoalbuminemia.[280] Plasma levels of factors II, VII, X, and XIII are often found to be increased.[281–283] There is no direct evidence that any of these changes are responsible for the hypercoagulable state. Indeed, the alterations in blood levels of these factors are often inconsistent and of minor degree. Therefore, these abnormalities may be of more biochemical than clinical interest. Most of the changes in concentration of these zymogen factors reverse with clinical remission of the nephrotic syndrome.

Inhibitors of Coagulation

The most well-studied biologic antagonist of coagulation, antithrombin III, is decreased in the plasma of nephrotic patients.[284–288] This is presumed to be due to urinary loss of antithrombin III, which has a relatively low molecular weight. Indeed, plasma antithrombin III levels in nephrotic syndrome correlate well with those of serum albumin and inversely with the renal clearance of antithrombin III. Because hereditary antithrombin III deficiency is associated with frequent thrombosis, it was hypothesized that the low plasma antithrombin III levels were insufficient to inactivate procoagulant factors and were the major cause for the hypercoagulable state and the development of thrombosis in nephrotic syndrome.[286] However, only patients with plasma albumin levels below 2 g per deciliter show significant reductions in plasma antithrombin III levels,[289] whereas hypercoagulability may be present in patients with albumin levels exceeding this value. Further, normal plasma levels of antithrombin III were found in nephrotic subjects who had loss of antithrombin III in the urine and who had thromboembolic complications.[290] Indeed, decreases in antithrombin III levels may be compensated for by increased plasma levels of α_2-macroglobulin,[283] leading to increased total antithrombin activity.[278]

A complex effect of nephrosis has been noted on the anticoagulation pathway by which protein C is activated by thrombin and thrombomodulin to aPC. Activated protein C and protein S combine to inhibit factor VIIIa (decreasing activation of factor X) and factor Va (decreasing activation of factor XI). Protein S exists in circulation in two forms: free and bound to C4b binding protein. Only the free protein S can serve as a cofactor with protein C to inactivate factors Va and VIIIa.[291] In nephrotic syndrome, although small amounts of protein C are lost in the urine, serum concentrations are normal,[292,293] indicating that hepatic synthesis is able to compensate. In contrast, although plasma levels of C4b binding protein–protein S complex are usually normal to elevated, free levels are markedly decreased.[294] This finding is consistent with the molecular sizes of the complex (640 kDa) and the free protein S (69 kDa). Acquired dysfunction of this system is a common cause of thrombotic diathesis.[291,295] Indeed, intractable deep vein thrombosis in an unusual nephrotic child with decreases in both protein S and C4b-binding protein concentrations[296] supports the notion that abnormalities of this system are clinically significant.

Fibrinolysis

Alterations in the concentrations of several of the components of the fibrinolytic system have been documented.[297] Decreased fibrinolytic activity has been associated with hypertriglyceridemia.[298] Of the individual components of the fibrinolytic system, decreased concentrations of plasminogen have been found[287,299]; levels of tissue-type plasminogen activator[277] and PAI-1[300] are elevated. Varying levels of α_2-antiplasmin have been reported,[277,278] possibly depending on whether thrombosis has occurred. Of the serine protease inhibitors that modulate both the fibrinolytic and thrombin systems, levels of α_2-macroglobulin are increased and those of α_1-antitrypsin are decreased.[283] Again, this probably reflects the effect of urinary loss on plasma concentrations. It also is possible that local vascular conditions affect fibrinolysis. The infusion of a variety of polyanions causes an immediate local increase in the release of plasminogen activator and PAI activity in the sow ear. The PAI activity immediately returns to normal but the increase in plasminogen activator activity is sustained,[301] suggesting that negative charges in the vascular tree are important for inducing the plasminogen activator pathway. If nephrosis is associated with a generalized reduction of fixed negative charge sites in the vascular space,[69] it is likely that decreased negative charges could have an impact on the induction of fibrinolysis. Coupled with increased α_2-antiplasmin concentrations, decreased tissue-type plasminogen activator activity would significantly impair fibrin degradation. However, the increase in circulating D-dimer cited previously indicates that at least some fibrinolysis occurs in nephrosis. It also is possible that fibrin polymerization is impaired in nephrotic patients. In one study of a broad spectrum of adults with nephrosis, most had prolonged thrombin times. Half of the patients showed decreased ability to polymerize fibrin monomer. There was no correlation of this finding with prothrombin time, partial thromboplastin time, fibrin degradation products, antithrombin III concentration, or platelet count.[302]

Physical Factors Affecting Coagulation

Physical factors such as increased blood viscosity also may contribute to the generation of thromboembolic complications.[303] Both children and adults with MCNS and well-preserved renal function may have marked hemoconcentration with elevated hematocrit and hemoglobin concentrations. Such changes are associated with disproportionate increases in viscosity and could be aggravated by the therapeutic use of diuretics, especially if these cause further hemoconcentration. In addition, when plasma fibrinogen levels increase, especially to values as high as 1 g per deciliter as can be seen in nephrotic syndrome, they cause increased erythrocyte aggregation and marked increases in plasma viscosity.[304] A role for physical factors is supported by the high incidence of renal vein thrombosis, because hemoconcentration of the blood and the effect of urinary inhibitor loss will be most pronounced in the radicles of the renal vein.[305]

Steroid administration increases the concentrations of several clotting factors and modifies coagulation mechanisms.[255] Moreover, a high incidence of thromboses was recorded after these drugs were first used to treat nephrotic syndrome.[306] Both arterial and venous thromboses, however, have been found in nephrotic subjects not receiving steroids. Furthermore, a hypercoagulable state is present in untreated MCNS patients, and levels of the coagulation factors do not change after steroid treatment is implemented.[278]

Except for the protein S data, the potential relationship between various biochemical findings and the clinical importance of thrombus formation remains largely theoretical. For example, the biochemical abnormalities in children may be more severe than in adults with the nephrotic syndrome, whereas the incidence of thromboembolic phenomena is worse in adults.[307] This may reflect the fact that MCN is more common in children, whereas membranous nephropathy (see Chapter 63) is more common in adults. Therefore, the underlying nature of the disease may be important in determining the occurrence of intravascular coagulation. Finally, it is important to consider the physiologic conditions within the circulatory tree. For example, one study suggested that although platelet aggregation is increased in nephrosis, fibrin conversion inhibits platelet interaction with the vessel wall extracellular matrix, actually decreasing the likelihood of platelet participation in thrombus formation. In this system, the data suggest that increased fibrin formation, but not increased platelet aggregation, contributes to the hypercoagulability of the nephrotic syndrome.[308] In support of a primary role for the coagulation cascade, nephrotic patients show biochemical evidence for endothelial injury.[309] The effects of negative-charge sites must also be considered. Like plasminogen activator activity, antithrombin III is active in association with vascular wall heparin sulfate proteoglycans. If MCNS involves a generalized decrease in negative-charge sites, antithrombin III activity may be impaired.

Infections

It has long been known that patients with MCNS have increased susceptibility to infection. This increase may be related to the prolonged presence of gross edema or ascites, which are composed of fluids that represent ideal culture media for bacterial growth. The infection risk may be potentiated by therapy with steroids or immunosuppressive drugs, although the high incidence of infections was noted in the era before these drugs were available. Humoral responses to bacteria may be defective. Plasma concentrations of IgG are markedly reduced during relapse,[310] and the ability of MCN patients to generate specific antibodies is impaired[311] between as well as during relapses. Although the role of these abnormalities in predisposing nephrotic subjects to infections remains to be elucidated, it may be significant that boys with MCN respond poorly to the hepatitis B vaccine.[312] This same population has a higher incidence of chronic hepatitis B surface antigenemia than that found in a control population.[313] Another factor that could contribute to a high rate of infections in patients with nephrosis is a decreased serum level of alternative complement pathway factor B. Absence of this factor has been linked to defective opsonization of *Escherichia coli* in nephrotic patients[314] and to defective neutrophil function.[315] Serum levels of hemolytic factor D also are decreased in patients during relapse and return to normal with remission.[316] Levels of both of these factors correlate strongly with serum albumin concentration, suggesting that decreased serum levels result from urinary loss. These concerns have led to recommendations that both pediatric and adult patients with nephrosis should receive the pneumococcal polysaccharide (23-valent) vaccine.[317,318] In addition, the use of penicillin prophylaxis may be required in children younger than 2 years of age, or in older patients who have low antibody titers or recurrent pneumococcal infections.[319] Immune system abnormalities more specifically associated with MCN are unlikely to result entirely from albuminuria, because they are specific for that disease; these will be considered in the section on MCN later in this chapter.

Consequences of Loss of Other Proteins

Numerous proteins in addition to albumin are lost in the urine. In most instances, these proteins are of a similar or smaller size than albumin. Such losses could alter function in the endocrine system or in metabolic pathways. Therefore, the loss of insulinlike growth factors could contribute to poor growth in some nephrotic children.[320] The urinary loss of thyroxin-binding globulin (TBG) correlates well with total urinary protein excretion.[321] In addition to TBG, losses of thyroxine (T_4) and triiodothyronine (T_3) in nephrotic urine are associated with decreased serum levels of T_3 and TBG. Most of the patients studied were clinically euthyroid and their serum levels of free T_4 and thyroid-stimulating hormone (TSH) did not differ from those in normal control subjects.[322] In addition, their values for T_3 uptake were normal. Another study documented urinary losses, but normal serum concentrations of TBG.[323] The patients had low or low-normal T_4 levels. Such differences in findings could relate to the underlying cause for nephrotic syndrome, whether it is associated with selective or nonselective proteinuria and whether it is accompanied by uremia. Children with MCNS have serum T_4 or free T_4 levels that are marginally low.[324] They have been interpreted as having mild thyroid failure based on increased baseline TSH levels and their response to thyrotropin-releasing hormone.[325] In patients who have congenital nephrotic syndrome, nephrectomy to eliminate proteinuria is associated with normalization of thyroid status, indicating that these abnormalities result from massive proteinuria rather than an intrinsic glandular defect.[326]

Total serum calcium is markedly reduced, primarily because of hypoalbuminemia and the consequent decrease in protein-bound calcium. Serum ionized calcium levels may be reduced as well,[327,328] even in nephrotic subjects with normal renal function; this may result in symptomatic hypocalcemia. At least some of the reduction in ionized calcium is the consequence of a loss of 25-hydroxyvitamin D (25-[OH]-D) in nephrotic urine[329,330]; normally bound to and absorbed via megalin, vitamin D–binding protein is lost as the protein reabsorptive capacity is saturated and exceeded due to proteinuria. Other metabolites of vitamin D may be lost as well.[331] Low plasma levels of 25-(OH)-D, 1,25$(OH)_2$-D, and 24,25-$(OH)_2$-D have been reported in patients with nephrotic syndrome,[330] and intestinal absorption of calcium is reduced[327]; serum parathyroid hormone levels are increased.[328] From these observations, it has been postulated[332] that urinary loss of vitamin D complex results in decreased absorption of intestinal calcium, skeletal resistance to parathyroid hormone, and reduced serum calcium levels. In turn, these changes cause increased parathyroid hormone (PTH) production and could result in defective bone mineralization. Although it has not been proved that the changes described cause significant bone disease,[333] ongoing steroid therapy may increase the likelihood of clinically significant problems.[334,335] In 60 children and adolescents with relapsing nephrotic syndrome, bone mineral density (BMD) was decreased, but whole-body bone mineral content was higher because of an increase in the body-metabolic index.[335] In patients with unremitting proteinuria and low 25-OH-D levels, supplementation with oral calcium and 25-OH-D should be considered.[336]

Carbohydrate metabolism also may be deranged. Of 38 adult nephrotic patients who had not received any drugs, including glucocorticoids, for at least 2 months, 14 had oral glucose tolerance test results that were similar to those found in diabetic patients.[337] Affected patients had increased insulin secretion that was thought to be secondary to increased growth hormone levels. The initiating event for these changes was not determined. There was no correlation of these findings with either serum albumin levels or renal histopathology. This observation raises the question of whether nephrotic hyperlipidemia could contribute to the development of noninsulin-dependent (type 2) diabetes mellitus.

Alterations in trace metal metabolism may be due to urinary losses of either the metals or their carrier proteins. Decreased serum levels of both iron and copper, associated with a low serum iron-binding capacity and low erythrocyte copper content, have been documented in nephrotic syndrome.[338] Serum levels of copper, but not iron, were improved by oral administration of the metal. Urinary iron and copper concentrations correlated with protein excretion. The intravenous infusion of albumin led to increased albuminuria and increased metal excretion. In each case, the abnormalities appeared to be related to urinary protein loss. Nephrotic children may develop anemia secondary to urinary loss of transferrin and iron.[339,340] Serum zinc levels are low in nephrotic syndrome, but urinary excretion of zinc is not elevated. Zinc binds to albumin so that serum zinc levels change with alterations in albumin levels, regardless of the etiology of the nephrotic syndrome. However, decreased zinc content in the hair of these patients suggests that other aspects of zinc metabolism also may be deranged.[341]

Many drugs are protein bound in the plasma. Hypoalbuminemia decreases the number of drug-binding sites and could result in increased toxicity of drugs that normally are bound to protein. For example, digoxin is 25% bound to proteins in the plasma, digitoxin is 90% bound, hydrochlorothiazide is 60% bound, and furosemide is 96% bound; hydralazine, prazosin, and diazoxide are all approximately 90% bound, whereas the binding of barbiturates varies from 5% to 80% depending on the molecular structure.[342]

General Approach to the Treatment of Nephrotic Syndrome

Based on the consequences of proteinuria described in the preceding text, symptomatic treatment regimens have been developed for the care of all nephrotic patients, even beyond those classified as having a form of primary nephrotic syndrome. These treatments, which are aimed at the physiology of nephrosis rather than the etiology of the disease, have implications beyond the reduction of nephrotic proteinuria and edema.

Diuretics and Fluid Management

Many patients with nephrotic syndrome respond to the acute use of diuretics with increased urinary losses of sodium and water. Although diuretics may be effective, there are limited indications for their use in the acute treatment of nephrotic subjects, especially children. The degree of diuresis and natriuresis they induce is small compared to that observed when the patient responds to treatment directed at the underlying cause. Furthermore, it is possible that diuretic use, by depleting intravascular as well as interstitial fluid volume, may contribute to the development of shock seen in some patients with MCNS.[173]

Nonetheless, oral or parenteral diuretics are effective and often are indicated in the management of persistent edema. Parenteral furosemide is more effective than an orally administered drug. Treatment may be initiated at 1 mg per kilogram (up to 40 mg) with judicious increases up to three to four times the usual dose[343] in an effort to elicit a response. Diuretic therapy may be less effective in patients with primary nephrotic syndrome than in most other patients, in part because of a combination of factors resulting in a physiologically decreased ability to excrete sodium. This is especially true of the loop diuretics such as furosemide, which also may be inhibited by its binding to albumin present in the tubular lumen.[344] Although spironolactone interferes with distal nephron sodium reabsorption and thus is a theoretically useful diuretic, in practice its delayed onset of action and relatively weak potency limit its usefulness to being a potentiating agent with loop diuretics. Metolazone, a thiazidelike drug that impedes both proximal and late distal nephron sodium absorption,[345] is a singularly effective oral diuretic in patients with sodium retention secondary to nephrotic syndrome. There is a possibility that diuretic therapy will deplete the intravascular volume without significantly reducing the tissue edema. Therefore, diuretics should be administered with care and withheld in patients for whom a rapid response to steroids is anticipated.

If the patient has anasarca, if respiratory embarrassment results from ascites or pleural effusion, if scrotal or vulval edema is sufficiently severe to threaten tissue breakdown,[346] or if peritonitis is present, then more aggressive therapy is warranted to decrease the amount of edema. A useful regimen consists of oral spironolactone, 1 mg per kilogram per day, and daily intravenous infusions of albumin, 0.5 g per kilogram initially and increasing, if well tolerated, to 1 g per kilogram per day. The albumin infusion should be preceded by the intravenous infusion of furosemide, 0.5 mg per kilogram. A repeated dose of diuretic is given toward the end of the albumin infusion. Blood pressure should be monitored throughout the albumin infusion to help avoid complications from rapid mobilization of edema fluid into the circulation, although the regimen usually is free from significant side effects when used in children and young adults. Some observations suggest that the administration of albumin may result in more severe glomerular epithelial changes, should raise the oncotic pressure of the tissue space, should delay the response to corticosteroid therapy, and should induce more frequent relapses after remission.[347] In view of the potential for complications of albumin infusion,[348] this treatment should be reserved for the specific indications of respiratory embarrassment, tissue breakdown, or the need to elicit urine output to confirm the diagnosis of nephrosis.

Management of the acute phase of nephrotic syndrome should include dietary sodium restriction. During relapse, dietary sodium intake optimally should be reduced to about 0.5 g per day, which is approximately equivalent to a 1-g salt diet or about 20 mEq of sodium per day. Such severe dietary restriction is difficult to accomplish even in a carefully controlled hospital setting. It is important to emphasize that severe restriction of sodium intake will not result in weight loss when nephrotic patients are in the sodium-retaining phase of their disease. In such patients, the normal extrarenal losses of sodium may amount to less than 10 mEq per day. Therefore, severe dietary sodium restriction is intended to prevent further accumulation of edema. Use of a salt substitute may facilitate compliance with the sodium-restricted diet, but in patients with renal insufficiency, it must be limited because these preparations consist of potassium and ammonium salts.

At home, most patients can rarely manage dietary restriction below that of a no-added-salt diet. This provides a sodium intake of 40 to 60 mEq per day depending on the patient's size. Even in remission, it should be employed not only to lessen the risk of edema formation if the patient has a relapse, but also to reduce side effects from steroid administration.

Although there is some debate regarding fluid management, we believe that fluid intake also should be restricted, at least initially. If intake equals insensible fluid losses plus urine output, the patient's weight will remain stable without further accumulation of edema. To accomplish a loss of weight, fluid intake must be reduced below this level. Some nephrotic patients experience intense thirst. If sodium intake is limited and fluid intake is great, the patient can become hyponatremic and will remain edematous.

Anecdotal experience suggests that bed rest may potentiate a diuresis, perhaps by redistributing fluid from the peripheral tissues to the vascular space, thereby increasing renal blood flow. Bed rest also may accelerate a response to steroids and, when practical, should be advised for patients with anasarca. Other therapies that may facilitate a diuresis in some patients by mobilizing tissue fluid include local pressure using surgical elastic stockings or immersion up to the neck in warm water.[135] After remission is induced, a high-protein diet may increase the rate at which plasma protein concentration returns to normal.[349]

Dietary Treatment

As already indicated, dietary sodium and water restriction is important in the management of the acute phase of nephrotic syndrome. Long-term reduction of dietary sodium intake in combination with diuretics can be most effective at controlling edema in patients resistant to steroids and other pharmacologic agents.

Other dietary manipulations have received attention. High-protein diets can be beneficial in special groups of patients such as those with congenital nephrotic syndrome.[350] The concept of increasing dietary protein in all nephrotic subjects has not proved to be beneficial. Although albumin synthesis increases with such diets, urinary protein excretion increases too, possibly due to an angiotensin II–induced increase in glomerular permeability. Therefore, it has been proposed that inhibitors of ACE should be used in conjunction with the high-protein intake.[100]

Conversely, low-protein diets will decrease albuminuria and will increase albumin mass.[351] This reflects conservation of essential amino acids in response to proteinuria.[352] The use of soy-based, low-protein, low-fat diets rich in polyunsaturated fats and supplemented with essential amino acids or keto analogs results in decreases in urinary protein excretion and in serum total and LDL cholesterol levels.[353–355] Supplementing diets with fish oils containing ω-3 fatty acids has not proved beneficial.[356] Concerns about such dietary manipulations include their cost, the lack of patient acceptance, and whether strict adherence might result in specific nutritional deficiencies.[351,357] Reducing dietary fat intake in hyperlipidemic but otherwise healthy children to the levels recommended by the National Cholesterol Education Program is safe and does not affect the children's growth or development.[358] The safety of more stringent restrictions in children with renal disease remains to be determined.

Lowering dietary fat intake has a limited effect on reducing serum lipids in the nephrotic patient. Therefore, attention has focused on whether there is a role for lipid-lowering drugs in managing hyperlipidemia in these patients (see the following paragraph). The efficacy of oligoantigenic diets or those that eliminate specific antigens has been tested in nephrotic subjects (see section on Atopy and Minimal Change Nephropathy). This approach is based on the possibility that some cases of nephrotic syndrome may be the consequence of food allergies, especially to milk and dairy products.

Lipid-Lowering Drugs

Long-term administration of HMG CoA reductase inhibitors in nephrotic patients will induce reductions of serum triglycerides as well as serum total and LDL cholesterol levels; HDL cholesterol values are maintained.[201,251,359,360] Long-term benefits from this therapy have yet to be proved, although anecdotal experience suggests that it may help to reduce proteinuria and maintain GFR,[361] as observed in experimental animals (see section on Hyperlipidemia).

Other Medical Therapy

Anticoagulation has been employed as indicated in patients with intravascular thromboses. Some clinicians use small doses of aspirin in an effort to prevent repeated thromboembolic episodes,[362] but there are no studies confirming the efficacy of this approach.

Although hypocalcemia is common in relapses of nephrotic syndrome, it is likely that most patients in relapse of brief duration do not require routine treatment with calcium or with vitamin D or one of its metabolites.[363] Supplementation with oral calcium (1 g per day) and 25-OH-vitamin D (25 μg per day) maintains normal bone status in steroid-dependent nephrotic patients.[336] Vitamin D treatment may be more routinely necessary in patients who are steroid-resistant[364] (see section on Consequences of Loss of Other Proteins previously in this chapter). Similarly, patients who develop other deficiencies secondary to renal losses, such as iron-deficiency anemia, will require appropriate treatment.

Medical Treatment to Reduce Proteinuria

In patients who prove to be unresponsive to therapy directed at the underlying cause of proteinuria, efforts have been employed to decrease protein loss by employing drugs that appear to be directed against the physiology of glomerular proteinuria. The intent behind this treatment is to facilitate general medical management by decreasing proteinuria, increasing serum albumin, and thereby lessening edema formation. Thus, indomethacin is effective at ameliorating intractable nephrosis.[365] Because of the association of nonsteroidal agents with renal failure in some nephrotic patients as described in the section on Complications, more recently, clinicians have emphasized the use of ACE inhibition.[103,366] Each of these treatments appears to reduce glomerular capillary hydraulic pressure, by different mechanisms. ACE inhibitors act by decreasing postglomerular arteriolar resistance, whereas nonsteroidal drugs enhance preglomerular capillary resistance.[367] Consistent with these mechanisms, Garini and colleagues[368] compared the effects of indomethacin, captopril, and the calcium-channel blocker, nifedipine, on the changes in renal hemodynamics and proteinuria induced by a high-protein mean. The increases in GFR and renal blood flow were not blocked by captopril or nifedipine, but were blocked by indomethacin. The increase in protein excretion was blocked by indomethacin and captopril but not by nifedipine.[368] Indeed, dihydropyridine calcium channel blockers do not decrease proteinuria[369] and may even increase it. Therefore, the effects on hemodynamics were different and the effect on proteinuria could be distinguished from both systemic effects on blood pressure and effects on GFR and RBF. In patients with membranous nephropathy, ACE inhibition may have a size-selective effect,[370] decreasing the fractional clearance of larger (>60 Å) molecules, suggesting an effect on the shunt pathway of macromolecular clearance. Such studies have supported efforts by clinicians to utilize ACE inhibitors to decrease proteinuria not only for symptomatic management but also in an effort to delay or prevent the progression of chronic kidney disease. Angiotensin-receptor blockade (ARB) has an equivalent effect to that of ACE inhibition, and the combination of ACE inhibition and ARB has been proposed to be more effective than either alone.[371] The efficacy of this treatment will be considered further in the section on FSGS.

It is possible that at least a part of the antiproteinuric effect of ACE inhibition is not mediated by the glomerulus. Angiotensin blockade enhances megalin expression and albumin reabsorption,[372] and indeed, the angiotensin antagonist, eplerenone, is synergistic with ACE inhibition in reducing nephrotic proteinuria.[373]

Nephrectomy. Unilateral nephrectomy has proved beneficial in some infants presenting with nephrotic syndrome in the first year of life,[374] and bilateral nephrectomy may be a useful part of the aggressive approach required in patients with congenital nephrotic syndrome if they are to survive to an age when transplantation is feasible[375,376] (see section on Nephrotic Syndrome in the First Year of Life, later in this chapter). Bilateral embolization of renal arteries can be an important therapeutic option in carefully selected patients with nephrotic syndrome who appear destined to progress to end-stage renal failure.[377]

MINIMAL CHANGE NEPHROPATHY

Although MCN is often thought of as a pediatric disease, it is the third most common cause of nephrosis in adults[9] and remains the most common cause of nephrotic syndrome in children younger than 16 years of age. Indeed, it is the second most common primary renal parenchymal disease in that age group. Two to 7 new cases occur annually per 100,000 children,[378] and the prevalence is about 15 cases per 100,000 children. Although most children with MCN achieve permanent remission of symptoms by the time they reach puberty, some cases persist into adulthood.[379] Furthermore, new cases have been reported in the eighth decade of life.[380] However, the relative incidence of MCN as the etiology of nephrotic syndrome decreases with age in both children and adults.[9,380–382] Although it is not clear that adult-onset disease represents the same entity as that found in childhood, or that all patients with the clinical picture of MCNS have an identical disease, the clinical course and outcome of pediatric and adult cases appear to be sufficiently similar[380] to consider all cases together.

Minimal change disease can appear in the first year of life, but it is more common later, with a peak incidence at 2 years of age. Most pediatric surveys report that it occurs twice as often in boys as in girls, whereas it has an equal sex incidence in adults.[383] Although no precipitating cause may be apparent in many children, it is not unusual for the development of edema and proteinuria to be preceded by an upper respiratory tract infection, an allergic reaction to an insect sting or other immunogenic stimuli, or the use of certain drugs (Table 52.4).[383–398,400–407,409–411,415] In both adult and pediatric patients, malignancies, especially Hodgkin disease, have been associated with the development of MCNS (see section on Nephrotic Syndrome and Malignancies).

Clinical Findings

Edema formation may begin within a few days of the inciting event. Facial edema usually is noted first, with few other indications of an ongoing disease process. This can be confused with allergic symptoms, especially if associated with an upper respiratory tract infection. Edema usually increases gradually. It becomes detectable in the adult only when several liters of fluid have accumulated; by the time medical advice is sought, the patient typically has pitting edema involving the sacrum and the lower extremities. When anasarca is present, periorbital edema can be so severe that the eyelids are swollen shut, scrotal or vulval edema may be marked, and there may be significant abdominal distension. Respiratory embarrassment may occur from accumulation of either pleural or ascitic fluid, although the infrequency of dyspnea or orthopnea in the setting of massive fluid retention is striking. This reflects the absence of increased pulmonary capillary wedge pressure needed to generate pulmonary edema. Headaches and irritability are common accompanying complaints of edema. The patient may note vague symptoms such as malaise, easy fatigability, irritability, and depression. Rarely, the development of cellulitis, peritonitis, or pneumonia may be the first indication of an underlying nephrotic syndrome. The pallor resulting from edema can be misinterpreted as indicating anemia.

On physical examination, dependent edema is the most prominent finding. The retina has a characteristic “wet” appearance. Subungual edema may reverse the usual color pattern on the fingernails—the normally white lunulae may be pink and the rest of the nail bed white. Horizontal white lines that may be seen on both the fingernails and the toenails are referred to as *Muehrcke bands*. Inguinal and umbilical hernias may be present, especially if the patient has had severe ascites for a prolonged period. The elasticity of the cartilage in the ear appears to be decreased.

Blood pressure in patients with MCN usually is normal, but elevated systolic pressure was recorded in 21% and elevated diastolic pressure in 14% of the children evaluated by the International Study of Kidney Disease in Children (ISKDC).[416] Hypertension is seen more commonly in adult patients with MCN.[417]

Growth failure occasionally may be found in children, most often in those who have had multiple relapses of MCNS.[418] Evidence for infection, especially peritonitis, cellulitis, or pneumonia, should be sought as part of the physical examination. These infections may be associated with septicemia and shock.

In MCNS, the chest radiograph usually shows a small or normal-sized heart; pleural effusions may be present, as may pneumonic infiltrates. The presence of an increased heart size and congestive changes in the hilar regions suggests that the nephrotic syndrome is secondary to glomerulonephritis.

TABLE 52.4 Factors Reported to Have Precipitated Minimal Change Nephropathy (MCN)

Gold[384] Penicillamine[385] Ampicillin[386] Mercury-containing compounds[387] Nonsteroidal anti-inflammatory agents[388–391] Trimethadione, paramethadione[392]
Atopy Pollen[393] Food allergy[394,395] House dust[396] Contact dermatitis (poison ivy and oak)[397] Bee[398] or wasp[399] stings
Tumors Lymphoma[400,401] Others[402]
Infections Various viral infections[403] Schistosomiasis[404] Ehrlichiosis[405]
Stimuli-associated with immune activation or inflammation Guillain-Barré syndrome[406] Still disease[407] Immunizations[408,409] Dermatitis herpetiformis[410] Epidermolysis bullosa[411] Autoimmune thyroiditis[412,413] Sclerosing cholangitis[414]

Laboratory Findings

Urinalysis

Clinicians who first characterized the nephrotic syndrome noted that the urine often foams excessively when voided and that it coagulates when heated. These findings result from marked proteinuria, now indicated by a dipstick reading of 3+. Other edema-forming, hypoalbuminemic states, such as malnutrition, milk protein sensitivity, and protein-losing enteropathy, can mimic nephrotic syndrome but do not manifest significant proteinuria. The amount of protein in the urine of nephrotic patients can range from less than 1 g to more than 25 g per day. The value for adult patients usually is between 3.5 and 16 g per day; that for children typically is lower than this amount, even when allowances are made for body size[419] and averages about 50 mg per kilogram of body weight per day.[420] Because urine protein is a function of plasma, and thus of filtrate, protein concentration,[421] children with MCNS, who may have serum albumin levels of 1 g per deciliter or less, may occasionally have amounts of urinary protein as low as 100 to 200 mg per day. This finding in patients with low plasma albumin concentrations also reflects the removal of much of the protein from the glomerular filtrate as it traverses the proximal convoluted tubule[422] (see previous section on Tubular Handling of Protein in Mechanisms for Proteinuria). As a consequence of proteinuria, the urine specific gravity in nephrosis usually is high, often exceeding 1.035. Exceptions include patients who are not in an edema-accumulating state (see section on Consequences of Proteinuria, earlier in this chapter) and the patient with nephrotic syndrome and renal failure or tubular dysfunction, in whom lower (but not isosthenuric) values of urine specific gravity are found. Physiologic responses of the kidney to the nephrotic state may cause further urine concentration.

The spectrum of excreted proteins depends on the renal disease responsible for the nephrotic syndrome. In primary nephrotic syndrome, most of the urine protein is albumin; in other diseases, such as glomerulonephritis, both albumin and globulins are lost in increased amounts. This occurrence has led to determination of "protein selectivity" being proposed as a noninvasive method to separate MCNS from other causes of nephrotic syndrome.[423] By comparing clearance of albumin to that of larger molecules such as IgG or transferrin, a curve can be generated, indicating whether the protein loss is *selective* and restricted to small molecules, or *nonselective*, consisting of both large and small molecules. Patients with MCNS tend to show more selective proteinuria, whereas those with nephrotic syndrome from other causes have nonselective proteinuria. Unfortunately, this generalization is limited by considerable overlap in results from patients in different diagnostic categories, so that the clinical determination of protein selectivity has limited value for individual patients. This limitation may reflect factors other than molecular size that also affect entry of proteins into the glomerular filtrate, and differences in tubular function, which modify the reabsorption of filtered protein.[424] A refined electrophoretic technique has been used to indicate protein selectivity and to predict outcomes. Patients with primarily albumin and transferrin in urine as determined by sodium dodecyl sulfate-polyacrylamide gel electrophoresis (SDS-PAGE) proved to be steroid sensitive, whereas patients who were steroid resistant also excreted considerable amounts of IgG, lysozyme, and other larger molecules.[425] Some of these larger molecules could be derived from tubular cells, reflecting tubulointerstitial injury rather than glomerular filtration, or from activation of the shunt pathway for filtration of macromolecules discussed earlier in this chapter. In analbuminemic rats with PAN nephrosis, fractional clearances of various macromolecules are similar to those in normoalbuminemic rats. The absence of competition for albumin implied by this finding suggests that the urinary loss of these proteins in nephrotic patients does not result from "overload" of tubular reabsorption by filtered albumin.[76]

The urine sediment from nephrotic subjects often contains oval fat bodies. Lipiduria is better diagnosed, however, using a microscope equipped with polarized light to demonstrate doubly refractile fat bodies ("Maltese crosses") in degenerative fatty vacuoles in the cytoplasm of desquamated renal epithelial cells or free in the urine as neutral fat droplets. Frequently, urine with large amounts of protein also contains hyaline casts.

Other urinary findings vary with the cause of the disease. Up to one third of patients with MCN may have microscopic hematuria. Gross hematuria may be seen in patients with uncomplicated MCN but is extremely rare.[426] By contrast, it is more common in patients with prominent mesangial proliferation. Hematuria is more likely to be seen with FSGS than MCN.[427] In patients with nephrotic syndrome secondary to glomerulonephritis, the urine shows more abnormalities, with cellular elements and granular, cellular, and mixed hyaline casts being present. However, patients with MCN cannot always be differentiated from those with glomerulonephritis on the basis of urine sediment abnormalities alone.

Blood Studies

Hypoproteinemia is common to all nephrotic patients and is caused, primarily, by hypoalbuminemia. Total serum protein is characteristically reduced to between 4.5 and 5.5 g per deciliter; serum albumin concentrations usually fall to below 2 g per deciliter, and, in children, may be less than 1 g per deciliter.[379] Although serum albumin concentrations are usually decreased, those of total globulins are remarkably well preserved in MCN despite massive proteinuria. Typically, serum α_1-globulin concentrations are normal or slightly decreased, whereas levels of serum α_2- and β-globulins are increased. Although the concentration of γ-globulin determined by electrophoresis is normal or reduced, the levels of individual components vary. In MCN,[310,403] serum IgG levels average approximately 20% of normal, whereas IgA levels are less severely reduced; IgM and in some cases IgE levels are increased. The changes in serum IgG and IgA concentrations are less pronounced in patients with nephrotic syndrome of other causes; IgM and IgE are typically normal in these subjects.[310,403]

Hyperlipidemia is one of the findings that define the nephrotic syndrome. Serum total cholesterol level is usually elevated, especially when the serum albumin level has fallen to 2 g per deciliter or less.[175] Values average 400 mg per deciliter, but levels in excess of 1,000 mg per deciliter have been recorded. Other changes in plasma lipids are summarized in the section on Consequences of Proteinuria.

Most often, serum electrolyte concentrations are within the normal range even when anasarca is present, indicating a proportionate retention of sodium and water. Factitiously low serum sodium concentrations (~130 mEq per liter) may be measured with marked hyperlipidemia. This pseudohyponatremia results from the nonaqueous, nonsodium-containing component of the serum or plasma (lipid) being increased. It does not require treatment, because the sodium concentration in the aqueous phase of blood is normal, as is plasma osmolality. This artifact is not observed when sodium levels are determined by techniques that measure sodium activity with ion-specific electrodes or after sample ultracentrifugation. Low serum sodium may be an accurate finding in the case of excess free water ingestion relative to dietary sodium intake,[428] compounded by potential effects of elevated plasma vasopressin.[429] This problem may be exacerbated by diuretic therapy. A decreased anion gap is associated with decreased total serum protein or albumin levels. This finding is common to all hypoalbuminemic states and does not directly reflect either renal dysfunction or altered serum lipid levels.[430] Serum calcium may be low, mainly as a result of the hypoalbuminemia. Normally, 40% of total serum calcium is bound to protein. A decrease in serum albumin concentration of 1 g per deciliter results in a decrease in total serum calcium of 0.8 mg per deciliter. In contrast, 1 g of globulin binds only 0.16 mg of calcium. In some cases, the hypocalcemia may be out of proportion to the hypoalbuminemia and is caused by a reduction of ionized calcium levels[431] by as much as 5% to 20%, possibly because of urinary loss of 25-OH-D (see section on Consequences of Proteinuria). Acute symptoms of hypocalcemia rarely occur. Total and ionized calcium levels return to normal with remission. Serum phosphorus is normal unless the nephrotic syndrome is associated with renal insufficiency.

Blood urea nitrogen (BUN) and serum creatinine values are usually close to normal in MCN, but may be mildly elevated if decreased intravascular volume from nephrosis causes prerenal azotemia. The BUN may be elevated because of either increased intrarenal urea circulation or increased protein catabolism if the patient has received steroids. The GFR measured by inulin clearance is reduced to an average of 80% of normal[157]; occasionally, values are reduced to 20% to 30% of normal. This may represent decreased renal perfusion secondary to hypovolemia. Reduced GFR at the onset of MCN is reversible and does not imply an unfavorable outcome.[110] The presence or absence of azotemia therefore cannot be used as a reliable indicator in the differential diagnosis of the nephrotic syndrome.

Hemoglobin levels and hematocrit values may be normal or even increased if there is hemoconcentration secondary to a loss of fluid into the peripheral tissues. This factor may help to differentiate azotemic patients with MCN from those who have severe renal insufficiency from parenchymal disease, in whom anemia is more typical. However, as noted previously, iron deficiency may cause nephrotic patients with normal renal function to become anemic.

Measured concentrations of serum complement and its components are generally considered to be normal in MCN. Although urinary losses cause decreases in low–molecular-weight complement components, serum concentrations of the components measured to detect activation of the complement cascade are unchanged.[432] Thus, reduced levels of the third component of complement (β-1-C globulin; C3) or C4 indicate that a glomerulonephritis underlies the nephrotic syndrome; conversely, such changes do not occur invariably with glomerulonephritis. Circulating immune complexes may be elevated in MCN or in FSGS.[433,434] Plasma renin activity may be increased in some patients who manifest physiologic changes consistent with decreased intravascular volume.

Histopathology

Minimal Change Nephropathy

The morphologic classification of nephrotic syndrome in childhood derives from classic papers by Churg and colleagues[435] and White and colleagues.[436] The term *minimal change nephrotic syndrome* was used to describe the pathologic appearance on light microscopy of biopsies from nephrotic patients in which there are no definitive changes from normal in glomeruli (Fig. 52.7). Here, we have chosen to use the term *minimal change nephropathy* because some adult patients have been reported with proteinuria but no nephrosis[9,10] and in order to describe a histologic entity in parallel to FSGS. The degree of change from normal histology that is considered significant remains the subject of some controversy. The spectrum of these changes is classified in Table 52.2 at the beginning of this chapter. Other terms that have been used to describe this general entity include *nil disease* and *steroid-sensitive nephrotic syndrome*. Changes in the proximal tubule cells reflect increased reabsorption of protein. Tubular cells may contain apparent vacuoles that are doubly refractile and are similar to the fine lipid droplets seen in oval fat bodies in the urine. This pathologic abnormality generated the term *lipoid nephrosis*, in which there is no tubular atrophy and the renal interstitium is normal. Older patients may show some globally fibrosed glomeruli with associated nephron loss. This finding is rare in children and should not involve more than 5% to 10% of glomeruli, even in elderly patients.[3] Staining for glomerular polyanion with Alcian blue, colloidal iron, or ruthenium red may be reduced in the glomerular tufts. No immunoglobulin or complement deposition is observed by immunofluorescence. Electron microscopy (Fig. 52.7) reveals only glomerular epithelial cell foot-process effacement (see next paragraph).[437] In some cases this finding may be visualized by high-resolution light microscopy.[438] The diffuse effacement of the podocytes that often contain protein-reabsorptive droplets typically results in the appearance of an almost continuous layer of cytoplasm on the urinary side of the GBM. Epithelial cells may appear detached in segments, producing denuded areas of the GBM. The GBM itself, however, appears normal. There

A
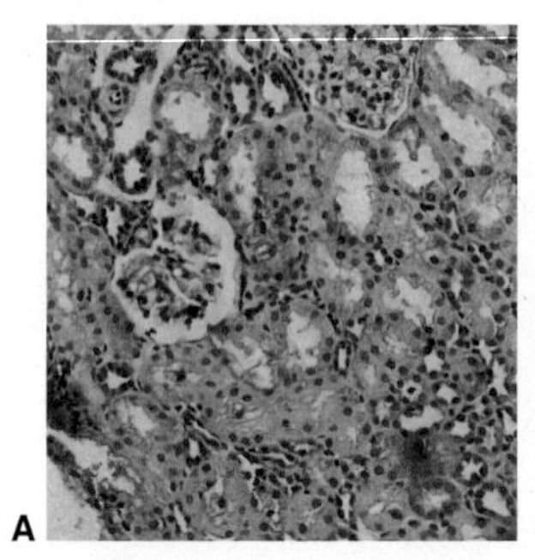

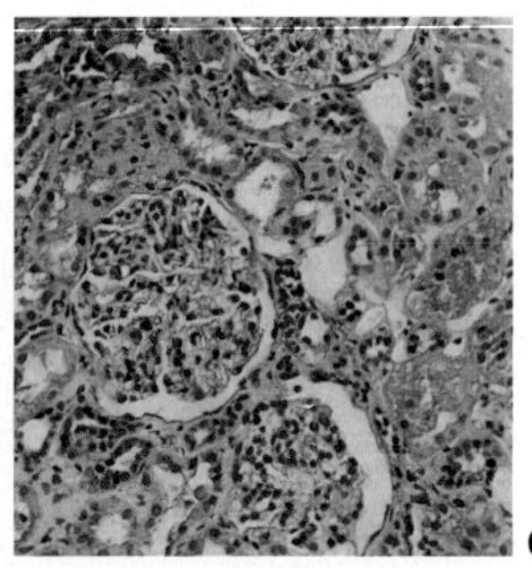
C

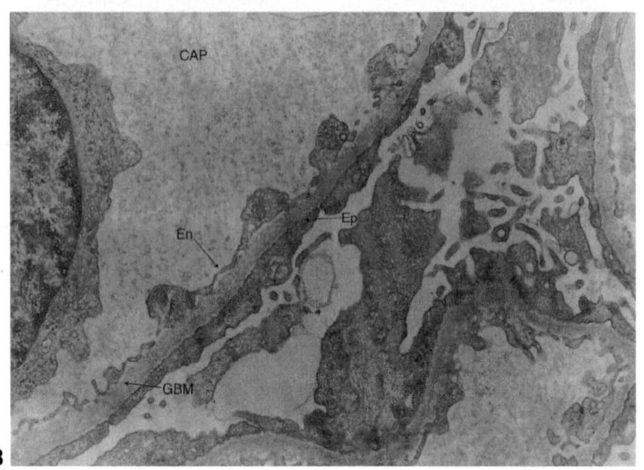

B

FIGURE 52.7 Findings on renal biopsies from three children with the clinical features of minimal change nephropathy. **A:** Light microscopy of a patient with MCN. Portions of two glomeruli are shown. Cellularity is normal and the capillary loops are patent. Tubular and interstitial structures are normal in appearance. (Magnification for all light microscopy ×350.) **B:** Electron microscopy from the same patient. The endothelial cells (En) lining the capillary loop show a normal fenestrated structure; the glomerular basement membrane (GBM) is uniform in thickness and structure. The epithelial cell (Ep) layer shows characteristic fusion of the epithelial foot processes, with the podocytes being in continuous contact with the GBM. Proteinaceous material and a nucleated cell are present in the capillary lumen (CAP). **C:** Light microscopy in a patient with mesangial hypercellularity. The tubular and glomerular capillary structures are normal, but an increased number of nuclei are present in the mesangial areas of the glomeruli. Immunofluorescent microscopy was negative for immunoglobulins and C3. The patient behaved clinically as one with MCNS. (Histology courtesy of Dr. John M. Kissane.)

are no electron-dense deposits adjacent to the GBM.[439] Historically, 65% to 85% of children with primary nephrotic syndrome have this lesion,[440] compared to a prevalence of about 30% of primary nephrotic syndrome and 15% of all nephrosis in adults.[9]

Podocyte Foot Process Effacement

Podocyte foot process effacement is due to retraction, widening, and shortening of foot processes and is not due to fusion.[441] With complete effacement, the GBM is covered by thin, sheetlike processes of podocyte cytoplasm, with gaps between the processes of adjacent cells (where protein filtration presumably occurs). Foot-process effacement is associated with a mild reduction in GFR, which is caused mainly by a reduction in the ultrafiltration coefficient K_f (see section on Physiologic and Anatomic Factors Affecting GFR in Consequences of Proteinuria, earlier in this chapter).

Podocyte effacement is accompanied by striking morphologic changes in the cytoskeleton. The continuous layer of podocyte cytoplasm that overlies the GBM shows an increase in microfilaments and the appearance of a dense cytoskeletal band located within the basal portion of the podocyte, adjacent to the GBM. The cytoskeletal band has regions of high density at regular intervals. En face views demonstrate that the filaments are distributed radially from these central densities, suggesting that they may function to distribute mechanical strain and thereby prevent glomerular capillary expansion.[442] Endlich et al.[443] exposed cultured podocytes to biaxial cyclic stress in order to model stress that might be experienced by podocytes in glomerulomegaly. Transverse stress fibers disappeared and were replaced by radial stress fibers connected to a single actin-rich center. The stress fibers were composed of myosin II, α-actinin, and synaptopodin. These findings differ in important ways from podocytes in vivo, where the actin-rich center is absent and actin is confined to the foot processes. Nevertheless, the results do suggest that podocyte response to stress consistently involves formation of radial cytoskeletal structures.

It appears likely that podocyte foot-process effacement arises by different mechanisms in different settings. Certain podocyte injury models (protamine infusion, reactive oxygen species infusion, PAN administration) are associated with a redistribution of α-dystroglycan from the basal surface of the podocyte, a process that occurs within as little as 15 minutes.[444] MCN but not FSGS is associated with loss of podocyte dystroglycan expression.[445] Kojima and Kerjaschki[446] have suggested that polycations compete with GBM laminin for binding to its receptor, dystroglycan; free dystroglycan is then internalized into podocyte endosomes. This process is dependent upon cellular ATP and participation of the actin cytoskeleton.

Related but distinct mechanisms may explain foot process effacement in FSGS, in particular, adaptive FSGS (see further, the section on Histopathology of FSGS, later in this chapter). Shirato[441] and Kriz et al.[447] have proposed that the podocyte supports the essential but contradictory functions of structural stability and leakiness (hydraulic conductivity). Cytoskeletal hypertrophy represents cellular adaptation to increased stress. The source of stress might be glomerular enlargement, increased glomerular P_{GC} (associated with the overload state), or increased GBM distensibility (due to GBM damage). Johnson[450] has pointed out that the transmembrane oncotic pressure gradient influences the net filtration pressure (P_{UF}) and thereby might also contribute to net hydraulic stress. P_{UF} is the difference between transmembrane hydraulic pressure and the transmembrane oncotic pressure gradient. In the setting of nephrotic-range proteinuria, plasma albumin is reduced, which reduces the transmembrane oncotic pressure gradient across the capillary wall and thereby increases P_{UF}. In the face of mechanical or hydraulic stress, the capillary wall has three defenses: the mesangial cell, the podocyte, and the GBM. The mesangial cell may undergo proliferation and hypertrophy. Little is known about how the GBM responds to stress. The podocyte cannot proliferate and adapts by elaborating a more complex cytoskeleton to defend the structural integrity of the capillary wall. This occurs, however, at the cost of a reduction in total slit diaphragm width, podocyte effacement, and reduced K_f.

An alternative consideration in FSGS is how a loss of specific podocyte structural proteins impairs cytoskeletal integrity, initiating foot-process effacement. This issue was discussed in the section on Molecular Mechanisms of Podocyte Effacement earlier in this chapter.

Variations in Histopathology

Immunoglobulin Deposition. Some patients with all the clinical features of MCN may have minor morphologic differences from those already described. A common variation is the presence of IgM in the glomerular mesangium. An early report[448] suggested that this variant represents a separate entity, which was termed mesangial IgM nephropathy. All of the patients, whose ages ranged from 1.5 to 59 years, showed a slight increase in the mesangial matrix, and in addition to the IgM deposits, some had C3 and rare IgA deposition. Dense mesangial deposits were noted by electron microscopy in 9 of the 12 subjects. Subsequent observations did not support this as being a separate entity. In one study, 40% of 149 consecutive patients with the clinical picture of primary nephrotic syndrome were found on biopsy to have mesangial IgM deposits. Of these, 20 had mostly or entirely IgM without complement. They could not be differentiated clinically from other MCN patients.[449] Because the presence of a mesangial IgM deposit in patients with clinical MCN does not appear to affect either the patient's response to treatment or the disease outcome,[450] it is now believed that this finding has little significance.

Mesangial IgM deposits in apparent MCN may, in some cases, be associated with immune complexes.[451] Because deposits are often found in patients who undergo biopsy after receiving a trial of corticosteroid therapy, it is of interest that experimental models of immune complex metabolism suggest that steroid administration may prolong the systemic half-life of larger complexes and increase and sustain their appearance in the mesangium.[452] The presence in the glomeruli of immunoglobulins in addition to IgM usually indicates a diagnosis of a disease other than MCN.[453] One group of patients with a clinical diagnosis of MCN showed some glomerular proliferation associated with immunoglobulin deposits, primarily IgG, in the glomeruli. This lesion was more often observed in African American children,[125] whereas a racial predilection may not be present in adults.[454] Although the patients described in this report responded to treatment with steroids initially, their subsequent course was one of frequent relapses or the development of resistance to treatment.

Mesangial Proliferation. Some patients with otherwise typical MCN have increased numbers of mesangial cells in the glomeruli. One study that correlated glomerular morphometry with the patient's clinical course found increased numbers of mesangial nuclei and smaller nuclear sizes in patients who had frequent relapses. The authors proposed that this indicated mesangial cell activation. They cautioned, however, that disease duration could play a role in the development of this finding, because the frequently relapsing patients had a 4-year course compared to 1.4 years in the population with infrequent relapses.[455] Mesangial hypercellularity may be associated with a decreased response to steroid therapy,[143,456,457] frequent relapse,[456] steroid dependency,[458] or a poorer prognosis.[458–460] The ISKDC found that approximately 2.5% of children with nephrotic syndrome had mesangial hypercellularity.[461]

Mechanisms of mesangial proliferation. Based on the finding of identical immunohistochemistry in patients with or without mesangial proliferation, it has been argued that mesangial IgM deposition does not appear to play a role in the induction of the mesangial cell response.[457] Intrinsic kidney cells and cells migrating into the kidney as part of the inflammatory response release factors that regulate mesangial cell proliferation. Mesangial cells produce platelet-derived growth factor (PDGF), a stimulant of mesangial and endothelial cell growth and wound healing.[462–464] Prostacyclin and thromboxane, produced by a variety of cells, are stimulatory cofactors for mesangial cell proliferation.[465] In addition, two autocrine growth mechanisms have been defined. The first involves interleukin (IL)-1. Mesangial cells in culture secrete a mesangial cell growth factor with characteristics identical to those of IL-1.[466] Indeed, these cells express messenger RNA (mRNA) for IL-1 in vivo.[467] The second autocrine system involves IL-6. Mesangial cell–derived IL-6 stimulates mesangial cell growth in vitro.[468] Moreover, mice transgenic for the human IL-6 gene show marked mesangial proliferation.[469] In human disease, urinary excretion of IL-6 and mesangial staining of biopsy material for IL-6 were associated with mesangial proliferation by some,[470] but not all[471] authors. Because mesangial proliferative changes are associated with steroid resistance, it is noteworthy that IL-6–induced cell activation is not inhibited by steroids.[472] Finally, negative regulation of mesangial cell growth may be provided by the GBM itself, because the proliferation of mesangial cells is decreased by heparin sulfate.[473]

Tip Lesion. A group of patients has been described as having steroid-responsive nephrotic syndrome with intercapillary foam cells adherent to the Bowman capsule in a tuft near the tubular origin (the glomerular tip lesion). Although this adhesion is irreversible, the patients appear to have a good prognosis closer to that of MCN than that of steroid-resistant nephrotic syndrome.[10,474] Tip lesion is considered more extensively in the section on Selected Clinical Variants of FSGS.

Disease Processes and Other Findings Associated with MCN

Several clinical findings have been associated with MCN, including specific malignancies, atopy, various human leukocyte antigen (HLA) haplotypes, and abnormalities in immune function. These associations, which could elucidate issues of both causality and treatment, will be considered here.

Malignancy. Several glomerulopathies, notably membranous glomerulopathy, have been associated with neoplasia. A significant number of patients with cancer-related nephrotic syndrome, however, have MCN. The relationship between MCN and lymphomatous disorders, particularly Hodgkin disease, is especially striking.[402] In a survey of the literature, 33 of 134 patients with cancer-related nephrotic syndrome had MCN, as determined by biopsy.[401] Of the patients with MCN, 26 had Hodgkin disease and an additional two had non-Hodgkin lymphoma. In another review,[400] 36 of 44 patients who had Hodgkin disease and the nephrotic syndrome had MCN and only 2 had membranous glomerulonephritis. There was a much higher incidence of nephritic diseases in patients with other types of neoplasia. Nonlymphomatous tumors that have been associated rarely with MCN include renal oncocytomas,[475] embryonic cell tumors,[401] pancreatic carcinoma,[476] nephroblastoma,[477] Waldenström macroglobulinemia,[478] bronchogenic carcinoma,[479] and cecal adenocarcinoma.[480]

Evidence suggests that in these cases the tumor may be directly involved in the pathogenesis of the MCN. MCN can be the initial presenting sign of a lymphomatous disorder[481] and may precede clinical evidence of lymphoma by several years.[482] With appropriate and successful antineoplastic therapy, either medical or surgical, the proteinuria in tumor-related MCN resolves, renal function remains normal, and the nephrotic syndrome remits.[401,475,479,482] The relationship between relapse of the tumor and of the nephrotic syndrome[483,484] also strongly suggests an etiologic role for the tumor in the pathogenesis of MCN in these patients. These observations indicate the importance of considering a malignancy as an underlying cause in any adult[483–486] and, rarely, in pediatric[487] patients who present with apparent primary nephrotic syndrome. If Hodgkin lymphoma is the cause, it is essential to treat the neoplasm rather than the renal disease.

Atopy and Minimal Change Nephropathy. A relationship between allergy and MCN has long been suspected. Anecdotal reports suggest that exposure to allergens may precipitate the nephrotic syndrome[393,394,487,488]; rhinorrhea and allergic skin reactivity frequently precede relapses,[489] and a high prevalence of allergic symptoms has been observed in nephrotic patients. Highly allergic patients who had a pathologic diagnosis of MCN based on renal biopsy experienced a decrease in urinary protein excretion when placed on an elemental diet and did not require treatment with corticosteroids. Challenge with milk led to a decrease in serum C3 and increased protein excretion, strongly suggesting that hypersensitivity was causally linked to proteinuria.[395] A human basophil degranulation test was positive in 16 of 28 adults with MCN and 14 of 18 adults with FSGS; in contrast, only 5 of 29 patients with glomerulonephritis and 1 of 11 healthy donors showed a positive response.[490] In addition, atopy and MCN were associated with increased frequency of expression of human leukocyte antigen (HLA)-B12 and -DRw7.[490–492]

Although values ranged widely, mean serum IgE levels were significantly elevated in patients with MCN compared to those with other renal problems[493]; elevated levels also are associated with frequent relapse in children.[494] In one study, the majority of adult MCN patients had serum IgE levels more than two standard deviations above the normal mean; of these, more than 70% had associated allergic symptoms.[495] Other investigators have made similar observations, but sought to draw a distinction between primary allergic disease and the elevated IgE levels found in nephrotic syndrome. They suggest that because IgE deposition in the glomerulus is rare,[496] elevated serum IgE levels could represent not the causal factor in MCN but rather evidence of more generalized derangement in the immune system.[497] A finding that increased serum IgE may persist even with remission supports this concept. If this view is correct, it could explain why attempts to treat MCN in atopic patients with inhaled disodium cromoglycate[498] or an orally administered analog[489] were unsuccessful.

These apparently conflicting observations may be resolved by the study of specific antigens. Therefore, a majority of adult nephrotic patients studied by Meadow et al.,[489] Lagrue and Laurent,[499] and Laurent et al.[500] had detectable elevations of specific IgE titers, with the most common sensitizing agent being house dust or dust mites. After remission, which was induced by the institution of specific desensitization and sodium cromolyn, several of these patients had a relapse on reexposure to the allergen.[489,499,500]

Immunogenetics. There may be a familial incidence of MCN. A survey from Europe, which excluded patients with the congenital nephrotic syndrome,[501] found that 63 of 1,877 nephrotic children had affected family members. This prevalence of 3.35% was higher than that predicted from the frequency with which MCN occurs in the general population. Siblings were most often affected. The similarity of pathologic findings and the clinical course for affected members within a family was striking,[502] although in at least one report, siblings showed differences in these features.[503] Familial nephrotic syndrome in children has been divided into two broad categories: (1) patients with an infantile onset and a poor prognosis regardless of renal morphology and (2) patients with a juvenile onset and a generally good response to conventional therapy, provided MCN is found by renal biopsy.

An indication of a possible genetic predisposition for the development of MCN is the reported association of MCN, and in some cases atopy,[492,504] with certain histocompatibility-complex antigens. The most commonly cited are HLA-B8[492,504–506] and -DRw7.[507,508] Not all studies have confirmed these associations. Indeed, a variety of HLA antigens have been associated with MCN[491,492,505–515] and negative associations have been reported, too. HLA-B8 was found frequently in families with more than one member having childhood nephrosis.[516] In one study, the combined occurrence of B8 with DR3 and DR7 produced a relative risk of 21.5.[514] In another study, DR7 was linked to steroid-sensitive disease and DR3 to steroid-resistant disease.[510] In French and German patients, specific DQB1 alleles have been associated with MCNS, most strongly in steroid-dependent or frequently relapsing patients.[517] German studies also suggested that patients with HLA-DR7/-DR3 together are less steroid sensitive,[518] and those with HLA-DR7 are less likely to respond permanently to alkylating agent treatment of frequent relapse.[519]

MCN was associated with HLA-DQB1*0601, -DRB1*01, and -DRB1*07011 in Egyptian children[509,520] and -DQA*0201 in German children.[511] Studies from Japan linked steroid-sensitive MCN in adult patients to HLA-DRw8 and -DQw3[512] and to specific DQB1 alleles.[521,522] Different results obtained in Singaporean[523] or Bengali[524] children are likely due in part to racial or geographic differences. The observation that two extended HLA haplotypes (HLA-A1, -B8, -DR3, -DRw52, SCO1; and HLA-B44, -DR7, -DRw53, and FC31) occurred with higher than expected frequency in children with steroid-sensitive, frequently relapsing MCN provided strong evidence for an immunogenetic predisposition to the disease.[513]

The association between HLA type and MCN has been made primarily in children, with some studies being unable to make similar correlations in adult patients. This finding suggests that MCN in adult and pediatric patients could represent different diseases that share common pathologic and clinical features. For example, HLA-DR7, which has been linked to MCN, was observed in only 18% of adult European MCN patients, a frequency not different from that of control subjects. If the data were analyzed according to age at onset of the nephrotic syndrome, 45% of patients in whom onset was before the age of 15 years were HLA-DR7, whereas the equivalent incidence in adult-onset patients was only 7%.[525] It remains unclear whether these associations represent linkage disequilibrium with another gene or reflect potential underlying immune influences on the development and response of MCN.

Disordered Immunity in Minimal Change Nephropathy. It has long been recognized that immunogenic stimuli may precipitate the presentation or relapse of MCN. In addition to the frequent association with atopy (discussed previously), episodes may follow upper respiratory tract infections, bee stings, or diseases linked with abnormal immune responses. The relationship of immunogenic events to the onset of disease and the finding of disordered immune responses in these patients led Shalhoub[526] to propose a unifying hypothesis relating MCN to the immune system. He cited four points: (1) evidence for abnormal humoral immune responsiveness; (2) marked sensitivity of the disease process to treatment with corticosteroids or immunosuppressive agents; (3) remission of MCN upon infection with measles, an inhibitor of cell-mediated immunity; and (4) the association of MCN with Hodgkin disease. In view of the lack of significant morphologic evidence of renal damage, Shalhoub suggested that MCN represents the renal manifestation of a systemic immunologic abnormality, perhaps a T-lymphocyte disorder, rather than a primary renal parenchymal disorder. Although subsequent investigation has not yet demonstrated a causal immunologic event, numerous abnormalities in both humoral and cellular immune responses[527] have been noted in nephrotic patients (Table 52.5).[528,529,549] These may, in time, provide a pathogenic mechanism.

Immunoglobulin synthesis. Clinical and in vitro assays show impaired immunoglobulin synthesis in MCN. Serum IgG levels are decreased significantly in children with MCNS, whereas IgM levels are markedly increased.[310,532–534] These values return toward normal with remission, although the IgM levels may remain elevated. Not all studies have found an equal tendency toward normalization with remission, nor is this abnormality confined to MCN in all cases.[575,576] Although nephrotic proteinuria may be associated with urinary loss of IgG,[577] such losses are insufficient to explain the very low serum IgG levels often found in MCN.[531] This pattern of increased IgM and decreased IgG levels in the serum also is associated with some other immune-deficient states, most notably X-linked immunodeficiency disease.[531]

Depression of specific antibody titers, such as those to the common streptococcal antigens endostreptosin, streptolysin O, and streptozyme, was observed in children and adults with idiopathic nephrotic syndrome.[535] Levels were low during active disease, remained low for up to 20 years afterward, and were not changed by steroid therapy. Patients who were nephrotic from chronic glomerulonephritis, systemic lupus erythematosus, membranous nephropathy, diabetes mellitus, or amyloidosis did not have depressed titers. These data suggest a chronic, specific impairment of response in patients with MCN. An inability to generate[311] or to maintain[536] specific titers against pneumococcal polysaccharide has been described in MCN, but not all studies confirmed this observation.[578] Thus, depression of specific antibody titers may be restricted to certain patients or certain antigens.

Several groups evaluated the in vitro secretion of immunoglobulins by lymphocytes activated with lectins. Consistent with the decrease in serum IgG levels, pokeweed mitogen-stimulated synthesis of IgG by patient lymphocytes

TABLE 52.5 **Immunologic Abnormalities in Minimal Change Nephropathy**

Immunologic Abnormalities in Minimal Change Nephropathy
Defective opsonization
Decreased factor B[314,315]
Decreased factor D[316]
Decreased neutrophil chemiluminescence[315]
Abnormal reticuloendothelial function[528]
Circulating immune complexes[433, 434, 529, 530]
Abnormal immunoglobulin production
Altered serum immunoglobulin concentrations[310,531–534]
Decreased specific antibody reactivity[311,535,536]
Decreased synthesis stimulated in vitro[537,538]
Increased spontaneous in vitro synthesis[531,537]
Alterations in cell-surface markers[538–542]
Altered cellular immunity
Cytotoxicity to renal tubular epithelium[543]
Proliferation in response to glomerular basement membrane[544]
Decreased delayed-type hypersensitivity[545–547]
Decreased experimental local graft-versus-host disease[548]
Decreased induced lymphocyte blast transformation[549,550]
Increased inducible suppressor cell activity[551]
Humoral immune abnormalities
Serum toxicity to lymphocytes[552]
Inhibition of rosette formation by serum[528,553,554]
Altered antibody-dependent cellular cytotoxicity[555]
Increased interleukin (IL) production[556]
Decreased IL production[557,558]
Suppressor lymphokines[559–561]
Monocyte migration inhibitory factor[544,562]
Vascular permeability factor[563,564]
Soluble immune-response suppressor[565,566]
Tumor necrosis factor[567]
Lymphocyte activation
Increased secretion of β_2-microglobulin[568]
Soluble IL-2 receptor production[569–572]
Increased production of IL-2, IL-4, and IFN-γ[573]; and IL-13[574]

IFN, interferon.

was decreased in MCN patients during the active stage of disease, returning toward normal with remission.[531,533,538] Unstimulated secretion of immunoglobulin may be increased,[531,537] suggesting spontaneous activation of lymphocytes in MCN. Studies of IgA and IgM synthesis by lymphocytes obtained from patients with nephrotic syndrome of other causes produced more variable results.[579] Decreased immunoglobulin production in vitro or in vivo could result from either abnormalities of lymphocytes or the presence of inhibitory agents systemically or on the cell surface. Evidence suggests that both mechanisms may be present in MCN.

Studies of lymphocyte surface marker expression. These studies were employed to determine whether the immunoglobulin abnormalities in MCN reflect some form of immune cell dysfunction. Cells infiltrating the renal interstitium are predominantly T lymphocytes.[580] The ratio of helper cells to suppressor cells in the glomerulus can be similar to that found in lymphocytes in the peripheral circulation[580] but may vary from one patient to another.[581] Immunostaining detects higher numbers of CD3-positive glomerular and interstitial T cells, but fewer FoxP3-positive cells, in biopsies from nephrotic patients than from controls. In contrast, there was no difference in CD4-positive or CD8-positive cells. Interstitial, CD68-positive macrophages were also higher in nephrotic patient biopsies.[582] Circulating lymphocyte subsets in MCN were initially reported to show no significant alterations in helper–suppressor cell ratios.[583] Studies of B-cell and T-cell subpopulations also produced conflicting data, regardless of whether patients with MCN or FSGS were studied.[538,540,542,584,585] A potential increase in the number of cells coexpressing B-cell and T-cell surface markers has been reported, comparable to findings in X-linked immunodeficiency.[541] However, in most studies of lymphocyte subpopulations in primary nephrotic syndrome, there are few significant changes. The meaning of the differences that were found remains to be determined. In general, studies showing alterations in lymphocyte subpopulations may be useful in suggesting the possible presence of immune derangement, but inferences of a potential role for these changes in disease pathogenesis should be made with caution unless corroborated by accompanying functional analysis. Some progress in this direction is provided by reports of two-color flow cytometry indicating that the counts for circulating activated total T cells and suppressor or suppressor/inducer T cells are increased, whereas those for activated helper T cells are decreased, during relapse.[539,586] Another study found that populations of activated suppressor-inducer cells and suppressor-effector cells are increased in patients whose nephrosis was sensitive to steroid treatment, accompanied by decreased memory T cells and decreased lymphocyte proliferation in response to tetanus toxoid. Lymphocytes of steroid-resistant patients also had increased suppressor-inducer cells, but decreased suppressor-effector cells and increased memory T cells, with increased responses to tetanus toxoid.[587]

Cellular immunity. In studies of delayed-type hypersensitivity to common antigens, MCN patients in relapse had decreased skin reactivity to purified protein derivative of tuberculin (PPD), *Candida*, live varicella vaccine, streptokinase–streptodornase, and topical dinitrochlorobenzene.[545–547] Reactivity returns when the patient enters remission.[545] In addition, the lymphocytes of patients with MCN manifest decreased local graft-versus-host activity when injected into rats, a finding that can be normalized by preincubation of the cells with a thymic factor.[588] These observations may not be restricted to MCN.[585]

In vitro studies also showed abnormal cellular responses in nephrotic patients. Lymphocytes from MCN patients, but not from normal control subjects or patients who were nephrotic secondary to proliferative glomerulonephritis, were toxic to cultured renal tubular epithelial cells.[543] Lymphocytes from some patients also proliferated on exposure to GBM.[544] It is not clear from these reports whether the findings represent a primary process or the result of immunologic sensitization after renal abnormality. Blast transformation of patient lymphocytes was decreased in the presence of control or nephrotic serum,[550] returning to normal after entry of the patient into remission.[547] Other results showed that MCN is associated with increased concanavalin A–activated suppressor cell activity. This finding demonstrates at least the potential for exaggerated suppressor lymphocyte responses and is not consistently found in other renal diseases.[551,589]

Evidence for abnormal lymphokine activity. Serum from adult nephrotic patients inhibits leukocyte migration in the presence of renal antigens[562] and serum monocyte migration inhibitory factor activity present during relapse of MCN disappears with remission of the disease.[543] Furthermore, serum from most patients with MCN as well as some with diffuse proliferative glomerulonephritis is lymphocytotoxic, whereas serum from patients with acute tubular necrosis or urologic disease is not.[552] These findings suggest that an immune inhibitory agent, or a series of such agents, is present in the circulation of patients with primary nephrotic syndrome. Sera from nephrotic patients may inhibit the ability of cells to form rosettes,[553,554] although this is not specific for MCN, and patient sera do not support in vitro antibody-dependent cell-mediated cytotoxicity (ADCC) assays.[555] Decreased splenic uptake of radiolabeled complexes was correlated with deficient Fc receptor function in nephrotic patients and could be due to the presence of an inhibitory protein that attaches to cell surfaces.[528] Finally, multiple studies demonstrate a suppressive effect of patient sera on blastogenesis by normal lymphocytes.[561,590–592] The specificity of this phenomenon for MCN varies from one study to another. Efforts to attribute suppressive activity in nephrotic sera to a lymphokine should attempt to exclude the possibility that the observed effects are caused by nonspecific toxicity to immune responses, resulting from the biochemical abnormalities that occur in nephrotic syndrome. For example, the suppressive activity in plasma from nephrotic children segregates in the lipid-rich fraction.[593] It could thus be derived from constituents of LDLs and VLDLs that are present in increased concentrations in nephrotic plasma and suppress in vitro cellular immune responses.[594,595] However, this finding also is consistent with the migration of an immunosuppressive agent with the lipid-rich fraction. Alternatively, oxidized LDL could itself affect lymphocyte function. In either case, it is noteworthy that a patient with refractory nephrotic syndrome entered remission after LDL apheresis.[596]

Several studies that partially characterized the suppressive activity suggested the production of a suppressor lymphokine. A heat-stable substance, present in the serum of nephrotic patients, inhibits lymphocyte proliferation. It binds to lymphocytes in the assay system and is not removed by washing.[560] One study found a heat-stable inhibitory substance in the plasma of 51 (76%) of 67 children with MCN and 6 of 9 children with FSGS.[559] Only 1 sample from 7 patients with membranous glomerulonephritis or 31 healthy adults and children showed similar activity. The factor was toxic to normal lymphocytes and was between 100 and 300 kDa. The presence of tumor necrosis factor,[567] IL-4,[574,597] and IL-13[576] in the serum of some patients may be related to suppressive activity.

Urine and serum samples from children and adults with steroid-sensitive nephrotic syndrome, but not other causes for proteinuria, contain the lymphokine soluble immune response suppressor (SIRS).[565] This factor, which inhibits antibody production[598] and delayed-type hypersensitivity responses,[599] is secreted by patient lymphocytes without a requirement for exogenous stimulating agents. SIRS production thus could account for the suppression of immune responses seen in nephrotic patients. Suppressive activity disappears from the urine after the initiation of corticosteroid therapy but before urinary protein loss decreases significantly. Patient serum activates normal lymphocytes to produce SIRS by a steroid-sensitive process,[566] and a regulatory mechanism has been proposed by which CD4+ T lymphocytes from patients in relapse secrete a protein that activates CD8+ T cells to produce SIRS.[600] Although the parallel between the sensitivity of SIRS production to steroids and steroid responsiveness of nephrotic proteinuria in patients who produce SIRS is striking, there is no evidence to indicate that SIRS itself causes nephrotic proteinuria. It is, however, a clear marker for steroid-sensitive mechanisms of proteinuria. The means by which SIRS acts on immune responses are not known. Although this issue remains intriguing, little recent progress has been made in this area.

Circulating immune complexes. A variety of glomerular diseases have been associated with soluble circulating immune complexes. The circulating complexes reflect immunoglobulins found in the kidney; patients with MCN had little or no IgG or IgA complexes but did have marked variation with regard to circulating IgM complexes.[601] Although circulating immune complexes have been documented in some patients with MCN or FSGS,[530] not all studies have confirmed this observation[529] and the relationship of this finding to mesangial immune complexes remains uncertain. A possible reason for varied results is the use of different assay systems.[433] In screening studies that employed liquid-phase and solid-phase C1q binding and Raji cell assays, at least one assay was positive in serum from 11 of 14 adults with MCN, 13 of 27 patients with FSGS, and 26 of 55 patients with membranous nephropathy. Prednisone treatment did not affect the prevalence of circulating immune complexes in this study.[602] In another report, 17 of 18 MCN patients had IgG immune complexes that did not bind to Clq; in 7 of 9 patients assessed longitudinally, immune complexes disappeared within 6 weeks of entry into remission.[434] This temporal relationship and the absence of glomerular IgG in patients with MCN suggest that circulating immune complexes could be a result rather than a cause of the disease. Although they may not cause the disease, some circulating immune complexes could account for the apparently nonspecific presence of IgM in the mesangium of some patients. In support of this is the finding that neutral, or anionic, large complexes show focal to diffuse mesangial localization.[603,604] Complexes containing IgM tend to be large. In contrast, low-avidity, polycationic, and small immune complexes tend to deposit in capillary or mesangiocapillary distribution.

Other findings related to immunity. Further evidence of a potential role for the immune system in MCN is the possible relationship between this disease and allergic phenomena, already discussed, as well as the unique association between MCN and tumors of immune cell origin. Impaired lymphocyte blast transformation was found in the presence of plasma from patients with MCN and Hodgkin disease[486,605]; in vitro responses improved significantly after antitumor therapy.[606] The strong association of lymphoid tumor, abnormal cellular immune responses, and MCN supports a role for deranged immunity. The nature of this derangement is unclear. Despite the clinical evidence of suppressed immune responses, the underlying abnormality paradoxically may be general immune system activation. In support of such an event, production of a number of specific cytokines and their regulators may be elevated. Increased IL-2 mRNA expression in patient lymphocytes,[607] increased IL-8 production in steroid-resistant patients,[608] and increased incidence of one polymorphism of IL-1 receptor antagonist[609] have been reported. Circulating soluble IL-2 receptor concentrations are increased in MCN.[569–572] Production of gamma interferon (IFN-γ) may also be increased in nephrotic children. Further, although various responses of stimulated patient lymphocytes are decreased, unstimulated cells from patients show, for example, increased immunoglobulin production relative to that of unstimulated control cells. Taken together, these findings suggest that in MCN, the immune system is generally activated, whereas the induction of responses to specific stimuli is impaired.[527] Consistent with this hypothesis are the recent data indicating that rituximab, which targets B lymphocytes, rather than the T cells implicated by Shalhoub, is effective in MCN (see section on Treatment of MCN).

Relationship of the immunologic abnormalities to disease pathogenesis. Despite all of these studies, Shalhoub's hypothesis has not yet been proved. There is strong support, however, for the concept that cellular immunity may be a mediator of proteinuria. Monocytes or macrophages are important in the pathogenesis of some forms of glomerulonephritis[610] and in the genesis of proteinuria.[611,612] CD34-positive immature lymphocytes from patients with MCN induce proteinuria upon their injection into non-obese diadbetic/severe combined immunodeficiency (NOD/SCID)-immunodeficient mice.[613] These studies imply a role for mononuclear cells but do not explain how they may act. One possibility is through release of the lymphokine, vascular permeability factor (VPF), which is produced by activated lymphocytes from some nephrotic patients and which, when injected intradermally, causes increased permeability of vessels to macromolecules.[563] This protein, usually referred to by its function as an endothelial cell stimulant called vascular endothelial cell growth factor (VEGF),[564] was detected in supernatants of unstimulated cultures of patients' cells but not those of normal controls.[614] A VEGF-like serine protease in patient serum decreased staining for polyanion when used to treat histologic sections of normal glomerular tissue.[615] However, the effect of VEGF does not appear to be specific for permeability of albumin, making it an unlikely cause of selective proteinuria. VEGF activates endothelial cells in numerous ways; by causing the cells to "round up," it disrupts tight cell–cell adhesions, promoting permeability of an endothelial monolayer.[616] It also promotes the formation of endothelial fenestrae.[617] However, because the glomerular capillary endothelium is not the final barrier to glomerular permeability, it is not clear how increased fenestration would cause albuminuria in primary nephrotic syndrome. Furthermore, a similar substance was described in IgA nephropathy, even in the absence of nephrotic syndrome,[618] indicating that VEGF activity could be secondary to renal disease rather than a cause of proteinuria. VEGF production could be enhanced by IL-12 or IL-15.[619] Substances produced by T-cell hybridomas derived from the lymphocytes of nephrotic patients,[620] or found in culture media conditioned by mononuclear cells from nephrotic children,[621] may prove to represent one or more selective permeability factors. One such factor could be IL-8, which is produced by lymphocytes from patients with steroid-responsive nephrosis and increases renal clearance of protein in an ex vivo model.[622] However, varied circulating levels have been reported in disease.[608,623] IL-2[573] and tumor necrosis factor alpha [TNFα][624] production by patient lymphocytes normalized after the patients entered remission. A single case report describes remission of steroid-resistant disease after infliximab anti-TNFα therapy.[625] Another potentially significant mediator is IL-13. This Th2 cytokine, which has been associated with allergy, is found in increased concentrations in serum from children with MCN.[626] In an animal model, overexpression of IL-13 caused nephrotic-range proteinuria in rats.[627]

Despite the absence of proof for Shalhoub's hypothesis, the indirect evidence of an immunogenic basis for many cases of MCN remains compelling. Onset is often preceded by an immunogenic stimulus. Measles, which induces remission, inhibits lymphokine production but not proliferation by lymphocytes.[628] Studies of MCN induced by NSAIDs[629] or cimetidine[630] indicated that these cases of disease may be associated with abnormal T-cell function. The relationship of disease to altered immunity is particularly striking with regard to suppressor cell activity. A good therapeutic response to cyclophosphamide was associated with decreased suppressor cell activity after treatment,[631] although others were unable to confirm this finding.[632] Furthermore, as described previously, cellular and humoral immune responses are suppressed in MCN. Thus, it is intriguing that recombinant leukocyte interferon A, an agent that induces production of SIRS, causes nephrotic syndrome with minimal glomerular changes in some patients with T-lymphocyte malignancy[633] and that the anthelminthic agent levamisole, which inhibits SIRS activity,[598] has been used successfully to treat MCN.[634,635] Despite evidence suggesting that cytokines may be involved in promoting vascular permeability,[636] the data regarding lymphokines do not address their role as a pathogenic agent in nephrosis and are equally consistent with the interpretation that production of these substances is an epiphenomenon of the derangement that causes albuminuria. In addition, the existence of differences between studies or even within a patient group in a given study suggest that multiple etiologies may exist for MCN, only one (or several) of which may be immunologic.

One explanation for the apparent role of the immune system and the sensitivity of disease to treatments that affect immune responses is that podocytes may have molecular signaling pathways that are analogous to those observed in lymphocytes. The molecule, B7-1, termed CD80 in humans, is found on activated B lymphocytes and monocytes and provides a costimulatory signal necessary for T-cell activation and survival. It also is expressed in the podocytes of patients with MCN in relapse.[91] When overexpressed in cultured podocytes, it disrupts the cytoskeleton, interfering with assembly of the slit-diaphragm complex.[90] In vivo, its expression in podocytes induces proteinuria in mice. Another immunologic signaling molecule, c-maf-interfering protein (c-mip), was previously found in lymphocytes of MCN patients in relapse. It is expressed in the podocytes of mice treated with lipopolysaccharide, an experimental stimulus for proteinuria, and disrupts podocyte architecture when it is expressed in those cells.[637] It also has been detected in Reed-Sternberg cells as well as in the podocytes of patients who have MCN related to Hodgkin disease.[638] Together, these results suggest a paradigm in which podocytes express signaling pathways analogous to those previously characterized in immunocytes. Rather than mediating immune responses, their activation is associated with proteinuria, perhaps with a teleogic purpose to clear circulating antigens. Because the podocyte and lymphocyte pathways are similar, the podocytes might respond in parallel to the immune system in the presence of systemic immunogenic stimuli that result from atopy or viral infection. These considerations provide a potential relationship between the immune abnormalities that have been associated with MCN and the pathogenesis of proteinuria in the disease.

Treatment of Minimal Change Nephropathy

Indications for Renal Biopsy

Although most older children and adults will undergo renal biopsy prior to starting treatment, the indications for and benefits of this procedure in patients with primary nephrotic syndrome remain somewhat controversial.[639] Children 1 to 9 years old with all the features of MCNS and no atypical features (Table 52.6) may be given a therapeutic

TABLE 52.6 **Features Suggesting that Nephrotic Syndrome Is Caused by a Disease Other than Minimal Change Nephropathy (MCN)**

Features
History Onset: before 1 year or after 9 years of age[a] History: skin rashes, joint pains, "nephritis," or hematuria[a] Family history: family member with Alport syndrome or development of end-stage renal disease[a]
Physical examination General: clinical features of collagen vascular disease Blood pressure: marked elevation or evidence of vascular changes in fundi[a] Skin: purpura[a] Subcutaneous tissue: lipodystrophy
Laboratory findings Urine: dilute urine sediment containing more than 10 red blood cells per high-power field; cylindruria[a]; nonselective proteinuria[a] Renal function: markedly decreased[a]
Chest X-ray: enlarged heart, vascular engorgement, pulmonary edema
Serology: decreased C3 or C4, antinuclear antibody or anti-DNA positive
Serum cholesterol: only mild increase[a]
Plasma protein: only mild decrease in albumin[a] markedly decreased or increased globulin

[a]Although these features are unusual for MCN, their presence does not exclude the lesion.

trial of steroids without prior histologic confirmation of the diagnosis. Induction of a complete remission by steroids in such patients is considered to be adequate confirmation of the diagnosis of MCN,[440] although other benign conditions may occasionally appear to respond to steroid therapy.[640] A histologic diagnosis by renal biopsy is recommended in all patients who present with nephrotic syndrome in the first year of life or after the age of 9 years. Risk–benefit analysis at one point suggested that a biopsy may not be diagnostically superior to a therapeutic trial of steroids, even in adults,[641] but the increasing incidence of FSGS in nephrotic adults has led most clinicians to perform a biopsy at the time of presentation. All patients who are steroid-resistant (see Table 52.7 for some commonly used descriptors of nephrotic patients and their responses) should undergo biopsy, although the timing of this decision remains uncertain. Although steroid resistance in children usually is defined by 8 weeks of nonresponse, many clinicians recognize that most children who respond do so by 4 weeks. Therefore, it may be appropriate to perform a biopsy after 4 weeks or less, because those who have not responded by then are more likely to have a different disease that might require an alternative treatment. Other pediatric patients who may require a biopsy include those who have frequent relapses, or who are candidates for therapy with immunosuppressive drugs. Some experts have suggested that any steroid-dependent pediatric patients who continue to be steroid sensitive are, statistically, so likely to have MCN[416,461] that biopsy is not indicated. Alternatively, response to steroids may itself be a more important determinant of disease process and outcome than is histopathology.[642]

A renal biopsy may be technically difficult to perform in the patient with anasarca; surrounding fluid allows the kidney to be balloted by the biopsy needle. In such subjects, it is preferable to delay the attempted biopsy until after a spontaneous or drug-induced diuresis has occurred and most of the ascites has resolved.

Treatment of Minimal Change Disease

The optimal treatment for MCN is based on corticosteroids but continues to evolve. It is noteworthy that in the era before current drugs were available, 25% of children with idiopathic nephrotic syndrome underwent a spontaneous remission.[643] Even today, a careful history will often suggest that prior to the presenting episode, the nephrotic patient has had one or more periods of edema that resolved without treatment. The association between MCN and both allergy and malignancy was reviewed earlier in this chapter. An occasional patient with frequently relapsing MCN may enter long-term remission only when a dietary allergen is withdrawn[394] or an underlying malignancy is identified and treated.[483,487] Therefore, the possibility that either of these conditions is responsible for the patient's symptoms should be considered before any drug therapy is instituted.

Prior to 1940, the mortality rate for nephrotic syndrome was 40%; the major cause of death was infection.[644] After the introduction of antibiotics, mortality was reduced by more

TABLE 52.7 **Some Definitions Used to Describe Patients with Primary Nephrotic Syndrome**

Nephrotic-range proteinuria Pediatric: Urine protein: creatinine ratio >2 g/g Adult: 24-hour protein excretion >3.5 g
Relapse Proteinuria (>1+ on dipstick or >4 mg/hr/m^2 surface area) for at least 1 week
Complete remission (CR) Pediatric: Protein-free urine ($<1^+$ on dipstick or <4 mg/hr/m^2 surface area) for at least 3 days Or, urine protein: creatinine ratio <0.2 Adult: 24-hour protein excretion <0.3 g
Partial remission (PR) Pediatric: ≥50% fall from baseline and/or <2.0 (or <0.3) and/or loss of edema and/or serum albumin >2.5 mg/dL with preserved GFR Adult: PR 50%: 50% fall from baseline and <3.5 g/day with preserved GFR Or, PR2: ≤2.0 g/1.73 m^2
Limited response (LR) Pediatric and Adult: Fall to ≤50% baseline but not PR
Steroid-sensitive nephrotic syndrome (SSNS) Response to prednisone (60 mg/m^2 surface area/day) within 8 weeks of starting treatment[a]
Steroid-resistant nephrotic syndrome (SRNS) Pediatric: No response to prednisone (60 mg/m^2 surface area/day) within 8 weeks of starting treatment (ISKDC)[a] Adult: No change or increased proteinuria compared to baseline
Frequent relapsing nephrotic syndrome Initially responsive to prednisone: At least two relapses in a subsequent 6-month period or five relapses in 18 months
Steroid-dependent nephrotic syndrome Initially responsive to prednisone Either two consecutive relapses during period of steroid taper, or two consecutive relapses, each occurring within 2 weeks of ending a course of corticosteroid therapy

Those responding between 5 and 8 weeks are referred to as late responders.
[a] Some studies define steroid-sensitive patients as those responding within 4 weeks of starting treatment.
ISKDC, International Study of Kidney Disease in Children.

than 50%. The development of corticosteroids has further reduced mortality to between 3% and 7%.[426,436,644] The major benefits of steroids, however, may well be the faster induction of a remission and a reduction of morbidity, although this has never been subjected to a controlled trial. In the older adult nephrotic patient, the risk of undesirable steroid side effects could outweigh the benefits of these drugs.[645] Despite these caveats, adrenocorticosteroids remain the therapeutic agent of choice for MCN in patients of all ages.

Corticosteroid Therapy. As stated in the preceding text, the cessation of urinary protein excretion in response to the oral administration of prednisone is virtually diagnostic of this entity in children.[646] The standard dosage regimen for inducing a remission is 2 mg per kilogram of body weight per day or 60 mg per square meter of body surface area per day (a maximum of 80 mg per day).[647] Although the initial ISKDC studies used the same daily dose but divided it into three equal parts, we prefer the alternative approach of giving the entire daily amount in a single dose. The Cochrane group has reported that the single daily dose is as effective as a more complex dosing schedule.[648] Furthermore, short-term side effects such as hunger and hypomania are more manageable with use of the single daily dose. In addition, a single dose is more convenient to administer, with a greater likelihood of patient adherence. The daily dose is rounded up to the nearest multiple of 20 mg. A tuberculin test should be administered, but because nephrotic patients may be anergic, a chest radiograph should be obtained to rule out the possibility of subclinical pulmonary tuberculosis before prednisone therapy is begun. Typically, patients respond with a diuresis[120] followed by resolution of proteinuria. In most instances, response can be considered to have occurred if the patient has had protein-free urine for at least 3 days (Table 52.7). There are as yet no universally agreed upon definitions for complete remission (CR) or partial remission (PR). Nevertheless, those presented in Table 52.7 represent a starting point for discussion. Among children, CR is commonly defined as the absence of proteinuria on dipstick or alternatively of random (or first-void) urine protein/creatinine ratio of <0.2. Among adults, where 24-hour urine collections remain the standard for definition, CR is commonly defined as <0.3 g per day (although the upper limits of normal protein excretion at various clinical laboratories may be 150 to 250 mg per day and some studies have used a >0.5 g per day to define CR). The definitions of PR are more problematic. Troyanov, Cattran et al.[649] have argued for a 50% decrease in proteinuria from baseline and becoming subnephrotic.

This definition has the merit of capturing the benefit of a substantial reduction in proteinuria, for example from 10 to 3 g per day, and has been shown recently to correlate with long-term preservation of kidney function. Others have used a more restrictive definition of PR, for example, proteinuria <2 g per day. There may be some utility to capturing lesser degrees of benefit (e.g., limited response [LR], defined as a 50% fall in proteinuria that does not reach subnephrotic levels) but such a utility has not been tested in longitudinal studies. In children, CR may occur within 1 week of starting treatment in 75% of responders, and by 4 weeks in more than 90% (Fig. 52.8).

According to the definitions derived by ISKDC and others (Table 52.7), patients who do not respond after 4 weeks of glucocorticoid therapy are considered to be steroid resistant. However, response may be delayed for up to 8 weeks or more in a small percentage of patients, so that approximately 95% of patients with MCNS eventually will prove to be steroid sensitive. Serum albumin levels may not return to normal for up to 3 months,[120] and serum lipid abnormalities may persist for protracted periods.[179]

The persistence of some proteinuria does not necessarily indicate steroid resistance. Postural proteinuria may persist in a minority of patients and, in others, contraction of blood volume consequent to a brisk diuresis may result in renin-mediated proteinuria.[650] In either case, the degree of proteinuria is modest, typically registering 1+ to 2+ on dipstick and being <1 g per day. This should not be misinterpreted as partial responsiveness and should not be used to justify continuing steroid therapy in high doses. Alternatively, failure to respond to steroids may indicate the presence of an occult infection[647] or malignancy.

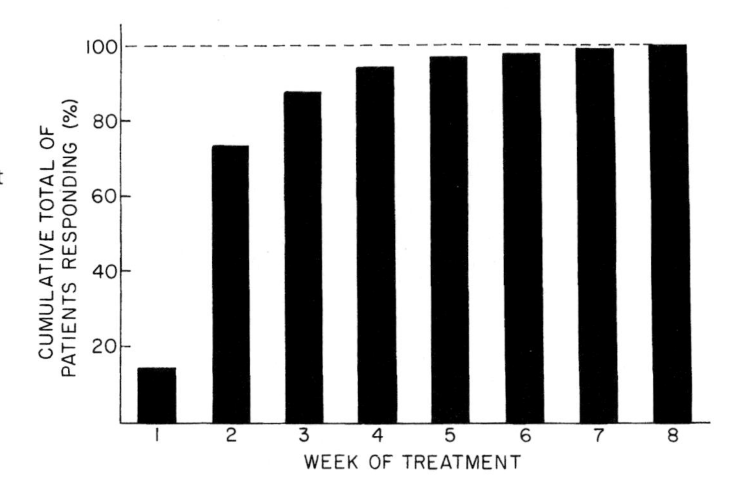

FIGURE 52.8 The cumulative rate of response to treatment with prednisone of children with primary nephrotic syndrome. Only steroid-sensitive patients are included in this analysis. The majority of patients respond in the 2nd or 3rd week of treatment. A small percentage, however, may take 7 or 8 weeks to respond. (Data derived from: International Study of Kidney Disease in Children. The primary nephrotic syndrome in children: identification of patients with minimal change nephrotic syndrome from initial response to prednisone. *J Pediatr.* 1981;98:561, with permission.)

Studies in children have demonstrated that, *for the initial episode only*, a prolonged period of treatment with a full dose of daily glucocorticoids decreases the incidence or frequency of subsequent relapses. After 6 weeks of daily treatment (rather than the standard 4 weeks of daily treatment) with prednisone, 60 mg per square meter, the patient is switched to 40 mg per square meter on alternate days.[651] Although some controlled studies may disagree,[652] meta-analysis by the Cochrane Group has determined that initial treatment with high-dose daily and then prolonged alternate-day oral prednisone decreases the likelihood of relapse over the first 12 to 24 months, and suggests that long-term continuation of alternate day steroids has increasing benefit for up to 7 months.[648] Most groups continue prednisone (total of daily and alternate day) for about 3 months and then discontinue the drug. For subsequent relapses, the steroids are tapered beginning with a switch to alternate day therapy only a few days after the response to treatment. The dose is then reduced in a stepwise fashion during the next 4 to 8 weeks. Longer tapering periods may decrease the likelihood of subsequent relapses.[651,653,654] For example, in a relapsed patient treated initially with prednisone, 60 mg per day, the dose is reduced to 40 mg daily after response (3 days of protein-free urine) for 2 weeks, then to 40 mg on alternate days. At 2-week intervals, the doses are reduced by 50%, with the final dose of 5 mg on alternate days being given for 3 weeks. It should be noted that this regimen is a matter of preference. The only regimen that has been established by a controlled trial as efficacious is the prolonged course for children of daily and then alternate day steroids in the initial episode. It is of interest that although prolonged treatment of the first episode seems to consolidate remission in children, those children who respond most rapidly to the initial course of corticosteroids tend to have longer remissions.[655] This relationship was not observed in adults.[656]

The presence of IgM deposits does not have an effect on response to steroids.[657] Although initial observations suggested that patients with mesangial hypercellularity respond to treatment in a manner similar to that seen with MCN,[658] subsequent studies indicated that a considerable proportion of these patients may be steroid resistant.[456,659] Conversely, an evaluation of large groups of children indicated that the persistence of proteinuria is only weakly predictive of mesangial hypercellularity on biopsy.[177,461]

Because bacterial peritonitis is a relatively common occurrence in patients with MCN (see Complications of Minimal Change Nephropathy later in this chapter), many clinicians support immunization with pneumococcal polysaccharide vaccines. Concern regarding possible poor response to immunogens in nephrotic patients, and the potential for an immunogenic stimulus to trigger a relapse, has made the issue of childhood immunization in nephrotic patients somewhat controversial. A survey of North American pediatric nephrologists indicated that many modified their approach to immunization but that there was little evidence upon which to base such modifications.[660] However, a British study suggests that the administration of meningococcal C conjugate vaccine may increase the likelihood of relapse.[408] Current recommendations on vaccination in children and adults and use of immunoglobulins[661] support the use of polyvalent pneumococcal vaccine[317,318] and (in the case of children) *Haemophilus influenzae* type B vaccine. Live virus vaccines should not be given to immunocompromised patients.

Frequent Relapse. Although earlier reports suggested that as high as 50% of steroid-sensitive children do not have a relapse after the initial episode of nephrotic syndrome, subsequent observations indicate that this figure approximates only 25%.[378] The difference could be due to an altering pattern of disease but also may reflect the types of patients being referred to reporting centers. Another 25% to 30% of children have infrequent relapses and usually respond well to further courses of steroids, as already described. The remaining patients have either frequently relapsing or steroid-dependent nephrotic syndrome (Table 52.7). Several attempts have been made to correlate pathology with response to steroids or with the pattern of relapses.[662] The frequency of relapse showed no correlation with histopathology in a study by the ISKDC,[663] but early relapse after the initial episode was predictive of more frequent relapses subsequently. Frequent relapse may be associated with earlier age presentation in children.[664]

Attempts to control frequent relapses with steroids may result in their protracted use and possible steroid toxicity. In an effort to minimize these side effects, alternative regimens have been proposed using smaller doses of steroids to treat relapses. Unfortunately, the lower response and higher relapse rates associated with most of these approaches usually result in higher cumulative doses of steroids and may not be justified.[654] One study suggested that for some frequently relapsing patients, maintenance on daily rather than alternate day steroids during the tapering regimen can result in a less frequent relapse rate and an equal or lesser cumulative steroid dose.[665]

Corticotropin (adrenocorticotropic hormone [ACTH]) stimulation tests suggest that prolonged postprednisone adrenocortical suppression may predispose one to frequent relapses. A normal response to ACTH predicted a remission for 6 months or longer; a subnormal response was associated with remissions of less than 6 months.[666] Early relapse in children with poor adrenal function can be prevented with low-dose maintenance hydrocortisone administration.[667]

Nitrogen mustard was found to prolong the duration of remission in patients with MCN,[668] but less toxic alternatives such as cyclophosphamide and related drugs are now used in frequently relapsing and steroid-dependent nephrotic patients, especially in those with marked steroid side effects.[669] Ideally, cyclophosphamide should not be used until a patient has been followed for 2 to 3 years to document a frequently relapsing course. Although some centers prefer histologic confirmation of MCN before the drug is used, steroid responsiveness may eliminate the need to obtain a biopsy specimen in children, because the disease remains overwhelmingly likely to be MCN.[670]

The original cyclophosphamide regimen used doses of 5 mg/kg/day, but it was associated with a high incidence of leukopenia, hair loss, and cystitis.[671] Most centers obtain satisfactory results with a dosage of 2 mg/kg/day for children (1.5 mg/kg/day for adults) given for no more than 90 consecutive days; others reported equally good results with 2.5 mg/kg/day for 8 weeks.[671–674] At 2 mg/kg/day, a course of cyclophosphamide limited to 8 weeks is followed by a higher relapse rate.[675] Most centers use cyclophosphamide in conjunction with steroids.[673] The induction of a remission with steroids before therapy with cyclophosphamide is instituted permits a liberal fluid intake to induce a high urine flow rate during treatment with the immunosuppressive agent, thereby reducing the risk of cystitis. The steroid taper is accomplished more rapidly, over a 6-week period.

Approximately 65% of frequently relapsing patients remain in remission for at least 5 years after a course of cyclophosphamide.[673,676,677] Response to cyclophosphamide may be predictable from the patterns of relapse after steroids. Of patients who have a relapse immediately after tapering of steroids, two-thirds also have a relapse quickly after cyclophosphamide treatment. Conversely, frequently relapsing patients who can maintain remission for more than 14 days after steroid therapy is discontinued have longer remissions and fewer relapses after cyclophosphamide treatment.[675]

It is rare to see acute side effects with the current cyclophosphamide regimens, although white blood cell counts should be monitored at least weekly, especially early in the course of therapy. The frequency of cystitis, alopecia, and leukopenia has been reduced markedly by the institution of smaller daily and cumulative doses of the drug, and is further minimized by encouraging fluid intake and frequent voiding for 4 hours after administration. The gonadal toxicity of cyclophosphamide also appears to be cumulative-dose related; testicular and ovarian toxicity is uncommon if the total dose is less than 200 mg per kilogram.[653,678,679] However, such doses do decrease sperm counts,[680] and some men experience gonadal toxicity even at low doses.[681] Higher doses lead to more significant testicular dysfunction.[682] In children, the drug is usually given well before puberty to minimize the risk of gonadal toxicity, although it has been suggested that prepubertal males are more sensitive than pubertal males.[683] Injection of slowly absorbed testosterone may protect against iatrogenic azoospermia.[684] Female patients treated with a mean total dose of 439 mg per kilogram at an average age of 8.7 years were followed for a mean of 12.3 years. All had normal pubertal development and regular menstrual patterns. Hormonal studies did not show obvious ovarian or pituitary–gonadal dysfunction, and two patients gave birth to normal children.[682] There are no data available to convincingly demonstrate a protective effect of ovarian suppression with oral contraceptives during alkylating agent therapy.[685] Concern has been expressed about the potential for cyclophosphamide to induce malignancies. It remains uncertain whether this is a major risk of therapeutic regimens currently used in nephrotic syndrome, although leukemia occurred in at least one child treated for nephrotic syndrome with prednisone and cyclophosphamide.[686] Furthermore, the use of cyclophosphamide may be associated with findings of increased sister chromatid exchange[687] and long-lasting immunosuppressive effects.[549]

Anecdotal experience in patients who are refractory to conventional therapies suggests that adding six monthly intravenous injections of cyclophosphamide, 0.5 g per square meter of body surface area per injection, to the oral steroid regimen may result in prolonged remission of the nephrotic syndrome even after discontinuation of the steroids.[688] This bolus therapy has potential advantages related to facilitated compliance and the availability of newer agents to counter drug toxicity.

An alternative alkylating agent, chlorambucil, shares many of the side effects seen with cyclophosphamide but does not induce cystitis. Unlike cyclophosphamide, however, it may produce seizures in some patients[689] and may induce electroencephalographic changes in the absence of seizures in others.[690] Malignancies have developed in at least three nephrotic children treated with this drug.[666,691,692] However, the overall incidence of serious complications with chlorambucil is low, especially when it is used in a dosage of 0.1 to 0.2 mg/kg/day for an 8-week course. It may produce a more stable remission than cyclophosphamide does[693,694] and be effective in some steroid-dependent and cyclophosphamide-resistant children with nephrotic syndrome.[695] A meta-analysis found that both cyclophosphamide and chlorambucil are effective in frequently relapsing patients and was unable to discern a difference between the two treatments.[696]

Cyclosporine and other calcineurin inhibitors can be beneficial in the management of patients with frequent relapses, especially in those who do not achieve a long-term remission with an alkylating agent. The usual dose of cyclosporine, 150 mg/m^2/day (7 mg/kg/day), is effective at inducing and sustaining remissions in these patients. An analysis of 129 children from nine studies showed complete remission in 84.5%.[697] With cessation of the cyclosporine, however, there is a high rate of relapse, the subsequent relapses possibly being more difficult to control than those prior to cyclosporine treatment. Although some reports have indicated that cyclosporine is a safe, steroid-sparing agent for treating steroid-dependent nephrotic syndrome,[698] others suggest that prolonged use can be associated with nephrotoxicity.[699,700] An alternative and successful approach to management is the long-term use of low-dose cyclosporine combined with low-dose, alternate day prednisone. Because of the potential for toxicity, serum creatinine should be monitored periodically in patients receiving cyclosporine.

Levamisole, an anthelminthic drug and immunopotentiating agent, can be used to treat children with MCN, especially those who have frequent relapses.[11,634] The usual dose is 2.5 mg per kilogram of body weight given by mouth on alternate days. The drug may be valuable as a steroid-sparing agent. In a controlled trial, 14 of 31 patients taking levamisole were able to discontinue steroids and remain in remission for the 112 days of the trial, compared to only 4 of the 30 control subjects taking placebo.[635] When the drug was added to the regimen of patients after a steroid-induced remission, the relapse rate fell from 5.2 episodes to less than 0.7 episodes per year during a 2-year period of treatment. The beneficial effect appeared to last beyond completion of the course of levamisole.[701] Side effects of levamisole include a decreased neutrophil count or transient granulocytopenia in two-thirds of patients. More severe complications such as skin rash, a flulike illness, vomiting, thrombocytopenia, and neurologic symptoms (insomnia, hyperactivity, and seizures) have been reported.[702]

Mycophenolate mofetil has been reported to successfully treat frequently relapsing minimal change disease in adults[703] and children.[704,705] In two prospective studies of children, mycophenolate (600 mg per square meter twice daily) was effective at decreasing corticosteroid dose and frequency of relapse[706] and was equally effective whether or not it was preceded by a trial of cyclosporine.[707] Side effects were minimal. Rituximab may be effective at decreasing or preventing relapses,[708] although the relative benefits of this therapy remains to be determined.

A Cochrane Report[709] analyzing 26 studies of frequently relapsing nephrotic syndrome covering 1173 children found no differences in efficacy among 8-week courses of cyclophosphamide or chlorambucil and extended courses of either levamisole or cyclosporine. The use of intravenous immunoglobulin as an adjunct to steroids has not resulted in any clinically important extension of the period of remission in patients with frequent relapses.[710]

Steroid-Dependent Patients. The management of these patients is similar in many respects to that of frequently relapsing patients. A minority of these individuals can be controlled with long-term, low-dose oral prednisone. Unfortunately, the dose of prednisone required to maintain a remission is usually sufficiently high to result in unacceptable side effects. Therefore, alternative approaches to management are required.

Methylprednisolone pulses have not been shown to be beneficial in this population of patients.[711] Some patients respond to cyclophosphamide and, as is the case with frequent relapses, the likelihood of a prolonged remission is increased if the course of drug is extended to 12 weeks.[712]

The results of using cyclosporine in steroid-dependent patients are similar to those in the frequently relapsing group. Some clinicians advocate a course of alkylating agents before resorting to cyclosporine.[713] Remissions can be maintained for 2 years or longer, especially if the cyclosporine is given continuously. However, 40% of these patients also require low-dose, alternate day steroids to stay in remission. Unfortunately, long-term remission after discontinuing the cyclosporine is relatively rare.[714] Treated patients show an average 20% decline in GFR after 3 months of therapy, but GFR stabilizes during subsequent therapy and has the potential to return toward normal with discontinuation of the drug.[715] Nonetheless, toxicity can be chronic.[716] A controlled multicenter study evaluating both pediatric and adult patients with either frequently relapsing or steroid-dependent nephrotic syndrome documented that cyclosporine and cyclophosphamide have a similar degree of efficacy but that more patients given cyclophosphamide have stable remissions.[717] One study has suggested that cyclosporine given concomitantly with cytotoxic agents may diminish the efficacy of the latter treatment.[718]

For most clinicians, when a steroid-dependent or frequently relapsing patient shows signs of steroid toxicity, the next drug to be used is cyclophosphamide, given for 12 weeks. If frequent relapses recur, cyclosporine in the lowest possible dose would be the next therapy used.[719] Levamisole is reserved for patients who continue to have relapses. However, recent studies showing the efficacy of mycophenolate in steroid-dependent disease[704,705,720,721] suggest the possibility that consideration should be given to using mycophenolate before these other drugs in view of its lesser toxicity.

A significant number of patients who are steroid-dependent are resistant to all alternative forms of treatment and must be controlled symptomatically on a chronic basis with dietary sodium restriction and diuretics. Oral furosemide or metolazone, used alone or in combination, or in conjunction with spironolactone, is usually effective. Most patients learn to individualize their dosage. Unless there is evidence for a progressive loss of renal function, this regimen probably is preferable to attempting control of the nephrotic syndrome with longer term steroid therapy because of the significant complication rate of this latter approach. However, progressive interstitial nephritis has occurred in nephrotic patients chronically treated with diuretics, especially furosemide.[722]

Treatment of Adult Patients with Minimal Change Nephropathy. Most of the recommendations made for pediatric patients are equally applicable to their adult counterparts because there are remarkable similarities of MCN in the different age groups. In general, the response rates to steroids in adult and pediatric patients with MCN are comparable.[673,723] Differences between pediatric and adult patients with MCN may include a less rapid response to corticosteroids in adults[724] and a more effective response in adults to cyclophosphamide used alone[725,726]; however, these differences may reflect technical or experimental design issues. For example, adults generally receive a lower dose of steroids on a per weight basis.

Adult patients may be somewhat more prone to steroid complications,[727] particularly in the skeleton. This has resulted in a philosophical debate about how aggressive one should be in the use of these drugs as well as immunosuppressants when treating nephrotic syndrome. However, given (1) the possibility of irreversible glomerular lesions from prolonged heavy proteinuria, (2) undesirable and potentially harmful effects of hyperlipidemia and protein deficiencies, and (3) the potential reduction of side effects from glucocorticoids and cytotoxic alkylating agents if the course of drugs is brief and the dosage not excessive,[728] most internists employ aggressive therapy in treating patients with MCN.

Treatment of Steroid-Resistant Minimal Change Nephropathy

Approximately 5% of children with MCN are unresponsive to a standard steroid regimen. Before considering a patient to be steroid resistant, infection or occult malignancy must be ruled out. A small but significant percentage of those who initially are steroid responsive will become steroid resistant after one or more subsequent relapses. This development is an indication for renal biopsy and often denotes the presence of FSGS.

Alternative steroid regimens have been attempted to improve the response to therapy. High-dose boluses of intravenous methylprednisolone induced remission in five of eight corticosteroid-resistant children.[711] In another experience, methylprednisolone pulses reduced proteinuria but did not result in remission.[729] One major problem in this group of patients is the development of severe side effects from protracted use of steroids. Therefore, regimens combining drugs in an attempt to reduce the amount of steroid administered, or alternative drugs to steroids, have been tried.

Occasionally, a patient with biopsy-confirmed MCN who does not respond to oral steroid therapy will respond to an equivalent dose of the drug given as methylprednisolone by intramuscular injection. In several patients, we have found that a tapered course of parenteral, sustained-release methylprednisolone in combination with prolonged chlorambucil (3 months at a dose sufficient to decrease the peripheral white blood count <5,000/mm^3) either induced remission or decreased proteinuria sufficiently that the patient was edema free with little or no additional diuretic therapy. The effects appear to be long lasting. This treatment must be employed cautiously after full consideration of its potential long-term side effects such as risk of neoplasm. It is not clear whether this improved response to injected steroids relates to the patient's compliance, to poor absorption of oral drugs, or to the metabolism of steroids by the liver. The routine measurement of prednisolone kinetics,[730] however, does not appear to help in the management of children with MCN.

Cyclosporine for steroid-resistant MCN has not been as effective as once anticipated. In a summary of nine studies, only 12 of 60 (20%) children had complete remission and many had a relapse with the cessation of therapy. Potential nephrotoxicity is of concern in any patient receiving cyclosporine for protracted periods. Tacrolimus has anecdotally been shown to be effective.[731] Mycophenolate mofetil was reported to induce a response in 8 of 19 children with biopsy-confirmed MCN who were resistant to both corticosteroids and cyclosporine.[732]

Therapy with NSAIDs also has produced variable results in patients with MCN.[733] Some patients with frequently relapsing or steroid-resistant MCNS who were treated with one of these drugs demonstrated a reduction in proteinuria, but all remained nephrotic and a high percentage had no response.[734] Thus, drugs such as indomethacin and meclofenamate may at best represent a useful adjunct in selected patients who are receiving symptomatic treatment only. One potential explanation for the disappointing results is that patients selected for this therapy typically are unresponsive to all standard forms of treatment and may represent a recalcitrant population.[734] NSAIDs should be used cautiously because of association with renal failure in nephrotic patients (see section on Consequences of Proteinuria).

Steroid-resistant patients who do not respond to alternative therapies often have to be maintained on a regimen of sodium and fluid restriction combined with judicious use of diuretics. Balancing the desire to minimize tissue edema against the importance of avoiding intravascular volume depletion is a rigorous challenge for the clinician (see section on Symptomatic Treatment of Nephrotic Syndrome).

Outcomes

Although late relapses of MCN have been reported,[735,736] the majority of children with MCN enter permanent remission either before or at puberty. Their long-term prognosis is good, with at least 70% entering adult life without renal or urinary abnormalities. This finding contrasts with the much less favorable outcome if the nephrotic syndrome is associated with glomerulonephritis.[737] A minority of pediatric patients who are initially steroid responsive eventually progress to renal failure. Most are found to have FSGS,[460,738] although this lesion is not always present.[739]

There have been many attempts to predict the long-term course either from renal histology or from patterns of response to treatment with steroids. For example, in one study of children, the presence of mesangial hypercellularity and immune complexes in the glomeruli was associated with an increased relapse rate.[456] In contrast, the ISKDC[663] was unable to correlate a frequency of relapse with (1) the histopathologic subgroups of MCN, (2) clinical or laboratory characteristics present at the time of diagnosis, (3) the timing of initial response, or (4) the interval between the initial response and the first relapse. Frequent relapses in the first 6 months, however, were highly predictive of frequent relapses subsequently. In contrast, children who present with minimal edema and are steroid sensitive follow an extremely favorable clinical course.[740] Another potential predictor of steroid dependence or resistance, or of frequent relapse, is low birth weight.[741,742]

Adult patients with MCN also have a good prognosis; in one series, more than 90% survived for 10 years or more without the development of end-stage renal disease (ESRD).[743,744]

Complications

The most common complications observed in patients with nephrotic syndrome are secondary to therapy. Steroid-induced side effects are well known and include the typical changes in facies, obesity, hirsutism, striae, and pseudotumor cerebri. Acutely, patients receiving large doses of corticosteroids may complain of difficulty sleeping or abdominal distress from high gastric acidity. Hypertension can occur but is seen less often in patients adhering to a sodium-restricted diet. Although growth retardation may be seen in children, especially if they receive high doses of steroids for protracted periods,[745] the incidence of significantly decreased height in prepubertal children is relatively low, even with repeated courses of corticosteroid therapy,[746] particularly when the prednisone is given on alternate days.[747] Catch-up growth often occurs when steroid therapy is discontinued.[748] Patients with steroid-responsive nephrotic syndrome who had received repeated courses of high-dose steroids during childhood and who had completed growth had a mean height equivalent to the 40th percentile[749]; total corticosteroid dose, however, correlated only weakly with the height scores. In another study, patients were slightly but not significantly shorter than their peers. More importantly, they had a higher body mass index (BMI) than controls.[418] This obesity could have mitigating effects on the impact of corticosteroids on growth.[750] Corticosteroid-induced cataracts were found in a high percentage of children,[751] although visual acuity was not impaired. The complications of cytotoxic drugs were discussed previously.

Peritonitis is a particularly important complication of nephrotic syndrome in children.[752] Patients who have one such episode are at increased risk for subsequent episodes. Peritonitis typically occurs during relapses of the disease associated with gross edema and ascites. Clinical evidence of peritoneal irritation usually is present even in patients receiving steroids. The most common infecting agent remains *Streptococcus pneumoniae*, which is found in approximately half of the affected patients[752]; *Escherichia coli* is cultured in an additional 25%; a variety of other organisms, including *Haemophilus influenzae*, may be found in a small percentage of patients, and the peritoneal fluid may be culture negative in some patients. Interestingly, this complication is far less common in adults; the basis for this disparity is not known.

Infections were responsible for the majority of deaths in nephrotic patients in the preantibiotic era. Although infections occur with much less frequency now, they continue to have serious implications. For example, in a report on long-term outcomes of treatment from the ISKDC in which 389 children with MCNS were followed for 5 to 15 years, 6 of the 10 deaths were due to infections. Other causes of death included one episode of dural sinus thrombosis and one incident of cardiorespiratory failure following the infusion of salt-poor albumin. One child died in chronic renal failure after the development of FSGS not seen in initial biopsy specimens, and one death was from uncertain causes. Five initially nonresponsive patients and four patients manifesting early relapse died. The number of fatalities among nonresponders was particularly striking; 20% of all initial nonresponders in the study died.[753] Nonrenal causes of death not mentioned in this study but that may be encountered include other thromboembolic phenomena, hemorrhagic pancreatitis,[420] and hypovolemic shock.

Nonfatal complications of MCNS include azotemia, hypovolemic shock, thrombosis, anemia, and effects of decreased vitamin D levels. These were discussed in the section on Consequences of Proteinuria.

FSGS, COLLAPSING GLOMERULOPATHY, AND DMS: THE PROGRESSIVE PODOCYTOPATHIES

FSGS is a common cause of nephrotic syndrome in infants, children, and adults. Synonyms for this lesion include *focal and segmental glomerulosclerosis with hyalinosis*, *focal sclerosing glomerulonephritis*, and *focal sclerosing glomerulopathy*. Some patients, particularly adults, may present with subnephrotic proteinuria or may lack other features of nephrotic syndrome. This is particularly true of adaptive FSGS, as compared with primary (idiopathic) FSGS.

FSGS should be distinguished from the finding of occasional globally sclerosed (obsolescent) glomeruli, a benign pattern that is seen in the United States in up to 1% to 3% of glomeruli until the age of 40 to 55 years and then rises steadily, reaching 30% in individuals 80 years of age.[754,755] Howie[756] makes the point that FSGS "cannot be defined in a sensible, useful, unambiguous way." The problem is that there are at least three meanings to the term and that definitions must include both pathologic description and clinical information: (1) idiopathic nephrotic syndrome with segmental glomerulosclerosis (which in this chapter will be termed *primary FSGS*), (2) FSGS arising as a consequence of structural and functional adaptation to various conditions, all of which are characterized by glomerular hypertrophy and hyperfiltration (which in this chapter will be termed *adaptive FSGS*), and (3) segmental glomerulosclerosis arising in the setting of other glomerular diseases, such as proliferative glomerulonephritis, membranous nephropathy, and diabetic nephropathy (which are not dealt with in this chapter, out of the belief that they should not be considered part of the spectrum of primary podocyte diseases).

A related histologic entity has been termed *collapsing focal segmental glomerulosclerosis* or *collapsing glomerulopathy* (as suggested by Detwiler et al.[757]). We have chosen the latter term because we believe that the histology, biology, and etiology of collapsing glomerulopathy are sufficiently distinct to merit a separate classification. Moreover, the glomerular lesions may be global rather than segmental and the defining lesions are podocyte hyperplasia and capillary collapse rather than sclerosis, all of which make the use of the term FSGS less than ideal. Nonetheless, the nephrology and pathology literature continues to most commonly include collapsing glomerulopathy within FSGS, and, therefore, in this chapter will follow that convention when necessary.

Another disorder is DMS, an uncommon syndrome generally restricted to the pediatric population. Many cases of DMS are associated with genetic mutations in podocyte genes, placing this syndrome within the spectrum of podocyte diseases. Furthermore, podocytes in these disorders manifest varying degrees of immaturity and exhibit a proliferation marker, which could either represent preserved proliferative potential or enhanced replacement by podocyte stem cells.

Presentation and Epidemiology

The clinical presentation of FSGS is highly variable. Nephrotic range proteinuria is seen in approximately 90% of children and 70% of adults,[758] although the fraction of nonnephrotic patients in a particular practice will clearly depend on the inclination of the nephrologist to perform a renal biopsy in the setting of subnephrotic proteinuria. Common associated features include microscopic hematuria (55% children, 45% adults) and renal insufficiency (20% children, 30% adults).[758]

FSGS is now the leading cause of primary nephrotic syndrome among adults, as shown by a review of renal biopsy archives from Chicago;[9] Springfield, Massachusetts; and New York.[381] Therefore, it has replaced membranous nephropathy as the leading cause of adult nephrotic syndrome in the United States, with a relative incidence of 30% to 40% among patients undergoing renal biopsy.

A similar pattern has been seen among children. In Houston, FSGS was present in 35% of renal biopsies in children with primary nephrotic syndrome prior to 1990, rising to 47% (and the leading diagnosis) among biopsies performed after 1990.[760] In India, the prevalence of FSGS on kidney biopsy rose from 20% to 47% during the 1990s.[761] In South Africa, over the period from 1970 to 1995, FSGS as a cause of nephrotic syndrome rose from 2% to 20% among Indian children and from 5% to 28% among African children.[762] Among children in Ontario (with a largely Caucasian population), who represent a closed population evaluated by a single pathology center, FSGS now represents 18% of the renal biopsies performed for nephrotic syndrome. This is a 2.5-fold increase in incidence, from 0.37 cases per 100,000 during 1985 to 1993 to 0.94 from 1993 to 2002.[763] Furthermore, FSGS remains a leading cause of ESRD in children aged 0 to 19.[764] Over the period from 1999 to 2002, 4,859 children progressed to ESRD; in 1,262 children, the cause was glomerulonephritis, of which 592 cases were FSGS (representing 47% of glomerulonephritis ESRD and 12% of all ESRD in children). By comparison, other major ESRD categories included "other cause" (including chiefly congenital renal and urologic abnormalities), 1,262 children; and "missing or unknown cause," 670 children.

To date, there has not been a population-based study of FSGS incidence in the United States, because incidence data have not been systematically acquired. Therefore, the increased relative incidence of FSGS could represent a decline in other diagnostic entities or an absolute increase in FSGS incidence (other possibilities, such as a change in biopsy practice or diagnostic classification, seem unlikely to account for more than a small fraction of the changes). However, as a proxy for incident FSGS trends, Kitiyakara and colleagues[765,766] examined the incidence of FSGS ESRD (excluding AIDS nephropathy) and found a steady increase over the last two decades. This was not unique to FSGS (e.g., there was a similar increase in the category, "other glomerular disease") but it contrasts with a more modest increase in membranous nephropathy ESRD and a drop in ESRD due to glomerular disease, "histologically not examined." Thus, it appears to be likely that there has been a true increase in incident FSGS cases in recent years. The reasons behind these trends are not understood.

Worldwide, there is considerable heterogeneity in the relative incidence of FSGS compared to other causes of adult nephrotic syndrome, ranging from 10% to 45% (Fig. 52.9). Factors contributing to this variability likely include population genetic differences, renal biopsy practices, and environmental factors including HIV-1 infection. There are also striking racial differences in the incidence of FSGS ESRD. In the United States, individuals of African descent are at an approximately fourfold increased risk for FSGS ESRD compared to Caucasians, Hispanics (who may be of any race), and Native Americans (Fig. 52.10). Recently, it has become apparent that much of this health disparity can be explained by variants on chromosome 22, particularly in *APOL1*[767] and *MYH9*.[768,769] With regard to the progression to ESRD, studies of adults[770] and children[771,772] have

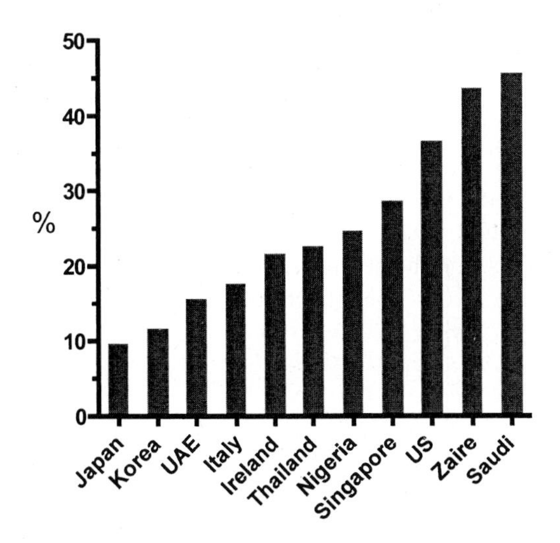

FIGURE 52.9 Relative incidence of focal segmental glomerulosclerosis (FSGS) as a cause of adult nephrotic syndrome. The fraction of adult nephrotic syndrome attributed to FSGS (which probably includes collapsing glomerulopathy in most or all series) is presented in select countries. *UAE*, United Arab Emirates; *US*, United States.

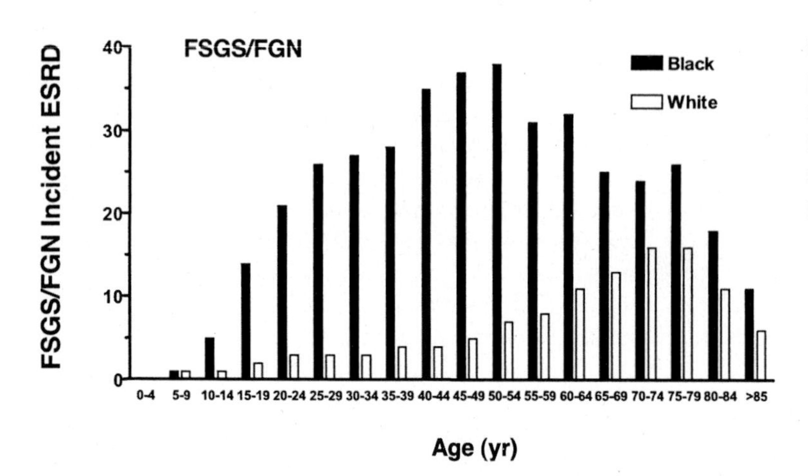

FIGURE 52.10 Racial differences (cases per million population per year) in focal segmental glomerulosclerosis (FSGS) end-stage renal disease (ESRD) in the United States. The annual incidence of ESRD attributed to FSGS for the years 1995 to 2000 are shown.

suggested that Africans are more likely to progress to ESRD than are those of other races by a factor of approximately two- to fourfold. Chromosome 22–associated FSGS progresses more quickly to ESRD.[773] The chromosome 22 variants are fairly common in the African American population, and most individuals with two risk copies do not develop CKD; this suggests that additional genetic and/or environmental factors contribute. The chromosome 22 findings are discussed further in the section on FSGS susceptibility genes later in this chapter.

Interestingly, there also is a racial difference in the age of onset of FSGS ESRD (Fig. 52.11). In Africans, the incidence peaks in the early 50s, whereas in Caucasians, the incidence peaks two decades later (when there is a second peak among Africans).

Histopathology

Fahr,[774] writing in 1925, first noted that patients with lipoid nephrosis who progress to renal failure showed focal glomerular damage. In 1957, Rich[775] examined autopsy tissues from 20 children with nephrotic syndrome and otherwise typical lipoid nephrosis and described progressive sclerosis of glomeruli, affecting first the juxtamedullary glomeruli. Heptinstall,[776] in the 1966 edition of his renal pathology textbook, confirmed that some patients with lipoid nephrosis had hyalinization of the glomerular tuft, particularly affecting the juxtamedullary glomeruli. McGovern[777] and Hayslett et al.[778] showed that in some patients whose initial renal biopsy was consistent with MCN, a later renal biopsy showed FSGS. In 1970, two reports demonstrated that FSGS was the second most common cause of nephrotic syndrome in children.[435,436] Thus, by 1970, it was clear that FSGS was a distinct and common glomerular disease.

Classically, the pathologic abnormalities affect only some glomeruli (focal), with only part of the glomerular tuft involved (segmental). There may be accumulation of acellular hyaline subendothelial deposits within glomerular capillaries; these represent the insudation of plasma protein below an injured endothelium. Tubular atrophy and interstitial inflammatory infiltrates are common.[435] The first glomeruli affected are those located near the medulla. As a consequence, an early or superficial renal biopsy may miss the lesion. Furthermore, an evaluation of sclerosis on the basis of one section or a few sections, as is typical of routine pathologic analysis, will significantly underestimate the fraction of glomeruli that are affected.[779,780]

Immunofluorescence microscopy may demonstrate IgM and C3 deposits in a granular pattern, particularly within affected sclerotic segments.[781] Unaffected glomerular areas also may reveal IgM and C3 in a mesangial distribution. Electron microscopy shows epithelial cell foot-process effacement that in patients with heavy proteinuria is diffuse and involves areas of the glomeruli that do not demonstrate sclerosis. Mesangial hypercellularity is present variably. In a patient with otherwise normal glomeruli, the presence of glomerular hypertrophy, focal interstitial fibrosis, or tubular atrophy may reflect FSGS that is not present in the glomeruli that are sampled in the renal biopsy.[782]

The incidence of FSGS in a subsequent biopsy when the original biopsy shows apparent MCN has varied from less than 10% to more than 40% in individual studies,[722] which may reflect whether each report presents a primary or referral population.

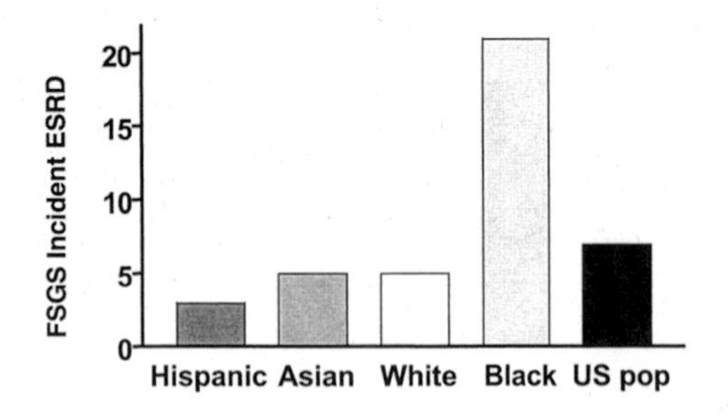

FIGURE 52.11 Incidence of focal segmental glomerulosclerosis (FSGS) end-stage renal disease (ESRD) by age and race in the United States. The incidence of ESRD (cases per million population per year) attributed to FSGS is presented by age and race; data from the USRDS. (Reprinted from: Kitiyakara C, Kopp JB, Eggers P, et al. Trends in the epidemiology of focal segmental glomerulosclerosis. *Semin Nephrol.* 2003;23:172, with permission.)

Histopathologic Variants: FSGS and Collapsing Glomerulopathy

It is now clear that the spectrum of primary podocyte diseases (MCN, DMS, FSGS, and collapsing glomerulopathy) represent several histopathologic patterns, each including multiple disease entities. The relationships among these entities remain enigmatic; we present one schema (Table 52.2). In that schema, we have excluded disorders that might otherwise be placed in the MCN/FSGS spectrum, such as idiopathic nodular sclerosis, which has been proposed to have a vascular etiology.[783] Others have presented parallel but distinct approaches.[784–786]

The existing classification schemes for the primary podocyte diseases, including the one presented here, rely on a mixture of morphologic, immunologic, genetic, and historical criteria in ways that are not ideally integrated. Importantly, the presence of a risk factor for a diagnostic entity in a particular case under investigation will not always mean that that particular factor has been responsible. Therefore, although obese patients are at increased risk to develop adaptive FSGS, they remain at some risk for other FSGS variants. Likewise, many patients with FSGS have hypertension, and distinguishing hypertension-associated FSGS from other variants can be problematic. As a practical matter, information about genetic history and the presence of relevant comorbid conditions may not be available to the pathologist at the time of diagnosis. All of these comments point out the limitations of relying on clinical factors in determining pathologic diagnosis, or conversely, determining disease based solely on histopathology. This issue may be successfully addressed by new molecular diagnostic techniques, which may improve the accuracy of a clinical diagnosis and may generate more useful classification schemes in the future. Immunostaining to evaluate protein expression is one approach. For example, dystroglycan, a podocyte membrane protein contributing to cellular adhesion to the GBM, is reduced in MCN but not in FSGS.[445] Another approach is quantitative analysis of RNA extracted from microdissected glomeruli. Schmid and colleagues[787] showed that the ratio of podocin/synaptopodin mRNA distinguished MCN from FSGS and predicted steroid responsiveness in cases where the distinction of MCN from FSGS was uncertain.

Columbia Classification

D'Agati and colleagues[786] have proposed a working classification (the Columbia classification) for primary FSGS, which comprises five categories: collapsing variant, tip lesion, cellular lesion, perihilar variant, plus a final category for those cases that do not have the diagnostic criteria for the other categories, not otherwise specified (NOS), corresponding to classic FSGS (Table 52.8, Fig. 52.12).

TABLE 52.8 Columbia Classification of the Morphologic Variants of Focal Segmental Glomerulosclerosis

Variant	Positive Criteria	Negative Criteria
FSGS, not otherwise specified	■ At least one glomerulus with segmental increase in matrix obliterating the capillary lumina ■ There may be segmental GBM collapse without podocyte hyperplasia	Exclude other defined variants that follow
Perihilar variant	■ At least one glomerulus with perihilar hyalinosis, with or without hyalinosis ■ Perihilar sclerosis and hyalinosis involving >50% of segmentally sclerotic glomeruli	Exclude cellular, tip, and collapsing variants
Cellular variant	■ At least one glomerulus with segmental endocapillary hypercellularity occluding lumina, with or without foam cells and karyorrhexis	Exclude tip and collapsing variants
Tip variant	■ At least one segmental lesion involving the tip domain (outer 25% of the tuft next to the origin of the proximal tubule) ■ The tubular pole must be identified in the defining lesion ■ The lesion must have either an adhesion or confluence of podocytes with parietal or tubular cells at the tubular lumen or neck ■ The tip lesion may be sclerosing or cellular	Exclude collapsing variant Exclude if any glomeruli show perihilar sclerosis
Collapsing variant	■ At least one glomerulus with segmental or global collapse and podocyte hypertrophy or hyperplasia	No exclusions

The flow of diagnostic decision making begins at the bottom, as the pathologist diagnoses or excludes collapsing variant, then tip variant, then cellular variant, then perihilar variant, and, finally, FSGS not otherwise specified.
FSGS, focal segmental glomerulosclerosis; GBM, glomerular basement membrane.
Adapted from D'Agati V. Pathologic classification of focal segmental glomerulosclerosis. *Semin Nephrol.* 2003;23:117; and D'Agati VD, Fogo AB, Bruijin JA, et al. Pathologic classification of focal segmental glomerulosclerosis: a working proposal. *Am J Kidney Dis.* 2004;43:368.

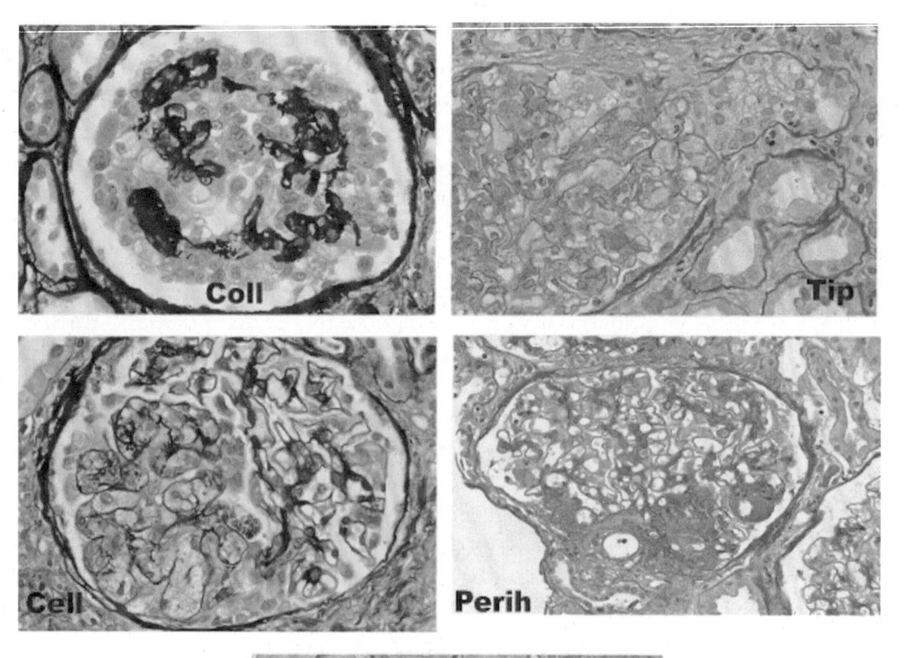

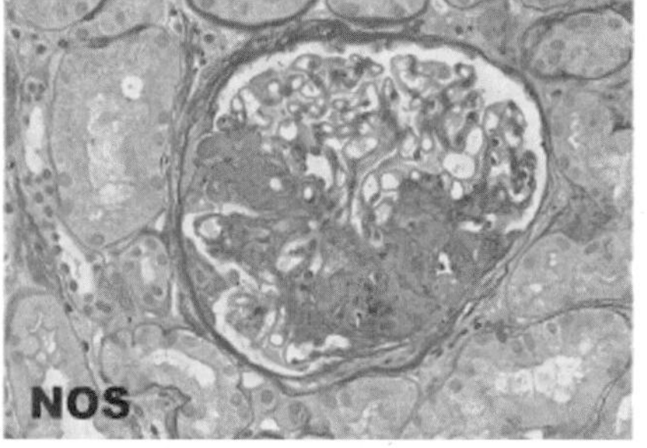

FIGURE 52.12 Variants of focal segmental glomerulosclerosis: the Columbia classification. This classification was developed for diagnostic purposes and involves the stepwise consideration of collapsing variant (coll), tip lesion (tip), cellular variant (cell), perihilar variant (perih), and FSGS not otherwise specified (NOS). (Figure reproduced from D'Agati V, Fogo AB, Bruijn JA, et al. Pathologic classification of focal segmental glomerulosclerosis: a working proposal. *Am J Kidney Dis.* 2004;368:43, with permission.)

An evaluation of the renal biopsy requires immunologic and ultrastructural studies to exclude other disease entities. The Columbia classification of FSGS variants is based solely on a semiquantitative analysis of morphology by light microscopy. There is no minimum glomerular number required in order to make a diagnosis, but obviously diagnostic accuracy will increase with a larger sample size. A single glomerulus with the defining characteristic findings is sufficient, as long as the other criteria are met. This classification scheme was not specifically designed to serve clinical or research purposes, but rather to address both needs.

The collapsing variant of primary FSGS is defined by the presence of at least one glomerulus with segmental or global collapse *and* with podocyte hypertrophy or hyperplasia. Thus, podocyte changes alone are insufficient to make the diagnosis (such findings would indicate cellular FSGS). This entity is termed primary collapsing glomerulopathy in Table 52.2. HIV-associated collapsing glomerulopathy has an identical histologic appearance, so that the appearance of classic or other forms of FSGS in a patient with HIV-1 infection is sufficiently unusual to raise the issue of coincidental primary FSGS. Both idiopathic collapsing FSGS and HIV-associated FSGS are frequently associated with tubulointerstitial injury and fibrosis that is out of proportion to the extent of glomerular involvement.

The glomerular tip variant of primary FSGS is defined by the presence of at least one glomerulus with a segmental scar involving the glomerular tuft adjacent to the proximal tubule. The collapsing variant must be excluded (it would take precedence over the diagnosis of the tip variant). Most tip variants have increased cellularity as well as the required sclerosis. Mesangial hypercellularity may be present. Perihilar sclerosis cannot be present but other peripheral (nontip, nonhilar) lesions containing IgM and C3 may be present within the tip lesion. Heavy proteinuria and extensive foot-process effacement is typically present.

The cellular variant of primary FSGS has had a complicated history. Grishman and Churg[788] described the ultrastructure of 16 patients with FSGS and found that 5 patients had podocyte abnormalities, including cellular degeneration and detachment, together with glomerular capillary collapse; 3 of these patients exhibited rapid clinical deterioration. Schwartz and Lewis[789] coined the term *cellular lesion of FSGS*. The original cellular definition included segmental or global hypercellularity (representing proliferation and/or infiltration, or hypercellularity within the Bowman space overlying a segmental scar or a capillary collapse). Thus, many of these cases meet the Columbia criteria for collapsing variant. In the Columbia framework, the diagnosis of a cellular variant requires the presence of endocapillary proliferation (segmental or global) in at least one glomerulus; these lesions include endothelial cells, macrophages, and foam cells. Podocyte hypertrophy and hyperplasia may be present. Mesangial hypercellularity may also be present but is uncommon. Consequently, the focus of the Columbia definition of cellular variant has shifted away from podocytes to endocapillary cells, although abnormalities of both cellular compartments may be present. A tubulopathy is present that may be disproportionate to the extent of glomerular involvement. This may include afocal microcystic dilation and tubular epithelial cells manifesting acute injury (including focal acute tubular necrosis), regeneration, and chronic injury (cellular atrophy and thickening of the tubular basement membrane). A tip variant and a collapsing variant must be excluded (these diagnoses would take precedence over the cellular variant).

The Columbia classification makes the perihilar variant a formal diagnostic entity. This variant is diagnosed when perihilar hyalinosis is present in one or more glomeruli and perihilar sclerosis and/or hyalinosis is present in at least 50% of segmentally sclerotic glomeruli. Hyalinosis represents the accumulation of glassy, homogeneous, eosinophilic material within the capillary wall and is believed to consist of plasma proteins. In the remnant rat model, hyalinosis appears first as the accumulation of periodic acid-Schiff (PAS)-positive and electron-dense material beneath damaged glomerular capillary endothelial cells, with later expansion and encroachment on the capillary lumen.[790] Glomerulomegaly is common, although approaches to quantify glomerular size in clinical samples are fraught with difficulty. The perihilar variant is commonly associated with *adaptive* FSGS (defined in subsequent text). Cellular variant, tip variant, and collapsing variants must be excluded (these diagnoses would take precedence over perihilar variant).

The most common variant of FSGS (NOS) may include features of any of the prior variants, but lacks sufficient criteria to make a more specific diagnosis. The term *classic FSGS* would include FSGS NOS.

Since the publication of the Columbia classification of FSGS, several groups have compared presentation and outcomes using these definitions in adults, including groups from Columbia[791] and Chapel Hill[792] and in children[793] these reports suggest that the classification does have some degree of clinical validity.

The Columbia classification represents a very important step forward in the process of developing a robust, consistent, and clinically useful diagnostic classification system for FSGS. By laying out consensus diagnostic criteria for FSGS for the first time, D'Agati and colleagues[786] have framed the issues that the field will address in the coming years. As the authors recognize, this is a working proposal that will almost certainly undergo revision. The next iteration might usefully address some of the following issues, and may well make use of molecular markers to refine the classification system.

First, the relationship between the cellular variant and the collapsing FSGS (collapsing glomerulopathy) remains controversial. Chun and colleagues[794] note that in their terminology, the cellular lesion includes collapsing FSGS, whereas the Columbia classification includes cellular lesion and collapsing FSGS as distinct entities. Stokes and colleagues[791] reported a series of 22 patients with cellular variants and suggested that both the response to treatment and the rate of progression to ESKD are intermediate between those for tip lesions and for collapsing variants.

Second, and related to the previous issue, the importance of different forms of podocyte injury has become apparent as we have developed a new understanding of the biologic processes underlying FSGS (podocyte depletion) and collapsing glomerulopathy (proliferation of podocytes, or more likely, podocyte precursors, but referred to as podocytes here for simplicity). Morphologically, podocyte proliferation is characteristic of the collapsing variant, but must be coupled with capillary loop collapse for the diagnosis to be determined. When capillary loop collapse is absent and podocyte changes are coupled with endothelial cell proliferation, the diagnosis of a cellular lesion is made. Thus, when podocyte hyperplasia is present, the diagnosis depends on whether capillary collapse or endocapillary proliferation is present.[795] The biologic rationale for this distinction is not immediately clear, because we do not understand the mechanisms responsible for glomerular collapse. If further studies indicate that the podocyte phenotype is similar in collapsing FSGS and those cases of cellular variant FSGS with podocyte hyperplasia, and that the responses to therapy and prognosis are also similar, it is probably more logical to combine these categories.

Third, the stability of classification when serial biopsies are performed needs to be defined by further research. The few studies available suggest that patients may change diagnostic categories on subsequent biopsies (discussed in the subsequent text). Future studies involving serial renal biopsies of FSGS patients would be an essential starting point. Careful consideration must be given as to whether these events represent disease evolution (category change) or disease progression (progressive scarring), and what the implication for the classification system might be.

Fourth, interrater reliability needs to be rigorously evaluated by practicing pathologists to ensure that the existing diagnostic framework yields reproducible results. Finally, the ability of diagnostic categories to make predictions as to etiology and prognosis, based solely on morphology and independent of clinical history, must be tested both retrospectively and prospectively on patient cohorts drawn from diverse ethnic and racial populations. Despite these considerations, the Columbia classification remains an excellent starting point, providing a common set of diagnostic criteria with which the field can advance.

A Revised Taxonomy for the Podocytopathies

Barisoni and colleagues[12,13] have proposed an alternative approach, based not only on morphology but also on our current understanding of disease pathogenesis. This taxonomy

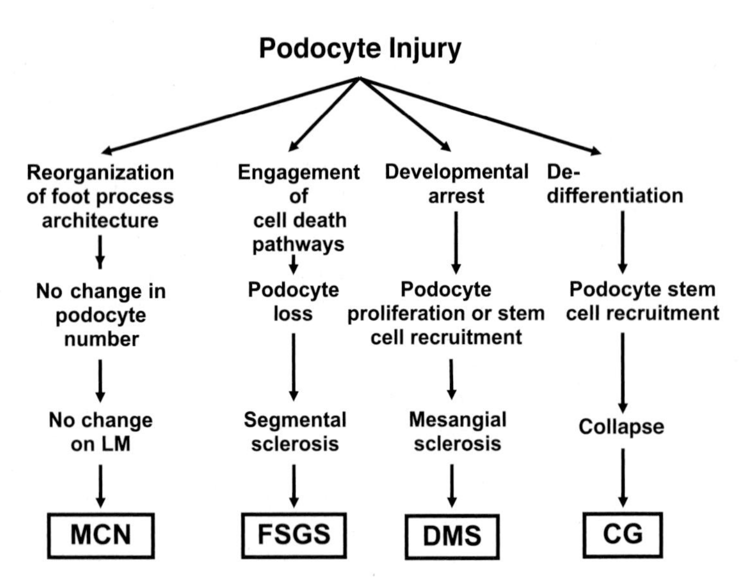

FIGURE 52.13 Different diagnoses among the primary podocytopathies are distinguished by the relative number of podocytes present in the lesion. These differences suggest that each one of these diseases represents a distinct pathogenic mechanism. *LM,* light microscopy; *MCN,* minimal change nephropathy; *FSGS,* focal segmental glomerulosclerosis; *DMS,* diffuse mesangial sclerosis; *CG,* collapsing glomerulopathy. Adapted with permission from Barisoni L, Schnaper HW, Kopp JB. (Advances in the biology and genetics of the podocytopathies: implications for diagnosis and therapy. *Arch Pathol Lab Med.* 2009;133:201–216.)

is influenced by clinical history, causal associations, and the potential presence of associated genetic mutations. Importantly, the disease categories outlined in Table 52.2 are determined by a relative podocyte number (Fig. 52.13). Because these are likely to reflect the podocyte response to injury, each category presumably represents a defined area of similar pathogenic mechanisms or cellular response to injury. Thus, in MCN, the podocyte number is relatively neutral, whereas FSGS is characterized by podocytopenia. Patients with diffuse mesangial sclerosis manifest mildly increased podocyte numbers, and collapsing glomerulopathy is characterized by a significant degree of podocyte (or podocyte precursor) proliferation, accompanied by markers of epithelial cell dedifferentiation and proliferation.[12,13] Recent data suggest that at least some of these epithelial cells may be derived from the parietal rather than the visceral epithelium.[796] Importantly, differences in pathogenesis would, in turn, suggest the need for mechanism-specific treatments.

Adaptive Focal Segmental Glomerulosclerosis

Adaptive *FSGS* includes those forms of FSGS that are believed to arise as a consequence of structural adaptation (glomerular hypertrophy) and functional adaptation (glomerular hyperperfusion and hyperfiltration) to either reduced nephron mass or particular disease states (obesity, sickle cell anemia, cyanotic congenital heart disease, and others). The term *secondary FSGS* has also been used to describe this form of FSGS, although the term sometimes has been extended to HIV-associated nephropathy, to drug-associated FSGS, and to segmental scarring arising in proliferative glomerulonephritis; these varied uses have diminished the use of the term.

The diagnosis of adaptive FSGS remains a challenge. Ideally, the diagnosis would be made on pathologic grounds alone. The problem with relying on clinical factors in reaching a diagnosis is that patients with obesity, hypertension, and other disorders might present with either primary FSGS or adaptive FSGS. Because these entities may have different responses to therapy, particularly immunosuppressive therapy, the distinction becomes important. Three approaches are available at present.

First, adaptive FSGS may manifest less foot-process effacement than primary FSGS. Chiang et al.[797] studied renal biopsies obtained from 30 children and found that the extent of foot-process effacement was similar in MCN (63% ± 21%), FSGS (70% ± 25%), and MCN that subsequently evolved into FSGS (56% ± 23%). The large standard deviation suggests that many patients in all three disease categories had <50% effacement. Furthermore, the extent of foot-process effacement did not correlate with proteinuria, although only 15 patients were included in the analysis. Kambham and colleagues[798] defined obesity-associated glomerulopathy as glomerulomegaly in the setting of BMI >30 kg per square meter, with or without FSGS. They found that obesity-associated glomerulomegaly cases had a mean foot-process effacement of 40% (range, 10% to 100%), whereas primary FSGS patients had mean foot-process effacement of 75% (range, 30% to 100%). Importantly, although there were significant differences in the group means, there was much overlap, so the use of particular diagnostic criteria (such as podocyte foot-process effacement >50% in the former and <50% in the latter) is limited.[786]

Second, the initial lesion in adaptive FSGS is preferentially localized to the hilum. Rat models of FSGS that are characterized by increased transcapillary hydraulic pressure are associated with predominant or exclusive perihilar sclerosis. This is probably explained by the observation that the first capillary branches of the afferent arteriole are the largest, and thus by Laplace's law, these branches would have the highest wall tension and would be the most susceptible to podocyte injury.[799,800] The problems in clinical use are that correctly identifying the location of the sclerosis, even with multiple sections, and the number of glomeruli available for study is limited. (It remains to be determined whether the perihilar variant of primary FSGS also arises as a consequence of glomerular overload from an unrecognized risk factor or biologic process. In this context, it would be interesting to see a detailed analysis of the clinical and physiologic characteristics of these patients.)

Third, glomerulomegaly can be demonstrated by direct measurement of glomerular size. D'Agati et al.[786] have proposed defining glomerulomegaly as 1.5-fold increase in glomerular diameter over controls (comparable to a 2.5-fold increase in glomerular area and 3.4-fold increase in glomerular volume, assuming that the glomerulus is a sphere). Kambham and colleagues[798] have also defined glomerulomegaly as average glomerular diameter >180 μm, based on a study of four biopsy levels and the measurement limited to glomeruli in which the hilus was identified. In normal controls, glomerular diameter averaged 168 μm (range, 138 to 186 μm), and in obese subjects with glomerulomegaly, glomerular diameter averaged 226 μm (range, 172 to 300 μm).

Therefore, presently available methods to identify adaptive FSGS include determining the fraction of glomeruli with perihilar sclerosis and measuring glomerular size. Needed are prospective studies evaluating each of these approaches, and defining the receiver-operating characteristic (ROC) curves for the diagnostic thresholds. Even with these data, a major limitation remains the requirement for sufficient numbers of intact glomeruli. An important research goal will be to identify molecular markers that reflect the glomerular adaptation; these might include proteins that are upregulated by podocytes or mesangial cells in response to mechanical stress.

Diffuse Mesangial Sclerosis and Related Disorders

Diffuse mesangial sclerosis represents a small fraction of pediatric renal biopsies (0.9% in India)[801] and all-age renal biopsies (0.45% in the United States).[802] In the pediatric population, many cases are associated with *WT1* and *LAMB2* mutations, as discussed elsewhere in this chapter. Some cases seen in children and adults are idiopathic. Unidentified genetic mutations may contribute. Two adult cases have been reported in association with multiple myeloma.[803] One note of diagnostic caution is that it may be difficult to exclude advanced FSGS in renal biopsies lacking glomeruli with segmental sclerosis.

Disease Mechanisms of FSGS and Collapsing Glomerulopathy

Animal Models

A number of animal models have been used to delineate the mechanisms of FSGS and collapsing glomerulopathy, as has been reviewed recently.[804] These models have been crucial for elucidating mechanisms, particularly for adaptive FSGS, HIV-associated collapsing glomerulopathy, and most recently, for genetic causes of FSGS. In particular, they have led the field to highlight the central role of podocytes in FSGS and collapsing glomerulopathy. A significant gap is the absence of generally accepted animal models for MCN, idiopathic classic FSGS, or recurrent FSGS after renal transplantation.

Available animal models include experimentally induced disease,[805–817] spontaneous genetic models,[799,818–827] null mutation animals,[828–838] and transgenic animals.[835,839–857] Each model has particular strengths and limitations and reflects a certain portion of the spectrum of human podocyte disease. The interested reader is referred to the provided references; here we will consider the pathogenesis of FSGS and collapsing glomerulopathy by considering the structural and functional processes involved, rather than a detailed review of particular molecular pathways.

A critical aspect of these models is disordered podocyte function. Direct injury to the podocyte underlies many of the animal models of glomerulosclerosis, including toxic injury (Adriamycin, puromycin aminonucleoside [PAN]), proliferation (fibroblast growth factor [FGF]-2 administration), viral gene expression (HIV-1 accessory genes, SV40 T antigen), and gene (*NPHS2*, *CD2AP*, *ACTN4*) deletion or modification. Podocyte stress likely contributes in models of adaptive FSGS associated with nephron loss (remnant nephron, aging plus uninephrectomy, bromo-ethylamine–induced papillary necrosis). The genetic rat models demonstrate the importance of systemic and glomerular hypertension and hyperlipidemia, although the restriction of these traits to particular strains suggests that particular genetic loci are required for the full interaction of the hypertension and lipids with renal injury.

Glomerular Adaptation: Glomerular Overload and Glomerulomegaly

A reduction in nephron mass is a well-established model of adaptive FSGS in experimental animal models. In 1952, Platt and colleagues[858] noted in rats subjected to 5/6 nephrectomy, creatinine clearance fell to a lesser degree than the reduction in renal mass would predict. Subsequently, Shimamura and Morrison[816] and Morrison and Howard[859] reported similar findings using inulin clearance and went on to suggest that hyperfiltration might play a role in glomerulomegaly, podocyte hypertrophy, and the subsequent appearance of glomerulosclerosis. In 1981, in a highly influential study, Hostetter et al.[810] demonstrated that the remnant nephron model is characterized by increased single nephron glomerular filtration rate (SNGFR), due to increased transcapillary hydraulic pressure. The glomerular overload (or glomerular hyperfiltration) hypothesis states that some feature of adaptation to reduced renal mass, including possibly hyperperfusion, hyperfiltration, glomerulomegaly, and/or podocyte mechanical stretch, underlies some forms of FSGS and accounts for the progressive nature of chronic kidney disease in general.

In human subject s, the removal of one kidney (e.g., donor nephrectomy) is not associated with an increased risk of renal disease after long-term follow-up. There is a poorly defined boundary of minimal renal mass, below which patients are at risk for progressive renal disease. It is quite possible that the boundary differs among patients based on various factors, including nephron endowment. Novick et al.[860] studied 14 patients who had a solitary kidney and then underwent partial nephrectomy for cancer, with 25% to 75% of the solitary kidney having been removed. Five patients subsequently developed proteinuria, including three with biopsy-proven FSGS.[861]

The Barker hypothesis proposes that prenatal programming influences fetal development in ways that influence adult susceptibility to diseases, including hypertension, coronary heart disease, and type 2 diabetes.[862] Considerable variability in nephron endowment has been noted, ranging from 200,000 to 2.5 million glomeruli per kidney, with the median value being around 1 million.[863] The Brenner corollary of the Barker hypothesis proposes that a reduced number of nephrons at birth predisposes one to hypertension and progressive renal disease during adult life.[864] Low birth weight may be a predictor of low nephron number,[865] although studies in various human populations have come to discrepant findings.[866,867] Studies support a relationship between low birth weight and essential hypertension[868] and between low birth weight and ESRD (odds ratio, 1.4 for birth weight <2.5 kg compared to birth weight 3 to 3.5 kg).[869] One small series has suggested an association of FSGS with low birth weight,[870] but this finding may represent a general tendency for increased chronic kidney disease (CKD) in adults who had low birth weight.[871–873] rather than a specific causal factor in FSGS.

Glomerulomegaly. Human glomeruli increase in size during childhood, with mean diameters increasing from 112 μm at birth to 167 μm at age 15, as assessed in an autopsy study where maximal glomerular diameter was measured.[874] In normal kidney donors aged 24 to 53, mean glomerular area was not correlated with age or sex.[875] When assessed by microdissection, mean glomerular diameter remains stable until about age 40 to 50, after which there is a modest decline.[876] The mechanism of age-associated decline in glomerular diameter is unknown, but could be due to an increasing fraction of obsolescent glomeruli. By contrast, children with FSGS have increased glomerular size and there is no correlation with age.[877]

Glomerulomegaly is a hallmark of adaptation to reduced nephron mass. Glomerular enlargement may arise as a consequence of widening of the glomerular capillaries, increasing glomerular capillary length, or some combination of both. Experimental rat models suggest that both mechanisms occur with adaptation to reduced renal mass at different ages. In *young rats*, there are large increases in capillary length and only small increases in capillary diameter.[878,879] In *older rats*, the major change is increased capillary diameter.[880,881] In *children* undergoing uninephrectomy in the setting of reflux nephropathy, the nephrectomized kidney shows glomerulomegaly without increased capillary diameters.[882] In *adults* with FSGS, glomerulomegaly is associated primarily with an increase in capillary diameter.[883] Kidneys showing greater numbers of sclerotic glomeruli (more advanced disease), however, showed greater capillary lengthening, whereas there was no relationship between extent of sclerosis and capillary diameter. In conclusion, (1) the results in rats and humans show similar age-dependent patterns, with capillary lengthening predominantly in the young individual and capillary lumen increase predominating in the mature individual, and (2) the results in adults with FSGS suggests that the increase in capillary lumen diameter may occur early (as a consequence of unknown mechanisms) and capillary lengthening may later occur in response to reduced functional nephron mass.

Glomerulomegaly is also present in experimental and clinical settings characterized by glomerular overload (defined as an increase in glomerular blood flow, or glomerular filtration, or both). These settings include obesity, sickle cell anemia, and cyanotic congenital heart disease. Thus, in obese patients with glomerular disease and proteinuria, the mean glomerular diameter has been reported as 226 μm (range, 172 to 300 μm), compared to a mean of 168 μm (range, 138 to 186 μm) in age-matched normal subjects,[798] and 256 μm (range, 192 to 280 μm).[884]

Glomerular Overload: Hyperperfusion and Hyperfiltration. Glomerular hyperperfusion and hyperfiltration are present at the *single nephron level* in animal models of reduced nephron mass. Under normal circumstances in the rat, the pressure gradient across the glomerular capillary wall (P_{GC}) is approximately 50 mm Hg and SNGFR is approximately 30 nL per minute; in the remnant nephron model P_{GC} exceeds 60 mm Hg and SNGFR exceeds 60 nL per minute.[810] Furthermore, glomerular hyperfiltration is present at the *whole kidney level* early in the disease course in experimental models of adaptive FSGS and most, if not all, human forms of adaptive FSGS.

Conversely, there are several experimental settings where glomerular hyperperfusion, glomerular hyperfiltration, glomerulomegaly, and FSGS are less closely correlated. Yoshida et al.[885] compared two rat models, both with 1/3 left nephrectomy; in one group, the right kidney was removed and in the other group, the right ureter was diverted into the peritoneum. SNGFR and P_{GC} increased to an equivalent degree in both models, but glomerulomegaly and glomerulosclerosis were blunted (although present) in the urinary diversion group. Thus, remnant nephrons in the left kidney acted differently in the presence of a filtering but nonexcreting right kidney. It remains unclear by what mechanism the remnant nephrons apparently sense total body functioning nephron mass; perhaps a circulating molecular product of glomerular cells contributes. In any case, although this experiment suggests caution in assuming that hyperfiltration will necessarily lead to glomerulomegaly and FSGS, the urinary diversion model has uncertain relevance to clinical situations involving glomerular adaptation.

Furthermore, glomerular hyperperfusion and hyperfiltration clearly are not essential for the development of all forms of FSGS. In rats with PAN nephrosis and rats with Adriamycin nephrosis, average P_{GC} values remain normal despite the subsequent appearance of sclerosis.[886] In the former model, increased SNGFR was uniformly absent, and in the latter model, although some glomeruli exhibit increased GFR, these glomeruli did not have elevated P_{GC} and did not subsequently develop sclerosis, at least within the time frame of the study. (Adriamycin causes DNA strand breaks, and murine renal susceptibility to Adriamycin is associated with mutations in genes affecting the mitochondrial genome,[887] pointing to a role for bioenergetics in this model.) Consequently, hyperperfusion and hyperfiltration appear to characterize most, if not all, adaptive FSGS models, but are absent from FSGS models that involve direct podocyte injury (presumably models of primary FSGS).

In obese human subjects, absolute GFR (without a correction for body size) has been reported to be increased by 25% to 60%,[888–890] and this is partially returned to normal values by weight loss.[888] Obese subjects have both increased GFR and increased filtration fraction, whereas even in nonobese subjects there is a positive correlation between BMI and filtration fraction (but not GFR).[891] Others have not found an increase in absolute GFR, despite similar levels of BMI, although the reasons for the discrepant findings are not apparent.[892] The increased GFR is more striking in central compared to peripheral obesity.[893] The mechanisms of obesity-related glomerular hyperfiltration are unknown but may include protein intake, various components of the metabolic syndrome (discussed in subsequent text), and possibly particular adipokines.

Most but not all studies suggest that early in the course of children with sickle cell anemia, GFR and renal plasma flow are increased.[894–896] Limited data available in children with cyanotic congenital heart disease suggest that glomerular filtration may be slightly impaired[897] or normal.[898] In the latter study, GFR was normal and renal plasma flow was decreased, indicating an increased filtration fraction. The authors proposed that increased blood viscosity associated with polycythemia increases renal vascular resistance and intraglomerular blood pressure.

There is at least one clinical situation in which the link between glomerulomegaly and glomerular overload is absent. Fogo et al.[782] studied 42 pediatric MCN patients, of whom 10 subsequently experienced renal functional decline and a repeat renal biopsy showed FSGS. In those patients who later developed FSGS, glomerular area was on average 76% larger (which would correspond to a 1.3-fold increased diameter, assuming the glomerulus was spherical). Although the data on creatinine clearances were not provided, there is no reason to suspect hyperfiltration, and these patients had no obvious clinical features that would suggest reduced renal mass. It remains uncertain what processes might account for glomerulomegaly in this setting.

Podocyte Depletion Hypothesis

The podocyte depletion hypothesis proposes that an absolute or relative reduction in podocyte number is a critical process in the initiation or progression of FSGS of all types. Also, it now appears that podocyte depletion also is present in other glomerular diseases, including diabetic nephropathy[899] and primary glomerulonephritis,[900] and may promote sclerosis in these settings.

Podocytes are postmitotic cells in the normal human kidney. In a study of 164 kidneys, podocyte mitoses were found in one kidney (the diagnosis was given as FSGS) and binucleate cells were found in four kidneys (FSGS, lupus nephritis, and IgA nephropathy).[901] In a seminal study, Fries et al.[902] noted that in rats subjected to 3/4 nephrectomy plus Adriamycin, the remnant nephrons undergo compensatory hypertrophy, more than doubling tuft volume. As part of this process, endothelial cells and mesangial cells proliferate but podocytes do not. As podocyte volume density declines, each podocyte must cover a larger capillary surface area. Areas of podocyte detachment were present, particularly in areas of segmental sclerosis. Extending these studies to human renal biopsies, Bhathena[903] found that the unit distance of GBM covered by podocytes increased in oligomeganephronia, unilateral renal agenesis with FSGS (but not unilateral renal agenesis without FSGS), uninephrectomy with FSGS (but not uninephrectomy without FSGS), and renal transplantation with late (nonrecurrent) FSGS (but not without FSGS). Together, these findings describe a model in which either a loss of podocytes (primary FSGS) or increased capillary length or size (adaptive FSGS) decreases the ratio of podocytes to capillary surface area, with podocyte hypertrophy in response. In support of this model, reduced podocyte numbers are present in children with FSGS compared to those with MCN.[877] More recently, evidence has been presented that there is a limited capacity for podocyte replenishment, with the source being stem cells located in the parietal epithelium (reviewed in Romagnani[904])

Evolution of Segmental Sclerosis: The Misdirected Filtration Hypothesis

Kriz and Lemley[800,905,906] have proposed an intriguing model of misdirected glomerular filtration to explain the propensity for segmental sclerotic scars of FSGS to expand, to progress to global sclerosis, and to be associated with tubular damage and interstitial inflammation. This model was developed from an intensive study of rat models of FSGS, including the hypertensive Fawn hooded rat and the normotensive Milan rat, with more limited studies of human FSGS.

The process begins when one or more podocytes undergo apoptosis or necrosis, or loses adhesion and is released into the Bowman space. Naked GBM tends to lie in apposition to the parietal cells lining the Bowman capsule, perhaps due to the ballooning of the glomerular capillary in response to the loss of mechanical restraint consequent to podocyte loss or perhaps due to a response on the part of the parietal cells to contact the GBM. This manifests as tuft adhesion (synechia). Tuft adhesion involves a loosening of contacts between parietal cells, allowing glomerular ultrafiltrate to penetrate between parietal cells. A loop of glomerular capillary also penetrates between parietal cells, leading to an expanding paraglomerular space located beneath the parietal cells or extending between layers of the Bowman capsule. These capillary loops remain perfused, at least for a time, and this allows the continued delivery of glomerular filtrate into the paraglomerular space. This filtrate, having passed through an abnormal capillary wall lacking podocytes, is likely enriched in growth factors, chemokines, and other inflammatory mediators. These mediators promote the recruitment and activation of fibroblasts and leukocytes, both within the paraglomerular space and in the surrounding interstitium.

Once the paraglomerular space has formed, there are several possible outcomes. First, the process may stabilize and a segmental scar may remain. Second, the enlarging paraglomerular space may engulf additional capillary loops, thereby compromising podocyte integrity in those loops and eventually leading to global sclerosis. Third, and overlapping with the preceding outcomes, the paraglomerular space may expand and encircle the proximal tubule. This has the potential of separating the tubule from the peritubular capillary, leading to tubular atrophy and the development of an atubular glomerulus. This model has considerable power to explain the pathology of FSGS. It remains to be determined which forms of human primary FSGS, adaptive FSGS, genetic FSGS, and medication-associated FSGS follow this model.

Cellular Injury and Response

A consensus has emerged that podocyte injury plays a central role in the pathogenesis of FSGS. This notion is supported by animal models and genetic mutations in human FSGS (all mutations identified to date are in genes that are exclusively expressed in the podocyte or that play critical roles in the podocyte). Several excellent reviews of podocyte biology are available. [907–909]

In vivo, podocyte abnormalities are most prominent in collapsing glomerulopathy, where podocyte dedifferentiation and proliferation are characteristic, but podocyte abnormalities are seen in FSGS as well (Table 52.9).[445,910–923] Podocyte proliferation and associated dedifferentiation are likely the critical biologic process in the pathogenesis of collapsing glomerulopathy. This striking distinction between podocyte depletion without proliferation in FSGS and podocyte hyperplasia in collapsing glomerulopathy provides the rationale for separating these diagnostic categories.

Contribution of Other Glomerular and Nonresident Cells. Mesangial cell injury and response is an important component of progressive glomerular injury in FSGS. There is extensive literature on the role of mesangial cells in elaborating the extracellular matrix. It remains unclear by what pathways podocyte injury stimulates mesangial cell activation. One possibility, relevant to adaptive FSGS, is that glomerulomegaly may lead to mechanical stretch being imposed on mesangial cells (reviewed in Riser et al.[924]). Cultured mesangial cells respond to stretch with an increase in expression of collagens, fibronectin, laminin, transforming growth factor (TGF)-β1, connective tissue growth factor (CTGF), macrophage chemotactic protein (MCP)-1, and intercellular adhesion molecule (ICAM)-1, of which the latter two are capable of promoting leukocyte immigration and attachment.[925–930] The role of mesangial cell proliferation in progressive scarring is less certain; it could simply be an index of mesangial cell activation. The mechanisms stimulating mesangial proliferation are discussed in the section on the histopathology of MCN.

Endothelial cell injury and response are also important components of progressive glomerular injury. In the remnant nephron model, the glomerular capillary endothelial cell manifests the first structural changes[790] and the first upregulation in mRNAs for extracellular matrix genes (fibronectin, laminin-β1) and TGF-β1, occurring 24 days after ablation.[931] In this model, there is an early and rapid increase in endothelial cell number and total capillary surface per glomerulus in parallel with glomerular hypertrophy; enalapril therapy partially reverses these established changes.[932]

Lymphocytes, particularly CD3+ and/or CD8+ T cells, and monocyte/macrophages may be present in human glomeruli affected by FSGS.[582,933] The latter may be recognized within capillary loops as lipid-laden foam cells. In the rat remnant nephron model, bone marrow suppression via X-irradiation is associated with a transient reduction in glomerular macrophage numbers and mesangial matrix scores, suggesting that macrophages might contribute to glomerular matrix expansion.[934] Conversely, a blockade of chemokine (C-C motif) receptor (CCR)-1 (the major receptor for macrophage inflammatory protein [MIP]-1α and regulated on activation, normal T cell expressed and secreted [RANTES]) in murine Adriamycin nephropathy reduced interstitial fibrosis but had no effect on proteinuria or glomerulosclerosis.[935] Therefore, the pathophysiologic role of infiltrating glomerular leukocytes in FSGS remains to be established. The potential role of infiltrating tubulointerstitial leukocytes in the progression of chronic renal disease is considered elsewhere in this text.

Cytokines and Other Mediators

Although many mediators have been implicated in glomerulosclerosis and progressive kidney disease, there are few data directly defining a role for these mediators. Experimental data indicate that they could play a role in regulating the balance between *extracellular matrix (ECM) synthesis and degradation* in the glomerulus. The most prominent of these mediators is TGF-β,[936] which both directly[937] and indirectly, through induction of the cytokine CTGF[938] and the generation of reactive oxygen species,[939] stimulates mesangial and additional cell types to produce collagens, laminin, and other ECM proteins. There are two parallel systems regulating ECM degradation.[940] The balance between the matrix

TABLE 52.9 Expression of Podocyte Differentiation, Injury, and Proliferation Markers in Human Disease

	Normal	MCN	Primary FSGS	Collapsing Glomerulopathy and/or Cellular FSGS	Reference
Nephrin	Present	Unchanged or irregular (LM) ↓ per μm (EM)[a]	Unchanged; lost in sclerotic areas	ND	910, 911
Podocin	Present	Unchanged or ↓	↓ In all glomeruli, absent from sclerotic areas	ND	912, 913
Synaptopodin	Present	↓	↓ Or absent from all glomeruli	Absent in abnormal podocytes; ↓ in some podocytes in unaffected glomeruli	913–918
Podocalyxin	Present	ND	Absent	Absent in abnormal podocytes	914
GLEPP 1 (PTPRO)	Present	ND		Absent in abnormal podocytes	914
αβ Dystroglycan	Present	Reduced	Normal	ND	445
α5 Integrin	Present	ND	↓, Lost with progressive sclerosis	ND	919
WT-1	Present	Unchanged	Absent in sclerotic areas	Absent in abnormal podocytes, ↓ in some podocytes in unaffected glomeruli	914, 918
Pax-2	Absent	Absent	Absent	Present in abnormal podocytes	918
Vimentin	Present	Present	Variably ↓ in sclerotic areas	↓	918
Cytokeratin	Absent	ND	ND	Present in abnormal podocytes	916, 920
Ki67	Absent	Absent	ND	Present in abnormal podocytes	914
Cyclin D1	Present	ND	ND	↓ in abnormal podocytes, ↓ in some unaffected glomeruli	915, 921
Cyclin E	Present	ND	ND	↑ in abnormal podocytes	921
p21	Absent	Unchanged	ND	↑ In abnormal podocytes	922
$p27^{kip1}$, $p57^{kip1}$	Present	Unchanged	ND	↓ In normal and abnormal glomeruli, absent in proliferating podocytes	915, 920, 922
$p57^{kip2}$	Present	Unchanged	ND	↓ in normal podocytes, absent in proliferating podocytes, ↓ in occasional podocytes, normal glomeruli	920, 922, 923

Podocyte proteins were localized by immunostaining or by ultrastructural labeling in human tissue. Diagnoses are shown as identified in the references; in some references the type of FSGS was not specified. For simplicity, details of altered subcellular distribution of proteins have been omitted. In some cases, discrepant findings were reported.

[a]Absent in congenital nephrotic syndrome due to nephrin mutations.

ND, not determined; LM, light microscopy; EM, electron microscopy; GLEPP, glomerular epithelial protein-1; PTPRO, protein tyrosine phosphatase, receptor type O; WT-1, Wilms tumor-1.

metalloproteinases and the tissue inhibitors of metalloproteinases (TIMPs) has been implicated in animal models of progressive kidney disease.[941,942] The plasmin system enhances glomerular ECM turnover[943] and is inhibited by the plasminogen activator inhibitor, PAI-1.[944] Biologic roles for these molecules in regulating cellular functions beyond matrix turnover also have been proposed.

Cytokine mediators play a role in *proliferative changes* in the glomerulus, although the data have been limited to effects on mesangial cells. Interestingly, despite the significance of podocyte proliferation in collapsing glomerulopathy, no data are available to convincingly link a particular mediator with this proliferation. Basic fibroblast growth factor (bFGF, FGF-2) has been linked with multiple podocyte abnormalities, including proliferation, in experimental membranous nephropathy.[945] Another important aspect of glomerulosclerosis is the possible loss of a continuous podocyte support structure for the glomerular capillaries. Cytokines have equally important and complex roles in podocyte *apoptosis and phenotypic changes*, as shown for TGF-β1[946] and endothelin-1 (ET-1).[947]

Other systems play a significant part in glomerulosclerosis. An important one is the multiple potential roles of the renin-angiotensin-aldosterone system (RAAS). Spironolactone decreases renal fibrosis in many animal models of glomerulosclerosis. Aldosterone stimulates the expression of TGF-β, PAI-1, endothelin, leptin, and other profibrotic molecules, and fibrotic changes mediated through the generation of reactive oxygen species.[948] A role for the RAAS is supported by the strong data demonstrating that ACE inhibition and ARB ameliorate progressive glomerulosclerosis and renal fibrosis in multiple diseases. These data support a role for the RAAS in altering glomerular cell phenotypes (e.g., angiotensin II stimulates mesangial cell TGF-β production[949]), as well as in hemodynamic mechanisms that relate to glomerular perfusion and filtration. Further, it is not clear the extent to which the RAAS stimulates glomerular hypertrophy through its effects on hemodynamics or via direct, growth factor-like effects on resident cells. Other systems regulating hemodynamics that also may have direct effects upon cellular fibrogenic activity include those representing the balance between nitric oxide and ET-1,[950] or those involving arachidonic acid metabolites.[951] Leptin also has multiple effects relevant to glomerulosclerosis.[952]

Recent studies demonstrated an interaction between putatively hemodynamic and sclerogenic mediators (Fig. 52.14). Angiotensin activation leads to the activation of the type I angiotensin receptor, which leads directly or indirectly to the production of aldosterone, ET-1, PAI-1, and TGF-β, with subsequent production of CTGF and reactive oxygen species, and extracellular matrix accumulation. This one system can thus contribute to glomerular hypertension/hyperfiltration, sodium retention, glomerular hypertrophy, podocyte dysfunction/apoptosis, and fibrosis—all of the manifestations of FSGS. Alternatively, there may be two waves of cytokine production: an initial wave that mediates

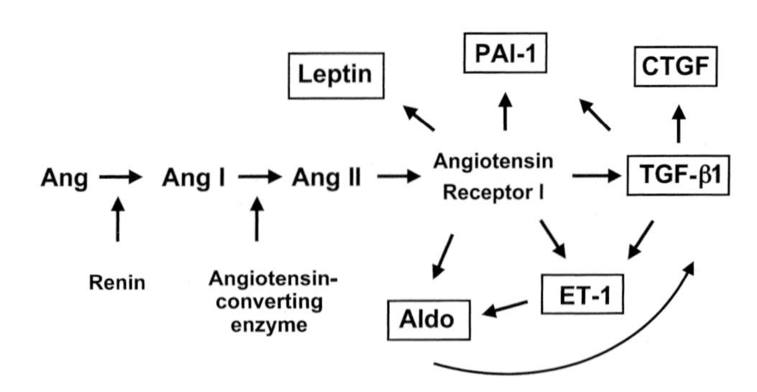

FIGURE 52.14 The renin–angiotensin system and interaction with profibrotic cytokines. In addition to the role of the renin–angiotensin–aldosterone system in regulating extracellular fluid volume and potassium homeostasis, it has been become clear that this system also influences vascular remodeling and tissue fibrosis. These vascular and profibrotic effects are mediated by at least five effector molecules (*shown within boxes*), which are present in the plasma and also produced locally in tissues. *Aldo,* aldosterone; *Ang,* angiotensinogen; *ET-1,* endothelin-1; *TGF-β1,* transforming growth factor β1; *CTGF,* connective tissue growth factor; *PAI-1,* plasminogen activator inhibitor-1.

podocyte injury and proteinuria, and a subsequent wave that, in a process of misdirected repair, causes scarring and a loss of nephron mass.[953]

Based on the data presented in this section, a pathogenic schema for FSGS and collapsing glomerulopathy can be proposed (Fig. 52.15). Both lesions begin with podocyte injury, resulting from a gene variant, adaptive glomerular hyperperfusion, or an unidentified stimulus. Depending on the nature of the injury, this may lead to podocyte dysregulation and proliferation, causing collapsing glomerulopathy or podocyte depletion in the case of FSGS. Podocyte depletion may be absolute or relative, in the latter case when glomerulomegaly increases capillary surface area. It is noteworthy that, despite significant differences in disease etiology and course for FSGS and collapsing glomerulopathy, both manifest decreased integrity of the glomerular filtration barrier and proteinuria. Misdirected glomerular filtrate, exposure of the podocyte to excess protein, and cellular stretch/stress lead to glomerular cellular activation, changes in perfusion, and extracellular matrix accumulation. Therefore, distinct pathways may use similar mechanisms that result in distinct diseases, with the critical difference being the presence or absence of podocyte proliferation.

Selected Clinical Variants of FSGS and Collapsing Glomerulopathy

Glomerular Tip Lesion: A Diagnostic Cluster

The glomerular tip lesion has been a controversial subject since its description by Howie and Brewer[954] in 1984. In the intervening years, as Howie has recently pointed out, the term *glomerular tip lesion* has been used in three senses,

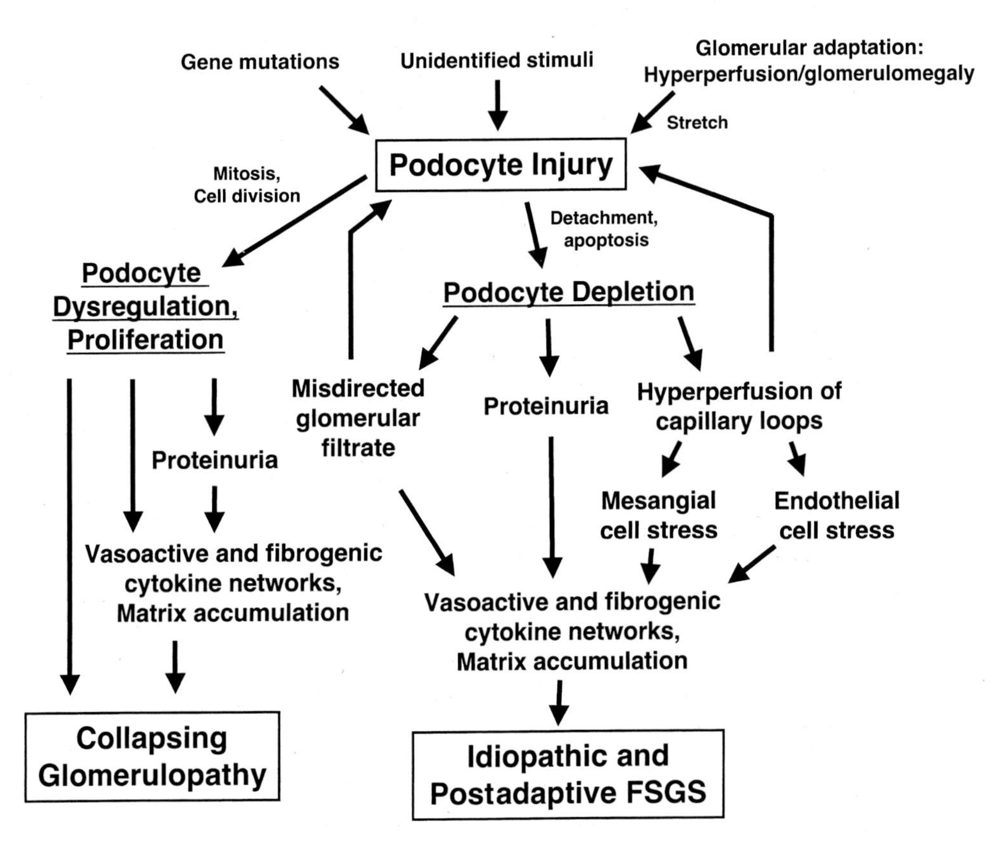

FIGURE 52.15 Proposed pathogenic schema for focal segmental glomerulosclerosis (FSGS) and collapsing glomerulopathy. Both lesions begin with podocyte injury, resulting from a mutated gene, glomerular hyperperfusion (adaptive FSGS), or an unidentified stimulus. Depending upon the nature of the injury, this may lead to podocyte dysregulation and proliferation, causing collapsing glomerulopathy; or relative podocyte depletion in the case of FSGS (note that podocyte depletion can be absolute, resulting from either decreased numbers of podocytes, or relative, when there are a fixed number of podocytes but a larger glomerular capillary surface area). In either FSGS or collapsing glomerulopathy, the result is a decrease in the integrity of the glomerular filtration barrier and proteinuria. Misdirected glomerular filtrate, exposure of the podocyte to excess protein, and cellular stretch/stress lead to glomerular cellular activation, changes in glomerular perfusion, and extracellular matrix accumulation. Thus, podocyte injury evolves into distinct glomerular diseases by various mechanisms, some of which are pathway specific and others are common.

which are given distinct names here.[955,956] Estimates of the incidence of glomerular tip lesion vary enormously by definition and population: 13% of FSGS patients in Chicago[794] and 66% of patients with segmental lesions (cellular or sclerosis) in Britain.[956]

First, the *glomerular tip lesion MCN variant* (term introduced here but with a definition that follows Howie's original description) is situated at the portion of the glomerular tuft located adjacent to the origin of the proximal convoluted tubule and consists of a localized collection of vacuolated podocytes and intracapillary foam cells. In some cases, the podocytes rest in apposition to tubular epithelial cells. The lesion may consist partly or predominantly of sclerosis. Importantly, other glomerular lesions must be absent, including mesangial hypercellularity and sclerosis located elsewhere in the glomerulus. IgM and C3 may be present within the tip lesion. Both affected and unaffected glomeruli typically show diffuse foot-process effacement.

Second, a *glomerular tip lesion FSGS variant* has been recognized and made part of the Columbia classification. There are several differences from the preceding entity: mesangial hypercellularity may be present and peripheral scars (nontip, nonhilar) can be present in other glomeruli. Stokes, D'Agati and colleagues[10] identified 49 cases (0.46% of their biopsy archive). There were 45 adults and 2 children. Cellular lesions (81% average per biopsy) were more typical than scarring lesions (19%). Twelve cases had glomerular tip lesion only, 18 had peripheral lesions, and 17 had associated indeterminate lesions (i.e., in some glomeruli the tip and the hilum could not be identified). Focal mild mesangial hypercellularity was present in 45%; no cases exhibited diffuse mesangial hyperplasia. At presentation, the clinical features of glomerular tip lesion were more like those of MCN than primary FSGS: Caucasian race 77% and 59% versus 52% (p = NS), mean age 48 and 48 versus 33 ($p < .001$ overall), and nephrotic syndrome in 89% and 97% versus 54% ($p < .001$ overall). Among those with the glomerular tip lesion, 59% of patients entered CR with steroids, in some cases supplemented with other therapies, and 14% of patients entered PR. Therefore, the response to therapy is much better than classic FSGS and worse than

MCN. Patients with glomerular tip lesion alone versus those with peripheral and/or indeterminate lesions had similar likelihood of CR versus PR versus nonresponse ($p = .88$), but this may be due to small numbers in this two-by-three group analysis. Importantly, those with other glomerular lesions had higher initial serum creatinine and higher likelihood of nonresponse ($P < .02$). The authors conclude that the glomerular tip lesion occupies an intermediate location along the MCN/FSGS spectrum and that the presence of sclerosis in a nontip location confers a worse prognosis. These data can be interpreted to argue for distinguishing between a glomerular tip lesion MCN variant (lacking nontip sclerosis) and a glomerular tip lesion FSGS variant (allowing peripheral and indeterminate scars but not perihilar scars), as these forms appear to have distinct outcomes.[10]

Another study of the outcome of the glomerular tip lesion published by Howie and colleagues[956] came to generally similar conclusions. Two biopsy series of adult nephrotic syndrome comprised of 108 patients with biopsies showed segmental lesions and lacked a non-FSGS diagnosis (e.g., classic MCN, collapsing glomerulopathy, or other glomerular disease). Segmental cellular or scarring lesions at first or only biopsy were divided into two categories: tip lesions (confined to the tubular pole) and multiple lesions (at least one nontip lesion, a lesion extending from the tubular pole to the hilum, and lesions at various sites). After 10 years, renal survival was 84% in those with tip lesions and 45% in those with multiple lesions ($P < .001$ by Cox proportional hazards analysis). The statistical significance of the beneficial effect of tip lesion was lost in multivariable analysis, when other variables (number of segmental lesions, extent of global sclerosis, and chronic tubular damage) were included in the model. No other factor showed an independent association with outcome; instead, all these variables showed correlation with each other. Therefore, the presence of a tip lesion conferred a favorable diagnosis when it was narrowly defined (no other segmental lesions). Forty patients underwent repeat biopsies, generally for declining renal function, but also in some cases when proteinuria recurred in an allograft. Tip lesions were frequently (perhaps always, given the uncertainty of localizing all lesions) the initial segmental lesions. With progressive loss of renal function, lesions at other glomerular locations appeared. These data are important, because they suggest that in some cases a tip lesion can evolve into classic FSGS. Like the preceding paper, these data can be read as supporting a glomerular tip lesion MCN variant and glomerular tip FSGS variant, although it is unclear whether the two can be reliably distinguished at the initial biopsy.

These findings support a third category, various nondiagnostic *glomerular tip changes* (Howie's suggested term), which have been described in other proteinuric conditions, including membranous nephropathy (present in 64% of cases),[957] an IgM variant of MCN,[958] postinfectious glomerulonephritis,[959] and diabetic nephropathy.[960] Experimentally, glomerular tip lesions develop in rats with crescentic glomerulonephritis; Howie showed that the initial change involves prolapse of injured podocytes into the tubule, followed by localization of macrophages to the adjacent capillary tuft and adhesion of the tuft to the Bowman capsule.[961] The predisposition to injury of the podocytes at the glomerular tip remains unexplained. Haas and Yousefzadeh[962] has argued that the tip lesion is a response to prolonged heavy proteinuria and does represent a specific disease entity. In autopsy cases of severe, untreated MCN from patients who died before 1950, they identified tip lesions in 5 of 8 cases. Among those with a tip lesion, the average number of affected glomeruli was 1.8% (range, 0.3% to 4.4%); there was no predilection for juxtamedullary glomeruli (unlike FSGS lesions). Thus, there is a consensus that proteinuric states are commonly associated with tip changes.

In conclusion, a consensus probably exists that there is a glomerular tip lesion MCN variant and a glomerular tip lesion FSGS variant, with the former having a distinctly better prognosis, but both exhibit some degree of steroid sensitivity. Some glomerular tip MCN variants appear to progress over time to glomerular tip FSGS variants or classic FSGS. Important questions, however, remain to be resolved. Is it clinically useful to identify a glomerular tip lesion MCN variant rather than identify this morphology as a consequence of heavy proteinuria? In other words, is the prognosis affected, independent of the degree of proteinuria? This question remains open, because there is no published case series that compares the outcome of typical MCN patients with the glomerular tip lesion to MCN patients lacking this feature. Can we distinguish glomerular tip FSGS variants that will progress to classic FSGS? Finally, what molecular diagnostic markers might help us to differentiate between forms of the tip lesion to improve our understanding, classification, and prognostication of these disorders?

Focal Segmental Glomerulosclerosis, Cellular Variant

As noted in the preceding text, the cellular variant of FSGS was first described by Schwartz and colleagues[789] to include segmental or global endocapillary proliferation, hypercellularity in the Bowman space, or podocytes manifesting a reactive phenotype. Clinically, these patients were more likely than were those with only segmental scars (90% versus 49%) to have nephrotic range proteinuria. Compared to patients with classic FSGS, patients with cellular lesion FSGS were more likely to be African (70% versus 49%), to have a higher likelihood of proteinuria >10 g per day (44% versus 11%), and to have a higher likelihood of progression to ESRD (40% versus 18%).[794,963] Steroid sensitivity (remission defined as CR or PR) was similar in cellular FSGS and classic FSGS (53% versus 52%). The fraction of glomeruli involved was an important predictor: >20% glomerular involvement involved a group that was almost exclusively African (94%), had heavier proteinuria (67% with >10 g per day), and were less responsive to treatment (23% remission), compared to those with a lesser degree of glomerular involvement.

It appears that most or all of these patients would be classified as collapsing glomerulopathy (collapsing FSGS in the Columbia classification). As stated previously, a published series of patients with the lesion as defined by the Columbia classification have an intermediate prognosis, with an anticipated outcome between that of tip lesion and the collapsing variant.[791]

Adaptive Focal Segmental Glomerulosclerosis

As detailed earlier in this chapter, data as disparate as the remnant kidney model of glomerulosclerosis and epidemiologic evidence for a relationship among low nephron number, hypertension, and progressive renal scarring support the notion that increased workload per nephron can lead to glomerulosclerosis. Some clinical criteria have been developed for identifying adaptive FSGS (Table 52.10). Here, we consider two clinical circumstances in which this can occur: a reduction of nephron number or increased workload with a fixed number of nephrons.

Adaptive Focal Segmental Glomerulosclerosis with Reduced Nephron Mass. There are characteristic features of FSGS associated with reduced nephron mass. First, glomerular enlargement is common in this setting.

TABLE 52.10 **Clinical Features that May Differentiate Between Primary FSGS and Adaptive FSGS**

	Primary FSGS Diagnosis Favored	Adaptive FSGS Diagnosis Favored
Birth weight		Birth weight <2 kg in full-term infants is suggestive; the role of low birth weight in premature infants is less clear
Body habitus		Morbid obesity or extreme muscular development is suggestive but the positive predictive value is probably low and the presence of these conditions does not exclude primary FSGS
Sickle cell anemia, cyanotic congenital heart disease, >50% renal mass reduction		These conditions are strongly associated with adaptive FSGS
Peripheral edema		Absence of edema despite nephrotic range proteinuria is suggestive
Serum albumin	Albumin <2 g/dL is suggestive	Normal serum albumin concentration despite nephrotic range proteinuria is suggestive[968]
Proteinuria	Massive proteinuria (>10 g/day) is suggestive	
Kidney biopsy features	Widespread podocyte foot process effacement is suggestive but does not exclude adaptive FSGS[798]	■ The presence of glomerulomegaly (glomerular diameter >186 μm) is suggestive but limited sample size may limit confidence in this finding[798] ■ Perihilar pattern of glomerulosclerosis is suggestive, although predictive characteristics remain to be determined
Response to RAS antagonist therapy		A >75% reduction in proteinuria is suggestive

When confronted with a renal biopsy that shows FSGS, no history suggesting a genetic cause of FSGS (onset in childhood, family history of FSGS, extrarenal manifestations) and no use of FSGS-associated medication, the pathologist and clinician must weigh the likelihood of primary FSGS versus adaptive FSGS. Multiple features must be considered in making this distinction.
FSGS, focal segmental glomerulosclerosis; RAS, renin-angiotensin system.

Bhathena[964] studied patients with FSGS appearing more than 2 years after renal transplantation in association with chronic allograft nephropathy and interstitial nephritis. These patients had larger glomeruli compared to those without FSGS or those with recurrent FSGS who were diagnosed within 2 years of transplantation. Subsequently, Bhathena[965] showed that glomeruli are larger in unilateral renal agenesis and following uninephrectomy when FSGS is present compared to patients with the same disorders when FSGS is lacking. Second, the segmental scars are preferentially located adjacent to the vascular hilum. In the rat nephrectomy model, the sclerosis preferentially affects the vascular pole.[966] When colloidal carbon is injected immediately after a nephrectomy, it is found preferentially within perihilar sclerotic lesions 4 months later.[967] These findings suggest that some feature of this glomerular zone, possibly related to hemodynamic stress, leads to increased uptake (presumably by mesangial cells) long before the appearance of sclerotic lesions. Third, podocyte effacement is modest, typically involving <50% of the interface between podocyte and GBM, as discussed previously. There is considerable variability, however, so this characteristic may be of limited value in clinical diagnosis. Fourth, hypoalbuminemia and edema are uncommon despite nephrotic range proteinuria.[968]

Adaptive Focal Segmental Glomerulosclerosis Associated with Increased Metabolic Workload. There are a number of examples in which increased circulatory demands or metabolic workload lead to the development of FSGS. Examples include patients with obesity, or with certain kinds of anemia such as sickle cell disease and congenital cyanotic heart disease. Obesity is the most well studied, and is associated with increased renal blood flow and glomerular filtration rate, and microalbuminuria, features that it shares with diabetes mellitus. The mechanisms for these renal abnormalities are not well understood (recently reviewed in Bagby[969]). Contributing factors may include increased renal venous pressure, hyperlipidemia, and increased production of vasoactive and fibrogenic substances by adipocytes, including angiotensin II, insulin, leptin, and TGF-β1. Dogs fed a high fat diet to produce a 60% increase in body weight manifested an increased blood pressure, plasma renin activity, and GFR, together with increased mesangial matrix and TGF-β expression (glomerular size was unchanged).[970] Obese, prediabetic monkeys manifest hyperinsulinemia and glomerulomegaly, suggesting that some feature of the insulin-resistant state may contribute to glomerular hypertrophy.[971] Leptin is of particular interest, because it acts on cultured glomerular endothelial cells to stimulate proliferation and production of TGF-β1 and collagen I, and it stimulates the expression of TGF-β type II receptor and collagen I by mesangial cells.[952] Furthermore, leptin also stimulates the production of angiotensin II. Therefore, leptin may initiate a profibrogenic circuit within the glomerulus.

Kambham and colleagues[798] reviewed their experience with obesity-related glomerular disease, including 14 patients with glomerulomegaly alone and 57 patients with glomerulomegaly plus FSGS. The combined prevalence of these disorders rose from 0.2% of all renal biopsies during the period from 1986 to 1990 to 2% during the period from 1996 to 2000; 53% had BMIs >40 kg per square meter (morbid obesity) and 47% had BMIs 30 to 40 kg per square meter. Therefore, morbid obesity is not required for the diagnosis. Compared to patients with primary FSGS, patients with obesity-associated glomerulopathy had lower levels of proteinuria (nephrotic-range proteinuria in 48% compared to 66%), less foot-process effacement, and a more indolent course (progression to ESRD 4% versus 42%). By contrast, Praga et al.[884] found that the outcome in obesity-related disease was almost as poor as that of primary FSGS. Over an 82-month observation period, 8 of 15 patients maintained stable renal function and 7 of 15 patients demonstrated progressive loss of GFR, with 5 reaching ESRD. Proteinuria was in the nephrotic range at presentation or on follow-up in 80% of patients. The level of proteinuria correlated with BMI ($R = 0.45$, $P < .05$). Despite heavy proteinuria (>10 g per day in three patients), edema and hypoalbuminemia were uniformly absent. With the epidemic of obesity spreading to adolescents in the United States, particularly in minority populations, obesity-associated FSGS is appearing in that age range also.[972] Case reports in both an adult[973] and a child[974] describe amelioration of the lesion after a reduction of BMI via bariatric surgery.

Recently, glomerular hypertrophy and FSGS also have been reported in patients with increased BMI associated with increased muscle mass but without increased body fat, suggesting that adiposity is not required.[975] Important questions remain. We do not know whether glomerulomegaly is a precursor lesion to FSGS, although that appears likely; we do not know whether there is a threshold BMI for the appearance of glomerulomegaly and FSGS; and we do not understand the molecular signals by which increased fat mass or BMI lead to glomerular hyperfiltration.

Hypertension and Focal Segmental Glomerulosclerosis

Hypertension is the attributed cause of approximately 15% of incident ESRD cases in Europe and approximately 30% of incident ESRD cases in the United States (discussed in depth in Chapter 51). Few of these patients, however, undergo renal biopsy and there remains doubt about the nature of the role of hypertension in initiating renal injury. It is undisputed that malignant hypertension can lead to ESRD; it is more controversial whether benign nephrosclerosis leads to ESRD. This controversy has been the subject of several thoughtful reviews in recent years.[976–978] Hypertensive nephrosclerosis (benign nephrosclerosis) is defined by the presence of arteriolar changes consisting of hyaline arteriosclerosis and myointimal hypertrophy, which particularly affect the afferent arteriole and small arterioles lacking an internal elastic lamina. The initial glomerular morphologic changes include thickening and wrinkling of the GBM, followed by contraction of the capillary tuft toward the vascular pole. As the tuft contracts, fibrotic material accumulates within the Bowman space. The glomerulus ultimately shrinks to a hyalinized mass at the vascular pole. In contrast to FSGS, glomerular tufts showing global glomerulosclerosis in hypertensive nephrosclerosis are not enlarged, but rather are shrunken.[979]

In recent biopsy series, a substantial fraction of patients with a diagnosis of hypertensive nephrosclerosis manifested segmentally sclerosed glomeruli. In a study from Brazil[980] of 90 hypertensive patients with renal insufficiency and subnephrotic proteinuria, 19% were found to have segmental sclerosis, most of whom also had vascular features of hypertensive injury. In a study from Japan,[981] 33% of patients with hypertensive nephrosclerosis had segmental sclerotic lesions; these patients also had significantly higher serum creatinine values. Patients who experienced a progressive loss of renal function during follow-up had larger glomeruli, but the authors did not state whether those with segmental sclerosis had larger glomeruli. In a study from Tennessee, Fogo and colleagues[982] found segmental sclerosis in 34% of patients with hypertensive nephrosclerosis. The authors excluded primary FSGS on the following grounds: lack of nephrotic range proteinuria, lack of extensive foot-process effacement, and glomerulosclerosis in proportion to vascular lesions. Segmental sclerosis was associated with global sclerosis and was more common in Africans than in Caucasians. Importantly, the authors found that the extent of vascular injury did not correlate with the extent of global and segmental glomerulosclerosis, and statistical modeling failed to identify a link between blood pressure and the severity of the glomerular lesions. The authors concluded that a simple causal pathway, whereby hypertension causes vascular sclerosis, which in turn causes glomerulosclerosis, is not supported by their data.

Kincaid-Smith[977] noted that the original description of hypertensive nephrosclerosis, made 50 years ago, did not include segmental sclerosis. She made the provocative proposal that many cases that are clinically diagnosed as hypertensive nephrosclerosis without renal biopsy, or pathologically diagnosed as hypertension-associated FSGS, may in fact be adaptive FSGS due to obesity and associated conditions, including insulin resistance associated with the metabolic syndrome and hyperuricemia. This hypothesis is testable, with closer attention to clinical factors (obesity, proteinuria, uric acid levels, and levels of insulin and other endocrine factors) and pathologic variables (glomerular size, podocyte number, and extent of foot-process effacement) in patients with FSGS arising in the setting of hypertension. In conclusion, it remains uncertain whether hypertension causes a form of adaptive FSGS, or whether hypertensive vascular changes coexist with segmental sclerosis lesions, which arise as a consequence of obesity and other clinical factors associated with hypertension.

C1q Nephropathy

Biopsies from some nephrotic patients show mesangial deposits of the complement component, C1q, despite the presence of normal serum complement levels and the absence of complement-activating diseases such as systemic lupus erythematosus. Accompanying pathologic findings can be protean,[983] including FSGS,[783] crescentic glomerulopathy,[984] or minimal changes.[985] Patients may present with congenital nephrotic syndrome,[986] steroid-sensitive disease,[985] or steroid resistance.[987] Whether C1q deposits represent a distinct entity or an incidental finding remains uncertain, because some patients have a benign course whereas others progress to CKD.

C1q nephropathy was first described by Jennette and Hipp[987] at Chapel Hill as the presence of mesangial C1q staining, either dominant or codominant with IgG, IgM, and/or C3 and the lack of serologic or clinical findings of lupus. The immune deposits were predominantly mesangial, although occasionally the deposits extended into glomerular capillary loops. In this series of 15 patients (2% of renal biopsies; age range, 14 to 27 years), the glomerular histology ranged from normal to mesangial proliferation to focal or diffuse proliferative glomerulonephritis.

Two subsequent series have suggested that the disease probably fits best in the MCN/FSGS/collapsing glomerulopathy spectrum. Iskandar et al.[988] at Winston-Salem, North Carolina reported on 15 children with prominent mesangial C1q staining and histology consistent with MCN (8 cases) and FSGS (7 cases). Markowitz et al.[783] in New York described 19 patients (9 children, 10 adults), representing 0.2% of all renal biopsies. Histologies ran the gamut of podocyte diseases, including MCN (2 patients), FSGS (2 patients with the cellular variant, 9 patients with the NOS variant), and collapsing glomerulopathy (6 patients). Mesangial hypercellularity was seen in 1 MCN case and in 10 of the other cases.

In the series from Chapel Hill, North Carolina; Winston-Salem, North Carolina; and New York, African Americans were generally overrepresented (60%, 27%, and 74%, respectively) compared to their presence in the local populations. Nephrotic-range proteinuria was common (71%, 80%, and 79%, respectively), although many patients (particularly adults) did not have nephrotic syndrome. The response to therapy was variable but has improved in the most recent series, with CR or PR seen in 0% (0/9 patients treated) in Chapel Hill, 44% (4/9 patients treated) in Winston-Salem, and 57% in New York (7/13 with available data; 2 additional patients progressed to ESRD during follow-up), respectively. In the New York series, CR or PR occurred in 2/2 patients with MCN, 4/11 with FSGS, and 1/6 with collapsing glomerulopathy, mirroring the steroid responses typical of other forms of these diseases. Other reports have also suggested that some patients with C1q nephropathy remit spontaneously or with therapy, but some of these patients had atypical features, such as prominent subendothelial or subepithelial deposits.[821,983]

C1q and other members of the newly recognized C1q/TNF superfamily share a structurally similar globular domain.[989] C1q, a portion of the tripartite C1 molecule, functions as a major link between innate and acquired immunity, because it binds a range of ligands via the globular domain and promotes apoptosis and phagocytosis of cells and cellular debris.[990–992] Human genetic C1q deficiency is associated with lupus, presumably by impairing apoptotic cell clearance and thereby exposing the immune system to nuclear and cytoplasmic antigens. Interestingly, the classical swine fever virus may provide an animal model of C1q nephropathy. Pigs experimentally infected with swine fever virus develop immune complex glomerulonephritis characterized by a viral infection of glomerular endothelial cells and podocytes, macrophage infiltration, and a deposition of IgG, IgM, and C1q in mesangial, subendothelial, and subepithelial locations.[993]

Therefore, by histology and clinical course, C1q nephropathy would appear to fit into the spectrum of MCN/FSGS/collapsing glomerulopathy, as Markowitz and colleagues[783] have proposed. The pathogenesis remains poorly understood; specifically, it is unclear how to link C1q mesangial deposits with podocyte injury.

Idiopathic Collapsing Glomerulopathy

HIV-associated nephropathy was the first recognized form of collapsing glomerulopathy, and this topic is covered in Chapter 59. Idiopathic collapsing glomerulopathy was first described in Ohio,[994] with subsequent reports from elsewhere within the United States and Europe.[757,995–998] A retrospective review of the renal biopsy archive at Columbia University found that the first case was seen in 1979, with a rapid increase to causing approximately 25% of primary FSGS by the early 1990s.[998] This epidemiologic pattern strongly suggests a new environmental agent, possibly a virus or a toxin, although little progress has been reported in identifying what that agent might be. De novo collapsing glomerulopathy also has been described following renal transplantation.[999,1000] Reviews are available for further consideration.[1001,1002]

Idiopathic collapsing glomerulopathy presents clinically as the sudden onset of heavy proteinuria, although some patients have subnephrotic proteinuria. Progression to ESRD may be rapid but this is not invariably the case. Some patients report a viral-like prodrome occurring prior to presentation, with symptoms that may include fever, cough, and diarrhea.

Collapsing glomerulopathy occurs in several distinct clinical settings. It has been associated with systemic diseases, particularly adult Still disease.[1003,1004] Parvovirus B19 infection has been linked with collapsing glomerulopathy,[1005] although controversy remains about the strength and specificity of the association.[1006] SV40 infection has been linked to both collapsing glomerulopathy and other forms of FSGS; these data await replication.[1007]

As discussed later in this chapter, podocytes in collapsing glomerulopathy express dedifferentiation markers and markers of proliferation. It now appears likely that the proliferating cells are derived from podocyte precursors rather than dedifferentiated podocytes.[796] Hattori et al.[1008] studied patients with cellular lesions, although it is likely that many or all of these had collapsing glomerulopathy. They noted that the glomerular expression of smooth muscle α-actin (a marker for activated mesangial cells exhibiting a myofibroblastic phenotype) was much greater in cellular FSGS compared to those with classic FSGS. Expression of collagen III was similar. Therefore, intense mesangial activation is part of the process and may account for the propensity to rapid progression.

Medication-Associated Focal Segmental Glomerulosclerosis and Collapsing Glomerulopathy

A number of medications have been associated with FSGS and collapsing glomerulopathy, as shown in Table 52.2. Cyclosporine is associated with FSGS in renal transplant patients and nonrenal organ transplant patients. In renal transplant recipients, cyclosporine contributes to the pathogenesis of chronic allograft nephropathy, but the role of other factors makes the specific role of these agents difficult to determine. The appearance of FSGS in nonrenal organ transplant recipients and its link to cyclosporine[1009–1011] makes the relationship more compelling. Tacrolimus likely has a very similar risk but fewer data are available. Cyclosporine induces FSGS following chronic administration to rats.[1012] The mechanism of glomerular toxicity may include increased matrix synthesis by glomerular cells and glomerular ischemia. The 5-year risk for chronic renal failure in nonrenal organ transplantation ranges from 7% to 21%.[1013] The use of a calcineurin inhibitor was significantly associated with increased risk, but the degree of relative risk was modest (1.25), probably due to the study design (only use on initial hospitalization was available) and the fact that 98% of patients used these agents.

Lithium has been associated with FSGS.[1014–1016] Chronic exposure to lithium causes tubulointerstitial injury in rats,[1017] which would be evidence in favor of a adaptive mechanism for FSGS. Conversely, some patients have extensive foot-process effacement,[1014] and nephrotic syndrome may resolve with the cessation of therapy.[1018] These findings suggest the alternate possibility of a direct toxicity to glomerular cells.

Interferon-α has been associated with both FSGS[1019–1023] and collapsing glomerulopathy.[1024] Pamidronate has been associated with collapsing glomerulopathy.[1002,1025] Very little is known about the mechanism of renal injury with these medications.

Nephrotic Syndrome in the First Year of Life

Nephrotic syndrome may occur in the first year of life and can result from MCN. Much more often, however, it is due to congenital nephrotic syndrome, and it is especially associated with infantile microcystic disease.[1026,1027] This lesion is most commonly found in Finland and in people of Finnish ancestry, but it has also been documented in many other ethnic groups throughout Europe and North America. The disease is inherited as an autosomal-recessive trait. Affected infants typically have a large placenta,[1027] with the placental–fetal weight ratio ranging from 0.25 to 0.43, compared to a normal ratio of 0.14. They often are born prematurely, may show signs of perinatal asphyxia, and may have a high perinatal mortality rate. Indeed, the incidence of early death from congenital nephrotic syndrome may be higher than that reported, because edema and failure to thrive may not become apparent for several weeks or months, even though proteinuria is present from birth. The natural course in infancy is usually one of progressive deterioration, with hypoalbuminemia, edema, and wasting dominating the clinical picture and being more significant than decreasing renal function. In the past, half of the patients died before the age of 6 months and few survived past 2 years. However, aggressive management has dramatically improved the outlook.[350,375]

The majority of patients with this disease have abnormal expression of the gene for nephrin, a putative cell–cell adhesion molecule that is expressed only by the glomerular podocytes.[1028] The gene is located on chromosome 19q13.1.[1029] Histologic changes of congenital nephrotic syndrome can be subtle in the newborn. They may include dilated cortical tubules (the origin of the term *microcystic*), mesangial hypercellularity, and glomerulosclerosis, none of which are pathognomonic for congenital nephrotic syndrome of the Finnish type. The Bowman capsule may be significantly enlarged, dwarfing the glomerulus within it, in a pattern described as being *glomerulocystic*. Extensive follow-up histologic studies of Finnish patients with nephrin mutations demonstrated some mesangial cell proliferation and ECM accumulation.[1030] Although this presentation was not associated with synechia formation, paraglomerular inflammation and fibrosis were frequently observed.[1031] Decreased glomerular and peritubular circulation, accompanied by rarefaction of peritubular capillaries and subsequent markedly increased tubulointerstitial expression of hypoxia-inducible factor (HIF)-1α,[1032] suggest that hypoxic injury is an important progression factor in this disease.

Prenatal diagnoses have been determined by finding increased α-fetoprotein levels in the amniotic fluid. However, levels may be high in amniotic fluid from pregnancies with a heterozygous (carrier) phenotype.[1033] Studies of patients and their families suggest that a direct analysis of the fetal nephrin gene can be used for prenatal diagnosis in many patients.[1034]

Other idiopathic types of congenital nephrotic syndrome have been described. These are not as well defined and probably represent a heterogeneous group of diseases, many of which do not appear to be inherited.[1028] They are distinguished from the Finnish type by the combination of clinical characteristics and histologic picture. Most have a poor prognosis, but the clinical course is often more protracted. Attempts have been made to classify these lesions according to the dominant pathologic findings. According to this approach, the presence of microcystic disease has been used to diagnose the Finnish type of congenital nephrotic syndrome. In the absence of microcystic tubules, the disease has been classified on the basis of the most prominent glomerular lesion, for example, mesangial proliferation, DMS, FSGS, or global glomerular sclerosis. Without such changes, the patient is diagnosed as having MCNS. A study that summarized the problems of this classification system emphasized that microcystic tubules are neither specific nor diagnostic for the Finnish lesion and may be acquired as a consequence of severe proteinuria in the immature kidney.[1035]

Increasingly, a diagnosis is made based on genetic testing. In one study of 89 children in 80 European families,[1036] mutations in four genes (*NPHS1*, *NPHS2*, *WT1*, and *LAMB2*) accounted for two-thirds of cases (see next section for further discussion of the nature of these mutations). The cases were largely monogenic in their involvement, and patients with nephrotic syndrome secondary to nephrin (NPHS1) mutations presented earliest. Another study of 117 cases in 107 families[1037] was able to identify a podocyte protein mutation in 80% of cases. The age of onset was a function of the specific mutation, with nephrin mutations presenting in 77% within the first week, over 90% in the first month, and the rest within the first 2 months.

In many cases of infantile nephrotic syndrome, DMS clearly is the dominant pathologic picture. Prognosis is poor, irrespective of whether the onset of disease is congenital or infantile. Congenital glomerulosclerosis characterized by hyalinized glomeruli in otherwise normal kidneys also has been found in infants developing nephrotic syndrome and renal failure early in life. Although such lesions could be the consequence of intrauterine infections,[1038] the development of DMS more frequently reflects a genetically determined metabolic or structural abnormality. It is found in a variety of syndromes associated with the gene for the WT-1 transcription factor (see discussion of *WT-1* and Denys-Drash and Frasier syndromes in the next section). Other entities that have been associated with the nephrotic syndrome in the first year of life[261,477,1035,1039–1047] are summarized in Table 52.11.

The age at presentation is an important factor in outcome. In one study,[1048] 97% of 177 patients died or subsequently required care for ESRD if they presented with nephrotic syndrome in the first 3 months of life. In contrast, death or end-stage disease occurred in only 31% of patients with an onset of nephrotic syndrome between the ages of 3 and 12 months. In an effort to identify children with the most severe, progressive disease, the ratio of urinary heparin

TABLE 52.11 **Nephrotic Syndrome in the First Year of Life: Causes and Associations**

Relatively common
Congenital nephrotic syndrome of the Finnish (inherited) type
Other congenital nephrotic syndromes
Less common
Diffuse mesangial sclerosis
Focal segmental glomerulosclerosis, congenital glomerulosclerosis, and hyalinosis
Minimal change nephrotic syndrome (MCNS)
AIDS
Rare
Cytomegalic inclusion disease1035
Hemolytic–uremic syndrome1039
Mercury intoxication1040
Nail–patella syndrome1041
Pseudohermaphroditism1042,1043
Renal vein thrombosis261
Syphilis1044,1045
Toxoplasmosis1046
Wilms tumor1047
XY Gonadal dysgenesis[1047]

sulfate to chondroitin sulfate was measured in 37 patients and 17 healthy controls. Patients with Finnish-type disease, DMS, and focal sclerosis had elevated ratios, whereas children with MCNS had results similar to those of normal subjects.[1049] Patients with nephrin mutations also tended to reach end-stage faster. Of all patients, 13.6% presented with syndromes (extrarenal manifestations).[1037]

An early diagnosis is essential, because early intervention is optimal. Congenital nephrotic syndrome is associated with profound malnutrition, dehydration, hypercoagulability, and hypothyroidism. All of these problems are amenable to medical therapy. Patients may be stabilized with daily or even more frequent albumin infusions, enteral hyperalimentation, anticoagulants, and thyroid replacement. In some cases, uninephrectomy or even bilateral nephrectomy is required to overcome the effects of severe protein loss. It is our practice to begin with albumin infusions and progress to at least a uninephrectomy in the hope that the child will be permitted to grow for as much as a year before entering into ESRD care.

Kidney transplantations for children with congenital nephrotic syndrome usually are effective, with the nephrotic syndrome rarely recurring in the recipient. The major exception is the child with Finnish-type congenital nephrotic syndrome. Children who have homozygous, large deletions in the nephrin gene (the defect is termed Fin-major) lack nephrin entirely and may recognize intact nephrin in the transplanted kidney as foreign, thus developing antinephrin antibodies.[1050] This problem is treated most effectively with a combination of plasmapheresis and alkylating agents.[1033]

Genetics of Focal Segmental Glomerulosclerosis and Collapsing Glomerulopathy

A major advance in the last decade has been the recognition of loci responsible for FSGS with Mendelian inheritance (Table 52.12). These advances have greatly furthered our understanding of the pathogenesis of FSGS. Moreover, the molecular diagnosis of mutations, particularly podocin (*NPHS2*) and *WT1*, has now become an important part of the evaluation of pediatric FSGS. Genotyping for *NPHS1* and *NPHS2* is commercially available and is rapidly becoming a routine part of clinical practice.

As shown in Tables 52.2 and 52.12, the age at presentation and renal histology help identify the most likely genetic causes:

- Congenital nephrotic syndrome: *NPHS1* homozygous mutations or *NPHS1* + *NPHS2* compound heterozygous mutations
- DMS, congenital presentation: *LAMB2*
- DMS, congenital presentation: *WT1*
- FSGS, congenital presentation: *ITGB4*
- FSGS, infancy/childhood presentation: *NPHS2, NPHS1* + *NPHS2, WT1, PAX2,* mtDNA, *COQ2, MYO1E, PLCE1, PTRO*
- FSGS, adult presentation: *INF2, ACTN4, CD2AP, TRPC6,* mtDNA

Collapsing glomerulopathy rarely presents with familial inheritance.[1051–1053] A single genetic syndrome has been reported, action-myoclonus-renal failure syndrome, in which renal failure occurred in 12 patients from 8 families of diverse European ethnic background; the gene responsible has not been identified.[1054]

NPHS2

In 2000, Boute and colleagues[1055] identified *NPHS2*, encoding podocin, by positional cloning in the evaluation of 14 of 16 families with autosomal-recessive steroid-resistant nephrotic syndrome. Subsequently, NPHS2 mutations have been identified in steroid-resistant nephrotic syndrome and FSGS from patients from a wide variety of racial and ethnic backgrounds.[1056–1069] Homozygous or compound heterozygous mutations have been found in 35% of familial autosomal recessive FSGS and 8% of sporadic FSGS.[1070,1071] To date, all patients have presented by age 25 and most patients present before age 10.

NPHS2 is a highly polymorphic gene. In Figure 52.16 is shown the location of 58 *NPHS2* sequence variants within the exon structure, including mutations (defined as variants associated with renal disease either in homozygosity or in

TABLE 52.12 Genetic Causes of Human Podocyte Diseases

Gene	Gene Product	Organelle/ Function	Inheritance	Renal Syndrome	Prevalence	Extrarenal Findings
NPHS1	Nephrin	Slit diaphragm complex	AR	Congenital nephrotic syndrome; infantile onset FSGS	Insufficient data	None
NPHS2	Podocin	Slit diaphragm complex	AR	FSGS onset <20 year	Up to 20% of familial or sporadic pediatric FSGS	None
CD2AP	CD2-associated protein	Slit diaphragm complex	AD	FSGS onset >20 year	Rare	None
INF2	Inverted formin 2	Cytoskeleton	AD	FSGS	Explains ~20% of AD FSGS families	Charcot-Marie-Tooth neuropathy
ACTN4	α-Actinin-4	Cytoskeleton	AD	FSGS onset >20 year	Rare	None
MYO1E	Myosin 1E	Cytoskeleton	AR	FSGS	Rare	None
WT1	Wilms tumor–1	Transcription factor	AD	DMS or less commonly FSGS (Denys-Drash syndrome) FSGS (Frasier syndrome)	Uncommon	Wilms tumor, gonadal abnormalities
PAX2	Pax2 homeobox protein	Transcription factor	AR	Renal dysplasia, oligomeganephronia	Uncommon	Ophthalmic defects (coloboma)
TRPC6	Transient receptor, cationic, 6	Calcium channel	AD		Rare	None
ITGB4	β-1 integrin	Matrix protein receptor	AR	Congenital FSGS	Rare	Epidermolysis bullosa, pyloric atresia
LAMB2	Laminin β2	Basement membrane protein	AR	Congenital mesangial sclerosis	Rare	Ophthalmic defects (Pierson syndrome)

(continued)

TABLE 52.12 **Genetic Causes of Human Podocyte Diseases *(continued)***

Gene	Gene Product	Organelle/ Function	Inheritance	Renal Syndrome	Prevalence	Extrarenal Findings
PLCE1	Phospholipase Cε1	Enzyme	AR	DMS, FSGS	Rare	None
mtDNA	Mitochondrial tRNA	Protein synthesis	Maternal	FSGS	Uncommon	MELAS syndrome, diabetes mellitus, cardiomyopathy
COQ2	COQ2 Synthetase	Enzyme	AR	FSGS, infantile or early childhood	Rare	Myopathy, central nervous system disorders
Galloway-Mowat syndrome	Unknown	Unknown	AR	DMS or FSGS, congenital, infancy, or early childhood	Rare	Microcephaly, hypotonia
SCARB2	Limp2	Lysosome	AR	Collapsing glomerulopathy	Rare	Myoclonus, seizures
PTPRO	Protein tyrosine phosphatase receptor type 0 (GLEPP1)	Receptor	AR	FSGS	Rare	None

AD, autosomal dominant; AR, autosomal recessive; DMS, diffuse mesangial sclerosis; FSGS, focal segmental glomerulosclerosis; MELAS syndrome, myopathy, encephalopathy, lactic acidosis, stroke. References are provided in the text.

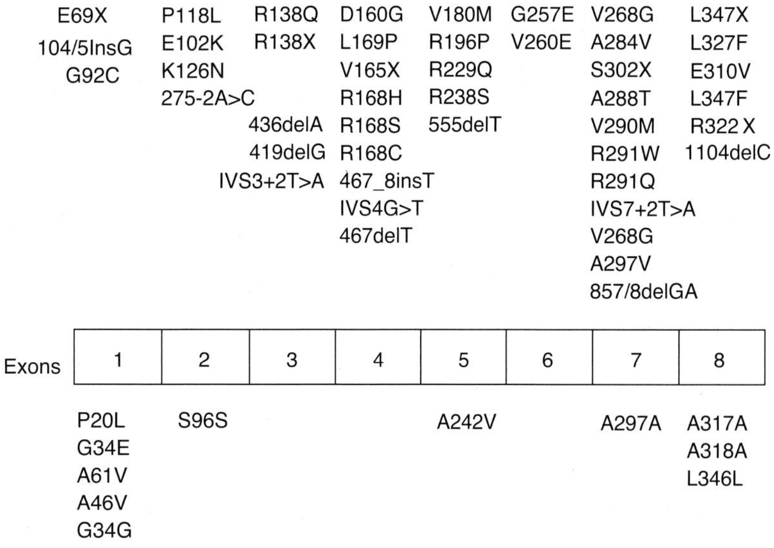

FIGURE 52.16 *NPHS2* (podocin) gene structure and variants. The eight exons of podocin are shown schematically, without portraying relative size. Mutations within the coding region (defined as variants that are associated with focal segmental glomerulosclerosis, when present in homozygosity or compound heterozygosity) are shown above the structure. Variants not associated with FSGS are shown below the structure. Missense mutations are shown by the change in amino acid at the given position, with *X* denoting a premature stop codon. Insertions, deletions, and splice site variants are also shown.

	E69X 104/5InsG G92C	P118L E102K K126N 275-2A>C	R138Q R138X 436delA 419delG IVS3+2T>A	D160G L169P V165X R168H R168S R168C 467_8insT IVS4G>T 467delT	V180M R196P R229Q R238S 555delT	G257E V260E	V268G A284V S302X A288T V290M R291W R291Q IVS7+2T>A V268G A297V 857/8delGA	L347X L327F E310V L347F R322 X 1104delC
Exons	1	2	3	4	5	6	7	8
	P20L G34E A61V A46V G34G	S96S			A242V		A297A	A317A A318A L346L

compound heterozygosity, which involves two distinct *NPHS2* mutations on different alleles) and sequence variants (nucleotide variants, which are present in healthy individuals and do not meet the criteria for mutations). Podocin is a transmembrane protein restricted to the podocyte that contributes to the maintenance of a normal slit diaphragm. Podocin is located within lipid rafts and interacts with other molecules that constitute the slit diaphragm complex, including nephrin and CD2AP.[1072,1073] Furthermore, podocin facilitates the signaling of nephrin and CD2AP via phosphatidylinositol and AKT.[1074,1075] *NPHS2* mutants are either retained within the endoplasmic reticulum or delivered to the plasma membrane but fail to associate with lipid rafts.[1076] *NPHS2* mutants that are retained within the endoplasmic reticulum are associated with an earlier onset of FSGS compared to those that are targeted to the plasma membrane.[1077] Recent studies in mice have shown that a mutation of this gene alone is sufficient to cause FSGS to develop.[1078]

In patients with *NPHS2* mutations, FSGS can recur following renal transplantation, but the risk appears to be lower than in patients with primary FSGS. Ruf et al.[1066] reported recurrence in 7 of 20 patients (35%) without *NPHS2* mutations and 2 of 24 patients (8%) with *NPHS2* mutations. In an update of an earlier publication that reported a surprisingly high rate of recurrence,[1079] Caridi and colleagues[1070] reported that 5 of 65 subjects (8%) with homozygous or compound heterozygous mutations had recurrence.

The *NPHS2 R229Q* variant is a common polymorphism, occurring in approximately 7% of European-derived populations and approximately 3% of African-derived populations.[1067, 1080] The pathologic significance of this variant remains unclear. FSGS has been associated with a homozygous *R229Q* mutation in only one individual[1066]; if this common polymorphism were sufficient to induce FSGS, one would expect more cases to have been identified. Tsukaguchi et al.[1067] found that 11 of 91 African Americans with primary FSGS were R229Q heterozygotes, of whom 2 were compound heterozygotes with A248V. The prevalence of a simple R229Q heterozygous was not statistically different from the control population. Conversely, two infants with congenital FSGS were found to have triallelic mutations (compound *NPHS1* heterozygotes with the *NPHS2* R229Q mutation), suggesting that the R229Q variant may modify the typical *NPHS1* presentation.[1064] This finding of gene interaction between *NPHS1* and *NPHS2* has been challenged.[1081] Finally, the R229Q variant may be associated with microalbuminuria in the Brazilian population (relative risk, 2.8-fold; $p < .01$).[1080] Therefore, it may be that the R229Q variant acts in concert with other genetic and environmental factors to compromise glomerular function, but the hypothesis will require further testing.

WT1

Mutations in *WT1*, the gene encoding the Wilms tumor suppressor gene 1, cause four syndromes: WAGR (Wilms tumor, aniridia, genitourinary malformations, retardation), Beckwith-Wiedemann syndrome, Denys-Drash syndrome, and Frasier syndrome.[1082] The rates of Wilms tumor among these syndromes are widely divergent, ranging from <5% in Beckwith-Wiedemann syndrome to >90% in Denys-Drash syndrome. Patients have a single mutant *WT1* allele; in XX female patients with heterozygous *WT1* mutations, Wilms tumors frequently have mutations in both alleles, suggesting that a loss of heterozygosity has occurred. The WT1 protein is a transcriptional regulator of genes important in renal development, including amphiregulin[1083] and *PAX2*, and genes important in maintaining the differentiated podocyte phenotype, including $p21^{Cip1}$, nephrin (*NPHS1*), and podocalyxin.[1084] As shown in Figure 52.17, the *WT1* gene is composed of 10 exons, with the last 5 exons encoding the 4 C_2H_2 fingers comprising the zinc finger domain responsible for transcriptional regulation.

As depicted in Figure 52.17, the *WT1* gene undergoes a complex pattern of alternate splicing, producing at least

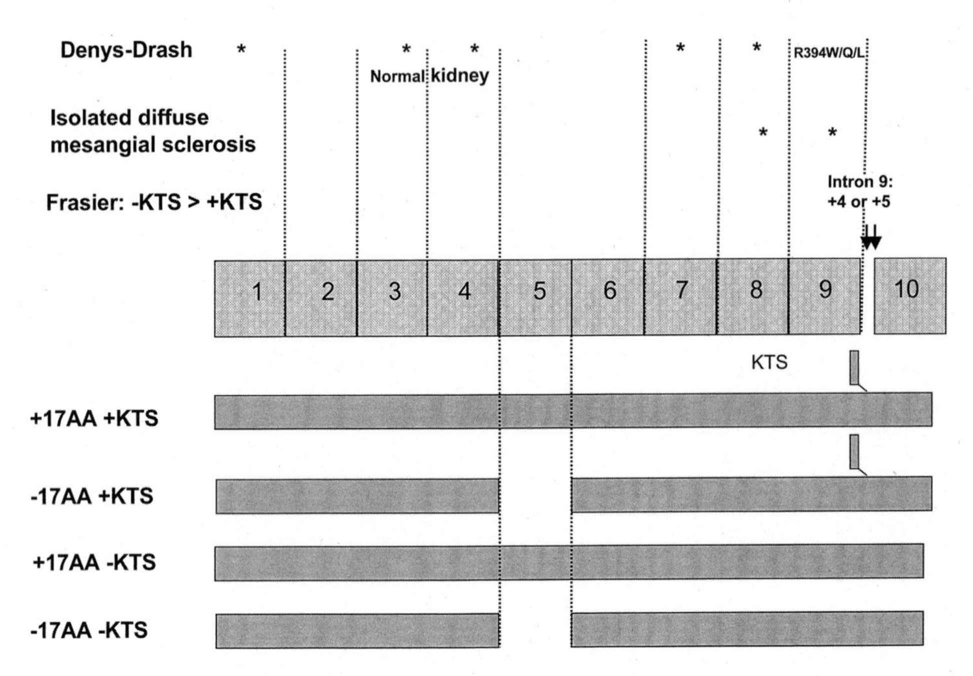

FIGURE 52.17 *WT1* gene structure, mRNA structure, and mutations associated with kidney disease. The *WT1* gene contains 10 exons (*shaded boxes*). At least 24 distinct mRNAs are generated, of which 4 predominate (*bottom*): these either do or do not contain the 17 amino acids encoded by exon 5, based on alternate splicing, and do or do not contain the three amino acids lysine-threonine-serine (KTS), based on the use of alternate splice acceptor sites located within intron 9. mRNAs lacking KTS generate more potent transcriptional activators. The Denys-Drash syndrome is associated with mutations in exons 3 and 4 (associated with normal kidneys) and in exons 7, 8, and 9 (especially the hotspot *R394W/Q/L* mutation; all are associated with DMS). Isolated diffuse mesangial sclerosis is also associated with mutations in exons 8 and 9. Frasier syndrome is associated with mutations in intron 9 at position +4 or +5, which disrupt the second splice acceptor site and lead to an excess of mRNAs that do not encode KTS (KTS-).

24 distinct mRNAs. Four mRNAs predominate: these do or do not contain the 17 amino acids encoded by exon 5, based on alternate splicing, and do or do not contain the 3 amino acids lysine-threonine-serine (KTS) located between zinc fingers 3 and 4, based on the use of alternate splice acceptor sites located within intron 9. mRNAs that do not encode KTS (KTS-) generate more potent transcriptional activators.[1085] In cells from normal individuals, the +KTS/-KTS ratio ranges from 1.5 to 2; in cells from Frasier syndrome patients with intron 9 splice-site mutations, the ratio falls below 1, which would increase transcriptional activity.[1086] By contrast, Denys-Drash syndrome is associated with point mutations and premature stop codon mutations, particularly involving zinc fingers 2 and 3. Many of the involved mutations disrupt the zinc finger structures, suggesting that the mutant protein might act in a dominant negative fashion to suppress or alter activation of target genes (although this has not been formally demonstrated).[1087]

The Denys-Drash syndrome is a triad composed of nephropathy (DMS or FSGS), male pseudohermaphroditism, and Wilms tumor, although many patients lack the full triad and some may have isolated DMS. Most patients have a 46,XY karyotype but a 46,XX karyotype can occur. Patients present commonly with ambiguous genitalia at birth, although up to 40% are phenotypically female and may present with primary amenorrhea. Rarely, patients are phenotypically male. Nephropathy typically presents in infancy or early childhood, and occasionally at birth. The renal biopsy shows focal or DMS, or less commonly, FSGS. Patients typically progress rapidly to ESRD, often within months and almost always by age 10. Importantly, because of the association with Wilms tumor, any phenotypical girl with diffuse mesangial sclerosis should be karyotyped and, especially if the result is an XY genotype, should be followed by serial renal ultrasound. Many clinicians advise native nephrectomy at the time of kidney transplantation in order to alleviate further concern about Wilms tumors, especially in anticipation of posttransplant immunosuppression.

Mutations in *WT1* are found in 90% of patients with Denys-Drash syndrome.[1088–1092] The locations of the mutations are either in the N-terminal domain (exons 1 through 3, often in patients lacking nephropathy) or the exons 7 through 9, disrupting the zinc finger domains (especially at R394). Podocyte proliferation has also been reported, with the development of pseudocrescents and shrunken glomeruli.[1093] The authors did not specifically describe capillary collapse, but these findings suggest that the Denys-Drash phenotype may occasionally extend to collapsing glomerulopathy. Slowly progressive FSGS has been reported with a *F392L* mutation.[1094]

The Frasier syndrome is a triad composed of nephropathy, male pseudohermaphroditism, and gonadoblastoma, although many patients lack the full triad. Patients are most often phenotypically female. Wilms tumors are not seen. Mutations in the intron 9 splice donor site are uniformly present.[1086,1090,1095,1096] The mutations are usually de novo, but in one case, maternal inheritance was been described.[1097] Onset of proteinuria is typically between 2 and 18 years of age, with ESRD reached between 8 and 20 years. FSGS is most common, and occasionally DMS is present. In one case, a patient with Wilms tumor was shown to have MCN with mild segmental hypercellularity.[1098] FSGS was not demonstrated in a sample that included more than 100 glomeruli; nevertheless, the patient progressed to ESRD.

WT1 mutations have not been identified in sporadic FSGS or collapsing glomerulopathy, but this genomic region may harbor susceptibility loci. Denamur et al.[1099] found only 1 of 37 children with steroid-resistant nephrotic syndrome (SRNS) or FSGS to have a *WT1* intron 9 mutation, and this child had other manifestations including genitourinary abnormalities. Orloff et al.[1100] studied 218 African American FSGS patients, mostly with adult-onset kidney disease, and found no pathogenic mutations. They studied two candidate genes, *WT1* and *WIT1,* which lie in close proximity on chromosome 11, by genotyping subjects for seven SNPs in *WT1* and one SNP in *WIT1*. Three SNPs were associated with primary FSGS or collapsing glomerulopathy (but not HIV-associated collapsing glomerulopathy): two SNPs in the *WT1* gene (odds ratio [OR] 1.7 and OR, 1.9) and one SNP in *WT1* (OR, 1.8). One SNP within a *WT1* intron was associated with HIV-associated collapsing glomerulopathy (OR, 4.3). Extending these analyses to haplotypes (particular allelic combinations at multiple loci along a chromosomal segment), they observed that a haplotype comprising one *WIT1* SNP and four *WT1* SNPs was associated with HIV-associated collapsing glomerulopathy, but not primary FSGS or collapsing glomerulopathy. These data suggest that genetic variation within *WT1*, *WIT1*, or nearby genes may contribute to susceptibility to both idiopathic and HIV-associated glomerular diseases in African Americans, but that the contributions of particular genetic variants are complex.

The mechanism(s) by which the WT1 transcription factor affects podocyte function leading to nephrotic syndrome and scarring is uncertain. Schumacher and colleagues[1101] reported that WT1 modulates vascular endothelial growth factor (VEGF)A and FGF2 signaling by increasing the expression of the 6-O-endosulfatases, Sulf1 and Sulf2, which regulate sulfation of the extracellular matrix. Genetic heterogeneity of disease expression could be accounted for in part by a WT1-interacting protein (WTIP) that appears to act as a chaperone or binding protein and shuttles to the nucleus after podocyte injury.[1102]

PLCE1

Hinkes and colleagues[1103] identified recessive mutations in *PLCE1*, encoding phospholipase Cε1, as a cause of DMS. It accounts for approximately one-third of cases[1104,1105] and appears to be a significant cause of FSGS as well.[1104,1105] The onset of nephrotic syndrome is often before 1 year of age, but it can present as late as 9 years. Although some patients progressed to ESKD, others responded to glucocorticoids or cyclosporine. Interestingly, one individual homozygous for *PLCE1* mutation, the father of two affected children, had normal kidney function, suggesting that other genetic or environmental factors may contribute.[1106]

OTHER GENES IN CHILDHOOD ONSET GENETIC FOCAL SEGMENTAL GLOMERULOSCLEROSIS

Two recent additions to the list of genes associated with FSGS are *MYO1E*, encoding myosin 1E[1107] and *PTPRO*, a tyrosine phosphatase initially described as a glomerular epithelial protein-1 (GLEPP1).[1108] Mutations in *SCARB2/LIMP2*, a gene encoding a lysosomal membrane protein, may lead to action myoclonus-renal failure syndrome that can involve collapsing glomerulopathy.[1109]

ACTN4

Pollak and colleagues[1110] identified *ACTN4* mutations in three families with FSGS showing autosomal dominant inheritance. The mutations (K228E, T232I, R235P, recently renumbered as K256E, T260E, S263P) were in exon 8 (out of 21 exons). Affected individuals showed a range of phenotypes, from microalbuminuria and subnephrotic proteinuria (including elderly individuals) to ESRD. Penetrance was incomplete, because some patients with mutations lack proteinuria. Importantly, in the cases identified to date, proteinuria does not develop until adulthood. The α-actinins are actin-binding and cross-linking proteins; α-actinin-4 is expressed in many tissues. Podocytes express α-actinin-4 in abundant amounts and the mutant α-actinin-4 variants were initially shown to bind actin more tightly than does the wild-type protein. Mutant proteins also have an increased propensity to form aggregates, which Yao and colleagues[835] suggest could explain the apparent increase in actin binding, and the mutant molecules have a greatly decreased half-life. Two models are proposed: the mutant protein is unavailable for cytoskeletal interactions or, alternatively, aggregates are cytotoxic.

ACTN4-null mice develop glomerular disease, consisting of foot-process effacement and GBM duplication, but in contrast to humans, two abnormal genes are required.[831] Interestingly, heterozygous transgenic mice expressing the mouse homolog of the human K256E *ACTN4* mutation develop proteinuria.[1111] Nephrin mRNA and protein expression, but not synaptopodin protein expression, were reduced in mouse podocytes in vivo, suggesting that cytoskeletal alterations affect the podocyte transcriptional program. By contrast, homozygous knockin mice bearing ACTN4 K228E manifested proteinuria and podocyte abnormalities but did not develop FSGS.[835] These discrepancies between the two mouse models may indicate the limitations of this model system, perhaps due to the short life of the rodents, to model a disease that takes decades to develop in humans.

CD2AP

CD2-associated protein (CD2AP) was first identified as an adaptor protein that interacts with the cytoplasmic tail of CD2. Surprisingly, homozygous *CD2AP* null mutation mice develop diffuse global glomerulosclerosis[834] and heterozygotes develop FSGS.[830] Subsequently, it was demonstrated that CD2AP is expressed in podocytes, colocalized with F-actin in lamellipodia of cultured podocytes[1112] and to the slit diaphragm in vivo.[1113] CD2AP interacts with F-actin[1114] and nephrin.[1074,1115] CD2AP interacts with phosphatidylinositol 3-kinase, stimulating the AKT signaling pathway and suppressing apoptosis.[1116] In a study of 45 African Americans with FSGS and collapsing glomerulopathy, six *CD2AP* variants were identified. One variant, affecting the splice effector site in exon 7, changes amino acid coding (P243S) and generates a truncated protein.[830] Two unrelated FSGS patients had the *P234S* variant; one patient lacked a family history of kidney disease and the other patient had two family members with kidney disease of uncertain cause. Family studies of these individuals have not been performed, and so it remains unclear whether the variant is truly pathogenic.

TRPC6

Winn et al.[1117] reported that a missense mutation (*P112G*) in *TRCP6* (a member of the transient receptor potential channel protein family) was responsible for autosomal dominant FSGS in a New Zealand family of British origin. Affected individuals presented in the third or fourth decades of life with heavy proteinuria and 60% progressed to ESRD. TRPC proteins are nonselective cation channels, which increase calcium flux in response to diacylglycerol. TRCP6 is expressed in the glomerular cells, probably including the podocyte, and the P112G mutant protein exhibits increased activity. TRCP6 participates in VEGF receptor signaling.[1118] Thus, it is possible that increased signaling via the VEGF or other receptors induces podocyte injury. Because TRPC6-deficient mice show decreased albuminuria in response to angiotensin II infusion,[1119] an activating mutation of TRPC6 could increase albuminuria. Patch-clamp studies in cultured podocytes[1119] and in podocytes in intact glomeruli ex vivo[1120] have confirmed TRPC6-mediated cation channel activity in these cells.

INF2

Boyer and colleagues[1121] identified mutations in inverted formin 2, a protein involved in the regulation of the actin cytoskeleton, a major cause of autosomal dominant FSGS, typically with adolescent and adult onset. *INF2* mutations were also found to be present in individuals with Charcot-Marie-Tooth disease, which is characterized by progressive distal motor neuropathy and hand and foot deformities, who also had glomerulopathy.[1122]

Mitochondrial Proteins: Mutations in Mitochondrial and Nuclear Genomes

The mitochondrial genome consists of a circular DNA molecule, approximately 16 kb in length. Mitochondrial DNA (mtDNA) encodes 13 essential subunits of the respiratory chain, 22 transfer RNA (tRNA) molecules, and 2 ribosomal RNA molecules. Cellular DNA replication is accompanied by mtDNA replication. mtDNA has a high rate of mutation when compared to nuclear DNA. Somatic cells possess 10 to 1,000 copies of mtDNA, whereas the oocyte has ~100,000 copies. When an mtDNA mutant arises or is inherited from a precursor cell, it exists in a pool of mtDNA that includes wild-type and mutant; this variety is termed *heteroplasmy*, and at least theoretically can range from near 0% to near 100%.

The mitochondrial encephalopathy, lactic acidosis and seizures (MELAS) syndrome involves children who present with mitochondrial encephalopathy, lactic acidosis, and stroke-like episodes. In 1990, Goto et al. identified an mtDNA mutation in 26 of 31 MELAS patients; this mutation is located at position 3243 of mtDNA (A3243G) and involves mitochondrial $tRNA^{Leu}$.[1123] MELAS has been associated with FSGS in both children and adults, with at least 14 reports describing patients with FSGS.[1124–1138] Of a total of 30 patients with FSGS described in these reports, 17 children had typical MELAS syndrome and FSGS and 13 pediatric and adult patients presented in an atypical fashion, either with isolated FSGS, or with deafness or type 2 diabetes, or both. Importantly, the extrarenal manifestations may become apparent only after renal disease has appeared, with a lag time in some cases of many years. The diagnosis requires an evaluation of mtDNA by resequencing or by other molecular techniques. Due to heteroplasmy, leukocyte DNA may or may not show the mutation, and it may be important to test urinary cells or kidney tissue. Of the 30 patients with FSGS, all but 2 patients had the *A3243G* mutation; single patients have been described with other tRNA mutations: $tRNA^{Ile}$ A269G[1136] and $tRNA^{Tyr}$ A5843G.[1135]

The mechanism of glomerular injury is not well understood, but giant (and presumably abnormal) mitochondria are present in podocytes and tubular epithelial cells.[1128] Some patients have isolated tubulointerstitial nephritis, raising the possibility that in some cases FSGS could arise as a consequence of the physiologic response to nephron loss.

A mutation in the nuclear gene encoding the enzyme coenzyme Q synthase 2 (COQ2) has been identified as the cause of at least some cases of autosomal recessive infantile encephalopathy and nephropathy syndrome, where the renal histology typically shows FSGS.[1139] COQ2 is an essential enzyme in the synthesis of COQ10, also known as ubiquinone. COQ10 plays an important role in electron transport within the mitochondrion, and also serves as an antioxidant. Children with the syndrome present as infants or, in some cases, as young children; they may also manifest with cerebellar ataxia, sensorineural deafness, and myopathy involving skeletal muscle and the heart. Other mutations in COQ10 synthetic enzymes may well exist and will likely present as phenocopies with similar syndromic features.

Oligomeganephronia

Oligomeganephronia is characterized by bilateral renal hypoplasia without dysplasia or urinary tract abnormalities. Pathologic findings include diminished nephron number and glomerulomegaly, leading ultimately to adaptive FSGS. Renal function is typically impaired from birth, rises as an absolute value during development, reaches a plateau in early childhood, and begins to decrease in middle or late childhood. By contrast, children and adults who present with a single kidney most commonly have renal aplasia rather than renal agenesis; the distinction lies in the fact that a small kidney is present at birth and subsequently undergoes regression.[1140] This is a common finding, affecting 1:1,300 newborns, and does not appear to be associated with oligomeganephronia or FSGS.

Oligomeganephronia occurs in the setting of several congenital syndromes. The *renal-coloboma syndrome* is due to mutations in *PAX2*, one of a family of homeobox genes, encoding paired-box–containing transcription factors.[1141] These children may present with syndromic oligomeganephronia, accompanied by ocular defects, or isolated oligomeganephronia.[1142,1143] The *acro-renal ocular syndrome* may include various urinary tract abnormalities, including renal hypoplasia[1144]; some cases overlap with syndromes associated with *SALL4* mutations.[1145] Patients with *branchio-oto-renal syndrome* present with mixed hearing loss, bilateral branchial cleft fistulas, and bilateral renal dysplasia; the genes responsible for the majority of cases are *EYA1* and for an associated protein family, *SIX*.[1146,1147] The *bilateral renal agenesis or dysplasia syndrome* may be familial, with dominant inheritance.[1148] The locus has not been identified.

Focal Segmental Glomerulosclerosis Susceptibility Genes

The mutations listed in Table 52.12 have been associated with FSGS that is inherited in typical Mendelian fashion, and additional genes are likely to be identified in the years ahead. As noted in the preceding text, there are striking racial discrepancies in the incidence of FSGS that may be due to genetic variation, but the loci responsible are not well understood. It is likely that there is a subtle interplay between genetic susceptibility factors (genes, nephron number), environmental factors (viruses, toxins), and risk factors (obesity, hypertension, dietary protein) that determines risk for both primary FSGS and adaptive FSGS. Therefore, FSGS likely fits the pattern of a complex genetic disease, like hypertension, type 2 diabetes, and asthma, in which multiple genes are believed to interact with each other and with environmental factors. The search for susceptibility genes is challenging and requires convincing evidence of association. The probability of false positive identification is high, given the many genes and the many polymorphisms that can be tested. A convincing case can be made that a polymorphism (or better, a haplotype covering most or all of a gene) is relevant and requires significant associations that are reproduced in multiple studies, ideally in geographically (and possibly racially) diverse populations.

An important recent advance has been the identification of a locus on chromosome 22 that explains much of the excess risk for FSGS and collapsing glomerulopathy that characterizes African Americans and certain African populations, particularly those of western Africa. Admixture mapping first identified this locus and noted the association between certain intronic single-nucleotide polymorphisms (SNPs) in *MYH9*, encoding myosin heavy chain 9 and primary FSGS, HIV-associated collapsing glomerulopathy, and hypertension-attributed end-stage kidney disease (generally lacking kidney biopsies).[768, 769] A weaker association was made with clinically diagnosed diabetic nephropathy.[1149] Genovese and coworkers[1150] subsequently carried out another admixture mapping study and noted a stronger signal in APOL1, encoding apolipoprotein 1. This signal was explained by two codon-changing alleles (termed G1 and G2), with dramatic effect sizes for primary FSGS (odds ratio, 17),[773] HIV-associated collapsing glomerulopathy (odds ratio, 29),[773,1151] HIV-associated FSGS,[1152] and hypertension-attributed end-stage renal disease (ESRD).[767] In normal human kidney tissue, apolipoprotein L1 is expressed in podocytes and glomerular arteriolar endothelial cells, whereas expression appears in glomerular arteriolar vascular cells in the FSGS.[1153]

Approximately 35% of African American *APOL1* risk alleles are G1 or G2 risk alleles (which confer quantitatively similar degrees of risk), and thus approximately 12% to 14% of African Americans have two risk alleles. The kidney risk is almost exclusively recessive in nature. The estimated lifetime risk for primary FSGS among African Americans with two risk alleles is estimated at approximately 4%, compared to approximately 0.8% in the general African American population. This relatively low penetrance suggests that other genetic and/or environmental factors interact with the *APOL1* risk genotype, but these factors remain to be identified. *APOL1*-associated FSGS is associated with a faster loss of kidney function but appears similarly responsive to glucocorticoid therapy, compared to other primary FSGS.

Many issues about this chromosome 22 locus remain to be addressed. Although the association between the *APOL1* variant and glomerular disease is strong, a causal relationship has not been established. After adjustment for the *APOL1* variants, intronic SNPs in *MYH9* remain associated with FSGS; the actual gene and mechanism underlying this effect remain to be determined. It is unclear if *APOL1* variants are also associated with susceptibility to adaptive FSGS. Finally, optimal therapy for *APOL1*-associated FSGS remains to be determined.

The *ACE* gene is highly polymorphic, but most published renal disease association studies have focused on a single polymorphism: the intron 16 *Alu* element insertion/

deletion polymorphism. This variant has not been shown to alter gene expression, but could conceivably be in linkage disequilibrium with pathogenic mutations.[1154,1155] Although the results are not consistent in all populations, some evidence suggests that the D allele is weakly associated with FSGS in Asian populations, and stronger evidence indicates that the D allele (or perhaps the DD genotype) may increase the risk for progressive loss of renal function.

Treatment of Focal Segmental Glomerulosclerosis and Collapsing Glomerulopathy

The goal of treatment of all podocyte diseases is to reduce proteinuria to normal or alternatively to the lowest level possible. There is clear-cut evidence that the level of proteinuria predicts long-term outcome. The definitions of response are presented in Table 52.7.

Treatment of Children

Approaches to pediatric FSGS show considerable heterogeneity. In 1997, Vehaskari[1156] surveyed 181 members of the American Society of Pediatric Nephrology to learn their therapeutic practices. Daily glucocorticoid therapy lasting more than 3 months was used often or sometimes by 50% of respondents (which the author found surprising, as there are no trials of this approach in children). Intravenous glucocorticoids were used often or sometimes by 52% of respondents. Oral cytotoxic therapy (cyclophosphamide or chlorambucil) were used often or sometimes by 85% of respondents. The combination of intravenous glucocorticoids plus oral cytotoxic therapy (the Tune-Mendoza protocol and variants) was used often or sometimes by 44% of respondents. Cyclosporine was used often or sometimes by 74% of respondents. ACE inhibitors were used often or sometimes by 92% of respondents.

Glucocorticoids. Because younger children undergo a therapeutic trial of corticosteroids prior to biopsy, they may be considered by the standard ISKDC nomenclature to be steroid resistant by the time they are diagnosed as having FSGS. However, most pediatricians do not wait for 8 to 12 weeks of nonresponse before performing a biopsy, and the ISKDC standard is sufficiently narrow that it does not preclude the possibility that patients will respond to some form of glucocorticoid therapy. Of those patients who are found to have FSGS, about 15% will respond to conventional oral steroid therapy and have a high likelihood of retaining kidney function long term. The remaining 85% of patients are steroid resistant and are at a substantial risk to progress to ESRD.[1157]

More commonly, however, a more aggressive regimen is necessary for steroids to be effective. In the Tune-Mendoza treatment regimen, patients receive high-dose, intravenous boluses of methylprednisolone[1158] with or without an accompanying alkylating agent.[1159] On this regimen, more than half of patients developed stable remission and the majority had normal renal function several years later.[1160,1161] However, treatment is accompanied by significant steroid toxicity, including neoplasms[1161] and serious infection.[1162] The frequent administration of high-dose, intravenous medications also is labor intensive, with significant toxicity, and has largely been abandoned.

Calcineurin Inhibitors. As an alternative to prolonged glucocorticoid therapy, cyclosporine has been the subject of several randomized trials in pediatric steroid-resistant nephrotic syndrome (SRNS). In one uncontrolled pediatric study, very high-dose cyclosporine was used in an effort to address the hyperlipidemia of unresponsive nephrotic patients.[1163] The New York–New Jersey Pediatric Nephrology study group randomized 25 patients to cyclosporine (3 mg per kilogram, to achieve a trough level of 300 to 500 ng per milliliter) or placebo treatment for 6 months.[1164] Proteinuria decreased by 71% in the cyclosporine group and was unchanged in the placebo group, although the CR and PR responses are not provided. Large, prospective studies have shown that cyclosporine may be at least as effective as high-dose methylprednisolone in treating FSGS.[1165,1166] Tacrolimus has been used in a small number of steroid-resistant nephrotic patients including some with FSGS. The drug helped to control the level of urinary protein loss in some of these patients.[1167] Given the positive results with cyclosporine and the potential benefits of tacrolimus data, calcineurin inhibitors are used frequently by the clinician treating steroid-resistant FSGS in children.

Cytotoxic Therapy. The response of children with FSGS to treatment with cytotoxic drugs has been extensively studied. A review of nine series involving children[722] revealed that 23% of 247 children with FSGS were steroid responsive; 70 of the patients were treated with cytotoxic drugs, and 21 (30%) of the 70 responded; at the time of their last examination, 19.5% of the 247 children were in remission. It was not possible to determine how many of these children had FSGS documented when they presented with nephrotic syndrome and how many were found to have this lesion only when they became steroid resistant after having previous episodes of steroid-responsive nephrotic syndrome. Although chlorambucil[1168] and intravenous boluses of cyclophosphamide[1169] have been reported to be effective, these agents have not been evaluated in a larger, prospective controlled trial.

Mycophenolate Mofetil. This drug induced complete or partial remission of proteinuria in over 50% of corticosteroid- and cyclophosphamide-resistant Brazilian children, whether given alone or in combination with other treatments.[732] This study was not a controlled trial and the length of follow-up varied considerably.

Rituximab. An international, multicenter report described an uncontrolled analysis of the treatment of children with frequently relapsing, steroid-resistant or transplant-recurrence nephrotic syndrome, using this B-cell–regulating antibody. There were 28 patients in the first group, 27 patients in the second group, and 15 patients in the third group; 82% of patients in group 1, 44% of patients in group 2, and 60% of patients in group 3 had a good initial response.[1170] In another report, rituximab was effective at inducing a sustained remission in 20 of 24 steroid-dependent nephrotic children and, in 33 steroid-resistant nephrotic children, induced complete remission in 9 and partial remission in 7. Response was sustained in 15 of these 16 patients after a mean time of 21.5 months.[708] Although a controlled trial remains to be performed and concerns regarding the mechanism of action and potential toxicity must be addressed, these initial findings are promising.

Other Therapies. Recently, the National Institutes of Health (NIH)-funded FSGS –Controlled Trial randomized 138 children and young adults with steroid-resistant FSGS to cyclosporine plus low-dose prednisone versus mycophenolate mofetil and pulse oral dexamethasone for 52 weeks, together with low-dose prednisone for the first 26 weeks.[1171] At the end of the study, the proteinuria class (primary outcome) was statistically similar between groups, although the cyclosporine arm had significantly lower proteinuria at 26 weeks and a numerically greater remission rate at 52 weeks. Relapse rates were statistically similar between groups, although they were numerically higher in the cyclosporine arm. Thus, these two treatment approaches were deemed comparable in efficacy and safety.

Treatment of Adults with Primary Focal Segmental Glomerulosclerosis and Collapsing Glomerulopathy

There is a wide range of therapeutic approaches to adults with FSGS and collapsing glomerulopathy. For simplicity, the following discussion will use the term FSGS for both conditions, because most references have not distinguished between the two disorders. Because collapsing glomerulopathy may follow a more aggressive course compared to primary FSGS, a common approach is to pursue more aggressive therapy, but there are no prospective data to support this approach.

Glucocorticoids. Glucocorticoids are widely accepted as an initial therapy for adult FSGS and collapsing glomerulopathy, although there is considerable controversy as to the dose and duration of therapy and no randomized controlled trials have been carried out. The mechanism of action is unclear. Possible mechanisms include immunosuppression, the activation of podocyte antioxidant enzymes,[1172] and stabilization of the podocyte cytoskeleton.[1173]

In Table 52.13 are summarized nine studies of glucocorticoid therapy for adult FSGS that have been reported in the last 20 years. Two studies included patients who received additional immunosuppressive therapy: 10% of patients in the Chicago study and 41% of patients in the Toronto study received such therapy; studies with more than 50% of patients treated with nonglucocorticoid therapy were excluded from this summary. Eight reports provide attained CR and PR rates, with relapse rates provided in four studies; the North Carolina study provided only sustained CR rates at follow-up. Two studies were prospective, uncontrolled trials, and seven studies were retrospective analyses. Entry criteria included nephrotic-range proteinuria in five studies. Exclusion criteria included collapsing glomerulopathy in the North Carolina study, adaptive FSGS, variously defined, in all but the Toronto study, and impaired GFR in the Italian study (patients with serum creatinine levels of >3 mg per deciliter). Although most patients in these studies likely had primary FSGS, diagnostic standards for adaptive FSGS have differed, so it is quite possible that some patients had adaptive FSGS. The mean or median duration of high-dose daily glucocorticoid therapy (generally prednisolone or prednisone 1 mg/kg/day) was 2 to 4 months, and the duration of total therapy was a mean and median of 3 to 9 months. Two studies used pulse therapy, either as initiation or as sole treatment.

Does glucocorticoid therapy increase the likelihood of remission? Spontaneous remission is rare, occurring with conservative treatment in 4% (two patients with CR)[1157] and 6% (two patients with PR).[1175] As shown in Table 52.13, with treatment, CR rates ranged from 0% to 44%, and combined remission rates (CR plus PR) ranged from 33% to 59% (with data on PR lacking from two studies). None of the studies were randomized, but three studies described the outcome in a comparison group that did not receive immunosuppressive treatment. Rydel et al.[1175] reported that remission rates were higher with treatment (CR, 33%; PR, 17%) than with conservative treatment (CR, 0%; PR, 7%). Conversely, Stiles et al.[1178] noted that remission rates were similar in patients receiving either prednisone (CR, 0%; PR, 42%) or conservative therapy including ACE inhibitors (CR, 0%; PR, 60%). Franceschini et al.[1180] found that CR rates at 18 months of observation were similar with prednisone (11%) and conservative therapy (11%), but they did not provide PR rates; it appears that CR is uncommon with ACE inhibitor and ARB therapy. One consideration is that the aggressive use of ACE inhibitors for proteinuric patients is a relatively recent phenomenon, becoming more common after the publication of the landmark captopril trial in diabetic nephropathy in 1993.[1182] This might explain the lower response rate in the conservative treatment group observed by Rydel and colleagues[1175] (patients diagnosed 1975 to 1993), compared to Stiles and colleagues[1178] (patients diagnosed from 1992 to 1999).

Does a longer total duration of glucocorticoid therapy improve the chance of remission (combined CR plus PR) or CR? Two intrastudy comparisons argue for and two argue against this hypothesis. In the Italian study,[1176] patients treated longer than 16 weeks were also more likely to reach CR than those treated less than 16 weeks (61% versus 15%;

TABLE 52.13 **Clinical Trials of Glucocorticoid Therapy for Adults with Focal Segmental Glomerulosclerosis (FSGS): Regimen, Remission, Relapse, and Long-Term Outcome**

First Author Location, Year	Design	N	Black Subjects	Nephrotic Proteinuria	Glucocorticoid Therapy	Total Prednisone Dose Equivalent
Agarwal, New Dehli, 1993	Prospective	65 (23 lost)	0%	100%	High dose 8–12 wk Taper to 6 m	ND
Rydel, Chicago, 1995	Retrospective	30	63%	100%	High dose ≥8 wk in 67%, total therapy mean 5 mo	ND
Cattran, Toronto, 1998	Retrospective	17	0%	100%	Total therapy median 5 mo range 2–50 mo	6.4 g
Ponticelli, Italy, 1999	Retrospective	53	0%	100%	A) High dose for 8 wk, total therapy mean of 6 mo B) High dose for 8 wk, total therapy mean of 5 mo	A) 6.4 g B) ND
Chitalia, New Zealand, 1999	Retrospective	28	0%	ND	High dose 6–8 wk, maximum duration 12 wk	ND
Stiles, Washington, DC, 2001	Retrospective	12	83%	100%	High dose prednisone mean 4 mo (alternate day in 17%)	8.4 g
Pokhariyal, Lucknow, India, 2003	Retrospective	83 (12 lost)	0%	59%	High dose prednisolone mean 3 mo	5.6 g
Franceschini, North Carolina, 2003	Retrospective	36	31%	ND	High dose daily or alternate day for mean of 9 mo	10.6 g
Nava Bethesda, 2012	Prospective	21	50%	100%	Pulse oral dexamethasone for 6 or 8 mo	9.6 g

The results of nine studies, describing 338 adult focal segmental glomerulosclerosis (FSGS) patients with nephrotic range proteinuria who were treated primarily with glucocorticoids, are presented in chronological order. The number (N) of patients with nephrotic range proteinuria who were treated with glucocorticoids is shown. Nephrotic range proteinuria was variously defined as >3 g/day, >3.5 g/day, or >3 g/day/1.73 m^2. High dose prednisone is defined as prednisone or prednisolone at a dose of ~1 mg/kg/day. In the Italian study, patients received either regimen A) prednisone 1 mg/kg/day for 8 weeks, followed by a taper to a mean of 24 weeks, or regimen B) 3 doses of intravenous methylprednisolone, followed by prednisolone 0.5 mg/kg/day for 8 weeks, and then a taper to a mean of 19 weeks. In the Bethesda study, patients received oral dexamethasone at a dose of 100 mg/m^2 monthly. For

Other Immunosuppressive Therapy	CR Definition	CR	PR Definition	PR	CR + PR	Relapse	Final Status (Duration Observation)	Reference
None	<0.3 g/day	18%	2 g/day	15%	33%	NS	ESRD 5% (34 mo)	1174
Cytotoxic therapy (10%)	<0.25 g/day	33%	<2.5 g/day	17%	50%	From CR or PR: 67%	CR 30%, PR 16% ESRD 20% (79 mo) (additional therapy used)	1175
Cyclophosphamide (41%)	<0.2 g/day	47%	ND	ND	ND	From CR: 38%	CR: 47% ESRD 29% (155 mo)	1157
None	<0.2 g/day	40%	<2 g/day	19%	58%	From CR or PR: 55%	ND	1176
None	<0.3 g/day	21%	ND	ND	ND	ND	ND	1177
None	<0.2 g/day	0%	<3 g/day	42%	42%	ND	ND	1178
None	<0.3 g/day	25%	<2 g/day or 50% decrease if subnephrotic	25%	50%	ND	ND	1179
Cyclophosphamide 3, cyclosporine 3 (17%)	<0.6 g/day	ND	ND	ND	ND	ND	CR 11% ESRD 18% (27 mo)	1180
None	<0.3 g/day	0%	<2 g/day	33%	33%	From CR or PR: 60%	CR 10%, PR: 32% ESRD 14% (5.4 yr)	1181 Nava, submitted

total mean prednisone dose, the value was provided by the reference or was calculated from the mean duration and assumes a mean weight of 70 kg if the reference described the total dose in mg/kg or a mean body size of 1.73 m^2 if the dosing was by body surface area. The definitions of complete remission (CR) and partial remission (PR) are shown. The two studies from India lacked complete follow-up for end-point determination; for the present analysis, calculation of outcome made here on the conservative intention to treat basis with the assumption that patients lost to follow-up were nonresponders. The mean duration of follow-up is shown and percent of patients who achieved remission are shown. ESRD, end-stage renal disease; ND, no data provided; NS, not specified.

relative risk, 4.0; $p < .01$). Multivariate analysis indicated that only the duration of glucocorticoid therapy (and not other clinical or histologic variables) predicted CR. These authors found that most responders entered remission after 6 months of therapy, although this observation derives from all treated patients (adults and children, glucocorticoids, and other immunosuppressive therapy). In the Lucknow study,[1179] patients treated for more than 16 weeks were more likely to remit than those treated for less than 16 weeks (p <.01); the relative risk of remission was similar in nephrotic and nonnephrotic patients (1.6 and 1.5, respectively), although treatment duration was not significantly different between remitters and nonremitters in either group studied alone. Conversely, in the Chicago study,[1175] the duration of daily prednisone therapy was similar in remitting patients and in nonremitting patients (5.7 versus 5.5 months). In the Toronto study,[1157] the median duration of daily prednisone was similar for those patients in CR at follow-up and those not in CR (5 months compared to 6 months). Furthermore, the median time to CR was 4 months, with a range of 0.5 to 6 months, which the authors interpreted to mean that therapy beyond 6 months is unlikely to add to the response rate.

Does a longer duration of high-dose daily therapy improve the chance of remission? Only one (retrospective) study, the one from Chicago,[1175] addresses this hypothesis. The duration of daily prednisone at a dose of ≥60 mg per day was greater in remitting patients than in nonremitting patients (mean 2.7 months versus mean 1.5 months, $p < .01$, and median 3 months versus median 1 month).

How do the high-response rate studies differ from the low-response rate studies? The studies can be arbitrarily dichotomized into four high-response studies (CR ≥25%) and four low-response studies (CR <25%). The North Carolina study[1180] is excluded because it did not provide attained response rates and provided sustained response rates at follow-up. The high-response studies[1157,1175,1176,1179] (Chicago, Toronto, Italy, and Lucknow) showed CR rates of 25% to 44% and combined response rates of 50% to 59% (PR data were not provided in the Toronto study). The low-response studies[1174,1177,1178,1181] (New Delhi, New Zealand, Washington DC, and Bethesda) showed attained CR rates of 0% to 21% and combined response rates of 33% to 42%. (The Lucknow study[1179] would have been classified as a high-response study [31% CR] if the analysis excluded lost patients, as the authors proposed.) A qualitative interstudy comparison of the high-response studies with the low-response studies follows:

- Similar prevalence of African Americans in high-response studies (0%, 0%, 0%, 63%) and low response studies (0%, 0%, 50%, 83%)
- Similar *mean duration of high-dose* daily glucocorticoid therapy (approximately 1 mg per kilogram) in high-response studies (8, 8, 12, 12 weeks) compared to low-response studies (7, 10, 16 weeks; not applicable in the Bethesda study)
- Similar *minimum duration of high-dose* daily glucocorticoid therapy (approximately 1 mg per kilogram), specified in only three studies: high-response studies (8 weeks in the Chicago study) versus low-response studies (6 weeks in the New Zealand study, 8 weeks in the New Delhi study)
- Similar use of *daily* glucocorticoid therapy (as opposed to alternate day or intermittent pulse therapy) in high-response studies (3 of 3 studies, excluding the Italian study which used both) and low-response studies (3 of 4 studies; the Washington DC study used alternate day therapy in 17% and the Bethesda study using pulse therapy in 100%)
- Similar *mean/median total duration* of glucocorticoid therapy in high-response studies (3, 5, 5.5, 5 months) compared to low-response studies (4, 6 months; not applicable in the Bethesda study and no data from the New Zealand study)
- Similar total prednisone equivalent doses in high-response studies, when data were provided (5.6, 6.4, 6.4 g) compared to low-response studies (8.4, 8.6 g)
- More use of other immunosuppressive therapy in high response studies (2 of 4 studies) than in the low-response studies (0 of 4 studies)

Although these interstudy comparisons are qualitative in nature, because of the limitations of varying study design and study reporting, they do not suggest any compelling hypotheses to explain the difference between high-response and low-response studies but do suggest that combination therapy may be superior.

Relapses were common, occurring in 38% to 67% of remitting patients. Often, patients who experienced relapse were brought back into remission with additional glucocorticoid therapy or other treatment. Surprisingly, the remission status at last follow-up was generally higher with a greater length of observation (duration from presentation or from initiation of therapy), ranging from 11% (CR only, mean 18 months observation) through 21% (CR plus PR, mean 20 months observation) to 46% (CR plus PR, mean 79 months observation) and 44% (CR only, 155 months).

Do children respond better than adults to therapy, including with glucocorticoids? In the only study that compared children and adults, Cattran and Rao[1157] suggested that CR rates were similar in children (47%) and adults (44%).

Can clinicians identify patients who are most likely to respond to glucocorticoid therapy? Shiiki et al.[1183] studied the likelihood of response to any immunosuppressive therapy in 35 adults with primary FSGS, of whom 66% experienced a CR or PR, and found the following were significant predictors of nonresponse on multivariate logistic regression analysis: larger mean glomerular diameter (OR, 2.93; CI, 1.07 to 7.92; $p = .04$) and more severe tubulointerstitial changes (OR, 8.86; CI, 1.06 to 43.9; $p = .04$). By contrast, other investigators studying 30 adult FSGS patients[1175] and 81 adult FSGS patients[1179] could not identify any clinical or histologic features that predicted a response to therapy on multivariate analysis.

What is the toxicity of a prolonged course of glucocorticoid therapy in adults? There are few published data on the toxicity of daily prednisone when used for FSGS. The Toronto study,[1157] with a mean observation time of 155 months, reported four deaths (two patients who received only glucocorticoids, one patient who had received glucocorticoids and cyclophosphamide, and one patient who received neither). The Washington, DC study,[1178] with a mean observation time of 18 months, reported that 41% of patients experienced severe adverse events (diabetes mellitus, hypertension exacerbation, cellulitis, and severe myopathy). In the Lucknow study,[1179] 16% of patients experienced significant adverse events (diabetes mellitus, infections, Cushingoid facies, and dyspepsia).

Is alternate day glucocorticoid therapy an effective option, with the prospect of less toxicity? This regimen is widely used, particularly for patients who are at an increased risk of adverse events, but the published data supporting this regimen are sparse. In 1977, Bolton et al.[1184] reported on the treatment of 81 adult patients with nephrotic syndrome, including 10 patients with FSGS, using prednisone 60 to 120 mg on alternate days for up to 10 years. In the FSGS group, CR or PR (defined as a >50% decrease and <3 g per day) occurred in three patients (30%). In the entire patient group, the regimen was well tolerated, being associated with one adverse event per 12 patient years of therapy. These adverse events included Cushingoid facies (10%), cataracts (6%), bone disease (5%), psychosis (1%), cytopenia (7%), infection (2%), and stroke (2%). Nagai et al.[1185] reported a case series of 17 patients older than age 60 with FSGS; 82% were nephrotic. Nine patients received 100 mg prednisone on alternate days, with 2 patients also receiving oral cyclophosphamide. Five patients entered remission (CR, 4; PR, 1), all of whom received prednisone only. A control group of 8 patients did not receive treatment and experienced only one PR. Two patients died during follow-up (of pancreatic cancer and stroke); other adverse events were not described. These limited data do support further studies of alternate day therapy. Some patients in the North Carolina study[1180] received alternate day prednisone, but there no data were presented comparing daily and alternate day therapy.

If the high response-rate studies suggest that total therapy duration in excess of 4 months is desirable, does intermittent pulse therapy for an extended duration offer similar efficacy with an acceptable safety profile? The Bethesda study[1181] was a small open-label study of oral pulse dexamethasone (25 mg per square meter, given on each of the first 4 days of each 4 week cycle), administered over 32 weeks to 14 patients. A distinguishing feature of the inclusion criteria was nephrotic proteinuria despite aggressive ACE inhibitor or ARB therapy, which might be expected to reduce the PR rate compared to studies that added these agents as part of the regimen. The efficacy outcomes would place this study in the low-response category: the CR response rate was 7% and the combined CR and PR response rates were 36%. A low rate of adverse events was observed, limited to bone loss exceeding 3% in one patient (7%) and no hypertension, diabetes mellitus, avascular necrosis, glaucoma, cataract, or adrenal suppression were observed.

Calcineurin Inhibitors and Cytotoxic Therapy. The literature on glucocorticoids is extensive due to the number of studies available and the controversies involved. By contrast, calcineurin inhibitors, and cyclosporine in particular, are generally accepted as standard therapy, although these agents do have significant limitations. Cyclosporine has been used to treat FSGS for approximately 20 years.[1186] Six studies have suggested combined CR and PR rates of 30% to 80%, CR rates of 0% to 25%, and relapse rates of 43% to 100%.[717,1165,1187–1190] Two of these trials were prospective trials. Ponticelli et al.[717] studied 28 adult patients and 19 pediatric patients with FSGS; of those receiving cyclosporine 57% experienced CR or PR and 40% of these remained in remission after 2 years. In the highest quality study, Cattran et al.[1165] studied 49 adult FSGS patients with steroid resistance, defined as nephrotic proteinuria despite ≥8 weeks of glucocorticoid therapy. Patients were randomized to cyclosporine or placebo, together with low-dose prednisone (0.15 mg/kg/day). At the end of the study, CR occurred in 12% of the treatment arm and 0% of the control arm, whereas PR (defined as a 50% decrease in proteinuria, becoming subnephrotic, and a preserved GFR) occurred in 57% of the treatment arm and 4% of the control arm. At 78 weeks and again at 104 weeks of follow-up, 50% of those with CR and PR had experienced relapse. Cyclosporine also significantly reduced the chance of doubling serum creatinine over a 2-year period. Taken together, these six studies show a consistent effect of cyclosporine to reduce proteinuria in patients with FSGS (and possibly collapsing glomerulopathy, although this diagnosis was not standard when these trials were carried out).

Current recommendations are typically to initiate cyclosporine therapy at a dose of 3.5 mg/kg/day in a divided dose, with dose adjustment to achieve trough levels of 125 to 225 ng per milliliter (some nephrologists might aim for the slightly lower level, perhaps 100 to 150 ng per milliliter).[1191] Prednisone is not generally added unless a patient is already receiving it. Given the high relapse rate, many nephrologists opt to extend therapy to 1 or 2 years, or in some cases for a longer duration. A note of caution about pursuing prolonged cyclosporine therapy was raised by Meyrier and colleagues,[1189] who noted that histologic injury progressed in some patients, including some patients who remained in CR. Risk factors for histologic progression included cyclosporine dose >5.5 mg per day, renal insufficiency prior to initiating cyclosporine therapy, and a high percentage of glomeruli with FSGS on initial renal biopsy. It seems prudent to taper cyclosporine over several months when a patient has been in CR or PR, rather than abrupt cessation of therapy, but there are no published data that support this recommendation.

There are limited data addressing the use of tacrolimus in FSGS. Three studies involving a total 29 patients have been published: one study in children[731] and two studies in adults.[1167,1192] There is no reason to predict that tacrolimus would be superior to cyclosporine in terms of nephrotoxicity, and the response rates appear to be similar to those seen with cyclosporine. The toxicity profile differs between cyclosporine and tacrolimus and this may influence the selection of medication for a particular patient.

The mechanisms by which cyclosporine and tacrolimus reduce proteinuria, in primary podocyte diseases and in other glomerular diseases, are unknown. The immunosuppressive action of these agents may contribute, but there is no certain evidence that this is the case. Sharma et al.[1193] demonstrated that cyclosporine antagonizes the permeability-enhancing properties of FSGS permeability factor on isolated rat glomeruli, suggesting that cyclosporine may have direct effects on glomerular cells. This hypothesis is supported by studies from Faul and colleagues,[1194] in which they found that cyclosporine blocks the calcineurin-dependent dephosphorylation of synaptopodin, protecting synaptopodin from cathepsin-mediated degradation and preserving cytoskeletal structure. Other direct effects on podocytes have been identified for glucocorticoids,[1195] thiazolidinediones,[1196] and aldosterone antagonists.[1197] These studies further support the notion that podocyte dysfunction occurs in parallel to, rather than as a result of, immune abnormalities in the primary podocytopathies (see Relationship of the Immunologic Abnormalities to Disease Pathogenesis, earlier in this chapter).

Cytotoxic therapy, including cyclophosphamide and chlorambucil, plays a very limited role in adults with steroid-resistant FSGS and collapsing glomerulopathy. Korbet et al.[1198] reviewed the literature and found that among 105 steroid-resistant patients, cytotoxic therapy was associated with CR in 11% and PR in 11%. By contrast, the responses were better among 33 steroid-responsive patients (CR, 52%; PR, 24%), suggesting that in patients with steroid-dependent or frequently relapsing FSGS, these agents may be a reasonable choice.

Mycophenolate Mofetil. Cyclosporine has demonstrated limited efficacy in the treatment of FSGS, and has the drawbacks of exacerbating hypertension and potential nephrotoxicity with prolonged therapy. Mycophenolate mofetil (MMF) is an appealing alternative therapy. In Baltimore, Choi et al.[1199] reported results with MMF used in clinical practice in 18 adults with FSGS (at least 1 of these patients had collapsing glomerulopathy). CR was defined as a urine protein/creatinine ratio of <0.3; PR was defined as a $\geq 50\%$ fall in the urine protein/creatinine ratio. MMF was administered for a mean of 8 months (range, 4 to 22 months) to 9 nephrotic patients, 7 of whom also received glucocorticoids. At the end of treatment, 1 patient was in CR, 3 in PR, and 5 did not respond (response rate 44%). At follow-up, 2 patients were in CR (MMF continued and 8 months after MMF withdrawal, respectively) and 1 patient was in PR (12 months after MMF withdrawal), for a sustained response rate of 33%.

Cattran et al.[1200] reported the results of a prospective, multicenter uncontrolled study of patients with glucocorticoid-resistant FSGS in Toronto, Baltimore, and New York; 18 patients participated, of whom only 22% were African American. Therapy consisted of 6 months of MMF (dosage, 1.5 g per day; actual duration, 3 to 18 months because two patients were noncompliant) combined with prednisone (0.25 mg/kg/day, tapered to a maximum of 10 mg per day over 6 weeks). Inclusion criteria included nephrotic range proteinuria and creatinine clearance ≥ 30 mL/min/1.73 m^2. Outcomes included 0 CR; 6 PR (defined as 50% fall, becoming subnephrotic, and stable GFR), 33%; 2 patients with proteinuria response (defined as 50% fall in proteinuria), 11%; and 10 patients with no response, 56%. Among the 6 PR, further follow-up included 1 CR on MMF plus cyclosporine, 1 continued PR on MMF, 2 sustained PR off MMF (duration of observation off therapy approximately 10 months) and 2 relapses off MMF. Therefore, the sustained PR off-therapy was 12% (2/16 patients, with 2 patients continuing therapy). These results are less favorable than those from the initial single-center report. Further studies are needed to examine efficacy—in particular, sustained remission rates—in additional populations.

Consistently, nephrotic patients who are sensitive to other therapies tend to respond to mycophenolate also. Thus, among 7 glucocorticoid-sensitive British adults with MCN or FSGS, all had a RR or PR in response to mycophenolate. 703 By contrast, Segarra Medrano et al.[1202] found that among 27 cyclosporine-resistant Spanish adults with primary FSGS, combined cyclosporine plus and mycophenolate treatment induced remission in only 15% of subjects. A similar pattern with mycophenolate response, tracking response to glucocorticoids, was seen in Spanish children.[1201]

A single randomized controlled trial has compared MMF for 6 months plus low-dose prednisolone (0.5 mg/kg/day for 2 to 3 months) versus prednisolone 1 mg/kg/day for 3 to 6 months in 33 Indian FSGS patients[1202]). Remission rates (~70%) and relapse rates (~30%) were similar in the two arms, but time to remission was faster with MMF.

Rituximab. Several case series of rituximab monotherapy for adult patients with FSGS, who were typically glucocorticoid resistant, have shown that a minority respond and most relapse.[1203,1204] If a place is to be found for rituximab, it will be in combination with other therapies or perhaps in well-defined patient subsets.

Effect of Immunosuppressive Therapy on Renal Survival. Does immunosuppressive therapy (glucocorticoids alone or glucocorticoids combined with other therapy) increase the likelihood of renal survival? There are no randomized controlled studies that address this question, and therefore, the possibility of treatment selection bias limits the use of the four nonrandomized studies that are available. Alexopoulos et al.,[1205] in a study from Greece, found improved survival in treated nephrotic patients compared with untreated nephrotic patients, with 5-year renal survival of 86% versus 65% ($p < .03$ by Kaplan Meier survival analysis). Four retrospective studies were identified that provided outcome analysis for immunosuppressive treatment and control groups, with separate identification of nephrotic and nonnephrotic patients (Table 52.14). A pooled analysis of

TABLE 52.14 **Effect of Immunosuppressive Treatment on Long-Term Renal Survival in FSGS**

Location, Year	Population	Immunosuppressive Treatment	Duration of Observation	Nephrotic, Treated	Nephrotic, Untreated	Relative Risk of ESRD in Treatment Group (CI)	Non-nephrotic, Treated	Non-nephrotic, Untreated	Relative Risk of ESRD in Treatment Group (CI)	Reference
Washington, DC, 2001	Adults	Prednisone	~20 F/U	ESRD 2 No ESRD 10	ESRD 3 No ESRD 7	0.55 (0.11–2.70)	ND	ND		1178
Greece, 2000	Adults	Prednisolone; CSA, CTX in some patients	57 mo	ESRD 0 No ESRD 11	ESRD 3 No ESRD 3	0.43 (0.12–1.5)	ESRD 2 No ESRD 5	ESRD 6 No ESRD 3	0.43 (0.12–1.51)	1205
Chicago, 1995	Adults	Prednisone; cytotoxic therapy in some patients	79 mo	ESRD 6 No ESRD 24	ESRD 10 No ESRD 20	0.80 (0.33–2.0)	ND	ND		1175
Ontario, 1998	Children, adults	Prednisone; cyclophosphamide in some patients	155 mo	ESRD 16 No ESRD 33	ESRD 15 No ESRD 15	0.65 (0.38–1.11)	ESRD 1 No ESRD 2	ESRD 4 No ESRD 7	0.92 (0.15–5.4)	1157
Total				ESRD 24 No ESRD 78	ESRD 31 No ESRD 45	0.58 (0.37–0.90) $P = .02$	ESRD 3 No ESRD 7	ESRD 10 No ESRD 10	0.60 (0.27–1.70) $P = .44$	

Four retrospective studies are presented in order of increasing mean duration of observation (months). All treatment regimens included glucocorticoids; other immunosuppressive agents were used in selected patients as shown. The relative risk of end-stage renal disease (ESRD) and the 95% confidence interval (CI) for the outcome data from each study are shown; none of the individual studies showed a significant treatment effect when analyzed by Fisher exact test (not shown). Although each study individually is underpowered, there is a consistent pattern favoring treatment in both nephrotic and nonnephrotic patients. Pooled analyses suggest a clinically and statistically significant treatment effect in nephrotic patients, with relative risk for ESRD of 0.58. The treatment effect was of the same magnitude in nonnephrotic patients, although the group size is smaller and the results were not statistically significant.

F/U, follow-up; ND, no data provided; CSA, cyclosporine; CTX, cyclophosphamide.

these studies shows that immunosuppressive therapy is associated with a relative risk of ESRD of 0.52 (CI, 0.32 to 0.84; P = .02) in nephrotic patients and 0.45 (CI, 0.11 to 1.84; P = NS) in nonnephrotic patients. Therefore, the treatment-effect size is similar in nephrotic and nonnephrotic patients, but only in nephrotic patients is the treatment effect statistically significant. The Greek study is an outlier in two respects: use of other immunosuppressive therapy (70% of patients, compared with 10% in the other three studies combined) and the effect size (no ESRD observed with treatment of nephrotic patients). If the Greek study is omitted from analysis, the relative risk of ESRD with treatment in the remaining three studies is 0.59 (CI, 0.36 to 0.97), which remains statistically significant (P = .02) and clinically significant.

Without randomized trials, the problem of treatment selection bias is a major concern and greatly limits the impact of these findings. In this regard, the authors of the North Carolina study carried out proportional hazards analysis and found that when controlling for relevant clinical factors (age, sex, race, smoking status, use of ACE inhibitors or ARB, entry serum creatinine level, and entry proteinuria), immunosuppressive therapy had no effect on renal survival.[1180]

Other Therapies. Several other therapeutic approaches have been tried for therapy-resistant FSGS patients. In an uncontrolled pilot study, the nonsteroidal anti-inflammatory agent meclofenamate reduced urinary protein loss by 40% without decreasing GFR in more than half of the 30 steroid-resistant nephrotic adults studied, 16 of whom had FSGS.[1206] The antioxidant vitamin E, 200 IU twice daily, was studied in an open-label study involving 11 therapy-resistant pediatric FSGS patients and was associated with a fall in the mean protein/creatinine ratio from 9.7 to 4.1 (P <.005).[1207] The antifibrotic agent pirfenidone was also studied in an open-label trial involving 20 adult FSGS patients and was found to slow the progressive loss of GFR by 35% (P <.03) without affecting proteinuria.[1208]

Although plasmapheresis has been used to treat recurrent FSGS in patients undergoing transplantation (see Transplantation section, later in this chapter), there is no evidence to support the routine use of this treatment in FSGS occurring in native kidneys.[1209]

CONSERVATIVE THERAPY AND THERAPY FOR ADAPTIVE FSGS

Therapy for primary FSGS aims for remission, typically with agents that are classed as immunosuppressive agents but likely have direct effects on the podocytes, whereas therapy for adaptive FSGS focuses on agents that have favorable effects on glomerular hemodynamics and on glomerular fibrosis. Although the latter therapy is commonly termed conservative, in certain settings, particularly adaptive FSGS, it can have a dramatic effect to reduce protein and slow the progressive loss of kidney function. These different approaches suggest that the pathologist and nephrologist should work together to assess the presence of features that can distinguish primary FSGS from adaptive FSGS (Table 52.10).

Conservative therapy for chronic kidney disease has several elements: blood pressure control, renin-angiotensin system (RAS) antagonism, dietary sodium restriction, smoking cession, and weight loss if indicated.

All patients with primary FSGS, whether they are receiving immunosuppressive therapy or not, should adhere to a conservative regimen if they have proteinuria (best evidence for this recommendation if proteinuria >1 g per day) or impaired GFR. This regimen is likely effective in genetic FSGS (few data are available) and, as noted, can be strikingly effective in adaptive FSGS.

Blood pressure should be controlled to <130/80 mm Hg as recommended by the Joint National Committee VII.[1210] Although certain ACE inhibitor trials have included FSGS among multiple diagnoses,[1211] few studies have provided data on substantial numbers of primary FSGS patients (reviewed in Korbet[1212]). Stiles et al.[1178] retrospectively compared the results in 22 nephrotic adults with primary FSGS, of whom 10 received prednisone at a dose of approximately 1 mg/kg/day for a mean of 4 months (range, 1 to 6 months) plus ACE inhibitors, and 10 received ACE inhibitors alone. Outcomes were similar, with no CR in 5 patients, and PR occurring in 6 patients. Proteinuria fell by 33% with glucocorticoids and 65% with ACE inhibitors. The patient population at the Walter Reed Army Medical Center was predominantly young and male and disproportionately (86%) African American. The authors concluded that although the study was too small for definitive conclusions, conservative therapy was not inferior to glucocorticoids in this population. In a small controlled trial, losartan reduced proteinuria from 3.6 to 1.9 g per day in 13 FSGS patients, whereas a control group experienced an increase in proteinuria.[1213] Conversely, a retrospective study[1214] of 42 African American patients treated with ACE inhibitors, glucocorticoids, both, or neither, was unable to demonstrate a protective effect of ACE inhibitors in delaying progression to ESRD compared to 6 untreated patients.

ACE inhibitors and ARBs have a major role to play in adaptive FSGS. Praga et al.[1215] showed that captopril therapy over 12 months reduced proteinuria to a greater extent in adaptive FSGS (associated with reduced nephron mass and reflux nephropathy) compared to primary FSGS. Next, Praga and colleagues studied 17 patients with obesity-associated proteinuria (>1 g per day); renal histology obtained from 5 patients documented FSGS in only 2 patients. Captopril therapy in 8 patients lowered proteinuria by 79% (mean, 3.4 g per day falling to 0.7 g per day); interestingly, weight loss in 9 patients (mean BMI falling from 37 kg per square meter to 33 kg per square meter) was associated with a similar fall in proteinuria by 86% (mean, 2.9 g per day falling to 0.4 g per day). Unfortunately, Praga and colleagues[884] subsequently reported that the proteinuria reduction induced by ACE inhibitors is lost after 12 months. Still, early treatment with ACE inhibitors appears to preserve renal function in obesity-associated FSGS, although appropriate controls are lacking.

Current Therapeutic Recommendations. Some experts propose that nephrotic adults with primary FSGS who have preserved renal function and lack prominent contraindications receive 4 to 6 months of daily therapy with glucocorticoids beginning with prednisone at a dose of 1 mg/kg/day (maximum 80 mg).[1212,1216,1217] Many experts would recommend a dose reduction after 3 to 4 months, particularly for those who have not shown a significant reduction in urine protein. Those who fail 4 to 6 months of daily glucocorticoid therapy are then labeled steroid resistant and progress to other therapies.

The Nephrology and Hypertension Medical Knowledge Self-Assessment Program[1218] expresses reluctance to endorse this aggressive approach in the absence of a controlled trial demonstrating efficacy and safety. Instead, the text recommends, for adults with FSGS and serum creatinine <2.5 mg per deciliter and <20% interstitial fibrosis area on renal biopsy, a trial of daily prednisone at a dose of 1 mg per kilogram of ideal body weight (to a maximum dose of 80 mg per day), until CR or *8 weeks* have been reached. In the case of a CR, the recommendation is to prescribe an ~20-week tapering schedule of prednisone on alternate days, tapering at a rate of 20 mg every month. If there is no CR, the recommendation is to reduce the dose to 0.5 mg per kilogram until a CR or PR or *another 8 weeks* have been reached. If there is a CR or PR, the recommendation is to prescribe an ~20-week tapering schedule of alternate day prednisone, which would require tapering at a rate of 10 mg every other month. If there is no response, the recommendation is a slow taper involving ~*40 weeks* of alternative day prednisone while adjunctive therapy (ACE inhibitors or ARBs) are initiated. Therefore, patients with steroid resistance would receive 16 weeks of daily prednisone and up to 40 weeks of alternate daily prednisone for a total dose of 7.7 g for an 80-kg person. Further options during the prolonged taper would include cyclosporine for 1 year or oral cyclophosphamide or chlorambucil for 8 to 12 weeks. A newer option that was not included would be mycophenolate mofetil.

Ruf and colleagues[1066] noted that pediatric patients with homozygous or compound heterozygous *NPHS2* mutations appear refractory to glucocorticoids (defined as 6 weeks of therapy) and have only limited responsiveness to cyclosporine. By contrast, *NPHS2* homozygous and compound heterozygous mutations were absent from 124 children with steroid-sensitive nephrotic syndrome. Although these data are not representative of all racial and ethnic groups, it would appear at the present time that immunosuppressive treatment is of limited benefit in children with *NPHS2* homozygous and compound heterozygous mutations.

We have few data about the adult patients with *ACTN4*, *CD2AP*, *TRPC6*, and mtDNA mutations, but it would seem prudent to withhold or limit the duration of some immunosuppressive therapy, particularly glucocorticoids. Similarly, FSGS or collapsing glomerulopathy associated with medication is probably best managed by withdrawing the implicated medication and instituting conservative therapy. The clinician selecting therapy for patients with genetic FSGS (i.e., patients with single-gene variants with high penetrance) should consider three approaches. First, a few genetic loci have been associated with complete or partial glucocorticoid sensitivity in some individuals (e.g., PLCE1[1103]). Second, RAS antagonist therapy, coupled with sodium restriction and diuretic therapy, reduces proteinuria in many such patients and may stabilize the podocyte phenotype, possibly retarding progressive glomerulosclerosis. Third, other agents with direct effects on the podocyte may be considered for a therapeutic trial in a given patient, particularly in the presence of nephrotic proteinuria. Thus, cyclosporine reduces proteinuria in selected individuals with NPHS2 mutations,[1066] and this may also prove to be the case with other agents used for nephrotic diseases.

It should be noted that there are significant parallels but some differences between the approach to pediatric and adult patients. In particular, the majority of nephrotic children (those age 1 to 9 years) will have received an empirical trial of corticosteroids for 4 to 8 weeks before biopsy, and already have been defined as being steroid resistant, albeit by ISKDC criteria rather than by response to the longer course used in adults. This may be appropriate given the relatively aggressive course of classical FSGS often observed in young children. There are many areas of uncertainty where there are no published data to determine the balance between the risks and benefits of immunosuppressive therapy, including in the following patient populations:

- Patients with subnephrotic proteinuria at presentation, especially those with proteinuria <2 g per day (most experts would not use immunosuppressive therapy)
- Patients who become subnephrotic with therapy with ACE inhibitors, ARBs, or the combination, coupled with sodium restriction and blood pressure control to <130/80 mm Hg, particularly in whom proteinuria falls to <2 g per day
- Patients with primary FSGS who are at a significantly increased risk of toxicity associated with glucocorticoid therapy, including those who are obese (in particular, BMI >35 kg per square meter), and those who have diabetes mellitus or a prediabetic state, severe osteoporosis, prominent peptic ulcer diathesis, or advanced age

Novel Therapies. New approaches to therapy may supplement existing medication in one of several ways: (1) agents that induce a durable CR with less toxicity than glucocorticoids and cyclosporine, (2) agents that reduce proteinuria to a greater extent than ACE inhibitors and ARBs, and (3) agents that slow progressive renal scarring in patients who have proven refractory to remittive therapy. Table 52.15 lists a number of agents that have been tested in phase I or II trials for primary FSGS.

TABLE 52.15 Novel Therapies Tested in Phase I/II Studies of Primary FSGS

Drug	Mode of Action	Phase and Design	Major Findings	Reference
Mizoribine	Inhibits T- and B-cell proliferation	Multiple phase II single arm studies	May potentiate the effects of other agents	1219, 1220
Pirfenidone	Not well defined; reduces production	Phase II, single arm, baseline phase versus treatment phase	Slows eGFR decline	1221
Sirolimus	Inhibits mammalian target of rapamycin (mTOR) pathway	Two phase II open label trials	Conflicting efficacy and safety results	1221, 1222
Galactose	May bind of recurrent FSGS plasma factor	Case reports	May reduce proteinuria	1223
Adalimumab	Anti-TNF monoclonal antibody	Phase I	Single dose appeared safe	1224
ACTH gel	Possibly role of alpha-melanocyte stimulating hormone	Phase II, single arm (1 patient with FSGS)	Uncertain	1225
Fresolimumab	Anti-TGF- β1 monoclonal antibody	Phase I	Single dose appeared safe	1226

eGFR, glomerular filtration rate; FSGS, focal segmental glomerulosclerosis; TNF, tumor necrosis factor; ACTH, adrenocorticotropic hormone.

Clinical Course and Outcome

FSGS and collapsing glomerulopathy have the worst prognosis of the common primary nephrotic diseases. Ten-year event rates for reaching a combined end point of ESRD or death are as follows: for children in a U.S. study,[427] 21% and in a Toronto study,[1157] 32%; and for adults in a Toronto study,[1157] ~28%, in a New Zealand study,[1177] 38%, in a Hong Kong study,[1227] 40%, and in a Chicago study,[1175] 43% (ESRD only) for nephrotic patients (compared with 8% for nonnephrotic patients) (Table 52.16).

It has been known for some time that FSGS patients who enter a CR, even if they experience a relapse, have an excellent chance of renal survival. Cattran et al.[1157] showed that patients who experience a PR (defined as a 50% fall in proteinuria and a fall to <3.5 g per day) have significantly improved renal survival (Fig. 52.18). These data provide justification for considering the combined response rate (CR plus PR) as well as CR alone in weighing the relative costs and benefits of particular therapeutic approaches.

What clinical factors predict a long-term prognosis for renal survival? The conflicting data on the impact of treatment on outcomes have been reviewed in the preceding text. In Table 52.17 the findings of 10 studies that have sought clinical and histologic variables that predict long-term renal function are summarized. The variables that consistently appear as significant predictors include baseline serum creatinine, baseline proteinuria, and tubulointerstitial damage/fibrosis score. The role of African race has been controversial. Ingulli and Tejani[772] found that among children, progression to ESRD occurred in 78% of Africans and in 33% of Caucasians, despite similar baseline serum creatinine and proteinuria values. Conversely, Rydel and colleagues[1175] found that in adults the progression rates are similar among Africans (64%) and Caucasians (55%). They did find that Africans were more likely to be nephrotic at presentation (88% versus 55%). Earlier in the chapter, data were reviewed from nonrandomized, controlled studies that treatment may improve renal survival. Thus, patients who enter CR have an excellent outcome, with few developing ESRD on follow-up.[1157,1165]

Recurrent Focal Segmental Glomerulosclerosis after Renal Transplantation

FSGS recurs following renal transplantation with a frequency that ranges from 15% to 50% depending upon the population, with the average figure cited typically being approximately 25%. When a prior allograft has manifested recurrent FSGS, the risk of recurrence rises anywhere from

TABLE 52.16 **Long-Term Outcomes in Focal Segmental Glomerulosclerosis (FSGS)**

Location, Year	Population	Average Observation (yr)	Complete Remission	Persistent Renal Abnormalities	CKD	ESRD	Nonrenal Death	Lost to Follow-Up	Reference
North Carolina, 1976	16 children	7 (children)	56%	24%	19%	0%	(6%)	0%	1228
	17 adults	3.8 (adults)	0%	0%	76%	24%	0%		
London, 1978	12 children	9.5	10%	18%	20%	50%	2%	0%	743
	28 adults								
Montreal, 1981	25 children	7.4	24%	40%	4%	20%	12%	0%	1229
United States, 1985	75 children	4.8	11%	37%	23%	21%	0%	8%	427
Hong Kong, 1991	2 children	6.8	9%	ND	ND	16%	ND	ND	1227
	30 adults								
Chicago, 1995	81 adults	5.1	ND	ND	ND	17%	ND	ND	1175
Toronto, 1998	38 children	11	42%	13%	11%	34%	0%	0%	1157
	55 adults		22%	24%	13%	42%	(4%)		
Christchurch, New Zealand, 2000	165 adults	6.9	29%	8%	16%	44%			1177

All reports that included at least 30 patients and provided group outcomes after average duration of >4 years are presented in chronologic order. Most patients appear to have had primary FSGS but some reports included a limited number of adaptive FSGS or focal global glomerulosclerosis. Children are variously defined as individuals <15–18 yr at the time of initial presentation, depending upon reference. When data are presented for children and adults separately, the data for children are presented first. Chronic kidney disease (CKD) is defined as impaired GFR. The percentage of patients experiencing nonrenal deaths is shown in parentheses when these patients are also included in another category. Empty cells indicate that no data were provided from the report.
ESRD, end-stage renal disease; ND, no data available.

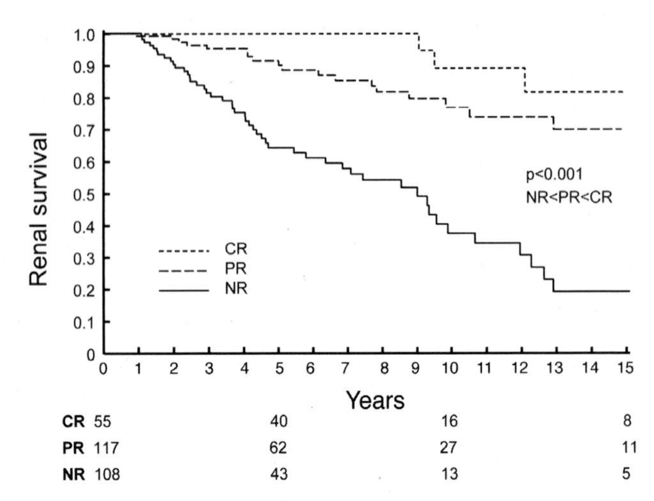

FIGURE 52.18 Long-term renal survival in focal segmental glomerulosclerosis by remission status. The fraction of patients with renal function is shown in nephrotic focal segmental glomerulosclerosis patients who enter complete remission (CR) (defined as <0.3 g/day) or partial remission (PR_ 50% (defined as a 50% fall in proteinuria and falling to <3.5 g/day), and those who never reach either remission (NR). (Adapted from Troyanov S, Wall CA, Miller JA, et al. Focal and segmental glomerulosclerosis: definition and relevance of a partial remission. *J Am Soc Nephrol.* 2005;16:1061, with permission.)

70% to 80%. Recurrence is heralded by the sudden appearance of heavy proteinuria, often within the first week after transplantation. Renal biopsy obtained within the first few weeks of recurrence uniformly shows extensive foot-process effacement without other changes. Subsequent biopsies commonly demonstrate FSGS. Most recurrent FSGS appears within the first 6 months following renal transplantation, as shown in the graphic depiction of data abstracted from 14 reports[1233–1246] and from unpublished data kindly provided by Dr. Alok Kalia (Fig. 52.19). An FSGS that appears more than 12 months after renal transplantation is typically not considered recurrent FSGS; alternative diagnoses include de novo FSGS and FSGS appearing as a manifestation of progressive chronic allograft nephropathy.

In patients with low-level proteinuria originating from their native kidneys, screening for recurrent FSGS may be done via urine dipstick testing performed by the patient (or parents). For those with significant proteinuria from their native kidneys, it is advisable to obtain monthly urine protein/creatinine ratios during the first 12 months, and particularly for the first 6 months following a renal transplantation. In either case, a significant worsening of proteinuria is an indication for immediate renal biopsy to establish the diagnosis. The response to therapy appears substantially greater if initiated within 2 to 4 weeks of clinical recurrence.

Pretransplantation risk factors for recurrent FSGS include the following: rapid progression of initial disease, typically defined as <3 years from diagnosis to ESRD; age of onset of FSGS between 6 and 15 years; mesangial hyperplasia; Caucasian race; and recurrent FSGS in a prior renal transplant.[1247] The risk of recurrence for individuals with FSGS associated with podocin mutations is controversial. Although an initial report suggested a higher rate of recurrence,[1248] there is now a consensus that the risk of recurrent FSGS in individuals with *NPHS2* mutations is lower than in other patients with FSGS, ranging from 0%[1055] to 8%.[1060,1066]

Older studies suggested that living donor transplants may be associated with a higher rate of FSGS recurrence, but recent data suggest that living donor transplants still retain an overall advantage in outcomes for the FSGS patient with ESRD. A review of data from the U.S. Renal Data System (USRDS) found a higher rate of allograft loss due to FSGS recurrence with living donor allografts (19% of graft loss due to recurrence) compared to cadaveric allografts (8% of graft loss due to recurrence), but overall allograft survival remained higher for living donor allografts.[1249] Recipient factors that contribute to increased FSGS recurrence risk include prior recurrence, younger age, and Caucasian race.[1249] Also, there was an increased FSGS recurrence risk with African donor kidneys and Caucasian recipients.

Posttransplantation risk factors for recurrent FSGS remain controversial; the studies are difficult to interpret in that none are controlled and many rely on historical controls. Some observers have suggested that recurrence has increased in recent years and this has been linked to particular lymphocyte-depletion therapies. Raafat et al.[1245] found that recurrence was greater in patients who receive antilymphocyte serum (53% compared to 11% in those who did not). The Miami group[1250] suggests that recurrence rose from 38% to 83% after the introduction of daclizumab.

Focal Segmental Glomerulosclerosis Permeability Factor

The rapid recurrence of FSGS following renal transplantation appears to be due to a circulating molecule. Molecular identification has been elusive and the activity has been referred to by various names. Here we will use the term FSGS permeability factor (FPF). A critical advance was the development by Savin and colleagues[1251] of an in vitro assay, which relies on the albumin permeability of isolated rat glomeruli as reflected by volume changes induced by an oncotic gradient. There is a correlation between the level of FPF and the likelihood of recurrent FSGS following renal transplantation.[1236,1252] FPF is unique to FSGS, being absent from patients with membranous nephropathy and with ESRD due to other causes. Godfrin and colleagues[1253] developed a variation on Savin's assay. In contrast to the findings of Savin and colleagues, they reported that although FPF levels were higher in FSGS patients with ESRD compared to patients with other causes of ESRD, FPF levels did not predict a recurrence of FSGS. The reasons for the discrepant findings might include subtle differences in assay conditions and differences in patient populations. Resolving these discrepancies may not be possible until the molecular identity of FPF is established. In summary, the FPF assay has important limitations: it is laborious; it lacks high specificity, sensitivity,

TABLE 52.17 **Clinical and Histologic Predictors of Renal Survival in Focal Segmental Glomerulosclerosis**

Location, Year	*N*	Population	Analytic Approach	Baseline Clinical Variables	Histologic Variables	Reference
London, 1978	40	Children, adults	Univariate analysis	■ Proteinuria	None tested	743
Rochester, Minnesota, 1983	64	Children, adults	Univariate analysis	■ Proteinuria ■ Serum creatinine	■ Tubulointerstitial damage (only severe)	1230
Tübingen, Germany, 1990	250	Adults	Multivariate analysis	■ Proteinuria	■ Tubulointerstitial damage (fibrosis, atrophy)	1231
New York, 1991	57	Children	Multivariate analysis	■ Serum creatinine ■ Serum cholesterol	None tested	772
Hong Kong, 1991	32	Children, adults	Multivariate analysis	■ Serum creatinine	None tested	1227
Chicago, 1995	81	Adults	Multivariate analysis	■ Serum creatinine ■ Proteinuria (only when those entering remission were excluded)	None predictive	1175
Columbus, Ohio, 1996	49	Adults	Multivariate analysis	■ Serum C3 (high normal levels are protective)	■ Combined glomerular, tubular, interstitial, and vascular score	1232
Christchurch, New Zealand, 1999	111	Children, adults	Multivariate analysis	■ Serum creatinine	■ Interstitial fibrosis	1177
Thessaloniki, Greece, 2000	33	Adult	Multivariate analysis	■ Serum creatinine (only nephrotic patients) ■ Age	■ Mesangial sclerosis (only nonnephrotic patients) ■ Interstitial infiltrates (only nonnephrotic patients)	1205
Jackson, Mississippi, 2000	42	Adults	Multivariate analysis	■ Serum creatinine	■ Interstitial fibrosis ■ Global glomerulosclerosis	1214

Each study shown tested either clinical variables alone or both clinical and histologic variables, using either univariate analysis or multivariate analysis (in the latter case only variables that contributed to the model are shown).

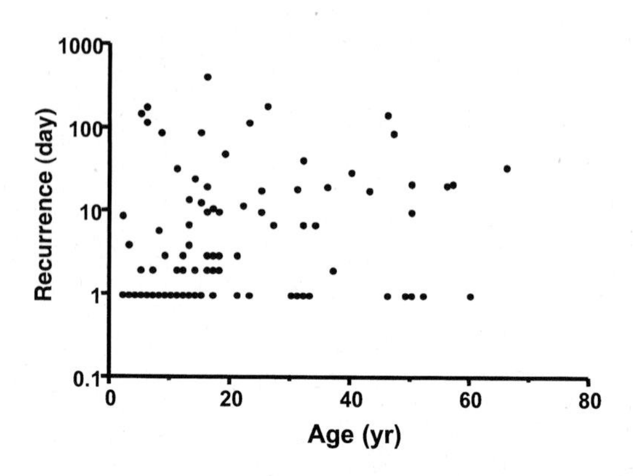

FIGURE 52.19 The timing of focal segmental glomerulosclerosis recurrence following renal transplant, correlated with age. Data on the timing of recurrent FSGS and patient age at renal transplantation were available for 101 patients, including 55 children <18 years of age and 46 adults. There was no relationship between age and time to focal segmental glomerulosclerosis recurrence (R = 0.01). In 63 cases (62%), recurrent FSGS was diagnosed within 1 week of renal transplantation.

and precision; and it has not been validated by all centers that work with it. Therefore, the assay must be viewed as a research tool, with limited clinical use to supplement clinical indicators of risk for recurrence of FSGS.

FPF is a protein, as shown by sensitivity to proteolytic enzymes and heat.[1254] Immunoadsorption of patient plasma using a protein A column reduces proteinuria in recurrent FSGS, which is a characteristic of immunoglobulin, but plasma fractionation to remove immunoglobulin does not remove FPF activity.[1255] McCarthy and colleagues[1223] and Sharma and colleagues[1256] have used sequential column chromatography to generate plasma fractions that have increased activity (10,000-fold purification) but these fractions remain complex, with multiple proteins and glycoproteins of <30 kDa. Some of these glycoproteins are absent from normal plasma and from sera following therapeutic plasma exchange. Musante and colleagues[1257] have taken a similar approach and identified a number of proteins (albumin isoforms, vitronectin, fibrinogen gamma chain, fibulin, and mannan-binding lectin-associated serine protease), but have not demonstrated activity in vivo. Partially purified fractions are able to induce proteinuria in rats.[1258,1259]

Wei and coworkers[93] made a seminal discovery, identifying elevated levels of suPAR in subjects with recurrent FSGSD following kidney transplant (although there is substantial overlap between recurrent FSGS and nonrecurrent FSGS, limiting the positive predictive value of an elevated plasma suPAR level). Furthermore, suPAR was shown to activate β3-integrin, suggesting a pathogenic pathway leading to podocyte activation and possibly injury, and indeed, the expression of suPAR in mice induced proteinuria and podocyte injury. This exciting development opens a pathway to new therapeutic approaches. Other molecules that may act as a permeability factor are cardiotrophinlike cytokine 1, as was identified in a proteomic screen[1223] and angiopoeitin-like-4.[1260]

There also may be plasma factors that antagonize FPF activity. Thus, normal serum blocks the activity in the rat glomerulus assay.[1261] Candiano and colleagues[1262] confirmed these findings and reported that inhibitory proteins include the apo allelic variants E2 and E4 and apo J. Nephrotic urine, but not normal urine, contains inhibitory activity.[1263] Pharmacologic inhibitors of FPF activity in vitro include cyclosporine, indomethacin, cyclic AMP (cAMP) analogs, 12-hydroxyeicosatetraenoic acid (HETE), and serine protease inhibitors.[1223,1263]

Therapy of Recurrent Focal Segmental Glomerulosclerosis

The recurrence of nephrotic syndrome after renal transplantation is particularly refractory to treatment, and none of the available therapies can be recommend without serious qualifications. Plasma exchange (using either plasma or albumin as a replacement solution) or immunoadsorption (using columns bearing ligands such as protein A, which bind immunoglobulins) have been used with limited success. A single course of plasma exchange or immunoadsorption is associated with response rates (CR and PR) of approximately 58% (Table 52.18).[1073,1233,1234,1237,1239,1243,1255,1264] The number of plasma exchange treatments has varied greatly among different centers, and has not been subjected to careful studies. Davenport[1265] reviewed the literature and identified 44 recurrent FSGS cases using a (liberal) definition of response as a 50% fall in proteinuria in 32 patients (73%). He concluded that the optimal apheresis dose was nine treatments, which he proposed should be delivered as three daily treatments followed by six treatments delivered on alternate days. Unfortunately, most patients relapse. In some patients, particularly children, a maintenance schedule of plasma modulating therapy may sustain a remission.

The limitations of this approach have led to the empiric use of cyclophosphamide, with or without plasma exchange, in four trials of pediatric patients (Table 52.19).[1235,1236,1240,1266] The long-term outcome appears to be markedly better than those studies using only plasma exchange or immunoadsorption. This approach has not been reported in adults. Clearly, randomized trials are needed before firm conclusions can be reached about either approach.

High-dose cyclosporine has been used in two pediatric trials. Salomon et al.[1267] administered intravenous cyclosporine, which was dose adjusted to achieve trough levels of 250 to 350 ng per milliliter, and achieved CR in 14 of 17 (82%) of consecutive patients with recurrent FSGS. Plasma exchange was also used in 4 patients. Sustained remission was noted in 11 of 17 (65%) of patients. Raafat et al.[1268] administered oral cyclosporine, with the dose increased until proteinuria resolved or nephrotoxicity (rising serum creatinine) was noted. They found that 13 of 16 patients (81%) entered remission, either CR (11 patients) or PR

TABLE 52.18 Plasma Exchange and Immunoadsorption Therapy for Recurrent Focal Segmental Glomerulosclerosis

Report	Location	Modality	*N*	Age (y)	Complete Response	Partial Response	Prolonged Response
Dantal et al., 1991[1237]	France	PE	9	A	4	1	1 PR
Artero et al., 1994[1234]	Italy	PE	9	P, A	3	3	3 CR/2 PR
Dantal et al., 1994[1255]	France	Adsorption	8	A	2	4	1 CR
Dantal et al., 1998[1238]	France	Adsorption	4	A	2	2	0
Andresdottir et al., 1999[1233]	The Netherlands	PE	7	A	5	0	3 CR
Greenstein et al., 2000[1239]	New York	PE	6	P	5	0	ND
Matalon et al., 2001[1243]	New York	PE	13	A	1	1	ND
Shariatmadar et al., 2002[1264]	Miami	PE	11	A	5	2	ND
Total			**67**		**27 (40%)**	**13 (19%)**	**10 CR (27%)** **3PR (8%)**

This table summarizes the studies that used plasma exchange or plasma absorption to treat recurrent FSGS, in studies that treated more than three patients. CR is defined as proteinuria <0.5 g/day and PR is defined as a fall in proteinuria to <2 g/day. Long-term outcome was at ≥1 year following recurrence. Chronic therapy includes that for patients who had subsequent repeat course of PE or who required intermittent, maintenance PE. PE, plasma exchange; A, adult; P, pediatric; CR, complete remission; PR, partial remission.

(2 patients). Cyclosporine doses ranged from 6 to 25 mg/kg/day and cyclosporine trough levels ranged from 200 to 1000 ng per milliliter. Remission was sustained in all patients with CR, with a conversion to tacrolimus in some patients. Toxicity included hirsutism and gingival hypertrophy in all patients. Although these are intriguing data, more experience is needed, especially in view of the potential toxicity of such high cyclosporine doses; whether adults would tolerate this approach without unacceptable adverse events is unclear.

A serendipitous finding that rituximab, administered to a renal transplant patient with lymphoma, induced the remission of recurrent FSGS[1269] has led to wider use of this agent.

Prophylactic Therapy to Prevent Recurrent Focal Segmental Glomerulosclerosis

Otsubu and colleagues[1270] assigned FSGS ESRD patients to undergo plasma exchange prior to or immediately after renal transplantation. Recurrent FSGS was seen in 4 of 19 treated patients and 9 of 19 untreated patients. Ohta et al.[1271] reported data from 21 patients and compared patients undergoing prophylactic plasma exchange (transplantations from 1991 to publication) with historical controls (transplantation prior to 1991). Recurrence was seen in 5 of 15 patients versus 4 of 6 patients. Neither study had sufficient power for a definitive result, and a prospective adequately powered trial remains to be done. If prophylactic plasma exchange is effective, the mechanism of benefit remains somewhat puzzling. Evidence suggests that the permeability factor returns following plasma exchange; therefore, any benefit from transient reduction would suggest that the factor is particularly injurious in the immediate peritransplantation period.

CONCLUSIONS

From the discussion in this chapter, several conclusions can be drawn regarding the group of diseases under consideration. First, the nephrotic syndrome represents a complex of symptoms resulting from urinary protein loss rather than a disease entity characterized by specific pathology. The abnormalities that were found include not only the hypoalbuminemia, edema, and hyperlipidemia classically associated with nephrotic syndrome, but also derangements of hemostasis, metabolism, and endocrine function. All of these findings can be attributed to the characteristics and effects of

TABLE 52.19 **Cyclophosphamide, with or without Plasma Exchange, for Recurrent Focal Segmental Glomerulosclerosis**

Report	Population	Treatment	*N*	Complete Response	Partial Response	No Response	Long-Term Response	Graft Preservation
Cochat et al., 1993[1235]	Children	PE + CTX 3 mo	3	3	0	0	3 CR (1 retreatment)	3
Kershaw et al., 1994[1240]	Children	CTX 2–3 mo	3	3	0	0	3 CR (1 relapse)	3
Dall'Amico et al., 1999[1236]	Children	PE + CTX 2 mo	11	9	0	2	7 CR	7
Cheong et al., 2000[1266]	Children	PE + CTX 3 mo	6	3	3	0	2 CR	5
Total			23	18 (78%)	3 (13%)	2 (9%)	15 CR (60%)	18 (78%)

N, number; PE, plasma exchange; CTX, cyclophosphamide; CR, complete remission.

nephrotic proteinuria. Second, we have defined a group of diseases in which the common attribute is that the lesion appears to initiate with the podocyte. In MCN, the restrictive component of the glomerular filtration barrier fails, yet podocyte effacement decreases the area of the GBM that is open to the urinary space, decreasing the effective filtration surface area. In FSGS, genetic, morphologic, and functional data all suggest that podocyte abnormality initiates the disease. Like MCN, there is massive proteinuria, but in contrast to the more benign condition, there is a disruption of podocyte architecture. FSGS is accompanied by podocyte injury and depletion, whereas collapsing glomerulopathy manifests podocyte proliferation and capillary collapse. In both cases, these changes are accompanied by the extracellular matrix accumulation that is a hallmark of this disease. Multiple cell types may serve as effector cells for fibrosis, but the common denominator of podocyte involvement suggests that a more appropriate appellation for these diseases might be *podocytopathies.*[1272]

A third conclusion relates to the observation that these conditions are characterized by heterogeneity of therapeutic response and prognosis. Although certain subgroups may be associated more often with specific patterns of response to treatment and outcome, such categorizations are not absolute. Most of the patients with MCN and some of those with FSGS are steroid sensitive. The remaining patients with MCN and a larger proportion of those with FSGS are steroid resistant. Of particular distinction is the group of patients who have collapsing glomerulopathy. Few of these patients respond to treatment, and the nature of their lesion is so distinctive that we have chosen to consider them as belonging to an entirely separate subgroup of primary nephrotic syndrome. It should be clear that all of the patients having a poor prognosis with regard to long-term renal function are steroid resistant. Moreover, a few patients with MCN and more with FSGS—particularly those with adaptive FSGS—may not have nephrotic syndrome. These findings suggest heterogeneity of pathogenic mechanisms, even within a given histopathologic subgroup.

In view of the differences among MCN, FSGS, and collapsing glomerulopathy, the assumption previously held by many clinicians that patients may move from one disorder to another should be revisited. Collapsing glomerulopathy, the rapidly progressing lesion, appears quite distinct. There are many features that also differentiate MCN from FSGS. These include (1) differences in permselectivity curves, where patients with FSGS demonstrate greater use of the shunt pathway[80]; (2) the association of FSGS with podocyte gene mutations, whereas mutations have not yet been defined for classical MCN (as opposed to congenital nephrotic syndrome); and (3) the more clearly defined and more likely irreversible podocyte abnormalities in FSGS. In particular, as technical capability for detecting subtle mutations or polymorphisms in podocyte-specific genes improves, it is likely that mutations will be associated with FSGS with increasing frequency.[1058] Therefore, although both MCN and FSGS initiate with a podocyte lesion, the abnormalities in FSGS appear more profound, either leading to or reflecting the pathogenic mechanism(s) of FSGS. Given these differences, it is likely that many (perhaps a great majority) of observations of progression from MCN to FSGS have represented sampling error or early lesions on biopsy.

The concept that different manifestations of the primary nephrotic syndrome may represent distinct podocyte disorders offers a paradigm shift from the thinking that was generally accepted at the beginning of this century. This new concept reflects the rapid growth of our knowledge of podocyte biology and reactions to injuries. We have gained significant insight into the mechanisms by which nephrotic proteinuria occurs and we are beginning to learn how subsequent events lead to nephron loss. The next challenge will be to translate this progress into strategies for intervening and preventing that loss.

ACKNOWLEDGMENTS

The authors wish to thank Dr. Laura Barisoni for her essential insights into the classification scheme for podocyte diseases, Dr. Nader Rifai for suggestions about hyperlipidemia, Dr. Gerard Soff for suggestions about coagulation abnormalities, and Dr. Alok Kalia for sharing unpublished data.

REFERENCES

1. Arneil GC. The nephrotic syndrome. *Pediatr. Clin. North Amer.*, 1971;18:547–559.

2. International Study of Kidney Disease in Children. A controlled therapeutic trial of cyclophosphamide plus prednisone vs. prednisone alone in children with focal segmental glomerulonephritis. *Pediatr. Res.*, 1980;14:1006 (Abstr.).

3. Glassock RJ. The nephrotic syndrome. *Hosp. Pract.*, 1979;14:105–129.

4. Adu D, Anin-Addo Y, Foli AK, et al. The nephrotic syndrome in Ghana: Clinical and pathological aspects. *Q. J. Med.*, 1981;50:297–306.

5. Hendrickse RG, Adenyi A, Edington GM, et al. Quartan malarial nephrotic syndrome. A collaborative clinicopathololic study in Nigerian children. *Lancet*, 1972;1:1143–1149.

6. Morgan AG, Shah DJ, Williams W, et al. Proteinuria and glomerular disease in Jamaica. *Clin. Nephrol.*, 1984;21:205–209.

7. Prathap K, Looi LM. Morphological patterns of glomerular disease in renal biopsies from 1,000 Malaysian patients. *Ann. Acad. Med. Singapore*, 1982;11:52–56.

8. Seggie J, Davies PG, Ninin D, et al. Patterns of glomerulonephritis in Zimbabwe: Survey of disease characterized by nephrotic syndrome. *Q. J. Med.*, 1984;53:109–118.

9. Haas M, Meehan SM, Karrison TG, et al. Changing etiologies of unexplained adult nephrotic syndrome: a comparison of renal biopsy findings from 1976–1979 and 1995–1997. *Am J Kidney Dis*, 1997;30:621–631.

10. Stokes MB, Markowitz GS, Lin J, et al. Glomerular tip lesion: a distinct entity within the minimal change disease/focal segmental glomerulosclerosis spectrum. *Kidney Int*, 2004;65:1690–1702.

11. Filler G. Treatment of nephrotic syndrome in children and controlled trials. *Nephrol Dial Transplant*, 2003;18 Suppl 6:vi75–78.

12. Barisoni L, Schnaper HW, Kopp JB. A proposed taxonomy for the podocytopathies: a reassessment of the primary nephrotic diseases. *Clin J Am Soc Nephrol*, 2007;2:529–542.

13. Barisoni L, Schnaper HW, Kopp JB. Advances in the biology and genetics of the podocytopathies: implications for diagnosis and therapy. *Arch Pathol Lab Med*, 2009;133:201–216.

14. Rennke HG, Venkatachalam MA. Glomerular permeability of macromolecules. Effect of molecular configuration on the fractional clearance of uncharged dextran and neutral horseradish peroxidase in the rat. *J. Clin. Invest.*, 1979;63:713.

15. Simpson LO. Glomerular permeability: An alternate to the pore theory. *Lancet*, 1981;ii:251.

16. Edwards A, Deen WM, Daniels BS. Hindered transport of macromolecules in isolated glomeruli. I. Diffusion across intact and cell-free capillaries. *Biophys J*, 1997;72:204–213.

17. Smithies O. Why the kidney glomerulus does not clog: a gel permeation/diffusion hypothesis of renal function. *Proc Natl Acad Sci U S A*, 2003;100:4108–4113.

18. Brenner BM, Hostetter TH, Humes HD. Glomerular permselectivity: Barrier function based on discrimination of molecular size and charge. *Am. J. Physiol.*, 1978;234:F455.

19. Schneeberger EE, Levey RH, McCluskey RT, et al. The isoporous substructures of the human glomerular slit diaphragm. *Kidney Int.*, 1975;8:48.

20. Gagliardini E, Conti S, Benigni A, et al. Imaging of the porous ultrastructure of the glomerular epithelial filtration slit. *J Am Soc Nephrol*, 2010;21:2081–2089.

21. Schneeberger EE. Glomerular permeability to protein molecules—its possible structural basis. *Nephron*, 1974;13:7.

22. Reiser J, Kriz W, Kretzler M, et al. The glomerular slit diaphragm is a modified adherens junction. *J. Am. Soc. Nephrol.*, 2000;11:1–8.

23. Patrakka J, Tryggvason K. Molecular make-up of the glomerular filtration barrier. *Biochem Biophys Res Commun*, 2010;396:164–169.

24. Rodewald R, Karnovsky M. Porous substructure of the glomerular slit diaphragm in the rat and mouse. *J. Cell Biol.*, 1974;60:423–433.

25. Deen WM, Myers BD, Brenner BM, The glomerular barrier to macromolecules: theoretical and experimental considerations, in *Contemporary Issues in Nephrology. IX. Nephrotic Syndrome*, Brenner BM, Stein JH, Editors. 1982, Churchill Livingstone: New York. p. 1.

26. Wallenius G. Renal clearance of dextran as a measure of glomerular permeability. *Acta. Soc. Med. Ups.*, 1954;[Suppl.] 4:1.

27. Bridges CR, Rennke HG, Deen WM, et al. Reversible hexadimethrine-induced alterations in glomerular structure and permeability. *J. Am. Soc. Neph.*, 1991;1:1095.

28. Deen WM, Bridges CR, Brenner BM, et al. Heteroporous model of glomerular size selectivity: application to normal and nephrotic humans. *Am J Physiol*, 1985;249:F374–389.

29. Shemesh O, Deen WM, Brenner BM, et al. Effect of colloid volume expansion on glomerular barrier size selectivity in humans. *Kidney Int.*, 1986;29:916–923.

30. Alfino PA, Neugarten J, Schacht RG, et al. Glomerular size-selective barrier dysfunction in nephrotoxic serum nephritis. *Kidney Int.*, 1988;34:151.

31. Loon N, Shemesh O, Morelli E, et al. Effect of angiotensin II infusion on the human glomerular filtration barrier. *Am. J. Physiol.*, 1989;257:F608.

32. Golbetz H, Black V, Shemesh O, et al. Mechanism of the antiproteinuric effect of indomethacin in nephrotic humans. *Am J Physiol*, 1989;256:F44–51.

33. Brenner BM, Hostetter TH, Humes HD. Molecular basis of proteinuria of glomerular origin. *N. Engl. J. Med.*, 1978;298:826.

34. Mohos SC, Skoza L. Glomerular sialoprotein. *Science*, 1967;164:1519.

35. Kanwar YS, Farquhar MG. Anionic sites in the glomerular basement membrane. In vivo and in vitro localization to the laminase rarae by cationic probes. *J. Cell Biol.*, 1979;81:137.

36. Latta H, Johnston WH. The glycoprotein inner layer of glomerular capillary basement membrane as a filtration barrier. *J. Ultrastruct. Res.*, 1976;57:65.

37. Latta H, Johnston WH, Stanley TM. Sialoglycoproteins and filtration barriers in the glomerular capillary wall. *J. Ultrastruct. Res.*, 1975;51:354.

38. Bohrer MP, Baylis C, Humes HD, et al. Permselectivity of the glomerular capillary wall. Facilitated filtration of circulating polycations. *J. Clin. Invest.*, 1978;61:72.

39. Chang RLS, Deen WM, Robertson CR, et al. Permselectivity of the glomerular capillary wall: III. Restricted transport of polyanion. *Kidney Int.*, 1975;8:212.

40. Salmon AH, Toma I, Sipos A, et al. Evidence for restriction of fluid and solute movement across the glomerular capillary wall by the subpodocyte space. *Am J Physiol Renal Physiol*, 2007;293:F1777–1786.

41. Hausmann R, Kuppe C, Egger H, et al. Electrical forces determine glomerular permeability. *J Am Soc Nephrol*, 2010;21:2053–2058.

42. Gudehithlu KP, Pegoraro AA, Dunea G, et al. Degradation of albumin by the renal proximal tubule cells and the subsequent fate of its fragments. *Kidney Int*, 2004;65:2113–2122.

43. Eppel GA, Osicka TM, Pratt LM, et al. The return of glomerular-filtered albumin to the rat renal vein. *Kidney Int*, 1999;55:1861–1870.

44. Wang SS, Devuyst O, Courtoy PJ, et al. Mice lacking renal chloride channel, CLC-5, are a model for Dent's disease, a nephrolithiasis disorder associated with defective receptor-mediated endocytosis. *Hum Mol Genet*, 2000;9:2937–2945.

45. Piwon N, Gunther W, Schwake M, et al. ClC-5 Cl-channel disruption impairs endocytosis in a mouse model for Dent's disease. *Nature*, 2000;408:369–373.

46. Norden AG, Scheinman SJ, Deschodt-Lanckman MM, et al. Tubular proteinuria defined by a study of Dent's (CLCN5 mutation) and other tubular diseases. *Kidney Int*, 2000;57:240–249.

47. Gekle M. Renal tubule albumin transport. *Annu Rev Physiol*, 2005;67:573–594.

48. Zhai XY, Nielsen R, Birn H, et al. Cubilin- and megalin-mediated uptake of albumin in cultured proximal tubule cells of opossum kidney. *Kidney Int*, 2000;58:1523–1533.

49. Amsellem S, Gburek J, Hamard G, et al. Cubilin is essential for albumin reabsorption in the renal proximal tubule. *J Am Soc Nephrol*, 2010;21:1859–1867.

50. Birn H, Fyfe JC, Jacobsen C, et al. Cubilin is an albumin binding protein important for renal tubular albumin reabsorption. *J Clin Invest*, 2000;105: 1353–1361.

51. Christensen EI, Birn H. Megalin and cubilin: synergistic endocytic receptors in renal proximal tubule. *Am J Physiol Renal Physiol*, 2001;280:F562–573.

52. Chaudhury C, Mehnaz S, Robinson JM, et al. The major histocompatibility complex-related Fc receptor for IgG (FcRn) binds albumin and prolongs its lifespan. *J Exp Med*, 2003;197:315–322.

53. Robson AM, Cole BR, Pathologic and functional correlations in the glomerulopathies, in *Immune Mechanisms in Renal Disease*, Cummings NB, Michael AF, Wilson CB, Editors. 1982, Plenum: New York. p. 109–127.

54. Robson AM, Vehaskari VM, The role of charge sites in vascular permeability. In *Pediatric Nephrology*, Brodehl J, Ehrich JHH, Editors. 1983, Springer-Verlag: New York.

55. Kelley VE, Cavallo T. Glomerular permeability. Ultrastructural studies in New Zealand black/white mice using polyanionic ferritin as a molecular probe. *Lab. Invest.*, 1977;37:265.

56. Scandling JD, Myers BD. Glomerular size-selectivity and microalbuminuria in early diabetic glomerular disease. *Kidney Int.*, 1992;41:840–846.

57. Blau EB, Haas JE. Glomerular sialic acid and proteinuria in human renal disease. *Lab Invest.*, 1973;38:447.

58. Carrie BJ, Salyer WR, Myers BD. Minimal change nephropathy: an electrochemical disorder of the glomerular membranes. *Am. J. Med.*, 1981;70:262–268.

59. Mahan JD, Sisson SP, Vernier RL. Altered glomerular basement membrane (GBM) anionic sites in the minimal change nephrotic syndrome (MCNS) in man. (Abstract). *Kidney Int.*, 1985;27:217.

60. Vernier RL, Klein DJ, Sisson SP, et al. Heparan sulfate-rich anionic sites in the human glomerular basement membrane. Decreased concentrations in congenital nephrotic syndrome. *N. Engl. J. Med.*, 1983;309:1001.

61. Bridges CR, Myers BD, Brenner BM, et al. Glomerular charge alterations in human minimal change nephropathy. *Kidney Int.*, 1982;22:677.

62. Michael AF, Blau E, Vernier RL. Glomerular polyanion: Alteration in aminonucleoside nephrosis. *Lab. Invest.*, 1970;23:649.

63. Blau EB, Michael AF. Rat glomerular glycoprotein composition and metabolism in aminonucleoside nephrosis. *Proc. Soc. Exp. Biol. Med.*, 1972;141:164.

64. Bohrer MP, Baylis C, Robertson CR, et al. Mechanism of the puromycin-induced defects in the transglomerular passage of water and macromolecules. *J. Clin. Invest.*, 1977;60:152.

65. Barnes JL, Radnik RA, Gilchrist EP, et al. Size and charge selective permeability defects induced in glomerular basement membrane by a polycation. *Kidney Int.*, 1984;25:11.

66. Hunsicker LG, Shearer TP, Shaffer SJ. Acute reversible proteinuria induced by infusion of the polycation hexadimethrine. *Kidney Int.*, 1981;20:7.

67. Vehaskari VM, Chang CTC, Stevens JK, et al. The effect of polycation on vascular permeability in the rat: A proposed role for charge sites. *J. Clin. Invest.*, 1984;73:1053.

68. Levin M, Gascoine P, Turner MW, et al. A highly cationic protein in plasma and urine of children with steroid-responsive nephrotic syndrome. *Kidney Int.*, 1989;36:867.

69. Levin M, Smith C, Walters MDS, et al. Steroid-responsive nephrotic syndrome: A generalised disorder of membrane negative charge. *Lancet*, 1985;ii:239.

70. Cheung PK, Klok PA, Baller JF, et al. Induction of experimental proteinuria in vivo following infusion of human plasma hemopexin. *Kidney Int*, 2000;57: 1512–1520.

71. Cheung PK, Stulp B, Immenschuh S, et al. Is 100KF an isoform of hemopexin? Immunochemical characterization of the vasoactive plasma factor 100KF. *J. Am. Soc. Nephrol.*, 1999;10:1700–1708.

72. Schaeffer RC, Jr., Gratrix ML, Mucha DR, et al. The rat glomerular filtration barrier does not show negative charge selectivity. *Microcirculation*, 2002;9: 329–342.

73. Peti-Peterdi J, Sipos A. A high-powered view of the filtration barrier. *J Am Soc Nephrol*, 2010;21:1835–1841.

74. Osicka TM, Comper WD. Tubular inhibition destroys charge selectivity for anionic and neutral horseradish peroxidase. *Biochim Biophys Acta*, 1998; 1381:170–178.

75. Koltun M, Comper WD. Retention of albumin in the circulation is governed by saturable renal cell-mediated processes. *Microcirculation*, 2004;11: 351–360.

76. Osicka TM, Strong KJ, Nikolic-Paterson DJ, et al. Renal processing of serum proteins in an albumin-deficient environment: an in vivo study of glomerulonephritis in the Nagase analbuminaemic rat. *Nephrol Dial Transplant*, 2004;19:320–328.

77. Russo LM, Bakris GL, Comper WD. Renal handling of albumin: a critical review of basic concepts and perspective. *Am J Kidney Dis*, 2002;39:899–919.

78. Deen WM, Lazzara MJ. Glomerular filtration of albumin: how small is the sieving coefficient? *Kidney Int Suppl*, 2004:S63–64.

79. Luke RL. Permselectivity: Relation between foot process simplification and macromolecular configuration. *Renal Physiol.*, 1984;7:129.

80. Winetz JA, Robertson CR, Golbetz HV, et al. The nature of the glomerular injury in minimal change and focal sclerosing glomerulopathies. *Am. J. Kidney Dis.*, 1981;1:91–98.

81. Drummond MC, Kristal B, Myers BD, et al. Structural basis for reduced glomerular filtration capacity in nephrotic humans. *J. Clin. Invest.*, 1994;94: 1187–1195.

82. Guasch A, Hashimoto H, Sibley RK, et al. Glomerular dysfunction in nephrotic humans with minimal changes or focal glomerulosclerosis. *Am. J. Physiol.*, 1991;260:F728–F737.

83. Yoshioka T, Shiraga H, Yoshida Y, et al. "Intact nephrons" as the primary origin of proteinuria in chronic renal disease. Study in the rat model of subtotal nephrectomy. *J Clin Invest*, 1988;82:1614–1623.

84. Robson AM, Mor J, Root ER, et al. Mechanism of proteinuria in nonglomerular renal disease. *Kidney Int.*, 1979;16:416–429.

85. Yoshioka T, Mitarai T, Kon V, et al. Role for angiotensin II in an overt functional proteinuria. *Kidney Int*, 1986;30:538–545.

86. Yoshioka T, Rennke HG, Salant DJ, et al. Role of abnormally high transmural pressure in the permselectivity defect of glomerular capillary wall: a study in early passive Heymann nephritis. *Circ Res*, 1987;61:531–538.

87. Remuzzi A, Puntorieri S, Battaglia C, et al. Angiotensin converting enzyme inhibition ameliorates glomerular filtration of macromolecules and water and lessens glomerular injury in the rat. *J. Clin Invest.*, 1990;85:541–549.

88. Smoyer WE, Mundel PE, Gupta A, et al. Podocyte alpha-actinin induction precedes foot process effacement in experimental nephrotic syndrome. *Am. J. Physiol.*, 1997;273:F150–F157.

89. Mundel P, Heid HW, Mundel TM, et al. Synaptopodin: an actin-associated protein in telencephalic dendrites and renal podocytes. *J. Cell Biol.*, 1997;139: 193–204.

90. Reiser J, von Gersdorff G, Loos M, et al. Induction of B7-1 in podocytes is associated with nephrotic syndrome. *J Clin Invest*, 2004;113:1390–1397.

91. Garin EH, Mu W, Arthur JM, et al. Urinary CD80 is elevated in minimal change disease but not in focal segmental glomerulosclerosis. *Kidney Int*, 2010;78:296–302.

92. Wei C, El Hindi S, Li J, et al. Circulating urokinase receptor as a cause of focal segmental glomerulosclerosis. *Nat Med*, 2011;17:952–960.

93. Gitlin D, Janeway CA, Farr LE. Studies on the metabolism of plasma proteins in the nephrotic syndrome. I. Albumin, γ-globulin and iron-binding globulin. *J. Clin. Invest.*, 1956;35:44.

94. Galaske RG, Baldamus CA, and Stolte H. Plasma protein handling in the rat kidney: Micropuncture experiments in the acute heterologous phase of anti-GBM nephritis. *Pfluegers Arch.*, 1978;375:269.

95. Jensen H, Rossing N, Andersen SB, et al. Albumin metabolism in the nephrotic syndrome in adults. *Clin. Sci.*, 1967;33:445.

96. Walker WA, Lowman JT, Hong RA. Measuring albumin turnover rates in patients with hypoproteinemia. *Am. J. Dis. Child.*, 1973;125:53.

97. Dulaney JT, Hatch FE, Jr. Peritoneal dialysis and loss of protein: a review. *Kidney Int.*, 1984;26:253.

98. Jaffa AA, Harvey JN, Sutherland SE, et al. Renal kallikrein responses to dietary protein: a possible mediator of hyperfiltration. *Kidney Int.*, 1989;36:1003.

99. Mizuiri S, Hayashi I, Ozawa T, et al. Effects of an oral protein load on glomerular filtration rate in healthy controls and nephrotic patients,. *Nephron*, 1986;48:101.

100. Kaysen GA, Gambertoglio J, Jimenez I, et al. Effect of dietary protein intake on albumin homeostasis in nephrotic patients. *Kidney Int.*, 1986;29:572.

101. Kaysen GA, Jones HJ, Hutchison FN. High protein diets stimulate albumin synthesis at the site of albumin mRNA transcription. *Kidney Int.*, 1989;36: S-168.

102. Kaysen GA, Jones HJ, Martin V, et al. A low-protein diet restricts albumin synthesis in nephrotic rats. *J. Clin Invest.*, 1990;83:1623.

103. Don BR, Wada L, Kaysen GA, et al. Effect of dietary protein restriction and angiotensin converting enzyme inhibition on protein metabolism in the nephrotic syndrome. *Kidney Int.*, 1989;36(suppl 27):S-163.

104. Hutchison FN, Martin VI, Jones HJ, et al. Differing actions of dietary protein and enalapril on renal function and proteinuria. *Am. J. Physiol.*, 1990;258:F126.
105. Hutchison FN, Schambelan M, Kaysen GA. Modulation of albuminuria by dietary protein and converting enzyme inhibition. *Am. J. Physiol*, 1987; 253:F719.
106. Starling EH. On the absorption of fluids from the connective tissue space. *J. Physiol. (Lond.)*, 1986;19:312.
107. Robson AM, Edema and edema-forming states, in *The Kidney and Body Fluids in Health and Disease*, Klahr S, Editor 1983, Plenum: New York. p. 119.
108. Landis EM, Pappenheimer JR, Exchange of substances through the capillary walls, in *Handbook of Physiology, Section Z, Circulation*, Hamilton WF, Dow P, Editors. 1963, American Physiological Society: Washington, D. C. p. 961.
109. Schrier RW, Fassett RG. A critique of the overfill hypothesis of sodium and water retention in the nephrotic syndrome. *Kidney Int.*, 1998;53:1111–1117.
110. Bohlin A-B. Clinical course and renal function in minimal change nephrotic syndrome. *Acta Paediatr. Scand.*, 1984;73:631.
111. Bohlin A-B, Berg U. Renal sodium handling in minimal change nephrotic syndrome. *Arch. Dis. Child.*, 1984;59:825.
112. Bohlin A-B, Berg U. Renal water handling in minimal change nephrotic syndrome. *Int. J. Pediatr. Nephrol.*, 1984;2:93.
113. Johnson AK, Mann JFE, Rascher W, et al. Plasma angiotensin II concentrations and experimentally induced thirst. *Am. J. Physiol.*, 1981;240:R229.
114. Kaysen GA, Paukert TT, Menke DJ, et al. Plasma volume expansion is necessary for edema formation in the rat with Heymann nephritis. *Am. J. Physiol.*, 1985;248:F247.
115. Keller H, Morell A, Noseda G, et al. Analbuminamie Pathophysiologische Untersuchungen an einem Fall. *Schweiz. Med. Wochenschr.*, 1972;102:72.
116. Usberti M, Federico S, Meccariello S, et al. Role of plasma vasopressin in the impairment of water excretion in nephrotic syndrome. *Kidney Int.*, 1984;25:422.
117. Eisenberg S. Blood volume in persons with the nephrotic syndrome. *Am. J. Med. Sci.*, 1968;255:320.
118. Geers AB, Koomans HA, Roos JC, et al. Functional relationships in the nephrotic syndrome. *Kidney Int.*, 1984;26:324.
119. Dorhout Mees EJ, Roos JC, Boer P, et al. Observations on edema formation in the nephrotic syndromes in adults with minimal lesion. *Am. J. Med.*, 1979;67:378.
120. Oliver WJ. Physiologic responses associated with steroid-induced diuresis in the nephrotic syndrome. *J. Lab. Clin. Med.*, 1963;62:449.
121. Lewis DM, Tooke JE, Beaman M, et al. Peripheral microvascular parameters in the nephrotic syndrome. *Kidney Int.*, 1998;54:1261–1266.
122. Meltzer JI, Keim HJ, Laragh JH, et al. Nephrotic syndrome: Vasoconstriction and hypervolemia types indicated by renin-sodium profiling. *Ann. Intern. Med.*, 1979;91:688.
123. Garnett ES, Webber CE. Changes in blood-volume produced by treatment of the nephrotic syndrome. *Lancet ii*, 1967;7:798.
124. Fleck A, Raines G, Hawker F. Increased vascular permeability: A major cause of hypoalbuminemia in disease and injury. *Lancet*, 1985;ii:781.
125. Vehaskari VM, Robson AM. The nephrotic syndrome in children. *Ann. Pediatr.*, 1981;10:42–62.
126. Koomans HA, Braam B, Geers AB, et al. The importance of plasma protein for blood volume and blood pressure homeostasis. *Kidney Int.*, 1986;30:730.
127. Vande Walle JG, Donckerwolcke RA, van Isselt JW, et al. Volume regulation in children with early relapse of minimal-change nephrosis with or without hypovolaemic symptoms. *Lancet*, 1995;346:148–152.
128. Warren JV, Merrill AJ, Stead EA, Jr. Role of extracellular fluid in maintenance of normal plasma volume. *J. Clin. Invest.*, 1943;22:635.
129. Luetscher JA, Jr.Johnson BB. Chromatographic separation of the sodium-retaining corticoid from the urine of children with nephrotic syndrome, compared with observations in normal children. *J. Clin. Invest.*, 1954;33:276.
130. Metcoff J, Janeway CA. Studies on the pathogenesis of nephrotic edema. *J. Pediatr.*, 1961;58:640.
131. Paller MS, Schrier RW. Pathogenesis of sodium and water retention in edematous disorders. *Am. J. Kidney Dis.*, 1982;2:241.
132. Shapiro M, Hasbargen J, Cosby R, et al. Role of aldosterone in the Na retention of patients with nephrotic syndrome. *Kidney Int.*, 1986;29:203.
133. Nochy D, Barres D, Camilleri JP, et al. Abnormalities of renin-containing cells in human glomerular and vascular renal diseases. *Kidney Int.*, 1983;23:375.
134. Brown EA, Markandu ND, Roulston JE. Is the renin-angiotensin system involved in the sodium retention in the nephrotic syndrome? *Nephron*, 1982;32:102.
135. Krishna GG, Danovitch GM. Effects of water immersion and renal function in the nephrotic syndrome. *Kidney Int.*, 1982;21:395.
136. Epstein EH. Underfilling vs. overflow in hepatic ascites. *N. Engl. J. Med.*, 1982;307:1577.
137. Kim SW, de Seigneux S, Sassen MC, et al. Increased apical targeting of renal ENaC subunits and decreased expression of 11betaHSD2 in HgCl2-induced nephrotic syndrome in rats. *Am J Physiol Renal Physiol*, 2006;290:F674–687.
138. de Seigneux S, Kim SW, Hemmingsen SC, et al. Increased expression but not targeting of ENaC in adrenalectomized rats with PAN-induced nephrotic syndrome. *Am J Physiol Renal Physiol*, 2006;291:F208–217.
139. Raij L, Keane WF, Leonard A, et al. Irreversible acute renal failure in idiopathic nephrotic syndrome. *Am. J. Med.*, 1976;61:207.
140. Oliver WJ, Kelsch RC, Chandler JP. Demonstration of increased catecholamine excretion in the nephrotic syndrome. *Proc. Soc. Exp. Biol. Med.*, 1967; 125:1176.
141. Apostol E, Ecelbarger CA, Terris J, et al. Reduced renal medullary water channel expression in puromycin aminonucleoside—induced nephrotic syndrome. *J Am Soc Nephrol*, 1997;8:15–24.
142. Fernandez-Llama P, Andrews P, Nielsen S, et al. Impaired aquaporin and urea transporter expression in rats with adriamycin-induced nephrotic syndrome. *Kidney Int*, 1998;53:1244–1253.
143. Garin EH, Donnelly WH, Geary D, et al. Nephrotic syndrome and diffuse mesangial proliferative glomerulonephritis in children. *Am. J. Dis. Child.*, 1983;137:109.
144. Arisz I, Donker AJM, Brentjens JRH, et al. The effect of indomethacin on proteinuria and kidney function in the nephrotic syndrome. *Acta Med. Scand.*, 1976;199:121.
145. Gutierrez Millet V, Ruilope LM, Alcazar JM, et al. Effect of indomethacin administration upon renal function, proteinuria, renin-angiogensin-aldosterone axis, and urinary prostaglandin E2 in nephrotic syndrome. *Kidney Int.*, 1982; 22:213.
146. Needleman P, Adams SP, Cole BR, et al. Atriopeptins as cardiac hormones. *Hypertension*, 1985;7:469.
147. Tulassay T, Rascher W, Lang RE, et al. Atrial natriuretic peptide and other vasoactive hormones in nephrotic syndrome. *Kidney Int.*, 1987;31:1391.
148. Rodriguez-Iturbe B, Colic D, Parra G, et al. Atrial natriuretic factor in the acute nephritic and nephrotic syndromes. *Kidney Int.*, 1990;38:512.
149. Perico N, Delaini F, Lupini C, et al. Blunted excretory response to atrial natriuretic peptide in experimental nephrosis. *Kidney Int.*, 1989;36:57.
150. Perico N, Delaini F, Lupini C, et al. Renal response to atrial peptides is reduced in experimental nephrosis. *Am. J. Physiol.*, 1987;252: F654.
151. Zietse R, Schalekamp MA. Effect of synthetic human atrial natriuretic peptide (102–126) in nephrotic humans. *Kidney Int.*, 1988;34:717.
152. Peterson C, Madsen B, Perlman A, et al. Atrial natriuretic peptide and the renal response to hypervolemia in nephrotic humans. *Kidney Int.*, 1988; 34:825.
153. Epstein M, Loutzenhiser R, Friedland E, et al. Relationship of increased plasma atrial natriuretic factor and renal sodium handling during immersion-induced central hypervolemia in normal humans. *J. Clin. Invest.*, 1987;79:738.
154. Rabelink TJ, Koomans HA, Boer P, et al. Role of ANP in natriuresis of head-out immersion in humans. *Am. J. Physiol.*, 1989;257:375.
155. Ichikawa I, Rennke HG, Hoyer JR, et al. Role for intrarenal mechanisms in the impaired salt excretion of experimental nephrotic syndrome. *J. Clin. Invest.*, 1983;71:91–103.
156. Berg U, Bohlin AB. Renal hemodynamics in minimal change nephrotic syndrome in childhood. *Int. J. Pediatr. Nephrol.*, 1982;3:187.
157. Robson AM, Giangiancomo J, Kienstra RA, et al. Normal glomerular permeability and its modification by minimal change nephrotic syndrome. *J. Clin. Invest.*, 1974;54:1190.
158. Bohman S-O, Jeremko G, Bohlin A-B, et al. Foot process fusion and glomerular filtration rate in minimal change nephrotic syndrome. *Kidney Int.*, 1984;25:696.
159. Kuroda S, Aynedjian HS, Bank N. A micropuncture study of renal sodium retention nephrotic syndrome in rats: Evidence for increases resistance to tubular fluid flow. *Kidney Int.*, 1979;16:561.
160. Sakai T, Harris FH, Jr, Marsh DJ, et al. Extracellular fluid expansion and autoregulation in nephrotoxic serum nephritis in rats. *Kidney Int.*, 1984; 25:619.
161. Lowenborg EK, Berg UB. Influence of serum albumin on renal function in nephrotic syndrome. *Pediatr Nephrol*, 1999;13:19–25.
162. Powell HR. Relationship between proteinuria and epithelial cell changes in minimal lesion glomerulopathy. *Nephron*, 1976;16:310–317.
163. Koop K, Eikmans M, Baelde HJ, et al. Expression of podocyte-associated molecules in acquired human kidney diseases. *J Am Soc Nephrol*, 2003;14: 2063–2071.
164. van den Berg JG, van den Bergh Weerman MA, Assmann KJ, et al. Podocyte foot process effacement is not correlated with the level of proteinuria in human glomerulopathies. *Kidney Int*, 2004;66:1901–1906.

165. Dash SC, Molhotra KK, Sharma RK, et al. Reversible acute renal failure in idiopathic nephrotic syndrome with minimal change nephropathy. *J. Assoc. Physicians India*, 1982;30:399.
166. Sjoberg RJ, McMillan VM, Bartram LS, et al. Renal failure with minimal change nephrotic syndrome: Reversal with hemodialysis. *Clin. Nephrol.*, 1983; 20:98.
167. Steele BT, Bacheyie GS, Baumal R, et al. Acute renal failure of short duration in minimal lesion nephrotic syndrome of childhood. *Int. J. Pediatr. Nephrol.*, 1982;3:59.
168. Vande Walle J, Mauel R, Raes A, et al. ARF in children with minimal change nephrotic syndrome may be related to functional changes of the glomerular basal membrane. *Am J Kidney Dis*, 2004;43:399–404.
169. Whelton A. Renal and related cardiovascular effects of conventional and COX-2-specific NSAIDs and non-NSAID analgesics. *Am J Ther*, 2000;7:63–74.
170. Hulter HN, Bonner EL, Jr. Lipoid nephrosis appearing as acute oliguric renal failure. *Arch. Intern. Med.*, 1980;140:403.
171. Editorial. More about minimal change. *Lancet*, 1981;1:1298.
172. Lowenstein J, Schacht RG, Baldwin DS. Renal failure in minimal change nephrotic syndrome. *Am. J. Med*, 1981;70:227–233.
173. Yamauchi H, Hopper J, Jr. Hypovolemic shock and hypotension as a complication in the nephrotic syndrome: Report of ten cases. *Ann. Intern. Med.*, 1964;60:242.
174. Epstein AA. The nature and treatment of chronic parenchymatous nephritis (nephrosis). *J.A.M.A.*, 1917;69:444.
175. Baxter JH, Goodman HC, Havel RJ. Serum lipid and lipoprotein alterations in nephrosis. *J. Clin. Invest.*, 1960;39:455, 1960:455.
176. Hu P, Lu L, Hu B, et al. Characteristics of lipid metabolism under different urinary protein excretion in children with primary nephrotic syndrome. *Scand J Clin Lab Invest*, 2009;69:680–686.
177. Bernard DB, Metabolic abnormalities in nephrotic syndrome: pathophysiology and complications, in *Contemporary Issues in Nephrology. IX. Nephrotic Syndrome*, Brenner BM, Stein JH, Editors. 1982, Churchill Livingstone: New York. p. 85.
178. Baxter JH. Hyperlipoproteinemia in nephrosis. *Arch. Intern. Med.*, 1962; 109:742.
179. Zilleruelo G, Hsia SL, Freundlich M, et al. Persistence of serum lipid abnormalities in children with ideopathic nephrotic syndrome. *J. Pediatr.*, 1984; 104:61.
180. Joven J, Vilella E. Hyperlipidaemia of the nephrotic syndrome—the search for a nephrotic factor. *Nephrol. Dial. Transplant.*, 1995;10:314–316.
181. Chopra JS, Mallick NP, Stone MC. Hyperlipoproteinemias in the nephrotic syndrome. *Lancet*, 1971;1:317.
182. Newmark SR, Anderson CF, Donadio JV, et al. Lipoprotein profiles in adult nephrotics. *Mayo Clin. Proc.*, 1975;50:359.
183. Michaeli J, Bar-On H, Shafrir EL. Lipoprotein profiles in a heterogeneous group of patients with nephrotic syndrome. *Isr. J. Med. Sci.*, 1981;17:1001.
184. Oetliker OH, Mordasini R, Lutschg J, et al. Lipoprotein metabolism in nephrotic syndrome in childhood. *Pediatr. Res.*, 1980;14:64.
185. Cameron JS, Wass V, Jarrett RJ, et al. Nephrotic syndrome and cardiovascular disease. *Lancet*, 1979;2:1017.
186. Ohta T, Matsuda I. Lipid and apolipoprotein levels in patients with nephrotic syndrome. *Clin. Chim. Acta*, 1981;117:133.
187. Chan MK, Persuad JW, Ramdial L, et al. Hyperlipidemia in untreated nephrotic syndrome, increased production or decreased removal? *Clin. Chim. Acta*, 1981;117:317.
188. Gherardi E, Rota E, Calandra S, et al. Relationship among the concentrations of serum lipoproteins and changes in their chemical composition in patients with untreated nephrotic syndrome. *Eur. J. Clin. Invest.*, 1977;7:563.
189. Kaysen GA. Hyperlipidemia in the nephrotic syndrome. *Am. J. Kid. Dis.*, 1988;12:548.
190. Rifai N. Lipoproteins and apolipoproteins: composition, metabolism, and association with coronary heart disease. *Arch. Pathol. Lab. Med.*, 1986;110:694.
191. Kekki M, Nikkila EA. Plasma triglyceride metabolism in the adult nephrotic syndrome. *Eur. J. Clin. Invest.*, 1971;1:345.
192. Marsh JB, Sparks CE. Hepatic secretion of lipoproteins in the rat and the effect of experimental nephrosis. *J. Clin. Invest.*, 1979;64:1229.
193. Marsh JB, Sparks CE. Lipoproteins in experimental nephrosis: Plasma levels and composition. *Metabolism*, 1979;28:1040.
194. Velden MGS, Kaysen GA, Barrett HA, et al. Increased VLDL in nephrotic patients results from decreased catabolism while increased LDL results from increased synthesis. *Kidney Int.*, 1998;53:994–1001.
195. Appel GB, Blum CB, Chien S, et al. The hyperlipidemia of the nephrotic syndrome. Relation to plasm albumin concentration, oncotic pressure and viscosity. *N. Engl. J. Med.*, 1985;312:1544.
196. deMendoza SG, Kashyap ML, Chen CY, et al. High density lipoproteinuria in nephrotic syndrome. *Metabolism*, 1976;25:1143.
197. Davis RA, Engelhorn SC, Weinstein DB, et al. Very low density lipoprotein secretion by cultured rat hepatocytes. Inhibition by albumin and other macromolecules. *J. Biol. Chem.*, 1980;255:2039.
198. Yedgar S, Weinstein DB, Patsch W, et al. Vicosity of culture medium as a regulation of synthesis and secretion of very low density lipoproteins by cultured hepatocytes. *J. Biol. Chem.*, 1982;257:2188.
199. Golper TA, Feingold KR, Fulford MH, et al. The role of circulating mevalonate in nephrotic hypercholesterolemia. *J. Lipid Res.*, 1976;27:1044.
200. Golper TA, Swartz SH. Impaired renal mevalonate metabolism in nephrotic syndrome: a stimulus for increased hepatic cholesterogenesis independent of GFR and hypoalbuminemia. *Metabolism*, 1982;31:471.
201. Grundy SM. Management of hyperlipidemia of kidney disease. *Kidney Int.*, 1990;37:847.
202. Warwick GL, Caslake MJ, Boulton-Jones JM, et al. Low-density lipoprotein metabolism in the nephrotic syndrome. *Metabolism*, 1990;34:10.
203. Moorehead JF, Wheeler DC, Varghese Z. Glomerular structures and lipids in progressive renal disease. *Am. J. Med.*, 1989;87: 5.12N–5.20N.
204. Vaziri ND, Gollapudi P, Han S, et al. Nephrotic syndrome causes upregulation of HDL endocytic receptor and PDZK-1-dependent downregulation of HDL docking receptor. *Nephrol Dial Transplant*, 2011;26:3118–3123.
205. Wanner C, Kramer-Guth A, Nauck M, et al. Cholesterol metabolism in glomerular cells: effect of lipoproteins from nephrotic patients. *Miner. Elect. Metab.*, 1996;22:39–46.
206. Joven J, Vilella E. The influence of apoportein epsilon 2 homozygosity on nephrotic hyperlipidemia. *Clin. Nephrol.*, 1997;48:141–145.
207. Cohen L, Cramp DG, Lewis AD, et al. The mechanism of hyperlipidemia in nephrotic syndrome—role of low albumin and the LCAT reaction. *Clin. Chim. Acta.*, 1980;104:393.
208. Yamada M, Matsuda I. Lipoprotein lipase in clinical and experimental nephrosis. *Clin. Chim. Acta*, 1970;30:787.
209. Garber DW, Gottleib BA, Marsh JB, et al. Catabolism of very low density lipoproteins in experimental nephrosis. *J. Clin. Invest.*, 1984;74:1375–1383.
210. Shearer GC, Kaysen GA. Endothelial bound lipoprotein lipase (LpL) depletion in hypoalbuminemia results from decreased endothelial binding, not decreased secretion. *Kidney Int*, 2006;70:647–653.
211. Sestak TL, Alavi N, Subbaiah PV. Plasma lipids and acyltransferase activities in experimental nephrotic syndrome. *Kidney Int.*, 1989;36:240.
212. Fielding CJ. Human lipoprotein lipase inhibition of activity by cholesterol. *Biochim. Biophys. Acta*, 1970;218:221.
213. Gitlin D, Cornwell DG, Nakasato D, et al. Studies on the metabolism of plasma proteins in the nephrotic syndrome. II. The lipoproteins. *J. Clin. Invest.*, 1958;37:172.
214. Fielding CJ, Shore VG, Fielding PE. Lecithin: cholesterol acyltransferase: Effects of substrate upon enzyme activity. *Biochim. Biophys. Acta*, 1972;270:513.
215. Dixit VM, Hettiaratchi ES. The mechanism of hyperlipidemia in the nephrotic syndrome. *Med. Hypotheses*, 1979;5:1327.
216. Rosenman RH, Byres SO, Friedman M. Plasma lipid interrelationships in experimental nephrosis. *J. Clin. Invest.*, 1957;36:1558.
217. Rosenman RH, Friedman M. In vivo studies of the roles of albumin in endogenous heparin-activated lipaemia clearing in nephrotic rats. *J. Clin. Invest.*, 1957;36:700.
218. Kaysen GA, Gambertoglio J, Felts J, et al. Albumin synthesis, albuminuria and hyperlipemia in nephrotic patients. *Kidney Int.*, 1987;31:1368.
219. Davies RW, Staprans I, Hutchison FN, et al. Proteinuria, not altered albumin metabolism, affects hyperlipidemia in the nephrotic rat. *J. Clin Invest.*, 1990;86:600.
220. Felts JM, Mayerle JA. Urinary loss of plasma high density lipoprotein: A possible cause of hyperlipidemia in the nephrotic syndrome. *Circulation*, 1974;49/50 (Suppl.III):263.
221. Gherardi E, Vecchia L, Calandra S. Experimental nephrotic syndrome in the rat induced by puromycin aminonucleoside. Plasma and urinary lipoproteins. *Exp. Mol. Pathol.*, 1980;32:128.
222. Lopes-Virella M, Virella G, Debeukelaer M, et al. Urinary high density lipoprotein in minimal change glomerular disease and chronic glomerulopathies. *Clin. Chim. Acta*, 1979;94:73.
223. Kashyap ML, Srivastava LS, Hynd BA. Apolipoprotein C-II and lipoprotein lipase in human nephrotic syndrome. *Atherosclerosis*, 1980;35:29.
224. Kallen RJ, Brynes RK, Aronson AJ, et al. Premature coronary atherosclerosis in a 5-year-old with corticosteroid-refractory nephrotic syndrome. *Am. J. Dis. Child.*, 1977;131:976.
225. Alexander JH, Schapel GJ, Edwards DG. Increased incidence of coronary heart disease associated with combined elevation of serum triglyceride and

cholesterol concentrations in the nephrotic syndrome in man. *Med. J. Aust.*, 1974;2:119.

226. Berlyne GM, Mallick NP. Ischaemic heart disease as a complication of nephrotic syndrome. *Lancet*, 1969;ii:399.

227. Wass VJ, Jarrett RJ, Chilvers C, et al. Does the nephrotic syndrome increase the risk of cardiovascular disease? *Lancet*, 1979;ii:664.

228. Kniazewska MH, Obuchowicz AK, Wielkoszynski T, et al. Atherosclerosis risk factors in young patients formerly treated for idiopathic nephrotic syndrome. *Pediatr Nephrol*, 2009;24:549–554.

229. Nakahara C, Kobayashi K, Hamaguchi H, et al. Plasma lipoprotein (a) levels in children with minimal lesion nephrotic syndrome. *Pediatr. Nephrol.*, 1999;13:657–661.

230. Bass JE, Fisher EA, Prack MM, et al. Macrophages from nephrotic rats regulate apolipoprotein E biosynthesis and cholesterol content independently. *J. Clin. Invest.*, 1991;87:470.

231. Newman JW, Kaysen GA, Hammock BD, et al. Proteinuria increases oxylipid concentrations in VLDL and HDL but not LDL particles in the rat. *J Lipid Res*, 2007;48:1792–1800.

232. Soyoral YU, Aslan M, Emre H, et al. Serum paraoxonase activity and oxidative stress in patients with adult nephrotic syndrome. *Atherosclerosis*, 2011; 218:243–246.

233. Gilboa N. Incidence of coronary heart disease associated with the nephrotic syndrome. *Med. J. Aust.*, 1976;1:207.

234. Vosnides G, Cameron JS. Hyperlipidemia in renal disease. *(Letter) Med. J. Aust.*, 1974;2:855.

235. Mallick NP, Short CD. The nephrotic syndrome and ischaemic heart disease. *Nephron*, 1981;27:54.

236. Wass VJ, Cameron JS. Cardiovascular disease and the nephrotic syndrome: The other side of the coin. *Nephron*, 1981;27:58.

237. Dalrymple LS, Kaysen GA. The effect of lipoproteins on the development and progression of renal disease. *Am J Nephrol*, 2008;28:723–731.

238. Diamond JR, Karnovsky MJ. Focal and segmental glomerulosclerosis: analogies to atherosclerosis. *Kidney Int.*, 1988;33:917–924.

239. Kasiske BL, O'Donnell MP, Garvis WJ, et al. Pharmacologic treatment of hyperlipidemia reduces glomerular injury in rat 5/6 nephrectomy model of chronic renal failure. *Circulation Res.*, 1988;62:367.

240. Kasiske BL, O'Donnell MP, Lee H, et al. Impact of dietary fatty acid supplementation in obese Zucker rats. *Kidney Int.*, 1991;39:1125–1134.

241. Harris KPG, Purkerson ML, Yates J, et al. Lovastatin ameliorates the development of glomerulosclerosis and uremia in experimental nephrotic syndrome. *Am. J. Kid. Dis.*, 1990;15:16.

242. Querfeld U. Should hyperlipidemia in children with the nephrotic syndrome be treated? *Pediatr. Nephrol.*, 1999;13:77–84.

243. Grundy SM, Vega GL. Rationale and management of hyperlipidemia of the nephrotic syndrome. *Am. J. Med.*, 1989;87;5-3N–5-8N.

244. Kaplan R, Aynedjian HS, Schlondorff D, et al. Renal vasoconstriction caused by short-term cholesterol feeding is corrected by thromboxane antagonist or probucol. *J. Clin. Invest.*, 1990;86:1707.

245. Querfeld U, Kohl B, Fiehn W, et al. Probucol for treatment of hyperlipidemia in persistent childhood nephrotic syndrome. Report of a prospective uncontrolled multicenter study. *Pediatr. Nephrol,*, 1999;13:7–12.

246. Groggel GC, Cheung AK, Ellis-Benigni K, et al. Treatment of nephrotic hyperlipoproteinemia with gemfibrozil. *Kidney Int.*, 1989;36:266.

247. Joven J, Villabona C, Vilella E, et al. Abnormalities of lipoprotein metabolism in patients with the nephrotic syndrome. *N. Engl. J. Med.*, 1990; 323:579.

248. Golper TA, Illingworth R, Morris CD, et al. Lovastatin in the treatment of multifactorial hyperlipidemia. *Am. J. Kid. Dis.*, 1989;13:312.

249. Vega GL, Grundy SM. Lovastatin therapy in nephrotic hyperlipidemia: effects on lipoprotein metabolism. *Kidney Int.*, 1988;33:1160.

250. Aguilar-Salinas CA, Barrett PHR, Kelber J, et al. Physiologic mechanisms of action of lovastatin in nephrotic syndrome. *J. Lipid Res.*, 1995;36:188–199.

251. Valdivielso P, Moliz M, Valera A, et al. Atorvastatin in dyslipidaemia of the nephrotic syndrome. *Nephrology (Carlton)*, 2003;8:61–64.

252. Addis T, Glomerular Nephritis, Diagnosis and Treatment, 1948, Macmillan: New York. p. 216.

253. Egli F, Eiminger P, Stalder G. Thromboembolism in the nephrotic syndrome. *Pediatr. Res.*, 1974;8:903.

254. Llach FH. Hypercoagulability, renal vein thrombosis, and thrombotic complications of nephrotic syndrome. *Kidney Int.*, 1985;28:429–439.

255. Cameron JS. Coagulation and thromboembolic complications in the nephrotic syndrome. *Adv. Nephrol.*, 1984;13:75.

256. Sung SF, Jeng JS, Yip PK, et al. Cerebral venous thrombosis in patients with nephrotic syndrome—case reports. *Angiology*, 1999;40:427–432.

257. Jones CL, Hebert D. Pulmonary thrombo-embolism in the nephrotic syndrome. *Pediatr. Nephrol.*, 1991;5:56.

258. Apostol EL, Kher KK. Cavitating pulmonary infarction in nephrotic syndrome. *Pediatr. Nephrol.*, 1994;8:347–348.

259. Wagoner RD, Stanson AW, Holley KE. Renal vein thrombosis in idiopathic membranous glomerulopathy and nephrotic syndrome. Incidence and significance. *Kidney Int.*, 1983;23:368.

260. Cade R, Spooner G, Juncos L, et al. Chronic renal vein thrombosis. *Am. J. Med.*, 1977;63:387.

261. Lewy PR, Jao W. Nephrotic syndrome in association with renal vein thrombosis in infancy. *J. Pediatr.*, 1974;85:359.

262. Llach F, Arieff AI, Massry SG. Renal vein thrombosis and nephrotic syndrome: A prospective study of 36 adult patients. *Ann. Intern. Med.*, 1975;83:8.

263. Kanfer A. Coagulation factors in nephrotic syndrome. *Am. J. Nephrol.*, 1990;10 (suppl 1):63–68.

264. De Mattia M, Penza R, Giordano P, et al. Throembolic risk in children with nephrotic syndrome. *Haemostasis*, 1991;21:300–304.

265. Tkaczyk M, Baj Z. Surface markers of platelet function in idiopathic nephrotic syndrome in children. *Pediatr Nephrol*, 2002;17:673–677.

266. Richman AV, Kasnic G, Jr. Endothelial and platelet reactions in the idiopathic nephrotic syndrome: An ultrastructural study. *Hum. Pathol.*, 1982;13:548.

267. Adler AJ, Lundin AP, Feinroth MV, et al. β-Thromboglobulin levels in the nephrotic syndrome. *Am. J. Med.*, 1980;69:551.

268. Andrassy K, Depperman D, Ritz E, et al. Different effects of renal failure on beta-thromboglobulin and high affinity platelet factor 4 (HA-PF4) concentrations. *Thromb. Res.*, 1980;18:469.

269. Svetlov SI, Moskaleva ES, Pinelas VG, et al. Decreased intraplatelet Ca^{2+} release and ATP secretion in pediatric nephrotic syndrome. *Pediatr. Neprhol.*, 1999;13:205–208.

270. Kuhlmann U, Steurer J, Rhyner K. Platelet aggregation and beta thromboglobulin levels in nephrotic patients with and without thrombosis. *Clin. Nephrol.*, 1981;15:229.

271. Carvalho A, Colman R, Lees R. Platelet function in hyperlipoproteinemia. *N. Engl. J. Med.*, 1974;290:434.

272. Jorgensen KA, Stofferson E. On the inhibitory effect of albumin on platelet aggregation. *Thromb. Res.*, 1980;17:13.

273. Yoshida A, Aoki N. Release of arachidonic acid from human platelets. A key role for the potentiation of platelet aggregating ability in normal subjects as well as in those with nephrotic syndrome. *Blood*, 1978;52:969.

274. Schieppati A, Dodesini P, Benigni A, et al. The metabolism of arachidonic acid by platelets in nephrotic syndrome. *Kidney Int.*, 1984;25:671.

275. Pepper DS, Jamieson GA. Studies on glycoproteins. III. Isolation of sialoglycopeptides from human platelet membranes. *Biochemistry*, 1969;8: 3362.

276. George JN, Nurden AT, Phillips DR. Molecular defects in interactions of platelets with the vessel wall. *N. Engl. J. Med.*, 1984;311:1084.

277. Vaziri ND, Gonzales EC, Shayestehfar B, et al. Plasma levels and urinary excretion of fibrinolytic and protease inhibitory proteins in nephrotic syndrome. *J. Lab. Clin. Med.*, 1994;124:118–124.

278. Alkjaersig N, Fletcher AP, Narayanan M, et al. Course and resolution of the coagulopathy in nephrotic children. *Kidney Int.*, 1987;31:772–780.

279. Vaziri ND, Ngo J-CT, Ibsen KH, et al. Deficiency and urinary loss of factor XII in nephrotic syndrome. *Nephron*, 1982;32:342.

280. Kanfer A, Kleinknecht D, Broyer M, et al. Coagulation studies in 45 cases of nephrotic syndrome without uremia. *Thromb. Diathes. Haemorrh.*, 1970;24: 562.

281. Coppola R, Guerra L, Ruggeri ZM, et al. Factor VIII/von Willebrand factor in glomerular nephropathies. *Clin. Nephrol.*, 1981;16:217.

282. Kendall AG. Nephrotic syndrome: A hypercoagulable state. *Arch. Intern. Med.*, 1971;127:1021.

283. Thomson C, Forbes CD, Prentice CR, et al. Changes in blood coagulation and fibrinolysis in the nephrotic syndrome. *Q. J. Med.*, 1974;43:399–407.

284. Boneu B, Boissou F, Abbal M, et al. Comparison of progressive antithrombin activity and the concentration of three thrombin inhibitors in nephrotic syndrome. *Thromb. Haemost.*, 1981;46:623.

285. Jorgensen KA, Stofferson E. Antithrombin III and the nephrotic syndrome. *Scand. J. Haematol.*, 1979;22:442.

286. Kauffman RH, Veltkamp JJ, van-Tilburg N. Acquired antithrombin III deficiency and thrombosis in the nephrotic syndrome. *Am. J. Med.*, 1978;65:607.

287. Lau SO, Tkachuck MT, Hasegawa DK, et al. Plasminogen and antithrombin III deficiencies in the childhood nephrotic syndrome associated with plasminogenuria and antithrombinuria. *J. Pediatr.*, 1980;96:390.

288. Thaler E, Balzar E, Kopsa H, et al. Acquired antithrombin III deficiency in patients with glomerular proteinuria. *Haemostasis*, 1978;7:257.

289. Andrassy K, Ritz E, Bommer J. Hypercoagulability in the nephrotic syndrome. *Klin. Wochenchr.*, 1980;58:1029–1036.

290. Panicucci F, Sagripanti A, Vispi M, et al. Comprehensive study of haemostasis in nephrotic syndrome. *Nephron*, 1983;33:9–13.

291. Dahlbeck B. Physiological anticoagulation. Resistance to protein C and venous thromboembolism. *J. Clin. Invest.*, 1994;94:923–927.

292. Cosio FG, Harker C, Batard MA, et al. Plasma concentrations of the natural anticoagulants protein C and protein S in patients with proteinuria. *J. Lab. Clin. Med.*, 1985;106:218–222.

293. Soff GA, Jackman RW, Rosenberg RD. Expression of thrombomodulin by smooth muscle cells in culture. *Blood*, 1991;77:515–518.

294. Vigano-D'Angelo S, D'Angelo A, Kaufman CEJ, et al. Protein S deficiency occurs in the nephrotic syndrome. *Ann. Intern. Med.*, 1987;107:42–47.

295. Kemkes-Matthes B. Acquired protein S deficiency. *Clin. Investig.*, 1992; 70:529–534.

296. Garbrecht F, Gardner S, Johnson V, et al. Deep venous thrombosis in a child with nephrotic syndrome associated with a circulating anticoagulant and acquired protein S deficiency. *Am. J. Pediatr. Hematol. Oncol.*, 1991;13:330–333.

297. Scheinman KI, Stiehm ER. Fibrinolytic studies in the nephrotic syndrome. *Pediatr. Res.*, 1971;5:206.

298. Simpson HCR, Mann JI, Meade IW, et al. Hypertriglyceridaemia and hypercoagulability. *Lancet*, 1983;i:786.

299. Shimamatsu K, Onoyama K, Maeda T, et al. Massive pulmonary embolism occurring with corticosteroid and diuretics therapy in a minimal-change nephrotic syndrome. *Nephron*, 1982;32:78.

300. Yoshida Y, Shiiki H, Iwano M, et al. Enhanced expression of plasminogen activator inhibitor 1 in patients with nephrotic syndrome. *Nephron*, 2001;88:24–29.

301. Klocking H-P, Hoffmann A, Fareed J. Influence of hypersulfated lactobionic acid amides on tissue plasminogen activator release. *Semin. Thrombosis Hemostasis*, 1991;17:379–384.

302. Mysliwiec M, Ralston A, Ackrill P, et al. A study of impaired fibrin polymerization in patients with the nephrotic syndrome. *Folia Haematol., Leipzig*, 1990;117:S. 73–78.

303. Llach F, Papper S, Massry SG. The clinical spectrum of renal vein thrombosis. Acute and chronic. *Am. J. Med.*, 1980;69:819.

304. Ozanne P, Francis RB, Meiselman HJ. Red blood cell aggregation in nephrotic syndrome. *Kidney Int.*, 1983;23:519.

305. Elliott GB, Grant-Tyrell J, Ringer G. Congenital lipoid nephrosis with left renal vein thrombosis and Chiari's syndrome. *J. Can. Assoc. Radiol.*, 1979;30:175.

306. Cosgriff SW. Thromboembolic complications associated with ACTH and cortisone therapy. *J.A.M.A.*, 1951;147:924.

307. Eldrissy ATH, Abdurrahman MB, Bahakim HM, et al. Haemostatic measurements in childhood nephrotic syndrome. *Eur. J. Pediatr.*, 1991;150:374–378.

308. Zwaginga JJ, Koomans HA, Sixma JJ, et al. Thrombus formation and platelet-vessel wall interaction in the nephrotic syndrome under flow conditions. *J. Clin. Invest.*, 1994;93:204–211.

309. Malyszko J, Malyszko JS, Mysliwiec M. Markers of endothelial cell injury and thrombin activatable fibrinolysis inhibitor in nephrotic syndrome. *Blood Coagul Fibrinolysis*, 2002;13:615–621.

310. Giangiacomo J, Cleary TG, Cole BR, et al. Serum immunoglobulins in the nephrotic syndrome. A possible cause of minimal change nephrotic syndrome. *N. Engl. J. Med.*, 1975;293:8.

311. Spika JS, Halsy NA, Fish AJ, et al. Serum antibody response to pneumococcal vaccine in children with nephrotic syndrome. *Pediatrics*, 1982;69:219.

312. La Manna A, Polito C, Foglia AC, et al. Reduced response to HBV vaccination in boys with steroid-sensitive nephrotic syndrome. *Pediatr. Nephrol.*, 1992; 6:251–253.

313. La Manna A, Polito C, Del Gado R, et al. Hepatitis B surface antigenaemia and glomerulopathies in children. *Acta Paediatr. Scand.*, 1985;74:122.

314. McLean RH, Forsgren A, Bjorksten B, et al. Decreased serum factor B concentration associated with decreased opsonization of Escherichia coli in the idiopathic nephrotic syndrome. *Pediatr. Res.*, 1977;11:910.

315. Anderson DC, York TL, Rose G, et al. Assessment of serum factor B, serum opsonins, granulocyte chemotaxis and infection in nephrotic syndrome of children. *J. Infect. Dis.*, 1979;140:1.

316. Ballow M, Kennedy TL, Gaudio KM, et al. Serum hemolytic factor D values in children with steroid-responsive idiopathic nephrotic syndrome. *J. Pediatr.*, 1982;100:192.

317. American Academy of Pediatrics, Active and passive immunization, in *Red Book: Report of the Committee on Infectious Diseases*, Peter G, Editor 1997, American Academy of Pediatrics: Elk Grove Village, IL. p. 50–53.

318. Centers for Disease Control and Prevention. Prevention of pneumococcal disease: recommendations fo the Advisory Committee on Immunization Practices (ACIP). *MMWR*, 1997;46 (No. RR-8):1–31.

319. McIntyre P, Craig JC. Prevention of serious bacterial infection in children with nephrotic syndrome. *J. Paediatr. Child Health*, 1998;34:314–317.

320. Garin EH, Grant MB, Silverstein JH. Insulinlike growth factors in patients with active nephrotic syndrome. *Am. J. Dis. Child.*, 1989;143:865.

321. Gavin LA, McMahon FA, Castle JN, et al. Alterations in serum hormones and serum thyroxine-binding globulin in patients with nephrosis. *J. Clin. Endocrinol. Metab.*, 1978;46:125.

322. Afrasiabi MA, Vaziri ND, Gwinup G, et al. Thyroid function studies in the nephrotic syndrome. *Ann. Intern. Med.*, 1979;90:335–338.

323. Musa BU, Seal US, Doe RP. Excretion of corticosteroid-binding globulin, thyroxine-binding globulin and total protein in adult males with nephrosis: Effect of sex hormones. *J. Clin. Endocrinol.*, 1967;27:768.

324. Ito S, Kano K, Ando T, et al. Thyroid function in children with nephrotic syndrome. *Pediatr. Nephrol.*, 1994;8:412–415.

325. DeLuca F, Gemelli M, Pandullo E, et al. Changes in thyroid function tests in infantile nephrotic syndrome. *Horm. Metab. Res.*, 1983;15:258.

326. Chadha V, Alon US. Bilateral nephrectomy reverses hypothyroidism in congenital nephrotic syndrome. *Pediatr. Nephrol.*, 1999;13:209–211.

327. Lim P, Jacob E, Tock EPC, et al. Calcium and phosphorus metabolism in nephrotic syndrome. *Q. J. Med.*, 1977;46:327.

328. Malluche HH, Goldstein DA, Massry SG. Osteomalacia and hyperparathyroid bone disease in patients with nephrotic syndrome. *J. Clin. Invest.*, 1979; 63:494.

329. Barragry JM, France MW, Carter ND, et al. Vitamin D metabolism in nephrotic syndrome. *Lancet*, 1977;2:629.

330. Goldstein DA, Oda Y, Kurokawa K, et al. Blood levels of 25-hydroxyvitamin D in nephrotic syndrome. *Ann. Intern. Med.*, 1977;86:664.

331. Chan YL, Mason RS, Parmentier M, et al. Vitamin D metabolism in nephrotic rats. *Kidney Int.*, 1983;24:336.

332. Goldstein DA, Haldimann B, Sherman D, et al. Vitamin D metabolites and calcium metabolism in patients with nephrotic syndrome and normal renal function. *J. Clin. Endocrinol. Metab.*, 1981;52:116.

333. Korkor A, Schwartz J, Bergfeld M, et al. Absence of metabolic bone disease in adult patients with nephrotic syndrome and normal renal function. *J. Clin. Endocrinol. Metab.*, 1983;56:496.

334. Freundlich M, Jofe M, Goodman WG, et al. Bone histology in steroid-treated children with non-azotemic nephrotic syndrome. *Pediatr Nephrol*, 2004;19: 400–407.

335. Lettgen B, Jeken C, Reiners C. Influence of steroid medication on bone mineral density in children with nephrotic syndrome. *Pediatr. Nephrol.*, 1994;8:667–670.

336. Polito C, LaManna A, Todisco N, et al. Bone mineral content in nephrotic children on long-term, alternate-day prednisone therapy. *Clin. Pediatr.*, 1995;34: 234–236.

337. Loschiavo C, Lupo A, Valvo E, et al. Carbohydrate metabolism in patients with nephrotic syndrome and normal renal function. *Nephron*, 1983;33:257.

338. Cartwright GE, Gubler CJ, Wintrobe MM. Studies on copper metabolism. XI. Copper and iron metabolism in the nephrotic syndrome. *J. Clin. Invest.*, 1954;33:685.

339. Ellis D. Anemia in the course of nephrotic syndrome secondary to transferrin depletion. *J. Pediatr.*, 1977;90:953.

340. Rifkind D, Kravetz HM, Knight V, et al. Urinary excretion of iron-binding protein in nephrotic syndrome. *N. Engl. J. Med.*, 1961;265:115.

341. Reimold EW. Changes in zinc metabolism during the course of nephrotic syndrome. *Am. J. Dis. Child.*, 1980;134:46.

342. Gilman AG, Goodman LS, Rall TW, et al. *Goodman and Gilman's, The Pharmacological Basis of Therapeutics, 7th Edition*New York: Macmillan. 1985.

343. Ellison DH. Diuretic drugs and the treatment of edema: from clinic to bench and back again. *Am. J. Kidney Dis.*, 1994;23:623–643.

344. Kirchner KA, Voelker JR, Brater DC. Binding inhibitors restore furosemide potency in tubule fluid containing albumin. *Kidney Int.*, 1991;40:418.

345. Bennett WM, Porter GA. Efficacy and safety of metolazone in renal failure and the nephrotic syndrome. *J. Clin. Pharmacol.*, 1973;13:357.

346. Welch TR, Gianis J, Sheldon CA. Perforation of the scrotum complicating nephrotic syndrome. *J. Pediatr.*, 1988;113:336.

347. Yoshimura A, Ideura T, Iwasaki S. Aggravation of minimal change nephrotic syndrome by administration of human albumin. *Clin. Nephrol*, 1992; 37:109–114.

348. Haws RM, Baum M. Efficacy of albumin and diuretic therapy in children with nephrotic syndrome. *Pediatrics*, 1993;91:1142.

349. Blainey JD, Brewer DB, Hardwicke J, et al. The nephrotic syndrome: Diagnosis by renal biopsy and biochemical and immunologic analyses related to the response to steroid therapy. *Am. J. Med.*, 1960;29:235.

350. Mahan JD, Mauer SM, Sibley RK, et al. Congenital nephrotic syndrome: Evaluation of medical management and results of renal transplantation. *J. Pediatr.*, 1984;105:549.

351. Mansy H, Goodship THJ, Tapson JS, et al. Effect of a high protein diet in patients with nephrotic syndrome. *Clin. Sci.*, 1989;77:445–451.
352. Maroni BJ, Staffeld C, Young VR, et al. Mechanisms permitting nephrotic patients to achieve nitrogen equilibration with a protein-restricted diet. *J. Clin. Invest.*, 1997;99:2479–2487.
353. Barsotti G, Morelli E, Cupisti A, et al. A special, supplemented 'vegan' diet for nephrotic patients. *Am. J. Nephrol.*, 1991;11:380–385.
354. D'Amico G, Gentile MG. Effect of dietary manipulation on the lipid abnormalities and urinary protein loss in nephrotic patients. *Miner. Elect. Metab.*, 1992;18:203–206.
355. Dwyer J. Vegetarian diets for treating nephrotic syndrome. *Nutrition Rev.*, 1993;51:44–46.
356. Hall AV, Parbtani A, Clark WF, et al. Omega-3 fatty acid supplementation in primary nephrotic syndrome: effects on plasma lipids and coagulopathy. *J. Am. Soc. Nephrol.*, 1992;3:1321–1329.
357. Feehally J, Baker F, Walls J. Dietary manipulation in experimental nephrotic syndrome. *Nephron*, 1988;50:247–252.
358. DISC Writing Group. Efficacy and safety of lowering dietary intake of fat and cholesterol in children with elevated low-density lipoprotein cholesterol: the dietary intervention study in children. *J. Am. Med. Assn. 1995*, 1995;273: 1429–1435.
359. Prata MM, Nogueira AE, Pinto JR, et al. Long-term effect of lovastatin on lipoprotein profile in patients with primary nephrotic syndrome. *Clin. Nephrol.*, 1994;41:277–283.
360. Wanner C, Bohler J, Eckardt HG, et al. Effects of simvastatin on lipoprotein (a) and lipoprotein composition in patients with nephrotic syndrome. *Clin. Nephrol.*, 1994;41:138–143.
361. Rabelink AJ, Hene RJ, Erkelens DW, et al. Partial remission of nephrotic syndrome in patients on long-term simvastatin. *Lancet*, 1990;1:1045–1046.
362. Hodson E. The management of idiopathic nephrotic syndrome in children. *Paediatr Drugs*, 2003;5:335–349.
363. Grymonprez A, Proesmans W, Van Dyck M, et al. Vitamin D metabolites in childhood nephrotic syndrome. *Pediatr. Nephrol.*, 1995;9:278–281.
364. Mehls O. Is it correct to supplement patients with nephrotic syndrome with vitamin D and calcium? *Pediatr. Nephrol.*, 1990;4:518.
365. Torres VE, Velosa JA, Holley KE, et al. Meclofenamate treatment of recurrent idiopathic nephrotic syndrome with focal segmental glomerulosclerosis after renal transplant. *Mayo. Clin. Proc.*, 1984;59:146–152.
366. Trachtman H, Gauthier B. Effect of angiotensin converting enzyme inhibitor therapy on proteinuria in children with renal disease. *J. Pediatr.*, 1988;112:295.
367. de Jong PE, Anderson S, de Zeeuw D. Glomerular preload and afterload reduction as a tool to lower urinary protein leakage: will such treatments also help to improve renal function outcome? *J. Am. Soc. Nephrol.*, 1993;3: 1333–1341.
368. Garini G, Mazzi A, Buzio C, et al. Renal effects of captopril, indomethacin and nifedipine in nephrotic patients after an oral protein load. *Nephrol Dial Transplant*, 1996;11:628–634.
369. Bakris GL, Weir MR, Secic M, et al. Differential effects of calcium antagonist subclasses on markers of nephropathy progression. *Kidney Int*, 2004;65: 1991–2002.
370. Ruggenenti P, Mosconi L, Vendramin G, et al. ACE inhibition improves glomerular size selectivity in patients with idiopathic membranous nephropathy and persistent nephrotic syndrome. *Am J Kidney Dis*, 2000;35:381–391.
371. Kunz R, Friedrich C, Wolbers M, et al. Meta-analysis: effect of monotherapy and combination therapy with inhibitors of the renin angiotensin system on proteinuria in renal disease. *Ann Intern Med*, 2008;148:30–48.
372. Tojo A, Onozato ML, Kurihara H, et al. Angiotensin II blockade restores albumin reabsorption in the proximal tubules of diabetic rats. *Hypertens Res*, 2003;26:413–419.
373. Nakhoul F, Khankin E, Yaccob A, et al. Eplerenone potentiates the antiproteinuric effects of enalapril in experimental nephrotic syndrome. *Am J Physiol Renal Physiol*, 2008;294:F628–637.
374. Mattoo TK, al-Sowallem AM, al-Harbi MS, et al. Nephrotic syndrome in first year of life and the role of bilateral nephrectomy. *Pediatr. Nephrol.*, 1992;6:16–18.
375. Holmberg C, Laine J, Ronnholm K, et al. Long-term results of active treatment of congenital nephrotic syndrome of the Finnish type. *J. Am. Soc. Nephrol.*, 1994;5:646 (Abstr.).
376. Kim MS, Primack W, Harmon WE. Congenital nephrotic syndrome: preemptive bilateral nephrectomy and dialysis before renal transplantation. *J. Am. Soc. Nephrol.*, 1992;3:260–263.
377. Olivero JJ, Frommer JP, Gonzalez JM. Medical nephrectomy: the last resort for intractable complications of the nephrotic syndrome. *Am. J. Kidney Dis.*, 1993;21:260–263.
378. Hoyer JR, Idiopathic nephrotic syndrome with minimal glomerular changes, in *Contemporary Issues in Nephrology. Nephrotic Syndrome*, Brenner BM, Stein JH, Editors. 1982, Churchill Livingstone: New York. p. 145.
379. Barnett HL, Schoeneman M, Bernstein J, et al., Minimal change nephrotic syndrome, in *Pediatric Kidney Disease*, Edelmann CM, Editor 1978, Little, Brown, and Co.: Boston. p. 695.
380. Cameron JS. Nephrotic syndrome in the elderly. *Semin Nephrol*, 1996;16: 319–329.
381. Dragovic D, Rosenstock JL, Wahl SJ, et al. Increasing incidence of focal segmental glomerulosclerosis and an examination of demographic patterns. *Clin Nephrol*, 2005;63:1–7.
382. Kari JA. Changing trends of histopathology in childhood nephrotic syndrome in western Saudi Arabia. *Saudi Med J*, 2002;23:317–321.
383. Cameron JS, Turner DR, Ogg CS, et al. The nephrotic syndrome in adults with "minimal change glomerular lesion". *Q. J. Med.*, 1974;43:461–488.
384. Francis KL, Jenis EH, Jensen GE. Gold-associated nephropathy. *Arch. Pathol. Lab. Med.*, 1984;108:234–238.
385. Falck HM, Tornroth T, Kock B, et al. Fatal renal vesculitis and minimal change glomerulonephritis complicating treatment with penicillamine. Report on two cases. *Acta Med. Scand.*, 1979;205:133–138.
386. Rennke HG, Roos PC, Wall SG. Drug-induced interstitial nephritis with heavy glomerular proteinuria. *N. Engl. J. Med.*, 1980;302:691–692.
387. Barr RD, Rees PH, Cordy PE, et al. Nephrotic syndrome in adult Africans in Nairobi. *Br. Med. J.*, 1972;2:131–134.
388. Curt GA, Kaldany A, Whitley LG, et al. Reversible rapidly progressive renal failure with nephrotic syndrome due to fenoprofen calcium. *Ann. Intern. Med.*, 1980;92:72–73.
389. Feinfeld DA, Olesnicky L, Pirani CL, et al. Nephrotic syndrome associated with use of the nonsteroidal anti-inflammatory drugs. Case report and reviews of the literature. *Nephron*, 1984;37:174–179.
390. Lomvardias S, Pinn VW, Wadhwa ML, et al. Nephrotic syndrome associated with sulindac. *N. Engl. J. Med.*, 1981;304:424.
391. Morgenstern SJ, Bruns FJ, Fraley DS, et al. Ibuprofen-associated lipoid nephrosis without interstitial nephritis. *Am. J. Kid. Dis.*, 1989;14:50–52.
392. Heymann W. Nephrotic syndrome after use of trimethadione and paramethadione in petit mal. *J.A.M.A.*, 1967;202:893–894.
393. Reeves WG, Cameron JS, Johansson SG, et al. Seasonal nephrotic syndrome. Description and immunological findings. *Clin. Allergy*, 1975;5:121–137.
394. Howanietz H, Lubec G. Idiopathic nephrotic syndrome, treated with steroids for five years, found to be allergic reaction to pork. *Lancet*, 1985;ii:450.
395. Sandberg DH, McIntosh RM, Bernstein CW, et al. Severe steroid-responsive nephrosis associated with hypersensitivity. *Lancet*, 1977;i:388–391.
396. Laurent J, Lagrue G, Belghiti D, et al. Is house dust allergen a possible causal factor for relapses in lipoid nephrosis? *Allergy*, 1984;39:231–236.
397. Rytand DA. Fatal anuria, the nephrotic syndrome and glomerular nephritis as sequels of the dermatitis of poison oak. *Am. J. Med.*, 1948;5:548.
398. Rytand DA. Onset of the nephrotic syndrome during a reaction to bee sting. *Stanford Med. Bull.*, 1955;13:224.
399. Zaman F, Saccaro S, Latif S, et al. Minimal change glomerulonephritis following a wasp sting. *Am J Nephrol*, 2001;21:486–489.
400. Cale WF, Ullrich IH, Jenkings JJ. Nodular sclerosing Hodgkin's disease presenting as nephrotic syndrome. *South. Med. J.*, 1982;75:604–606.
401. Eagen JW, Lewis EJ. Glomerulopathies of neoplasia. *Kidney Int.*, 1977;11: 297–306.
402. Gagliano RG, Costanzi JJ, Beathard GA, et al. The nephrotic syndrome associated with neoplasia: An unusual paraneoplastic syndrome. *Am. J. Med.*, 1976;60:1026–1031.
403. Grupe WE. Childhood nephrotic syndrome: Clinical associations and response to therapy. *Postgrad. Med.*, 1979;65:229–231.
404. Magalhaes-Filho AG, Barbosa AB, Ferreira TC. Glomerulonephritis in schistosomiasis with mesangial IgM deposits. *Mem Inst. Oswaldo Cruz*, 1981;76:181–188.
405. Scaglia F, Vogler LB, Hymes LC, et al. Minimal change nephrotic syndrome: a possible complication of erlichosis. *Pediatr. Nephrol.*, 1999;13:600–601.
406. Froelich CJ, Searles RP, Davis LE, et al. A case of Guillain-Barre syndrome with immunologic abnormality. *Ann. Intern. Med.*, 1980;93:563–565.
407. Jassim A, Kumar N, Kelly C. Adult Still's disease with nephrotic syndrome at presentation. *Rheumatology (Oxford)*, 1999;38:283.
408. Abeyagunawardena AS, Goldblatt D, Andrews N, et al. Risk of relapse after meningococcal C conjugate vaccine in nephrotic syndrome. *Lancet*, 2003;362:449–450.
409. Habib R, Bois E. Heterogeneite des syndromes nephrotiques a debut precoce du nourisson (syndrome nephrotique "infantile"). *Helv. Paediatr. Acta*, 1973;28:91–107.

410. Gaboardi F, Perletti L, Cambie M, et al. Dermatitis herpetiformis and nephrotic syndrome. *Clin. Nephrol.*, 1983;20:49–51.
411. Khambam N, Tanji N, Seigle RL, et al. Congenital focal segmental glomerulosclerosis associated with b4 integrin mutation and epidermolysis bullosa. *Am. J. Kid. Dis.*, 2000;36:190–196.
412. Kuzmanovska DB, Shahpazova EM, Kocova MJ, et al. Autoimmune thyroiditis and vitiligo in a child with minimal change nephrotic syndrome. *Pediatr Nephrol*, 2001;16:1137–1138.
413. Tanwani LK, Lohano V, Broadstone VL, et al. Minimal change nephropathy and Graves' disease: report of a case and review of the literature. *Endocr Pract*, 2002;8:40–43.
414. Fracchia M, Manganaro M, Poccardi G, et al. Minimal change nephropathy presenting in a patient with primary sclerosing cholangitis. *Ital J Gastroenterol Hepatol*, 1997;29:267–269.
415. Jennette JC, Charles L, Grubb W. Glomerulomegaly and focal segmental glomerulosclerosis associated with sleep-apnea syndrome. *Am. J. Kid. Dis.*, 1987;10:470–472.
416. International Study of Kidney Disease in Children. Nephrotic syndrome in children: Prediction of histopathology from clinical and laboratory characteristics at time of diagnosis. *Kidney Int.*, 1978;13:159–165.
417. Danielsen H, Kornerup HJ, Olsen S, et al. Arterial hypertension in chronic glomerulonephritis. An analysis of 310 cases. *Clin. Nephrol.*, 1983;19:284–287.
418. Leonard MB, Feldman HI, Shults J, et al. Long-term, high-dose glucocorticoids and bone mineral content in childhood glucocorticoid-sensitive nephrotic syndrome. *N Engl J Med*, 2004;351:868–875.
419. Dennis VW, Robinson RR, Proteinuria, in *Pediatric Kidney Disease*, Edelmann CM, Editor 1978, Little, Brown,: Boston. p. 306.
420. Habib R, Kleinknecht C, The primary nephrotic syndrome in childhood. Classification and clinicopathologic study of 406 cases, in *Pathology Annual*, Somers SC, Editor 1971, Appleton-Century Crofts: New York. p. 417–474.
421. Chinard FP, Lauson HD, Eder HA, et al. A study of the mechanism of proteinuria in patients with the nephrotic syndrome. *J. Clin. Invest.*, 1954;33:621.
422. Cortney MA, Sawin LL, Weiss DD. Renal tubular protein absorption int the rat. *J. Clin. Invest.*, 1970;49:1.
423. Cameron JS, Blandford G. The simple assessment of selectivity in heavy proteinuria. *Lancet*, 1966;ii:242.
424. Pesce AJ, Gaizutis M, Pollak VE. Selectivity of proteinuria: An evaluation of the immunochemical gel filtration techniques. *J. Lab. Clin. Med.*, 1970;75:586.
425. Ramjee G, Coovadia HM, Adhikari M. Sodium dodecyl sulfate polyacrylamide gel electrophoresis of urine proteins in steroid-responsive and steroid-resistant nephrotic syndrome in children. *Pediatr. Nephrol.*, 1994;8:653–656.
426. Habib R. Focal glomerulosclerosis. *Kidney Int.*, 1973;4:355–361.
427. Southwest Pediatric Nephrology Study Group. Focal segmental glomerulosclerosis in children with idiopathic nephrotic syndrome in children. A report of the southwest pediatric nephrology study group. *Kidney Int.*, 1985;27:442–449.
428. Pedersen EB, Danielsen H, Sorenson SS, et al. Renal water excretion before and after remission of nephrotic syndrome: relationship between free water clearance and kidney function, arginine vasopressin, angiotensin II and aldosterone in plasma before and after water loading. *Clin. Sci.*, 1986;71:97–104.
429. Trachtman H, Gauthier B. Platelet vasopressin levels in childhood idiopathic nephrotic syndrome. *Am. J. Dis. Child.*, 1988;142:1313.
430. Sheth KJ, Kher KK. Anion gap in nephrotic syndrome. *Int. J. Pediatr. Nephrol.*, 1984;2:89.
431. Alon U, Chan JCM. Calcium and vitamin D metabolism in nephrotic syndrome. *Int. J. Pediatr. Nephrol.*, 1983;4:115.
432. Strife CF, Jackson EC, Forristal J, et al. Effect of the nephrotic syndrome on the concentration of serum complement components. *Am. J. Kid. Dis.*, 1986;8:37–42.
433. Cairns SA, London RA, Mallick NP. Circulating immune complexes in idiopathic glomerular disease. *Kidney Int.*, 1982;21:507.
434. Levinsky RJ, Malleson PN, Barratt TM, et al. Circulating immune complexes in steroid-responsive nephrotic syndrome. *N. Engl. J. Med.*, 1978;298:126.
435. Churg J, Habib R, White RHR. Pathology of the nephrotic syndrome in children. A report for the International Study of Kidney Disease in Children. *Lancet*, 1970;1:1299–1302.
436. White RHR, Glasgow EF, Mills RJ. Clinicopathologic study of nephrotic syndrome in children. *Lancet*, 1970;i:1353–1359.
437. Farquhar MG, Vernier RL, Good RA. An electron microscope study of the glomerulus in nephrosis, glomerulonephritis, and lupus erythematosus. *J. Exp. Med.*, 1957;106:649.
438. Hoffmann EO. The detection of effaced podocytes by high resolution light microscopy. *Am. J. Clin. Pathol.*, 1982;78:508.
439. Churg J, Grishman E, Goldstein MH, et al. Idiopathic nephrotic syndrome in adults. *N. Engl. J. Med.*, 1965;272:165.
440. International Study of Kidney Disease in Children. The primary nephrotic syndrome in children. Identification of patients with minimal change nephrotic syndrome from initial response to prednisone. *J. Pediatr.*, 1981;98:561.
441. Shirato I. Podocyte process effacement in vivo. *Microsc Res Tech*, 2002;57:241–246.
442. Shirato I, Hosser H, Kimura K, et al. The development of focal segmental glomerulosclerosis in masugi nephritis is based on progressive podocyte damage. *Virchows Arch*, 1996;429:255–273.
443. Endlich K, Kriz W, Witzgall R. Update in podocyte biology. *Curr Opin Nephrol Hypertens*, 2001;10:331–340.
444. Kojima K, Davidovits A, Poczewski H, et al. Podocyte flattening and disorder of glomerular basement membrane are associated with splitting of dystroglycan-matrix interaction. *J Am Soc Nephrol*, 2004;15:2079–2089.
445. Regele HM, Fillipovic E, Langer B, et al. Glomerular expression of dystroglycans is reduced in minimal change nephrosis but not in focal segmental glomerulosclerosis. *J Am Soc Nephrol*, 2000;11:403–412.
446. Kojima K, Kerjaschki D. Is podocyte shape controlled by the dystroglycan complex? *Nephrol Dial Transplant*, 2002;17 Suppl 9:23–24.
447. Kriz W, Kretzler M, Provoost AP, et al. Stability and leakiness: opposing challenges to the glomerulus. *Kidney Int*, 1996;49:1570–1574.
448. Cohen AH, Border WA, Glassock RJ. Nephrotic syndrome with glomerular mesangial IgM deposits. *Lab Invest.*, 1978;38:610.
449. Murphy MJ, Bailey RR, McGiven AR. Is there an IgM nephropathy? *Aust. N.Z. J. Med.*, 1983;13:35.
450. Pardo V, Reisgo I, Zilleruello G, et al. The clinical significance of mesangial IgM deposits and mesangial hypercellularity in minimal change nephrotic syndrome. *Am. J. Kidney Dis.*, 1984;3:264.
451. Cavallo T, Johnson MP. Immunopathologic study of minimal change of glomerular disease with mesangial IgM depositsNephron 27:281, 1981. *Nephron*, 1981;27:281–284.
452. Haakenstad AO, Case JB, Mannik M. Effect of cortisone on the disappearance kinetics and tissue localization of soluble immune complexes. *J. Immunol.*, 1975;114:1153–1160
453. Larsen S. Immunofluorescent microscopy findings in minimal or no change disease and slight generalized mesangioproliferative glomerulonephritis. Fluorescent microscopy results correlated to symptoms and clinical cause. *Acta Pathol. Microbiol. Scand.*, 1978;86A:531.
454. Korbet SM, Genchi RM, Borok RZ, et al. The racial prevalence of glomerular lesions in nephrotic adults. *Am. J. Kidney Dis.*, 1996;27:647–651.
455. Fydryk J, Waldherr R, Mall G, et al. Mesangial alterations in steroid-responsive minimal change nephrotic syndrome. *Virchow's Arch. [Pathol. Anat.]*, 1982;397:193.
456. Allen WR, Travis LB, Cavallo T, et al. Immune deposits and mesangial hypercellularity in minimal change nephrotic syndrome: Clinical relevance. *J. Pediatr.*, 1982;100:188.
457. Ji-Yun Y, Melvin T, Sibley R, et al. No evidence for a specific role of IgM in mesangial proliferation of idiopathic nephrotic syndrome. *Kidney Int.*, 1984;25:100.
458. Vangelista A, Frasca G, Biagini G, et al. Long-term study of mesangial proliferative glomerulonephritis with IgM deposits. *Proc. Eur. Dial. Transplant. Assoc.*, 1981;18:503–507.
459. Hirszel P, Yamase HT, Carney WR, et al. Mesangial proliferative glomerulonephritis with IgM deposits. Clinicopathologic analysis and evidence for morphologic transitions. *Nephron*, 1984;38:100–108.
460. Waldherr R, Gubler MC, Levy M, et al. The significance of pure diffuse mesangial proliferation in idiopathic nephrotic syndrome. *Clin. Nephrol.*, 1978;10:171–179.
461. International Study of Kidney Disease in Children. Primary nephrotic syndrome in children: Clinical significance of histopathologic variants of minimal change and of diffuse mesangial hypercellularity. *Kidney Int.*, 1981;20:765.
462. Abboud HE, Poptic E, DiCorleto P. Production of platelet-derived growth factorlike protein by rat mesangial cells in culture. *J. Clin. Invest.*, 1987; 80:675–683.
463. Floege J, van Roeyen C, Boor P, et al. The role of PDGF-D in mesangioproliferative glomerulonephritis. *Contrib Nephrol*, 2007;157:153–158.
464. Hudkins KL, Gilbertson DG, Carling M, et al. Exogenous PDGF-D is a potent mesangial cell mitogen and causes a severe mesangial proliferative glomerulopathy. *J Am Soc Nephrol*, 2004;15:286–298.
465. Mene P, Abboud HE, Dunn MJ. Regulation of human mesangial cell growth in culture by thromboxane A_2 and prostacyclin. *Kidney Int.*, 1990;38: 232–239.
466. Lovett DH, Szamel M, Ryan JL, et al. Interleukin 1 and the glomerular mesangium: I. Purification and characterization of a mesangial cell-derived autogrowth factor. *J. Immunol.*, 1986;136:3700–3705.
467. Werber HI, Emancipator SN, Tykocinski ML, et al. The interleukin 1 gene is expressed by rat glomerular mesangial cells and is augmented in immune complex glomerulonephritis. *J. Immunol.*, 1987;138:3207.

468. Ruef C, Budde K, Lacy J, et al. Interleukin 6 is an autocrine growth factor for mesangial cells. *Kidney Int.*, 1990;38:249–257.
469. Suematsu S, Matsuda T, Aozasa K, et al. IgG1 plasmacytosis in interleukin 6 transgenic mice. *Proc. Natl. Acad. Sci. USA*, 1989;86:7547–7551.
470. Horii Y, Muraguchi A, Iwano M, et al. Involvement of IL–6 in mesangial proliferative glomerulonephritis. *J. Immunol.*, 1989;143:3949–3955.
471. Gordon C, Richards N, Howie AJ, et al. Urinary IL–6: a marker for mesangial proliferative glomerulonephritis? *Clin Exp Immunol*, 1991;86:145–149.
472. Jevnikar AM, Singer GG, Brennan DC, et al. Dexamethasone prevents autoimmune nephritis and reduces renal expression of Ia but not costimulatory signals. *Am J Pathol*, 1992;141:743–751.
473. Groggel GC, Marinides GN, Hovingh P, et al. Inhibition of rat mesangial cell growth by heparan sulfate. *Am. J. Physiol.*, 1990;259:F259.
474. Howie AJ. Pathology of minimal change nephropathy and segmental sclerosing glomerular disorders. *Nephrol Dial Transplant*, 2003;18 Suppl 6:vi33–38.
475. Forland M, Bannayan GA. Minimal-change lesion nephrotic syndrome with renal oncocytoma. *Am. J. Med.*, 1983;75:715–720.
476. Whelan TV, Hirszel P. Minimal-change nephropathy associated with pancreatic carcinoma. *Arch. Intern. Med.*, 1988;148:975–976.
477. Lines DR. Nephrotic syndrome and nephroloblastoma. Report of a case. *J. Pediatr.*, 1968;72:264–265.
478. Hory B, Saunier F, Wolff R, et al. Waldenstrom macroglobulinemia and nephrotic syndrome with minimal change lesion. *Nephron*, 1987;45:68–70.
479. Moorthy AV. Minimal change glomerular disease: A paraneoplastic syndrome in two patients with bronchogenic carcinoma. *Am. J. Kidney Dis.*, 1983;3:58–62.
480. Gandini E, Allaria P, Castilioni A, et al. Minimal change nephrotic syndrome with cecum adenocarcinoma. *Clin. Nephrol.*, 1996;45:268–270.
481. Ghosh L, Muehrcke RC. The nephrotic syndrome: A prodrome to lymphoma. *Ann. Intern. Med.*, 1970;72:379–382.
482. Huisman RM, deJong PE, de Zeeuw D, et al. Nephrotic syndrome preceding Hodgkin's disease by 42 months. *Clin. Nephrol.*, 1986;26:311–313.
483. Delmez JA, Safdar SH, Kissane JM. The successful treatment of recurrent nephrotic syndrome with the MOPP regimen in a patient with remote history of Hodgkin's disease. *Am. J. Kid. Dis.*, 1994;23:743–746.
484. Hyman LR, Burkholder PM, Joo PA, et al. Malignant lymphoma and nephrotic syndrome. A clinicopathologic analysis with light, immunofluorescence and electron microscopy of the renal lesion. *J. Pediatr.*, 1973;82:207–212.
485. Kiely JM, Wagoner RD, Holley KE. Renal complications of lymphoma. *Ann. Intern. Med.*, 1969;71:1159–1175.
486. Moorthy AV, Zimmerman SW, Burkholder PM. Nephrotic syndrome in Hodgkin's disease: Evidence for pathogenesis alternative to immune complex deposition. *Am. J. Med.*, 1976;61:471–477.
487. Mori T, Yabuhara A, Nakayama J, et al. Frequently relapsing minimal change nephrotic syndrome with natural killer cell deficiency prior to the overt relapse of Hodgkin's disease. *Pediatr. Nephrol.*, 1995;9:619–620.
488. Richards W, Olson D, Church JA. Improvement of idiopathic nephrotic syndrome following allergy therapy. *Ann. Allergy*, 1977;39:332.
489. Meadow SR, Brocklebank JT, Wainscott G. Anti-allergic drugs in idiopathic nephrotic syndrome of childhood. *Lancet*, 1978;i:1200.
490. Pirotzky E, Hieblot C, Benveniste J, et al. Basophil sensitization in idiopathic nephrotic syndrome. *Lancet*, 1982;1:358.
491. deMouzon-Cambon A, Bouissou F, Dutau G, et al. HLA-DR7 in children with idiopathic nephrotic syndrome. Correlation with atopy. *Tissue Antigens*, 1981;17:518.
492. Thomson PD, Barratt TM, Stokes CR, et al. HLA antigens and atopic features in steroid-responsive nephrotic syndrome of childhood. *Lancet*, 1976;ii:765.
493. Groshong T, Mendelson L, Mendoza S, et al. Serum IgE in patients with minimal-change nephrotic syndrome. *J. Pediatr.*, 1973;83:767.
494. Meadow SR, Sarsfield JK. Steroid-responsive nephrotic syndrome and allergy: Clinical studies. *Arch. Dis. Child.*, 1981;56:509.
495. Lagrue G, Laurent G, Hirbec G, et al. Serum IgE in primary glomerular disease. *Nephron*, 1984;36:5.
496. Gerber MA, Paronetto F. IgE in glomeruli of patients with nephrotic syndrome. *Lancet*, 1971;i:1097.
497. Schulte-Wisserman H, Gortz W, Straub E. IgE in patients with glomerulonephritis and minimal-change nephrotic syndrome. *Eur. J. Pediatr.*, 1979;131:105.
498. Trompeter RS, Thomson PD, Barratt TM, et al. Controlled trial of disodium cromoglycate in prevention of relapse of steroid-responsive nephrotic syndrome of childhood. *Arch. Dis. Child.*, 1978;53:430.
499. Lagrue G, Laurent J. Allergy and lipoid nephrosis. *Adv. Nephrol.*, 1983;12:151.
500. Laurent J, Rostoker G, Robeva R, et al. Is adult idiopathic nephrotic syndrome food allergy? Value of oligoantigenic diets. *Nephron*, 1987;47:7.
501. White RHR. The familial nephrotic syndrome. I. A European survey. *Clin. Nephrol.*, 1973;1:215.
502. Moncrieff MW, White RHR, Glasgow EF, et al. The familial nephrotic syndrome: II. A clinicopathologic study. *Clin. Nephrol.*, 1973;1:220–229.
503. Kleinknecht C, Gonzales G, Gubler MC. Familial nephrosis. *Pediatr. Res.*, 1980;14:1003 (Abstr.).
504. Chandra M, Mouradian J, Hoyer FR. Familial nephrotic syndrome and focal segmental glomerulosclerosis. *J. Pediatr.*, 1981;98:556–560.
505. Noss G, Bachmann HJ, Olbing H. Association of minimal change nephrotic syndrome (MCNS) with HLA-B8 and B–13. *Clin. Nephrol.*, 1981;15:172–174.
506. O'Regan D, O'Callaghan U, Dundon S, et al. HLA antigens and steroid responsive nephrotic syndrome of childhood. *Tissue Antigens*, 1980;16:147–151.
507. Alfiler CA, Roy LP, Doran T, et al. HLA-DRw7 and steroid-responsive nephrotic syndrome of childhood. *Clin. Nephrol.*, 1980;14:71.
508. Nunez-Roldan A, Villechenous E, Fernandez-Andrade C, et al. Increased HLA-DR7 and decreased DR2 in steroid-responsive nephrotic syndrome. *N. Engl. J. Med.*, 1982;306:366.
509. Bakr AM, El-Chenawy F. HLA-DQB1 and DRB1 alleles in Egyptian children with steroid-sensitive nephrotic syndrome. *Pediatr. Nephrol.*, 1998;12: 234–237.
510. Cambon-Thomsen A, Boissou F, Abbal M, et al. HLA et Bf dans le syndrome nephrotique idiopathique de l'enfant: differences entre les formes corticosensibles et corticoresistantes. *Path. Biol.*, 1986;34:725.
511. Haeffner A, Abbal M, Mytilineos J, et al. Oligotyping for HLA-DQA, -DQB, and -DPB in idiopathic nephrotic syndrome. *Pediatr. Nephrol.*, 1997;11:291–295.
512. Kobayashi Y, Chen X-M, Hiki Y, et al. Association of HLA-DRw8 and DQw3 with minimal change nephrotic syndrome in Japanese adults. *Kidney Int.*, 1985;28:193.
513. Lagueruela CC, Buettner TL, Cole BR, et al. HLA extended haplotypes in steroid-sensitive nephrotic syndrome of childhood. *Kidney Int.*, 1990;38: 145–150.
514. Ruder H, Scharer K, Opelz G, et al. Human leukocyte antigens in idiopathic nephrotic syndrome in children. *Pediatr. Nephrol.*, 1990;4:478–481.
515. Trompeter RS, Barratt TM, Kay R, et al. HLA, atopy and cyclophosphamide in steroid-responsive childhood nephrotic syndrome. *Kidney Int.*, 1980;17:113.
516. McEnery PT, Welch TE. Major histocompatibility complex antigens in steroid-responsive nephrotic syndrome. *Pediatr. Nephrol.*, 1989;3:33.
517. Konrad M, Mytilineos J, Bouissou F, et al. HLA class II associations with idiopathic nephrotic syndrome in children. *Tissue Antigens*, 1994;43:275–280.
518. Bouissou F, Meissner I, Konrad M, et al. Clinical implications from studies of HLA antigens in idiopathic nephrotic syndrome in children. *Clin Nephrol*, 1995;44:279–283.
519. Konrad M, Mytilineos J, Ruder H, et al. HLA-DR7 predicts the response to alkylating agents in steroid-sensitive nephrotic syndrome. *Pediatr. Nephrol.*, 1997;11:16–19.
520. Bakr AM, El-Chenawi F, Al-Husseni F. HLA alleles in frequently relapsing steroid-dependent and -resistant nephrotic syndrome in Egyptian children. *Pediatr Nephrol*, 2005;20:159–162.
521. Abe KK, Michinaga I, Hiratsuka T, et al. Association of DQB1*0302 alloantigens in Japanese pediatric patients with steroid-sensitive nephrotic syndrome. *Nephron*, 1995;70:28–34.
522. Kobayashi T, Ogawa A, Takahashi K, et al. HLA-DQB1 allele associates with idiopathic nephrotic syndrome in Japanese children. *Acta Paediatr Jpn*, 1995;37:293–296.
523. Cheung W, Ren EC, Chan SH, et al. Increased HLA- A*11 in Chinese children with steroid-responsive nephrotic syndrome. *Pediatr Nephrol*, 2002;17: 212–216.
524. Kari JA, Sinnott P, Khan H, et al. Familial steroid-responsive nephrotic syndrome and HLA antigens in Bengali children. *Pediatr Nephrol*, 2001;16:346–349.
525. Laurent J, Ansquer JC, deMouzon-Cambon A, et al. Adult onset lipoid nephrosis is not DR7 associated. *Tissue Antigens*, 1983;22:229.
526. Shalhoub RJ. Pathogenesis of lipoid nephrosis: A disorder of T-cells function. *Lancet*, 1976;ii:556.
527. Schnaper HW. The immune system in minimal change nephrotic syndrome. *Pediatric Nephrol.*, 1989;3:101.
528. Davin JC, Foidart JB, Mahieu PR. Fc receptor function in minimal change nephrotic syndrome of childhood. *Clin. Nephrol.*, 1983;20:280.
529. Madalinski K, Wyszynska T, Mikulska B, et al. Immune complexes in children with different forms of glomerulonephritis. *Arch. Immunol. Ther. Exp. (Warsz.)*, 1984;7:129.
530. Sølling J. Molecular weight of immune complexes in patients with glomerulonephritis. *Nephron*, 1982;30:137.

531. Brouhard BH, Goldblum RM, Bunce H III, et al. Immunoglobulin synthesis and urinary IgG excretion in the idiopathic nephrotic syndrome of children. *Int. J. Pediatr. Nephrol.*, 1981;2:163.
532. Ganguly NK, Singhal PC, Tewari SC, et al. Serum immunoglobulins in glomerulonephritis with special reference to minmal lesion glomerulonephritis. *J. Assoc. Physicians India*, 1979;27:1003.
533. Heslan JM, Lautie JP, Intrator L, et al. Impaired IgG synthesis in patients with the nephrotic syndrome. *Clin. Nephrol.*, 1982;18:144.
534. Rashid H, Skillen AW, Morley AR, et al. Serum immunoglobuins in minimal change nephrotic syndrome—A possible defect in T-cell function. *Bangladesh Med. Res. Council Bull.*, 1982;8:15.
535. Lange K, Ahmed U, Seligson G, et al. Depression of endostreptosin, streptolysin O and streptozyme antibodies in patients with idiopathic nephrosis with and without nephrotic syndrome. *Clin. Nephrol.*, 1981;15:279.
536. Moore DH, Shackelford PG, Robson AM, et al. Recurrent pneumococcal sepsis and defective opsonization after pneumococcal capsular polysaccharide vaccine in a child with nephrotic syndrome. *J. Pediatr.*, 1980;96:882–885.
537. Beale MG, Nash GS, Bertovich MJ, et al. Immunoglobulin synthesis by peripheral blood mononuclear cells in minimal change nephrotic syndrome. *Kidney Int.*, 1983;23:380.
538. Dall'Aglio P. Minimal change glomerulonephritis and focal glomerulosclerosis markers and 'in vitro' activity of peripheral blood mononuclear cells. *Proc. Eur. Dial. Transplant. Assoc.*, 1982;19:673.
539. Fiser RT, Arnold WC, Charlton RW, et al. T-lymphocyte subsets in nephrotic syndrome. *Kidney Int.*, 1991;40:913–916.
540. Herrod HG, Stapleton FB, Trouy RL, et al. Evaluation of T lymphocyte subpopulations in children with nephrotic syndrome. *Clin. Exp. Immunol.*, 1983;52:581.
541. Kerpen HO, Bhat JG, Kantor R, et al. Lymphocyte subpopulations in minimal change nephrotic syndrome. *Clin. Immunol. Immunopathol.*, 1979;14:130.
542. Tani Y, Kida H, Abe T, et al. B-lymphocyte subset patterns and their significance in idiopathic glomerulonephritis. *Clin. Exp. Immunol.*, 1982;48:201.
543. Eyres K, Mallick NP, Taylor G. Evidence for cell-mediated immunity to renal antigens in minimal-change nephrotic syndrome. *Lancet*, 1976;1:1158.
544. Eyres K, Mallick NP, Taylor G. Studies of cellular immune responses in patients with minimal change nephropathy. *Dial. Transplant. Nephol.*, 1976;11:533.
545. Fodor P, Saitua MT, Rodriguez E, et al. T-cell dysfunction in minimal-change nephrotic syndrome of childhood. *Am. J. Dis. Child.*, 1982;136:713.
546. Lin T-Y, Wang YM, Lin S-T. Application of a live varicella vaccine in children with acute leukemia or nephrotic syndrome. *J. Formosan Med. Assoc.*, 1981;70:683.
547. Matsumoto K, Osakabe K, Harada M, et al. Impaired cell-mediated immunity in lipoid nephrosis. *Nephron*, 1981;29:190.
548. Matsumoto K, Katayama H, Hatano M. Effect of thymic humoral factor on a local graft-versus-host reaction of lymphocytes in patients with lipoid nephrosis. (Letter). *Nephron*, 1982;32:279.
549. Chapman S, Taube D, Brown Z, et al. Impaired lymphocyte transformation in minimal change nephropathy in remission. *Clin. Nephrol.*, 1982;18:34.
550. Minchin MA, Turner KJ, Bower GD. Lymphocyte blastogenesis in nephrotic syndrome. *Clin. Exp. Immunol.*, 1980;42:241.
551. Osakabe K, Matsumoto K. Concanavalin A-induced suppressor cell activity in lipoid nephrosis. *Scand. J. Immunol.*, 1981;14:161.
552. Ooi BS, Orlina AR, Masaitis L. Lymphocytotoxins in primary renal disease. *Lancet*, 1974;ii:1348.
553. Smith MD, Barratt TM, Hayward AR, et al. The inhibitions of complement-dependent lymphocyte rosette formation by the sera of children with steroid-sensitive nephrotic syndrome and other renal diseases. *Clin. Exp. Immunol.*, 1975;21:236.
554. Tomizawa S, Suzuki S, Oguri M, et al. Studies of T lymphocyte function and inhibitory factors in minimal change nephrotic syndrome. *Nephron*, 1979;24:179.
555. Lin C-Y. Decreased antibody-dependent cellular cytotoxicity in minimal change nephrotic syndrome. *Pediatric Nephrol.*, 1988;2:224.
556. Saxena S, Mittal A, Andal A. Pattern of interleukins in minimal-change nephrotic syndrome of childhood. *Nephron*, 1993;65:56–61.
557. Hinoshita F, Noma T, Tomura S, et al. Decreased production and responsiveness of interleukin 2 in lymphocytes of patients with nephrotic syndrome. *Nephron*, 1990;54:122–126.
558. Matsumoto K. Decreased production of interleukin-1 by monocytes from patients with lipoid nephrosis. *Clin. Nephrol.*, 1989:292–296.
559. Barna BP, Makker S, Kallen R, et al. A lymphocytotoxic factor(s) in plasma of patients with minimal change nephrotic syndrome: partial characterization. *Clin. Immunol. Immunopathol.*, 1983;27:272.
560. Iitaka K, West CD. A serum inhibitor of blastogenesis in idiopathic nephrotic syndrome transferred by lymphocytes. *Clin. Immunol. Immunopathol.*, 1979;12:62.
561. Martini A, Vitiello MA, Siena S, et al. Multiple serum inhibitors of lectin-induced lymphocyte proliferation in nephrotic syndrome. *Clin. Exp. Immunol.*, 1981;45:178.
562. Mallick NP, Williams RJ, McFarlane H, et al. Cell-mediated immunity in nephrotic syndrome. *Lancet*, 1972;i:507.
563. Lagrue G, Branellec A, Blanc C, et al. A vascular permeability factor in lymphocyte culture supernatants from patients with nephrotic syndrome. II. Pharmacological and physicochemical properties. *Biomedicine*, 1975;23:73.
564. Monacci WT, Merrill MJ, Oldfield EH. Expression of vascular permeability factor/vascular endothelial growth factor in normal rat tissues. *Am. J. Physiol.*, 1993;264:C995–C1002.
565. Schnaper HW, Aune TM. Identification of the lymphokine soluble immune response suppressor in urine of nephrotic children. *J. Clin. Invest.*, 1985;76:341.
566. Schnaper HW, Aune TM. Steroid-sensitive mechanism of soluble immune response suppressor production in patients with steroid-responsive nephrotic syndrome. *J. Clin. Invest.*, 1987;79:254.
567. Suranyi MG, Gausch A, Hall BM, et al. Elevated levels of tumor necrosis factor-alpha in the nephrotic syndrome in humans. *Am. J. Kidney Dis.*, 1993;21:251–259.
568. Robeva R, Heslan JM, Branellec A, et al. Enhanced β2-microglobulin levels in lymphocyte culture supernatants from patients with idiopathic nephrotic syndrome; inhibition of lymphocyte activation by cyclosporine. *Clin. Nephrol.*, 1988;30:211–215.
569. Bock GH, Ongkingco JR, Patterson LT, et al. Serum and urine soluble interleukin-2 receptor in idiopathic nephrotic syndrome. *Pediatr. Nephrol.*, 1993;7:523–528.
570. Hulton SA, Shah V, Byrne MR, et al. Lymphocyte subpopulations, interleukin-2 and interleukin-2 receptor expression in childhood nephrotic syndrome. *Pediatr. Nephrol.*, 1994;8:135–139.
571. Mandreoli M, Beltrandi E, Casadei-Maldini M, et al. Lymphocyte release of soluble IL-2 receptors in patients with minimal change nephropathy. *Clin. Nephrol.*, 1992;37:177–182.
572. Ohno I, Gomi H, Matsuda H, et al. Soluble IL-2 receptor in patients with primary nephrotic syndrome. *Nippon Jinzo Gakkai Shi.*, 1991;33:483–489.
573. Neuhaus JT, Wadhwa M, Callard R, et al. Increased IL-2, IL-4 and interferon gamma (IFN-γ) in steroid-sensitive nephrotic syndrome. *Clin. Exp. Immunol.*, 1995;100:475–479.
574. Yap HK, Cheung W, Murugasu B, et al. Th1 and Th2 cytokine mTNA profiles in childhood nephrotic syndrome: evidence for increased IL-13 mRNA expression in relapse. *J. Am. Soc. Nephrol.*, 1999;10:529–537.
575. Chan MK, Chan KW, Jones B. Immunoglobulins (IgG, IgA, IgM, IgE) and complement components (C_3, C_4) in nephrotic syndrome due to minimal change and other forms of glomerulonephritis, a clue for steroid therapy? *Nephron*, 1987;47:125.
576. Harris HW, Umetsu D, Geha R, et al. Altered immunoglobulin status in congenital nephrotic syndrome. *Clin. Nephrol.*, 1986;25:308.
577. Al-Bander HA, Martin VI, Kaysen GA. Plasma IgG pool is not defended from urinary loss in nephrotic syndrome. *Am J. Physiol.*, 1992;262:F333-F337.
578. Tejani A, Fikrig S, Schiffman G, et al. Persistence of protective pneumococcal antibody following vaccination in patients with nephrotic syndrome. *Am. J. Nephrol.*, 1984;4:32.
579. Lin C-Y, Chen C-H, Lee P-P. In vitro B-lymphocyte switch disturbance from IgM into IgG in IgM mesangial nephropathy. *Pediatric Nephrol.*, 1989;3:254.
580. Stachura I, Si L, Madan E, et al. Mononuclear cell subsets in human renal disease. Enumeration in tissue sections with monoclonal antibody. *Clin. Immunol. Immunopathol.*, 1984;30:362.
581. Nagata K, Platt JL, Michael AF. Interstitial and glomerular immune cell populations in idiopathic nephrotic syndrome. *Kidney Int.*, 1984;25:88.
582. Benz K, Buttner M, Dittrich K, et al. Characterisation of renal immune cell infiltrates in children with nephrotic syndrome. *Pediatr Nephrol*, 2010;25:1291–1298.
583. Cagnoli L, Tabacchi P, Pasquali S, et al. T cell subset alterations in idiopathic glomerulonephritis. *Clin. Exp. Immunol.*, 1982;50:70.
584. Kemper MJ, Meyer-Jark T, Lilova M, et al. Combined T- and B-cell activation in childhood steroid-sensitive nephrotic syndrome. *Clin Nephrol*, 2003;60:242–247.
585. Matsumoto K, Osakabe K, Hatano M. Impaired cell-mediated immunity in idiopathic membranous nephropathy mediated by suppressor cells. *Clin. Nephrol.*, 1983;19:213.
586. Kobayashi K, Yoshikawa N, Nakamura H. T-cell subpopulations in childhood nephrotic syndrome. *Clin. Nephrol.*, 1994;41:253–258.
587. Stachowski J, Barth C, Michalkiewicz J, et al. Th1/Th2 balance and CD45-positive T cell subsets in primary nephrotic syndrome. *Pediatr Nephrol*, 2000;14:779–785.

588. Matsumoto K. Impaired local graft-versus host reaction in lipoid nephrosis. (Letter). *Nephron*, 1982;31:281.
589. Wu MJ, Moorthy AV. Suppressor cell function in patients with primary glomerular disease. *Clin. Immunol. Immunopathol.*, 1982;22:442.
590. Beale MG, Hoffsten PE, Robson AM, et al. Inhibitory factors of lymphocyte transformation in sera from patients with minimal change nephrotic syndrome. *Clin. Nephrol.*, 1980;13:271.
591. Moorthy AV, Zimmerman SW, Burkholder PM. Inhibition of lymphocyte blastogenesis by plasma of patients with minimal-change nephrotic syndrome. *Lancet*, 1976;i:1160.
592. Taube D, Chapman S, Brown Z, et al. Depression of normal lymphocyte transformation by sera of patients with minimal change nephropathy and other forms of nephrotic syndrome. *Clin. Nephrol.*, 1981;15:286.
593. Lenarsky C, Jordan SC, Ladisch S. Plasma inhibition of lymphocyte proliferation in nephrotic syndrome: Correlation with hyperlipidemia. *J. Clin. Immunol.*, 1982;2:276.
594. Chisari FV. Immunoregulatory properties of human plasma in very low density lipoproteins. *J. Immunol.*, 1977;119:2129.
595. Curtiss LK, Edgington TS. Regulatory serum lipoproteins: Regulation of lymphocyte stimulation by a species of low density lipoprotein. *J. Immunol.*, 1976;118:1452.
596. Faucher C, Albert C, Beaufils H, et al. Remission of a refractory nephrotic syndrome after low-density lipoprotein apheresis based on dextrane sulphate adsorption. *Nephrol. Dial. Transpl.*, 1997;12:1037–1039.
597. Cho B-S, Yoon S-R, Jang J-Y, et al. Up-regulation of interleukin-4 and CD23/FcϵRII in minimal change nephrotic syndrome. *Pediatr. Neprhol.*, 1999;13:199–204.
598. Schnaper HW, Pierce CW, Aune TM. Identification and initial characterization of concanavalin A- and interferon-induced human suppressor factors: Evidence for a human equivalent of murine soluble immune response suppressor (SIRS). *J. Immunol.*, 1984;132:2429.
599. Schnaper HW, Aune TM. Suppression of immune responses to sheep erythrocytes by the lymphokine soluble immune response suppressor (SIRS) in vivo. *J. Immunol.*, 1986;137:863.
600. Schnaper HW. A regulatory system for soluble immune response suppressor production in steroid-responsive nephrotic syndrome. *Kidney Int.*, 1990;38:151.
601. Doi T, Kanatsu K, al e. Circulating immune complexes of IgG, IgA and IgM classes in various glomerular diseases. *Nephron.*, 1982;32:335.
602. Abrass CK. Circulating immune complexes in adults with idiopathic nephrotic syndrome. *Kidney Int.*, 1980;17:545.
603. Isaacs KL, Miller F. Antigen size and charge in immune complex glomerulonephritis. *Am. J. Pathol.*, 1983;111:298.
604. Iskandar SS, Jennette JC. Influence of antibody avidity on glomerular immune complex localization. *Am J Pathol*, 1983;112:155–159.
605. Sherman RL, Susin M, Wexler ME. Lipoid nephrosis in Hodgkin's disease. *Am. J. Med.*, 1972;52:699.
606. Crowley JP, Ree HJ, Esparza A. Monocyte-dependent serum suppression of lymphcyte blastogenesis in Hodgkin's disease: An association with nephrotic syndrome. *J. Clin. Immunol.*, 1982;2:270.
607. Shimoyama H, Nakajima M, Naka H, et al. Up-regulation of interleukin-2 mRNA in children with idiopathic nephrotic syndrome. *Pediatr Nephrol*, 2004;19:1115–1121.
608. Sakurai M, Muso E, Matushima H, et al. Rapid normalization of interleukin-8 production after low-density lipoprotein apheresis in steroid-resistant nephrotic syndrome. *Kidney Int Suppl*, 1999;71:S210–212.
609. Kim SD, Park JM, Kim IS, et al. Association of IL-1beta, IL-1ra, and TNF-alpha gene polymorphisms in childhood nephrotic syndrome. *Pediatr Nephrol*, 2004;19:295–299.
610. Kawasaki K, Yaoita E, Yamamoto T, et al. Antibodies against intercellular adhesion molecule-1 and lymphocyte function-associated antigen-1 prevent glomerular injury in rat experimental crescentic glomerulonephritis. *J. Immunol.*, 1993;150:1074–1083.
611. Holdsworth SR, Neale TJ, Wilson CB. Abrogation of macrophage-dependent injury in experimental glomerulonephritis in the rabbit. *J. Clin. Invest.*, 1981;68:686.
612. Kreisberg JE, Wayne DB, Karnovsky MJ. Rapid and focal loss of negative charge associated with mononuclear cell infiltration early in nephrotoxic serum nephritis. *Kidney Int.*, 1979;16:290.
613. Sellier-Leclerc AL, Duval A, Riveron S, et al. A humanized mouse model of idiopathic nephrotic syndrome suggests a pathogenic role for immature cells. *J Am Soc Nephrol*, 2007;18:2732–2739.
614. Tomizawa S, Maruyama K, Nagasawa N, et al. Studies of vascular permeability factor derived from T lymphocytes and inhibitory effect of plasma on its production in minimal change nephrotic syndrome. *Nephron*, 1985;41:157.
615. Bakker WW, Baller JFW, vanLuijk WHJ, et al. A kallikrein-like molecule and vasoactivity in minimal change disease. Increased turnover in relapse vs. remission. *Contr. Nephrol.*, 1988;67:31.
616. Dejana E, Lampugnani MG, Martinez-Estrada O, et al. The molecular organization of endothelial junctions and their functional role in vascular morphogenesis and permeability. *Int J Dev Biol*, 2000;44:743–748.
617. Risau W. Development and differentiation of endothelium. *Kidney Int Suppl*, 1998;67:S3–6.
618. Bakker WW, Beukhof JR, VanLuijh WH, et al. Vascular permeability increasing factor (VPF) in IgA nephropathy. *Clin. Nephrol.*, 1982;18:165.
619. Matsumoto K, Kanmatsuse K. Interleukin-15 and interleukin 12 have an additive effect on the release of vascular permeability factor by peripheral blood mononuclear cells in normals and in patients with nephrotic syndrome. *Clin. Nephrol.*, 1999;52:10–18.
620. Koyama A, Fuijisak M, Kobayashi M, et al. A glomerular permeability factor produced by human Tcell hybridomas. *Kidney Int.*, 1991;40:453.
621. Tanaka R, Yoshikawa N, Nakamura H, et al. Infusion of peripheral blood mononuclear cell products from nephrotic children increases albuminuria in rats. *Nephron*, 1992;60:35–41.
622. Garin EH, Laflam P, Chandler L. Anti-interleukin 8 antibody abolishes effects of lipoid nephrosis cytokine. *Pediatr. Nephrol.*, 1998;12:381–385.
623. Daniel V, Trautmann Y, Konrad M, et al. T-lymphocyte populations, cytokines and other growth factors in serum and urine of children with idiopathic nephrotic syndrome. *Clin. Nephrol.*, 1997;47:289–297.
624. Bakr A, Shokeir M, El-Chenawi F, et al. Tumor necrosis factor-alpha production from mononuclear cells in nephrotic syndrome. *Pediatr Nephrol*, 2003;18:516–520.
625. Raveh D, Shemesh O, Ashkenazi YJ, et al. Tumor necrosis factor-alpha blocking agent as a treatment for nephrotic syndrome. *Pediatr Nephrol*, 2004;19:1281–1284.
626. Cheung W, Wei CL, Seah CC, et al. Atopy, serum IgE, and interleukin-13 in steroid-responsive nephrotic syndrome. *Pediatr Nephrol*, 2004;19:627–632.
627. Lai KW, Wei CL, Tan LK, et al. Overexpression of interleukin-13 induces minimal-change-like nephropathy in rats. *J Am Soc Nephrol*, 2007;18:1476–1485.
628. Joffe MI, Rabson AR. Dissociation of lymphokine production and blastogenesis in children with measles infection. *Clin. Immunol. Immunopathol.*, 1978;10:335.
629. Finkelstein A, Fraley DS, Stachura I. Fenprofen nephropathy: Lipoid nephrosis and interstitial nephritis. A possible T-lymphocyte disorder. *Am. J. Med.*, 1982;72:81.
630. Watson AJS, Dalbow MH, Stachura I, et al. Immunologic studies in cimetidine-induced nephropathy and polymyositis. *N. Engl. J. Med.*, 1983;308:142.
631. Taube D, Brown Z, Williams DG. Longterm impairment of suppressor-cell function by cyclophosphamide in minimal-change nephropathy and its association with therapeutic response. *Lancet*, 1981;1:235.
632. Feehally J, Beattie TJ, Brenchley PEC, et al. Modulation of cellular immune function by cyclophosphamide in children with minimal change nephropathy. *N. Engl. J. Med.*, 1984;310:415.
633. Averbuch SD, Austin HA III, Sherwin SA, et al. Acute interstitial nephritis with the nephrotic syndrome following recombinant leukocyte A interferon therapy for mycosis fungoides. *N. Engl. J. Med.*, 1984;310:32.
634. Niaudet P, Drachman R, Gagnadoox MF, et al. Treatment of idiopathic nephrotic syndrome with levamisole. *Acta Paediatr. Scand.*, 1984;76:637.
635. Nephrology BAfP. Levamisole for corticosteroid dependent nephrotic syndrome in childhood. *Lancet*, 1991;337:1555–1557.
636. Abe Y, Sekiya S, Yamasita T, et al. Vascular hyperpermeability induced by tumor necrosis factor and its augmentation by IL-1 and IFN-γ is inhibited by selective depletion of neutrophils with a monoclonal antibody. *J. Immunol.*, 1990;145:2902.
637. Zhang SY, Kamal M, Dahan K, et al. c-mip impairs podocyte proximal signaling and induces heavy proteinuria. *Sci Signal*, 2010;3:ra39.
638. Audard V, Zhang SY, Copie-Bergman C, et al. Occurrence of minimal change nephrotic syndrome in classical Hodgkin lymphoma is closely related to the induction of c-mip in Hodgkin-Reed Sternberg cells and podocytes. *Blood*, 2010;115:3756–3762.
639. Gault MH, Muehrcke RC. Renal biopsy: Current views and controversies. (Editorial). *Nephron*, 1983;34:1.
640. Thompson AL, Durrett RR, Robinson RR. Fixed and reproducible orthostatic proteinuria. VI. Results of a 10-year follow-up evaluation. *Ann Intern Med*, 1970;73:235–244.
641. Lau J, Levey AS, Kassirer JP, et al. Idiopathic nephrotic syndrome in a 53 year old woman. Is a kidney biopsy necessary? *Med. Decision Making*, 1982;2:497–519.
642. Webb NJA, Lewis MA, Iqbal J, et al. Childhood steroid-sensitive nephrotic syndrome: does histology matter? *Am. J. Kidney Dis.*, 1996;27:484–488.

643. Cornfeld D, Schwartz MW. Nephrosis: A long-term study of children treated with corticosteroids. *J. Pediatr.*, 1966.;68:507.
644. Barness LA, Moll GH, Janeway CA. Nephrotic syndrome. I. Natural history of the disease. *Pediatrics*, 1949;5:486.
645. Coggins CH, Minimal change nephrosis in adults, in *Proceedings of the Eighth International Congress of Nephrology: Advances in Basic and Clinical Nephrology*, Zurukzoglu W, Papadimitriou M, Pyrpasopoulis M, et al., Editors. 1981, S. Karger: Basel. p. 336.
646. Moxey-Mims MM, Stapelton FB, Feld LD. Applying decision analysis to management of adolescent idiopathic nephrotic syndrome. *Pediatr. Nephrol.*, 1994;8:660–664.
647. McEnery PT, Strife CF. Nephrotic syndrome in childhood. Management and treatment in patients with minimal change disease, mesangial proliferation, or focal glomerulosclerosis. *Prediatr. Clin. North Am.*, 1982;29:875–894.
648. Hodson EM, Knight JF, Willis NS, et al. Corticosteroid therapy for nephrotic syndrome in children. *Cochrane Database Syst Rev*, 2004:CD001533.
649. Troyanov S, Wall CA, Miller JA, et al. Focal and segmental glomerulosclerosis: definition and relevance of a partial remission. *J Am Soc Nephrol*, 2005;16:1061–1068.
650. Bohrer MP, Deen WM, Robertson C, et al. Mechanism of angiotensin II-induced proteinuria in the rat. *Am. J. Physiol.*, 1977;233:F13.
651. Ehrich JH, Brodehl J. Long versus standard prednisone therapy for initial treatment of idiopathic nephrotic syndrome. Arbeitsgemeinschaft fur Padiatrische Nephrologie. *European J. Pediatr.*, 1993;152:357–361.
652. Lande MB, Gullion C, Hogg RJ, et al. Long versus standard initial steroid therapy for children with the nephrotic syndrome. A report from the Southwest Pediatric Nephrology Study Group. *Pediatr Nephrol*, 2003;18:342–346.
653. International Study of Kidney Disease in Children. Nephrotic syndrome in children: A randomized trial comparing two prednisone regimens in steroid-responsive patients who relapse early. *J. Pediatr.*, 1979;95:239.
654. Arbeitsgemeinschaft fur Padiatrische Nephrologie. Short versus standard prednisone therapy for initial treatment of idiopathic nephrotic syndrome in children. *Lancet*, 1988;i:380.
655. Constantinescu AR, Shah HB, Foote EF, et al. Predicting first-year relapses in children with nephrotic syndrome. *Pediatrics*, 2000;105:492–495.
656. Nakayama M, Katafuchi R, Yanase T, et al. Steroid responsiveness and frequency of relapse in adult-onset minimal change nephrotic syndrome. *Am J Kidney Dis*, 2002;39:503–512.
657. Kim PK, Kim NA, Kim KS, et al. Steroid effects on minimal lesion nephrotic syndrome with and without immune deposits. *Int. J. Pediatr. Nephrol.*, 1983;3:257.
658. Brown EA, Upadhyaya K, Hayslett JP, et al. The clinical course of mesangial proliferative glomerulonephritis. *Medicine (Baltimore)*, 1979;58:295.
659. Hopper J, Jr., Ryan P, Lee JC. Lipoid nephrosis in 31 adult patients: Renal biopsy study by light, electron and fluorescent microscopy with experience in treatment. *Medicine*, 1970;49:321.
660. Schnaper HW. Immunization practices in childhood nephrotic syndrome: a survey of North American pediatric nephrologists. *Pediatr. Nephrol.*, 1994;8:4–6.
661. Steele RW. Current status of vaccines and immune globulins in children with renal disease. *Pediatr. Nephrol.*, 1994;8:7–10.
662. Koskimies O, Vilska J, Rapola J, et al. Long-term outcome of primary nephrotic syndrome. *Arch. Dis. Child.*, 1982;57:544.
663. International Study of Kidney Disease in Children. Early identification of frequent relapsers among children with minimal change nephrotic syndrome. *J. Pediatr.*, 1982;101:514.
664. Andersen RF, Thrane N, Noergaard K, et al. Early age at debut is a predictor of steroid-dependent and frequent relapsing nephrotic syndrome. *Pediatr Nephrol*, 2010;25:1299–1304.
665. Wingen A-M, Muller-Wiefel DE, Scharer K. Comparison of different regimens of prednisone therapy in frequently relapsing nephrotic syndrome. *Acta Paediatr. Scand.*, 1990;79:305.
666. Leisti S, Vilska J, Hallman N. Adrenocortical insufficiency and relapsing in the idiopathic nephrotic syndrome of childhood. *Pediatrics*, 1977;60:334.
667. Schoeneman MJ. Minimal change nephrotic syndrome: Treatment with low doses of hydrocortisone. *J. Pediatr.*, 1983;102:791.
668. West CD. Use of combined hormone and mechlorethamine (nitrogen mustard) therapy in lipoid nephrosis. *Am. J. Dis. Child.*, 1958;95:498.
669. Lewis EJ. Chlorambucil for childhood nephrotic syndrome. A word of caution. *N. Engl. J. Med.*, 1980;302:963.
670. Schulman SL, Kaiser BA, Polinsky MS, et al. Predicting the response to cytotoxic therapy for childhood nephrotic syndrome: superiority of response to corticosteroid therapy over histopathologic patterns. *J. Pediatr.*, 1988;113:996.
671. McCrory WW, Shibuya M, Lu W-H, et al. Therapeutic and toxic effects observed with different dosage programs of cyclophosphamide in treatment of steroid-responsive but frequently relapsing nephrotic syndrome. *J. Pediatr.*, 1973;82:614.
672. Barratt TM, Soothill JF. Controlled trial of cyclophosphamide in steriod-sensitive relapsing nephrotic syndrome of childhood. *Lancet*, 1970;2:479.
673. Cameron JS, Chantler C, Ogg CS, et al. Long-term remission in nephrotic syndrome after treatment with cyclophosphamide. *Br. Med. J.*, 1974;4:7.
674. International Study of Kidney Disease in Children. Prospective, controlled trial of cyclophosphamide therapy in children with the nephrotic syndrome. *Lancet*, 1974;ii:423.
675. Arbeitsgemeinschaft fur Padiatrische Nephrologie. Effect of cytoxic drugs in frequently relapsing nephrotic syndrome with and without steroid dependence. *N. Engl. J. Med.*, 1982;306:451.
676. Dundon S, O'Callaghan U, Raftery J. Stability of remission in minimal lesion nephrotic syndrome after treatment with prednisone and cyclophosphamide. *Int. J. Pediatr. Nephrol.*, 1980;1:22.
677. McDonald J, Murphy AV, Arneil GC. Long-term assessment of cyclophosphamide therapy for nephrosis in children. *Lancet.*, 1974;ii:980.
678. Etteldorf JN, West CD, Pitcock JA, et al. Gonadal function, testicular histology and meiosis following cyclophosphamide. *J. Pediatr.*, 1976;88:206.
679. Lentz RD, Bergstein J, Steffes MW, et al. Postpubertal evaluation of gonadal function following cyclophosphamide therapy before and during puberty. *J. Pediatr.*, 1977;91:385.
680. Trompeter RS, Evans PR, Barratt TM. Gonadal function in boys with steroid-responsive nephrotic syndrome treated with cyclophosphamide for short periods. *Lancet*, 1981;i:1177.
681. Rivkees SA, Crawford JD. The relationship of gonadal activity and chemotherapy-induced gonadal damage. *J. Am. Med. Assn.*, 1988;259:2123–2125.
682. Bogdanovic R, Banicevic M, Cvoric A. Pituitary-gonadal function in women following cyclophosphamide treatment for childhood nephrotic syndrome: long -term follow-up study. *Pediatr. Nephrol.*, 1990;4:455.
683. Parra A, Santos D, Cervantes C, et al. Plasma gonadotropins and gonadal steroids in children treated with cyclophosphamide. *J. Pediatr.*, 1978;92:117.
684. Masala A, Faedda R, Alagna S, et al. Use of testosterone to prevent cyclophosphamide-induced azoospermia. *An. Intern. Med.*, 1997;126:292–295.
685. Blumenfeld Z, Haim N. Prevention of gonadal damage during cytotoxic therapy. *Ann. Med.*, 1997;29:199–206.
686. Kuis W, DeKraker J, Kuijten RH, et al. Acute lymphoblastic leukemia after treatment of nephrotic syndrome with immunosuppressive drugs. *Helv. Paediatr. Acta*, 1976;31:91.
687. Elzouki AY, Al-Nassar K, Al-Ali M, et al. Sister chromatid exchange analysis in monitoring chlorambucil therapy in primary nephrotic syndrome of childhood. *Pediatr. Nephrol.*, 1991;5:59.
688. Jones BF. Cyclophosphamide pulse therapy in frequently relapsing nephrotic syndrome. *Nephron*, 1993;63:472.
689. Williams SA, Makker SP, Grupe WE. Seizures: A significant side effect of chlorambucil therapy in children. *J. Pediatr.*, 1978;93:516.
690. Matsui A, Takezawa N, Suzuki K, et al. Neurotoxicity of chlorambucil and cyclophosphamide therapy in steroid-dependent and/or frequently relapsing nephrotic syndrome. *Pediatric Nephrol.*, 1989;3:C167.
691. Kleinknecht C, Guesry P, Lenoir G, et al. High-cost benefit of chorambucil in frequently relapsing nephrotic syndrome. *N. Engl. J. Med.*, 1977;296:48.
692. Muller W, Brandis Mx. Acute leukemia after cytotoxic treatment for nonmalignant disease in childhood. A case report and review of the literature. *Eur. J. Pediatr.*, 1981;136:105.
693. Grupe WE, Makker SP, Ingelfinger IR. Chlorambucil treatment of frequently relapsing nephrotic syndrome. *N. Engl. J. Med.*, 1976;295:746.
694. Williams SA, Makker SP, Inglefinger JR, et al. Long-term evaluation of chlorambucil plus prednisone in the idiopathic nephrotic syndrome of childhood. *N. Engl. J. Med.*, 1980;302:929.
695. Elzouki AT, Jaiswal OP. Evaluation of chlorambucil therapy in steroid-dependent and cyclophosphamide-resistant children with nephrosis. *Pediatr. Nephrol.*, 1990;4:459.
696. Durkan AM, Hodson EM, Willis NS, et al. Immunosuppressive agents in childhood nephrotic syndrome: a meta-analysis of randomized controlled trials. *Kidney Int*, 2001;59:1919–1927.
697. Niaudet P, Habib R. Cyclosporine in the treatment of idiopathic nephrosis. *J. Am. Soc. Nephrol.*, 1994;5:1049–1056.
698. Rinaldi S, Sesto A, Barsotti P, et al. Cyclosporine therapy monitored with abbreviated area under curve in nephrotic syndrome. *Pediatr Nephrol*, 2005;20:25–29.
699. Gregory MJ, Smoyer WE, Sedman A, et al. Long-term cyclosporine therapy for pediatric nephrotic syndrome: a clinical and histologic analysis. *J. Am. Soc. Nephrol.*, 1996;7:543–549.

700. Hymes LC. Steroid-resistant, cyclosporine-responsive, relapsing nephrotic syndrome. *Pediatr Nephrol*, 1995;9:137–139.
701. Ginevri F, Trivelli A, Ciardi MR, et al. Protracted levamisole in children with frequently relapsing nephrotic syndrome. *Pediatr. Nephrol.*, 1996;10:550.
702. Palcoux JB, Niaudet P, Goumy P. Side effects of levamisole in children with nephrosis. *Pediatr. Nephrol.*, 1994;8:263–264.
703. Day CJ, Cockwell P, Lipkin GW, et al. Mycophenolate mofetil in the treatment of resistant idiopathic nephrotic syndrome. *Nephrol Dial Transplant*, 2002;17:2011–2013.
704. Bagga A, Hari P, Moudgil A, et al. Mycophenolate mofetil and prednisolone therapy in children with steroid-dependent nephrotic syndrome. *Am J Kidney Dis*, 2003;42:1114–1120.
705. Barletta GM, Smoyer WE, Bunchman TE, et al. Use of mycophenolate mofetil in steroid-dependent and -resistant nephrotic syndrome. *Pediatr Nephrol*, 2003;18:833–837.
706. Hogg RJ, Fitzgibbons L, Bruick J, et al. Mycophenolate mofetil in children with frequently relapsing nephrotic syndrome: a report from the Southwest Pediatric Nephrology Study Group. *Clin J Am Soc Nephrol*, 2006;1:1173–1178.
707. Dorresteijn EM, Kist-van Holthe JE, Levtchenko EN, et al. Mycophenolate mofetil versus cyclosporine for remission maintenance in nephrotic syndrome. *Pediatr Nephrol*, 2008;23:2013–2020.
708. Gulati A, Sinha A, Jordan SC, et al. Efficacy and safety of treatment with rituximab for difficult steroid-resistant and -dependent nephrotic syndrome: multicentric report. *Clin J Am Soc Nephrol*, 2010;5:2207–2212.
709. Hodson EM, Craig JC. Therapies for steroid-resistant nephrotic syndrome. *Pediatr Nephrol*, 2008;23:1391–1394.
710. Rowe PC, McLean RH, Ruley EJ, et al. Intravenous immunoglobulin in minimal change nephrotic syndrome: a crossover trial. *Pediatr. Nephrol.*, 1990;4:32–35.
711. Murnaghan K, Vasmant D, Bensman A. Pulse methylprednisolone therapy in severe idiopathic childhood nephrotic syndrome. *Acta Paediatr. Scand.*, 1984;73:733.
712. Arbeitsgemeinschaft fur Padiatrische Nephrologie. Cyclophosphamide treatment of steroid dependent nephrotic syndrome: comparison of eight week with 12 week course. *Arch. Dis. Child.*, 1987;62:1102.
713. Niaudet P. Comparison of cyclosporine and chlorambucil in the treatment of steroid dependent idiopathic nephrotic syndrome: a multicenter randomized controlled trial. The French Society of Paediatric Nephrology. *Pediatr. Nephrol.*, 1992;6:1–3.
714. Hulton. Long-term cyclosporin A treatment of minimal-change nephrotic syndrome of childhood. *Pediatr. Nephrol.*, 1994;8:401–403.
715. Hulton. Effect of cyclosporin A on glomerular filtration rate in children with minimal change nephrotic syndrome. *Pediatr. Nephrol.*, 1994;8:404–407.
716. Inoue Y, Iijima K, Nakamura H, et al. Two-year cyclosporin treatment in children with steroid-dependent nephrotic syndrome. *Pediatr. Nephrol.*, 1999;13:33–38.
717. Ponticelli C, Rissoni G, Edefonti A, et al. A randomized trial of cyclosporin in steroid-resistant nephrotic syndrome. *Kidney Int.*, 1993;43:1377–1384.
718. Takeda A, Ohgushi H, Niimura F, et al. Long-term effects of immunosuppresants in steroid-dependent nephrotic syndrome. *Pediatr. Nephrol.*, 1998;12:746–750.
719. Brodehl J. In what order should one introduce cyclophosphamide, or chlorambucil, cyclosporine or levamisole in a child with steroid-dependent, frequently relapsing nephrotic syndrome? *Pediatr. Nephrol.*, 1993;7:514.
720. Baudouin V, Alberti C, Lapeyraque AL, et al. Mycophenolate mofetil for steroid-dependent nephrotic syndrome: a phase II Bayesian trial. *Pediatr Nephrol*, 2011;27:389–396.
721. Sinha A, Bagga A, Gulati A, et al. Short-term efficacy of rituximab versus tacrolimus in steroid-dependent nephrotic syndrome. *Pediatr Nephrol*, 2012;27:235–241.
722. Melvin T, Sibley R, Michael AF, Nephrotic syndrome, in *Contemporary Issues in Nephrology. Pediatric Nephrology*, Tune BM, Mendoza SA, Editors. 1984, Churchill Livingstone: New York. p. 191–230.
723. Zech P, Colon S, Pointet P, et al. The nephrotic syndrome in adults aged over 60: Etiology, evolution, and treatment of 76 cases. *Clin. Nephrol.*, 1982;17:232–236.
724. Yeung CK, Wong KL, Ng WL. Intravenous methylprednisolone pulse therapy in minimal change nephrotic syndrome. *Aust. N.Z. J. Med.*, 1983;13:349.
725. Alkhader AA, Lien JW, Aber GM. Cyclophosphamide alone in the treatment of adult patients with minimal change glomerulonephritis. *Clin. Nephrol.*, 1979;11:26.
726. Nolasco F, Cameron JS, Heywood EF, et al. Adult-onset minimal change nephrotic syndrome: a long-term follow-up. *Kidney Int.*, 1986;29:1215–1223.
727. Black DAK. Controlled trial of prednisone in adult patients with the nephrotic syndrome. *Br. Med. J.*, 1970;3:421.
728. Glassock RJ. Therapy of idiopathic nephrotic syndrome in adults: a conservative or aggressive therapeutic approach. *Amer. J. Nephrol.*, 1993;13:422–428.
729. Rose GM, Cole BR, Robson AJ. The treatment of renal glomerulopathies in children using high dose intravenous methylprednisolone pulses. *Am. J. Kidney Dis.*, 1981;1:148.
730. Rostin M, Barthe P, Houin G, et al. Pharmacokinetics of prednisolone in children with the nephrotic syndrome. *Pediatr. Nephrol.*, 1990;4:470.
731. Loeffler K, Gowrishankar M, Yiu V. Tacrolimus therapy in pediatric patients with treatment-resistant nephrotic syndrome. *Pediatr Nephrol*, 2004;19:281–287.
732. de Mello VR, Rodrigues MT, Mastrocinque TH, et al. Mycophenolate mofetil in children with steroid/cyclophosphamide-resistant nephrotic syndrome. *Pediatr Nephrol*, 2010;25:453–460.
733. Bergstein JM. Prostaglandin inhibitors in the treatment of nephrotic syndrome. *Pediatr. Nephrol.*, 1991;5:335.
734. Garin EH, Williams RL, Rennell RS III, et al. Indomethacin in the treatment of idiopathic minimal lesion nephrotic syndrome. *J. Pediatr.*, 1978;93:138.
735. Cuoghi D, Evangelista A, Baraldi A, et al. Relapse of nephrotic syndrome following remission for 20 years. *Int. J. Pediatr. Nephrol*, 1983;4:211.
736. Pru C, Kjellstrand CM, Cohn RA, et al. Late recurrence of minimal lesion nephrotic syndrome. *Ann. Intern. Med.*, 1984;100:69.
737. Scharer K, Minges U. Long-term prognosis of the nephrotic syndrome in childhood. *Clin. Nephrol.*, 1973;1:182.
738. Trainin EB, Gomez-Leon G. Development of renal insufficiency after long-standing steroid-responsive nephrotic syndrome. *Int. J. Pediatr. Nephrol.*, 1982;3:55–58.
739. Mauer SM, Hellerstein S, Cohen RA, et al. Recurrence of steroid-responsive nephrotic syndrome after renal transplantation. *J. Pediatr.*, 1979;95:261.
740. Hiraoka M, Takeda N, Tsukahara H, et al. Favorable course of steroid-responsive nephrotic children with mild attack. *Kidney Int.*, 1995;47:1392–1393.
741. Plank C, Ostreicher I, Dittrich K, et al. Low birth weight, but not postnatal weight gain, aggravates the course of nephrotic syndrome. *Pediatr Nephrol*, 2007;22:1881–1889.
742. Teeninga N, Schreuder MF, Bokenkamp A, et al. Influence of low birth weight on minimal change nephrotic syndrome in children, including a meta-analysis. *Nephrol Dial Transplant*, 2008;23:1615–1620.
743. Cameron JS, Turner DR, Ogg CS, et al. The long-term prognosis of patients with focal segmental glomerulosclerosis. *Clin. Nephrol.*, 1978;10:213–218.
744. Idelson BA, Smithline N, Smith GW. Prognosis in steroid-treated idiopathic nephrotic syndrome in adults. *Arch. Intern. Med.*, 1977;137:891.
745. Hyams JS, Carey DE. Corticosteroids and growth. *J. Pediatr.*, 1988;113:249.
746. Saha MT, Laippala P, Lenko HL. Normal growth of prepuberatal nephrotic children during long-term treatment with repeated courses of prednisone. *Acta Paed.*, 1998;87:545–548.
747. Polito C, Oporto MR, Totino SF, et al. Normal growth of nephrotic children during long-term alternate-day prednisone therapy. *Acta. Pediatr. Scand.*, 1986;75:245–250.
748. Fleisher DS, McCrory WW, Rapoport M. The effects of intermittent doses of adrenocortical steroids on the statural growth of nephrotic children. *J. Pediatr.*, 1960;57:192.
749. Foote KD, Brocklebank JT, Meadow SR. Height attainment in children with steroid-responsive nephrotic syndrome. *Lancet*, 1985;ii:917.
750. Foster BJ, Shults J, Zemel BS, et al. Interactions between growth and body composition in children treated with high-dose chronic glucocorticoids. *Am J Clin Nutr*, 2004;80:1334–1341.
751. Brockelbank JT, Harcourt RB, Meadow SR. Corticosteroid-induced cataracts in idiopathic nephrotic syndrome. *Arch. Dis. Child.*, 1982;53:30.
752. Krensky AM, Inglefinger JR, Grupe WE. Peritonitis in childhood nephrotic syndrome. *Am. J. Dis. Child.*, 1982;136:732–736.
753. International Study of Kidney Disease in Children. Minimal change nephrotic syndrome in children: Deaths during the first 5 to 15 years' observation. *Pediatrics*, 1984;73:497–501.
754. Kappel B, Olsen S. Cortical interstitial tissue and sclerosed glomeruli in the normal human kidney, related to age and sex. A quantitative study. *Virchows Arch A Pathol Anat Histol*, 1980;387:271–277.
755. Smith SM, Hoy WE, Cobb L. Low incidence of glomerulosclerosis in normal kidneys. *Arch Pathol Lab Med*, 1989;113:1253–1255.
756. Howie AJ, Kizaki T. Glomerular tip lesion in the 1962–66 Medical Research Council trial of prednisone in the nephrotic syndrome. *Nephrol. Dial. Transplant.*, 1993;8:1059–1063.
757. Detwiler RK, Falk RJ, Hogan SL, et al. Collapsing glomerulopathy: A clinically and pathologically distinct variant of focal segmental glomerulosclerosis. *Kidney Int.*, 1994;45:1416–1424.
758. Korbet SM. Clinical picture and outcome of primary focal segmental glomerulosclerosis. *Nephrol Dial Transplant*, 1999;14 Suppl 3:68–73.

759. Braden GL, Mulhern JG, O'Shea MH, et al. Changing incidence of glomerular diseases in adults. *Am J Kidney Dis*, 2000;35:878–883.
760. Bonilla-Felix M, Parra C, Dajani T, et al. Changing patterns in the histopathology of idiopathic nephrotic syndrome in children. *Kidney Int.*, 1999;55:1885–1890.
761. Gulati S, Sharma AP, Sharma RK, et al. Changing trends of histopathology in childhood nephrotic syndrome. *Am J Kidney Dis*, 1999;34:646–650.
762. Adhikari M, Bhimma R, Coovadia HM. Focal segmental glomerulosclerosis in children from KwaZulu/Natal, South Africa. *Clin Nephrol*, 2001;55:16–24.
763. Filler G, Young E, Geier P, et al. Is there really an increase in non-minimal change nephrotic syndrome in children? *Am J Kidney Dis*, 2003;42:1107–1113.
764. United States Renal Data System. *2004 Annual Data Report: Atlas of End-Stage Renal Disease in the United States*Bethesda: National Institutes of Health, National Institute of Diabetes and Digestive and Kidney Diseases, Department of Health and Human Services. 2004.
765. Kitiyakara C, Eggers P, Kopp JB. Twenty-one-year trend in ESRD due to focal segmental glomerulosclerosis in the United States. *Am J Kidney Dis*, 2004;44:815–825.
766. Kitiyakara C, Kopp JB, Eggers P. Trends in the epidemiology of focal segmental glomerulosclerosis. *Semin Nephrol*, 2003;23:172–182.
767. Genovese G, Tonna SJ, Knob AU, et al. A risk allele for focal segmental glomerulosclerosis in African Americans is located within a region containing APOL1 and MYH9. *Kidney Int*, 2010;78:698–704.
768. Kao WH, Klag MJ, Meoni LA, et al. MYH9 is associated with nondiabetic end-stage renal disease in African Americans. *Nat Genet*, 2008;40:1185–1192.
769. Kopp JB, Smith MW, Nelson GW, et al. MYH9 is a major-effect risk gene for focal segmental glomerulosclerosis. *Nat Genet*, 2008;40:1175–1184.
770. Korbet SM. Primary focal segmental glomerulosclerosis. *J Am Soc Nephrol*, 1998;9:1333–1340.
771. Dixit M, Mansur A, Dixit N, et al. The role of ACE gene polymorphism in rapidity of progression of focal segmental glomerulosclerosis. *J Postgrad Med*, 2002;48:266–269; discussion 269.
772. Ingulli E, Tejani A. Racial differences in the incidence and renal outcome of idiopathic focal segmental glomerulosclerosis in children. *Pediatr. Nephrol.*, 1991;5:393–397.
773. Kopp JB, Nelson GW, Sampath K, et al. APOL1 genetic variants in focal segmental glomerulosclerosis and HIV-associated nephropathy. *J Am Soc Nephrol*, 2011;22:2129–2137.
774. Fahr T, Pathologische anatomie des morbus brightii, in *Handbuch*, Henke F, Editor 1925: Berlin.
775. Rich AR. A hitherto undescribed vulnerability of the juxtamedullary glomeruli in lipoid nephrosis. *Bull. Johns Hopkins Hosp.*, 1957;100:173–180.
776. Heptinstall RH, Nephrotic Syndrome, in *Pathology of the Kidney*1966, Little Brown: Boston. p. 355.
777. McGovern VJ. Persistent nephrotic syndrome: a renal biopsy study. *Australas Int Med*, 1964.;13:306.
778. Hayslett JP, Krasser LS, Bensch KG, et al. Progression of "lipid nephrosis" to renal insufficiency. *N. Engl. J. Med.*, 1969;281:181–187.
779. Fogo A, Glick AD, Horn SL, et al. Is focal segmental glomerulosclerosis really focal? Distribution of lesions in adults and children. *Kidney Int.*, 1995;47:1690–1696.
780. Remuzzi A, Pergolizzi R, Mauer MS, et al. Three-dimensional morphometric analysis of segmental glomerulosclerosis in the rat. *Kidney Int.*, 1990;38:851–856.
781. Morel-Maroger L, Leathem A, Richet G. Glomerular abnormalities in nonsystemic diseases. Relationship between findings by light microscopy and immunofluorescence in 433 renal biopsy specimens. *Am. J. Med.*, 1972;53:170–184.
782. Fogo A, Hawkins EP, Berry PL, et al. Glomerular hypertrophy in minimal change disease predicts subsequent progression to focal glomerular sclerosis. *Kidney Int.*, 1990;38:115–123.
783. Markowitz GS, Schwimmer JA, Stokes MB, et al. C1q nephropathy: a variant of focal segmental glomerulosclerosis. *Kidney Int*, 2003;64:1232–1240.
784. Barisoni L, Kopp JB. Modulation of podocyte phenotype in collapsing glomerulopathies. *Microsc Res Tech*, 2002;57:254–262.
785. Jennette JC, Mandal AK, The nephrotic syndrome, in *Diagnosis and Management of Renal Disease and Hypertension*, Mandal AK, Jennette JC, Editors. 1994, Carolina Academic Press: Durham, NC. p. 235.
786. D'Agati VD, Fogo AB, Bruijn JA, et al. Pathologic classification of focal segmental glomerulosclerosis: a working proposal. *Am J Kidney Dis*, 2004;43:368–382.
787. Schmid H, Henger A, Cohen CD, et al. Gene expression profiles of podocyte-associated molecules as diagnostic markers in acquired proteinuric diseases. *J Am Soc Nephrol*, 2003;14:2958–2966.
788. Grishman E, Churg J. Focal glomerular sclerosis in nephrotic patients: an electron microscopic study of glomerular podocytes. *Kidney Int*, 1975;7:111–122.
789. Schwartz MM, Lewis EJ. Focal segmental glomerular sclerosis: the cellular lesion. *Kidney Int*, 1985;28:968–974.
790a. D'Agati V. Pathologic classification of focal segmental glomerulosclerosis. *Semin Nephrol.* 2003;23:117.
790b. D'Agati VD, Fogo AB, Bruijin JA, et al. Pathologic classification of focal segmental glomerulosclerosis: a working proposal. *Am J Kidney Dis.* 2004;43:368.
790. Olson JL, de Urdaneta AG, Heptinstall RH. Glomerular hyalinosis and its relation to hyperfiltration. *Lab Invest*, 1985;52:387–398.
791. Stokes MB, Valeri AM, Markowitz GS, et al. Cellular focal segmental glomerulosclerosis: Clinical and pathologic features. *Kidney Int*, 2006;70:1783– 1792.
792. Thomas DB, Franceschini N, Hogan SL, et al. Clinical and pathologic characteristics of focal segmental glomerulosclerosis pathologic variants. *Kidney Int*, 2006;69:920–926.
793. Silverstein DM, Craver R. Presenting features and short-term outcome according to pathologic variant in childhood primary focal segmental glomerulosclerosis. *Clin J Am Soc Nephrol*, 2007;2:700–707.
794. Chun MJ, Korbet SM, Schwartz MM, et al. Focal segmental glomerulosclerosis in nephrotic adults: presentation, prognosis, and response to therapy of the histologic variants. *J Am Soc Nephrol*, 2004;15:2169–2177.
795. Meyrier A. E pluribus unum: The riddle of focal segmental glomerulosclerosis. *Semin Nephrol*, 2003;23:135–140.
796. Romagnani P. Parietal epithelial cells: their role in health and disease. *Contrib Nephrol*, 2011;169:23–36.
797. Chiang ML, Hawkins EP, Berry PL, et al. Diagnostic and prognostic significance of glomerular epithelial cell vacuolization and podocyte effacement in children with minimal lesion nephrotic syndrome and focal segmental glomerulosclerosis: an ultrastructural study. *Clin Nephrol*, 1988;30:8–14.
798. Kambham N, Markowitz GS, Valeri AM, et al. Obesity-related glomerulopathy: An emerging epidemic. *Kidney Int*, 2001;59:1498–1509.
799. Kriz W, Hosser H, Hahnel B, et al. Development of vascular pole-associated glomerulosclerosis in the Fawn-hooded rat. *J Am Soc Nephrol*, 1998;9:381–396.
800. Kriz W, Lemley KV. The role of the podocyte in glomerulosclerosis. *Curr Opin Nehprol Hypertens*, 1999;8:489–497.
801. Gulati S, Sharma AP, Sharma RK, et al. Do current recommendations for kidney biopsy in nephrotic syndrome need modifications? *Pediatr Nephrol*, 2002;17:404–408.
802. Markowitz GS, Lin J, Valeri AM, et al. Idiopathic nodular glomerulosclerosis is a distinct clinicopathologic entity linked to hypertension and smoking. *Hum Pathol*, 2002;33:826–835.
803. Au WY, Chan KW, Lui SL, et al. Focal segmental glomerulosclerosis and mesangial sclerosis associated with myeloproliferative disorders. *Am. J. Kidney Dis.*, 1999;34:889–893.
804. Fogo AB. Animal models of FSGS: lessons for pathogenesis and treatment. *Semin Nephrol*, 2003;23:161–171.
805. Backman L, Sundelin B, Bohman SO. Focal glomerulosclerosis and nephron atrophy in rats on long-term cyclosporine treatment. *APMIS Suppl*, 1988;4:27–36.
806. Cahill MM, Ryan GB, Bertram JF. Biphasic glomerular hypertrophy in rats administered puromycin aminonucleoside. *Kidney Int*, 1996;50:768–775.
807. Chen A, Sheu LF, Ho YS, et al. Experimental focal segmental glomerulosclerosis in mice. *Nephron*, 1998;78:440–452.
808. Diamond JR, Karnovsky MJ. Focal and segmental glomerulosclerosis following a single intravenous dose of puromycin aminonucleoside. *Am J Pathol*, 1986;122:481– 487.
809. Garber SL, Mirochnik Y, Arruda JA, et al. Evolution of experimentally induced papillary necrosis to focal segmental glomerulosclerosis and nephrotic proteinuria. *Am J Kidney Dis*, 1999;33:1033–1039.
810. Hostetter TH, Olson JL, Rennke HG, et al. Hyperfiltration in remnant nephrons: a potentially adverse response to renal ablation. *Am J Physiol*, 1981;241:F85–93.
811. Kriz W, Hahnel B, Rosener S, et al. Long-term treatment of rats with FGF-2 results in focal segmental glomerulosclerosis. *Kidney Int*, 1995;48:1435–1450.
812. Ma LJ, Fogo AB. Model of robust induction of glomerulosclerosis in mice: importance of genetic background. *Kidney Int*, 2003;64:350–355.
813. Meyer TW, Rennke HG. Progressive glomerular injury after limited renal infarction in the rat. *Am. J. Physiol.*, 1988;254:F856-F862.
814. O'Donnell MP, Michels L, Kasiske B, et al. Adriamycin-induced chronic proteinuria: a structural and functional study. *J Lab Clin Med*, 1985;106:62–67.
815. Okuda S, Motomura K, Sanai T, et al. Influence of age on deterioration of the remnant kidney in uninephrectomized rats. *Clin Sci (Lond)*, 1987;72:571–576.
816. Shimamura T, Morrison AB. A progressive glomerulosclerosis occurring in partial five-sixths nephrectomized rats. *Am J Pathol*, 1975;79:95–106.
817. Zheng F, Plati AR, Potier M, et al. Resistance to glomerulosclerosis in B6 mice disappears after menopause. *Am J Pathol*, 2003;162:1339–1348.
818. Kondo S, Yoshizawa N, Wakabayashi K. Natural history of renal lesions in spontaneously hypercholesterolemic (SHC) male rats. *Nippon Jinzo Gakkai Shi*, 1995;37:91–99.

819. Le Berre L, Godfrin Y, Perretto S, et al. The Buffalo/Mna rat, an animal model of FSGS recurrence after renal transplantation. *Transplant Proc*, 2001;33: 3338–3340.
820. Nakamura T, Oite T, Shimizu F, et al. Sclerotic lesions in the glomeruli of Buffalo/Mna rats. *Nephron*, 1986;43:50–55.
821. Nishida E, Yamanouchi J, Ogata S, et al. Age-related histochemical and ultrastructural changes in renal glomerular mesangium of APA hamsters. *Exp Anim*, 1996;45:339–345.
822. O'Donnell MP, Kasiske BL, Keane WF. Risk factors for glomerular injury in rats with genetic hypertension. *Am J Hypertens*, 1989;2:9–13.
823. Remuzzi A, Puntorieri S, Alfano M, et al. Pathophysiologic implications of proteinuria in a rat model of progressive glomerular injury. *Lab Invest*, 1992;67:572–579.
824. Shimamura T. Focal glomerulosclerosis in obese zucker rats and prevention of its development. *Kidney Int Suppl*, 1983;16:S259–262.
825. Yagil C, Sapojnikov M, Katni G, et al. Proteinuria and glomerulosclerosis in the Sabra genetic rat model of salt susceptibility. *Physiol Genomics*, 2002;9:167–178.
826. Yoshida F, Matsuo S, Fujishima H, et al. Renal lesions of the FGS strain of mice: a spontaneous animal model of progressive glomerulosclerosis. *Nephron*, 1994;66:317–325.
827. Yoshikawa Y, Yamasaki K. Renal lesions of hyperlipidemic Imai rats: a spontaneous animal model of focal glomerulosclerosis. *Nephron*, 1991;59:471–476.
828. Gao F, Maiti S, Sun G, et al. The Wt1+/R394W mouse displays glomerulosclerosis and early-onset renal failure characteristic of human Denys-Drash syndrome. *Mol Cell Biol*, 2004;24:9899–9910.
829. Gassler N, Elger M, Inoue D, et al. Oligonephronia, not exuberant apoptosis, accounts for the development of glomerulosclerosis in the bcl-2 knockout mouse. *Nephrol Dial Transplant*, 1998;13:2509–2518.
830. Kim JM, Wu H, Green G, et al. CD2-associated protein haploinsufficiency is linked to glomerular disease susceptibility. *Science*, 2003;300:1298–1300.
831. Kos CH, Le TC, Sinha S, et al. Mice deficient in alpha-actinin-4 have severe glomerular disease. *J Clin Invest*, 2003;111:1683–1690.
832. Patek CE, Little MH, Fleming S, et al. A zinc finger truncation of murine WT1 results in the characteristic urogenital abnormalities of Denys-Drash syndrome. *Proc Natl Acad Sci U S A*, 1999;96:2931–2936.
833. Powell DR, Desai U, Sparks MJ, et al. Rapid development of glomerular injury and renal failure in mice lacking p53R2. *Pediatr Nephrol*, 2005;20:432–440.
834. Shih N-Y, Li J, Karpitskii V, et al. Congenital nephrotic syndrome in mice lacking CD2-associated protein. *Science*, 1999;286:312–315.
835. Yao J, Le TC, Kos CH, et al. Alpha-actinin-4-mediated FSGS: an inherited kidney disease caused by an aggregated and rapidly degraded cytoskeletal protein. *PLoS Biol*, 2004;2:e167.
836. Lambert G, Sakai N, Vaisman BL, et al. Analysis of glomerulosclerosis and atherosclerosis in lecithin cholesterol acyltransferase-deficient mice. *J Biol Chem*, 2001;276:15090–15098.
837. O'Bryan T, Weiher H, Rennke HG, et al. Course of renal injury in the Mpv17-deficient transgenic mouse. *J Am Soc Nephrol*, 2000;11:1067–1074.
838. Roselli S, Heidet L, Sich M, et al. Early glomerular filtration defect and severe renal disease in podocin-deficient mice. *Mol Cell Biol*, 2004;24:550–560.
839. Brantley JG, Sharma M, Alcalay NI, et al. Cox-1 transgenic mice develop glomerulosclerosis and interstitial fibrosis. *Kidney Int*, 2003;63:1240–1248.
840. Clouthier DE, Comerford SA, Hammer RE. Hepatic fibrosis, glomerulosclerosis, and a lipodystrophy-like syndrome in PEPCK-TGF-beta1 transgenic mice. *J Clin Invest*, 1997;100:2697–2713.
841. Doi T, Striker LJ, Quaife C, et al. Progressive glomerulosclerosis develops in transgenic mice expressing growth hormone and growth hormone releasing factor but not in those expressing insulinlike growth factor-1. *Am. J. Pathol.*, 1988;131:398–403.
842. Godley LA, Kopp JB, Eckhaus M, et al. Wild-type p53 transgenic mice exhibit altered differentiation of the ureteric bud and possess small kidneys. *Genes Dev*, 1996;10:836–850.
843. Hocher B, Thone-Reineke C, Rohmeiss P, et al. Endothelin-1 transgenic mice develop glomerulosclerosis, interstitial fibrosis, and renal cysts but not hypertension. *J Clin Invest*, 1997;99:1380–1389.
844. Hoffmann S, Podlich D, Hahnel B, et al. Angiotensin II type 1 receptor overexpression in podocytes induces glomerulosclerosis in transgenic rats. *J Am Soc Nephrol*, 2004;15:1475–1487.
845. Kopp JB, Factor VM, Mozes M, et al. Transgenic mice with increased plasma levels of TGF-beta 1 develop progressive renal disease. *Lab Invest*, 1996;74:991–1003.
846. Kopp JB, Klotman ME, Adler SH, et al. Progressive glomerulosclerosis and enhanced renal accumulation of basement membrane components in mice transgenic for human immunodeficiency virus type 1 genes. *Proc. Natl. Acad. Sci. USA*, 1992;89:1577–1581.
847. MacKay K, Striker LJ, Pinkert CA, et al. Glomerulosclerosis and renal cysts in mice transgenic for the early region of SV40. *Kidney Int*, 1987;32:827–837.
848. Mervaala E, Muller DN, Park JK, et al. Cyclosporin A protects against angiotensin II-induced end-organ damage in double transgenic rats harboring human renin and angiotensinogen genes. *Hypertension*, 2000;35:360–366.
849. Michaud JL, Lemieux LI, Dube M, et al. Focal and segmental glomerulosclerosis in mice with podocyte-specific expression of mutant alpha-actinin-4. *J Am Soc Nephrol*, 2003;14:1200–1211.
850. Mullins JJ, Peters J, Ganten D. Fulminant hypertension in transgenic rats harbouring the mouse Ren-2 gene. *Nature*, 1990;344:541–544.
851. Reid W, Sadowska M, Denaro F, et al. An HIV-1 transgenic rat that develops HIV-related pathology and immunologic dysfunction. *Proc Natl Acad Sci U S A*, 2001;98:9271–9276.
852. Sasaki S, Nishihira J, Ishibashi T, et al. Transgene of MIF induces podocyte injury and progressive mesangial sclerosis in the mouse kidney. *Kidney Int*, 2004;65:469–481.
853. Smeets B, Te Loeke NA, Dijkman HB, et al. The parietal epithelial cell: a key player in the pathogenesis of focal segmental glomerulosclerosis in Thy-1.1 transgenic mice. *J Am Soc Nephrol*, 2004;15:928–939.
854. Takayama H, LaRochelle WJ, Sabnis SG, et al. Renal tubular hyperplasia, polycystic disease, and glomerulosclerosis in transgenic mice overexpressing hepatocyte growth factor/scatter factor. *Lab Invest*, 1997;77:131–138.
855. Trudel M, De Paepe ME, Chretien N, et al. Sickle cell disease of transgenic SAD mice. *Blood*, 1994;84:3189–3197.
856. Wagner J, Klotz S, Haufe CC, et al. Progression of renal failure after subtotal nephrectomy in transgenic rats carrying an additional renin gene [TGR(mREN2)27]. *J Hypertens*, 1997;15:441–449.
857. Dickie P, Felser J, Eckhaus M, et al. HIV-associated nephropathy in transgenic mice expressing HIV-1 genes. *Virology*, 1991;185:109–119.
858. Platt R, Roscoe MH, Smith FW. Experimental renal failure. *Clin Sci (Lond)*, 1952;11:217–231.
859. Morrison AB, Howard RM. The functional capacity of hypertrophied nephrons. Effect of partial nephrectomy on the clearance of inulin and PAH in the rat. *J Exp Med*, 1966;123:829–844.
860. Novick AC, Gephardt G, Guz B, et al. Long-term follow-up after partial removal of a solitary kidney. *N Engl J Med*, 1991;325:1058–1062.
861. Howie AJ, Kizaki T, Beaman M, et al. Different types of segmental sclerosing glomerular lesions in six experimental models of proteinuria. *J Pathol*, 1989;157:141–151.
862. Barker DJ, Osmond C, Golding J, et al. Growth in utero, blood pressure in childhood and adult life, and mortality from cardiovascular disease. *Bmj*, 1989;298:564–567.
863. Bertram JF, Douglas-Denton RN, Diouf B, et al. Human nephron number: implications for health and disease. *Pediatr Nephrol*, 2011;26:1529–1533.
864. Brenner BM, Mackenzie HS. Nephron mass as a risk factor for progression of renal disease. *Kidney Int Suppl*, 1997;63:S124–127.
865. Kwinta P, Klimek M, Drozdz D, et al. Assessment of long-term renal complications in extremely low birth weight children. *Pediatr Nephrol*, 2011;26: 1095–1103.
866. Manalich R, Reyes L, Herrera M, et al. Relationship between weight at birth and the number and size of renal glomeruli in humans: a histomorphometric study. *Kidney Int*, 2000;58:770–773.
867. Jones SE, Nyengaard JR, Flyvbjerg A, et al. Birth weight has no influence on glomerular number and volume. *Pediatr Nephrol*, 2001;16:340–345.
868. Keller G, Zimmer G, Mall G, et al. Nephron number in patients with primary hypertension. *N Engl J Med*, 2003;348:101–108.
869. Lackland DT, Bendall HE, Osmond C, et al. Low birth weights contribute to high rates of early-onset chronic renal failure in the Southeastern United States. *Arch Intern Med*, 2000;160:1472–1476.
870. Hodgin JB, Rasoulpour M, Markowitz GS, et al. Very low birth weight is a risk factor for secondary focal segmental glomerulosclerosis. *Clin J Am Soc Nephrol*, 2009;4:71–76.
871. Franke D, Volker S, Haase S, et al. Prematurity, small for gestational age and perinatal parameters in children with congenital, hereditary and acquired chronic kidney disease. *Nephrol Dial Transplant*, 2010;25:3918–3924.
872. Li S, Chen SC, Shlipak M, et al. Low birth weight is associated with chronic kidney disease only in men. *Kidney Int*, 2008;73:637–642.
873. White SL, Perkovic V, Cass A, et al. Is low birth weight an antecedent of CKD in later life? A systematic review of observational studies. *Am J Kidney Dis*, 2009;54:248–261.
874. Moore L, Williams R, Staples A. Glomerular dimensions in children under 16 years of age. *J Pathol*, 1993;171:145–150.
875. Ellis EN, Mauer SM, Sutherland DE, et al. Glomerular capillary morphology in normal humans. *Lab Invest*, 1989;60:231–236.

876. Cortes P, Zhao X, Dumler F, et al. Age-related changes in glomerular volume and hydroxyproline content in rat and human. *J Am Soc Nephrol*, 1992;2:1716–1725.
877. Yoshikawa N, Cameron AH, White RH. Glomerular morphometry I: nephrotic syndrome in childhood. *Histopathology*, 1981;5:239–249.
878. Olivetti G, Anversa P, Melissari M, et al. Morphometry of the renal corpuscle during postnatal growth and compensatory hypertrophy. *Kidney Int*, 1980;17:438–454.
879. Nyengaard JR. Number and dimensions of rat glomerular capillaries in normal development and after nephrectomy. *Kidney Int*, 1993;43:1049–1057.
880. Bidani AK, Mitchell KD, Schwartz MM, et al. Absence of glomerular injury or nephron loss in a normotensive rat remnant kidney model. *Kidney Int*, 1990;38:28–38.
881. Daniels BS, Hostetter TH. Adverse effects of growth in the glomerular microcirculation. *Am J Physiol*, 1990;258:F1409–1416.
882. Akaoka K, White RHR, Raafat F. Glomerular morphometry in childhood reflux nephropathy, emphasizing the capillary changes. *Kidney Int.*, 1995;47:1108–1114.
883. Matsumae T, Fukuzaki M, Takebayashi S, et al. Two different pathways of glomerular enlargement in adults with focal and segmental glomerulosclerosis: a morphometric study. *Am J Nephrol*, 1998;18:21–27.
884. Praga M, Hernandez E, Morales E, et al. Clinical features and long-term outcome of obesity-associated focal segmental glomerulosclerosis. *Nephrol Dial Transplant*, 2001;16:1790–1798.
885. Yoshida Y, Fogo A, Ichikawa I. Glomerular hemodynamic changes vs. hypertrophy in experimental glomerular sclerosis. *Kidney Int.*, 1989;35:654–660.
886. Fogo A, Yoshida Y, Glick AD, et al. Serial micropuncture analysis of glomerular function in two rat models of glomerulosclerosis. *J. Clin. Invest.*, 1988;82:322–330.
887. Papeta N, Zheng Z, Schon EA, et al. Prkdc participates in mitochondrial genome maintenance and prevents Adriamycin-induced nephropathy in mice. *J Clin Invest*, 2010;120:4055–4064.
888. Chagnac A, Weinstein T, Herman M, et al. The effects of weight loss on renal function in patients with severe obesity. *J Am Soc Nephrol*, 2003;14:1480–1486.
889. Chagnac A, Weinstein T, Korzets A, et al. Glomerular hemodynamics in severe obesity. *Am J Physiol Renal Physiol*, 2000;278:F817–822.
890. Stokholm KH, Brochner-Mortensen J, Hoilund-Carlsen PF. Increased glomerular filtration rate and adrenocortical function in obese women. *Int J Obes*, 1980;4:57–63.
891. Bosma RJ, van der Heide JJ, Oosterop EJ, et al. Body mass index is associated with altered renal hemodynamics in non-obese healthy subjects. *Kidney Int*, 2004;65:259–265.
892. Anastasio P, Spitali L, Frangiosa A, et al. Glomerular filtration rate in severely overweight normotensive humans. *Am J Kidney Dis*, 2000;35:1144–1148.
893. Scaglione R, Ganguzza A, Corrao S, et al. Central obesity and hypertension: pathophysiologic role of renal haemodynamics and function. *Int J Obes Relat Metab Disord*, 1995;19:403–409.
894. Morgan AG, Serjeant GR. Renal function in patients over 40 with homozygous sickle-cell disease. *Br Med J (Clin Res Ed)*, 1981;282:1181–1183.
895. Guasch A, Cua M, Mitch WE. Early detection and the course of glomerular injury in patients with sickle cell anemia. *Kidney Int*, 1996;49:786–791.
896. Herrera J, Avila E, Marin C, et al. Impaired creatinine secretion after an intravenous creatinine load is an early characteristic of the nephropathy of sickle cell anaemia. *Nephrol Dial Transplant*, 2002;17:602–607.
897. Passwell J, Orda S, Modan M, et al. Abnormal renal functions in cyanotic congenital heart disease. *Arch Dis Child*, 1976;51:803–805.
898. Burlet A, Drukker A, Guignard JP. Renal function in cyanotic congenital heart disease. *Nephron*, 1999;81:296–300.
899. Pagtalunan ME, Miller PL, Jumping-Eagle S, et al. Podocyte loss and progressive glomerular injury in type II diabetes. *J Clin Invest*, 1997;99:342–348.
900. Lemley KV, Lafayette RA, Safai M, et al. Podocytopenia and disease severity in IgA nephropathy. *Kidney Int*, 2002;61:1475–1485.
901. Nagata M, Yamaguchi Y, Komatsu Y, et al. Mitosis and the presence of binucleate cells among glomerular podocytes in diseased human kidneys. *Nephron*, 1995;70:68–71.
902. Fries JW, Sandstrom DJ, Meyer TW, et al. Glomerular hypertrophy and epithelial cell injury modulate progressive glomerulosclerosis in the rat. *Lab Invest*, 1989;60:205–218.
903. Bhathena DB. Glomerular basement membrane length to podocyte ratio in human nephronopenia: implications for focal segmental glomerulosclerosis. *Am J Kidney Dis*, 2003;41:1179–1188.
904. Romagnani P. Family portrait: renal progenitor of Bowman's capsule and its tubular brothers. *Am J Pathol*, 2011;178:490–493.
905. Kriz W. The pathogenesis of 'classic' focal segmental glomerulosclerosis-lessons from rat models. *Nephrol Dial Transplant*, 2003;18 Suppl 6:vi39–44.
906. Kriz W, Kretzler M, Nagata M, et al. A frequent pathway to glomerulosclerosis: deterioration of tuft architecture-podocyte damage-segmental sclerosis. *Kidney Blood Press Res*, 1996;19:245–253.
907. Greka A, Mundel P. Cell biology and pathology of podocytes. *Annu Rev Physiol*, 2012;74:299–323.
908. Welsh GI, Saleem MA. The podocyte cytoskeleton—key to a functioning glomerulus in health and disease. *Nat Rev Nephrol*, 2012;8:14–21.
909. Tryggvason K, Patrakka J, Wartiovaara J. Hereditary proteinuria syndromes and mechanisms of proteinuria. *N Engl J Med*, 2006;354:1387–1401.
910. Hingorani SR, Finn LS, Kowalewska J, et al. Expression of nephrin in acquired forms of nephrotic syndrome in childhood. *Pediatr Nephrol*, 2004;19:300–305.
911. Huh W, Kim DJ, Kim MK, et al. Expression of nephrin in acquired human glomerular disease. *Nephrol Dial Transplant*, 2002;17:478–484.
912. Guan N, Ding J, Zhang J, et al. Expression of nephrin, podocin, alpha-actinin, and WT1 in children with nephrotic syndrome. *Pediatr Nephrol*, 2003;18:1122–1127.
913. Horinouchi I, Nakazato H, Kawano T, et al. In situ evaluation of podocin in normal and glomerular diseases. *Kidney Int*, 2003;64:2092–2099.
914. Barisoni L, Kriz W, Mundel P, et al. The dysregulated podocyte phenotype: a novel concept in the pathogenesis of collapsing idiopathic focal segmental glomerulosclerosis and HIV-associated nephropathy. *J. Am. Soc. Nephrol.*, 1999;10:51–61.
915. Barisoni L, Mokrzycki M, Sablay L, et al. Podocyte cell cycle regulation and proliferation in collapsing glomerulopathies. *Kidney Int*, 2000;58:137–143.
916. Kihara I, Yaoita E, Kawasaki K, et al. Origin of hyperplastic epithelial cells in idiopathic collapsing glomerulopathy. *Histopathology*, 1999;34:537–547.
917. Srivastava T, Garola RE, Whiting JM, et al. Synaptopodin expression in idiopathic nephrotic syndrome of childhood. *Kidney Int*, 2001;59:118–125.
918. Yang Y, Gubler MC, Beaufils H. Dysregulation of podocyte phenotype in idiopathic collapsing glomerulopathy and HIV-associated nephropathy. *Nephron*, 2002;91:416–423.
919. Kemeny E, Mihatsch MJ, Durmuller U, et al. Podocytes lose their adhesive phenotype in focal segmental glomerulosclerosis. *Clin Nephrol*, 1995;43:71–83.
920. Nagata M, Horita S, Shu Y, et al. Phenotypic characteristics and cyclin-dependent kinase inhibitors repression in hyperplastic epithelial pathology in idiopathic focal segmental glomerulosclerosis. *Lab Invest*, 2000;80:869–880.
921. Wang S, Kim JH, Moon KC, et al. Cell-cycle mechanisms involved in podocyte proliferation in cellular lesion of focal segmental glomerulosclerosis. *Am J Kidney Dis*, 2004;43:19–27.
922. Shankland SJ, Eitner F, Hudkins KL, et al. Differential expression of cyclin-dependent kinase inhibitors in human glomerular disease: role in podocyte proliferation and maturation. *Kidney Int*, 2000;58:674–683.
923. Hiromura K, Haseley LA, Zhang P, et al. Podocyte expression of the CDK-inhibitor p57 during development and disease. *Kidney Int*, 2001;60:2235–2246.
924. Riser BL, Cortes P, Yee J. Modelling the effects of vascular stress in mesangial cells. *Curr Opin Nephrol Hypertens*, 2000;9:43–47.
925. Riser BL, Varani J, Cortes P, et al. Cyclic stretching of mesangial cells up-regulates intercellular adhesion molecule-1 and leukocyte adherence: a possible new mechanism for glomerulosclerosis. *Am J Pathol*, 2001;158:11–17.
926. Yasuda T, Kondo S, Homma T, et al. Regulation of extracellular matrix by mechanical stress in rat glomerular mesangial cells. *J. Clin. Invest.*, 1996;98:1991–2000.
927. Suda T, Osajima A, Tamura M, et al. Pressure-induced expression of monocyte chemoattractant protein-1 through activation of MAP kinase. *Kidney Int*, 2001;60:1705–1715.
928. Hishikawa K, Oemar BS, Nakaki T. Static pressure regulates connective tissue growth factor expression in human mesangial cells. *J Biol Chem*, 2001;276:16797–16803.
929. Riser BL, Cortes P, Zhao X, et al. Intraglomerular pressure and mesangial stretching stimulate extracellular matrix formation in the rat. *J Clin Invest*, 1992;90:1932–1943.
930. Riser BL, Cortes P, Heilig C, et al. Cyclic stretching force selectively up-regulates transforming growth factor-β isoforms in cultured rat mesangial cells. *Am J Pathol*, 1996;148:1915–1923.
931. Lee LK, Meyer TM, Pollock AS, et al. Endothelial cell injury initiates glomerular sclerosis in the rat remnant kidney. *J. Clin. Invest.*, 1995;96:953–964.
932. Adamczak M, Gross ML, Amann K, et al. Reversal of glomerular lesions involves coordinated restructuring of glomerular microvasculature. *J Am Soc Nephrol*, 2004;15:3063–3072.
933. Markovic-Lipkovski J, Muller CA, Risler T, et al. Mononuclear leukocytes, expression of HLA class II antigens and intercellular adhesion molecule 1 in focal segmental glomerulosclerosis. *Nephron*, 1991;59:286–293.
934. van Goor H, van der Horst ML, Fidler V, et al. Glomerular macrophage modulation affects mesangial expansion in the rat after renal ablation. *Lab Invest*, 1992;66:564–571.

935. Vielhauer V, Berning E, Eis V, et al. CCR1 blockade reduces interstitial inflammation and fibrosis in mice with glomerulosclerosis and nephrotic syndrome. *Kidney Int*, 2004;66:2264–2278.
936. Branton MH, Kopp JB. TGF-beta and fibrosis. *Microbes Infect*, 1999;1: 1349–1365.
937. Poncelet A-C, Schnaper HW. Regulation of mesangial cell collagen turnover by transforming growth factor-β1. *Am. J. Physiol.*, 1998; 275 (Renal Physiol. 44):F458–F466.
938. Leask A, Abraham DJ. The role of connective tissue growth factor, a multifunctional matricellular protein, in fibroblast biology. *Biochem Cell Biol*, 2003;81:355–363.
939. Diamond JR. The role of reactive oxygen species in animal models of glomerular disease. *Am J Kidney Dis*, 1992;19:292–300.
940. Schnaper HW. Balance between matrix synthesis and degradation: a determinant of glomerulosclerosis. *Pediatr. Nephrol.*, 1995;9:104–111.
941. Eddy AA. Molecular basis of renal fibrosis. *Pediatr Nephrol*, 2000;15:290–301.
942. Lovett DH, Johnson RJ, Marti H-P, et al. Structural characterization of the mesangial cell type IV collagenase and enhanced expression in a model of immune complex-mediated glomerulonephritis. *Am. J. Pathol.*, 1992;141:85–98.
943. Baricos WH, Cortez SL, El-Dahr SS, et al. ECM degradation by cultured human mesangial cells is mediated by a plasminogen activator/plasmin/matrix metalloproteinase 2 cascade. *Kidney Int.*, 1995;47:1039–1047.
944. Ma LJ, Fogo AB. Angiotensin as inducer of plasminogen activator inhibitor-1 and fibrosis. *Contrib Nephrol*, 2001:161–170.
945. Floege J, Kriz W, Schulze M, et al. Basic fibroblast growth factor augments podocyte injury and induces glomerulosclerosis in rats with experimental membranous nephropathy. *J Clin Invest*, 1995;96:2809–2819.
946. Schiffer M, Bitzer M, Roberts IS, et al. Apoptosis in podocytes induced by TGF-beta and Smad7. *J. Clin. Invest.*, 2001;108:807–816.
947. Ortmann J, Amann K, Brandes RP, et al. Role of podocytes for reversal of glomerulosclerosis and proteinuria in the aging kidney after endothelin inhibition. *Hypertension*, 2004;44:974–981.
948. Hollenberg NK. Aldosterone in the development and progression of renal injury. *Kidney Int*, 2004;66:1–9.
949. Weigert C, Brodbeck K, Klopfer K, et al. Angiotensin II induces human TGF-beta 1 promoter activation: similarity to hyperglycaemia. *Diabetologia*, 2002;45:890–898.
950. Sorokin A, Kohan DE. Physiology and pathology of endothelin-1 in renal mesangium. *Am J Physiol Renal Physiol*, 2003;285:F579–589.
951. Sraer JD, Kanfer A, Rondeau E, et al. Mechanisms of glomerular injury: overview and relation with hemostasis. *Ren Fail*, 1993;15:343–348.
952. Wolf G, Chen S, Han DC, et al. Leptin and renal disease. *Am J Kidney Dis*, 2002;39:1–11.
953. Schnaper HW, Hubchak SC, Runyan CE, et al. A conceptual framework for the molecular pathogenesis of progressive kidney disease. *Pediatr Nephrol*, 2010;25:2223–2230.
954. Howie AJ, Brewer DB. The glomerular tip lesion: a previously undescribed type of segmental glomerular abnormality. *J Pathol*, 1984;142:205–220.
955. Haas M. The glomerular tip lesion: what does it really mean? *Kidney Int*, 2005;67:1188–1189.
956. Howie AJ, Pankhurst T, Sarioglu S, et al. Evolution of nephrotic-associated focal segmental glomerulosclerosis and relation to the glomerular tip lesion. *Kidney Int*, 2005;67:987–1001.
957. Howie AJ. Changes at the glomerular tip: a feature of membranous nephropathy and other disorders associated with proteinuria. *J Pathol*, 1986;150:13–20.
958. Thomsen OF, Ladefoged J. Glomerular tip lesions in renal biopsies with focal segmental IgM. *Apmis*, 1991;99:836–843.
959. Howie AJ, Ferreira MA, Majumdar A, et al. Glomerular prolapse as precursor of one type of segmental sclerosing lesions. *J Pathol*, 2000;190:478–483.
960. Najafian B, Kim Y, Crosson JT, et al. Atubular glomeruli and glomerulotubular junction abnormalities in diabetic nephropathy. *J Am Soc Nephrol*, 2003;14:908–917.
961. Howie AJ, Lee SJ, Sparke J. Pathogenesis of segmental glomerular changes at the tubular origin, as in the glomerular tip lesion. *J Pathol*, 1995;177:191–199.
962. Haas M, Yousefzadeh N. Glomerular tip lesion in minimal change nephropathy: a study of autopsies before 1950. *Am J Kidney Dis*, 2002;39:1168–1175.
963. Schwartz MM, Evans J, Bain R, et al. Focal segmental glomerulosclerosis: prognostic implications of the cellular lesion. *J. Am. Soc. Nephrol.*, 1999;10: 1900–1907.
964. Bhathena DB. Glomerular size and the association of focal glomerulosclerosis in long-surviving human renal allografts. *J Am Soc Nephrol*, 1993;4: 1316–1326.
965. Bhathena DB. Focal glomerulosclerosis and maximal glomerular hypertrophy in human nephronopenia. *J Am Soc Nephrol*, 1996;7:2600–2603.
966. Elema JD, Arends A. Focal and segmental glomerular hyalinosis and sclerosis in the rat. *Lab. Invest.*, 1975;33:554–561.
967. Grond J, Koudstaal J, Elema JD. Mesangial function and glomerular sclerosis in rats with aminonucleoside nephrosis. *Kidney Int.*, 1985;27:405–410.
968. Praga M, Morales E, Herrero JC, et al. Absence of hypoalbuminemia despite massive proteinuria in focal segmental glomerulosclerosis secondary to hyperfiltration. *Am J Kidney Dis*, 1999;33:52–58.
969. Bagby SP. Obesity-initiated metabolic syndrome and the kidney: a recipe for chronic kidney disease? *J Am Soc Nephrol*, 2004;15:2775–2791.
970. Henegar JR, Bigler SA, Henegar LK, et al. Functional and structural changes in the kidney in the early stages of obesity. *J Am Soc Nephrol*, 2001;12:1211–1217.
971. Cusumano AM, Bodkin NL, Hansen BC, et al. Glomerular hypertrophy is associated with hyperinsulinemia and precedes overt diabetes in aging rhesus monkeys. *Am J Kidney Dis*, 2002;40:1075–1085.
972. Adelman RD, Restaino IG, Alon US, et al. Proteinuria and focal segmental glomerulosclerosis in severely obese adolescents. *J Pediatr*, 2001;138:481–485.
973. Huan Y, Tomaszewski JE, Cohen DL. Resolution of nephrotic syndrome after successful bariatric surgery in patient with biopsy-proven FSGS. *Clin Nephrol*, 2009;71:69–73.
974. Fowler SM, Kon V, Ma L, et al. Obesity-related focal and segmental glomerulosclerosis: normalization of proteinuria in an adolescent after bariatric surgery. *Pediatr Nephrol*, 2009;24:851–855.
975. Schwimmer JA, Markowitz GS, Valeri AM, et al. Secondary focal segmental glomerulosclerosis in non-obese patients with increased muscle mass. *Clin Nephrol*, 2003;60:233–241.
976. Freedman BI, Isakander SS, Appel RG. The link between hypertension and nephrosis. *Am. J. Kidney Dis.*, 1995;25:207–221.
977. Kincaid-Smith P. Hypothesis: obesity and the insulin resistance syndrome play a major role in end-stage renal failure attributed to hypertension and labelled 'hypertensive nephrosclerosis'. *J Hypertens*, 2004;22:1051–1055.
978. Udani S, Lazich I, Bakris GL. Epidemiology of hypertensive kidney disease. *Nat Rev Nephrol*, 2011;7:11–21.
979. Hughson MD, Johnson K, Young RJ, et al. Glomerular size and glomerulosclerosis: relationships to disease categories, glomerular solidification, and ischemic obsolescence. *Am J Kidney Dis*, 2002;39:679–688.
980. Caetano ER, Zatz R, Saldanha LB, et al. Hypertensive nephrosclerosis as a relevant cause of chronic renal failure. *Hypertension*, 2001;38:171–176.
981. Takebayashi S, Kiyoshi Y, Hisano S, et al. Benign nephrosclerosis: incidence, morphology and prognosis. *Clin Nephrol*, 2001;55:349–356.
982. Marcantoni C, Ma LJ, Federspiel C, et al. Hypertensive nephrosclerosis in African Americans versus Caucasians. *Kidney Int*, 2002;62:172–180.
983. Davenport A, Maciver AG, Mackenzie JC. C1q nephropathy: do C1q deposits have any prognostic significance in the nephrotic syndrome? *Nephrol Dial Transplant*, 1992;7:391–396.
984. Srivastava T, Chadha V, Taboada EM, et al. C1q nephropathy presenting as rapidly progressive crescentic glomerulonephritis. *Pediatr Nephrol*, 2000;14:976–979.
985. Hashimoto S, Ogawa Y, Ishida T, et al. Steroid-sensitive nephrotic syndrome associated with positive C1q immunofluorescence. *Clin Exp Nephrol*, 2004;8: 266–269.
986. Kuwano M, Ito Y, Amamoto Y, et al. A case of congenital nephrotic syndrome associated with positive C1q immunofluorescence. *Pediatr Nephrol*, 1993;7:452–454.
987. Jennette JC, Hipp CG. C1q nephropathy: a distinct pathologic entity usually causing nephrotic syndrome. *Am J Kidney Dis*, 1985;6:103–110.
988. Iskandar SS, Browning MC, Lorentz WB. C1q nephropathy: a pediatric clinicopathologic study. *Am J Kidney Dis*, 1991;18:459–465.
989. Kishore U, Gaboriaud C, Waters P, et al. C1q and tumor necrosis factor superfamily: modularity and versatility. *Trends Immunol*, 2004;25:551–561.
990. Cortes-Hernandez J, Fossati-Jimack L, Carugati A, et al. Murine glomerular mesangial cell uptake of apoptotic cells is inefficient and involves serum-mediated but complement-independent mechanisms. *Clin Exp Immunol*, 2002;130:459–466.
991. Navratil JS, Watkins SC, Wisnieski JJ, et al. The globular heads of C1q specifically recognize surface blebs of apoptotic vascular endothelial cells. *J Immunol*, 2001;166:3231–3239.
992. Sato T, van Dixhoorn MG, Heemskerk E, et al. C1q, a subunit of the first component of complement, enhances antibody-mediated apoptosis of cultured rat glomerular mesangial cells. *Clin Exp Immunol*, 1997;109:510–517.
993. Ruiz-Villamor E, Quezada M, Bautista MJ, et al. Classical swine fever: pathogenesis of glomerular damage and immunocharacterization of immunocomplex deposits. *J Comp Pathol*, 2001;124:246–254.
994. Weiss MA, Daquioag E, Margolin EG, et al. Nephrotic syndrome, progressive irreversible renal failure, and glomerular "collapse": a new clinicopathologic entity? *Am J Kidney Dis*, 1986;7:20–28.

995. Grcevska L, Polenakovik M. Collapsing glomerulopathy: clinical characteristics and follow-up [see comments]. *Am J Kidney Dis*, 1999;33:652–657.
996. Laurinavicius A, Hurwitz S, Rennke HG. Collapsing glomerulopathy in HIV and non-HIV patients: a clinicopathological and follow-up study. *Kidney Int*, 1999;56:2203–2213.
997. Singh HK, Baldree LA, McKenney DW, et al. Idiopathic collapsing glomerulopathy in children. *Pediatr Nephrol*, 2000;14:132–137.
998. Valeri A, Barisoni L, Appel GB, et al. Idiopathic collapsing focal segmental glomerulosclerosis: a clinicopathologic study. *Kidney Int*, 1996;50:1734–1746.
999. Meehan SM, Pascual M, Williams WW, et al. De novo collapsing glomerulopathy in renal allografts. *Transplantation*, 1998;65:1192–1197.
1000. Stokes MB, Davis CL, Alpers CE. Collapsing glomerulopathy in renal allografts: a morphological pattern with diverse clinicopathologic associations. *Am J Kidney Dis*, 1999;33:658–666.
1001. Laurinavicius A, Rennke HG. Collapsing glomerulopathy—a new pattern of renal injury. *Semin Diagn Pathol*, 2002;19:106–115.
1002. Schwimmer JA, Markowitz GS, Valeri A, et al. Collapsing glomerulopathy. *Sem Nephrol*, 2003;23:209–218.
1003. Bennett AN, Peterson P, Sangle S, et al. Adult onset Still's disease and collapsing glomerulopathy: successful treatment with intravenous immunoglobulins and mycophenolate mofetil. *Rheumatology (Oxford)*, 2004;43:795–799.
1004. Kumar S, Sheaff M, Yaqoob M. Collapsing glomerulopathy in adult Still's disease. *Am J Kidney Dis*, 2004;43:e4–10.
1005. Moudgil A, Nast CC, Bagga A, et al. Association of parvovirus B19 infection with idiopathic collapsing glomerulopathy. *Kidney Int*, 2001;59: 2126–2133.
1006. Tanawattanacharoen S, Falk RJ, Jennette JC, et al. Parvovirus B19 DNA in kidney tissue of patients with focal segmental glomerulosclerosis. *Am J Kidney Dis*, 2000;35:1166–1174.
1007. Li RM, Branton MH, Tanawattanacharoen S, et al. Molecular Identification of SV40 infection in human subjects and possible association with kidney disease. *J Am Soc Nephrol*, 2002;13:2320–2330.
1008. Hattori M, Horita S, Yoshioka T, et al. Mesangial phenotypic changes associated with cellular lesions in primary focal segmental glomerulosclerosis. *Am J Kidney Dis*, 1997;30:632–638.
1009. Falkenhain ME, Cosio FG, Sedmak DD. Progressive histologic injury in kidneys from heart and liver transplant recipients receiving cyclosporine. *Transplantation*, 1996;62:364–370.
1010. Griffiths MH, Crowe AV, Papadaki L, et al. Cyclosporin nephrotoxicity in heart and lung transplant patients. *Qjm*, 1996;89:751–763.
1011. Paller MS, Cahill B, Harmon KR, et al. Glomerular disease and lung transplantation. *Am J Kidney Dis*, 1995;26:527–531.
1012. Ghiggeri GM, Altieri P, Oleggini R, et al. Cyclosporine enhances the synthesis of selected extracellular matrix proteins by renal cells "in culture". Different cell responses and phenotype characterization. *Transplantation*, 1994;57: 1382–1388.
1013. Ojo AO, Held PJ, Port FK, et al. Chronic renal failure after transplantation of a nonrenal organ. *N Engl J Med*, 2003;349:931–940.
1014. Markowitz GS, Radhakrishnan J, Kambham N, et al. Lithium nephrotoxicity: a progressive combined glomerular and tubulointerstitial nephropathy. *J Am Soc Nephrol*, 2000;11:1439–1448.
1015. Santella RN, Rimmer JM, MacPherson BR. Focal segmental glomerulosclerosis in patients receiving lithium carbonate. *Am J Med*, 1988;84:951–954.
1016. Schreiner A, Waldherr R, Rohmeiss P, et al. Focal segmental glomerulosclerosis and lithium treatment. *Am J Psychiatry*, 2000;157:834.
1017. Christensen S, Marcussen N, Petersen JS, et al. Effects of uninephrectomy and high protein feeding on lithium-induced chronic renal failure in rats. *Ren Physiol Biochem*, 1992;15:141–149.
1018. Sakarcan A, Thomas DB, O'Reilly KP, et al. Lithium-induced nephrotic syndrome in a young pediatric patient. *Pediatr Nephrol*, 2002;17:290–292.
1019. Coroneos E, Petrusevska G, Varghese F, et al. Focal segmental glomerulosclerosis with acute renal failure associated with alpha-interferon therapy. *Am J Kidney Dis*, 1996;28:888–892.
1020. Haas M, Jager U, Mayer G. Interferon alfa-2c and proteinuria in a patient with focal and segmental glomerulosclerosis. *Lancet*, 1997;349:1147–1148.
1021. Jadoul M. Interferon-alpha-associated focal segmental glomerulosclerosis with massive proteinuria in patients with chronic myeloid leukemia following high dose chemotherapy. *Cancer*, 1999;85:2669–2670.
1022. Shah M, Jenis EH, Mookerjee BK, et al. Interferon-alpha-associated focal segmental glomerulosclerosis with massive proteinuria in patients with chronic myeloid leukemia following high dose chemotherapy. *Cancer*, 1998;83:1938–1946.
1023. Bremer CT, Lastrapes A, Alper AB, Jr., et al. Interferon-alpha-induced focal segmental glomerulosclerosis in chronic myelogenous leukemia: a case report and review of the literature. *Am J Clin Oncol*, 2003;26:262–264.
1024. Stein DF, Ahmed A, Sunkhara V, et al. Collapsing focal segmental glomerulosclerosis with recovery of renal function: an uncommon complication of interferon therapy for hepatitis C. *Dig Dis Sci*, 2001;46:530–535.
1025. Kunin M, Kopolovic J, Avigdor A, et al. Collapsing glomerulopathy induced by long-term treatment with standard-dose pamidronate in a myeloma patient. *Nephrol Dial Transplant*, 2004;19:723–726.
1026. Habib R. Nephrotic syndrome in the first year of life. *Pediatr. Nephrol.*, 1993;7:347–353.
1027. Huttunen NP. Congenital nephrotic syndrome of the Finnish type: Study of 75 patients. *Arch. Dis. Child.*, 1976;51:344–348.
1028. Kestila M, Lenkkeri U, Mannikko M, et al. Positionally cloned gene for a novel glomerular protein—nephrin—is mutated in congenital nephrotic syndrome. *Mol. Cell*, 1998;1:575–582.
1029. Lenkkeri U, Mannikko M, McCready P, et al. Structure of the gene for congenital nephrotic syndrome of the finnish type (NPHS1) and characterization of mutations. *Am. J. Hum. Gen.*, 1999;64:51–61.
1030. Kaukinen A, Kuusniemi AM, Helin H, et al. Changes in glomerular mesangium in kidneys with congenital nephrotic syndrome of the Finnish type. *Pediatr Nephrol*, 2010;25:867–875.
1031. Kuusniemi AM, Merenmies J, Lahdenkari AT, et al. Glomerular sclerosis in kidneys with congenital nephrotic syndrome (NPHS1). *Kidney Int*, 2006;70:1423–1431.
1032. Kaukinen A, Lautenschlager I, Helin H, et al. Peritubular capillaries are rarefied in congenital nephrotic syndrome of the Finnish type. *Kidney Int*, 2009;75:1099–1108.
1033. Patrakka J, Martin P, Salonen R, et al. Proteinuria and prenatal diagnosis of congenital nephrosis in fetal carriers of nephrin gene mutations. *Lancet*, 2002;359:1575–1577.
1034. Kestila M, Jarvela I. Prenatal diagnosis of congenital nephrotic syndrome (CNF, NPHS1). *Prenat Diagn*, 2003;23:323–324.
1035. DeLuca G, Delinid N, D'Andrea S. Un raro caso di nefrosi congenita e malattia de inclusioni citomegalicho. *Minerva Pediatr.*, 1964;16:1164.
1036. Hinkes BG, Mucha B, Vlangos CN, et al. Nephrotic syndrome in the first year of life: two thirds of cases are caused by mutations in 4 genes (NPHS1, NPHS2, WT1, and LAMB2). *Pediatrics*, 2007;119:e907–919.
1037. Machuca E, Benoit G, Nevo F, et al. Genotype-phenotype correlations in non-Finnish congenital nephrotic syndrome. *J Am Soc Nephrol*, 2010;21: 1209–1217.
1038. Beale MG, Strayer DS, Kissane JM, et al. Congenital glomerulosclerosis and nephrotic syndrome in two infants. *Am. J. Dis. Child.*, 1979;133:842.
1039. Gianantonio C, Vitacco M, Mendilaharzu F, et al. The hemolytic uremic syndrome. *J. Pediatr.*, 1964;64:478.
1040. Wilson VK, Thomson ML, Hohlzel A. Mercury nephrosis in young children. *Br. Med. J.*, 1952;1:359.
1041. Simila S, Vesa L, Wasz-Hockert O. Hereditary onycho-osteodysplasia (nail-patella syndrome) with nephrosis-like renal disease in a newborn boy. *Pediatrics*, 1970;46:61.
1042. Gottloib L, London R, Rosenmann E. Infantile nephrotic syndrome due to glomerulonephritis in a male pseudohermaphrodite. *Isr. J. Med. Sci.*, 1976;12:52.
1043. Spear GS, Hyde TP, Gruppo RA, et al. Pseudohermaphroditism, glomerulonephritis with the nephrotic syndrome, and Wilms' tumor in infancy. *J. Pediatr.*, 1971;79:677.
1044. Kaplan BS, Wiglesworth FW, Marks MI, et al. The glomerulopathy of congenital syphilis: An immune deposit disease. *J. Pediatr.*, 1972;81:1154.
1045. Taitz LS, Isaacson C, Stein H. Acute nephritis associated with congenital syphilis. *Br. Med. J.*, 1961;2:152.
1046. Shahin B, Papadopulous ZL, Jenis EH. Congenial nephrotic syndrome associated with congenial toxoplasmosis. *J. Pediatr.*, 1974;85:366.
1047. Gentner JM, Kauschowsky A, Gresher DW, et al. XY gonadal dysgenesis associated with the congenital nephrotic syndrome. *Obstet. Gynecol.*, 1980; 35:655.
1048. Sibley RK, Mahan J, Mauer SM, et al. A clinicopathologic study of forty-eight infants with nephrotic syndrome. *Kidney Int.*, 1985;27:544.
1049. Jadresic LP, Filler G, Barratt TM. Urine glycosaminoglycans in congenital and acquired nephrotic syndrome. *Kidney Int.*, 1991;40:280.
1050. Patrakka J, Ruotsalainen V, Reponen P, et al. Recurrence of nephrotic syndrome in kidney grafts of patients with congenital nephrotic syndrome of the Finnish type: role of nephrin. *Transplantation*, 2002;73:394–403.
1051. Aucella F, De Bonis P, Gatta G, et al. Molecular analysis of NPHS2 and ACTN4 genes in a series of 33 Italian patients affected by adult-onset nonfamilial focal segmental glomerulosclerosis. *Nephron Clin Pract*, 2005;99:c31–36.
1052. Ekim M, Ozcakar ZB, Acar B, et al. Three siblings with steroid-resistant nephrotic syndrome: new NPHS2 mutations in a Turkish family. *Am J Kidney Dis*, 2004;44:e22–24.

1053. Weber S, Gribouval O, Esquivel EL, et al. NPHS2 mutation analysis shows genetic heterogeneity of steroid-resistant nephrotic syndrome and low post-transplant recurrence. *Kidney Int*, 2004;66:571–579.
1054. Badhwar A, Berkovic SF, Dowling JP, et al. Action myoclonus-renal failure syndrome: characterization of a unique cerebro-renal disorder. *Brain*, 2004;127:2173–2182.
1055. Boute N, Gribouval O, Roselli S, et al. *NPHS2*, encoding the glomerular protein podocin, is mutated in autosomal recessive steroid-resistant nephrotic syndrome. *Nature Genetics*, 2000;24:349–354.
1056. Caridi G, Berdeli A, Dagnino M, et al. Infantile steroid-resistant nephrotic syndrome associated with double homozygous mutations of podocin. *Am J Kidney Dis*, 2004;43:727–732.
1057. Caridi G, Bertelli R, Carrea A, et al. Prevalence, genetics, and clinical features of patients carrying podocin mutations in steroid-resistant nonfamilial focal segmental glomerulosclerosis. *J Am Soc Nephrol*, 2001;12:2742–2746.
1058. Caridi G, Bertelli R, Di Duca M, et al. Broadening the spectrum of diseases related to podocin mutations. *J Am Soc Nephrol*, 2003;14:1278–1286.
1059. Caridi G, Bertelli R, Perfumo F, et al. Heterozygous NPHS1 or NPHS2 mutations in responsive nephrotic syndrome and the multifactorial origin of proteinuria. *Kidney Int*, 2004;66:1715–1716.
1060. Caridi G, Bertelli R, Scolari F, et al. Podocin mutations in sporadic focal-segmental glomerulosclerosis occurring in adulthood. *Kidney Int*, 2003; 64:365.
1061. Frishberg Y, Rinat C, Megged O, et al. Mutations in NPHS2 encoding podocin are a prevalent cause of steroid-resistant nephrotic syndrome among Israeli-Arab children. *J Am Soc Nephrol*, 2002;13:400–405.
1062. Fuchshuber A, Gribouval O, Ronner V, et al. Clinical and genetic evaluation of familial steroid-responsive nephrotic syndrome in childhood. *J Am Soc Nephrol*, 2001;12:374–378.
1063. Karle SM, Uetz B, Ronner V, et al. Novel mutations in NPHS2 detected in both familial and sporadic steroid-resistant nephrotic syndrome. *J Am Soc Nephrol*, 2002;13:388–393.
1064. Koziell A, Grech V, Hussain S, et al. Genotype/phenotype correlations of NPHS1 and NPHS2 mutations in nephrotic syndrome advocate a functional inter-relationship in glomerular filtration. *Hum Mol Genet*, 2002;11:379–388.
1065. Lowik MM, Levtchenko EN, Monnens LA, et al. WT-1 and NPHS2 mutation analysis in patients with non-familial steroid-resistant focal-segmental glomerulosclerosis. *Clin Nephrol*, 2003;59:143–146.
1066. Ruf RG, Lichtenberger A, Karle SM, et al. Patients with mutations in NPHS2 (podocin) do not respond to standard steroid treatment of nephrotic syndrome. *J Am Soc Nephrol*, 2004;15:722–732.
1067. Tsukaguchi H, Sudhakar A, Le TC, et al. NPHS2 mutations in late-onset focal segmental glomerulosclerosis: R229Q is a common disease-associated allele. *J Clin Invest*, 2002;110:1659–1666.
1068. Wu MC, Wu JY, Lee CC, et al. Two novel polymorphisms (c954T>C and c1038A>G) in exon8 of NPHS2 gene identified in Taiwan Chinese. *Hum Mutat*, 2001;17:237.
1069. Wu MC, Wu JY, Lee CC, et al. A novel polymorphism (c288C>T) of the NPHS2 gene identified in a Taiwan Chinese family. *Hum Mutat*, 2001;17:81–82.
1070. Caridi G, Perfumo F, Ghiggeri GM. NPHS2 (Podocin) mutations in nephrotic syndrome. Clinical spectrum and fine mechanisms. *Pediatr Res*, 2005;57:54R–61R.
1071. Ruf RG, Schultheiss M, Lichtenberger A, et al. Prevalence of WT1 mutations in a large cohort of patients with steroid-resistant and steroid-sensitive nephrotic syndrome. *Kidney Int*, 2004;66:564–570.
1072. Roselli S, Gribouval O, Boute N, et al. Podocin localizes in the kidney to the slit diaphragm area. *Am J Pathol*, 2002;160:131–139.
1073. Schwarz K, Simons M, Reiser J, et al. Podocin, a raft-associated component of the glomerular slit diaphragm, interacts with CD2AP and nephrin. *J Clin Invest*, 2001;108:1621–1629.
1074. Huber TB, Hartleben B, Kim J, et al. Nephrin and CD2AP associate with phosphoinositide 3-OH kinase and stimulate AKT-dependent signaling. *Mol Cell Biol*, 2003;23:4917–4928.
1075. Huber TB, Kottgen M, Schilling B, et al. Interaction with podocin facilitates nephrin signaling. *J Biol Chem*, 2001;276:41543–41546.
1076. Huber TB, Simons M, Hartleben B, et al. Molecular basis of the functional podocin-nephrin complex: mutations in the NPHS2 gene disrupt nephrin targeting to lipid raft microdomains. *Hum Mol Genet*, 2003;12:3397–3405.
1077. Roselli S, Moutkine I, Gribouval O, et al. Plasma membrane targeting of podocin through the classical exocytic pathway: effect of NPHS2 mutations. *Traffic*, 2004;5:37–44.
1078. Mollet G, Ratelade J, Boyer O, et al. Podocin inactivation in mature kidneys causes focal segmental glomerulosclerosis and nephrotic syndrome. *J Am Soc Nephrol*, 2009;20:2181–2189.
1079. Carraro M, Caridi G, Bruschi M, et al. Serum glomerular permeability activity in patients with podocin mutations (NPHS2) and steroid-resistant nephrotic syndrome. *J Am Soc Nephrol*, 2002;13:1946–1952.
1080. Pereira AC, Pereira AB, Mota GF, et al. NPHS2 R229Q functional variant is associated with microalbuminuria in the general population. *Kidney Int*, 2004;65:1026–1030.
1081. Schultheiss M, Ruf RG, Mucha BE, et al. No evidence for genotype/phenotype correlation in NPHS1 and NPHS2 mutations. *Pediatr Nephrol*, 2004;19:1340–1348.
1082. Wagner KD, Wagner N, Schedl A. The complex life of WT1. *J Cell Sci*, 2003;116:1653–1658.
1083. Lee SB, Huang K, Palmer R, et al. The Wilms tumor suppressor WT1 encodes a transcriptional activator of amphiregulin. *Cell*, 1999;98:663–673.
1084. Palmer RE, Kotsianti A, Cadman B, et al. WT1 regulates the expression of the major glomerular podocyte membrane protein Podocalyxin. *Curr Biol*, 2001;11:1805–1809.
1085. Hammes A, Guo JK, Lutsch G, et al. Two splice variants of the Wilms' tumor 1 gene have distinct functions during sex determination and nephron formation. *Cell*, 2001;106:319–329.
1086. Barbaux S, Niaudet P, Gubler MC, et al. Donor splice-site mutations in WT1 are responsible for Frasier syndrome. *Nat Genet*, 1997;17:467–470.
1087. Little MH, Williamson KA, Mannens M, et al. Evidence that WT1 mutations in Denys-Drash syndrome patients may act in a dominant-negative fashion. *Hum Mol Genet*, 1993;2:259–264.
1088. Jadresic L, Leake J, Gordon I, et al. Clinicopathologic review of twelve children with nephropathy, Wilms tumor, and genital abnormalities (Drash syndrome). *J Pediatr*, 1990;117:717–725.
1089. Jeanpierre C, Denamur E, Henry I, et al. Identification of constitutional WT1 mutations, in patients with isolated diffuse mesangial sclerosis, and analysis of genotype/phenotype correlations by use of a computerized mutation database. *Am J Hum Genet*, 1998;62:824–833.
1090. McTaggart SJ, Algar E, Chow CW, et al. Clinical spectrum of Denys-Drash and Frasier syndrome. *Pediatr Nephrol*, 2001;16:335–339.
1091. Pelletier J, Bruening W, Kashtan CE, et al. Germline mutations in the Wilms' tumor suppressor gene are associated with abnormal urogenital development in Denys-Drash syndrome. *Cell*, 1991;67:437–447.
1092. Schumacher V, Scharer K, Wuhl E, et al. Spectrum of early onset congenital nephrotic syndrome associated with WT1 missense mutations. *Kidney Int.*, 1998;53:1594–1600.
1093. Yang AH, Chen JY, Chen BF. The dysregulated glomerular cell growth in Denys-Drash syndrome. *Virchows Arch*, 2004;445:305–314.
1094. Kaltenis P, Schumacher V, Jankauskiene A, et al. Slow progressive FSGS associated with an F392L WT1 mutation. *Pediatr Nephrol*, 2004;19:353–356.
1095. Kikuchi H, Takata A, Akasaka Y, et al. Do intronic mutations affecting splicing of WT1 exon 9 cause Frasier syndrome? *J Med Genet*, 1998;35:45–48.
1096. Klamt B, Koziell A, Poulat F, et al. Frasier syndrome is caused by defective alternative splicing of WT1 leading to an altered ratio of WT1 +/-KTS splice isoforms. *Hum Mol Genet*, 1998;7:709–714.
1097. Denamur E, Bocquet N, Mougenot B, et al. Mother-to-child transmitted WT1 splice-site mutation is responsible for distinct glomerular disease. *J. Am. Soc. Nephrol.*, 1999;10:2219–2223.
1098. Loirat C, Andre JL, Champigneulle J, et al. WT1 splice site mutation in a 46,XX female with minimal-change nephrotic syndrome and Wilms' tumour. *Nephrol Dial Transplant*, 2003;18:823–825.
1099. Denamur E, Bocquet N, Baudouin V, et al. WT1 splice-site mutations are rarely associated with primary steroid-resistant focal and segmental glomerulosclerosis. *Kidney Int*, 2000;57:1868–1872.
1100. Orloff MS, Iyengar SK, Winkler CA, et al. Variants In The Wilms Tumor Gene Are Associated With Focal Segmental Glomerulosclerosis In The African American Population. *Physiol Genomics*, 2005;21:212–221.
1101. Schumacher VA, Schlotzer-Schrehardt U, Karumanchi SA, et al. WT1-dependent sulfatase expression maintains the normal glomerular filtration barrier. *J Am Soc Nephrol*, 2011;22:1286–1296.
1102. Srichai MB, Konieczkowski M, Padiyar A, et al. A WT1 co-regulator controls podocyte phenotype by shuttling between adhesion structures and nucleus. *J Biol Chem*, 2004;279:14398–14408.
1103. Hinkes B, Wiggins RC, Gbadegesin R, et al. Positional cloning uncovers mutations in PLCE1 responsible for a nephrotic syndrome variant that may be reversible. *Nat Genet*, 2006;38:1397–1405.
1104. Boyer O, Benoit G, Gribouval O, et al. Mutational analysis of the PLCE1 gene in steroid resistant nephrotic syndrome. *J Med Genet*, 2010;47:445–452.
1105. Gbadegesin R, Hinkes BG, Hoskins BE, et al. Mutations in PLCE1 are a major cause of isolated diffuse mesangial sclerosis (IDMS). *Nephrol Dial Transplant*, 2008;23:1291–1297.

1106. Gilbert RD, Turner CL, Gibson J, et al. Mutations in phospholipase C epsilon 1 are not sufficient to cause diffuse mesangial sclerosis. *Kidney Int*, 2009;75:415–419.
1107. Mele C, Iatropoulos P, Donadelli R, et al. MYO1E mutations and childhood familial focal segmental glomerulosclerosis. *N Engl J Med*, 2011;365: 295–306.
1108. Ozaltin F, Ibsirlioglu T, Taskiran EZ, et al. Disruption of PTPRO causes childhood-onset nephrotic syndrome. *Am J Hum Genet*, 2011;89:139–147.
1109. Berkovic SF, Dibbens LM, Oshlack A, et al. Array-based gene discovery with three unrelated subjects shows SCARB2/LIMP-2 deficiency causes myoclonus epilepsy and glomerulosclerosis. *Am J Hum Genet*, 2008;82:673–684.
1110. Kaplan JM, Kim S-H, North KN, et al. Mutations in ACTN4, encoding α-actinin-4, cause familial focal segmental glomerulosclerosis. *Nature Genetics*, 2000;24:251–256.
1111. Henderson JM, Al-Waheeb S, Weins A, et al. Mice with altered alpha-actinin-4 expression have distinct morphologic patterns of glomerular disease. *Kidney Int*, 2008;73:741–750.
1112. Welsch T, Endlich N, Kriz W, et al. CD2AP and p130Cas localize to different F-actin structures in podocytes. *Am J Physiol Renal Physiol*, 2001;281: F769–777.
1113. Shih NY, Li J, Cotran R, et al. CD2AP localizes to the slit diaphragm and binds to nephrin via a novel C-terminal domain. *Am J Pathol*, 2001;159:2303–2308.
1114. Lehtonen S, Zhao F, Lehtonen E. CD2-associated protein directly interacts with the actin cytoskeleton. *Am J Physiol Renal Physiol*, 2002;283:F734–743.
1115. Palmen T, Lehtonen S, Ora A, et al. Interaction of endogenous nephrin and CD2-associated protein in mouse epithelial M-1 cell line. *J Am Soc Nephrol*, 2002;13:1766–1772.
1116. Schiffer M, Mundel P, Shaw AS, et al. A novel role for the adaptor molecule CD2-associated protein in transforming growth factor-beta-induced apoptosis. *J Biol Chem*, 2004;279:37004–37012.
1117. Winn MP, Conlon PJ, Lynn KL, et al. A mutation in the TRPC6 cation channel causes familial focal segmental glomerulosclerosis. *Science*, 2005;308:1801–1804.
1118. Pocock TM, Foster RR, Bates DO. Evidence of a role for TRPC channels in VEGF-mediated increased vascular permeability in vivo. *Am J Physiol Heart Circ Physiol*, 2004;286:H1015–1026.
1119. Eckel J, Lavin PJ, Finch EA, et al. TRPC6 enhances angiotensin II-induced albuminuria. *J Am Soc Nephrol*, 2011;22:526–535.
1120. Ilatovskaya DV, Levchenko V, Ryan RP, et al. NSAIDs acutely inhibit TRPC channels in freshly isolated rat glomeruli. *Biochem Biophys Res Commun*, 2011;408:242–247.
1121. Boyer O, Benoit G, Gribouval O, et al. Mutations in INF2 are a major cause of autosomal dominant focal segmental glomerulosclerosis. *J Am Soc Nephrol*, 2011;22:239–245.
1122. Boyer O, Nevo F, Plaisier E, et al. INF2 mutations in Charcot-Marie-Tooth disease with glomerulopathy. *N Engl J Med*, 2011;365:2377–2388.
1123. Goto Y, Nonaka I, Horai S. A mutation in the tRNA(Leu)(UUR) gene associated with the MELAS subgroup of mitochondrial encephalomyopathies. *Nature*, 1990;348:651–653.
1124. Ban S, Mori N, Saito K, et al. An autopsy case of mitochondrial encephalomyopathy (MELAS) with special reference to extra-neuromuscular abnormalities. *Acta Pathol Jpn*, 1992;42:818–825.
1125. Cheong HI, Chae JH, Kim JS, et al. Hereditary glomerulopathy associated with a mitochondrial tRNA(Leu) gene mutation. *Pediatr Nephrol*, 1999;13: 477–480.
1126. Dinour D, Mini S, Polak-Charcon S, et al. Progressive nephropathy associated with mitochondrial tRNA gene mutation. *Clin Nephrol*, 2004;62:149–154.
1127. Doleris LM, Hill GS, Chedin P, et al. Focal segmental glomerulosclerosis associated with mitochondrial cytopathy. *Kidney Int*, 2000;58:1851–1858.
1128. Guery B, Choukroun G, Noel LH, et al. The spectrum of systemic involvement in adults presenting with renal lesion and mitochondrial tRNA(Leu) gene mutation. *J Am Soc Nephrol*, 2003;14:2099–2108.
1129. Hotta O, Inoue CN, Miyabayashi S, et al. Clinical and pathologic features of focal segmental glomerulosclerosis with mitochondrial tRNALeu(UUR) gene mutation. *Kidney Int*, 2001;59:1236–1243.
1130. Inui K, Fukushima H, Tsukamoto H, et al. Mitochondrial encephalomyopathies with the mutation of the mitochondrial tRNA(Leu(UUR)) gene. *J Pediatr*, 1992;120:62–66.
1131. Jansen JJ, Maassen JA, van der Woude FJ, et al. Mutation in mitochondrial tRNA(Leu(UUR)) gene associated with progressive kidney disease. *J Am Soc Nephrol*, 1997;8:1118–1124.
1132. Kobayashi Y, Momoi MY, Tominaga K, et al. A point mutation in the mitochondrial tRNA(Leu)(UUR) gene in MELAS (mitochondrial myopathy, encephalopathy, lactic acidosis and stroke-like episodes). *Biochem Biophys Res Commun*, 1990;173:816–822.
1133. Kurogouchi F, Oguchi T, Mawatari E, et al. A case of mitochondrial cytopathy with a typical point mutation for MELAS, presenting with severe focal-segmental glomerulosclerosis as main clinical manifestation. *Am J Nephrol*, 1998;18:551–556.
1134. Mochizuki H, Joh K, Kawame H, et al. Mitochondrial encephalomyopathies preceded by de-Toni-Debre-Fanconi syndrome or focal segmental glomerulosclerosis. *Clin Nephrol*, 1996;46:347–352.
1135. Scaglia F, Vogel H, Hawkins EP, et al. Novel homoplasmic mutation in the mitochondrial tRNATyr gene associated with atypical mitochondrial cytopathy presenting with focal segmental glomerulosclerosis. *Am J Med Genet A*, 2003;123:172–178.
1136. Taniike M FH, Yanagihara I, Tsukamoto H, Tanaka J, Fujimori H, Nagai T, Sano T, Yamaoka K, Inui K, Okada S. Mitochondrial rRNA Ile mutations in fatal cardiomyopathy. *Biochem Biophys Res Commun*, 1992;186:47–53.
1137. Ueda Y, Ando A, Nagata T, et al. A boy with mitochondrial disease: asymptomatic proteinuria without neuromyopathy. *Pediatr Nephrol*, 2004;19:107–110.
1138. Yamagata K, Muro K, Usui J, et al. Mitochondrial DNA mutations in focal segmental glomerulosclerosis lesions. *J Am Soc Nephrol*, 2002;13:1816–1823.
1139. Quinzii C, Naini A, Salviati L, et al. A mutation in para-hydroxybenzoate-polyprenyl transferase (COQ2) causes primary coenzyme Q10 deficiency. *Am J Hum Genet*, 2006;78:345–349.
1140. Hiraoka M, Tsukahara H, Ohshima Y, et al. Renal aplasia is the predominant cause of congenital solitary kidneys. *Kidney Int*, 2002;61:1840–1844.
1141. Favor J, Sandulache R, Neuhauser-Klaus A, et al. The mouse Pax2(1Neu) mutation is identical to a human PAX2 mutation in a family with renal-coloboma syndrome and results in developmental defects of the brain, ear, eye, and kidney. *Proc Natl Acad Sci U S A*, 1996;93:13870–13875.
1142. Salomon R, Tellier AL, Attie-Bitach T, et al. PAX2 mutations in oligomeganephronia. *Kidney Int*, 2001;59:457–462.
1143. Nishimoto K, Iijima K, Shirakawa T, et al. PAX2 gene mutation in a family with isolated renal hypoplasia. *J Am Soc Nephrol*, 2001;12:1769–1772.
1144. Miltenyi M, Balogh L, Schmidt K, et al. A new variant of the acrorenal syndrome associated with bilateral oligomeganephronic hypoplasia. *Eur J Pediatr*, 1984;142:40–43.
1145. Kohlhase J, Schubert L, Liebers M, et al. Mutations at the SALL4 locus on chromosome 20 result in a range of clinically overlapping phenotypes, including Okihiro syndrome, Holt-Oram syndrome, acro-renal-ocular syndrome, and patients previously reported to represent thalidomide embryopathy. *J Med Genet*, 2003;40:473–478.
1146. Abdelhak S, Kalatzis V, Heilig R, et al. A human homologue of the Drosophila eyes absent gene underlies branchio-oto-renal (BOR) syndrome and identifies a novel gene family. *Nat Genet*, 1997;15:157–164.
1147. Krug P, Moriniere V, Marlin S, et al. Mutation screening of the EYA1, SIX1, and SIX5 genes in a large cohort of patients harboring branchio-oto-renal syndrome calls into question the pathogenic role of SIX5 mutations. *Hum Mutat*, 2011;32:183–190.
1148. McPherson E, Carey J, Kramer A, et al. Dominantly inherited renal adysplasia. *Am J Med Genet*, 1987;26:863–872.
1149. Freedman BI, Hicks PJ, Bostrom MA, et al. Non-muscle myosin heavy chain 9 gene MYH9 associations in African Americans with clinically diagnosed type 2 diabetes mellitus-associated ESRD. *Nephrol Dial Transplant*, 2009;24:3366–3371.
1150. Genovese G, Friedman DJ, Ross MD, et al. Association of trypanolytic ApoL1 variants with kidney disease in African Americans. *Science*, 2010;329:841–845.
1151. Atta MG, Estrella MM, Kuperman M, et al. HIV-associated nephropathy patients with and without apolipoprotein L1 gene variants have similar clinical and pathologic characteristics. *Kidney International*, 2012;in press.
1152. Fine DM, Wasser WG, Estrella MM, et al. APOL1 Risk Variants Predict Histopathology and Progression to ESRD in HIV-Related Kidney Disease. *J Am Soc Nephrol*, 2012;23:343–350.
1153. Madhavan SM, O'Toole JF, Konieczkowski M, et al. APOL1 localization in normal kidney and nondiabetic kidney disease. *J Am Soc Nephrol*, 2011;22: 2119–2128.
1154. Hori C, Hiraoka M, Yoshikawa N, et al. Significance of ACE genotypes and medical treatments in childhood focal glomerulosclerosis. *Nephron*, 2001;88:313–319.
1155. Lee DY, Kim W, Kang SK, et al. Angiotensin-converting enzyme gene polymorphism in patients with minimal-change nephrotic syndrome and focal segmental glomerulosclerosis. *Nephron*, 1997;77:471–473.
1156. Vehaskari VM. Treatment practices of FSGS among North American pediatric nephrologists. *Pediatr. Nephrol.*, 1999;13:301–303.
1157. Cattran DC, Rao P. Long-term outcome in children and adults with classic focal segmental glomerulosclerosis. *Am J Kidney Dis*, 1998;32:72–79.

1158. Griswold WR, Tune BM, Reznik VM, et al. Treatment of childhood prednisone-resistant nephrotic syndrome and focal segmental glomerulosclerosis with intravenous methylprednisolone and oral alkylating agents. *Nephron*, 1987;46:73–77.
1159. Tune BM, Lieberman E, Mendoza SA. Steroid-resistant nephrotic focal segmental glomerulosclerosis: a treatable disease. *Pediatr. Nephrol.*, 1996;10: 772–778.
1160. Mendoza SA, Reznik VM, Griswold WR, et al. Treatment of steroid-resistant focal segmental glomerulosclerosis with pulse methylprednisolone and alkylating agents. *Pediatr. Nephrol.*, 1990;4:303–307.
1161. Waldo FB, Benfield MR, Kohaut EC. Therapy of focal and segmental glomerulosclerosis with methylprednisolone, cyclosporine A and prednisone. *Pediatr. Nephrol.*, 1998;12:397–400.
1162. Murphy JL, Kano HL, Chenaille PJ, et al. Fatal *Pneumocystis* pneumonia in a child treated for focal segmental glomerulosclerosis. *Pediatr. Nephrol.*, 1993;7:444–445.
1163. Ingulli E, Baqi N, Ahmad H, et al. Aggressive, long-term cyclosporine therapy for steroid-resistant focal segmental glomerulosclerosis. *J. Am. Soc. Nephrol.*, 1995;5:1820–1825.
1164. Lieberman KV, Tejani A. A randomized double-blind placebo-controlled trial of cyclosporine in steroid-resistant idiopathic focal segmental glomerulosclerosis in children. *J. Am. Soc. Nephrol.*, 1995;7:56–63.
1165. Cattran DC, Appel GB, Hebert LA, et al. A randomized trial of cyclosporine in patients with steroid-resistant focal segmental glomerulosclerosis. *Kidney Int.*, 1999;56:2220–2226.
1166. Singh A, Tejani C, Tejani A. One-center experience with cyclosporine in refractory nephrotic syndrome in children. *Pediatr. Nephrol.*, 1999;13:26–32.
1167. McCauley J, Shapiro R, Ellis D. Pilot trial of FK 506 in the management of steroid-resistant nephrotic syndrome. *Nephrol. Dial. Transplant.*, 1993;8: 1286–1290.
1168. Baluarte HJ, Gruskin AB, Polinsky MS, et al., Chlorambucil therapy in the nephrotic syndrome, in *Pediatric Nephrology*, Gruskin AB, Norman M, Editors. 1981, Martinus Nijhoff: Boston. p. 429.
1169. Rennert WP, Kala UK, Jacobs D, et al. Pulse cyclophosphamide for steroid-resistant focal segmental glomerulosclerosis. *Pediatr. Nephrol.*, 1999;13:113–116.
1170. Prytula A, Iijima K, Kamei K, et al. Rituximab in refractory nephrotic syndrome. *Pediatr Nephrol*, 2010;25:461–468.
1171. Gipson DS, Trachtman H, Kaskel FJ, et al. Clinical trial of focal segmental glomerulosclerosis in children and young adults. *Kidney Int*, 2011;80:868–878.
1172. Kawamura T, Yoshioka T, Bills T, et al. Glucocorticoid activates glomerular antioxidant enzymes and protects glomeruli from oxidant injuries. *Kidney Int*, 1991;40:291–301.
1173. Smoyer WE, Ransom RF. Hsp27 regulates podocyte cytoskeletal changes in an in vitro model of podocyte process retraction. *FASEB J*, 2002; 16:315–326.
1174. Agarwal SK, Dash SC, Tiwari SC, et al. Idiopathic adult focal segmental glomerulosclerosis: a clinicopathological study and response to steroids. *Nephron*, 1993;63:161–171.
1175. Rydel JJ, Korbet SM, Borok RZ, et al. Focal segmental glomerulosclerosis in adults: presentation, course and response to treatment. *Am. J. Kid. Dis.*, 1995;25:534–542.
1176. Ponticelli C, Villa M, Banfi G, et al. Can prolonged treatment improve the prognosis in adults with focal segmental glomerulosclerosis? *Am J Kidney Dis*, 1999;34:618–625.
1177. Chitalia VC, Wells JE, Robson RA, et al. Predicting renal survival in primary focal glomerulosclerosis from the time of presentation. *Kidney Int*, 1999;56:2236–2242.
1178. Stiles KP, Abbott KC, Welch PG, et al. Effects of angiotensin-converting enzyme inhibitor and steroid therapy on proteinuria in FSGS: a retrospective study in a single clinic. *Clin Nephrol*, 2001;56:89–95.
1179. Pokhariyal S, Gulati S, Prasad N, et al. Duration of optimal therapy for idiopathic focal segmental glomerulosclerosis. *J Nephrol*, 2003;16:691–696.
1180. Franceschini N, Hogan SL, Falk RJ. Primum non nocere: Should adults with idiopathic FSGS receive steroids? *Semin Nephrol*, 2003;23:229–233.
1181. Smith D, Branton M, Fervenza F, et al. Pulse dexamethasone for focal segmental glomerulosclerosis. *J Am Soc Nephrol*, 2003;14.
1182. Lewis EJ, Hunsicker LG, Bain RP, et al. The effect of angiotensin-converting-enzyme inhibition on diabetic nephropathy. The Collaborative Study Group. *N. Engl. J. Med.*, 1993;329:1456–1462.
1183. Shiiki H, Nishino T, Uyama H, et al. Clinical and morphological predictors of renal outcome in adult patients with focal and segmental glomerulosclerosis (FSGS). *Clin Nephrol*, 1996;46:362–368.
1184. Bolton WK, Atuk NO, Sturgill BC, et al. Therapy of the idiopathic nephrotic syndrome with alternate day steroids. *Am J Med*, 1977;62:60–70.
1185. Nagai R, Cattran DC, Pei Y. Steroid therapy and prognosis of focal segmental glomerulosclerosis in the elderly. *Clin Nephrol*, 1994;42:18–21.
1186. Cattran DC. Cyclosporine in the treatment of idiopathic focal segmental glomerulosclerosis. *Semin Nephrol*, 2003;23:234–241.
1187. Ittel TH, Clasen W, Fuhs M, et al. Long-term ciclosporine A treatment in adults with minimal change nephrotic syndrome or focal segmental glomerulosclerosis. *Clin Nephrol*, 1995;44:156–162.
1188. Lee HY, Kim HS, Kang CM, et al. The efficacy of cyclosporine A in adult nephrotic syndrome with minimal change disease and focal-segmental glomerulosclerosis: a multicenter study in Korea. *Clin Nephrol*, 1995;43:375–381.
1189. Meyrier A, Noel LH, Auriche P, et al. Long-term renal tolerance of cyclosporin A treatment in the adult idiopathic nephrotic syndrome. *Kidney Int.*, 1994;45:1446–1456.
1190. Walker RG, Kincaid-Smith P. The effect of treatment of corticosteroid-resistant idiopathic (primary) focal and segmental hyalinosis and sclerosis (focal glomerulosclerosis) with ciclosporin. *Nephron*, 1990;54:117–121.
1191. Matalon A, Valeri A, Appel GB. Treatment of focal segmental glomerulosclerosis. *Semin Nephrol*, 2000;20:309–317.
1192. Duncan N, Dhaygude A, Owen J, et al. Treatment of focal and segmental glomerulosclerosis in adults with tacrolimus monotherapy. *Nephrol Dial Transplant*, 2004;19:3062–3067.
1193. Sharma R, Sharma M, Ge X, et al. Cyclosporine protects glomeruli from FSGS factor via an increase in glomerular cAMP. *Transplantation*, 1996;62:1916–1920.
1194. Faul C, Donnelly M, Merscher-Gomez S, et al. The actin cytoskeleton of kidney podocytes is a direct target of the antiproteinuric effect of cyclosporine A. *Nat Med*, 2008;14:931–938.
1195. Guess A, Agrawal S, Wei CC, et al. Dose- and time-dependent glucocorticoid receptor signaling in podocytes. *Am J Physiol Renal Physiol*, 2010;299:F845–853.
1196. Agrawal S, Guess AJ, Benndorf R, et al. Comparison of direct action of thiazolidinediones and glucocorticoids on renal podocytes: protection from injury and molecular effects. *Mol Pharmacol*, 2011;80:389–399.
1197. Fukuda A, Fujimoto S, Iwatsubo S, et al. Effects of mineralocorticoid and angiotensin II receptor blockers on proteinuria and glomerular podocyte protein expression in a model of minimal change nephrotic syndrome. *Nephrology (Carlton)*, 2010;15:321–326.
1198. Korbet SM, Schwartz MM, Lewis EJ. Primary focal segmental glomerulosclerosis: clinical course and response to therapy. *Am J Kidney Dis*, 1994;23:773–783.
1199. Choi MJ, Eustace JA, Gimenez LF, et al. Mycophenolate mofetil treatment for primary glomerular diseases. *Kidney Int*, 2002;61:1098–1114.
1200. Cattran DC, Wang MM, Appel G, et al. Mycophenolate mofetil in the treatment of focal segmental glomerulosclerosis. *Clin Nephrol*, 2004;62:405–411.
1201. Mendizabal S, Zamora I, Berbel O, et al. Mycophenolate mofetil in steroid/cyclosporine-dependent/resistant nephrotic syndrome. *Pediatr Nephrol*, 2005;20:914–919.
1202. Senthil Nayagam L, Ganguli A, Rathi M, et al. Mycophenolate mofetil or standard therapy for membranous nephropathy and focal segmental glomerulosclerosis: a pilot study. *Nephrol Dial Transplant*, 2008;23:1926–1930.
1203. Fernandez-Fresnedo G, Segarra A, Gonzalez E, et al. Rituximab treatment of adult patients with steroid-resistant focal segmental glomerulosclerosis. *Clin J Am Soc Nephrol*, 2009;4:1317–1323.
1204. Kisner T, Burst V, Teschner S, et al. Rituximab Treatment for Adults with Refractory Nephrotic Syndrome: A Single-Center Experience and Review of the Literature. *Nephron Clin Pract*, 2012;120:c79-c85.
1205. Alexopoulos E, Stangou M, Papagianni A, et al. Factors influencing the course and the response to treatment in primary focal segmental glomerulosclerosis. *Nephrol Dial Transplant*, 2000;15:1348–1356.
1206. Velosa JA, Torres VE, Donadio JV, et al. Treatment of severe nephrotic syndrome with meclofenamate: An uncontrolled pilot study. *Mayo Clin. Proc.*, 1985;60:586–592.
1207. Tahzib M, Frank R, Gauthier B, et al. Vitamin E treatment of focal segmental glomerulosclerosis: results of an open-label study. *Pediatr Nephrol*, 1999;13:649–652.
1208. Cho M, Smith D, Branton M, et al. Pirfenidone slows progressive loss of renal function in focal segmental glomerulosclerosis. *J Am Soc Nephrol*, 2004;15:906–913.
1209. Feld SM, Figueroa P, Savin V, et al. Plasmapheresis in the treatment of steroid-resistant focal segmental glomerulosclerosis in native kidneys. *Am. J. Kidney Dis.*, 1998;32:230–237.
1210. Chobanian AV, Bakris GL, Black HR, et al. Seventh report of the Joint National Committee on Prevention, Detection, Evaluation, and Treatment of High Blood Pressure. *Hypertension*, 2003;42:1206–1252.
1211. GISEN. Randomised placebo-controlled trial of effect of ramipril on decline in glomerular filtration rate and risk of terminal renal failure in proteinuric, non-diabetic nephropathy. *Lancet*, 1997;349:1857–1863.

1212. Korbet SM. Angiotensin antagonists and steroids in the treatment of focal segmental glomerulosclerosis. *Semin Nephrol*, 2003;23:219–228.
1213. Usta M, Ersoy A, Dilek K, et al. Efficacy of losartan in patients with primary focal segmental glomerulosclerosis resistant to immunosuppressive treatment. *J Intern Med*, 2003;253:329–334.
1214. Crenshaw G, Bigler S, Salem M, et al. Focal segmental glomerulosclerosis in African Americans: effects of steroids and angiotensin converting enzyme inhibitors. *Am J Med Sci*, 2000;319:320–325.
1215. Praga M, Hernandez E, Montoyo C, et al. Long-term beneficial effects of angiotensin-converting enzyme inhibition in patients with nephrotic proteinuria. *Am J Kidney Dis*, 1992;20:240–248.
1216. Burgess E. Management of focal segmental glomerulosclerosis: evidence-based recommendations. *Kidney Int.*, 1999;(Suppl. 70):S26–S32.
1217. Ponticelli C, Passerini P. Alternative treatments for focal and segmental glomerular sclerosis. *Clin Nephrol*, 2001;55:345–348.
1218. Kunau RT, ed. *Nephrology and Hypertension Medical Knowledge Self-Assessment Program*. 1998, American College of Physicians: Philadelphia. 6–9.
1219. Aizawa-Yashiro T, Tsuruga K, Watanabe S, et al. Novel multidrug therapy for children with cyclosporine-resistant or -intolerant nephrotic syndrome. *Pediatr Nephrol*, 2011;26:1255–1261.
1220. Fujinaga S, Hirano D, Nishizaki N, et al. Single daily high-dose mizoribine therapy for children with steroid-dependent nephrotic syndrome prior to cyclosporine administration. *Pediatr Nephrol*, 2011;26:479–483.
1221. Cho ME, Hurley JK, Kopp JB. Sirolimus therapy of focal segmental glomerulosclerosis is associated with nephrotoxicity. *Am J Kidney Dis*, 2007; 49:310–317.
1222. Tumlin JA, Miller D, Near M, et al. A prospective, open-label trial of sirolimus in the treatment of focal segmental glomerulosclerosis. *Clin J Am Soc Nephrol*, 2006;1:109–116.
1223. McCarthy ET, Sharma M, Savin VJ. Circulating permeability factors in idiopathic nephrotic syndrome and focal segmental glomerulosclerosis. *Clin J Am Soc Nephrol*, 2010;5:2115–2121.
1224. Joy MS, Gipson DS, Powell L, et al. Phase 1 trial of adalimumab in Focal Segmental Glomerulosclerosis (FSGS): II. Report of the FONT (Novel Therapies for Resistant FSGS) study group. *Am J Kidney Dis*, 2010;55:50–60.
1225. Bomback AS, Tumlin JA, Baranski J, et al. Treatment of nephrotic syndrome wth adrenocorticotropic hormone (ACTH) gel. *Drug Design, Development and Therapy*, 2011;5:147–153.
1226. Trachtman H, Fervenza FC, Gipson DS, et al. A phase 1, single-dose study of fresolimumab, an anti-TGF-beta antibody, in treatment-resistant primary focal segmental glomerulosclerosis. *Kidney Int*, 2011;79:1236–1243.
1227. Chan PC, Chan KW, Cheng IK, et al. Focal sclerosing glomerulopathy. Risk factors of progression and optimal mode of treatment. *Int Urol Nephrol*, 1991;23:619–629.
1228. Newman WJ, Tisher CC, McCoy RC, et al. Focal glomerular sclerosis: Contrasting clinical patterns in children and adults. *Medicine*, 1978;55: 67–87.
1229. Mongeau JG, Corneille L, Robitaille P, et al. Primary nephrosis in childhood associated with focal glomerulosclerosis: Is long-term prognosis that severe? *Kidney Int.*, 1981;20:743–746.
1230. Velosa JA, Holley KE, Torres VE, et al. Significance of proteinuria on the outcome of renal function in patients with focal segmental glomerulosclerosis. *Mayo Clin Proc*, 1983;58:568–577.
1231. Wehrmann M, Bohle A, Held H, et al. Long-term prognosis of focal sclerosing glomerulonephritis. An analysis of 250 cases with particular regard to tubulointerstitial changes. *Clin. Nephrol.*, 1990;33:115–122.
1232. Cosio FG, Hernandez RA. Favorable prognostic significance of raised serum C3 concentration in patients with idiopathic focal glomerulosclerosis. *Clin Nephrol*, 1996;45:146–152.
1233. Andresdottir MB, Ajubi N, Croockewit S, et al. Recurrent focal glomerulosclerosis: natural course and treatment with plasma exchange. *Nephrol Dial Transplant*, 1999;14:2650–2656.
1234. Artero ML, Sharma R, Savin VJ, et al. Plasmapheresis reduces proteinuria and serum capacity to injure glomeruli in patients with recurrent focal glomerulosclerosis. *Am J Kidney Dis*, 1994;23:574–581.
1235. Cochat P, Kassir A, Colon S, et al. Recurrent nephrotic syndrome after transplantation: early treatment with plasmaphaeresis and cyclophosphamide. *Pediatr. Nephrol.*, 1993;7:50–54.
1236. Dall'Amico R, Ghiggeri G, Carraro M, et al. Prediction and treatment of recurrent focal segmental glomerulosclerosis after renal transplantation in children. *Am J Kidney Dis*, 1999;34:1048–1055.
1237. Dantal J, Baatard R, Hourmant M, et al. Recurrent nephrotic syndrome following renal transplantation in patients with focal glomerulosclerosis. A one-center study of plasma exchange effects. *Transplantation*, 1991;52:827–831.
1238. Dantal J, Godfrin Y, Koll R, et al. Antihuman immunoglobulin affinity immunoadsorption strongly decreases proteinuria in patients with relapsing nephrotic syndrome. *J. Am. Soc. Nephrol.*, 1998;9:1709–1715.
1239. Greenstein SM, Delrio M, Ong E, et al. Plasmapheresis treatment for recurrent focal sclerosis in pediatric renal allografts. *Pediatr Nephrol*, 2000;14: 1061–1065.
1240. Kershaw DB, Sedman AB, Kelsch RC, et al. Recurrent focal segmental glomerulosclerosis in pediatric renal transplant recipients: successful treatment with oral cyclophosphamide. *Clin Transplant*, 1994;8:546–549.
1241. Kooijmans-Coutinho MF, Tegzess AM, Bruijn JA, et al. Indomethacin treatment of recurrent nephrotic syndrome and focal segmental glomerulosclerosis after renal transplantation. *Nephrol Dial Transplant*, 1993;8:469–473.
1242. Marcen R, Matesanz R, Quereda C, et al. [Immediate recurrence of segmental and focal hyalinosis postrenal transplant [letter]]. *Med Clin (Barc)*, 1986;86:778.
1243. Matalon A, Markowitz GS, Joseph RE, et al. Plasmapheresis treatment of recurrent FSGS in adult renal transplant recipients. *Clin Nephrol*, 2001;56: 271–278.
1244. Pradhan M, Petro J, Palmer J, et al. Early use of plasmapheresis for recurrent post-transplant FSGS. *Pediatr Nephrol*, 2003;18:934–938.
1245. Raafat R, Travis LB, Kalia A, et al. Role of transplant induction therapy on recurrence rate of focal segmental glomerulosclerosis. *Pediatr Nephrol*, 2000;14:189–194.
1246. Saleem MA, Ramanan AV, Rees L. Recurrent focal segmental glomerulosclerosis in grafts treated with plasma exchange and increased immunosuppression. *Pediatr Nephrol*, 2000;14:361–364.
1247. Seikaly MG. Recurrence of primary disease in children after renal transplantation: an evidence-based update. *Pediatr Transplant*, 2004;8:113–119.
1248. Bertelli R, Ginevri F, Caridi G, et al. Recurrence of focal segmental glomerulosclerosis after renal transplantation in patients with mutations of podocin. *Am J Kidney Dis*, 2003;41:1314–1321.
1249. Abbott KC, Sawyers ES, Oliver JD III, et al. Graft loss due to recurrent focal segmental glomerulosclerosis in renal transplant recipients in the United States. *Am J Kidney Dis*, 2001;37:366–373.
1250. Hubsch H, Montane B, Abitbol C, et al. Recurrent focal glomerulosclerosis in pediatric renal allografts: the Miami experience. *Pediatr Nephrol*, 2005;20:210–216.
1251. Savin VJ, Sharma R, Lovell HB, et al. Measurement of albumin reflection coefficient with isolated rat glomeruli. *J. Am. Soc. Nephrol.*, 1992;3:1260.
1252. Savin VJ, Sharma R, Sharma M, et al. Circulating factor in recurrent focal segmental glomerular sclerosis. *N. Engl. J. Med.*, 1996;334:878–883.
1253. Godfrin Y, Dantal J, Perretto S, et al. Study of the in vitro effect on glomerular albumin permselectivity of serum before and after renal transplantation in focal segmental glomerulosclerosis. *Transplantation*, 1997;64: 1711–1715.
1254. Sharma M, Sharma R, McCarthy ET, et al. "The FSGS factor:" enrichment and in vivo effect of activity from focal segmental glomerulosclerosis plasma. *J Am Soc Nephrol*, 1999;10:552–561.
1255. Dantal J, Bigot E, Bogers W, et al. Effect of plasma protein adsorption on protein excretion in kidney-transplant recipients with recurrent nephrotic syndrome. *N. Engl. J. Med.*, 1994;330:7–14.
1256. Sharma M, Sharma R, McCarthy ET, et al. The focal segmental glomerulosclerosis permeability factor: biochemical characteristics and biological effects. *Exp Biol Med (Maywood)*, 2004;229:85–98.
1257. Musante L, Candiano G, Bruschi M, et al. Characterization of plasma factors that alter the permeability to albumin within isolated glomeruli. *Proteomics*, 2002;2:197–205.
1258. Le Berre L, Godfrin Y, Lafond-Puyet L, et al. Effect of plasma fractions from patients with focal and segmental glomerulosclerosis on rat proteinuria. *Kidney Int*, 2000;58:2502–2511.
1259. Sharma M, Sharma R, Reddy SR, et al. Proteinuria after injection of human focal segmental glomerulosclerosis factor. *Transplantation*, 2002;73: 366–372.
1260. Clement LC, Avila-Casado C, Mace C, et al. Podocyte-secreted angiopoietin-like-4 mediates proteinuria in glucocorticoid-sensitive nephrotic syndrome. *Nat Med*, 2011;17:117–122.
1261. Sharma R, Sharma M, McCarthy ET, et al. Components of normal serum block the focal segmental glomerulosclerosis factor activity in vitro. *Kidney Int*, 2000;58:1973–1979.
1262. Candiano G, Musante L, Carraro M, et al. Apolipoproteins prevent glomerular albumin permeability induced in vitro by serum from patients with focal segmental glomerulosclerosis. *J Am Soc Nephrol*, 2001;12:143–150.
1263. Carraro M, Zennaro C, Artero M, et al. The effect of proteinase inhibitors on glomerular albumin permeability induced in vitro by serum from patients

with idiopathic focal segmental glomerulosclerosis. *Nephrol Dial Transplant*, 2004;19:1969–1975.
1264. Shariatmadar S, Noto TA. Therapeutic plasma exchange in recurrent focal segmental glomerulosclerosis following transplantation. *J Clin Apheresis*, 2002;17:78–83.
1265. Davenport RD. Apheresis treatment of recurrent focal segmental glomerulosclerosis after kidney transplantation: re-analysis of published case-reports and case-series. *J Clin Apheresis*, 2001;16:175–178.
1266. Cheong HI, Han HW, Park HW, et al. Early recurrent nephrotic syndrome after renal transplantation in children with focal segmental glomerulosclerosis. *Nephrol Dial Transplant*, 2000;15:78–81.
1267. Salomon R, Gagnadoux MF, Niaudet P. Intravenous cyclosporine therapy in recurrent nephrotic syndrome after renal transplantation in children. *Transplantation*, 2003;75:810–814.
1268. Raafat RH, Kalia A, Travis LB, et al. High-dose oral cyclosporin therapy for recurrent focal segmental glomerulosclerosis in children. *Am J Kidney Dis*, 2004;44:50–56.
1269. Pescovitz MD. Rituximab, an anti-cd20 monoclonal antibody: history and mechanism of action. *Am J Transplant*, 2006;6:859–866.
1270. Otsubo S, Tanabe K, Tokumoto T, et al. Long-term outcome in renal transplant recipients with focal and segmental glomerulosclerosis. *Transplant Proc*, 1999;31:2860–2862.
1271. Ohta T, Kawaguchi H, Hattori M, et al. Effect of pre-and postoperative plasmapheresis on posttransplant recurrence of focal segmental glomerulosclerosis in children. *Transplantation*, 2001;71:628–633.
1272. Pollak MR. Inherited podocytopathies: FSGS and nephrotic syndrome from a genetic viewpoint. *J Am Soc Nephrol*, 2002;13:3016–3023.

CHAPTER 53

Renal Involvement in Systemic Lupus Erythematosus

Brad H. Rovin • Daniel J. Birmingham • Tibor Nadasdy

The kidney is affected in a clinically important way in about 38% of patients with systemic lupus erythematosus (SLE), although renal involvement varies considerably by race and ethnicity. Caucasians (European, European Americans) have an incidence of renal lupus of 12% to 33%, whereas black (African American, Afro-Caribbean), Hispanic, or Asian patients have a 50% or greater incidence.[1–4] Of the patients who eventually have clinical renal involvement, 40% to 60% have overt findings of kidney disease at the time of initial diagnosis of SLE.[1,2,4]

Kidney damage in SLE is most often due to lupus nephritis (LN) in which glomerular immune complex accumulation leads to an inflammatory response that damages glomeruli and eventually the renal interstitium. LN is associated with a worse outcome in SLE, in part due to the development of chronic kidney disease (CKD) or end-stage renal disease (ESRD).[5,6] The incidence of ESRD attributed to LN in adults from 1996 to 2004 was 4.4 to 4.9 cases per million in the general population according to the United States Renal Data Service.[7] However, in blacks and Hispanics, the incidence of ESRD was 6 to 20 per million compared to Caucasians (2.5 per million). Similarly, in the United Kingdom 19% of Caucasians versus 62% of blacks with LN progressed to ESRD.[3] The prevalence of CKD in patients with SLE is difficult to estimate, but because current therapies induce complete remission in 50% or fewer LN patients, CKD is likely to be high in the lupus population.

LN is generally treatable. Presently this requires intense, nonspecific immunosuppression, which confers considerable risk of severe infection and other morbidities. Efforts are under way to develop new LN therapies that have greater efficacy and less toxicity. These new therapies are based on our current understanding of the pathogenesis of LN.

THE PATHOGENESIS OF LUPUS NEPHRITIS

Overview

SLE occurs when there is a loss of tolerance to self-antigens, and autoantibodies to these antigens are produced. Although the exact etiology of SLE remains unknown, a number of pathogenic mechanisms are thought to be involved. These include defects in the clearance of cellular debris and immune complexes (IC) that lead to enhanced self-antigen presentation, HLA-based polymorphisms that reduce the tolerogenic presentation of self-antigen, defects in B and T lymphocytes that facilitate their activation, and overproduction of cytokines that affect lymphocyte activation. In addition to their role in breaking tolerance, many of these pathways also directly contribute to the clinical manifestations of SLE.

The pathogenesis of LN mirrors, in many respects, the pathogenesis of systemic lupus, particularly immune complex (IC)-driven inflammation. Inflammatory kidney injury occurs following intrarenal IC accumulation. However, there appears to be qualitative differences between the 30% and 40% of the SLE patients who develop LN and those who do not. Most patients without kidney involvement in the first few years of the disease will never develop LN, and younger age has been shown to be a risk factor for LN. Thus, certain aspects of the pathogenic pathways of SLE are manifested only in the subset of SLE patients that develop LN. The following discussion will highlight some of these aspects, focusing in particular on what is known about human LN, with animal models of LN cited for support where appropriate.

Autoantibodies and Immune Complexes

One of the earliest demonstrations of loss of tolerance in SLE was the discovery of autoantibodies in lupus, in particular antinuclear and anti–double-stranded (ds)DNA antibodies.[8] Antinuclear antibodies (ANAs) are the most prevalent, appearing in over 95% of SLE patients. However, over 100 self-antigens have been identified in SLE patients that are targets of autoantibodies, including dsDNA, single-stranded (ss)DNA, nucleoproteins, RNA-protein complexes, ribosomes, phospholipids, carbohydrates, cell cytoplasm and cell surface molecules, blood components, and endothelial cells.[9] The fact that autoantibodies to all of these antigens are not present in every patient suggests that autoantibody specificities may define which organs are affected. Two antibody specificities seem to be particularly relevant to LN pathogenesis, those against dsDNA and those against the complement component C1q.

Two lines of evidence have historically suggested a specific role for anti-dsDNA in the development of LN. First, numerous studies found an association of high titer anti-dsDNA with active LN.[10] Second, anti-dsDNA antibodies can be isolated from the glomeruli of LN patients.[11] Why these antibodies, and IC containing these antibodies, target renal tissue is not completely clear, although two main mechanisms are proposed that focus on the nature of the dsDNA antigen. One mechanism involves nucleosomes, which are composed of DNA in association with a core of positively charged histone proteins. Nucleosomes are released by cells undergoing apoptosis, and can be trapped in the glomeruli, perhaps facilitated by interactions between the positively charged histones and the negatively charged glomerular basement membrane.[12] Anti-dsDNA can recognize the DNA in nucleosomes, and the binding of anti-dsDNA in lupus renal tissue occurs at the site of glomerular nucleosome deposition.[13] Another mechanism is based on cross-reactivity between anti-DNA and one or more renal tissue antigens. Many potential tissue antigens have been implicated, and two of the more relevant candidates are alpha-actinin expressed in both glomerular podocytes and mesangial cells,[14] and annexin II on mesangial cells.[15] Regardless of which mechanism predominates, the result is localized anti-dsDNA-containing IC with the potential to drive local tissue inflammation. Anti-dsDNA autoantibodies appear to be predominantly immunoglobulin G1 (IgG1)[16] which is an inflammatory IgG subtype due to its ability to activate complement and engage Fc receptors for IgG.

Antibodies to C1q, the first component of the classical complement pathway, have been strongly associated with LN in so many studies[17] that some investigators feel they are required for active nephritis.[18] However, this does not seem to be true in all cases.[19] Nevertheless, the high prevalence of anti-C1q antibodies in active LN patients suggests an important pathogenic role. Anti-C1q does not appear to cause an acquired deficiency of circulating C1q because anti-C1q binding requires a neoepitope formed when it becomes fixed to its target substrate. Rather, injury is likely related to interaction of anti-C1q with C1q already present in the kidney, such as in IC bound to nucleosomes.[20,21] The resulting C1q/anti-C1q IC could focus on inflammatory response to renal tissue, similar to anti-dsDNA/nucleosome IC, leading to nephritis. It should be noted, however, that unlike anti-dsDNA antibodies, most anti-C1q antibodies appear to be IgG2,[22] which is a poor activator of complement and binds Fc receptors with low affinity. Other IgG subtypes (mainly IgG1) can be present in these IC, so the role of anti-C1q in LN pathogenesis may depend on the relative amounts of each anti-C1q IgG subtype.

The Complement and Fcγ Receptor Systems

The formation of IC leads to the activation of both the complement cascade and cells bearing Fc receptors for IgG (known as Fcγ receptors, or FcγR). The activation of complement and FcγR by IC can provide protective effects against SLE, mainly by promoting proper clearance of circulating IC. However, once IC are deposited in tissue, both of these pathways can drive tissue inflammation and damage, either through direct effects on tissue (complement membrane attack complex) or by activating cells to produce proinflammatory cytokines and toxic mediators.

Complement is thought to provide *protection* from SLE in a few different ways. First, classical complement activation by IC results in a more soluble, less phlogistic form of IC that is less likely to be trapped in tissue.[23] Second, complement contributes to clearance of apoptotic debris through opsonization by C1q, thus removing a highly immunogenic source of self-antigen.[24] Third, IC opsonization by other complement components (C4b and C3b/bi) that result from complement activation promotes IC clearance through C4b/C3b/C3bi receptors.[25] The type one complement receptor (CR1, CD35), which binds C4b, C3b and C3bi and acts as a regulator of complement activation, is expressed in the circulation predominantly on erythrocytes (E-CR1), and mediates the binding of complement-opsonized IC to erythrocytes (a process known as immune adherence).[26] This binding allows erythrocytes to shuttle IC through the circulation, minimizing glomerular trapping of IC, and promoting IC delivery to the liver and spleen for safe removal.[26] The evidence that all of these complement functions protect against SLE include studies showing that individuals with homozygous deficiencies of classical pathway components have an increased risk for developing SLE and SLE-like diseases,[27] and that E-CR1 levels are decreased in SLE and fluctuate in chronically active disease.[28,29]

In contrast, several observations suggest complement-mediated inflammation and direct tissue damage contribute to the pathogenesis of LN:

- Circulating levels of C3 and C4 are lower in active LN compared to inactive LN or nonrenal SLE, indicating ongoing complement activation.[30,31]
- Complement components, including the membrane attack complex, are deposited in LN kidneys.[30,32,33]
- Longitudinal assessment of circulating C3 and C4 levels during SLE flare showed that levels decrease significantly at the time of a renal flare, but not at nonrenal flare, even if the nonrenal flare occurred in patients with a history of LN.[29]
- Renal tubular production of C3 and complement factor B occurs in LN patients but not healthy controls.[34,35]
- The inflammatory receptor for C3a (C3aR), absent from healthy kidneys, becomes expressed in glomerular endothelium in association with IC deposits in LN, and the expression level correlates with LN severity.[36]
- The inflammatory receptor for C5a (C5aR), although present in normal kidneys, is greatly upregulated in the mesangium and podocytes of LN kidneys.[37]
- The expression of CR1 is decreased in LN glomeruli, compared to its normal expression on podocytes.[38]

- The expression of another complement regulator, decay accelerating factor (DAF, CD55), is also reduced in LN patients from its normal expression in the juxtaglomerular apparatus, and appears de novo in the renal vasculature, interstitium, and mesangium.[39]

Although there have been no human studies of complement inhibition in LN to verify its pathogenic role, such experiments have been done in experimental animals. For instance, in the NZB/NZW murine lupus model, anti-C5 antibody blocks the development of glomerulonephritis, suggesting C5a and/or the membrane attack complex are critical nephritic factors.[40] In the MRL/lpr mouse model of SLE, the administration of a rodent inhibitor of complement activation (Crry) was effective at protecting against glomerulonephritis.[41] Interestingly, nephritis in the MRL/lpr model appears to be dependent on the alternative pathway of complement activation, as deleting either the factor B or factor D genes significantly reduced the degree of renal injury.[42,43] The alternative complement pathway is an amplification pathway that is tightly regulated, suggesting that renal damage in LN is due to amplified complement activation occurring in the face of inadequate or overwhelmed complement regulation.

The role of FcγR in the pathogenesis of LN, although perhaps not as complex as complement, is similarly confounding. Like complement, IC activation of FcγR can provide protection by mediating IC phagocytosis and clearance, but can also induce inflammatory responses by activating the cells expressing FcγR.[44] Studies of polymorphic forms of FcγR have clarified which role has the most influence in SLE pathogenesis. There are three classes of FcγR (FcγRI, FcγRII, and FcγRIII), with different genes that produce full length products for FcγRII (FcγRIIA, FcγRIIB, FcγRIIC) and FcγRIII (FcγRIIIA and FcγRIIIB). Single nucleotide polymorphisms (SNPs) that affect the peptide sequence have been identified in some of these genes that influence binding affinity for IgG, including the FcγRIIA 491G>A SNP (amino acid 131R>H) and the FcγRIIIA 559T>G SNP (amino acid 158F>V).[45,46] Although not unequivocal, most studies have reported that the lower affinity forms of FcγRIIa (R131) and FcγRIIIa (F158) are associated with SLE, and particularly with LN.[47,48] The fact that the forms of these receptors that bind IC more efficiently are associated with protection against SLE suggest that their overall function is to promote IC clearance rather than drive tissue inflammation, and that relative deficiencies in this function contribute to LN.

It should be noted that there is an extensive body of work in mouse models of SLE that suggests IC inflammation is mainly FcγR-mediated, with little contribution from the complement system.[49] This includes nephritis in the NZB/NZW model, where deleting the signaling unit of FcγRI and FcγRIII, which also prevents expression of these FcγR, significantly reduces proteinuria, and increases survival time.[50] Although these studies support the potential of FcγR to drive inflammation, they do not negate the contributions of complement to this process. Caution must also be taken in their interpretation, as the relative contribution of complement and FcγR to mouse models of IC inflammation, including LN, depends on the mouse strain that is being tested.[51,52] Finally, if the role of FcγR, particularly FcγRIIIa, in lupus and LN is mainly to drive inflammation, higher affinity forms of the receptor should be associated with worse IC inflammation and LN. However, the studies in human lupus discussed previously demonstrate the opposite; higher affinity forms of FcγRIIIa and FcγRIIa are associated with protection against SLE and LN. Thus the extent to which these models recapitulate the complex nature of human SLE and LN must be considered.

Renal Chemokines, Cytokines, and Cellular Infiltrates

The presence of IC and the activation of the complement system are key initiators of inflammation that define LN. One consequence of complement activation is the deposition of the membrane attack complex, which directly induces cell membrane damage through the formation of transmembrane pores.[33] Another consequence of IC and complement activation is more indirect, and is mediated by the induction of chemokines and cytokines that induce infiltration and activation of proinflammatory cells. These chemokines and cytokines can be initially produced by renal parenchymal tissue, including glomerular endothelial cells, mesangial cells, podocytes, and tubular epithelium.[53] Once leukocytes containing chemokine receptors are drawn into the kidney, inflammation is accelerated through leukocyte secretion of additional chemokines and inflammatory cytokines. Some notable examples of upregulated chemokines and cytokines in kidneys of LN patients include monocyte chemoattractant protein-1 (MCP-1), and macrophage inflammatory protein-1-alpha (MIP-1α); interleukin (I)L-6, IL-10, IL-12, IL-17, IL-18; interferon (IFN)-gamma (IFN-γ); tumor necrosis factor (TNF)-alpha (TNF-α); and Eta-1/osteopontin.[53–57]

In support of a role for chemokines and cytokines in the pathogenesis of LN, deletion or inhibition of their expression substantially reduces kidney injury in mouse models of lupus. For example, deletion of the genes for MCP-1 or its receptor (CCR2) in the MRL/lpr mouse,[58,59] or predisease treatment of the mouse with a MCP-1 antagonist,[60] reduced infiltration of macrophages and T cells and attenuated clinical and histologic measures of injury, despite accumulation of renal IC comparable to wild-type animals. In both MRL/lpr and NZB/NZW mice, anti-IL-6 antibody treatment reduced anti-dsDNA antibodies and glomerulonephritis, as reflected by near normal renal function and glomerular histology.[61,62] Anti-IL-18 antibodies, induced in MRL/lpr mice through IL-18 cDNA vaccination, attenuated LN.[63] Anti-TNF-α treatment of NZB/NZW mice reduced proteinuria, renal inflammatory infiltrates, and glomerulosclerosis, despite increasing circulating anti-dsDNA levels.[64] These data suggest that the renal expression of proinflammatory chemokines and cytokines is an integral step in the pathogenesis of LN.

Some of these may specifically mediate kidney damage (e.g., MCP-1 and TNF-α), whereas others may predispose to kidney injury through general effects on autoimmunity.

Infiltrating neutrophils and monocytes/macrophages can cause direct renal tissue damage by secreting mediators like reactive oxygen species and proteolytic enzymes. The effect of infiltrating T cells is less direct, and is reflected by the cytokine profile of these T cells. During proliferative LN the intrarenal production of Th1 cytokines appears to predominate over Th2 cytokines and correlates with histologic activity. Th1 responses are associated with activated macrophages, and with the production of IgG capable of activating complement and FcγR pathways. Specifically, relatively high levels of IL-12, IFN-γ, and IL-18 are present, although IL-10, a Th2 cytokine, has also been shown to increase. This leads to an overall higher Th1/Th2 cytokine ratio.[55,56,65,66] Th1-dominant expression can also be observed in serum, urine, and circulating T cells of LN patients.[66] The Th1 dominance displayed in LN patients, both locally in the kidney and systemically in the circulation, suggests that this may be an important prerequisite for developing LN.

IL-17 may also play a particularly important role in the pathogenesis of LN. As mentioned previously, IL-17 is found in the kidney in LN, and two major cell sources of IL-17, Th17 cells and CD4-CD8 T cells, have been observed in renal biopsies of LN patients.[57] Local production of IL-17 may drive inflammatory cytokine and chemokine expression by resident glomerular and tubular cells having the IL-17 receptor,[67] leading to activation of neutrophils and monocytes.[68] The presence of IL-17-producing cells in the LN kidney may also represent a shift away from natural regulatory T cells capable of suppressing immune responses.[69] The role of regulatory T cells is discussed later.

Although not usually prevalent, infiltrating B cells have also been described in LN kidneys. Their presence may directly target autoantibodies to the kidney, as has been shown in NZB/NZW mice.[70] B cells in renal tissue may also present kidney antigens to intrarenal T cells. Recent work has shown that intrarenal B and T cells associate with various degrees of organization, including structures resembling germinal centers with central follicular dendritic cells.[71] Interestingly, these structures appear to occur mainly outside of the glomeruli, and are associated with tubular basement membrane IC.[71] These may contribute specifically to tubulointerstitial inflammation in LN.

Intrinsic Regulatory T Cells

Human regulatory T cells (Treg), characterized as $CD4^+$ $CD25^{hi}FoxP3^+$, inhibit immune responses through effects on T and B cells, and particularly autoantibody production.[72,73] Studies in the NZB/NZW mouse suggest a role for Tregs in lupus pathogenesis, with an inverse correlation between circulating Treg numbers and circulating anti-dsDNA levels,[74] and suppression of lupus-like disease activity, including glomerulonephritis by adoptive transfer of Tregs.[75] More than 25 studies have been done on human SLE and the majority of these indicate lower circulating levels of Tregs in SLE, although there is no clear consensus.[76] With regard to the role of Tregs in human LN, one study demonstrated an increase in Treg markers following rituximab-induced B cell depletion in LN patients ($n = 7$) that correlated with clinical remission,[77] whereas a second study showed no relationship between circulating Treg numbers or function and active LN.[78] Although Tregs are likely involved in SLE pathogenesis, the specific nature of that involvement, especially with respect to LN, remains to be determined.

Interferon-α and Plasmacytoid Dendritic Cells

IFN-α has recently taken a central role in the proposed paradigms of SLE pathogenesis.[79] This pathway is initiated when IFN-α is produced in response to a variety of stimuli, most involving nucleic acids. Plasmacytoid dendritic cells (pDCs) are the major sources of IFN-α following engagement of their endosomal toll-like receptors 7 and 9 (TLR7, TLR9) by ssRNA and unmethylated CpG in DNA, respectively.[80,81] Both TLRs are intracellular. Other cell types can produce IFN-α following engagement of different receptors, such as TLR3 in myeloid dendritic cells, or non-TLR pattern recognition receptors such as the helicases RIG-I and MDA5 in a variety of cells.[82] All these receptors sense various viral and bacterial nucleic acids and activate signaling cascades that end in the production of IFN-α. The effects of IFN-α on the immune response includes driving maturation of conventional dendritic cells into potent antigen presenting cells,[83] inducing B cell differentiation to plasma cells,[84] and contributing to the development of CD4 helper T cells[85] and CD8 central memory T cells.[86]

The IFN-α response receptors theoretically are important in discriminating between self and nonself. For example, TLR7 shows specificity for guanosine/uridine rich ssRNA such as viral ssRNA, whereas TLR9 shows specificity for unmethylated CpG that occurs mainly in nonmammalian DNA. Both receptors also can recognize mammalian nucleic acid in the form of IC containing RNA/protein (e.g., anti-RNP IC) or anti-dsDNA containing IC.[87] The presence of autoantibody may be crucial for this recognition, as RNA and DNA in the form of IC allow phagocytosis of the nucleic acids via FcγRIIa expressed on pDCs.[88] By generating increased IFN-α through this mechanism, an enhanced immune response can occur that may break tolerance to RNA and DNA-containing antigens, resulting in the types of autoantibody that are prevalent in SLE. Initiation of SLE strictly by this mechanism would require a baseline level of IgG against nucleic acids, which is reasonable as ANA positivity occurs in $>1\%$ of the general population.[89] Whether the IFN-α /pDC pathway initiates SLE or not, evidence suggests that the pathway is important to the pathogenesis of SLE. This evidence includes the observation that patients treated with IFN-α can develop a lupuslike disease,[90,91] the identification of a number of IFN-α-related genes as susceptibility genes for SLE onset,[79] an increase in IFN-α induced gene expression (the IFN-α signature) associated with active SLE,[92] and the number of known SLE autoantigens that can drive IFN-α secretion.

There is also evidence that IFN-α may be particularly involved in the pathogenesis of LN. Serum levels of IFN-α correlate directly with anti-dsDNA and inversely with C3 levels,[93,94] markers that are associated with LN. Peripheral blood cell levels of the IFN-α signature are associated with LN patients.[92,95] IFN-α-inducible chemokines, including MCP-1, correlate negatively with C3 levels, and are associated with active LN,[94] and with risk for renal flare.[96] During severe LN pDC disappear from the circulation and accumulate in glomeruli, due in part to glomerular expression of IL-18 and pDC expression of the IL-18 receptor.[97] It is plausible that the presence of renal IC containing dsDNA (e.g., nucleosomes) could drive glomerular pDCs to produce IFN-α, thus amplifying the autoimmune response to local glomerular antigens and contributing to the formation of local germinal centers. Studies in mouse models also generally support a role for IFN-α in LN pathogenesis. Experimental LN is reduced by deletion of the IFN-α receptor or by administration of TLR7 or TLR9 antagonists, whereas LN is worsened by administration of an IFN-α-producing vector or an agonist of TLR7 or 9.[98] One exception is seen in the MRL/lpr model, in which LN is significantly worsened following deletion of the IFN-α receptor,[99] suggesting that IFN-α protects against LN in this mouse strain.

The realization of the importance of the IFN-α pathway in SLE pathogenesis has reinvigorated the concept of microbial pathogen involvement in SLE pathogenesis. The activation of TLRs and other sensors that stimulate IFN-α by viral and bacterial nucleic acids may be important in initiating the break in tolerance, or in accelerating the autoimmune response.

The Genetics of Lupus Nephritis

Much effort has gone into identifying the basis for genetic susceptibility to SLE, using genomewide and candidate gene studies.[100] Over 30 genes have been identified that appear to be related to specific pathogenic pathways in SLE. These include IC clearance/inflammatory pathway genes, immune response genes, and IFN-α signaling and response genes. A number of these impart particular susceptibility to LN.[101] Examples include genetic variation in the FcγRIIA and FcγRIIIA genes described previously, in which the higher affinity variants are associated with protection against LN.[47,48] Two cytokines previously discussed as important for cell infiltration into the kidney, the chemokine MCP-1 for monocytes/T cells and IL-18 for pDCs, have promoter polymorphisms that influence expression levels. The MCP-1 variant that results in higher expression levels is associated with LN.[102] Similarly, the IL-18 variant that causes higher expression is associated with diffuse proliferative LN.[103] Also of interest, the HLA DR3 allele (DRB1*0301) correlates with renal disease,[104] and with anti-dsDNA antibodies,[104] supporting a genetic contribution to a type of autoantibody that may target renal tissue. For the IFN-α pathway, STAT4, which is important for transmitting the IFN-α signal, has a genetic variant that is associated with increased STAT4 RNA levels, and with SLE, particularly LN.[105]

Genome studies have identified six quantitative trait loci (QTLs) that are linked to LN, supporting the fact that LN has a specific genetic component.[106,107] Three of these regions are linked to LN in European Americans, and three are linked to LN in African Americans. One of the loci for European Caucasians occurs on chromosome 4, at q13.1, a region that contains the gene for IL-18. This may account for the relationship between this QTL and LN.

A Composite Picture of Lupus Nephritis Pathogenesis

Considering all of the LN-specific "traits" of the various pathways that contribute to SLE pathogenesis, a picture emerges as to what may be the important steps that culminate in clinical LN (Fig. 53.1). Clinically active LN is always associated with IC accumulation and complement deposition in the kidneys, and often with corresponding evidence of systemic complement activation. The IC that are perhaps most relevant to LN are those containing nuclear antigens. These can arise due to deficiencies in clearance of IC containing nuclear antigens from microbes or apoptotic debris. Deficiencies in the clearance of apoptotic debris may also lead to glomerular accumulation of self-antigen, such as nucleosomes, that can target autoantibody directly to renal tissue. Initial accumulation of glomerular IC sets the stage for an escalating cascade of events that includes local complement activation and chemokine/cytokine production, leading to infiltration and activation of inflammatory (monocytes, neutrophils) and immune cells (pDCs, T cells), and a heightened intrarenal Th1-dominant immune response with significant Th17 contributions. This then leads to an escalation of autoantibody production targeted to the kidney, and inflammation driven primarily by complement and FcγR activation. Many of the mediators derived from this activation contribute to kidney injury, including direct tissue damage by complement proteins and toxic factors produced by inflammatory sells, such as reactive oxygen species and proteolytic enzymes. Continued inflammation can lead to matrix expansion, fibrosis, scarring, and eventually ESRD.

Why LN occurs only in some SLE patients remains an unknown, although the data discussed previously point to the existence of specific LN genes, including those that favor inefficient IC clearance, exuberant chemokine/cytokine production, and loss of tolerance and activation of T and B cells. Environmental contributions such as exposure to certain microbial infections may also be involved in the development of LN. As the specifics of how genetic

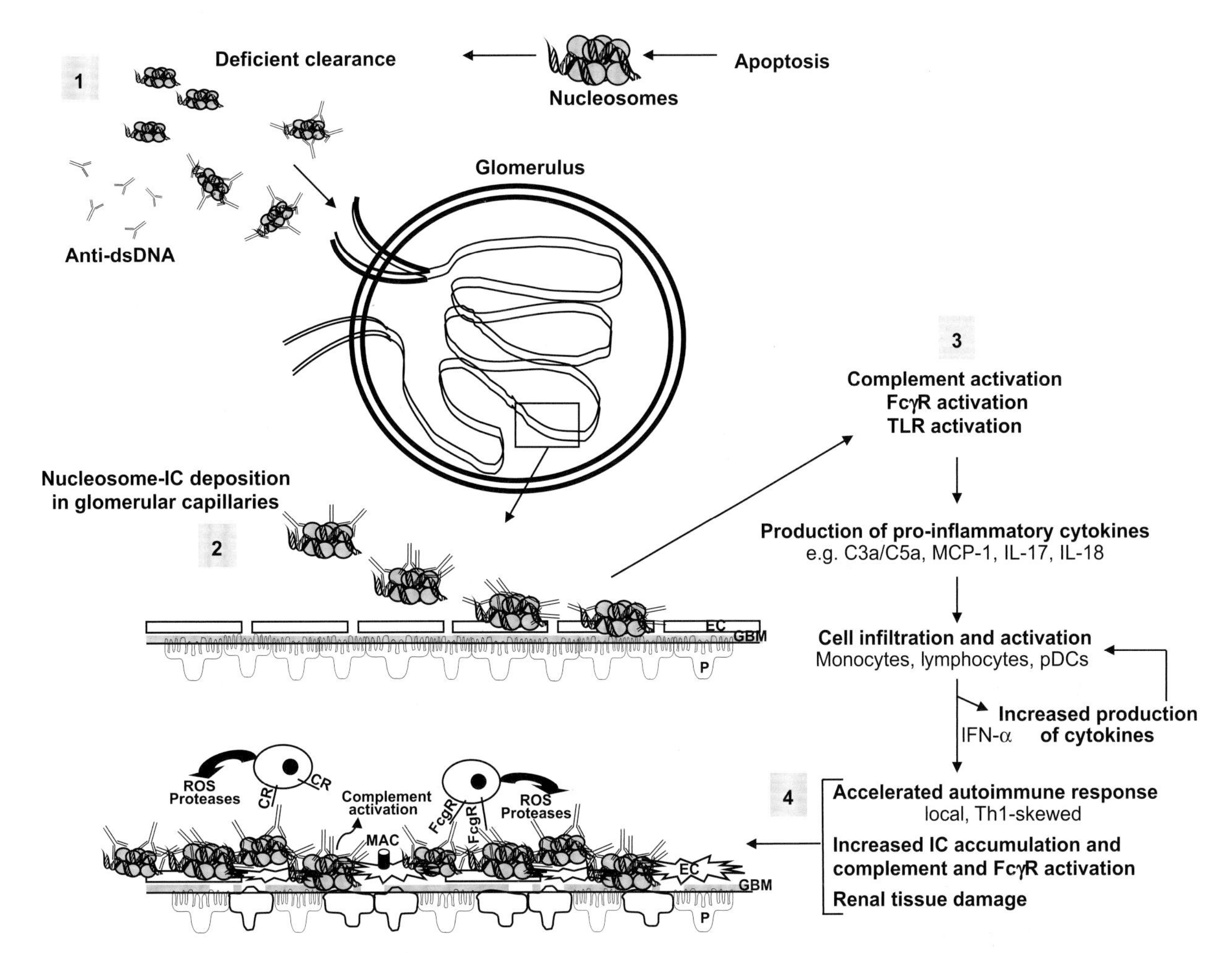

FIGURE 53.1 A paradigm for lupus nephritis pathogenesis. The onset of lupus nephritis likely begins with initial accumulation of self-antigen and immune complexes. In the model presented in the figure, the self-antigens are nucleosomes that can persist due to deficient clearance or overwhelming production, and which in turn can drive anti-dsDNA production (step 1, in shaded box). The resulting immune complexes (IC) are prone to deposit in the renal vascular beds (step 2), in part due to the positively charged core histones of the nucleosome. Once deposited, the IC can activate the complement system, activate circulatory leukocytes via expressed FcγR, and activate resident cells expressing TLRs (step 3). This establishes a cascade of inflammatory cytokine and chemokine production that recruits and activates inflammatory cells, lymphocytes, and pDCs. These infiltrating cells further amplify the production of cytokines and chemokines in the kidney microenvironment. The result is a locally driven and accelerated autoimmune response with Th1 characteristics, and increased IC accumulation and accompanying complement and FcγR activation. This response culminates in the production of inflammatory mediators of tissue damage (step 4). One immediate consequence is destruction of the glomerular filtration barrier through the damaging effects on glomerular endothelial cells (EC), glomerular basement membrane (GBM), and podocytes (P), which leads to proteinuria and hematuria, the hallmark clinical manifestations of active lupus nephritis. *CR,* complement receptor; *MAC,* complement membrane attack complex.

and environmental factors interact and contribute to LN become clearer, so too will our understanding of the pathogenesis of LN.

DIAGNOSIS OF LUPUS NEPHRITIS

Preservation of kidney function in patients with LN is best achieved with early diagnosis and treatment.[108–110] This requires a high index of suspicion for renal involvement in all patients with SLE. Although some patients may present with overt clinical signs of renal disease, such as edema secondary to nephrotic syndrome, or severe hypertension, it is more likely that the initial evidence of kidney involvement will be an abnormality of serum creatinine and/or the urinalysis. An approach for evaluating the SLE patient for kidney involvement is presented in Figure 53.2. Considering serum creatinine, it is important to recognize that a normal range value may be abnormally high for a woman with small-moderate muscle mass and low rates of creatinine production. Also, hypoalbuminemic patients with severe nephrotic syndrome may have increased tubular creatinine secretion, lowering serum creatinine, and leading to an impression of better renal function than in actuality.[111] Finally, in addition to LN, SLE patients may develop acute renal insufficiency because

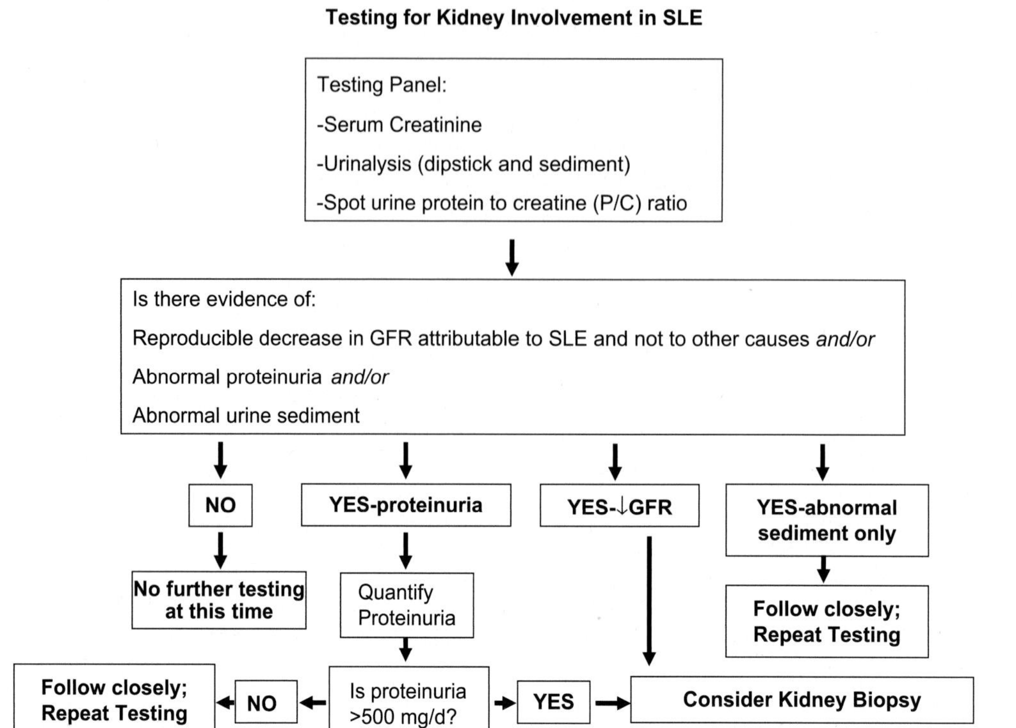

FIGURE 53.2 An algorithm for the evaluation of the kidney in patients with systemic lupus nephritis. Note that patients with a history of lupus nephritis and previous kidney biopsy may not need a repeat biopsy (see text). Kidney biopsy should be done for all new diagnoses of kidney involvement.

of infection, medications, nephrotoxins, hemolysis, thrombosis, and cardiac failure.

Urinalysis is a useful screening test for patients with SLE. A urine dipstick positive for blood and/or protein suggests possible LN; however, a systematic study of the accuracy of the urine dipstick as a screening tool found a false-negative rate in up to 30% of SLE patients and a false-positive rate in about 40% of patients.[112] Therefore the urine sediment should be evaluated for evidence of glomerulonephritis. Glomerular bleeding is suggested by acanthocytes and/or red blood cell (RBC) casts. White blood cells (WBCs) and white blood cell casts in the absence of infection are indicative of renal inflammation, and support a diagnosis of glomerulonephritis.

Proteinuria is a key indicator of kidney injury in SLE. It has prognostic importance because proteinuria may injure the kidney, and it is used as a clinical biomarker of relapse, remission, and successful treatment. Therefore accurate measurement of protein excretion is crucial to the ongoing management of LN.

Random spot urine protein-to-creatinine (P/C) ratios can be used in addition to urine dipsticks to screen patients, but are not accurate enough to be used to make therapeutic decisions or to follow changes in proteinuria magnitude in response to therapy. The most reliable method to quantify proteinuria is to measure the P/C ratio of a 24-hour urine collection, or an intended 24-hour collection that is at least 50% complete.[113] Measuring the P/C ratio reduces confounding the assessment of proteinuria by errors in collecting the 24-hour urine. A 12-hour overnight urine collection that includes the first morning void urine also provides an accurate measure of proteinuria magnitude, and may be easier for patients to collect.[114]

Ultimately a kidney biopsy is essential for the optimal diagnosis and management of most cases of LN. A biopsy is not necessarily required if the only abnormalities are isolated hematuria, or low level proteinuria in the absence of hematuria and an active urine sediment. A biopsy should be considered when proteinuria is above 500 mg per day, as this degree of proteinuria has been associated with significant renal injury.[115–117]

There is some controversy surrounding the utility of kidney biopsies in LN. The main argument against biopsy is a prevalent notion that most patients can be treated with mycophenolate mofetil (see later), and biopsy information would not change the approach to therapy.[118] There are, however, several important reasons to obtain a biopsy:

- Not all kidney disease in SLE patients is classic, IC-mediated glomerulonephritis (LN), so one therapy does not fit all patients. For example non-LN glomerular diseases have been reported in SLE patients.[119–121] This literature is mostly case reports, but in a series of 252 patients, 5% were found to have changes consistent with focal segmental glomerulosclerosis, minimal change disease, thin glomerular basement membrane disease, hypertensive nephrosclerosis, and amyloidosis.[119] The incidence of podocytopathies in lupus patients appears to be greater than in the general population, suggesting a causal link to the immune dysregulation of SLE.[122,123] Amyloid A (AA) amyloidosis has also been reported frequently in some series.[120,121] Finally, there are other important kidney lesions found in SLE patients that are treated differently than LN, such as interstitial nephritis without glomerulonephritis[121] and thrombotic microangiopathy with or without LN.[124,125]

- The kidney biopsy, especially if performed serially, assesses the degree of chronic kidney injury, and therefore the risk of progressive renal failure that is not related to active LN. If extensive scarring is the dominant process found on biopsy even with some areas of active inflammation, the risk of immunosuppression may outweigh its benefits in terms of renal survival. Such patients may be more appropriately treated with kidney-protective therapies alone.
- In the context of LN therapeutics, kidney biopsies can and should be exploited in novel ways to better inform future drug development. For example, leukocyte subsets can be analyzed by specific staining in lupus kidneys and may yield new insights on renal inflammation.[126] Proteomic techniques can be used to look for patterns of protein expression in LN.[127,128] Gene expression in biopsies can be analyzed with microarray techniques.[128,129] These technologies are just being applied to kidney biopsies, but have the potential to greatly enhance the amount of information available from renal tissue.

KIDNEY PATHOLOGY IN SYSTEMIC LUPUS ERYTHEMATOSUS

Although the gold standard for the exact diagnosis and classification of LN is the renal biopsy, it should be emphasized that LN is not a renal biopsy diagnosis. Renal biopsy changes, although characteristic, are not specific and the diagnosis of LN cannot be made unless the patient fulfills the American College of Rheumatology criteria for SLE. In the absence of a concurrent clinical diagnosis of SLE, only a diagnosis of immune complex glomerulonephritis can be made, with the suggestion that the glomerulonephritis, in the appropriate clinical setting, could be associated with SLE.

The clinical utility of the kidney biopsy depends on obtaining an adequate sample of renal cortex (at least 10 glomeruli) and examination by a renal pathologist.[130] In as much as every biopsy is a clinicopathologic correlation, the nephropathologist must be given all relevant clinical information in order to properly interpret the tissue and integrate the microscopic findings with the clinical data. Furthermore, it is essential that the clinician and pathologist review the findings together before initiation of therapy to ensure that specific clinical concerns have been addressed and that the lesions have been contextualized appropriately.

The first renal biopsy of a patient with LN, although important diagnostically and therapeutically, has somewhat limited prognostic value because most of the active lesions are reversible with treatment. However, a follow-up biopsy performed after several months or years may provide important prognostic information.[131–133] If the degree of chronic injury in the follow-up biopsy does not change substantially, and the patient had a good response to treatment, outcome is likely to be favorable. In contrast, if the degree of chronic injury is substantially more prominent in a follow-up biopsy, a progressive decline in the disease course can be anticipated.

Classification Schemes for Lupus Nephritis

Renal biopsy findings in LN involve the entire spectrum of renal pathology. Therefore, it became necessary to develop a pathologic classification of LN. A first attempt was made in 1974 by a group of pathologists under the auspices of the World Health Organization (WHO), and was later designated as the WHO classification. This was further modified in 1982 and 1995.[134] The original WHO classification was relatively simple, with five classes of LN (Table 53.1). Subsequent modifications made the WHO classification more complicated and cumbersome to use, leading a group of nephrologists and pathologists to develop a new classification of LN (Table 53.1) in 2003 under the auspices of the International Society of Nephrology (ISN) and the Renal Pathology Society (RPS).[135]

Similar to the previous WHO classification, the ISN/RPS classification is based primarily on characteristic light microscopic patterns of glomerular injury:

- Mesangial hypercellularity. Mesangial hypercellularity is almost always present in LN, except in Class I (Fig. 53.3), and is the basic, and probably the earliest LN lesion which is later combined with other pathologic patterns of injury.
- Endocapillary hypercellularity. Endocapillary hypercellularity is the hallmark lesion in forms of proliferative LN (Figs. 53.4 and 53.5). Intracapillary cells usually are infiltrating inflammatory cells (including monocytes/macrophages, polymorphonuclear leukocytes, lymphocytes, and rarely eosinophils or basophils). There may also be a component of endothelial cell proliferation.
- Extracapillary hypercellularity. Extracapillary proliferation results in crescent formation (Fig. 53.6), and is common in proliferative forms of LN. It is frequently associated with glomerular capillary rupture, Bowman's capsular basement membrane rupture, fibrin in Bowman's space, and fibrinoid necrosis of the glomerular capillary tuft.
- Karyorrhexis with or without associated fibrinoid necrosis of the glomerular capillary tuft (Figs. 53.7 and 53.8). Karyorrhexis in glomeruli usually reflects apoptosis, a common finding in LN. The apoptotic cells may be infiltrating inflammatory cells or native glomerular cells. Hematoxylin bodies (Fig. 53.9), seen occasionally in

TABLE 53.1 **Classification of Lupus Nephritis**

	Original World Health Organization Classification	Simplified ISN/RPS Classification
Class I	Normal: No pathologic findings, no glomerular IC	Minimal mesangial LN: Mesangial IC
Class II	Mesangial LN: Mesangial IC, normal or hypercellular mesangium	Mesangial proliferative LN: Mesangial IC, hypercellular mesangium
Class III	Focal LN (<50% of glomeruli) Glomerular lesions mainly segmental	Focal LN (<50% of glomeruli) – III (A): active lesions – III (A/C): active and chronic lesions – III (C): chronic lesions
Class IV	Diffuse LN (>50% of glomeruli) Glomerular lesions mainly global	Diffuse LN (≥50% of glomeruli involved, lesions may be segmental [S] or global [G]) – IV (A): active lesions IV-S(A); IV-G(A) – IV (A/C): active and chronic lesions – IV-S(A/C); IV-G(A/C) – IV (C): chronic lesions IV-S(C); (IV-G(C)
Class V	Membranous LN	Membranous LN
Class VI		Advanced sclerosing LN

IC, immune complex; LN, lupus nephritis.

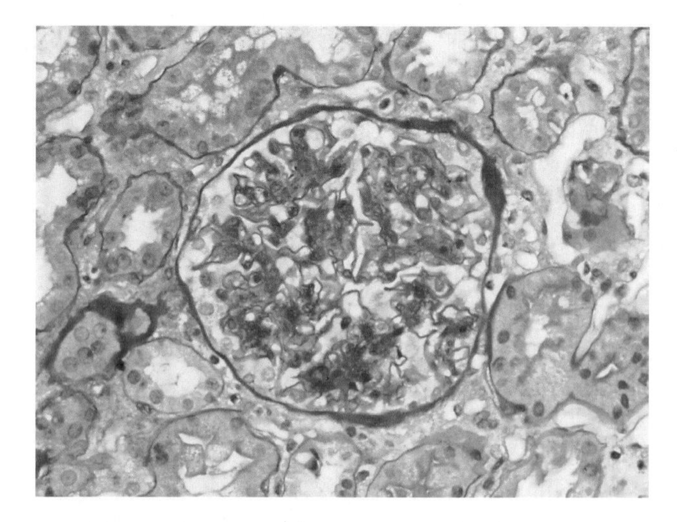

FIGURE 53.3 Mesangial hypercellularity in a case of class II lupus nephritis. Note that the glomerular capillaries are patent. (Periodic acid-Schiff [PAS] ×400.)

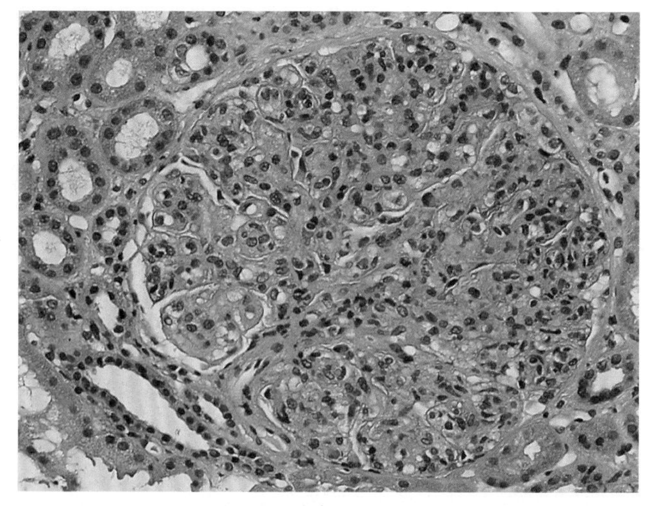

FIGURE 53.4 Global endocapillary hypercellularity with obliteration of the glomerular capillaries in a case of class IV lupus nephritis. The hypercellularity is the result of infiltrating inflammatory cells, including occasional polymorphonuclear leukocytes, as well as proliferating glomerular cells, including endothelial cells and mesangial cells. (Hematoxylin and eosin [H&E] ×400.)

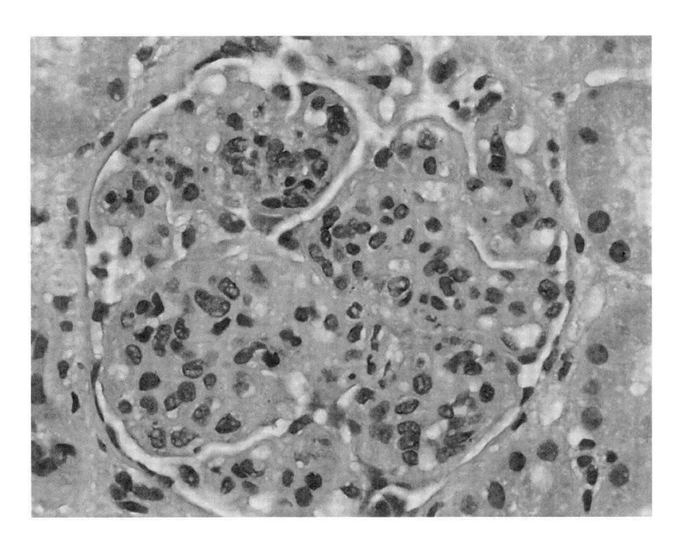

FIGURE 53.5 Global endocapillary hypercellularity with accented lobularization of the glomerular capillary tuft, resembling a membranoproliferative glomerulonephritis in a case of class IV lupus nephritis. (H&E, ×400.)

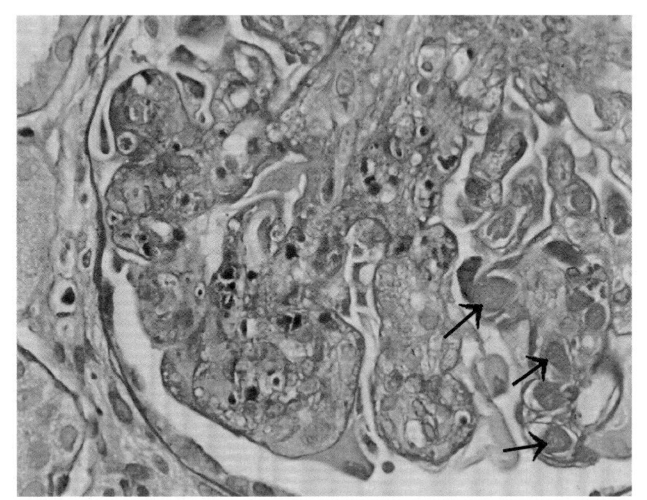

FIGURE 53.7 Apoptotic debris (karyorrhectic nuclei) in the glomerular capillaries in a case of class IV lupus nephritis. In this glomerulus, large subendothelial deposits ("wire loop" lesions) and intracapillary hyalin thrombi (*arrows*) are also present. (PAS ×600.)

biopsies, most likely represent a tissue equivalent of the LE cell phenomenon.

- Wire loop lesions. These lesions are due to large subendothelial immune complex deposits, visible even with light microscopy (Fig. 53.10). If these subendothelial deposits are large enough, they may occlude the entire glomerular capillary lumen and appear as "hyalin thrombi" (Figs. 53.7 and 53.10). Wire loop lesions are positive for periodic acid-Schiff (PAS), negative with methenamine silver stain, and red with Masson's trichrome stain. Wire loop lesions are much more common in LN with global glomerular hypercellularity than with biopsies showing mainly segmental hypercellularity and/or necrosis.
- Spikes. Diffuse uniform glomerular capillary loop thickening with "spike" formation on methenamine silver stain (Figs. 53.11 and 53.12) is the main light microscopic pattern of injury if the immune complex deposits are subepithelial in membranous lupus nephritis.

The ISN/RPS classification (Table 53.1) retained the main subclasses of the modified WHO classification, but introduced several modifications: The ISN/RPS classification

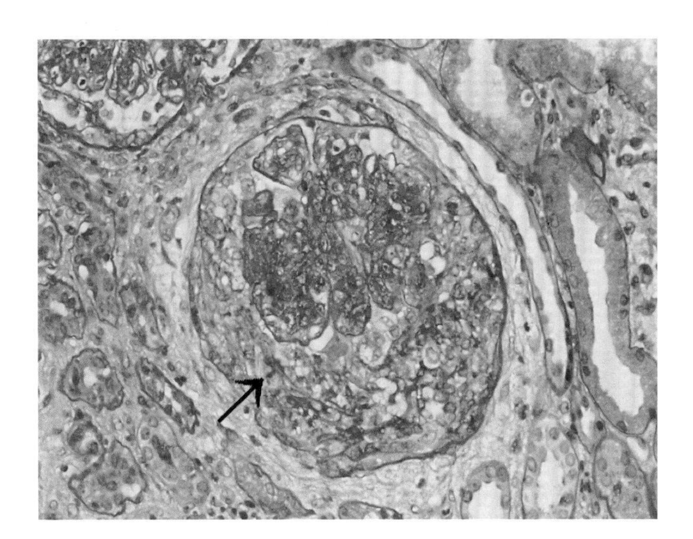

FIGURE 53.6 A cellular crescent in a case of class IV lupus nephritis. Note the compressed glomerular capillary tuft and the rupture in the Bowman's capsule (*arrow*). (PAS ×400.)

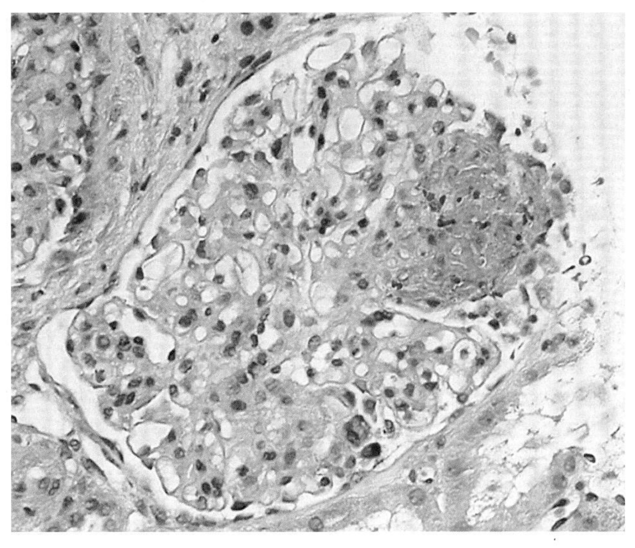

FIGURE 53.8 Segmental glomerular capillary tuft necrosis associated with karyorrhectic/apoptotic debris in a case of focal lupus nephritis. (H&E ×400.)

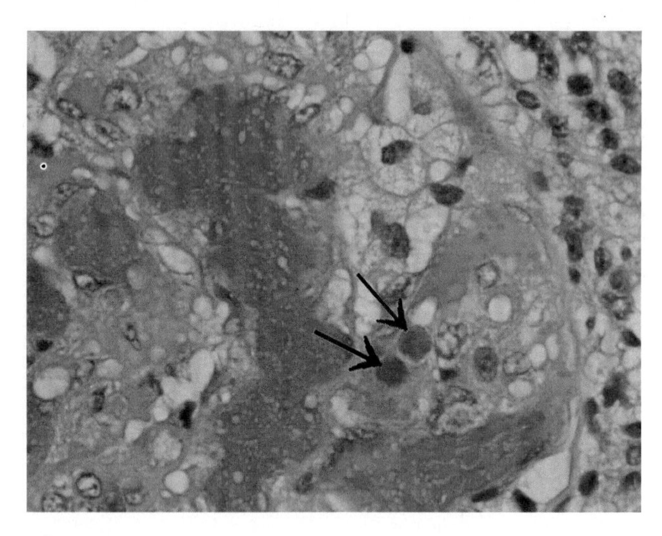

FIGURE 53.9 Hematoxylin bodies in a glomerular capillary (*arrows*) in a case of active class IV lupus nephritis. (H&E ×1000.)

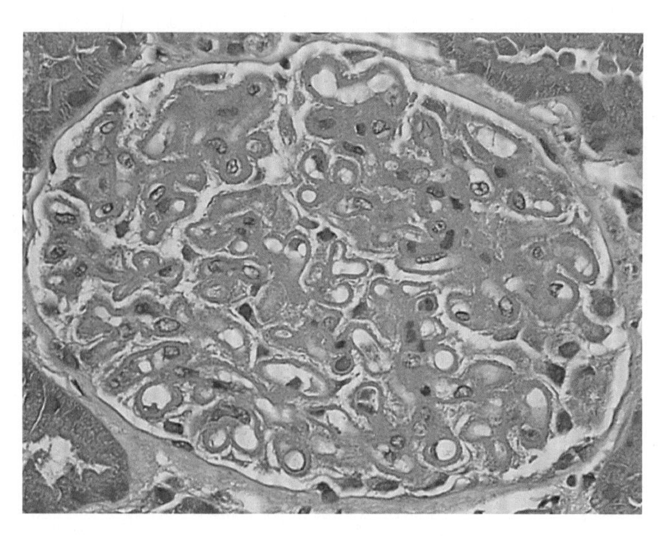

FIGURE 53.11 Diffuse uniform glomerular capillary thickening without hypercellularity in a case of membranous class V lupus nephritis. (H&E ×400.)

differentiates active (A) and chronic (C), and segmental (S) and global (G) glomerular lesions. Active glomerular lesions include glomerular endocapillary hypercellularity with or without leukocyte infiltration and with substantial luminal reduction, karyorrhexis, fibrinoid necrosis, rupture of the glomerular basement membrane, cellular or fibrocellular crescents, wire loop lesions, and large intraluminal immune complexes (hyalin thrombi) (Figs. 53.4 to 53.8 and 53.10). Chronic lesions include glomerular sclerosis (segmental or global), fibrous adhesions, and fibrous crescents (Figs. 53.13 to 53.15). Segmental lesions involve less than half of the glomerular capillary tuft area; global lesions involve more than 50% of the glomerular capillary tuft area.

Class I: Minimal Mesangial Lupus Nephritis

In class I LN, the glomeruli appear entirely normal by light microscopy. However, immunofluorescence and electron microscopy reveal obvious mesangial immune complex deposits (Fig. 53.16).

Class II: Mesangial Proliferative Lupus Nephritis

In class II LN, there is pure mesangial hypercellularity (Fig. 53.3) without glomerular endocapillary hypercellularity or crescents. Immunofluorescence and electron microscopy reveal mesangial deposits (Figs. 53.17 and 53.18) as in class I LN. By electron microscopy a few isolated glomerular capillary deposits may be seen. If many peripheral

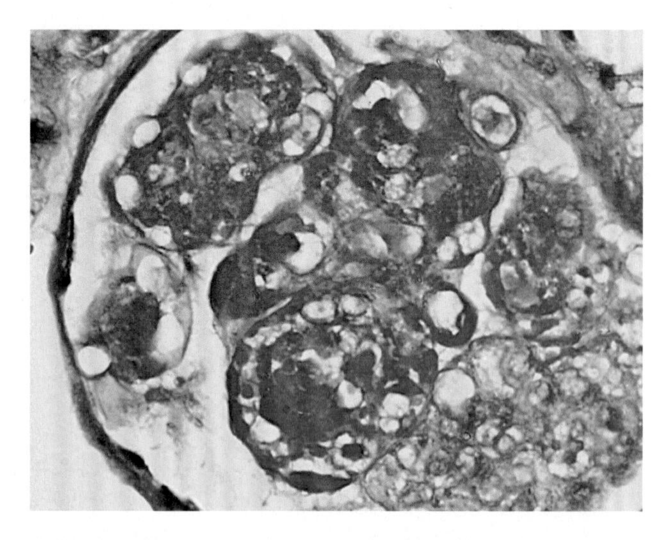

FIGURE 53.10 Large PAS positive deposits along the glomerular capillary loops ("wire loop" lesions) as well as extensive mesangial deposits and glomerular capillary hyalin thrombi in a case of class IV lupus nephritis. (PAS ×600.)

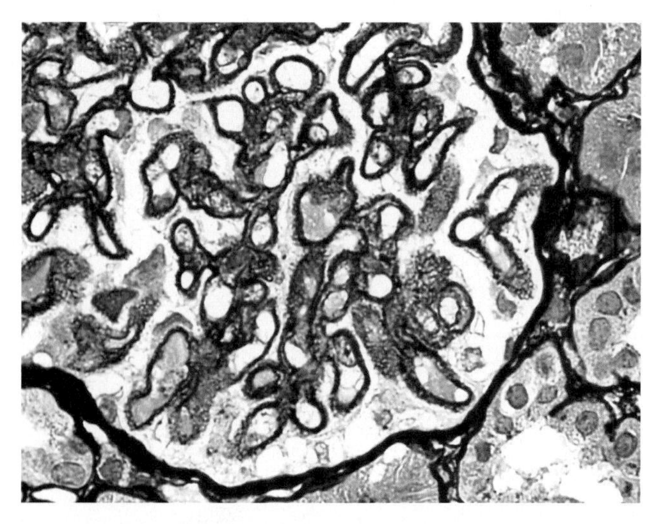

FIGURE 53.12 Methenamine silver stain reveals extensive spike formation along the glomerular capillary loops in the same biopsy shown in Figure 53.11. (Jones' methenamine silver ×600.)

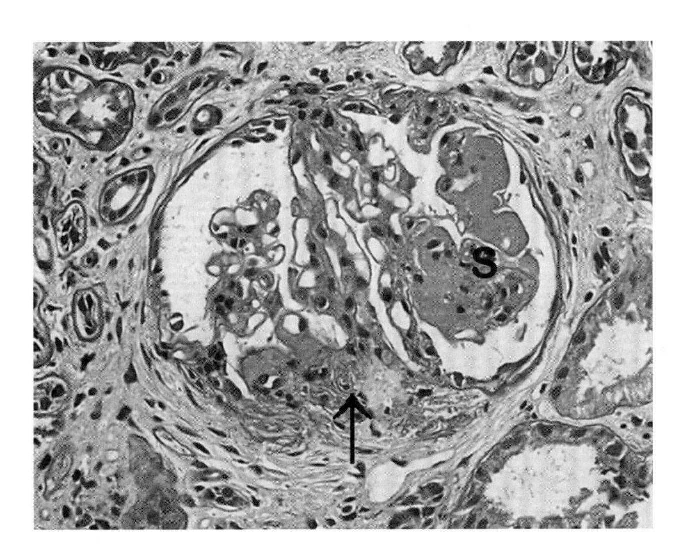

FIGURE 53.13 Segmental sclerosis (*S*) and glomerular capillary adhesion (*arrow*) in a glomerulus from a biopsy with class III lupus nephritis. (PAS ×400.)

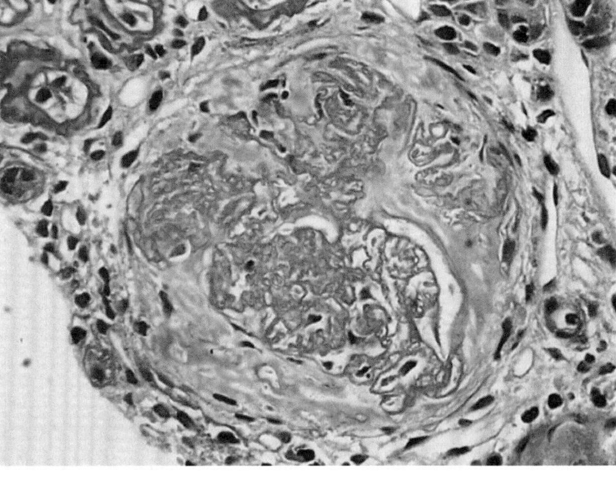

FIGURE 53.15 A fibrous crescent from biopsy with class IV lupus nephritis with moderate to advanced chronicity and mild activity. Note the disrupted Bowman's capsule and the separation of sclerosing glomerular lobules by faintly PAS positive interstitial type collagen. (PAS ×400.)

glomerular capillary immune complex deposits are present, the diagnosis of class II LN should not be made.

Class III: Focal Lupus Nephritis

In class III LN, obvious endocapillary or extracapillary (crescents) proliferative lesions are seen (Figs. 53.7, 53.8, and 53.19), but in less than 50% of all glomeruli, including sclerotic glomeruli, which are also taken into account. Glomerular lesions in focal LN are almost always segmental (Fig. 53.8). By immunofluorescence and electron microscopy, abundant mesangial immune complex deposits are seen, usually associated with segmental glomerular capillary deposits (Fig. 53.20). There are three possible subclasses of focal LN.

- In class III (A) there are only active lesions (focal proliferative LN).
- In class III (A/C) both active and chronic lesions are present (focal proliferative and sclerosing LN). In such cases, focal or segmental sclerosing glomeruli coexist with glomeruli with active proliferative/necrotizing lesions.

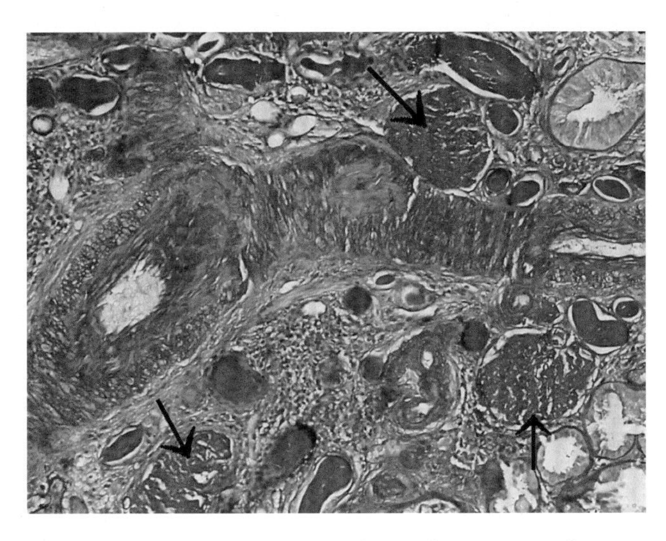

FIGURE 53.14 Globally sclerotic glomeruli (arrows) in a biopsy with advanced sclerosing (class VI) lupus nephritis. (PAS ×200.)

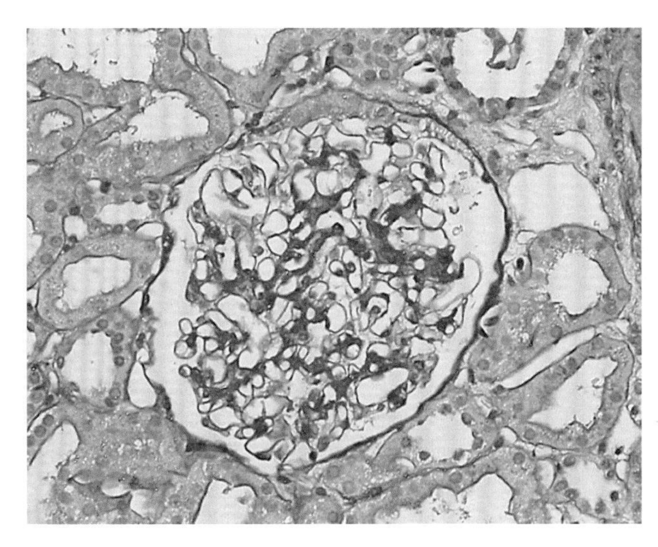

FIGURE 53.16 A light microscopically unremarkable glomerulus in a biopsy with class I lupus nephritis. Immunofluorescence and electron microscopy revealed mesangial immune complex deposits. (PAS ×400.)

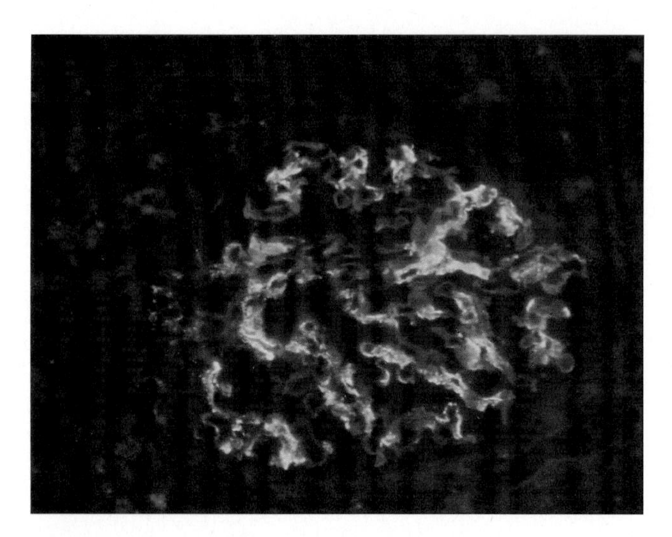

FIGURE 53.17 Mesangial immune complex deposits in a case of class II lupus nephritis. (Direct immunofluorescence with an antibody to IgA, ×400.)

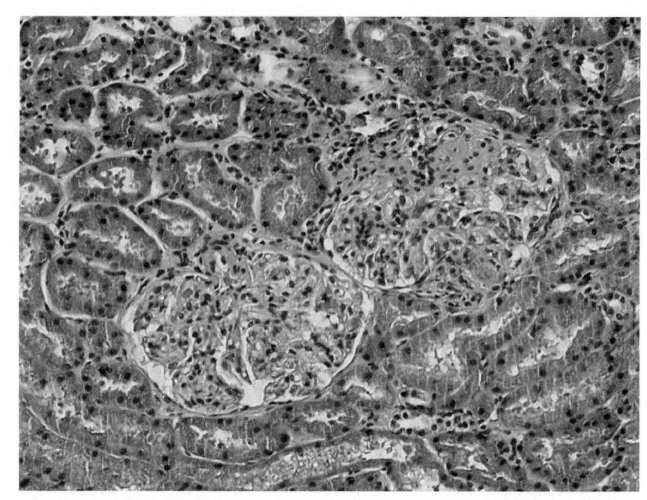

FIGURE 53.19 Two glomeruli from a biopsy with class III lupus nephritis. Note that the left lower glomerulus is light microscopically unremarkable whereas the right upper glomerulus reveals segmental proliferative lesions. (H&E, ×200.)

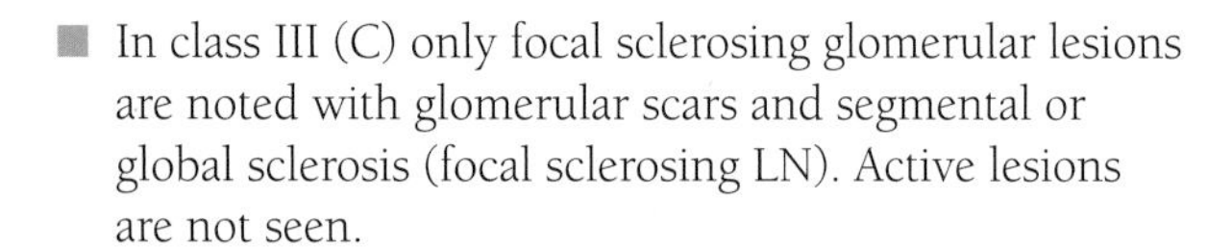

- In class III (C) only focal sclerosing glomerular lesions are noted with glomerular scars and segmental or global sclerosis (focal sclerosing LN). Active lesions are not seen.

Class IV: Diffuse Lupus Nephritis

In this class of LN, segmental or global endo- or extracapillary glomerular proliferative lesions are seen in more than 50% of all glomeruli (Figs. 53.4 to 53.8). Large subendothelial deposits, visible under the light microscope (wire loop lesions) (Figs. 53.7 and 53.10), are common. In class IV LN, the glomerular lesions can be global or segmental. Also, active and chronic glomerular lesions are evaluated separately. Immunofluorescence and electron microscopy reveal abundant glomerular mesangial and capillary loop deposits. The glomerular capillary loop deposits are mainly subendothelial, and frequently quite large (Figs. 53.21 and 53.22). Scattered intramembranous and subepithelial deposits are common. Therefore, there are six possible subclasses of diffuse LN.

- Class IV-S(A) indicates active diffuse segmental endocapillary or extracapillary proliferative glomerular lesion or necrosis involving more than 50% of the glomeruli.
- Class IV-G(A) shows diffuse global LN with active endocapillary or extracapillary proliferative glomerular

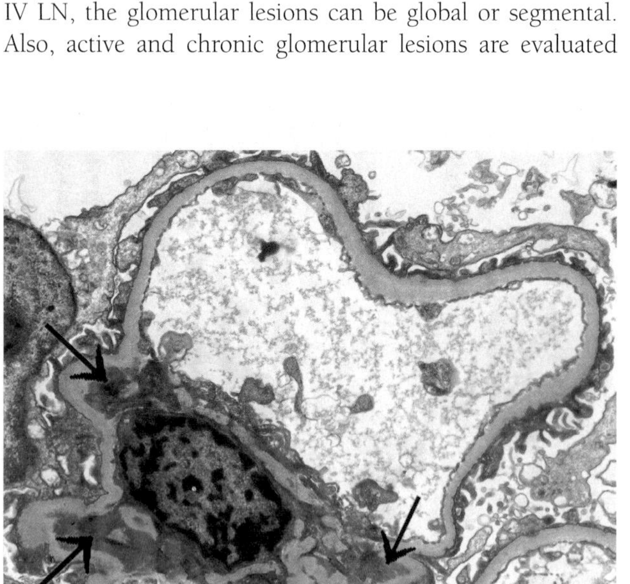

FIGURE 53.18 Mesangial electron dense immune type deposits (*arrows*) in a case of class II lupus nephritis. (Uranyl acetate, lead citrate ×8000.)

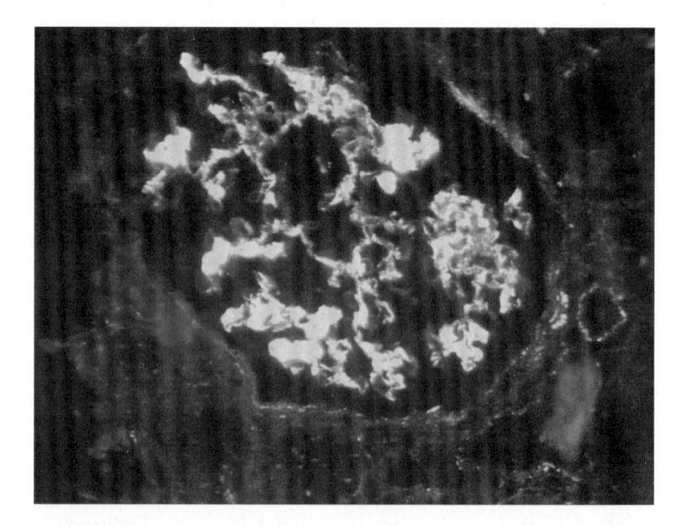

FIGURE 53.20 Granular mesangial and segmental glomerular capillary loop deposits in a case of class III lupus nephritis. Also note the subtle granular tubulointerstitial staining. (Direct immunofluorescence with an antibody to IgG, ×400.)

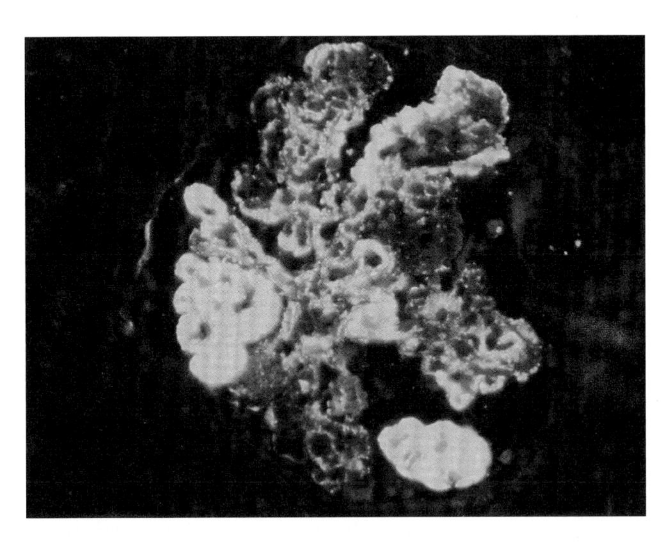

FIGURE 53.21 Diffuse granular glomerular deposits with large subendothelial deposits ("wire loop" lesions) in a case of class IV lupus nephritis. (Direct immunofluorescence with an antibody to IgG, ×400.)

lesions and/or necrosis involving more than 50% of glomeruli.

- Class IV-S(A/C) indicates diffuse segmental proliferative and sclerosing LN. In such biopsies, active segmental proliferative lesions coexist with chronic sclerosing glomerular lesions.
- Class IV-G(A/C) indicates diffuse global proliferative and sclerosing LN. These biopsies show active global proliferative lesions with chronic sclerosing glomerular lesions.
- Class IV-S(C) indicates diffuse segmental sclerosing LN. In this subclass, no active lesions are present; only inactive, mainly segmental glomerular lesions are seen, such as segmental sclerosis/scarring.
- Class IV-G(C) shows diffuse global sclerosing LN. In such biopsies, glomeruli reveal global sclerosis or scarring with or without fibrous crescents, involving more than 50% of all glomeruli, in the absence of active proliferative lesions.

Class V: Membranous Lupus Nephritis

In class V LN the glomeruli do not reveal endocapillary hypercellularity; the mesangium may be normocellular or hypercellular. The glomerular capillaries are uniformly and diffusely thickened (Fig. 53.11), except in very early stages of the disease. Spike formation on methenamine silver stain is common, just like in idiopathic membranous glomerulonephritis (Fig. 53.12). Glomerular subepithelial immune complex deposits involve over 50% of the glomerular capillary tufts (Figs. 53.23 and 53.24). In contrast to idiopathic membranous glomerulonephritis, in class V LN the immunofluorescence frequently, shows a "full house" pattern (see later text), and the IgG deposits contain mainly IgG1 and IGg3 as opposed to IgG2 and IgG4 (see later). However, we encountered several cases of class V LN with IgG4 predominant glomerular capillary deposits. Mesangial immune complex deposits are almost invariably present. A few small subendothelial deposits are possible. Electron microscopy usually reveals endothelial tubuloreticular inclusions (TRIs) (Fig. 53.25).

Class VI: Advanced Sclerosing Lupus Nephritis

In class VI LN over 90% of the glomeruli are globally sclerosed without residual activity (Fig. 53.14). There has to be clinical or morphologic evidence that the advanced glomerular

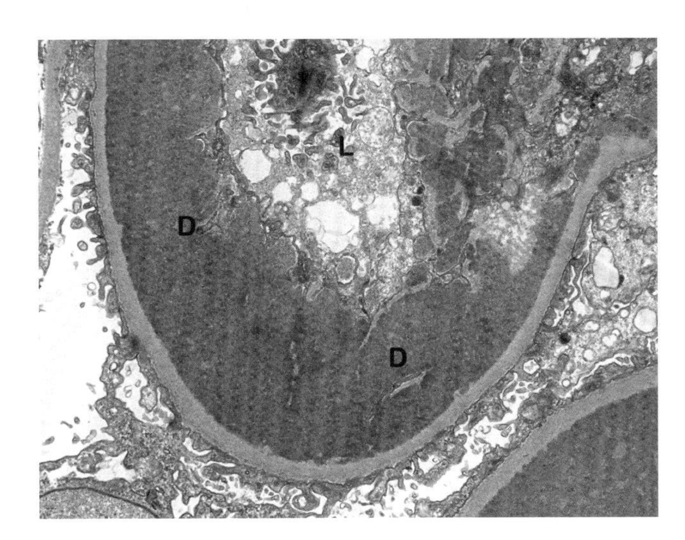

FIGURE 53.22 This electron micrograph shows a large subendothelial electron dense deposit (*d*) in the same biopsy shown in Figure 53.21. *L*, glomerular capillary lumen. (Uranyl acetate, lead citrate, ×8,000.)

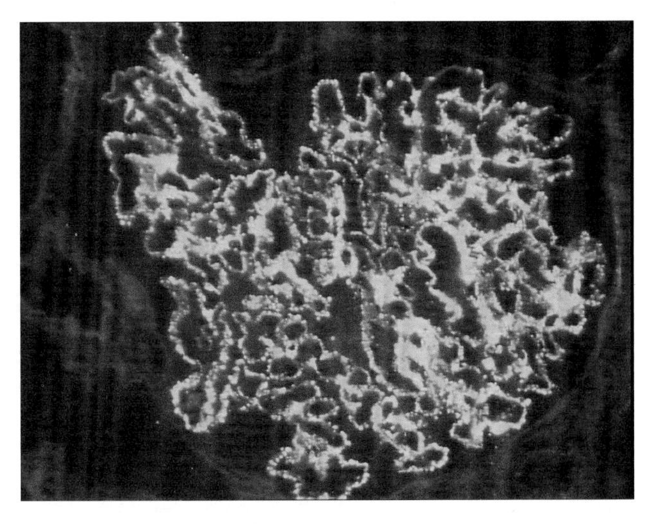

FIGURE 53.23 Granular mesangial and glomerular capillary fluorescence with an antibody to IgG in a case of membranous (class V) lupus nephritis. Note that over 50% of the glomerular capillaries contain granular deposits. (Direct immunofluorescence, ×400.)

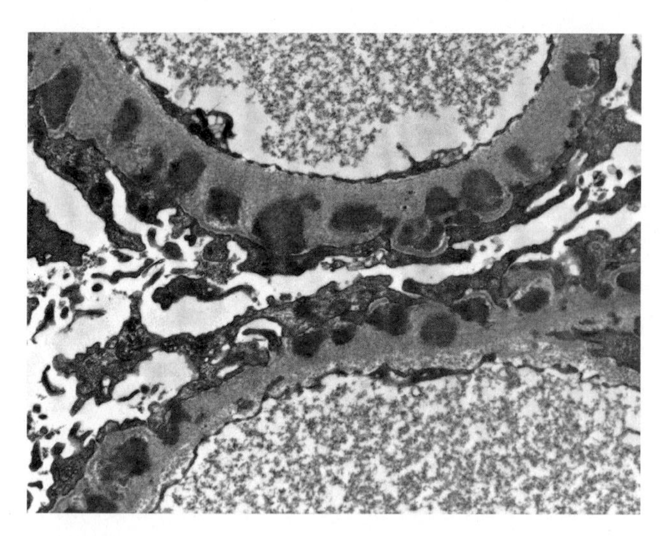

FIGURE 53.24 Subepithelial electron dense immune type deposits along the glomerular basement membrane in a case of class V (membranous) lupus nephritis. Note that occasional deposits are already completely incorporated into the glomerular basement membrane. (Uranyl acetate, lead citrate ×15,000.)

sclerosis is secondary to LN. Immunofluorescence and electron microscopy still frequently reveal mild glomerular immune complex deposits in the few nonsclerotic glomeruli.

Controversies with the ISN/RPS Classification

Although several follow-up studies emphasize the benefits of the ISN/RPS classification of LN,[136,137] not all investigators share this enthusiasm.[138,139] The classification is based purely on morphologic findings and arbitrary definitions. For example, the classification of proliferative LN into focal and diffuse forms is based on an arbitrary cut off value of 50% glomerular involvement. It is hard to imagine that a patient with LN and 40% glomerular involvement would be treated and respond differently than a patient with 60% glomerular involvement.

The definitions of segmental and global lesions are even more controversial. A segmental lesion is defined by involvement of less than 50% of the glomerular surface area in the tissue section. In contrast, a global lesion is defined as involvement of more than 50% of the glomerular surface area. The degree of involvement in a given tissue section depends on the plane of the section through the glomerular tuft. Thus, depending on the level of the cut, a segmental lesion could appear to involve more or less than 50% of the glomerular capillary surface area.

Furthermore, some investigators argue that the pathogenesis of LN with true global lesions is different from LN with segmental glomerular lesions, and that this affects outcomes, and may require different treatment.[139–142] Class IV LN cases with segmental lesions involving more than 50% of the glomerular tuft area (classified as class IV-G) appear to have a worse outcome than true global proliferative LN with 100% involvement of the glomerular capillary tuft area (also classified IV-G by ISN/RPS), and class IV-S with less than 50% glomerular tuft involvement.[139] In contrast, others did not find any difference in outcome between patients with class IV-S and class IV-G LN,[143–146] but this may be because cases of class IV-G with segmental lesions involving more than 50% of the glomerular tuft were generally not separated out from class IV-G with 100% tuft involvement.[139,142,147] At the present time, these concerns remain unresolved.

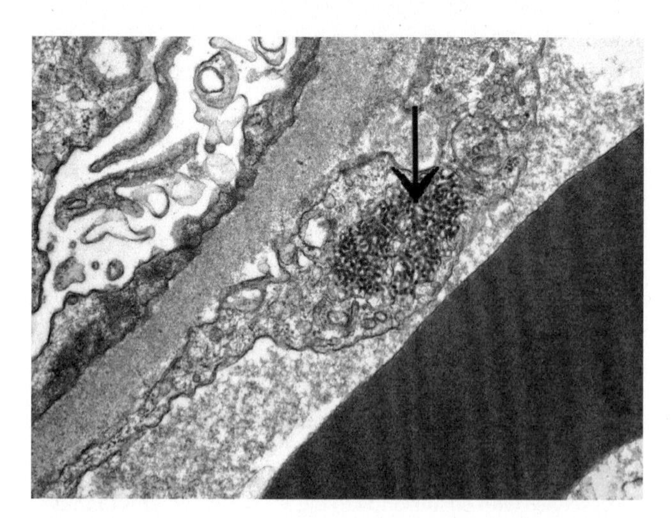

FIGURE 53.25 A large, tubuloreticular inclusion in a glomerular capillary endothelial cell (*arrow*). (Uranyl acetate, lead citrate, ×20,000.)

Immunofluorescence Findings in Lupus Nephritis

Most renal pathology laboratories perform immunofluorescence with a panel of antibodies to IgG, IgA, IgM, kappa and lambda light chains, complement components C1q, C3, C4, fibrinogen, and albumin. The distribution of glomerular immune complexes in the various classes of LN was addressed previously. Interestingly, glomerular immune complex deposits in LN often show a "full house" pattern, meaning that all or almost all immunoreactants (IgG, IgA, IgM, kappa and lambda light chains, C1q, C3) are present. This is unusual in other forms of glomerulonephritis. However, the absence of full house immunofluorescence does not exclude LN. In membranous LN the full house pattern may be absent, and even in proliferative LN, it is not always evident. C1q staining is usually quite prominent in LN and may show the most intense staining among all antigens. Such strong C1q staining is rare in other forms of glomerulonephritis. Another characteristic immunofluorescence feature in LN biopsies is the frequent deposition of extraglomerular immune complexes (Fig. 53.26). Extraglomerular immune complexes are most commonly seen along the tubular basement membrane, but they are also common in the interstitium, particularly along the basement membranes of peritubular capillaries. Bowman's capsule immune complexes are also common. In our experience, if

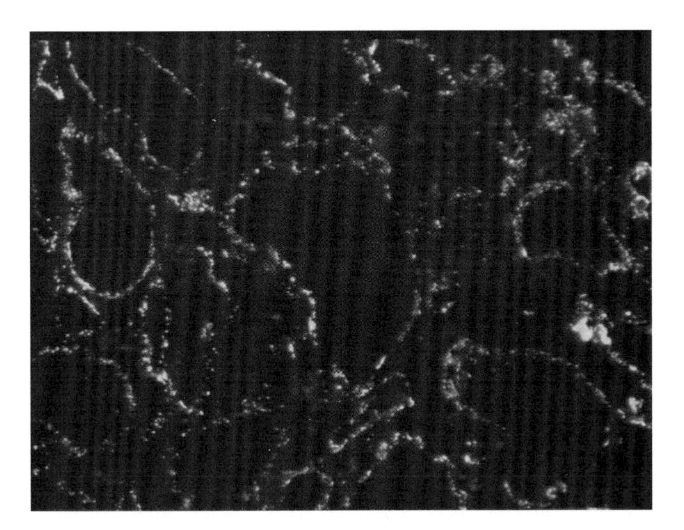

FIGURE 53.26 Prominent granular tubular basement membrane and interstitial immune complex deposits in a case of class IV lupus nephritis. (Direct immunofluorescence with an antibody to C1q, ×400.)

there are tubulointerstitial immune complex deposits, it is quite common to see vascular (arterial/arteriolar) immune complex deposits as well (Fig. 53.27). Superficially, the composition of glomerular and extraglomerular immune complex deposits appears similar; however, we found that glomerular and extraglomerular deposits frequently have different IgG subclass distributions.[148] In general, most cases of LN immune complexes contain IgG1 and IgG3, less IgG2, and minimal IgG4. The differences in IgG subclass distribution in different renal compartments raise the possibility that glomerular and extraglomerular immune complex deposits have a different pathogenesis.

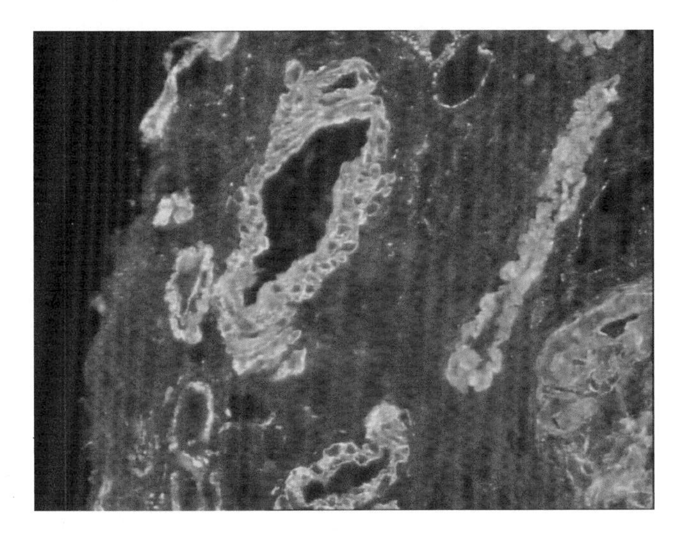

FIGURE 53.27 Arterial and arteriolar staining with an antibody to IgG in a biopsy with class IV lupus nephritis. (Indirect immunofluorescence ×200.)

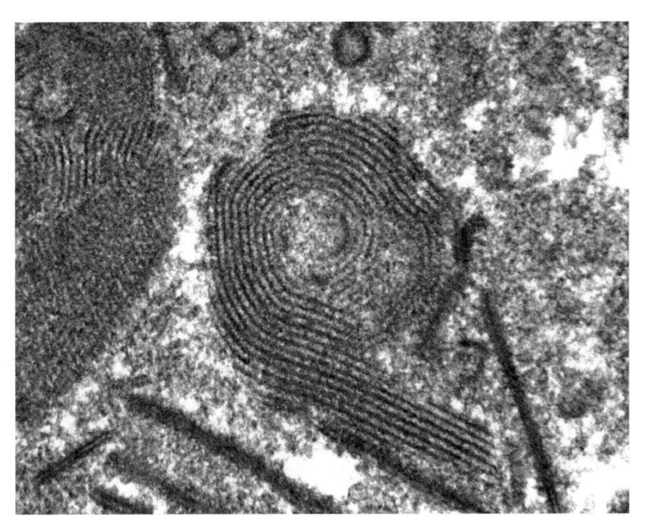

FIGURE 53.28 Subendothelial electron dense deposits with so-called fingerprint substructure. Such fingerprint substructure in the deposit is quite characteristic of lupus nephritis (LN). (Uranyl acetate-lead citrate, ×50,000.)

Electron Microscopy in Lupus Nephritis

Ultrastructural examination practically always reveals mesangial immune complex deposits in any form of LN (Fig. 53.18). Sometimes, the electron dense deposits may have a "fingerprint" substructure (Fig. 53.28). TRIs seen mainly in endothelial cells are a very common ultrastructural finding in LN (Fig. 53.25). Although not diagnostic of LN, TRIs reflect high interferon levels in patients with active SLE; therefore, they are also called interferon footprints. TRIs are present all over the body, not only in renal endothelial cells.

Tubulointerstitial Lesions in Lupus Nephritis

Light microscopic lesions in the tubulointerstitium are nonspecific. Interstitial inflammatory cell infiltrates may or may not be present in biopsies with LN (Fig. 53.29). They are more common in patients with proliferative LN (class III or IV) and indicate an active disease process. Interestingly, the degree of interstitial inflammatory cell infiltrate does not correlate with the degree of tubulointerstitial immune complex deposition.[148,149] In later stages of LN, interstitial fibrosis and tubular atrophy appear and indicate progressive chronic injury (Fig. 53.30). Interstitial fibrosis and tubular atrophy may or may not be associated with active inflammatory cell infiltrate in the same biopsy specimen.

Arterial/Arteriolar Lesions in Lupus Nephritis

Although any type of vascular pathology may occur in a patient with SLE, there are four basic vascular patterns of injury that are attributed to SLE.[150]

- Uncomplicated arterial/arteriolar immune complex deposits (Fig. 53.27). This is the most common pattern of vascular pathology related to SLE and is frequently

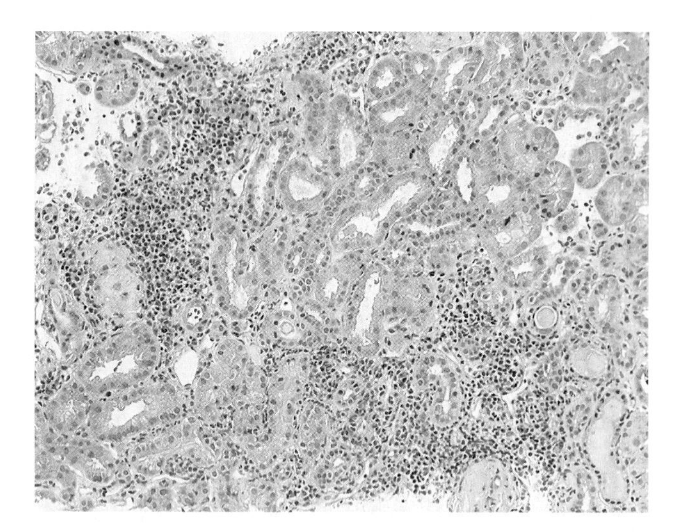

FIGURE 53.29 Interstitial inflammatory cell infiltrate in a case of class III lupus nephritis. The interstitial inflammatory cells are mainly mononuclear cells, but scattered eosinophils are also present. Occasional polymorphonuclears may also be seen. (H&E ×200.)

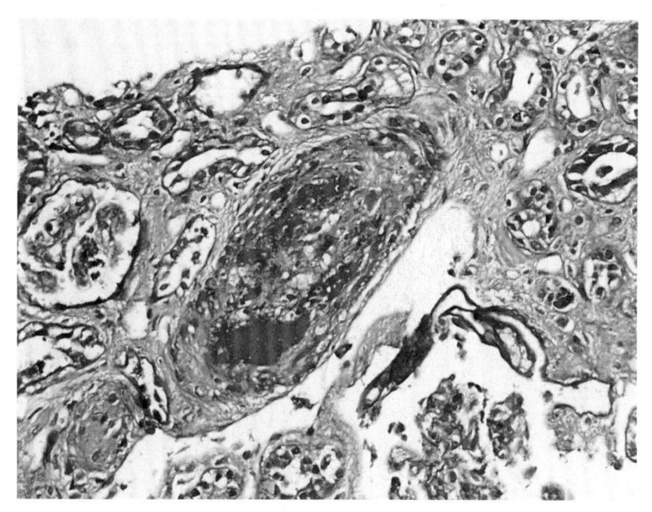

FIGURE 53.31 A small interlobular artery occluded by amorphous material, including fibrin (*bright red color*), in a patient with systemic lupus erythematosus, antiphospholipid antibodies, elevated d-dimers, and thrombotic microangiopathy. Immune complex deposits were not seen in this biopsy. (Masson's trichrome, ×400.) (See Color Plate.)

seen in biopsies with LN. There is no correlation between vascular inflammation and the degree of arterial/arteriolar immune complex deposition; by light microscopy, the arterial/arteriolar walls are usually normal.

- Thrombotic microangiopathy (TMA). TMA is a rare but serious complication of SLE and is particularly common in patients who have circulating antiphospholipid antibodies and high d-dimer levels.[151] The biopsy findings are similar to those seen in other forms of TMA (Fig. 53.31), and include arterial/arteriolar fibrin thrombi with or without fibrinoid necrosis of the vessel wall, fragmented RBCs in the fibrin thrombi or embedded in the thickened loosened arterial/arteriolar walls, and mucoid subendothelial widening of the arteries/arterioles. In more chronic stages, concentric thickening (onion skinning) of the arterial/arteriolar walls may develop. Arterial/arteriolar immune complex deposits may or may not be present. The glomerular changes include fibrin thrombi and/or prominent thickening of the glomerular capillaries, secondary to subendothelial electron lucent widening between the glomerular capillary basement membrane and the swollen endothelium (seen on electron microscopy). Because of the capillary wall thickening, the glomerular capillary lumen is narrowed and many of these glomeruli appear "bloodless." Fragmented RBCs are not unusual in the glomerular capillaries. In some glomeruli, the dominant feature is ischemic wrinkling of the capillaries, particularly if there is severe obliteration of arterial/arteriolar lumen.

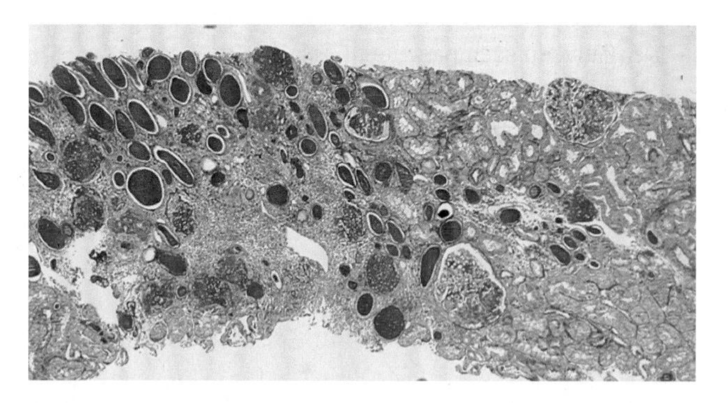

FIGURE 53.30 Zonal renal cortical scarring in a patient with class III lupus nephritis. This patient also had antiphospholipid antibodies. Note that the left part of the image shows completely scarred renal parenchyma with thyroidization of the tubules. Such zonal renal cortical scarring with tubular thyroidization is not unusual in patients with antiphospholipid antibodies, in our experience. (PAS ×100.)

- Noninflammatory necrotizing lupus vasculopathy (Fig. 53.32). This is a somewhat controversial vascular pattern of injury in patients with SLE. In such cases, there is necrosis of the wall of the small arteries/arterioles without obvious thrombus formation and inflammatory cell reaction. The lesion is thought to be related to abundant vascular immune complex deposits and is very difficult to differentiate from TMA.
- True lupus vasculitis. It is very rare to see true lupus vasculitis in a renal biopsy specimen, probably because of sampling issues. The morphology of lupus vasculitis is similar to other forms of vasculitis and includes fibrinoid necrosis of the wall of arteries with an associated active mixed inflammatory cell infiltrate (Fig. 53.33). This vascular wall necrosis/inflammation may or may not be associated with secondary thrombus formation.

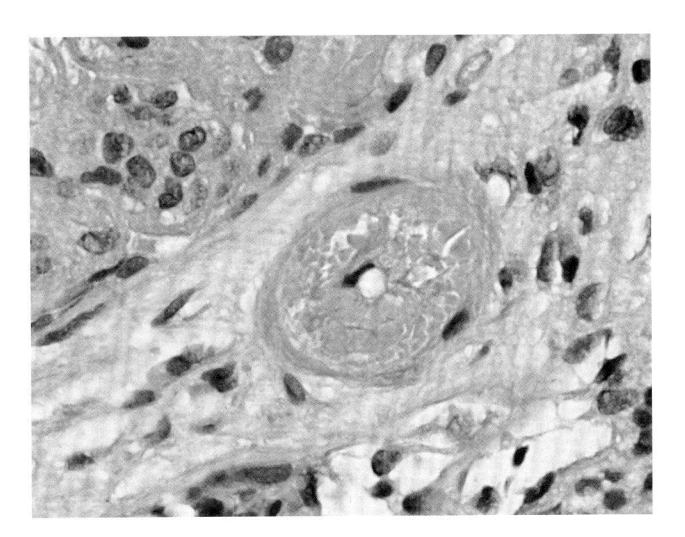

FIGURE 53.32 An arteriole with extensive subendothelial deposition of eosinophilic material (immune complexes) in a biopsy with noninflammatory necrotizing lupus vasculopathy. Interestingly, inflammatory cell infiltrate is usually absent in such arteries. (H&E ×600.)

Combination of Different Classes of Lupus Nephritis

Mild LN with only mesangial deposits (classes I and II) is the basic lesion of LN; therefore, we do not diagnose combinations of classes III, IV, or V + class I or II. By ISN/RPS definition, classes III and IV cannot combine. Class V LN is common in combination with class III or class IV LN. In these combined patterns of injury the proliferative component is listed first (such as classes III+V or classes IV+V).

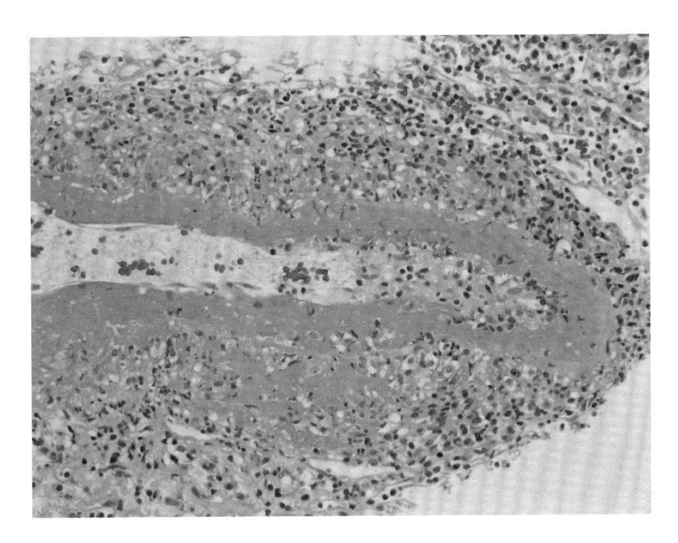

FIGURE 53.33 An arcuate artery with widespread fibrinoid change of the media and transmural inflammatory cell infiltrate. Such true vasculitic lesions are rare in kidney biopsies with lupus nephritis. (H&E ×200.)

Class Transformation in Lupus Nephritis

Follow-up biopsies of LN often show a class different from the initial biopsy.[133,134] If the initial biopsy reveals class I or II LN, the follow-up biopsy commonly shows focal, diffuse proliferative, or membranous LN. Another common transformation is for focal proliferative LN (class III) to evolve into diffuse proliferative LN (class IV). Classes I, II, III, or IV may transform into membranous (class V) LN. In cases of proliferative LN this transition usually reflects a combination of proliferative and membranous LN. Any class can turn into class VI (advanced sclerosing) LN eventually. It is less common for a higher class LN to turn into a lower class LN in a renal biopsy because this kind of transformation usually reflects a good response to treatment and most centers would not perform a repeat biopsy in this situation. Membranous (class V) LN on initial biopsy may turn into combined proliferative and membranous LN.

Less Common Patterns of Glomerular Injury Associated with Systemic Lupus Erythematosus

- Minimal change disease. Occasional patients with SLE develop acute onset nephrotic syndrome and kidney biopsy reveals only minimal change disease without immune complex deposits or with only mild mesangial immune complex deposits. Considering the autoimmune nature of lupus, it is likely that immunologic podocyte damage can occur and induce minimal change-like disease responsive to corticosteroids.[122]
- Collapsing glomerulopathy. It has been reported that occasionally glomerular changes of collapsing glomerulopathy may develop in patients with SLE.[152] The pathogenesis is unclear.
- Pauci-immune proliferative glomerulonephritis. This may rarely occur in patients with SLE.[153,154] Biopsies show active proliferative lesions, including occasional crescents, in the absence of relevant glomerular immune complex deposits. Antineutrophil cytoplasmic antibody (ANCA) is negative in such patients. If ANCA is positive and necrotizing proliferative lesions are present, it is likely that the patient with SLE also developed ANCA-associated crescentic and necrotizing glomerulonephritis.[140]
- Lupus patients rarely can develop renal diseases not related to SLE, such as diabetic nephropathy, hypertensive nephrosclerosis, or infection-related glomerulonephritis.

Activity and Chronicity Indices in Lupus Nephritis

Because renal biopsy findings provide important guidance to treatment of patients with LN, but the renal biopsy interpretation can be quite individual, an attempt was made to standardize the scoring of active and chronic lesions in biopsies with LN.[154a] The value of the activity and chronicity indices is debated, but they provide guidelines as to what to look for while evaluating renal biopsies (Table 53.2).

TABLE 53.2 **Active and Chronic Lesions in Lupus Nephritis**

Activity (score: 0–24)
• Crescents[a]
• Glomerular necrosis/karyorrhexis[a]
• Glomerular polymorphonuclear leukocytes
• Endocapillary hypercellularity
• Large subendothelial deposits ("wire loops")
• Interstitial inflammation
Chronicity (score: 0–12)
• Glomerular sclerosis
• Fibrous crescents
• Tubular atrophy
• Interstitial fibrosis

[a]The scores for renal lesions are doubled.
Lesions are scored on a semiquantitative scale from 0–3 (0 absent, 1 mild, 2 moderate, 3 severe).

Clinicopathologic Correlations

There is a reasonable correlation between clinical presentation and the class of LN in many patients (Table 53.3). Usually patients with active proliferative forms of LN have severe proteinuria, hematuria, and low complement levels. However, these clinicopathologic correlations are far from perfect and the degree of activity and chronicity cannot be determined based on clinical presentation alone. As mentioned earlier, the prognostic value of active lesions in the biopsy is poor; however, a follow-up biopsy may reveal important prognostic information. For example, advanced chronic injury in a biopsy specimen, just as in any other renal disease condition, indicates poor renal outcome. Follow-up biopsies in LN are not yet universally done, but many clinicians are beginning to think of these as part of the standard of care for LN patients.

TABLE 53.3 **Clinicopathologic Correlations in Lupus Nephritis, Simplified**

Class I:	Usually no clinical kidney abnormalities; often normal serum complement
Class II:	Normal kidney function, mild hematuria and/or proteinuria, often normal serum complement
Class III:	Normal or impaired kidney function, nephritic sediment, proteinuria (may be nephrotic), often low serum complement
Class IV:	Normal or impaired kidney function, nephritic sediment, proteinuria (may be nephrotic), often low serum complement
Class V:	Normal kidney function, often nephrotic syndrome, microscopic hematuria, often normal serum complement
Class VI:	Chronic renal failure

MANAGEMENT OF LUPUS NEPHRITIS

The treatment of LN should be based on biopsy findings, and historically has been tied to the pathologic class of the kidney lesion. However, within each ISN/RPS lupus class there is considerable clinical variation (severity of proteinuria and renal dysfunction) and severity of kidney injury (proliferation, necrosis, crescents, fibrosis/sclerosis). These variations should be taken into account to individualize the application of the aggressive immunosuppressive regimens outlined later.

In addition to the protocols described subsequently, all patients receiving moderate to high dose immunosuppression should be treated with a sulfa antibiotic or dapsone if sulfa-allergic for *Pneumocystis* prophylaxis. All LN patients should be treated with hydroxychloroquine unless there is a contraindication. Anti-malarials have activity against TLR7 and 9, which may be important in the pathogenesis of SLE and LN.[155a] Hydroxychloroquine may protect against vascular thrombosis,[155] kidney damage,[156] renal flares,[157] ESRD,[158] and has a favorable impact on lipid profiles. Finally, the renoprotective measures discussed elsewhere in this book should be used in LN patients at risk of progressive kidney injury, including control of blood pressure with antiproteinuric antagonists of the renin-angiotensin-aldosterone system.

Most of the evidence-based protocols for LN were designed to treat proliferative or membranous LN (classes III, IV, V). An overview of generally accepted approaches to management of LN is shown in Figure 53.34. Class I is rarely diagnosed because there are no or few clinical renal manifestations that would warrant a biopsy. Patients with class II LN may have glomerular hematuria and proteinuria (usually nonnephrotic), but kidney function is normal.[159] The immunomodulatory regimens used to treat extrarenal SLE are generally sufficient for class II (and I), along with renoprotective measures for hypertension and proteinuria as clinically indicated. At the other end of the spectrum of kidney function, inactive sclerosing LN, such as class VI, and advanced stage sclerosing class III (C) or class IV (C) are clinically associated with severe chronic kidney disease (CKD). When LN has reached this stage, the therapeutic strategy should shift from an immunosuppression focus, except as needed for extrarenal SLE, to a renal protection focus. The goal of renoprotection in inactive sclerosing LN is to prolong kidney function and avoid ESRD requiring renal replacement therapies for as long as possible.

Proliferative Lupus Nephritis

Proliferative LN (class III or IV) can be an aggressive disease that requires intense therapy. Corticosteroids have historically been the backbone of all approaches to class III and IV

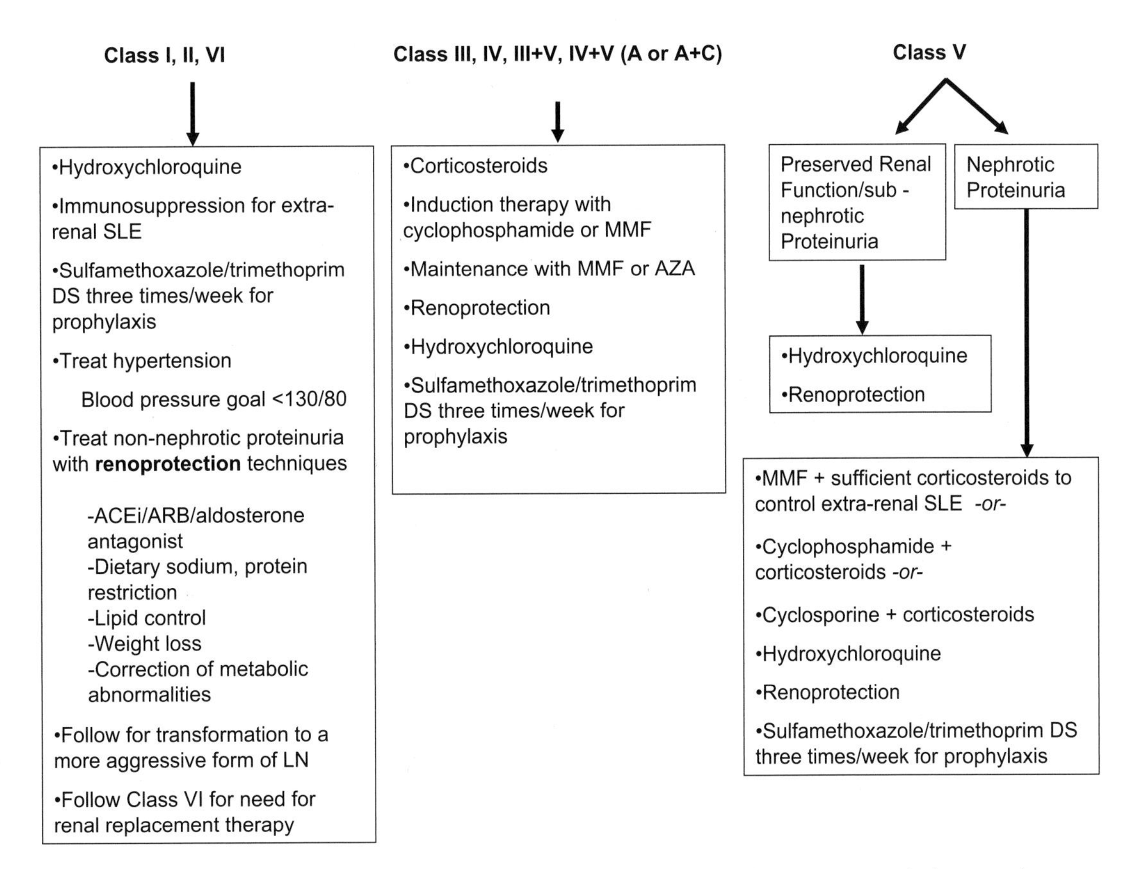

FIGURE 53.34 An approach to the treatment of lupus nephritis. See text for details of the recommended approaches.

LN. Pioneering randomized clinical trials at the National Institutes of Health (NIH) showed that, although corticosteroids were effective in controlling proliferative LN, combination with cytotoxic agents at treatment initiation decreased the frequency of renal relapse and the development of future CKD or ESRD.[160,161] Importantly, the beneficial effect of cytotoxic agents to preserve kidney function was only apparent after 5 years of follow-up.[160–162] This finding has implications for assessing the benefits of new therapies.

As a result of the NIH trials, high-dose corticosteroids and cyclophosphamide, given intravenously every month, followed by quarterly boluses for an extended time (18 months or more), became the prevalent practice. Because of associated toxicities, trials were done limiting cyclophosphamide to 6 months, but this resulted in an increase in renal relapses.[161] These findings were consistent with a need for maintenance therapy after initial treatment with steroids and cyclophosphamide. The role of cyclophosphamide as maintenance was successfully challenged by a prospective study of proliferative LN that compared six to seven monthly pulses of cyclophosphamide followed by maintenance azathioprine (AZA) or mycophenolate mofetil (MMF), to six monthly pulses of cyclophosphamide followed by quarterly cyclophosphamide pulses for 1 year after remission.[163] Over 72 months patients treated with maintenance AZA or MMF were significantly less likely to reach the composite endpoint of death or CKD than the cyclophosphamide-only group, and experienced fewer adverse side effects. Thus the prevalent treatment strategy for proliferative LN became an *initial* (also called *induction*) treatment phase of high-dose corticosteroids plus cyclophosphamide for 6 months, followed by substitution of an antimetabolite, usually AZA or MMF for cyclophosphamide, for a prolonged *maintenance* phase (Fig. 53.35).

Intravenous cyclophosphamide has dominated proliferative LN protocols, although oral cyclophosphamide shows comparable efficacy along with ease of administration and generally less cost.[160,164–168] Oral cyclophosphamide was originally associated with increased toxicity, especially cystitis,[160] but many of the early studies were done using very high doses (up to 2.5 mg/kg/day) for 6 or more months. However lower dose, shorter duration oral cyclophosphamide (Fig. 53.35) is effective, well-tolerated, and results in a cumulative cyclophosphamide exposure similar to 6 months of pulse therapy.[169]

Important caveats with any cyclophosphamide regimen include dose reduction by 20% to 30% in patients with moderate-severe renal insufficiency,[170] and dose-adjustment to keep the neutrophil count ≥2000 cells per μl. To protect fertility women should be offered prophylaxis with leuprolide and men testosterone while cyclophosphamide is being given.[171,172] Sperm banking and ovarian tissue cryopreservation are additional options. To avoid increasing risk of future malignancy, lifetime cumulative exposure to cyclophosphamide should be limited to 36 grams or less.[173,174]

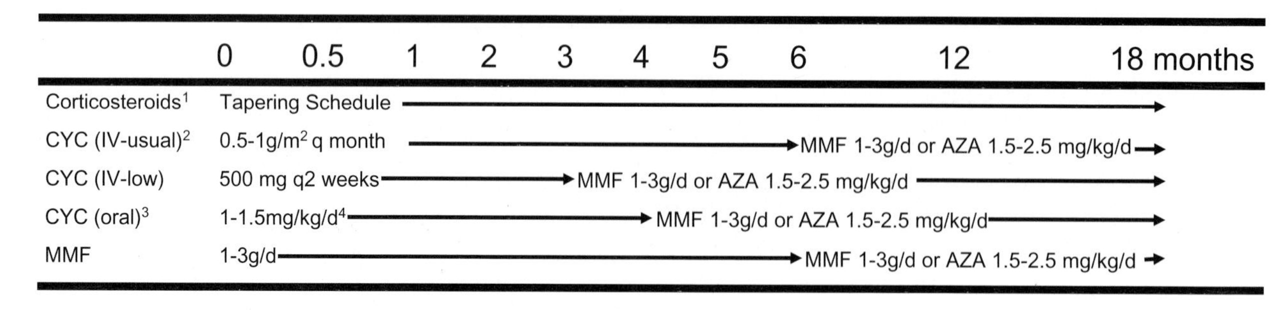

[1]An Example of a Prednisone Tapering Schedule

Week	Prednisone Dose-Severe Disease
0-2	1 mg/kg/day Ideal Body Weight (IBW, maximum 80 mg/d, 2 divided doses)In very severe disease this may be preceded by 500-1000 mg/d methylprednisolone intravenously for 3 days
2-4	0.6 mg/kg/d
4-8	0.4 mg/kg/d
8-10	30 mg/d
10-11	25 mg/d
11-12	20 mg/d
12-13	17.5 mg/d
13-14	15 mg/d
14-15	12.5 mg/d
15-16	10 mg/d
16-	IBW < 70 kg: 7.5 mg/d IBW 70 kg: 10 mg/d

Week	Prednisone Dose-Moderate Disease
0-2	0.4-0.6 mg/kg/day (IBW, maximum 50 mg/d, 2 divided doses)
2-4	0.3-0.4 mg/kg/d
4-6	20 mg/d
6-7	15 mg/d
7-8	12.5 mg/d
8-9	10 mg/d
9-	IBW: <70 kg: 7.5 mg/d IBW: 70 kg: 10 mg/d

[2]Cyclophosphamide, intravenous
[3]Treat for 2-4 months, depending on response
[4]Maximum dose 150 mg/d

FIGURE 53.35 Induction and maintenance regimens for proliferative lupus nephritis.

In an effort to reduce cyclophosphamide exposure in LN, a low-dose cyclophosphamide induction regimen (Fig. 53.35) was designed and compared to six monthly pulses followed by two quarterly pulses of cyclophosphamide.[175,176] This low-dose regimen was termed "Euro-lupus," and after 10 years of follow-up the endpoints of death, ESRD, and doubling of the serum creatinine were similar in both groups, suggesting that low-dose cyclophosphamide can be used successfully in proliferative LN. Importantly, the Euro-lupus patient population was mostly Caucasian, and the proliferative LN was of mild-moderate severity.

To completely eliminate the undesirable side effects of cyclophosphamide, non-cyclophosphamide containing protocols have been evaluated. The regimen that has achieved widespread utilization used MMF for both initial treatment and maintenance of LN (Fig. 53.35). The Aspreva Lupus Management Study (ALMS) prospectively compared MMF + corticosteroids to intravenous pulse cyclophosphamide + corticosteroids, looking for superiority in response at the end of a 6-month induction period.[177] This endpoint was not achieved. The ALMS induction trial showed the response to MMF and pulse cyclophosphamide was equivalent at 6 months. There was a similar incidence of adverse events, serious infections, and deaths for both MMF and cyclophosphamide, and although not statistically significant, withdrawals due to adverse events were almost double in the MMF arm. A provocative result from the ALMS trial was found in a post hoc analysis after stratifying response by race and ethnicity. Black or mixed-race patients who received intravenous cyclophosphamide did worse than those who received MMF, and the response rate among Hispanic patients was greater with MMF. These findings suggest that black and Hispanic patients, generally considered to have more resistant LN,[178] may respond better to MMF than intravenous cyclophosphamide. This will need to be verified in an independent prospective trial.

Other alternatives to cyclophosphamide induction have been tried. Intravenous cyclophosphamide was compared prospectively to AZA plus corticosteroids. Repeat biopsy showed more chronic damage in the AZA group, and those treated with AZA had a higher incidence of renal relapse and doubling of the serum creatinine.[179] However, in some areas of the world AZA may be the only option because of cost or availability, and at least some large retrospective studies have shown long-term responses similar to initial treatment with cyclophosphamide.[180]

Calcineurin inhibitors have recently been tested as an alternative to cyclophosphamide for initial therapy in proliferative and mixed proliferative plus membranous LN. In a prospective, randomized noninferiority trial, 81 patients were treated either with pulse intravenous cyclophosphamide and corticosteroids, or tacrolimus (TAC) and corticosteroids.[181] At 6 months there was no difference between groups in terms of complete or complete plus partial remissions, but long-term follow-up was not available. Nine patients with class IV LN, refractory to treatment with prolonged cyclophosphamide, received TAC and corticosteroids and 78% showed improvement with two complete remissions.[182] Another small ($n = 40$) randomized, controlled study compared 9 months of cyclosporin A (CSA) followed by a 9-month taper to an unusual 9-month course/dosing regimen of intravenous cyclophosphamide followed by 9 months of maintenance with oral cyclophosphamide.[183] At the end of 18 months there were no differences between the two treatments. Long-term follow-up (40 months) continued to show no difference between treatments; however, this was determined retrospectively, and maintenance therapy after 18 months was not protocol-prescribed. Additionally, patients had only mild renal insufficiency because of concern over reductions in glomerular filtration rate (GFR) by CSA, but had rather high renal biopsy chronicity scores. In summary, calcineurin inhibitors may have a role in treating proliferative LN, but that role remains to be determined based on long-term prospective randomized trials.

Leflunomide is a drug that blocks lymphocyte proliferation, T cell activation, and suppresses production of cytokines such as interleukin-2. It is currently used to treat rheumatoid arthritis. There have been two small trials from China using leflunomide to treat LN.[184,185] Response rates were similar to those of cyclophosphamide. Interestingly, in one study repeat biopsies at 6 months showed a large increase in the chronicity index,[184] but this was not seen in repeat biopsies from the second study.[185] Thus long-term trials will be required to determine if leflunomide preserves kidney function over time as well as cyclophosphamide.

Because the renal response rate for class III and IV LN with any of the initial therapies discussed is only about 60% at 6 to 12 months (see later), an add-on strategy was employed in a randomized controlled trial to determine if rituximab *plus* MMF and corticosteroids could improve this outcome.[186] This was based on several small, open-label, uncontrolled trials that suggested rituximab may be effective in proliferative LN, either for refractory disease or as initial therapy.[187–190] At 12 months, however, there were no differences between the rituximab and placebo groups in terms of complete or partial remissions. Thus rituximab cannot be recommended as adjunctive initial therapy.

The choice of initial therapy for proliferative LN is currently between a cyclophosphamide-containing regimen and an MMF-only regimen. The patients in the two largest studies of MMF versus cyclophosphamide generally had less severe LN, according to the level of proteinuria and kidney function,[191,192] than the patients in some of the randomized clinical trials of cyclophosphamide.[162] Thus, in severe class III/IV LN, a cyclophosphamide-containing protocol for initial therapy may be preferred. Low-dose cyclophosphamide could be considered in Caucasians with moderate LN.

The goal of long-term preservation of kidney function should also be considered when choosing an initial therapy. As mentioned earlier, the superiority of cyclophosphamide plus corticosteroids versus corticosteroids alone on preservation of kidney function was only apparent after 3 to 5 years of follow-up.[160–162] In a long-term study of initial therapy with MMF compared to initial therapy with cyclophosphamide, there were no significant differences in renal function between the groups after a median of 64 months.[168] However, more patients in the MMF group had relapses, prolonged proteinuria >1 g per day, and persistent serum creatinine >2 mg per dL. These combined clinical findings have been associated in other studies with deterioration of kidney function over time. Similarly, after the initial 6 month treatment period, the ALMS trial was extended (see later) for 3 years to evaluate maintenance therapy with either MMF or AZA.[193] Although not designed to compare the long-term efficacy of initial therapy on kidney function, there was a (nonsignificant) trend toward fewer treatment failures in those who received cyclophosphamide as initial therapy as opposed to MMF. This result was independent of whether maintenance therapy was AZA or MMF. Thus it cannot yet be stated with certainty that initial therapy with MMF is equivalent to cyclophosphamide for proliferative LN with respect to long-term preservation of kidney function.

Maintenance therapies after the initial treatment of proliferative LN are outlined in Figure 53.28. AZA and MMF have received the most evaluation as maintenance agents. The MAINTAIN trial prospectively compared MMF to AZA as maintenance therapy in a predominantly Caucasian population after initial treatment with the low-dose Euro-lupus cyclophosphamide protocol, regardless of whether patients had achieved remission.[194] The primary endpoint was time to renal relapse, and after at least 3 years of follow-up, MMF and AZA were found to be statistically equivalent, although MMF was numerically better.

The ALMS trial Extension Phase[193] prospectively compared MMF and AZA as maintenance therapies after the 6-month initial treatment period with either MMF or cyclophosphamide. Patients entered this extension phase only if they achieved a complete or partial remission with initial therapy. Over 3 years the composite treatment failure endpoint (death, ESRD, renal flare, sustained doubling of serum creatinine, or requirement for rescue therapy) was reached in 16% of maintenance MMF-treated patients compared to 32% of maintenance AZA-treated patients ($P = .003$). The superiority of MMF over AZA was not dependent on initial therapy (MMF or cyclophosphamide) or race of the patient.

A pilot randomized clinical trial in 69 patients with class III/IV LN suggested that 2 years of CSA may be as effective as 2 years of AZA for maintenance after initial treatment with prednisone and oral CYC, in terms of relapse prevention and reduction of proteinuria.[195] Another randomized clinical trial showed CSA was as effective as AZA in terms of tapering maintenance corticosteroids in severe systemic lupus, but only 29% of the patients had LN.[196]

From these studies it is difficult to make a definitive recommendation for a maintenance drug. Individualizing by patient-specific factors such as desire for pregnancy or occurrence of side effects may be considered when making this choice.

Few patients reach complete remission by 6 months, and kidney biopsies after 6 months of initial therapy have shown that although active inflammation tends to improve, complete resolution of pathologic changes is unusual.[197–200] Consistent with this, clinical improvement in class III/IV LN continues well beyond 6 months and into the maintenance phase of therapy.[166,169,175,201,202] Thus, unless there is clear evidence for deterioration of renal status (rising serum creatinine, worsening proteinuria, increased activity of the urine sediment) at 6 months, the initial treatment plan should be maintained. A recent reanalysis of the ALMS data showed that for patients treated with MMF or cyclophosphamide, a reduction in proteinuria of ≥25%, or a normalization of complement components C3 and/or C4 by week 8 of therapy was prognostic of a renal response by 6 months.[203] The positive predictive value of these variables was about 70%, and therefore they could be helpful in guiding treatment decisions.

There are no specific guidelines for duration of maintenance therapy. In seven randomized clinical trials, immunosuppression was continued for an average of 3.5 years.[160,161,165,168,175,176,201] A repeat biopsy study found that after 2 years of immunosuppressive therapy only 40% of patients with class III/IV reverted to class II, consistent with the need for a prolonged maintenance phase.[179] It is reasonable to consider slowly tapering immunosuppressive therapy after patients have been in complete remission for a year. If a patient has a history of renal relapses it may be prudent to extend maintenance therapy. Although there is no standard definition of complete remission for LN in the literature, for preservation of kidney function the most important clinical variable currently available is proteinuria. Proteinuria less than 0.5 g per day should be the target for complete remission.[204] Serum creatinine should improve to a patient's pre-LN baseline if known. A caveat is that serum creatinine may be increased (acceptably) by renoprotective therapies. Thus, a stable serum creatinine should be the minimum requirement for complete remission. Urine sediment should not have any RBC or WBC casts, but hematuria may persist for months.[205] Finally, at remission normalization of serologic markers of lupus activity, such as complement and double-stranded DNA antibodies is expected, but there are several caveats regarding lupus serologies (see later).

Immunosuppression should be continued indefinitely for patients who achieve only a partial remission, and renoprotective therapies intensified. This is supported by the finding of continued activity in biopsies taken 2 or more years after initial therapy when significant proteinuria or an abnormal serum creatinine is still present.[206] Although the strategy of trying to convert a partial remission to a complete remission by increasing corticosteroids or using alternative immunosuppressive agents is not supported by evidence, it is often tried. A repeat kidney biopsy may be useful to determine the level of pathologic activity, which if severe could provide a rationale for re-induction therapy.

Membranous Lupus Nephritis

Membranous LN (class V) is a nonproliferative glomerulopathy that can be seen alone or with superimposed proliferative LN. Patients with mixed membranous and proliferative LN are treated as for the proliferative component, but may have a less favorable prognosis.[207] Alternatively, in a small randomized, controlled trial from China in patients with mixed class IV and V LN, the combination of TAC (4 mg per day), MMF (1 g per day), and oral corticosteroids was compared to pulse monthly intravenous CYC (0.75 g per m^2 for 6 months) plus oral corticosteroids. At 6 months 90% of patients treated with this lower dose, "multitarget" therapy and 45% of patients treated with CYC achieved either complete or partial remission ($P = .002$).[208]

Pure membranous LN occurs in 8% to 20% of patients with LN.[207,209,210] It is generally regarded as a less aggressive form of LN but long-term follow-up suggests a 20% incidence of chronic kidney disease, and ESRD develops in about 8% to 12% of patients.[207,209–211] In addition to renal insufficiency, the heavy proteinuria characteristic of membranous LN, if chronically present, predisposes to hyperlipidemia and atherosclerosis, contributing to cardiovascular morbidity and mortality.[212,213] Heavy proteinuria can also lead to a hypercoagulable state and arterial and venous thromboses.[213,214] Thrombotic events occur in 13% to 23% of lupus patients, and have been linked to the presence of antiphospholipid antibodies, and/or the nephrotic syndrome.[207,209,215] Spontaneous remission of heavy proteinuria occurs in only a minority of membranous LN patients.[216,217] Thus, membranous LN, although indolent compared to proliferative LN, can be associated with important morbidities and therefore warrants therapy.

Renoprotective and antiproteinuric therapies should be used for pure membranous LN with low level proteinuria. In addition to renoprotective and antiproteinuric measures, class V LN patients with nephrotic-range proteinuria and/or renal insufficiency should be considered for immunosuppression. A single prospective, randomized clinical trial showed that the addition of cyclophosphamide (six intravenous pulses of 0.5 to 1 g per m^2 every other month) or cyclosporin A (5 mg/kg/day for 11 months) to corticosteroids was superior to corticosteroids (prednisone 1 mg per kg every other day for 8 weeks, then taper) alone, but within a year of finishing treatment 40% of the cyclosporin group had relapsed.[218] Relapses were not seen in the cyclophosphamide group for 48 months posttreatment.[218] MMF (2 to 3 g per day) was found to be as efficacious as cyclophosphamide when subgroup analysis of class V LN was performed on data collected prospectively in two trials of MMF versus cyclophosphamide for classes III, IV, and V LN.[219] This is consistent with a number of smaller, nonrandomized, retrospective, or open-label studies of MMF and AZA (1 to 2 mg/kg/day) with or without corticosteroids in class V LN.[215,220–222]

Therefore, MMF plus corticosteroids may be tried initially to induce remission and, if that fails, a switch in immunosuppression to cyclophosphamide or cyclosporin A plus corticosteroids in patients with membranous LN and heavy proteinuria appears justified (Fig. 53.34).

TREATMENT OUTCOMES IN LUPUS NEPHRITIS

Treatment objectives for LN include remission in the short term, and prevention of relapse, CKD, ESRD, or death in the long term. The first 6 months of LN treatment is generally considered induction.[177,223] Although the term induction carries an expectation of remission, the number of complete responses at 6 and 12 months is low.

It is difficult to make direct comparisons of short-term outcomes among studies because treatment regimens differ, and the definitions of response and complete remission are not uniform. To generalize, a complete response requires normalization, improvement, improvement to baseline, or stabilization of serum creatinine and a reduction of proteinuria to ≤0.5 g per day. A partial response requires a stable or improved serum creatinine and a reduction of proteinuria by 50% and to below nephrotic range. Individual studies applied these criteria more or less rigorously, and some included improvement in the urinalysis in the definition of response. A survey of six studies of class III and IV LN[163,169,175,177,192,224] showed a median (range) 6-month complete response rate of 8.6% (7.4% to 25%), and an overall (complete plus partial) response rate of 53.5% (18% to 85%). The median (range) response 12 months after initiation of therapy was 60.5% (32% to 85%). These studies were done in black, Hispanic, and Caucasian patients, and used corticosteroids plus low or usual-dose intravenous cyclophosphamide, oral cyclophosphamide, or MMF. Interestingly, in four studies of Chinese SLE patients,[164–167] the median complete response at 12 to 24 months was 71% (57% to 81%), and the median overall response was 90% (73% to 95%). It is not known why Chinese patients respond so much better than most groups to initial therapy. These patients were, however, more often treated with oral cyclophosphamide than intravenous cyclophosphamide, and their genetic and environmental differences may have contributed to response rates.

For membranous LN, treatment trials suggest that the addition of an immunosuppressive to background corticosteroid will yield a complete response in the neighborhood of 40% to 60% of the patients within 6 to 12 months.[215,218,221,222,225] Response may be more rapid with calcineurin inhibitors, but the risk of relapse is high.

The long-term outcomes for proliferative LN in most studies were death, doubling of serum creatinine, ESRD, and renal relapse. Considering five studies[163,164,166,224,226] that included black, Hispanic, Caucasian, and Chinese patients, observed for a median (range) of 6 years (3 to 10 years), the rate of mortality and ESRD were 5% (0% to 20%) and 4% (0% to 10%), respectively. Doubling of serum creatinine occurred in 7.2% (0.04% to 18.2%) of patients, and renal relapse in 23% (0.04% to 42%). Similarly, 25% of patients reached a composite endpoint of death, doubling serum creatinine, or ESRD in 10 years of follow-up after treatment with the low-dose (Eurolupus) cyclophosphamide protocol.[176]

In univariate analyses, a large number of risk factors for treatment outcomes of proliferative LN have been reported. However, multivariate analyses demonstrated that many were not independent risk factors. Independent risk factors for LN outcomes from several multivariate analyses.[164–166,178,179,202,203,226–228] are shown in Table 53.4. Among these studies, only serum creatinine at the beginning of treatment appears to reach consensus as a biomarker of future remission, renal relapse, CKD, or ESRD. It is interesting that failure to achieve a complete remission was identified by only a few investigations to be a significant risk factor for relapse, CKD, ESRD, or mortality,[166,229,230] especially considering that for most proteinuric kidney diseases resolution of proteinuria is the strongest predictor of renal survival.[213,231,232] It is possible that if a more rigorous definition of complete remission had been applied, more studies would have found achieving a complete remission to be an important factor in long-term renal preservation. Finally, few studies included socioeconomic status in their analyses, which may have affected the strength of race and ethnicity as independent risk factors.

There is far less information on risk factors for the outcome of membranous LN after treatment. By multivariate analysis, the only independent predictor of failure to achieve remission was initial proteinuria over 5 g per day, and failure to achieve sustained remission was a risk factor for decline in kidney function.[218] Race or ethnicity did not appear to affect response.

FOLLOWING PATIENTS WITH LN

After successful initial treatment of LN, patients must be carefully followed because LN relapses. Renal flares in LN patients who had participated in randomized clinical trials occurred in 40% of complete responders within a median of 41 months of remission, and 63% of partial responders within a median of 11.5 months of response.[233] Putative risk factors for renal relapse are listed in Table 53.4, but there is no consensus on what predisposes patients to flare. It is important to recognize and treat flares because, with each episode of active LN, the kidney sustains chronic damage as demonstrated by repeat biopsy studies that showed an increase in the renal chronicity index at the second biopsy.[179,197,199,200,208,234] LN relapses may thus culminate in CKD or, eventually, ESRD.

Renal flare is diagnosed by increases in activity of the urine sediment, amount of proteinuria, and serum creatinine. Consensus definitions for SLE and LN flares have

TABLE 53.4 **Risk Factors[a] for Renal Outcomes in Proliferative LN**

Achieve Remission			Renal Flare			Doubling SCr[b]			ESRD			Double SCr, ESRD, Death			ESRD or Death		
	HR/RR[c]	Type[d]		HR/RR	Type		HR/RR	Type		HR/RR	Type		HR/RR	Type		HR/RR	Type
Proteinuria	0.86 / ↑ g/d	R	Time to remit	1.03/mo	R	SCr > 1 mg/dL	4.1	R	SCr	2.8/↑ 1mg/dL	R	SCr	1.26/↑ 1 mg/dL	R	Age >50	3.3	R
Delay therapy >3 months	0.58	R	CNS SLE	8.41	R	Hispanic	3.6	R	No remit	6.8	R	Chronicity index	1.18/point		SCr	2.32	
White race	2.63	R	Class IV LN	.28	R	Poverty[i]	3.5	R	Class III ≥50% LN[k]	2.77	R	Mean BP	1.02/mm Hg		Non-white race	2.28	
SCr	0.21/↑ g/d	R	Chronicity index[f]	1.22/ point	R	Government insurance[j]	3.0	R	Anti-R0 positive	2.35	R						
Class IV lupus nephritis	2.05	R	Persistently + DS-DNA	2.94	R	Nephritic flare	17.7	R	None		R						
SCr	0.96/μmol/l	P	Activity index[g]	1.13/ point	P	Chronicity index	2.1/point	P									
None[e]		P	No CR[h]	6.2	P	None		P									
			None		P												

[a]All clinical variables are taken at baseline before systemic lupus erythematosus lupus nephritis treatment.
[b]SCr, serum creatinine.
[c]Hazard ratio (HR) or relative risk (RR).
[d]Retrospective or prospective study.
[e]No variables were predictive in multivariate analysis.
[f]Chronicity index on kidney biopsy.
[g]Activity index on kidney biopsy.
[h]Complete remission not achieved.
[i]Living in a neighborhood where >10% of residents are below federal poverty line.
[j]Medicare, Medicaid as opposed to private insurance.
[k]Class III with active and/or necrotizing lesions in ≥50% of nonsclerotic glomeruli.
BP, blood pressure; CNS, central nervous system; ESRD, end-stage renal disease; LN, lupus nephritis.

TABLE 53.5 **Criteria for Diagnosis and Classification of Severity of SLE Renal Flare**[a]

Mild Renal Flare	Moderate Renal Flare	Severe Renal Flare
↑ in glomerular hematuria from <5 to >15 RBC/hpf, with ≥2 acanthocytes/hpf	If baseline creatinine is: <2.0 mg/dL, an ↑ of 0.20–1.0 mg/dL ≥2.0 mg/dL, an ↑ of 0.40–1.5 mg/dL	If baseline creatinine is: <2 mg/dL, an ↑ of >1.0 mg/dL ≥2 mg/dL, an ↑ of >1.5 mg/dL
and/or	*and/or*	*and/or*
recurrence of ≥ 1 RBC cast, WBC cast (no infection), or both	If baseline Pr/Cr is: <0.5, an ↑ to ≥1.0 0.5–1.0, an ↑ to ≥2.0, but < absolute ↑ of 5.0 >1.0, an ↑ of ≥ twofold with absolute Pr/Cr <5.0	an absolute ↑ Pr/Cr >5.0

[a]Remission of nephritis is defined as stabilization or improvement of serum creatinine to baseline or better, and a return of proteinuria to baseline or better. hpf, high-power field; Pr/Cr, protein/creatinine; RBC, red blood cell; WBC, white blood cell.

recently been published,[235,236] and one way of operationalizing these as criteria is shown in Table 53.5.[237] Other findings that support a diagnosis of renal flare, but are not necessarily always present (see later) include a fall in serum complement levels and a rise in anti–double-stranded DNA antibody titers. Flares are less likely to occur in patients who have been highly immunosuppressed. Depressed serum immunoglobulin levels may indicate overt immunosuppression; however, in severe nephrotic syndrome due to LN flare, serum immunoglobulins can also be low. Non-LN causes of an increase in creatinine or an increase in proteinuria must be excluded (see also page 1528). Increases in proteinuria can occur with pregnancy, uncontrolled hypertension, and increased sodium intake. An approach to flare therapy based on flare severity is given in Figure 53.36.

Complement components 3 and 4 (C3, C4) and anti–double-stranded DNA antibodies have been used to support the diagnosis of renal flare and also to anticipate impending flare. However, these serologies have low sensitivity (49% to 79%) and specificity (51% to 74%) for concurrent renal flare, and do not reliably predict impending flare even when measured serially, with sensitivities and specificities around 50% and 70%, respectively.[238–240] In one cohort the positive predictive values for C3 and C4 to forecast impending flare were 7.4% and 5.5%, respectively.[238]

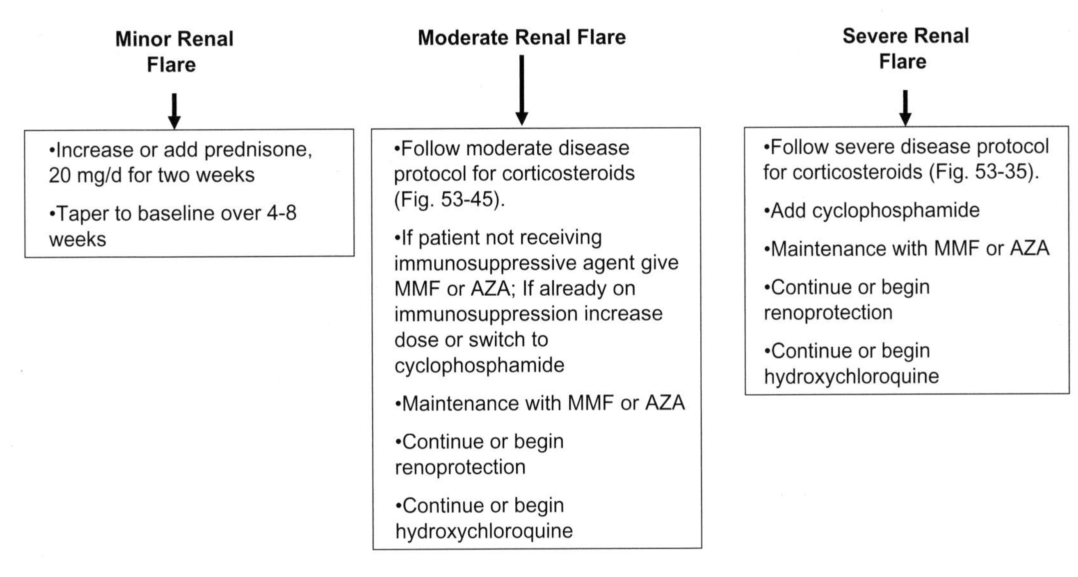

FIGURE 53.36 Severity-based approach to renal flare therapy.

Being able to anticipate imminent renal flare and potentially start therapy preemptively could attenuate the development of chronic kidney injury and minimize exposure to cytotoxic agents. Similarly, modification of drug dose and duration of therapy based on biomarkers that predict outcome of a flare would be expected to improve treatment efficacy and reduce toxicity. Finally, because kidney biopsies are not repeated at every flare, a noninvasive surrogate of renal pathology would be very useful in choosing therapy. This approach to LN treatment represents a fundamental change from a reactive to a proactive paradigm, and will require biomarkers that accurately predict SLE nephritis activity, pathology, and prognosis to guide therapeutic decisions. Efforts are under way to identify such novel biomarkers. A major focus has been on developing urine markers[241,249a] because urine generally reflects intrarenal events. Several urine biomarker candidates[237,242–249,249a] have been found (Table 53.6). None of these candidates has, to date, been validated in a large, independent, prospectively followed lupus cohort, although such studies are anticipated.

THROMBOTIC INJURY TO THE KIDNEY IN SYSTEMIC LUPUS ERYTHEMATOSUS

The most common clotting events that affect the kidney in SLE occur as a manifestation of the antiphospholipid syndrome (APS). The incidence of renal APS is about 30% in SLE, usually in conjunction with LN, but also alone.[125,250] Serologic studies show that lupus anticoagulant is present in 30% to 52% of cases of renal APS, anticardiolipin antibodies in 72% to 95% of patients, but up to 15% had neither.[124,125] Thrombi or evidence of past clotting may be found in any of the kidney blood vessels. The term APS nephropathy describes renal injury due to thrombi or their consequences in glomeruli and small intrarenal blood vessels, and characteristically presents a histologic picture of a thrombotic microangiopathy.[251] Although renal artery occlusion and renal vein thrombosis due to APS can be diagnosed with imaging studies, APS nephropathy requires a kidney biopsy. Failure to treat APS, and especially APS nephropathy, can lead to insidious CKD or ESRD despite adequate treatment of LN with immunosuppression, because APS results in noninflammatory occlusions of renal blood vessels and renal ischemia. Renal APS is treated with chronic anticoagulation therapy plus hydroxychloroquine.

Thrombotic thrombocytopenic purpura (TTP) may also occur in the setting of SLE and is associated with a high mortality.[252] TTP is treated with plasma exchange in addition to high-dose steroids. Because of the high associated mortality, it is important to consider this diagnosis and treat early.

PREGNANCY AND LUPUS NEPHRITIS

SLE affects women during their reproductive years, so pregnancy concerns are very common. In several retrospective analyses the risk of fetal loss in SLE patients with LN was not higher than SLE patients with no history of LN.[253,254] If LN is in remission, fetal losses of 8% to 25% have been reported,[254–257] but in active LN, fetal loss can be considerably higher, around 35% to 59%.[254,257] In addition to the clinical activity of LN, hypocomplementemia appears to be a risk factor for fetal loss, whereas the use of low-dose aspirin may be protective.[255]

TABLE 53.6 **Novel Candidate Biomarkers for Monitoring LN**

Forecast Impending LN Flare	Predict Development of CKD	Predict Renal Pathologies
uMCP-1[a]	uLFABP[c]	uGlycoproteins[f]
uNGAL[b]	mEPCR staining on kidney biopsy[d]	uCXCL10 mRNA[g]
uTransferrin	uFOXP3 mRNA[e]	CD29 on T cells[h]
uHepcidin		uMCP-1 + serum creatinine[i]

[a]MCP-1, monocyte chemoattractant protein-1, a proinflammatory chemokine upregulated in lupus nephritis; u, urine as the source.
[b]NGAL, neutrophil gelatinase-associated lipocalin, an antibacterial protein, that also transports iron and is an epithelial growth factor.
[c]LFABP, liver-type fatty-acid binding protein, produced by human proximal tubular cells.
[d]mEPCR, membrane endothelial protein C receptor, found on cortical peritubular capillaries in lupus nephritis kidney biopsies.
[e]FOXP3, forkhead transcription factor, important in development of regulatory T cells.
[f]Serum glycoproteins excreted in urine; for example, α-1 acid glycoprotein, α1 microglobulin, and zinc α-2 glycoprotein.
[g]CXCL10, a TH-1 chemokine upregulated in lupus nephritis.
[h]CD29, a T-cell β1 integrin.
[i]A composite biomarker of interstitial inflammation.
CKD, chronic kidney disease; LN, lupus nephritis.

There is also risk to the kidneys in patients with LN who become pregnant. One study noted that renal flares and progressive renal dysfunction were not different between pregnant and nonpregnant patients with LN.[253] In other studies, renal flares were found to be higher in patients who became pregnant and had only achieved partial remission of the LN, or who had more than 1 g per day proteinuria or renal insufficiency.[255,257] Renal flare rates of 10% to 69% have been reported during or directly following pregnancy.[253,255–257] Hydroxychloroquine may be protective again SLE flares in general, and/or in the setting of pregnancy.[254]

To protect the kidneys and the fetus, it is recommended that SLE patients with kidney involvement be advised to wait at least 6 months after complete renal remission before trying to become pregnant. Cytotoxic drugs such as cyclophosphamide and MMF, and anti-hypertensive/renoprotective agents like angiotensin-converting enzyme (ACE) inhibitors and angiotensin receptor blockers (ARBs) should not be used during pregnancy. Hydroxychloroquine should be continued, and corticosteroids and AZA may be used if needed to control SLE activity.

RENAL REPLACEMENT THERAPIES IN SYSTEMIC LUPUS ERYTHEMATOSUS

ESRD occurring as a result of SLE requires renal replacement therapy with either dialysis or transplantation. There has been concern that SLE patients do not do as well as other patients with renal replacement therapies; however, available evidence, although limited and mainly retrospective, does not suggest this is completely warranted.

SLE patients receiving hemodialysis were found to have similar outcomes as patients with other causes of ESRD,[258] but SLE patients on peritoneal dialysis appeared to have a higher mortality and more infectious complications.[259,260] In contrast, a small study suggested 5-year survivals were similar for the two modalities.[258,261]

There is no consensus on extrarenal SLE activity in patients receiving renal replacement therapy. This may be due, in part, to lack of a consistent definition of flare. Consequently, some investigations have shown significant improvement in extrarenal lupus and reduced need for immunosuppression, whereas in other investigations, despite 3 or more years of dialysis, SLE activity remained prevalent (40% to 50%), or worsened in peritoneal dialysis recipients.[258,259,262,263]

Kidney allograft survival in transplant recipients with SLE appears to be close to that of non-SLE ESRD patients, according to multivariate analyses of the United States Renal Data Service (USRDS) and the United Network for Organ Sharing (UNOS) databases.[264,265] These large studies looked at information from 43,000 to 93,000 transplant recipients, 2,000 to 3,000 having been transplanted for ESRD due to LN. Analysis of the USRDS lupus patients who received deceased donor kidneys showed lower allograft and patient survival rates than a diabetic ESRD reference group, but the hazard ratios were small at 1.14 and 1.3, respectively.[264] The analysis of UNOS showed that compared to non-SLE recipients in general, recipients with SLE had the same rate of patient and allograft survival.[265] Additionally, in smaller studies SLE recipients did not seem to have a higher frequency of acute rejection episodes,[264] except in one study where the hazard ratio for acute rejection in recipients of living (but not deceased donor) kidneys was slightly increased at 1.19.[265] Posttransplant treatment with MMF reduced allograft loss in lupus patients who received deceased donor kidneys and improved patient survival.[265,266] Finally, a common finding was that SLE recipients had a higher rate of thrombotic events than non-SLE recipients.

The recurrence of LN in transplanted kidneys was found to be in the range of 2.4% to 11%.[266–270] One surveillance biopsy study found a 54% recurrence rate, but most of these were class II, and only 12% were class III, IV, or V.[271] Although some studies did not find recurrent LN to affect allograft loss,[268–270] in the largest investigation,[267] which examined 6,850 SLE recipients, recurrent LN was independently associated with allograft loss (hazard ratio 4.09; 95% CI 3.41–4.92). The attributable risk for allograft loss was low, however, because the recurrence rate of LN was so low (2.4%). Recurrent LN did not affect patient survival.[266,267]

In summary, lupus patients who come to ESRD should be offered the option of a kidney transplant. Before transplantation SLE should be quiescent. Additionally, because of the higher incidence of cardiovascular disease in lupus, patients need to be carefully evaluated for this before surgery. Living donor transplants and an MMF-containing antirejection regimen are preferred. There are no data regarding prophylaxis for thrombotic events—a high index of suspicion is warranted. If dialysis is needed before transplantation, hemodialysis may be the preferred modality. While on dialysis, even though lupus can become quiescent, vigilance for extrarenal flares is appropriate, and treatment for active lupus with immunosuppression may be necessary.

THE FUTURE DIRECTION OF LUPUS NEPHRITIS TREATMENT

The need for new approaches to the treatment of LN is highlighted by the low complete remission rate, the modest overall remission rate, and the high occurrence of side effects from current therapies. The therapeutics now under development and in various phases of clinical trial assessment attempt to target cytokines or cells specifically involved in the pathogenesis of SLE. This will presumably result in less overall immunosuppression but increased efficacy.

Figure 53.37 summarizes the relationship of these novel biologic agents to pathogenic mediators in SLE and LN. Targeted B cell therapies have received the most attention because the B cell has such a wide array of relevant functions including autoantibody production, antigen presentation, and regulation of T and dendritic cells.

The most widely studied anti-B cell agent is rituximab, a monoclonal antibody to the B cell antigen CD20. Rituximab

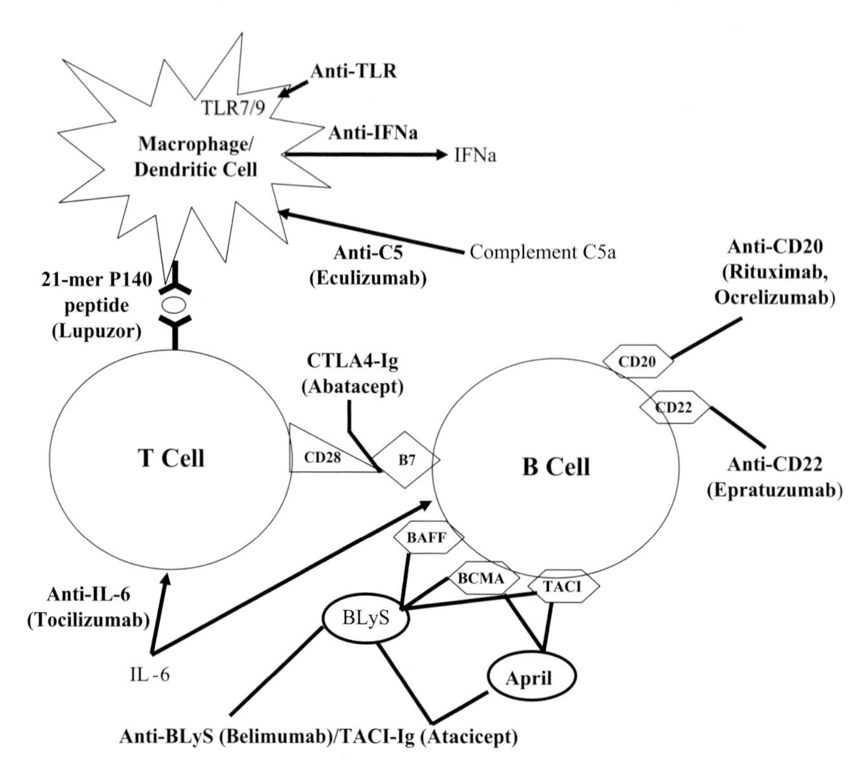

FIGURE 53.37 Novel therapies for lupus nephritis that are being developed or are in clinical trials.

causes profound depletion of circulating B cells that lasts for several months. A number of small, open-label, uncontrolled trials have suggested that rituximab is effective in proliferative LN, either for refractory disease or as induction therapy.[188–190,272] An equally small ($n = 8$) longer term study of refractory LN treated with rituximab suggested poor efficacy, but half of the patients did achieve complete or partial remission.[273] However, in a large, prospective, double-blind controlled study of rituximab versus placebo added to MMF plus corticosteroids for proliferative LN, there was no difference in complete or partial responses at 12 months between groups.[186] The niche for rituximab in the therapy of LN thus remains unclear.

Epratuzumab is a humanized monoclonal antibody that targets the B cell antigen receptor coreceptor, CD22. Epratuzumab partially depletes B cells, but may also interfere with their proliferation and activation in lupus. Although few LN patients ($n = 4$, published) have been treated with epratuzumab, 75% showed some improvement in BILAG scores.

B cells require the cytokines BLyS and APRIL for survival and proliferation. Drugs that inhibit these factors including belimumab, an anti-BLyS monoclonal antibody and atacicept, a soluble receptor that binds to BLyS and APRIL, are being evaluated in SLE. Although belimumab has not been used specifically for LN, two phase III trials in SLE were recently completed and at 12 months successfully met the composite endpoint of improvement in the Systemic Lupus Erythematosus Disease Activity Index, no worsening of physician's global assessment of disease activity, and no new BILAG organ occurrences.[274,275]

Autoreactive B cells communicate with and activate T cells through interaction of B7.1/B7.2 receptors with CD28 on T cells. Recombinant CTLA4 fused to IgG heavy chain components (abatacept) blocks the interaction between CD28 and B7.1/B7.2, and has been shown to reduce proteinuria in a rodent model of LN.[276] Abatacept is currently approved for rheumatoid arthritis and is being tested in human LN.

Autoreactive T cells from SLE patients bind and proliferate to a peptide containing residues 131 to 151 of the 70K spliceosomal protein within the U1 small nuclear RNP. A phosphorylated analog called P140 (lupuzor) prevents T cell proliferation and induces secretion of the anti-inflammatory cytokine interleukin-10. This peptide may tolerize T cells, and in a human SLE phase II trial had minimal side effects and a reduction in anti–double-stranded DNA antibody levels by over 20%, suggesting possible utility in treatment.[277]

As previously discussed, a number of cytokines have been implicated in the pathogenesis and/or tissue damage of SLE and LN. Of these, antagonists of IFN-α, IL-6, complement component C5, and TLR7 and 9 or their receptors have been developed, and are at various stages of preclinical or clinical testing.[274]

REFERENCES

1. Seligman VA, Lum RF, Olson JL, et al. Demographic differences in the development of lupus nephritis: A retrospective analysis. *Am J Med.* 2002;112: 726–729.

2. Bastian HM, Roseman JM, McGwin G Jr, et al. Systemic lupus erythematosus in three ethnic groups. XII. Risk factors for lupus nephritis after diagnosis. *Lupus.* 2002;11(3):152–160.

3. Adler M, Chambers S, Edwards C, et al. An assessment of renal failure in an SLE cohort with special reference to ethnicity, over a 25-year period. *Rheumatol.* 2006;45:1144–1147.

4. Arfaj AS, Khalil N. Clinical and immunological manifestations in 624 SLE patients in Saudi Arabia. *Lupus.* 2009;18:465–473.

5. Campbell R Jr, Cooper GS, Gilkeson GS. Two aspects of the clinical and humanistic burden of systemic lupus erythematosus: mortality risk and quality of life early in the course of disease. *Arthritis Rheum.* Apr 15 2008;59(4): 458–464.

6. Danila MI, Pons-Estel GJ, Zhang J, et al. Renal damage is the most important predictor of mortality within the damage index: data from LUMINA LXIV, a multiethnic US cohort. *Rheumatology (Oxford).* 2009;48(5):542–545.

7. Ward MM. Changes in the incidence of endstage renal disease due to lupus nephritis in the United States, 1996–2004. *J Rheumatol.* 2009;36:63–67.

8. Holman HR, Kunkel HG. Affinity between the lupus erythematosus serum factor and cell nuclei and nucleoprotein. *Science.* 1957;126(3265):162–163.

9. Sherer Y, Gorstein A, Fritzler MJ, et al. Autoantibody explosion in systemic lupus erythematosus: more than 100 different antibodies found in SLE patients. *Semin Arthritis Rheum.* 2004;34(2):501–537.

10. Hahn BH. Antibodies to DNA. *N Engl J Med.* 1998;338(19):1359–1368.

11. Krishnan C, Kaplan MH. Immunopathologic studies of systemic lupus erythematosus. II. Antinuclear reaction of gamma-globulin eluted from homogenates and isolated glomeruli of kidneys from patients with lupus nephritis. *J Clin Invest.* 1967;46(4):569–579.

12. Schmiedeke TM, Stockl FW, Weber R, et al. Histones have high affinity for the glomerular basement membrane. Relevance for immune complex formation in lupus nephritis. *J Exp Med.* 1989;169(6):1879–1894.

13. Kalaaji M, Fenton KA, Mortensen ES, et al. Glomerular apoptotic nucleosomes are central target structures for nephritogenic antibodies in human SLE nephritis. *Kidney Int.* 2007;71(7):664–672.

14. Mason LJ, Ravirajan CT, Rahman A, et al. Is alpha-actinin a target for pathogenic anti-DNA antibodies in lupus nephritis? *Arthritis Rheum.* 2004;50(3): 866–870.

15. Yung S, Cheung KF, Zhang Q, et al. Anti-dsDNA antibodies bind to mesangial annexin II in lupus nephritis. *J Am Soc Nephrol.* 2010;21(11):1912–1927.

16. Winkler TH, Henschel TA, Kalies I, et al. Constant isotype pattern of anti-dsDNA antibodies in patients with systemic lupus erythematosus. *Clin Exp Immunol.* 1988;72(3):434–439.

17. Sinico RA, Rimoldi L, Radice A, et al. Anti-C1q autoantibodies in lupus nephritis. *Ann N Y Acad Sci.* 2009;1173:47–51.

18. Trendelenburg M, Lopez-Trascasa M, Potlukova E, et al. High prevalence of anti-C1q antibodies in biopsy-proven active lupus nephritis. *Nephrol Dial Transplant.* 2006;21(11):3115–3121.

19. Marto N, Bertolaccini ML, Calabuig E, et al. Anti-C1q antibodies in nephritis: correlation between titres and renal disease activity and positive predictive value in systemic lupus erythematosus. *Ann Rheum Dis.* 2005;64(3):444–448.

20. Trouw LA, Groeneveld TW, Seelen MA, et al. Anti-C1q autoantibodies deposit in glomeruli but are only pathogenic in combination with glomerular C1q-containing immune complexes. *J Clin Invest.* 2004;114(5):679–688.

21. Flierman R, Daha MR. Pathogenic role of anti-C1q autoantibodies in the development of lupus nephritis—a hypothesis. *Mol Immunol.* 2007;44(1–3): 133–138.

22. Prada AE, Strife CF. IgG subclass restriction of autoantibody to solid-phase C1q in membranoproliferative and lupus glomerulonephritis. *Clin Immunol Immunopathol.* 1992;63(1):84–88.

23. Schifferli JA, Peters DK. Complement, the immune-complex lattice, and the pathophysiology of complement-deficiency syndromes. *Lancet.* 1983; 2(8356):957–959.

24. Pickering MC, Botto M, Taylor PR, et al. Systemic lupus erythematosus, complement deficiency, and apoptosis. *Adv Immunol.* 2000;76:227–324.

25. Hebert LA. The clearance of immune complexes from the circulation of man and other primates. *Am J Kidney Dis.* 1991;17:352–361.

26. Birmingham DJ, Hebert LA. CR1 and CR1-like: The primate immune adherence receptors. *Immunol Rev.* 2001;180:100–111.

27. Navratil JS, Korb LC, Ahearn JM. Systemic lupus erythematosus and complement deficiency: clues to a novel role for the classical complement pathway in the maintenance of immune tolerance. *Immunopharmacology.* 1999;42 (1–3):47–52.

28. Walport MJ, Ross GD, Mackworth YC, et al. Family studies of erythrocyte complement receptor type 1 levels: reduced levels in patients with SLE are acquired, not inherited. *Clin Exp Immunol.* 1985;59(3):547–554.

29. Birmingham DJ, Gavit KF, McCarty SM, et al. Consumption of erythrocyte CR1 (CD35) is associated with protection against systemic lupus erythematosus renal flare. *Clin Exp Immunol.* 2006;143(2):274–280.

30. Koffler D, Agnello V, Carr RI, et al. Variable patterns of immunoglobulin and complement deposition in the kidneys of patients with systemic lupus erythematosus. *Am J Pathol.* 1969;56:305–316.

31. Ricker DM, Hebert LA, Rohde R, et al. Serum C3 levels are diagnostically more sensitive and specific for systemic lupus erythematosus activity than are serum C4 levels. The Lupus Nephritis Collaborative Study Group. *Am J Kidney Dis.* 1991;18(6):678–685.

32. Verroust PJ, Wilson CB, Cooper NR, et al. Glomerular complement components in human glomerulonephritis. *J Clin Invest.* 1974;53(1):77–84.

33. Biesecker G, Katz S, Koffler D. Renal localization of the membrane attack complex in systemic lupus erythematosus nephritis. *J Exp Med.* 1981;154(6): 1779–1794.

34. Welch TR, Beischel LS, Witte DP. Differential expression of complement C3 and C4 in the human kidney. *J Clin Invest.* 1993;92(3):1451–1458.

35. Welch TR, Beischel LS, Frenzke M, et al. Regulated expression of complement factor B in the human kidney. *Kidney Int.* 1996;50(2):521–525.

36. Mizuno M, Blanchin S, Gasque P, et al. High levels of complement C3a receptor in the glomeruli in lupus nephritis. *Am J Kidney Dis.* 2007;49(5): 598–606.

37. Abe K, Miyazaki M, Koji T, et al. Enhanced expression of complement C5a receptor mRNA in human diseased kidney assessed by in situ hybridization. *Kidney Int.* 2001;60(1):137–146.

38. Kazatchkine MD, Fearon DT, Appay MD, et al. Immunohistochemical study of the human glomerular C3b receptor in normal kidney and in seventy five cases of renal diseases. *J Clin Invest.* 1982;69:900–912.

39. Cosio FG, Sedmak DD, Mahan JD, et al. Localization of decay accelerating factor in normal and diseased kidneys. *Kidney Int.* 1989;36(1):100–107.

40. Wang Y, Hu Q, Madri JA, et al. Amelioration of lupus-like autoimmune disease in NZB/WF1 mice after treatment with a blocking monoclonal antibody specific for complement component C5. *Proc Natl Acad Sci U S A.* 1996; 93(16):8563–8568.

41. Bao L, Haas M, Kraus DM, et al. Administration of a soluble recombinant complement C3 inhibitor protects against renal disease in MRL/lpr mice. *J Am Soc Nephrol.* 2003;14(3):670–679.

42. Watanabe H, Garnier G, Circolo A, et al. Modulation of renal disease in MRL/lpr mice genetically deficient in the alternative complement pathway factor B. *J Immunol.* 2000;164(2):786–794.

43. Elliott MK, Jarmi T, Ruiz P, et al. Effects of complement factor D deficiency on the renal disease of MRL/lpr mice. *Kidney Int.* 2004;65(1):129–138.

44. Li X, Ptacek TS, Brown EE, et al. Fc gamma receptors: structure, function and role as genetic risk factors in SLE. *Genes Immun.* 2009;10(5):380–389.

45. Warmerdam PAM, van de Winkle JGJ, Vlug J, et al. A single amino acid in the second Ig-like domain of the human Fcγ receptor II plays a critical role in human IgG2 binding. *J. Immunol.* 1991;144:1338–1343.

46. Koene HR, Kleijer M, Algra J, et al. Fc gammaRIIIa-158V/F polymorphism influences the binding of IgG by natural killer cell Fc gammaRIIIa, independently of the Fc gammaRIIIa-48L/R/H phenotype. *Blood.* 1997;90(3):1109–1114.

47. Karassa FB, Trikalinos TA, Ioannidis JP. Role of the Fc gamma receptor IIa polymorphism in susceptibility to systemic lupus erythematosus and lupus nephritis: a meta-analysis. *Arthritis Rheum.* 2002;46(6):1563–1571.

48. Karassa FB, Trikalinos TA, Ioannidis JP. The Fc gamma RIIIA-F158 allele is a risk factor for the development of lupus nephritis: a meta-analysis. *Kidney Int.* 2003;63(4):1475–1482.

49. Ravetch JV, Clynes RA. Divergent roles for Fc receptors and complement in vivo. *Annu Rev Immunol.* 1998;16:421–432.

50. Clynes R, Dumitru C, Ravetch JV. Uncoupling of immune complex formation and kidney damage in autoimmune glomerulonephritis. *Science.* 1998; 279:1052–1054.

51. Heller T, Gessner JE, Schmidt RE, et al. Cutting edge: Fc receptor type I for IgG on macrophages and complement mediate the inflammatory response in immune complex peritonitis. *J Immunol.* 1999;162(10):5657–5661.

52. Matsumoto K, Watanabe N, Akikusa B, et al. Fc receptor-independent development of autoimmune glomerulonephritis in lupus-prone MRL/lpr mice. *Arthritis Rheum.* 2003;48(2):486–494.

53. Rovin BH. The chemokine network in systemic lupus erythematosus nephritis. *Frontiers in Bioscience.* 2007;13:904–922.

54. Peterson KS, Huang JF, Zhu J, et al. Characterization of heterogeneity in the molecular pathogenesis of lupus nephritis from transcriptional profiles of laser-captured glomeruli. *J Clin Invest.* 2004;113(12):1722–1733.

55. Chan RW, Lai FM, Li EK, et al. Intrarenal cytokine gene expression in lupus nephritis. *Ann Rheum Dis.* 2007;66(7):886–892.

56. Masutani K, Akahoshi M, Tsuruya K, et al. Predominance of Th1 immune response in diffuse proliferative lupus nephritis. *Arthritis Rheum.* 2001;44(9): 2097–2106.

57. Crispin JC, Oukka M, Bayliss G, et al. Expanded double negative T cells in patients with systemic lupus erythematosus produce IL-17 and infiltrate the kidneys. *J Immunol.* 2008;181(12):8761–8766.
58. Tesch GH, Maifert S, Schwarting A, et al. Monocyte chemoattractant protein 1–dependent leukocytic infiltrates are responsible for autoimmune disease in MRL-faslpr mice. *J Exp Med.* 1999;190:1813–1824.
59. Perez de Lema G, Maier H, Franz TJ, et al. Chemokine receptor CCR2 deficiency reduces renal disease and prolongs survival in MRL/lpr lupus-prone mice. *J Am Soc Nephrol.* 2005;16:3592–3601.
60. Hasegawa H, Kohno M, Sasaki M, et al. Antagonist of monocyte chemoattractant protein 1 ameliorates the initiation and progression of lupus nephritis and renal vasculitis in MRL/lpr mice. *Arthritis Rheum.* 2003;48(9):2555–2566.
61. Kiberd BA. Interleukin-6 receptor blockage ameliorates murine lupus nephritis. *J Am Soc Nephrol.* 1993;4(1):58–61.
62. Liang B, Gardner DB, Griswold DE, et al. Anti-interleukin-6 monoclonal antibody inhibits autoimmune responses in a murine model of systemic lupus erythematosus. *Immunology.* 2006;119(3):296–305.
63. Bossu P, Neumann D, Del Giudice E, et al. IL-18 cDNA vaccination protects mice from spontaneous lupus-like autoimmune disease. *Proc Natl Acad Sci U S A.* 2003;100(24):14181–14186.
64. Venegas-Pont M, Manigrasso MB, Grifoni SC, et al. Tumor necrosis factor-alpha antagonist etanercept decreases blood pressure and protects the kidney in a mouse model of systemic lupus erythematosus. *Hypertension.* 2010;56(4):643–649.
65. Uhm WS, Na K, Song GW, et al. Cytokine balance in kidney tissue from lupus nephritis patients. *Rheumatology (Oxford).* 2003;42(8):935–938.
66. Tucci M, Lombardi L, Richards HB, et al. Overexpression of interleukin-12 and T helper 1 predominance in lupus nephritis. *Clin Exp Immunol.* 2008;154(2):247–254.
67. Ge D, You Z. Expression of interleukin-17RC protein in normal human tissues. *Int Arch Med.* 2008;1(1):19.
68. Qiu Z, Dillen C, Hu J, et al. Interleukin-17 regulates chemokine and gelatinase B expression in fibroblasts to recruit both neutrophils and monocytes. *Immunobiology.* 2009;214(9–10):835–842.
69. Bettelli E, Carrier Y, Gao W, et al. Reciprocal developmental pathways for the generation of pathogenic effector TH17 and regulatory T cells. *Nature.* 2006; 441(7090):235–238.
70. Cassese G, Lindenau S, de Boer B, et al. Inflamed kidneys of NZB / W mice are a major site for the homeostasis of plasma cells. *Eur J Immunol.* 2001;31(9): 2726–2732.
71. Chang A, Henderson SG, Brandt D, et al. In situ B cell-mediated immune responses and tubulointerstitial inflammation in human lupus nephritis. *J Immunol.* 2011;186(3):1849–1860.
72. Baecher-Allan C, Brown JA, Freeman GJ, et al. CD4+CD25 high regulatory cells in human peripheral blood. *J Immunol.* 2001;167(3):1245–1253.
73. Lim HW, Hillsamer P, Banham AH, et al. Cutting edge: direct suppression of B cells by CD4+ CD25+ regulatory T cells. *J Immunol.* 2005;175(7):4180–4183.
74. Hsu WT, Suen JL, Chiang BL. The role of CD4CD25 T cells in autoantibody production in murine lupus. *Clin Exp Immunol.* 2006;145(3):513–519.
75. Scalapino KJ, Tang Q, Bluestone JA, et al. Suppression of disease in New Zealand Black/New Zealand White lupus-prone mice by adoptive transfer of ex vivo expanded regulatory T cells. *J Immunol.* 2006;177(3):1451–1459.
76. Gerli R, Nocentini G, Alunno A, et al. Identification of regulatory T cells in systemic lupus erythematosus. *Autoimmun Rev.* 2009;8(5):426–430.
77. Sfikakis PP, Souliotis VL, Fragiadaki KG, et al. Increased expression of the FoxP3 functional marker of regulatory T cells following B cell depletion with rituximab in patients with lupus nephritis. *Clin Immunol.* 2007;123(1):66–73.
78. Yates J, Whittington A, Mitchell P, et al. Natural regulatory T cells: number and function are normal in the majority of patients with lupus nephritis. *Clin Exp Immunol.* 2008;153(1):44–55.
79. Ronnblom L, Alm GV, Eloranta ML. The type I interferon system in the development of lupus. *Semin Immunol.* 2011;23(2):113–121.
80. Diebold SS, Kaisho T, Hemmi H, et al. Innate antiviral responses by means of TLR7–mediated recognition of single-stranded RNA. *Science.* 2004; 303(5663):1529–1531.
81. Hemmi H, Takeuchi O, Kawai T, et al. A Toll-like receptor recognizes bacterial DNA. *Nature.* 2000;408(6813):740–745.
82. Kato H, Takeuchi O, Sato S, et al. Differential roles of MDA5 and RIG-I helicases in the recognition of RNA viruses. *Nature.* 2006;441(7089):101–105.
83. Gao Y, Majchrzak-Kita B, Fish EN, et al. Dynamic accumulation of plasmacytoid dendritic cells in lymph nodes is regulated by interferon-beta. *Blood.* 2009;114(13):2623–2631.
84. Jego G, Palucka AK, Blanck JP, et al. Plasmacytoid dendritic cells induce plasma cell differentiation through type I interferon and interleukin 6. *Immunity.* 2003;19(2):225–234.
85. Gallagher KM, Lauder S, Rees IW, et al. Type I interferon (IFN alpha) acts directly on human memory CD4+ T cells altering their response to antigen. *J Immunol.* 2009;183(5):2915–2920.
86. Ramos HJ, Davis AM, Cole AG, et al. Reciprocal responsiveness to interleukin-12 and interferon-alpha specifies human CD8+ effector versus central memory T-cell fates. *Blood.* 2009;113(22):5516–5525.
87. Bave U, Alm GV, Ronnblom L. The combination of apoptotic U937 cells and lupus IgG is a potent IFN-alpha inducer. *J Immunol.* 2000;165(6):3519–3526.
88. Means TK, Latz E, Hayashi F, et al. Human lupus autoantibody-DNA complexes activate DCs through cooperation of CD32 and TLR9. *J Clin Invest.* 2005;115(2):407–417.
89. Tan EM, Feltkamp TE, Smolen JS, et al. Range of antinuclear antibodies in "healthy" individuals. *Arthritis Rheum.* 1997;40(9):1601–1611.
90. Wandl UB, Nagel-Hiemke M, May D, et al. Lupus-like autoimmune disease induced by interferon therapy for myeloproliferative disorders. *Clin Immunol Immunopathol.* 1992;65(1):70–74.
91. Ronnblom LE, Alm GV, Oberg KE. Possible induction of systemic lupus erythematosus by interferon-alpha treatment in a patient with a malignant carcinoid tumour. *J Intern Med.* 1990;227(3):207–210.
92. Baechler EC, Batliwalla FM, Karypis G, et al. Interferon-inducible gene expression signature in peripheral blood cells of patients with severe lupus. *Proc Natl Acad Sci U S A.* 2003;100(5):2610–2615.
93. Dall'era MC, Cardarelli PM, Preston BT, et al. Type I interferon correlates with serological and clinical manifestations of SLE. *Ann Rheum Dis.* 2005; 64(12):1692–1697.
94. Fu Q, Chen X, Cui H, et al. Association of elevated transcript levels of interferon-inducible chemokines with disease activity and organ damage in systemic lupus erythematosus patients. *Arthritis Res Ther.* 2008;10(5): R112.
95. Feng X, Wu H, Grossman JM, et al. Association of increased interferon-inducible gene expression with disease activity and lupus nephritis in patients with systemic lupus erythematosus. *Arthritis Rheum.* 2006;54(9):2951–2962.
96. Bauer JW, Petri M, Batliwalla FM, et al. Interferon-regulated chemokines as biomarkers of systemic lupus erythematosus disease activity: A validation study. *Arthritis Rheum.* 2009;60(10):3098–3107.
97. Kaser A, Kaser S, Kaneider NC, et al. Interleukin-18 attracts plasmacytoid dendritic cells (DC2s) and promotes Th1 induction by DC2s through IL-18 receptor expression. *Blood.* 2004;103(2):648–655.
98. Anders HJ, Lichtnekert J, Allam R. Interferon-alpha and -beta in kidney inflammation. *Kidney Int.* 2010;77(10):848–854.
99. Hron JD, Peng SL. Type I IFN protects against murine lupus. *J Immunol.* 2004;173(3):2134–2142.
100. Harley IT, Kaufman KM, Langefeld CD, et al. Genetic susceptibility to SLE: new insights from fine mapping and genome-wide association studies. *Nat Rev Genet.* 2009;10(5):285–290.
101. Matsumoto M, Seya T. TLR3: interferon induction by double-stranded RNA including poly(I:C). *Adv Drug Deliv Rev.* 2008;60(7):805–812.
102. Tucci M, Barnes EV, Sobel ES, et al. Strong association of a functional polymorphism in the monocyte chemoattractant protein 1 promoter gene with lupus nephritis. *Arthritis Rheum.* 2004;50:1842–1849.
103. Chen DY, Hsieh CW, Chen KS, et al. Association of interleukin-18 promoter polymorphisms with WHO pathological classes and serum IL-18 levels in Chinese patients with lupus nephritis. *Lupus.* 2009;18(1):29–37.
104. Taylor KE, Chung SA, Graham RR, et al. Risk alleles for systemic lupus erythematosus in a large case-control collection and associations with clinical subphenotypes. *PLoS Genet.* 2011;7(2):e1001311.
105. Taylor KE, Remmers EF, Lee AT, et al. Specificity of the STAT4 genetic association for severe disease manifestations of systemic lupus erythematosus. *PLoS Genet.* 2008;4(5):e1000084.
106. Quintero-Del-Rio AI, Kelly JA, Kilpatrick J, et al. The genetics of systemic lupus erythematosus stratified by renal disease: linkage at 10q22.3 (SLEN1), 2q34–35 (SLEN2), and 11p15.6 (SLEN3). *Genes Immun.* 2002;3 Suppl 1:S57–62.
107. Quintero-del-Rio AI, Kelly JA, Garriott CP, et al. SLEN2 (2q34–35) and SLEN1 (10q22.3) replication in systemic lupus erythematosus stratified by nephritis. *Am J Hum Genet.* 2004;75(2):346–348.
108. Faurschou M, Starklint H, Halbert P, et al. Prognosis factors in lupus nephritis: Diagnostic and therapeutic delay increases the risk of terminal renal failure. *J Rheumatol.* 2006;33(8):1563–1569.
109. Fiehn C. Early diagnosis and treatment in lupus nephritis: How we can influence the risk for terminal renal failure. *J Rheumatol.* 2006;33(8): 1464–1466.
110. Fiehn C, Hajjar Y, Mueller K, et al. Improved clinical outcome of lupus nephritis during the past decade: importance of early diagnosis and treatment. *Ann Rheum Dis.* 2003;62:435–439.

111. Branten AJW, Vervoort G, Wetzels JFM. Serum creatinine is a poor marker of GFR in nephrotic syndrome. *Nephrol Dial Transplant.* 2005;20:707–711.
112. Siedner MJ, Gelber AC, Rovin BH, et al. Diagnostic accuracy study of urine dipstick in relation to 24–hour measurement as a screening tool for proteinuria in lupus nephritis. *J Rheumatol.* 2008;35(1):84–90.
113. Birmingham DJ, Rovin BH, Shidham G, et al. Spot urine protein/creatinine ratios are unreliable estimates of 24 h proteinuria in most systemic lupus erythematosus nephritis flares. *Kidney Int.* 2007;72:865–870.
114. Fine DM, Ziegenbein M, Petri M, et al. A prospective study of 24–hour protein excretion in lupus nephritis: Adequacy of short-interval timed urine collections. *Kidney Int.* 2009;76:1284–1288.
115. Christopher-Stine L, Siedner MJ, Lin J, et al. Renal biopsy in lupus patients with low levels of proteinuria. *J Rheumatol.* 2007;34:332–335.
116. Zoja C, Morigi M, Remuzzi G. Proteinuria and phenotypic change of proximal tubular cells. *J Am Soc Nephrol.* 2003;14:S36–S41.
117. Remuzzi G, Ruggenenti P, Benigni A. Understanding the nature of renal disease progression: In proteinuric nephropathies enhanced glomerular protein traffic contributes to interstitial inflammation and renal scarring. *Kidney Int.* 1997;51:2–15.
118. Rovin BH. Treatment of lupus nephritis: Are we beyond cyclophosphamide yet? *Nat Rev Nephrol.* 2009;5(9):492–494.
119. Baranowska-Daca E, Choi Y-J, Barrios R, et al. Non-lupus nephrritides in patients with systemic lupus erythematosus: A comprehensive clinicopathologic study and review of the literature. *Hum Pathol.* 2001;32:1125–1135.
120. Ellington KT, Truong L, Olivero JJ. Renal amyloidosis in systemic lupus erythematosus. *Am J Kidney Dis.* 1993;21(6):676–678.
121. Mori Y, Kishimoto N, Yamahara H, et al. Predominant tubulointerstitial nephritis in a patient with systemic lupus nephritis. *Clin Exp Nephrol.* 2005; 9(1):79–84.
122. Kraft SW, Schwartz MM, Korbet SM, et al. Glomerular podocytopathy in patients with systemic lupus erythematosus. *J Am Soc Nephrol.* 2005;16(1): 175–179.
123. Mok CC, Cheung TT, Lo WH. Minimal mesangial lupus nephritis: a systematic review. *Scand J Rheumatol.* 2010;39:181–189.
124. Tektonidou MG, Sotsiou F, Moutsopoulos HM. Antiphospholipid syndrome nephropathy in catastrophic, primary, and systemic lupus erythematosus-related APS. *J Rheumatol.* 2008;35:1983–1988.
125. Daugas E, Nochy D, Huong DL, et al. Antiphospholipid syndrome nephropathy in systemic lupus erythematosus. *J Am Soc Nephrol.* 2002;13(1): 42–52.
126. Hill GS, Delahousse M, Nochy D, et al. Predictive poawer of the second renal biopsy in lupus nephritis: Significance of macrophages. *Kidney Int.* 2001;59:304–316.
127. Sedor JR. Tissue proteomics: a new investigative tool for renal biopsy analysis. *Kidney Int.* 2009;75:876–879.
128. Yasuda Y, Cohen CD, Henger A, et al. Gene expression profiling analysis in nephrology: towards molecular definition of renal disease. *Clin Exp Nephrol.* 2006;10:91–98.
129. Peterson KS, Huang J-F, Zhu J, et al. Characterization of heterogeneity in the molecular pathogenesis of lupus nephritis from transciptional profiles of laser-captured glomeruli. *J Clin Invest.* 2004;113(12):1722–1733.
130. Walker PD. The renal biopsy. *Arch Pathol Lab Med.* 2009;133(2):181–188.
131. Moroni G, Pasquali S, Quaglini S, et al. Clinical and prognostic value of serial renal biopsies in lupus nephritis. *Am J Kidney Dis.* 1999;34:530–539.
132. Bajaj S, Albert L, Gladman DD, et al. Serial renal biopsy in systemic lupus erythematosus. *J Rheumatol.* 2000;27(12):2822–2826.
133. Daleboudt GMN, Bajema IM, Goemaere NNT, et al. The clinical relevance of a repeat biopsy in lupus nephritis flares. *Nephrol Dial Transplant.* 2009; 24(12):3712–3717.
134. Seshan SV, Jennette JC. Renal disease in systemic lupus erythematosus with emphasis on classification of lupus glomerulonephritis: advances and implications. *Arch Pathol Lab Med.* 2009;133(2):233–248.
135. Weening JJ, D'Agati VD, Schwartz MM, et al. The classification of glomerulonephritis in systemic lupus erythematosus revisited. *J Am Soc Nephrol.* 2004; 15(2):241–250.
136. Markowitz GS, D'Agati VD. The ISN/RPS 2003 classification of lupus nephritis: an assessment at 3 years. *Kidney Int.* 2007;71(6):491–495.
137. Sada KE, Makino H. Usefulness of ISN/RPS classification of lupus nephritis. *Journal of Korean Medical Science.* 2009;24 Suppl:S7–10.
138. Grootscholten C, Bajema IM, Florquin S, et al. Interobserver agreement of scoring of histopathological characteristics and classification of lupus nephritis. *Nephrol Dial Transplant.* 2008;23(1):223–230.
139. Schwartz MM, Korbet SM, Lewis EJ. The prognosis and pathogenesis of severe lupus glomerulonephritis. *Nephrol Dial Transplant.* 2008;23:1298–1306.
140. Nasr SH, D'Agati VD, Park HR. Necrotizing and crescentic lupus nephritis with antineutrophil cytoplasmic antibody seropositivity. *Clin J Am Soc Nephrol.* 2008;3:682–690.
141. Najafi CC, Korbet SM, Lewis EJ, et al. Significance of histologic patterns of glomerular injury upon long-term prognosis in severe lupus glomerulonephritis. *Kidney Int.* 2001;59(6):2156–2163.
142. Schwartz MM, Korbet SM, Katz RS, et al. Evidence of concurrent immunopathological mechanisms determining the pathology of severe lupus nephritis. *Lupus.*2009;18(2):149–158.
143. Mittal B, Hurwitz S, Rennke H, et al. New subcategories of class IV lupus nephritis: are there clinical, histologic, and outcome differences? *Am J Kidney Dis.* 2004;44(6):1050–1059.
144. Hill GS, Delahousse M, Nochy D, Bariety J. Class IV-S versus class IV-G lupus nephritis: clinical and morphologic differences suggesting different pathogenesis. *Kidney Int.* 2005;68(5):2288–2297.
145. Yokoyama H, Wada T, Hara A, et al. The outcome and a new ISN/RPS 2003 classification of lupus nephritis in Japanese. *Kidney Int.* 2004;66(6): 2382–2388.
146. Hiramatsu N, Kuroiwa T, Ikeuchi H, et al. Revised classification of lupus nephritis is valuable in predicting renal outcome with an indication of the proportion of glomeruli affected by chronic lesions. *Rheumatology (Oxford).* 2008; 47(5):702–707.
147. Behara VY, Whittier WL, Korbet SM, et al. Pathogenetic features of severe segmental lupus nephritis. *Nephrol Dial Transplant.* 2010;25(1):153–159.
148. Satoskar A, Brodsky S, Nadasdy G, et al. Discrepancies in IgG subtype composition between glomerular and tubulointerstitial immune complex deposits in proliferative lupus nephritis. *Lupus.* 2011;20(13):1396–1403.
149. Park MH, D'Agati V, Appel GB, et al. Tubulointerstitial disease in lupus nephritis: relationship to immune deposits, interstitial inflammation, glomerular changes, renal function, and prognosis. *Nephron.* 1986;44(4):309–319.
150. Appel GB, Pirani CL, D'Agati V. Renal vascular complications of systemic lupus erythematosus. *J Am Soc Nephrol.* 1994;4(8):1499–1515.
151. Wu H, Birmingham DJ, Rovin B, et al. D-dimer level and the risk for thrombosis in systemic lupus erythematosus. *Clin J Am Soc Nephrol.* 2008;3(6): 1628–1636.
152. Gupta R, Sharma A, Bhowmik DM, et al. Collapsing glomerulopathy occurring in HIV-negative patients with systemic lupus erythematosus: Report of three cases and brief review of the literature. *Lupus.* 2011;20(8):866–870.
153. Schwartz MM, Roberts JL, Lewis EJ. Necrotizing glomerulitis of systemic lupus erythematosus. *Human pathology.* 1983;14(2):158–167.
154. Charney DA, Nassar G, Truong L, et al. "Pauci-Immune" proliferative and necrotizing glomerulonephritis with thrombotic microangiopathy in patients with systemic lupus erythematosus and lupus-like syndrome. *Am J Kidney Dis.* 2000;35(6):1193–1206.
154a. Austin HA III, Muenz LR, et al. Diffuse proliferative lupus nephritis: identification of specific pathologic features affecting renal outcome. *Kidney Int.* 1984 Apr;25(4):689–695.
155. Kaiser R, Cleveland CM, Criswell LA. Risk and protective factors for thrombosis in systemic lupus erythematosus: results from a large, multi-ethnic cohort. *Ann Rheum Dis.* 2009;68(2):238–241.
155a. Sun S, Rao NL, Venable J, et al. TLR7/9 antagonists as therapeutics for immune-mediated inflammatory disorders. *Inflamm Allergy Drug Targets.* 2007 Dec;6(4):223–235.
156. Pons-Estel GJ, Alarcon GS, McGwin G Jr, et al. Protective effect of hydroxychloroquine on renal damage in patients with lupus nephritis: LXV, data from a multiethnic US cohort. *Arthritis Rheum.* 2009;61(6):830–839.
157. Tsakonas E, Joseph L, Esdaile JM, et al. A long-term study of hydroxychloroquine withdrawal on exacerbations in systemic lupus erythematosus. The Canadian hydroxychloroquine study group. *Lupus.* 1998;7:80–85.
158. Siso A, Ramos-Casals M, Bove A, et al. Previous antimalarial therapy in patients diagnosed with lupus nephritis: influence on outcomes and survival. *Lupus.* 2008;17(4):281–288.
159. Flanc RS, Roberts MA, Strippoli GFM, et al. Treatment for lupus nephritis. *Cochrane Database of Systematic Reviews.* 2004;(1):1–75.
160. Austin HA, Klippel JH, Balow JE, et al. Therapy of lupus nephritis. Controlled trial of prednisone and cytotoxic drugs. *N Engl J Med.* 1986;314:614–619.
161. Boumpas DT, Austin HA, Vaughn EM, et al. Controlled trial of pulse methylprenisolone versus two regimens of pulse cyclophosphamide in severe lupus nephritis. *Lancet.* 1992;340:741–745.
162. Donadio JV, Holley KE, Ferguson RH, et al. Treatment of diffuse proliferative lupus nephritis with prednisone and combined prednisone and cyclophosphamide. *N Engl J Med.* 1978;23:1151–1155.
163. Contreras G, Pardo V, Leclercq B, et al. Sequential therapies for proliferative lupus nephritis. *N Engl J Med.* 2004;350:971–980.

164. Mok CC, Ho CTK, Chan KW, et al. Outcome and prognostic indicators of diffuse proliferative lupus glomerulonephritis treated with sequential oral cyclophosphamide and azathioprine. *Arthritis Rheum.* 2002;46:1003–1013.
165. Mok CC, Ho CTK, Siu YP, et al. Treatment of diffuse proliferative lupus glomerulonephritis: A comparison of two cyclophosphamide-containing regimens. *Am J Kidney Dis.* 2001;38:256–264.
166. Chan TM, Tse KC, Tang CSO, et al. Long-term outcome of patients with diffuse proliferative lupus nephritis treated with prednisolone and oral cyclophosphamide followed by azathioprine. *Lupus.* 2005;14:265–272.
167. Chan TM, Li FK, Tang CSO, et al. Efficacy of mycophenolate mofetil in patients with diffuse proliferative lupus nephritis. *N Engl J Med.* 2000;343: 1156–1162.
168. Chan TM, Tse KC, Tang CSO, et al. Long-term study of mycophenolate mofetil as continuous induction and maintenance treatment for diffuse proliferative lupus nephritis. *J Am Soc Nephrol.* 2005;16:1076–1084.
169. McKinley A, Park E, Spetie DN, et al. Oral cyclophosphamide for lupus glomerulonephritis: An under-utilized therapeutic option. *Clin J Am Soc Nephrol.* 2009;4:1754–1760.
170. Haubitz M, Bohnenstengel F, Brunkhorst R, et al. Cyclophosphamide pharmacokinetics and dose requirements in patients with renal insufficiency. *Kidney Int.* 2002;61:1495–1501.
171. Pendse S, Ginsburg E, Singh AK. Strategies for preservation of ovarian and testicular function after immunosuppression. *Am J Kidney Dis.* 2004;43: 772–781.
172. Sommers EC, Marder W, Christman GM, et al. Use of a gonadotropin-releasing hormone analog for protection against premature ovarian failure during cyclophosphamide therapy in women with severe lupus. *Arthritis Rheum.* 2005;52:2761–2767.
173. Philibert D, Cattran D. Remission of proteinuria in primary glomerulonephritis: we know the goal but do we know the price? *Nat Clin Pract Nephrol.* 2008;4(10):550–559.
174. Faurschou M, Sorensen IJ, Meliemkjaer L, et al. Malignancies in Wegener's granulomatosis: Incidence and relation to cyclophosphamide therapy in a cohort of 293 patients. *J Rheumatol.* 2008;35:100–105.
175. Houssiau FA, Vasconcelos C, D'Cruz D, et al. Immunosuppressive therapy in lupus nephritis: the Euro-Lupus Nephritis Trial, a randomized trial of low-dose versus high-dose intravenous cyclophosphamide. *Arthritis Rheum.* 2002;46(8):2121–2131.
176. Houssiau FA, Vasconcelos C, D'Cruz D, et al. The 10–year follow-up data of the Euro-Lupus Nephritis Trial comparing low-dose versus high-dose intravenous cyclophosphamide. *Ann Rheum Dis.* 2010;69:61–64.
177. Appel GB, Contreras G, Dooley MA, et al. Mycophenolate mofetil versus cyclophosphamide for induction treatment of lupus nephritis. *J Am Soc Nephrol.* 2009;20:1103–1112.
178. Korbet SM, Schwartz MM, Evans J, et al. Severe lupus nephritis: Racial differences in presentation and outcome. *J Am Soc Nephrol.* 2007;18:244–254.
179. Grootscholten C, Bajema IM, Florquin S, et al. Treatment with cyclophosphamide delays the progression of chronic lesions more effectively than does treatment with azathioprine plus methylprednisolone in patients with proliferative lupus nephritis. *Arthritis Rheum.* 2007;56(3):924–937.
180. Urowitz M, Ibanez D, Ali Y, et al. Outcomes in patients with active lupus nephritis requiring immunosuppressives who never received cyclophosphamide. *J Rheumatol.* 2007;34:1491–1496.
181. Chen W, Tang X, Liu Q, et al. Short-term outcomes of induction therapy with tacrolimus versus cyclophosphamide for active lupus nephritis: A multicenter randomized clinical trial. *Am J Kidney Dis.* 2011;57(2):235–244.
182. Lee T, Oh KH, Joo KW, et al. Tacrolimus is an alternative therapeutic option for the treatment of refractory lupus nephritis. *Lupus.* 2010;19(8):974–980.
183. Zavada J, Pesickova S, Rysava R, et al. Cyclosporine A or intravenous cyclophosphamide for lupus nephritis: the Cyclofa-Lune study. *Lupus.* 2010;19(11):1281–1289.
184. Wang HY, Cui TG, Hou FF, et al. Induction treatment of proliferative lupus nephritis with leflunomide combined with prednisone: a prospective multicentre observational study. *Lupus.* 2008;17(7):638–644.
185. Zhang FS, Nie YK, Jin XM, et al. The efficacy and safety of leflunomide therapy in lupus nephritis by repeat kidney biopsy. *Rheumatol Int.* 2009; 29(11):1331–1335.
186. Rovin BH, Furie RA, Lantinis K, et al. Efficacy and safety of rituximab in patients with active proliferative lupus nephritis: The LUpus Nephritis Assessment with Rituximab (LUNAR) study. *Arthritis Rheum.* 2012 Jan 9 [Epub ahead of print].
187. Ramos-Casals M, Soto MJ, Cuadrado MJ, et al. Rituximab in systemic lupus erythematosus: A systematic review of off-label use in 188 cases. *Lupus.* 2009;18:767–776.
188. Lu TY, Ng KP, Cambridge G, et al. A retrospective seven-year analysis of the use of B cell depletion therapy in systemic lupus erythematosus at University College London Hospital: the first fifty patients. *Arthritis Rheum.* 2009; 61(4):482–487.
189. Li EK, Tam LS, Zhu TY, et al. Is combination rituximab with cyclophosphamide better than rituximab alone in the treatment of lupus nephritis? *Rheumatology (Oxford).* 2009;48(8):892–898.
190. Gunnarsson I, Sundelin B, Jonsdottir T, et al. Histopathologic and clinical outcome of rituximab treatment in patients with cyclophosphamide-resistant proliferative lupus nephritis. *Arthritis Rheum.* 2007;56:1263–1272.
191. Appel GB, Contreras G, Dooley MA, et al. Mycophenolate mofetil versus cyclophosphamide for induction treatment of lupus nephritis. *J Am Soc Nephrol.* 2009;20(5):1103–1112.
192. Ginzler EM, Dooley MA, Aranow C, et al. Mycophenolate mofetil or intravenous cyclophosphamide for lupus nephritis. *N Engl J Med.* 2005;353:2219–2228.
193. Dooley MA, Jayne D, Ginzler EM, et al. ALMS Group. Mycophenolate versus azathioprine as maintenance therapy for lupus nephritis. *N Engl J Med.* 2011;365(20):1886–1895.
194. Houssiau FA, D'Cruz D, Sangle S, et al. Azathioprine versus mycophenolate mofetil for long-term immunosuppression in lupus nephritis: results from the MAINTAIN Nephritis Trial. *Ann Rheum Dis.* 2010;69(12):2083–2089.
195. Moroni G, Doria A, Mosca M, et al. A randomized pilot trial comparing cyclosporine and azathioprine for maintenance in diffuse lupus nephritis over four years. *Clin J Am Soc Nephrol.* 2006;1:925–932.
196. Griffiths B, Emery P, Ryan V, et al. The BILAG multicentre open randomized controlled trial comparing ciclosporin vs azathioprine in patients with severe SLE. *Rheumatology (Oxford).* 2010;49(4):723–732.
197. Ong LM, Hooi LS, Lim TO, et al. Randomized controlled trial of pulse intravenous cyclophosphamide versus mycophenolate mofetil in the induction therapy of proliferative lupus nephritis. *Nephrology (Carlton).* 2005;10(5): 504–510.
198. Hill GS, Delahousse M, Nochy D, et al. Predictive power of the second renal biopsy in lupus nephritis: significance of macrophages. *Kidney Int.* 2001; 59(1):304–316.
199. Gunnarsson I, Sundelin B, Heimburger M, et al. Repeated renal biopsy in proliferative lupus nephritis—predictive role of serum C1q and albuminuria. *J Rheumatol.* 2002;29(4):693–699.
200. Traitanon O, Avihingsanon Y, Kittikovit V, et al. Efficacy of enteric-coated mycophenolate sodium in patients with resistant-type lupus nephritis: a prospective study. *Lupus.* 2008;17(8):744–751.
201. Venkataseshan VS, Marquet E. Heat shock protein 72/73 in normal and diseased kidneys. *Nephron.* 1996;73:442–449.
202. Ioannidis JPA, Boki KA, Katsorida ME, et al. Remission, relapse, and re-remission of proliferative lupus nephritis treated with cyclophosphamide. *Kidney Int.* 2000;57:258–264.
203. Dall'era M, Stone D, Levesque V, et al. Identification of biomarkers that predict response to treatment of lupus nephritis with mycophenolate mofetil or pulse cyclophosphamide. *Arthritis Care Res.* 2011;63(3):351–357.
204. Jafar TH, Schmid CH, Landa M, et al. Angiotensin-converting enzyme inhibitors and progression of nondiabetic renal disease. A meta-analysis of patient-level data. *Ann Intern Med.* 2001;135(2):73–87.
205. Hill GS, Delahousse M, Nochy D, et al. Outcome of relapse in lupus nephritis: roles of reversal of renal fibrosis and response of inflammation to therapy. *Kidney Int.* 2002;61:2176–2186.
206. Howie AJ, Turhan N, Adu D. Powerful morphometric indicator of prognosis in lupus nehpritis. *Q J Med.* 2003;96:411–420.
207. Pasquali S, Banfi G, Zucchelli A, et al. Lupus membranous nephropathy: long-term outcome. *Clin Nephrol.* 1993;39:175–182.
208. Bao H, Liu Z-H, Xie H-L, et al. Successful treatment of class V+IV lupus nephritis with multitarget therapy. *J Am Soc Nephrol.* 2008;19:2001–2010.
209. Mercadal L, Montcel ST, Nochy D, et al. Factors affecting outcome and prognosis in membranous lupus nephropathy. *Nephrol Dial Transplant.* 2002; 17(10):1771–1778.
210. Mok CC. Membranous nephropathy in systemic lupus erythematosus: a therapeutic enigma. *Nat Rev Nephrol.* 2009;5:212–220.
211. Sloan RP, Schwartz MM, Korbet SM, et al. Long-term outcome in systemic lupus erythematosus membranous glomerulonephritis. *J Am Soc Nephrol.* 1996; 7:299–305.
212. Ordonez JD, Hiatt RA, Killebrew EJ, et al. The increased risk of coronary heart disease associated with the nephrotic syndrome. *Kidney Int.* 1993;44:638–642.
213. Wilmer WA, Rovin BH, Hebert CJ, et al. Management of glomerular proteinuria: a commentary. *J Am Soc Nephrol.* 2003;14:3217–3232.
214. Font J, Ramos-Casals M, Cervera R, et al. Cardiovascular risk factors and the long-term outcome of lupus nephritis. *Q J Med.* 2001;94:19–26.

215. Mok CC, Ying KY, Lau CS, et al. Treatment of pure membranous lupus nephropathy with prednisone and azathioprine: an open-label trial. *Am J Kidney Dis.* 2004;43(2):269–276.
216. Donadio JV, Burgess JH, Holley KE. Membranous lupus nephropathy: A clinicopathologic study. *Medicine.* 1977;56:527–536.
217. Gonzalez-Dettoni H, Tron F. Membranous glomerulonephropathy in systemic lupus erythematosus. *Adv. Nephrol.* 1985;14:347–364.
218. Austin HA, Illei GG, Braun MJ, et al. Randomized, controlled trial of prednisone, cyclophosphamide, and cyclosporine in lupus membranous nephropathy. *J Am Soc Nephrol.* 2009;20:901–911.
219. Radhakrishnan J, Moutzouris DA, Ginzler EM, et al. Mycophenolate mofetil and intravenous cyclophosphamide are similar as induction therapy for class V lupus nephritis. *Kidney Int.* 2010;77(2):152–160.
220. Mok C, Ying K, Yim C, et al. Very long-term outcome of pure membranous nephropathy treated with glucocorticoid and azathioprine. *Lupus.* 2009; 18:1091–1095.
221. Kasitanon N, Petri M, Haas M, et ak. Mycophenolate mofetil as the primary treatment of membranous lupus nephritis with and without concurrent proliferative disease: a retrospective study of 29 cases. *Lupus.* 2008;17:40–45.
222. Spetie DN, Tang Y, Rovin BH, et al. Mycophenolate therapy of SLE membranous nephropathy. *Kidney Int.* 2004;66:2411–2415.
223. Houssiau FA, Vasconcelos C, D'Cruz D, et al. Early response to immunosuppressive therapy predicts good renal outcome in lupus nephritis: lessons from long-term followup of patients in the Euro-Lupus Nephritis Trial. *Arthritis Rheum.* 2004;50(12):3934–3940.
224. Grootscholten C, Ligtenberg G, Hagen EC, et al. Azathioprine/methylprednisolone versus cyclophosphamide in proliferative lupus nephritis. A randomized, controlled trial. *Kidney Int.* 2006;70:732–742.
225. Szeto CC, Kwan BC-H, Lai FM-M, et al. Tacrolimus for the treatment of systemic lupus erythematosus with pure class V nephritis. *Rheumatol.* 2008;47:1678–1681.
226. Marshall T, Williams K. Two-dimensional electrophoresis of human urinary proteins following concentration by dye precipitation. *Electrophoresis.* 1996; 17:1256–1272.
227. Barr RG, Seliger S, Appel GB, et al. Prognosis in proliferative lupus nephritis: the role of socio-economic status and race/ethnicity. *Nephrol Dial Transplant.* 2003;18(10):2039–2046.
228. Contreras G, Pardo V, Cely C, et al. Factors associated with poor outcomes in patients with lupus nephritis. *Lupus.* 2005;14(11):890–895.
229. Moroni G, Quaglini S, Gallelli B, et al. The long-term outcome of 93 patients with proliferative lupus nephritis. *Nephrol Dial Transplant.* 2007;22:2531–2539.
230. Chen YE, Korbet SM, Katz RS, et al. Value of a complete or partial remission in severe lupus nephritis. *Clin. J Am Soc Nephrol.* 2008;3:46–53.
231. Hebert LA, Wilmer WA, Falkenhain ME, et al. Renoprotection: One or many therapies. *Kidney Int.* 2001;59:1211–1226.
232. Reich HN, Troyanov S, Scholey JW, et al. Remission of proteinuria improves prognosis in IgA nephropathy. *J Am Soc Nephrol.* 2007;18(12):3177–3183.
233. Illei GG, Takada K, Parkin D, et al. Renal flares are common in patients with severe proliferative lupus nephritis treated with pulse immunosuppressive therapy: long-term followup of a cohort of 145 patients participating in randomized controlled studies. *Arthritis Rheum.* 2002;46(4):995–1002.
234. Birmingham DJ, Nagaraja HN, Rovin BH, et al. Fluctuation in self-perceived stress increases risk of flare in patients with lupus nephritis carrying the serotonin receptor1A-1019G allele. *Arthritis Rheum.* 2006;54:3291–3299.
235. Ruperto N, Hanrahan L, Alarcon G, et al. International consensus for a definition of disease flare in lupus. *Lupus.* 2011;20(5):453–462.
236. Gordon C, Jayne D, Pusey C, et al. European consensus statement on the terminology used in the management of lupus glomerulonephritis. *Lupus.* 2009;18(3):257–263.
237. Rovin BH, Song H, Birmingham DJ, et al. Urine chemokines as biomarkers of human systemic lupus erythematosus activity. *J Am Soc Nephrol.* 2005;16:467–473.
238. Rovin BH, Birmingham DJ, Nagaraja HN, et al. Biomarker discovery in human SLE nephritis. *Bull NYU Hosp Jt Dis.* 2007;65(3):187–193.
239. Moroni G, Radice A, Giammarresi G, et al. Are laboratory tests useful for monitoring the activity of lupus nephritis? A 6–year prospective study in a cohort of 228 patients with lupus nephritis. *Ann Rheum Dis.* 2009;68(2):234–237.
240. Coremans IEM, Spronk PE, Bootsma H, et al. Changes in antibodies to C1q predict renal relapse in systemic lupus erythematosus. *Am J Kidney Dis.* 1995;26:595–601.
241. Rovin BH, Zhang X. Biomarkers for lupus nephritis: The quest continues. *Clin. J Am Soc Nephrol.* 2009;4:1858–1865.
242. Chan RW-Y, Lai FM-M, Li EK-M, et al. The effect of immunosuppressive therapy on the messenger RNA expression of target genes in the urinary sediment of patients with active lupus nephritis. *Nephrol Dial Transplant.* 2006;21(6): 1534–1540.
243. Avihingsanon Y, Phumesin P, Benjachat T, et al. Measurement of urinary chemokine and growth factor messenger RNAs: A noninvasive monitoring in lupus nephritis. *Kidney Int.* 2006;69:747–753.
244. Hinze CH, Suzuki M, Klein-Gitelman M, et al. Neutrophil gelatinase-associated lipocalin (NGAL) anticipates the course of global and renal childhood-onset systemic lupus erythematosus disease activity. *Arthritis Rheum.* 2009;60(9):2772–2781.
245. Suzuki M, Wiers K, Brooks EB, et al. Initial validation of a novel protein biomarker panel for active pediatric lupus nephritis. *Pediatr Res.* 2009;65:530–536.
246. Izmirly PM, Barisoni L, Buyon JP, et al. Expression of endothelial protein C receptor in cortical peritubular capillaries associates with a poor clinical response in lupus nephritis. *Rheumatology (Oxford).* 2009;48(5):513–519.
247. Wang G, Lai FM, Tam LS, et al. Urinary FOXP3 mRNA in patients with lupus nephritis—relation with disease activity and treatment response. *Rheumatology (Oxford).* 2009;48(7):755–760.
248. Oates JC, Varghese S, Bland AM, et al. Prediction of urinary protein markers in lupus nephritis. *Kidney Int.* 2005;68:2588–2592.
249. Nakayamada S, Saito K, Nakano K, et al. Activation signal transduction by beta1 integrin in T cells from patients with systemic lupus erythematosus. *Arthritis Rheum.* 2007;56(5):1559–1568.
249a. Zhang X, Nagaraja HN, Nadasdy T, et al. A composite urine biomarker reflects interstitial inflammation in lupus nephritis kidney biopsies. *Kidney Int.* 2012;81(4):401–406.
250. Tektonidou MG. Renal involvement in the antiphospholipid syndrome (APS)-APS nephropathy. *Clin Rev Allergy Immunol.* 2009;36(2–3):131–140.
251. Alchi B, Griffiths M, Jayne D. What nephrologists need to know about antiphospholipid syndrome. *Nephrol Dial Transplant.* 2010;25(10):3147–3154.
252. Kwok SK, Ju JH, Cho CS, et al. Thrombotic thrombocytopenic purpura in systemic lupus erythematosus: risk factors and clinical outcome: a single centre study. *Lupus.* 2009;18(1):16–21.
253. Tandon A, Ibanez D, Gladman D, et al. The effect of pregnancy on lupus nephritis. *Arthritis Rheum.* 2004;50:3941–3946.
254. Al Arfaj AS, Khalil N. Pregnancy outcome in 396 pregnancies in patients with SLE in Saudi Arabia. *Lupus.* 2010;19(14):1665–1673.
255. Imbasciati E, Tincani A, Gregorini G, et al. Pregnancy in women with pre-existing lupus nephritis: predictors of fetal and maternal outcome. *Nephrol Dial Transplant.* 2009;24(2):519–525.
256. Carvalheiras G, Vita P, Marta S, et al. Pregnancy and systemic lupus erythematosus: review of clinical features and outcome of 51 pregnancies at a single institution. *Clin Rev Allergy Immunol.* 2010;38(2–3):302–306.
257. Wagner SJ, Craici I, Reed D, et al. Maternal and foetal outcomes in pregnant patients with active lupus nephritis. *Lupus.* 2009;18(4):342–347.
258. Rietveld A, Berden JH. Renal replacement therapy in lupus nephritis. *Nephrol Dial Transplant.* 2008;23(10):3056–3060.
259. Siu YP, Leung KT, Tong MK, et al. Clinical outcomes of systemic lupus erythematosus patients undergoing continuous ambulatory peritoneal dialysis. *Nephrol Dial Transplant.* 2005;20(12):2797–2802.
260. Huang JW, Hung KY, Yen CJ, et al. Systemic lupus erythematosus and peritoneal dialysis: outcomes and infectious complications. *Perit Dial Int.* 2001; 21(2):143–147.
261. Nossent HC, Swaak TJ, Berden JH. Systemic lupus erythematosus: analysis of disease activity in 55 patients with end-stage renal failure treated with hemodialysis or continuous ambulatory peritoneal dialysis. Dutch Working Party on SLE. *Am J Med.* 1990;89(2):169–174.
262. Ribeiro FM, Leite MA, Velarde GC, et al. Activity of systemic lupus erythematosus in end-stage renal disease patients: study in a Brazilian cohort. *Am J Nephrol.* 2005;25:596–603.
263. Goo YS, Park HC, Choi HY, et al. The evolution of lupus activity among patients with end-stage renal disease secondary to lupus nephritis. *Yonsei Med J.* 2004;45(2):199–206.
264. Chelamcharla M, Javaid B, Baird BC, et al. The outcome of renal transplantation among systemic lupus erythematosus patients. *Nephrol Dial Transplant.* 2007;22(12):3623–3630.
265. Bunnapradist S, Chung P, Peng A, et al. Outcomes of renal transplantation for recipients with lupus nephritis: analysis of the Organ Procurement and Transplantation Network database. *Transplantation.* 2006;82(5):612–618.
266. Burgos PI, Perkins EL, Pons-Estel GJ, et al. Risk factors and impact of recurrent lupus nephritis in patients with systemic lupus erythematosus undergoing renal transplantation: data from a single US institution. *Arthritis Rheum.* 2009;60(9):2757–2766.
267. Contreras G, Mattiazzi A, Guerra G, et al. Recurrence of lupus nephritis after kidney transplantation. *Clin J Am Soc Nephrol.* 2010;21:1200–1207.
268. Ghafari A, Etmadi J, Ardralan MR. Renal transplantation in patients with lupus nephritis: A single-center experience. *Transplant Proc.* 2008;40:143–144.

269. Moroni G, Tantardini F, Gallelli B, et al. The long-term prognosis of renal transplantation in patients with lupus nephritis. *Am J Kidney Dis.* 2005; 45(5):903–911.
270. Lionaki S, Kapitsinou PP, Iniotaki A, et al. Kidney transplantation in lupus patients: a case-control study from a single centre. *Lupus.* 2008;17(7):670–675.
271. Norby GE, Strom EH, Midtvedt K, et al. Recurrent lupus nephritis after kidney transplantation: a surveillance biopsy study. *Ann Rheum Dis.* 2010; 69(8):1484–1487.
272. Ramos-Casals M, Soto MJ, Cuadrado MJ, et al. Rituximab in systemic lupus erythematosus: A systematic review of off-label use in 188 cases. *Lupus.* 2009;18(9):767–776.
273. Arce-Salinas CA, Rodriguez-Garcia F, Gomez-Vargas JI. Long-term efficacy of anti-CD20 antibodies in refractory lupus nephritis. *Rheumatol Int.* 2011 Jan 22 [Epub ahead of print].
274. Wallace DJ. Advances in drug therapy for systemic lupus erythematosus. *BMC Med.* 2010;8:77.
275. Wiglesworth AK, Ennis KM, Kockler DR. Belimumab: a BLyS-specific inhibitor for systemic lupus erythematosus. *Ann Pharmacother.* 2010;44(12):1955–1961.
276. Daikh DI, Wofsy D. Cutting edge: reversal of murine lupus nephritis with CTLA4Ig and cyclophosphamide. *J Immunol.* 2001;166(5):2913–2916.
277. Muller S, Monneaux F, Schall N, et al. Spliceosomal peptide P140 for immunotherapy of systemic lupus erythematosus: results of an early phase II clinical trial. *Arthritis Rheum.* 2008;58(12):3873–3883.

CHAPTER

54 Systemic Sclerosis, Rheumatoid Arthritis, Sjögren Syndrome, and Polymyositis and Dermatomyositis

Meryl Waldman • James E. Balow • Howard A. Austin III

SYSTEMIC SCLEROSIS (SCLERODERMA)

Scleroderma is a broad, often confusing, term that encompasses a subset of chronic connective tissue diseases resulting from the overproduction and accumulation of collagen and other extracellular matrix proteins. Derived from the Greek word *sklēros,* meaning hard, and *derma,* meaning skin, scleroderma describes the hardened skin that is the hallmark clinical feature of this disorder. However, the disease is far more complex than this term implies. As such, scleroderma is now classified into two accepted disease subsets, morphea and systemic sclerosis (SSc), which more accurately reflect the broad range of clinical features seen in this disease.[1,2] Morphea, the localized form of scleroderma, is limited to the skin and generally carries a favorable prognosis with normal life expectancy. On the other hand, SSc, a widespread disorder with internal organ involvement, is generally associated with a worse prognosis and significant disability and mortality.

SSc is characterized by intense uncontrolled fibrosis of the skin, subcutaneous tissues, and organs (most notably the kidneys, lungs, gastrointestinal tract, and heart), accompanied by a proliferative and obliterative vasculopathy. There is considerable heterogeneity in the clinical manifestations and severity of SSc. Two well-recognized clinical subsets of SSc, the limited cutaneous (lcSSc) and diffuse cutaneous (dcSSc) forms, are used to further subclassify patients based on the extent and distribution of skin involvement. Autoantibody profiles, patterns of internal organ involvement, and prognosis differ considerably between the groups. The limited form, which primarily affects the skin distal to the elbows and knees, is typically associated with Raynaud phenomenon, telangiectasia, and gastrointestinal involvement as part of the CREST syndrome (calcinosis cutis, Raynaud phenomenon, esophageal dysmotility, sclerodactyly, and telangiectasia). Pulmonary hypertension and anticentromere antibodies are more common in this disease subset. Diffuse SSc is associated with more extensive sclerosis involving the skin proximal to the elbow and knee flexures or the trunk and earlier onset of internal organ involvement. Antitopoisomerase I and anti-RNA polymerase III antibodies are frequently present. Patients with dcSSc are at increased risk of developing the devastating complication, scleroderma renal crisis, discussed in the following paragraphs.

Epidemiology

Although there are conflicting estimates of prevalence and incidence of SSc, it is known that it is relatively uncommon compared to other connective tissue diseases. Prevalence estimates range from 7 to 489 cases per million persons and an incidence range from 0.6 to 122 cases per million persons per year (for comparison, prevalence of lupus ranges from 200 to 1500 cases per million persons).[3,4] The wide range in reported estimates between studies reflects a multitude of factors including different diagnostic definitions, inclusion of different subtypes of disease, data acquisition strategies, geographic variation, and study methods and design. The average disease onset is between the fourth and fifth decades. There is a female predominance with a female to male ratio ranging from 3:1 to 8:1, and it is almost twice as common in blacks as in whites.

Pathogenesis

The events that lead to the systemic fibrosis, microvascular damage, and immune dysregulation that are characteristic of SSc are only partially understood. Collectively, the body of evidence supports a multistep process involving a complex interplay between the vascular system, the immune system, and the extracellular matrix. This occurs in the context of a unique genetic susceptibility[5] and possible environmental stimuli.[6,7] Although a detailed discussion of disease pathogenesis is beyond the scope of this chapter, important concepts will be highlighted here. For a more detailed discussion, we refer the reader to several recent excellent reviews.[8–11]

Injury to the vascular endothelium, primarily of small vessels, is an important proximal event preceding the development of fibrosis.[12] The inciting factor remains unknown, though numerous environmental and infectious agents have been suggested. There is significant evidence that mechanisms of vascular remodeling, needed to restore vessel integrity and function after this initial injury, are abnormal in SSc. This adverse remodeling leads to pathologic intimal proliferation and medial hypertrophy, culminating in luminal narrowing (or obliteration) and tissue ischemia.[13] The abnormally thickened vessel walls promote intravascular thrombosis from platelet aggregation and further contribute to luminal narrowing. Angiogenesis and vasculogenesis also appear dysregulated in SSc, leading to vascular malformations and an impaired ability to generate new functional microvessels.[10]

Functional abnormalities of the vascular system are superimposed on structural abnormalities.[13] Vascular instability and altered vasoreactivity are prominent features in SSc and further compromise the vascular compartment.[10] An imbalance between vasoconstrictive and vasodilating mediators plays a role. Endothelin 1 (ET-1), released by injured endothelial cells, has received much attention in this regard. ET-1 is not only a potent vasoconstrictor but is also known to be profibrogenic, enhancing fibroblast proliferation and collagen synthesis. Thus, ET-1 may be an important link between the observed vasculopathy and pathologic fibrosis.

Tissue fibrosis dominates the second phase of this disease.[8] Persistent and uncontrolled upregulation of collagen gene expression by recruited fibroblasts and myofibroblasts leads to excessive deposition of collagen and other extracellular matrix (ECM) proteins. Complex autocrine and paracrine signaling loops sustain and amplify the abnormal fibrogenic response. Some of the relevant mediators in the signaling loops include the cytokines interleukin (IL)-1, IL-2, IL-4, and IL-6, activating factors such as transforming growth factor beta (TGF-β), platelet-derived growth factor and connective tissue growth factor, and monocyte chemotactic protein-1.[9] There is also increasing recognition that tissue hypoxia, which occurs in the context of the aforementioned vascular abnormalities, perpetuates the cycle of fibrosis and vascular pathology. Several mechanisms have been postulated: (1) hypoxia stimulates the production of extracellular matrix proteins via hypoxia-inducible factor-1 α-dependent and α-independent pathways; (2) hypoxia is also a potent inducer of vascular endothelial growth factor (VEGF), which when chronically overexpressed, leads to the formation of chaotic vessels with decreased blood flow.[14,15] Thus, hypoxia may be another link between vasculopathy and fibrosis in SSc.

Although it is generally accepted that autoimmunity has a role in disease pathogenesis, many issues remain unresolved.[8,12] It is unclear whether immune dysfunction is involved in initiation and/or disease maintenance. It is also not clear how the pathways of vascular pathology, fibrosis, and autoimmunity intersect. Numerous disturbances of both the humoral and cell-mediated immune systems have been described in different subsets of SSc patients at varying stages of the disease with different clinical manifestations.[9] Conflicting and inconsistent reports regarding these immune abnormalities (related in part to the heterogeneity of the populations studied) have led to difficulty with the interpretation of such findings and uncertainty regarding their relevance. Nevertheless, considerable evidence indicates that a skewed balance between type 1 and type 2 helper T cells toward Th2 activation is important for development of fibrosis. Emerging data also suggest that IL-17–producing T cells (Th17) may be relevant in pathogenesis.[9]

Numerous autoantibodies are also detected in the sera of SSc patients.[16] These include antinuclear antibodies such as antitopoisomerase 1 (anti-Scl 70) and anticentromere, as well as antinuclear antibodies (i.e., anti-RNA polymerase III and anti-U3-fibrillarin). Much is known about the associations of these antibodies with clinical subsets and patterns of organ involvement in SSc (i.e., anticentromere with limited SSc; anti-Scl 70 with diffuse SSs). However, to date, evidence that these autoantibodies are pathogenic has not been firmly established. More recently, several additional autoantibodies directed against nonnuclear antigens have been detected. These include antiendothelial cell antibodies, antifibrillin-1 antibodies, antimatrix metalloproteinase antibodies, and antiplatelet-derived growth factor receptor antibodies.[17] Experimental evidence suggests that these antibodies may be relevant in disease pathogenesis by initiating and/or propagating tissue damage. However, confirmatory studies are needed.

Scleroderma Renal Crisis

Scleroderma renal crisis (SRC) is one of the most devastating and life-threatening complications of systemic sclerosis. It develops in 5% to 10% of SSc patients and is seen almost exclusively in patients with diffuse systemic sclerosis. Two large cohort studies reviewed the clinical characteristics of SSc patients who develop this renal complication.[2,18] Penn et al.[18] described the course of 1997 SSc patients seen at a single institution between 1990 and 2005 and reported that 110 (5.5%) developed SRC. Of these, 86 patients (78%) had diffuse disease and 24 (22%) had limited disease. These data are comparable to those of other studies.

Scleroderma renal crisis usually develops early in the course of the disease. Approximately two thirds of affected patients carry the diagnosis of SSc for less than 1 year and almost all SRC cases are diagnosed within 5 years of the onset of SSc. Patients typically present with a precipitous onset of severe hypertension and rapid deterioration of renal function with oliguria or anuria. This is often accompanied by signs of microangiopathic hemolysis. Clinical manifestations of SRC are mainly those of malignant hypertension (e.g., headache and/or seizures from hypertensive encephalopathy and visual disturbances from hypertensive retinopathy). Dyspnea may be due to acute left ventricular failure and pulmonary edema due to the effects of malignant hypertension on the myocardium and volume overload from oliguria. Associated laboratory findings include elevated serum creatinine that progressively and rapidly rises and may be accompanied by proteinuria, which is usually in the subnephrotic range (<2.5 g per 24 hours). Nephrotic range proteinuria is uncommon. Urine sediment may be normal or may reveal microscopic hematuria with few cells or casts but a nephritic sediment is unusual. Anemia, thrombocytopenia, and schistocytes in the peripheral blood smear support the presence of a microangiopathic hemolytic process along with other markers of intravascular hemolysis such as elevated lactate dehydrogenase (LDH) and low haptoglobin.

Atypical presentations may make the syndrome more difficult to recognize, leading to missed diagnoses. Normotensive renal crisis occurs in 10% of cases of SRC.[19] Although blood pressures are normal or only modestly elevated in this variant of renal crisis, they are often higher than the patient's baseline blood pressure. This subtle change can serve as an important clue to the diagnosis and underscores the need to closely monitor blood pressures in SSc patients (particularly those at a high risk of SRC). Thrombotic microangiopathy is often present in normotensive SRC and its presence should also raise suspicion of this syndrome.[20] Renal crisis can also occur rarely in a subset of patients who have no significant dermal sclerosis (referred to as sclerosis sine scleroderma). These patients have characteristic internal organ involvement but an absence of detectable skin features. Finally, in one quarter of patients, the diagnosis of SRC will precede a formal diagnosis of systemic sclerosis.[18,21]

One of the challenges in diagnosing SRC, in both typical and atypical presentations, is distinguishing it from other forms of thrombotic microangiopathy (i.e., thrombotic thrombocytopenic purpura/hemolytic uremic syndrome [TTP/HUS]) given the similarities in presentation and laboratory abnormalities. This distinction is important as therapies differ. A renal biopsy does not reliably distinguish between these disorders. Rather, the clinical diagnosis relies on a compatible history, an evaluation of appropriate serologies, and a careful assessment of risk factors. Several factors may help to identify patients at a greater risk of developing SRC.[22] These include early diffuse systemic sclerosis, rapidly progressive skin thickening, new onset anemia, and new cardiac events (such as heart failure or pericardial effusion). Use of glucocorticoids (≥15 mg per day or the equivalent) in the preceding 6 months have long been considered a potential precipitant in SRC. In a case control study, Steen and Medsger[23] reported that high dose corticosteroids were administered more frequently in SRC patients (36%) than in controls (12%) (odds ratio [OR], 4.37). Although this association has also been reported by other investigators, causality is difficult to prove.[21] Rather, corticosteroids may have a confounding role because patients who are most likely to receive corticosteroids are also those at the highest risk for SRC. Nevertheless, the avoidance of corticosteroids in patients at risk is prudent. Autoantibody profiles may also provide clues regarding the risk of SRC. Anti-RNA polymerase III antibodies are associated with the development of SRC. Antifibrillarin or anti-U3-RNP antibodies may also identify patients at risk of developing internal organ manifestations, including SRC.[24] Conversely, patients with anticentromere antibodies are less likely to develop SRC.[18]

Pathophysiology of Scleroderma Renal Crisis

Injury to vascular endothelial walls, which underlies the pathophysiology of SSc in general, is considered a primary event in SRC. The vascular insult in SRC occurs in the interlobular and arcuate arteries of the renal cortex. The resulting thickening and proliferation of the intima, the deposition of glycoproteins and mucopolysaccharides, and the formation of platelet microthrombi lead to luminal narrowing and reduced renal perfusion. Chronic renal cortical ischemia leads to hyperplasia of the juxtaglomerular apparatus, stimulation of renin release, and activation of the renin-angiotensin-aldosterone system (RAAS). Hyperreninemia and ongoing activation of the RAAS is well recognized as playing a pivotal role in SRC by perpetuating intrarenal vasoconstriction, exacerbating renal ischemia, and inducing hypertension.[25] However, RAAS activation alone appears insufficient to initiate the full expression of SRC. Indeed, investigators have found that plasma renin levels can be markedly elevated for some time prior to the onset of SRC and may even be seen in patients that do not develop SRC.[26] Thus, an additional trigger(s), superimposed on a system "primed" by renin excess, is believed necessary to set in motion the explosive cascade of events of SRC. This trigger is unknown, but it has been proposed that conditions or stimuli that acutely compromise renal perfusion such as dehydration, sepsis, cardiac dysfunction, or intense vasospasm of intrarenal arterioles (possibly from cold exposure or other stressors) may contribute.[26–28]

Dysregulation in the endothelin system has also been implicated in the pathophysiology of SRC. Levels of ET-1 are increased in SSc patients with renal crisis.[29,30] One pathology study compared the distribution of ET-1 (by immunohistochemistry) in renal biopsies from SRC patients and patients with other vascular diseases involving the kidney.[31] Increased expression of both ET-1 and ET-1 receptors was detected in the small renal arteries of SRC patients, and the pattern of endothelial staining for ET-1 in both glomeruli and arteriolar lesions appeared specific for renal crisis.

The Role of a Renal Biopsy

A renal biopsy is usually not required to establish the diagnosis of SRC. Histologic changes are not pathognomonic for SRC and can be seen in other conditions that share endothelial injury as an underlying mechanism, such as malignant hypertension, TTP/HUS, and antiphospholipid syndrome. A renal biopsy is warranted when there is diagnostic uncertainty and/or to exclude other pathologies that warrant different management, such as crescentic glomerulonephritis or other inflammatory glomerular diseases.

The pathologic changes of SRC are evident in the small interlobular and arcuate arteries.[32,33] There is edema and thickening of the intima from mucin accumulation, and the characteristic onion skin lesion is due to concentrically arranged myointimal cellular proliferation and fibrosis, as shown in Figure 54.1. Both contribute to a luminal occlusion. Thrombosis and fibrinoid necrosis may be seen. The juxtaglomerular apparatus may appear particularly prominent, which is consistent with hyperreninemia from a reduced renal perfusion. Glomerular changes are variable and may be related to renal ischemia or direct glomerular endothelial injury. There may be a collapse of capillary loops or a thickening of

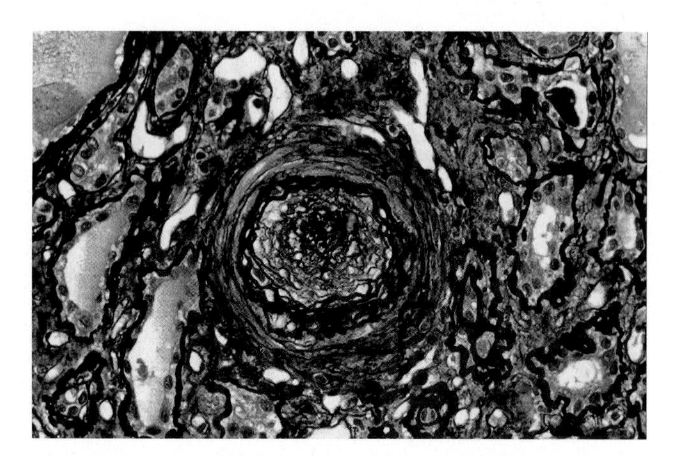

FIGURE 54.1 Scleroderma renal crisis, advanced stage. A methenamine silver stain of severe vasculopathy in a small arcuate artery compromised by luminal narrowing resulting from endothelial damage and the formation of concentric rings of myointimal fibrosis (onion skinning). (Biopsy specimen provided by Dr. Mark Haas, Renal Pathology Service, Cedars-Sinai Medical Center, Los Angeles, CA.)

capillary walls with a double contour appearance (on silver or periodic acid Schiff [PAS] staining), which are due to fibrin thrombi. Immune complexes are not present.

Treatment of Scleroderma Renal Crisis

Early diagnosis and prompt, aggressive treatment with ACE inhibitors (ACE-I) is crucial to prevent irreversible renal damage and a potentially fatal course. The effectiveness of ACE-I in halting progression and even reversing the process may be attributed to the interruption of the renin-angiotensin system, and AT-II–induced vasoconstriction. The angiotensin-converting enzyme also degrades bradykinin, a potent vasodilator. Interfering with this degradation of bradykinin may also contribute to the positive effects of ACE-I.

Most experience in SRC is with captopril, the agent used in early studies. There are fewer data available regarding the efficacy of other ACE-I in this setting, but they likely provide comparable benefit. Nevertheless, advantages of captopril in the acute setting include a rapid onset of action and a short duration of action, which provide more flexibility for dose titration. Captopril is usually initiated at 6.25 to 12.5 mg every 8 hours. The dose is titrated up (to 50 mg three times daily) to achieve gradual but steady blood pressure reduction. The goal is to return the patient to baseline blood pressures within 72 hours. Some recommend that blood pressure reductions should not exceed 20 mm Hg per 24 hours because this may compromise renal perfusion and should increase the risk of acute tubular necrosis. Even with judicious control of blood pressure, serum creatinine may rise with ACE-I therapy because of the associated decrease in efferent arteriolar resistance and intraglomerular pressure. However, this is not an indication for the discontinuation of therapy. Treatment with ACE-I is also indicated for patients with normotensive renal crisis, but escalation should be done carefully to avoid hypotension.

Data regarding the efficacy of AT-II receptor blockers (ARB) for the initial management of SRC are less clear. Some have reported benefit; others suggest suboptimal blood pressure control and greater rates of renal failure in patients with SRC treated with ARBs alone and subsequent improvement in renal function with the substitution of ACE-I.[34] The reason for such differences is unknown, but a possible explanation may be that ARBs, unlike ACE-I, do not inhibit the degradation of bradykinin.

If ACE inhibitors (at maximum recommended doses) are not sufficient to lower the blood pressure, other antihypertensive agents should be added. There are no studies that address which agents are most effective in this setting. Diuretics are best avoided (unless there is a strong clinical indication) because they may stimulate renin level. β-Blockers have the theoretic potential to worsen Raynaud phenomenon. Thus avoidance, if possible, might be prudent. Calcium channel blockers and vasodilators are reasonable options. Blocking the RAAS at multiple sites is an attractive approach in SRC. Aliskiren, a direct renin inhibitor, has theoretic benefit to further attenuate the RAAS in SRC and lower blood pressure. By blocking the catalytic activity of renin at the point of activation of the RAAS, aliskiren blocks the synthesis of all angiotensin peptides. This prevents the compensatory increase in renin that can be seen with ACE-I and ARB. At present, no studies have explored direct renin inhibition for therapy of SRC.

Despite the overall impressive impact of ACE-I on disease course, individual responses vary and many patients still suffer the full expression of SRC. The extent of this problem is highlighted in studies by Steen and Medsger[35] and Penn et al.,[18] which reviewed the course of SRC patients treated immediately (and aggressively) with ACE inhibitors. Permanent dialysis was required in 20% and 41% of these patients, respectively. This underscores the need for additional therapeutic strategies (beyond blockade of the RAAS) for this devastating complication. Intravenous prostacyclin and its analog, iloprost, have been used at some centers during the hypertensive phase of the renal crisis based on anecdotal observations of benefit.[36,37] Prostacyclin mediates vasodilation and has been reported to increase renal perfusion. There are no formal trials addressing the role of prostanoids as adjunctive therapy to angiotensin converting enzyme [ACE-I] in SRC.[37] HMG-CoA reductase inhibitors (statins) have been proposed for the treatment of SRC and possible prophylaxis.[38] This is based on evidence suggesting that statins may have a direct protective effect on endothelium, in addition to their well-known cholesterol lowering effect. ET is also a potential target of interest. The use of ET receptor antagonists in SRC is a particularly compelling idea in light of the possible role of ET in this disorder. Apart from their vasodilating effects, ET receptor antagonists may also reduce the profibrotic effects of endothelin. Data regarding the use of ET-receptor antagonism in SRC are limited. In a small pilot study, six patients with SRC were treated with bosentan, a nonselective ET-receptor antagonist, within 6 weeks of their diagnosis.[38a] All patients were also receiving ACE-I at full therapeutic doses. The treatment regimen consisted of bosentan at 62.5 mg for 1 month and then 125 mg twice daily for 5 months. Bosentan was well tolerated. Overall, mortality and dialysis rates were not significantly different compared to a historic cohort receiving standard therapy. Rebound phenomena (i.e., Raynaud phenomenon, hypertension), occurred in half of the patients upon the withdrawal of therapy. A larger, open label trial using bosentan is currently recruiting in France to more fully assess efficacy of this drug in SRC. (clinical trials.gov: Effect of Bosentan in Scleroderma Renal Crisis/ScS-REINBO)

Prognosis

Prior to the availability and aggressive use of ACE inhibitors, the prognosis of SRC was abysmal with progression to end stage kidney disease (ESKD) over a period of 1 to 2 months and death usually within 1 year. The benefits of ACE-I in SRC were supported in an early single center study by Steen et al.,[39] which compared outcomes before and after the availability of ACE-I. One-year survival improved from 15% to 76% after the introduction of ACE-I therapy. Five-year survival improved from 10% to 65% with treatment. No randomized controlled trials have performed a head-to-head comparison of other therapies versus ACE-I and, given the evidence, there likely will never be.

In patients who do not require dialysis during their course of SRC, improvements in renal function are detectable for several years, suggesting that recovery is a slow, prolonged process that likely includes vascular remodeling.[18] Among patients who require renal replacement therapy during the acute episode of SRC, more than half may recover sufficient renal function to permanently discontinue dialysis within 12 to 18 months.[35] The continuation of ACE inhibitors is recommended during dialysis while monitoring for signs of renal recovery. Long-term survival of patients who never require dialysis or only need temporary dialysis seems to be comparable to patients with diffuse disease without a renal crisis. In contrast, long-term survival is less favorable for patients who remain dialysis dependent. These patients appear to have a higher mortality compared to those with end-stage kidney disease for other reasons.

It is noteworthy that the prognosis of patients with normotensive SRC appears worse than in hypertensive patients.[20] The basis for this is unclear, but hypotheses have been proposed. Difficulty in recognizing SRC in an atypical form may lead to a delay in diagnosis and management, allowing ongoing subclinical injury that may be irreversible. Alternatively, different pathogenetic mechanisms may underlie this form of SRC, which may be less dependent on the activation of the RAAS and thus, less responsive to ACE inhibitors. Other risk factors associated with a poor outcome in SRC include male sex, older age, the presence of congestive heart failure, serum creatinine levels greater than 3 mg per deciliter at the initiation of treatment, and a time period of more than 3 days to control blood pressure.[35,39]

Renal Transplant

A renal transplant is an acceptable option for those who progress to end-stage kidney disease and who fail to recover renal function due to SRC. Transplantation may offer a survival advantage compared to patients who remain on dialysis.[40] However, in light of the potential for delayed renal recovery, decisions regarding renal transplantation should be deferred for at least 2 years. Renal allograft outcomes are reasonable, although they may be reduced compared to the general renal transplant population.[40,41]

Recurrence of SRC is a concern but is uncommon. It is estimated to occur in less than 5% of cases.[42] Most of the reported cases recurred relatively early in the posttransplant course within 2 years. Establishing the diagnosis of recurrent SRC in the allograft can be particularly challenging because other processes such as acute antibody mediation rejection, chronic transplant vasculopathy, and acute calcineurin inhibitor nephrotoxicity produce a similar histologic appearance. To reduce the risk of recurrent disease, high dose glucocorticoids should be used judiciously given their potential role in precipitating a renal crisis. When unavoidable, limiting the dose and duration is recommended. Calcineurin inhibitors have also been associated with precipitating renal crises in case reports. Thus, it may be prudent to consider alternative immunosuppressants.

Monitoring and Prevention

The unpredictable onset of SRC and the importance of a prompt diagnosis underscores the necessity of careful monitoring of SSc patients, particularly those considered at the highest risk for this complication. Educating patients about symptoms and signs of SRC is important, and consistent home blood pressure monitoring should be encouraged.

Prophylactic use of ACE-I or ARB do not appear to protect against the development of SRC.[21,23] Retrospective and case control studies have found neither benefit nor harm with ACE inhibitors related to the development of SRC,[23] although some investigators have noted a trend toward worse renal outcomes.[18,21] Further investigations are needed to clarify these findings.

Antineutrophil Cytoplasmic Antibody–Associated Renal Disease

Antineutrophil cytoplasmic antibody (ANCA)–associated vasculitis (AAV) is another distinct cause of rapidly progressive renal failure in SSc patients. The concurrence of AAV and SSc is a relatively rare complication described only in case reports and small cases series.[43–46] Nevertheless, AAV is an important entity to consider in the differential diagnosis of acute kidney injury in SSc patients and needs to be distinguished from SRC, which may have a similar clinical presentation but a completely different therapeutic approach.

AAV can occur in both the diffuse and limited variants of SSc, and it has also been reported in patients with systemic sclerosis sine scleroderma.[47,48] It is most common in the fifth and sixth decade of life and has a similar gender distribution as all SSC patients (female to male ratio, 4:1). Nearly all SSc patients with concurrent AAV have ANCAs with a perinuclear staining pattern (p-ANCA) directed against myeloperoxidase (MPO-ANCA). Clinical manifestations are more consistent with microscopic polyangiitis rather than granulomatosis with polyangiitis (Wegener granulomatosis). ANCAs directed against PR3 ANCA are rarely detected in this population.[49]

Certain presenting clinical and laboratory features may help to distinguish AAV from SRC (Table 54.1).[44,46] ANCA-associated kidney disease tends to occur later in the course of SSc, whereas SRC generally occurs earlier. The average duration of SSc prior to the onset of AAV and SRC is 7.8 years and 3.2 years, respectively. In contrast to SRC, which is associated with severe hypertension, blood pressure in ANCA-related acute kidney injury tends to be normal, although mild-to-moderate hypertension may be present in up to one third of patients. As such, AAV may be confused with and misdiagnosed as normotensive SRC. Patients with AAV in the context of SSc may present with other manifestations of vasculitis including limb ischemia, cutaneous lesions, and neuromuscular involvement (i.e., mononeuritis multiplex). The presence of such findings favors a diagnosis of AAV over SRC. Also, the vasculitis of AAV is an inflammatory vasculitis, whereas SSc is a noninflammatory vasculopathy. Thus, evidence of inflammation such as fever and elevated acute phase reactants (erythrocyte sedimentation rate [ESR], C-reactive protein [CRP]) favors a diagnosis of AAV rather than SRC. Pulmonary hemorrhage is a frequent vasculitic manifestation leading to respiratory distress in this setting (pulmonary renal syndrome). Distinguishing an alveolar hemorrhage from a pulmonary edema, which may occur in SRC, is often difficult because the symptoms and radiologic imaging may be similar. Anemia can be present in both, but is usually normochromic normocytic in AAV and microangiopathic in SRC. The urine sediment is active and nephritic in AAV but typically is bland in SRC.

If AAV is suspected, tests for ANCA and for anti-MPO and anti-PR3 by enzyme-linked immunosorbent assay (ELISA) are warranted, but results are usually not available in a timely manner. A kidney biopsy should be performed expeditiously

TABLE 54.1 **Differentiating Etiologies of Rapidly Progressive Kidney Injury in Systemic Sclerosis: Scleroderma Renal Crisis Versus Antineutrophil Cytoplasmic Antibody (ANCA)–Associated Vasculitis**

	Scleroderma Renal Crisis	ANCA-Associated Crescentic Glomerulonephritis
Timing during disease course	Early	Late
Blood pressure	Usually malignant, uncommon: normotensive	Normal-to-moderate elevation
Anemia	Microangiopathic	Normochromic
Urine sediment	Bland	Nephritic
Acute phase reactants	Normal	Elevated
Acute respiratory issues	Pulmonary edema, congestive heart failure	Alveolar hemorrhage
Renin levels	Markedly elevated	Normal
Histology	Intimal edema and thickening; onion skin lesion, narrowing of vascular lumens	Pauci-immune necrotizing and crescentic glomerulonephritis
Treatment	ACE inhibitors	Immunosuppression

ACE, angiotensin converting enzyme.

to confirm the diagnosis. A histology is consistent with pauci-immune necrotizing and crescentic glomerulonephritis.

The treatment of AAV requires aggressive immunosuppression consisting of induction with high dose corticosteroids and cyclophosphamide with or without plasma exchange, followed by maintenance immunosuppressive therapy. B-cell depletion with rituximab might also be considered. Although data are limited, there are no reported cases of steroids promoting the development of SRC during the treatment of AAV despite the theoretic risk. Because prognosis is so poor without therapy, intensive immunosuppression, including steroids, is recommended.

What predisposes some SSc patients to the development of a superimposed vasculitis is not known. In some cases, a hypersensitivity reaction to the medication, D-penicillamine, has been considered to be a trigger, but in the vast majority, a cause is not identified. ANCAs have also been detected (rarely) in the sera of unselected SSc patients during screening evaluations.[44,46,49–51] The significance of ANCA in SSc patients without clinically evident vasculitis is controversial. Some authors suggest that this finding is considered a red flag, indicating an inflammatory component to the underlying disease, whereas others have found no increased risk of renal disease or other vasculitic complications.[50]

Other Renal Manifestations in Systemic Sclerosis

Other renal abnormalities may occur in SSc patients that are not as overt or as dramatic as SRC or ANCA vasculitis. Estimates of kidney involvement in SSc vary widely based on different definitions of kidney injury and the markers of renal disease that are examined.[52–58] One report identified abnormal renal function (defined as creatinine ≥1.2 mg per deciliter) or proteinuria (defined as 3 or 4+ proteinuria on dipstick on two occasions) in 16% and 13%, respectively, of patients with dcSSc (without a history of SRC).[57] Over a mean follow-up of 10 years, only 2 of 546 patients in this cohort reached end-stage kidney disease, suggesting a benign clinical course for the vast majority. A greater percentage of patients are considered to be affected if more sensitive measures of GFR are used.[53] One study measured GFR using technetium 99mDTPA in 31 patients with normal serum creatinine and showed a reduction of GFR in 55% of patients, with 32% categorized as stage II chronic kidney disease (CKD) (60 to 89 mL per minute) and 23% as stage III (30 to 59 mL per minute).[55] When pathologic renal change at an autopsy is used as the criterion, approximately 60% of patients will have histologic evidence of kidney involvement, indicating that subclinical disease is relatively common in SSc.[52,58]

Renal involvement in SSc patients may be related or unrelated to the underlying disease process, other organ involvement (i.e., heart failure, pulmonary hypertension), or associated therapies (Table 54.2). Treatment with D-penicillamine, which had been used for years for the management of skin involvement in dcSSc, has been associated with renal injury and proteinuria.[59] Up to 20% of treated patients develop membranous nephropathy, which resolves with drug cessation.[60] Diffuse proliferative glomerulonephritis, pulmonary renal syndrome, drug-induced lupus syndrome, and ANCA-related vasculitis have also been reported to be associated with D-penicillamine treatment.[61,62] Due to its high rate of side effects, including renal toxicity and questionable therapeutic effect, penicillamine is now rarely used in the treatment of SSc.

TABLE 54.2 Renal Manifestations in Systemic Sclerosis

- Prerenal associated with cardiac or pulmonary artery involvement (heart failure, pulmonary hypertension), diuretics, NSAIDs
- Scleroderma renal crisis
- Glomerulonephritis
  - ANCA-associated crescentic glomerulonephritis
  - Penicillamine-induced renal injury
  - Overlap syndrome (i.e., with lupus or other connective tissue diseases)
- Chronic hypertension
- Decreased renal plasma flow,[54] higher renal vascular resistance[56]

NSAIDs, nonsteroidal anti-inflammatory drugs; ANCA, antineutrophil cytoplasmic antibody.

An important association exists between the presence of pulmonary hypertension and a reduced glomerular filtration rate. Campo et al.[63] evaluated 76 SSc patients with pulmonary arterial hypertension and reported that 45.6% had renal dysfunction (estimated glomerular filtration rate [eGFR] <60 mL/min/1.73 m^2) at the time of diagnosis.[63] Only 6.5% of these patients had a prior episode of renal crisis. eGFR was a strong predictor of survival in this cohort, with an eGFR less than 60 mL/min/1.73 m^2 associated with a threefold risk of mortality. The reduction in GFR may reflect simultaneous structural damage to both the pulmonary and the renal vascular beds, or may be related to the prerenal effects of severe pulmonary hypertension.

Other studies have identified proteinuria as an independent risk factor for death in SSc patients with a hazard ratio of 3.34.[64–66] Although the mechanism for this association is not clear, it has been proposed that the presence of proteinuria may be a marker of more severe underlying endothelial dysfunction, which could portend a worse prognosis.

Novel Therapies for Systemic Sclerosis and the Potential for Renal Injury

Nonselective immunosuppressive medications (i.e., cyclophosphamide, azathioprine, prednisone, methotrexate) are frequently used to treat the complications of SSc despite a lack of convincing data that these therapies reverse the natural disease progression.[67] Therapeutic attempts at selectively blocking fibrotic pathways have not met with much success, probably because of the complexity of the fibrotic process with its multiple layers of regulation. A number of newer biologic agents targeting other molecular pathways, cellular effectors, and signaling molecules believed to be operative in SSc are now available and are under clinical investigation.[68]

Autologous hematopoietic stem cell transplantation (HSCT) has also been applied for selected SSc patients with a poor prognosis (predominantly with diffuse cutaneous disease and severe internal organ involvement).[69] The rationale for HSCT in SSc is to reset the dysregulated immune system. Phase I/II trials of HSCT have demonstrated a reversal of skin fibrosis, improved functionality and quality of life, and stabilization of the internal organ function in SSc patients.[70–74] Experience is still limited and toxicity remains a concern. The potential for renal complications in SSc patients deserves special consideration.

Acute kidney injury (AKI) is not an uncommon complication after HSCT irrespective of the transplant indication. Kidney injury may manifest as thrombotic microangiopathy, radiation nephritis, glomerular disease, and acute tubular necrosis (ATN) (among others) and may be attributed to such factors as conditioning regimens, total body irradiation (TBI), nephrotoxic drugs (i.e., calcineurin inhibitors), and infections. Whether having SSc, with the associated underlying vasculopathy, conveys a higher risk of kidney injury after HSCT, particularly if exposed to radiation (which has effects on vascular endothelium), glucocorticoids, or calcineurin inhibitors, is unclear. Furthermore, both TMA and radiation nephritis can clinically mimic SRC. Distinguishing among these causes of AKI can be particularly challenging in SSc patients after HSCT. Until further data are available, measures to minimize nephrotoxicity will be important. These include aggressive control of blood pressure, the restricted use of glucocorticoids and calcineurin inhibitors, the avoidance of TBI or renal shielding, and close monitoring of renal function.

Presently, there are three ongoing randomized trials investigating the safety and efficacy of autologous HSCT for SSc: Autologous Stem Cell Transplantation International Scleroderma (ASTIS), American Systemic Sclerosis Immune Suppression Versus Transplant (ASSIST), and Scleroderma Cyclophosphamide Versus Transplant (SCOT). ASSIST and ASTIS use a nonmyeloablative regimen and SCOT uses a myeloablative regimen with total body irradiation. Hopefully, results from these trials will clarify the role of HSCT in SSc and will address the risk of kidney injury in these patients.

RHEUMATOID ARTHRITIS

Rheumatoid arthritis (RA) is an inflammatory polyarthritis with a peak age of onset between 40 and 60 years and with a greater than twofold increased prevalence in women. RA is generally considered to represent an autoimmune disorder because of its characteristic laboratory profile of autoantibodies to cyclic citrullinated peptides (anti-CCP), to immunoglobulin G (rheumatoid factor), and to nuclear antigens (antinuclear antibodies [ANA]). There are numerous defects in cytokine production and cell-mediated immunoregulatory pathways that are integral components of the pathogenic inflammation and autoreactivity. Some investigators hypothesize, based on animal models and on epidemiologic evidence, that certain infections can be the triggering event, which in a susceptible person with genetically determined or otherwise acquired defects in immunoregulatory circuits leads to RA.[75]

Clinical Features of Rheumatoid Arthritis

RA is characterized by symmetrical stiffness and painful swellings (inflammation and effusions), typically of multiple joints of the upper and lower extremities; if these findings persist for more than 6 weeks, they fulfill a key diagnostic criterion for RA. Because RA typically progresses to a chronic disease, persistent or recurring synovitis leads to joint effusions and the destruction of cartilage and erosions of periarticular bone, eventuating in deforming arthropathies. Fatigability, malaise, anorexia, and weight loss are common debilitating features of RA, reflecting high circulating levels of immune complexes, acute phase reactants, and cytokines. The protracted inflammatory state, when not interdicted by effective disease remitting treatment, appears to be a major contributor to accelerated atherosclerotic cardiovascular disease, which in turn leads to increased rates of debilitating morbidity and premature mortality in patients with RA.[76]

General Treatment Strategies for Rheumatoid Arthritis

Multiple studies have shown definitively that destructive pathologic processes start very early in the course of RA, and that there are long-term benefits of aggressive therapy on the natural history of RA. In the acute stage of the disease, the clinical and laboratory manifestations of RA typically respond dramatically to corticosteroids. However, because it is unusual to find a nontoxic dose of corticosteroid that can provide sustained control of RA, alternative therapies have been intensely pursued. Historically, there has been a succession of agents used adjunctively with corticosteroids for the treatment of RA, including general anti-inflammatory drugs (e.g., salicylates, nonsteroidal anti-inflammatory drugs [NSAIDs], antimalarials, gold salts, penicillamine, sulfasalazine), as well as more potent and directly immunosuppressive agents (e.g., methotrexate, cyclophosphamide, azathioprine, leflunomide). These agents, categorized as disease-modifying antirheumatic drugs (DMARDs), have shown objective salutary effects on clinical manifestations and long-term complications of RA; however, none of these agents predictably or consistently induces complete remissions and most have had excessive adverse side effects when used as maintenance therapy. For example, gold salts and penicillamine have been largely abandoned as treatment for RA due to suboptimal efficacy and their propensity to cause secondary membranous nephropathy.

Weekly doses of oral methotrexate have been the stalwart therapy for long-term management of RA for the past 3 decades. Methotrexate and low dose corticosteroid combination therapy produces satisfactory remissions in a substantial majority of cases. However, for patients with refractory or relapsing disease, biologic agents that antagonize tumor necrosis factor (e.g., etanercept, infliximab, adalimumab) are added to the basal methotrexate regimen. Other agents under active investigation as adjuncts to methotrexate include rituximab, anti-IL6-receptor (tocilizumab), and the costimulation inhibitor, CTLA4-Ig.[77,78]

Kidney Involvement in Rheumatoid Arthritis

Abnormalities of kidney function (e.g., abnormal urinalysis, proteinuria, diminished glomerular filtration rate [GFR], abnormal pathology) were recognized several decades ago in up to half of patients with RA. These clinical laboratory abnormalities were attributed to poorly controlled RA (e.g., secondary amyloidosis) or to the complications of the limited options for symptomatic treatment of RA (e.g., interstitial nephritis due to the protracted use of high dose aspirin).[79,80] With subsequent availability of disease-modifying therapeutic strategies that provided more effective management of RA, the frequency of renal abnormalities has dramatically decreased and types of clinically significant renal complications have substantively changed over the past 2 to 3 decades. For example, both drug-induced interstitial nephritis and secondary amyloidosis have become increasingly rare due to the more effective treatment of RA. On the other hand, some types of glomerulonephritis do occur sporadically during the course of RA. The impacts on renal and patient survival of the different forms of glomerular disease vary from minor, in patients with isolated hematuria and low grade pathology, to major, in those with complicated nephritic and nephrotic syndromes and high grade pathology.[81]

Table 54.3 shows the range and weighted mean frequency of the main forms of kidney pathology occurring in renal biopsies from patients with RA as reported in four relatively large case series.[82–85] In rank order, mesangial proliferative glomerulonephritis, membranous nephropathy, and AA amyloidosis are the most frequent diagnoses, but there are several other nephropathies observed in patients undergoing a renal biopsy for clinical indications, including a very imposing and ominous form of renal vasculitis.

Mesangial Glomerulonephritis

Although mesangial proliferative glomerulonephritis accounts for approximately one third of cases, this may be an underestimate of its frequency, because isolated hematuria, following negative imaging studies of the upper and lower urinary tracts, is not universally considered an indication for a renal biopsy. Mesangial glomerulonephritis is associated with mesangial deposits of immune complexes. Because the mesangium is considered to be a normal channel of egress for at least some fraction of immune complexes from the circulation, it is likely that this pathway is simply overloaded in RA where there is an extremely heavy burden of circulating immune complexes (even if the immune complexes, per se, are characteristically of low intrinsic nephritogenicity). The mesangial proliferative glomerulonephritis associated with RA tends to be mild and has been shown in long-term follow-up studies to have a benign prognosis.[86]

Membranous Nephropathy

The emergence of proteinuria, particularly into the nephrotic range, heralds more clinically challenging glomerular diseases, most commonly membranous nephropathy or secondary AA amyloidosis. Mixed nephritic, nephrotic, and azotemic syndromes in the patient with RA may also indicate overlap-

TABLE 54.3 **Renal Biopsy Series in Patients with Rheumatoid Arthritis**

Author, yr [Ref]	# Cases	Percentage			
		Mes	MN	AA	Other
Sellers et al., 1983[85]	30	43	30	3	23%
Adu et al., 1993[82]	10	20	50		30%
Helin et al., 1995[83]	110	36	17	30	7%
Nakano et al., 1998[84]	158	34	31	19	16%
Weighted mean (total # cases = 308)		35	27	21	14%

yr, year; Mes, mesangial glomerulonephritis; MN, membranous nephropathy; AA, amyloidosis. Other category includes lupus nephritis, renal vasculitis, IgA nephropathy, and interstitial nephritis.

ping rheumatic diseases. For example, some patients with RA have diagnostic features of both RA and systematic lupus erythematosus (SLE) (sometimes called rhupus). In this case, the manifestations and prognostic implications of SLE and lupus nephritis are likely to be of pre-eminent importance in the management of the patient with underlying RA. Patients with RA may also have features of a mixed connective tissue disease (MCTD), including Sjögren syndrome. However, the concurrence with RA of either MCTD or Sjögren syndrome rarely increases the likelihood of serious renal disease, aside from membranous nephropathy.

The etiopathogenesis of membranous nephropathy in any of the rheumatic diseases has not been determined, but it is likely to be related to the emergence of polyclonal antibodies with particular autoreactivity (or cross-reactivity) to constitutive antigens of the podocytes of the glomerular epithelial cell. An alternative hypothesis is based on the historical impression of a modestly increased frequency of membranous nephropathy in the context of sustained treatment of RA with gold salts[87] and penicillamine.[60] Based on experimental models, this hypothesis holds that exogenous agents may create autoreactivity after being bound or "planted" in the glomerular basement membrane or on the visceral epithelial cell. Thus, although there are numerous case series suggesting an association between the use of gold, penicillamine, or bucillamine and the emergence of membranous nephropathy in RA, it is clear that the risk of membranous nephropathy is associated with RA, per se.[61,88–92] The pathogenic role of these drugs to amplify the risk of membranous nephropathy in RA has never been fully resolved and, indeed, has become moot, because gold salts, penicillamine, or bucillamine are rarely used for the treatment of RA in current medical practice.

Initial approaches to membranous nephropathy discovered during the course of RA should be examined to discover whether there are cofactors (e.g., SLE, syphilis, hepatitis B, occult malignancy) that could be modified, as well as substituting alternative antirheumatic drugs for those that have been suspected to incite membranous nephropathy. Examining whether inadequate treatment for RA may also foster secondary membranous nephropathy is another consideration and may lead to modification of the treatment regimen for better control of RA. If no other contributing factors are identified, the treatment of membranous nephropathy occurring in the context of RA is basically governed by the same principles that apply to the treatment of idiopathic membranous nephropathy.

AA Amyloidosis

Patients with persistently active, unremitting RA are burdened with protracted inflammation and have high levels of acute phase reactants, including elevations of the serum amyloid A (SAA) protein, which predispose them to secondary or AA amyloidosis (Fig. 54.2).[93] Some autopsy surveys have shown that AA amyloidosis can be subclinical and that small amounts of amyloid deposits may be detectable in more than one quarter of the autopsies of RA patients.[94] Risks of developing amyloidosis associated with RA also increases in the setting of poor access to medical care, as well as the historical inclination of many physicians to administer disease-modifying agents for RA in a "go low and go slow" fashion. Older age of onset of RA also predisposes a patient to an increased risk of AA amyloidosis.[95]

AA amyloidosis characteristically affects the kidney where glomerular deposits of amyloid produce proteinuria and arterial deposits further contribute to decreased renal function. Gastrointestinal tract involvement is equally frequent, and debilitating gut malabsorption syndromes may precede or emerge concurrently with manifestations of renal amyloidosis. AA amyloidosis of the kidney has a significant impact on patient survival.[81]

Numerous studies over the past few years have demonstrated the long-term benefits of aggressive early treatment of RA both in *preventing* deforming arthropathy and systemic complications such as AA amyloidosis, as well as decreasing the rates of progression to end-stage renal disease[96] and mortality from accelerated cardiovascular disease.[78] Fortunately, the incidence of AA amyloidosis as a complication of uncontrolled RA has been steadily decreasing in the setting of early intervention with the armamentarium of modern treatment options for RA.

The development of amyloidosis during the course of RA should prompt a critical reassessment of whether the treatment regimen has been on goal based on objective measures of the disease activity of RA because interdiction of the dire consequences of AA amyloid depends mostly on comprehensive therapeutic measures to induce a complete remission of RA. Thus, new onset amyloidosis usually warrants intensification of standard treatments for RA and/or the addition of newer experimental options (e.g., rituximab, tocilizumab, abatacept), several of which have shown the potential to ameliorate amyloidosis emerging in the context of RA.[97–99] One unusual feature of AA amyloid occurring in the context of RA is the finding in some cases of numerous cellular crescents, a feature that seems to auger a particularly dire outcome of the glomerular disease.[100,101] Finally, it is noteworthy that nonamyloidotic fibrillary glomerulonephritis has been reported as a rare association with RA.[102,103]

Renal Vasculitis

One of the more ominous late-stage complications of RA is the development of systemic (rheumatoid) vasculitis. The emergence of small- and/or medium-sized arteritis usually produces multisystem and visceral complications with their attendant high risks of morbidity and mortality. Renal vasculitis is a relatively rare component of rheumatoid vasculitis, but its development is associated with an ominous prognosis. Like secondary AA amyloidosis, patients with RA at risk for systemic vasculitis are those with protracted high levels of rheumatoid factor and persistently active disease, usually with cutaneous vasculitis and rheumatoid nodules occurring late in the course of joint destructive RA.

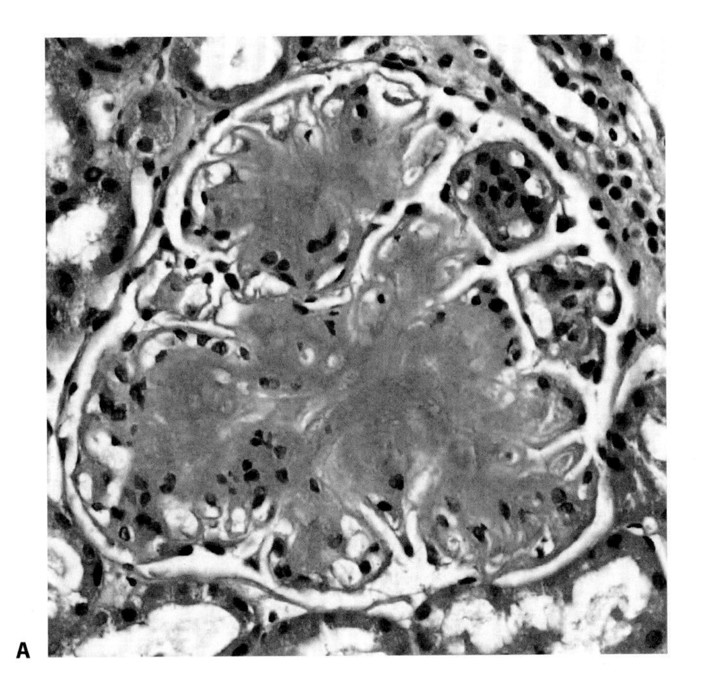

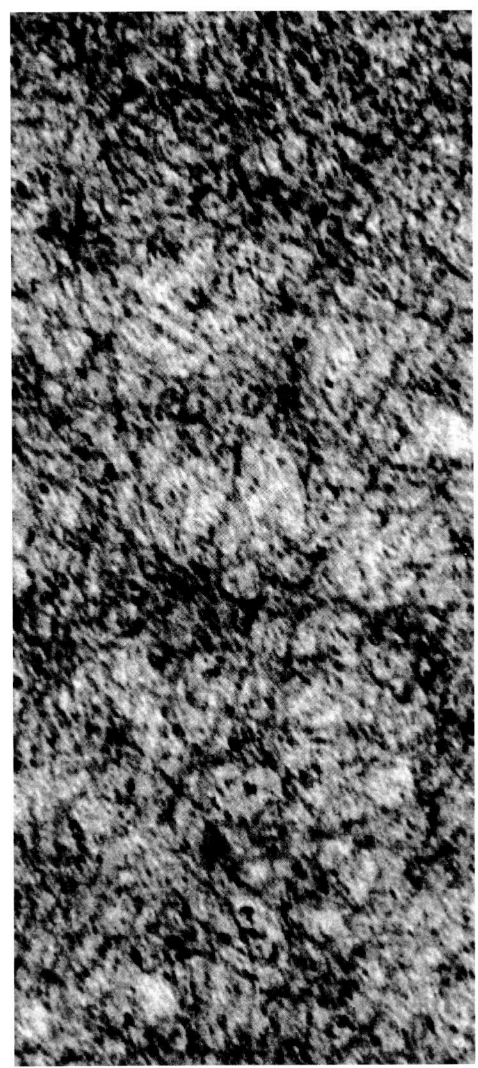

FIGURE 54.2 AA amyloidosis in a patient with severe chronic rheumatoid arthritis. Panel **A** shows characteristic acellular, nodular deposits of amyloid within the glomeruli. Taken with a hematoxylin and eosin stain. Panel **B** shows the characteristic ultrastructure of the tangled array of amyloid fibrils (approximately 10 nm in diameter).

Renal vasculitis is usually manifested by severe hypertension, nephritic syndrome, and often rapidly progressive renal failure.[104,105] ANCA, mostly antimyeloperoxidase autoantibodies, are usually (though not invariably) present.[106–108] Necrotizing, crescentic glomerulonephritis can be seen on a renal biopsy, as illustrated in Figure 54.3.[109] Aggressive therapy with high dose corticosteroids and cytotoxic drugs are indicated to counter the otherwise ominous prognosis of this form of renal vasculitis (see Chapter 48 on the treatment of vasculitis).

One perplexing aspect of the relationship between RA and systemic vasculitis is that anti-tumor necrosis factor (TNF) therapies have been recently recognized to have the potential to augment autoantibody production. This has been well documented for increments in titers of anti-dsDNA and flares of SLE and lupus nephritis.[110] Similar observations have been reported in patients with RA treated with anti-TNF therapies, which paradoxically appear to have precipitated the onset or flares of ANCA-associated renal vasculitis.[111–113] A detailed

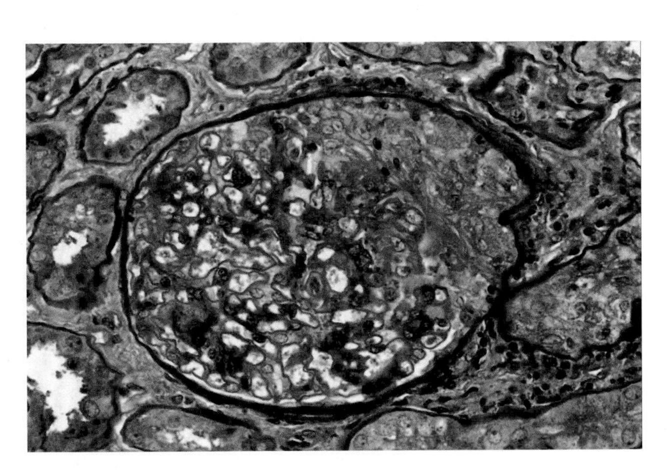

FIGURE 54.3 Antineutrophil cytoplasmic antibody (ANCA)–associated renal vasculitis in a patient with rheumatoid arthritis. A segmental necrotizing glomerulonephritis is present with fibrinoid necrosis, karyorrhexis, and a developing cellular crescent. Taken with a hematoxylin and eosin stain.

perspective on the role of anti-TNF therapies on autoantibody production and flares of autoimmune diseases remains a substantive challenge and the subject of ongoing research.

PRIMARY SJÖGREN SYNDROME

Sjögren syndrome is a relatively common autoimmune disease characterized by chronic inflammation and dysfunction of the exocrine glands. Lymphocytic infiltrates of salivary and lacrimal glands lead to typical clinical manifestations, including dry mouth, dry eyes, and parotid enlargement. The involvement of other exocrine glands can lead to dry skin, dryness of the upper respiratory tract, hypochlorhydria, pancreatic dysfunction, and vaginal dryness.[114,115] This autoimmune disorder can occur alone, as primary Sjögren syndrome, or in association with other autoimmune conditions, such as systemic lupus erythematosus, rheumatoid arthritis, and progressive systemic sclerosis (secondary Sjögren syndrome). This chapter will focus on renal abnormalities associated with primary Sjögren syndrome.

Similar to SLE, primary Sjögren syndrome predominantly affects women with a female to male ratio of 9:1. Although this condition is most frequently diagnosed in middle-aged individuals, children and elderly patients have been identified as well.[116–118] It may be difficult to recognize the diagnosis because the presenting signs and symptoms are typically nonspecific and mimic those seen in other conditions. In two large studies,[119,120] average delays of 4 and 6 years have been observed between the first symptom attributable to primary Sjögren syndrome and the diagnosis. This is of importance to the nephrologist who may encounter a patient with an unusual renal manifestation of primary Sjögren syndrome, before the underlying condition has been recognized.

Comparable to other autoimmune rheumatic disorders, the diagnosis of primary Sjögren syndrome requires the presence of a constellation of clinical, laboratory, and/or histologic features; the individual criteria are characteristic but not specifically diagnostic, because each can be attributed to alternative conditions. In 1993, a European Study Group published preliminary criteria for the classification of Sjögren syndrome to promote consistency in clinical studies of this condition.[121] In 2002, an American–European Consensus Group revised the rules to enhance the specificity of the criteria. Table 54.4 shows the widely accepted American–European classification criteria for Sjögren syndrome[122] published in 2002. The classification rules underscore the importance of the objective criteria (#3 to 6). The diagnosis of primary Sjögren syndrome can be based on the presence of three of four objective criteria or on the presence of any four of the six criteria as long as either the pathology or the autoantibody criteria (or both) are fulfilled. The diagnosis of secondary Sjögren syndrome requires symptoms of dry eyes and/or dry mouth (criteria #1 and/or 2) and any two items from the objective criteria #3, 4, or 5. The classification criteria exclude conditions and medications that may mimic features of Sjögren syndrome.

TABLE 54.4 American–European Classification Criteria for Sjögren Syndrome

1.	**Ocular symptoms** – A positive response to at least one of three specific questions about dry eyes, sand, or gravel in the eyes or the use of tear substitutes >3 times a day
2.	**Oral symptoms** – A positive response to at least one of three specific questions about dry mouth for >3 months, swollen salivary glands as an adult, or drinking liquids to swallow dry foods.
3.	**Objective evidence of ocular involvement** – A positive Schirmer I test or positive Rose Bengal score (or other ocular dye score).
4.	**Histopathology** – A minor salivary gland biopsy that shows focal lymphocytic sialadenitis according to specific criteria.
5.	**Objective evidence of salivary gland involvement** – Specific abnormalities on at least one of the following tests: unstimulated whole salivary flow, parotid sialography, or salivary scintigraphy.
6.	**Autoantibodies** – Anti-SSA and/or anti-SSB[56]

SSA, Sjögren's syndrome-A; SSB, Sjögren's syndrome-B

It is important to emphasize that primary Sjögren syndrome is a systemic autoimmune condition that is frequently associated with constitutional symptoms and major organ dysfunction.[114,115,119,120,123] Constitutional symptoms commonly include fatigue and low-grade fever. Articular involvement is typically symmetric and nonerosive. Skin manifestations include Raynaud phenomenon, purpura, and vasculitis. Sensory neuropathies are the most common neurologic complications of primary Sjögren syndrome.[124,125] Patients may experience severe neuropathic pain before the systemic condition has been recognized. The lungs may be affected by a broad range of conditions including proximal and distal airway disease, interstitial pneumonitis, diffuse lymphoid hyperplasia of the lungs, and lymphoma.[126,127]

Approximately 4% of patients with Sjögren syndrome develop non-Hodgkin lymphoma.[115,128,129] Frequently, they are indolent mucosa-associated lymphoid tissue (MALT) lymphomas that predominantly involve the salivary glands; however, major organs including the kidneys, lungs, liver, and stomach may be affected as well. Less often, patients develop aggressive lymphomas that may arise de novo or from preexisting low-grade lymphomas. Skopouli and colleagues[120] found that among their patients with primary Sjögren syndrome, those with glomerulonephritis were at increased risk for lymphoma as well as peripheral neuropathy.

They observed that the development of glomerulonephritis and lymphoproliferative disorders was associated with purpura (especially palpable purpura), low levels of C4 complement, and mixed monoclonal cryoglobulinemia; they recommended vigilant monitoring of these patients.

Kidney Disorders in Patients with Primary Sjögren Syndrome

Table 54.5 shows the results of several relatively large, recently published studies that illustrate the broad range of kidney disorders that have been associated with primary Sjögren syndrome[119,130–135]. The patients fulfilled consensus criteria for the classification of primary Sjögren syndrome that were current at the time of the study—the European criteria[121] prior to 2002 and the American–European criteria,[122] subsequently. Goules et al.,[132] Ren et al.,[135] and Maripuri et al.[133] studied patients with primary Sjögren syndrome who were known to have kidney disease. Goules et al.[132] described 20 patients with overt kidney disease that the investigators felt called for a renal biopsy; 2 patients declined. Maripuri et al.[133] reported clinical and kidney pathology observations from 24 patients who had undergone a renal biopsy. Pertovaara et al.,[134] Aasarod et al.,[130] Bossini et al.,[131] and Lin et al.[119] sought to identify patients with renal involvement among cohorts of patients who had not been preselected for the presence of kidney disease. Pertovaara et al.,[134] Aasarod et al.,[130] and Bossini et al.[131] performed provocative tests to detect subclinical, latent kidney disorders that are frequently seen in patients with primary Sjögren syndrome; their studies included ammonium chloride loading tests to detect incomplete distal renal tubular acidosis (RTA) and water deprivation tests followed by the administration of l-deamino, 8-D arginine-vasopressin (DDAVP) to diagnose nephrogenic diabetes insipidus. It is unclear how often Lin and colleagues[119] used provocative tests to identify latent kidney disease in their patients. Overall, investigators have found that approximately a third of unselected patients with primary Sjögren syndrome have evidence of overt or latent renal involvement. A small fraction of those typically have overt kidney disease, which has a substantial impact on the patient's health. For example, Bossini et al.[131] found that 16 of 60 patients (27%) had laboratory abnormalities consistent with tubular and/or glomerular dysfunction. Only 4 presented with overt manifestations of kidney disease—2 patients had nephrotic syndrome, 1 had hypokalemic quadriparesis, and 1 had recurrent renal calculi and nephrocalcinosis associated with complete distal RTA.

Distal Renal Tubular Acidosis

Distal RTA (often incomplete distal RTA) has been reported in approximately 10% to 70% of patients with primary Sjögren syndrome.[119,130,132,134–142] Particularly high incidence rates are seen in cohorts that include substantial numbers of Sjögren patients with previously recognized kidney disease and/or a history of urolithiasis.[132,135,136] Patients with complete or incomplete distal RTA are at increased risk for nephrolithiasis or nephrocalcinosis. Hypocitraturia has been observed frequently among these patients[130,136] and increases the risk of forming calcium stones. Screening for hypocitraturia may be useful when evaluating patients with primary Sjögren syndrome, because this may facilitate the recognition of complete or incomplete distal RTA and may underscore the need for citrate supplementation to decrease the risk of nephrolithiasis, nephrocalcinosis, and bone disease observed in these patients.

Several investigators have sought to identify other clinical features that predict the occurrence of distal RTA among patients with primary Sjögren syndrome. Pertovaara and colleagues[134] found by multivariate logistic regression analysis that hypertension, proteinuria ($<$0.5 g per day in all) and the duration of xerostomia were each independently associated with the occurrence of distal RTA among their patients with primary Sjögren syndrome. On the other hand, Ren and colleagues[135] found that their Sjögren patients with RTA were significantly younger and were significantly more likely to have hypergammaglobulinemia than those without RTA. An association of hypergammaglobulinemia with distal RTA has been noted in some,[143,144] but not all[137,140] studies of Sjögren syndrome. The occurrence of several autoantibodies commonly detected in patients with primary Sjögren syndrome (antinuclear antibody [ANA], anti-Sjögren's syndrome-A [SSA], and anti-Sjögren's syndrome-B [SSB]) has not been consistently linked with the presence of distal RTA.[130,134,135,137,140] Furthermore, increased urinary excretion of β-2 microglobulin, N-acetyl-β-amino-glucosidase (NAG), or retinol binding protein (RBP) has been observed among patients with distal RTA in some,[130] but not all[135] recent studies of primary Sjögren syndrome. Thus, it appears that hypergammaglobulinemia, serum levels of ANA, anti-SSA, and anti-SSB autoantibodies, as well as the urinary excretion rate of β-2 microglobulin, NAG, or RBP are not reliable predictors of the occurrence of distal RTA in patients with primary Sjögren syndrome.

Clinical and pathologic studies offer insights into the pathogenesis of distal RTA in patients with primary Sjögren syndrome. Patients have been diagnosed functionally to have secretory defect distal RTA, based on a failure to acidify urine (spontaneously or after the administration of ammonium chloride or furosemide), a positive urinary anion gap despite systemic acidosis (suggesting impaired urinary ammonium excretion), normal or low serum potassium values, and an abnormally low urine–blood pCO_2 difference during a bicarbonate infusion.[145–148] Apical H^+-ATPase and basolateral anion exchanger 1 (AE1) mediate H^+ secretion from α-intercalated cells in the collecting ducts. Several studies of primary Sjögren patients with distal RTA have shown little or no immunoreactive H^+-ATPase in collecting duct cells despite the presence of normal appearing α-intercalated cells by light and electron microscopy.[145–151] Absent AE1 immunoreactivity has been observed in some of these patients as well.[146,148,150,151] Pathogenic mechanisms underlying the absence of H^+-ATPase and AE1 have not been fully elucidated. For example, it is unclear to what degree cellular and/

TABLE 54.5 **Recent Studies of Renal Involvement in a Series of Patients with Primary Sjögren Syndrome**

	Pertovaara et al.[134]	Aasarod et al.[130]	Goules et al.[132]	Bossini et al.[131]	Ren et al.[135]	Maripuri et al.[133]	Lin et al.[119]
Year published	1999	2000	2000	2001	2008	2009	2010
Number of patients	78	62	471	60	130	7276	573
# w/renal involvement			20 (4%) overt	16 (27%)	130	24 (renal bx)	34%
Abnormal renal function	19%	21%	9/18 (50%)	8/60 (13%)	27%	18/24 (75%)	41/573 (7%)
Hypertension			3/20 (15%)	25%	5%	12/24 (50%)	
Proteinuria	44% (<0.5 g/d)	1 microalb	10/20 (50%)	12/60 (20%)		16/24 (67%)	126/573 (22%)
Tubular proteinuria				6/9 by UPEP	21%		
Nephrotic proteinuria				2/60	6%	2/24 (8%)	
Distal RTA	18/55 (33%)		12/20 (60%)		70%	7/24 (29%)	88/ 573 (15%)
Complete	2	7%		3/60 (5%)	51%		
Incomplete	16	5%			19%		
Renal calculi	2/78 (3%)	8%	4/20 (20%)	2/60 (3%)		17%	45/481 (9%[a])
Nephrocalcinosis		2		1			
Proximal RTA						1/24 (4%)	8/573 (1%)
Fanconi syndrome					3%	1/24 (4%)	
Hypokalemia		1/62		4/60 (7%)	47%	1/24 (4%)	
Hypokalemic paralysis				1/60	7%		
Nephrogenic DI		21%	12/20 (60%)	10/48 (21%)	2%		
Interstitial nephritis (IN)	1/3 biopsied		9/18 (50%)	6/9	31/41	71%	21/64
Glomerulonephritis (GN)	2/3		8/18 (44%)	3/9	8/41	29%	23/64
IN + GN			1/18 (6%)				18/64

[a] Kidney stones ± renal calcification.
bx, biopsy; microalb, microalbuminuria; UPEP, urine protein electrophoresis; RTA, renal tubular acidosis; DI, diabetes insipidus.

or autoantibody-mediated mechanisms are involved. A cell-mediated inflammatory process could disrupt key transporters in α-intercalated cells, but several investigators have pointed out that inflammatory tubulointerstitial infiltrates have not been seen consistently in Sjögren patients with distal RTA.[140,148] This could represent a kidney biopsy sampling artifact, or humoral mechanisms may be involved. Autoantibodies directed against α-intercalated cells have been detected in a Sjögren patient with secretory defect distal RTA.[147]

Furthermore, Takemoto and colleagues[152,153] have recently shown that high titers of autoantibody against carbonic-anhydrase-II may contribute to the pathogenesis of RTA in primary Sjögren syndrome. Carbonic anhydrase II is found in proximal and distal renal tubular epithelial cells where it plays an important role in the bicarbonate reabsorption and regeneration. Takemoto and colleagues[152] found significantly higher serum anti–carbonic-anhydrase-II levels in 13 patients with primary Sjögren syndrome diagnosed with distal RTA (that was confirmed by the ammonium chloride loading test in 7), compared to 33 Sjögren patients without RTA and 19 normal controls. By multivariate logistic regression analysis, anti–carbonic-anhydrase-II antibody levels and the duration of disease were each independently associated with the presence of RTA. This group of investigators has also shown that mice immunized to produce high titers of anti–carbonic-anhydrase-II antibody develop a urinary acidification defect that is consistent with incomplete distal RTA.[153] These observations raise the interesting possibility that autoantibodies to H^+-ATPase, AE1, and/or carbonic-anhydrase-II may contribute to RTA observed in these patients.

Proximal Renal Tubular Acidosis and Fanconi Syndrome

As illustrated in Table 54.5, proximal RTA and Fanconi syndrome are reported much less often among patients with primary Sjögren syndrome compared to distal RTA. It is interesting to speculate whether autoantibodies against anti–carbonic-anhydrase-II or membrane proteins, such as β-fodrin,[154] as well as cell-mediated injury, might contribute to the development of proximal RTA and Fanconi syndrome in these patients. Recent reviews have identified approximately a dozen case reports of primary Sjögren syndrome with features of proximal tubular dysfunction consistent with Fanconi syndrome and proximal RTA (in most).[155,156] Of note, many of these patients also manifested abnormalities in distal tubular function, compatible with distal RTA and/or nephrogenic diabetes insipidus. Phosphaturia was observed frequently among these cases and in other series of patients with Sjögren syndrome,[136,138] and may contribute to the development of osteomalacia, which is seen in some patients with primary Sjögren syndrome.[157,158] Supportive treatment for Fanconi syndrome includes supplements to correct metabolic acidosis, hypokalemia, and hypophosphatemia. Five of the 10 patients reviewed by Wang et al.[156] were also treated with Immunosuppressants (low-to-intermediate dose prednisolone in 4 patients and mycophenolate mofetil [1g per day] in 1 patient). Although many of these patients showed signs of improved tubular (and glomerular) function following immunosuppression, no studies have compared the value of immunosuppression to supportive therapy. Furthermore, it is important to weigh the risks of immunosuppression, including the risk that corticosteroids may aggravate the bone disease that may occur in Sjögren patients with renal tubular acidosis and Fanconi syndrome.[157,158]

Hypokalemic Paralysis

Patients with primary Sjögren syndrome are at risk for developing hypokalemia as a complication of immune-mediated interstitial nephritis and RTA.[159] It is noteworthy that a substantial number of these patients have presented with severe hypokalemia complicated by paralysis, respiratory failure, and/or cardiac arrest.[135,160,161] For example, in Ren et al.'s[135] study of 130 Sjögren patients with previously recognized renal involvement, 61 (47%) had hypokalemia and 9 consulted a nephrologist because of hypokalemic paralysis; 1 died following a cardiac arrest. Soy and colleagues[161] identified 18 cases of hypokalemic periodic paralysis associated with Sjögren syndrome in a Medline search of the literature between 1966 and 2004; 3 experienced respiratory arrest. Seven patients, including the 3 who experienced respiratory arrest, were treated with glucocorticoids. Although electrolyte and alkali replacement therapy was successful in many patients, corticosteroids (occasionally in combination with another immunosuppressant) have been recommended for patients with severe, persistent, or recurring manifestations of profound hypokalemia.[160,161]

Bartter Syndrome and Gitelman Syndrome

Small numbers of Sjögren patients have been described who have these rare tubular disorders.[162–167] In two cases, sequencing of the Na^+/Cl^- cotransporter (NCCT) gene showed that Gitelman syndrome was acquired, not inherited.[163,165] In the kidney biopsy sample of one of those patients, NCCT could not be detected in the distal convoluted tubules by immunohistochemical staining.[165] Incubation of that patient's serum with a normal mouse kidney showed a pattern of reactivity, which suggested that she had developed circulating autoantibodies to NCCT.[165]

Nephrogenic Diabetes Insipidus

Aasarod et al.[130] and Bossini et al.[131] studied cohorts of patients with primary Sjögren syndrome who were not specifically selected because they were previously known to have kidney disease. Each found that about 20% of their Sjögren patients had urinary concentrating abnormalities consistent with nephrogenic diabetes insipidus. In many of these cases, the urine was concentrated after water deprivation and the administration of DDAVP, but urine osmolality failed to reach normal maximum age-adjusted values. Consequently, for these patients, the urine concentrating defect was mild and asymptomatic. Other patients with primary Sjögren syndrome may experience symptomatic nephrogenic diabetes insipidus due to immune-mediate tubular dysfunction or protracted profound hypokalemia. Alternatively, Sjögren patients may induce polyuria by drinking large volumes of fluids to quench their symptoms associated with xerostomia.

Kidney Biopsy Findings

Maripuri and colleagues[133] described the clinical data and the renal pathology of 24 patients with primary Sjögren syndrome who underwent a kidney biopsy at the Mayo Clinic from 1967 to 2007. The predominant lesion was acute or chronic tubulointerstitial nephritis (TIN) in 17 patients (71%) as illustrated in Figure 54.4. Eleven of these patients had chronic TIN, making that the most common kidney biopsy diagnosis. Acute TIN with tubulitis was seen in 6 patients, 4 of whom had RTA. Diverse glomerular lesions were the predominant histologic change in 7 patients. Two had cryoglobulinemic membranoproliferative glomerulonephritis (MPGN); 2 had focal segmental glomerulosclerosis (FSGS), 1 had membranous glomerulonephritis (MGN), 1 had minimal change, and 1 had global glomerulosclerosis. Finally, 1 had chronic TIN and FSGS.

Goules et al.[132] found TIN in 10 patients, MPGN in 5, and mesangial proliferative GN in 4. The tubulointerstitial infiltrates included lymphocytes, plasma cells, and monocytes. The lymphocytes were predominantly CD4+, comparable to those seen in Sjögren salivary gland infiltrates. Many of the patients in the study with GN had mixed monoclonal cryoglobulinemia IgM kappa (IgMκ) and low levels of C4 complement. Two patients with glomerular disease, but none of their patients with isolated TIN, developed end-stage renal failure.

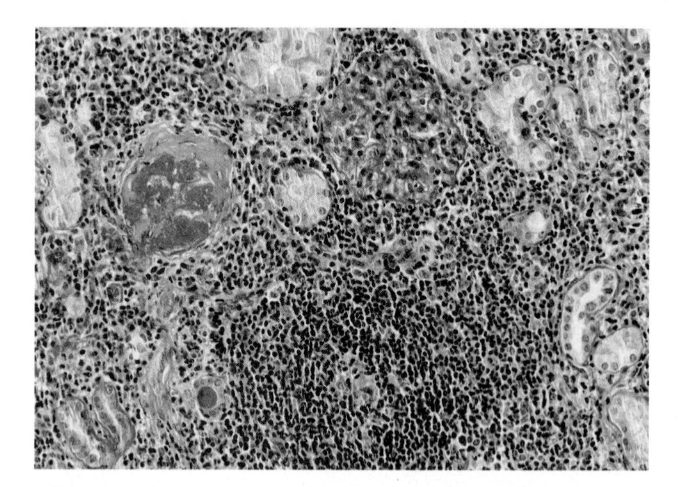

FIGURE 54.4 Severe chronic interstitial nephritis in a patient with Sjögren syndrome. The mononuclear lymphoid cells have infiltrated the interstitium causing extensive tubular atrophy; an obsolescent glomerulus is present indicating the associated nephron damage, but the other viable glomerulus shows no evidence of substantive pathology. Taken using a periodic acid Schiff stain.

Other relatively large studies of kidney biopsies in patients with primary Sjögren syndrome have also shown a diverse range of glomerular lesions, including mesangial proliferative GN, MGN, FSGS, and diffuse or focal proliferative GN.[119,135] The range of glomerular disease possibly associated with primary Sjögren syndrome has been expanded further by case reports of ANCA-positive necrotizing crescentic GN, immunoglobulin A (IgA) nephropathy, amyloidosis, hemolytic uremic syndrome, and thrombotic thrombocytopenic purpura.[168–173] However, the causal relationship of these glomerular lesions with primary Sjögren syndrome is unknown.

Treatment

Ren and colleagues[135] noted that 96 of their 130 primary Sjögren patients with clinically evident renal involvement were treated with immunosuppressants. Approximately two thirds of those treated received corticosteroids alone; the others received an additional immunosuppressive agent, frequently oral or intravenous cyclophosphamide. Although detailed information about the clinical and histologic characteristics of the patients treated with these regimens was not provided, they do specify that renal function improved or normalized following treatment in 25 of 35 patients with an elevated serum creatinine. Four patients progressed to end-stage renal failure, and 4 died (2 from infection, 1 from a cerebrovascular accident, and 1 from lymphoma). They concluded that immunosuppressive therapy may be beneficial for some patients with primary Sjögren syndrome, especially those with major organ system involvement.

Maripuri et al.[133] reported that 20 of their 24 patients were treated with prednisone, often alone and occasionally with cyclophosphamide, mycophenolate mofetil, rituximab, or plasma exchange (for cryoglobulinemia). Immunosuppression was associated with statistically significant improvements in estimated glomerular filtration rate and proteinuria among 17 patients who had more than 3 months of follow-up. Consequently, the authors recommended a course of corticosteroids as first-line therapy for all primary Sjögren patients with active glomerular and/or tubulointerstitial disease. Because this and other studies have not been designed to determine which immunosuppressive regimen has the most favorable risk/benefit ratio, the authors suggested that further immunosuppressive treatments need to be individualized based on clinical and pathology observations as well as the impact of the initial treatment regimen.

Goules et al.[132] indicated that most patients with primary Sjögren syndrome followed at the universities of Ioannina and Athens, Greece were treated according to a somewhat different strategy. Goules and colleagues noted that 9 of 10 patients with glomerular disease (confirmed by kidney biopsy in all but 1) received immunosuppression with methylprednisolone alone in 2 cases, methylprednisolone and azathioprine in 1 case, and methylprednisolone and cyclophosphamide in 6 cases. On the other hand, only 3 of 10 patients with TIN received immunosuppression. The authors have observed that the clinical course of TIN in their primary Sjögren patients has been relatively favorable and suggest that kidney biopsy and immunosuppression may not be necessary for many of those patients. On the other hand, they are concerned that the prognosis of primary Sjögren patients with glomerular disease is less favorable. Consequently, kidney biopsy assessment and immunosuppressive treatments should be considered for many of these patients.

POLYMYOSITIS AND DERMATOMYOSITIS

Polymyositis (PM) and dermatomyositis (DM) are part of a heterogeneous group of rare inflammatory myopathies, characterized by muscle weakness and inflammation.[174–177] Among patients with DM and PM, the female to male ratio is approximately 2:1.[178] DM can occur at any age, but PM is rarely seen in children. Muscle biopsies show evidence of autoimmune pathogenesis, mediated predominantly by cytotoxic T lymphocytes in PM and complement-associated microangiopathy in DM. Although DM and PM are often idiopathic conditions, they may be seen in association with various cancers or other autoimmune conditions.[179] Patients with PM and DM typically present with symmetric proximal muscle weakness that evolves over several weeks to months and causes difficulty with a range of activities including climbing stairs, getting out of a chair, and performing tasks overhead. Distal muscles may be affected late in the course of the disease. In contrast to myasthenia, extraocular muscles are spared. Sensation is normal, and deep tendon reflexes are intact unless the relevant muscles are extremely weak.

Recognition of DM is often facilitated by characteristic cutaneous manifestations that are typically seen before or coincident with the development of muscle weakness. The heliotrope rash (a purplish discoloration of the eyelids) and Gottron papules (a scaly erythematous eruption on the extensor surfaces of the hands and fingers) are considered pathognomonic for DM.[177] Lacking a pathognomonic clinical sign, the diagnosis of PM may be more difficult. Muscle biopsy is needed to establish a definitive diagnosis of DM or PM and to rule out conditions that mimic myositis, including a broad range of muscular dystrophies, metabolic diseases, mitochondrial disorders, and neurologic diseases.[174] Infectious, endocrine, and drug-induced etiologies must be considered as well.

PM and DM are systemic autoimmune conditions that often affect extramuscular systems including the lungs, heart, and gastrointestinal tract, as well as the skin and joints. Pulmonary manifestations (including interstitial lung disease, respiratory muscle weakness, and aspiration pneumonia) are common causes of morbidity and mortality among patients with PM and DM.[180,181] Antibodies against amino-tRNA-synthetases (e.g., anti-Jo-1) are strongly associated with interstitial lung disease, as well as fever, arthritis, characteristic hyperkeratotic lesions along the fingers called mechanic's hands, and Raynaud phenomenon; this constellation constitutes antisynthetase syndrome.[174,177] Cardiac involvement may cause conduction abnormalities, arrhythmias, or congestive heart failure in some cases. Gastrointestinal manifestations include dysphagia, aspiration, delayed gastric emptying, and rarely, intestinal vasculitis. Joint involvement typically leads to nondeforming symmetric arthritis.

Kidney Disorders in Patients with Polymyositis and Dermatomyositis

In general, two types of renal involvement have been described among patients with DM or PM. If severe, myositis may cause myoglobinemia, myoglobinuria, and acute kidney injury.[182–184] Furthermore, various glomerular diseases have been reported, though rarely (particularly, mesangial proliferative GN in PM and membranous nephropathy as well as mesangial proliferative GN in DM).[184–189] The presence of glomerular disease in patients with DM and PM should prompt careful, serial evaluations to rule out the concurrence of another collagen vascular disease or a malignancy that may underlie the development of glomerulopathy in these patients.

It is difficult to describe the scope and frequency of renal involvement in patients with DM and PM because there are very few studies that have examined renal parameters in a cohort of myositis patients who were not selected for the presence of kidney disease. A recent study of 65 Taiwanese patients with DM or PM (admitted to the Chang Gung Memorial Hospital in Taipei, Taiwan between 1992 and 2002) provides an interesting perspective.[184] Yen and colleagues[184] found that 14 of 65 patients (22%) had evidence of renal involvement. Five of these patients had PM; 1 had moderate proteinuria and was considered to have SLE as well. Four PM patients died suddenly because of severe hyperkalemia due to rhabdomyolysis and myoglobinuric acute renal failure. Of the 9 DM patients with renal involvement, 3 had a concurrent autoimmune condition (SLE +/or rheumatoid arthritis), and 1 had cancer. Five DM patients developed myoglobinuric acute renal failure; 4 required hemodialysis.

Myoglobinuric Acute Renal Failure

Overall, Yen and colleagues[184] observed acute tubular necrosis due to rhabdomyolysis in 9 of their 65 patients (14%) with DM or PM; 4 died suddenly because of hyperkalemia and metabolic acidosis. The incidence of these adverse events was surprisingly high and underscores the importance of careful monitoring and preventive measures. Several clinical features may increase the risk of these complications, including an unusually acute presentation of myositis, a poor response to immunosuppressive therapy, and comorbid conditions that impair renal perfusion and the clearance of myoglobin. Treatment typically includes immunosuppression to quell immune-mediated muscle injury and hydration to optimize renal blood flow and maintain a dilute diuresis. Alkalinization of the urine to inhibit pigment cast formation should be considered as well. Hemodialysis may be required to manage acute renal failure, hyperkalemia, hyperphosphatemia, and/or metabolic acidosis if standard medical interventions are not effective.

Glomerular Disease

Several reviews of the literature have found very small numbers of patients with DM or PM who had glomerular disease without evidence of an associated systemic autoimmune condition or a malignancy.[185–188] There are case reports of approximately a dozen patients with PM who had mesangial proliferative glomerulonephritis and about a half dozen patients with DM who had membranous nephropathy. Smaller numbers of patients with PM were noted to have membranous nephropathy, crescentic glomerulonephritis, or focal glomerulosclerosis. A few patients with DM were reported to have mesangial proliferative glomerulonephritis, diffuse proliferative glomerulonephritis, or IgA nephropathy.

Given the small number of patients with DM or PM who have developed glomerular disease, it is important to look for a concurrent systemic autoimmune disease, such as SLE, Sjögren syndrome, vasculitis, rheumatoid arthritis, systemic sclerosis, and MCTD. Patients with MCTD typically have anti-U1 ribonucleoprotein (RNP) antibodies and overlapping features of SLE, PM, and systemic sclerosis, but this constellation of characteristic findings may evolve slowly over several years before the diagnosis is evident. Renal involvement has been described in 10% to 50% of MCTD patients. Membranous nephropathy has been the most common glomerular lesion, but mesangial proliferative GN, MPGN, SRC, vasculitis, and collapsing glomerulopathy have been reported as well.[190,191]

A number of studies have shown that patients with DM and PM are at an increased risk for a broad range of malignancies.[192] Buchbinder and colleagues[193] studied the risk of cancer in a large cohort of patients with biopsy-proven DM or PM; they found a sixfold increased risk among patients with DM and a twofold increased risk among those with PM compared to the general population after adjusting for age and gender. The risk of malignancy gradually declined over 5 years after the diagnosis of myositis, but remained statistically elevated for colorectal and pancreatic cancer beyond more than 5 years of follow-up among patients with DM in a pooled analysis of three large Scandinavian studies.[194] These observations underscore the diagnostic challenge presented by patients with DM or PM, who may also have one of the glomerular diseases that have been associated with an increased risk of malignancy. Several cancer-screening strategies have been proposed, but additional studies are needed to refine our approach to the evaluation of these patients.[174,195]

ACKNOWLEDGMENTS

This work was supported in part by the Intramural Research Program of the National Institutes of Health (NIH) and the National Institute of Diabetes and Digestive and Kidney Diseases (NIDDK).

REFERENCES

1. LeRoy EC, Black C, Fleischmajer R et al. Scleroderma (systemic sclerosis): classification, subsets and pathogenesis. *J Rheumatol.* 1988;15(2):202–205.

2. Walker JG, Ahern MJ, Smith MD, et al. Scleroderma renal crisis: poor outcome despite aggressive antihypertensive treatment. *Intern Med J.* 2003;33(5–6):216–220.

3. Chifflot H, Fautrel B, Sordet C, Chatelus E, Sibilia J. Incidence and prevalence of systemic sclerosis: a systematic literature review. *Semin Arthritis Rheum.* 2008;37(4):223–235.

4. Ranque B, Mouthon L. Geoepidemiology of systemic sclerosis. *Autoimmun Rev.* 2010;9(5):A311–A318.

5. Granel B, Bernard F, Chevillard C. Genetic susceptibility to systemic sclerosis from clinical aspect to genetic factor analyses. *Eur J Intern Med.* 2009;20(3):242–252.

6. Radic M, Martinovic KD, Radic J. Infectious disease as aetiological factor in the pathogenesis of systemic sclerosis. *Neth J Med.* 2010;68(11):348–353.

7. Romano E, Manetti M, Guiducci S, et al. The genetics of systemic sclerosis: an update. *Clin Exp Rheumatol.* 2011;29(2 Suppl 65):S75–S86.

8. Hunzelmann N, Krieg T. Scleroderma: from pathophysiology to novel therapeutic approaches. *Exp Dermatol.* 2010;19(5):393–400.

9. Katsumoto TR, Whitfield ML, Connolly MK. The pathogenesis of systemic sclerosis. *Annu Rev Pathol.* 2011;6:509–537.

10. Manetti M, Guiducci S, Ibba-Manneschi L, Matucci-Cerinic M. Mechanisms in the loss of capillaries in systemic sclerosis: angiogenesis versus vasculogenesis. *J Cell Mol Med.* 2010;14(6A):1241–1254.

11. Yamamoto T. Scleroderma—pathophysiology. *Eur J Dermatol.* 2009;19(1):14–24.

12. Kahaleh MB, LeRoy EC. Autoimmunity and vascular involvement in systemic sclerosis (SSc). *Autoimmunity.* 1999;31(3):195–214.

13. Fleming JN, Schwartz SM. The pathology of scleroderma vascular disease. *Rheum Dis Clin North Am.* 2008;34(1):41–55.

14. Distler JH, Jungel A, Pileckyte M, et al. Hypoxia-induced increase in the production of extracellular matrix proteins in systemic sclerosis. *Arthritis Rheum.* 2007;56(12):4203–4215.

15. Higgins DF, Kimura K, Bernhardt WM, et al. Hypoxia promotes fibrogenesis in vivo via HIF-1 stimulation of epithelial-to-mesenchymal transition. *J Clin Invest.* 2007;117(12):3810–3820.

16. Bosello S, De LG, Tolusso B, et al. B cells in systemic sclerosis: a possible target for therapy. *Autoimmun Rev.* 2011;10(10):624–630.

17. Baroni SS, Santillo M, Bevilacqua F, et al. Stimulatory autoantibodies to the PDGF receptor in systemic sclerosis. *N Engl J Med.* 2006;354(25):2667–2676.

18. Penn H, Howie AJ, Kingdon EJ, et al. Scleroderma renal crisis: patient characteristics and long-term outcomes. *QJM.* 2007;100(8):485–494.

19. Haviv YS, Safadi R. Normotensive scleroderma renal crisis: case report and review of the literature. *Ren Fail.* 1998;20(5):733–736.

20. Helfrich DJ, Banner B, Steen VD, Medsger TA Jr. Normotensive renal failure in systemic sclerosis. *Arthritis Rheum.* 1989;32(9):1128–1134.

21. Teixeira L, Mouthon L, Mahr A, et al. Mortality and risk factors of scleroderma renal crisis: a French retrospective study of 50 patients. *Ann Rheum Dis.* 2008;67(1):110–116.

22. Steen VD. Scleroderma renal crisis. *Rheum Dis Clin North Am.* 2003;29(2):315–333.

23. Steen VD, Medsger TA Jr. Case-control study of corticosteroids and other drugs that either precipitate or protect from the development of scleroderma renal crisis. *Arthritis Rheum.* 1998;41(9):1613–1619.

24. Tormey VJ, Bunn CC, Denton CP, Black CM. Anti-fibrillarin antibodies in systemic sclerosis. *Rheumatology (Oxford).* 2001;40(10):1157–1162.

25. Gavras H, Gavras I, Cannon PJ, Brunner HR, Laragh JH. Is elevated plasma renin activity of prognostic importance in progressive systemic sclerosis? *Arch Intern Med.* 1977;137(11):1554–1558.

26. Steen VD, Medsger TA Jr, Osial TA Jr, et al. Factors predicting development of renal involvement in progressive systemic sclerosis. *Am J Med.* 1984;76(5):779–786.

27. Clements PJ, Lachenbruch PA, Furst DE, et al. Abnormalities of renal physiology in systemic sclerosis. A prospective study with 10-year followup. *Arthritis Rheum.* 1994;37(1):67–74.

28. Fleischmajer R, Gould AB. Serum renin and renin substrate levels in scleroderma. *Proc Soc Exp Biol Med.* 1975;150(2):374–379.

29. Kadono T, Kikuchi K, Sato S, et al. Elevated plasma endothelin levels in systemic sclerosis. *Arch Dermatol Res.* 1995;287(5):439–442.

30. Kobayashi H, Nishimaki T, Kaise S, et al. Immunohistological study endothelin-1 and endothelin-A and B receptors in two patients with scleroderma renal crisis. *Clin Rheumatol.* 1999;18(5):425–427.

31. Mouthon L, Mehrenberger M, Teixeira L, et al. Endothelin-1 expression in scleroderma renal crisis. *Hum Pathol.* 2011;42(1):95–102.

32. Batal I, Domsic RT, Medsger TA, Bastacky S. Scleroderma renal crisis: a pathology perspective. *Int J Rheumatol.* 2010;2010:543704.

33. Donohoe JF. Scleroderma and the kidney. *Kidney Int.* 1992;41(2):462–477.

34. Caskey FJ, Thacker EJ, Johnston PA, Barnes JN. Failure of losartan to control blood pressure in scleroderma renal crisis. *Lancet.* 1997;349(9052):620.

35. Steen VD, Medsger TA Jr. Long-term outcomes of scleroderma renal crisis. *Ann Intern Med.* 2000;133(8):600–603.

36. Denton CP, Black CM. Scleroderma—clinical and pathological advances. *Best Pract Res Clin Rheumatol.* 2004;18(3):271–290.

37. Scorza R, Rivolta R, Mascagni B, et al. Effect of iloprost infusion on the resistance index of renal vessels of patients with systemic sclerosis. *J Rheumatol.* 1997;24(10):1944–1948.

38. Shor R, Halabe A. New trends in the treatment of scleroderma renal crisis. *Nephron.* 2002;92(3):716–718.

38a. 2009 Abstracts of the American College of Rheumatology, Annual Scientific Meeting, October 16–21, 2009, Philadelphia, PA. Arthritis & Rheumatism, 60:1. Suppl 10:451.

39. Steen VD, Costantino JP, Shapiro AP, Medsger TA Jr. Outcome of renal crisis in systemic sclerosis: relation to availability of angiotensin converting enzyme (ACE) inhibitors. *Ann Intern Med.* 1990;113(5):352–357.

40. Tsakiris D, Simpson HK, Jones EH, et al. Report on management of renal failure in Europe, XXVI, 1995. Rare diseases in renal replacement therapy in the ERA-EDTA Registry. *Nephrol Dial Transplant.* 1996;11(Suppl 7):4–20.

41. Bleyer AJ, Tell GS, Evans GW, Ettinger WH Jr, Burkart JM. Survival of patients undergoing renal replacement therapy in one center with special emphasis on racial differences. *Am J Kidney Dis.* 1996;28(1):72–81.

42. Pham PT, Pham PC, Danovitch GM, et al. Predictors and risk factors for recurrent scleroderma renal crisis in the kidney allograft: case report and review of the literature. *Am J Transplant.* 2005;5(10):2565–2569.

43. Anders HJ, Wiebecke B, Haedecke C, et al. MPO-ANCA-Positive crescentic glomerulonephritis: a distinct entity of scleroderma renal disease? *Am J Kidney Dis.* 1999;33(4):e3.

44. Arad U, Balbir-Gurman A, Doenyas-Barak K, et al. Anti-neutrophil antibody associated vasculitis in systemic sclerosis. *Semin Arthritis Rheum.* 2011 [Epub ahead of print].

45. Arnaud L, Huart A, Plaisier E, et al. ANCA-related crescentic glomerulonephritis in systemic sclerosis: revisiting the "normotensive scleroderma renal crisis". *Clin Nephrol.* 2007;68(3):165–170.

46. Endo H, Hosono T, Kondo H. Antineutrophil cytoplasmic autoantibodies in 6 patients with renal failure and systemic sclerosis. *J Rheumatol.* 1994;21(5):864–870.

47. Katrib A, Sturgess A, Bertouch JV. Systemic sclerosis and antineutrophil cytoplasmic autoantibody-associated renal failure. *Rheumatol Int.* 1999;19(1–2):61–63.

48. Tomioka M, Hinoshita F, Miyauchi N, et al. ANCA-related crescentic glomerulonephritis in a patient with scleroderma without marked dermatological change and malignant hypertension. *Intern Med.* 2004;43(6):496–502.

49. Ruffatti A, Sinico RA, Radice A, et al. Autoantibodies to proteinase 3 and myeloperoxidase in systemic sclerosis. *J Rheumatol.* 2002;29(5):918–923.

50. Akimoto S, Ishikawa O, Tamura T, Miyachi Y. Antineutrophil cytoplasmic autoantibodies in patients with systemic sclerosis. *Br J Dermatol.* 1996;134(3):407–410.

51. Locke IC, Worrall JG, Leaker B, Black CM, Cambridge G. Autoantibodies to myeloperoxidase in systemic sclerosis. *J Rheumatol.* 1997;24(1):86–89.

52. D'Angelo WA, Fries JF, Masi AT, Shulman LE. Pathologic observations in systemic sclerosis (scleroderma). A study of fifty-eight autopsy cases and fifty-eight matched controls. *Am J Med.* 1969;46(3):428–440.

53. Kingdon EJ, Knight CJ, Dustan K, et al. Calculated glomerular filtration rate is a useful screening tool to identify scleroderma patients with renal impairment. *Rheumatology (Oxford).* 2003;42(1):26–33.

54. Livi R, Teghini L, Pignone A, et al. Renal functional reserve is impaired in patients with systemic sclerosis without clinical signs of kidney involvement. *Ann Rheum Dis.* 2002;61(8):682–686.

55. Mohamed RH, Zayed HS, Amin A. Renal disease in systemic sclerosis with normal serum creatinine. *Clin Rheumatol.* 2010;29(7):729–737.

56. Rivolta R, Mascagni B, Berruti V, et al. Renal vascular damage in systemic sclerosis patients without clinical evidence of nephropathy. *Arthritis Rheum.* 1996;39(6):1030–1034.

57. Steen VD, Syzd A, Johnson JP, Greenberg A, Medsger TA Jr. Kidney disease other than renal crisis in patients with diffuse scleroderma. *J Rheumatol.* 2005;32(4):649–655.

58. Trostle DC, Bedetti CD, Steen VD, et al. Renal vascular histology and morphometry in systemic sclerosis. A case-control autopsy study. *Arthritis Rheum.* 1988;31(3):393–400.

59. Steen VD, Blair S, Medsger TA Jr. The toxicity of D-penicillamine in systemic sclerosis. *Ann Intern Med.* 1986;104(5):699–705.

60. Hall CL. The natural course of gold and penicillamine nephropathy: a longterm study of 54 patients. *Adv Exp Med Biol.* 1989;252:247–256.

61. Hall CL, Jawad S, Harrison PR, et al. Natural course of penicillamine nephropathy: a long term study of 33 patients. *Br Med J (Clin Res Ed).* 1988;296(6629): 1083–1086.

62. Karpinski J, Jothy S, Radoux V, Levy M, Baran D. D-penicillamine-induced crescentic glomerulonephritis and antimyeloperoxidase antibodies in a patient with scleroderma. Case report and review of the literature. *Am J Nephrol.* 1997; 17(6):528–532.

63. Campo A, Mathai SC, Le PJ, et al. Hemodynamic predictors of survival in scleroderma-related pulmonary arterial hypertension. *Am J Respir Crit Care Med.* 2010;182(2):252–260.

64. Bryan C, Knight C, Black CM, Silman AJ. Prediction of five-year survival following presentation with scleroderma: development of a simple model using three disease factors at first visit. *Arthritis Rheum.* 1999;42(12):2660–2665.

65. Seiberlich B, Hunzelmann N, Krieg T, Weber M, Schulze-Lohoff E. Intermediate molecular weight proteinuria and albuminuria identify scleroderma patients with increased morbidity. *Clin Nephrol.* 2008;70(2):110–117.

66. Tyndall AJ, Bannert B, Vonk M, et al. Causes and risk factors for death in systemic sclerosis: a study from the EULAR Scleroderma Trials and Research (EUSTAR) database. *Ann Rheum Dis.* 2010;69(10):1809–1815.

67. Manno R, Boin F. Immunotherapy of systemic sclerosis. *Immunotherapy.* 2010;2(6):863–878.

68. Asano Y. Future treatments in systemic sclerosis. *J Dermatol.* 2010;37(1): 54–70.

69. Milanetti F, Bucha J, Testori A, Burt RK. Autologous hematopoietic stem cell transplantation for systemic sclerosis. *Curr Stem Cell Res Ther.* 2011; 6(1):16–28.

70. Farge D, Passweg J, van Laar JM, et al. Autologous stem cell transplantation in the treatment of systemic sclerosis: report from the EBMT/EULAR Registry. *Ann Rheum Dis.* 2004;63(8):974–981.

71. McSweeney PA, Nash RA, Sullivan KM, et al. High-dose immunosuppressive therapy for severe systemic sclerosis: initial outcomes. *Blood.* 2002; 100(5):1602–1610.

72. Nash RA, McSweeney PA, Crofford LJ, et al. High-dose immunosuppressive therapy and autologous hematopoietic cell transplantation for severe systemic sclerosis: long-term follow-up of the US multicenter pilot study. *Blood.* 2007;110(4):1388–1396.

73. Oyama Y, Barr WG, Statkute L, et al. Autologous non-myeloablative hematopoietic stem cell transplantation in patients with systemic sclerosis. *Bone Marrow Transplant.* 2007;40(6):549–555.

74. Tsukamoto H, Nagafuji K, Horiuchi T, et al. A phase I-II trial of autologous peripheral blood stem cell transplantation in the treatment of refractory autoimmune disease. *Ann Rheum Dis.* 2006;65(4):508–514.

75. McInnes IB, O'Dell JR. State-of-the-art: rheumatoid arthritis. *Ann Rheum Dis.* 2010;69(11):1898–1906.

76. Myasoedova E, Davis JM III, Crowson CS, Gabriel SE. Epidemiology of rheumatoid arthritis: rheumatoid arthritis and mortality. *Curr Rheumatol Rep.* 2010;12(5):379–385.

77. Klarenbeek NB, Kerstens PJ, Huizinga TW, Dijkmans BA, Allaart CF. Recent advances in the management of rheumatoid arthritis. *BMJ.* 2010;341:c6942.

78. Tak PP, Kalden JR. Advances in rheumatology: new targeted therapeutics. *Arthritis Res Ther.* 2011;13(Suppl 1):S5.

79. Brun C, Olsen TS, Raaschou F, Sorensen AW. Renal biopsy in rheumatoid arthritis. *Nephron.* 1965;2(2):65–81.

80. Bulger RJ, Healey LA, Polinsky P. Renal abnormalities in rheumatoid arthritis. *Ann Rheum Dis.* 1968;27(4):339–344.

81. Karstila K, Korpela M, Sihvonen S, Mustonen J. Prognosis of clinical renal disease and incidence of new renal findings in patients with rheumatoid arthritis: follow-up of a population-based study. *Clin Rheumatol.* 2007;26(12):2089–2095.

82. Adu D, Berisa F, Howie AJ, et al. Glomerulonephritis in rheumatoid arthritis. *Br J Rheumatol.* 1993;32(11):1008–1011.

83. Helin HJ, Korpela MM, Mustonen JT, Pasternack AI. Renal biopsy findings and clinicopathologic correlations in rheumatoid arthritis. *Arthritis Rheum.* 1995;38(2):242–247.

84. Nakano M, Ueno M, Nishi S, et al. Analysis of renal pathology and drug history in 158 Japanese patients with rheumatoid arthritis. *Clin Nephrol.* 1998;50(3):154–160.

85. Sellars L, Siamopoulos K, Wilkinson R, Leohapand T, Morley AR. Renal biopsy appearances in rheumatoid disease. *Clin Nephrol.* 1983;20(3):114–120.

86. Kelly CA, Mooney P, Hordon LD, Griffiths ID. Haematuria in rheumatoid arthritis: a follow up study. *Ann Rheum Dis.* 1988;47(12):993–994.

87. Katz WA, Blodgett RC Jr, Pietrusko RG. Proteinuria in gold-treated rheumatoid arthritis. *Ann Intern Med*. 1984;101(2):176–179.

88. Honkanen E, Tornroth T, Pettersson E, Skrifvars B. Membranous glomerulonephritis in rheumatoid arthritis not related to gold or D-penicillamine therapy: a report of four cases and review of the literature. *Clin Nephrol*. 1987;27(2):87–93.

89. Hoshino J, Ubara Y, Hara S, et al. Outcome and treatment of bucillamine-induced nephropathy. *Nephron Clin Pract*. 2006;104(1):c15–c19.

90. Obayashi M, Uzu T, Harada T, et al. Clinical course of bucillamine-induced nephropathy in patients with rheumatoid arthritis. *Clin Exp Nephrol*. 2003;7(4):275–278.

91. Samuels B, Lee JC, Engleman EP, Hopper J Jr. Membranous nephropathy in patients with rheumatoid arthritis: relationship to gold therapy. *Medicine (Baltimore)*. 1978;57(4):319–327.

92. Yoshida A, Morozumi K, Takeda A, Koyama K, Oikawa T. Membranous glomerulonephritis in patients with rheumatoid arthritis. *Clin Ther*. 1994;16(6):1000–1006.

93. Cohen AS. Amyloidosis associated with rheumatoid arthritis. *Med Clin North Am*. 1968;52(3):643–653.

94. Koivuniemi R, Paimela L, Suomalainen R, Tornroth T, Leirisalo-Repo M. Amyloidosis is frequently undetected in patients with rheumatoid arthritis. *Amyloid*. 2008;15(4):262–268.

95. Okuda Y, Yamada T, Matsuura M, Takasugi K, Goto M. Ageing: a risk factor for amyloid A amyloidosis in rheumatoid arthritis. *Amyloid*. 2011; 18(3):108–111.

96. Immonen K, Finne P, Gronhagen-Riska C, et al. A marked decline in the incidence of renal replacement therapy for amyloidosis associated with inflammatory rheumatic diseases - data from nationwide registries in Finland. *Amyloid*. 2011;18(1):25–28.

97. Chevrel G, Jenvrin C, McGregor B, Miossec P. Renal type AA amyloidosis associated with rheumatoid arthritis: a cohort study showing improved survival on treatment with pulse cyclophosphamide. *Rheumatology (Oxford)*. 2001;40(7):821–825.

98. Nakamura T, Higashi S, Tomoda K, Tsukano M, Baba S. Efficacy of etanercept in patients with AA amyloidosis secondary to rheumatoid arthritis. *Clin Exp Rheumatol*. 2007;25(4):518–522.

99. Nakamura T, Higashi S, Tomoda K, Tsukano M, Shono M. Etanercept can induce resolution of renal deterioration in patients with amyloid A amyloidosis secondary to rheumatoid arthritis. *Clin Rheumatol*. 2010;29(12):1395–1401.

100. Harada A, Tomita Y, Yamamoto H, et al. Renal amyloidosis associated with crescentic glomerulonephritis. *Am J Nephrol*. 1984;4(1):52–55.

101. Nagata M, Shimokama T, Harada A, Koyama A, Watanabe T. Glomerular crescents in renal amyloidosis: an epiphenomenon or distinct pathology? *Pathol Int*. 2001;51(3):179–186.

102. Alonso R, Novoa D, Alonso MC, et al. Nonamyloidotic fibrillar glomerulopathy and rheumatoid arthritis. *Nephron*. 1993;63(1):120–121.

103. Rosenstock JL, Markowitz GS, Valeri AM, et al. Fibrillary and immunotactoid glomerulonephritis: distinct entities with different clinical and pathologic features. *Kidney Int*. 2003;63(4):1450–1461.

104. Breedveld FC, Valentijn RM, Westedt ML, Weening JJ. Rapidly progressive glomerulonephritis with glomerular crescent formation in rheumatoid arthritis. *Clin Rheumatol*. 1985;4(3):353–359.

105. Kuznetsky KA, Schwartz MM, Lohmann LA, Lewis EJ. Necrotizing glomerulonephritis in rheumatoid arthritis. *Clin Nephrol*. 1986;26(5):257–264.

106. Goto A, Mukai M, Notoya A, Kohno M. Rheumatoid arthritis complicated with myeloperoxidase antineutrophil cytoplasmic antibody (MPO-ANCA)-associated vasculitis: a case report. *Mod Rheumatol*. 2005;15(2):118–122.

107. Messiaen T, M'bappe P, Boffa JJ, et al. MPO-ANCA necrotizing glomerulonephritis related to rheumatoid arthritis. *Am J Kidney Dis*. 1998;32(5):E6.

108. Mustila A, Korpela M, Mustonen J, et al. Perinuclear antineutrophil cytoplasmic antibody in rheumatoid arthritis: a marker of severe disease with associated nephropathy. *Arthritis Rheum*. 1997;40(4):710–717.

109. Harper L, Cockwell P, Howie AJ, et al. Focal segmental necrotizing glomerulonephritis in rheumatoid arthritis. *QJM*. 1997;90(2):125–132.

110. Zhu LJ, Yang X, Yu XQ. Anti-TNF-alpha therapies in systemic lupus erythematosus. *J Biomed Biotechnol*. 2010;2010:465898.

111. Kaneko K, Nanki T, Hosoya T, Mizoguchi F, Miyasaka N. Etanercept-induced necrotizing crescentic glomerulonephritis in two patients with rheumatoid arthritis. *Mod Rheumatol*. 2010;20(6):632–636.

112. Simms R, Kipgen D, Dahill S, Marshall D, Rodger RS. ANCA-associated renal vasculitis following anti-tumor necrosis factor alpha therapy. *Am J Kidney Dis*. 2008;51(3):e11–e14.

113. Stokes MB, Foster K, Markowitz GS, et al. Development of glomerulonephritis during anti-TNF-alpha therapy for rheumatoid arthritis. *Nephrol Dial Transplant*. 2005;20(7):1400–1406.

114. Fox RI. Sjögren's syndrome. *Lancet*. 2005;366(9482):321–331.

115. Tzioufas AG, Voulgarelis M. Update on Sjögren's syndrome autoimmune epithelitis: from classification to increased neoplasias. *Best Pract Res Clin Rheumatol*. 2007;21(6):989–1010.

116. Mavragani CP, Moutsopoulos HM. The geoepidemiology of Sjögren's syndrome. *Autoimmun Rev*. 2010;9(5):A305–A310.

117. Ng KP, Isenberg DA. Sjögren's syndrome: diagnosis and therapeutic challenges in the elderly. *Drugs Aging*. 2008;25(1):19–33.

118. Singer NG, Tomanova-Soltys I, Lowe R. Sjögren's syndrome in childhood. *Curr Rheumatol Rep*. 2008;10(2):147–155.

119. Lin DF, Yan SM, Zhao Y, et al. Clinical and prognostic characteristics of 573 cases of primary Sjögren's syndrome. *Chin Med J (Engl)*. 2010;123(22): 3252–3257.

120. Skopouli FN, Dafni U, Ioannidis JP, Moutsopoulos HM. Clinical evolution, and morbidity and mortality of primary Sjögren's syndrome. *Semin Arthritis Rheum*. 2000;29(5):296–304.

121. Vitali C, Bombardieri S, Moutsopoulos HM, et al. Preliminary criteria for the classification of Sjögren's syndrome. Results of a prospective concerted action supported by the European Community. *Arthritis Rheum*. 1993;36(3):340–347.

122. Vitali C, Bombardieri S, Jonsson R, et al. Classification criteria for Sjögren's syndrome: a revised version of the European criteria proposed by the American-European Consensus Group. *Ann Rheum Dis*. 2002;61(6):554–558.

123. Seror R, Ravaud P, Bowman SJ, et al. EULAR Sjögren's syndrome disease activity index: development of a consensus systemic disease activity index for primary Sjogren's syndrome. *Ann Rheum Dis*. 2010; 69(6):1103–1109.

124. Birnbaum J. Peripheral nervous system manifestations of Sjögren syndrome: clinical patterns, diagnostic paradigms, etiopathogenesis, and therapeutic strategies. *Neurologist*. 2010;16(5):287–297.

125. Chai J, Logigian EL. Neurological manifestations of primary Sjögren's syndrome. *Curr Opin Neurol*. 2010;23(5):509–513.

126. Hatron PY, Tillie-Leblond I, Launay D, et al. Pulmonary manifestations of Sjögren's syndrome. *Presse Med*. 2011;40(1Pt2):e49–e64.

127. Papiris SA, Tsonis IA, Moutsopoulos HM. Sjögren's syndrome. *Semin Respir Crit Care Med*. 2007;28(4):459–471.

128. Voulgarelis M, Skopouli FN. Clinical, immunologic, and molecular factors predicting lymphoma development in Sjögren's syndrome patients. *Clin Rev Allergy Immunol*. 2007;32(3):265–274.

129. Voulgarelis M, Tzioufas AG, Moutsopoulos HM. Mortality in Sjögren's syndrome. *Clin Exp Rheumatol*. 2008;26(5 Suppl 51):S66–S71.

130. Aasarod K, Haga HJ, Berg KJ, Hammerstrom J, Jorstad S. Renal involvement in primary Sjögren's syndrome. *QJM*. 2000;93(5):297–304.

131. Bossini N, Savoldi S, Franceschini F, et al. Clinical and morphological features of kidney involvement in primary Sjögren's syndrome. *Nephrol Dial Transplant* 2001;16(12):2328–2336.

132. Goules A, Masouridi S, Tzioufas AG, et al. Clinically significant and biopsy-documented renal involvement in primary Sjögren syndrome. *Medicine (Baltimore)*. 2000;79(4):241–249.

133. Maripuri S, Grande JP, Osborn TG, et al. Renal involvement in primary Sjögren's syndrome: a clinicopathologic study. *Clin J Am Soc Nephrol*. 2009;4(9):1423–1431.

134. Pertovaara M, Korpela M, Kouri T, Pasternack A. The occurrence of renal involvement in primary Sjögren's syndrome: a study of 78 patients. *Rheumatology (Oxford)*. 1999;38(11):1113–1120.

135. Ren H, Wang WM, Chen XN, et al. Renal involvement and followup of 130 patients with primary Sjögren's syndrome. *J Rheumatol*. 2008;35(2):278–284.

136. Eriksson P, Denneberg T, Larsson L, Lindstrom F. Biochemical markers of renal disease in primary Sjögren's syndrome. *Scand J Urol Nephrol*. 1995; 29(4):383–392.

137. Pokorny G, Sonkodi S, Ivanyi B et al. Renal involvement in patients with primary Sjögren's syndrome. *Scand J Rheumatol*. 1989;18(4):231–234.

138. Shiozawa S, Shiozawa K, Shimizu S, Nakada M, Isobe T, Fujita T. Clinical studies of renal disease in Sjögren's syndrome. *Ann Rheum Dis*. 1987;46(10): 768–772.

139. Siamopoulos KC, Mavridis AK, Elisaf M, Drosos AA, Moutsopoulos HM. Kidney involvement in primary Sjögren's syndrome. *Scand J Rheumatol Suppl*. 1986;61:156–160.

140. Siamopoulos KC, Elisaf M, Drosos AA, Mavridis AA, Moutsopoulos HM. Renal tubular acidosis in primary Sjögren's syndrome. *Clin Rheumatol*. 1992;11(2):226–230.

141. Viergever PP, Swaak TJ. Renal tubular dysfunction in primary Sjögren's syndrome: clinical studies in 27 patients. *Clin Rheumatol*. 1991;10(1):23–27.

142. Vitali C, Tavoni A, Sciuto M, et al. Renal involvement in primary Sjögren's syndrome: a retrospective-prospective study. *Scand J Rheumatol*. 1991;20(2): 132–136.

143. Pertovaara M, Korpela M, Pasternack A. Factors predictive of renal involvement in patients with primary Sjögren's syndrome. *Clin Nephrol*. 2001;56(1):10–18.
144. Talal N, Zisman E, Schur PH. Renal tubular acidosis, glomerulonephritis and immunologic factors in Sjögren's syndrome. *Arthritis Rheum*. 1968;11(6):774–786.
145. Cohen EP, Bastani B, Cohen MR, et al. Absence of H(+)-ATPase in cortical collecting tubules of a patient with Sjögren's syndrome and distal renal tubular acidosis. *J Am Soc Nephrol*. 1992;3(2):264–271.
146. DeFranco PE, Haragsim L, Schmitz PG, Bastani B. Absence of vacuolar H(+)-ATPase pump in the collecting duct of a patient with hypokalemic distal renal tubular acidosis and Sjögren's syndrome. *J Am Soc Nephrol*. 1995;6(2):295–301.
147. Devuyst O, Lemaire M, Mohebbi N, Wagner CA. Autoantibodies against intercalated cells in Sjögren's syndrome. *Kidney Int*. 2009;76(2):229.
148. Han JS, Kim GH, Kim J, et al. Secretory-defect distal renal tubular acidosis is associated with transporter defect in H(+)-ATPase and anion exchanger-1. *J Am Soc Nephrol*. 2002;13(6):1425–1432.
149. Bae EH, Han CW, Lee JH, et al. The case. Hypokalemia associated with nephrocalcinosis. Distal renal tubular acidosis associated with Sjögren's syndrome. *Kidney Int*. 2009;75(4):443–444.
150. Bastani B, Haragsim L, Gluck S, Siamopoulos KC. Lack of H-ATPase in distal nephron causing hypokalaemic distal RTA in a patient with Sjögren's syndrome. *Nephrol Dial Transplant*. 1995;10(6):908–909.
151. Walsh S, Turner CM, Toye A, et al. Immunohistochemical comparison of a case of inherited distal renal tubular acidosis (with a unique AE1 mutation) with an acquired case secondary to autoimmune disease. *Nephrol Dial Transplant*. 2007;22(3):807–812.
152. Takemoto F, Hoshino J, Sawa N, et al. Autoantibodies against carbonic anhydrase II are increased in renal tubular acidosis associated with Sjögren syndrome. *Am J Med*. 2005;118(2):181–184.
153. Takemoto F, Katori H, Sawa N, et al. Induction of anti-carbonic-anhydrase-II antibody causes renal tubular acidosis in a mouse model of Sjögren's syndrome. *Nephron Physiol*. 2007;106(4):63–68.
154. Kuwana M, Okano T, Ogawa Y, Kaburaki J, Kawakami Y. Autoantibodies to the amino-terminal fragment of beta-fodrin expressed in glandular epithelial cells in patients with Sjögren's syndrome. *J Immunol*. 2001;167(9):5449–5456.
155. Bridoux F, Kyndt X, bou-Ayache R et al. Proximal tubular dysfunction in primary Sjögren's syndrome: a clinicopathological study of 2 cases. *Clin Nephrol*. 2004;61(6):434–439.
156. Wang CC, Shiang JC, Huang WT, Lin SH. Hypokalemic paralysis as primary presentation of Fanconi syndrome associated with Sjögren syndrome. *J Clin Rheumatol*. 2010;16(4):178–180.
157. Kawashima M, Amano T, Morita Y, Yamamura M, Makino H. Hypokalemic paralysis and osteomalacia secondary to renal tubular acidosis in a case with primary Sjögren's syndrome. *Mod Rheumatol*. 2006;16(1):48–51.
158. Yang YS, Peng CH, Sia SK, Huang CN. Acquired hypophosphatemia osteomalacia associated with Fanconi's syndrome in Sjögren's syndrome. *Rheumatol Int*. 2007;27(6):593–597.
159. Wrong OM, Feest TG, MacIver AG. Immune-related potassium-losing interstitial nephritis: a comparison with distal renal tubular acidosis. *Q J Med*. 1993;86(8):513–534.
160. Kaufman I, Schwartz D, Caspi D, Paran D. Sjögren's syndrome - not just Sicca: renal involvement in Sjögren's syndrome. *Scand J Rheumatol*. 2008;37(3):213–218.
161. Soy M, Pamuk ON, Gerenli M, Celik Y. A primary Sjögren's syndrome patient with distal renal tubular acidosis, who presented with symptoms of hypokalemic periodic paralysis: report of a case study and review of the literature. *Rheumatol Int*. 2005;26(1):86–89.
162. Casatta L, Ferraccioli GF, Bartoli E. Hypokalaemic alkalosis, acquired Gitelman's and Bartter's syndrome in chronic sialoadenitis. *Br J Rheumatol*. 1997;36(10):1125–1128.
163. Chen YC, Yang WC, Yang AH, et al. Primary Sjögren's syndrome associated with Gitelman's syndrome presenting with muscular paralysis. *Am J Kidney Dis*. 2003;42(3):586–590.
164. Higashi K, Kawaguchi Y, Suzuki K, Nakamura H. Sjögren's syndrome associated with hypokalemic myopathy due to Bartter's syndrome. *J Rheumatol*. 1997;24(8):1663–1664.
165. Kim YK, Song HC, Kim WY, et al. Acquired Gitelman syndrome in a patient with primary Sjögren syndrome. *Am J Kidney Dis*. 2008; 52(6):1163–1167.
166. Pedro-Botet J, Tomas S, Soriano JC, Coll J. Primary Sjögren's syndrome associated with Bartter's syndrome. *Clin Exp Rheumatol*. 1991;9(2):210–212.
167. Schwarz C, Barisani T, Bauer E, Druml W. A woman with red eyes and hypokalemia: a case of acquired Gitelman syndrome. *Wien Klin Wochenschr*. 2006;118(7–8):239–242.
168. Abe H, Tsuboi N, Yukawa S, et al. Thrombotic thrombocytopenic purpura complicating Sjögren's syndrome with crescentic glomerulonephritis and membranous nephritis. *Mod Rheumatol*. 2004;14(2):174–178.
169. Chen HA, Chen CH, Cheng HH. Hemolytic uremic syndrome and pericarditis as early manifestations of primary Sjögren's syndrome. *Clin Rheumatol*. 2009;28(Suppl 1):S43–S46.
170. Chen Y, Zhao X, Tang D, et al. IgA nephropathy in two patients with Sjögren's syndrome: one with concomitant autoimmune hepatitis. *Intern Med*. 2010;49(1):37–43.
171. Guillot X, Solau-Gervais E, Coulon A, Debiais F. Sjögren's syndrome with ANCA-associated crescentic extramembranous glomerulonephritis. *Joint Bone Spine*. 2009;76(2):188–189.
172. Ooms V, Decupere M, Lerut E, Vanrenterghem Y, Kuypers DR. Secondary renal amyloidosis due to long-standing tubulointerstitial nephritis in a patient with Sjögren syndrome. *Am J Kidney Dis*. 2005;46(5):e75–e80.
173. Tsai TC, Chen CY, Lin WT, Lee WJ, Chen HC. Sjögren's syndrome complicated with IgA nephropathy and leukocytoclastic vasculitis. *Ren Fail*. 2008;30(7):755–758.
174. Christopher-Stine L, Plotz PH. Adult inflammatory myopathies. *Best Pract Res Clin Rheumatol*. 2004;18(3):331–344.
175. Dalakas MC. Review: an update on inflammatory and autoimmune myopathies. *Neuropathol Appl Neurobiol*. 2011;37(3):226–242.
176. Dimachkie MM. Idiopathic inflammatory myopathies. *J Neuroimmunol*. 2011;231(1–2):32–42.
177. Mammen AL. Dermatomyositis and polymyositis: clinical presentation, autoantibodies, and pathogenesis. *Ann NY Acad Sci* 2010;1184:134–153.
178. Prieto S, Grau JM. The geoepidemiology of autoimmune muscle disease. *Autoimmun Rev*. 2010;9(5):A330–A334.
179. Dalakas MC, Hohlfeld R. Polymyositis and dermatomyositis. *Lancet*. 2003;362(9388):971–982.
180. Connors GR, Christopher-Stine L, Oddis CV, Danoff SK. Interstitial lung disease associated with the idiopathic inflammatory myopathies: what progress has been made in the past 35 years? *Chest*. 2010;138(6):1464–1474.
181. Labirua A, Lundberg IE. Interstitial lung disease and idiopathic inflammatory myopathies: progress and pitfalls. *Curr Opin Rheumatol*. 2010;22(6):633–638.
182. Kim HW, Choi JR, Jang SJ, et al. Recurrent rhabdomyolysis and myoglobinuric acute renal failure in a patient with polymyositis. *Nephrol Dial Transplant*. 2005;20(10):2255–2258.
183. Lewington AJ, D'Souza R, Carr S, O'Reilly K, Warwick GL. Polymyositis: a cause of acute renal failure. *Nephrol Dial Transplant*. 1996;11(4):699–701.
184. Yen TH, Lai PC, Chen CC, Hsueh S, Huang JY. Renal involvement in patients with polymyositis and dermatomyositis. *Int J Clin Pract*. 2005;59(2):188–193.
185. Akashi Y, Inoh M, Gamo N, et al. Dermatomyositis associated with membranous nephropathy in a 43-year-old female. *Am J Nephrol*. 2002;22(4):385–388.
186. Frost NA, Morand EF, Hall CL, Maddison PJ, Bhalla AK. Idiopathic polymyositis complicated by arthritis and mesangial proliferative glomerulonephritis: case report and review of the literature. *Br J Rheumatol*. 1993;32(10):929–931.
187. Takizawa Y, Kanda H, Sato K, et al. Polymyositis associated with focal mesangial proliferative glomerulonephritis with depositions of immune complexes. *Clin Rheumatol*. 2007;26(5):792–796.
188. Xie Q, Liu Y, Liu G, Yang N, Yin G. Diffuse proliferative glomerulonephritis associated with dermatomyositis with nephrotic syndrome. *Rheumatol Int*. 2010;30(6):821–825.
189. Yen TH, Huang JY, Chen CY. Unexpected IgA nephropathy during the treatment of a young woman with idiopathic dermatomyositis: case report and review of the literature. *J Nephrol*. 2003;16(1):148–153.
190. Pope JE. Other manifestations of mixed connective tissue disease. *Rheum Dis Clin North Am*. 2005;31(3):519–533, vii.
191. Rifkin SI, Gutta H, Nair R, McFarren C, Wheeler DE. Collapsing glomerulopathy in a patient with mixed connective tissue disease. *Clin Nephrol*. 2011;75(Suppl 1):32–36.
192. Madan V, Chinoy H, Griffiths CE, Cooper RG. Defining cancer risk in dermatomyositis. Part I. *Clin Exp Dermatol*. 2009;34(4):451–455.
193. Buchbinder R, Forbes A, Hall S, Dennett X, Giles G. Incidence of malignant disease in biopsy-proven inflammatory myopathy. A population-based cohort study. *Ann Intern Med*. 2001;134(12):1087–1095.
194. Hill CL, Zhang Y, Sigurgeirsson B, et al. Frequency of specific cancer types in dermatomyositis and polymyositis: a population-based study. *Lancet*. 2001;357(9250):96–100.
195. Selva-O'Callaghan A, Trallero-Araguas E, Grau-Junyent JM, Labrador-Horrillo M. Malignancy and myositis: novel autoantibodies and new insights. *Curr Opin Rheumatol*. 2010;22(6):627–632.

Hemolytic Uremic Syndrome, Thrombotic Thrombocytopenic Purpura, and Acute Cortical Necrosis

Marina Noris • Giuseppe Remuzzi • Piero Ruggenenti

HEMOLYTIC UREMIC SYNDROME AND THOMBOTIC THROMBOCYTOPENIC PURPURA

The term thrombotic microangiopathy (TMA) defines a lesion of arteriolar and capillary vessel wall thickening with intraluminal platelet thrombosis and a partial or complete obstruction of the vessel lumina. Laboratory features of thrombocytopenia and microangiopathic hemolytic anemia are almost invariably present in patients with TMA lesions and reflect the consumption and disruption of platelets and erythrocytes in the microvasculature. Depending on whether renal or brain lesions prevail, two pathologically indistinguishable but somehow clinically different entities have been described: hemolytic uremic syndrome (HUS) and the thrombotic thrombocytopenic purpura (TTP). Because HUS can involve extrarenal manifestations and TTP can sometimes involve severe renal disease, the two can be difficult to distinguish on clinical grounds only.[1] Newly identified pathophysiologic mechanisms, however, have allowed for the differentiation of the two syndromes on a molecular basis (Table 55.1). Independent of the initial cause, all different forms of HUS and TTP share a similar trend of circulating blood to form thrombi in the microvasculature because of primary endothelial damage, as in Shiga toxin–associated HUS; uncontrolled complement activation, as in atypical HUS; or abnormal cleavage of von Willebrand factor, as inTTP.

Clinical Features

Hemolytic Uremic Syndrome

The term HUS was introduced in 1955 by Gasser and coworkers[2] in their description of an acute fatal syndrome in children characterized by hemolytic anemia, thrombocytopenia, and severe renal failure. HUS occurs most frequently in children under the age of 5 years (incidence, 5 to 6 children/100,000/year compared to an overall incidence of 0.5 to 1/100,000/year. Most cases (over 90% of those in children) are associated with infection by Shigalike toxin (Stx), producing *Escherichia coli* (Stx-HUS).[3] In 90% of cases, Stx-HUS is preceded by diarrhea, which is often bloody. Usually patients are afebrile. *Streptococcus pneumoniae* causes a distinctive form of HUS, accounting for 40% of cases not associated with Stx-producing bacteria.[4]

Approximately 10% of HUS cases are classified as atypical, caused neither by Stx-producing bacteria nor by *Streptococcus*.[5] Atypical HUS occurs at any age, can be familial or sporadic, and has a poor outcome; 50% progress to end-stage renal disease (ESRD) and 25% may die in the acute phase.[4,6] Neurologic symptoms and fever can occur in 30% of patients. Pulmonary, cardiac, and gastrointestinal manifestations can also occur.[4,6]

Thrombotic Thrombocytopenic Purpura

TTP was first described in 1925 by Moschcowitz[7] in a 16-year-old female patient with a fulminant febrile attack, hemolytic anemia, bleeding, renal failure, and neurologic involvement. Pathologic changes were characterized by widespread hyaline thrombosis of small vessels. It is a rare disease, with an incidence of approximately 2 to 4 cases per 1 million persons per year.[8,9] It is more common in women (female to male ratio, 3:2 to 5:2) and in whites (white to black ratio, 3:1). Although the peak incidence is in the third and fourth decades of life, TTP can affect any age group.[9–11] Thrombotic thrombocytopenic purpura classically presents with the pentad of thrombocytopenia, microangiopathic hemolytic anemia, fever, and neurologic and renal dysfunction.[7] Thrombocytopenia is essential for the diagnosis; most patients present with values below 60,000 per microliter.[9,11] Purpura is minor and can be absent. Retinal hemorrhages can be present; however, bleeding is rare. Neurologic symptoms can be seen in over 90% of patients during the entire course of the disease. Central nervous system involvement mainly represents thrombo-occlusive disease of the grey matter, but can also include headache, cranial nerve palsies, confusion, stupor, and coma. These features are transient but recurrent. Up to half of patients who present with neurologic involvement may be left with sequelae. Renal insufficiency may occur. One group has reported 25% of patients with creatinine clearance of less than 40 mL per minute. Low-grade

TABLE 55.1 **Classification of Hemolytic Uremic Syndrome (HUS) and Thrombotic Thrombocytopenic Purpura (TTP) According to Clinical Presentation and Underlying Etiology**

Clinical Presentation			Etiology
Hemolytic Uremic Syndrome			
- Stx-associated			Infections by Stx-producing bacteria
- Neuraminidase associated			Infections by *Streptococcus pneumoniae*
- Atypical	***Familial***		*Mutations*: *CFH*, 40%–45%; *CFI*, 5%–10%; *C3*, 8%–10%; *MCP*, 7%–15%; *THBD*, 9%; *CFB*, 1%–2%
	Sporadic	Idiopathic	*Mutations*: *CFH*, 15%–20%; *CFI*, 3%–6%; *C3*, 4%–6%; *MCP*, 6%–10%; *THBD*, 2%; *CFB*, 2 cases *Anti-CFH antibodies*: 6%–10%
		- Pregnancy-associated	*Mutations*: *CFH*, 20%; *CFI*, 15%
		- HELLP syndrome	*Mutations*: *CFH*, 10%; *CFI*, 20%; *MCP*, 10%
		- Drugs	*Mutations*: rare CFH mutations, the large majority unknown
		- Transplantation (de novo aHUS)	*Mutations*: *CFH*, 15%; *CFI*, 16%
		- HIV	Unknown[a]
		- Malignancy	Unknown[a]
Thrombotic Thrombocytopenic Purpura			
- Congenital			Homozygous or compound heterozygous mutations in ADAMTS13 gene
- Idiopathic			Anti-ADAMTS13 autoantibodies
- Secondary		- Ticlopidine clopidogrel	Anti-ADAMTS13 autoantibodies (ticlopidine, 80%–90%, clopidogrel, 30%)
		- HSC transplantation	Unknown, rarely low ADAMTS13 levels
		- Malignancies	Unknown, rarely low ADAMTS13 levels
		- HIV	HIV virus, rarely low ADAMTS13 levels
		SLE, APL, and other autoimmune disease	Depends on the specific primary diseases

[a]No published data on frequency of complement gene mutations or anti-CFH autoantibodies.
Stx, Shiga toxin; CFH, complement factor H; CFI, complement factor I; HELLP, hemolytic anemia, elevated liver enzymes, and low platelet count; MCP, membrane cofactor protein; THBD, thrombomodulin; aHUS, atypical hemolytic uremic syndrome; HSC, hematopoietic stem cell transplantation; SLE, systemic lupus erythematosus; APL, antiphospholipid syndrome.

fever is present in one-quarter of patients at the diagnosis, but can often be seen as a consequence of plasma exchange. Less common manifestations include acute abdomen, pancreatitis, and sudden death.[11]

Laboratory Findings

Laboratory features of thrombocytopenia and microangiopathic hemolytic anemia are almost invariably present in patients with TMA lesions and reflect consumption and disruption of platelets and erythrocytes in the microvasculature.[5,11,12] Hemoglobin levels are low (less than 10 g per deciliter in more than 90% of patients). Reticulocyte counts are uniformly elevated. The peripheral smear reveals an increased schistocyte number (Fig. 55.1), with polychromasia, and often, nucleated red blood cells. The latter may represent not only a compensatory response, but also may represent damage to the bone marrow–blood barrier resulting from intramedullary vascular occlusion. Detection of fragmented

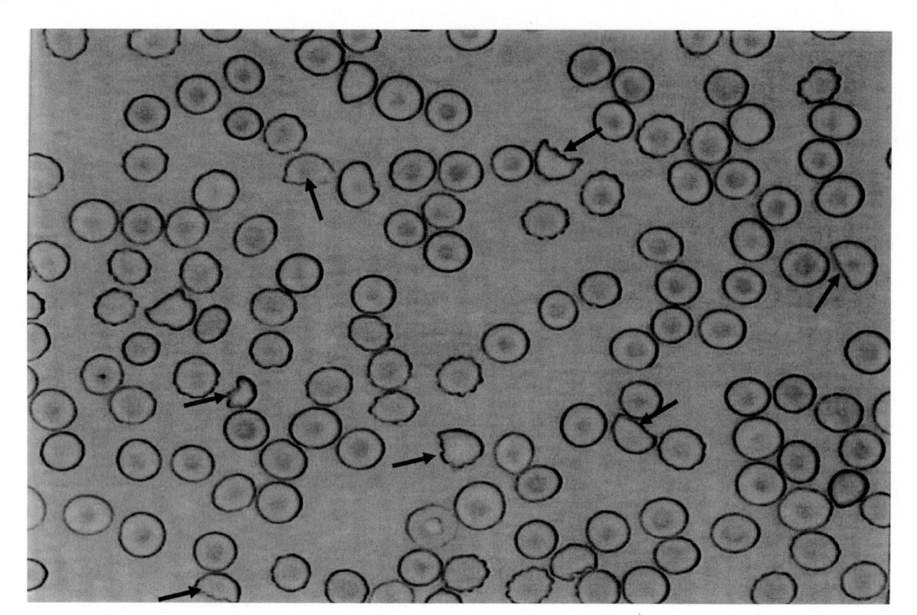

FIGURE 55.1 A peripheral blood smear from a patient with thrombotic microangiopathy. The presence of fragmented red blood cells that may acquire the appearance of a helmet (fragmented erythrocytes with the shape of a helmet are identified by the *black arrows*) is pathognomonic for microangiopathic hemolysis in patients with no evidence of heart valvular disease.

erythrocytes is crucial to confirm the microangiopathic nature of the hemolytic anemia, provided that heart valvular disease and other anatomic artery abnormalities that may cause erythrocyte fragmentation are excluded. Other indicators of intravascular hemolysis include elevated lactate dehydrogenase (LDH), increased indirect bilirubin, and low haptoglobin levels.[5,11,12] The Coombs test is negative. Moderate leukocytosis may accompany the hemolytic anemia. Thrombocytopenia is uniformly present in HUS and TTP. It may be severe, but is usually less so in patients with predominant renal involvement.[13] The presence of giant platelets in the peripheral smear or reduced platelet survival time (or both) is consistent with peripheral consumption. In children with Stx-HUS, the duration of thrombocytopenia is variable and does not correlate with the course of renal disease.[14] Bone marrow biopsy specimens usually show erythroid hyperplasia and an increased number of megakaryocytes. Prothrombin time (PT), partial thromboplastin time (PTT), the fibrinogen level, and coagulation factors are normal, thus differentiating HUS and TTP from disseminated intravascular coagulation (DIC). Mild fibrinolysis with minimal elevation in fibrin degradation products, however, may be observed.

Evidence of renal involvement is present in all patients with HUS (by definition) and in about 25% of patients with TTP.[1,12,15] Microscopic hematuria and subnephrotic proteinuria are the most consistent findings. In a retrospective study of 216 patients with a clinical picture of TTP, hematuria was detected in 78% and proteinuria in 75% of cases.[15] Sterile pyuria and casts were present in 31% and 24% of cases, respectively. Gross hematuria was rare.[15]

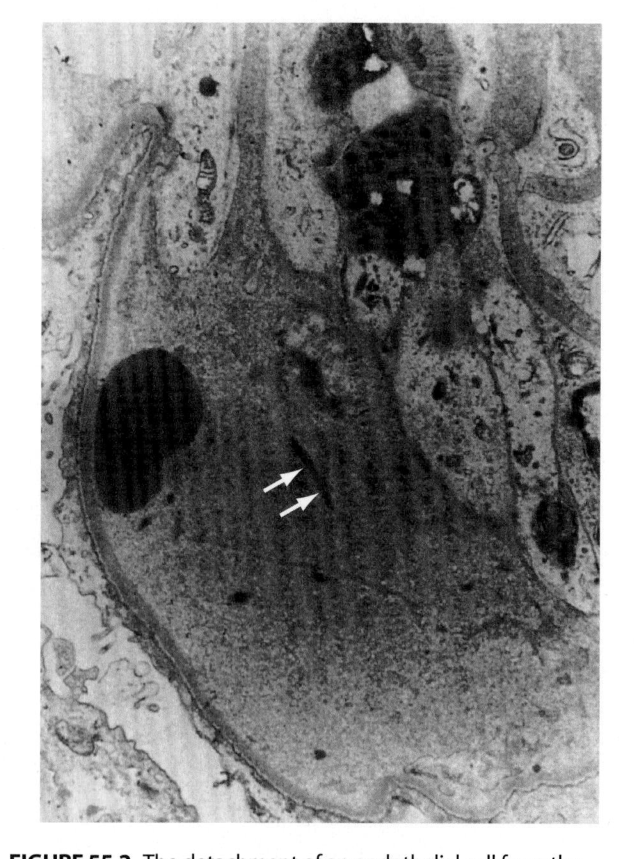

FIGURE 55.2 The detachment of an endothelial cell from the underlying glomerular basement membrane in a case of hemolytic–uremic syndrome. A red blood cell is in close contact with the glomerular basement membrane. Electron-lucent "fluffy" material and a few strands of fibrin (*arrows*) are present in the subendothelial space (×7,000). (Courtesy of Drs. C. L. Pirani and V. D'Agati.)

Pathology

The diagnostic histologic lesions of TMA consist of widening of the subendothelial space and microvascular thrombosis. Electron microscopy best identifies the characteristic lesions of swelling and detachment of the endothelial cells from the basement membrane and the accumulation of fluffy material in the subendothelium (Figs. 55.2 and 55.3), intraluminal platelet thrombi, and a partial or complete obstruction of the vessel lumina (Fig. 55.4).[16–18] These lesions are similar to those seen in other renal diseases such as scleroderma, malignant nephrosclerosis, chronic transplant rejection, and calcineurin inhibitor nephrotoxicity. In HUS, microthrombi are present primarily in the kidneys, whereas in TTP they mainly involve the brain, where thrombi may repeatedly form and resolve, producing intermittent neurologic deficits. In pediatric patients, particularly in those younger than 2 years of age, and in those with HUS secondary to gastrointestinal infection with Stx-producing strains of *E. coli*, the glomerular injury is predominant.[16]

Thrombi and infiltration by leukocytes are common in the early phases of the disease and usually resolve after 2 to 3 weeks. Patchy cortical necrosis may be present in severe cases; crescent formation is uncommon. In idiopathic and familial forms and in adults, the injury mostly involves arteries and arterioles with thrombosis and intimal thickening (Figs. 55.5 and 55.6), and secondary glomerular ischemia and retraction of the glomerular tuft (Fig. 55.7). The prognosis is good in patients with predominant glomerular involvement, but it is more severe in those with predominant preglomerular injury. Focal segmental glomerulosclerosis may be a long-term sequela of acute cases of HUS and is usually seen in children with long-lasting hypertension and progressive chronic renal function deterioration.[16–18]

The typical pathologic changes of TTP are the thrombi that occlude capillaries and arterioles in many organs

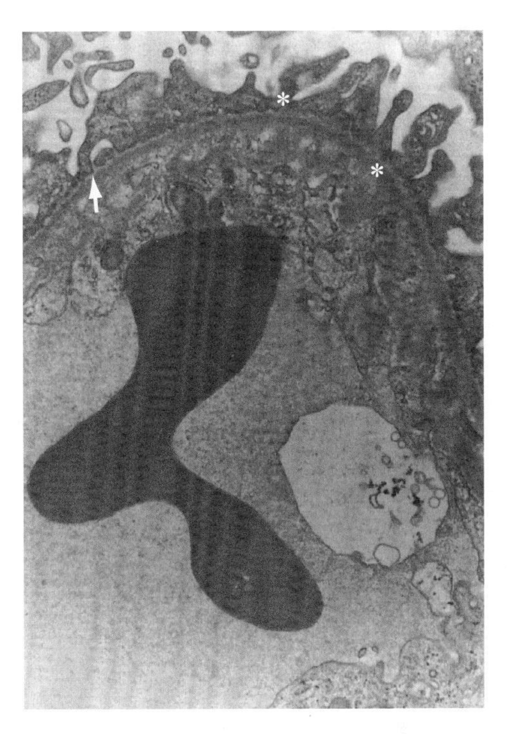

FIGURE 55.3 Electron-lucent "fluffy" material (*arrow*) with some electron-dense deposits (*asterisks*) are located between the cytoplasm of an endothelial cell and the glomerular basement membrane in a segment of glomerular capillary from a patient with hemolytic–uremic syndrome (×12,000). (Courtesy of Drs. C. L. Pirani and V. D'Agati.)

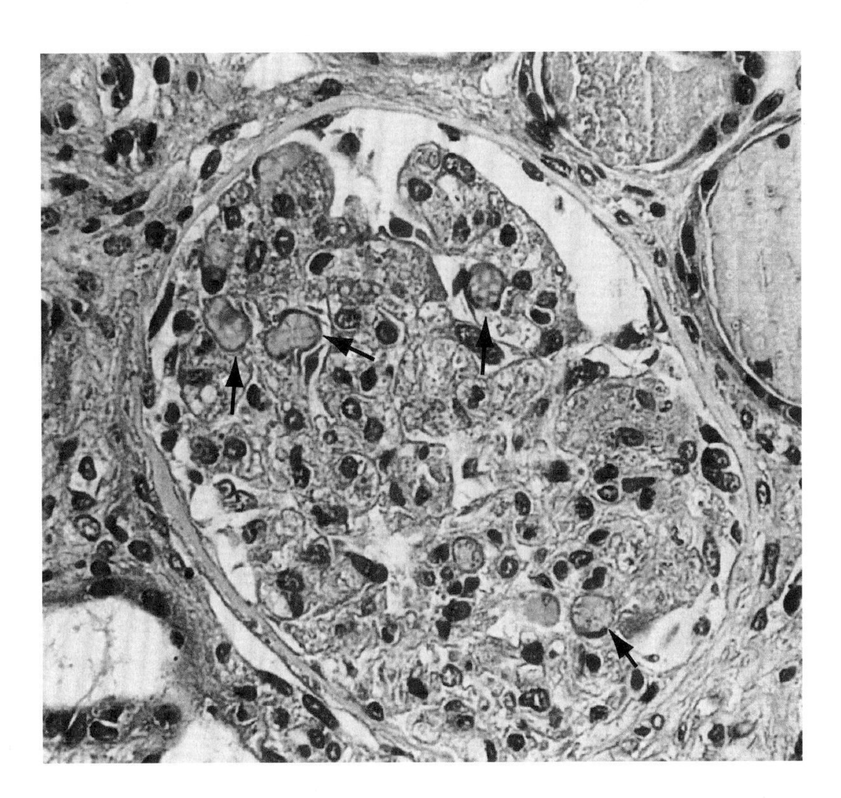

FIGURE 55.4 Swelling of the glomerular endothelial cells and occlusion of almost all capillary lumens packed with red blood cells (*arrows*) in a case of hemolytic–uremic syndrome (Trichrome, ×250).

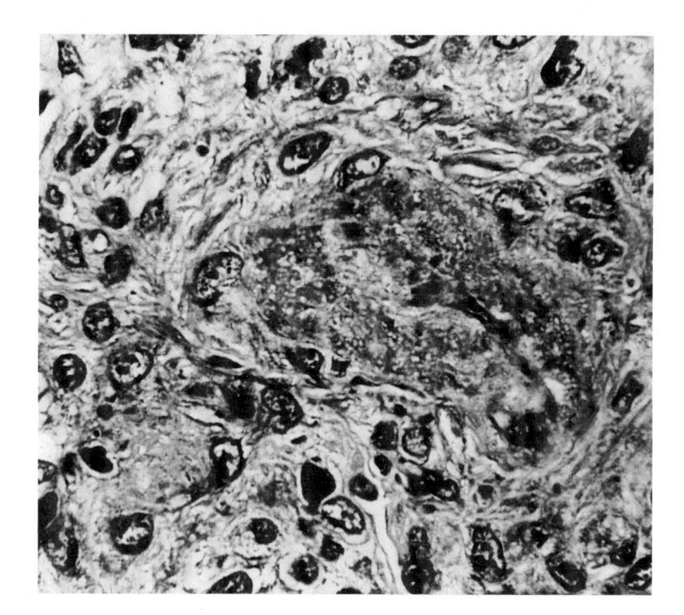

FIGURE 55.5 Thrombotic and necrotic changes in a small artery from an adult patient with hemolytic–uremic syndrome. (Trichrome, ×375.)

and tissues (Fig. 55.8). These thrombi consist of fibrin and platelets, and their distribution is widespread. They are most commonly detected in the kidneys, the pancreas, the heart, the adrenals, and the brain. Compared to HUS, pathologic changes of TTP are more extensively distributed, probably reflecting the more systemic nature of the disease.[16–18]

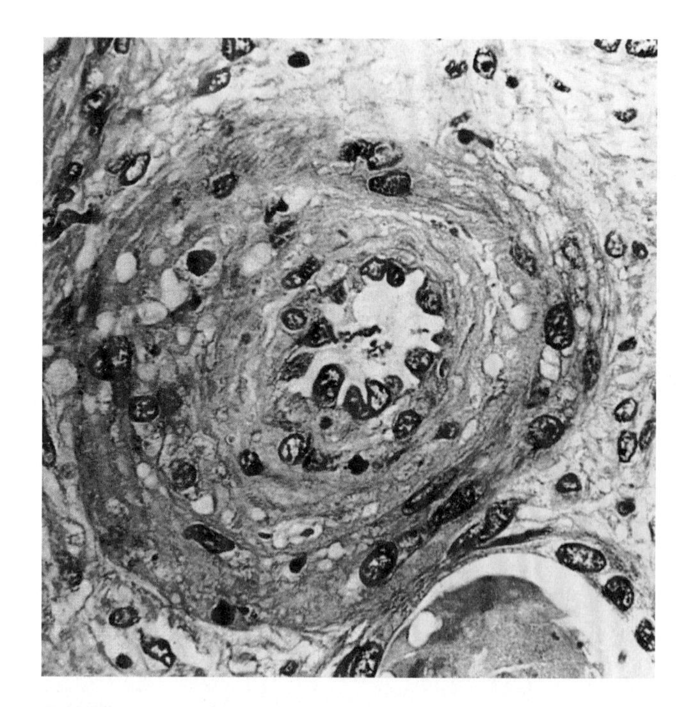

FIGURE 55.6 Occlusion of an interlobular artery with intimal swelling and myointimal proliferation in a case of adult hemolytic–uremic syndrome. (Trichrome, ×375.)

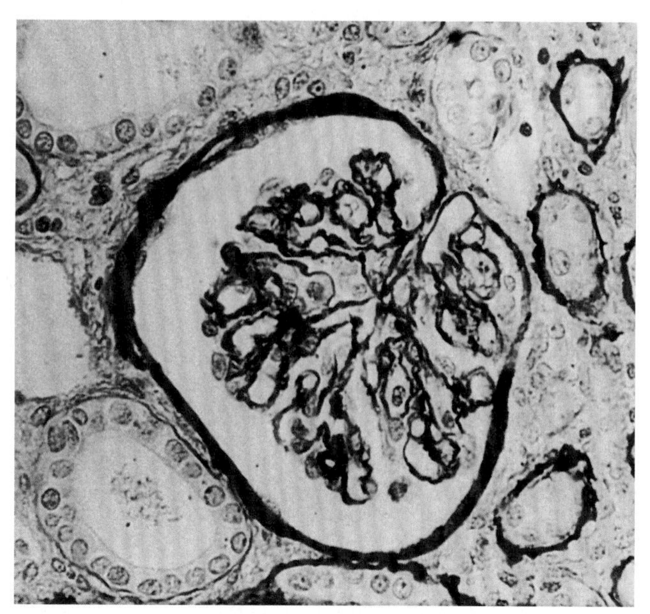

FIGURE 55.7 Ischemic glomerular lesions characterized by thickening and wrinkling of glomerular capillary walls and atrophy of the glomerular tuft in a case of adult hemolytic–uremic syndrome. (Silver, ×250.)

Mechanisms, Clinical Course, and Therapy According to Different Forms of Thrombotic Microangiopathy

Hemolytic Uremic Syndrome

Shiga Toxin–Associated Hemolytic Uremic Syndrome

Mechanisms. Stx-HUS, the most frequent form of TMA, may follow infection by certain strains of *E. coli or Shigella dysenteriae*, which produce powerful exotoxins (Stx).[3,19] The term Shiga toxin was initially used to describe the exotoxin produced by *S. dysenteriae* type 1. Then, some strains of *E. coli* (mostly the serotype 0157:H7, but also other serotypes

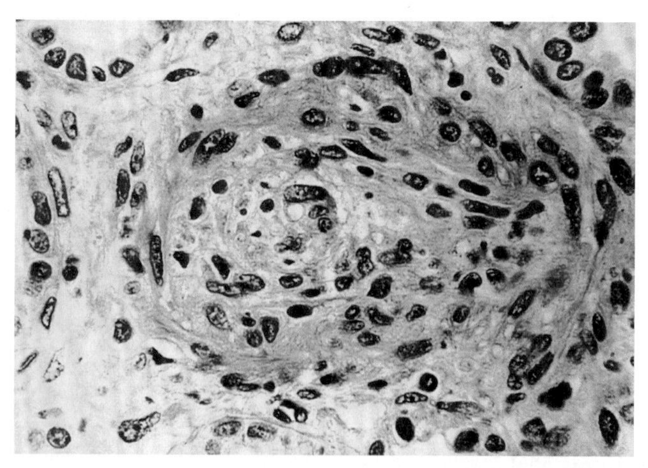

FIGURE 55.8 Marked endothelial and myointimal cell proliferation with occlusion of the lumen of an interlobular artery in a case of thrombotic thrombocytopenic purpura (Trichrome, ×375.)

such as O111:H8, O103:H2, O123, O26, and the O104:H4 strain isolated in the recent German outbreak)[20,21] isolated from human cases with diarrhea were found to produce a toxin similar to the one of *S. dysenteriae*. After food contaminated by Stx-producing *E. coli* or *S. dysenteriae* is ingested, the toxin is released into the gut and may cause watery or, most often, bloody diarrhea because of a direct effect on the intestinal mucosa. Stx-producing *E. coli* closely adhere to the epithelial cells of the gastrointestinal mucosa causing the destruction of the brush border villi.[22] Stxs are picked up by polarized gastrointestinal cells via transcellular pathways and translocate into the circulation,[23] probably facilitated by the transmigration of neutrophils,[24] which increase paracellular permeability. Circulating human blood cells, such as erythrocytes,[25] platelets,[26,27] and monocytes,[28] express Stx receptors on their surface and have been suggested to serve as Stx carriers from the intestine to the kidney and other target organs.

The disease is caused by two distinct exotoxins, Stx-1 and Stx-2, which are almost identical to the toxin produced by *S. dysenteriae* type 1.[29] Both Stx-1 and Stx-2 are 70-kDa AB5 holotoxins comprising a single A subunit of 32 kDa and five 7.7-kDa B subunits. Interestingly, an AB5 toxin comprising a single 35-kDa A subunit and a pentamer of 13-kDa B subunits have been isolated from a highly virulent *E. coli* strain (O113:H21) responsible for an outbreak of HUS, which may represent the prototype of a new class of toxins, accounting for HUS associated with strains of *E. coli* that do not produce Stxs.[30] Despite their similar sequences, Stx-1 and Stx-2 cause different degrees and types of tissue damage, as documented by the higher pathogenicity of strains of *E. coli* that produce only Stx-2 than of those that produce Stx-1 alone.[31–33] In a study in children who became infected by Stx *E. coli*, *E. coli* strains producing Stx-2 were most commonly associated with HUS, whereas most strains isolated from children with diarrhea alone or from those who remained asymptomatic only produced Stx-1.[34] This is also true in mice and in baboons.[35]

Stx-1 and Stx-2 bind to different epitopes on the Gb3 molecules and they also differ in binding affinity and kinetics.[36] Surface plasmon resonance analysis showed that Stx-1 easily binds to and detaches from Gb3, in contrast to Stx-2, which binds slowly but also dissociates very slowly, thus leaving time enough for the cell's incorporation.[36] After binding to endothelial cell receptors, the toxin is internalized in the cytosol by endocytosis[37] within 2 hours[38] and inhibits protein synthesis within 30 minutes (Fig. 55.9). The number of high-affinity receptors is a major determinant of susceptibility of cells to Stx.[39] Therefore, cell viability and protein synthesis of endothelial cells of the kidney were reduced by 50% upon exposure to 1 pM Stx, unlike endothelial cells of the umbilical vein that were viable up to greater than 1 nM exposure to the toxin. These findings are consistent with basal levels of Stx receptors 50 times higher in the renal endothelium than in the umbilical cord endothelium.[40] During internalization, the alpha subunit of the toxin dissociates from the beta subunits. Approximately 10% of the alpha subunit protein is removed in a trypsinlike process, resulting in a maximally active 27-kDa subunit enzyme. It is well established that this fragment is a direct inhibitor of protein synthesis and is responsible for the cytotoxic action of the toxin. Stx selectively inactivates 60S ribosomal subunits by removing one nucleotide in the 28S ribosomal RNA in a nucleotide-specific manner (Fig. 55.9).[40]

For many years it was assumed that the only relevant biologic activity of Stx was the block of protein synthesis and destruction of endothelial cells. However, the treatment of endothelial cells with sublethal doses of Stx—exerting minimal influence on protein synthesis—leads to increased mRNA levels and protein expression of chemokines, such as interleukin (IL)-8 and monocyte chemoattractant protein-1 (MCP-1) and cell adhesion molecules, a process preceded by nuclear factor-kappa B (NF-κB) activation.[41] Adhesion molecules seem to play a critical role in mediating the binding of inflammatory cells to endothelium. Indeed, Stx-2 treatment enhanced the number of leukocytes adhering and migrating across a monolayer of human endothelial cells.[42] Moreover, preventing IL-8 and MCP-1 overexpression by adenovirus-mediated NF-κB blocking, inhibited adhesion and the transmigration of leukocytes.[41]

Therefore, it can be inferred that Stx, by altering endothelial cell adhesion properties and metabolism, favor leukocyte-dependent inflammation and induce the loss of thromboresistance in endothelial cells, leading to microvascular thrombosis. Evidence for such a sequence of events has been obtained in experiments of whole blood flowing on human microvascular endothelial cells preexposed to Stx-1 at high shear stress.[43] In these circumstances, early platelet activation and adhesion occurs, followed by the formation of organized endothelial P-selectin and platelet-endothelial cell adhesion molecule (PECAM)-1–dependent thrombi. This offers a likely pathophysiologic pathway for microvascular thrombosis in HUS.

Evidence is also emerging that complement activation at the renal endothelial level may contribute to microangiopathic lesions in Stx-HUS. High plasma levels of complement activation products Bb and C5b-9 were recently measured in 17 children with Stx-HUS, indicating complement activation via an alternative pathway.[44] Another study reported that Stx2 binds to the plasma complement regulatory protein, factor H, and may activate complement in the fluid phase in vitro.[45] In a recent study, Stx-induced complement activation via P-selectin was identified as a key mechanism of microvascular thrombosis in Stx-HUS. Stx induced the expression of P-selectin on a cultured human microvascular endothelial cell surface, and P-selectin bound and activated C3 via the alternative pathway, leading to thrombus formation under flow.[46] In a murine model of HUS obtained by the coinjection of Stx2 and LPS and characterized by thrombocytopenia and renal dysfunction, the upregulation of glomerular endothelial P-selectin was associated with C3 and fibrin(ogen) deposits and platelet clumps. Treatment with anti–P-selectin Ab limited glomerular C3 accumulation. Factor B deficient mice after Stx2/LPS exhibited less thrombocytopenia and

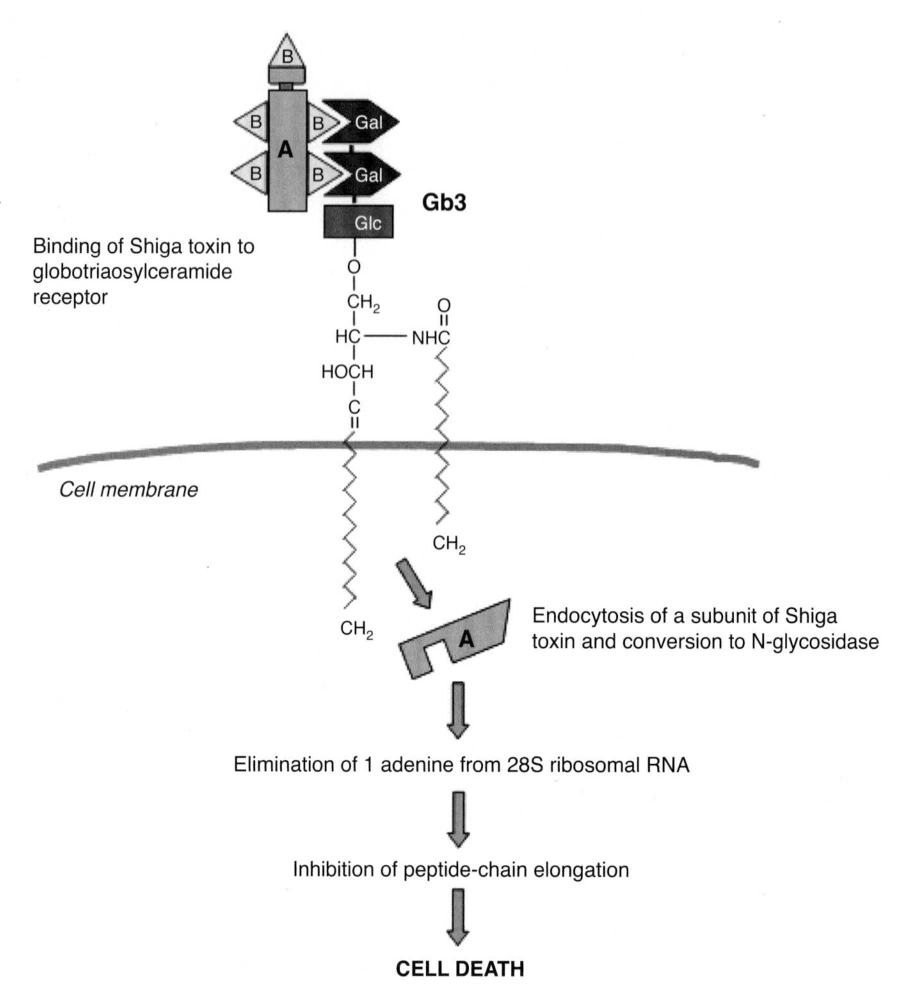

FIGURE 55.9 The binding and mechanism of action of Shigalike toxin. The B subunits of Shiga toxin molecules attach to galactose (*Gal*) disaccharides of globotriaosylceramide (*Gb3*) receptors on the membrane of monocytes, polymorphonuclear cells, platelets, glomerular endothelial cells, and tubular epithelial cells. The toxin is internalized via retrograde transport through the Golgi complex. Then the A and B subunits dissociate, and the A subunit is translocated to the cytosol. The A subunit blocks peptide chain elongation by eliminating one adenine from the 28S ribosomal RNA.

were protected against glomerular abnormalities and renal function impairment, indicating the involvement of complement activation, via the alternative pathway, in the glomerular thrombotic process in HUS mice.[46]

Diagnosis. Diagnosis rests on the detection of *E. coli* O157:H7 and other Stx-producing bacteria in sorbitol-MacConkey stool cultures. Unlike most other *E coli*, serotype O157:H7 and other Stx-producing bacteria do not ferment sorbitol rapidly and thus form colorless colonies on sorbitol containing MacConkey agar (SMAC). Suspect colonies can be assayed for the O157 antigen with commercially available antiserum or latex agglutination kits. Newer protocols that use SMAC that contains cefixime tellurite, other selective culture media, immunomagnetic separation, and enzyme-linked immunosorbent assays to detect O157 lipopolysaccharide or Shiga toxins can further enhance detection.[19] In regions where sorbitol-fermenting strains have been identified,[19] the use of tests that identify Shiga toxins or the genes encoding them (by PCR) is helpful for diagnosis.

Over the last 2 decades *E. coli* 0157:H7 and, although less frequently, other Stx-producing *E. coli* strains, have been responsible for multiple outbreaks throughout the world, becoming a public health problem in both developed and developing countries.[19] Contaminated undercooked ground beef, meat patties, raw vegetables, fruit, milk, and recreational or drinking water have all been implicated in the transmission of *E. coli*. A widespread outbreak associated with spinach in North America had dramatically higher than typical rates of both hospitalization (52%) and HUS (16%), due to the emergence of a new variant of the 0157:H7 serotype that has acquired several gene mutations that likely contributed to more severe disease.[47] From May through June 2011, a very large outbreak of HUS occurred in Germany and was caused by an unusual Shiga toxin–producing *E. coli* (STEC) strain O104:H4 through the ingestion of contaminated sprouts.[48]

Secondary person-to-person contact is an important way of spread in institutional centers, particularly day care centers and nursing homes. Infected patients should be excluded from day care centers until two consecutive stool cultures are negative for Stx-producing *E. coli* in order to prevent further transmission. However, the most important preventive measure in child care centers is supervised hand washing.

Clinical course. Following exposure to Stx *E. coli*, 38% to 61% of individuals develop hemorrhagic colitis and 3% to 9% (in sporadic infections) to 20% (in epidemic forms) progress to overt HUS.[19,49] Stx *E. coli* hemorrhagic colitis not

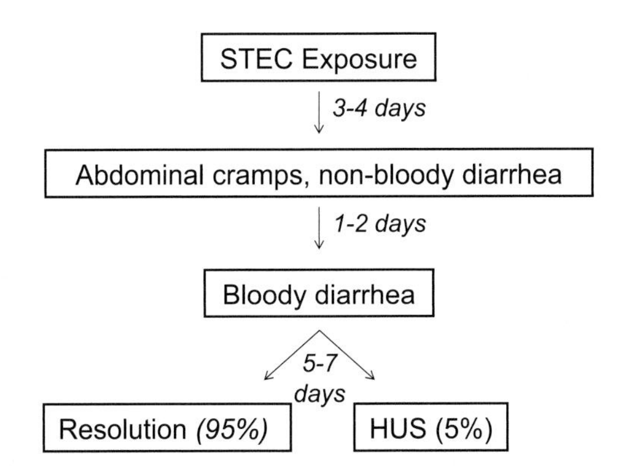

FIGURE 55.10 Timing of the events that may follow exposure to Shiga toxin–producing *E. coli*. *HUS*, hemolytic uremic syndrome.

complicated by HUS is self-limiting and is not associated with an increased long-term risk of high blood pressure or renal dysfunction, as shown by a 4-year follow-up study in 951 children who were exposed to a drinking water outbreak of *E. coli* O157:H7.[50]

Stx-HUS is characterized by prodromal diarrhea, followed by acute renal failure. The average interval between *E. coli* exposure and illness is 3 days. Illness typically begins with abdominal cramps and nonbloody diarrhea; diarrhea may become hemorrhagic in 70% of cases, usually within 1 or 2 days.[51] Vomiting occurs in 30% to 60% of cases and fever in 30%. Leukocyte count is usually elevated, and a barium enema may demonstrate "thumb-printing," suggestive of edema and submucosal hemorrhage, especially in the region of the ascending and transverse colon. HUS is usually diagnosed 6 to 10 days after the onset of diarrhea (Fig. 55.10).[3] After infection, Stx *E. coli* may be shed in the stools for several weeks after the symptoms are resolved, particularly in children $<$5 years of age.[3]

Bloody diarrhea, fever, vomiting, elevated leukocyte count, extremes of age, and female sex, as well as the use of antimotility agents,[52] have been associated with an increased risk of HUS following an *E. coli* infection.[19] Stx-HUS is not a benign disease. Of patients who develop HUS, 70% require red blood cell transfusions, 50% need dialysis, and 25% have neurologic involvement, including stroke, seizure, and coma.[19,53,54] Although mortality for infants and young children in industrialized countries decreased when dialysis became available, as well as after the introduction of intensive care facilities, still 3% to 5% of patients die during the acute phase of Stx-HUS.[53] A meta-analysis of 49 published studies (3,476 patients, mean follow-up of 4.4 years) describing the long-term prognoses of patients who survived an episode of Stx-HUS, reported death or permanent ESRD in 12% of patients and GFR below 80 mL/min/1.73m^2 in 25%.[54] The severity of acute illness, particularly central nervous system symptoms, the need for initial dialysis, and microalbuminuria in the first 6 to 8 months were strongly associated with a worse long-term prognosis.[54–56]

Disease presentation and outcome were particularly unusual during the STEC O104:H4 German outbreak, which since May 1, 2011 had involved more than 4,000 people in Germany, of whom 800 had progressed to HUS and 50 had died in Germany and 15 in other countries by July 20.[48] The outbreak was foodborne in contaminated sprouts.[21] The chain of transmission appeared to have started in Egypt with fecal contamination of fenugreek seeds by either humans or farm animals. During sprout germination, bacteria multiplied and produced large amounts of toxin and were then diffused with food provided to restaurants and consumers. Almost 90% of affected patients were adults and, compared to previous enterohemorragic *E. coli* (EHEC) epidemics, there was a higher prevalence of affected young and middle-aged women and an extremely high incidence of dialysis-dependent kidney failure (20% versus 6%) and death (6% versus 1%), respectively.[20] The predominance of women among the case patients has been suggested to be explained by the food vehicle if women are more health conscious and thus more likely to eat sprouts.[20] Conversely, severe outcome was in part explained by a lack of previous immunity to this novel phenotype and, most likely, by the exceptional virulence of the strain.[57] The involved O104:H4 *E. coli* shared 93% of the genomic sequence of enteroaggregative *E. coli* (EAEC), microbes that form fimbriae that help sticking to the intestinal wall, but was also able to produce the same Shiga toxin of EHEC.[20,58] Thus, this *E. coli* is likely the result of an acquisition of Shiga toxin–encoding phage from a preexisting Shiga toxin–producing EHEC pathogen (Fig. 55.11). Blending the two virulence factors would lead to stronger gut colonization and more toxin being released into the circulation. Moreover, although EHEC are found in the gastrointestinal tract of ruminants, EAEC have adapted to the human gut and appear to have their reservoir in humans.[59] This might explain why this strain has now acquired a host of new resistances to antibiotics most commonly used in human disease that are in large part mediated by extended-spectrum beta-lactamases (ESBL).[20]

Therapy. The typical Stx-associated HUS treatment for children is based on supportive management of anemia, renal failure, hypertension, and electrolyte and water imbalance. Intravenous isotonic volume expansion as soon as an *E. coli* O157:H7 infection is suspected—that is, within the first 4 days of illness, even before culture results are available—may limit the severity of kidney dysfunction and the need for renal replacement therapy.[60] Bowel rest is important for the enterohemorrhagic colitis associated with Stx-HUS. Antimotility agents should be avoided because it may prolong the persistency of *E. coli* in the intestinal lumen and therefore increase patient exposure to its toxin. The use of antibiotics should be restricted to the very limited number of patients presenting with bacteremia[61] because, in children with gastroenteritis, the risk of HUS increases by 17-fold.[62] A possible explanation is that antibiotic-induced injury to the bacterial membrane might favor the acute release of large amounts of preformed toxin. Alternatively, antibiotic therapy might give

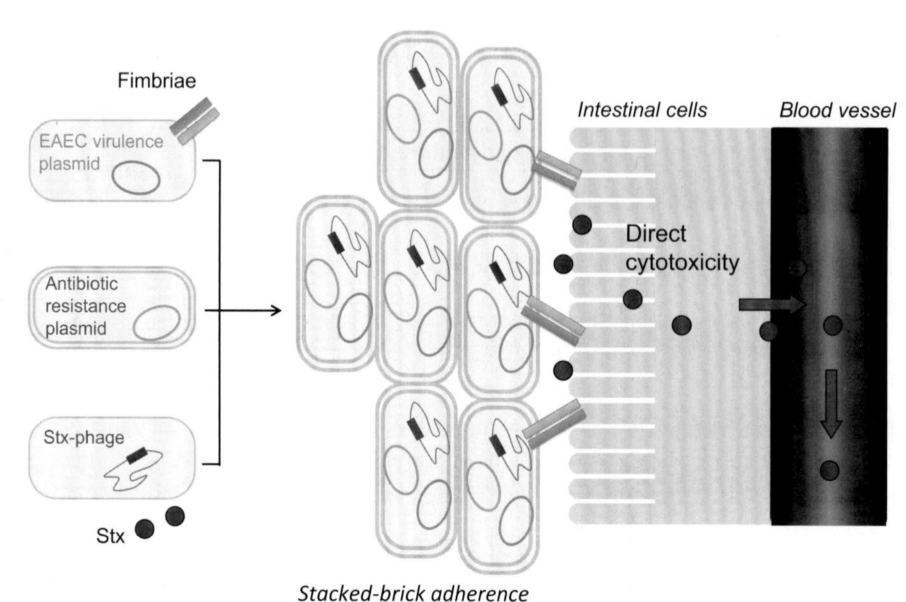

FIGURE 55.11 The hypothetical origin of the O104:H4 *E. coli* strain isolated from the German outbreak. An ancestral enteroaggregative *E. coli* (EAEC) strain with plasmids encoding for different virulence factors, including fimbriae that help stick to the intestinal cell, might have acquired the Shiga toxin phage (Stx-phage) characteristic of enterohemorragic *E. coli* (EHEC) and plasmids encoding for expanded-spectrum beta-lactamases. Close adhesion to the intestinal cell would facilitate the uptake of the Shiga toxin into the bloodstream, whereas resistance to most commonly used antibiotics would offer selective advantage over the normal intestinal flora upon antibiotic exposure.

E. coli O157:H7 a selective advantage if these organisms are not as readily eliminated from the bowel as are the normal intestinal flora. This might specifically apply to the O104:H4 strain, which has acquired a host of new resistances to antibiotics most commonly used in human diseases, such as cephalosporins, monobactams, fluoroquinolones, cotrimoxazole, tetracyclines, and aminoglycosides, which are in large part mediated by ESBL.[20,63] Actually, ESBL-mediated resistances might offer to this strain a selective advantage over the normal intestinal flora upon exposure to one or more of the previous antimicrobials administered at the onset of gastrointestinal symptoms.[57] Moreover, several antimicrobial drugs, particularly the quinolones, trimethoprim, and furazolidone, are potent inducers of the expression of the Stx2 gene and may increase the level of toxin in the intestine. Although the possibility of a cause-and-effect relationship between antibiotic therapy and an increased risk of HUS has been challenged by a recent meta-analysis of 26 reports,[64] there is no reason to prescribe antibiotics because they do not improve the outcome of colitis, and bacteremia is only exceptionally found in Stx-associated HUS. However, when hemorrhagic colitis is caused by *Shigella* dysentery type 1, early and empirical antibiotic treatment shortens the duration of diarrhea, decreases the incidence of complications, and reduces the risk of transmission by shortening the duration of bacterial shedding. Thus, in developing countries where *Shigella* is the most frequent cause of hemorrhagic colitis, antibiotic therapy should be started early and even before the involved pathogen is identified. Whether early treatment with carbapenems or antimicrobials, such as fosfomycin, which are electively effective against ESBL-producing bacteria,[65] may help prevent progression from enterocolitis to HUS in patients with evidence or suspicion of gastrointestinal infection with *E. coli* O104:H4 or other ESBL-producing strains may merit formal investigation.

Careful blood pressure control and renin–angiotensin system blockade may be particularly beneficial in the long term for those patients who suffer chronic renal disease after an episode of Stx-HUS. A study in 45 children with renal sequelae of HUS followed for 9 to 11 years documented that the early restriction of proteins and the use of ACE inhibitors may have a beneficial effect on the long-term renal outcome, as documented by a positive slope of 1/Cr values over time in treated patients.[66] In another study, an 8- to 15-year treatment with ACE inhibitors after severe Stx-HUS normalized blood pressure, reduced proteinuria, and improved GFR.[67]

An oral Shiga toxin–binding agent that may compete with endothelial and epithelial receptors for Shiga toxin in the gut (SYNSORB Pk) has been developed with the rationale of limiting target organs' exposure to the toxin (Table 55.2). However, a prospective, randomized, double-blind, placebo-controlled clinical trial of 145 children with diarrhea-associated HUS failed to demonstrate any beneficial effect of treatment on disease outcome.[68] Among newer treatments for Stx-HUS, the development of Stx-neutralizing monoclonal antibodies, including dual antibodies against Stx 1 and 2 (SHIGATEC, NCT0152199) to be given at the time of gastrointestinal infection, is the most advanced.[69] Peptides impairing the ability of EHEC to survive under the acidic conditions of the gastric system could halt the disease process at even earlier stages by preventing bacterial intrusion into the gut.[70] Heparin and antithrombotic agents may increase the risk of bleeding and should be avoided.

Efficacy of specific treatments in adult patients is difficult to evaluate because most information is derived by uncontrolled series that may also include atypical HUS cases. In particular, no prospective, randomized trials are available to definitely establish whether plasma infusion or exchange may offer some specific benefit as compared to supportive treatment alone. However, comparative analyses of two large series of patients treated[71] or not[72] with plasma suggest that plasma therapy may dramatically decrease the overall mortality of Stx *E. coli* 0157:H7–associated HUS. These findings

TABLE 55.2 **Specific Therapies Used in Thrombotic Microangiopathy, Dosing, and Efficacy**

Therapy	Dosing	Efficacy
Antiplatelet		Anecdotal efficacy in TTP.
-Aspirin	325–1,300 mg/day	
-Dipyridamole	400–600 mg/day	
-Dextran 70	500 mg twice/day	
-Prostacyclin	4-20 mg/kg/min	
Antithrombotic		Anecdotal efficacy in HUS.
- Heparin	5000 U bolus followed by 750–1000 U/hr infusion	
- Streptokinase	250,000 U bolus followed by 100,000 U/hr infusion	
Shiga toxin-binding *(Synsorb)*	500 mg/kg per day for 7 days	Not effective in preventing or treating Stx-associated HUS.
Antioxidant *(Vitamin E)*	1,000 mg/sqm/day	Anecdotal efficacy in HUS.
Immunosuppressive		Probably effective in addition to plasma exchange in patients with TTP and anti-ADAMST13 autoantibodies or in aHUS with antifactor H autoantibodies and in forms associated with autoimmune diseases. Lack of evidence from controlled trials in immune-mediated HUS or TTP.
-Prednisone	200 mg tapered to 60 mg/day then 5 mg reduction per week	
-Prednisolone	200 mg tapered to 60 mg/day then 5 mg reduction per week	
-Immunoglobulins	400 mg/kg/day	
-Vincristine	1.4 mg/sqm followed by 1 mg every 4 days	
CD20 Cell-depleting *(Rituximab)*	375 mg/sqm per week up to CD20 depletion	Effective in treatment or prevention of TTP associated with immune-mediated ADAMTS13 deficiency resistant to, or relapsing after, immunosuppressive therapy.
Fresh frozen plasma		
- Exchange	1–2 plasma volumes/day	First-line therapy for aHUS and TTP. Unproven efficacy in childhood Stx- HUS.
- Infusion	20–30 mL/kg followed by 10–20 mL/kg/day	To be considered if plasma exchange not available.
- Cryosupernatant	See plasma infusion/exchanges	To replace whole plasma in case of plasma resistance or sensitization.
- Solvent-detergent treated plasma	See plasma infusion/exchanges	To limit the risk of infections.
Liver-kidney transplant		To prevent CFH-associated HUS recurrence posttransplant. About 30% mortality risk.
Complement inhibition *(Eculizumab)*	600 mg weekly for the first 4 weeks 900 mg every 14 days up to 6 months	Reported efficacy in aHUS, STEC O104:H4-associated HUS, and in occasional cases of STEC O157:H7 childhood HUS.

TTP, thrombotic thrombocytopenic purpura; HUS, hemolytic uremic syndrome; Stx, Shiga toxin; aHUS, atypical hemolytic uremic syndrome; CFH, complement factor H; STEC, shiga toxin-producing E. coli.

lead us to consider plasma infusion or exchange suitable for adult patients, in particular in those with severe renal insufficiency and central nervous system involvement.

Kidney transplants should be considered as an effective and safe treatment for those children who progress to ESRD. Indeed, recurrence rates range from 0% to 10%,[73,74] and graft survival at 10 years is even better than in control children with other diseases.[75]

Evidence that uncontrolled complement activation may contribute to microangiopathic lesions of Stx-HUS[44–46] provided the background for complement inhibitor therapy in three children with severe EHEC-associated typical HUS who fully recovered with the anti-C5 monoclonal antibody eculizumab.[76] These encouraging results prompted nephrologists to use eculizumab therapy in HUS patients involved in the STEC O104:H4 outbreak in Germany (Table 55.2). In the setting of a controlled multicenter clinical study (EudraCT, 2011-002691-17; Clinicaltrials.gov ID: NCT01410916) 148 patients with bloody diarrhea and/or evidence of STEC/EHEC infection, microangiopathic hemolysis, thrombocytopenia, renal insufficiency, and/or central nervous system complications or thrombosis received at least an 8-week eculizumab treatment. At the inclusion, 94 patients were on dialysis therapy, 22 required ventilatory support, and 129 were receiving plasma exchange or infusion. Outcome data were reported by Dr. Rolf Stahl from the Hamburg University Medical Center during the 43rd Annual Meeting of the American Society of Nephrology held in Denver in November 2011. No patient died. At 8 weeks, platelet count and serum creatinine levels normalized in 123 and 82 patients, respectively, and no patient had persistent seizures. Dialysis, ventilatory support, and plasma therapy were no longer required. Treatment was well tolerated in all patients and no case of meningococcal infection was reported. Comparative analyses versus 108 patients who had been treated with plasma exchange but without eculizumab showed remarkably larger and faster recovery in platelet count and kidney function in those receiving eculizumab therapy. Even better outcomes were observed in patients maintained on eculizumab therapy also after the completion of the originally planned 8-week treatment period. Altogether, the data clearly showed that complement inhibition by eculizumab therapy was lifesaving and almost fully prevented the risk of renal or neurologic sequelae in patients with severe diarrhea-associated HUS secondary to O104:H4 *E. coli* infection. Whether and to what extent these findings can be generalized to patients with more severe forms of typical HUS associated with gastrointestinal infections with other strains of Shiga toxin–producing *E. coli* remains to be addressed.

Neuraminidase-Associated Hemolytic Uremic Syndrome

Mechanisms. This is a rare but potentially fatal disease that may complicate pneumonia, or less frequently, meningitis caused by *Streptococcus pneumoniae*.[77] Neuraminidase produced by *S. pneumoniae* cleaves N-acetylneuraminic acid from the glycoproteins on the cell membrane of erythrocytes, platelets, and glomerular cells.[78,79] Removing the N-acetylneuraminic acid exposes the normally hidden Thomsen-Friedenreich antigen (T-antigen),[80] which can then react with anti-T immunoglobulin M (IgM) antibody naturally present in human plasma. This antigen–antibody reaction occurs more frequently in infants and children and causes polyagglutination of red blood cells in vitro. This is the reason why, unlike in other forms of HUS, in neuraminidase-associated HUS there is a positive Coombs test. T-anti–T interaction on red cells, platelets, and the endothelium was thought to explain the pathogenesis, whereas the pathogenic role of the anti-T cold antibody in vivo is uncertain.[81] T-antigen exposure on red cells is detected using the lectin hypogaea.

Clinical course and therapy. Patients, usually less than 2 years old, present with severe microangiopathic hemolytic anemia. The clinical picture is severe, with respiratory distress, neurologic involvement, and coma. The acute mortality is about 25%. The outcome is strongly dependent on the effectiveness of antibiotic therapy. In theory, plasma either infused or exchanged, is contraindicated, because adult plasma contains antibodies against the T-antigen that may accelerate polyagglutination and hemolysis.[80] Thus, patients should be treated only with antibiotics and washed red cells. In some cases, however, plasma therapy, occasionally in combination with steroids, has been associated with recovery.

Atypical Hemolytic Uremic Syndrome. Atypical HUS (aHUS) includes a number of associations and presentations. It can occur sporadically or within families. Research in the last 10 years has linked aHUS to uncontrolled activation of the complement system (Fig. 55.12 and Table 55.1).[5]

Familial atypical hemolytic uremic syndrome. Fewer than 20% of aHUS cases are familial. Reports date back to 1965, when Campbell and Carré described hemolytic anemia and azotemia in concordant monozygous twins.[82] Since then, familial HUS has been reported in children and, less frequently, in adults. Although some were in siblings, suggesting autosomal recessive transmission, others were across two to three generations, suggesting an autosomal dominant mode.[83,84] The prognosis is poor (cumulative incidence of death or ESRD, 50% to 80%).

Sporadic atypical hemolytic uremic syndrome. Sporadic aHUS encompasses cases without a family history of the disease. Triggering conditions for sporadic aHUS[85] include HIV infection, anticancer drugs (e.g., mitomycin, cisplatin, bleomycin, gemcitabine), immunotherapeutic agents (e.g., cyclosporine, tacrolimus, OKT3, interferon, quinidine), antiplatelet agents (ticlopidine and clopidogrel), malignancies, transplantation, and pregnancy.[12,86]

De novo posttransplant HUS has been reported in patients receiving renal transplants or other organs, due to calcineurin inhibitors or humoral rejection. It occurs

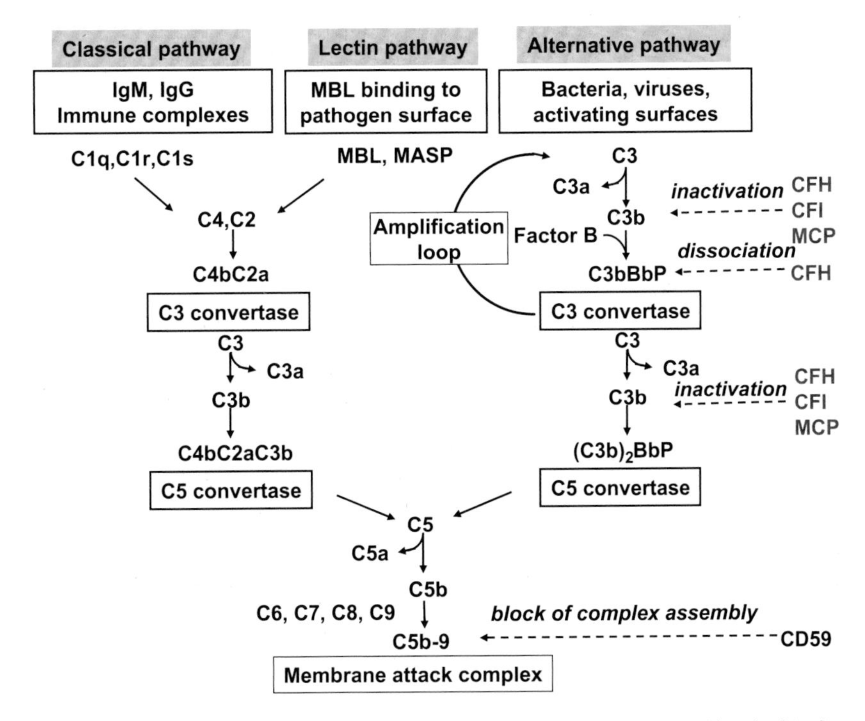

FIGURE 55.12 The three activation pathways of complement. The classical pathway is initiated by the binding of the C1 complex to antibodies bound to an antigen on the surface of a bacterial cell, leading to the formation of a C4b2a enzyme complex, the C3 convertase of the classical pathway. The mannose-binding lectin pathway is initiated by binding of the complex of mannose-binding lectin (MBL) and the serine proteases mannose-binding lectin–associated proteases 1 and 2 (MASP1 and MASP2) to mannose residues on the surface of a bacterial cell, which leads to the formation of the C3 convertase enzyme C4bC2a. The alternative pathway is initiated by the covalent binding of a small amount of C3b generated by spontaneous hydrolysis in plasma to hydroxyl groups on cell-surface carbohydrates and proteins. This C3b binds factor B to form the alternative pathway C3 complex C3bBb. The C3 convertase enzymes cleave many molecules of C3 to form the anaphylatoxin C3a and C3b, which binds covalently around the site of complement activation. Some of this C3b binds to C4b and C3b in the convertase enzymes of the classical and alternative pathways, respectively, forming C5 convertase enzymes that cleave C5 to form the anaphylatoxin C5a and C5b, which initiates the formation of the membrane-attack complex. The human complement system is highly regulated as to prevent nonspecific damage to host cells and to limit the deposition of complement to the surface of pathogens. This fine regulation occurs through a number of membrane-anchored and fluid phase regulators that inactivate complement products formed at various levels in the cascade and that protect host tissues. (See Color Plate.) *CFB,* complement factor B; *CFI,* complement factor I; *CFH,* complement factor H; *MCP,* membrane cofactor protein; *CD59,* protectin (prevents the terminal polymerization of the membrane attack complex).

in 5% to 10% of renal transplant patients who receive cyclosporine and in approximately 1% of those who are given tacrolimus.[87–89] TMA usually develops in the first weeks posttransplant when patients are treated with high doses of the immunosuppressant. Plasma exchange, combined with dose reduction or the withdrawal of calcineurin inhibitors, achieved remission in up to 80% of patients with de novo posttransplant HUS.[88]

In 10% to 15% of female patients, aHUS manifests during pregnancy or postpartum.[6,85] aHUS may present at any time during pregnancy but mostly in the last trimester and about the time of delivery. It is sometimes difficult to distinguish it from preeclampsia. HELLP syndrome (HEmolytic anemia, elevated Liver enzymes, and Low Platelets) is a life-threatening disorder of the last trimester or parturition with severe thrombocytopenia, microangiopathic hemolytic anemia, renal failure, and liver involvement. These forms are always an indication for prompt delivery that is usually followed by complete remission.[85] Postpartum HUS manifests within 3 months of delivery in most cases. The outcome is usually poor.

About 50% of sporadic aHUS cases show no clear trigger (idiopathic HUS).

Mechanisms.

Complement abnormalities. Reduced serum levels of C3 with normal C4 in HUS patients were known since 1974.[90,91] In cases of familial aHUS, serum C3 was low even during remission, hinting at genetic defects.[90,92] Low C3 reflected complement activation and consumption with high levels of activated products, C3b, C3c, and C3d.[93]

The complement system is part of innate immunity and consists of several plasma and membrane-bound proteins that protect against invading organisms.[94] Three activation pathways—classical, lectin, and alternative pathways—produce protease complexes, termed C3 and C5 convertases that cleave C3 and C5, respectively, eventually leading to the membrane attack complex (MAC or C5b-9) that causes cell lysis (Fig. 55.12). The alternative pathway is initiated spontaneously in plasma by C3 hydrolysis, which is responsible for covalent deposition of a low amount of C3b onto practically all plasma-exposed surfaces. On the bacterial surface, C3b leads to opsonization for phagocytosis by neutrophils and macrophages. Without regulation, a small initiating stimulus is quickly amplified to a self-harming response until the consumption of complement components. On host cells, such a dangerous cascade is controlled by membrane-anchored and fluid-phase regulators (Fig. 55.12). They both favor the cleavage of C3b to inactive iC3b by the plasma serine–protease factor I (CFI, cofactor activity) and dissociate the multicomponent C3 and C5 convertases (decay acceleration activity). Foreign targets and injured cells that either lack membrane-bound regulators or cannot bind soluble regulators are attacked by complement.

The C3 convertases of classic/lectin pathways are formed by C2 and C4 fragments, whereas the alternative pathway convertase requires the cleavage of C3 only (Fig. 55.12).[94] Thus, low serum C3 levels in aHUS with normal C4 indicated selective alternative pathway activation.[92]

Genetic abnormalities. A variety of genetic abnormalities in members of the alternative pathway of complement have been described in aHUS, which account for about 60% of cases (Table 55.1). Of note, different genetic abnormalities account for different patterns of dysfunction of the complement system with a different outcome, response to therapy, and risk of recurrence after kidney transplantation (Table 55.3).

- **Complement factor H.** Complement factor H (CFH) regulates the alternative pathway by competing with complement factor B (CFB) for C3b recognition, by acting as a cofactor for CFI, and by enhancing the dissociation of C3 convertase.[95] In 1998, Goodship and coworkers[96] demonstrated a linkage of aHUS to the chromosome 1q32 locus, containing genes for CFH

TABLE 55.3 **Outcome of Atypical Hemolytic Uremic Syndrome According to the Associated Genetic Abnormality**

Affected Gene	Affected Protein and Main Effect	Frequency in aHUS	Rate of Remission with Plasma Exchange[a]	5- to 10-yr Rate of Death or ESRD	Rate of Recurrence after Kidney Transplant
CFH	Factor H (no binding to endothelium)	20%–30%	60% (Dose and timing dependent)	70%–80%	80%–90%
CFHL1/3	Factor HR1, R3 (antifactor H antibodies)	6%	70%–80% (combined with immunosuppression)	30%–40%	20%
MCP	Membrane cofactor protein (no surface expression)	10%–15%	No indication to plasma exchange	<20%	15%–20%
CFI	Factor I (low levels/low cofactor activity)	4%–10%	30%–40%	60%–70%	70%–80%
CFB	Factor B (C3 convertase stabilization)	1%–2%	30%	70%	One case reported
C3	Complement C3 (resistance to C3b inactivation)	5%–10%	40%–50%	60%	40%–50%
THBD	Thrombomodulin (reduced C3b inactivation)	5%	60%	60%	One case reported

[a]Complete remission or hematologic remission with renal sequelae. aHUS, atypical hemolytic uremic syndrome; ESRD, end-stage renal disease; CFH, complement factor H; MCP, membrane cofactor protein; CFI, complement factor I; THBD, thrombomodulin.

and other complement regulators. Since then, over 100 *CFH* mutations (interactive FH-HUS mutations database, http://www.FH-HUS.org) have been identified in aHUS patients (mutation frequency, familial forms: 40% to 45%, sporadic forms: 10% to 20%).[97–103] These mutations most commonly do not result in a quantitative deficiency in CFH, but instead result in normal levels of a protein that is unable to bind to and regulate complement on endothelial cells and platelets.[104,105] A high degree of sequence identity between *CFH* and the genes *CFHR1-5* for five factor H-related proteins (CFHR) located in tandem to *CFH* may predispose one to nonallelic recombinations.[106,107] In 3% to 5% of patients with aHUS, a heterozygous hybrid gene deriving from an uneven cross-over between *CFH* and *CFHR1* contained the first 21 *CFH* exons and the last two *CFHR1* exons,[107] resulting in a gene product with decreased complement regulatory activity on endothelial surfaces. Additional forms of CFH/CFHRs hybrid genes have been recently described.[108]

- **Membrane Cofactor Protein.** Membrane cofactor protein (MCP) is pivotal against C3 activation on the glomerular endothelium. Indeed, the anti-MCP antibody completely blocked cofactor activity in cell extracts.[109] In 2003, two groups[110,111] described mutations in *MCP*, encoding the widely expressed transmembrane regulator, the membrane cofactor protein, in affected individuals of four families. MCP serves as a cofactor for CFI to cleave C3b and C4b on cell surface.[112] *MCP* mutations account for 10% to 15% of aHUS cases.[101] Most are heterozygous, and about 25% are either homozygous or compound heterozygous (http://www.FH-HUS.org). The majority cluster in critical extracellular modules for regulation. Expression on blood leukocytes was reduced for about 75% of mutants, causing a quantitative defect. Others have low C3b-binding capability and decreased cofactor activity.[101,113]

- **Complement Factor I.** CFI is a plasma serine protease that regulates the three complement pathways by cleaving C3b and C4b in the presence of cofactor proteins. *CFI* mutations affect 4% to 10% of aHUS patients.[101,114–116] All mutations are heterozygous, and 80% cluster in the serine–protease domain. Approximately 50% of mutations result in low CFI levels. Others disrupt C3b and C4b cleavage.[101,114–116]

- **Complement Factor B and C3.** Gain-of-function mutations can affect genes encoding the alternative pathway C3 convertase components, CFB and C3.[117,118] *CFB* mutations are rare in aHUS (1% to 2%).[118] Patients have chronic alternative pathway activation with low C3 and, usually, normal C4.[118] CFB mutants have excess C3b-affinity and form a hyperactive C3 convertase resistant to dissociation. C3b formation is thereby enhanced in vivo.[118] About 4% to 10% of aHUS patients have heterozygous mutations in *C3*, usually with low C3 levels.[117] Most mutations reduce C3b binding to CFH and MCP, severely impairing degradation of mutant C3b.[117]

- **Thrombomodulin.** Mutations in the gene *THBD* encoding thrombomodulin, a membrane-bound glycoprotein with anticoagulant properties that modulates complement activation on cell surfaces, have been very recently associated to aHUS.[119] About 5% of aHUS patients carry heterozygous *THBD* mutations. Cells expressing these variants inactivate C3b less efficiently than cells expressing wild-type thrombomodulin.[119] These data document a functional link between complement and coagulation, opening new perspectives for candidate gene research in aHUS.

Acquired abnormalities. Acquired defects of CFH function are also seen in the form of inhibitory antibodies that are reported in 5% to 10% of aHUS patients.[120–123] Analogous to the genetic defect seen in CFH, these autoantibodies also predominantly target the C-terminal end of the protein, thereby impairing complement regulation on host cell surfaces. The development of CFH autoantibodies in aHUS has a genetic predisposition, being strongly associated with a genomic deletion of the *CFHR1* and *CFHR3* genes. More detailed analysis subsequently suggested that the association between *CFHR1/CFHR3* deletion and autoantibodies in aHUS is probably related to the absence of CFHR1 protein.[121,124] CFH and CFHR1 share a high degree of homology with the two C-terminal SCR of CFHR1 almost identical to SCR 19 to 20 of CFH. It is not surprising therefore that autoantibodies to CFH also bind to CFHR1.[121]

Clinical Course. Irrespective of mutation type, 60% to 70% of patients are affected during childhood,[101,125] and almost all patients with anti-CFH antibodies developed the disease before 16 years of age.[126] Acute episodes manifest with severe hemolytic anemia, thrombocytopenia, and acute renal failure. Extrarenal involvement (central nervous system or multivisceral) occurs in 20% of cases.[5,101,125]

Short- and long-term outcomes vary according to the underlying complement abnormality (Table 55.3). About 60% to 70% of patients with *CFH, CFI,* and *C3* mutations and one-third of children with anti-CFH autoantibodies lose renal function or die during the presenting episode, or develop ESRD following relapses.[5,101,125] *CFB* mutations are associated with poor renal outcome (renal function loss in seven out of eight patients).[118]

Chronic complement dysregulation may lead to atheromalike lesions. About 20% of patients with *CFH* mutations have cardiovascular complications (e.g., coronary or cerebrovascular disease, myocardial infarction) and excess mortality. Long-term survival is worse in patients with *CFH* mutations (50% at 10 years) than in those with *CFI* and *C3* mutations or anti-CFH autoantibodies (80% to 90% at 10 years).[5,101,125,127]

MCP-mutation carriers have a good prognosis (complete remission, 80% to 90%). Recurrences are frequent, but long-term outcome is good; 80% of patients remain dialysis free.[5,101,125] However, rarely, patients with *MCP* mutations had severe disease, immediate ESRD, intractable hypertension, and coma,[101,128] possibly because of concurrent genetic abnormalities.

Therapy

Fresh frozen plasma. Guidelines suggest that plasma therapy (plasma-exchange, 1 to 2 plasma volumes/day, plasma infusion, 20 to 30 mL/kg/day) should be started within 24 hours of diagnosis.[5] Plasma exchange allows for supplying larger amounts of plasma than would be possible with infusion while avoiding fluid overload (Table 55.2). Trials of plasma therapy in HUS are scanty and not current. The only two published trials in HUS comparing supportive therapy alone with supportive therapy plus plasma infusion did not demonstrate significant benefit of plasma in inducing remission. However, neither trial[129,130] examined outcomes separately for Stx-HUS versus aHUS, which invariably weakened potential benefits of plasma in aHUS.[131,132] Because CFH is a plasma protein, plasma infusion or exchange provided normal CFH to patients carrying *CFH* mutations.[101,125,133,134] Long-term treatment, however, may fail due to the development of plasma resistance.[135] Heterozygous *CFH* mutation carriers usually have normal levels of CFH, half of which is dysfunctional. The beneficial effect of plasma is strongly dependent on the amount, frequency, and modality of administration, with plasma exchange being superior to plasma infusion for remission and the prevention of recurrences by removal of mutant CFH that could antagonize the normal protein.[136,137] Overall published data[5,101,125] in patients with *CFH* mutations show either complete or partial (hematologic normalization with renal sequelae) remission of 60% of plasma-treated episodes (Table 55.3).[127] Plasma exchange is used to remove anti-CFH antibodies,[120,125] but the effect is usually transient. Immunosuppressants (corticosteroids and azathioprine or mycophenolate-mofetil) and rituximab, an anti-CD20 antibody, combined with plasma exchange allowed for long-term dialysis-free survival in 60% to 70% of patients.[120,122,126,138]

Patients with *CFI* mutations show only a partial response with remission in about 30% to 40% of plasma-treated episodes.[5,101,125,139] As MCP is a cell-associated protein, effects of plasma are unlikely in patients with *MCP* mutations. Indeed, 80% to 90% of patients undergo remission independently of plasma treatment (Table 55.3).[5,101,125,127,139]

Thirty-forty percent of patients with *CFB* mutations and 50% of those with *C3* mutations responded to plasma infusion or exchange.[5,117,118] These patients possibly need abundant and frequent plasma exchanges to clear the hyperfunctional mutant CFB and C3.[5]

Transplantation. Whether kidney transplantation is appropriate for aHUS patients with ESRD has been long debated. Disease recurred in about 50% of transplanted patients with CFH, CFI, CFB, and C3 mutations, and graft failure occurred in 80% to 90% of them.[114,117,118,125,140–142] A live-related donation is contraindicated by a high risk of recurrences[142,143] and may be risky to donors. An adult male with a heterozygous *CFH* mutation developed de novo HUS after donating a kidney to his child.[143] Most studies have shown that plasma exchange therapy fails to prevent graft loss in patients with recurrent posttransplant HUS.[144,145] Use of intensive plasma prophylaxis has been proposed for patients with aHUS-related ESRD undergoing kidney transplantation. According to this proposal, plasma exchange should be initiated just before transplantation, continued as a daily treatment, and then progressively tapered according to the posttransplant course.[145] Use of a preemptive plasma strategy has been successful in preventing recurrent aHUS in eight renal transplant recipients.[145,146] However, in some of the patients, delayed recurrence occurred when plasma therapy was tapered.[136,147,148]

Simultaneous kidney and liver transplant was performed in two children with aHUS and *CFH* mutations with the rationale of correcting the genetic defect and preventing recurrences.[149,150] However, both cases were complicated by premature liver failure. The first child recovered after a second liver transplantation. The child had no symptoms of HUS for 3 years but died by sequelae of hepatic encephalopathy.[149] This case offered the proof-of-concept that transplant could cure HUS associated with *CFH* mutations by correcting the genetic defect. The second case was also complicated by liver failure with widespread microvascular thrombosis and complement deposition.[150] It was reasoned that the surgical stress with ischemia/reperfusion induced complement activation in liver that could not be regulated because of functional *CFH* deficiency. A modified approach to the combined transplant was applied to eight cases,[151–153] including extensive plasma exchange before surgery to provide timely enough normal CFH until the liver graft recovered synthetic functions. This procedure was successful in seven patients. However, another child developed severe hepatic thrombosis and fatal encephalopathy. The risks of kidney and liver transplantation require a careful assessment of benefits for candidate patients.

The risk of posttransplant aHUS recurrence in patients with anti-CFH autoantibodies is not well known, because available reports only describe a total of 12 renal transplants in 8 patients.[145] The assessment of risk is further complicated by the recent finding that almost 40% of patients with anti-CFH antibodies also carried a mutation in genes encoding complement proteins.[121] A reduction in autoantibody levels with plasmapheresis, steroids, and/or rituximab enabled the successful renal transplantation in a few patients,[138,154] suggesting that high anti-CFH antibody titers positively correlated with a risk of aHUS recurrence. Thus, it is reasonable to recommend that titers of anti-CFH antibody are regularly monitored in an attempt to evaluate the risk of posttransplant aHUS recurrence.

The outcome of kidney transplant is favorable in patients with *MCP* mutations. More than 80% did not experience HUS recurrence, with long-term graft survival comparable with that of patients transplanted for other causes.[5,125,140,141]

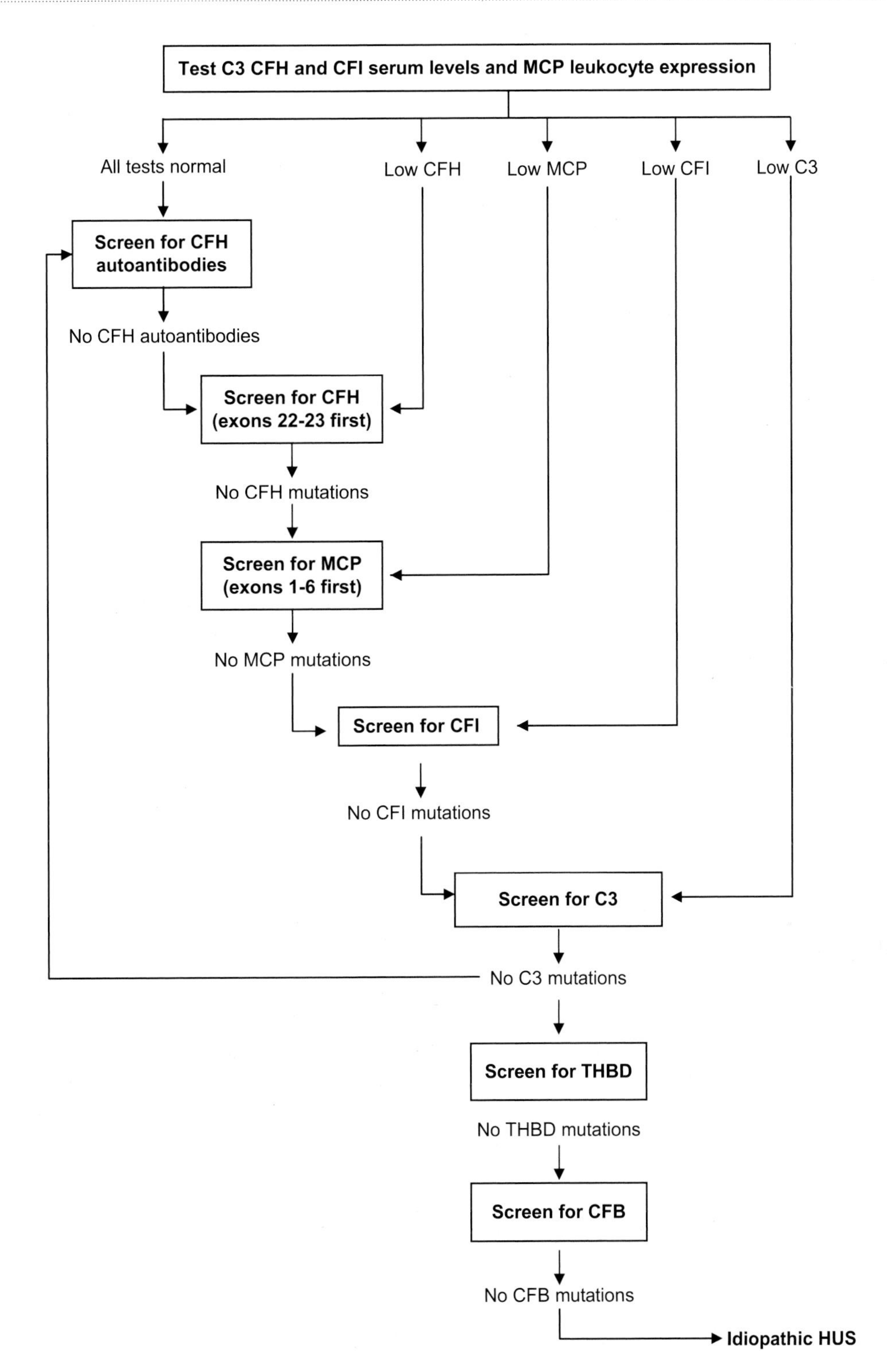

FIGURE 55.13 A flow diagram of the steps suggested to optimize the cost-effectiveness of screening for genetic defects in patients with atypical hemolytic uremic syndrome (aHUS) and suspected genetically determined abnormalities in complement regulatory proteins. A preliminary screen for serum C3 levels by nephelometry, complement factor H (CFH), and complement factor I (CFI) levels by either enzyme-linked immunosorbent assay (ELISA) or radial immune diffusion (RID), and of membrane cofactor protein (MCP) expression in peripheral blood leukocytes by fluorescence-activated cell sorting (FACS), is recommended to identify which is the candidate gene to evaluate. If no abnormalities are detected, we suggest to screen for anti-CFH autoantibodies and then, if no autoantibodies are detected, to look for mutations of candidate genes beginning with evaluating the CFH gene, which is more frequently affected by pathogenic mutations, followed by MCP, CFI genes, C3, thrombomodulin (THBD), and complement factor B (CFB) respectively. Within each gene, the exons where the mutations tend to localize more frequently should be studied first.

The theoretical rationale is strong. MCP is a transmembrane protein highly expressed in the kidney. A kidney graft, not surprisingly, corrects the defect of *MCP*-mutated recipients.

Screening for mutations should allow patients and clinicians to make informed decisions regarding listing for transplantation based on the risk of recurrence. Algorithms have been developed to optimize the cost-effectiveness of screening programs for genetic defects in patients with aHUS based on prevalence of the mutations (Figure 55.13). A position paper[151] has defined the groups of patients in which isolated kidney transplantation is risky, whereas a combined kidney-liver transplant is recommended, and those eligible for isolated kidney transplantation.

Complement inhibitors. Identifying complement genetic abnormalities has paved the way for tailored treatments aimed at specifically tuning down complement activation. A human plasma–derived CFH concentrate is being developed following the European Orphan drug designation (http://www.emea.europa.eu/pdfs/human/comp/opinion/52123506en.pdf). Currently, a number of drug companies have complement inhibitors under preclinical and clinical development. Phase III clinical trials showed efficacy and tolerance of the humanized anti-C5 monoclonal antibody eculizumab in paroxysmal nocturnal hemoglobinuria.[155] More than 20 aHUS patients treated with eculizumab have been reported in the literature thus far.[156–169] Some patients were treated for aHUS on the native kidneys, whereas others received eculizumab to treat or to prevent posttransplant aHUS recurrences. The efficacy of eculizumab in aHUS has been definitely proven in two open label controlled trials (ClinicalTrials.gov Identifier: NCT1410916) of adult and adolescent patients over the age of 12 years with plasma therapy–sensitive or plasma therapy–resistant aHUS.[170,171] All of the patients with plasma-dependent HUS did not require plasma infusion or exchange any longer over 26 to 52 weeks of eculizumab therapy. Platelet count persistently normalized in all cases with the exception of transient fluctuations in four patients without any other evidence of disease activity. Consistently, the platelet count normalized in 13 patients with plasma-resistant HUS over 26 to 64 weeks of eculizumab therapy, and renal function improved in 11 cases. Eculizumab was well tolerated and quality of life improved in all patients. At the end of 2011, eculizumab has been approved by the U.S. Food and Drug Administration (FDA) and by the European Commission (EC) for the treatment of adult and pediatric patients with aHUS.

How long eculizumab therapy should be continued and what is the ideal treatment regimen to be administered, however, remains to be established. Conceivably, chronic, lifetime treatment with eculizumab at doses able to persistently block the alternative pathway of the complement cascade might be indicated to prevent disease recurrence in genetic forms. However, whether and to what extent this applies to all patients with atypical HUS and complement intrinsic abnormalities is unknown. Reasonably, different underlying genetic defects, different clinical courses before eculizumab therapy, and different residual complement activity while on eculizumab therapy, should be taken into consideration when strategies of chronic eculizumab therapy are planned. In this regard, the case of a 42-year-old woman with a heterozygous gain of function mutation in the C3 gene and posttransplant plasma-dependent recurrent aHUS may be informative.[159] This woman received four 900 mg IV doses every 7 days followed by a maintenance regimen of 1,200 mg every 2 weeks. With this regimen, the disease fully recovered and no plasma exchange session was required any longer. However, 7 months later, as soon as the time elapsing between two infusions was prolonged just by 6 days because of an intercurrent disease, hemolysis recurred in parallel with an acute worsening of kidney function. Disease again recovered with blood transfusions and with the reintroduction of the every other week 1,200 mg eculizumab regimen. These findings suggest that chronic treatment with regimens able to persistently inhibit the complement system may be required in at least some patients. On the other hand, the risk of sensitization associated with chronic drug exposure and the enormous costs that could be unbearable in resource-limited settings suggest that a careful treatment tapering up to withdrawal whenever possible should be attempted in most cases under a tight control of disease and complement activity.

HUS Associated with Inborn Abnormal Cobalamin Metabolism

Mechanisms. This is a rare autosomal recessive form of HUS associated with an inborn abnormality of cobalamin-C metabolism.[172] The biochemical characteristics of cobalamin-C deficiency are hyperhomocysteinemia and methylmalonic aciduria.

Clinical course. Patients with cobalamin-C deficiency usually present in the early days and months of life with a failure to thrive, poor feeding, and vomiting.[85,172] Rapid deterioration occurs due to metabolic acidosis, gastrointestinal bleeding, hemolytic anemia, thrombocytopenia, severe respiratory and hepatic failure, and renal insufficiency. Children may present neurologic symptoms of fatigue, delirium, psychosis, and seizures. In cases with early onset, the disease has a fulminant evolution and occasionally involves the pulmonary vasculature, but when it ensues later in childhood, it may follow a more chronic course. The hallmarks of defective cobalamin metabolism are hyperhomocysteinemia and methylmalonic aciduria, and the extremely high homocysteine levels (up to tenfold higher than normal) have been suggested to have a role in the pathogenesis of the vascular lesions. Without treatment, the disease is fatal and some children likely die undiagnosed.

Therapy. Daily intramuscular administrations of hydroxycobalamin may reduce both homocysteine levels and methylmalonic aciduria, whereas oral hydroxycobalamin and cyanocobalamin are ineffective. Oral betaine contributes to further reduce serum homocysteine levels by activating betaine-homocysteine methyltransferase. The supplementation of folic acid to avoid folate deficiency induced by methyltetrahydrofolate trapping, and of L-carnitine to increase propionylcarnitine excretion have been suggested, but their role in improving disease outcome is unclear.[173]

Despite treatment, the majority of children with early onset disease die or have severe neurologic sequelae. Intensified treatment in older children with less acute disease may achieve remission of the microangiopathic process and amelioration of the other clinical manifestations of the metabolic disorder. Whether plasma therapy has a role in improving disease outcome is unknown.

Thrombotic Thrombocytopenic Purpura

In the microvasculature of patients with TTP, systemic platelet thrombi are developed, mainly formed by platelets and von Willebrand factor (vWF). This protein plays a major role in primary hemostasis, forming platelet plugs at sites of vascular injury under high shear stress. VWF is a large glycoprotein synthesized in vascular endothelial cells and megakaryocytes. Upon stimulation, vWF is secreted by endothelial cells as ultralarge (UL) multimers that form stringlike structures attached to the endothelial cells, possibly through interaction with P-selectin.[174] Under fluid shear stress, the UL-vWF strings are cleaved to generate the range of vWF multimer sizes that normally circulate in the blood, from approximately 500 kDa to 20 million Da.[175] The proteolytic cleavage of vWF multimers appears to be critical to prevent thrombosis in the microvasculature (Fig. 55.14, upper panel).

ADAMST13 is the protease deputed to cleave vWF, which is deficient in the majority of patients with TTP leading to the accumulation of UL-vWF multimers that are highly reactive with platelets (Fig. 55.14, lower panel).[176–178] ADAMTS13 is encoded by the homonymous gene located on chromosome 9q34. ADAMTS13 is expressed predominantly in liver and consists of a N-terminal signal peptide, a propeptide, a reprolysinlike metalloprotease domain, a disintegrinlike domain, a first thrombospondin type-1 motif (TSP1), a cysteine-rich domain, a spacer domain, seven additional TSP1 repeats, and two complement unit binding (CUB) domains. Two mechanisms for deficiency of the ADAMTS13 activity have been identified in patients with idiopathic TTP, an acquired deficiency due to the formation of anti-ADAMTS13 autoantibodies (acquired TTP), and a genetic deficiency due to homozygous or compound heterozygous mutations in *ADAMTS13* gene (congenital TTP) (Table 55.1).

TTP Associated with Immune-Mediated Deficiency of ADAMTS13

Mechanisms. This is an immune-mediated, nonfamilial form of TTP that most likely accounts for the majority of cases (from 60% to 90%) reported to date as acute idiopathic or sporadic TTP (Table 55.1). The disease is characterized by a severe deficiency of ADAMTS13,[179] the activity of which is inhibited by specific autoantibodies that develop transiently and tend to disappear during remission.[9,176,177,180]

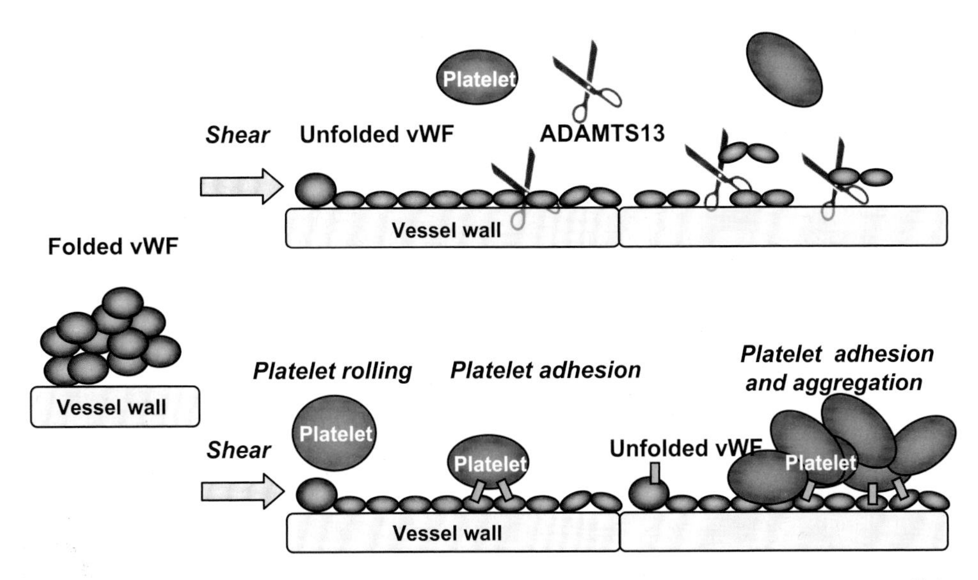

FIGURE 55.14 The pathophysiology of platelet aggregation in thrombotic thrombocytopenic purpura. von Willebrand factor (vWF) is synthesized and stored as ultralarge (UL) multimers in endothelial cells and megakaryocytes. Upon stimulation, UL-vWF multimers are secreted by endothelial cells into the circulation in a folded structure. Upon exposure to enhanced shear stress, UL multimers form stringlike structures that adhere to endothelial cells. Normally, UL-vWF strings are cleaved by ADAMTS13 to generate vWF multimers from 500 kDa to 20 million Da in molecular weight to prevent thrombosis in the microvasculature *(upper panel)*. When the ADAMTS13 proteolytic activity is defective because of the inhibitory effect of anti-ADAMTS13 autoantibodies or congenital defective synthesis of the protease, UL-vWF multimers accumulate and interact with activated platelets to facilitate platelet adhesion and aggregation, with thrombi formation and occlusion of the vascular lumen *(lower panel)*.

These inhibitory anti-ADAMTS13 antibodies are mainly IgG,[176,177,181] although IgM and IgA anti-ADAMTS13 antibodies have also been described.[181]

Patients with TTP secondary to hematopoietic stem cell transplantation, malignancies, or HIV infection rarely have severe ADAMTS13 deficiency and inhibitory IgG antibodies.[182–184] TTP associated with ticlopidine and clopidogrel (thienopyridine drugs that inhibit platelet aggregation) represent interesting exceptions of secondary TTP, which is consistent with a drug-induced autoimmune disorder. Severe ADAMTS13 deficiency and ADAMTS13 inhibitory antibodies were detected in 80% to 90% of patients with ticlopidine-associated TTP[184] and in two patients with clopidogrel-induced TTP.[184] The deficiency resolved after the drugs were discontinued.

The ADAMTS13 epitopes recognized by autoantibodies have been mapped and, so far, all plasmas contain at least some antibodies directed against the Cys-rich/spacer domain.[185,186] In some cases, the antibodies were directed only against these epitopes, but in the majority of patients combinations of antibodies were found, including antibodies against CUB domains, the TSP1 repeats, and the ADAMTS13 propeptide.[186] When cloned and prepared as monoclonal antibodies, many of these antibodies inhibit ADAMTS13 activity in vitro and in vivo in mice.[184]

Evidence of the pathogenic role of TTP-associated anti-ADAMTS13 autoantibodies is derived by finding that they usually disappear from the circulation when remission is achieved by effective treatment; this occurs in parallel with the normalization of ADAMTS13 activity. In patients with acquired ADAMTS13 deficiency, a risk as high as 50% to develop relapses has been reported, and undetectable ADAMTS13 activity and the persistence of anti-ADAMTS13 inhibitors during remission predict recurrences.[181]

Clinical course. Patients with anti-ADAMTS13 inhibitors experience a more severe manifestation of the disease and have a higher mortality rate than patients without antibodies.[187] Neurologic symptoms usually dominate the clinical picture and may be fleeting and fluctuating, probably because of continuous thrombi formation and dispersion in the brain microcirculation. Coma and seizures complicate the most severe forms. The detection of high titers of anti-ADAMTS13 autoantibodies is correlated with relapsing disease and a poor prognosis.

TTP has been reported in 1 of every 1,600 to 5,000 patients treated with ticlopidine. Eleven cases have been reported during treatment with clopidogrel, a new anti-aggregating agent that has achieved widespread clinical use for its safety profile. Most patients with TTP associated with ticlopidine or clopidogrel had neurologic involvement. The overall survival rate is 67% and is improved by early treatment withdrawal and plasma therapy.

Therapy. Plasma manipulation is a cornerstone in the therapy of the acute episode (Table 55.2). Plasma may serve to induce remission of the disease by replacing defective protease activity. As compared to an infusion, an exchange may offer the advantage of also rapidly removing anti-ADAMTS-13 antibodies. This, however, needs to be proven in controlled trials. Corticosteroids might be of benefit in autoimmune forms of TTP by inhibiting the synthesis of anti-ADAMTS13 autoantibodies. In a series of 33 patients with undetectable ADAMTS-13 activity and anti-ADAMTS13 antibodies, a combined treatment with plasma exchange and prednisone was associated with disease remission in around 90% of cases.[181] The rationale of using the combined treatment is that plasma exchange will have only a temporary effect on the presumed autoimmune basis of the disease and additional immunosuppressive treatment may cause a more durable response. Thirty out of 108 patients with either TTP or HUS were reported to have recovered after treatment with corticosteroids alone. All of them, however, had mild forms and none of them were tested for ADAMTS13 activity.[188]

Prospective studies have successfully and safely used rituximab in patients who had failed to respond to standard daily plasma exchanges and methylprednisolone and in patients with relapsed acute TTP who had previously demonstrated antibodies to ADAMTS13 (Table 55.2).[189,190] Treatment was associated with clinical remission in all patients, the disappearance of anti-ADAMTS13 antibodies, and with an increase of ADAMTS13 activity to levels >10%. Rituximab has been also used electively to prevent relapses in patients with autoantibodies and recurrent disease.[9,190–192] In a study, five patients with persistent undetectable ADMTS13 activity and high titers of autoantibody were treated with rituximab as preemptive therapy during remission. ADAMTS13 activity ranged from 15% to 75% and the disappearance of inhibitors was achieved after 3 months in all patients, and activity was still >20% at 6 months. Three patients maintained in a disease-free status after 29, 24, and 6 months, respectively.[192,193] Relapses were documented at 13 and 51 months in the remaining two patients during follow-up. A longitudinal evaluation of ADAMTS13 activity and autoantibody levels may help in monitoring a patient's response to treatment. Retreatment with rituximab should be considered when ADAMTS13 activity decreases and inhibitors reappear into the circulation in order to prevent a relapse (Table 55.2).

TTP Associated with Congenital Deficiency of ADAMTS-13

Mechanisms. This rare form is associated with a genetic defect of ADAMTS13 and accounts for about 5% of all cases of TTP (Table 55.2).[193] Emerging data also indicate that patients with a clinical diagnosis of HUS[180,194] may have a complete lack of ADAMTS13 activity, albeit less frequently. Thus, on clinical grounds, a possible congenital defect of ADAMTS13 cannot be excluded only on the basis of predominant renal localization of disease manifestation. TTP associated with congenital ADAMTS13 deficiency presented either in families or in patients with no familial history of the disease.[176,178,180] In both cases the disease is inherited as a recessive trait, as documented by the fact that ADAMTS13 levels in unaffected relatives of patients fell into a bimodal distribution with a group with half normal levels, consistent with carriers of a heterozygous mutation, and the other with normal values.

To date more than 80 *ADAMTS13* mutations have been identified in patients with TTP.[178,193,195] Approximately 60% of these mutations are missense, causing single amino acid substitutions, and the remaining are nonsense deletions or insertions causing frameshifts or splice site mutants leading to a truncated protein. Most patients are carriers of compound heterozygous mutations; only 15 mutations have been observed in homozygous forms. Studies on secretion and activity of the mutated forms of the protease showed that most of these mutations led to an impaired secretion from the cells, and, when the mutated protein is secreted, the proteolytic activity is greatly reduced.[195]

Clinical course. Approximately 60% of patients with a congenital deficiency of ADAMTS13 experience their first acute episode of disease in the neonatal period or during infancy, but a second group (10% to 20%) manifests the disease after the third decade of life. TTP recurrences are common, but their frequency varies widely. Although some patients with congenital ADAMTS13 deficiency depend on frequent chronic plasma infusions to prevent recurrences, many patients who achieved clinical remission after plasma treatment remain in a disease-free status for long periods of time after plasma discontinuation, despite the absence of protease activity.[193]

Emerging data suggest that the type and location of *ADAMTS13* mutations may influence the age of onset of TTP and the penetrance of the disease in mutation carriers.[193] One of the most frequently reported *ADAMTS13* mutations, the 4143-4144insA in the second CUB domain, leading to a frameshift and loss of the last 49 amino acids of the protein, is associated with neonatal-childhood onset; indeed only 1 out of 16 reported carriers, either homozygous or compound heterozygous with other *ADAMTS13* mutations, reached the adult age without developing TTP.[193,196] In vitro expression studies revealed that the mutation causes a severe impairment of protein secretion combined with a strongly reduced specific protease activity. On the other hand, mutations in the sixth and the seventh TSP1[193,197] appear to lead to an adult onset and a milder course of TTP. Expression studies revealed that these mutations result in severe defects in the secretion of the metalloprotease, although a small fraction of the mutant protein is released in the supernatant, but the mutants maintain normal specific protease activity.[193,198] It is possible that in carriers of these mutations, small ADAMTS13 activity may be present in the circulation, which is enough to prevent the onset of the disease in childhood or even in adulthood. The latter possibility is supported by descriptions of asymptomatic carriers of such mutations who never developed TTP.[193,195,197]

Environmental factors may contribute to induce a full-blown manifestation of the disease. According to this "two hit model," deficiency of ADAMTS13 predisposes one to microvascular thrombosis, and thrombotic microangiopathy supervenes after a triggering event that activates microvascular endothelial cells and causes the secretion of UL-vWF multimers and P-selectin expression. Potential triggers of this phenomena are infections and pregnancy. Six women with congenital ADAMTS13 deficiency developed late onset TTP during pregnancy.[195,199] Also, genetic modifiers may be implicated in susceptibility to develop thrombotic microangiopathy in the condition of ADAMTS13 deficiency, which may include gene-encoding proteins involved in the regulation of the coagulation cascade, vWF, or platelet function, or components of the endothelial vessel surface or of the complement cascade.

Therapy. At the moment, therapy of TTP associated with congenital ADAMTS13 deficiency involves plasma infusion or exchange to replenish the active protease (Table 55.2). Actually, providing just a 5% normal enzymatic activity may be sufficient to degrade large vWF multimers, which may be relevant to induce remission of the microangiopathic process, and this effect is sustained over time due to the relatively long half-life (2 to 4 days) of the protease. In two brothers with a complete deficiency of the protease and relapsing TTP, disease remission was achieved by plasmapheresis and was concurrent with an almost full recovery of the ADAMTS13 activity. Both patients achieved a long lasting remission, although protease activity decreased to less than 20% over 20 days after plasma therapy withdrawal.[200] Although individual attacks usually respond to treatment, long-term prognosis is invariably poor if therapy fails to achieve lasting remission.

ACUTE CORTICAL NECROSIS

Acute bilateral cortical necrosis affects no more than 2% of patients with acute renal failure (ARF),[201] and has been mainly related to obstetrical causes in the 1970s.[202] The disease is caused by the destruction of the renal cortex except for a thin rim of tissue under the capsule and usually a thicker layer under the corticomedullary junction. This phenomenon likely reflects a disturbed blood flow to the interlobular and afferent arterioles, whereas the arcuate arteries, which supply blood to the juxtamedullary nephrons, are usually spared. The lack of necrosis in subcapsular nephrons is due to the presence of anastomoses with extrarenal vessels that allow for a minimal perfusion to the superficial nephrons—just enough to prevent necrotic changes. In 50% to 70% of the series considered, acute cortical necrosis is a complication of pregnancy (especially in multiparous women older than 30 years of age). Abruptio placentae is the most common prior complication of ARF.[201,203] Preexisting toxemia seems to be an important predisposing factor,[204–206] but there is no general agreement on this issue.[201] Intrauterine death, hemorrhage from placenta previa, septic abortion, postpartum hemorrhage, and, occasionally hyperemesis, are other conditions that may be complicated by acute cortical necrosis.[201,207–210] Bacterial and postoperative shock, pancreatitis, dissecting aneurysms, gastrointestinal hemorrhage, trauma, burns, phosphorus and diethylene glycol poisoning, snake venom bites, and sometimes TTP and HUS are other conditions that can be complicated by acute cortical necrosis.[203,211–222] In recent years, cases have also been reported in patients with paraneoplastic antiphospholipid syndrome[223] or with antiphospholipid syndrome associated with systemic lupus erythematosus.[224] In children, cases of cortical necrosis have been reported, most frequently after protracted vomiting and diarrhea with marked dehydration. Moreover, as in adults, the disease has been seen concomitantly with infections such as peritonitis, septicemia, pharyngitis, transfusion reactions, and phosphorus poisoning.[221,225–229]

Mechanisms

According to Sheehan and Moore,[203] who studied specimens from patients who died after abruptio placentae, vasospasm is the primary event causing cortical necrosis. Acute vascular injury is then followed by the activation of coagulation and thrombosis with consequent tissue necrosis.[230,231] Consistent with this hypothesis is evidence that cortical necrosis can be produced by prolonged clamping of the renal pedicle[232] or by the infusion of a large amount of vasoactive substances such as epinephrine and oxytocin.[233–235] The same lesions, however, can be observed in rabbits following two intravenous injections of endotoxin from gram-negative bacteria, spaced 18 to 24 hours apart—a phenomenon known as an acute Shwartzman reaction.[230] Of note, in pregnant rabbits or rats[236,237] or in animals pretreated with corticosteroids,[230] sympathomimetics (α-agonists),[238] or synthetic acid polymers,[230] the same reaction can be triggered by a single endotoxin injection. Thus, vasospasm and toxic damage to the vascular endothelium may both play a role in the pathogenesis of human disease.[239]

Experimental Shwartzman reactions produced in pregnant rabbits after a single injection of bacterial toxin supports the theory that vascular injury is the major etiologic event in cortical necrosis.[240] In all the previous models, acute cortical necrosis is preceded by intravascular coagulation, an event that appears to play a central pathogenic role as suggested by the fact that cortical necrosis is prevented when heparin is administered to nonpregnant rabbits with a Shwartzman reaction.[241] However, the main difference between an experimental Shwartzman reaction and cortical necrosis in humans is that, in animals, the necrotic process also involves the renal medulla and organs other than the kidney. Probably in humans, selective damage of the cortical vasculature predisposes one to the subsequent development of localized damage as soon as a "trigger event" (e.g., abruptio placentae) occurs. In this context, recent experimental data are particularly relevant. A unilateral Shwartzman phenomenon confined to a single kidney has been produced by the local perfusion of a low-dose endotoxin before the systemic injection of an endotoxin.[242] Cortical necrosis in experimental animals has also been obtained using diethylene glycol.[213,243] The mechanisms by which these toxic agents lead to cortical necrosis are far from being understood, but these agents are known to cause endothelial damage. Another intriguing issue is the significance of glomerular fibrin thrombi. Early reports have focused on the possible crucial role of glomerular thrombosis in the pathogenesis of the disease.[207,244] However, a detailed analysis of the most representative series reported in the literature revealed that glomerular fibrin thrombi are relatively rare in cortical necrosis. Only occasionally have extensive intraglomerular thrombi been documented.[201,209] Altogether, the available data do not support the idea that cortical necrosis is the consequence of a mechanical blockage of glomeruli by fibrin thrombi. Moreover, in the two largest series[209,245] reported so far of patients affected by DIC with glomerular fibrin thrombi, the majority of whom had bacterial sepsis, cortical necrosis was found in only 4 of the 63 cases studied.

Diagnosis and Clinical Course

The most typical clinical sign of acute cortical necrosis is sudden oliguria, with the amount of urine ranging from zero to 100 mL per day.[246] Sometimes this is preceded by gross hematuria. Lumbar pain, if present, constitutes a rather nonspecific symptom and may be associated with fever and leukocytosis. Urine contains protein, red blood cells, white blood cells, epithelial cells, and various types of casts. Hypertension may occur, but generally the blood pressure is only slightly elevated. A picture of acute renal failure with hyperazotemia, metabolic acidosis, and hyperkalemia emerges from laboratory data. LDH and glutamic oxaloacetic transaminases in the serum are elevated during the first days of the disease.[243] DIC is frequent, especially in obstetric patients. Fibrinogen and platelet counts fall very low, prothrombin time is prolonged, and fibrinogen degradation products (FDPs) in serum are often elevated.[239]

Acute cortical necrosis must be suspected when oliguria or anuria tends to persist for a long period. A renal biopsy provides the definitive diagnosis. However, the patient's clinical condition may not always permit the performance of a biopsy, and in some cases, the diagnosis may be missed because, especially in the incomplete form of disease, the specimen does not allow for the detection of the typical changes. Radiologic techniques are very useful in the evaluation of the diagnosis of acute cortical necrosis.[201,247,248] Renal echography may exclude obstruction. Selective arteriography may provide information about the extent of lesions, permitting a distinction between the complete and incomplete forms. The most typical radiologic sign of acute cortical necrosis is the renal cortical calcification, which, however, is uncommon and does not occur in the early phases of the disease.[243]

Pathology

The earliest histologic lesion of the generalized Shwartzman reaction is the deposition of a homogeneous, eosinophilic material with the staining properties of fibrinoid within the lumen of the glomerular capillaries of the kidneys.[249]

Similar material is deposited in the vessels in other visceral organs in association with necrotizing and hemorrhagic lesions.[230,249] In humans with massive or complete cortical necrosis, almost the whole cortex is affected by necrosis except the corticomedullary junction and a thin rim of cortical tissue under the capsule.[203] On gross examination, the kidneys are enlarged and weigh 200 to 300 g. The cortex has a yellowish-white appearance, but congested areas are detected in the periphery. Moreover, the columns of Bertin are necrosed. The main renal arteries—the lobar and the arciform—are generally spared. A microscopic examination shows pathologic changes appearing 48 to 72 hours after the initial injury. Glomeruli and tubules show extensive necrotic changes, whereas the afferent arterioles are occluded by thrombi extending to the interlobular arteries. At the periphery of the necrosis, a large-scale infiltration of polymorphonuclear leukocytes fully develops after 3 to 4 days.

In addition to the pattern of complete cortical necrosis, Sheehan and Moore[203] described other forms of acute cortical necrosis characterized by more limited necrotic changes, the so-called incomplete acute cortical necrosis. The latter includes the focal form, in which the necrotic lesion can reach a diameter ranging from 0.5 to 3.0 mm, and the patchy form, with much larger necrotic areas. The authors described an additional variant of acute cortical necrosis called confluent focal cortical necrosis, which differs from the forms previously described in the following aspects: (1) The focal lesions are so numerous that they merge with one another; (2) the typical changes are present in tubules and glomeruli but not in the arterioles and arteries, and appear at different stages in the course of the disease; and (3) the pattern is not associated with abruptio placentae.

Histologically, the lesions of incomplete cortical necrosis are essentially the same as those in the complete form. The edge of the necrotic area forms a sharp border with normal renal tissue. In the late phases of the disease, kidneys are reduced in size, interstitial fibrosis occurs in the injured areas, and sclerotic substitutions occur in the glomeruli and in vessels. Calcium deposits detected by a von Kossa stain can be found in the glomeruli or in arteries.

In addition to the kidney, other organs are sometimes injured too, though to a lesser extent and more mildly, such as the adrenals, spleen, liver, large intestine, and particularly, the pituitary gland sinusoids.[201,250–252]

Prognosis and Therapy

The course of acute cortical necrosis is characterized by prolonged oliguria and death during the first days of the disease unless dialysis treatment is available. After a period of 1 to 3 months, renal function may partially recover, so that patients become dialysis independent. Urine output progressively increases, and renal function may improve over a period of 1 to 2 years, to a final plateau of 20 to 25 mL per minute.[239,243] Hypertrophy of the juxtamedullary nephrons has been suggested as a factor contributing to the partial restoration of renal function.[239] After the initial renal function recovery, however, most patients eventually progress to ESRD, possibly because of progressive failure of the few nephron units surviving the acute phase of the disease.

No specific therapeutic approaches in addition to supportive maneuvers commonly employed in ARF are available for acute cortical necrosis. Renal replacement therapy must be started as early as possible, and daily dialytic therapy may be necessary considering the high catabolic rate often present in these patients. Many patients have received renal transplants, and the prognosis of such patients has greatly improved during the last few years.[243]

ACKNOWLEDGMENTS

The authors are grateful to Manuela Passera for help in preparing the manuscript.

REFERENCES

1. Remuzzi G. HUS and TTP: variable expression of a single entity. *Kidney Int.* 1987;32(2):292–308.
2. Gasser C, Gautier E, Steck A, et al. [Hemolytic-uremic syndrome: bilateral necrosis of the renal cortex in acute acquired hemolytic anemia]. *Schweiz Med Wochenschr.* 1955;85(38–39):905–909.
3. Ruggenenti P, Noris M, Remuzzi G. Thrombotic microangiopathy, hemolytic uremic syndrome, and thrombotic thrombocytopenic purpura. *Kidney Int.* 2001;60(3):831–846.
4. Constantinescu AR, Bitzan M, Weiss LS, et al. Non-enteropathic hemolytic uremic syndrome: causes and short-term course. *Am J Kidney Dis.* 2004; 43(6):976–982.
5. Noris M, Remuzzi G. Atypical hemolytic-uremic syndrome. *N Engl J Med.* 2009;361(17):1676–1687.
6. Noris M, Remuzzi G. Hemolytic uremic syndrome. *J Am Soc Nephrol.* 2005;16(4):1035–1050.
7. Moschcowitz E. An acute febrile pleiochromic anemia with hyaline thrombosis of the terminal arterioles and capillaries: an undescribed disease. 1925. *Mt Sinai J Med.* 2003;70(5):352–355.
8. Crowther MA, George JN. Thrombotic thrombocytopenic purpura: 2008 update. *Cleve Clin J Med.* 2008;75(5):369–375.
9. Galbusera M, Noris M, Remuzzi G. Thrombotic thrombocytopenic purpura—then and now. *Semin Thromb Hemost.* 2006;32(2):81–89.
10. George JN. The thrombotic thrombocytopenic purpura and hemolytic uremic syndromes: overview of pathogenesis (Experience of The Oklahoma TTP-HUS Registry, 1989-2007). *Kidney Int Suppl.* 2009;(112):S8–S10.
11. George JN. Clinical practice. Thrombotic thrombocytopenic purpura. *N Engl J Med.* 2006;354(18):1927–1935.
12. Ruggenenti P, Galli M, Remuzzi G. Hemolytic uremic syndrome, thrombotic thrombocytopenic purpura, and antiphospholipid antibody syndromes. In: Neilson EG, Couser WG, eds. *Immunologic Renal Diseases*, 2nd ed. Philadelphia: Lippincott Williams & Wilkins; 2001: 1173–1201.
13. Rock G, Kelton JG, Shumak KH, et al. Laboratory abnormalities in thrombotic thrombocytopenic purpura. Canadian Apheresis Group. *Br J Haematol.* 1998;103(4):1031–1036.
14. Kaplan BS, Proesmans W. The hemolytic uremic syndrome of childhood and its variants. *Semin Hematol.* 1987;24(3):148–160.
15. Eknoyan G, Riggs SA. Renal involvement in patients with thrombotic thrombocytopenic purpura. *Am J Nephrol.* 1986;6(2):117–131.
16. Richardson SE, Karmali MA, Becker LE, et al. The histopathology of the hemolytic uremic syndrome associated with verocytotoxin-producing *Escherichia coli* infections. *Hum Pathol.* 1988;19(9):1102–1108.
17. Remuzzi G, Ruggenenti P. Thrombotic microangiopathies. In: Tisher C, Brenner B, (eds). *Renal Pathology*, 2nd ed. Philadelphia: J.B. Lippincott; 1994: 1154–1184.
18. Remuzzi G, Ruggenenti P. The hemolytic uremic syndrome. *Kidney Int.* 1995;48:2–19.
19. Mead PS, Griffin PM. *Escherichia coli* O157:H7. *Lancet.* 1998;352(9135): 1207–1212.
20. Frank C, Werber D, Cramer JP, et al. Epidemic profile of shiga-toxin-producing *Escherichia coli* O104:H4 outbreak in Germany - preliminary report. *N Engl J Med.* 2011;365(19):1771–1780.

21. Buchholz U, Bernard H, Werber D, et al. German outbreak of *Escherichia coli* O104:H4 associated with sprouts. *N Engl J Med.* 2011;365(19):1763–1770.
22. Donnenberg MS, Tacket CO, James SP, et al. Role of the eaeA gene in experimental enteropathogenic *Escherichia coli* infection. *J Clin Invest.* 1993; 92(3):1412–1417.
23. Acheson DW, Moore R, De Breucker S, et al. Translocation of Shiga toxin across polarized intestinal cells in tissue culture. *Infect Immun.* 1996;64(8): 3294–3300.
24. Hurley BP, Thorpe CM, Acheson DW. Shiga toxin translocation across intestinal epithelial cells is enhanced by neutrophil transmigration. *Infect Immun.* 2001;69(10):6148–6155.
25. Bitzan M, Richardson S, Huang C, et al. Evidence that verotoxins (Shiga-like toxins) from *Escherichia coli* bind to P blood group antigens of human erythrocytes in vitro. *Infect Immun.* 1994;62(8):3337–3347.
26. Cooling LL, Walker KE, Gille T, et al. Shiga toxin binds human platelets via globotriaosylceramide (Pk antigen) and a novel platelet glycosphingolipid. *Infect Immun.* 1998;66(9):4355–4366.
27. Stahl AL, Svensson M, Morgelin M, et al. Lipopolysaccharide from enterohemorrhagic *Escherichia coli* binds to platelets through TLR4 and CD62 and is detected on circulating platelets in patients with hemolytic uremic syndrome. *Blood.* 2006;108(1):167–176.
28. van Setten PA, Monnens LA, Verstraten RG, et al. Effects of verocytotoxin-1 on nonadherent human monocytes: binding characteristics, protein synthesis, and induction of cytokine release. *Blood.* 1996;88(1):174–183.
29. O'Brien AD, Lively TA, Chang TW, et al. Purification of *Shigella dysenteriae* 1 (Shiga)-like toxin from *Escherichia coli* O157:H7 strain associated with haemorrhagic colitis. *Lancet.* 1983;2(8349):573.
30. Paton AW, Srimanote P, Talbot UM, et al. A new family of potent AB(5) cytotoxins produced by Shiga toxigenic *Escherichia coli*. *J Exp Med.* 2004; 200(1):35–46.
31. Scotland SM, Willshaw GA, Smith HR, et al. Properties of strains of *Escherichia coli* belonging to serogroup O157 with special reference to production of Vero cytotoxins VT1 and VT2. *Epidemiol Infect.* 1987;99(3):613–624.
32. Ostroff SM, Kobayashi JM, Lewis JH. Infections with *Escherichia coli* O157:H7 in Washington State. The first year of statewide disease surveillance. *JAMA.* 1989;262(3):355–359.
33. Cimolai N, Carter JE, Morrison BJ, et al. Risk factors for the progression of *Escherichia coli* O157:H7 enteritis to hemolytic-uremic syndrome. *J Pediatr.* 1990;116(4):589–592.
34. Jenkins C, Willshaw GA, Evans J, et al. Subtyping of virulence genes in verocytotoxin-producing *Escherichia coli* (VTEC) other than serogroup O157 associated with disease in the United Kingdom. *J Med Microbiol.* 2003;52(Pt 11): 941–947.
35. Siegler RL, Obrig TG, Pysher TJ, et al. Response to Shiga toxin 1 and 2 in a baboon model of hemolytic uremic syndrome. *Pediatr Nephrol.* 2003; 18(2):92–96.
36. Nakajima H, Kiyokawa N, Katagiri YU, et al. Kinetic analysis of binding between Shiga toxin and receptor glycolipid Gb3Cer by surface plasmon resonance. *J Biol Chem.* 2001;276(46):42915–42922.
37. Sandvig K, Olsnes S, Brown JE, et al. Endocytosis from coated pits of Shiga toxin: a glycolipid-binding protein from Shigella dysenteriae 1. *J Cell Biol.* 1989;108(4):1331–1343.
38. Obrig TG, Del Vecchio PJ, Brown JE, et al. Direct cytotoxic action of Shiga toxin on human vascular endothelial cells. *Infect Immun.* 1988;56(9):2373–2378.
39. Lingwood CA. Verotoxin-binding in human renal sections. *Nephron.* 1994; 66(1):21–28.
40. Zoja C, Buelli S, Morigi M. Shiga toxin-associated hemolytic uremic syndrome: pathophysiology of endothelial dysfunction. *Pediatr Nephrol.* 2010; 25(11):2231–2240.
41. Zoja C, Angioletti S, Donadelli R, et al. Shiga toxin-2 triggers endothelial leukocyte adhesion and transmigration via NF-kappaB dependent up-regulation of IL-8 and MCP-1. *Kidney Int.* 2002;62(3):846–856.
42. Morigi M, Micheletti G, Figliuzzi M, et al. Verotoxin-1 promotes leukocyte adhesion to cultured endothelial cells under physiologic flow conditions. *Blood.* 1995;86(12):4553–4558.
43. Morigi M, Galbusera M, Binda E, et al. Verotoxin-1-induced up-regulation of adhesive molecules renders microvascular endothelial cells thrombogenic at high shear stress. *Blood.* 2001;98(6):1828–1835.
44. Thurman JM, Marians R, Emlen W, et al. Alternative pathway of complement in children with diarrhea-associated hemolytic uremic syndrome. *Clin J Am Soc Nephrol.* 2009;4(12):1920–1924.
45. Orth D, Khan AB, Naim A, et al. Shiga toxin activates complement and binds factor H: evidence for an active role of complement in hemolytic uremic syndrome. *J Immunol.* 2009;182(10):6394–6400.
46. Morigi M, Galbusera M, Gastoldi S, et al. Alternative pathway activation of complement by Shiga toxin promotes exuberant C3a formation that triggers microvascular thrombosis. *J Immunol.* 2011;187(1):172–180.
47. Manning SD, Motiwala AS, Springman AC, et al. Variation in virulence among clades of *Escherichia coli* O157:H7 associated with disease outbreaks. *Proc Natl Acad Sci USA.* 2008;105(12):4868–4873.
48. Blaser MJ. Deconstructing a lethal foodborne epidemic. *N Engl J Med.* 2011;365(19):1835–1836.
49. Banatvala N, Griffin PM, Greene KD, et al. The United States National Prospective Hemolytic Uremic Syndrome Study: microbiologic, serologic, clinical, and epidemiologic findings. *J Infect Dis.* 2001;183(7):1063–1070.
50. Garg AX, Clark WF, Salvadori M, et al. Absence of renal sequelae after childhood *Escherichia coli* O157:H7 gastroenteritis. *Kidney Int.* 2006;70(4): 807–812.
51. Chandler WL, Jelacic S, Boster DR, et al. Prothrombotic coagulation abnormalities preceding the hemolytic-uremic syndrome. *N Engl J Med.* 2002; 346(1):23–32.
52. Beatty ME, Griffin PM, Tulu AN, et al. Culturing practices and antibiotic use in children with diarrhea. *Pediatrics.* 2004;113(3 Pt 1):628–629.
53. Milford D. The hemolytic uremic syndromes in the United Kingdom. In: Kaplan BS, Trompeter RS, Moake JL, eds. *Hemolytic Uremic Syndrome and Thrombotic Thrombocytopenic Purpura.* New York: Marcel Dekker Inc.; 1992:39–59.
54. Garg AX, Suri RS, Barrowman N, et al. Long-term renal prognosis of diarrhea-associated hemolytic uremic syndrome: a systematic review, meta-analysis, and meta-regression. *JAMA.* 2003;290(10):1360–1370.
55. Tönshoff B, Sammet A, Sanden I, et al. Outcome and prognostic determinants in the hemolytic uremic syndrome of children. *Nephron.* 1994;68(1):63–70.
56. Lou-Meda R, Oakes RS, Gilstrap JN, et al. Prognostic significance of microalbuminuria in postdiarrheal hemolytic uremic syndrome. *Pediatr Nephrol.* 2007;22(1):117–120.
57. Ruggenenti P, Remuzzi G. A German outbreak of haemolytic uraemic syndrome. *Lancet.* 2011;378(9796):1057–1058.
58. Cui Y, Qin J, Zhao X, et al. Identification of the hybrid strain responsible for Germany food-poisoning outbreak by polymerase chain reaction. *J Clin Microbiol.* 2011;49(10):3714–3716.
59. Uber AP, Trabulsi LR, Irino K, et al. Enteroaggregative *Escherichia coli* from humans and animals differ in major phenotypical traits and virulence genes. *FEMS Microbiol Lett.* 2006;256(2):251–257.
60. Ake JA, Jelacic S, Ciol MA, et al. Relative nephroprotection during *Escherichia coli* O157:H7 infections: association with intravenous volume expansion. *Pediatrics.* 2005;115(6):e673–680.
61. Chiurchiu C, Firrincieli A, Santostefano M, et al. Adult nondiarrhea hemolytic uremic syndrome associated with Shiga toxin *Escherichia coli* O157:H7 bacteremia and urinary tract infection. *Am J Kidney Dis.* 2003;41(1):E4.
62. Wong CS, Jelacic S, Habeeb RL, et al. The risk of the hemolytic-uremic syndrome after antibiotic treatment of *Escherichia coli* O157:H7 infections. *N Engl J Med.* 2000;342(26):1930–1936.
63. Colic E, Dieperink H, Titlestad K, et al. Management of an acute outbreak of diarrhoea-associated haemolytic uraemic syndrome with early plasma exchange in adults from southern Denmark: an observational study. *Lancet.* 2011;378(9796):1089–1093.
64. Safdar N, Said A, Gangnon RE, et al. Risk of hemolytic uremic syndrome after antibiotic treatment of *Escherichia coli* O157:H7 enteritis: a meta-analysis. *JAMA.* 2002;288(8):996–1001.
65. Falagas ME, Kastoris AC, Kapaskelis AM, et al. Fosfomycin for the treatment of multidrug-resistant, including extended-spectrum beta-lactamase producing, Enterobacteriaceae infections: a systematic review. *Lancet Infect Dis.* 2010;10(1):43–50.
66. Caletti MG, Lejarraga H, Kelmansky D, et al. Two different therapeutic regimes in patients with sequelae of hemolytic-uremic syndrome. *Pediatr Nephrol.* 2004;19(10):1148–1152.
67. Van Dyck M, Proesmans W. Renoprotection by ACE inhibitors after severe hemolytic uremic syndrome. *Pediatr Nephrol.* 2004;19(6):688–690.
68. Trachtman H, Cnaan A, Christen E, et al. Effect of an oral Shiga toxin-binding agent on diarrhea-associated hemolytic uremic syndrome in children: a randomized controlled trial. *JAMA.* 2003;290(10):1337–1344.
69. Bitzan M, Schaefer F, Reymond D. Treatment of typical (enteropathic) hemolytic uremic syndrome. *Semin Thromb Hemost.* 2010;36(6):594–610.
70. Lino M, Kus JV, Tran SL, et al. A novel antimicrobial peptide significantly enhances acid-induced killing of Shiga toxin-producing *Escherichia coli* O157 and non-O157 serotypes. *Microbiology.* 2011;157(Pt 6):1768–1775.
71. Dundas S, Murphy J, Soutar RL, et al. Effectiveness of therapeutic plasma exchange in the 1996 Lanarkshire *Escherichia coli* O157:H7 outbreak. *Lancet.* 1999;354(9187):1327–1330.

72. Carter AO, Borczyk AA, Carlson JA, et al. A severe outbreak of *Escherichia coli* O157:H7—associated hemorrhagic colitis in a nursing home. *N Engl J Med.* 1987;317(24):1496–1500.

73. Artz MA, Steenbergen EJ, Hoitsma AJ, et al. Renal transplantation in patients with hemolytic uremic syndrome: high rate of recurrence and increased incidence of acute rejections. *Transplantation.* 2003;76(5):821–826.

74. Loirat C, Niaudet P. The risk of recurrence of hemolytic uremic syndrome after renal transplantation in children. *Pediatr Nephrol.* 2003;18(11):1095–1101.

75. Ferraris JR, Ramirez JA, Ruiz S, et al. Shiga toxin-associated hemolytic uremic syndrome: absence of recurrence after renal transplantation. *Pediatr Nephrol.* 2002;17(10):809–814.

76. Lapeyraque AL, Malina M, Fremeaux-Bacchi V, et al. Eculizumab in severe Shiga-toxin-associated HUS. *N Engl J Med.* 2011;364(26):2561–2563.

77. Brandt J, Wong C, Mihm S, et al. Invasive pneumococcal disease and hemolytic uremic syndrome. *Pediatrics.* 2002;110(2 Pt 1):371–376.

78. Cochran JB, Panzarino VM, Maes LY, et al. Pneumococcus-induced T-antigen activation in hemolytic uremic syndrome and anemia. *Pediatr Nephrol.* 2004;19(3):317–321.

79. Martinot A, Hue V, Leclerc F, et al. Haemolytic-uraemic syndrome associated with *Streptococcus pneumoniae* meningitis. *Eur J Pediatr.* 1989;148(7): 648–649.

80. McGraw ME, Lendon M, Stevens RF, et al. Haemolytic uraemic syndrome and the Thomsen Friedenreich antigen. *Pediatr Nephrol.* 1989;3(2):135–139.

81. Eder AF, Manno CS. Does red-cell T activation matter? *Br J Haematol.* 2001;114(1):25–30.

82. Campbell S, Carré IJ. Fatal haemolytic uraemic syndrome and idiopathic hyperlipaemia in monozygotic twins. *Arch Dis Child.* 1965;40(214):654–658.

83. Kaplan BS, Chesney RW, Drummond KN. Hemolytic uremic syndrome in families. *N Engl J Med.* 1975;292(21):1090–1093.

84. Kaplan BS, Leonard MB. Autosomal dominant hemolytic uremic syndrome: variable phenotypes and transplant results. *Pediatr Nephrol.* 2000;14(6):464–468.

85. Besbas N, Karpman D, Landau D, et al. A classification of hemolytic uremic syndrome and thrombotic thrombocytopenic purpura and related disorders. *Kidney Int.* 2006;70(3):423–431.

86. Zakarija A, Bennett C. Drug-induced thrombotic microangiopathy. *Semin Thromb Hemost.* 2005;31(6):681–690.

87. Ruggenenti P. Post-transplant hemolytic-uremic syndrome. *Kidney Int.* 2002;62(3):1093–1104.

88. Karthikeyan V, Parasuraman R, Shah V, et al. Outcome of plasma exchange therapy in thrombotic microangiopathy after renal transplantation. *Am J Transplant.* 2003;3(10):1289–1294.

89. Zarifian A, Meleg-Smith S, O'Donovan R, et al. Cyclosporine-associated thrombotic microangiopathy in renal allografts. *Kidney Int.* 1999;55(6): 2457–2466.

90. Carreras L, Romero R, Requesens C, et al. Familial hypocomplementemic hemolytic uremic syndrome with HLA-A3,B7 haplotype. *JAMA.* 1981; 245(6):602–604.

91. Stühlinger W, Kourilsky O, Kanfer A, et al. Letter: Haemolytic-uraemic syndrome: evidence for intravascular C3 activation. *Lancet.* 1974;2(7883): 788–789.

92. Noris M, Ruggenenti P, Perna A, et al. Hypocomplementemia discloses genetic predisposition to hemolytic uremic syndrome and thrombotic thrombocytopenic purpura: role of factor H abnormalities. Italian Registry of Familial and Recurrent Hemolytic Uremic Syndrome/Thrombotic Thrombocytopenic Purpura. *J Am Soc Nephrol.* 1999;10(2):281–293.

93. Kim Y, Miller K, Michael AF. Breakdown products of C3 and factor B in hemolytic-uremic syndrome. *J Lab Clin Med.* 1977;89(4):845–850.

94. Walport MJ. Complement. First of two parts. *N Engl J Med.* 2001;344(14): 1058–1066.

95. Zipfel PF, Skerka C. Complement factor H and related proteins: an expanding family of complement-regulatory proteins? *Immunol Today.* 1994;15(3): 121–126.

96. Warwicker P, Goodship TH, Donne RL, et al. Genetic studies into inherited and sporadic hemolytic uremic syndrome. *Kidney Int.* 1998;53(4):836–844.

97. Richards A, Buddles MR, Donne RL, et al. Factor H mutations in hemolytic uremic syndrome cluster in exons 18-20, a domain important for host cell recognition. *Am J Hum Genet.* 2001;68(2):485–490.

98. Dragon-Durey MA, Frémeaux-Bacchi V, Loirat C, et al. Heterozygous and homozygous factor h deficiencies associated with hemolytic uremic syndrome or membranoproliferative glomerulonephritis: report and genetic analysis of 16 cases. *J Am Soc Nephrol.* 2004;15(3):787–795.

99. Caprioli J, Bettinaglio P, Zipfel PF, et. al. The molecular basis of familial hemolytic uremic syndrome: mutation analysis of factor H gene reveals a hot spot in short consensus repeat 20. *J Am Soc Nephrol.* 2001;12(2):297–307.

100. Caprioli J, Castelletti F, Bucchioni S, et al. Complement factor H mutations and gene polymorphisms in haemolytic uraemic syndrome: the C-257T, the A2089G and the G2881T polymorphisms are strongly associated with the disease. *Hum Mol Genet.* 2003;12(24):3385–3395.

101. Caprioli J, Noris M, Brioschi S, et al. Genetics of HUS: the impact of MCP, CFH, and IF mutations on clinical presentation, response to treatment, and outcome. *Blood.* 2006;108(4):1267–1279.

102. Pérez-Caballero D, Gonzalez-Rubio C, Gallardo ME, et al. Clustering of missense mutations in the C-terminal region of factor H in atypical hemolytic uremic syndrome. *Am J Hum Genet.* 2001;68(2):478–484.

103. Saunders RE, Abarrategui-Garrido C, Fremeaux-Bacchi V, et al. The interactive Factor H-atypical hemolytic uremic syndrome mutation database and website: update and integration of membrane cofactor protein and Factor I mutations with structural models. *Hum Mutat.* 2007;28(3):222–234.

104. Ferreira VP, Herbert AP, Cortes C, et al. The binding of factor H to a complex of physiological polyanions and C3b on cells is impaired in atypical hemolytic uremic syndrome. *J Immunol.* 2009;182(11):7009–7018.

105. Manuelian T, Hellwage J, Meri S, et al. Mutations in factor H reduce binding affinity to C3b and heparin and surface attachment to endothelial cells in hemolytic uremic syndrome. *J Clin Invest.* 2003;111(8):1181–1190.

106. Heinen S, Sanchez-Corral P, Jackson MS, et al. De novo gene conversion in the RCA gene cluster (1q32) causes mutations in complement factor H associated with atypical hemolytic uremic syndrome. *Hum Mutat.* 2006;27(3): 292–293.

107. Venables JP, Strain L, Routledge D, et al. Atypical haemolytic uraemic syndrome associated with a hybrid complement gene. *PLoS Med.* 2006;3(10):e431.

108. Maga TK, Meyer NC, Belsha C, et al. A novel deletion in the RCA gene cluster causes atypical hemolytic uremic syndrome. *Nephrol Dial Transplant.* 2011;26(2):739–741.

109. Nakanishi I, Moutabarrik A, Hara T, et al. Identification and characterization of membrane cofactor protein (CD46) in the human kidneys. *Eur J Immunol.* 1994;24(7):1529–1535.

110. Noris M, Brioschi S, Caprioli J, et al. Familial haemolytic uraemic syndrome and an MCP mutation. *Lancet.* 2003;362(9395):1542–1547.

111. Richards A, Kemp EJ, Liszewski MK, et al. Mutations in human complement regulator, membrane cofactor protein (CD46), predispose to development of familial hemolytic uremic syndrome. *Proc Natl Acad Sci USA.* 2003;100(22): 12966–12971.

112. Liszewski MK, Leung M, Cui W, et al. Dissecting sites important for complement regulatory activity in membrane cofactor protein (MCP; CD46). *J Biol Chem.* 2000;275(48):37692–37701.

113. Fremeaux-Bacchi V, Moulton EA, Kavanagh D, et al. Genetic and functional analyses of membrane cofactor protein (CD46) mutations in atypical hemolytic uremic syndrome. *J Am Soc Nephrol.* 2006;17(7):2017–2025.

114. Kavanagh D, Kemp EJ, Mayland E, et al. Mutations in complement factor I predispose to development of atypical hemolytic uremic syndrome. *J Am Soc Nephrol.* 2005;16(7):2150–2155.

115. Kavanagh D, Richards A, Noris M, et al. Characterization of mutations in complement factor I (CFI) associated with hemolytic uremic syndrome. *Mol Immunol.* 2008;45(1):95–105.

116. Fremeaux-Bacchi V, Dragon-Durey MA, Blouin J, et al. Complement factor I: a susceptibility gene for atypical haemolytic uraemic syndrome. *J Med Genet.* 2004;41(6):e84.

117. Frémeaux-Bacchi V, Miller EC, Liszewski MK, et al. Mutations in complement C3 predispose to development of atypical hemolytic uremic syndrome. *Blood.* 2008;112(13):4948–4952.

118. Goicoechea de Jorge E, Harris CL, Esparza-Gordillo J, et al. Gain-of-function mutations in complement factor B are associated with atypical hemolytic uremic syndrome. *Proc Natl Acad Sci USA.* 2007;104(1):240–245.

119. Delvaeye M, Noris M, De Vriese A, et al. Mutations in thrombomodulin in hemolytic-uremic syndrome. *N Engl J Med.* 2009;361(4):345–357.

120. Dragon-Durey MA, Loirat C, Cloarec S, et al. Anti-Factor H autoantibodies associated with atypical hemolytic uremic syndrome. *J Am Soc Nephrol.* 2005;16(2):555–563.

121. Moore I, Strain L, Pappworth I, et al. Association of factor H autoantibodies with deletions of CFHR1, CFHR3, CFHR4, and with mutations in CFH, CFI, CD46, and C3 in patients with atypical hemolytic uremic syndrome. *Blood.* 2010;115(2):379–387.

122. Józsi M, Strobel S, Dahse HM, et al. Anti factor H autoantibodies block C-terminal recognition function of factor H in hemolytic uremic syndrome. *Blood.* 2007;110(5):1516–1518.

123. Zipfel PF, Edey M, Heinen S, et al. Deletion of complement factor H-related genes CFHR1 and CFHR3 is associated with atypical hemolytic uremic syndrome. *PLoS Genet.* 2007;3(3):e41.

124. Abarrategui-Garrido C, Martínez-Barricarte R, López-Trascasa M, et al. Characterization of complement factor H-related (CFHR) proteins in plasma reveals novel genetic variations of CFHR1 associated with atypical hemolytic uremic syndrome. *Blood.* 2009;114(19):4261–4271.

125. Loirat C, Noris M, Fremeaux-Bacchi V. Complement and the atypical hemolytic uremic syndrome in children. *Pediatr Nephrol.* 2008;23(11):1957–1972.

126. Skerka C, Józsi M, Zipfel PF, et al. Autoantibodies in haemolytic uraemic syndrome (HUS). *Thromb Haemost.* 2009;101(2):227–232.

127. Noris M, Caprioli J, Bresin E, et al. Relative role of genetic complement abnormalities in sporadic and familial aHUS and their impact on clinical phenotype. *Clin J Am Soc Nephrol.* 2010;5(10):1844–1859.

128. Fremeaux-Bacchi V, Sanlaville D, Menouer S, et al. Unusual clinical severity of complement membrane cofactor protein-associated hemolytic-uremic syndrome and uniparental isodisomy. *Am J Kidney Dis.* 2007;49(2):323–329.

129. Loirat C, Sonsino E, Hinglais N, et al. Treatment of the childhood haemolytic uraemic syndrome with plasma. A multicentre randomized controlled trial. The French Society of Paediatric Nephrology. *Pediatr Nephrol.* 1988;2(3): 279–285.

130. Rizzoni G, Claris-Appiani A, Edefonti A, et al. Plasma infusion for hemolytic-uremic syndrome in children: results of a multicenter controlled trial. *J Pediatr.* 1988;112(2):284–290.

131. Noris M, Remuzzi G. Thrombotic microangiopathy: what not to learn from a meta-analysis. *Nat Rev Nephrol.* 2009;5(4):186–188.

132. Michael M, Elliott EJ, Craig JC, et al. Interventions for hemolytic uremic syndrome and thrombotic thrombocytopenic purpura: a systematic review of randomized controlled trials. *Am J Kidney Dis.* 2009;53(2):259–272.

133. Cho HY, Lee BS, Moon KC, et al. Complete factor H deficiency-associated atypical hemolytic uremic syndrome in a neonate. *Pediatr Nephrol.* 2007;22(6):874–880.

134. Licht C, Weyersberg A, Heinen S, et al. Successful plasma therapy for atypical hemolytic uremic syndrome caused by factor H deficiency owing to a novel mutation in the complement cofactor protein domain 15. *Am J Kidney Dis.* 2005;45(2):415–421.

135. Nathanson S, Frémeaux-Bacchi V, Deschênes G. Successful plasma therapy in hemolytic uremic syndrome with factor H deficiency. *Pediatr Nephrol.* 2001;16(7):554–556.

136. Davin JC, Strain L, Goodship TH. Plasma therapy in atypical haemolytic uremic syndrome: lessons from a family with a factor H mutation. *Pediatr Nephrol.* 2008;23(9):1517–1521.

137. Lapeyraque AL, Wagner E, Phan V, et al. Efficacy of plasma therapy in atypical hemolytic uremic syndrome with complement factor H mutations. *Pediatr Nephrol.* 2008;23(8):1363–1366.

138. Kwon T, Dragon-Durey MA, Macher MA, et al. Successful pre-transplant management of a patient with anti-factor H autoantibodies-associated haemolytic uraemic syndrome. *Nephrol Dial Transplant.* 2008;23(6):2088–2090.

139. Sellier-Leclerc AL, Fremeaux-Bacchi V, Dragon-Durey MA, et al. Differential impact of complement mutations on clinical characteristics in atypical hemolytic uremic syndrome. *J Am Soc Nephrol.* 2007;18(8):2392–2400.

140. Bresin E, Daina E, Noris M, et al. Outcome of renal transplantation in patients with non-Shiga toxin-associated hemolytic uremic syndrome: prognostic significance of genetic background. *Clin J Am Soc Nephrol.* 2006;1(1):88–99.

141. Loirat C, Fremeaux-Bacchi V. Hemolytic uremic syndrome recurrence after renal transplantation. *Pediatr Transplant.* 2008;12(6):619–629.

142. Chan MR, Thomas CP, Torrealba JR, et al. Recurrent atypical hemolytic uremic syndrome associated with factor I mutation in a living related renal transplant recipient. *Am J Kidney Dis.* 2009;53(2):321–326.

143. Donne RL, Abbs I, Barany P, et al. Recurrence of hemolytic uremic syndrome after live related renal transplantation associated with subsequent de novo disease in the donor. *Am J Kidney Dis.* 2002;40(6):E22.

144. Noris M, Remuzzi G. Thrombotic microangiopathy after kidney transplantation. *Am J Transplant.* 2010;10(7):1517–1523.

145. Zuber J, Le Quintrec M, Sberro-Soussan R, et al. New insights into postrenal transplant hemolytic uremic syndrome. *Nat Rev Nephrol.* 2011;7(1): 23–35.

146. Olie KH, Goodship TH, Verlaak R, et al. Posttransplantation cytomegalovirus-induced recurrence of atypical hemolytic uremic syndrome associated with a factor H mutation: successful treatment with intensive plasma exchanges and ganciclovir. *Am J Kidney Dis.* 2005;45(1):e12–15.

147. Hirt-Minkowski P, Schaub S, Mayr M, et al. Haemolytic uraemic syndrome caused by factor H mutation: is single kidney transplantation under intensive plasmatherapy an option? *Nephrol Dial Transplant.* 2009;24(11):3548–3551.

148. Olie KH, Florquin S, Groothoff JW, et al. Atypical relapse of hemolytic uremic syndrome after transplantation. *Pediatr Nephrol.* 2004;19(10): 1173–1176.

149. Remuzzi G, Ruggenenti P, Codazzi D, et al. Combined kidney and liver transplantation for familial haemolytic uraemic syndrome. *Lancet.* 2002;359 (9318):1671–1672.

150. Remuzzi G, Ruggenenti P, Colledan M, et al. Hemolytic uremic syndrome: a fatal outcome after kidney and liver transplantation performed to correct factor h gene mutation. *Am J Transplant.* 2005;5(5):1146–1150.

151. Jalanko H, Peltonen S, Koskinen A, et al. Successful liver-kidney transplantation in two children with aHUS caused by a mutation in complement factor H. *Am J Transplant.* 2008;8(1):216–221.

152. Saland JM, Emre SH, Shneider BL, et al. Favorable long-term outcome after liver-kidney transplant for recurrent hemolytic uremic syndrome associated with a factor H mutation. *Am J Transplant.* 2006;6(8):1948–1952.

153. Wilson C, Torpey N, Jaques B, et al. Successful simultaneous liver-kidney transplant in an adult with atypical hemolytic uremic syndrome associated with a mutation in complement factor H. *Am J Kidney Dis.* 2011;58(1): 109–112.

154. Le Quintrec M, Zuber J, Noel LH, et al. Anti-Factor H autoantibodies in a fifth renal transplant recipient with atypical hemolytic and uremic syndrome. *Am J Transplant.* 2009;9(5):1223–1229.

155. Brodsky RA, Young NS, Antonioli E, et al. Multicenter phase 3 study of the complement inhibitor eculizumab for the treatment of patients with paroxysmal nocturnal hemoglobinuria. *Blood.* 2008;111(4):1840–1847.

156. Gruppo RA, Rother RP. Eculizumab for congenital atypical hemolytic-uremic syndrome. *N Engl J Med.* 2009;360(5):544–546.

157. Nürnberger J, Philipp T, Witzke O, et al. Eculizumab for atypical hemolytic-uremic syndrome. *N Engl J Med.* 2009;360(5):542–544.

158. Davin JC, Gracchi V, Bouts A, et al. Maintenance of kidney function following treatment with eculizumab and discontinuation of plasma exchange after a third kidney transplant for atypical hemolytic uremic syndrome associated with a CFH mutation. *Am J Kidney Dis.* 2010;55(4):708–711.

159. Chatelet V, Frémeaux-Bacchi V, Lobbedez T, et al. Safety and long-term efficacy of eculizumab in a renal transplant patient with recurrent atypical hemolytic-uremic syndrome. *Am J Transplant.* 2009;9(11):2644–2645.

160. Mache CJ, Acham-Roschitz B, Frémeaux-Bacchi V, et al. Complement inhibitor eculizumab in atypical hemolytic uremic syndrome. *Clin J Am Soc Nephrol.* 2009;4(8):1312–1316.

161. Al-Akash SI, Almond PS, Savell VH Jr, et al. Eculizumab induces long-term remission in recurrent post-transplant HUS associated with C3 gene mutation. *Pediatr Nephrol.* 2011;26(4):613–619.

162. Prescott HC, Wu HM, Cataland SR, et al. Eculizumab therapy in an adult with plasma exchange-refractory atypical hemolytic uremic syndrome. *Am J Hematol.* 2010;85(12):976–977.

163. Zimmerhackl LB, Hofer J, Cortina G, et al. Prophylactic eculizumab after renal transplantation in atypical hemolytic-uremic syndrome. *N Engl J Med.* 2010;362(18):1746–1748.

164. Lapeyraque AL, Frémeaux-Bacchi V, Robitaille P. Efficacy of eculizumab in a patient with factor-H-associated atypical hemolytic uremic syndrome. *Pediatr Nephrol.* 2011;26(4):621–624.

165. Larrea CF, Cofan F, Oppenheimer F, et al. Efficacy of eculizumab in the treatment of recurrent atypical hemolytic-uremic syndrome after renal transplantation. *Transplantation.* 2010;89(7):903–904.

166. Weitz M, Amon O, Bassler D, et al. Prophylactic eculizumab prior to kidney transplantation for atypical hemolytic uremic syndrome. *Pediatr Nephrol.* 2011;26(8):1325–1329.

167. Nester C, Stewart Z, Myers D, et al. Pre-emptive eculizumab and plasmapheresis for renal transplant in atypical hemolytic uremic syndrome. *Clin J Am Soc Nephrol.* 2011;6(6):1488–1494.

168. Hadaya K, Ferrari-Lacraz S, Fumeaux D, et al. Eculizumab in acute recurrence of thrombotic microangiopathy after renal transplantation. *Am J Transplant.* 2011;11(11):2523–2527.

169. Tschumi S, Gugger M, Bucher BS, et al. Eculizumab in atypical hemolytic uremic syndrome: long-term clinical course and histological findings. *Pediatr Nephrol.* 2011;26(11):2085–2088.

170. Licht C, Muus P, Legendre C, et al. Ph II study of eculizumab (ECU) in patients (PTS) with atypical hemolytic uremic syndrome (aHUS) receiving chronic plasma exchange/infusion (PE/PI). *J Am Soc Nephrol.* 2011;22:197A.

171. Greenbaum LA, Babu S, Furman R, et al. Continued improvements in renal function with sustained eculizumab (ECU) in patients (PTS) with atypical hemolytic uremic syndrome (aHUS) resistant to plasma exchange/infusion (PE/PI). 2011;22:197A.

172. Baumgartner ER, Wick H, Maurer R, et al. Congenital defect in intracellular cobalamin metabolism resulting in homocysteinuria and methylmalonic aciduria. I. Case report and histopathology. *Helv Paediatr Acta.* 1979;34(5): 465–482.

173. Van Hove JL, Van Damme-Lombaerts R, Grünewald S, et al. Cobalamin disorder Cbl-C presenting with late-onset thrombotic microangiopathy. *Am J Med Genet.* 2002;111(2):195–201.
174. Padilla A, Moake JL, Bernardo A, et al. P-selectin anchors newly released ultralarge von Willebrand factor multimers to the endothelial cell surface. *Blood.* 2004;103(6):2150–2156.
175. Sadler JE. Von Willebrand factor, ADAMTS13, and thrombotic thrombocytopenic purpura. *Blood.* 2008;112(1):11–18.
176. Furlan M, Robles R, Galbusera M, et al. von Willebrand factor-cleaving protease in thrombotic thrombocytopenic purpura and the hemolytic-uremic syndrome. *N Engl J Med.* 1998;339:1578–1584.
177. Tsai HM, Lian EC. Antibodies to von Willebrand factor-cleaving protease in acute thrombotic thrombocytopenic purpura. *N Engl J Med.* 1998;339(22): 1585–1594.
178. Levy GG, Nichols WC, Lian EC, et al. Mutations in a member of the ADAMTS gene family cause thrombotic thrombocytopenic purpura. *Nature.* 2001;413(6855):488–494.
179. Furlan M, Robles R, Lämmle B. Partial purification and characterization of a protease from human plasma cleaving von Willebrand factor to fragments produced by in vivo proteolysis. *Blood.* 1996;87(10):4223–4234.
180. Veyradier A, Obert B, Houllier A, et al. Specific von Willebrand factor-cleaving protease in thrombotic microangiopathies: a study of 111 cases. *Blood.* 2001;98(6):1765–1772.
181. Ferrari S, Scheiflinger F, Rieger M, et al. Prognostic value of anti-ADAMTS 13 antibody features (Ig isotype, titer, and inhibitory effect) in a cohort of 35 adult French patients undergoing a first episode of thrombotic microangiopathy with undetectable ADAMTS 13 activity. *Blood.* 2007;109(7): 2815–2822.
182. Zheng XL, Kaufman RM, Goodnough LT, et al. Effect of plasma exchange on plasma ADAMTS13 metalloprotease activity, inhibitor level, and clinical outcome in patients with idiopathic and nonidiopathic thrombotic thrombocytopenic purpura. *Blood.* 2004;103(11):4043–4049.
183. Vesely SK, George JN, Lämmle B, et al. ADAMTS13 activity in thrombotic thrombocytopenic purpura-hemolytic uremic syndrome: relation to presenting features and clinical outcomes in a prospective cohort of 142 patients. *Blood.* 2003;102(1):60–68.
184. Zheng XL, Sadler JE. Pathogenesis of thrombotic microangiopathies. *Annu Rev Pathol.* 2008;3:249–277.
185. Soejima K, Matsumoto M, Kokame K, et al. ADAMTS-13 cysteine-rich/spacer domains are functionally essential for von Willebrand factor cleavage. *Blood.* 2003;102(9):3232–3237.
186. Klaus C, Plaimauer B, Studt JD, et al. Epitope mapping of ADAMTS13 autoantibodies in acquired thrombotic thrombocytopenic purpura. *Blood.* 2004; 103(12):4514–4519.
187. Mannucci PM, Peyvandi F. TTP and ADAMTS13: when is testing appropriate? *Hematology Am Soc Hematol Educ Program.* 2007;2007:121–126.
188. Ruggenenti P, Noris M, Remuzzi G. Thrombotic microangiopathies. In: C Wilcox, ed. *Therapy in Nephrology & Hypertension. A Companion to Brenner & Rector's The Kidney*, 3rd ed. Philadelphia: Saunders Elsevier; 2008: 294–312.
189. Scully M, Cohen H, Cavenagh J, et al. Remission in acute refractory and relapsing thrombotic thrombocytopenic purpura following rituximab is associated with a reduction in IgG antibodies to ADAMTS-13. *Br J Haematol.* 2007;136(3):451–461.
190. Fakhouri F, Vernant JP, Veyradier A, et al. Efficiency of curative and prophylactic treatment with rituximab in ADAMTS13-deficient thrombotic thrombocytopenic purpura: a study of 11 cases. *Blood.* 2005;106(6):1932–1937.
191. Galbusera M, Bresin E, Noris M, et al. Rituximab prevents recurrence of thrombotic thrombocytopenic purpura: a case report. *Blood.* 2005;106(3): 925–928.
192. Bresin E, Gastoldi S, Daina E, et al. Rituximab as pre-emptive treatment in patients with thrombotic thrombocytopenic purpura and evidence of anti-ADAMTS13 autoantibodies. *Thromb Haemost.* 2009;101(2):233–238.
193. Galbusera M, Noris M, Remuzzi G. Inherited thrombotic thrombocytopenic purpura. *Haematologica.* 2009;94(2):166–170.
194. Remuzzi G, Galbusera M, Noris M, et al. von Willebrand factor cleaving protease (ADAMTS13) is deficient in recurrent and familial thrombotic thrombocytopenic purpura and hemolytic uremic syndrome. *Blood.* 2002;100(3): 778–785.
195. Donadelli R, Banterla F, Galbusera M, et al. In-vitro and in-vivo consequences of mutations in the von Willebrand factor cleaving protease ADAMTS13 in thrombotic thrombocytopenic purpura. *Thromb Haemost.* 2006;96(4): 454–464.
196. Schneppenheim R, Kremer Hovinga JA, Becker T, et al. A common origin of the 4143insA ADAMTS13 mutation. *Thromb Haemost.* 2006;96(1):3–6.
197. Palla R, Lavoretano S, Lombardi R, et al. The first deletion mutation in the TSP1-6 repeat domain of ADAMTS13 in a family with inherited thrombotic thrombocytopenic purpura. *Haematologica.* 2009;94(2):289–293.
198. Tao Z, Anthony K, Peng Y, et al. Novel ADAMTS-13 mutations in an adult with delayed onset thrombotic thrombocytopenic purpura. *J Thromb Haemost.* 2006;4(9):1931–1935.
199. Camilleri RS, Cohen H, Mackie IJ, et al. Prevalence of the ADAMTS-13 missense mutation R1060W in late onset adult thrombotic thrombocytopenic purpura. *J Thromb Haemost.* 2008;6(2):331–338.
200. Furlan M, Robles R, Morselli B, et al. Recovery and half-life of von Willebrand factor-cleaving protease after plasma therapy in patients with thrombotic thrombocytopenic purpura. *Thromb Haemost.* 1999;81(1):8–13.
201. Kleinknecht D, Grünfeld JP, Gomez PC, et al. Diagnostic procedures and long-term prognosis in bilateral renal cortical necrosis. *Kidney Int.* 1973; 4(6):390–400.
202. Kim HJ. Bilateral renal cortical necrosis with the changes in clinical features over the past 15 years (1980–1995). *J Korean Med Sci.* 1995;10(2): 132–141.
203. Sheehan HL, Moore HD. *Renal Cortical Necrosis and the Kidney of Concealed Accidental Haemorrhage.* Oxford: Blackwell Scientific Publications; 1952.
204. Chugh KS, Singhal PC, Sharma BK, et al. Acute renal failure of obstetric origin. *Obstet Gynecol.* 1976;48(6):642–646.
205. Ferris TF. The kidney and pregnancy. In: Earley LE, Gottschalk CW, eds. *Strauss and Welt's Diseases of the Kidney.* Boston: Little, Brown; 1979: 1321.
206. Merrill JP, Ober WE, Reid DE, et al. Renal lesions and acute renal failure in pregnancy. *Am J Med.* 1956;21(5):781–810.
207. McKay DG. *Disseminated Intravascular Coagulation: An Intermediary Mechanism of Disease.* New York: Hoeber Medical Division, Harper&Row; 1965.
208. Mookerjee BK, Bilefsky R, Kendall AG, et al. Generalized Shwartzman reaction due to gram-negative septicemia after abortion: recovery after bilateral cortical necrosis. *Can Med Assoc J.* 1968;98(12):578–583.
209. Solez K. Acute renal failure ('Acute tubular necrosis' infarction and cortical necrosis). In: Heptinstall RH, ed. *Pathology of the Kidney.* Boston: Little, Brown; 1983: 1069.
210. Yoshikawa T, Tanaka KR, Guze LB. Infection and disseminated intravascular coagulation. *Medicine (Baltimore).* 1971;50(4):237–258.
211. Brown CE, Crane GL. Bilateral cortical necrosis following severe burns. *JAMA.* 1943;122(13):871–873.
212. da Silva OA, López M, Godoy P. Bilateral cortical necrosis and calcification of the kidneys following snakebite: a case report. *Clin Nephrol.* 1979;11(3): 136–139.
213. Geiling EMK, Cannon PR. Pathologic effects of elixir of sulfanilamide (diethylene glycol) poisoning. A clinical and experimental correlation: final report. *JAMA.* 1938;111(10):919–926.
214. Godwin B, McCall AJ. Cortical necrosis complicating perforated gastric ulcer. *Lancet.* 1941;238(6166):512–513.
215. Lauler DP, Schreiner GE. Bilateral renal cortical necrosis. *Am J Med.* 1958;24(4):519–529.
216. Matlin RA, Gary NE. Acute cortical necrosis. Case report and review of the literature. *Am J Med.* 1974;56(1):110–118.
217. Moss SW, Gary NE, Eisinger RP. Renal cortical necrosis following Streptococcal infection. *Arch Intern Med.* 1977;137(9):1196–1197.
218. Oram S, Ross G, Pell L, et al. Renal cortical calcification after snake-bite. *Br Med J.* 1963;1(5346):1647–1648.
219. Rosello SG, Piulats EL, Gomez I, et al. Renal cortical necrosis and right nephrectomy, with survival, in a man. *Am J Med.* 1968;45(2):309–311.
220. Sporn IN. Renal cortical necrosis. *Arch Intern Med.* 1978;138(12):1866.
221. Walls J, Schorr WJ, Kerr DN. Prolonged oliguria with survival in acute bilateral cortical necrosis. *Br Med J.* 1968;4(5625):220–222.
222. Woods JW, Williams TF. Hypertension due to renal vascular diseases, renal infarction and renal cortical necrosis. In: Strauss MB, Welt LG, eds. *Diseases of the Kidney.* Boston: Little, Brown; 1971: 769.
223. Vigneau C, Daugas E, Maury E, et al. Renal cortical necrosis related to paraneoplastic antiphospholipid syndrome. *Am J Kidney Dis.* 2006;47(6): 1072–1074.
224. Kim JO, Kim GH, Kang CM, et al. Bilateral acute renal cortical necrosis in SLE-associated antiphospholipid syndrome. *Am J Kidney Dis.* 2011;57(6): 945–947.
225. Campbell AC, Henderson JL. Symmetrical cortical necrosis of the kidneys in infancy and childhood. *Arch Dis Child.* 1949;24(120):269–285, illust.
226. Groshong TD, Taylor AA, Nolph KD, et al. Renal function following cortical necrosis in childhood. *J Pediatr.* 1971;79(2):267–275.
227. Perry JW. Phosphorus poisoning with cortical necrosis of the kidney; a report of two fatal cases. *Australas Ann Med.* 1953;2(1):94–98.

228. Wahle GH Jr, Muirhead EE. Bilateral renal cortical necrosis in a child associated with an incompatible blood transfusion. *Tex State J Med.* 1953;49(10): 770–775.
229. Zuelzer WW, Charles S, Kurnetz R, et al. Circulatory diseases of the kidneys in infancy and childhood. *AMA Am J Dis Child.* 1951;81(1):1–46.
230. Thomas L, Good RA. Studies on the generalized Shwartzman reaction: I. General observations concerning the phenomenon. *J Exp Med.* 1952;96(6): 605–624.
231. Rohrer H. Kidney necrosis in acute hog cholera. *Virchowos Arch Pathol Anat.* 1983;284:203.
232. Sheehan HL, Davis JC. Renal ischaemia with failed reflow. *J Pathol Bacteriol.* 1959;78:105–120.
233. Byrom FB. Morbid effects of vasopressin in the organs and vessels of rats. *J Pathol Bacteriol.* 1937;45:1–16.
234. Byrom FB, Pratt OE. Oxytocin and renal cortical necrosis. *Lancet.* 1959;1: 753–754.
235. Penner A. Acute ischaemic necrosis of the kidney: a clinico pathologic and experimental study. *Arch Pathol.* 1940;30:465–480.
236. Galton M, Wong TC, McKay DG. Vasomotor changes in the pregnant rabbit induced by bacterial endotoxin. *Fed Proc.* 1960;19:246.
237. Fontaine A, Arondel J, Sansonetti PJ. Role of Shiga toxin in the pathogenesis of bacillary dysentery, studied by using a Tox-mutant of Shigella dysenteriae 1. *Infect Immun.* 1988;56(12):3099–3109.
238. Whitaker AN. Acute renal failure in disseminated intravascular coagulation. Experimental studies of the induction and prevention of renal fibrin deposition. *Prog Biochem Pharmacol.* 1974;9:45–64.
239. Donohoe JF. Acute bilateral cortical necrosis. In: Brenner BM, Lazarus JM, eds. *Acute Renal Failure*. Philadelphia: Saunders; 1983: 252.
240. Shwartzman G. *Phenomenon of Local Tissue Reactivity, and Its Immunological, Pathological and Clinical Significance*. New York: P.B.Hoeber, Inc.; 1937.
241. Corrigan JJ Jr. Effect of anticoagulating and non-anticoagulating concentrations of heparin on the generalized Shwartzman reaction. *Thromb Diath Haemorrh.* 1970;24(1):136–145.
242. Raij L, Keane WF, Michael AF. Unilateral Shwartzman reaction: cortical necrosis in one kidney following in vivo perfusion with endotoxin. *Kidney Int.* 1977;12(2):91–95.
243. Schreiner GE. La necrose corticale bilaterale des reins. In: Hamburger J, Crosnier J, eds. *Nephrologie*. Paris: Editions Medicale Flammarion; 1979.
244. Marcussen H, Asnaes S. Renal cortical necrosis. An evaluation of the possible relation to the Shwartzman reaction. *Acta Pathol Microbiol Scand A.* 1972;80(3):351–356.
245. Robboy SJ, Major MC, Colman RW, et al. Pathology of disseminated intravascular coagulation (DIC). Analysis of 26 cases. *Hum Pathol.* 1972;3(3):327–343.
246. Levinsky NG, Alexander EA. Acute renal failure. In: Brenner BM, Rector FC, eds. *The Kidney*. Philadelphia: Saunders; 1981: 1181.
247. Moell H. Gross bilateral renal cortical necrosis during long periods of oliguria-anuria; roentgenologic observations in two cases. *Acta Radiol.* 1957;48(5):355–360.
248. Whelan JG Jr, Ling JT, Davis LA. Antemortem roentgen manifestations of bilateral renal cortical necrosis. *Radiology.* 1967;89(4):682–689.
249. Brunson JG, Thomas L, Gamble CN. Morphologic changes in rabbits following the intravenous administration of meningococcal toxin. II. Two appropriately spaced injections; the role of fibrinoid in the generalized Shwartzman reaction. *Am J Pathol.* 1955;31(4):655–667.
250. Duff GL, Murray EGD. Bilateral cortical necrosis of the kidneys. *Am J Med Sci.* 1941;201:428.
251. MacGillivray I. Combined renal and anterior pituitary necrosis. *J Obstet Gynaecol Br Emp.* 1950;57:924–930.
252. Sheldon WH, Hertig AT. Bilateral cortical necrosis of the kidney: a report of 2 cases. *Arch Pathol.* 1942;34:866.

CHAPTER

56 Renal Artery Thrombosis, Thromboembolism, Aneurysms, Atheroemboli, and Renal Vein Thrombosis

John W. O'Bell • George P. Bayliss • Lance D. Dworkin

This chapter focuses on vascular complications of the main renal arteries and veins. The chapter is divided into the following subsections: (1) acute thrombosis of the renal artery from trauma; (2) nontraumatic renal arterial occlusive disease; (3) renal artery aneurysms, including ruptured aneurysm; (4) renal artery dissecting aneurysms; (5) atheroembolic renal disease; and (6) acute and chronic renal vein thrombosis. Because renal vein thrombosis occurs primarily in patients with nephrotic syndrome, particular attention will be paid to the discussion of the hypercoagulability of nephrotic syndrome. Although some of the conditions described may participate in the pathophysiology of renovascular hypertension, they are listed for purposes of a differential diagnosis, as renovascular hypertension is discussed in detail elsewhere.

ACUTE THROMBOSIS OF THE RENAL ARTERY FROM TRAUMA

Blunt abdominal trauma such as that occurring after a motor vehicle accident is the most common cause of renal artery thrombosis.[1,2] The mechanism of injury is felt to be acute deceleration injury causing intimal tears, subintimal dissection, and resultant thrombosis.[3] Increased mobility of the left kidney and a more acute angle of attachment to the aorta are felt to explain the observation that the left renal artery is more frequently involved than the right[3] although in some series this pattern is not observed.[4] Injuries to other abdominal viscera are commonly reported due to the severity of the abdominal trauma.[3–6] In a review of 250 cases of traumatic renal artery injury requiring surgical exploration, the following patterns were observed: thrombosis (52%) was the most common finding followed by avulsion (12%), branch injury, and lacerations (3%).[6] Bilateral renal artery findings were noted in 9% and injury to other abdominal organs was present 45% of the time.[6] Renal artery dissection with resultant thrombosis has also been reported after vigorous exercise such as prolonged cycling,[7] marathon running,[8] and aerobics.[9] Isolated cases of traumatic dissection due to seat belt related injury[10] and shock wave lithotripsy[11] have also been reported in the literature.

The major concern with renal arterial thrombosis is renal infarction and permanent loss of function. Although the maximal duration of warm ischemia tolerated by human kidneys is uncertain, warm ischemia time as short as 1 to 2 hours may be sufficient to cause irreversible loss of renal function.[12] Animal studies have helped further understanding of the importance of even low amounts of blood flow in maintaining renal viability. In dog models of unilateral renal artery occlusion by clamping, warm ischemia times of 1, 2, and 3 hours resulted in irreversible loss of viability in the occluded kidney in 40%, 62%, and 100%, respectively.[12–14] In contrast, animals subjected to a partial occlusion of the suprarenal aorta (mean arterial pressures downstream of 17 to 30 mm Hg) tolerated up to 2 hours of reduced perfusion with good recovery in all the animals. For these reasons, the extent of occlusion and presence or absence of collateral circulation may have a major impact on viability of the affected kidney.

Clinical Features

Anuria or oliguria are likely to be present in bilateral renal arterial thrombosis, or unilateral thrombosis in patients with a solitary kidney, but are uncommon features in patients with unilateral thrombosis. Laboratory abnormalities may include hematuria, elevations in lactate dehydrogenase (LDH), creatinine kinase (CK), aspartate aminotransferase (AST), and alkaline phosphatase.[1] Flank pain or abdominal pain are common, but considering most cases are related to trauma, may not be reliable indicators as there may be alternate explanations for pain.

Diagnosis

Because of the short duration of warm ischemia time that can be tolerated by the kidneys, timely diagnosis is critical. Computed tomography (CT) with intravenous contrast is a useful study in patients with abdominal trauma and compares favorably to angiography, the gold standard for renal artery injury or thrombosis.[14] Characteristic CT findings are a lack of renal parenchymal contrast uptake and excretion.

The "cortical rim sign" or contrast enhancement of the peripheral renal cortex may be noted and is attributed to collateral or capsular perfusion.[15] Angiography remains the gold standard study, and may provide information about collateral circulation (which may indicate better chance for preserved renal viability).[16] Use of digital subtraction angiography or imaging with carbon dioxide and/or gadolinium can reduce or eliminate the need for contrast if there are concerns about contrast-induced nephrotoxicity.[17] Concerns about exposure to gadolinium and its link to nephrogenic systemic fibrosis in patients with acute or chronic kidney failure may limit its utility in some patients. In patients too unstable for extensive preoperative imaging, even a "one shot" excretory urogram following a bolus injection of contrast may provide useful information to the surgeon as a normal urogram would exclude the presence of major trauma to that kidney. This could be of use in predicting renal outcome in a patient requiring unilateral nephrectomy to control hemorrhage as normal imaging of the contralateral kidney suggests a better outcome.[18]

Treatment

Treatment for unilateral traumatic renal artery occlusion can be supportive, surgical, or endovascular. Early surgical intervention has been attempted in an effort to salvage renal function, but with mixed results. Factors influencing surgical outcomes include duration of warm ischemia, severity of occlusion (complete or partial), and degree of collateral circulation.[18–25] Case series suggest better results with earlier intervention. Maggio and Brosman reported 80% success of renal salvage when revascularization occurred within 12 hours of injury, 57% success for repairs performed between 12 and 18 hours, and 0% for later attempts.[25] Clark et al. reported substantially lower success rates despite earlier revascularization attempts (17% success rate for revascularization performed 3–18 hours after the injury).[6] Haas et al. reviewed cases from their own institution and from the literature and reported surgical outcomes of 20 cases of bilateral occlusion and 34 cases of unilateral renal arterial occlusion.[4,5] In these cases surgical revascularization was successful in 56% of the bilateral cases and 26% of the unilateral cases.

More recently, an endovascular, rather than surgical approach has been attempted in order to salvage renal function. Good outcomes have been reported in isolated cases of traumatic renal artery occlusion following endovascular stenting procedures, in some cases as long as 24 hours following the injury.[2,26,27] Even following a successful endovascular procedure, the presence of more peripheral thrombi may still limit recovery of renal function.[28] Considering these cases are related to trauma, the decision regarding an endovascular versus a surgical approach may be dictated by the presence of other injuries and need for other abdominal surgery to address those injuries or to control hemorrhage.

In general, surgical or endovascular intervention is reserved for patients with bilateral renal artery occlusion, or unilateral occlusion in patients with a solitary kidney. It is not clear that revascularization of a unilateral occlusion offers advantages over medical management when there is normal function of the contralateral kidney. Although reports in the literature raise significant concerns about viability of the ischemic kidney when thrombosis is prolonged, there are still scattered reports of successful revascularization long after the injury.[23–25,29,30] Other factors such as collateral circulation or incomplete occlusion may have played a role in some of the reported successes.

In cases of surgical revascularization, it is advised not to perform isolated thrombectomy.[4] Resection of the occluded segment with reattachment to the aorta, or placement of an aortorenal graft is advised.[29] In surgical cases with substantial hemorrhage, urgent nephrectomy may be required.

NONTRAUMATIC RENAL ARTERY OCCLUSIVE DISEASE

In addition to traumatic injury resulting in renal arterial thrombosis, there are a variety of nontraumatic causes for renal arterial occlusion. These may be related to thromboembolic disease from a cardiac or other source, or thrombotic disease, for example from local endothelial damage such as that seen in atherosclerosis, or systemic hypercoagulable states. A number of causes for nontraumatic renal artery thrombosis are listed in Table 56.1.

Any disease process that disrupts the arterial endothelial surface can cause acute thrombosis. Most common among these is atherosclerotic renovascular disease. Other possible causes include fibromuscular dysplasia,[31,32] inflammation/vasculitis, infection, aneurysms, or dissection. Renal arterial thrombosis has been reported in the medium and large vessel vasculitides, including Takayasu arteritis,[33,34] polyarteritis nodosum,[35,36] and Behçet disease.[37–40] Other unusual causes include syphilis,[41] cocaine use,[42–44] phycomycosis,[45,46] neurofibromatosis,[47] and urothelial carcinoma of the renal pelvis.[48] Sickle cell anemia typically leads to microscopic infarcts and progressive loss of renal function, but large vessel thrombosis with resulting infarction has been reported as well.[49] Congenital disorders of collagen structure such as Ehlers-Danlos syndrome are also associated with renal artery thrombosis.[50,51]

Hypercoagulable states are much more commonly associated with venous thrombosis, including renal vein thrombosis, which is discussed elsewhere in this chapter. Notable exceptions include antiphospholipid antibody syndrome (APS), particularly catastrophic APS, and heparin-induced thrombocytopenia.[52] Primary or secondary (lupus-related) APS have been implicated in renal artery thrombosis and reported extensively.[53–63] Renal infarct was a common finding in a recent review of abdominal CT scans for patients with APS, occurring in 22 of the 215 patients and accounting for over 50% of the intra-abdominal thromboses.[64] Renal arterial thrombosis has also been reported in antithrombin 3 deficiency[65] and has been reported rarely in patients with

TABLE 56.1 Nontraumatic Causes of Acute Occlusive Renovascular Disease

Renal Artery Thrombosis
Endothelial damage
Atherosclerotic disease
Fibromuscular dysplasia
Renal artery aneurysms and dissecting aneurysms
Polyarteritis nodosum
Takayasu arteritis
Kawasaki disease
Thromboangiitis obliterans
Behçet disease
Syphilis
Cocaine
Ehlers-Danlos syndrome
Hypercoagulable state
Antiphospholipid antibody syndrome
Heparin-induced thrombocytopenia
Factor V Leiden mutation
Nephrotic syndrome
Renal Artery Thromboembolism
Cardiac origin
Atrial fibrillation
Endocarditis
Myocardial infarction
Cardiomyopathy
Paradoxical emboli through patent septal defect
Aortic or renal artery source
Severe atherosclerosis/thrombosis

nephrotic syndrome.[66–68] Factor V Leiden deficiency, again a much more common cause of venous thrombosis, has been associated with renal arterial thrombosis in native and transplanted kidneys.[69]

Thromboembolic Disease

Emboli to the renal arteries are typically of cardiac origin. These may be arrhythmia associated, particularly with atrial fibrillation.[70–72] Mural thrombi as can be seen in acute myocardial infarction or severe cardiomyopathy may also be the source. Thrombi may also occur on diseased or prosthetic heart valves. Septic emboli in the setting of bacterial endocarditis may also be a cause of embolic occlusion and renal infarct, up to 31% in one retrospective series looking at renal biopsy and necropsy results.[73] Renal artery embolism may also be seen in cases of atrial or ventricular myxoma.[74,75] Paradoxical arterial emboli in the setting of a venous thrombosis and an atrial or ventricular septal defect have also been reported.[76] Sources of noncardiac emboli include clots developing elsewhere in arterial circulation and embolizing the renal arteries, or thrombi that originate within aneurysms of the suprarenal aorta or renal artery.

With the advent of increased numbers of endovascular procedures, including angioplasty and stent treatment for aortic and renal artery lesions, iatrogenic causes of renal artery thromboembolism are an increasing concern. Major complications such as thrombosis, dissection, rupture, and atheroembolic showering have been reported to complicate as many as 7% to 10% of endovascular aortic and renovascular procedures.[77,78] Morris et al. in 2001 reported renal artery rupture or occlusion from acute thrombosis in 4.2% of 308 renal artery angioplasties with and without stenting.[79] In a more recent retrospective analysis of 203 renal artery angioplasty with and without stenting procedures, Eklof et al. reported a rate of distal embolization of 2.5% and renal artery occlusion occurred in only a single patient (0.5%).[80] Another concern is the possibility for in-stent thrombus formation in patients following renal artery stenting.[81,82] Renal infarction may also occur as a complication of aortic procedures. In two series of 775 thoracic and abdominal aortic aneurysm repairs using a variety of endografts and techniques, the incidence of renal infarction (diagnosed by postprocedure CT scan) was around 10%.[83,84] Most were small and asymptomatic, but one of the two series reported a 2.6% incidence of total unilateral renal arterial occlusion.[83]

A variety of devices have been manufactured to limit the impact of distal emboli following endovascular procedures. Limited studies have demonstrated efficacy in capturing embolic debris,[85] but it remains unclear whether such devices will be shown to decrease or prevent distal embolic complications.[86] A combination of antiplatelet therapy (abciximab) and distal embolic protection device was found to have improved 1-month outcomes in one randomized controlled trial of distal protection devices, but neither the device alone nor antiplatelet therapy alone had this benefit.[87] Further study is warranted to determine the role of distal protection therapies and devices.

Pathology of Renal Infarction

Renal infarction is a relatively infrequent clinical diagnosis, but common finding at autopsy. In a review of over 14,000 autopsies from Los Angeles County Hospital in the 1930s, renal infarctions were noted in 1.4%, and were most often postmortem diagnoses.[88] Renal infarctions most commonly occur with arterial occlusions, but may occur in venous thrombosis. The size of the infarct depends on the size of the occluded artery and may be a small wedge-shaped infarct or may involve the entire kidney. The gross appearance of the infarct depends on the size of the occluded artery, age of the infarct, and presence or absence of infection. In the first few hours the infarct is red and pyramidal, and subsequently becomes gray with a narrow red rim of congested parenchyma. The area shrinks, leaving behind a V-shaped scar. Infarctions typically involve only the renal cortex, sparing the medulla.[89]

TABLE 56.2 Clinical and Laboratory Features of Thromboembolic Diseases of the Kidney

Feature	Approximate Incidence
History and Physical Findings	
Pain and tenderness (flank, abdomen, chest, back)	75%
Nausea and vomiting	50%
Gross hematuria	20%
Cardiac disease (myocardial infarction, atrial fibrillation, valvular heart disease)	90%
Laboratory Features	
Leukocytosis (11,000–32,000/μL)	95%
Microscopic hematuria (>15 erythrocytes per high-power field)	90%
Pyuria (>10 leukocytes per high-power field)	80%
Proteinuria (1+ to 4+)	95%
Increased enzymes (LDH, AST, ALT, alkaline phosphatase)	95–100%
Special Diagnostic Procedures	**Finding**
Computed tomography (with contrast material)	Area of decreased attenuation, "wedge-shaped" infarct; possible cortical rim of enhancement
Nuclear medicine renal flow scan	Decreased flow to all or part of the kidney
Intravenous urogram	Decreased or absent function, delayed appearance
Renal ultrasonography	No obstruction; rarely, wedge-shaped mass

LDH, lactic acid dehydrogenase; AST, aspartate transaminase; ALT, alanine transaminase.

On microscopic examination, sterile infarcts have the classical picture of coagulative necrosis.[89] The initial findings of marked congestion are followed by cytoplasmic and nuclear degenerative changes, with gradual loss of viable cytologic structure. The cytoplasm becomes homogeneous and eosinophilic, and the nuclei undergo condensation and karyorrhexis. Surrounding this necrotic area is a transitional zone of sublethal injury with findings similar to acute tubular necrosis. This peripheral area becomes infiltrated with polymorphonuclear leukocytes. Eventually the central necrotic area becomes smaller, with eventual collapse, and is replaced by a collagenous scar.[89]

Clinical Features and Diagnosis of Acute Occlusive Renal Arterial Disease

There are no definitive signs or symptoms specific for arterial occlusion (Table 56.2). The most common presenting symptom for arterial occlusion of the kidney is pain, which may be flank and/or abdominal pain. Other nonspecific symptoms may include nausea, vomiting, or fever and chills. Anuria or oliguria is usually suggestive of bilateral arterial occlusion, or unilateral occlusion in patients with a solitary kidney, but transient oliguria lasting a few days may occur in unilateral occlusion as well. This oliguria has been attributed to arteriolar spasm of the contralateral kidney. The size of the infarct may impact the severity of pain as in one small series of iatrogenic renal infarcts following endovascular procedures, the patients were all asymptomatic, with the infarctions being discovered by routine CT imaging.[84] Because of the relative infrequency with which it occurs compared to more common intra-abdominal pathology such as gastroenteritis, pancreatitis, pyelonephritis, and nephrolithiasis, renal infarction may not be among diagnostic considerations in the initial workup, and diagnosis may be delayed. Unfortunately this may lead to irreversible loss of renal function. With increasing reliance on abdominal imaging by CT scan as part of initial diagnostic evaluations for patients presenting to emergency departments with abdominal pain, this pattern may change in the future with more events being discovered earlier in the evaluation. Figure 56.1 demonstrates transverse and coronal CT images of a renal infarction.

Other physical findings may be elevated blood pressure. Bowel sounds may be diminished. Abdominal and/or flank tenderness are often present on physical examination. With smaller infarcts, there may be no signs or symptoms.

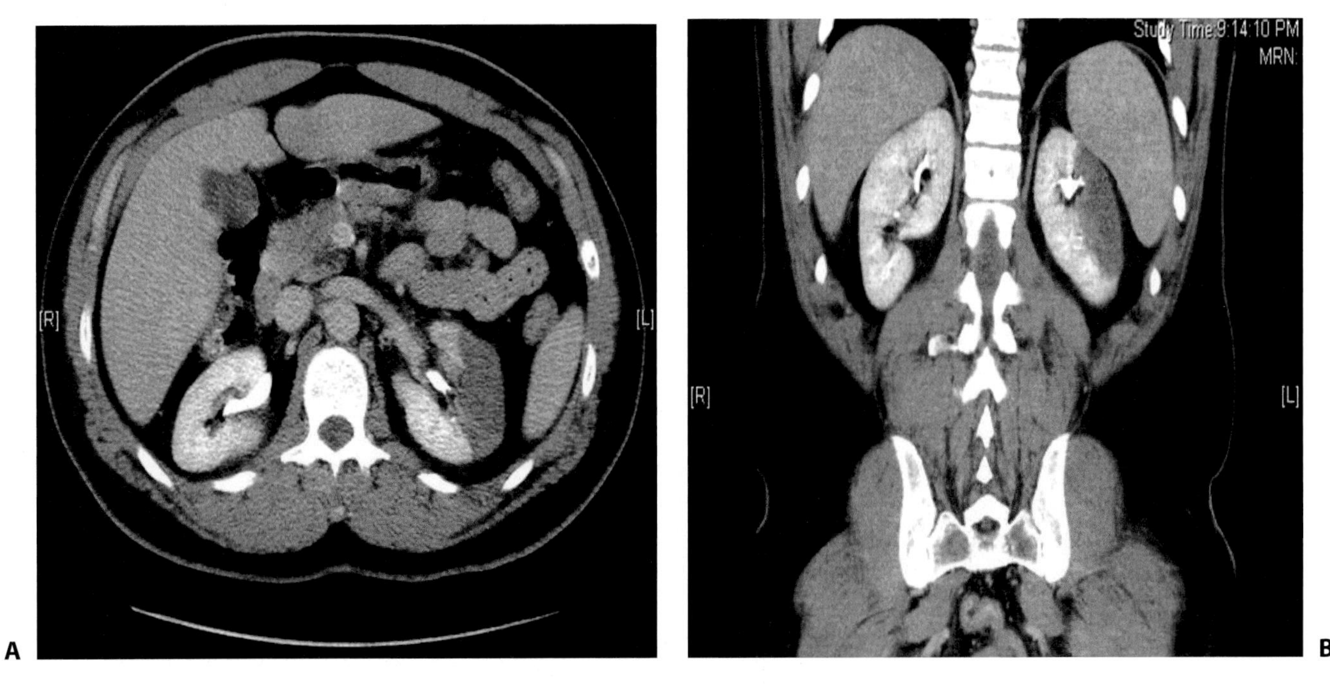

FIGURE 56.1 Computed tomography with contrast. Transverse **(A)** and coronal **(B)** images demonstrate a wedge-shaped embolic infarct localized to the lateral midpole of the left kidney.

The most common laboratory abnormality is elevation in LDH, with levels that reach as high as 2,000 IU per L. Other associated laboratory abnormalities include elevation in serum AST, ALT, and alkaline phosphatase, but these are typically less dramatic and are not universally noted. Microscopic hematuria, leukocytosis, and mild proteinuria are common findings.[90] Reduced urinary excretion of sodium, as is commonly noted in renal hypoperfusion, is also noted at times.[91] The course of changes in LDH, AST, ALT, and alkaline phosphatase in a patient are noted in Figure 56.2, with changes in urine volume, serum creatinine, and urine sodium noted in Figure 56.3.[92]

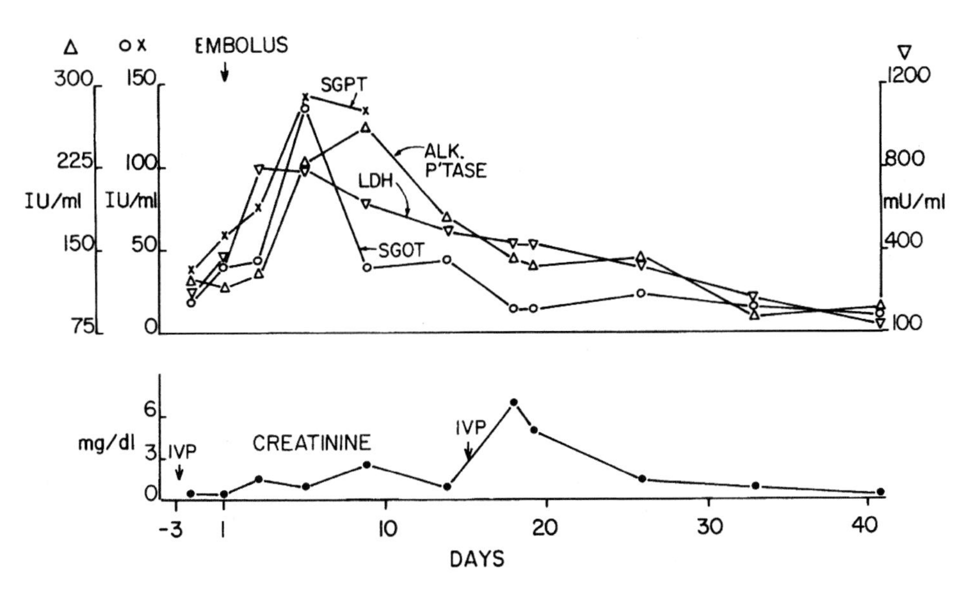

FIGURE 56.2 Serial serum levels of glutamic-oxaloacetic transaminase (SGOT, ○)glutamic-pyruvic transaminase (SGPT, X), lactic dehydrogenase (LDH, ▽), alkaline phosphatase (ALK P TASE, △), and creatinine (●) in a 62-year-old man with thromboembolism to a single kidney 10 days after a myocardial infarction. Right flank and chest pain and lower abdominal tenderness appeared on day 1. The patient also exhibited an increase in serum creatinine level following the second intravenous pyelogram (IVP). (From Lessman RK, Johnson SF, Coburn JW, et al. Renal artery embolism: clinical features and long-term follow-up in 17 cases. *Ann Intern Med.* 1978;89:477, with permission.)

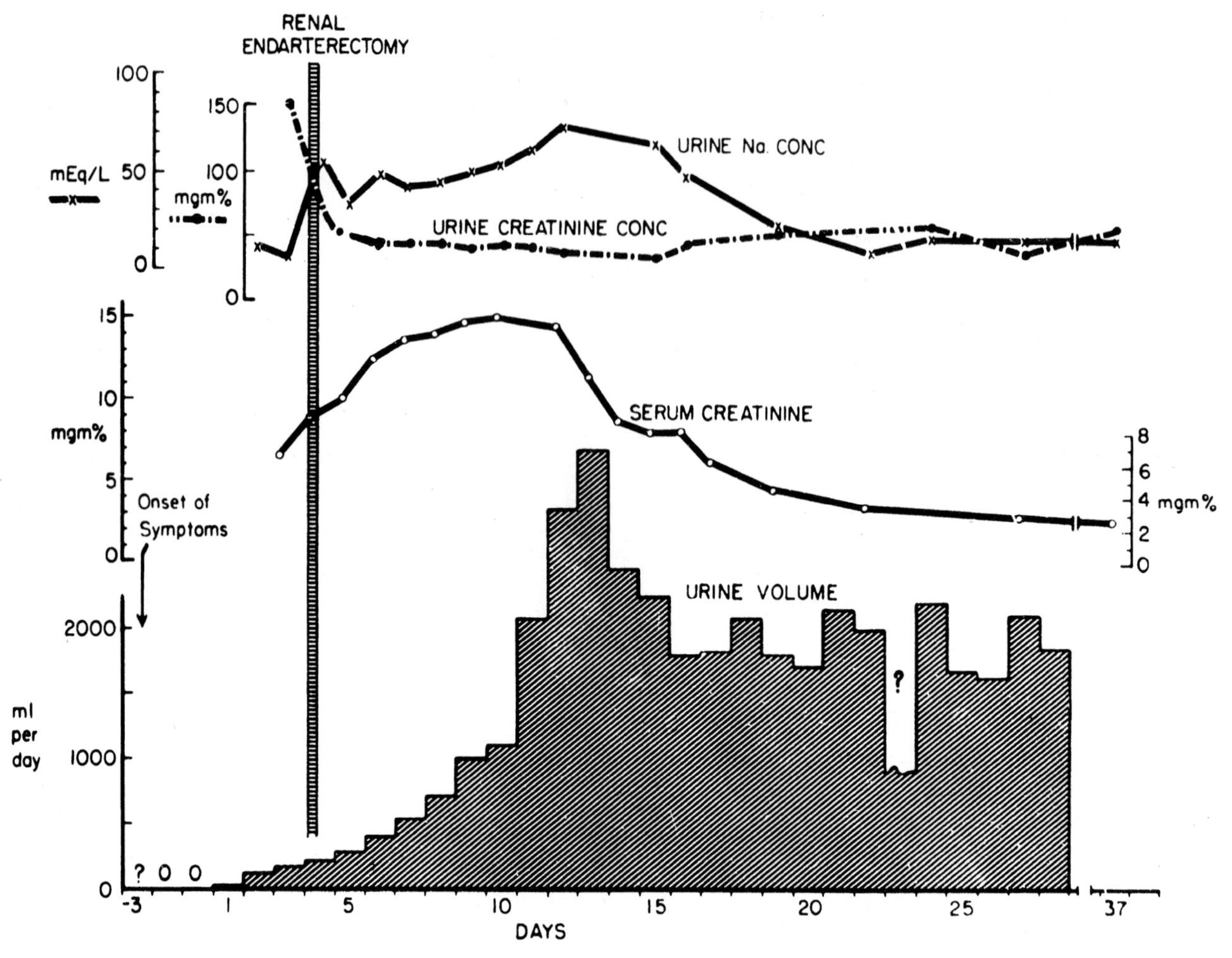

FIGURE 56.3 Course of a 56-year-old woman with abrupt onset of anuria and right lower quadrant and low back pain; she had atrial fibrillation and mitral stenosis owing to rheumatic heart disease. One year earlier she had undergone a left nephrectomy for malignant hypertension. (Earlier, she had had a stroke and blindness of the left eye owing to an embolism.) A diagnosis of thromboembolism to the renal artery was confirmed by aortography (Fig. 56.4), and surgery was performed with removal of the embolus and endarterectomy. The fractional excretion of sodium was 0.36% before surgery and increased to 7.3% after removal of the thrombus. There was ultimate recovery from acute tubular necrosis, as indicated. (From Lessman RK, Johnson SF, Coburn JW, et al. Renal artery embolism: clinical features and long-term follow-up in 17 cases. *Ann Intern Med.* 1978;89:477, with permission.)

CT scan with contrast is probably the most rapid, widely available, and reliable imaging modality. Magnetic resonance angiography may also be useful, but may take longer and is not as widely available. Angiography is of course the most accurate diagnostic method, and holds the additional advantage of allowing rapid endovascular intervention or thrombolytic therapy for an acute occlusion, and should be considered as a first line test if clinical suspicion is high. A characteristic angiographic image of renal infarct is shown in Figure 56.4. Nuclear medicine renal flow scans can also be used to identify isolated perfusion defects (Figure 56.5), but if isotope uptake is globally reduced (as can be seen in acute kidney injury) it may fail to identify an area of hypoperfusion. Ultrasonography of the renal arteries is of limited value as it is time consuming, operator-dependent, and difficult to image the entire renal artery, although for cases of transplant renal artery thrombosis or for thrombosis of the main renal artery, it may have some utility.[93]

Therapy for Nontraumatic Acute Occlusive Renal Arterial Disease

Similar to traumatic renal arterial occlusion, the major concern is irreversible loss of renal function, and likewise the response to therapy depends on the duration of warm ischemia, location, and severity of the occlusion and presence or absence of collateral circulation. Acute thromboembolic events may be amenable to intraarterial thrombolytic therapy, and a timely diagnosis is crucial to preserve renal function.

Blum et al. published a series of 14 patients with acute embolic renal artery occlusion treated with thrombolytic therapy.[94] The estimated ischemic time varied from 12 hours

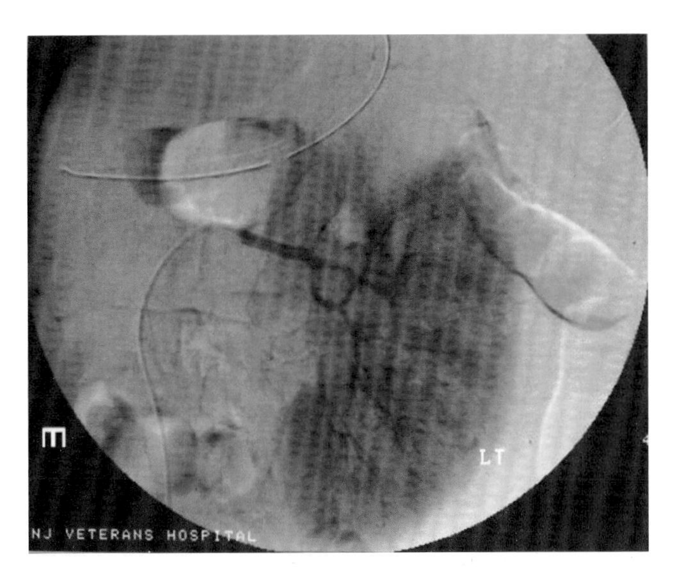

FIGURE 56.4 Left renal angiogram shows a wedge-shaped perfusion defect involving the upper pole of the kidney due to a thromboembolism.

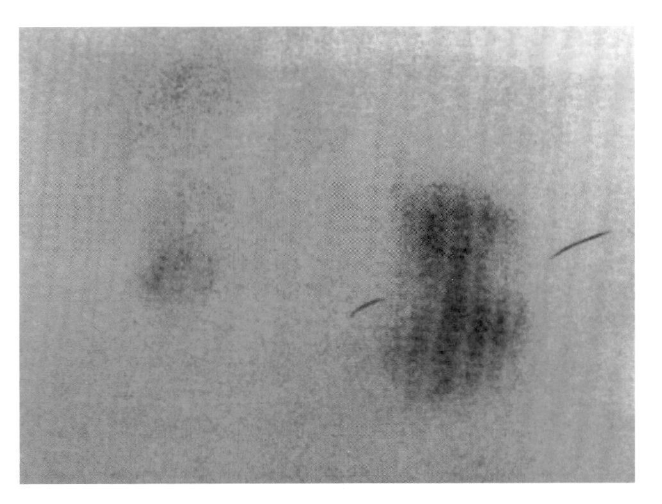

FIGURE 56.5 Renal scan with technetium 99m-labeled dimercaptosuccinic acid (DMSA) showing evidence of segmental renal infarcts of the left kidney of a 74-year-old man who was hospitalized with abrupt appearance of a supraventricular tachycardia. There was a progressive rise in serum creatinine from a baseline value of 2.2 to 4.4 mg/dL over 5 successive days. He was never oliguric; urinalysis showed 2+ proteinuria. His white blood cell count rose from 10,200/μL on admission to 15,400/μL after 4 days; there was no eosinophilia. The serum alanine aminotransferase level rose from 33 to 42 U/L and lactate dehydrogenase, from 49 to 173 U/L. A technetium-labeled "flow" scan disclosed markedly reduced flow bilaterally that was more marked on the left than the right. There was a history of emboli to his feet, with the serum creatinine level increasing from 1.2 to 2.2 mg/dL in association with an acute myocardial infarction several years earlier. On the basis of DMSA scan, a diagnosis of thromboembolism to the kidney was made; the patient received anticoagulants and his serum creatinine level gradually fell to 2.4 mg/dL.

to 8 days. Although renal perfusion was restored in 13 of the patients, this did not translate into recovery of renal function. None of the patients with complete occlusion had restoration of renal function, but the patients with partial occlusion were stabilized. Their review of 50 cases of complete renal artery occlusion suggested a warm ischemia duration of 3 hours or less in order to preserve renal function without permanent injury.[94] This "critical ischemia time" has been refuted by a number of isolated case reports who achieved good clinical outcomes even after delayed restoration of renal perfusion.[95–99] Several of the cases described duration of ischemia longer than 20 hours and in one case of an elderly patient with solitary functioning kidney, satisfactory renal recovery occurred despite a 4-day history of occlusion with anuria and a temporary dialysis requirement.[97]

Surgical treatment of acute occlusive renal arterial disease has produced mixed results. Lacombe described a series of 20 patients (5 with acute embolism, and 15 with acute thrombosis) who underwent surgical revascularization between 18 hours and 68 days after the occlusion. Kidney salvage rate was 64%, but postoperative mortality was 15%. A number of these patients may have had underlying renal artery stenosis with development of collateral circulation that may have led to a better rate of renal preservation.[100] Another series reported by Ouriel et al. describes 13 patients in whom renal artery embolectomy failed to restore renal function.[101]

Much as is the case for traumatic thrombosis, the decision to intervene on patients with acute nontraumatic thrombosis or thromboembolism should be based on duration and extent of ischemia and identification of patients most likely to benefit. Patients with substantial risk of significant loss of renal function, such as those with bilateral occlusion, or unilateral occlusion of a solitary kidney, should be considered for revascularization. Patients with a normal contralateral kidney or smaller infarctions may be better served by more conservative therapy. Another clinical decision is the need for short- or long-term systemic anticoagulation. There are no guidelines specifically oriented toward anticoagulation for renal arterial thrombosis or thromboembolic disease. A decision for systemic anticoagulation should be based on subsequent risk of further embolic events, such as with atrial fibrillation or severe ventricular dysfunction.

RENAL ARTERY ANEURYSMS

Renal artery aneurysms (RAAs) are uncommon in the general population. Autopsy studies report a prevalence in the general population of around 0.01%.[102,103] In patients undergoing renal arterial angiography (to evaluate hypertension for example) the prevalence is between 0.3% and 1.3%.[104–107] One series of 8525 renal angiograms identified RAAs in 83 patients (0.97%).[102] Of these, 80% were saccular, 61% were right-sided, and 7% were bilateral.

Renal artery aneurysms can be classified as saccular, fusiform, dissecting, and intrarenal.[106,108] Saccular aneurysms are the most common and account for 80% of renal artery aneurysms. They are typically located at the first-order bifurcation of the main renal artery. Less than 10% are within the renal parenchyma.

Fusiform aneurysms are less common, and most commonly noted in an area following stenosis, giving the appearance of poststenotic dilatation.[32,109–112] Fusiform aneurysms are responsible for the "string of beads" appearance of some cases of fibromuscular dysplasia, where several stenotic areas are followed by dilatations.

Intrarenal aneurysms make up 10% to 15% of RAAs. They may be congenital, posttraumatic (e.g., following renal biopsy), or associated with polyarteritis nodosa.[110,113]

Histologic findings of RAAs resemble medial fibromuscular dysplasia. In the arterial wall, degeneration of the internal elastic lamina with fragmentation, increased collagen, and a lack of elastic tissue are observed. Atherosclerotic lesions may be the cause of the aneurysm or, more likely, may be a secondary factor.[114] Calcification of the arterial walls may occur.

Table 56.3 shows demographic and clinical data of 277 patients undergoing surgical correction of renal aneurysms from three published series.[114–116] The mean age was 50 years (range 13 to 78). Women outnumbered men by 65% to 35% and hypertension was common, in >70% of the patients. Medial fibromuscular dysplasia was considered the major cause (34% to 54%) and was the presumed reason for the female gender preference. Atherosclerosis was noted in 25% to 35%. Small numbers of patients had renal artery aneurysms due to polyarteritis nodosum, giant cell arteritis, Marfan syndrome, dissection, mycotic aneurysms, and trauma.[114–118]

The most serious complication of renal artery aneurysms is rupture, which can quickly lead to hemorrhagic shock, loss of renal function, and death.[119] Other complications may include dissection (discussed later in this section) and thrombosis with distal embolization. Embolization can further result in formation of an arteriovenous fistula with resultant high-output heart failure.[108,109] Most patients with RAAs are asymptomatic, although some may complain of nonspecific flank or abdominal pain, and there may be hematuria or abdominal bruit on assessment.

Rupture of renal artery aneurysms is a potentially catastrophic event and may quickly lead to hemorrhagic shock, irreversible loss of kidney function, and death. It is typically accompanied by severe flank pain and flank ecchymoses. For unclear reasons rupture of RAAs occurs disproportionately in pregnancy. Because of the relative infrequency

TABLE 56.3 **Data from Three Large Studies Reporting Their Surgical Outcomes of Renal Artery Aneurysms in 277 Patients**

Author	English[a]	Pfeiffer[b]	Henke[c]
No. patients	62	94	121
No. RAAs repaired	72	107	168
Time period of surgery (yr)	1987–2003	1980–2002	1965–2000
Mean patient age (yr)	46	51	51
Male/female (%)	70/30	61/39	60/40
Hypertension (%)	89	80	73
Pathogenesis			
Fibromuscular dysplasia (%)	54	51	34
Atherosclerosis (%)	35	30	25
Outcomes			
Perioperative mortality	1 (1.6%)	0	0
Perioperative morbidity (%)	12	17	?
Hypertension improved (%)	54	22	?
Hypertension cured (%)	21	25	?
Long-term artery patency (%)	91	81	98

[a]English WP, Pearce JD, Craven TE, et al. Surgical management of renal artery aneurysms. *J Vasc Surg.* 2004;40:53–60.
[b]Pfeiffer T, Reiher L, Grabitz K, et al. Reconstruction for renal artery aneurysm: operative techniques and long-term results. *J Vasc Surg.* 2003;37:293–300.
[c]Henke PK, Cardneau JD, Welling TH, 3rd, et al. Renal artery aneurysms: a 35-year clinical experience with 252 aneurysms in 168 patients. *Ann Surg.* 2001;234:454–462; discussion 62–63.
RAA, renal artery aneurysm.

of renal artery aneurysm, there are no prospective data regarding risk of rupture, but individuals at higher risk are felt to be those with larger aneurysms (particularly those >4.0 cm) and with aneurysms during pregnancy. There have been some prospective data regarding natural history of smaller aneurysms. Two-hundred patients, mostly with RAAs less than 2.0 cm, were managed conservatively for up to 17 years.[102,104,114,120–122] None of them ruptured during follow-up and very few caused symptoms or increased substantially in size. Henriksson et al. reported a series of 34 patients with RAAS undergoing periodic angiographic surveillance.[120] Twenty-eight of the patients experienced no change in the size, five had slight enlargement, and one patient underwent surgical repair to address a worrisome dilation. These observational data suggest that, for smaller aneurysms, conservative management with interval imaging studies is a reasonable management approach.

Pregnant women with RAAs represent a unique group in which conservative therapy may not be appropriate. In a review of 43 cases of RAA rupture, 18 (42%) occurred in pregnant women.[122] Most ruptures occur during the third trimester, but there have been case reports of rupture earlier in pregnancy and also in the postpartum period.[119,123–125] There has also been a report during pregnancy of a ruptured renal artery aneurysm involving a transplanted kidney.[126] The explanation for increased risk of rupture during pregnancy is not clear. Most of the pregnant women who experienced rupture did not have hypertension before or during the pregnancy.[123,127,128] Some of the proposed contributing factors include increased renal blood flow, particularly during the third trimester, steroid hormone effects, and increased intra-abdominal pressure.[127] Pressure on the pelvic vasculature, which may be positional, is also felt to be a potential contributor.[123,128,129] Cases of RAA rupture during pregnancy typically require emergent nephrectomy to control hemorrhage. Maternal mortality is 6% and fetal mortality 25% if the pregnancy has reached the third trimester.[130] Fetal mortality approaches 100% in cases before the third trimester.

The most sensitive imaging study for renal artery aneurysm is angiogram. Magnetic resonance angiography (MRA) may be a useful technique depending on the size and location of the aneurysm. CT may be useful as a screening tool as well. For detection of smaller, more distal or intrarenal aneurysms, angiogram may be the only useful imaging modality.

Patients undergoing surgical repair of RAAs in one of three large published series have demonstrated good surgical outcomes. In a combined number of 277 patients undergoing repair of aneurysms with a mean size of 1.6 to 2.6 cm, primary surgical success was 97% and long-term arterial patency ranged from 81% to 91%.[114–116] One of the centers reported a rate of unplanned nephrectomy of 6.6% (8 of 121 surgeries). Two of the series reported data about hypertension outcomes and reported improvement in hypertension in 20% to 50% and "cure" in 20% to 25%.[115,116] Perioperative death rate was 0% to 1.6% and morbidity 12% to 17%. Because of the complexity of the surgery, referral to an experienced surgical team is recommended for successful outcome.

The following should be considered in the decision whether to proceed with surgical repair of a renal artery aneurysm: the low risk of rupture of small aneurysms, but increased risk with large ones, the increased risk in pregnancy, and the potential contribution of the aneurysm to renovascular hypertension. Risks of the surgery including mortality and need for nephrectomy should be considered. Although there are no strict guidelines for who should be referred for surgery, the following are recommendations from the published studies[110,114–116]:

1. RAA diameter greater than 1.5 to 2.0 cm in a healthy, normotensive person
2. RAA greater than 1.0 cm in women of child-bearing age, since risk of rupture during pregnancy is increased
3. RAAs with associated renal artery stenosis or evidence of distal embolization
4. RAA showing significant expansion during follow-up imaging studies

Endovascular procedures to treat renal artery aneurysms have also been reported, but long-term outcomes remain unclear. Treatment with coil embolization has been reported,[131] although with incomplete success and potential long-term complications including renal infarction and hypertension.[132] Use of liquid embolic agent to address RAAs has also been reported.[133–135] Arterial stenting of aneurysms has also been reported, including in an emergent case of acute ruptured renal artery aneurysm.[136] A recent survey of surgical and endovascular repair of renal artery aneurysms in New York State demonstrates an increasing number of patients undergoing endovascular procedures while the number of surgical repairs has been relatively stable—because the analysis was retrospective and database driven, no specific conclusions about outcomes could be drawn.[137] Depending on the clinical scenario, an endovascular approach may be appropriate in some patients but there are no current recommendations as there are for surgical intervention.

Dissecting Aneurysms of the Renal Artery

Tears of the arterial intima and medial necrosis lead to dissection of the arterial wall. Predisposing factors include atherosclerosis and fibromuscular dysplasia. Dissection may follow vascular trauma, for example due to guidewire, catheters, or balloon angioplasty procedures.[138] It may also follow blunt abdominal trauma.[139,140] Renal artery dissection is occasionally noted at autopsy, presumably with no apparent manifestations during life.

Dissecting aneurysms of the renal artery can cause occlusion and resulting ischemia, infarction, or renovascular hypertension,[117] and should be considered during an evaluation for a patient with an otherwise unexplained renal infarct. Chronic dissection can result in renovascular hypertension in much the same way that other causes of renal artery stenosis or narrowing can.[141]

Symptoms of acute dissection may include new-onset or worsening hypertension, or flank pain. Malignant hypertension is a less common complication, and may be related to aggressive stimulation of the renin-angiotensin system.[142] Headache may occur, possibly related to hypertension. For patients with iatrogenic dissection following an angiography, there may be no signs or symptoms.

Renal artery dissection occurs three times more often in men than women.[117,141] The typical age range is between 40 and 60, but dissection may occur in younger patients when fibromuscular dysplasia and hypertension are present. Dissecting aneurysms are more commonly right-sided, but may be bilateral in 20% to 30% of cases.[117,141]

Other findings may include proteinuria, hematuria (20% to 35% of cases), and renal impairment (serum creatinine >1.5 mg per dL in 9% to 33% of cases).[117,141]

Angiogram or MRA can be used to diagnose dissection. Arteriography typically reveals an abrupt narrowing of the lumen (Fig. 56.6). Less often, both the true lumen and false lumen fill with contrast, giving the appearance of a double lumen separated by an intimal flap. Dissection may extend from the main renal artery, distally to the first bifurcation, and into the branch arteries. Follow-up arteriography may show persistent dissection, but there have also been reports of a degree of reversibility, gradual improvement in renal function, and improvement of hypertension.[140,141]

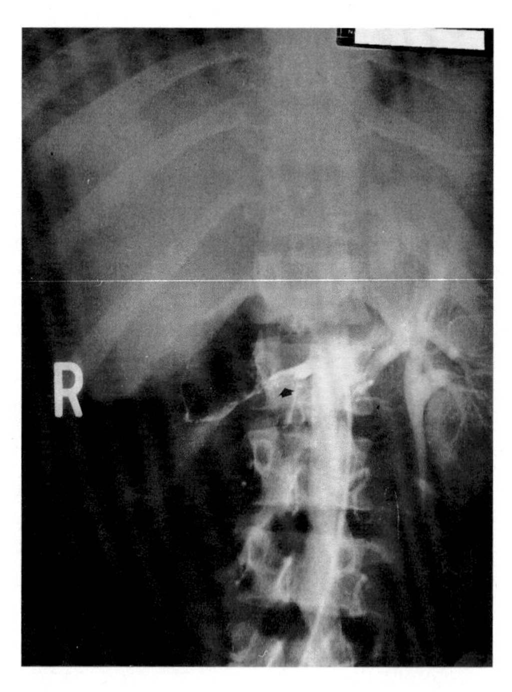

FIGURE 56.6 Aortogram demonstrates an intimal flap and dissection with thrombosis of the right renal kidney. Note the absence of enhancement of the right kidney. (From Lang EK. *Radiology of the Upper Urinary Tract.* Heidelberg: Springer; 1991, with permission.)

Therapy for dissection depends on the severity of hypertension and response to medical management. Surgical revascularization or even nephrectomy have been performed in patients with poor response to therapy or renal infarction, in some cases with good outcomes.[143,144] Patients have also been successfully managed with medical therapy, and may improve gradually over time.[141]

ATHEROEMBOLIC RENAL DISEASE

Atheroembolic renal disease, also known as cholesterol embolic disease, predominantly strikes older men with severe atherosclerotic disease, smokers, and people with hypertension.[145] Renal damage can be abrupt or insidious, and the disease itself has been described as "the great masquerader"[146] and the "Cinderella" of renal disease.[147]

Pathology

As distinct from acute renal ischemia and large thromboemboli to the renal artery and moderate-sized arteries, atheroembolic renal disease occurs when cholesterol-containing plaques with fibrin slough off from the aorta and shower distal arteries, occluding those of 150 to 200 micrometers.[148] Cholesterol crystals provoke infiltration by giant cells (Riesenzell arteritis), which later disappear and leave the cholesterol emboli encased by connective tissue.[149] Handler described the pathologic changes sequentially as granulomatous endarteritis followed by intimal fibrosis with sequestration of the cholesterol crystals and marked decrease in the diameter of the vessel lumen. Tissue distal to the lesion becomes ischemic with impaired function progressing to atrophy and necrosis.[150]

The most common organs involved in atheroembolic disease are the skin, kidneys, gastrointestinal tract, and central nervous system. Autopsy studies cited in the literature describe renal cholesterol emboli in 5% of men and 3% of women over the age of 50.[148] Flory[151] found vascular occlusions in 9 of 267 autopsies of patients with advanced arteriosclerosis of the aorta, or 3.4%. Flory later produced similar lesions in the lungs of rabbits by injecting atheromatous material from human aortas into the animals to demonstrate that the cholesterol crystals did not develop in situ. Fukumoto and colleagues found an incidence of 1.4% for "cholesterol embolization syndrome" in a series of patients who underwent cardiac catheterization (25/1,786).[152] Twelve of 25 patients (48%) had cutaneous manifestations whereas 16/25 (64%) had signs of renal dysfunction. Flory also described lesions in the spleen and pancreas.

Angiography and aortic surgery increase the risk of cholesterol embolization. In a series of 755 men age 49 to 72 who had not undergone recent surgical or diagnostic procedures, cholesterol emboli were found in only 8 (1%) on renal biopsy performed because of an unexplained loss of kidney function.[153] This is in contrast to a rate of 77.3% for atheromatous emboli to the kidneys after aortic surgery described in one early series.[7] The same authors found rates of

31% for embolization of the kidney by atheromatous material in patients with large aneurysms and 15.8% in patients with severe aortic atherosclerosis, ulceration, and mural thrombosis.

Cholesterol crystal embolization often presents with nonspecific findings that mimic other systemic diseases. A review of 221 biopsy proven cases of cholesterol crystal embolization found that affected patients were older men (average age 66) with a history of hypertension (61%), atherosclerotic cardiovascular disease (44%), renal failure (34%), and aortic aneurysms (25%) at presentation.[154] Skin findings and renal failure, 34% and 50%, respectively, were the most common findings. Other nonspecific signs and symptoms include fever (7%), weight loss (7%), myalgias (4%), and headache (3%). Mortality was 81%, due to multifactorial, cardiac, and renal causes.

Fragments of atheroembolic material become embedded in small arteries, arterioles, and sometimes in the glomerular capillaries. Autopsy series demonstrate crystalline clefts in arterial lumens with fresh emboli or embedded in thickened intima of older lesions, which show an intense intimal proliferation with giant cell and histiocytic aggregates and crystals. Thrombosis is not a characteristic feature. On ultrastructural examination, early findings included crystals without reaction or endothelial damage and early histiocytic response. The intermediate stage included histiocyte and giant cell reaction with some intimal reaction and edema of the arterial wall. The late phase showed more intimal proliferation, histiocytic reaction, and exclusion of the crystals from the lumen and embedding in the intima.[152] Cholesterol is dissolved during the processing of specimens for pathologic exam, leaving characteristic clefts.

In experimental models using rats and rabbits, cholesterol emboli in suspension were introduced intravenously. Early lesions included thrombosis and a focal inflammatory reaction in the vessel wall. Leukocytes are promptly replaced by neutrophils and giant cells within the first 24 hours. By the end of the first week, endothelium has overgrown the crystals, which become encased in fibrous tissue and slowly penetrate the arterial wall.[155–157]

Renal impairment results from chronic ischemic damage as a result of repeated small injuries. Vessels are not able to autoregulate. Reduced perfusion leads to apoptosis and atrophy as well as upregulation of the renin-angiotensin-aldosterone system with increased oxidative stress leading to interstitial fibrosis.[8] Debris and cholesterol crystals at the site occlusion are identical to material found in severe atheromatous lesions of the aorta, with some authors noting a correlation between the severity of atherosclerosis and atheroembolic disease.[149,158]

A form of secondary focal segmental glomerulosclerosis (FSGS) with heavy proteinuria has also been attributed to atheroembolic disease. Greenberg and colleagues[159] described 24 patients thought to have atheroembolic embolic disease with heavy proteinuria. Eight of the patients had renal biopsies for proteinuria and four to exclude rapidly progressive glomerulonephritis. All shared risk factors for atheroembolic disease. FSGS was observed in 15 (63%) of the biopsies. FSGS did not occur more frequently in the proteinuric group than in the nonnephrotic group, but the number of sclerosed lesions was greater. A variant of FSGS, cellular lesions with epithelial cell prominence and capillary collapse, was seen in 7 of 9 patients with nephritic range proteinuria but only 3 of 12 patients with lesser degrees of proteinuria. The authors attributed the association to ischemic damage and hyperfiltration.

Others have reported an association between cholesterol crystal embolic disease and necrotizing glomerulonephritis that is antineutrophil cytoplasmic antibody positive with pauci-immune extracapillary glomerulonephritis. In the small number of cases reported, treatment has involved steroids and cytotoxic therapy with mixed success.[160–165]

Clinical Features

Atheroembolic disease primarily affects adults older than 60. It appears to be diagnosed more frequently in whites than in blacks, possibly because of the difficulty of recognizing skin lesions.[166] The incidence is unknown.[167] Autopsy studies cited in the literature describe atheroemboli in anywhere from 0.31% to 2.4% with the number increasing to 4% to 6.5% in patients over the age of 65[168] and has high as 77% in patients who have had aortic surgery, as noted previously. Estimates on the incidence of atheroembolic disease in clinical practice range from 3% of all patients admitted to a tertiary renal intensive care unit to 5% to 10% of all cases of acute renal failure.[169,170]

In addition to age and race, risk factors for atheroembolic and cholesterol crystal disease include male gender, tobacco use, hypertension, diabetes, and atherosclerotic vascular disease.[171] Cigarette smoking was found in 79% to 92% of patients. Hypertension was found in as low 61% in a large literature review, but in 81% to 91% of patients in several cases series from single centers.[153,164,166,172] Coronary artery disease was found in 54% to 73%, peripheral vascular disease in 54% to 69%, and cerebrovascular disease in 32% to 46% of the patients in the three case series. Aortic abdominal aneurysm was present in 42% to 67% of the patients in those series.

The proximal cause of atheroembolic and cholesterol crystal disease appears to be largely iatrogenic. Although most of the case series report anywhere from 0% to 69% spontaneous atheroembolic events, the majority of cases reported in the literature are a result of angiography (18%–96%), cardiovascular surgery (5%–36%), and anticoagulation (13%–37%).[153,164,166,173,174] Less frequently, atheroembolic and cholesterol crystal disease can arise from blunt abdominal trauma, aortic balloon placement, cardiopulmonary resuscitation, and percutaneous renal angioplasty.[167,175]

The time course from precipitating events to clinically evident disease is variable from one day to a month. In their study of 52 patients with atheroembolic and cholesterol crystal disease and renal failure, Thadhani and colleagues reported that at least 50% of patients had some sign of atheroembolic disease within 24 hours of the initial insult although no particular finding predominated. Only 21% of patients had a skin finding within 24 hours whereas 50% did within 30 days. Hollenhorst retinal plaques were noted in 4/16 patients.[166] Skin findings include purpura, petechia, violaceous mottling of toes, livedo reticularis, ulcers, and gangrene. The lower extremities are most commonly involved, frequently bilaterally. Scrotal and penile necrosis due to cholesterol crystal emboli has also been described.[176–178]

Renal failure may present acutely, although the initial presentation acute renal failure may also be attributable to contrast nephropathy. More frequently renal involvement follows a subacute time course of days to weeks with renal impairment occurring in a stepwise fashion. Finally, renal impairment can present as chronic, stable ischemic damage. In one series of 52 patients, 35% were found to have presented with sudden acute renal failure 3 to 7 days after the inciting event, in this case, angiography. Fifty-six percent of patients presented with a subacute, insidious deterioration in renal function over 2 to 6 weeks. Finally, 9% of patients had stable, chronic, renal disease at the time of diagnosis.[179] Renal failure requiring renal replacement therapy, hemodialysis, or peritoneal dialysis has been reported in anywhere from 17% to 44% of patients with atheroembolic disease with recovery of renal function reported in 10% to 20% of those patients.[145,153,166,174] Hypertension and preexisting renal disease were predictors of progression to end-stage renal disease (ESRD). Use of statins was independently associated with reduced risk of ESRD. Age, diabetes, and ESRD are independent risk factors for patient mortality.[167] Atheroembolic disease has also been reported in donor kidneys after transplantation, possibly as result of accepting older donor kidneys, although the recipients could not be eliminated as the source in some of the case reports.[180–182]

Gastrointestinal involvement from cholesterol crystal emboli has been reported in as few as 8% to 10% of patients to 29% to 33% and as many as 48% in various series.[153,164,166,169,174,183–185] Embolization can occur at any point along the length of the gut. The most common presentation is hemorrhage and abdominal pain. GI bleeding can often result from superficial mucosal ulcerations, erosions, or infarcts. Clinical presentation may range from occult blood loss and melena to bloody diarrhea.[174,179,186–188]

Central nervous system involvement from cholesterol embolization can manifest itself as transient ischemic attacks, cerebral infarction, amaurosis fugax, paralysis, confusion, and gradual deterioration of neurologic function.[174] Hollenhorst described the phenomena of cholesterol emboli to the retina giving rise to the characteristic yellow plaques at the bifurcation of retinal arterioles that bear his name.[189,190]

Finally, pulmonary involvement with hemoptysis and renal failure has been described, giving rise to the suggestion that cholesterol crystal atheroembolic disease should also be considered in the differential diagnosis of pulmonary-renal syndromes.[191–193]

Laboratory findings in cholesterol crystal atheroembolic disease are nonspecific. Urinalysis is nonspecific with evidence of hematuria and proteinuria, on rare occasions in the nephrotic range. Dysmorphic red blood cells and red blood cell casts are rare, and may be a result of accelerated hypertension.[164,174] Eosinophiluria is variously reported in 8 of 9 patients with Hansel stain in one series but only 2 of 37 patients with Wright stain in another.[166,194]

Peripheral eosinophilia has been reported in as few as 14% of 37 patients in one study to as many as 59% to 71% of patients in other series.[164,166,174,195,196] The erythrocyte sedimentation rate can be elevated. Low complement levels have been noted in several studies, although the significance of complement is not clear. Others have reported normal complement levels. Depending on the site of crystal embolization, liver enzymes, lipase, amylase, or creatinine kinase may also be elevated.

Acute renal failure in an elderly patient with diffuse atherosclerotic disease should raise suspicion for atheroembolic disease, particularly after a vascular procedure. Tissue diagnosis may be necessary in cases of spontaneously occurring disease. Skin biopsies are the safest and diagnostic in 90% of cases.[145,172,197] Renal biopsies are also diagnostic, but may miss the characteristic lesions because of their patchy distribution. Muscle, bone marrow, prostate, stomach, and lung tissue may also show evidence of crystal embolization on biopsy, depending on the pattern of crystal showering.[186,187,198]

Treatment for atheroembolic disease is largely supportive. Belenfant and colleagues developed a treatment protocol, which they applied to 67 consecutive patients admitted to their facility with renal failure and evidence of cholesterol embolization. Causes included angiographic procedure (85%), anticoagulation (76%), and cardiovascular surgery (33%). To prevent further embolization, they stopped all anticoagulation and proscribed further aortic catheterization or surgery. They also instituted a regimen of intensive vasodilation with angiotensin-converting enzyme inhibitors and loop diuretics. If volume overload persisted and was refractory to medical management, hemodialysis was initiated, with minimal or no anticoagulation. Enteral or parenteral nutritional support was provided. Patients were treated with corticosteroids if there was evidence of further decline of function or cholesterol embolization. In-hospital mortality was 16%; among survivors, 32% remained in hemodialysis. Survival at 1 year was 87% compared to 1-year mortality cited in the literature of 64% to 81%.[164] Others have recommended cessation of antiplatelet therapy and anticoagulation as well as initiation of statins to help improve glomerular filtration.[199–202]

Several authors have suggested surgical revascularization as a possible treatment for atheroembolic renal disease, particularly where there is association with renal artery stenosis. In one series of 12 patients who underwent surgical revascularization of the renal artery, five patients experienced improvement in renal function, five had stable renal function, and renal function worsened in one (no information was provided about the 12th patient).[203] Others have looked at surgery for limb salvage. In one series of 100 cases in which the infrarenal aorta or ileac arteries were the source of the atheroemboli, long-term prognosis was good, whereas outcomes were poor if the suprarenal aorta was the source of ateroemboli.[204] In another series of 62 patients with atheroembolic disease, 42 patients underwent surgical revascularization with bypass grafting. Limb salvage was possible in 86 of 88 limbs. Thirty-day mortality was 5%.[205]

RENAL VEIN THROMBOSIS

Our understanding of the etiology and pathophysiology of renal vein thrombosis (RVT) has advanced considerably since the 18th century when Hunter first described renal vein thrombosis in Lady Beauchamp, which he attributed to complications of osteomyelitis.[206] In 1840, Rayer made the first association of RVT with the nephrotic syndrome. [207] In the 1940s, Abeshouse reviewed the literature on RVT up to that point. Infectious suppuration, malignancy, and trauma were cited among the most important causes.[208] Llach and Yudd in their previous edition of this chapter noted that Abeshouse's cases were all diagnosed postmortem before the development of more advanced angiographic and radiologic techniques made antemortem diagnosis more feasible.[209]

Early descriptions of RVT emphasized lumbar pain with flank tenderness, edema, and lumbar masses. Indeed case reports still discuss flank pain and hematuria as presenting symptoms of RVT. Harrison in 1956 described RVT in 11 patients, with the condition detected radiologically in four patients. Three patients presented with nephritic syndrome.[210] The etiology of RVT was divided into several groups. In two groups RVT occurred secondarily as a result of primary occlusion of the inferior vena cava or secondary occlusion as result of invasion of the renal vein by malignant neoplasm. In a third group, RVT occurred as a secondary result of primary renal disease, including amyloidosis, glomerulonephritis, and malignant hypertension. More recently, RVT as a subset of deep venous thrombosis (DVT) has come to be understood as a complication of the nephrotic syndrome, particularly membranous and membranoproliferative glomerulonephritis.[211,212]

Etiology

The incidence of thromboembolic events in nephritic syndrome has been reported anywhere from less than 10% to 45%.[213] A review of 29,280 autopsies between 1920 and 1961 found 17 cases of bilateral renal vein thrombosis. Only two of the 17 patients had nephrotic syndrome.[214] Prospective studies published between 1979 and 1988 cite an incidence of RVT in nephrotic syndrome overall of anywhere from 2% to 42% and in membranous nephropathy of 5% to 60%.[215,216]

Recently, Lionaki and colleagues published results of a retrospective review of 898 patients in two cohorts with biopsy proven membranous glomerulonephritis. They concluded that clinically evident venous thromboembolic events (VTEs) occur in 65 (7.2%) of patients with membranous nephropathy. Renal vein thrombosis accounted for 30% of the cases of venous thrombolic events.[217] They cited a serum albumin equal to or less than 2.8 g per dL as a risk factor for VTE in membranous nephropathy. Mahmoodi and colleagues found a high absolute risk of VTE in the first 6 months of nephrotic syndrome, which they found strongly associated with the ratio of proteinuria to serum albumin.[218] The reason for the wide discrepancy in incidence may be related to some of the studies including patients who were asymptomatic as well as differences in the underlying immunologic causes of nephrotic syndrome and persistence and magnitude of hypoalbuminemia.[209] The notion that RVT causes the nephrotic syndrome, once widely held, has been largely disproved.[219–223]

Pathophysiology

The causative link between RVT and the nephrotic syndrome is the hypercoagulable state. Llach and Yudd reviewed the coagulation cascade in their earlier review of the subject, which is summarized here, and abnormalities found in patients with nephrotic syndrome.[209] The coagulation cascade is broken into five functional classes: zymogens (factors II, V, IX, XI, and XII), which are activated by enzymes and cofactors (factors V and VIII); fibrinogen and products from the conversion of fibrinogen to fibrin; the fibrinolytic system; clotting inhibitors; and components of platelet reaction and thrombogenisis.[224–233]

Several studies have noted a loss of factor XII in the urine, and others have reported normal levels of factor XII in the blood but decreased levels of active factor XII. Saito and colleagues,[231] for example, noted that the ratio of immunoreactive factor XII to functional factor XII activity was significantly higher in patients with nephrotic syndrome than in normal controls. They failed to detect circulating inhibitors to factor XII and noted no difference in prekallikrein levels in the plasma of patients with nephrotic syndrome. They argued that urinary losses did not seem to account for decreased factor XII activity and suggested that there were changes to functional sites in factor XII in patients with nephrotic syndrome.

Others have suggested that the drop in functional factor XII activity may result from an inability of biosynthetic capacity to keep up with urinary losses of factor XII.[232] Green and colleagues found both factor IX and XII in the urine of a woman with heavy proteinuria.[225] Several studies showed a correlation between increases in factors V and VIII and a fall in the level of serum albumin.[234,235] The alterations in levels of cofactors are a result of increased synthesis of these proteins by the liver.[236] Llach and Yudd argued in an earlier edition of this chapter that elevated levels of cofactors do not lead to hypercoagulability because the level of cofactors in circulation is generally in excess of the activated amount at any given time in normal patients. Furthermore, high levels of cofactors are present in the inflammatory state because they are acute phase reactant proteins, and there is no evidence to suggest that this leads to increased thromboembolic phenomena.[211]

Elevated plasma fibrinogen levels have been observed consistently in nephrotic patients. Using ^{131}I labeled fibrinogen, researchers have found a normal rate of fibrinogen catabolism but increased liver fibrinogen synthesis that is proportional to urinary protein loss.[237] There is also a significant correlation between fibrinogen and cholesterol levels, and both are related inversely to levels of serum albumin. The level of fibrinogen may be as high as 1 g per dL.[237] Llach and Yudd suggested that high fibrinogen levels by increasing blood viscosity play a role in the hypercoagulable state of the nephrotic syndrome.[209]

Some researchers have observed an increase in fibrinogen degradation products in the urine of patients with nephrotic syndrome although they are not generally observed in the serum.[238–241] And yet this is not necessarily evidence of increased fibrinolysis in the vasculature but may in fact represent filtered fibrinogen that has been degraded in the tubules.[240]

A number of studies have demonstrated alterations in the fibrinolytic system of nephrotic patients in the conversion of plasminogen by plasminogen activators to the serine protease plasmin.[235,242] In the nephrotic syndrome, researchers have observed a decrease in general levels of plasminogen, which in turn correlates with low levels of albumin, although the clinical significance is not clear and cause and effect relationship has not been established.[215,243–245] One group demonstrated elevated levels of a plasmin inhibitor, alpha 2-antiplasmin, in 13 or 14 patients with nephrotic syndrome and RVT and only 12 of 30 patients with nephrotic syndrome and no RVT. They suggested that elevated levels of the plasmin inhibitor may be a factor in determining susceptibility to the development and persistence of RVT in patients with nephrotic syndrome.[246]

Nephrotic patients have also been found to have alterations in coagulation inhibitors, particularly antithrombin III, the main inhibitor of thrombin and activated factors XII, IX, X, and XI and plasmin. Case reports and case series noted the relationship between nephrotic syndrome, low levels of antithrombin III, and RVT.[247,248] The molecular weight of antithrombin III is similar to that of albumin and these researchers found a significant correlation in the plasma levels of the two proteins as well as between renal clearance of antithrombin III and antithrombin III deficiency with antithrombin III deficiency associated with albumin levels of less than 2 g per dL. And yet other studies have found normal or increased antithrombin III activity in nephrotic children, although this may have been due to nonspecific in vitro inhibition of thrombin by two other clotting inhibitors.[249,250] Some researchers have demonstrated that plasma levels of antithrombin III correlate well with albumin but not with proteinuria, whereas urinary antithrombin III levels correlate well with proteinuria,[251,252] suggesting that increased antithrombin III synthesis compensated for urinary losses.[252] Other investigators noticed a significant decrease in plasma antithrombin III concentration and activity in 20 nephrotic patients compared with normal patients.[253] They also saw heavy losses of antithrombin III in the urine. Although the rate of synthesis and breakdown of antithrombin III may not be known, renal losses likely contribute to antithrombin III deficiency in nephrotic patients, especially when the losses are abrupt before hepatic synthesis has had a chance to increase. Indeed, increased levels of antithrombin III have been noted in nephrotic children treated with steroids.[252]

Protein C and S play an important role in inhibiting coagulation, and data about the role of deficiencies in these two proteins in nephrotic syndrome has been reported. Yermiahu and colleagues reported on 15 children with proteinuria, including 13 with nephrotic syndrome and two with subnephrotic range proteinuria. Plasma levels of proteins C and S were normal, but protein C antigenicity was increased in the urine of five out of 14 children, whereas protein S antigenicity was noted in the urine of 7 out of 12 children. No thromboembolic events were noted.[254] Hanevold and colleagues, on the other hand, found evidence of protein S deficiency in five children with steroid-resistant nephrotic syndrome.[255] Other investigators have also noted a role for functional protein S deficiency in nephrotic syndrome.[256] Some investigators have reported normal levels of protein C in the nephrotic syndrome, with decreased activity in late renal disease.[257] Others have reported elevated levels of proteins C and S in nephrotic syndrome and suggested a general increase in vitamin-K dependent anticoagulation factors in nephrotic sydrome.[258]

Thrombocytosis has been reported in the nephrotic syndrome.[259,260] Increased platelet aggregation with collagen and adenosine diphosphate but not with epinephrine has been noted.[261,262] Remuzzi et al. reported that the degree of platelet function abnormalities correlates with the degree of hypoalbuminemia and severity of proteinuria. Levels of beta-thromboglobulin, a specific protein released by platelets aggregation, have reported to be elevated in nephrotic patients but to return to normal levels upon clinical remission, suggesting that nephrotic patients have increased levels of platelet aggregation.[261] And yet, other studies have reported normal levels of beta thromboglobulin in nephrotic patients.[262] One study of nephrotic patients showed that thrombotic complications occurred only in patients with increased platelet aggregation and elevated beta-thromboglobulin levels.[263] These researchers noted an inverse relationship between beta-thromboglobulin levels and serum albumin, with increased risk of thrombosis at serum albumin levels less than 2 g per dL, suggesting a regulatory role for albumin in platelet aggregation.

Other factors that may contribute to RVT beyond hypercoagulability include a persistent reduction in plasma volume. Llach and Yudd postulated that a sustained reduction in blood volume could lead to decreased renal venous blood flow and thereby potentiate RVT.[209] Others have suggested that intensive diuretic therapy is associated with increased risk of RVT.[264] The nature of immunologic injury in nephrotic syndrome may also play a role in a subpopulation of patients with membranous nephropathy and RVT.[265] Indeed, in one study, factor XII and prekallikrein were found in subepithelial deposits in 29 patients with membranous nephropathy, suggesting that such deposits triggered the coagulation cascade.[266,267] A tendency toward greater coagulability in nephrotic patients may be behind reports of peripheral vascular thrombosis and RVT following placement of central catheters.[268] Finally, although steroids have become a mainstay of therapy in the treatment of proteinuric renal disease, reports in the literature suggest a relationship between steroids and the hypercoagulable state.[269–271]

In summary, the pathogenesis of RVT is a complex interplay of increased glomerular permeability leading to urinary losses of clotting inhibitors (zymogens, plasminogen, and albumin), leading to hypoalbuminemia, with resultant increased hepatic production of fibrinogen and cofactors and increased platelet aggregation—urinary losses and hypoalbuminemia together result in hypercoagulability. At the same time, the loss of oncotic pressure leads to hemoconcentration and reduced renal blood flow. Finally, diuretics, steroid therapy, and immunologic injury, particularly in membranous nephropathy, round out the underlying causes of RVT.

Clinical Manifestations

As noted in the introduction to this section, the clinical presentation of RVT varies from patient to patient.[210,223] In general, the mode of presentation can be either acute or chronic, which is observed more frequently and is usually asymptomatic. Acute RVT is characterized by sudden onset and usually occurs in younger patients complaining of persistent, at times colicky, flank pain; marked costovertebral angle tenderness and macroscopic hematuria are usually present. Acute RVT may on occasion be bilateral, resulting in oliguric renal failure and flank pain.[209]

Other causes of RVT include trauma, oral contraceptives, volume depletion, and steroids, as previously mentioned. Oral contraceptives have been reported as an isolated cause of RVT in case reports. In a recent one, a 35-year-old woman was awoken from sleep by acute flank pain. CT showed thrombus extending from the right renal vein into the inferior vena cava. Her sole risk factor was chronic ingestion of oral contraceptives. In an earlier case, the patient presented with accelerated hypertension and RVT and underwent nephrectomy.[272,273] A cause-and-effect relationship could not be established in the earlier case, but a meta-analysis of studies on the risk of VTE and oral contraceptive use concluded that the connection is valid, particularly in women with a previous history of VTE.[274]

Volume depletion is associated with RVT in infants.[275] Thrombosis develops in the small renal veins, predominantly the arcuate or the intralobular vein. In children without the nephrotic syndrome or proteinuria, this syndrome develops in the clinical setting of diarrhea, vomiting, or shock. Oliguria and hematuria rapidly ensue. The common clinical presentation is a hyperosmolar hypovolemic state. An enlarged palpable kidney may be found in 60% of affected infants. Mortality is high.

Acute RVT has been reported in transplant kidneys with increased frequency.[276–278] Predisposing factors included OKT3 and cyclosporine.[279] Some researchers have argued that cyclosporine increased the risk of transplant thrombosis by exacerbating hypercoagulability.[280] Other authors, however, saw the risk of thrombosis in the transplanted kidney related more to a previous history of thrombosis and diabetes than to warm or cold ischemic time or whether cyclosporine or OKT3 was used as an induction agent.[281] A search for reports of RVT related to newer induction and maintenance immunosuppressive agents at the time of writing did not reveal any reports of RVT caused by these agents. It did, however, reveal case reports of membranous nephropathy with RVT treated with the newer calcineurin inhibitor tacrolimus.[282] Nor was there an increased risk of postoperative thromboembolic events in transplant patients who were treated with sirolimus in addition to cyclosporine.[283]

Radiologic manifestations of acute RVT are well defined compared to chronic RVT in which the signs on imaging are often minimal. In an experimental model of complete occlusion of the renal vein, the organ experiences a sudden increase in size within the first 24 hours of occlusion.[284] There is then a progressive decline in size over the next 2 months resulting in an atrophic kidney. Plain film of the abdomen with intravenous pyelogram may reveal an enlarged kidney; if the obstruction is sudden and complete, the collecting system may not be visualized at all in which case retrograde pyelography may be useful. When visualized, the renal pelvis can be stretched, distorted, and blurred as a result of interstitial edema. Notching of the ureter is a frequent radiographic finding in RVT and likely represents indentation of the ureters by collateral venous circulation.[285,286] Notching of the ureter occurs only infrequently in patients with chronic RVT as in nephrotic syndrome.[285]

Diagnosis of RVT on ultrasonogram is made by direct visualization of thrombi within the renal vein and inferior vena cava, dilation of the renal vein proximal to the point of occlusion, loss of normal renal structure, and an increase in renal size in the acute phase.[286] Doppler ultrasonography may be useful in the evaluation of RVT in the transplanted kidney.

CT has become the imaging modality of choice for noninvasive evaluation of acute RVT. Gatewood and colleagues reviewed CT findings in 50 patients with nephrotic syndrome. The diagnosis of RVT was confirmed in four patients who presented with acute clinical manifestations. All four had thrombus in the inferior vena cava at the level of the renal veins. In the remaining 46 asymptomatic patients, one had bilateral RVT, two had left RVT, and five had isolated IVC thrombus. Radiographic findings on CT included enlargement and distention of the affected renal vein as well as persistent parenchymal opacification, thickening of Gerota fascia, pericapsular stranding, and capsular venous collaterals are also observed.[287] Magnetic resonance imaging (MRI) has become increasingly useful as a tool for evaluating renal pathology. In a review of published literature on renal vein thrombosis, Asghar and colleagues concluded that CT angiography remains the investigation of choice although MRA and renal venography would also be useful in selected patients.[288]

Clinical Course and Treatment

RVT represents a distinct clinical entity, with malignancy the underlying cause in 66% of cases and nephrotic syndrome the cause of 20% in one relatively recent series.[289] Older series looked at the prognosis and treatment of RVT in nephrotic syndrome. Kowal and colleagues reviewed 65 cases of RVT in nephrotic syndrome of whom only 14 were alive at 2 years. Data was available only for the 14 surviving patients, of whom 10 had acute RVT.[285] Rosenmann and colleagues followed 15 nephrotic patients with RVT. Only four of the patients had symptoms suggestive of acute RVT. Seven patients had one or more episodes of pulmonary embolism and four had repeated thrombosis of the renal venous system. Seven patients died, and the authors suggested that recurrent thromboembolic events portended a worse outcome.[290] Richet and Meyrier reviewed 112 cases of RVT cited in the literature, and of those 112, 72 had died for a mortality rate of around 64%.[291] McCarthy et al. estimated the average survival after the onset of RVT at around 9 months.[214] But that may overestimate mortality since kidney failure was a cause of death in some of the patients, and dialysis therapy was not readily available.[209]

In the 1980s, Laville and colleagues reviewed the cases of 27 patients with RVT to assess their long-term prognosis.[292] Twenty-four patients had nephrotic syndrome, and 15 had renal impairment. Ten patients were treated with anticoagulation alone. Eleven patients died within the first 6 months, mainly from hemorrhagic complications or sepsis. Among the survivors, nephrotic syndrome improved or went away in 12 patients, and renal function did not worsen in any of the survivors. Patients with membranous nephropathy had significantly better renal function and a lower mortality rate than patients with other types of nephropathy. Initial renal insufficiency portended a poor outcome. There was no survival advantage to thrombectomy over anticoagulation alone.

Wysokinski and colleagues reviewed the files of 218 patients with RVT followed from the Mayo Clinic between 1980 and 2000, comparing then with patients who suffered DVT and normal controls.[289] During a mean follow-up of 42 ± 57 months there were 8 recurrent RVTs, significantly fewer than in the DVT group. Survival was also lower on an age- and sex-matched basis for patients in the RVT group than for patients in the DVT group. Active malignancy and infection were also associated with poor outcomes. Patients on warfarin therapy had a survival advantage.

Other studies have noted treatment with anticoagulation therapy reduced the risk of recurrent RVT and reversed the deterioration in renal function that occurred with RVT.[212,293] For patients receiving warfarin anticoagulation, heparin is the initial drug of choice with the aim to maintain a clotting time of 2 to 2.5 times normal. Once oral anticoagulation therapy is established, the prothrombin time should be around 1.5 to 2 times normal. Llach recommends that the patients should be treated with anticoagulants as long as the albumin is less than 2.5 g per dL.[209]

Several cases reports have been published in which the authors used low-molecular weight heparin to treat RVT. Renal function was reported as normal.[294,295] But use of low-molecular-weight heparin, which is cleared by the kidneys, is not recommended in patients with creatinine clearance less than 30 mL per min because of increased risk of bleeding.[296] Some have suggested a possible role for the newer class of direct thrombin inhibitors in treatment of venous thromboembolism.[297] But a search of the U.S. National Library of Medicine online database at the time of this writing did not reveal any articles specifically on the use of direct thrombin inhibitors in the treatment of RVT.

Both streptokinase and urokinase have been used either systemically or with selective infusion.[67,298,299] Selective infusion has been used selectively in RVT of transplanted kidneys.[300,301] Surgical treatment for RVT is rarely used because the role for thrombectomy has not been established as beneficial.

REFERENCES

1. Stables DP, Fouche RF, de Villiers van Niekerk JP, et al. Traumatic renal artery occlusion: 21 cases. *J Urol.* 1976;115:229–233.
2. Vidal E, Marrone G, Gasparini D, et al. Radiological treatment of renal artery occlusion after blunt abdominal trauma in a pediatric patient: is it never too late? *Urology.* 2011;77:1220–1222.
3. Barlow B, Gandhi R. Renal artery thrombosis following blunt trauma. *J Trauma.* 1980;20:614–617.
4. Haas CA, Dinchman KH, Nasrallah PF, et al. Traumatic renal artery occlusion: a 15-year review. *J Trauma.* 1998;45:557–561.
5. Haas CA, Spirnak JP. Traumatic renal artery occlusion: a review of the literature. *Tech Urol.* 1998;4:1–11.
6. Clark DE, Georgitis JW, Ray FS. Renal arterial injuries caused by blunt trauma. *Surgery.* 1981;90:87–96.
7. Thurlbeck WM, Castleman B. Atheromatous emboli to the kidneys after aortic surgery. *N Engl J Med.* 1957;257:442–447.
8. Textor SC. Ischemic nephropathy: where are we now? *J Am Soc Nephrol.* 2004;15:1974–1982.
9. Montgomery JH, Moinuddin M, Buchignani JS, et al. Renal infarction after aerobics. *Clin Nucl Med.* 1984;9:664–665.
10. Hornez E, Bourgouin S, Baudoin Y, et al. [Management of seat-belt aorta in severe polytrauma: a review]. Journal des maladies vasculaires 2011;36:237–242.
11. Orhan O, Kultigin T, Osman K, et al. An exceedingly rare cause of secondary hypertension: bilateral renal artery dissection possibly secondary to extracorporeal shock-wave lithotripsy (ESWL). *Intern Med.* 2011;50:2633–2636.
12. Handley C, Heider C, Morris GC Jr, et al. Renal failure. I. The effect of complete renal artery occlusion for variable periods of time as compared to exposure to sub-filtration arterial pressures below 30 mm Hg for similar periods. *Annal Surg.* 1957;145:41–58.
13. Vollmar J, Helmstadter D, Hallwachs O. Complete occlusion of the renal artery: nephrectomy or revascularization? *J Cardiol Surg.* 1971;12:441–446.
14. Lang EK, Sullivan J, Frentz G. Renal trauma: radiological studies. Comparison of urography, computed tomography, angiography, and radionuclide studies. *Radiology.* 1985;154:1–6.
15. Kamel IR, Berkowitz JF. Assessment of the cortical rim sign in posttraumatic renal infarction. *J Comput Assit Tomogr.* 1996;20:803–806.
16. Lang EK. Arteriography in the assessment of renal trauma. The impact of arteriographic diagnosis on preservation of renal function and parenchyma. *J Trauma.* 1975;15:553–566.

17. Spinosa DJ, Matsumoto AH, Angle JF, et al. Renal insufficiency: usefulness of gadodiamide-enhanced renal angiography to supplement CO2-enhanced renal angiography for diagnosis and percutaneous treatment. *Radiology.* 1999;210:663–672.

18. Spirnak JP, Resnick MI. Revascularization of traumatic thrombosis of the renal artery. *Surg Gynecol Obstet.* 1987;164:22–26.

19. Cass AS. Renovascular injuries from external trauma. Diagnosis, treatment, and outcome. *Urol Clin N Am.* 1989;16:213–220.

20. Munoz D, Gutierrez C, Hidalgo F, et al. Traumatic renal artery thrombosis. *Scand J Urol Nephrol.* 1998;32:296–298.

21. Peterson NE. Traumatic bilateral renal infarction. *J Trauma.* 1989;29: 158–167.

22. Weimann S, Flora G, Dittrich P, et al. Traumatic renal artery occlusion: is late reconstruction advisable? *J Urol.* 1987;137:727–729.

23. Letsou GV, Gusberg R. Isolated bilateral renal artery thrombosis: an unusual consequence of blunt abdominal trauma—case report. *J Trauma.* 1990;30:509–511.

24. Fort J, Camps J, Ruiz P, et al. Renal artery embolism successfully revascularized by surgery after 5 days' anuria. Is it never too late? *Nephrol Dial Transplant.* 1996;11:1843–1845.

25. Maggio AJ Jr, Brosman S. Renal artery trauma. *Urology.* 1978;11:125–130.

26. Dowling JM, Lube MW, Smith CP, et al. Traumatic renal artery occlusion in a patient with a solitary kidney: case report of treatment with endovascular stent and review of the literature. *Am Surg.* 2007;73:351–353.

27. Chabrot P, Cassagnes L, Alfidja A, et al. Revascularization of traumatic renal artery dissection by endoluminal stenting: three cases. *Acta Radiol.* 2010; 51:21–26.

28. Kushimoto S, Shiraishi S, Miyauchi M, et al. Traumatic renal artery occlusion treated with an endovascular stent—the limitations of surgical revascularization: report of a case. *Surg Today.* 2011;41:1020–1023.

29. van der Wal MA, Wisselink W, Rauwerda JA. Traumatic bilateral renal artery thrombosis: case report and review of the literature. *Cardiovasc Surg.* 2003;11:527–529.

30. Adovasio R, Pancrazio F. Acute thrombosis of renal artery: restoration of renal function after late revascularization. *Vasa.* 1989;18:239–241.

31. Vuong PN, Desoutter P, Mickley V, et al. Fibromuscular dysplasia of the renal artery responsible for renovascular hypertension: a histological presentation based on a series of 102 patients. *Vasa.* 2004;33:13–18.

32. Stinchcombe SJ, Manhire AR, Bishop MC, et al. Renal arterial fibromuscular dysplasia: acute renal infarction in three patients with angiographic evidence of medial fibroplasia. *Br J Radiol.* 1992;65:81–84.

33. Teoh MK. Takayasu's arteritis with renovascular hypertension: results of surgical treatment. *Cardiovasc Surg.* 1999;7:626–632.

34. Dardik A, Ballermann BJ, Williams GM. Successful delayed bilateral renal revascularization during active phase of Takayasu's arteritis. *J Vasc Surg.* 1998;27:552–554.

35. Hoover LA, Hall-Craggs M, Dagher FJ. Polyarteritis nodosa involving only the main renal arteries. *Am J Kidney Dis.* 1988;11:66–69.

36. Templeton PA, Pais SO. Renal artery occlusion in PAN. *Radiology.* 1985;156:308.

37. El Ramahi KM, Al Dalaan A, Al Shaikh A, et al. Renal involvement in Behcet's disease: review of 9 cases. *J Rheumatol.* 1998;25:2254–2260.

38. Sherif A, Stewart P, Mendes DM. The repetitive vascular catastrophes of Behcet's disease: a case report with review of the literature. *Ann Vasc Surg.* 1992;6:85–89.

39. Sueyoshi E, Sakamoto I, Hayashi N, et al. Ruptured renal artery aneurysm due to Behcet's disease. *Abdom Imaging.* 1996;21:166–167.

40. Akpolat T, Akkoyunlu M, Akpolat I, et al. Renal Behcet's disease: a cumulative analysis. *Semin Arthritis Rheum.* 2002;31:317–337.

41. Price RK, Skelton R. Hypertension due to syphilitic occlusion of the main renal arteries. *Br Heart J.* 1948;10:29–33.

42. Heng MC, Haberfeld G. Thrombotic phenomena associated with intravenous cocaine. *J Am Acad Dermatol.* 1987;16:462–468.

43. Goodman PE, Rennie WP. Renal infarction secondary to nasal insufflation of cocaine. *Am J Emerg Med.* 1995;13:421–423.

44. Kramer RK, Turner RC. Renal infarction associated with cocaine use and latent protein C deficiency. *South Med J.* 1993;86:1436–1438.

45. Sane SY, Deshmukh SS. Total renal infarct and peri-renal abscess caused by phycomycosis (a case report). *J Postgrad Med.* 1988;34:44B–7.

46. Vesa J, Bielsa O, Arango O, et al. Massive renal infarction due to mucormycosis in an AIDS patient. *Infection.* 1992;20:234–236.

47. Lam J, Henriquez R, Cruzat C. [Pheochromocytoma and von Recklinghausen neurofibromatosis: postpartum crisis and renal artery thrombosis]. Revista medica de Chile 1998;126:1367–1371.

48. Hitti IF, Celmer EJ, Rapuano J. Hemorrhagic infarction of the kidney. An uncommon presentation of infiltrating urothelial carcinoma of the renal pelvis. *Urol Int.* 1986;41:212–215.

49. Granfortuna J, Zamkoff K, Urrutia E. Acute renal infarction in sickle cell disease. *Am J Hematol.* 1986;23:59–64.

50. Penn DE, Gist A, Axon RN. Spontaneous renal artery thrombosis and common iliac artery dissection in a previously healthy young adult. *South Med J.* 2008;101:1263–1265.

51. Conway R, Bergin D, Coughlan RJ, et al. Renal infarction due to spontaneous renal artery dissection in Ehlers-Danlos syndrome type IV. *J Rheumatol.* 2012;39:199–200.

52. Chevalier J, Ducasse E, Dasnoy D, et al. Heparin-induced thrombocytopenia with acute aortic and renal thrombosis in a patient treated with low-molecular-weight heparin. *Eur J Vasc Endovasc Surg.* 2005;29:209–212.

53. Sa H, Freitas L, Mota A, et al. Primary antiphospholipid syndrome presented by total infarction of right kidney with nephrotic syndrome. *Clin Nephrol.* 1999;52:56–60.

54. Klein O, Bernheim J, Strahilevitz J, et al. Renal colic in a patient with antiphospholipid antibodies and factor V Leiden mutation. *Nephrol Dial Transplant.* 1999;14:2502–504.

55. Karassa FB, Avdikou K, Pappas P, et al. Late renal transplant arterial thrombosis in a patient with systemic lupus erythematosus and antiphospholipid syndrome. *Nephrol Dial Transplant.* 1999;14:472–474.

56. Remondino GI, Mysler E, Pissano MN, et al. A reversible bilateral renal artery stenosis in association with antiphospholipid syndrome. *Lupus.* 2000;9: 65–67.

57. Ostuni PA, Lazzarin P, Pengo V, et al. Renal artery thrombosis and hypertension in a 13 year old girl with antiphospholipid syndrome. *Ann Rheum Dis.* 1990;49:184–187.

58. Poux JM, Boudet R, Lacroix P, et al. Renal infarction and thrombosis of the infrarenal aorta in a 35-year-old man with primary antiphospholipid syndrome. *Am J Kidney Dis.* 1996;27:721–725.

59. Sonpal GM, Sharma A, Miller A. Primary antiphospholipid antibody syndrome, renal infarction and hypertension. *J Rheumatol.* 1993;20:1221–1223.

60. Hernandez D, Dominguez ML, Diaz F, et al. Renal infarction in a severely hypertensive patient with lupus erythematosus and antiphospholipid antibodies. *Nephron.* 1996;72:298–301.

61. Kleinknecht D, Bobrie G, Meyer O, Noel LH, Callard P, Ramdane M. Recurrent thrombosis and renal vascular disease in patients with a lupus anticoagulant. *Nephrol Dial Transplant.* 1989;4:854–858.

62. Arnold MH, Schrieber L. Splenic and renal infarction in systemic lupus erythematosus: association with anti-cardiolipin antibodies. *Clin Rheumatol.* 1988;7:406–410.

63. Dasgupta B, Almond MK, Tanqueray A. Polyarteritis nodosa and the antiphospholipid syndrome. *Br J Rheumatol.* 1997;36:1210–1212.

64. Kaushik S, Federle MP, Schur PH, Krishnan M, Silverman SG, Ros PR. Abdominal thrombotic and ischemic manifestations of the antiphospholipid antibody syndrome: CT findings in 42 patients. *Radiology.* 2001;218:768–771.

65. Miura K, Takahashi T, Takahashi I, et al. Renovascular hypertension due to antithrombin deficiency in childhood. *Pediatr Nephrol.* 2004;19:1294–1296.

66. Nakamura M, Ohnishi T, Okamoto S, et al. Abdominal aortic thrombosis in a patient with nephrotic syndrome. *Am J Nephrol.* 1998;18:64–66.

67. Temes Montes XL, Almaraz Jimenez MA, Lorenzo Aguiar MD, et al. Renal artery thrombosis occurring in an adult with the idiopathic nephrotic syndrome: results of local treatment with streptokinase. *Clin Nephrol.* 1979;12:90–92.

68. Pochet JM, Bobrie G, Basile C, Grunfeld JP. [Renal arterial thrombosis complicating nephrotic syndrome]. *Presse Med.* 1988;17:2139.

69. Guirguis N, Budisavljevic MN, Self S, et al. Acute renal artery and vein thrombosis after renal transplant, associated with a short partial thromboplastin time and factor V Leiden mutation. *Ann Clin Lab Sci.* 2000;30:75–78.

70. Morris D, Kisly A, Stoyka CG, Provenzano R. Spontaneous bilateral renal artery occlusion associated with chronic atrial fibrillation. *Clin Nephrol.* 1993;39:257–259.

71. Argiris A. Splenic and renal infarctions complicating atrial fibrillation. *Mt Sinai J Med.* 1997;64:342–349.

72. Cheng KL, Tseng SS, Tarng DC. Acute renal failure caused by unilateral renal artery thromboembolism. *Nephrol Dial Transplant.* 2003;18:833–835.

73. Majumdar A, Chowdhary S, Ferreira MA, et al. Renal pathological findings in infective endocarditis. *Nephrol Dial Transplant.* 2000;15:1782–1787.

74. Blackmon SH, Kassis ES, Ge Y, et al. Left atrial myxoma embolus to the renal artery: should a nephrectomy be advised? *Ann Thorac Surg.* 2010;90:289–292.

75. Young RD, Hunter WC. Primary myxoma of the left ventricle with embolic occlusion of the abdominal aorta and renal arteries. *Arch Pathol (Chic).* 1947;43:86–91.

76. Gill TJ III, Dammin GJ. Paradoxical embolism with renal failure caused by occlusion of the renal arteries. *Am J Med.* 1958;25:780–787.

77. Isles CG, Robertson S, Hill D. Management of renovascular disease: a review of renal artery stenting in ten studies. *QJM.*1999;92:159–167.

78. Textor SC. Managing renal arterial disease and hypertension. *Curr Opin Cardiol.* 2003;18:260–267.

79. Morris CS, Bonnevie GJ, Najarian KE. Nonsurgical treatment of acute iatrogenic renal artery injuries occurring after renal artery angioplasty and stenting. *AJR Am J Roentgenol.* 2001;177:1353–1357.

80. Eklof H, Bergqvist D, Hagg A, et al. Outcome after endovascular revascularization of atherosclerotic renal artery stenosis. *Acta Radiol.* 2009;50:256–264.

81. Torre J, Hashisho M, Lo C, et al. Acute renal artery stent thrombosis with a solitary functioning kidney. *Ann Vasc Surg.* 2010;24:953 e13–19.

82. Dobbeleir N, Vermeersch P, Agostoni P. Late renal stent thrombosis. *Cardiovasc Revasc Med.* 2010;11:170–171.

83. Bockler D, Krauss M, Mansmann U, et al. Incidence of renal infarctions after endovascular AAA repair: relationship to infrarenal versus suprarenal fixation. *J Endovasc Ther.* 2003;10:1054–1060.

84. Kramer SC, Seifarth H, Pamler R, et al. Renal infarction following endovascular aortic aneurysm repair: incidence and clinical consequences. *J Endovasc Ther.* 2002;9:98–102.

85. Laird JR, Tehrani F, Soukas P, et al. Feasibility of FiberNet(R) embolic protection system in patients undergoing angioplasty for atherosclerotic renal artery stenosis. *Catheter Cardiovasc Interv.* 2012;79(3):430–436.

86. Roberts M, Kumar SK, MacGinley R, et al. The CARI guidelines. Role of distal protection devices. *Nephrology (Carlton).* 2010;15 Suppl 1:S227–233.

87. Cooper CJ, Haller ST, Colyer W, et al. Embolic protection and platelet inhibition during renal artery stenting. *Circulation.* 2008;117:2752–2760.

88. Hoxie HJ, Coggin CB. Renal infarction: statistical study of 255 cases and detailed report of an unusual case. *Arch Intern Med.* 1940;65:587–594.

89. Jennette JC, Olson JL, Schwartz MM, Silva FG, eds. *Heptinstall's Pathology of the Kidney*, 6th ed. New York: Lippincott Williams and Wilkins; 2006.

90. Abuelo JG. Diagnosing vascular causes of renal failure. *Ann Intern Med.* 1995;123:601–614.

91. Blakely P, Cosby RL, McDonald BR. Nephritic urinary sediment in embolic renal infarction. *Clin Nephrol.* 1994;42:401–403.

92. Lessman RK, Johnson SF, Coburn JW, Kaufman JJ. Renal artery embolism: clinical features and long-term follow-up of 17 cases. *Ann Intern Med.* 1978;89:477–482.

93. Cai S, Ouyang YS, Li JC, et al. Evaluation of acute renal artery thrombosis or embolism with color Doppler sonography. *Clin Imaging.* 2008;32:367–371.

94. Blum U, Billmann P, Krause T, et al. Effect of local low-dose thrombolysis on clinical outcome in acute embolic renal artery occlusion. *Radiology.* 1993;189:549–554.

95. Mesnard L, Delahousse M, Raynaud A, et al. Delayed angioplasty after renal thrombosis. *Am J Kidney Dis.* 2003;41:E9–12.

96. Pilmore HL, Walker RJ, Solomon C, et al. Acute bilateral renal artery occlusion: successful revascularization with streptokinase. *Am J Nephrol.* 1995;15:90–91.

97. Skinner RE, Hefty T, Long TD, et al. Recovery of function in a solitary kidney after intra-arterial thrombolytic therapy. *J Urol.* 1989;141:108–110.

98. Marron B, Ubeda I, Gallego J, et al. Functional renal recovery after spontaneous renal embolization in a sole kidney. *Nephrol Dial Transplant.* 1997;12:2417–2419.

99. Syed MI, Shaikh A, Ullah A, et al. Acute renal artery thrombosis treated with t-PA power-pulse spray rheolytic thrombectomy. *Cardiovasc Revasc Med.* 2010;11:264 e1–7.

100. Lacombe M. Acute non-traumatic obstructions of the renal artery. *J Cardiol Surg.* 1992;33:163–168.

101. Ouriel K, Andrus CH, Ricotta JJ, et al. Acute renal artery occlusion: when is revascularization justified? *J Vasc Surg.* 1987;5:348–355.

102. Tham G, Ekelund L, Herrlin K, et al. Renal artery aneurysms. Natural history and prognosis. *Annal Surg.* 1983;197:348–352.

103. Abeshouse BS. Aneurysm of the renal artery; report of two cases and review of the literature. *Urol Cutaneous Rev.* 1951;55:451–463.

104. Hageman JH, Smith RF, Szilagyi E, et al. Aneurysms of the renal artery: problems of prognosis and surgical management. *Surgery.* 1978;84:563–572.

105. Silver PR, Budin JA. Unusual manifestations of renal artery aneurysms. *Urol Radiol.* 1990;12:80–83.

106. Cummings KB, Lecky JW, Kaufman JJ. Renal artery aneurysms and hypertension. *J Urol.* 1973;109:144–148.

107. Eskandari MK, Resnick SA. Aneurysms of the renal artery. *Semin Vasc Surg.* 2005;18:202–208.

108. Edsman G. Angionephrography and suprarenal angiography; a roentgenologic study of the normal kidney, expansive renal and suprarenal lesions and renal aneurysms. *Acta Radiol.* 1957:1–141.

109. Poutasse EF. Renal artery aneurysms. *J Urol.* 1975;113:443–449.

110. Cinat M, Yoon P, Wilson SE. Management of renal artery aneurysms. *Semin Vasc Surg.* 1996;9:236–244.

111. Kincaid OW, Davis GD, Hallermann FJ, et al. Fibromuscular dysplasia of the renal arteries. Arteriographic features, classification, and observations on natural history of the disease. *Am J Roentgenol Radium Ther Nucl Med.* 1968;104:271–282.

112. Barth RA. Fibromuscular dysplasia with clotted renal artery aneurysm. *Pediatr Radiol.* 1993;23:296–297.

113. Smith JN, Hinman F Jr. Intrarenal arterial aneurysms. *J Urol.* 1967;97:990–996.

114. Henke PK, Cardneau JD, Welling TH III, et al. Renal artery aneurysms: a 35-year clinical experience with 252 aneurysms in 168 patients. *Annal Surg.* 2001;234:454–62; discussion 62–63.

115. English WP, Pearce JD, Craven TE, et al. Surgical management of renal artery aneurysms. *J Vasc Surg.* 2004;40:53–60.

116. Pfeiffer T, Reiher L, Grabitz K, et al. Reconstruction for renal artery aneurysm: operative techniques and long-term results. *J Vasc Surg.* 2003;37:293–300.

117. Sicard GA, Reilly JM, Picus DD, et al. Alternatives in renal revascularization. *Curr Probl Surg.* 1995;32:571–652.

118. Henke PK, Stanley JC. Renal artery aneurysms: diagnosis, management and outcomes. *Minerva Chir.* 2003;58:305–311.

119. Hidai H, Kinoshita Y, Murayama T, et al. Rupture of renal artery aneurysm. *Eur Eurol.* 1985;11:249–253.

120. Henriksson C, Lukes P, Nilson AE, Pettersson S. Angiographically discovered, non-operated renal artery aneurysms. *Scand J Urol Nephrol.* 1984;18:59–62.

121. Hubert JP Jr, Pairolero PC, Kazmier FJ. Solitary renal artery aneurysm. *Surgery.* 1980;88:557–565.

122. Martin RS III, Meacham PW, Ditesheim JA, Mulherin JL, Jr., Edwards WH. Renal artery aneurysm: selective treatment for hypertension and prevention of rupture. *J Vasc Surg.* 1989;9:26–34.

123. Cohen JR, Shamash FS. Ruptured renal artery aneurysms during pregnancy. *J Vasc Surg.* 1987;6:51–59.

124. Schoon IM, Seeman T, Niemand D, et al. Rupture of renal arterial aneurysm in pregnancy. Case report. *Acta Chir Scand.* 1988;154:593–597.

125. Smith JA, Macleish DG. Postpartum rupture of a renal artery aneurysm to a solitary kidney. *Aust NZ J Surg.* 1985;55:299–300.

126. Richardson AJ, Liddington M, Jaskowski A, et al. Pregnancy in a renal transplant recipient complicated by rupture of a transplant renal artery aneurysm. *Br J Surg.* 1990;77:228–229.

127. Rijbroek A, van Dijk HA, Roex AJ. Rupture of renal artery aneurysm during pregnancy. *Eur J Vasc Surg.* 1994;8:375–376.

128. Love WK, Robinette MA, Vernon CP. Renal artery aneurysm rupture in pregnancy. *J Urol.* 1981;126:809–811.

129. Milsom I, Forssman L. Factors influencing aortocaval compression in late pregnancy. *Am J Obstet Gynecol.* 1984;148:764–771.

130. Yang JC, Hye RJ. Ruptured renal artery aneurysm during pregnancy. *Ann Vasc Surg.* 1996;10:370–372.

131. Klein GE, Szolar DH, Breinl E, et al. Endovascular treatment of renal artery aneurysms with conventional non-detachable microcoils and Guglielmi detachable coils. *Br J Urol.* 1997;79:852–860.

132. Seo JM, Park KB, Kim KH, et al. Clinical and multidetector CT follow-up results of renal artery aneurysms treated by detachable coil embolization using 3D rotational angiography. *Acta Radiol.* 2011;52:854–859.

133. Lupattelli T, Abubacker Z, Morgan R, et al. Embolization of a renal artery aneurysm using ethylene vinyl alcohol copolymer (Onyx). *J Endovasc Ther.* 2003;10:366–370.

134. Jahan R, Murayama Y, Gobin YP, et al. Embolization of arteriovenous malformations with Onyx: clinicopathological experience in 23 patients. *Neurosurgery.* 2001;48:984–95; discussion 95–97.

135. Garcia-Roig M, Gorin MA, Castellan M, et al. OMNEX surgical sealant in the extracorporeal repair of renal artery aneurysms. *Ann Vasc Surg.* 2011;25:1141 e5–8.

136. Krokidis M, Amer H, Key S, et al. Acute rupture of a fibromuscular dysplasia related renal artery aneurysm: emergency treatment with a covered stent. *Hellenic J Cardiol.* 2011;52:541–544.

137. Hislop SJ, Patel SA, Abt PL, et al. Therapy of renal artery aneurysms in New York State: outcomes of patients undergoing open and endovascular repair. *Ann Vasc Surg.* 2009;23:194–200.

138. Smith BM, Holcomb GW III, Richie RE, Dean RH. Renal artery dissection. *Annal Surg.* 1984;200:134–146.

139. Gewertz BL, Stanley JC, Fry WJ. Renal artery dissections. *Arch Surg.* 1977;112:409–414.

140. Alamir A, Middendorf DF, Baker P, et al. Renal artery dissection causing renal infarction in otherwise healthy men. *Am J Kidney Dis.* 1997;30:851–855.

141. Edwards BS, Stanson AW, Holley KE, et al. Isolated renal artery dissection, presentation, evaluation, management, and pathology. *Mayo Clin Proc.* 1982;57:564–571.
142. Esayag-Tendler B, Yamase H, Ramsby G, et al. Accelerated hypertension with encephalopathy due to an isolated dissection of a renal artery branch vessel. *Am J Kidney Dis.* 1994;23:869–873.
143. Slavis SA, Hodge EE, Novick AC, et al. Surgical treatment for isolated dissection of the renal artery. *J Urol.* 1990;144:233–237.
144. Reilly LM, Cunningham CG, Maggisano R, et al. The role of arterial reconstruction in spontaneous renal artery dissection. *J Vasc Surg.* 1991;14:468–477; discussion 477–479.
145. Vidt DG. Cholesterol emboli: a common cause of renal failure. *Ann Rev Med.* 1997;48:375–385.
146. Lie JT. Cholesterol atheromatous embolism. The great masquerader revisited. *Pathol Annu.* 1992;27 Pt 2:17–50.
147. Scoble JE, O'Donnell PJ. Renal atheroembolic disease: the Cinderella of nephrology? *Nephrol Dial Transplant.* 1996;11:1516–1517.
148. Eliot RS, Kanjuh VI, Edwards JE. Atheromatous embolism. *Circulation.* 1964;30:611–618.
149. Meyer WW. Cholesterinkrystallembolie kleiner Organarterien und ihre Folgen. *Virch Arch.*1947;314:616–638.
150. Handler FP. Clinical and pathologic significance of atheromatous embolization, with emphasis on an etiology of renal hypertension. *Am J Med.* 1956;20:366–373.
151. Flory CM. Arterial occlusions produced by emboli from eroded aortic atheromatous plaques. *Am J Pathol.* 1945;21:549–565.
152. Fukumoto Y, Tsutsui H, Tsuchihashi M, et al. The incidence and risk factors of cholesterol embolization syndrome, a complication of cardiac catheterization: a prospective study. *J Am Coll Cardiol.* 2003;42:211–216.
153. Jones DB, Iannaccone PM. Atheromatous emboli in renal biopsies. An ultrastructural study. *Am J Pathol.* 1975;78:261–276.
154. Fine MJ, Kapoor W, Falanga V. Cholesterol crystal embolization: a review of 221 cases in the English literature. *Angiology.* 1987;38:769–784.
155. Gore I, McCombs HL, Lindquist RL. Observations on the fate of cholesterol emboli. *J Atheroscler Res.* 1964;4:527–535.
156. Gore I, Collins DP. Spontaneous atheromatous embolization. Review of the literature and a report of 16 additional cases. *Am J Clin Pathol.*1960;33:416–426.
157. Otken LB Jr. Experimental production of atheromatous embolization. *Arch Pathol.* 1959;68:685–689.
158. Sayre GP, Campbell DC. Multiple peripheral emboli in atherosclerosis of the aorta. *Arch Intern Med.* 1959;103:799–806.
159. Greenberg A, Bastacky SI, Iqbal A, et al. Focal segmental glomerulosclerosis associated with nephrotic syndrome in cholesterol atheroembolism: clinicopathological correlations. *Am J Kidney Dis.* 1997;29:334–344.
160. Aviles B, Ubeda I, Blanco J, et al. Pauci-immune extracapillary glomerulonephritis and atheromatous embolization. *Am J Kidney Dis.* 2002;40:847–851.
161. Kaplan-Pavlovcic S, Vizjak A, Vene N, et al. Antineutrophil cytoplasmic autoantibodies in atheroembolic disease. *Nephrol Dial Transplant.* 1998;13:985–987.
162. Maeshima E, Yamada Y, Mune M, et al. A case of cholesterol embolism with ANCA treated with corticosteroid and cyclophosphamide. *Ann Rheum Dis.* 2001;60:726.
163. Hannedouche T, Godin M, Courtois H, et al. Necrotizing glomerulonephritis and renal cholesterol embolization. *Nephron.* 1986;42:271–272.
164. Ballesteros AL, Bromsoms J, Valles M, et al. Vasculitis look-alikes: variants of renal atheroembolic disease. *Nephrol Dial Transplant.* 1999;14:430–433.
165. Goldman M, Thoua Y, Dhaene M, et al. Necrotising glomerulonephritis associated with cholesterol microemboli. *Br Med J (Clin Res Ed).* 1985;290:205–206.
166. Saklayen MG. Atheroembolic renal disease: preferential occurrence in whites only. *Am J Nephrol.* 1989;9:87–88.
167. Scolari F, Ravani P. Atheroembolic renal disease. *Lancet.* 2010;375: 1650–1660.
168. Preston RA, Stemmer CL, Materson BJ, et al. Renal biopsy in patients 65 years of age or older. An analysis of the results of 334 biopsies. *J Am Geriatr Soc.* 1990;38:669–674.
169. Belenfant X, Meyrier A, Jacquot C. Supportive treatment improves survival in multivisceral cholesterol crystal embolism. *Am J Kidney Dis.* 1999;33:840–850.
170. Mayo RR, Swartz RD. Redefining the incidence of clinically detectable atheroembolism. *Am J Med.* 1996;100:524–529.
171. Thadhani RI, Camargo CA Jr. Xavier RJ, et al. Atheroembolic renal failure after invasive procedures. Natural history based on 52 histologically proven cases. *Medicine.* 1995;74:350–358.
172. Scolari F, Ravani P, Pola A, et al. Predictors of renal and patient outcomes in atheroembolic renal disease: a prospective study. *J Am Soc Nephrol.* 2003;14:1584–1590.
173. Scolari F, Ravani P, Gaggi R, et al. The challenge of diagnosing atheroembolic renal disease: clinical features and prognostic factors. *Circulation.* 2007;116:298–304.
174. Lye WC, Cheah JS, Sinniah R. Renal cholesterol embolic disease. Case report and review of the literature. *Am J Nephrol.* 1993;13:489–493.
175. Scolari F, Bracchi M, Valzorio B, et al. Cholesterol atheromatous embolism: an increasingly recognized cause of acute renal failure. *Nephrol Dial Transplant.* 1996;11:1607–1612.
176. Frock J, Bierman M, Hammeke M, et al. Atheroembolic renal disease: experience with 22 patients. *Nebr Med J.* 1994;79:317–321.
177. Falanga V, Fine MJ, Kapoor WN. The cutaneous manifestations of cholesterol crystal embolization. *Arch Dermatol.* 1986;122:1194–1198.
178. Quintart C, Treille S, Lefebvre P, Pontus T. Penile necrosis following cholesterol embolism. *Br J Urol.* 1997;80:347–348.
179. Scolari F, Tardanico R, Zani R, et al. Cholesterol crystal embolism: A recognizable cause of renal disease. *Am J Kidney Dis.* 2000;36:1089–1109.
180. Scolari F, Tardanico R, Pola A, et al. Cholesterol crystal embolic disease in renal allografts. *J Nephrol.* 2003;16:139–143.
181. Aujla ND, Greenberg A, Banner BF, et al. Atheroembolic involvement of renal allografts. *Am J Kidney Dis.* 1989;13:329–332.
182. Singh I, Killen PD, Leichtman AB. Cholesterol emboli presenting as acute allograft dysfunction after renal transplantation. *J Am Soc Nephrol.* 1995;6:165–170.
183. Jimenez-Heffernan JA, Martinez-Garcia CM, Sanchez MA, et al. Small bowel perforation due to cholesterol atheromatous embolism. *Digest Dis Sci.* 1995;40:481–484.
184. Moolenaar W, Lamers CB. Cholesterol crystal embolization and the digestive system. *Scand J Gastroenterol Suppl.* 1991;188:69–72.
185. Probstein JG, Joshi RA, Blumenthal HT. Atheromatous embolization; an etiology of acute pancreatitis. *Arch Surg.* 1957;75:566–71; discussion 71–72.
186. Moolenaar W LC. Gastrointestinal blood loss due to cholesterol crystal embolization. *J Clin Gastroenterol.* 1995 21:220–223.
187. Moolenaar W, Lamers CB. Cholesterol crystal embolisation to the alimentary tract. *Gut* 1996;38:196–200.
188. Moolenaar W, Lamers CB. Cholesterol crystal embolization to liver, gallbladder, and pancreas. *Digest Dis Sci.* 1996;41:1819–1822.
189. Hollenhorst RW. Significance of bright plaques in the retinal arterioles. *Trans Am Ophthalmol Soc.* 1961;59:252–273.
190. Hollenhorst RW. Significance of bright plaques in the retinal arterioles. *JAMA.* 1961;178:23–29.
191. Sabatine MS, Oelberg DA, Mark EJ, et al. Pulmonary cholesterol crystal embolization. *Chest.* 1997;112:1687–1692.
192. Vacher-Coponat H, Pache X, Dussol B, et al. Pulmonary-renal syndrome responding to corticosteroids: consider cholesterol embolization. *Nephrol Dial Transplant.* 1997;12:1977–1979.
193. Stanton R. Case records of the Massachusetts General Hospital. *N Engl J Med.* 1996;334:973–979.
194. Wilson DM, Salazer TL, Farkouh ME. Eosinophiluria in atheroembolic renal disease. *Am J Med.* 1991;91:186–189.
195. Kasinath BS, Corwin HL, Bidani AK, et al. Eosinophilia in the diagnosis of atheroembolic renal disease. *Am J Nephrol.* 1987;7:173–177.
196. Levine J, Rennke HG, Idelson BA. Profound persistent eosinophilia in a patient with spontaneous renal atheroembolic disease. *Am J Nephrol.* 1992;12:377–379.
197. McGowan JA, Greenberg A. Cholesterol atheroembolic renal disease. Report of 3 cases with emphasis on diagnosis by skin biopsy and extended survival. *Am J Nephrol.* 1986;6:135–139.
198. Knechtges TC, Defever BA. Cholesterol emboli in transurethral curettings: report of 4 cases. *J Urol.* 1975;114:102–106.
199. Bruns FJ, Segel DP, Adler S. Control of cholesterol embolization by discontinuation of anticoagulant therapy. *Am J Med Sci.* 1978;275:105–108.
200. Drost H, Buis B, Haan D, et al. Cholesterol embolism as a complication of left heart catheterisation. Report of seven cases. *Br Heart J.* 1984;52:339–342.
201. Vidt DG, Harris S, McTaggart F, et al. Effect of short-term rosuvastatin treatment on estimated glomerular filtration rate. *Am J Cardiol.* 2006;97: 1602–1606.
202. Smyth JS, Scoble JE. Atheroembolism. *Curr Treat Options Cardiovasc Med.* 2002;4:255–265.
203. Vidt DG, Eisele G, Gephardt GN, et al. Atheroembolic renal disease: association with renal arterial stenosis. *Cleve Clin J Med.* 1989;56:407–413.
204. Keen RR, McCarthy WJ, Shireman PK, et al. Surgical management of atheroembolization. *J Vasc Surg.* 1995;21:773–780; discussion 80–81.
205. Baumann DS, McGraw D, Rubin BG, et al. An institutional experience with arterial atheroembolism. *Ann Vasc Surg.* 1994;8:258–265.
206. Keele KD. John Hunter's contribution to cardio-vascular pathology. *Ann R Coll Surg Engl.* 1966;39:248–259.

207. Rayer P. *Traite des Maladies des Reins et des Alterations de la Secretion urinaire.* Paris: JB Bailliere; 1840.
208. Abeshouse BS. Thrombosis and thrombophlebitis of the renal veins. *Urol Cutaneous Rev.* 1945;49:661–675.
209. Llach F, Yudd, M. Renal artery thrombosis, thromboembolism, aneurysms, atheroemboli and renal vein thrombosis. In: Schrier RW, ed. *Diseases of the Kidney & Urinary Tract.* 8th ed. Philadelphia: Wolters Kluwer/Lippincott Williams & Wilkins; 2007:1787–1810.
210. Harrison CV, Milne MD, Steiner RE. Clinical aspects of renal vein thrombosis. *Q J Med.* 1956;25:285–298.
211. Llach F, Arieff AI, Massry SG. Renal vein thrombosis and nephrotic syndrome. A prospective study of 36 adult patients. *Ann Intern Med.* 1975;83:8–14.
212. Llach F, Koffler A, Finck E, et al. On the incidence of renal vein thrombosis in the nephrotic syndrome. *Arch Intern Med.* 1977;137:333–336.
213. Bellomo R, Atkins RC. Membranous nephropathy and thromboembolism: is prophylactic anticoagulation warranted? *Nephron.* 1993;63:249–254.
214. McCarthy LJ, Titus JL, Daugherty GW. Bilateral renal-vein thrombosis and the nephrotic syndrome in adults. *Ann Intern Med.* 1963;58:837–857.
215. Llach F. Hypercoagulability, renal vein thrombosis, and other thrombotic complications of nephrotic syndrome. *Kidney Int.* 1985;28:429–439.
216. Velasquez Forero F, Garcia Prugue N, Ruiz Morales N. Idiopathic nephrotic syndrome of the adult with asymptomatic thrombosis of the renal vein. *Am J Nephrol.* 1988;8:457–462.
217. Lionaki S, Derebail VK, Hogan SL, et al. Venous thromboembolism in patients with membranous nephropathy. *Clin J Am Soc Nephrol.* 2012;7:43–51.
218. Mahmoodi BK, ten Kate MK, Waanders F, et al. High absolute risks and predictors of venous and arterial thromboembolic events in patients with nephrotic syndrome: results from a large retrospective cohort study. *Circulation.* 2008;117:224–230.
219. Fisher ER, Sharkey D, Pardo V, et al. Experimental renal vein constriction. Its relation to renal lesions observed in human renal vein thrombosis and the nephrotic syndrome. *Lab Invest.* 1968;18:689–699.
220. Deodhar KP, Bhalerao RA, Kelkar MD, et al. Inferior vena cava obstruction. Study of 26 cases. *J Postgrad Med.* 1969;15:64–68.
221. Jackson BT, Thomas ML. Post-thrombotic inferior vena caval obstruction. A review of 24 patients. *BMJ.* 1970;1:18–22.
222. Thoenes W, Anders D, Gekle D. Glomerulonephritis - Nephrotisches Syndrom - Nierenvenenthrombose. *J Mol Med.* 1971;49:1323–1329.
223. Llach F, Papper S, Massry SG. The clinical spectrum of renal vein thrombosis: acute and chronic. *Am J Med.* 1980;69:819–827.
224. Hruby MA, Honig GR, Shapira E. Immunoquantitation of Hageman factor in urine and plasma of children with nephrotic syndrome. *J Lab Clin Med.* 1980;96:501–510.
225. Green D, Arruda J, Honig G, et al. Urinary loss of clotting factors due to hereditary membranous glomerulopathy. *Am J Clin Pathol.*1976;65:376–383.
226. Berger J, Yaneva H. Hageman factor deposition in membranous glomerulopathy. *Transplant Proc.* 1982;14:472–473.
227. Handley DA, Lawrence JR. Factor-IX deficiency in the nephrotic syndrome. *Lancet.* 1967;1:1079–1081.
228. Honig GR, Lindley A. Deficiency of Hageman factor (factor XII) in patients with the nephrotic syndrome. *Pediatrics.* 1971;78:633–637.
229. Lange LG III, Carvalho A, Bagdasarian A, et ak. Activation of Hageman factor in the nephrotic syndrome. *Am J Med.* 1974;56:565–569.
230. Natelson EA, Lynch EC, Hettig RA, et al. Acquired factor IX deficiency in the nephrotic syndrome. *Ann Intern Med.* 1970;73:373–378.
231. Saito H, Goodnough LT, Makker SP, et al. Urinary excretion of Hageman factor (factor XII) and the presence of nonfunctional Hageman factor in the nephrotic syndrome. *Am J Med.* 1981;70:531–534.
232. van Royen EA, de Boer JE, Wilmink JM, et al. Acquired factor XII deficiency in a patient with nephrotic syndrome. *Acta Med Scand.* 1979;205:535–539.
233. Kanfer A, Kleinknecht D, Broyer M, et al. Coagulation studies in 45 cases of nephrotic syndrome without uremia. *Thrombosis Diath Haemorrh.* 1970; 24:562–571.
234. Kendall AG, Lohmann RC, Dossetor JB. Nephrotic syndrome. A hypercoagulable state. *Arch Intern Med.* 1971;127:1021–1027.
235. Thomson C, Forbes CD, Prentice CR, et al. Changes in blood coagulation and fibrinolysis in the nephrotic syndrome. *Q J Med.* 1974;43:399–407.
236. Earley LE, Havel RJ, Hopper J Jr, et al. Nephrotic syndrome. *California medicine* 1971;115:23–41.
237. Takeda Y, Chen AY. Fibrinogen metabolism and distribution in patients with the nephrotic syndrome. *J Lab Clin Med.* 1967;70:678–685.
238. Clarkson AR, MacDonald MK, Petrie JJ, et al. Serum and urinary fibrin-fibrinogen degradation products in glomerulonephritis. *BMJ.* 1971;3:447–451.
239. Cade R, Spooner G, Juncos L, et al. Chronic renal vein thrombosis. *Am J Med.* 1977;63:387–397.
240. Hall CL, Pejhan N, Terry JM, et al. Urinary fibrin-fibrinogen degradation products in nephrotic syndrome. *BMJ.* 1975;1:419–422.
241. Wu KK, Hoak JC. Urinary plasminogen and chronic glomerulonephritis. *Am J Clin Pathol.*1973;60:915–919.
242. Edward N, Young DP, Macleod M. Fibrinolytic activity in plasma and urine in chronic renal disease. *J Clin Pathol.* 1964;17:365–368.
243. Hedner U, Nilsson IM. Antithrombin-3 in a clinical material. *Bibl Anat.* 1973;12:267–271.
244. Scheinman JI, Stiehm ER. Fibrinolytic studies in the nephrotic syndrome. *Pediatr Res.* 1971;5:206–212.
245. Lau SO, Tkachuck JY, Hasegawa DK, et al. Plasminogen and antithrombin III deficiencies in the childhood nephrotic syndrome associated with plasminogenuria and antithrombinuria. *Pediatrics.* 1980;96:390–392.
246. Du XH, Glas-Greenwalt P, Kant KS, et al. Nephrotic syndrome with renal vein thrombosis: pathogenetic importance of a plasmin inhibitor (alpha 2-antiplasmin). *Clin Nephrol.* 1985;24:186–191.
247. Kauffmann RH, de Graeff J, de la Riviere GB, et al. Unilateral renal vein thrombosis and nephrotic syndrome. Report of a case with protein selectivity and antithrombin III clearance studies. *Am J Med.* 1976;60:1048–1054.
248. Kauffmann RH, Veltkamp JJ, Van Tilburg NH, et al. Acquired antithrombin III deficiency and thrombosis in the nephrotic syndrome. *Am J Med.* 1978;65:607–613.
249. Thaler E, Balzar E, Kopsa H, et al. Acquired antithrombin III deficiency in patients with glomerular proteinuria. *Haemostasis.* 1978;7:257–272.
250. Ellis D. Recurrent renal vein thrombosis and renal failure associated with antithrombin-III deficiency. *Pediatr Nephrol.* 1992;6:131–134.
251. Jorgensen KA, Stoffersen E. Antithrombin III and the nephrotic syndrome. *Scand J Haematol.* 1979;22:442–448.
252. Panicucci F, Sagripanti A, Vispi M, et al. Comprehensive study of haemostasis in nephrotic syndrome. *Nephron.* 1983;33:9–13.
253. Vaziri ND, Paule P, Toohey J, et al. Acquired deficiency and urinary excretion of antithrombin III in nephrotic syndrome. *Arch Intern Med.* 1984;144:1802–1803.
254. Yermiahu T, Shalev H, Landau D, et al. Protein C and protein S in pediatric nephrotic patients. *Sangre (Barc).* 1996;41:155–157.
255. Hanevold CD, Lazarchick J, Constantin MA, et al. Acquired free protein S deficiency in children with steroid resistant nephrosis. *Ann Clin Lab Sci.* 1996;26:279–282.
256. Vigano-D'Angelo S, D'Angelo A, Kaufman CE Jr, et al. Protein S deficiency occurs in the nephrotic syndrome. *Ann Intern Med.* 1987;107:42–47.
257. Sorensen PJ, Knudsen F, Nielsen AH, et al. Protein C activity in renal disease. *Thromb Res.* 1985;38:243–249.
258. Cosio FG, Harker C, Batard MA, et al. Plasma concentrations of the natural anticoagulants protein C and protein S in patients with proteinuria. *J Lab Clin Med.* 1985;106:218–222.
259. Bang NU, Trygstad W, Schroeder JE, et al. Enhanced platelet function in glomerular renal disease. *J Lab Clin Med.* 1973;81:651–660.
260. Remuzzi G, Mecca G, Marchesi D, et al. Platelet hyperaggregability and the nephrotic syndrome. *Thromb Res.* 1979;16:345–354.
261. Adler AJ, Lundin AP, Feinroth MV, et al. Beta-thromboglobulin levels in the nephrotic syndrome. *Am J Med.* 1980;69:551–554.
262. Andrassy K, Ritz E, Bommer J. Hypercoagulability in the nephrotic syndrome. *Klinische Wochenschrift.* 1980;58:1029–1036.
263. Kuhlmann U, Steurer J, Rhyner K, et al. Platelet aggregation and beta-thromboglobulin levels in nephrotic patients with and without thrombosis. *Clin Nephrol.* 1981;15:229–235.
264. Cheng H. [Mechanism of renal vein thrombosis in patients with nephrotic syndrome: a prospective study]. *Zhonghua Yi Xue Za Zhi.* 1992;72:416–419, 447.
265. Ooi BS, Ooi YM, Pollak VE. Identification of circulating immune complexes in a subpopulation of patients with membranous glomerulonephropathy. *Clin Immunol Immunopathol.* 1980;16:447–453.
266. Lohmann RC, Kendall AG, Dossetor JB, et al. The fibrinolytic system in the nephrotic syndrome. *Clin Res.* 1969;17:333.
267. Makino Mea. A fulminant case of renal vain thrombosis in a patient with autoimmnune disorder and membranous nephropathy. *Intern Med.* 2008;47: 969–973.
268. Harms K, Speer CP. [Thrombosis: an underestimated complication of central catheters? Subclavian vein, vena cava and renal vein thrombosis after silastic catheters]. *Monatsschrift Kinderheilkunde: Organ der Deutschen Gesellschaft fur Kinderheilkunde.* 1993;141:21–25.
269. Mukherjee AP, Toh BH, Chan GL, et al. Vasculas complications in nephrotic syndrome: relationship to steroid therapy and accelerated thromboplastin generation. *BMJ.* 1970;4:273–276.
270. Luetscher JA Jr, Deming QB. Treatment of nephrosis with cortisone. *J Clin Invest.* 1950;29:1576–1587.

271. Cosgriff SW, Diefenbach AF, Vogt W Jr. Hypercoagulability of the blood associated with ACTH and cortisone therapy. *Am J Med.* 1950;9:752–756.
272. Ajmera A, Joshi A, Kamat B, et al. Idiopathic acute renal vein thrombosis in a young healthy woman with no hypercoagulable state taking oral contraceptives. *Am J Med Sci.* 2010;339:380–382.
273. Slick GL, Schnetzler DE, Kaloyanides GJ. Hypertension, renal vein thrombosis and renal failure (occurring in a patient on an oral contraceptive agent). *Clin Nephrol.* 1975;3:70–74.
274. Douketis JD, Ginsberg JS, Holbrook A, et al. A reevaluation of the risk for venous thromboembolism with the use of oral contraceptives and hormone replacement therapy. *Arch Intern Med.* 1997;157:1522–1530.
275. Arneil GC, MacDonald AM, Sweet EM. Renal venous thrombosis. *Clin Nephrol.* 1973;1:119–131.
276. Gomez E, Aguado S, Gago E, et al. Main graft vessels thromboses due to conventional-dose OKT3 in renal transplantation. *Lancet.* 1992;339:1612–1613.
277. Hollenbeck M, Westhoff A, Bach D, et al. Doppler sonography and renal graft vessel thromboses after OKT3 treatment. *Lancet.* 1992;340:619–620.
278. Richardson AJ, Higgins RM, Jaskowski AJ, et al. Spontaneous rupture of renal allografts: the importance of renal vein thrombosis in the cyclosporin era. *Br J Surg.* 1990;77:558–560.
279. Brown Z, Neild GH, Willoughby JJ, et al. Increased factor VIII as an index of vascular injury in cyclosporine nephrotoxicity. *Transplantation.* 1986;42:150–153.
280. Brown Z, Neild GH. Cyclosporine inhibits prostacyclin production by cultured human endothelial cells. *Transplant Proc.* 1987;19:1178–1180.
281. Bakir N, Sluiter WJ, Ploeg RJ, et al. Primary renal graft thrombosis. *Nephrol Dial Transplant.* 1996;11:140–147.
282. Chang CT, Wu MS. Successful treatment of idiopathic membranous glomerulonephritis complicated with renal vein thrombosis with FK506. *Ren Fail.* 2002;24:523–528.
283. Langer RM, Kahan BD. Sirolimus does not increase the risk for postoperative thromboembolic events among renal transplant recipients. *Transplantation.* 2003;76:318–323.
284. Koehler PR, Bowles WT, McAlister WH. Renal arteriography in experimental renal vein occlusion. *Radiology.* 1966;86:851–855.
285. Kowal J, Figur A, Hitzig WM. Renal vein thrombosis and the nephrotic syndrome with complete remission. *J Mt Sinai Hosp NY.* 1963;30:47–58.
286. Scanlon GT. The radiographic changes in renal vein thrombosis. *Radiology.* 1963;80:208–211.
287. Gatewood OM, Fishman EK, Burrow CR, et al. Renal vein thrombosis in patients with nephrotic syndrome: CT diagnosis. *Radiology.* 1986;159:117–122.
288. Asghar M, Ahmed K, Shah SS, et al. Renal vein thrombosis. Eur *J Vasc Endovasc Surg.* 2007;34:217–223.
289. Wysokinski WE, Gosk-Bierska I, Greene EL, et al. Clinical characteristics and long-term follow-up of patients with renal vein thrombosis. *Am J Kidney Dis.* 2008;51:224–232.
290. Rosenmann E, Pollak VE, Pirani CL. Renal vein thrombosis in the adult: a clinical and pathologic study based on renal biopsies. *Medicine.* 1968;47:269–335.
291. Liposclerose retroperitoneal. Thrombose des veines renales. Deux syndromes retroperitoneaux. In: Richet G, Meyrier A, ed. Saint Germain: Masson & Cie; 1970.
292. Laville M, Aguilera D, Maillet PJ, et al. The prognosis of renal vein thrombosis: a re-evaluation of 27 cases. *Nephrol Dial Transplant.* 1988;3:247–256.
293. Briefel GR, Manis T, Gordon DH, et al. Recurrent renal vein thrombosis consequent to membranous glomerulonephritis. *Clin Nephrol.* 1978;10:32–37.
294. Yang SH, Lee CH, Ko SF, et al. The successful treatment of renal-vein thrombosis by low-molecular-weight heparin in a steroid-sensitive nephrotic patient. *Nephrol Dial Transplant.* 2002;17:2017–2019.
295. Wu CH, Ko SF, Lee CH, et al. Successful outpatient treatment of renal vein thrombosis by low-molecular weight heparins in 3 patients with nephrotic syndrome. *Clin Nephrol.* 2006;65:433–440.
296. Lai S, Barbano B, Cianci R, et al. [The risk of bleeding associated with low molecular weight heparin in patients with renal failure]. *G Ital Nefrol.* 2010;27:649–654.
297. Combe S, Buller HR. [New treatments for venous thromboembolic disease]. *Journal des maladies vasculaires.* 2011;36 Suppl 1:S16–19.
298. Vogelzang RL, Moel DI, Cohn RA, et al. Acute renal vein thrombosis: successful treatment with intraarterial urokinase. *Radiology.* 1988;169:681–682.
299. Kennedy JS, Gerety BM, Silverman R, et al. Simultaneous renal arterial and venous thrombosis associated with idiopathic nephrotic syndrome: treatment with intra-arterial urokinase. *Am J Med.* 1991;90:124–127.
300. Chiu AS, Landsberg DN. Successful treatment of acute transplant renal vein thrombosis with selective streptokinase infusion. *Transplant Proc.* 1991;23:2297–2300.
301. Schwieger J, Reiss R, Cohen JL, et al. Acute renal allograft dysfunction in the setting of deep venous thrombosis: a case of successful urokinase thrombolysis and a review of the literature. *Am J Kidney Dis.* 1993;22:345–350.

CHAPTER 57

Chronic Tubulointerstitial Nephritis

Allison A. Eddy • Ikuyo Yamaguchi

Chronic tubulointerstitial nephritis (TIN) encompasses a vast array of chronic kidney diseases that share a primary pathologic process that begins at the level of the tubules and their surrounding interstitial space. In addition, it is now recognized that chronic tubulointerstitial disease is the final common pathway that causes progressive renal functional loss in all chronic kidney disease (CKD), whether it begins in the tubulointerstitium or in other renal compartments. Due to the importance and unique clinicopathologic features of many diseases that cause chronic TIN, many are discussed in greater detail in other chapters. The present chapter provides a general overview and discussion of this entire group of disorders, with an effort to highlight shared and unique features of each. For the purpose of presentation, chronic TIN is divided into subcategories (Table 57.1). One of the most common causes of chronic TIN in developed countries is chronic renal allograft rejection, which is discussed in Chapter 81.

NORMAL TUBULOINTERSTITIAL ARCHITECTURE

Renal tubules constitute the largest component of the renal parenchyma, estimated at 80% to 90%, which explains why disrupted tubular integrity and function plays such an important role in renal functional decline. Most of the tubules in the renal cortex are proximal tubules. The peritubular region is occupied by the vasculature and the interstitial space. The glomerular efferent arterioles branch to form the peritubular capillary network, which serves the vital role of delivering oxygen to support tubular cell metabolic and transport functions. The extravascular peritubular compartment, known as the interstitium, is typically inconspicuous, especially in the renal cortex. However, stromal cells and extracellular matrix proteins residing in the interstitium play a key role during renal development and in polarizing the renal response to injury toward regeneration or chronic sequelae. Residing within the interstitium are two important cell populations. The most abundant are fibroblasts, well recognized for their role of synthesizing extracellular matrix proteins. These proteins (primarily fibronectin; fibrillar; collagens I, III, and VI; and proteoglycans) provide a structural framework for nephrons and the vascular network. The functional heterogeneity of interstitial fibroblasts is increasingly recognized, even within normal kidneys.[1] A subset is specialized to synthesize erythropoietin (Fig. 57.1),[2] whereas others are pericytes closely opposed to peritubular capillaries.[3] Present within the medulla is a unique population of lipid-laden interstitial cells which are thought to be a source of prostaglandins involved in blood pressure control.[4] The second interstitial cell population consists of myeloid cells that are derived from bone marrow cells and are slowly and continuously replenished. This group of cells also has functional heterogeneity. The majority appear to be MCH class II positive dendritic cells, whereas others are scavenger-type macrophages. In normal kidneys the myeloid cells are thought to serve surveillance functions to protect the kidney from noxious materials and foreign invaders. They become actively engaged in renal responses to injury. Interstitial myeloid cells rarely proliferate in situ; the interstitial inflammatory response that characterizes many acute and chronic kidney diseases is dependent upon the recruitment of lymphohematopoietic cells from the circulation.

Ongoing studies are attempting to answer the question of whether a pluripotent stem cell also resides within the renal interstitium.[5] It has been suggested that the renal medulla is a niche for kidney stem cells. These slowing dividing cells can be identified as "label-retaining cells" using detectable thymidine markers. There are conflicting data about the ability of these cells to proliferate and migrate to the site of injury and participate in renal regeneration.[6,7] It has also been proposed that specialized progenitor cells may reside within tubules, but this remains unproven.

HISTOPATHOLOGIC FEATURES OF CHRONIC TIN

The histologic hallmark of chronic TIN is an increase in the fractional volume of the interstitial space caused by an expansion of extracellular matrix proteins—the defining feature

TABLE 57.1 **Chronic Tubulointerstitial Nephritis Classification**

PRIMARY TUBULOINTERSTITIAL KIDNEY DISEASES		
Genetic diseases	Familial TIN (MCKD2)	Uromodulin mutations Renin mutations Unknown mutations
	Nephronophthisis (NPHP)	Isolated kidney disease Associated with extrarenal manifestations
	Polycystic kidney diseases (PKD)	Autosomal dominant Autosomal recessive Syndromic Others
	Metabolic disorders	Cystinosis Oxalosis Mitochondrial cytopathies Methylmalonic acidemia
Immunologic diseases	TIN most common kidney manifestation	Sjögren syndrome IgG4-related disease Sarcoidosis TINU Renal allograft rejection Anti-TBM nephritis
	TIN usually associated with glomerulonephritis	Systemic lupus erythematosus ANCA+ vasculitis Anti-GBM nephritis Cryoglobulinemia Membranoproliferative glomerulonephritis IgA nephropathy Others
Chronic nephrotoxicity	Drugs	Calcineurin inhibitors Analgesic nephropathy Lithium
	Herbs	Aristolochic acid Others
	Heavy metals	Lead Cadmium
Chronic metabolic disorders	Hypercalcemia/hypercalciuria Hyperphosphatemia/hyperphosphaturia Hyperuricemia/hyperuricosuria Hypokalemia	
Congenital abnormalities	Dysplasia Obstruction	
CHRONIC KIDNEY DISEASE-ASSOCIATED TIN		
Proteinuria-associated TIN		
Chronic kidney disease universal progression pathway		

(continued)

TABLE 57.1 Chronic Tubulointerstitial Nephritis Classification *(continued)*

SEQUELAE TO ACUTE TUBULOINTERSTITIAL INJURY		
Acute kidney injury	Ischemia-reperfusion injury	
Acute interstitial nephritis/ nephrotoxicity	Infections	Bacterial (systemic, pyelonephritis, xanthogranulomatous pyelonephritis)
		Mycobacteria
		Viral
		Fungal
		Parasitic
	Drugs	Proton pump inhibitors
		Chemotherapeutic drugs
		Antimicrobial drugs
		NSAIDs
	Hematologic disorders	Leukemia
		Lymphoma
		Multiple myeloma
		Sickle cell disease

MCKD2, medullary cystic kidney disease type 2, familial juvenile hyperuricemic nephropathy; TINU, tubulointerstitial nephritis with uveitis; anti-TBM, anti-tubular basement membrane; anti-GBM, anti-glomerular basement membrane; NSAIDs, nonsteroidal anti-inflammatory drugs.

of interstitial fibrosis or scarring. This abnormal matrix is comprised of both a greater abundance of normal interstitial matrix proteins and the de novo appearance of additional matrix proteins. Interstitial fibrosis is accompanied by irreversible tubular damage, ranging from abnormally dilated (ectatic) tubules to atrophic tubules surrounded by abnormally thickened and wrinkled tubular membranes to complete tubular drop-out (often leaving behind the signature "atubular" glomeruli). In parallel, peritubular capillaries are also lost. In some diseases such as chronic allograft rejection, an abnormal process of interstitial lymphangiogenesis has been described, but its specificity and functional significance remain unclear.

The other important histopathologic feature that typifies chronic TIN is a significant change in interstitial cellularity. Unlike normal kidneys, the interstitial space becomes populated by transformed fibroblasts that are recognized by their expression of α-smooth muscle actin (α-SMA), a protein typically associated with smooth muscle cells. Known as "myofibroblasts," these cells are considered the primary source of extracellular matrix proteins that generate the fibrotic or scarred interstitium. The second important

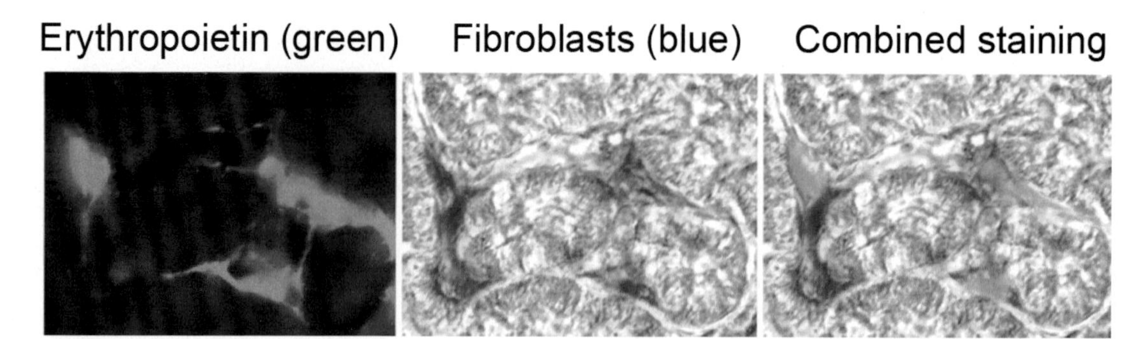

FIGURE 57.1 Peritubular fibroblasts produce erythropoietin. Using a mouse line that was genetically engineered to express green fluorescent protein-labeled erythropoietin, and kidney *Cre*-labeled fibroblasts that are detectable by beta galactosidase staining (blue), peritubular fibroblasts are identified as the source of erythropoietin. Loss of this function explains why anemia may be more severe in patients with chronic kidney disease due to chronic tubulointerstitial nephritis. (From Asada N, Takase M, Nakamura J, et al. Dysfunction of fibroblasts of extrarenal origin underlies renal fibrosis and renal anemia in mice. *J Clin Invest.* 2011;121:3981, with permission.) (See Color Plate.)

TABLE 57.2 Histopathologic Features of Acute and Chronic Tubulointerstitial Nephritis

Features	Acute	Chronic
Tubules		
Epithelium	Necrosis	Atrophy
Basement membrane	Disrupted	Thickened
Shape	Preserved	Dilated
Interstitium[a]		
Cell infiltrates	Lymphocytes (CD4$^+$ T cell dominant) Eosinophils in early stage	Monocytes and macrophages Lymphocytes
Myofibroblasts	Minimum	Increased
Edema	+++	+
Fibrosis	+	+++ (Collagen and other matrix protein deposits)
Vasculature		
Peritubular capillaries	Preserved	Reduced density De novo lymphatic vessels
Large vessels	Minimum	Varies[b]
Glomeruli	None to minimal change	Periglomerular fibrosis Focal or global glomerulosclerosis

[a]The severity of the changes is given as an estimate with + for minimal to +++ as severe.
[b]Pathologic changes may suggest a primary process such as atherosclerosis, scleroderma, thromboembolic disease, vasculitis, or chronic allograft rejection.

change in interstitial cellularity is the appearance of an infiltrate of mononuclear cells. These cells are primarily of bone marrow origin.

A frequent challenge of a new histopathologic diagnosis of chronic TIN is the lack of clarity of the initiating disease process. For some disease entities, specific diagnoses are made using other criteria: imaging for cystic kidney disease and anatomic genitourinary anomalies, the presence of extrarenal manifestations (autoimmune diseases, metabolic disorders, hematologic diseases, and congenital hepatic fibrosis), a positive family history, or history of exposure to a drug or toxin that is known to cause chronic TIN. In the absence of these diagnostic clues, it may not be possible to determine the primary etiology, as the renal histologic findings of many chronic TINs overlap. When more specific diagnostic criteria are available, they are discussed under the specific disease entities that are reviewed later.

Another potential diagnostic dilemma is the difficulty of differentiating acute and reversible TIN from chronic progressive TIN. Early diagnosis is important for certain disease etiologies, such as an exposure to nephrotoxins or development of treatable autoimmune diseases, for which a delayed diagnosis may be too late for injury reversal. Many of the tubulointerstitial disorders have a variable clinical course that spans the spectrum from acute to chronic and reversible to progressive. The tissue repair process itself may lead to pathologic fibrosis. Frequent regional variations in the TIN process mean that the degree of acute and chronic TIN may vary considerably from one tissue sample to another. The primary histologic findings that are used in an effort to differentiate acute from chronic TIN are summarized in Table 57.2.

CLINICAL MANIFESTATIONS AND LABORATORY ABNORMALITIES

Clinical manifestations of chronic TIN tend to be subtle. Patients with TIN may present with symptoms related to their primary diseases. They often also have nonspecific constitutional symptoms of chronic kidney disease such as fatigue, loss of appetite, nausea, vomiting, and sleep disturbance. In general, tubular dysfunction develops proportionally as glomerular filtration rate (GFR) declines. However, primary TIN diseases may present more prominent tubular dysfunction in the early stage compared to glomerular or vascular diseases. Proximal tubule dysfunction is characterized by inability to reabsorb filtered bicarbonate, glucose, amino acids, and phosphate in varying combinations, resulting in acidosis, glucosuria, phosphaturia, and aminoaciduria, as in

Fanconi syndrome. Low molecular weight proteins such as β_2-microglobulin may not be properly reabsorbed, leading to tubular proteinuria. Distal tubular dysfunction manifests as renal sodium wasting, hyperkalemia, and nonanion gap metabolic acidosis. Collecting duct dysfunction leads to renal concentrating defects including features of diabetes insipidus and countercurrent exchange washout resulting in polyuria. Most TIN affects multiple sites of the nephron simultaneously, but to varying degrees. Hypertension, severe proteinuria, and edema are not usually characteristic of TIN in the early stage, but may develop later as progressing chronic kidney disease (CKD) with glomerular sclerosis. In addition to tubular dysfunction, anemia may be found disproportionally compared to the change in GFR if erythropoietin-producing peritubular cells (Fig. 57.1) are damaged early in the disease. Bone disease may also be prominent, as a result of chronic phosphate wasting caused by proximal tubular dysfunction.

INTERSTITIAL FIBROSIS: THE FINAL COMMON PATHWAY TO CHRONIC KIDNEY DISEASE

In both native and transplanted kidneys, progressive fibrosis of the renal interstitium is the predominant final common pathway of renal destruction, regardless of the etiology of the original kidney disease.[8] Fibrotic injury is not limited to extracellular matrix accumulation, but also results in the subsequent loss of tubules and peritubular capillaries. Histopathologically, interstitial volume and reduced tubular epithelial cell density closely correlate with the loss of renal function and predict long-term outcomes (Fig. 57.2). The pathogenic process leading to fibrosis can be initiated by a variety of insults, including chronic tubular, glomerular, and vascular disease. Chemokines and chemoattractants such as monocyte chemoattractant protein 1 (MCP-1), complement

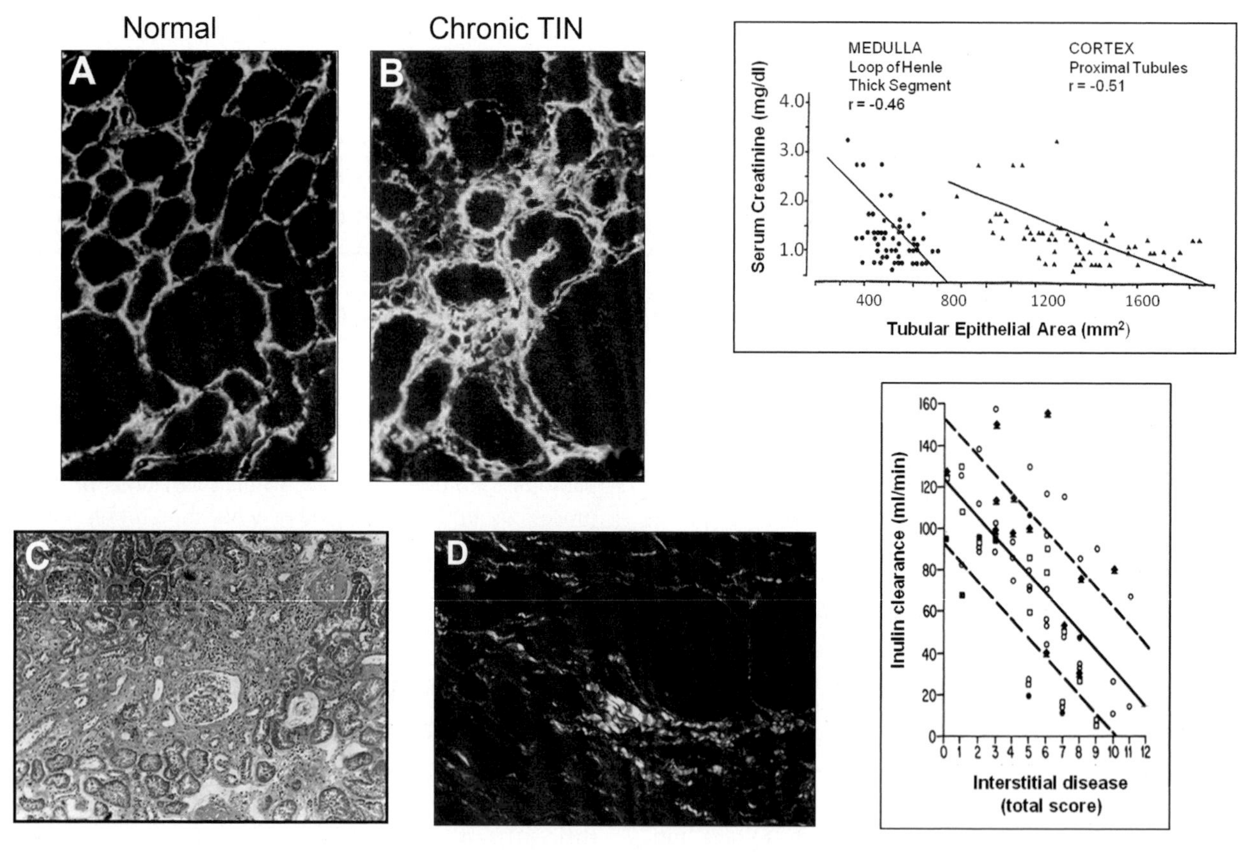

FIGURE 57.2 Interstitial fibrosis: detection and correlation with renal functional loss. The fibrotic or scarred interstitium contains several extracellular matrix proteins, the most abundant being fibrillar collagens such as collagen III **(A,B)**. Routine renal biopsy staining with Masson trichrome reacts with collagen to produce a green-blue color **(C)**. Quantitative pathologic research studies often use picrosirius red staining, which is specific for cross-linked collagen fibrils (polarized image shown in **D**). The key structural change that underlies the loss of renal function in all chronic kidney diseases is tubular atrophy (upper graph) which is closely associated with interstitial fibrosis severity (lower graph). (A and B are from Jones CL, Buch S, Post M, et al. Pathogenesis of interstitial fibrosis in chronic purine aminonucleoside nephrosis. *Kidney Int.* 1991;40:1020. Upper graph is from Mackensen-Haen S, Bohle A, Christensen J, et al. The consequences for renal function of the interstitium and changes in the tubular epithelium of the cortex and medulla in various diseases. *Clin Nephrol.* 1992;37;70. Lower graph is from Schainuck LI, Striker GE, Cutler RE, et al. Structural-functional correlations in renal diseases: Part II: the correlations. *Human Pathol.* 1970;1:631. All are reproduced with permission.) (See Color Plate.)

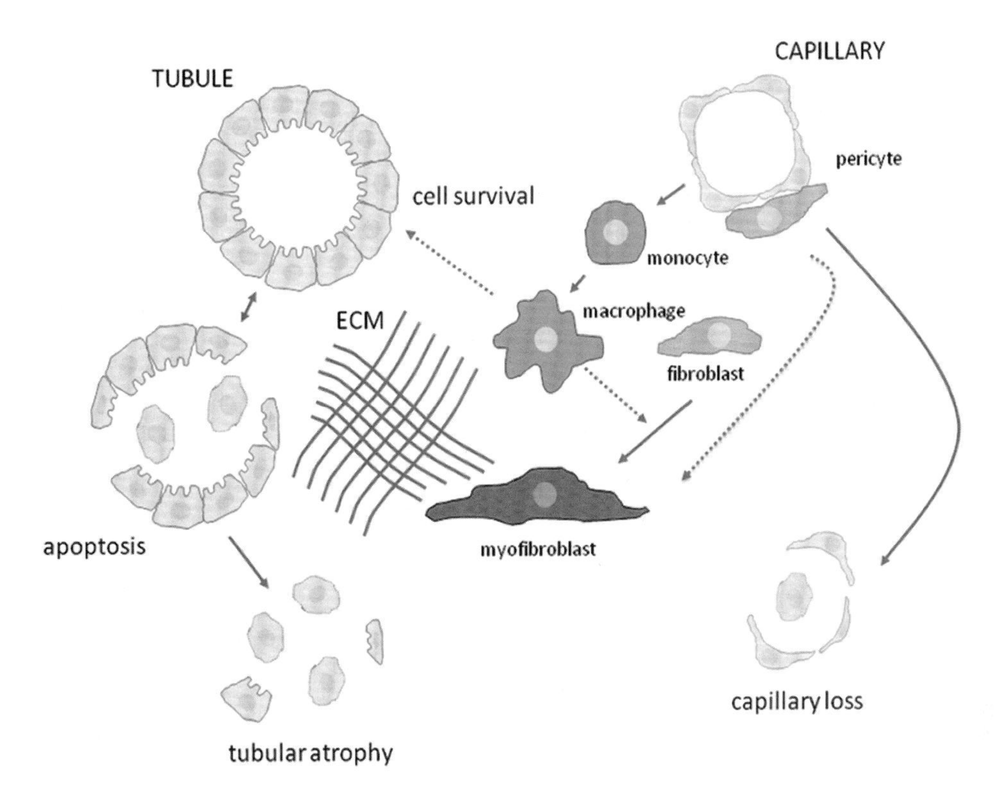

FIGURE 57.3 Schematic summary of the key cellular events contributing to the pathogenesis of chronic tubulointerstitial nephritis. Inflammatory macrophages are primarily recruited from the circulating pool of peripheral blood monocytes, under the direction of chemotactic signals derived from endothelial cells and damaged tubules and facilitated by increased capillary permeability. Functionally distinct macrophage subpopulations either propagate injury or promote tissue repair (including fibrosis) by releasing a variety of cytokines, growth factors, and other soluble products. A population of myofibroblasts appears de novo in the interstitium where they synthesize the majority of the extracellular matrix (ECM) proteins responsible for interstitial scarring. The primary origin of the myofibroblasts is still controversial; resident interstitial fibroblasts and capillary pericytes are considered most likely during active fibrogenesis. Through a variety of mechanisms, including hypoxia and oxidant stress, interstitial capillaries disappear and tubular epithelia undergo apoptotic death in parallel with progressive fibrosis.

component C3, and osteopontin (OPN) activate capillary endothelial cells, leading to increased capillary permeability, recruitment of leukocytes into the interstitium, and activation of myofibroblast precursors. Inflammatory macrophages secrete diverse proinflammatory and profibrotic products that perpetuate injury and promote scarring. This process unleashes a cascade of inflammatory and fibrogenic signals within the interstitium. Some key molecules including fibrinogen, complement components C3a and C5a, tissue plasminogen activator (tPA), and oxidized albumin may arrive by leakage from the plasma, whereas others, such as the major fibrogenic factor transforming growth factor β (TGF-β), connective tissue growth factor (CTGF), platelet-derived growth factor (PDGF), tumor necrosis factor α (TNF-α), endothelin-1, angiotensin-II, placental growth factor, and angiopoietin-2, appear to be produced locally. Together, these factors activate fibroblasts, and promote their transformation into α-SMA positive myofibroblasts. The activated myofibroblasts produce collagen I, collagen III, fibronectin, and other matrix proteins, which accumulate in the interstitial space. The fibrotic process culminates in death of tubular cells and peritubular capillaries, leading to ablation of the entire nephron (Fig. 57.3).[9–12]

Key Mechanisms

Tubular Epithelial Cells

The renal tubules account for approximately 80% of the total kidney volume. Tubular epithelial cells may be injured by immunologic, mechanical, chemical, genetic, or ischemic insults, which stimulate synthesis of inflammatory cytokines, cause functional perturbations, and/or lead to necrotic or apoptotic cell death. In acute kidney injury (AKI), tubular epithelial cells proliferate and replace damaged cells, restoring the architecture of the tubules. However, in CKD, complete tubular regeneration fails due to incomplete repair and persistent inflammation, leading to endoplasmic reticulum (ER) stress, loss of cytoskeletal integrity and polarity, and tubular barrier dysfunction, ultimately resulting in irreversible atrophic changes. The failure of tubular restoration is a critical turning point for CKD. Tubular atrophy may leave behind intact, atubular glomeruli, which are nonfunctional nephrons.[13]

Injured tubular epithelial cells often play a direct role in renal inflammation by secreting proinflammatory cytokines and growth factors including TNF-α, MCP-1, TGF-β, and RANTES. The production of growth factors may be cell cycle stage–specific, as it has been shown that acute kidney injury induced by ischemia/reperfusion leads to cell cycle arrest in the G2/M phase, followed by the release of growth factors such as TGFβ-1 and CTGF. These factors activate c-Jun N-terminal kinase (JNK) signaling, which promotes fibrosis.[14]

The fate of tubular epithelial cells is a critical determinant of nephron regeneration, and several mechanisms can direct each cell toward death by necrosis or apoptosis, or toward survival and proliferation. Tubular cell apoptosis is a common feature of CKD, and is known to be triggered by TGF-β1, TNF-α, Fas, p53, caspases, ceramide, and reactive oxygen species. Apoptosis can also be stimulated by the downregulation of survival factors such as epidermal growth factor (EGF) and vascular endothelial growth factor (VEGF). An important step in cell survival following injury is the removal of damaged proteins and organelles by cell-mediated autophagy. In this process, an autophagosome is formed from the ER membrane, engulfs intracellular deposits, and delivers the contents to lysosomes for degradation. There is evidence of enhanced autophagy in obstructed tubules and AKI, which is thought to promote recovery; failure of autophagy may lead to apoptosis and prevent recovery of tubular epithelial cells.[15,16]

When the tubular damage is controlled, the tubules can regenerate. The origin of the new tubular epithelial cells has been a topic of debate. The current prevailing view is that proliferation of surviving tubular cells is sufficient to account for the recovery, without compelling evidence that renal and/or extrarenal progenitor cells are incorporated. However, soluble factors released by bone marrow–derived cells are thought to facilitate the repair process.[7,17,18]

Inflammatory Cells

Infiltration of the interstitium by inflammatory cells is an integral component of the fibrogenic response (Fig. 57.4). One of the most important inflammatory cell types is the macrophage, which primarily originates from circulating monocytes. Resident dendritic cells have limited proliferative capacity. Macrophages are functionally heterogeneous and have the potential to secrete a vast repertoire of soluble mediators, including proinflammatory and profibrotic cytokines. Inflammatory monocytes undergo differentiation in response to cytokines and typically become polarized into one of two distinct phenotypes.[19–21] This polarization process has been extensively investigated in mice, where classically activated "M1" macrophages are generated by exposure to interferon-γ and lipopolysaccharide. The M1 cells produce proinflammatory cytokines that propagate tissue injury. Alternatively activated "M2" macrophages are generated by exposure to interleukin-4 (IL-4) and IL-13. The M2 cells synthesize anti-inflammatory cytokines that promote tissue repair; however, this repair response may also lead to fibrosis. These differential functions have mainly been characterized using in vitro studies. In vivo, macrophage phenotypes are more diverse, and macrophages appear to switch phenotypes in response to different stimuli and microenvironments.[19,21,22] The role of the lymphocytes (which are typically present and may even outnumber interstitial macrophages) and the resident dendritic cells in renal fibrosis is still not clear.[23] It has been hypothesized that chronic

Macrophages

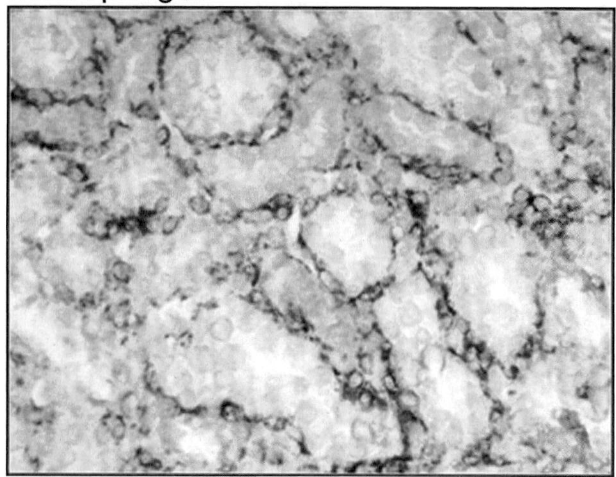

Myofibroblasts

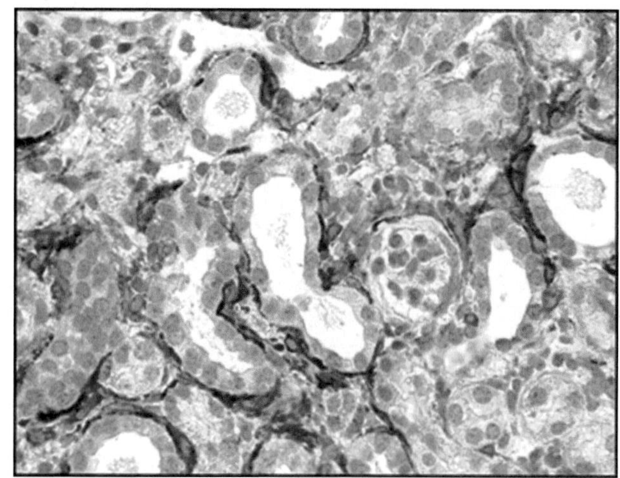

FIGURE 57.4 Interstitial cell mediators of chronic tubulointerstitial nephritis (TIN). Interstitial hypercellularity is a feature of chronic TIN, characterized by the presence of two distinct cell populations: lymphohematopoietic cells, with macrophages in particular (shown by CD68 staining in the upper photomicrograph) known to play an important pathogenic role, and myofibroblasts (shown by alpha smooth muscle actin staining in the lower photomicrograph). Limited human biopsy data show a significant relationship between interstitial myofibroblast density and renal prognosis. (The upper image is from Yamaguchi I, Tchao BN, Burger NL, et al. Vascular endothelial cadherin modulates renal interstitial fibrosis. *Nephron Exp Nephrol.* 2011;120:e20, with permission.)

renal injury may expose neoantigens that trigger a secondary antigen-driven immune response to propagate injury, but this hypothesis has been difficult to test using experimental models. Candidate neoantigens have not been identified, and thus this paradigm remains hypothetical.

Myofibroblasts

Interstitial myofibroblasts serve a pivotal role in renal fibrosis by synthesizing extracellular matrix (ECM) proteins such as collagen I, collagen III, and fibronectin that accumulate within the renal interstitium. Myofibroblasts contain contractile stress fibers and express α-SMA (Fig. 57.4). Myofibroblasts are essential for wound healing and tissue remodeling. During wound healing, they are activated, migrate within the damaged tissue, proliferate, and secrete ECM in response to inflammatory factors such as TGF-β1. Once healing is complete, myofibroblasts disappear by apoptosis. However, in chronic fibrosis myofibroblasts persist and lead to pathologic tissue remodeling, ultimately impairing organ function.[24]

The origin of renal interstitial myofibroblasts is a topic of great interest and some controversy. Myofibroblasts are functionally heterogeneous, depending to some extent on their local environment and perhaps on their origin. Most myofibroblasts appear to be derived from intrarenal cells, which may include resident interstitial fibroblasts, pericytes, or perivascular cells within the adventitia of arterioles and arteries.[3,25] Myofibroblasts might also be derived from epithelial-mesenchymal transition (EMT)[26] and endothelial-mesenchymal transition (EndMT),[27] although both of these events appear to be delayed until the advanced phase of renal fibrosis when basement membranes are destroyed. Other origins could include bone marrow-derived circulating fibroblasts or fibrocytes. Recent cell lineage tracing studies in genetically engineered mice support the view that myofibroblasts are rarely derived from tubular epithelial cells or fibrocytes; rather, they represent transformed interstitial fibroblasts, perivascular progenitor cells, and pericytes.[3] TGF-β and CTGF produced by injured tubular cells and inflammatory interstitial cells not only stimulate fibroblast proliferation and transformation to myofibroblasts, but also induce fibroblast epigenetic changes that influence cell survival. For example, TGFβ-induced hypermethylation of RASAL1, an inhibitor of the Ras oncoprotein, results in prolonged fibroblast activation and kidney fibrosis.[28]

Multiple growth factors such as TGF-β1, PDGF, fibroblast growth factor 2, and CTGF are known to stimulate fibroblast activation and extracellular matrix production, whereas hepatocyte growth factor and bone morphogenetic protein 7 are antifibrogenic. Numerous studies have investigated the downstream signaling cascades leading to fibrogenesis, which are too numerous to describe here.[8,11,12,29,30] Epigenetic mechanisms of regulation such as inhibition of DNA methylation and control of mRNA stability and translation by microRNA are also thought to play important roles in renal fibrosis.[28]

The processes of myofibroblast activation and apoptosis are of considerable interest as potential targets for antifibrotic therapy. TGF-β inhibition would appear to be an ideal strategy, but the complex effects of this multifunctional growth factor have presented challenges. Recent studies have focused on its downstream intracellular signals such as SMAD3, which activates microRNA-21, stimulating matrix production and fibrosis.[31] The renoprotective effects of renin-angiotensin system (RAS) blockade are thought to be mediated at least in part by TGF-β inhibition. Other cell-targeted strategies currently under investigation are aimed at inhibiting the formation of scar-forming myofibroblasts by profibrotic cytokines, promoting myofibroblast apoptosis, and/or inhibiting myofibroblast function (e.g., cell contraction or interactions via specific integrins).[32,33]

Capillary Changes, Hypoxia, and Oxidant Stress

The renal interstitium is perfused by an intricate network of peritubular capillaries that serve the vital role of oxygen delivery to metabolically active tubular epithelial cells. Peritubular capillary endothelial cells (ECs) undergo apoptosis during CKD, leading to capillary loss, and propagation of tissue hypoxia and oxidant stress. Based on several studies in animal models and human chronic kidney diseases, it is known that peritubular capillaries disappear in association with progressive interstitial fibrosis and tubular atrophy (Fig. 57.5).[34–37] Although the sequence of events connecting capillary loss to fibrosis and impaired tubular function is poorly characterized, it has been suggested that interstitial hypoxia caused by arteriolar vasoconstriction and/or peritubular capillary regression is a primary event in CKD.[38]

Under normal conditions, ECs are quiescent and turn over slowly. Vessel stability depends on cell–cell and cell–matrix interactions, normal levels of growth and angiogenic factors, and shear stress from blood flow. However, during kidney injury shear stress is altered, interactions between ECs change, cell–matrix interactions are disrupted, and growth and angiogenic factors are produced, including TGF-β, angiopoietin 2, and in some models VEGF.[39] As a consequence, ECs enter an activated state characterized by hyperpermeability, expression of leukocyte adhesion molecules, release of cytokines and growth factors, and enhanced cell migration and proliferation. EC activation is crucial for host defense and repair but may lead to dysfunctional changes including reduced production of nitric oxide (NO), a chronic proinflammatory state, and apoptotic EC cell death leading to capillary rarefaction.[40,41] Chronic hypoxia is a significant component of the pathogenetic process in interstitial fibrosis, in part because oxygen demand is actually increased above the high basal level during inflammation and tubular epithelial cell regeneration. The distortion and loss of peritubular capillaries establishes a vicious cascade, with worsening hypoxia propagating inflammation and fibrosis, with further nephron loss and renal functional decline.

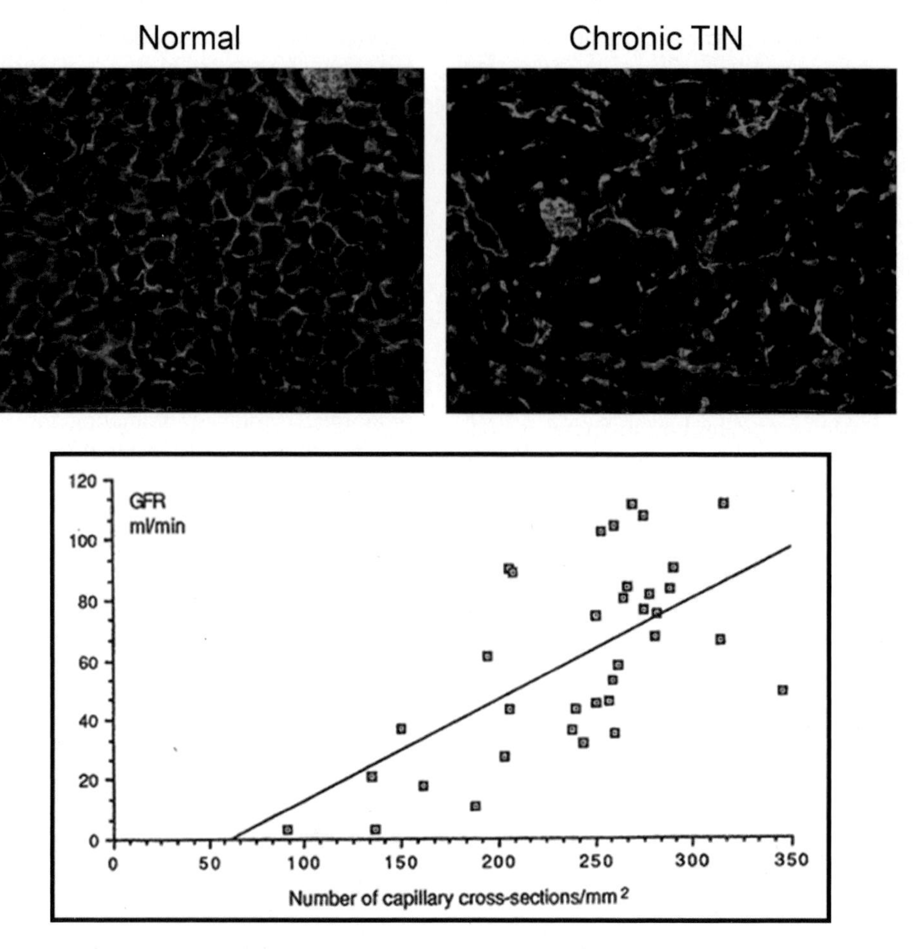

FIGURE 57.5 Interstitial capillary rarefaction is a feature of chronic tubulointerstitial nephritis (TIN). Using CD31 as an endothelial cell marker, the decrease in interstitial capillary cell density in chronic TIN is illustrated by the photomicrographs. In a study of human kidney biopsies, the extent of capillary loss was shown to correlate with the decline in glomerular filtration rate. (The photomicrographs are from Yamaguchi I, Tchao BN, Burger NL, et al. Vascular endothelial cadherin modulates renal interstitial fibrosis. *Nephron Exp Nephrol.* 2011;120:e20 and the graph is from Serón D, Alexopoulos E, Raftery MJ, et al. Number of interstitial capillary cross-sections assessed by monoclonal antibodies: relation to interstitial damage. *Nephrol Dial Transplant.* 1990;5:889, both with copyright permission.)

Matrix Accumulation

During fibrosis, the interstitial space is expanded by the accumulation of native and novel extracellular matrix (ECM) proteins. Expansion of the interstitial matrix appears to be the consequence of both increased matrix protein synthesis by myofibroblasts and decreased degradation by intracellular and extracellular connective tissue proteases. The expanded interstitium may include a gelatinous matrix of glycosaminoglycans (heparan sulfate, dermatan sulfate, chondroitin sulfate) and hyaluronic acid, an early scaffold rich in fibronectin, a fibrillar network of collagens (mainly types I, III and VI), and the presence of a variety of other extracellular matrix proteins (basement membrane collagens IV and V, collagens VII and XV, tenascin), laminin, proteoglycans (aggrecan, versican, decorin, fibromodulin, biglycan, perlecan), and various glycoproteins (thrombospondin, tenascin, hensin, vitronectin, secreted protein acidic and rich in cysteine [SPARC]). In addition to their structural effects, many of these matrix proteins elicit important effects on neighboring cells and molecules. For example, SPARC may inhibit cellular adhesion and proliferation, and also stimulates TGF-β expression and collagen I and fibronectin synthesis. Thrombospondin also activates TGF-β expression.

An unresolved question is the identity of the matrix-degrading proteases that maintain the status quo in normal kidneys despite ongoing collagen synthesis; it is also unclear why these mechanisms are perturbed during fibrogenesis.[42] For example, in normal mouse kidneys, approximately 20% of the kidney collagen is newly synthesized over a 2-week period yet total kidney collagen content does not increase, indicating that a similar rate of collagen degradation is going on at the same time.[43] The metalloproteinases (MMPs) are known to be important for extracellular matrix degradation and were long considered lead candidates for renal matrix homeostasis. MMP-2 and MMP-9 are abundant in the kidney and degrade collagen IV. However, paradoxically, MMP-2 and MMP-9 do not attenuate but accelerate interstitial fibrosis in experimental models. The serine proteases urokinase-type plasminogen activator (uPA), tPA, and plasmin have been investigated as alternative candidates, but tPA and plasmin were found to promote fibrosis and uPA had no effect, despite the fact that the inhibitor PAI-1 is a potent fibrosis-promoting molecule. The latter effect may best be explained by PAI's ability to enhance macrophage and myofibroblast recruitment in the interstitium. The urokinase receptor (uPAR) attenuates myofibroblast recruitment and fibrosis, and acts in conjunction with its coreceptor LDL receptor-related protein (LRP) to regulate fibroblast proliferation and extracellular signal-regulated kinase (ERK) signaling.[44] Recent studies have focused on the role of an uPAR coreceptor, uPAR-associated protein (uPARAP), also known as the mannose receptor 2 (Mrc2) and Endo180. This receptor is expressed by interstitial macrophages and myofibroblasts and serves as a collagen endocytic receptor that delivers interstitial collagens to lysosomes for degradation by cathepsins.[43] Renal fibrosis is significantly worse in mice with genetic Mrc2 deficiency.

PRIMARY DISEASES ASSOCIATED WITH CHRONIC TIN

Genetic Renal Diseases

Familial Juvenile Hyperuricemic Nephropathy/ Medullary Cystic Disease Type 2

Medullary cystic disease type 2 (MCKD2) is a rare form of autosomal-dominant chronic TIN that is now known to be caused by a mutation on chromosome 16p12 involving the gene that encodes uromodulin (UMOD) (also known as Tamm-Horsfall protein).[45–47] Approximately 60 distinct mutations have been identified. UMOD expression is restricted to the thick ascending limb of the loop of Henle and the early distal convoluted tubule. UMOD is the most abundant normal urinary protein, with levels reported in the range of 50 mg per day. Although its function is still under active investigation, UMOD is known to form a water-impermeable barrier on the surface of these cells. It may also regulate cell membrane function, based on recent evidence that it associates with cilia, lipid rafts, and sodium transporters such as ROMK2.[48] It is also thought to inhibit stone formation. The *UMOD* mutation results in the production of a misfolded, aberrantly trafficking protein that is trapped in the endoplasmic reticulum (ER), leading to reduced urinary levels (hence the description of MCKD2 as a "UMOD storage disease") (Fig. 57.6). Such accumulation is thought to cause ER stress, which leads to renal tubular cell death. Most patients first seek medical attention with gout symptoms between 15 and 40 years of age, caused by hyperuricemia (present in ~70% of the patients) due to a reduced fractional excretion of uric acid—these patients are found to also have CKD.[47] Some patients have mild urinary concentrating deficits, which may contribute to the genesis of hyperuricemia. The renal biopsy shows nonspecific changes of tubular atrophy, interstitial fibrosis, and mild interstitial inflammation but no unique diagnostic features. Small cysts are detected by renal ultrasound in one third of the patients. Treatment with allopurinol may slow the progression of kidney disease, and RAS blockade may decrease production of the abnormal UMOD protein. Although most patients develop end-stage renal disease (ESRD), the rate of progression is highly variable, with ESRD developing between 30 and 60 years of age.

Familial juvenile hyperuricemic nephropathy type 2 has been reported as a distinct genetic entity (autosomal dominant) caused by a mutation in the *REN* gene encoding renin.[46,49] The mutations impair translocation of the nascent preprorenin protein into the ER, resulting in reduced or abolished renin biosynthesis and secretion. It has been suggested the mutant preprorenin may be toxic to juxtaglomerular

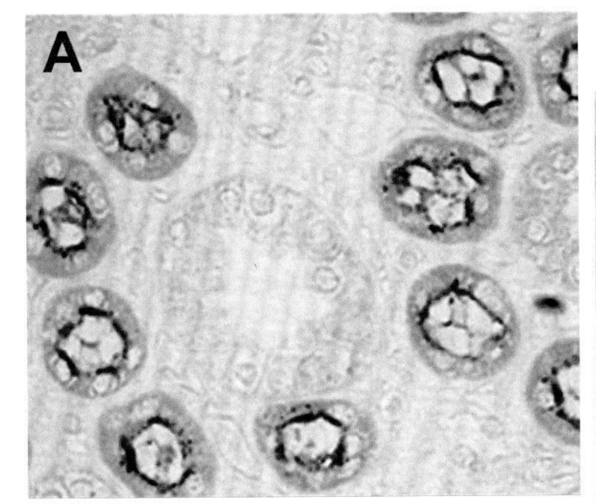

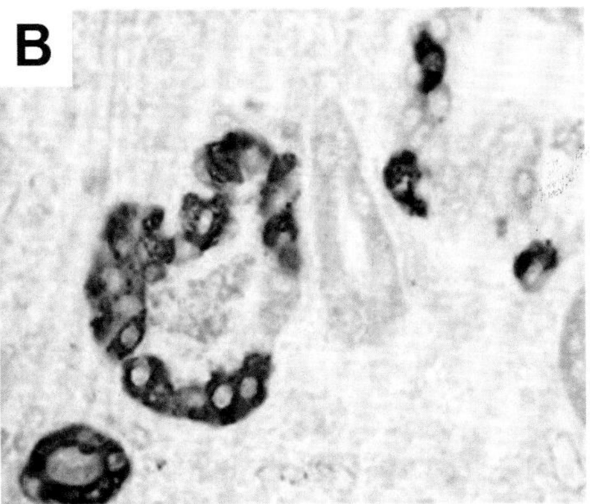

FIGURE 57.6 Familial chronic tubulointerstitial nephritis associated with mutations in the uromodulin (*UMOD*) gene, which encodes a protein normally expressed on the apical membrane of the thick ascending limb of the loop of Henle (shown on left). These mutations result in an abnormal UMOD protein that is trapped within the endoplasmic reticulum (right photograph). (From Dahan K, Devuyst O, Smaers M, et al. A cluster of mutations in the UMOD gene causes familial juvenile hyperuricemic nephropathy with abnormal expression of uromodulin. *J Am Soc Nephrol.* 2003;14:2883, with permission.)

cells, causing additional damage to the RAS and leading to nephron dropout and progressive renal failure. Patients typically present with early-onset anemia due to low erythropoietin production, mild hyperkalemia, and low-normal blood pressure. A history of gout in some affected family members should raise the suspicion of this disorder. Plasma renin, aldosterone, and erythropoietin levels are low; fractional urate excretion is reduced; and kidney biopsies show chronic TIN, although none of these findings alone confirms the diagnosis. Mutational analysis of the *REN* gene is required. Treatment is supportive. CKD typically develops in the third or fourth decade and progresses slowly.

Nephronophthisis: Associated Ciliopathies

Nephronophthisis (NPHP) is a group of autosomal-recessive disorders that share chronic progressive TIN and genetic mutations in genes encoding proteins that localize to primary tubular cell cilia (reviewed in greater detail in Chapter 15).[50–52] Clinically the patients have been subdivided into four groups based on the presence or absence of extrarenal manifestations and the causative genetic mutation. All patients with renal involvement share a form of chronic tubulointerstitial disease that typically progresses to ESRD before adulthood (median age 13 years). It is estimated that NPHP may account for 5% to 10% of pediatric patients with ESRD. The name nephronophthisis means "disintegration of nephrons" and epitomizes the histologic findings, which include nonspecific tubular atrophy with tubular basement membrane thickening and/or disruption, interstitial inflammation, and fibrosis. Small corticomedullary cysts may be present, especially with more advanced disease. These cysts and small echogenic kidneys may be detected by renal ultrasonography. Clinically, most patients have polyuria, polydipsia, and anemia but are otherwise asymptomatic until manifestations of renal failure develop in the second decade of life. The causative gene has been identified in ~30% of cases, the most common (20%) being a homozygous deletion in nephrocystin 1 (*NPHP1*), which encodes a protein involved in ciliary function in collecting duct cells. An estimated 10% to 15% of the NPHP patients have extrarenal involvement. The most common is retinitis pigmentosa (Senior-Loken syndrome). Others include cerebellar ataxia (Joubert syndrome) and oculomotor apraxia (Cogan syndrome), as well as several rarer genetic syndromes. Treatment of the kidney disease is symptomatic. The kidney disease does not recur after kidney transplantation.

Polycystic Kidney Diseases

Genetic disorders associated with polycystic kidney disease (PKD) are reviewed in Chapter 16. They are mentioned here to emphasize the importance of interstitial inflammation and fibrosis to disease progression. The progression of CKD is not simply a matter of total cyst volume expanding to mechanically compress adjacent renal parenchyma; the disease is also associated with damage to otherwise normal noncystic nephrons as a consequence of chronic TIN. The degree of renal fibrosis in patients with PKD is closely associated with the rate of progression to ESRD, just as it is in all CKD.[53] Studies by Grantham et al.[54]in the 1990s first suggested a potential pathogenetic link between renal cysts and interstitial inflammation and fibrosis. Many macrophage innate immune response genes are upregulated in cystic mouse kidneys.[55] Polycystin-1-deficient tubular cells have been shown to stimulate macrophage migration and to secrete monocyte chemoattractant protein-1 and the chemokine CXCL16.[56] Inflammatory cytokines are also present in cystic fluid. This inflammatory cell response has been implicated in both cystogenesis and interstitial fibrosis. Anti-inflammatory therapy such as corticosteroids or depletion of monocytes significantly attenuates interstitial inflammation and the rate of renal functional decline in animal cystic kidney disease models (Fig. 57.7).[56,57] Taken together, these data suggest that epithelial cell changes precede and drive the interstitial inflammatory response in patients with PKD.[58] Possible protective tubulointerstitial effects should be taken into consideration as potential beneficial mechanisms when evaluating new drug therapies such as mammalian target of rapamycin inhibitors and vasopressin receptor antagonist.

Genetic Metabolic Disorders

Several severe metabolic disorders that present during infancy and childhood are known to cause CKD via disease processes that primarily involve the tubulointerstitial compartment.

Cystinosis. Cystinosis is an autosomal recessive disorder caused by a mutation in the lysosomal membrane protein cystinosin (CTNS).[59] The estimated incidence is 1 in 100,000 to 200,000 live births. Affected children are normal at birth but develop clinical complications due to renal Fanconi syndrome, which typically brings them to medical attention before 2 years of age with failure to thrive and a history of excessive thirst, polyuria, recurrent vomiting, constipation, and episodes of dehydration. The children may already have evidence of rickets due to renal phosphate wasting. Although this is a systemic disorder, the kidney is the first organ affected and CKD progresses rapidly over the first decade if untreated. In addition to this classical presentation in infancy (nephropathic infantile form), a less aggressive renal disease has been reported but is much less common, accounting for <5% of cases (nephropathic juvenile form). Cystine is a dimeric amino acid formed by the oxidation of two cysteine residues, which become linked by a disulfide bond. Cysteine is a product of normal protein turnover, and the cystine dimer is normally recycled via the lysosomal cystinosin transporter (Fig. 57.8). In its absence, abnormal levels of cystine accumulate within lysosomes, often forming cystine crystals and leading to significant cellular damage. It is thought that the renal proximal tubules are an early target of injury due to their high rate of urinary protein uptake and processing. By 1 year of age, pathognomonic ocular corneal crystals can be detected by slit lamp examination. The

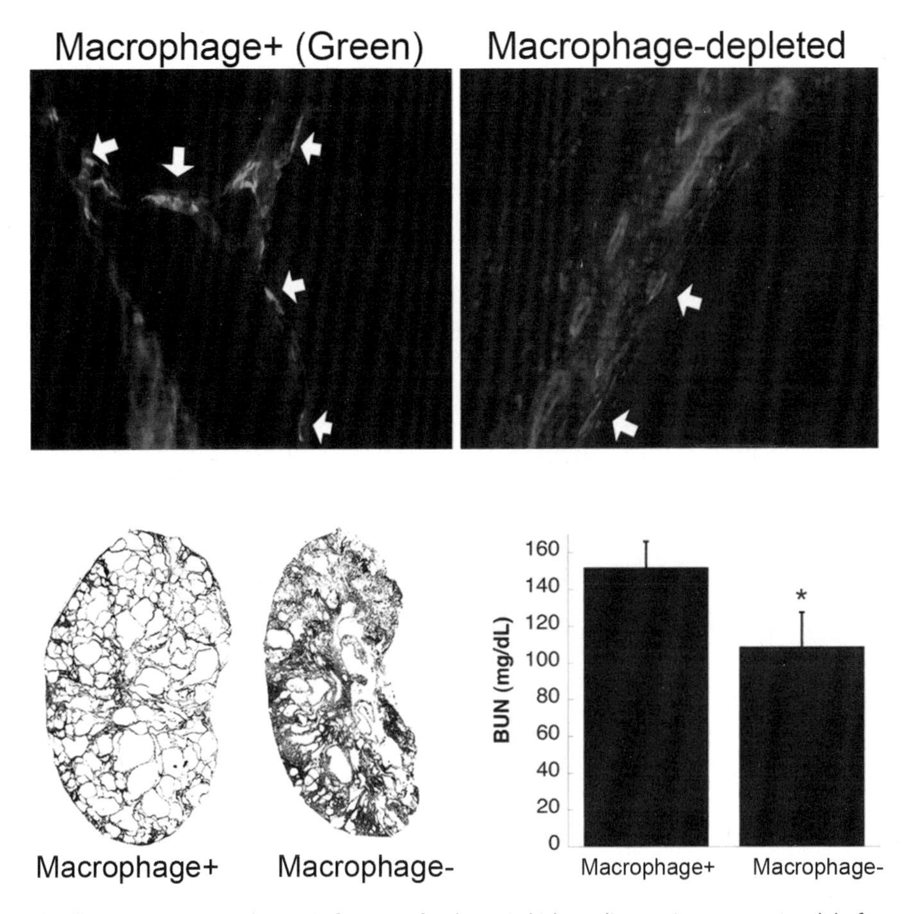

FIGURE 57.7 Interstitial inflammation is a pathogenic feature of polycystic kidney disease. In a mouse model of autosomal dominant polycystic kidney disease, macrophages (green) are seen lining cystic spaces (*upper left*). When macrophages were experimentally depleted (*upper right*), renal parenchyma was better preserved (*lower left*), and kidney function estimated by blood urea nitrogen levels was significantly better in the macrophage depleted (−) mice, shown in the lower right graph. (From Karihaloo A, Koraishy F, Huen SC, et al. Macrophages promote cyst growth in polycystic kidney disease. *J Am Soc Nephrol.* 2011;22:1809, with permission.) (See Color Plate.)

diagnosis is typically confirmed by the presence of elevated cystine levels in peripheral blood leukocytes, measured in a reference laboratory. Since the cystinosis gene (*CTNS*) was cloned in 1998, over 90 mutations have been reported in the United States and northern Europe—approximately 40% have a homozygous 57 kb deletion.

Human renal pathologic studies and recent studies in a mouse model indicate universal changes in renal tubules. The classical findings of a "swan neck deformity" occur as a consequence of proximal tubular cell atrophy, emphasizing the early and severe involvement of this nephron segment in cystine-associated injury. Progressive CKD is characterized by chronic TIN together with nonspecific chronic glomerular changes. The primary pathogenesis of target organ injury is thought to be due to lysosomal cystine accumulation, which perturbs several cellular functions, leading to altered energy metabolism, oxidant stress, and tubular cell death by apoptosis. However, many aspects of the kidney injury are not completely understood, such as the failure of the early and severe tubular transport defects to improve with cysteamine therapy.[60] In the cystinosin knockout mice, a mild renal phenotype despite high kidney cystine levels and the benefit of bone marrow transplantation suggest that mechanisms beyond renal tubular toxicity are involved.[61]

Medical therapy includes a combination of water, mineral, and electrolyte replacement therapy; nutritional support; and specific therapy with the amino thiol drug cysteamine. Cysteamine lowers lysosomal cystine levels via a disulfide exchange reaction with cystine, generating a cysteine-cysteamine product that can exit via an alternative transport system (Fig. 57.8). If therapy is started at a young age and leukocyte cysteine levels are maintained in the target range, kidney survival can be significantly prolonged; however, most patients still develop ESRD by the second or third decade of life.[62] The disease does not recur in a renal allograft. Most children require a gastrostomy tube in order to maintain fluid and electrolyte balance and to achieve normal growth. A minority of the patients may also require growth hormone therapy. Extrarenal manifestations are universal and may include skin and hair hypopigmentation, hypothyroidism (70% within the first decade), and eye involvement

Cystinosis

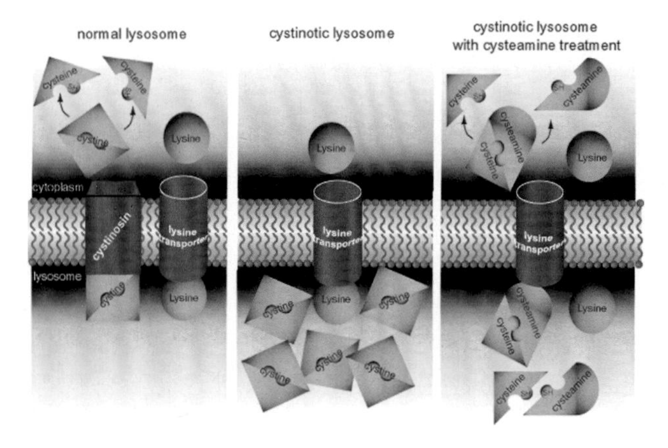

Oxalosis

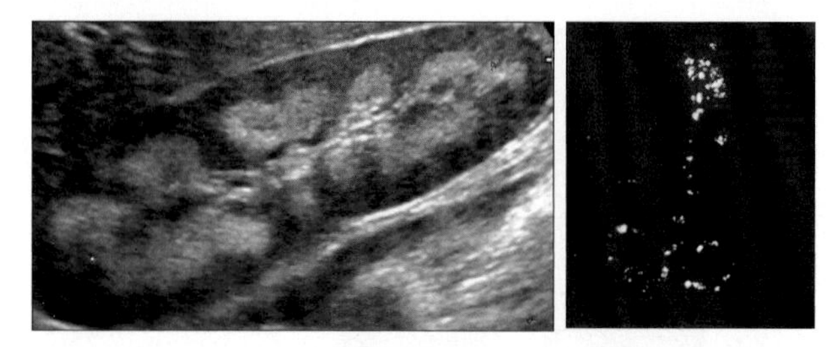

FIGURE 57.8 Inherited metabolic diseases cause chronic tubulointerstitial nephritis. The upper drawing illustrates the abnormal function of the lysosomal membrane in patients with autosomal recessive cystinosis due to a mutation in the *CTNS* gene that encodes the cystine transporter cystinosin. In the absence of cystinosin, cystine accumulates in lysosomes and contributes to some of the associated tissue pathologies. An elevated peripheral blood leukocyte cystine level is diagnostic. The drug cysteamine provides an alternative pathway for cystine exit from lysosomes by forming a cysteine-cysteamine dimer that is transported by an alternative (system c) lysosomal transporter. Though not yet definitively identified, it has been suggested that system c is the lysine transporter. (From Wilmer MJ, Schoeber JP, van den Heuvel P, et al. Cystinosis: practical tools for diagnosis and treatment. *Pediatr Nephrol.* 2011;26:205, with permission.) Primary infantile oxalosis is associated with aggressive chronic tubulointerstitial nephritis due to the deposition of calcium oxalate in renal tubules and the interstitium, which may be detected as nephrocalcinosis on the renal ultrasound (*lower left*) or the actual deposits can be visualized by polarized light microscopic examination of kidney tissue (*lower right*). (See Color Plate.)

with photophobia that requires treatment with topical cysteamine. Neuromuscular involvement and pancreatic insufficiency often develop in the older patients.

Methylmalonic Acidemia. Methylmalonic acidemia (MMA) is an autosomal recessive inborn error of organic acid metabolism.[63,64] Methylmalonic acid, which is normally generated via the metabolism of isoleucine, methionine, threonine, valine, and certain odd-chain fatty acids, accumulates in MMA patients due to a deficiency in its degrading enzyme methylmalonyl-CoA mutase (primarily expressed in the liver). Deficiency of the enzymatic cofactor cobalamin (vitamin B12) can also lead to MMA. The incidence of MMA may be as high as 1:48,000 based on newborn screening data. Although the timing of the clinical diagnosis ranges from the neonatal period to adulthood, the most common form of the disease begins in infancy with clinical manifestations caused by metabolic decompensation: lethargy, vomiting, dehydration, hypotonia, encephalopathy, ketoacidosis, and hyperammonemia. Rarely, infants may present with a hemolytic uremic syndrome. A definitive diagnosis requires measurement of plasma or urine organic acids. Genetic testing is currently available for some of the mutations. In addition to a variety of neurologic complications, many of the patients develop CKD due to TIN.[65] The pathogenesis is unclear but is presumed to result from tubular cell injury due to altered energy metabolism and MMA toxicity.[64] Treatment of the primary metabolic disorder involves dietary control of protein catabolism with a low protein/high carbohydrate diet and cobalamin therapy for patients whose disease is shown to be vitamin B12 responsive. Patients frequently require hospitalization to manage metabolic complications during periods of decompensation. Several patients have undergone successful kidney transplantation, but the primary genetic defect persists due to uncorrected systemic enzyme deficiency. Liver transplantation and combined kidney–liver transplantation have been performed but remain controversial, as liver transplantation only partially corrects the enzyme deficiency due to MMA production by skeletal muscle.[66]

Primary Hyperoxaluria. Hyperoxaluria can be inherited or acquired. The primary diseases are rare autosomal recessive inborn errors of metabolism that are characterized by very high urinary oxalate levels and the development of nephrocalcinosis (Fig. 57.8) and/or recurrent kidney stones leading to progressive renal parenchymal damage.[67] Histopathologically, the kidneys are characterized by the presence of calcium oxalate crystals in tubular lumina, tubular epithelial cells, and interstitial cells (Fig. 57.8), together with interstitial inflammation and fibrosis. Symptoms due to recurrent stone formation typically begin in childhood—approximately 50% progress to ESRD by adulthood. Approximately one quarter of the patients with primary hyperoxaluria present with a severe, life-threatening infantile disease with rapid progression to renal failure. Mutations have been identified in three separate genes encoding enzymes in the pathway that regulates oxalate metabolism. The most common deficit (~80%) is due to a deficiency of the hepatic enzyme pyridoxal phosphate-dependent enzyme alanine glyoxylate aminotransferase (AGT). The second type is caused by a deficiency of glyoxylate reductase/hydroxypyruvate reductase (GRHPR), and the third has been linked to an as yet uncharacterized gene, *DHDPSL*. The diagnosis of primary hyperoxaluria is suggested by significantly elevated urinary oxalate levels; elevated urinary glycolate suggests an *AGT* mutation, whereas elevated urinary L-glyceric acid suggests a *GRHPR* mutation. A definitive diagnosis requires either molecular genetic studies or documented low enzyme activity in a liver biopsy specimen.

Because the large oxalate burden is primarily excreted by the kidney, treatment is based on strategies to decrease production (~30% of the patients respond to the AGT cofactor pyridoxine) and to decrease urinary oxalate concentration (fluids), together with inhibitors of calcium oxalate crystallization (pyrophosphate, citrate, magnesium). As renal function declines, plasma oxalate levels rise and lead to extrarenal deposits in many tissues—especially bones, heart, vessels, joints, retina, thyroid, and soft tissue. Patients with *AGT* mutations are most likely to develop ESRD and are now being treated with combined liver–kidney transplants, although variations in this approach are still considered. After transplantation the heavy burden of extrarenal calcium oxalate (especially in bones) is slowly released, leading to persistent hyperoxaluria for a significant period of time posttransplantation.

Mitochondrial Cytopathies. The primary mitochondrial cytopathies are a heterogeneous group of rare genetic disorders caused by mutations in maternally inherited mitochondrial DNA (mtDNA) or nuclear-encoded mitochondrial genes that share common functional defects in the mitochondrial respiratory chain. Multiple organ systems are typically involved, especially in tissues with high metabolic activity. Neurologic and myopathic features are common, although more than 40 clinical syndromes have been reported. Most of the published reports of CKD due to TIN come from children who presented with clinical manifestations before 2 years of age.[68] However, it has been suggested that the prevalence of mitochondrial cytopathies in the adult population with CKD is underestimated.[69,70] From a renal perspective, proximal tubular dysfunction is the most common finding (~50% of the mitochondrial cytopathy patients), often leading to Fanconi syndrome. However, several patients developed chronic TIN in the absence of features of the renal Fanconi syndrome. Other reported renal manifestations include cystic renal disease and glomerulopathies (especially focal segmental glomerulosclerosis in adults). By electron microscopy, a variety of abnormalities have been described in tubular epithelial cell mitochondria, including changes in both morphology and number. Because a detailed analysis of tubular cell mitochondria has only been performed in very few chronic tubulointerstitial diseases, it is unclear whether any of the reported findings are specific to patients with primary mitochondrial cytopathies. Because mitochondria are involved secondarily in many pathways of CKD in association with oxidant stress and apoptosis, acquired morphologic changes might be anticipated. Primary mitochondrial disorders are being recognized with increasing frequency in adults with a variety of clinical manifestations, including chronic TIN. An elevated serum lactate level may be an initial diagnostic clue, but is not universally present in patients with renal mitochondrial cytopathies. Making a definitive diagnosis can be difficult for a variety of reasons, including the lack of a unique clinical phenotype and challenges pertaining to the interpretation of genetic studies. In particular, because spontaneous acquired mutations in the multiple copies of circular mtDNA that are present in each cell (~71,000) are common, it is first necessary to establish the pathogenetic significance of any novel mutations that are detected. Treatment is primarily symptomatic. Coenzyme Q10 therapy is recommended for patients with CoQ10 deficiency, although it is not clear that this treatment improves renal outcomes.

Chronic TIN in Primary Immunologic Disorders

Many of the disorders reviewed in this section are traditionally considered causes of acute TIN, but due to the insidious nature of the clinical manifestations, significant chronic changes are often present by the time that a renal biopsy is performed. TIN is typically one manifestation of a multisystem disorder, and the extrarenal manifestations often attract greater attention initially. From a renal perspective, the disease entities can be arbitrarily divided into two groups: (1) TIN is the primary renal manifestation and (2) TIN occurs in conjunction with glomerulonephritis. It is not clear whether primary humoral mechanisms ever cause TIN as they only target organs involved in the disease process. Studies in the 1990s characterized a circulating antibody in a small number of patients with TIN that bound to a unique 48–54 kd glycoprotein present in tubular basement membranes (especially proximal) and Bowman's capsule but not in the glomerular basement membrane.[71] Some of these patients also had membranous nephropathy. Antitubular basement membrane (TBM) antibodies are most likely to be associated with chronic TIN in patients with antiglomerular basement membrane (GBM) nephritis or Goodpasture syndrome (see Chapter 48). Chronic TIN associated with deposition of immune complexes along the TBM is most likely to occur as a manifestation of systemic lupus erythematosus. However, most TIN that occurs in association with systemic autoimmune disorders is not associated with pathologic evidence of antibody deposition and is presumed to be caused by cell-mediated mechanisms. Although beyond the scope of this chapter, another important immune-mediated cause of chronic TIN is chronic allograft nephropathy (see Chapter 81).

Primary Sjögren Syndrome

Primary Sjögren syndrome (SS) is a systemic autoimmune disease associated with autoantibodies to Ro/SSA and/or La/SSB that principally targets salivary and lacrimal glands. Many patients also have a positive rheumatoid factor, ANA antibodies, and hypergammaglobulinemia. Maripuri et al.[72] recently summarized findings in 24/7,276 patients (0.3%)

with SS and kidney involvement that was confirmed by renal biopsy over a 40-year period. The most common renal finding was TIN (70%), which was chronic in 46%; the severity of chronic TIN identified patients with estimated GFRs of less than 30 mL/min/1.73 m^2. The prevalence of renal involvement in SS is highly variable and likely underrecognized. Because both systemic and renal disease may be effectively controlled with corticosteroids and immunosuppressive therapy, the importance of early diagnosis is evident. Proximal or distal renal tubular acidosis, which is present in ~75% of the TIN patients, often associated with hypokalemia and polyuria, may prove to be a sensitive early indicator of TIN in this patient group.[73] Dysfunctions of the H-ATPase pump and carbonic anhydrase II have been implicated as potential mechanisms. Periodic paralysis due to severe hypokalemia is not uncommon in primary SS patients with severe TIN. Although the inciting antigen and specific pathogenetic mechanisms remain unclear, the TIN is characterized by interstitial infiltrates of lymphohematopoietic cells similar to those in extrarenal target organs. There do not appear to be unique serologic abnormalities that predict the risk of TIN. Tubulointerstitial immune deposits are not typically found by IF or EM. Antibodies to the extractable nuclear antigens Ro and La and perhaps other more recently described antigens (α-fodrin and the muscarinic receptor M3) may ultimately be shown to serve a specific pathogenic role.[74] Treatment is usually guided by the extrarenal manifestations and may include corticosteroids, hydroxychloroquine, and possibly one of the newer anti-TNF or anti-CD20 biologic agents. Patients with primary SS have an increased risk of lymphoma, which should be taken into consideration in the treatment plan. The renal outcome typically depends on the degree of interstitial fibrosis at the time of diagnosis.

IgG4-related Disease

IgG4-related disease was first recognized as a cause of autoimmune pancreatitis in 2001. It is now known to be a cause of TIN (first reported in 2004) as well as a variety of other extrarenal manifestations, including cholangitis, sialadenitis, pneumonitis, pseudotumor, and periarthritis. Although many patients have clinical factors that overlap with SS, serologic findings appear to be unique. In patients with IgG4-related disease, total serum IgG and IgG4 levels are elevated, antibodies to double-stranded DNA, SSA, and SSB are typically negative (although ANA may be positive), and hypocomplementemia is common (~70%). Although SS is a disease of middle-aged women, IgG4-related disease primarily affects older men. Abnormal renal imaging studies suggestive of a mass have been reported in ~30% of patients, manifest as multifocal, low attenuation lesions, or diffuse nephromegaly. On histologic examination, these lesions correspond to areas of TIN. Two recent studies focusing on IgG4-related TIN, from Japan and the United States respectively, reported renal involvement in 20% to 30% of the patients.[75,76] Within this combined cohort, ~50% had documented pancreatic involvement. Histologically, the lesions were characterized by an interstitial infiltrate of plasma cells, many expressing IgG4, together with variable degrees of interstitial fibrosis and tubular atrophy—interstitial eosinophils were also common. Excluding the interstitial inflammatory lesions that were observed in patients with ANCA-associated vasculitis (31% IgG4 positive), only 12% of the patients with other causes of TIN had IgG4+ interstitial cells. Detection of granular TBM immune deposits varied between the two studies: 7% in the first series and 83% in the second. Minor glomerular abnormalities were also observed in a few of the patients. Most patients were treated with corticosteroids with or without immunosuppressive drugs. Short-term outcomes appear to be good—three patients (5%) with renal failure at diagnosis had developed ESRD at last follow-up.

Sarcoidosis

Sarcoidosis is a multisystem disease of unknown etiology that primarily affects the 10- to 40-year age group and is characterized by organ injury associated with noncaseating epithelioid giant cell granulomas.[77] A rare familial form of the disease has been reported to be associated with mutations in nucleotide-binding oligomerization domain 2/caspase activation recruitment domain 15 (*NOD2/CARD15*), a gene involved in inflammation and apoptosis. In the absence of diagnostic serologic markers, elevated serum angiotensin-converting enzyme (ACE) and lysozyme levels suggest a diagnosis of sarcoidosis.[78] Other characteristic features include hypercalcemia, interstitial lung disease, and hilar adenopathy. Many of the patients (>50%) develop renal insufficiency, which has largely been ascribed to perturbations in calcium metabolism that develop in association with elevated 1,25-dihydroxy vitamin D levels, hypercalcemia, hypercalciuria, and nephrocalcinosis. However, a subset of patients develops a unique form of TIN that is characterized by the presence of interstitial granulomas.[79] Recent studies of granulomatous TIN have identified sarcoidosis as the primary etiology in almost 30% of cases. Like many types of TIN, this lesion is often unrecognized clinically and may be associated with significant chronic TIN when tissue is obtained for histologic analysis typically when patients develop CKD. Autopsy studies have reported granulomatous TIN in ~13% of sarcoidosis patients. Rarely, TIN may be the initial manifestation of the disease. Recurrent disease has been reported in renal allografts. Corticosteroids with or without immunosuppressive therapy are beneficial, although recovery is often incomplete due to the presence of irreversible chronic TIN.

Tubulointerstitial Nephritis with Uveitis Syndrome

The recognition of TIN with uveitis (TINU) syndrome as a distinct clinical entity was first reported in 1995. The syndrome can occur as an isolated entity of unknown etiology or as a manifestation of specific autoimmune disorders (SS, sarcoidosis, systemic lupus erythematosus [SLE], ANCA+

vasculitis, Behçet disease) and certain infectious diseases (tuberculosis, brucellosis, toxoplasmosis, histoplasmosis, Epstein-Barr virus, HIV, chlamydia, mycoplasma). In the absence of a diagnostic serologic marker, the diagnosis of idiopathic TINU is based on the exclusion of other possibilities. The disease is considered an autoimmune disease mediated by a cellular immune response to an antigen that is expressed by renal tubules and the uveal tract of the eye. Modified C-reactive protein has recently been suggested as an antigenic candidate based on the presence of circulating anti-CRP antibodies.[80] Unlike many of the other disorders discussed in this section, idiopathic TINU primarily affects adolescents and young adults and is usually associated with acute systemic manifestations such as fever, weight loss, and general malaise. Flank pain is not uncommon. Although the kidney disease is thought to be self-limited, many patients are treated with corticosteroids with or without immunosuppressive drugs due to severe ocular involvement that may follow a relapsing course and lead to chronic eye disease. The renal disease is typically acute TIN with a good prognosis, but fibrotic sequelae including both ESRD and disease recurrence in a renal allograft have been reported, although these outcomes are considered rare. A recent study of 26 Finnish children with TINU reported that 15% had permanent renal insufficiency and 31% had persistent low molecular weight proteinuria, which suggests that sequelae due to chronic TIN may become evident with longer term follow-up.[81]

TIN ASSOCIATED WITH PRIMARY GLOMERULAR DISEASES

With the exception of steroid-responsive nephrotic syndrome, virtually all glomerular diseases are accompanied by an interstitial inflammatory response, although its severity varies widely. The subsequent progression to interstitial fibrosis and tubular atrophy is an important prognostic indicator, as first shown by the studies of Risdon[82] and Schainuck[83] and their respective colleagues more than 40 years ago. The pathogenetic mechanisms of acute TIN associated with primary glomerular disease have not been clearly elucidated. For immune complex-associated disease such as lupus nephritis, TBM immune deposits may be present and associated with interstitial inflammation, but TIN more commonly occurs in their absence. Occasionally TIN is the primary renal lesion in lupus nephritis. Similarly, anti-TBM antibodies are observed in a subset of patients with anti-GBM nephritis/Goodpasture syndrome, but the tubulointerstitial inflammation is disproportionately severe and its relationship to anti-TBM antibodies is unclear. T-cell mediated immune responses are likely involved, although specific antigens and effector cell pathways remain unknown. For some diseases, such as ANCA-positive vasculitis, interstitial inflammation may be severe and associated with noncaseating granulomas. Crescentic glomerular diseases may be characterized by impressive periglomerular interstitial inflammation, often in association with breaks in Bowman's capsule that allow chemotactic factors, fibrinogen, and other inflammatory mediators to leak directly into the interstitium to trigger TIN. Irrespective of the inciting mechanisms, delayed diagnosis or inadequate therapy means that patients with severe glomerular disease may develop chronic TIN, which has important prognostic implications. This relationship has been well established in patients with lupus nephritis. For example, in a recent study of 313 patients with lupus nephritis, Yu et al.[84] graded the severity of interstitial inflammation, tubular atrophy, and interstitial fibrosis and showed that these changes were a significant predictor of renal survival (Fig. 57.9).

Proteinuria as a Mediator of Progressive Kidney Damage

A series of observations over the last two decades support a pathogenetic connection between severe proteinuria and chronic TIN that underlies progressive functional deterioration, and may explain at least in part why patients with primary glomerular disease develop TIN. The basis of this hypothesis derives from an extensive literature indicating that the degree of proteinuria is one of the strongest predictors of renal outcome (Fig. 57.10),[85,86] coupled with plausible mechanistic paradigms derived from in vitro models, animal models, and careful analytic studies of human kidney tissue. Two distinct (but not mutually exclusive) possibilities have emerged: (1) inflammatory and fibrogenic responses may be triggered by tubular cells reacting to abnormal quantities and/or composition of filtered proteins, and (2) a tubulointerstitial response may be stimulated by a proteinuric glomerular ultrafiltrate that is misdirected to periglomerular and peritubular spaces.

The first hypothesis, summarized in Fig. 57.11, posits that receptors on the apical membrane of proximal tubular cells interact with luminal urinary proteins, triggering responses that lead to basolateral secretion of proinflammatory or fibrosis-promoting factors into the interstitial space.[87] Also plausible are similar effects due to paracellular leakage between tubular epithelial cells directly into interstitial spaces, and the involvement of distal nephron segments, especially if they are distended by obstructing proteinaceous casts. Supporting evidence derives from the observation that animals with "overload" proteinuria develop acute and chronic TIN, and from findings that cultured tubular cells exposed to high concentrations of albumin in particular respond by activating the NF-κB, ERK1/2, and STAT signaling pathways, which stimulate production of a variety of inflammatory mediators (MCP-1, RANTES, IL-6, TNF, fractalkine, complement proteins) and fibrogenic molecules (TGF-β, endothelin-1, extracellular matrix proteins) and activate the RAS.[88]

The identity of the detrimental urinary protein(s) is unclear. Although many of the cell culture studies have used albumin, it is argued that because patients with highly "selective" proteinuria, such as those with steroid-responsive

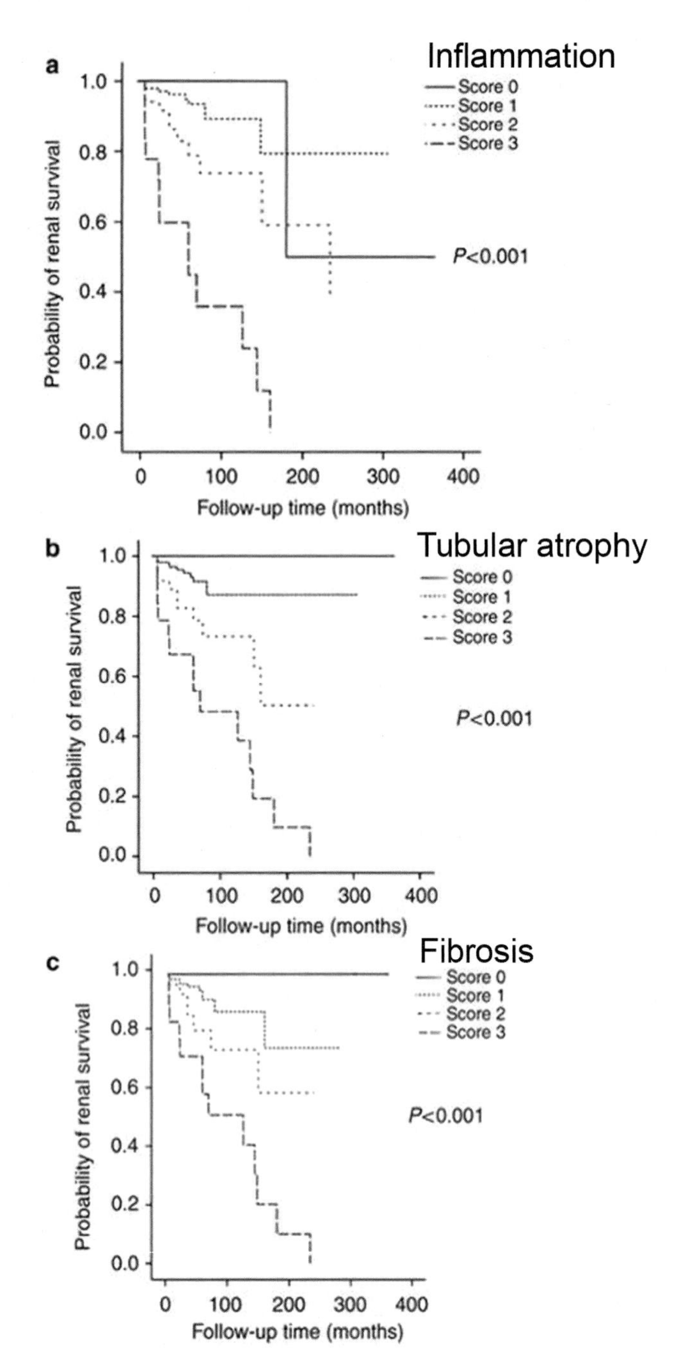

FIGURE 57.9 Severity of chronic tubulointerstitial nephritis predicts renal outcome in primary glomerular diseases. As a representation of several studies, which show similar findings, in this Chinese study of 313 patients with lupus nephritis, the severity of the tubulointerstitial inflammation (a), tubular atrophy (b), and fibrosis (c), graded on a scale from 0 to 3+ based on the area involved, were significant predictors of kidney survival rates. (From Yu F, Wu LH, Tan Y, et al. Tubulointerstitial lesions of patients with lupus nephritis classified by the 2003 International Society of Nephrology and Renal Pathology Society system. *Kidney Int.* 2010;77:820, with permission.)

nephrotic syndrome, do not develop TIN, native albumin is probably not the culprit. However, albumin is known to be a carrier for numerous molecules, making it possible for modified albumin (or its conjugates) to trigger these responses. Alternatively, other urinary proteins may be the primary stimulus—inflammatory cytokines generated within damaged glomeruli, iron-binding proteins such as transferrin and apoferritin, and high molecular weight proteins not normally present in the glomerular ultrafiltrate such as immunoglobulin have been suggested as candidates.

Assuming that the damaging effects of proteinuria are the consequence of a receptor-dependent process, the low affinity albumin receptor megalin has been considered a lead candidate. Expressed on the apical brush border membrane, this scavenger receptor and member of the LDL receptor family internalizes multiple protein ligands by endocytosis and may initiate intracellular signaling after phosphorylation of its cytoplasmic tail. Megalin may engage the nonsignaling receptors cubilin and amnion less in this pathway. Cubilin is also implicated by the finding that a polymorphic variant of the cubilin gene is associated with albuminuria in a large European ancestry cohort.[89] However, a central role for megalin has been challenged by the finding that megalin-deficient mice are not protected from TIN associated with anti-GBM nephritis.[90] The apical membrane of proximal tubules is a rich source of several other receptors that could be activated by abnormal or excessive urinary proteins. Candidates that have already been considered are CD36, complement receptors, Toll-like receptors, chemokine receptors, and growth factor receptors. As genomewide association studies (GWAS), urinary biomarker studies, and genomic and proteomic kidney tissue studies identify new CKD-associated molecules, it is likely that new proteinuria–tubular cell–TIN pathways will emerge. A study by Reich et al.[91] identified 11 genes induced by exposing human tubular cells to albumin, which were also upregulated in the tubulointerstitial compartment of kidney biopsies from human IgA nephropathy patients and correlated with the severity of proteinuria. GWAS studies have identified uromodulin as a pathway of great interest.

To link these early tubular responses to chronic TIN and progressive kidney disease, several plausible pathways have been proposed.[88]

1. Basolateral secretion of proinflammatory mediators may trigger the recruitment and activation of the interstitial fibroblasts that synthesize interstitial collagens and a variety of other extracellular matrix proteins leading to fibrosis, either directly or indirectly as a consequence of inflammatory cell recruitment (Fig. 57.11).
2. Tubular cells may synthesize collagen proteins that directly contribute to the expanding pool of fibrotic interstitial matrix proteins.
3. Tubular cell death, a recognized consequence of interstitial fibrosis, may occur as a consequence of severe proteinuria. Evidence includes a study reporting Fas pathway activation leading to tubular cell apoptosis

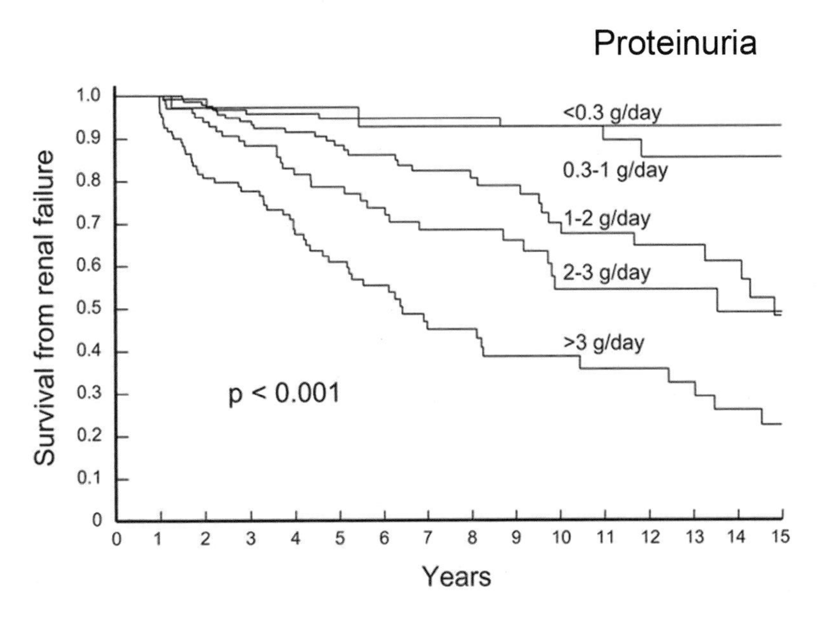

FIGURE 57.10 Proteinuria severity predicts outcomes in chronic kidney disease. An observation that has been made for virtually all chronic glomerular diseases, this representative study of 542 patients with biopsy-proven IgA nephropathy shows that time-averaged 24-hour urinary protein levels predict renal survival rates. Although this association does not establish causality, data from several experimental studies suggest that high levels of proteinuria can trigger tubular injury and the release of several inflammatory mediators. (Data from Reich HN, Troyanov S, Scholey JW, et al. Remission of proteinuria improves prognosis in IgA nephropathy. *J Am Soc Nephrol.* 2007;18:3177, with permission.)

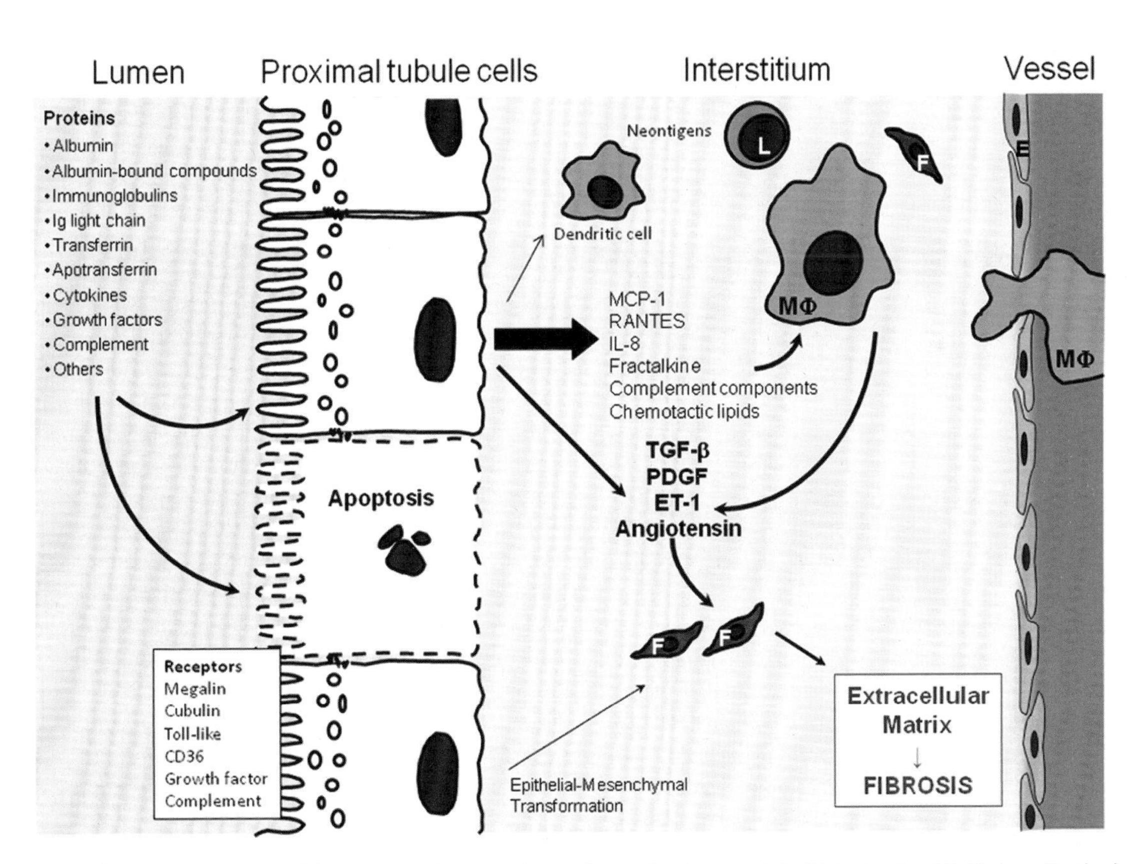

FIGURE 57.11 Schematic summary of the proposed mechanisms of proteinuria-associated tubulointerstitial injury. On the luminal side, a variety of proteins in the glomerular ultrafiltrate may interact with apical receptors on proximal tubular cells. Although megalin has been the receptor of greatest interest, others are likely to be involved. These interactions may trigger the synthesis and release of a variety of proinflammatory and profibrotic molecules across the basolateral membrane, leading to interstitial inflammation and fibrosis. In vitro studies have also reported tubular cell apoptosis and epithelial-mesenchymal transition. A more challenging mechanism to confirm, MCH class II receptors can be upregulated on tubular cells, preparing them to serve as antigen-presenting cells to activate immunologic responses. An important question is the identity of proteinuria-associated neoantigen(s) that might activate such a cascade. (From Zandi-Nejad K, Eddy AA, Glassock RJ, et al. Why is proteinuria an ominous biomarker of progressive kidney disease? *Kidney Int.* 2004;66:S76, with permission.)

following exposure to high albumin concentrations.[92] Oxidant stress triggered by proteinuria may participate in tubular cell death.

4. Following receptor-mediated uptake, urinary proteins are delivered to lysosomes to be recycled as amino acids.[93] It has been proposed that excessive demands on this system may lead to lysosomal rupture and release of cytotoxic contents into the tubular cell cytoplasm, with damaging consequences such as autolysis or autophagy.
5. Proteinuria may trigger the process of epithelial-to-mesenchymal transdifferentiation (EMT), which has been proposed as a mechanism by which tubular cells ultimately become collagen-producing interstitial myofibroblasts after their tight connections with adjacent tubular cells are disassembled and they migrate into the interstitium through breaks in tubular basement membranes.[94]
6. Urinary proteins may be a source of antigenic peptides that are processed by renal dendritic cells to initiate T-cell mediated injury.[95]

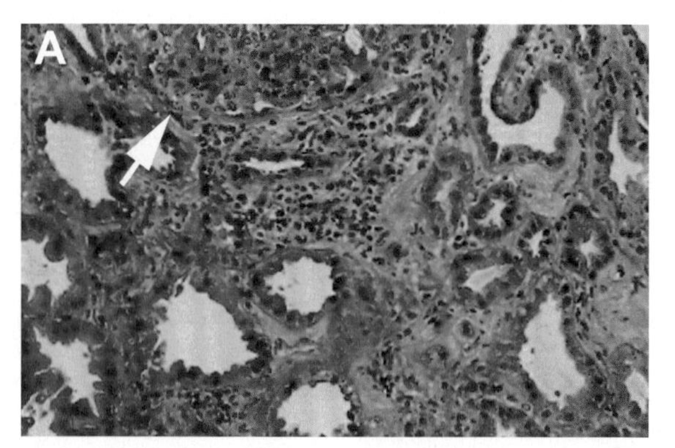

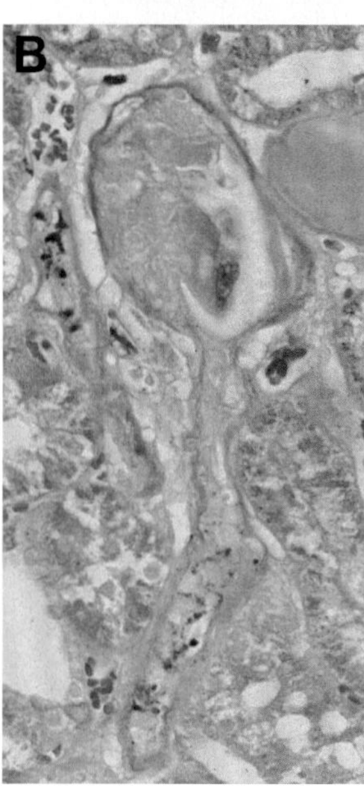

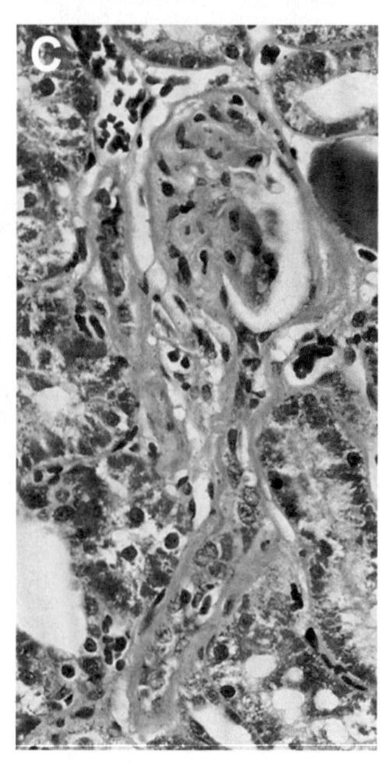

FIGURE 57.12 The misdirected filtration theory of proteinuria-associated chronic tubulointerstitial nephritis (TIN). This paradigm is based on the view that the triggering event is a disruption of the integrity of Bowman's capsule by encroachment of a damaged glomerular tuft (arrow) **(A)**. This change allows some of the glomerular ultrafiltrate to be redirected from the proximal tubule directly into the periglomerular interstitial space. It may also leak out of glomerulotubular junctions at the urinary pole and travel along the outer aspect of tubules. The presence of the ultrafiltrate in these unusual sites triggers chronic TIN. Support for this mechanism is based on the tracer studies that Kriz et al. performed in nephrotic rats. Serial sections of the same nephron illustrate the blue ferritin tracer **(B)** and trichrome-positive fibrosis in the peritubular interstitium **(C)** in an identical distribution pattern. (From Kriz W, Hartmann I, Hosser H, et al. Tracer studies in the rat demonstrate misdirected filtration and peritubular filtrate spreading in nephrons with segmental glomerulosclerosis. *J Am Soc Nephrol.* 2001;12:496, with permission.)

The theory of "misdirected filtration," championed by Kriz and colleagues based on careful histomorphologic studies that were enhanced by tracing the fate of exogenous markers in rat proteinuria models, suggest an alternative mechanistic link between proteinuria and interstitial fibrosis.[96] The theory is based on the premise that proteins derived from the glomerular ultrafiltrate are not delivered to the interstitial space from either tubular lumina or interstitial capillaries. Rather, this theory proposes that damaged podocytes, which are the primary cause of proteinuria, can adhere to Bowman's capsule to create a conduit between parietal epithelial cells through which the glomerular ultrafiltrate leaks into the periglomerular interstitial space (Fig. 57.12). The process then extends to involve the tubules, beginning at the urinary pole of glomeruli, where the ultrafiltrate next appears within the subepithelial peritubular space surrounding proximal tubules. This misdirected glomerular ultrafiltrate is thought to elicit a fibroblast response within the interstitium and cause progressive tubular cell degeneration, beginning with the proximal tubule and extending distally. Ultimately, the affected nephron degenerates, leaving behind a fibrotic interstitial space. Alternatively, the process may obstruct proximal tubules, leading to downstream tubular atrophy and formation of "atubular" glomeruli.

SEQUELAE TO ACUTE TUBULOINTERSTITIAL DISEASES

Acute Kidney Injury

Several recently published studies in adult patients with acute kidney injury (AKI) presumed to be caused by tubular necrosis have reported that surviving patients are at a significantly increased risk of developing advanced CKD. This is true whether patients had normal baseline kidney function or preexisting CKD. A recent meta-analysis of 13 cohort studies reported a pooled adjusted hazard rate of 8.8 for CKD and 3.1 for ESRD compared to a matched patient cohort without AKI (Fig. 57.13).[97] Significant predictors of CKD

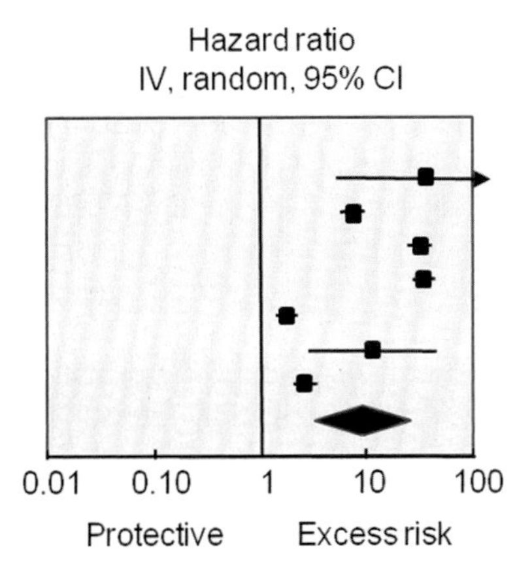

FIGURE 57.13 Severe acute kidney injury (AKI) is a risk factor for chronic tubulointerstitial nephritis. In a review of 13 published cohort studies (>3,000 patients), the pooled adjusted hazard ratio (HR) for chronic kidney disease after AKI was 8.8. *IV*, inverse variance weighted averages of logarithmic HRs. (From Coca SG, Singanamala S, Parikh CR, et al. Chronic kidney disease after acute kidney injury: a systematic review and meta-analysis. *Kidney Int.* 2012;81(5):442–448, with permission.)

risk included the severity of the acute injury (based on need for dialysis or not, mean serum creatinine level), diabetes, and hypoalbuminemia.[98,99] There are few data evaluating renal outcomes in children who survived severe AKI, although relevant studies are now in progress. The best pediatric data come from long-term follow-up of children with diarrhea-positive hemolytic uremic syndrome. A meta-analysis of 49 studies reported combined renal sequelae (CKD, ESRD, proteinuria, hypertension) in 25% of survivors.[100]

Although renal biopsies are rarely performed in this patient group to evaluate findings and potential pathogenetic mechanisms, informative animal models of ischemia-reperfusion injury have been extensively investigated and provide insights that are likely relevant to humans.[101] These data support the view that chronic injury is a consequence of AKI. The acute phase of ischemia-reperfusion injury is characterized by microvascular changes and tubular cell production of a variety of proinflammatory and chemotactic cytokines that recruit lymphohemopoietic cells to the renal interstitium. It is now recognized that specific subsets of interstitial cells (especially neutrophils, macrophages, and B cells) promote kidney injury whereas others (T-regulatory cells, alternatively actuated macrophages) facilitate kidney repair. The studies in animal models have shown that the interstitial inflammation persists for several weeks, even after a single 60-minute ischemic event, and is associated with areas of interstitial capillary rarefaction, tubular atrophy, interstitial fibrosis, and irreversible nephron loss.[102] The specific cellular and molecular mechanisms that are involved in the transition of AKI to chronic TIN are under active investigation. A transformational switch of the interstitial macrophages to an alternatively activated ("M2") phenotype is likely involved.[20] Although M2 cells characterize tissue repair responses, part of the repair response is fibrosis, and when it is "maladaptive," irreversible parenchymal injury ensues. When the rate of replacement of damaged tubular cells by proliferation of surviving tubular cells fails to keep pace with tubular cell death, tubular recovery is incomplete and sets the stage for CKD. To some extent this reparative response could be considered an antecedent event that accelerates normal kidney aging. Glomerular filtration rates decline slowly and progressively with advancing age. It has been reported that the "normal" mean glomerular filtration rates is 60 mL/min/1.73 m^2 in octogenarians (Fig. 57.14).[103] Histopathologically, this decline in renal function is associated with progressive tubular loss and interstitial fibrosis. It is likely that residual damage after severe AKI compromises renal parenchymal reserve, setting that stage for faster aging-associated functional decline.

Acute Interstitial Nephritis

Primary acute interstitial nephritis (see Chapter 35) has multiple etiologies and outcomes. Many of the acute pathogenic immunologic reactions are triggered by exposure to offending

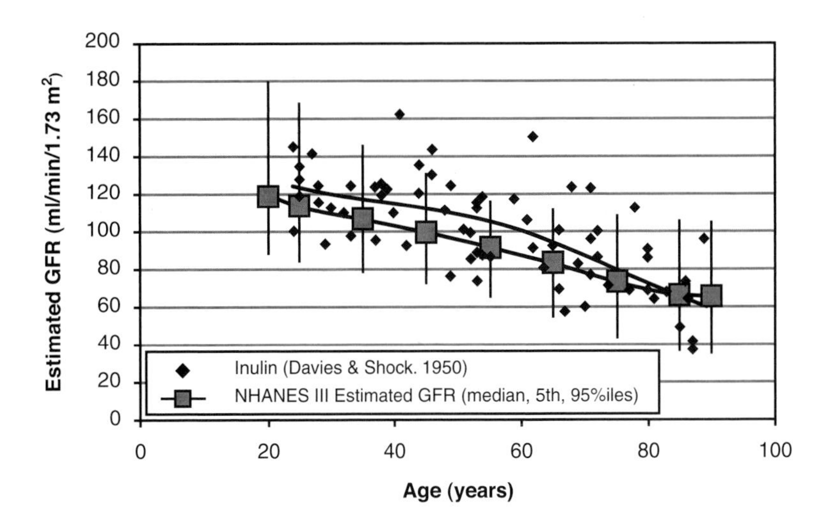

FIGURE 57.14 Decline in estimated glomerular filtration rate with age. Data are derived from the U.S. population using National Health and Nutrition Examination Survey (NHANES) III data and inulin clearances among 70 healthy men. (Abstracted from Davies DF, Shock NW. Age changes in glomerular filtration rate, effective renal plasma flow, and tubular excretory capacity in adult males. *J Clin Invest.* 1950;29:496.) Aging studies in animal models have established aging-related glomerulosclerosis and chronic tubulointerstitial nephritis as the histopathologic correlate of this progressive functional loss. (Figure from Part 4. Definition and classification of stages of chronic kidney disease. *Am J Kidney Dis.* 2002;39:S46, with permission.)

drugs (~70%) or microorganisms (~15%) and subside once the offending agent is identified and eliminated. With normalization of the serum creatinine level and urine sediment, it has traditionally been thought that tubulointerstitial architecture had been restored to normal. Although there are few long-term follow-up data, a study by Rossert et al.[104] reported evidence of renal functional impairment in 40% of patients after drug-induced interstitial nephritis. Additional studies are needed to determine whether patients with reversible kidney injury due to acute interstitial nephritis are predisposed to future CKD and if early steroid therapy can significantly reduce this risk, as suggested by the study of Gonzalez et al.[105]

Bacterial Infection-Associated Chronic TIN

TIN associated with scarlet fever was the first type of interstitial nephritis recognized as a unique clinical entity—dating back to 1860, with Councilman's classic histologic description following in 1898. The incidence of renal parenchymal invasion by bacteria greatly declined after antibodies became available. Indeed, since the 1960s, drugs have become the primary cause of acute TIN. Two mechanisms of bacteria-associated TIN are recognized. In the first, the renal parenchyma is directly invaded and the infected region is characterized by a neutrophil-rich interstitial infiltrate (pyelonephritis).[106] A delay in treatment may lead to abscess formation and/or interstitial scarring. The second pattern is considered an immune-mediated response, characterized by an interstitial infiltrate of mononuclear cells and absence of bacteria within the renal parenchyma.

The association between pyelonephritis and chronic TIN has been most extensively investigated in young children with primary vesicoureteral reflux (VUR). In children less than 5 years of age, serial imaging studies have established a relationship between VUR and renal parenchymal deficits and between febrile urinary tract infection (UTI) and renal scarring. For many years, it was assumed that pyelonephritis caused chronic TIN and that medical interventions designed to reduce UTIs would reduce the risk of new scar formation. This therapeutic approach has been validated for girls less than 5 years of age with high-grade reflux (III-V), but current evidence strongly supports the view that most of the renal parenchymal defects detected in patients with primary VUR predate infections and represent congenital lesions of hypodysplasia (primary renal scarring).[107] Now, with the frequent use of antenatal ultrasound, recent prospective clinical studies have reported low rates of new scar formation after febrile UTIs. In addition, the high prevalence (~50%) of renal parenchymal deficits detected in children with febrile UTIs in the absence of VUR and the presence of renal parenchymal deficits associated with VUR in the absence of infection provide further supporting evidence that many of the renal parenchymal deficits are congenital. This would also explain why the incidence of ESRD due to "reflex nephropathy" has not changed over the past 40 years despite earlier diagnosis and efforts to reduce the frequency of urinary tract infections. It has also become clear that genetic factors play a major role in the risk of VUR even though specific genes have not yet been identified. It is estimated that 30% of the siblings of a child with VUR and 60% of the offspring of parents with VUR also have VUR.[108]

Mycobacterium tuberculosis is an important infectious microorganism that can directly invade the renal parenchyma and cause severe chronic tubulointerstitial destruction and fibrosis when the diagnosis and treatment are delayed. Both caseating and noncaseating interstitial granulomas should always raise suspicion of renal tuberculosis.[109] Despite the fact that the kidney is the extrapulmonary organ most commonly involved in tuberculosis (15% to 20%), there are few data on the role of tuberculosis as a cause of chronic TIN and ESRD, although this outcome has been reported. For example, in a report of 25 patients with chronic granulomatous TIN due to tuberculosis (17 confirmed by biopsy), 20% developed ESRD within 6 months.[110] Although much less common, immune-mediated TIN without direct renal parenchymal invasion by mycobacteria is a well-documented entity.

Several bacterial infections have been reported to cause acute TIN, presumably as a consequence of an immunologic response to a systemic infection. There are few data available on the risk of progression to chronic TIN and CKD, even though recent follow-up data for other causes of AKI suggest that these patients should also be monitored long-term for evidence of CKD. The most commonly implicated microorganisms are *Escherichia coli*, *Enterococcus*, *Leptospirosis*, *Mycobacteria*, *Actinobacteria*, *Legionella*, *Streptococci*, *Campylobacter*, *Brucella*, *Staphylococci*, *Corynebacterium diphtheria*, *Yersinia*, *Treponema pallidum*, and *Mycoplasma*.

Xanthogranulomatous Pyelonephritis

Xanthogranulomatous pyelonephritis is a unique and uncommon infection-mediated cause of CKD that affects patients of all ages and is typically unilateral.[111] Histopathologically, the disease is chronic TIN with the hallmark feature of numerous interstitial lipid-laden xanthomatous macrophages with variable degrees of chronic tubular damage and interstitial fibrosis (Fig. 57.15). Because of the insidious nature of the clinical presentation, with nonspecific symptoms such as fever, abdominal or flank pain, and weight loss, it is not uncommon for the normal renal parenchyma to be severely damaged and the kidney nonfunctional by the time the diagnosis is made. These changes are often associated with hydronephrosis, renal stones, and an enlarged kidney. Nephrectomy is the usual treatment for patients with advanced disease. The most commonly implicated bacteria are *E. coli*, *Proteus mirabilis*, *Pseudomonas*, *Streptococcus faecalis*, and *Klebsiella*. The urine culture is negative ~25% of the time, despite evidence of renal parenchymal infection. The primary pathogenesis of the abnormal immune response that leads to this unusual chronic inflammatory response remains unknown.

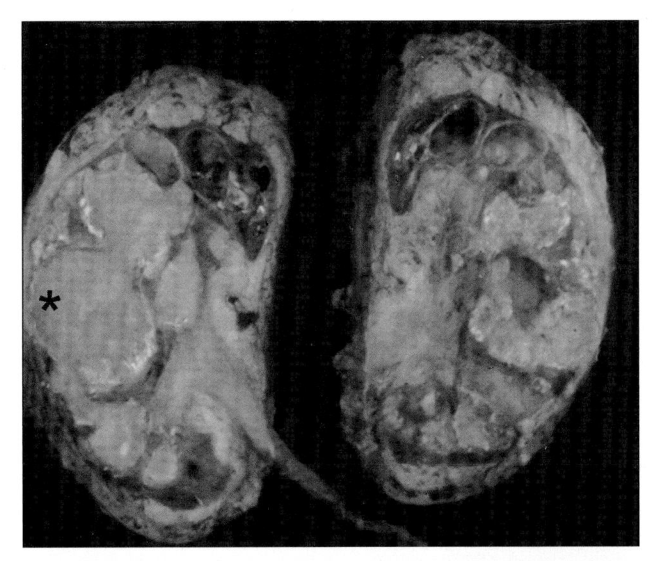

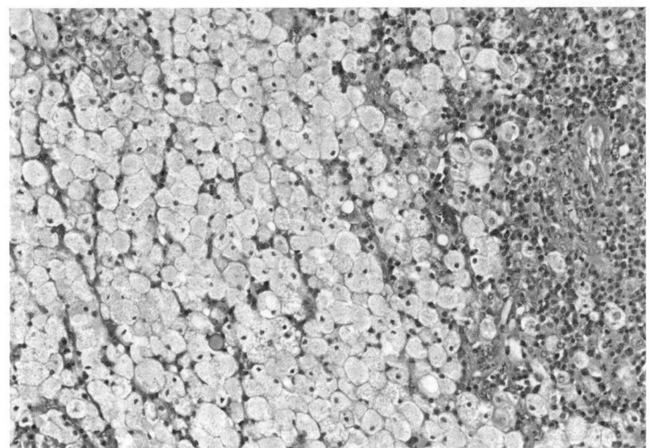

FIGURE 57.15 Xanthogranulomatous pyelonephritis is a bacteria-associated cause of chronic tubulointerstitial nephritis. The nephrectomy specimen shows extensive destruction of the renal parenchyma by cystic cavities, stones, and xanthogranulomas (*). Histopathology shows a plasma cell infiltrate to the right and a dense interstitial foam cell infiltrate which has destroyed the surrounding parenchyma. (From Levy M, Baumal R, Eddy AA, et al. Xanthogranulomatous pyelonephritis in children. Etiology, pathogenesis, clinical and radiologic features and management. *Clin Pediatr.* 1994;33:360, with permission.)

Viral Infections

The recognition of viral infections as a potential cause of chronic TIN is likely to occur with increasing frequency as the use of molecular diagnostics continues to expand. In 1999, Becker et al.[112] provided evidence for the presence of the Epstein-Barr virus genome in the proximal tubules in kidney biopsy specimens from patients with idiopathic chronic TIN and suggested that EBV was involved in disease pathogenesis.

BK polyomavirus is recognized as an important cause of chronic TIN in immunologically compromised individuals, especially renal transplant recipients.[113] Most normal adults have had a prior asymptomatic BK polyomavirus infection and harbor the virus in a latent form in the genitourinary epithelium. Plasma polymerase chain reaction (PCR) surveillance studies suggest that the virus is reactivated in 27% of renal transplant recipients. Without appropriate reduction in immunosuppressive therapy, the virus may invade renal tubular epithelial cells (especially in the medulla) with cytopathic effects that lead to interstitial inflammation and subsequent fibrosis, which is estimated to occur in 5% of renal transplant recipients. In patients with BK virus-associated nephropathy, viral inclusions may be present in tubular epithelia and the presence of the BK virus within nuclei can be confirmed by polyomavirus-specific immunostaining (Fig. 57.16). If renal dysfunction and BK viremia do not improve after a reduction in immunosuppression therapy, other efforts to reduce the viral load are often considered, using intravenous IgG, ciprofloxacin, leflunomide and/or cidofovir, but the efficacy of this therapy remains unclear.[114] Recipients of nonrenal solid organ transplants are also at risk for BK nephropathy, although the incidence is much lower than in kidney transplant recipients. The nephropathy has also been reported in hematopoietic stem cell transplant recipients.[115]

Adenovirus infections are increasingly recognized in kidney transplant recipients, often causing hemorrhagic cystitis.[116] However, granulomatous TIN has also been reported among kidney transplant recipients using in situ hybridization to identify adenoviral DNA within tubular epithelial cells.

Another viral infection that has been shown to infect renal epithelia and trigger chronic interstitial inflammation is HIV-1.[117] Although most patients with HIV-associated nephropathy have significant glomerular pathologic changes, coexistent chronic TIN is more severe than would be anticipated on the basis of the glomerular pathology alone and may be associated with microcystic and/or tubular changes. Although it is often impossible to exclude drugs as a factor contributing to the pathogenesis of TIN in HIV-infected patients, there is experimental evidence that the HIV-1 *Vpr* gene induces tubular cell apoptosis, suggesting one relevant pathogenetic mechanism of HIV-associated chronic TIN.[118] Similar findings have been reported in patients with hepatitis C virus (HCV)-associated nephropathy. In particular, when patients with membranous nephropathy were matched for the stage of glomerular disease, TIN was more severe in the HVC-positive group and HCV peptide and/or RNA was identified in both tubular and interstitial cells.[119] Several other viruses have also been associated with TIN, including cytomegalovirus, Hantaan, hepatitis B, rubeola, herpes simplex, and mumps viruses. Among this latter group, hemorrhagic fever with renal syndrome (HFRS) caused by Hantavirus is associated with a higher risk of CKD.[120] Humans acquire this infection from infected rodents, primarily in Asia and Europe. A renal biopsy performed during the acute illness shows acute TIN together with widespread tubular necrosis. Patients may also develop hematuria and proteinuria due to glomerular pathology.

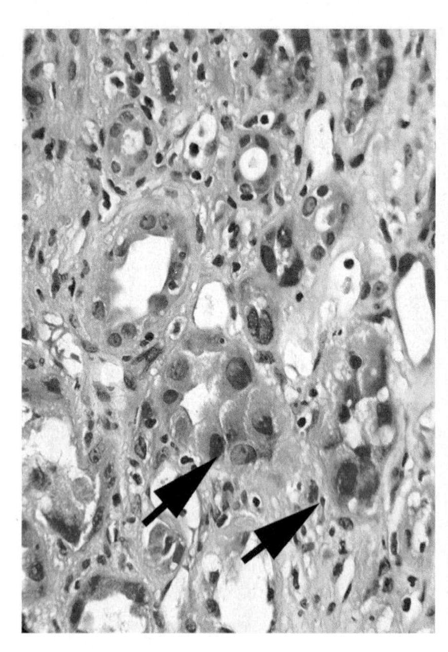

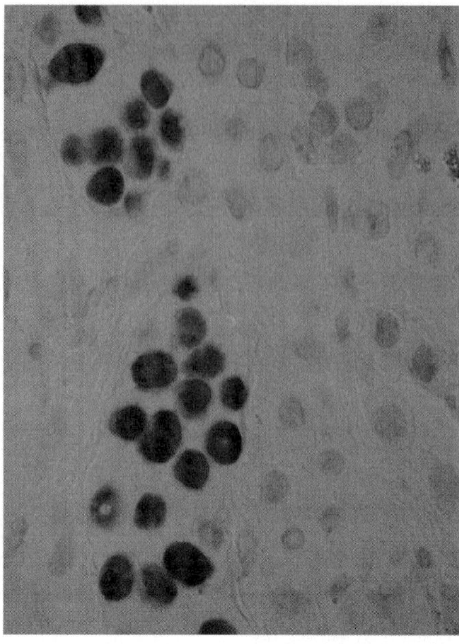

FIGURE 57.16 BK virus nephropathy is a cause of chronic tubulointerstitial nephritis in renal allograft recipients. The presence of intranuclear viral inclusions within tubular epithelial cells (highlighted by *arrows* in left photomicrograph), often more evident in the medulla, should raise suspicion of this diagnosis, which can be confirmed by SV40 T antigen immunostaining (nuclear reaction product in the right photomicrograph). (Photomicrographs were provided by Dr. Laura Finn, University of Washington and Seattle Children's Hospital.)

Other Infections Associated with Chronic TIN

Basically any microbial pathogen known to cause acute TIN has the potential to progress to chronic disease. This list includes certain fungi (histoplasmosis, *Candida*, and *Cryptococcus*) and parasites (toxoplasmosis, leishmaniasis, and *Rickettsia*).

Drugs

Drugs may cause chronic TIN through a variety of mechanisms that can be subdivided into groups.

1. *Idiosyncratic immune-mediated TIN.* This mechanism is thought to cause most drug-induced acute TIN. There is increasing evidence that chronic TIN may ensue after severe acute injury. Most patients with drug-induced TIN do not present clinically with the classical triad of fever, rash, and eosinophilia that was originally associated with methicillin-induced interstitial nephritis. There are likely many patients who remain asymptomatic without a diagnosis of acute TIN ever being made. Drug exposure then continues for the recommended duration and recovery from TIN may be incomplete, although this concern is impossible to validate. Follow-up studies of patients with an established diagnosis of drug-induced acute TIN have reported that early drug cessation is important for full renal recovery. Both acute and chronic changes may be evident in those with biopsy-confirmed drug-induced TIN. In a case series reported by Schwartz et al.,[121] 31% had permanent loss of renal function. Further studies are needed to determine whether corticosteroid therapy reduces the risk of CKD for those presenting with severe AKI.[105] The spectrum of drugs most likely to cause acute TIN is changing. In particular, protein pump inhibitors have emerged as a leading cause, as shown in a study of biopsy-confirmed cases of TIN between 1995 and 1999, which concluded that 35% were associated with protein pump inhibitor drugs.[122] Given the widespread use of these drugs, often over prolonged time periods without routine kidney function surveillance, there is reason for concern about the risk of unrecognized chronic TIN.
2. *Tubular cell nephrotoxicity.* Several drugs or their metabolites are known to damage renal tubular cells, often in a dose-dependent fashion. The specific mechanisms are multiple, but they often share in common the generation of oxidant stress and tubular cell death. Depending on the primary cellular target, specific patterns of tubular cell dysfunction may be observed and may be the only manifestation of nephrotoxicity. However, a reduced GFR is not uncommon as a consequence of acute tubular cell death by apoptosis or necrosis and the associated interstitial inflammatory response. Beyond direct tubular cell cytotoxicity, some drugs trigger chemokine and cytokine release that initiates a peritubular inflammatory response that may progress to fibrosis.
3. *Tubulointerstitial hypoxia.* The primary effect of some nephrotoxins is thought to be mediated by alterations in tubular cell oxygenation due to effects on the vasculature.
4. *Crystalline nephropathy.* Poorly soluble drugs or their metabolites that are primarily excreted in the urine may precipitate in tubular lumina and cause injury by obstruction, leading to secondary effects on the tubules and interstitial spaces. Such a mechanism has been reported in patients receiving high doses of methotrexate and with antiretroviral drugs.

The classes of drugs most commonly associated with both acute and chronic TIN are summarized in the following text.

Chemotherapeutic Agents

Cisplatinum is the classic chemotherapeutic nephrotoxin.[123] A hydrolyzed intracellular metabolite appears to be the primary mediator of cytotoxicity, which only affects the S3 segment of proximal tubules. Renal magnesium wasting is an early manifestation in more than half of the patients and may be accompanied by salt wasting and features of the renal Fanconi syndrome. Studies in animal models have identified vasoconstriction and interstitial inflammatory responses (neutrophils and T cells in particular) as important pathogenetic features. Long-term follow-up studies of cancer survivors suggest that the nephrotoxic injury persists after treatment is finished.[124]

Ifosfamide, a synthetic analogue of cyclophosphamide, is metabolized to chloroacetaldehyde, which is directly toxic to proximal tubular cells. Energy depletion via mitochondrial damage is thought to be an important pathogenetic mechanism. Disease severity is related to the dose and duration of therapy. Most patients develop tubular transport dysfunction that leads to hypophosphatemia, hypokalemia, metabolic acidosis, and polyuria in addition to reduced GFRs. Limited histologic data highlight tubular cell damage. Long-term follow-up studies have reported variable outcomes depending on the severity of the acute nephrotoxicity. The degree of the tubular dysfunction often improves, but impaired glomerular filtration often persists. Ten-year follow-up studies report a GFR $<$90 mL per minute in 21% and $<$60 mL per minute in 13% of patients.[125]

The nitrosoureas are a class of alkylating agents that have been associated with an insidious form of chronic TIN that develops slowly over 3 to 5 years in patients on long-term therapy. Histologically, the lesion is characterized by tubular atrophy and interstitial fibrosis.

Antimicrobials

Antibiotics are frequently implicated as causes of drug-induced and immunologically mediated TIN, the most common being the beta-lactams, cephalosporins, and sulfonamides. In addition, certain antimicrobials are known to be tubular cell nephrotoxins, especially aminoglycosides and amphotericin B. Gentamicin may cause AKI in as many as 10% to 20% of treated patients, despite drug level monitoring.[126] This high nephrotoxicity rate relates to drug uptake by megalin-mediated endocytosis in the proximal tubules, leading to intracellular levels that may be considerably higher than blood levels. The primary mechanism of injury is tubular cell death due to apoptosis and necrosis. There is histologic evidence from both humans and animal models that interstitial inflammation commonly occurs and is a mechanism of injury propagation.[127] Emerging evidence suggests that single daily dosing in patients with normal renal function may be therapeutically effective and reduce the risk of nephrotoxicity. Although the injury is thought to be reversible, chronic TIN may develop, especially with prolonged use. Long-term follow-up data are not yet available to address the possibility of gentamicin-induced nephrotoxicity as a CKD risk factor.

Amphotericin B reduces GFR in as many as 80% of treated patients. The newer lysosomal preparations are less nephrotoxic for reasons that are not entirely clear—absence of the deoxycholate moiety may be a partial explanation. Renal injury is targeted to distal nephrons within the medullary rays and the outer medulla. In experimental models, tubular injury is associated with evidence of tubulitis, interstitial inflammation, and fibrosis.[128] In addition to directly damaging tubular cells, amphotericin is thought to insert into tubular cell membranes, where it creates pores that may explain renal electrolyte wasting—potassium, magnesium, and bicarbonate in particular. Amphotericin also has direct vascular effects that induce vasoconstriction and hypoxia. In a retrospective review of 494 adults treated with amphotericin, 28% developed renal insufficiency; it was classified as moderate-to-severe (defined as doubling of baseline serum creatinine to $\geq$2.0 mg per dL) in 12%.[129] In the latter group, 70% had a serum creatinine $\geq$0.5 mg per dL above baseline at the time of discharge or death, illustrating the need for long-term follow-up studies to establish the risk of chronic TIN and CKD.

Antiretroviral medications used in combination (highly active antiretroviral therapy or HAART) have been associated with an overall decline in the incidence of CKD in patients with HIV-1 infection.[130] Nonetheless, several of these drugs are nephrotoxic and occasionally cause severe kidney injury. In a retrospective review of 7,378 patients in France, 4.7% had chronic kidney disease (eGFR $\leq$60 mL/min/1.73 m^2); recent exposures to indinavir, tenofovir, and abacavir were associated with an increased CKD risk.[131] Histopathologically, chronic TIN was most common, although different triggering mechanisms may be involved. Indinavir is a protease inhibitor that is known to cause a unique form of TIN associated with intratubular deposition of indinavir crystals, especially when high doses of the medication are used. Formation of renal stones has also been reported. Other protease inhibitors appear to be less nephrotoxic, although there are case reports of TIN and AKI. Now that lower doses are prescribed, protease inhibitor nephrotoxicity is rarely encountered. The nephrotoxic effects of the nucleotide reverse-transcriptase inhibitors, especially tenofovir, are well-established and most common when used in conjunction with protease inhibitor drugs ($\sim$12% incidence). The proximal tubule, where the drug accumulates via the organic anion transporter 1, is the primary target of injury. Evidence of tubular dysfunction (proteinuria, glycosuria, urinary phosphate washing) often precedes measurable changes in GFR. Ultrastructural changes in tubular mitochondria have been highlighted. Evidence of chronic TIN on biopsy and outcome studies suggests that renal injury does not reverse in a significant number of patients ($\sim$25%) after the drug is discontinued.[132]

Nonsteroidal Anti-inflammatory Drugs

The nonsteroidal anti-inflammatory drugs (NSAIDs) have renal effects that can cause chronic TIN by at least three distinct mechanisms. Through effects on prostaglandin metabolism, NSAIDs may alter renal hemodynamics in vulnerable patient groups. These renal effects are generally reversible, but may lead to acute tubular necrosis and its sequelae. Via an idiosyncratic dose-independent mechanism, the NSAIDs may also cause acute interstitial nephritis, typically without fever or rash, but with eosinophilia reported in 40% of cases. A unique feature of NSAID-induced TIN is its frequent association with nephrotic syndrome due to a minimal change-like disease or, rarely, due to membranous nephropathy. This entity has been reported with virtually all of the nonselective NSAIDs, although most commonly with fenoprofen.[133] Schwarz et al.[121] reported that 56% of patients with biopsy-confirmed NSAID-induced TIN had permanent renal functional impairment after the offending agent was discontinued. The third entity, known as analgesic nephropathy, was an important cause of CKD until the disease was recognized and prevention strategies implemented. This slowly progressive kidney disease, characterized by chronic TIN that is often associated with papillary necrosis (25% to 40%), is caused by prolonged daily consumption of combinations of analgesics, usually in conjunction with centrally acting, dependency-inducing substances such as caffeine, codeine, or barbiturates. The damage is most severe in the medulla, often leading to calcification of the medullary pyramids. CT scans have been diagnostically useful in advanced cases, as the small kidneys often have bumpy renal contours and medullary calcifications (Fig. 57.17). It has been suggested that the primary target is capillary endothelial cells that become sclerosed and that the primary offending agent is phenacetin and its metabolites, although

Analgesic nephropthy

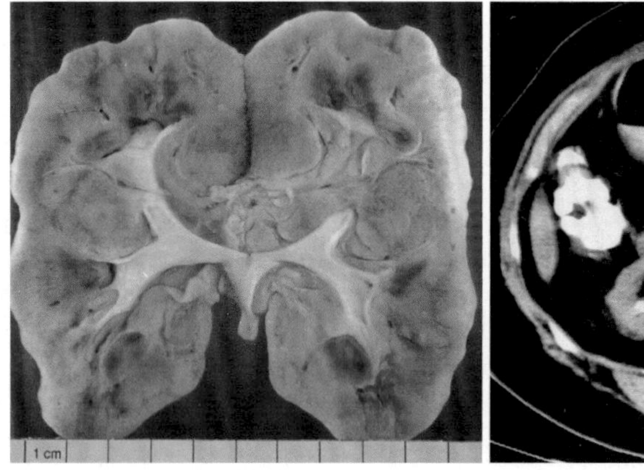

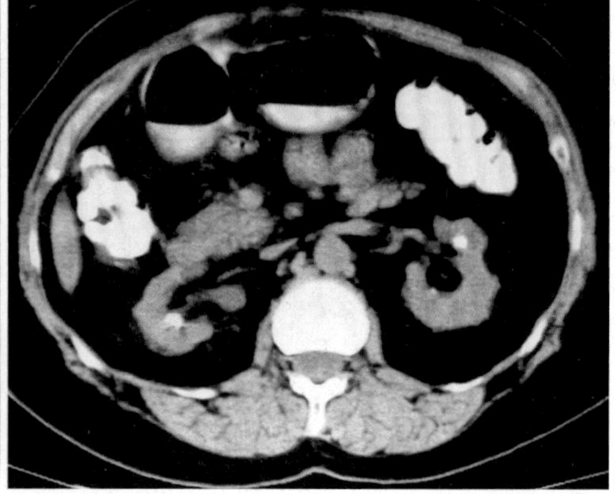

Calcineurin inhibitor nephrotoxicity

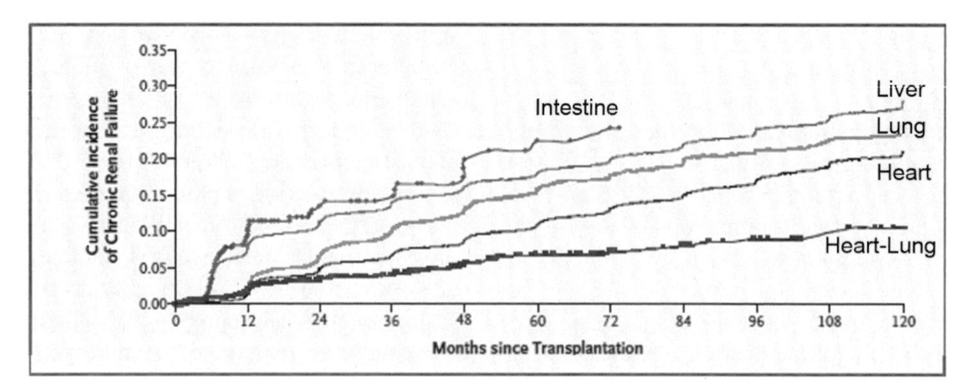

FIGURE 57.17 Drug-induced chronic tubulointerstitial nephritis (TIN). Prolonged ingestion of analgesic combinations may cause analgesic nephropathy. The prototypic disease is characterized by small kidneys with bumpy contours (shown in macroscopic view of an end-stage kidney on the upper left), which is apparent on a computed tomography scan (upper right). (From De Broe ME, Elseviers MM. Over-the-counter analgesic use. *J Am Soc Nephrol.* 2009;20:2103, with permission.) The calcineurin inhibitors have well-recognized dose-related nephrotoxic effects that are characterized by arteriolar vasculopathy and chronic TIN. The high incidence of end-stage renal disease in nonrenal solid organ transplant recipients highlights the potential severity of this nephrotoxicity, even after taking into consideration that multiple factors likely contribute to chronic kidney disease in this complex patient cohort. (From Ojo AO, Held PJ, Port FK, et al. Chronic renal failure after transplantation of a nonrenal organ. *N Engl J Med.* 2003;349:931, with permission.)

neither hypothesis has been definitely proven. Once an important cause of ESRD in countries where these combination analgesics products were available, the incidence of analgesic nephropathy has declined since many of the combined analgesics have been discontinued.

Calcineurin Inhibitors

Although cyclosporine and tacrolimus are structurally unrelated, they both inhibit calcineurin as its primary immunosuppressive mechanism, and this effect appears to account for their shared nephrotoxicity.[134,135] Although still a topic of some debate, tacrolimus appears to be slightly less nephrotoxic. The classic histopathologic lesion of chronic calcineurin inhibitor (CNI) nephropathy is chronic TIN that develops in association with a progressive arteriopathy, characterized by nodular hyaline deposits and eventual vascular occlusion. This arteriolar lesion is considered the primary CNI-induced renal lesion, which causes ischemic changes and secondary chronic TIN. However, CNI can directly activate other cellular pathways that likely lead to renal injury, including activation of the RAS, TGF-β production, and tubular cell apoptosis. The risk and severity of chronic TIN are related to drug levels and duration of therapy. Given the overlap between histologic features of CNI nephropathy and other causes of renal allograft dysfunction, including rejection, the undisputed recognition of CNI nephropathy as a distinct entity came from studies of extrarenal transplant recipients and from patients with autoimmune disease. In the early years of CNI therapy, a significant number of nonrenal transplant patients on CNI therapy eventually developed ESRD, highlighting the potent nephrotoxic potential of these drugs (Fig. 57.17).[136] The cornerstone of prevention remains dose optimization to control the primary disease process (such as rejection prevention) with the lowest possible drug doses. It has been reported that kidney CNI drug levels are higher than blood levels, which likely explains the specific vulnerability of this organ to drug toxicity.

The CNI drugs are also known to induce functional renal hemodynamic changes as a result of vasoconstriction of the afferent and efferent arterioles. These effects are considered reversible, but they may lead to significant acute changes in glomerular filtration rates. When this occurs in the face of preexisting renal ischemia and acute tubular necrosis, renal recovery may be delayed, leading to long-term fibrotic TIN sequelae. Calcium channel blockers have been used as a strategy to counteract these vasoconstrictive effects. Evidence of CNI nephrotoxicity may also be suggested by the presence of tubular dysfunction, which leads to hyperkalemia, metabolic acidosis, hyperuricemia, and urinary phosphate and magnesium wasting.

Herbal Medicines

The nephrotoxicity of plant-derived herbal medications is increasingly recognized.[137] The kidney is thought to be particularly vulnerable because it is responsible for excretion of most herbal substances. Chronic TIN has been reported as a complication of long-term use of certain herbal products, the best documented being aristolochic acid (AA). The entity of AA nephropathy was first reported in Belgium in 1991 when women taking AA as part of a weight loss regimen developed CKD. Eventually 300 cases were identified in Belgium, 70% progressing to ESRD within a relatively short time.[138] The histopathology is unique for the intensity of the interstitial fibrotic reaction in the cortex, often with relatively sparse interstitial inflammation. A high proportion of these patients (40% to 45%) also developed urothelial malignancies. AA nephropathy has now been identified worldwide. Despite the fact that AA has been banned in many countries, it is still present in several herbal products. Animal models of AA nephropathy have been developed. Although the disease pathogenesis is not completely understood, arterioles and proximal tubular cells appear to be the primary targets of injury. AA is also considered the leading candidate as the environmental trigger of Balkan endemic nephropathy (BEN). This familial but not inherited type of CKD was first reported in the late 1950s in individuals living in rural communities near branches of the Danube River in Bosnia, Bulgaria, Croatia, Romania, and Serbia.[138,139] By histopathology, BEN is chronic TIN with tubular atrophy and interstitial fibrosis but modest interstitial inflammation that is more severe in the outer cortex. A series of epidemiologic studies support the hypothesis that contamination of the wheat fields in the endemic region by AA is the primary environmental cause of the endemic nephropathy. A unique clinical feature of this group of patients is their high risk of developing urothelial cancer. Many of the identified patients with BEN have developed ESRD.

Lithium

Patients with bipolar disorders who are treated with long-term lithium therapy (10 to 20 years) may develop chronic TIN. The overall incidence is unclear, the onset is insidious, and the rate of disease progression is typically slow, although a small number do develop ESRD.[140] The only predictive factors are duration of therapy and cumulative lithium dose; daily doses and drug levels have not differed between the chronic TIN and unaffected patients. The primary susceptible kidney cell is the principal cell of the collecting duct, where apical sodium channels (ENaC) transport lithium into the cells.[141] Based on this physiology, a hypothetical consideration is the possibility that ENaC inhibition by concomitant use of amiloride might reduce the risk of chronic TIN. Once the disease is well established, discontinuing lithium may not alter the rate of subsequent renal functional decline. Lithium has other effects that may reversibly compromise renal function. Up to 40% of treated patients develop nephrogenic diabetes due to lithium-induced alterations in the expression and trafficking of the vasopressin-regulated water channel aquaporin 2. A significant number of patients (25% to 35%) develop hyperparathyroidism and hypercalcemia that may contribute to chronic TIN.

Heavy Metals

Through a series of unfortunate environmental and occupational exposures, heavy metal-induced kidney disease has been well documented. Because of its ability to reabsorb and store divalent metals, the kidney is typically the primary target organ of toxicity. Lead and cadmium are most commonly implicated as the cause of chronic TIN.[142] Both of these heavy metals primarily target proximal tubular cells, with exposure over many years leading to insidious-onset chronic TIN and renal insufficiency.

Two of the best documented examples of lead nephropathy derive from a cohort of Australian patients with ESRD who shared in common childhood lead poisoning due to exposure to lead-based paints and adults exposed to illegal moonshine whiskey made in lead containers such as radiators. Animal models of lead-induced nephropathy have been developed. Legislation has greatly reduced environmental lead exposure in developed countries by eliminating lead-based paints and lead-containing gasoline, but exposure risk still occurs, especially in poor urban areas, with certain industrial occupations, and in certain unregulated import products. The diagnosis can be inferred by evidence of chronic TIN and an appropriate exposure history. Although the half-life of plasma lead is short (30 days), it extends to 10 to 30 years once lead is deposited in bone. For this reason, plasma levels are not reliable predictors of the total body lead burden. When a definitive diagnosis is desired, the bioavailable pool has been estimated by measuring plasma lead levels after calcium disodium ethylenediaminetetraacetic acid (EDTA) infusion or by bone imaging studies. Although the entity of classic lead nephropathy is now considered rare, recent public health studies have focused on the effects of low-dose lead exposure as an accelerating factor for patients with other causes of CKD.[143] There is ongoing interest in a possible pathologic relationship between lead-related nephrotoxicity, impaired uric acid excretion, and hyperuricemia and its associated complications.

Cadmium occurs naturally in combination with zinc. Following ingestion, it complexes with the low molecular weight protein metallothionein and is efficiently reabsorbed by proximal tubular cells. At this site, metallothionein appears to serve a protective role; when the complex is degraded and cadmium ions are released into the cytosol, tubular cell toxicity ensues. With chronic cadmium exposure, chronic TIN may develop. The urinary cadmium-to-creatinine ratio has been used to estimate the cadmium burden. Numerous household, environmental, and occupational sources of exposure have been identified. One of the best characterized environmental epidemics occurred in Japan as a consequence of soil contamination by an upstream mine, leading to high cadmium levels in rice fields. Affected individuals developed severe bone pain due to associated osteomalacia—"itai-itai-byo" or "ouch-ouch" disease—that was associated with chronic TIN in patients with the most severe disease.

ABNORMALITIES IN MINERAL METABOLISM

Hypercalcemia/Hypercalciuria

In addition to the risk of prerenal azotemia due to afferent arteriolar vasoconstriction, sustained hypercalcemia and/or hypercalciuria can impair renal function due to recurrent nephrolithiasis and nephrocalcinosis. The latter is characterized by calcium phosphate or calcium oxalate deposition in tubular lumina and the renal interstitium in association with parenchymal damage due to chronic TIN. Calcification typically involves the medulla (97%), although cortical nephrocalcinosis has been reported, especially in conjunction with severe cortical diseases, renal allograft rejection, and oxalosis. Hypercalciuria is the primary etiology in most patients. Why some people develop stones and others develop nephrocalcinosis remains unknown—they may occur together. Hypercalcemia may be a predisposing factor, but several renal tubular disorders are associated with nephrocalcinosis in the absence of hypercalcemia. The most common are distal renal tubular acidosis, medullary sponge kidney, premature kidneys, use of loop diuretics, vitamin D therapy, certain inherited tubular disorders, sarcoidosis (less than 50% are hypercalcemic), and conditions associated with increased urinary excretion of phosphate or oxalate. Histopathology may identify calcium deposits within tubular lumina (likely adherent to apical membrane osteopontin or hyaluronan), within tubular epithelial cells, and/or in the interstitium. Interstitial inflammation and fibrosis are usually present and associated with evidence of tubular cell injury and/or atrophy. Clinical manifestations usually relate to the underlying disorder; nephrocalcinosis itself is generally asymptomatic except for polyuria due to impaired urinary concentrating mechanism.[144] The diagnosis of nephrocalcinosis is typically made by renal imaging (Fig. 57.8). The renal prognosis depends on the underlying etiology and the ability to reverse hypercalciuria and the associated conditions that promote renal calcification. For example, in premature infants with nephrocalcinosis, renal ultrasounds are normal in 75% to 90% by age 7.5 years, whereas progressive kidney disease is the rule in children with primary hyperoxaluria.[145] For many, nephrocalcinosis is not reversible but specific medical interventions to reduce further calcification can effectively preserve renal function. ESRD due to nephrocalcinosis-associated chronic TIN is unusual.

Hyperphosphatemia/Hyperphosphaturia

The entity of acute phosphate nephropathy reported in association with the use of oral sodium phosphate bowel purgatives has refocused attention on the importance of hyperphosphaturia as a mediator of acute TIN, which may progress to chronic TIN and irreversible renal functional impairment. Renal histologic data were obtained from a cohort of 21 patients who underwent renal biopsies 2 to 8 months (mean 3.8 months) after a phosphate enema was used as preparation for a colonoscopy and associated with subsequent AKI;

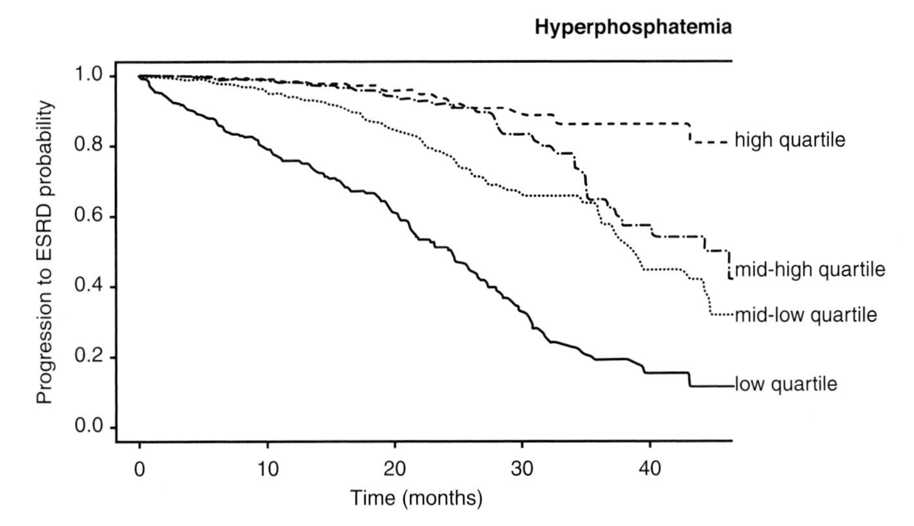

FIGURE 57.18 Hyperphosphatemia as an acquired metabolic cause of chronic tubulointerstitial nephritis (TIN). In addition to the well-known nephrotoxic effects of acute severe hyperphosphatemia, there is a growing body of evidence suggesting that hyperphosphatemia may also play a pathogenetic role in the genesis of the chronic TIN that characterizes all progressive kidney diseases. The graph is from an Italian study of 1,716 patients with chronic kidney disease, which showed a significant relationship between serum phosphorus levels (divided into quartiles) and the rate of progression to end-stage renal disease. (From Bellasi A, Mandreoli M, Baldrati L, et al. Chronic kidney disease progression and outcome according to serum phosphorus in mild-to-moderate kidney dysfunction. *Clin J Am Soc Nephrol.* 2011;6:883, with permission.)

the results showed widespread von Kossa positive calcium phosphate deposits in tubular lamina, tubular epithelial cells, and the peritubular interstitium.[146,147] These changes were associated with evidence of chronic injury—tubular atrophy and interstitial fibrosis. Despite a mean serum creatinine level of 1.0 mg per dL (0.6–1.7 range) pre-colonoscopy, only four patients had a creatinine level less than 2.0 mg per dL at the time of renal biopsy and four patients progressed to ESRD. Although this study is biased to patients with severe AKI following acute oral phosphate loading, it highlights the potential for extreme hyperphosphaturia to cause both acute and chronic TIN. Because the primary pathogenetic mechanisms have not been fully elucidated, it remains possible that hyperphosphatemia also plays a direct role, as suggested by clinical epidemiologic evidence for a significant relationship between the degree of hyperphosphatemia and the rate of CKD progression (Fig. 57.18).[148,149]

Acute, severe hyperphosphatemia caused by the sudden release of endogenous intracellular phosphate can also cause AKI due to calcium phosphate deposition and tubulointerstitial injury. This is a well-recognized complication of acute rhabdomyolysis and tumor lysis syndrome. With the routine use of optimal hydration and rasburicase, the incidence of acute urate nephropathy in patients at risk for tumor lysis has declined substantially, and hyperphosphatemia has become the primary metabolic complication associated with AKI in patients with tumor lysis syndrome. In light of the recent recognition of the risk of chronic TIN following acute phosphate nephropathy, all of these patients deserve long-term follow-up for evidence of CKD.

Hyperuricemia/Hyperuricosuria

In addition to uric acid nephrolithiasis, hyperuricemia may induce tubulointerstitial injury by alternative mechanisms. Best characterized is the entity of acute uric acid nephropathy that frequently developed as a complication of tumor lysis syndrome in the era before effective prevention strategies were employed. Renal failure was associated with acute tubular injury due to the deposition of undissociated uric acid within tubules. A chronic form of TIN is also thought to occur as a result of monosodium urate crystal deposition in medullary tubules, where the crystals induce tubular injury, interstitial inflammation, and fibrosis.[150] However, the prevalence of the entity of chronic crystal–associated uric acid nephropathy has been difficult to establish, due to the frequent presence of potentially confounding variables. For example, many of the earlier studies of chronic urate nephropathy are now thought to represent lead nephrotoxicity. A form of autosomal-dominant chronic TIN associated with hyperuricemia is now known to be caused by a mutation in the gene that encodes the urinary protein uromodulin—the hyperuricemia is no longer believed to serve a primary pathogenetic role. Many of the patients thought to have "gouty nephropathy" also have hypertension and metabolic syndrome but rarely undergo renal biopsy to establish a diagnosis of chronic urate TIN. Perhaps one of the most compelling arguments in support of the existence of chronic urate nephropathy in humans derives from boys with Lesch-Nyhan syndrome, who have been reported to develop increased echogenicity of the medullary pyramids visualized by renal ultrasound.

Rodent models of urate nephropathy have been developed; these models have taken advantage of the fact that hyperuricemia can be induced by inhibiting the uric acid-degrading enzyme uricase.[151] However, the relevance of this model to humans has been questioned, as humans lack uricase and normally have serum uric acid levels that are considerably higher than the rats with nephropathy. Studies based on the rodent models suggest that the primary pathogenic mechanism is not related to crystal-induced injury. Rather, it is proposed that soluble uric acid induces renal microvascular injury and arteriolopathy, with chronic TIN developing as a consequence of hypoxic injury.[152,153] Building on this potential mechanistic paradigm, human epidemiologic studies are now investigating the role of serum uric acid as a pathogenetic factor in patients with hypertension, diabetes-associated vascular disease, and CKD. In several studies of healthy individuals with normal renal function, such as the one reported by Obermayr et al.,[154] the risk for incident kidney disease is higher in those with elevated uric acid levels.

Hypokalemia

Potassium depletion may lead to acute, reversible changes in renal tubular function, especially impaired urinary concentration. Longstanding hypokalemia has been reported to cause chronic, irreversible TIN in both humans and animal models, an entity referred to as "hypokalemia nephropathy."[155] Histopathologically, it is characterized by early renal tubular cell hyperplasia and late tubular atrophy, interstitial inflammation, and fibrosis. The changes are greatest in the outer medulla and may be associated with formation of small cysts. This entity is most commonly reported in patients with severe and prolonged hypokalemia, typically caused by malnutrition or the abuse of laxatives or diuretics in patients with eating disorders. CKD and ESRD have been reported. The early tubular functional changes associated with shorter duration hypokalemia are reversible with potassium repletion. Although the pathogenesis of hypokalemia nephropathy is incompletely understood, studies in animal models have identified renal vasoconstriction, interstitial capillary rarefaction, ammonia-mediated complement activation, and growth factor and cytokine activity as features of this chronic TIN process. In some patients it may be challenging to differentiate between hypokalemia as consequence or a cause of chronic TIN.

CHRONIC TIN IN ONCO-HEMATOLOGIC DISORDERS

AKI is a relatively common complication in patients with malignancies, and a variety of potential mechanisms have been identified.[156,157] Long-term renal sequelae in cancer survivors is a topic of current interest, but very little is known about the specific risk of CKD due to chronic TIN. Efforts to determine this risk are complicated by the fact that many of the patients have comorbidities, including several that could be risk factors for AKI. The most important include exposure to nephrotoxic agents (especially chemotherapeutic agents and antimicrobial drugs), infectious processes, and sepsis syndromes with renal hypoperfusion. Each of these imposes a small potential risk of residual chronic TIN.

Malignant cells may also invade the renal parenchyma (Fig. 57.19). Leukemia and lymphoma are well-established causes of TIN. Autopsy-based studies suggest that such involvement is relatively common, but is typically silent clinically, occurring in as many as one third of patients with Hodgkin lymphoma and 60% with acute leukemia. In a series of adults with acute lymphoblastic leukemia, 10% had enlarged kidneys whereas only 0.4% had clinical evidence of renal disease.[158] Although there are case reports of severe AKI in patients presenting with enlarged kidneys due to leukemic or lymphomatous infiltrates, superimposed tumor lysis syndrome may be a significant contributing factor. Overall, the risk of chronic TIN due to malignant-cell associated acute TIN appears to be low.

The unique malignancy-associated tubulointerstitial disease that carries a risk of progression to chronic TIN occurs in patients with multiple myeloma.[159,160] Almost 50% of newly diagnosed patients have evidence of renal functional impairment, a complication that significantly reduces survival rates (less than 1 year in patients with severe kidney injury). Tubulointerstitial disease is the primary pattern of injury, with a propensity to progress rapidly to chronic TIN. At least four distinct patterns of TIN have been identified, sharing a common primary pathogenetic mechanism pertaining to the plasma cell dyscrasia that leads to the overproduction of free immunoglobulin light chains (kappa or lambda). These light chains appear to owe their nephrotoxic potential to unique physiochemical properties that differ from normal immunoglobulins.

1. *Proximal tubular dysfunction.* Low molecular weight (~22 kDa) light chains are freely filtered by the glomerulus and reabsorbed in the proximal tubule by megalin-cubilin-dependent endocytosis. Certain abnormal light chains appear to resist intralysosomal degradation and may even form intracellular crystals. These features are thought to be associated with cytotoxic effects, characterized by the production of inflammatory cytokines, TGF-β, interstitial inflammation, tubular cell apoptosis, and interstitial fibrosis.
2. *Myeloma cast nephropathy* (Fig. 57.19). This classical pattern of tubulointerstitial injury is characterized by the formation of obstructing intratubular casts that contain aggregates of the abnormal light chain together with uromodulin (Tamm-Horsfall protein). Disease risk is correlated with the level of light chain excretion. The severity of the chronic TIN correlates with the degree of renal functional impairment.
3. *Interstitial nephritis.* A less common pattern of injury, acute TIN may be a consequence of light chain deposition along tubular basement membranes.

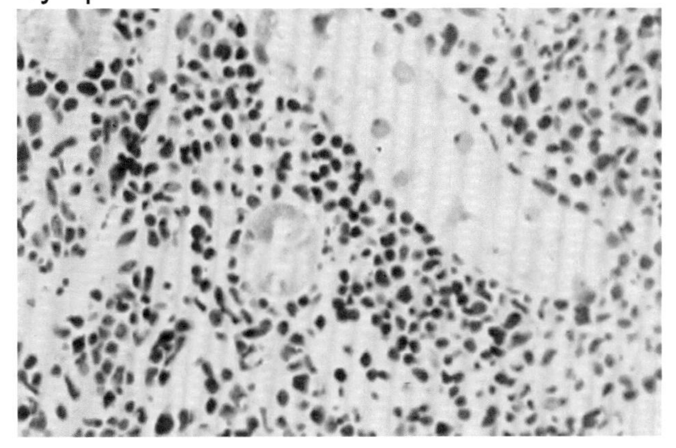

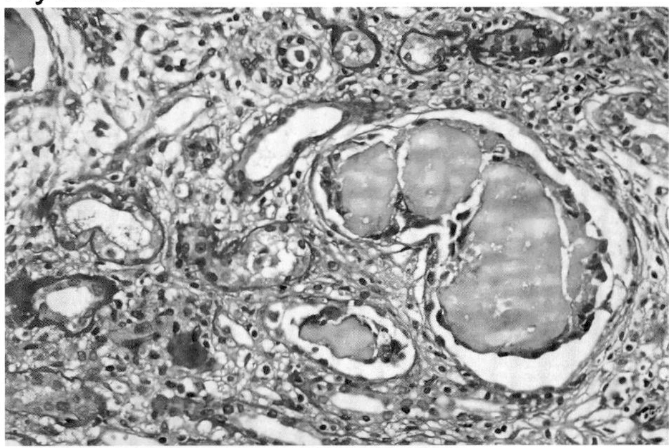

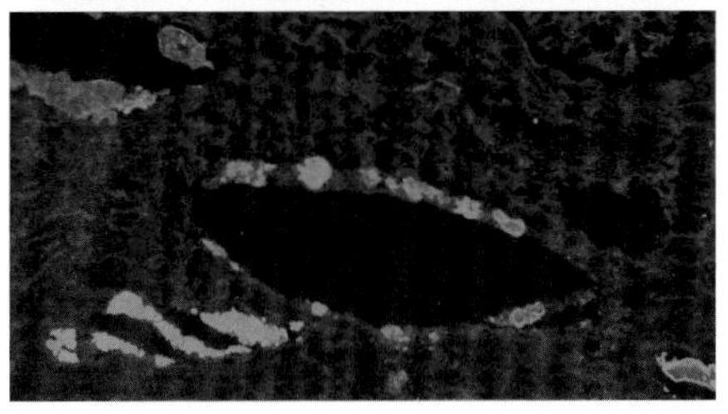

FIGURE 57.19 Hematologic malignancies as a cause of chronic tubulointerstitial nephritis (TIN). The renal interstitium can be directly infiltrated by malignant cells, as shown in the upper photomicrograph of a diagnostic renal biopsy performed on a patient who presented with renal failure and enlarged kidneys of unknown etiology. It revealed a monomorphic interstitial infiltrate of lymphoma cells. The middle photomicrograph shows an example of myeloma cast nephropathy, which is characterized by obstructing tubular casts with a characteristic fractured appearance and evidence of chronic TIN. The lower immunofluorescence photomicrograph illustrates lambda light chains in tubular casts and protein reabsorption droplets. As expected, staining for kappa light chains was negative. (Multiple myeloma photomicrographs were provided by Dr. Agnes Fogo, Department of Pathology, Vanderbilt University.)

4. *Plasma cell infiltration.* A rare cause of TIN is direct interstitial invasion by the abnormal plasma cells. Other types of myeloma-associated kidney disease involve the glomeruli, associated with variable degrees of chronic TIN depending on disease severity. The latter group of diseases typically cause glomerular proteinuria and include amyloidosis, cryoglobulinemia, and monoclonal immunoglobulin deposition diseases. The specific properties that render myeloma-derived light chains nephrotoxic remain unclear but may be related to their ability to form aggregates, bind to uromodulin, resist lysosomal degradation, and/or mediate tubular cell toxicity. There is considerable variability in the nephrotoxic effects of various free light chains. Early initiation of chemotherapy to eradicate the dysplastic plasma cells and stop free light chain production before severe TIN has developed is the most effective strategy to prevent progressive kidney damage. Although still a debated topic, current data suggest that therapeutic apheresis adds no additional benefit to current immunotherapy.

The classic nonmalignant hematologic disorder known to cause CKD is sickle cell disease, which is reviewed in greater detail in Chapter 62.[161,162] It is estimated that 5% to 18% of patients with sickle cell disease will develop ESRD, typically between 30 and 40 years of age. Proteinuria, an early marker of renal dysfunction, is reported in 40% of patients. In addition to a higher incidence of certain glomerular diseases, a unique renal disorder termed "sickle cell nephropathy" is the most common etiology. Its pathogenesis remains unproven, but the current prevailing view is one of hypoxia-induced chronic tubular damage as a consequence of erythrocyte sickling and sludging in the vasa recta within the hypoxic, acidemic, and hypertonic environment of the renal medulla. During this early phase, deficits in urinary concentration are common. Severe ischemic injury may also lead to papillary necrosis. The unproven but presumed essential secondary step is glomerular hyperperfusion, as a consequence of the production of vasodilating substances such as prostaglandins and nitric oxide. Early glomerular hypertrophy, with a high GFR, progresses to glomerulosclerosis and CKD due to interstitial inflammation and fibrosis. The presence of tubular hemosiderin deposits suggests a potential role for iron-related nephrotoxicity.

SUMMARY

Recent advances in the understanding of the cellular and molecular biology of chronic TIN as the final common pathway of all CKD—whether they start in the glomerular, tubulointerstitial, or vascular compartments—offer new opportunities to identify and treat patients at risk for kidney disease progression. Future genetic studies are likely to identify a series of genetic determinants of kidney fibrosis, and new therapeutics directed at specific molecular targets offer promise of the ability to attenuate fibrosis severity and enhance renal parenchymal repair and protection. Advances in the field of stem cell and regenerative medicine offer hope that one day we will have the tools to reverse fibrosis and regenerate intact nephrons within regions of renal parenchymal scarring. An increasing number of ongoing research studies are making creative use of human kidney biopsy material to identify distinct molecular and cellular profiles that characterize high-risk patients who would benefit from such therapies.

REFERENCES

1. Pan X, Suzuki N, Hirano I, et al. Isolation and characterization of renal erythropoietin-producing cells from genetically produced anemia mice. *PLoS One*. 2011;6:e25839.
2. Asada N, Takase M, Nakamura J, et al. Dysfunction of fibroblasts of extrarenal origin underlies renal fibrosis and renal anemia in mice. *J Clin Invest*. 2011;121:3981.
3. Humphreys BD, Lin SL, Kobayashi A, et al. Fate tracing reveals the pericyte and not epithelial origin of myofibroblasts in kidney fibrosis. *Am J Pathol*. 2010;176:85.
4. Pitcock JA, Brown PS, Brooks B, et al. The morphology and antihypertensive effect of renomedullary interstitial cells derived from Dahl sensitive and resistant rats. *Exp Mol Pathol*. 1985;42:29.
5. Reule S, Gupta S. Kidney regeneration and resident stem cells. *Organogenesis*. 2011;7:135.
6. Oliver JA, Klinakis A, Cheema FH, et al. Proliferation and migration of label-retaining cells of the kidney papilla. *J Am Soc Nephrol*. 2009;20:2315.
7. Humphreys BD, Czerniak S, DiRocco DP, et al. Repair of injured proximal tubule does not involve specialized progenitors. *Proc Natl Acad Sci U S A*. 2011;108:9226.
8. Eddy AA. Molecular basis of renal fibrosis. *Pediatr Nephrol*. 2000;15:290.
9. Eddy AA. Progression in chronic kidney disease. *Adv Chronic Kidney Dis*. 2005;12:353.
10. Schlondorff DO. Overview of factors contributing to the pathophysiology of progressive renal disease. *Kidney Int*. 2008;74:860.
11. Boor P, Ostendorf T, Floege J. Renal fibrosis: novel insights into mechanisms and therapeutic targets. *Nat Rev Nephrol*. 2010;6:643.
12. Liu Y. Cellular and molecular mechanisms of renal fibrosis. *Nat Rev Nephrol*. 2011;7:684.
13. Kaissling B, Le Hir M. The renal cortical interstitium: morphological and functional aspects. *Histochem Cell Biol*. 2008;130:247.
14. Yang L, Besschetnova TY, Brooks CR, et al. Epithelial cell cycle arrest in G2/M mediates kidney fibrosis after injury. *Nat Med*. 2010;16:535.
15. Li L, Zepeda-Orozco D, Black R, et al. Autophagy is a component of epithelial cell fate in obstructive uropathy. *Am J Pathol*. 2010;176:1767.
16. Kimura T, Takabatake Y, Takahashi A, et al. Autophagy protects the proximal tubule from degeneration and acute ischemic injury. *J Am Soc Nephrol*. 2011;22:902.
17. Togel F, Hu Z, Weiss K, et al. Administered mesenchymal stem cells protect against ischemic acute renal failure through differentiation-independent mechanisms. *Am J Physiol Renal Physiol*. 2005;289:F31.
18. Duffield JS, Bonventre JV. Kidney tubular epithelium is restored without replacement with bone marrow-derived cells during repair after ischemic injury. *Kidney Int*. 2005;68:1956.
19. Ricardo SD, van Goor H, Eddy AA. Macrophage diversity in renal injury and repair. *J Clin Invest*. 2008;118:3522.
20. Lee S, Huen S, Nishio H, et al. Distinct macrophage phenotypes contribute to kidney injury and repair. *J Am Soc Nephrol*. 2011;22:317.
21. Duffield JS. Macrophages in kidney repair and regeneration. *J Am Soc Nephrol*. 2011;22:199.
22. Anders HJ, Muruve DA. The inflammasomes in kidney disease. *J Am Soc Nephrol*. 2011;22:1007.
23. Snelgrove SL, Kausman JY, Lo C, et al. Renal dendritic cells adopt a pro-inflammatory phenotype in obstructive uropathy to activate T cells but do not directly contribute to fibrosis. *Am J Pathol*. 2012;180:91.
24. Hinz B, Phan SH, Thannickal VJ, et al. The myofibroblast: one function, multiple origins. *Am J Pathol*. 2007;170:1807.
25. Lin SL, Kisseleva T, Brenner DA, et al. Pericytes and perivascular fibroblasts are the primary source of collagen-producing cells in obstructive fibrosis of the kidney. *Am J Pathol*. 2008;173:1617.
26. Iwano M, Plieth D, Danoff TM, et al. Evidence that fibroblasts derive from epithelium during tissue fibrosis. *J Clin Invest*. 2002;110:341.
27. Zeisberg EM, Potenta SE, Sugimoto H, et al. Fibroblasts in kidney fibrosis emerge via endothelial-to-mesenchymal transition. *J Am Soc Nephrol*. 2008; 19:2282.
28. Bechtel W, McGoohan S, Zeisberg EM, et al. Methylation determines fibroblast activation and fibrogenesis in the kidney. *Nat Med*. 2010;16:544.
29. Ferenbach D, Kluth DC, Hughes J. Inflammatory cells in renal injury and repair. *Semin Nephrol*. 2007;27:250.
30. Wynn TA. Common and unique mechanisms regulate fibrosis in various fibroproliferative diseases. *J Clin Invest*. 2007;117:524.
31. Zhong X, Chung AC, Chen HY, et al. Smad3-mediated upregulation of miR-21 promotes renal fibrosis. *J Am Soc Nephrol*. 2011;22:1668.
32. Prunotto M, Gabbiani G, Pomposiello S, et al. The kidney as a target organ in pharmaceutical research. *Drug Discov Today*. 2011;16:244–259.
33. Boor P, Sebekova K, Ostendorf T, et al. Treatment targets in renal fibrosis. *Nephrol Dial Transplant*. 2007;22:3391.
34. Choi YJ, Chakraborty S, Nguyen V, et al. Peritubular capillary loss is associated with chronic tubulointerstitial injury in human kidney: altered expression of vascular endothelial growth factor. *Hum Pathol*. 2000;31:1491.
35. Ishii Y, Sawada T, Kubota K, et al. Loss of peritubular capillaries in the development of chronic allograft nephropathy. *Transplant Proc*. 2005;37:981.
36. Ohashi R, Shimizu A, Masuda Y, et al. Peritubular capillary regression during the progression of experimental obstructive nephropathy. *J Am Soc Nephrol*. 2002;13:1795.
37. Yamaguchi I, Tchao BN, Burger ML, et al. Vascular endothelial cadherin modulates renal interstitial fibrosis. *Nephron Exp Nephrol*. 2011;120:e20.
38. Mimura I, Nangaku M. The suffocating kidney: tubulointerstitial hypoxia in end-stage renal disease. *Nat Rev Nephrol*. 2010;6:667.
39. Mayer G. Capillary rarefaction, hypoxia, VEGF and angiogenesis in chronic renal disease. *Nephrol Dial Transplant*. 2011;26:1132.
40. Goligorsky MS, Rabelink T. Meeting report: ISN forefronts in nephrology on endothelial biology and renal disease: from bench to prevention. *Kidney Int*. 2006;70:258.
41. Pober JS, Min W, Bradley JR. Mechanisms of endothelial dysfunction, injury, and death. *Annu Rev Pathol*. 2009;4:71.
42. Eddy AA, Fogo AB. Plasminogen activator inhibitor-1 in chronic kidney disease: evidence and mechanisms of action. *J Am Soc Nephrol*. 2006;17:2999.
43. Lopez-Guisa JM, Cai X, Collins SJ, et al. Mannose receptor 2 attenuates renal fibrosis. *J Am Soc Nephrol*. 2012;23:236.
44. Eddy AA. Serine proteases, inhibitors and receptors in renal fibrosis. *Thromb Haemost*. 2009;101:656.
45. Vyletal P, Bleyer AJ, Kmoch S. Uromodulin biology and pathophysiology - an update. *Kidney Blood Press Res*. 2010;33:456.
46. Bleyer AJ, Zivna M, Kmoch S. Uromodulin-associated kidney disease. *Nephron Clin Pract*. 2011;118:c31.
47. Bollee G, Dahan K, Flamant M, et al. Phenotype and outcome in hereditary tubulointerstitial nephritis secondary to UMOD mutations. *Clin J Am Soc Nephrol*. 2011;6:2429.
48. Eddy AA. Scraping fibrosis: UMODulating renal fibrosis. *Nat Med*. 2011;17:553.
49. Zivna M, Hulkova H, Matignon M, et al. Dominant renin gene mutations associated with early-onset hyperuricemia, anemia, and chronic kidney failure. *Am J Hum Genet*. 2009;85:204.
50. Hildebrandt F, Attanasio M, Otto E. Nephronophthisis: disease mechanisms of a ciliopathy. *J Am Soc Nephrol*. 2009;20:23.
51. Salomon R, Saunier S, Niaudet P. Nephronophthisis. *Pediatr Nephrol*. 2009; 24:2333.
52. Simms RJ, Eley L, Sayer JA. Nephronophthisis. *Eur J Hum Genet*. 2009;17:406.
53. Zeier M, Fehrenbach P, Geberth S, et al. Renal histology in polycystic kidney disease with incipient and advanced renal failure. *Kidney Int*. 1992;42:1259.
54. Grantham JJ. The etiology, pathogenesis, and treatment of autosomal dominant polycystic kidney disease: recent advances. *Am J Kidney Dis*. 1996;28:788.
55. Mrug M, Zhou J, Woo Y, et al. Overexpression of innate immune response genes in a model of recessive polycystic kidney disease. *Kidney Int*. 2008;73:63.
56. Karihaloo A, Koraishy F, Huen SC, et al. Macrophages promote cyst growth in polycystic kidney disease. *J Am Soc Nephrol*. 2011;22:1809.
57. Gattone VH II, Cowley BD Jr, Barash BD, et al. Methylprednisolone retards the progression of inherited polycystic kidney disease in rodents. *Am J Kidney Dis*. 1995;25:302.
58. Norman J. Fibrosis and progression of autosomal dominant polycystic kidney disease (ADPKD). *Biochim Biophys Acta*. 2011;1812:1327.
59. Wilmer MJ, Schoeber JP, van den Heuvel LP, et al. Cystinosis: practical tools for diagnosis and treatment. *Pediatr Nephrol*. 2011;26:205.

60. Wilmer MJ, Emma F, Levtchenko EN. The pathogenesis of cystinosis: mechanisms beyond cystine accumulation. *Am J Physiol Renal Physiol.* 2010;299:F905.
61. Yeagy BA, Harrison F, Gubler MC, et al. Kidney preservation by bone marrow cell transplantation in hereditary nephropathy. *Kidney Int.* 2011;79:1198.
62. Greco M, Brugnara M, Zaffanello M, et al. Long-term outcome of nephropathic cystinosis: a 20-year single-center experience. *Pediatr Nephrol.* 2010;25:2459.
63. Tanpaiboon P. Methylmalonic acidemia (MMA). *Mol Genet Metab.* 2005;85:2.
64. Chandler RJ, Venditti CP. Genetic and genomic systems to study methylmalonic acidemia. *Mol Genet Metab.* 2005;86:34.
65. Cosson MA, Benoist JF, Touati G, et al. Long-term outcome in methylmalonic aciduria: a series of 30 French patients. *Mol Genet Metab.* 2009;97:172.
66. Lubrano R, Elli M, Rossi M, et al. Renal transplant in methylmalonic acidemia: could it be the best option? Report on a case at 10 years and review of the literature. *Pediatr Nephrol.* 2007;22:1209.
67. Harambat J, Fargue S, Bacchetta J, et al. Primary hyperoxaluria. *Int J Nephrol.* 2011;2011:864580.
68. Emma F, Bertini E, Salviati L, et al. Renal involvement in mitochondrial cytopathies. *Pediatr Nephrol.* 2012;27(4):539–550.
69. Yanagihara C, Oyama A, Tanaka M, et al. An autopsy case of mitochondrial encephalomyopathy with lactic acidosis and stroke-like episodes syndrome with chronic renal failure. *Intern Med.* 2001;40:662.
70. Hall AM, Unwin RJ, Hanna MG, et al. Renal function and mitochondrial cytopathy (MC): more questions than answers? *QJM.* 2008;101:755.
71. Butkowski RJ, Langeveld JP, Wieslander J, et al. Characterization of a tubular basement membrane component reactive with autoantibodies associated with tubulointerstitial nephritis. *J Biol Chem.* 1990;265:21091.
72. Maripuri S, Grande JP, Osborn TG, et al. Renal involvement in primary Sjogren's syndrome: a clinicopathologic study. *Clin J Am Soc Nephrol.* 2009;4:1423.
73. Pessler F, Emery H, Dai L, et al. The spectrum of renal tubular acidosis in paediatric Sjogren syndrome. *Rheumatology (Oxford).* 2006;45:85.
74. Routsias JG, Tzioufas AG. Sjogren's syndrome—study of autoantigens and autoantibodies. *Clin Rev Allergy Immunol.* 2007;32:238.
75. Saeki T, Nishi S, Imai N, et al. Clinicopathological characteristics of patients with IgG4-related tubulointerstitial nephritis. *Kidney Int.* 2010;78:1016.
76. Raissian Y, Nasr SH, Larsen CP, et al. Diagnosis of IgG4-related tubulointerstitial nephritis. *J Am Soc Nephrol.* 2011;22:1343.
77. Berliner AR, Haas M, Choi MJ. Sarcoidosis: the nephrologist's perspective. *Am J Kidney Dis.* 2006;48:856.
78. Birnbaum AD, Oh FS, Chakrabarti A, et al. Clinical features and diagnostic evaluation of biopsy-proven ocular sarcoidosis. *Arch Ophthalmol.* 2011;129:409.
79. Mahevas M, Lescure FX, Boffa JJ, et al. Renal sarcoidosis: clinical, laboratory, and histologic presentation and outcome in 47 patients. *Medicine (Baltimore).* 2009;88:98.
80. Tan Y, Yu F, Qu Z, et al. Modified C-reactive protein might be a target autoantigen of TINU syndrome. *Clin J Am Soc Nephrol.* 2011;6:93.
81. Jahnukainen T, Ala-Houhala M, Karikoski R, et al. Clinical outcome and occurrence of uveitis in children with idiopathic tubulointerstitial nephritis. *Pediatr Nephrol.* 2011;26:291.
82. Risdon RA, Sloper JC, De Wardener HE. Relationship between renal function and histological changes found in renal-biopsy specimens from patients with persistent glomerular nephritis. *Lancet.* 1968;2:363.
83. Schainuck LI, Striker GE, Cutler RE, et al. Structural-functional correlations in renal disease. II. The correlations. *Hum Pathol.* 1970;1:631.
84. Yu F, Wu LH, Tan Y, et al. Tubulointerstitial lesions of patients with lupus nephritis classified by the 2003 International Society of Nephrology and Renal Pathology Society system. *Kidney Int.* 2010;77:820.
85. Jafar TH, Stark PC, Schmid CH, et al. Proteinuria as a modifiable risk factor for the progression of non-diabetic renal disease. *Kidney Int.* 2001;60:1131.
86. Reich HN, Troyanov S, Scholey JW, et al. Remission of proteinuria improves prognosis in IgA nephropathy. *J Am Soc Nephrol.* 2007;18:3177.
87. Zandi-Nejad K, Eddy AA, Glassock RJ, et al. Why is proteinuria an ominous biomarker of progressive kidney disease? *Kidney Int Suppl.* 2004:S76.
88. Abbate M, Zoja C, Remuzzi G. How does proteinuria cause progressive renal damage? *J Am Soc Nephrol.* 2006;17:2974.
89. Boger CA, Chen MH, Tin A, et al. CUBN is a gene locus for albuminuria. *J Am Soc Nephrol.* 2011;22:555.
90. Theilig F, Kriz W, Jerichow T, et al. Abrogation of protein uptake through megalin-deficient proximal tubules does not safeguard against tubulointerstitial injury. *J Am Soc Nephrol.* 2007;18:1824.
91. Reich HN, Tritchler D, Cattran DC, et al. A molecular signature of proteinuria in glomerulonephritis. *PLoS One.* 2010;5:e13451.
92. Erkan E, Garcia CD, Patterson LT, et al. Induction of renal tubular cell apoptosis in focal segmental glomerulosclerosis: roles of proteinuria and Fas-dependent pathways. *J Am Soc Nephrol.* 2005;16:398.
93. Park CH, Maack T. Albumin absorption and catabolism by isolated perfused proximal convoluted tubules of the rabbit. *J Clin Invest.* 1984;73:767.
94. Zeisberg M, Neilson EG. Mechanisms of tubulointerstitial fibrosis. *J Am Soc Nephrol.* 2010;21:1819.
95. Macconi D, Chiabrando C, Schiarea S, et al. Proteasomal processing of albumin by renal dendritic cells generates antigenic peptides. *J Am Soc Nephrol.* 2009;20:123.
96. Kriz W, Hartmann I, Hosser H, et al. Tracer studies in the rat demonstrate misdirected filtration and peritubular filtrate spreading in nephrons with segmental glomerulosclerosis. *J Am Soc Nephrol.* 2001;12:496.
97. Coca SG, Singanamala S, Parikh CR. Chronic kidney disease after acute kidney injury: a systematic review and meta-analysis. *Kidney Int.* 2012;81(5):442–448.
98. Lo LJ, Go AS, Chertow GM, et al. Dialysis-requiring acute renal failure increases the risk of progressive chronic kidney disease. *Kidney Int.* 2009;76:893.
99. Chawla LS, Amdur RL, Amodeo S, et al. The severity of acute kidney injury predicts progression to chronic kidney disease. *Kidney Int.* 2011;79:1361.
100. Garg AX, Suri RS, Barrowman N, et al. Long-term renal prognosis of diarrhea-associated hemolytic uremic syndrome: a systematic review, meta-analysis, and meta-regression. *JAMA.* 2003;290:1360.
101. Bonventre JV, Yang L. Cellular pathophysiology of ischemic acute kidney injury. *J Clin Invest.* 2011;121:4210.
102. Burne-Taney MJ, Yokota N, Rabb H. Persistent renal and extrarenal immune changes after severe ischemic injury. *Kidney Int.* 2005;67:1002.
103. Part 4. Definition and classification of stages of chronic kidney disease. *Am J Kidney Dis.* 2002;39:S46.
104. Rossert J. Drug-induced acute interstitial nephritis. *Kidney Int.* 2001;60:804.
105. Gonzalez E, Gutierrez E, Galeano C, et al. Early steroid treatment improves the recovery of renal function in patients with drug-induced acute interstitial nephritis. *Kidney Int.* 2008;73:940.
106. Montini G, Tullus K, Hewitt I. Febrile urinary tract infections in children. *N Engl J Med.* 2011;365:239.
107. Craig JC, Simpson JM, Williams GJ, et al. Antibiotic prophylaxis and recurrent urinary tract infection in children. *N Engl J Med.* 2009;361:1748.
108. Puri P, Gosemann JH, Darlow J, et al. Genetics of vesicoureteral reflux. *Nat Rev Urol.* 2011;8:539.
109. Eastwood JB, Corbishley CM, Grange JM. Tuberculosis and the kidney. *J Am Soc Nephrol.* 2001;12:1307.
110. Chapagain A, Dobbie H, Sheaff M, et al. Presentation, diagnosis, and treatment outcome of tuberculous-mediated tubulointerstitial nephritis. *Kidney Int.* 2011;79:671.
111. Li L, Parwani AV. Xanthogranulomatous pyelonephritis. *Arch Pathol Lab Med.* 2011;135:671.
112. Becker JL, Miller F, Nuovo GJ, et al. Epstein-Barr virus infection of renal proximal tubule cells: possible role in chronic interstitial nephritis. *J Clin Invest.* 1999;104:1673.
113. Dall A, Hariharan S. BK virus nephritis after renal transplantation. *Clin J Am Soc Nephrol.* 2008;3 Suppl 2:S68.
114. Gabardi S, Waikar SS, Martin S, et al. Evaluation of fluoroquinolones for the prevention of BK viremia after renal transplantation. *Clin J Am Soc Nephrol.* 2010;5:1298.
115. Lekakis LJ, Macrinici V, Baraboutis IG, et al. BK virus nephropathy after allogeneic stem cell transplantation: a case report and literature review. *Am J Hematol.* 2009;84:243.
116. Storsley L, Gibson IW. Adenovirus interstitial nephritis and rejection in an allograft. *J Am Soc Nephrol.* 2011;22:1423.
117. Parkhie SM, Fine DM, Lucas GM, et al. Characteristics of patients with HIV and biopsy-proven acute interstitial nephritis. *Clin J Am Soc Nephrol.* 2010;5:798.
118. Medapalli RK, He JC, Klotman PE. HIV-associated nephropathy: pathogenesis. *Curr Opin Nephrol Hypertens.* 2011;20:306.
119. Kasuno K, Ono T, Matsumori A, et al. Hepatitis C virus-associated tubulointerstitial injury. *Am J Kidney Dis.* 2003;41:767.
120. Pergam SA, Schmidt DW, Nofchissey RA, et al. Potential renal sequelae in survivors of hantavirus cardiopulmonary syndrome. *Am J Trop Med Hyg.* 2009;80:279.
121. Schwarz A, Krause PH, Kunzendorf U, et al. The outcome of acute interstitial nephritis: risk factors for the transition from acute to chronic interstitial nephritis. *Clin Nephrol.* 2000;54:179.
122. Torpey N, Barker T, Ross C. Drug-induced tubulo-interstitial nephritis secondary to proton pump inhibitors: experience from a single UK renal unit. *Nephrol Dial Transplant.* 2004;19:1441.
123. Skinner R. Nephrotoxicity—what do we know and what don't we know? *J Pediatr Hematol Oncol.* 2011;33:128.
124. Skinner R, Parry A, Price L, et al. Persistent nephrotoxicity during 10-year follow-up after cisplatin or carboplatin treatment in childhood: relevance of age and dose as risk factors. *Eur J Cancer.* 2009;45:3213.

125. Oberlin O, Fawaz O, Rey A, et al. Long-term evaluation of Ifosfamide-related nephrotoxicity in children. *J Clin Oncol.* 2009;27:5350.

126. Lopez-Novoa JM, Quiros Y, Vicente L, et al. New insights into the mechanism of aminoglycoside nephrotoxicity: an integrative point of view. *Kidney Int.* 2011;79:33.

127. Houghton DC, English J, Bennett WM. Chronic tubulointerstitial nephritis and renal insufficiency associated with long-term "subtherapeutic" gentamicin. *J Lab Clin Med.* 1988;112:694.

128. Heyman SN, Stillman IE, Brezis M, et al. Chronic amphotericin nephropathy: morphometric, electron microscopic, and functional studies. *J Am Soc Nephrol.* 1993;4:69.

129. Harbarth S, Pestotnik SL, Lloyd JF, et al. The epidemiology of nephrotoxicity associated with conventional amphotericin B therapy. *Am J Med.* 2001; 111:528.

130. Izzedine H, Harris M, Perazella MA. The nephrotoxic effects of HAART. *Nat Rev Nephrol.* 2009;5:563.

131. Flandre P, Pugliese P, Cuzin L, et al. Risk factors of chronic kidney disease in HIV-infected patients. *Clin J Am Soc Nephrol.* 2011;6:1700.

132. Zimmermann AE, Pizzoferrato T, Bedford J, et al. Tenofovir-associated acute and chronic kidney disease: a case of multiple drug interactions. *Clin Infect Dis.* 2006;42:283.

133. De Broe ME, Elseviers MM. Over-the-counter analgesic use. *J Am Soc Nephrol.* 2009;20:2098.

134. Naesens M, Kuypers DR, Sarwal M. Calcineurin inhibitor nephrotoxicity. *Clin J Am Soc Nephrol.* 2009;4:481.

135. Gaston RS. Chronic calcineurin inhibitor nephrotoxicity: reflections on an evolving paradigm. *Clin J Am Soc Nephrol.* 2009;4:2029.

136. Ojo AO, Held PJ, Port FK, et al. Chronic renal failure after transplantation of a nonrenal organ. *N Engl J Med.* 2003;349:931.

137. Jha V. Herbal medicines and chronic kidney disease. *Nephrology (Carlton).* 2010;15 Suppl 2:10.

138. Debelle FD, Vanherweghem JL, Nortier JL. Aristolochic acid nephropathy: a worldwide problem. *Kidney Int.* 2008;74:158.

139. Grollman AP, Jelakovic B. Role of environmental toxins in endemic (Balkan) nephropathy. October 2006, Zagreb, Croatia. *J Am Soc Nephrol.* 2007; 18:2817.

140. Bendz H, Schon S, Attman PO, et al. Renal failure occurs in chronic lithium treatment but is uncommon. *Kidney Int.* 2010;77:219.

141. Grunfeld JP, Rossier BC. Lithium nephrotoxicity revisited. *Nat Rev Nephrol.* 2009;5:270.

142. Gonick HC. Nephrotoxicity of cadmium and lead. *Indian J Med Res.* 2008; 128:335.

143. Ekong EB, Jaar BG, Weaver VM. Lead-related nephrotoxicity: a review of the epidemiologic evidence. *Kidney Int.* 2006;70:2074.

144. Vervaet BA, Verhulst A, D'Haese PC, et al. Nephrocalcinosis: new insights into mechanisms and consequences. *Nephrol Dial Transplant.* 2009;24:2030.

145. Habbig S, Beck BB, Hoppe B. Nephrocalcinosis and urolithiasis in children. *Kidney Int.* 2011;80:1278.

146. Markowitz GS, Stokes MB, Radhakrishnan J, et al. Acute phosphate nephropathy following oral sodium phosphate bowel purgative: an underrecognized cause of chronic renal failure. *J Am Soc Nephrol.* 2005;16:3389.

147. Markowitz GS, Perazella MA. Acute phosphate nephropathy. *Kidney Int.* 2009;76:1027.

148. Bellasi A, Mandreoli M, Baldrati L, et al. Chronic kidney disease progression and outcome according to serum phosphorus in mild-to-moderate kidney dysfunction. *Clin J Am Soc Nephrol.* 2011;6:883.

149. Tangri N, Stevens LA, Griffith J, et al. A predictive model for progression of chronic kidney disease to kidney failure. *JAMA.* 2011;305:1553.

150. Moe OW. Posing the question again: does chronic uric acid nephropathy exist? *J Am Soc Nephrol.* 2010;21:395.

151. Kang DH, Nakagawa T, Feng L, et al. A role for uric acid in the progression of renal disease. *J Am Soc Nephrol.* 2002;13:2888.

152. Heinig M, Johnson RJ. Role of uric acid in hypertension, renal disease, and metabolic syndrome. *Cleve Clin J Med.* 2006;73:1059.

153. Feig DI, Kang DH, Johnson RJ. Uric acid and cardiovascular risk. *N Engl J Med.* 2008;359:1811.

154. Obermayr RP, Temml C, Gutjahr G, et al. Elevated uric acid increases the risk for kidney disease. *J Am Soc Nephrol.* 2008;19:2407.

155. Reungjui S, Roncal CA, Sato W, et al. Hypokalemic nephropathy is associated with impaired angiogenesis. *J Am Soc Nephrol.* 2008;19:125.

156. Buemi M, Fazio MR, Bolignano D, et al. Renal complications in oncohematologic patients. *J Investig Med.* 2009;57:892.

157. Lameire N, Van Biesen W, Vanholder R. Electrolyte disturbances and acute kidney injury in patients with cancer. *Semin Nephrol.* 2010;30:534.

158. Suh WM, Wainberg ZA, de Vos S, et al. Acute lymphoblastic leukemia presenting as acute renal failure. *Nat Clin Pract Nephrol.* 2007;3:106.

159. Hutchison CA, Batuman V, Behrens J, et al. The pathogenesis and diagnosis of acute kidney injury in multiple myeloma. *Nat Rev Nephrol.* 2012;8:43.

160. Korbet SM, Schwartz MM. Multiple myeloma. *J Am Soc Nephrol.* 2006;17:2533.

161. da Silva GB Jr, Liborio AB, Daher Ede F. New insights on pathophysiology, clinical manifestations, diagnosis, and treatment of sickle cell nephropathy. *Ann Hematol.* 2011;90:1371.

162. Becker AM. Sickle cell nephropathy: challenging the conventional wisdom. *Pediatr Nephrol.* 2011;26:2099.

CHAPTER 58

Clinical Aspects of Diabetic Nephropathy

Jamie P. Dwyer • Julia B. Lewis

The term "diabetic nephropathy" (DN) refers to the classic pathologic structural and functional changes seen in the kidneys of subjects with diabetes mellitus (DM) (either type 1 or type 2). Some differences exist in DN in patients with type 1 or 2 diabetes and may be clinically relevant, particularly with respect to their onset, natural history, and treatment.

In this chapter, we review the natural history and stages of DN, discuss the treatment of DN as it pertains to slowing its progression, and consider the future of the treatment of DN.

DEFINITIONS AND MEASUREMENT OF URINARY ALBUMIN EXCRETION

In order to consider the stages of DN, we must first define what is meant by the commonly encountered terms normoalbuminuria, microalbuminuria, and overt proteinuria (also known as macroalbuminuria). In the absence of kidney disease, the average amount of albumin excreted in the urine is 8 to 10 mg per day. Normoalbuminuria is arbitrarily defined as <30 mg per day. Microalbuminuria (MA) is defined as 30 to 299 mg per day, an amount sufficiently low enough often not to be detected by standard colorimetric test-strip (dipstick) methodologies. In order to measure MA, specialized immunoassays are required, including turbidimetric, nephelometric, and two-site immunometric tests.[1] Typically, these assays have a lower limit of detection of 2 to 10 mg per L.[2] A variety of clinical situations can increase urinary albumin excretion (UAE), including physical exercise, hyperglycemia, water loading, fever, seizure, and heart failure. Because the absolute magnitude of these increases in UAE are small, this can lead to temporary increases in UAE sufficient enough to misclassify a patient as having MA or not, but represent trivial changes in a patient with overt proteinuria. MA is considered persistent and clinically significant if it is present on two of three assays performed over a specified time period (usually 2 weeks), which helps to avoid the misclassification of a patient on the basis of the inherent variability in daily UAE. Overt proteinuria is so-named because the proteinuria is sufficient enough to activate the standard urinalysis dipstick, and corresponds to an albumin excretion of >300 mg per day. Once a patient has this level of proteinuria, there is little reason to measure the more expensive tests specifically for UAE. Albumin in general represents anywhere from 20% to 60% of total urinary protein excretion. The standard urinary dipstick actually measures all negatively charged proteins, rather than only albumin concentration. Because albumin is the most abundantly negatively charged protein found in urine, it is the principal urinary protein that is measured. In the presence of other conditions in which positively charged proteins are the principal proteins excreted in the urine (e.g., positively charged immunoglobulins), the standard dipstick may not be activated. Additionally, the dipstick is sensitive to the concentration of, but not the absolute amount of, albumin in a random or spot specimen.[3] A patient may have normal albumin excretion over the course of the day, but the concentration of charge in that spot specimen may be great enough to activate the dipstick.

To circumvent these issues with dipstick measurements of albuminuria, various other laboratory measures to specifically measure albumin or total protein excretion have been developed. Twenty-four-hour urinary collection, an overnight collection, or a random or first-morning void can be assayed. Total albumin concentration, total protein concentration, an albumin-to-creatinine ratio (ACR), or a protein-to-creatinine ratio (PCR) can be measured in any of these collections. The 24-hour collection is difficult and cumbersome for the patient to do, and is prone to both over- and under-collections. Collection errors can be partially corrected for by measuring an ACR or PCR in a 24-hour urine collection, and this may best reflect the patient's albuminuria or proteinuria. ACR or PCR in a random spot or first-morning urine is less cumbersome to the patient

*Disclosures: Dr. Dwyer reports research support from Keryx Biopharmaceuticals, Inc., Eli Lilly, Inc., and ChemoCentryx, Inc. Dr. Lewis reports research support from Keryx Biopharmaceuticals, Eli Lilly, Inc., Bristol-Myers-Squibb, Inc., Sanofi-Aventis, Inc., and Nephrogenix, Inc.

than a 24-hour collection, but are subject to error and variation, because albumin excretion increases in the upright versus prone position, or with exercise. An ACR or PCR in a first-morning urine will be more reproducible than a random spot urine, but will represent about 30% to 50% lower albumin excretion than an upright daytime urine. Due to its consistency, the first-morning void ACR may be the best method among these to predict renal events in type 2 diabetes and DN.[4]

NATURAL HISTORY OF DIABETIC NEPHROPATHY

The natural history of DN in type 1 diabetes was characterized by Kussman et al. in 1976.[5] They examined the death records of patients with juvenile-onset diabetes who were classified as having died from renal failure between 1962 and 1972, and characterized the time of onset of type 1 diabetes, onset of dipstick-positive proteinuria, onset of "early" and "late" renal failure (here defined as serum creatinine [SCr] >2.0 mg per dL and >5.0 mg per dL, respectively) in the 40% of subjects destined to develop DN, and death. Following the onset of type 1 diabetes, the onset of proteinuria occurred at 17.3 ± 6.0 years (mean ± standard deviation), early renal failure at 19.4 ± 5.4 years, late renal failure at 21.6 ± 6.3 years, and death at 22.1 ± 6.4 years. It should be emphasized that this was prior to the advent of the therapies discussed later to delay the progression of DN, and thus represents the true, untreated natural history of DN due to type 1 diabetes. With the development of assays capable of detecting lower amounts of UAE, MA was demonstrated to precede proteinuria in most patients 5 to 10 years after the onset of type 1 diabetes.[6] Figure 58.1 summarizes the natural history of DN due to type 1 diabetes, including the functional and structural changes which are described later (see Risk section, later).

The natural history of DN due to type 2 diabetes is nearly the same, but because the onset of type 2 diabetes cannot be pinpointed, patients may present for medical care at any stage of DN. Perhaps the most important difference in DN between types 1 and 2 diabetes stems from the fact that the onset of type 2 diabetes confers cardiovascular (CV) risk upon a patient that is equivalent to that risk conferred

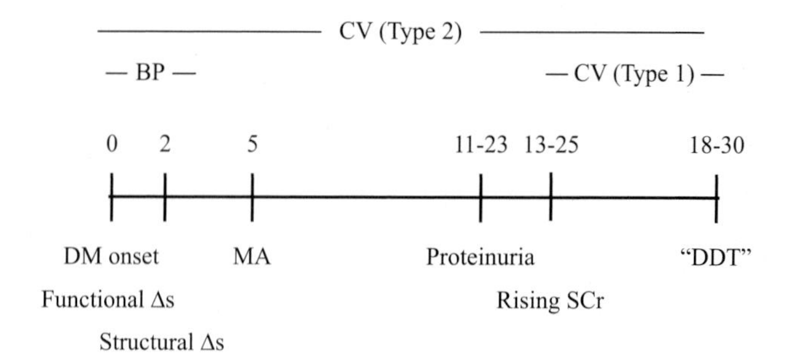

FIGURE 58.1 The natural history of untreated diabetic nephropathy due to type 1 diabetes. In the case of type 2 diabetes, the onset of diabetes is often unknown, and cardiovascular death may occur at any time point, censoring the patient's progression to end-stage renal disease. *BP*, deranged systemic blood pressure; *MA*, microalbuminuria; *DM*, diabetes mellitus; *DDT*, death, dialysis, or transplantation.

by having had a prior myocardial infarction (MI).[7] In other words, type 2 diabetes is an "MI equivalent." Thus, there is a risk of CV death at any stage along the natural history of DN due to type 2 diabetes[8,9] (Fig. 58.1), and death censors many patients with DN from progression to end-stage renal disease (ESRD). However, in patients with type 1 diabetes, the excess CV risk is not apparent until they have advanced renal disease, so most patients with type 1 diabetes and DN will reach ESRD.

STAGES OF DIABETIC NEPHROPATHY

DN has been characterized according to its traditional stages—glomerular hyperfiltration, MA, overt proteinuria, abnormal renal clearance, and renal failure—which have been derived from the natural history of DN described previously. These stages can really be considered a continuum of injury to the kidney (Fig. 58.2). There is evidence that there are markers for the risk of developing nephropathy which occur prior to the onset of MA. This alternative scheme for classifying DN allows us to consider the risk of developing nephropathy, clinicopathologic injury, and renal failure. These terms and a similar classification construct are in use for acute kidney injury (AKI).[10]

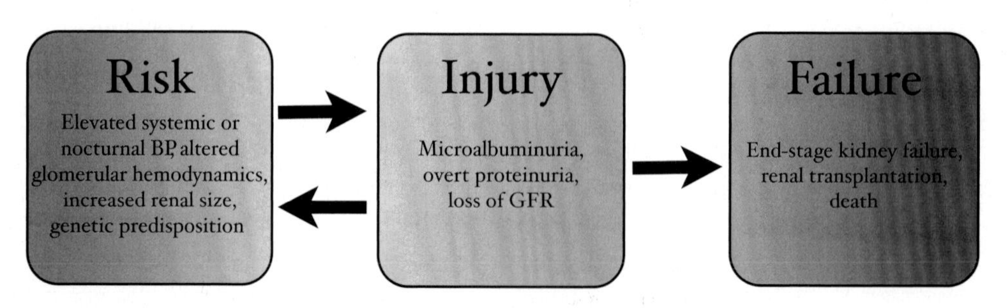

FIGURE 58.2 Classification scheme for diabetic nephropathy.

Risk

Approximately 40% of patients with diabetes develop clinically significant DN.[8,11–26] A variety of clinical, epidemiologic, familial, and genetic factors predict the risk of the development of DN (Table 58.1). Longer prepubertal duration of type 1 diabetes and prepubertal hyperglycemia increase the risk of postpubertal MA.[24] Older age at the time of diagnosis of type 1 and type 2 diabetes appears to increase the risk of DN,[19,27,28] but specifically in Pima Indians, it seems that the onset of type 2 diabetes prior to the age of 20 years confers a fivefold risk for ESRD in middle age as compared to onset after age 20.[22] A longer duration of diabetes is associated with an increased risk of DN,[29] but a majority of patients with diabetes (60%) do not ever develop clinically significant DN. Even slight elevations in body mass index (BMI) are associated with a higher risk of DN in patients with type 2 diabetes.[30] Very mild elevations of UAE (even within the normoalbuminuric range) predict a greater risk of development of DN.[30–34] In a 10-year prospective observational cohort, baseline UAE was 9 mg per 24 hours in those subjects who remained normoalbuminuric, but was 13 mg per 24 hours in those who ultimately developed MA or overt proteinuria.[31]

TABLE 58.1 Risk Factors for the Development of Diabetic Nephropathy

Older age of diabetes onset[19,25,27] (type 1); younger age of onset in Pima Indians[22] (type 2)
Elevated systemic BP[6,25,30,32] (type 1 and type 2)
Nocturnal systolic BP elevation[36] (type 1)
Elevated 24-hour ambulatory systolic and diastolic BP[35] (type 1)
Increased body mass index[26] (type 1 and type 2)
Increased waist-to-hip ratio[26] (type 1 and type 2)
Longer diabetes duration[25,29] (type 1 and type 2)
Increased baseline albumin excretion rate[30–34] (type 1 and type 2)
Poor glycemic control[6,25,26,30,31] (type 1 and type 2)
High level of low-density lipoprotein[25,26] (type 1 and type 2)
Male sex[6] (type 1)
African Americans, Polynesian, Maori, and Hispanic American race[13,54,61] (type 1 and type 2)
Retinopathy, any diabetic, presence of[31] (type 1, less so type 2)
Smoking[31] (type 2)
High triglycerides, fasting[25,26] (type 1 and type 2)
Genetic factors[70–72] (type 1 and type 2)
Family history of diabetic nephropathy[63–68] (type 1 and type 2)

In the earliest stages of the changes to the kidney in diabetes there are both elevations in systemic blood pressure (BP) and glomerular hyperfiltration, which portend more serious injury. The earliest detectable marker of deranged BP regulation in type 1 diabetes is elevated nocturnal systolic BP. An early study demonstrated this correlation with systolic and diastolic BP obtained via 24-hour ambulatory BP monitoring (ABPM).[35] Elevation of nocturnal systolic BP was demonstrated in a prospective longitudinal cohort analysis of 75 adolescents and young adults with type 1 diabetes and normal urinary albumin excretion,[36] in which nocturnal systolic BP elevation by ABPM preceded and predicted the onset of MA. The risk of development of MA was 70% lower in those subjects with a normal nocturnal dipping status, even in those subjects with poor metabolic control (a known predictor of MA, see later text).

Elevated systemic BP at the time of diagnosis of diabetes is associated with the later development of DN, in both types 1 and 2 diabetes. In a cohort of patients with type 1 diabetes followed for 20 years after the onset of diabetes, those patients who were ultimately destined to develop DN (20 years later) had statistically significantly higher systolic and diastolic BP at the time of diagnosis of diabetes compared to those who never developed DN (mean BP 122/76 mm Hg in those subjects who did not develop MA, as compared to 128/80 mm Hg in those who did).[6] Further supporting the role of elevated systemic BP as a risk factor for the development of DN, Parving et al.[12] characterized the prevalence of hypertension (HTN) (defined, at the time, as >160/95 mm Hg or on antihypertensive medications) in 982 subjects with type 1 diabetes attending a diabetes clinic, stratified according to albumin excretion. The presence of HTN strongly correlated with DN, such that HTN was present in 19%, 30%, and 65% of subjects with normo-, micro-, and overt proteinuria. Due to this high prevalence of hypertension at the time of diagnosis of type 2 diabetes, the presence of HTN is less predictive of the risk of developing DN in the future in type 2 rather than type 1 diabetes.[37–39]

Glomerular filtration rate (GFR) is higher at the onset of diabetes as compared to weight- and age-matched controls, both in types 1[40–42] and 2 diabetes.[43] In their study of 13 males with type 1 diabetes of short duration (mean duration 2.4 years), Christiansen et al.[42] demonstrated that iothalamate-GFR was increased in diabetes (144 vs. 113 mL per min), as were renal plasma flow and kidney volume (assessed by hippuran and ultrasound, respectively). Glomerular function was investigated in type 2 diabetic Pima Indians,[43] which demonstrated that iothalamate-GFR was 140 versus 122 mL per min in diabetic subjects as compared to nondiabetic controls, and was higher in subjects with impaired versus normal glucose tolerance (before the onset of diabetes).[44] Although glomerular hyperfiltration is common at the time of diagnosis of diabetes, those patients destined to develop DN have, on average, higher GFR than those patients with diabetes who never develop DN.[45,46] Despite the correlation between higher GFR at the onset of DM and the risk of developing DN, there is no absolute cut-off level of GFR above which DN develops with certainty in the future. Various mediators of hyperfiltration[47–49] have been postulated, including alterations in eicosanoids, nitric oxide, atrial natriuretic peptide, and transforming growth factor-beta. Treatment with continuously infused insulin for 2 years (via insulin pump) moderates the hyperfiltration in type 1 diabetes.[50]

Renal size is also increased in early diabetes.[51] Christiansen et al.[42] demonstrated that males with type 1 diabetes had mean renal volume of 278 mL per 1.73 m^2 versus 224 mL per 1.73 m^2 for nondiabetic control males, a significant increase of 24%. Treatment with insulin for 3 months was shown to reduce kidney size in newly diagnosed men with type 1 diabetes.[52] Interestingly, kidney size remains larger at ESRD in those patients with ESRD due to diabetes than from other causes.[53] In one study, renal length was estimated using ultrasonography, and mean right renal length was 9.9 versus 8.8 cm (DN vs. no DN); mean left renal length was 10.0 versus 9.1 cm.

African Americans, Asians, Polynesians, Maori, Native Americans, and Hispanic Americans with diabetes all have an increased risk of developing DN as compared to Caucasians with diabetes.[13,54–61] The overall incidence of diabetes-related ESRD in Jefferson County, Alabama, was 3.4 times higher in African Americans than in Caucasians[56]; similarly, the incidence was 4.4 times higher among African Americans with ESRD reported to the Michigan Kidney Registry from 1974 to 1983.[13] In Mexican Americans studied in the Texas Kidney Health Program over the period 1978 to 1984, the incidence of diabetes-related ESRD was six times higher than in non-Hispanic whites.[59] The prevalence of DN (as estimated by a single dipstick assessment of MA) in a global cohort of type 2 diabetes was nearly 40% higher in Asians, and 30% higher in Hispanics, than in Caucasians.[54] In addition to certain groups having an increased risk of developing DN, it appears that some have an accelerated rate of decline of renal function once DN is established.[62]

In those families in which multiple members have diabetes, the presence of DN in one member predicts an increased risk of DN in other family members.[63–68] An early report demonstrated that there was evidence of DN in 83% of the siblings of probands who had undergone renal transplantation for DN.[63] In this study, the presence of nephropathy in the proband was the only significant predictor of the presence of it in the sibling. These clinical observations have led to studies[69] to identify genetic markers that predict the development of DN. Candidate genes span many gene classes, and were recently summarized,[70] but include glucose transporter 2, kininogen, adiponectin, transforming growth factor-beta II and III, catalase, endothelial nitric oxide synthase, apolipoprotein E, tissue inhibitor of metalloproteinase 3,[71] and angiotensin-I converting enzyme.[72] Identification of genes involved in the pathogenesis of DN will likely help direct the development of novel agents to treat it.

Injury

Albuminuria (from MA to overt proteinuria) and loss of GFR represent a spectrum of pathologic diabetic injury to the kidneys. We review these forms of diabetic kidney injury in turn.

MA has traditionally been considered the hallmark of DN, and the earliest clinical feature of it. MA occurs in patients with either type 1 or type 2 diabetes. Approximately 10% to 20% of patients with type 1 diabetes develop MA after 5 to 15 years of diabetes.[11] It is important to note, however, that not all patients with type 1 diabetes develop DN. The cumulative incidence of MA was approximately 30% to 40% at 20 years in a cohort of subjects characterized from the onset of type 1 diabetes,[6] but there appears to be an upper limit of nearly 55%, after 40 years of type 1 diabetes.[29]

The prevalence of MA in type 2 diabetes ranges in large trials and a global cohort from 25% to 45% after approximately 10 years of diabetes, but may be present at the time of diagnosis of diabetes.[8,37,54,73] The presence of MA, or even overt proteinuria, at the time of diagnosis of diabetes in patients with type 2 DM may reflect the delay in diagnosis of DM, in type 2 as compared to type 1 diabetes. The prevalence of MA varies by age, with older adults more likely to have MA at the time of diagnosis of diabetes,[74] and race; it is highest in Asians and Hispanics and lowest in Caucasians.[54,75] It was estimated that 2.0% of patients will transition to persistent MA from normoalbuminuria per year (based on data from the United Kingdom Prospective Diabetes Study [UKPDS]).[8] MA is associated with increased CV mortality compared to patients with type 2 diabetes and no MA,[8] with a relative risk for all-cause mortality (which is driven predominantly by CV mortality) of 1.9.[76]

The majority of patients with MA who survive progress to overt proteinuria, and the presence of MA is the single most important risk factor for progression to overt proteinuria.[6,11,29,31,77–80] In type 1 diabetes, risk factors for progression to overt proteinuria include higher baseline urinary albumin excretion rate, poor glycemic control, the presence of diabetic retinopathy, smoking,[31] higher systemic blood pressure, and dyslipidemia.[6]

In type 2 diabetes, the transition rate from MA to overt proteinuria in newly diagnosed patients with diabetes was 2.8% per year in the UKPDS. The observed prevalence of overt proteinuria was 5.3% at 10 years, and 7.1% at 15 years.[8] The rates of conversion are likely higher in certain ethnicities, and have been well characterized in Pima Indians, in whom they are highest.[44]

However, not every patient with MA will progress to overt proteinuria, and some patients may spontaneously regress from MA to normoalbuminuria,[6,76] or they may do so after effective treatment (see later text, Therapy of Diabetic Nephropathy). In an individual patient, this regression from MA to normoalbuminuria may be a reflection of misclassification of the patient as having MA in the first place, because the method used to measure MA has an inherent insensitivity, and there is variability in albumin excretion during the course of the day or with intercurrent illness or exercise (see previous section, Definitions and Measurement of Urinary Albumin Excretion). Regression in a cohort more likely reflects a true clinical phenomenon in a subgroup of diabetic patients. This regression from persistent MA to normoalbuminuria was characterized in type 1 diabetes in a study of 386 subjects in a single center in which the cumulative incidence of regression was 58% over 6 years.[81] Factors associated with regression included younger absolute age, MA of shorter duration, better lipid status, better glycemic control, and lower systolic BP. Intervention in the care of these patients likely contributed to the regression. Regression of MA is associated with a reduced risk of subsequent CV events,[82] and may therefore be a treatment goal in and of itself.

Once proteinuria is established, renal function inevitably declines (see section later, Failure), with faster rates of decline in renal function seen with higher amounts of proteinuria.[83,84] It is important to note that in the classic study by Kussman et al. (see previous), overt proteinuria begins before GFR has begun to decline. In general, MA and overt proteinuria precede the decrease in GFR in type 1 diabetes; indeed, albuminuria is practically a prerequisite for loss of GFR. In a study of nearly 600 subjects with type 1 diabetes and normoalbuminuria or MA,[85] the risk of loss of GFR over 8 to 12 years was 9% with normal albumin excretion, 16% with MA regression (MA at least halved), 32% with stable MA, and 68% with progressive MA (MA at least doubled). The single most important predictor of the loss of renal function in patients with diabetes is the degree of proteinuria. However, small studies and a global cross-sectional cohort of patients with type 2 diabetes[54,86–92] have reported small subpopulations of patients with normoalbuminuria or MA and reduced GFR, such that 17% of subjects with normoalbuminuria and 27% of subjects with MA had significant kidney dysfunction.[86] The design of the global cohort study[54] precludes exact clarification of the causes for this decreased GFR. Many possibilities exist to explain these subpopulations of patients—including misclassification, treatments that decreased albuminuria and slowed, but did not halt, the loss of renal function, and renal injury not related to DN, such as unresolved AKI. In patients with type 1 diabetes, the presence of decreased GFR in the absence of MA has been associated with worse glomerular histology than in those patients with MA.[93] Alternately, other biopsy studies in patients with type 2 diabetes have demonstrated higher amounts of proteinuria associated with worse glomerular lesions.[94] Overall, in both patients with type 1 and type 2 diabetes, the worse the proteinuria, the faster the rate of decline of renal function, leading many to argue that decreasing proteinuria should be a goal or clinical endpoint of therapy.

Failure

Once loss of GFR has begun, the patient with DN begins a near inexorable decline toward dialysis, renal transplant, or death. Untreated, the rate of loss of GFR in type 1 diabetes may be as high as 7 to 12 mL/min/1.73 m^2 per year.[95,96] In type 2 diabetes in Pima Indians, the average decline was 11 mL/min/1.73 m^2 per year.[44] This rate of decline in GFR can also be quantified as transition rates along the spectrum of diabetic injury, which were estimated in the UKPDS. The annual rate of transition from overt proteinuria to renal failure was 2.3%, from overt proteinuria to death 4.6%, and from renal failure to death was 19.2%.[8] Additionally, the UKPDS, not designed as a renal study, and with infrequent (yearly) measurement of renal function, suggested that there was a greater incidence of CV death than progression of DN, at every stage of DN under consideration in the study.[8] However, analysis of a large cohort of well-characterized patients with DN, proteinuria, and low GFR, obtained from two large multinational renal clinical trials with frequent (quarterly) measurement of renal function (see later), showed that the risk of ESRD was significantly more common than CV death in the whole cohort, with an incidence rate ratio (IRR) of 4.92, and more common than all-cause mortality (IRR 2.61).[9] Finally, the renal prognosis of type 1 diabetes has improved, as estimated by the decreasing incidence of ESRD over time, characterized in a very large prospective cohort of patients with type 1 diabetes.[19] These data highlight the variability of the competing risks of progression, failure, and death.

DIAGNOSIS AND CLINICAL MANAGEMENT OF DIABETIC NEPHROPATHY

We discussed the factors that predict the development of the various stages of DN, and presented a framework to consider the likelihood of progression from one stage of DN to another. However, the clinician, faced with a patient with diabetes and markers of chronic kidney disease (e.g., proteinuria, hematuria, or decreased GFR), must assign some likelihood that the disease under consideration is actually DN. In type 1 diabetes, the epidemiology of DN and the presence of proliferative diabetic retinopathy help determine the likelihood that DN is present. For example, if massive proteinuria is present within 5 years of the diagnosis of type 1 diabetes, it is unlikely to be due to DN; conversely, the onset of proteinuria more than 25 years after the diagnosis of type 1 diabetes makes DN less likely (Fig. 58.1). Additionally, because 95% of patients with type 1 diabetes and DN also have diabetic retinopathy,[15] the absence of retinopathy may imply some kidney lesion other than DN.

These epidemiologic findings are not as useful in type 2 diabetes, however. The concordance rate of DN and diabetic retinopathy is only about 60% to 65% in type 2 diabetes,[94,97–101] thus the absence of retinopathy is not as strong a predictor of other nondiabetic renal diseases. Additionally, because the onset of diabetes is less reliably known in type 2 than in type 1, one cannot readily rely on the natural history to exclude DN. Thus, a systematic evaluation for other causes of kidney disease (a thorough history and physical examination, and selected laboratory and imaging tests) must be utilized to distinguish which patients may benefit from a renal biopsy.

It is incumbent on the practicing nephrologist to assess whether something other than diabetes is the cause of kidney disease. Such an approach was undertaken in a prospective biopsy study,[94] in which patients were carefully screened for history, physical, or serologic evidence of a disease other than DN. Diabetic glomerulosclerosis was responsible for the renal clinical findings in 94% of patients with type 2 diabetes. Two distinct glomerular lesions were found, classical Kimmelstiel-Wilson (KW) nodules and mesangial sclerosis; proliferative retinopathy was associated with KW glomerulopathy, and patients with mesangial sclerosis more frequently had no evidence of retinopathy, or retinal microaneurysms only. Importantly, there was no cut-off level for proteinuria above which DN was not found to be the cause for the underlying glomerular lesion, since the range of proteinuria reported in this study was 700 mg per day to 18 g per day.

The presence of hematuria is also not sufficient to suggest the presence of a renal lesion other than DN. In a study of 68 subjects with the clinical diagnosis of DN, 62% of them had hematuria, as assessed on a single urine examination.[102] Dysmorphic red blood cells (acanthocytes), indicative of glomerular hematuria, however, were only present in 4% of subjects with clinical DN, but were present in 40% of subjects with known glomerular lesions.

Hence, if a patient with diabetes has diabetic retinopathy (type 1 diabetes), the onset of proteinuria in the expected time frame (type 1), and no history, physical, or serologic evidence to support another disease (type 1 and 2) such as systemic lupus erythematosus, a renal biopsy is rarely indicated because an alternate diagnosis that would be treated differently is rarely found.

Once the diagnosis of DN is established, there are some unique features to the clinical management of the patient with renal insufficiency and diabetes. Thirty to 45% of insulin is metabolized by the kidney. As GFR decreases, any available insulin lasts longer, and patients are thus at greater risk for hypoglycemic episodes if doses of hypoglycemic medications are not reduced. Furthermore, most oral hypoglycemic agents are metabolized by the kidney, and if hypoglycemia does develop, it is prolonged far longer than it would be in a patient with diabetes and normal renal function, necessitating hospitalization for observation in many cases. Metformin is contraindicated in patients with SCr ≥1.5 mg per dL due to its association with severe metabolic acidosis (lactic acidosis) in these patients.

The most common cause of type IV renal tubular acidosis (RTA) or hyperkalemic hyperchloremic metabolic acidosis is diabetes. Thus, at any level of kidney function, these patients are at risk for hyperkalemia and metabolic acidosis. Treating this specific tubular transport defect with a low potassium diet, diuretics (often requiring high-dose loop or very potent thiazide agents), and base supplementation can be critical and allow these patients to receive continuous, uninterrupted therapy with renin angiotensin system (RAS) inhibitors (see later text) which would otherwise be limited by hyperkalemia.

The presence of diabetes is a risk factor for developing acute kidney injury (AKI) due to intravenous iodinated contrast, volume depletion, and nonsteroidal anti-inflammatory agent use. Because unresolved AKI can hasten a patient's course to ESRD, all patients with diabetes and their physicians should be educated to avoid these potential nephrotoxic exposures. Lastly, due to advanced vascular disease often present in patients with diabetes, early access planning for dialysis is prudent.

TREATMENT OF DIABETIC NEPHROPATHY

Few therapies exist to treat DN, and treatment focuses on slowing the progression of DN from each stage to the next. Here we summarize the major clinical findings that direct DN treatment and outline the progress of ongoing trials, the results of which will likely direct future care.

Glycemic Control

The role of poor glycemic control in the progression of DN was first demonstrated in epidemiologic studies. The effect of improved glycemic control on the progression of DN has been tested in large clinical trials in both type 1 and type 2 diabetes. The definitive evidence in type 1 diabetes that intensive therapy with insulin delays the onset and slows the progression of diabetic nephropathy comes from the Diabetes Control and Complications Trial (DCCT).[103] Conducted from 1983 to 1993 in the United States and Canada, the DCCT randomized 1441 subjects aged 13 to 39 with type 1 diabetes to conventional versus intensive insulin control (goal hemoglobin A1c in the intensive arm <6.05%) and followed them for a mean of 6.5 years. The median A1c was 9.1% versus 7.3% for conventional versus intensive control. Intensive control demonstrated a relative risk reduction (RRR) of 39% for the development of MA, and a RRR of 56% for the development of overt proteinuria. Intensive blood sugar control was also associated with a reduction in the development of retinopathy and neuropathy. The tradeoff for improved renal outcomes was an increased incidence of severe hypoglycemic events (62 vs. 19 events/100 patient-years in the intensive vs. conventional control). Despite these successes, there was no reduction in CV events in DCCT (probably as a result of the very few events due to the relative youth of the cohort).

After the trial was ended, 1,375 subjects volunteered to participate in the Epidemiology of Diabetes Interventions and Complications (EDIC) study.[104] Note that all subjects had been advised to either remain at or convert to intensive control at the closeout period of DCCT. Not unsurprisingly, glucose control "converged" in each former treatment arm, and remained in alignment with one another (overall mean A1c 7.8% vs. 7.9% for former conventional vs. former intensive control, at EDIC year 11[105]). Despite the convergence of glycemic control, the development of MA and overt proteinuria were reduced (53% and 86%, respectively) by intensive control, in those subjects who did not experience a renal outcome in DCCT, after 4 (additional) years of follow-up in

EDIC. After 8 years of follow-up, the prevalence of HTN was greater in the conventional versus intensive arm (40.3% vs. 29.9%, $P < 0.001$).[106] There were no statistically significant differences in subjects requiring dialysis or transplantation, but there were more episodes of SCr >2 mg per dL in the conventional arm through year 8 of EDIC. Interestingly, there was a 42% reduction in the cumulative incidence of a first CV event after 10 years of EDIC follow-up. This CV benefit (of 6.5 years of intensive glucose control) was not apparent at 10 years (the end of DCCT), but by 20 years (corresponding to 10 years' follow-up in EDIC) it was, despite the fact that glycemic control was no longer different between the two groups.

In type 2 diabetes, the UKPDS tested the same hypothesis.[107] A total of 3,867 patients with newly diagnosed type 2 diabetes were randomized to intensive glucose control with oral agents or insulin, or to conventional therapy (dietary therapy). The mean achieved A1c was 7.0% in the intensive control arm as compared to 7.9% for the conventional arm. Subjects randomized to intensive control had a reduction in any diabetes-related endpoint, but no reduction in the renal outcomes of interest (development of MA, overt proteinuria, or a doubling of serum creatinine). Since UKPDS, three large trials (Action in Diabetes and Vascular Disease: Preterax and Diamicron Modified Release Controlled Evaluation [ADVANCE], Action to Control Cardiovascular Risk in Diabetes [ACCORD], and the VA Diabetes Trial [VADT])[73,108,109] have collectively studied nearly 25,000 subjects to try to elucidate any benefit of intensive glucose control in type 2 diabetes. Table 58.2 summarizes the findings of these three trials. The CV effects ranged from no benefit to increased CV risk associated with intensive glycemic control, and there was either no renal benefit or, in one study, a reduction in albuminuria. There was a significant increase in hypoglycemia in all the intensive groups. Thus, it seems that intensive control is of demonstrated benefit in type 1 diabetes, but is of unproven benefit in type 2 diabetes. Currently, the American Diabetes Association recommends an A1c goal for nonpregnant adults of <7% for microvascular risk reduction.[110]

Blood Pressure Control

Numerous large well-designed clinical trials across many populations of patients have demonstrated that systolic BP on average below 140 mm Hg reduces the incidence of CV events compared to systolic BP ≥140 mm Hg.[111–114] Unfortunately, most of these trials excluded patients with chronic kidney disease. However, observational studies have linked the presence of HTN to the development of MA or overt proteinuria in patients with diabetes.[54,115–117] Finally, there is a strong and continuous correlation between higher achieved blood pressures and worse renal outcomes in numerous epidemiologic and longitudinal cohort studies in patients with diabetes.

In newly diagnosed patients with diabetes, the UKPDS compared the impact of randomization to one of two levels of blood pressure control on the development of micro- and

TABLE 58.2 There is No Compelling Benefit of Intensive Glucose Control in Type 2 Diabetes

	ACCORD	ADVANCE	VADT
Population	n = 10,251 with CV event or risk	n = 11,140 with CV event or risk factor	n = 1,791 with poor BP control
Age (years, mean)	62	66	60
Duration of diabetes (years)	10	8	11.5
On insulin at baseline (%)	39/8.1%	1.5/7.2%	54/9.4%
Hemoglobin A1c, baseline	8.1%	7.2%	9.4%
A1c target (%)	<6.0% vs. 7–7.9	<6.5% vs. routine care (achieved 6.3% vs. 7.0%)	6.9% vs. 8.4% (1.5% difference)
Primary outcome	Increased total and CV mortality in intensive group	No benefit on CV outcomes, reduction in microvascular events	No benefit
Renal outcome	No benefit	Albuminuria reduced 21%	No benefit
Hypoglycemia (%)	16.2	2.7	21.2

ADVANCE, Action in Diabetes and Vascular Disease: Preterax and Diamicron Modified Release Controlled Evaluation; ACCORD, Action to Control Cardiovascular Risk in Diabetes; VADT, VA Diabetes Trial; CV, cardiovascular; BP, blood pressure.

macrovascular complications.[118] Over a mean of 8.4 years of follow-up, with achieved BP control of 144/82 versus 154/87 in the two arms, the risk of any complication of diabetes or death from diabetes, adverse CV events, and the composite of microvascular complications were dramatically decreased in the lower BP arm.[119] The study did not demonstrate any benefit of lower BP on the renal endpoints, namely proteinuria or doubling of SCr, but it was not designed as a renal study, and renal outcomes were tested only yearly.

Additionally, early studies on small numbers of diabetic subjects suggested that BP control could reduce the rate of loss of GFR in patients with established DN.[120,121] However, the intensive systolic BPs achieved were far higher than 140 mm Hg. The benefits of systolic BP goals below 140 mm Hg in patients with diabetes with or without kidney disease have been more difficult to demonstrate. The Appropriate Blood Pressure in Diabetes (ABCD) trial[122] randomized 480 normotensive subjects with type 2 diabetes to intensive (mean achieved BP approximately 128/75) versus moderate BP control (mean achieved BP approximately 137/81). After 5 years of follow-up, the development of MA or overt proteinuria was measured. There was a reduction in the development of MA and overt proteinuria in the group randomized to the intensive BP control, but there was no difference in the primary outcome of the study (creatinine clearance).

Similarly, a small study in type 1 diabetes[123] and advanced DN randomized subjects to a mean arterial pressure (MAP) of 92 mm Hg versus 100 to 107 mm Hg (treated with ramipril) and followed them for 2 years. In this case, proteinuria again improved in the lower BP arm, but increased in the higher.

The landmark study which addressed the issue of intensive BP control in type 2 diabetes is the ACCORD trial.[108] All subjects in ACCORD were randomized to intensive or standard glycemic control, and 4,733 of the participants were also randomized to intensive (systolic <120 mm Hg) or standard (systolic <140 mm Hg) BP control.[124] At 1 year, mean systolic BP was 119.3 mm Hg versus 133.5 mm Hg in the two groups, respectively. There was no reduction in the rate of the primary composite outcome of fatal and nonfatal major CV events (Fig. 58.3). Intensive BP control was associated with

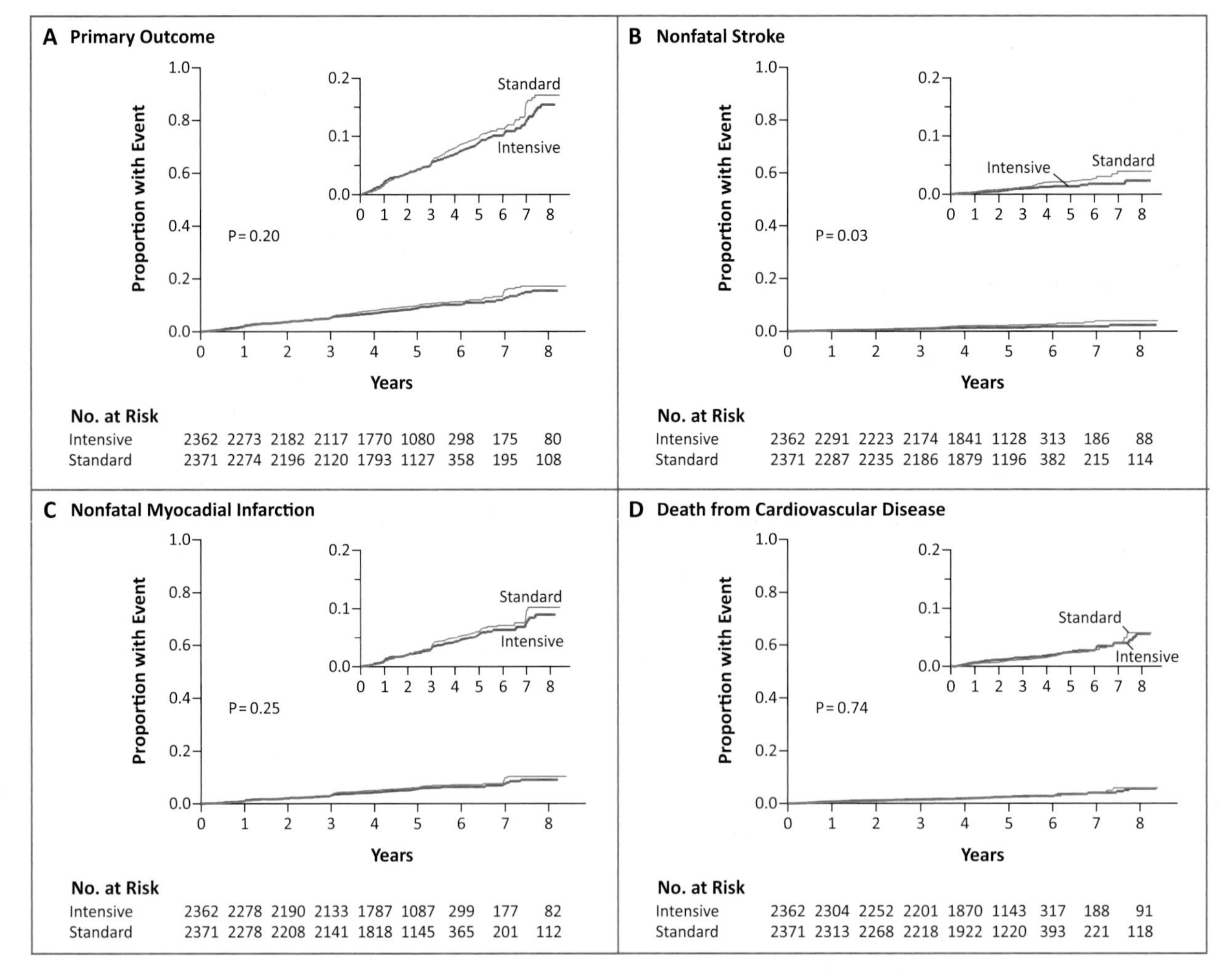

FIGURE 58.3 Targeting a systolic blood pressure of 120 mm Hg does not reduce the rate of cardiovascular events in type 2 diabetes, as compared to 140 mm Hg. (Cushman WC, Evans GW, Byington RP, et al. Effects of intensive blood-pressure control in type 2 diabetes mellitus. *N Engl J Med.* 2010;362:1575–1585.)

a reduction in albuminuria, but no difference in ESRD, and an increased risk of AKI requiring dialysis. There were nearly three times more adverse events attributed to antihypertensive therapies in the intensive control arm, including more episodes of hypotension, bradycardia, hyper-, and hypokalemia. Not unsurprisingly, lower systolic BP reduced the risk of stroke, but this study was not powered to detect a cerebrovascular outcome. It took nearly 3.5 versus 2.3 BP medications to control BP in the intensive versus standard arms, respectively.

The Irbesartan Diabetic Nephropathy Trial (IDNT) and Reduction in End-Points in Non-Insulin Dependent Diabetes Mellitus with the Angiotensin II Antagonist Losartan (RENAAL) trial convincingly demonstrated that the use of the angiotensin receptor blockers (ARBs) reduce the rate of loss of renal function in type 2 diabetes and DN (see later text, Inhibition of the Renin-Angiotensin System).[125,126] Although the patients were not randomized to different levels of BP control, it was clear that patients who entered with more poorly controlled BP were more likely to develop renal failure. However, in both the RENAAL and IDNT studies, achieved BP had a more profound effect on the primary outcome than did the baseline BP.[127–129] In other words, achieving BP control is important, even in the face of prior uncontrolled BP. Those patients who had a reduction in their systolic BP at month 6 or 12 (from baseline) had reduced risk of ESRD as compared to those who did not.[129] It took an average of three other antihypertensive agents to achieve BP control, however. When the effect of BP control was analyzed in IDNT, it appeared that there was a J-curve to the CV risk, as the risk of renal outcomes plateaued at systolic BP $<$130 mm Hg, but more importantly, all-cause mortality increased at systolic BP $<$120 mm Hg.[128]

Thus, it is clear that across the continuum of blood pressure in patients with diabetes, risks for CV events and progression of renal disease are high at the high end of the continuum, and are reduced progressively by lowering BP, but there may be a point beyond which further reductions in BP may be harmful. Below this point, although there may be less proteinuria, there is no difference in CV risk (save for stroke), or the risk of renal failure, and there are increased renal adverse events. Current guidelines recommend $<$130/80 for most patients with type 2 diabetes and DN, but with individualization.

Inhibition of the Renin-Angiotensin System

Drugs which block the RAS (i.e., angiotensin converting enzyme [ACE] inhibitors, ARBs, direct renin inhibitors, and mineralocorticoid antagonists) have demonstrated benefits to block the deleterious effects of angiotensin II on the kidney in animal models of DN, across the full spectrum of diabetic injury. These agents have been studied at each stage of DN, starting with the prevention of the development of MA.

Drugs which block the RAS have been studied in type 1 and type 2 diabetes in patients with normoalbuminuria to delay or prevent the development of MA. In type 1 diabetes, the Renin-Angiotensin System Study (RASS) evaluated losartan versus enalapril versus placebo for 5 years in subjects with normal BP and normoalbuminuria.[130] The 5-year cumulative incidence of MA was 17 versus 4.0 versus 6.0 (losartan vs. enalapril vs. placebo), thus, neither losartan nor enalapril prevented the development of MA in type 1 diabetes. The ARB candesartan was tested in the Diabetic Retinopathy Candesartan Trials (DIRECT) Program,[131] of which the DIRECT-Prevent 1 and the DIRECT-Protect 1 trials randomized patients with type 1 diabetes and normoalbuminuria to candesartan versus placebo and followed them for 5 years. The 5-year cumulative incidence of MA was 2.56% versus 2.32% (candesartan vs. placebo) in DIRECT-Prevent 1, and 7.36% versus 7.26% in DIRECT-Protect 1. Taken together, RASS and the DIRECT program suggest that the use of RAS inhibition is ineffective in the prevention of microalbuminuria in patients with type 1 diabetes.

In type 2 diabetes, the use of ramipril[132] in the Heart Outcomes Prevention Evaluation (HOPE) trial did not statistically significantly prevent the development of MA in type 2 diabetes. A trial in the DIRECT Program (see previous text), the DIRECT-Protect 2, studied candesartan in subjects with type 2 diabetes, normoalbuminuria, and either normal BP or controlled HTN. In the 725 normotensive subjects, MA developed in 13.9% versus 16.7% of subjects (candesartan vs. placebo), but in the 1,180 subjects with HTN, there was no difference in the development of MA over 5 years (15.34% vs. 15.30% of subjects, candesartan vs. placebo). The DIRECT Program was not powered for this renal endpoint, but the primary analysis suggested that candesartan did not prevent MA in type 2 diabetes. The Bergamo Nephrologic Diabetes Complications Trial (BENEDICT)[133] randomized 1,204 subjects to one of four arms (placebo, trandolapril, verapamil, or trandolapril plus verapamil) for at least 3 years, with a goal BP of 120/80 mm Hg. The use of trandolapril and trandolapril plus verapamil reduced the development of MA, but verapamil alone was similar to placebo. A post-hoc analysis suggested that trandolapril and BP reduction both independently reduce the risk of development of MA.[134] The Randomized Olmesartan and Diabetes Microalbuminuria Prevention (ROADMAP) trial studied the ARB olmesartan, following 4,449 subjects for a median of 3.2 years. There was a statistically significant baseline and follow-up BP difference between the olmesartan and placebo arms, but in the primary analysis, olmesartan prevented or delayed the onset of MA, with MA developing in 8.2% versus 9.8% of subjects (olmesartan vs. placebo) (Fig. 58.4). The trial was not designed to assess for CV outcomes, but there were more fatal CV events in the olmesartan group.[135] Thus it appears that use of RAS inhibition may prevent the development of MA in type 2 diabetes, but this intermediate outcome may be of uncertain value for the prevention of hard renal endpoints, and the value to the health care system has not been proven for these interventions as they have been for other stages of DN (see later text).

Many small clinical studies demonstrated that inhibition of the renin-angiotensin system reduced the number of patients with type 1 diabetes and MA who progressed to overt proteinuria,[136–142] in both hypertensive and normotensive subjects.

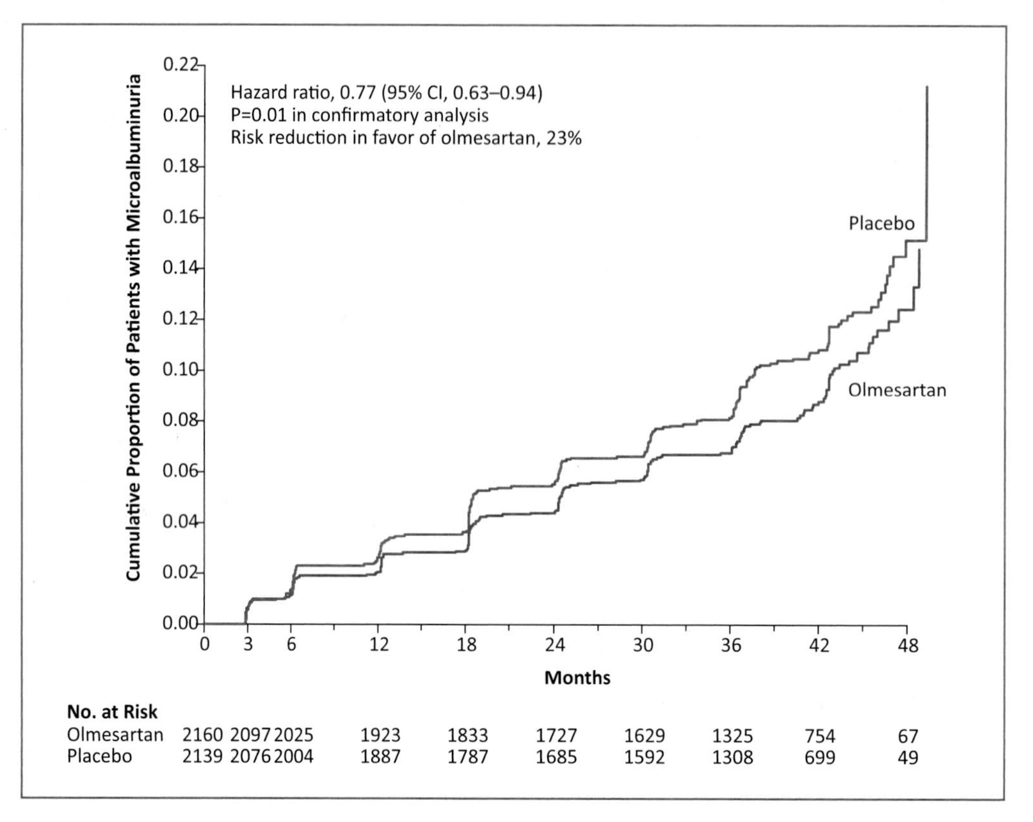

FIGURE 58.4 Olmesartan delays or prevents the development of microalbuminuria in type 2 diabetes, in the ROADMAP trial. (Haller H, Ito S, Izzo JL, et al. Olmesartan for the delay or prevention of microalbuminuria in Type 2 diabetes. *N Engl J Med.* 2011;364:907–917.)

In type 2 diabetes, therapy with the ARB irbesartan was studied to assess its impact on the development of overt proteinuria in subjects with established MA. The Effect of Irbesartan in the Development of Diabetic Nephropathy in Patients with Type 2 Diabetes (IRMA-2) trial[143] randomized 590 subjects with type 2 diabetes and MA to placebo, irbesartan 150 mg daily, or irbesartan 300 mg daily, for 2 years. Irbesartan reduced the risk of the development of overt proteinuria (defined here as >200 mg per day) as compared to placebo, with the 300 mg daily dose further reducing the number of patients who progressed from MA to overt proteinuria (Fig. 58.5). This trial demonstrates the importance of dose on efficacy.

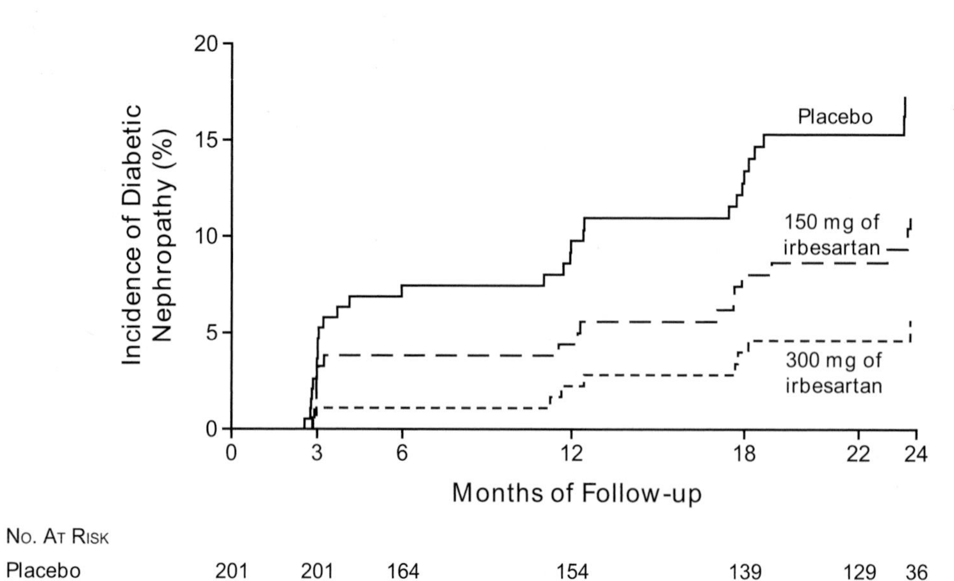

FIGURE 58.5 Irbesartan delays the progression from microalbuminuria to overt proteinuria in type 2 diabetes. Note there is a dose effect. (Parving HH, Lehnert H, Brochner-Mortensen J, et al. The effect of irbesartan on the development of diabetic nephropathy in patients with type 2 diabetes. *N Engl J Med.* 2001;345:870–878.)

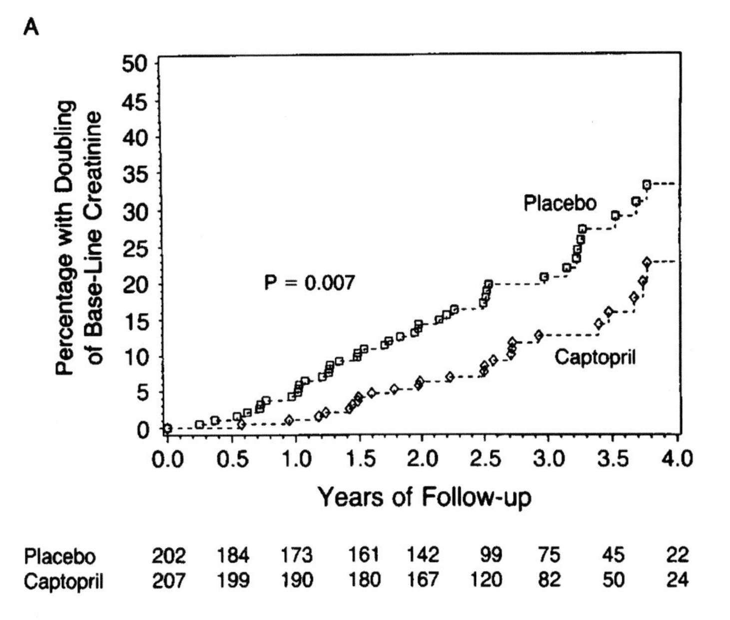

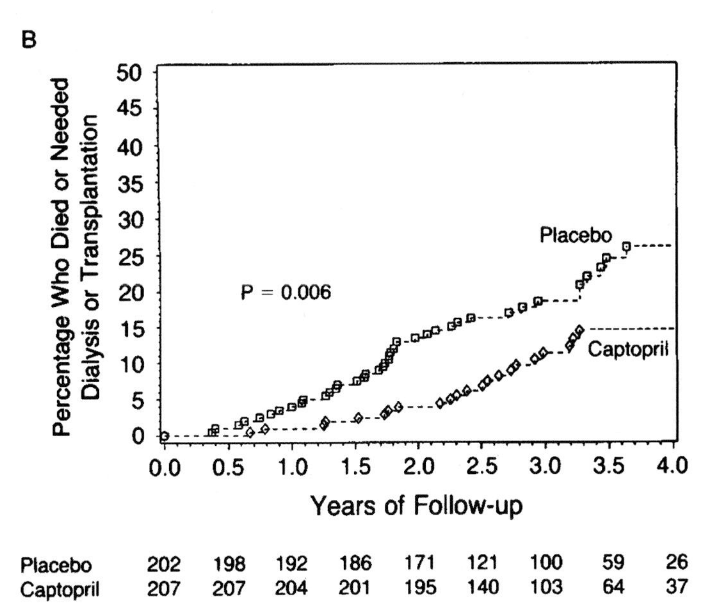

FIGURE 58.6 Captopril reduces the risk of the progression of diabetic nephropathy due to type 1 diabetes, as measured by doubling of serum creatinine **(A)** and by death or the need for dialysis or renal transplantation **(B)**. (Lewis EJ, Hunsicker LG, Bain RP, et al. The effect of angiotensin-converting-enzyme inhibition on diabetic nephropathy. The Collaborative Study Group. *N Engl J Med.* 1993;329:1456–1462.)

The first large trial to examine the role of ACE inhibitors in renoprotection in advanced DN[144] studied 409 subjects with type 1 diabetes, overt proteinuria (≥500 mg per day), and renal insufficiency (SCr ≤2.5 mg per dL). Subjects were randomized to captopril 25 mg three times daily or placebo, and could receive other antihypertensive agents to achieve BP control. There was a 48% reduction in the risk of doubling of SCr, as well as a similar reduction (50%) in the time to the composite endpoint of death, dialysis, or transplantation (Fig. 58.6). This trial confirmed the renoprotective effect of ACE inhibition in patients with type 1 diabetes and overt proteinuria, and was superior to BP control alone with other classes of antihypertensives.

In patients with type 2 diabetes and advanced nephropathy, the IDNT and RENAAL studies examined the effect of ARBs in type 2 diabetes, overt proteinuria, and renal failure. The IDNT randomized 1,715 subjects with HTN to irbesartan 300 mg daily, amlodipine 10 mg daily, or placebo, and followed them for 2.6 years. BP was targeted to <135/85 mm Hg and was obtained with agents other than calcium-channel blockers, ACE inhibitors, or ARBs. Irbesartan reduced the risk of the primary outcome of the composite of doubling of SCr, development of ESRD, or death, as compared to placebo or amlodipine (Fig. 58.7A). BP was similar in all three groups and not significantly different in the irbesartan and amlodipine groups.

Further supporting the efficacy of therapeutic intervention with an ARB, the RENAAL trial studied 1,513 subjects with type 2 diabetes and overt proteinuria for a mean of 3.4 years, and showed that treatment with losartan 100 mg daily was superior to placebo to reduce the risk of the composite endpoint doubling of SCr, ESRD, or death (Fig. 58.7B).

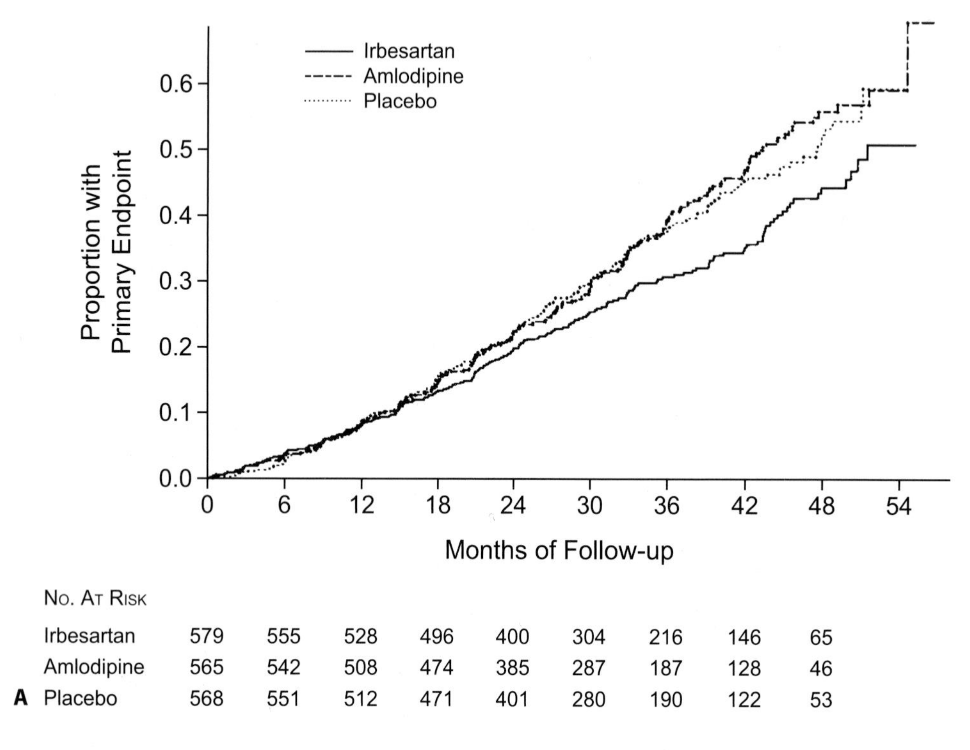

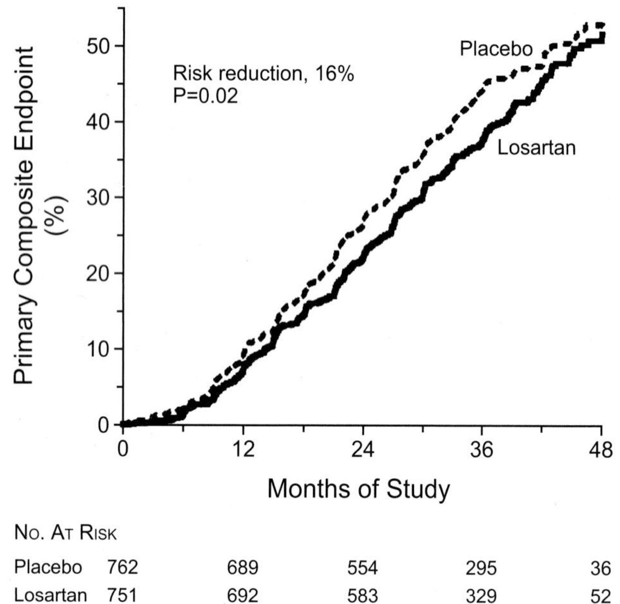

FIGURE 58.7 Both irbesartan in IDNT **(A)** and losartan in RENAAL **(B)** have been shown to delay the progression of diabetic nephropathy in type 2 diabetes. (**A** from Lewis EJ, Hunsicker LG, Clarke WR, et al. Renoprotective effect of the angiotensin-receptor antagonist irbesartan in patients with nephropathy due to type 2 diabetes. *N Engl J Med.* 2001;345:851–860. **B** from Brenner BM, Cooper ME, de Zeeuw D, et al. Effects of losartan on renal and cardiovascular outcomes in patients with type 2 diabetes and nephropathy. *N Engl J Med.* 2001;345:861–869.)

Taken together, IRMA2, IDNT, and RENAAL form a robust data set that convincingly show that ARBs reduce the progression of DN; the data from the IDNT and RENAAL were combined to form the Diabetes Mellitus Treatment for Renal Insufficiency Consortium (DIAMETRIC) database. Analysis of this dataset demonstrated robustly a strong beneficial effect of treatment with ARBs to delay or prevent doubling of SCr or ESRD (personal communication).[145]

The effect of an ARB on delaying the progression of DN from type 2 diabetes is independent yet additive to its effect on BP. This was demonstrated in post-hoc analyses of IDNT[128] and RENAAL[129] in which lower achieved systolic BP was associated with improved renal outcomes (Fig. 58.8).

In both the IDNT and RENAAL trials, baseline proteinuria was a predictor of the development of a renal endpoint.[84,125] More predictive, however, was what happened to the proteinuria at 6 to 12 months after randomization; a reduction in proteinuria during the course of these trials was associated with improved renal outcomes, particularly if it occurred early after randomization.[83,84] Arguably, medical therapy with RAS inhibition should be maximized to achieve the lowest amount of proteinuria possible.

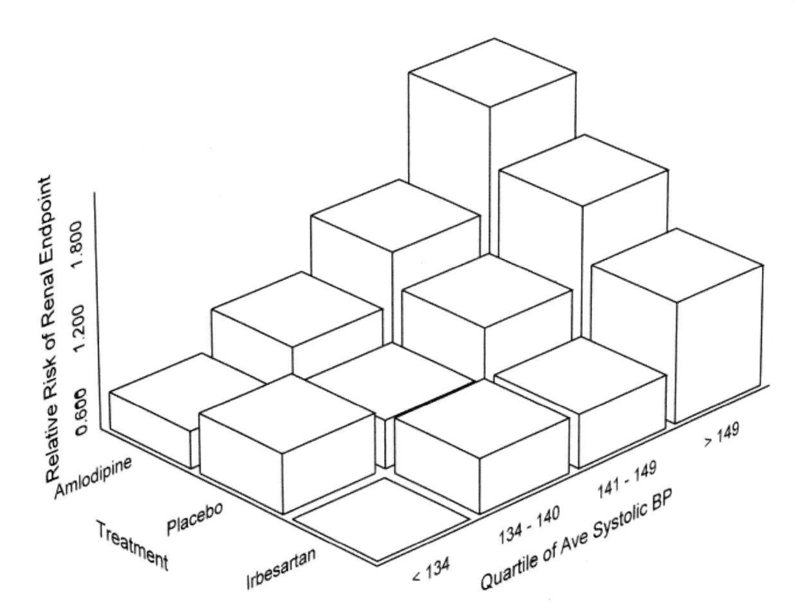

FIGURE 58.8 There is benefit to the use of irbesartan beyond its ability to control blood pressure on the relative risk of reaching a renal endpoint. In this case, the renal endpoint was defined as a doubling of serum creatinine (SCr) or end-stage renal disease (considered present when SCr ≥ 6.0 mg per dL or renal replacement therapy commenced). (Pohl MA, Blumenthal S, Cordonnier DJ, et al. Independent and additive impact of blood pressure control and angiotensin II receptor blockade on renal outcomes in the irbesartan diabetic nephropathy trial: clinical implications and limitations. *J Am Soc Nephrol.* 2005;16:3027–3037.)

Additionally, supratherapeutic doses (i.e., higher than the maximum approved dose) of ARB have shown improvement in proteinuria in small clinical studies, as opposed to the above-noted large clinical trials.[146–148] Irbesartan 900 mg daily reduced proteinuria more than 300 mg daily when administered over 2 months.[146] Similar studies have been conducted with telmisartan and valsartan as well. However, use of this approach to therapy has not yet been tested in large clinical trials with ESRD as an outcome.

Use of More Than One Inhibitor of the Renin Angiotensin System

A variety of clinical studies have examined the efficacy of combining inhibitors of the RAS but have often been limited by small sample size, submaximal doses of drugs, or surrogate renal outcomes, such as decreased proteinuria. These studies have employed dual therapy of ACE inhibitor plus ARB, the mineralocorticoid antagonists spironolactone and eplerenone, or the direct renin inhibitor (DRI) aliskiren, in combination with ACE inhibitor or ARB. In general, these small studies have shown a benefit to combination therapy.[149–161] The Aliskiren in the eValuation Of proteinuria In Diabetes (AVOID) trial[162] studied the effect on proteinuria of adding aliskiren versus placebo to losartan in type 2 diabetic nephropathy. Five hundred and ninety-nine subjects with type 2 diabetes, HTN, albuminuria 300 to 3,500 mg per g creatinine (200 to 3,500 mg per g if on RAS blocking agents), and eGFR >30 mL/min/1.73 m^2 were studied. Aliskiren reduced albuminuria at 24 weeks, but subjects treated with this combination therapy developed hyperkalemia more often (4.7% vs. 1.7%). The trial, although large and appropriately powered for a surrogate outcome of the change in UAE, could not assess the effect of aliskiren on the clinically significant outcome of ESRD.

The largest trial performed to date which utilized a combination of RAS agents is The ONgoing Telmisartan Alone and in combination with Ramipril Global EndpoinT (ONTARGET) trial.[163] ONTARGET studied 25,260 patients with CV risk (coronary, peripheral, or cerebrovascular vascular disease or diabetes with end-organ damage) with ramipril, telmisartan, or both, for the effect on the composite primary CV outcome, namely death from a CV cause, myocardial infarction, stroke, or hospitalization for heart failure. There was no difference in the primary outcome among the three arms. Although not designed primarily as a renal trial, ONTARGET enrolled 9,612 subjects with diabetes and 2,781 subjects with MA. The renal post-hoc analyses[164] showed less worsening of proteinuria with combination therapy, but GFR decreased more in the combination arm as compared to the single-agent arms (by about 2 mL/min/1.73 m^2). Additionally, there was a significant increase in the renal endpoint (dialysis, doubling of serum creatinine, or death) in the combination arm as compared to single-agent arms. This suggested the possibility that combination therapy might actually be harmful to renal function in some patient populations. The biggest contributor to this endpoint was the need for acute dialysis. It is important to note that this trial was not designed to test the renal outcomes, and its interpretation must be treated with caution; a trial designed specifically to answer this question is ongoing (see later text).

Lipid-Lowering Therapy

Many small studies have tested the use of lipid-lowering medications for their ability to delay the progression of DN, along with a meta-analysis which included these DN trials, suggested that treatment of dyslipidemia may help preserve GFR.[165] The largest trial performed on the role of aggressive lipid reduction in diabetes is the ACCORD Lipid trial,[166] which was embedded within the main ACCORD trial. As described previously, all subjects of the ACCORD trial were randomized to either intensive or standard glycemic control, but half (5,518 subjects) were also randomized (in a 2 × 2 factorial design) to intensive lipid lowering with simvastatin and fenofibrate versus simvastatin and placebo. The addition of fenofibrate did not affect the primary CV outcome of the trial, nor was there a difference in the incidence of ESRD or dialysis. There was, however, a reduction in both MA and overt proteinuria in the intensive group. Thus, intensive lipid lowering with simvastatin and fenofibrate may reduce proteinuria but may not prevent death or dialysis in type 2 diabetes. This trial was not designed to detect these renal endpoints, but the results are hypothesis-generating nonetheless. With the well-described CV risk conferred by the presence of diabetes, and specifically DN, treatment of dyslipidemia is indicated to reduce CV risk, irrespective of its specific impact on renal outcomes.

Multi-Intervention Treatments

The value of multiple-intervention risk reduction in patients with type 2 diabetes has been well studied, but most trials excluded subjects with DN. These are the very subjects who are at the highest risk for CV complications and death. The Steno-2 study[167] tested the hypothesis that a multifactorial intervention (consisting of lifestyle modification, smoking cessation, tight glucose control, and the use of RAS agents, aspirin, and lipid-lowering therapies) would affect the risk of death (from any cause and CV death) in patients with DN. One hundred sixty subjects with type 2 diabetes and persistent MA were studied for a mean of 7.8 years, and those who received intensive therapy had a significant reduction in CV death, peripheral vascular disease, urinary albumin excretion, retinopathy, and neuropathy. Although this study was not designed to detect which of the interventions was responsible for what proportion of effect, it is clear that a multitargeted approach was beneficial for the endpoints studied. There are no large trials which test the value of cessation of smoking, a specific component on the multiple-intervention study above, on the progression of DN. Epidemiologic studies associate smoking with a faster rate of loss of renal function. A small study suggests that smokers are more likely to progress to overt proteinuria and lose kidney function at a faster rate than nonsmokers or those who quit.[168] We recommend smoking cessation for all our patients, including those with DN.

ONGOING AND RECENTLY COMPLETED TRIALS

Several ongoing and recently completed trials should address current uncertainties in the landscape of the progression of DN, particularly with respect to combination therapies. The Department of Veterans' Affairs NEPHROpathy iN Diabetes (VA NEPHRON-D) Study[169] is testing whether the combination of lisinopril and losartan is superior to losartan alone to delay the progression of DN in type 2 diabetes. Approximately 1,900 subjects will be recruited until 2013. The ALiskiren Trial In Type 2 Diabetes Using Cardio-Renal Endpoints (ALTITUDE) study[170] tested whether dual RAS blockade with aliskiren and an ACE inhibitor or ARB reduces CV and renal morbidity and mortality. It was recently terminated early after there was an increase in adverse events and no apparent benefit to dual RAS blockade.[171] These trials were designed to assess if use of more than one agent that blocks that RAS affects clinically meaningful outcomes such as CV death or ESRD.

FUTURE DIRECTIONS

The future of DN perhaps centers around the prevention of it, and of diabetes, entirely. Once DN has begun, the few currently available therapies are limited in that they slow but do not prevent progression completely. Agents that are aimed at modulating physiologic inflammatory networks, or inhibiting cell proliferation, transforming growth factor beta (TGF-beta), matrix metalloproteinases, the accumulation of advanced glycosylation end-products, or interstitial fibrosis are currently under study for their ability to prevent or delay the progression of DN. Reversal of the lesions of DN[172] with a cure for diabetes (e.g., in the case of pancreas or islet-cell transplantation in type 1 diabetes) is unlikely to be successful for patients with type 2 diabetes. Large, well-powered, and properly designed clinical trials will be necessary to test the effect of these novel interventions and their combinations on clinically relevant and intermediate endpoints.

REFERENCES

1. Miller WG, Bruns DE, Hortin GL, et al. Current issues in measurement and reporting of urinary albumin excretion. *Clin Chem.* 2009;55:24–38.
2. Giampietro O, Penno G, Clerico A, et al. Which method for quantifying "microalbuminuria" in diabetics? Comparison of several immunological methods (immunoturbidimetric assay, immunonephelometric assay, radioimmunoassay and two semiquantitative tests) for measurement of albumin in urine. *Acta Diabetol.* 1992;28:239–245.
3. Constantiner M, Sehgal AR, Humbert L, et al. A dipstick protein and specific gravity algorithm accurately predicts pathological proteinuria. *Am J Kidney Dis.* 2005;45:833–841.
4. Lambers Heerspink HJ, Gansevoort RT, Brenner BM, et al. Comparison of different measures of urinary protein excretion for prediction of renal events. *J Am Soc Nephrol.* 2010;21:1355–1360.
5. Kussman MJ, Goldstein H, Gleason RE. The clinical course of diabetic nephropathy. *JAMA.* 1976;236:1861–1863.
6. Hovind P, Tarnow L, Rossing P, et al. Predictors for the development of microalbuminuria and macroalbuminuria in patients with type 1 diabetes: inception cohort study. *BMJ.* 2004;328:1105.
7. Haffner SM, Lehto S, Ronnemaa T, et al. Mortality from coronary heart disease in subjects with type 2 diabetes and in nondiabetic subjects with and without prior myocardial infarction. *N Engl J Med.* 1998;339:229–234.
8. Adler AI, Stevens RJ, Manley SE, et al. Development and progression of nephropathy in type 2 diabetes: the United Kingdom Prospective Diabetes Study (UKPDS 64). *Kidney Int.* 2003;63:225–232.
9. Packham DK, Alves TP, Dwyer JP, et al. Greater frequency of end stage renal disease than cardiovascular mortality in proteinuric type 2 diabetic nephropathy: results from the DIAMETRIC Database, 2010. *Am J Kidney Dis.* 2012;59(1):75–83.
10. Bellomo R, Ronco C, Kellum JA, et al. Acute renal failure - definition, outcome measures, animal models, fluid therapy and information technology needs: the Second International Consensus Conference of the Acute Dialysis Quality Initiative (ADQI) Group. *Crit Care.* 2004;8:R204–212.
11. Krolewski AS, Warram JH, Christlieb AR, et al. The changing natural history of nephropathy in type I diabetes. *Am J Med.* 1985;78:785–794.
12. Parving HH, Hommel E, Mathiesen E, et al. Prevalence of microalbuminuria, arterial hypertension, retinopathy and neuropathy in patients with insulin dependent diabetes. *Br Med J (Clin Res Ed).* 1988;296:156–160.

13. Cowie CC, Port FK, Wolfe RA, et al. Disparities in incidence of diabetic end-stage renal disease according to race and type of diabetes. *N Engl J Med.* 1989; 321:1074–1079.
14. Nelson RG, Knowler WC, Pettitt DJ, et al. Diabetic kidney disease in Pima Indians. *Diabetes Care.* 1993;16:335–341.
15. Orchard TJ, Dorman JS, Maser RE, et al. Prevalence of complications in IDDM by sex and duration. Pittsburgh Epidemiology of Diabetes Complications Study II. *Diabetes.* 1990;39:1116–1124.
16. Ismail N, Becker B, Strzelczyk P, et al. Renal disease and hypertension in non-insulin-dependent diabetes mellitus. *Kidney Int.* 1999;55:1–28.
17. Krolewski M, Eggers PW, Warram JH. Magnitude of end-stage renal disease in IDDM: a 35 year follow-up study. *Kidney Int.* 1996;50:2041–2046.
18. Bojestig M, Arnqvist HJ, Hermansson G, et al. Declining incidence of nephropathy in insulin-dependent diabetes mellitus. *N Engl J Med.* 1994;330:15–18.
19. Finne P, Reunanen A, Stenman S, et al. Incidence of end-stage renal disease in patients with type 1 diabetes. *JAMA.* 2005;294:1782–1787.
20. Rossing P, Rossing K, Jacobsen P, et al. Unchanged incidence of diabetic nephropathy in IDDM patients. *Diabetes.* 1995;44:739–743.
21. Costacou T, Ellis D, Fried L, et al. Sequence of progression of albuminuria and decreased GFR in persons with type 1 diabetes: a cohort study. *Am J Kidney Dis.* 2007;50:721–732.
22. Pavkov ME, Knowler WC, Bennett PH, et al. Increasing incidence of proteinuria and declining incidence of end-stage renal disease in diabetic Pima Indians. *Kidney Int.* 2006;70:1840–1846.
23. Nathan DM, Zinman B, Cleary PA, et al. Modern-day clinical course of type 1 diabetes mellitus after 30 years' duration: the diabetes control and complications trial/epidemiology of diabetes interventions and complications and Pittsburgh epidemiology of diabetes complications experience (1983-2005). *Arch Intern Med.* 2009;169:1307–1316.
24. Schultz CJ, Konopelska-Bahu T, Dalton RN, et al. Microalbuminuria prevalence varies with age, sex, and puberty in children with type 1 diabetes followed from diagnosis in a longitudinal study. Oxford Regional Prospective Study Group. *Diabetes Care.* 1999;22:495–502.
25. Coonrod BA, Ellis D, Becker DJ, et al. Predictors of microalbuminuria in individuals with IDDM. Pittsburgh Epidemiology of Diabetes Complications Study. *Diabetes Care.* 1993;16:1376–1383.
26. Chaturvedi N, Bandinelli S, Mangili R, et al. Microalbuminuria in type 1 diabetes: rates, risk factors and glycemic threshold. *Kidney Int.* 2001;60:219–227.
27. Svensson M, Nystrom L, Schon S, et al. Age at onset of childhood-onset type 1 diabetes and the development of end-stage renal disease: a nationwide population-based study. *Diabetes Care.* 2006;29:538–542.
28. Tapp RJ, Shaw JE, Zimmet PZ, et al. Albuminuria is evident in the early stages of diabetes onset: results from the Australian Diabetes, Obesity, and Lifestyle Study (AusDiab). *Am J Kidney Dis.* 2004;44:792–798.
29. Warram JH, Gearin G, Laffel L, et al. Effect of duration of type I diabetes on the prevalence of stages of diabetic nephropathy defined by urinary albumin/creatinine ratio. *J Am Soc Nephrol.* 1996;7:930–937.
30. Predictors of the development of microalbuminuria in patients with Type 1 diabetes mellitus: a seven-year prospective study. The Microalbuminuria Collaborative Study Group. *Diabet Med.* 1999;16:918–925.
31. Rossing P, Hougaard P, Parving HH. Risk factors for development of incipient and overt diabetic nephropathy in type 1 diabetic patients: a 10-year prospective observational study. *Diabetes Care.* 2002;25:859–864.
32. Mathiesen ER, Ronn B, Jensen T, et al. Relationship between blood pressure and urinary albumin excretion in development of microalbuminuria. *Diabetes.* 1990;39:245–249.
33. Effect of intensive therapy on the development and progression of diabetic nephropathy in the Diabetes Control and Complications Trial. The Diabetes Control and Complications (DCCT) Research Group. *Kidney Int.* 1995;47:1703–1720.
34. Near-normal urinary albumin concentrations predict progression to diabetic nephropathy in Type 1 diabetes mellitus. *Diabet Med.* 2000;17:782–791.
35. Poulsen PL, Hansen KW, Mogensen CE. Ambulatory blood pressure in the transition from normo- to microalbuminuria. A longitudinal study in IDDM patients. *Diabetes.* 1994;43:1248–1253.
36. Lurbe E, Redon J, Kesani A, et al. Increase in nocturnal blood pressure and progression to microalbuminuria in type 1 diabetes. *N Engl J Med.* 2002;347:797–805.
37. Hypertension in Diabetes Study (HDS): I. Prevalence of hypertension in newly presenting type 2 diabetic patients and the association with risk factors for cardiovascular and diabetic complications. *J Hypertens.* 1993;11:309–317.
38. Hypertension in Diabetes Study (HDS): II. Increased risk of cardiovascular complications in hypertensive type 2 diabetic patients. *J Hypertens.* 1993; 11:319–325.
39. UK Prospective Diabetes Study (UKPDS). VIII. Study design, progress and performance. *Diabetologia.* 1991;34:877–890.
40. Ditzel J, Schwartz M. Abnormally increased glomerular filtration rate in short-term insulin-treated diabetic subjects. *Diabetes.* 1967;16:264–267.
41. Mogensen CE. Glomerular filtration rate and renal plasma flow in normal and diabetic man during elevation of blood sugar levels. *Scand J Clin Lab Invest.* 1971;28:177–182.
42. Christiansen JS, Gammelgaard J, Frandsen M, et al. Increased kidney size, glomerular filtration rate and renal plasma flow in short-term insulin-dependent diabetics. *Diabetologia.* 1981;20:451–456.
43. Myers BD, Nelson RG, Williams GW, et al. Glomerular function in Pima Indians with noninsulin-dependent diabetes mellitus of recent onset. *J Clin Invest.* 1991;88:524–530.
44. Nelson RG, Bennett PH, Beck GJ, et al. Development and progression of renal disease in Pima Indians with non-insulin-dependent diabetes mellitus. Diabetic Renal Disease Study Group. *N Engl J Med.* 1996;335:1636–1642.
45. Mogensen CE. Early glomerular hyperfiltration in insulin-dependent diabetics and late nephropathy. *Scand J Clin Lab Invest* 1986;46;201–206.
46. Rudberg S, Persson B, Dahlquist G. Increased glomerular filtration rate as a predictor of diabetic nephropathy—an 8-year prospective study. *Kidney Int.* 1992;41:822–828.
47. Christiansen JS. On the pathogenesis of the increased glomerular filtration rate in short-term insulin-dependent diabetes. *Dan Med Bull.* 1984;31:349–361.
48. Hostetter TH. Hyperfiltration and glomerulosclerosis. *Semin Nephrol.* 2003;23:194–199.
49. Sharma K, Deelman L, Madesh M, et al. Involvement of transforming growth factor-beta in regulation of calcium transients in diabetic vascular smooth muscle cells. *Am J Physiol Renal Physiol.* 2003;285:F1258–1270.
50. Dahl-Jorgensen K, Brinchmann-Hansen O, Hanssen KF, et al. Effect of near normoglycaemia for two years on progression of early diabetic retinopathy, nephropathy, and neuropathy: the Oslo study. *Br Med J (Clin Res Ed).* 1986;293:1195–1199.
51. Mogensen CE, Andersen MJ. Increased kidney size and glomerular filtration rate in early juvenile diabetes. *Diabetes.* 1973;22:706–712.
52. Mogensen CE, Andersen MJ. Increased kidney size and glomerular filtration rate in untreated juvenile diabetes: normalization by insulin-treatment. *Diabetologia.* 1975;11:221–224.
53. Yang CC, Chen TC, Wu CS, et al. Sex differences in kidney size and clinical features of patients with uremia. *Gend Med.* 2010;7:451–457.
54. Parving HH, Lewis JB, Ravid M, et al. Prevalence and risk factors for microalbuminuria in a referred cohort of type II diabetic patients: a global perspective. *Kidney Int.* 2006;69:2057–2063.
55. Easterling RE. Racial factors in the incidence and causation of end-stage renal disease (ESRD). *Trans Am Soc Artif Intern Organs.* 1977;23:28–33.
56. Rostand SG, Kirk KA, Rutsky EA, et al. Racial differences in the incidence of treatment for end-stage renal disease. *N Engl J Med.* 1982;306:1276–1279.
57. Eggers PW, Connerton R, McMullan M. The Medicare experience with end-stage renal disease: trends in incidence, prevalence, and survival. *Health Care Financ Rev.* 1984;5:69–88.
58. Sugimoto T, Rosansky SJ. The incidence of treated end stage renal disease in the eastern United States: 1973-1979. *Am J Public Health.* 1984;74:14–17.
59. Pugh JA, Stern MP, Haffner SM, et al. Excess incidence of treatment of end-stage renal disease in Mexican Americans. *Am J Epidemiol.* 1988;127:135–144.
60. Young BA, Maynard C, Boyko EJ. Racial differences in diabetic nephropathy, cardiovascular disease, and mortality in a national population of veterans. *Diabetes Care.* 2003;26:2392–2399.
61. Burden AC, McNally PG, Feehally J, et al. Increased incidence of end-stage renal failure secondary to diabetes mellitus in Asian ethnic groups in the United Kingdom. *Diabet Med.* 1992;9:641–645.
62. Earle KK, Porter KA, Ostberg J, et al. Variation in the progression of diabetic nephropathy according to racial origin. *Nephrol Dial Transplant.* 2001;16: 286–290.
63. Seaquist ER, Goetz FC, Rich S, et al. Familial clustering of diabetic kidney disease. Evidence for genetic susceptibility to diabetic nephropathy. *N Engl J Med.* 1989;320:1161–1165.
64. Bleyer AJ, Sedor JR, Freedman BI, et al. Risk factors for development and progression of diabetic kidney disease and treatment patterns among diabetic siblings of patients with diabetic kidney disease. *Am J Kidney Dis.* 2008;51:29–37.
65. Quinn M, Angelico MC, Warram JH, et al. Familial factors determine the development of diabetic nephropathy in patients with IDDM. *Diabetologia.* 1996;39:940–945.
66. Harjutsalo V, Katoh S, Sarti C, et al. Population-based assessment of familial clustering of diabetic nephropathy in type 1 diabetes. *Diabetes.* 2004;53: 2449–2454.
67. Canani LH, Gerchman F, Gross JL. Familial clustering of diabetic nephropathy in Brazilian type 2 diabetic patients. *Diabetes.* 1999;48:909–913.

68. Satko SG, Langefeld CD, Daeihagh P, et al. Nephropathy in siblings of African Americans with overt type 2 diabetic nephropathy. *Am J Kidney Dis.* 2002;40:489–494.

69. Genetic determinants of diabetic nephropathy: The family investigation of nephropathy and diabetes (FIND). *J Am Soc Nephrol.* 2003;14:S202–204.

70. Freedman BI, Bostrom M, Daeihagh P, et al. Genetic factors in diabetic nephropathy. *Clin J Am Soc Nephrol.* 2007;2:1306–1316.

71. Ewens KG, George RA, Sharma K, et al. Assessment of 115 candidate genes for diabetic nephropathy by transmission/disequilibrium test. *Diabetes.* 2005;54:3305–3318.

72. Fujisawa T, Ikegami H, Kawaguchi Y, et al. Meta-analysis of association of insertion/deletion polymorphism of angiotensin I-converting enzyme gene with diabetic nephropathy and retinopathy. *Diabetologia.* 1998;41:47–53.

73. Patel A, MacMahon S, Chalmers J, et al. Intensive blood glucose control and vascular outcomes in patients with type 2 diabetes. *N Engl J Med.* 2008;358:2560–2572.

74. Mykkanen L, Haffner SM, Kuusisto J, et al. Microalbuminuria precedes the development of NIDDM. *Diabetes.* 1994;43:552–557.

75. Young BA, Katon WJ, Von Korff M, et al. Racial and ethnic differences in microalbuminuria prevalence in a diabetes population: the pathways study. *J Am Soc Nephrol.* 2005;16:219–228.

76. Newman DJ, Mattock MB, Dawnay AB, et al. Systematic review on urine albumin testing for early detection of diabetic complications. *Health Technol Assess.* 2005;9:iii–vi, xiii–163.

77. Viberti GC, Hill RD, Jarrett RJ, et al. Microalbuminuria as a predictor of clinical nephropathy in insulin-dependent diabetes mellitus. *Lancet.* 1982;1:1430–1432.

78. Mogensen CE, Christensen CK. Predicting diabetic nephropathy in insulin-dependent patients. *N Engl J Med.* 1984;311:89–93.

79. Mogensen CE. Microalbuminuria as a predictor of clinical diabetic nephropathy. *Kidney Int.* 1987;31:673–689.

80. Messent JW, Elliott TG, Hill RD, et al. Prognostic significance of microalbuminuria in insulin-dependent diabetes mellitus: a twenty-three year follow-up study. *Kidney Int.* 1992;41:836–839.

81. Perkins BA, Ficociello LH, Silva KH, et al. Regression of microalbuminuria in type 1 diabetes. *N Engl J Med.* 2003;348:2285–2293.

82. Ruggenenti P, Fassi A, Ilieva AP, et al. Effects of verapamil added-on trandolapril therapy in hypertensive type 2 diabetes patients with microalbuminuria: the BENEDICT-B randomized trial. *J Hypertens.* 2011;29:207–216.

83. Atkins RC, Briganti EM, Lewis JB, et al. Proteinuria reduction and progression to renal failure in patients with type 2 diabetes mellitus and overt nephropathy. *Am J Kidney Dis.* 2005;45:281–287.

84. de Zeeuw D, Remuzzi G, Parving HH, et al. Proteinuria, a target for renoprotection in patients with type 2 diabetic nephropathy: lessons from RENAAL. *Kidney Int.* 2004;65:2309–2320.

85. Perkins BA, Ficociello LH, Ostrander BE, et al. Microalbuminuria and the risk for early progressive renal function decline in type 1 diabetes. *J Am Soc Nephrol.* 2007;18:1353–1361.

86. Dwyer JP, Lewis JB, Parving HH, et al. Renal dysfunction in the presence of normoalbuminuria in type 2 diabetes: results from the DEMAND cohort: International Society of Nephrology Nexus: Diabetes and the Kidney. Dublin, Ireland, 2008.

87. Cirillo M, Laurenzi M, Mancini M, et al. Low glomerular filtration in the population: prevalence, associated disorders, and awareness. *Kidney Int.* 2006; 70:800–806.

88. Leitao CB, Canani LH, Kramer CK, et al. Masked hypertension, urinary albumin excretion rate, and echocardiographic parameters in putatively normotensive type 2 diabetic patients. *Diabetes Care.* 2007;30:1255–1260.

89. MacIsaac RJ, Tsalamandris C, Panagiotopoulos S, et al. Nonalbuminuric renal insufficiency in type 2 diabetes. *Diabetes Care.* 2004;27:195–200.

90. Kramer HJ, Nguyen QD, Curhan G, et al. Renal insufficiency in the absence of albuminuria and retinopathy among adults with type 2 diabetes mellitus. *JAMA.* 2003;289:3273–3277.

91. Retnakaran R, Cull CA, Thorne KI, et al. Risk factors for renal dysfunction in type 2 diabetes: U.K. Prospective Diabetes Study 74. *Diabetes.* 2006;55:1832–1839.

92. So WY, Kong AP, Ma RC, et al. Glomerular filtration rate, cardiorenal end points, and all-cause mortality in type 2 diabetic patients. *Diabetes Care.* 2006; 29:2046–2052.

93. Caramori ML, Fioretto P, Mauer M. Low glomerular filtration rate in normoalbuminuric type 1 diabetic patients: an indicator of more advanced glomerular lesions. *Diabetes.* 2003;52:1036–1040.

94. Schwartz MM, Lewis EJ, Leonard-Martin T, et al. Renal pathology patterns in type II diabetes mellitus: relationship with retinopathy. The Collaborative Study Group. *Nephrol Dial Transplant.* 1998;13:2547–2552.

95. Walker JD, Bending JJ, Dodds RA, et al. Restriction of dietary protein and progression of renal failure in diabetic nephropathy. *Lancet.* 1989;2:1411–1415.

96. Zeller K, Whittaker E, Sullivan L, et al. Effect of restricting dietary protein on the progression of renal failure in patients with insulin-dependent diabetes mellitus. *N Engl J Med.* 1991;324:78–84.

97. Parving HH, Gall MA, Skott P, et al. Prevalence and causes of albuminuria in non-insulin-dependent diabetic patients. *Kidney Int.* 1992;41:758–762.

98. Christensen PK, Larsen S, Horn T, et al. Causes of albuminuria in patients with type 2 diabetes without diabetic retinopathy. *Kidney Int.* 2000;58:1719–1731.

99. Olsen S, Mogensen CE. How often is NIDDM complicated with non-diabetic renal disease? An analysis of renal biopsies and the literature. *Diabetologia.* 1996;39:1638–1645.

100. Schmitz A, Vaeth M. Microalbuminuria: a major risk factor in non-insulin-dependent diabetes. A 10-year follow-up study of 503 patients. *Diabet Med.* 1988;5:126–134.

101. Marshall SM, Alberti KG. Comparison of the prevalence and associated features of abnormal albumin excretion in insulin-dependent and non-insulin-dependent diabetes. *Q J Med.* 1989;70:61–71.

102. Heine GH, Sester U, Girndt M, et al. Acanthocytes in the urine: useful tool to differentiate diabetic nephropathy from glomerulonephritis? *Diabetes Care.* 2004;27:190–194.

103. The effect of intensive treatment of diabetes on the development and progression of long-term complications in insulin-dependent diabetes mellitus. The Diabetes Control and Complications Trial Research Group. *N Engl J Med.* 1993;329:977–986.

104. Writing Team for the Diabetes Control and Complications Trial/Epidemiology of Diabetes Interventions and Complications Research Group. Effect of intensive therapy on the microvascular complications of type 1 diabetes mellitus. *JAMA.* 2002;287:2563–2569.

105. Nathan DM, Cleary PA, Backlund JY, et al. Intensive diabetes treatment and cardiovascular disease in patients with type 1 diabetes. *N Engl J Med.* 2005;353:2643–2653.

106. Sustained effect of intensive treatment of type 1 diabetes mellitus on development and progression of diabetic nephropathy: the Epidemiology of Diabetes Interventions and Complications (EDIC) study. *JAMA.* 2003;290:2159–2167.

107. Intensive blood-glucose control with sulphonylureas or insulin compared with conventional treatment and risk of complications in patients with type 2 diabetes (UKPDS 33). UK Prospective Diabetes Study (UKPDS) Group. *Lancet.* 1998;352:837–853.

108. Gerstein HC, Miller ME, Byington RP, et al. Effects of intensive glucose lowering in type 2 diabetes. *N Engl J Med.* 2008;358:2545–2559.

109. Reaven PD, Moritz TE, Schwenke DC, et al. Intensive glucose-lowering therapy reduces cardiovascular disease events in veterans affairs diabetes trial participants with lower calcified coronary atherosclerosis. *Diabetes.* 2009;58:2642–2648.

110. Executive Summary: Standards of Medical Care in Diabetes-2010. *Diabetes Care.* 2010;33:S4–S10.

111. Prevention of stroke by antihypertensive drug treatment in older persons with isolated systolic hypertension. Final results of the Systolic Hypertension in the Elderly Program (SHEP). SHEP Cooperative Research Group. *JAMA.* 1991;265:3255–3264.

112. Dahlof B, Lindholm LH, Hansson L, et al. Morbidity and mortality in the Swedish Trial in Old Patients with Hypertension (STOP-Hypertension). *Lancet.* 1991;338:1281–1285.

113. Multiple risk factor intervention trial. Risk factor changes and mortality results. Multiple Risk Factor Intervention Trial Research Group. *JAMA.* 1985;248:1465–1477.

114. Five-year findings of the hypertension detection and follow-up program. I. Reduction in mortality of persons with high blood pressure, including mild hypertension. Hypertension Detection and Follow-up Program Cooperative Group. *JAMA.* 1979;242:2562–2571.

115. Barzilay J, Warram JH, Bak M, et al. Predisposition to hypertension: risk factor for nephropathy and hypertension in IDDM. *Kidney Int.* 1992;41:723–730.

116. Krolewski AS, Canessa M, Warram JH, et al. Predisposition to hypertension and susceptibility to renal disease in insulin-dependent diabetes mellitus. *N Engl J Med.* 1988;318:140–145.

117. Savage S, Nagel NJ, Estacio RO, et al. Clinical factors associated with urinary albumin excretion in type II diabetes. *Am J Kidney Dis.* 1995;25:836–844.

118. Tight blood pressure control and risk of macrovascular and microvascular complications in type 2 diabetes: UKPDS 38. UK Prospective Diabetes Study Group. *BMJ.* 1998;317:703–713.

119. Adler AI, Stratton IM, Neil HA, et al. Association of systolic blood pressure with macrovascular and microvascular complications of type 2 diabetes (UKPDS 36): prospective observational study. *BMJ.* 2000;321:412–419.

120. Mogensen CE. Long-term antihypertensive treatment inhibiting progression of diabetic nephropathy. *Br Med J (Clin Res Ed).* 1982;285:685–688.

121. Parving HH, Andersen AR, Smidt UM, et al. Effect of antihypertensive treatment on kidney function in diabetic nephropathy. *Br Med J (Clin Res Ed).* 1987;294:1443–1447.

122. Schrier RW, Estacio RO, Esler A, et al. Effects of aggressive blood pressure control in normotensive type 2 diabetic patients on albuminuria, retinopathy and strokes. *Kidney Int.* 2002;61:1086–1097.
123. Lewis JB, Berl T, Bain RP, et al. Effect of intensive blood pressure control on the course of type 1 diabetic nephropathy. Collaborative Study Group. *Am J Kidney Dis.* 1999;34:809–817.
124. Cushman WC, Evans GW, Byington RP, et al. Effects of intensive blood-pressure control in type 2 diabetes mellitus. *N Engl J Med.* 2010;362:1575–1585.
125. Lewis EJ, Hunsicker LG, Clarke WR, et al. Renoprotective effect of the angiotensin-receptor antagonist irbesartan in patients with nephropathy due to type 2 diabetes. *N Engl J Med.* 2001;345:851–860.
126. Brenner BM, Cooper ME, de Zeeuw D, et al. Effects of losartan on renal and cardiovascular outcomes in patients with type 2 diabetes and nephropathy. *N Engl J Med.* 2001;345:861–869.
127. Berl T, Hunsicker LG, Lewis JB, et al. Impact of achieved blood pressure on cardiovascular outcomes in the Irbesartan Diabetic Nephropathy Trial. *J Am Soc Nephrol.* 2005;16:2170–2179.
128. Pohl MA, Blumenthal S, Cordonnier DJ, et al. Independent and additive impact of blood pressure control and angiotensin II receptor blockade on renal outcomes in the irbesartan diabetic nephropathy trial: clinical implications and limitations. *J Am Soc Nephrol.* 2005;16:3027–3037.
129. Eijkelkamp WB, Zhang Z, Remuzzi G, et al. Albuminuria is a target for renoprotective therapy independent from blood pressure in patients with type 2 diabetic nephropathy: post hoc analysis from the Reduction of Endpoints in NIDDM with the Angiotensin II Antagonist Losartan (RENAAL) trial. *J Am Soc Nephrol.* 2007;18:1540–1546.
130. Mauer M, Zinman B, Gardiner R, et al. Renal and retinal effects of enalapril and losartan in type 1 diabetes. *N Engl J Med.* 2009;361:40–51.
131. Bilous R, Chaturvedi N, Sjolie AK, et al. Effect of candesartan on microalbuminuria and albumin excretion rate in diabetes: three randomized trials. *Ann Intern Med.* 2009;151:11–20, W13–14.
132. Effects of ramipril on cardiovascular and microvascular outcomes in people with diabetes mellitus: results of the HOPE study and MICRO-HOPE substudy. Heart Outcomes Prevention Evaluation Study Investigators. *Lancet.* 2000;355:253–259.
133. Ruggenenti P, Fassi A, Ilieva AP, et al. Preventing microalbuminuria in type 2 diabetes. *N Engl J Med.* 2004;351:1941–1951.
134. Ruggenenti P, Perna A, Ganeva M, et al. Impact of blood pressure control and angiotensin-converting enzyme inhibitor therapy on new-onset microalbuminuria in type 2 diabetes: a post hoc analysis of the BENEDICT trial. *J Am Soc Nephrol.* 2006;17:3472–3481.
135. Haller H, Ito S, Izzo JL, et al. Olmesartan for the delay or prevention of microalbuminuria in type 2 diabetes. *N Engl J Med.* 2011;364:907–917.
136. Viberti G, Mogensen CE, Groop LC, et al. Effect of captopril on progression to clinical proteinuria in patients with insulin-dependent diabetes mellitus and microalbuminuria. European Microalbuminuria Captopril Study Group. *JAMA.* 1994;271:275–279.
137. Marre M, Chatellier G, Leblanc H, et al. Prevention of diabetic nephropathy with enalapril in normotensive diabetics with microalbuminuria. *BMJ.* 1988;297:1092–1095.
138. Mathiesen ER, Hommel E, Hansen HP, et al. Randomised controlled trial of long term efficacy of captopril on preservation of kidney function in normotensive patients with insulin dependent diabetes and microalbuminuria. *BMJ.* 1999;319:24–25.
139. O'Donnell MJ, Rowe BR, Lawson N, et al. Placebo-controlled trial of lisinopril in normotensive diabetic patients with incipient nephropathy. *J Hum Hypertens.* 1993;7:327–332.
140. Crepaldi G, Carta Q, Deferrari G, et al. Effects of lisinopril and nifedipine on the progression to overt albuminuria in IDDM patients with incipient nephropathy and normal blood pressure. The Italian Microalbuminuria Study Group in IDDM. *Diabetes Care.* 1998;21:104–110.
141. Randomised placebo-controlled trial of lisinopril in normotensive patients with insulin-dependent diabetes and normoalbuminuria or microalbuminuria. The EUCLID Study Group. *Lancet.* 1997;349:1787–1792.
142. Comparison between perindopril and nifedipine in hypertensive and normotensive diabetic patients with microalbuminuria. Melbourne Diabetic Nephropathy Study Group. *BMJ.* 1991;302:210–216.
143. Parving HH, Lehnert H, Brochner-Mortensen J, et al. The effect of irbesartan on the development of diabetic nephropathy in patients with type 2 diabetes. *N Engl J Med.* 2001;345:870–878.
144. Lewis EJ, Hunsicker LG, Bain RP, et al. The effect of angiotensin-converting-enzyme inhibition on diabetic nephropathy. The Collaborative Study Group. *N Engl J Med.* 1993;329:1456–1462.
145. Lambers Heerspink HJ, 2010
146. Rossing K, Schjoedt KJ, Jensen BR, et al. Enhanced renoprotective effects of ultrahigh doses of irbesartan in patients with type 2 diabetes and microalbuminuria. *Kidney Int.* 2005;68:1190–1198.
147. Hollenberg NK, Parving HH, Viberti G, et al. Albuminuria response to very high-dose valsartan in type 2 diabetes mellitus. *J Hypertens.* 2007;5:1921–1926.
148. Makino H, Haneda M, Babazono T, et al. Prevention of transition from incipient to overt nephropathy with telmisartan in patients with type 2 diabetes. *Diabetes Care.* 2007;30:1577–1578.
149. Bianchi S, Bigazzi R, Campese VM. Long-term effects of spironolactone on proteinuria and kidney function in patients with chronic kidney disease. *Kidney Int.* 2006;70:2116–2123.
150. Bianchi S, Bigazzi R, Campese VM. Antagonists of aldosterone and proteinuria in patients with CKD: an uncontrolled pilot study. *Am J Kidney Dis.* 2005;46:45–51.
151. Chrysostomou A, Pedagogos E, MacGregor L, et al. Double-blind, placebo-controlled study on the effect of the aldosterone receptor antagonist spironolactone in patients who have persistent proteinuria and are on long-term angiotensin-converting enzyme inhibitor therapy, with or without an angiotensin II receptor blocker. *Clin J Am Soc Nephrol.* 2006;1:256–262.
152. Kuriyama S, Sugano N, Ueda H, et al. Successful effect of triple blockade of renin-angiotensin-aldosterone system on massive proteinuria in a patient with chronic kidney disease. *Clin Exp Nephrol.* 2009;13:663–666.
153. Rachmani R, Slavachevsky I, Amit M, et al. The effect of spironolactone, cilazapril and their combination on albuminuria in patients with hypertension and diabetic nephropathy is independent of blood pressure reduction: a randomized controlled study. *Diabet Med.* 2004;21:471–475.
154. Saklayen MG, Gyebi LK, Tasosa J, et al. Effects of additive therapy with spironolactone on proteinuria in diabetic patients already on ACE inhibitor or ARB therapy: results of a randomized, placebo-controlled, double-blind, crossover trial. *J Investig Med.* 2008;56:714–719.
155. Sato A, Hayashi K, Saruta T. Antiproteinuric effects of mineralocorticoid receptor blockade in patients with chronic renal disease. *Am J Hypertens.* 2005;18:44–49.
156. Schjoedt KJ, Rossing K, Juhl TR, et al. Beneficial impact of spironolactone on nephrotic range albuminuria in diabetic nephropathy. *Kidney Int.* 2006;70:536–542.
157. Sengul E, Sahin T, Sevin E, et al. Effect of spironolactone on urinary protein excretion in patients with chronic kidney disease. *Ren Fail.* 2009;31:928–932.
158. van den Meiracker AH, Baggen RG, Pauli S, et al. Spironolactone in type 2 diabetic nephropathy: Effects on proteinuria, blood pressure and renal function. *J Hypertens.* 2006;24:2285–2292.
159. Persson F, Rossing P, Reinhard H, et al. Renal effects of aliskiren compared with and in combination with irbesartan in patients with type 2 diabetes, hypertension, and albuminuria. *Diabetes Care.* 2009;32:1873–1879.
160. Persson F, Rossing P, Schjoedt KJ, et al. Time course of the antiproteinuric and antihypertensive effects of direct renin inhibition in type 2 diabetes. *Kidney Int.* 2008;73:1419–1425.
161. Epstein M, Williams GH, Weinberger M, et al. Selective aldosterone blockade with eplerenone reduces albuminuria in patients with type 2 diabetes. *Clin J Am Soc Nephrol.* 2006;1:940–951.
162. Parving HH, Persson F, Lewis JB, et al. Aliskiren combined with losartan in type 2 diabetes and nephropathy. *N Engl J Med.* 2008;358:2433–2446.
163. Yusuf S, Teo KK, Pogue J, et al. Telmisartan, ramipril, or both in patients at high risk for vascular events. *N Engl J Med.* 2008;358:1547–1559.
164. Mann JF, Schmieder RE, McQueen M, et al. Renal outcomes with telmisartan, ramipril, or both, in people at high vascular risk (the ONTARGET study): a multicentre, randomised, double-blind, controlled trial. *Lancet.* 2008;372:547–553.
165. Fried LF, Orchard TJ, Kasiske BL. Effect of lipid reduction on the progression of renal disease: a meta-analysis. *Kidney Int.* 2001;59:260–269.
166. Ginsberg HN, Elam MB, Lovato LC, et al. Effects of combination lipid therapy in type 2 diabetes mellitus. *N Engl J Med.* 2010;362:1563–1574.
167. Gaede P, Lund-Andersen H, Parving HH, et al. Effect of a multifactorial intervention on mortality in type 2 diabetes. *N Engl J Med.* 2008;358:580–591.
168. Phisitkul K, Hegazy K, Chuahirun T, et al. Continued smoking exacerbates but cessation ameliorates progression of early type 2 diabetic nephropathy. *Am J Med Sci.* 2008;335:284–291.
169. Fried LF, Duckworth W, Zhang JH, et al. Design of combination angiotensin receptor blocker and angiotensin-converting enzyme inhibitor for treatment of diabetic nephropathy (VA NEPHRON-D). *Clin J Am Soc Nephrol.* 2009;4:361–368.
170. Parving HH, Brenner BM, McMurray JJ, et al. Aliskiren Trial in Type 2 Diabetes Using Cardio-Renal Endpoints (ALTITUDE): rationale and study design. *Nephrol Dial Transplant.* 2009;24:1663–1671.
171. Novartis. Novartis Press Release. Retrieved January 19, 2012, from http://www.novartis.com/newsroom/media-releases/en/2011/1572562.shtml.
172. Fioretto P, Steffes MW, Sutherland DE, et al. Reversal of lesions of diabetic nephropathy after pancreas transplantation. *N Engl J Med.* 1998;339:69–75.

CHAPTER

59 The Normal and Diseased Kidney in Pregnancy

Michelle A. Hladunewich • Ayodele Odutayo • Ravi Thadhani

Of all medical disorders that add risk to pregnancy, renal disease is ranked among one of the most feared by physicians. Kidney disease during pregnancy, even when mild, can considerably increase both the maternal and fetal risk necessitating close follow-up by both specialists in nephrology and high-risk obstetrics. Risk increases with the degree of renal dysfunction and is further heightened by comorbid conditions like diabetes and hypertension, which are often now present for many years given the societal trends in developed countries to delay childbearing. In addition to advanced maternal age, risk is further exacerbated by the expanded use of reproductive technologies that often results in multigestational births. Thus, the role of the nephrologist must begin prior to conception to stabilize a woman's condition and provide an appropriate risk assessment. During pregnancy, close monitoring by both subspecialties likely improves outcome by providing early identification of both renal and fetal compromise.

The goal of this chapter is to provide practical clinical guidance to physicians consulted when such patients contemplate conceiving or are already pregnant. First, we briefly review the normal gestational anatomic and physiologic renal changes, as such knowledge permits early detection of abnormalities. We subsequently discuss an approach to risk stratification and optimization during prepregnancy counselling and, finally, management of renal disease in pregnancy including acute compromise secondary to preeclampsia and other causes of acute kidney injury specific to pregnancy.

PREGNANCY-INDUCED CHANGES IN RENAL ANATOMY AND FUNCTION

Anatomy

It is classically taught that kidney size increases in a normal human pregnancy likely due to a combination of increased renal weight, dilatation of the renal collecting system, and perhaps increased glomerular volume. Contemporary data utilizing imaging techniques or the assessment of human biopsy or autopsy tissue carefully delineating healthy renal accommodation to pregnancy, however, are truly limited. Older data that included 97 women dying during or shortly after pregnancy from causes other than preeclampsia suggested that the increased combined renal weight of "normal" kidneys to be greater than in nonpregnant women, but data for age-matched nonpregnant females was not presented.[1]

Radiologic estimation of kidney length shows an approximate 1-cm increase in renal size and notes dilatation of the collecting system—calyces, renal pelvis, and ureters—that is significantly more pronounced on the right side (Fig. 59.1).[2,3] In the largest study in the literature wherein over 1,000 women were followed serially during pregnancy, dilatation in the right kidney began in the sixth week of gestation and maximal dilatation progressed at a rate of 0.5 mm per week until week 24 to 26 and then slowed to 0.3 mm per week until term.[4] Dilatation on the left was less marked as in earlier studies. Although the majority of gravid women (>50%) demonstrate some degree of dilatation,[4–6] there is significant variability between patients and even serial variability within the same patient making the diagnosis of true obstruction challenging.[7] Resolution begins immediately postpartum, but return to the prepregnancy state likely takes a number of weeks.[6]

The mechanism of this dilatation of the urinary tract is not entirely clear and is most likely a combination of pregnancy-related hormonal factors and mild obstruction. Support for hormonal factors includes the evidence of early dilatation before the uterus has enlarged sufficiently to become an obstructive factor as well as persistence into the postpartum period after delivery.[4,6] One study, however, found no correlation between dilatation and either serum estradiol, serum progesterone, or urinary estradiol excretion, but perhaps other hormonal factors that have not been studied in relation to dilatation may be important.[5] The best evidence for the obstructive theory comes from studies in which intraureteral pressure was monitored in third trimester gravid patients utilizing a fluid-filled catheter connected to a strain gauge transducer.[8] Pressure was greatest in the supine or standing position, but decreased markedly in a lateral decubitus or knee-to-chest position as well as immediately

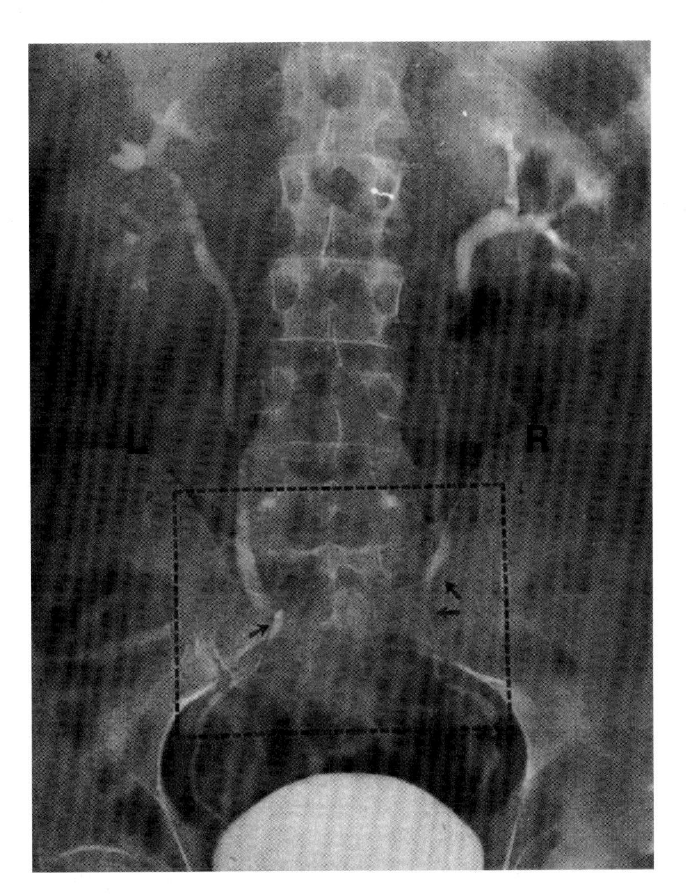

FIGURE 59.1 Normal physiologic dilatation of the urinary collecting system. Note the increased dilatation on the right side.

after cesarian delivery of the fetus, implying that the gravid uterus can obstruct the ureters. In addition, the increased pressure was present only above the pelvic brim where the ureters and the iliac arteries cross. Although this is consistent with the dilatation pattern in most gravid women,[9] the largest study to date did note at least some degree of dilatation in 10% to 15% of women in both kidneys before the uterus reached the pelvic rim. Thus, a combination of hormonal factors as well as obstruction is likely of physiologic importance.

In healthy pregnant subjects, the anatomic changes that occur at the level of the glomerulus are even less well described. There is data from 27 autopsy cases[1] and more recently from 12 third trimester biopsies[10] to suggest that glomerular diameter is greater than that measured in nonpregnant subjects. As already mentioned, the autopsy series conducted within 2 hours of death by the celebrated pathologist H.L. Sheehan between 1935 and 1946 at the Glasgow Royal Maternity Hospital did not include age-matched nonpregnant controls, but instead compared their data to even older autopsy studies wherein the timing and effect of autolysis was not clearly described.[1] The more recent biopsy series also failed to utilize careful stereologic techniques to carefully assess the glomerulus, but noted endotheliosis, albeit to a lesser degree, in healthy pregnant controls as well as in patients with preeclampsia.

Renal Function

Healthy pregnant women exhibit marked hyperfiltration. Both the glomerular filtration rate (GFR) and renal plasma flow (RPF) increase markedly during gestation. Unfortunately, however, there are few studies in which inulin or iothalamate and p-aminohippurate (PAH) clearance were measured serially and simultaneously throughout gestation in a sizable study population. Therefore, this knowledge comes from a synthesis of a small number of available studies that assessed renal physiology with proper clearance methodology at different time points during gestation (Fig. 59.2).

Hyperfiltration begins as early as the sixth week of gestation.[11] By the second half of pregnancy, GFR is elevated by

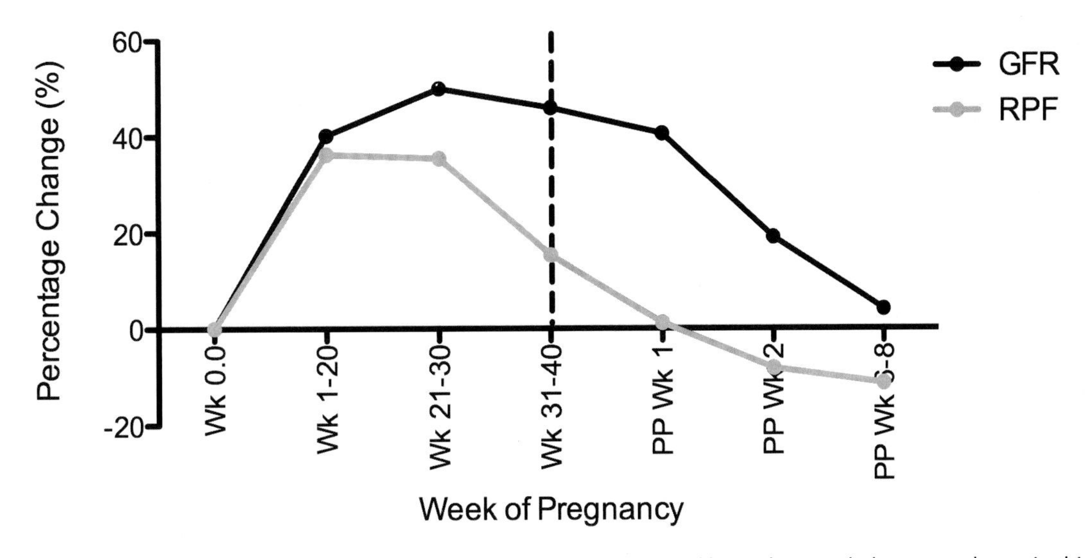

FIGURE 59.2 Glomerular filtration rate (GFR) and renal plasma flow (RPF) measured by inulin or iothalamate and p-aminohippurate clearance methodology, respectively, at different time points during gestation.[11,17,20,22,387]

40% to 60% above normal, nongravid levels, whereas the increase in RPF at least during the first trimester surpasses that of GFR with an increase in the order of 50% to as high as 80% in one study.[11–19] Thus, the filtration fraction is thought to fall in a pattern consistent with renal vasodilation. These high levels are maintained through gestational week 36, after which there is a decrease in GFR and a more pronounced decrease in RPF returning the filtration fraction to normal or a slightly elevated value compared to values observed in nonpregnant populations.[17,20,21] Despite normalization of RPF, the GFR remains elevated by approximately 41% on the first postpartum day[20] and by approximately 20% in the second postpartum week,[22] returning to baseline within the first postpartum month.[17,23]

The relationship between GFR and its determinants can be assessed using the following equation:

$$GFR = (\Delta P - \pi_{GC}) \chi K_f$$

where ΔP is the transcapillary hydraulic pressure difference or the pressure generated across the glomerulus; π_{GC} is the mean glomerular intracapillary oncotic pressure, the force that opposes the formation of glomerular filtration; and K_f is the glomerular ultrafiltration coefficient—that is, the product of the surface area available for filtration and the hydraulic permeability (*k*), which is the permeability to ultrafiltrate across the three layers of the glomerulus. As not all of these individual determinants can be directly measured in humans, and are instead inferred from complex mathematical modeling and theoretical analysis, the mechanisms of hyperfiltration during human pregnancy are not fully understood.[24]

The hyperfiltration that accompanies human pregnancy, however, appears to result primarily from depression of the oncotic pressure (π_{GC}) in the plasma that flows axially along the glomerular capillaries. The reduction of π_{GC} in pregnancy is attributable to two phenomena. The first is a hypervolemia-induced hemodilution that lowers the protein concentration and oncotic pressure of plasma entering the glomerular microcirculation.[25–28] The second is the elevated rate of RPF.[11,12,15,16] Hyperperfusion of glomeruli blunts the extent to which the axial protein concentration and oncotic pressure can increase along the glomerular capillaries during filtrate formation.[29]

Alternative explanations for increased GFR might include an increase in either K_f or ΔP. Utilizing a mathematical modeling of neutral dextran sieving coefficients to examine the determinants of the GFR in 13 healthy women late in pregnancy, investigators confirmed hyperfiltration was accomplished by an increase in RPF, but suggested perhaps a slight increase in K_f without any alteration in ΔP.[30] Our study that assessed determinants of GFR in the early postpartum period could not, with certainty, exclude a role for increased ΔP as an increment in either ΔP of 16% or an approximate increase in K_f of 50% would be necessary to account for the increased GFR in the postpartum period given the normalization of RPF and hence π_{GC}.[22] However, one must underscore the theoretical nature of these approaches in pregnant women, as direct micropuncture studies of the determinants of ultrafiltration are obviously not possible in humans. In rodent models, micropuncture studies consistently demonstrate a marked and parallel decrease in afferent and efferent vascular resistance resulting in an increased RPF without intraglomerular hypertension (increased ΔP).[31–33] Even following repeated pregnancies[34] or after a five-sixths reduction in renal mass[35] (an extreme example of compromised kidney function), the mechanism of renal accommodation to gestation did not change and there was no potential explanation for the pregnancy-associated renal damage often noted in young women with kidney disease. Further, no adequate human physiologic studies have been performed in diseased states and studies in humans that have utilized protein loading to assess potential renal reserve for accommodation have proven equivocal.[36,37] Thus, one cannot state with absolute certainty that the accommodation to pregnancy in a woman with advanced underlying renal disease does not involve an increase in intraglomerular pressure (ΔP) that could potentially have a long-term damaging effect on kidney function, and this is an area of renal physiology worthy of future study.

Tubular Function

Although precise mechanisms are not completely understood, the enhanced GFR that accompanies healthy pregnancy along with altered tubular reabsorption may be responsible for increased urinary levels of glucose, amino acids, uric acid, and protein. This classic teaching, however, is based on sparse data that in many scenarios lacks obvious clinical relevance.

In the nonpregnant state, healthy kidneys efficiently reabsorb glucose (>90%) and glycosuria is a clinical indicator of a filtered load that exceeds the maximal tubular reabsorption capacity (T_m). Despite the increased GFR that accompanies pregnancy, studies that utilized a continuous intravenous glucose challenge with inulin clearance techniques did not document a difference in GFR between women who displayed glycosuria and those who did not, suggesting instead that T_m was significantly decreased in pregnant women who displayed glycosuria.[38–40] The endogenous mechanism responsible is unclear, but the increased cortisol levels that accompany pregnancy have been postulated as a potential etiology based on observations in nonpregnant diabetic patients.[41]

The precise incidence of glycosuria in pregnancy is unclear with extensive variability noted between women and even in the same woman at different times during pregnancy.[40,42] During an oral glucose tolerance test, 26.9% of 104 patients in the second trimester and 42.8% of 205 patients in the third trimester developed glycosuria,[43] but a subsequent retrospective chart assessment of 17,647 pregnancies with normal carbohydrate screening noted an incidence of only 1.6% on routine clinical screening.[44] Further, no relationship of glycosuria to clinical diabetes has been demonstrated, as the majority of women who demonstrate glycosuria have normal glucose tolerance, and even obviously diabetic patients do not consistently demonstrate glycosuria. A theoretical risk of the altered proximal tubular glucose reabsorption might apply to pregnant diabetic patients demonstrating increased susceptibility to hypoglycemia,[45] but this has never been proven.

A similarly confusing pattern has emerged for increased urinary excretion of amino acids and water soluble vitamins.[42,46] The few studies designed to determine mechanisms were inconclusive and noted patterns of excretion were not related to the biologic function or chemical structure of the compound.[46] However, it is likely that alterations in both GFR and tubular reabsorption would be needed to account for the magnitude of the some of the excretion rates noted.

Serum uric acid has been documented to be decreased in the first trimester, reach a nadir in the second trimester, and then gradually increase as pregnancy progresses and high renal clearance is necessary to clear the increased production that accompanies fetal and/or placental growth.[47,48] Uric acid has been noted to be elevated in pregnancies complicated by preeclampsia,[49] and even first trimester uric acid levels have been shown to be elevated prior to the diagnosis of preeclampsia.[50,51] In one study, uric acid levels in the highest quartile (>3.56 mg per dL) compared to the lowest three quartiles were associated with an increased risk of developing preeclampsia (aOR [adjusted odds ratio] 1.82; 95% CI [confidence interval], 1.03–3.21), but not gestational hypertension.[51] Thus, it is not clear if the noted increase in serum uric acid during pregnancies complicated by preeclampsia is solely due to decreased renal clearance secondary to glomerular endotheliosis or increased production caused by trophoblast breakdown. Cytokine release and ischemia might also contribute to increased serum levels.

In healthy adults, proteinuria is typically defined as a protein excretion rate two standard deviations above the mean or greater than 150 mg per day. Due to the aforementioned physiologic changes that accompany the gravid state, the upper limit for proteinuria in pregnancy has been increased and most obstetric guidelines define significant protein excretion as ≥300 mg in a 24-hour period.[52] To date, there have been limited efforts to carefully assess serial urine protein or albumin excretion. One of the largest studies wherein the primary attempt was to establish a range for proteinuria in normal pregnancy included 270 healthy women and noted a mean 24-hour urine protein excretion of 116.9 mg with a 95% upper confidence limit of 259.4 mg.[53] These levels corresponded to an albumin excretion rate of 11.8 mg with a 95% upper confidence limit of 28.7 mg with no participants exceeding 30 mg per L. Further, the increase in proteinuria did not mirror the increase in filtration, as it typically increased after 20 weeks' gestation. This later increase in urine protein was also noted in a study that followed protein-to-creatinine ratios in healthy singleton and twin pregnancies, noting a rise in the mean ratio between 34 to 38 weeks that was more pronounced in the twin pregnancies albeit still not impressively elevated (150 and 220 mg per g creatinine in the singleton and twin pregnancies, respectively).[54]

Of interest, other studies assessing only urine albumin suggest, in fact, no glomerular leak in the vast majority of healthy pregnancies.[55–57] In a study that assayed 193 consecutive uncomplicated pregnancies, an upward trend in the albumin-to-creatinine ratio was noted as the pregnancy progressed, but only six women had a ratio in excess of 15 mg per g creatinine.[55] A similar study that assayed 95 healthy pregnant women between 16 and 20 weeks' gestation demonstrated only four women with an albumin/creatinine (A/C) ratio greater than 17 mg per g creatinine, of which two proceeded to develop preeclampsia.[56] Another study confirmed the slightly higher levels of urine albumin in late pregnancy that further increased in labor, but again noted that the vast majority of the values did not exceed the upper limit of normoalbuminuria.[57] The presence of an alternative proteinaceous material is also possible, as one study did demonstrate the protein-to-creatinine ratio exceeded the albumin-to-creatinine ratio more than might be expected.[49] In summary, data establishing this well-subscribed higher upper limit for normal proteinuria in pregnancy is suspect at best by the sheer paucity of large, carefully conducted studies with serial measurements, and the presence of significant proteinuria cannot simply be ascribed to the hyperfiltration that accompanies the gravid state.

Electrolytes and Acid-Base Balance

An intricate balance of natriuretic and antinatriuretic factors governs gestational changes in electrolytes (Table 59.1). During pregnancy, total body sodium levels increase significantly by an average of 3 to 4 mEq per day to ultimately peak at an increase of approximately 900 to 1,000 mEq.[58] Elevations in GFR cause an increase in sodium filtration from 20,000 to 30,000 mEq per day, whereas increments in progesterone[59] and atrial natriuretic peptide (ANP)[60,61] levels blunt tubular reabsorption. Other factors that may promote natriuresis include decrements in serum albumin concentration and increments in prostaglandins and melanocyte stimulating hormone.[62] These changes are counteracted by the antinatriuretic effect of aldosterone and deoxycorticosterone, which increase drastically in the third trimester of pregnancy. Of interest, aldosterone is particularly responsive to volume levels, and volume expansion with saline has been shown to suppress aldosterone.[63] In contrast, deoxycorticosterone is produced through extra-adrenal hydroxylation of progesterone[64] and is not suppressible with dexamethasone.[65] Therefore, aldosterone may play a more important role in sodium homeostasis whereas deoxycorticosterone might represent an important mechanism to attenuate the natriuretic effects of progesterone. Glomerulotubular changes may also facilitate sodium resorption through increased reabsorption in the proximal and distal tubules.[66] Some authors have suggested that this may be mediated by

TABLE 59.1 **Major Physiologic Changes Associated with Sodium and Potassium Balance in Healthy Human Pregnancy**

Physiologic Change	Effect During Pregnancy	Change During Pregnancy
Atrial natriuretic peptide	Natriuretic	Increased at 12 weeks/still elevated at 36 weeks
Progesterone	Natriuretic/Antikaliuretic	Increased after LH surge during ovulation/peak at 4 weeks before delivery
Glomerular filtration rate	Natriuretic	Increased in early pregnancy and sustained until delivery
Aldosterone	Antinatriuretic	Increased by 6 weeks gestation and sustained until delivery
Deoxycorticosterone	Antinatriuretic	Increased in first trimester/peak in third trimester
Na^+/K^+ transporters	Antinatriuretic	Increased in pregnancy

LH, luteinizing hormone.

increments in number of renal Na^+/K^+ ATPase,[67] but this is controversial.[68] Overall, the interplay of natriuretic and antinatriuretic factors is complex and varies during different periods of gestation.

Given the mineralocorticoid-induced retention of sodium, it is surprising that total body potassium increases by up to 320 mEq,[58] while serum potassium decreases.[47,69] Potassium balance was preserved in studies involving mineralocorticoid administration to gravidas,[70] while a similar maneuver in males produced decrements in potassium suggesting pregnancy may be responsible for attenuating the kaliuretic effects of mineralocorticoids.[70] These authors went on to identify progesterone as the key factor in facilitating potassium retention.[70] Pregnancy-induced alterations in potassium handling have important ramifications for the management of diseases associated with potassium processing. For instance, increments in potassium that are noted in sickle-cell anemia may be amplified in pregnancy.[71] Of interest, this amplification may not be secondary to potassium retention, but instead due to alterations in aldosterone release. It has also been hypothesized that the net potassium retention in pregnancy may attenuate the hypokalemia induced by diseases such as Bartter syndrome.[72] However, exacerbation of Bartter syndrome is more likely given the decrements in serum potassium that characterize normal pregnancy. In fact, complicated pregnancies with an increased need for potassium supplementation have been consistently reported in women with Bartter syndrome.[73,74] Altogether, it is imperative that health care providers consider pregnancy-induced alterations in electrolytes during clinical decision making. A recent report by Larsson et al. that details biochemical reference values in normal pregnancy can facilitate this process.[75]

Acid-base balance is also altered during pregnancy.[76] Respiratory alkalosis is induced by an increase in tidal volume[77,78] and a concomitant decrease in arterial partial pressure of carbon dioxide ($PaCO_2$).[79] A compensatory decrease in plasma bicarbonate is noted along with decrements in hydrogen ion levels.[79] Pregnancy-induced elevations in estrogen and progesterone have been implicated as the key factors in elevating minute ventilation, and therefore initiating these downstream changes.[80]

Blood Pressure and Volume Status in Pregnancy

In parallel with these absolute elevations in electrolytes, body water increases by approximately 8 L[81] and plasma volume increases by 1.2 L,[82] whereas plasma osmolality falls.[47,60,69,82] Such physiologic adjustments are in stark contrast to the nonpregnant state where sustained hypervolemia and decrements in plasma osmolality would result in high blood pressure and remarkable diuresis. Instead, blood pressure begins to decrease early in the first trimester and reaches a nadir between 18 and 24 weeks of gestation[11,83] due to significant systemic vasodilatation likely mediated through an altered balance of an array of vasodilatory and vasoconstricting hormones including, but not limited to, nitric oxide and endothelin, prostacyclin and prostaglandin, relaxin, as well as insensitivity to components of the renin angiotensin system (RAS).

The events initiating these changes are not completely understood, but human chorionic gonadotropin (HCG)-induced increased production of relaxin by the corpus luteum may facilitate vasodilation in normal pregnancy.[84] In animal models, relaxin upregulates vascular gelatinase activity, thereby contributing to vasodilation and reduced myogenic reactivity of small arteries through activation of the endothelial endothelin B receptor–nitric oxide (NO) pathway.[84] A recent study noted a similar effect in small subcutaneous human arteries incubated with relaxin that was shown to be mediated through vascular endothelial growth factor (VEGF).[85] Thus, angiogenic factors may also have an important function in the increased production of NO and prostacyclin in pregnancy via pathways involving phospholipase C (PLC), mitogen-activated protein kinase (MAPK), and protein kinase C (PKC).[86] The importance of NO-mediated vasodilatation in the normal vascular adaptation to pregnancy has also been demonstrated in studies that utilize flow-mediated vasodilatation (FMD). In healthy pregnant women, an endothelial NO synthase Glu298Asp polymorphism was noted to be associated with differences in endothelium-dependent dilation at 12 weeks' gestation[87] and the concentration of l-homoarginine, another substrate for NO, has been shown to positively correlate with FMD ($r = 0.362$, $P = 0.006$).[88]

With respect to the RAS, it is the lack of vascular response that is integral for achieving decrements in blood pressure during pregnancy. In normal pregnancy, components of the RAS are upregulated. Prorenin, released from the ovaries, parallels the increase of β-HCG peaking at 10 times the usual blood level.[89] Angiotensinogen also increases gradually throughout pregnancy in response to increasing estrogen levels, as does plasma renin activity, possibly in response to progesterone. Increased plasma renin activity results in increased levels of ANG II,[90,91] but, as in the luteal phase of the normal menstrual cycle, resistance to its pressor effects characterizes normal pregnancy.[92] Vascular insensitivity to ANG II infusion has been demonstrated in healthy pregnant women[93,94] and reduced sensitivity of the renal circulation has been demonstrated in pregnant rats.[95] Although the mechanism of resistance to the effects of ANG II remains elusive, increased plasma levels and urinary excretion rates of ANG^{1-7} have been documented in human pregnancy.[90,96] The increased ANG^{1-7}-to-ANG II ratio may be critical for maintaining the decreased blood pressure that is characteristic of healthy human pregnancy.

Maintenance of hypervolemia is another important deviation from the nonpregnant state. The initial shift toward volume retention is dependent on the lowering of the osmotic threshold for AVP release thereby allowing for continued secretion of the hormone.[97] In mid to late pregnancy, AVP levels increase[97] in order to compensate for increments in vasopressinase-mediated clearance of the hormone.[98] Altogether the preservation of equilibrium is not a static process. Instead, there is a complex and dynamic interplay of increments and decrements in hormone control systems. It is, therefore, not surprising that three major hypotheses have emerged to explain the hypervolemia that attends the gravid state.[99] The "underfill" hypothesis is founded on the drastic depression in systematic vascular tone that is noted in early gestation.[60] This reduction in pressure results in a transient state of hypovolemia or underfill and the induction of compensatory hormones such as the RAS and vasopressin. Accordingly, there is a subsequent shift toward increased thirst and volume retention. In addition, investigators suggest that the threshold for AVP secretion is also lowered in an attempt to correct underfill. In contrast, the "normal fill" hypothesis suggests that hypervolemia is recognized as the new hemodynamic set point in pregnancy. Increments in β-HCG have been implicated as an initial and independent trigger for reductions in the AVP threshold,[100,101] and water intake and retention would increase until plasma osmolality decreases in parallel. Lastly, the "overfill" hypothesis stipulates that the primary change in pregnancy is fluid retention as opposed to decreased vascular tone and intravascular expansion.[99,102] The aforementioned elevations in natriuretic factors would, therefore, be consistent with an overfilled state.[99] Of interest, some authors have suggested that each of the three hypotheses are correct and all occur in gestation,[99] but the temporality of these events has not been clearly established.

A particularly important aberration in volume homeostasis during pregnancy is diabetes insipidus (DI). DI frequently occurs in the third trimester of pregnancy and is characterized by polydipsia and dilute polyuria. At a clinical level, DI during gestation can present as a resurgence of preexisting central or nephrogenic DI, transient DI of pregnancy, or a sequelae of Sheehan syndrome. Given the pregnancy-induced increments in vasopressinase, it is conceivable that AVP levels will further decrease and DI would be exacerbated by pregnancy. In fact, the resurgence of latent DI is documented in the literature.[103] Similarly, DI may be subclinical prior to gestation, but become symptomatic during pregnancy. As the increase in vasopressinase correlates with the timing of increments in trophoblastic mass,[98] it has been also speculated that women with multigestational pregnancies may have higher vasopressinase levels and therefore be at increased risk for DI.[104–106] However, this hypothesis has not been directly examined in the literature.

Accumulation or increased activity of vasopressinase may also underlie the development of a transient form of DI during pregnancy.[107] Although vasopressinase normally undergoes hepatic clearance during pregnancy, impairments in liver function increase circulating levels of the enzyme thereby leading to decrements in AVP, ultimately resulting in DI.[103] Of interest, the hepatic dysfunction noted in HELLP syndrome,[106,108] and acute fatty liver of pregnancy[109] may be associated with transient DI of pregnancy. Therefore, the diagnosis of DI should also prompt increased vigilance for preeclampsia and hepatic dysfunction. Current treatment for resurgence of latent DI, or transient DI of pregnancy, involves administration of desmopressin (DDAVP), a vasopressinase resistant analogue of AVP. DDAVP can be safely used in pregnancy[110] and its transfer to breast milk is limited.

Lastly, an uncommon, but important cause of DI is Sheehan syndrome, characterized by postpartum hemorrhage leading to avascular necrosis of the pituitary gland. It can also produce diabetes insipidus if the posterior pituitary is affected.[111–113] However, the independent blood supply of the anterior and posterior pituitary may be protective.[112] Nevertheless, polyuria and polydipsia postpartum following significant hemorrhage should raise the appropriate suspicion.[112]

MONITORING RENAL FUNCTION DURING PREGNANCY

Glomerular Filtration Rate

The gold standard for determining GFR in pregnancy remains a carefully timed clearance utilizing either inulin or iothalamate plasma disappearance techniques or carefully timed urine clearances through a Foley catheter, but even in research settings these methodologies have become scarce. Further, clearance methodology, including a timed creatinine clearance, is hampered by the dilated urinary system and the potential bladder retention that accompanies the gravid state, resulting in an underestimation of the true GFR even when creatinine clearance is measured.[114] GFR equations, including the Cockcroft-Gault and the MDRD, can substantially overestimate or underestimate GFR and cannot be recommended for use in clinical practice.[114–116] A recent study that utilized Bland and Altman methodology noted the Cockcroft-Gault equation to underestimate GFR by 25% in 23% of the cases studied and to overestimate GFR by 25% in 16% of the cases studied.[114] The MDRD equation, on the other hand, underestimated GFR by 25% in 61% of the cases studied without any cases wherein there was a significant overestimation.[114] The newer CKD-EPI equation, which has been deemed superior to the MDRD when assessing patients with higher rates of GFR,[117] remains to be assessed in pregnancy.

Thus, trends in the serum creatinine are typically used to assess for renal insufficiency in pregnant women, but the inverse hyperbolic relationship between serum creatinine and GFR is blunted in the elevated range of the latter that is typically associated with pregnancy. A comparison of the serum creatinine and GFR as measured by inulin clearance revealed that the often profound depression in K_f that accompanies preeclampsia could not be appreciated by evaluation of the serum creatinine.[118] Although statistically significantly different, the serum creatinine remained in the normal range for both groups with a value of 0.85 ± 0.22 mg per dL in preeclamptic patients and 0.60 ± 0.10 mg per dL in healthy gravid controls, despite a loss of GFR in excess of 50%.

Cystatin C is a potential assay to detect subtle changes in GFR during pregnancy. However, to date, no serial longitudinal studies, spanning all three trimesters and utilizing a gold standard technique for GFR measurement, have been done to determine the value of cystatin C to reflect early changes in GFR. Further, there is evidence to suggest a placental source also exists and cystatin C may be released in response to placental ischemia. Cysteine-proteases are felt to be important for trophoblast invasion and are controlled by inhibitors such as cystatin C. Increases in placental expression of cystatin C at the mRNA and protein level have been noted in women with preeclampsia compared to women with normal pregnancies suggesting that an increase in placental production of cystatin C may contribute to the higher maternal levels seen in women with preeclampsia.[119] Although the process is not fully understood, an increase in the synthesis and secretion of cystatin C may be associated with poor placentation, consequently complicating interpretation of cystatin C as a marker of GFR.

Proteinuria

As in the nonpregnant population, issues exist with all the methods used to quantify urine protein. The accuracy of the urine dipstick for predicting meaningful proteinuria is poor with numerous false-negative and false-positive results due to either dilute or concentrated samples, respectively. A systematic review identified only six studies of adequate methodologic quality producing a pooled positive likelihood ratio of 3.48 (95% CI 1.66–7.27) and a negative likelihood ratio of 0.6 (CI 0.45–0.8) for predicting 300 mg per day of urine protein at the 1+ or greater threshold on urinalysis.[120] Despite this lack of accuracy, urinalysis as an initial screen is still frequently utilized by the obstetrical community to assess for abnormal proteinuria.

To date, a multitude of studies have correlated either the protein-to-creatinine or the albumin-to-creatinine ratio to the 24-hour urine collection or shorter timed collections typically demonstrating highly positive correlations as might be expected[121–123] and larger systematic reviews do confirm the ability of ratios to identify clinically meaningful urine protein,[124] irrespective of the time of collection,[125] making it a tool that can be utilized in the outpatient clinic setting. Correlation, however, would not be the optimal assessment tool to compare two obviously related measures. To date, only a single study utilized the appropriate Bland Altman test to confirm agreement between the 24-hour urine protein and the protein-to-creatinine ratio.[126] These authors confirmed the correlation between the two measures and examination of the plots suggests (like the systematic reviews) that at lower levels of urine protein, there is a high level of agreement, but the ratio is less precise at higher levels of urine protein not unlike the nonpregnant state.

Thus, a carefully timed urine protein collection along with an assessment of creatinine excretion to ensure adequacy of the collection remains the most commonly used test for the quantification of urine protein in pregnancy. The potential for inadequate collection due to significant dilatation of the urinary tract system, however, is an issue that remains to be adequately addressed and clarified. One study noted a high error rate (13%–54%) when the adequacy of the collection was assessed based on the predicted creatinine excretion for prepregnancy maternal weight.[127] In a recent excellent review on the topic, the author recommended adequate hydration and maintaining the lateral recumbent position for an hour prior to initiating and completing the collection to reduce the potential errors from retention.[128] Although rarely practiced clinically, such techniques should at least be utilized in future studies wherein the careful assessment of proteinuria is required.

Kidney Biopsy

As mentioned, significant proteinuria in a pregnant woman should not simply be attributed to the hyperfiltration of pregnancy. If the clinical presentation includes nephrotic syndrome or deterioration in renal function early in pregnancy without an established diagnosis, a kidney biopsy can be done to assist with the diagnosis and guide treatment. Data is limited with respect to the safety of kidney biopsy in pregnant women. An early study noted bleeding complications to be almost three times more common in pregnant women with serious complications arising including a patient death.[129] However, this study predated ultrasound guidance and the diagnosis on a number of the biopsies was preeclampsia with significant hypertension that should have precluded the procedure. The only sizable series was published in 1987 reporting a low complication rate of 4.5% based on 111 renal biopsies in 104 women over 20 years.[130] A smaller subsequent case series confirmed safety in women <30 weeks' gestation.[131] Most guidelines, therefore, come from expert opinion recommending a cutoff of approximately 32 weeks' gestation,[132] as the further along in gestation, the more likely that preeclampsia may be factoring into the presentation. In the presence of possible preeclampsia, a kidney biopsy should not be applied indiscriminately, given that the safety of the procedure can be further compromised by evolving hypertension, abnormal coagulation indices, and a low hemoglobin.[129] On the other hand, the initiation of steroid or immunosuppressive therapy on the speculation of a potential glomerular-based disease is also not without risk.

PREPREGNANCY RISK STRATIFICATION AND OPTIMIZATION

Prognostication of an individual woman's pregnancy-associated risk in the setting of chronic kidney disease (CKD) remains profoundly challenging. The literature is complicated and incomplete, and therefore divergent opinions arise with respect to the impact of kidney disease on pregnancy outcome as well as the impact of pregnancy on future CKD progression. The many issues including nonhomogeneity in the classification of the maternal condition (renal function, proteinuria, and hypertension), the frequent absence of preconception baseline data, and the many different definitions of relevant pregnancy outcomes—particularly the nearly impossible task of diagnosing preeclampsia superimposed on CKD wherein hypertension and proteinuria are often already present—are beautifully summarized in a recent excellent systematic review of the literature.[133] Suffice to say, prepregnancy renal insufficiency, proteinuria, and hypertension all likely factor toward untoward maternal and fetal outcomes in an additive manner.

Early studies tended to utilize the serum creatinine to stratify pregnancy risk. A typical stratification schema defined mild renal insufficiency as a serum creatinine less than 123 μmol per L (1.4 mg per dL), moderate renal insufficiency as 124–220 μmol per L (1.4–2.4 mg per dL), and severe renal insufficiency as a serum creatinine exceeding 221 μmol per L (2.5 mg per dL). As the grade of renal insufficiency increased, the healthy accommodation to pregnancy (GFR increase with a simultaneous drop in the serum creatinine) was documented to occur in only approximately 50% of women within the moderate category and in none in the severe renal insufficiency category.[134,135] In a classic paper by Jones and Hayslett published over two decades ago, they assessed pregnancy outcome in women with mild, moderate, and severe renal insufficiency as defined above and noted pregnancy-related loss of kidney function in a staggering 43% of pregnancies of which 10% rapidly progressed to end-stage renal disease (ESRD).[136] Of interest, not all the accelerated loss occurred only in those with the most severe renal compromise (Fig. 59.3). Both proteinuria and hypertension

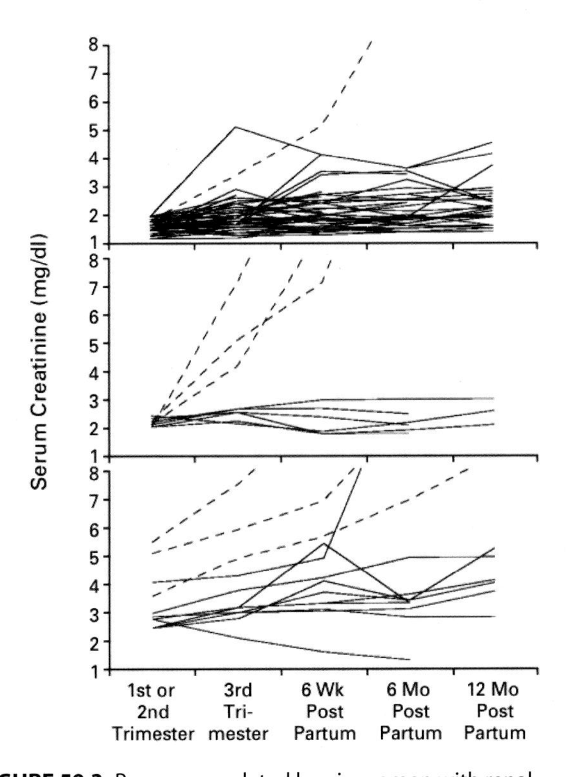

FIGURE 59.3 Pregnancy-related loss in women with renal insufficiency as determined by the serum creatinine level where mild renal insufficiency is <123 μmol/L (1.4 mg/dL), moderate renal insufficiency is 124 to 220 μmol/L (1.4 to 2.4 mg/dL), and severe renal insufficiency is >221 μmol/L (2.5 mg/dL), respectively. (Reprinted with permission from Jones DC, Hayslett JP. Outcome of pregnancy in women with moderate or severe renal insufficiency. *N Engl J Med.* 1996;335:226–232.)

are also important factors with respect to the risk for progression that are difficult to examine simultaneously in small single center experiences.[135] Further, the serum creatinine is likely too imprecise to be utilized to stratify women prior to pregnancy as it does not take into account patient size and muscle mass, and in young women serum creatinine is often inadequately reflective of the actual degree of histologic renal damage. Tubulointerstitial changes involving in excess of 20% of the cortical area, glomerulosclerosis, and severe arteriolar hyalinosis have all been deemed important with respect to pregnancy outcome.[137,138]

More recently, therefore, studies have prognosticated pregnancy outcome on the basis of a calculated GFR, which has served to increase the reported prevalence of CKD in pregnancy significantly from $<1\%$ to 3% as women with more subtle renal insufficiency are identified.[133,139] A recent study assessed pregnancy outcome in women with stage 3–5 CKD, excluding women with diabetes and lupus.[140] They utilized the MDRD formula to calculate the GFR and stratified women into four groups based on GFR (>40 or ≤ 40 mL/min/1.73 m^2) and the baseline level of proteinuria (<1 or ≥ 1 g per d). In women with a GFR in excess of 40 mL/min/1.76 m^2, there was no change in the rate of progression before and after pregnancy irrespective of the degree of urine protein. In women with a GFR ≤ 40 mL/min/1.73 m^2, the change in the rate of the postpartum decline in renal function was governed by the presence or absence of proteinuria, wherein the rate of progression increased from -0.55 mL/min/month to -1.17 mL/min/month. Gestational age decreased across the four groups as did birth weight. They concluded that only women with advanced kidney dysfunction and proteinuria need be counselled aggressively with respect to pregnancy, but their study overall was small ($n = 49$) and requires confirmation specifically in the group with GFR >40 mL/min/1.73 m^2 and with significant proteinuria as there were only six women in this group. Further, a subsequent study did note adverse outcomes even at early stages of CKD that associated with the degree of proteinuria and hypertension, but was limited by the fact that a first trimester serum creatinine was utilized in quite a number of cases, which could have served to reclassify more severe renal insufficiency to stage I CKD following accommodation to pregnancy.[133] The most recent study utilized the CKD-EPI equation to calculate eGFR from a preconception serum creatinine and noted an odds ratio for a composite maternal complication (worsening kidney function or preeclampsia) to be 6.75 (95% CI 1.8–24.8) and an odds ratio for a fetal complication (intrauterine growth restriction [IUGR], preterm birth, and fetal death) to be 2.91 (95% CI 1.19–7.09) when eGFR ranged between 60 and 89 mL/min/1.73 m^2.[141] A large study that utilized data from the HUNT II cohort, however, noted that the increased risk of preeclampsia in women with an eGFR between 60 and 89 mL/min/1.73 m^2 occurred only in women who also had hypertension and that there was a significant interaction between reduced kidney function and hypertension.[142] Although interesting, only a fraction of these women had microalbuminuria and therefore this is not the population likely to present to a renal clinic for prepregnancy consultation. Instead, women with identified kidney disease of various histologic types along with varying degrees of renal insufficiency, proteinuria, and hypertension will deserve guidance with respect to preconception planning and existent data suggests caution be exercised in women with established kidney disease. Multicenter efforts with larger numbers of patients will be necessary to refine counselling strategies particularly in the large group of women with moderate disease and to better understand the impact of different types of kidney disease along with current available treatment regimens. Available data for specific disease entities, as well as ESRD, are discussed in later text.

Diabetic Nephropathy

Due to increasing rates of obesity, diabetes mellitus is becoming a growing public health concern. Prepregnancy assessment and optimization can be effective[143] and it is, therefore, mandatory to improve pregnancy outcomes. Adequate prepregnancy optimization includes achieving a glycosylated hemoglobin (HbA1c) of $\leq 7.0\%$[144] and is typically achieved with multiple daily injections of insulin or an insulin pump. In addition to minimizing potential congenital abnormalities,[145] meticulous glycemic control improves pregnancy outcomes. In fact, for each 1% increment in HbA1c the adjusted odds ratio for preeclampsia is 1.6 (95% CI 1.3–2.0) whereas it is 0.6 (95% CI 0.5–0.8) for every 1% decrement during the first half of pregnancy.[146] The trend to delay childbirth, however, is resulting in more end-organ damage, including diabetic nephropathy, even prior to the consideration of pregnancy, thereby mandating early involvement of nephrology as well as endocrinology in prepregnancy counselling and optimization. The exact manner in which to counsel and optimize a young woman with significant nephropathy, however, is remarkably less clear based on the sparse and often controversial existing literature. Although most series note approximately a 90% live birth rate,[147–149] risks inherent to a pregnancy complicated by diabetic kidney disease are twofold. Significant fetal risks include poor growth and preterm delivery. Frequent maternal complications include acceleration of hypertension and preeclampsia as well as the potential to hasten progression of underlying nephropathy.

Like other forms of kidney disease, pregnancy outcome is affected by the prepregnancy kidney function, proteinuria, and blood pressure, but the rates of untoward outcomes are likely higher than described in other forms of kidney disease. One study assessing pregnancy outcome categorized women according to their urinary albumin excretion rate.[150] Compared to women with normal albumin excretion wherein the rate of preeclampsia was 6%, the rate increased to 42% and 64% in women with microalbuminuria and diabetic nephropathy, respectively. A similar pattern emerged for extreme preterm delivery (<34 weeks' gestation) wherein the rate was 6% in women with normal urine albumin excretion, 23% in women with microalbuminuria, and finally

45% in women with diabetic nephropathy, defined as urine protein excretion >500 mg daily. However, there were also differences between the groups in both baseline HbA1c and blood pressure. Irrespective, the strong relationship between microalbuminuria and preeclampsia has been noted in other studies,[151–154] including one that noted no additive predictive value of blood pressure[151] and in another that adjusted for both baseline hypertension and glycemic control.[153] Unfortunately, baseline serum creatinine was rarely reported and never adjusted for as a potential contributor to untoward pregnancy outcome in any of these studies, but has been shown to be an independent predictor of delivery before 32 weeks' gestation and very low birth weight independent of proteinuria and glycemic control in any trimester.[155] Although microalbuminuria and proteinuria are a reflection of established endothelial dysfunction, a well-described correlate of preeclampsia and preterm delivery,[156] HbA1c, blood pressure, and baseline kidney function are likely additive with respect to adverse pregnancy outcomes.

In addition to pregnancy-related complications, the potential for progression of nephropathy and accelerated loss of kidney function is serious and deserves careful consideration given the poor outcome of patients with ESRD secondary to diabetes mellitus. Proteinuria has been described to increase throughout pregnancy with nephrotic syndrome (>3 g per day) developing in the vast majority (>70%) who enter pregnancy with diabetic nephropathy (>500 mg per day) and tends to occur along with some increase in blood pressure in the third trimester.[157–160] In those studies that followed urine protein well into the postpartum period significant improvements were noted and in many women the value returned to prepregnancy levels.[157,158] The rates of late gestation nephrotic range proteinuria being higher than the quoted rate of preeclampsia in this population reflects the difficulty of diagnosing the syndrome in a population that already has significant proteinuria as well as lack of understanding of the pathophysiologic mechanisms of preeclampsia in this particularly high risk population (see later section, Pathophysiology of Preeclampsia).

Despite the almost uniform worsening of urine protein during pregnancy in women with diabetes mellitus, the literature has been conflicting with respect to pregnancy impact on progression of renal dysfunction. Early studies concluded that pregnancy did not hasten disease progression in diabetes,[147,157,158,161–163] but these early studies were small with variable follow-up periods and included a spectrum of baseline kidney function with the majority of patients having well preserved kidney function at conception. Those with significant renal insufficiency and nephropathy certainly did deteriorate during pregnancy, but the overall slope toward ESRD, which was already steep, did not change significantly reflecting the overall poor outcome of diabetic nephropathy prior to more widespread use of blockade of the RAS. Studies that more effectively stratified women based on baseline renal function noted that women with well-preserved kidney function at conception had better outcomes whereas moderate to severe renal insufficiency predicted more rapid deterioration in kidney function during and after pregnancy.[159,160,164,165] One such study noted a baseline creatinine clearance of 70 mL per min to be a potentially meaningful value with respect to outcome.[164] Women who entered pregnancy with a creatinine clearance >70 mL per min were more likely to have an appropriate early pregnancy renal accommodation and stable kidney function after pregnancy whereas women with lower baseline clearance values had a significant decline in renal function at 3 months postpartum (36% lower). Another study that assessed women with more significant baseline renal dysfunction (mean creatinine 1.8 mg per dL) found a significant deterioration in kidney function that was transient in 27% and permanent in 45%.[159] It is distinctly possible that superimposed preeclampsia manifesting as worsening proteinuria and kidney function during pregnancy is damaging over the long term. A health administrative study from the Norwegian Renal Registry that identified 2,204 women with pregestational diabetes whose pregnancy was complicated by either preeclampsia, preterm delivery, or a low birth weight baby and noted higher future rates of nephropathy, ESRD, and death.[166] Another study noted the median age of children to be 9 (3–17) when the mother expired secondary to complications of renal or cardiac disease,[167] reminding us that this is a very vulnerable, high-risk group that is not to be taken lightly.

Despite the great potential for both untoward maternal and fetal outcome, there are precious little data to guide prepregnancy preparation outside of optimization of HbA1c. In one study, for example, hypertension was not treated unless the diastolic blood pressure exceeded 105 mm Hg.[157] There is, however, some data to suggest that adequate blood pressure control is important. Although no randomized data exists, one retrospective cohort study compared outcomes in women with a mean arterial pressure either ≥100 mm Hg or <100 mm Hg and noted patients with higher blood pressures were significantly more likely to deliver before 32 weeks' gestation (38.1% versus 4.6%, $P = .007$) even after adjusting for duration of diabetes and glycemic control.[168] A second prospective study targeted a blood pressure of <135/85 mm Hg in 117 pregnant women with type 1 diabetes mellitus and noted a trend toward longer gestation and higher birth weight as compared to historical data published prior to theirs from the same geographical region in Europe.[169] However, it is difficult to draw comparisons between these small single-centered studies, and the vast majority of the women included in their study did not have even microalbuminuria, a group one might overall expect to do better. Only one group has assessed the potential for prepregnancy optimization in women with significant diabetic nephropathy. They have published two articles advocating for aggressive prepregnancy blockade of the RAS with captopril to lower proteinuria prior to pregnancy along with aggressive glycemic control.[170,171] They recommend stopping captopril at the time of conception and effectively demonstrated the ability to lower proteinuria from a mean value in excess of a gram to a mean value <300 mg. Although proteinuria still increased throughout pregnancy, the rate of increase was not as dramatic as what might be expected from the previous literature and kidney function was stable at 2 years postpartum. Of note, the patients in these two small series had well-preserved kidney function, which likely also factored into favorable long-term outcomes. Irrespective, there are data outside of pregnancy that speak to the potential for prolonged renoprotective effect after cessation of RAS blockade.[172]

Of course, anyone prescribing RAS blockade to a woman of child-bearing potential needs to be cognizant of the potential for teratogenicity.[173] Second and third trimester teratogenicity secondary to angiotensin-converting enzyme (ACE) inhibition is well described and includes oligohydramnios, neonatal anuria and renal failure, limb contractures, craniofacial abnormalities, pulmonary hypoplasia, and patent ductus arteriosus. Children that survive ACE inhibition/angiotensin receptor blocker (ARB) fetopathy are left with renal insufficiency and profound impairment in the urine concentrating ability likely due to papillary atrophy and disturbed formation of the medullary concentration gradient.[174] A more recent publication, however, suggests the potential as well for first trimester teratogenicity.[175] This study has a number of issues such as the inclusion of defects not previously described in risk estimates as well as the inability to control for other potential confounders including maternal age, obesity, and diet-controlled diabetes. ARBs may very well be more teratogenic with case reports of significant malformations emerging after first trimester exposure.[176–178] There are no case reports as yet of teratogenicity after exposure to the newer direct renin inhibitors, but there is no reason to expect they will not be equally or even more teratogenic, and this class of medication also should be used with extreme caution in young women. The risk of teratogenicity must be carefully balanced against the need to prevent progression of diabetic nephropathy. It is, therefore, imperative that physicians educate young diabetic women as to the risks of an unplanned pregnancy as opposed to denying them a potentially renoprotective therapy. Unintentional first trimester exposure does not require termination, but careful fetal imaging is recommended.[179] In the postpartum period, there is also no need to deny RAS blockade while breastfeeding. Captopril, enalapril, and quinapril have all been tested and noted to be absent in breast milk and, therefore, can be used if necessary to treat diabetic nephropathy in the early postpartum period.[180,181]

IgA Nephropathy

Although IgA nephropathy is the most common glomerular-based disease diagnosed in women of childbearing age, there is a remarkable paucity of data in the literature to assist with prepregnancy counselling and management. Most studies, being small and decades old, could not simultaneously assess the impact of kidney function, blood pressure, and proteinuria on pregnancy outcome or potential impact of treatment prior to conception with either immunosuppression or blockade of the RAS.[137,182–184] Due to the slow insidious nature of the disease, a large proportion of women first come to medical attention during pregnancy without a careful prepregnancy assessment of blood pressure, proteinuria, and kidney function to assist with the understanding of the impact of these variables on the prognostication of pregnancy outcome. The follow-up time used to determine if pregnancy ultimately has an impact on progression is likely inadequate with only 5 years of long-term follow-up in most studies.[182,183,185–187] Finally, in studies that attempt to assess the impact of histology, older classification systems were used and the baseline clinical correlates of disease were not consistently reported, therefore making this area of literature very difficult to interpret.[188,189]

Early data would suggest that even mild disease associated with preserved renal function might significantly increase the risks of untoward pregnancy outcomes and worsening maternal condition. In a large analysis of 116 pregnancies, the fetal loss was noted to be 22%.[190] Maternal renal function declined transiently in 26%, and was progressive and irreversible in 2%. Proteinuria and hypertension increased in 52% and 62% of women, respectively, and did not resolve after delivery in 13% and 10%, respectively. This study, however, was retrospective with the vast majority of women formally diagnosed by biopsy either during or after pregnancy limiting the collection of careful prepregnancy data.

Also supporting the notion that even mild disease may have consequences in pregnancy are studies that assessed women with isolated hematuria, a marker perhaps of even milder glomerular disease. A study that assessed 276 women, of which 44 had isolated hematuria on their first prenatal visit, noted significantly increased rates of preeclampsia (OR 9.1, 95% CI 2.5–33.7).[191] That odds ratio was mitigated albeit still statistically significant in a larger dataset wherein the same authors utilized data from the trial of Calcium for Preeclampsia Prevention (CPEP) noting idiopathic hematuria in 132/4307 (3%) of participants. An almost twofold increased risk was observed for the development of preeclampsia after adjustment for blood pressure, race/ethnicity, and medical center (aOR = 1.89; 95% CI 1.12–3.18).[192] However, the most recent and largest study to date ($n = 1{,}000$) noted that dipstick positive hematuria was common (20%) and typically did not signify any meaningful renal disease, as 60% of these patients were carefully assessed in the nephrology clinic.[193] In this more comprehensive study, microscopic hematuria did not increase the likelihood of preeclampsia, gestational hypertension, or delivery of a small for gestational age baby. Further, a sizable study that assessed women with known thin basement membrane disease, another potential explanation for hematuria, also failed to note rates of pregnancy-related complications that differed significantly from those of the general population.[194]

The absence of prepregnancy baseline data and the use of serum creatinine to determine baseline renal function likely hampered the interpretation of pregnancy risk in many of the early studies. In studies wherein the creatinine clearance was calculated, a better understanding of pregnancy risks emerged. Women with preserved kidney function as defined by a creatinine clearance over 70 mL per min were demonstrated to have reasonable pregnancy outcomes.[137,186,195] Exceptions were noted in women with difficult to control prepregnancy hypertension (blood pressure [BP] >140/90 mm Hg)[66,69,77] or worsening of hypertension early in pregnancy[183,196] as well as in women with significant renal scarring on biopsy that perhaps was not appropriately reflected by clinical measures of renal function. Specifically, worse pregnancy outcomes have been noted in women with sclerosed glomeruli,[188,189,195] tubulointerstitial damage that involves in excess of 20% of the cortical area,[137,195] or significant arteriosclerosis.[137] Whether the biopsy findings might be better reflected in the baseline proteinuria is not known as the impact of that variable on pregnancy outcome cannot be assessed without much larger multicenter efforts due to the inherent variability and issues with quantifying urine protein that are not unique to the pregnancy literature.

Although, as mentioned, the literature does note exceptions, in general, pregnancy does not hasten progression of renal dysfunction as long as kidney function prepregnancy is well preserved. A recent study that compared 136 pregnant women with IgA to 87 matched controls noted an overall rate of progression of 1.31 (95% CI, 0.99–1.63) mL/min/year that was impacted by levels of proteinuria, but not affected by pregnancy.[187] Of note, all women in this study had well-preserved kidney function with a creatinine clearance of 92 ± 17 mL/min/1.73 m^2 in the pregnancy group. Although not as high as quoted in the earlier studies, pregnancy complications still exceeded what might be expected in the general population including a perinatal death rate of 3%, premature delivery rate of 10%, low birth weight in 11%, and 21% of the pregnancies were complicated by hypertension. Data with respect to more moderate or severe disease with renal dysfunction was poorly addressed in this study due to inadequate numbers, but the limited existing data does suggest these women should approach pregnancy with due caution as both poor fetal and maternal outcomes have been noted.[182,195,196] As women delay childbearing and are more likely to approach pregnancy with more moderate degrees of renal impairment, this is an area in need of further study.

Urinary Tract Infections, Pyelonephritis, and Reflux Nephropathy

Urinary tract infections (UTIs) are among the most common complications noted in pregnancy and *Escherichia coli* is the most frequently cultured bacterial organism.[197,198] Patients commonly present with asymptomatic bacteriuria that can progress to cystitis or even pyelonephritis if not promptly treated given the dilation of the urinary tract that accompanies the gravid state.[199] The classification of patients into either of these clinical categories has implications for medical management, which must be hastened in pregnancy due to the risk of progression to more severe maternal complications such as septicemia[200] and renal insufficiency.[200,201]

With respect to asymptomatic bacteriuria, current guidelines support the screening for bacteriuria using urine dipstick followed by urine culture when positive.[197] Subsequent initiation of antibiotic therapy based on culture sensitivity is also recommended as this practice reduces progression to cystitis and, more importantly, to pyelonephritis and its associated complications.[202] Safe, empiric antibiotic choices in pregnancy include trimethoprim-sulfamethoxazole, nitrofurantoin, and cephalexin.[197] However, controversy currently exists regarding the duration of antibiotic administration. Recent meta-analyses comparing the 1-day to 4- and 7-day regimens demonstrated that 1-day regimens resulted in fewer side effects and increased compliance at the expense of a decreased cure rate.[198,203] Accordingly, current guidelines support the use of a 3-day regimen in healthy women[197] or a 7-day regimen to increase the likelihood of definitive cure in women with comorbidities.[198] Successful treatment must also be assured by the acquisition of a negative follow-up urine culture after completion of the antibiotic regimen and periodic screening throughout the remainder of the pregnancy.[197]

Cystitis or symptomatic bacteriuria resides further along the continuum of UTI severity. Cystitis is a clinical diagnosis based on the presence of bacteriuria and the clinical symptoms of dysuria, frequency, lower abdominal or suprapubic pain, but not fever.[199] In contrast to asymptomatic bacteriuria, urine culture and sensitivity results are often unavailable at the time of diagnosis and empiric therapy is required.[197] Selection of the appropriate antibiotic regimen was previously a contentious issue, but a recent *Cochrane Review* found few significant differences in cure rates and recurrence between the various empiric antibiotic regimens examined in the literature.[199] Similar to asymptomatic bacteriuria, a follow-up urine culture and periodic re-screening must occur throughout the pregnancy.

Pyelonephritis is the most severe manifestation of a UTI and is significantly more prevalent in young nulliparous women.[200] Clinically, patients often present in the third trimester of pregnancy with irritative urologic symptoms as well as fever and costovertebral tenderness,[199] but an increasing prevalence of pyelonephritis has recently been noted in earlier trimesters.[200] As such, health care providers must be vigilant for pyelonephritis at all stages of pregnancy and administer prompt empiric treatment until culture and sensitivity results are available. The importance of aggressively managing pyelonephritis cannot be overstated. Recent data from a cohort of 440 inpatients with antepartum pyelonephritis demonstrated a decrease in the prevalence of renal dysfunction (20% to 2%)—a finding the authors attribute to early treatment.[200] However, respiratory insufficiency within the context of pyelonephritis remained common in this cohort (10%), and one in five women with pyelonephritis were diagnosed with septicemia based on blood culture results.[200] It has been suggested that pyelonephritis can be managed in the outpatient setting,[204] but this decision should be individualized based on the patient and available outpatient resources. Based on available data,[244,250] current recommendations for chronic suppressive prophylactic antibiotics include women with frequent prepregnancy UTIs, persistent asymptomatic or symptomatic infection despite two courses of antibiotics, and women who have recovered from pyelonephritis or may be at particular risk for pyelonephritis (e.g., diabetic patients or immunosuppressed patients). Emergence of resistance in the face of decreased safe antibiotic options remains a theoretical concern.

Reflux nephropathy is a common condition with a female preponderance that is typically diagnosed in childhood and, therefore, is another condition that can affect young women of childbearing age. Reflux nephropathy can be an incidental finding during standard pregnancy screens for bacteruria, UTI, or pyelonephritis (17%–28%).[205–208] However, the impact of reflux nephropathy on maternal and fetal health is certainly not benign and, like other renal conditions, complications include preeclampsia, deterioration of renal function, and fetal loss.[206,207,209] Unique to this condition, however, is the predisposition to UTIs (17%–65%) and pyelonephritis (3%–37%) that can cause significant maternal morbidity.[210] Further, the genetic preponderance of the condition necessitates assessment of the newborn for vesicoureteral reflux.[211] Pregnancy outcome can be largely prognosticated by prepregnancy renal function and hypertension as a reflection of the degree renal parenchymal scarring. A recent systematic review noted primary vesicoureteral reflux without renal scarring was not associated with an increased incidence of gestational hypertension, preeclampsia, and fetal morbidity,[210] but persistent reflux during pregnancy does increase the likelihood of pyelonephritis.[205]

The majority of data on reflux nephropathy in pregnancy comes from three older, but sizable retrospective case series[205,206,209] and a more recent prospective series,[211] examining just over 1,000 pregnancies in women with reflux nephropathy. All studies assessed the prognostic value of prepregnancy renal function as a reflection of parenchymal scarring, typically utilizing a serum creatinine cutoff of 110 μmol per L (1.3 mg per dL) to distinguish preserved kidney function from renal impairment. An increased serum creatinine of ≥110 μmol per L (>1.3 mg per dL) significantly increased the risk of maternal complications including preclampsia and loss of kidney function as well as fetal loss. Preeclampsia, in one series, was 36% in women with renal insufficiency compared to 13% in women with preserved kidney function and the presence of parenchymal scarring was noted to be positively correlated with prevalence of preeclampsia.[206] Further, in another study, preeclampsia was noted to be higher in women with bilateral as opposed to unilateral scarring (24 versus 7%; $P < .001$).[205] The difference was more dramatic in a second series at 56.7% compared to 6.4%, respectively,[209] and preexisting hypertension has been noted to further increase the risk.[211]

Similarly, at a prepregnancy serum creatinine threshold of ≥110 μmol per L (>1.3 mg per dL), 8% of women with reflux nephropathy experienced a decline in renal function whereas only 2% of women with preserved renal function exhibited a similar deterioration.[206] Again, the results were more striking in the second series wherein an increase in serum creatinine above the preconception value was observed in all cases with renal insufficiency, reversing partially in most with the exception of cases also complicated by hypertension and increased proteinuria that proved progressive.[205,209] Thus, the relative risk of renal function deterioration was determined to be 12.7 (95% CI 1.6–98.5) in women with mild renal insufficiency (90–120 μmol per L or 1.0–1.4 mg per dL) and 19.8 (95% CI 2.6–155) in women with moderate to severe renal insufficiency (130–350 μmol per L or 1.5–4.0 mg per dL).[211] The large confidence intervals reflect the small number of patients assessed in the prospective cohort ($n = 54$ pregnancies).[211]

Fetal outcomes are also governed by the degree of renal impairment, and, likely to be of even more significance, the presence of significant first trimester hypertension. In the series published by Jungers et al.,[208] maternal blood pressure at early gestation was the only significant prognostic marker for adverse fetal outcomes after adjustment for covariates, including serum creatinine and proteinuria, with the relative risk of fetal loss in hypertensive patients being 4.8 times higher than in normotensive patients wherein there were no fetal losses.[209] Of note, there was no correlation between the degree of renal dysfunction and hypertension. Moreover, in the subset of women with early gestational hypertension, adequate control of blood pressure resulted in significantly lower rates of fetal loss (11% vs. 74%) and no fetal deaths occurred in late-gestational hypertension.[208,209] Although serum creatinine was noted to be a significant predictor of fetal outcome in this study, fetal loss has been demonstrated to be significantly more likely in women with impaired renal function (serum creatinine ≥110 μmol per L or 1.3 mg per dL).[205,209] Similarly, the birth weight of living neonates was significantly lower in this cohort.[209]

Given these risks, women with reflux nephropathy and diminished renal function require careful coordinated nephrologic and obstetric care such that manageable renal complications such as UTIs can be immediately diagnosed and treated and hypertension can be aggressively controlled. Efforts toward this endeavor have been successful as the prevalence of UTIs has been documented to be lower in women with reflux nephropathy and diminished renal function as compared to women with preserved function presumably due to differences in the intensity of follow-up.[206,208] Further, fetal outcomes have been demonstrated to be more favorable in planned and carefully monitored pregnancies despite the presence of renal insufficiency and hypertension.[208]

Lupus Nephritis and Other Connective Tissue Diseases

Because of the female preponderance and the typical young age of onset, lupus is another disease that frequently requires management during a woman's reproductive years. Even prior to considering a pregnancy, treatment of the condition requires mindfulness of the reproductive potential of this patient population while imparting an understanding to the patient that an unplanned pregnancy can be hazardous. Lupus itself does not impact female fertility, but some of the medications frequently prescribed to treat the renal manifestations of the disease may impact fertility and have proven teratogenicity. Thus, sexually active women initiating either cyclophosphamide or mycophenolate mofetil should have a negative pregnancy test prior to starting these therapies, and young women initiating cyclophosphamide need to be informed that fertility may be compromised. Amenorrhea secondary to cyclophosphamide use is related to the age of the patient and the number of prescribed treatment cycles. Rates of sustained amenorrhea have been documented to be 12% in women ≤25 years old, 27% in women between the age of 26 and 30, and rise sharply to 62% in women ≥31 ($P = 0.04$).[212] There are limited data to suggest a gonadotropin-releasing hormone analog (GnRH-a) may provide ovarian protection, decreasing the rates of premature ovarian failure from 30% to 5% in one study.[213]

Historically, lupus patients did poorly in pregnancy, but outcomes have improved over time, presumably as new treatment strategies for the disease emerge to induce remission prior to a pregnancy attempt. As in all chronic kidney diseases, renal insufficiency and chronic hypertension cause poor pregnancy outcomes. However, lupus is unique in that active nephritis predicts a particularly poor pregnancy outcome, and pregnancy itself has been demonstrated by some to increase the potential of a disease flare during any trimester or in the early postpartum.[214] The literature on maternal and fetal outcomes has been recently summarized in a systematic review and meta-analysis that included 2,751 pregnancies in women with lupus from 37 studies wherein adequate outcome data was reported.[215] Significant study heterogeneity was noted due to variable definitions of active lupus nephritis and a disease flare. Twenty-two cited studies did not meet study validity criteria. Irrespective, useful outcome data was synthesized and reported, and areas in need of future study were elucidated. Overall, 23.4% (95% CI 19.5–27.3%) of pregnancies were unsuccessful. The most frequent maternal complications included a disease flare in 26% that included nephritis in 16% of cases along with hypertension (16%) and preeclampsia (8%). Fortunately, severe maternal complications, including stroke, ESRD, and death, were rare (approximately 1%). Fetal complications included spontaneous abortion (16%), premature birth rate (37%), IUGR (13%), stillbirth (4%), and neonatal death (2.5%). Active lupus nephritis and positive antiphospholipid antibodies were significantly associated with maternal hypertension and premature birth. Antiphospholipid antibodies also correlated with an increased risk of spontaneous pregnancy loss. Of interest, there was no statistically significant association between antiphospholipid antibodies and active nephritis. A history of nephritis predicted maternal hypertension and preeclampsia and this finding was confirmed by a recent Toronto study comparing pregnancy outcomes in patients with renal involvement within 6 months prior to pregnancy to those without renal involvement.[216]

This study also confirmed disease flares during pregnancy to be more common in patients with active nephritis.[216] Therefore, 6 months of sustained disease quiescence prior to considering a pregnancy has been recommended based on studies that show the disease flared in 7% of patients with inactive disease as compared to 61% of patients wherein there was active disease at the time of conception.[217] Despite the knowledge that an unequivocal clinical remission is necessary prior to consideration of a pregnancy, judging disease activity in a clinical setting can prove very challenging for the practicing clinician. Although, for example, hypocomplementemia and abnormal serology have been demonstrated to be associated with poor pregnancy outcomes,[218] many patients' clinical presentations are not concordant with their serology. In many studies >500 mg of proteinuria was defined as active nephritis, but available data are inadequate to definitely determine the impact of histologic subtype or level of kidney function and degree of proteinuria on outcome.[215] Thus, further study is needed to assist the many young women with lupus who attain a partial remission to make an informed choice with respect to pregnancy.

A reasonable approach based on current data includes treatment with appropriate immunosuppression to attain remission for at least 6 months prior to converting a young woman to pregnancy safe treatment, which can include prednisone, azathioprine, and the calcineurin inhibitors (see section on Renal Transplantation). Hydroxychloroquine does not appear to be associated with any increased risk of congenital defects, spontaneous abortions, prematurity, or fetal death, and therefore can be used safely in pregnancy.[219] A repeat biopsy may prove necessary in select cases wherein it is difficult to clinically confirm absence of active nephritis in pregnant women receiving safe immunosuppression therapy. Baseline laboratory assessment of serology including antiphospholipid antibody levels and lupus anticoagulant as well as anti-Ro and La antibodies can help predict the rate of spontaneous fetal loss with pregnancy complications[220] and the rate neonatal lupus, respectively. Women with positive antiphospholipid antibody titers in conjunction with a history of thrombosis, fetal loss, or untoward pregnancy complications require assessment and management by physicians who are expert in the area of thromboprophylaxis and pregnancy. Even in the presence of positive anti-Ro and La antibodies, fetal heart block is rare. Recent studies suggest that the titer is more predictive than just simply the presence of antibodies and should guide referral for serial fetal echocardiography. Cardiac complications were diagnosed in the presence of moderate to high maternal anti-Ro levels (50–100 U/mL or 15%–85%) independent of anti-La levels.[221]

Other connective tissue diseases of relevance to the practicing nephrologist include renal ANCA-associated vasculitis, Goodpasture syndrome, and scleroderma renal disease. Of these, ANCA-associated vasculitis will be encountered most frequently, but there is still inadequate data from which to provide definitive pregnancy counseling with the exception that women conceiving while their disease is active do poorly.[222] The literature notes a number of cases either presenting in pregnancy or relapsing during pregnancy to suggest the possibility that, like lupus, pregnancy might result in disease activation.[222] Even in the presence of inactive disease, approximately 25% of patients have been noted to relapse irrespective of the presence or absence of maintenance immunosuppression.[223] Despite an approximate 75% live birth rate, there are numerous complications with preeclampsia complicating approximately 25% of the reported cases in the literature and preterm delivery occurring is just over 40%.[222] Outcome will depend on severity of the presentation and nephrologists will likely be involved in the most severe presentations necessitating treatment decisions. Steroids remain first line therapy, but will likely be inadequate as a single agent. Azathioprine can be used safely, but in at least one case proved inadequate and resulted in maternal death,[224] and in another there were a number of relapses during pregnancy.[222] Intravenous immunoglobulin and plasmapheresis are safe options in pregnancy for this disease and have been used with some success.[225–227] Cyclophosphamide has rarely been used with success,[228] and as a rule is contraindicated at least in the first trimester wherein it has been noted to cause spontaneous pregnancy loss, growth deficiency, developmental delay, craniosynostosis, blepharophimosis, flat nasal bridge, abnormal ears, and distal limb defects including hypoplastic thumbs and oligodactyly.[229] At present, there are some limited data on the use of rituximab primarily from the oncology literature, which might be an option. To date, no fetal malformations have been noted, but CD19 B cells were either undetectable or severely decreased in exposed neonates returning to normal levels by 3 to 6 months' gestation without documented serious infections.[230] Also of interest to the neonate is the report of placental transport of myeloperoxidase-antineutrophil cytoplasmic antibodies (MPO-ANCA) resulting in neonatal pulmonary hemorrhage.[231]

Goodpasture syndrome is a rare disease wherein anti-glomerular basement membrane (GBM) antibodies result in pulmonary hemorrhage and crescentic renal disease. There are only a handful of cases presented in the literature and those suggest overall poor maternal and fetal outcomes.[232–236] Given that women diagnosed and treated prior to conception have better outcomes,[232,236] one can postulate that the infrequency of the condition likely delays appropriate diagnosis and expeditious treatment when it presents during pregnancy.[234,235] Further, in some cases, the anti-GBM antibody was negative until the postpartum period and it has been postulated that the placenta might act as an absorbent.[233,235] Overall, there is inadequate data in the literature to make any formal recommendations short of having high clinical suspicion in women presenting with symptoms suggestive of pulmonary-renal syndrome.

Fortunately, scleroderma is rare and presents in older age groups. However, as women delay childbearing, there is more potential for a pregnancy to be affected by this disease. Although women whose disease is limited to the skin may do reasonably well with the exception of increased rates of preeclampsia (22.9%) and IUGR (5.3%) compared with the general population,[237] those with underlying vascular involvement can have devastating outcomes with maternal morbidity and mortality due to accelerated hypertension, renal failure, and pulmonary hypertension.[238–240] Thus women with progressive disease complicated by renal involvement and/or significantly increased pulmonary pressures should be cautioned against pregnancy. Of interest, prompt institution of captopril in the postpartum period resulting in partial renal recovery and cessation of hemodialysis has been described.[240]

Other Glomerular-Based Diseases

There are limited published data with respect to the pregnancy outcomes for less frequently encountered glomerular-based diseases including minimal change disease (MCD), focal segmental glomerular sclerosis (FSGS), membranous nephropathy (MN), and hereditary nephritis or Alport disease. Trends have emerged to suggest perhaps pregnancy outcomes are best in MN and the worst in MPGN and FSGS,[185] but the study numbers are too small and too varied with respect to the definition of a poor outcome and timing of biopsy in relation to the pregnancy to definitively make these conclusions. If one examines studies wherein hard outcomes including spontaneous abortion and fetal or neonatal death were reported independently then the live birth rates for MCD, FSGS, MN, MPGN, and hereditary nephritis are approximately 74%, 71%, 96%, 80%, and 85%, respectively (Table 59.2).[183,185,241–244] These live birth rates may be dependent on the status of the disease and may vary significantly in treated as compared to untreated disease. Further, issues with respect to potential side effects from nephrotic syndrome in pregnancy, including difficult to manage edema and potential thrombosis, are not adequately reported in the literature. Suffice to say, treatment and maintenance of nephrotic syndrome with pregnancy safe immunosuppression where indicated and possible should be the prepregnancy goal.

Polycystic Kidney Disease

Despite the potential presence for ovarian cysts in women with polycystic kidney disease, fertility is not impaired, but there are data to suggest ectopic pregnancies might be more common and should be considered in the differential of abdominal pain in young women.[245] Unlike other forms of kidney disease, women with autosomal dominant polycystic kidney disease (ADPKD) need to be educated that there is a 50% chance of transmission of their renal disease to their offspring. Prenatal diagnosis is possible, but not always readily available and typically not desired by a patient who is

TABLE 59.2 Pregnancy Outcome in Glomerular-Based Disease

Disease	Cases	Spontaneous Loss	Fetal/Neonatal Death	Live Birth Rate (%)
MCD[137,183]	19	3	2	74
FSGS[137,183,241,244]	74	5	16	72
MN[137,183,241,242]	51	1	1	96
MPGN[137,183,241]	40	4	4	80
Alport disease[183]	33	2	3	85

MCD, minimal change disease; FSGS, focal segmental glomerulosclerosis; MN, membranous nephropathy; MPGN, membranoproliferative glomerulonephritis.

otherwise well.[245,246] For the most part, pregnancy outcomes in young women with ADPKD are quite good largely because kidney function is still well preserved with minimal proteinuria during the reproductive stage of life, but there are notable exceptions.

The largest series to date compared 605 pregnancies in women with ADPKD to 244 pregnancies in their unaffected family members.[245] No significant differences were noted in the live birth rate between women with ADPKD and unaffected controls: 77% of 605 pregnancies and 82% of 244 pregnancies, respectively. However, age >30 years predicted increased fetal complications and preexisting hypertension predicted both increased fetal and maternal complications in women with ADPKD. Maternal complications occurred in 35% of women with ADPKD compared to 19% of unaffected controls ($P < .001$) and included new or worsening hypertension (25%) and superimposed preeclampsia (11%) complicated by placental abruption and acute kidney injury (AKI) (0.8%). Similar to other forms of kidney disease, prepregnancy renal impairment (serum creatinine > 106 μmol per L or 1.2 mg per dL) may hasten progression to ESRD as these women progressed to ESRD on average 15 years earlier than the general female ADPKD population, but the numbers were too small to assess for a potential independent effect of pregnancy-induced hypertension or preeclampsia. Of interest, normotensive women with ADPKD who developed either pregnancy-induced hypertension or preeclampsia were at greater risk for the later development of chronic hypertension.

Finally, in this same study,[245] mean renal volume measurements did not differ in women with four or more pregnancies compared to age-adjusted measurements for women with fewer than three pregnancies suggesting that the hormonal changes that occur during pregnancy do not promote cyst growth in the kidneys as has been demonstrated in the liver.[247] Liver cysts, fortunately, are rarely of clinical significance, but should be mentioned during counselling of these young women prior to pregnancy.

End-Stage Renal Disease

Pregnancy, once on dialysis, is difficult due to the decreased fertility that accompanies ESRD and is historically associated with poor outcomes. Data are emerging, however, to suggest that pregnancy while on intensive renal replacement therapy may result in better outcomes for both mother and baby and, therefore, may prove a viable option for a large number of young women whose reproductive years are lost to ESRD.

The ovulatory menstrual cycle reflects normal function and physiology of the hypothalamic-pituitary-gonadal axis, which is known to be affected on multiple levels in women with advanced renal disease. Menstrual irregularities, infertility, and sexual dysfunction are known to occur in patients with ESRD and worsen in parallel with the renal disease. Even in those dialysis patients who menstruate, their cycles are often anovulatory.[248] There are numerous documented endocrine abnormalities that affect fertility in young women with ESRD. During the follicular phase, FSH levels are comparable or slightly lower than nonuremic controls, whereas luteinizing hormone (LH) levels are elevated.[249,250] Despite the elevated baseline LH levels, women on hemodialysis fail to have the luteal surge in LH.[250] Both progesterone and estradiol levels are extremely low[249] and prolactin levels are higher due to prolonged plasma half-life from decreased clearance.[251,252] In fact, levels have been found to correlate with serum creatinine.[252] Compounding the hormonal alterations, which can render these women infertile, medications, anemia, fatigue, and depression can contribute to a lack of libido.[253,254]

Given the many reasons for impaired fertility and sexual dysfunction in patients with ESRD on dialysis, it is not surprising that conception is uncommon. There is, however, emerging data that does suggest the conception rate might be improving over time. Representing approximately 10% of the U.S. dialysis population, a slightly higher rate of 2.4% of hemodialysis patients became pregnant over a 4-year period (1992 and 1995)[255] in contrast to earlier data from the same group wherein a 1.5% rate of pregnancy in hemodialysis patients was described over a 2-year period (1990–1992).[256] In the last decade, higher pregnancy rates of 5% to 7.9% were noted on questionnaire data collected from dialysis units in Saudi Arabia.[257,258] Most recently, clearance augmented by intensive nocturnal hemodialysis has resulted in higher conception rates. Seven pregnancies occurred in 45 women of childbearing age on nocturnal hemodialysis for a pregnancy rate of 15.9%.[259] All these women were previously on conventional hemodialysis, but none conceived, suggesting fertility can be improved with more intensive clearance.

With fewer case reports of pregnancy occurring in peritoneal dialysis as compared to hemodialysis patients, the potential to conceive actually appears significantly lower on peritoneal dialysis. However, to date, there are very few studies that attempted to systematically collect this data. In Saudi Arabia, wherein the highest rates of conception were noted in conventional hemodialysis patients, data was also collected on peritoneal dialysis and no patients conceived.[257] In the U.S. dialysis registry that reported data from 930 dialysis centers including 1,699 women of child-bearing age on peritoneal dialysis, the pregnancy rate was only 1.1%.[255] In addition to the hormonal and functional causes of infertility described in ESRD patients, experts in the field have hypothesized additional etiologies for decreased conception rates in peritoneal dialysis patients might include damage to fallopian tubes from peritonitis or interference with ovum transport from the ovaries to the fallopian tubes from the presence of hypertonic solutions in the intraperitoneal space.[260]

The first successful pregnancy reported in a patient on chronic hemodialysis occurred in 1970.[261] However, initial enthusiasm was tempered following the first registry report from the European Dialysis and Transplant Association published a decade later.[262] Of the original 115 reported pregnancies, 45 were electively terminated and there were only 16 viable pregnancies of the remaining 70 women for a live birth rate of 23%. The majority of those whose pregnancies succeeded were noted to have residual renal function and four pregnancies occurred prior to the initiation of hemodialysis. They described very difficult to manage hypertension in most cases, and note a mean birth weight of 1,900 g with a mean gestational age of 33.2 weeks.

One might presume the high rates of termination influenced the poor live birth rate, but subsequent data from the United States[256] and the Saudi Arabian Registry,[263] wherein termination was unlikely, did not reflect a much better outcome with a live birth rate of only 37%. However, even in this early data, the relationship between time on dialysis and outcome began to emerge. Those cases that progressed beyond 28 weeks had their weekly dialysis time increased from an average of 9.4 ± 2.3 to 12.0 ± 2.6 hours, whereas unsuccessful pregnancies did not have their dialysis time increased after conception. The importance of enhanced clearance was also noted in the second registry study from the United States wherein infant survival was 40.2% in women who conceived on hemodialysis compared to 73.6% in women who conceived prior to initiating hemodialysis.[255] Still, overall maternal and fetal outcomes were poor with documented maternal deaths, high rates of severe uncontrolled hypertension, and prematurity. A similar discrepancy in outcome between established dialysis patients (live birth rate 50%) and those who started dialysis after conception (live birth rate 80%) was noted in the Belgian registry.[264] In addition, this study also noted a correlation between birth weight and dose of dialysis. Still, the incidence of prematurity was 100% with high rates of complications adding growth restriction and polyhydramnios to the list of potential adverse outcomes.

More recently, however, live birth rates have improved as it has become standard practice to increase the dose of delivered dialysis after conception. In 2005, Haase and colleagues described a systematic approach wherein intensive hemodiafiltration 6 days a week was prescribed for five pregnant patients with ESRD.[265] They received an average of 28.6 ± 6.3 hours per week and were able to maintain urea levels consistently <50 mg per dL. All had a live birth and the mean gestational age was 32.8 ± 3.3 weeks with a mean birth weight of 1,765 ± 554 g. The authors felt convective clearance was important to outcome by enhancing both the clearance of large and small solutes. However, in another study wherein intensified clearance was provided by increasing the amount of nocturnal hemodialysis from a weekly mean of 36 ± 10 to 48 ± 5 hours, six live births after seven pregnancies (one pregnancy was electively terminated) were documented with a mean gestational age of 36.2 ± 3 weeks and a mean birth weight of 2,417.5 ± 657 g.[259] Complications were minimal and included two babies that were small for gestational age, a single preterm birth (<32 weeks), and a single shortened cervix. Hypertension was either absent or easily managed.

The success of intensified regimens appears to be directly related to enhanced clearance of urea and likely other solutes. An early study prior to the use of widespread dialysis noted fetal mortality to be directly related to the blood urea nitrogen (BUN) level with no documented successful pregnancies once the BUN exceeded 21.4 μmol per L (60 mg per dL).[266] More recently, in a series of 28 pregnant women receiving hemodialysis with 18 surviving infants, a significant negative relationship was noted between BUN and birth weight ($r = -0.533$, $P = .016$) as well as gestational age ($r = -504$, $P = .023$).[267] A birth weight of at least 1,500 g was achieved at a BUN <17.9 μmol per L (49 mg per dL) and a gestational age of at least 32 weeks was achieved at a BUN <17.1 μmol per L (48 mg per dL). Thus, the authors recommended adequately intensified dialysis to maintain the BUN <48 mg per dL. In the most recent and largest series to date wherein dialysis was increased from three to four

TABLE 59.3 Series Reporting on Greater than 20 Pregnancies in Hemodialysis Patients

Year	Geographic Region	Terminations	Losses	Live Births
1980[262]	Europe	39%	38%	23 %
1992[263]	Saudi Arabia	0%	63%	37%
1994[256]	United States	8%	52%	37%
1998[255]	United States	11%	46%	42%
1999[386]	Japan	19%	24%	49%
2009[267]	Japan	–	36%	64%
2010[268]	Brazil	–	13%	87%

to six times weekly, 52 pregnancies with an 87% overall successful birth rate was described.[268] Mean gestational age was noted to be 32.7 ± 3.1 weeks and birth weight was 1,554 ± 663 g. A summary of pregnancy outcomes from studies with >20 pregnancies is displayed in Table 59.3. Obvious trends include the decreased rate of therapeutic abortions likely reflecting a change in counselling practices over time secondary to an observed improved live birth rate as the decades pass and dialysis is routinely intensified.

In the early 1980s, the first reported outcomes of pregnant women on chronic ambulatory peritoneal dialysis (CAPD) were mixed with a successful pregnancy delivering at 33 weeks' gestation[269] as well as a reported intrauterine fetal death at 30 weeks' gestation.[270] The largest, early series by Redrow et al. concluded peritoneal dialysis to be superior to hemodialysis, and therefore, the preferred option for young pregnant women, but their own data did not clearly support that conclusion.[271] They described 14 pregnancies of which four ended in spontaneous abortion. The spontaneous losses occurred in one woman on established CAPD and in another woman on established hemodialysis, but the other two losses occurred in hemodialysis patients who were switched to peritoneal dialysis to potentially improve their pregnancy outcome. Another patient had three failed attempts to switch from hemodialysis to peritoneal dialysis due to drainage failure, eventually delivering a preterm, small for gestational age baby weighing 780 g. Of the remaining nine pregnancies, four were patients approaching ESRD who were started on either peritoneal dialysis ($n = 2$) or hemodialysis ($n = 2$), and therefore had significant residual renal function whereas established peritoneal and hemodialysis patients accounted for only five patients. Of interest, the three established peritoneal dialysis patients delivered babies weighing 1,065 to 1,720 grams between 32 and 34 weeks' gestation whereas the hemodialysis patients delivered at 35 and 36 weeks' gestation babies weighing 2,044 and 2,218 g, respectively. Subsequent case reports and series continued to demonstrate mixed results with the vast majority of patients conceiving prior to the initiation of peritoneal dialysis, and therefore having residual renal function.[272–283] Although early registry data from the United States did not document a statistically significant live birth rate in peritoneal versus hemodialysis patients,[255,284] a later single-center series noted worse outcomes in peritoneal versus hemodialysis patients.[285] Numbers of peritoneal dialysis patients, however, are typically few in single-center experiences.[285,286]

In addition to the potential maternal and fetal complications already described in hemodialysis patients, a number of maternal complications are unique to peritoneal dialysis. Abdominal fullness, discomfort, catheter drainage difficulties, and polyhydramnios necessitating a progressive decline in fill volumes have been described.[287] Bloody dialysate can herald an obstetrical catastrophe including placental abruption[275] or can be secondary to trauma to the expanding uterus from the peritoneal dialysis catheter,[282,288] and has been documented to be severe resulting in significant maternal morbidity with fetal demise.[288,289] Preterm delivery, premature rupture of membranes, and stillbirth have also been documented to occur secondary to acute peritonitis.[278,280,290]

A pregnant woman on either intensive hemodialysis or peritoneal dialysis requires meticulous follow-up. Fetal follow-up includes careful screening for congenital anomalies and follow-up of fetal growth. Amniotic fluid and cervical status also need careful assessment and follow-up. Issues for maternal care include the careful follow-up and supplementation of electrolytes, vitamins, and minerals as well as the management of anemia, volume status, and blood pressure.

Thus, care is best delivered by a dedicated team including nephrologists, obstetricians, and a full multidisciplinary staff.

Renal Transplantation

The first successful pregnancy in a renal transplant recipient occurred in 1958 with the birth of a 3,300-g, term, male infant.[291] Since that first successful pregnancy, there have been over 15,000 more reported in the literature. Similar to native kidneys, allografts accommodate to pregnancy with an increase in kidney volume[292] as well as an increase in GFR and enhanced creatinine clearance, 34% on average ranging from 10% to 60% with better allograft function prepregnancy predicting more robust pregnancy accommodation.[293] The anatomic increase in renal size is also associated with a better pregnancy outcome.[292] Pregnancy outcomes in women with renal allografts, therefore, are also dependent on baseline kidney function, the degree of proteinuria, and the frequent coexistence of hypertension and diabetes, which governs the kidney's ability to accommodate to pregnancy. Other additional issues that must also be carefully considered to ensure a successful outcome include the timing of pregnancy to minimize the risk of rejection, the careful management of various immunosuppressive agents, and the careful monitoring and treatment of potential infectious complications.

Outcome data, by and large, come from a multitude of single-center experiences that span the globe[294–301] along with a number of sizable registries including the National Transplantation Pregnancy Registry (NTPR),[302] the United Kingdom (UK) Transplant Pregnancy Registry,[303] and the Australian and New Zealand Dialysis and Transplant (ANZDATA) Registry.[304] Each has their own potential sources of bias and is incomplete with respect to capturing the entire population and/or relevant variables. The National Transplantation Pregnancy Registry includes data from over 1,200 subjects. Although the largest of the three registries, the data is self-reported. The other two registries are smaller, but are reported by health care practitioners and therefore are more complete and less prone to reporting errors of possible adverse outcomes. Regardless, as summarized in Table 59.4, all three report a similar live birth rate ranging from 73% to 79%, and pregnancy-related complications remain more common than the general population with the UK Transplant Pregnancy Registry reporting approximately half of all pregnancies ending preterm (<37 weeks' gestation) with a low birth weight (<2.5 g). The vast majority of untoward outcomes are secondary to superimposed preeclampsia with rates that range from approximately 25% to 30%.

Risk factors for poor outcome do not differ drastically from those that hamper a favorable outcome in women with native kidney disease. Further, the literature is similarly flawed by the use of serum creatinine to predict pregnancy outcome and cognizance is required to counsel women who may have more significant renal dysfunction than evident from serum creatinine alone. Regardless, the worst pregnancy outcomes are noted in women with poor

TABLE 59.4 **Pregnancy Outcome Data from Transplant Registries**

	NTPR	UK	ANZDATA
Live births	882 (73%)	149 (79%)	444 (76%)
Spontaneous abortions	NA	21 (11%)	52 (9%)
Stillbirths	NA	6 (4%)	14 (2%)
Mean gestational age	36.5 ± 2.7	35.6 ± 0.3	NA
Birth weight	2668 ± 784	2316 ± 80	NA
Preterm delivery (<37 weeks)	NA	61 (50%)	NA
Preeclampsia	≈29%	18 (36%)	27%
Deterioration in SCr	NA	14 (24%)	NA
Low birth weight (<2.5 g)	NA	53 (52%)	NA
Rejection	2%–4%	NA	NA

NTPR, National Transplantation Pregnancy Registry[302]; UK, United Kingdom Transplant Pregnancy Registry[303]; ANZDATA, Australian and New Zealand Dialysis and Transplant Registry[304]; NA, not available; SCr, serum creatinine.

allograft function prior to conception as defined by a serum creatinine >150 μmol per L (>1.7 mg per dL) and urine protein >500 mg per day.[302–304] Further, comorbidities, including hypertension, that necessitate more than a single therapeutic agent, and diabetes can further compromise outcome. A recent acute rejection episode is deemed a relative contraindication to pregnancy. These same risk factors that compromise pregnancy outcomes also predict accelerated postpartum deterioration in graft function, but prepregnancy baseline graft function and a rising serum creatinine during pregnancy appear to be the most important predictors of accelerated postpartum graft loss after adjustment for immunosuppressive therapy, hypertension before and during pregnancy, and preeclampsia.[302] In women who experienced postpartum graft loss, the mean prepregnancy serum creatinine was 1.5 ± 0.6 mg per dL and the creatinine during pregnancy was 1.7 ± 0.9 mg per dL compared to 1.3 ± 0.4 mg per dL and 1.2 ± 0.4 mg per dL, respectively, among women who did not have postpartum graft loss.[302] Thus, these women need to thoroughly understand the potential for both a poor pregnancy outcome along with the potential for graft compromise if pregnancy is considered in the presence of compromised graft function.

Repeated pregnancies in healthy women with a well-functioning graft do not hasten graft loss and can be encouraged.[302] At present, there is very limited data with respect to in vitro fertilization in renal transplant recipients and preliminary results are not encouraging, but this is gathered from self-reported data and therefore poor outcomes might be over-represented.[302]

Similar to intensive hemodialysis, successful kidney transplantation restores ovarian function and fertility. However, a recent report from USRDS data detailing 16,195 female transplant recipients noted decreasing pregnancy rates, and therefore live birth rates, over time that did not parallel the general population.[305] A variety of potential explanations for this finding exist including the introduction of mycophenolate mofetil and the realization of its teratogenic potential, prompting both physicians and patients to use appropriate contraception. Another possibility is the longer waiting times for cadaveric transplantation that could result in the loss of a woman's reproductive window or damage from other underlying comorbidities like hypertension and diabetes. In this same study, risk factors for increased rates of fetal loss included African American race, diabetes, and a lower socioeconomic status. An aging female recipient population with other comorbidities, therefore, has important implications for pregnancy timing.

Historically, the optimal timing for pregnancy post-transplantation was stated to be 2 years. This allowed for stabilization of graft function and the lowering of immunosuppression doses. However, the data from the USRDS noted only a borderline increase in pregnancy loss during the first as compared to the third year after transplantation, suggesting the historical 2-year waiting period might be overly conservative.[305] Another small study of 74 patients compared pregnancy outcomes in women who conceived within the first year after transplantation ($n = 11$) and compared them to women conceiving after 1 year ($n = 63$) noting no difference in the live birth rate.[306] In fact, there was a trend toward higher rates of preterm delivery and smaller babies in the women further out from transplantation suggesting that timing of pregnancy has to be carefully balanced by maternal age and comorbidities. We typically recommend women wait a year after transplantation prior to initiating a switch to pregnancy safe immunosuppression, but this warrants careful case by case consideration. Pregnancy itself does not cause acute rejection, but changing to pregnancy-safe immunosuppression requires cautious surveillance. Although there are no immunosuppressive medications adequately tested in pregnancy to be designated by the U.S. Food and Drug Administration (FDA) as pregnancy category A, there are a number of medications wherein the risk-benefit ratio is appropriate for use in pregnant women. These include prednisone, azathioprine, and the calcineurin inhibitors, but not mycophenolate mofetil.[307]

Only a fraction of the oral dose of prednisone reaches the fetus and, therefore, at the low doses that one would expect to be using in a stable transplant recipient, prednisone is considered a safe option. Higher doses, however, may not be completely without risk, as first trimester exposure may be associated with an increased risk of cleft palate (approximately 3/1,000 compared to 1/1,000 in the general population) and exposure later in pregnancy can be associated with an increased potential for the development of gestational diabetes and exacerbation of hypertension. Azathioprine requires the enzyme inosinate pyrophosphorylase for conversion to its active metabolite, an enzyme lacking by the fetal liver. Both cyclosporine and tacrolimus can be safely used in pregnant women, but the metabolism of these medications can change, necessitating close follow-up of blood levels. Cyclosporine metabolism tends to increase and therefore higher doses may be required whereas tacrolimus metabolism may be decreased by inhibition of hepatic cytochrome P450 enzymes. Although smaller babies have been reported in conjunction with use of these medications, it is not clear if this is a direct drug effect or secondary to the underlying disease state that necessitated use of these medications. The calcineurin inhibitors do have the potential to exacerbate hypertension and can be nephrotoxic even at therapeutic levels in our experience. Mycophenolate mofetil has now clearly emerged as a human teratogen with an identifiable pattern of malformations—craniofacial (microtia or anotia, absent auditory canal, cleft palate, hypertelorism) and limb anomalies (Fig. 59.4).[308] In pregnant transplant recipients ($n = 48$) exposed to a wide range of doses of mycophenolate mofetil, birth defects were noted in 11 women resulting in an incidence of 22.9%.[302] Thus it is recommended women initiating mycophenolate mofetil have a negative pregnancy test and utilize appropriate contraception. Those who desire pregnancy should be off mycophenolate mofetil at least 6 weeks prior to conception. Although human data

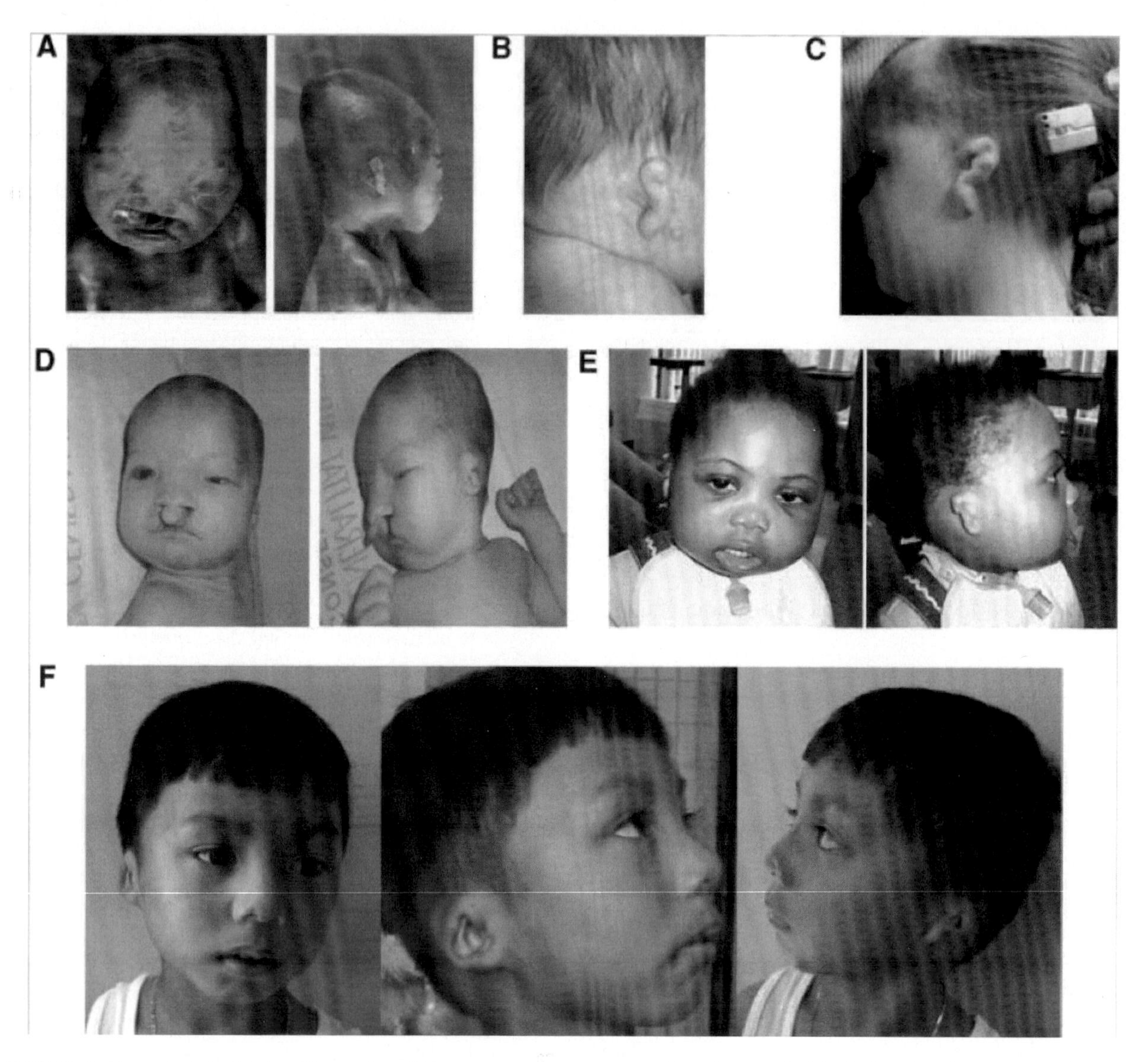

FIGURE 59.4 Characteristic fetal malformations following exposure to mycophenolate mofetil include microtia or anotia, absent auditory canal, cleft palate, hypertelorism, and limb anomalies. (Reprinted with permission from Anderka MT, Lin AE, Abuelo DN, et al. Reviewing the evidence for mycophenolate mofetil as a new teratogen: case report and review of the literature. *Am J Med. Genet A* 2009;149A:1241–1248.)

are lacking, rapamycin is highly teratogenic in animals and is therefore contraindicated in pregnancy.

Typically, drugs that can be used safely during pregnancy can also be used during breastfeeding. Minimal amounts of prednisone and azathioprine are actually found in breast milk. Thus, the potential for neonatal immunosuppression and future carcinogenesis is largely theoretical. Cyclosporine is now deemed compatible with breastfeeding as a completely breastfed infant would likely receive no more than 2% of the mother's weight-adjusted dose.[309] Although breastfeeding on tacrolimus is often discouraged, even less is passed to the infant (0.5% of the mother's weight adjusted dose).[310] Regardless, there are rare case reports that describe detectable and even therapeutic levels in the neonate.[311] Not surprisingly, there are no data to guide the safety of mycophenolate mofetil or rapamycin use during breastfeeding and therefore this practice should be avoided.

The mandated immunosuppressed state of pregnant women with renal allografts places these women at increased risk for infections. Ongoing close surveillance for bacterial infections, including regular urine cultures, for example, along with prompt treatment is necessary. A number of potential infectious complications can also result in serious neonatal compromise, the most common and significant of which is primary or reactivated cytomegalovirus (CMV) infection during pregnancy.[312] Primary maternal infection has a 30% to 40% risk of intrauterine transmission and a 20% to 25% risk for the development of fetal sequelae including microcephaly, hearing loss, visual impairment, mental retardation, as well as more subtle learning disabilities.[313]

The transmission rate to the fetus is significantly lower in reactivated CMV disease. The diagnosis of primary maternal CMV infection is based on the de novo appearance of viral specific IgM or IgG if previously known to be IgG seronegative. The prenatal diagnosis of fetal infection should be based on presence of the virus in amniotic fluid. The diagnosis of secondary infection is based on a significant rise in IgG antibody titre and the risk–benefit ratio of amniocentesis in cases of secondary infection must be considered more carefully given the lower rate of transmission. The incidence of primary or reactivated infections in transplant recipients, however, is largely unknown with very few cases reported to the National Transplant Registry.[302] Further, it is not clear if rates of transmission perhaps are higher given the immunosuppressed state of these patients. It is our practice to establish antibody status at the outset of pregnancy and follow titers during each trimester and in women who develop an influenza-like infection during pregnancy. Ganciclovir has been noted to be teratogenic in high doses in animal studies and to date there are only case reports to guide its use in humans.[314]

Renal Donation

Although renal donation is universally encouraged as a safe and altruistic endeavor, confusing data has emerged with respect to future pregnancy complications in young female donors that warrants further investigation. In a study utilizing the Norwegian Birth Registry, 326 kidney donors were identified and pregnancy outcome before (n = 620) and after (n = 106) were compared.[315] Although no significant difference was noted in the incidence of preeclampsia between the groups, a generalized linear mixed model demonstrated a significantly higher incidence of preeclampsia in postdonation pregnancies compared to predonation pregnancies (5.7% versus 2.6%, P =.026). A second study that collected survey data from 1,769 female donors identified 98 donors with pregnancies both before and after donation.[316] They noted that postdonation pregnancies were significantly less likely to have gone to term (73.7% versus 84.6%, P = .0004) and significantly more likely to have resulted in fetal loss (19.2% versus 11.3%, P <.0001) likely due to increased rates of gestational hypertension (5.7% versus 0.6%, P <.0001) and preeclampsia (5.5% versus 0.8%, P <.0001). As these studies are not without limitations, such as the confounder of advancing age between pregnancies, kidney donation in young women of childbearing potential warrants further research.

ACUTE KIDNEY INJURY IN PREGNANCY

The approach to and assessment of AKI should not differ from the nonpregnant population with attention paid to potential prerenal, renal, and postrenal etiologies. However, there are conditions that can impair kidney function that are either unique to pregnancy or worsened by the gravid state, and therefore, warrant further discussion. The main etiologies of AKI in a recent assessment of 55 obstetric cases requiring dialysis included pregnancy-related hypertensive conditions and the thrombotic microangiopathies.[317] Other potential pregnancy-specific etiologies of AKI include acute fatty liver of pregnancy and rarely acute cortical necrosis secondary to shock from obstetrical hemorrhage, severe sepsis, or an amniotic fluid embolus.

Preeclampsia

Affecting 5% to 7% of pregnancies, preeclampsia is easily the most common glomerular-based disease and remains the leading cause of infant and maternal morbidity and mortality worldwide.[318] Preeclampsia is a disease of the glomerular endothelial cell characterized by decreased GFR, proteinuria, and hypertension that can evolve to include coagulopathies and affect liver function (HELLP syndrome) as well as cause seizures (eclampsia). The pathophysiology of preeclampsia is best understood at the level of the kidney wherein novel insights into the release of antiangiogenic factors from an abnormal placenta that are injurious to the maternal endothelium as well as abnormalities in the RAS have elucidated the mechanisms responsible for the clinical syndrome. With very rare exceptions, preeclampsia is limited to the second half of the gestation and the early postpartum period. Hypertension, GFR depression, and proteinuria typically resolve rapidly after delivery of the placenta.

As compared to the healthy gravid state, preeclampsia presents with variable degrees of renal insufficiency. A study that utilized precise physiologic measurements in conjunction with morphometric analysis of postpartum biopsies to examine the determinants of the GFR in 13 women with preeclampsia and 12 healthy gravid controls noted GFR to be significantly depressed in women with preeclampsia compared to healthy controls (91 versus 149 mL/min/1.73 m^2, respectively; P <.0001) without detected differences in either RPF or π_{GC}.[319] As compared to tissue obtained from healthy female kidney transplant donors, the morphometric analysis revealed numerous significant ultrastructural differences including swelling of the endothelial cells, the presence of subendothelial fibrinoid deposition, and mesangial cell interposition (Fig. 59.5). Scanning electron microscopy was utilized to characterize the endothelial fenestral dimensions wherein a substantial decrease in endothelial permeability was noted (Fig. 59.6). The authors concluded that a reduction in density and size of the endothelial fenestrae and subendothelial accumulation of fibrinoid deposits lowered glomerular hydraulic permeability whereas mesangial cell interposition also likely decreased available surface area for filtration in patients with preeclampsia compared to controls, resulting in a depression of K_f that was proportional to the decrease in GFR without a hemodynamic basis.

These findings were confirmed by a more recent study that used a semiquantitative scale to grade the endotheliosis present on biopsy specimens taken from women with

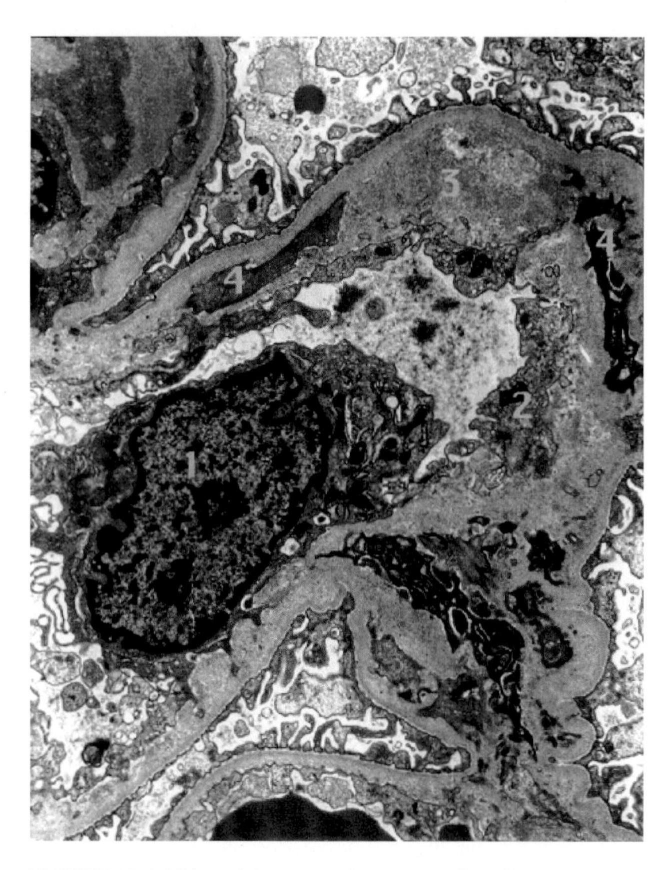

FIGURE 59.5 Kidney biopsy specimen revealing the characteristic findings associated with preeclampsia including swelling of the endothelial cells, the presence of subendothelial fibrinoid deposition, and mesangial cell interposition. (Reprinted with permission from Lafayette RA, Druzin M, Sibley R, et al. Nature of glomerular dysfunction in pre-eclampsia. *Kidney Int.* 1998;54(4):1240–1249.)

preeclampsia approximately 1 week prior to delivery.[10,320] The authors noted moderate to severe endotheliosis in all women with significant hypertension and proteinuria prior to delivery and found a strong linear trend between the degree of endotheliosis and cystatin C. Although, as discussed, issues do exist with the use of cystatin C as a marker for GFR in pregnancy, this study also supports the notion that the basis for hypofiltration in preeclampsia is largely secondary to structural changes in the glomerulus as opposed to renal vasoconstriction. Others, however, have suggested a modest decrease in renal plasma flow in women with preeclampsia compared to normotensive women in the third trimester.[321,322]

Given preeclampsia is largely understood as an endothelial disease, the mechanism of nephrotic range proteinuria was difficult to reconcile prior to the discovery of soluble antiangiogenic factors released from an ischemic placenta, as well as the understanding of crosstalk between the glomerular endothelial cell and the podocyte. Recent studies have described the release of soluble fms-like tyrosine kinase 1 (sFlt-1), which binds placental growth factor (PlGF) and vascular endothelial growth factor (VEGF), potent angiogenic factors that play critical roles in the maintenance of a healthy vascular endothelium, preventing their interaction with receptors located on the vascular endothelial cells.[323]

In the kidney, podocytes have been shown to be the site of VEGF production in vivo. VEGF receptors are expressed on the endothelial cells suggesting that the VEGF produced by the podocyte travels against the flow of filtrate to its receptor. More recently, VEGFR-1 and neuropilin-1 have been shown to be present on podocytes, both in vitro and in vivo. Thus, paracrine and autocrine pathways could very well exist that promote fenestration formation and govern the integrity of the glomerular filtration barrier,[324,325] and tight regulation of VEGF signalling is necessary to maintain a healthy glomerulus. Mice with a homozygous deletion in podocyte specific VEGF fail to develop a filtration barrier, a uniformly lethal condition.[326] Podocyte-specific heterozygosity, on the other hand, resulted in glomerular endotheliosis and proteinuria, a lesion reminiscent of human preeclampsia. In another rat model wherein adenoviral overexpression of sFlt-1 produced hypertension, proteinuria, and glomerular endotheliosis, VEGF121 treatment improved the clinical symptoms as well as renal histology.[327] Human data linking endothelial injury with enhanced glomerular permeability in preeclampsia includes two studies. The first study noted decreased glomerular expression of podocyte-specific proteins, nephrin, and synaptopodin in renal tissue from autopsies of women who died from preeclampsia compared to women who died from trauma.[328] The same authors then went on to demonstrate that podocyturia was associated with preeclampsia and correlated with the degree of proteinuria.[329] One can therefore postulate that in preeclamptic women,

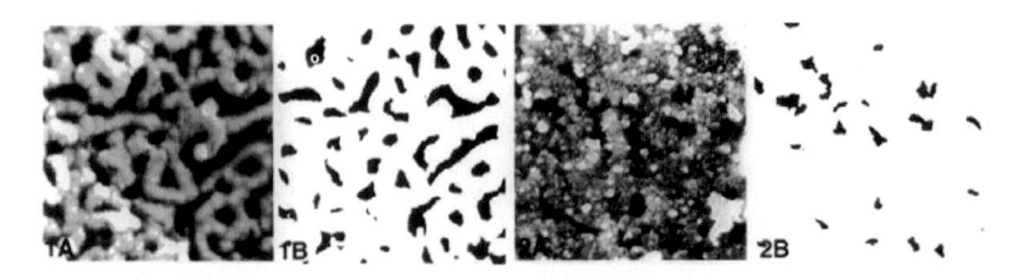

FIGURE 59.6 Scanning electron microscopy comparing the endothelial fenestral dimensions in a healthy transplant donor and a woman with severe preeclampsia. (Reprinted with permission from Lafayette RA, Druzin M, Sibley R, et al. Nature of glomerular dysfunction in pre-eclampsia. *Kidney Int.* 1998;54(4):1240–1249.)

high levels of circulating sFlt-1 systematically deprive the glomeruli of local VEGF signalling. sFlt-1 molecules displace locally derived VEGF produced by the podocyte reducing both size and density of fenestrations to cause endotheliosis and damage the fenestral glycocalyx, a potentially important part of the barrier to albumin permeability.

The hypertension associated with preeclampsia can also certainly be explained by the presence of soluble antiangiogenic factors. Abnormally increased levels of sFlt-1 have been demonstrated in women with gestational hypertension albeit with levels not as high as in women with preeclampsia.[330] Further, soluble Endoglin (sEng), also released from an ischemic placenta, deleteriously affects vascular tone by blocking the activation of endothelial nitric oxide synthase.[331] Recently, the role of the RAS in blood pressure control in pregnancy has received more attention. In contrast to the healthy gravid state, RAS components in preeclampsia are depressed, yet enhanced vascular sensitivity to angiotensin has been noted. Angiotensin infusions have resulted in a more dramatic hemodynamic response in women destined to develop preeclampsia as compared to healthy pregnant controls.[332,333] The exact mechanism underlying the angiotensin resistance in normal pregnancy is still unclear, but studies have shown that plasma and urine levels of ANG(1-7) are increased in pregnancy.[90,334] This potential counter regulator of angiotensin is also significantly decreased in preeclamptic women as compared to healthy gravid women.[90] Alternatively, upregulation of the AT1 receptor has been demonstrated on the decidual or maternal side of the placenta.[335] Finally, recent studies in women with preeclampsia have also identified circulating autoantibodies belonging to the fraction of IgG antibodies that are capable of stimulating the angiotensin 1 receptor.[336,337] In preeclamptic women, they may induce heterodimerization between the angiotensin I receptor for the vasopressor angiotensin II and the bradykinin 2 receptor for the vasodilator bradykinin. Expression of these heterodimers may result in an increased responsiveness to angiotensin II.[338]

New insights into the pathogenesis of disease also provide novel diagnostic opportunities (Fig. 59.7). Both the soluble antiangiogenic factors and the AT1 autoantibody have been shown to predate the clinical syndrome, but the

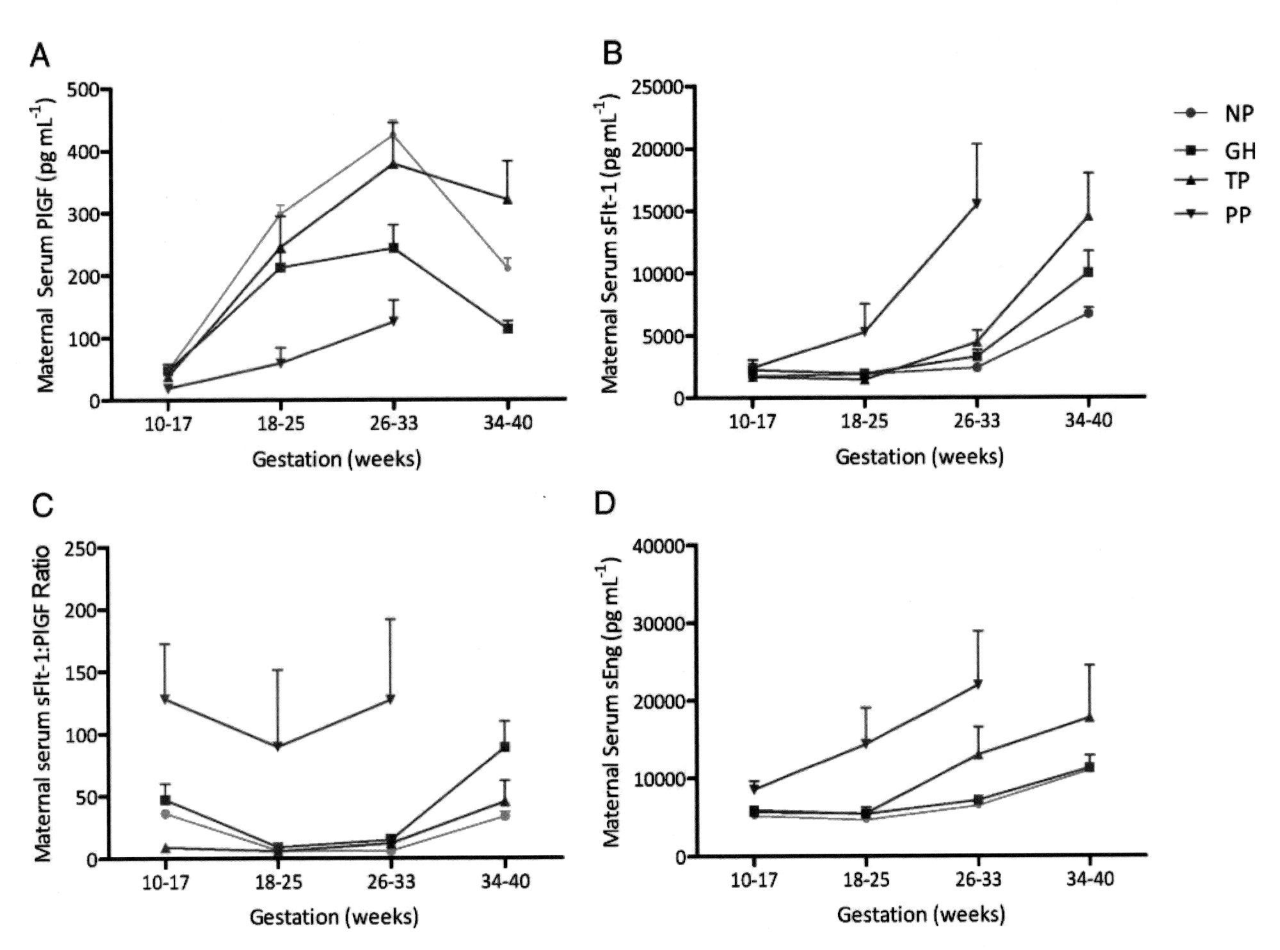

FIGURE 59.7 Gestational changes of maternal serum PlGF, sFlt-1, Flt-1/PlGF ratio, and sEng in normotensive pregnancies (NP), gestational hypertension (GH), term preeclampsia (TP), and preterm preeclampsia (PP). (Reprinted with permission from Noori M, Donald AE, Angelakopoulou A, et al. Prospective study of placental angiogenic factors and maternal vascular function before and after preeclampsia and gestational hypertension. *Circulation.* 2010;122(5):478–487.)

soluble antiangiogenic factors provide more accurate discrimination between cases and healthy gravid controls.[339] Increased sFlt-1 and sEng along with decreased serum and urine PlGF and VEGF levels results in an adjusted odds ratio of 31.6; 95% CI 10.7–93.4 for the development of early onset preeclampsia.[340] The antiangiogenic factor assays can be used to discriminate preeclampsia from other etiologies of renal compromise and have proven useful in a variety of clinical scenarios including presumed glomerulonephritis,[341] lupus,[342] and in patients on hemodialysis.[343] Most recently, a small pilot study utilized dextran sulfate cellulose apheresis treatments to reduce circulating sFlt-1 levels in a dose-dependent fashion.[344] Treatments in three women with severe early onset preeclampsia lowered circulating sFlt-1 levels, reduced proteinuria, and stabilized blood pressure without apparent adverse events to mother or fetus. Further studies will determine the feasibility of using clearance techniques to possibly prolong pregnancy and improve fetal outcomes.

Chronic kidney disease is a risk factor for the development of preeclampsia. Further, preeclampsia may be the disorder revealing the existence of underlying renal disease that is often diagnosed when proteinuria and hypertension fail to subside postpartum, and has been noted to be as high as 20% in some series wherein women developed preeclampsia prior to 30 weeks' gestation.[345] Abnormalities in glomerular VEGF expression have been linked to glomerular diseases other than preeclampsia and may specifically increase susceptibility in diseased populations. Di Marco and colleagues assayed sFlt1 levels in 130 patients with CKD, stages 3 to 5, and in 56 age and gender matched controls.[346] The sFlt1 levels were higher in patients with CKD and exclusively associated with renal function. A reverse transcription/polymerase chain reaction assessment of glomerular and tubular VEGF expression in patients with type II diabetes revealed progressive decline in VEGF expression with more severe glomerular and tubulointerstitial disease.[347] One can easily conceptualize based on such data why women with diabetic nephropathy are at a substantially increased risk for the development of preeclampsia. However, the levels of VEGF expression likely vary between different glomerulopathies and can vary with the stage of progression. Further, a distinction has to be made between circulating VEGF levels and glomerular VEGF bioactivity. Moreover, regulation of the bioactivity of glomerular VEGF may be dependent on other factors such as TGF-beta, NO, mechanical strain, and hyperglycemia.[348] Future research should attempt to elucidate the levels of angiogenic and antiangiogenic factors that underlie the complex interaction between preeclampsia and kidney disease as these interactions are necessary to better understand the physiologic basis for the increased risk of preeclampsia noted in women with kidney disease, and may allow for the measurement of antiangiogenic factors to play a role in the often complex diagnostic dilemmas that practicing clinicians regularly face.

The clinical syndrome of preeclampsia resolves with delivery of the placenta, but recently is has become clear that placental disease is associated with long-term health consequences. The first study to describe the relationship between preeclampsia and cardiovascular disease utilized the Norwegian Medical Birth Registry.[349] Although this study did not show an increased risk of death among women with preeclampsia who delivered at term, it did show almost a threefold increased risk of death with an eightfold increased risk of cardiovascular death in women who delivered prior to 37 weeks, interpreted as a surrogate marker for more severe disease. These findings have been confirmed and expanded by other studies where, in addition to an increased risk of cardiovascular disease, an increased risk of cerebrovascular disease, peripheral vascular disease, and ESRD was also noted.[350,351] Of interest to nephrologists is the concept of whether preeclampsia as a secondary insult hastens the progression of underlying glomerular-based disease. The variable etiologies of kidney disease preceding ESRD in the aforementioned study suggests that it might,[351] but a subsequent study did not confirm this hypothesis.[351] Clearly further data that examine the impact of expectant management in women with kidney disease and superimposed preeclampsia prior to delivery is necessary.

Thrombotic Microangiopathies

The thrombotic microangiopathies include thrombotic thrombocytopenic purpura (TTP) and hemolytic uremic syndrome (HUS), disorders characterized by disseminated occlusion of arterioles and capillaries by agglutinated platelets with resultant ischemia. Both disorders present with hemolytic anemia, thrombocytopenia, and renal insufficiency, whereas neurologic abnormalities and fever may also accompany TTP. With recent insights into the pathophysiology, TTP is becoming well understood in the context of pregnancy and, more recently, the pregnancy outcomes in atypical HUS associated complement gene mutations have been described.

TTP is a rare condition with incidence rates across the globe ranging from 2.2 to 6.5 per million in the United Kingdom and the United States, respectively.[352] It is more common in women who represent approximately 70% of cases.[353] Black race and obesity also appear to be risk factors, and pregnancy is a well-described precipitant[353] with TTP occurring in approximately 1 in 25,000 pregnancies.[354] As pregnancy in some way incites the cascade of endothelial disruption resulting in microthrombi, a significant percentage of young women present for the first time during pregnancy even in the presence of congenital or familial disease.[355,356]

It is now understood that the pathophysiology involves either a congenital absence of, or an immunoglobulin G (IgG) autoantibody inhibitor to ADAMTS13 (A Disintegrin And Metalloproteinase with ThromboSpondin type 1 motifs 13) normally produced by the liver, platelets, vascular endothelial cells, and the renal podocytes. This metalloproteinase specifically cleaves unusually large multimers of von Willebrand factor (ULVWF) preventing interaction of these large multimers with platelets and the subsequent vascular occlusion characteristic of the syndrome. Plasmapheresis inhibits platelet aggregation, replenishes absent ADAMTS13, and/or removes pathogenic antibodies. There are a number of theories why pregnancy might pose a heightened risk for the development of TTP including the procoagulant state that accompanies pregnancy as well as the potential effect of estrogen on the level of ADAMTS13, which progressively decreases throughout pregnancy to a nadir in the early postpartum period. In the largest, most complete patient registry of TTP-HUS from Oklahoma City, pregnancy accounted for 26 of the 352 cases collected over approximately 15 years and the vast majority presented in the third trimester and early postpartum period.[353]

Establishing a diagnosis of TTP with rapid initiation of treatment is critical to decrease morbidity and mortality. Its typical presentation in the later stages of pregnancy and the early postpartum period can result in a diagnostic dilemma as preeclampsia complicated by the HELLP syndrome presents with similar features. Further, the two entities are not mutually exclusive and may very well coexist. A systematic review of the literature that summarized the outcome in 166 reported cases spanning 1955 to 2006 noted the coexistence of TTP with preeclampsia/HELLP syndrome in 28 cases without obvious laboratory discriminants[357] and other careful case series reported a true association as opposed to a mistaken diagnosis.[358] Further, placental pathology in cases of TTP describes similar features as noted in preeclampsia including small placental size, vascular thrombosis, infarction, and accelerated villous maturation in conjunction with zones of vascular dilatation and constriction consistent with aneurysmal dilatation of the spiral arteries on the maternal side of the placenta, a finding distinctive of TTP.[359] Finally, ADAMST13 levels do fluctuate significantly between and within patients,[360] levels have been demonstrated to be lower in patients with HELLP syndrome than in healthy gravid patients[361] and severe deficiency (<5%), wherein one is confident with respect to the diagnosis, is certainly not uniform in reported pregnancy cases.[74,358,362] Thus, without useful laboratory assays to definitively diagnose these entities it is difficult to definitively distinguish them and it is not entirely clear how often they coexist. Although more common in the later stages of pregnancy, TTP can certainly occur at any stage of pregnancy as fatal and nonfatal cases in the first trimester have been documented,[353,363] as have cases following a molar pregnancy[364] and first trimester therapeutic abortion.[365] Thus, a high level of clinical acumen with mindfulness of this rare disease as a possibility is necessary irrespective of the timing in pregnancy as misdiagnosis is common and improved outcome has been demonstrated with the shortest latency from diagnosis to therapy.[366]

Prior to modern treatment with plasmapheresis mortality approached 100%. Despite better outcomes with treatment, TTP remains a serious condition with significant potential morbidity and mortality for both mother and fetus. Maternal morbidity has been documented in case reports and case series, but the exact incidence is unclear. In the systematic review that spanned six decades, maternal morbidity decreased over time, but remained substantially higher in women experiencing an initial TTP compared to women with recurrent disease (26% versus 10.7%, respectively) as well as in women diagnosed with coexistent preeclampsia/HELLP syndrome.[357] Maternal morbidity is also not negligible with significant renal insufficiency and even subtle cognitive deficits noted in survivors.[354,367] The stillbirth rate was not significantly different in patients with a first presentation of TTP compared to recurrent disease (32 versus 44%, respectively),[357] and both fetal growth restriction and preterm delivery are common.[354] However, documented successful outcomes with therapy have been documented even with congenital[356] and early onset disease.[363] Thus, clinicians are often in the position of counselling with respect to risk of pregnancy flare in idiopathic disease and recurrence in cases where the first presentation occurred during pregnancy.

The most comprehensive study with respect to the potential occurrence during pregnancy comes from the Oklahoma TTP-HUS Registry wherein they compared their data to the existing literature.[362] In women who recovered from idiopathic TTP, recurrences were reported, but none in association with a subsequent pregnancy. In women with pregnancy-associated TTP, the overall risk of recurrent TTP is reported to be infrequent (14%).[368] The risk of recurrence in congenital TTP, on the other hand, is reported to be 100%,[362] and therefore the detection of severe deficiency of ADAMTS13 levels may assist with pregnancy planning.[369] Overall, the rates in the Oklahoma TTP-HUS Registry are more optimistic than the older literature in general, and differences could be explained by misdiagnosis or a bias to the publication of more severe and complicated cases. There are insufficient data in the literature to comment on the benefit or lack thereof associated with the prophylactic use of maintenance plasmapheresis, immunosuppression, antiplatelet agents, or anticoagulation with respect to pregnancy outcomes.[361,362]

Although more often seen secondary to acute infection (Shigatoxin-producing *Escherichia coli* O157), HUS can rarely be induced by genetic mutations involving the activation or regulation of the alternative complement pathway triggered by pregnancy. These disorders present clinically with low serum complement levels and predominant renal involvement. Currently, data are limited, but overall maternal outcome appears to be quite poor. Documented HUS cases most frequently present in the postpartum period with severe renal involvement, necessitating dialysis during the acute phase of the disease in 81% with 62% reaching ESRD within a month despite therapy.[370] However, given the late onset of disease, fetal outcomes are reasonable with the vast majority proving uneventful (74.7%). Preeclampsia and fetal loss complicated 7.7% and 4.8% of pregnancies, respectively. Further studies will be needed to better understand these rare presentations of atypical HUS.

Acute Fatty Liver of Pregnancy

Acute fatty liver of pregnancy (AFLP) is a serious, but rare complication with an estimated incidence between 1 in 7,000 and 1 in 13,000 births.[371,372] With respect to pathophysiology, AFLP is characterized by accumulation of lipids in hepatocytes.[373] Recently, investigators have demonstrated that the fetus may be the source of increased fatty acids due to inherited autosomal recessive genetic mutations from heterozygous parents.[374] Clinically, the management of AFLP must be swift and decisive given the risk of fetal and maternal mortality, 19% and 12% respectively.[375] Yet, a common challenge in prompt identification of AFLP is distinguishing it from preeclampsia or HELLP syndrome. Recently, investigators have highlighted important clinical findings that can aid in clinical decision-making.[376] Although epigastric pain, nausea/vomiting, and jaundice were noted in 60% of women in AFLP, these signs and symptoms were only identified in 5% of women with HELLP syndrome.[376] Furthermore, albumin phosphatase, total bilirubin, and white blood cell count were significantly more elevated in the context of AFLP, whereas glucose, cholesterol, triglycerides, fibrinogen, and antithrombin III were significantly more elevated in the context of HELLP syndrome. However, the conditions were similar with respect to the presence of hypertension and proteinuria.[376] The syndromes can also be distinguished based on complications associated with the disease course. In particular, renal failure is a common complication in AFLP (>70%) and tends to present earlier.[376–378] Altogether, prompt termination of pregnancy (which is the treatment of choice for HELLP syndrome as well) is an important aspect of the management of AFLP as time to termination can affect maternal outcomes.[379] Further interventions including liver transplantation may also be required.[375,380]

Renal Cortical Necrosis

Renal cortical necrosis is an uncommon complication of pregnancy that is primarily noted in developing countries.[381,382] Recently, decrements in the prevalence were reported by investigators in India, citing improvements in medical management of obstetrical complications.[381,383] Commonly reported causes of renal cortical necrosis include septic abortion and hemorrhage from placental abruption.[381,384] The exact pathophysiology is not known, but it is widely accepted that the final common pathway involves renal ischemia. In particular, disseminated intravascular coagulation, a potential source of ischemic injury, has been reported to occur concurrently with renal cortical necrosis.[385] However, previous studies suggest that DIC does not predispose to renal cortical necrosis.[244] Given the low incidence, it is not surprising that there are no recent studies examining this relationship. Although mortality from renal cortical necrosis has decreased,[381] outcomes are still not favorable. In a general cohort of patients with obstetrical and nonobstetrical causes, mortality was 19%, whereas partial recovery of renal function and ESRD occurred in 33% and 50%, respectively.[381]

CONCLUSION

The kidney and its many functions undergo profound physiologic alterations to support a healthy pregnancy so women with significant renal disease may prove higher risk as impaired renal function, proteinuria, and hypertension can compromise this healthy accommodation. Thus, these women require meticulous prepregnancy assessment and effective optimization by nephrologists along with careful pregnancy follow-up by both nephrology and a high risk obstetrician. Further research is necessary to better understand the diseased kidney's ability to accommodate pregnancy and to better understand disease-specific risks. Intensive dialysis regimens may make possible pregnancy in a subset of patients wherein previously that was most unlikely. Finally, recent insights into the pathophysiology of preeclampsia should yield novel diagnostic and treatment opportunities for the most common pregnancy-related complications experienced by women with underlying renal disease.

REFERENCES

1. Sheenan H, Lynch J, eds. *Pathology of Toxemia and Pregnancy*. Essex, UK: Longman Group Limited; 1973.
2. Rasmussen PE, Nielsen FR. Hydronephrosis during pregnancy: a literature survey. *Eur J Obstet Gynecol. Reprod Biol.* 1988;27(3):249–259.
3. Cietak KA, Newton JR. Serial qualitative maternal nephrosonography in pregnancy. *Br J Radiol.* 1985;58:399–404.
4. Faundes A, Bricola-Filho M, Pinto e Silva JL. Dilatation of the urinary tract during pregnancy: proposal of a curve of maximal caliceal diameter by gestational age. *Am J Obstet Gynecol.* 1998;178:1082–1086.
5. Au KK, Woo JS, Tang LC, et al. Aetiological factors in the genesis of pregnancy hydronephrosis. *Aust N Z J Obstet Gynaecol.* 1985;25:248–251.
6. Woo JS, Wan CW, Ma HK. Pregnancy hydronephrosis—a longitudinal ultrasonic evaluation. *Aust N Z J Obstet Gynaecol.* 1984;24:9–13.
7. Fried AM, Woodring JH, Thompson DJ. Hydronephrosis of pregnancy: a prospective sequential study of the course of dilatation. *J Ultrasound Med.* 1983;2:255–259.
8. Rubi RA, Sala NL. Ureteral function in pregnant women. 3. Effect of different positions and of fetal delivery upon ureteral tonus. *Am J Obstet Gynecol.* 1968;101:230–237.
9. Dure-Smith P. Pregnancy dilatation of the urinary tract. The iliac sign and its significance. *Radiology.* 1970;96:545–550.
10. Strevens H, Wide-Swensson D, Hansen A, et al. Glomerular endotheliosis in normal pregnancy and pre-eclampsia. *BJOG.* 2003;110:831–836.
11. Chapman AB, Abraham WT, Zamudio S, et al. Temporal relationships between hormonal and hemodynamic changes in early human pregnancy. *Kidney Int.* 1998;56:2056–2063.
12. Roberts M, Lindheimer MD, Davison JM. Altered glomerular permselectivity to neutral dextrans and heteroporous membrane modeling in human pregnancy. *Am J Physiol.* 1996;270:F338–343.
13. Davison JM, Dunlop W. Renal hemodynamics and tubular function normal human pregnancy. *Kidney Int.* 1980;18(2):152–161.
14. Milne JE, Lindheimer MD, Davison JM. Glomerular heteroporous membrane modeling in third trimester and postpartum before and during amino acid infusion. *Am J Physiol Renal Physiol.* 2002;282(1):F170–175.
15. de Alvarez RR. Renal glomerular tubular mechanisms during normal pregnancy. I. Glomerular filtration rate, renal plasma flow and creatinine clearance. *Am J Obstet Gynecol.* 1958;11(20):931–944.
16. Assali NS, Dignam WJ, Dasgupta K. Renal function in human pregnancy. II. Effects of venous pooling on renal hemodynamics and water, electrolyte and aldosterone excretion during normal gestation. *J Lab Clin Med.* 1959;54:394–408.
17. Sims EA, Krantz KE. Serial studies of renal function during pregnancy and the puerperium in normal women. *J Clin Invest.* 1958;37(12):1764–1774.

18. Ezimokhai M, Davison JM, Philips PR, et al. Non-postural serial changes in renal function during the third trimester of normal human pregnancy. *Br J Obstet Gynaecol.* 1981;88(5):465–471.
19. Dunlop W. Serial changes in renal haemodynamics during normal human pregnancy. *Br J Obstet Gynaecol.* 1981;88(1):1–9.
20. Lafayette RA, Malik T, Druzin M, et al. The dynamics of glomerular filtration after Caesarean section. *J Am Soc Nephrol.* 1999;10(7):1561–1565.
21. Duvekot JJ, Cheriex EC, Pieters FA, et al. Early pregnancy changes in hemodynamics and volume homeostasis are consecutive adjustments triggered by a primary fall in systemic vascular tone. *Am J Obstet Gynecol.* 1993;169(6):1382–1392.
22. Hladunewich MA, Lafayette RA, Derby GC, et al. The dynamics of glomerular filtration in the puerperium. *Am J Physiol Renal Physiol.* 2004;286(3): F496–503.
23. Krutzen E, Olofsson P, Back SE, et al. Glomerular filtration rate in pregnancy: a study in normal subjects and in patients with hypertension, preeclampsia and diabetes. *Scand J Clin Lab Invest.* 1992;52(5):387–392.
24. Deen WM, Robertson CR, Brenner BM. A model of glomerular ultrafiltration in the rat. *Am J Physiol.* 1972;223(5):1178–1183.
25. Honger PE. Albumin metabolism in normal pregnancy. *Scand J Clin Lab Invest.* 1968:3–9.
26. Nguyen HN, Clark SL, Greenspoon J, et al. Peripartum colloid osmotic pressures: correlation with serum proteins. *Obstet Gynecol.* 1986;68(6):807–810.
27. Olufemi OS, Whittaker PG, Halliday D, et al. Albumin metabolism in fasted subjects during late pregnancy. *Clin Sci (Lond).* 1991;81(2):161–168.
28. Paaby P. Changes in serum proteins during pregnancy. *J Obstet Gynaecol Br Emp.* 1960;67:43–55.
29. Brenner BM, Troy JL, Daugharty TM, et al. Dynamics of glomerular ultrafiltration in the rat. II. Plasma-flow dependence of GFR. *Am J Physiol.* 1972;223(5):1184–1190.
30. Moran P, Baylis PH, Lindheimer MD, et al. Glomerular ultrafiltration in normal and preeclamptic pregnancy. *J Am Soc Nephrol.* 2003;14(3):648–652.
31. Baylis C. The mechanism of increased glomerular filtration rate during pregnancy in the rat [proceedings]. *J Physiol.* 1979;295:101P.
32. Baylis C. The mechanism of the increase in glomerular filtration rate in the twelve-day pregnant rat. *J Physiol.* 1980;305:405–414.
33. Baylis C. Glomerular ultrafiltration in the pseudopregnant rat. *Am J Physiol.* 1982;243(3):F300–305.
34. Baylis C, Rennke HG. Renal hemodynamics and glomerular morphology in repetitively pregnant aging rats. *Kidney Int.* 1985;28(2):140–145.
35. Deng A, Baylis C. Glomerular hemodynamic responses to pregnancy in rats with severe reduction of renal mass. *Kidney Int.* 1995;48(1):39–44.
36. Heguilen RM, Liste AA, Bellusci AD, et al. Renal response to an acute protein challenge in pregnant women with borderline hypertension. *Nephrology (Carlton).* 2007;12(3):254–260.
37. Ronco C, Brendolan A, Bragantini L, et al. Renal functional reserve in pregnancy. *Nephrol Dial Transplant.* 1988;3(2):157–161.
38. Welsh GW III, Sims EA. The mechanisms of renal glucosuria in pregnancy. *Diabetes.* 1960;9:363–369.
39. Drexel H, Sailer S. Kinetics of glucose handling in renal glucosuria during pregnancy. *Klin Wochenschr* 1980;58(23):1299–1306.
40. Davison JM, Hytten FE. The effect of pregnancy on the renal handling of glucose. *Br J Obstet Gynaecol.* 1975;82(5):374–381.
41. Oltmanns KM, Dodt B, Schultes B, et al. Cortisol correlates with metabolic disturbances in a population study of type 2 diabetic patients. *Eur J Endocrinol.* 2006;154(2):325–331.
42. Hytten FE. The renal excretion of nutrients in pregnancy. *Postgrad Med J.* 1973;49(575):625–629.
43. Zarowitz H, Newhouse S. Renal glycosuria in normoglycemic glysoduric pregnancy: a quantitative study. *Metabolism.* 1973;22(5):755–761.
44. Chen WW, Sese L, Tantakasen P, et al. Pregnancy associated with renal glucosuria. *Obstet Gynecol.* 1976;47(1):37–40.
45. Landon MB, Spong CY, Thom E, et al. A multicenter, randomized trial of treatment for mild gestational diabetes. *N Engl J Med.* 2009;361(14):1339–1348.
46. Hytten FE, Cheyne GA. The aminoaciduria of pregnancy. *J Obstet Gynaecol Br Commonw.* 1972;79(5):424–432.
47. van Buul EJ, Steegers EA, Jongsma HW, et al. Haematological and biochemical profile of uncomplicated pregnancy in nulliparous women; a longitudinal study. *Neth J Med.* 1995;46(2):73–85.
48. Boyle JA, Campbell S, Duncan AM, et al. Serum uric acid levels in normal pregnancy with observations on the renal excretion of urate in pregnancy. *J Clin Pathol.* 1966;19(5):501–503.
49. Hayashi M, Ueda Y, Hoshimoto K, et al. Changes in urinary excretion of six biochemical parameters in normotensive pregnancy and preeclampsia. *Am J Kidney Dis.* 2002;39(2):392–400.
50. Powers RW, Bodnar LM, Ness RB, et al. Uric acid concentrations in early pregnancy among preeclamptic women with gestational hyperuricemia at delivery. *Am J Obstet Gynecol.* 2006;194(1):160.
51. Laughon SK, Catov J, Powers RW, et al. First trimester uric acid and adverse pregnancy outcomes. *Am J Hypertens.* 2011;24(4):489–495.
52. Brown MA, Lindheimer MD, de Swiet M, et al. The classification and diagnosis of the hypertensive disorders of pregnancy: statement from the International Society for the Study of Hypertension in Pregnancy (ISSHP). *Hypertens Pregnancy.* 2001;20(1):IX-XIV.
53. Higby K, Suiter CR, Phelps JY, et al. Normal values of urinary albumin and total protein excretion during pregnancy. *Am J Obstet Gynecol.* 1994;171(4): 984–989.
54. Smith NA, Lyons JG, McElrath TF. Protein:creatinine ratio in uncomplicated twin pregnancy. *Am J Obstet Gynecol.* 2010;203(4);381.e1–381.e4.
55. Beunis MH, Schweitzer KJ, van Hooff MH, et al. Midtrimester screening for microalbuminuria in healthy pregnant women. *J Obstet Gynaecol.* 2004;24(8): 863–865.
56. Konstantin-Hansen KF, Hesseldahl H, Pedersen SM. Microalbuminuria as a predictor of preeclampsia. *Acta Obstet Gynecol Scand.* 1992;71(5):343–346.
57. Erman A, Neri A, Sharoni R, et al. Enhanced urinary albumin excretion after 35 weeks of gestation and during labour in normal pregnancy. *Scand J Clin Lab Invest.* 1992;52(5):409–413.
58. Hytten FE, Leitch I. *The Physiology of Human Pregnancy.* Oxford: Blackwell; 1971.
59. Mishina T, Scholer DW, Edelman IS. Glucocorticoid receptors in rat kidney cortical tubules enriched in proximal and distal segments. *Am J Physiol.* 1981;240(1):F38–45.
60. Chapman AB, Abraham WT, Zamudio S, et al. Temporal relationships between hormonal and hemodynamic changes in early human pregnancy. *Kidney Int.* 1998;54(6):2056–2063.
61. Irons DW, Baylis PH, Davison JM. Effect of atrial natriuretic peptide on renal hemodynamics and sodium excretion during human pregnancy. *Am J Physiol.* 1996;271:F239–242.
62. Davison JM, Lindheimer MD. Volume homeostasis and osmoregulation in human pregnancy. *Baillieres Clin Endocrinol Metab.* 1989;3(2):451–472.
63. Bentley-Lewis R, Graves SW, Seely EW. The renin-aldosterone response to stimulation and suppression during normal pregnancy. *Hypertens Pregnancy.* 2005;24(1):1–16.
64. Winkel CA, Milewich L, Parker CR Jr, et al. Conversion of plasma progesterone to deoxycorticosterone in men, nonpregnant and pregnant women, and adrenalectomized subjects. *J Clin Invest.* 1980;66(4):803–812.
65. Nolten WE, Lindheimer MD, Oparil S, et al. Desoxycorticosterone in normal pregnancy. I. Sequential studies of the secretory patterns of desoxycorticosterone, aldosterone, and cortisol. *Am J Obstet Gynecol.* 1978;132(4): 414–420.
66. Atherton JC, Bielinska A, Davison JM, et al. Sodium and water reabsorption in the proximal and distal nephron in conscious pregnant rats and third trimester women. *J Physiol.* 1988;396:457–470.
67. Lindheimer MD, Katz AI. Kidney function in the pregnant rat. *J Lab Clin Med.* 1971;78(4):633–641.
68. Mahaney J, Felton C, Taylor D, et al. Renal cortical Na1-K1-ATPase activity and abundance is decreased in normal pregnant rats. *Am J Physiol.* 1998; 275:F812–817.
69. Newman RL. Serum electrolytes in pregnancy, parturition, and puerperium. *Obstet Gynecol.* 1957;10(1):51–55.
70. Ehrlich EN, Lindheimer MD. Effect of administered mineralocorticoids or ACTH in pregnant women. Attenuation of kaliuretic influence of mineralocorticoids during pregnancy. *J Clin Invest.* 1972;51(6):1301–1309.
71. Lindheimer MD, Richardson DA, Ehrlich EN, et al. Potassium homeostasis in pregnancy. *J Reprod Med.* 1987;32(7):517–522.
72. Luqman A, Kazmi A, Wall BM. Bartter's syndrome in pregnancy: review of potassium homeostasis in gestation. *Am J Med Sci.* 2009;338(6):500–504.
73. Li IC, To WW. Bartter's syndrome in pregnancy: a case report and review. *J Obstet Gynaecol Res.* 2000;26(2):77–79.
74. Deruelle P, Dufour P, Magnenant E, et al. Maternal Bartter's syndrome in pregnancy treated by amiloride. *Eur J Obstet Gynecol Reprod Biol.* 2004; 115(1):106–107.
75. Larsson A, Palm M, Hansson LO, et al. Reference values for clinical chemistry tests during normal pregnancy. *BJOG.* 2008;115(7):874–881.
76. Jensen D, Webb KA, O'Donnell DE. Chemical and mechanical adaptations of the respiratory system at rest and during exercise in human pregnancy. *Appl Physiol Nutr Metab.* 2007;32(6):1239–1250.
77. Knuttgen HG, Emerson K Jr. Physiological response to pregnancy at rest and during exercise. *J Appl Physiol.* 1974;36(5):549–553.

78. Pernoll ML, Metcalfe J, Kovach PA, et al. Ventilation during rest and exercise in pregnancy and postpartum. *Respir Physiol.* 1975;25(3):295–310.
79. Machida H. Influence of progesterone on arterial blood and CSF acid-base balance in women. *J Appl Physiol.* 1981;51(6):1433–1436.
80. Jensen D, Duffin J, Lam YM, et al. Physiological mechanisms of hyperventilation during human pregnancy. *Respir Physiol Neurobiol.* 2008;161(1):76–86.
81. Lukaski HC, Siders WA, Nielsen EJ, et al. Total body water in pregnancy: assessment by using bioelectrical impedance. *Am J Clin Nutr.* 1994;59(3): 578–585.
82. Hytten F. Blood volume changes in normal pregnancy. *Clin Haematol.* 1985;14(3):601–612.
83. Halligan A, O'Brien E, O'Malley K, et al. Twenty-four-hour ambulatory blood pressure measurement in a primigravid population. *J Hypertens.* 1993; 11(8):869–873.
84. Jeyabalan A, Novak J, Danielson LA, et al. Essential role for vascular gelatinase activity in relaxin-induced renal vasodilation, hyperfiltration, and reduced myogenic reactivity of small arteries. *Circ Res.* 2003;93(12):1249–1257.
85. McGuane JT, Debrah JE, Sautina L, et al. Relaxin induces rapid dilation of rodent small renal and human subcutaneous arteries via PI3 kinase and nitric oxide. *Endocrinology.* 2011;152(7):2786–2796.
86. He H, Venema VJ, Gu X, et al. Vascular endothelial growth factor signals endothelial cell production of nitric oxide and prostacyclin through flk-1/KDR activation of c-Src. *J Biol Chem.* 1999;274(35):25130–25135.
87. Savvidou MD, Vallance PJ, Nicolaides KH, et al. Endothelial nitric oxide synthase gene polymorphism and maternal vascular adaptation to pregnancy. *Hypertension.* 2001;38(6):1289–1293.
88. Valtonen P, Laitinen T, Lyyra-Laitinen T, et al. Serum L-homoarginine concentration is elevated during normal pregnancy and is related to flow-mediated vasodilatation. *Circ J.* 2008;72(11):1879–1884.
89. Sealey JE, McCord D, Taufield PA, et al. Plasma prorenin in first-trimester pregnancy: relationship to changes in human chorionic gonadotropin. *Am J Obstet Gynecol.* 1985;153(5):514–519.
90. Merrill DC, Karoly M, Chen K, et al. Angiotensin-(1–7) in normal and preeclamptic pregnancy. *Endocrine.* 2002;18(3):239–245.
91. Weir RJ, Doig A, Fraser R, et al. Studies of the renin-angiotension-aldosterone system, cortisol, DOC, and ADH in normal and hypertensive pregnancy. *Perspect Nephrol Hypertens.* 1976;5:251–261.
92. Benjamin N, Rymer J, Todd SD, et al. Sensitivity to angiotensin II of forearm resistance vessels in pregnancy. *Br J Clin Pharmacol.* 1991;32(4):523–525.
93. Bowyer L, Brown MA, Jones M. Forearm blood flow in pre-eclampsia. *BJOG.* 2003;110(4):383–391.
94. Magness RR, Cox K, Rosenfeld CR, et al. Angiotensin II metabolic clearance rate and pressor responses in nonpregnant and pregnant women. *Am J Obstet Gynecol.* 1994;171(3):668–679.
95. Novak J, Reckelhoff J, Bumgarner L, et al. Reduced sensitivity of the renal circulation to angiotensin II in pregnant rats. *Hypertension.* 1997;30:580–584.
96. Valdes G, Germain AM, Corthorn J, et al. Urinary vasodilator and vasoconstrictor angiotensins during menstrual cycle, pregnancy, and lactation. *Endocrine.* 2001;16(2):117–122.
97. Brown MA, Crawford GA, Horgan EA, et al. Arginine vasopressin in primigravid human pregnancy. A prospective study. *J Reprod Med.* 1988;33(1):35–40.
98. Davison JM, Sheills EA, Barron WM, et al. Changes in the metabolic clearance of vasopressin and in plasma vasopressinase throughout human pregnancy. *J Clin Invest.* 1989;83(4):1313–1318.
99. Lindheimer MD, Roberts JM, Cunningham FG, et al. *Chesley's Hypertensive Disorders in Pregnancy.* Amsterdam ; Boston: Academic Press; 2009.
100. Davison JM, Shiells EA, Philips PR, et al. Influence of humoral and volume factors on altered osmoregulation of normal human pregnancy. *Am J Physiol.* 1990;258:F900–907.
101. Davison JM, Gilmore EA, Durr J, et al. Altered osmotic thresholds for vasopressin secretion and thirst in human pregnancy. *Am J Physiol.* 1984;246:F105–109.
102. Schrier RW, Durr JA. Pregnancy: an overfill or underfill state. *Am J Kidney Dis.* 1987;9(4):284–289.
103. Soule SG, Monson JP, Jacobs HS. Transient diabetes insipidus in pregnancy—a consequence of enhanced placental clearance of arginine vasopressin. *Hum Reprod.* 1995;10(12):3322–3324.
104. Ichaliotis SD, Lambrinopoulos TC. Serum oxytocinase in twin pregnancy. *Obstet Gynecol.* 1965;25:270–272.
105. Aleksandrov N, Audibert F, Bedard MJ, et al. Gestational diabetes insipidus: a review of an underdiagnosed condition. *J Obstet Gynaecol Can.* 2010;32(2): 225–231.
106. Yamanaka Y, Takeuchi K, Konda E, et al. Transient postpartum diabetes insipidus in twin pregnancy associated with HELLP syndrome. *J Perinat Med.* 2002;30(3):273–275.
107. Durr JA, Hoggard JG, Hunt JM, et al. Diabetes insipidus in pregnancy associated with abnormally high circulating vasopressinase activity. *N Engl J Med.* 1987;316(17):1070–1074.
108. Ferrara JM, Malatesta R, Kemmann E. Transient nephrogenic diabetes insipidus during toxemia in pregnancy. *Diagn Gynecol Obstet.* 1980;2(3):227–230.
109. Cammu H, Velkeniers B, Charels K, et al. Idiopathic acute fatty liver of pregnancy associated with transient diabetes insipidus. Case report. *Br J Obstet Gynaecol.* 1987;94(2):173–178.
110. Kallen BA, Carlsson SS, Bengtsson BK. Diabetes insipidus and use of desmopressin (Minirin) during pregnancy. *Eur J Endocrinol.* 1995;132(2):144–146.
111. Wang HY, Chang CT, Wu MS. Postpartum hemorrhage complicated with irreversible renal failure and central diabetes insipidus. *Ren Fail.* 2002;24(6): 849–852.
112. Weston G, Chaves N, Bowditch J. Sheehan's syndrome presenting post-partum with diabetes insipidus. *Aust N Z J Obstet Gynaecol.* 2005;45(3): 249–250.
113. Kan AK, Calligerous D. A case report of Sheehan syndrome presenting with diabetes insipidus. *Aust N Z J Obstet Gynaecol.* 1998;38(2):224–226.
114. Koetje PM, Spaan JJ, Kooman JP, et al. Pregnancy reduces the accuracy of the estimated glomerular filtration rate based on Cockroft-Gault and MDRD formulas. *Reprod Sci.* 2011;18(5):456–462.
115. Cote AM, Lam EM, von Dadelszen P, et al. Monitoring renal function in hypertensive pregnancy. *Hypertens Pregnancy.* 2010;29(3):318–329.
116. Smith MC, Moran P, Ward MK, et al. Assessment of glomerular filtration rate during pregnancy using the MDRD formula. *BJOG.* 2008;115(1):109–112.
117. Stevens LA, Schmid CH, Greene T, et al. Comparative performance of the CKD Epidemiology Collaboration (CKD-EPI) and the Modification of Diet in Renal Disease (MDRD) Study equations for estimating GFR levels above 60 mL/min/1.73 m^2. *Am J Kidney Dis.* 2010;56(3):486–495.
118. Hladunewich MA, Myers BD, Derby GC, et al. Course of preeclamptic glomerular injury after delivery. *Am J Physiol Renal Physiol.* 2008;294(3):F614–620.
119. Kristensen K, Larsson I, Hansson SR. Increased cystatin C expression in the pre-eclamptic placenta. *Mol Hum Reprod.* 2007;13(3):189–195.
120. Waugh JJ, Clark TJ, Divakaran TG, et al. Accuracy of urinalysis dipstick techniques in predicting significant proteinuria in pregnancy. *Obstet Gynecol.* 2004;103(4):769–777.
121. Haas DM, Sabi F, McNamara M, et al. Comparing ambulatory spot urine protein/creatinine ratios and 24–h urine protein measurements in normal pregnancies. *J Matern Fetal Neonatal Med.* 2003;14(4):233–236.
122. Kyle PM, Fielder JN, Pullar B, et al. Comparison of methods to identify significant proteinuria in pregnancy in the outpatient setting. *BJOG.* 2008;115(4): 523–527.
123. Leanos-Miranda A, Marquez-Acosta J, Romero-Arauz F, et al. Protein: creatinine ratio in random urine samples is a reliable marker of increased 24–hour protein excretion in hospitalized women with hypertensive disorders of pregnancy. *Clin Chem.* 2007;53(9):1623–1628.
124. Cote AM, Brown MA, Lam E, et al. Diagnostic accuracy of urinary spot protein:creatinine ratio for proteinuria in hypertensive pregnant women: systematic review. *BMJ.* 2008;336(7651):1003–1006.
125. Gonsales Valerio E, Lopes Ramos JG, Martins-Costa SH, et al. Variation in the urinary protein/creatinine ratio at four different periods of the day in hypertensive pregnant women. *Hypertens Pregnancy.* 2005;24(3):213–221.
126. Evans W, Lensmeyer JP, Kirby RS, et al. Two-hour urine collection for evaluating renal function correlates with 24–hour urine collection in pregnant patients. *J Matern Fetal Med.* 2000;9(4):233–237.
127. Cote AM, Firoz T, Mattman A, et al. The 24–hour urine collection: gold standard or historical practice? *Am J Obstet Gynecol.* 2008;199(6):625.e1–625.e 6.
128. Lindheimer MD, Kanter D. Interpreting abnormal proteinuria in pregnancy: the need for a more pathophysiological approach. *Obstet Gynecol.* 2010; 115:365–375.
129. Schewitz LJ, Friedman IA, Pollak VE. Bleeding after renal biopsy in pregnancy. *Obstet Gynecol.* 1965;26:295–304.
130. Packham D, Fairley KF. Renal biopsy: indications and complications in pregnancy. *Br J Obstet Gynaecol.* 1987;94(10):935–939.
131. Chen HH, Lin HC, Yeh JC, et al. Renal biopsy in pregnancies complicated by undetermined renal disease. *Acta Obstet Gynecol Scand.* 2001;80(10):888–893.
132. Lindheimer MD, Davison JM. Renal biopsy during pregnancy: 'to b . . . or not to b . . .?'. *Br J Obstet Gynaecol.* 1987;94(10):932–934.
133. Piccoli GB, Conijn A, Attini R, et al. Pregnancy in chronic kidney disease: need for a common language. *J Nephrol.* 2011;24(3):282–299.
134. Cunningham FG, Cox SM, Harstad TW, et al. Chronic renal disease and pregnancy outcome. *Am J Obstet Gynecol.* 1990;163(2):453–459.
135. Jungers P, Chauveau D, Choukroun G, et al. Pregnancy in women with impaired renal function. *Clin Nephrol.* 1997;47(5):281–288.

136. Jones DC, Hayslett JP. Outcome of pregnancy in women with moderate or severe renal insufficiency. *N Engl J Med*. 1996;335(4):226–232.
137. Abe S, Amagasaki Y, Konishi K, et al. The influence of antecedent renal disease on pregnancy. *Am J Obstet Gynecol*. 1985;153(5):508–514.
138. Packham DK, North RA, Fairley KF, et al. Primary glomerulonephritis and pregnancy. *Q J Med*. 1989;71(266):537–553.
139. Piccoli GB, Attini R, Vasario E, et al. Pregnancy and chronic kidney disease: a challenge in all CKD stages. *Clin J Am Soc Nephrol*. 2010;5(5):844–855.
140. Imbasciati E, Gregorini G, Cabiddu G, et al. Pregnancy in CKD stages 3 to 5: fetal and maternal outcomes. *Am J Kidney Dis*. 2007;49(6):753–762.
141. Alsuwaida A, Mousa D, Al-Harbi A, et al. Impact of early chronic kidney disease on maternal and fetal outcomes of pregnancy. *J Matern Fetal Neonatal Med*. 2011;24(12):1432–1436.
142. Munkhaugen J, Lydersen S, Romundstad PR, et al. Kidney function and future risk for adverse pregnancy outcomes: a population-based study from HUNT II, Norway. *Nephrol Dial Transplant*. 2009;24(12):3744–3750.
143. Anwar A, Salih A, Masson E, et al. The effect of pre-pregnancy counselling for women with pre-gestational diabetes on maternal health status. *Eur J Obstet Gynecol Reprod Biol*. 2011;155(2):137–139.
144. Ali S, Dornhorst A. Diabetes in pregnancy: health risks and management. *Postgrad Med J*. 2011;81(1028):417–427.
145. Ray JG, O'Brien TE, Chan WS. Preconception care and the risk of congenital anomalies in the offspring of women with diabetes mellitus: a meta-analysis. *QJM*. 2001;94(8):435–444.
146. Hiilesmaa V, Suhonen L, Teramo K. Glycaemic control is associated with pre-eclampsia but not with pregnancy-induced hypertension in women with type I diabetes mellitus. *Diabetologia*. 2000;43(12):1534–1539.
147. Bar J, Ben-Rafael Z, Padoa A, et al. Prediction of pregnancy outcome in subgroups of women with renal disease. *Clin Nephrol*. 2000;53(6):437–444.
148. Dunne F, Brydon P, Smith K, et al. Pregnancy in women with Type 2 diabetes: 12 years outcome data 1990–2002. *Diabet Med*. 2003;20(9):734–738.
149. Dunne FP, Chowdhury TA, Hartland A, et al. Pregnancy outcome in women with insulin-dependent diabetes mellitus complicated by nephropathy. *QJM*. 1999;92(8):451–454.
150. Ekbom P, Damm P, Feldt-Rasmussen B, et al. Pregnancy outcome in type 1 diabetic women with microalbuminuria. *Diabetes Care*. 2001;24(10):1739–1744.
151. Ekbom P, Damm P, Nogaard K, et al. Urinary albumin excretion and 24–hour blood pressure as predictors of pre-eclampsia in Type I diabetes. *Diabetologia*. 2000;43(7):927–931.
152. Howarth C, Gazis A, James D. Associations of Type 1 diabetes mellitus, maternal vascular disease and complications of pregnancy. *Diabet Med*. 2007; 24(11):1229–1234.
153. Combs CA, Rosenn B, Kitzmiller JL, et al. Early-pregnancy proteinuria in diabetes related to preeclampsia. *Obstet Gynecol*. 1993;82(5):802–807.
154. Schroder W, Heyl W, Hill-Grasshoff B, et al. Clinical value of detecting microalbuminuria as a risk factor for pregnancy-induced hypertension in insulin-treated diabetic pregnancies. *Eur J Obstet Gynecol Reprod Biol*. 2000;91(2):155–158.
155. Khoury JC, Miodovnik M, LeMasters G, et al. Pregnancy outcome and progression of diabetic nephropathy. What's next? *J Matern Fetal Neonatal Med*. 2002;11(4):238–244.
156. Yinon Y, Kingdom JC, Odutayo A, et al. Vascular dysfunction in women with a history of preeclampsia and intrauterine growth restriction: insights into future vascular risk. *Circulation*. 2010;122(18):1846–1853.
157. Reece EA, Coustan DR, Hayslett JP, et al. Diabetic nephropathy: pregnancy performance and fetomaternal outcome. *Am J Obstet Gynecol*. 1988;159(1): 56–66.
158. Kitzmiller JL, Brown ER, Phillippe M, et al. Diabetic nephropathy and perinatal outcome. *Am J Obstet Gynecol*. 1981;141(7):741–751.
159. Purdy LP, Hantsch CE, Molitch ME, et al. Effect of pregnancy on renal function in patients with moderate-to-severe diabetic renal insufficiency. *Diabetes Care*. 1996;19(10):1067–1074.
160. Irfan S, Arain TM, Shaukat A, et al. Effect of pregnancy on diabetic nephropathy and retinopathy. *J Coll Physicians Surg Pak*. 2004;14(2):75–78.
161. Mackie AD, Doddridge MC, Gamsu HR, et al. Outcome of pregnancy in patients with insulin-dependent diabetes mellitus and nephropathy with moderate renal impairment. *Diabet Med*. 1996;13(1):90–96.
162. Miodovnik M, Rosenn BM, Khoury JC, et al. Does pregnancy increase the risk for development and progression of diabetic nephropathy? *Am J Obstet Gynecol*. 1996;174(4):1180–1189; discussion 1189–1191.
163. Kaaja R, Sjoberg L, Hellsted T, et al. Long-term effects of pregnancy on diabetic complications. *Diabet Med*. 1996;13(2):165–169.
164. Biesenbach G, Grafinger P, Stoger H, et al. How pregnancy influences renal function in nephropathic type 1 diabetic women depends on their pre-conceptional creatinine clearance. *J Nephrol*. 1999;12(1):41–46.
165. Bagg W, Neale L, Henley P, et al. Long-term maternal outcome after pregnancy in women with diabetic nephropathy. *N Z Med J*. 2003;116(1180):U566.
166. Sandvik MK, Iversen BM, Irgens LM, et al. Are adverse pregnancy outcomes risk factors for development of end-stage renal disease in women with diabetes? *Nephrol Dial Transplant*. 2010;25(11):3600–3607.
167. Rossing K, Jacobsen P, Hommel E, et al. Pregnancy and progression of diabetic nephropathy. *Diabetologia*. 2002;45(1):36–41.
168. Carr DB, Koontz GL, Gardella C, et al. Diabetic nephropathy in pregnancy: suboptimal hypertensive control associated with preterm delivery. *Am J Hypertens*. 2006;19(5):513–519.
169. Nielsen LR, Damm P, Mathiesen ER. Improved pregnancy outcome in type 1 diabetic women with microalbuminuria or diabetic nephropathy: effect of intensified antihypertensive therapy? *Diabetes Care*. 2009;32(1):38–44.
170. Hod M, van Dijk DJ, Karp M, et al. Diabetic nephropathy and pregnancy: the effect of ACE inhibitors prior to pregnancy on fetomaternal outcome. *Nephrol Dial Transplant*. 1995;10(12):2328–2333.
171. Bar J, Chen R, Schoenfeld A, et al. Pregnancy outcome in patients with insulin dependent diabetes mellitus and diabetic nephropathy treated with ACE inhibitors before pregnancy. *J Pediatr Endocrinol Metab*. 1999;12(5):659–665.
172. Andersen S, Brochner-Mortensen J, Parving HH. Kidney function during and after withdrawal of long-term irbesartan treatment in patients with type 2 diabetes and microalbuminuria. *Diabetes Care*. 2003;26(12):3296–3302.
173. How HY, Sibai BM. Use of angiotensin-converting enzyme inhibitors in patients with diabetic nephropathy. *J Matern Fetal Neonatal Med*. 2002;12(6):402–407.
174. Miura K, Sekine T, Iida A, et al. Salt-losing nephrogenic diabetes insipidus caused by fetal exposure to angiotensin receptor blocker. *Pediatr Nephrol*. 2009;24(6):1235–1238.
175. Cooper WO, Hernandez-Diaz S, Arbogast PG, et al. Major congenital malformations after first-trimester exposure to ACE inhibitors. *N Engl J Med*. 2006;354(23):2443–2451.
176. Boix E, Zapater P, Pico A, et al. Teratogenicity with angiotensin II receptor antagonists in pregnancy. *J Endocrinol Invest*. 2005;28(11):1029–1031.
177. Schaefer C. Angiotensin II-receptor-antagonists: further evidence of fetotoxicity but not teratogenicity. *Birth Defects Res A Clin Mol Teratol*. 2003;67(8):591–594.
178. Enzensberger C, Eskef K, Schwarze A, et al. Course and outcome of pregnancy after maternal exposure to angiotensin-II-receptor blockers - case report and review of the literature. *Ultraschall Med*. 2011 May 31 [Epub ahead of print].
179. Diav-Citrin O, Shechtman S, Halberstadt Y, et al. Pregnancy outcome after in utero exposure to angiotensin converting enzyme inhibitors or angiotensin receptor blockers. *Reprod Toxicol*. 2011;31(4):540–545.
180. Beardmore KS, Morris JM, Gallery ED. Excretion of antihypertensive medication into human breast milk: a systematic review. *Hypertens Pregnancy*. 2002; 21(1):85–95.
181. Begg EJ, Robson RA, Gardiner SJ, et al. Quinapril and its metabolite quinaprilat in human milk. *Br J Clin Pharmacol*. 2001;51(5):478–481.
182. Kincaid-Smith PS, Whitworth JA, Fairley KF. Mesangial IgA nephropathy in pregnancy. *Clin Exp Hypertens*. 1980;2(5):821–838.
183. Surian M, Imbasciati E, Cosci P, et al. Glomerular disease and pregnancy. A study of 123 pregnancies in patients with primary and secondary glomerular diseases. *Nephron*. 1984;36(2):101–105.
184. Nagai Y, Waschizawa Y, Suzuki T, et al. Influence of gestation on renal function in gravida with IgA nephropathy. *Nippon Jinzo Gakkai Shi*. 1989;31(6):635–641.
185. Abe S. An overview of pregnancy in women with underlying renal disease. *Am J Kid Dis*. 1991;17(2):112–115.
186. Abe S. The influence of pregnancy on the long-term renal prognosis of IgA nephropathy. *Clin Nephrol*. 1994;41(2):61–64.
187. Limardo M, Imbasciati E, Ravani P, et al. Pregnancy and progression of IgA nephropathy: results of an Italian multicenter study. *Am J Kidney Dis*. 2010; 56(3):506–512.
188. Packham D, Whitworth JA, Fairley KF, et al. Histological features of IgA glomerulonephritis as predictors of pregnancy outcome. *Clin Nephrol*. 1988;30(1):22–26.
189. Koido S, Makino H, Iwazaki K, et al. IgA nephropathy and pregnancy. *Tokai J Exp Clin Med*. 1998;23(1):31–37.
190. Packham DK, North RA, Fairley KF, et al. IgA glomerulonephritis and pregnancy. *Clin Nephrol*. 1988;30(1):15–21.
191. Stehman-Breen C, Miller L, Fink J, et al. Pre-eclampsia and premature labour among pregnant wowen with haematuria. *Paediatr Perinat Epidemiol*. 2000;14(2):136–140.
192. Stehman-Breen CO, Levine RJ, Qian C, et al. Increased risk of preeclampsia among nulliparous pregnant women with idiopathic hematuria. *Am J Obstet Gynecol*. 2002;187(3):703–708.
193. Brown MA, Holt JL, Mangos GJ, et al. Microscopic hematuria in pregnancy: relevance to pregnancy outcome. *Am J Kidney Dis*. 2005;45(4):667–673.

194. Packham D. Thin basement membrane nephropathy in pregnancy. *Semin Nephrol.* 2005;25(3):180–183.

195. Abe S. Pregnancy in IgA nephropathy. *Kidney Int.* 1991;40(6):1098–1102.

196. Jungers P, Forget D, Houillier P, et al. Pregnancy in IgA nephropathy, reflux nephropathy, and focal glomerular sclerosis. *Am J Kidney Dis.* 1987;9(4): 334–338.

197. ACOG educational bulletin. Antimicrobial therapy for obstetric patients. Number 245, March 1998 (replaces no. 117, June 1988). American College of Obstetricians and Gynecologists. *Int J Gynaecol Obstet.* 1998;61(3):299–308.

198. Lumbiganon P, Villar J, Laopaiboon M, et al. One-day compared with 7–day nitrofurantoin for asymptomatic bacteriuria in pregnancy: a randomized controlled trial. *Obstet Gynecol.* 2009;113:339–345.

199. Vazquez JC, Abalos E. Treatments for symptomatic urinary tract infections during pregnancy. *Cochrane Database Syst Rev.* 2011;(1):CD002256.

200. Hill JB, Sheffield JS, McIntire DD, et al. Acute pyelonephritis in pregnancy. *Obstet Gynecol.* 2005;105(1):18–23.

201. Whalley PJ, Cunningham FG, Martin FG. Transient renal dysfunction associated with acute pyelonephritis of pregnancy. *Obstet Gynecol.* 1975;46(2):174–177.

202. Smaill F, Vazquez JC. Antibiotics for asymptomatic bacteriuria in pregnancy. *Cochrane Database Syst Rev.* 2007;(2):CD000490.

203. Villar J, Lydon-Rochelle MT, Gulmezoglu AM, et al. Duration of treatment for asymptomatic bacteriuria during pregnancy. *Cochrane Database Syst Rev.* 2000;(2):CD000491.

204. Millar LK, Wing DA, Paul RH, et al. Outpatient treatment of pyelonephritis in pregnancy: a randomized controlled trial. *Obstet Gynecol.* 1995;86:560–564.

205. el-Khatib M, Packham DK, Becker GJ, et al. Pregnancy-related complications in women with reflux nephropathy. *Clin Nephrol.* 1994;86:50–55.

206. Kincaid-Smith P, Fairley KF. Renal disease in pregnancy. Three controversial areas: mesangial IgA nephropathy, focal glomerular sclerosis (focal and segmental hyalinosis and sclerosis), and reflux nephropathy. *Am J Kidney Dis.* 1987;86:328–333.

207. Zucchelli P, Gaggi R. Reflux nephropathy in adults. *Nephron.* 1991;57(1):2–9.

208. Jungers P. Reflux nephropathy and pregnancy. *Baillieres Clin Obstet Gynaecol.* 1994;8(2):425–442.

209. Jungers P, Houillier P, Chauveau D, et al. Pregnancy in women with reflux nephropathy. *Kidney Int.* 1996;50(2):593–599.

210. Hollowell JG. Outcome of pregnancy in women with a history of vesico-ureteric reflux. *BJU Int.* 2008;102(7):780–784.

211. North RA, Taylor RS, Gunn TR. Pregnancy outcome in women with reflux nephropathy and the inheritance of vesico-ureteric reflux. *Aust N Z J Obstet Gynaecol.* 2000;40(3):280–285.

212. Boumpas DT, Austin HA, Vaughan EM, et al. Risk for sustained amenorrhea in patients with systemic lupus erythematosus receiving intermittent pulse cyclophosphamide therapy. *Ann Intern Med.* 1993;119(5):366–369.

213. Somers EC, Marder W, Christman GM, et al. Use of a gonadotropin-releasing hormone analog for protection against premature ovarian failure during cyclophosphamide therapy in women with severe lupus. *Arthritis Rheum.* 2005;52(9):2761–2767.

214. Petri M, Howard D, Repke J. Frequency of lupus flare in pregnancy. The Hopkins Lupus Pregnancy Center experience. *Arthritis Rheum.* 1991;34(12): 1538–1545.

215. Smyth A, Oliveira GH, Lahr BD, et al. A systematic review and meta-analysis of pregnancy outcomes in patients with systemic lupus erythematosus and lupus nephritis. *Clin J Am Soc Nephrol.* 2010;5(11):2060–2068.

216. Gladman DD, Tandon A, Ibanez D, et al. The effect of lupus nephritis on pregnancy outcome and fetal and maternal complications. *J Rheumatol.* 2010; 37(4):754–758.

217. Bobrie G, Liote F, Houillier P, et al. Pregnancy in lupus nephritis and related disorders. *Am J Kidney Dis.* 1987;9(4):339–343.

218. Clowse ME, Magder LS, Petri M. The clinical utility of measuring complement and anti-dsDNA antibodies during pregnancy in patients with systemic lupus erythematosus. *J Rheumatol.* 2011;38(6):1012–1016.

219. Abarientos C, Sperber K, Shapiro DL, et al. Hydroxychloroquine in systemic lupus erythematosus and rheumatoid arthritis and its safety in pregnancy. *Expert Opin Drug Saf.* 2011;10(5):705–714.

220. Simchen MJ, Dulitzki M, Rofe G, et al. High positive antibody titers and adverse pregnancy outcome in women with antiphospholipid syndrome. *Acta Obstet Gynecol Scand.* 2011;90(12):1428–1433.

221. Jaeggi E, Laskin C, Hamilton R, et al. The importance of the level of maternal anti-Ro/SSA antibodies as a prognostic marker of the development of cardiac neonatal lupus erythematosus: a prospective study of 186 antibody-exposed fetuses and infants. *J Am Coll Cardiol.* 2010;55(24):2778–2784.

222. Koukoura O, Mantas N, Linardakis H, et al. Successful term pregnancy in a patient with Wegener's granulomatosis: case report and literature review. *Fertil Steril.* 2008;89(2):457.e1–457.e5.

223. Auzary C, Huong DT, Wechsler B, et al. Pregnancy in patients with Wegener's granulomatosis: report of five cases in three women. *Ann Rheum Dis.* 2000;59(10):800–804.

224. Milford CA, Bellini M. Wegener's granulomatosis arising in pregnancy. *J Laryngol Otol.* 1986;100(4):475–476.

225. Harber MA, Tso A, Taheri S, et al. Wegener's granulomatosis in pregnancy—the therapeutic dilemma. *Nephrol Dial Transplant.* 1999;14(7):1789–1791.

226. Bellisai F, Morozzi G, Marcolongo R, et al. Pregnancy in Wegener's granulomatosis: successful treatment with intravenous immunoglobulin. *Clin Rheumatol.* 2004;23(6):533–535.

227. Kim SY, Linton JM, Kolasinski SL. Successful treatment of new onset Wegener's granulomatosis with IVIG (intravenous immunoglobulin) during pregnancy: a case report. *Mod Rheumatol.* 2008;18(2):177–180.

228. Dayoan ES, Dimen LL, Boylen CT. Successful treatment of Wegener's granulomatosis during pregnancy: a case report and review of the medical literature. *Chest.* 1998;113(3):836–838.

229. Enns GM, Roeder E, Chan RT, et al. Apparent cyclophosphamide (cytoxan) embryopathy: a distinct phenotype? *Am J Med Genet.* 1999;86(3):237–241.

230. Azim HA Jr, Azim H, Peccatori FA. Treatment of cancer during pregnancy with monoclonal antibodies: a real challenge. *Expert Rev Clin Immunol.* 2010;6(6):821–826.

231. Bansal PJ, Tobin MC. Neonatal microscopic polyangiitis secondary to transfer of maternal myeloperoxidase-antineutrophil cytoplasmic antibody resulting in neonatal pulmonary hemorrhage and renal involvement. *Ann Allergy Asthma Immunol.* 2004;93(4):398–401.

232. Hatfield T, Steiger R, Wing DA. Goodpasture's disease in pregnancy: case report and review of the literature. *Am J Perinatol.* 2007;24(10):619–621.

233. Al-Harbi A, Malik GH, Al-Mohaya SA, et al. Anti-glomerular basement membrane antibody disease presenting as acute renal failure during pregnancy. *Saudi J Kidney Dis Transpl.* 2003;14(4):516–521.

234. Vasiliou DM, Maxwell C, Shah P, et al. Goodpasture syndrome in a pregnant woman. *Obstet Gynecol.* 2005;106:1196–1199.

235. Deubner H, Wagnild JP, Wener MH, et al. Glomerulonephritis with anti-glomerular basement membrane antibody during pregnancy: potential role of the placenta in amelioration of disease. *Am J Kidney Dis.* 1995;25(2): 330–335.

236. Yankowitz J, Kuller JA, Thomas RL. Pregnancy complicated by Goodpasture syndrome. *Obstet Gynecol.* 1992;79:806–808.

237. Chakravarty EF, Khanna D, Chung L. Pregnancy outcomes in systemic sclerosis, primary pulmonary hypertension, and sickle cell disease. *Obstet Gynecol.* 2008;111(4):927–934.

238. Mok CC, Kwan TH, Chow L. Scleroderma renal crisis sine scleroderma during pregnancy. *Scand J Rheumatol.* 2003;32(1):55–57.

239. Younker D, Harrison B. Scleroderma and pregnancy. Anaesthetic considerations. *Br J Anaesth.* 1985;57(11):1136–1139.

240. Altieri P, Cameron JS. Scleroderma renal crisis in a pregnant woman with late partial recovery of renal function. *Nephrol Dial Transplant.* 1988;3(5): 677–680.

241. Barcelo P, Lopez-Lillo J, Cabero L, et al. Successful pregnancy in primary glomerular disease. *Kidney Int.* 1986;30(6):914–919.

242. Malik GH, Al-Harbi AS, Al-Mohaya S, et al. Repeated pregnancies in patients with primary membranous glomerulonephritis. *Nephron.* 2002;91(1): 21–24.

243. Matsubara S, Ueda Y, Takahashi H, et al. Pregnancy complicated with Alport syndrome: a good obstetric outcome and failure to diagnose an infant born to a mother with Alport syndrome by umbilical cord immunofluorescence staining. *J Obstet Gynaecol Res.* 2009;35(6):1109–1114.

244. Packham DK, North RA, Fairley KF, et al. Pregnancy in women with primary focal and segmental hyalinosis and sclerosis. *Clin Nephrol.* 1988;29(4): 185–192.

245. Chapman AB, Johnson AM, Gabow PA. Pregnancy outcome and its relationship to progression of renal failure in autosomal dominant polycystic kidney disease. *J Am Soc Nephrol.* 1994;5(5):1178–1185.

246. Torra Balcells R, Ars Criach E. Molecular diagnosis of autosomal dominant polycystic kidney disease. *Nefrologia.* 2011;31(1):35–43.

247. Gabow PA, Johnson AM, Kaehny WD, et al. Risk factors for the development of hepatic cysts in autosomal dominant polycystic kidney disease. *Hepatology.* 1990;11(6):1033–1037.

248. Holley JL, Schmidt RJ, Bender FH, et al. Gynecologic and reproductive issues in women on dialysis. *Am J Kidney Dis.* 1997;29(5):685–690.

249. Mantouvalos H, Metallinos C, Makrygiannakis A, et al. Sex hormones in women on hemodialysis. *Int J Gynaecol Obstet.* 1984;22(5):367–370.

250. Lim VS, Henriquez C, Sievertsen G, et al. Ovarian function in chronic renal failure: evidence suggesting hypothalamic anovulation. *Ann Intern Med.* 1980; 93(1):21–27.

251. Gomez F, de la Cueva R, Wauters JP, et al. Endocrine abnormalities in patients undergoing long-term hemodialysis. The role of prolactin. *Am J Med.* 1980;68(4):522–530.
252. Hou SH, Grossman S, Molitch ME. Hyperprolactinemia in patients with renal insufficiency and chronic renal failure requiring hemodialysis or chronic ambulatory peritoneal dialysis. *Am J Kidney Dis.* 1985;68(4):245–249.
253. Bailie GR, Elder SJ, Mason NA, et al. Sexual dysfunction in dialysis patients treated with antihypertensive or antidepressive medications: results from the DOPPS. *Nephrol Dial Transplant.* 2007;22(4):1163–1170.
254. Steele TE, Wuerth D, Finkelstein S, et al. Sexual experience of the chronic peritoneal dialysis patient. *J Am Soc Nephrol.* 1996;7(8):1165–1168.
255. Okundaye I, Abrinko P, Hou S. Registry of pregnancy in dialysis patients. *Am J Kidney Dis.* 1998;31(5):766–773.
256. Hou SH. Frequency and outcome of pregnancy in women on dialysis. *Am J Kidney Dis.* 1994;32(1):60–63.
257. Malik GH, Al-Harbi A, Al-Mohaya S, et al. Pregnancy in patients on dialysis—experience at a referral center. *J Assoc Physicians India.* 2005;53:937–941.
258. Bahloul H, Kammoun K, Kharrat M, et al. Pregnancy in chronic hemodialysis women: outcome of multicentric study. *Saudi J Kidney Dis Transpl.* 2003;14(4):530–531.
259. Barua M, Hladunewich M, Keunen J, et al. Successful pregnancies on nocturnal home hemodialysis. *Clin J Am Soc Nephrol.* 2008;3(2):392–396.
260. Hou S. Conception and pregnancy in peritoneal dialysis patients. *Perit Dial Int.* 2001;21 Suppl 3:S290–294.
261. Confortini P, Galanti G, Ancona G, et al. Full term pregnancy and successful delivery in a patient on chronic hemodialysis. *Proc Eur Dial Transplant Assoc.* 1971:74–80.
262. Successful pregnancies in women treated by dialysis and kidney transplantation. Report from the Registration Committee of the European Dialysis and Transplant Association. *Br J Obstet Gynaecol.* 1980;87(10):839–845.
263. Souqiyyeh M, Huraib O, Abdul Ghayoum M, et al. Pregnancy in chronic hemodialysis patients in the kingdom of Saudi Arabia. *Am J Kidney Dis.* 1992;19(3):235–238.
264. Bagon JA, Vernaeve H, De Muylder X, et al. Pregnancy and dialysis. *Am J Kidney Dis.* 1998;31(5):756–765.
265. Haase M, Morgera S, Bamberg C, et al. A systematic approach to managing pregnant dialysis patients—the importance of an intensified haemodiafiltration protocol. *Nephrol Dial Transplant.* 2005;20(11):2537–2542.
266. Mackay EV. Pregnancy and renal disease: a ten-year survey. *Aust NZ J Obstet Gynaecol.* 1963;3:21–34.
267. Asamiya Y, Otsubo S, Matsuda Y, et al. The importance of low blood urea nitrogen levels in pregnant patients undergoing hemodialysis to optimize birth weight and gestational age. *Kidney Int.* 2009;75(11):1217–1222.
268. Luders C, Castro MC, Titan SM, et al. Obstetric outcome in pregnant women on long-term dialysis: a case series. *Am J Kidney Dis.* 2010;56(1):77–85.
269. Kioko EM, Shaw KM, Clarke AD, et al. Successful pregnancy in a diabetic patient treated with continuous ambulatory peritoneal dialysis. *Diabetes Care.* 1983;6(3):298–300.
270. Cattran DC, Benzie RJ. Pregnancy in a continuous ambulatory peritoneal dialysis patient. *Perit Dial Int.* 1983;3(1):13–14.
271. Redrow M, Cherem L, Elliott J, et al. Dialysis in the management of pregnant patients with renal insufficiency. *Medicine (Baltimore).* 1988;67(4):199–208.
272. Bennett-Jones DN, Aber GM, Baker K. Successful pregnancy in a patient treated with continuous ambulatory peritoneal dialysis. *Nephrol Dial Transplant.* 1989;4(6):583–585.
273. Melendez R, Franquero C, Gill P, et al. Successful pregnancy with CAPD. *ANNA J.* 1988;15(5):280–281, 312.
274. Lew SQ, Watson JA. Urea and creatinine generation and removal in a pregnant patient receiving peritoneal dialysis. *Adv Perit Dial.* 1992;8:131–135.
275. Elliott JP, O'Keeffe DF, Schon DA, et al. Dialysis in pregnancy: a critical review. *Obstet Gynecol Surv.* 1991;46(6):319–324.
276. Dunbeck D, Klopstein K, Heroux J, et al. Peritoneal dialysis patient completes successful pregnancy. *ANNA J.* 1992;19(3):269, 272.
277. McLigeyo SO, Swao JO, Wairagu SG, et al. Pregnancy in a patient on continuous ambulatory peritoneal dialysis (CAPD): a case report. *East Afr Med J.* 1992;69(5):294–295.
278. Gadallah MF, Ahmad B, Karubian F, et al. Pregnancy in patients on chronic ambulatory peritoneal dialysis. *Am J Kidney Dis.* 1992;20(4):407–410.
279. Irish AB, Garland TJ, Hayes JM, et al. Supplementing renal function with CAPD in a patient with chronic renal failure and pregnancy. *Perit Dial Int.* 1993;13(2):155–156.
280. Jakobi P, Ohel G, Szylman P, et al. Continuous ambulatory peritoneal dialysis as the primary approach in the management of severe renal insufficiency in pregnancy. *Obstet Gynecol.* 1992;79:808–810.
281. Jefferys A, Wyburn K, Chow J, et al. Peritoneal dialysis in pregnancy: a case series. *Nephrology (Carlton).* 2008;13(5):380–383.
282. Smith WT, Darbari S, Kwan M, et al. Pregnancy in peritoneal dialysis: a case report and review of adequacy and outcomes. *Int Urol Nephrol.* 2005;37(1):145–151.
283. Gomez Vazquez JA, MartinezCalva IE, Mendiola Fernandez R, et al. Pregnancy in end-stage renal disease patients and treatment with peritoneal dialysis: report of two cases. *Perit Dial Int.* 2007;27(3):353–358.
284. Okundaye I, Hou S. Management of pregnancy in women undergoing continuous ambulatory peritoneal dialysis. *Adv Perit Dial.* 1996;12:151–155.
285. Chou CY, Ting IW, Lin TH, et al. Pregnancy in patients on chronic dialysis: a single center experience and combined analysis of reported results. *Eur J Obstet Gynecol Reprod Biol.* 2008;136(2):165–170.
286. Romao JE Jr, Luders C, Kahhale S, et al. Pregnancy in women on chronic dialysis. A single-center experience with 17 cases. *Nephron.* 1998;78(4):416–422.
287. Schneider K, Ferenczi S, Vas S, et al. Pregnancy and successful full-term delivery in a patient on peritoneal dialysis: one center's experience and review of the literature. *Dialysis & Transplantation.* 2007;36(8):438–444.
288. Chou CY, Ting IW, Hsieh FJ, et al. Haemoperitoneum in a pregnant woman with peritoneal dialysis. *Nephrol Dial Transplant.* 2006;21(5):1454–1455.
289. Lew SQ. Persistent hemoperitoneum in a pregnant patient receiving peritoneal dialysis. *Perit Dial Int.* 2006;26(1):108–110.
290. Tison A, Lozowy C, Benjamin A, et al. Successful pregnancy complicated by peritonitis in a 35-year old CAPD patient. *Perit Dial Int.* 1996;16 Suppl 1:S489–491.
291. Murray J, Reid D, Harrison J, et al. Successful pregnancies after human renal transplantation. *N Engl J Med.* 1963;269:341–343.
292. Absy M, Metreweli C, Matthews C, et al. Changes in transplanted kidney volume measured by ultrasound. *Br J Radiol.* 1987;60(714):525–529.
293. Davison JM. The effect of pregnancy on kidney function in renal allograft recipients. *Kidney Int.* 1985;27(1):74–79.
294. Sgro MD, Barozzino T, Mirghani HM, et al. Pregnancy outcome post renal transplantation. *Teratology.* 2002;65(1):5–9.
295. Pour-Reza-Gholi F, Nafar M, Farrokhi F, et al. Pregnancy in kidney transplant recipients. *Transplant Proc.* 2005;37(7):3090–3092.
296. Salmela KT, Kyllonen LE, Holmberg C, et al. Impaired renal function after pregnancy in renal transplant recipients. *Transplantation.* 1993;56(6):1372–1375.
297. Tan PK, Tan A, Koon TH, et al. Effect of pregnancy on renal graft function and maternal survival in renal transplant recipients. *Transplant Proc.* 2002;34(4):1161–1163.
298. Yildirim Y, Uslu A. Pregnancy in patients with previous successful renal transplantation. *Int J Gynaecol Obstet.* 2005;90(3):198–202.
299. Galdo T, Gonzalez F, Espinoza M, et al. Impact of pregnancy on the function of transplanted kidneys. *Transplant Proc.* 2005;37(3):1577–1579.
300. Oliveira LG, Sass N, Sato JL, et al. Pregnancy after renal transplantation—a five-yr single-center experience. *Clin Transplant.* 2007;21(3):301–304.
301. Gutierrez MJ, Acebedo-Ribo M, Garcia-Donaire JA, et al. Pregnancy in renal transplant recipients. *Transplant Proc.* 2005;37(9):3721–3722.
302. Coscia LA, Constantinescu S, Moritz MJ, et al. Report from the National Transplantation Pregnancy Registry (NTPR): outcomes of pregnancy after transplantation. *Clin Transpl.* 2009;37(9):103–122.
303. Sibanda N, Briggs JD, Davison JM, et al. Pregnancy after organ transplantation: a report from the UK Transplant pregnancy registry. *Transplantation.* 2007;83(10):1301–1307.
304. Levidiotis V, Chang S, McDonald S. Pregnancy and maternal outcomes among kidney transplant recipients. *J Am Soc Nephrol.* 2009;20(11):2433–2440.
305. Gill JS, Zalunardo N, Rose C, et al. The pregnancy rate and live birth rate in kidney transplant recipients. *Am J Transplant.* 2009;9(7):1541–1549.
306. Kim HW, Seok HJ, Kim TH, et al. The experience of pregnancy after renal transplantation: pregnancies even within postoperative 1 year may be tolerable. *Transplantation.* 2008;85(10):1412–1419.
307. Rubin P, Ramsay M, eds. *Prescribing in Pregnancy*, 4th ed. London: Blackwell Publishing; 2008.
308. Anderka MT, Lin AE, Abuelo DN, et al. Reviewing the evidence for mycophenolate mofetil as a new teratogen: case report and review of the literature. *Am J Med Genet A.* 2009;149A(6):1241–1248.
309. Nyberg G, Haljamae U, Frisenette-Fich C, et al. Breast-feeding during treatment with cyclosporine. *Transplantation.* 1998;65(2):253–255.
310. Gardiner SJ, Begg EJ. Breastfeeding during tacrolimus therapy. *Obstet Gynecol.* 2006;107:453–455.
311. Moretti ME, Sgro M, Johnson DW, et al. Cyclosporine excretion into breast milk. *Transplantation* 2003;75(12):2144–2146.
312. Yinon Y, Farine D, Yudin MH. Screening, diagnosis, and management of cytomegalovirus infection in pregnancy. *Obstet Gynecol Surv.* 2010;65(11):736–743.

313. McCarthy FP, Giles ML, Rowlands S, et al. Antenatal interventions for preventing the transmission of cytomegalovirus (CMV) from the mother to fetus during pregnancy and adverse outcomes in the congenitally infected infant. *Cochrane Database Syst Rev.* 2011:CD008371.

314. Puliyanda DP, Silverman NS, Lehman D, et al. Successful use of oral ganciclovir for the treatment of intrauterine cytomegalovirus infection in a renal allograft recipient. *Transpl Infect Dis.* 2005;7(2):71–74.

315. Reisaeter AV, Roislien J, Henriksen T, et al. Pregnancy and birth after kidney donation: the Norwegian experience. *Am J Transplant.* 2009;9(4):820–824.

316. Ibrahim HN, Akkina SK, Leister E, et al. Pregnancy outcomes after kidney donation. *Am J Transplant.* 2009;9(4):825–834.

317. Silva GB Jr, Monteiro FA, Mota RM, et al. Acute kidney injury requiring dialysis in obstetric patients: a series of 55 cases in Brazil. *Arch Gynecol Obstet.* 2009;279(2):131–137.

318. Duley L. The global impact of pre-eclampsia and eclampsia. *Semin Perinatol.* 2009;33(3):130–137.

319. Lafayette RA, Druzin M, Sibley R, et al. Nature of glomerular dysfunction in pre-eclampsia. *Kidney Int.* 1998;54(4):1240–1249.

320. Strevens H, Wide-Swensson D, Grubb A, et al. Serum cystatin C reflects glomerular endotheliosis in normal, hypertensive and pre-eclamptic pregnancies. *BJOG.* 2003;110(9):825–830.

321. Moran P, Baylis PH, Lindheimer MD, et al. Glomerular ultrafiltration in normal and preeclamptic pregnancy. *J Am Soc Nephrol.* 2003;14(3):648–652.

322. Jeyabalan A, Conrad KP. Renal function during normal pregnancy and preeclampsia. *Front Biosci.* 2007;12:2425–2437.

323. Maynard SE, Min JY, Merchan J, et al. Excess placental soluble fms-like tyrosine kinase 1 (sFlt1) may contribute to endothelial dysfunction, hypertension, and proteinuria in preeclampsia. *J Clin Invest.* 2003;111(5):649–658.

324. Foster RR, Saleem MA, Mathieson PW, et al. Vascular endothelial growth factor and nephrin interact and reduce apoptosis in human podocytes. *Am J Physiol Renal Physiol.* 2005;288(1):F48–57.

325. Foster RR, Hole R, Anderson K, et al. Functional evidence that vascular endothelial growth factor may act as an autocrine factor on human podocytes. *Am J Physiol Renal Physiol.* 2003;284(6):F1263–1273.

326. Eremina V, Sood M, Haigh J, et al. Glomerular-specific alterations of VEGF-A expression lead to distinct congenital and acquired renal diseases. *J Clin Invest.* 2003;111(5):707–716.

327. Li Z, Zhang Y, Ying Ma J, et al. Recombinant vascular endothelial growth factor 121 attenuates hypertension and improves kidney damage in a rat model of preeclampsia. *Hypertension.* 2007;22(4):686–692.

328. Garovic VD, Wagner SJ, Petrovic LM, et al. Glomerular expression of nephrin and synaptopodin, but not podocin, is decreased in kidney sections from women with preeclampsia. *Nephrol Dial Transplant.* 2007;22(4):1136–1143.

329. Garovic VD, Wagner SJ, Turner ST, et al. Urinary podocyte excretion as a marker for preeclampsia. *Am J Obstet Gynecol.* 2007;196(4):320 e–e7.

330. Hirashima C, Ohkuchi A, Takahashi K, et al. Gestational hypertension as a subclinical preeclampsia in view of serum levels of angiogenesis-related factors. *Hypertens Res.* 2011;34(2):212–217.

331. Venkatesha S, Toporsian M, Lam C, et al. Soluble endoglin contributes to the pathogenesis of preeclampsia. *Nat Med.* 2006;12(6):642–649.

332. Brown CE, Gant NF, Cox K, et al. Low-dose aspirin. II. Relationship of angiotensin II pressor responses, circulating eicosanoids, and pregnancy outcome. *Am J Obstet Gynecol.* 1990;163:1853–1861.

333. Sanchez-Ramos L, Briones DK, Kaunitz AM, et al. Prevention of pregnancy-induced hypertension by calcium supplementation in angiotensin II-sensitive patients. *Obstet Gynecol.* 1994;84(3):349–353.

334. Valdes G, Germain AM, Corthorn J, et al. Urinary vasodilator and vasoconstrictor angiotensins during menstrual cycle, pregnancy, and lactation. *Endocrine.* 2001;16(2):117–122.

335. Herse F, Dechend R, Harsem NK, et al. Dysregulation of the circulating and tissue-based renin-angiotensin system in preeclampsia. *Hypertension.* 2007; 49(3):604–611.

336. Wallukat G, Homuth V, Fischer T, et al. Patients with preeclampsia develop agonistic autoantibodies against the angiotensin AT1 receptor. *J Clin Invest.* 1999;103(7):945–952.

337. Wallukat G, Neichel D, Nissen E, et al. Agonistic autoantibodies directed against the angiotensin II AT1 receptor in patients with preeclampsia. *Can J Physiol Pharmacol.* 2003;81(2):79–83.

338. AbdAlla S, Lother H, el Massiery A, et al. Increased AT(1) receptor heterodimers in preeclampsia mediate enhanced angiotensin II responsiveness. *Nat Med.* 2001;7(9):1003–1009.

339. Herse F, Verlohren S, Wenzel K, et al. Prevalence of agonistic autoantibodies against the angiotensin II type 1 receptor and soluble fms-Like tyrosine kinase 1 in a gestational age-matched case study. *Hypertension.* 2009;53(2):393–398.

340. Levine RJ, Lam C, Qian C, et al. Soluble endoglin and other circulating antiangiogenic factors in preeclampsia. *N Engl J Med.* 2006;355(10):992–1005.

341. Hladunewich MA, Steinberg G, Karumanchi SA, et al. Angiogenic factor abnormalities and fetal demise in a twin pregnancy. *Nat Rev Nephrol.* 2009;5(11): 658–662.

342. Williams WW, Ecker JL, Thadhani RI, et al. Case records of the Massachusetts General Hospital. Case 38–2005. A 29-year-old pregnant woman with the nephrotic syndrome and hypertension. *N Engl J Med.* 2005;353(24): 2590–2600.

343. Shan HY, Rana S, Epstein FH, et al. Use of circulating antiangiogenic factors to differentiate other hypertensive disorders from preeclampsia in a pregnant woman on dialysis. *Am J Kidney Dis.* 2008;51(6):1029–1032.

344. Thadhani R, Kisner T, Hagmann H, et al. Pilot study of extracorporeal removal of soluble fms-like tyrosine kinase 1 in preeclampsia / clinical perspective. *Circulation.* 2011;124(8):940–950.

345. Murakami S, Saitoh M, Kubo T, et al. Renal disease in women with severe preeclampsia or gestational proteinuria. *Obstet Gynecol.* 2000;96(6):945–949.

346. Di Marco GS, Reuter S, Hillebrand U, et al. The soluble VEGF receptor sFlt1 contributes to endothelial dysfunction in CKD. *J Am Soc Nephrol.* 2009;20(10):2235–2245.

347. Bortoloso E, Del Prete D, Gambaro G, et al. Vascular endothelial growth factor (VEGF) and VEGF receptors in diabetic nephropathy: expression studies in biopsies of type 2 diabetic patients. *Ren Fail.* 2001;23(3–4):483–493.

348. Foster RR. The importance of cellular VEGF bioactivity in the development of glomerular disease. *Nephron Exp Nephrol.* 2009;113(1):e8–e15.

349. Irgens HU, Reisaeter L, Irgens LM, et al. Long term mortality of mothers and fathers after pre-eclampsia: population based cohort study. *BMJ.* 2001; 323(7323):1213–1217.

350. Ray JG, Vermeulen MJ, Schull MJ, et al. Cardiovascular health after maternal placental syndromes (CHAMPS): population-based retrospective cohort study. *Lancet.* 2005;366(9499):1797–1803.

351. Vikse BE, Hallan S, Bostad L, et al. Previous preeclampsia and risk for progression of biopsy-verified kidney disease to end-stage renal disease. *Nephrol Dial Transplant.* 2010;25(10):3289–3296.

352. Miller DP, Kaye JA, Shea K, et al. Incidence of thrombotic thrombocytopenic purpura/hemolytic uremic syndrome. *Epidemiology.* 2004;15(2):208–215.

353. George JN, Vesely SK, Terrell DR. The Oklahoma Thrombotic Thrombocytopenic Purpura-Hemolytic Uremic Syndrome (TTP-HUS) Registry: a community perspective of patients with clinically diagnosed TTP-HUS. *Semin Hematol.* 2004;41(1):60–67.

354. Dashe JS, Ramin SM, Cunningham FG. The long-term consequences of thrombotic microangiopathy (thrombotic thrombocytopenic purpura and hemolytic uremic syndrome) in pregnancy. *Obstet Gynecol.* 1998;91:662–668.

355. Wiznitzer A, Mazor M, Leiberman JR, et al. Familial occurrence of thrombotic thrombocytopenic purpura in two sisters during pregnancy. *Am J Obstet Gynecol.* 1992;166:20–21.

356. Meti S, Paneesha S, Patni S. Successful pregnancy in a case of congenital thrombotic thrombocytopenic purpura. *J Obstet Gynaecol.* 2010;30(5): 519–521.

357. Martin JN Jr, Bailey AP, Rehberg JF, et al. Thrombotic thrombocytopenic purpura in 166 pregnancies: 1955–2006. *Am J Obstet Gynecol.* 2008;199(2): 98–104.

358. He Y, Chen Y, Zhao Y, et al. Clinical study on five cases of thrombotic thrombocytopenic purpura complicating pregnancy. *Aust N Z J Obstet Gynaecol.* 2010;50(6):519–522.

359. Jamshed S, Kouides P, Sham R, et al. Pathology of thrombotic thrombocytopenic purpura in the placenta, with emphasis on the snowman sign. *Pediatr Dev Pathol.* 2007;10(6):455–462.

360. Epp A, Larochelle A, Lovatsis D, et al. Recurrent urinary tract infection. *J Obstet Gynaecol Can.* 2010;32(11):1082–1101.

361. Ezra Y, Rose M, Eldor A. Therapy and prevention of thrombotic thrombocytopenic purpura during pregnancy: a clinical study of 16 pregnancies. *Am J Hematol.* 1996;51(1):1–6.

362. Vesely SK, Li X, McMinn JR, et al. Pregnancy outcomes after recovery from thrombotic thrombocytopenic purpura-hemolytic uremic syndrome. *Transfusion.* 2004;44(8):1149–1158.

363. Rozdzinski E, Hertenstein B, Schmeiser T, et al. Thrombotic thrombocytopenic purpura in early pregnancy with maternal and fetal survival. *Ann Hematol.* 1992;64(5):245–248.

364. Meng H, Kumar NS, Nannapaneni J, et al. Thrombotic thrombocytopenic purpura with complete molar pregnancy: a case report. *J Reprod Med.* 2011;56(3–4): 169–171.

365. Vosti KL. Recurrent urinary tract infections. Prevention by prophylactic antibiotics after sexual intercourse. *JAMA.* 1975;231(9):934–940.

366. Stella CL, Dacus J, Guzman E, et al. The diagnostic dilemma of thrombotic thrombocytopenic purpura/hemolytic uremic syndrome in the obstetric triage and emergency department: lessons from 4 tertiary hospitals. *Am J Obstet Gynecol.* 2009;200(4):381.e1–381.e6.
367. George JN. The thrombotic thrombocytopenic purpura and hemolytic uremic syndromes: evaluation, management, and long-term outcomes experience of the Oklahoma TTP-HUS Registry, 1989–2007. *Kidney Int Suppl.* 2009;(112):S52–54.
368. George JN. The thrombotic thrombocytopenic purpura and hemolytic uremic syndromes: overview of pathogenesis (Experience of The Oklahoma TTP-HUS Registry, 1989–2007). *Kidney Int Suppl.* 2009;(112):S8–S10.
369. Raman R, Yang S, Wu HM, et al. ADAMTS13 activity and the risk of thrombotic thrombocytopenic purpura relapse in pregnancy. *Br J Haematol.* 2011 Jan 31 [Epub ahead of print].
370. Fakhouri F, Roumenina L, Provot F, et al. Pregnancy-associated hemolytic uremic syndrome revisited in the era of complement gene mutations. *J Am Soc Nephrol.* 2010;21(5):859–867.
371. Castro MA, Goodwin TM, Shaw KJ, et al. Disseminated intravascular coagulation and antithrombin III depression in acute fatty liver of pregnancy. *Am J Obstet Gynecol.* 1996;174:211–216.
372. Pockros PJ, Peters RL, Reynolds TB. Idiopathic fatty liver of pregnancy: findings in ten cases. *Medicine (Baltimore).* 1984;63(1):1–11.
373. Varner M, Rinderknecht NK. Acute fatty metamorphosis of pregnancy. A maternal mortality and literature review. *J Reprod Med.* 1980;24(4):177–180.
374. Ko H, Yoshida EM. Acute fatty liver of pregnancy. *Can J Gastroenterol.* 2006;20(1):25–30.
375. Fesenmeier MF, Coppage KH, Lambers DS, et al. Acute fatty liver of pregnancy in 3 tertiary care centers. *Am J Obstet Gynecol.* 2005;192(5):1416–1419.
376. Vigil-De Gracia P. Acute fatty liver and HELLP syndrome: two distinct pregnancy disorders. *Int J Gynaecol Obstet.* 2001;73(3):215–220.
377. Lau HH, Chen YY, Huang JP, et al. Acute fatty liver of pregnancy in a Taiwanese tertiary care center: a retrospective review. *Taiwan J Obstet Gynecol.* 2010;49(2):156–159.
378. Davies MH, Wilkinson SP, Hanid MA, et al. Acute liver disease with encephalopathy and renal failure in late pregnancy and the early puerperium—a study of fourteen patients. *Br J Obstet Gynaecol.* 1980;87(11):1005–1014.
379. Aso K, Hojo S, Yumoto Y, et al. Three cases of acute fatty liver of pregnancy: postpartum clinical course depends on interval between onset of symptoms and termination of pregnancy. *J Matern Fetal Neonatal Med.* 2010;23(9):1047–1049.
380. Ockner SA, Brunt EM, Cohn SM, et al. Fulminant hepatic failure caused by acute fatty liver of pregnancy treated by orthotopic liver transplantation. *Hepatology.* 1990;11(1):59–64.
381. Prakash J, Vohra R, Wani IA, et al. Decreasing incidence of renal cortical necrosis in patients with acute renal failure in developing countries: a single-centre experience of 22 years from Eastern India. *Nephrol Dial Transplant.* 2007;22(4):1213–1217.
382. Liano F, Pascual J. Epidemiology of acute renal failure: a prospective, multicenter, community-based study. Madrid Acute Renal Failure Study Group. *Kidney Int.* 1996;50(3):811–818.
383. Prakash J, Kumar H, Sinha DK, et al. Acute renal failure in pregnancy in a developing country: twenty years of experience. *Ren Fail.* 2006;28(4):309–313.
384. Prakash J, Tripathi K, Pandey LK, et al. Spectrum of renal cortical necrosis in acute renal failure in eastern India. *Postgrad Med J.* 1995;72(834):208–210.
385. Matlin RA, Gary NE. Acute cortical necrosis. Case report and review of the literature. *Am J Med.* 1974;56(1):110–118.
386. Toma H, Tanabe K, Tokumoto T, et al. Pregnancy in women receiving renal dialysis or transplantation in Japan: a nationwide survey. *Nephrol Dial Transplant.* 1999;14(6):1511–1516.
387. Bucht H. Studies in renal function in man. *Scand J Clin Lab Invest.* 1951; 3 Suppl. 3:1–55.
388. Lafayette RA, Druzin M, Sibley R, et al. Nature of glomerular dysfunction in pre-eclampsia. *Kidney Int.* 1998;54(4):1240–1249.
389. Noori M, Donald AE, Angelakopoulou A, et al. Prospective study of placental angiogenic factors and maternal vascular function before and after preeclampsia and gestational hypertension. *Circulation.* 2010;122(5):478–487.

CHAPTER

Monoclonal Gammopathies: Multiple Myeloma, Amyloidosis, and Related Disorders

Pierre Ronco • Frank Bridoux • Pierre Aucouturier

Monoclonal proliferations of the B cell lineage, often referred to as plasma cell dyscrasias, are characterized by abnormal and uncontrolled expansion of a single clone of B cells at different maturation stages, with a variable degree of differentiation to immunoglobulin (Ig)-secreting plasma cells. Therefore, they are usually associated with the production and secretion in blood of a monoclonal Ig and/or a fragment thereof. An ominous consequence of secretion of monoclonal Ig products is their deposition in tissues. These proteinaceous deposits can take the form of casts (in myeloma cast nephropathy [CN]), crystals (in myeloma-associated Fanconi syndrome [FS]), fibrils (in light-chain [LC] and exceptional heavy-chain [HC] amyloidosis), or granular precipitates (in monoclonal Ig deposition disease [MIDD]) (Table 60.1). They may disrupt organ structure and function, inducing life-threatening complications. In a large proportion of patients with crystals, fibrils, or granular deposits of Ig products, major clinical manifestations and mortality are related to visceral Ig deposition rather than to expansion of the B cell clone. Indeed, except for myeloma CN, which is generally associated with a large tumor mass malignancy, Ig precipitation or deposition diseases often occur in the course of a benign B cell proliferation or of a smoldering or low-mass myeloma.[1]

The presence of abnormal urine components in a patient with severe bone pain and edema was first recognized in the 1840s by Henry Bence Jones and William MacIntyre, who described unusual thermal solubility properties of urinary proteins, far later attributed to Ig LCs. To perpetuate this discovery, monoclonal LC proteinuria is often referred to as *Bence Jones proteinuria*. This term is not appropriate because less than 50% of LCs do show thermal solubility. Renal damage characterized by large protein casts surrounded by multinucleated giant cells within distal tubules was identified in the early 1900s and termed *myeloma kidney*. This term must, however, be abandoned because CN with acute renal failure may occasionally occur in conditions other than myeloma and because other patterns of renal injury were subsequently found in patients with myeloma. The first of these was amyloidosis, wherein tissue deposits are characterized by Congo red binding and fibrillar ultrastructure. In 1971, Glenner et al.[2] showed that the amino acid sequence of amyloid fibrils extracted from tissue was identical to the variable region of a circulating Ig LC, thereby providing the first demonstration that an Ig component could be responsible for tissue deposition. The spectrum of renal diseases due to monoclonal Ig deposition has expanded dramatically with the advent of routine staining of renal biopsy specimens with specific anti-κ and anti-λ LC antibodies, and of electron and immunoelectron microscopy (Table 60.1). These morphologic techniques associated with more sensitive and sophisticated analyses of blood and urine monoclonal components have led to the description of new entities, including nonamyloid monoclonal LC deposition disease (LCDD),[3] HC (or AH) amyloidosis,[4] nonamyloid HC deposition disease (HCDD),[5,6] glomerulopathies with organized microtubular monoclonal Ig deposits,[7,8] and proliferative glomerulonephritis with non-organized monoclonal IgG deposits.[9] All of these pathologic entities principally involve the kidney, which appears as the main target for deposition of monoclonal Ig components. This is not only explained by the high levels of renal plasma flow and glomerular filtration rate (GFR), but also by the sieving properties of the glomerular capillary wall and by the prominent role of the renal tubule in LC handling and catabolism.[10,11]

Polymorphism of renal lesions may be due to specific properties of Ig components influencing their precipitation, their interaction with renal tissue, or their processing after deposition. Alternatively, the type of renal lesions may be driven by the local response to Ig deposits, which may vary from one patient to another. That intrinsic properties of Ig components are responsible for the observed renal alterations was first suggested by in vitro biosynthesis of abnormal Ig by bone marrow cells from patients with lymphoplasmacytic disorders and visceral LC deposition[12] and by recurrence of nephropathy in renal grafts.[13] A further demonstration of the specificity of Ig component pathogenicity was provided by Solomon et al.[14] They showed that the pattern of human renal lesions associated with the production of monoclonal LC, that is, myeloma CN, LCDD, and LC (or AL) amyloidosis,

TABLE 60.1 **Pathologic Classification of Diseases Featuring Tissue Deposition or Precipitation of Monoclonal Immunoglobulin-Related Material**

	Organized		Nonorganized	
Crystals	**Fibrillar**	**Microtubular**	**MIDD ("Randall type")**	**Other**
Myeloma cast nephropathy[a]	Amyloidosis (AL, AH)	Cryoglobulinemia kidney	LCDD	GN with monoclonal IgG
Fanconi's syndrome	Nonamyloid	Immunotactoid	LHCDD	Crescentic GN (IgA or IgM)
Other (extrarenal)			HCDD	

[a]Crystals are predominantly localized within casts in the lumen of distal tubules and collecting ducts, but may also occasionally be found in the cytoplasm of proximal tubule epithelial cells.
AH, heavy-chain amyloidosis; AL, light-chain amyloidosis; GN, glomerulonephritis; HCDD, LCDD, LHCDD, MIDD, heavy-chain, light-chain, light- and heavy-chain, monoclonal immunoglobulin deposition disease.
Adapted from Preud'homme JL, Aucouturier P, Touchard G, et al. Monoclonal immunoglobulin deposition disease (Randall type): relationship with structural abnormalities of immunoglobulin chains. *Kidney Int.* 1994;46:965, with permission.

could be reproduced in mice injected intraperitoneally with large amounts of LCs from patients. The good correlation between experimental findings and human lesions led to the conclusion that physicochemical or structural properties of LCs might be responsible for the specificity of renal lesions.

A normal Ig is composed of two LCs and two HCs, which are themselves made up of so-called constant (C) and variable (V) globular domains. Whereas a limited number of genes encode the constant region, multiple gene segments are rearranged to produce a variable domain unique to each chain. Diversity is further amplified by junctional molecular events that affect the third hypervariable zone (CDR3), and then by the hypermutation process that occurs in the germinal centers of lymphoid follicles. Consequently, although LCs (and HCs) have many structural similarities, they also possess a unique sequence that may be responsible for physicochemical peculiarities, hence their deposition in tissue or interaction with tissue constituents. A number of structural and physicochemical abnormalities of Ig have already been described. They include deletions of C_H domains in HCDD[5,6] and HC amyloidosis,[4] shortened or lengthened LCs and abnormal LC glycosylation in LCDD,[12,15] and resistance to proteolysis of the V_L fragment in FS.[16] Moreover, overrepresentation of certain V_L gene subgroups was also reported in amyloidosis[17,18] and LCDD.[19] The mechanisms generating Ig diversity may randomly create HCs or LCs with peculiar properties such as proneness to deposition, whereas mistakes in the rearrangement or hypermutation processes may result in altered genes encoding truncated Ig. It must be stressed, however, that some abnormal Ig chains produced in immunoproliferative disorders are not associated with any special clinical features. Conversely, structural abnormalities of LCs are not a constant feature of diseases associated with LC deposition. These observations suggest the need to increase the number of nephritogenic Ig components to be analyzed at the complementary DNA (cDNA) and protein levels.

Myeloma- and AL amyloidosis-induced renal failure accounts for less than 2% of the patients admitted to a chronic dialysis program each year.[20] This is due in part to the relative rarity of these immunoproliferative diseases, but also to a deteriorated clinical condition of patients at the time of end-stage renal disease. A substantial effort of prevention must therefore be carried out, relying in part on a better understanding of the structural and physicochemical properties of Ig components leading to deposition or precipitation in tissues. Any progress in this field may also enlighten the pathogenesis of immunologically mediated renal diseases, especially glomerulonephritides, because properties of monoclonal Ig components favoring their deposition may apply as well to polyclonal Ig involved in the formation of immune complexes.

We have classified the various forms of renal involvement in monoclonal gammopathies according to the lesions observed in renal biopsy specimens. The majority of patients (63% in a series of 87) with serum and/or urine monoclonal gammopathy who undergo renal biopsy have disease unrelated to monoclonal gammopathy deposition.[21] Therefore, the diagnosis of virtually all of the entities to be discussed is critically dependent on the inclusion of κ and λ in the standard of immunofluorescence stains. In some of the rarer entities, a more refined and precise diagnosis can be made with immunofluorescence staining for the subclasses of IgG. Collectively these stains may demonstrate light chain isotype restriction and γ-heavy chain subclass restriction, which strongly favors, but does not definitely prove, the presence of a monoclonal Ig. Demonstration of monoclonality requires serum and urine studies by immunoelectrophoresis or immunofixation.

MYELOMA-ASSOCIATED TUBULOPATHIES

The prevalence of tubular lesions in patients with myeloma is difficult to assess because most patients do not undergo a renal biopsy, but it is most likely high. In Ivanyi's necropsy study including immunofluorescence, 18 of 57 patients (32%) had CN, whereas 6 (11%) had renal amyloidosis and 3 (5%) had κ-LCDD.[22] The higher prevalence of CN (30%) was confirmed in the more recent autopsy series of Herrera.[23] Tubular alterations are also demonstrated by increased urinary concentrations of the low molecular weight proteins normally reabsorbed by the proximal tubule, increased urinary elimination of the tubular lysosomal enzyme β-acetyl-D-glucosaminidase, and frequent abnormalities in renal tubular acidifying and concentrating ability[24] in patients with LC proteinuria. However, myeloma-associated FS remains an exception.

CN is not only the most frequent lesion in myeloma patients, it is also the major cause of renal failure, which is observed in about 25% of patients with multiple myeloma. In nephrology departments that usually receive only myeloma patients with severe renal abnormalities, the prevalence of CN assessed histologically varies from 63% to 87%[25–28] among the myeloma patients with renal failure. This prevalence is most likely underestimated because patients with presumed CN do not systematically undergo a renal biopsy, whereas those exhibiting significant albuminuria or a fortiori the nephrotic syndrome do. In myeloma patients with an albumin urinary output of less than 1 g per day, there is a good correlation between the diagnosis of CN and renal failure. Of note, CN may occur in other immunoproliferative disorders featuring urinary LC excretion including Waldenström macroglobulinemia[29] and μ-HC disease.[30] In a case of μ-HC disease, the urinary secretion of large amounts of free κ-chain was responsible for acute renal failure with a typical histologic presentation of "myeloma kidney."[30]

Myeloma Cast Nephropathy

Pathophysiology of Myeloma Cast Nephropathy

CN occurs mainly in patients with myeloma with a high LC secretion rate. That LCs are the main culprits is supported also by the following clinical, pathologic, and experimental data:

1. Renal lesions may recur on grafted kidneys.
2. Similar crystals may occasionally be seen within casts, proximal tubule cells, and plasma cells. Their usual lack of staining with anti-LC antibody is most likely due to degradation or masking of the relevant epitopes.
3. Mice injected with LC purified from patients with CN developed extensive cast formation in the distal renal tubules.[14]

However, a number of patients produce large amounts of LCs and yet fail to present significant signs of renal involvement throughout the course of the disease. This may be related to the absence of enhancing factors (see later text), but this also suggests that some LCs may be particularly prone to induce renal lesions, especially cast formation.

LCs are directly toxic to epithelial cells, resulting in decreased proximal reabsorption of the LCs and increased delivery to the distal tubule in which they coprecipitate with Tamm-Horsfall protein (THP). Tubular obstruction by large and numerous casts may also contribute to the development of tubular lesions. For clarity, we will analyze separately the pathogenesis of proximal tubule lesions that result from renal metabolism of LCs, the mechanisms of cast formation, and the respective role of tubular obstruction and tubular lesions in the genesis of renal failure (Fig. 60.1).

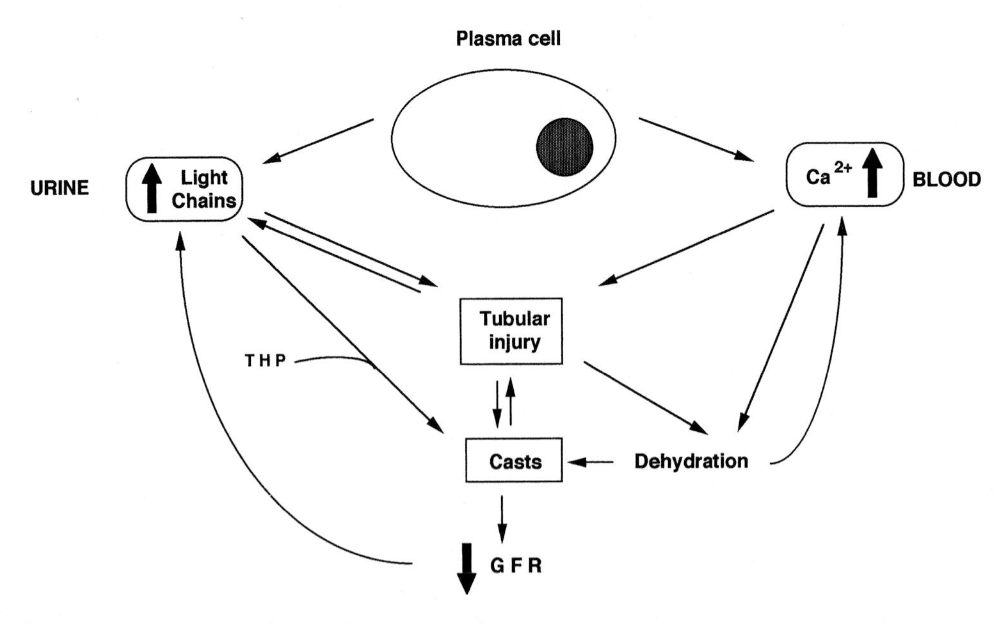

FIGURE 60.1 Schematic representation of the pathogenesis of myeloma cast nephropathy. *GFR*, glomerular filtration rate; *THP*, Tamm-Horsfall protein. (Adapted from Winearls CG. Nephrology forum: acute myeloma kidney. *Kidney Int.* 1995;48:1347.)

Renal Metabolism of Light Chains and Pathogenesis of Proximal Tubule Lesions. Normal as well as malignant plasma cells can secrete free LC, in addition to complete Ig molecules; the amount of free LC secretion is highly variable, depending on the variable (V_L) domain structure. The LCs are normally filtered by the glomerulus and then reabsorbed by the proximal tubule. Lambda and, to a lesser extent, κ-LCs circulate mainly as covalently linked dimers that have a mass-restricted glomerular filtration. In normal individuals, several hundred milligrams per day of circulating free polyclonal LCs are filtered by glomeruli and more than 90% of these are reabsorbed and catabolized by proximal tubular cells. LCs bind to a single class of low affinity, high capacity noncooperative binding sites on both rat and human kidney brush-border membranes. These sites exhibit relative selectivity for LCs compared with albumin and β-lactoglobulin. It has been shown that LCs could bind to the tandem receptor cubilin[10] and megalin,[11] a multiligand receptor belonging to the large family of low density lipoprotein receptors, located in the intermicrovillar areas of the brush border. After binding to the luminal domain of proximal tubular epithelial cells, LCs are incorporated in endosomes that fuse with primary lysosomes where proteases, mainly cathepsin B, degrade the proteins into amino acids, which are returned to the circulation by the basolateral route.

When the concentration of filtered LCs is increased as in myeloma patients, profound functional and morphologic alterations of proximal tubule epithelial cells may occur. The functional disturbances include low molecular weight proteinuria and inhibition of sodium-dependent uptake of amino acids and glucose by brush-border preparations. Furthermore, in human proximal tubule cells, endocytosis of LCs was shown to induce activation of redox pathways,[31,32] NF-κB,[33] and mitogen activated protein kinases (MAPK),[34] resulting in cytokine production including interleukin (IL)-6, IL-8, transforming growth factor (TGF)-β, and monocyte chemoattractant protein-1 (MCP-1). Part of these effects may be mediated by megalin itself because megalin possesses intrinsic signaling properties. Moreover, excessive LC endocytosis may promote apoptosis[35] and induce epithelial-mesenchymal transition of tubular cells.[36,37] Increased cytokine production may be a major mechanism mediating tubulointerstitial injury and progressive kidney disease in some patients with myeloma. Suppression of proinflammatory cytokine production using inhibition of p38 MAPK and translocation of NF-κB by pituitary adenylate cyclase-activating polypeptide with 38 residues (PACAP38) was shown to dramatically prevent injury of cultured renal proximal tubule cells caused by myeloma LCs.[38]

Morphologically, some of the LCs infused in mice or rats or perfused in rat nephrons in vivo accumulated in enlarged, distorded endosomes and lysosomes of the proximal convoluted tubule with frequent crystalloid formations. This was associated with mitochondrial alterations, focal loss of the microvillus border, and epithelial cell exfoliation.

Pathogenesis of Cast Formation. Because myeloma casts are composed principally of the monoclonal LC and THP/uromodulin, it has long been hypothesized that interaction of these two proteins was a key event in cast formation. THP is a highly glycosylated and acidic protein (isoelectric point [pI] = 3.2) synthesized exclusively by the cells of the ascending limb of the loop of Henle. It is the major protein constituent of normal urine, and an almost universal component of casts. This 80-kDa protein is also remarkable for its ability to form reversibly high-molecular-size aggregates of about 7×10^6 daltons at high but physiologic concentrations of sodium and calcium, and at low urinary pH. The role of THP in cast formation has prompted a wealth of studies on its interactions with LCs. These studies were performed with the aim of defining a population of myeloma patients at risk of developing renal damage. The role of LC pI has long been suggested. It was proposed that LC with a high pI (greater than 5.6) and THP could bear opposite charges in the normal urine pH range, and undergo polar interaction and precipitation. However, this hypothesis was not confirmed in further experimental and clinical studies.[25,39]

In a rat model, development of casts and injury to proximal tubule cells in renal tubules microperfused with human nephritogenic LC were not correlated with LC pI, molecular form, or isotype.[40] Intranephronal obstruction was aggravated by decreasing extracellular fluid volume or adding furosemide. In perfused loop segments, cast-forming LCs reduced chloride absorption directly, thereby increasing tubule fluid [Cl^-] and promoting their own aggregation with THP.[41] Pretreatment of rats with colchicine, which prevents addition of sialic acid to the protein, completely prevented obstruction and cast formation in perfused nephrons, and THP from those rats did not aggregate with LCs in vitro, contrary to THP purified from control rats. In vitro studies suggest that THP can undergo both self (homotypic) aggregation and heterotypic aggregation with LCs. Homotypic aggregation is enhanced by calcium, furosemide, and low pH, and is dependent on THP sialic-acid content. Heterotypic aggregation requires previous binding of LC to the THP protein backbone. A 9-residue sequence of the THP was identified as a binding site of LCs, including a histidine at position 226, which explains, at least partially, the pH dependence of molecular interactions.[42] LCs bind to THP through their third complementary determining region (CDR3).[43] The sugar moiety is also essential for coaggregation of LC and THP. THP from normal volunteers treated with colchicine had a lower sialic acid content and a decreased aggregation potential in the presence of pathogenic LCs. These findings suggest that colchicine may be useful in the treatment of cast nephropathy and that it is conceivable to design peptides or analogs that would inhibit interactions of LCs with THP and theoretically prevent myeloma CN.

Cast formation may not rely only on interactions between LC and THP. First, 5 of 12 LCs purified from the urine of patients with CN failed to react with THP.[16] Second, myeloma casts occasionally do not stain for THP in human biopsies, and casts induced in mice by LC injection do not seem to contain THP during the first 24 hours, indicating that some LCs may undergo aggregation or precipitation in the absence of THP. This hypothesis is supported by studies showing that the deposition of certain LCs in vivo may be related to their capability to aggregate in vitro.[44] Resistance of LCs to renal and macrophage-released proteases may also contribute to cast formation and persistence.[16]

Role of Tubular Obstruction by Casts in the Genesis of Renal Failure. The role of casts as plugs obstructing the tubules has been clearly shown in micropuncture studies. In myeloma patients, the correlation between severity of renal insufficiency and the number of casts remains controversial.[24,25,45] This may be explained partly by the prominent medullary localization of casts, the count of which is underestimated in superficial kidney cortex biopsy specimens. The first indication that antibodies to THP could serve as probes of tubular obstruction was provided by Cohen and Border,[46] who identified the protein in glomerular urinary spaces of two myeloma patients. This finding is indicative of intratubular urinary backflow. We detected THP in glomerular urinary spaces in 16 of 18 biopsies of patients with myeloma CN (Ronco and Mougenot, personal data) (Fig. 60.2). The proportion of obstructed tubules is too small to account by itself for renal failure. Renal failure induced by CN is multifactorial, implicating also tubular epithelial cell and interstitial lesions. Tubule obstruction by casts may explain the slow recovery of renal function noted in many patients.[25]

Interstitial deposits of THP were also found in 8 (44%) of the 18 biopsies (Ronco and Mougenot, personal data). They probably result from a leakage of the protein through gaps in the tubular basement membrane favored by tubular obstruction. Clinical and experimental models have implicated the protein in the pathogenesis of tubulointerstitial nephritis. Thomas et al.[47] identified a single class of sialic acid–specific cell surface receptors for THP on polymorphonuclear leukocytes, and further showed that in vitro activation of human mononuclear phagocytes by particulate THP led to the release of gelatinase and reactive oxygen metabolites, both probably contributing to tissue damage.

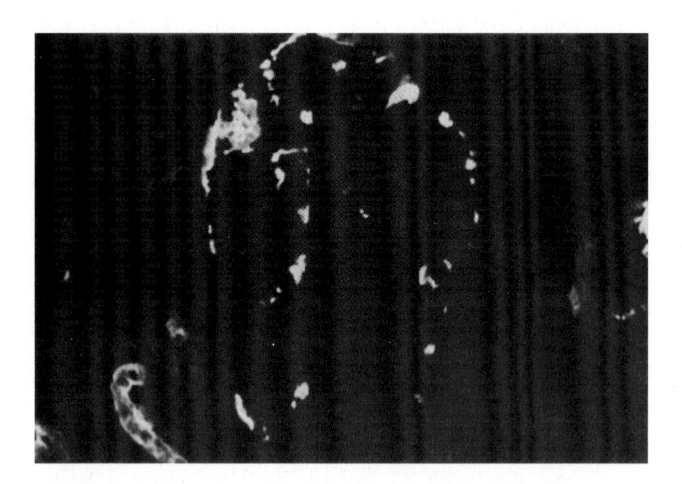

FIGURE 60.2 Myeloma cast nephropathy. Immunofluorescence stain with anti–Tamm-Horsfall protein (THP) monoclonal antibody. Glomerular deposits in Bowman's space delineate the inner aspect of Bowman's capsule and penetrate between lobules of the capillary tuft. Identification of THP in the urinary spaces of glomeruli supports the obstructive role of casts with reflux of tubular urine. (Magnification, ×312.)

Clinical Presentation

Changing Presentation of Patients with Myeloma-Induced Renal Failure. When DeFronzo et al. reported the first series of 14 myeloma patients with acute renal failure in 1960,[48] it was established that renal failure occurred at some time during the illness in approximately half of the patients, but that the mode of presentation was usually chronic with a slow progression over a period of several months to years.

The mode of presentation of renal failure in myeloma has changed dramatically over the years. In their review of 141 patients treated in Nottingham between 1960 and 1988, Rayner et al.[49] showed that the absence of severe renal impairment at presentation predicted a low probability of developing renal failure subsequently. In only 5 of 34 patients of our own renal series[25] did the diagnosis of myeloma antedate the discovery of renal failure by more than 1 month. In three patients, the presence of a monoclonal Ig was known for 10 to 18 years, but it only showed criteria of malignancy for less than 9 months. Two-thirds of the 107 patients referred to the Oxford Kidney Unit from 1987 to 2006[50] had myeloma diagnosed after their admission with acute kidney injury (AKI). More aggressive treatment of myeloma and higher awareness of the conditions that induce CN in the last two decades may have prevented LC precipitation within the tubule lumen in the patients with an established diagnosis of myeloma.

Demographic and Hematologic Characteristics of Patients with Cast Nephropathy-Related Renal Failure. Table 60.2 summarizes the clinical and pathologic data in four large series of myeloma patients with acute renal failure in which a renal biopsy was performed in at least 40% of the patients. A diagnosis of myeloma CN was established histologically in 81 of 99 (82%) renal biopsies, and lesions compatible with this diagnosis were found in 10 further biopsy specimens (10%). In comparison with the Mayo Clinic series of 869 unselected myeloma cases[52] in which the mean age was 62 years and the male–female ratio was 1.55, patients with acute renal failure did not show any demographic particularity. Myeloma patients with renal failure are characterized by high tumor mass and virtually constant urinary LC loss, often of high output.

More than 70% of patients in the renal series have a high tumor burden (Table 60.2). This is confirmed by the

TABLE 60.2 **Clinical and Pathologic Characteristics of Patients with Myeloma-Induced Renal Failure of Presumed or Established Tubulointerstitial Origin**

Series	No. of Patients	Age (yr)	Male–Female Ratio	Tumor Mass		Serum Creatinine (μmol/L)	Urinary Light Chain >2 g/day	Renal Lesions in Biopsy Specimen
				IIB	IIIB			
Rota et al.[25]	34	66 (33–90)	0.88	15%	73%	960 (164–2000)	53%	26 MCN 2 ATN 2 CIN
Pozzi et al.[26]	50	63 (47–60)	1.38	12%	82%	798 (273–1518)	41%[a]	16 "Myeloma kidney"[b] 8 other
Pasquali et al.[27]	25	60 (48–74)	2.12	24%	72%	891 (455–1391)	72%	25 MCN
Irish et al.[51]	56	67 (42–82)	1.33	22%	78%	811 (302–2600)	NA	16 MCN, 5 AIN[c]

[a]Total proteinuria, including light chains.
[b]Presumably myeloma cast nephropathy.
[c]"Compatible with myeloma."
AIN, acute interstitial nephritis; ATN, acute tubular necrosis; CIN, chronic interstitial nephritis; MCN, myeloma cast nephropathy; NA, not available; IIB, intermediate tumor mass; IIIB, high tumor mass.

Alexanian series, which included 494 consecutive patients referred to an oncology center (Table 60.3).[53] Only 3% of patients with myeloma of low tumor mass had renal failure, whereas 40% of those with high tumor burden had a serum creatinine greater than 180 μmol/L. These data contrast with the hematologic characteristics of patients with other renal complications of dysproteinemia including FS, amyloidosis, and MIDD, in whom the monoclonal B lymphocyte or plasma cell proliferation is either malignant but usually of low magnitude, or often benign from a hematologic point of view.

TABLE 60.3 **Relation Between Tumor Mass and Renal Function**

Tumor Mass	No. of Patients[a]	% of Patients with Serum Creatinine (μmol/L)		
		<180	180–270	>270
Low	151	97	1	2
Intermediate	183	89	5	6
High	160	60	17	23

[a]This series included 494 consecutive, previously untreated patients with multiple myeloma.
From Alexanian R, Barlogie B, Dixon D. Renal failure in multiple myeloma: pathogenesis and prognostic implications. *Arch Intern Med.* 1990;150:1693, with permission.

Another salient feature of myeloma associated with renal failure is the high prevalence of pure LC myelomas. Although they represent only about 20% of all myelomas, they are found in between 37% and 64% of patients with renal failure of presumed or established tubulointerstitial origin. Development of CN in two studies in which this diagnosis was established histologically[25,27] was associated with urinary excretion of LCs exceeding 2 g per day in 53% and 72% of the patients (Table 60.2). LC protein excretion emerges as a highly significant independent factor of renal failure on multivariate analysis (Table 60.4). The risk of developing renal failure is twice as high in patients with pure LC myeloma, and five to six times greater in patients with LC proteinuria greater than 2.0 g per day compared to those with proteinuria less than 0.05 g per day. This indicates that in patients producing complete Ig molecules, CN essentially occurs in those synthetizing an excess of LCs. The frequency of renal failure is identical in patients excreting κ or λ LCs. IgD myeloma has the greatest potential for causing renal disease.[50] Hypercalcemia also is a prominent independent pathogenetic factor on multivariate analysis, with a risk of renal failure five times greater in those patients with corrected calcium greater than 2.87 mmol/L.[53]

TABLE 60.4 **Features Associated with Renal Failure in Myeloma**

	No. of Patients[a]	% with Renal Failure	P
All patients	494	18	
Urinary LC (g/day)			
>2.0	123	39	0.00001
0.05–2.00	149	17	
<0.05	222	7	
Myeloma protein type			
Only LC protein	93	31	0.0003
Other	401	15	
Serum calcium (mmol/L)[b]			
>2.87	104	49	0.00001
≤2.87	390	10	

[a]Same series of patients as in Table 60.3.
[b]Corrected calcium (mmol/L).
LC, light chain.
From Alexanian R, Barlogie B, Dixon D. Renal failure in multiple myeloma: pathogenesis and prognostic implications. *Arch Intern Med.* 1990;150:1693, with permission.

The Clinical and Urinary Syndrome of Myeloma Cast Nephropathy. CN-induced renal failure is remarkably silent. Clinical signs are due to myeloma (or to hypercalcemia), including weakness, weight loss, bone pain, and infection. Because of their nonspecificity and their frequency in older patients, they often do not lead patients to take medical advice or physicians to prescribe serum and urinary electrophoreses, which are the key laboratory investigations for the diagnosis of myeloma. Peaks visible on serum or urine electrophoresis are then identified by immunoelectrophoresis or immunofixation. A preserved corrected calcium at presentation in patients with unexplained renal failure should alert clinicians to the possibility of myeloma.

The main urinary feature is the excretion of a monoclonal LC, which accounts for 70% or more of total proteinuria in 80% of patients.[25] LC proteinuria is usually not detected by urinary dipsticks, but only by techniques measuring total proteinuria. Certain LCs fail to react or react weakly in some widely used precipitation assays, such as the sulfosalicylic acid method, leading to falsely negative or underestimated results. The remaining proteins are composed of albumin and low molecular weight globulins that have failed to be reabsorbed by proximal tubule cells. In the rare patients with albuminuria greater than 1 g per day, CN is usually associated with glomerular lesions due to amyloidosis or MIDD. There is no hematuria in pure CN.

Precipitants of Cast Nephropathy. These are of paramount importance because of measures to prevent precipitation (Table 60.5). It is often difficult to identify a particular event responsible for precipitating renal failure, as these patients experience many of the complications of the disease at once, a common thread of which seems to be an effect on renal perfusion.

Hypercalcemia is an important precipitant found in 16% to 44% of the renal series (Table 60.5), and in 57% of the patients with renal failure in Alexanian nonrenal series.[53] Presumably, hypercalcemia acts by inducing dehydration as a result of emesis and a nephrogenic diabetes insipidus. It may also enhance LC toxicity and cause nephrocalcinosis.

TABLE 60.5 **Precipitants of Acute Renal Failure in Myeloma**

Series	No. of Patients	Dehydration	Sepsis	Hypercalcemia	Contrast Medium	NSAIDs	None
Rota et al.[25]	34[a]	65%	44%	44% (>2.60 mmol/L)	0%	24%	—
Pozzi et al.[26]	50[a]	24%	10%	34% (≥2.60 mmol/L)	4%	0%	44%
Ganeval et al.[28]	80[b]	10%	9%	30%	11%	—	35%
Irish et al.[51]	56[a]	4%	4%	23%	0%	11%	57%
Haynes et al.[50]	107	6%	5%	16% (> 2.90 mmol/L)	—	18%	65%

[a]Renal lesions are described in Table 60.2.
[b]Includes 19 patients with myeloma cast nephropathy, two with amyloidosis, and eight with LCDD (light- and heavy-chain deposition disease).
NSAIDs, nonsteroidal anti-inflammatory drugs.

Dehydration, with or without hypercalcemia, and infection are other major risk factors for acute renal failure. Rota et al.[25] found a high rate of urinary infections (10/34, 29%), which were associated in three cases with an increased proportion of polymorphonuclear leukocytes in the renal biopsy, suggesting an etiologic link between infection and deterioration of renal function. Infection also operates by causing dehydration and prompting the use of nephrotoxic antibiotics.

Contrast media have hitherto been considered an important precipitant of acute renal failure. It was hypothesized that the contrast medium bound to intratubular proteins, especially the LC and THP, causing them to precipitate and obstruct tubular flow. Contrast media also have vasoconstrictive effects, decreasing GFR and urinary output. McCarthy and Becker[54] reviewed seven retrospective studies of myeloma patients receiving contrast media, involving 476 patients who had undergone a total of 568 examinations. The prevalence of acute renal failure (which was not defined) was 0.6% to 1.25%, compared to 0.15% in the general population. This is a low risk and contradicts the dogma that contrast media should not be used in myeloma patients. This change may reflect awareness of the risk and care taken to hydrate patients actively with alkaline solutes before and during the administration of contrast media. No clinical data currently support the preferential use of nonionic agents in myeloma patients to decrease the risk of acute renal failure.

A number of drugs are noxious in myeloma patients. They include antibiotics, particularly aminoglycosides, and nonsteroidal anti-inflammatory drugs (NSAIDs).[25,50] NSAIDs reduce the production of vasodilatory prostaglandins that help to maintain an appropriate GFR in patients with renal hemodynamics compromised by dehydration. Angiotensin-converting enzyme (ACE) inhibitors can also precipitate renal failure because they reduce GFR dramatically in dehydrated patients. Their use as that of angiotensin type-1 receptor antagonists should be avoided as long as a risk of decreased renal perfusion persists.

Recently introduced therapies including bisphosphonates may also induce toxic tubular injury. Renal failure secondary to acute tubular necrosis was reported with zoledronate, a potent bisphosphonate that is in widespread use for the treatment of hypercalcemia of malignancy,[55] and with short-term, high-dose pamidronate.[56] Doses should be adapted to GFR to avoid toxicity.

Renal Pathology and the Value of Kidney Biopsy

A kidney biopsy should not be routinely performed in patients with a presumed diagnosis of myeloma CN. However, it is useful in three circumstances:

1. To establish the cause of renal failure in anuric patients with clinically silent myeloma without evidence of serum monoclonal component on electrophoresis;
2. To analyze tubulointerstitial lesions and predict the reversibility of renal failure in patients with presumed CN but multiple precipitating factors;
3. To identify glomerular lesions in patients with urinary albumin greater than 1 g per day and no evidence of amyloid deposits in "peripheral" biopsies (accessory salivary glands, rectum, abdominal fat).

A kidney biopsy should be systematically performed in patients enrolled in therapeutic protocols because renal lesions should be precisely identified.[57]

Myeloma Casts. Myeloma CN is characterized by the presence of specific casts associated with severe alterations of the tubule epithelium. Myeloma casts are large and usually numerous. Their prevailing localization is the distal tubule and the collecting duct, but they may also be found in the proximal tubule and even in the glomerular urinary space. They often have a "hard" and "fractured" appearance, and show polychromatism upon staining with Masson's trichrome (Fig. 60.3). Casts may also have a stratified or laminated appearance. They may stain with Congo red, but only exceptionally do they show the typical yellow-green dichroism of amyloid under polarized light.

An important diagnostic feature of myeloma casts is the presence of crystals, which may be suspected by light microscopy.[58] Such casts are often angular or heterogeneous because they contain multiple rhomboid or needle-shaped crystals surrounded by amorphous material and cell debris.

Casts are frequently surrounded by mononuclear cells, exfoliated tubular cells, and, more characteristically, by multinucleated giant cells whose macrophagic origin has been established by specific antibodies. These cells are often seen engulfing the casts and at times actually phagocytizing fragments. In some cases, the cellular reaction is made

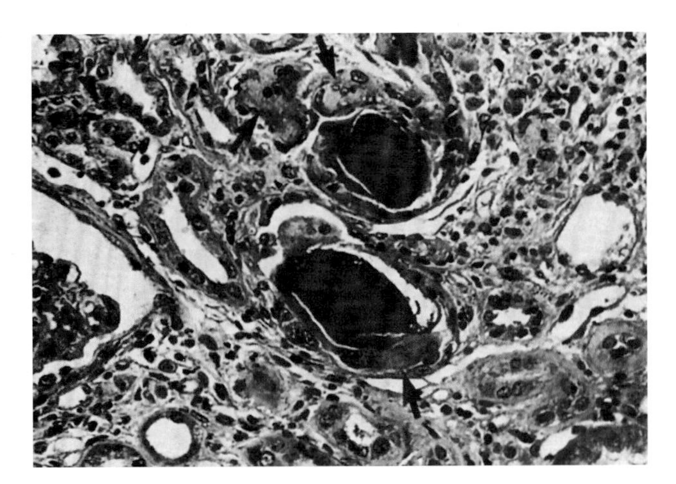

FIGURE 60.3 Myeloma cast nephropathy. Typical myeloma casts with fractured appearance are surrounded by multinucleated macrophagic cells (*arrows*) in a patient with λ-light-chain myeloma. (Masson's trichrome, ×312.)

of polymorphonuclear leukocytes in the absence of urinary tract infection. Typical myeloma casts with a giant, multinucleated cell reaction (Fig. 60.3) can be very occasionally detected in other hemopathies including μ-HC disease[30] and Waldenstöm's macroglobulinemia.[29] In myeloma CN, there is a great variability in the respective percentage of typical myeloma casts and of nonspecific hyaline casts. In some instances, most casts have nonspecific characteristics by light microscopy, even if by immunofluorescence the vast majority consists predominantly of one of the two LC types. The search for typical casts has to be conducted on all available sections if necessary.

By immunofluorescence, myeloma casts are essentially composed of the monoclonal LC excreted by the patient, together with THP. In most cases, casts are stained exclusively or predominantly with either the anti-κ or the anti-λ antibody. However, in about 25% of myeloma biopsies, casts stain for both antibodies because they contain polyclonal LCs, together with albumin and fibrinogen.[58] Staining of "angular" casts is often irregular, and more intense at the periphery (Fig. 60.4). In heterogeneous casts, the crystals themselves fail to stain, whereas the matrix of the cast and the surrounding cellular debris and amorphous material often stain positively for one of the LC isotypes.

Cast ultrastructure was studied by electron microscopy in 24 biopsies of myeloma CN by Pirani et al.[58] Crystals were detected in 14 biopsy specimens and suspected in another 4. The authors have identified four major categories of casts, according to their content and ultrastructural appearance. One category characterized by large rectangular crystals, or fragments thereof, with a pentagonal or hexagonal cross-section, is found only in myeloma CN. It seems to be closely linked to the development of a giant cell reaction around the cast. A second category also frequently contains crystals, but they are small, electron-dense, and needle-shaped, and seemingly not associated with a cellular reaction. Similar large rectangular and small, needle-shaped crystals can be found within plasma cells. They are also seen occasionally within the cytoplasm of either proximal or distal tubular cells (Fig. 60.5), surrounded by a single smooth membrane, which suggests that they are located within lysosomes.

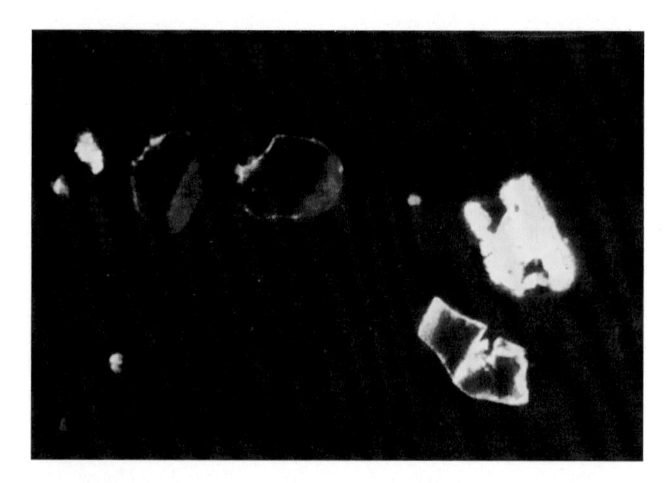

FIGURE 60.4 Myeloma cast nephropathy. Several tubules contain large casts, one of which has an angular and fractured aspect. The stain with anti-κ antibody is more intense at the periphery of most casts. (Immunofluorescence, ×312.)

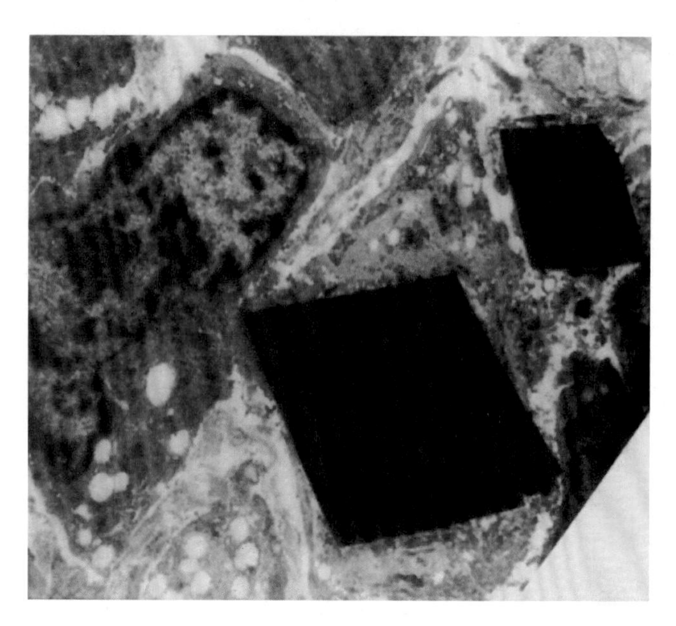

FIGURE 60.5 Myeloma cast nephropathy. Rectangular crystals presumably composed of λ-light chains in tubular cells. (Electron micrograph, uranyl acetate, and lead citrate, ×7,000.)

Tubules and Interstitium. Considerable tubular damage is almost always present in myeloma CN. Epithelial tubular lesions are not only seen in the distal tubules where casts are principally located, but also in proximal convoluted tubules, where the epithelium undergoes atrophy and degenerative changes. Frank tubular necrosis may also be seen, with or without typical myeloma CN.[25] By immunofluorescence, a variable number of tubule sections contain numerous "protein reabsorption droplets" staining for the monoclonal LC.[46]

Interstitial lesions are often associated with the tubular damage. They may be mild and consist of inflammatory infiltrates and fibroedema, but fibrosis and its correlate, tubular atrophy, may also be fairly extensive. In severe cases with epithelial denudation and gaps in the continuity of the tubular basement membrane, often in close contact with myeloma casts, granulomatouslike formations containing macrophages and histiocytes develop around the ruptured tubules (Fig. 60.6).[46]

Glomeruli and Vessels. The glomeruli are usually normal, except for small clusters of globally sclerotic glomeruli and a mild thickening of the mesangial matrix. When mesangial thickening is more prominent, the possibility of an associated

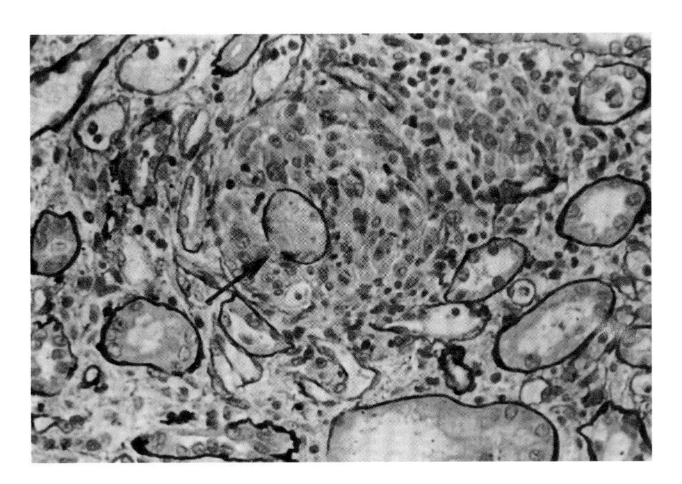

FIGURE 60.6 Myeloma cast nephropathy. Interstitial granulomatous-like formations with macrophages surrounding disrupted tubular basement membrane (*arrow*) were numerous in this λ-chain cast nephropathy. (Silver stain, ×312.)

MIDD should be considered. Rarely, amorphous deposits reminiscent of myeloma casts can be seen in capillary loops or in the glomerular urinary space. In younger patients, severe chronic vascular lesions are sometimes observed, which may contribute to progression of sclerosis.

Outcome and Prognosis of Myeloma Cast Nephropathy

Until the 1980s, myeloma-induced renal failure was associated with a very poor prognosis, with a median survival of less than 1 year.[48] In recent years, the outcome of patients with myeloma, including those with renal impairment, has improved with the introduction of novel therapies, including high dose therapy followed by autologous stem cell support, and development of new drugs with a strong anti-myeloma effect (bortezomib, thalidomide, lenalidomide).[59] However, because patients with elevated serum creatinine levels were excluded from most randomized controlled studies, optimal treatment of multiple myeloma with renal failure remains to be defined. The establishment of consensus criteria for the assessment of renal function and renal response in multiple myeloma, and the use of modern sensitive tests to evaluate hematologic response, such as as nephelometric assays for serum free LC,[60] should help to improve renal and patient outcomes in the future.[61]

Renal Outcome and Prognostic Factors. Renal prognosis in patients with myeloma who present with renal failure remains poor, as complete or partial renal recovery occurs in half of patients after weeks to months,[62] and in only 20% to 40% of those with dialysis-dependent renal failure.[63–66] Elevated plasma creatinine concentration or decreased estimated GFR (calculated using the MDRD equation) have been quoted as markers of poor renal prognosis in most studies,[26,28,62,65,67] implying that renal functional impairment of any degree should be treated as a medical emergency. In the study by Rota et al.,[25] main prognostic indicators were provided by renal histology. Renal response was seen in patients with typical cast nephropathy and/or tubular necrosis without interstitial damage. Global tubular atrophy and interstitial fibrosis were associated with partially or totally irreversible renal failure, whereas the number of casts has a controversial predictive value.[25,26,68]

The rapid achievement of sustained hematologic response appears as a key factor for renal prognosis.[57,65,69,70] In three recent studies a minimum of 50% reduction in serum free LC concentration was required for recovery of renal function in patients with biopsy proven CN.[57,70,71] Recent data indicate that outcome of severe renal failure may be substantially improved by bortezomib plus dexamethasone-based chemotherapy[61,65,66,72] and, in patients requiring dialysis, by extended hemodialysis using a high-cut off dialyzer that allows effective removal of LCs.[70,73]

Survival and Predictors. Myeloma patients with renal failure have a shorter survival than those with normal renal function. In the presence of renal failure, mortality in the first 3 months is about 30%,[26,28,67] and median survival ranges from 9 to 22 months. However, several studies have indicated that recovery of renal function is associated with improved survival, close to that of patients who do not develop renal failure.[25–28,50,67,62,69] A response to chemotherapy is a key predictor of renal outcome and patient survival.

Treatment

Myeloma patients with renal failure should be treated with chemotherapy just as those without renal failure, and any measures that may contribute to improved renal function should be undertaken from the day of diagnosis.

Decreasing Precipitability of the Urinary LC by Immediate Symptomatic Measures. Because co-precipitation in renal tubules of free LC and THP is the main nephritogenic event, measures to reduce concentration and precipitability of both partners are essential and urgent. These include rehydration, correction of hypercalcemia, stopping administration of NSAIDs and ACE inhibitors, and treatment of infections with nonnephrotoxic antibiotics. Despite controversy about the role of LC pI in cast formation, alkalinization of urine remains recommended because solubility of THP is reduced at low pH. Therefore, a daily urine output greater than 3 L and a urine pH greater than 7.0 should be reached in all patients whose cardiac and renal function can tolerate a deliberate expansion of the extracellular fluid volume. These measures alone are sufficient to improve renal function in the majority of patients with renal impairment at presentation, especially in those with hypercalcemia.[53] However, they must be completed by therapeutic means aimed at decreasing the amount of urinary LCs filtered by glomeruli.

Reducing the Production Rate (and Concentration) of the Monoclonal Light Chains

Conventional Chemotherapy. The goal of chemotherapy is to obtain a rapid and profound reduction in the rate of production of monoclonal LC in order to induce a renal response, which is a main prognostic factor for patient survival. Therefore, chemotherapy should be initiated without delay, as soon as the diagnosis of myeloma is confirmed. The choice of first-line chemotherapy in patients with multiple myeloma and inaugural renal failure is still under investigation. Because of their anti-inflammatory properties, high-dose steroids are considered as mandatory. A retrospective review from a single institution demonstrated reversal of renal insufficiency in 73% of patients treated with high-dose dexamethasone, either alone or combined with other agents.[69] Renal elimination of some agents may limit their use in patients with reduced GFR. Melphalan containing regimens in general should be avoided, as they have slow antimyeloma effect, and because clearance of melphalan is partly dependent on renal function. As the risk of severe hematologic side effects increases with reduced creatinine clearance, melphalan dose should be adapted in patients with impaired renal function.[74] The vincristine, doxorubicin, dexamethasone (VAD) regimen, which induces earlier responses compared to the melphalan plus prednisone combination and has the advantage of being used without dose adaptation in renal failure, has been widely employed, despite cardiac toxicity of doxorubicin and peripheral nerve complications of vincristine.

New Agents. The recent introduction of novel agents, such as the immunomodulatory drugs thalidomide and lenalidomide, and, above all, the proteasome-inhibitor bortezomib, has transformed the strategy of initial chemotherapy in multiple myeloma with renal failure. Pharmacokinetics of thalidomide are not modified in patients with impaired renal function. However, due to the risk of central nervous system side effects, including seizures, thalidomide dose in patients with impaired renal function should not exceed 200 mg per day. Moreover, serum potassium levels should be closely monitored, as severe hyperkalemia has been described in thalidomide-treated patients on dialysis.[60] Little information is available on the efficacy of thalidomide in myeloma patients with renal failure. In a recent series of 31 patients with newly diagnosed myeloma and a creatinine clearance ≤50 mL per min (seven of whom required chronic hemodialysis), thalidomide plus dexamethasone therapy induced hematologic response in 74% of patients, of whom 82% showed improvement in renal function.[76] In a previous retrospective study, the median time for renal response was significantly lower (0.8 versus 2 months) in patients treated with thalidomide plus dexamethasone compared to those who received dexamethasone alone or combined with other agents.[69]

Lenalidomide, which is mainly eliminated through the kidney, should be used with reduced dose depending on the value of creatinine clearance. A subgroup analysis of two phase 3 trials (MM-009 and MM010) using lenalidomide and dexamethasone found that 68% of the patients with renal failure had at least one level of improvement in renal function according to chronic kidney disease stages. The incidence of severe thrombocytopenia was higher in patients with severe renal failure, who required more frequent reductions of lenalidomide dose and had a shorter overall survival.[77]

Because of its potent inhibitory effect on the NF-κB mediated production of pro-inflammatory cytokines, which is likely to play a central role in the pathogenesis of CN, bortezomib appears as a molecule of choice in association with high-dose dexamethasone, in first-line therapy of myeloma with renal failure. Moreover, bortezomib is devoid of nephrotoxicity and may be used without dose adaptation, whatever the degree of renal impairment, including in patients requiring dialysis, with a safety and efficacy similar to those observed in myeloma patients with preserved renal function.[64,78,79] Side effects related to bortezomib therapy mainly involve the gastrointestinal tract, bone marrow (thrombocytopenia), and peripheral nerves.

In several retrospective studies, bortezomib plus dexamethasone-based regimens (combined or not with other agents) appeared to be safe and effective in myeloma patients with renal failure. They induced rapid hematologic responses (usually in less than 2 months) in more than two thirds of patients, with a complete reponse rate of around 30%, close to that of patients with preserved renal function,[65,66,72] and an overall survival of 50% to 60% at 2 years.[66,72] Renal response occurred in 40% to 60% of patients in a median time of 2 months in most series, with a complete renal response (as defined by improvement of creatinine clearance from lower than 50 mL per min at baseline to ≥60 mL per min) rate around 40%.[65,66,72] In a recent prospective phase III trial, hematologic response rates, overall survival, and time to progression were higher in patients with renal failure who received a combination of bortezomib, melphan, and prednisone (VMP), compared to those treated with melphalan plus prednisone (MP). Complete renal responses were 44% in the VMP group and 34% in the MP group.[80] In the VMP group, the incidence of severe hematologic side effects was increased in patients with renal failure, as in patients treated with bortezomib, dexamethasone, and doxorubicin in another study.[81] The impact on renal function and survival of bortezomib-based regimens, and their tolerance in patients with severe renal failure, remain to be investigated in prospective controlled studies. In patients requiring dialysis, bortezomib-based regimens have also shown similar rates of hematologic responses, with an incidence of severe side effects comparable to that observed in patients with preserved renal function. However, the rate of discontinuation of renal replacement therapy was low, ranging from 17% to 33% suggesting that, in this situation, other measures should be undertaken in combination with chemotherapy to rapidly decrease the burden of circulating free LCs.

High-Dose Therapy with Autologous Blood Stem Cell Transplantation. High-dose therapy with autologous blood stem cell transplantation (ASCT) is currently considered as standard therapy in patients aged less than 65 years, with good performance status. In 1996, a randomized controlled trial first demonstrated the benefits of high-dose therapy over conventional chemotherapy in terms of complete remission rate, event-free survival, and overall survival in patients with normal renal function.[82] High-dose therapy with ASCT can lead to a median overall survival exceeding 5 years.[83] In patients with preserved renal function, it is usually based on a single dose of melphalan 200 mg per m^2, given after hematologic response has been obtained with few cycles of chemotherapy (generally based on bortezomib-containing regimens), and peripheral stem cell collection. Several studies have demonstrated that the procedure is feasible in patients with renal failure, but with increased melphalan-related toxicity.[84–86] Despite a 5-year event-free and overall survival of 24% and 36%, respectively, treatment-related mortality (TRM; i.e., in the first 3 months) was high, reaching up to 19% in a series of 59 patients, mainly related to mucosal, infectious, and cerebral complications.[85] However, renal function improved in 24% of patients with dialysis-dependent renal failure, after a median of 4 months following high-dose therapy. Reduction of melphalan dose reduced TRM and did not affect the efficacy of the procedure. In patients less than 65 years old with creatinine clearance lower than 60 mL per min, high-dose therapy may thus be considered; however it is recommended to reduce melphalan dose to 140 mg per m^2,[61,84,85] although the place of high-dose therapy with ASCT in patients with myeloma and renal failure has not been established in prospective controlled studies.

Removal of Circulating Free LCs. Rapid sustained reduction in circulating free LC is the goal of therapy in multiple myeloma. Beside rapid introduction of effective chemotherapy, free LC removal from the serum should be considered. Ig LCs can be directly removed from the circulation by either plasma exchange or intensive haemodialysis using high cut-off membranes. Plasmapheresis has been used in this indication for 30 years and is very effective at reducing LC concentration rapidly. However, its efficacy has not been established, except in patients with hyperviscosity syndrome. Three randomized controlled trials have been published to date[63] and did not support evidence for a benefical effect of plasmapheresis in improving the rate of renal recovery in patients with myeloma-associated renal failure. As the distribution of Ig LCs is predominately extravascular, a short duration treatment as plasmapheresis might be inappropriate to significantly reduce the burden of LCs.[87]

Recently an extended hemodialysis technique, using a new generation dialyser with very high permeability to proteins that allows reduction of 35% to 70% in serum free LC levels after 2 hours of dialysis, has shown encouraging results.[73] Hutchison et al. reported a series of 19 patients with biopsy-proven myeloma CN and dialysis-dependent renal failure, who received extended high cut-off hemodialysis (using two dialyzers in series, with a dialysis schedule of daily 8 hour sessions for 5 days, then progressively tapered), combined with conventional chemotherapy (mostly based on high-dose dexamethasone plus thalidomide). Treatment resulted in a median reduction of 85% in serum free LC concentration in 13 patients, in whom hemodialysis was withdrawn after a median time of 27 days. Survival of patients free of dialysis was significantly improved.[70] Clinical tolerance of extended high cut-off dialysis appears to be good, although due to the high membrane permeability to large molecules, an infusion of albumin is required after each dialysis session.[73] Preliminary reports indicate that online high-efficiency hemodiafitration is another interesting option to rapidly remove circulating free LCs.[88] Wether these novel strategies may improve prognosis in myeloma cast nephropathy remains to be evaluated in randomized prospective studies.

Supportive Therapy. Blood transfusion, analgesia, erythropoietin, and bisphosphonates are important adjuncts to therapy. Beyond delaying the onset of skeletal events, the new generation of bisphosphonates, pamidronate and zoledronate, also exert antimyeloma effects indirectly by inducing osteoclast apoptosis, thereby reducing a major source of the antiapoptotic IL-6 molecule, or directly by inducing myeloma cell apoptosis. Bisphosphonates were shown to reduce skeletal events in myeloma patients with bone disease, but their use in the absence of bone disease needs to be further evaluated in the context of potential nephrotoxicity. Cases of acute renal failure[55,56] and nephrotic proteinuria with focal segmental glomerulosclerosis and its collapsing variant were indeed reported in patients receiving zoledronate and pamidronate.[89] Therefore, pamidronate (90 mg intravenously over at least 2 hours monthly) and zoledronate (4 mg intravenously over at least 15 minutes monthly) should be given at the appropriate doses, with careful monitoring of renal function and albuminuria.

Dialysis and Renal Transplantation. Dialysis is clearly indicated for the treatment of acute renal failure and end-stage renal disease, except in patients with refractory myeloma.[90] It should be started early to avoid the complications of uremia and to compensate for the hypercatabolic state induced by the use of high doses of corticosteroids. If peritoneal dialysis is chosen, the early placement of a permanent indwelling dialysis catheter is recommended to avoid infectious peritonitis, the risk of which is increased by chemotherapy-induced leukopenia.[50] Residual renal function must be carefully monitored because of possible improvement after several months of dialysis. Two early reports from Great Britain[91] and the United States[92] suggested that chronic dialysis could be a worthwhile treatment in patients with myeloma and renal failure. Survival at 1 year was 45% in the British study (23 patients) and 54% in the American study (731 patients). At 30 months, survival declined to 25% compared with 66%

in nondiabetic ESRD patients without myeloma.[92] In the United States Renal Data System registry, the 2-year all-cause mortality of patients with myeloma during the period 1992 to 1997 was 58% versus 31% in all other patients.[93] In the ERA-EDTA Registry study which gathered patients with CN and LCDD,[20] the median patient survival was 0.91 years, compared to 4.46 years for nonmyeloma patients. Myeloma patients requiring long-term dialysis live as long as those with less severe renal failure,[90] with little difference between hemodialysis and peritoneal dialysis,[51,91,94] although most authors insist on the serious risk of infection in continuous ambulatory peritoneal dialysis (CAPD) patients.[91] However, median survival was less in patients on hemodialysis with myeloma CN (12 months) than in those with AL amyloidosis (24 months) or with LCDD (48 months), most likely because of higher tumor burden.[95] Nevertheless, recent data from the ERA-EDTA Registry[50] showed that the incidence of renal replacement therapy for end-stage renal disease due to myeloma (including cast nephropathy and LCDD) has progressively increased over the past 20 years in Europe, probably because of increased acceptance and improved treatment of myeloma as shown by a 5-year event-free survival in 25% of 59 myeloma patients on dialysis treated with high-dose melphalan and ASCT.[85]

The experience with renal transplantation in myeloma is extremely limited, as the risk of infectious complications and exacerbation of the disease with immunosuppression is usually regarded as prohibitive and myeloma-related lesions may occur.[96,97] Recent data suggest that combined HLA-matched donor bone marrow and renal allotransplantation result in sustained renal allograft tolerance and prolonged antimyeloma response, with acceptable toxicity.[98] However, very few patients are eligible for the procedure. The place of renal transplantation in myeloma, which should be limited to carefully selected patients with an inactive hematologic disease, remains to be defined.

Finally, if most cases of severe renal failure cannot be prevented because they occur simultaneously with the finding of myeloma, it is necessary to avoid or correct all precipitating factors of renal failure in patients with established myeloma. It is particularly important to reduce the use of NSAIDs as analgesic drugs, to detect and control hypercalcemia as soon as possible, and to correct dehydration.

Fanconi Syndrome

Fanconi syndrome (FS) is characterized by renal glycosuria, generalized aminoaciduria, hypophosphatemia, and, frequently, by chronic acidosis, hypouricemia, and hypokalemia. It often includes osteomalacia, with pseudofractures. These manifestations result from functional impairment of the renal proximal tubule. The first association of FS with myeloma was reported by Sirota and Hamerman,[99] although these authors considered FS and myeloma as two separate diseases. Engle and Wallis[100] identified crystal-like inclusions in both tumor cells and renal tubule epithelial cells, and suggested that FS and myeloma could be related. Costanza and Smoller[101] described the cytoplasmic inclusions as round or rodlike electron–opaque structures with longitudinally oriented fibrils. Lee et al.[102] established clearly that myeloma was a cause of adult FS. Maldonado et al.[103] reported 17 cases of FS associated with plasma cell dyscrasia, and two more recent studies described the clinicopathologic features of the disease in two series of 11 and 32 patients.[104,105] The disease is most likely underdiagnosed. The rarity of FS in patients with myeloma contrasts, however, with the high prevalence of tubule alterations in myeloma autopsy series. This suggests that unusual specific properties of LCs, mostly κ, are involved in the pathophysiology of FS.

Pathophysiology of Plasma Cell Dyscrasia-Associated Fanconi Syndrome

The peculiar propensity of certain LCs to form crystals in vivo is attested by experimental studies in mice[14] and rats.[40] It is remarkable that the κ LCs that induced crystallization in vivo, also significantly reduced the glucose, chloride, and volume fluxes.

Crystal composition was analyzed in a patient with myeloma-associated FS and hexagonal crystals in kidney proximal tubular cells, bone marrow plasma cells, and phagocytes.[106] N-terminal sequencing and mass spectrometry studies showed that a 107-amino acid fragment corresponding to the variable domain of the κ-LC (Vκ) was the essential component of crystals forming spontaneously from the patient's urine (Fig. 60.7A). Vκ was also crystallized alone using the hanging drop technique (Fig. 60.7B). Crystals were hexagonal bipyramids and had the same 6.0-nm periodicity on electron micrographs as those found in the cells. The V domain (12-kDa) resisted proteolysis by trypsin, pepsin, and cathepsin B, self-reacted, and formed crystals in vitro, which may explain its accumulation in plasma cells and proximal tubular cells. The resistance of LC V domains to proteolytic enzymes including cathepsin B was confirmed in further studies,[16,104] except in a few patients with a high-mass myeloma or Waldenström's macroglobulinaemia[107] and FS. At variance with the observations made in patients with CN,[16] LCs from patients with FS did not bind THP, except in one case where both syndromes were associated.

The unusual physicochemical behavior of FS κ-chains was tentatively correlated with their structure in a number of cases.[108] Sequence analyses showed that 90% of LCs belonged to the VκI variability subgroup, whereas this subgroup only accounts for 56% of all monoclonal κ-LCs.[104,109] The VκI appeared to originate from only two germline genes, IGKV1-39 in five cases and IGK1-33 in four. Analyses of the DNA sequence suggested that all structure peculiarities arose from somatic mutations in the proliferating clone.[110] In the 10 available sequences, residues had never or rarely been reported among VκI subgroup LCs. The unusual presence of nonpolar or hydrophobic amino acids in the complementary determining region (CDR)-L1

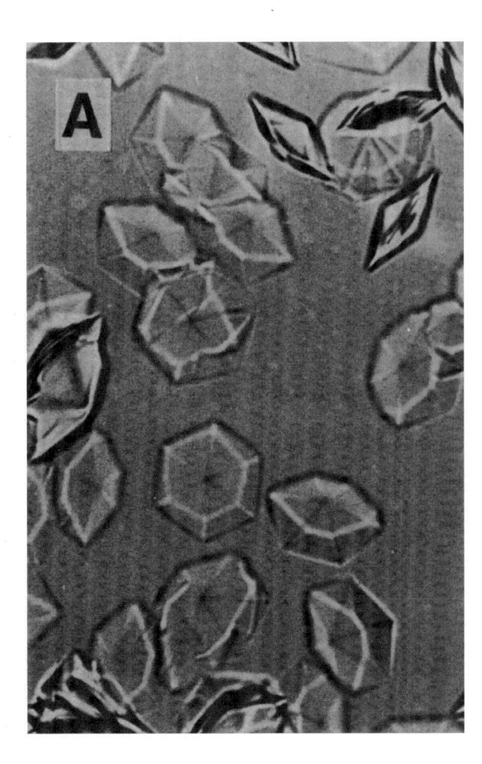

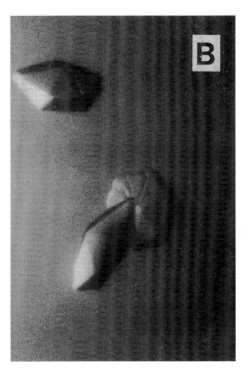

FIGURE 60.7 Plasma cell dyscrasia-associated Fanconi syndrome. Crystals spontaneously obtained in vitro from a Sephadex G100 fraction of the patient's urinary proteins **(A)** and by the hanging drop technique from purified Vκ fragment **(B)**. (**A**, magnification, ×400; **B**, size of these crystals, 0.25 mm.) (From Aucouturier P, Bauwens M, Khamlichi AA, et al. Monoclonal Ig L chain and L chain V domain fragment crystallization in myeloma-associated Fanconi's syndrome. *J Immunol.* 1993;150:3561, with permission.)

loop at position 30, together with a nonpolar amino acid at position 50, seems to be specific for FS LCs derived from gene IGKV1-39. These hydrophobic residues are exposed to the LC surface[108] and may be involved in the pathophysiology of FS, as is suggested by site-directed mutagenesis in an experimental model for FS.[111] Recently, a transgenic mouse model with overexpression of human FS κ LC (CHEB) was generated through insertion of the V domain from CHEB LC in the Igκ locus of the mouse. This resulted in the expression of a hybrid κ LC made up of the human V domain and the mouse constant (C) region. Despite the replacement of the human C region, animals exhibited characteristic LC crystals within proximal tubular cells. This model confirmed that LC aggregation in FS is promoted by the V domain structure. The extent of tubular inclusions was proportional to the production rate and serum levels of CHEB LC. Using an inducible CRE mediated deletion of the CHEB V domain, tubular lesions were shown to recover after a few weeks when the LC production was stopped.[112]

After endocytosis, LCs are processed in the endosomal and lysosomal compartment where "normal" LCs are degraded. In FS, accumulation of the protease-resistant V domain fragment generated by lysosomal enzymes may induce crystal formation. Clogging of the endolysosomal system may subsequently alter apical membrane recycling and/or adenosine triphosphate (ATP) production (hence, Na^+-K^+-ATPase functioning) as suggested by mitochondrial injury,[102] and lead to progressive impairment of sodium-dependent apical transporters. However, in a few cases of FS, crystalline inclusions were not observed within proximal tubular cells.[104,107,108] In two patients, LCs, which belonged to the VkIII subgroup, showed no common substitution with previously described FS VκI LC and did not display resistance to proteolysis, suggesting that other mechanisms of toxicity may be involved in the pathogenesis of the disease.[107,108] Furthermore, why FS does not occur in patients with apparently the same degree of distortion of the lysosomal compartment as can be seen in certain myeloma patients with or without CN is unclear. The molecular mechanisms responsible for glycosuria, phosphaturia, generalized aminoaciduria, and uric acid loss remain poorly understood. An impairment of the megalin-cubilin system might be involved.

Clinical Presentation

The clinical features are summarized in Table 60.6.[104] The median age at diagnosis is 57 years. Most common initial manifestations are bone pain and weakness, principally due to osteomalacia. The major cause of this osteomalacia is hypophosphatemia, which results from increased urinary clearance of phosphate. Chronic acidosis and abnormal renal vitamin D metabolism further contribute to the development of bone lesions. Bone pain may also be the consequence of lytic lesions in patients with a high-mass myeloma. Other revealing signs are essentially due to the proximal tubule impairment, including hypokalemia. Renal failure occurs more frequently than one would expect in a disease of the proximal tubule.

Criteria for the diagnosis of FS may not all be present together, especially in patients with renal failure.[109] The diagnosis of FS is often unrecognized for several years in patients presenting with proteinuria, bone pain, or renal failure. The mean time from onset to diagnosis of FS is about 3 years.[104] Typically, the diagnosis of FS precedes that of the plasma cell dyscrasia, most often a κ-LC-excreting multiple

TABLE 60.6 **Clinical Characteristics of Patients with Plasma Cell Dyscrasia-Associated Fanconi Syndrome[a]**

Total No. of Patients	Age Mean/ Extremes	Gender	Initial Manifestations	Bone Lesions	Renal Failure[c]	Plasma Cell Dyscrasia	Light-Chain Isotype
68	57 22–81	30 males 38 females	Bone pain (25)[b] Weakness, fatigue (16) Weight loss (7) Polyuria–polydipsia(7) Hypokalemia-related signs (4) Proteinuria (18) Renal failure (16) Renal glycosuria (13)	Osteomalacia (25) High-mass myeloma (12) Plasmacytoma (1)	54	Myeloma (36)[d] MGUS (21)[e] MGUS/ myeloma (4)[f] Lymphoma/ CLL (4)[g] “Atypical” plasma cell dyscrasia (1)	49κ 7λ

[a]Figures in parentheses indicate number of patients.
[b]Related to osteomalacia.
[c]Serum creatinine >130 μmol/L, or creatinine clearance
[d]Including 12 patients with a high-mass myeloma.
[e]Monoclonal gammopathy of undetermined significance (MGUS).
[f]Undetermined diagnosis, mostly due to cytoplasmic inclusions in plasma cells making interpretation of cytology difficult.
[g]Chronic lymphocytic leukemia (CLL).
From Messiaen T, Deret S, Mougenot B, et al. Adult Fanconi's syndrome secondary to light-chain gammopathy: clinicopathologic heterogeneity and unusual features in 11 patients. *Medicine (Baltimore)*. 2000;79:135, with permission.

myeloma, because the hematologic disease has a low tumor burden and a slow progression. In 35 of 98 (36%) published cases,[104,105] even criteria for the diagnosis of myeloma were lacking, and patients were classified initially as having a benign monoclonal gammopathy of undetermined significance (MGUS). In some patients, the diagnosis of the plasma cell dyscrasia remained undetermined between myeloma and MGUS because it may be difficult to recognize the cytologic characteristics of myeloma cells when their cytoplasm is stuffed with crystals. Three patients of 99 had Waldenström's macroglobulinemia.[104,105,107]

Conversely, the metabolic disorders of FS may be overseen in the context of myeloma, and FS-related bone lesions should not be interpreted as the consequence of high-mass myeloma.

Pathologic Data

Typically there are prominent crystals in enlarged proximal tubular cells and degenerative changes of proximal tubules.[104] Proximal tubular cells are stuffed with microcrystals that stain red or green with Masson's trichrome and are periodic acid-Schiff negative. In the most severely affected tubules, crystal-containing exfoliated cells are seen in the tubular lumen, whereas intracytoplasmic crystals are still present in atrophic tubules. In other cases, crystals can only be suspected by the presence of a finely granular material of glassy appearance in an enlarged proximal tubular epithelium (Fig. 60.8A). Their presence is more easily demonstrated by toluidine-blue staining of semi-thin sections and by hematoxylin and eosin staining of cryostat sections. In the same tubule sections, all the cells are not equally affected; cells with a normal aspect coexist with those stuffed with crystals.

A universal feature is the additional presence of severe lesions of the proximal tubule epithelium apparently devoid of crystals. These lesions include vacuolization, loss of the luminal brush border, and focal cell sloughing, with cell fragments in the lumen of the tubules. Interstitial cellular infiltrate, including plasma cells, may contain crystalline inclusion bodies. Patchy tubular atrophy and focal interstitial fibrosis, together with a variable number of obsolescent glomeruli, are often observed.

In several cases, attempts to characterize the crystal proteins with anti-Ig conjugates, including anti-LC antibodies, have failed. When immunohistochemical studies are positive, crystals stain only (or predominantly) for the monoclonal LC, most often κ (Fig. 60.8B).

By electron microscopy, crystals of various size and shape (rectangular, rhomboid, round, or needle-shaped) are detected within the cytoplasm of proximal tubule cells

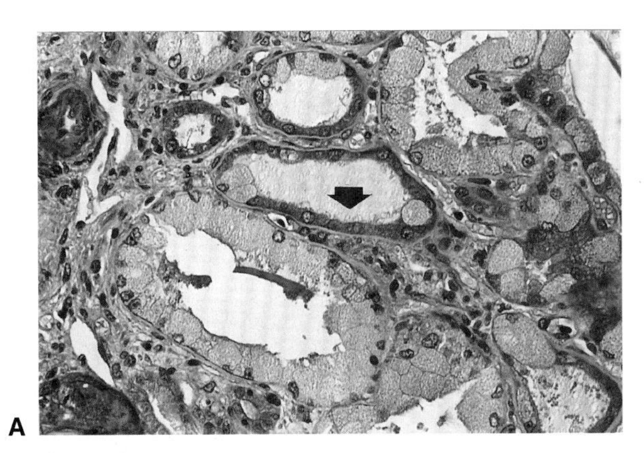

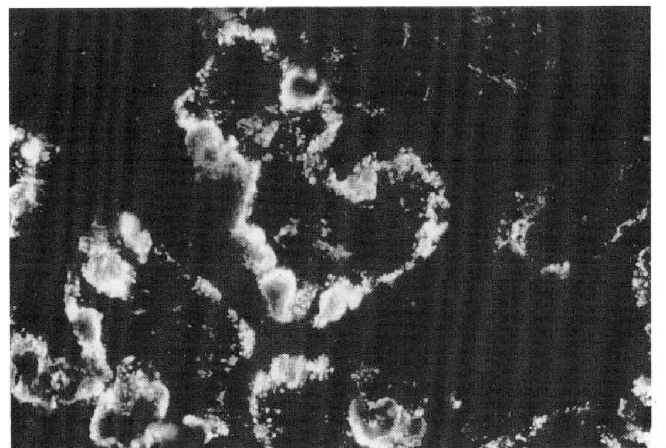

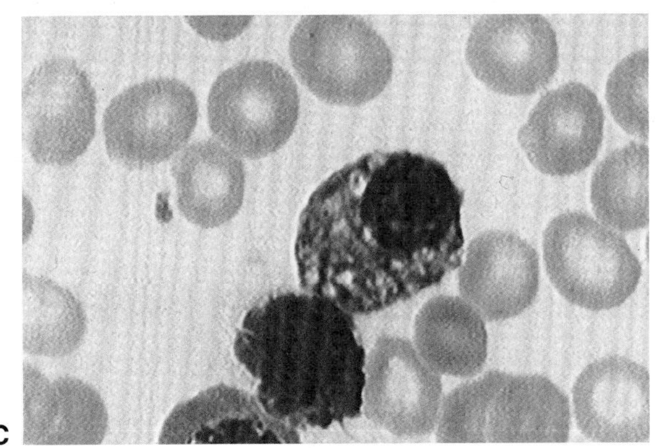

FIGURE 60.8 Plasma cell dyscrasia-associated Fanconi syndrome. **A,B:** Renal biopsy. **A:** Glassy appearance of the epithelium of several proximal convoluted tubules. Crystals were not evident by light microscopy, but were demonstrated by electron microscopy. Note also the severe lesions of the epithelial cells lining some tubules (*arrow*), and mild interstitial fibrosis. (Masson's trichrome, ×312.) **B:** Immunofluorescence stain of the same tubules with anti-κ monoclonal antibody. (Magnification, ×312.) **C:** Bone marrow smear from the same patient. The cytoplasm of a plasma cell shows a vacuolated aspect, suggesting the presence of crystals. (May-Grünwald-Giemsa stain, ×1,000.)

(Fig. 60.8C). Intracytoplasmic crystals are surrounded by a single smooth membrane, likely of lysosomal origin.[58,106] In rare cases, crystals are also seen in distal tubule cells. In other cases, crystals are not found by light microscopy, but electron microscopy shows enlarged vesicular bodies containing dense tubular and rod-like structures[101–103] or fibrils and needle-shaped deposits very close to crystalline structures.

Crystal formation in plasma cell dyscrasia–associated FS is not limited to renal tubule epithelium but also occurs in bone marrow and tissue-infiltrating plasma cells, and in macrophages (Figs. 60.8C and 60.9).[103,106] In plasma cells, crystals are localized not only in lysosomes, but they are also frequently found inside the granular endoplasmic reticulum. Crystal formation in these organelles therefore suggests incomplete proteolysis of LCs. The slow progression of myeloma disease in typical FS associated with crystal formation may be explained by the deleterious effects on cell growth of the accumulation of crystalline inclusions in the tumor plasma cells. A peculiar accumulation of LC crystals may be observed within lysosomes of macrophages in the bone marrow and other organs, defining "crystal-storing histiocytosis" (CSH). In CSH, invariably associated with κ LC monoclonal gammopathy, crystals appear to be mostly made up of monoclonal κ LC, and more rarely of entire IgG. Renal manifestations in CSH are mostly represented by chronic tubulointerstitial nephritis and FS with accumulation of monoclonal κ LC crystals within proximal tubular cells. Perirenal and interstitial infiltration by histiocytes containing eosinophilic crystalline inclusions (pseudo-pseudo Gaucher cells) is suggestive of the disease. Specific molecular peculiarities in the V domains of CSH monoclonal κ LCs may account for crystal accumulation within histiocytes and multiple organ involvement.[113]

Although crystals are a salient feature of the plasma cell dyscrasia–associated FS, they are neither specific nor absolutely constant. Crystals were found in 16 of 28 (57%) patients in the two largest series published so far.[104,105] They may also be found, albeit in low amounts, in proximal tubule epithelial cells of patients with CN,[16,58] and occasionally in myeloma patients with isolated tubular lesions, that is, in the absence of myeloma casts.

Outcome and Treatment

As expected, patients with multiple myeloma have shorter survival time than those with MGUS. In the Mayo Clinic's series, only one of the 14 patients with MGUS developed multiple myeloma, and at the end of follow-up, only 5 of 32 patients had evolved to end-stage renal disease.[105]

In patients with osteomalacia, considerable improvement can be obtained with 1α-hydroxyvitamin D, calcium, and phosphorus supplementation. The effect of chemotherapy on the proximal tubule impairment is much more debated. It was reported that the treatment of underlying myeloma improved urinary signs and tubular transport abnormalities. However, no significant change in renal function was observed in the two largest series.[104,105] It has been suggested that the presence of crystals within plasma cells should be added to the list of criteria against chemotherapy in

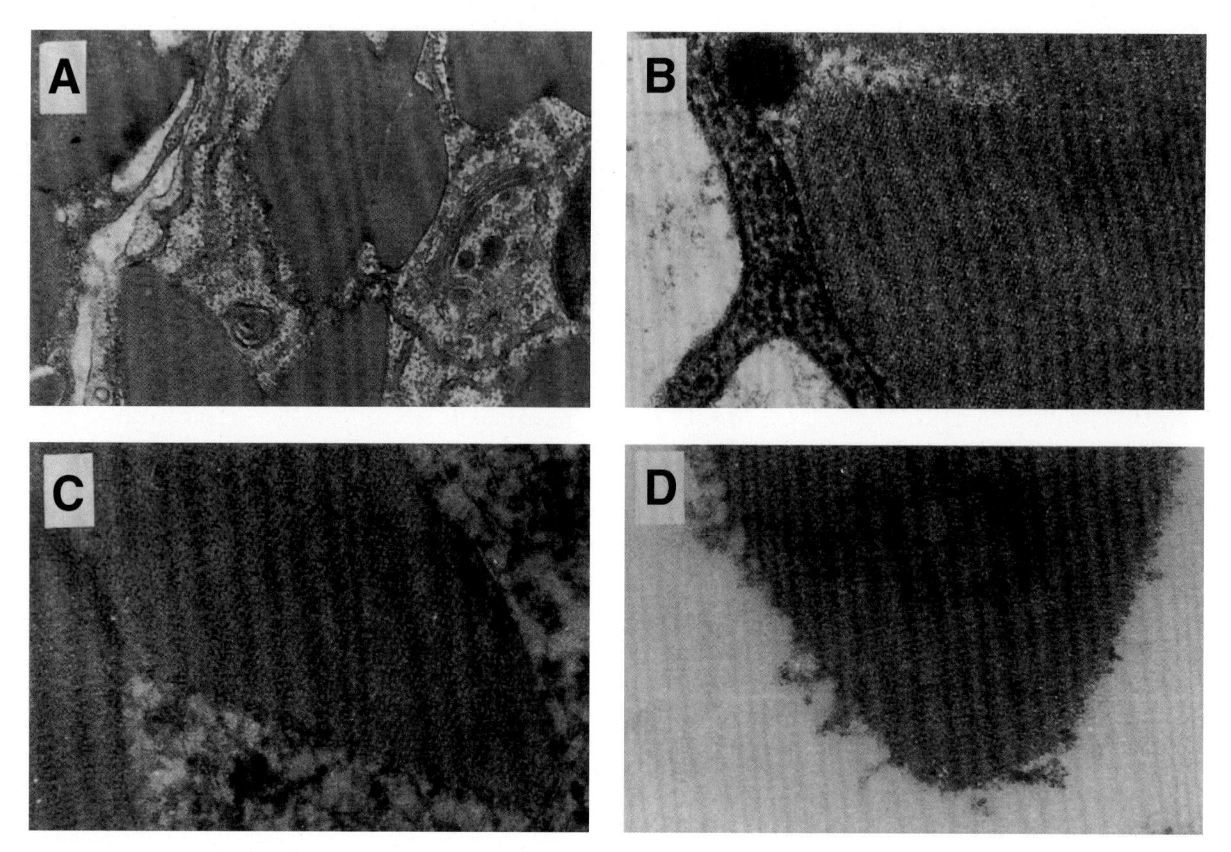

FIGURE 60.9 Plasma cell dyscrasia-associated Fanconi syndrome in same patient as in Figure 60.7. Electron microscopic study of intracellular (*A, B,* and *C*) and in vitro-formed crystals in the same patient. **A:** Bone marrow plasma cell (and a macrophage on the left). (Magnification, ×8,000.) **B:** Bone marrow macrophage. (Magnification, ×50,000.) **C:** Proximal convoluted tubular epithelial cell. (Magnification, ×50,000.) **D:** Crystal obtained in vitro from Sephadex G100 fraction C from the patient's urine. (From Aucouturier P, Bauwens M, Khamlichi AA, et al. Monoclonal Ig L chain and L chain V domain fragment crystallization in myeloma-associated Fanconi's syndrome. *J Immunol.* 1993;150:3561, with permission.)

myeloma. Because chemotherapy, especially with alkylating agents, carries a significant risk of complications but without much benefit for kidney function, and because patients who do not have an overt malignancy show a relatively benign course, the risks and benefits of chemotherapy should be weighed carefully. Whether novel antimyeloma agents might improve renal prognosis in FS remains to be established.

AMYLOIDOSIS

Amyloidosis has been known to be associated with or to cause renal disease for more than 100 years. Amyloid was originally identified as a waxy substance by Rokitansky in 1842, but the term *amyloid* was coined by Virchow in 1854 because the substance stained with iodine in a way that was similar to starch and cellulose. Although the protein content of amyloid was recognized subsequently, the term *amyloid* persisted. The diversity of amyloidotic disease was rapidly suspected on clinical grounds, but chemical studies in the late 1960s actually provided the basis of the present classification of amyloid (Table 60.7). In 1968, Pras et al.[114] isolated and purified amyloid fibrils, which opened the way to further chemical analyses. In 1971, Glenner et al.[2] found that the amyloid fibril proteins from two patients had an N-terminal sequence identical to Ig LCs, which was the first demonstration of a relation between amyloidosis and Ig. They also generated "amyloidlike" fibrils by proteolytic digestion of some human LCs, thereby demonstrating their propensity for forming amyloid.[115]

AL amyloidosis is certainly among the most severe complications of plasma cell proliferative disorders. The only efficient therapeutic tools to date are chemotherapeutic drugs against B cell proliferations. However, pathophysiologic considerations and advances in the treatment of other types of amyloidosis may open new therapeutic avenues (Table 60.7).

General Characteristics of Amyloidosis

A Common Ultrastructural Molecular Organization Defining a Morphologic Entity

Amyloidosis is the general term for a morphologic entity, defined by visceral, extracellular deposition of protein material with unique tinctorial properties and ultrastructural characteristics. After Congo red staining, amyloid deposits exhibit

TABLE 60.7 **Classification of Amyloidoses**

Amyloid Protein	Precursor	Distribution	Type	Syndrome or Main Involved Tissues
AA	**Serum amyloid A**	**Systemic**	**Acquired**	**Secondary amyloidosis, reactive to chronic infection or inflammation including hereditary periodic fever (FMF, TRAPS, HIDS, FCU, and MWS)**
AApoAI	**Apolipoprotein A-I**	**Systemic**	**Hereditary**	**Liver, kidney, heart, skin, larynx**
AApoAII	**Apolipoprotein A-II**	**Systemic**	**Hereditary**	**Kidney, liver, adrenal glands, spleen, skin**
Aβ	Aβ protein precursor	Localized Localized	Acquired Hereditary	Sporadic Alzheimer disease, aging Prototypical hereditary cerebral amyloid angiopathy, Dutch type
Aβ2M	β_2-microglobulin	Systemic	Acquired	Chronic hemodialysis
ABri	Abri protein precursor	Localized or systemic?	Hereditary	British familial dementia
ACys	Cystatin C	Systemic	Hereditary	Icelandic hereditary cerebral amyloid angiopathy
AFib	**Fibrinogen Aα chain**	**Systemic**	**Hereditary**	**Kidney**
AGel	**Gelsolin**	**Systemic**	**Hereditary**	**Finnish hereditary amyloidosis**
AH	**Immunoglobulin heavy chain**	**Systemic or localized**	**Acquired**	**Primary amyloidosis, myeloma-associated**
AL	**Immunoglobulin light chain**	**Systemic or localized**	**Acquired**	**Primary amyloidosis, myeloma-associated**
ALys	**Lysozyme**	**Systemic**	**Hereditary**	**Kidney, liver, spleen, adrenal glands**
APrP	Prion protein	Localized Localized	Acquired Hereditary	Sporadic (iatrogenic CJD, new variant CJD) (alimentary?) Familial CJD, GSSD, FFI
ATTR	**Transthyretin**	**Systemic**	**Hereditary** **Acquired**	**Prototypical FAP** **Senile heart, vessels**
ALECT2	**Leukocyte chemotactic factor 2**	Systemic	**Acquired?**	Kidneys, liver, adrenal glands

Lines in bold characters indicate amyloid types with kidney involvement.

The following proteins may also cause amyloidosis: calcitonin, islet-amyloid polypeptides, atrial natriuretic factor, prolactin, insulin, lactadherin, keratoepithelin, and Danish amyloid protein (which comes from the same gene as ABri and has an identical *N*-terminal sequence).

CJD, denotes Creutzfeldt-Jakob disease; FAP, familial amyloidotic polyneuropathy; FCU, familial cold urticaria; FFI, fatal familial insomnia; FMF, familial Mediterranean fever; GSSD, Gerstmann-Strüassler-Scheinker disease; HIDS, hyper-IgD syndrome; MWS, Muckle-Wells syndrome; TRAPS, tumor necrosis factor receptor-associated periodic syndrome.

Adapted from Westermark G, Benson MD, Buxbaum JN, et al. Amyloid fibril protein nomenclature—2002. *Amyloid* 2002;9:97; Merlini G, Bellotti V. Molecular mechanisms of amyloidosis. *N Engl J Med.* 2003;349:583.

birefringence under polarized light, which indicates the presence of highly ordered structures. These deposits have been extensively studied at the ultrastructural level by electron microscopy, infrared spectroscopy, and X-ray diffraction. Glenner[116] clustered all amyloidoses under the denomination of β-fibrilloses on the basis of the highly similar organization of the amyloid deposits. These are "typically composed of a felt-like array of 7.5- to 10-nm wide rigid, linear, nonbranching, aggregated fibrils of indefinite length." One amyloid fibril is made of two twisted 3-nm–wide filaments, each having a regular antiparallel β-pleated sheet configuration; the β-sheets are perpendicular to the filament axis. A regular packing of peptides or proteins with a β-sheet conformation results in the elongation of amyloid fibrils. The numerous hydrogen bonds between virtually all amide functions of the peptide backbones make such a structure highly stable. Other components, described in subsequent text, are supposed to stabilize the fibrils.

Amyloid Protein Precursors and Classification of Amyloidoses

Amyloid protein precursors share the property of either a native β-pleated conformation or a high propensity to form β-sheets. All are globular structures, clearly distinct from fibrillar proteins such as collagen, which are proline-rich polymers with a longitudinal arrangement.

The International Committee for Amyloidosis recommended a nomenclature essentially based on the nature of amyloid proteins[117]; the abbreviated name of each amyloid protein is preceded by the letter A. The list provided in Table 60.7 is not exhaustive. Twenty-seven different amyloid protein precursors have been identified to date. It is worth noting that hereditary and secondary forms of the same disease exist and should be distinguished; for instance, normal transthyretin is responsible for senile systemic amyloidosis, whereas certain mutations are the cause of familial amyloidotic polyneuropathy (Fig. 60.10A). Multiple different factors, either intrinsic (structural) or external (concentration of the precursor proteins, tissue factors, etc.), may influence the pathogenicity of a variety of potentially amyloidogenic proteins.

Other Constituents of Amyloid

In addition to the unique "pseudocrystalline" stacking of β-sheets, a few structural features are shared by all types of amyloid, and might help the understanding of some aspects

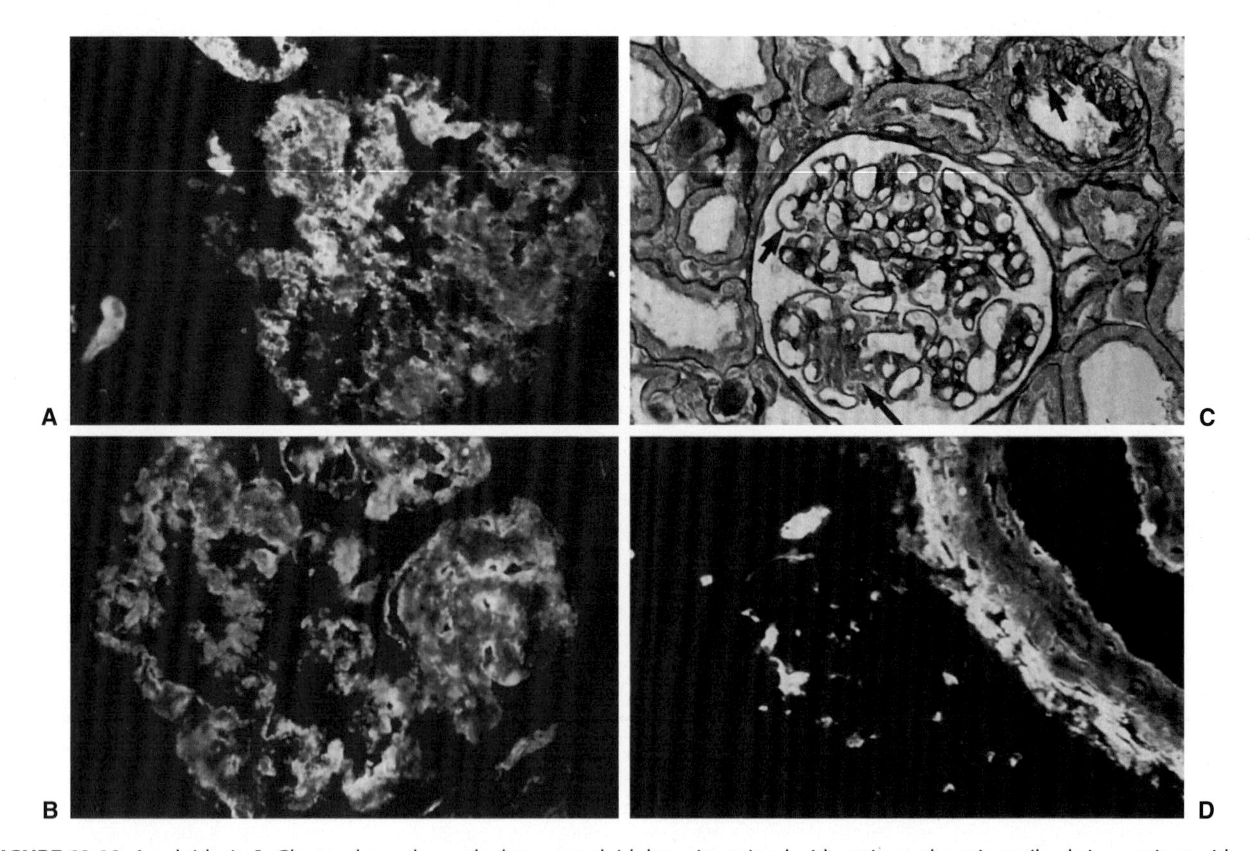

FIGURE 60.10 Amyloidosis. **A:** Glomerular and vascular heavy amyloid deposits stained with antitransthyretin antibody in a patient with Portuguese-type hereditary amyloidosis. (Immunofluorescence, ×312.) **B:** Co-deposition of amyloid P (AP) component in a glomerulus from the same patient as in **(A)**. (Immunofluorescence stain with anti-AP component antibody, ×312.) **C:** Glomerulus with early amyloid deposits in mesangium, capillary walls, and arteriolar wall (*arrows*) from a patient with AA amyloidosis. (Light microscopy, periodic acid-Schiff, ×312.) **D:** Glomerulus from a patient with AL amyloidosis. Scanty glomerular deposits contrast with almost complete replacement of arterial walls by amyloid. (Immunofluorescence stain with anti-κ antibody, ×312.)

of the pathophysiology. Glycosaminoglycans (GAGs) have been found tightly associated with all isolated amyloid fibrils. GAGs are polysaccharide chains made of repeating uronic acid–hexosamine units of several types and normally linked to a protein core, thus constituting proteoglycans, which are important constituents of extracellular matrices. The invariable presence of GAGs in amyloid fibrils raises two suggestions:

1. Proteoglycans might interact with amyloidogenic precursors during the nucleation steps of amyloidogenesis; indeed, most GAGs associated with fibrils are of the heparan sulfate type, and heparan sulfate proteoglycans are essential components of the basement membranes, which are preferential sites of amyloid deposition. Recent data indicate that specific interactions occur between motifs within heparan sulfate and properly modified AL LCs.[118]
2. Sulfated GAGs might be important for inducing and stabilizing the β-pleated structure of the amyloid fibrils.[119]

Another constituent of all amyloid deposits is a protein of the pentraxin family, the serum amyloid P component (SAP) (Fig. 60.10B). SAP is a plasma glycoprotein made up of two noncovalently linked pentamers of identical subunits. The β-pleated structure of SAP[120] is strongly homologous to that of legume lectins such as concanavalin A. It shows no allelic polymorphism and displays striking interspecies homology. Furthermore, no occurrence of SAP deficiency has yet been described, which suggests that it has essential physiologic functions. SAP is a calcium-dependent lectin, with binding affinities toward DNA, C4-binding protein, and the collagenlike region of C1q, and several constituents of extracellular matrices such as fibronectin and proteoglycans. SAP was shown to bind apoptotic cells and nuclear debris, and mice with targeted deletion of the SAP genes spontaneously develop anti-DNA antibody and a syndrome resembling human systemic lupus erythematosus.[121] Two calcium sites are involved in carbohydrate binding. In the presence of calcium, SAP is remarkably resistant to proteolytic digestion, suggesting a physiologic role in maintaining extracellular matrix structures. Coating of amyloid fibrils with unaltered SAP is a constant feature that could result in their protection from catabolism. It is probable that SAP binding to amyloid deposits is mediated by GAGs through the formation of multicomponent complexes. The high affinity of SAP toward all types of amyloid is used for diagnosing and monitoring the extent of systemic amyloidosis using scintigraphy with ^{123}I-labeled SAP.[122] SAP binding to all ligands is inhibited by specific sugars such as β-D-galactose cyclic pyruvate acetal. Moreover, the knowledge of SAP structure offers the opportunity of designing competitive inhibitors as potential drugs for the treatment of amyloidoses. Recently, CPHPC, a compound that specifically binds to SAP allowing a rapid decrease in serum SAP levels, has been developed.[123] The combination of CPHPC with an antibody specific for SAP, which targets amyloid deposits and enables their elimination by recruiting phagocytic cells, has shown impressive results in an experimental mouse model of systemic AA amyloidosis.[124]

General Mechanisms of Fibrillogenesis

The amyloidoses are diseases of protein conformation in which a particular soluble innocuous protein transforms and aggregates into an insoluble fibrillar structure that deposits in extracellular spaces of certain tissues. Fibrillogenesis may be the consequence of several mechanisms of processing the amyloid precursor, including partial proteolysis and conformational modifications. In systemic AA amyloidosis, removing of the C-terminal part of an apolipoprotein acute-phase reactant, SAA, yields a 5- to 10-kDa fibril-forming fragment. Phagocytic cells, in particular macrophages, supposedly play a central role in this disease by providing the intralysosomal processing of the precursor. In other forms of amyloidosis, such as those involving transthyretin and Ig LCs, partial proteolysis has been demonstrated but may as well occur after fibrillogenesis, as shown in AA amyloidosis. The demonstration of small fragments from the LC constant domain in deposited fibrils also argues in favor of a postfibrillogenic proteolysis in AL amyloidosis.

In certain types of hereditary amyloidoses due to mutations in the genes coding for the precursor protein,[125] amyloid formation seems to occur via a conformational change leading to a soluble partially folded intermediate. The property shared by these amyloidogenic variants is a native conformation that is thermodynamically less stable than that of the normal counterpart. A reduction in the stability of the variant was shown to favor the formation of partially folded conformers (alternative spatial arrangements of the same polypeptide) that have a strong propensity to self-aggregate and assemble into fibrils. Whether conclusions from structural studies of transthyretin or lysozyme mutants may be extended to other amyloidoses, including AL and AA amyloidoses, remains questionable.

Amyloidogenesis seems to be a nucleation-dependent polymerization process. Unlike other protein deposition diseases, in which amorphous aggregates are the consequence of insolubility of the pathogenic protein in the tissues, amyloid may result from a "one-dimensional crystallization." Formation of an ordered nucleus is the initial and limiting step, followed by a thermodynamically favorable addition of monomers leading to elongation of the fibrils. As shown in Alzheimer and prion diseases, the nucleation step can be overrun by adding a preformed nucleus to a supersaturated solution of the amyloidogenic protein. A similar "seeding" phenomenon may explain the "amyloid-enhancing factor" activity of extracts from amyloid-containing tissues in AA amyloidosis animal models. Recent data indicate that this activity can reside in macrophages.[126]

Distribution of Amyloid: Localized Versus Systemic Amyloidosis

Tissue localization of the deposits is characteristic of many amyloidoses (Table 60.7). Single-organ involvement may reflect either local secretion or particular tropism of the amyloid precursor. Systemic amyloidoses are derived from circulating precursors, which either display unusual structural features or are present at abnormally high plasma levels, or both. Although most cases of LC amyloidosis are due to systemic organ deposition of LCs, localized forms of LC amyloidosis have also been reported mostly in the orbit, larynx, nasopharynx, lung, skin, and the genitourinary tract. A local infiltration of plasma cells is then usually found in proximity to the amyloid deposits, and may be responsible for the secretion of an amyloidogenic LC.

Pathologic Data with Special Emphasis on Renal Involvement

Despite the diversity of amyloidogenic proteins, they all deposit in tissue as fibrils constituted by the stacking of β-pleated sheets as identified by X-ray crystallography and diffraction studies. This unique protein conformation is responsible for the tinctorial and optical properties revealed by Congo red staining of tissue sections, and for the relative resistance of the fibrils to solution in physiologic solvents and to normal proteolytic digestion, which leads to their implacable accumulation in tissues.[116]

By light microscopy, the deposits are extracellular, eosinophilic, and metachromatic. After Congo red staining, they appear faintly red and show the characteristic apple-green birefringence under polarized light. This light microscopic method is the most reliable to detect amyloid because it yields virtually no false-positive findings. Sections thicker than those usually recommended for renal pathologic examination (i.e., $>5\mu m$ in thickness) may be necessary to produce sufficient color density. Metachromasia is also observed with crystal violet, which stains the deposits in red. The use of other stains such as thioflavine T has been proposed, but the results lack specificity. The permanganate method may help to discriminate AA from AL fibrils if the sections are treated with permanganate before the Congo red procedure. AL amyloid is resistant, whereas AA amyloid is sensitive to permanganate oxidation. However, this method has been supplanted by immunohistochemical analysis of the deposits.

In the kidney, the earliest lesions are located in the mesangium, along the glomerular basement membrane, and in the blood vessels (Fig. 60.10C). Within the mesangium, deposits are associated primarily with the mesangial matrix, and subsequently irregularly increase by spreading from lobule to lobule and then invading the whole mesangial area. Amyloid deposits may also infiltrate the capillary basement membrane or be localized on both sides of it. When subepithelial deposits predominate, spikes recalling those seen in membranous glomerulopathy may be observed. It was shown that the severity of proteinuria correlated with the presence of spicules and podocyte destruction rather than with the amount of amyloid in the glomerulus. Glomerular cell proliferation is infrequent. Advanced amyloid typically produces a nonproliferative, noninflammatory glomerulopathy, responsible for a marked enlargement of the kidney. The amyloid deposits replace normal glomerular architecture with loss of cellularity. When glomeruli become massively sclerotic, the deposits may be difficult to demonstrate by Congo red staining, and electron microscopy may then be helpful. The latter may also be required at very early stages, which may not be detected by light microscopy examination in patients presenting with the nephrotic syndrome. Except in fibrinogen A α-chain amyloidosis, which characteristically does not affect renal vessels, the media of the blood vessels is prominently involved at early stages. Vascular involvement may predominate, and occasionally occur alone, particularly in AL amyloidosis (Fig. 60.10D). Deposits may also affect the tubules and the interstitium, leading to atrophy and disappearance of the tubular structures and to interstitial fibrosis. In apolipoprotein AI amyloidosis related to the Leu160Pro variant, deposits markedly predominate in the interstitium, whereas glomeruli are not or are occasionally involved.[127]

Because of the heterogeneity of amyloidotic diseases, which results in specific diagnostic and therapeutic strategies adapted to the type of protein deposited within tissues, immunofluorescence examination of snap-frozen biopsy specimens with specific antisera should be routinely performed.[128–130] In the first series published by Gallo et al.,[129] immunohistochemical classification of amyloid type was possible for 44 (88%) of 50 patients using anti-LC and anti-AA antisera. However, Noel et al.[128] pointed out that immunofluorescence with sera directed against HCs and LCs of Ig might be more difficult to interpret than with anti-AA antiserum. This is likely due to the frequent loss of LC constant domains in fibrils, accounting for the absence of epitopes normally recognized by antibodies. It is also possible that the pseudocrystalline structure of the fibrils makes these epitopes poorly accessible to antibodies. In a more recent series, 12 of 34 patients (35.3%) with proven AL-amyloidosis had negative immunofluorescence staining for κ and λ light chains, which confirms the relatively low sensitivity of immunofluorescence microscopy in the detection of AL amyloidosis in the kidney and underscores the need to pursue additional diagnostic studies to identify the plasma cell dyscrasia.[131] A genetic cause should be sought in all patients with amyloidosis that is not the reactive systemic amyloid AA type and in whom confirmation of the AL type cannot be obtained. Indeed in 350 patients with systemic amyloidosis, in whom a diagnosis of the AL type of the disorder had been suggested by clinical and laboratory findings and by the absence of a family history, amyloid mutations were present in 34 cases, most often in the genes encoding fibrinogen A α-chain (18 patients) and transthyretin (13 patients).[130] A low-grade monoclonal gammopathy was detected in 8 of the 34 patients (24%), but none of these patients had free LC identified in the urine. When the nature of the amyloid deposits remains undetermined using conventional immunohistochemical methods, novel sensitive and specific techniques, such as laser microdissection of deposits followed by mass spectrometric-based proteomic analysis, should be used, as it allows accurate typing of amyloid in most cases.[132,133]

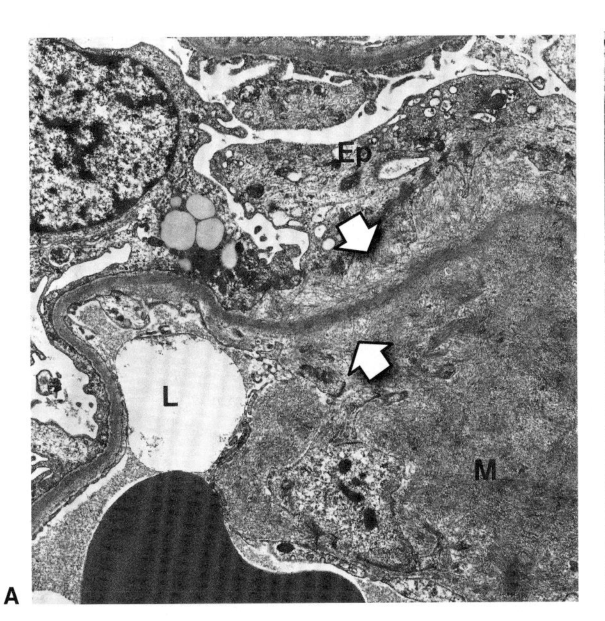

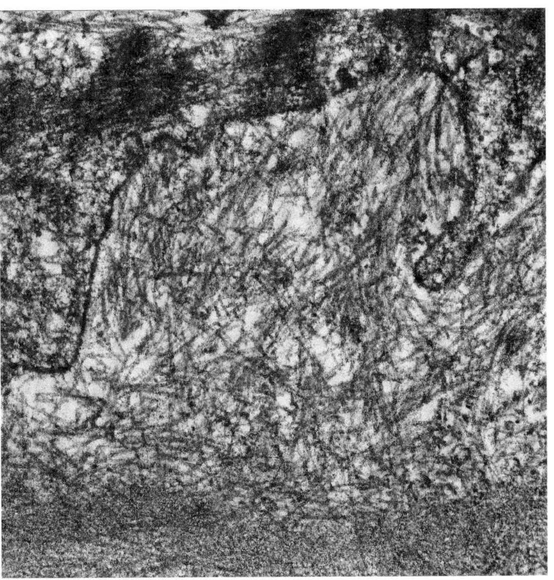

FIGURE 60.11 Amyloidosis. **A:** Electron micrograph of glomerular deposits of amyloid. Fibrils are seen in the basement membrane on both sides of the lamina densa (*arrows*). The lamina densa is attenuated. *Ep*, epithelium; *L*, capillary lumen; *M*, mesangium. (Magnification, ×5,000.) **B:** High magnification view of the randomly oriented fibrils on the epithelial aspect of the basement membrane. (Magnification, ×30,000.)

By electron microscopy, amyloid deposits are characterized by randomly oriented, nonbranching fibrils with an 8- to 10-nm diameter (Fig. 60.11). Early deposits can be found in close connection with mesangial cells that undergo important changes, and in the capillary walls distant from the mesangium on both sides of the basement membrane SAP has been found in all chemical types of amyloid thus far examined. In studies using double-label immunogold staining of AL and AA amyloid deposits, Yang and Gallo[134] showed that SAP represented 1.5% and 6.5% of the total gold label in AL and AA, respectively. SAP occurred as widely separated single units while the major fibril protein was labeled in single rows, similar to beads on a string. Immunoelectron microscopy can also be useful for the correct identification of amyloid fibril type in the fat tissue.[135]

Pathophysiologic Considerations of AL Amyloidosis

Studies on the mechanisms of AL amyloidogenesis are made particularly difficult by the unique degree of structural heterogeneity of the precursor. Each monoclonal LC is different from all others. An Ig LC typically includes two globular domains of 105 to 110 amino acids, strongly homologous to each other, that exhibit the classic conformation of all domains belonging to the "Ig superfamily" of proteins. The COOH-terminal domain (constant domain, C) is encoded by a single gene segment with very little allelic polymorphism in κ-chains and by no more than four different gene segments in λ-chains. Conversely, the NH_2-terminal domain structure (variable domain, V) results from complex somatic rearrangement and mutation events occurring in the course of B-cell differentiation, and leads to a high degree of diversity. The antiparallel β-pleated ("β-barrel") structure of Ig domains seems particularly adapted to amyloid formation. It is worth noting that another protein of the Ig superfamily, β_2-microglobulin, may form amyloid fibrils.

The implication of Ig HC in amyloidosis is exceptional. In the first case of AH amyloidosis almost entirely documented at the molecular level, the pathogenic IgG HC had an internal deletion of half the molecule, so that the V domain was directly joined to the COOH-terminal C domain C_H3, thus strikingly resembling an LC.[7] Other AH-amyloidosis cases related to deposition of IgA-related α-heavy chain,[136] or of V domains only,[137,138] or of γ3 heavy chain.[133] A case of γ-HC amyloidosis was also reported in a patient whose nephrotic syndrome recurred 6 years after autologous peripheral blood stem cell transplantation for a λ-LCDD.[139]

Not All Light Chains are Amyloidogenic

Despite predisposing conformation, a majority of Ig chains are not amyloidogenic, even at long-lasting high secretion rates. Several LC characteristics are considered amyloidogenic, particularly the LC isotype. First, the λ–κ ratio is between 2:1 and 4:1, depending on the series. Second, a homology family of LC V region, the $V_{\lambda VI}$ variability subgroup, was shown to be overrepresented in AL amyloidosis.[17] This rare subgroup is expressed exclusively in amyloid-associated monoclonal Ig and represents 41% (17/41) of amyloidogenic λ-chains.[18] A study of 55 consecutive unselected cases of primary amyloidosis showed a very skewed repertoire, as only two germline genes belonging to the λIII and λVI families, namely 3r (22% of cases, λIII) and 6a (20%, λVI), contributed equally to encode 42% of amyloid $V_\lambda$regions.[140] Furthermore, there was a significant correlation between the use of the $V_{\lambda VI}$ germline donor, IGLV6-57, and renal involvement[141,142] and that of the$V_{\lambda III}$ gene, IGLV3-1, with soft-tissue AL.[142] The use of a biased V_L gene repertoire also correlated with clinical outcome; the use of $V_{\lambda II}$ germline genes was associated with cardiac amyloidosis and affected survival adversely.[142] In contrast, no significant imbalance of the variability subgroups of κ-chains was found, but patients with κLCs were more likely to have dominant hepatic involvement.[141]

Empirical studies also show that amyloidogenicity is often associated with some physicochemical features such as the presence of low molecular mass LC fragments in the urine, and low pI; together with LC isotypy, these parameters allow the prediction of the amyloidogenic/nonamyloidogenic character of a monoclonal LC, with a correct allocation in 81% of tested cases.[143]

Comparison of Structures of Amyloid Light-Chain Precursors and Deposited Light Chains: A Role for Proteolysis?

After the demonstration by Glenner et al. that an LC was the predominant constituent of amyloid fibrils,[2] the possibility that a mutant form or a molecular variant of the soluble LC could be the amyloid precursor still remained, and only 20 years later the complete sequence identity between a circulating and a deposited LC was established.[144] Analyses of LC precursor primary structures were performed either at the protein or at the cDNA levels. All cases had an overall normal structure, including a normal C domain sequence.

The essential role of the V domain in fibrillogenesis is supported by analyses of fibrils extracted using adaptations of the method of Pras et al.,[114] which showed it to always be the main amyloid constituent. The C domain is often partially or totally absent from the fibrils after extraction. In a few cases, intact LC was present together with fragments; such heterogeneity might have been present but unrecognized in other cases. These results raise the hypothesis of a possible role of proteolysis, as already demonstrated in other forms of amyloidosis. Bellotti et al.[145] showed the disappearance of a conformational LC idiotope in the course of fibril formation, and suggested that polymerization results from the loss of the dimer conformation, possibly due to proteolysis of the C domain.

The question of a role of LC proteolysis in the amyloidogenic process has been addressed in different ways, but has not yet received a fully satisfactory answer. Abnormally low molecular mass LCs were secreted in in vitro biosynthesis experiments on bone marrow cells from AL amyloidosis subjects, but they might result from either abnormal synthesis or proteolytic processing, or both.[146,147] In vitro digestion experiments using pepsin, trypsin, and kidney lysosomes yielded fibrils resembling amyloid by electron microscopy and displaying typical Congo red binding and green polarization birefringence.[148] However, most tested LCs were from patients without amyloidosis, and the in vitro fibrils generally contained smaller fragments than those found in vivo. Another intriguing matter of all in vitro fibrillogenesis experiments is the absence of GAGs and SAP, which are invariable constituents in vivo. Although these studies contribute to the general understanding of the molecular mechanisms of fibril formation, their validity as models is questionable. In bone marrow cell culture from an AL amyloidosis patient, Durie et al.[149] found amyloidlike material immediately adjacent to macrophages, and concluded that a processing of the LCs by these cells, similar to that observed in AA amyloidosis, might lead to amyloid formation. Conversely, several observations point to the amyloidogenic potential of intact LCs; specifically, experimental mouse amyloid fibrils are made essentially of the entire injected human LC[150]; in vitro fibrils with characteristic properties of amyloid can be generated after simple reduction of the interchain disulfide bond of an intact LC dimer. Considering the sensitivity of C domains to proteases, it is conceivable that they are digested after constitution of the fibrils and tissue deposition, or during the purification process. Several recent studies have also highlighted a previously underestimated role for the LC constant domains in amyloid fibril formation, by initiating aggregation and providing a template for the V domain deposition.[151,152]

Amyloidogenic Light Chains: Light Chains with Peculiar Sequence or with Affinity for Extracellular (Matrix) Constituents?

The search for primary sequence peculiarities of the LC V domains first led to disappointing conclusions. Several unusual features such as N-glycosylations, insertion of acidic residues, and changes charged to hydrophobic residues have been noted. Infrequent amino acids at certain positions have been considered to affect the secondary structure of the framework regions or the LC dimerization. This led Stevens et al.[153] to determine amyloid-associated LC residues from the comparison of 52 pathogenic sequences with a bank of 128 other LCs. In a further report that collected 100 LCs of the VκI variability subgroup, including 37 amyloidosis cases, Stevens defined a limited number of structural risk factors, based on three sites of amino acid substitution and the occurrence of N-glycosylation.[154] A study with LC mutants bearing certain amino acids found in amyloidogenic precursors suggested that an unfolding step facilitated by these substitutions could be required for fibril formation[155]; however, the in vitro conditions were clearly nonphysiologic, and such models with single replacements have an essentially theoretical interest. Mutations in specific structural regions of LCs seem to be associated with free LC levels and amyloidogenic propensity.[156]

Environmental factors may also play some role. For example, the kidney contains high concentrations of urea that were shown to enhance fibril formation by reducing the nucleation lag time.[157] The same LC can assemble into fibrils or form granular aggregates upon exposure to various environmental conditions.[158]

One AL amyloidosis-associated LC, protein Mcg, has been extensively studied at the three-dimensional level by X-ray crystallography.[159] The dimer Mcg is strikingly "normal" and similar to other known mouse and human LCs and antigen-binding (Fab) fragments. The combination of hypervariable regions (CDRs) from both monomers mimics a normal antigen-binding site with affinities toward haptenlike compounds such as dinitrophenyl (DNP)-lysine and opioid peptides.[160] The number of contact residues and consequent binding affinity are decreased after reduction of the disulfide bond between COOH-terminal cysteinyls of the C domains.[161] Because DNP-lysine can bind specifically amyloidogenic dimers, it is possible that covalent binding between LCs influences their pathogenicity. The hypothesis that specific recognition by amyloidogenic LCs plays a pathogenic role is enforced by the demonstration of their higher dimerization constants,[162] and by the finding of high rates of somatic mutations clustered in the CDRs, suggesting antigen-driven selection.[163,164] Specific affinity of an LC toward an extracellular structure might create a nucleus that could lead to elongation of a fibril, in accordance with proposed mechanisms of other forms of amyloidogenesis.

Mechanisms of Tissue Injury

Tissue injury is mostly the consequence of extensive deposition of amyloid. However, at least in some tissues such as the heart, the infiltration alone did not correlate well with the degree of heart failure or survival. Infusion of LCs from patients with cardiac amyloidosis caused diastolic dysfunction in isolated mouse hearts.[165] Amyloid LC proteins isolated from patients with amyloid cardiomyopathy specifically provoke oxidative stress, cellular dysfunction, and apoptosis in isolated adult cardiomyocytes through activation of p38 mitogen-activated protein kinase (MAPK).[166,167] Amyloid LCs may thus contribute directly to the pathogenesis of amyloid cardiomyopathy, independent of extracellular fibril deposition. This is illustrated by the dramatic improvement in cardiac symptoms, with pararallel decrease in serum levels of sensitive markers of amyloid heart disease (NT-proBNP and troponin) whereas cardiac deposits are unchanged, that is sometimes observed after clonal response to chemotherapy. Along the same line, LCs from AL amyloid patients incubated with cultured human mesangial cells induced a macrophage-like phenotype, whereas those from LCDD patients induced a myofibroblastic phenotypic transformation.[168]

Epidemiology and Clinical Features of AL Amyloidosis

Epidemiology

The incidence of primary AL amyloidosis in the United States is 9 per million per year and has remained stable during the last four decades.[169] The male-to-female ratio varies from 1 to 2 according to series.[170–172] The median age at diagnosis is between 60 and 65 years. About two thirds of patients are between 50 and 70 years of age at diagnosis, and only 1% to 4% are younger than age 40 years.[171,173]

Amyloid deposits are found in approximately 10% of myeloma cases,[22] and this incidence reaches 20% in patients with pure LC myeloma. The high frequency of amyloidosis associated with myeloma (56%) in Alexanian's series[174] was attributed to the referral of more myeloma patients for chemotherapy to the authors' institution. Conversely, a minority (probably less than one of four) of patients with AL amyloidosis are considered to bear a patent immunoproliferative disease, which usually is a multiple myeloma, although other forms such as Waldenström macroglobulinemia and non-Hodgkin lymphoma[160] may occur. AL amyloidosis without overt immunoproliferative disease is usually referred to as *primary amyloidosis*. If multiple myeloma is not present at the diagnosis of AL amyloidosis, it is unlikely to develop.

Clinical and Laboratory Features of AL Amyloidosis

In a series of 474 patients with biopsy-proved amyloidosis, 99% of the patients were 40 years of age or older; 69% were men and 31% were women. Seventy-one patients (15%) had a myeloma. Two hundred and nineteen (56%) of 391 patients had an increased number (≥6%) of plasma cells in the bone marrow.[173]

The clinical and laboratory features at presentation and at diagnosis are summarized in Tables 60.8 and 60.9.[173,176] The main clinical symptoms at presentation are weakness and weight loss. Except for bone pain, there is no difference in the incidence of initial symptoms in patients with and without myeloma. Nephrotic syndrome, orthostatic hypotension, and peripheral neuropathy are, however, more common at diagnosis in patients with AL amyloidosis without myeloma than in those with associated myeloma (Table 60.9).

Proteinuria mainly composed of albumin is noted in 55% of the patients, indicating that glomerular involvement is a common feature of AL amyloidosis. There is a poor correlation between the extent of amyloid deposits seen on a kidney biopsy specimen and the extent of proteinuria. Even small amyloid deposits have been associated with severe nephrotic syndrome.[177] Microscopic hematuria is an exception, and, therefore, should prompt the search of a bleeding lesion of the urinary tract. Renal manifestations may also include renal tubular acidosis (mostly as a part of Fanconi syndrome) and polyuria-polydipsia (resulting from urinary concentration defect), when amyloid deposits occur around proximal tubules and Henle's loops or collecting ducts, respectively. High urinary protein excretion and high serum creatinine at diagnosis are pejorative renal predictors.[178,179] Renal insufficiency occurs usually in the presence of marked kidney enlargement and is usually not associated with hypertension.

Restrictive cardiomyopathy is found at presentation in up to one third of patients and causes death in about half.

TABLE 60.8 **Clinical and Laboratory Features at Presentation in 474 Patients with Proven AL Amyloidosis**

Initial Symptoms	
Fatigue	62%
Weight loss	52%
Pain	5%
Purpura	15%
Gross bleeding	3%
Physical Findings[a]	
Palpable liver	24%
Palpable spleen	5%
Lymphadenopathy	3%
Macroglossia	9%
Laboratory Findings	
Increased plasma cells (bone marrow ≥6%)	56%
Anemia (hemoglobin <10 g/dL)	11%
Elevated serum creatinine (≥1.3 mg/dL)	45%
Elevated alkaline phosphatase	26%
Hypercalcemia (>11 mg/dL)	2%
Proteinuria (≥1.0 g/24 hours)	55%
Urine light chain	73%[b]
κ chain	23%
λ chain	50%

[a]A comparison of the prevalence of clinical syndromes according to the presence or the absence of myeloma is given in Table 60.10.
[b]Of 429 patients. All other figures refer to all 474 cases.
Data from Kyle RA, Gertz MA. Primary systemic amyloidosis: clinical and laboratory features in 474 cases. *Semin Hematol.* 1995;32:45.

Characteristic features of amyloid on ECG include low voltages and a pattern suggestive of myocardial infarction without evidence of ischemic damage on echocardiography. Infiltration of the ventricular walls and the septum may be recognized by echocardiography. The ejection fraction is frequently normal or even increased. Doppler flow studies are required to identify diastolic dysfunction frequently missed in routine studies. Amyloid may also induce dysrhythmias and the sick sinus syndrome. Amyloid deposits in the coronary arteries may result in angina pectoris and myocardial infarction. Blood levels of cardiac troponins (including high-sensitivity cardiac troponin T) and N-terminal pro-brain natriuretic peptide (NT-proBNP) are sensitive markers of myocardial dysfunction and powerful predictors of overall survival in patients with AL amyloidosis.[180–184]

Involvement of the gastrointestinal tract is also common and can cause motility disturbances, malabsorption, hemorrhage, or obstruction. Macroglossia occurs in about one fifth of these patients. It may interfere with eating and obstruct airways. Hepatomegaly occurs initially in one third of the patients, but abnormalities of hepatic function remain generally mild. Hyposplenism, usually associated with splenomegaly, is occasionally found. Peripheral neuropathy occurs in one fifth of cases and is usually responsible for a painful sensory polyneuropathy followed later by motor deficits. Autonomic neuropathy causing orthostatic hypotension, lack of sweating, gastrointestinal disturbances, bladder dysfunction, and impotence may occur alone or together with peripheral neuropathy. Orthostatic hypotension is one of the major hampering complications of AL amyloidosis, causing some patients to be bedridden. Skin involvement may take the form of purpura, characteristically around the eyes, as well as ecchymoses, papules, nodules, and plaques, usually on the face and upper trunk. AL amyloidosis may also infiltrate articular structures and mimic rheumatoid or an asymmetric seronegative synovitis. Infiltration of the shoulders may produce severe pain and swelling ("shoulder-pad" sign). A rare but potentially serious manifestation of AL amyloidosis is an acquired bleeding diathesis that may be associated with deficiency of factor X and sometimes also factor IX, or with increased fibrinolysis.[185] It should be systematically sought before any biopsy of a deep organ. Actually, AL amyloidosis may infiltrate almost any organ other than the brain and thus be responsible for a wide variety of clinical manifestations.

On average, monoclonal LCs can be detected by immunoelectrophoresis in 73% of the urine samples, and the λ-isotype is twice as common as the κ-isotype, contrasting with the 1:2 λ-to-κ ratio observed in patients with multiple

TABLE 60.9 **Syndromes at Diagnosis in 229 Patients with Proven AL Amyloidosis**

Syndromes	Without Myeloma (182 patients)	With Myeloma (47 patients)
Nephrotic syndrome	37%	13%
Carpal tunnel syndrome	21%	38%
Congestive heart failure	23%	23%
Peripheral neuropathy	20%	6%
Orthostatic hypotension	16%	4%

Data from Kyle RA, Greipp PR. Amyloidosis (AL): clinical and laboratory features in 229 cases. *Mayo Clin Proc.* 1983;58:665.

myeloma alone. With the use of more sensitive immunochemical techniques, a serum and/or urine monoclonal Ig and/or a dysbalanced concentration of serum free LCs is found in more than 90% of patients.[186,187] It is, however, worth noting that, even under such conditions, there is no detectable monoclonal Ig in the serum and urine of some patients.

"Primary" Amyloidosis: A True Plasma Cell Dyscrasia

It is now well established that "primary" amyloidosis (i.e., AL amyloidosis without myeloma) is a true plasma cell dyscrasia. This concept, introduced by Osserman et al.,[188] was elegantly confirmed by immunofluorescence and biosynthetic studies of bone marrow cells. Preud'homme et al.[146] identified, by immunofluorescence, monoclonal plasma cell populations in 12 of 14 patients with "primary" amyloidosis, even in those without detectable serum and urine monoclonal Ig and with a normal percentage of bone marrow plasma cells. Moreover, the synthesis and excretion of large amounts of free monoclonal LCs by plasma cells were demonstrated in every patient studied by Buxbaum[147] and Preud'homme et al.,[146] together with the presence of LC fragments in almost all patients. This contrasted with nonmyelomatous secondary amyloidosis, which was characterized by normal distribution of bone marrow plasma cells by immunofluorescence and by synthesis of normal-sized Ig, without free LC secretion and fragments.[146]

From a pathophysiologic point of view, myeloma-associated and "primary" AL amyloidoses represent two ends of a single entity. The intrinsic pathogenicity of the precursor free LC is probably highly variable from one patient to another, so that expression of the disease occurs in the context of very different tumor masses and LC secretion rate. AL amyloidosis is typical of these forms of plasma cell dyscrasias in which malignancy is conferred by the pathogenic LC rather than the underlying hematologic disease.

Diagnostic Procedures in AL Amyloidosis

AL amyloidosis should be considered in any patient who presents with nephrotic range proteinuria with or without renal insufficiency, nondilated cardiomyopathy, peripheral neuropathy, hepatomegaly, or autonomic neuropathy, whether or not a paraprotein can be detected in the serum or urine. Particular vigilance should be maintained in patients with multiple myeloma or MGUS, especially of the λ isotype. Initial investigation should confirm the diagnosis of amyloidosis on tissue biopsy and this should be followed by investigations to establish the type of amyloid present and the extent of organ involvement.

All patients require immunofixation of serum and urine in an attempt to demonstrate the presence of a monoclonal LC. A bone marrow specimen is necessary because 10% of patients will not have a demonstrable monoclonal LC by immunofixation, and a clone of plasma cells detected in the bone marrow by immunofluorescence or immunohistochemistry is strong supportive evidence of AL. Immunonephelometric quantitation of free LCs is a useful complement to immunofixation, because it shows remarkable specificity and sensitivity. The assay gives a positive result (raised level of either κ or λ together with an altered ratio of free κ to free λ LC) in >90% of patients with systemic AL amyloidosis.[187,189]

Histologic diagnosis may be achieved by biopsies of various tissues. Biopsy of an affected organ is usually diagnostic, but less invasive alternatives should be preferred first. As indicated in Table 60.10, the less invasive procedures yield positive results in up to 90% of cases.[173,190] Rectal biopsy is diagnostic in greater than 80% of cases, provided that the biopsy specimen contains submucosal vessels in which early deposits are located. Bone marrow biopsy should also be stained with Congo red for the presence of amyloid, and involvement of the bone marrow is strongly suggestive of the AL type. Evaluation of adequate specimens in experienced laboratories is necessary to maintain high diagnostic sensitivity and specificity. Both false-positive and false-negative interpretations are not uncommon.

TABLE 60.10 Diagnostic Yield of Biopsies in 100 Patients with AL Amyloidosis According to the Site of Biopsy

Site of Biopsy	No. Tested	Sensitivity of the Diagnostic Procedure
Bone marrow	44	52.3
Gingiva	6	83.3
Rectal mucosa	21	85.7
Small bowel	8	87.5
Subcutaneous abdominal fat	97	88.7
Kidney[a]	21	100
Heart[a]	14	100
Liver[a]	11	100
Skin[a]	3	100
Nerve[a]	2	100
All other	22	

[a]Organ biopsy was performed because of clinical manifestations.
Data from Skinner M, Anderson J, Simms R, et al. Treatment of 100 patients with primary amyloidosis: a randomized trial of melphalan, prednisone, and colchicine versus colchicine only. *Am J Med.* 1996;100:290.

It is not always easy to be certain that amyloidosis is of the AL type because immunohistochemical staining for Ig LCs is not fully reliable, and the presence of a monoclonal component is strong but not conclusive evidence of AL. Caution is required when patients have an intact monoclonal Ig in the serum without evidence of circulating free LCs in the serum or in the urine. In those cases, hereditary forms of amyloidosis should be considered because they may produce clinical syndromes indistinguishable from AL and coexist with MGUS.[130] In cases of doubt, DNA analysis and/or amyloid fibril typing by mass spectrometric-based analysis may be necessary. Imaging using SAP scanning may be helpful in demonstrating bone marrow involvement.

A consensus panel has established criteria that define organ involvement, organ response, and organ disease progression (Table 60.11).[191] Particularly, elevation of NT-proBNP,[181] and cardiac troponins[180] are markers of myocardial dysfunction in AL amyloidosis that strongly correlate

TABLE 60.11 **Criteria for Organ Involvement, Organ Response, and Organ Disease Progression in Patients with AL Amyloidosis**

	Organ Involvement	Organ Response	Organ Disease Progression
Kidney	24-hour urine protein >0.5 g, predominantly albumin	50% decrease (at least 0.5 g/day) of 24-hour urine protein (urine protein must be >0.5 g/day pretreatment); in the absence of a reduction in eGFR ≥25% and an increase in serum creatinine ≥0.5 mg/dL (2010 consensus opinion)	50% increase (at least 1 g/day) of urine protein to greater than 1 g/day
Heart	Echo: mean wall thickness >12 mm, no other cardiac cause; or an elevated (> 332 ng/L) concentration of NT-proBNP in the absence of renal failure or atrial fibrillation (2010 consensus opinion)	Mean interventricular septal thickness decreased by 2 mm, 20% improvement in ejection fraction, improvement by two NYHA[a] classes without an increase in diuretic use, or improvement by one NYHA class associated with a 50% reduction in diuretic requirements and no increase in wall thickness; reduction (≥30% and ≥300 ng/L) of NT-proBNP concentration (2010 consensus opinion)	Interventricular septal thickness increased by 2 mm, increase in NYHA class by 1 grade with a decreasing ejection fraction of ≥10%
Liver	Total liver span >15 cm in the absence of heart failure or alkaline phosphatase >1.5 times upper limit of normal	50% decrease in abnormal alkaline phosphatase, decrease in liver size radiographically of at least 2 cm	50% increase of alkaline phosphatase above the lowest value
Nerve	P[b] (clinical): symmetric lower extremity sensorimotor neuropathy	Improvement in electromyogram nerve conduction velocity (rare)	Progressive neuropathy by electromyography or nerve conduction velocity
	A[c]: gastric-emptying disorder, pseudo-obstruction, voiding dysfunction		

[a]NYHA: New York Heart Association.
[b]P: peripheral.
[c]A: autonomic.
[d]Not related to direct organ infiltration.
Data from Gertz M, Comenzo R, Falk RH, et al. Definition of organ involvement and treatment response in primary systemic amyloidosis AL. *Am J Hematol.* 2005;79:319.

with prognosis and should be used for risk assessment staging.[182] A new consensus panel has recently updated these criteria: an elevated concentration of NT-proBNP in the absence of renal failure or atrial fibrillation, or a mean left ventricular wall thickness >12 mm by echocardiography provide criteria for cardiac involvement.[192]

Outcome and Treatment of AL Amyloidosis

"Natural" History and Markers of Prognosis

AL amyloidosis is among the most severe complications of plasma cell proliferative disorders, with a median survival of only 12 months in patients not treated or with refractory disease.[173] The natural history varies with the extent and nature of organ involvement (Table 60.12). Heart involvement is a main predictive factor of prognosis that represents more than 30% of all causes of death and is associated with a median survival of less than 6 months in patients with symptomatic heart failure.[193,194] Cardiac troponins, B natriuretic peptide (BNP), or its N-terminal fraction (NT-proBNP) have all been recognized as reliable prognostic markers in AL amyloidosis. A prognostic score based on the serum levels of troponin T and NT-proBNP has been proposed, with three stages defined by normal serum levels of troponin T and NT-proBNP (stage 1), increased level in one marker level (stage 2), or in both (stage 3).[182] The rapid achievement of hematologic response (i.e., a 50% or more reduction in serum free LC levels) is a key determinant of prognosis in AL amyloidosis,[130] particularly when serum NT-proBNP levels decrease simultaneously.[196] Recent studies suggest that treatment should aim at obtaining normal serum free LC levels and kappa/lambda ratio to improve overall and renal survival.[172,197]

TABLE 60.12 **Prognostic Factors in Patients with AL Amyloidosis**

Pejorative Prognostic Indicators
Symptomatic or substantial echocardiographic evidence of cardiac amyloid (median survival of about 6 months)
Autonomic neuropathy
Liver involvement with hyperbilirubinemia
Associated multiple myeloma
A large whole-body amyloid load on SAP scintigraphy and evidence of accumulation of amyloid on serial SAP scans when available
Better Prognostic Indicators
Proteinuria or peripheral neuropathy (without autonomic neuropathy) as the dominant clinical feature
Substantial suppression of underlying clonal disease by chemotherapy
Decrease in serum troponin and NT-proBNP levels
Regression of amyloid deposits on serial SAP scintigraphy when available

Adapted from guidelines Working Group of UK Myeloma Forum; British Committee for Standards in Haematology, British Society for Haematology. Guidelines on the diagnosis and management of AL amyloidosis. *Br J Haematol.* 2004;125:681.

Monitoring AL Amyloidosis and Assessing Response

As tissue catabolism of amyloid fibrils is a slow process, results of chemotherapy in amyloidosis may be difficult to document clinically, because organ response is often delayed after the achievement of hematologic response. Scintigraphy after the injection of ^{123}I-labeled SAP component is helpful for monitoring the extent of systemic amyloidosis,[122,189] but this technique is not readily available. Therefore, the goal of treatment in AL amyloidosis is to rapidly and efficiently suppress the underlying plasma cell, lymphoplasmacytic, or lymphoproliferative disorder that is responsible for the secretion of the amyloid precursor. As the assessment of treatment efficacy is primarily based on the evaluation of hematologic response,[191] routine measurements of serum free LC levels and markers of cardiac disease are mandatory to evaluate the effects of treatment and to rapidly modify chemotherapy if required. New criteria for hematologic response have been proposed in 2010, based on the evaluation of the difference between involved and uninvolved FLC (dFLC), the measurable absolute concentration of the involved FLC being defined by a dFLC >50 mg per L. A complete hematologic response is defined by negativity of serum and urine for a monoclonal protein by immunofixation, with normal serum free LC ratio, and less than 5% plasma cells in the bone marrow. Partial and very good partial responses are defined by a ≥50% decrease in dFLC, and by a dFLC <40 mg per L, respectively.[192] Criteria for organ response and organ disease progression are depicted in Table 60.11.

Principles of Treatment

As therapy is aimed at annihilating the plasma cell clone, all treatment strategies which have shown efficiency in multiple myeloma or in lymphoproliferative disorders can be used in AL amyloidosis, providing that they are adapted to the type of the causal hematologic disease, to the nature and number of affected organs, and bearing in mind their potential toxicity. Supportive measures to preserve organ function are essential adjuncts to therapy.

Chemotherapy and High-Dose Therapy with Stem Cell Support

MP (melphalan and prednisone) has been used for years as first-line therapy in AL amyloidosis (Table 60.13). In the 1990s two randomized controlled clinical trials showed that MP was superior to colchicine alone in terms of response and survival. However, the beneficial effect was limited, with a

TABLE 60.13 **Outcome in Previously Untreated AL Amyloidosis**

Regimen	Series	No. of Patients	Response (% all patients)[a]	TRM[b]	Overall Survival (Median)	Comments
MP	Kyle et al.[193]	77	28	Not reported	18 months	Risk of MDS
	Gertz et al.[198]	52	27	Not reported	29 months	
VAD	Lachmann et al.[199]	98	54 (63% of evaluable)	7%	50 months (projected)	Selected patients
IDM	Lachmann et al.[199]	33	46	18%	Not reached	Poor risk group
M-Dex	Palladini et al.[200]	46	67	None	Not reached	Patients ineligible for PBSCT
	Jaccard et al.[201]	50	68 (ITT: 52%)	2%	56.9 months	Selected patients
PBSCT	Comenzo and Gertz[202]	148	39 (62% of evaluable)	21%–39%	60%–70% at 1 year	Selected patients
	Skinner et al.[203]	312	40	13%	54 months	Selected patients
	Jaccard et al.[201]	50	67 (ITT: 36%)	19%	22.2 months	Selected patients

[a]Response criteria have varied but generally include response of either plasma cell dyscrasia and/or organ dysfunction.
[b]Treatment-related mortality (TRM) is defined as death during treatment or within 100 days from completing treatment. Note that the reported TRM in PBSCT studies did not include deaths during mobilization and reinfusion of peripheral blood progenitor cells.
[c]21% average of four single center studies; 39% average of two multicenter studies.
IDM, intermediate dose melphalan; ITT, intent to treat; MDS, myelodysplastic syndrome; M-HDD, melphalan and high-dose pulsed dexamethasone; MP, melphalan and prednisone; PBSCT, peripheral blood stem cell transplantation; VAD, vincristine, Adriamycin, dexamethasone.
Adapted from guidelines Working Group of UK Myeloma Forum; British Committee for Standards in Haematology, British Society for Haematology. Guidelines on the diagnosis and management of AL amyloidosis. *Br J Haematol.* 2004;125:681.

median overall survival of 18 months, compared to 12 months in patients who received no treatment or colchicine therapy alone. The poor efficacy of MP is related to a hematologic response rate of less than 30%, with a median time to response of about 12 months, far too long in patients with severe disease, particularly in those with heart involvement.

In the past 10 years, tremendous advances have been made in the treatment of AL amyloidosis. They have consisted of three major steps.

High-Dose Chemotherapy with Stem Cell Support. Ray Comenzo and colleagues first demonstrated the feasibility and efficacy of high-dose mephalan followed by ASCT (Table 60.13).[204,205] The protocol includes a step of stem cell collection after mobilization through injections of G-CSF-type growth factor, followed by high-dose melphalan of 100 to 200 mg per m^2, depending on the patient's age and disease extension. In highly experienced centers, this strategy results in a hematologic response (defined by a ≥50% reduction in sFLCs) rate of more than 60%, including 40% complete responses (CR) (defined by the absence of detectable monoclonal Ig with normal sFLCs and kappa/lambda ratio) and a median survival around 4.5 years.[203] However, the toxicity of ASCT is such that only certain patients benefit. The 100-day TRM is substantially higher among patients with AL amyloid than among those with multiple myeloma: it initially comprised between 13% and 39% mortality[202,203,206–208] and now approaches 10% even in the largest centers after careful patient selection.[209] ASCT is not recommended in patients with any of the following: age older than 70 years; symptomatic cardiac amyloid; symptomatic autonomic neuropathy; history of gastrointestinal bleeding due to amyloid; dialysis-dependent renal failure; and more than two organ systems involved.[171] In highly selected patients, the benefits of high-dose therapy with ASCT over conventional treatment are questionable. Dispenzieri et al.[210] examined data from patients with AL amyloid treated at the Mayo Clinic from 1983 to 1997, and identified 229 patients who would now have been eligible for ASCT based on age younger than 70 years and well-preserved cardiac, renal, and hepatic function. At a median follow-up of 52 months, their median survival was 42 months and 5- and 10-year survival rates were 36% and 15%, respectively. Although more than 50 studies have confirmed its efficacy over the last 10 years, ASCT in AL amyloidosis remains restricted to selected patients as previously defined.

High-Dose Dexamethasone-Based Chemotherapy. In parallel, several investigators have shown the efficacy of high-dose dexamethasone-based regimens at inducing hematologic responses and prolonging survival. Unexpected efficacy, close to that of ASCT, was obtained with the vincristine-Adriamycin-dexamethasone (VAD) and melphalan dexamethasone (MDex) regimens (Table 60.13).[189,200] MDex consists of melphalan 10 mg/m^2/day and dexamethasone 40 mg per day, 4 days per month for 6 to 12 months. MDex, which needs to be dose-adapted according to GFR and age, is more rapidly effective than the MP regimen, allowing a 60% hematologic response rate, including 25% CR and clinical responses among 50% of patients.[200] In 2007, a French multicenter randomized prospective trial showed that, compared to ASCT, MDex had similar efficacy with less toxicity, resulting in better survival (56.9 vs. 22.2 months).[201] The place of ASCT is currently debated, and to date, there is no evidence that ASCT is superior to conventional chemotherapy in improving overall survival in AL amyloidosis. Due to a low toxicity profile, with a TRM between 2% and 7%, dexamethasone-based regimens may be used even in patients with advanced disease. However, among patients with advanced amyloid cardiomyopathy, mortality remains substantial and alternative strategies are required.

Novel Antimyeloma Agents. Recently, several preliminary studies have shown encouraging results with newer antimyeloma drugs such as thalidomide, lenalidomide, and the proteasome inhibitor bortezomib. Combined with dexamethasone, these agents induce rapid hematologic responses in most patients, even in those with refractory or relapsing disease. The cyclophosphamide, thalidomide, and dexamethasone regimen appears to produce similar results as MDex alone,[211] whereas the combination of MDex with lenalidomide slightly increases hematologic response rates.[212] A striking difference has been observed with the introduction of bortezomib, which results in clonal response rates of 70% tp 90%, including around 40% of CR. Furthermore, the bortezomib plus dexamethasone regimen has shown remarkable efficacy in previously treated patients with refractory disease. These high hematologic response rates are achieved with manageable toxicity and within a relatively short time span.[213–216] In a recent phase II study, MDex plus bortezomib induced a 94% hematologic response rate, with 60% CR.[217] This combination will soon be compared to MDex in an international randomized trial. Bortezomib has to be used with caution in patients with advanced amyloid heart disease, who may occasionally develop abrupt reduction in left ventricular ejection fraction. Nevertheless, due to their superior tolerability and efficacy compared to ASCT and MDex, bortezomib-based regimens will probably become first-line therapy in systemic AL amyloidosis in the near future.

Treatment of AL Amyloidosis with Underlying Lymphoplasmacytic Proliferation

In patients with underlying lymphoplasmacytic proliferation (usually associated with an IgM monoclonal gammopathy), treatment regimens should be similar to those used in Waldenström disease (i.e., based on rituximab combined with fludarabine-cyclophosphamide) or dexamethasone plus cyclophosphamide or bortezomib.[218] Intensive therapy with high dose of melphalan followed by autologous stem cell transplantation also appears to be effective.[219]

Renal Supportive Care and Kidney Transplantation

Organ function in amyloid is precarious, and renal or cardiac failure is easily precipitated, even in individuals with apparently normal organ function by factors such as intravascular fluid depletion or intercurrent infection.

End-stage renal disease occurs in 13% to 40% of patients with AL amyloidosis,[172,219,220] after a median time that has progressed from 14 months[95,221] to about 30 months over the past 20 years,[172,220] with improved treatment strategies. Impaired renal function, and, in some series, proteinuria above 2 g per day at diagnosis, are predictive of poor renal outcome.[220–222] Above all, the achievement of hematologic response is the main factor that influences renal prognosis. In a cohort of 36 patients requiring dialysis, median time to end-stage renal disease was 6.9 months in those who did not achieve a clonal response, versus 92 months in responders.[220] The depth of clonal response also influences renal outcome: in a series of 923 patients with renal AL amyloidosis, achieving more than 90% FLC response at 6 months was associated with a fourfold increase in the chance of renal response ($P < 0.001$) and a 68% reduction in the risk of renal progression ($P < 0.001$).[172]

Median survival in patients on chronic dialysis has also progressed from 8 to 10 months to 26 to 39 months in recent series.[172,222] The survival rate of patients treated with chronic ambulatory peritoneal dialysis (CAPD) is similar to that of patients on hemodialysis.

Cardiac amyloid is the most important predictor of poor survival in patients with AL amyloidosis undergoing dialysis, and cardiac deaths represent the main cause of mortality in such patients.[220–222] Congestive heart failure, atrioventricular or intraventricular conduction defects, and dysrhythmias due to amyloid myocardial involvement often occur. The management of patients with AL amyloid on hemodialysis is also often complicated by permanent hypotension, gastrointestinal hemorrhage, chronic diarrhea, and difficulties in the creation and maintenance of vascular accesses. It has, therefore, been suggested that CAPD could have several advantages over hemodialysis in the management of end-stage renal amyloidosis, including avoiding vascular access and deleterious effect on blood pressure; however, CAPD may induce protein loss in the dialysate fluid and thereby enhance malnutrition.

AL amyloidosis is usually considered a relative contraindication to renal transplantation, even among patients with isolated renal involvement, due to organ shortage and the lack of effective therapy to prevent disease recurrence in the allograft and/or progressive extrarenal amyloidosis. The same limitations were also applied to cardiac transplantation in patients with dominant cardiac disease. Furthermore, risk of death from infectious complications of kidney transplantation was reportedly high.[223] As survival of patients on chronic dialysis has progressively improved in recent years, an increasing number of patients are candidates for kidney transplantation. Recent studies suggest that renal transplantation may be a valid option in patients with limited extrarenal manifestations, and whose underlying clonal plasma cell disease has remitted following chemotherapy. In a series of 22 renal transplant recipients with AL amyloidosis, 1- and 5-year patient survival was 95% and 67%, respectively. Nineteen patients had received chemotherapy or ASCT before renal transplantation, which induced clonal response in 14 of 15 evaluable patients. No transplant failed due to amyloid recurrence, despite evidence of amyloid within the allografts of five patients.[224] In another recent study of 19 patients, 11 underwent renal transplantation after a hematologic response had been achieved either with ASCT (six patients) or conventional chemotherapy (mostly MDex-based, five cases). In the remaining patients kidney transplantation was performed prior to ASCT. Twelve patients had limited extrarenal disease, including heart involvement in nine. Hematologic treatment resulted in clonal CR in all but one patient. After a median follow-up time of 41.4 months, 15 patients (79%) were alive. Recurrence of LC amyloid deposits on the renal allograft occurred in two cases. All allograft losses were the result of patient death, mainly related to infectious or cardiovascular events.[225] New drugs, particularly bortezomib, which are effective and well tolerated in patients with ESRD, will probably enable more patients with AL amyloidosis to be eligible for solid organ transplantation by inducing deep and sustained hematologic responses.

Epidemiology and Specific Features of AA Amyloidosis

Although AA amyloidosis does not involve deposition of Ig fragments and thus should not be classified within the group of monoclonal gammopathies, it shares with AL amyloidosis pathogenetic pathways, high prevalence of renal involvement, and some therapeutic aspects that deserve further consideration.

AA amyloidosis develops in 5% of patients with sustained elevation of serum amyloid A protein (SAA). Patients at risk are those with long duration of chronic inflammatory disease (median, about 10 years), high magnitude of acute phase SAA response, homozygosity for SAA1 isotype, familial Mediterranean fever (FMF) trait (heterozygosity for variant pyrin), and family history of AA amyloidosis (50% risk).

An important epidemiologic aspect of AA amyloidosis is the changing spectrum of underlying diseases (Table 60.14).

TABLE 60.14 Changing Spectrum of Underlying Diseases in Secondary AA Amyloidosis[a]

	Dahlin[226] (n = 30)	Brownstein et al.[227] (n = 100)	Browning et al.[228] (n = 60)	Gertz and Kyle[229] (n = 64)	Joss et al.[230] (n = 43)	Gillmore et al.[231] (n = 80)	Lachmann et al.[232] (n = 374)
Rheumatic disease	2 (7)	15 (15)	55 (73)	42 (66)	30 (70)	60 (60)	224 (60)
Granulomatous infection (tuberculosis, fungus, leprosy)	9 (30)	28 (28)	8 (11)	0	6 (14)	0	3 (1)
Pyogenic infection	10 (33)	35 (35)	5 (7)	11 (17)	0	7 (9)	53 (14)
Inflammatory bowel disease	2 (7)	4 (4)	3 (4)	6 (9)	1 (2)	2 (3)	17 (4)
Malignancy/Castleman	7 (23)	18 (18)	3 (4)	2 (3)	1 (2)	2 (3)	11 (3)
Other[b]	—	—	2 (3)	3 (5)	5 (12)	9 (11)	34 (9)

[a]Data are number of patients (percentage).
[b]Including hereditary recurrent fevers and unknown.

Pyogenic and granulomatous infections, especially tuberculosis, account for far fewer cases than in the older series. This is because of the efficacy of antibiotic treatments for bacteria, which shows that amyloidosis can be efficiently prevented when its cause is suppressed. In contrast, the prevalence of amyloid linked to autoimmune inflammatory diseases, such as rheumatoid arthritis and juvenile chronic arthritis, has increased dramatically, reaching 60% in the largest series published to date.[232] AA amyloidosis in patients with Hodgkin disease has virtually disappeared with more efficient treatment of the hematologic disease. In contrast, hereditary AA amyloidoses associated with familial recurrent fever syndromes are claiming an increasing portion of about 10% of cases in recent series.

There are a number of clinical manifestations of AA amyloidosis (Table 60.15).[228,229] The main target organ by far is the kidney, affected in almost all patients with AA amyloidosis. Renal dysfunction may be acute with nephrotic syndrome, or very insidious. Proteinuria is absent in about 5% of cases. Gastrointestinal disturbances (including diarrhea, constipation, and malabsorption) and hepatosplenomegaly are the most common after kidney manifestations. In contrast with AL amyloidosis, congestive heart failure, peripheral neuropathy, macroglossia, and carpal tunnel syndrome occur in less than 10% of patients. Peripheral or autonomic neuropathy is rare, as well as involvement of adrenal glands and thyroid. The reason for the differential distribution of AA and AL tissue deposits is not understood.

The optimal method for diagnosing AA amyloidosis remains controversial. Although kidney biopsy is positive in about 100% of symptomatic patients, less invasive biopsy procedures should be preferred first (Table 60.15). Biopsies of accessory salivary glands, abdominal fat, and rectal mucosa yield positive results in 50% to 80% of patients. Immunohistochemical staining using antibodies to SAA is required to confirm that Congo red positive amyloid deposits are of AA type. SAP scintigraphy, when available, shows early accumulation of amyloid in spleen, kidneys, and adrenal glands whereas bones are not affected (contrary to AL amyloid).

Survival time of patients with AA amyloidosis is usually longer than in AL amyloidosis (Table 60.15). Elevated serum creatinine or end-stage renal disease at baseline, older age, and a low serum albumin are strong adverse prognostic indicators. Main causes of death are infections and dialysis complications, but not cardiac complications. Estimated survival was about 40% at 3 years, and median survival time was approximately 2 years, in older series.[228,229] In a recent series, estimated median survival from diagnosis was 133 months, indicating that prognosis of systemic AA has improved over the years.[232]

Amyloid load and clinical outcome in AA amyloidosis are dependent on circulating concentrations of SAA.[231] In a cohort of 374 patients who were followed for a median of 86 months, Lachmann et al. showed that amyloid burden increased in 12%, was unchanged in 48%, and decreased in 39%; SAA values were significantly lower (median, 7 mg per L) in patients in whom amyloid regressed, than in those in whom the amyloid burden increased (median, 54 mg per L) ($P < 0.001$). The median SAA concentration during each year of follow-up was strongly associated with survival: the relative risk of death among patients with a SAA level <4 mg per L was 18 times lower than among patients in whom SAA level was ≥155 mg per L. Similarly, median SAA values were 6 mg per L in patients in whom renal function improved, and 28 mg per L in those who showed progression of chronic kidney disease (CKD).[232] These data emphasize the fact that underlying inflammatory diseases responsible for amyloid must be treated as vigorously as possible and SAA (preferentially to C reactive protein [CRP]) levels must be monitored monthly and maintained at a target value of less than 5 to 10 mg per L. In patients with inflammatory arthritis, antitumor necrosis factor-*α* therapy may help to achieve this goal.[233]

Other factors promote progression of CKD in systemic AA amyloidosis, including the amount of proteinuria, and associated cardiac or hepatic disease.[220,230] Kidney biopsy may also provide indicators of pejorative renal outcome, such as predominant glomerular pattern of deposits, glomerular inflammation,[234] quantity of amyloid deposition, extent of tubulointerstitial and vascular damage.[235] End-stage renal disease, that occurs in 23% to 47% of patients within variable median time (18 to 245 months) after diagnosis is a factor of poor patient survival.[220,230,232] Median survival of patients with SAA amyloidosis on renal replacement therapy is 37 months, whatever the method used, hemodialysis or peritoneal dialysis, with amyloid heart involvement being the major cause of death.[220] A few studies have shown encouraging results with renal transplantation in patients with AA amyloidosis, close to that of the general population of transplant recipients.[223,236–238] In a series of 62 renal transplantations including 29 grafts from related living donors,[223] the 1-year actuarial patient survival rate was 79%, decreasing to 65% after 5 years. Recently, in 59 renal recipients with AA amyloidosis, 5- and 10-year patient survival rates were 82.5% and 61.7%, respectively, significantly lower when compared with a control group of 177 renal transplant recipients. However, no statistical difference was observed in the 5- and 10-year graft survival censored for death between the two groups.[239] Amyloid deposits recur in about 10% of the grafts.[223,236,239] There is a high risk of infection that is the main cause of early deaths. As with dialysis, cardiac involvement is a major threat for patients receiving renal transplants. Efforts should be made to control SAA levels in these patients to improve both graft and patient outcomes.

Familial Mediterranean Fever and Other Hereditary Recurrent Fever Syndromes

Familial Mediterranean fever (FMF) is both a particular type of AA amyloidosis and the most common cause of familial amyloidosis. Colchicine has proved to be efficient both in the prevention and treatment of this type of

TABLE 60.15 **Characteristics of Patients with Secondary AA Amyloidosis**

	No. of Patients	Age (yrs)	Male–Female Ratio	Presenting Clinical Syndrome—no. (%)	Source of Tissue for Diagnosis—no. (%)	Causes of Death—no./totals (%)	Survival
Browning, et al.[228]	60	57 (18–81)	0.8	Proteinuria/renal failure—49 (65) Gastrointestinal disturbance—4 (5) Hepatosplenomegaly—3 (4)	Rectum—45 (60) Kidney—11 (15)	Renal failure—18/37 (49) Bronchopneumonia—7/37 (19) Cardiac—4/37 (11)	~40% at 3 years
Gertz and Kyle[229]	64	56 (14–80)	1.5	Proteinuria/renal failure—58 (91) Gastrointestinal disturbance—14 (22) Goiter—6 (9) Neuropathy/carpal tunnel—2 (3)	Rectum—32 (50) Kidney—24 (38) Stomach/small bowel—15 (23) Marrow—12 (19)	Uremia/dialysis complications—32/47 (68) Sepsis—4/47 (9) Cardiac—4/47 (9)	~40% at 3 years Median = 24.5 mos
Lachmann[232]	374	50 (9–87)	1.3	Proteinuria/renal failure—363 (97) Gastrointestinal disturbance—NA Hepatomegaly—35 (9) (hepatic amyloidosis on SAP scintigraphy = 85) (23%) Cardiac amyloid = 2/224 (1%)* Adrenal deposits on SAP scintigraphy = 153 (41)	NA	NA	56% after median follow-up time of 86 months (range: 2–47) Median survival: 133 months

amyloidosis.[240] FMF is usually transmitted as an autosomal recessive disorder and occurs most commonly in Sephardic Jews and Armenians.[241] Mutations of the gene for proteins called pyrin or marenostrin have been demonstrated.[242,243] Clinically, there are two independent phenotypes. In the first, brief episodic febrile attacks of peritonitis, pleuritis, or synovitis occur in childhood or adolescence and precede the renal manifestations. In the second, renal symptoms precede and may be the only manifestation of the disease for a long time. The attacks are accompanied by dramatic elevations of acute phase reactants, including SAA. Amyloid deposits of the AA type are responsible for severe renal lesions with prominent glomerular involvement leading to end-stage renal disease at a young age, and early death. Zemer et al.[240] showed that in a cohort of 1,070 patients with FMF, colchicine, an agent effective in preventing attacks,[244] could prevent the appearance of proteinuria and deterioration of renal function (in patients with amyloidosis who had proteinuria but not the nephrotic syndrome or renal insufficiency). Life-table analysis showed that the cumulative rate of proteinuria was 1.7% after 11 years in the compliant patients and 48.9% after 9 years in the noncompliant patients ($P < .0001$). In 1992, the authors further showed that colchicine reversed the nephrotic syndrome in three patients.[245] They insisted on the importance of a dosage adapted to the clinical situation. The minimum daily dose of colchicine for prevention of amyloidosis is 1 mg even if attacks are suppressed by a smaller dose. Patients with clinical evidence of amyloidotic kidney disease and kidney transplant recipients should receive daily doses of between 1.5 and 2.0 mg. The recombinant IL-1 receptor antagonist anakinra and potentially other IL-1 targeting drugs may represent an effective treatment in the 10% of patients who are resistant to colchicine therapy,[246] or develop severe side effects with colchicine.

Next to FMF, there is a growing family of hereditary autoinflammatory disorders that bear the significant risk of developing AA amyloidosis (Table 60.16). Recent advances into their pathogenesis with the identification of susceptibility genes and characterization of pathways involved in raised acute phase response have resulted in new therapeutic approaches. Among these, Il-1 blockade with anakinra and anti-TNF agents have shown variable results in the treatment of TNF receptor-associated periodic syndrome (TRAPS) and hyper IgD syndrome. Remarkably, Il-1 blockade with either anakinra,[247] rinolacept,[248] or canakinumab (a human anti-IL1β monoclonal antibody)[249] was shown to produce rapid and complete clinical and inflammatory responses in most patients with cryopirin-asociated periodic syndrome (CRAPS), an entity that comprises three different diseases: familial cold autoinflammatory syndrome (FCAS), Muckle-Wells syndrome (MWS), and chronic infantile neurologic, cutaneous, and articular (CINCA) syndrome. Anakinra is also effective in the treatment of the newly described autoinflammatory disease due to deficiency of the IL-1 receptor antagonist.[250]

Therapeutic Prospects

New therapeutic strategies should be directed at the three steps of the amyloidogenic process: synthesis of the precursor, deposition of amyloid fibrils, and removal or dissolution of amyloid fibrils.

Prevention of Amyloid Precursor Synthesis

Curing the underlying disease has proved to be extremely effective, as shown in inflammation-related AA amyloidosis. This objective must be envisioned in all forms of amyloidosis. The possibility of immunotargeting against precursor synthesis is also worth exploring.

Prevention of Amyloid Fibril Deposition

A potential therapeutic strategy is blockade of RAGE (receptor for advanced glycation end-products), a multiligand receptor of the immunoglobulin superfamily that also is a receptor for the amyloidogenic form of serum amyloid A. Antagonizing RAGE with a soluble form of the receptor or with blocking antibodies inhibits amyloid deposition in the spleen of mice injected with amyloid-enhancing factor and silver nitrate.[251]

Rapidly growing data on the nucleation process might lead to the synthesis of nucleation inhibitors for all types of amyloid. Low-molecular-weight (135 to 1,000) anionic sulfate or sulfate compounds were shown to interfere with heparan sulfate-stimulated β-peptide fibril aggregation in vitro.[252] When administered orally, these compounds by inhibiting polymerization and tissue deposition of amyloid fibrils substantially reduced murine splenic AA amyloid progression. In a prospective randomized trial in patients with AA amyloidosis and kidney involvement, one of these compounds, eprodisate, reduced by 30% the mean rate of decline in creatinine clearance, compared to placebo.[253] Further studies are needed to evaluate whether such agents (that may theoretically apply to other types of amyloid), will have a major impact on patients with AA amyloidosis who do not respond to therapy for the underlying disorder.

Removal or Dissolution of Amyloid Fibrils and Immunotherapeutic Perspectives

The regression of amyloid deposits under effective treatment of the underlying disease as well as the finding that amyloid deposits may undergo redistribution strongly suggest that amyloid fibrils can be catabolized and removed from tissues. This process is most likely restrained by proteinase inhibitors that have been detected in amyloid deposits of various types, and by fibril coating with the calcium-dependent lectin SAP.[120] A potential approach, therefore, would be to block these inhibitors to target proteolytic enzymes at the amyloid deposition site or to dissociate SAP with competitive ligands.

At present, most attempts to use dimethylsulfoxide (DMSO) as an amyloid solvent have been disappointing because of lack of efficacy and bad odor from the patient's breath. Similarly the clinical efficacy of the iodinated anthracycline, (4′-iodo-4′-deoxydoxorubicin) that binds

TABLE 60.16 **Main Autoinflammatory Syndromes**

	FMF	TRAPS	MWS	FCAS	CINCA/NOMID	HIDS	DIRA
Ethnic geographic background	Sephardic Jews Armenians Turkish	Europe	Europe	Northern Europe	Northern Europe	Northern Europe	Northern Europe, Canada, Lebanon
Inheritance	Autosomal recessive	Autosomal dominant	Autosomal dominant	Autosomal dominant	Sporadic	Autosomal recessive	Autosomal recessive
Gene	MEFV (16p13)	TNFRSF1A (12p13)	NRLP3/CIAS1 (1q44)	NRLP3/CIAS1 (1q44)	NRLP3/CIAS1 (1q44)	MVK (12q24)	IL1RN (2q14.2)
Protein	Pyrin/marenostrin	55 kDa TNF receptor	Cryopyrin	Cryopyrin	Cryopyrin	Mevalonate kinase	IL-1 receptor antagonist
Age at onset	Childhood	Variable	Variable	Childhood	Neonatal	Childhood	Childhood
Duration of attacks (days)	±3–4	± 7–21	± continuous (worse in the evenings)	± 1–2 (cold-induced)	Continuous	3–7	Continuous
Abdominal pain	++	++	+	+	−	+	−
Articular symptoms	Arthritis ++	Arthritis +	Arthritis +	Arthritis +	Deforming arthropathy	+	Sterile osteomyelitis, periostitis
Skin	+/− Rash	++ Erysipeloid	++ Urticaria	++ Urticaria	Urticaria	+ Rash	+ Pustulosis
Deafness	−	−	+	−	+	−	−
			Conjunctivitis	Conjunctivitis			
Other	Sephardic Jews		Europe	Northern Europe	Aseptic meningitis	Diarrhea, lymphadenopathy	Mental retardation

FMF, familial Mediterranean fever; TRAPS, TNF receptor-associated periodic syndrome; MWS, Muckle-Wells syndrome; FCAS, familial cold autoinflammatory syndrome, CINCA/NOMID, chronic infantile neurologic cutaneous and articular syndrome/neonatal-onset multisystem inflammatory disease; HIDS, hyperimmunoglobulin-D syndrome; DIRA, deficiency of the IL-1 receptor antagonist.
Adapted from Lachmann HJ, Hawkins PN. Developments in the scientific and clinical understanding of autoinflammatory disorders. *Arthritis Res Ther*. 2009;11:212.

specifically and with high affinity to all the natural amyloid fibrils and promotes the disaggregation of fibrils both in vitro and in vivo,[254] is not established.[123,255]

A competitive inhibitor of SAP binding to amyloid fibrils has been developed by Pepys et al.[123] This palindromic compound, referred to as *R*-1-[6-[*R*-2-carboxy-pyrrolidin-1-yl]-6-oxo-hexanoyl] pyrrolidine-2-carboxylic acid (CPHPC), also crosslinks and dimerizes SAP molecules, leading to their very rapid clearance by the liver, and thus produces a marked depletion of circulating human SAP. Preliminary studies of the therapeutic effect of CPHPC in mice and humans were unsuccessful, because despite efficient depletion in circulating SAP, significant amounts of SAP remained in the amyloid deposits. Recently, the same group elegantly demonstrated the validity of this approach. In an experimental model of AA amyloidosis in mice transgenic for human SAP, depletion of circulating SAP with oral CPHPC, followed by a single injection of polyclonal antihuman SAP antibodies, efficiently removed massive visceral amyloid deposits, without adverse effects. Elimination of tissue deposits was related to a potent complement-dependent macrophage-derived giant cell reaction, triggered by human anti-SAP antibodies.[124] Clinical evaluation based on a fully humanized anti-SAP antibody is planned.

The immune system might be manipulated in order to recognize amyloid fibrils as harmful foreign entities. In AL amyloidosis, Hrncic et al. demonstrated that a monoclonal antibody specific for a conformational determinant could accelerate the clearing of amyloid.[256] This antibody recognizes an epitope contained within the first N-terminal amino acids of misfolded LCs.[257] Although we are still far from applicable human immunotherapy, such experimental approaches might lead to future developments.

MONOCLONAL IMMUNOGLOBULIN DEPOSITION DISEASE

History and Nomenclature

It has been known since the late 1950s that nonamyloidotic forms of glomerular disease can occur in multiple myeloma. Kobernick and Whiteside[258] and Sanchez and Domz[259] first described glomerular nodules "resembling the lesion of diabetic glomerulosclerosis," lacking the staining features and fibrillar organization of amyloid. The monoclonal LC content of these lesions was confirmed by Randall et al.,[3] who published the first description of LCDD in 1976.

Monoclonal HCs were found together with LCs in the tissue deposits from certain patients, and the term light and heavy chain deposition disease (LHCDD) was proposed.[260] Deposits containing monoclonal HCs only, that is, in the absence of detectable LCs, were first observed in 1993 in patients affected with otherwise typical Randall disease (HC deposition disease [HCDD]),[5] and three series of similar patients were published later.[6,261,262] More than 30 cases of HCDD have been reported so far, but this disease is most likely underdiagnosed. In two further cases, termed "pseudo-γ HCDD," predominant $\gamma 4$ chain deposits were demonstrated with similar pathologic aspects; the authors suggested that misfolding or denaturation of the LC was responsible for its nonreactivity with specific antibodies.[263]

In clinical and pathologic terms, LCDD, LHCDD, and HCDD are essentially similar and are now gathered under the generic term of monoclonal Ig deposition disease (MIDD). They differ from amyloidosis by the lack of affinity for Congo red and lack of fibrillar organization. The distinction also relates to different pathophysiology of amyloid, which implicates one-dimensional elongation of a pseudocrystalline structure, and of MIDD, which would rather involve a one-step precipitation of Ig chains.

Pathophysiology

The pathogenetic mechanisms leading to MIDD remain entirely hypothetical because circulating or urinary monoclonal immunoglobulin chain precursors are frequently not detected, or present at very low levels, making their purification and analysis particularly difficult, and data on the precise nature of the visceral deposits remains speculative. In LCDD, there is a modest but significant overrepresentation of κ chains occurring in approximately 80% of cases (versus approximately two-thirds among polyclonal Ig), which contrasts with the increased λ to κ ratio observed in AL-amyloidosis. The rare $V\kappa_{IV}$ variability subgroup is frequent,[19] which is worth noting because this subgroup features a strikingly long complementarity-determining region 1 (CDR1) loop that contains several hydrophobic residues; however, contrary to the $V\lambda_{VI}$ subgroup, which was found exclusively on monoclonal LCs from AL amyloidosis patients,[18] $V\kappa_{IV}$ LCs may be encountered in myeloma without renal involvement.

That immunoglobulin chain deposition involves unusual immunoglobulin chain properties is supported by the absence of detectable monoclonal component in the serum and urine in 10% to 20% of patients with MIDD, the recurrence of the disease in the transplanted kidney, and the biosynthesis of abnormal LCs by bone marrow plasma cells.[12,260]

Abnormal Glycosylation and Structure of MIDD LCs

Structural abnormalities of immunoglobulins in MIDD have long been suggested by empirical studies of in vitro bone marrow cell biosynthesis products.[12,260] In a study of immunoglobulin biosynthesis by bone marrow plasma cells in eight consecutive patients, LCs were of normal size in two cases, and short or apparently large in the other six patients. These short or large LCs showed a striking ability to polymerize when secreted in vitro. Abnormal glycosylation may be responsible for an increase in apparent molecular weight of the corresponding LC.

When pathogenic LCs could not be detected in the serum and urine, they were N-glycosylated in all tested cases.[19,263] In vitro biosynthetic labeling experiments on short-term plasma cell cultures showed that LCs which were absent in the urine actually were secreted by the bone marrow plasma cells.[12,15,260] Together with the presence of exposed hydrophobic residues, LC glycosylation might increase the propensity of LCs to precipitate in tissues and displace the equilibrium from soluble toward deposited forms so that they are no more detectable in the body fluids.

Sequence Analysis

The first complete primary structure of an LC in LCDD was determined by Cogné et al. in 1991.[15] The 30-kDa κ chain found in the kidney was presumably identical to that secreted by the malignant plasma cells, since they shared the same apparent molecular mass and 13-amino acid N-terminal sequence. It was encoded by a normal-sized κ mRNA and was *N*-glycosylated. The C region was entirely normal and the V region belonged to the $V\kappa_{IV}$ subgroup. Eight mutations were observed, including replacement of Pro95 (considered as essential for the conformation of the third hypervariable region). Replacement of Asp70 by Asn determined a *N*-glycosylation site.

The primary structures of a few further LCDD precursors were analysed at the complementary DNA and protein levels. Most peculiarities are clustered in peptide loops corresponding to CDRs, that is, parts of the molecules normally implicated in antigen binding, suggesting that a first step of the pathogenesis could be an LC tropism for extracellular components behaving as antigenlike structures. The most remarkable observations were unusual hydrophobic residues at positions where they could either be exposed to the solvent or strongly modify the conformation, potentially leading to LC aggregation or interaction with other hydrophobic molecules.[265] A role for V domain in renal tissue deposition was demonstrated in a mouse experimental model, in which the injection of hybridoma cells transfected with the human LCCD Vκ4 FRA LC resulted in diffuse granular glomerular deposits, identical to those observed in the patient's kidney biopsy. Injection of cells that secreted a control Vκ4 LC, with the same C domain, but which differed from FRA by few residues in the hypervariable region, did not induce LC glomerular deposition.[266]

In a recent study, it was shown that LCDD LCs are characterized by cationic isoelectric points (pIs), whereas pI profile of AL amyloid LCs is heterogeneous, suggesting that fibrillar amyloid deposits form by electrostatic interaction between oppositely charged polypeptides, whereas granular deposits in LCDD result from binding of cationic polypeptides to anionic basement membranes.[267]

However, as in AL amyloidosis, extrinsic conditions may also contribute to aggregation of the LC. The same LC can form granular aggregates or amyloid fibrils depending on the environment, and different partially folded intermediates of this protein may be responsible for amorphous or fibrillar aggregation pathways.[268]

Heavy-Chain Deposition Disease: A Disease Featuring Heavy-Chain Deletions

A deletion of the first constant domain C_H1 was found in the deposited or circulating HC in all patients with γ-HC deposition disease where this deletion was searched for (Table 60.17).[5,6,262,269–272] It also was suggested in a patient

TABLE 60.17 **Immunologic Characteristics of Patients with Heavy-Chain Deposition Disease (HCDD) According to IG Subtype**[a]

	No. of Patients	C_H1 Deletion	Complement Deposition	Complement Activation
γ1	10	7/7[b]	7/10	9/10
γ2	1	NS	1 (weak)	0/1
γ3	6	4/4	4/4	4/4
γ4	3	2/2	1 (weak)	NS
γ (isotype not specified)	4	NS	1/1	0/1
α	2	NS	1/2	0/2
μ	1	NS	1/1	0/1

[a]Cases are from references 8, 9, 352, 359, and 360.
[b]In one patient, C_H1 and C_H2 were deleted.[8]
NS, not specified.

with α HCDD.[273] A larger deletion also including the C_H1 domain, the hinge, and the C_H2 domain was found in one case.[5] In the blood, the deleted HC was associated with LCs, mostly of the λ isotype, or circulated in small amounts as a free unassembled subunit.[6] It is likely that the C_H1 deletion facilitates the secretion of free HCs that are rapidly cleared from the circulation by organ deposition.[274] Deletion of the C_H1 is also found in HC disease, a lymphoproliferative disorder with free HC secretion without corresponding renal tissue deposition, and in AH amyloidosis in which deposits have a fibrillar organization. In heavy chain disease, however, the variable domain also is partially or completely deleted, which suggests that the V_H domain is required for tissue precipitation. Sequence analysis of two HCDD proteins did show unusual amino acid substitutions in the V_H, which might change their physicochemical properties, including charge and hydrophobicity.[375]

Deposition Does Not Mean Pathogenicity

The finding by Solomon et al.[14] of unexpectedly frequent (14 of 40) deposition of human monoclonal LCs along basement membranes in a mouse experimental model raises the question of the relationship between tissue precipitation and pathogenic effects. Although approximately 80% of MIDDs are caused by κ chains, human LCs that deposited along basement membranes in mice were predominantly of the λ type (9 of 14). In addition, LC deposition similar in aspect to LCDD by immunofluorescence but with only scanty granular electron-dense deposits in the tubular basement membrane may occur in the absence of glomerular lesions and tubular basement membrane thickening.[262] Whether the diagnosis of MIDD should be restricted to the patients with extracellular matrix accumulation, remains debated. However, follow-up data indicate that the subgroup of patients with evidence of LC deposition by immunofluorescence and negative electron microscopy is not characterized by a milder course.[261]

Pathophysiology of Extracellular Matrix Accumulation

A striking feature of MIDD is the dramatic associated accumulation of extracellular matrix.[277] Nodules are made of normal constituents and of tenascin-C. They stain weakly for the small proteoglycans, decorin and biglycan. A role for transforming growth factor-β (TGF-β) is supported by its strong expression in glomeruli of MIDD patients, and by in vitro experiments using cultured mesangial cells.[278] In a series of 36 patients with LC-related renal diseases including AL amyloidosis, CN, fibrillary glomerulopathy, and LCDD, transforming growth factor-β (TGF-β) was detected only in glomeruli of the three patients with LCDD and nodular glomerular lesions.[279] In the control series, TGF-β was essentially found in nodular diabetic glomerulosclerosis, which may suggest that distinct initial insults to the glomerular mesangium may trigger similar fibrogenetic pathways. Because of the similarities between MIDD- and diabetes-induced nodular glomerulosclerosis, including the strong reactivity of lesions with the periodic acid-Schiff (PAS) reagent, it has been suggested that immunoglobulin chains might stimulate mesangial cells in a similar manner to advanced glycation end-products (AGEs). Recent experiments[280] showed that monoclonal LCs responsible for LCDD or AL amyloidosis are endocytosed by cultured mesangial cells through a yet unidentified caveolae-associated receptor, and that different pathologic actions probably result from distinct cellular trafficking. Indeed, mesangial cells incubated with LCs from patients with MIDD or AL amyloidosis undergo either a myofibroblastic or a macrophagelike phenotypic transformation after incubation with LCDD or AL LCs, respectively. LCCD LCs, when incubated with mesangial cells, induce cell changes, production of PDGF-β, TGF-β, and MCP-1, as well as increased expression of Ki-67, a proliferation marker. This results in increased synthesis of extra-cellular matrix proteins (particularly tenascin-C), that, combined with decreased production and activity of metalloproteases, is likely to be involved in the development of glomerulosclerosis.[168,281,282]

Pathologic Features

Light Microscopy

MIDD should not be considered a pure glomerular disease. In fact, tubular lesions may be more conspicuous than the glomerular damage. Tubular lesions are characterized by the deposition of a refractile, eosinophilic, PAS-positive, ribbon-like material along the outer part of the tubular basement membrane in virtually all patients with MIDD. The deposits predominate around the distal tubules, Henle's loops, and in some instances the collecting ducts, the epithelium of which is flattened and atrophied. Typical myeloma casts are only occasionally seen. In advanced stages, a marked interstitial fibrosis including refractile deposits is frequently associated with tubular lesions. In rare cases, inflammatory infiltrates composed predominantly of lymphocytes and plasma cells and associated with tubulitis, are observed in the absence of glomerular lesions.[283]

Glomerular lesions are much more heterogeneous.[274] Nodular glomerulosclerosis is the most characteristic (Fig. 60.12A), being found in 30% to 100% of patients with LCDD.[262,274] Kappa-LC deposition is more likely than λ-LC deposition to be associated with nodular glomerulosclerosis and granular electron-dense deposits (see subsequent text).[261] Expansion of the mesangial matrix was observed in all cases of HCDD, with nodular glomerulosclerosis in almost all of them.[6,262] Mesangial nodules are composed of PAS-positive membranelike material and are often accompanied by mild mesangial hypercellularity. The capillary loops stretch at the periphery of florid nodules and may undergo aneurysmal dilation. The Bowman's capsule may contain a material identical to that present in the center of the nodules. These lesions resemble nodular diabetic glomerulosclerosis,

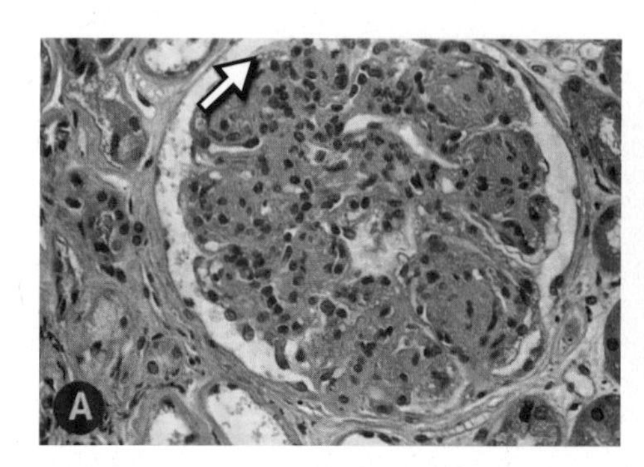

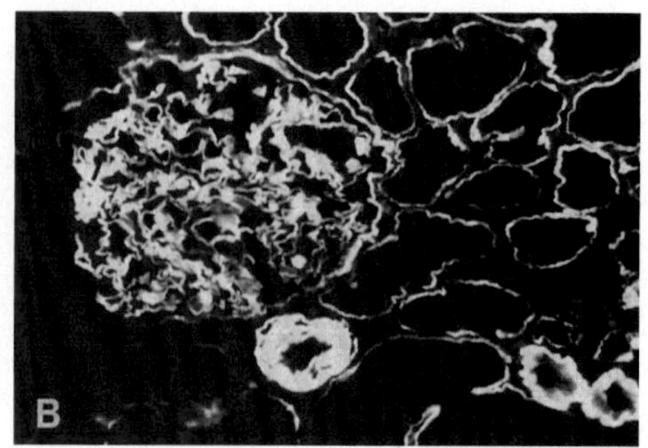

FIGURE 60.12 Monoclonal immunoglobulin deposition disease. **A:** Typical nodular glomerulosclerosis. Note membranelike material in the center of the nodules and nuclei at the periphery. Some glomerular capillaries show double contours (*arrow*). Note also thickening of the basement membrane of atrophic tubules. (Light microscopy, Masson's trichrome, ×312.) **B:** Bright staining of tubular and glomerular basement membranes, and of mesangium and arteriolar wall with anti-κ antibody in a patient with κ–light-chain deposition disease without nodular glomerular lesions. (Immunofluorescence, ×312.)

but some characteristics are distinctive: The distribution of the nodules is fairly regular in a given glomerulus, the nodules are often poorly argyrophilic, and exudative lesions as "fibrin caps" and extensive hyalinosis of the efferent arterioles are not observed. In occasional cases with prominent endocapillary cellularity and mesangial interposition, the glomerular features mimic a lobular glomerulonephritis.

Milder forms simply show an increase in mesangial matrix and sometimes in mesangial cells, and a modest thickening of the basement membranes appearing abnormally bright and rigid. Glomerular lesions may not be detected by light microscopy but require ultrastructural examination. These lesions may represent early stages of glomerular disease or be induced by LCs with a weak pathogenic potential. Their diagnosis would be unrecognized without the immunostaining results.

Arteries, arterioles, and peritubular capillaries all may contain LC deposits in close contact with their basement membranes.

Immunofluorescence

A key step in the diagnosis of the various forms of MIDD is immunofluorescence examination of the kidney. All biopsy specimens show evidence of monotypic LC and/or HC fixation along tubular basement membranes (Fig. 60.12B). This criterion is requested for the diagnosis of MIDD. In contrast with AL amyloidosis, the κ-isotype is markedly predominant.

The tubular deposits stain strongly and predominate along the loops of Henle and the distal tubules, but they are also often detected along the proximal tubules. In contrast, the pattern of glomerular immunofluorescence displays marked heterogeneity. In patients with nodular glomerulosclerosis, deposits of monotypic Ig chains are usually found along the peripheral glomerular basement membranes and, to a lesser extent, in the nodules themselves. The staining in glomeruli is typically weaker than that observed along the tubular basement membranes. This may not be a function of the actual amount of deposited material, since several cases have been reported in which glomerular immunofluorescence was negative despite the presence of large amounts of granular glomerular deposits by electron microscopy.[58] Local modifications of deposited LCs might thus change their antigenicity.[264] In patients without nodular lesions, glomerular staining occurs along the basement membrane, but it may involve the mesangium in some cases (Fig. 60.12B). Linear Ig-chain staining is usually present along Bowman's capsule basement membrane. Deposits of Ig chains are constantly found in vascular walls (Fig. 60.12B). Focal staining of tubular basement membranes was seen in interstitial forms.[283]

In patients with HCDD, immunofluorescence with anti-LC antibodies is negative, despite typical nodular glomerulosclerosis. Monotypic deposits of γ-, α-, or μ-HC may be identified. Any γ-subclass may be observed. Analysis of the kidney biopsies with monoclonal antibodies directed to the various constant domains of the γ-HC showed that C_H1 domain determinants were undetectable in all tested cases (Table 60.17 and Fig. 60.13). In addition, monoclonal antibodies to the $\gamma 1$ C_H2 domain also failed to react with the renal deposits of one patient, due to a combined deletion of C_H1 and C_H2 domains (5). In most cases of HCDD (Table 60.17) and in LHCDD,[284] especially when a $\gamma 1$ or $\gamma 3$ chain was involved, complement components could be demonstrated in a granular or pseudolinear pattern. Complement deposits were often associated with signs of complement activation in serum.

Electron Microscopy

The most characteristic ultrastructural feature is the presence of finely or coarsely granular electron-dense deposits that delineate the outer aspect of the tubular basement membranes (Fig. 60.14). They appear to be in contact with a well-preserved basal lamina. The deposits are usually quite large and may protrude into the adjacent part of the interstitium.

Ultrastructural glomerular lesions are characterized by the deposition of a nonfibrillar, electron-dense material

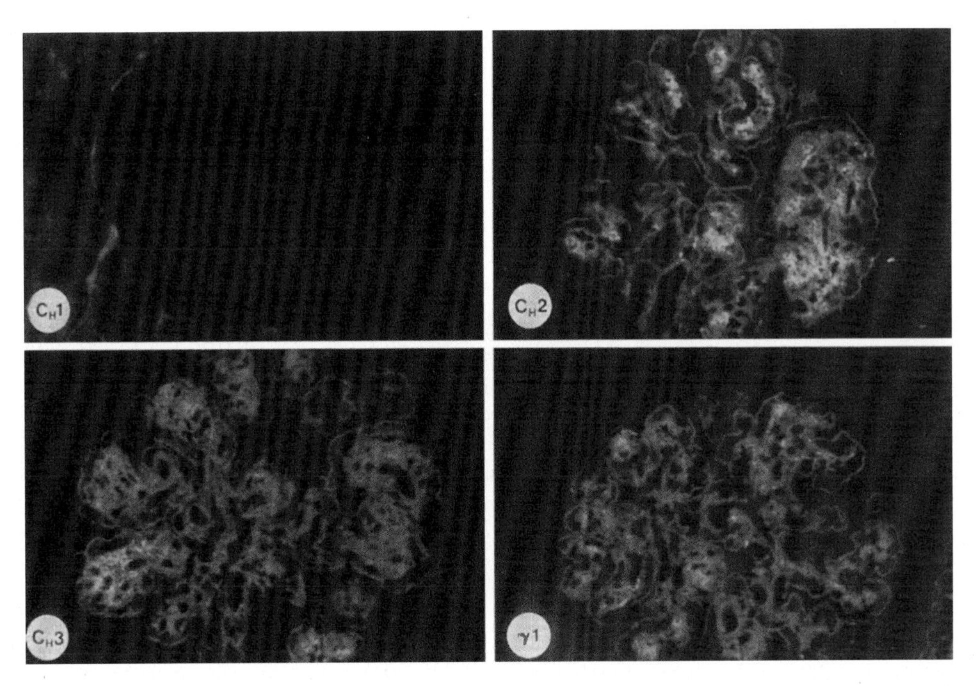

FIGURE 60.13 Heavy-chain deposition disease in a patient presenting with nodular glomerulosclerosis. Mesangial and parietal deposits stain with a monoclonal antibody specific for the $\gamma 1$-isotype in the absence of detectable light chain (*bottom right*). Immunofluorescence with a panel of monoclonal antibodies directed to the various constant domains of the γ-heavy chain shows that the glomerular deposits are stained with anti-C_H2 and -C_H3, but not with anti-C_H1 antibodies. (Magnification, ×312.) (From Moulin B, Deret S, Mariette X. et al. Nodular glomerulosclerosis with deposition of monoclonal immunoglobulin heavy chains lacking C_H1. *J Am Soc Nephrol.* 1999;10:519, with permission.)

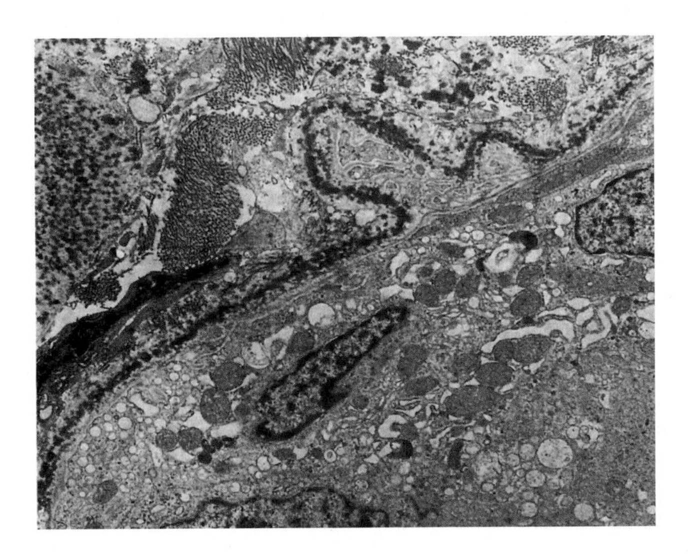

FIGURE 60.14 Light-chain deposition disease. Coarsely granular dense deposits lining the outer aspect of the tubular basement membrane. (Electron microscopy, uranyl acetate and lead citrate, ×6,000.) (From Ganeval D, Mignon F, Preud'homme JL, et al. Visceral deposition of monoclonal light chains and immunoglobulins: a study of renal and immunopathologic abnormalities. *Adv Nephrol Necker Hosp.* 1982;11:25, with permission.)

in the mesangial nodules and along the glomerular basement membrane. The mesangial material is usually finely granular with a membranoid appearance (Fig. 60.15), but in some cases, it may contain strongly electron-dense granules identical to the peritubular deposits. The deposits along the glomerular basement membrane appear as a prominent, but thin, continuous band delineating the endothelial aspect of the basement membrane. The limits between the deposits and the basement membrane may be difficult to distinguish. In rare cases the deposits invade the lamina densa. Glomerular endothelial cells are separated from this material by areas of electron-lucent fluffy material. Deposits can also be found in Bowman's capsules and in the wall of small arteries between the myocytes.[274]

Ultrastructural immunogold labeling may aid the demonstration of monotypical LCs along basement membranes in some cases.[285]

Clinical Presentation

In Tables 60.18 and 60.19 are summarized the main data from five large series.[260,261,262,286,287] They show an unexpectedly wide range of affected ages (28 to 94 years), with a male preponderance. MIDD is a systemic disease with Ig-chain deposition in a variety of organs leading to various clinical manifestations,[274] but visceral Ig-chain deposits may be totally asymptomatic and found only at autopsy.

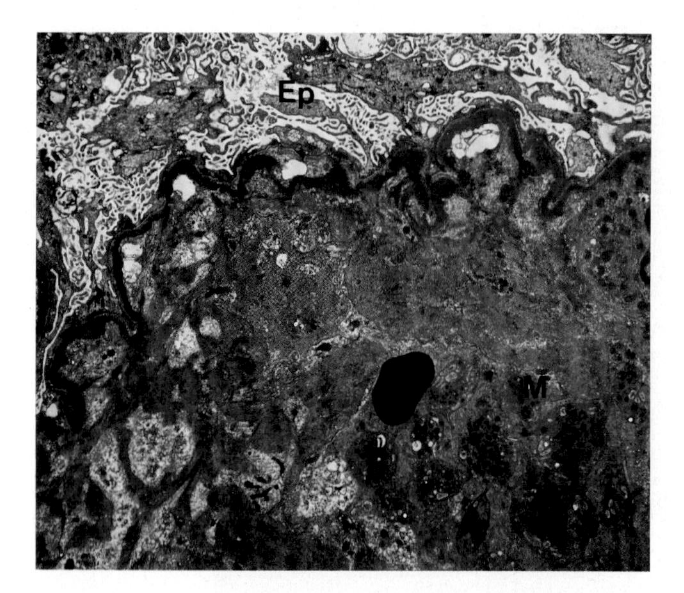

FIGURE 60.15 Light-chain deposition disease. A heavy layer of dense granular deposit lies along the inner part of the basement membrane lining a large mesangial nodule. *Ep*, epithelium; *M*, mesangium. (Electron microscopy, uranyl acetate and lead citrate, ×2,500.)

Renal Features

Renal involvement is a constant feature of MIDD, and renal symptoms, mostly proteinuria and renal failure, often dominate the clinical presentation (Table 60.18). In 23% to 53% of the patients, albuminuria is associated with the nephrotic syndrome. However, in about 20% of the cases, it is less than 1 g per day, and these patients exhibit mainly a tubulointerstitial syndrome.[283] Albuminuria is not correlated with the existence of nodular glomerulosclerosis, at least initially, and may occur in the absence of significant glomerular lesions by light microscopy. Hematuria is more frequent than one would expect for a nephropathy in which cell proliferation is usually modest, with a few exceptions.

The high prevalence, early appearance, and severity of renal failure are other salient features of MIDD.[3,261,262,274,288] In most cases, renal function declines rapidly, which is a main reason for referral. It occurs with comparable frequency in patients with either low or heavy proteinuria,[264] and thus presents in the form of a subacute tubulointerstitial nephritis or a rapidly progressive glomerulonephritis, respectively. The prevalence of hypertension is variable, but must be interpreted according to associated medical history.

TABLE 60.18 **Renal Manifestations at Presentation in Patients with Light-Chain Deposition Disease (LCDD) and Light-and Heavy-Chain Deposition Disease (LHCDD)**

Series (ref. no.)	Age (yrs)	Male–Female Ratio	Proteinuria >1 g/d	Nephrotic Syndrome	Hematuria	Renal Failure	Hypertension
Ganeval et al.[286] (*n* = 17)	57 (38–73)	11/6	13 (76%)	5 (29%)	5 (29%)	15 (88%)	3 (23%)[d]
Buxbaum et al.[260] (*n* = 13)	NS (35–71)	9/4	10 (77%)	3 (23%)	NS	12 (92%)	8 (61%)
Heilman et al.[287] (*n* = 19)	51 (37–77)	12/7	NS	10 (53%)	11 (58%)	17 (89%)	12 (63%)
Lin et al.[262,a] (*n* = 17)	57 (NS)	9/8	NS	3 (18%)	8 (47%)	16 (94%)	12 (71%)
Pozzi et al.[261,b] (*n* = 63)	58 (28–94)	40/23	53 (84%)	25 (40%)	NS	60 (96%)	NS
Masai et al.[284] (*n* = 12)	57 (39–60)	9/12	9/10 (90%)	3 (25%)	NS	8 (67%)[c]	NS
Total (*n* = 129)	57	1.5/1	83%	35%	45%	93%	53%

[a]Cases of LCDD with MCN (*n* = 11) are not included.
[b]Including 10 cases with MCN that could not be distinguished from those without MCN.
[c]Defined by serum creatinine >1.2 mg/dL.
[d]Plus three patients with past history of hypertension.
NS, not specified.

TABLE 60.19 **Hematologic Features, Extrarenal Manifestations, and Outcomes of Patients with Light-Chain Deposition Disease (LCDD) and Light- and Heavy-Chain Deposition Disease (LHCDD)**

Series (ref. no)	Plasma Cell Dyscrasia	Monoclonal Component in Blood or Urine	Extrarenal Manifestations	Survival
Ganeval et al.[286] (n = 17)	Myeloma—9 Waldenström—1	12/17 (71%)(8κ)	Liver—10 Heart—4 Lung—2 Spleen—3 Nervous system—4	1–46 mos 8/16 deceased
Buxbaum et al.[260] (*n* = 13)	Myeloma—4	10/12 (83%) (6κ)	Heart—6 Liver—3	1 mo to 10 yrs 9/13 deceased
Heilman et al.[287] (*n* = 19)	Myeloma—6 Malignant LPD—1	16/19 (84%) (15κ)	Heart—4 Nervous system—2	89% : 1 yr 70% : 5 yrs
Lin et al.[262] (*n* = 17)	Myeloma—8	15/17 (88%)[a]	NS	LCDD, 69 mos[b] LHCDD, 13 mos[b] 9/17 deceased
Pozzi et al.[261] (n = 63)	Myeloma—41 LPD—2	59/63 (94%) (43κ)	Heart—13 Liver—12 Spleen—5 Nervous system—5	66%: 1 yr 31%: 8 yrs 37/63 deceased
Masai et al.[284] (*n* = 12)	Myeloma—5	6/12 (50%) (5κ)	Heart—4 Liver—2	8/12 deceased (time to death: 81 mos) 7/12 hemodialysis
Total (*n* = 129)	Myeloma—52%	84% (κ65%)	Heart—25% Liver—22%	71/121 (59%) deceased

[a]14 κ chains in 17 kidney biopsies.
[b]Mean patient survival time.
LPD, lymphoproliferative disease.

Renal features of patients with HCDD are basically similar to those seen in LCDD and LHCDD although hypertension, nephrotic syndrome, and hematuria may be more common (Table 60.20).

Extrarenal Manifestations

Liver and cardiac manifestations occur in about one-fourth of patients (Table 60.19).[286] Liver deposits were constant in patients whose liver was examined. They were either discrete, confined to sinusoids and basement membranes of biliary ductules without associated parenchymal lesions, or massive with marked dilation and multiple ruptures of sinusoids resembling peliosis. Hepatomegaly with mild alterations of liver function tests was the most usual symptom, but several patients developed hepatic insufficiency and portal hypertension, and some of them died because of hepatic failure.[264]

Cardiac involvement is also frequent and may be responsible for cardiomegaly and severe renal failure. Dysrhythmias, conduction disturbances, and congestive heart failure are seen. Echocardiography and catheterization may reveal diastolic dysfunction and reduction in myocardial compliance similar to that seen in cardiac amyloid. As in the kidney and liver, immunofluorescence showed monotypic LC deposits in the vascular walls and perivascular areas of the heart, in all autopsy cases.[264]

Deposits may also occur along the nerve fibers and in the choroid plexus, as well as in the lymph nodes, bone marrow, spleen, pancreas, thyroid gland, submandibular glands, adrenal glands, gastrointestinal tract, abdominal vessels, lungs, and skin.[274] They may be responsible for peripheral neuropathy (20% of the reported cases), gastrointestinal disturbances, pulmonary nodules, amyloidlike

TABLE 60.20 **Comparison of Clinical Manifestations, Renal Lesions, and Hematologic Features in Patients with Monoclonal Immunoglobulin Deposition Disease (MIDD)**

Characteristics	LCDD/HCDD[a] (n = 129)	HCDD[b] (n = 27)
Male–female ratio	1.5	0.7
Age (y)	57 (28–94)	56 (26–79)
Hypertension (%)	53	90
Renal failure (serum creatinine ≥130 μmol/L) (%)	93	85
Nephrotic syndrome[c] (%)	35	50
Hematuria (%)	45	88
Nodular glomerulosclerosis (%)	31–100	96
Multiple myeloma (%)	52	22
M component (blood or urine) (%)	84	56[d]

[a]Patients are from the series of Tables 60.19 and 60.20.
[b]Cases are from references 5, 6, 261, 268–272, 283, 288–295.
[c]Proteinuria ≥3 g/day.
[d]Including two cases with only free κ chain.

arthropathy, and sicca syndrome. In some patients, nonamyloidotic, localized nodules, termed "aggregomas," developed in the lung or as a cervical mass without systemic LCDD.[297,298] It is not certain whether they are truly localized or they represent an initial expression of a silent, systemic LCDD. In some cases, LCDD present as isolated bilateral cystic lung disease with emphysematous-like changes, dilatations, and rapidly progressive chronic obstructive respiratory insufficiency. In all patients, a lung monoclonal B cell population was found that shared an unmutated antigen receptor variable region sequence, suggestive of an antigen-driven process. Bilateral lung transplantation is the only effective therapy.[299,300]

Extrarenal deposits are less common in patients with HCDD. They have been reported in the heart,[269] synovial tissue,[269,301] skin,[293] striated muscles,[293] pancreas,[5] around the thyroid follicles,[5] and in Disse's spaces in the liver.

Hematologic Findings

The most common underlying disease in MIDD is myeloma, which accounts for about 50% of pure MIDD (Table 60.19) and greater than 90% of LC deposits associated with myeloma CN. MIDD was found at postmortem examination in 5% of myeloma cases.[22] MIDD, like AL amyloidosis, often is the presenting disease that leads to the discovery of myeloma at an early stage. In some patients who first presented with common myeloma and with normal-sized monoclonal Ig without kidney disease, LCDD occurred when the disease relapsed after chemotherapy, together with Ig structural abnormalities.[264,302] Because melphalan was shown to induce Ig gene mutations, the disease in these patients might result from the emergence of a variant clone induced by the alkylating agent. Apart from myeloma, MIDD may complicate Waldenström macroglobulinemia, chronic lymphocytic leukemia, and nodal marginal-zone lymphoma.[302,303] It often occurs in the absence of detectable malignant process, even after prolonged (more than 10 years) follow-up (Tables 60.19 and 60.20). In such "primary" forms, a monoclonal bone marrow plasma cell population can be documented easily by immunofluorescence examination.

Diagnostic Procedures in MIDD

The diagnosis of MIDD must be suspected in any patient with the nephrotic syndrome or rapidly progressive tubulointerstitial nephritis, or with echocardiographic findings indicating diastolic dysfunction, and the presence of a monoclonal Ig component in the serum and/or the urine. The same combination is also seen in AL amyloidosis, but the latter is more often associated with the λ LC isotype. Sensitive techniques including immunofixation and free light chain assay fail to identify a monoclonal Ig component in up to 20% of patients with LCDD/HCDD[304] and about 40% of patients with HCDD (Table 60.20). Renal biopsy plays an essential role in the diagnosis of MIDD and of the associated dysproteinemia.

The definitive diagnosis is made according to the immunohistologic analysis of tissue from an affected organ, in most cases the kidney, using a panel of Ig chain-specific antibodies, including anti-κ and anti-λ LC antibodies to stain the non-Congophilic deposits. When the biopsy stains for a single heavy chain isotype and does not stain for light chain isotypes, the diagnosis of HCDD should be suspected, and antibodies specific for the three constant HC domains (CH) should be applied to detect deletion of the CH1.

The diagnosis of the plasma cell dyscrasia relies on bone marrow aspiration and bone marrow biopsy with cell morphologic evaluation and, if necessary, immunophenotyping with anti-κ and anti-λ antisera to demonstrate monoclonality. Diagnostic criteria for a multiple myeloma are present in about half of the patients with LCDD, and in one-fourth of those with HCDD.

Outcome and Treatment

The outcome of MIDD remains uncertain, mainly because extrarenal deposits of LCs can be totally asymptomatic or cause severe organ damage leading to death. Survival from onset of symptoms varies from 1 month to 10 years (Table 60.19). In the largest series as yet reported of patients with LCDD,[276] 36 of the 63 (57%) patients reached uremia, 37 of those patients (59%) died during follow-up (mean, 27.5 months), and patient survival was only 66% at 1 year and 31% at 8 years, although 54 patients (86%) were treated by chemotherapy. Multivariate analysis showed that the only variables independently associated with renal survival were age and degree of renal insufficiency at presentation[276] or at the time of renal biopsy.[262] Those independently associated with a worse patient survival were age, associated multiple myeloma, and extrarenal LC deposition,[276] or initial serum creatinine.[262] The survival of the uremic patients treated with dialysis was not different from that of the patients not reaching uremia.[276] Renal and patient survivals were significantly better in patients with "pure" MIDD (mean, 22 and 54 months, respectively), compared with those who presented with myeloma CN (mean, 4 and 22 months).[262]

As in AL amyloidosis, treatment should be aimed at reducing Ig production. Whether appropriate treatment can result in sustained remission has long remained unclear. Clearance of the LC deposits has been unequivocally demonstrated in some patients after intensive chemotherapy with syngeneic bone marrow transplantation or blood stem cell autografting.[305–307] Disappearance of nodular mesangial lesions and LC or γ3 HC deposits was also reported after conventional long-term chemotherapy.[271,308] These observations demonstrate that fibrotic nodular glomerular lesions are reversible, and they argue for intensive chemotherapy in patients with severe visceral involvement.

In a retrospective study of 11 young (<65 years) patients with LHCDD treated by high-dose therapy (HDT) with the support of autologous blood stem cell transplantation (ASCT), no treatment-related death occurred.[309] A decrease in the monoclonal Ig level was observed in eight patients, with complete disappearance from serum and urine in six cases. Improvement in manifestations related to deposits was observed in six patients, and histologic regression was documented in cardiac, hepatic, and skin biopsies. No manifestation related to deposits occurred or recurred in any patient. Other groups have recently confirmed that HDT with ASCT is a valid option in young patients (aged less than 65 years) with LCDD, in whom it provides prolonged hematologic reponse and survival.[310–313] Reversal of dialysis dependency and sustained improvement in renal function was also noted in one patient with LCDD by Firkin et al.[314] Novel antimyeloma agents might further improve renal and patient outomes, but their efficacy remains to be established. In four patients with LCDD and renal failure, renal and hematologic response (including complete clonal response in two patients) was obtained after six cycles of bortezomib plus dexamethasone in all cases. Two patients developed peripheral neuropathy that regressed with bortezomib dose adaptation. Three patients relapsed and were later succesfully treated with HDT and ASCT.[315]

As in AL amyloidosis, monitoring of LC production should rely on free LC assay, particularly in the patients without a blood and urine monoclonal component.

Kidney transplantation has been performed in a few patients with MIDD. Recurrence of the disease is usually observed, with an overall median allograft survival of only 33.3 months. Therefore, kidney transplantation should not be an option for LCDD patients unless measures have been taken to reduce LC production.[13] A prerequisite to kidney transplantation is hematologic complete remission as defined by normalization of κ : λ free LC ratio.

COMBINED GLOMERULAR AND TUBULAR LESIONS

Tubular Lesions Associated with Glomerular and Tubular Light-Chain Deposits

The association of monoclonal LC deposits, mostly along renal tubular basement membranes, with typical myeloma CN is more frequent than reported initially. Myeloma casts were found in 11 of 34 (32%) patients with MIDD.[262] Nodular glomerulosclerosis is, however, infrequent (<10%), and some ribbonlike tubular basement membranes are seen in less than one half of the patients. One third of the patients do not have granular-dense deposits by electron microscopy. The lack of matrix accumulation in most of these patients who present with acute renal failure in the setting of a true myeloma may relate to insufficient time for the development of fibrosis or to a weaker sclerogenic effect of the LC, if any.[274] As discussed in the preceding text, the presence of LC deposits along the tubular basement membrane is not sufficient to make a diagnosis of MIDD. The pattern of renal lesions may change with time under chemotherapy. In three patients with typical myeloma cast nephropathy on initial biopsy, casts were replaced by massive tissue deposits of LCs (κ chains in two, amyloid in one),[45] suggesting chemotherapy-induced mutation of the LCs.[302]

More exceptional is the association of AL amyloidosis with a Fanconi syndrome unrelated to massive amyloid infiltration of the kidney.[103,316,317] Finkel et al.[318] noticed that nodular amyloid deposits were surrounded by atypical lymphoid cells containing numerous needle-shaped crystals, and suggested that "a product" from these cells "may have been involved with both crystal formation and amyloid production." Since the nucleation processes initiating amyloid and crystal formation may share similarities, it is tempting to speculate that the responsible LC bore unusual physicochemical properties, inducing both pathologic conditions.

Combined AL or AH Amyloidosis and Monoclonal Immunoglobulin Deposition Disease

Since the description of MIDD, it was expected that the two types of deposits might coexist at different sites in a single patient. A review by Gallo et al.[319] indicated that in approximately 7% of 135 cases of light-chain deposition disease, amyloid was found in one or more organs. Because amyloid deposits were focal, the true incidence of the association may be markedly underestimated. In patients with both types of deposits, amyloid P component was found in the fibrillar, but not the nonfibrillar, LC deposits by immunohistochemical methods. The pathophysiologic significance of this association remains controversial. Some light chains may possess intrinsic properties, which make them prone to form both fibrillar and nonfibrillar deposits, depending on the tissue microenvironment,[268] although in the absence of structural analysis of the deposited LCs, one cannot exclude that they are generated by different variant clones. In a patient with IgD myeloma, MIDD and amyloidosis were associated with cast nephropathy.[320]

Late development of systemic λ-LC amyloidosis was reported in a patient with γ-HCDD during long-term follow-up.[321] Copeland et al.[139] reported the metachronous development of nonamyloidogenic λ-LCDD and γ-HC amyloidosis in the same patient. Given the length of time between the development of the two diseases (6 years) and the apparent success of stem cell transplantation in treating the first, it is most likely that the patient produced two different plasma cell clones.

OTHER DYSPROTEINEMIA-ASSOCIATED GLOMERULAR LESIONS

Glomerulopathies Associated with IgM-Secreting Monoclonal Proliferations

Glomerulonephritis with intracapillary thrombi of IgM is almost specific of Waldenström's macroglobulinemia (WM).[322] In the series of 16 autopsy and biopsy cases published by Morel-Maroger et al.,[322] this lesion was found in six cases and was associated with a variable degree of proteinuria and normal or slightly altered renal function. It was characterized by PAS-positive, non-Congophilic endomembranous deposits in a variable number of capillary loops. Deposits were sometimes so voluminous as to occlude the capillary lumens partially or completely, thereby forming thrombi. By immunofluorescence, thrombi and deposits were stained with anti-IgM (three cases studied) and with anti-κ (one case studied) antibodies. Two of the six patients had cryoglobulinemia and slight glomerular cell proliferation. In the remaining four, the amount of circulating IgM was higher than in the other patients of the series with amyloidosis or no detectable renal lesion, which suggested that hyperviscosity could favor IgM deposition in glomerular capillaries where ultrafiltration further increases the protein concentration.

However, recent data indicate that the spectrum of renal lesions associated with IgM monoclonal gammopathies has changed over the years, due to early management and development of effective chemotherapy in WM and other IgM secreting lymphoproliferative disorders. In 2008, Audard et al. showed that out of 14 patients with a circulating monoclonal IgM (including seven patients with WM) and renal disease, only five patients had typical granular intracapillary IgM thrombi occluding capillary lumens. In the remaining patients, renal disease was related to atypical membranoproliferative glomerulonephritis with IgMκ deposits (three cases), lambda LC amyloidosis (two cases), or CD20+ lymphomatous infiltration.[323] These findings strongly suggest that kidney biopsy should be performed to ascertain the nature of renal lesions in patients with WM and evidence of renal disease. Because renal biopsy may be hazardous in patients with Waldenström macroglobulinemia with frequently increased bleeding time, it is wise to search for amyloid deposits first by a less invasive tissue biopsy.

Recent studies have focused on AL amyloidosis associated with IgM monoclonal gammopathy, which appears as a distinct entity with frequent lymph node involvement. Variable outcomes have been reported, related to variable hematologic response rates to alkylating agents. Therefore, appropriately tailored chemotherapeutic regimens that specifically target the underlying clonal disorder (mostly lymphoid), based on purine analogs, HDT with ASCT, or new antimyeloma agents, should be considered to improve prognosis (see chapter Treatment of AL amyloidosis).[325,326]

Glomerulonephritis with Nonamyloid Organized Monotypic Deposits

These entities are characterized by fibrillar or microtubular deposits in mesangium and glomerular capillary loops that are readily distinguishable from amyloid because fibrils are thicker and are not stained by Congo red. They were termed "fibrillary glomerulonephritis" (FGN) by Alpers et al.[327] and immunotactoid glomerulopathy (IT) by Korbet et al.[328] There has been considerable debate about the relationship of FGN to IT, and most authors suggested that the two denominations might cover partly different morphologic entities as defined by the size and aspect of organized structures. For Alpers,[329] the distinguishing morphologic features of IT are the presence of organized deposits of large, thick-walled microtubules, usually greater than 30 nm in diameter, which are often hollow and arranged in parallel or stacked arrays, whereas FGN is characterized by more amyloidlike deposits with smaller fibrils (12 to 22 nm).

Although these criteria remain controversial,[330–333] distinguishing IT from FGN may be of great clinical and pathophysiologic interest because the former seemed to be more often associated with monotypic Ig deposits. However, until 2002, it was difficult to assess precisely from the literature, the respective prevalence in each entity of monotypic deposits and of circulating monoclonal Ig because studies of biopsies with anti-LC antibodies were often incomplete, urine and blood data uncertain, and, even more, patients with dysproteinemias were excluded a priori from several series.[328–330] This issue has been settled in three studies,[333–335] which confirmed that IT has a significant association with underlying dysproteinemia whereas FGN has a wide spectrum of etiologies. Therefore, differentiation of IT from FGN appears justified on immunopathologic and clinical grounds, and this has important therapeutic consequences.

Epidemiology and Clinical Manifestations

The incidence of glomerulopathies with nonamyloid deposition of fibrillary or microtubular material in a nontransplant adult biopsy population is estimated to be about 1% (equivalent to that of antiglomerular basement membrane [anti-GBM] disease). Despite a growing number of case reports, this is most likely underestimated because of the insufficient attention given to atypical reactions with histochemical stains for amyloid and the lack of immunohistochemical and ultrastructure studies of most biopsy specimens.

The characteristics of fibrillary and immunotactoid glomerulopathies are described in Table 60.21 by comparison with AL amyloid. Patients with IT and FGN have a mean age of 53 to 60 years (extreme: 19 to 86 years) with a male-to-female ratio that varies from one series to another.[8,333–335] They usually present with the nephrotic syndrome, microscopic hematuria, and mild-to-severe renal failure. In most recent series,[333–335] there was no significant difference between IT and FGN patients in serum creatinine level, incidence of nephrotic syndrome, microscopic hematuria, hypertension, and renal failure.

TABLE 60.21 **Immunologic and Clinical Characteristics of Fibrillary and Immunotactoid Glomerulopathies**

Characteristics	Amyloidosis (AL-type)	Fibrillary Glomerulonephritis (FGN)	Immunotactoid Glomerulopathy (IT)
Congo red staining	Yes	No	No
Composition	Fibrils	Fibrils	Microtubules
Fibril or microtubule size	8–15 nm	12–22 nm	>30 nm[a]
Organization in tissues	Random (β-pleated sheet)	Random	Parallel arrays
Immunoglobulin deposition	Monoclonal LC (mostly λ)	Usually polyclonal (mostly IgG4), occasionally monoclonal (IgG1, IgG4)	Usually monoclonal (IgGκ or IgGλ)
Glomerular lesions	Deposits spreading from the mesangium	MPGN, CGN, MP	Atypical MN, MPGN
Renal presentation	Severe NS, absence of hypertension and hematuria	NS with hematuria, hypertension; RPGN	NS with microhematuria and hypertension
Extrarenal manifestations (fibrillar deposits)	Systemic deposition disease	Pulmonary hemorrhage	Microtubular inclusions in leukemic lymphocytes
Association with LPD	Yes (myeloma)	Uncommon	Common (CLL, NHL, MGUS)
Treatment	Melphalan + prednisone; intensive therapy with blood stem cell autograft	Corticosteroids ± cyclophosphamide (crescentic GN)	Treatment of the associated LPD

[a]Mean diameter of the substructures did not differ between fibrillary glomerulonephritis (15.8 ± 3.5 nm) and immunotactoid glomerulopathy (15.2 ± 7.3 nm) in Bridoux's series.[333]

CGN, crescentic glomerulonephritis; CLL, chronic lymphocytic leukemia; GN, glomerulonephritis; LC, light chain; LPD, lymphoproliferative disorder; MN, membranous nephropathy; MP, mesangial proliferation; MPGN, membranoproliferative glomerulonephritis; NHL, non-Hodgkin lymphoma; NS, nephrotic syndrome; RPGN, rapidly progressive glomerulonephritis.

Pathologic Features

Immunotactoid Glomerulopathy. In IT, renal biopsy shows either membranous glomerulonephritis (often associated with segmental mesangial proliferation) or lobular membranoproliferative glomerulonephritis.[333] By immunofluorescence, coarse granular deposits of IgG and C3 are observed along capillary basement membranes and in mesangial areas. In a series of 23 patients based on ultrastructural appearance of the deposits, IgG deposits were monotypic in 13 of 14 patients with IT (κ, seven cases; λ, six cases), and in only one of nine patients with FGN.[333] However, a circulating monoclonal Ig was detected by immunoelectrophoresis or immunoblotting in only 6 of the 14 patients with IT.[333] Among the five cases of IT available for IgG subtype analysis reported by Rosenstock and associates,[334] four cases featured monotypic deposits of IgG1 subclass, whereas deposits composed of a single gamma subtype (two IgG1 and two IgG4) but with equivalent staining for the κ and λ LCs were found in four of 19 FGN cases.

By electron microscopy, the distinguishing morphologic features of IT are the presence of organized deposits of large, thick-walled microtubules, usually greater than 30 nm in diameter, at times arranged in parallel arrays (Fig. 60.16). However, the mean diameter of the substructures did not differ with their ultrastructural fibrillar or microtubular appearance in Bridoux's series,[333] with the mean external diameter of the microtubules ranging from 9 to 45 nm in patients with IT.

Of the 14 patients with IT reported by Bridoux et al.,[333] six had a chronic lymphocytic leukemia, one a small lymphocytic B cell lymphoma, and three a MGUS. Intracytoplasmic crystal-like Ig inclusions were found in four patients with chronic lymphocytic leukemia and in the lymphoma patient.[333] They showed the same microtubular organization and contained the same IgG subclass and LC isotype as renal deposits. Whether crystallization in lymphocytes and the glomerulus results from unusual intrinsic physicochemical properties of the monoclonal Ig, or from reactivity with a shared epitope, remains to be established. These properties may also account for rapid disappearance of the Ig from the blood and its recurrence on renal graft noted in several patients.[336–339]

Fibrillary Glomerulonephritis. Mesangial proliferation and aspects of membranoproliferative glomerulonephritis are predominantly reported in series of FGN. Glomerular crescents are present in 17% to 30% of the biopsies.[334,335] Immunofluorescence studies mainly show IgG deposits of the γ4-isotype[333,341] with a predominant mesangial localization and along the GBM. Monotypic deposits containing mostly IgGκ are detected in no more than 15% of patients. In a recent series of 66 patients with FGN,[335] seven of 61 biopsies (11%) showed monotypic deposits including five IgGλ and two IgGκ. By electron microscopy, fibrils are randomly arranged and their diameter varies between 9 and 26 nm. Of note, the fibril size alone is not sufficient to distinguish nonamyloidotic fibrillary glomerulonephritis from amyloid.

Although fibril deposition is almost always confined to the kidney, similar fibrillary deposits have been reported in the alveolar capillary membrane in patients presenting with a pulmonary–renal syndrome and in the skin of a patient with a leukocytoclastic vasculitis. In a patient with IT who suffered from severe mononeuritis multiplex of the lower limbs, peripheral nerve biopsy showed a similar ultrastructural microtubular organization to the glomerular deposits.[333]

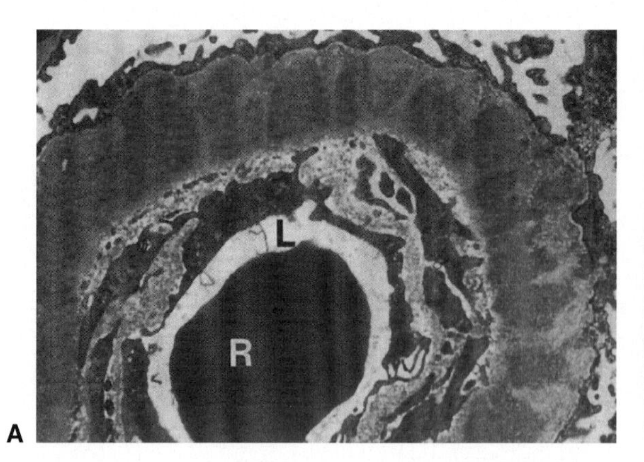

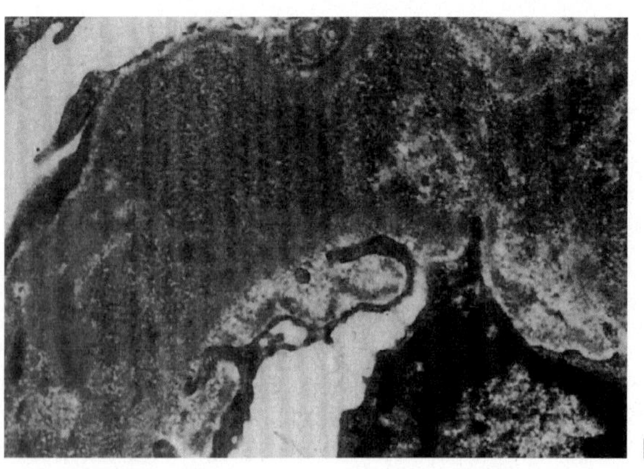

FIGURE 60.16 Immunotactoid glomerulopathy. Atypical membranous glomerulonephritis showing exclusive staining of the deposits with anti-immunoglobulin G and anti-κ–light-chain antibodies, in a patient with chronic lymphocytic leukemia. **A:** Electron microscopy of a glomerular capillary showing subepithelial deposits with effacement of the foot processes and mesangial interposition. *L*, capillary lumen; *R*, red blood cell. (Uranyl acetate and lead citrate, ×4,400.) **B:** Higher magnification of the capillary wall showing microtubular structure of the deposits. (Magnification, ×12,000.) (From Moulin B, Ronco PM, Mougenot B, et al. Glomerulonephritis in chronic lymphocytic leukemia and related B-cell lymphomas. *Kidney Int.* 1992;42:127, with permission.)

Pathogenesis

The cause of FGN is not known. The exclusive or prevailing presence of IgG4 in the immune deposits of patients with FGN is of great interest. Although not monoclonal, this isotype-restricted homogeneous material made of highly anionic Ig may facilitate fibril formation. Amyloid P component has also been found in the fibrils. The description of fibrillar cryoprecipitates consisting of Ig-fibronectin complexes in the serum of patients with FGN without evidence of systemic disease indicates that serum precursors can lead to the formation of fibrillary deposits.[341]

The mechanisms of Ig deposition in lymphocytes and kidney of patients with IT are also poorly understood. Analysis of monoclonal Ig both at the protein and mRNA levels has not disclosed size abnormalities in two patients.[342]

Treatment and Outcome

Patients with FGN usually respond poorly to corticosteroids and cytotoxic drugs, with an incidence of end-stage renal disease of 40% to 50%.[328,331,335,340,343] By contrast, in those with IT, corticosteroid and/or chemotherapy were associated with partial or complete remission of the nephrotic syndrome in most cases, with a parallel improvement of the hematologic parameters.[331,333]

After a mean follow-up period of 54 months for the IT group and 56 months for the FGN group, patient survival (71.4% vs. 88.8%, respectively) was found to be similar for the two groups.[333] The incidence of chronic renal failure (IT: 8/14, 57.1%; FGN: 8/9, 88.8%) and end-stage renal failure (IT: 2/14, 14.3%; FGN: 4/9, 55.8%) tended to be lower in the IT group, but the difference was not statistically significant. In the largest series of FGN published so far,[335] persistent renal dysfunction and end-stage renal failure occurred in 43% and 44% of patients, respectively. Renal transplantation has been performed in only a few patients, and recurrent disease occurred in several.[336–339]

IT (microtubular) glomerulopathies must now be added to the list of glomerulopathies caused by B cell chronic lymphocytic leukemia and related lymphomas, including AL amyloidosis and the larger cohort of cryoglobulinemia-associated membranoproliferative glomerulonephritis (Table 60.22).

TABLE 60.22 **Renal Lesions Observed in B-Cell Proliferations**

Renal Lesions	Multiple Myeloma	Waldenström Macroglobulinemia	Chronic Lymphocytic Leukemia and Related Lymphomas
Tubular lesions			
Cast nephropathy	+++	−	−
(Proximal) tubule lesions[a]	+	−	−
Fanconi syndrome	+ (smoldering)	−	−
Glomerular lesions[b]			
AL amyloidosis	++	+	+
MIDD (nodular, membranoproliferative, minimal change)	++	+	−
Nonamyloid organized deposits[c]	−	−	+
Type I and type II	+	++	++
cryoglobulinemia	−	+	−
IgM capillary thrombi	+	+	+
Other (crescentic, minimal change, etc.)			
Interstitial lesions			
B cell infiltrate	+[d]	++	++
Nephrocalcinosis	+	−	−
Pyelonephritis (infections)	+	−	−

[a]Without detectable myeloma casts, sometimes acute tubular necrosis.
[b]Glomerular involvement is usually but not always preponderant.
[c]Usually atypical membranous (or membranoproliferative) glomerulonephritis.
[d]Exceptionally, plasmacytoma.
−, not or exceptionally observed; + to +++, semiquantitative rating of the prevalence of renal lesions; MIDD, monoclonal immunoglobulin deposition disease

Proliferative Glomerulonephritis with Nonorganized Monoclonal Ig Deposits

Recently, it has been shown that in the absence of detectable cryoglobulin, glomerular deposition of monoclonal IgG could produce a proliferative glomerulonephritis that mimics immune complex glomerulonephritis by light and electron microscopy.[9] Proper recognition of this entity requires confirmation of monoclonality by staining for the γ-heavy chain subclasses and the LC isotypes. In the largest series to date,[344] that included 37 patients, clinical presentation included renal insufficiency in 68%, proteinuria in 100%, nephrotic syndrome in 49%, and microhematuria in 77%. None of the patients had significant extrarenal symptoms. A monoclonal serum protein with the same heavy and light chain isotype as that of the glomerular deposits (mostly IgG1 or IgG2) was identified in 30% of cases. Most patients displayed membranoproliferative or endocapillary proliferative patterns with membranous features. Glomerular monotypic deposits were made up of IgG3 (mostly κ) in two thirds of the cases. By electron microscopy, granular nonorganized deposits were mostly subendothelial and mesangial, and, by contrast with MIDD, were confined to the glomerular compartment. Tissue fixation of complement was observed in virtually all cases, wherears around 30% of patients had hypocomplementemia.

Treatment with steroids alone or combined with immunosuppressive drugs with or without renin-angiotensin sytem blockade was given in 56% of patients, half of whom achieved complete or partial renal recovery. During an average 30 months of follow-up, 38% of patients had at least partial renal recovery, whereas 38% had persistent renal dysfunction and 22% progressed to end-stage renal disease. Only one patient had myeloma at presentation, and none developed hematologic malignancy over the course of follow-up.[344]

Since the first description of the disease,[345] an increasing number of endocapillary proliferative or membranoproliferative glomerulonephritis cases characterized by monoclonal nonorganized granular IgG or IgM deposits (mostly associated with κ LC) have been reported.[346,354] Similarly with Nasr's series, the disease appears as a renal-limited condition mostly associated with monoclonal IgG3, without C_H1 deletion and systemic monoclonal Ig deposition. MGUS is the most commonly associated clonal disorder, but some patients have evidence of myeloma, chronic lymphocytic laukemia, or other non-Hodgkin B cell lymphomas. As with other renal diseases associated with monoclonal gammopathy, it is likely to recur after kidney transplantation.[347] Whether or not specific treatment aimed at suppressing the underlying clonal disease may reverse or halt progression of chronic kidney disease remains to be confirmed in further studies. Recent studies indicate that treatment with anti-CD20 antibody alone may be very efficient in patients with no overt hematologic malignancy.[348]

Other Types of Glomerulonephritis

Additional histologic forms of glomerulonephritis have been described in monoclonal gammopathies. In type I cryoglobulinemia, a membranoproliferative glomerulonephritis (MPGN) with macrophage infiltration is the most characteristic histologic pattern and the deposits are typically, but not invariably, organized into fibrillary or microtubular structures at the ultrastructural level.[349] Type II cryoglobulinemias are much more common.

Few cases of nonorganized monoclonal Ig deposition disease with a membranous pattern have been reported.[9,346,350,351] Guiard et al. recently reviewed the cases of 26 patients with non-cryoglobulinemic glomerulonephritis and monoclonal Ig deposits. Patients were almost equally divided in two distinct histologic patterns with 14 patients having a membranous nephropathy and the 12 remaining ones having a membranoproliferative glomerulonephritis.[348]

There was a striking relationship between the type of glomerulopathy and the subclass of deposited IgG. As previously reported,[348] IgG3 was the predominant deposited subclass in patients with membranoproliferative glomerulonephritis (80% of cases) whereas IgG1 was identified in 64% of those with a membranous pattern. The κ LC isotype was largely predominant (21/26 cases). A circulating monoclonal Ig could be detected in only 8 of 26 patients. Ultrastructural studies showed that immune deposits were not organized in the majority of patients (78%). In a similar case with a membranous pattern and nonorganized IgG1λ deposits, the circulating monoclonal IgG1λ deposits showed unusual in vitro aggregation properties, including dependence on low ionic strength and neutral pH, which suggest that electrostatic interactions had a role in the precipitation process.[352]

Renal manifestations may also occur in POEMS syndrome (polyneuropathy, organomegaly, endocrinopathy, M protein, and skin changes), although they are not related to deposition of the monoclonal immunoglobulin.[353] Finally, rare observations of dense deposit disease[354] and glomerulonephritis with isolated C3 deposits[355] have been recently reported in patients with monoclonal gammopathy or smoldering myeloma. Patients usually present with hematuria, proteinuria, nephrotic syndrome, and severe renal failure. Systemic activation of the complement alternative pathway (CAP) is found in most cases, with autoantibodies against complement factor H in some patients. Kidney biopsy shows glomerular electron-dense C3 deposits without concomitant monoclonal immunoglobulin deposition. Isolated glomerular C3 deposits probably represent an unusual complication of plasma cell dyscrasia related to systemic or local complement activation, through an autoantibody activity of the monoclonal immunoglobulin against a CAP regulatory protein.[356]

REFERENCES

1. Merlini G, Stone MJ. Dangerous small B-cell clones. *Blood.* 2006;108:2520.
2. Glenner GG, Terry W, Harada M, et al. Amyloid fibril proteins: proof of homology with immunoglobulin light chains by sequence analyses. *Science.* 1971;172:1150.

3. Randall RE, Williamson WC Jr, Mullinax F, et al. Manifestations of systemic light chain deposition. *Am J Med.* 1976;60:293.

4. Eulitz M, Weiss DT, Solomon A. Immunoglobulin heavy-chain-associated amyloidosis. *Proc Natl Acad Sci U S A.* 1990;87:6542.

5. Aucouturier P, Khamlichi AA, Touchard G, et al. Brief report: heavy-chain deposition disease. *N Engl J Med.* 1993;329:1389.

6. Moulin B, Deret S, Mariette X, et al. Nodular glomerulosclerosis with deposition of monoclonal immunoglobulin heavy chains lacking C_H1. *J Am Soc Nephrol.* 1999;10:519.

7. Touchard G, Preud'homme JL, Aucouturier P, et al. Nephrotic syndrome associated with chronic lymphocytic leukemia: an immunological and pathological study. *Clin Nephrol.* 1989;31:107.

8. Moulin B, Ronco PM, Mougenot B, et al. Glomerulonephritis in chronic lymphocytic leukemia and related B-cell lymphomas. *Kidney Int.* 1992;42:127.

9. Nasr SH, Markowitz GS, Stokes MB et al. Proliferative glomerulonephritis with monoclonal IgG deposits: a distinct entity mimicking immune-complex glomerulonephritis. *Kidney Int.* 2004;65:85.

10. Batuman V, Verroust PJ, Navar GL, et al. Myeloma light chains are ligands for cubilin (gp280). *Am J Physiol.* 1998;260:F246.

11. Klassen RB, Allen PL, Batuman V, et al. Light chains are a ligand for megalin. *J Appl Physiol.* 2005;98:257.

12. Preud'homme JL, Morel-Maroger L, Brouet JC, et al. Synthesis of abnormal immunoglobulins in lymphoplasmacytic disorders with visceral light chain deposition. *Am J Med.* 1980;69:703.

13. Leung N, Lager DJ, Gertz MA, et al. Long-term outcome of renal transplantation in light-chain deposition disease. *Am J Kidney Dis.* 2004;43:147.

14. Solomon A, Weiss DT, Kattine AA. Nephrotoxic potential of Bence Jones proteins. *N Engl J Med.* 1991;324:1845.

15. Cogné M, Preud'homme JL, Bauwens M, et al. Structure of a monoclonal kappa chain of the $V_{\kappa IV}$ subgroup in the kidney and plasma cells in light chain deposition disease. *J Clin Invest.* 1991;87:2186.

16. Leboulleux M, Lelongt B, Mougenot B, et al. Protease resistance and binding of Ig light chains in myeloma-associated tubulopathies. *Kidney Int.* 1995;48:72.

17. Solomon A, Frangione B, Franklin EC. Bence Jones proteins and light chains of immunoglobulins: preferential association of the $V_{\lambda VI}$ subgroup of human light chains with amyloidosis AL (λ). *J Clin Invest.* 1982;70:453.

18. Ozaki S, Abe M, Wolfenbarger D, et al. Preferential expression of human λ-light chain variable region subgroups in multiple myeloma, AL amyloidosis, and Waldenström's macroglobulinemia. *Clin Immunol Immunopathol.* 1994;71:183.

19. Denoroy L, Déret S, Aucouturier P. Overrepresentation of the $V_{\kappa IV}$ subgroup in light chain deposition disease. *Immunol Lett.* 1994;42:63.

20. Tsakiris DJ, Stel VS, Fine P, et al. Incidence and outcome of patients starting renal replacement therapy for end-stage renal disease due to myeloma or light-chain deposition disease: an ERA-EDTA Registry study. *Nephrol Dial Transplant.* 2010;25:1200.

21. Paueksakon P, Revelo MP, Horn RG, et al. Monoclonal gammopathy: significance and possible causality in renal disease. *Am J Kidney Dis.* 2003;42:87.

22. Ivanyi B. Frequency of light chain deposition nephropathy relative to renal amyloidosis and Bence Jones cast nephropathy in a necropsy study of patients with myeloma. *Arch Pathol Lab Med.* 1990;114:986.

23. Herrera GA, Joseph L, Gu X, et al. Renal pathologic spectrum in an autopsy series of patients with plasma cell dyscrasia. *Arch Pathol Lab Med.* 2004;128:860.

24. DeFronzo RA, Cooke CR, Wright JR, et al. Renal function in patients with multiple myeloma. *Medicine (Baltimore).* 1978;57:151.

25. Rota S, Mougenot B, Baudouin B, et al. Multiple myeloma and severe renal failure: a clinicopathologic study of outcome and prognosis in 34 patients. *Medicine (Baltimore).* 1987;66:126.

26. Pozzi C, Pasquali S, Donini U, et al. Prognostic factors and effectiveness of treatment in acute renal failure due to multiple myeloma: a review of 50 cases. Report of the Italian Renal Immunopathology Group. *Clin Nephrol.* 1987;28:1.

27. Pasquali S, Casanova S, Zucchelli A, et al. Long-term survival patients with acute and severe renal failure due to multiple myeloma. *Clin Nephrol.* 1990;34:247.

28. Ganeval D, Rabian C, Guerin V, et al. Treatment of multiple myeloma with renal involvement. *Adv Nephrol Necker Hosp.* 1992;21:347.

29. Isaac J, Herrera GA. Cast nephropathy in a case of Waldenström's macroglobulinemia. *Nephron.* 2002;91:512.

30. Preud'homme JL, Bauwens M, Dumont G, et al. Cast nephropathy in μ heavy chain disease. *Clin Nephrol.* 1997;48:118.

31. Wang PX, Sanders PW. Immunoglobulin light chains generate hydrogen peroxide. *J Am Soc Nephrol.* 2007;18:1239.

32. Basnayake K, Ying WZ, Wang PX, et al. Immunoglobulin light chains activate tubular epithelial cells through redox signaling. *J Am Soc Nephrol.* 2010;21:1165.

33. Ying WZ, Wang PX, Aaron KJ, et al. Immunoglobulin light chains activate NF-{kappa}B in renal epithelial cells through a Src-dependent mechanism. *Blood.* 2011;117:1301.

34. Sengul S, Zwizinski C, Batuman V. Role of MAPK pathways in light chain-induced cytokine production in human proximal tubule cells. *Am J Physiol Renal Physiol.* 2003;284:F1245.

35. Pote A, Zwizinski C, Simon EE, et al. Cytotoxicity of myeloma light chains in cultured human kidney proximal tubule cells. *Am J Kidney Dis.* 2000;36:735.

36. Li M, Hering-Smith KS, Simon EE et al. Myeloma light chains induce epithelial-mesenchymal transition in human renal proximal tubule epithelial cells. *Nephrol Dial Transplant.* 2008;23:860.

37. Hertig A, Bonnard G, Ulinski T, et al. Tubular nuclear accumulation of Snail and epithelial phenotypic changes in human myeloma cast nephropathy. *Hum Pathol.* 2011;42(8):1142–1148.

38. Arimura A, Li M, Batuman V. Potential protective action of pituitary adenylate cyclase-activating polypeptide (PACAP38) on in vitro and in vivo models of myeloma kidney injury. *Blood.* 2006;107:661.

39. Melcion C, Mougenot B, Baudouin B, et al. Renal failure in myeloma: relationship with isoelectric point of immunoglobulin light chains. *Clin Nephrol.* 1984;22:138.

40. Sanders PW, Herrera GA, Chen A, et al. Differential nephrotoxicity of low molecular weight proteins including Bence Jones proteins in the perfused rat nephron in vivo. *J Clin Invest.* 1988;82:2086.

41. Sanders PW, Booker BB, Bishop JB, et al. Mechanisms of intranephron. al proteinaceous cast formation by low molecular weight proteins. *J Clin Invest.* 1990;85:570.

42. Huang ZQ, Sanders PW. Localization of a single binding site for immunoglobulin light chains on human Tamm-Horsfall glycoprotein. *J Clin Invest.* 1997;99:732.

43. Ying WZ, Sanders PW. Mapping the binding domain of immunoglobulin light chains for Tamm-Horsfall protein. *Am J Pathol.* 2001;158:1859.

44. Myatt EA, Westholm FA, Weiss DT, et al. Pathogenic potential of human monoclonal immunoglobulin light chains: relationship of in vitro aggregation to in vivo organ deposition. *Proc Natl Acad Sci U S A.* 1994;91:3034.

45. Hill GS, Morel-Maroger L, Mery JP, et al. Renal lesions in multiple myeloma: Their relationship to associated protein abnormalities. *Am J Kidney Dis.* 1983;2:423.

46. Cohen AH, Border WA. Myeloma kidney: an immunomorphogenetic study of renal biopsies. *Lab Invest.* 1980;42:248.

47. Thomas DB, Davies M, Williams JD. Release of gelatinase and superoxide from human mononuclear phagocytes in response to particulate Tamm Horsfall protein. *Am J Pathol.* 1993;142:249.

48. DeFronzo RA, Humphrey RL, Wright JR, et al. Acute renal failure in multiple myeloma. *Medicine (Baltimore).* 1960;54:209.

49. Rayner HC, Haynes AP, Thompson JR, et al. Perspectives in multiple myeloma: survival, prognostic factors and disease complications in a single centre between 1960 and 1988. *Q J Med.* 1991;290:517.

50. Haynes RJ, Read S, Collins GP, et al. Presentation and survival of patients with severe acute kidney injury and multiple myeloma: a 20-year experience from a single centre. *Nephrol Dial Transplant.* 2010;25:419.

51. Irish AB, Winearls CG, Littlewood T. Presentation and survival of patients with severe renal failure and myeloma. *Q J Med.* 1997;90:773.

52. Kyle RA. Multiple myeloma: review of 869 cases. *Mayo Clin Proc.* 1960; 50:29.

53. Alexanian R, Barlogie B, Dixon D. Renal failure in multiple myeloma: pathogenesis and prognostic implications. *Arch Intern Med.* 1990;150:1693.

54. McCarthy CS, Becker JA. Multiple myeloma and contrast media. *Radiology.* 1992;183:519.

55. Markowitz GS, Fine PL, Stack JI, et al. Toxic acute tubular necrosis following treatment with zoledronate (Zometa). *Kidney Int.* 2003;64:281.

56. Banerjee D, Asif A, Striker L, et al. Short-term, high-dose pamidronate-induced acute tubular necrosis: the postulated mechanisms of bisphosphonate nephrotoxicity. *Am J Kidney Dis.* 2003;41:E18.

57. Leung N, Gertz MA, Zeldenrust SR, et al Improvement of cast nephropathy with plasma exchange depends on the diagnosis and on reduction of serum free light chains. *Kidney Int.* 2008;73:1282.

58. Pirani CL, Silva F, D'Agati V, et al. Renal lesions in plasma cell dyscrasias: ultrastructural observations. *Am J Kidney Dis.* 1987;10:208.

59. Kumar SK, Rajkumar SV, Dispenzieri A, et al. Improved survival in multiple myeloma and the impact of novel therapies. *Blood.* 2008;111:2516.

60. Bradwell AR, Carr-Smith HD, Mead GP, et al. Serum test for assessment of patients with Bence Jones myeloma. *Lancet.* 2003;361:489.

61. Dimopoulos MA, Terpos E, Chanan-Khan A, et al. Renal impairment in patients with multiple myeloma: a consensus statement on behalf of the International Myeloma Working Group. *J Clin Oncol.* 2010;28:4976.

62. Knudsen LM, Hjorth M, Hippe E. Renal failure in multiple myeloma: reversibility and impact on the prognosis. Nordic Myeloma Study Group. *Eur J Haematol.* 2000;65:160.

63. Clark WF, Stewart AK, Rock GA, et al. Plasma exchange when myeloma presents as acute renal failure. *Ann Intern Med.* 2005;143:777.

64. Chanan-Khan AA, Kaufman JL, Mehta J, et al. Activity and safety of bortezomib in multiple myeloma patients with advanced renal failure: a multicenter retrospective study. *Blood.* 2007;109:2604.

65. Dimopoulos MA, Roussou M, Gavriatopoulou M, et al. Reversibility of renal impairment in patients with multiple myeloma treated with bortezomib-based regimens: identification of predictive factors. *Clin Lymphoma Myeloma.* 2009;9:302.

66. Morabito F, Gentile M, Ciolli S, et al. Safety and efficacy of bortezomib-based regimens for multiple myeloma patients with renal impairment: a retrospective study of Italian Myeloma Network GIMEMA. *Eur J Haematol.* 2010;84:223.

67. Blade J, Fernandez-Llama P, Bosch F, et al. Renal failure in multiple myeloma: presenting features and predictors of outcome in 94 patients from a single institution. *Arch Intern Med.* 1998;158:1889.

68. Johnson WJ, Kyle RA, Pineda AA, et al. Treatment of renal failure associated with multiple myeloma. *Arch Intern Med.* 1990;150:863.

69. Kastritis E, Anagnostopoulos A, Roussou M, et al. Reversibility of renal failure in newly diagnosed multiple myeloma patients treated with high dose dexamethasone-containing regimens and the impact of novel agents. *Haematologica.* 2007;92:546.

70. Hutchison CA, Bradwell AR, Cook M, et al. Treatment of acute renal failure secondary to multiple myeloma with chemotherapy and extended high cut-off hemodialysis. *Clin J Am Soc Nephrol.* 2009;4:745.

71. Hutchison CA, Cockwell P, Stringer S, et al. Early reduction of serum-free light chains associates with renal recovery in myeloma kidney. *J Am Soc Nephrol.* 2011;22:1129.

72. Ludwig H, Adam Z, Hajek R, et al. Light chain-induced acute renal failure can be reversed by bortezomib-doxorubicin-dexamethasone in multiple myeloma: results of a phase II study. *J Clin Oncol.* 2010;28:4635.

73. Hutchison CA, Cockwell P, Reid S, et al. Efficient removal of immunoglobulin free light chains by hemodialysis for multiple myeloma: in vitro and in vivo studies. *J Am Soc Nephrol.* 2007;18:886.

74. Carlson K, Hjorth M, Knudsen LM. Nordic Myeloma Study Group. Toxicity in standard melphalan-prednisone therapy among myeloma patients with renal failure—a retrospective analysis and recommendations for dose adjustment. *Br J Haematol.* 2005;128:631.

75. Fakhouri F, Guerraoui H, Presne C, et al. Thalidomide in patients with multiple myeloma and renal failure. *Br J Haematol.* 2004;125:96.

76. Tosi P, Zamagni E, Tacchetti P, et al. Thalidomide-dexamethasone as induction therapy before autologous stem cell transplantation in patients with newly diagnosed multiple myeloma and renal insufficiency. *Biol Blood Marrow Transplant.* 2010;16:1115.

77. Dimopoulos M, Alegre A, Stadtmauer EA, et al. The efficacy and safety of lenalidomide plus dexamethasone in relapsed and/or refractory multiple myeloma patients with impaired renal function. *Cancer.* 2010;116:3807.

78. Jagannath S, Barlogie B, Berenson JR et al. Bortezomib in recurrent and/or refractory multiple myeloma. Initial clinical experience in patients with impaired renal function. *Cancer.* 2005;103:1195.

79. San Miguel JF, Richardson PG, Sonneveld P, et al. Efficacy and safety of bortezomib in patients with renal impairment: results from the APEX phase 3 study. *Leukemia.* 2008;22:842.

80. Dimopoulos MA, Richardson PG, Schlag R, et al. VMP (Bortezomib, Melphalan, and Prednisone) is active and well tolerated in newly diagnosed patients with multiple myeloma with moderately impaired renal function, and results in reversal of renal impairment: cohort analysis of the phase III VISTA study. *J Clin Oncol.* 2009;27:6086.

81. Bladé J, Sonneveld P, San Miguel JF, et al. Pegylated liposomal doxorubicin plus bortezomib in relapsed or refractory multiple myeloma: efficacy and safety in patients with renal function impairment. *Clin Lymphoma Myeloma.* 2008;8:352.

82. Attal M, Harousseau JL, Stoppa AM, et al. A prospective, randomised trial of autologous bone marrow transplantation and chemotherapy in multiple myeloma. *N Engl J Med.* 1996;35:91.

83. Fermand JP, Ravaud P, Chevret S, et al. High dose therapy and autologous peripheral blood stem cell transplantation in multiple myeloma: up-front or rescue treatment? Results of a multicenter sequential randomized clinical trial. *Blood.* 1998;92:3131.

84. Badros A, Barlogie B, Siegel E, et al. Results of autologous stem cell transplant in multiple myeloma patients with renal failure. *Br J Haematol.* 2001;114:822.

85. Lee CK, Zangari M, Barlogie B, et al. Dialysis-dependent renal failure in patients with myeloma can be reversed by high-dose myeloablative therapy and autotransplant. *Bone Marrow Transplant.* 2004;33:823.

86. Knudsen LM, Nielsen B, Gimsing P, et al. Autologous stem cell transplantation in multiple myeloma: outcome in patients with renal failure. *Eur J Haematol.* 2005;60:27.

87. Hutchison CA, Harding S, Mead G, et al. Serum free-light chain removal by high cutoff hemodialysis: optimizing removal and supportive care. *Artif Organs* 2008:32:910.

88. Granger Vallée A, Chenine L, Leray-Moragues H, et al. Online high-efficiency hemodiafiltration achieves higher serum free light chain removal than high flux hemodialysis in multiple myeloma patients: preliminary quantitative study. *Nephrol Dial Transplant.* 2011;26(11):3627–3633.

89. Desikan R, Veksler Y, Raza S, et al. Nephrotic proteinuria associated with high-dose pamidronate in multiple myeloma. *Br J Haematol.* 2002;119:496.

90. Sharland A, Snowdon L, Joshua DE, et al. Hemodialysis: an appropriate therapy in myeloma-induced renal failure. *Am J Kidney Dis.* 1997;30:786.

91. Iggo N, Palmer AB, Severn A, et al. Chronic dialysis in patients with multiple myeloma and renal failure: a worthwhile treatment. *Q J Med.* 1989; 270:903.

92. Port FK, Nissenson AR. Outcome of end-stage renal disease in patients with rare causes of renal failure. II. Renal or systemic neoplasms. *Q J Med.* 1989;272:1161.

93. Abbott KC, Agodoa LY. Multiple myeloma and light chain-associated nephropathy at end-stage renal disease in the United States: patient characteristics and survival. *Clin Nephrol.* 2001;56:207.

94. Shetty A, Oreopoulos DG. Myeloma patients do well on CAPD too! *Br J Haematol.* 1997;96:654.

95. Montseny JJ, Kleinknecht D, Meyrier A, et al. Long-term outcome according to renal histological lesions in 118 patients with monoclonal gammopathies. *Nephrol Dial Transplant.* 1998;13:1438.

96. van Bommel EF. Multiple myeloma treatment in dialysis-dependent patients: to transplant or not to transplant? *Nephrol Dial Transplant.* 1996;11:1486.

97. Dagher F, Sammett D, Abbi R, et al. Renal transplantation in multiple myeloma. Case report and review of the literature. *Transplantation.* 1996;62:1577.

98. Spitzer TR, Sykes M, Tolkoff-Rubin N, et al. Long-term follow-up of recipients of combined human leukocyte antigen-matched bone marrow and kidney transplantation for multiple myeloma with end-stage renal disease. *Transplantation.* 2011;91:672.

99. Sirota JH, Hamerman D. Renal function studies in an adult subject with the Fanconi syndrome. *Am J Med.* 1954;16:138.

100. Engle RL, Wallis LA. Multiple myeloma and the adult Fanconi syndrome. *Am J Med.* 1957;22:5.

101. Costanza DJ, Smoller M. Multiple myeloma with the Fanconi syndrome. Study of a case, with electron microscopy of the kidney. *Am J Med.* 1963;34:125.

102. Lee DB, Drinkard JP, Rosen VJ, et al. The adult Fanconi syndrome. Observations on etiology, morphology, renal function and mineral metabolism in three patients. *Medicine (Baltimore).* 1972;51:107.

103. Maldonado JE, Velosa JA, Kyle RA, et al. Fanconi syndrome in adults. A manifestation of a latent form of myeloma. *Am J Med.* 1960;58:354.

104. Messiaen T, Deret S, Mougenot B, et al. Adult Fanconi syndrome secondary to light chain gammopathy: clinicopathologic heterogeneity and unusual features in 11 patients. *Medicine.* 2000;79:135.

105. Ma CX, Lacy MQ, Rompala JF, et al. Acquired Fanconi syndrome is an indolent disorder in the absence of overt multiple myeloma. *Blood.* 2004; 104:40.

106. Aucouturier P, Bauwens M, Khamlichi AA, et al. Monoclonal Ig L chain and L chain V domain fragment crystallization in myeloma-associated Fanconi's syndrome. *J Immunol.* 1993;150:3561.

107. Bridoux F, Sirac C, Hugue V, et al. Fanconi's syndrome induced by a monoclonal Vkappa3 light chain in Waldenstrom's macroglobulinemia. *Am J Kidney Dis.* 2005;45:749.

108. Deret S, Denoroy L, Lamarine M, et al. Kappa light chain-associated Fanconi's syndrome: molecular analysis of monoclonal immunoglobulin light chains from patients with and without intracellular crystals. *Protein Eng.* 1999;12:363.

109. Decourt C, Bridoux F, Touchard G, et al. A monoclonal V kappa l light chain responsible for incomplete proximal tubulopathy. *Am J Kidney Dis.* 2003; 41:497.

110. Vidal R, Goni F, Stevens F, et al. Somatic mutations of the L12a gene in V-kappa(1) light chain deposition disease: potential effects on aberrant protein conformation and deposition. *Am J Pathol.* 1999;155:2009.

111. Decourt C, Rocca A, Bridoux F, et al. Mutational analysis in murine models for myeloma-associated Fanconi's syndrome or cast myeloma nephropathy. *Blood.* 1999;94:3559.

112. Sirac C, Bridoux F, Carrion C, et al. Role of the monoclonal kappa chain V domain and reversibility of renal damage in a transgenic model of acquired Fanconi syndrome. *Blood.* 2006;108:536.

113. El Hamel C, Thierry A, Trouillas P, et al. Crystal-storing histiocytosis with renal Fanconi syndrome: pathological and molecular characteristics compared with classical myeloma-associated Fanconi syndrome. *Nephrol Dial Transplant.* 2010;25:2982.

114. Pras M, Schubert M, Zucker-Franklin D, et al. The characterization of soluble amyloid prepared in water. *J Clin Invest.* 1968;47:924.

115. Glenner GG, Ein D, Eanes ED, et al. Creation of "amyloid" fibrils from Bence Jones proteins in vitro. *Science.* 1971;174:712.

116. Glenner GG. Amyloid deposits and amyloidosis: the β-fibrilloses (first of two parts). *N Engl J Med.* 1980;302:1283.

117. Sipe JD, Benson MD, Buxbaum JN, et al. Amyloid fibril protein nomenclature: 2010 recommendations from the nomenclature committee of the International Society of Amyloidosis. *Amyloid.* 2010;17:101.

118. Ren R, Hong Z, Gong H, et al. Role of glycosaminoglycan sulfation in the formation of immunoglobulin light chain amyloid oligomers and fibrils. *J Biol Chem.* 2010;285:37672.

119. Kisilevsky R. Proteoglycans, glycosaminoglycans, amyloid-enhancing factor, and amyloid deposition. *J Intern Med.* 1992;232:515.

120. Emsley J, White HE, O'Hara BP, et al. Structure of pentameric human serum amyloid P component. *Nature.* 1994;367:338.

121. Bickerstaff MC, Botto M, Hutchinson WL, et al. Serum amyloid P component controls chromatin degradation and prevents antinuclear autoimmunity. *Nature Med.* 1999;5:694.

122. Hawkins PN, Lavender JP, Pepys MB. Evaluation of systemic amyloidosis by scintigraphy with ^{123}I-labeled serum amyloid P component. *N Engl J Med.* 1990;323:508.

123. Pepys MB, Herbert J, Hutchinson WL, et al. Targeted pharmacological depletion of serum amyloid P component for treatment of human amyloidosis. *Nature.* 2002;417:254.

124. Bodin K, Ellmerich S, Kahan MC et al. Antibodies to human serum amyloid P component eliminate visceral amyloid deposits. *Nature.* 2010;468:93.

125. Merlini G, Bellotti V. Molecular mechanisms of amyloidosis. *N Engl J Med.* 2003;349:583.

126. Sponarova J, Nyström SN, Westermark GT. AA-amyloidosis can be transferred by peripheral blood monocytes. *PLoS One.* 2008;3:e3308.

127. Gregorini G, Izzi C, Obici L et al. Renal apolipoprotein A-I amyloidosis: a rare and usually ignored cause of hereditary tubulointerstitial nephritis. *J Am Soc Nephrol.* 2005;16:3680.

128. Noel LH, Droz D, Ganeval D. Immunohistochemical characterization of renal amyloidosis. *Am J Clin Pathol.* 1987;87:606.

129. Gallo GR, Feiner HD, Chuba JV, et al. Characterization of tissue amyloid by immunofluorescence microscopy. *Clin Immunol Immunopathol.* 1986;39:479.

130. Lachmann HJ, Booth DR, Booth SE, et al. Misdiagnosis of hereditary amyloidosis as AL (primary) amyloidosis. *N Engl J Med.* 2002;346:1786.

131. Novak L, Cook WJ, Herrera GA, et al. AL-amyloidosis is underdiagnosed in renal biopsies. *Nephrol Dial Transplant.* 2004;19:3050.

132. Vrana JA, Gamez JD, Madden BJ et al. Classification of amyloidosis by laser microdissection and mass spectrometry-based proteomic analysis in clinical biopsy specimens. *Blood.* 2009;114:4957.

133. Sehti S, Theis JD, Leung N et al. Mass spectrometry-based proteomic diagnosis of renal immunoglobulin heavy chain amyloidosis. *Clin J Am Soc Nephrol.* 2010;5:2180.

134. Yang GC, Gallo GR. Protein A-gold immunoelectron microscopic study of amyloid fibrils, granular deposits, and fibrillar luminal aggregates in renal amyloidosis. *Am J Pathol.* 1990;137:1223.

135. Arbustini E, Verga L, Concardi M, et al. Electron and immuno-electron microscopy of abdominal fat identifies and characterizes amyloid fibrils in suspected cardiac amyloidosis. *Amyloid.* 2002;9:108.

136. Nasr SH, Lobritto SJ, Lauring BP, et al. A rare complication of monoclonal gammopathy. *Am J Kidney Dis.* 2002;40:867.

137. Solomon A, Weiss DT, Murphy C. Primary amyloidosis associated with a novel heavy-chain fragment (AH amyloidosis). *Am J Hematol.* 1994;45:171.

138. Yazaki M, Fushimi T, Tokuda T, et al. A patient with severe renal amyloidosis associated with an immunoglobulin gamma-heavy chain fragment. *Am J Kidney Dis.* 2004;43:e23.

139. Copeland JN, Kouides PA, Grieff M, et al. Metachronous development of nonamyloidogenic lambda light chain deposition disease and IgG heavy chain amyloidosis in the same patient. *Am J Surg Pathol.* 2003;27:1477.

140. Perfetti V, Casarini S, Palladini G, et al. Analysis of V(lambda)-J(lambda) expression in plasma cells from primary (AL) amyloidosis and normal bone marrow identifies 3r (lambdaIII) as a new amyloid-associated germline gene segment. *Blood.* 2002;100:948.

141. Comenzo RL, Zhang Y, Martinez C, et al. The tropism of organ involvement in primary systemic amyloidosis: contributions of Ig V(L) germ line gene use and clonal plasma cell burden. *Blood.* 2001;98:714.

142. Abraham RS, Geyer SM, Price-Troska TL, et al. Immunoglobulin light chain variable (V) region genes influence clinical presentation and outcome in light chain-associated amyloidosis (AL). *Blood.* 2003;101:3801.

143. Bellotti V, Merlini G, Bucciarelli E, et al. Relevance of class, molecular weight and isoelectric point in predicting human light chain amyloidogenicity. *Br J Haematol.* 1990;74:65.

144. Klafki HW, Kratzin HD, Pick AI, et al. Complete amino acid sequence determinations demonstrate identity of the urinary Bence Jones protein (BJP-DIA) and the amyloid fibril protein (AL-DIA) in a case of AL-amyloidosis. *Biochemistry.* 1992;31:3265.

145. Bellotti V, Stoppini M, Perfetti V, et al. Use of an anti-idiotypic monoclonal antibody in studying amyloidogenic light chains in cells, urine and fibrils: pathophysiology and clinical implications. *Scand J Immunol.* 1992;36:607.

146. Preud'homme JL, Ganeval D, Grünfeld JP, et al. Immunoglobulin synthesis in primary and myeloma amyloidosis. *Clin Exp Immunol.* 1988;73:389.

147. Buxbaum J. Aberrant immunoglobulin synthesis in light chain amyloidosis: free light chain and light chain fragment production by human bone marrow cells in short-term tissue culture. *J Clin Invest.* 1986;78:798.

148. Linke RP, Tischendorf RW, Zucker-Franklin D, et al. The formation of amyloid-like fibrils in vitro from Bence Jones proteins of the Vλ1 subclass. *J Immunol.* 1973;111:24.

149. Durie BG, Persky B, Soehnlen BJ, et al. Amyloid production in human myeloma stem-cell culture, with morphologic evidence of amyloid secretion by associated macrophages. *N Engl J Med.* 1982;307:1689.

150. Solomon A, Weiss DT, Pepys MB. Induction in mice of human light-chain-associated amyloidosis. *Am J Pathol.* 1992;140:629.

151. Klimtchuk ES, Gursky O, Patel RS, et al. The critical role of the constant region in thermal stability and aggregation of amyloidogenic immunoglobulin light chain. *Biochemistry.* 2010;49: 9848.

152. Yamamoto, Yagi H, Lee YH, et al. The amyloid fibrils of the constant domain of immunoglobulin light chain. *FEBS Lett.* 2010;584:3348.

153. Stevens FJ, Myatt EA, Chang CH, et al. A molecular model for self-assembly of amyloid fibrils: immunoglobulin light chains. *Biochemistry.* 1995;34:10697.

154. Stevens FJ. Four structural risk factors identify most fibril-forming kappa light chains. *Amyloid.* 2000;7:200.

155. Hurle MR, Helms LR, Li L, et al. A role for destabilizing amino acid replacements in light-chain amyloidosis. *Proc Natl Acad Sci U S A.* 1994;91:5446.

156. Poshusta TL, Sikkink LA, Leung N, et al. Mutations in specific structural regions of immunoglobulin light chains are associated with free light chain levels in patients with AL amyloidosis. *PLoS One.* 2009;4:e5169.

157. Kim YS, Cape SP, Chi E, et al. Counteracting effects of renal solutes on amyloid fibril formation by immunoglobulin light chains. *J Biol Chem.* 2001; 276:1626.

158. Davis DP, Gallo G, Vogen SM, et al. Both the environment and somatic mutations govern the aggregation pathway of pathogenic immunoglobulin light chain. *J Mol Biol.* 2001;313:1021.

159. Schiffer M, Girling RL, Ely KR, et al. Structure of a λ-type Bence-Jones protein at 3.5-Å resolution. *Biochemistry.* 1973;12:4620.

160. Edmundson AB, Ely KR, Herron JN, et al. The binding of opioid peptides to the Mcg light chain dimer: flexible keys and adjustable locks. *Mol Immunol.* 1987;24:915.

161. Edmundson AB, Ely KR, He XM, et al. Cocrystallization of an immunoglobulin light chain dimer with bis(dinitrophenyl) lysine: tandem binding of two ligands, one with and one without accompanying conformational changes in the protein. *Mol Immunol.* 1989;26:207.

162. Stevens PW, Raffen R, Hanson DK, et al. Recombinant immunoglobulin variable domains generated from synthetic genes provide a system for in vitro characterization of light-chain amyloid proteins. *Protein Sci.* 1995;4:421.

163. Perfetti V, Ubbiali P, Vignarelli MC, et al. Evidence that amyloidogenic light chains undergo antigen-driven selection. *Blood.* 1998;91:2948.

164. Abraham RS, Geyer SM, Ramirez-Alvarado M, et al. Analysis of somatic hypermutation and antigenic selection in the clonal B cell in immunoglobulin light chain amyloidosis (AL). *J Clin Immunol.* 2004;24:340.

165. Liao R, Jain M, Teller P, et al. Infusion of light chains from patients with cardiac amyloidosis causes diastolic dysfunction in isolated mouse hearts. *Circulation.* 2001;104:1594.

166. Brenner DA, Jain M, Pimentel DR, et al. Human amyloidogenic light chains directly impair cardiomyocyte function through an increase in cellular oxidant stress. *Circ Res.* 2004;94:1008.

167. Shi J, Guan J, Jiang B, et al. Amyloidogenic light chains induce cardiomyocyte contractile dysfunction and apoptosis via a non-canonical p38alpha MAPK pathway. *Proc Natl Acad Sci U S A.* 2010;107:4188.

168. Keeling J, Teng J, Herrera GA. AL-amyloidosis and light-chain deposition disease light chains induce divergent phenotypic transformations of human mesangial cells. *Lab Invest.* 2004;84:1322.

169. Kyle RA, Linos A, Beard CM, et al. Incidence and natural history of primary systemic amyloidosis in Olmsted County, Minnesota, 1950 through 1989. *Blood.* 1992;79:1817.
170. Gertz MA, Lacy MQ, Dispenzieri A. Immunoglobulin light chain amyloidosis and the kidney. *Kidney Int.* 2002;61:1.
171. Guidelines Working Group of UK Myeloma Forum; British Committee for Standards in Haematology, British Society for Haematology. Guidelines on the diagnosis and management of AL amyloidosis. *Br J Haematol.* 2004;125:681.
172. Pinney JH, Lachmann HJ, Bansi L et al. Outcome in renal AL amyloidosis after chemotherapy. *J Clin Oncol.* 2011;29:674.
173. Kyle RA, Gertz MA. Primary systemic amyloidosis: clinical and laboratory features in 474 cases. *Semin Hematol.* 1995;32:45.
174. Alexanian R, Fraschini G, Smith L. Amyloidosis in multiple myeloma or without apparent cause. *Arch Intern Med.* 1984;144:2158.
175. Cohen AD, Zhou P, Xiao Q, et al. Systemic AL amyloidosis due to non-Hodgkin's lymphoma: an unusual clinicopathologic association. *Br J Haematol.* 2004;124:309.
176. Kyle RA, Greipp PR. Amyloidosis (AL): clinical and laboratory features in 229 cases. *Mayo Clin Proc.* 1983;58:665.
177. Hetzel GR, Uhlig K, Mondry A, et al. AL-amyloidosis of the kidney initially presenting as minimal change glomerulonephritis. *Am J Kidney Dis.* 2000;36:630.
178. Leung N, Dispenzieri A, Lacy MQ, et al. Severity of baseline proteinuria predicts renal response in immunoglobulin light chain-associated amyloidosis after autologous stem cell transplantation. *Clin J Am Soc Nephrol.* 2007;2:440.
179. Gertz MA, Leung N, Lacy MQ, et al. Clinical outcome of immunoglobulin light chain amyloidosis affecting the kidney. *Nephrol Dial Transplant.* 2009;24:3132.
180. Dispenzieri A, Kyle RA, Gertz MA, et al. Survival in patients with primary systemic amyloidosis and raised serum cardiac troponins. *Lancet.* 2003; 361:1787.
181. Palladini G, Campana C, Klersy C, et al. Serum N-terminal pro-brain natriuretic peptide is a sensitive marker of myocardial dysfunction in AL amyloidosis. *Circulation.* 2003;107:2440.
182. Dispenzieri A, Gertz MA, Kyle RA, et al. Serum cardiac troponins and N-terminal pro-brain natriuretic peptide: a staging system for primary systemic amyloidosis. *J Clin Oncol.* 2004;22:3601.
183. Dispenzieri A, Gertz MA, Kyle RA, et al. Prognostication of survival using cardiac troponins and N-terminal pro-brain natriuretic peptide in patients with primary systemic amyloidosis undergoing peripheral blood stem cell transplantation. *Blood.* 2004;104:1881.
184. Palladini G, Barassi A, Klersy C, et al. The combination of high-sensitivity cardiac troponin T (hs-cTnT) at presentation and changes in N-terminal natriuretic peptide type B (NT-proBNP) after chemotherapy best predicts survival in AL amyloidosis. *Blood.* 2010;116:3426.
185. Sucker C, Hetzel GR, Grabensee B, et al. Amyloidosis and bleeding: pathophysiology, diagnosis, and therapy. *Am J Kidney Dis.* 2006 47;947.
186. Alyanakian MA, Abbas A, Delarue R, et al. Free immunoglobulin light-chain serum levels in the follow-up of patients with monoclonal gammopathies: correlation with 24-hr urinary light-chain excretion. *Am J Hematol.* 2004;60:246.
187. Palladini G, Russo P, Bosoni T, et al. Identification of amyloidogenic light chains requires the combination of serum-free light chain assay with immunofixation of serum and urine. *Clin Chem.* 2009;55:499.
188. Osserman EF, Takatsuki K, Talal N. Multiple myeloma. I. The pathogenesis of "amyloidosis." *Semin Hematol.* 1964;1:3.
189. Lachmann HJ, Gallimore R, Gillmore JD, et al. Outcome in systemic AL amyloidosis in relation to changes in concentration of circulating free immunoglobulin light chains following chemotherapy. *Br J Haematol.* 2003;122:78.
190. Skinner M, Anderson JJ, Simms R, et al. Treatment of 100 patients with primary amyloidosis: a randomized trial of melphalan, prednisone, and colchicine versus colchicine only. *Am J Med.* 1996;100:290.
191. Gertz MA, Comenzo R, Falk RH, et al. Definition of organ involvement and treatment response in primary systemic amyloidosis AL. *Am J Hematol.* 2005;79:319.
192. Gertz MA, Merlini G. Definition of organ involvement and response to treatment in AL amyloidosis: a consensus opinion. *Amyloid.* 2010;17:48.
193. Kyle RA, Gertz MA, Greipp PR, et al. A trial of three regimens for primary amyloidosis: colchicine alone, melphalan and prednisone, and melphalan, prednisone, and colchicine. *N Engl J Med.* 1997;336:1202.
194. Falk RH. Diagnosis and management of the cardiac amyloidoses. *Circulation.* 2005;112:2047.
195. Hawkins PN, Lachmann HJ, McDermott MF. Interleukin-1-receptor antagonist in the Muckle-Wells syndrome. *N Engl J Med.* 2003;348:2583.
196. Palladini G, Lavatelli F, Russo P, et al. Circulating amyloidogenic free light chains and serum N-terminal natriuretic peptide type B decrease simultaneously in association with improvement of survival in AL. *Blood.* 2006;107:3854.
197. Sanchorawala V, Skinner M, Quillen K, et al. Long-term outcome of patients with AL amyloidosis treated with high-dose melphalan and stem-cell transplantation. *Blood.* 2007;110:3561.
198. Gertz MA, Lacy MQ, Lust JA, et al. Prospective randomized trial of melphalan and prednisone versus vincristine, carmustine, melphalan, cyclophosphamide, and prednisone in the treatment of primary systemic amyloidosis. *J Clin Oncol.* 1999;17:262.
199. Lachmann HJ, Gillmore JD, Pepys MB, et al. Outcome in systemic AL amyloidosis following stem cell transplantation or infusional chemotherapy. *Blood.* 2002;100:210a.
200. Palladini G, Perfetti V, Obici L, et al. Association of melphalan and high-dose dexamethasone is effective and well tolerated in patients with AL (primary) amyloidosis who are ineligible for stem cell transplantation. *Blood.* 2004;103:2936.
201. Jaccard A, Moreau P, Leblond V, et al. High-dose melphalan versus melphalan plus dexamethasone for AL amyloidosis. *N Engl J Med.* 2007;357:1083.
202. Comenzo RL, Gertz MA. Autologous stem cell transplantation for primary systemic amyloidosis. *Blood.* 2002;99:4276.
203. Skinner M, Sanchorawala V, Seldin DC, et al. High-dose melphalan and autologous stem-cell transplantation in patients with AL amyloidosis: an 8-year study. *Ann Intern Med.* 2004;140:85.
204. Comenzo RL, Vosburgh E, Simms RW, et al. Dose-intensive melphalan with blood stem cell support for the treatment of AL amyloidosis: one-year ollow-up in five patients. *Blood.* 1996;88:2801–2806.
205. Comenzo RL, Vosburgh E, Falk RH, et al. Dose-intensive melphalan with blood stem-cell support for the treatment of AL (amyloid light-chain) amyloidosis: survival and responses in 25 patients. *Blood.* 1998;91:3662–3670.
206. Moreau P, Leblond V, Bourquelot P, et al. Prognostic factors for survival and response after high-dose therapy and autologous stem cell transplantation in systemic AL amyloidosis: a report on 21 patients. *Br J Haematol.* 1998;101:766.
207. Sanchorawala V, Wright DG, Seldin DC, et al. An overview of the use of high dose melphalan with autologous stem cell transplantation for the treatment of AL amyloidosis. *Bone Marrow Transplant.* 2001;28:637.
208. Gertz MA, Lacy MQ, Gastineau DA, et al. Blood stem cell transplantation as therapy for primary systemic amyloidosis (AL). *Bone Marrow Transplant.* 2000;26:963.
209. Gertz MA, Lacy MQ, Dispenzieri A, et al. Trends in day 100 and 2-year survival after auto-SCT for AL amyloidosis: outcomes before and after 2006. *Bone Marrow Transplant.* 2011;46(7):970–975.
210. Dispenzieri A, Lacy MQ, Kyle RA, et al. Eligibility for hematopoietic stem-cell transplantation for primary systemic amyloidosis is a favorable prognostic factor for survival. *J Clin Oncol.* 2001;19:3350.
211. Wechalekar AD, Goodman HJ, Lachmann HJ, et al. Safety and efficacy of risk-adapted cyclophosphamide, thalidomide, and dexamethasone in systemic AL amyloidosis. *Blood.* 2007;109:457–464.
212. Moreau P, Jaccard A, Benboubker L, et al. Lenalidomide in combination with melphalan and dexamethasone in patients with newly diagnosed AL amyloidosis: a multicenter phase 1/2 dose-escalation study. *Blood.* 2010;116:4777.
213. Wechalekar AD, Lachmann HJ, Offer M, et al. Efficacy of bortezomib in systemic AL amyloidosis with relapsed/refractory clonal disease. *Haematologica.* 2008;93:295.
214. Reece DE, Sanchorawala V, Hegenbart U, et al. Weekly and twice-weekly bortezomib in patients with systemic AL amyloidosis: results of a phase 1 dose-escalation study. *Blood.* 2009;114:1489.
215. Kastritis E, Wechalekar AD, Dimopoulos MA, et al. Bortezomib with or without dexamethasone in primary systemic (light chain) amyloidosis. *J Clin Oncol.* 2010;28:1031–1037.
216. Lamm W, Willenbacher W, Lang A, et al. Efficacy of the combination of bortezomib and dexamethasone in systemic AL amyloidosis. *Ann Hematol.* 2011;90:201.
217. Zonder JA, Snyder RM, Matous J, et al. Melphalan and dexamethasone plus bortezomib induces hematologic and organ responses in AL-amyloidosis with tolerable neurotoxicity. *Blood (ASH Annual Meeting Abstracts).* 2009;114:746.
218. Palladini G, Foli A, Russo P, et al. Treatment of IgM-associated AL amyloidosis with the combination of rituximab, bortezomib, and dexamethasone. *Clin Lymphoma Myeloma Leuk.* 2011;11:143.
219. Gertz MA, Hayman SR, Buadi FK. Transplantation for IgM amyloidosis and IgM myeloma. *Clin Lymphoma Myeloma.* 2009;9:77.
220. Bergesio F, Ciciani AM, Manganaro M, et al. Renal involvement in systemic amyloidosis: an Italian collaborative study on survival and renal outcome. *Nephrol Dial Transplant.* 2008;23:941.
221. Gertz MA, Kyle RA, O'Fallon WM. Dialysis support of patients with primary systemic amyloidosis. A study of 211 patients. *Arch Intern Med.* 1992;152:2245.

222. Bollee G, Guery B, Joly D, et al. Presentation and outcome of patients with systemic amyloidosis undergoing dialysis. *Clin J Am Soc Nephrol.* 2008;3:360.
223. Hartmann A, Holdaas H, Fauchald P et al. Fifteen years' experience with renal transplantation in systemic amyloidosis. *Transplant Int.* 1992;5:15.
224. Sattianayagam PT, Gibbs SD, Pinney JH, et al. Solid organ transplantation in AL amyloidosis. *Am J Transplant.* 2010;10:2124.
225. Herrmann SMS, Gertz MA, Stegall MD, et al. Long-term outcomes of patients with light chain amyloidosis (AL) after renal transplantation with or without stem cell transplantation. *Nephrol Dial Transplant.* 2011;26(6):2032–2036.
226. Dahlin DC. Amyloidosis. *Mayo Clin Proc.* 1949;24:637.
227. Brownstein MH, Helwig EB. Secondary systemic amyloidosis: analysis of underlying disorders. *South Med J.* 1971;64:491.
228. Browning MJ, Banks RA, Tribe CR, et al. Ten years' experience of an amyloid clinic - a clinicopathological survey. *Q J Med.* 1985;54:213.
229. Gertz MA, Kyle RA. Secondary systemic amyloidosis: response and survival in 64 patients. *Medicine (Baltimore).* 1991;70:246.
230. Joss N, McLaughlin K, Simpson K, et al. Presentation, survival and prognostic markers in AA amyloidosis. *Q J Med.* 2000;93:535.
231. Gillmore JD, Lovat LB, Persey MR, et al. Amyloid load and clinical outcome in AA amyloidosis in relation to circulating concentration of serum amyloid A protein. *Lancet.* 2001;358:24.
232. Lachmann H, Goodman HJB, Gilbertson JA, et al. Natural history and outcome in systemic AA amyloidosis. *N Engl J Med.* 2007;356:2361.
233. Gottenberg JE, Merle-Vincent F, Bentaberry F, et al. Anti-tumor necrosis factor alpha therapy in fifteen patients with AA amyloidosis secondary to inflammatory arthritides: a followup report of tolerability and efficacy. *Arthritis Rheum.* 2003;48:2019.
234. Verine J, Mourad N, Desseaux K, et al. Clinical and histological characteristics of renal AA amyloidosis: a retrospective study of 68 cases with a special interest to amyloid-associated inflammatory response. *Hum Pathol.* 2007;38:1798.
235. Sasatomi Y, Sato H, Chiba Y, et al. Prognostic factors for renal amyloidosis: a clinicopathological study using cluster analysis. *Intern Med.* 2007;46:213.
236. Pasternack A, Ahonen J, Kuhlböck B. Renal transplantation in 45 patients with amyloidosis. *Transplantation.* 1986;42:598.
237. Isoniemi H, Eklund B, Höckerstedt K, et al. Renal transplantation in amyloidosis. *Transplant Proc.* 1989;21:2039.
238. Sherif AM, Refaie AF, Sobh MA, et al. Long-term outcome of live donor kidney transplantation for renal amyloidosis. *Am J Kidney Dis.* 2003;42:370.
239. Kofman T, Grimbert P, Canouï-Poitirine F, et al. Renal transplantation in patients with AA amyloidosis nephropathy: results from a French multicenter study. *Am J Transplant* 2011;11: 2423.
240. Zemer D, Pras M, Sohar E, et al. Colchicine in the prevention and treatment of the amyloidosis of familial Mediterranean fever. *N Engl J Med.* 1986;314:1001.
241. Tunca M, Akar S, Onen F, et al. Familial Mediterranean fever (FMF) in Turkey: results of a nationwide multicenter study. *Medicine (Baltimore).* 2005;84:1.
242. The International FMF Consortium. Ancient missense mutations in a new member of the *Roret* gene family are likely to cause familial Mediterranean fever. *Cell.* 1997;90:797.
243. The French FMF Consortium. A candidate gene for familial Mediterranean fever. *Nat Genet.* 1997;17:25.
244. Zemer D, Revach M, Pras M, et al. A controlled trial of colchicine in preventing attacks of familial Mediterranean fever. *N Engl J Med.* 1974;291:932.
245. Zemer D, Livneh A, Langevitz P. Reversal of the nephrotic syndrome by colchicine in amyloidosis of familial Mediterranean fever. *Ann Intern Med.* 1992;116:426.
246. Moser C, Pohl G, Haslinger I, et al. Successful treatment of familial Mediterranean fever with anakinra and outcome after renal transplantation. *Nephrol Dial Transplant.* 2009;24:676.
247. Leslie KS, Lachmann HJ, Bruning E, et al. Phenotype, genotype, and sustained response to anakinra in 22 patients with autoinflammatory disease associated with CIAS-1/NALP3 mutations. *Arch Dermatol.* 2006;142:1591.
248. Hoffman HM, Throne ML, Amar NJ, et al. Efficacy and safety of rilonacept (interleukin-1 Trap) in patients with cryopyrin-associated periodic syndromes: results from two sequential placebo-controlled studies. *Arthritis Rheum.* 2008;58:2443.
249. Lachmann HJ, Kone-Paut I, Kuemmerle-Deschner JB, et al. Use of canakinumab in the cryopyrin-associated periodic syndrome. *N Engl J Med.* 2009;360:2416.
250. Aksentijevich I, Masters SL, Ferguson PJ, et al. An autoinflammatory disease with deficiency of the interleukin-1-receptor antagonist. *N Engl J Med.* 2009;360:2426.
251. Yan SD, Zhu H, Zhu A, et al. Receptor-dependent cell stress and amyloid accumulation in systemic amyloidosis. *Nat Med.* 2000;6:643.
252. Kisilevsky R, Lemieux LJ, Fraser PE, et al. Arresting amyloidosis in vivo using small-molecule anionic sulphonates or sulphates: implications for Alzheimer's disease. *Nat Med.* 1995;1:143.
253. Dember L, Hawkins PM, Hazenberg BPC, et al. Eprodisate for the treatment of renal disease in AA amyloidosis. *N Engl J Med.* 2007;356:2349.
254. Merlini G, Ascari E, Amboldi N, et al. Interaction of the anthracycline 4′-iodo-4′-deoxydoxorubicin with amyloid fibrils: inhibition of amyloidogenesis. *Proc Natl Acad Sci U S A.* 1995;92:2959.
255. Gertz MA, Lacy MQ, Dispenzieri A, et al. Multicenter phase II trial of 4′-iodo-4′deoxydoxorubicin (IDOX) in primary amyloidosis (AL). *Amyloid.* 2002;9:24.
256. Hrncic R, Wall J, Wolfenbarger DA, et al. Antibody-mediated resolution of light chain-associated amyloid deposits. *Am J Pathol.* 2000;157:1239.
257. O'Nuallain B, Allen A, Kennel SJ, et al. Localization of a conformational epitope common to non-native and fibrillar immunoglobulin light chains. *Biochemistry.* 2007;46:1240.
258. Kobernick SD, Whiteside JH. Renal glomeruli in multiple myeloma. *Lab Invest.* 1957;6:478.
259. Sanchez LM, Domz CA. Renal patterns in myeloma. *Ann Intern Med.* 1960;52:44.
260. Buxbaum JN, Chuba JV, Hellman GC, et al. Monoclonal immunoglobulin deposition disease: light chain and light and heavy chain deposition diseases and their relation to light chain amyloidosis. Clinical features, immunopathology, and molecular analysis. *Ann Intern Med.* 1990;112:455.
261. Kambham N, Markowitz GS, Appel GB, et al. Heavy chain deposition disease: the disease spectrum. *Am J Kidney Dis.* 1999;33:954.
262. Lin J, Markowitz GS, Valeri AM, et al. Renal monoclonal immunoglobulin deposition disease: the disease spectrum. *J Am Soc Nephrol.* 2001;12:1482.
263. Tubbs RR, Berkley V, Valenzuela R, et al. Pseudo-γ heavy chain ($IgG_4\lambda$) deposition disease. *Mod Pathol.* 1992;5:185.
264. Ganeval D, Noël LH, Preud'homme JL, et al. Light-chain deposition disease: its relation with AL-type amyloidosis. *Kidney Int.* 1984;26:1.
265. Deret S, Chomilier J, Huang DB, et al. Molecular modeling of immunoglobulin light chains implicates hydrophobic residues in non-amyloid light chain deposition disease. *Protein Eng.* 1997;10:1191.
266. Khamlichi AA, Rocca A, Touchard G, et al. Role of light chain variable region in myeloma with light chain deposition disease: evidence from an experimental model. *Blood.* 1995;86:3655.
267. Kaplan B, Livneh A, Gallo G. Charge differences between in vivo deposits in immunoglobulin light chain amyloidosis and non-amyloid light chain deposition disease. *Br J Haematol.* 2007;136:723.
268. Khurana R, Gillespie JR, Talapatra A, et al. Partially folded intermediates as critical precursors of light chain amyloid fibrils and amorphous aggregates. *Biochemistry.* 2001;40:3525.
269. Husby G, Blichfeldt P, Brinch L, et al. Chronic arthritis and γ heavy chain disease: coincidence or pathogenic link? *Scand J Rheumatol.* 1998;27:257.
270. Soma J, Sato K, Sakuma T, et al. Immunoglobulin gamma3-heavy-chain deposition disease: report of a case and relationship with hypocomplementemia. *Am J Kidney Dis.* 2004;43:E10.
271. Soma J, Tsuchiya Y, Sakuma T, et al. Clinical remission and histopathological resolution of nodular lesions in a patient with gamma3 heavy-chain deposition disease. *Clin Nephrol.* 2008;69:383.
272. Oe Y, Nakaya I, Yahata M, et al. A case of γ1-heavy chain deposition disease successfully treated with melphalan and prednisolone therapy. *Intern Med.* 2010;49:1411.
273. Cheng IK, Ho SK, Chan DT, et al. Crescentic nodular glomerulosclerosis secondary to truncated immunoglobulin alpha heavy chain deposition. *Am J Kidney Dis.* 1996;28:283.
274. Ronco P, Plaisier E, Mougenot B, et al. Immunoglobulin light (heavy)-chain deposition disease: from molecular medicine to pathophysiology-driven therapy. *Clin J Am Soc Nephrol.* 2006;1:1342.
275. Khamlichi AA, Aucouturier P, Preud'homme JL, et al. Structure of abnormal heavy chains in human heavy chain deposition disease. *Eur J Biochem.* 1995;229:54.
276. Pozzi C, D'Amico M, Fogazzi GB, et al. Light chain deposition disease with renal involvement: clinical characteristics and prognostic factors. *Am J Kidney Dis.* 2003;42:1154.
277. Ronco P, Plaisier E, Aucouturier P. Monoclonal immunoglobulin light and heavy chain deposition diseases: molecular models of common renal diseases. *Contrib Nephrol.* 2011;169:221.
278. Zhu L, Herrera GA, Murphy-Ullrich JE, et al. Pathogenesis of glomerulosclerosis in light chain deposition disease: role of transforming growth factor-β. *Am J Pathol.* 1995;147:360.
279. Herrera GA, Shultz JJ, Soong SJ, et al. Growth factors in monoclonal light-chain-related renal diseases. *Hum Pathol.* 1994;25:883.

280. Teng J, Russell WJ, Gu X, et al. Different types of glomerulopathic light chains interact with mesangial cells using a common receptor but exhibit different intracellular trafficking patterns. *Lab Invest.* 2004;84:440.
281. Russell WJ, Cardelli J, Harris E, et al. Monoclonal light chain—mesangial cell interactions: early signaling events and subsequent pathologic effects. *Lab Invest.* 2001;81:689.
282. Keeling J, Herrera GA. An in vitro model of light chain deposition disease. *Kidney Int.* 2009;60:634.
283. Gu X, Herrera GA. Light-chain-mediated acute tubular interstitial nephritis: a poorly recognized pattern of renal disease in patients with plasma cell dyscrasia. *Arch Pathol Lab Med.* 2006;130:165.
284. Masai R, Wakui H, Togashi M, et al. Clinicopathological features and prognosis in immunoglobulin light and heavy chain deposition disease. *Clin Nephrol.* 2009;71:9.
285. Herrera GA, Turbat-Herrera EA. Ultrastructural immunolabeling in the diagnosis of monoclonal light-and heavy-chain-related renal diseases. *Ultrastruct Pathol.* 2010;34:161.
286. Ganeval D, Mignon F, Preud'homme JL, et al. Visceral deposition of monoclonal light chains and immunoglobulins: a study of renal and immunopathologic abnormalities. *Adv Nephrol Necker Hosp.* 1982;11:25.
287. Heilman RL, Velosa JA, Holley KE, et al. Long-term follow-up and response to chemotherapy in patients with light-chain deposition disease. *Am J Kidney Dis.* 1992;20:34.
288. Tubbs RR, Gephardt GN, McMahon JT, et al. Light chain nephropathy. *Am J Med.* 1981;71:263.
289. Strom EH, Fogazzi GB, Banfi G, et al. Light chain deposition disease of the kidney: morphological aspects in 24 patients. *Virchows Arch.* 1994;425:271.
290. Katz A, Zent R, Bargman JM. IgG heavy-chain deposition disease. *Mod Pathol.* 1994;7:874.
291. Yasuda T, Fujita K, Imai H, et al. Gamma-heavy chain deposition disease showing nodular glomerulosclerosis. *Clin Nephrol.* 1995;44:394.
292. Herzenberg AM, Lien J, Magil AB. Monoclonal heavy chain (immunoglobulin G3) deposition disease: report of a case. *Am J Kidney Dis.* 1996;28:128.
293. Rott T, Vizjak A, Lindic J, et al. IgG heavy-chain deposition disease affecting kidney, skin, and skeletal muscle. *Nephrol Dial Transplant.* 1998;13:1825.
294. Polski JM, Galvin N, Salinas-Madrigal L. Non-amyloid fibrils in heavy chain deposition disease. *Kidney Int.* 1999;56:1601.
295. Liapis H, Papadakis I, Nakopoulou L. Nodular glomerulosclerosis secondary to μ heavy chain deposits. *Hum Pathol.* 2000;31:122.
296. Vedder AC, Weening JJ, Krediet RT. Intracapillary proliferative glomerulonephritis due to heavy chain deposition disease. *Nephrol Dial Transplant.* 2004;19:1302.
297. Rostagno A, Frizzera G, Ylagan L, et al. Tumoral non-amyloidotic monoclonal immunoglobulin light chain deposits ('aggregoma'): presenting feature of B-cell dyscrasia in three cases with immunohistochemical and biochemical analyses. *Br J Haematol.* 2002;119:62.
298. Khoor A, Myers JL, Tazelaar HD, et al. Amyloid-like pulmonary nodules, including localized light-chain deposition: clinicopathologic analysis of three cases. *Am J Clin Pathol.* 2004;121:200.
299. Colombat M, Stern M, Groussard O, et al. Pulmonary cystic disorder related to light chain deposition disease. *Am J Respir Crit Care Med.* 2006;173:777.
300. Colombat M, Mal H, Copie-Bergman C, et al. Primary cystic lung light chain deposition disease: a clinicopathologic entity derived from unmutated B cells with a stereotyped IGHV 34/IGKV1 receptor. *Blood.* 2008;112:2004.
301. Husby G. Is there a pathogenic link between gamma heavy chain disease and chronic arthritis? *Curr Opin Rheumatol.* 2000;12:65.
302. Preud'homme JL, Morel-Maroger L, Brouet JC, et al. Synthesis of abnormal heavy and light chains in multiple myeloma with visceral deposition of monoclonal immunoglobulin. *Clin Exp Immunol.* 1980;42:545.
303. Went P, Ascani S, Strom E, et al. Nodal marginal-zone lymphoma associated with monoclonal light-chain and heavy-chain deposition disease. *Lancet.* 2004;5:381.
304. Katzmann JA, Kyle RA, Benson J, et al. Screening panels for detection of monoclonal gammopathies. *Clin Chem.* 2009;55:1517.
305. Mariette X, Clauvel JP, Brouet JC. Intensive therapy in AL amyloidosis and light-chain deposition disease. *Ann Intern Med.* 1995;123:553.
306. Petrakis I, Stylianou K, Mavroeidi V, et al. Biopsy-proven resolution of renal light-chain deposition disease after autologous stem cell transplantation. *Nephrol Dial Transplant.* 2010;25:2020.
307. Harada K, Akai Y, Sakan H, et al. Resolution of mesangial light chain deposits 3 years after high-dose melphalan with autologous peripheral blood stem cell transplantation. *Clin Nephrol.* 2010;74:384.
308. Komatsuda A, Wakui H, Ohtani H, et al. Disappearance of nodular mesangial lesions in a patient with light chain nephropathy after long-term chemotherapy. *Am J Kidney Dis.* 2000;35:E9.
309. Royer B, Arnulf B, Martinez F, et al. High dose chemotherapy in light chain or light and heavy chain deposition disease. *Kidney Int.* 2004;65:642.
310. Weichman K, Dember LM, Prokaeva T, et al. Clinical and molecular characteristics of patients with non-amyloid light chain deposition disorders, and outcome following treatment with high-dose melphalan and autologous stem cell transplantation. *Bone Marrow Transplant.* 2006;38:339.
311. Hassoun H, Flombaum C, D'Agati VD, et al. High-dose melphalan and auto-SCT in patients with monoclonal Ig deposition disease. *Bone Marrow Transplant.* 2008;42:405.
312. Lorenz EC, Gertz MA, Fervenza FC, et al. Long-term outcome of autologous stem cell transplantation in light chain deposition disease. *Nephrol Dial Transplant.* 2008;23:2052.
313. Telio D, Shepherd J, Forrest D, et al. High-dose melphalan followed by ASCT has favorable safety and efficacy in selected patients with light chain deposition disease and light and heavy chain deposition disease. *Bone Marrow Transplant.* 2011;47:453–455.
314. Firkin F, Hill PA, Dwyer K, et al. Reversal of dialysis-dependent renal failure in light-chain deposition disease by autologous peripheral blood stem cell transplantation. *Am J Kidney Dis.* 2004;44:551.
315. Kastritis E, Migkou M, Gavriatopoulou M, et al. Treatment of light chain deposition disease with bortezomib and dexamethasone. *Haematologica.* 2009; 94:300.
316. Sanders PW, Herrera GA, Lott RL, et al. Morphologic alterations of the proximal tubules in light-chain related renal disease. *Kidney Int.* 1988; 33:881.
317. Short IA, Smith JP. Myelomatosis associated with glycosuria and aminoaciduria. *Scot Med J.* 1959;4:89.
318. Finkel PN, Kronenberg K, Pesce AJ, et al. Adult Fanconi syndrome, amyloidosis and marked kappa light chain proteinuria. *Nephron.* 1973;10:1.
319. Gallo G, Picken M, Buxbaum J, et al. The spectrum of monoclonal immunoglobulin deposition disease associated with immunocytic dyscrasias. *Semin Hematol.* 1989;26:234.
320. Lam KY, Chan KW. Unusual findings in a myeloma kidney: a light- and electron-microscopic study. *Nephron.* 1993;65:133.
321. Komatsuda A, Maki N, Wakui H, et al. Development of systemic λ-light chain amyloidosis in a patient with γ–heavy deposition disease during long-term follow-up. *Nephrol Dial Transplant.* 2005;20:434.
322. Morel-Maroger L, Basch A, Danon F, et al. Pathology of the kidney in Waldenström's macroglobulinemia. Study of sixteen cases. *N Engl J Med.* 1970;283:123.
323. Audard V, Georges B, Vanhille P, et al. Renal lesions associated with IgM-secreting monoclonal proliferations: revisiting the disease spectrum. *Clin J Am Soc Nephrol.* 2008;3:1339.
324. Terrier B, Jaccard A, Harousseau JL, et al. The clinical spectrum of IgM-related amyloidosis: a French nationwide retrospective study of 72 patients. *Medicine (Baltimore).* 2008;87:99.
325. Wechalekar AD, Lachmann HJ, Goodman HJ, et al. AL amyloidosis associated with IgM paraproteinemia: clinical profile and treatment outcome. *Blood.* 2008;112:4009.
326. Palladini G, Russo P, Bosoni T, et al. AL amyloidosis associated with IgM monoclonal protein: a distinct clinical entity. *Clin Lymphoma Myeloma.* 2009;9:80.
327. Alpers CE, Rennke HG, Hopper J, et al. Fibrillary glomerulonephritis. An entity with unusual immunofluorescence features. *Kidney Int.* 1987;31:781.
328. Korbet SM, Schwartz MM, Rosenberg BF, et al. Immunotactoid glomerulopathy. *Medicine (Baltimore).* 1985;64:228.
329. Alpers CE. Immunotactoid (microtubular) glomerulopathy: an entity distinct from fibrillary glomerulonephritis? *Am J Kidney Dis.* 1992;19:185.
330. Schwartz MM, Korbet SM, Lewis EJ. Immunotactoid glomerulopathy. *J Am Soc Nephrol.* 2002;13:1390.
331. Fogo A, Qureshi N, Horn RG. Morphologic and clinical features of fibrillary glomerulonephritis versus immunotactoid glomerulopathy. *Am J Kidney Dis.* 1993;22:367.
332. Alpers CE. Fibrillary glomerulonephritis and immunotactoid glomerulopathy: two entities, not one. *Am J Kidney Dis.* 1993;22:448.
333. Bridoux F, Hugue V, Coldefy O, et al. Fibrillary glomerulonephritis and immunotactoid (microtubular) glomerulopathy are associated with distinct immunologic features. *Kidney Int.* 2002;62:1764.
334. Rosenstock JL, Markowitz GS, Valeri AM, et al. Fibrillary and immunotactoid glomerulonephritis: distinct entities with different clinical and pathologic features. *Kidney Int.* 2003;63:1450.
335. Nasr SH, Valeri AM, Cornell LD, et al. Fibrillary glomerulonephritis: a report of 66 cases from a single institution. *Clin J Am Soc Nephrol.* 2011; 6:760.

336. Pronovost PH, Brady HR, Gunning ME, et al. Clinical features, predictors of disease progression and results of renal transplantation in fibrillary immunotactoid glomerulopathy. *Nephrol Dial Transplant.* 1996;11:837.
337. Markowitz GS, Cheng JT, Colvin RB, et al. Hepatitis C viral infection is associated with fibrillary glomerulonephritis and immunotactoid glomerulopathy. *J Am Soc Nephrol.* 1998;9:2244.
338. Samaniego M, Nadasdy GM, Laszik Z, et al. Outcome of renal transplantation in fibrillary glomerulonephritis. *Clin Nephrol.* 2001;55:159.
339. Carles X, Rostaing L, Modesto A, et al. Successful treatment of recurrence of immunotactoid glomerulopathy in a kidney allograft recipient. *Nephrol Dial Transplant.* 2000;15:897.
340. Iskandar SS, Falk RJ, Jennette JC. Clinical and pathologic features of fibrillary glomerulonephritis. *Kidney Int.* 1992;42:1401.
341. Rostagno A, Vidal R, Kumar A, et al. Fibrillary glomerulonephritis related to serum fibrillar immunoglobulin–fibronectin complexes. *Am J Kidney Dis.* 1996;28:676.
342. Touchard G, Bauwens M, Goujon JM, et al. Glomerulonephritis with organized microtubular monoclonal immunoglobulin deposits. *Adv Nephrol. Necker Hosp.* 1994;23:149.
343. Brady HR. Nephrology forum: fibrillary glomerulopathy. *Kidney Int.* 1998; 53:1421.
344. Nasr SH, Satoskar A, Markowitz GS, et al. Proliferative glomerulonephritis with monoclonal IgG deposits. *J Am Soc Nephrol.* 2009;20:2055.
345. Alpers CE, Tu WH, Hopper J Jr, et al. Single light chain subclass (kappa chain) immunoglobulin deposition in glomerulonephritis. *Hum Pathol.* 1985;16:294.
346. Bridoux F, Zanetta G, Vanhille P, et al. Glomerulopathy with non-organized and non-Randall type monoclonal immunoglobulin deposits: a rare entity [Abstract]. *J Am Soc Nephrol.* 2001;12:94A.
347. Lorenz EC, Sethi S, Leung N, et al. Recurrent membranoproliferative glomerulonephritis after kidney transplantation. *Kidney Int.* 2010;77:721.
348. Guiard E, Karras A, Plaisier E, et al. Patterns of non-cryoglobulinemic glomerulonephritis with monoclonal Ig deposits : correlation with IgG subclass and response to rituximab. *Clin J Am Soc Nephrol.* 2011;6(7):1609–1616.
349. Karras A, Noel LH, Droz D, et al. Renal involvement in monoclonal (type I) cryoglobulinemia: two cases associated with IgG3 kappa cryoglobulin. *Am J Kidney Dis.* 2002;40:1091.
350. Evans DJ, Macanovic M, Dunn MJ, et al. Membranous glomerulonephritis associated with follicular B-cell lymphoma and subepithelial deposition of IgG1-kappa paraprotein. *Nephron Clin Pract.* 2003;93:c112.
351. Komatsuda A, Masai R, Ohtani H, et al. Monoclonal immunoglobulin deposition disease associated with membranous features. *Nephrol Dial Transplant.* 2008;23:3888.
352. de Seigneux S, Bindi P, Debiec H, et al. Immunoglobulin deposition disease with a membranous pattern and a circulating monoclonal immunoglobulin G with charge-dependent aggregation properties. *Am J Kidney Dis.* 2010;56:117.
353. Dispenzieri A, Kyle RA, Lacy MQ, et al. POEMS syndrome: definitions and long-term outcome. *Blood.* 2003;101:2496.
354. Sethi S, Zand L, Leung N, et al. Membranoproliferative glomerulonephritis secondary to monoclonal gammopathy. *Clin J Am Soc Nephrol* 2010:5:770
355. Bridoux F, Desport E, Frémeaux-Bacchi V, et al. Glomerulonephritis with isolated C3 deposits and monoclonal gammopathy: a fortuitous association? *Clin J Am Soc Nephrol* 2011;6:2165.
356. Sethi S, Fervenza FC, Zhang Y, et al. Proliferative glomerulonephritis secondary to dysfunction of the alternative pathway of complement. *Clin J Am Soc Nephrol.* 2011;6(5):1009–1017.

CHAPTER

61 Hyperuricemia, Gout, and the Kidney

Duk-Hee Kang • Mehmet Kanbay • Richard Johnson

Uric acid is a weak acid trioxopurine with a molecular weight of 168 that is composed of a pyrimidine and imidazole substructure with oxygen molecules ($C_5H_4N_4O_3$). It is produced during the metabolism of purines, and specifically is generated by the degradation of xanthine by the enzyme xanthine oxidase or its isoform, xanthine dehydrogenase. In most mammals uric acid is oxidized to 5-hydroxyisourate by the hepatic enzyme, urate oxidase (uricase), which is then further hydrolyzed to allantoin.[1] However, during early hominoid evolution (12 to 20 million years ago) a series of mutations occurred, first affecting the promoter region and then the actual gene, eventually rendering uricase nonfunctional.[2,3] As a consequence, serum uric acid levels in humans are higher (3 to 15 mg per dL, 180 to 900 μM) and less regulatable than in most mammals (1 to 3 mg per dL, 60 to 180 μM).[4] Great apes (such as the chimpanzee, gorilla, and orangutan) share the same uricase mutation as humans, and lesser apes (gibbons and siamangs) have a different uricase mutation, but these apes have lower serum uric acid levels (2 to 4 mg per dL, 120 to 240 μM),[4] primarily due to diets relatively low in purines and fructose.

The most well-known consequence of an elevated uric acid in humans is the disease gout, due to the deposition of urate crystals in synovial joints, occasionally with tophi formation. However, there are also a number of renal manifestations associated with elevated uric acid, including the formation of uric acid kidney stones (urate nephrolithiasis), acute urate nephropathy (due to intratubular crystal formation with obstruction), and chronic urate ("gouty") nephropathy. The latter has been historically viewed as occurring as a consequence of interstitial urate crystal deposition with local inflammation; however, there is increasing evidence suggesting this entity may also result from crystal-independent effects of uric acid. There is also the entity of familial juvenile hyperuricemic nephropathy (FJHN), for which the gene responsible has been identified. Recent studies also suggest that uric acid may have a role in other renal diseases and may also have a direct role in mediating intrarenal vascular disease, hypertension, and even the metabolic syndrome. These are all discussed in subsequent text of this chapter.

URATE METABOLISM AND HOMEOSTASIS

Generation of Uric Acid

Uric acid is produced from metabolic conversion of either dietary or endogenous purines, primarily in the liver, muscle, and intestine (Fig. 61.1).[5] Uric acid can also be produced de novo from glycine, glutamine, and other precursors. The immediate precursor of uric acid is xanthine, which is degraded to uric acid by either xanthine oxidase, which generates superoxide anion in the process, or by its isoform, xanthine dehydrogenase, which generates the reduced form of nicotinamide-adenine dinucleotide. Both exogenous purines (such as is present in fatty meat, organ meats, and seafood) and endogenous purines are major sources of uric acid in humans. Approximately two thirds of total body urate is produced endogenously, whereas the remaining one third is accounted for by dietary purines. Purine-rich foods include beer and other alcoholic beverages, anchovies, sardines in oil, fish roes, herring, organ meat (liver, kidneys, sweetbreads), legumes (dried beans, peas), meat extracts, consommé, gravies, mushrooms, spinach, asparagus, and cauliflower.[6] In healthy men, the urate pool averages about 1,200 mg with a mean turnover rate of 700 mg per day.

Excretion of Uric Acid

The primary site of excretion of uric acid is the kidney, with normal urinary urate excretion in the range of 250 to 750 mg per day. Although urate (the form of uric acid at blood pH of 7.4) is freely filtered in the glomerulus, there is evidence that there is both reabsorption and secretion in the proximal tubule, and as a consequence the fractional urate excretion is only 8% to 10% in the normal adult because urate reabsorption dominates oversecretion in the kidney. Some adaptation occurs with renal disease, in which the fractional excretion will increase to the 10% to 20% range. In addition, uric acid is also removed by the gut, where uric acid is degraded by uricolytic bacteria, and this may account for one third of the elimination of uric acid in the setting of renal failure.

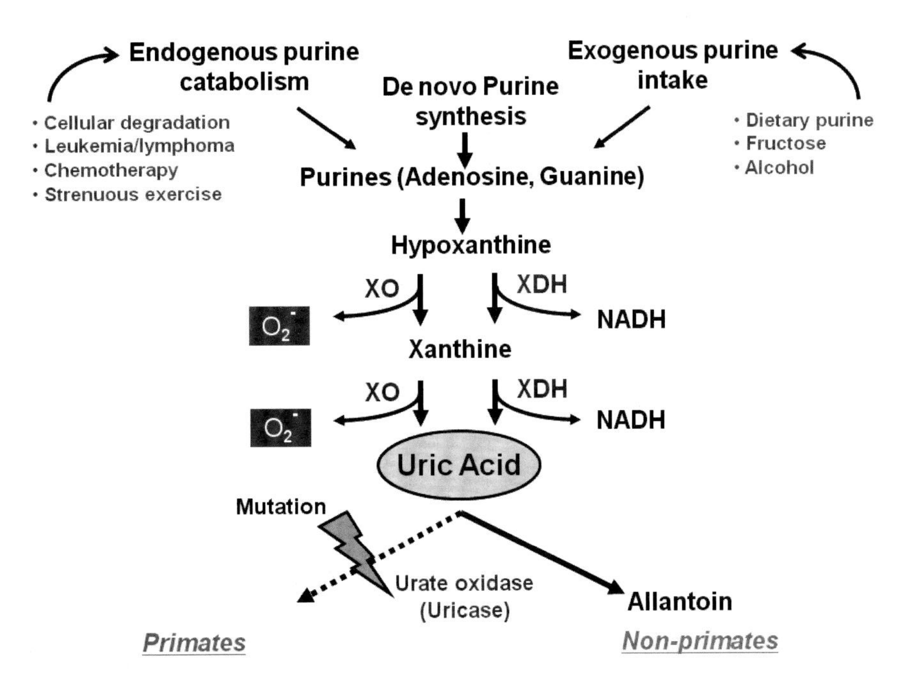

FIGURE 61.1 Urate metabolism.

The historic paradigm of uric acid excretion consists of a four-step model with glomerular filtration, followed by reabsorption, secretion, and postsecretory reabsorption, the latter three processes all occurring in the proximal convoluted tubule.[7,8] However, ideas of the handling of uric acid by the kidney have changed greatly during the last decades, with characterization and isolation of transporters and channels mainly or exclusively restricted to urate transport (Fig. 61.2).[9,10] Membrane vesicle studies have suggested the existence of two major mechanisms modulating urate reabsorption and secretion, consisting of a voltage-sensitive pathway and a urate/organic anion exchanger. Recently several of these transporters/channels have been identified. Organic anion transporters 1–10 (OAT1-10) and the urate transporter-1 (URAT-1) belong to the SLC22A gene family and accept a huge variety of chemically unrelated endogenous and exogenous organic anions including uric acid. Endou's group identified URAT-1, which is encoded by SLC22A12, as the major organic anion exchanger for uric acid on the apical (luminal brush border) side of the proximal tubular cell.[9] In the human kidney, urate is transported via URAT-1 across the apical membrane of proximal tubular cells, in exchange for anions being transported back into the tubular lumen to maintain electrical balance. URAT-1 has a high affinity for urate together with lactate, ketones, a-ketoglutarate, and related compounds. Pyrazinamide, probenecid, losartan, and benzbromarone all inhibit urate uptake in exchange for chloride at the luminal side of the cell by competition with the urate exchanger. OAT-4 exhibits 53% amino acid homology with URAT1.

Urate then moves across the basolateral membrane into the blood by other organic anion transporters, of which the most important is SLC2A9 (also known as GLUT9).[11,12] GLUT-9 is highly expressed in the kidney and liver. GLUT-9L (long isoform) is localized to basolateral membranes in proximal tubule epithelial cells, whereas the splice variant GLUT-9S (short isoform) localizes to apical membranes (Fig. 61.2).[13] Vitart et al.[14] showed that GLUT-9 transports urate and fructose, using a *Xenopus* oocyte expression system. GLUT-9 deficiency resulted in renal hypouricemia and is consistent with GLUT-9 being an efflux transporter of intracellular urate from the tubular cell to the interstitium/blood space.[15] Efflux transport of urate at basolateral membranes appears to depend principally on GLUT-9L whereas URAT-1 mainly acts as an influx transporter for urate at apical membranes.

OAT-4 and OAT-10 function as an organic anion/dicarboxylate exchanger and are responsible for the reabsorption of organic anions driven by an outwardly directed dicarboxylate gradient.[16] In addition, OAT1 and OAT3 may have a role in the transport of urate from the blood into the proximal tubule.[17,18]

Urate secretion appears to be mediated principally by a voltage-sensitive urate transporter, which is expressed ubiquitously and localizes to the apical side of the proximal tubule in the kidney. Genomewide association studies revealed the region which is related to serum urate concentration.[19] Recently, a novel human renal apical organic anion efflux transporter, called MRP4, has been identified.[20] MRP4 is a member of the ATP-binding cassette transporter family. It is proposed to mediate secretion of urate and other organic anions such as cAMP, cGMP, and methotrexate across the apical membrane of human renal proximal tubular cells. Human MRP4 is an ATP-dependent unidirectional efflux pump for urate with multiple allosteric substrate binding sites.[21] Renal sodium-dependent phosphate transport protein-1 (NPT-1),[22] which was first cloned as a phosphate transporter, is located in the proximal

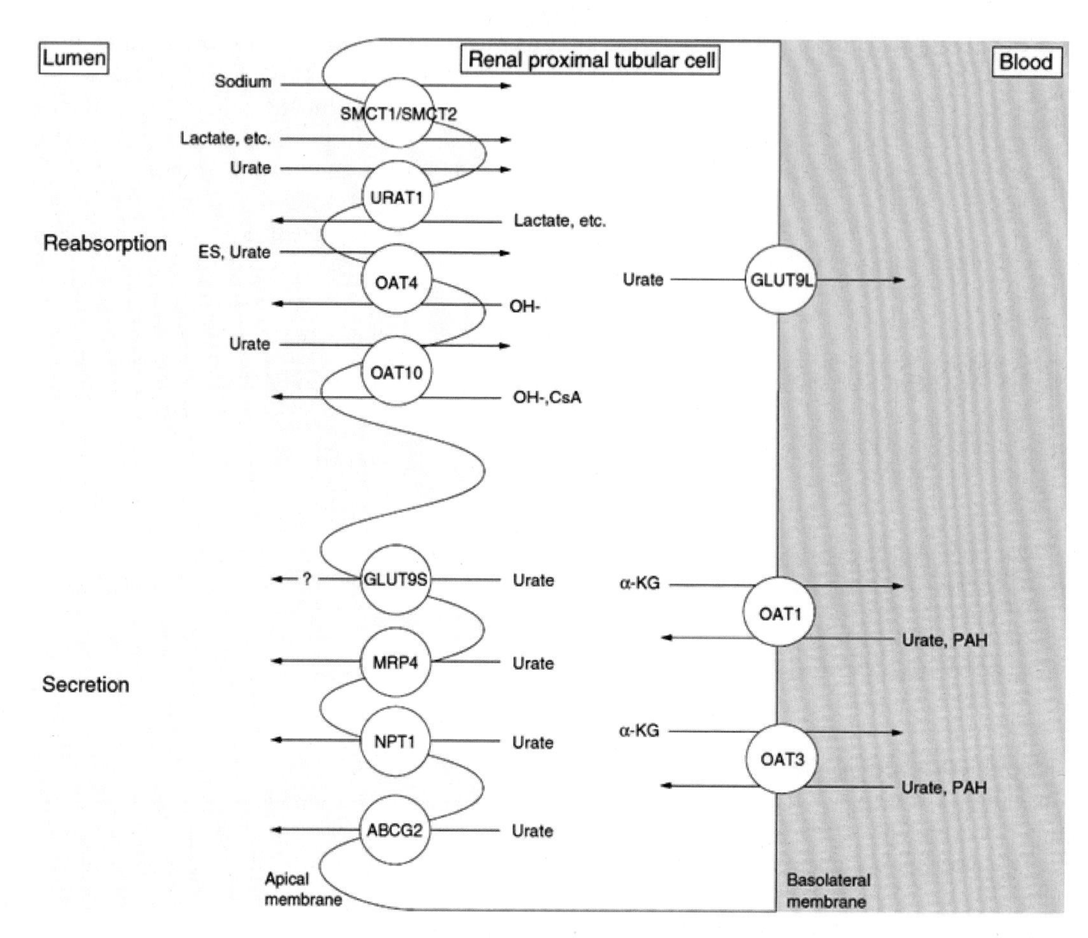

FIGURE 61.2 Urate transport. (From Ichida K. What lies behind serum urate concentration? Insights from genetic and genomic studies. *Genome Med.* 2009;1(12):118.)

convoluted renal tubule (Fig. 61.2). NPT1 mediates voltage-sensitive transport of organic anions, including urate, and is suggested to function as a urate secretor.[23] Another transporter located at the apical membrane of proximal tubules is ATP-binding cassette, sub-family G, member 2 (ABCG2). The ability of ABCG2 to transport urate was recently confirmed by measuring urate efflux from ABCG2-expressing *Xenopus* oocytes.[24]

Another gene involved in renal transport of urate is Tamm-Horsfall protein (THP), also known as uromodulin. THP is exclusively expressed and secreted by epithelial cells of the thick ascending limb, where it has been shown to have antibacterial effects. THP also co-localizes with the Na-K-2Cl transporter in lipid rafts in the apical cell membrane, suggesting a functional interaction.[25] Mutations in the human uromodulin gene have been identified in subjects with medullary cystic kidney disease type 2 and in patients with familial juvenile hyperuricemic nephropathy (see subsequent text).[26,27] It is not yet known how the THP mutation leads to hyperuricemia, as most evidence suggests that uric acid handling is restricted to the proximal tubule. However, there is some evidence that some urate secretion in the rat can occur distal to the proximal tubule.[28] Furthermore, there is also some evidence that the THP mutation may lead to sodium and water wasting, possibly resulting in stimulating urate reabsorption proximally (see following section on Familial Juvenile Hyperuricemic Nephropathy).

Causes of Hyper- and Hypouricemia

Hyperuricemia has been arbitrarily defined as >7.0 mg per dL in men and >6.5 mg per dL in women. "Normal" serum uric acid levels in the population appear to be rising throughout the last century, likely as a consequence of changes in diet, and mean levels in men in the United States are now in the 6.0 to 6.5 mg per dL range.[4] Uric acid levels tend to be higher in certain populations (e.g., African American and Pacific Islanders), with certain phenotypes (obesity, metabolic syndrome) and with special diets (meat eaters).[4] Uric acid also has a circadian variation, with the highest levels in the early morning.[29]

The serum urate concentration reflects the balance between urate production and elimination. Hyperuricemia may occur from excessive production of urate (overproduction) or decreased elimination (underexcretion), and frequently a combination of both processes occur in the same patient. Furthermore, uric acid levels may vary in the same individual by as much as 1 to 2 mg per dL during the course of a day, due to the effects of diet and exercise.

Genetic mechanisms mediating hyperuricemia include overproduction due to mutations of two enzymes: hypoxanthine–guanine phosphoribosyltransferase (HGPRT) and phosphoribosyl pyrophosphate synthetase (PRPPS) (Table 61.1). Subjects with Lesch-Nyhan syndrome (due to a mutation of HGPRT on the X chromosome) present in childhood with neurologic manifestations (mental retardation, choreoathetosis, and dystonia) and have an increased risk for nephrolithiasis, renal failure, and gout. A partial deficiency of HGPRT may manifest later in life as recurrent gout and/or nephrolithiasis (partial HGPRT deficiency (Kelley-Seegmiller syndrome).[30] Other genetic mechanisms include subjects with the uromodulin mutation, who develop hyperuricemia (due to underexcretion) with early and progressive renal disease (see subsequent text). Certain populations such as indigenous peoples living in Oceania also have higher uric acid levels than Caucasian populations.[31] Finally, African Americans also have higher uric acid levels and a twofold higher incidence of gout compared to Caucasian or Asian populations[32]; however, this could also reflect diets higher in fructose-containing sugars (see subsequent text) rather than genetic mechanisms.

TABLE 61.1 Major Causes of Hyperuricemia

Genetic causes
- Familial hyperuricemic nephropathy (mutation of uromodulin)
- Lesch-Nyhan syndrome (HGPRT mutation)
- Phosphoribosyl pyrophosphate synthetase mutation (PRPPS)

Dietary causes
- Diet high in purines (organ meats, shellfish, fatty meats)
- Diet high in fructose (high fructose corn syrup, table sugar, honey)
- Ethanol
- Low salt diet

Drugs
- Thiazides
- Loop diuretics
- Calcineurin inhibitors (cyclosporine > tacrolimus)
- Pyrazinamide
- Low dose aspirin

Volume depletion
Hypoxia (systemic or tissue)
Increased cell turnover (myeloproliferative disorders, polycythemia vera)
Conditions associated with higher uric acid levels
Renal failure
Obesity metabolic syndrome
Untreated hypertension
African-American race
Preeclampsia
Vigorous exercise

Hyperuricemia may also result from diets high in purines, from ethanol, and from fructose. The effect of alcohol is in part related to increased urate synthesis, which is due to enhanced turnover of ATP during the conversion of acetate to acetyl-CoA as part of the metabolism of ethanol.[33] In addition, acute alcohol consumption causes lactate production, and because lactate is an antiuricosuric agent, it will reduce renal urate excretion and exacerbate hyperuricemia.[34] Fructose (a simple sugar present in sucrose, table sugar, high fructose corn syrup, honey, and fruits) can also induce a rapid rise in serum uric acid, due in part to its rapid phosphorylation in hepatocytes with the stimulation of AMP deaminase and ATP consumption.[35] Chronic fructose consumption also stimulates uric acid synthesis.[35] It has been proposed that the marked increase in fructose intake may have a role in the rising levels of serum uric acid and obesity worldwide.[36]

Uric acid may also be affected by exercise, with moderate exercise reducing urate levels (probably by increasing renal blood flow) and severe exercise causing a rise in uric acid (probably due to ATP consumption with adenosine and xanthine formation). Urate levels vary among gender, in that premenopausal women have lower uric acid, a fact attributed to the uricosuric effect of estrogen.[37] The mechanism may relate to gender effects on URAT-1 expression, as recent studies suggest that male mice have higher URAT-1 expression in their proximal tubules compared to female mice.[38] Androgens also increase xanthine oxidase levels that might contribute to the higher uric acid levels observed in men.[39] Uric acid also tends to increase in the setting of low blood volume and/or low salt diet (due to increased proximal reabsorption), and following the administration of catecholamines or angiotensin II (due to renal vasoconstriction resulting in increased reabsorption). Urate production also relates to body size and weight, so that larger persons produce more urate than those who are smaller. Hyperuricemia is particularly common in the obesity and metabolic syndrome (thought to be secondary to the effect of insulin to stimulate uric acid reabsorption)[40] and in untreated hypertension (thought to be due to reduced renal blood flow).[41] Thiazides also increase uric acid reabsorption by decreasing blood volume and via direct interaction with the organic anion exchanger.

Other drugs (cyclosporine, pyrazinamide, low dose aspirin) also increase uric acid, primarily by interfering with renal excretion. In addition, the generation of organic anions such as lactate, β-hydroxybutyrate, and others may interfere with urate secretion in the proximal tubule and cause a rise in serum uric acid. Chronic lead ingestion can also cause hyperuricemia by reducing urate excretion, whereas high concentrations tend to cause proximal tubular injury with no rise in uric acid.

Uric acid is also increased in the setting of tissue hypoxia[42] or with cell turnover.[43] With tissue hypoxia, ATP is consumed and the isoform, xanthine oxidase, is induced, resulting in increased local uric acid concentrations. Uric acid levels are thus high in subjects with congestive heart failure, high altitude hypoxia, congenital cyanotic heart disease, and with obstructive sleep apnea. Uric acid levels are commonly elevated with certain malignancies, especially leukemias and lymphomas, and levels may sharply rise following chemotherapy (see acute urate nephropathy in the following text).[44] Finally, uric acid has a tendency to be elevated in polycythemia vera and other myeloproliferative disorders.[45]

In the setting of reduced renal function, the fractional excretion of urate increases but is not enough to fully compensate for the reduction in glomerular filtration rate (GFR), and as a consequence serum uric acid levels rise. Conversely, uric acid excretion via the gastrointestinal tract is also enhanced,[46] and therefore serum uric acid levels tend to be only mildly elevated in patients with chronic renal disease, and gout is relatively rare.

Low uric acid levels (levels <2.0 mg per dL) can occur via a variety of mechanisms, including with liver disease (due to decreased production), Fanconi syndrome (due to impaired proximal tubular function), and with diabetic glycosuria (due to proximal tubular dysfunction) (Table 61.2). Drugs such as probenecid, high-dose salicylates, sulfinpyrazone, benziodarone, benzbromarone, and losartan are all uricosuric, whereas allopurinol, febuxostat, and oxypurinol lower uric acid by blocking xanthine oxidase. Statins also lower uric acid,[47] and recombinant uricase (rasburicase) can markedly reduce serum uric acid and is approved for use in children with tumor lysis syndrome (in which marked hyperuricemia may develop).[48] There is also a hereditary hypouricemia syndrome that has been observed, and is particularly common in Japan, where it has been shown to be due to a mutation in the URAT-1 gene.[49] A similar hypouricemia syndrome has also been observed with mutations in SLC2A9.[50] These patients are particularly prone to develop acute renal failure following vigorous exercise, in which it is postulated to be due to massive uricosuria following ATP consumption in the muscle.

TABLE 61.2 Major Causes of Hypouricemia

Major Causes of Hypouricemia
Liver disease
Fanconi syndrome
Diabetes (with glycosuria)
Inappropriate secretion of vasopressin
Familial hypouricemia (due to URAT1 mutation)
Total parenteral hyperalimentation
Medications with uricosuric property including aspirin (>2.0 g/day), X-ray contrast materials, ascorbic acid, calcitonin, outdated tetracycline, and glyceryl guaiacolate

URIC ACID AND RENAL DISEASE

In the following section, we discuss the major associations of uric acid with renal disease.

Acute Kidney Injury Associated with Hyperuricemia

Acute urate nephropathy is a form of acute renal failure that may occur when serum uric acid rapidly rises, such as in patients with malignancies following chemotherapy ("tumor lysis" syndrome).[44] Typically the patient has a hematologic malignancy in which rapid tumor lysis occurs, resulting in the release of DNA and RNA and their rapid metabolism to uric acid by the liver and other tissues. Serum uric acid levels may increase to greater than 14 mg per dL (>840 μM), resulting in a marked increase in urinary urate excretion that exceeds its solubility. Uric acid crystals form within the tubules, leading to obstruction and sometimes rupturing into the interstitium (Fig. 61.3). Monocytes and T cells are attracted to the site, and form giant cell reactions with tubular

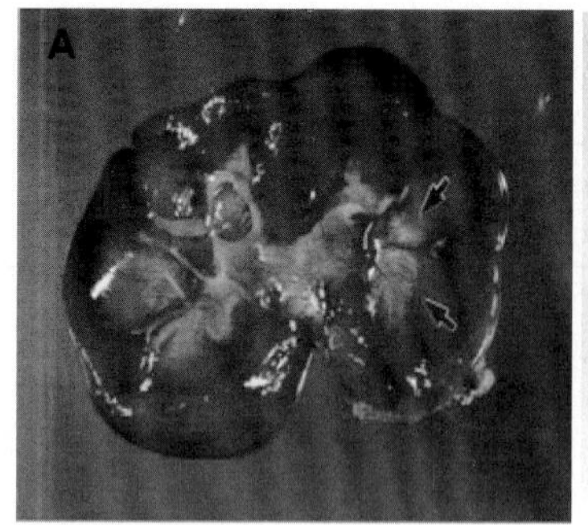

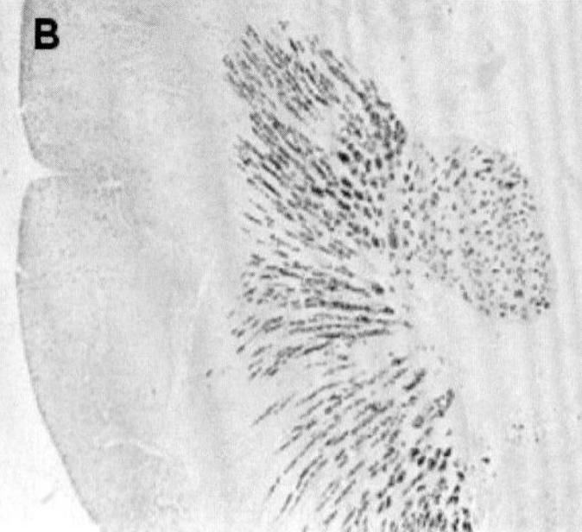

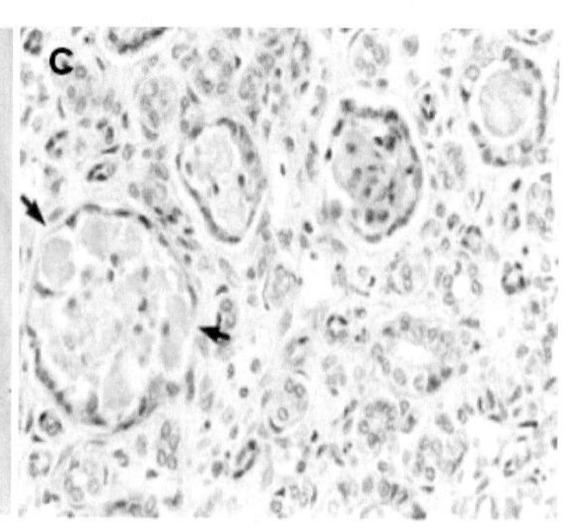

FIGURE 61.3 Pathology of acute uric acid nephropathy. **A:** Yellow/white streaks in the pyramids represent intratubular urate deposition (*arrows*). **B:** Intratubular urate deposition (Schultz stain, ×6). **C:** Urate precipitation in ducts of renal medulla with a denuded tubular basement membrane (*arrows*, H&E, ×125). (From Nickeleit V, Mihatsch MJ. Uric acid nephropathy and end-stage renal disease—review of a non-disease. *Nephrol Dial Transplant.* 1997;12(9):1832–1838.) (See Color Plate.)

proliferation and extracellular matrix deposition.[51] Diagnosis is facilitated by the characteristic clinical syndrome and with a urinary uric acid/urinary creatinine ratio of >1 mg per mg (or >0.66 mM/mM),[52] and by the presence of urate crystals in the urinary sediment. Historically, treatment consisted of forced alkaline diuresis (to facilitate solubilizing the urate) and large doses of xanthine oxidase inhibitors (typically allopurinol 300 to 600 mg per day). Recently, recombinant uricase (rasburicase) has become available, which can be administered intravenously and effectively lowers serum uric acid levels and corrects renal dysfunction more rapidly than allopurinol.[48] Dialysis can also be used to acutely lower the serum uric acid levels. The natural course is one similar to that for acute renal failure of any etiology with a period of oliguria, followed by partial or complete clinical recovery. However, some degree of residual renal injury/damage is common.

Hyperuricemia may also act as an independent risk factor for acute kidney injury in other settings such as following cardiovascular surgery or in association with the administration of nephrotoxic agents such as contrast or cisplatin.[53,54] Experimentally raising uric acid has also been shown to exacerbate acute kidney injury from cisplatin.[55] The mechanism is not due to crystals but rather appears to be secondary to the induction of local inflammation by uric acid. These observations have led to renewed interest that uric acid may be a potentially modifiable risk factor for preventing acute kidney injury.

Hyperuricemia as a Primary Cause of Chronic Kidney Disease

Hyperuricemia is common in subjects with chronic kidney disease. Some cases are due to specific entities, such as lead nephropathy or familial juvenile hyperuricemic nephropathy (discussed later). Uric acid is also retained with a reduction in GFR, so in many cases the rise in uric acid is likely secondary to chronic kidney disease (CKD). However, there remains the possibility that the uric acid may still have a role in modifying progression of renal disease.

Originally the entity of "gouty nephropathy" was attributed to the progressive renal disease seen commonly in subjects with gout. Natural history studies prior to the availability of uric acid–lowering drugs reported that as much as 25% of gouty subjects developed proteinuria, 50% developed renal insufficiency, and 10% to 25% developed end-stage renal disease (ESRD).[52,56] Histologic changes consist of arteriolosclerosis, glomerulosclerosis, and tubulointerstitial fibrosis, similar to the findings one observes in patients with hypertensive renal disease (nephrosclerosis) or with aging (Fig. 61.4).[56,57] In addition, subjects with chronic gout often have focal deposition of monosodium urate in interstitial areas, especially the outer

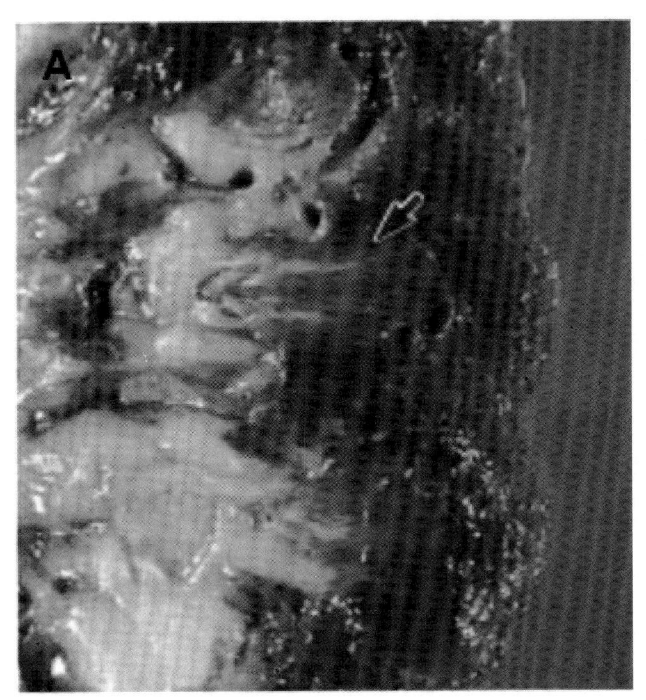

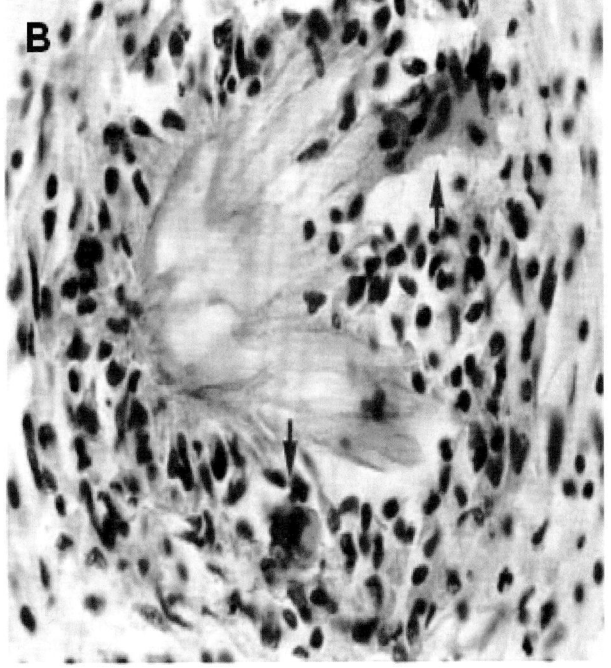

FIGURE 61.4 Pathology of chronic uric acid nephropathy. **A:** Gout tophi in renal pyramid (*arrow*) representing fibrosis and urate deposit. **B:** Typical gouty tophus in renal medulla surrounded by mononuclear inflammatory cells and giant cells (*arrow*, H&E, ×160). (From Nickeleit V, Mihatsch MJ. Uric acid nephropathy and end-stage renal disease—review of a non-disease. *Nephrol Dial Transplant.* 1997;12(9):1832–1838.)

medulla. Although intrarenal crystal deposition was originally thought to be mediating the renal injury,[57] this was later dispelled due to the focal deposition of crystals despite diffuse disease[58] and the fact that the renal disease was commonly associated with hypertension or aging, both conditions associated with the development of microvascular disease, glomerulosclerosis, and tubulointerstitial fibrosis.[59–61] Finally, although some studies suggested that lowering uric acid could improve the renal disease in gout,[62,63] other studies could not demonstrate any significant improvement of renal function with allopurinol.[64] Therefore, many authorities considered the term "gouty nephropathy" a misnomer, and concluded that uric acid had little to do with the renal disease present in these subjects.[65]

New Insights on the Entity of Primary Hyperuricemic Nephropathy

Renewed interest on the role of gout and/or asymptomatic hyperuricemia in CKD was sparked by the recognition that it seemed inappropriate to use the presence of hypertension to explain every case of renal insufficiency in the gouty patient, because most subjects with essential hypertension have relatively preserved renal function.[66] Another implicit assumption was that gouty nephropathy had to be due to crystal deposition, and the possibility that uric acid might mediate effects through crystal-independent mechanisms was not considered. Furthermore, the analysis also assumed that the presence of hypertension was a separate cause of renal disease and that it had to be independent of the uric acid. This led to a proposal to reinvestigate the role of uric acid in chronic renal disease.[66]

Subsequently numerous epidemiologic studies have shown that serum uric acid is an independent risk factor for developing CKD. In one Japanese study, hyperuricemia conferred a 10.8-fold increased risk in women and a 3.8-fold increased risk in men for the development of CKD compared to those with normal uric acid levels.[67] This higher relative risk in subjects with hyperuricemia was independent of age, body mass index, systolic blood pressure, total cholesterol, serum albumin, glucose, smoking, alcohol use, exercise habits, proteinuria, and hematuria. An elevated uric acid was also independently associated with a markedly increased risk of renal failure in another study of more than 49,000 male railroad workers.[68] A second insight came from experimental studies in which chronic mild hyperuricemia was induced in rats.[69,70] Because rats have functional uricase, the model of hyperuricemia was induced by administering the uricase inhibitor, oxonic acid, to the diet.[69,70] This resulted in serum uric acid levels that were only 1.5- to 3.0-fold greater than in the normal rat, levels which did not result in intratubular or interstitial urate crystal deposition. Over time, however, rats developed hypertension and progressive renal disease. Early in the course the rats developed arteriolar thickening and rarely hyalinosis of the preglomerular arterioles, often accompanied by glomerular hypertrophy.[70,71] Proteinuria appeared subsequently with the development of worsening vascular disease, glomerulosclerosis, and interstitial fibrosis.[70] The lesion was identical to that observed with nephrosclerosis of hypertension, with aging-associated glomerulosclerosis, and with gouty nephropathy, except for the absence of crystal deposition that had been observed in the latter condition. This led the authors to suggest that chronic hyperuricemia may cause renal disease and hypertension via a crystal-independent pathway.

Further studies showed that uric acid was able to induce endothelial dysfunction in vitro, and that it could inhibit endothelial release of nitric oxide, block endothelial cell proliferation, and induce senescence via an activation of the local renin-angiotensin system and an induction of oxidative stress.[72–74] Uric acid also stimulated vascular smooth muscle cell proliferation via uptake of urate into the cell with activation of MAP kinases, nuclear transcription factors (including NF-κB and AP-1), and inflammatory mediators (including monocyte chemoattractant protein-1 and C-reactive protein).[71–73,75,76] An induction of COX-2 with thromboxane production was also shown.[77] Uric acid can also inhibit tubular cell proliferation in vitro.[78] Hyperuricemic rats displayed evidence of endothelial dysfunction (with low serum nitrites reflecting low NO) and increased intrarenal renin expression.[69–72] The in vivo renal changes could be reversed by lowering uric acid with allopurinol. In addition, micropuncture studies performed on the hyperuricemic rats demonstrated that the rats developed glomerular hypertension with a reduction in renal plasma flow, both mechanisms that could lead to renal injury.[79,80]

Clinical Manifestations of Hyperuricemic Nephropathy

Most subjects with longstanding gout have asymptomatic renal involvement with either normal or only mild renal insufficiency, and with the majority having hypertension.[59–61] Renal blood flow is usually disproportionately low for the degree of renal insufficiency.[59–61,81] Fractional excretion of uric acid is usually less than 10%. Proteinuria occurs in the minority of cases and, when present, is usually in the nonnephrotic range. The urinary sediment is also usually benign. However, hypertension is frequent, occurring in 50% to 60% of subjects and increasing in prevalence as renal function worsens. Renal biopsy when performed may show chronic changes indistinguishable from chronic hypertensive nephropathy, with chronic glomerulosclerosis, tubulointerstitial fibrosis, and renal microvascular disease. Intrarenal crystals may occasionally be observed using ethanol fixed tissue with the De Galantha stain, but as discussed previously their presence or absence may not rule out a role for uric acid in the kidney disease. Nonetheless, a disproportionately elevated serum uric acid in relation to impaired renal function (such as a uric acid level of >9 mg per dL for a serum creatinine of <1.5 mg per dL, a uric acid of >10 mg per dL for a serum creatinine of 1.5 to 2.0 mg per dL, and a serum uric acid of >12 mg per dL when serum creatinine is >2.0 mg per dL) should make one consider the possibility that uric acid may have a role in the process.

Management of Primary Hyperuricemic Nephropathy

Historically hyperuricemic or gouty nephropathy was not thought to be due to gout, and hence management was focused on classical treatment strategies for CKD. The role of lowering uric acid still remains controversial in primary hyperuricemic nephropathy, and no definitive studies have been performed to resolve this important issue. Based on the experimental studies, it may be reasonable to lower serum uric acid in subjects with hyperuricemia, particularly in individuals in which it is markedly elevated (>10 mg per dL). In the setting of CKD most uricosuric agents are relatively ineffective, although some success with benziodarone has been reported in Europe.[82] The most effective way to lower uric acid chronically is with the use of xanthine oxidase inhibitors, but allopurinol can be associated rarely with the allopurinol hypersensitivity syndrome in which subjects develop a Stevens Johnson–like syndrome with fever, abnormal liver function tests, and worsening renal failure.[83] Recent studies suggest that subjects who develop the allopurinol hypersensitivity syndrome are usually HLA-B58 positive, and hence screening for HLA-B58 is recommended prior to initiating treatment.[84] In addition, high doses of allopurinol may lead to either xanthine or allopurinol intratubular crystal deposition and worsening of renal function. Thus, if allopurinol is to be used, one should start with 50 mg daily and then slowly increase the dose. The usual dose is 100 mg for each 30 mL per minute of GFR. An alternative choice is febuxostat, a non-purine-analogue inhibitor of xanthine oxidase; it may be preferential to allopurinol as there is no indication for dose adjustment in renal disease and to date it has not been associated with the hypersensitivity syndrome.[85] Finally, one should consider having the subject reduce ingestion of foods that can raise uric acid, such as foods with high-purine content, ethanol, and fructose.

Chronic Lead Nephropathy

Chronic lead ingestion may also lead to the triad of renal disease, hypertension, and hyperuricemia. In the 1800s some cases of lead nephropathy were observed in England where large amounts of fortified port wine that had been contaminated with lead was consumed. More recently chronic lead-induced renal disease has been observed in individuals exposed to lead as a consequence of working in or near foundries or individuals who drink moonshine prepared with lead distilling equipment.[86] Emmerson also reported a large number of subjects from Queensland who developed lead toxicity as a consequence of ingesting lead paint chips when they were children.[87] Some subjects provide no history of known exposure to lead, and in certain populations (such as in Taiwan), a substantial number of subjects with CKD may have low level lead toxicity.[88]

The etiology of lead nephropathy is complex. Experimentally lead-induced hypertension is observed only with low-dose ingestion of lead acetate, and this results in hypertension and mild renal injury that can be shown to be mediated by oxidants.[89] In contrast, high doses of lead cause proximal tubular injury with intranuclear inclusions, and a Fanconi-like picture in which serum uric acid levels are low and blood pressure is normal.[90] Acute lead toxicity in humans is also associated with development of Fanconi syndrome secondary to direct tubular toxicity.

Subjects present with hypertension, slowly progressive CKD, with hyperuricemia and/or gout (termed "saturnine" gout when it is secondary to lead). The renal excretion of uric acid is reduced, and this correlates with elevated blood lead levels.[91] The renal sediment is benign, similar to the findings observed with gouty nephropathy and/or arteriolosclerosis. Histologically, the renal lesion also appears like chronic hypertension, and is characterized by prominent vascular changes of arteriolosclerosis, often with variable degrees of glomerulosclerosis and tubulointerstitial fibrosis.[92] The strong association of lead intoxication with renal microvascular disease led Huchard, the French academician of the 1800s, to declare that lead intoxication was the second common cause of arteriolosclerosis.[93]

Diagnosis should be suspected when one observes hyperuricemia and/or gout in the presence of CKD and hypertension. Definitive diagnosis requires the EDTA challenge test. Ethylene diamine tetraacetic acid (EDTA, 1 gram) is administered intravenously and the total urinary lead excretion determined over the subsequent 72 hours. A urinary lead excretion over 600 μg per 72 hours is considered positive.[94] The differential diagnosis should include primary gouty nephropathy, familial juvenile hyperuricemic nephropathy (FJHN), and hyperuricemia accompanying other renal disorders.

Treatment consists of standard regimens for CKD of any etiology, ideally with the avoidance of drugs that can further raise serum uric acid levels (see previous section on treatment of gouty nephropathy). The role of lowering uric acid levels in this population is unknown. More recently, double-blind and prospective studies have shown that intravenous EDTA treatment can chelate the lead and improve renal function over time.[95] The dose used in the study consisted of 1 g calcium disodium EDTA in 200 mL of normal (0.9%) saline given over 2 hours on a weekly basis for 3 months with reassessment of lead burden, and if the urinary excretion continued to be greater than 600 μg per 72 hours, then the course was repeated.[95]

Familial Juvenile Hyperuricemic Nephropathy

A rare form of hereditary renal disease is familial juvenile hyperuricemic nephropathy (FJHN). This is an autosomal-dominant disorder typically present in children and/or young adults with slowly progressive CKD and marked hyperuricemia.[27,96,97] Renal histology shows glomerulosclerosis, tubulointerstitial fibrosis, and arteriolosclerosis, but urate crystal deposition is rare. Gout may or may not occur in the individual. A characteristic feature is a very low fractional excretion of urate, typically < 5%.[96] Subjects often are normotensive initially, but hypertension is common as the CKD progresses. Hemodynamic studies have shown that there is severe renal vasoconstriction, with marked depression in renal plasma flow relative to the GFR.[97]

FJHN is due to a mutation in uromodulin, also known as the gene encoding the THP.[26] THP is produced only by the thick ascending limb tubular epithelial cells in the kidney, raising questions of how this mutation could result in hyperuricemia and renal failure. Interestingly, mutations in uromodulin have also been shown to be the cause of autosomal-dominant medullary cystic kidney disease type 2.[27] Indeed, a recent study also suggests that this latter entity is commonly associated with severe hyperuricemia and clinically mimics the phenotype of familial hyperuricemic nephropathy.[27] Therefore, these two conditions should be viewed as the same disease.

The pathogenesis of the renal injury remains unclear. Medullary cystic kidney disease is associated with salt wasting, but it remains uncertain if patients with FJHN also have a salt or water wasting defect. However, preliminary studies in such patients suggest that they have a defect in salt and water concentration, and this correlated inversely with the serum uric acid levels.[27] Mice with the uromodulin mutation also show a mild water and sodium wasting phenotype, and have evidence for upregulation of sodium transporters in their proximal tubules, as well as a relative defect in urinary urate excretion when factored for the sodium excretion.[98,99] This raises the possibility that the hyperuricemia in FJHN is due to increased proximal sodium and urate reabsorption secondary to renal salt loss. Moreover, the THP mutant mouse does not develop either hyperuricemia or renal disease. Again, it is tempting to speculate that this may be due to the presence of uricase in these mice that maintains serum uric acid within normal levels.

Diagnosis is suggested by a positive family history, the early onset of CKD in the setting of elevated uric acid levels (often >9 mg per dL), and by a fractional urinary urate excretion of <5%.[96] Confirmation is now possible by having leukocyte DNA analyzed for the mutation (available commercially by Athena Diagnostics [www.AthenaDiagnostics.com]).[100] Treatment is largely supportive. Controversy exists over whether lowering uric acid slows renal progression, but one group has suggested a benefit using this approach if treatment is started early.[96]

Hyperuricemia in Subjects with CKD of Other Etiologies

Patients with established renal diseases may also develop hyperuricemia, mainly in the setting of reduced renal clearance of uric acid associated with progressive decline of GFR. As discussed earlier, there is some retention of uric acid with CKD of other causes, despite compensatory increases in the fractional excretion of uric acid and an increase in enteric excretion in the gut.[46] Indeed, gouty arthritis is uncommon in CKD. This may relate to the fact that uric acid levels are often not that elevated and to the fact that uremia inhibits neutrophil chemotaxis and function,[101] and hence the inflammatory response may be partially subdued.

The role of uric acid in the progression of established CKD remains controversial (Table 61.3). Experimentally uric acid has been shown to be a risk factor for renal progression.[77] Hyperuricemic rats with CKD induced by surgical removal (remnant kidney model) show accelerated progression with worsening hypertension, proteinuria, renal function, and glomerulosclerosis. These hyperuricemic rats also developed severe preglomerular vascular disease, with vascular smooth muscle cell proliferation in the interlobular and afferent arterioles.[77] All of these changes could be reversed by allopurinol, and partially by benziodarone (a uricosuric drug used in Europe). Similarly, the lowering of uric acid in a model of type 2 diabetic renal disease was also associated with a reduction in albuminuria and less tubulointerstitial injury.[102]

There is also compelling evidence that hyperuricemia is an independent risk factor for CKD in the general population.[67,103] Hyperuricemia has also been reported to be an independent risk factor for renal disease progression in patients with glomerular diseases,[104–106] and in subjects with essential hypertension.[107] Subjects with type 1 diabetes who have higher serum uric acid levels are also at increased risk for the development of diabetic nephropathy.[108,109] To date only a few studies have examined if lowering uric acid can slow renal progression in subjects with CKD. Siu et al. randomly assigned 54 hyperuricemia CKD patients to allopurinol or placebo for 1 year. Allopurinol treatment resulted in a decrease in serum uric acid associated with a significant slowing of renal disease progression.[48] A recent randomized, prospective study in 113 CKD patients also found that allopurinol administration decreased C-reactive protein and slowed down the progression of CKD.[110] A small Iranian study also found that allopurinol could reduce proteinuria in type 2 diabetic subjects.[111]

Treatment Guideline of Hyperuricemia in CKD

Asymptomatic hyperuricemia in patients with CKD appears to be a risk factor for CKD, but larger studies are necessary before routine treatment should be recommended. Allopurinol and febuxostat are currently not indicated for treatment of CKD, and can be associated with toxicities.[112] Although screening for HLA-B58 appears to reduce the risk for allopurinol hypersensitivity syndrome,[84] more studies are needed to determine the safety and efficacy of uric acid lowering therapies in subjects with CKD.

Management of Hyperuricemia

Lifestyle modification with low purine diet and low fructose diets are the first option for treating hyperuricemia in CKD patients. Careful monitoring of nutritional status is necessary to avoid malnutrition. Dietary purines make a substantial

TABLE 61.3 **Epidemiology of Uric Acid and Chronic Kidney Disease**

1st Author	Year	Subjects	Major Findings
Hsu	2009	177,570, USRDS	Higher uric acid quartile conferred 2.14-fold increased risk of ESRD over 25 years (+)
Obermayr	2008	21,457 Vienna Health Screening Project	Uric acid >7 mg/dL increased risk of CKD 1.74-fold in men, 3.12-fold in women (+)
Weiner	2008	13,338, ARIC	Each 1 mg/dL increase in uric acid increased risk of CKD 7%-11%
Iseki	2001	6403, Okinawa General Health	Uric acid >8 mg/dL increased CKD risk 3-fold in men and 10-fold in women (+)
Borges	2009	385, hypertensive women	Elevated uric acid associated with 2.63 fold increased risk of CKD in hypertensive women (+)
Chen, N	2009	2596, Ruijin Hospital, China	Linear correlation between uric acid and degree of CKD (+)
Chen, Y	2009	5722, Taipei University Hospital	Uric acid associated wtih prevalent CKD in elderly (+)
Park	2009	134, Yonsei University	Uric acid >7 mg/dL correlates with more rapid decline in residual renal function in peritoneal dialysis patients (+)
Sturm	2008	227, MMKD Study	Uric acid predicted progression of CKD only in unadjusted sample (+)
Chonchol	2007	5808, Cardiovascular Health Study	Uric acid strongly associated with prevalent but weakly with incident CKD (−)
See	2009	28,745, Chang Gung University	Uric acid >7.7 md/dL in men and >6.6 mg/dL in women only weakly associated with prevalent renal impairment (−)
Madero	2009	840, Instituto Nacional de Cariologia, Mexico	Patients with CKD 3-4 and uric acid correlates with death but not to ESRD (−)

+Supports the hypothesis that uric acid contributes to CKD progression.
−Does not support the hypothesis that uric acid contributes to CKD.
From Feig DI. Uric acid: a novel mediator and marker of risk in chronic kidney disease? *Curr Opin Nephrol Hypertens.* 2009;18(6):526–530.

contribution to serum uric acid levels, and a low purine diet can reduce serum uric acid levels by approximately 1 to 2 mg per dL.[113] Low fructose diets can also reduce uric acid and improve inflammatory markers and blood pressure in subjects with CKD.[114] In addition, the reduction of alcohol, and especially beer, is recommended to help lower uric acid levels.[115]

Medications that raise plasma uric acid levels, such as loop and thiazide diuretics, cyclosporine, aspirin (low dose), pyrazinamide, ethambutol, or nicotinic acid should also be discontinued if possible. In contrast, the angiotensin II receptor antagonist losartan has been reported to have a uricosuric effect[116] and the calcium channel blocker amlodipine increases uric acid clearance and reduces uric acid concentrations in comparison with perindopril.[117] In patients with primary hyperlipidemias, atorvastatin, but not simvastatin, has been shown to reduce uric acid concentrations.[118] Fenofibrate, but not other fibrates, has been shown to enhance renal uric acid clearance and reduce uric acid concentrations.[119] However, it should be noted that the fibrates have also been associated with an increase in serum urea and creatinine.[120] Sevelamer can also lower serum uric acid levels.[121] In summary, clinicians should carefully consider the therapeutic options for conditions associated with hyperuricemias such as hypertension and hyperlipidemia. In patients with difficult-to-control hyperuricemia, use of an agent that assists in reducing serum uric acid (or at least that does not increase serum uric acid) may be beneficial.

Antihyperuricemic Treatment: Old and New Drugs

Currently available options for reducing serum uric acid include either reducing uric acid production by the use of xanthine oxidase inhibitors (allopurinol) or increasing the renal excretion of uric acid through the use of uricosuric agents (probenecid, benzbromarone).

Allopurinol is the most commonly used hypouricemic agent because of its ability to lower serum uric acid regardless of the cause of hyperuricemia and the convenience of once daily dosing. It reduces the production of uric acid at its rate-limiting step through inhibition of xanthine oxidase. Allopurinol is rapidly metabolized to oxypurinol, which is responsible for most of the xanthine oxidase inhibition. The half-life of allopurinol is 1 to 2 hours, and that of oxypurinol is 18 to 30 hours in those with normal renal function, but its action is prolonged in CKD extending to a week in those with a creatinine clearance (CrCL) of <3 mL per minute.[122] Approximately 20% of patients experience side effects with allopurinol, with up to 5% ultimately discontinuing therapy.[123] The most serious side effect is a rare hypersensitivity syndrome, which results in fever, rash, eosinophilia, hepatitis, renal failure, and in some cases death. The exact mechanism of the allopurinol hypersensitivity syndrome is unclear, but it has been postulated to be related to elevated serum oxypurinol levels as well as to immunologic processes.[124]

Careful dosing of allopurinol is necessary in patients with renal impairment (Table 61.2).[112] However, such dosing regimens are often ineffective in controlling hyperuricemia and gout.[124] Furthermore, the ability of such dosing regimens to reduce allopurinol hypersensitivity syndrome remains unclear.[125] The net result is often undertreatment of a potentially curable disorder. Although there are multiple reports of clinicians using higher than recommended doses of allopurinol,[126] there is a lack of evidence as to the benefit of such therapy in controlling hyperuricemia.[125]

Uricosuric agents, such as probenecid and benzbromarone, lower serum uric acid by increasing renal uric acid excretion. One potential complication is the deposition of uric acid crystals within the kidney, which can result in urate nephropathy and/or the formation of uric acid stones. The risk of these complications can be reduced by gradual increases in drug dose, ensuring urine volume is ≥1,500 mL per day and maintaining an alkaline urine (pH 6.4 to 6.8). Probenecid was the first uricosuric drug available. Its use is limited as efficacy of probenecid declines as renal function declines, and it is ineffective when CrCL is <60 mL per minute. Probenecid is usually well tolerated at the recommended doses of 1 to 3 g per day. Of note, the uricosuric effect of probenecid is blocked by the simultaneous administration of aspirin.

Benzbromarone is a potent uricosuric agent, which lowers serum uric acid by inhibiting postsecretory tubular resorption of uric acid.[127] Low-dose benzbromarone (50 to 100 mg per day) has been reported to be more potent than 300 mg per day of allopurinol[82] and equipotent to 1 to 1.5 g per day of probenecid.[128] Benzbromarone appears to have only slightly impaired efficacy in patients with impaired renal function,[82] and in renal transplant recipients, it has been reported to be beneficial in patients with a CrCL >25 mL per minute. Benzbromarone therapy has also been associated with a faster tophus reduction than has allopurinol therapy.[129] Hepatic toxicity, rarely leading to death, has been reported in patients taking high doses of benzbromarone.[130] Benzbromarone is unavailable in the United States because of concerns over the potential for hepatotoxicity. However, in the largest series published there was no significant liver toxicity in 200 patients treated for a mean of 5 years with 75 to 125 mg per day of benzbromarone.[131] Benzbromarone remains a therapeutic option particularly for patients with significant renal impairment or with intolerance to allopurinol, or in transplant recipients who are taking azathioprine.

In the last few years, several new hypouricemic agents have emerged. One of them is febuxostat, a non-purine-selective inhibitor of xanthine oxidase. Unlike allopurinol, febuxostat does not resemble purines or pyrimidines structurally. In comparison to allopurinol, which only weakly inhibits the oxidized form of xanthine oxidase, febuxostat inhibits both the oxidized and reduced forms of xanthine oxidase.[132] Febuxostat has been shown to be safe and effective in lowering uric acid concentrations in randomized double-blind studies. Importantly, there is no need for dose adjustment in renal disease. In patients with normal (CrCL 80 mL/min/1.73 m^2), mild (CrCL 50–80 mL/min/1.73 m^2), moderate (CrCL 30–59 mL/min/1.73 m^2), or severe (CrCL 10–20 mL/min/1.73 m^2) impairment in renal function, 80 mg febuxostat daily for 7 days has been reported to be safe without requirement for dose adjustment.[133] General recommendations for the management of hyperuricemia in CKD patients are summarized in Table 61.3.[134]

Hyperuricemia in Renal Transplantation

Hyperuricemia commonly occurs following renal transplantation, and in particular has been associated with the use of cyclosporine, and to a lesser extent, tacrolimus.[135] Indeed, several studies suggest that hyperuricemia occurs in greater than 50% of subjects and gout develops in 10% to 15%.[135] The mechanism has been shown to be due to decreased renal excretion, driven in part by increased net tubular reabsorption as well as decreased glomerular filtration.[136]

Although the primary complication of hyperuricemia in renal transplant patients has classically been thought to be gout, again there has been recent concern that the rise in serum uric acid may contribute to the renal vasoconstriction and renal injury that occurs with chronic calcineurin inhibitors. Thus, Mazzali et al. reported that cyclosporine-treated rats developed mild hyperuricemia with the classic lesions of arteriolar hyalinosis and tubulointerstitial fibrosis, but this lesion was markedly exacerbated if uric acid levels were further increased by administering a uricase inhibitor.[137] Kobelt et al. also reported that allopurinol lowers blood pressure and improves renal blood flow in rats administered cyclosporine,[138] and Assis et al. also demonstrated that allopurinol improved GFR (inulin clearances) in cyclosporine-treated rats.[139] Most notably, Neal et al. recently reported that allopurinol therapy lowered uric acid and improved renal function in liver transplant patients receiving cyclosporine.[140]

At this time insufficient evidence has been provided to recommend uric acid-lowering therapy in renal transplant subjects. However, if a subject has repeated episodes of gout, or if serum uric acid levels are excessively elevated (>9 mg per dL), we would consider pharmacologic therapy to lower uric acid. Because allopurinol interacts with azathioprine, the latter should be reduced to 25% to 50% of its original dose. In addition, we recommend initiating low doses of allopurinol (50 to 100 mg per day) with slow increases to minimize the risk for precipitating a gout attack (which is common on initiating allopurinol).

URIC ACID AND CARDIOVASCULAR DISEASE

In addition to its controversial role in renal disease, there has also been reawakened interest in the role of uric acid in cardiovascular disease, and in particular its role in hypertension. Although it had been known for over 100 years that hyperuricemic and/or gouty individuals are at increased risk for cardiovascular events and or mortality, this had historically been attributed to the fact that patients with gout frequently are obese or have other features associated with cardiovascular risk. Studies such as the Framingham analysis published in 1999 reported that this relationship of uric acid with cardiovascular disease was not independent when it was controlled for other accepted cardiovascular risk factors, such as hypertension, diuretic use, obesity, and renal disease.[141] Most societies concluded that there is insufficient evidence to support uric acid as a true cardiovascular risk factor.

However, recent studies have provided provocative data that uric acid may be a true risk factor for hypertension. Thus, a meta-analysis concluded that elevated serum uric acid is an independent risk factor for the development of hypertension.[142] Furthermore, an elevated serum uric acid is common in subjects with new onset hypertension. In one study of new onset hypertension in adolescents, 89% of subjects had a serum uric acid >5.5 mg per dL whereas this was not observed in any of 63 controls (including 22 subjects with white coat hypertension).[143] Furthermore, in a recent pilot study, treatment with allopurinol resulted in reduction in blood pressure in 30 adolescents with newly diagnosed hypertension.[144] Hyperuricemia has also been found to be an independent factor for mortality in subjects with normal renal function as well as in stage 3 and 4 CKD patients.[145,146] A recent prospective study in 294 newly diagnosed patients with CKD stage 5 followed for an average of 6 years revealed that subjects with markedly increased serum uric acid levels (≥9.0 mg per dL) had a twofold increased risk for mortality after adjusting for numerous comorbidities.[147] Although high uric acid levels were associated with lipid levels, calcium/phosphate metabolism, and levels of inflammation markers, an elevated uric acid level itself may represent a true risk factor for cardiovascular disease and mortality in CKD patients.[148] Few clinical studies have examined the effect of lowering uric acid on cardiovascular disease in subjects with CKD. However, in the randomized study by Goicoechea et al., the use of allopurinol was associated with a 70% reduction in cardiovascular events.[110]The mechanism by which uric acid may cause cardiovascular disease has been explored using both cell culture and animal models. It appears that uric acid must enter the endothelial and vascular smooth muscle cell via a specific organic anion exchanger, where it activates a variety of intracellular signaling molecules involved in inflammation and proliferation. In the endothelial cell there is a decrease in nitric oxide levels and an inhibition of endothelial proliferation, whereas in the vascular smooth muscle cell there is activation of proliferative and inflammatory pathways.[69–73,75,76] Local activation of the renin angiotensin system could also be shown.[73,75,76] Uric acid may also have direct effects on cardiac fibroblasts.[149] Experimental studies have further demonstrated that the mechanism by which uric acid causes hypertension is via a decrease in endothelial-derived nitric oxide, activation of the renin-angiotensin system, and the induction of preglomerular vascular disease. The latter may promote continued salt sensitivity even after the serum uric acid is corrected.[73]

URIC ACID AND METABOLIC SYNDROME

Hyperuricemia may also have a role in obesity and metabolic syndrome. A number of observational and cross-sectional studies showed an unequivocal association of high serum uric acid with metabolic syndrome.[150–153] Some reports have suggested that serum uric acid may be directly related to components of metabolic syndrome such as insulin resistance,[154] hypertension, abdominal adiposity,[155,156] and hypertriglyceridemia.[157] Hyperuricemia is also associated with increased risk of myocardial infarction and sudden cardiac death in patients with metabolic syndrome.[158] In a small prospective, open label study, Shelmadine et al.[159] demonstrated that 3 months administration of allopurinol in ESRD patients with gout led to significant reductions in serum uric acid levels and LDL cholesterol, although serum triglycerides increased. Ogino et al. also reported that lowering uric acid with benzbromarone can improve insulin resistance and markers of inflammation in subjects with congestive heart failure.[160] In addition, recent studies in which rats were fed fructose to induce metabolic syndrome found that lowering uric acid with allopurinol could significantly prevent the development of hypertension, hyperinsulinemia, hypertriglyceridemia, and obesity.[36]

Kidney

- Increases Glomerular Pressure
- Reduces Renal Blood Flow
- Induces Afferent Arteriolopathy (arteriolosclerosis)
- Causes Albuminuria, Glomerular Hypertrophy and Glomerulosclerosis
- Causes Renal Inflammation and Interstitial Disease

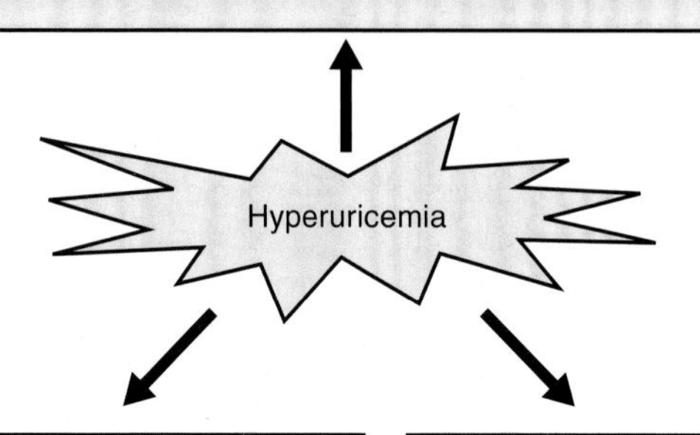

Vascular Effects

- Causes Endothelial Dysfunction and Reduces Nitric Oxide
- Stimulates Vascular Smooth Muscle Cell Proliferation
- Induces Afferent Arteriolopathy (arterioloclerosis)
- Causes Vasoconstriction (Stimulates Ang II and Oxidants)
- Causes Hypertension in Animal Models

Metabolic Effects

- Induces Insulin Resistance and Dyslipidemia
- Induces Oxidative Stress and Injury in Pancreatic Islet Cells
- Induces Systemic Inflammation
- Induces Adipocyte Activation and Inflammation

FIGURE 61.5 Proposed effects of uric acid on the kidney, vasculature, and metabolic state.

CONCLUSION

In conclusion, uric acid is emerging as a potential contributing factor to kidney disease, vascular disease, and metabolic disorders (Fig. 61.5). There is a strong relationship of uric acid with both acute and chronic kidney disease. Emerging evidence suggests that it may not only cause acute kidney injury as a consequence of crystal formation within the tubular lumina, but that both acute and chronic hyperuricemia may also cause renal disease via crystal-independent pathways. Indeed, uric acid may not only be a primary cause of chronic renal disease (gouty nephropathy), but could be a contributory factor in lead nephropathy, primary renal diseases, diabetic nephropathy, cyclosporine nephropathy, and the progression of CKD. Uric acid may also be an unrecognized contributor to cardiovascular risk as evidenced by recent studies linking it pathogenetically to hypertension and metabolic syndrome. An adequately powered randomized controlled trial is required to determine whether uric acid–lowering therapy prevents or ameliorates renal, cardiovascular, and metabolic diseases associated with hyperuricemia in order to better inform clinical practice and public health policy for the optimal management of hyperuricemia.

REFERENCES

1. Sarma AD, Serfozo P, Kahn K, et al. Identification and purification of hydroxyisourate hydrolase, a novel ureide-metabolizing enzyme. *J Biol Chem.* 1999;274(48):33863–33865.

2. Oda M, Satta Y, Takenaka O, et al. Loss of urate oxidase activity in hominoids and its evolutionary implications. *Mol Biol Evol.* 2002;19(5):640–653.

3. Wu XW, Muzny DM, Lee CC, et al. Two independent mutational events in the loss of urate oxidase during hominoid evolution. *J Mol Evol.* 1992;34(1):78–84.

4. Johnson RJ, Titte S, Cade JR, et al. Uric acid, evolution and primitive cultures. *Semin Nephrol.* 2005;25(1):3–8.

5. Hediger MA, Johnson RJ, Miyazaki H, et al. Molecular physiology of urate transport. *Physiology (Bethesda).* 2005;20:125–133.

6. Schlesinger N. Dietary factors and hyperuricaemia. *Curr Pharm Des.* 2005;11(32):4133–4138.

7. Roch-Ramel F, Werner D, Guisan B. Urate transport in brush-border membrane of human kidney. *Am J Physiol.* 1994;266(5 Pt 2):F797–805.

8. Roch-Ramel F, Guisan B, Diezi J. Effects of uricosuric and antiuricosuric agents on urate transport in human brush-border membrane vesicles. *J Pharmacol Exp Ther.* 1997;280(2):839–845.

9. Enomoto A, Kimura H, Chairoungdua A, et al. Molecular identification of a renal urate anion exchanger that regulates blood urate levels. *Nature.* 2002;417(6887):447–452.

10. Lipkowitz MS, Leal-Pinto E, Rappoport JZ, et al. Functional reconstitution, membrane targeting, genomic structure, and chromosomal localization of a human urate transporter. *J Clin Invest.* 2001;107(9):1103–1115.

11. Bibert S, Hess SK, Firsov D, et al. Mouse GLUT9: evidences for a urate uniporter. *Am J Physiol Renal Physiol.* 2009;297(3):F612–619.

12. Anzai N, Ichida K, Jutabha P, et al. Plasma urate level is directly regulated by a voltage-driven urate efflux transporter URATv1 (SLC2A9) in humans. *J Biol Chem.* 2008;283(40):26834–26838.

13. Augustin R, Carayannopoulos MO, Dowd LO, et al. Identification and characterization of human glucose transporter-like protein-9 (GLUT9): alternative splicing alters trafficking. *J Biol Chem.* 2004;279(16):16229–16236.

14. Vitart V, Rudan I, Hayward C, et al. SLC2A9 is a newly identified urate transporter influencing serum urate concentration, urate excretion and gout. *Nat Genet.* 2008;40(4):437–442.

15. Matsuo H, Chiba T, Nagamori S, et al. Mutations in glucose transporter 9 gene SLC2A9 cause renal hypouricemia. *Am J Hum Genet.* 2008;83(6):744–751.

16. Ekaratanawong S, Anzai N, Jutabha P, et al. Human organic anion transporter 4 is a renal apical organic anion/dicarboxylate exchanger in the proximal tubules. *J Pharmacol Sci.* 2004;94(3):297–304.

17. Ichida K, Hosoyamada M, Kimura H, et al. Urate transport via human PAH transporter hOAT1 and its gene structure. *Kidney Int.* 2003;63(1):143–155.

18. Cha SH, Sekine T, Fukushima JI, et al. Identification and characterization of human organic anion transporter 3 expressing predominantly in the kidney. *Mol Pharmacol.* 2001;59(5):1277–1286.

19. Ho KY, Tay HH, Kang JY. A prospective study of the clinical features, manometric findings, incidence and prevalence of achalasia in Singapore. *J Gastroenterol Hepatol.* 1999;14(8):791–795.

20. van Aubel RA, Smeets PH, Peters JG, et al. The MRP4/ABCC4 gene encodes a novel apical organic anion transporter in human kidney proximal tubules: putative efflux pump for urinary cAMP and cGMP. *J Am Soc Nephrol.* 2002;13(3):595–603.

21. Van Aubel RA, Smeets PH, van den Heuvel JJ, et al. Human organic anion transporter MRP4 (ABCC4) is an efflux pump for the purine end metabolite urate with multiple allosteric substrate binding sites. *Am J Physiol Renal Physiol.* 2005;288(2):F327–333.

22. Chong SS, Kristjansson K, Zoghbi HY, et al. Molecular cloning of the cDNA encoding a human renal sodium phosphate transport protein and its assignment to chromosome 6p21.3-p23. *Genomics.* 1993;18(2):355–359.

23. Uchino H, Tamai I, Yamashita K, et al. p-aminohippuric acid transport at renal apical membrane mediated by human inorganic phosphate transporter NPT1. *Biochem Biophys Res Commun.* 2000;270(1):254–259.

24. Woodward OM, Kottgen A, Coresh J, et al. Identification of a urate transporter, ABCG2, with a common functional polymorphism causing gout. *Proc Natl Acad Sci U S A.* 200923;106(25):10338–10342.

25. Welker P, Bohlick A, Mutig K, et al. Renal Na1-K1-Cl- cotransporter activity and vasopressin-induced trafficking are lipid raft-dependent. *Am J Physiol Renal Physiol.* 2008;295(3):F789–802.

26. Hart TC, Gorry MC, Hart PS, et al. Mutations of the UMOD gene are responsible for medullary cystic kidney disease 2 and familial juvenile hyperuricaemic nephropathy. *J Med Genet.* 2002;39(12):882–892.

27. Scolari F, Caridi G, Rampoldi L, et al. Uromodulin storage diseases: clinical aspects and mechanisms. *Am J Kidney Dis.* 2004;44(6):987–999.

28. Podevin R, Ardaillou R, Paillard F, et al. [Study in man of the kinetics of the appearance of uric acid 2-14C in the urine]. *Nephron.* 1968;5(2):134–140.

29. Kanabrocki EL, Third JL, Ryan MD, et al. Circadian relationship of serum uric acid and nitric oxide. *JAMA.* 2000;283(17):2240–2241.

30. Augoustides-Savvopoulou P, Papachristou F, Fairbanks LD, et al. Partial hypoxanthine-guanine phosphoribosyltransferase deficiency as the unsuspected cause of renal disease spanning three generations: a cautionary tale. *Pediatrics.* 2002;109(1):E17.

31. Merriman TR, Dalbeth N. The genetic basis of hyperuricemia and gout. *Joint Bone Spine.* 2011;78(1):35–40.

32. Hochberg MC, Thomas J, Thomas DJ, Merriman TR, Dalbeth N. The genetic basis of hyperuricemia and gout. Racial differences in the incidence of gout. The role of hypertension. *Arthritis Rheum.* 1995;38(5):628–632.

33. Faller J, Fox IH. Ethanol-induced hyperuricemia: evidence for increased urate production by activation of adenine nucleotide turnover. *N Engl J Med.* 1982;307(26):1598–1602.

34. Lieber CS, Jones DP, Losowsky MS, Davidson CS. Interrelation of uric acid and ethanol metabolism in man. *J Clin Invest.* 1962;41:1863–1870.

35. Emmerson BT. Effect of oral fructose on urate production. *Ann Rheum Dis.* 1974;33(3):276–280.

36. Nakagawa T, Hu H, Zharikov S, et al. A causal role for uric acid in fructose-induced metabolic syndrome. *Am J Physiol Renal Physiol.* 2006;290(3):F625–631.

37. Nicholls A, Snaith ML, Scott JT. Effect of oestrogen therapy on plasma and urinary levels of uric acid. *Br Med J.* 1973;1(5851):449–451.

38. Hosoyamada M, Ichida K, Enomoto A, et al. Function and localization of urate transporter 1 in mouse kidney. *J Am Soc Nephrol.* 2004;15(2):261–268.

39. Levinson DJ, Chalker D. Rat hepatic xanthine oxidase activity: age and sex specific differences. *Arthritis Rheum.* 1980;23(1):77–82.

40. Quinones Galvan A, Natali A, Baldi S, et al. Effect of insulin on uric acid excretion in humans. *Am J Physiol.* 1995;268(1 Pt 1):E1–5.

41. Messerli FH, Frohlich ED, Dreslinski GR, et al. Serum uric acid in essential hypertension: an indicator of renal vascular involvement. *Ann Intern Med.* 1980;93(6):817–821.

42. Friedl HP, Till GO, Trentz O, et al. Role of oxygen radicals in tourniquet-related ischemia-reperfusion injury of human patients. *Klin Wochenschr.* 1991;69(21–23):1109–1112.

43. Conger JD. Acute uric acid nephropathy. *Med Clin North Am.* 1990;74(4):859–871.

44. Tsimberidou AM, Keating MJ. Hyperuricemic syndromes in cancer patients. *Contrib Nephrol.* 2005;147:47–60.

45. Denman M, Szur L, Ansell BM. Hyperuricaemia in polycythaemia vera. *Ann Rheum Dis.* 1966;25(4):340–344.

46. Sorensen LB. Role of the intestinal tract in the elimination of uric acid. *Arthritis Rheum.* 1965;8(5):694–706.

47. Athyros VG, Elisaf M, Papageorgiou AA, et al. Effect of statins versus untreated dyslipidemia on serum uric acid levels in patients with coronary heart disease: a subgroup analysis of the GREek Atorvastatin and Coronary-heart-disease Evaluation (GREACE) study. *Am J Kidney Dis.* 2004;43(4):589–599.

48. Ronco C, Inguaggiato P, Bordoni V, et al. Rasburicase therapy in acute hyperuricemia and renal dysfunction. *Contrib Nephrol.* 2005;147:115–123.

49. Iwai N, Mino Y, Hosoyamada M, et al. A high prevalence of renal hypouricemia caused by inactive SLC22A12 in Japanese. *Kidney Int.* 2004;66(3):935–944.

50. Dinour D, Gray NK, Campbell S, et al. Homozygous SLC2A9 mutations cause severe renal hypouricemia. *J Am Soc Nephrol.* 2010;21(1):64–72.

51. Kim YG, Huang XR, Suga S, et al. Involvement of macrophage migration inhibitory factor (MIF) in experimental uric acid nephropathy. *Mol Med.* 2000;6(10):837–848.

52. Brochner-Mortensen K. Gout. *Ann Rheum Dis.* 1958;17(1):1–8.

53. Ejaz AA, Mu W, Kang DH, et al. Could uric acid have a role in acute renal failure? *Clin J Am Soc Nephrol.* 2007;2(1):16–21.

54. Ejaz AA, Beaver TM, Shimada M, et al. Uric acid: a novel risk factor for acute kidney injury in high-risk cardiac surgery patients? *Am J Nephrol.* 2009;30(5):425–429.

55. Roncal CA, Mu W, Croker B, et al. Effect of elevated serum uric acid on cisplatin-induced acute renal failure. *Am J Physiol Renal Physiol.* 2007;292(1):F116–122.

56. Talbott JH, Terplan KL. The kidney in gout. *Medicine (Baltimore).* 1960;39:405–467.

57. Greenbaum D, Ross JH, Steinberg VL. Renal biopsy in gout. *Br Med J.* 1961;1(5238):1502–1504.

58. Linnane JW, Burry AF, Emmerson BT. Urate deposits in the renal medulla. Prevalence and associations. *Nephron.* 1981;29(5–6):216–222.

59. Yu TF, Berger L, Dorph DJ, et al. Renal function in gout. V. Factors influencing the renal hemodynamics. *Am J Med.* 1979;67(5):766–771.

60. Yu TF, Berger L. Impaired renal function in gout: its association with hypertensive vascular disease and intrinsic renal disease. *Am J Med.* 1982;72(1):95–100.

61. Berger L, Yu TF. Renal function in gout. IV. An analysis of 524 gouty subjects including long-term follow-up studies. *Am J Med.* 1975;59(5):605–613.

62. Patial RK, Sehgal VK. Non-oliguric acute renal failure in gout. *Indian J Med Sci.* 1992;46(7):201–204.

63. Briney WG, Ogden D, Bartholomew B, et al. The influence of allopurinol on renal function in gout. *Arthritis Rheum.* 1975;18(6 Suppl):877–881.

64. Rosenfeld JB. Effect of long-term allopurinol administration on serial GFR in normotensive and hypertensive hyperuricemic subjects. *Adv Exp Med Biol.* 1974;41:581–596.

65. Nickeleit V, Mihatsch MJ. Uric acid nephropathy and end-stage renal disease—review of a non-disease. *Nephrol Dial Transplant.* 1997;12(9):1832–1838.

66. Johnson RJ, Kivlighn SD, Kim YG, et al. Reappraisal of the pathogenesis and consequences of hyperuricemia in hypertension, cardiovascular disease, and renal disease. *Am J Kidney Dis.* 1999;33(2):225–234.

67. Iseki K, Ikemiya Y, Inoue T, et al. Significance of hyperuricemia as a risk factor for developing ESRD in a screened cohort. *Am J Kidney Dis.* 2004;44(4):642–650.

68. Tomita M, Mizuno S, Yamanaka H, et al. Does hyperuricemia affect mortality? A prospective cohort study of Japanese male workers. *J Epidemiol.* 2000;10(6):403–409.

69. Mazzali M, Hughes J, Kim YG, et al. Elevated uric acid increases blood pressure in the rat by a novel crystal-independent mechanism. *Hypertension.* 2001;38(5):1101–1106.

70. Nakagawa T, Mazzali M, Kang DH, et al. Hyperuricemia causes glomerular hypertrophy in the rat. *Am J Nephrol.* 2003;23(1):2–7.

71. Mazzali M, Kanellis J, Han L, et al. Hyperuricemia induces a primary renal arteriolopathy in rats by a blood pressure-independent mechanism. *Am J Physiol Renal Physiol.* 2002;282(6):F991–997.

72. Khosla UM, Zharikov S, Finch JL, et al. Hyperuricemia induces endothelial dysfunction. *Kidney Int*. 2005;67(5):1739–1742.

73. Watanabe S, Kang DH, Feng L, et al. Uric acid, hominoid evolution, and the pathogenesis of salt-sensitivity. *Hypertension*. 2002;40(3):355–360.

74. Yu MA, Sanchez-Lozada LG, Johnson RJ, et al. Oxidative stress with an activation of the renin-angiotensin system in human vascular endothelial cells as a novel mechanism of uric acid-induced endothelial dysfunction. *J Hypertens*. 2010;28(6):1234–1242.

75. Kanellis J, Watanabe S, Li JH, et al. Uric acid stimulates monocyte chemoattractant protein-1 production in vascular smooth muscle cells via mitogen-activated protein kinase and cyclooxygenase-2. *Hypertension*. 2003;41(6): 1287–1293.

76. Kaiser AM, Kang JC, Chan LS, et al. Laparoscopic-assisted vs. open colectomy for colon cancer: a prospective randomized trial. *J Laparoendosc Adv Surg Tech A*. 2004;14(6):329–334.

77. Kang DH, Nakagawa T, Feng L, et al. A role for uric acid in the progression of renal disease. *J Am Soc Nephrol*. 2002;13(12):2888–2897.

78. Han HJ, Lim MJ, Lee YJ, et al. Uric acid inhibits renal proximal tubule cell proliferation via at least two signaling pathways involving PKC, MAPK, cPLA2, and NF-kappaB. *Am J Physiol Renal Physiol*. 2007;292(1):F373–381.

79. Sanchez-Lozada LG, Tapia E, Avila-Casado C, et al. Mild hyperuricemia induces glomerular hypertension in normal rats. *Am J Physiol Renal Physiol*. 2002;283(5):F1105–1110.

80. Sanchez-Lozada LG, Tapia E, Santamaria J, et al. Mild hyperuricemia induces vasoconstriction and maintains glomerular hypertension in normal and remnant kidney rats. *Kidney Int*. 2005;67(1):237–247.

81. Coombs FS, Pecora LJ, Thorogood E, et al. Renal function in patients with gout. *J Clin Invest*. 1940;19(3):525–535.

82. Perez-Ruiz F, Alonso-Ruiz A, Calabozo M, et al. Efficacy of allopurinol and benzbromarone for the control of hyperuricemia. A pathogenic approach to the treatment of primary chronic gout. *Ann Rheum Dis*. 1998;57(9):545–549.

83. Anderson BE, Adams DR. Allopurinol hypersensitivity syndrome. *J Drugs Dermatol*. 2002;1(1):60–62.

84. Jung JW, Song WJ, Kim YS, et al. HLA-B58 can help the clinical decision on starting allopurinol in patients with chronic renal insufficiency. *Nephrol Dial Transplant*. 2011;26(11):3567–3572.

85. Becker MA, Schumacher HR Jr, Wortmann RL, et al. Febuxostat, a novel nonpurine selective inhibitor of xanthine oxidase: a twenty-eight-day, multicenter, phase II, randomized, double-blind, placebo-controlled, dose-response clinical trial examining safety and efficacy in patients with gout. *Arthritis Rheum*. 2005;52(3):916–923.

86. Bennett WM. Lead nephropathy. *Kidney Int*. 1985;28(2):212–220.

87. Emmerson BT. Chronic lead nephropathy: the diagnostic use of calcium Edta and the association with gout. *Australas Ann Med*. 1963;12:310–324.

88. Yu CC, Lin JL, Lin-Tan DT. Environmental exposure to lead and progression of chronic renal diseases: a four-year prospective longitudinal study. *J Am Soc Nephrol*. 2004;15(4):1016–1022.

89. Vaziri ND, Sica DA. Lead-induced hypertension: role of oxidative stress. *Curr Hypertens Rep*. 2004;6(4):314–320.

90. Wilson VK, Thomson ML, Dent CE. Amino-aciduria in lead poisoning; a case in childhood. *Lancet*. 1953;265(6776):66–68.

91. Lin JL, Tan DT, Ho HH, et al. Environmental lead exposure and urate excretion in the general population. *Am J Med*. 2002;113(7):563–568.

92. Inglis JA, Henderson DA, Emmerson BT. The pathology and pathogenesis of chronic lead nephropathy occurring in Queensland. *J Pathol*. 1978;124(2): 65–76.

93. Arteriosclerosis. *Cal State J Med*. 1909;7(4):121–123.

94. Lin JL, Ho HH, Yu CC. Chelation therapy for patients with elevated body lead burden and progressive renal insufficiency. A randomized, controlled trial. *Ann Intern Med*. 1999;130(1):7–13.

95. Lin JL, Lin-Tan DT, Hsu KH, et al. Environmental lead exposure and progression of chronic renal diseases in patients without diabetes. *N Engl J Med*. 2003;348(4):277–286.

96. Fairbanks LD, Cameron JS, Venkat-Raman G, et al. Early treatment with allopurinol in familial juvenile hyerpuricaemic nephropathy (FJHN) ameliorates the long-term progression of renal disease. *QJM*. 2002;95(9):597–607.

97. Puig JG, Miranda ME, Mateos FA, et al. Hereditary nephropathy associated with hyperuricemia and gout. *Arch Intern Med*. 1993;153(3):357–365.

98. Bachmann S, Mutig K, Bates J, et al. Renal effects of Tamm-Horsfall protein (uromodulin) deficiency in mice. *Am J Physiol Renal Physiol*. 2005;288(3): F559–567.

99. Gersch MS, Sautin YY, Gersch CM, et al. Does Tamm-Horsfall protein-uric acid binding play a significant role in urate homeostasis? *Nephrol Dial Transplant*. 2006;21(10):2938–2942.

100. Bleyer AJ, Woodard AS, Shihabi Z, et al. Clinical characterization of a family with a mutation in the uromodulin (Tamm-Horsfall glycoprotein) gene. *Kidney Int*. 2003;64(1):36–42.

101. Horl WH. Neutrophil function in renal failure. *Adv Nephrol Necker Hosp*. 2001;31:173–192.

102. Kosugi T, Nakayama T, Heinig M, et al. Effect of lowering uric acid on renal disease in the type 2 diabetic db/db mice. *Am J Physiol Renal Physiol*. 2009; 297(2):F481–488.

103. Iseki K, Oshiro S, Tozawa M, et al. Significance of hyperuricemia on the early detection of renal failure in a cohort of screened subjects. *Hypertens Res*. 2001;24(6):691–697.

104. Ohno I, Hosoya T, Gomi H, et al. Serum uric acid and renal prognosis in patients with IgA nephropathy. *Nephron*. 2001;87(4):333–339.

105. Myllymaki J, Honkanen T, Syrjanen J, et al. Uric acid correlates with the severity of histopathological parameters in IgA nephropathy. *Nephrol Dial Transplant*. 2005;20(1):89–95.

106. Syrjanen J, Mustonen J, Pasternack A. Hypertriglyceridaemia and hyperuricaemia are risk factors for progression of IgA nephropathy. *Nephrol Dial Transplant*. 2000;15(1):34–42.

107. Johnson RJ, Segal MS, Srinivas T, et al. Essential hypertension, progressive renal disease, and uric acid: a pathogenetic link? *J Am Soc Nephrol*. 2005;16(7): 1909–1919.

108. Hovind P, Rossing P, Tarnow L, et al. Serum uric acid as a predictor for development of diabetic nephropathy in type 1 diabetes: an inception cohort study. *Diabetes*. 2009;58(7):1668–1671.

109. Jalal DI, Rivard CJ, Johnson RJ, et al. Serum uric acid levels predict the development of albuminuria over 6 years in patients with type 1 diabetes: findings from the Coronary Artery Calcification in Type 1 Diabetes study. *Nephrol Dial Transplant*. 2010;25(6):1865–1869.

110. Goicoechea M, de Vinuesa SG, Verdalles U, et al. Effect of allopurinol in chronic kidney disease progression and cardiovascular risk. *Clin J Am Soc Nephrol*. 2010;5(8):1388–1393.

111. Momeni A, Shahidi S, Seirafian S, et al. Effect of allopurinol in decreasing proteinuria in type 2 diabetic patients. *Iran J Kidney Dis*. 2010;4(2):128–132.

112. Hande KR, Noone RM, Stone WJ. Severe allopurinol toxicity. Description and guidelines for prevention in patients with renal insufficiency. *Am J Med*. 1984; 76(1):47–56.

113. Fam AG. Gout, diet, and the insulin resistance syndrome. *J Rheumatol*. 2002;29(7):1350–1355.

114. Brymora A, Flisińsk M, Johnson RJ, et al. Low-fructose diet lowers blood pressure and inflammation in patients with chronic kidney disease. *Nephrol Dial Transplant*. 2012;27(2):608–612.

115. Choi HK, Atkinson K, Karlson EW, et al. Alcohol intake and risk of incident gout in men: a prospective study. *Lancet*. 2004;363(9417):1277–1281.

116. Burnier M, Roch-Ramel F, Brunner HR. Renal effects of angiotensin II receptor blockade in normotensive subjects. *Kidney Int*. 1996;49(6):1787–1790.

117. Sennesael JJ, Lamote JG, Violet I, et al. Divergent effects of calcium channel and angiotensin converting enzyme blockade on glomerulotubular function in cyclosporine-treated renal allograft recipients. *Am J Kidney Dis*. 1996;27(5): 701–708.

118. Milionis HJ, Kakafika AI, Tsouli SG, et al. Effects of statin treatment on uric acid homeostasis in patients with primary hyperlipidemia. *Am Heart J*. 2004;148(4):635–640.

119. Desager JP, Hulhoven R, Harvengt C. Uricosuric effect of fenofibrate in healthy volunteers. *J Clin Pharmacol*. 1980;20(10):560–564.

120. Lipscombe J, Lewis GF, Cattran D, et al. Deterioration in renal function associated with fibrate therapy. *Clin Nephrol*. 2001;55(1):39–44.

121. Garg JP, Chasan-Taber S, Blair A, et al. Effects of sevelamer and calcium-based phosphate binders on uric acid concentrations in patients undergoing hemodialysis: a randomized clinical trial. *Arthritis Rheum*. 2005;52(1):290–295.

122. Murrell GA, Rapeport WG. Clinical pharmacokinetics of allopurinol. *Clin Pharmacokinet*. 1986;11(5):343–353.

123. Wortmann RL. Recent advances in the management of gout and hyperuricemia. *Curr Opin Rheumatol*. 2005;17(3):319–324.

124. Young JL Jr, Boswell RB, Nies AS. Severe allopurinol hypersensitivity. Association with thiazides and prior renal compromise. *Arch Intern Med*. 1974; 134(3):553–558.

125. Vazquez-Mellado J, Morales EM, Pacheco-Tena C, et al. Relation between adverse events associated with allopurinol and renal function in patients with gout. *Ann Rheum Dis*. 2001;60(10):981–983.

126. Stamp L, Gow P, Sharples K, et al. The optimal use of allopurinol: an audit of allopurinol use in South Auckland. *Aust N Z J Med*. 2000;30(5):567–572.

127. Sinclair DS, Fox IH. The pharmacology of hypouricemic effect of benzbromarone. *J Rheumatol*. 1975;2(4):437–445.

128. Heel RC, Brogden RN, Speight TM, et al. Benzbromarone: a review of its pharmacological properties and therapeutic use in gout and hyperuricaemia. *Drugs*. 1977;14(5):349–366.
129. Perez-Ruiz F, Calabozo M, Pijoan JI, et al. Effect of urate-lowering therapy on the velocity of size reduction of tophi in chronic gout. *Arthritis Rheum*. 2002;47(4):356–360.
130. Arai M, Yokosuka O, Fujiwara K, et al. Fulminant hepatic failure associated with benzbromarone treatment: a case report. *J Gastroenterol Hepatol*. 2002; 17(5):625–626.
131. Masbernard A, Giudicelli CP. Ten years' experience with benzbromarone in the management of gout and hyperuricaemia. *S Afr Med J*. 1981;59(20):701–706.
132. Takano Y, Hase-Aoki K, Horiuchi H, et al. Selectivity of febuxostat, a novel non-purine inhibitor of xanthine oxidase/xanthine dehydrogenase. *Life Sci*. 2005; 76(16):1835–1847.
133. Mayer MD, Khosravan R, Vernillet L, et al. Pharmacokinetics and pharmacodynamics of febuxostat, a new non-purine selective inhibitor of xanthine oxidase in subjects with renal impairment. *Am J Ther*. 2005;12(1):22–34.
134. El-Zawawy H, Mandell BF. Managing gout: how is it different in patients with chronic kidney disease? *Cleve Clin J Med*. 2010;77(12):919–928.
135. Abdelrahman M, Rafi A, Ghacha R, et al. Hyperuricemia and gout in renal transplant recipients. *Ren Fail*. 2002;24(3):361–367.
136. Marcen R, Gallego N, Orofino L, et al. Impairment of tubular secretion of urate in renal transplant patients on cyclosporine. *Nephron*. 1995;70(3): 307–313.
137. Mazzali M, Kim YG, Suga S, et al. Hyperuricemia exacerbates chronic cyclosporine nephropathy. *Transplantation*. 2001;71(7):900–905.
138. Kobelt V, Hess T, Matzkies F, et al. Does allopurinol prevent side effects of cyclosporine-A treatment? *Transplant Proc*. 2002;34(5):1425–1427.
139. Assis SM, Monteiro JL, Seguro AC. L-Arginine and allopurinol protect against cyclosporine nephrotoxicity. *Transplantation*. 1997;63(8):1070–1073.
140. Neal DA, Tom BD, Gimson AE, et al. Hyperuricemia, gout, and renal function after liver transplantation. *Transplantation*. 2001;72(10):1689–1691.
141. Culleton BF, Larson MG, Kannel WB, et al. Serum uric acid and risk for cardiovascular disease and death: the Framingham Heart Study. *Ann Intern Med*. 1999;131(1):7–13.
142. Grayson PC, Kim SY, LaValley M, et al. Hyperuricemia and incident hypertension: a systematic review and meta-analysis. *Arthritis Care Res (Hoboken)*. 2011; 63(1):102–110.
143. Feig DI, Johnson RJ. Hyperuricemia in childhood primary hypertension. *Hypertension*. 2003;42(3):247–252.
144. Feig DI, Soletsky B, Johnson RJ. Effect of allopurinol on blood pressure of adolescents with newly diagnosed essential hypertension: a randomized trial. *JAMA*. 2008;300(8):924–932.
145. Madero M, Sarnak MJ, Wang X, et al. Uric acid and long-term outcomes in CKD. *Am J Kidney Dis*. 2009;53(5):796–803.
146. Enriquez R, Abad R, Salcedo C, et al. Nalidixic acid disk for laboratory detection of ciprofloxacin resistance in Neisseria meningitidis. *Antimicrob Agents Chemother*. 2009;53(2):796–797.
147. Suliman ME, Johnson RJ, Garcia-Lopez E, et al. J-shaped mortality relationship for uric acid in CKD. *Am J Kidney Dis*. 2006;48(5):761–771.
148. Johnson RJ, Feig DI, Herrera-Acosta J, et al. Resurrection of uric acid as a causal risk factor in essential hypertension. *Hypertension*. 2005;45(1):18–20.
149. Cheng TH, Lin JW, Chao HH, et al. Uric acid activates extracellular signal-regulated kinases and thereafter endothelin-1 expression in rat cardiac fibroblasts. *Int J Cardiol*. 2010;139(1):42–49.
150. Kim ES, Kwon HS, Ahn CW, et al. Serum uric acid level is associated with metabolic syndrome and microalbuminuria in Korean patients with type 2 diabetes mellitus. *J Diabetes Complications*. 2011;25(5):309–313.
151. Feig DI, Kang DH, Johnson RJ. Uric acid and cardiovascular risk. *N Engl J Med*. 2008;359(17):1811–1821.
152. Franse LV, Pahor M, Di Bari M, et al. Serum uric acid, diuretic treatment and risk of cardiovascular events in the Systolic Hypertension in the Elderly Program (SHEP). *J Hypertens*. 2000;18(8):1149–1154.
153. Meshkani R, Zargari M, Larijani B. The relationship between uric acid and metabolic syndrome in normal glucose tolerance and normal fasting glucose subjects. *Acta Diabetol*. 2011;48(1):79–88.
154. Yoo TW, Sung KC, Shin HS, et al. Relationship between serum uric acid concentration and insulin resistance and metabolic syndrome. *Circ J*. 2005;69(8): 928–933.
155. Chedid R, Zoghbi F, Halaby G, et al. Serum uric acid in relation with the metabolic syndrome components and adiponectin levels in Lebanese university students. *J Endocrinol Invest*. 2011;34(7):153–157.
156. Onat A, Uyarel H, Hergenc G, et al. Serum uric acid is a determinant of metabolic syndrome in a population-based study. *Am J Hypertens*. 2006;19(10): 1055–1062.
157. Gagliardi AC, Miname MH, Santos RD. Uric acid: A marker of increased cardiovascular risk. *Atherosclerosis*. 2009;202(1):11–17.
158. Brodov Y, Behar S, Boyko V, et al. Effect of the metabolic syndrome and hyperuricemia on outcome in patients with coronary artery disease (from the Bezafibrate Infarction Prevention Study). *Am J Cardiol*. 2010;106(12):1717–1720.
159. Shelmadine B, Bowden RG, Wilson RL, et al. The effects of lowering uric acid levels using allopurinol on markers of metabolic syndrome in end-stage renal disease patients: a pilot study. *Anadolu Kardiyol Derg*. 2009;9(5):385–389.
160. Ogino K, Kato M, Furuse Y, et al. Uric acid-lowering treatment with benzbromarone in patients with heart failure: a double-blind placebo-controlled crossover preliminary study. *Circ Heart Fail*. 2010;3(1):73–81.
161. Feig DI. Uric acid: a novel mediator and marker of risk in chronic kidney disease? *Curr Opin Nephrol Hypertens*. 2009;18(6):526–530.
162. Ichida K. What lies behind serum urate concentration? Insights from genetic and genomic studies. *Genome Med*. 2009;1(12):118.

CHAPTER 62

Sickle Cell Disease

Vimal K. Derebail • Abhijit V. Kshirsagar

Although reports suggestive of the disease that would come to be known as sickle cell anemia were published in the 1800s,[1,2] Dr. James B. Herrick is credited with the first modern description in 1910. Herrick and his intern Ernest E. Irons described the case of Walter Clement Noel, a male dental student from Grenada (West Indies), who originally sought care for a cough and fever and whose blood film revealed what Irons described as "peculiar elongated and sickle-shaped red blood corpuscles."[3,4] In this first report, Herrick went on to describe isosthenuria, now recognized as one of the most common manifestations of sickle nephropathy.

Current understanding of sickle cell disease reveals it to be a genetic disorder that follows a pattern of Mendelian autosomal co-dominant inheritance[5,6] and affects numerous organ systems. Molecular studies have demonstrated the defect to be with the hemoglobin molecule,[7] specifically, the result of a substitution of the amino acid valine for glutamic acid at position 6 of the β chain.[8–10] A high prevalence of sickle cell disease and heterozygous sickle hemoglobin exists in areas with a high burden of malaria, including sub-Saharan Africa, the Arabian peninsula, and parts of the Indian subcontinent. The presence of hemoglobin S (HbS) has long been postulated to confer a protective benefit to infection by *Plasmodium falciparum*, making carriers less susceptible to malarial morbidity and mortality. This characteristic offers possible explanation for the global distribution and persistence of the mutation.

This chapter focuses on renal abnormalities caused by the presence of sickle hemoglobin. Since Herrick's initial description of isosthenuria, a greater understanding of the clinical effects of sickle hemoglobin on kidney morbidity has been gained. The chapter also includes a discussion of the rare but lethal cancers seen among individuals with sickle cell disease. In addition, the chapter describes the potential role of heterozygote inheritance of hemoglobin S in renal disease.

GENETICS

Several decades following Herrick's description, Linus Pauling noted differing electrophoretic properties of hemoglobin taken from individuals with sickle cell anemia in 1949.[7] With this discovery, it became known as the first "molecular disease." Shortly thereafter, Vernon Ingram and James Hunt identified the exact nature of the molecular alteration—the substitution of valine for glutamic acid at the sixth residue of the β chain of hemoglobin.[9–11]

The genetic mutation responsible for the single amino acid substitution occurs on the short arm of chromosome 11, and asserts as an autosomal recessive pattern of inheritance. The mutation itself results from a single nucleotide substitution from a GAG to GTG codon mutation. Because of incomplete recessive inheritance, those with a single mutation (i.e., carriers with sickle cell trait), produce a measurable quantity of hemoglobin S.

The hemoglobin S mutation seems to have arisen in at least two separate occurrences, one in Africa and the other in Asia. In fact, there are four African specific β-globin gene haplotypes—the Benin, Cameroon, Senegal, and Central African Republic (CAR) haplotypes—and one specific to Asia–the Arab-Indian haplotype.[12,13] These several variations in the β-globin gene mutation do seem to confer variance in the observed phenotype. Those individuals with the Senegal haplotype seem to have the least severe disease course, whereas those with the CAR haplotype have the worst disease manifestations.[13] Worldwide, sickle cell disease is estimated to affect over 275,000 live births annually, and over 300 million individuals are carriers of the gene for sickle hemoglobin. In North America and Europe, 2,600 and 1,300 individuals, respectively, are born yearly with these disorders, whereas in southeast Asian regions and Africa these numbers reach 26,000 and 230,000, respectively.[14] These disease frequencies closely parallel the distribution of malaria, prior to the interventions to control its spread.[12]

PATHOPHYSIOLOGY

Normal adult hemoglobin (HbA) is a 68 kilodalton molecule composed of two pairs of α and β polypeptide chains folded around an iron-containing heme ring. Fetal hemoglobin (HbF), consisting of α and γ chains, predominates during in utero development. The β chain synthesis overtakes γ chain production shortly after birth and the hemoglobin tetramer takes on adult form.

The result of the point mutation in the β chain is a modest change in the three-dimensional spatial configuration but a profound change in the solubility of hemoglobin. Glutamic acid is a charged amino acid and as a polar molecule, highly soluble in water. Valine is uncharged, making it poorly soluble in water. The entire sickle hemoglobin molecule takes on the property of the valine amino acid, becoming nonpolar and poorly soluble in water. The loss of charge, incidentally, explains the altered migration of sickle cell hemoglobin during electrophoresis.

The clinical sequelae of sickle cell disease, including kidney manifestations, arise from the properties of the hemoglobin resulting from the glutamine to valine amino acid substitution of the β subunit. The key steps that lead to organ injury include (1) polymerization of the sickle hemoglobin; (2) adhesion of affected red blood cells; and (3) ischemic/oxidative injury to the vasculature. The degree of injury to any organ system, including the kidney, depends on a number of factors that promote or inhibit these key steps.

Left unimpeded, the uncharged, poorly soluble valine residues allow the hemoglobin molecules to adhere to one another. Polymerization of the hemoglobin S results from the continued aggregation the insoluble molecules. Classically, seven pairs of sickle hemoglobin chains aggregate to form large, insoluble polymers.[15] The rate of sickle hemoglobin polymerization has been proposed to determine the ultimate morphology of the red blood cell[16]; slow polymerization results in long sickle hemoglobin fibers with classic sickle shape whereas rapid polymerization leads to shorter, more granular fibers. Once polymerized, sickle hemoglobin forms a highly viscous, semisolid "gel"[16] with a solubility much less than hemoglobin A and forms elongated structures that distort the red cells into their characteristic sickle and other abnormal shapes (Fig. 62.1).

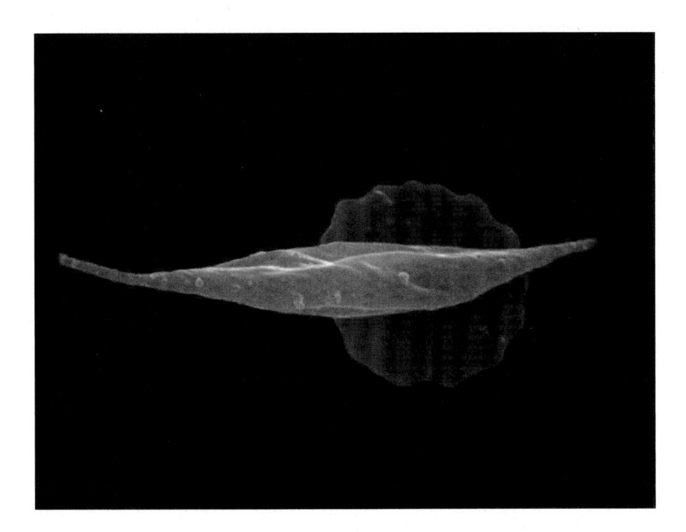

FIGURE 62.1 Normal red blood cell (*background*) and red blood cell affected by sickle-cell anaemia (*foreground*). Wellcome Library, London, "Sickle Cell Anemia" under Creative Commons by-nc-nd 2.0 UK: England & Wales, with permission from the Wellcome Trust. (See Color Plate.)

The polymerization of sickle hemoglobin leads to mechanical deformation of the red blood cell. Acquired red blood cell membrane abnormalities result, including a loss of phospholipids, asymmetry, increased fragility, and abnormal integrin–protein interactions.[17] This injury, in addition to the retention of adhesion molecules, promotes sickle red blood cell adhesion to vascular endothelium.[18,19] Furthermore, the presence of hemoglobin S accentuates red cell endothelial adhesion,[20,21] potentially producing stasis and occlusion in slow-flowing renal vessels under even mild physiologic stress. Clinical disease severity has been correlated with red blood cell adhesivity.[22]

Oxidative injury related to free heme exposure is a notable feature of the pathology of renal injury. Heme oxygenase (HO), the rate-limiting enzyme in heme degradation, serves as a measure of oxidative stress. Studies in transgenic murine models and in humans have demonstrated renal induction of heme-oxygenase-1 (HO-1), the isozyme induced by oxidative stress (Fig. 62.2). Inhibition of glutathione synthesis in the same transgenic murine model to produce acute oxidative stress precipitated acute vaso-occlusive episodes in the kidney, further demonstrating the role of oxidative stress to renal pathology.[23]

Physiologic, metabolic, and genetic conditions promote and mitigate the polymerization process and may help to explain the variability of clinical disease. In vitro studies have demonstrated that decreased oxygen concentration, increased hydrogen ion concentration, rapid deoxygenation, low temperature, advanced red blood cell age, high osmolality, and high intracellular HbS concentration promote the formation of the sickle polymers.[24–29]

Two well-established genetic modifiers of phenotypic severity are fetal hemoglobin concentrations and coinheritance of α-thalassemia. Fetal hemoglobin concentration may range between 1% and 30% and is determined by at least three different genetic loci.[12] With higher levels of fetal hemoglobin, the concentration of hemoglobin S in the erythrocyte is reduced. Nearly 30% to 50% of patients with sickle cell disease have coexistent α-thalassemia trait, which leads to an overall reduction in the concentration of total erythrocyte hemoglobin and reduced hemoglobin S polymerization.[12] Both of these modifying genetic factors have been shown to modulate the severity of clinical manifestations.[12]

Normal physiologic functions of the kidney include excretion of acid and solute. Gradients of acid and solute occur as a result of counter-current transport, and render the medulla with especially high concentrations of both. Furthermore, the renal medulla has a very low partial pressure of oxygen (10–20 mm Hg),[30] sufficient to induce sickling.[31] In aggregate, the conditions of the renal medulla—relative hypoxia, hyperosmolarity, acidity, and sluggish blood flow (Fig. 62.3)—represent an environment primed for sickling of red blood cells containing hemoglobin S. Angiographic studies have demonstrated significant renal vascular disruption and vessel dropout in individuals with HbSS and HbAS compared to individuals with normal hemoglobin

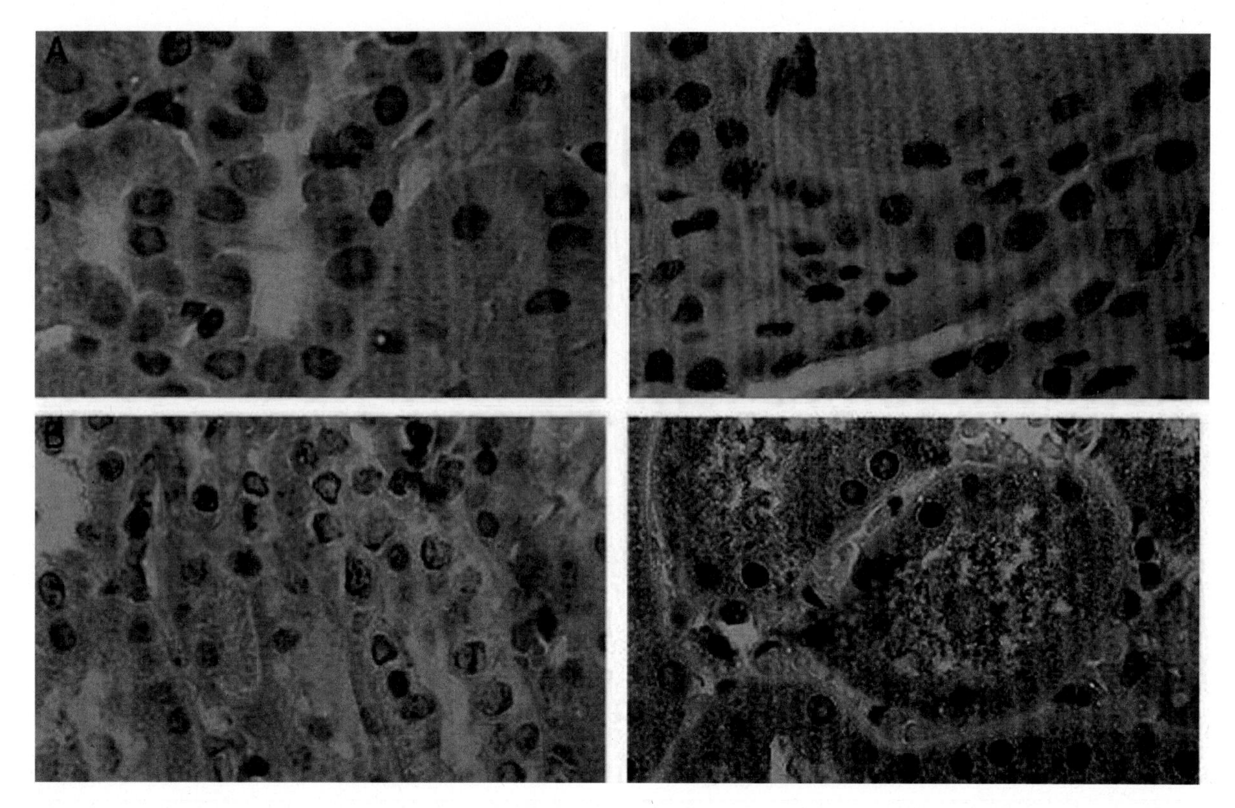

FIGURE 62.2 Immunoperoxidase staining for HO-1 in normal human kidney **(A)** and in the kidney of a patient with sickle cell disease **(B)**. In **A** and **B**, immunoperoxidase studies were undertaken in the absence (*left*) and presence (*right*) of HO-1 antibody. **B:** Positive staining with the HO-1 antibody in renal proximal tubules in the kidney of the patient with sickle cell disease (*right*). Original magnification, ×400. (From Nath KA, Grande JP, Haggard JJ, et al. Oxidative stress and induction of heme oxygenase-1 in the kidney in sickle cell disease. *Am J Pathol.* 2001;158:893–903, with permission from Elsevier at the courtesy of the editors.)

(HbAA)—likely the result of repeated episodes of red blood cell sickling with resultant ischemia (Fig. 62.4).[32] Experimental mouse models of sickle cell anemia have demonstrated an exquisite sensitivity to ischemic injury.[33,34] Chronic hypoxia may mediate the development of focal segmental glomerular scarring and subsequent proteinuria notable in sickle cell disease.

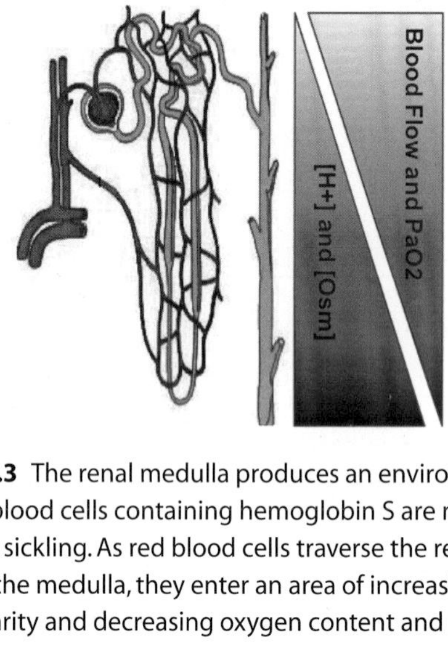

FIGURE 62.3 The renal medulla produces an environment in which red blood cells containing hemoglobin S are more likely to undergo sickling. As red blood cells traverse the renal vasculature into the medulla, they enter an area of increasing acidity and osmolarity and decreasing oxygen content and blood flow.

Recent investigations into the pathophysiology have also demonstrated a role for endothelial dysfunction. Patients with sickle cell disease demonstrate high levels of soluble fms-lke tyrosine kinase-1 (sFlt-1), which is a member of the vascular endothelial growth factor (VEGF) receptor family. High levels of sFlt-1 are felt to promote endothelial dysfunction by binding to the receptor-binding domains of circulating VEGF and preventing the normal interaction with endothelial cell receptors. A recent cohort study of 73 patients with sickle cell disease demonstrated statistically higher values of sFLT-1 among those patients with albuminuria, suggesting it may induce glomerular endothelial dysfunction.[35]

Additional investigations into the pathophysiology of chronic kidney disease (CKD) have gone beyond previous understanding of genetic modifiers as mentioned previously and have focused on the role of coinherited gene polymorphisms in the development of kidney disease.[36] Specifically, investigators have focused on the transforming growth factor beta and bone morphogenetic protein (TGF-β/BMP) pathway, implicated in the development of diabetic nephropathy and also associated with other organ involvement in sickle cell anemia.[37–42] In a longitudinal analysis of over 1,000 individuals with sickle cell anemia, the authors found that

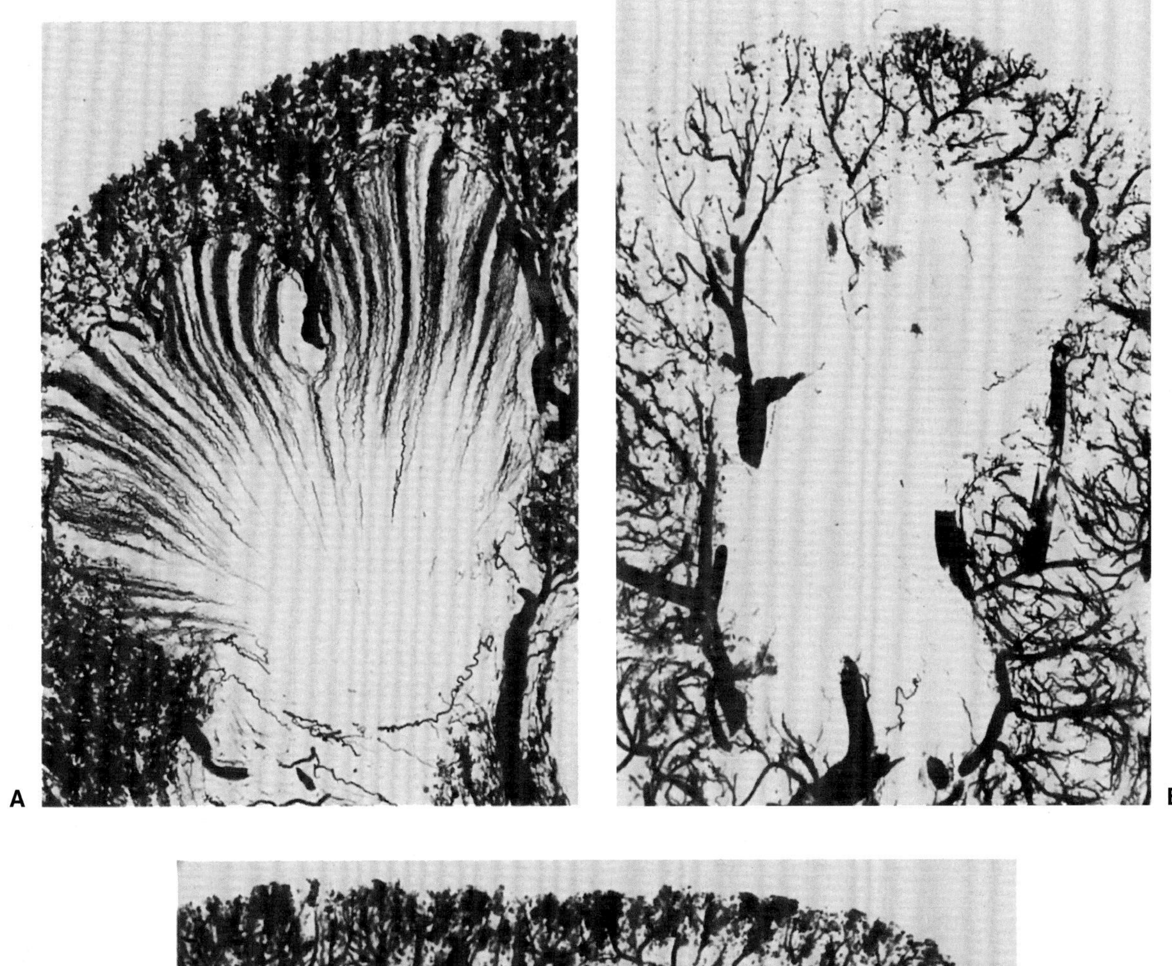

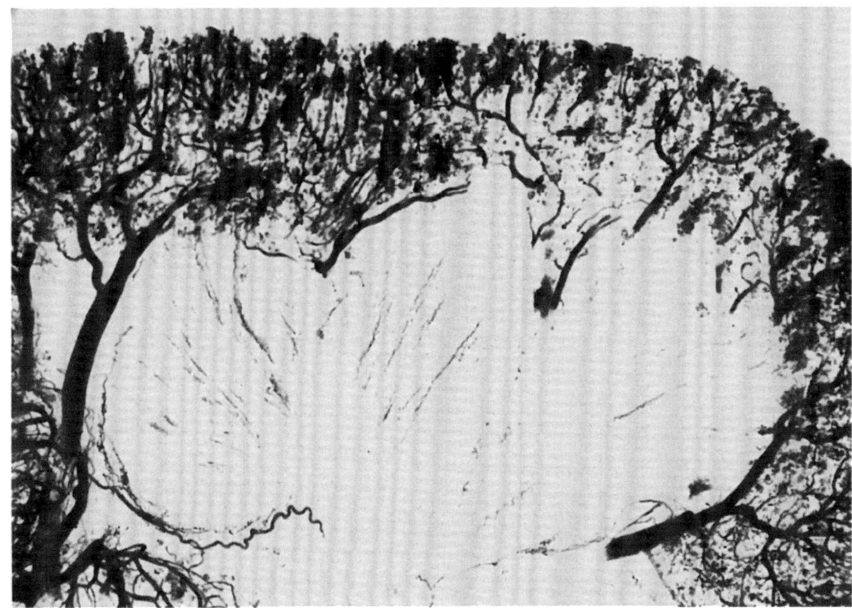

FIGURE 62.4 Injection microradioangiographs of kidneys from a subject without hemoglobinopathy **(A)**, a patient with sickle cell disease **(B)**, and a patient with sickle cell–hemoglobin C disease **(C)**. In the normal kidney **(A)**, vasa recta are visible radiating into the renal papilla; in sickle cell anemia **(B)**, vasa recta are virtually absent. Those vessels that are present are abnormal, are dilated, form spirals, and end bluntly, and many appear to be obliterated. The patient with Hb-SC **(C)** shows changes intermediately between the Hb-SS patients and the normal subjects. (Reprinted from Statius van Eps LW, et al. Nature of concentrating defect in sickle cell nephropathy, microradioangiographic studies. *Lancet*. 1970;1:450, with permission from Elsevier at the courtesy of the editors.)

four distinct single nucleotide polymorphisms (SNPs) in the BMPR1B, a receptor gene, were significantly associated with GFR. Utilization of genomewide association studies (GWAS) has identified further SNPs that may be important to explaining the phenotypic heterogeneity of sickle cell disease.[43] Additional analyses are needed to confirm promising exploratory studies that demonstrate modulation of renal morbidity among individuals with sickle cell anemia.

RENAL MANIFESTATIONS

Structural Changes

Renal Size

The kidneys of patients with sickle cell disease typically vary in size with age. Infants and young children have kidneys of near-normal size.[44] The kidneys increase in length and weight in older children and young adults—on average the kidneys growing by 5 to 8 mm per year by ultrasound imaging in patients with Hb-SC and Hb-SS disease as compared with age-matched controls.[45] After age 40 years, the size decreases.[46]

Other structural changes are commonly seen on radiographic imaging. These findings increase with advancing age and likely reflect the cumulative effect of repeated episodes of "sickling." Cortical scarring is seen on intravenous pyelography among 8% of individuals aged 16 to 25 years, and rising to 45% among those over 35 years.[47] Calyceal abnormalities such as blunting, cysts, and clubbing are seen among 28% of youths and among 57% of individuals over 35 years.[47] Papillary necrosis among adults is seen at high frequency, ranging from 15% to 65%.[48–50] B-mode ultrasound imaging can reveal increased echogenicity of the kidneys in up to 25% of individuals with sickle cell anemia.[51,52]

Kidneys removed due to severe hematuria may demonstrate submucosal hemorrhages in the pelvis, medulla, and cortex.[53] Radiographic changes suggesting papillary necrosis, medullary cavitations, ring shadows, and calcifications in the pyramids have also been observed.[54,55] Occasionally, minimal papillary necrosis is apparent only on microscopic examination. Renal vein thrombosis is also an occasional finding in Hb-SS disease. Finally, the macroscopic appearance of kidneys of affected individuals may show irregularity and granularity of the surface.

Vasculature

Microradioangiographic studies (Fig. 62.4) have been performed on kidneys removed at autopsy from patients with normal hemoglobin, patients with Hb-SS disease, and patients with Hb-AS and Hb-SC disease.[32] A significantly reduced number of vasa recta are seen in kidneys from Hb-SS patients. The vessels that remain are abnormal as they are dilated, show spiral formation, and end bluntly. Patients with Hb-AS and Hb-SC disease show changes intermediate between those of the Hb-SS patients and normal subjects. In patients with Hb-AS, sparse bundles of vasa recta are surrounded by a chaotic pattern of dilated capillaries, with loss of the original bundle architecture. The changes presumptively result from occlusion of vasa recta and represent the structural basis for the development of functional changes. The loss of the highly specialized structure of parallel running loops of Henle and vasa recta disrupts the normal countercurrent multiplication and exchange.

Histology

Glomerular

Enlargement of the glomeruli is a common finding in patients with sickle cell disease. The glomeruli may be visible by the naked eye and have been described as red "pinheads."[27,56] Individuals with homozygous sickle hemoglobin have both an increase in glomerular diameter and size compared to normal controls.[57,58] Glomerular enlargement and congestion are more common in children beyond the age of 2 years and are most marked in juxtamedullary glomeruli.[57,59] When the size of juxtamedullary glomeruli is systemically measured, there is a distinct difference between those of children with sickle cell disease and normal children. In older patients, this glomerular enlargement and congestion may lead to progressive ischemia and fibrosis with obliteration of glomeruli.[46,60]

Histology of the enlarged glomeruli is notable for the marked hypercellularity and lobulation of the glomerular tuft. Other changes include replication of the basement membrane and mesangial proliferation.[57,61,62] Aggregates of sickled red blood cells may pack and distend the glomerular capillaries and the afferent and efferent arterioles. Electron microscopy of glomeruli may reveal foot process effacement and local thickening of the basement membrane,[61] although an exact prevalence is difficult to ascertain.

Clinical syndromes resulting from glomerular pathology, including glomerulonephritis, have been described among individuals with sickle cell disease. These conditions are discussed later in the chapter.

Medullary

The major components of the medulla are the vasa recta and renal tubules. As noted earlier, physiologic factors favoring sickling are routinely found in the medulla and, as such, medullary lesions are among the earliest and most prominent renal abnormalities. Initial changes consist of edema, focal scarring, and interstitial fibrosis. Progressive scarring leads to tubular atrophy and infiltration of mononuclear cells. Iron deposition has been observed in proximal tubules and pigmented casts may be seen.[55,57,61] Defective iron metabolism, as suggested by decreased renal cortical spin echo with magnetic resonance imaging (MRI), may contribute to the nephrotic syndrome.[63] All these changes could be the result of the observed obliteration or attenuation of the medullary circulation.[32]

Functional Changes

Renal Hemodynamics and Function

Renal hemodynamics are thought to be either normal or supernormal in homozygous (Hb-SS) patients younger than 30 years of age.[64–66] In Hb-SS infants, increased values have been observed for both GFR and effective renal blood flow (ERBF), as well as for the tubular transport maximum of *para*-aminohippurate (Tm_{PAH}). A recent study of a cohort of infants with sickle cell disease has demonstrated similar findings of increased GFR.[67,68] ERBF has been reported to be normal or elevated, although less elevated than effective renal plasma flow (ERPF) because of the typically very low hematocrit, while the extraction ratio of *para*-aminohippurate (E_{PAH}) was decreased. Filtration fraction (GFR/ERPF) has been found to be decreased (mean 14% to 18%; normal 19% to 22%).[64,65,69] Selective damage of the juxtamedullary glomeruli might result in a lower filtration fraction because these nephrons have the highest filtration fractions.[70,71] Microradioangiographic studies lend support to this suggestion.[32]

In sickle cell trait, Hb-SC disease, Hb-CC disease, hemoglobin C trait, and Hb-Sβ^+thalassemia, GFR, and ERPF have been reported to be within the range of normal.[72] As compared to patients with Hb-SS, studies in individuals with sickle cell trait do not appear to demonstrate significant age-related increases in GFR or microalbuminuria.[73]

Several mechanisms have been postulated for the increase in renal hemodynamics in patients with sickle cell disease. With severe anemia, peripheral vascular resistance decreases and cardiac output increases, possibly causing blood to be preferentially shunted to the renal circulation. However, in studies with short follow-up, correction of the anemia does not alter the GFR or ERBF.[64,74] Multiple transfusions with Hb-AA blood to patients with Hb-SS result in significant, although temporary, increases in hemoglobin concentration, with gradual and almost complete replacement of Hb-S by Hb-A. Because this procedure does not reduce the supernormal GFR and ERPF,[64] the cause of the supernormal renal clearances in sickle cell nephropathy cannot be explained by the anemia per se or by the presence of the abnormal hemoglobin. Altered nitric oxide production and renin secretion as seen in transgenic sickle cell mouse models may play a role in hyperfiltration.[75,76] (See section entitled "Pathophysiology.") The ischemic damage to the medulla could also be a stimulus for increased prostaglandin synthesis that may drive hyperfiltration.[66,69,77] Administration of indomethacin, an inhibitor of prostaglandin synthesis, to individuals with sickle cell anemia results in a significant fall in GFR, ERPF, creatinine clearance, and urea clearance supporting this contention.[69]

A number of possible mechanisms may be responsible for the decline in renal hemodynamics with aging, sometimes ending in renal failure with shrunken end-stage kidneys at necropsy. Although advancing age has an effect on renal hemodynamics and overall kidney function in all individuals, these effects may be heightened in individuals with sickle cell anemia because of the disruption of the medullary vasa recta. Support for the idea of a reduction in medullary blood flow in sickle cell disease can be found in the microradioangiographic examination of Hb-SS kidneys (Fig. 62.4).[32] In these studies of kidneys obtained at autopsy, perfusion of the vasa recta by contrast medium is virtually absent, suggesting an almost complete absence of vasa recta in Hb-SS. Supernormal hemodynamics and hyperfiltration have been proposed as causative mechanisms of glomerulosclerosis,[78] which may lead to the chronic renal failure seen in sickle cell disease. Increased apoptosis, stimulated by ischemic and/or oxidative injury, may also contribute to progressive renal dysfunction.[79–81] Over a number of years, continued loss of medullary circulation, interstitial fibrosis, and possibly superimposed pyelonephritis may lead to a progressive decline in GFR and advanced renal insufficiency in the patient with Hb-SS disease. Thus, there is a progressive decline in ERBF, ERPF, and GFR,[65,82] although there are rare individuals with apparently normal kidney function.

Clinically, the progressive loss of GFR is used to stage CKD. Stages 1 and 2 capture a GFR range above 60 mL/min/1.73 m^2 with proteinuria whereas stages 3 to 5 include a GFR range less than 60 mL/min/1.73 m^2 and stage 6 denotes those receiving renal replacement therapy or dialysis. Although advanced renal failure—that which requires renal replacement therapy, or that which is ascribed as a cause of death—is well documented,[83–86] estimates of earlier stages of renal failure vary widely[87,88] and should be interpreted with caution. Death from nonrenal causes (infection, pulmonary disease, etc.) may be a competing risk, limiting detection of CKD or end-stage renal disease (ESRD). Determining CKD prevalence is further complicated by the fact that serum creatinine, derived from muscle tissue and routinely used to estimate GFR in a variety of formulas,[89–91] may actually overestimate GFR determined by gold standard radionucleotide excretion studies in individuals with sickle cell anemia.[92,93]

Generation of Negative Solute-Free Water

The capacity to generate negative solute-free water (Tc_{H2O}) has been studied in patients with sickle cell disease using different protocols of mannitol loading with conflicting results. Although Whitten and Younes found normal Tc_{H2O} in Hb-SS children,[94] Levitt et al. describe two patients with a Tc_{H2O} of 3.2 mL/min/100 mL glomerular filtrate.[95] Hatch et al. similarly noted a mean Tc_{H2O} of 4.2 ± 0.9 SD mL/min/100 mL glomerular filtrate in 11 Hb-SS patients compared to a mean Tc_{H2O} of 5.7 ± 1.2 SD mL/min/100 mL glomerular filtrate in 7 control subjects.[96] These results suggest that Tc_{H2O} after mannitol loading is impaired in sickle cell anemia.

Studies following the response to saline infusion[96,97] demonstrate impaired Tc_{H2O} in Hb-SS patients. From these studies, sickle cell anemia patients were concluded to have a defect in the water impermeable medullary loops of Henle that transports solute. The normal solute-free water clearance under standard conditions argues against such impairment in sodium chloride reabsorption from the ascending limb of the loop of Henle. However, in comparison to normal solute-free water clearance, a normal Tc_{H2O} depends on adequate function of the portion of the loop of Henle that is localized in the *inner medulla*. Sickle cell anemia patients are able to increase urinary osmolality generally to 450 mOsm per kg H_2O or higher, to the level that can be generated in the outer medulla. As shown in Figure 62.4, the capillary plexus surrounding short loops of Henle in the outer zone does not necessarily penetrate into the inner medullary zone.

Urinary Diluting Capacity

Patients with sickle cell anemia are capable of diluting their urine normally.[74,96,98] Under conditions of water diuresis, the fall in urinary osmolality and percentage of filtered water excreted (C_{H2O}/GFR) has been found to be the same in Hb-SS patients when compared to[99,100] controls. Therefore, the capacity to reabsorb solute in the thick portion of the medullary ascending limb of the loop of Henle apparently is intact in sickle cell anemia.

This combination of a defect in renal concentrating capacity with a normal diluting capacity is quite characteristic for sickle cell anemia. However, unlike control subjects, the normal diluting capacity of sickle cell patients may be particularly dependent on prostaglandins. In one series, administration of indomethacin, an inhibitor of prostaglandins, led to a greater fall in C_{H2O}/GFR in sickle cell subjects and a rise in urinary osmolality from 42 to 125 mOsm per kg H_2O (Fig. 62.5).[99,100] These results suggest that impairment of renal prostaglandins may hamper the normal diluting capacity in sickle cell anemia.

Urinary Acidification

Although systemic acidosis is generally not a feature of sickle cell disease in the absence of advanced renal failure, patients with Hb-SS or Hb-SC may demonstrate an incomplete form of renal tubular acidosis.[101–104] In response to a short-duration acid load, between 29% and 100% of patients with Hb-SS [101–104] are unable to decrease urine pH below 5.3, whereas normal subjects can achieve a urinary pH of 5.0 or lower. Titratable acid and total hydrogen ion excretion are lower in patients with Hb-SS and Hb-SC, but ammonia excretion is appropriate for the coexisting urine pH in most cases. The increased ammonia excretion induced by acid loading is also impaired by indomethacin,[101] suggesting the assumed enhanced prostaglandin synthesis in sickle cell disease[105] may also be important to maintaining normal ammoniagenesis in sickle cell disease. When a maximal acidifying stimulus is employed, such as infusion of sodium sulfate, patients with Hb-SS may lower urine pH and increase net acid excretion to the same degree as normal subjects. Thus, the distal tubule of Hb-SS patients apparently requires a greater-than-normal stimulus to generate a normal urine-to-blood hydrogen ion gradient. In contrast, renal acidification has been found to be normal in patients with sickle cell trait.[106]

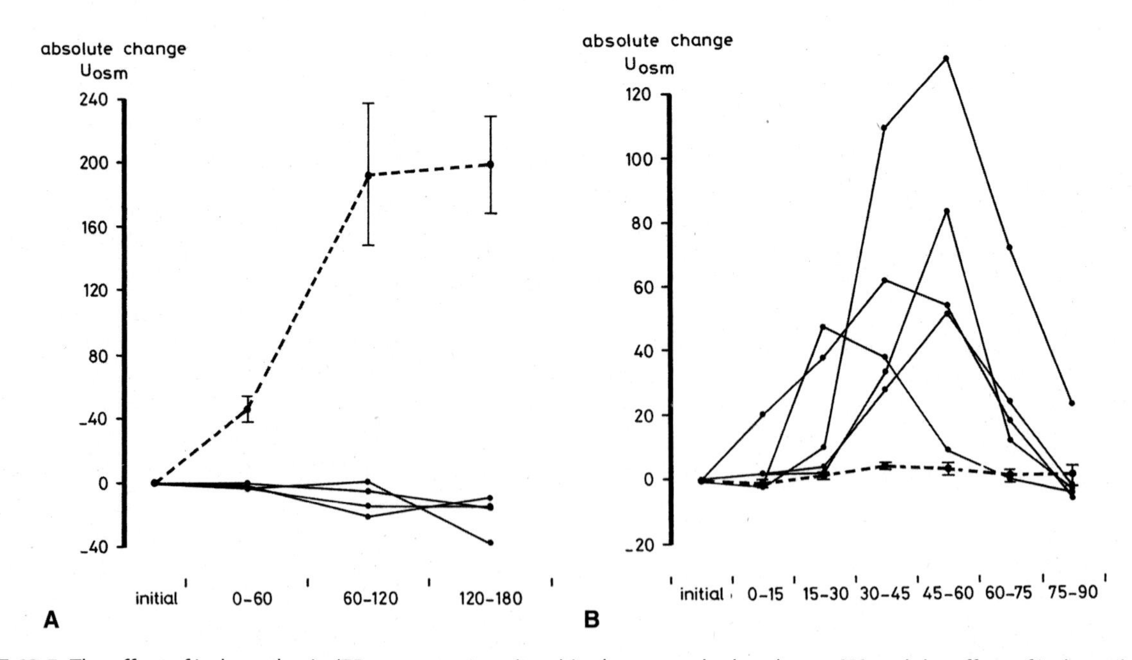

FIGURE 62.5 The effect of indomethacin (75 mg as a suppository) in the water-depleted state **(A)** and the effect of indomethacin (0.25 mg/kg body weight intravenously) in the water-loaded state **(B)**. The *broken lines* represent the mean ± standard error of the mean in control subjects, and the *continuous lines* represent the individual data in patients with sickle cell anemia. (Reproduced with permission from De Jong PE, et al. The influence of indomethacin on renal concentrating and diluting capacity in sickle cell nephropathy. *Clin Sci.* 1982;63:53, © the Biochemical Society.)

The acidification defect has been classified as distal rather than proximal[103] and is characterized by failure to achieve a normal minimal urinary pH with acid loading but is not associated with bicarbonate wasting. Because patients studied not were acidemic or hyperchloremic before acid loading and no generalized proximal tubular reabsorptive defect was observed, the acidification defect was consistent with an incomplete distal renal tubular acidosis.[106] Speculatively, alterations in microcirculation of the renal papillae may impair maintenance of the normally steep hydrogen ion gradients in the collecting ducts. This very subtle defect in renal acidification generally does not cause a systemic metabolic acidosis, which could increase sickling. Several studies globally[102,104,107,108] have been unable to demonstrate evidence of metabolic acidosis in the absence of a sickle cell crisis, but do exhibit changes consistent with a mild chronic respiratory alkalosis.

Potassium Metabolism

In addition to the defect in hydrogen ion excretion, potassium excretion may also be impaired in sickle cell patients.[109–111] Following potassium chloride, sodium sulfate, or furosemide administration, potassium excretion was found to be subnormal in patients with sickle cell disease. Hypoaldosteronism does not appear to explain these findings as both plasma renin activity and plasma aldosterone concentration were normal, both during normovolemia and after volume contraction. Additionally, despite impaired renal potassium excretion, hyperkalemia did not develop in these patients during acute potassium chloride loading. Although administration of angiotensin-converting enzyme (ACE) inhibitors and other agents may elevate plasma potassium concentration,[112] significant alterations in plasma potassium concentration has not been seen with ACE inhibitor therapy for proteinuria in sickle cell disease.[113]

As with the defect in water and hydrogen ion excretion, the disturbance in potassium excretion could be due to an abnormality resulting from ischemic injury to the collecting duct; potassium excretion is known to reflect primarily secretion in the distal nephron. Potassium excretion in sickle cell trait appears to be normal.[114]

A hyperkalemic, hyperchloremic metabolic acidosis in sickle cell nephropathy has been reported.[109] Among six patients—three with Hb-SS, two with Hb-AS, and one with Hb-SC—all had impaired renal potassium excretion. Five of these patients had a moderate-to-severe decrease of GFR and all patients had spontaneous metabolic acidosis. Selective aldosterone deficiency was found in three patients, two with normal and one with low plasma renin activity.

Other reports describe hyporeninemic hypoaldosteronism in patients with sickle cell disease.[110,114] Diminished renin secretion may result in impaired function of the adrenal glomerulosa cells, reduced aldosterone secretion, and subsequently impaired ability to excrete potassium loads. In these cases, the hyperkalemia responded favorably to treatment with mineralocorticosteroids.

Proximal Tubular Secretion

Although severe disturbances in medullary transport occur in patients with sickle cell anemia, proximal tubular activity, both secretory and reabsorptive, appears to be supernormal. The tubular transport maximum of *para*-aminohippurate is elevated in sickle cell anemia, particularly in children.[66] Other evidence of an increased proximal tubular secretory capacity has been obtained from studies regarding uric acid excretion. Despite the increased red cell turnover and consequent uric acid overproduction, most patients with sickle cell anemia are normouricemic due to augmented urate clearance[62,115] from increased pyrazinamide-suppressible urate.[115,116] Hyperuricemia in Hb-SS patients may occur with decreased urate clearance, but these patients often have some decrement in renal function or proteinuria.[62,117,118] Urate clearance decreases with age and the incidence of hyperuricemia increases as renal function deteriorates.[62] Attacks of gout can occur[118–120] and sometimes be clinically difficult to differentiate from vasoocclusive crises or sickle cell arthropathy.[121]

As previously mentioned, the tubular secretion of creatinine can be elevated, with a 20% to 29% rise in fractional creatinine excretion in Hb-SS patients compared to controls.[69,77] However, one study demonstrated that following an intravenous load of creatinine to adults with sickle cell disease, most without proteinuria, creatinine clearance did not increase as expected. Compared to controls, GFR remained the same.[122] The investigators suggested that reduced tubular secretion of creatinine in response to a creatinine load may be an early indicator of renal dysfunction. Importantly, this abnormal tubular function may adversely impact the utility of creatinine clearance measurements to estimate GFR in sickle cell disease.

Proximal Tubular Reabsorption

Relative tubular reabsorption of phosphate is also increased in sickle cell anemia. Consequent to this higher phosphate reabsorption, serum phosphate can be elevated in some subjects.[123,124] High phosphate reabsorption may reflect increased reabsorptive activity of the proximal tubule.[123] In contrast, children with sickle cell anemia have lower serum phosphate levels than normal children[125] that is associated with significantly lower renal tubular resorption of phosphate. This contrast may be due to increased parathyroid levels reported in children with sickle cell disease[126] or may simply indicate the absence of sickle cell renal injury early in life.

Sodium reabsorption in the proximal tubule parallels phosphate reabsorption and may also be enhanced in HbSS patients. Indeed some studies report increased plasma volume in the steady-state Hb-SS patients.[96,127,128] Conversely, increased proximal tubular sodium reabsorption may be a secondary mechanism to correct for defects in salt reabsorption in the more distal nephron. One might expect patients to develop volume depletion as a consequence of defects in medullary water and sodium conservation. However, such distal compensatory mechanisms would not increase plasma volume.

Increased tubular uptake of β_2 microglobulin has also been described in sickle cell anemia.[129] Resorption of β_2 microglobulin positively correlates with the reabsorption of phosphate, providing further evidence of increased proximal tubule activity. However, estimates of GFR are comparable among ^{51}Cr-EDTA, creatinine clearance, and β_2 microglobulin determinations in sickle cell patients older than 40 years of age.[130] Zinc excretion has also been found to be abnormal in Hb-SS patients, exceeding the filtered load as compared to controls whose excretion is lower than the filtered load.[131]

Therefore, Hb-SS patients have a defect in renal medullary functions with a tendency to lose water and sodium, whereas ERPF, GFR, and proximal tubular activity are increased. In general, under typical conditions of health, the ultimate result of this compensation is normal homeostasis of fluid and electrolytes.

Renal Hormones

Erythropoietin

Data on plasma erythropoietin (EPO) levels in sickle cell anemia are conflicting. EPO levels strongly correlate with red cell mass in sickle cell disease patients.[132] Increased values have been reported during infectious episodes and in asymptomatic patients.[133] However, when comparing plasma EPO concentrations in sickle cell anemia to other causes of anemia, Hb-SS patients have been shown to have similar or decreased values.[134] EPO titers in patients with pure red cell aplasia, for instance, may be 10-fold higher than those in Hb-SS patients.

Other observations have shown patients with sickle cell anemia produce less EPO at a given hemoglobin concentration than do patients with non–sickle cell anemias.[135,136] Notably, pediatric patients with sickle cell anemia have significantly higher EPO levels than do adults.[136]

In a study of patients older than 40 years, a fall in the Hb concentration was observed that correlated with declining renal function. The investigators postulated that lower Hb concentrations may be due to reduced EPO production. In sickle cell disease patients with renal failure, supplementation with erythropoietin using doses of 100 to 150 U per kg three times a week,[137–139] up to 30,000 U per week,[140] result in increased reticulocyte counts, but may not increase the absolute hemoglobin value.

Renal transplantation may correct the erythropoietin-resistant anemia in Hb-SS patients with ESRD.[140,141] This improvement may reflect decreased uremic and other toxins or reduced inflammation that may suppress erythropoiesis or even enhance hemolysis.[141] Hydroxyurea therapy in some patients with sickle cell disease may increase erythropoietin levels 5 to 10 days after starting therapy[142] but this increase is not necessarily sustained.

Potential mechanisms for the low EPO levels observed in sickle cell disease include interference with the renal synthesis of EPO, as a result of renal damage by the sickling process, and the displacement to the right of the oxygen equilibrium curve. Circulating red blood cell progenitors from patients with sickle cell disease have increased expression of erythropoietin receptors, which correlated with increased stimulated and autocrine erythroid colony development.[143] This may be a compensatory mechanism, in the absence of renal disease, for relatively lower erythropoietin levels in sickle cell disease.

Renin–Angiotensin–Aldosterone System

Plasma renin activity and aldosterone concentration are generally normal in patients with Hb-SS disease during steady-state conditions[69,111] despite lower mean arterial pressure than controls.[144] After volume depletion, normal or increased values may occur,[145] and both supine and upright plasma renin activities for different sodium intakes always were higher in Hb-SS patients than in control subjects.[146] Upregulation of renin has been demonstrated in the kidneys of transgenic sickle cell mice exposed to hypoxia.[75] As mentioned previously, some patients may exhibit hyporeninemic hypoaldosteronism and hyperkalemia.[110,114] Interestingly, high plasma renin activity has been described in a patient with intermittent hypertension occurring during a painful crisis. When the crisis had subsided, blood pressure normalized again.[147] Typically, though, hypertension seldom occurs in Hb-SS patients, even during crisis.

Renal Prostaglandins

Prostaglandin production occurs in renal interstitial medullary cells and collecting duct cells[148] and is promoted by various vasoconstrictor stimuli.[149] The interstitial cells of the medulla in patients with sickle cell anemia contain aggregates of granular electron-dense material,[61] likely representative of prostaglandin production. Speculatively, ischemic and/or oxidative insult to the inner medulla in sickle cell anemia may induce synthesis of vasodilator prostaglandins. The role of renal prostaglandins in sickle cell anemia has been studied in several ways: indirectly using indomethacin as a prostaglandin synthesis inhibitor, directly measuring urinary prostaglandin E_2 and $F_{2\alpha}$ (PGE_2 and $PGF_{2\alpha}$) excretion, and via assessment of gene regulation in the transgenic sickle cell mouse model.

As already discussed, indomethacin administration does not change GFR and ERPF in controls, but a significant fall in both were found after indomethacin administration to Hb-SS patients.[69,76] These findings suggest prostaglandins maintain the supernormal or normal GFR and ERPF in sickle cell anemia and may play a role in hyperfiltration and subsequent rise in GFR seen in young sickle cell patients. The rise in renal blood flow and glomerular filtration may also explain the increased proximal tubular activity in these patients.

In normal subjects, indomethacin causes sodium and water retention and a rise in body weight. In Hb-SS patients,

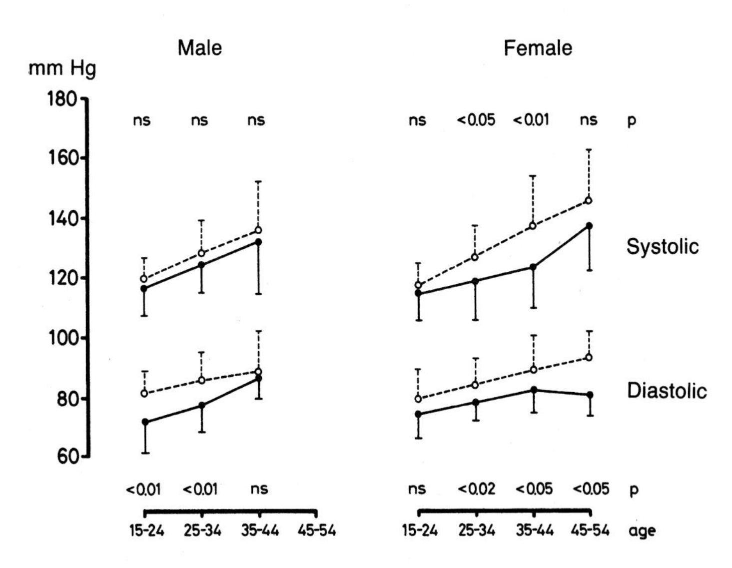

FIGURE 62.6 Mean ± standard deviation of systolic and diastolic blood pressure in control subjects (*dotted lines*) and patients with sickle cell anemia (*closed lines*) who are age- and sex-matched. (From De Jong PE, et al. Blood pressure in sickle cell disease. *Arch Intern Med.* 1982;142:1239; and reprinted by permission from Macmillan Publishers Ltd. De Jong PE, Statius van Eps LW. Sickle cell nephropathy. New insights into its pathophysiology. [Editorial review]. *Kidney Int.* 1985;27:711, through courtesy of the editors.)

similar sodium retention occurs after indomethacin administration, but without water retention or an increase in weight. Rather, serum osmolality increased in these patients.[66]

Indomethacin administration to water-deprived normal subjects leads to a rise in urinary osmolality of 836 to 1,027 mOsm per kg H_2O, whereas the defect in urinary concentration in sickle cell anemia does not improve after indomethacin[100] (Fig. 62.5). This result supports a diminished solute gradient in the inner medulla of patients with Hb-SS that is not modulated by prostaglandins. During a water load, however, a rise in urinary osmolality in sickle cell subjects occurs after indomethacin administration, but not in controls. Normal diluting capacity in sickle cell patients therefore appears to be dependent on adequate renal prostaglandin synthesis.[77,100]

Both in the dehydrated and in the water-loaded state, PGE_2 excretion is normal in patients with sickle cell disease. $PGF_{2\alpha}$ excretion, however, is decreased; therefore, the $PGE_2/PGF_{2\alpha}$ ratio is higher than in healthy persons.[105] Because PGE_2 and $PGF_{2\alpha}$ have different and sometimes opposite effects on renal hemodynamics, renin release, and sodium and water excretion,[150,151] an abnormal balance between these two prostaglandins may contribute to some characteristics of sickle cell nephropathy. For example, the relative excess of vasodilating PGE_2 could explain the rise in renal blood flow and GFR, particularly in juxtamedullary nephrons.

In the transgenic sickle cell mouse, cytochrome P450 4a14 is upregulated in renal tissue.[75] This enzyme catalyzes arachidonic acid to 20-hydroxyeicosatetraenoic acid (20–HETE), which regulates renal vascular tone, tubular resorption, arterial pressure, and natriuresis.[75]

Atrial Natriuretic Peptide

In normal subjects, atrial natriuretic peptide (ANP) exerts its effects in several nephron segments dependent on prevailing ANP levels. Infusion of a low-dose ANP induces natriuresis in normal individuals but not in matched patients with sickle cell disease.[152] This observation suggests that low-dose ANP inhibits sodium reabsorption in the long loops of Henle, possibly by increasing medullary blood flow and renal interstitial pressure. Natriuresis under supraphysiologic plasma levels of ANP appears to be multifactorial, by an increase in GFR and a decrease in both proximal and distal tubular sodium reabsorption. Infusion of high-dose ANP in patients with sickle cell disease and normal subjects induces a similar degree of natriuresis.[152]

Hypertension and Sickle Cell Disease

The incidence of hypertension in the adult black population in the United States is 32%, contrasting sharply with its incidence in sickle cell disease. Reports from both the Caribbean,[153,154] the United States,[146,155] and Europe[144] demonstrate hypertension in only 2% to 6% of Hb-SS patients overall (Fig. 62.6) and in 15% of patients older than 55 years of age. The explanation for these findings remains unclear. Renal salt losing has been suggested as an etiology,[114] but these data are not convincing. Hb-SS patients are able to conserve sodium adequately on a severely restricted sodium diet.[145,146] Moreover, the demonstration of an increased, rather than lowered, plasma volume[127,128,146] does not support the hypothesis that these lower blood pressures are related to volume loss. Altered systemic vasoreactivity also has been postulated, but with limited study. One study demonstrating decreased forearm vascular resistance that does not increase with cold-induced, sympathetic-mediated stimulation or angiotensin II suggests altered vascular reactivity protects patients from hypertension.[146]

CLINICAL MANIFESTATIONS

Hematuria

In 1948, Abel and Brown were the first to discover a relationship between sickle cell disease and hematuria.[156] They described a young black soldier who underwent nephrectomy because of severe and persistent unilateral hematuria. A renal neoplasm was suspected, but histopathology of the excised kidney demonstrated only sickled red blood cells in medullary vessels.

Hematuria is a very dramatic manifestation of sickle cell nephropathy. Gross hematuria in affected patients can occur at any age, including young children, and may be more common in males than in females.

The pathologic abnormalities causing hematuria have not yet been elucidated. Kimmelsteil[157] describes the changes as temporary capillary stasis after spasm. As a consequence, plugging of capillaries by sickled cells results in vessel wall injury and, rarely, in true capillary thrombi with ischemia and necrosis. In a study of 21 kidneys from Hb-SS patients removed due to massive blood loss and possible renal neoplasm,[53] the absence of significant gross alterations emphasize that these lesions are inconspicuous and may be easily missed. The most striking change noted was severe stasis in peritubular capillaries in the cortex and most markedly in the medulla. Extravasation of blood, mainly into the collecting tubules, was also observed. Hb-SS erythrocytes traversing the hyperosmotic inner renal medulla have been shown to undergo instant sickling resulting from an increase in intracellular hemoglobin concentration.[158] Moreover, the acidic and hypoxic environment of the renal medulla promotes sickling and red cell adhesion in the vasa recta. Vasoocclusion and increased blood viscosity may result in microthrombi, ischemia, oxidative/reperfusion injury, and/or necrosis, which could cause structural changes leading to hematuria.

Hematuria is generally unilateral in 90% of cases, and interestingly involves the left kidney four times more often than the right kidney. Increased pressure in the left renal vein due to its length and course between the aorta and superior mesenteric artery[159] may explain this observation.

In almost half of all such patients with gross hematuria, blood clots produce filling defects by intravenous urography in the renal pelvis that may be confused with neoplasm, calculus, or hemangioma. Such findings have led to unnecessary nephrectomy in the past. Computed tomography (CT) can generally exclude the presence of a renal neoplasm.[160]Although hematuria can be massive and life threatening, the treatments of choice are conservative measures including bed rest, urinary alkalinization, and maintenance of high urine flow rates. Intravenous triglycyl vasopressin has been successful in two cases of persistent hematuria.[157,161] Epsilon aminocaproic acid (EACA) may have a therapeutic effect in the control of hematuria associated with hemoglobinopathies.[162] Complete inhibition of fibrinolytic activity normally occurs with 8 g of EACA daily. Urinary levels of EACA reach 50 to 100 times those of plasma. With repeated oral dosage, gradual sustained renal excretion occurs so that adequate urinary levels are maintained. The reported results of EACA for hematuria of sickle cell nephropathy have been successful, although therapeutic regimens have varied in dose and frequency.[162–165] Thrombotic complications may occur in patients receiving large doses of EACA, usually in excess of 12 g per day. Control of hemorrhage often can be obtained with doses as low as 2 or 3 g per day.[165] Therefore, EACA should be administered on a short-term basis at the lowest dosage required to inhibit urinary fibrinolytic activity. Surgical intervention (i.e., nephrectomy) should be considered in the presence of life-threatening hemorrhage that does not improve with conservative therapy. If bleeding can be localized to a distinct part of the kidney, one should consider embolization. Other causes of hematuria should also be considered, including mild bleeding disorders (e.g., von Willebrand disease), other forms of kidney disease such as polycystic kidney disease, and renal medullary carcinoma.

Urinary Tract Infections

In a review of 321 children with sickle cell disease, 7% have had urinary tract infections, 60% of which were associated with a febrile illness.[166] The incidence of asymptomatic bacteriuria during pregnancy and the puerperium appears to be twofold higher in women with sickle cell disease or sickle cell trait than in nonpregnant women or women without sickle cell disease or trait.[167] The rate of pyelonephritis is approximately 1%, similar to that in non–sickle cell pregnant populations.[168] An increased incidence of "pyelonephritis" found at autopsy in Hb-AS patients[169] may reflect the pathologic changes due to Hb-S nephropathy (medullary ischemia and fibrosis). Pyelonephritis or urosepsis, like other infections, may precipitate a crisis. Most episodes of gram-negative sepsis in sickle cell patients are due to urinary tract infections.[170] Patients with painful crises should be evaluated for infection, including the urinary tract.

Papillary Necrosis and Caliectasis

Renal papillary necrosis and caliectasis are frequent occurrences in sickle cell disease, in both homozygotes and heterozygotes. Renal papillary necrosis in sickle cell nephropathy has an incidence ranging from 15% to 36%.[55] As in sickle cell nephropathy, the distinctive abnormalities of the renal medulla and papillae are obliteration of the vasa recta and medullary necrosis and fibrosis; papillary necrosis is a logical consequence of these processes.[54]

Gross, painless hematuria[171] is a common symptom reported. Renal colic from passage of blood clots or ruptured particles of necrotic papillae is less frequent. Intravenous pyelography is the method of choice to diagnose papillary necrosis.[54,171] Most commonly a medullary type of partial papillary necrosis is found, appearing as cavitation within one or more of renal papillae (SS). Multiphasic helical CT may permit early detection of medullary and papillary necrosis and allows visualization of the entire kidney, facilitating the identification of other conditions.[160] Treatment is supportive and similar to the management of hematuria. Ureteral obstruction by thrombus or necrotic material should be relieved by stenting if required.[171] Renal papillary necrosis has not been associated with an increased risk of renal failure.[87]

Microalbuminuria, Proteinuria, and the Nephrotic Syndrome

As in other disease states, microalbuminuria may indicate early glomerular injury and renal dysfunction. Although most often attributed to hyperfiltration, early permselectivity pore defects may occur in glomerular capillaries.[172,173] As assessed by urine albumin/creatinine ratio (U Alb/Cr), the prevalence of microalbuminuria increases with age and is uncommon before age 7, but is present in up to 20% to 40% of children between ages 10 and 18.[174,175] The presence and amount of albuminuria correlates with age and hemoglobin levels, but not consistently with other clinical manifestations of sickle cell disease, such as pain or other acute sickling events,[175] although one recent study demonstrated a correlation with pulmonary hypertension.[35] The prevalence of microalbuminuria in adolescents and young adults with sickle cell disease ranges from 9% to 40%, depending on the type of sickle cell disease.[176,177] In one study of 72 adult sickle cell disease patients estimates of urinary albumin excretion found using a spot U Alb/Cr to be highly variable and inconsistently correlated with 12-hour urine samples to quantitate albumin excretion.[178] Furthermore, the spot U Alb/Cr did not demonstrate the reduction in albumin excretion achieved by ACE inhibitor therapy, which was detected using 12-hour collections.[178]

Reduction in microalbuminuria with ACE inhibitor therapy has been demonstrated. In eight adult sickle cell patients treated with enalapril over 120 days, albuminuria normalized or was markedly reduced without changes in sodium, potassium, or lithium excretion or in mean arterial blood pressure.[179] Two years after stopping enalapril, four of six patients still had normal albumin excretion. A placebo-controlled randomized trial of captopril in 22 adult sickle cell patients demonstrated a mean 37% reduction in albumin excretion with captopril over placebo after 6 months of therapy,[180] and was associated with a 5 mm Hg drop in diastolic blood pressure in the treatment group. To date, no long-term trial data exist to demonstrate whether ACE inhibitor therapy reduces prevalence or progression of chronic renal disease in sickle cell patients.

Overt proteinuria is a frequent finding in sickle cell disease, occurring in about 30% of patients when observed over a prolonged period. Nephrotic range proteinuria has been reported in children and adults with sickle cell disease,[181,182] although its prevalence is not well studied. From a review of 386 patients with sickle cell anemia,[183] 78 patients (20.4%) had proteinuria and 17 (4.6%) had renal insufficiency. Both renal insufficiency and proteinuria increased with age, reaching rates of 33% and 56%, respectively, in patients 40 years and older. In some series, proteinuria occurs in 40% of patients with sickle nephropathy[184] and is associated with progression to chronic renal failure and early mortality.[87,113,184,185]

Falk et al. investigated 381 patients with sickle cell disease for proteinuria and renal insufficiency.[113] Twenty-six (7%) had serum creatinine concentrations above the normal range and 101 (26%) had proteinuria of at least 1+ by urinalysis. Among 44 patients with a complete 24-hour urine collection, protein excretion ranged from 28 mg per 24 hours to 10.8 g per 24 hours, with a mean of 1.7 g per 24 hours and SD of ±2.4 g. Twelve patients excreted more than 2.5 g of protein per 24 hours, associated with other features of the nephrotic syndrome. In 10 biopsied patients with proteinuria, administration of enalapril decreased 24-hour urinary protein excretion by 57% (range 23% to 79%), which then increased to 25% below baseline after discontinuation of enalapril. No significant change in GFR, ERPF, filtration fraction, or decrease in arterial pressure occurred. Other causes of proteinuria and nephrotic syndrome should be considered including primary and secondary renal diseases before one assumes sickle cell nephropathy is present.

Postinfectious and membranoproliferative glomerulonephritis[61,186–190] are among the more common case reports. Whether a mechanism specific to sickle cell anemia is responsible for the glomerular diseases or whether these result from the increased susceptibility to encapsulated bacterial organisms remains unclear.

Nephrotic syndrome, rather than just proteinuria, has been described among individuals with sickle cell disease. The causes of nephrotic syndrome have been varied, and include focal segmental glomerular sclerosis,[113,177,191] and mesangioproliferative glomerulonephritis (and is usually associated with albuminuria). Mechanistic theories for these lesions include iron deposition,[192] mesangial phagocytosis of fragmented and sickled red cells,[58,185] hyperfiltration,[191] or infection with parvovirus B19.[193,194]

Acute Renal Failure

Despite the underlying functional and structural changes in the kidney, reports of acute renal failure in sickle cell disease are rare. Some reports describe reversible acute oliguric renal failure in the setting of sickle cell crisis.[195,196] In both studies rhabdomyolysis was suggested to be the cause of acute renal failure. In another study of 12 sickle cell patients with acute renal failure, volume depletion in the setting of crisis was the most common cause.[183] Of the 12 patients, 10 survived and had recovery of renal function.

A syndrome of acute multiorgan failure has been described in 14 sickle cell patients (10 Hb-SS, 4 Hb-SC) occurring during an unusually severe sickle cell crisis event.[197] At least two of three organs (lung, liver, or kidney) demonstrated acute injury. Acute renal insufficiency developed in 13 episodes, with a rapid, reversible elevation of serum creatinine concentration above 2.0 mg per dL over 24 to 36 hours. Acute liver abnormalities and pulmonary infiltrates were observed. All but one patient recovered after treatment with multiple blood transfusions.

RENAL MEDULLARY CARCINOMA

Renal medullary carcinoma is a rare tumor that occurs among individuals with sickle hemoglobinopathy. The vast majority of individuals with the tumor have been shown to have sickle trait rather than homozygous sickle hemoglobin. To date, there are about 137 cases reported in the literature.[198,199]

The pathogenesis of renal medullary carcinoma is not known. Like much of the morbidity associated with sickle disease, the pathogenesis is felt to be medullary ischemia. One study with a small number of patients demonstrated an amplification of the known oncogene, ABL.[200] Structurally, the tumors are believed to arise in the renal medulla, possibly from the renal papillae.[198] They grow rapidly in an infiltrative pattern into the renal sinus. Histologically, renal medullary carcinoma has glandular and squamoid features along with inflammatory and desmoplastic elements, findings that suggest origination from transitional epithelium.

The typical age of presentation is among individuals less than 40 years of age. Diagnosis of the tumor is difficult as it is rapidly growing and has a nonspecific presentation. Renal medullary carcinoma is often found unexpectedly during evaluation of hematuria. The tumor often has grown extensively in the kidney, and has produced local nodal metastases. Diagnosis is made by biopsy and histologic examination. Treatment options such as chemotherapy or surgery are limited because of the advanced stage of presentation.

TREATMENT

General treatment of sickle cell anemia has focused on the use of antibiotic prophylaxis in childhood and support of management of acute vasoocclusive crises. Hydroxyurea has been used as well in patients to induce hemoglobin F (fetal hemoglobin) and reduce the overall percentage of hemoglobin S and subsequently sickling episodes. Bone marrow transplantation in severe cases may provide more definitive therapy. Specific therapies related to renal manifestations of sickle cell disease are discussed in the following text.

Chronic Kidney Disease

Intervention for proteinuria has been the most well-studied intervention for CKD associated with sickle cell disease. The previously described series by Falk et al. demonstrated a reduction in proteinuria by approximately 60% with the use of ACE inhibitors.[113] Subsequent data have reiterated this effect of ACE inhibitors. Present management of renal disease in sickle cell disease primarily involves screening for the development of macroalbuminuria (≥300 mg per day of urinary albumin excretion) as the earliest manifestation of chronic kidney disease. Once detected blockade of the renin-angiotensin-aldosterone systems (RAAS) via ACE inhibitors or angiotensin receptor blockers (ARBs) should be initiated. Hydroxyurea, used commonly for other manifestations of sickle cell disease as above, may also play a role in the management of proteinuria. A small case series of pediatric patients had demonstrated that the addition of hydroxyurea to patients with proteinuria already on ACE inhibitor therapy led to further reductions in proteinuria.[12,201] Another small study involving nine patients with microalbuminuria who were treated with hydroxyurea for other indications demonstrated resolution in four patients. Furthermore those without microalbuminuria who were treated with hydroxyurea failed to develop proteinuria in follow-up.[202,203] A recent report from the BABY HUG cohort,[204] a study of infants with sickle cell disease evaluating use of hydroxyurea in infancy, failed to demonstrate a difference in the increase in GFR between the treatment and placebo groups.[68,203] However, the very young age of the group at enrollment (9 to 19 months) with only 2 years of follow-up may have precluded the investigators' ability to predict longer term effects of hydroxyurea on eGFR. However, the optimal use of this agent in management of sickle cell renal disease remains to be determined.

Concomitant hypertension is predictive of progressive loss of renal function, and is therefore a target for intervention. With management of hypertension, further progression of disease may be allayed.[205] Apart from the use of RAAS blockade for proteinuria, no other specific antihypertensive therapy has been indicated. Some have advocated for the avoidance of diuretics as they may exacerbate the tendency for dehydration.[205]

End-Stage Renal Disease

As a whole, patients with sickle cell disease represent less than 1% of the total ESRD population in the United States.[86] Either peritoneal or hemodialysis present viable options although these patients are more likely to choose hemodialysis.[184] Management of these patients while receiving dialysis is similar to that of others with the exception of the use of erythropoietin-stimulating agents (ESAs). These agents should be reserved only for those with profound anemia, and sickle cell disease patients should not be assigned to the same hemoglobin targets as other ESRD patients. Unfortunately, little data and no consensus exist to further guide ESA dosing although many suggest hemoglobin goals should not exceed 10 mg per dL. Sickle cell disease patients receiving dialysis in early reports were suggested to have a 2-year mortality of 60% although a more recent series has suggested mortality up to 40% in the first year alone.[86] Additionally, McClellan et al. also demonstrated that sickle cell disease patients were more likely to have disparities in care when entering dialysis. More sickle cell disease patients are likely to have had prior stroke and heart failure at the time of dialysis initiation. Importantly, a trend to less arteriovenous fistula use and less pre-dialysis nephrology care was seen.[86] These disparities in entry care may represent later than needed nephrology referral and may be a point of intervention to improve care.

Renal Transplantation

Renal transplant is also a viable option of renal replacement therapy for those with sickle cell disease. Unique complications at the time of transplantation do exist including allograft vein thrombosis and recurrent sickle cell crises.[206]

The use of hydroxyurea and exchange transfusion has been explored at the time of transplantation to prevent these complications. Sickle cell disease transplant patients do not fare as well as African Americans in the general transplant population, with 67% surviving for 7 years following transplantation (compared to 83%). However, allograft transplantation is still preferable, with 56% surviving at 10 years compared to only 14% on dialysis.[206] Recurrence of sickle cell nephropathy has been reported as early as 3.5 years following transplantation.[206,207] Simultaneous bone marrow transplantation may be explored in the future as an included measure to "cure" sickle cell disease.[206]

SICKLE CELL TRAIT

Although sickle cell trait (SCT; i.e., heterozygous inheritance of the HbS mutation) has generally been regarded as a benign carrier state, renal abnormalities are perhaps the best-acknowledged complications of SCT. The renal medulla presents an ideal environment to promote dehydration and sickling of erythrocytes containing hemoglobin S. As a result, some of the same features seen in sickle cell disease present among carriers of the disease, although perhaps as less severe manifestations.

Hematuria is thought to be the most common manifestation of SCT, having first been reported more than 50 years ago.[208] From a large Veterans Administration series, hematuria was the reason for hospitalization in 4% of African American patients with SCT, nearly twice the rate of those with normal hemoglobin phenotypes.[209] The true prevalence of hematuria among the general population of those with sickle cell trait remains undetermined. Bleeding, typically painless, may present as either microscopic or gross hematuria and can occur with or without frank renal papillary necrosis. The left kidney is involved more commonly due to its slightly larger size and its higher venous pressure due to compression of the left renal vein by the aorta and superior mesenteric vein.[210,211] As with sickle cell disease, bedrest and aggressive hydration is usually all that is needed to manage urinary bleeding. In cases that remain refractory to conservative management, use of desmopressin or epsilon aminocaproic acid (EACA), and even invasive intervention via ureteroscopy and angiography, have been advocated.

Impaired urinary concentration is also a common occurring characteristic of those with SCT and likely results from the same vascular abnormalities that cause hematuria via ischemia and microinfarction. Microradiographs performed at autopsy in those with SCT demonstrate reduction in the number of vasa recta and disruption of the remaining medullary vascular architecture.[32] While these changes are not as severe as those seen in sickle cell disease, they likely account in part for the observed impairment of urinary concentration in patients with SCT.[32] Furthermore, this loss of maximal concentration capacity is thought to predispose these patients to dehydration, which is thought to play a role in the higher rates of rhabdomyolysis and sudden death related to extreme exercise observed in SCT.[212–215]

Urinary concentration has also been found to be variable among subjects with SCT, and relates to the percentage of hemoglobin S expressed as determined by the coinheritance of the α-globin gene deletion(s).[216] In one series of SCT individuals, maximal achievable concentration of urine following administration of intranasal desmopressin acetate ranged between 530 and 845 mOsm. The range observed correlated inversely with the number of α-globin gene deletions.[98] With two α-globin gene deletions, HbS concentration averaged 29% of total hemoglobin expressed and urine concentration was only moderately reduced. In those with no α-globin gene deletions, mean HbS concentration was 42% and impairment of urinary concentration was highest.

With the various structural and functional abnormalities noted to occur in the kidney, some have posited that SCT may represent a risk factor for CKD.[217–219] Microalbuminuria, thought to be a marker of early renal injury, has been reported by some to be more common in those with SCT, particularly among diabetic men.[73,220] Other studies in diabetics, however, have shown no association.[221,222] In the ESRD population, SCT has been reported more commonly among African American patients with polycystic kidney disease (PCKD), and those with SCT and PCKD appear to progress more quickly to ESRD and perhaps have more frequent bleeding episodes.[223–225] A recent study utilizing systematic screening of African American ESRD patients demonstrated a twofold prevalence of SCT, as identified by hemoglobin phenotyping, compared to that of the background population.[217] In contradistinction, analysis of genotyping results of African American ESRD patients recruited into a large genetic cohort study with both diabetic and nondiabetic nephropathy failed to demonstrate a similar association.[226] Yet the data remain preliminary in nature and the potential role of sickle trait in CKD needs further investigation. These studies, furthermore, have not addressed the potential contribution of SCT to progression of established CKD.

The presence of sickle trait may also affect the comorbidity associated with ESRD. One study has demonstrated SCT patients on hemodialysis may be more likely to receive higher doses of ESAs, although again, the data for this is relatively preliminary.[227] Additionally, other potential morbidities associated with SCT, such as venous thromboembolism,[228,229] may have particular importance in the ESRD population.

Presently the association between SCT and CKD remains speculative, albeit biologically plausible, and warrants further evaluation via larger, prospective studies. Furthermore, no data exist as to whether detection of SCT in early CKD would allow meaningful intervention to modify disease progression (i.e., RAAS blockade). Although the effect size at an individual level may be modest or only contributory to renal disease, due to its relative commonality (7%–9% among African Americans in the United States), the population effect could be relatively large.

REFERENCES

1. Lebby R. Case of the absence of the spleen. *Southern J. Med. Pharm.* 1846;1: 481–483.

2. Hodenpyl E. A case of apparent absence of the spleen, with general compensatory lymphatic hyperplasia. *Med Record.* 1898;54:695–698.

3. Herrick J. Peculiar elongated and sickle shaped red blood corpuscles in a case of severe anemia. *Arch Intern Med.* 1910;6:517.

4. Savitt TL, Goldberg MF. Herrick's 1910 case report of sickle cell anemia. The rest of the story. *JAMA.* 1989;261(2):266–271.

5. Emmel VE. A study of the erythrocytes in a case of severe anemia with elongated and sickle-shaped cells. *Arch Intern Med.* 1917;20:586–598.

6. Cook JE, Meyer, J. Severe anemia with remarkable elongated and sickle-shaped red blood cells and chronic leg ulcer. *Arch Intern Med.* 1915;16:644–651.

7. Pauling L, Itano HA, et al. Sickle cell anemia a molecular disease. *Science.* 1949;110(2865):543–548.

8. Ingram VM. Abnormal human haemoglobins. I. The comparison of normal human and sickle-cell haemoglobins by fingerprinting. *Biochim Biophys Acta.* 1958;28(3):539–545.

9. Ingram VM. Gene mutations in human haemoglobin: the chemical difference between normal and sickle cell haemoglobin. *Nature.* 1957;180(4581): 326–328.

10. Ingram VM. A specific chemical difference between the globins of normal human and sickle-cell anaemia haemoglobin. *Nature.* 1956;178(4537):792–794.

11. Hunt JA, Ingram VM. Allelomorphism and the chemical differences of the human haemoglobins A, S and C. *Nature.* 1958;181(4615):1062–1063.

12. Rees DC, Williams TN, Gladwin MT. Sickle-cell disease. *Lancet.* 2010;376(9757):2018–2031.

13. Powars DR, Meiselman HJ, Fisher TC, et al. Beta-S gene cluster haplotypes modulate hematologic and hemorheologic expression in sickle cell anemia. Use in predicting clinical severity. *Am J Pediatr Hematol Oncol.* 1994;16(1):55–61.

14. Modell B, Darlison M. Global epidemiology of haemoglobin disorders and derived service indicators. *Bull World Health Organ.* 2008;86(6):480–487.

15. Vekilov PG. Sickle-cell haemoglobin polymerization: is it the primary pathogenic event of sickle-cell anaemia? *Br J Haematol.* 2007;139(2):173–184.

16. Eaton WA, Hofrichter J. Hemoglobin S gelation and sickle cell disease. *Blood.* 1987;70(5):1245–1266.

17. Platt OS. *Sickle Cell Disease: Basic Principles and Clinical Practice.* New York: Raven Press; 1994.

18. Bunn HF. Pathogenesis and treatment of sickle cell disease. *N Engl J Med.* 1997;337(11):762–769.

19. Harlan JM. Introduction: anti-adhesion therapy in sickle cell disease. *Blood.* 2000;95(2):365–367.

20. Barabino GA, Wise RJ, Woodbury VA, et al. Inhibition of sickle erythrocyte adhesion to immobilized thrombospondin by von Willebrand factor under dynamic flow conditions. *Blood.* 1997;89(7):2560–2567.

21. Hebbel RP. Perspectives series: cell adhesion in vascular biology. Adhesive interactions of sickle erythrocytes with endothelium. *J Clin Invest.* 1997; 99(11):2561–2564.

22. Hebbel RP, Boogaerts MA, Eaton JW, Steinberg MH. Erythrocyte adherence to endothelium in sickle-cell anemia. A possible determinant of disease severity. *N Engl J Med.* 1980;302(18):992–995.

23. Nath KA, Grande JP, Haggard JJ, et al. Oxidative stress and induction of heme oxygenase-1 in the kidney in sickle cell disease. *Am J Pathol.* 2001;158(3):893–903.

24. Hahn EV, Gillespie, EB. Sickle cell anemia. Report of a case greatly improved by splenectomy. Experimental study of sickle cell formation. *Arch Intern Med.* 1927;39:233–254.

25. Lange RD, Minnich V, Moore CV. Effect of oxygen tension and of pH on the sickling and mechanical fragility of erythrocytes from patients with sickle cell anemia and the sickle cell trait. *J Lab Clin Med.* 1951;37(5):789–802.

26. Allison AC. Observations on the sickling phenomenon and on the distribution of different haemoglobin types in erythrocyte populations. *Clin Sci (Lond).* 1956;15(4):497–510.

27. Sydenstricker VP, Mulherin WA, Houseal R. W. Sickle cell anemia. Report of two cases in children, with necropsy in one case. *Am J Dis Child.* 1923;26: 132–154.

28. Diggs LW, Bibb J. The erythrocyte in sickle cell anemia. Morphology, size, hemoglobin content, fragility and sedimentation rate. *JAMA.* 1939;112:695–701.

29. Itoh T, Chien S, Usami S. Effects of hemoglobin concentration on deformability of individual sickle cells after deoxygenation. *Blood.* 1995;85(8): 2245–2253.

30. Brezis M, Rosen S. Hypoxia of the renal medulla—its implications for disease. *N Engl J Med.* 1995;332(10):647–655.

31. Noguchi CT, Torchia DA, Schechter AN. Polymerization of hemoglobin in sickle trait erythrocytes and lysates. *J Biol Chem.* 1981;256(9):4168–4171.

32. Statius van Eps LW, Pinedo-Veels C, de Vries GH, de Koning J. Nature of concentrating defect in sickle-cell nephropathy. Microradioangiographic studies. *Lancet.* 1970;1(7644):450–452.

33. Juncos JP, Grande JP, Croatt AJ, et al. Early and prominent alterations in hemodynamics, signaling, and gene expression following renal ischemia in sickle cell disease. *Am J Physiol Renal Physiol.* 2010;298(4):F892–899.

34. Nath KA, Grande JP, Croatt AJ, et al. Transgenic sickle mice are markedly sensitive to renal ischemia-reperfusion injury. *Am J Pathol.* 2005;166(4): 963–972.

35. Ataga KI, Brittain JE, Moore D, et al. Urinary albumin excretion is associated with pulmonary hypertension in sickle cell disease: potential role of soluble fms-like tyrosine kinase-1. *Eur J Haematol.* 2010;85(3):257–263.

36. Nolan VG, Ma Q, Cohen HT, et al. Estimated glomerular filtration rate in sickle cell anemia is associated with polymorphisms of bone morphogenetic protein receptor 1B. *Am J Hematol.* 2007;82(3):179–184.

37. Baldwin C, Nolan VG, Wyszynski DF, et al. Association of klotho, bone morphogenetic protein 6, and annexin A2 polymorphisms with sickle cell osteonecrosis. *Blood.* 2005;106(1):372–375.

38. Nolan VG, Adewoye A, Baldwin C, et al. Sickle cell leg ulcers: associations with haemolysis and SNPs in Klotho, TEK and genes of the TGF-beta/BMP pathway. *Br J Haematol.* 2006;133(5):570–578.

39. Sebastiani P, Ramoni MF, Nolan V, Baldwin CT, Steinberg MH. Genetic dissection and prognostic modeling of overt stroke in sickle cell anemia. *Nat Genet.* 2005;37(4):435–440.

40. Chen S, Jim B, Ziyadeh FN. Diabetic nephropathy and transforming growth factor-beta: transforming our view of glomerulosclerosis and fibrosis build-up. *Semin Nephrol.* 2003;23(6):532–543.

41. Nicholas SB. Advances in pathogenetic mechanisms of diabetic nephropathy. *Cell Mol Biol (Noisy-le-grand).* 2003;49(8):1319–1325.

42. Ziyadeh FN. Mediators of diabetic renal disease: the case for tgf-Beta as the major mediator. *J Am Soc Nephrol.* 2004;15 Suppl 1:S55–57.

43. Sebastiani P, Solovieff N, Hartley SW, et al. Genetic modifiers of the severity of sickle cell anemia identified through a genome-wide association study. *Am J Hematol.* 2010;85(1):29–35.

44. Coppoletta JM, Wolbach SB. Body length and organ weights of infants and children: a study of the body length and normal weights of the more important vital organs of the body between birth and twelve years of age. *Am J Pathol.* 1933;9(1):55–70.

45. Walker TM, Beardsall K, Thomas PW, et al. Renal length in sickle cell disease: observations from a cohort study. *Clin Nephrol.* 1996;46(6):384–388.

46. Morgan AG, Shah DJ, Williams W. Renal pathology in adults over 40 with sickle-cell disease. *West Indian Med J.* 1987;36(4):241–250.

47. McCall IW, Moule N, Desai P, et al. Urographic findings in homozygous sickle cell disease. *Radiology.* 1978;126(1):99–104.

48. Pandya KK, Koshy M, Brown N, et al. Renal papillary necrosis in sickle cell hemoglobinopathies. *J Urol.* 1976;115(5):497–501.

49. Minkin SD, Oh KS, Sanders RC, et al. Urologic manifestations of sickle hemoglobinopathies. *South Med J.* 1979;72(1):23–28.

50. Odita JC, Ugbodaga CI, Okafor LA, et al. Urographic changes in homozygous sickle cell disease. *Diagn Imaging.* 1983;52(5):259–263.

51. Zinn D, Haller JO, Cohen HL. Focal and diffuse increased echogenicity in the renal parenchyma in patients with sickle hemoglobinopathies—an observation. *J Ultrasound Med.* 1993;12(4):211–214.

52. Walker TM, Serjeant GR. Increased renal reflectivity in sickle cell disease: prevalence and characteristics. *Clin Radiol.* 1995;50(8):566–569.

53. Mostofi FK, Vorder Bruegge CF, Diggs LW. Lesions in kidneys removed for unilateral hematuria in sickle-cell disease. *AMA Arch Pathol.* 1957;63(4):336–351.

54. Harrow BR, Sloane JA, Liebman NC. Roentgenologic demonstration of renal papillary necrosis in sickle-cell trait. *N Engl J Med.* 1963;268:969–976.

55. Vaamonde CA. Renal papillary necrosis in sickle cell hemoglobinopathies. *Semin Nephrol.* 1984;4:48–64.

56. Yater WM, Mollari M. The pathology of sickle-cell anemia. *JAMA.* 1931; 96(20):1671–1675.

57. Bernstein J, Whitten CF. A histologic appraisal of the kidney in sickle cell anemia. *Arch Pathol.* 1960;70:407–418.

58. Elfenbein IB, Patchefsky A, Schwartz W, et al. Pathology of the glomerulus in sickle cell anemia with and without nephrotic syndrome. *Am J Pathol.* 1974;77(3):357–374.

59. Buckalew VM Jr, Someren A. Renal manifestations of sickle cell disease. *Arch Intern Med.* 1974;133(4):660–669.

60. Walker BR, Alexander F, Birdsall TR, et al. Glomerular lesions in sickle cell nephropathy. *JAMA.* 1971;215(3):437–440.

61. Pitcock JA, Muirhead EE, Hatch FE, et al. Early renal changes in sickle cell anemia. *Arch Pathol.* 1970;90(5):403–410.
62. Walker BR, Alexander F. Uric acid excretion in sickle cell anemia. *JAMA.* 1971;215(2):255–258.
63. Lande IM, Glazer GM, Sarnaik S, et al. Sickle-cell nephropathy: MR imaging. *Radiology.* 1986;158(2):379–383.
64. Statius van Eps LW, Schouten H, La Porte-Wijsman LW, et al. The influence of red blood cell transfusions on the hyposthenuria and renal hemodynamics of sickle cell anemia. *Clin Chim Acta.* 1967;17(3):449–461.
65. Etteldorf JN, Smith JD, Tuttle AH, et al. Renal hemodynamic studies in adults with sickle cell anemia. *Am J Med.* 1955;18(2):243–248.
66. de Jong PE, Statius van Eps LW. Sickle cell nephropathy: new insights into its pathophysiology. *Kidney Int.* 1985;27(5):711–717.
67. Ware RE, Rees RC, Sarnaik SA, et al. Renal function in infants with sickle cell anemia: baseline data from the BABY HUG trial. *J Pediatr.* 2010;156(1): 66–70 e61.
68. Wang WC, Ware RE, Miller ST, et al. Hydroxycarbamide in very young children with sickle-cell anaemia: a multicentre, randomised, controlled trial (BABY HUG). *Lancet.* 2011;377(9778):1663–1672.
69. de Jong PE, de Jong-Van Den Berg TW, Sewrajsingh GS, et al. The influence of indomethacin on renal haemodynamics in sickle cell anaemia. *Clin Sci (Lond).* 1980;59(4):245–250.
70. Hollenberg NK, Adams DF. Hypertension and intrarenal perfusion patterns in man. *Am J Med Sci.* 1971;261(5):232–239.
71. Horster M', Thurau K. Micropuncture studies on the filtration rate of single superficial and juxtamedullary glomeruli in the rat kidney. *Pflugers Arch Gesamte Physiol Menschen Tiere.* 1968;301(2):162–181.
72. Statius van Eps LW, Schouten H, Haar Romeny-Wachter CC, et al. The relation between age and renal concentrating capacity in sickle cell disease and hemoglobin C disease. *Clin Chim Acta.* 1970;27(3):501–511.
73. Sesso R, Almeida MA, Figueiredo MS, et al. Renal dysfunction in patients with sickle cell anemia or sickle cell trait. *Braz J Med Biol Res.* 1998;31(10): 1257–1262.
74. Itano HA, Keitel HG, Thompson D. Hyposthenuria in sickle cell anemia: a reversible renal defect. *J Clin Invest.* 1956;35(9):998–1007.
75. Rybicki AC, Fabry ME, Does MD, et al. Differential gene expression in the kidney of sickle cell transgenic mice: upregulated genes. *Blood Cells Mol Dis.* 2003;31(3):370–380.
76. Bank N, Aynedjian HS, Qiu JH, et al. Renal nitric oxide synthases in transgenic sickle cell mice. *Kidney Int.* 1996;50(1):184–189.
77. Allon M, Lawson L, Eckman JR, et al. Effects of nonsteroidal antiinflammatory drugs on renal function in sickle cell anemia. *Kidney Int.* 1988;34(4):500–506.
78. Hostetter TH, Olson JL, Rennke HG, et al. Hyperfiltration in remnant nephrons: a potentially adverse response to renal ablation. *Am J Physiol.* 1981; 241(1):F85–93.
79. Osarogiagbon UR, Choong S, Belcher JD, et al. Reperfusion injury pathophysiology in sickle transgenic mice. *Blood.* 2000;96(1):314–320.
80. Bank N, Kiroycheva M, Ahmed F, et al. Peroxynitrite formation and apoptosis in transgenic sickle cell mouse kidneys. *Kidney Int.* 1998;54(5):1520–1528.
81. Kiroycheva M, Ahmed F, Anthony GM, et al. Mitogen-activated protein kinase phosphorylation in kidneys of beta(s) sickle cell mice. *J Am Soc Nephrol.* 2000;11(6):1026–1032.
82. Levin WC, Gregory R, Bennett A. The effect of chronic anemia on renal function as measured by inulin and diodrast clearances. *Proc Annu Meet Cent Soc Clin Res U S.* 1947;20:42.
83. Platt OS, Brambilla DJ, Rosse WF, et al. Mortality in sickle cell disease. Life expectancy and risk factors for early death. *N Engl J Med.* 1994;330(23): 1639–1644.
84. Darbari DS, Kple-Faget P, Kwagyan J, et al. Circumstances of death in adult sickle cell disease patients. *Am J Hematol.* 2006;81(11):858–863.
85. System USRD. USRDS 2010 Annual Data Report: Atlas of Chronic Kidney Disease and End-Stage Renal Disease in the United States. *National Institutes of Health, National Institute of Diabetes and Digestive and Kidney Diseases.* Bethesda, MD:2010.
86. McClellan AC, Guasch A, Gilbertson D, McClellan W, et al. Characteristics of Pre-ESRD Care and Early Mortality among Incident ESRD Patients with Sickle Cell Disease (SCD) [abstract]. Presented at the 42nd Annual Meeting of the American Society of Nephrology; 2009 Oct 27–Nov 1; San Diego, CA: ASN; 2009. p 7. F-PO1493.
87. Powars DR, Elliott-Mills DD, Chan L, et al. Chronic renal failure in sickle cell disease: risk factors, clinical course, and mortality. *Ann Intern Med.* 1991; 115(8):614–620.
88. Morgan AG, Serjeant GR. Renal function in patients over 40 with homozygous sickle-cell disease. *Br Med J (Clin Res Ed).* 1981;282(6271):1181–1183.
89. Cockcroft DW, Gault MH. Prediction of creatinine clearance from serum creatinine. *Nephron.* 1976;16(1):31–41.
90. Levey AS, Bosch JP, Lewis JB, et al. A more accurate method to estimate glomerular filtration rate from serum creatinine: a new prediction equation. Modification of Diet in Renal Disease Study Group. *Ann Intern Med.* 1999;130(6):461–470.
91. Levey AS, Stevens LA, Schmid CH, et al. A new equation to estimate glomerular filtration rate. *Ann Intern Med.* 2009;150(9):604–612.
92. Thompson J, Reid M, Hambleton I, et al. Albuminuria and renal function in homozygous sickle cell disease: observations from a cohort study. *Arch Intern Med.* 2007;167(7):701–708.
93. Barros FB, Lima CS, Santos AO, et al. 51Cr-EDTA measurements of the glomerular filtration rate in patients with sickle cell anaemia and minor renal damage. *Nucl Med Commun.* 2006;27(12):959–962.
94. Whitten CF, Younes AA. A comparative study of renal concentrating ability in children with sickle cell anemia and in normal children. *J Lab Clin Med.* 1960;55:400–415.
95. Levitt MF, Hauser AD, Levy MS, et al. The renal concentrating defect in sickle cell disease. *Am J Med.* 1960;29:611–622.
96. Hatch FE, Culbertson JW, Diggs LW. Nature of the renal concentrating defect in sickle cell disease. *J Clin Invest.* 1967;46(3):336–345.
97. Forrester TE, Alleyne GA. Excretion of salt and water by patients with sickle-cell anaemia: effect of a diuretic and solute diuresis. *Clin Sci Mol Med.* 1977;53(6):523–527.
98. Gupta AK, Kirchner KA, Nicholson R, et al. Effects of alpha-thalassemia and sickle polymerization tendency on the urine-concentrating defect of individuals with sickle cell trait. *J Clin Invest.* 1991;88(6):1963–1968.
99. Alleyne GA. The kidney in sickle cell anemia. *Kidney Int.* 1975;7(6):371–379.
100. De Jong PE, De Jong-van den Berg LT, De Zeeuw D, et al. The influence of indomethacin on renal concentrating and diluting capacity in sickle cell nephropathy. *Clin Sci (Lond).* 1982;63(1):53–58.
101. de Jong PE, de Jong-van den Berg LT, Schouten H, et al. The influence of indomethacin on renal acidification in normal subjects and in patients with sickle cell anemia. *Clin Nephrol.* 1983;19(5):259–264.
102. Kong HH, Alleyne GA. Studies on acid excretion in adults with sickle-cell anaemia. *Clin Sci (Lond).* 1971;41(6):505–518.
103. Goossens JP, Statius van Eps LW, Schouten H, et al. Incomplete renal tubular acidosis in sickle cell disease. *Clin Chim Acta.* 1972;41:149–156.
104. Oster JR, Lespier LE, Lee SM, et al. Renal acidification in sickle-cell disease. *J Lab Clin Med.* 1976;88(3):389–401.
105. de Jong PE, Saleh AW, de Zeeuw D, et al. Urinary prostaglandins in sickle cell nephropathy: a defect in 9–ketoreductase activity? *Clin Nephrol.* 1984;22(4):212–213.
106. Buckalew VM Jr, McCurdy DK, Ludwig GD, et al. Incomplete renal tubular acidosis. Physiologic studies in three patients with a defect in lowering urine pH. *Am J Med.* 1968;45(1):32–42.
107. Kong HH, Alleyne GA. Acid-base status of adults with sickle-cell anaemia. *Br Med J (Clin Res Ed).* 1969;3(5665):271–273.
108. Oduntan SA. Blood gas studies in some abnormal haemoglobin syndromes. *Br J Haematol.* 1969;17(6):535–541.
109. Batlle D, Itsarayoungyuen K, Arruda JA, et al. Hyperkalemic hyperchloremic metabolic acidosis in sickle cell hemoglobinopathies. *Am J Med.* 1982;72(2):188–192.
110. DeFronzo RA. Hyperkalemia and hyporeninemic hypoaldosteronism. *Kidney Int.* 1980;17(1):118–134.
111. DeFronzo RA, Taufield PA, Black H, et al. Impaired renal tubular potassium secretion in sickle cell disease. *Ann Intern Med.* 1979;90(3):310–316.
112. Allon M. Renal abnormalities in sickle cell disease. *Arch Intern Med.* 1990;150(3):501–504.
113. Falk RJ, Scheinman J, Phillips G, et al. Prevalence and pathologic features of sickle cell nephropathy and response to inhibition of angiotensin-converting enzyme. *N Engl J Med.* 1992;326(14):910–915.
114. Yoshino M, Amerian R, Brautbar N. Hyporeninemic hypoaldosteronism in sickle cell disease. *Nephron.* 1982;31(3):242–244.
115. Diamond HS, Meisel A, Sharon E, et al. Hyperuricosuria and increased tubular secretion of urate in sickle cell anemia. *Am J Med.* 1975;59(6):796–802.
116. Diamond HS, Meisel AD, Holden D. The natural history of urate overproduction in sickle cell anemia. *Ann Intern Med.* 1979;90(5):752–757.
117. De Ceulaer K, Morgan AG, Choo-Kang E, et al. Serum urate concentrations in homozygous sickle cell disease. *J Clin Pathol.* 1981;34(9):965–969.
118. Ball GV, Sorensen LB. The pathogenesis of hyperuricemia and gout in sickle cell anemia. *Arthritis Rheum.* 1970;13(6):846–848.
119. Leff RD, Aldo-Benson MA, Fife RS. Tophaceous gout in a patient with sickle cell-thalassemia: case report and review of the literature. *Arthritis Rheum.* 1983;26(7):928–929.

120. Rothschild BM, Sienknecht CW, Kaplan SB, et al. Sickle cell disease associated with uric acid deposition disease. *Ann Rheum Dis.* 1980;39(4):392–395.
121. Espinoza LR, Spilberg I, Osterland CK. Joint manifestations of sickle cell disease. *Medicine (Baltimore).* 1974;53(4):295–305.
122. Herrera J, Avila E, Marin C, et al. Impaired creatinine secretion after an intravenous creatinine load is an early characteristic of the nephropathy of sickle cell anaemia. *Nephrol Dial Transplant.* 2002;17(4):602–607.
123. De Jong PE, de Jong-van Den Berg LT, Statius van Eps LW. The tubular reabsorption of phosphate in sickle-cell nephropathy. *Clin Sci Mol Med.* 978;55(5):429–434.
124. Smith EC, Valika KS, Woo JE, et al. Serum phosphate abnormalities in sickle cell anemia. *Proc Soc Exp Biol Med.* 1981;168(2):254–258.
125. Al-Harbi N, Annobil SH, Abbag F, et al. Renal reabsorption of phosphate in children with sickle cell anemia. *Am J Nephrol.* 1999;19(5):552–554.
126. Mohammed S, Addae S, Suleiman S, et al. Serum calcium, parathyroid hormone, and vitamin D status in children and young adults with sickle cell disease. *Ann Clin Biochem.* 1993;30 (Pt 1):45–51.
127. Barreras L, Diggs LW, Lipscomb A. Plasma volume in sickle cell disease. *South Med J.* 1966;59(4):456–458.
128. Wilson WA, Alleyne GA. Total body water, extracellular and plasma volume compartments in sickle cell anemia. *West Indian Med J.* 1976;25(4):241–250.
129. de Jong PE, de Jong-van den Berg LT, Sewrajsingh GS, et al. Beta-2–microglobulin in sickle cell anaemia. Evidence of increased tubular reabsorption. *Nephron.* 1981;29(3–4):138–141.
130. Aparicio SA, Mojiminiyi S, Kay JD, et al. Measurement of glomerular filtration rate in homozygous sickle cell disease: a comparison of 51Cr-EDTA clearance, creatinine clearance, serum creatinine and beta 2 microglobulin. *J Clin Pathol.* 1990;43(5):370–372.
131. Yuzbasiyan-Gurkan VA, Brewer GJ, Vander AJ, et al. Net renal tubular reabsorption of zinc in healthy man and impaired handling in sickle cell anemia. *Am J Hematol.* 1989;31(2):87–90.
132. Serjeant G, Serjeant B, Stephens A, et al. Determinants of haemoglobin level in steady-state homozygous sickle cell disease. *Br J Haematol.* 1996;92(1):143–149.
133. Haddy TB, Lusher JM, Hendricks S, et al. Erythropoiesis in sickle cell anaemia during acute infection and crisis. *Scand J Haematol.* 1979;22(4):289–295.
134. de Klerk G, Rosengarten PC, Vet RJ, et al. Serum erythropoietin (EST) titers in anemia. *Blood.* 1981;58(6):1164–1170.
135. Morgan AG, Gruber CA, Serjeant GR. Erythropoietin and renal function in sickle-cell disease. *Br Med J (Clin Res Ed).* 1982;285(6356):1686–1688.
136. Sherwood JB, Goldwasser E, Chilcote R, et al. Sickle cell anemia patients have low erythropoietin levels for their degree of anemia. *Blood.* 1986;67(1):46–49.
137. Tomson CR, Edmunds ME, Chambers K, et al. Effect of recombinant human erythropoietin on erythropoiesis in homozygous sickle-cell anaemia and renal failure. *Nephrol Dial Transplant.* 1992;7(8):817–821.
138. Steinberg MH. Erythropoietin for anemia of renal failure in sickle cell disease. *N Engl J Med.* 1991;324(19):1369–1370.
139. Roger SD, Macdougall IC, Thuraisingham RC, et al. Erythropoietin in anemia of renal failure in sickle cell disease. *N Engl J Med.* 1991;325(16):1175–1176.
140. Thuraisingham RC, Roger SD, Macdougall IC, et al. Improvement in anaemia following renal transplantation but not after erythropoietin therapy in a patient with sickle-cell disease. *Nephrol Dial Transplant.* 1993;8(4):371–372.
141. Breen CP, Macdougall IC. Improvement of erythropoietin-resistant anaemia after renal transplantation in patients with homozygous sickle-cell disease. *Nephrol Dial Transplant.* 1998;13(11):2949–2952.
142. Papassotiriou I, Voskaridou E, Stamoulakatou A, et al. Increased erythropoietin level induced by hydroxyurea treatment of sickle cell patients. *Hematol J.* 2000;1(5):295–300.
143. Perlingeiro RC, Costa FF, Saad ST, et al. Early circulating erythroid progenitor cells and expression of erythropoietin receptors in sickle cell disease. *Eur J Haematol.* 1998;60(4):226–232.
144. Karayaylali I, Onal M, Yildizer K, et al. Low blood pressure, decreased incidence of hypertension, and renal cardiac, and autonomic nervous system functions in patients with sickle cell syndromes. *Nephron.* 2002;91(3):535–537.
145. Matustik MC, Carpentieri U, Corn C, et al. Hyperreninemia and hyperaldosteronism in sickle cell anemia. *J Pediatr.* 1979;95(2):206–209.
146. Hatch FE, Crowe LR, Miles DE, et al. Altered vascular reactivity in sickle hemoglobinopathy. A possible protective factor from hypertension. *Am J Hypertens.* 1989;2(1):2–8.
147. Sellers BB Jr. Intermittent hypertension during sickle cell crisis. *J Pediatr.* 1978;92(6):941–943.
148. Nissen HM, Andersen H. On the localization of a prostaglandin-dehydrogenase activity in the kidney. *Histochemie.* 1968;14(2):189–200.
149. Zins GR. Renal prostaglandins. *Am J Med.* 1975;58(1):14–24.
150. Levenson DJ, Simmons CE Jr, Brenner BM. Arachidonic acid metabolism, prostaglandins and the kidney. *Am J Med.* 1982;72(2):354–374.
151. Tannenbaum J, Splawinski JA, Oates JA, et al. Enhanced renal prostaglandin production in the dog. I. Effects on renal function. *Circ Res.* 1975;36(1):197–203.
152. ter Maaten JC, Serne EH, van Eps WS, et al. Effects of insulin and atrial natriuretic peptide on renal tubular sodium handling in sickle cell disease. *Am J Physiol Renal Physiol.* 2000;278(3):F499–505.
153. de Jong PE, Landman H, van Eps LW. Blood pressure in sickle cell disease. *Arch Intern Med.* 1982;142(6):1239–1240.
154. Grell GA, Alleyne GA, Serjeant GR. Blood pressure in adults with homozygous sickle cell disease. *Lancet.* 1981;2(8256):1166.
155. Johnson CS, Giorgio AJ. Arterial blood pressure in adults with sickle cell disease. *Arch Intern Med.* 1981;141(7):891–893.
156. Abel MS, Brown CR. Sickle cell disease with severe hematuria simulating renal neoplasm. *JAMA.* 1948;136(9):624.
157. Kimmelsteil P. Vascular occlusion and ischemic infarction in sickle cell disease. *Am J Med Sci.* 1948;216(1):11–19.
158. Perillie PE, Epstein FH. Sickling phenomenon produced by hypertonic solutions: a possible explanation for the hyposthenuria of sicklemia. *J Clin Invest.* 1963;42:570–580.
159. Bruno D, Wigfall DR, Zimmerman SA, et al. Genitourinary complications of sickle cell disease. *J Urol.* 2001;166(3):803–811.
160. Lang EK, Macchia RJ, Thomas R, et al. Multiphasic helical CT diagnosis of early medullary and papillary necrosis. *J Endourol.* 2004;18(1):49–56.
161. John EG, Schade SG, Spigos DG, et al. Effectiveness of triglycyl vasopressin in persistent hematuria associated with sickle cell hemoglobin. *Arch Intern Med.* 1980;140(12):1589–1593.
162. Immergut MA, Stevenson T. The use of epsilon amino caproic acid in the control of hematuria associated with hemoglobinopathies. *J Urol.* 1965;93:110–111.
163. Statius van Eps LW, Leeksma OC. Sickle cell nephropathy and haemostasis. In: Remuzzi G, Rossi EC, eds. *Haemostasis and the Kidney*. London: Butterworth; 1989.
164. Black WD, Hatch FE, Acchiardo S. Aminocaproic acid in prolonged hematuria of patients with sicklemia. *Arch Intern Med.* 1976;136(6):678–681.
165. Deysine M, Cliffton EE. Mechanism of action of epsilon aminocaproic acid in the control of hemorrhage. *Ann N Y Acad Sci.* 1964;115:291–297.
166. Tarry WF, Duckett JW Jr, Snyder HM III. Urological complications of sickle cell disease in a pediatric population. *J Urol.* 1987;138(3):592–594.
167. Whalley PJ, Martin FG, Pritchard JA. Sickle cell trait and urinary tract infection during pregnancy. *JAMA.* 1964;189:903–906.
168. Smith JA, Espeland M, Bellevue R, et al. Pregnancy in sickle cell disease: experience of the Cooperative Study of Sickle Cell Disease. *Obstet Gynecol.* 1996;87(2):199–204.
169. Amin UF, Ragbeer MM. The prevalence of pyelonephritis among sicklers and nonsicklers in an autopsy population. *West Indian Med J.* 1972;21:166.
170. Zarkowsky HS, Gallagher D, Gill FM, et al. Bacteremia in sickle hemoglobinopathies. *J Pediatr.* 1986;109(4):579–585.
171. Molitierno JA, Jr., Carson CC, 3rd. Urologic manifestations of hematologic disease sickle cell, leukemia, and thromboembolic disease. *Urol Clin North Am.* 2003;30(1):49–61.
172. Guasch A, Cua M, Mitch WE. Early detection and the course of glomerular injury in patients with sickle cell anemia. *Kidney Int.* 1996;49(3):786–791.
173. Guasch A, Cua M, You W, et al. Sickle cell anemia causes a distinct pattern of glomerular dysfunction. *Kidney Int.* 1997;51(3):826–833.
174. Dharnidharka VR, Dabbagh S, Atiyeh B, et al. Prevalence of microalbuminuria in children with sickle cell disease. *Pediatr Nephrol.* 1998;12(6):475–478.
175. McBurney PG, Hanevold CD, Hernandez CM, et al. Risk factors for microalbuminuria in children with sickle cell anemia. *J Pediatr Hematol Oncol.* 2002;24(6):473–477.
176. Aoki RY, Saad ST. Microalbuminuria in sickle cell disease. *Braz J Med Biol Res.* 1990;23(11):1103–1106.
177. Abdu A, Emokpae MA, Uadia PO, et al. Proteinuria among adult sickle cell anemia patients in Nigeria. *Ann Afr Med.* 2011;10(1):34–37.
178. Lima CS, Bottini PV, Garlipp CR, et al. Accuracy of the urinary albumin to creatinine ratio as a predictor of albuminuria in adults with sickle cell disease. *J Clin Pathol.* 2002;55(12):973–975.
179. Aoki RY, Saad ST. Enalapril reduces the albuminuria of patients with sickle cell disease. *Am J Med.* 1995;98(5):432–435.
180. Foucan L, Bourhis V, Bangou J, et al. A randomized trial of captopril for microalbuminuria in normotensive adults with sickle cell anemia. *Am J Med.* 1998;104(4):339–342.

181. Berman LB, Tublin I. The nephropathies of sickle-cell disease. *AMA Arch Intern Med.* 1959;103(4):602–606.
182. Sweeney MJ, Dobbins WT, Etteldorf JN. Renal disease with elements of the nephrotic syndrome associated with sickle cell anemia: A report of 2 cases. *J Pediatr.* 1962;60(1):42–51.
183. Sklar AH, Campbell H, Caruana RJ, et al. A population study of renal function in sickle cell anemia. *Int J Artif Organs.* 1990;13(4):231–236.
184. Saborio P, Scheinman JI. Sickle cell nephropathy. *J Am Soc Nephrol.* 1999; 10(1):187–192.
185. Bakir AA, Hathiwala SC, Ainis H, et al. Prognosis of the nephrotic syndrome in sickle glomerulopathy. A retrospective study. *Am J Nephrol.* 1987;7(2):110–115.
186. Susmano S, Lewy JE. Sickle cell disease and acute glomerulonephritis. *Am J Dis Child.* 1969;118(4):615–618.
187. Strauss J, Pardo V, Koss MN, et al. Nephropathy associated with sickle cell anemia: an autologous immune complex nephritis. I. Studies on nature of glomerular-bound antibody and antigen identification in a patient with sickle cell disease and immune deposit glomerulonephritis. *Am J Med.* 1975;58(3):382–387.
188. Roy S, Murphy WM, Pitcock JA, et al. Sickle-cell disease and poststreptococcal acute glomerulonephritis. *Am J Clin Pathol.* 1976;66(6):986–990.
189. Nicholson GD. [Post-streptococcal glomerulonephritis in adult Jamaicans with and without sickle cell anaemia]. *West Indian Med J.* 1977;26(2):78–84.
190. Assar R, Pitel PA, Lammert NL, et al. Acute poststreptococcal glomerulonephritis and sickle cell disease. *Child Nephrol Urol.* 1988;9(3):176–179.
191. Tejani A, Phadke K, Adamson O, et al. Renal lesions in sickle cell nephropathy in children. *Nephron.* 1985;39(4):352–355.
192. McCoy RC. Ultrastructural alterations in the kidney of patients with sickle cell disease and the nephrotic syndrome. *Lab Invest.* 1969;21(2):85–95.
193. Wierenga KJ, Pattison JR, Brink N, et al. Glomerulonephritis after human parvovirus infection in homozygous sickle-cell disease. *Lancet.* 1995;346(8973): 475–476.
194. Tolaymat A, Al Mousily F, MacWilliam K, et al. Parvovirus glomerulonephritis in a patient with sickle cell disease. *Pediatr Nephrol.* 1999;13(4):340–342.
195. Devereux S, Knowles SM. Rhabdomyolysis and acute renal failure in sickle cell anaemia. *Br Med J (Clin Res Ed).* 1985;290(6483):1707.
196. Kelly CJ, Singer I. Acute renal failure in sickle-cell disease. *Am J Kidney Dis.* 1986;8(3):146–150.
197. Hassell KL, Eckman JR, Lane PA. Acute multiorgan failure syndrome: a potentially catastrophic complication of severe sickle cell pain episodes. *Am J Med.* 1994;96(2):155–162.
198. Davis CJ Jr, Mostofi FK, Sesterhenn IA. Renal medullary carcinoma. The seventh sickle cell nephropathy. *Am J Surg Pathol.* 1995;19(1):1–11.
199. Dimashkieh H, Choe J, Mutema G. Renal medullary carcinoma: a report of 2 cases and review of the literature. *Arch Pathol Lab Med.* 2003;127(3):e135–138.
200. Simpson L, He X, Pins M, et al. Renal medullary carcinoma and ABL gene amplification. *J Urol.* 2005;173(6):1883–1888.
201. Fitzhugh CD, Wigfall DR, Ware RE. Enalapril and hydroxyurea therapy for children with sickle nephropathy. *Pediatr Blood Cancer.* 2005;45(7):982–985.
202. McKie KT, Hanevold CD, Hernandez C, et al. Prevalence, prevention, and treatment of microalbuminuria and proteinuria in children with sickle cell disease. *J Pediatr Hematol Oncol.* 2007;29(3):140–144.
203. Becker AM. Sickle cell nephropathy: challenging the conventional wisdom. *Pediatr Nephrol.* 2011;26(12):2099–2109.
204. Thompson BW, Miller ST, Rogers ZR, et al. The pediatric hydroxyurea phase III clinical trial (BABY HUG): challenges of study design. *Pediatr Blood Cancer.* 2010;54(2):250–255.
205. Wong WY, Elliott-Mills D, Powars D. Renal failure in sickle cell anemia. *Hematol Oncol Clin North Am.* 1996;10(6):1321–1331.
206. Scheinman JI. Sickle cell disease and the kidney. *Nat Clin Pract Nephrol.* 2009;5(2):78–88.
207. Ataga KI, Orringer EP. Renal abnormalities in sickle cell disease. *Am J Hematol.* 2000;63(4):205–211.
208. Chapman AZ, Reeder PS, Friedman IA, et al. Gross hematuria in sickle cell trait and sickle cell hemoglobin-C disease. *Am J Med.* 1955;19(5):773–782.
209. Heller P, Best WR, Nelson RB, et al. Clinical implications of sickle-cell trait and glucose-6–phosphate dehydrogenase deficiency in hospitalized black male patients. *N Engl J Med.* 1979;300(18):1001–1005.
210. Sears DA. The morbidity of sickle cell trait: a review of the literature. *Am J Med.* 1978;64(6):1021–1036.
211. Kiryluk K, Jadoon A, Gupta M, Radhakrishnan J. Sickle cell trait and gross hematuria. *Kidney Int.* 2007;71(7):706–710.
212. Kark JA, Posey DM, Schumacher HR, et al. Sickle-cell trait as a risk factor for sudden death in physical training. *N Engl J Med.* 1987;317(13):781–787.
213. Tsaras G, Owusu-Ansah A, Boateng FO, et al. Complications associated with sickle cell trait: a brief narrative review. *Am J Med.* 2009;122(6):507–512.
214. Connes P, Reid H, Hardy-Dessources MD, et al. Physiological responses of sickle cell trait carriers during exercise. *Sports Med.* 2008;38(11):931–946.
215. Mitchell BL. Sickle cell trait and sudden death—bringing it home. *J Natl Med Assoc.* 2007;99(3):300–305.
216. Embury SH, Dozy AM, Miller J, et al. Concurrent sickle-cell anemia and alpha-thalassemia: effect on severity of anemia. *N Engl J Med.* 1982;306(5):270–274.
217. Derebail VK, Nachman PH, Key NS, et al. High prevalence of sickle cell trait in African Americans with ESRD. *J Am Soc Nephrol.* 2010;21(3):413–417.
218. Key NS, Derebail VK. Sickle-cell trait: novel clinical significance. *Hematology Am Soc Hematol Educ Program.* 2010;2010:418–422.
219. Shaw C, Sharpe CC. Could sickle cell trait be a predisposing risk factor for CKD? *Nephrol Dial Transplant.* 2010;25(8):2403–2405.
220. Ajayi AA, Kolawole BA. Sickle cell trait and gender influence type 2 diabetic complications in African patients. *Eur J Intern Med.* 2004;15(5):312–315.
221. Oli JM, Watkins PJ, Wild B, et al. Albuminuria in Afro-Caribbeans with Type 2 diabetes mellitus: is the sickle cell trait a risk factor? *Diabet Med.* 2004; 21(5):483–486.
222. Bleyer AJ, Reddy SV, Sujata L, et al. Sickle cell trait and development of microvascular complications in diabetes mellitus. *Clin J Am Soc Nephrol.* 2010; 5(6):1015–1020.
223. Kimberling WJ, Yium JJ, Johnson AM, et al. Genetic studies in a black family with autosomal dominant polycystic kidney disease and sickle-cell trait. *Nephron.* 1996;72(4):595–598.
224. Yium J, Gabow P, Johnson A, et al. Autosomal dominant polycystic kidney disease in blacks: clinical course and effects of sickle-cell hemoglobin. *J Am Soc Nephrol.* 1994;4(9):1670–1674.
225. Peces R, Peces C, Cuesta-Lopez E, et al. [Co-inheritance of autosomal dominant polycystic kidney disease and sickle cell trait in African Americans]. *Nefrologia.* 2011;31(2):162–168.
226. Hicks PJ, Langefeld CD, Lu L, et al. Sickle cell trait is not independently associated with susceptibility to end-stage renal disease in African Americans. *Kidney Int.* 2011;80(12):1339–1343.
227. Derebail VK, Nachman PH, Key NS, et al. Variant hemoglobin phenotypes may account for differential erythropoiesis-stimulating agent dosing in African-American hemodialysis patients. *Kidney Int.* 2011;80(9):992–999.
228. Austin H, Key NS, Benson JM, et al. Sickle cell trait and the risk of venous thromboembolism among blacks. *Blood.* 2007;110(3):908–912.
229. Austin H, Lally C, Benson JM, et al. Hormonal contraception, sickle cell trait, and risk for venous thromboembolism among African American women. *Am J Obstet Gynecol.* 2009;200(6):620e1–3.

CHAPTER

63 Tropical Nephrology

Rashad S. Barsoum • Tarek Fayad •
Kearkiat Praditpornsilpa • Visith Sitprija

As its name implies, the tropical zone is the region of earth lying between the tropics of Cancer and Capricorn (23.5 degrees north and south) (Fig. 63.1). This zone has unique characteristics that significantly modify the profile of kidney disease with regard to etiology, clinical features, and management. Three major factors interact in this respect, namely the population genetics, environment, and prevailing socioeconomic conditions (Fig. 63.2).

Of the great human races, first described in the 1839 Meyers Konversations-Lexikon German encyclopedia, two are well expressed in the tropics. These are the "Negroid," hallmarked by grades of dark skin, and the "Mongoloid," mainly identified by typical facial features. It is obvious that neither skin color nor facial configuration is a modifier of any disease process; it is the associated genetic polymorphism that is truly incriminated, such as the ACE, MYH9, and a few Nephrin genes in blacks[1–3] and the gene polymorphisms associated with increased susceptibility to immunoglobulin (Ig)A nephropathy in the Chinese.[4] Genetic factors are amplified by the tendency of tropical populations to live in closed communities, sharing the same lifestyle and exposure to the same environment, for many decades. These are called "indigenous populations" of which over 5,000 groups are recognized in 72 countries, according to recent World Bank data.

The tropical environment is quite variable. Although commonly perceived as warm and rainy with a rich bioecology, which, indeed, is true for many areas as sub-Saharan Africa, Southeast Asia, and Central America, it may be hot, dry, and void of any significant natural cultivation as in the Arab Gulf countries and the great African Sahara, or icy-cold as in the great glaciers of Argentina. Each of these and other environmental conditions reflect on the animal and plant life in these regions, which reflects on the etiology of kidney as well as other diseases.

Despite considerable improvement over the past few decades, the average socioeconomic standards are suboptimal in the majority of tropical countries. The deadly vicious circle of poverty, illiteracy, and chronic disease remains escalating in many populations. Nearly 70% of the world's population live in the tropics, almost coinciding with the World Bank's map of "low" (≤US$ 995/year) and "lower-middle" (US$ 996–3,945/year) income categories. Expenditure on health is even more limited, with single digit annual expenditure per capita in many tropical countries in Africa and Asia. The highest rates of illiteracy are reported from the tropics, with numbers as high as 82.4% in Niger, compared to the world weighted average of 20.1%. All this translates into a distressingly high prevalence of malnutrition, chronic infection, and malignancy.

Kidney disease shares in this scenario in many ways. Acute kidney injury (AKI) is often caused by viral (e.g., HIV), bacterial (e.g., leptospirosis), or parasitic (e.g., malaria) infections; snake bites; or herbal medications. Chronic kidney disease (CKD) is caused by a parallel list of infectious and chemical agents, in addition to the increasing burden of diabetes and hypertension. The typical fast progression of CKD seems to be related to late medical attention, poor blood pressure control, obesity, smoking, lower nephron number attributed to low birth weights associated with malnutrition, and other factors. End-stage kidney disease (ESKD) treatment is quite modestly available. Survival on dialysis and the success of transplantation are strikingly low in most tropical countries, expectedly inversely related to national income.[5]

In this chapter, an overview is given on the epidemiology of common renal diseases in the tropics that are also present in the West but with different prevalence and nephropathy due to tropical infection and toxin poisoning, which is uniquely tropical. This is followed by descriptions of specific diseases including diseases related to chemical toxins and the environment. Finally, the issue of ESKD and its management in different tropical regions is reviewed.

OVERVIEW

Epidemiology of Common Kidney Diseases in the Tropics

Acute Kidney Injury

The incidence of AKI in the tropics is unknown, owing to the lack of reliable registries and unified definitions. It was only during the past decade that the RIFLE or AKIN definitions

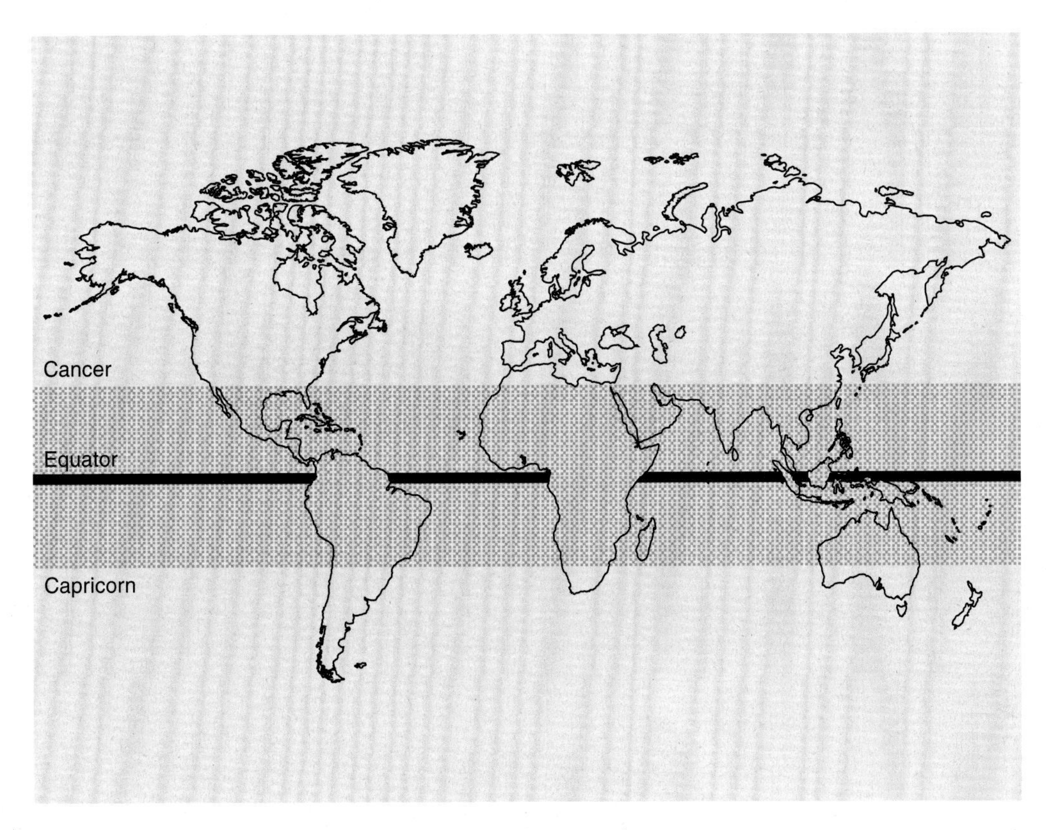

FIGURE 63.1 The tropical zone.

were adopted in the northern hemisphere, and less than a handful of studies reported from the tropics.[6,7] However, considering the reported incidence of AKI in the prevailing spectrum of primary causes, and referring it to the known prevalence of these conditions in the tropical environment, suggests extremely high figures, at least 10-fold higher than those reported in the north.

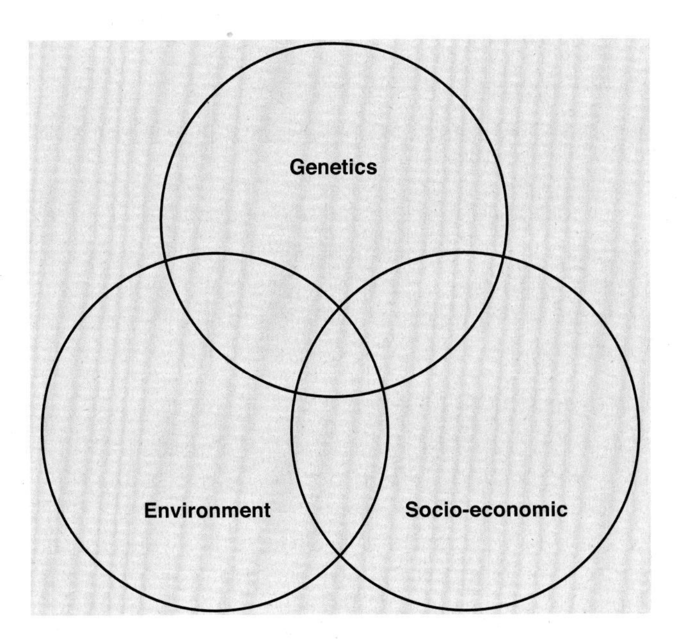

FIGURE 63.2 Major factors in the pathogenesis of tropical diseases.

Much of the recent literature distinguishes hospital-acquired from community-acquired AKI. The former constitutes the majority of cases in the north, which are related to surgical complications, administration of radiocontrast material, and sepsis. A similar profile is noticed in urban tropical communities, although constituting a small fraction of the overall burden of AKI.[6] On the other hand, at least 80% of AKI in the tropics is community-acquired, and occurs in the rural areas. Infection, intoxication with animal and plant poisons, and obstetric complications are the main causes. Breakdown of the different etiologies yields a remarkable geographical variation, depending on the predominant primary health problems and medical care. Falciparum malaria, scrub typhus, leptospirosis, snake bites, and toxic plants are the leading causes of AKI in different tropical communities.

The risk factors for developing AKI in the tropics are similar to those in the north. Those who are older, diabetic, or having CKD, etc. are more vulnerable. Yet there are additional risk factors in the tropics such as the nature of the causative agent (Fig. 63.3); severity of host response; multiple systemic effects involving the liver, lung, or heart; preexisting undernutrition or chronic illness; and drug nephrotoxicity.[8] Many such risk factors may coexist in the same patient, hence the high frequency of AKI.

End-Stage Kidney Disease

The incidence of ESKD in the tropics is commonly reported in between 150 and 200 patients per million population

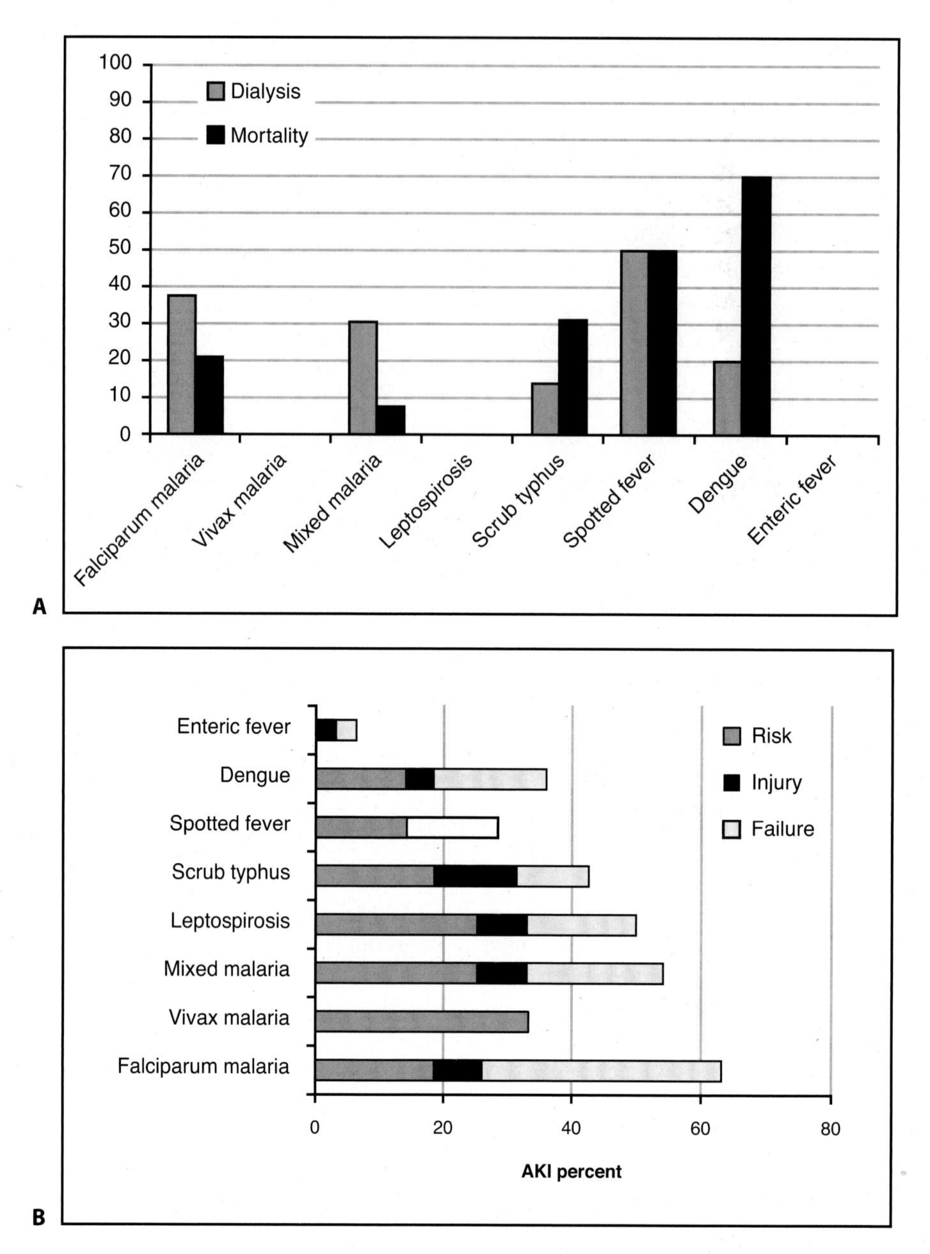

FIGURE 63.3 A: Incidence of acute kidney injury (AKI) in a study on tropical infections in India.[7] **B:** Outcome of AKI (percent) in tropical infections.[7] (See Color Plate.)

(pmp), which seems to be an underestimate when compared with recent data from the United States (averaging 350 pmp). It may be argued, though, that a relatively low incidence in the tropics is expected owing to the currently low rate of diabetes, which accounts for the majority of cases in the United States. This privilege alone seems to "overcorrect" for the additional burden of ESKD due to unique etiologies in the tropics, such as chronic infection and exogenous intoxication.[9] If this is true, the incidence of ESKD should progressively increase in the coming three decades, in parallel with the anticipated increase in diabetes.[10]

Prevalence, on the other hand, is far lower than in Japan, Europe, and the United States, owing to the low acceptance rates and the poor outcomes of renal replacement therapies. Prevalence rates typically exhibit the correlation with national income,[5] as observed in other countries with gross domestic products (GDPs) less than US$10,000 per capita.[11]

Chronic Kidney Disease

Only a few screening studies for the prevalence of CKD have been conducted in the tropics. The pioneering study of Remuzzi's group[12] in Bolivia shows evidence of CKD in 20% of 14,082 screened individuals. Other contemporary studies in other tropical countries have come up with different figures, ranging from 1.39% in the east of India[13] to 50% in north Australian Aboriginals.[14] Much of these differences are attributed to inconsistent definitions and methodology,

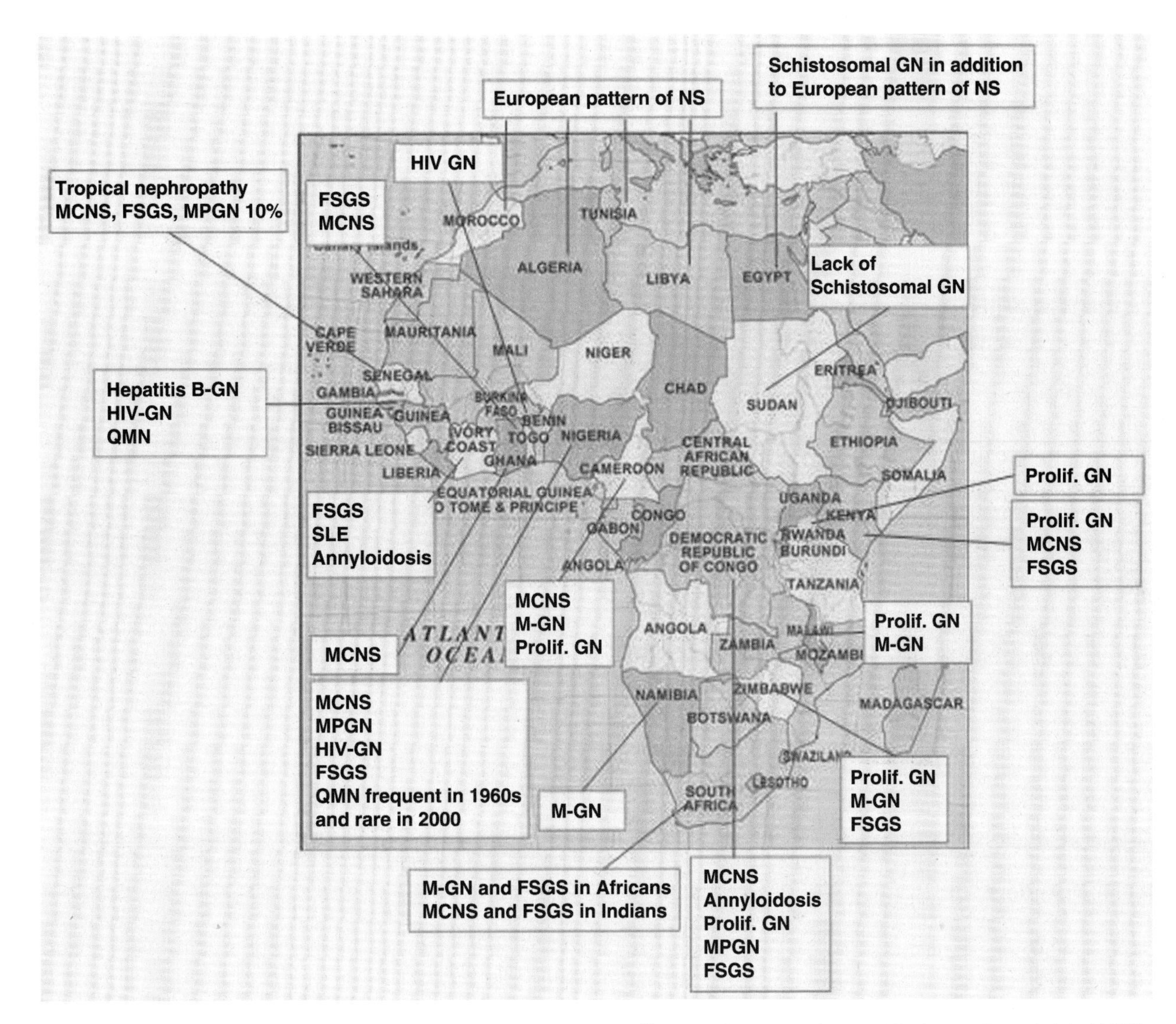

FIGURE 63.4 Glomerulonephritis profiles in different African countries.[26] *NS*, nephrotic syndrome; *GN*, glomerulonephritis; *MCGN*, mesangiocapillary GN; *FSGS*, focal/segmental glomerulosclerosis; *MPGN*, mesangioproliferative GN; *MCNS*, minimal change nephrotic syndrome; *HIV GN*, human immunodeficiency virus-associated GN; *QMN*, quartan malarial nephropathy; *Prolif. GN*, proliferative GN; *SLE*, systemic lupus erythematosus; *M-GN*, membranous nephropathy.

although true variation due to genetic, environmental, and socioeconomic factors undoubtedly exist.

Although the nature of CKD varies in different regions, there are gross similarities that distinguish the tropics from other parts of the world.

Glomerulonephritis. The prevalence of glomerulonephritis (GN) in the tropics has been estimated to be 1 in 10,000, which is 2.5 times the rate in Western countries. In most reports from the tropics, GN remains as the leading cause of ESKD to date.[15–19]

It is remarkable that secondary forms of GN are far more common in the tropics as compared with the rest of the world, reaching up to 34% in a report from Brazil.[20] This includes both genders and all age groups, being noticed as steroid-resistant nephrotic syndrome in children, aggressive lupus nephritis in young black women,[23] or focal segmental glomerulosclerosis (FSGS) in elderly men (Fig. 63.4).[24]

FSGS (15%–45% of all GNs) and various forms of proliferative GN (25%–35%) are notoriously common in the tropical zone.[15,19,25] It is likely that the former lesion is the result of genetic predisposition as explained earlier. Proliferative GNs are the typical lesions associated with most "nephritogenic" infections as described later. The distinction between primary and secondary forms of these lesions is sometimes difficult, when a primary cause is not identified.

IgA nephropathy has a high prevalence in the Far East and Southeast Asia (35%–45%) although it is rare in Africa (3%–4%).[19] Membranous nephropathy is less common in these regions as well as in South America and the Caribbean,[27] yet is notoriously common in others such as South Africa, where it is associated with hepatitis B viral infection in children.[22]

Mixed pathology is common in tropical GN, reflecting the multiplicity of causes and complexity of pathogenesis. The persistent antigenic load of chronic infection may lead to amyloid deposits, which may confound the glomerular lesions as in schistosomiasis, leprosy, and leishmaniasis (see later).

Interstitial Nephritis. The prevalence of interstitial nephritis in the tropics is generally higher than in the northern hemisphere, amounting to one quarter of incident dialysis patients in Pakistan.[19] Its etiology differs across individual tropical countries, depending on local ecology. It includes specific infection as tuberculosis, leprosy and leishmaniasis, "nonspecific" infection in association with stones or schistosomal urinary obstruction, and exposure to environmental or occupational nephrotoxins.

Diabetes. The contribution of diabetes to CKD varies from 9.1% to 29.9% in different reports.[19] More than 80% of cases are type 2 insulin-resistant. End-stage diabetic nephropathy exhibits a constantly rising trend, attributed to increasing incident cases as well as improved survival on renal replacement therapy (RRT). In a single center experience in Egypt, diabetic patients constituted 8% of patients on chronic dialysis in 1980, a figure that multiplied fourfold over 30 years (Barsoum, unpublished data).

Vascular Disorders. The lack of general agreement on the role of primary hypertension in causing ESKD is evident in the statistical reports from most tropical countries. Upon standardization of the definition of this disease entity, the prevalence of hypertensive nephrosclerosis among ESKD patients in the tropics was reported between 13% and 21%.[19]

Even more uncertain is the prevalence of renovascular hypertension, which requires a level of diagnostic sophistication that is often beyond availability in many tropical countries. In the many reports on this condition from India[28] and also from Southeast Asia, China, and South Africa, Takayasu's arteritis was a major underlying cause.

Nephrolithiasis. The overall prevalence of urolithiasis (3%–5%) does not seem to be different in the tropics when compared to the rest of the world.[29] A notable exception is in South Asia, where nephrolithiasis was reported to account for 40% of renal disorders in what is known as the "stone belt" in India, Pakistan, the Arabian Peninsula, and adjacent countries.[30] Most of these stones are formed of calcium oxalate, without significant changes in respective urinary concentration. It is presumable that dehydration may be a causative factor in most of these countries, whereas a high protein intake may contribute in the richer population strata, such as those in the northern hemisphere. In a small fraction of patients, as shown in South Africa and Thailand,[31] low urinary citrate may be the underlying defect.

Nephrolithiasis in the tropics is often secondary to urinary bacterial or parasitic infection (see later). Subsequent obstruction and ascending infection are responsible for renal damage, constituting up to 10% of ESKD in a country where schistosomiasis is endemic, such as Egypt.[32]

Other Conditions. Other "traditional" causes of CKD such as cystic disease and dysproteinemias seem to occur in the same frequency as in the rest of the world, yet they have a relatively limited impact on the overall prevalence.

Clinicopathologic Profile of Tropical Nephropathies

Etiology

Exposure to infection or toxins is responsible for the vast majority of kidney disease in the tropics. While these agents are frequent causes of AKI, their incrimination in CKD is often transient and spontaneously reversible. Exceptions to this rule are the chronic nephropathies associated with schistosomiasis, onchocercosis, possibly quartan malaria, and exposure to certain mycotoxins.

Infection. Of the principal bacterial infections, tuberculosis ranks quite high in India and the Arabian Peninsula, and is associated with ureteric strictures, back pressure, and chronic interstitial nephritis. Streptococcal infections of the throat and skin (complicating scabies) are responsible for chronic glomerular disease in a large number of African children. Of the viral infections, hepatitis C is currently the most important cause of progressive mesangiocapillary (membranoproliferative) glomerulonephritis in many countries, particularly Egypt, whereas HIV is responsible for a large spectrum of renal disorders, particularly in sub-Saharan Africa. Several parasitic infections cause ESKD through ureteric obstruction (e.g., schistosomiasis in most of Africa), interstitial nephritis (e.g., Kala-azar in many African and Asian countries), and glomerulonephritis (e.g., malaria in West Africa, schistosomiasis in Africa and Latin America, filariasis in Nigeria) (see Table 63.1).

Toxins. Several studies in North Africa have documented a fairly high prevalence of serum antibodies to ochratoxins in patients with "idiopathic" interstitial nephritis. However, a cause-and-effect relationship could not be established. The disease burden due to occupational exposure to lead, mercury, or cadmium; environmental exposure to various pollutants (see later); or the inadvertent use of nephrotoxic drugs or traditional medicines remains to be elucidated.

Pathophysiology

Being a highly vascularized organ, the kidney is vulnerable to a variety of tropical infections and toxins (Fig. 63.5). Nephropathy is attributed to either hemodynamic changes, immune responses, or direct nephrotoxicity.

TABLE 63.1 **Reported Clinical Spectrum of Parasitic Nephropathies**

	Acute Renal Failure	Asymptomatic Urinary Abnormalities	Acute Nephritic Syndrome	Nephrotic Syndrome	Chronic Tubulointerstitial	Ureteral Obstruction	Other Features	Chronic Renal Failure
Caused by Protozoa								
Malaria								
Quartan		++		++	+			+++
Falciparum	+++	++	+	+				
Babesiosis	++[a]							
Visceral leishmaniasis		++		+[b]	+			
Trypanosomiasis—African	++							
Toxoplasmosis				+				
Congenital				+				
Acquired								
Caused by Cestoda								
Echinococcosis		+					+[c]	
Caused by Trematoda								
Schistosomiasis								
Hematobium		+	+	+[b]	+	+++		+++
Mansoni		+		+++		+		+++
Opisthorchiasis	++	+					+[b,e]	
Caused by Nematoda								
Filariasis								
Wuchereria bancrofti		+	+	+			+[d]	
Onchocerca volvulus		++		+				+
Loa loa		+		+				
Strongyloidiasis		+		+				
Trichinosis		+						

Note: +, occasionally reported; ++, infrequently reported; +++, commonly reported.
[a]Usually with asplenia.
[b]Usually with amyloidosis.
[c]Mass effect of renal cysts.
[d]Chyluria.
[e]Jaundice.

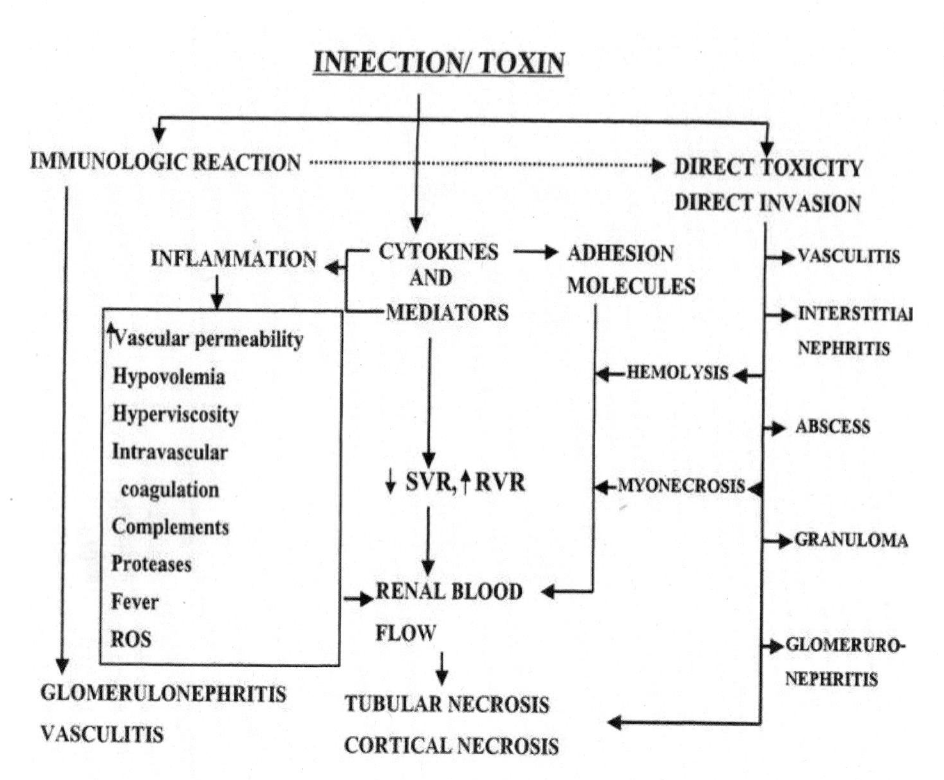

FIGURE 63.5 Pathogenetic mechanisms in infection/toxin related kidney injury.

Hemodynamic Alterations. Hemodynamic alterations in tropical infection are similar to those observed in sepsis. In mild and moderate infection, systemic vascular resistance is decreased, accompanied by increased cardiac output and increased renal vascular resistance. The renal blood flow and the glomerular filtration rate (GFR) are decreased. In severe infection systemic vascular resistance is either normal or slightly increased whereas the cardiac output is either normal or decreased. Renal vascular resistance is further increased with marked diminution of renal blood flow and GFR. In toxin envenoming the cardiac output is initially decreased, followed by the same hemodynamic pattern as in infection.

In uncomplicated febrile illnesses transient hypervolemia is associated with pyrexia.[33] The rise in blood volume may be attributed to vasodilatation due to vasodilatory mediators such as nitric oxide, prostaglandins, and kinins, as well as to the fluid-retaining hormones antidiuretic hormone (ADH) and aldosterone. Hypovolemia is observed in severe infection due to increased vascular permeability with fluid leakage from the intravascular compartment. This is further confounded by the increased insensible loss and sweating due to pyrexia. Among the most common causes of severe hypovolemia in the tropics are diarrheal diseases, dengue hemorrhagic fever, and intestinal anthrax.

Hemorheologic changes may be induced by increased plasma viscosity, increased erythrocyte viscosity in malaria and babesiosis, and erythrocyte swelling due to snake venoms and pore-forming toxins.[34] Cyto-adherence in between the vascular endothelium and the leukocytes in many infections, or parasitized erythrocytes in falciparum malaria, is a common phenomenon. Hemoglobinuria, myoglobinuria, intravascular coagulation, free radical release, bile acids, complement, and protease activation are among the nonspecific effects of infection and toxins.[35] These factors, in addition to hypovolemia, hemorheologic changes, and cyto-adherence, further contribute to decreased renal blood flow. Ischemic renal failure is therefore common in severe infection. The effect of toxin on ion channels on the vascular endothelium and smooth muscle cells can also alter hemodynamics in toxin envenomation.

Immunologic Perturbation. Both innate and acquired immunity are involved in the pathogenesis of renal injury in tropical infection. The major players in this context are the toll-like receptors (TLRs), which are expressed in all glomerular cells, the proximal tubule cells, and the interstitial monocytes and dendritic cells.[36] The ligands for these receptors include bacterial and viral peptides, lipopolysaccharides, necrotic cells, and other mediators associated with infection. Activation of TLRs utilizes the same signaling molecules as for interleukin (IL)-1 receptors (IL-1Rs) which include MyD88, IL-1R-associated protein kinase, and tumor necrosis factor (TNF) receptor-activated factor.[37]

Adaptive immune response takes further steps in antibody production. Both Th_1 and Th_2 subsets of T cells are in operation (Fig. 63.6). Th_1 cytokines, consisting of IL_2, interferon (IFN)-γ, and TNFα, are effective against bacteria and viruses. Th_2 cytokines, comprising IL_4, IL_5, and IL_{10}, defend

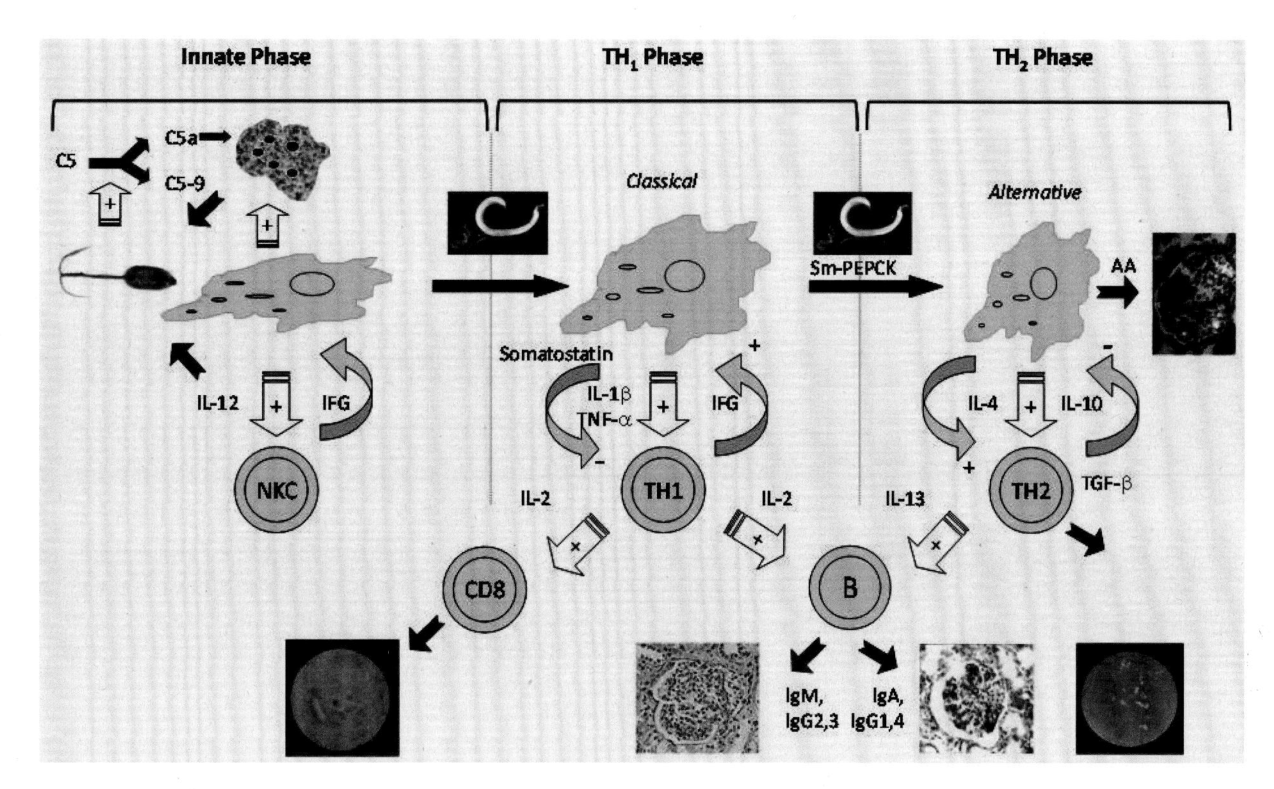

FIGURE 63.6 Broad immunologic pathways involved in infection: the schistosomiasis scenario. The cercaria (infective stage) provokes the innate immune pathways including the macrophages, neutrophils, natural killer cells, and complement. Adult worm and oval antigens are presented by the same cells, now serving as antigen-presenting cells (APCs), to the helper T cells (TH1) and B lymphocytes. The former activate CD8 cells, which are crucial for the formation of granulomata, aggregates of which form bladder pseudotubercles. B lymphocytes form antigen-specific IgM and IgG2,3 which are responsible for proliferative glomerular lesions. Under the influence of adult worm proteins (smPEPCK) the APCs transform into plasmoid cells which activate TH2 cells that secrete modulating and profibrotic cytokines which favor bladder fibrosis and "sandy patches." The B lymphocytes are "switched" under these cytokines to produce IgA, IgG1, and IgG4, which are associated with mesangiocapillary glomerulonephritis. Persistent commitment of the plasmoid cells in the immune process impairs their ability to remove the chemoattractant amyloid-A protein, leading to amyloidosis. Most infections utilize these pathways to a greater or lesser extent with variable emphasis on individual components.

against parasitic or mucosal infection. Glomerulonephritis, usually immune complex mediated, is the classic finding in most infectious diseases. Because IgM antibodies are produced early in infection and fix complement efficiently, granular immune complex deposition in the glomeruli with IgM and C_3 is commonly observed. Through the release of cytokines and chemokines, leukocytes are recruited and interstitial cells proliferate. In certain infections such as leptospirosis and schistosomiasis, tubulointerstitial lesions and granulomata may be observed. Persistent antigen load may result in secondary amyloidosis as seen in leprosy, leishmaniasis, schistosomiasis, and opisthorchiasis.

Direct Invasion and Nephrotoxicity. Direct cytotoxicity may be a significant pathogenetic mechanism in tropical nephropathies. Viruses such as HIV, parvovirus, and possibly hepatitis C virus (HCV)[38] may directly invade the podocytes. Bacterial toxins such as the Shiga toxin, the outer membrane proteins of leptospires, and the exotoxins of cyanobacteria have a selective affinity to membrane receptors of different renal cells.

Microbial invasion of the kidney, urinary tract, and lymphatics can provoke injury through a local inflammatory reaction in the form of cellular proliferation, infiltration, cystic, and granulomatous changes.[39] Renal lesions in leptospirosis, echinococcosis, filariasis, schistosomiasis, and tuberculosis represent injury by this mechanism.

Raw bile, impila (Callilepis laureola), toxic mushroom, and cotton seed oil are toxic to renal tubules.[40] Djenkolic acid, the main composition of djenkol bean, obstructs renal tubules in the presence of acid and concentrated urine.[40] Drinking star fruit juice causes renal failure through tubular obstruction by oxalate crystals.[41] Russell's viper venom and green pit viper venom have direct toxicity to the vascular and glomerular endothelial and renal tubular cells.[42] It has been postulated that venoms and toxins exert direct toxicity through phospholipase A_2 and metalloproteases.

Clinical Manifestations

Nonspecific urinary sediment changes consisting of few erythrocytes, leukocytes, and granular casts are often observed in febrile infectious diseases. Significant microscopic hematuria may be seen in a hematotoxic snake bite. These findings resolve when the disease is under control.

Proteinuria is transient and often mild with a protein-to-creatinine ratio of less than one. Significant proteinuria, even at the nephrotic range, may be seen, but disappears when the disease resolves. Persistent proteinuria with abnormal urinary sediment has been observed in certain infectious diseases that run a progressive clinical course, such as schistosomiasis, or are associated with superimposed infection or autoimmune reaction.

Hemoglobinuria is one of the common findings in venom or toxin poisoning.[43] Bites by vipers and hornet or wasp stings can cause significant intravascular hemolysis.[44] Glucose-6-phosphate dehydrogenase (G6PD) deficiency is common in tropical countries because deficient cells resist malarial parasitization, and it may account for intravascular hemolysis in the patient with infection or with use of certain drugs.[45] Myoglobinuria is observed in several infectious diseases with rhabdomyolysis such as leptospirosis, trichinosis, malaria, typhoid fever, viral infection, and septicemia.[46] Sea-snake bite and insect stings also cause rhabdomyolysis and myoglobinuria by direct effect on respective cell membranes.

Hyponatremia is common in the patients with febrile diseases. The causes are multiple including increased ADH, low sodium intake, sodium loss, sodium influx into the cells, and osmoreceptor resetting.[47] Response to water load may be delayed. Hypokalemia attributed to respiratory alkalosis due to high fever is noted in 38% of the patients with febrile illness. Potassium loss due to diarrhea is a common cause of hypokalemia. Interestingly, cotton seed oil ingestion[48] and leptospirosis[47] can cause kaliuresis and hypokalemia. Intravascular hemolysis and rhabdomyolysis are important causes of hyperkalemia. Hypocalcemia and hypophosphatemia are seen in severe infection.

AKI, often caused by tubular necrosis, either ischemic or toxic, is observed in 0.5% to 4% of patients with infection and toxin poisoning. Renal failure is hypercatabolic in 68% of the patients, characterized by rapid rises of blood urea nitrogen (BUN) and serum creatinine (SCr). AKI may be accompanied by jaundice, myoglobinuria, or hemoglobinuria. Cholestatic jaundice is a common complication, noted in 60% of the cases. Prognosis of AKI is usually good unless complicated by multiorgan failure, cortical necrosis, or papillary necrosis. The clinical course may be prolonged in severe acute diffuse interstitial nephritis.

TROPICAL INFECTIONS

Bacterial Infections

Several bacterial infections are known to cause AKI. Based on the evidence that most clinical features of severe infection reflect response to a large quantity of microorganism load, it is not surprising that in severe infection renal injury can occur.

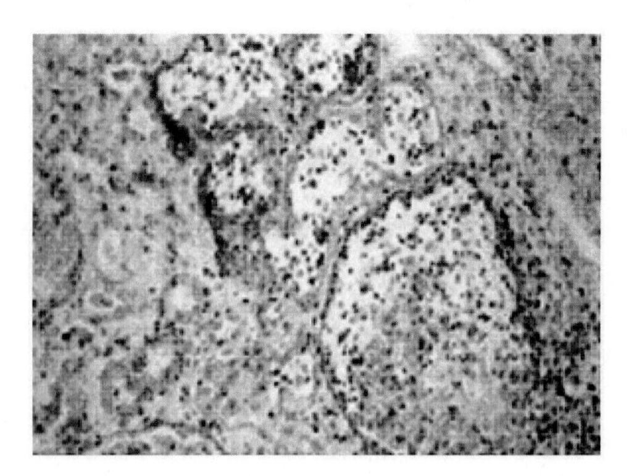

Figure 63.7 Typhoid interstitial nephritis with abscess formation.

Typhoid Fever and *Salmonella* Infections

Typhoid fever is a common disease in tropical countries. Clinically, renal disease due to typhoid fever is uncommon. However, with careful and repeated urinalysis, more than 50% of the patients are found to have definite findings of renal involvement.[49] The spectrum of renal disease in typhoid fever includes mild to severe glomerular involvement, interstitial nephritis (Fig. 63.7), and acute tubular necrosis.[49,50]

Hematuria and proteinuria are quite frequent during the febrile phase. The urinary protein loss is less than 1 g per 24 hours in the majority of patients, but can exceed this in occasional patients. The glomerular disease usually has a benign course, with complete recovery occurring in a 1- to 2-week period.[49] Less commonly, fever, generalized edema, and hypertension mimicking acute poststreptococcal glomerulonephritis have been reported. Recovery was usually complete with appropriate antimicrobial treatment. Renal histology, reported in several series, shows large glomeruli with mild to moderate mesangial proliferation. Immunofluorescence staining has shown variable amounts of C3, IgG, and IgM deposits. IgA deposition in the mesangial area has been described.[50] The pathogenesis of typhoid glomerulonephritis is of an immunologic nature. *Salmonella* Vi antigen has been demonstrated in the glomerular capillary wall.[51] The complement level is usually low during the acute phase in patients with renal involvement and normal in those without renal involvement.[51] However, this has not been a consistent finding, especially in experimental typhoid. AKI has occurred with typhoid fever associated with intravascular hemolysis due to G6PD deficiency, disseminated intravascular coagulation, severe jaundice,[49] and rhabdomyolysis.[52] An interesting syndrome reported from Egypt is the nephrotic syndrome, which occurs in patients with chronic salmonellosis associated with schistosomiasis (see later text).[53] A similar combination of *Salmonella* and schistosomal infection has been reported in Brazil without nephrotic syndrome.[54]

Leptospirosis

Leptospirosis, an infectious disease caused by several serotypes of pathogenic leptospires, is worldwide in distribution. The disease is transmitted through contact of abraded skin or mucous membrane with blood, tissue, or urine of infected animals or through exposure to contaminated environments. It is an unusual cause of AKI in Western countries; however, it plays an important role in certain tropical regions. In Southeast Asia and Sri Lanka, leptospirosis is one of the important causes of AKI, accounting for 24% and 32% of all reported cases, respectively. The kidney is invariably involved in leptospirosis, and AKI of variable severity occurs in the majority of the patients (Fig. 63.8).

Clinically, patients present with sudden onset of chills, fever, generalized muscle pain, and variable degrees of jaundice. Urinary abnormality consists of mild proteinuria, a variable number of erythrocytes, occasional hemoglobinuria, granular casts, and bile-pigmented casts. Leptospiruria is demonstrated by dark-field illumination. Renal failure, occurring in 60% of the patients, may be mild and nonoliguric. Oliguric renal failure with hyperbilirubinemia occurs in severe cases. In severe leptospirosis hypotension is frequently observed and can lead to AKI and pulmonary complications if not promptly treated.[55] Hypokalemia secondary to kaliuresis has been observed. Kaliuresis in leptospirosis is due to inhibition of potassium reabsorption in the medullary thick ascending limb of Henle loops and increased sodium delivery to the principal cells of the collecting ducts, due to decreased sodium reabsorption in the proximal tubules resulting in potassium excretion.[56] Renal bicarbonate wasting similar to proximal renal tubular acidosis may be observed. Hypocalcemia and hypomagnesemia are common. In severe cases (Weil syndrome), marked renal failure with a rapid rise in SCr and uric acid occurs in association with jaundice. Jaundice is usually cholestatic. Hepatocellular jaundice may be observed when associated with shock. In rare cases, hemolytic-uremic syndrome may be seen.

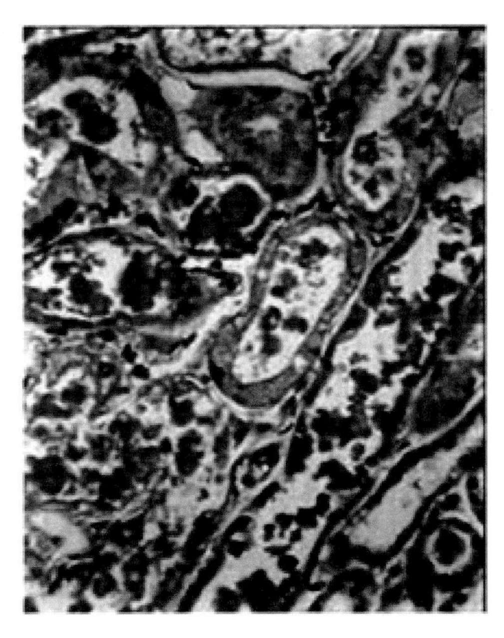

FIGURE 63.8 Leptospirosis. Acute tubular necrosis, with blood and pigment intratubular deposits and interstitial edema.

Thrombocytopenia is common and renal failure may be associated with significant thrombocytopenia. Full-blown disseminated intravascular coagulopathy is rare. Infection with different leptospiral serotypes does not seem to explain the marked variability in renal involvement.[47]

Although leptospirosis involves every structure of the kidney, the primary lesion is interstitial in nature, with local or diffuse mononuclear cell infiltration. Renal function can be normal. In AKI, cellular degeneration of both proximal and distal tubules is seen. Glomerular changes are quite mild and limited to mild mesangial hypercellularity. On immunofluorescent staining, nonspecific C3 and IgM uptake is seen in the mesangial area and occasionally in the afferent arterioles. On electron microscopy, occasional dense deposits are seen in mesangial, paramesangial, and intramembranous locations. The organism itself is rarely seen in human biopsy studies. However, in hamster models, leptospires can be seen initially in the glomeruli and then in the interstitium and renal tubules a few hours following inoculation.[57]

The pathogenesis of renal changes in leptospirosis is multifactorial. Through monocyte activation and TLRs, the outer membrane proteins of leptospires can cause a release of nitric oxide, TNF-α, and monocyte chemoattractant protein from the medullary thick ascending limb of Henle loops. Peptidoglycans and lipopolysaccharide also induce monocytes to release proinflammatory cytokines and vasoactive mediators causing hemodynamic changes. The renal blood flow is decreased through the effects of cytokines, mediators, and nonspecific inflammatory factors. Decreased cardiac function, attributed either to myocarditis or myocardial depressant factor or jaundice, further contributes to decreased renal blood flow leading to AKI. Intercalation of leptospire glycolipid in the host cell membrane and inhibition of membrane Na-K ATPase can cause cellular injury. Interaction between leptospire outer membrane proteins and extracellular receptors on the host cell membrane activates innate immune response with leukocyte infiltration resulting in interstitial nephritis.[58] The humoral immune mechanism plays a major role in leptospire elimination. However, it plays a minor role in leptospire nephropathy. An increased number of B lymphocytes have been observed in a patient with leptospirosis, along with a decrease in the number of CD3+ and CD4+ cells.[59]

Management of renal failure in patients with leptospirosis should focus on treatment of the underlying abnormality. Penicillin, including its derivatives, is the drug of choice. Hypotension should be promptly treated with vasopressor agents. Intravenous fluid should be given cautiously because of decreased response to fluid load. A small dose of dopamine increases blood pressure and urine flow[60] although its impact on survival or need for dialysis is questionable.[61] Hemodialysis and peritoneal dialysis have been used successfully in patients with renal failure. Plasma exchange coupled with hemodialysis is advocated for patients with marked hyperbilirubinemia. In most patients who recover from acute illness, renal function returns to normal. Prognosis is generally good. Bad prognostic indices include hyperbilirubinemia, hyperkalemia, and pulmonary complications of either pulmonary edema, adult respiratory distress syndrome (ARDS), or hemorrhage. Continuous hemofiltration, either arteriovenous or venovenous form, plasmapheresis, and blood exchange are useful in these clinical settings.

Leprosy

Leprosy is a common infectious disease in tropical regions including Africa, Asia, and South America. It has been estimated that of 12 million cases of leprosy in the world, 3 million are in India. Renal involvement is frequent among patients with lepromatous leprosy, although it can also be seen in those with tuberculoid or borderline types. The prevalence of glomerulonephritis in leprosy varies from 6% to 50% in biopsy studies.[62]

The clinical spectrum covers asymptomatic proteinuria and hematuria, nephrotic syndrome, nephritic syndrome, and renal failure.[63] Circulating immune complexes and cryoglobulinemia are detectable in the majority of patients. Serum complement levels may be low. The cell-mediated immune response is depressed in the lepromatous type. Nephrotic syndrome is common in patients with amyloidosis, but may be observed in patients with membranous and diffuse proliferative glomerulonephritis. Urinary concentration and acidification defects have been described.[64] Chronic renal failure often results from complicated amyloidosis. AKI is mostly observed in lepromatous leprosy with a prevalence of 63%, whereas only 2% of nonlepromatous patients have impaired renal function.[65] AKI may also be a complication of the multidrug treatment of leprosy. Treatment should concentrate on the leprosy; management of the renal involvement is only supportive.

Pathologically, diffuse proliferative glomerulonephritis and mesangial proliferative glomerulonephritis are common. Focal proliferative glomerulonephritis, membranous nephropathy, mesangiocapillary glomerulonephritis, crescentic glomerulonephritis, focal glomerulosclerosis, and interstitial nephritis have been reported.[65] Immunofluorescence study shows granular deposition of IgM, IgG, IgA, and C3 in the mesangial areas and along the glomerular capillary walls. Deposition of IgA alone has been occasionally demonstrated. There is electron-dense deposition in the mesangial, subendothelial, intramembranous, and subepithelial areas.[66] The findings are compatible with immune complex glomerulonephritis. The nature of the antigen has not been identified. Glomerulonephritis may be only a nonspecific reaction. The possibilities exist among mycobacterial antigens, other microbial antigens, and autoantigen. Secondary amyloidosis is noted in 2.4% to 8.4% of patients, predominantly with lepromatous and borderline lepromatous leprosy, although it may be observed occasionally in tuberculoid leprosy.[62]

Melioidosis

Melioidosis is an infectious disease caused by a gram-negative bacillus, *Burkholderia pseudomallei*. The disease is prevalent in the tropics, especially in India, Thailand, Myanmar, Cambodia, Laos, Vietnam, Malaysia, the Philippines, and Papua New Guinea. Melioidosis was an important health problem during the Vietnam War when many soldiers became the victims of this deadly disease. Antibodies to *B. pseudomallei* were detected in 39.5% of the people in northeastern Thailand. There are a few reports on melioidosis of the urinary tract. The data on renal involvement are scanty, and according to a few reports the rate varies from 2.4% to 35%.[67] Renal abscess diagnosed by ultrasonography is noted in 12% of the patients.[68] AKI can occur in the septicemic form of the disease. In a series of 220 patients with melioidosis in northeastern Thailand, renal failure was noted in 35%.[69] There were associated morbidities in 56% of the patients including diabetes mellitus, renal stone, cirrhosis, and glomerulonephritis. Hypoproteinemia was present in 60% of the patients. Hyponatremia was observed in 90% of the patients. The duration of renal failure varied from 1 week to 6 weeks, averaging 3 weeks. The mortality rate was close to 90%.

Renal pathologic changes include multiple renal abscesses, tubular necrosis, and interstitial nephritis. The bacteria are seen in the suppurative lesions. In an animal model, thrombi have been demonstrated in blood vessels and cortical necrosis has been observed. These have not been shown in human melioidosis. Renal changes are attributed to severe sepsis, which causes renal ischemia and inflammatory reactions to bacterial invasion. Recently, nephritic syndrome has been observed in a patient with melioidosis, and spontaneously resolved following antimicrobial treatment.[70]

Tetanus

Tetanus is capable of causing AKI through stimulation of the sympathetic nervous system[71] and rhabdomyolysis.[72] In a report from Brazil where the condition is not uncommon,[73] proteinuria was noted in 50% of the patients and impaired renal function was observed in 39% of patients in whom serum myoglobin levels were found to be elevated. There is no correlation between the serum level of myoglobin or creatine phosphokinase (CPK) and renal failure. AKI is usually nonoliguric and mild.

Scrub Typhus

Scrub typhus, caused by *Orientia tsutsugamushi*, is widely distributed in the tropics and can involve the kidney. As with the other infectious diseases, mild proteinuria with abnormal urine sediment is not uncommon. In the majority of patients, renal function is normal. AKI can be observed with severe infection associated with either jaundice, intravascular coagulation, or hemolysis.[7] According to recent reports, AKI occurred in 7.7% of the patients in Taiwan and in 25% of the patients with hypotension in Thailand. ARDS has been described. The usual renal changes are those of mild mesangial proliferative glomerulonephritis. Deposition of IgM and C3 is seen in the mesangial area. In severe cases, platelet thrombi may be seen in the glomeruli, with focal thickening of the basement membrane. Tubular necrosis is observed in the presence of AKI. Interstitial nephritis may be present.[7] The infiltrate often occurs in the corticomedullary region and consists of mononuclear cells. Perivascular infiltration and thrombophlebitis may be seen in the interlobular veins.

Diphtheria

Diphtheria can occasionally cause AKI in children. In a review of 155 patients,[74] renal failure was observed in only two patients. This could be attributed to decreased cardiac output due to myocarditis. Yet, diphtheria toxin may be nephrotoxic because it inhibits protein synthesis when it is added to the basolateral side of the renal tubular cells.[75] Diphtheria toxin enters the cell by endocytosis through receptors. The process is inhibited by methylamine. Renal histologic changes in those with AKI are consistent with tubular necrosis. The patients on renal replacement therapy are at high risk of developing diphtheria if they have not been vaccinated.

Cholera

Cholera remains a global threat. The number of cases in Africa greatly exceeds the number reported from other countries. Cholera is still endemic in Asian countries. The A subunit of cholera toxin enters the intestinal epithelial cells and activates adenylate cyclase with generation of cAMP and opening of chloride channels.[75] This results in diarrhea due to chloride and water hypersecretion. Renal failure is attributed to fluid and electrolyte loss. Isolated renal perfusion by cholera toxin resulted in reduction of GFR and urine flow, as mediated by platelet-activating factor.[76] Acidosis in cholera is associated with an increased anion gap due to hyperproteinemia, hyperphosphatemia, and increased serum lactate levels. Hypokalemia can be striking. Interestingly, the ratio between BUN and SCr may be lower than normal because of the larger loss of urea than creatinine through diarrhea and perhaps rhabdomyolysis due to hypokalemia. In addition to tubular necrosis, vacuolation of the proximal convoluted tubules due to hypokalemia may be present. Cortical necrosis has been described.

Shigellosis

Shigellosis can be caused by any of the four species of *Shigella*: *Shigella dysenteriae*, *S. flexneri*, *S. boydii*, and *S. sonnei*. Among these species *S. dysenteriae* is most virulent. Bacterial AB exotoxin known as Shiga toxin is composed of subunit A and subunit B. Subunit B binds to glycolipids Gb3 on the host vascular endothelium, renal epithelium, and neurons, thereby stimulating internalization of subunit A which binds to ribosomes and inhibits protein synthesis.[77] Therefore, in addition to diarrhea caused by colonic inflammation due to bacteria, renal injury and vascular injury can occur. Shigellosis can cause renal failure through volume depletion induced by diarrhea and direct renal injury. In a series of 2,018 patients,[78] renal failure occurred in 26%. By multivariate analysis, younger age, decreased serum protein, altered consciousness, and thrombocytopenia were indices of a poor prognosis. Because shigella toxin causes endothelial injury, hemolytic-uremic syndrome may occur.[79] In this setting there may be cortical necrosis and diffuse fibrin deposition in the glomeruli. Srivastava et al.[80] reported an incidence of hemolytic-uremic syndrome of 34% in patients with AKI mostly related to shigellosis. Renal histology showed cortical necrosis in 40% of the patients.[80] The mortality rate was 60%.

Vibrio vulnificus Infection

Vibrio vulnificus is a gram-negative bacillus found in coastal and brackish waters. Infection by *V. vulnificus* usually occurs in immunocompromised or chronic alcoholic hosts following consumption of contaminated seafood or injury to the skin in a marine environment. *V. vulnificus* infection in man can be expressed as primary sepsis, wound infection, or gastrointestinal manifestation. The presenting symptoms consist of fever with chills, abdominal pain, vomiting, diarrhea, and lower extremity pain. Disseminated intravascular coagulation can occur. AKI is common with tubular necrosis as a significant pathologic change.[81] Renal failure is ischemic in origin. Yet, cellular injury can be induced by bacterial cytolysin, collagenase, protease, metalloprotease, and phospholipases.[82] The disease may be confused with leptospirosis, scrub typhus, malaria, and other forms of sepsis. *V. vulnificus* requires iron for growth. Therefore, the patients on long-term hemodialysis who receive intravenous iron infusion may be at risk of *V. vulnificus* infection if exposed to the bacteria.[83]

Viral Infections

Many viral diseases can cause mild glomerular involvement. Rhabdomyolysis may be seen with viral infection and can be responsible for AKI. It is, however, interesting that several viruses harbored in the kidney produce viruria without renal function changes.

Dengue

The disease is caused by any of four serotypes of dengue virus and is characterized by flulike symptoms with headache, muscular pains, arthralgia, flushing of the face, conjunctival injection, and skin rashes. The disease, presented either as dengue fever, dengue hemorrhagic fever, or dengue shock syndrome, is common in Southeast Asia and is transmitted by the mosquito *Aedes aegypti*. *Aedes albopictus*, *A. scutellaris*, and *A. polynesiensis* may be important vectors in certain areas. Dengue hemorrhagic fever often occurs in a dengue-immune person reinfected by the virus of different serotype. The preexisting nonneutralizing antibodies, through antibody-dependent enhancement, increase the virus uptake and replication in the macrophage resulting in high viral loads, T cell activation, and apoptosis. Hypotension may occur during the second phase of the disease, a few days after the onset when fever declines. Complement activation, increased vascular permeability, thrombocytopenia, and prolonged bleeding time and prothrombin time are the main pathophysiologic changes of the disease that lead to hypovolemia and bleeding.[84] Immune complexes play an important part in complement activation. Anaphylatoxins C3a and C5a, cytokines, and mediators are elevated and result in plasma leakage from the intravascular space. Usual renal manifestations in dengue hemorrhagic fever include mild urinary sediment changes, mild proteinuria, and hyponatremia. Renal failure in children is often mild and usually prerenal due to hypotension. In adults, renal failure can be severe and associated with cerebral symptoms, liver dysfunction, intravascular hemolysis due to G6PD deficiency, rhabdomyolysis, or superimposed infection.[85] Hypotension may or may not be present. As in sepsis, hemodynamic alteration plays a key role in the pathogenesis. It is not clear why the disease is more severe in adults. It could be related to virus virulence, associated infection, drugs used, and late hospitalization. Also, the disease may not be recognized earlier in adults. Jaundice is hepatocellular, with marked elevation of liver enzyme levels. Renal failure is oliguric with a prolonged clinical course. Mortality of adult AKI can be as high as 60%.

Renal histologic changes include mesangial proliferation with IgM and C3 deposition, endothelial cell swelling, and perivascular infiltration by mononuclear cells.[86] Tubules show degeneration along with interstitial edema. The diseases can be confused with Hantavirus infection, which can produce almost similar pathophysiology and symptoms.

Hantavirus Infection

Hantavirus is an RNA virus in the family Bunyaviridae. The disease is seen worldwide throughout Asia, Europe, North and South America, Australia, and Africa. It is considered a rare disease in tropical Asian countries. In Korea, Hantaan and Seoul serotypes are common. Hantaan virus causes severe disease with a renal syndrome. Seoul virus causes a disease of moderate severity, and Puumala virus produces the least severe disease. The epidemiologic significance of Prospect Hill serotype is not well understood. Belgrade virus is associated with severe disease in the Balkans. Sin nombre serotype causes the most severe disease with a pulmonary syndrome in the United States. Thottapalayam virus is found in India without clinical significance. Rodents, especially rats, mice, and voles, are the important reservoirs. Infection is acquired mostly by inhalation of rodent excreta, although direct inoculation by abrasion or cuts of the skin is also possible. The virus replicates in macrophages and endothelial cells of small blood vessels of several organs, especially the kidney and the lung. Increased vascular permeability is the main pathophysiology of the disease, owing to the effects of various mediators, cytokines, complement activation, and vascular endothelial injury which finally result in hypovolemia, decreased renal perfusion, and AKI.[87]

The symptoms of Hantavirus infection with different serotypes vary greatly. Even in the same serotype, the symptoms can vary from mild to severe. The description of Hantaan virus infection with renal syndrome is classic. Clinically, after the incubation period of 2 to 5 weeks, the disease is manifested by flulike symptoms with fever, headache, flushed face, myalgia, abdominal pain, nausea, and vomiting. Periorbital edema, conjunctival hemorrhage, and palatal and axillary petechiae may be present. The clinical course can be divided into five phases: febrile, hypotensive, oliguric, diuretic, and convalescent. The febrile phase lasts for 3 to 7 days and is followed by the hypotensive phase due to hypovolemia, which develops with lysis of fever. The hypotensive phase lasts from 3 hours to 3 days and is followed by the oliguric phase, which may be prerenal or renal in origin. The duration of the oliguric phase, therefore, varies from a few days to longer. The diuretic and convalescent phases follow. In infection with other serotypes or in mild cases these five phases may not be apparent. Hypotension and oliguria may not be present.

Renal involvement is common in Hantaan virus infection. Proteinuria, hematuria, and pyuria are usually observed. Renal failure is more common in Hantaan virus infection than in infections with the other serotypes, and may be associated with pulmonary edema. Thrombocytopenia may occur in severe cases. Disseminated intravascular coagulation has been shown.

Renal pathologic changes are consistent with tubular necrosis. Medullary vessels are dilated and congested. Marked interstitial changes with edema and hemorrhage, with later infiltration by mononuclear cells, can be seen. The interstitial changes are pronounced in Puumala infection. Glomerular changes are not remarkable. Mild glomerular hypercellularity may be found. IgM, IgG, and C3 deposition in the glomeruli and interstitium may be observed. Residual renal dysfunction including proteinuria, impaired urinary concentration, hypertension, and CKD have been reported.[88]

Hepatitis B

Hepatitis B virus (HBV) infection is worldwide in distribution, with a low carrier rate in Western countries. The prevalence of the hepatitis B surface antigen (HBsAg) carrier varies from 0.3% to 1.0% in North America to 1% in western Europe; 5% in South America, eastern Europe, Japan, and western Asia; 7% in Africa; and 10% to 20% in China, Taiwan, and Southeast Asia. The observations of a high incidence of HBsAg carriers among patients with various forms of glomerulonephritis when compared with the general population tend to support the role of HBV in the pathogenesis of glomerulonephritis. In Hong Kong, 22% of patients with glomerulonephritis are HBsAg positive, which is higher than the carrier rate in the general population. In South Africa 20% of the patients with glomerulonephritis are HBsAg positive. In Zimbabwe, Japan, and Taiwan, HBV antigenemia has been found in 80% to 100% of children with membranous glomerulonephritis. Focal segmental glomerulosclerosis associated with chronic HBV infection has been observed. However, in Thailand and South Korea, the renal pathologic spectrum of HBV does not differ from that of the general population. In the Thai population, the most common glomerulopathy in chronic HBV infection is IgA nephropathy followed by membranous nephropathy, focal segmental glomerulosclerosis, and membranoproliferative glomerulonephritis.[89] The findings are not different from the pathologic spectrum of glomerulopathy in general Thai population.

Clinical presentations vary from asymptomatic proteinuria and hematuria to nephrotic syndrome and impaired renal function with hypertension. Nephrotic syndrome is common in membranous and mesangiocapillary glomerulonephritis, whereas hematuria and asymptomatic proteinuria are present in mesangial proliferative glomerulonephritis. In about 33% of patients the serum complement level is decreased. Patients with HBV may present with the clinical picture of essential cryoglobulinemia with purpura, arthralgia, and splenomegaly.[90] AKI may occur with fulminant hepatitis, but may occasionally develop with uncomplicated HBV.[91]

The natural history of HBV-associated glomerulonephropathy is not well understood. Spontaneous remission has been reported to occur in 50% of membranous nephropathy patients. Seroconversion to positive antihepatitis B e antibody (anti-HBeAb) is associated with remission of proteinuria. In children the disease may run a benign course and the pathology is mainly membranous. Among patients with IgA deposition, 19% had deterioration of renal function in 40 months. Clearance of HbsAg from blood has been associated with remission of polyarteritis. The use of steroids as treatment for glomerulonephritis should be discouraged. Corticosteroid therapy has been associated with active virus replication and hepatic dysfunction with an appearance of virus-like particles in the glomeruli.[92] IFN-α administration has been shown to suppress HBV expression with clearing of HbeAg, and decrease proteinuria in HBV associated glomerulonephritis with short duration of infection. The use of adenine arabinoside and thymic extract reduced proteinuria in 87% of membranous nephropathy patients, with a reduction of HBV DNA in T cells, B cells, and macrophages along with seroconversion from HBeAg positive to anti-HBe positive. The use of antiviral agents such as lamivudine can be beneficial. Lamivudine may resolve HBV-associated membranous nephropathy.[93]

Renal pathologic changes include membranous glomerulonephritis, mesangial proliferative glomerulonephritis, mesangiocapillary glomerulonephritis, and polyarteritis nodosa. Among these, membranous nephropathy is usually associated with deposition of HBeAg in the immune complexes whereas mesangial proliferative glomerulonephritis is associated with HBsAg complexes.[94] Hepatitis B core antigen (HBcAg) has been found in membranous nephropathy patients when polyclonal anti-HBcAg antiserum was used. Glomerular deposition of HBeAg and HBsAg is demonstrable in mesangiocapillary glomerulonephritis. The pathogenetic association between IgA nephropathy and HBV has attracted attention, as the geographic area with the highest endemicity of HBV infection has also the highest incidence of IgA nephropathy. Glomerular HBsAg deposition similar in distribution to that of IgA immune staining is detected in 21% to 40% of patients.[95] There is no HBeAg deposition.

Hepatitis C

The incidence of hepatitis C virus (HCV) carrier in the tropics is less than 5%. HCV is classified into six genotypes. The preponderance of distribution of HCV genotype varies globally. In North America, genotype 1a predominates followed by 1b, 2a, and 2b. In Europe, genotype 1b is predominant followed by 2a, 2b, and 2c. Genotypes 4 and 5 are found almost exclusively in Africa whereas genotype 3 is endemic in Southeast Asia. The genotype is clinically important in determining potential response to IFN-based therapy and the required duration of such therapy. Genotypes 1 and 4 are less responsive to IFN-based treatment than are the other genotypes. Chronic HCV infection can be associated with mesangiocapillary or diffuse proliferative glomerulonephritis, membranous or IgA nephropathy, and, rarely, crescentic, fibrillary, or immunotactoid glomerulonephritis.[38]

Mesangiocapillary GN with mixed cryoglobulinemia is the most common pattern. Glomerular immune complex deposits consist of HCV, anti-HCV IgG, and IgM rheumatoid factor. The cryoprecipitate containing HCV RNA and HCV antibody can be seen in the subendothelial glomerular deposits. Core antigen was demonstrated in the glomeruli of patients with HCV, even in the absence of circulating cryoglobulins. Electron microscopy shows cryoglobulin-like structures, virus-like particles, and viral RNA in the renal tissue.[96] The patients have proteinuria, hematuria, decreased renal function and hypocomplementemia, rheumatoid factor, and circulating cryoglobulin. Nephrotic syndrome is a common presentation.

Treatment with IFN-α improves liver function and decreases urinary protein excretion with disappearance of HCV RNA. Exacerbation of glomerulonephritis with proteinuria and hematuria during IFN administration has been reported. It was suggested that renal damage was either a direct or indirect effect of IFN on the glomerular endothelial and epithelial cells. The result of treatment by IFN therefore varies. The viral genotype and titer may be important determinants in response. Antiviral therapy with IFN-α and ribavirin may be beneficial.[96] However, ribavirin is contraindicated in the presence of renal failure, and only IFN is recommended in dialysis patients. In comparing with the other causes of secondary glomerulonephritis in the tropics, HCV is a rather uncommon cause. However, it is an important cause of morbidity and mortality among recipients of renal transplantation and chronic dialysis patients. Pretransplant IFN may reduce the occurrence of posttransplant HCV-related de novo glomerulonephritis.[97]

Hepatitis A

Fulminant hepatitis A can produce renal failure in a similar fashion to hepatorenal syndrome. Viral hepatitis associated with G6PD deficiency may present with massive intravascular hemolysis and AKI. Recently, there have been several reports of AKI developing in patients with hepatitis A in the nonfulminant form.[98] The mechanism of renal failure is not well understood. In some patients, there are no apparent renal histologic changes whereas in the others tubular necrosis is seen. Perhaps various nonspecific factors in inflammation that lead to renal ischemia superimposing on hepatic dysfunction produce the renal failure. IgA-dominant immune complex glomerulonephritis with nephrotic syndrome has been reported.[99]

Severe Acute Respiratory Syndrome Virus

The SARS virus is a coronavirus that causes severe acute respiratory syndrome (SARS). The outbreak of SARS started in Asia in 2003 and then expanded elsewhere in the world. SARS manifests by systemic symptoms of muscle pain, headache, lymphopenia, and fever, followed in 2 to 10 days by the onset of respiratory tract symptoms, namely cough, dyspnea, and pneumonia. The overall mortality rate was 9%. In patients over 50 years old, the mortality rate approaches 50%. Apart from respiratory syndrome, AKI has been observed in some patients, especially those with rhabdomyolysis and associated diseases. A study in Hong Kong in 2003 showed that 6.7% of cases developed acute renal impairment occurring at a median duration of 20 days (range 5 to 48 days) after the onset of disease. The mortality rate was higher among SARS patients with renal impairment (91.7% vs. 8.8%). Kidney tissue by postmortem examination revealed predominantly acute tubular necrosis with no evidence of glomerular pathology.[100]

H1N1 Virus Infection

H1N1 virus, a subtype of influenza A virus, is the cause of swine flu declared by the World Health Organization in 2009. This novel virus infection spread worldwide and had caused about 17,000 deaths by 2010. Symptoms of zoonotic swine flu in humans are similar to those of influenza and of influenza-like illness in general, namely chills, fever, sore throat, muscle pains, severe headache, coughing, and weakness. The virus infected lung cells with overstimulation of the immune system through cytokine release. There is extensive leukocyte migration toward the lungs, causing destruction of lung tissue and secretion of fluid into the organ. The pandemic killed mostly young adults, possibly due to their healthy immune systems and damaging response with cytokine storm. In recent studies, 53% of H1N1 infected patients developed AKI and one third of cases required hemodialysis.[101] Factors associated with AKI in H1N1-infected patients were vasopressor use, mechanical ventilation, high Acute Physiology and Chronic Health Evaluation II (APACHE II) scores, severe acidosis, high C-reactive protein, and lactic dehydrogenase level. The mortality rate of AKI-associated H1N1 infection was 19%. The renal histopathologic findings were typical of acute tubular necrosis. There was no evidence of viral infiltration on kidney biopsy. Although the antibody response in postkidney transplant recipients is reduced, inactivated influenza vaccine is strongly recommended for kidney transplantation recipients. H1N1-infected kidney transplant recipients who received prompt oseltamivir have a good prognosis with scarce complications.[102]

HIV Infection

HIV-associated nephropathy (HIVAN) refers to kidney disease developing in association with HIV infection. The most common, or classical, type of HIV-associated nephropathy is a collapsing FSGS, although other forms of kidney disease may also occur with HIV.[103] Typical findings are that of collapsing FSGS and microcystic tubular dilatation. HIVAN may be caused by direct infection of the renal cells with the HIV-1 virus, with resulting renal damage through the viral gene products. It could also be caused by changes in the release of cytokines during HIV infection. Approximately 80% of patients with HIVAN have a CD4 count of less than 200. HIVAN presents with nephrotic syndrome and progressive renal failure. The kidney size is usually normal or large. HIVAN is much more common in African patients with HIV. In a series of 99 consecutive kidney biopsies in HIV-infected black South Africans, 27% were diagnostic of HIVAN.[104] Among black adults in the United States, HIVAN is the third most common cause of ESKD. Although the large number of HIV-infected cases overwhelm the Asian countries, HIVAN in Asians is uncommon. A kidney biopsy study[105] in Thai HIV-infected patients with proteinuria greater than 1.5 g per day showed that mesangial proliferative glomerulonephritis was the most common renal histopathology. No HIVAN cases were identified. None of the patients were treated with antiretroviral drugs at the time of renal biopsy. Racial differences, and familial clustering of kidney disease, strongly suggest the existence of HIVAN-specific genetic susceptibility factors that are unmasked in the setting of HIV infection.[106]

HIV infection is risk factor for development of CKD especially in black patients with CD4 count <200 cells per mm^3, HIV RNA levels >4,000 copies per mL, family history of CKD and presence of diabetes mellitus, hypertension, or hepatitis C coinfection. The prevalence of CKD with HIV infection was 3.5% to 4.7% in European countries, 27% in India, and 12.3% in Iran.[107] Reported prevalence of CKD in HIV-infected patients in sub-Saharan Africa ranges from 6% to 48.5%. In HIV-infected Asians, prevalence and predictors of CKD have not been well defined. A cohort study in Asia revealed a high prevalence of advanced CKD among Thai HIV-infected patients, particularly those with older age, prior indinavir exposure, diabetes mellitus, and tenofovir nephrotoxicity. In a large cohort, increasing exposure to tenofovir was associated with a higher incidence of CKD.[108] Despite the efficacy of highly active antiretroviral therapy (HAART) in reducing the risk of HIV-related renal disease, the incidence of ESKD continues to increase among patients with HIV infection.

Mycotic Infections

Mycotic infections constitute an important part of tropical nephrology. Kidney involvement may be a part of the disease or a complication of treatment using drugs with nephrotoxic potential. Because no particular features distinguish such infections in the tropics from those in other parts of the world, this chapter does not include detailed accounts, which can be found elsewhere. For easy reference, however, the important mycotic infections of clinical significance in tropical countries are highlighted.

Mycotic Nephropathies in the Immunocompetent Individual

Coccidioidomycosis. The disease is widely distributed over the globe, but endemic foci are identified in the tropical zone of the American continent, particularly Central America and Argentina. Infection is acquired through inhalation of dust containing the fungal hyphae, leading to predominantly pulmonary disease. The kidneys are involved in the rare disseminated form of the disease, particularly in black patients.[109] The lesions are interstitial, either granulomatous or suppurative, usually multiple, and often associated with lung cavities.

Paracoccidioidomycosis. This is a chronic granulomatous disease, also endemic in Central and South America. It is characterized by mucocutaneous manifestations, in addition to foci of granulomatous inflammation in different viscera including the kidneys.[110]

Fungal Toxins

Ochratoxin. These fungal products may contaminate stored cereals. They are documented to induce a form of interstitial nephritis in pigs that resembles and has been incriminated in the pathogenesis of Balkan nephropathy in humans. However, this theory has been recently challenged as evidence accumulated in favor of exposure to aristolochic acid. Ochratoxins are also potent carcinogens that induce renal adenocarcinoma in small laboratory animals, but the relevance of this observation to humans is unknown.

Chronic interstitial nephritis associated with serum antibodies against ochratoxin-A has been reported from the tropical zone, including Egypt[111] and northwest Africa.[112] The pathogenetic link in this observation remains questionable.

Aflatoxin. Aflatoxins B_1 and B_2—produced by *Aspergillus flavus*, which contaminates many foods, particularly cereals—have been associated with hepatomas in humans and in experimental animals. They can also induce changes in GFR and the development of adenocarcinoma and pelvic neoplasms in experimental models.[113]

Although aflatoxins are present worldwide, they have recently attracted a lot of interest in the tropics. They have been incriminated in the remarkable increase in the incidence of hepatomas in most of Africa, particularly in association with persistent HBV-antigenemia. It is unknown whether aflatoxins are also responsible for a higher incidence of renal malignancy in the same continent. Although high contamination levels have been documented in mothers and infants in an Egyptian cohort there was no evidence of kidney damage.[114]

Opportunistic Mycotic Infections in the Immunocompromised

Fungi are well-known opportunistic organisms worldwide. Fungal infections are even more prevalent in tropical countries because of the uncontrolled use of antibiotics and immunosuppressive agents, poor general hygienic standards, and the high prevalence of AIDS in certain areas.

The principal opportunistic fungi[115] encountered in the tropics are described in the following text.

Candidiasis. Candidiasis is, by far, the most common. Urethritis, cystitis, and pyelonephritis are usually ascending infections. Oropharyngeal candidiasis is less common. It may spread to involve the upper gastrointestinal tract or respiratory passages. Local colonic candidiasis may spread from perianal or vaginal infection. Disseminated candidiasis may follow any of these localized forms, often being a terminal event in patients with AIDS and over-immunosuppressed transplant recipients.

Invasive Aspergillosis. This is a serious infection in renal transplant recipients, particularly after bacterial infection in neutropenic patients and those with active cytomegaloviral (CMV) infection. The disease is characterized by interstitial pneumonia or consolidation with or without cavitation, often accompanied by intracranial, gastrointestinal, hepatic, cardiac, and osseous lesions. Interstitial renal disease may also occur, presenting as proteinuria, pyuria, and hematuria, with rapid loss of function. Fungal "balls" have been observed in the urine of such patients.

Cryptococcosis. Infection is acquired by inhalation of bird droppings. Current data suggest that 20% to 60% of the cases of cryptococcosis in HIV-negative patients occur in organ transplant recipients, usually encountered 6 months after grafting. However, of the solid organs, renal transplant recipients have the lowest incidence. The usual manifestations are meningoencephalitic, pulmonary, and cutaneous. Infection of the graft is rare unless involved in disseminated infection. The renal lesion is interstitial with persistent graft pyelonephritis in most cases.[116]

***Pneumocystis jiroveci* Pneumonia.** This infection causes serious pneumonia and occasional extrapulmonary manifestations in patients with AIDS, and less often in those receiving immunosuppressive therapy including renal transplant recipients.

Disseminated Histoplasmosis. This is an important risk to renal transplant recipients in Central and South America. Both primary infection and reactivation of dormant infection seem to occur. The disease is characterized by focal necrotic lesions in different viscera, bones, joints, meninges, endocardium, skin, and oral mucosa.

Mucormycosis. The rhinocerebral, pulmonary, and renal forms of this infection are rare. Renal involvement may be silent, or associated with local pain and urinary symptoms. AKI is increasingly recognized in these patients due to fungal interstitial nephritis.[117]

Disseminated disease may be encountered in patients with uncontrolled diabetes, particularly with ketoacidosis or CKD. It often complicates desferrioxamine therapy in patients on dialysis and is occasionally seen in renal transplant recipients, being strongly associated with the use of purine inhibitors. The kidney is involved in about 50% of these patients, affected by vascular thrombosis, suppuration, and granuloma formation with renal failure supervening in the majority.

Parasitic Infections

Parasitic infestations influence the practice of clinical nephrology in the tropics in three ways: (1) they are the causative agents of certain renal diseases, usually referred to as parasitic nephropathies (Table 63.1); (2) they are among the important agents that may infect immunocompromised patients (Table 63.2); and (3) they often modify the typical clinical picture, prognosis, and management of renal disorders at large.

Parasitic Nephropathies

Renal lesions have been described with many parasitic infections. However, the incidence seems to be relatively low relative to the global prevalence of parasitic diseases. Only two of those have been associated with epidemiologically significant kidney disease, namely malaria and schistosomiasis. Other parasitic nephropathies are either too mild to achieve clinical significance (e.g., trichinosis) or geographically too restricted to be of epidemiologic importance (e.g., onchocercosis).

Parasitic Infections in the Immunocompromised

The list of agents known to affect the immunocompromised host in the tropics involves some 20 parasitic species.[118] These may be (1) acquired de novo, due to impairment of immunity to primary infection (e.g., cryptosporidiosis); (2) reactivated, having been dormant due to a balanced host–parasite concomitant immunity (e.g., leishmaniasis); or (3) transmitted with a transplanted organ (e.g., trypanosomiasis). Unfortunately, the mode of acquisition of clinical disease remains uncertain in most posttransplantation parasitic infections. Such knowledge is important because it will settle the debate about the need for prophylaxis in transplanted travelers, pretransplantation chemotherapy, and specific screening of potentially infective donors.

Although some of these infections produce insignificant morbidity, others may be associated with severe disease that may be fatal (e.g., strongyloides hyperinfection).

There are several interesting considerations regarding therapy because several antiparasitic drugs may interact with immunosuppressive agents (e.g., quinine or chloroquine with cyclosporine),[119,120] or they may acquire a specific toxicity profile in transplant recipients (e.g., antimony-induced pancreatitis).[121] Conversely, immunosuppressive agents may have antiparasitic properties (e.g., cyclosporine and strongyloidiasis, malaria, or leishmaniasis[122]; and tacrolimus or rapamycin and malaria[123]).

Impact on the Clinical Patterns and Management of Renal Disease

The clinical patterns of renal diseases in the tropics may be modified in different ways by associated parasitic infestations. Many infestations cause, or are associated with, malnutrition, which, in addition to reflecting on the severity of the infestation per se (malaria, schistosomiasis, strongyloidiasis), augments nephrotic edema, increases anemia and bone disease in CKD, superimposes skin and peripheral nerve complications, and increases the risk of bacterial infection.

The associated chronic activation of the immune system is often blamed for increasing the incidence of secondary amyloidosis as in schistosomiasis.[124] The same was also attributed to impairment of macrophage function in leishmaniasis.[125] Immune activation may be expressed by hyperglobulinemia, which often poses diagnostic difficulties in the interpretation of false-positive results on serologic tests.

Most parasitic diseases are characterized by multisystem involvement, which confounds the clinical picture, prognosis, and management of the associated renal disorder. Common examples are the extensive microcirculatory disturbance in malarial AKI, the chronic hepatic and lower urinary tract pathology in schistosomiasis, and the chyluria of filariasis. Such elements in the scenario may have a considerable impact on treatment strategies, use of medications, and choice of acute and chronic dialysis modalities as well as on the safety and efficacy of dialysis. They often influence the donor selection, the recipient's immunosuppression, and the eventual outcome of renal transplantation.

Individual Parasitic Diseases and the Kidney

Malaria. Malaria is a parasitic disease of great epidemiologic importance in the tropics, largely because of the warmth and humidity that favor the multiplication of mosquitoes, of which the anopheline species is the principal vector for malarial transmission. The incidence of malaria in the world is of the order of 300 to 500 million clinical cases each year, with mortality averaging 2 million per year. The disease is caused by a protozoan, *Plasmodium*, of which five species are pathogenic to humans, namely, *Plasmodium vivax*, *P. malariae*, *P. ovale*, *P. falciparum*, and *P. knowlesi*. The clinical pattern of the disease, incidence of acute and chronic complications, and, consequently, the outcome are influenced by certain differences among the infective species. These include inherent features in their own life cycles as well as their selective adhesion to specific red blood cell and hepatocyte receptors. The age of infected erythrocytes is an important factor. Thus, whereas *P. vivax* and *P. ovale* infect only young red blood cells, and *P. malariae* infects only aging cells, *P. falciparum* and *P. knowlesi* infect erythrocytes at any age, explaining the heavy parasitemia associated with them.

TABLE 63.2 **Important Parasitic Infections in the Immunocompromised**

		De novo Infection	Recrudescence	Transmission with Graft	Disease	Clinical Presentation
Circulatory parasites	*Plasmodium falciparum, Plasmodium vivax, Plasmodium malariae*	Natural in endemic and indigenous areas (travelers, expatriates, exposure in airports); parenteral	Vivax, malariae, ? Falciparum	Kidney, liver, bone marrow, multiorgan	Malaria	Fever, anemia, thrombocytopenia, acute renal graft dysfunction, hepatosplenic γ–δ lymphoma
	Babesia microti	Transfusion			Babesiosis	Fever, anemia, arthralgia, hemolytic uremic syndrome
	Schistosoma haematobium, mansoni	Reinfection	*S. mansoni* glomerulopathy		Schistosomiasis	Hematuria, proteinuria
Tissue parasites	*Leishmania donovani*		Kidney, bone marrow, heart, lung	Possible, not documented	Kala azar	Fever, splenomegaly, pancytopenia, acute renal graft dysfunction
	Trypanosoma cruzi	Possible, not documented	Heart	Debated	Chagas disease	Fever, subcutaneous nodules, cardiomyopathy
	Toxoplasma gondii	Possible, not documented	Heart, bone marrow, liver, kidney, multiorgan	Heart, bone marrow	Toxoplasmosis	Fever, lymphadenopathy, hemophagic syndrome, encephalopathy, Guillain Barré syndrome, hepatitis, pneumonia
Alimentary parasites	*Strongyloides stercoralis*		Heart, kidney, stem cells	Possible, not documented	Strongyloidiasis hyperinfection	Fever, gastrointestinal symptoms, pneumonia, ARDS, eosinophilia
	Capillaria philippinensis		Debated	Possible, not documented	Capillaria hyperinfection	Fever, eosinophilia
Protozoa	*Cryptosporidium parvum*		All solid organs		Cryptosporidiosis	Diarrhea
	Acanthamoeba castellani		Bone marrow, kidney, lung		Acanthamebiasis	Keratitis, encephalitis, osteomyelitis, cutaneous ulceration
	Encephalitozoon cuniculi		Kidney, bone marrow,		Microsporidiosis	Conjunctivitis, encephalitis, pneumonia

ARDS, acute respiratory distress syndrome.

The type and severity of clinical disease depends on the parasite's ability to modify the physical properties of parasitized red blood cells such as deformability, fragility, and adhesiveness, as well as on the host's immune response to the parasite's antigens.

Clinical Features. The disease is characterized by recurrent pyrexia with chills, the frequency of which varies according to the infective species. Constitutional features such as headache, malaise, and muscle and joint aches are usually encountered, more often with the first infection episode and in expatriates. Diarrhea, pulmonary edema, jaundice, coma, and circulatory failure may complicate falciparum infection, hence the term malignant malaria. The spleen is usually enlarged, particularly with relapsing disease. Anemia and neutrophil leukocytosis are prominent laboratory findings. The diagnosis is confirmed by direct visualization of the parasite in Giemsa-stained peripheral blood smears. Fluorescent staining with acridine orange enhances the diagnostic accuracy of peripheral blood examination. Routine serology was once of limited diagnostic value, particularly in endemic areas where old infection is highly prevalent. However, the recent introduction of synthetic peptides for the detection of epitopes on infected red blood cell membranes has opened a new diagnostic dimension. The use of polymerase chain reaction (PCR) technology can detect very low parasite levels as well as mixed infections; however, its use is still limited.

Renal Involvement in Malaria. Clinically significant renal disease may typically complicate infection with three malarial species, namely, *P. malariae*, *P. falciparum,* and *P. vivax*. The former is believed to be associated with progressive CKD, whereas infection with either of the latter two species may lead to an acute kidney disease that is more often than not reversible by adequate management.

Chronic Malarial Nephropathy. The causative link between *P. malariae* infection and glomerulonephritis is based on epidemiologic, experimental, and some immunologic evidence.[126–129] Epidemiologic evidence is based on the overlap of geographical distribution of quartan malaria with that of steroid-resistant nephritic syndrome,[130] and regression of the latter's incidence with the successful implementation of malaria control campaigns.[131] Glomerular disease was experimentally induced by the closely related species *Plasmodium berghei*[132] and *Plasmodium brazilianum*,[133] yielding ultrastructural changes similar to those seen clinically. Parasite-specific circulating immune complexes[129] and glomerular deposits were detected both in the mentioned experimental models and patients, thereby providing an immunologic basis for the syndrome.

Extrapolation of these observations into a distinct clinical entity is controversial,[26] mainly because of three issues. Firstly, there is no consistent histopathologic pattern of what is called quartan malarial nephropathy. For example, the typical glomerular lesion described in West Africa is pseudomembranous,[128] with the formation of intramembranous "lacunae" (Fig. 63.9) and frequently associated with FSGS, whereas that in East Africa was mesangioproliferative.[26] It is noteworthy, though, that variation in

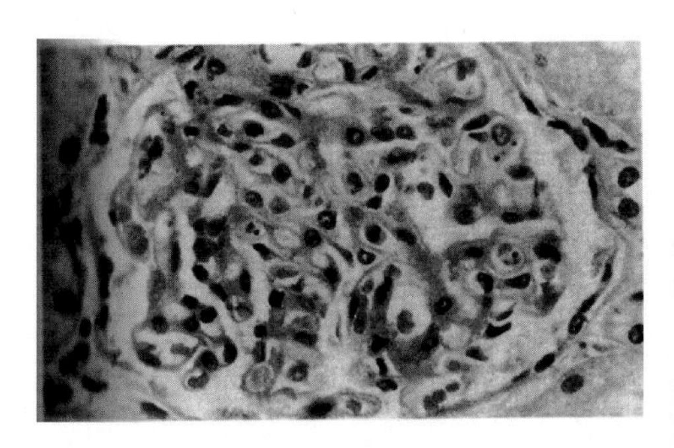

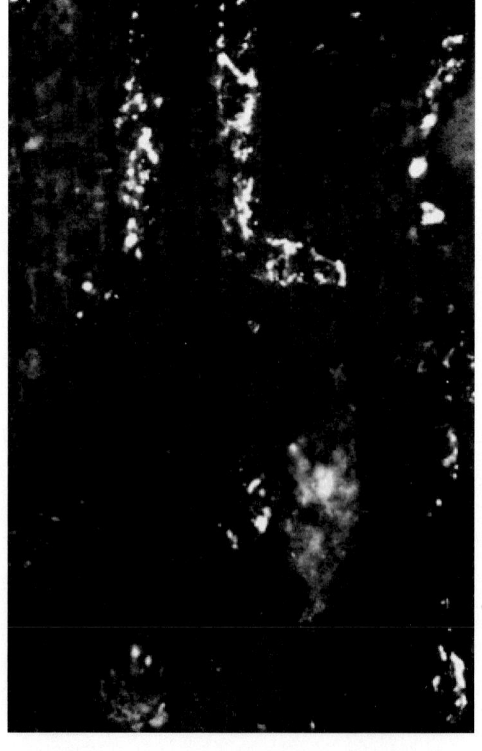

FIGURE 63.9 Glomerular lesion associated with quartan malaria (*left*). Peritubular malaria antigen deposits by immunofluorescence (*right*).

the glomerular response to the same infection may vary according to differences in the agent's strains or host's genetic factors and concomitant diseases.[19] The second controversy concerns the inconsistency and paucity of malarial antigen deposits in different cohorts.[134,135] It is unclear if some of this discrepancy is attributable to technical factors, differences in the timing of biopsy, or the presence of associated endemic diseases, known to confound the immune response as seen in marmosets.[133] Finally, although the incidence of secondary glomerulonephritis in endemic areas has truly regressed with the control of malaria, the question remains whether this would be alternatively attributed to overall improvement of primary healthcare and control of other primary causes of kidney disease.

As described in the original reports,[126–129] the clinical renal syndrome ascribed to quartan malaria is nonspecific, apart from its association with the features of the parasitic infection. Most patients are children, with a mean age of 5 years. Proteinuria is encountered in a variable proportion of patients, up to 46% in the first published series. Microhematuria is occasionally noticed, particularly in the older age groups. Overt nephrotic syndrome develops in a yet-undefined fraction, and hypertension is a late encounter. Serum complement levels are normal, and blood cholesterol values are usually not elevated, owing to the associated nutritional deficiency. Renal biopsy shows one or another of the patterns described here. Mesangial deposits of malarial antigens are occasionally demonstrated by immunohistochemistry. The disease progressively leads to chronic renal failure over 3 to 5 years regardless of any treatment.[126]

Acute Malarial Nephropathy. Acute kidney disease (AKD) may occur in patients with *P. falciparum*[136–138] or, less frequently, *P. vivax*[139–142] infection. This includes AKI, glomerulonephritis, and a number of superimposed characteristic metabolic disturbances.

Acute Kidney Injury. This is, by far, the most important malarial complication in the kidneys, being relatively frequent and potentially fatal.[136–142] The reported incidence is 1% to 4%, but it may reach up to 60% in high-risk individuals. AKI usually occurs in patients with heavy parasitemia (infected erythrocytes, more than 5%), particularly in pregnant women, HIV-infected individuals, children with cerebral malaria, and foreigners visiting endemic areas. It also occurs in almost all cases of blackwater fever secondary to hemolysis.

Patients developing malarial AKI (MARF) have the typical *clinical features* of severe systemic illness with profound disturbances of the microcirculation, multiorgan involvement (particularly the liver with falciparum malaria[138] and the lungs with vivax infection[140]), and prominent metabolic disturbances including hypoglycemia, lactic acidosis, and hyponatremia (see later).

MARF is usually oliguric and hypercatabolic. Hyperkalemia can be profound in patients with intravascular hemolysis. Hyperuricemia, disproportionate to the nonprotein nitrogen retention, is frequently seen. The oliguric phase usually lasts for a few days to several weeks. Mortality is usually within the range of 30%, but it may vary from 10% to 50%, depending on the severity of infection,[137] pregnancy,[143] response to antiparasitic treatment,[140] availability of dialysis, and the predominant pathogenetic factors involved.[144]

Therapy usually poses challenging problems because of the complexity of the syndrome. Quinine remains the drug of choice, particularly in Africa and other economically compromised regions. Intravenous artemisinin derivatives are

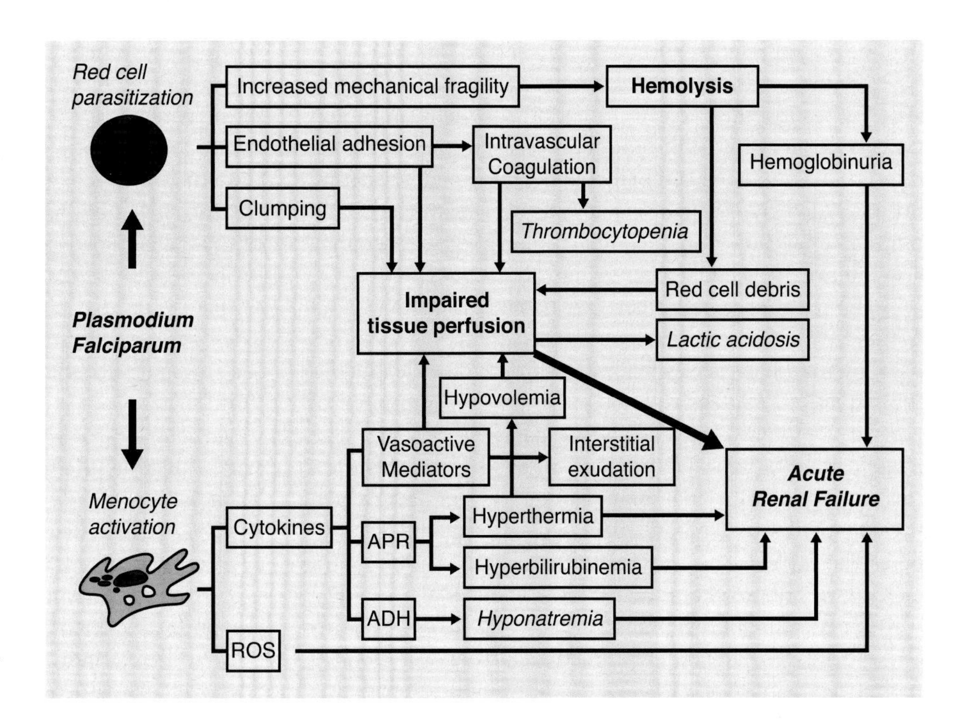

FIGURE 63.10 Pathogenetic mechanisms in acute malarial nephropathy.

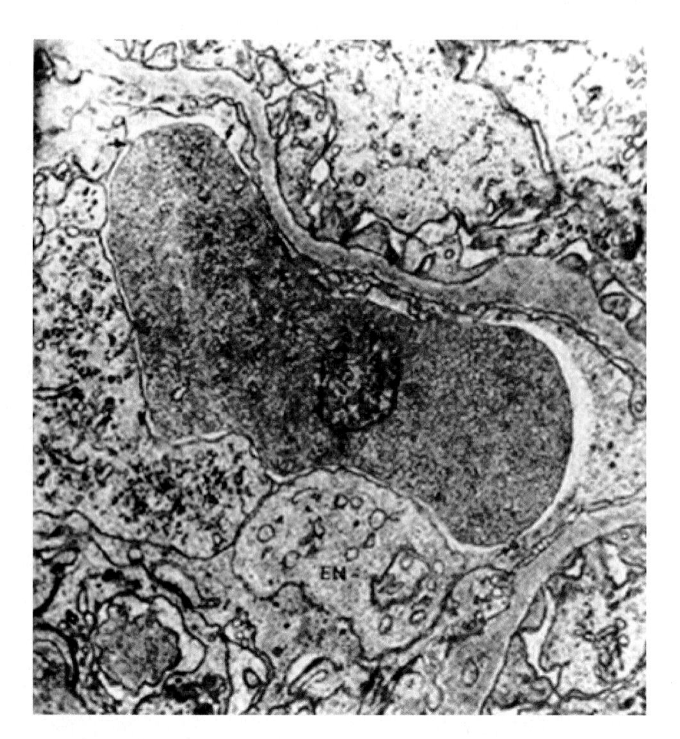

FIGURE 63.11 Parasitized red cell showing the sticky knobs (*arrows*).

recommended as first choice when affordable, and may be the only choice in quinine-resistant patients. Early dialysis is often needed to treat the hypercatabolic state. Although peritoneal dialysis is less effective because of the supervening circulatory disturbances, it becomes more effective as the flow in microcirculation is improved by treatment. It is often the only available dialysis modality available in underdeveloped communities. In some cases, continuous peritoneal dialysis may be indicated. Exchange transfusion is helpful in patients with heavy parasitemia and those with severe jaundice.

MARF is basically an ischemic acute tubular necrosis (ATN), attributed to shock, endothelial activation, and capillary congestion with red blood cell and platelet sludging. Yet, in contrast to cerebral malaria, the blood vessels are not occluded by the parasitized cells. The pathogenesis is multifactorial, involving a complex interaction of rheologic and immunologic components (Fig. 63.10).

The parasitized red blood cell is the cornerstone of all events.[136–138] Characteristic of *P. falciparum* infection are particular red blood cell membrane abnormalities leading to the formation of adhesive knobs (Fig. 63.11), composed of abnormal proteins encoded by the parasite's genome. The major family of adhesive proteins is called *Plasmodium falciparum* erythrocyte membrane proteins (PfEMPs), which includes several members identified by sequential numbers. The PfEMP-1 appears to be the major determinant of erythrocyte adhesiveness and subsequent malarial morbidity. A striking feature of this protein is variability, being structurally and antigenically different in consecutive generations of parasitized red blood cells. This is attributed to switching in-between alleles in the "Major Var Gene" in successive merozoite generations. Switching is largely a spontaneous process but is also influenced by host factors, as shown by the effect of splenectomy in experimental models. This "cross-talk" between the parasite and the host keeps the balance that permits both to survive.

Other adhesive protein families have been identified in the erythrocyte knobs including the histidine-rich proteins, rifins, rosettins, and others. Most of these are also variable proteins of importance in the host–parasite relationship, but their relative pathogenetic significance seems to be less prominent than that of the PfEMP-1.

The main red blood cell receptors for PfEMP-1 are the erythrocyte complement receptor (CR1) and glycosaminoglycans (GAGs). There are many platelet and endothelial receptors. Although some are constitutively expressed, as CD36, PECAM-1/CD31, thrombomodulin, and chondroitin-4-sulfate, many are induced by the host's immune response as a part of widespread endothelial activation including E-selectin, P-selectin, ICAM-1, and VCAM-1.

The physiologic deformability of parasitized red blood cells is impaired and their mechanical fragility increased, which leads to hemolysis. Although this is usually extravascular, intravascular hemolysis may also occur, particularly in patients with G6PD deficiency who are receiving quinidine or pyrimethamine therapy. In extreme forms, massive intravascular hemolysis leads to the frank hemoglobinuria characteristic of blackwater fever. Red cell debris and their free products exert their hemodynamic and toxic ill effects, which include vasoconstriction, renal tubular toxicity, and activation of intravascular coagulation. Activation of coagulation factors, thrombocytopenia, and increased plasma fibrin degradation products have been well documented. However, glomerular capillary thrombosis is uncommon, and fibrin deposits have not been consistently seen by immunofluorescence.

Antigenic proteins are expressed on the cell membranes of the parasite as well as the parasitized host cells. However, owing to the intracellular residence of the sporozoan during most of its life cycle in humans, it is the antigen expression on the parasitized red blood cells that constitutes the major part of the antigen load. In addition to the adhesive proteins described earlier, other antigenic proteins have been identified on parasitized red blood cells, monocytes, and hepatocytes. These include "var" gene products other than the PfEMP-1, the ring-infected erythrocyte surface antigen (RESA), Pf332, 70-kDa and 78-kDa heat shock proteins, and others.[137]

There is evidence that different antigens may provoke different immune responses. For example, glycosylphosphatidylinositol moieties covalently linked to the surface antigens of falciparum malarial parasites appear to act like endotoxin that interacts with upregulated monocyte CD14 receptors, thereby provoking a Th_1 pro-inflammatory response. Conversely, the Pf332 antigen appears to interact with a different monocyte receptor that favors Th2 proliferation, which is associated with immunity to reinfection.[145–147]

The hallmark of pro-inflammatory monocyte activation is the release of TNF-α, which plays a pivotal role in the pathogenesis of acute malarial morbidity. Of equal significance is the release of IL-6, which is the main proliferative signal for Th_1 cells. The latter secrete IFN-α which amplifies the monocyte response by a positive feedback mechanism. The observed increase in neopterin serum levels in malignant malaria is the consequence of this augmented release of IFG-1.

Th_1 activation also leads to B lymphocyte proliferation, with IL-2–induced switching to IgG2 synthesis. This often leads to autoantibody formation that is usually associated with *P. falciparum* and *P. vivax* infections. Anticardiolipin, antiphospholipid, and antineutrophil cytoplasmic antibody (ANCA) have been suggested to have a role in the pathogenesis of microvascular complications. Antibodies to triosephosphate isomerase have been associated with prolonged complement-dependent hemolytic anemia following acute malaria.[137]

Th_2 activation has an immune modulatory function and is associated with immunity to reinfection. The release of IL-4 induces B lymphocyte proliferation, favoring IgE and IgG4 synthesis. Together with IL-10, IL-4 downregulates the monocytes and inhibits the release of IL-8. However, Th_2 lymphocytes have been recently shown to behave as pro-inflammatory cells. This is particularly manifest in cerebral malaria, where IgE antibody levels are considerably elevated. Malarial antigen–IgE antibody complexes are identified by CD23 monocyte receptors, leading to increased TNF-α generation through an NO-transduction mechanism. The interaction of TNF-α and IL-5 leads to eosinophil activation, which seems to be crucial in cerebral malaria.

Peripheral gamma-delta T lymphocytes are strongly upregulated in malaria. They seem to have a mandatory role in the regulation of the early immune response and the elimination of chronic infection. However, their exact role in this respect is not yet understood.

As a consequence of early increase in pro-inflammatory cytokines, the peripheral blood capillaries, mainly in the skeletal muscles, are dilated, leading to decreased peripheral resistance. Blood volume is consequently increased, being associated with increased cardiac output. In severe infection, blood tends to pool in the peripheral capillaries, with fluid transudation into the interstitial tissues, owing to increased permeability. The slow circulation is further impeded by the previously mentioned rheologic abnormalities, leading to impaired cardiac filling. Together with the frequently associated drug-induced left ventricular dysfunction, or, rarely, parasite-induced pericardial tamponade, this leads to a critically low cardiac output and impaired renal perfusion. The latter is augmented by the supervening nonspecific humoral imbalance, endothelial cell activation, and sludging of red blood cells and platelets. Free hemoglobin and myoglobin add their independent ill effects to the renal hemodynamics and tubular cell integrity, leading to ATN.

Glomerulonephritis. Glomerular lesions have been described with *P. falciparum* infection since the early 1970s.[146] Similar lesions were observed later in experimental models infected with the closely related *P. brasilianum.*[133] Subsequent reports, mainly from Africa, have substantiated this clinical entity with both *P. falciparum* and *P. vivax*. These included all ages, although children were the main target of vivax infection. It is impossible to estimate the true incidence because the disease is essentially mild, transient, and overshadowed by other complications. Mild proteinuria, microhematuria, and red blood cell casts were found in 20% to 50% of patients. Nephrotic and acute nephritic syndromes were occasionally seen, but hypertension was unusual. Serum C3 and C4 levels were occasionally reduced during the acute phase. The disease was very rarely progressive. Falciparum glomerulopathy was reversible within 1 to 6 weeks after eradication of the infection.

The typical falciparum glomerular lesion is characterized by prominent mesangial proliferation with many transit cells. Mesangial matrix expansion is modest, and basement membrane changes are unusual. Deposition of an eosinophilic granular material has been noticed along the capillary walls, within the mesangium, and in Bowman's capsule. The glomerular capillaries are often empty, but they may contain a few parasitized red cells or giant nuclear masses in patients with intravascular coagulation. Immunofluorescence shows finely granular IgM and C3 deposits along the capillary walls and in the mesangium. Malarial antigens are occasionally seen, analogous with an animal model,[134] along the glomerular endothelium and the medullary capillaries. ICAM-1 is expressed in the glomerular mesangium, vascular endothelium, and proximal tubular cells. The tubules and the vascular endothelium show expression of TNFα IL-1, IL-6, and granulocyte–macrophage colony-stimulating factor.[147,148] Electron microscopy shows subendothelial and mesangial electron-dense deposits along with granular, fibrillar, and amorphous material.

There is general agreement that the glomerular lesion in falciparum malaria, like that associated with quartan malaria, is immune-complex mediated. Yet, there is an ill-defined proportion of cases in which the glomerular lesions are attributed to direct activation of the alternative complement pathway, thereby explaining the paucity of immune-complex deposits.[137]

Metabolic Abnormalities. The metabolic abnormalities associated with, and often contributing to acute malarial nephropathies are the consequence of: (1) perturbation of the host's red and other cell membranes, (2) the parasite's consumption of nutrients and cofactors, (3) repercussions of the described hemodynamic and immunologic disturbances, and (4) side effects of treatment.

In addition to the de novo synthesis of antigenic and adhesive polypeptides encoded by the parasite's DNA, changes in the parasitized cell membrane structure may lead to important functional abnormalities. Most notorious in falciparum malaria is the inhibition of the erythrocyte magnesium-activated ATPase. This impairs the sodium pump in a "sick-cell syndrome" fashion, leading to internal dilutional hyponatremia. Secondary calcium influx alters the calmodulin-dependent erythrocyte kinetics,[149] reduces hemoglobin–cell wall interaction, and curtails red blood cell deformability. This further augments the peripheral hemodynamic derangement and increases the erythrocyte mechanical fragility. Shortened red blood cell survival is, therefore, almost invariable in malaria.

Even nonparasitized red blood cells undergo membrane changes that lead to rosette formation. Many factors have been implicated in this phenomenon including parasite-derived rosettins, immunoglobulins, and other plasma protein abnormalities. As mentioned previously, rosette formation is an important contributor to the disturbed peripheral blood rheology in malaria.

It is not clear whether the same or other factors, or the abnormal cytokine profile supervening in malaria, are responsible for the hepatocyte membrane abnormality that leads to cholestatic jaundice in the majority of cases.[150] The same question applies to leaky muscle membranes associated with malarial rhabdomyolysis.[151]

Plasmodia consume large quantities of glucose for their metabolism. This seems to overwhelm the host's compensatory mechanisms, often leading to clinically overt hypoglycemia. A recent study has also shown an increase of the serum transketolase activity in patients with falciparum malaria. This indicates thiamine depletion, which is attributed to the increased demand for the parasite's glycolytic pathway. Because thiamine is an essential cofactor for coenzyme A, its depletion may be an additional factor in depressing the host's aerobic glycolysis, causing increased anaerobic glycolysis (Pasteur effect) and lactic acid accumulation. However, none of the clinical manifestations of severe malaria, particularly the neurologic aspects, could be statistically correlated to measurable biochemical parameters of thiamine deficiency.[137]

Other factors contributing to hypoglycemia in malaria include hyperinsulinemia associated with quinine or sulfadoxine-pyrimethamine[152] therapy and possibly the impaired glucogenesis in patients with significant hepatic complications.

The disturbed peripheral blood rheology, the release of local cytokines, and the immune-mediated systemic inflammatory response integrate in the pathogenesis of peripheral pooling leading to impaired tissue oxygenation.

The metabolic sequelae of tissue hypoxia and potential impairment of glucose availability include increased lactic acid production with increased lactate-to-pyruvate ratio,[153] depressed mitochondrial respiration, and increased generation of reactive oxygen molecules.[154] Inducible NO generation and abnormal lipid peroxidation are documented consequences of the increased oxidative stress in falciparum malaria.[155]

A lot of secondary humoral changes are seen in falciparum malaria.[136] These include hypercatecholaminemia; increased levels of circulating plasma renin activity, kinins, and prostaglandins; ADH secretion; and hyperinsulinemia in quinine-treated patients. Most of these effects are nonspecific, being attributed to the severe acute infection. However, they seem to have a significant impact on the final target of all pathogenetic factors in malignant malaria, namely, the microcirculation.

Fluid and electrolyte changes in malaria are of clinical and physiologic interest.[47] Hyponatremia, usually asymptomatic, is observed in 67% of patients. Hyponatremic patients have a higher parasitemia than those with normal serum sodium levels. There are multiple causes including increased nonosmotic ADH release, low sodium intake, sodium loss, cellular sodium influx, and resetting of osmoreceptors. Hypernatremia, usually associated with hypothalamic injury, is rare. Hypokalemia, attributed to augmented tubular loss, is common. Hyperkalemia is seen in patients with intravascular hemolysis, rhabdomyolysis, or renal failure. As in sepsis, hypocalcemia and hypophosphatemia are seen in severe malaria. Hypocalcemia without renal failure may be caused by unexplained hypoparathyroidism. Phosphate shift into the cells induced by respiratory alkalosis accounts for hypophosphatemia. Both hypocalcemia and hypophosphatemia are transient and resolve with clinical improvement. Of clinical importance is the decreased response to water load, which can be observed in moderate and severe malaria. In this clinical setting, hemodynamic changes include hypervolemia, decreased peripheral vascular resistance, increased cardiac output, elevated plasma renin activity, and increased plasma norepinephrine levels, ADH, and renal vascular resistance. Hyponatremia is an important clinical marker in these patients. A decreased response to water load occurs in 20% of hyponatremic patients. Fluid administration to the patient with moderate or severe malaria should be cautiously done to avoid fluid overload. Furosemide should be given when there is decreased response to fluid load.

Babesiosis. This rare febrile disease is closely related to falciparum malaria.[156] It is not strictly tropical, as most cases have been described in Eastern Europe and the United States. However, it is often confused with falciparum malaria in patients returning from the tropics. Either *Babesia microti* or *Babesia divergens* is responsible for infection. The disease manifests with fever, chills, and malaise associated with nausea and arthralgias. It is particularly severe in asplenic patients, who are more likely to develop AKI as a result of hypotension, intravascular hemolysis, and disseminated intravascular coagulation. Mesangial proliferative glomerulonephritis with deposition of IgG and C3 is observed.[157,158] Babesiosis has been reported in a renal transplant recipient due to transfusion with contaminated blood.[159] Diagnosis is made by finding the intraerythrocytic parasite in a blood smear or by a serologic test. Therapy with quinine sulfate and clindamycin is usually effective in eradicating the parasite. Pentamidine is effective in resistant cases.

Visceral Leishmaniasis. This disease, also known as Kala azar (or black sickness), is one of three forms of human leishmaniasis with worldwide distribution, being highly

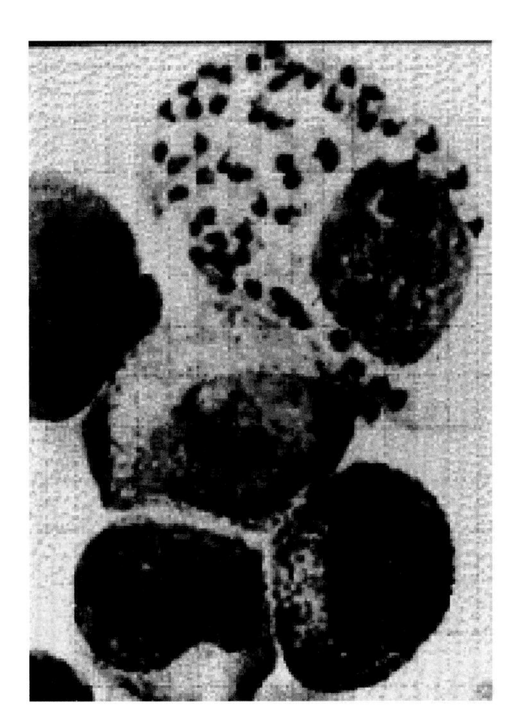

FIGURE 63.12 *Leishmania donovani*. Amastigotes in a monocyte.

prevalent in east and north Africa, northeastern China, Iran, the Mediterranean region, and Brazil. It is caused *by Leishmania donovani* or *L. infantum*, protozoa that infect humans through a sandfly bite. The parasite lives and multiplies in the monocytes (Fig. 63.12), being protected by a peculiar host–parasite interaction that involves depression of cell-mediated immunity.

Most patients remain asymptomatic, often with spontaneous cure. Leishmaniasis can occur in the immunocompromised individual, including an increasing frequency in HIV infected subjects.[160] Overt disease ushers in with pyrexia, chills, sweating, asthenia, weight loss, and hepatosplenomegaly. Lymphadenopathy is often noticed but is seldom striking. Skin nodules containing the parasite may be seen, particularly at the inoculation site. If untreated, the disease may end fatally, usually due to intercurrent infections. Liposomal amphotericin B is the current treatment of choice because the response to the commonly used pentavalent antimony is slow, often incomplete, and may be challenged with primary resistance in about 10% of cases.[161]

The main renal lesions in Kala azar are interstitial. In the immunocompetent patient, the parasite induces a chronic inflammatory lesion[162] (Fig. 63.13) that is usually asymptomatic and rarely progresses to fibrosis. On the other hand, infection in immunocompromised kidney transplant recipients may lead to a more severe acute interstitial graft inflammation with pyrexia and impaired graft function.[118] This has often been confused with a cellular rejection, but the proper diagnosis was made upon spotting the characteristic macrophage-laden amastigotes (Fig. 63.12).

Glomerular lesions have rarely been described in Kala azar, mesangioproliferative glomerulonephritis being the most common pattern (Fig. 63.13). IgM and C3 deposits were detected in the capillary walls and mesangium. Leishmanial antigens have been detected in experimental models with similar lesions,[163] which have been attributed to activation of humoral as well as cellular pathways.[164] Glomerular amyloid deposits have been described in patients with concomitant HIV infection,[125] presumably attributed to critical impairment of monocyte AA protein scavenger functions.

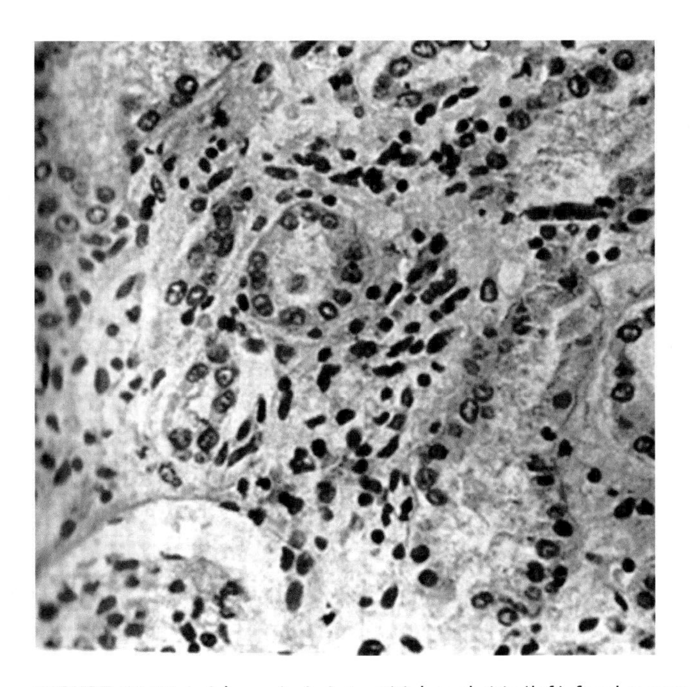

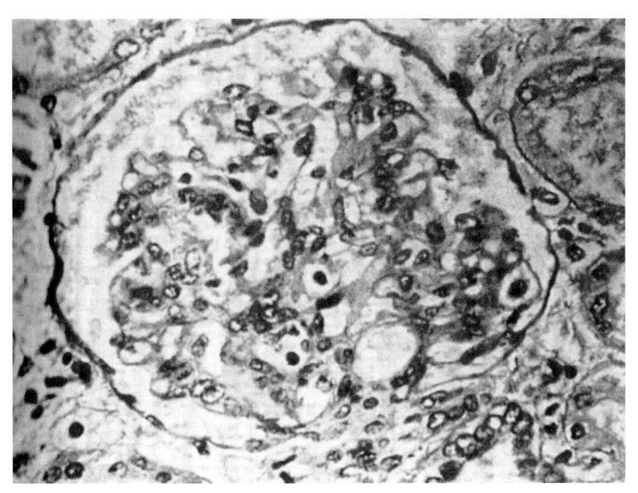

FIGURE 63.13 Leishmaniasis. Interstitial nephritis (*left*); focal mesangial proliferation (*right*).

Trypanosomiasis. African trypanosomiasis, caused by *Trypanosoma brucei* and transmitted by the tsetse fly, is the cause of sleeping sickness. The Rhodesian version is an acute febrile illness with neurologic and cardiac manifestations, anemia, and disseminated intravascular coagulation that often ends fatally within a few weeks. AKI may be encountered during the terminal phases as a component of multiorgan failure.

The Gambian type is more chronic, initially presenting with pyrexia, lymphadenopathy, and a skin eruption, followed several months or even years later by progressive meningoencephalitic manifestations.

Experimental infection in monkeys by *T. brucei* leads to proliferative glomerulonephritis,[165] with IgM and C3 deposits in the mesangium and along the capillary walls. Serologic studies in this model showed high levels of circulating immune complexes and a reduction of serum C3 levels with normal C4 levels, suggestive of direct alternative complement activation by the parasitic antigens. Similar observations were made in a seminal murine model, in which electron-dense deposits were also found in the mesangium and subendothelial space.[166] Whether similar lesions also occur in humans is unknown. Clinically relevant renal complications have not been reported.

South American trypanosomiasis, known as Chagas disease, has attracted considerable recent attention in view of its potential role in organ transplantation (see later text).

Toxoplasmosis. *Toxoplasma gondii* infection is common worldwide, with a current estimate of 500 million infected humans. It is acquired through contact with cats and certain birds, by ingestion of cysts or oocysts. It can also occur through transplacental transmission (congenital toxoplasmosis). In most instances, the infection is dormant, with a few cysts lying in the lymph nodes, muscle, heart, or brain and little or no inflammatory response.

Overt clinical disease is rare in the immunocompetent individual. It usually manifests by cervical lymphadenopathy associated with pyrexia and malaise. The disease is self-limiting in most patients. Progressive chorioretinitis is the notorious expression of congenital toxoplasmosis in the immunocompetent individual.

In the immunocompromised, the disease is much more disseminated, presenting with pyrexia, hepatosplenomegaly, pneumonitis, maculopapular rash, myositis, myocarditis, meningoencephalitis, or central nervous system mass lesions. The course is rapidly fatal.

Renal involvement in the immunocompetent or the immunocompromised host has been rarely described. The lesion was mainly glomerular, with a mesangioproliferative pattern. Mesangial IgM and toxoplasma antigen deposits have been detected by immunofluorescent study. Renal disease was subclinical, although the nephrotic syndrome has been described in association with chorioretinitis in congenital toxoplasmosis.[167] In more recent reports, however, the potential etiology of glomerular injury was mixed and the precise role of toxoplasmosis remained questionable.

Cryptosporidiosis. The causative protozoan, *Cryptosporidium*, belongs to the same family as *T. gondii*. The disease is also acquired through contact with infected domestic animals. It has recently emerged as an important opportunistic infection in immunocompromised patients in the tropics and in the West, causing severe watery diarrhea, abdominal cramps, and occasional infection of the biliary system, leading to ascending cholangitis and rarely gangrene of the gallbladder. It is not surprising that renal involvement can occur through nonspecific inflammatory factors resulting in proteinuria and urinary sediment changes. There is currently no effective therapy for cryptosporidiosis.[168]

Echinococcosis. Humans act as an intermediate host for *Echinococcus granulosus*, a parasite of worldwide distribution, mainly encountered among sheep-herding populations and those in close contact with dogs. Infection is acquired by ingestion of eggs contaminating the environment through the feces of infected dogs. The ova hatch in the gut, and larvae migrate into the liver, lungs, brain, kidneys, muscles, and other tissues where they eventually yield cysts. The cysts contain and reproduce protoscoleces, which have the potential of completing the life cycle if ingested by a dog.

Echinococcosis (hydatid disease) in humans is characterized by multiorgan infection. Involvement of the kidneys may be silent, being discovered only during routine imaging. Hilar cysts have been described to cause calyceal back pressure and to stretch the arteries, leading to renovascular hypertension.[169]

Immune-mediated glomerular injury has also been described in several case reports. The disease was usually mild or subclinical. It affected young adults and presented with mild-to-moderate proteinuria and an increase in the urinary cellular elements. Renal biopsy revealed minimal change, membranous or mesangioproliferative glomerulonephritis with IgM and C3 deposits.[170] IgA nephropathy has been reported in Europe, in patients with hepatic cysts.[171] Parasitic antigens have not pursued in the glomeruli, but they are readily detected in circulating immune complexes, particularly after mebendazole treatment or surgical intervention.[169]

Schistosomiasis. Schistosomiasis is among the most widely spread of parasitic diseases, with an estimated 500 to 600 million people at risk, 200 million actually infested, 20 million with serious morbidity, and 20,000 annual deaths attributed directly to the disease. There are many strains of schistosomes, of which only five infect humans: *Schistosoma haematobium*, mainly in Africa; *Schistosoma mansoni* in Africa and South America; *Schistosoma japonicum* in China, Southeast Asia, and Japan; *Schistosoma intercalatum*, related to *S. mansoni* and found mainly in central Africa; and *Schistosoma mekongi*, related to *S. japonicum* and found in a few foci in Southeast Asia.

Infection is acquired through contact with fresh water harboring the specific snails, which act as the intermediate hosts and define the prevalence and density of infestation in different geographic areas. The infective agent is the cercaria, a fishlike organism with a bifid tail, 400 to 600 μm in length; the organism penetrates the skin or mucous membranes, loses its tail, and becomes a schistosomula. The latter gains access to the bloodstream through lymphatics and circulates in different capillary beds until it randomly reaches the portal or perivesical venous plexus. These sites contain trophic factors that promote the rapid growth of the schistosomula, which soon matures into an adult worm in the downstream veins. The adult worm is bisexual, the male being stronger and larger. The female stays in almost continuous copulation with the male in a special groove called the gynecophoral canal. It only leaves to travel against the bloodstream to lay eggs in the submucosa of the urinary bladder (*S. haematobium*), colon, or rectum (*S. mansoni* and *S. japonicum*). During its active sexual life, the female *S. haematobium* or *S. mansoni* lays about 300 ova per day, whereas *S. japonicum* may lay up to 3,000 ova per day. Most ova find their way to the exterior by virtue of spines in their shells, aided by the muscle contractions of their habitat. Contact with fresh water leads to swelling and rupture of the shells, and release of miracidia, the infective stage to the snail, which completes the cycle.

Ova that fail to be exteriorized are the principal cause of pathogenicity. They cause a delayed hypersensitive reaction and granuloma formation that heals with fibrosis. The resulting functional consequences depend on the strategic anatomic sites of such fibrosis. Ova may be driven back along the bloodstream to deposit in different organs, where they also form granulomas. Most notorious are the hepatic granulomas, leading to periportal fibrosis and portal hypertension, and the pulmonary granulomas, which result in arteriolar occlusion and pulmonary hypertension. Other metastatic lesions include cerebral granulomas, often seen with *S. japonicum* infestations, subcutaneous nodules, and ocular granulomas, which are occasionally mistaken for other clinically similar conditions.[172]

Renal Disorders Associated with Schistosomiasis

Schistosomiasis Haematobium. The deposited ova form small tubercles that superficially resemble those of tuberculosis, hence, the name pseudotubercles. These coalesce to form nodules, which often get secondarily infected. With the evolution of the lesions, the underlying bladder wall becomes fibrotic and the trapped ova become calcified. A thin mucosal layer may cover these lesions, which appear as pale granular areas called sandy patches. Other late lesions include mucosal cysts and fibrotic nodules, cystitis cystica, and cystitis glandularis. Bladder malignancy often supervenes—a slowly growing squamous cell carcinoma being the predominant histopathologic pattern.

Functional consequences often complicate urinary schistosomiasis, depending on the site and extent of fibrosis. At the lower ends of the ureters, this leads to partial obstruction; at the bladder neck, it results in chronic outflow obstruction; and in the detrusor, it impairs contractility, resulting in an atonic viscus, which is often associated with vesicoureteric reflux. Upstream repercussions are attributed to ureteric obstruction, reflux, and chronic infection.

The clinical features of *Schistosomiasis haematobium* are encountered soon after the establishment of infection. Painful terminal hematuria is the time-honored presentation. It often affects children, more frequently men, reflecting the variance in exposure imposed by social constraints. The diagnosis is confirmed by finding the characteristic ova, with terminal spines, seen with routine urine microscopy. Pyuria and bacilluria are also detected in the presence of secondary infection. If untreated, hematuria persists for many years, although its intensity declines as the process of bladder fibrosis progresses. Eventually the patient is left with the symptoms of chronic cystitis, and upstream complications may develop.

Renal morbidity (Fig. 63.14) is reported in different endemic areas to vary from 2% to 52% of patients with lower urinary tract *S. haematobium*, depending on the infective

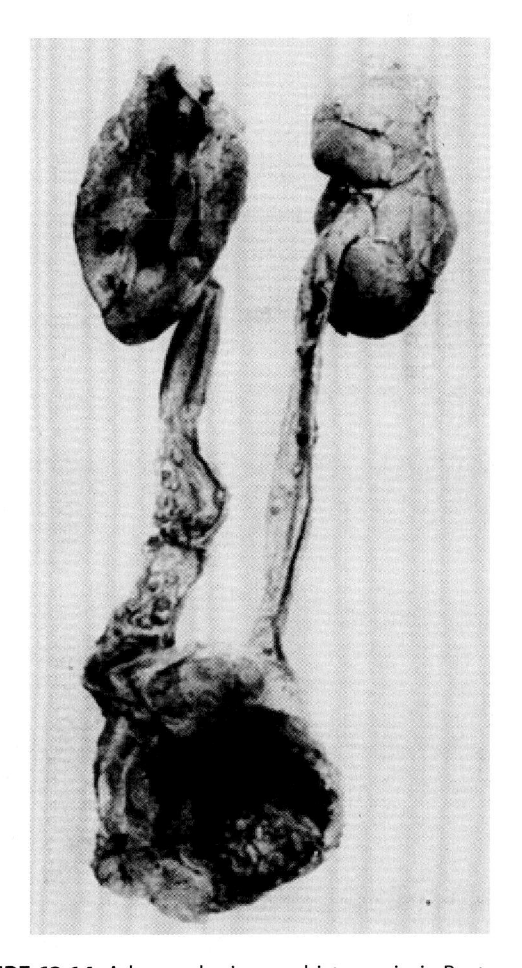

FIGURE 63.14 Advanced urinary schistosomiasis. Postmortem specimen showing chronic cystitis, a bladder carcinoma, bilateral ureteric dilatation with inflammatory cystic lesions (cystic ureteritis), and bilateral hydronephrosis with cortical scarring.

strain, intensity of infestation, availability of therapy, and probably genetic predisposition.[172]

Because the disease is usually localized in the submucosa of the lower ureteric sites, the proximal healthy part often undergoes significant hypertrophy, which allows adequate urodynamic compensation without any back-pressure sequelae. However, hydronephrosis develops in 9.7% to 48% of patients who fail to maintain this compensatory mechanism. Ascending infection is common, usually after instrumentation performed for various reasons. It is particularly common in patients with vesicoureteric reflux, again frequently induced by surgical or instrumental interventions. In addition to the regular features of acute and chronic pyelonephritis, infection often leads to the formation of stones. The proportion of patients with *S. haematobium* who ultimately progress to end-stage is unknown; a broad estimate in Egypt is 1 per 1,000.[32] With the high prevalence of infestation, even this small proportion amounts to 40 patients per million of the total population.

Early haematobium infestation is easy to cure. Several drugs have been used through the years, starting with the old-fashioned antimony preparations and ending up with the more modern, highly effective, and safe compounds niridazole and praziquantel. Surgical treatment is needed occasionally for the relief of obstruction or repair of reflux. ESKD management is classic, although often modified because of the problems imposed by active chronic pyelonephritis and bladder fibrosis.

S. Mansoni. This organism is principally an inhabitant of the portal venous tributaries, with colorectal disease and periportal hepatic fibrosis being the major consequences of infestation. During the 1970s, experimental and clinical studies from Brazil and Egypt established that an immune-mediated glomerular injury may complicate this disease. Of the more than 100 antigens identified in the parasite, those of the adult worm's gut were incriminated in the pathogenesis of renal lesions. Particularly interesting are a proteoglycan and a glycoprotein, often referred to as cathodal and anodal antigens, respectively, found by immunofluorescence in the early glomerular lesions associated with schistosomiasis.[173]

The initial glomerular response in humans and in large and small experimental animals is essentially mesangial, with focal or diffuse axial cellular proliferation and no matrix expansion (Fig. 63.15). IgM and C3 deposits are detected by immunofluorescence, often along with parasitic antigens.[124] This lesion is not specific for *S. mansoni*, being also observed in humans with *S. haematobium* infection and in experimental

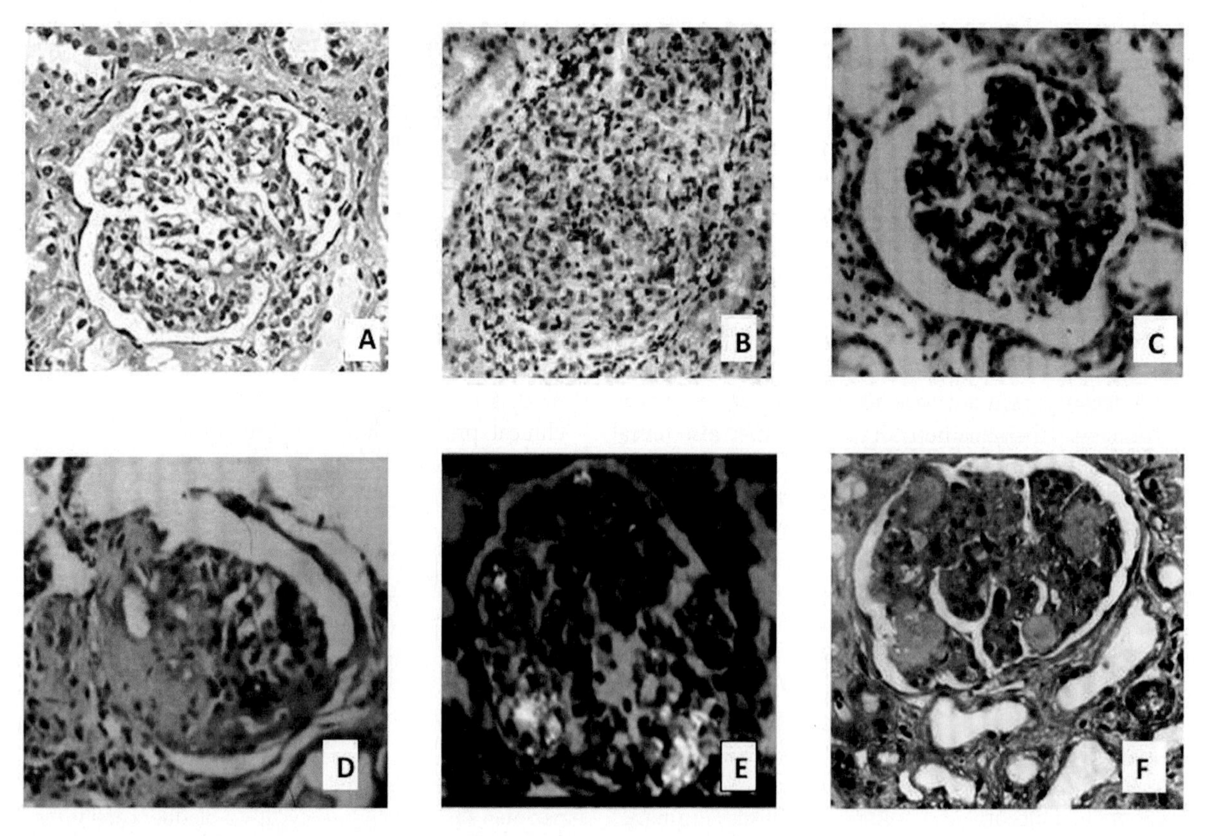

FIGURE 63.15 Schistosoma-associated glomerular lesions. **A:** Class I (axial mesangioproliferative glomerular nephritis [GN]); **(B)** class II (exudative GN); **(C)** class III (mesangiocapillary) GN; **(D)** class IV (focal segmental glomerulosclerosis); **(E)** class V (amyloidosis); and **(F)** class VI (mixed amyloidosis and cryoglobulinemic GN).

animals infected with *S. japonicum*. Apart from the nature of the antigen deposits, this condition is morphologically similar to that seen with many other parasitic glomerulopathies.[174]

Only mild clinical manifestations, usually limited to subnephrotic proteinuria and increased cellular excretion in urine, are associated with this lesion (class I). There are considerable doubts whether the lesion progresses in the absence of other factors. However, the reported response to treatment with antiparasitic agents, steroids, and immunosuppressive agents has not been confirmed.[175]

The initial glomerular lesions may subsequently progress into three distinct clinicopathologic syndromes.

Exudative glomerulonephritis (class II) often complicates concomitant *Salmonella* infection, a frequent association in endemic areas, which leads to an acute, reversible nephrotic syndrome.[124]

Progression into either *type III mesangiocapillary (membranoproliferative) glomerulonephritis (class III)* or *focal segmental sclerosis (class IV)* seems to occur mainly in the presence of significant hepatic disease. The crucial role of the liver has been documented in experimental models, postmortem, and clinical studies.[124] When associated with significant impairment of macrophage function, liver disease seems to permit a high worm antigen load to escape from the portal into the systemic circulation, thereby contributing to the formation of pathogenic immune complexes. Hepatic fibrosis has also been blamed for the defective clearance of IgA, originating in the gut in response to the parasite's antigenic products.[176] On the other hand, data suggest switching of B lymphocytes in favor of IgA synthesis under the effect of IL-10 which supervenes in late stages of parasitic infection.[53] Superimposed on the initial glomerular injury, IgA may be crucial in the progression of glomerular lesions into an overt nephropathy, and further on into ESKD. Autoimmunity may also have a potential role in disease progression.[53]

The classic clinical presentation is the development of nephrotic edema and hypertension (50%) in a patient with typical hepatosplenic schistosomiasis. The diagnosis is supported by finding living schistosomal ova in the stools or rectal snips or by acquiring serologic evidence of active infestation. Liver biopsy results reveal the characteristic periportal fibrosis mostly sparing the hepatocytes, and may also reveal deposited ova or worm pigments. This histopathologic pattern is reflected on conventional liver function tests, which are usually nearly normal unless HBV or HCV infection is associated, which is fairly common. Endoscopic examination usually shows lower esophageal or fundal varices.

Examination of renal biopsy specimens usually reveals either of the two described patterns of glomerular injury, probably depending on genetic factors.[124] Immunofluorescence shows IgG and IgA deposits, and occasionally IgM and C3 deposits. Worm antigens are seldom seen at this stage. Variable degrees of nonspecific tubulointerstitial lesions have been observed, particularly with concomitant *S. haematobium* infection.

Both glomerular lesions are progressive. They do not respond to treatment. ESKD ultimately develops in those who survive the risks of ruptured esophageal varices or hepatocellular failure when the disease is compounded by viral hepatitis.

The epidemiologic importance of classes III and IV schistosomal glomerulopathy as a cause of ESKD is not accurately quantitated; certain estimates suggest the figures of 10 per million of the general population[32] and 15% of those with schistosomal hepatic fibrosis.[124]

Renal amyloidosis (class V) is the third potential outcome of schistosomal glomerulopathy, based on experimental findings in small laboratory animals[177] and epidemiologic evidence in endemic areas.[124]

It is suggested that the chronic parasitic antigen load of either *S. mansoni* or *S. haematobium* may lead to increased synthesis and/or impaired uptake of amyloid-A (AA protein) by the monocytes, and that local glomerular changes enhance deposition of this protein in the characteristic fibrillar structure.[124] The clinical presentation of *Schistosoma*-associated amyloidosis resembles that of mesangiocapillary glomerulonephritis and focal segmental sclerosis, yet hepatosplenic disease may be less prominent and hypertension is less frequent. However, the disease progresses more rapidly to ESKD.

With the increasing encounter of HCV-associated *Schistosoma mansoni* hepatic fibrosis, a peculiar renal syndrome *(class VI)* was recently identified.[178] This consists of a mixture of glomerular amyloidosis, IgM mesangial deposits, and macroglobulinemic vasculitis and tubular casts. It is attributed to the ambiguous activation of the classical and the alternative activation of the antigen presenting cells by the virus and the parasite respectively. In addition, the T lymphocyte response may be modified by the direct invasion of HCV via the CD80 ligands.

S. japonicum. This infestation is similar to that with *S. mansoni* in causing hepatic fibrosis, portal hypertension, and splenomegaly. Metastatic lesions, particularly those in the central nervous system, are more common and more serious. Although most of the experimental background on schistosomal glomerulopathy is based on *S. japonicum* models, the impact of this infection is extremely limited in clinical practice. Early mesangioproliferative lesions have been described, but overt disease is seldom reported and even denied.[179] The reasons for this discrepancy are unclear; the nature of parasitic antigens, host genetic factors, limited hepatic involvement, and other factors may be involved. The high prevalence of IgA nephropathy in areas where *S. japonicum* infection is endemic may mask the identity of *S. japonicum* glomerulopathy as a distinct disease.

Filariasis. Filariasis is highly prevalent in Africa, Asia, and South America. Of the eight filarial strains that infect humans, *Wuchereria bancrofti*, *Brugia malayi*, *Onchocerca volvulus*, and *Loa loa* are most frequently encountered in clinical practice. All species are transmitted by insect bites. The infective larvae migrate into the lymphatic vessels and slowly mature into adult worms over 3 to 18 months.

Adult *W. bancrofti* and *B. malayi* reside in the lymph nodes or afferent lymphatic vessels for decades. They mate and deliver the microfilariae, which either circulate in the bloodstream or migrate by way of the lymphatic channels to the dermis, awaiting their vector to complete the life cycle. *W. bancrofti* and *B. malayi* infections may be entirely dormant (asymptomatic microfilaremia) and are usually identified by the accidental discovery of eosinophilia. Infected subjects with a pronounced immunologic response may present with hypereosinophilia and pulmonary involvement. The classic presentation, however, is recurrent pyrexia with chills and lymphangitis caused by the local immune-mediated granulomatous response against the adult worms. In *B. malayi* infection, this reaction often leads to the formation of local abscesses that rupture and subsequently heal with characteristic scars. With *W. bancrofti*, the local reaction usually leads to lymphatic obstruction, gross upstream dilation, and distortion. Elephantiasis of the extremities and genitalia is the usual consequence (Fig. 63.16). Rupture of the dilated lymphatic vessels may lead to chylous effusions, usually in the form of hydrocele or ascites. Rupture of the dilated retroperitoneal lymphatics into the renal pelvis leads to chyluria.

Adult *O. volvulus* coil into spherical bundles in subcutaneous tissues and deep fascia, leading to characteristic nodules called onchocercomas. Regional lymph nodes may be enlarged. The worms deliver millions of microfilariae, which migrate into the skin and ocular tissues. In the latter tissues, microfilariae may cause keratitis, anterior uveitis, and less often chorioretinitis. Blindness (river blindness) supervenes in 1% to 4% of patients.

Adult *L. loa* worms live wandering in the subcutaneous and subconjunctival tissues. They may induce a peculiar hypersensitivity skin reaction, the Calabar swellings, which are localized erythematous and angioedematous lesions. Generalized angioedema may be encountered in expatriates and undernourished native individuals.

Renal Involvement in Filariasis. The best-documented renal lesion in filariasis is that associated with *O. volvulus*. In a large epidemiologic study in Cameroon, where this strain is hyperendemic, proteinuria was significantly more frequent among infected subjects.[180] Minimal change, mesangioproliferative, mesangiocapillary, and chronic sclerosing glomerulonephritis lesions are most often encountered (Fig. 63.17). Subendothelial and mesangial immune complexes containing IgM, IgG, C3, and onchocercal antigens[181] were detected by immunofluorescence and mesangial electron-dense deposits,[182] by electron microscopy. Onchocercal glomerulonephritis is known to recur in transplanted kidneys.

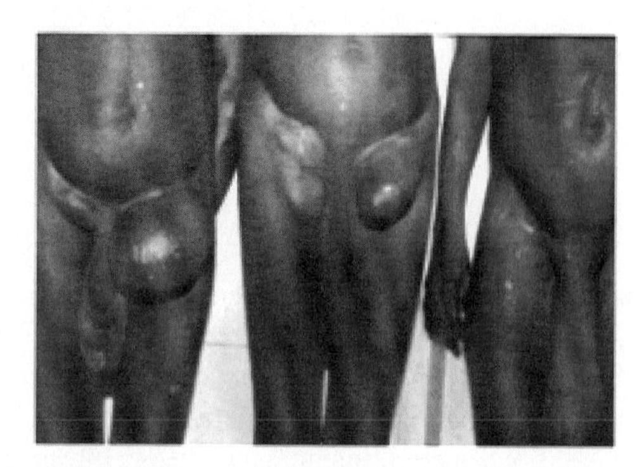

FIGURE 63.16 Filariasis: hanging scrotum with massive inguinal lymphadenopathy.

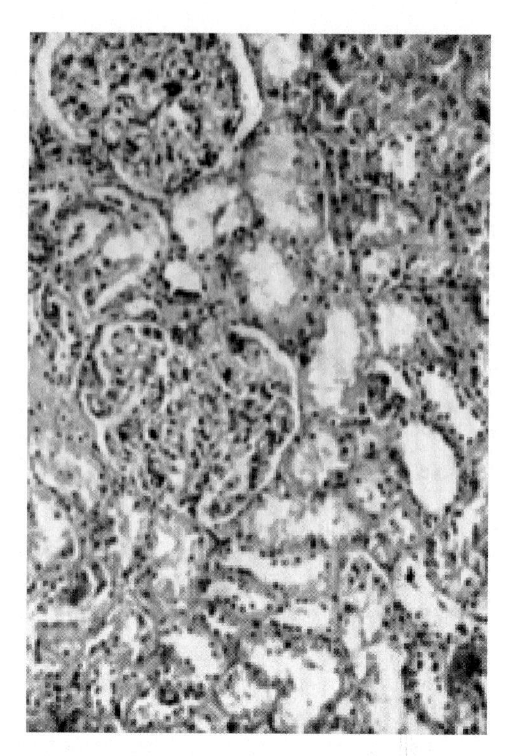

FIGURE 63.17 Filaria-associated mesangioproliferative glomerulonephritis.

Similar lesions have also been described in bancroftiasis[183] and loiasis.[184] Bancrofti specific immune complexes were detected in urine of 34% of infected subjects in one series.[185] In addition, an exudative eosinophilic glomerulonephritis has been documented in patients with *W. bancrofti* infection,[186] and collapsing FSGS in those with *L. loa*[187] infections. Microfilariae may be seen in the glomerular capillaries.

The clinical spectrum of filarial glomerulonephritis ranges from asymptomatic proteinuria to ESKD. Nephrotic syndrome is often ascribed to such infections in endemic areas. Acute nephritic syndrome in patients with bancroftiasis has been reported. Treatment with diethylcarbamazine (DEC) or ivermectin (IVM), alone or in combination with albendazole, may help to resolve early glomerular lesions, but it usually fails when the nephrotic syndrome is manifested.[188] Renal disease may be aggravated by treatment with either DEC or IVM in heavily infested patients, which is attributed to further release of filarial antigens.

Trichinosis. Trichinosis is a nematodal infection of worldwide distribution, being particularly prevalent in communities where raw, smoked, or undercooked meat, especially pork, is eaten. It is fairly common in Southeast Asia and Latin America but, for obvious reasons, is rare in countries with large Muslim and Jewish populations.

Infection is acquired by ingestion of infective larvae encysted in striated muscles. Excystation occurs by acid-pepsin digestion in the stomach; parasites mature in the upper small intestine. The adult female produces larvae, which penetrate the blood and lymphatic vessels and migrate into different host organs. Those reaching the muscles become encysted and remain viable for many years.

Although trichinosis is often associated with nonspecific gastrointestinal symptoms, its main clinical impact is related to the eosinophilic granulomatous reaction that the encysted larvae provoke in different organs, including skeletal and cardiac muscles, lungs, and the central nervous system. Proptosis and periorbital edema associated with pyrexia and myalgia are the usual clinical clues to the diagnosis.

Renal involvement in trichinosis was vaguely reported as early as 1916.[189] It became more firmly established in recent years as more elaborate diagnostic criteria became established. The lesions are mainly glomerular, in the form of mesangial proliferation associated with immunoglobulin, C3, and occasionally fibrin deposits.[190] Trichinella-specific immune complexes were detected in the glomeruli of infected rats.[191]

Renal involvement is usually subclinical, with mild proteinuria and microhematuria. Blood pressure is not elevated, and renal function is usually preserved or only mildly impaired. Hypoalbuminemia is occasionally noted, leading to contraction of the blood volume with a mild reduction of p-aminohippurate and creatinine clearances. Circulating immune complexes associated with a decrease in serum C3 level have been described. All clinical abnormalities are reversible by thiabendazole treatment (50 mg per kg of body weight per day for 2 days).[190]

Opisthorchiasis. The disease is caused by *Opisthorchis felineus* and *Opisthorchis viverrini* through the ingestion of raw or undercooked fish. *O. felineus* is common in the Philippines, Vietnam, and India, whereas *O. viverrini* is prevalent in Thailand, Laos, and Kampuchea. The liver is the target organ where the parasites lodge in the biliary tract. The incidence of cholangiocarcinoma is high in opisthorchiasis. Renal failure can occur in the patients with opisthorchiasis.[192] AKI is seen in 49% of the patients with cholangiocarcinoma and severe jaundice. Hyponatremia and hypokalemia secondary to natriuresis and kaliuresis are frequently observed.[193] The causes of renal failure are multiple and include hypovolemia, endotoxemia, cardiac dysfunction, effects of vasoactive mediators, hypotension, hyperbilirubinemia, and hyperuricosuria.

Renal pathologic changes[194] include tubular degeneration with bile staining and vacuolation of proximal tubules in the potassium-depleted patients. IgA deposition in the mesangium may be observed. In Syrian golden hamsters infected with *O. viverrini*, immune complex glomerulonephritis with deposition of IgG antibody specific to the integumental membrane of the adult worm has been shown. Renal amyloidosis with AA protein deposition was observed in the glomeruli and interstitium.[195]

Strongyloidiasis. Infestation by *Strongyloides stercoralis* is endemic worldwide, particularly in the warm climates of the tropics. Infection is acquired by skin contact with soil containing the free filariform larvae. The larvae migrate into the pulmonary capillaries where they break into the alveolar spaces, ascend through the airways to the pharynx, are then swallowed, and eventually mature in the duodenum into adult worms. In most infested subjects, only female worms are found in the small intestine. They reproduce by parthenogenesis, forming eggs that hatch in the gut and release rhabditiform larvae, which eventually transform into the infective filariform larvae in the soil. This transformation can also occur in the gut of an immunocompromised host.

Strongyloidiasis is a mild disease in the immunocompetent individual, being either asymptomatic or associated with vague abdominal symptoms. In the immunocompromised, however, reinfection with filariform larvae can occur through the intestinal walls or the perianal skin. As this process is repeated, hyperinfection occurs, leading to a potentially fatal disseminated disease. As the infective larvae migrate through the lungs, they can induce pulmonary hemorrhage and acute respiratory complications that mimic the adult respiratory distress syndrome. The larvae can also disseminate into various organs including the brain, eyes, pancreas, peritoneum, kidneys, and skin where they form creeping eruptions.[118] Minimal change disease[196] and mesangial proliferative glomerulonephritis with nephrotic syndrome have been observed in association with strongyloidiasis. The nephrotic syndrome resolved after treatment of the disease.[197] The response to thiabendazole treatment is remarkable, with parasitologic cure in more than 90% of patients.

Other Parasitic Diseases. Renal lesions rarely occur in visceral larva migrans caused by the migration of larval stages of *Toxocara canis* or *Toxocara cati*.[198] Granulomatous changes consisting of eosinophils and histiocytes with giant cells may be observed. Hematuria and eosinophiluria may be noted.

Immune complex–mediated glomerulonephritis has been reported in amebiasis.[199] However, ameba antigen was not demonstrated in the immune deposits.

TOXIC NEPHROPATHIES IN THE TROPICS

Animal Toxins

The kidney, as a highly vascularized and excretory organ, is vulnerable to toxin poisoning. Release of proinflammatory cytokines and vasoactive mediators leading to decreased renal blood flow is fundamental in the development of renal failure. Renal injury can also be induced by toxin enzymes, especially phospholipases and metalloproteases. Other associated factors including hemorrhage, hypovolemia, intravascular coagulation, intravascular hemolysis, and rhabdomyolysis are additional insults.[46]

Snake Bites

Snake bites are a worldwide problem. The vast majority occur in the tropical countries of Africa, south and Southeast Asia, and Latin America.

Renal involvement in snake bites has been observed following bites by snakes from the families Elapidae, Viperidae, and Colubridae. Renal failure complicates in 1.2% to 70% of all snake envenomations.[43,200,201] Most cases are due to the snake venoms with hemotoxicity or myotoxicity,[46] whereas direct nephrotoxicity has also been shown in experimental models.[202] Commonly reported are patients with AKI due to bites of rattlesnake, Russell's viper, saw scale viper, *Bothrops jararaca*, puff adder, brown snakes, and sea snakes.[46,201]

Clinically, the victim shows either local symptoms with pain, swelling, local bleeding at the site of bite, or systemic symptoms with generalized bleeding, hypotension, or oliguria. Oliguria usually occurs 24 to 72 hours following the bite. Patients can be hypotensive at presentation, but often are normotensive. With viper bites, renal failure is usually associated with intravascular hemolysis and disseminated intravascular coagulation. Those patients with renal failure have higher urinary fibrin degradation product than those with normal renal function, suggesting the role of intravascular coagulation in the pathogenesis of renal failure.[203] In sea snake bites, renal failure is associated with rhabdomyolysis. Sepsis can be a complicating factor at presentation. Nephrotic syndrome has been reported in a rare patient following snake bite.[204] However, transient heavy proteinuria can occur in patients bitten by Russell's viper.

In the majority of the patients, histologic findings are compatible with acute tubular necrosis.[46,201] Acute cortical necrosis is seen in a significant minority of the patients. Electron microscopic study in Russell's viper envenoming complicated by AKI has shown glomerular mesangial hypercellularity, vascular endothelial swelling, tubular epithelial necrosis, and interstitial infiltrates. Interstitial nephritis, proliferative glomerulonephritis, and arteritis of interlobular vessels have been reported. Granular deposition of IgM and C3 in the mesangium has been observed. There is evidence of deposition of immune complex in situ.[43] In sea snake envenoming, rhabdomyolysis is the primary event leading to myoglobinuric renal failure.[205] Renal histology shows tubular necrosis while muscle shows diffuse hyaline lesions of its fibers.

Pathogenesis. Snake venom contains many proteolytic enzymes and phospholipases capable of triggering hemolysis, disseminated intravascular coagulopathy, fibrinolysis, complement activation, rhabdomyolysis, and tissue necrosis. Hypotension can result from blood loss, anaphylaxis, myocardial depression, and generalized vasodilatation due to nitric oxide, bradykinin, and prostaglandins. Systemic and renal hemodynamics in snake envenomation bear resemblance to those observed in infection and in fact share the same cytokines and mediators triggered by phospholipase A2 and metalloproteases.[206,207] Given the protein nature of snake venom, AKI is rarely due to one factor but rather multiple factors. In an isolated perfused kidney, Russell's viper venom decreased the renal blood flow and GFR and increased the fractional excretion of sodium in dose-dependent fashion.[208] Russell's viper venom decreases renal cortical mitochondrial oxygen consumption and increases P/O ratio.[42] Toxicity to glomeruli and tubular epithelial cells has been shown.[202] Immune mechanism plays a minor role in the pathogenesis of glomerulonephritis in some patients. Therefore, there is evidence of hemodynamic changes, direct nephrotoxicity, and immunologic mechanism in snake bite nephropathy.

Treatment and Prognosis. Treatment of renal failure caused by snake envenoming is complicated by other systemic complications of the venom. Standard treatment consists of local care, use of antivenom, generalized support, and early dialysis. Dialysis in patients with a sea snake bite can improve muscular symptoms. Early administration of sodium bicarbonate to alkalinize urine in the patient who has intravascular hemolysis or rhabdomyolysis prevents the development of AKI.[219] With early dialysis, prognosis for patients with renal failure in general is favorable except for those with cortical necrosis. Residual renal damage can occur in those with severe pathologic changes and old age.

Insect Stings

Proteinuria, nephrotic syndrome, and AKI have been reported in association with bee, wasp, and hornet stings. In a study of 20 healthy subjects stung by bees or wasps, pathologic albuminuria was found in three patients. The urine albumin excretion normalized in 2 months in two of those patients.[209]

Nephrotic Syndrome. An association between bee stings and nephrotic syndrome has long been described.[210] A relapse of nephrotic syndrome following a bee sting has been reported.[211] The onset of nephrotic syndrome varies from 2 to 14 days after the sting. Serum immunoglobulin and complement levels and renal function are usually normal. The response to steroid treatment is favorable in 50% of the patients.

Renal pathologic changes vary. Minimal change lesions, mesangial proliferative glomerulonephritis, membranous glomerulonephritis, and glomerulosclerosis are among the changes described. Deposition of C3, IgM, and IgG is demonstrable. However, no report has demonstrated the presence of bee venom antigens in the glomeruli. Although such a finding would indicate a role for an immunologic mechanism in the pathogenesis of glomerulonephritis, the cause-and-effect relationship between the bee venom and glomerulonephritis has not been substantiated. The association between the bee sting and nephrotic syndrome with minimal lesions, erythema of the skin, and eosinophilia described in one report could be related to basophil sensitization.[212]

The mechanism responsible for the development of glomerulonephritis is therefore not understood. The role of the bee venom (*Apis mellifera*) in inducing the alteration of T cell function in mice might link with the development of glomerulonephritis.[213]

Acute Kidney Injury. Renal failure has occurred in patients stung by wasps and bees.[46,214] Stings are usually multiple. A single sting does not cause renal failure, but can cause anaphylactic shock in the previously sensitized patient. Bee venoms decrease the renal blood flow and GFR. Glomerular filtration remains low despite the return of renal blood flow to normal.[215] Renal failure in insect stings is often associated with rhabdomyolysis or intravascular hemolysis which develops within 24 hours. Thrombocytopenia may be present with or without disseminated intravascular coagulation. Hepatocellular jaundice may be observed. Pancreatitis has been reported. Laboratory findings include hyperkalemia, hyperuricemia, hyperphosphatemia, hypocalcemia, hemoglobinuria, myoglobinuria, and elevation of muscle enzyme levels. Nonoliguric renal failure is not uncommon. Oligoanuria is often observed in the elderly. The mechanisms of renal injury are believed to be decreased renal blood flow, myoglobinuria, hemoglobinuria, and direct tubular toxicity. The duration of renal failure varies from one week to several weeks. The course of renal failure is prolonged in the elderly. Recovery of renal function is usual; however, residual renal damage can occur. The elderly and children are at high risk for a fatal outcome.

Renal pathologic changes include tubular necrosis and interstitial lesions with edema and mononuclear infiltration. The proximal, distal, and collecting tubules are affected. Acute interstitial nephritis with renal failure presumably due to hypersensitivity has been reported.[216] Increased calcium uptake in the proximal tubule cells by melittin may enhance renal tubular injury.[217]

Raw Carp Bile

Ingestion of raw carp bile—traditionally believed to improve visual acuity, stop coughing, decrease body temperature, and lower blood pressure—can result in renal failure. The problem is well known in Southeast Asia, Taiwan, China, and Korea. The raw bile of carp, belonging to the order of Cypriniformes, including *Ctenopharyngodon idellus*, *Cyprinus carpio*, *Hypophthalmichthys molitrix*, *Mylopharyngodon piceus*, and *Aristichthys nobilis*, is nephrotoxic.[218] Clinical manifestations, which start from gastrointestinal symptoms, consist of abdominal pain, nausea, vomiting, and diarrhea occurring 10 minutes to 12 hours after the ingestion of raw bile.[218] Seizure and bradycardia may be observed.[219] The amount of bile ingested varies from 15 to 30 mL. The gastrointestinal symptoms are followed by hepatitis and AKI. The onset of oliguria varies from 2 to 48 hours after ingestion. Oliguria renal failure is noted in 54% of patients. Hematuria occurs in 77% and jaundice in 62%. The duration of renal failure varies from 2 to 3 weeks.

Renal pathologic changes are those of tubular necrosis. Glomeruli show no remarkable changes. The pathogenesis of renal failure is not well understood and perhaps is due to multiple factors. Nonspecific factors including diarrhea and jaundice leading to renal ischemia cannot be excluded. In rats, nephrotoxicity developed after the ingestion of carp raw bile but not hog raw bile. Cyprinol, a bile alcohol, has been suggested to be nephrotoxic.[220,221] Lin and associates[221] showed that the toxic compound exists in the ethanol-soluble fraction of bile, which has bile acids. Of interest is hepatic and renal injury following ingestion of raw sheep bile as a traditional medicine for diabetes mellitus in Saudi Arabia.

Jellyfish Stings

Box jellyfish (*Chironex* and *Chiropsalmus*), the Portuguese Man of War (*Physalia physalis*), the Irukandi jellyfish (*Carukia barnesi*), and Nomura's jellyfish (*Nemopilema nomurai*) are poisonous. Jellyfish venom has myotoxin, hemolysin, and peptides that activate sodium channels and voltage dependent calcium channels and form pores on the cell membrane.[46] Cellular sodium and calcium influx leads to the release of catecholamines, 5-hydroxytryptamine, tetramine, prostaglandins, and kinins resulting in hemodynamic changes. Severe poisoning can cause nausea, diarrhea, blood pressure changes, intravascular hemolysis, rhabdomyolysis, convulsion, and renal failure.

Scorpion Stings

Odontobuthus, *Mesobuthus*, *Hemiscorpius*, *Androctonus*, *Buthotus*, *Buthus*, *Tityus*, *Leiurus*, and *Centruroides* are medically important scorpions. Scorpion venom consists of mucopolysaccharides, lipids, amino acids, hyaluronidase, phospholipase, 5-hydroxytryptamine, and neurotoxic peptides. Through activation of sodium and calcium channels and pore formation, the venom can cause the release of acetylcholine, catecholamines, and various mediators, with toxic effects to the neuromuscular system. Scorpion charybdotoxin and iberiotoxin close calcium-activated potassium channels in the distal nephron.[222] Among the clinical features following severe reaction to a scorpion sting are symptoms of autonomic nervous system stimulation, disseminated intravascular coagulation, myocarditis, cardiac failure, pancreatitis, pulmonary edema, convulsions, and hypotension.[223] Renal involvement including proteinuria, hematuria, hemoglobinuria, and impaired renal function is observed in 70% of the patients with severe complications.[224] Renal failure has been described in association with disseminated intravascular coagulation and massive hemorrhage in various organs. Hemolytic-uremic syndrome has been reported.[225]

Spider Bites

Atrax, *Harpactirella*, *Loxosceles*, *Latrodectus*, *Lycosa,* and *Phoneutria* are among venomous spiders. Spider venom contains histamine, 5-hydroxytryptamine, hyaluronidase, phospholipase D, collagenase, proteases, and polypeptides. In most cases the symptoms of spider bite are mild. Yet, severe reaction can occur from the bite of certain spiders. Venom polypeptides slow sodium channel inactivation, suppress activation of P type calcium channels, and inhibit glutamate uptake by synaptosomes. Interestingly, *Latrodectus* venom activates calcium channels causing massive neurotransmitter release. *Latrodectus* venom can cause severe pain at the site of the bite, nausea, vomiting, salivation, sweating, headache, muscular twitching, hypertension, respiratory paralysis, myocardial damage, rhabdomyolysis, compartment syndrome, and renal dysfunction.[226] Brown spider (*Loxoceles*) bites can cause local dermonecrosis and hemorrhage at the site of bite. Systemic manifestations including intravascular hemolysis, disseminated intravascular coagulation, thrombocytopenia, and renal failure have been reported.[227] The venom has metalloproteases that cause degradation of extracellular matrix such as fibronectin, fibrinogen, entactin, heparan sulfate proteoglycan, and basement membrane.[227]

Centipede Bites

A centipede bite usually causes local reactions. Severe systemic symptoms including proteinuria can occur.[228] The venom contains histamine, hyaluronidase, proteases, phospholipase A_2, serotonin, and cardiotoxic protein. Nausea, vomiting, headache, rhabdomyolysis, and AKI have been reported following the bite of the giant desert centipede, *Scolopendra heros*, which is found in the southern part of the United States and Mexico.[229]

Lonomia Caterpillar Contact

The hemolymph and hair extract of caterpillar of moths in the genus *Lonomia* have phospholipase A_2, procoagulant serine and cysteine proteases which activate factor X, factor XIII, prothrombin, and fibrinolysis. Contact with *Lonomia obliqua* can cause both fibrinolysis and disseminated intravascular coagulation.[230] Severe AKI with a hemorrhagic syndrome resembling disseminated intravascular coagulation following contact with *Lonomia* caterpillars has been described.[231] Contact with several caterpillars, delayed treatment, thrombocytopenia, and old age are risk factors for development of chronic kidney disease.[232]

Beetles

Beetles can cause vesicular lesions when crushed against the skin. Spanish fly (*Lytta vesicatoria*) produces cantharidin, a protein-phosphatase inhibitor, which is nephrotoxic. Consumption of cantharidin in aphrodisiac preparations or Spanish fly contamination in the fried cricket food (popular for Southeast Asians) causes hematuria and AKI with tubular necrosis.[233] Mesangial proliferative glomerulonephritis with IgA deposition has been observed.

Plant Toxins

Several kinds of plants exert pharmacologic effects on the body. Certain effects are harmful and may directly or indirectly cause nephropathy. The subject has recently been reviewed.[40,200]

Djenkol Bean

Djenkol beans (*Pithecolobium lobatum, Pithecolobium jiringa*) are consumed by people in Indonesia, Malaysia, and southern Thailand.[40,234] The beans are eaten as food, either raw, fried, or roasted. Toxicity, due to djenkolic acid, follows ingestion of the raw bean in large amounts (more than five beans) although there are different susceptibilities among individuals. Poisoning may be caused by a single bean in some individuals, whereas it may take 20 beans to cause toxicity in others.[234] Ingestion of the boiled beans does not cause toxicity because the toxic substance, djenkolic acid, is removed from the bean. The amount of djenkolic acid may vary among beans from various sources. Poisoning is characterized by abdominal discomfort, loin pains, severe colic, nausea, vomiting, dysuria, gross hematuria, and oliguria occurring 2 to 6 hours after the beans were ingested. The patient may be anuric. Hypertension may be present. In a report of 22 patients with djenkol bean poisoning, dysuria was noted in 17 (77%), hematuria in 15 (68%), proteinuria in 10 (45%), hypertension in 8 (36%), and renal failure in 12 (55%) patients.[235]

Urine analysis reveals erythrocytes, epithelial cells, protein, and the needle-like crystals of djenkolic acid. The symptoms are due to mechanical irritation of the renal tubules and urinary tract by the djenkolic acid crystals. Precipitation of djenkolic acid causing tubular obstruction occurs in acid and concentrated urine. Urolithiasis has been reported, with djenkolic acid as the nucleus. The majority of patients recover within a few days.

Diagnosis can easily be made by the history of bean ingestion and occasional sulfurous fetor in the breath. Treatment requires hydration to increase urine flow and alkalinization of urine by sodium bicarbonate. When the urine pH is increased from 5.0 to 7.4, the solubility of djenkolic acid is increased by 43%, and at a pH of 8.1 the solubility increases to 92%.[40]

Callilepis Laureola

Callilepis laureola (Impila) is a perennial herb with a tuberous rootstock found widely in South Africa, Zambia, Zaire, Zimbabwe, and the neighboring countries. The plant is used in the form of infusion for coughs, constipation, intestinal worms, and many other illnesses. An alkaloid, atractyloside, found in the tuber of the plant is believed to have nephrotoxic and hypoglycemic effects. It has an inhibitory effect on oxidative phosphorylation. After medication, toxic symptoms usually occur in less than 24 hours in 40% of the patients and within a few days in 72%.[236] Clinically, the patient has abdominal pain, vomiting, and diarrhea. Hypoglycemia is observed in 81% of patients. Convulsions and coma are common. Hepatocellular jaundice is present. Renal failure ensues in the majority of patients. Treatment is supportive. The mortality rate is more than 50%.

The kidney shows tubular necrosis involving the proximal tubules and the ascending loops of Henle. Interstitial edema and cellular infiltration are present.

Semecarpus Anacardium

Semecarpus anacardium is the name for the marking nut tree in India and tropical forests. The bark and the pericarp of the fruit have a black caustic juice that is irritating to the skin, causing eruptions and blisters. Prolonged exposure to the sap can cause abdominal pain, vomiting, fever, and renal failure.[237] Cortical necrosis has been reported. Nephrotoxicity is attributed to the phenolic substance in the sap.

Star Fruit

Star fruit (*Averrhoa carambola*) is a popular fruit among Asians. The fruit has high oxalate content. Ingestion of large quantities of pure fresh juice can cause within hours nausea, vomiting, abdominal pain, and back ache, followed by acute oliguric renal failure, due to acute oxalate nephropathy. Pure fresh star fruit juice should not be consumed in large amounts, especially on an empty stomach or in a state of dehydration. Apoptosis is the mode of renal tubular cell death.[238]

Mangosteen

Mangosteen (*Garcinia mangostana*) is among the tasty fruits in Southeast Asia. The fruit has several xanthone compounds. Alpha mangostin, one of these compounds, causes depolarization of mitochondrial membrane, disrupting the electron transport chain.[239] Cytochrome c is released into the cytosol. Production of adenosine triphosphate is decreased and there is apoptosis.[240] Consumption of large quantities of mangosteen juice for a long period of time has been reported to cause severe lactic acidosis.[241]

Mushrooms

Toxic mushroom poisoning leads to a variety of clinical presentations ranging from gastrointestinal symptoms to fulminant liver failure and renal failure. The *Amanita, Cortinarius,* and *Galerina* species of mushrooms are nephrotoxic. Amatoxin, phallotoxin, and orellanine are toxic ingredients.[242] Amatoxin inhibits DNA-dependent RNA polymerase II. Phallotoxin binds with F actin and polymerizes G actin. Orellanine is toxic to proximal tubular cells. Toxic symptoms occur within 10 to 14 hours after ingestion and consist of abdominal pain, nausea, vomiting, and diarrhea, followed by jaundice, renal failure, convulsions, and coma.[243] Renal failure is severe, with a mortality rate of more than 50%. In an animal model of *Cortinarius orellanus* mushroom poisoning, renal dysfunction occurred within 48 hours.[244] The pattern of renal impairment included decreased GFR, proteinuria, glycosuria, and decreased tubular reabsorption of sodium, potassium, and water. Renal pathologic changes are those of tubular necrosis, with prominent necrosis of the proximal tubules and interstitial edema. There are no glomerular changes. Given early in the course of disease penicillin G, silymarin, silibinin, or *N*-acetylcysteine can be useful. Mushroom poisoning with liver and renal failure has high mortality despite optimal medical therapy including plasmapheresis, charcoal hemoperfusion, and hemodiafiltration. Molecular absorbent regenerating system (MARS), which removes albumin-bound toxins, has been reported to favor recovery.[245]

Cotton Seed Oil

The principal ingredient of cotton seed oil is gossypol. Gossypol can cause kaliuresis and hypokalemia. The mechanism is not well understood. In central and southern China, where the dietary potassium is low, the incidence of gossypol-induced hypokalemia is between 4% and 5%.[48] It has also been reported to cause distal renal tubular acidosis in Chinese people who consume cotton seed oil.

Herbal Medicines

Traditional herbs as alternative medicinal drugs are commonly used in the tropics. A number of Chinese herbs are nephrotoxic. The use of *Taxus celebica* for diabetes mellitus can cause hemolysis and renal failure due to flavonoid sciadopitysin.[246] Consumption of rhubarb leaves can cause oxalate renal stones due to high oxalic acid content.

Several plants including *Securidaca longipedunculata, Euphorbia matabelensis,* and *Crotalaria laburnifolia* have been listed as being nephrotoxic.[247] Yet, there is no supporting scientific evidence. These plants are usually used as traditional medicine for the treatment of many illnesses, and may cause renal failure through their side effects. For example, infusion of the leaves, bark, and root of *S. longipedunculata* can cause severe gastroenteritis with diarrhea and vomiting, which can result in AKI through volume depletion without evidence of direct nephrotoxicity. *Thiloa glaucocarpa* is tubulotoxic due to toxic tannins. *Solanum malacoxylon*[248] and *Cestrum diurnum*[249] can cause hypercalcemia due to 1,25 dihydroxycholecalciferol in the plant. Ingestion of the essential oil of wormwood (*Artemisia absinthium*) has been reported to cause seizures, rhabdomyolysis, and AKI.[250] The toxic ingredient is thujone, an aromatic hydrocarbon.

An association between the use of Chinese herbal medicine containing aristolochic acid and chronic renal disease has been described. Renal pathologic changes include tubular atrophy, interstitial fibrosis, glomerulosclerosis, and thickening of the wall of the interlobular artery and glomerular afferent arteriole. Tubular dysfunction, including Fanconi-like syndrome, is commonly manifested. Uroepithelial malignancy has been observed. Multifocal atypia of the medullary collecting ducts, the pelvis, and ureter with overexpression of p53 has been shown. On the positive side, traditional Chinese herbal medicine (Sairei-to) with the active principle saikosaponin-d has been shown to prevent glomerulosclerosis in uninephrectomized rats with anti-thy-1 antibody injection.[251]

Chemical Toxins

Accidental exposure to certain chemical toxins is well documented as a cause of AKI in the tropics, as it is in the

West. Chemical intoxication may also be associated with certain occupational hazards, involving exposure to industrial poisons such as lead, mercury, cadmium, uranium, and asbestos. This is highly prevalent in tropical countries, owing to the inadequacy of environmental protection measures in industrial plants.

Certain chemical hazards of particular importance in the tropics deserve mentioning, namely, paraquat, copper sulfate, and diethylene glycol.

Paraquat Poisoning

This is mainly reported in Southeast Asia. Paraquat is an herbicide, widely used in agriculture, to which humans are exposed by ingestion (including suicidal intake), inhalation of sprays, or contact with skin abrasions. Pulmonary, hepatic, and renal manifestations attributed to the massive generation of reactive oxygen radicals commonly occur.[253] Nephrotoxicity expressed as acute tubular necrosis[254] further leads to accumulation of the poison and increases its systemic toxicity. Fanconi syndrome has been described in paraquat poisoning.[255] Plasma paraquat levels higher than 2 mg per L at 24 hours and 1 mg per L at 48 hours are of grave prognostic significance.

Like many other chemical intoxications, the first line of treatment is to reduce absorption by gastric lavage and the administration of adsorbing substances such as fuller's earth. If renal function permits, forced diuresis should be attempted. Hemodialysis and charcoal hemoperfusion are effective, whereas peritoneal dialysis is too inefficient. Reduction of oxygen radical load by suppressing leukocytic function with corticosteroids and cyclophosphamide has been used.[256]

Copper Sulfate Poisoning

Until recently, this hazard used to be of considerable epidemiologic significance in India. Copper sulfate is used in the leather industry. Exposure occurs through accidental or intentional ingestion. Acute toxicity ushers in with prominent gastrointestinal manifestations, intravascular hemolysis, rhabdomyolysis, hepatic injury, and renal failure.[257]

Renal injury is the result of massive intravascular hemolysis, induced by the action of the poison on intracellular enzyme systems including G6PD, glutathione reductase, and catalase.[257] The associated hypovolemia, due to gastrointestinal fluid losses, further aggravates the renal insult. Acute tubular necrosis with rupture of the tubular basement membrane, copper deposits in the tubule cells, and hemoglobin casts in the tubule lumens are characteristic histopathologic features.

In addition to the conventional methods for reducing the absorption of the poison, fluid replacement and induction of diuresis, dimercaprol and D-penicillamine are effectively used for chelation in copper sulfate poisoning.[258] Dialysis is often necessary during the critical hypercatabolic phase, and also to assist in eliminating the toxin.

Diethylene Glycol Poisoning

Diethylene glycol is a known nephrotoxic agent. Poisoning with diethylene glycol in the tropics has frequently been associated with contamination of ingestible pharmaceutical products. Outbreaks of AKI by diethylene glycol contaminated acetaminophen have been reported in Nigeria[259] and Bangladesh.[260] Recently there was a large outbreak of AKI with deaths in children consuming diethylene glycol contaminated acetaminophen syrup in Haiti.[261] Renal failure was severe and associated with hepatitis, pancreatitis, and central nervous system involvement with high mortality. It has been postulated that acetaminophen could provide additive or potentiating effects for diethylene glycol toxicity. Hypovolemia due to vomiting could be another contributing factor.

TROPICAL ENVIRONMENTAL POLLUTION

A wide spectrum of CKD is attributed to environmental pollution, [262] which has been implicated in the pathogenesis of glomerulonephritis (e.g., heavy metals, hydrocarbons), tubulointerstitial disease (e.g., lead), and renal and urothelial malignancies (cigarette smoking, cadmium, and aflatoxins).

Much of the available information is based on animal models. Extrapolation to humans is often hypothetical, and may indeed be inappropriate owing to differences in body size, relevant metabolic pathways, and duration of exposure. Apart from occupational exposure, it is difficult to ascertain the duration and exposure, pollutant dose, and confounding factors that may alter its toxicity.

The epidemiologic significance of environmental pollution in the tropics is unknown, yet it is often blamed for the high prevalence of CKD at large, and particularly for the progressive increase in the incidence of tubulointerstitial disease in the recently industrialized tropical countries that lack effective safety control measures.

Smoke, Dust, and Fumes

Tobacco smoking is well recognized as a major risk factor in cardiovascular morbidity and mortality in patients with CKD, progression of renal damage particularly among diabetic patients, and in the pathogenesis of bladder cancer. This problem is particularly relevant in tropical countries where more than 80% of the world's 1 billion smokers live.

Compared with the rest of the world, the major cities in tropical countries have the highest levels of pollution from car, motorcycle, and other engine exhausts. There is unequivocal evidence that the combustion products of diesel fuel and unleaded gasoline are nephrotoxic to adult male rats.[263] This effect is mediated by proximal tubular accumulation of $\alpha_{2\mu}$-globulin, which is deficient in man, hence the uncertainty of human pathogenicity. Other hydrocarbons such as paint, mineral spirits, and aromatic solvents have a similar nephrotoxic potential.

Most of the gasoline used in the tropics is leaded. Although lead nephrotoxicity has been recognized for decades, most information is not evidence-based,[264] and it is unclear if the level of environmental contamination generated by fuel combustion is enough to induce kidney disease in humans.

Chronic exposure to cadmium[265] and asbestos,[266] which in addition to industrial intoxication are often ingested with contaminated water or inhaled with dust, also carries a potential risk for the development of renal cell carcinoma.

Food Additives

Many artificial flavors, colors, thickening substances, solvents, and even wrapping material to which tropical inhabitants are extensively exposed, owing to the lack of effective safety regulations, have documented nephrotoxic effects in experimental animals. These include limonene, carotenes, β-cyclodextrin, 1,2-dichloroethane, dichloromethane, α-methyl-benzyl alcohol, and diethylene glycol monoethyl ether. Although no clinical nephrotoxicity has been attributed to most of these agents, AKI was reported to complicate the accidental ingestion of large quantities of 1,2-dichloroethane or diethylene glycol monoethyl ether, or inhalation of dichloromethane.[267]

Renal adenomas and adenocarcinomas have been induced in rats and hamsters by long-term ingestion of potassium bromide, which is often used as a flour-treatment agent. Accidental or suicidal administration in humans may be associated with AKI, tubulointerstitial nephritis, interstitial fibrosis, and glomerulosclerosis.[268]

Food Contaminants

Exogenous food contaminants may induce human nephrotoxicity in the tropics where agriculture remains the predominant occupation. These include mycotoxins, pesticides, and veterinary drug residues.

Mycotoxins are discussed elsewhere in this and in other chapters, where reference is made to ochratoxin-associated interstitial renal disease and aflatoxin-associated neoplasias.

Pesticides are ingested with drinking water, plants, fish, poultry, and meat. Adequate control is beyond the capacity of most tropical countries because of problems with analytical methodology, standardization, and so on. Large amounts, therefore, may be inevitably ingested by tropical inhabitants for lifelong periods.

Most pesticides are organophosphates; their main toxicity is on the red blood cells, thyroid gland, and nervous system. Weight loss, anemia, hepatic adenomas, esophageal and other gastrointestinal tract tumors, skin allergy, and teratogenicity are the principal toxic manifestations. There is some experimental evidence of toxicity to the liver and kidney, but no clinically significant renal disease has been ascribed to pesticides in the developed world. It is unknown if this also applies to the tropics.

Veterinary drug residues constitute an important source of pollution in an agricultural environment where close contact between humans and animals is inevitable. These residues are ingested with vegetables, fruits, and meat. Some residues, including certain anthelmintics, antimicrobial agents, and production aids, are nephrotoxic to experimental animals.

Of particular concern is tetracycline, which is excreted largely unmetabolized in animal manure leading to increasing environmental contamination.[269] This has been associated with direct toxicity to plants and farm animals as well as to unwanted effects on soil bioecology. The impact on humans is currently under investigation in the tropical environment.

The Environment and Electrolyte and Acid–Base Disorders

Hypokalemia in northeastern Thailand is endemic and reflects the effects of the environment. Northeastern Thailand is a plateau in the arid area of the country, where the weather is dry and hot. The soil, therefore, has low levels of potassium and is infertile. The people in the villages are of low socioeconomic status and consume the products of the land. Therefore, 38% of them have hypokalemia and are potassium depleted. The erythrocyte membranes of the villagers are found to have decreased Na-K-ATPase activity. The urine has a low citrate concentration. Both potassium depletion and decreased Na-K-ATPase activity lead to low urine citrate through intracellular acidosis, which enhances citrate reabsorption. Intracellular sodium concentration is increased, whereas intracellular potassium concentration is decreased. The basic abnormalities of these northeastern Thai villagers are, therefore, potassium depletion, decreased Na-K-ATPase activity, and low urinary citrate levels.[249] These abnormalities resolved when they migrated to the capital city. Besides renal stones, sudden unexplained death and distal renal tubular acidosis are also important health problems of the region.

Sudden unexplained nocturnal death has received much attention within recent years. The incidence is 38 per 100,000 men between 20 and 49 years old.[270] The victims are usually muscular young men of low socioeconomic class who die in their sleep without apparent organic lesion. Ventricular fibrillation has been observed and hypokalemia has been reported in some patients. They have decreased Na-K-ATPase activity of the erythrocyte membrane.[271] It has been postulated that hypokalemia, the possible decrease in myocardial Na-K-ATPase, and sympathetic stimulation due to stress could lead to cardiac arrhythmias and death. The causes are likely multiple and could involve genetic variations. Recent evidence indicates mutation of the sodium channel (SCN5A) in the cardiac muscle resembling Brugada syndrome.[272]

The prevalence of distal renal tubular acidosis in northeastern Thailand is approximately 3.6%, with a female preponderance.[273] The patients are usually admitted in the hospital during the midsummer because of muscular weakness or paralysis; nephrocalcinosis or renal stones, or both, are noted in 27% of the patients. Interestingly, the patients have low urinary potassium levels, a finding different from Western reports. In addition, gastric acidity is low,[274] suggestive of decreased H-K-ATPase (HKα1) activity or decreased chloride bicarbonate exchange (AE2). Whether this is on a genetic or environmental basis remains unknown. Because of hypokalemia, aldosterone secretion is likely suppressed, and this would in turn decrease H-ATPase activity. In Southeast Asian ovalocytosis with distal renal tubular acidosis AE1 gene mutation has been reported.[275] Two novel compound heterozygous SLC4A1 mutations have been identified in Thai patients with autosomal recessive distal renal tubular acidosis.[276] Despite the genetic evidence the role of the environment is still a missing link required to explain the whole problem.

END-STAGE RENAL DISEASE IN TROPICAL COUNTRIES

Epidemiology

Prevalence

With the progressive improvement of renal replacement therapy (RRT) worldwide, prevalence curves continue to rise in most countries. The reported prevalence is currently highest in Japan, exceeding 2,000 patients per million population (pmp), which is attributed to the strikingly high survival on dialysis. The respective figure in the tropics ranges from less than 100 to about 600 pmp, being proportionate to the national economy (Fig. 63.18).[5] Because there are no significant differences in incidence between individual countries, the major determinants of prevalence are the capacity and competence of RRT programs, both of which are financially demanding.

Incidence

The incidence of new cases of ESKD in the tropics is generally within the range of 100 to 150 pmp.[28] There is no point in focusing on minor differences between individual countries or regions because the available information is only approximate, being based on questionnaires to leaders, small samples, official governmental reports, and, very occasionally, registries with doubtful credibility. These numbers are lower than those reported in the West, with figures up to threefold as much. Although underreporting may be responsible for this discrepancy, it has been estimated that the lower incidence of diabetes[9,10] in the tropics can account for the difference. This is quite alarming given that the incidence of diabetes is expected to boom in tropical countries during the coming two decades, which will undoubtedly reflect on the incidence of ESKD.

Clinical Patterns

The usual clinical syndrome of ESKD is modified in the tropics by three factors: (1) associated manifestations of the primary disease, (2) manifestations of concomitant disorders, and (3) late diagnosis and poor management.

Manifestations of the Primary Disease. As described previously in this chapter, renal disease in the tropics is often secondary to an endemic infection, is attributed to environmental pollution, or is caused by a drug or traditional medication. The associated features of the primary etiology frequently modify the clinical picture of ESKD. Examples include the concomitant hepatic disease in schistosomal glomerulopathy; severe hypertension, arthropathy, and polyneuropathy with chronic exposure to lead; and persistent hyperkalemia with certain herbal intoxications.

Concomitant Disorders. Many patients have a concomitant illness, the features of which may overlap with or modify those of conventional ESKD. Such disorders reflect the general health status of the community, often dominated by endemic infections and infestations, malnutrition, and certain malignancies.

Endemic Infections and Infestations. Acute and chronic bacterial infections often complicate renal disease in the

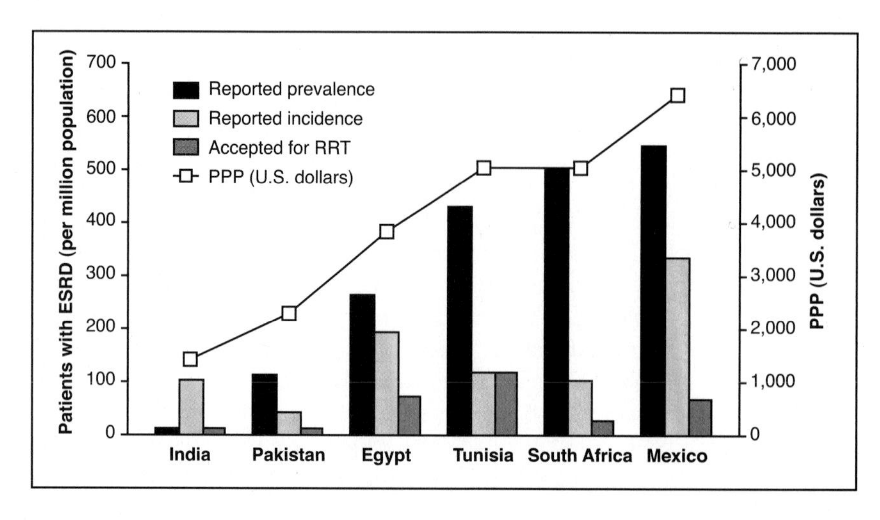

FIGURE 63.18 Impact of wealth on the prevalence of end-stage kidney disease. Data for 2005.[5]

tropics. In addition to those causing renal disease (see preceding text) and those acquired during dialysis (see subsequent text), certain infectious agents may have an independent impact. One of the most outstanding infections is tuberculosis, which is encountered in 4.1% to 11.5% of the Saudi Arabian population on hemodialysis,[277] Gulf countries, India, Bangladesh, and Indonesia. Tuberculous peritonitis has been reported in patients on chronic ambulatory peritoneal dialysis, wherein it poses notorious diagnostic difficulties.[278] Evidence of previous *Salmonella* infection was detected in 42% of patients on regular hemodialysis in Egypt. *Salmonella* infection–associated acute graft rejections has been observed in renal transplant recipients (unpublished data). The list includes many other infections, the most common being scabies, HBV, HCV, HIV infection (see the following), and intestinal parasitic infections. In addition to imposing their specific symptomatology, these infections generally tend to induce a catabolic state that augments such uremic manifestations as asthenia, anemia, and bone disease.

Malnutrition. Protein-energy malnutrition is often a major problem in dealing with renal disease in the tropics. This may be attributed to starvation, catabolic disorders, or physicians' instructions. It is unfortunate that general practitioners are still advising their patients to restrict protein intake to exceedingly low levels. Even nephrologists maintain this trend in patients on dialysis, as shown in a meta-analysis of European Dialysis and Transplant Association (EDTA) data, where 73.5% of uremic patients in developing countries were instructed to receive a daily protein intake of less than 0.6 g per kg, compared with 31.3% in Western Europe.

Specific nutritional deficiencies of iron, calcium, vitamin D, other vitamins, and trace elements are also frequently encountered. The effects of these on anemia, bone, and peripheral nerve disease are obvious.

Malignancies. Infection-related malignancies are notoriously common in the tropics. Examples include Burkitt lymphoma and Kaposi sarcoma.[279] These often become a significant epidemiologic risk in immunocompromised patients.

Late Diagnosis and Inadequate Management. Owing to the prevailing standards of medical care, renal disease may not be suspected, may be neglected, or may be poorly managed for a long time before adequate nephrologic care is provided. Advanced uremic manifestations, of almost historic interest according to present-day Western standards, remain fairly common in the tropical glossary. It is not unusual to see a patient with extensive uremic frost on his or her cheeks or finger creases, or with multiple soft tissue swellings of metastatic calcification, or another crippled with bone deformities or motor polyneuropathy. Many patients are first seen in coma, in convulsions, or with a hematocrit level of 8% to 10%. The clinical picture is often further complicated by the use of medications without any dose adjustment in consideration of residual renal function.

Dialysis in the Tropics

Acute Dialysis

Hemodialysis is available for the management of AKI in most of the major hospitals in the tropics, even in those countries with the lowest gross national products (GNPs).[28] The efficiency of such units is widely variable, ultimately depending on socioeconomic development. For obvious reasons, acute peritoneal dialysis is more widely used. It is often implemented where limited or no specialized nephrologic care is available, at least as a first-line therapy. Unfortunately, the prevailing hygienic conditions in many tropical hospitals yield a high incidence of peritonitis.

Chronic Dialysis

The number of patients treated by chronic dialysis in the tropics cannot be precisely defined because of the scarcity of reliable registries. Data generated from sporadic publications (which are, unfortunately, mostly found in the nonindexed local literature), national registries (by personal communication with colleagues in charge), and supranational (African, Arabian, Latin American, and Asian Pacific registries) and international (ERA, USRDS) registries suggest that the chronic dialysis activity in the tropics is fairly extensive. Prevalent chronic dialysis varies from less than 5 pmp in most sub-Saharan African countries (e.g., Sudan, Tanzania, Ethiopia, Uganda, Nigeria, Ghana); 100 to 200 pmp in Paraguay, the Philippines, Bangladesh, and Pakistan; 200 to 500 pmp in India, Southern and Northern Africa, Thailand, and most South American countries; and close to 1000 pmp in Singapore, Saudi Arabia, and Chile.[28,280–284]

The Dialysis Environment

The Patient. Young adults in their 20s or early 30s constitute 70% to 80% of the dialysis population in the tropics, which is attributed to the nature of the prevailing primary diseases. Children constitute less than 10%. There is a male preponderance, which is partly explained by cultural factors and possibly the increased exposure to noxious environmental factors (see later text). Most patients are poor, uneducated, and suffering from chronic endemic diseases, malnutrition, and advanced uremic state, which has a significantly negative impact on the outcome of dialysis treatment (see later text). They do not adequately comply with the regularity of dialysis, diet, intake of medications, or rehabilitation. Although this is partly attributed to improper patient information, the lack of motivation and financial shortcomings certainly have a considerable influence.

Human Resources. Shortage of adequately trained medical and paramedical local staff is the rule in most tropical countries. Dramatic examples are vast countries like Kenya, Sudan, and Nigeria, where the proportion of nephrologists to the general population is around 0.5 pmp.[285] Despite such shortage, many qualified nephrologists emigrate from such deprived areas to the West. For example, it has been estimated that 20% of Indian nephrologists have been permanently installed in the United States and even more Nigerian and Ghanaian nephrologists practice in foreign countries.[286]

The majority of countries do not have a structured program for training physicians, nurses, and technicians. Yet recent years have witnessed an increasing regional and international collaboration for such training. Training guidelines have been developed by the International Society of Nephrology and several supranational societies of nephrology; and many have launched mechanisms for bilateral collaboration between well-developed dialysis units in the West and developing units in the tropics.

Dialysis Centers. The reported number of dialysis centers varies, in different tropical countries, from less than 1 to 12 units pmp.[28] When detailed figures are compared with the respective numbers of patients actually receiving regular dialysis, it can be appreciated that the units are not kept sufficiently busy. The reasons for nonfunctional equipment are many and include lack of personnel, shortage of funds, poor maintenance, and inefficient organization.[285]

Most units are located in hospitals, with a few satellite units in the better-developed countries. State-sponsored, insurance-sponsored, and private units are available in most countries, in proportions that differ according to the political systems and GNPs. Excellent state-sponsored units comprise most dialysis units in the economically better-off countries. However, the standard of service in state-sponsored units in most tropical countries with low GNPs is modest, which invites active participation of the private sector. Political system permitting—as in India, Egypt, Latin America, and most of Southeast Asia—private units tend to take the technical lead. Governments generally provide partial reimbursement for private dialysis in these countries. Insurance-sponsored units are also growing where health insurance systems are strong enough to support the cost. Unique models of charity-sponsored programs have emerged in recent years, notably in Singapore and Pakistan.

Standard equipment is the rule, including nonvolumetric hemodialysis machines, acetate-based dialysate, cuprophane membrane hollow fibers, and so on. Peritoneal dialysis fluid is often locally manufactured, although at a very high cost (see later text). A few units accept children and older adults, but almost none is specialized in pediatric or geriatric dialysis.

Chronic Dialysis Modalities. With a few exceptions, hemodialysis is the predominant dialysis modality in most tropical countries, constituting 80% to 90% of the population on dialysis. In countries with the lowest GNPs, however, intermittent peritoneal dialysis (IPD) is the inevitable alternative. The implementation of continuous ambulatory peritoneal dialysis (CAPD) is widely variable, from sporadic experiences[287] to a national policy (Mexico, about 60%[284]; Hong Kong, 70%[288]; South Africa, 40%[28]). Certain countries, as Sudan since the 1970s[289] and Thailand since 2002,[281] have adopted a policy of "PD First" leading to progressive increase of patients on CAPD.

Most other countries refrain from using CAPD because of the high cost (see later text), high incidence of infection, and poor patient compliance. Accordingly, CAPD is offered only as a second choice to selected patients of the higher social classes.

IPD is still used for high-risk patients such as those with severe ischemic heart disease or complicated diabetes. On the whole, it accounts for at least 60% of all chronic peritoneal dialysis treatment in the tropics. Because adequate urea kinetics can only be achieved by an impossible number of dialysis hours, IPD is associated with an extremely poor median survival time, 1 year, and modest quality of life. Although IPD is usually carried out in hospitals, the incidence of infection remains high, up to one episode per 4.3 patient years in a recent series.[290]

The Cost of Regular Dialysis. Calculating dialysis costs is a difficult and complex procedure. Besides the direct costs including the prices of consumable items, overhead expenses, salaries, and fees, one must include the costs of interdialytic therapy, transfusions, hospital admissions, transportation, and so on. In even broader terms, one should also consider the days missed from work and the reduced productivity of some patients.

The items of typical annual direct dialysis cost per capita in a tropical country are essentially the same, with the differences being mainly influenced by the proportion of imported versus locally manufactured materials, prevailing dialyzer reuse policy, and the standards of salaries and professional fees, which vary from 10% to 35% of the total cost.[28]

Peritoneal dialysis is generally the most expensive modality of ESKD therapy in most tropical countries, even when locally manufactured solutions are used. This is attributed to the high overhead expenses entailed in small-scale production lines. When the scale of PD is expanded enough to reduce such cost, substantial health and socioeconomic benefits are achieved, as in a recent study in Thailand.[291]

Results and Limitations of Chronic Dialysis Treatment. The reported annual mortality rate after the first year for all dialysis modalities, for all ages, and regardless of the primary renal disease in different tropical countries varies from 15% to 35%. The first-year mortality is about 25% to 45% higher. When considered separately, the mortality for IPD is much higher, whereas CAPD has yielded impressive results in several series. There is a remarkable "center effect," in favor of economically privileged units that can afford recruiting better equipment and staff and that tend to attract those in the higher socioeconomic category of patients.

Attention to the quality of life is proportionate to an individual nation's GNPs. In the poorer countries, which constitute the majority in the tropical zone, this issue is not even raised. Patients are often content just to be alive, even though they are disabled. The incidence of complications is quite high, mainly because of inadequate dialysis, poor water quality, undernutrition, dialysis-acquired infections, and deficient interdialytic care.

Dialysis-acquired infections are extremely common, mainly including the hepatitis viruses, HIV, and CMV. HBV infection, with a prevalence approaching 90% among dialysis patients in certain countries a couple of decades ago, has now considerably regressed to a rate of less than 20% in most tropical countries and even to less than 6% in wealthier countries. This decline is at least partly attributed to vaccination of the populations at risk. Unfortunately, HBV infection has been largely replaced by infection with HCV, antibodies to which have been reported in 35% to 65% of populations from different tropical countries. The outcome of HCV-positive patients on dialysis is poor, with a 5-year survival of less than 20% in several series.[292]

With the recognition of methicillin-resistant staphylococcal infection as an important threat in dialysis units, an increasing number of reports have confirmed the major negative impact of this infection in the tropics. The precise incidence of this infection is unknown, but it has been certainly responsible for major outbreaks such as that reported from China in 2004.[293]

As a rule, interdialytic medical care is extremely modest in tropical countries. Even such basic goals as blood pressure control, correction of anemia, and maintenance of the calcium and acid–base balance are often overlooked. Access to active vitamin D and erythropoietin (EPO) is a matter of affordability. In the majority of tropical countries, 10% to 20% of dialysis patients receive regular EPO therapy. Exceptions to this are reported from Saudi Arabia and Argentina (60% and 64%, respectively).[28] The subsequent need for multiple transfusions obviously facilitates the spread of dialysis-associated viral infections.

Renal Transplantation in the Tropics

Availability

Renal transplantation is widely available in many tropical countries. The precise data about different countries obtained from local, supranational, or different international registries are controversial. The number of transplantations per million population ranges from less than 1 (in sub-Saharan Africa) to more than 100 patients (in South America).[18] Besides the availability of human and financial resources, the major factor that determines this variation is cultural, and depends on whether prevailing religions and heritage accept the concepts of brain death, removal of organs from the dead, and transplanting them into strangers.

The Transplantation Environment

Donors for renal transplantation are either deceased, living related, or living unrelated.

Deceased Donor Transplantation. The most active tropical countries in this respect are South Africa (82.5%), Venezuela (63%), and Thailand (46%). Despite earlier difficulties in harvesting and transporting donor kidneys, most of these programs are prosperous, expanding, and progressively limiting the growth of the dialysis pools. Recipients are generally selected according to standard rules and put on waiting lists with waiting times varying between 1 and 6 months.

Living Donor Transplantations. Living related donors constitute 15% to 85% of the overall transplant activity in different tropical countries, depending on the availability of a national deceased donor program, and the popularity of unrelated donor transplantation.[294] The latter is particularly flourishing in Pakistan, Egypt, India, and Mexico, accounting for 50% to 80% of all transplants. It is difficult for nonnationals to understand the moral aspects of this practice in countries where patients with ESKD have no alternatives, and donors are left in extreme need without any kind of social support. Nevertheless, this rationale has opened the door to foreigners to seek transplantation in these countries, leading to a highly unethical international trade. This issue has been addressed by a consortium of several physician associations and the World Health Organization, who issued a set of regulations to limit organ trafficking and commercialism through what is known as the "Declaration of Istanbul."[295] Following this firm stand, most countries no longer permit free unrelated donor transplantation; some require a formal permit of an independent ethics committee, and one country, Iran, has legalized and organized the procedure of unrelated donor transplantation through a central agency.[294]

Transplantation Centers. Most transplantations are performed in general hospitals. There are very few independently standing specialized transplantation centers. As with the dialysis activity and according to the same rules (see later text), private transplantation teams share in providing the service in living donor programs.

The hygienic standards are variable. In some areas, they are far below average and are responsible for high postoperative morbidity and mortality rates, as well as for the transmission of infections such as HIV, hepatitis, malaria, and others.

Results and Limitations of Renal Transplantation

Data obtained from national registries suggest that the outcome of renal transplantation in tropical countries is in accordance with international standards. However, it is presumable that most transplantations are not registered at all, because, for example, some countries do not have registries. It is therefore impossible to know the precise outcomes of those thousands of grafts transplanted in patients in tropical countries.

However, the published sporadic data suggest that the recipient morbidity and mortality rates are relatively high, mainly due to postoperative wound and systemic infections. The latter include activation of dormant disease as well as de novo infections. Notorious for the tropics are such infections as tuberculosis, salmonellosis, certain parasitic infections (see later text), and others. As outlined previously, the high incidence of certain malignancies such as Kaposi sarcoma and Burkitt lymphoma also accounts for the increased recipient mortality rate.

The Cost of Transplantation

The ultimate burden of renal transplantation on a national economy is less than that of dialysis. Despite the high initial expenses and the cost of expensive medications such as cyclosporine and monoclonal antibodies, the ultimate analysis shows that transplantation is both less expensive and more cost effective. A local study in which cumulative survival rates were taken into consideration estimated that the annual steady-state budget for accepting 100 new patients for dialysis would be approximately $7.5 million U.S. dollars, compared with $6.2 million U.S. dollars for transplantation. The median survival times would be 2.0 and 7.1 years, respectively.

Socioeconomic Impact of ESKD in the Tropics

ESKD is imposing a distinct socioeconomic strain on the economy, social integrity, and even morals of tropical communities at large. The financial burden in certain countries seems impossible to meet, whether by individuals or by the state. It is important to know that the cost of keeping one patient alive but partially rehabilitated on dialysis may literally exceed the average GNP per capita generated by 10 citizens. Yet, it is also important to realize the facts about the expenditures made by the same countries on such issues as political security, cigarette imports, and the purchase of weapons.

A few tropical countries have established independent national kidney foundations that take care of the organization and funding of ESKD therapy, promote research and development, and support staff training. This positive trend has gained success in some tropical countries.

REFERENCES

1. Lee DY, Kim W, Kang SK, et al. Angiotensin-converting enzyme gene polymorphism in patients with minimal-change nephrotic syndrome and focal segmental glomerulosclerosis. *Nephron.* 1997;77(4):471–473.
2. Kopp JB, Smith MW, Nelson GW, et al. MYH9 is a major-effect risk gene for focal segmental glomerulosclerosis. *Nat Genet.* 2008;40(10):1175–1184.
3. Andreoli SP. Racial and ethnic differences in the incidence and progression of focal segmental glomerulosclerosis in children. *Adv Ren Replace Ther.* 2004;11(1):105–109.
4. Huang W, Gu H, Li R, et al. Association of -27T>C and its haplotype at the putative promoter for IgA-specific receptor gene with IgA nephropathy among the Chinese Han population. *Nephrol Dial Transplant* 2011;26(8):2537–2544.
5. Barsoum RS. Chronic kidney disease in the developing world. *N Engl J Med.* 2006;354(10):997–999.
6. Cerdá J, Bagga A, Kher V, et al. The contrasting characteristics of acute kidney injury in developed and developing countries. *Nat Clin Pract Nephrol.* 2008;4:138–153.
7. Basu G, Chrispal A, Boorugu H, et al. Acute kidney injury in tropical acute febrile illness in a tertiary care centre—RIFLE criteria validation. *Nephrol Dial Transplant.* 2011;26(2):524–531.
8. Kellum J, Lameire N, et al. KDIGO guideline on Acute Kidney Injury-Kidney Disease: Improvement of Global Outcomes. Clinical practice guideline on Acute Kidney Injury. . Retrieved February 9, 2011, from http://www.kdigo.org/clinical_practice_guidelines_3.php.
9. Barsoum R. Epidemiology of ESRD: a world-wide perspective. In: El-Nahas AM, Barsoum RS, Dirks J, et al, eds. *Kidney Diseases in the Developing World and Ethnic Minorities.* London: Taylor and Francis; 2005:1.
10. Wild S, Roglic G, Green A, et al. Global prevalence of diabetes: Estimates for the year 2000 and projections for 2030. *Diabetes Care.* 2004;27:1047.
11. Grassmann A, Gioberge S, Moeller S, et al. ESRD patients in 2004: global overview of patient numbers, treatment modalities and associated trends. *Nephrol Dial Transplant.* 2005;20:2587.
12. Plata R, Silva C, Yahuita J, et al. The first clinical and epidemiological programme on renal disease in Bolivia: a model for prevention and early diagnosis of renal diseases in the developing countries. *Nephrol Dial Transplant.* 1998;13(12):3034–3036.
13. Mani MK. Experience with a program for prevention of chronic renal failure in India. *Kidney Int.* 2005;67:S75–S78.
14. Hoy WE, Mathews JD, McCredie DA, et al. The multidimensional nature of renal disease: rates and associations of albuminuria in an Australian Aboriginal community. *Kidney Int.* 1998;54(4):1296–1304.
15. Seedat YK. Glomerular disease in the tropics. *Semin Nephrol.* 2003;23(1):12–20.
16. Woo KT, Chan CM, Mooi CY, et al. The changing pattern of primary glomerulonephritis in Singapore and other countries over the past 3 decades. *Clin Nephrol.* 2010;74(5):372–383.
17. Abdelraheem MB, Ali el-TM, Mohamed RM, et al. Pattern of glomerular diseases in Sudanese children: a clinico-pathological study. *Saudi J Kidney Dis Transpl.* 2010;21(4):778–783.
18. Barsoum RS. Overview: end-stage renal disease in the developing world. *Artif Organs.* 2002;26:737.
19. Barsoum RS. Glomerulonephritis in disadvantaged populations. *Clin Nephrol.* 2010;74Suppl1:S44–50.
20. Malafronte P, Mastroianni-Kirsztajn G, Betônico GN, et al. Paulista Registry of glomerulonephritis: 5-year data report. *Nephrol Dial Transplant.* 2006;21(11):3098–3105.
21. Banerjee S. Steroid resistant nephrotic syndrome. *Indian J Pediatr.* 2002;69(12):1065–1069.
22. Bhimma R, Coovadia HM, Adhikari M. Nephrotic syndrome in South African children: Changing perspectives over 20 years. *Pediatr Nephrol.* 1997;11:429–434.
23. Borchers AT, Naguwa SM, Shoenfeld Y, et al. The geoepidemiology of systemic lupus erythematosus. *Autoimmun Rev.* 2010;9(5):A277–287.
24. Kanjanabuch T, Lewsuwan S, Kitiyakara C, et al. Update in pathophysiology and histopathology of focal segmental glomerulosclerosis. *J Med Assoc Thai.* 2006;89Suppl2:S262–279.
25. El-Refaey AM, Bakr A, Hammad A, et al. Primary focal segmental glomerulosclerosis in Egyptian children: a 10-year single-centre experience. *Pediatr Nephrol.* 2010;25(7):1369–1373.
26. Ehrich HH, Eke FU. Malaria-induced renal dmage: facts and myths. *Pediatr Nephrol.* 2007;22:626–637.
27. Morgan AG, Shah DJ, Williams W, et al. Proteinuria and glomerular disease in Jamaica. *Clin Nephrol.* 1984;21:205.
28. Panja M, Mondal PC. Current status of aortoarteritis in India. *J Assoc Physicians India.* 2004;52:48–52.
29. Trinchieri A. Epidemiology of urolithiasis: an update. *Clin Cases Miner Bone Metab.* 2008;5(2):101–106.
30. Naqvi SA. Regional problems in Pakistan—most prevalent kidney diseases and related problems. Proceedings 8th Colloquium in Nephrol. Jakarta; 1989:283.
31. Tosukhowong P, Tungsanga K, Eiam-Ong S, et al. Environmental distal renal tubular acidosis in Thailand: an enigma. *Am J Kidney Dis.* 1999;33:1180.
32. Egyptian Society of Nephrology. Registry report 2008. Retrieved February 25, 2011, from http://esntonline.com/content/downloads/registry/2008.pdf.
33. Choovichian P, Luvira U, Moolla-or P, et al. Renal function in acute febrile disease. *Intern Med.* 1988;4:105.
34. Arthur CK, McCallum D, Loveday DJ, et al. Effects of taipan (Oxyuranus scutellatus) venom on erythrocyte morphology and blood viscosity in a human victim in vivo and in vitro. *Trans R Soc Trop Med Hyg.* 1991;85(3):401–403.
35. Sitprija V. Overview of tropical nephrology. *Semin Nephrol.* 2003;23:3–11.
36. Anders HJ, Banas B, Schlöndorff D. Signaling danger: toll-like receptors and their potential roles in kidney disease. *J Am Soc Nephrol.* 2004;15(4):854–867.
37. Akira S, Takeda K, Kaisho T. Toll-like receptors: critical proteins linking innate and acquired immunity. *Nat Immunol.* 2001;2(8):675–680.
38. Barsoum RS. Hepatitis C virus: from entry to renal injury—facts and potentials. *Nephrol Dial Transplant.* 2007;22(7):1840–1848.
39. Sitprija V, Boonpucknavig V. Renal involvement in parasitic diseases. In: Tisher CC, Brenner BM, ed. *Renal Pathology.* Philadelphia: Lippincott; 1989:575.
40. Eiam-Ong S, Sitprija V. Tropical plant-associated nephropathy. *Nephrology.* 1998;4:313.
41. Chen CL, Fang HC, Chou KJ, et al. Acute oxalate nephropathy after ingestion of star-fruit. *Am J Kidney Dis.* 2001;37:418.

42. Chaiyabutr N, Sitprija V. Pathophysiological effects of Russell's viper venom on renal function. *J Nat Toxicol.* 1999;8:351–358.

43. Sitprija V. Snakebite nephropathy. *Nephrology.* 2006;11:442.

44. Paudel B, Paudel K. A study of wasp bites in a tertiary hospital of western Nepal. *Nepal Med Coll J.* 2009;11(1):52–56.

45. Sarkar S, Biswas NK, Dey B, et al. A large, systematic molecular-genetic study of G6PD in Indian populations identifies a new non-synonymous variant and supports recent positive selection. *Infect Genet Evol.* 2010;10(8):1228–1236.

46. Sitprija V. Animal toxins and the kidney. *Nat Clin Pract Nephrol.* 2008; 4(11):616–627.

47. Sitprija V. Altered fluid, electrolyte and mineral status in tropical disease, with an emphasis on malaria and leptospirosis. *Nat Clin Pract Nephrol.* 2008;4(2):91–101.

48. Yu ZH, Chan HC. Gossypol and hypokalemia: a critical review. *Adv Contracept Deliv Syst.* 1994;10(1–2):23–33.

49. Khajehdehi P, Tastegar A, Kharazmi A. Immunological and clinical aspects of kidney disease in typhoid fever in Iran. *Q J Med.* 1984;53:101.

50. Hayashi M, Kouzu H, Nishihara M, et al. Acute renal failure likely due to acute nephritic syndrome associated with typhoid fever. *Intern Med.* 2005;44(10):1074–1077.

51. Sitprija V, Pipantanagul V, Boonpucknavig V, et al. Glomerulitis in typhoid fever. *Ann Intern Med.* 1974;81(2):210–213.

52. Khan FY, Al-Ani A, Ali HA. Typhoid rhabdomyolysis with acute renal failure and acute pancreatitis: a case report and review of the literature. *Int J Infect Dis.* 2009;13(5):e282–285.

53. Barsoum RS. Schistosomiasis and the kidney. *Semin Nephrol.* 2003;23 (1):34–41.

54. Muniz-Junqueira MI, Tosta CE, Prata A. Schistosoma-associated chronic septicemic salmonellosis: evolution of knowledge and immunopathogenic mechanisms. *Rev Soc Bras Med Trop.* 2009;42(4):436–445.

55. Niwattayakul K, Homvijitkul J, Niwattayakul S, et al. Hypotension, renal failure and pulmonary complications in leptospirosis. *Ren Fail.* 2002;24(3):297–305.

56. Andrade L, Rodrigues AC Jr, Sanches TR, et al. Leptospirosis leads to dysregulation of sodium transporters in the kidney and lung. *Am J Physiol Renal Physiol.* 2007;292(2):F586–592.

57. Sitprija V, Pipatanagul V, Mertowidjojo K, et al. Pathogenesis of renal disease in leptospirosis: Clinical and experimental studies. *Kidney Int.* 1980;17(6):827–836.

58. Breiner DD, Fahey M, Salvador R, et al. Leptospira interrogans binds to human cell surface receptors including proteoglycans. *Infect Immun.* 2009; 77(12):5528–5536.

59. Yamash iro-Kanashiro EH, Benard G, Sato MN, et al. Cellular immune response analysis of patients with leptospirosis. *Am J Trop Med Hyg.* 1991;45:138.

60. Losuwanrak K, Sitprija V. Fluid administration in leptospirosis: the potential use of dopamine. *Intern Med J Thai.* 2003;19:180.

61. Ruel O, Teaño MD, Efren M, et al. Leptospirosis with acute renal failure: the role of conservative management. *Phi J Microbiol Infect Dis.* 2001;30(2):51–55.

62. da Silva Júnior GB, Daher Ede F. Renal involvement in leprosy: retrospective analysis of 461 cases in Brazil. *Braz J Infect Dis.* 2006;10(2):107–112.

63. Lomonte C, Chiarulli G, Cazzato F, et al. End-stage renal disease in leprosy. *J Nephrol.* 2004;17(2):302–305.

64. Oliveira RA, Silva GB Jr, Souza CJ, et al. Evaluation of renal function in leprosy: a study of 59 consecutive patients. *Nephrol Dial Transplant.* 2008;23(1):256–262.

65. Nigam P, Pant KC, Kapoor KK, et al. Histo-functional status of kidney in leprosy. *Indian J Lepr.* 1986;58(4):567–575.

66. Cöloğblu AS. Immune complex glomerulonephritis in leprosy. *Lepr Rev.* 1979;50(3):213–222.

67. Paveenkittiporn W, Apisarnthanarak A, Dejsirilert S, et al. Five-year surveillance for Burkholderia pseudomallei in Thailand from 2000 to 2004: prevalence and antimicrobial susceptibility. *J Med Assoc Thai.* 2009;92 Suppl 4:S46–52.

68. Wibulpolprasert B, Dhiensiri T. Visceral organ abscesses in meliodosis: sonographic findings. *Clin Ultrasound.* 1999;27:29.

69. Susaengrat W, Dhiensiri T, Sinavatana P, Sitprija V. Renal failure in melioidosis. *Nephron.* 1987;46(2):167–169.

70. Northfield J, Whitty CJM, MacPhee IAM. Burkholderia pseudomallei infection, or melioidosis, and nephritic syndrome. *Nephrol Dial Transplant.* 2002;17:137.

71. Daher EF, Abdulkader RC, Motti E, et al. Prospective study of tetanus-induced acute renal dysfunction: role of adrenergic overactivity. *Am J Trop Med Hyg.* 1997;57(5):610–614.

72. Weiss MF, Badalamenti J, Fish E. Tetanus as a cause of rhabdomyolysis and acute renal failure. *Clin Nephrol.* 2010;73:64.

73. Martinelli R, Matos CM, Rocha H. Tetanus as a cause of acute renal failure: possible role of rhabdomyolysis. *Rev Soc Bras Med Trop.* 1993;26(1):1–4.

74. Singh M, Saidali A, Bakhtiar A, et al. Diphtheria in Afghanistan. Review of 155 cases. *J Trop Med Hyg.* 1985;88:373.

75. Melby EL, Jacobsen J, Olsnes S, et al. Entry of protein toxins in polarized epithelial cells. *Cancer Res.* 1993;53:1755.

76. Monteiro HS, Lima AA, Fonteles MC. Glomerular effects of cholera toxin in isolated perfused rat kidney: a potential role for platelet activating factor. *Pharmacol Toxicol.* 1999;85:105.

77. Sandvig K, Bergan J, Dyve AB, et al. Endocytosis and retrograde transport of Shiga toxin. *Toxicon.* 2010;56(7):1181–1185.

78. Bennish ML, Harris JR, Wojtyniak BJ, et al. Death in shigellosis: incidence and risk factors in hospitalized patients. *J Infect Dis.* 1990;162:573.

79. Olotu AI, Mithwani S, Newton CR. Haemolytic uraemic syndrome in children admitted to a rural district hospital in Kenya. *Trop Doct.* 2008;38(3):165–167.

80. Srivastava RN, Moudgil A, Bagga A, et al. Hemolytic-uremic syndrome in children in northern India. *Pediatr Nephrol.* 1991;5:284.

81. Lerstloompleephunt N, Tantawichien T, Sitprija V. Renal failure in vibrio vulnificus infection. *Ren Fail.* 2000;22(3):337–343.

82. Miyoshi S, Hirata Y, Tomochika K, et al. Vibrio vulnificus may produce a metalloproteinase causing an edematous skin lesion in vivo. *FEMS Microbiol Lett.* 1994;121(3):321–325.

83. Barton JC, Coghlan ME, Reymann MT, et al. Vibrio vulnificus infection in a hemodialysis patient receiving intravenous iron therapy. *Clin Infect Dis* 2003;37(5):e63–67.

84. Malik A, Earhart K, Mohareb E, et al. Dengue hemorrhagic fever outbreak in children in Port Sudan. *J Infect Public Health.* 2011;4(1):1–6.

85. Gunasekera HH, Adikaram AV, Herath CA, et al. Myoglobinuric acute renal failure following dengue viral infection. *Ceylon Med J.* 2000;45:181.

86. Boonpucknavig V, Bhamaraparavati N, Boonpucknavig S, et al. Glomerular changes in dengue hemorrhagic fever. *Arch Pathol Lab Med.* 1976;100:206.

87. Cosgriff TM, Levis RM. Mechanisms of disease in hemorrhagic fever with renal syndrome. *Kidney Int.* 1991;35:S72.

88. Ferluga D, Vizjak A. Hantavirus nephropathy. *J Am Soc Nephrol.* 2008;19:1653.

89. Panomsak S, Lewsuwan S, Eiam-Ong S, et al. Hepatitis-B virus-associated nephropathies in adults: a clinical study in Thailand. *J Med Assoc Thai.* 2006;89 Suppl 2:S151–156.

90. Han SH. Extrahepatic manifestations of chronic hepatitis B. *Clin Liver Dis.* 2004;8(2):403–418.

91. Alam S, Azam G, Mustafa G, et al. Natural course of fulminant hepatic failure: the scenario in Bangladesh and the differences from the west. *Saudi J Gastroenterol.* 2009;15(4):229–233.

92. Lai KN, Lai FM. Clinical features and the natural course of hepatitis B virus-related glomerulopathy in adults. *Kidney Int. Suppl.* 1991;35:S40–45.

93. Chan TM. Hepatitis B and renal disease. *Curr Hepat Rep.* 2010;9(2):99–105.

94. Jiang W, Liu LQ. Effect of content of hepatitis B virus DNA in the serum on the pathologic change in hepatitis B virus associated-glomerulonephritis. *Zhong Nan Da Xue Xue Bao Yi Xue Ban.* 2008;33(9):857–860.

95. Lai KN, Lai FM, Tam JS. IgA nephropathy associated with chronic hepatitis B virus infection in adults: the pathogenetic role of HBsAg. *J Pathol.* 1989;157:321.

96. Sabry AA, Sobh MA, Irving WL, et al. A comprehensive study of the association between hepatitis C virus and glomerulopathy. *Nephrol Dial Transplant.* 2002;17(2):239–245.

97. KDIGO. Clinical practice guidelines for the prevention, diagnosis, evaluation, and treatment of hepatitis C in chronic kidney disease. *Kidney Int.* 2008;73(Suppl 109):S1–S2.

98. Lee JH, Choi MS, Gwak GY, et al. Clinical features and predictive factors of acute hepatitis A complicated with acute kidney injury. *Korean J Gastroenterol.* 2010;56(6):359–364.

99. Cheema SR, Arif F, Charneg D, et al. IgA-dominant glomerulonephritis associated with hepatitis A. *Clin Nephrol.* 2004;62:138.

100. Chu KH, Tsang WK, Tang CS, et al. Acute renal impairment in coronavirus-associated severe acute respiratory syndrome. *Kidney Int.* 2005;67(2):698–705.

101. Bellomo R, Pettilä V, Webb SA, et al. Acute kidney injury and 2009 H1N1 influenza-related critical illness. *Contrib Nephrol.* 2010;165:310–314.

102. Trimarchi H, Greloni G, Campolo-Girard V, et al. H1N1 infection and the kidney in critically ill patients. *J Nephrol.* 2010;23(6):725–731.

103. Kimmel PL. HIV-associated nephropathy: virologic issues related to renal sclerosis. *Nephrol Dial Transplant.* 2003;18 Suppl 6:vi59–63.

104. Gerntholtz TE, Goetsch SJ, Katz I. HIV-related nephropathy: a South African perspective. *Kidney Int.* 2006;69(10):1885–1891.

105. Praditpornsilpa K, Napathorn S, Yenrudi S, et al. Renal pathology and HIV infection in Thailand. *Am J Kidney Dis.* 1999;33(2):282–286.

106. Kiryluk K, Martino J, Gharavi AG. Genetic susceptibility, HIV infection, and the kidney. *Clin J Am Soc Nephrol.* 2007;2 Suppl 1:S25–35.

107. Naicker S, Fabian J. Risk factors for the development of chronic kidney disease with HIV/AIDS. *Clin Nephrol.* 2010;74 Suppl 1:S51–56.

108. Mocroft A. The difficulties of classifying renal disease in HIV-infected patients. *HIV Med.* 2011;12(1):1–3.
109. Ruddy BE, Mayer AP, Ko MG, et al. Coccidioidomycosis in African Americans. *Mayo Clin Proc.* 2011;86(1):63–69.
110. Ferreira MS. Paracoccidioidomycosis. *Paediatr Respir Rev.* 2009;10(4): 161–165.
111. Wafa EW, Yahya RS, Sobh MA, et al. Human ochratoxicosis and nephropathy in Egypt: a preliminary study. *Hum Exp Toxicol.* 1998;17(2):124–129.
112. Hmaissia Khlifa K, Ghali R, Mazigh C, et al. Serum levels of ochratoxin A in healthy subjects and in nephropathic patients in Tunisia. *Ann Biol Clin (Paris).* 2008;66(6):631–636.
113. Epstein SM, Bartus B, Farber E. Renal epithelial neoplasm induced in male Wistar rats by oral aflatoxin B1. *Cancer Res.* 1969;29:1045.
114. Hassan AM, Sheashaa HA, Abdel Fatah MF, et al. Does aflatoxin as an environmental mycotoxin adversely affect the renal and hepatic functions of Egyptian lactating mothers and their infants? A preliminary report. *Int Urol Nephrol.* 2006;38(2):339–342.
115. Ascioglu S, Rex JH, de Pauw B, et al. Defining opportunistic invasive fungal infections in immunocompromised patients with cancer and hematopoietic stem cell transplants: an international consensus. *Clin Infect Dis.* 2002,34(1): 7–14.
116. Baer S, Baddlet JW, Gnann JW, et al. Cryptococcal disease presenting as necrotizing cellulitis in transplant recipients. *Transplant Infect Dis.* 2009;11: 353–358.
117. Gupta KL, Joshi K, Sud K, et al. Renal zygomycosis: an under-diagnosed cause of acute renal failure. *Nephrol Dial Transplant.* 1999;14:2720.
118. Barsoum RS. Parasitic infections in transplant recipients. *Nat Clin Pract Nephrol.* 2006;2:490–503.
119. Tan HW, Ch'ng SL. Drug interaction between cyclosporine A and quinine in a renal transplant patient with malaria. *Singapore Med J.* 1991;32:89.
120. Nampoory MR, Nessim J, Gupta RK, et al. Drug interaction of chloroquine with ciclosporin. *Nephron.* 1992;62:108.
121. Llorente S, Gimeno L, Navarro MJ, et al. Therapy of visceral leishmaniasis in renal transplant recipients intolerant to pentavalent antimonials. *Transplantation.* 2000;70:800.
122. Bell A, Roberts HC, Chappell LH. The antiparasite effect t of cyclosporine A: Possible drug target and clinical application. *Gen Pharmacol.* 1996;27: 963–971.
123. Monaghan P, Bell A. A Plasmodium falciparum FK506–binding protein (FKBP) with peptidyl-prolyl cis-trans isomerase and chaperone activities. *Mol Biochem Parasitol.* 2005;139(2):185–195.
124. Barsoum RS. Schistosomal glomerulopathies. *Kidney Int.* 1993;44:1.
125. de Vallière S, Mary C, Joneberg JE, et al. AA-Amyloidosis caused by visceral leishmaniasis in a human immunodeficiency virus-infected patient. *Am J Trop Med Hyg.* 2009;81(2):209–212.
126. Gilles HM, Hendrichse RG. Nephrosis in Nigerian children. Role of malaria and effect of antimalarial treatment. *Br Med J (Clin Res).* 1963;5348:27.
127. Powell KC, Meadows R. The nephrotic syndrome in New Guinea. A clinical and histological spectrum. *Aust N Z J Med.* 1971;1:363.
128. Morel-Maroger L, Saimot AG, Sloper JC, et al. Topical nephropathy and tropical extramembranous glomerulonephritis of unknown aetiology in Senegal. *Br Med J.* 1975;1:541.
129. Hendrickse RG, Adeniyi A. Quartan malarial nephrotic syndrome in children. *Kidney Int.* 1979;16:64.
130. Atkinson LE. Bright's disease of Malarial origin. *Am J Med Sci.* 1884;88:149.
131. Olowu WA, Adelusola KA, Adefehinti O, et al. Quartan malaria-associated childhood nephrotic syndrome: now a rare clinical entity in malaria endemic Nigeria. *Nephrol Dial Transplant.* 2010;25(3):794–801.
132. Boonpucknavig V, Boonpucknavig S, Bhamarapravati N. Plasmodium berghei infection in mice: an ultrastructural study of immune complex nephritis. *Am J Pathol.* 1973;70:89.
133. Wedderburn N, Davies DR, Mitchell GH, et al. Glomerulonephritis in common marmosets infected with Plasmodium brasilianum and Epstein-Barr virus. *J Infect Dis.* 1988;158:789.
134. Pakasa M, Van Damme B, Desmet VJ. Free intraglomerular malarial antigens. *Br J Exp Pathol.* 1985;66:493.
135. Houba V. Immunologic aspects of renal lesions associated with malaria. *Kidney Int.* 1979;16:3.
136. Sitprija V. Nephrology forum: nephropathy in falciparum malaria. *Kidney Int.* 1988;34:866.
137. Barsoum RS. Malarial acute renal failure. *J Am Soc Nephrol.* 2000;11:2147.
138. Eiam-Ong S. Malarial nephropathy. *Semin Nephrol.* 2003;23:21.
139. Bircan Z, Kervancioglu M, Soran M, et al. Two cases of nephrotic syndrome and tertian malaria in south-eastern Anatolia. *Pediatr Nephrol.* 1997;11:78.
140. Price RN, Douglas NM, Anstey NM. New developments in Plasmodium vivax malaria: severe disease and the rise of chloroquine resistance. *Curr Opin Infect Dis.* 2009;22(5):430–435.
141. Prakash J, Singh AK, Kumar NS, et al. Acute renal failure in Plasmodium vivax malaria. *J Assoc Physicians India.* 2003;51:265.
142. Das BS. Renal failure in malaria. *J Vector Borne Dis.* 2008;45(2):83–97.
143. Singh N, Shukla MM, Sharma VP. Epidemiology of malaria in pregnancy in central India. *Bull World Health Organ.* 1999;77:567.
144. Naqvi R, Ahmad E, Akhtar F, et al. Outcome in severe acute renal failure associated with malaria. *Nephrol Dial Transplant.* 2003;18:1820.
145. Eiam-Ong S, Sitprija V. Falciparum malaria and the kidney: a model of inflammation. *Am J Kidney Dis.* 1998;32:361.
146. Rui-Mei L, Kara AU, Sinniah R. Dysregulation of cytokine expression in tubulointerstitial nephritis associated with murine malaria. *Kidney Int.* 1998; 53:845.
147. Sinniah R, Rui-Mei L, Kara A. Up-regulation of cytokines in glomerulonephritis associated with murine malaria infection. *Int J Exp Pathol.* 1999;80:87.
148. Hartenbower DL, Kantor GL, Rosen VJ. Renal failure due to acute glomerulonephritis during falciparum malaria: case report. *Mil Med.* 1972;137:74.
149. Tromans A. Malaria. The calcium connection. *Nature.* 2004;429:253.
150. Dash SC, Bhuyan UN, Gupta A, et al. Falciparum malaria complicating cholestatic jaundice and acute renal failure. *J Assoc Physicians India.* 1994;42:1012.
151. Reynaud F, Mallet L, Lyon A, Rodolfo JM. Rhabdomyolysis and acute renal failure in Plasmodium falciparum malaria. *Nephrol Dial Transplant.* 2005;20(4):847.
152. Fairhurst RM, Sadou B, Guindo A, et al. Case report: life-threatening hypoglycaemia associated with sulfadoxine-pyrimethamine, a commonly used antimalarial drug. *Trans R Soc Trop Med Hyg.* 2003;97:595.
153. Odeh M. Lactic acidosis and falciparum malaria. *Q J Med.* 1993;86:619.
154. Uyemura SA, Luo S, Moreno SN, et al. Oxidative phosphorylation, Ca(2+) transport, and fatty acid-induced uncoupling in malaria parasites mitochondria. *J Biol Chem.* 2000;275:9709.
155. Arun-Kumar C, Das UN. Lipid peroxides, nitric oxide and essential fatty acids in patients with Plasmodium falciparum malaria. *Prostaglandins Leukot Essent Fatty Acids.* 1999;61(4):255–258.
156. Krause PJ, Daily J, Telford SR, et al. Shared features in the pathobiology of babesiosis and malaria. *Trends Parasitol.* 2007;23(12):605–610.
157. Annable CR, Ward PA. Immunopathology of the renal complications of babesiosis. *J Immunol.* 1974;112:1.
158. Itturri GM, Cox HW. Glomerulonephritis associated with acute haemosporidian infection. *Mil Med (Special Issue).* 1969;134:1119.
159. Perdrizet GA, Olson NH, Krause PJ, et al. Babesiosis in a renal transplant recipient acquired through blood transfusion. *Transplantation.* 2000;70:205.
160. Alex S, Criado C, Fernandez-Guerrero ML, et al. Nephrotic syndrome complicating chronic visceral leishmaniasis re-emergence in patients with AIDS. *Clin Nephrol.* 2008;70(1):65–68.
161. Veerareddy PR, Vobalaboina V, Ali N. Antileishmanial activity, pharmacokinetics and tissue distribution studies of mannose –grafted amphotericin B lipid nanospheres. *J Drug Target.* 2009;17(2):140–147.
162. Efstratiadis G, Boura E, Giamalis P, et al. Renal involvement in a patient with visceral leishmaniasis. *Nephrol Dial Transplant.* 2006;21(1):235–236.
163. Prianti MG, Yokoo M, Saldanha LC, et al. Leishmania (Leishmania) chagasi-infected mice as a model for the study of glomerular lesions in visceral leishmaniasis. *Braz J Med Biol Res.* 2007;40(6):819–823.
164. Costa FA, Prianti MG, Silva TC, et al. T cells, adhesion molecules and modulation of apoptosis in visceral leishmaniasis glomerulonephritis. *BMC Infect Dis.* 2010;10:112.
165. van Velthuysen ML, Mayen AE, van Rooijen N, et al. T cells and macrophages in Trypanosoma brucei-related glomerulopathy. *Infect Immun.* 1994;62(8): 3230–3235.
166. Nagle RB, Ward PA, Lindsley HB, et al. Experimental infections with African trypanosomiasis. VI. Glomerulonephritis involving the alternate pathway of complement activation. *Am J Trop Med Hyg.* 1974;23:15.
167. Ginsburg BE, Wasserman J, Huldt G, et al. Case of glomerulonephritis associated with acute toxoplasmosis. *Br Med J.* 1974;3:664.
168. Crawford FG, Vermund SH. Human cryptosporidiosis. *CRC Crit Rev Microbiol.* 1988;16:113.
169. Schantz PM, Okelo GB. Echinococcosis (Hydatidosis). In: Warren KS, Mahmoud AA, eds. *Tropical and Geographic Medicine.* 2nd ed. New York: McGraw Hill; 1990:505.
170. Aziz F, Pandy T, Patel HV, et al. Nephrotic presentation in hydatid cyst disease with predominant tubulointerstital disease. *Int J Nephrol Renovasc Dis.* 2009;2:23–26.
171. Covic A, Mititiuc I, Caruntu L, et al. A reversible nephrotic syndrome due to mesangiocapillary glomerulonephritis secondary to hepatic hydatid disease. *Nephrol Dial Transplant.* 1996;11:2074–2076.

172. Barsoum RS. Schistosomiasis. In: Davison AM, Cameron JS, Gruenfeld JP, eds, et al. *Oxford Textbook of Clinical Nephrology*. London: Oxford University Press; 2005:1173–1195.
173. De Water R, Van Marck EA, Fransen JA, et al. Schistosoma mansoni: ultrastructural localization of the circulating anodic antigen and the circulating cathodic antigen in the mouse kidney glomerulus. *Am J Trop Med Hyg.* 1988;38:118.
174. Barsoum RS. Tropical parasitic nephropathies. *Nephrol Dial Transplant.* 1999;14 Suppl 3:79.
175. Martinelli R, Nobiat AC, Brito E, et al. Schistosoma mansoni induced mesangiocapillary glomerulonephritis: influence of therapy. *Kidney Int.* 1989;35:1227.
176. Barsoum RS, Nabil M, Saady G, et al. Immunoglobulin-A and the pathogenesis of schistosomal glomerulopathy. *Kidney Int.* 1996;50:920.
177. Sobh M, Moustafa F, Ramzy R, et al. Schistosomal mansoni nephropathy in Syrian golden hamsters. Effect of dose and duration of infection. *Nephron.* 1991;59:121.
178. Barsoum R. The changing face of schistosomal glomerulopathy. *Kidney Int.* 2004;66:2472.
179. Watt G, Long GW, Calubaquib C, et al. Prevalence of renal involvement in Schistosoma japonicum infection. *Trans R Soc Trop Med Hyg.* 1987;81:339.
180. Ngu JL, Chatelanat F, Leke R, et al. Nephropathy in Cameroon: evidence for filarial derived immune complex pathogenesis in some cases. *Clin Nephrol.* 1985;24:128.
181. Waugh DA, Alexander JH, Ibels LH. Filarial chyluria–associated glomerulonephritis and therapeutic consideration in the chyluric patient. *Aust N Z J Med.* 1980;10:559.
182. Ormerod AD, Petersen J, Hussey JK, et al. Immune complex glomerulonephritis and chronic anaerobic urinary tract infection; complication of filariasis. *Postgrad Med J.* 1983;59:730.
183. Chugh KS, Singhal PC, Tewari SC, et al. Acute glomerulonephritis associated with filariasis. *Am J Trop Med Hyg.* 1978;27:630.
184. Lukiana T, Mandina M, Situakibanza NH, et al. A possible case of spontaneous Loa loa encephalopathy associated with a glomerulopathy. *Filaria Journal.* 2006;5:6–13.
185. Dixit V, Subhadra AV, Bisen PS, et al. Antigen-specific immune complexes in urine of patients with lymphatic filariasis. *J Clin Lab Anal.* 2007;21(1):46–48.
186. Date A, Gunasekaran V, Kirubakaran MG, et al. Acute eosinophilic glomerulonephritis with bancroftian filariasis. *Postgrad Med J.* 1979;55:905.
187. Pakasa NM, Nseka NM, Nyimi LM. Secondary collapsing glomerulopathy associated with Loa loa filariasis. *Am J Kidney Dis.* 1997;30(6):836–839.
188. Fernando SD, Rodrigo C, Rajapakse S. Current evidence on the use of antifilarial agents in the management of bancroftian filariasis. *J Trop Med.* 2011;2011:175941.
189. Cummins WT, Carson GR. Human trichinosis. A study of 15 cases. *JAMA.* 1916;67:806.
190. Sitprija V, Keoplung M, Boonpucknavig V, et al. Renal involvement in human trichinosis. *Arch Intern Med.* 1980;140:544.
191. Todorova V, Krustev L, Svilenov D, et al. Antigen-antibody complexes in experimental infection with Trichinella spiralis and their role in the development of kidney lesions. *Angew Parasitol.* 1990;31(1):35–42.
192. Koompirochana C, Sonakul D, Chinda K, et al. Opisthorchiasis. A clinicopathologic study of 154 autopsy cases. *Southeast Asian J Trop Med Public Health.* 1978;9:60.
193. Sitprija V, Kashemsant U, Sriratanaban A, et al. Renal function in obstructive jaundice in man: cholangiocarcinoma model. *Kidney Int.* 1990;38:948.
194. Sripa B. Pathobiology of opisthorchiasis: an update. *Acta Trop.* 2003;88(3):209–220.
195. Boonpucknavig S, Boonpucknavig V, Tanvanich S, et al. Opisthorchis viverrini: development of immune complex glomerulonephritis and amyloidosis in infected Syrian golden hamsters. *J Med Assoc Thai.* 1992;75(Suppl):7.
196. Hsieh YP, Wen YK, Chen ML. Minimal change nephrotic syndrome in association with strongyloidiasis. *Clin Nephrol.* 2006;66(6):459–463.
197. Wong TY, Szeto CC, Lai FF, et al. Nephrotic syndrome in strongyloidiasis: remission after eradication with anthelmintic agents. *Nephron.* 1998;79(3):333–336.
198. Sasmal NK, Acharya S, Laha R. Larval migration of Toxocara canis in piglets and transfer of larvae from infected porcine tissue to mice. *J Helminthol.* 2008;82(3):245–249.
199. Westendorp RG, Doorenbos CJ, Thompson J, et al. Immune complex glomerulonephritis associated with an amebic liver abscess. *Trans R Soc Trop Med Hyg.* 1990;84:385.
200. Jha V, Chugh KS. Nephropathy associated with animal, plant, and chemical toxins in the tropics. *Semin Nephrol.* 2003;23(1):49–65.
201. Chugh KS. Snake bite induced renal failure in India. *Kidney Int.* 1989;35:891.
202. Collares-Buzato CB, Le Sueur LP, Cruz-Hofling MA. Impairment of the cell-to-matrix adhesion and cytotoxicity induced by Bothrops moojeni snake venom in cultured renal tubular epithelia. *Toxicol Appl Pharmacol.* 2002;181:124.
203. Han HE, Than T, Lwin M, et al. Urinary fibrinogen degradation products in Russell's viper (Daboia russelli siamensis) bite victims. *Southeast Asian J Trop Med Public Health.* 1993;24:198.
204. Steinbeck VW. Nephrotic syndrome developing after snake bite. *Med J Aust.* 1960;1:543.
205. Sitprija V, Gopalakrishnakone P. Snake bite, rhabdomyolysis, and renal failure. *Am J Kidney Dis.* 1998;31(6):l-lii.
206. Thamaree S, Sitprija V, Leepipatpaiboon S, et al. Mediators and renal hemodynamics in Russell's viper envenomation. *J Nat Toxicol.* 2000;9:43.
207. Suwansrinon K, Khow O, Mitmoonpitak C, et al. Effects of Russell's viper venom fractions on systemic and renal hemodynamics. *Toxicon.* 2007;49(1):82–88.
208. Ratcliff PJ, Pukrittayakamee S, Ledingham JG, et al. Direct nephrotoxicity of Russell's viper venom demonstrated in the isolated perfused rat kidney. *Am J Trop Med Hyg.* 1987;40:312.
209. Elming H, Sølling K. Urine protein excretion after Hymenoptera sting. *Scand J Urol Nephrol.* 1994;28(1):13–15.
210. Barss P. Renal failure and death after multiple stings in Papua New Guinea. Ecology, prevention and management of attacks by vespid wasps. *Med J Aust.* 1989;151:659.
211. Cuoghi D, Venturi P, Cheli E. Bee sting and relapse of nephrotic syndrome. *Child Nephrol Urol.* 1988;9:82.
212. Pirotzky E, Hieblot C, Benveniste J, et al. Basophil sensitization in idiopathic nephrotic syndrome. *Lancet.* 1982;319:358–361.
213. Hyre HM, Smith RA. Immunological effects of honey bee (Apis mellifera) venom using BALB/c mice. *Toxicon.* 1986;24(5):435–440.
214. Brosolin NL, Carvalho LC, Goes EC, et al. Acute renal failure following massive attack by Africanized bee stings. *Pediatr Nephrol.* 2002;17:625.
215. Grisotto LS, Mendes GE, Castro I, et al. Mechanisms of bee venom-induced acute renal failure. *Toxicon.* 2006;48(1):44–54.
216. Zhang R, Meleg-Smith S, Batuman V. Acute tubulointerstitial nephritis after wasp stings. *Am J Kidney Dis.* 2001;38:E33.
217. Han Hj, Lee JH, Park SH, et al. Effect of bee venom and its melittin on apical transporters of renal proximal tubule cells. *Kidney Blood Pres Res.* 2000;23:393.
218. Park SK, Kim DG, Kang SK, et al. Toxic acute renal failure and hepatitis after ingestion of raw carp bile. *Nephron.* 1990;56:188.
219. Xuan BH, Thi TX, Nguyen ST, et al. Ichthyotoxic ARF after fish gall-bladder ingestion: a large case series from Vietnam. *Am J Kidney Dis.* 2003;41:220.
220. Hwang DF, Yeh YH, Lai YS, Deng JF. Identification of cyprinol and cyprinol sulfate from grass carp bile and their toxic effects in rats. *Toxicon.* 2001;39(2–3):411–414.
221. Lin CT, Huang PC, Yen TS, et al. Partial purification and some characteristic nature of a toxic fraction of the grass carp bile. *Chin Biochem Soc.* 1977;6:1.
222. Harvey AL, Rowan EG, Vatanpour H, et al. Potassium channel toxins and transmitter release. *Ann N Y Acad Sci.* 1994;710:1–10.
223. Waterman JA. Some notes on scorpion poisoning in Trinidad. *Trans R Soc Trop Med Hyg.* 1993;32:607.
224. Pipelzadeh MH, Jalali A, Taraz M, et al. An epidemiological and a clinical study on scorpionism by the Iranian scorpion Hemiscorpius lepturus. *Toxicon.* 2007;50(7):984–992.
225. Bahloul M, Ben Hmida M, Belhoul W, et al. Hemolytic uremic syndrome secondary to scorpion envenomation. *Nephrologie.* 2004;25:49.
226. Ramialiharisoa A, de Haro L, Jouglard J, et al. Latrodectism in Madagascar (French). *Med Trop (Mars).* 1994;54(2):127–130.
227. Veiga SS, Zaanetti VC, Braz A, et al. Extracellular matrix molecules as targets for brown spider venom toxins. *Braz J Med Biol Res.* 2001;34:843.
228. Hasan S, Hassan K. Proteinuria associated with centipede bite. *Pediatr Nephrol.* 2005;20(4):550–551.
229. Logan JL, Ogden DA. Rhabdomyolysis and acute renal failure following the bite of the giant desert centipede Scolopendra heros. *West J Med.* 1985;142(4):549–550.
230. Arocha-Pinango CL, de Bosch NB, Torres A, et al. Six new cases of a caterpillar-induced bleeding disorder. *Thromb Haemost.* 1992;67:402.
231. Burdmann EA, Antunes I, Saldanha LB, et al. Severe acute renal failure induced by the venom of Lonomia caterpillars. *Clin Nephrol.* 1996;40:337.
232. Gamborgi GP, Metcalf EB, Barros EJ. Acute renal failure provoked by toxin from caterpillars of the species Lonomia obliqua. *Toxicon.* 2006;47(1):68–74.
233. Mallari RQ, Saif M, Elbualy MS, Sapru A. Ingestion of a blister beetle (Mecoidae family). *Pediatrics.* 1996;98(3 Pt 1):458–459.
234. H'ng PK, Nayar SK, Lau WM, et al. Acute renal failure following jering ingestion. *Singapore Med J.* 1991;32:148.
235. Eiam-Ong S, Sitprija V, Saetang P, et al. Djenkol bean nephrotoxicity in Southern Thailand. Proceedings First Asian Pacific Congress Animal, Plant and Microbial Toxins. Singapore; 1987:628.

236. Stewart MJ. The cytotoxic effects of a traditional Zulu remedy, impila (Callilepis laureola). *Hum Exp Toxicol.* 2002;21(12):643–647.
237. Matthai TP, Date A. Renal cortical necrosis following exposure to sap of the marking-nut tree (Semecarpus anacardium). *Am J Trop Med Hyg.* 1979;28:773.
238. Fang HC, Lee PT, Lu PJ, et al. Mechanisms of star fruit-induced acute renal failure. *Food Chem Toxicol.* 2008;46(5):1744–1752.
239. Sato A, Fujiwara H, Oku H, et al. Alpha-mangostin induces Ca2+-ATPase-dependent apoptosis via mitochondrial pathway in PC12 cells. *J Pharmacol Sci.* 2004;95(1):33–40.
240. Matsumoto K, Akao Y, Yi H, et al. Preferential target is mitochondria in alpha-mangostin-induced apoptosis in human leukemia HL60 cells. *Bioorg Med Chem.* 2004;12(22):5799–5806.
241. Wang LR, Klemmer PJ. Severe lactic acidosis associated with juice of the mangosteen fruit. Garcinia mangostana. *Am J Kidney Dis.* 2008;51:879.
242. Vetter J. Toxins of Amanita phalloides. *Toxicon.* 1997;63:13.
243. McClain JL, Hause DW, Clark MA. Amanita phalloides mushroom poisoning : A cluster of four fatalities. *J Forensic Sci.* 1989;34:83.
244. Prast H, Pfaller W. Toxic properties of the mushroom Cortinarius orellanus (Fries) II. Impairment of renal function in rats. *Arch Toxicol.* 1988;62:89.
245. Covic A, Goldsmith DJ, Gusbeth-Tatomir P, et al. Successful use of Molecular Absorbent Regenerating System (MARS) dialysis for the treatment of fulminant hepatic failure in children accidentally poisoned by toxic mushroom ingestion. *Liver Int.* 2003;23 Suppl 3:21–27.
246. Lin JL, Ho YS. Flavonoid-induced acute nephropathy. *Am J Kidney Dis.* 1994;23(3):433–440.
247. Gold CH. Acute renal failure from herbal and patent remedies in Blacks. *Clin Nephrol.* 1980;14:128.
248. Lowenthal MN, Jones IG, Mohelsky V. Acute renal failure in Zambia women using traditional herbal medicine. *J Trop Med Hyg.* 1974;77:190.
249. Tokarnia CH, Dobereiner J, Peixoto PV. Poisonous plants affecting livestock in Brazil. *Toxicon.* 2002;40:1635.
250. Prema TP, Raghuramulu N. Vitamin D—like activity in Cestrum diurnum grown in Hyderabad, India. *J Sci Food Agr.* 1993;62(1):21–27.
251. Weisbord SD, Soule JB, Kimel PL. Poison on line—acute renal failure caused by oil of wormwook purchased through internet. *N Engl J Med.* 2010;337:825.
252. Li P, Kawachi H, Suzuki Y, et al. The prevention of glomerulosclerosis in rats using traditional Chinese medicine, Sairei-to. *Nephrology.* 2000;5:83.
253. Dinis-Oliveira RJ, Duarte JA, Sánchez-Navarro A, et al. Paraquat poisonings: mechanisms of lung toxicity, clinical features, and treatment. *Crit Rev Toxicol.* 2008;38(1):13–71.
254. Kim SJ, Gil HW, Yang JO, et al. The clinical features of acute kidney injury in patients with acute paraquat intoxication. *Nephrol Dial Transplant.* 2009;24(4):1226–1232.
255. Gil HW, Yang JO, Lee EY, et al. Paraquat-induced Fanconi syndrome. *Nephrology.* 2005;10(5):430–432.
256. Lin JL, Lin-Tan DT, Chen KH, et al. Repeated pulse of methylprednisolone and cyclophosphamide with continuous dexamethasone therapy for patients with severe paraquat poisoning. *Crit Care Med.* 2006;34(2):368–373.
257. Faure A, Mathon L, Poupelin JC, et al. Acute cupric sulfate intoxication: pathophysiology and therapy about a case report. *Ann Fr Anesth Reanim.* 2003;22(6):557–559.
258. Takeda T, Yukoka T, Shimazaki S. Cupric sulfate intoxication with rhabdomyolysis, treated with chelating agents and blood purification. *Intern Med.* 2000;39:253.
259. Okuonghae HO, Ighogboja IS, Lawson JO, et al. Diethylene glycol poisoning in Nigerian children. *Ann Trop Pediatr.* 1992;12:235.
260. Hanif M, Mobarak MR, Ronan A, et al. Fatal renal failure caused by diethylene glycol in paracetamol elixir: the Bangladesh epidemic. *BMJ.* 1995;311:88.
261. O'Brien KL, Selanikio JD, Hecdivert C, et al. Epidemic of pediatric deaths from acute renal failure caused by diethylene glycol poisoning. *JAMA.* 1998;279:1175.
262. Soderland P, Lovekar S, Weiner DE, et al. Chronic kidney disease associated with environmental toxins and exposures. *Adv Chronic Kidney Dis.* 2010;17(3):254–264.
263. Hard GC, Rodgers IS, Baetcke KP, et al. Hazard evaluation of chemicals that cause accumulation of alpha 2u-globulin, hyaline droplet nephropathy, and tubule neoplasia in the kidneys of male rats. *Environ Health Perspect.* 1993;99:313–349.
264. Evans M, Elinder CG. Chronic renal failure from lead: myth or evidence-based fact?. *Kidney Int.* 2011;79(3):272–279.
265. Nawrot TS, Staessen JA, Roels HA, et al. Cadmium exposure in the population: from health risks to strategies of prevention. *Biometals.* 2010;23(5):769–782.
266. Lipworth L, Tarone RE, McLaughlin JK. The epidemiology of renal cell carcinoma. *J Urol.* 2006;176(6 Pt 1):2353–2358.
267. Silva FG. Chemical-induced nephropathy: a review of the renal tubulo-interstitial lesions in humans. *Toxicol Pathol.* 2004;32 Suppl 2:71–84.
268. Gultekin F, Hicyilmaz H. Renal deterioration caused by carcinogens as a consequence of free radical mediated tissue damage: a review of the protective action of melatonin. *Arch Toxicol.* 2007;81(10):675–681.
269. Popowska M, Miernik A, Rzeczycka M, et al.The impact of environmental contamination with antibiotics on levels of resistance in soil bacteria. *J Environ Qual.* 2010;39(5):1679–1687.
270. Tungsanga K, Sriboonlue P. Sudden unexplained death syndrome in northeast Thailand. *Int J Epidemiol.* 1993;22:81.
271. Tosukhowong P, Tungsanga K, Kittinantavorakoon C, et al. Low erythrocyte Na/K pump activity and number in northeast Thailand adults: evidence suggesting an acquired disorder. *Metabolism.* 1996;45:804.
272. Sangwatanaroj S, Prechawat S, Sunsaneewitayakul B, et al. New electrocardiographic leads and the procainamide test for the detection of the Brugada sign in sudden unexplained death syndrome survivors and their relatives. *Eur Heart J.* 2001;22:2290.
273. Nilwarangkur S, Nimmannit S, Chaovakul V, et al. Endemic primary distal renal tubular acidosis in Thailand. *Q J Med.* 1990;74(275):289–301.
274. Robertson WG. The role of environment in the pathogeneses of renal stones. In: Mochizuki M, Sugino N, Sitprija V, eds. *Geographic Nephrology*. Kobe: International Center for Medical Research; 1990.
275. Vasuvattakul S, Yenchitsomanus PT, Vachuanichsanong P, et al. Autosomal recessive distal renal tubular acidosis associated with Southeast Asian ovalocytosis. *Kidney Int.* 1999;56(5):1674–1682.
276. Sritippayawan S, Sumboonnanonda A, Vasuvattakul S, et al. Novel compound heterozygous SLC4A1 mutations in Thai patients with autosomal recessive distal renal tubular acidosis. *Am J Kidney Dis.* 2004;44:64.
277. Shohaib SA, Scringeour EM, Shaerya F. Tuberculosis in active dialysis patients in Jeddah. *Am J Nephrol.* 1999;19:34.
278. Thanaletchuml K, Lee GS, Woo KT. TB peritonitis in patients on continuous ambulatory peritoneal dialysis (CAPD). Clinical features (abstract). 1st Int Congress Dial Develop Countries. Singapore; 1994:59.
279. Krown SE, Metroka C, Wernz J. Kaposi sarcoma in the acquired immune deficiency syndrome. A proposal for uniform evaluation response and staging criteria. AIDS Clinical Trials Group Oncology Committee. *J Clin Oncol.* 1989;7:1201.
280. Naicker S. End-stage renal disease in sub-Saharan Africa. *Ethn Dis.* 2009;19:S1.
281. Praditpornsilpa K. Thailand renal replacement therapy year 2008. Annual Report of The Nephrology Society of Thailand; 2010.
282. Lugon JR, Strogoff de Matos JP. Disparities in end stage renal disease care in South America. *Clin Nephrol.* 2010;74(S1):66.
283. Jha V. Current status of end-stage renal disease care in South Asia. *Ethn Dis.* 2009;19(1 Suppl 1):S1–27.
284. U.S. Renal Data System, USRDS 2010 Annual Data Report : Atlas of Chronic Kidney Disease and End Stage Renal Disease in the United States, National Institutes of Health, National Institute of Diabetes and Digestive and Kidney Diseases, Bethesda, MD; 2010.
285. Katz IJ, Gerntholtz T, Naicker S. Africa and nephrology: the forgotten continent. *Nephron Clin Pract.* 2010;117(4):c320.
286. Eastwood JB, Conroy RE, Naicker S, et al. Loss of health professionals from sub-Saharan Africa: the pivotal role of the UK. *Lancet.* 2005;365(9474):1893–1900.
287. Finkelstein FO, Abdallah TB, Pecoits-Filho R. Peritoneal dialysis in the developing world: lessons from the Sudan. *Perit Dial Int.* 2007;27(5):529.
288. Yu AW, Chau KF, Ho YW, et al. Development of the "peritoneal dialysis first" model in Hong Kong. *Perit Dial Int.* 2007;27 Suppl 2:S53–55.
289. Abu-Aisha H, Elamin S. Peritoneal dialysis in Africa. *Perit Dial Int.* 2010;30:23.
290. Raaijmakers R, Gajjar P, Schröder C, et al. Peritonitis in children on peritoneal dialysis in Cape Town, South Africa : epidemiology and risks. *Pediatr Nephrol.* 2010;25(10):2149.
291. Teerawattananon Y, Mugford M, Tangcharoensathien V. Economic evaluation of palliative management versus peritoneal dialysis and hemodialysis for end-stage renal disease: evidence for coverage decisions in Thailand. *Value Health.* 2007;10:61–72.
292. Sezer S, Ozdemir FN, Akcay A, et al. Renal transplantation offers a better survival in HCV-infected ESRD patients. *Clin Transplant.* 2004;18:619.
293. Lee SC, Chen KS, Tsai CJ, et al. An outbreak of methicillin-resistant Staphylococcus aureus infections related to central venous catheters for hemodialysis. *Infect Control Hosp Epidemiol.* 2004;25:678.
294. Barsoum RS. Trends in unrelated-donor kidney transplantation in the developing world. *Pediatr Nephrol.* 2008;23(11):1925–1929.
295. Participants in the International Summit on Transplant Tourism and Organ Trafficking Convened by the Transplantation Society and International Society of Nephrology in Istanbul, Turkey, April 30–May 2, 2008. The Declaration of Istanbul on organ trafficking and transplant tourism. *Transplantation.* 2008;86(8):1013–1018.

CHAPTER

A Clinical Approach to Kidney Disease in Infants, Children, and Adolescents

Craig B. Langman • Gal Finer • Neziha Celebi

THE EXPRESSION OF "KIDNEY DISEASE" IN CHILDREN

This chapter is intended for medical professionals who are not pediatric nephrologists or pediatricians but who may be called on to evaluate the infant, child, or adolescent patient for the possible presence of kidney disease. Therefore, it is not possible to include an in-depth discussion of all diseases of the specialty and, in particular, the chapter avoids discussions of therapy in most because confirmation of a certain diagnosis of childhood kidney disease would lead the concerned practitioner to consult with a pediatric nephrologist for definitive and ongoing care.

The fundamental difference between pediatric and adult patients is the capacity and, indeed, the expectation of somatic growth and development from infancy through late adolescence, as compared to homeostasis of body mass in the adult. The appearance of kidney disease in childhood interferes with the normalcy of those pediatric processes leading to undisturbed growth (failure to thrive). The pattern of growth from birth through first consultation, plotted formally on available charts of normal patterns of gain in height, height velocity, body mass, and, in children less than 36 months, head circumference, must be a high-ranking task in evaluation of the patient for possible chronic kidney disease (CKD). Absence of changes do not rule out all causes of kidney disease, as discussed throughout the chapter by category of disease, but its presence may help the astute clinician in differential diagnosis.

For ease, and as we teach and practice, children present with a limited, but understandable, series of specific features that alert the clinician to the presence of "kidney disease." Table 64.1 encompasses all topics discussed in this chapter. Understanding the limitations of the chapter, it is hoped the reader will still find the text useful in everyday consultation and practice.

There are common elements to a history and physical examination of the infant, child, and adolescent when thinking about the presence of kidney disease, and those are summarized in Table 64.2.

Measurement of Kidney Filtering Function[1,2]

Assessment of glomerular filtration rate (GFR) is the single most important test of renal function required in clinical practice. The 24-hour endogenous creatinine clearance is used in adults, but such urine collections can be difficult to obtain in infants and young children, particularly those who are outpatients. The 24-hour urine excretion of creatinine is a measure of creatinine production that is related to muscle mass, and in turn correlates with the cube of height in boys and girls from the age of 6 months to maturity. Because GFR correlates with body surface area (BSA) or the square of height, it follows that GFR corrected for BSA is related to height. Thus,

$$\text{GFR} = \frac{\text{UcrV}}{\text{Pcr}} \tag{1}$$

$$\text{UcrV}\ \alpha\ \text{height}^3 \tag{2}$$

$$\text{GFR}\ \alpha\ \text{height}^2 \tag{3}$$

$$\frac{\text{GFR}}{\text{BSA}}\ \alpha\ \frac{\text{height}}{\text{Pcr}} \text{ or } \frac{\text{GFR}}{\text{BSA}} = \frac{\text{height}}{\text{Pcr}} \tag{4}$$

where *V* is urine flow rate and *Ucr* and *Pcr* are the urine and plasma concentrations of creatinine, respectively. The value for the constant k has been empirically based on measured GFR from iohexol-based GFR studies, and reinterpreted as the creatinine assay itself is now standardized around the world (bedside Chronic Kidney Disease in Children Prospective Cohort Study [CKiD]).

$$\text{GFR (mL/minute/1.73 m}^2) = 0.413 \times \text{height (cm)/Pcr (mg/dL)} \tag{5}$$

With the newer assays for serum creatinine in infants younger than age 1 year, and in adolescents older than 18 years, Equation 64.5 has not been validated. Due to the difficulty associated with 24-hour urine collection in young children, estimates of GFR from the height and plasma creatinine may be more reliable than the 24-hour endogenous clearance in

TABLE 64.1 **Major Features of the Presentation of Kidney Disease in Childhood**

Failure to thrive	Nephrolithiasis
Chronic metabolic acidosis	Rickets
Chronic metabolic alkalosis	Recurrent volume depletion
Kidney Fanconi syndrome	Polyuria
Hyponatremia	Oliguria
Hypokalemia	Recurrent urinary infection
Hyperkalemia	Abdominal masses
Edema	Dysuria, frequency
Hematuria	Disorders of sexual differentiation
Proteinuria	Hypercalcemia
Hypertension	Hypocalcemia
Hypophosphatemia	Hypomagnesemia
Hyperphosphatemia	Thrombotic microangiopathy
Hypocomplementemia	

children and obviously are more convenient. It is important to note that this method is likely unreliable when the normal relation between muscle mass and height is altered, as in malnutrition or muscular dystrophy, or in severe renal failure when tubular secretion of creatinine is increased.

Plasma creatinine concentration averages 0.88 mg per dL at birth, when the level is largely determined by the mother's plasma creatinine concentration. It falls to a nadir of 0.32 mg per dL at 2 years as GFR increases and then rises with the increase in muscle mass. From age 2 weeks to 5 years, a normal blood creatinine level is between 0.11 and 0.35 mg per dL. From 5 to 10 years, a normal blood creatinine level is between 0.28 and 0.55 mg per dL. Normal serum creatinine may be as high as 0.84 to 0.93 mg per dL in older teenagers or adult men. However, a serum creatinine concentration greater than 1.10 to 1.20 mg per dL should raise concern for underlying renal disease. Clinical paradigms for measured GFR (mGFR) using iohexol are evolving quickly in the pediatric nephrology clinics.

The addition of other agents such as cystatin C into the estimated GFR (eGFR) equation may improve precision, but not offer substantial important information when the mGFR is above 75 mL/min/1.73 m^2. Adolescents of adult size may benefit from the MDRD equation used in adults for determination of eGFR.

Genetics and Pediatric Kidney Diseases[3]

The expression of monogenic mutations is not infrequent in a variety of chronic kidney diseases in pediatrics, and encompasses the entire clinical spectrum of such disorders, from congenital anomalies of the kidney and urinary tract (CAKUT), glomerular and tubular disorders, through specific transport defects of single, selected ions, minerals, or other substances. As a result of the sequencing of the human genome, and the use of advanced techniques including high throughput technologies, rapid discoveries are made daily. As a result of the rapidity of mutational gene discoveries linked to pediatric kidney disease expression in patients, a comprehensive listing is immediately out of date. However, up-to-date knowledge of such findings can be learned from Online Mendelian Inheritance in Man (OMIM; http://www.omim.org/). Currently known mutations for monogenic disorders and CAKUT are shown in Tables 64.3 and 64.4, respectively. Throughout this chapter, diseases referred to may be found in this listing with a hyperlink about them.

Embryogenesis of the kidney and urinary tract has been advanced at the molecular level considerably in the recent past, and explains, in part, many of the well-recognized malformation complexes seen in patients ranging from infancy (e.g., aplasia, hypoplasia, dysplasia, cystic diseases) through later adolescence (e.g., autosomal-dominant polycystic kidney disease, autosomal-recessive nephrolithiasis with kidney failure/Dents disease). Alternatively, sporadic urologic malformations, the third most common birth defect overall in live-born neonates (e.g., posterior urethral valves, hydronephrosis), may not have easy to decipher molecular pathophysiology, but must be remembered not only in infancy, but during the entire spectrum of pediatrics, as their consequences may only be revealed in the older child or adolescent with the appearance of progressive CKD.

As in adult CKD, polygenic factors play a role in the expression of other disorders, or in their severity of expression. Little information that is different for pediatric CKD when compared to adult disease is available now, and the reader is referred to other chapters in this volume for a discussion of the topic.

HEMATURIA

Hematuria is one of the most common urinary symptoms in children, and may represent a benign condition such as hematuria resulting from strenuous exercise or from a life threatening illness such as Wilms tumor. Hematuria originating from glomerulonephritis (GN) is often signified by coco-cola- or tea-colored urine, red blood cell casts, and/or dysmorphic red blood cells (RBCs), whereas bleeding distal to the glomerulus, such as from urologic issues or infections, are more likely to be associated with red urine and end of void hematuria.

History

Abdominal, flank, or groin pain is suggestive of nephrolithiasis. Dysuria, foul smelling urine, urgency, and increased voiding frequency with or without fever may denote a urinary tract infection (UTI) that is usually caused by gram-negative bacteria or adenovirus in children outside of infancy

TABLE 64.2 **Common Elements of the Pediatric History and Physical Examination**

History	Physical Examination
Birth History: complete maternal obstetric history; birth weight, length, and head circumference; gestational age; placental abnormalities; neonatal history of illness and medications; malformations outside the kidney	Growth percentiles for length, body mass (weight), head circumference (through 2 years of age; http://www.cdc.gov/growthcharts/)
Feeding and Dietary History: source of protein intake (breast, formula); food allergies; food avoidances; urination pattern (frequency, stream appearance); defecation pattern	Blood pressure with appropriate size cuff, and if concern over hypertension, four extremity blood pressure at first consultation; plot normative values for measured arm blood pressure for boys and girls, respectively: http://www.cc.nih.gov/ccc/pedweb/pedsstaff/bptable1.PDF http://www.cc.nih.gov/ccc/pedweb/pedsstaff/bptable2.PDF
Family History: chronic kidney diseases, kidney rransplantation; hypertension; cystic kidney diseases; kidney stones; infant deaths; fractures in young adults; early onset osteoporosis; "unusual diseases"; early onset myocardial infarction, stroke	Complete Physical Examination, with special emphasis depending on the reason for consultation to: skin lesions, rashes, or purpura; peripheral edema; retinal examination for pigmentary changes, anterior chamber for crystal deposits, abnormalities of the eye; alterations of ears (location on the skull relative to the palpebral fissures; size and/or malformations); vascular bruits including abdominal aorta, renal artery locations; abdominal masses; organomegaly; sexual development, feminization, or masculinization of the opposite gender, Tanner sexual maturity rating; presence of arthritis or arthralgias; muscle tone; numbers of fingers and toes; scoliosis; rachitic changes of the extremities, chest and/or skull
Complete Review of Ten Systems	
Social History: developmental milestone achievements; school performance	A listing of relevant milestones by age can be accessed here: http://www.cdc.gov/ncbddd/actearly/milestones/
Immunization History	Schedules and recommendations by age can be accessed here: http://www.healthychildren.org/english/tips-tools/pages/default.aspx?nfstatus=401&nftoken=00000000–0000–0000–0000–000000000000&nfstatusdescription=ERROR:+No+local+token - immunization-schedules

or, alternatively, may represent the presence of hypercalciuria. Abdominal trauma may induce hematuria especially in abnormally shaped kidneys of polycystic or hydronephrotic nature. In postinfectious GN there is a window of at least a week between the occurrence of the febrile disease, most commonly streptococcal pharyngitis or impetigo, to the onset of tea-colored urine, whereas in immunoglobulin A (IgA) nephropathy, another common cause of acute glomerulonephritis in children, a febrile prodrome precedes renal symptoms by only 2 to 3 days. The review of systems is imperative in a child with hematuria as the differential diagnosis includes systemic lupus erythematosus (SLE) and other vasculitides. Alport syndrome, sickle cell disease, and benign familial hematuria are examples of hereditary conditions associated with microscopic hematuria. It is very unlikely for coagulopathic states to manifest as hematuria alone, although a history of bleeding disorder should be sought.

Physical Exam

Periorbital and facial edema are suggestive of GN. The joints and skin should be examined for involvement in vasculitis. Intravascular volume contraction, especially in infancy, can predispose to renal vein thrombosis that may present with gross or microscopic hematuria.

TABLE 64.3 **Selected Monogenic Kidney Disorders**

Disorder	Inheritance	OMIM	Gene(s)
Congenital nephrotic syndrome	AR	256300	*NPHS1, LAMB2, PLCE1*
WT-1 related disorders	AR	256370	*WT1*
Steroid-resistant nephrotic syndrome	AR	600995	*NPHS2, LAMB2*
FSGS1	AD	603278	*ACTN4*
FSGS2	AD	603965	*TRPC6*
FSGS3	AD	607832	*CD2AP*
Alport syndrome	X-linked	301050	*COL4A5*
	AR	203780	*COL4A3, COL4A4*
	AD	104200	*COL4A3, COL4A4*
ADPKD	AD	173900	*PKD1, PKD2*
ARPKD	AR	263200	*PKHD1*
NPHP	AR		
NPHP1		256100	*NPHP1*
NPHP2		602088	*NPHP2/INVS*
NPHP3		604387	*NPHP3*
NPHP4		606966	*NPHP4*
NPHP5–7			*NPHP5,NPHP6/CEP290, NPHP7/GLIS2*
MCKD	AD	603860	*UMOD (MCKD2)*
Cystinosis	AR	219800	*CTNS*
Lowe syndrome	X-linked	309000	*OCRL*
Dents disease	X-linked	300009	*CLCN5, OCRL*
Cystinuria	AR	220100	*SLC3A1, SLC7A9*
Bartter syndrome	AR		
Type I		601678	*SLC12A1/CLCNKB*
Type II		241200	*KCNJ1*
Type III		607364	*CLCNKB*
Type IV		602522	*BSND*
Gitelman syndrome	AR	263800	*SLC12A3*
Liddle syndrome	AD	177200	*SCNN1B, SCNN1G*
GRA	AD	103900	*CYP11B2, CYP11B1*
Apparent mineralocorticoid excess	AR	218030	*HSD11B2*
Distal RTA	AD	179800	*SLC4A1*
	AR	602722	*ATP6V0A4, SLC4A1*
. . .with progressive deafness	AR	267300	*ATP6V0A4, ATP6V1B1*
Osteopetrosis with RTA	AR	259730	*CA2*

(continued)

TABLE 64.3 **Selected Monogenic Kidney Disorders *(continued)***

Disorder	Inheritance	OMIM	Gene(s)
Nephrogenic diabetes insipidus			
	X-linked	304800	*AVPR2*
	AR, AD	125800	*AQP2*
Primary hyperoxaluria			
Type 1	AR	259900	*AGXT*
Type 2	AR	260000	*GRHPR*
Type 3	AR	613616	*DHDPSL (HOGA1)*

AD, autosomal dominant; AR, autosomal recessive; ADPKD, autosomal-dominant polycystic kidney disease; FSGS, focal and segmental glomerulosclerosis; GRA, glucocorticoid-remediable aldosteronism; MCKD, medullary cystic kidney disease; NPHP, nephronophthisis; OMIM, On-line Mendelian inheritance in man (http://www.ncbi.nlm.nih.gov/sites/entrez?db=omim); RTA, renal tubular acidosis.

TABLE 64.4 **Monogenic Disorders Producing CAKUT**

Type of Malformation	Cause	Anatomic and Histologic Charateristics	Gene
Renal agenesis	No interactions between the UB and MM	Absence of the ureter and kidney	*Ret, GDNF*
Renal hypoplasia	Aberrant interactions among the UB, MM, or stroma	Reduced number of UB branches and nephrons that are fully formed, small kidney size	*Pax2, Sall1* *Six2, BMP4* *HNF1β* *UMOD*
Renal dysplasia	Aberrant interactions among the UB, MM, or stroma	Reduced number of UB branches and nephrons. Presence of undiffrentiated stromal and mesenchymal cells, cysts, or cartilage. Frequently associated with kidney hypoplasia	*Pax2* *HNF1β* *UMOD* *Nphp1* *BMP4, Six2* *XPNPEP3*
Polycystic kidneys	Aberrant tubular and collecting duct patterning	Cysts in tubules and collecting ducts Normally formed glomeruli	*Pkd1, Pkd2* *HNF1β* *HPHP1*
Multicystic dysplastic kidneys	Aberrant interactions among the UB, MM, or stroma	Absence of glomeruli and tubules Presence of large cysts Aberrant patterning Poorly formed atretic ureters Small remnant kidney (if organ involutes)	*HNF1β* *UPIIIA*
Medullary cystic kidney disease 2	Aberrant tubular and collecting-duct patterning	Tubular atrophy, interstitial fibrosis, cysts in distal tubules and medullary collecting ducts	*UMOD*
Duplex ureters	Supernumerary UB budding from the ND	Duplex ureters and kidneys or duplex ureters and collecting systems May be associated with VUR or obstruction if UB budding is ectopic	*Robo2* *FoxC1* *FoxC2* *BMP4*
Horseshoe kidney	Defects in renal capsule	Kidneys are fused at inferior lobes and located lower than usual	*HNF1β*

UB, ureteric bud; MM, metanephric mesenchyme; ND, nephric duct.

Laboratory

In evaluation of hematuria, the urine should be examined both by dipstick and under a microscope. A positive urine dipstick for blood in the absence of RBC under the microscope suggests other causes of pigmenturia, such as hemoglobinuria or myoglobinuria. The presence of proteinuria (the dipstick is qualitative) is consistent with GN. Hematuria with low complement levels should raise the diagnosis of postinfectious GN, atypical hemolytic uremic syndrome, membranoproliferative GN, and GN associated with ventricular-peritoneal shunt infection and endocarditis. Increased calcium to creatinine ratio (>0.4) may signify the presence of hypercalciuria, a common condition leading to microscopic hematuria in childhood, and prompt an evaluation discussed in that section of this chapter.

Imaging

A kidney ultrasound is mandatory in the evaluation of hematuria, and further imaging should be ordered as required by the working diagnosis. As a general rule, intravenous pyelography has been replaced by other imaging modalities. Care should be taken in ordering imaging beyond the kidney ultrasound because all the side effects seen in adults with kidney disease (e.g., contrast nephropathy; nephrogenic systemic fibrosis) may occur in the pediatric population as well. Lifetime exposure to radiation factors into the decision as well for the pediatric patient undergoing such imaging. Rare causes of hematuria in children include abdominal tumors (neuroblastoma and rhabdomyosarcoma), or arteriovenous malformations of the kidney vasculature. Red urine with negative dipstick can be encountered in neonates as a result of urate crystals excretion ("brick dust" urine), and at all ages as the result of medications (e.g., rifampin, phenazopyridine), foods such as beets, or aniline dyes.

Figures 64.1 and 64.2 give a reasonable approach to the evaluation of microscopic and gross hematuria, respectively.

PROTEINURIA

Quantitative assessment of proteinuria in children is affected by the unreliability of extended urine collections. However, its main purpose is to detect damage to the glomerular filter leading to increased permeability, and for this purpose the most sensitive parameter is the sieving coefficient (the relative concentration in glomerular filtrate and plasma water) of a molecule of a size that normally is just restrained by the glomerular filter. The urinary protein to urinary creatinine ratio provides a suitable approximation for use in clinical practice; being a ratio, it is independent of urine flow rate and can be estimated from a random urine sample. A value of less than 0.2 is considered normal and greater than 2.0 is considered nephrotic range proteinuria in children. The use of this ratio is preferred for children rather than the commonly performed 24-hour urine excretion for which more than 200 mg or 5 mg per kg per day usually is regarded as abnormal in children.

Normal urine contains a minimal amount of protein and is physiologic. Increased urine protein can be an isolated finding in a benign condition such as orthostatic proteinuria, or associated with significant kidney disease as nephrotic syndrome or CKD.

Definition

The urine dipstick is a sensitive screening tool for albuminuria and the presence of >1+ indicates a further diagnostic workup is prudent. A 24-hour urine collection is considered the gold standard method to quantify protein excretion, but is very difficult to achieve in children. When collected, values above indexed to body surface area (m^2). Values above 4 mg/m^2/h are pathologic. Values above 40 mg/m^2/h signify nephrotic range proteinuria. Because of the difficulty in performing the 24-hour urinary collection for protein, a random urine sample for protein (mg/dL) and creatinine (mg/dL) ratio (unitless), preferably on the first morning void, is commonly obtained. A ratio above 0.2, beyond the first year of life, is abnormal and warrants evaluation. Neonatal urine contains higher levels of albumin and lower molecular weight proteins, so an albumin/creatinine ratio is more commonly obtained.

History and Physical Exam

Febrile illness, strenuous exercise, and severe dehydration are commonly associated with transient proteinuria that has no long-term renal consequences. The presence of facial, periorbital, pedal, and/or scrotal edema are suggestive of low serum albumin and nephrotic syndrome. A thorough review of systems and a family history of kidney diseases are always important in the face of proteinuria.

Laboratory

The nature of the protein found in the patient's urine may imply the location of the renal lesion; glomerular diseases usually result in albuminuria whereas tubular pathology often leads to low molecular weight proteinuria such as beta-2-microglobulin. The finding of tubular proteinuria may be seen in the setting of generalized proximal tubular disorders that can also lead to aminoaciduria, phosphaturia, glucosuria, and/or bicarbonaturia (Fanconi syndrome). Low-molecular-weight proteinuria has also been linked to renal interstitial damage related to reflux nephropathy, obstructive nephropathy, or acute and chronic pyelonephritis. In orthostatic proteinuria the first morning urine protein to creatinine ratio is normal. In this condition a timed 24-hour urine collection will result in elevated protein excretion when the subject is upright with normal urine protein in recumbency. Nephrotic range proteinuria in the setting of peripheral edema, hypoalbuminemia, and hypercholesterolemia are diagnostic of nephrotic syndrome (see section on nephrotic syndrome for further evaluation). Many of the conditions leading to CKD are associated with proteinuria. In CKD, proteinuria itself is thought to be a perpetuating factor, leading to further damage by various mechanisms

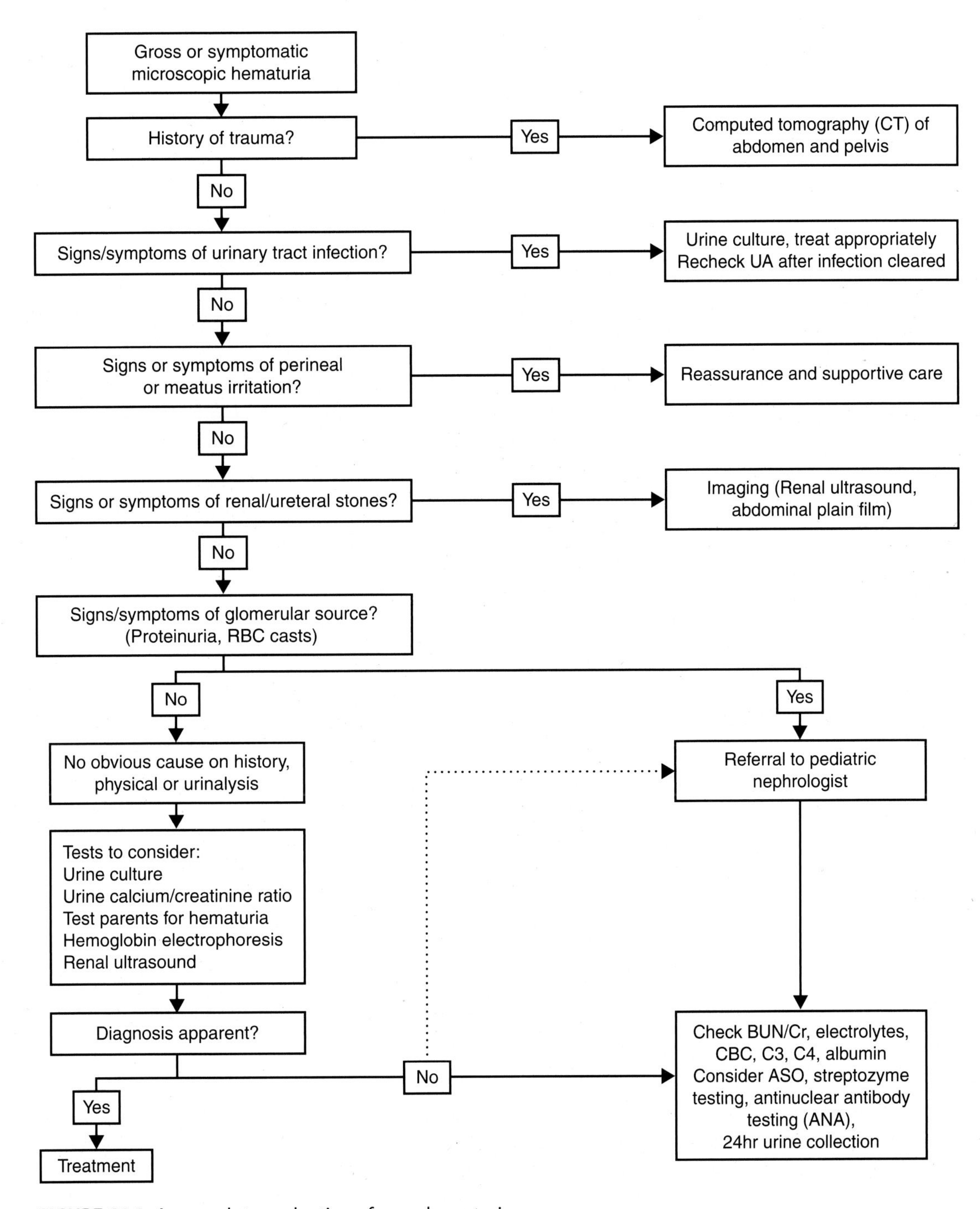

FIGURE 64.1 Approach to evaluation of gross hematuria.

including induction of apoptosis, cell atrophy, and epithelial to mesenchymal transformation. Isolated proteinuria in repeated urine samples over time is always an index of renal abnormality and should be further investigated. In addition to urinalysis, kidney function and serum electrolytes are required measurements in almost all cases of proteinuria. Persistent proteinuria of unclear etiology warrants the consideration of a kidney biopsy.

Table 64.5 lists a classification and some of the many causes of proteinuria in children.

ACUTE GLOMERULONEPHRITIS

The sudden onset of gross hematuria, proteinuria, azotemia, edema, and hypertension is a classic description of acute glomerulonephritis (AGN) in children and adolescents (Table 64.6). An important nodal point in the differential diagnosis is the level of serum complement factors, C3 and C4, which when depressed, suggest postinfectious (poststreptococcal disease most commonly) AGN, membranoproliferative GN, subacute bacterial endocarditis, shunt nephritis (plastic

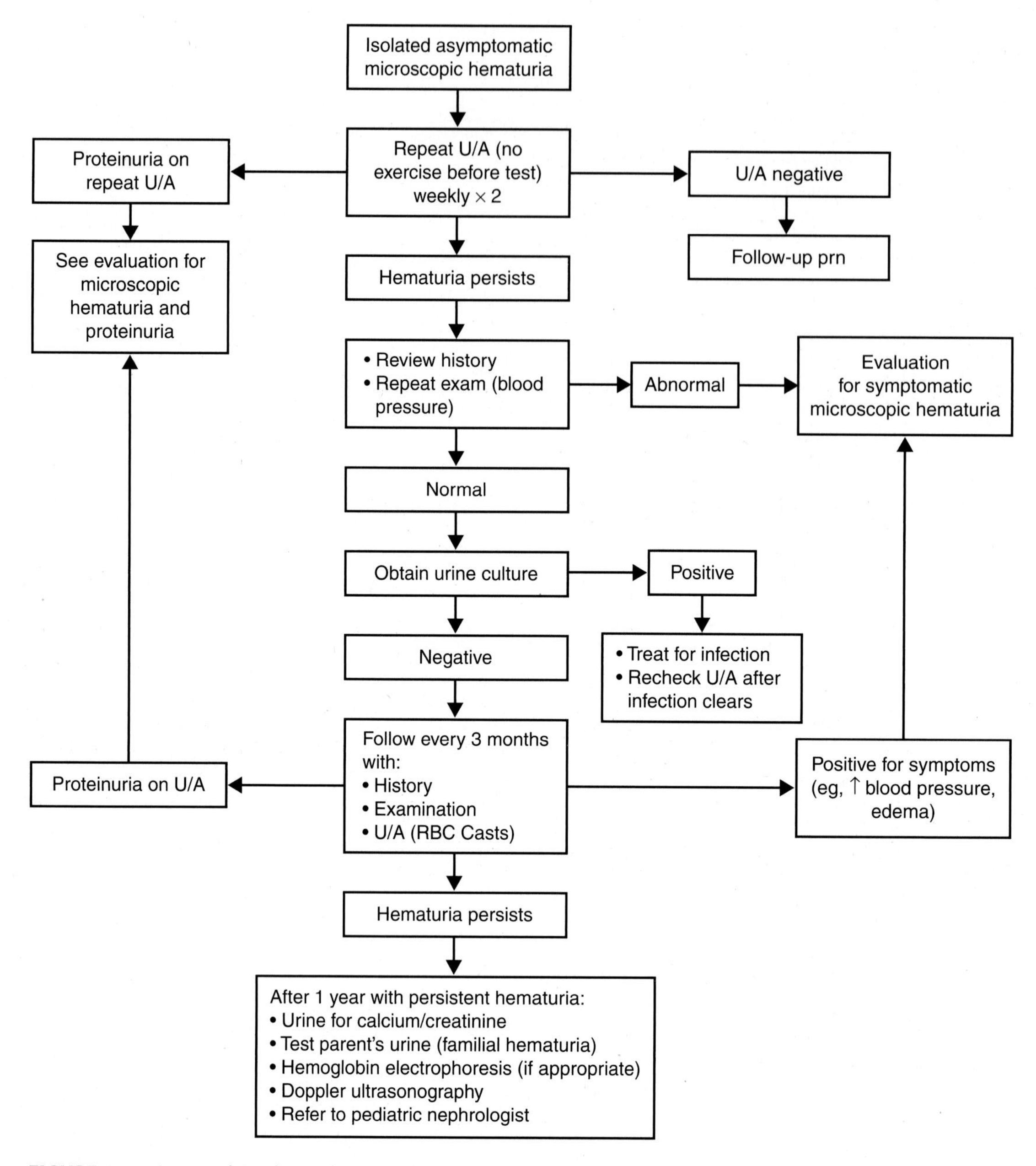

FIGURE 64.2 Approach to the evaluation of microscopic hematuria.

devices such as drains for cerebrospinal fluid placed into the vascular space), or, rarely, quartan malarial GN. Normocomplementemic postinfectious AGN, although occurring in up to 10% of those with biopsy-proven postinfectious AGN, suggests other etiologies that include IgA GN, Henoch-Schönlein purpura (when accompanied by a purpuric, lower extremity rash), vasculitides that include collagen-vascular diseases such as SLE, granulomatosis with polyangiitis (Wegeners), Goodpasture syndrome, or pauci-immune vasculitis.

Postinfectious AGN when associated with other components of thrombotic microangiopathies, including anemia, thrombocytopenia, and other wide-ranging organ dysfunctions, may connote diseases such as thrombotic thrombocytopenic purpura (TTP), shiga-toxin associated enterocolitis hemolytic uremic syndrome (STEC-HUS), or atypical HUS, a disease of complement regulatory protein mutational abnormalities, or in combination with autoantibodies to some of those proteins, in which the alternative complement pathway is constitutively activated and unregulated, leading to overactivity and resultant disease.

As in adults, a presentation with rapidly advancing kidney failure may be associated with a crescentic presentation on kidney biopsy that defines rapidly progressive glomerulonephritis (RPGN), most commonly associated in children with postinfectious AGN from postinfectious GN or one of the vasculitides noted.

TABLE 64.5 Classification and Causes of Proteinuria in Children

Transient Proteinuria, associated with fever, vigorous exercise, volume depletion, or prolonged seizures
Orthostatic Proteinuria, in which the first morning urine is devoid of pathologic levels of protein but subsequent urines throughout the day reveal excess protein levels
Glomerular Proteinuria, arising from any form of infantile or childhood nephrotic syndrome, or as part of a glomerulonephritis of any etiology
Tubular Proteinuria, associated with primary or acquired diseases of the proximal tubule, obstructive uropathy, or tubulointerstitial nephritis (including pyelonephritis)

TABLE 64.6 Common Causes of Acute Glomerulonephritis in Children and Adolescents

Associated with Hypocomplementemia	Associated with Normal Levels of Complement
Postinfectious AGN	GPA (granulomatosis with polyangiitis); MPA (microscopic polyangiitis); PAN (polyarteritis nodosa)
Collagen vascular disease (e.g., systemic lupus erythematosus)	Goodpasture
Membranoproliferative GN	IgA nephropathy
Shunt nephritis	Henoch-Schönlein purpura
Subacute bacterial endocarditis	Thrombotic thrombocytopenic purpura
Falciparum (quartan) malaria	STEC-HUS (commonly)
Atypical HUS (rarely)	Pauci-immune nephritis
STEC-HUS (rarely)	Atypical HUS (commonly) Alports syndrome

AGN, acute glomerulonephritis; GN, glomerulonephritis; HUS, hemolytic uremic syndrome; STEC, Shiga toxin-producing *Escherichia coli*.

Diagnostic evaluation of postinfectious AGN in children and adolescents should include evaluation for recent streptococcal infection of the throat (anti-streptolysin O titer), skin (anti-DNaseB titer), collagen-vascular disease, ANCA titers, complement levels, and a search for thrombotic microangiopathy (complete blood count [CBC], peripheral blood smear for schistocytes, reticulocyte count, platelet count, lactate dehydrogenase [LDH], haptoglobin level), and imaging of the kidneys by ultrasound to evaluate size and echo texture.

A percutaneous kidney biopsy in children and adolescents is a safe procedure performed by those with biopsy skills and the ability to provide proper anesthetic management. The biopsy is processed routinely for light, immunologic, and electron microscopic examinations and should be interpreted in collaboration with a pathologist skilled in pediatric kidney diseases.

As a general rule, the diagnosis of hypocomplementemic, postinfectious AGN in the child or adolescent does not mandate a kidney biopsy, as the hypocomplementemia resolves in 6 weeks in the overwhelming majority of cases, and the disease carries an excellent prognosis overall. Other causes of postinfectious AGN may indeed warrant a kidney biopsy early in its course for diagnostic, prognostic, and therapeutic decisions.

POSTINFECTIOUS GLOMERULONEPHRITIS[8]

From young childhood (older than three years) through late adolescence, the sudden appearance of gross hematuria with microscopic RBC casts, proteinuria, edema, and hypertension approximately 1 week to 1 month following a streptococcal pharyngitis or skin-based infection have defined the occurrence of postinfectious (poststreptococcal) postinfectious AGN. Documentation of a positive throat or skin culture for group A β-hemolytic streptococcus, or serologic evidence of elevated antistreptolysin O or DNaseB titers is commonly found and strengthens the diagnosis of postinfectious AGN. In developing areas of the world, many additional causative agents have been identified including other bacteria, viruses, fungi, and parasitic infectious agents.

The differential diagnosis of postinfectious AGN includes any kidney disease in which there is a nephritic picture, including IgA nephropathy, Henoch-Schönlein purpura, Goodpasture syndrome, systemic vasculitis related to ANCA, SLE, forms of hemolytic uremic syndrome, membranoproliferative glomerulonephritis, or an acute presentation of other chronic glomerular diseases.

Group A β-hemolytic streptococcus of the M-type is most commonly associated with the occurrence of postinfectious AGN, and type 12 is commonly isolated in cases of postinfectious AGN related to pharyngitis, and type 49 is commonly isolated in postinfectious AGN after skin-based infections. These are termed nephritogenic, although other types may produce postinfectious AGN too.

Postinfectious AGN is a prototypic hypocomplementemic disease in which there appears to be passive antigen-antibody complex deposition within the glomerulus in a characteristic subepithelial location, although many variants have been described that may mimic either membranoproliferative glomerulonephritis type I or, C3-glomerulopathy on kidney biopsy. The exact mechanisms whereby the circulating immune complexes deposit within the glomerulus remain uncertain, but may involve the alternative complement pathway (low C3, normal C4, and no C1q deposition in the kidney), rather than the classical complement pathway.

The hypocomplementemia is of short duration, with over 95% of patients recovering normal levels of complement C3 6 weeks after presentation. Postinfectious AGN may present with an RPGN clinical picture as well, with intense crescent formation found in the kidney biopsy. The depth of C3 depression does not correlate with disease severity or course. Up to 10% of patients with postinfectious AGN have normal C3 levels, depending on the time at which it is measured.

A kidney biopsy is rarely performed for postinfectious AGN related to group A β-hemolytic streptococcus, but is reserved for RPGN, uncertain assignment of postinfectious AGN as to etiology, or cases in which systemic manifestations suggest another cause of the postinfectious AGN.

More subtle cases of postinfectious AGN may be seen when the streptococcal disease is of a more epidemic nature, and in which gross hematuria is often absent and azotemia is minimal. We recommend a screening urinalysis of family members of index cases of postinfectious AGN, looking for hematuria and proteinuria, whether the case is epidemic or isolated.

No specific therapy has been shown to change the course of the typical child with postinfectious AGN, but we recommend looking for group A β-hemolytic streptococcus by culture, since treatment is warranted to prevent rheumatic fever if infection is present. The child with postinfectious AGN must be evaluated and managed for the potential complications of AGN that include malignant hypertension and its systemic sequelae, oligoanuria with hyperkalemia, dilutional hyponatremia, and acidosis. Rarely such management includes the use of iterative dialysis, unless a rapidly progressive picture is present and severe.

The prognosis of the overwhelming majority of isolated cases of postinfectious AGN that are related to an antecedent group A β-hemolytic streptococcal infection and without a picture of RPGN is uniformly excellent, with full recovery of normal kidney function and no long-term sequelae in over 95%. In developing countries, and in cases where prolonged dialysis is needed for RPGN, the prognosis is less well established, and continuation into ESRD or death may occur.

HENOCH-SCHÖNLEIN PURPURA GLOMERULONEPHRITIS[9]

The triadic finding of a predominant lower extremity and buttocks purpuric rash, abdominal pain, and fever in children and adolescents is prototypic for Henoch-Schönlein purpura (HSP). The disease is classified as a small vessel vasculitis of unknown etiology and, in addition to the organs involved above, may involve the kidney, the lower urinary tract, the joints, and, less commonly, the central nervous system or other organs. The disease is self-limited, may be recurrent, and the long-term morbidity is related to the degree, if any, of kidney involvement.

There is a literature that HSP is related to an antecedent infection, but no specific ones are implicated. Prior drug exposures have been noted rarely, and do not explain the overwhelming majority of such cases. Despite the presence of IgA deposition in the kidney, when kidney involvement is detected, circulating IgA levels are normal. Some evidence for circulating immune-complexes directed against altered moieties of IgA with subsequent mesangial deposition appears.

Kidney involvement is variable, and case series for frequency of involvement may reflect selection and referral biases. Even when initially absent as demonstrated by a normal urinalysis and serum creatinine initially, the kidney may become involved with a subsequent recurrence of the disease rash, but the exact frequency of such involvement subsequently ranges from infrequent to frequent for the biases cited. A good rule of thumb is that the absence of kidney involvement 2 months after clinical presentation of HSP (and without HSP recurrence) is generally associated with long-term sparing of kidney disease at all. Therefore, monitoring the child with HSP in those first 8 weeks after presentation with HSP, including a urinalysis, kidney function, and blood pressure measurement, seems warranted.

Kidney involvement, when present, ranges from low-grade proteinuria and hematuria, to AGN, or a nephrotic syndrome with heavy hematuria. A kidney biopsy is warranted for the latter three presentations for diagnosis, where a large range of findings may occur, from very little light microscopic abnormalities through focal and segmental proliferative GN and, at the worst, a crescentic GN. IgA is found commonly in association with IgG, C3, and fibrin in a granular, mesangial pattern that is indistinguishable from primary IgA nephropathy. HSP requires, therefore, the presence of the extrarenal system involvement as noted previously.

There is no specific treatment for HSP in general, and even the use of corticosteroids for the extrarenal manifestations remains unproven. In general, with general supportive measures the extrarenal disease improves and has no long-term sequelae in most.

In literature case series, the absence of kidney involvement 6 months after presentation is associated with a uniformly good outcome for normal kidney function. If severe manifestations of kidney involvement in HSP should occur the prognosis for good outcome diminishes, and should be followed for the appearance and/or management of CKD.

THROMBOTIC MICROANGIOPATHY[7]

Infants, children, and adolescents may present with a thrombotic microangiopathy (TMA) involving the kidney. TMA-based syndromes (Table 64.7) are microvascular occlusive disorders that result from aggregation of platelets, thrombocytopenia, and mechanical injury to erythrocytes, ultimately leading to organ dysfunction. A more specific definition of TMA is the activation of the endothelium due to various insults followed by a cascade of pathologic responses, including among others, platelet and/or complement activation of the terminal (C5b-9) complex, microthrombi formation, thrombocytopenia, and microangiopathic hemolytic anemia. Atypical hemolytic uremic syndrome (HUS) occurs both in the pediatric and adult populations; severe kidney impairment is a prominent but not an essential feature of the disease.

The most common cause of TMA and HUS is that associated with shiga-toxin producing infections (now termed *STEC-HUS*), including *Escherichia coli* serotype 0157:H7 and *Shigella dysenteriae* serotype 1, accounting for more than 90% of HUS cases. Recently, an outbreak in adults was linked to a unique serotype of *E. coli*, O4:H4. New evidence points to complement activation in STEC-HUS. The term atypical HUS has been used to describe cases of TMA not caused by shiga-toxin associated microorganisms and bacterial infections in general, and in which thrombotic thrombocytopenic purpura (TTP) has been excluded in the differential diagnosis by demonstrating levels of ADAMTS13 activity above 5% to 10%.

Atypical hemolytic uremic syndrome is a rare, life-threatening, chronic, genetic disease of uncontrolled alternative pathway complement activation. The understanding of the pathophysiology and genetics of this disease has expanded over recent decades and promising new developments in the management of atypical HUS have emerged.

In 50% to 60% of cases of atypical HUS, a genetic mutation in complement regulatory proteins and/or autoantibodies against these proteins has been found as an explanation for constitutive complement activation. Mutations have been described in complement factor H (CFH), complement factor I (CFI), Membrane Cofactor Protein (MCP), complement factor B (CFB), myosin binding protein C3 gene (C3), and thrombomodulin. In addition, autoantibodies to CFH can cause atypical HUS and are commonly associated with deletions of complement factor H-related proteins CFHR1 and CFHR3. Mutations in either CFH, CFI, MCP, thrombomodulin, and/or CFHR1/3 with autoantibodies to CFH are associated with loss of regulatory control of the alternative pathway of the complement cascade. Mutations in CFB and C3 are gain of function mutations leading to complement over-activation. A very rare cause of atypical HUS is genetic deficiency of cobalamimase activity.

However, this leaves another 40% to 50% of patients in whom a mutation or autoantibody cannot be demonstrated but for whom atypical HUS is the diagnosis. Thus, the ultimate diagnosis of atypical HUS does not require a formal demonstration of its underlying genetic cause. Less than 20% of atypical HUS cases are familial, with both autosomal-dominant and autosomal-recessive inheritance reported. Autosomal-recessive cases tend to present in childhood whereas autosomal-dominant cases more typically present in adulthood—prognosis is poor regardless of inheritance. Identification of a genetic mutation, although not required for an individual's diagnosis or management of atypical HUS, may be helpful for identifying and monitoring disease carriers and for providing genetic counseling.

Loss of function mutations in CFH are most common and have the worst prognosis based on registry data, with 60% to 70% of patients progressing to end-stage renal disease (ESRD) or death within a year of disease onset. The ultimate kidney and patient-based prognoses for patients with CFI mutations appears slightly better, followed by patients with MCP mutations, of whom 20% require renal replacement therapy. Patients without demonstrated mutations have similar dire outcomes, however, raising the idea that the presence or absence of a given mutation may have limited prognostic value, except for the MCP mutation that may not recur after kidney transplantation.

TABLE 64.7 TMA-Based Diseases

TMA-Based Diseases
■ Thrombotic thrombocytopenic purpura ■ Congenital *ADAMTS13* deficiency ■ Antibody-mediated *ADAMTS12* deficiency
■ Hemolytic uremic syndrome ■ STEC-HUS ■ Pneumococcal HUS ■ Atypical HUS (atypical HUS)
■ TMA associated with ■ Medications ■ Hypertension ■ Pregnancy/HELLP syndrome ■ Solid organ transplantation ■ Stem cell transplantation ■ Malignant solid tumors ■ HIV ■ Vasculitis, such as systemic lupus erythematosus

TMA, thrombotic microangiopathy; HUS, hemolytic uremic syndrome; STEC, Shiga toxin-producing *Escherichia coli*; HELLP: hemolysis, elevated liver enzymes, low platelet count

Until recently, there have been no specific therapies for atypical HUS. Therapeutic plasma exchange or plasma infusion has generally been the initial approach to disease management, although there are no randomized controlled trials of plasma therapy in atypical HUS to establish its effectiveness. Plasma exchange may only be beneficial for atypical HUS in the short term, because long-term kidney outcomes are uniformly poor with a varying short-term response in hematologic parameters. Plasma exchange would not be expected to be effective for patients with mutations in MCP, a transmembrane protein. Patients who do respond to plasma exchange frequently become plasma dependent, requiring long-term therapy to maintain remission.

Kidney transplantation can be successful for patients with MCP mutations. MCP is cell membrane-bound and highly expressed in the kidney; kidney transplant, then, would be expected to halt the disease process. Other mutations or unknown ones have led to high relapse rates of atypical HUS in the transplanted kidney. CFH and CFI mutations have been studied more extensively. These circulating proteins are primarily synthesized in the liver. Not unexpectedly, atypical HUS recurs in 80% of patients with CFH mutations and 90% of patients with CFI mutations after an isolated kidney transplant. Living-donor kidney transplantation is contraindicated in patients with atypical HUS due to mutations in CFH, CFI, C3, and CFB without other therapies concomitantly.

Combined liver-kidney transplantation has been attempted for patients with CFH and CFI mutations to address the abnormal protein synthesis in the liver and its downstream effect on the kidney. Simultaneous liver-kidney transplantation with prophylactic use of plasma therapy has been successful in patients with CFH mutations. However, liver-kidney transplantation is associated with a higher mortality rate than kidney transplantation alone. In the absence of a noted mutation, comprising a sizable fraction of patients with atypical HUS, liver-kidney transplantation should be avoided.

A pathophysiologic-based treatment in atypical HUS is available now with eculizumab, through inhibiting the formation of the common terminal complement complex (C5b-9). Its recent approval for atypical HUS in adults and in children represents its first approved use for pediatric patients. Due to the impaired capacity for opsonization and clearance of encapsulated organisms, meningococcal disease is a risk with the use of eculizumab and has been reported among patients given eculizumab for paroxysmal nocturnal hemoglobinuria (PNH). Patients must receive the meningococcal vaccine prior to treatment initiation.

NEPHROTIC SYNDROME IN THE FIRST YEAR OF LIFE[4,5]

The classic triad of findings in nephrotic syndrome in children, adolescents, and adults—hypoalbuminemia, high-degree proteinuria, and edema—are found in infants with nephrotic syndrome too. Congenital nephrotic syndrome has been used to describe the disease in utero through the first 3 months of life, whereas infantile nephrotic syndrome has referred to the development of the disease in months 4 through 12. We find this an arbitrary division, as there is great overlap in the causes between the two groupings, and prefer nephrotic syndrome in the first year of life (NSFL).

The differential diagnosis of NSFL includes disease secondary to congenital maternal infections (e.g., syphilis, cytomegalovirus) or from genetic causes. The majority of the genetic causes involve mutations in kidney morphogens such as WT-1, or mutations in genes related to the integrity of the tri-partite glomerular filtration barrier (the podocyte foot processes, the fenestrated glomerular endothelium, and the glomerular basement membrane). After exclusion of infection-related NSFL, NSFL is now considered a monogenic disease, with one of four genetic mutations (nephrin, podocin, WT1, LAMB2) accounting for over 66% of the cases in a recent Western European series. The disease is not responsive to corticosteroids or immunosuppressive medications as a general principle. Prompt referral to a center skilled in management of infantile nephrosis is recommended.

NSFL may be seen in syndromic diseases of newborns as well, and the clinician should evaluate the patient for extrakidney malformations including disorders of sexual differentiation (see below). For a comprehensive listing, the reader can access: http://www.ncbi.nlm.nih.gov/omim?term=nephrotic%20syndrome%20in%20infancy.

NEPHROTIC SYNDROME IN CHILDHOOD[6]

Primary nephrotic syndrome in children from 15 months through 8 to 10 years of age includes minimal change nephrotic syndrome (MCNS), focal segmental glomerulosclerosis (FSGS), membranoproliferative glomerulonephritis (MPGN; types I, II, III), and membranous nephropathy (MN). The overwhelming majority of children will have MCNS when the patient has normal kidney filtering function, is nonazotemic, normotensive, and with normocomplementemic. To date, the initial response to a course of oral corticosteroids, 2 mg/kg/day or 60 mg/m^2 BSA/day, defines the disease as steroid-responsive or resistant. Initial corticosteroid resistance mandates a biopsy for histologic diagnosis.

Steroid responsiveness is further delineated by frequency of relapse, into no further episodes (~10%–15% of cases) or recurrent (relapse) nephrotic syndrome, which is either infrequent (less than three times in 1 year) or frequent (three or more relapses per year). Treatment algorithms have evolved for relapsing disease. Frequently relapsing corticosteroid responsive disease may become corticosteroid-resistant as well, and treatment algorithms have evolved for these cases too. Kidney biopsy is indicated for corticosteroid resistance, and often when contemplating institution of potent immunosuppressive therapy with or without corticosteroids for the frequently relapsing course.

Genetic mutations in the components of the glomerular filtration barrier are increasingly recognized as a cause of FSGS in childhood nephrotic syndrome, and other such mutations can be expected. Additionally, mutations in many other genes have been linked to corticosteroid-resistant nephrotic syndrome as well, either occurring alone or as part of other diseases. A listing to date can be accessed at: http://www.ncbi.nlm.nih.gov/omim?term=Genetic%20causes%20of%20nephrotic%20syndrome.

Mutations in regulatory proteins of the alternative complement pathway involved in innate immunity have been linked to childhood MPGN, especially type II (dense deposit disease) or a recently described C3 nephropathy. Membranous nephropathy has been linked to the M-type phospholipase A(2) receptor (PLA(2)R) as a candidate antigen in 70% of cases of idiopathic membranous nephropathy. Recently, the presence of cationic bovine albumin, or circulating antibodies to it, was demonstrated in the serum of other children with idiopathic MN.

So-called secondary causes of nephrotic syndrome in this age grouping are much less common than in the adolescent patient, but may include the emergence of nephrotic syndrome in collagen vascular diseases represented by SLE; in infections represented by hepatitis B, HIV, or quartan malaria; from effects of drugs, represented by chemotherapy agents used for treatment of childhood malignancy or immunosuppressive drugs represented by sirolimus; or in systemic metabolic diseases represented by Fabry disease. A careful history and physical examination generally brings secondary causes to light in this age grouping.

NEPHROTIC SYNDROME IN ADOLESCENTS

The frequency of MCNS in children older than 10 years and in adolescents drops dramatically when compared to the younger age group described previously, and the other primary forms therefore assume a greater importance in the differential diagnosis. The emergence of the more usual causes of adult-onset nephrotic syndrome is common in the differential diagnosis as well (e.g., malignancy associated nephrotic syndrome), with the exception of the nodular sclerosis of advanced type 1 diabetes mellitus unless the disease has been present for >10 years in the adolescent patient. Almost uniformly, a kidney biopsy is performed for accurate diagnosis in the adolescent patient with nephrotic syndrome.

METABOLIC ACIDOSIS[10,11]

Definition

Chronic metabolic acidosis is defined by the presence of a reduced blood [HCO_3^-] as well as a reduced pCO_2 level resulting from compensatory hyperventilation. Importantly, there is developmental regulation of bicarbonate handling by the kidney. The normal range for serum bicarbonate is lower for preterm infants (16 to 20 mmol per L) and full-term infants (19 to 21 mEq per L) than for children and adults (24 to 28 mmol per L). This is explained by both the inability to excrete the byproducts of growth and metabolism on the one hand in infants, and the higher level of endogenous acid generated by protein metabolism and bone growth in the infant when compared to the older child or adolescent.

Additionally, the lowered bicarbonate concentration in preterm and term infants, compared to older children and adolescents, reflects the reduced bicarbonate threshold of nephron heterogeneity and a reduced fractional bicarbonate resorption, perhaps related to an expanded extracellular water volume in infants.

Postnatal maturation of the proximal tubular capacity for bicarbonate resorption results from increases in activities of the sodium-hydrogen exchanger (NHE) and H+-ATPase. Low carbonic anhydrase activity further exacerbates the limited bicarbonate resorption.

Developmentally, the capacity to respond to acid loading increases with advancing gestational and postnatal ages. In response to acid loading with ammonium chloride, urinary pH values of less than 6 are rarely observed in premature infants until the second month of life. In contrast, by the end of the second postnatal week, term infants can generate minimal urinary pH values of 5.0 or lower, comparable to those in the adult. The immaturity of the collecting duct intercalated cells may further lessen the ability of the neonatal kidney to eliminate an acid load.

Secondary to the developmental changes noted, up to 10% of preterm infants develop a hyperchloremic metabolic acidosis during weeks 1 to 3 of life, and this has been termed "late metabolic acidosis of infancy," despite an otherwise healthy appearance but with subnormal weight gains. Typically, spontaneous remission occurs in the subsequent 2 weeks.

History and Physical Examination

Chronic metabolic acidosis uniformly affects somatic growth in a negative way, with reduced body mass and linear height. Additionally, anorexia, nausea, emesis, and diarrhea are not uncommon gastrointestinal manifestations of a kidney disease–mediated metabolic acidosis. Apathy, listlessness, and reduced activity may be ascertained as well.

Patients generally have reduced growth parameters, especially when followed longitudinally with prior values. Patients with chronic metabolic acidosis may have a pallor, reduced skin perfusion, and, if from a primary disorder of organic acid metabolism, hepatomegaly. CKD and its attendant acidosis from obstructive uropathies may produce an abdominal mass (kidney). Chronic metabolic acidosis impairs normal bone mineralization, so the presence of rickets should be sought for as well (see Rickets, later). Rarer disorders of adrenal hormone metabolism produce incomplete masculinization of genotypic males and masculinization of genotypic females.

Laboratory

As in the adult with chronic metabolic acidosis, the serum anion gap should be measured, remembering that until later childhood, normal values for the calculation are 12 to 15 mEq per L, and decreasing to 10 to 12 mEq per L thereafter. An elevated serum anion gap metabolic acidosis has an expanded differential in infants and children, as it includes inborn errors of metabolism of organic acids and amino acids; an increased likelihood of poisoning with salicylates, methanol, or ethylene glycol; lactic acidosis; diabetic ketoacidosis; as well as hypermetabolic states such as leukemias or solid tumors. In younger children, acute and chronic kidney failure may result in an elevated anion gap metabolic acidosis too.

A normal anion gap metabolic acidosis demands measurement of the urinary anion gap (the sum of [Na + K] − Cl). Metabolic acidosis associated with a negative urinary anion gap implies an intact distal tubule acidification process, and may be seen with intestinal bicarbonate losses, proximal renal tubular acidosis (RTA, type II), the use of acetazolamide (often used to reduce cerebral spinal fluid production in infants and children), or, very rarely, exogenous acid administration.

Metabolic acidosis associated with a positive urinary anion gap demands measurement of the urinary pH by a pH meter-based method. When the measured urinary pH is >5.8, distal renal tubular acidosis (RTA) is present, as either type I (hypokalemia) or type IV (hyperkalemia). The latter may be seen with obstructive uropathy in infants and children. When the urinary pH is measured at ≤5.8, a type IV RTA is present, and the plasma renin activity (PRA) should be measured. When the PRA is elevated, the plasma aldosterone level should be determined, and if high, either pseudohypoaldosteronism type I (genetic, occurring in a kidney-limited, autosomal-dominant form due to mutations in the mineralocorticoid receptor, or as a widely disseminated, multiple organ form causing widespread aldosterone resistance due to one of several mutations in the subunits of the epithelial Na-channel) or type III (observed in infants and children with obstructive uropathy, acute pyelonephritis, or bilateral vesicoureteral reflux) diagnosed. Alternatively, when the PRA is elevated but the plasma aldosterone is reduced, a plasma cortisol must be determined. When that cortisol is normal and shows circadian rhythmicity, primary hypoaldosteronism is defined, and when that cortisol is low and shows the absence of circadian rhythmicity, concern over congenital adrenal hyperplasia (look also for disorders of sexual differentiation) or Addison disease may be present.

In this diagnostic pathway, if the PRA is reduced, and the patient is hypertensive, Gordon syndrome (chloride shunt) should be considered, whereas if the blood pressure is normal, conventional causes of hyporeninemic hypoaldosteronism seen in adults can be considered for children and adolescents too. Such disorders are associated with mutations of the WNK1 and WNK4 protein kinases.

TABLE 64.8 **Elevated Anion Gap**

Category of Acidosis	Specific Clinical States or Diseases
Lactic acidosis	Hypoperfusion Mitochondrial myopathies Inborn errors of carbohydrate metabolism
Ketoacidosis	Diabetic ketoacidosis
Organic acidemias	
Fatty acid oxidation defects	
Ingestions	Methanol, ethanol, ethylene glycol, salicylate intoxication
Advanced end-stage renal disease	
Rhabdomyolysis	
Normal Anion Gap (Hyperchloremic) Acidosis	
Loss of bicarbonate	
Loss through the gastrointestinal tract	Diarrhea, laxative abuse, enteric fistulae, ureteral-sigmoid connections
Kidney loss	Proximal (type 2) RTA
Reduced hydrogen secretion	Distal (type 1) RTA Type 3 RTA
Early end-stage renal disease	

RTA, renal tubular acidosis.

Some of the general causes of chronic metabolic acidosis are listed in Table 64.8.

RENAL FANCONI SYNDROME

The term refers to a complex and generalized proximal tubulopathy that has many different etiologies. In its complete form, there is a generalized disorder of brush border transport mechanisms leading to excessive loss of water (urine osmolality ≤300 mOsm per kg H_2O), salt wasting (fractional sodium excretion >1%), potassium wasting (TTKG >12), bicarbonaturia (FE >15%), phosphate (TRP below 85%), amino acids, glucose, and uric acid into the final urine—such that a chronic metabolic acidosis with hyponatremia, hypokalemia, hypophosphatemia, and reduced serum uric acid level, often in concert with volume depletion, occurs. Almost all causes of a renal Fanconi syndrome have excessive tubular proteinuria (e.g., increased excretions of B2-microglobulin, retinol-binding protein). Additionally, reduced production of the active vitamin D metabolite may occur as well, leading in concert with the other parts of the disorder to rickets and secondary hyperparathyroidism. Hypercalciuria is an inconsistent finding in all forms of renal Fanconi syndrome.

Partial forms of the renal Fanconi syndrome have been described in some diseases, such as those associated with mutations in the *CLCN5* or *OCRL-1* gene that goes by several names (Dents syndrome 1, hereditary X-linked nephrolithiasis with renal failure, Dents syndrome-2, respectively.), or in hereditary hypercalciuria with hypophosphatemia (HHRH) due to *Npt2* gene mutations, or severe nutrient vitamin D deficiency.

A renal Fanconi syndrome must be distinguished from single molecule transport disorders of the proximal tubule such as in patients with X-linked dominant hypophosphatemic rickets, autosomal-dominant hypophosphatemic rickets, cystinuria (the generalized dibasic aminoaciduria is only clinically relevant due to the insolubility of cystine in normal urine), isolated renal glycosuria, lysinuric protein intolerance (a cause of hypoglycemia in young children), or proximal bicarbonate loss in isolated proximal renal tubular acidosis.

Fanconi syndrome from inherited causes generally produces growth failure and often, rickets. Inherited causes of renal Fanconi syndrome include cystinosis (mutation in cystinosin), Dents disease (*CLCN5* or *OCRL* mutation), Lowe oculocerebrorenal syndrome (*OCRL* mutation, Fanconi Bickel glycogenosis [*Glut2* mutation]), tyrosinemia, Wilson disease, hereditary fructose intolerance, mitochondrial myopathies of diverse nature, galactosemia, or in an idiopathic form.

Acquired forms of renal Fanconi syndrome in children may result from toxic effects of therapeutic agents such as chemotherapy (ifosfamide, cisplatin), valproic acid, or aminoglycosides, or result from poisonings from heavy metals (lead, mercury, cadmium, uranium) or from glue sniffing, use of paraquat, or as a result of tubular injury associated with kidney transplantation.

CYSTINOSIS[12–14]

Cystinosis is the most common cause of an inherited Fanconi syndrome in children. It is an autosomal-recessive disease characterized by the abnormal accumulation of the amino acid cystine in lysosomes of all tissues due to a defective cystine transporter protein, cystinosin. The gene responsible for nephropathic cystinosis, *CTNS* on chromosome 17p, encodes for a 367-amino acid transmembrane protein called cystinosin. A common major deletion underlies most affected patients in Europe; other mutations have been reported.

Typically, cystinosis is a multisystem disease causing failure to thrive, recurrent volume depletion, polyuria and polydipsia, vomiting, constipation, Fanconi syndrome, and CKD in infancy or early childhood. Affected children may be erroneously diagnosed with nephrogenic diabetes insipidus or diabetes mellitus due to polyuria and recurrent episodes of volume depletion. Chronic metabolic acidosis contributes to failure to thrive. Phosphaturia can result in a form of hypophosphatemic rickets.

The hallmark of nephropathic cystinosis is the accumulation of cystine in nearly all tissues, including kidneys. Corneal accumulation of cystine crystals leads to photophobia beginning in mid-childhood. Crystal storage in the thyroid causes hypothyroidism at an average age of 10 years. Feeding dysfunction including reflux, dysmotility, and swallowing abnormalities is common, further contributing to impaired growth in this condition. Limited and specific cognitive dysfunction with impaired visual and spatial abilities is common, even in heterozygous siblings who do not manifest other features of the disease. The eGFR is only mildly impaired in infancy and early childhood. However, untreated, the disease progresses to chronic interstitial disease and glomerular necrosis with ESRD occurring at a median age of 9.2 years in untreated patients.

The diagnosis is made by measurement of an elevated leukocyte cystine content. Prenatal diagnosis is available through testing of amniotic fluid or chorionic villus samples. Supportive treatment includes replacement of tubular fluid and solute losses, and affected patients require increased water intake as well as supplementation with sodium-potassium citrate or sodium bicarbonate, sodium phosphate, 1,25-dihydroxyvitamin D., and possibly L-carnitine. Close attention to growth and nutritional needs is critical from an early age, and many centers now recommend placement of a gastrostomy tube in infancy to ensure adequate nutritional intake and compliance with the multiple required medications. Hypothyroidism should be treated appropriately. Although the linear growth failure in cystinosis is not associated with growth hormone deficiency, the administration of recombinant growth hormone to affected children has been shown to be of benefit.

Specific treatment involves depletion of intralysosomal cystine with cysteamine bitartrate, administered every 6 hours around the clock for the life of the patient, to form mixed disulfides that are capable of being transported out of the lysosome. Such treatment has been shown to slow the progression of renal insufficiency and thyroid disease in this condition. Specifically, chronic cysteamine therapy has shifted the point at which serum creatinine reaches 10 mg per dL from around 10 to 23 years of age. The search for newer agents that deplete intracellular accumulation of cystine but with a reduced frequency of administration is sought. Corneal crystal accumulation does not respond to oral cysteamine but instead requires topical treatment.

Patients with renal failure are candidates for peritoneal dialysis, hemodialysis, or renal transplantation. Cystine accumulates in renal allografts but does not cause functional abnormalities. It has been suggested that posttransplantation diabetes mellitus occurs at increased frequency in patients with cystinosis. Ongoing cysteamine treatment posttransplantation is indicated to prevent other systemic manifestations of this disease. With improved survival due to advancements in renal replacement therapy, it has become apparent that cystinosis is associated with severe neurologic sequelae, including cerebral atrophy, pyramidal signs, difficulties with speech, cerebellar ataxia, and pseudobulbar palsy. Further studies are needed to determine whether such neurologic deficits can be prevented with lifelong cysteamine-based therapies.

METABOLIC ALKALOSIS[15–18]

Definition

Metabolic alkalosis is characterized by an elevated serum bicarbonate level, in association with an elevated pCO_2 level as a compensatory change.

History and Physical Examination

Growth parameters should be determined, as well as the pattern of growth historically. Feeding disturbances are not uncommon, and stool and urinary outputs can be ascertained historically. The presence of edema may be sought, and determination of the state of volume repletion from the usual findings on examination should be made.

Laboratory

The major differential in determining the etiology of a chronic metabolic alkalosis must include the urinary chloride level, which when low ($\leq$20 mEq per L) defines an extra-kidney generation of the metabolic alkalosis, or when high (>20 mEq per L) defines a kidney-generated metabolic alkalosis.

Extra-kidney generated metabolic alkalosis includes some diarrheal states, low chloride intake from improperly made infant formulas, loss of gastric fluid such as with emesis, prolonged nasogastric suction, or congenital pyloric stenosis, cystic fibrosis, or a rare congenital chloride diarrhea or villous colonic adenoma. Hypoparathyroidism has been associated with this form of metabolic alkalosis, as have other rare conditions such as glucose infusions after starvation and inappropriate alkali administration.

Kidney-generated metabolic alkalosis demands an evaluation of the blood pressure of the patient, and when high, further determination of the plasma renin activity (PRA). A high PRA is seen in cases of renal artery stenosis from any cause, often bilateral, or in rare cases, renin-secreting tumors. When PRA is low, plasma aldosterone levels must be evaluated. When elevated, consideration for glucocorticoid-remediable hypertension (genetic mutational condition in which aldosterone comes under control of ACTH) or, less commonly, primary hyperaldosteronism should be entertained. When the plasma aldosterone is reduced, syndromes including Liddle syndrome, apparent mineralocorticoid excess (AME), 11α-hydroxylase deficiency, and true licorice ingestion should be entertained.

In kidney-generated metabolic alkalosis in which the blood pressure is normal, and the use of loop diuretics has been eliminated by history, hereditary potassium-losing tubulopathies such as Bartter syndrome (associated with hypercalciuria) or Gitelman syndrome (associated with hypocalciuria) should be entertained.

DISORDERS OF SODIUM HOMEOSTASIS

History and Physical Examination

Central to understanding the mechanism of disorders of serum sodium (Na) in either direction is the determination of the patient's intravascular volume status, ranging from reduced, normal, or increased, by conventional means of weights, and signs and symptoms well known to clinicians including skin turgor, the presence of tears, the moistness of the mucous membranes, the presence of orthostatic blood pressure changes, resting tachycardia, and alterations of skin perfusion/capillary refill time.

Laboratory

A complete picture of the blood electrolytes, blood osmolality, and kidney function should be obtained initially, and monitored at frequent intervals to assure patient safety. If at all possible, relatively simultaneous determinations of urinary Na, potassium (K), and chloride (Cl) excretions, the creatinine and urea nitrogen, and the urinary osmolality, should be obtained in the diagnostic evaluation of the disorder.

Hypernatremia

Algorithms for evaluation of hypernatremia (serum Na $\geq$150 mEq per L) based on the intravascular volume status of the patient and the urinary Na response have been published extensively for adults and do not need much additional comments when applied to children and adolescents. However, it should be remembered that very premature infants in the first weeks to months of life often lose substantial water through their exposed skin, producing hypernatremia, and infants and children with various causes of renal dysplasia or hypoplasia may have substantial natriuresis, leading to hypernatremia in the very young. Diarrheal diseases alone are likely the most common cause of hypernatremic volume depletion in infants and young children, and are ascertained easily with a careful history. An important point to remember is that the very premature infant can generate a urinary osmolality only about 20% of the maximal one in the adolescent and adult, or about 200 mOsm per kg H_2O.

Chronic disorders of water metabolism (outside of the first month of life and especially in premature infants, as disturbances in this time frame may represent immature kidney development alone) may result in hypernatremia and hypoosmotic urine, including central or nephrogenic diabetes insipidus. The differentiation of these disorders requires a formal water deprivation test under most circumstances, and must be performed in infants and children in the inpatient setting. The reader is encouraged to obtain consultation with a pediatric nephrologist or endocrinologist before studying water metabolism in this population. Normative data for interpretation of the various portions of the water deprivation test have been established.

Hyponatremia

Algorithms for evaluation of hyponatremia (serum Na ≤130 mEq per L) based on the intravascular volume status of the patient and the urinary Na response have been published extensively for adults and do not need much additional comment when applied to children and adolescents. Some hyponatremic diseases more unique to pediatrics include hypovolemic urinary salt conservation in cystic fibrosis and pancreatitis (from congenital malformations), whereas the hypovolemic urinary salt loss diseases more unique to pediatrics include genetic salt-losing nephropathies (Bartter syndrome, Gitelman syndrome, pseudohypoaldosteronism, salt-losing forms of congenital adrenal hyperplasia, and adrenoleukodystrophy). A not uncommon form of euvolemic hyponatremia associated with Na conservation by the kidney is the use of an inappropriately mixed infant powdered formula (excess water intake producing dilutional hyponatremia).

DISORDERS OF POTASSIUM HOMEOSTASIS

Hypokalemia

By definition, hypokalemia is present when the plasma K is <3.5 mEq per L in a patient. The urinary K response to hypokalemia is critical for the differential diagnosis. Potassium conservation (urinary [K] <20 mEq per L) is commonly seen when the dietary potassium intake is normal, but there are excessive extra-renal losses in the gastrointestinal (GI) tract, skin, or from increased intracellular localization of potassium. Rarely, prolonged parenteral fluid administration in the absence of potassium may be the reason for hypokalemia, but should be obvious from inspection of the hospital record.

GI losses may be associated with concomitant acidosis (diarrhea, malabsorption syndromes, intestinal or biliary fistulae, enterostomy losses, or the presence of an ureterosigmoidostomy), or with concomitant alkalosis (gastric drainage, pyloric stenosis, emesis, congenital chloride diarrhea), or variable acid-base abnormalities, such as with laxative or enema abuse or a villous adenoma. Cutaneous losses may be seen in cystic fibrosis or burn states. In hospitalized patients, hypokalemia is most commonly observed in children from altered intracellular distribution, including administration of insulin or beta-sympathomimetic medications. At all ages, consideration for the genetic disease, familial hypokalemic periodic paralysis, should be entertained.

When the hypokalemic patient has a urinary K >20 mEq per L, the response of the blood pressure allows an accurate differential diagnosis. When the blood pressure is normal or reduced, as in Fanconi syndrome, Bartter syndrome, or Gitelman syndrome, the use of diuretics or a postobstructive diuresis may be considered.

In the kaluretic hypokalemic patient with a high blood pressure, the plasma renin activity (PRA) should be determined, and if high, renovascular disease or rarely, a renin-secreting tumor should be entertained. In the patient with a low PRA, the plasma aldosterone must be measured to proceed with the differential diagnosis. When reduced or normal, diseases such as Liddle syndrome, AME, true licorice ingestion, or glucocorticoid or mineralocorticoid administration should be entertained. When the plasma aldosterone level is high, glucocorticoid remediable hypertension or rarely in children, primary hyperaldosteronism, should be entertained.

Hyperkalemia

By definition hyperkalemia is present when the plasma K is >5.5 mEq per L in a patient. It is important to remember that a markedly elevated platelet or white blood cell count may lead to test tube hemolysis and hyperkalemia that is not present in the patient (pseudohyperkalemia). The urinary K response to hypokalemia is critical for the differential diagnosis.

When the urinary K >20 mEq per L, the clinician should look for sources of exogenous potassium administration, such as from the diet or from blood transfusions in patients with reduced GFR (a unit of blood has <4 mEq of K). Without an identified exogenous source of potassium, altered K distribution (reduced intracellular localization) and hyperkalemia may result from chronic metabolic acidosis, insulin deficiency, familial hyperkalemic periodic paralysis, hyperthyroidism, or from specific drugs such as beta-blockers, succinylcholine, or digoxin overdosage.

When the urinary K is ≥20 mEq per L, and the GFR is reduced, generally to below 30 mL/min/1.73 m^2 body surface area, acute kidney injury (AKI) or CKD may be the culprit. In the absence of a reduced GFR to such levels, the plasma aldosterone helps provide a critical differential point. Elevated plasma aldosterone levels define pseudohypoaldosteronism types I and III (see above). Normal plasma aldosterone levels define defective kidney secretion of potassium, as in sickle cell disease, SLE, or type IV RTA associated with obstructive uropathy, or the effects of drugs which include spironolactone, triamterene, amiloride, angiotensin-converting enzyme inhibitors, angiotensin receptor blockers, calcineurin inhibitors, nonsteroidal anti-inflammatory agents, or trimethoprim. Low plasma aldosterone levels require measurement of the plasma renin activity, which when high suggest congenital adrenal hyperplasia, causes of adrenal failure, or rarely, specific defects in aldosterone biosynthesis (CMO 1 or 3), and when plasma renin activity is reduced, suggest Gordon syndrome (PHA type 2) or other causes of hyporeninemic hypoaldosteronism.

DISORDERS OF CALCIUM, PHOSPHORUS, AND MAGNESIUM

Disorders of Calcium

Hypocalcemia[19,20]

Definition

When the serum albumin is normal, hypocalcemia is defined as a decrease in serum total calcium to <8.3 mg per dL, or as a decrease in blood ionized calcium <4.4 mg per dL. Formulas for correction of serum total calcium based on a reduced blood albumin have not been validated in infants and children, but likely apply to adolescents.

History and Physical Examination

Clinical symptoms of hypocalcemia are protean and include altered neuromuscular function (tetany, generalized or focal seizures), altered sensorium and psychological disturbances, intracranial calcium deposits, bradyarrthymias, cataracts, constipation, dental enamel hypoplasia, neurodermatosis, and alopecia, among others.

Laboratory

Classification of hypocalcemia is best done by evaluation of a simultaneous serum phosphorus and level of alkaline phosphatase activity. If serum phosphorus is reduced, and the activity of alkaline phosphatase elevated, and the level of parathyroid hormone is elevated too, the differential should proceed for that of calcipenic rickets (see below).

Alternatively, if the serum phosphorus is not reduced and the activity of alkaline phosphatase is not elevated, then the level of serum magnesium should next be measured. If the serum magnesium level is markedly reduced (usually to levels below 1 mg per dL), the function of the extracellular calcium-sensing receptor can be so inhibited as to reduce both synthesis and secretion of parathyroid hormone, producing hypocalcemia. If the serum magnesium is not markedly reduced, the measurement of the blood level of parathyroid hormone should be performed.

An inappropriately normal or reduced parathyroid hormone level in the face of hypocalcemia suggests hypoparathyroidism, which may be familial (autosomal-recessive, -dominant, or X-linked), associated with the DiGeorge anomaly (most commonly part of a contiguous 22q11 syndrome including congenital heart disease and thymic hypoplasia), be a part of other syndromes such as Kearns-Sayre syndrome, other mitochondrial cytopathies, autoimmune endocrinopathy type I, and Kenney-Caffey syndrome, among others) secondary to either surgical removal of the glands, or from infiltrative diseases such as hemosiderosis, Wilson disease, or thalassemia. Alternatively, if the serum parathyroid hormone is elevated, the measurement of the serum creatinine provides a differential diagnostic nodal point. With normal kidney function, one of several types of pseudohypoparathyroidism (PHP) is entertained, dependent on the urinary cyclic AMP level (low: PHP-1a or -1c; PHP-1b or elevated: PHP-2). When the kidney function is not normal, concern over CKD–metabolic bone disorder is raised.

Hypocalcemia may be seen in any form of altered vitamin D metabolism, ranging from simple nutritional deficiency in which the measured 25-hydroxyvitamin D blood levels are low through end-organ resistance to the active vitamin D metabolite, 1,25-dihydroxyvitamin D, because of a mutation in the para-nuclear vitamin D receptor.

Hypercalcemia[21,22]

Definition

Hypercalcemia is defined as an increase in serum total calcium >10.2 mg per dL after the first 3 months of life, and within the first 3 months of life, >11 mg per dL.

History and Physical Examination

Symptoms of hypercalcemia include anorexia; weight loss; emesis; altered sensorium; hypertension; extraskeletal calcium deposits in the kidneys (nephrocalcinosis), heart, lungs, and skin among others; bone pain; subcutaneous nodules; and vasopressin resistant polyuria. Radiographs may reveal subperiosteal resorption if the hypercalcemia is mediated by parathyroid hormone excess, and imaging studies may reveal nephrocalcinosis or other extraskeletal deposits of calcium.

Laboratory

In children with hypercalcemia, the level of serum parathyroid hormone provides a differential diagnosis nodal point. If the parathyroid hormone level is elevated or in the normal range in the face of hypercalcemia, and the urinary calcium is increased (normal 24-hour urine calcium excretion is below 4 mg/kg/day), primary hyperparathyroidism should be considered (isolated adenoma, or syndromic in multiple endocrine neoplasia types 1 or 2). Alternatively, if the urinary calcium excretion is reduced in children older than 2 years, or at the lower limits of normal excretion in those younger than 2 years, the entity of familial hypocalciuric hypercalcemia (FHH; due to an inactivating mutation in the extracellular calcium-sensing receptor) should be entertained, and genetic testing considered.

In the child with hypercalcemia and a low level of parathyroid hormone, the level of circulating vitamin D metabolites (25-hydroxyvitamin D; 1,25-dihydroxyvitamin D_3) should be measured, and if markedly elevated, consider either exogenous vitamin D intoxication, or the recently described cause of infantile hypercalcemia associated with a mutation in the vitamin D-24-hydroxylase enzyme, leading to absent inactivation of the active vitamin D metabolite, 1,25-dihydroxyvitamin D and resultant elevated levels.

When the child with hypercalcemia, low level of parathyroid hormone, and normal values for circulating vitamin D metabolites presents to the clinician, the level of PTH-related protein (PTHrp) should be measured, and if elevated, consideration for tumor-associated hypercalcemia or the presence of dysplastic kidneys, which may make the hormone, should be entertained. When PTHrp levels are not elevated, the differential diagnosis revolves around the presence of a recognized syndrome (Jansen osseous dysplasia, Williams syndrome, infantile idiopathic hypercalcemia, hypophosphatasia) or the absence of one (consider phosphate depletion, vitamin A intoxication, adrenal insufficiency, immobilization, sarcoidosis [adolescent age], among others).

Disorders of Phosphorus

Hypophosphatemia[23,24]

Definition

The normal serum phosphorus declines continuously from infancy through adolescence, when it achieves the adult normal values, and a serum phosphorus <2.5 mg per dL defines hypophosphatemia. For reference for other age groups, the normal serum phosphorus is: infants, mean 6.5 mg per dL (range: 4.8–7.4 mg per dL); toddlers, mean 5.0 mg/dL (range: 4.5–5.8 mg per dL); and children, mean 4.4 mg/dL (range: 3.5–5.5 mg per dL).

History and Physical Examination

There may be no symptoms or signs of hypophosphatemia, or the condition may be very symptomatic as intracellular ATP levels decline with impaired oxygen delivery to tissues, producing anorexia, emesis, paresthesias, hyporeflexia, proximal myopathy, rickets, osteomalacia, cardiac failure, respiratory failure, hypotension, rhabdomyolysis, and coma.

Laboratory

Because 99% of the body's phosphorus stores are intracellular, small shifts in extracellular phosphorus can produce profound hypophosphatemia. Such shifts commonly explain hypophosphatemia in hospitalized infants and children, and include infusions of glucose or amino acids in total parenteral nutrition prescriptions, re-feeding in starvation, respiratory alkalosis, and administration of drugs such as insulin, glucagon, androgens, or beta-sympathomimetic agents.

In the absence of a likely redistributional cause of hypophosphatemia, the kidney's ability to reclaim filtered phosphorus becomes an important nodal point in the differential diagnosis. When the kidney reabsorptive capacity is high in the face of hypophosphatemia (calculated tubular reabsorption >90%), primary phosphorus deprivation should be entertained, such as in intestinal malabsorptive diseases, with the use of dietary phosphate binders, alcoholism, or in recovery from vitamin D deficient states (hungry bone syndrome). Alternatively, when the kidney does not reclaim filtered phosphorus in the presence of hypophosphatemia (calculated tubular reabsorption <90%), it is useful to consider measurement of the level of parathyroid hormone (at the time of this writing, the measurement of serum fibroblast growth factor-23 [FGF23] remains a research tool), which when high, indicates hyperparathyroidism. When the level of parathyroid hormone is normal or even suppressed, there may be nonselective kidney wasting of phosphorus, as in Fanconi syndrome, chronic metabolic acidosis, relief from urinary obstruction, or from the effects of glucocorticoids. Selective kidney wasting of phosphorus may occur in one of several forms of hypophosphatemic rickets (see below), oncogenic osteomalacia from PTHrp excess, Jansen osseous dysplasia, or post-kidney transplant tubular dysfunction.

Hyperphosphatemia[25]

Definition

The normal serum phosphorus declines continuously from infancy through adolescence, when it achieves the adult normal values, and a serum phosphorus >4.5 mg per dL defines hyperphosphatemia. For reference for other age groups, the normal serum phosphorus is: infants, mean 6.5 mg per dL (range: 4.8–7.4 mg per dL); toddlers, mean 5.0 mg per dL (range: 4.5–5.8 mg per dL); and children, mean 4.4 mg per dL (range: 3.5–5.5 mg per dL).

History and Physical Examination

Hyperphosphatemia is often asymptomatic when chronic in nature. Acute rises of serum phosphorus may precipitate hypocalcemia with its many associated symptoms (see Hypocalcemia). Chronic hyperphosphatemia may be associated with progressive extraosseous calcifications, or an acute calciphylaxis syndrome with rapid subcutaneous and small blood vessel calcification leading to painful necrosis of the skin and subcutaneous tissues.

Laboratory

The kidney can excrete phosphorous when in excess, so the kidney's excretory response becomes a nodal point for differential diagnosis. When the urine phosphorus is high (tubular reabsorption of phosphorus <85%), either acute redistribution into the intravascular volume (acute metabolic acidosis) or increased enteral absorption (enemas containing phosphate salts, vitamin D intoxication) should be entertained. More commonly, the child with hyperphosphatemia has a reduced excretion of phosphorus (tubular reabsorption ≥85%), and a search for reduced filtering function (GFR) should be done, as AKI or CKD may be present. If the GFR is normal, and the serum calcium is normal too, acromegaly, tumoral calcinosis, hyperthyroidism, or hyperostosis should be considered. If the calcium is reduced (hypocalcemia), either hypoparathyroidism or pseudohypoparathyroidism can be entertained, depending on finding a reduced or normal/elevated value for parathyroid hormone, respectively.

Disorders of Magnesium[26]

Hypomagnesemia

Definition

Serum magnesium below 1.5 mg per dL defines hypomagnesemia.

History and Physical Examination

Hypomagnesemia is often asymptomatic. Any signs and symptoms may be nonspecific and include nausea, emesis, muscle weakness, and constipation. When serum magnesium levels are below 1.0 mg per dL, signs and symptoms of neuromuscular irritability increase, including tremor, seizures, and altered sensorium. Cardiac signs include tachycardia, premature atrial or ventricular contractions, and prolonged QTc interval that may lead to a fatal torsade de pointes. Hypomagnesemia may lead to hypocalcemia and hypokalemia too (see above for each).

Laboratory

The kidney response to hypomagnesemia provides the initial nodal point in differential diagnosis. When the calculated fractional excretion of magnesium is <2%, either a primary decrease in dietary intake (malnutrition, alcoholism, prolonged parenteral fluid use), gastrointestinal losses (malabsorptive syndromes, diarrheal states, short bowel syndrome, laxative abuse, or a primary and selective lack of magnesium absorption in the intestine), or redistribution of blood magnesium (hungry bone syndrome, diabetic ketoacidosis, or re-feeding after starvation) should be entertained.

Alternatively, if the calculated fractional excretion of magnesium is >2%, indicating a renal-generated hypomagnesemia, specific genetic defects (Gitelman syndrome, one of several known mutations in magnesium-transport proteins, or autosomal-dominant hypoparathyroidism) may be entertained, or acquired disorders, such as from drugs (loop diuretics, thiazide diuretics, calcineurin inhibitors, aminoglycoside antibiotics, amphotericin B, or cisplatinum), during a postobstructive diuresis, recovery from AKI, or following kidney transplantation should be entertained.

Hypermagnesemia

Hypermagnesemia is often asymptomatic, as evidenced by women infused with magnesium during premature labor, in whom levels of 4 to 6 mg per dL are well tolerated. Symptoms attributable to hypermagnesemia include lethargy and confusion, muscle weakness, and cardiac irritability with arrhythmias.

There are no primary genetic abnormalities that result in hypermagnesemia, which is, therefore, almost always from excessive intake and diminished kidney excretion. Excessive intake in children may result from the use of magnesium-based laxatives, antacids, or herbal supplements that contain the mineral. In patients treated with lithium for psychiatric disorders, mild hypermagnesemia may occur due to the lithium ion interference with renal magnesium excretion. AKI, CKD, or ESRD, accompanied by increased magnesium intake and/or volume depletion, may predispose to the development of hypermagnesemia. Generally, cessation of the offending agent and restoration of circulating blood volume is sufficient for relief of hypermagnesemia. Severe cardiac instability with hypermagnesemia may require acute dialysis or chronic renal replacement therapy (CRRT).

RICKETS[27]

Rickets (see also disorders of serum calcium and phosphorus) is a term used to note the inability to mineralize osteoid in the growth plates of growing infants, children, and adolescents. As such, the term does not connote a unique disease entity, but is associated with many diseases that impair some critical aspect of healthy bone mineralization. In the past, it has been synonymous with vitamin D deficiency, and although this produces much rachitic disease, the clinician is urged to separate the two entities so that a more complete differential is available.

Rickets may present with hypercalcemia, normocalcemia, or hypocalcemia, and as such, the clinician may be asked to consult upon a patient with a disorder of serum calcium, in which rickets appears as well. Thus, we discuss rickets based on the concurrent levels of blood calcium. Radiographic similarities to rickets but in which other disease processes have been identified as primary abnormalities have been termed pseudorickets, but in general, are very hard to differentiate based on radiographic findings alone.

Regardless of etiology of the rachitic process, there are some general features that are worth noting (Table 64.9). The inability to mineralize bony tissue normally leads to a softening of bone (the original meaning of the word, rickets), and thus, unusual deformities. Such deformities occur most commonly in the bones that are growing the most at a given age. In the neonate, the skull mineralizes after birth, and neonatal rickets may produce a unique softening called the ping-pong ball skull in which gentle pressure against the skull can produce an indentation similar to that seen in ping-pong balls with such pressure. MacEwen crackpot sound has been ascribed to this indentation with pressure, but we discourage the attempt to produce the phenomenon, as brain injury may be induced. In younger infants who may not be walking, angular deformities of the wrists and a heaping up of the osteoid at the costochondral junction (rachitic rosary) are features that can be assessed by the astute clinician. In the toddler with rickets, a bowing out of the legs at the knees is quite common (valgus deformity), whereas in the older child and adolescent, the opposite changes (varus deformity, knock-knee) may be seen. As a general rule, rachitic bone is not a fracturing disease, but many fracturing diseases of childhood may have concomitant vitamin D deficiency–associated rickets.

When confronted with a patient with rickets, the diagnostic scheme should include the blood levels of calcium (and consideration for ionized calcium), phosphorus, magnesium, parathyroid hormone, 25-hydroxyvitamin D (the nutrient

TABLE 64.9 **Classification of Rickets Based on Serum Calcium Levels**[a]

Hypercalcemia	Normocalcemia or Hypocalcemia
Neonatal severe primary hyperparathyroidism (homozygous activating mutation of the extracellular Ca-sensing receptor)	Vitamin D nutritional deficiency (seen commonly in exclusively breastfed infants, or in infants and young children with extended absence of sunlight exposure, or infants born to vitamin D deficient mothers)
Hypophosphatasia	Renal Fanconi syndrome (resulting from a primary proximal tubular transport disorder most commonly in pediatrics, and including cystinosis, Dents disease, among many others)
Jansen metaphyseal chondrodysplasia	Hypophosphatemic rickets (due to either a *Phex* mutation [X-linked dominant hypophosphatemic rickets], *DMP-1* mutation [autosomal-recessive hypophosphatemic rickets], *FGF23* mutation with active hormone [autosomal-dominant hypophosphatemic rickets], among others)
Idiopathic infantile hypercalcemia due to PTHrp excess	Malabsorption of vitamin D (including cystic fibrosis, celiac sprue, primary disorder of bile salt metabolism, among others)
Idiopathic infantile hypercalcemia due to genetic absence of the vitamin D-24 hydroxylase	Genetic absence of the liver vitamin D-25-hydroxylase
	Genetic absence of the kidney 25-hydroxyvitamin D-1-α-hydroxylase (once termed vitamin D–dependent rickets, type I)
	Genetic mutations in the vitamin D receptor protein, leading to lack of signaling (once termed vitamin D–dependent rickets, type II)
	Chronic kidney disease mineral bone disorder

[a]The list is not an exhaustive one, but lists more commonly seen causes, even if considered "rare."

form of the parent compound vitamin D), and, in selected circumstances, the blood level of 1,25-dihydroxyvitamin D, the kidney-produced active hormone of the vitamin D endocrine system. Prompt attention to severe hypocalcemia is warranted to prevent life-threatening muscle failure, including respiratory failure or heart failure. Conduction system abnormalities should be evaluated with a formal electrocardiogram as well, and the patient monitored if indicated based on those findings.

Treatment of specialized forms of rickets is beyond the scope of our task, but simple nutritional rickets from insufficient dietary vitamin D intake and lack of production of vitamin D by the skin, responds easily to vitamin D replacement alone.

POLYURIA[28–32]

Definition

Polyuria is arbitrarily defined as urine output exceeding 2 L per m^2 in children. Polyuria can be discussed according to the measured urine osmolarity, and can be divided into:

1. Conditions in which there is a primary defect in the ability to maximally concentrate the urine, as reflected by a urine osmolarity of less than 250 to 300 mOsm per kg H_2O (hyposthenuric urine; "dilute polyuria") leading to solute-free water loss and hypernatremia.
2. Kidney diseases associated with tubular salt wasting and relatively fixed urine concentration of about 300 mOsm per kg H_2O (isosthenuric urine). Increased urine output that approaches the degree consistent with polyuria can be observed with the alleviation of urinary tract obstruction and is termed postobstructive diuresis.
3. Excessive renal solute load with a secondary increase in urinary water excretion, producing a urine of greater than 300 mOsm per kg H_2O (concentrated urine initially, but if prolonged, can be associated with isosthenuria, as the hypertonic medullary interstitial gradient is reduced or eliminated). This condition is also referred to as an osmotic diuresis and can be seen in the context of uncontrolled diabetes mellitus, or result from high protein feedings (increased urea load) in neonates or very young infants.

Dilute Polyuria: Differential Diagnosis

Excessive water consumption as in *primary polydipsia* may occur in children as in adults, but may result also from inappropriate water intake when powder-based infant formulas are mixed improperly, or inappropriate water is fed to infants on purpose by caretakers (termed Munchausen syndrome-by-proxy).

Inappropriately dilute urine can reflect complete or partial antidiuretic hormone (ADH) deficiency, a condition known as central diabetes insipidus (CDI). This condition is most often idiopathic (possibly due to autoimmune injury to the ADH-producing cells in the posterior hypophysis), familial with autosomal-dominant inheritance, or can be induced by pituitary tumor or surgery, head trauma, or hypoxic or ischemic encephalopathy.

Impaired responsiveness of the collecting duct to ADH action is referred to as nephrogenic diabetes insipidus (NDI). NDI is characterized by normal ADH secretion, but varying degrees of renal resistance to the water-retaining effect of the hormone. There are numerous conditions that have been associated with ADH resistance and may lead to symptomatic polyuria as a result of acquired NDI, although generally presenting later in childhood and adolescence compared to hereditary forms.

A variety of renal diseases have been associated with loss of ability to concentrate urine, including release of bilateral urinary tract obstruction,[41] sickle cell disease or trait, inherited renal cystic diseases collectively termed nephronophthises or ciliopathies, renal amyloidosis, hypodysplasia, and Sjögren syndrome.

Common Causes of Acquired NDI

The most common causes of ADH resistance severe enough to produce polyuria are hereditary NDI in children, and chronic lithium ingestion and hypercalcemia in adults. Acquired causes, particularly lithium and other drugs, are at least partially reversible with cessation of therapy or hypercalcemia.

There are also several congenital polyuric-polydipsic Bartter-like syndromes associated with urinary concentrating defects of varying severity.

Lithium

Polyuria due to impaired urinary concentrating ability occurs in up to 20% of patients chronically treated with lithium; an additional 30% have a subclinical impairment in concentrating ability. These adverse effects are mediated by lithium entry into the principal cells in the collecting tubule via the epithelial sodium channel (ENaC).

Hypercalcemia

A renal concentrating defect may become clinically apparent if the plasma calcium concentration is persistently above 11 mg per dL (2.75 mmol per L). This defect, which is generally reversible with correction of the hypercalcemia, may be associated with reductions both in sodium chloride reabsorption in the thick ascending limb of the loop of Henle, thereby interfering with the countercurrent mechanism, and in the ability of ADH to increase collecting tubule water permeability.

Hypokalemia

Persistent, severe hypokalemia (< 3 mEq per L) can impair urinary concentrating ability. As with hypercalcemia, both decreased collecting tubule responsiveness to ADH (which may be mediated by decreased expression of aquaporin-2) and diminished sodium chloride reabsorption in the thick ascending limb have been demonstrated in experimental animals.

History

Age of onset of polyuria may suggest the nature of the underlying disorder. Most hereditary forms of NDI present with severe polyuria during the first weeks to months of life. In familial central DI, usually an autosomal-dominant disease, polyuria may present only after the first year of life, and sometimes in young adulthood, due to preservation of function of the normal allele. The new onset of nocturia or secondary enuresis may be the first clue to DI. The urine is normally most concentrated in the morning due to lack of fluid ingestion overnight; as a result, the first manifestation of a loss of concentrating ability is often nocturia. Family history can be important to demonstrate familial forms of both central and nephrogenic DI. Measurement of urine output by obtaining a timed urine collection of 24 hours—or even a mid-day, 8-hour collection—may be helpful in confirming the presence of polyuria in children.

Laboratory

Comparing plasma sodium concentration and osmolarity to urine osmolarity is key in distinguishing between the three common causes of hyposthenuric polyuria: primary polydipsia, central DI, or nephrogenic DI. A low plasma sodium concentration (less than 135 mEq per L) with a low urine osmolality (e.g., less than one-half the plasma osmolality) is usually indicative of water overload due to primary polydipsia. A high-normal plasma sodium concentration (greater than 142 mEq per L, due to water loss) points toward DI, particularly if the urine osmolality is less than the plasma osmolality. A normal plasma sodium concentration is not helpful in diagnosis but, if associated with a urine osmolality more than 600 mOsmol per kg H_2O excludes a diagnosis of any form of DI.

Diagnosis

Water Deprivation Test

Water restriction can be helpful in confirming the concentration defect and in distinguishing NDI from CDI. It should only be undertaken under careful medical supervision by a physician familiar with its performance and interpretation. The water deprivation test is not necessary to perform if the plasma sodium concentration is greater than 145 mEq per L and the urine osmolality is less than the plasma osmolality.[7] Water restriction is also important to differentiate CDI from primary polydipsia. Once the plasma osmolality reaches 295 to 300 mOsmol per kg H_2O (normal 275 to 290 mOsmol per kg H_2O) or the plasma sodium is 145 mEq per L or higher, the effect of endogenous ADH on the kidney is maximal. At this point, administering desmopressin will not further elevate the urine osmolality unless endogenous ADH release is impaired as in CDI. Administration of 1-desamino-8-D-arginine vasopressin (DDAVP), a synthetic analogue of the natural arginine vasopressin, is expected to produce a high and prolonged antidiuretic effect in patients with impaired secretion of ADH. Withholding water (e.g., for diagnostic or surgical procedures) can result in severe dehydration. For safety reasons water deprivation should be discontinued in children once 3% of total body weight has been achieved irrespective of plasma osmolarity and sodium levels. After DDAVP administration, patients with NDI are unable to increase urinary osmolality, which remains below 200 mOsm per kg H_2O (normal $\geq$807 mOsm per kg H_2O) and such patients cannot reduce urine volume or free-water clearance. Plasma vasopressin levels are normal or only slightly increased in affected children.

Exceptions to this general rule for performance of a water deprivation test are patients with a dilute urine (i.e., urine osmolality well below that of the plasma) who are strongly suspected of having NDI (e.g., long-term lithium use), and newborns and young infants who are thought to have hereditary NDI. In these patients who are resistant to ADH, the response to desmopressin can be evaluated without prior water restriction.

RENAL DISEASE

Oliguria and Anuria[33–35]

Oliguria occurs when the urine output is below 400 mL/m^2/day, whereas anuria is the complete cessation of urine output. Either may be the initial manifestation of kidney disease in infants and children.

The anuric child must be evaluated for complete urinary obstruction (postrenal kidney failure) and appropriately managed by determining the etiology. The absence of a radiographic demonstration of urinary obstruction leads to the diagnosis of AKI, and management that is not different than the adult with AKI. The majority of neonates urinate in the first 48 hours of life, although a substantial number of infants who urinate at delivery are missed as having made urine. Therefore, consideration of anuria in the newborn should take this into account, especially when kidney function is normal.

Oliguric children should be evaluated based on the history and physical examination evidence of their intravascular volume status. The majority of children who are oliguric have a recognized cause of volume depletion that is extrarenal, and rehydration will produce urine above the oliguric level in the first 12 to 24 hours. The absence of such urine output, and perhaps the absence of response to a potent loop-active diuretic, defines AKI in this situation too. Euvolemic children with oliguria who have a fluid challenge with or without loop-active diuretics and do not resolve the oliguria have AKI as well. Most children with oliguria do not have a hypervolemic state that is not easily explained by aggressive fluid administration often in the hospital setting. Diuretic management of the hypervolemic, oliguric child should be initiated, and if unsuccessful, extracorporeal therapy for AKI should be considered strongly.

In some infants or young children, acute urinary retention may produce oliguria or anuria, but with normal kidney filtering function. The key finding on an ultrasound examination of the abdomen is a full but normal urinary bladder, and in such cases, placing the patient in a warm bath with supervision often leads to a spontaneous diuresis.

The differential diagnosis of AKI in the neonate involves extrarenal diseases such as volume depletion from perinatal issues of blood loss (hemorrhage, twin-twin transfusion), inadequate fluid intake due to environmental stressors such as phototherapy, high environmental temperatures, or any known cause of extrarenal volume depletion. Ischemia from perinatal asphyxia, aortic cross-clamping during cardiac surgery to repair a congenital heart defect, or severe respiratory distress syndrome of infancy may also produce the symptom. Severe congestive heart failure or cyanotic heart diseases without congestive failure may also produce AKI.

Intrinsic causes of AKI in neonates include bilateral renal agenesis, autosomal-recessive polycystic kidney disease, cortical necrosis, nephrotoxicity from drugs, renal vein thrombosis, renal artery thrombosis (often associated with prior or current use of indwelling umbilical artery catheters and the presence of systemic hypertension), acute pyelonephritis, obstructive uropathies, abdominal masses compressing the renal vessels, or, rarely, complete imperforate penile prepuce.

AKI in the older child and adolescent assume the differential diagnostic categories of the adult too and include, in addition to the previously mentioned causes, vasculitis, thrombotic microangiopathy of STEC-hemolytic uremic syndrome (HUS), atypical HUS, all forms of AGN and rapidly progressive glomerulonephritis, tubule-interstitial nephritis from any cause, kidney stones, obstructive fungal balls, retroperitoneal masses, hematoma, or fibrosing conditions, among others.

HYPERTENSION[36–37]

Diagnostic Approach to Hypertension in Childhood

The notion that hypertension in children is related most commonly to an identifiable abnormality in a specific organ system (i.e., secondary hypertension) has been challenged recently by finding an increasing prevalence of essential hypertension in the childhood years. Nevertheless, the finding of elevated blood pressure (BP) in children warrants careful evaluation for a specific diagnosis before essential hypertension is assigned.

Definitions

BP increases from infancy through adolescence, and generally is thought to track along given percentiles based on genetic and environmental influences. It is based on observational data and adjusted for the patient's age, gender, and statural height. Measurement of BP should take into account appropriate cuff sizes, as a smaller than appropriate cuff size may elevate normal BP falsely.

Normal BP is defined as values below the 90th percentile for age, gender, and height, in the absence of CKD. Prehypertension is average BP values that are ≥90th but <95th percentile. Stage 1 hypertension is systolic and/or diastolic BP ≥95th percentile and stage 2 hypertension is BP >99th percentile.

Hypertensive urgency is severe hypertension with possible end-organ damage in the heart, eye, or kidney, and with a high potential of progressing to a malignant hypertension phase. Hypertensive emergency/malignant hypertension is severe hypertension with symptoms such as headache, vomiting, encephalopathy, or evidence of pulmonary edema, AKI, stroke, or myocardial ischemia.

Technique of Measurement

Obtaining an accurate BP reading using an appropriate size cuff, comprising two thirds of the arm length, is critical in children. Ausculatory BP measurement taken on the upper extremity is considered the preferred method in pediatrics, but on finding an elevated BP, four extremity BP recordings are recommended to evaluate for a coarctation of the aorta, a secondary cause of hypertension in children of any age.

Diagnosis

The findings of at least three abnormal BP readings are often sufficient to establish the diagnosis of hypertension, especially if accompanied by evidence of end-organ damage. Ambulatory BP monitoring (ABPM) is a valuable tool in the diagnosis of "white coat" hypertension or masked hypertension and data regarding the normal values in children are available.

Differential Diagnosis

Secondary hypertension in childhood may be attributed to kidney pathology and accompanied renal parenchymal damage (e.g., polycystic kidney disease, GN, or Wilms tumor), or impaired renal perfusion, also known as renovascular hypertension, as in fibromuscular dysplasia, neurofibromatosis, and systemic vasculitides (e.g., Takayasu arteritis, Moyamoya, Kawasaki). Endocrinopathies such as pheochromocytoma, Cushing syndrome, hyperthyroidism, hyperaldosteronism, and hypercalcemia from various mechanisms are known causes of hypertension in children. Of the cardiovascular causes of secondary hypertension coarctation of the aorta (thoracic and abdominal) is the most recognizable condition. Not uncommon as a group are monogenic disorders (autosomal-dominant [AD] or -recessive [AR]) that may result in hereditary or sporadic hypertension and include Liddle syndrome (AD), apparent mineralocorticoid excess (AR), glucocorticoid remediable aldosteronism (AD), pseudohypoaldosteronism type 2 (AD), and congenital adrenal hyperplasia (11–β hydroxylase deficiency and 17–α hydroxylase deficiency).

Other secondary causes of elevated blood pressure in pediatrics include obstructive sleep apnea, or drug-induced hypertension (e.g., sympathomimetics, cocaine).

Essential hypertension has been increasingly recognized in children and has been linked to the high prevalence of the metabolic syndrome (i.e., hypertension, insulin resistance, hyperlipidemia and obesity), but surely occurs in its absence, too. Traditionally, essential hypertension can be diagnosed only after a thorough evaluation for secondary hypertension.

History should include family history and comprehensive review of systems directed at secondary and symptomatic hypertension. Four extremity BP measurments, as noted previously, and performance of a careful physical exam with particular attention to the presence of bruits over carotid, aorta, and renal arteries; funduscopic examination; and palpation of femoral pulses is an integral part of evaluating a child with elevated BP. Skin examination can lead to a diagnosis, as with the findings of café au lait spots (neurofibromatosis), adenoma sebaceum (tuberous sclerosis), and acanthosis nigricans (insulin resistance).

Laboratory evaluation of a child with newly diagnosed hypertension should follow the clinical suspicion raised by the history and physical exam, but baseline laboratory studies should include a serum creatinine, blood urea nitrogen (BUN), electrolytes, CBC with differential, platelet count, and reticulocyte count, thyroid-stimulating hormone (TSH), thyroxine (FT4), renin, aldosterone, urinalysis, and determination of the first morning random urine protein, creatinine, and level microalbumin excretion.

Imaging

Kidney ultrasound may be valuable for demonstration of an underlying condition such as enlarged kidneys in polycystic kidney disease, small kidneys in advanced CKD from any cause, and size discrepancy in long-standing unilateral renovascular lesions. Doppler studies of the renal vessels have low sensitivity and specificity in diagnosing renal vascular stenosis, and MRA and/or formal contrast-injected radiologic angiography (gold standard) are indicated based on clinical suspicion. An echocardiogram is important in the diagnosis of cardiovascular anomalies (e.g., thoracic coarctation), and in evaluating left ventricular (LV) hypertrophy or LV mass index. The finding of posterior reversible encephalopathy syndrome (PRES) on brain MRI is diagnostic of hypertensive-induced central nervous system injury.

Further diagnostic evaluations should be tailored to the individual patient based on the clinical suspicion and might include plasma metanephrines/catecholamines (pheochromocytoma), for example.

ABDOMINAL MASSES

A common approach to abdominal masses includes a careful history and physical examination, and multimodal kidney imaging including ultrasound, abdominal CT, MRI, and others as indicated. Care should be taken with the use of MR-contrast agents in children with diminished filtration, as the risk of systemic sclerosing nephropathy may occur during the childhood years too. A skilled pediatric urologist and pediatric surgeon are required almost always for surgical intervention in neonates and children with kidney masses. When malignancy is proven, consultation with a major pediatric center for cancer is required as well.

In the newborn, abdominal masses may include the kidney, where unilateral or bilateral kidney masses may occur. Cystic diseases of the newborn kidney that may produce such masses include autosomal-recessive polycystic kidney disease with large hyperechoic kidneys (and a history of oligohydramnios), autosomal-dominant polycystic kidney disease (large hyperechoic kidneys with or without demonstrable cysts, and often, unilateral in infancy), unilateral multicystic dysplastic kidney (in which the ureter is atretic or absent, the parenchyma is without any function, and other kidney abnormalities are common [vesicoureteral reflux, contralateral uteropelvic junction obstruction]), and rarely, glomerulocystic kidney disease (cortical cysts and CKD). Outside the newborn period, additional cystic kidney diseases include tuberous sclerosis with angiomyolipoma formation, neurofibromatosis, or cystic nephromas.

Tumors of the kidney that produce kidney masses may occur at all ages within pediatrics, and include Wilms tumor, mesoblastic nephromas, clear cell cancer, malignant rhabdoid tumor, nephroblastomatosis (residual metanephrogenic tissue in the mature kidney), hematologic malignancies of leukemia or lymphoma that invade one or both kidneys, neuroblastoma that involves the kidney by extension, and rare tumors of kidney adenomatoid malformation, histiocytic medullary reticulocytosis, or Castleman disease (a form of a lymphoproliferative disorder).

Obstructive lesions of the kidney may produce nephromegaly, including obstruction at the level of the ureteropelvic junction, the uterovesical junction, the presence of posterior urethral valves, or in prune belly syndrome, in which the abdominal musculature is extremely lax, and the peristaltic functions of the ureter is diminished to absent.

Congenital kidney malformations that produce nephromegaly include those in Beckwith-Wiedemann syndrome, horseshoe kidney, duplex kidney, pelvic kidney location, and crossed-fused renal ectopia. Kidney masses associated with infection may produce nephromegaly too, including abscess or urinoma. Hematomas from any etiology may produce a mass and enlargement. Rarely, children may have xanthogranulomatous pyelonephritis and kidney enlargement.

NEPHROLITHIASIS[38–42]

Kidney stones occur about one tenth less frequently in children than in adults, representing from 1 in 1000 to 1 in 7600 pediatric hospital admissions. They are most common in white children, and overall, tend to affect boys and girls equally. This differs from the adult disease, in which there is a male preponderance (3:1). Within subtypes of stone disease, however, male children do have a slightly higher incidence of stones related to hypercalciuria and urinary tract abnormalities. Predisposing factors for nephrolithiasis can be determined in the majority of children affected. These include metabolic abnormalities, UTI in 14% to 75%, and coexisting structural urinary tract abnormalities in about 40%. The recurrence rate of kidney stones in children has been reported as anywhere from 6.5% to 54%, and children with metabolic disorders are nearly five times more likely to have a recurrence. Calcium oxalate stones are the most common found in children, with a frequency of 45%. These are followed by calcium phosphate (14%–30%), struvite (13%), cystine (5%), uric acid (4%), and mixed stones (4%).

Clinical Evaluation

The clinical presentation of urinary tract stones in children may differ from that in adults. Urinary tract stones may present with abdominal, flank, or pelvic pain in only 50% of children with nephrolithiasis. Gross or microscopic hematuria (occurring in 33% to 90% of affected children), dysuria, frequency, emesis, and UTIs are additional common presenting signs in younger patients. A detailed history and physical should guide evaluation of kidney stones. Family history should focus on members with kidney stones (positive in greater than one third of affected children), gout, arthritis, or CKD. The presence of a concomitant UTI must be sought but should not be accepted as the cause of the stone. Patients should also be advised to submit any passed stones or stone fragments for analysis by polarization microscopy or X-ray diffraction but not by simple chemical analysis.

Useful imaging studies may include plain abdominal radiology, ultrasonography, and helical CT. Conventional abdominal radiographs may show only radiopaque but not radiolucent stones, whereas ultrasound of the urinary tract may show both radiolucent and radiopaque stones, in addition to the presence of urinary obstruction or nephrocalcinosis. Ultrasound has largely taken the place of intravenous pyelography (IVP) as an initial study for stone presence, secondary to concerns about radiation and contrast exposure with the latter procedure. Noncontrast helical CT has been found to have high sensitivity and specificity in identifying even small stones without requiring intravenous contrast administration. It may precisely localize stones, detect obstruction and hydronephrosis, and is much more sensitive than the previously mentioned imaging modalities.

Because the majority of children with stones may have a metabolic problem that is discoverable and generally amenable to therapy, diagnostic urinary and blood tests for stone evaluation should be obtained while the patient is on their routine activity schedule and diet. At least two 24-hour urine collections should be performed, waiting at least 2 weeks after any acute stone event. This time frame allows for the resumption of the child's normal intake of food and fluids after recovery from pain and/or surgical intervention, which is critical for correct assignment of metabolic disturbances. These collections can assess urinary volume as a reflection of fluid intake and creatinine excretion for completeness of the 24-hour collection (at least 10–15 mg/kg/d in children >2 years of age; 6–9 mg/kg/d <2 years of age) and measurement of levels of lithogenic substances such as calcium, oxalate, uric acid, and cystine. The collections can evaluate for the decreased stone inhibitor levels as well, such as citrate and magnesium. Normal values of these substances are shown in Table 64.10. Serum levels of uric acid, potassium, calcium, phosphorus, creatinine, bicarbonate (total CO), and biointact PTH (if hypercalcemia is present) should be obtained as well at the end of the urinary collections. Consultation with an expert in pediatric stone disorders is encouraged if questions arise about the results of these diagnostic studies.

Metabolic Abnormalities in Children with Nephrolithiasis

Hypercalciuria

Calcium oxalate and calcium phosphate stones in children are most frequently caused by hypercalciuria, defined as a urinary calcium excretion of >4 mg/kg/d. Patients with hypercalciuria may present with microscopic or gross hematuria, dysuria, or urgency, even in the absence of any stones. Such children often have a positive family history of kidney stones and may have up to a 17% chance of subsequently developing urolithiasis. Familial idiopathic hypercalciuria is the most common subset of hypercalciuria. Although the genetic basis of this condition is unknown, it seems to be inherited in an autosomal-dominant pattern with incomplete penetrance. The pathophysiology of familial idiopathic hypercalciuria (FIH) is not yet well defined but may include any combination of the following, to varying degrees: a primary kidney tubular reduction in calcium resorption, increased dietary calcium absorption in the gastrointestinal tract secondary to excessive 1,2S-dihydroxy-vitamin D action, and increased bone resorption. The contribution of bone resorption to this disorder has important clinical implications, because restricting calcium intake in these patients may worsen their propensi-ty toward significant osteoporosis.

Causes of hypercalciuria are listed in Table 64.11. Dents disease is an X-linked recessive condition of nephrolithiasis

TABLE 64.10 Normative Data for Urinary Solute Excretion

Substance	Reference Range
Calcium	≤4 mg/kg/day
Citrate	>400 mg/g creatinine spot citrate/ creatinine ratio >0.51 g/g
Oxalate	≤0.5 mmol/1.73 m^2 BSA/day <40 mg/1.73 m^2 BSA/day
Uric acid	Varies with age in pediatrics, rising to 815 mg/1.73 m^2 BSA/day by adolescence
Cystine	<60 mg/1.73 m^2 BSA/day

BSA, body surface area.

TABLE 64.11 Causes of Hypercalciuria

Associated with Hypercalcemia	Associated with Normal Levels of Blood Calcium
Primary hyperparathyroidism	Familial idiopathic hypercalciuria (FIH)
Idiopathic infantile hypercalcemia	Bartter syndrome
Vitamin D-24-hydroxylase deficiency	Dents disease
Immobilization	Familial hypomagnesemia-hypercalciuria
Thyrotoxicosis	Immobilization
Addison disease	Prematurity ± furosemide
Williams syndrome	Ketogenic diet
PTHrp excess	Distal (type 1) RTA
Osteolytic bone metastases	Medullary sponge kidney
Extra-renal production of calcitriol (Sarcoid, cat-scratch disease, hematologic malignancies)	Systemic inflammatory diseases (e.g., inflammatory bowel disease, juvenile arthritis)
Vitamin D intoxication	Corticosteroid therapy
Jansen metaphyseal chondrodysplasia	Activating mutation of the extracellular calcium-sensing receptor, often associated with hypocalcemia

and subsequent kidney failure, linked to mutations in the *CLCN5* gene. This gene is responsible for the transduction of a voltage-gated chloride channel in the kidney, the lack of which leads to hypercalciuria, low molecular weight proteinuria, nephrolithiasis, nephrocalcinosis, and varying degrees of glycosuria, aminoaciduria, and phosphaturia. Bartter syndrome occurs with one of a series of mutations of genes coding for transporters in the thick ascending limb of the loop of Henle. These genes include *NKCC2*, which transduces the Na-K-2CI transporter (type I Bartter syndrome); *ROMK*, which transduces the potassium channel (type 11); and *CLCNKB*, which transduces the chloride channel (type 111). There is also a type IV Bartter syndrome, or Bartter syndrome with sensorineural deafness, which is caused by a mutation in the gene for *barttin*, a P-subunit of the chloride channel. Type V has a similar phenotype as type IV but is caused by defects in one or both of the chloride channels that co-localize with barttin: C1C-Ka and C1C-Kb.

Distal renal tubular acidosis (dRTA) is a condition of metabolic acidosis, growth retardation, hypercalciuria, and nephrocalcinosis. When associated with a mutation in the *ATP6Bl* gene responsible for a vacuolar H+-ATPase, it is associated with deafness and an autosomal-dominant inheritance. Familial hypomagnesemia-hypercalciuria is associated with a mutation in the *PLCN-1* gene for the tight junction protein paracellin-1. Pseudohypoaldosteronism type I1 is seen with mutations in WNK kinases expressed in the distal nephron and presents with hypertension, hyperkalemia, and metabolic acidosis in addition to hypercalciuria. Other causes of hypercalciuria with normocalcemia include medullary sponge kidney, systemic inflammatory diseases, and iatrogenic resulting from medications such as loop diuretics and corticosteroids. If hypercalcemia is detected, primary hyperparathyroidism, sarcoidosis, immobilization, thyroid disease, osteolytic metastases, hypervitaminosis D, and Williams syndrome should be considered on the differential.

Hypocitraturia

Hypocitraturia is a contributory cause of nephrolithiasis, because citrate is necessary for the formation of a soluble calcium salt to prevent calcium stone crystallization. Most commonly it is seen in RTA, but it is also present in a subset of patients with familial idiopathic hypercalciuria. Hypocitraturia can also occur in concert with other forms of hypercalciuria, hyperuricosuria, or hyperoxaluria. Chronic diarrhea, a high protein diet, and hypokalemia can also induce low urinary citrate levels and a predisposition to stone formation, because citrate absorption in the proximal tubule is stimulated by intracellular acidosis and potassium depletion.

Hyperoxaluria

Oxalate is a human metabolic product made in the liver and excreted by the kidney, but can also be ingested and absorbed from dietary sources. Type 1 primary hyperoxaluria (PH1) is an autosomal-recessive reduction in or absence of alanine glyoxylate aminotransferase (AGT) activity, leading to increased conversion of glyoxylate to oxalate. Excessive urinary oxalate excretion may lead to crystallization and deposition in the urinary tract and kidney parenchyma. This in turn can result in kidney failure and systemic oxalosis, a clinical situation in which calcium oxalate precipitates in multiple organs and joints. Disease severity in PH1 varies widely. The course may be mild and fully responsive to medical therapy such as vitamin B_6 (pyridoxine) or may present aggressively in infancy with rapid kidney failure and severe systemic manifestations. Because AGT is predominantly expressed in the liver, diagnosis has in the past relied solely on liver biopsy to assess AGT presence and activity. The gene encoding AGT (*AGXT*), located on chromosome 2q37.3, to date has at least 83 mutations that have been described that either eliminate, or decrease substantially, enzyme activity. The relative ease in modern laboratory medicine at performance of sequence analysis, and the delineation of the molecular basis of many of the mutations behind PH1, has led to the proposal of molecular diagnostic algorithms that may obviate the need for invasive biopsy procedures. A recently reported comprehensive mutation screening across the entire *AGXT* coding region in 55 probands with PH1 showed a 96% to 98% sensitivity in this population. When limited to sequencing of exons 1, 4, and 7, the sensitivity was 77%. Given the relatively small size of the gene, complete molecular analysis should not be at a prohibitive expense. An algorithm beginning with limited sequencing of exons 1, 4, and 7, followed by direct sequencing of the entire gene if inconclusive, would make intuitive sense and would eliminate the need for liver biopsy in most patients. Type 2 primary hyperoxaluria (PH2) results from a deficiency of activity in the enzyme glyoxylate reductase/hydroxypyruvate reductase (GRHPR), which is more widely distributed in the human than AGTl, with a predominance in muscle, liver, and kidney. As a group, patients with PH2 seem to have less morbidity and mortality than those with PH1, with a lower incidence of ESRD and an older age at onset of symptoms. Unfortunately, up to one third of patients with PH in some case series present at end stage, when uremia develops. For this reason, PH should be considered in patients with recurrent calcium oxalate nephrolithiasis, unexplained nephrocalcinosis, or unexplained CKD in which the kidneys are echodense with calcium.

Secondary (enteric) hyperoxaluria can result from increased oxalate absorption in the colon caused by small bowel malabsorption of fatty and bile acids. These substances increase colonic permeability to oxalate by binding luminal calcium, freeing unbound oxalate to be absorbed. Epithelial damage in these states also increases colonic absorption, and low dietary calcium intake can exacerbate the condition. Depletion of *Oxalobacter formigenes*, an enteric oxalate-degrading bacterium, can also contribute to enteric hyperoxaluria. Other rare secondary causes are pyridoxine deficiency (a cofactor for AGT activity) and excessive intake of oxalate-containing foods (rhubarb gluttony) or oxalate precursors (ascorbic acid, ethylene glycol).

Hyperuricosuria

Uric acid is the end product of purine metabolism. Hyperuricosuria may occur either in the face of uric acid overproduction or with normal serum uric acid concentrations and can predispose to both uric acid stones and calcium oxalate nephrolithiasis, acting as a heterotopic nucleation factor. Lesch-Nyhan syndrome (complete deficiency of hypoxanthine-guanine phosphoribosyltransferase) and type 1 glycogen storage disease (glucose-6–phosphatase deficiency) are both inborn errors of metabolism that may present with hyperuricemia and hyperuricosuria/urolithiasis. Gout caused by a partial hypoxanthine-guanine phosphoribosyltransferase deficiency can also cause uric acid nephrolithiasis in older children. Myeloproliferative disorders and other causes of cell breakdown are other secondary causes of uric acid stones. Ketogenic diets, excessive protein intake, and uricosuric drugs such as high-dose aspirin, probenecid, and ascorbic acid can also cause hyperuricosuria. Normal or low serum uric acid levels may be associated with uricosuria secondary to proximal renal tubular defects. These may be caused by a single defect in the renal urate exchanger URAT1 or disorders of generalized proximal tubule dysfunction. Insulin resistance, as seen in type 2 diabetes mellitus and metabolic syndrome, may also predispose to uric acid stones and an overly acidic urine by decreasing renal ammonia excretion and impairing hydrogen ion buffering. In another perturbation of uric acid metabolism, xanthine stones are formed in an autosomal-recessive disorder of the gene for xanthine dehydrogenase, whereby uric acid cannot be formed from xanthine precursors, and the serum uric acid is commonly undetectable or below 0.2 mg/dL.

Cystinuria

Cystinuria is an autosomal-recessive disease of disordered dibasic amino acid transport in the kidney and may occasionally be diagnosed by the discovery of flat hexagonally shaped cystine crystals in the urine. Children with this condition have elevated urinary cystine, ornithine, arginine, and lysine levels, because all of these amino acids share transporters. Mutations of the *SLC3AI* gene on chromosome 2 and the *SLC7A9* gene on chromosome 19 have been identified, and patients may be either homozygous or compound or obligate heterozygotes. Affected homozygous children usually excrete >l000 pmol per g creatinine of cystine by the age of 1 year, with a mean excretion of 4500 pmol per g creatinine, exceeding its solubility and leading to lifelong recurrent nephrolithiasis.

Other Causes of Kidney Stones

Additional clinical situations in which patients are predisposed to forming kidney stones include patients with cystic fibrosis (who may have an absence of the oxalate-degrading bacterium *O. formigenes*), hyperoxaluria, hypercalciuria, and/or hypocitraturia. Patients taking protease inhibitors, especially the poorly soluble indinavir, may have urinary excretion of crystallized drug product. Patients on a ketogenic diet for seizure control are predisposed to hypercalciuria and/or hypocitraturia.

Surgical Management

The goals of the management of patients with kidney stones are to remove existing stones and prevent stone recurrence, with preservation of kidney function. Pediatric patients usually pass ureteral stones up to 5 mm in size. In the absence of infection or persistent pain, such stones can be safely observed for up to 6 weeks. Larger stones and kidney-located stones, however, require the consideration of surgical intervention, with a goal of achieving and maintaining a stone-free state. Choice of surgical modality depends on stone composition, size, and location along the urinary tract. Shock wave lithotripsy (SWL) uses the generation and focusing of shock wave energy toward the stone. Pulverized fragments are subsequently passed, and multiple treatment sessions are sometimes required. One large pediatric series (n = 344) showed a 92% stone-free rate for renal pelvis stones <1 cm, a 68% rate for stones 1 to 2 cm, and a 50% rate for stones >2 cm. Calyceal stone clearance rates were lower. Overall, stone-free rates in children treated using this procedure have ranged from 67% to 99% in various studies, the highest success rates appearing to be in the youngest children. This procedure seems to be safe in young children and infants, with no evidence of long-term changes in GFR or in functional renal parenchymal scarring before and after treatment in the affected area. Minor complications such as bruising, renal colic, and hematuria may occur with SWL treatment. Small children may require the use of lung shielding to prevent pulmonary contusion, as well as reduced power settings to avoid injury. Ureteral stenting may also be required for larger stone burdens.

In general, large stone burden (>2 cm) and anatomic abnormalities are risk factors for unsuccessful SWL, and alternative urologic approaches should be considered in these cases. Struvite, calcium oxalate dehydrate, and uric acid stones are especially amenable to fragmentation with SWL, whereas cystine, brushite, and calcium oxalate monohydrate stones are all resistant to SWL treatment.

Percutaneous nephrolithotomy is an alternative procedure that may be used alone or in conjunction with SWL in patients with large stone burden, significant renal obstruction, and/or staghorn calculi. It is also commonly used to remove lower pole calculi >1 cm in size. Percutaneous access to the collecting system of the kidney is achieved, and a wire is advanced to dilate the tract to accommodate a nephroscope. Stones may be removed or pulverized under direct visualization, making this approach ideal for complex upper tract stones. A nephrostomy tube is often placed postoperatively, although a small series in adults did show a decrease in pain and recovery time, with no increase in complications. Smaller nephroscopes have made percutaneous nephrolithotomy available for children, with stone-free rates ranging from 83% to 98%. Ureteroscopy is most ideally used for the removal and/or fragmentation of distal ureteral stones. Whereas SWL has good efficacy for some smaller ureteral stones, stone-free rates in those with stones >10 mm in size have been found to be markedly higher with ureteroscopy (93%) than with SWL (50%). Smaller rigid and flexible ureteroscopes have made this procedure an option for pediatric patients and have made the need for concomitant ureteral balloon dilation (and possible risks of stricture and vesicoureteral reflux) less frequent. Once the ureteroscope is passed, laser energy is used to fragment any visualized stones, and flexible wire baskets can be used to remove fragments. Postoperative stenting may be used to facilitate passage of residual fragments or to prevent ureteral obstruction in the face of edema caused by trauma to the ureteral wall. Stenting is not usually done in uncomplicated procedures, with easy passage of the scope.

Medical Management

Nonspecific management of urolithiasis includes an increase in fluid intake to increase urinary volume, urinary dilution, and induce stone particle motion through the urinary tract. Other specific measures depend on the underlying predisposing diagnosis. Hypercalciuria may be treated with a low sodium diet, thiazide diuretics, and adequate potassium intake. Thiazide therapy (e.g., hydrochlorothiazide 1 mg/kg/d, maximum of 25 mg/d) in FIH significantly decreases urinary calcium excretion and rate of stone formation. A decrease in urinary calcium excretion with thiazide treatment in children with FIH has also been shown. In a population with hypercalciuria from immobilization, 18 of 42 children were found to be hypercalciuric, with a higher rate of fracture. A 3-week course of hydrochlorothiazide and amiloride reduced the mean urinary calcium to creatinine ratio by 57.7%. Dietary calcium intake should not be limited. Citrate therapy (e.g., potassium citrate 2 mmol per kg once daily) is also appropriate in cases of documented hypocitraturia.

Another important issue for some patients is that of bone mineral density in FIH. One study of 40 girls with FIH and their premenopausal mothers showed that bone mass density lumbar spine Z-scores were significantly lower in these patients compared with controls. Others have shown that thiazide treatment, in addition to decreasing urinary calcium excretion, can also improve bone mass density scores in children. Average Z-score improved from −1.3 to +0.22 over 1 year of treatment with hydrochlorothiazide and potassium citrate in one study of 18 children.

The treatment of struvite stones rests on the eradication of stones, correction of any urinary obstruction, and treatment/prevention of UTIs. Urinary acidification could theoretically be used to prevent crystallization, but evidence for such an approach is thus far lacking. The urease inhibitor acetohydroxamic acid may have some clinical use, but its use is limited by a high incidence of neurologic and gastrointestinal side effects.

Hyperuricosuria may be treated with dietary sodium limitation, oral bicarbonate or citrate supplementation, or addition of allopurinol if increased uric acid production and hyperuricemia are present.

Patients with suspected primary hyperoxaluria should be given a therapeutic course of vitamin B_6 (pyridoxine), and urinary oxalate levels should be used to monitor success or to suggest the need for dose escalation. For patients with reduced kidney function, intensive dialysis followed by liver-kidney transplant can be curative, because a new liver replaces the enzymatic defect in PHl. While awaiting transplant, hemodialysis for five to six times per week, and perhaps with additional nightly peritoneal dialysis, is needed to lessen the systemic oxalate burden and prevent recurrence of disease in the transplant kidney. Prompt referral to a pediatric center with expertise in this disorder is suggested.

Secondary hyperoxaluria that results from enteric hyperoxaluria may be treated with a low sodium/low fat diet, high fluid intake, and a dietary calcium intake at the upper end of the daily recommended intake. Limitation of oxalate-containing foods such as chocolate, rhubarb, nuts, and spinach should be advised, as well as possible supplementation with magnesium, phosphorus, and citrate salts.

Cystinuria is treated with fluids (minimum of 3 L/1.73 m^2/d) and provision of alkali salts, such as citrate. Low sodium intake can also decrease urinary excretion of cystine. Chelating agents such as D-penicillamine, or more recently, alpha-mercapto propionylglycine (Thiola; Mission Pharmacal, San Antonio, TX) may also be prescribed by someone skilled in pediatric stone disease. D-penicillamine may cause a severe serum sickness–like reaction, but side effects are less severe with Thiola. Angiotensin converting enzyme inhibition with captopril therapy has been found beneficial in some patients with cystinuria (captopril-cystine complexes are 200 times more soluble than cystine alone) resistant to alkalinization and fluid therapy alone, and perhaps with less bothersome side effects. Captopril, however, is not as effective as thiol compound therapy.

DISORDERS OF SEXUAL DIFFERENTIATION[43,44]

Infants with a congenital discrepancy between external genitalia, gonadal, and chromosomal sex are classified as having a disorder of sex development (DSD). A 2006 consensus conference suggested that the potentially pejorative terms pseudohermaphroditism and intersex be replaced by the diagnostic category disorders of sex development (Table 64.12).

Kidney disease is associated with patients who have DSD. The diseases are those of kidney tumors such as Wilms tumor (Table 64.13) and forms of steroid-resistant nephrotic syndrome, generally leading to ESRD. The role of prophylactic bilateral nephrectomy to prevent the development of the Wilms tumor remains problematic and controversial, but frequent screening with an ultrasound examination is warranted. Newborns with DSD should be promptly referred to a center specializing in the multidisciplinary treatment of such disorders.

TABLE 64.12 **Proposed Revised Nomenclature for Disorders of Sex Differentiation**

Previous	Proposed, Current
Intersex	DSD
Male pseudohermaphrodite, undervirilization of an XY male, and undermasculinzation of an XY male	46 XY DSD
Female pseudohermaphrodite, overvirilization of an XX female, and masculinization of an XX female	46 XX DSD
True hermaphrodite	Ovotesticular DSD
XY male or XX sex reversal	46 XX testicular DSD
XY sex reversal	46 XY complete gonadal dysgenesis

DSD, disorders of sex differentiation.

Frasier syndrome is characterized as a DSD in which nephrotic syndrome (mostly FSGS) develops, and gonadoblastomas, but not Wilms tumors, predominate.

URINARY TRACT INFECTION[45–47]

UTI can occur in children of all ages. It has been estimated that UTI is diagnosed in 3% of prepubertal girls and 1% of prepubertal boys, with an even higher incidence in pubertal girls. The relative risk of UTI in girls and boys ages 2 months to 2 years is 2.27; this pattern is even more apparent in older children. Few children or adults who have recurrent UTI progress to serious renal disease, but chronic pyelonephritis may cause ESRD. The epidemiology of chronic pyelonephritis is complicated by the virulence of the infecting organism and the specific susceptibility of the child. Investigation of children with UTI has shown that vesicoureteral reflux (VUR) is present in 25% to 33% and that the degree of VUR correlates well with the prevalence of renal scarring. Numerous urinary pathogens possess fimbrial or nonfimbrial (type 1 fimbriae and P-fimbriae) adhesins for mucosal attachment and colonization. P-fimbriated *Escherichia coli* are associated with the development of renal scars, and inappropriate antibiotic therapy may favor colonization with such organisms. The understanding of UTI and its epidemiology with regard to congenital, genetic, and environmental aspects suggests that early diagnosis and treatment should lead to a reduction in morbidity and mortality rates.

The role of the pediatrician caring for children with UTI is to prevent recurrent UTI and new renal scar formation and consequently renal impairment by facilitating prompt diagnosis of UTI and identifying children with existing renal scars, underlying renal tract anomalies, or known complications of UTI or VUR. Indeed, without an underlying renal tract abnormality, progressive renal damage is rare in children with UTI. Population screening is not cost effective, but early diagnosis by primary health care workers, urgent treatment of acute pyelonephritis to minimize scar formation, and prevention of infection by long-term low-dose prophylactic antibiotics or the surgical correction of reflux in selected children can all contribute to an improved prognosis. Successful management of UTI in childhood by routine urine culture in all febrile infants and toddlers in Sweden has reduced the prevalence of reflux nephropathy/chronic pyelonephritis causing ESRD in pediatric transplant recipients from 20% in the 1970s to less than 5% in the 1990s in that country.

Reflux nephropathy or scarring in the presence of VUR may arise by two main independent mechanisms. Severe antenatal VUR causes segmental renal dysplasia or hypoplasia in the fetal kidney, whereas postnatal VUR with intrarenal reflux and urinary infection causes segmental renal pyelonephritic scars in both infants and older children. The presence of compound renal papillae, which allow the backflow of infected urine from the calyces into the collecting ducts (intrarenal reflux), is important in the generation of renal scars with VUR in animal models; however, the relevance of this mechanism in reflux nephropathy in children has been debated due to the rarity of such papillae in human kidneys. The increased frequency of UTI in infants, the presence of congenital segmental renal dysplasia, the increased risk of true infective pyelonephritic scars developing in infants, and renal impairment at presentation all demonstrate that the target population in which to detect UTI and renal "scars" is children under 18 months of age.

TABLE 64.13 **DSD Syndromes Associated with Wilms Tumor (site of chromosomal aberration)**

Denys-Drash (11p13)	Beckwith-Wiedeman (11p15)
WAGR (11p13)	Perlman syndrome
Hemi-hypertrophy	Sotos syndrome (5q35)
Blooms syndrome (15q26)	Simpson-Golabi-Behemel (Xp26)

WAGR, Wilms tumor, aniridia, genital abnormalities, mental retardation.

The clinical presentation of UTI varies with the age of the child. In young children, classic symptoms of UTI such as dysuria, frequency, urgency, and flank pain are uncommon. Instead, vague symptoms such as fever, abdominal pain, irritability, lethargy, poor feeding, or incontinence are frequent. Fever is a common symptom, and the American Academy of Pediatrics advises that UTI be excluded in any child between 2 months and 2 years of age with unexplained fever.

It is critical to obtain an uncontaminated urine sample for diagnosis. Bladder catheterization provides a sterile sample in the infant or incontinent child. Suprapubic aspiration, although providing definitive results in young infants, is difficult to perform in children older than 1 year of age and is becoming less popular. Bag urine specimens often are contaminated and should not be used for diagnosis of UTI. In older continent children, a clean-catch urine specimen can be obtained, but both clean-catch urine and midstream urine specimens can be difficult to acquire, particularly if parents are given the responsibility of obtaining them. A frequent mistake is to diagnose UTI from a significant growth of organisms after culture of a contaminated or improperly transported urine specimen. The specimen should be cultured within 2 hours or transported in a medium such as boric acid that prevents bacterial multiplication.

Most truly infected urines contain an excess of white blood cells and yield a pure growth of a single organism. Fresh urine without cells or visible organisms on microscopy is unlikely to be infected. Although more than 10^5 organisms per milliliter of urine is the standard criterion for UTI in girls, $>10^4$ organisms/mL in boys is highly indicative of a UTI. In infants a moderate growth of 10,000 to 100,000 organisms per milliliter of urine may represent an infection, and further specimens should be obtained. A detailed history about fever accompanying the illness, the adequacy of the urinary stream in boys, and the presence of functional bladder problems, followed by careful palpation of the abdomen for renal masses and bladder enlargement, thorough examination of the genitalia, and assessment of perineal sensation and neurologic function in the lower limbs, should be carried out.

Appropriate investigations depend on the age of the child and the clinical assessment. Several medical committees have published guidelines on appropriate protocols to investigate UTI in children. However, there is significant controversy in the literature regarding the extent and timing of evaluation in children with UTI and the impact that such evaluation has on the development of reflux nephropathy. What is needed is appropriate investigation of all children with UTI if outcomes of children who present in middle or late childhood with ESRD due to reflux nephropathy are to be avoided. At our institution, we recommend renal and bladder ultrasonography in boys of any age with UTI, all girls younger than 5 years of age, and all with pyelonephritis or recurrent UTI. A functional study such as ^{99m}Tc-DMSA renal isotope scan and or voiding cystourethrography can be performed to detect segmental renal dysplasia or scarring in selected cases, including infants, in which an ultrasound study is abnormal. Voiding contrast cystourethrography, if indicated by an abnormal ultrasound examination, is preferred to radionuclide cystography for the initial study, particularly in boys, due to the former's ability to exclude structural anomalies of the urethra including posterior urethral valves. Failure to make the diagnosis, investigate thoroughly, and follow guidelines remain the major obstacles in identifying those children at risk of renal impairment or hypertension.

Management of Urinary Tract Infection

There is little evidence that older children with normal urinary tracts without renal scars who have recurrent UTI will sustain renal damage, and for such children, attention to hygiene, prevention of constipation, and an adequate fluid intake with regular bladder emptying are important. Mild or moderate reflux without upper tract dilation in young children is likely to disappear in a reasonably short time so that, if the kidneys are not scarred, medical management seems appropriate, whereas severe reflux, especially with scarred kidneys, requires longer term follow-up, and surgery may be advisable if the quality of the surgery can be guaranteed. However, the single most important action required to reduce the morbidity and mortality of chronic pyelonephritis is the diagnosis and treatment of UTI in infants with fever.

Management of UTI involves early administration of appropriate antibiotics to treat the infection and reduce the risk of renal scarring, attention to the voiding habits of children and avoidance of constipation, encouragement of good fluid intake and good personal hygiene of the perineum and genitalia, and diagnosis of any underlying renal tract abnormality. Incontinence predisposes to infection, and the treatment of enuresis by bladder training is important. VUR of a significant grade may be treated medically with prophylactic antibiotics at night or surgical reimplantation of the ureter. Nightly prophylactic antibiotics should also be considered for children in the absence of VUR or other renal structural anomalies when attention to fluid intake, hygiene, and other intervention is not successful in prevention of recurrent infection. The International Reflux Study has shown that medical management of VUR is equivalent to surgery in reducing the number of new renal scars. No advantage between medical vs. surgical management has been shown after 5 years of follow-up. Prophylactic antibiotics reduce the incidence of UTI, but doubt has been cast on whether regular prophylactic antibiotics or even surgery significantly alter the rate of new scar formation—most authors agree that making an early diagnosis of UTI is most important in this regard. In those children who continue to reflux, cessation of prophylactic antibiotics after 8 years of age was associated with only 12% risk of another UTI. Antibiotic prophylaxis or surgery alone does not influence the number of children reaching ESRD.

Because most infections are caused by organisms from the bowel, at least in girls, successful antibiotic prophylaxis depends on the prevention of antibiotic resistance in the bowel flora. Suitable medicines are trimethoprim, 1 mg per kg, or trimethoprim/sulfamethoxazole; nitrofurantoin, 1 to 2 mg per kg; or nalidixic acid, 15 mg per kg, all given as a single dose at night.

The complications of UTI in children include renal scarring and renal calculi. *Proteus* infections more commonly cause renal calculi than any other infection because of the organism's ability to produce alkaline urine by degrading urea. In long-term follow-up studies of up to 41 years, hypertension was observed in young adults in approximately 10% of cases, with people in the higher percentile range for blood pressure being more at risk than others. Approximately 10% have significant renal impairment and may reach renal failure as young people. UTI, preeclampsia, fetal death, and low-birth-weight infants are more common in women with renal scarring.

REFERENCES

1. Schwartz GJ, Work DF. Measurement and estimation of GFR in children and adolescents. *Clin J Am Soc Nephrol.* 2009;4(11):1832–1843.
2. Ng DK, Schwartz GJ, Jacobson LP, et al. Universal GFR determination based on two time points during plasma iohexol disappearance. *Kidney Int.* 2011;80(4):423–430.
3. Guay-Woodford LM, Knoers NV. Genetic testing: considerations for pediatric nephrologists. *Semin Nephrol.* 2009;29(4):338–348.
4. Benoit G, Machuca E, Antignac C. Hereditary nephrotic syndrome: a systematic approach for genetic testing and a review of associated podocyte gene mutations. *Pediatr Nephrol.* 2010;25(9):1621–1632.
5. Hinkes BG, Mucha B, Vlangos CN, et al. Nephrotic syndrome in the first year of life: two thirds of cases are caused by mutations in 4 genes (NPHS1, NPHS2, WT1, and LAMB2). *Pediatrics.* 2007;119(4):e907–919.
6. Gipson DS, Massengill SF, Yao L, et al. Management of childhood onset nephrotic syndrome. *Pediatrics.* 2009;124(2):747–757.
7. Hodgkins KS, Langman CB. Clinical Grand Rounds: atypical hemolytic uremic syndrome. *Am J Nephrol.* 2012;35:394–400.
8. Eison TM, Ault BH, Jones DP, et al. Post-streptococcal acute glomerulonephritis in children: clinical features and pathogenesis. *Pediatr Nephrol.* 2011;26(2):165–180.
9. Kawasaki Y. The pathogenesis and treatment of pediatric Henoch-Schönlein purpura nephritis. *Clin Exp Nephrol.* 2011;15(5):648–657.
10. Manz F, Kalhoff H, Remer T. Renal acid excretion in early infancy. *Pediatr Nephrol.* 1997;11(2):231–243.
11. Kraut JA, Madias NE. Consequences and therapy of the metabolic acidosis of chronic kidney disease. *Pediatr Nephrol.* 2011;26(1):19–28.
12. Wilmer MJ, Emma F, Levtchenko EN, et al. The pathogenesis of cystinosis: mechanisms beyond cystine accumulation. *Am J Physiol Renal Physiol.* 2010;299(5):F905–916.
13. Wilmer MJ, Schoeber JP, van den Heuvel LP, et al. Cystinosis: practical tools for diagnosis and treatment. *Pediatr Nephrol.* 2011;26(2):205–215.
14. Nesterova G, Gahl W. Nephropathic cystinosis: late complications of a multisystemic disease. *Pediatr Nephrol.* 2008;23(6):863–878.
15. Seyberth HW, Schlingmann KP. Bartter- and Gitelman-like syndromes: salt-losing tubulopathies with loop or DCT defects. *Pediatr Nephrol.* 2011; 26(10):1789–1802.
16. Nimkarn S. Apparent mineralocorticoid excess - update. *Adv Exp Med Biol.* 2011;707:47–48.
17. Uchida S. Pathophysiological roles of WNK kinases in the kidney. *Pflugers Arch.* 2010;460(4):695–702.
18. Vehaskari VM. Heritable forms of hypertension. *Pediatr Nephrol.* 2009; 24(10):1929–1937.
19. Malloy PJ, Feldman D. Genetic disorders and defects in vitamin D action. *Endocrinol Metab Clin North Am.* 2010;39(2):333–346.
20. Shaw N. A practical approach to hypocalcaemia in children. *Endocr Dev.* 2009;16:73–92.
21. Lietman SA, Germain-Lee EL, Levine MA. Hypercalcemia in children and adolescents. *Curr Opin Pediatr.* 2010;22(4):508–515.
22. Hendy GN, Guarnieri V, Canaff L. Calcium-sensing receptor and associated diseases. *Prog Mol Biol Transl Sci.* 2009;89:31–95.
23. Gattineni J, Baum M. Regulation of phosphate transport by fibroblast growth factor 23 (FGF23): implications for disorders of phosphate metabolism. *Pediatr Nephrol.* 2010;25(4):591–601.
24. Bastepe M, Jüppner H. Inherited hypophosphatemic disorders in children and the evolving mechanisms of phosphate regulation. *Rev Endocr Metab Disord.* 2008;9(2):171–180.
25. Bergwitz C, Jüppner H. FGF23 and syndromes of abnormal renal phosphate handling. *Adv Exp Med Biol.* 2012;728:41–64.
26. San-Cristobal P, Dimke H, Hoenderop JG, et al. Novel molecular pathways in renal Mg2+ transport: a guided tour along the nephron. *Curr Opin Nephrol Hypertens.* 2010;19(5):456–462.
27. Mughal MZ. Rickets. *Curr Osteoporos Rep.* 2011;9(4):291–299.
28. Noda Y, Sohara E, Ohta E, et al. Aquaporins in kidney pathophysiology. *Nat Rev Nephrol.* 2010;6(3):168–178.
29. Bichet DG. V2R mutations and nephrogenic diabetes insipidus. *Prog Mol Biol Transl Sci.* 2009;89:15–29.
30. Loonen AJ, Knoers NV, van Os CH, et al. Aquaporin 2 mutations in nephrogenic diabetes insipidus. *Semin Nephrol.* 2008;28(3):252–265.
31. Babey M, Kopp P, Robertson GL. Familial forms of diabetes insipidus: clinical and molecular characteristics. *Nat Rev Endocrinol.* 2011;7(12):701–714.
32. Bockenhauer D, van't Hoff W, Dattani M, et al. Secondary nephrogenic diabetes insipidus as a complication of inherited renal diseases. *Nephron Physiol.* 2010;116(4):p23–29.
33. Askenazi D. Evaluation and management of critically ill children with acute kidney injury. *Curr Opin Pediatr.* 2011;23(2):201–207.
34. Twombley K, Baum M, Gattineni J. Accidental and iatrogenic causes of acute kidney injury. *Curr Opin Pediatr.* 2011;23(2):208–214.
35. Goldstein SL. Advances in pediatric renal replacement therapy for acute kidney injury. *Semin Dial.* 2011;24(2):187–191.
36. Feber J, Ahmed M. Hypertension in children: new trends and challenges. *Clin Sci (Lond).* 2010;119(4):151–161.
37. Meyers K, Falkner B. Hypertension in children and adolescents: an approach to management of complex hypertension in pediatric patients. *Curr Hypertens Rep.* 2009;11(5):315–322.
38. Langman CB. The molecular basis of kidney stones. *Curr Opin Pediatr.* 2004;16(2):188–193.
39. Bergsland KJ, Coe FL, White MD, et al. Urine risk factors in children with calcium kidney stones and their siblings. *Kidney Int.* 2012 [Epub ahead of print].
40. Bobrowski AE, Langman CB. The primary hyperoxalurias. *Semin Nephrol.* 2008;28(2):152–162.
41. Chillarón J, Font-Llitjós M, Fort J, et al. Pathophysiology and treatment of cystinuria. *Nat Rev Nephrol.* 2010;6(7):424–434.
42. Murphy C, Allen L, Jamieson MA. Ambiguous genitalia in the newborn: an overview and teaching tool. *J Pediatr Adolesc Gynecol.* 2011;24(5):236–250.
43. Cools M, Wolffenbuttel KP, Drop SL, et al. Gonadal development and tumor formation at the crossroads of male and female sex determination. *Sex Dev.* 2011;5(4):167–180.
44. Fallat ME, Donahoe PK. Intersex genetic anomalies with malignant potential. *Curr Opin Pediatr.* 2006;18(3):305–311.
45. Urinary Tract Infection: Clinical Practice Guideline for the Diagnosis and Management of the Initial UTI in Febrile Infants and Children 2 to 24 Months. Subcommittee on Urinary Tract Infection, Steering Committee on Quality Improvement and Management. *Pediatrics.* 2011;128(3):595–610.
46. Mattoo TK. Vesicoureteral reflux and reflux nephropathy. *Adv Chronic Kidney Dis.* 2011;18(5):348–354.
47. Wan J, Skoog SJ, Hulbert WC, et al. Section on urology response to new guidelines for the diagnosis and management of UTI. *Pediatrics.* 2012;129(4):e1051–1053.

CHAPTER

65 Renal Function and Disease in the Aging Kidney

Ramesh Saxena • Andrew Fenves • Xueqing Yu •
Nosratola D. Vaziri • Fred G. Silva • Xin J. Zhou

INTRODUCTION

The growth of an aging population in the world is on an explosive path and the cost of care for the elderly could overwhelm the budget of many countries in the next 40 years. The worldwide population of persons aged 65 years or more is estimated to be 420 million, or about 7% of the population, and is projected to increase to more than 1.5 billion by 2050.[1–4,2a,2b] In the United States, the percentage of people over 65 years of age has more than tripled since 1900 and continues to grow. The number of elderly has increased almost 15% (from 35 million to 40.5 million) from 2000 to 2009.[1] The growing number of older adults has drastically increased healthcare costs. In fact, healthcare cost per capita for persons over 65 years is three to five times greater than those under 65 years of age.[5]

Aging is a complex process driven by diverse molecular pathways and biochemical events culminating in profound anatomic and functional changes in the kidneys. Additionally, older individuals have diverse chronic diseases that can accelerate the age-related renal changes. In particular, the prevalence of chronic kidney disease (CKD) is greatest in the elderly and they have the fastest growth of end-stage renal disease (ESRD) at 11% for age 65 to 74 and 14% for age 75 and older.[6] This is a pressing problem that contributes substantially to disability, diminished quality of life, and enormous healthcare costs and begs for a massive effort to study the effect of aging on the kidney and the predisposing factors for nephropathy in the elderly population. This chapter provides an overview of the recent advances in the understanding of age-related changes in renal structure and function, the molecular pathways mediating these changes, and possible therapeutic interventions to mitigate age-related renal changes.

STRUCTURAL CHANGES OF THE AGING KIDNEY

Many studies have described the progressive structural and functional deterioration of kidneys with aging. Most of these studies are old and did not exclude patients with confounding comorbidities that might affect renal structures. Nevertheless, it appears that renal masses (i.e., weight of the kidney) progressively regress with advancing age.[7] The average kidney weight increases from ~50 g at birth to ~200 g during the fourth decade, after which it progressively declines (about 20% to 30%) by the ninth decade.[7,8] This loss of kidney mass is primarily cortical with relative sparing of the medulla, leading to thinning of the renal cortical parenchyma.[7,8] Although many morphologic changes are observed in the aging kidney, none is specific or pathognomonic.

The Aging Glomerulus

With aging, a number of morphologic changes emerge in the human glomerulus (Table 65.1). These include a decrease in the number of identifiable glomeruli and an escalation in the proportion of globally sclerotic glomeruli, which is associated with a progressive increase in the size of intact glomeruli (Fig. 65.1).

The number of glomeruli is extremely variable in individuals, ranging from 333,000 to 1,100,000 in each kidney and vary with age (inversely), gender (15% lower in females), and race (lower in Australian Aboriginals).[7–9] As renal cortical mass decreases with increasing age, the glomeruli decrease in number. There seems to be a direct correlation between the number/percentage of globally sclerotic glomeruli and increasing age and with intrarenal vascular disease, especially outer cortical vascular disease.[10] In general, globally sclerotic glomeruli comprise less than 10% of the total glomeruli under the age of 40 years and increase thereafter so that by the eighth decade as much as 30% of glomeruli may be globally sclerotic. However, the estimation of "normal" sclerosed glomeruli is difficult in the elderly due to confounding effects of comorbid conditions such as diabetes and hypertension. In such situations, "pathologic" glomerulosclerosis should be considered when the number of globally sclerosed glomeruli exceeds the number calculated by the formula: (patient's age/2) −10.[7,11,11a]

The pathogenesis of aging-associated global glomerulosclerosis is not completely understood and is likely multifactorial. Increasing oxidative stress that accompanies

TABLE 65.1 **Morphological Changes of the Aging Kidney**

Glomerulus
Increased number of globally sclerotic glomeruli; initially the glomeruli in the outer cortical regions
Progressive decline in the number of intact/normal glomeruli
Abnormal glomeruli with shunts between the afferent and efferent arterioles, especially those in the juxtamedullary region
Progressive decrease, and then later increase, in the size of intact glomeruli with higher filtration surface area
Tubulointerstitium
Decreased tubular volume, length, and number
Increased number of tubular diverticula, especially the distal convoluted tubules
Tubular atrophy, often with simplification of the tubular epithelium and thickening of the tubular basement membranes
Increased interstitial volume with interstitial fibrosis and, sometimes, inflammatory cells
Decreased peritubular capillary density
Vasculature
"Fibroelastic hyperplasia" of the arcuate and subarcuate arteries
Tortuous/spiraling interlobar arteries with thickening of the medial muscle cell basement membrane
Intimal fibroplasia of the interlobular arteries
"Hyaline" change/plasmatic insudation of the afferent arterioles
Vascular "simplification" with direct channels forming between the afferent and efferent arterioles

Modified from: Zhou XJ, Rakheja D, Silva FG. The aging kidney. In: Zhou XJ, Laszik Z, et al., eds. *Silva's Diagnostic Renal Pathology*. Cambridge, UK: Cambridge University Press; 2009.

aging can result in endothelial dysfunction and changes in vasoactive mediators resulting in atherosclerosis, hypertension, and glomerulosclerosis.[12] Furthermore, age-related changes in cardiovascular hemodynamics, such as reduced cardiac output and systemic hypertension, may contribute to glomerular changes.[13] Moreover, dysautoregulation of the afferent and efferent arterioles may increase glomerular plasma flow, glomerular capillary pressure, and "hyperfiltration," leading to mesangial matrix accumulation.[14] A morphometric study showed dilatation of the afferent arterioles, increased glomerular capillary lumens (especially hilar), and enlarged glomeruli, which suggested a discordance between the afferent and efferent arterioles.[15] The vascular adaptations to functional or structural nephron loss may help preserve glomerular filtration rate (GFR) by producing hyperperfusion and hyperfiltration in the surviving nephrons. This local glomerular hypertension and hypertrophy may lead to cytokine-mediated mesangial matrix expansion and, eventually, glomerulosclerosis. Such hyperperfusion-associated glomerular injury is seen with oligomeganephronia, diabetic nephropathy, morbid obesity, sickle cell anemia, and reflux nephropathy. It has been suggested that the vascular/ischemic changes seen in aging kidneys first cause cortical glomerulosclerosis and consequent juxtamedullary glomerular hypertrophy, followed by juxtamedullary glomerulosclerosis.[16]

The Aging Tubules and Interstitium

Several tubulointerstitial alterations parallel glomerular changes in the aging kidney. Three types of tubular atrophy can be seen in the aging kidney (Fig. 65.1). These include the *classic form* with wrinkling and thickening of the tubular basement membranes and simplification of the tubular epithelium; the *endocrine form* with simplified tubular epithelium, thin basement membranes, and numerous mitochondria in the tubular epithelial cells; and the *thyroidization form* with hyaline cast-filled dilated tubules.[17] Although there is an overlap, the endocrine form is classically seen with vascular ischemia, and the thyroidization form is considered to be characteristic but not pathognomonic of chronic pyelonephritis. With tubular atrophy, the distal renal tubules develop diverticula that increase in number with increasing age. These diverticula in distal and collecting tubules may be precursors of simple cysts that are increasingly observed in the aging kidney.[18] The diverticula may promote bacterial growth and contribute to the frequent renal infections in the elderly.

The Aging Renal Vasculature

Several changes in the renal vasculature have been documented in the aging human kidney, none of which are specific for aging (Fig. 65.1). Arterial sclerosis denotes thickening of the

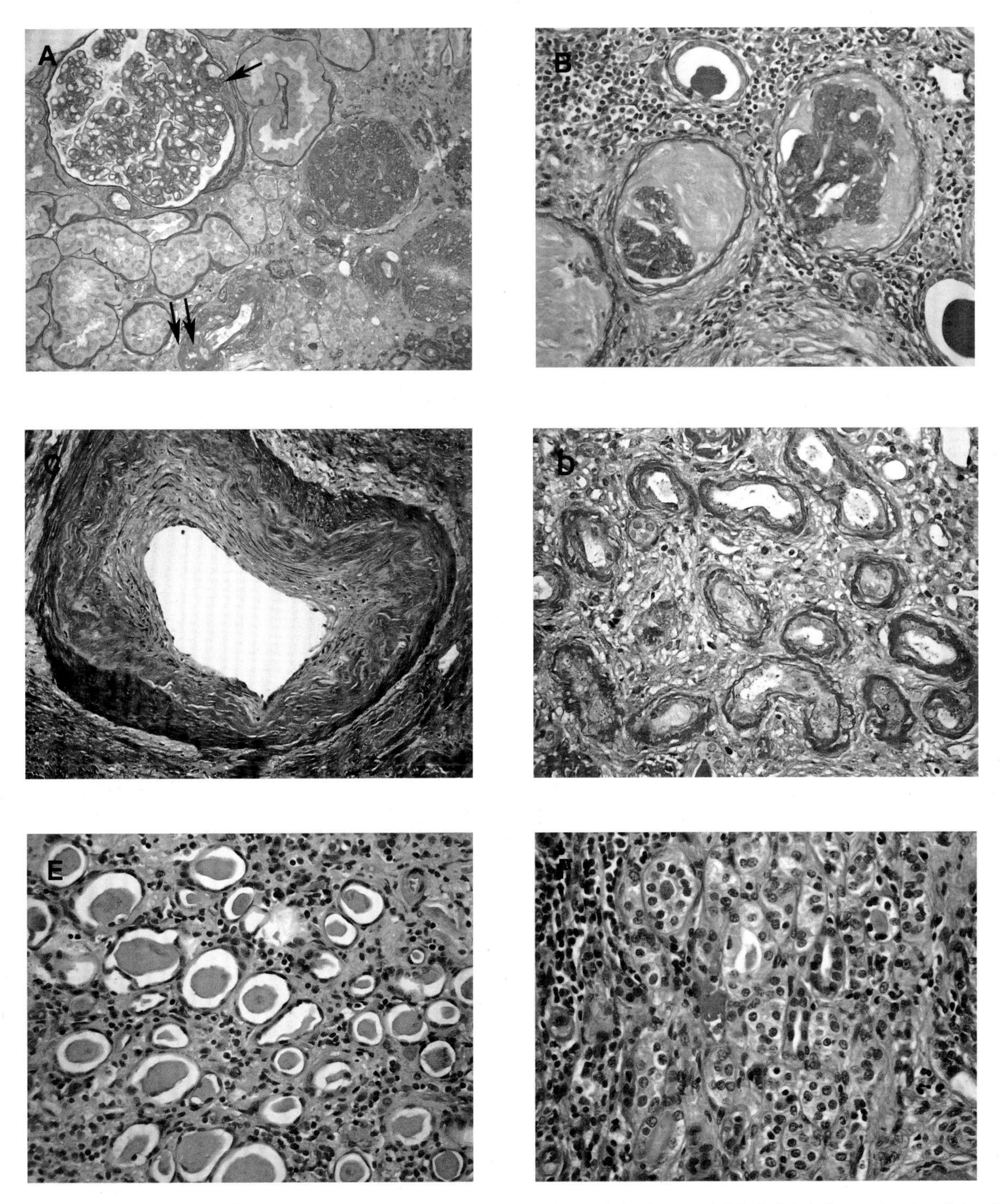

FIGURE 65.1 Morphological changes in the aging kidney. **A:** There are two glomeruli displaying solidified global glomerulosclerosis in which the sclerotic tufts fill the entirety of the Bowman space, often representing the sclerosis caused by focal segmental glomerulosclerosis. The nonsclerotic glomerulus shows ischemic changes with a segmental adhesion to the Bowman capsule (*arrow*). Significant tubular atrophy and interstitial fibrosis are also noted. A few arterioles demonstrate significant hyalinosis (*double arrows*, PAS, periodic acid-Schiff; × 200). **B:** The two glomeruli show ischemic obsolescence characterized by shrunken and globally wrinkled and thickened capillary tufts with the loss of most cells. The Bowman space is filled with collagenous material that stains less intensely than the capillary tuft (PAS; × 400). This type of global glomerulosclerosis is often secondary to ischemic vascular disease. **C:** An interlobular artery shows intimal fibrosis (arteriosclerosis) characterized by fibrous thickening and migration of medial muscle cells into the intima with an atrophic muscle layer (Trichrome; × 400). **D:** Classic type tubular atrophy: There is severe tubular atrophy with thickening and lamellation of the tubular basement membranes (PAS; × 400). **E:** A thyroidization type tubular atrophy: The atrophic tubules have a thin epithelium and contain homogeneous casts resembling thyroid tissue (H&E, hematoxylin and easin; × 400). **F:** An endocrine type tubular atrophy: The small tubules reveal cuboidal cells with pale-staining cytoplasma (containing abundant mitochondria) and virtually no lumens, reminiscent of endocrine glands (H&E; × 400). (See Color Plate.)

wall and narrowing of the arterial lumen produced by thickening of the medial smooth muscle layer, fibrosis of the media, and/or intimal thickening. These changes may be seen with hypertension, diabetes, and aging, with the prevalence of arterial sclerosis increasing with advancing age.[7,19,20] Intimal fibroplasia or collagenous fibrosis of the arterial intima may be associated with thinning of the media and is found uniformly in older kidneys with or without underlying cardiovascular disease. Intimal fibroplasia is seen primarily in arteries that are 80 to 300 μm in diameter, such as the interlobular arteries. The regional heterogeneity of intimal hyperplasia may account for the heterogeneity of ischemic nephrons. Although the etiology of aging-associated intimal fibroplasia is not entirely clear, it starts early in life and is accelerated by hypertension. Intimal hyperplasia in the interlobular arteries may allow the transmission of the pulse wave into the smaller distal branches leading to arteriolar hyaline changes, which may in turn accelerate the proximal intimal fibrosis. Global glomerulosclerosis appears to be associated with arterial intimal fibrosis rather than with arteriolar hyaline change.[21]

In aging kidneys, the thickening and folding/wrinkling of glomerular basement membrane (GBM) is accompanied by glomerular simplification and the formation of anastomoses between glomerular capillary loops. Frequently, afferent arteriole dilatation near the hilum is observed at this stage. The afferent arterioles commonly develop hyalinosis (accumulation of plasma proteins in the intima and/or media of small arteries and arterioles), a change that is less well correlated with systemic hypertension than with arterial intimal fibrosis in most, but not all studies. It may also be seen with diabetes mellitus; in fact, it is most severe and pronounced in patients with uncontrolled diabetes mellitus with or without hypertension.[17]

In the aging kidneys, the sclerosis and eventual loss of the glomerular tuft is often associated with a direct communication between afferent and efferent arterioles ("aglomerular arterioles"), particularly the juxtamedullary glomeruli.[19] These aglomerular arterioles are rarely seen in the kidneys of healthy adults but are observed with increased frequency both in aging and CKD kidneys.[19] The age-related vascular changes of intimal fibrosis and hyaline arteriolosclerosis are accentuated by hypertension, and probably diabetes mellitus as well. On the other hand, it has been suggested that aging-related interlobular arterial sclerosis may precede rather than follow systemic hypertension. Mean blood pressure rises by 1.6 mm Hg for each 1 μm increase in intimal thickness in a 100 μm diameter artery because of microischemia in scattered nephrons. This source of hypertension may account for the rise of blood pressure with age. The rate of decrease of renal plasma flow is accelerated by hypertension. Mean arterial blood pressure is directly proportional to the rate of decline of creatinine clearance. An increase in hypertension is a strong independent risk factor for ESRD, especially in African Americans. Thus, hypertension and morphologic vascular changes are not easily separable at this time.[20–22]

FUNCTIONAL CHANGES OF THE AGING KIDNEY

Aging is commonly associated with a decline in renal function. Unfortunately, most studies showing a diminished renal function with aging are confounded by comorbidities such as diabetes, hypertension, obesity, and smoking. It is therefore nearly impossible to separate the effect of physiologic (aging, per se) from pathologic (due to comorbidities) aging on renal function.[23] This section summarizes our current understandings of the effects of aging on renal function (Table 65.2).

Renal Hemodynamics

The morphologic changes of aging are accompanied by parallel changes in renal function and hemodynamics. Using various techniques, several studies conducted in elderly individuals without significant renal disease have demonstrated that renal blood flow (RBF) decreases with advancing age. In a review of 38 renal hemodynamic studies including 634 healthy subjects with wide age range, Wessen[24] described that total RBF was well maintained through approximately the fourth decade and progressively declined by approximately 10% per decade thereafter. In a study of 207 healthy kidney donors, Hollenberg et al.[25] demonstrated an explicit and progressive reduction in mean blood flow per

TABLE 65.2 Altered Glomerular, Tubular, and Vascular Functions in the Aging Kidney

Glomerulus
Decreased renal blood flow
Decreased glomerular filtration rate
Higher single-nephron ultrafiltration coefficient
Tubulointerstitium
Impaired urine concentrating and diluting ability
Impaired ability to maintain fluid and electrolyte balance
Reduced activity of the renin-angiotensin-aldosterone system (RAAS)
Reduced erythropoietin production
Reduced level/activation of 1,25 vitamin D
Increased renal calcium loss
Vasculature
Loss of compliance and increased stiffness of major arteries
Impaired angiogenesis
Impaired endothelial function

unit kidney mass with advancing age, suggesting that the decrease in RBF does not simply reflect the decline in the renal mass with aging. In addition, they demonstrated that the fall in renal perfusion with aging is most profound in the cortex, with relative sparing of flow to the medulla. This redistribution of blood flow from the cortex to the medulla may explain the slight increase in filtration fraction observed in the elderly population. Studies on the morphology and histology of the renal vasculature by postmortem angiograms and histologic sections demonstrate increased irregularity and tortuosity of the preglomerular vessels and tapering of afferent arterioles. However, no characteristic histologic lesion of aging has yet been identified in the renal vasculature.

The precise mechanisms of reduced RBF with aging are not yet known. Aging is associated with changes in vascular tone, which is determined by the balance between vasoconstrictors and vasodilators. In aging, there is an attenuated response to vasodilators such as nitric oxide (NO), endothelial-derived hyperpolarizing factor (EDHF), and prostacyclin, and an enhanced responsiveness to vasoconstrictors such as angiotensin II (Ang-II).[26] This may result in enhanced vasoconstrictive responses in aging, which can potentially cause renal damage and an ultimate fall in GFR. Although the renin-angiotensin system (RAS) is suppressed in aging, the intrarenal RAS may be relatively spared. In fact, the pharmacologic blockade of RAS has been shown to slow the progression of age-related CKD in experimental animals.[27] In addition to the suppression of RAS, there is significant decrease in NO production and availability that leads to renal vasoconstriction and sodium retention. Several potential mechanisms contribute to the reduction of NO with aging. Chief among them is oxidative stress that can reduce NO availability by the inactivation of NO; the inhibition of NO synthase (NOS) via the depletion of the NOS cofactor, tetrahydrobiopterin; the uncoupling of endothelial NOS; the accumulation of the endogenous NOS inhibitor, asymmetric dimethyl arginine; and by limiting uptake of NOS substrate, L-arginine, by endothelial cells via down-regulation of cationic amino acid transporter-1.[28]

There is also evidence that angiogenesis is attenuated in aging. In this context, vascular endothelial growth factor (VEGF) and angiopoietin-1 are altered both systemically and in the kidney with the aging process. Although levels of VEGF[29] have been shown to be reduced in the aging rat, a profound upregulation in protein levels of angiopoietin-1 in the kidney cortex has been observed in aged versus young rats.[30] Because angiopoietin-1 can stabilize blood vessels, its increase in aging may serve to counter the mechanisms leading to impaired angiogenesis and endothelial dysfunction. Taken together, these data indicate that strategies aimed at protecting the endothelium may help to mitigate the adverse renal effects of aging.

Recently, the role of arterial aging or arteriosclerosis in the pathogenesis of senescent changes in various organs, including the kidney, has become a major focus of interest. It has been observed that elastic arteries undergo two distinct physical changes, namely, dilation and stiffness with age.[31,32] This is due to fatigue and fracture of the medial elastin, mainly of the elastic arteries, with little aging change occurring in the distal muscular arteries.[33] Thus, dilation and stiffening are most marked in the proximal aorta and its major branches, namely, the brachiocephalic, carotid, and subclavian arteries. Increased arterial stiffening results in an increase in pulse wave velocity (PWV).[31,34] Aortic PWV is the speed with which pulse waves travel along the artery. A typical value is 5 m per second in a 20 year old and 12 m per second in an 80-year-old person, representing a 2.5-fold increase in 60 years.[31] The elastic properties of the aorta in the young serves to partially maintain blood volume and pressure during systole and then release them during diastole via the recoil process. This phenomenon helps to protect the vital organs by sustaining blood flow during diastole and blunting the damaging effects of high pressure waves during systole. In addition, the microcirculation, which comprises small arteries, arterioles, and the capillaries and constitutes the greatest resistance to blood flow, participates in transforming pulsatile flow to steady flow by reflecting the pulsations that enter from the larger arteries. With aortic stiffening and the consequent increase in aortic PWV, the transmission of flow pulsations downstream into various organs, principally the brain and kidney, can damage microvessels.[35,36] This mechanism may account for asymptomatic cerebral microvascular disease associated with microaneurysms and infarcts. The lesions comprise damage to the medial smooth muscle and the endothelium (which is not attributable to atherosclerosis), and in their chronic form are described as lipohyalinosis.[37] More recent studies have shown that amyloid plaques in older persons are probably a consequence of medial damage to small vessels and hemorrhage from damaged vessels.[38,39] It is thought that the neurofibrillary tangles of dementia may have a similar microvascular etiology.[40] Less data on pulsatile microvascular damage are available for the kidney, but one can expect this to emerge. The kidney afferent arterioles and glomeruli are exposed to the same high pulsatile microvascular stress and strain as in the brain. Recent studies have shown that independent of conventional brachial systolic and diastolic pressure values, measures of arterial stiffness are closely related to outcomes attributable to microvascular damage to vital organs, particularly the brain and the kidney.[35,36] Furthermore, measures of large artery stiffness are closely related to effects of microvascular changes in the kidney, including albuminuria.[35,36] Interventions aimed at reducing the ill effects of arterial stiffening by reducing the extent and frequency of the stretch cycles in order to minimize fatigue and fracture of the medial elastin of aorta can reverse or delay progression of cerebral and renal damage. These maneuvers entail a reduction in early wave reflection achieved through regular exercise, and the use of drugs such as angiotensin-converting enzyme inhibitors

(ACEI), angiotensin receptor blockers (ARB), calcium channel blockers, and nitrates, which relax smooth muscle in large and small conduit arteries throughout the body, thus resulting in arterial dilation.[37,41]

Glomerular Filtration Rate

GFR gradually increases after birth, approaching adult levels by the end of the second decade. It remains stable until the age of 30 to 40 years and then declines linearly at an average rate of about 8 mL per minute per decade, a phenomenon that can be partially explained by age-associated glomerulopenia.[7,8,42] However, about one-third of elderly individuals show no change in GFR.[43] This variability suggests that factors other than aging may be responsible for the apparent reduction in renal function. For instance, an increase in blood pressure, still within the normotensive range, is associated with an accelerated age-related loss of renal function.

The use of creatinine clearance in a timed urinary sample is commonly used as an estimate of GFR. Inulin and iothalamate clearance are very accurate measurements of GFR, but are clinically cumbersome to perform.[44] To obviate the need for a timed urine collection, various equations have been developed and are increasingly used to estimate GFR (Table 65.3). In adults, creatinine clearance is often estimated by the Cockcroft-Gault (CG) equation, and GFR is estimated by the Modification of Diet in Renal Disease (MDRD) formula.[45,46] It is important to point out that the CG equation estimates GFR in milliliters per minute, whereas the MDRD formula expresses GFR in milliliters per minute per 1.73 meters squared.

However, neither MDRD nor the CG equation was developed for elderly individuals, and reduced reliability would be expected when used in this population. In a study involving 100 individuals aged 65 to 111 years, GFR values calculated with the MDRD formula were much higher than those obtained with the CG equation. Moreover, no correlation was observed between these two predictions. Additionally, the difference in GFR values between MDRD and CG increased dramatically with aging and decreased with higher body mass index and serum creatinine values. Thus, the precision and accuracy of these formulas in estimating GFR in very old patients remain arguable.[47] Furthermore, a study in patients over 65 years old showed more than 60% discordance in GFR estimation by the two equations. The MDRD equation generally yielded higher estimates of GFR than the CG equation.[48] This has important implications, especially when calculating drug dosages in the elderly. It was recommended that the CG equation should be used in preference to the MDRD equation to estimate GFR for drug dosage calculations in the elderly. Recently, a new creatinine-based equation was developed by the Chronic Kidney Disease Epidemiology Collaboration (CKD-EPI). It reported a more accurate estimation of GFR than the MDRD equation, particularly at higher levels of estimated GFR (eGFR).[49] In a recent prospective observational study of 439 patients aged 65 and older admitted to 11 acute care medical

TABLE 65.3 **Formulas to Estimate Glomerular Filtration Rate**

Formula	Strengths	Weakness
1. Cockcroft-Gault	Simple	Estimates Ccr, not GFR Estimates lower value in older subjects Falsely elevated in chronic kidney disease Not validated for elderly population
2. MDRD	Simple with use of calculators Estimates GFR and not Ccr	Estimates higher GFR in the elderly Not validated for elderly population Not validated for higher levels of GFR Not validated to measure normal kidney function
3. CKD-EPI	Simple with use of calculators Estimates GFR and not Ccr More accurate estimates of high GFR Better estimation of GFR in elderly than 1& 2	May still overestimate GFR in the elderly
4. Cystatin C	Less dependent on muscle mass Better GFR estimate in elderly Better predictor of adverse outcomes in CKD	Not available readily Clinical role yet unclear

Ccr, creatinine clearance; GFR, glomerular filtration rate; MDRD, Modification of Diet in Renal Disease; CKD-EPI, Chronic Kidney Disease Epidemiology Collaboration.

wards in Italy, the relative risk of mortality in patients with eGFR = 30 to 59.9 or < 30 mL/min/1.73 m^2 was compared to subjects with eGFR ≥ 60 mL/min/1.73 m^2 using the body surface area–adjusted CG (CG-BSA), the MDRD, and the CKD-EPI formulas. Participants with reduced GFR showed an increased mortality regardless of the equation used, and CKD-EPI–derived GFR outperformed to some extent MDRD- and CG-BSA–derived GFR in a multivariable predictive model, suggesting its usefulness in the elderly population.[50] However, the performance of the serum creatinine–based estimating equations still remains insufficiently evaluated in older patients, in whom there may be a high prevalence of chronic disease associated with alterations in muscle mass and diet, resulting in an overestimation of the measured GFR and an underestimation of the severity of CKD. Lately, cystatin C has emerged as an alternative marker for the measurement of kidney function.[51] Cystatin C, a filtration marker that is less related to muscle mass than creatinine, may have a particular advantage in the estimation of GFR in the elderly population. However, the clinical role of cystatin C measurement remains unclear. In a recent study involving 11,909 patients, the risk of death, cardiovascular events, and kidney failure was compared in patients with GFR < 60 mL/min/1.73 m^2 (CKD) to those with GFR > 60 mL/min/1.73 m^2, as estimated by creatinine and cystatin C measurements. The survey showed that cystatin-based estimates were better predictors of adverse outcomes among adults with CKD, suggesting that cystatin C may be useful in identifying patients with CKD who have high risks of complications.[52]

Tubular Functions

Urine Concentrating Ability in the Aging Kidney

The urine concentrating phenomenon is a complex process that depends on many factors such as RBF, GFR, solute load, presence of vasopressin, functionality of vasopressin receptors, urea transporters, sodium transporters, and water channels (aquaporins), as well as the presence of an intact medullary countercurrent system. The Baltimore Longitudinal Study of Aging evaluated urine concentrating ability in healthy people aged between 20 to 79 years by assessing maximum urine osmolality, minimal urine flow rate over a period of 12 hours, and ability to concentrate solutes (or reabsorb sodium and urea). Compared to younger age groups, individuals aged 60 to 79 years had an approximately 20% reduction in maximal urine osmolality, a 100% increase in minimal urine flow rate, and a 50% decrease in the ability to conserve solutes.[53] These changes could not be explained by the reduction in GFR. A decrease in the abundance of aquaporin and urea transporter proteins, as observed with aging in the kidneys of animals, likely accounts for the reduced urinary concentrating capacity in the elderly. Interestingly, no significant differences in antidiuretic hormone (ADH) levels have been observed between the elderly and the younger cohorts, suggesting that the defect is likely due to ADH resistance as opposed to ADH deficiency.[54] Experimental studies suggest that an abundance of aquaporins-2 and -3 is reduced by 80% and 50%, respectively, in the aged rat's renal medullary collecting ducts.[55] Besides the decrease in aquaporin-2, there is impairment of its phosphorylation, which may interfere with trafficking and the insertion of aquaporin-2 in the apical membrane of the collecting duct. Together, these defects diminish urine concentrating ability by decreasing water reabsorption in the collecting ducts. In addition, aging results in decreased abundance of the major urea transporters (UT-A1 and A2) in the inner medullary collecting duct[55,56] and reduced NaCl transporter NKCC2/BSC1 in the thick ascending limb of loop of Henle.[57] These changes can reduce urine concentrating ability in the elderly by limiting urea and sodium reabsorption and, hence, inner medullary osmolality.

Although the reduction of water-conserving capacity in the elderly is mild and does not have significant clinical implications under normal conditions of water abundance, it becomes important when access to water is limited; for instance, in cases of inability to grasp fluid or communicate thirst as in stroke patients or in cases of nursing home neglect. Under such conditions, old patients might develop serious hypernatremia that may impair central nervous system function or prove fatal. Prompt treatment with intravenous hypotonic solutions may prove lifesaving in these situations.

Renal Diluting Ability

Although much less data are available on renal diluting capacity, existing studies suggest a mild impairment of renal diluting ability in the elderly. Clearance studies in water-loaded old rats have demonstrated free water formation at each level of the distal diluting segment, indirectly suggesting that the function of the limb of the Henle loop is not impaired.[58] The mild renal diluting defect seems to be a result of the reduced GFR. The increase in solute load in the remaining functioning nephrons combined with a decrease in NaCl reabsorption increases solute delivery to the collecting duct and decreases free water excretion. There is no evidence for impaired function of the diluting segment or altered suppressibility of vasopressin in the pathogenesis of this disorder.

Reduced renal diluting capacity renders the older subjects more susceptible to the development of dilutional hyponatremia in the setting of excess water load, stress situations such as surgery, fever, acute illness, or administration of drugs such as diuretics, or those that enhance vasopressin production and action. These events may act alone or in concert to impair renal diluting ability and render the elderly patients susceptible to water intoxication. In fact, hyponatremia is the most common electrolyte abnormality in hospitalized geriatric patients.[59] Hyponatremia usually develops insidiously and presents with nonspecific clinical findings including confusion, lethargy, anorexia, nausea, weakness, and seizures. Like hypernatremia, hyponatremia may impair central nervous system function or may prove fatal. In such situations, prompt treatment with free water restriction alone or with the concurrent administration of hypertonic solutions or vasopressin V2-receptor antagonists is warranted.[60,61]

Fluid and Electrolyte Balance

Ordinarily, age has no effect on basal plasma electrolyte concentrations or the ability to maintain normal extracellular fluid volume. However, structural changes in the elderly kidney have an impact on the adaptive mechanisms responsible for maintaining homeostasis of extracellular fluid volume and composition. Consequently, acute illnesses in geriatric patients are often complicated by the development of fluid and electrolyte abnormalities, which are associated with increased morbidity and mortality and prolonged hospitalization. In the elderly, the capacity to conserve sodium in response to reduced sodium intake is impaired.[62] The exact mechanism is not known, but a reduction in the number of functioning nephrons with increased sodium load per each remaining nephron as well as reduced aldosterone secretion in response to sodium depletion are plausible. Nevertheless, the inability to conserve sodium may predispose the elderly patient to hemodynamic instability in the setting of sodium loss. This, along with other structural and functional changes, make older patients more prone to develop acute kidney injury.[63]

In addition to the impairment in sodium conservation, the elderly are also prone to volume expansion when challenged with a sodium load. This is due to a diminished capacity of renal sodium excretion in the elderly.[64] Additionally, the elderly seem to have more sodium excretion at night compared to the daytime, suggesting an impaired circadian variation.[65] Impaired pressure natriuresis and altered response to Ang-II are apparent mechanisms involved.[66] Notwithstanding the mechanisms, geriatric patients may develop an expanded extracellular fluid volume in the setting of a sodium load. It will usually lead to modest weight gain and the appearance of mild peripheral edema in the absence of significant comorbidities. However, the geriatric patients with preexisting cardiac or renal disease may develop life-threatening pulmonary edema, necessitating aggressive emergency therapy with loop diuretics or dialysis.[66] Elderly subjects also show abnormalities in renal potassium and calcium handling, which are discussed in the ensuing section.

Endocrine and Metabolic Function

Renin-Angiotensin-Aldosterone System

Age-related changes in the RAS in healthy humans are well documented.[67] In elderly subjects at baseline, plasma renin activity is 40% to 60% lower than those of a young adult population.[68] This difference becomes even more pronounced under conditions that stimulate renin release because of the blunted renal response in the elderly.[69] This decrease may act to lower baseline intrarenal Ang-II levels, an adaptation that may contribute to the changes of intrarenal vascular tone and tubular function in the aging kidney.

The lower renin levels in the elderly results in 30% to 50% reductions in plasma aldosterone levels.[70] The age-related decrease in renin and aldosterone levels contributes to the development of various fluid and electrolyte abnormalities. For instance, elderly persons on salt restricted diets have a decreased ability to conserve sodium.[62] Decreased Ang-II production has been reported to impair urinary concentrating ability. Together, these conditions contribute to increased susceptibility of elderly persons to develop volume depletion and hypernatremia.[63] The loss of thirst in response to dehydration further contributes to hypernatremia in the elderly. Age-related decrease in renin and aldosterone also contributes to an increased risk of hyperkalemia in various clinical settings and is reflected by a reduced transtubular potassium gradient in the elderly population.[71]

Through action on distal tubules, aldosterone increases sodium reabsorption and facilitates potassium excretion, thereby protecting against hyperkalemia after a potassium load.[67] A decrease in the production of renin-angiotensin-aldosterone and reduced GFR impair the ability of the elderly to handle large potassium loads. Potassium levels can be seriously elevated after a potassium-loading event such as gastrointestinal bleeding, transfusion reaction, or the administration of oral or intravenous potassium. The tendency toward hyperkalemia can be further enhanced by certain inorganic metabolic acidosis or by the administration of medications that inhibit potassium excretion (such as potassium sparing diuretics, ACEI, ARB, nonsteroidal anti-inflammatory agents, direct renin inhibitors, or beta blockers). Given their higher susceptibility to hyperkalemia, caution should be exercised in prescribing such medications to the elderly.

Although the circulating RAS is suppressed in aging, the intrarenal RAS may be relatively intact. Ang-II has several hemodynamic and nonhemodynamic effects on the kidney, affecting not only filtration pressure and proximal tubular sodium and water transport but also tubular and glomerular cell growth, NO synthesis, immunomodulation, growth factor induction, production of reactive oxygen species (ROS), inflammation, cell migration, apoptosis, as well as extracellular matrix protein accumulation, which can work in concert to accelerate age-related glomerulosclerosis and tubulointerstitial fibrosis.[72,73] Preferential Ang-II–dependent efferent arteriolar vasoconstriction of older nephrons maintains adequate filtration pressure. However, this may also promote intraglomerular hypertension and glomerulosclerosis.[74] Furthermore, Ang-II activates proinflammatory and profibrotic pathways, including transforming growth factor (TGF-β), collagen IV transcription, monocyte-macrophage influx, mRNA, and protein expression of chemokine regulated upon activation, normal T-cell expressed, and secreted (RANTES) promoting fibrosis, as well as stimulating endothelial plasminogen activator inhibitor-1(PAI-1) to increase matrix accumulation.[75,76] Interestingly, physiologic intrarenal downregulation of both renin mRNA and ACE in the elderly may be protective toward long-term sclerosis, and the processes that increase Ang-II response with age can hasten kidney aging.[77]

Use of ACEI in aging animals has been shown to decrease glomerular and vascular sclerosis as well as tubulointerstitial fibrosis associated with a reduction in α smooth muscle cell actin.[75,78] Angiotensin antagonists (ACEI and ARB) may protect age-related renal sclerosis by additional mechanisms such as the prevention of age-associated oxidative stress, advanced glycation end products (AGEs) accumulation, and downregulation of endothelial nitric oxide synthase (eNOS), and Klotho.[79,80]

Erythropoietin

The prevalence of anemia increases with age. Although there are many causes of anemia in the elderly, normocytic normochromic anemia may be related to reduced erythropoietin (EPO) production by the kidney.[81] The InCHIANTI study showed an association between advancing age, declining renal function, reduced EPO production, and anemia. After adjusting for confounding variables, the subjects with a creatinine clearance of 30 mL per minute or lower had a higher prevalence of anemia and lower plasma EPO levels compared with those with a creatinine clearance higher than 90 mL per minute. Additionally, a trend toward an increase in the prevalence of anemia with decreasing renal function was observed in subjects with creatinine clearance > 30 mL per minute.[82] Serum EPO levels rise with age in healthy subjects, perhaps a compensation for aging-related subclinical blood loss, increased red blood cell turnover, or increased erythropoietin resistance of red cell precursors.[83] On the other hand, the serum EPO levels are unexpectedly lower in the elderly with anemia compared to young subjects with anemia, suggesting a blunted response to low hemoglobin.[84]

Erythropoiesis-stimulating agents (ESAs) are often used for the treatment of anemia in patients with CKD. However, several recent studies on the treatment of anemia with ESA, including CHOIR (correction of hemoglobin and outcomes in renal insufficiency), CREATE (the cardiovascular risk reduction by early anemia treatment with epoetin beta), and TREAT (trial to reduce cardiovascular events with Aranesp therapy), have caused concerns about the safety of ESA in CKD, including the elderly.[85–87] The major findings of these studies reveal an increased risk of adverse cardiovascular outcomes with a more aggressive treatment of anemia with ESA. The adverse effects observed in trials of anemia correction are primarily due to the nonerythropoietic actions of ESA given at high doses to overcome erythropoietin-resistant anemia.[88,89] Thus, caution should be exercised in using ESA to treat anemia in the elderly, and a rise in hemoglobin of greater than 12 g per deciliter should be avoided.

Calcium and Vitamin D

A creatinine clearance less than 65 mL per minute is reported to be an independent risk factor for falls and associated fractures in the elderly with osteoporosis.[90] In a recent study, elderly women with osteoporosis and a decreased creatinine clearance (< 60 mL per minute) had lower calcium absorption, lower serum 1,25-dihydroxyvitamin D, and normal serum 25-hydroxyvitamin D, suggesting a reduced conversion of 25-hydroxyvitamin D to 1,25-dihydroxyvitamin D by the aging kidney. Furthermore, calcitriol therapy reduced the number of falls by 50%, which was postulated to be related to an increase in serum 1,25-dihydroxyvitamin D, upregulation of vitamin D receptors (VDR) in muscle, and improvement in muscle strength.[91] Levels of 1,25 dihydroxyvitamin D3 and its receptor, VDR, which are highly expressed in the kidney, decrease with age. Evidence suggests that vitamin D3 and its analogs suppress renin, and the absence of the VDR gene results in a predisposition for high renin hypertension, cardiac hypertrophy, and thromobogencity.[92] Recent studies also demonstrate that VDR stimulation can decrease renal fibrosis.[93] Vitamin D and its analogs can also attenuate glomerulosclerosis and tubulointerstitial fibrosis mediated by proinflammatory, profibrotic, and oxidant stress via the suppression of nuclear factor kappaB (NF-κB).[94] Vitamin D deficiency in those with CKD appears to be an independent predictor of renal disease progression.[95] Results of ongoing clinical trials will help clarify the clinical benefit of vitamin D in renoprotection.[96]

In addition to reduced levels and an impaired activation of vitamin D, elderly individuals demonstrate increased renal calcium loss due to reduced calcium reabsorption in the distal convoluted and connecting tubules.[97] Distal calcium reabsorption is facilitated by the transient receptor potential ion channel, transient receptor potential cation channel subfamily V member 5 (TRPV5), in the tubular apical membrane.[98] TRPV5 gene expression is regulated by 1,25-dihydroxyvitamin D and parathyroid hormone (PTH).[99] Recently, the antiaging hormone, Klotho, has been shown to play a role in the regulation of distal calcium reabsorption by deglycosylating N-glycans on the surface of TRPV5.[100] Klotho deficiency is associated with a phenotype resembling aging in experimental animals.[101] Thus, impaired Klotho activity in the elderly may well be responsible for reduced calcium reabsorption via TRPV5.

MOLECULAR EVENTS IN AGING KIDNEYS

Over the last decade, significant advances have been made in identifying the molecular mechanisms associated with renal senescence. The key mechanisms are discussed in this section (Fig. 65.2).

Telomeres

Telomeres are the nucleoprotein structures constituting the physical ends of linear chromosomes. They prevent chromosomal ends from being recognized as double-strand breaks and protect them from end-to-end fusion and degradation.[102] Telomeres in somatic cells shorten with each cell division and this progressive attrition leads to critically short telomeres and cellular senescence, a state characterized by the absence of replication and biochemical changes.[102] This phenomenon was observed in earlier in vitro studies showing that cultured fibroblasts could only undergo a limited number of population doublings, the so-called Hayflick limit.[103] It is

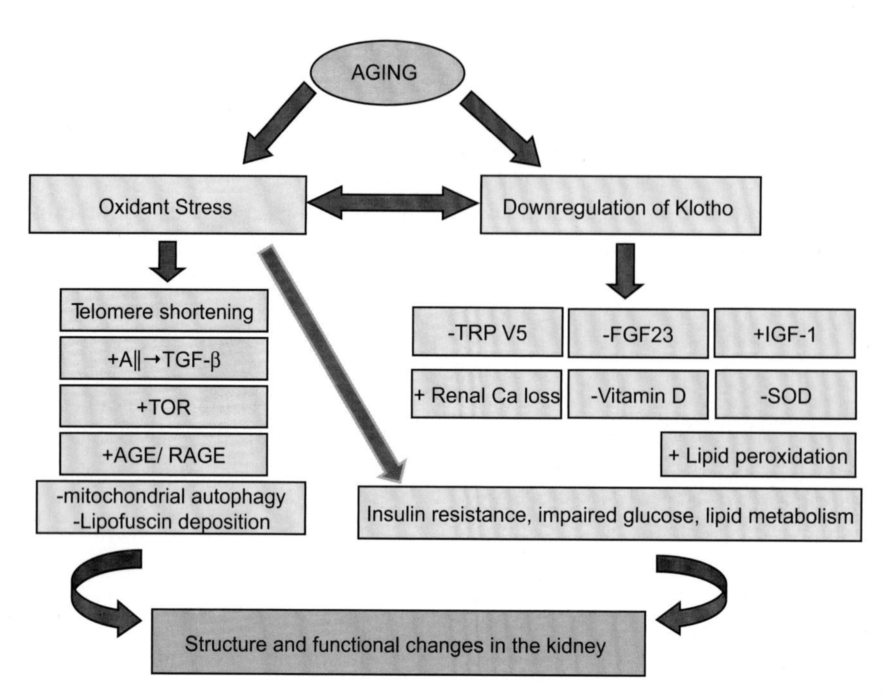

FIGURE 65.2 The pathogenesis of renal aging. As detailed in the chapter, the aging process is associated with oxidant stress and downregulation of the Klotho gene. The downregulation of Klotho begets several downstream events such as the inhibition of FGF23, TRPV5, and impaired vitamin D activation, leading to increased urinary calcium loss. Furthermore, the downregulation of Klotho increases susceptibility to oxidant stress via the stimulation of the IGF-1 pathway and the inhibition of SOD. Increased oxidant stress, in turn, causes the downregulation of the Klotho gene. In addition, oxidative stress leads to the activation of the angiotensin II (Ang-II) pathway, enhancement of AGE formation, shortening of telomeres by the inhibition of telomerase, as well as the accumulation of malignant mitochondria in cells due to the activation of TOR. All these pathways ultimately lead to increased lipid peroxidation, insulin resistance, as well as impaired glucose and lipid metabolism. Final results of the cascade of these intertwined pathways are the age-related structural and functional changes in various organs. In kidneys, there is a progressive regression of renal mass associated with glomerulosclerosis, tubular atrophy, interstitial fibrosis, arterial sclerosis, and hyalinosis. These structural changes are associated with a progressive decline in GFR, myriad tubular abnormalities, and a reduction in renal blood flow. *AGE,* advanced glycation end product; *RAGE,* receptor for advanced glycation end product; *FGF23,* fibroblast growth factor 23; *GFR,* glomerular filtration rate; *IGF-1,* insulin-like growth factor 1; *SOD,* superoxide dismutase; *TOR,* target for rapamycin; *TRPV5,* transient receptor potential ion channel. Modified from Zhou XJ, Saxena R, Liu Z, et al. Renal senescence in 2008: progress and challenges. *Int Urol Nephrol.* 2008;40:823–839.

believed that telomeres act as a mitotic clock, initiating replicative senescence when telomeres become critically short after a certain number of cell divisions. Melk et al.[104] have demonstrated that telomere shortening progresses with advancing age in the human kidney, and this phenomenon is more important in the cortical than the medullary area.[104]

The enzyme telomerase is required for the maintenance of the length and stability of telomeres. An overexpression of telomerase induces an artificial lengthening of the telomeres and markedly increases the proliferative potential of cells. The antiproliferative effect of aging appears to be governed by two signaling pathways activated by the cellular replication clock: one involves p53, which induces p21 overexpression, and the other stimulates the expression of the cell cycle inhibitor, p16. In vitro studies have shown that senescent cells express p16 and p21, which inhibit cellular proliferation by inhibiting cyclin-dependent kinases.[105] In vivo studies have demonstrated low levels of p16 in kidneys from young individuals. There is an overall increase in $p16^{INK4a}$ expression with age, particularly in the renal cortex, although this expression varies from individual to individual.[106] Furthermore, in age-related histologic changes, a strong correlation is found between glomerulosclerosis, interstitial fibrosis, tubular atrophy, and $p16^{INK4a}$ and p53 expression.[107] In a recent study, Westoff showed that telomerase-deficient mice were more vulnerable to ischemic–reperfusion injury due to reduced tubular regeneration.[108]

The pharmacologic activation of telomerase could be an appropriate therapy for aging diseases associated with replicative senescence. On the other hand, telomerase inhibitors have been proposed as a new option for chemotherapy, illustrating the trade-off between accelerated biologic aging and increased cancer risk.[102,109]

The Klotho Gene

The discovery of antiaging gene Klotho has extensively enhanced the understanding of the genetic bases of senescence. Klotho-deficient mice exhibited a syndrome resembling a premature aging phenotype with soft tissue and vascular calcification, hyperphosphatemia, muscle and skin atrophy, and early death. In contrast, overexpression of the Klotho gene extended the life span in the mouse.[110] In addition, several single-nucleotide polymorphisms in the human Klotho gene are associated with a shortened life span, osteoporosis, stroke, and coronary artery diseases, suggesting that Klotho may be involved in the regulation of human aging and age-related diseases.[111]

The Klotho gene encodes a single-pass transmembrane protein with two homologous extracellular domains, each having a weak homology to the β-glucosidase of bacteria and plants.[112] Although the Klotho gene is expressed in limited tissues, notably the kidney, the parathyroid, and the brain, a defect in Klotho gene expression leads to multiple aging-like phenotypes involving almost all organ systems. This effect of the Klotho protein is mediated by its hormonal action via its binding to a cell-surface receptor and repressing the intracellular signals of insulin and insulinlike growth factor 1 (IGF-1). It appears that the antiaging effect of the Klotho-induced inhibition of insulin/IGF-1 signaling is associated with increased resistance to oxidative stress.[113] It has been shown that the Klotho protein induces the expression of manganese superoxide dismutase, a mitochondrial antioxidant enzyme that facilitates the removal of superoxide, thereby conferring protection against oxidative stress.[114] On the other hand, hydrogen peroxide–induced oxidative stress has been shown to reduce Klotho expression in a mouse inner medullary collecting duct (mIMCD3) cell line.[115] Interestingly, the beneficial effects of peroxisome proliferator activated receptor-gamma (PPAR-γ) agonists on age-related glomerulosclerosis are mediated by intrarenal Klotho expression.[116]

Klotho also plays a central role in calcium and phosphorus homeostasis and the inhibition of active vitamin D synthesis.[117] Ang-II has been shown to downregulate Klotho expression, which may, in part, contribute to Ang-II–induced renal damage.[117] Klotho polymorphisms are associated with osteopenia in postmenopausal women. Klotho-deficient mice develop calcification of small arteries in the kidney and show increased serum levels of 1,25-dihydroxyvitamin D, which, along with increased calcium phosphate product, may be responsible for severe vascular and soft tissue calcification.[117] Interestingly, the abnormalities in bone and phosphate metabolism observed in Klotho-deficient mice are very similar to those observed in fibroblast growth factor (FGF)-23 knockout mice suggesting that Klotho and FGF23 function in a common signal transduction pathway.[118] Further studies indicate that Klotho acts as a cofactor by binding to FGF receptors and is essential for the signaling of FGF23 and related FGFs.[119] Studies have shown that FGFs play important roles, not only in mitosis and development but also in various metabolic processes including the regulation of insulin sensitivity, glucose/lipid/energy metabolism, and oxidative stress, all of which potentially affect the aging processes.[120,121] Klotho may regulate aging processes, partly through controlling the FGF-signaling pathways. The presence of any abnormality in either Klotho or FGF23 leads not only to phosphate retention but to premature aging in mice.[122] A recent study by Hu et al.[123] suggests that Klotho deficiency may have a direct effect on the rat vascular smooth muscle cell (VSMC) and promote VSMC calcification independent of FGF23 signaling.[123]

Klotho protein also regulates ion channel activity in renal tubular cells. Recently, Klotho was shown to activate transient receptor potential ion channel (TRPV)5, an epithelial calcium channel expressed on the apical membrane of the distal convoluted tubules and the connecting tubular cells.[100] TRPV5 functions as an entry gate for transcellular calcium reabsorption in these cells and participates in renal calcium reabsorption, thus countering the effects of low phosphate on bone.[124] Additionally, Klotho decreases cell surface abundance of the TRPC6 channel, the upregulation of which is associated with glomerulosclerosis.[125]

It has been shown that renal Klotho mRNA is downregulated under sustained circulatory or metabolic stress and in chronic kidney disease.[121] Mitani et al.[126] have demonstrated that Ang-II, which may be involved in age-related organ damage, plays a pivotal role in reducing renal Klotho gene expression in experimental animals. Conversely, induction of the Klotho gene by an adenovirus vector might protect against Ang-II–induced renal damage, such as tubulointerstitial injury and vascular wall thickening.[126] The Ang-II–induced downregulation of the Klotho gene expression may be mediated by promoting intrarenal iron deposition and ROS production.[120] In fact, treatment with a free radical scavenger and an iron chelator attenuated Ang-II–induced renal injury. Further investigations are required into other mechanisms involved in the regulation of the Klotho gene expression and senescence.

Oxidative Stress

Cumulative oxidative injury is believed to play a major role in the cellular aging process. Oxidative stress and the generation of free radicals increase with aging.[127] Persistent oxidative damage to cytosolic structures leads to the cross-linking of oxidized proteins, the deposition of lipofuscin, and impaired mitochondrial function and structure.[128] Lipofuscin (cross-linked proteins), which is insoluble and not degradable by either lysosomal enzymes or the proteasomal system, and giant mitochondria are taken up by lysosomes, wherein they bind additional material and eventually cause lysosomal rupture. The released lipofuscin and lysosomal contents cause cell damage and dysfunction.[128] In rats of different ages (2, 11, and 29.5 months) there was up to a 28-fold increase in lipofuscin deposition in kidneys and other organs in older compared to the 2-month-old animals.[129] Furthermore, increased oxidant stress (elevated serum lipoperoxides) and a reduced antioxidant activity (erythrocyte superoxide dismutase and glutathione peroxidase) were observed in the elderly in a cross-sectional study involving 249 healthy subjects.[127] The magnitude of oxidative stress and lipid peroxidation in the aging kidney correlates with an elevation of the advanced glycosylation end products and their receptors (AGE and RAGE) that can cross-link adjacent proteins. This, along with the ROS that can activate ubiquitin-proteasome, may degrade hypoxia-inducible factor-1alpha (HIF-1α) and limit the capacity of the aging cells to form HIF-1–DNA hypoxia-responsive recognition element (HRE) complexes (HIF-1-HRE complexes).[130,131] In the kidney, the subsequent decrease in the ability of the cells to respond to hypoxia could explain the attenuated anemia-induced secretion of erythropoietin as well as the decreased hypoxia-induced production of vascular endothelial growth factor leading, respectively, to reduced erythropoiesis and angiogenesis.[130] In a rat model, renal aging was associated with a 60% decline in GFR, a threefold increase in renal F2 isoprostanes (a marker of oxidative stress), an increase in oxidant-sensitive heme oxygenase, as well as increased AGEs and RAGE. Furthermore, a diet rich in vitamin E attenuated the age-related upregulation of heme oxygenase and RAGE, suppressed the production of F2 isoprostanes, lessened measured markers of oxidative stress, reduced glomerulosclerosis, and improved renal plasma flow and GFR by 50%.[132] In cultured rabbit proximal tubular epithelial cells, AGEs and even the early glycosylation end products (Amadori products) directly inhibited NOS activity and AGEs quenched the released NO.[133] Immunohistochemical studies of the aging rat kidneys have revealed a reduction of endothelial NOS (eNOS) in the peritubular capillaries and the presence of eNOS immunoreactivity in renal tubular epithelial cells, infiltrating mononuclear cells and foci of tubulointerstitial injury, suggesting that the aging-related renal tubulointerstitial fibrosis may be secondary to the ischemia caused by peritubular capillary injury and impaired eNOS expression.[134] Via activation of the angiotensin receptor AT1, the tissue RAS may promote the production of ROS and TGF-β1, events that can promote fibrosis. Indeed, the administration of ACEI and ARB in rats ameliorated the aging-related renal damage and attenuated glomerular sclerosis, mesangial expansion, tubular atrophy, interstitial fibrosis, and mononuclear cell infiltration.[135] The salutary effect of RAS blockade may be, in part, mediated by the ability to limit the impact of aging on the structure and function of mitochondria and other cellular organelles involved in energy metabolism and ROS production.[136]

In addition to the mechanisms described previously, recent data suggest that chronic oxidant stress contributes to the telomere shortening and thus senescent changes.[106] Furthermore, by downregulating Klotho gene expression, chronic oxidant stress can mediate the aging-associated changes.[137] Oxidative stress also activates the target of rapamycin (TOR) pathway, which plays an important role in the aging process by inhibiting mitochondrial autophagy (see the following).[138] Thus, interventions aimed at reducing ROS production, enhancing antioxidant capacity, increasing NO availability, and suppressing fibrogenic pathways may be effective in retarding aging-related renal damage.[139] In addition, calorie restriction via mechanisms described elsewhere in this chapter can decrease age-related oxidant stress, mitochondrial lipid peroxidation, and membrane damage.[140] Thus, dietary caloric restriction may be another approach to reduce age related renal damage.

Mitochondria and Autophagy

Mutations in mitochondrial DNA (mtDNA) accrue in various tissues of aging mammals. These mtDNA mutations may provide selective advantage among fast replicating mitochondrial variants, even if they are deleterious to the cell in which they reside. This leads to an accumulation of predominantly large defective mitochondria that resist autophagy, a process that plays an important role in the degradation of excess, defective, or injured mitochondria. It has been shown that autophagy influences susceptibility to glomerular disease in aging mice and in humans. Glomerular diseases are associated with a decreased expression of proteins involved in autophagy.[141] The inhibition of autophagy, as happens with aging, might create a permissive environment for the accumulation of giant, nonactive, malignant mitochondria in various organs. This permissive intracellular environment is TOR dependent. TOR inhibits autophagy, thus potentially allowing malignant mitochondria to accumulate and clonally expand. The inhibition of TOR by agents such as rapamycin or metformin may reverse the accumulation of defective mitochondria, and simultaneously retard the aging process.[142]

MicroRNAs

Lately, the role of microRNAs (miRNAs) in regulating various cellular processes, including aging, has evoked considerable interest. The miRNAs were first described 16 years ago in *Caenorhabditis elegans* as a 22 nucleotide RNA transcript (miRNA) of lin-4 with antisense RNA–RNA interaction. This miRNA/target relationship was later proven to determine the nematode's life span.[143] This initial discovery of miRNA was followed by an explosion in identifying not only new miRNAs in *C. elegans*, but also in a wide variety of species, including humans.[144] miRNAs are a major category among the noncoding small RNA fraction that negatively regulate gene expression at the posttranscriptional level. They have an ability to degrade the target gene or repress its expression without completely silencing it. Mature miRNAs are formed by cleaving off one arm of a stem-loop precursor miRNA (pre-miRNA), by the cytoplasmic RNaseIII, Dicer. Functionally, mature miRNAs are complexed together with catalytic protein, argonaute (Ago), forming RNA-induced silencing complexes (RISC).[145] RISC binds to the target complementary messenger RNA site, either perfectly for mRNA degradation, or imperfectly to inhibit translation, thereby achieving the posttranscriptional suppression of gene expression in either scenario.[145,146] miRNAs are now believed to play a pivotal role in various cellular processes such as cell proliferation, differentiation, and apoptosis through upregulation of specific groups of miRNAs to suppress unwanted gene expressions, or by downregulation of other miRNAs whose target genes' expression is necessary for cellular function. The equilibrium between these two groups of miRNA expressions largely determines the function of particular cell types. Recent data suggest that during aging, there is a trend of upregulation of unwanted miRNA expressions, which in turn downregulate their target gene products, such as proteins mediating the insulin/IGF1 and TOR signaling in *C. elegans*, both of which play a crucial role in the aging process.[147] Understanding age-dependent changes of miRNA expression and their target genes may open new vistas to understanding the mechanism of the aging process and may help identify new therapeutic targets to delay aging and extend healthy life spans.

Lipids

There is increasing evidence from animal and human studies suggesting that lipids play an important role in the pathogenesis and progression of renal disease.[148–151] Various changes in lipid metabolism have been recognized in aging subjects. These changes are associated with alterations in the expression and activities of several transcription factors and nuclear receptors. There are age-related increases in the sterol regulatory element binding proteins (SREBPs), SREBP-1 and SREBP-2, which are master regulators of fatty acid, triglyceride, and cholesterol metabolism.[152,153] In addition, there is an increase in the carbohydrate response element binding protein (ChREBP), which plays an important role in lipid metabolism.[152] A decrease in the peroxisome proliferator activated receptor-α (PPAR-α) activity, which is a major regulator of fatty acid oxidation, further augments the age-related alterations in lipid metabolism.[154] Interestingly, these changes are associated with an age-related decrease in the activity of the bile acid activated nuclear hormone receptor called farnesoid X receptor (FXR).[155] Activation of FXR has been demonstrated to reduce renal SREBP expression and renal lipid accumulation and to prevent renal disease in animal models of type 2 diabetes and diet-induced obesity and insulin resistance.[156] Whether pharmacologic activation of FXR will have beneficial effects in age-related renal disease needs further exploration.

Advanced Glycosylation End Products

With advancing age, renal and vascular accumulation of cross-linked glycosylated proteins, lipids, and nucleic acid is observed. It results in mesangial expansion, basement membrane thickening, and increased vascular permeability.[157] AGEs stimulate platelet-derived growth factor and TGF-β, leading to sclerosis of the tubulointerstitium and glomeruli.[157] A greater incidence of insulin resistance, hyperglycemia, and oxidative stress can predispose an elderly patient to AGE deposition and RAGE expression, particularly in the face of decreased GFR.[158] The newly identified mesangial cell receptor, AGER1, may be important in countering the proinflammatory mesangial cell response to AGE deposition, although a high AGE burden may mitigate the protective effects of this receptor.[159] Studies in human embryonic kidney cells suggest that AGER1 promotes the inactivation of FKHRL1 and prevents manganese superoxide dismutase (MnSOD) suppression, thus countering AGE-mediated cellular oxidant stress.[160] AGE-induced ROS production via nicotinamide adenine dinucleotide phosphate (NADPH) oxidase is also countered by AGER1.[161] Interestingly, less glomerular scarring and proteinuria is noted in mice chronically fed a low AGE diet that had a lower RAGE and higher AGER1 levels.[162] Furthermore, suppressed levels of AGER1 in human subjects with chronic kidney disease are restored with lower dietary AGE intake.[163] In addition, treatment of aged animals with amino guanidine has been shown to reverse the abnormal vascular permeability and to improve vasodilatory capacity, prevent mononuclear cell migration, decrease glomerulosclerosis, and lower proteinuria.[162,164] Calorie restriction also decreases the burden of AGE in aged rats and may be important in preventing age-associated nephrosclerosis.[164,165]

Calorie Restriction, Sirtuins, and Target of Rapamycin Signaling

The favorable effect of calorie restriction on longevity is well established in various animals. Several potential mechanisms have been proposed to account for the beneficial effects of calorie restriction. Among them are an increase in the activity of sirtuins and adenine monophosphate (AMP)-activated protein kinase (AMPK) signaling, and a decrease in mTOR and S6K1 signaling.[166–168] One of the compelling findings has been the association between increased level of sirtuins and the extension of life span in response to calorie restriction. Sirtuins are members of the silent information regulator 2 (Sir2) family (a family of class III histone/protein deacetylases). There are several mammalian sirtuins, of which sirtuins 1 has been extensively studied. Sirtuins 1 (SIRT1), silent hormone regulator 1, are present in subcellular compartments and regulate the expression of various genes and proteins involved in cell survival, differentiation, metabolism, DNA repair, inflammation, and longevity.[169] They can mediate nicotiramide adenine dinucleotide (NAD^+)-dependent histone deacetylase activity. Calorie restriction appears to increase SIRT1 activity in most tissues, including the kidney. This is based on the observations that SIRT1 knockout mice are resistant to beneficial effects of calorie restriction and that transgenic SIRT1 mice exhibit the same phenotype as calorie-restricted mice on unrestricted calorie intake.[170–172] Interestingly, a plant polyphenol, resveratrol, is a potent activator of SIRT1 activity and has been shown to have renoprotective effects in several models of nephrotoxic and ischemic renal injury.[173] More recent findings suggest SIRT1 induces Foxo3 deacetylation, resulting in increase in Bnip3, mitochondrial autophagy, and the prevention of age-dependent decline in kidney function.[174] Other metabolic regulatory actions of SIRT1 include activation of liver X receptor (LXR)[175] to promote reverse cholesterol transport and inhibit inflammation, as well as the activation of FXR,[176] which may prevent the development and progression of proteinuria and glomerulosclerosis by modulating renal lipid metabolism.[156] Further work is needed to determine whether the use of SIRT1 activators may prove useful in protecting the aging kidney.

Other interesting pathways associated with an increased life span in mice involve mTOR inhibition.[177] Decreased mTOR signaling is found in long-lived Ames dwarf mice.[178] In addition, the deletion of ribosomal protein S6 kinase 1 (S6K1), a factor in nutrient-responsive mTOR signaling, has been shown to improve insulin resistance, increase longevity, and simulate the gene expression patterns seen with calorie restriction and AMPK activation.[179]

Functional Genomics in Aging

A majority of the studies exploring molecular pathways involved in aging had focused on a single or a limited number of pathways. However, aging is a complex process involving a myriad of intimately related molecular pathways. In an attempt to understand the intricate relationship among diverse pathways, a whole genome analysis of gene expression in kidney samples from 74 patients ranging from 27 to 92 years of age was performed.[180] Not surprisingly, the study revealed that age-regulated genes are broadly expressed in the kidney and that the expression profiles of age-regulated genes correlate with the morphologic and physiologic state of the kidney in old age. More than 900 age-related genes could be identified. Interestingly, the transcriptional differences between young and old individuals involve small changes in the expression of many genes, rather than large changes in the expression of a few genes. These findings indicate that functional decline in old age is not the result of the complete failure of a small number of cellular processes. Rather, it is due to the slight decline of many pathways that collectively causes a significant decrease in cell function. Studying aging by analyzing one pathway at a time is difficult, because any single pathway might show only a small change with respect to age and might contribute only to a small extent of the overall functional decline in old age. By contrast, functional genomics is a powerful approach to study aging because it can simultaneously detect small changes in the expression of many genes. This could provide invaluable information on the underlying mechanisms and clinical course of the aging process in the kidney.

STRATEGIES TO RETARD AGE-RELATED RENAL CHANGES

The biologic causes of aging are incompletely understood, with many questions awaiting clarification. The understanding of the variability of the aging process among humans and animals may improve our fundamental knowledge of disease mechanisms and the possibility of preventing the decline in renal function and structure with aging. A number of interventions are presently available that may slow down the deterioration of renal function and structure in the elderly person with an otherwise intact kidney function. These interventions are described in the following sections.

Renin-Angiotensin-Aldosterone System Blockade

The renin-angiotensin-aldosterone system (RAAS) plays an important role in the renal aging process. Although circulating RAS is suppressed in aging, the intrarenal RAS may be relatively intact or even elevated. Ang-II has several hemodynamic and nonhemodynamic effects on the kidney that can accelerate age-related renal glomerulosclerosis and tubulointerstitial fibrosis.[72,73] Therefore, the use of RAAS blockers (renin inhibitors, ACEI, ARB, or aldosterone inhibitors) is a logical strategy in elderly patients with a high risk for progressive deterioration of renal function. Available data suggest that the administration of ACEI and ARB may slow the rate of the decline in GFR in elderly patients with diabetic and nondiabetic proteinuric kidney disease.[181–183] Studies evaluating the reversibility of renal parenchymal changes have been less conclusive given the need for prolonged observation to confirm reversibility.[184] Similarly, a RAAS blockade using a combination of aldosterone inhibitors and ACEI or ARB appears to improve proteinuria and lower urinary TGF-β in patients with nondiabetic chronic kidney disease.[185] However, the use of combination RAAS blockade is associated with an increased risk of hyperkalemia, particularly in the elderly population, thus requiring careful monitoring of serum potassium in such patients. Likewise, RAAS blockade with the renin inhibitor (aliskiren) and an ARB (losartan) has been shown to lower urinary protein excretion in patients with type 2 diabetic renal disease, but the effect on renal structure and function remains to be investigated.[186]

Treatment of Comorbidities

Many older individuals also have associated chronic diseases such as hypertension, diabetes mellitus, dyslipidemia, and other metabolic abnormalities that could accelerate the age-related decline in renal function. Treatment of these comorbidities may decrease the rate of decline in renal function in elderly subjects.

Blood Pressure Control in the Elderly

As described previously, elderly individuals have stiffened vasculature that increases PWV and leads to systolic hypertension and widening of the pulse pressure. This makes blood pressure (BP) control in the elderly difficult with a goal to maintain appropriate perfusion, yet decrease glomerular hyperfiltration and thus glomerular sclerosis. Recent data suggest that blood pressure reduction to $<150/80$ with achieved BP 140/80 mm Hg even in the very elderly improves cardiovascular outcome,[187] suggesting perhaps an improved vascular effect translating to decreased glomerular hypertension. Although a variety of medications can decrease BP, ACEI, diuretics, and dihydropyridine calcium channel blockers may be more useful in decreasing glomerular hypertension and proteinuria than other agents, and should be used preferentially if there are no contraindications.[188,189]

In addition to antihypertensive agents, lifestyle changes such as diet modification and exercise can help to improve BP control. The Canadian Hypertensive Education program recommends sodium restriction of 1200 mg (52 mmol) per day for individuals >70 years and 1300 mg (57 mmol) daily for those between 51 to 70 years, in addition to 30 to 60 minutes of moderate aerobic exercise 4 to 7 days per week.[188] Furthermore, it recommends limiting alcohol consumption, ceasing smoking, and increasing the consumption of fruits, vegetables, fiber, low fat dairy, whole grains, and plant proteins.[188]

Control of Blood Glucose, Lipid, and Other Metabolic Factors

A sedentary lifestyle is not uncommon, particularly in light of other comorbidities, including arthritis in the elderly, and can be associated with weight gain and especially central adiposity. In fact, according to the U.S. National Health and Nutritional Examination Survey, nearly half of the elderly over 65 years of age are obese and qualify for dietary intervention.[138,189,190] Central adiposity is associated with a greater prevalence of the metabolic syndrome (insulin resistance, elevated blood pressure, and lipid abnormalities characterized by low high density lipoprotein (HDL) but higher levels of triglycerides and low density lipoprotein (LDL)).[189,190] Weight loss, diet, and exercise have been shown to improve these metabolic abnormalities and retard the progression of CKD.[191–193] Lifestyle changes as described previously, along with decreased saturated and increased poly- and monounsaturated fats, may be the best approach in elderly persons with metabolic syndrome.[191,192] A low calorie diet not only decreased weight but serum AGEs and triglycerides in middle-aged Japanese men and women, supporting the benefit of calorie restriction in control of other inflammatory factors that can affect renal senescence.[194] In individuals with a predisposition to insulin resistance, hypertension, and hyperlipidemia, the use of statins can be beneficial.[188] Similarly, adequate glycemic control in the older adults with type 2 diabetes significantly lowers the incidence of nephropathy.[195] The combination of low calorie diet and exercise resulted in significant weight loss and improvements in serum lipids and insulin sensitivity.[196] These studies suggest that the early recognition of insulin resistance and initiation of lifestyle modification and/or medical therapy may help reduce age-related renal and cardiovascular disorders.

Natural Antioxidants

Low calorie, low saturated fat diets rich in antioxidants, such as the Okinawan diet, are associated with longevity and, given their salutary effects on AGEs, may be effective in preventing age-associated renal sclerosis.[196,197] The incorporation of leafy vegetables and vegetables rich in natural antioxidants in the diet may further help to prevent long-term vascular and renal aging.[196]

Drug Usage in the Elderly

Old age is associated with a high prevalence of many diseases that necessitate the use of multiple medications. Older people use, on average, two to five prescription drugs on a regular basis, and polypharmacy (the use of five or more medications) occurs in 20% to 40% of this age group.[197] This increases the risks of adverse outcomes from medication-related side effects including the progression of CKD, urinary retention or incontinence, neuropsychiatric symptoms, gastrointestinal problems (constipation), insomnia, falls, and Parkinsonism. In fact, as many as one in five hospital admissions in older people are medication-related and adverse drug reactions are the cause of death in 18% of hospitalized elderly patients.[198,199]

The impairment in kidney function in the elderly may affect the risks and may modify the potential benefits from medications that are cleared by the kidney (e.g., many antibiotics), have nephrotoxic potential (e.g., aminoglycosides, nonsteroidal anti-inflammatory agents [NSAIDs]), or affect glomerular hemodynamics (e.g., ACE inhibitors, ARB, NSAIDs). Combinations of these and other medications may pose even greater risks to those with impaired kidney function. Additionally, the use of over-the-counter (OTC) medications is quite common in the elderly. In one Canadian study, about 25% of patients used OTC and alternative medicines, adding to the polypharmacy.[200] Analgesics are among the most common OTC medications and their use is frequently underreported. There is substantial evidence that NSAIDs are associated with progressive kidney disease and acute kidney injury (AKI).[201]

Thus, an older population with a high burden of comorbid disease can both benefit from and be harmed by various prescribed and OTC medications. A careful consideration of the safety profile and drug–drug interactions is essential when treating these patients. Communication between treating subspecialists, geriatricians, and primary care physicians is imperative to minimize negative outcomes from drug-related side effects in this vulnerable population.

CLINICAL RENAL DISEASES IN THE ELDERLY

A myriad of diseases can affect the aging kidney. Although some are more prevalent in the elderly, none are exclusively confined to the aging population. These disorders are discussed elsewhere in this book and summarized in Table 65.4. However, some characteristic features pertaining to the aging population are briefly described in the following sections.

Acute Kidney Injury in the Elderly

It is well known that the elderly population is at a high risk of developing AKI. Using the new Risk-Injury-Failure-Loss-End stage renal disease (RIFLE) and AKI network (AKIN) classifications of AKI,[202] Joannidis et al.[203] found the incidence of AKI to be between 28.5% and 35.5% among 16,784 patients with a mean age of 63 years admitted to

TABLE 65.4 **Diseases that Commonly Affect the Aging Kidney**

Systemic diseases Hypertension Diabetes mellitus Dyslipidemia Atherosclerosis Atheroemboli Dysproteinemia-related renal diseases Vasculitides
Glomerular diseases Membranous nephropathy Mesangial proliferative GN (including IgA nephropathy) Pauci-immune crescentic GN Anti-GBM disease Minimal change disease Focal segmental glomerulosclerosis
Acute kidney injury Hypovolemic and cardiovascular shock Septic shock Nephrotoxic injury Nonsteroidal anti-inflammatory agents (NSAIDS) Antibiotics (penicillins, cephalosporins, sulfonamides, rifampin, ciprofloxacin) Diuretics (furosemide, potassium-sparing diuretics) Contrast media Cancer chemotherapy Allopurinol Cimetidine Captopril
Interstitial nephritis
Urinary tract infection
Renal stones
Obstructive uropathy Benign causes Nodular hyperplasia of prostate Neurogenic bladder Renal stones Obstructive pyelonephritis/papillary necrosis Urethral stricture Malignant causes Prostate cancer Bladder cancer Pelvic tumors Colonic tumors Retroperitoneal tumors
Renal tumors Primary Metastatic
Simple renal cysts

GN, glomerulonephritis; IgA, immunoglobulin A; GBM, glomerular basement membrane.
Modified from Zhou XJ, Rakheja D, Yu XQ, et al. The aging kidney. *Kidney Int.* 2008;74:710–720.

an intensive care unit. The high risk of AKI in the elderly population is due to the age-associated functional and structural changes in kidneys, a high prevalence of comorbidities, and reduced capability to metabolize drugs in these patients. Furthermore, compared to the younger individuals, the elderly patients are more frequently subjected to invasive procedures, exposed to multiple potentially nephrotoxic medications and radiocontrast agents and more commonly develop sepsis events that can raise the risk of AKI.[204]

AKI is traditionally diagnosed by an abrupt rise in serum creatinine, with or without a fall in urine output. However, because of decreased muscle mass, the rate and magnitude of the rise in serum creatinine may be blunted in the elderly, making it an unsatisfactory biomarker for AKI in this population. Consequently, even a small rise in serum creatinine may reflect a significant decline in GFR in elderly patients. To overcome the difficulties with serum creatinine, several novel biomarkers for the early diagnosis of AKI including cystatin C, kidney injury molecule 1 (KIM1), neutrophil gelatinase–associated lipocalin (NGAL), and interleukin (IL)-18 have been developed.[205] The validity of these biomarkers for the diagnosis of AKI in the elderly remains to be established.

The development of AKI in elderly patients has a strong impact on morbidity and mortality. Notwithstanding recent reports suggesting decreased mortality rates, both short- and long-term AKI-associated mortality remains high in the elderly population.[206,207] Even small changes in serum creatinine levels are associated with long-term death, and greater changes are associated with greater risks.[207] In addition to an increased risk of mortality, AKI in the elderly may be prolonged or may never recover and progress to CKD and ESRD. Several clinical observations described elsewhere in this chapter support these possibilities in elderly patients and highlight the need for preventive strategies and close monitoring of elderly patients after AKI.

Avoiding situations that could damage the kidney is the best strategy to avert the development and adverse consequences of AKI. Given that a major risk factor for AKI is impaired baseline renal function (i.e., CKD), a careful assessment of baseline renal function in the elderly at the time of hospital admission is critical. Close attention needs to be paid to avoid potential nephrotoxic substances and polypharmacy, prescribing the lowest desired dose of drugs and adjusting drug doses to the estimated or measured GFR of the patient. The purpose of these maneuvers is to provide an adequate renal perfusion and oxygenation. Once developed, the strategies to treat established AKI are limited. Because older patients are more prone to volume contraction and because it is often hard to distinguish between prerenal and parenchymal AKI, cautious volume repletion is a crucial step in the management of AKI in the elderly. Conversely, because these patients are unable to handle an excessive fluid load, they can easily develop salt and water overload leading to CHF, pulmonary edema, and increased mortality.[208,209] Close monitoring of volume status is imperative and an early transition from volume expansion to fluid restriction might be necessary in elderly patients with AKI. In addition to volume status, providing adequate nutrition to patients with AKI, particularly older individuals, is critical to improve outcomes. The indications and use of renal replacement therapy (RRT) in the elderly are not different from other age groups because the outcomes with these modalities in the elderly are similar to those of other age groups.[207]

Glomerular Diseases in the Elderly

With a soaring population of older patients with kidney disease, increasing numbers of these patients are referred for nephrologic assessment. Consequently, the number of elderly patients undergoing kidney biopsy has been escalating over the years.[210] Reports of renal biopsy findings in the elderly[211–214] indicate that glomerular diseases are common in these patients. The pattern of glomerular pathology, however, differs in the elderly compared with that in younger individuals. For instance, the prevalence of secondary forms of glomerular disease increases, whereas that of primary forms decreases with age.[210,215,216] In a recent study composed of 235 renal biopsies performed in patients aged 80 to 99 years, Moutzouris et al.[213] observed a common occurrence of pauci-immune crescentic glomerulonephritis (PICGN), membranous nephropathy (MN), minimal change disease (MCD), and renal amyloidosis in this very elderly population. Some of the commonly occurring forms of glomerulonephritis (GN) in the elderly population are reviewed here.

Postinfectious Glomerulonephritis

The epidemiology of postinfectious glomerulonephritis (PIGN) is shifting as the population ages. PIGN is becoming a growing cause of kidney disease in older individuals, particularly those with diabetes or malignancy, and the sites of infection and causative organisms differ from the typical childhood disease.[217] In a recent study of 109 patients 65 years or older with PIGN, more than 60% of the patients had diabetes or were immunocompromised as a result of malignancy.[218] The most common site of infection was skin, followed by pneumonia, and urinary tract infection. The most common causative agent was staphylococcus (46%), rather than group A beta-hemolytic streptococcal pharyngeal infections, as seen in children. AKI, fluid overload, and signs of congestive heart failure were quite common and 46% of patients required dialysis. Low serum complement values were seen in 72% of patients. A proliferative form of GN was seen by light microscopy on a renal biopsy. Immunopathology revealed an immunoglobulin A (IgA)-dominant pattern of Ig deposition in 17% of cases. Electron microscopy often showed electron-dense subepithelial deposits (humps) and subendothelial electron-dense deposits. The outcome, in general, was poor, with 33% of the patients progressing to ESRD, 44% with persistent renal dysfunction, and only 22% achieving complete recovery. The presence of diabetes, higher serum creatinine at biopsy, dialysis at presentation, the presence of diabetic glomerulosclerosis, and greater tubular atrophy and interstitial fibrosis were poor prognostic factors.

The treatment of PIGN is largely preventative. Early recognition and prompt antimicrobial treatment of the offending infection may prevent or modify the course of the disease. Late treatment may have little effect on outcome. In patients who present with a rapidly progressive course, high-dose steroids and immunosuppressants have been used with variable results. However, serious adverse events can occur from this therapeutic approach in this high-risk population.

Membranous Nephropathy

Nephrotic syndrome (NS) is a common glomerular disease in the elderly. In a series of 1368 patients aged 60 years or more, NS was found to be most frequently associated with MN comprising 36.6% of all cases of NS.[210] However, MN is observed less commonly in the very elderly population (>80 years).[219] MN in the elderly patient can be primary (idiopathic) or can be secondary to systemic illnesses, the most common being malignancies.[210] Conversely, the incidence of cancer is much higher among patients with MN than in the general population, especially with advancing age. No difference in clinical presentation of MN is observed between those without and with malignancy. The histologic picture of MN with or without associated neoplasia is fairly similar. However, certain features such as the presence of infiltrating inflammatory cells in the glomeruli, the pattern of IgG subclass deposition (IgG4 predominates in idiopathic MN whereas IgG1 and IgG3 are associated with secondary form), and the absence of antibodies to phospholipase 2 receptor may help to distinguish primary from secondary forms of MN.[221,222] In the majority of patients with secondary MN, the diagnosis of cancer is made long after the diagnosis of MN. In a recent study,[223] the median time from the diagnosis of MN to the diagnosis of cancer was found to be about 60 months. Thus, when MN is diagnosed in an elderly patient, appropriate cancer screening including colonoscopy, chest X-ray, stool for occult blood, hemogram, prostate-specific antigen (in men), and mammography (in women) should be performed.

Treatment of MN in the elderly is the same as that in younger adult patients.[219] As spontaneous remission can occur in approximately 30% of patients with idiopathic MN, conservative therapy for 6 to 9 months with observation is a reasonable option. If the NS is severe or if renal function is steadily deteriorating, initial therapy commonly employs the use of alkylating agents (cyclophosphamide or chlorambucil). Notably, these agents can be associated with serious adverse effects such as infections and bone marrow suppression in the elderly. Therefore, lower dosage of these drugs and close monitoring for infection and leukopenia is warranted. Alternatives to alkylating agents include calcineurin inhibitors, mycophenolate, or rituximab, but there is little experience with the use of these agents in the elderly population with MN.[219,224,225]

Minimal Change Disease

MCD was found to be the second most common glomerular abnormality presenting as nephrotic syndrome in a series of 1368 patients aged 60 years or older.[210] The clinical course of MCD in the elderly is different and unlike that in children; almost 40% of the elderly patients with MCD may develop AKI (Fig 65.3).[226] The risk factors for the development of AKI include heavy proteinuria (10 g per day or more), profound hypoalbuminemia, and the use of nonsteroidal anti-inflammatory agents. The majority of cases with AKI superimposed on MCD will remit with appropriate treatment, although in some cases, the course may be progressive and irreversible. The diagnosis of MCD by renal biopsy can be difficult in the elderly because of concomitant age-related changes of nephrosclerosis. An electron microscopic examination showing diffuse foot process effacement may be helpful to suggest the diagnosis of MCD.

The treatment of MCD in the elderly is the same as in children, but elderly patients may need more prolonged treatment to achieve a complete remission.[224,225] Oral prednisone given for 6 to 12 weeks is often the initial treatment of choice and usually results in a complete remission. However, the response in the elderly is not as robust as that observed in children. Available data suggest a complete remission occurs in approximately 50% of patients by 2 to 4 months of treatment and in approximately 75% of patients by 6 months of treatment. Relapses of NS do occur, but are less frequent in the elderly.[227] Partial remissions or a lack of response often indicates an underlying fecal segmental glomerulosclerosis (FSGS) lesion that may be missed on the initial renal biopsy. Elderly patients are quite prone to develop side effects from the prolonged use of steroids. Patients who do not tolerate or respond to steroid treatment may be candidates for alternative therapies such as calcineurin inhibitors, cyclophosphamide, mycophenolate, or rituximab. However, the efficacy and safety of these latter approaches have not been validated in the elderly.[228,229]

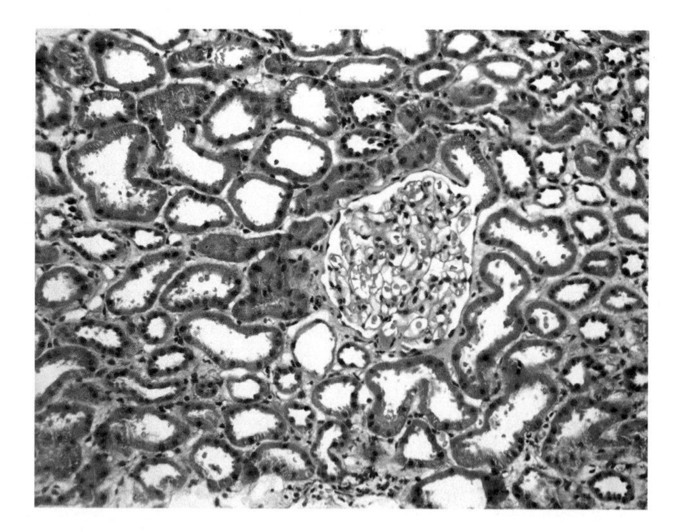

FIGURE 65.3 Minimal change disease with acute renal failure. The glomerulus appears normal. The tubular epithelium reveals diffuse simplification with flattening of epithelium and dilated lumens. There is also mild interstitial edema (H&E, hematoxylin and eosin; ×200). (See Color Plate.)

Crescentic Glomerulonephritis

Crescentic GN is commonly observed in elderly patients presenting with hematuria, proteinuria, and progressive impairment of renal function.[211,214,230] Among the subsets of crescentic GN, antineutrophil cytoplasmic antibody (ANCA)-associated small vessel vasculitis is most frequently seen.[211,214,230] Some of these patients will have a systemic form of vasculitis, either Wegener granulomatosis, microscopic polyangiitis, or Churg-Strauss syndrome, whereas others will have "renal-limited" disease. The other causes of crescentic GN, including anti-GBM GN or immune complex-mediated crescentic GN, are uncommon in the elderly population. Cyclophosphamide (oral or intravenous) plus high-dose glucocorticoids are the treatment of choice for most patients with ANCA-associated GN.[231] The addition of intensive plasma exchange for those with severe AKI has been shown to be effective.[232] However, the elderly patient with crescentic GN may not tolerate immunosuppression and may experience serious complications leading to a fatal outcome, particularly during the first 6 to 12 months of treatment with combined cyclophosphamide and glucocorticoids.[233,234] Advanced age and low GFR on presentation are independent predictors of mortality from immunosuppressive treatment in patients with ANCA-associated GN. Newer treatment regimens using rituximab show promise, but the available data pertaining to their safety and efficacy in the elderly with ANCA-associated vasculitis are limited.[235] Anti-GBM antibody nephritis (alone or in combination with ANCA) should be treated aggressively and promptly with combined immunosuppression and intensive plasma exchange, especially when life-threatening pulmonary hemorrhage is present.[236]

Monoclonal Immunoglobulin Deposition Disease

The monoclonal Ig deposition diseases (MIDD) are an important cause of renal disease and are much more common in the elderly than in younger individuals.[215,237,238] These disorders include amyloid and nonamyloid MIDD. Amyloidosis encompasses a group of diseases that result from the abnormal deposition of protein complexes, called amyloids, in various tissues including the kidneys. The amyloid deposits organize into fibrils that stain positive with Congo red and thioflavin dyes and exhibit birefringence in polarized light. Amyloid deposition can be localized to the kidneys alone, but more commonly, it is widespread and can involve virtually any organ in the body. Amyloidosis can be primary (AL) or secondary (AA) to systemic diseases such as chronic infections (like tuberculosis or osteomyelitis), or chronic inflammatory diseases (like rheumatoid arthritis and ankylosing spondylitis).

Amyloidosis is a cause of NS in approximately 10% of elderly patients.[237] It is usually associated with systemic symptoms such as postural hypotension, carpal tunnel syndrome, easy bruising, organomegaly, macroglossia, congestive heart failure, and diarrhea. Systemic amyloidosis is most commonly due to the deposition of monoclonal lambda light chains or their fragments (primary AL amyloid), but heavy-chain amyloid can also occur (AH amyloidosis). Approximately 10% to 15% of patients with multiple myelomas develop systemic amyloidosis. The diagnosis of amyloidosis is made by detecting the characteristic Congo red–positive amyloid deposition in a biopsy specimen of involved tissue such as kidney, fat pad, or rectum. The diagnosis of primary amyloidosis will further be supported by the presence of monoclonal free light chains/Ig on serum and urine protein electrophoresis (SPEP, UPEP), whereas they are normal in secondary amyloidosis. The prognosis for primary systemic (AL or AH) amyloidosis is very poor in the elderly, but it is improving as a result of advances in treatment.[239,240] Patients with amyloidosis presenting with NS often develop ESRD within a few years. Cardiac involvement, particularly the presence of congestive heart failure (CHF), portends poor outcome. Therapeutic approaches including melphalan, bortezomid, lenalindomide, and autologous bone marrow and peripheral stem cell transplant have improved outcomes of primary (AL/AH) amyloidosis, but their efficacy and tolerability in the elderly have not been accurately established.[241]

Disorders associated with the nonamyloid (Congo red–negative) deposition of monoclonal Igs or their fragments are also common in the elderly.[215,238] They include light-chain deposition disease (LCDD) and immunotactoid GN, among others. LCDD typically presents as NS and progressive renal impairment. SPEP and UPEP typically are positive for monoclonal light chains (usually kappa).[242] Renal biopsies often reveal a nodular intercapillary glomerulosclerosis (resembling the Kimmelstiel-Wilson lesion of diabetic nephropathy) with monoclonal light chain. An electron microscopy may show subendothelial or intramembranous powdery electron-dense deposits in glomeruli. Prognosis is poor in the elderly, most of whom progress to ESRD. Chemotherapy, including chlorambucil, melphalan, and bortezomid, may improve the outcome, but elderly patients may not tolerate them well.[243]

Hypertension in the Elderly

Hypertension (HTN) is one of the most prevalent disorders in the elderly population. By age 75, 75% of men and almost 90% of women will meet the definition of stage 1 HTN as defined by the Joint National Committee on Prevention, Detection, Evaluation, and Treatment of High Blood Pressure (JNC 7).[244] Several physiologic characteristics of aging contribute to this age-related increase in BP, including decreased vascular compliance, impaired baroreceptor sensitivity, increased sympathetic activity, and α-adrenergic receptor sensitivity, increased total and central adiposity, salt sensitivity, and metabolic changes including insulin resistance.[245,246] Changes in renal function with aging play an important role in the development of HTN and, in turn, the control of HTN can delay or prevent progression of renal disease. In the vast majority of the older patients, HTN is primary (so-called essential HTN). Secondary forms of HTN should be suspected if malignant HTN, resistant HTN, or a sudden increase in diastolic blood pressure (DBP) is found. Common causes of secondary HTN are renovascular disease, primary hyperaldosteronism, medications (e.g., NSAIDs, corticosteroids) and obstructive sleep apnea.

Given the rapid growth of the elderly population and their high prevalence of HTN, treatment of HTN in this population has become a global priority. Treatment of HTN in the elderly population has been demonstrated to reduce the relative risk (RR) of stroke by 25%, congestive heart failure (CHF) by 50%, and cardiovascular disease (CVD) mortality and events by 20%.[247,248] Because patients aged 80 years and older have been generally excluded from many HTN trials, the recent Hypertension in the Very Elderly Trial (HYVET) sought to establish the risks and benefits of treatment in this population.[249] HYVET was a multicenter, randomized, placebo-controlled trial comparing placebo with indapamide (and perindopril if needed), in hypertensive patients aged 80 years or older. The trial was prematurely halted when a significant reduction in mortality (28%), fatal and nonfatal strokes (34%), and CHF (72%) was found in the treated group. On the basis of the data from this and other HTN trials, the current treatment goals in the elderly population (those between 65 and 80 years of age) should be the same (i.e., 140/90 mm Hg) as those for younger patients unless diabetes and/or chronic kidney disease are present, in which case a lower target (130/80 mm Hg) is recommended. For those people aged 80 years or older who meet the criteria of HYVET, a goal BP of 150/80 mm Hg may be reasonable.

In addition to pharmacologic treatment, the inclusion of lifestyle changes is highly beneficial in the management of HTN. Systolic BP can be reduced by 5 to 20 mm Hg with a 10 kg weight loss, 8 to 14 mm Hg by adopting the Dietary Approaches to Stop Hypertension (DASH)-type diet, 2 to 8 mm Hg with sodium restriction, 4 to 9 mm Hg with increased physical activity, and 2 to 4 mm Hg with moderation in alcohol use.[250,251]

Although thiazide diuretics are often the first line of treatment for HTN, their efficacy is markedly reduced in the presence of significant renal dysfunction (serum creatinine [Cr] 2 mg per deciliter and/or glomerular filtration rate [GFR] < 50 mL per minute). Under these circumstances, loop diuretics may be more appropriate. Direct vasodilators and centrally acting α-adrenergic drugs should be avoided because of their contribution to orthostatic hypotension and central nervous system side effects. Drug selection should be individualized to the patient, taking existing comorbidities into account. In most patients, the level of BP reduction achieved is more important than the drug used. However, one can argue that the results of the Avoiding Cardiovascular Events through Combination Therapy in Patients Living with Systolic Hypertension (ACCOMPLISH) trial challenge this statement.[252] This trial compared benazepril-amlodipine with benazepril hydrochlorothiazide in an older population at high risk for CVD. As compared with the angiotensin converting enzyme inhibitor-hydrochlorothiazide (ACEI-HCTZ) group, the ACEI-CCB (calcium channel blocker) group showed a relative risk reduction of 20% in the primary end point of illness and death from cardiovascular causes. A similar benefit was observed with the secondary end point of death from cardiovascular (CV) causes and nonfatal MI and stroke. Most previous trials comparing drugs from different classes have not shown a difference in primary outcomes when the level of BP achieved was comparable. The benefits of the BP level achieved must be weighed against potential adverse effects such as orthostatic hypotension, metabolic/ electrolyte abnormalities, development of AKI, and possible drug–drug interactions given the high prevalence of polypharmacy in the elderly population.

Chronic Kidney Disease

A recent survey of the U.S. population has shown that the prevalence rate of CKD has increased from 10% between 1988 and 1994 to 13.1% in the 1999 to 2004 period.[253] Aging of the U.S. population is one of the main factors that accounts for the rising prevalence of CKD. CKD is defined by a reduction in GFR below 60 mL/min/1.73 m^2 and/or the evidence of kidney damage for 3 or more months. Many cases of CKD in the elderly population manifest without a readily apparent cause; this is particularly true for CKD defined only by reduced GFR. Controversy abounds in calling a moderate reduction in eGFR without other evidence of kidney damage in the elderly population a disease.[254] Notwithstanding this debate, there is consistent evidence that reduced eGFR and albuminuria, either separately or in combination in elderly individuals, are associated with a higher risk of adverse outcomes including ESRD, CVD, cognitive impairment, and all-cause mortality, providing support for the current definition of CKD in the elderly population.[255–258]

Regardless of the underlying cause of the CKD, elderly patients are at a high risk for further kidney injury, and therefore the progression of CKD. Analysis of data in over 10,000 Canadian patients aged ≥66 years with CKD revealed that approximately 40% of people with eGFR between 30 and 59 mL/min/1.73 m^2 experienced a decline in eGFR of >5 mL/min/1.73 m^2 over a 2-year period.[259] Similarly, a study of U.S. subjects aged ≥65 years showed that a substantial proportion of elderly people experienced the progression of CKD and 16% to 25% of the CKD cohort had an annual decline of eGFR of greater than 3 mL/min/1.73 m^2.[260] Major risk factors for the progression of CKD, including hypertension and diabetes, are rife in elderly people. Additionally, older patients are at a high risk for the development of AKI, which, as noted previously, is a major risk factor for the progression to CKD and ESRD.

In general, elderly people with CKD are far less likely to progress to ESRD than to die of other causes, primarily vascular disease. A recent study[261] of 386 patients with stage 4 CKD showed that subjects over 80 years of age were more likely to die than to reach ESRD, and that early preparation for RRT can be futile in this subgroup of patients. Coronary artery disease is highly prevalent among elderly in all stages of CKD and is associated with significantly greater hospitalization rates for myocardial infarction, stroke, and arrhythmia.[6,253,256,257] Likewise, cognitive impairment is associated with kidney disease in elderly individuals. Several studies have demonstrated relationships between albuminuria and both cognitive function and small vessel cerebrovascular disease.[255,262,263] Similar findings have been reported in the dialysis population, in whom small vessel cerebrovascular disease and cognitive impairment are common.[264]

The presence of CKD in the elderly may shape diagnostic and treatment decisions for comorbid conditions. Knowledge of the level of eGFR is important for decisions such as the use of iodinated contrast compounds and gadolinium for imaging studies as well as the selection and dosing of various medications.[265,266] The use of inappropriate medications or drug doses increases the risk for drug–drug interactions, adverse drug reactions, complications of routine procedures, progression of CKD, development of AKI, electrolyte disturbances, hospitalizations, and death.[267] For example, commonly used medications, including NSAIDs and oral phosphate purgatives, are associated with GFR declines in the elderly.[201,268] Moreover, patients with CKD are at a higher risk for adverse iatrogenic outcomes such as postsurgical complications, AKI, hypoglycemia, hyperkalemia, and other electrolyte abnormalities.[269,270] Given the high prevalence of comorbidities, the frequent use of multiple medications in complex regimens, and the often aberrant and ambiguous metabolism of medications in elderly individuals with CKD, treatment decisions require a meticulous balance of risks and benefits to achieve a therapeutic goal.

END-STAGE RENAL DISEASE AND MANAGEMENT IN THE ELDERLY

End-Stage Renal Disease

The new data on trends in CKD prevalence, as discussed previously, mirror the United States Renal Data System (USRDS) data on the ESRD population that showed a 42% increase in the ESRD population between 1991 and 2001. With extensive efforts made to prevent renal disease progression, there has been stabilization of the overall ESRD incidence recently.[6] However, the incidence of ESRD among elderly patients continues to grow. Since 2000, there has been a 9.4% growth in the incidence rate of ESRD in patients over 75 years of age. Moreover, as of 2008, the incidence rate was four times higher in patients over 65 years of age compared to the overall incidence rate of ESRD in the U.S. population.[6] Furthermore, since 2000, the total number of prevalent elderly patients with ESRD has increased by 25% in patients between 65 to 74 years of age and by 31% in patients 75 years or older.[6] Currently, one in four patients starting dialysis in the United States is over the age of 75 years.[6] An increase in prevalence of the associated comorbidities such as diabetes and hypertension as well as improved survival from cardiovascular disease may explain the increase in the incidence of ESRD among the elderly.[271] Moreover, broader access to ESRD care and an earlier initiation of dialysis may have further contributed to the disproportionate increase in treated ESRD incidence among the elderly. There is increasing interest in the role of AKI as a contributor to the ESRD epidemic.[272] This assumption is supported by a meta-analysis of 17 AKI studies, which demonstrated that patients 65 years or older had a 28% higher risk of nonrecovery of kidney function following an episode of AKI than younger patients.[273] A recent study of elderly Medicare beneficiaries (>67 years of age) with a discharge diagnosis of AKI were found to have a 7% cumulative incidence of ESRD in the first 2 years after hospitalization. The risk of ESRD was 13-fold higher in patients with AKI alone and 41-fold higher in those with AKI superimposed on CKD.[274] Data from a large healthcare system demonstrate that, on average, patients developing AKI are approximately 10 years older than those who do not, and that elderly patients developing AKI are less likely to recover kidney function.[273]

There are two RRT options for ESRD patients: renal transplantation and dialysis including hemodialysis (HD: in-center and home HD) and peritoneal dialysis (PD). Although renal transplantation remains the RRT of choice, the proportion of ESRD patients receiving transplants has not changed in the past decade.[6] The majority of ESRD patients require different dialysis modalities for sustenance of life. As expected, the mortality of elderly patients undergoing dialysis treatment is high. For this reason, the role of maximum conservative management among elderly ESRD patients has been explored. Various RRT options for the management of ESRD among elderly patients are discussed in the following sections.

Renal Transplant in the Elderly

Although the number of patients on the waiting list for kidney transplantation increases by about 10% annually, the annual increase in the number of transplants is only 4%.[275,276] Furthermore, because of the aging population, there is an increasing need for kidney transplants among older adults. Although during the last decade the number of patients added to the waiting list for kidney transplantation has remained constant among those younger than 50 years of age, it has tripled in patients aged 65 years or older. At present, 57% of the 73,000 candidates currently on the active waiting list for kidney transplantation are older than 50 years of age. The growing number of elderly patients with ESRD has resulted in a rise in the number of elderly patients receiving kidney transplants, increasing the disparity between organ supply and demand. Consequently, the criteria for accepting kidneys for transplantation have recently been extended to allow the use of organs from less ideal donors that may not have been accepted for transplantation in the past.[277] These expanded criteria donor (ECD) kidneys are from donors over the age of 60 years without comorbidities or donors over the age of 50 years with two comorbidities, such as hypertension, death from cerebrovascular accident, or terminal serum creatinine levels greater than 1.5 mg per deciliter.[278] Although ECD kidneys may have a greater risk of delayed graft function, primary nonfunction, and shortened graft survival, outcomes associated with these organs have been generally favorable.[279,280]

In order to optimize the use of ECD kidneys, appropriate donor and recipient profiling and selection is necessary. The report from the United Network for Organ Sharing (UNOS) database showed a graft survival of 78% at 1 year, supporting the use of organs from elderly donors for elderly recipients.[281] Several subsequent studies[282,283] have indicated that when appropriately used, ECD kidneys do not represent an inferior resource and excellent short- and medium-term outcomes can be achieved. The United States currently has two renal transplant lists: one for standard criteria donors and the other for ECDs. Most centers in the United States recommend that older patients, patients with diabetic ESRD, and patients with difficult vascular access issues be listed on the expanded criteria list. ECD kidneys now comprise 17% of the deceased donor transplants in the United States.[284] A recent analysis of the USRDS database showed that elderly patients were twice as likely to undergo transplantation in 2006 compared to 1995. This is due to a threefold increase in living donor and ECD transplantation and a 26% reduction in the risk for death while on the waiting list.[285] Similarly, the Eurotransplant Senior Program (ESP), established in January 1999, allows for the local allocation of kidneys from donors over 65 years of age to recipients over the age of 65 years.[286] Since its inception, the availability of elderly donors has doubled, and the waiting time for ESP patients has decreased.[287]

Several new strategies have been proposed more recently to further improve ECD allograft outcomes. [288–291] These include dual renal transplants that allow for the use of two marginal kidneys into one recipient to increase the number of functioning nephrons, a pretransplant histologic evaluation of the ECD kidneys, use of pulsatile pump perfusion for allograft preservation, and genomewide gene expression profile determination of the donor kidneys. Although an older recipient age has been shown to be an independent risk factor for graft loss because of a higher incidence of death with a functioning graft, death-censored analyses have demonstrated comparable graft survival rates between older and younger recipient age groups. Wolfe et al.[292] determined that renal transplantation doubles the life expectancy of 60- to 74-year-old dialysis patients listed for transplantation in the United States. More recent European data indicate that in patients aged >65 years, transplantation doubled the life expectancy compared to dialysis.[293] Subsequent studies[294–298] clearly document that excellent outcomes can be attained in elderly recipients from kidney transplantations. Regardless of age, patients derive a survival benefit from transplantation compared with dialysis. After transplantation, the immunosuppression protocols are similar to those for younger transplant recipients. Most studies suggest a lower incidence of acute rejections, but 20% to 40% higher morbidity and mortality from serious infections in the elderly.[299,300] From an allocation perspective, one might argue against the merits of transplanting in elderly patients, particularly because younger patients might derive a greater lifetime survival benefit. However, with the concept of age matching becoming more accepted as a method of optimizing the use of organs in elderly donors and recipients, it is becoming more evident that an absolute age limit cannot be set for transplantation and that kidney transplantation in the elderly is equally valuable.

Dialysis Therapy in the Elderly

With the rising population of elderly ESRD patients, an increasing number of older patients are accepted into dialysis programs. Although dialysis may offer a longer life span compared to conservative management, the quality of life may not always improve or may even deteriorate. No randomized controlled trials have been conducted in this area and only a small number of observational studies provide guidance; hence, predicting which patients will have poor outcomes remains a challenging task. The morbidity and mortality in the elderly ESRD population with or without dialysis is very high.[301] In a USRDS registry study, 1-year mortality for octogenarians and nonagenarians after dialysis initiation was 46%. Patients with two to three comorbidities had a 31% increased risk of death as compared to patients with fewer or no comorbidities. Mortality in ESRD is mainly a consequence of cardiovascular disease, which may be 10- to 100-fold greater than age- and gender-matched controls in the general population, or may be due to a higher prevalence of other causes such as pneumonia.[6,302] Available studies suggest that dialysis is still life extending in many elderly patients.[303,304] Older dialysis patients differ from younger patients in some important ways, typically initiating dialysis at higher eGFR levels and lower body mass indexes, having more comorbid conditions and higher mortality rates, and being less likely to be treated with peritoneal dialysis.[6] Not surprisingly, PD is frequently viewed as unfeasible in elderly patients, perhaps due to a negative image on the part of physicians and nurses in some dialysis centers. Many patients who have no contraindications for PD or HD are not adequately informed about home-based therapies. When patients with advanced kidney disease are adequately informed, the number of patients starting on PD increases.[305] In a large Dutch prospective multicenter study, entitled the Netherlands Cooperative Study of the Adequacy of Dialysis (NECOSAD), out of the 64% of patients who were given a choice, 27% of patients older than 70 years of age chose PD.[306] Therefore, an important cause of PD underuse may be the biased views of some physicians and nurses. These health professionals may exaggerate the relative contraindications for PD (i.e., obesity, impaired vision, poor hygiene, limited ability for self-care, and living alone),[307,308] which can be overcome in motivated patients after appropriate counseling.

Data comparing outcomes and quality of life in elderly patients treated by HD or PD are sparse but may serve to optimally allocate these modalities to all patient groups, who may sometimes benefit from consecutive use of both modalities. In some studies, a higher mortality was found in PD patients older than 80 years, in older PD patients with CHF, as well as in older (>65 years) diabetic PD patients.[309–311] The North Thames Dialysis study specifically examined outcomes and quality of life in dialysis patients older than 70 years of age who were starting dialysis.[312] The 1-year survival of 71% of patients was influenced by age but not by dialysis modality. No difference in survival, hospitalization rate, or quality of life was observed between the two modalities. The Broadening Options for Long-term Dialysis in the Elderly (BOLDE) study[313] compared quality of life, depression, symptoms, and illness intrusion in older (> 65 years) patients in PD and demographically matched HD patients. Although HD and PD patients did not differ in the unadjusted quality of life, PD patients had marginally but significantly better mental component scores. PD patients also had a lower number of symptoms and significantly less depression, suggesting that this modality may provide elderly ESRD patients with at least the same quality of life as HD.[313] A recent retrospective study based on the data from the French Language Peritoneal Dialysis Registry (RDPLF) analyzed the outcome of 1613 patients older than 75 years of age who started PD between January 2000 and December 2005. The majority of them were on assisted PD. Excellent median patient survival of 27.1 months and technique survival of 21.4 months were observed,[314] suggesting that PD is a suitable RRT modality for elderly patients.

Older patients with advanced CKD should be provided with adequate and unbiased information about the available dialysis modalities, the advantages and relative contraindications, and the impact of both PD and HD on outcomes and quality of life. These discussions should ideally occur several months before the commencement of dialysis. However, even in patients who present late to the nephrologists, PD as a RRT option of choice should not be entirely excluded. All elderly patients should have opportunities to choose a dialysis modality that will suite their lifestyle and improve their quality of life, irrespective of physician prejudices.

Conservative Management of End-Stage Renal Disease in the Elderly

Although dialysis therapy in older individuals confers prolonged survival, the quality-of-life benefits of dialysis therapy in the elderly remain unclear. An unpalatable diet, the time commitment for dialysis therapy, depression, and fatigue greatly impact the quality of life of these patients. Moreover, many elderly patients starting RRT have numerous comorbidities at the initiation of dialysis, which may affect their survival on dialysis, as observed in the retrospective study by Murtagh et al.[304] Older age is frequently associated with a loss of physical functions such as strength, dexterity, vision, or hearing.[315] Furthermore, elderly patients may present with cognitive dysfunction at the start of dialysis, which may then progress, leading to significant decline in their functional status.[316,317] The quality of life of elderly nursing home residents in the United States on dialysis is extremely poor. Within the first year after the initiation of dialysis, 58% of the residents die and 29% experience decreased functional status, whereas only 13% maintain functional status.[317] Moreover, vascular access failure rate is higher in older HD patients.[318] Not infrequently, elderly patients experience arrhythmias and hypotension during the HD sessions that may further curtail quality of life. Travel time to and from the HD center has a negative impact on a patient's quality of life.[319,320] Likewise, a recent study examined 206 individuals with kidney failure requiring dialysis who were discharged to a long-term care hospital and noted that only 31% returned home; older age was an independent predictor of failing to be discharged home.[321] These poor outcomes strongly suggest that alternative paths, such as a decision for conservative management (nondialysis therapy), should be incorporated into discussions in the predialysis setting.[316] In a small observational study in ESRD patients over 75 years of age, conservative therapy was associated with a quality of life similar to hemodialysis.[322] Murtagh et al.[304] reported results of a study of 129 patients aged 75 years or older with an eGFR of 15 mL/min/1.73 m^2 or less. Of those patients, 40% were recommended for dialysis and 60% were recommended for nondialytic management. In intention to treat analyses, 1-year survival rates were 84% in the group choosing dialysis and 68% in the group choosing nondialytic management. However, among those with high comorbidities or among those with ischemic heart disease, survival did not differ between the two groups. This was further supported by a recent study extending over an 18-year period in which 689 (82%) of 844 patients were treated by RRT and 155 (18%) were treated with conservative management (CM).[323] Overall the median survival was less in CM than in RRT (21.2 versus 67.1 months: $P<.001$). However, in patients aged >75 years when corrected for age, high comorbidity, and diabetes, the survival advantage from RRT was only about 4 months, which was not statistically significant. Increasing age, the presence of a high comorbidity, and the presence of diabetes were independent determinants of poorer survival in RRT patients. This suggests that an individualized approach is necessary when choosing management options in the elderly ESRD patient. RRT is likely to be beneficial in many patients, especially those with a low comorbidity and in those with rapidly declining renal function. Conversely, CM may have a role in those elderly patients with a high comorbidity and a more slowly declining renal function.[323] The role of conservative management in older ESRD patients was further suggested by a recent observational study[324] of a single-center cohort in the United Kingdom. In this study evaluating 202 elderly patients (>70 years of age) who had ESRD and had chosen either maximum conservative management or RRT, the median survival was 37.8 months for RRT patients and 13.9 months for maximum CM patients. However, RRT patients had significantly higher rates of hospitalization compared with maximum CM patients. RRT patients spent 47.5% of their survival days in hospitals and were more likely to die in the hospital. On the other hand, maximum CM patients spent only 4.3% of their survival time in the hospital and were significantly more likely to die at home or in a hospice. This study illustrates that although dialysis prolongs survival for elderly patients with ESRD and a significant comorbidity by approximately 2 years, patients who choose maximum CM can survive a substantial length of time, achieving similar numbers of hospital-free days compared to patients who choose hemodialysis.

Accordingly, maximal CM, including a rigorous effort to alleviate symptoms and improve quality of life, may be reasonable in many elderly patients with advanced CKD. Strategies including a low protein diet, the preservation of residual renal function, and the management of comorbidities may be effective for those opting for CM.[325] Comprehensive interdisciplinary care including nephrology and geriatric and palliative care services with frequent provider visits may play a considerable role in providing maximal conservative management to enhance the quality of life and survival of elderly individuals with advanced CKD.

REFERENCES

1. U.S. Census Bureau. International database. Table NC EST 2009 01. Midyear population, by age and sex. http://www.census.gov/population/www/projections/natdet-D1A.html. Accessed, February 22, 2011.

2. Zhou XJ, Saxena R, Liu Z, Vaziri ND, Silva FG. Renal senescence in 2008: progress and challenges. *Int Urol Nephrol*. 2008;40:823–839.

2a. Silva FG. The aging kidney: a review–part I. *Int Urol Nephrol*. 2005;37: 185–205.

2b. Silva FG. The aging kidney: a review–part I. *Int Urol Nephrol*. 2005;37: 419–432.

3. Zhou XJ, Rakheja D, Silva FG. The aging kidney. In: Zhou XJ, et al., eds. *Silva's Diagnostic Renal Pathology*. Cambridge, UK: Cambridge University Press; 2009:488–501.

4. *World Population Ageing, 1950–2050*. New York, NY: Department of Economic and Social Affairs; 2006.

5. Levit K, Smith C, Cowan C, et al. Trends in U.S. health care spending, 2001. *Health Affairs*. 2003;22:154–164.

6. *2010 Annual Data Report*. Bethesda, MD: United States Renal Data System; 2010.

7. Zhou XJ, Rakheja D, Vaziri ND, et al. The aging kidney. *Kidney Int*. 2008;74:710–720.

8. Tan JC, Busque S, Workeneh B, et al. Effects of aging on glomerular function and number in living kidney donors. *Kidney Int*. 2010;78:686–692.

9. Hughson MD, Douglas-Denton R, Bertram JF, Hoy WE. Hypertension, glomerular number, and birth weight in African Americans and white subjects in the southeastern United States. *Kidney Int*. 2006;69(4):671–678.

10. Kasiske BL. Relationship between vascular disease and age-associated changes in the human kidney. *Kidney Int*. 1987;31:1153–1159.

11. Kaplan C, Pasternack B, Shah H, et al. Age-related incidence of sclerotic glomeruli in human kidneys. *Am J Pathol*. 1995;80:227–234.

11a. Smith SM, Hoy WE, Cobb L. Law incidence of glomerulosclerosis in normal kidney. *Arch Path Lab Med*. 1989;113:1253–1255.

12. Barton M. Ageing as a determinant of renal and vascular disease: role of endothelial factors. *Nephrol Dial Transplant*. 2005;20:485–490.

13. Wei JY. Age and the cardiovascular system. *N Engl J Med.* 1992;327: 1735–1739.

14. Brenner BM. Hemodynamically mediated glomerular injury and the progressive nature of kidney disease. *Kidney Int.* 1983;23(4):647–655.

15. Hill GS, Heudes D, Bariéty J. Morphometric study of arterioles and glomeruli in the aging kidney suggests focal loss of autoregulation. *Kidney Int.* 2003;63(3):1027–1036.

16. Newbold KM, Sandison A, Howie AJ. Comparison of size of juxtamedullary and outer cortical glomeruli in normal adult kidney. *Virchows Arch A Pathol Anat Histopathol.* 1992;420(2):127–129.

17. Zhou XJ, Laszik ZG, Silva FG. Anatomical changes in the aging kidney. In: Macias-Nunez JF, Cameron JS, Oreopoulos DG, eds. *The Aging Kidney in Health and Disease*. New York, NY: Springer; 2008:39–54.

18. Baert L, Steg A. Is the diverticulum of the distal and collecting tubules a preliminary stage of the simple cyst in the adult? *J Urol.* 1977;118(5):707–710.

19. Takazakura E, Sawabu N, Handa A, et al. Intrarenal vascular changes with age and disease. *Kidney Int.* 1972;2(4):224–230.

20. Rule AD, Amer H, Cornell LD, et al. The association between age and nephrosclerosis on renal biopsy among healthy adults. *Ann Intern Med.* 2010;152(9): 561–567.

21. Tracy RE, Parra D, Eisaguirre W, Torres Balanza RA. Influence of arteriolar hyalinization on arterial intimal fibroplasia in the renal cortex of subjects in the United States, Peru, and Bolivia, applicable also to other populations. *Am J Hypertens.* 2002;15(12):1064–1073.

22. Fogo A, Breyer JA, Smith MC, et al. Accuracy of the diagnosis of hypertensive nephrosclerosis in African Americans: a report from the African American Study of Kidney Disease (AASK) Trial. AASK Pilot Study Investigators. *Kidney Int.* 1997;51(1):244–252.

23. Abdelhafiz AH, Brown SH, Bello A, El Nahas M. Chronic kidney disease in older people: physiology, pathology or both? *Nephron Clin Pract.* 2010;116:c19–c24.

24. Wesson LG Jr. Renal hemodynamics in physiological states. In: *Physiology of the Human Kidney.* New York, NY: Grune & Stratton; 1969:96–108.

25. Hollenberg NK, Adams DF, Solomon HS, et al. Senescence and the renal vasculature in normal man. *Circ Res.* 1974;34:309–316.

26. Long DA, Mu W, Price KL, Johnson RJ. Blood vessels and the aging kidney. *Nephron Exp Nephrol.* 2005;101:e95–e99.

27. Ferder LF, Inserra F, Basso N. Effects of renin angiotensin system blockade in the aging kidney. *Exp Gerontol.* 2003;38:237–244.

28. Delp MD, Behnke BJ, Spier SA, et al. Ageing diminishes endothelium-dependent vasodilatation and tetrahydrobiopterin content in rat skeletal muscle arterioles. *J Physiol.* 2008;586:1161–1168.

29. Kang DH, Anderson S, Kim YG, et al. Impaired angiogenesis in the aging kidney: vascular endothelial growth factor and thrombospondin-1 in renal disease. *Am J Kidney Dis.* 2001;37:601–611.

30. Long DA, Price KL, Mu W, et al. Angiopoietin-1, a vascular growth factor with a potentially novel role in aging (abstract). *J Am Soc Nephrol.* 2004;15:477A.

31. Nichols WW, O'Rourke MF. *McDonald's Blood Flow in Arteries: Theoretical, Experimental and Clinical Principles*, 5th ed. London, England: Hodder Arnold Publishers; 2005.

32. Virmani R, Avolio AP, Mergner WJ, et al. Effect of aging on aortic morphology in populations with high and low prevalence of hypertension and atherosclerosis. *Am J Pathol.* 1991;139:1119–1129.

33. Boutouyrie P, Laurent S, Benetos A, et al. Opposing effects of aging on distal and proximal large arteries of hypertensives. *J Hypertens.* 1992;10(suppl 6): S87–S91.

34. Laurent S, Cockcroft J, van Bortel L, et al. European Network for Non-invasive Investigation of Large Arteries. Expert consensus document on arterial stiffness: methodological issues and clinical applications. *Eur Heart J.* 2006;27:2588–2605.

35. Verhave JC, Fesler P, du Cailar G, et al. Elevated pulse pressure is associated with low renal function in elderly patients with isolated systolic hypertension. *Hypertension.* 2005;45:586–591.

36. O'Rourke MF. Arterial aging: pathophysiological principles. *Vasc Med.* 2007;12:329–341.

37. Fisher CM. Lacunar strokes and infarcts: a review. *Neurology.* 1982;32: 871–876.

38. Cullen KM, Kocsi Z, Stone J. Pericapillary haem-rich deposits: evidence for microhaemorrhages in aging human cerebral cortex. *J Cereb Blood Flow.* 2005;25: 1656–1667.

39. Cullen KM, Kocsi Z, Stone J. Microvascular pathology in the aging human brain: evidence that senile plaques are sites of microhemorrhages. *Neurobiol Aging.* 2006;27:1786–1796.

40. Buee L, Hof PR, Delacourte A. Brain microvascular changes in Alzheimer's disease and other dementias. *Ann N Y Acad Sci.* 1997;826:7–24.

41. Nichols W, O'Rourke M. Principles of measurement, preventing and treating arterial stiffness. In: Safar ME, O'Rourke MF, eds. *Arterial Stiffness, Vol 23: Handbook of Hypertension*. Philadelphia, PA: Elsevier 2006: 137–160,503–516.

42. Morrissey PE, Yango AF. Renal transplantation: older recipients and donors. *Clin Geriatr Med.* 2006;22(3):687–707.

43. Lindeman RD, Tobin J, Shock NW. Longitudinal studies on the rate of decline in renal function with age. *J Am Geriatr Soc.* 1985;33(4):278–285.

44. Maher FT, Nolan NG, Elveback LR. Comparison of simultaneous clearances of 125-I-labeled sodium iothalamate (Glofil) and of inulin. *Mayo Clin Proc.* 1971;46:690–691.

45. Cockcroft DW, Gault MH. Prediction of creatinine clearance from serum creatinine. *Nephron.* 1976;16:31.

46. Levey AS, Bosch JP, Lewis JB, et al. A more accurate method to estimate glomerular filtration rate from serum creatinine: a new prediction equation. Modification of Diet in Renal Disease Study Group. *Ann Intern Med.* 1999;130:461.

47. Wieczorowska-Tobis K, Niemir ZI, Guzik P, Breborowicz A, Oreopoulos DG. Difference in estimated GFR with two different formulas in elderly individuals. *Int Urol Nephrol.* 2006;38:381–385.

48. Berman N, Hostetter TH. Comparing the Cockcroft Gault and MDRD equations for calculation of GFR and drug doses in the elderly. *Nat Clin Pract Nephrol.* 2007;3:644–645.

49. Levey AS, Stevens LA, Schmid CH, et al. A new equation to estimate glomerular filtration rate. *Ann Intern Med.* 2009;150:604–612.

50. Corsonello A, Pedone C, Lattanzio F, et al. Chronic kidney disease and 1-year survival in elderly patients discharged from acute care hospitals: a comparison of three glomerular filtration rate equations. *Nephrol Dial Transplant.* 2010;26:360–364.

51. Ognibene A, Mannucci E, Caldini A, et al. Cystatin C reference values and aging. *Clin Biochem.* 2006;39(6):658–661.

52. Peralta CA, Katz RK, Sarnak MJ, et al. Cystatin C identifies chronic kidney disease patients at higher risk for complications. *J Am Soc Nephrol.* 2011;22:147–155.

53. Rowe JW, Shock NW, DeFronzo RA. The influence of age on the renal response to water deprivation in man. *Nephron.* 1976;17:270–278.

54. Preisser L, Teillet L, Aliotti S, et al. Downregulation of aquaporin-2 and -3 in aging kidney is independent of V_2 vasopressin receptor. *Am J Physiol Renal Physiol.* 2000;279: F144–F152.

55. Combet S, Teillet L, Geelen G, et al. Food restriction prevents age-related polyuria by vasopressin-dependent recruitment of aquaporin-2. *Am J Physiol Renal Physiol.* 2001;281:F1123–F1131.

56. Combat S, Geffroy N, Berthonaud V, et al. Correction of age related polyuria by dDAVP: molecular analysis of aquaporins and urea transporters. *Am J Physiol Renal Physiol.* 2003;284:F199–F208.

57. Tian Y, Riazi S, Khan O, et al. Renal ENaC subunit, Na-K-2Cl and Na-Cl cotransporter abundances in aged, water-restricted F344 × Brown Norway rats. *Kidney Int.* 2006;69:304–312.

58. Bengele HH, Mathias RS, Perkins JH, et al. Urinary concentrating defect in the aged rat. *Am J Physiol.* 1981;240:F147–F150.

59. Sunderam SG, Mankikar GD. Hyponatraemia in the elderly. *Age Aging.* 1983;12:77–80.

60. Adrogue HJ, Madias NE. Hyponatremia. *N Engl J Med.* 2000;342:1581–1589.

61. Ellison DH, Berl T. The syndrome of inappropriate antidiuresis. *N Engl J Med.* 2007;356:2064–2072.

62. Epstein M, Hollenberg NK. Age as a determinant of renal sodium conservation in normal man. *J Lab Chin Med.* 1976;87(3):411–417.

63. Musso CG, Liakopoulos V, Ioannidis I, Eleftheriadis T, Stefanidis I. Acute renal failure in the elderly: particular characteristics. *Int Urol Nephrol.* 2006;38:787–793.

64. Luft FC, Grim CE, Fineberg N, et al. Effects of volume expansion and contraction in normotensive whites, blacks and subjects of different ages. *Circulation.* 1979;59:644–650.

65. Luft FC, Weinberger MH, Fineberg NS, et al. Effects of age on renal sodium homeostasis and its relevance to sodium sensitivity. *Am J Med.* 1987; 82(1B):9–15.

66. Baylis C. Renal responses to acute angiotensin II inhibition and administered angiotensin II in the aging, conscious. chronically catheterized rat. *Am J Kidney Dis.* 1993;22:842–850.

67. Weidmann P, Demyttenaere-Bursztein S, Maxwell MH, et al. Effect of aging on plasma renin and aldosterone in normal man. *Kidney Int.* 1975;8:325–333.

68. Tsunoda K, Abe K, Goto T. Effect of age on the renin-angiotensin-aldosterone system in normal subjects: Simultaneous measurement of active and inactive renin, renin substrate and aldosterone in plasma. *J Chin Endocrinol Metab.* 1986;62: 384–389.

69. Weidman P, Beretta-Piccohl C, Ziegler WH, et al. Age versus urinary sodium for judging renin, aldosterone, and catecholamine levels: Studies in normal subjects and patients with essential hypertension. *Kidney Int.* 1978;14:619–628.

70. Skott P, Ingersbev J, Damkjaer Niebseon M, et al. The renin-angiotensin-aldosterone system in normal 85-year old people. *Scand J Chin Lab Invest.* 1987;47:6974.
71. Musso C, Liakopoulos V, De Miguel R, Imperiali N, Algranati L. Transtubular potassium concentration gradient: comparison between healthy old people and chronic renal failure patients. *Int Urol Nephrol.* 2006;38:387–390.
72. Maric C, Aldred GP, Antoine AM, et al. Effects of angiotensin II on cultured rat renomedullary interstitial cells are mediated by AT1A receptors. *Am J Physiol.* 1996; 271: F1020–1028.
73. Wolf G, Ziyadeh FN, Zahner G, Stahl RA. Angiotensin II is mitogenic for cultured rat glomerular endothelial cells. *Hypertension.* 1996;27:897–905.
74. Anderson S, Brenner BM. Effects of aging on the renal glomerulus. *Am J Med.* 1986;80:435–442.
75. Inserra F, Romano LA, de Cavanagh EM, et al. Renal interstitial sclerosis in aging: effects of enalapril and nifedipine. *J Am Soc Nephrol.* 1996;7:676–680.
76. Vaughan DE, Lazos SA, Tong K. Angiotensin II regulates the expression of plasminogen activator inhibitor-1 in cultured endothelial cells. A potential link between the renin-angiotensin system and thrombosis. *J Clin Invest.* 1995;95:995–1001.
77. Jung FF, Kennefick TM, Ingelfinger JR, Vora JP, Anderson S. Dow regulation of the intrarenal renin-angiotensin system in aging rat. *J Am Soc Nephrol.* 1995;5:1573–1580.
78. Ma LJ, Nakamura S, Aldigier JC, et al. Regression of glomerulosclerosis with high-dose angiotensin inhibition is linked to decreased plasminogen activator inhibitor-1. *J Am Soc Nephrol.* 2005;16:966–976.
79. Thomas MC, Tikellis C, Burns WM, et al. Interactions between renin angiotensin system and advanced glycation in the kidney. *J Am Soc Nephrol.* 2005; 16:2976–2984.
80. Baumann M, Bartholome R, Peutz-Kootstra CJ, Smits JF, Struijker-Boudier HA. Sustained tubulo-interstitial protection in SHRs by transient losartan treatment; an effect of decelerated aging? *Am J Hypertens.* 2008;21:177–182.
81. Eisenstaedt R, Penninx BW, Woodman RC. Anemia in the elderly: current understanding and emerging concepts. *Blood Rev.* 2006;20:213–226.
82. Ble A, Fink JC, Woodman RC, et al. Renal function, erythropoietin, and anemia of older persons: the InCHIANTI study. *Arch Intern Med.* 2005;165: 2222–2227.
83. Ershler WB, Sheng S, McKelvey J, et al. Serum erythropoietin and aging: a longitudinal analysis. *J Am Geriatr Soc.* 2005;53:1360–1365.
84. Ferrucci L, Guralnik JM, Bandinelli S, et al. Unexplained anaemia in older persons is characterised by low erythropoietin and low levels of pro-inflammatory markers. *Br J Haematol.* 2007;136:849–855.
85. Drueke TB, Locatelli F, Clyne N, et al. Normalization of hemoglobin level in patients with chronic kidney disease and anemia. *N Engl J Med.* 2006; 355:2071–2084.
86. Singh AK, Szczech L, Tang KL, et al. Correction of anemia with epoetin alfa in chronic kidney disease. *N Engl J Med.* 2006; 355:2085–2098.
87. Pfeffer MA, Burdmann EA, Chen CY, et al. A trial of darbepoetin alfa in type 2 diabetes and chronic kidney disease. *N Engl J Med.* 2009;361:2019–2032.
88. Vaziri ND, Zhou XJ. Potential mechanisms of adverse outcomes in trials of anemia correction with erythropoietin in chronic kidney disease. *Nephrol Dial Transplant.* 2009; 24:1082–1088.
89. Vaziri ND. Anemia and anemia correction: surrogate markers or causes of mortality in chronic kidney disease. *Nat Clin Pract Nephrol.* 2008;4:436–445.
90. Dukas L, Schacht E, Stähelin HB. In elderly men and women treated for osteoporosis a low creatinine clearance of <65 ml/min is a risk factor for falls and fractures. *Osteoporos Int.* 2005;16:1683–1690.
91. Gallagher JC, Rapuri P, Smith L. Falls are associated with decreased renal function and insufficient calcitriol production by the kidney. *J Steroid Biochem Mol Biol.* 2007;103:610–613.
92. Arnaud CD, Sanchez SD. The role of calcium in osteoporosis. *Annu Rev Nutr.* 1990;10:397–414.
93. Zhang Z, Sun L, Wang Y, et al. Renoprotective effects of vitamin D receptor in diabetic nephropathy. *Kidney Int.* 2008;73:163–171.
94. Zhang Y, Kong J, Deb DK, Chang A, Li LY. Vitamin D receptor attenuates renal fibrosis by suppressing renin-angiotensin system. *J Am Soc Nephrol.* 2010;21:966–973.
95. Ravani P, Malberti F, Tripepi G, et al. Vitamin D levels and patient outcome in chronic kidney disease. *Kidney Int.* 2009;75:88–95.
96. Lambers-Heerspink HJ, Agarwal R, Coyne DW, et al. The selective vitamin D receptor activator for albuminuria lowering (VITAL) study; study design and baseline characteristics. *Am J Nephrol.* 2009;30:280–286.
97. Mensenkamp AR, Hoenderop JG, Bindels RJ. Recent advances in renal tubular calcium reabsorption. *Curr Opin Nephrol Hypertens.* 2006;15:524–529.
98. Clapham DE, Julius D, Montell C, et al. International Union of Pharmacology XLIX Nomenclature and Structure-Function Relationships of Transient Receptor Potential Channels. *Pharmacol Rev.* 2005;57:427–450.
99. Hoenderop JG, Muller D, van der Kemp AW, et al. Calcitriol controls the epithelial calcium channel in kidney. *J Am Soc Nephrol.* 2001;12:1342–1349.
100. Chang Q, Hoefs S, van der Kemp AW, et al. The beta-glucuronidase Klotho hydrolyzes and activates the TRPV5 channel. *Science.* 2005;310:490–493.
101. Kuro-OM, Matsumura Y, Aizawa H, et al. Mutation of the mouse Klotho gene leads to a syndrome resembling ageing. *Nature.* 1997;390:45–51.
102. Jiang H, Ju Z, Rudolph KL. Telomere shortening and ageing. *Z Gerontol Geriat.* 2007; 40:314–324.
103. Hayflick L, Moorhead PS. The serial cultivation of human diploid cell strains. *Exp Cell Res.* 1961;25:585–621.
104. Melk A, Schmidt BM, Takeuchi O, et al. Expression of p16INK4a and other cell cycle regulator and senescence-associated genes in aging human kidney. *Kidney Int.* 2004;65:510–520.
105. Chkhotua AB, Gabusi E, Altimari A, et al. Increased expression of p16(INK4a) and p27(Kip1) cyclin-dependent kinase inhibitor genes in aging kidney and chronic allograft nephropathy. *Am J Kidney Dis.* 2003;41(6): 1303–1313.
106. Houben JM, Moonen HJ, van Schooten FJ, Hageman GJ. Telomere length assessment: Biomarker of chronic oxidative stress? *Free Radic Biol Med.* 2008;44:235–246.
107. Blackburn EH. Switching and signaling at telomere. *Cell.* 2001;106:661–673.
108. de Meyer T, Rietzschel ER, de Buyzere ML, et al. Studying telomeres in a longitudinal population based study. *Front Biosci.* 2008;13:2960–2970.
109. Westhoff JH, Schildhorn C, Jacobi C, et al. Telomere shortening reduces regenerative capacity after acute kidney injury. *J Am Soc Nephrol.* 2010;21:327–336.
110. Kuroso M, Matsumura Y, Aizawa H, et al. Mutation of the mouse Klotho gene leads to a syndrome resembling ageing. *Nature.* 1997;390:45–51.
111. Arking DE, Krebsova A, Macek M Sr, et al. Association of human aging with a functional variant of Klotho. *Proc Natl Acad Sci USA.* 2002;99:856–861.
112. Tohyama O, Imura A, Iwano A, et al. Klotho is a novel beta-glucuronidase capable of hydrolyzing steroid beta-glucuronides. *J Biol Chem.* 2004;279: 9777–9784.
113. Kurosu H, Yamamoto M, Clark JD, et al. Suppression of aging in mice by the hormone Klotho. *Science.* 2005;309:1829–1833.
114. Kuro-o M. Klotho as a regulator of oxidative stress and senescence. *Biol Chem.* 2008;389:233–241.
115. Mitobe M, Yoshida T, Sugiura H, et al. Oxidative stress decreases Klotho expression in a mouse kidney cell line. *Nephron Exp Nephrol.* 2005;101:e67–74.
116. Zhang H, Li YY, Fan YB, et al. Klotho is a target gene of PPAR-gamma. *Kidney Int.* 2008;74:732–739.
117. Razzaque MS, Sitara D, Taguchi T, et al. Premature aging-like phenotype in fibroblast growth factor 23 null mice is a vitamin D-mediated process. *FASEB J.* 2006;20:720–722.
118. Kurosu H, Ogawa Y, Miyoshi M, et al. Regulation of fibroblast growth factor-23 signaling by Klotho. *J Biol Chem.* 2006;281:6120–6123.
119. Kharitonenkov A, Shiyanova TL, Koester A, et al. FGF-21 as a novel metabolic regulator. *J Clin Invest.* 2005;115:1627–1635.
120. Saito K, Ishizaka N, Mitani H, et al. Iron chelation and free radical scavenger suppress angiotensin II–induced downregulation of Klotho, an anti-aging gene, in rat. *FEBS Lett.* 2003;551:58–62.
121. Koh N, Fujimori T, Nishiguchi S, et al. Severely reduced production of Klotho in human chronic renal failure. *Biochem Biophys Res Commun.* 2001;280:1015–1020.
122. Kuro-o M. A potential link between phosphate and aging—lessons from Klotho-deficient mice. *Mech Ageing Dev.* 2010;131:270–275.
123. Hu MC, Shi M, Zhang J, et al. Klotho deficiency causes vascular calcification in chronic kidney disease. *J Am Soc Nephrol.* 2011;22:124–136.
124. Huang CL. Regulation of ion channels by secreted Klotho: mechanisms and implications. *Kidney Int.* 2010;77:855–860.
125. Haruna Y, Kashihara N, Satoh M, et al. Amelioration of progressive renal injury by genetic manipulation of Klotho gene. *Proc Natl Acad Sci U S A.* 2007;104: 2331–2336.
126. Mitani H, Ishizaka N, Aizawa T, et al. In vivo Klotho gene transfer ameliorates angiotensin II-induced renal damage. *Hypertension.* 2002;39:838.
127. Mendoz-Nunez VM, Ruiz-Ramos M, Sanchez-Rodriguez MA, et al. Aging related oxidative stress in healthy humans. *Tohoku J Exp Med.* 2007;213:261–268.
128. Jung T, Bader N, Grune T. Lipofuscin: Formation, distribution and metabolic consequences. *Ann N Y Acad Sci.* 2007;1119:97–111.
129. Melk A, Kittikowit W, Sandhu I, et al. Cell senescence in rat kidneys in vivo increases with growth and age despite lack of telomere shortening. *Kidney Int.* 2003;63: 2134–2143.
130. Frenkel-Denkberg G, Gershon D, Levy AP. The function of hypoxia-inducible factor 1 (HIF-1) is impaired in senescent mice. *FEBS Lett.* 1999;462:341–344.
131. Zou AP, Cowley AW Jr. Reactive oxygen species and molecular regulation of renal oxygenation. *Acta Physiol Scand.* 2003;179:233–241.

132. Reckelhoff JF, Kanji V, Racusen LC, et al. Vitamin E ameliorates enhanced renal lipid peroxidation and accumulation of F2-isoprostanes in aging kidneys. *Am J Physiol.* 1998;274:R767–774.
133. Verbeke P, Perichon M, Friguet B, Bakala H. Inhibition of nitric oxide synthase activity by early and advanced glycation end products in cultured rabbit proximal tubular epithelial cells. *Biochim Biophys Acta.* 2000;1502:481–494.
134. Thomas SE, Anderson S, Gordon KL, et al. Tubulointerstitial disease in aging: evidence for underlying peritubular capillary damage, a potential role for renal ischemia. *J Am Soc Nephrol.* 1998;9:231–242.
135. Basso N, Paglia N, Stella I, et al. Protective effect of the inhibition of the renin-angiotensin system on aging. *Regul Pept.* 2005;128:247–252.
136. de Cavanagh EM, Piotrkowski B, Basso N, et al. Enalapril and losartan attenuate mitochondrial dysfunction in aged rats. *FASEB J.* 2003;17:1096–1098.
137. Mitobe M, Yoshida T, Sugiura H, et al. Oxidative stress decreases Klotho expression in a mouse kidney cell line. *Nephron Exp Nephrol.* 2005;101:e67–e74.
138. Huang C, Li J, Ke Q, et al. Ultraviolet-induced phosphorylation of p70(S6K) at Thr(389) and Thr(421)/Ser(424) involves hydrogen peroxide and mammalian target of rapamycin but not Akt and atypical protein kinase C. *Cancer Res.* 2002;62:5689–5697.
139. Adler S, Huang H, Wolin MS, Kaminski PM. Oxidant stress leads to impaired regulation of renal cortical oxygen consumption by nitric oxide in the aging kidney. *J Am Soc Nephrol.* 2004;15:52–60.
140. Kim HJ, Jung KJ, Yu BP, Cho CG, Chung HY. Influence of aging and calorie restriction on MAPKs activity in rat kidney. *Exp Gerontol.* 2002;37:1041–1053.
141. Hartleben B, Gödel M, Meyer-Schwesinger C, et al. Autophagy influences glomerular disease susceptibility and maintains podocyte homeostasis in aging mice. *J Clin Invest.* 2010;120:1084–1096.
142. Blagosklonny MV. Program-like aging and mitochondria: instead of random damage by free radicals. *J Cell Biochem.* 2007;102:1389–1399.
143. Lee RC, Feinbaum RL, Ambros V. The *C. elegans* heterochronic gene lin-4 encodes small RNAs with antisense complementarity to lin-14. *Cell.* 1993;75: 843–854.
144. Griffiths-Jones S, Saini HK, van Dongen S, Enright AJ. miRBase: tools for microRNA genomics. *Nucleic Acids Res.* 2008;3:D154–158.
145. Kim VN, Han J, Siomi MC. Biogenesis of small RNAs in animals. *Nat Rev Mol Cell Biol.* 2009;10:126–139.
146. Brodersen P, Voinnet O. Revisiting the principles of microRNA target recognition and mode of action. *Nat Rev Mol Cell Biol.* 2009;10:141–148.
147. Grillari J, Grillari-Voglauer R. Novel modulators of senescence, aging, and longevity: Small non-coding RNAs enter the stage. *Exp Gerontol.* 2010;45:302–311.
148. Ruan XZ, Varghese Z, Moorhead JF. An update on the lipid nephrotoxicity hypothesis. *Nat Rev Nephrol.* 2009;5:713–721.
149. Jiang T, Wang Z, Proctor G, et al. Diet-induced obesity in C57BL/6J mice causes increased renal lipid accumulation and glomerulosclerosis via a sterol regulatory element-binding protein-1c-dependent pathway. *J Biol Chem.* 2005;280:32317–32325.
150. Kim HJ, Moradi H, Vaziri ND. Renal mass reduction results in accumulation of lipids and dysregulation of lipid regulatory proteins in the remnant kidney. *Am J Physiol Renal Physiol.* 2009; 296(6):F1297–1306.
151. Vaziri ND. Lipotoxicity and impaired HDL-mediated reverse cholesterol/lipid transport in chronic kidney disease. *J Ren Nutr.* 2010;20:S35–S43.
152. Erhuma A, Salter AM, Sculley DV, Langley-Evans SC, Bennett AJ. Prenatal exposure to a low-protein diet programs disordered regulation of lipid metabolism in the aging rat. *Am J Physiol Endocrinol Metab.* 2007;292:E1702–1714.
153. Jiang T, Liebman SE, Lucia MS, Li J, Levi M. Role of altered renal lipid metabolism and the sterol regulatory element binding proteins in the pathogenesis of age-related renal disease. *Kidney Int.* 2005;68:2608–2620.
154. Cha DR, Han JY, Su DM, et al. Peroxisome proliferator-activated receptor-alpha deficiency protects aged mice from insulin resistance induced by high fat diet. *Am J Nephrol.* 2007;27:479–482.
155. Vila L, Roglans N, Alegret M, et al. Hepatic gene expression changes in an experimental model of accelerated senescence: the SAM-P8 mouse. *J Gerontol A Biol Sci Med Sci.* 2008;63:1043–1052.
156. Wang XX, Jiang T, Shen Y, et al. The farnesoid X receptor modulates renal lipid metabolism and diet-induced renal inflammation, fibrosis, and proteinuria. *Am J Physiol Renal Physiol.* 2009;297:F1587–1596.
157. Vlassara H. Advanced glycosylation in nephropathy of diabetes and aging. *Adv Nephrol Necker Hosp.* 1996;25:303–315.
158. He C, Sabol J, Mitsuhashi T, Vlassara H. Dietary glycotoxins: inhibition of reactive products by aminoguanidine facilitates renal clearance and reduces tissue sequestration. *Diabetes.*1999;48:1308–1315.
159. Lu C, He JC, Cai W, et al. Advanced glycation end product (AGE) receptor 1 is a negative regulator of the inflammatory response to AGE in mesangial cells. *Proc Natl Acad Sci U S A.* 2004;101:11767–11772.
160. Cai W, He JC, Zhu L, et al. AGE-receptor-1 counteracts cellular oxidant stress induced by AGEs via negative regulation of p66shc-dependent FKHRL1 phosphorylation. *Am J Physiol Cell Physiol.* 2008;294:C145–152.
161. Cai W, Torreggiani M, Zhu L, et al. AGER1 regulates endothelial cell NADPH oxidase-dependent oxidant stress via PKC-delta: implications for vascular disease. *Am J Physiol Cell Physiol.* 2010;298:C624–634.
162. Cai W, He JC, Zhu L, et al. Reduced oxidant stress and extended lifespan in mice exposed to a low glycotoxin diet: association with increased AGER1 expression. *Am J Pathol.* 2007;170:1893–1902.
163. Li YM, Steffes M, Donnelly T, et al. Prevention of cardiovascular and renal pathology of aging by the advanced glycation inhibitor aminoguanidine. *Proc Natl Acad Sci U S A.* 1996;93:3902–3907.
164. Vlassara H, Cai W, Goodman S, et al. Protection against loss of innate defenses in adulthood by low advanced glycation end products (AGE) intake: role of the anti inflammatory AGE receptor-1. *J Clin Endocrinol Metab.* 2009;94: 4483–4491.
165. Teillet L, Verbeke P, Gouraud S, et al. Food restriction prevents advanced glycation end product accumulation and retards kidney aging in lean rats. *J Am Soc Nephrol.* 2000;11:1488–1497.
166. Russell SJ, Kahn CR. Endocrine regulation of ageing. *Nat Rev Mol Cell Biol.* 2007; 8:681–691.
167. Mair W, Dillin A. Aging and survival: the genetics of life span extension by dietary restriction. *Annu Rev Biochem.* 2008;77:727–754.
168. Masoro EJ. Caloric restriction-induced life extension of rats and mice: a critique of proposed mechanisms. *Biochim Biophys Acta.* 2009;1790:1040–1048.
169. Finkel T, Deng CX, Mostoslavsky R. Recent progress in the biology and physiology of sirtuins. *Nature.* 2009;460:587–591.
170. Imai S. SIRT1 and caloric restriction: an insight into possible trade-offs between robustness and frailty. *Curr Opin Clin Nutr Metab Care.* 2009;12:350–356.
171. Cohen HY, Miller C, Bitterman KJ, et al. Calorie restriction promotes mammalian cell survival by inducing the SIRT1 deacetylase. *Science.* 2004;305: 390–392.
172. Pfluger PT, Herranz D, Velasco-Miguel S, Serrano M, Tschop MH. Sirt1 protects against high-fat diet-induced metabolic damage. *Proc Natl Acad Sci U S A.* 2008;105:9793–9798.
173. Lagouge M, Argmann C, Gerhart-Hines Z, et al. Resveratrol improves mitochondrial function and protects against metabolic disease by activating SIRT1 and PGC-1alpha. *Cell.* 2006;127:1109–1122.
174. Kume S, Uzu T, Horiike K, et al. Calorie restriction enhances cell adaptation to hypoxia through Sirt1-dependent mitochondrial autophagy in mouse aged kidney. *J Clin Invest.* 2010;120:1043–1055.
175. Li X, Zhang S, Blander G, et al. SIRT1 deacetylates and positively regulates the nuclear receptor LXR. *Mol Cell.* 2007;28:91–106.
176. Kemper JK, Xiao Z, Ponugoti B, et al. FXR acetylation is normally dynamically regulated by p300 and SIRT1 but constitutively elevated in metabolic disease states. *Cell Metab.* 2009;10:392–404.
177. Sharp ZD, Bartke A. Evidence for down-regulation of phosphoinositide 3 kinase/Akt/mammalian target of rapamycin (PI3K/Akt/mTOR)-dependent translation regulatory signaling pathways in Ames dwarf mice. *J Gerontol A Biol Sci Med Sci.* 2005;60:293–300.
178. Stanfel MN, Shamieh LS, Kaeberlein M, Kennedy BK. The TOR pathway comes of age. *Biochim Biophys Acta.* 2009;1790:1067–1074.
179. Selman C, Tullet JM, Wieser D, et al. Ribosomal protein S6 kinase 1 signaling regulates mammalian life span. *Science.* 2009;326:140–144.
180. Rodwell GE, Sonu R, Zahn JM, et al. A transcriptional profile of aging in the human kidney. *PLoS Biol.* 2004;2:e427.
181. Ruggenenti P, Perna A, Gherardi G, et al. Renoprotective properties of ACE inhibition in non-diabetic nephropathies with non-nephrotic proteinuria. *Lancet.* 1999;354:359–364.
182. Hou FF, Zhang X, Zhang GH, et al. Efficacy and safety of benazepril for advanced chronic renal insufficiency. *N Engl J Med.* 2006;354:131–140.
183. Parving HH, Lehnert H, Brochner-Mortensen J, et al. The effect of irbesartan on the development of diabetic nephropathy in patients with type 2 diabetes. *N Engl J Med.* 2001;345:870–878.
184. van der Meer IM, Cravedi P, Remuzzi G. The role of renin angiotensin system inhibition in kidney repair. *Fibrogenesis Tissue Repair.* 2010;3:7.
185. Guney I, Selcuk NY, Altintepe L, et al. Antifibrotic effects of aldosterone receptor blocker (spironolactone) in patients with chronic kidney disease. *Ren Fail.* 2009;31:779–784.
186. Parving HH, Persson F, Lewis JB, Lewis EJ, Hollenberg NK. Aliskiren combined with losartan in type 2 diabetes and nephropathy. *N Engl J Med.* 2008;358:2433–2446.
187. Beckett NS, Peters R, Fletcher AE, et al. Treatment of hypertension in patients 80 years of age or older. *N Engl J Med.* 2008;358:1887–1898.

188. Miyagawa K, Dohi Y, Nakazawa A, et al. Renoprotective effect of calcium channel blockers in combination with an angiotensin receptor blocker in elderly patients with hypertension. A randomized crossover trial between benidipine and amlodipine. *Clin Exp Hypertens*. 2010;32:1–7.
189. Ford ES, Giles WH, Dietz WH. Prevalence of the metabolic syndrome among US adults: findings from the third National Health and Nutrition Examination Survey. *JAMA*. 2002;287:356–359.
190. Windler E, Schoffauer M, Zyriax BC. The significance of low HDL-cholesterol levels in an ageing society at increased risk for cardiovascular disease. *Diab Vasc Dis Res*. 2007;4:136–142.
191. Ben-Avraham S, Harman-Boehm I, Schwarzfuchs D, Shai I. Dietary strategies for patients with type 2 diabetes in the era of multi-approaches; review and results from the Dietary Intervention Randomized Controlled Trial (DIRECT). *Diabetes Res Clin Pract*. 2009;86(Suppl 1):S41–48.
192. Kelly RB. Diet and exercise in the management of hyperlipidemia. *Am Fam Physician*. 2010;81:1097–1102.
193. Tonelli M, Isles C, Craven T, et al. Effect of pravastatin on rate of kidney function loss in people with or at risk for coronary disease. *Circulation*. 2005; 112:171–178.
194. Gugliucci A, Kotani K, Taing J, et al. Short-term low calorie diet intervention reduces serum advanced glycation end products in healthy overweight or obese adults. *Ann Nutr Metab*. 2009;54:197–201.
195. Patel A, MacMahon S, Chalmers J, et al. Intensive blood glucose control and vascular outcomes in patients with type 2 diabetes. *N Engl J Med*. 2008;358: 2560–2572.
196. Blumenthal JA, Babyak MA, Sherwood A, et al. Effects of the dietary approaches to stop hypertension diet alone and in combination with exercise and caloric restriction on insulin sensitivity and lipids. *Hypertension*. 2010;55:1199–1205.
197. Willcox DC, Willcox BJ, Todoriki H, Suzuki M. The Okinawan diet: health implications of a low-calorie, nutrient-dense, antioxidant-rich dietary pattern low in glycemic load. *J Am Coll Nutr*. 2009;28(Suppl):500S–516S.
198. Kennerfalk A, Ruigomez A, Wallander MA, Wilhelmsen L, Johansson S. Geriatric drug therapy and healthcare utilization in the United Kingdom. *Ann Pharmacother*. 2002;36:797–803.
199. Ebbesen J, Buajordet I, Erikssen J, et al. Drug-related deaths in a department of internal medicine. *Arch Intern Med*. 2001;161:2317–2323.
200. Laliberte MC, Normandeau M, Lord A, et al. Use of over-the-counter medications and natural products in patients with moderate and severe chronic renal insufficiency. *Am J Kidney Dis*. 2007;49:245–256.
201. Gooch K, Culleton BF, Manns BJ, et al. NSAID use and progression of chronic kidney disease. *Am J Med*. 2007;120:280.e1–e7.
202. Bagshaw SM, George C, Bellomo R. A comparison of the RIFLE and AKIN criteria for acute kidney injury in critically ill patients. *Nephrol Dial Transplant*. 2008;23:1569–1574.
203. Joannidis M, Metnitz B, Bauer P, et al. Acute kidney injury in critically ill patients classified by AKIN versus RIFLE using the SAPS 3 database. *Intensive Care Med*. 2009;35:1692–1702.
204. Jerkic M, Vojvodic S, Lopez-Novoa JM. The mechanism of increased renal susceptibility to toxic substances in the elderly. *Int Urol Nephrol*. 2001;32: 539–547.
205. Rosner MH. Urinary biomarkers for the detection of renal injury. *Adv Clin Chem*. 2009;49:73–97.
206. Xue JL, Daniels F, Star RA, et al. Incidence and mortality of acute renal failure in Medicare beneficiaries, 1992 to 2001. *J Am Soc Nephrol*. 2006;17:1135–1142.
207. Coca SG. Acute kidney injury in elderly persons. *Am J Kidney Dis*. 2010;56:122–131.
208. Bouchard J, Soroko SB, Chertow GM, et al. Fluid accumulation, survival and recovery of kidney function in critically ill patients with acute kidney injury. *Kidney Int*. 2009;76:422–427.
209. Prowle JR, Echeverri JE, Ligabo EV, Ronco C, Bellomo R. Fluid balance and acute kidney injury. *Nat Rev Nephrol*. 2010;6:107–115.
210. Davison AM, Johnston PJ. Idiopathic glomerulonephritis in the elderly. *Contr Nephrol*. 1993;105:38–48.
211. Bomback AS, Appel GB, Radhakrishnan J, et al. ANCA-associated glomerulonephritis in the very elderly. *Kidney Int*. 2011;79:757–764.
212. Haas M, Spargo BH, Wit EJ, Meehan SM. Etiologies and outcome of acute renal insufficiency in older adults: A renal biopsy study of 259 cases. *Am J Kidney Dis*. 2000;35:433–447.
213. Moutzouris DA, Herlitz L, Appel GB, et al. Renal biopsy in the very elderly. *Clin J Am Soc Nephrol*. 2009;4:1073–1082.
214. Uezono S, Hara S, Sato Y, et al. Renal biopsy in elderly patients: A clinicopathological analysis. *Ren Fail*. 2006;28:549–555.
215. Glassock RJ. Glomerular disease in the elderly. *Clin Geriatr Med*. 2009; 25:413–422.
216. Vendemia F, Gesualdo L, Schena FP, D'Amico G. Epidemiology of primary glomerulonephritis in the elderly: Report from the Italian Registry of Renal Biopsy. *J Nephrol*. 2001;14:340–352.
217. Rogers T, Rakheja D, Zhou XJ. Glomerular diseases associated with nephritic syndrome and/or rapidly progressive glomerulonephritis. In: Zhou XJ, et al., eds. *Silva's Diagnostic Renal Pathology*. Cambridge, UK: Cambridge University Press; 2009: 178–228.
218. Nasr SH, Fidler ME, Valeri AM, et al. Postinfectious glomerulonephritis in the elderly. *J Am Soc Nephrol*. 2011;22:187–195.
219. Deegens JK, Wetzels JF. Membranous nephropathy in the older adult: epidemiology, diagnosis and management. *Drugs Aging*. 2007;24:717–732.
220. Lefaucheur C, Stengel B, Nochy D, et al. Membranous nephropathy and cancer: Epidemiologic evidence and determinants of high-risk cancer association. *Kidney Int*. 2006;70:1510–1517.
221. Beck LH, Salant DJ. Membranous nephropathy: Recent travels and new roads ahead. *Kidney Int*. 2010;77:765–770.
222. Ohtani H, Wakui H, Komatsuda A, et al. Distribution of glomerular IgG subclass deposits in malignancy-associated membranous nephropathy. *Nephrol Dial Transplant*. 2004;19:574–579.
223. Bjornklett R, Vikse BE, Svarstad E, et al. Long-term risk of cancer in membranous nephropathy patients. *Am J Kidney Dis*. 2007;50:396–403.
224. Lindskog A, Ebefors K, Johansson ME, et al. Melanocortin 1 receptor agonists reduce proteinuria. *J Am Soc Nephrol*. 2010;21:1290–1298.
225. Segarra A, Praga M, Ramos N, et al. Successful treatment of membranous glomerulonephritis with rituximab in calcineurin inhibitor dependent patients. *Clin J Am Soc Nephrol*. 2009;4:1083–1088.
226. Waldman M, Crew RJ, Valeri A, et al. Adult minimal-change disease: Clinical characteristics, treatment and outcomes. *Clin J Am Soc Nephrol*. 2007; 2:445–453.
227. Tse K-C, Lam M-F, Yip P-S, et al. Idiopathic minimal change nephrotic syndrome in older adults: Steroid responsiveness and pattern of relapses. *Nephrol Dial Transplant*. 2003;18:1316–1320.
228. Eguchi A, Takei T, Yoshida T, Tsuchiya K, Nitta K. Combined cyclosporine and prednisolone therapy in adult patients with the first relapse of minimal-change nephrotic syndrome. *Nephrol Dial Transplant*. 2010;25:124–129.
229. Haffner D, Fischer DC. Nephrotic syndrome and Rituximab: facts and perspectives. *Pediatr Nephrol*. 2009;24:1433–1438.
230. Higgins RM, Goldsmith DJ, Connolly J, et al. Vasculitis and rapidly progressive glomerulonephritis in the elderly. *Postgrad Med J*. 1996;72:41–44.
231. Mukhtyar C, Guillevin L, Cid MC, et al. EULAR recommendations for the management of primary small and medium vessel vasculitis. *Ann Rheum Dis*. 2009;68:310–317.
232. Jayne DR, Gaskin G, Rasmussen N, et al. European Vasculitis Study Group: Randomized trial of plasma exchange or high-dosage methylprednisolone as adjunctive therapy for severe renal vasculitis. *J Am Soc Nephrol*. 2007;18: 2180–2188.
233. Little MA, Nightingale P, Verburgh CA, et al. European Vasculitis Study Group: Early mortality in systemic vasculitis: Relative contributions of adverse events and active vasculitis. *Ann Rheum Dis*. 2010;69:1036–1043.
234. Little MA, Nazar L, Farrington K. Outcome in glomerulonephritis due to small vessel vasculitis: Effect of functional status and nonvasculitic morbidity. *Nephrol Dial Transplant*. 2004;19:356–364.
235. Stone JH, Merkel PA, Spiera R, et al. Rituximab versus cyclophosphamide for ANCA-associated vasculitis. *N Engl J Med*. 2010;363:221–232.
236. Lindic J, Vizjak A, Ferluga D, et al. Clinical outcome of patients with coexistent antineutrophil cytoplasmic antibodies and antibodies against glomerular basement membrane. *Ther Apher Dial*. 2009;13:278–281.
237. Dember LM. Amyloidosis-associated kidney diseases. *J Am Soc Nephrol*. 2006;17:3458–3471.
238. Lin J, Markowitz GA, Valeri AM, et al. Renal immunoglobulin deposition diseases: The clinical spectrum. *J Am Soc Nephrol*. 2001;12:1482–1492.
239. Kastritis E, Wechalekar AD, Dimopoulos MA, et al. Bortezomib with or without dexamethasone in primary (light chain) amyloidosis. *J Clin Oncol*. 2010;28:1031–1037.
240. Dimopoulos MA, Kastritis E, Rajkumar SV. Treatment of plasma cell dyscrasias with lenalidomide. *Leukemia*. 2008;22:1343–1353.
241. Dember LM. Modern treatment of amyloidosis: unresolved questions. *J Am Soc Nephrol*. 2009;20:469–472.
242. Davern S, Tang LX, Williams TK, et al. Immunodiagnostic capabilities of anti-free immunoglobulin light chain monoclonal antibodies. *Am J Clin Pathol*. 2008;130:702–711.
243. Hassoun H, Flombaum D, D'Agati VD, et al. High-dose melphalan and auto-SCT in patients with monoclonal Ig deposition disease. *Bone Marrow Transplant*. 2008;42:405–412.

244. Chobanian AV, Bakris GL, Black HR, et al. The Seventh Report of the Joint National Committee on prevention, detection, evaluation, and treatment of high blood pressure. *Hypertension.* 2003;42:1206–1252.
245. Supiano MA, Hogikyan RV, Sidani MA, et al. Sympathetic nervous system activity and alpha-adrenergic responsiveness in older hypertensive humans. *Am J Physiol.* 1999;276:E519–E528.
246. Sowers JR, Whaley-Connell A, Epstein M. Narrative review: the emerging clinical implications of the role of aldosterone in the metabolic syndrome and resistant hypertension. *Ann Intern Med.* 2009;150:776–783.
247. SHEP Cooperative Research Group. Prevention of stroke by antihypertensive drug treatment in older persons with isolated systolic hypertension. Final results of the Systolic Hypertension in the Elderly Program (SHEP). *JAMA.* 1991;265:3255–3264.
248. Psaty BM, Lumley T, Furberg CD, et al. Health outcomes associated with various antihypertensive therapies used as first-line agents: a network metaanalysis. *JAMA.* 2003;289:2534–2544.
249. Beckett NS, Peters R, Fletcher AE, et al. Treatment of hypertension in patients 80 years of age or older. *N Engl J Med.* 2008;358:1887–1898.
250. Sacks FM, Svetkey LP, Vollmer WM, et al. Effects on blood pressure of reduced dietary sodium and the Dietary Approaches to Stop Hypertension (DASH) diet. *N Engl J Med.* 2001;344:3–10.
251. Whelton PK, Appel LJ, Espeland MA, et al. Sodium reduction and weight loss in the treatment of hypertension in older persons: a randomized controlled trial of non-pharmacologic interventions in the elderly (TONE). *JAMA.* 1998;279:839–846.
252. Jamerson K, Weber MA, Bakris GI, et al. Benazepril plus amlodipine or hydrochlorothiazide for hypertension in high-risk patients. *N Engl J Med.* 2008; 359:2417–2428.
253. Coresh J, Selvin E, Stevens LA, et al. Prevalence of chronic kidney disease in the United States. *JAMA.* 2007; 298:2038–2047.
254. Eckardt KU, Berns JS, Rocco MV, et al. Definition and classification of CKD: The debate should be about patient prognosis—a position statement from KDOQI and KDIGO. *Am J Kidney Dis.* 2009;53:915–920.
255. Kurella TM, Wadley V, Yaffe M, et al. Kidney function and cognitive impairment in US adults: The Reasons for Geographic and Racial Differences in Stroke (REGARDS) study. *Am J Kidney Dis.* 2008;52:227–234.
256. Manjunath G, Tighiouart H, Coresh J, et al. Level of kidney function as a risk factor for cardiovascular outcomes in the elderly. *Kidney Int.* 2003;63: 1121–1129.
257. Shlipak MG, Sarnak MJ, Katz R, et al. Cystatin C and the risk of death and cardiovascular events among elderly persons. *N Engl J Med.* 2005;352:2049–2060.
258. Hallan SI, Astor B, Romundstad S, et al. Association of kidney function and albuminuria with cardiovascular mortality in older compared to younger individuals: The HUNT II study. *Arch Intern Med.* 2007;167:2490–2496.
259. Hemmelgarn BR, Zhang J, Manns BJ, et al. Progression of kidney dysfunction in the community-dwelling elderly. *Kidney Int.* 2006;69:2155–2161.
260. Shlipak MG, Katz R, Kestenbaum B, et al. Rate of kidney function decline in older adults: A comparison using creatinine and cystatin C. *Am J Nephrol.* 2009;30:171–178.
261. Demoulin N, Beguin C, Labriola L, Jadoul M. Preparing renal replacement therapy in stage 4 CKD patients referred to nephrologists: a difficult balance between futility and insufficiency. A cohort study of 386 patients followed in Brussels. *Nephrol Dial Transplant.* 2011;26:220–226.
262. Weiner DE, Bartolomei K, Scott T, et al. Albuminuria, cognitive functioning, and white matter hyperintensities in homebound elders. *Am J Kidney Dis.* 2009;53:438–447.
263. Barzilay JI, Fitzpatric AL, Luchsinger J, et al. Albuminuria and dementia in the elderly: A community study. *Am J Kidney Dis.* 2008;52:216–226.
264. Murray AM, Tupper PR, Knopman DS, et al. Cognitive impairment in hemodialysis patients is common. *Neurology.* 2006;67:216–223.
265. O'Hare AM. The management of older adults with a low eGFR: Moving toward an individualized approach. *Am J Kidney Dis.* 2009;53:925–927.
266. Steinman MA, Landefeld CS, Rosenthal GE, et al. Polypharmacy and prescribing quality in older people. *J Am Geriatr Soc.* 2006;54:516–523.
267. Fink JC, Brown J, Hsu VD, et al. CKD as an underrecognized threat to patient safety. *Am J Kidney Dis.* 2009;53:681–688.
268. Khurana A, McLean L, Atkinson S, et al. The effect of oral sodium phosphate drug products on renal function in adults undergoing bowel endoscopy. *Arch Intern Med.* 2008;168:593–597.
269. Einhorn LM, Zhan M, Hsu VD, et al. The frequency of hyperkalemia and its significance in chronic kidney disease. *Arch Intern Med.* 2009;169: 1156–1162.
270. Moen MF, Zhan M, Hsu VD, et al. Frequency of hypoglycemia and its significance in chronic kidney disease. *Clin J Am Soc Nephrol.* 2009;4:1121–1127.
271. Muntner P, Coresh J, Powe NR, Klag MJ. The contribution of increased diabetes prevalence and improved myocardial infarction and stroke survival to the increase in treated end-stage renal disease. *J Am Soc Nephrol.* 2003;14:1568–1577.
272. Waikar SS, Liu KD, Chertow GM. The incidence and prognostic significance of acute kidney injury. *Curr Opin Nephrol Hypertens.* 2007;16:227–236.
273. Schmitt R, Coca S, Kanbay M, et al. Recovery of kidney function after acute kidney injury in the elderly: a systematic review and meta-analysis. *Am J Kidney Dis.* 2008;52:262–271.
274. Ishani A, Xue JL, Himmelfarb J, et al. Acute kidney injury increases risk of ESRD among elderly. *J Am Soc Nephrol.* 2009;20:223–228.
275. Cecka JM. The UNOS scientific renal transplant registry. In: Cecka JM, Terasaki PI, eds. *Clinical Transplants 1996.* Los Angeles, CA: UCLA Tissue Typing Laboratory; 1997:1–14.
276. Saxena R, Yu X, Giraldo M, et al. Renal transplantation in the elderly. *Int Urol Nephrol.* 2009;41:195–210.
277. Perico N, Ruggenenti P, Scalamogna M, et al. Tackling the shortage of donor kidneys: how to use the best that we have. *Am J Nephrol.* 2003;23:245–259.
278. Metzger RA, Delmonico FL, Feng S, et al. Expanded criteria donors for kidney transplantation. *Am J Transplant.* 2003;3(Suppl 4):114–125.
279. Collini A, De Bartolomeis C, Ruggieri G, et al. Long-term outcome of renal transplantation from marginal donors. *Transplant Proc.* 2006;38:3398–3399.
280. Greenstein SM, Schwartz G, Schechner R, et al. Selective use of expanded criteria donors for renal transplantation with good results. *Transplant Proc.* 2006;38:3390–3392.
281. Cecka JM, Terasaki PI. Optimal use for older donor kidneys: older recipients. *Transplant Proc.* 1995;27:801–802.
282. Waiser J, Schreiber M, Budde K, et al. Age matching in renal transplantation. *Nephrol Dial Transplant.* 2000;15:696–700.
283. Stratta RJ, Rohr MS, Sundberg AK, et al. Intermediate-term outcomes with expanded criteria deceased donors in kidney transplantation: a spectrum or specter of quality? *Ann Surg.* 2006;243:594–603.
284. Schold JD, Kaplan B, Baliga RS, Meier-Kriesche HU. The broad spectrum of quality in deceased donor kidneys. *Am J Transplant.* 2005;5:757–765.
285. Schaeffner ES, Rose C, Gill JS. Access to kidney transplantation among the elderly in the United States: A glass half full, not half empty. *Clin J Am Soc Nephrol.* 2010;5:2109–2114.
286. Smits JM, Persijn GG, van Houwelingen HC, et al. Evaluation of the Eurotransplant Senior Program. The results of the first year. *Am J Transplant.* 2002;2:664–670.
287. Freia U, Noeldeke J, Machold-Fabriziic V, et al. Prospective age-matching in elderly kidney transplant recipients, a 5-year analysis of the Eurotransplant Senior Program. *Am J Transplant.* 2008;8:50–57.
288. Tan JC, Alfrey EJ, Dafoe DC, Millan MT, Scandling JD. Dual-kidney transplantation with organs from expanded criteria donors: a long-term follow-up. *Transplantation.* 2004;78:692–696.
289. Remuzzi G, Cravedi P, Perna A, et al. Long-term outcome of renal transplantation from older donors. *N Engl J Med.* 2006;354:343–352.
290. Kainz A, Perco P, Mayer B, et al. Gene-expression profiles and age of donor kidney biopsies obtained before transplantation distinguish medium term graft function. *Transplantation.* 2007;83:1048–1054.
291. Sung RS, Christinsen LL, Leichtman AB, et al. Determinants of discard of expanded criteria donor kidneys: impact of biopsy and machine perfusion. *Am J Transplant.* 2008;8:783–792.
292. Wolfe RA, Ashby VB, Milford EL, et al. Comparison of mortality in all patients on dialysis, patients on dialysis awaiting transplantation, and recipients of a first cadaveric transplant. *N Engl J Med.* 1999;341:1725–1730.
293. Oniscu GC, Brown H, Forsythe JL. Impact of cadaveric renal transplantation on survival in patients listed for transplantation. *J Am Soc Nephrol.* 2005; 16:1859–1865.
294. Moore PS, Farney AC, Hartmann EL, et al. Experience with deceased donor kidney transplantation in 114 patients over age 60. *Surgery.* 2007;142:514–523.
295. Debska-Slizien A, Jankowska MM, Wołyniec W, et al. A single-center experience of renal transplantation in elderly patients: a paired-kidney analysis. *Transplantation.* 2007;83:1188–1192.
296. Rao PS, Merion RM, Ashby VB, et al. Renal transplantation in elderly patients older than 70 years of age: results from the Scientific Registry of Transplant Recipients. *Transplantation.* 2007;83:1069–1074.
297. Wu C, Shapiro R, Tan H, et al. Kidney transplantation in elderly people: The influence of recipient comorbidity and living kidney donors. *J Am Geriatr Soc.* 2008;56:231–238.
298. Heldal K, Leivestad T, Hartmann A, et al. Kidney transplant in the elderly—the Norwegian experience. *Nephrol Dial Transplant.* 2008;23:1026–1031.
299. Schold JD, Srinivas TR, Kayler LK, Meier-Kriesche HU. The overlapping risk profile between dialysis patients listed and not listed for renal transplantation. *Am J Transplant.* 2008;8:58–68.

300. Snyder JJ, Israni AK, Peng Y, et al. Rates of first infection following kidney transplant in the United States. *Kidney Int.* 2009;75:317–326.
301. Poppel DM, Cohen LM, Germain MJ. The renal palliative care initiative. *J Palliat Med.* 2003;6:321–326.
302. Coresh J. CKD prognosis: Beyond the traditional outcomes. *Am J Kid Dis.* 2009;54:1–3.
303. Joly D, Anglicheau D, Alberti C, et al. Octogenarians reaching end-stage renal disease: Cohort study of decision-making and clinical outcomes. *J Am Soc Nephrol.* 2003;14:1012–1021.
304. Murtagh FE, Marsh JE, Donohoe P, et al. Dialysis or not? A comparative survival study of patients over 75 years with chronic kidney disease stage 5. *Nephrol Dial Transplant.* 2007;22:1955–1962.
305. Goovaerts T, Jadoul M, Goffin E. Influence of a pre-dialysis education programme (PDEP) on the mode of renal replacement therapy. *Nephrol Dial Transplant.* 2005;20:1842–1847.
306. Jager KJ, Korevaar JC, Dekker FW, et al. The effect of contraindications and patient preference on dialysis modality selection in ESRD patients in the Netherlands. *Am J Kidney Dis.* 2004;43:891–899.
307. van Biesen W, Veys N, Lameire N, et al. Why less success of the peritoneal dialysis programmes in Europe? *Nephrol Dial Transplant.* 2008;23:1478–1481.
308. Brown EA. Peritoneal dialysis for older people: overcoming the barriers. *Kidney Int.* 2008;73:S68–S71.
309. Couchoud C, Moranne O, Frimat L, et al. Associations between comorbidities, treatment choice and outcome in the elderly with end-stage renal disease. *Nephrol Dial Transplant.* 2007;22:3246–3254.
310. Winkelmayer WC, Glynn RJ, Mittleman MA, et al. Comparing mortality of elderly patients on hemodialysis versus peritoneal dialysis: a propensity score approach. *J Am Soc Nephrol.* 2002;13:2353–2362.
311. Tamura MK. Incidence, management, and outcomes of end-stage renal disease in the elderly. *Curr Opin Nephrol Hypertens.* 2009;18:252–257.
312. Lamping DL, Constantinovici N, Roderick P, et al. Clinical outcomes, quality of life, and costs in the North Thames Dialysis Study of elderly people on dialysis: a prospective cohort study. *Lancet.* 2000;356:1543–1550.
313. Brown EA, Johansson L, Farrington K, et al. Broadening Options for Long-term Dialysis in the Elderly (BOLDE): differences in quality of life on peritoneal dialysis compared to haemodialysis for older patients. *Nephrol Dial Transplant.* 2010;25:3755–3763.
314. Castrale C, Evans D, Verger C, et al. Peritoneal dialysis in elderly patients: report from the French Peritoneal Dialysis Registry (RDPLF). *Nephrol Dial Transplant.* 2010;25:255–262.
315. Kurella M, Covinsky KE, Collins AJ, et al. Octogenarians and nonagenarians starting dialysis in the United States. *Ann Intern Med.* 2007;146:177–183.
316. Jassal SV, Chiu E, Hladunewich M. Loss of independence in patients starting dialysis at 80 years of age or older. *N Engl J Med.* 2009;361:1612–1613.
317. Kurella Tamura M, Covinsky KE, Chertow GM, et al. Functional status of elderly adults before and after initiation of dialysis. *N Engl J Med.* 2009;361: 1539–1547.
318. Lazarides MK, Georgiadis GS, Antoniou GA, et al. A meta-analysis of dialysis access outcome in elderly patients. *J Vasc Surg.* 2007;45:420–426.
319. Moist LM, Bragg-Gresham JL, Pisoni RL, et al. Travel time to dialysis as a predictor of health-related quality of life, adherence, and mortality: the Dialysis Outcomes and Practice Patterns Study (DOPPS). *Am J Kidney Dis.* 2008;51:641–650.
320. Loos-Ayav C, Frimat L, Kessler M, et al. Changes in health-related quality of life in patients of self-care vs. in-center dialysis during the first year. *Qual Life Res.* 2008;17:1–9.
321. Thakar CV, Quate-Operacz M, Leonard AC, et al. Outcomes of hemodialysis patients in a long-term care hospital setting: A single-center study. *Am J Kidney Dis.* 2010;55:300–306.
322. De Biase V, Tobaldini O, Boaretti C, et al. Prolonged conservative treatment for frail elderly patients with end-stage renal disease: The Verona experience. *Nephrol Dial Transplant.* 2008;23:1313–1317.
323. Chandna SM, Sa Silva-Gane MD, Marshall C, et al. Survival of elderly patients with stage 5 CKD: comparison of conservative management and renal replacement therapy. *Nephrol Dial Transplant.* 2011;26(5):1608–1614.
324. Carson RC, Juszczak M, Davenport A, Burns A. Is maximum conservative management an equivalent treatment option to dialysis for elderly patients with significant comorbid disease? *Clin J Am Soc Nephrol.* 2009;4:1611–1619.
325. Brunori G, Viola BF, Parrinello G, et al. Efficacy and safety of a very-low-protein diet when postponing dialysis in the elderly: A prospective randomized multicenter controlled study. *Am J Kidney Dis.* 2007;49:569–580.

CHAPTER 66

Mechanisms of Diuretic Action

David H. Ellison • Ewout J. Hoorn • Robert W. Schrier

The term *diuretic* derives from the Greek *diouretikos*, which means, "to promote urine."* Even though many substances promote urine flow, the term *diuretic* is usually taken to indicate a substance that can reduce the extracellular fluid volume by increasing urinary solute and water excretion. In 1553, Paracelsus recorded the first truly effective medical treatment for dropsy (edema), namely inorganic mercury (calomel). Inorganic mercury remained the mainstay of diuretic treatment until the first part of the 20th century. In 1919, the ability of organic mercurial antisyphilitics to affect diuresis was discovered by Vogl, then a medical student. This observation led to the development of effective organic mercurial diuretics that continued to be used through the 1960s. In 1937, the antimicrobial sulfanilamide was found to cause metabolic acidosis. This drug was soon thereafter shown to inhibit the enzyme carbonic anhydrase, which had been discovered in 1932. Pitts then showed that sulfanilamide inhibited sodium (Na) bicarbonate reabsorption in dogs and Schwartz showed that sulfanilamide could induce diuresis when administered to patients with congestive heart failure. Soon, more potent sulfonamide-based carbonic anhydrase inhibitors were developed, but these drugs suffered from side effects and limited potency. Nevertheless, a group at Sharp & Dohme Inc. was stimulated by these developments to explore the possibility that modification of sulfonamide-based drugs could lead to small molecules that enhanced Na excretion with *chloride* rather than *bicarbonate*, thus better enhancing depletion of the extracellular fluid, which is composed primarily of sodium chloride (NaCl) and water. The result of this program was the synthesis of chlorothiazide and its marketing in 1957. This drug ushered in the modern era of diuretic therapy and revolutionized the clinical treatment of edema.

The search for more potent classes of diuretics led to the development of ethacrynic acid and furosemide in the United States and Germany, respectively. The safety and efficacy of these drugs led them to replace the organic mercurials as drugs of choice for severe and resistant edema. Spironolactone, marketed in 1961, was developed after the properties and structure of aldosterone had been discovered and steroidal analogues of aldosterone were found to have aldosterone-blocking activity. Triamterene was initially synthesized as a folic acid antagonist, but was found to have diuretic and potassium (K)-sparing activity. The identification of the arginine vasopressin (AVP) receptor subtypes led to the more recent development of vasopressin antagonists, which have recently entered clinical practice. The identification and cloning of natriuretic peptides led to the development of drugs with similar effects.

The availability of safe, effective, and relatively inexpensive diuretic drugs has made it possible to treat edematous disorders and hypertension effectively. Incidentally, driven by clinical drug development, specific ligands that interact with discrete Na and Cl transport proteins in the kidney were developed, permitting these transport proteins to be identified. Subsequently, these ligands were used to clone the Na and Cl transport proteins that mediate the bulk of renal Na and Cl reabsorption. The diuretic-sensitive transport proteins that have been cloned include the sodium hydrogen exchanger (NHE3; gene symbol *SLC9A3*), the bumetanide-sensitive Na-K-2Cl cotransporter (NKCC2; gene symbol *SLC12A1*), the thiazide-sensitive Na-Cl cotransporter (NCC; gene symbol *SLC12A3*), and the epithelial Na channel (ENaC; gene symbols *SCNN1A, SCNN1B, SCNN1G*). The information derived from molecular cloning has also permitted identification of inherited human diseases that are caused by mutations in these diuretic-sensitive transport proteins. The phenotypes of several of these disorders resemble the manifestations of chronic diuretic administration. Thus, the development of clinically useful diuretics permitted identification and later cloning of specific ion transport pathways. The molecular cloning is now helping to define mechanisms of diuretic action and diuretic side effects. The use of animals in which diuretic-sensitive transport pathways have been "knocked out" permits a clearer understanding of which diuretic effects result directly or secondarily from actions of the drugs on specific ion transport pathways and which effects result from actions on other pathways or other organ systems.

*Many older and historical references have been omitted for brevity. These references can be found in prior editions of this text.

NORMAL RENAL NaCl HANDLING

The normal human kidneys filter approximately 23 moles of NaCl in 150 liters of fluid each day. According to data from NHANES III, typical dietary sodium consumption in the United States is 4.3 g daily for men and 2.9 g daily for women.[1] The sex difference reflects differences in caloric intake, not differential food choices. As 17 mEq of Na is 1 g of table salt and 43 mEq of Na is in 1 g of sodium, men typically consume 100 mEq of Na and women typically consume 67 mEq on a daily basis. To maintain balance, renal NaCl excretion must equal this, ignoring the modest losses in feces and sweat. Under normal circumstances, approximately 99.2% of the filtered NaCl is reabsorbed by kidney tubules generating a normal fractional sodium excretion of <1% (100 mEq in urine per 23,000 mEq filtered = 0.4%). Sodium, chloride, and water reabsorption by the nephron is driven by the metabolic energy provided by ATP. The ouabain-sensitive Na/K ATPase is expressed at the basolateral cell membrane of all Na transporting epithelial cells along the nephron. This pump maintains large ion gradients across the plasma membrane, with the intracellular Na concentration maintained low and the intracellular K concentration maintained high. Because the pump is electrogenic and associates with a K channel in the same membrane, renal epithelial cells have a voltage across the plasma membrane oriented with the inside negative relative to the outside.

The combination of the low intracellular Na concentration and the plasma membrane voltage generates a large electrochemical gradient favoring Na entry from lumen or interstitium. Specific diuretic-sensitive Na transport pathways are expressed at the apical (luminal) surface of cells along the nephron, permitting vectorial transport of Na from lumen to blood. Along the proximal tubule, where approximately 50% to 60% of filtered Na is reabsorbed, an isoform of the Na/H exchanger is expressed at the apical membrane. Along the thick ascending limb, where approximately 20% to 25% of filtered Na is reabsorbed, an isoform of the Na-K-2Cl cotransporter is expressed at the apical membrane. Along the distal convoluted tubule, where approximately 5% of filtered Na is reabsorbed, the thiazide-sensitive Na-Cl cotransporter is expressed. Along the connecting tubule (CNT) and cortical collecting duct (CCD), where approximately 3% of filtered Na is reabsorbed, the amiloride-sensitive epithelial Na channel is expressed. These apical Na transport pathways are the primary targets for diuretic drug action.

This chapter discusses the molecular and physiologic bases for diuretic action in the kidney. Although some aspects of clinical diuretic usage are discussed, physiologic principles and mechanisms of action are emphasized. Several recent texts provide detailed discussions of diuretic treatment of clinical conditions.[2] Extensive discussions of diuretic pharmacokinetics are also available.[3,4]

A rational classification of diuretic drugs (Table 66.1) is based on the primary nephron site of action. Such a scheme emphasizes that different chemical classes of drugs can affect the same ion transport mechanism and exhibit many of the same clinical effects and side effects. Furthermore, although

TABLE 66.1 **Effects of Diuretics on Electrolyte Excretion**

	Na	Cl	K	Pi	Ca	Mg
Osmotic diuretics[6,205,388–390]	⇑(10%–25%)	⇑(15%–30%)	⇑ (6%)	⇑(5%–10%)	⇑(10%–20%)	⇑(>20%)
Carbonic anhydrase inhibitors[57,98,205]	⇑(6%)	⇑(4%)	⇑(60%)	⇑(>20%)	⇑ or ⇔ (<5%)	⇑(<5%)
Loop diuretics[98,177,205,344,391,392]	⇑(30%)	⇑(40%)	⇑(60%–100%)	⇑(>20%)	⇑(>20%)	⇑(>20%)
DCT diuretics[177,205,391,393]	⇑(6%–11%)	⇑(10%)	⇑(200%)	⇑(>20%)	⇓	⇑(5–10%)
Collecting duct diuretics[177,205,344]	⇑(1%–5%)	⇑(6%)	⇓(8%)	⇔	⇔	⇓

Figures indicate approximate maximal fractional excretions of ions following acute diuretic administration in maximally effective doses. ⇑ indicates that the drug increases excretion; ⇓ indicates that the drug decreases excretion; ⇔ indicates that the drug has little or no direct effect on excretion. During chronic treatment, effects often wane (Na excretion), may increase (K excretion during distal convoluted tubule diuretic treatment), or may reverse as with uric acid (not shown).

Na, sodium; Cl, chloride; K, potassium; Pi, phosphate; Ca, calcium; Mg, magnesium.

most diuretic drugs affect transport processes along several nephron segments, most owe their clinical effects primarily to their ability to inhibit Na transport by one particular nephron segment. An exception is the osmotic diuretics. Although these drugs were initially believed to inhibit solute and water flux primarily along the proximal tubule, subsequent studies have revealed effects in multiple segments. Other diuretics, however, are classified according to their primary site of action.

OSMOTIC DIURETICS

Osmotic diuretics are substances that are freely filtered at the glomerulus, but are poorly reabsorbed (Fig. 66.1). The pharmacologic activity of drugs in this group depends entirely on the osmotic pressure exerted by the drug molecules in solution. It does not depend on interaction with specific transport proteins or enzymes. Mannitol is the prototypical osmotic diuretic.[5] Because the relationship between the magnitude of diuretic effect and concentration of osmotic diuretic in solution is linear, all osmotic diuretics are small molecules. Other agents considered in this class include urea, sorbitol, and glycerol.

Urinary Electrolyte Excretion

Although osmotic agents do not act directly on transport pathways, ion transport is affected. Following mannitol infusion, sodium, potassium, calcium, magnesium, bicarbonate, and chloride excretion rates increase (see Table 66.1). Rates of sodium and water fractional reabsorption are reduced by 27% and 12%, respectively, following the infusion of mannitol.[6] Reabsorption of magnesium and calcium is also reduced in the proximal tubule and loop of Henle. In contrast, phosphate reabsorption is only inhibited slightly by mannitol in the presence of parathyroid hormone.[7]

Mechanism of Action

The functional consequences that result from intravenous infusion of mannitol include an increase in cortical and medullary blood flow; a variable effect on glomerular filtration rate; an increase in sodium, water, calcium, magnesium, phosphorus, and bicarbonate excretion; and a decrease in medullary concentration gradient. The most pronounced effect observed with mannitol is a brisk diuresis and natriuresis. The mechanisms by which mannitol produces a diuresis include: (1) an increase in osmotic pressure in the lumens of the proximal tubule and loop of Henle, thereby retarding the passive reabsorption of water and (2) an increase in renal blood flow and washout of medullary tonicity.

Mannitol is freely filtered at the glomerulus and its presence in tubule fluid minimizes passive water reabsorption. Normally, within the proximal tubule, sodium reabsorption creates an osmotic gradient for water reabsorption. When an osmotic diuretic is administered, however, the osmotic force of the nonreabsorbable solute in the lumen opposes the osmotic force produced by sodium reabsorption. Isosmolality of tubule fluid is preserved because molecules of mannitol replace sodium ions reabsorbed. However, sodium reabsorption eventually stops because the luminal sodium concentration is reduced to a point where a limiting gradient is reached and net transport of sodium and water ceases. The validity of this mechanistic explanation has been confirmed by stationary micropuncture studies. Quantitatively, mannitol has a greater effect on inhibiting Na and water reabsorption in the loop of Henle than in the proximal tubule. Free-flow micropuncture studies following mannitol infusion in dogs demonstrated a modest decrease in fractional reabsorption of sodium and water by the proximal tubule, but a much larger effect by the loop of Henle.[7] Within the loop of Henle, the site of action of mannitol appears to be restricted to the thin descending limb, decreasing water reabsorption.[8] In the thick ascending limb, Na reabsorption continues, in proportion to its delivery to this segment. The sum of net transport in the thin and thick limbs determines the net effect of mannitol in the loop of Henle. Further downstream in the collecting duct, mannitol reduces sodium and water reabsorption.[9]

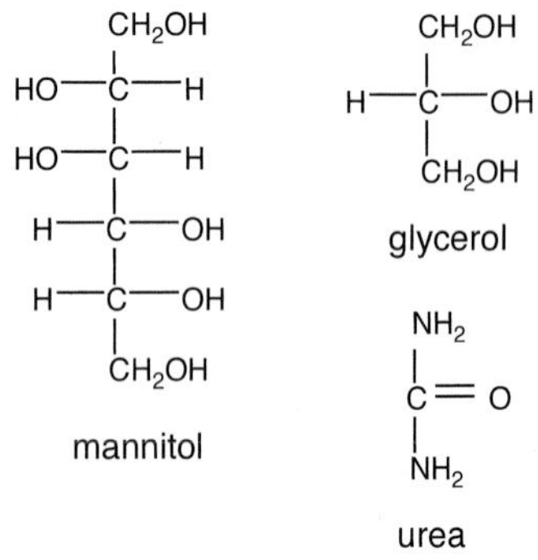

mannitol

glycerol

urea

FIGURE 66.1 Structures of osmotic diuretics.

Renal Hemodynamics

During the administration of mannitol, its molecules diffuse from the bloodstream into the interstitial space. In the interstitial space, the increased osmotic pressure draws water from the cells to increase extracellular fluid volume. This effect increases total renal plasma flow.[9] Cortical and medullary blood flow rates both increase following mannitol infusion.[9] Single nephron glomerular filtration rate (GFR), on the other hand, increases in cortex but decreases in medulla.[8] The mechanisms by which mannitol reduces the GFR of deep nephrons are not known, but it has been postulated that mannitol reduces efferent arteriolar pressure. Micropuncture studies examining the determinants of GFR in superficial nephrons have demonstrated that the increase in single nephron GFR results from an increase in single nephron plasma flow and a decrease in oncotic pressure.[10] The net effect of mannitol on total kidney GFR has been variable, but most studies indicate that the overall effect is to increase GFR.[10]

The combination of enhanced renal plasma flow and reduced medullary GFR washes out the medullary osmotic gradient by reducing papillary sodium and urea content. Experimental studies indicate that the osmotic effect of mannitol to increase water movement from intracellular to extracellular space leads to a decrease in hematocrit and in blood viscosity. This fact contributes to a decrease in renal vascular resistance and increase in renal blood flow. In addition, secretion of vasodilatory substances is stimulated by mannitol infusion. Both prostacyclin (PGI_2)[11] and atrial natriuretic peptide[12] could mediate the effect of mannitol on renal blood flow. The vasodilatory effect of mannitol is reduced when the recipient is pretreated with indomethacin or meclofenamate, suggesting that PGI_2 is involved in the vasodilatory effect. Alterations in renal hemodynamics contribute to the diuresis observed following administration of mannitol. An increase in medullary blood flow rate reduces medullary tonicity primarily by decreasing papillary sodium and urea content[13] and increasing urine flow rate.[14]

Pharmacokinetics

Mannitol is not readily absorbed from the intestine[5]; therefore, it is routinely administered intravenously. Following infusion, mannitol distributes in extracellular fluid with a volume of distribution of approximately 16 liters[15]; its excretion is almost entirely by glomerular filtration.[16] Of the filtered load, less than 10% is reabsorbed by the renal tubule, and a similar quantity is metabolized, probably in the liver. With normal glomerular filtration rate, plasma half-life is approximately 2.2 hours.

Clinical Use

Mannitol is used prophylactically to prevent acute kidney injury.[17] In the past, it was administered to patients with established acute kidney injury, but it has proven ineffective in this situation. Mannitol improves renal hemodynamics in a variety of situations of impending or incipient acute kidney injury. Mannitol (along with hydration and sodium bicarbonate) has been recommended by some,[18,19] but not all[20] investigators for the early treatment in myoglobinuric acute kidney injury and to prevent posttransplant acute kidney injury.[21] Mannitol is frequently used perioperatively to treat patients undergoing cardiopulmonary bypass surgery. The beneficial effects may relate to its osmotic activity thereby reducing intravenous fluid requirement[22] and its ability to act as a free radical antioxidant.[23] Although some studies have shown a beneficial effect when used prophylactically to treat patients at risk for contrast nephropathy,[24] most prospective controlled studies have not found mannitol beneficial in preventing acute kidney injury and it is not currently recommended.[25,26]

Mannitol is used for short-term reduction of intraocular pressure.[27] By increasing the osmotic pressure, mannitol reduces the volume of aqueous humor and the intraocular pressure by extracting water. Mannitol also decreases cerebral edema and the increase in intracranial pressure associated with trauma, tumors, and neurosurgical procedures,[22,23,28] although hypertonic saline appears more effective for this purpose.[29]

Mannitol and other osmotic agents have been used to treat dialysis disequilibrium.[30,31] This syndrome is characterized by acute symptoms during or immediately following hemodialysis, and is especially common when dialysis is first initiated. Most significant symptoms are attributable to disorders of the central nervous system such as headache, nausea, blurred vision, confusion, seizure, coma, and death. Rapid removal of small solutes such as urea during dialysis of patients who are markedly azotemic is associated with the development of an osmotic gradient for water movement into brain cells producing cerebral edema and neurologic dysfunction. Dialysis disequilibrium syndrome can be minimized by slow solute removal, using low blood flow and short treatment times; raising plasma osmolality with saline or mannitol can also be employed.

Adverse Effects

Patients who have a reduced cardiac output may develop pulmonary edema when mannitol is infused. Intravenous mannitol administration increases cardiac output and pulmonary capillary wedge pressures.[15] Acute and prolonged administration of mannitol leads to different electrolyte disturbances. Acute overzealous use or the accumulation of mannitol leads to dilutional metabolic acidosis and hypertonic hyponatremia (as mannitol shifts sodium-free water from cells to the extracellular space). Accumulation of mannitol also produces hyperkalemia[32] as a result of the same osmotic forces. An increase in plasma osmolality increases potassium movement from intracellular to extracellular fluid from bulk solute flow and increase in the electrochemical gradient for potassium secretion. Prolonged administration of mannitol generates urinary losses of sodium and potassium potentially leading to volume depletion, hypernatremia (as urinary loss of sodium is invariably less than water), and hypokalemia.[33] Although mannitol is sometimes used to induce hypernatremia to reduce intracranial pressure, studies have shown that the adverse effects of hypernatremia outweigh the benefits of reduced intracranial pressure, especially when serum sodium exceeds 160 mmol/l.[34]

Marked accumulation of mannitol in patients can lead to reversible acute kidney injury that appears to be caused by vasoconstriction and tubular vacuolization.[35,36] Mannitol-induced acute kidney injury usually occurs when large cumulative doses of ~295 g are given to patients with previously compromised renal function.[35]

PROXIMAL TUBULE DIURETICS (CARBONIC ANHYDRASE INHIBITORS)

Through the development of carbonic anhydrase inhibitors, important compounds were discovered that have utility as therapeutic agents and as research tools. Carbonic anhydrase

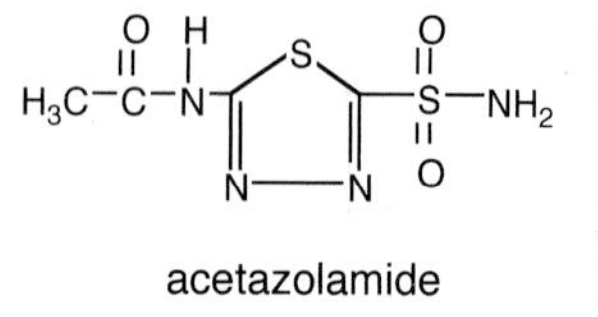

acetazolamide

FIGURE 66.2 Structure of a carbonic anhydrase inhibitor.

inhibitors have a limited therapeutic role as diuretic agents, however, because they are only weakly natriuretic when employed chronically. They are used primarily to reduce intraocular pressure in glaucoma, to enhance bicarbonate excretion in metabolic alkalosis or chronic hypercapnia, and to prevent mountain sickness. Structures of carbonic anhydrase inhibitors are shown in Figure 66.2.

Urinary Electrolyte Excretion

Through their effects on carbonic anhydrase in the proximal tubule, carbonic anhydrase inhibitors increase bicarbonate excretion by 25% to 30% (see Table 66.1). The increase in sodium and chloride excretion is smaller than might be expected, because these ions are reabsorbed by more distal segments of the nephron.[37] However, a residual small but variable amount of sodium is excreted along with bicarbonate (Table 66.1). Calcium and phosphate reabsorption are also inhibited along the proximal tubule by carbonic anhydrase inhibitors. Because distal calcium reabsorption is stimulated by increased distal delivery, fractional calcium excretion does not increase. In contrast, phosphate appears to escape distal reabsorption resulting in an increase in fractional excretion of phosphate by ~3%. Although proximal tubule magnesium transport is inhibited by carbonic anhydrase inhibitors, fractional excretion of magnesium is either unchanged or increased as a result of variable distal reabsorption.[38]

Carbonic anhydrase inhibitors increase potassium excretion. It is likely that several indirect effects contribute to the observed kaliuresis. Carbonic anhydrase inhibition could block proximal tubule potassium reabsorption and increase delivery to the distal tubule, but this has not been established clearly. Whereas carbonic anhydrase inhibitors decrease proximal tubule sodium, bicarbonate, and water absorption during both free flow micropuncture and microperfusion, the effects of carbonic anhydrase inhibitors on proximal tubule potassium transport have been less consistent. In free flow micropuncture studies, carbonic anhydrase inhibition did not affect proximal tubule potassium reabsorption,[39] whereas it did reduce net reabsorption by microperfused proximal tubules.[40] The effect of carbonic anhydrase inhibitors on the proximal tubule ion transport does, however, facilitate an increase in tubular fluid flow rate and sodium and bicarbonate but not chloride delivery to the distal nephron. This effect is thought to increase the concentration of bicarbonate in the distal tubule lumen, which increases lumen negative voltage[41] and increases flow rate,[42] factors known to increase potassium secretion by the distal tubule. Carbonic anhydrase inhibitors can also produce a luminal composition that is low in chloride and high in bicarbonate. This luminal fluid composition has been demonstrated to stimulate potassium secretion by the distal nephron independent of a change in lumen negative voltage.[43]

Mechanism of Action

In the kidney, carbonic anhydrase inhibitors act primarily on proximal tubule cells to inhibit bicarbonate absorption.[44] Carbonic anhydrase, a metalloenzyme containing one zinc atom per molecule, is important in sodium bicarbonate reabsorption and hydrogen ion secretion by renal epithelial cells. The biochemical, morphologic, and functional properties of carbonic anhydrase have been reviewed.[45] Carbonic anhydrase isoforms (CA) can be categorized into four groups: (1) cytosolic, I, II, III, VII; (2) mitochondrial, V; (3) membrane associated IV, IX, XII, XIV; and (4) secreted, VI.[45] Carbonic anhydrases regulate cellular H ion secretion through catalyzing the formation of HCO_3 from OH and CO_2 and by binding to transporters and directly regulating activity. There are three major renal carbonic anhydrases. Type II carbonic anhydrase (CAII) is distributed widely comprising more than 95% of the overall activity in kidney and is sensitive to inhibition by sulfonamides. CAII is expressed in the cytoplasm and facilitates the secretion of H ions by catalyzing the formation of HCO_3 from OH and CO_2 (see equation 66.3). In addition, CAII binds to the C-terminal region of NHE1 and likely regulates the transport efficiency of Na/H exchange. CAIV is bound to renal cortical membranes, comprising up to 5% of the remaining overall activity in rodent kidney, and is also sensitive to sulfonamides. Carbonic anhydrase activity at basolateral and luminal plasma membranes of proximal tubule cells and luminal membrane of intercalated cells catalyzes the dehydration of intraluminal carbonic acid generated from secreted protons. The carbonic anhydrase activity at the basolateral and luminal plasma membranes of proximal tubule cells is thought to be due in part to CAIV.[46] CAIV has been shown to also bind to the extracellular loop of $NaHCO_3$ transporter 1 (NBC1) regulating its transport activity.[47] Evidence for the physiologic importance for carbonic anhydrase is apparent as a deficiency of CAII leads to a renal acidification defect resulting in renal tubular acidosis. Furthermore, metabolic acidosis leads to an adaptive increase in both CAII and IV carbonic anhydrase mRNA expression in kidney[48] suggesting the importance of both carbonic anhydrase isoforms in this disorder. CAXII is also expressed in proximal tubules and collecting ducts and may contribute to the carbonic anhydrase activity in these segments.[49–51]

Normally the proximal tubule reabsorbs 80% of the filtered load of sodium bicarbonate and 60% of the filtered load of sodium chloride. Early studies by Pitts and micropuncture studies by DuBose and others indicated that hydrogen ion secretion is responsible for bicarbonate absorption and renal acidification. The cellular mechanism by which proximal

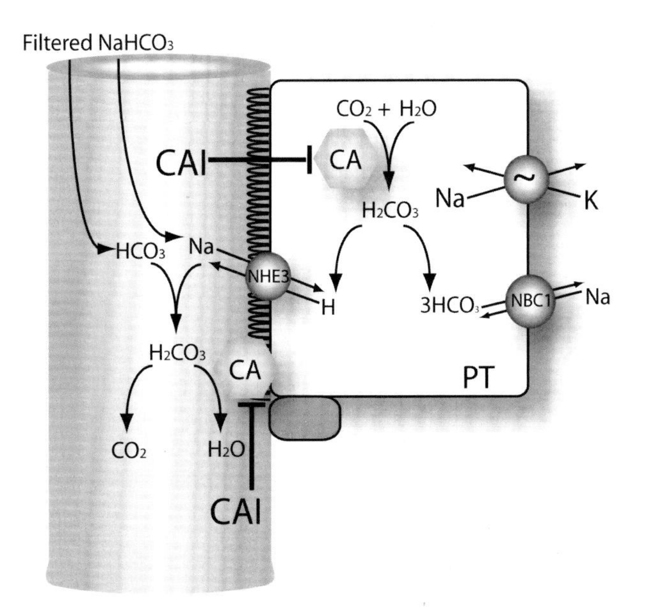

FIGURE 66.3 Mechanisms of diuretic action in the proximal tubule. The figure shows functional model of proximal tubule (PT) cells. Many transport proteins are omitted from the model, for clarity. Carbonic anhydrase (CA) catalyzes inside the cell the formation of HCO_3 from H_2O and CO_2. This is the result of the two-step process (please see equations in the text for additional details). Bicarbonate leaves the cell via the Na, HCO_3, cotransporter.[186,187] A second pool of carbonic anhydrase is located in the brush border (CA). This participates in disposing of carbonic acid, formed from filtered bicarbonate and secreted H^+. Both pools of carbonic anhydrase are inhibited by acetazolamide and other carbonic anhydrase inhibitors (see text for details).

tubules reabsorb bicarbonate is depicted in Figure 66.3. The effect of carbonic anhydrase to accelerate bicarbonate is a result of the reactions that occur in both luminal fluid and in the cell. The mechanism of carbonic anhydrase action in luminal fluid,[52] is shown here, where *E* represents the carbonic anhydrase enzyme:

Luminal Fluid

$$EH_2O + HCO_3{}_- \Leftrightarrow H_2O + CO_2 + EOH \quad (1)$$

$$EOH + H^+ \Leftrightarrow EH_2O \quad (2)$$

$$HCO_3{}_- + H^+ \Leftrightarrow CO_2 + H_2O \quad (3)$$

Note that the addition of reactions 1 and 2 leads to the classic reaction 3. In this scheme, the enzyme is viewed as a superhydroxylator.

Luminal carbonic anhydrase prevents H from accumulating in tubule fluid, which would eventually stop all Na/H exchange. Once formed, carbon dioxide diffuses rapidly from the lumen into the cell across the apical membrane.

The mechanism by which intracellular carbonic anhydrase participates in net H^+ secretion is functionally the reverse of the reactions shown previously.

Intracellular Fluid

$$EH_2O \Leftrightarrow EOH + H^+ \quad (2R)$$

$$EOH + H_2O + CO_2 \Leftrightarrow EH_2O + HCO_3{}_- \quad (1R)$$

$$CO_2 + H_2O \Leftrightarrow HCO_3{}_- + H^+ \quad (3R)$$

In this case, the enzyme splits water, thereby providing an hydroxyl ion to form bicarbonate. The bicarbonate ions then exit the basolateral membrane via $Na(HCO_3)_3$ cotransport.[53] Thus, in the early proximal tubule, the net effect of the process described results in the isosmotic reabsorption of $NaHCO_3$. The lumen chloride concentration increases because water continues to be reabsorbed, thereby producing a lumen positive potential. These axial changes provide an electrochemical gradient for transport of chloride, via paracellular and transcellular pathways. The latter pathway for chloride likely involves an exchange of Cl with anions, including oxalate and formate, operating in parallel with a Na/H proton exchanger. The dual operation of these parallel exchangers results in net NaCl absorption.[54]

Carbonic anhydrase inhibitors act primarily on proximal tubule cells, where approximately 60% of the filtered load of sodium chloride is reabsorbed. Despite the magnitude of sodium chloride reabsorption in the proximal tubule segment, the natriuretic potency of carbonic anhydrase inhibitors is relatively weak. Several factors explain this observation. First, proximal sodium reabsorption is mediated by carbonic anhydrase-independent as well as carbonic anhydrase-dependent pathways. Second, the increased sodium delivery to distal nephron segments is largely reabsorbed by these distal nephron segments. Third, carbonic anhydrase inhibitors generate a hyperchloremic metabolic acidosis further reducing the effects of subsequent doses of carbonic anhydrase inhibitor. Metabolic acidosis also produces resistance to carbonic anhydrase action. Following the induction of metabolic acidosis, the K_i for bicarbonate absorption by membrane impermeant carbonic anhydrase inhibitors was increased by a factor of 100 to 500, suggesting that metabolic acidosis is associated with changes in the physical properties of the carbonic anhydrase protein.[55] For these reasons, carbonic anhydrase inhibitors alone are rarely used as diuretic agents.

Following carbonic anhydrase inhibitor administration, proximal tubule bicarbonate reabsorption declines between 35% and 85%. Additional sites of action of carbonic anhydrase inhibitors include proximal straight tubule or loop of Henle, distal tubule, and the collecting and papillary collecting ducts. Yet, despite the effect of carbonic anhydrase inhibitors on proximal tubules as well as other nephron segments, compensatory reabsorption of bicarbonate at other downstream tubular sites limits net fractional excretion of bicarbonate to ~25% to 30%, even during acute administration.[56,57]

The relative contributions of membrane-bound and intracellular components of cellular carbonic anhydrase have been examined. Both species contribute to bicarbonate absorption. The role of membrane-bound carbonic anhydrase was addressed in studies that employed carbonic anhydrase inhibitors with different abilities to penetrate proximal tubule cell membranes. Benzolamide is charged at normal pH and does not penetrate cell membranes well, whereas acetazolamide enters the cell relatively easily.[58] Proximal tubular perfusion of benzolamide inhibits bicarbonate reabsorption by 90%[59] indicating that luminal carbonic anhydrase inhibition contributes importantly to bicarbonate absorption. Inhibition of luminal carbonic anhydrase causes lumen pH to decrease because of the continued secretion of hydrogen ions into the tubule lumen.[59] The conclusion that tubular fluid is in direct contact with membrane carbonic anhydrase was substantiated by the use of dextran-bound carbonic anhydrase inhibitors.[60,61] In proximal tubules perfused in vivo, Lucci et al. determined that dextran-bound inhibitors, which inhibit only luminal carbonic anhydrase, decreased proximal tubule bicarbonate absorption by approximately 80% and reduced lumen pH.[61]

Although these studies establish the importance of luminal carbonic anhydrase, they also support an important role for intracellular and basolateral carbonic anhydrase. Both acetazolamide and benzolamide inhibit proximal tubule bicarbonate reabsorption to a similar degree yet they produce opposite effects on tubule fluid pH, suggesting that intracellular carbonic anhydrase contributes to proximal tubule luminal acidification. Furthermore, inherited deficiency of the predominant renal carbonic anhydrase, CAII, causes proximal renal tubular acidosis.[62]

The expression of carbonic anhydrase in the basolateral membrane of proximal tubule cells suggests that this membrane-bound enzyme also has an important role in basolateral bicarbonate transport. Although it is well known that carbonic anhydrase inhibitors inhibit intracellular generation of substrate for the transporter,[63,64] the direct interaction between CAIV and NBC1, the sodium/bicarbonate cotransporter,[47] suggests the possibility that carbonic anhydrase inhibitors may also directly regulate anion transport activity. Functional studies using an impermeant carbonic anhydrase inhibitor, *p*-fluorobenzyl-aminobenzamide, that is 1% as permeable as acetazolamide, demonstrated the importance of basolateral membrane-bound carbonic anhydrase. *p*-Fluorobenzyl-aminobenzamide reduced fluid and bicarbonate absorption when applied to the basolateral membrane of rabbit proximal tubules perfused in vitro.[50]

In the collecting duct, carbonic anhydrase facilitates acid secretion that is mediated by a vacuolar H adenosine triphosphatase (H-ATPase)[65] and a P-type gastric H-K-ATPase.[66–68] Luminal administration of acetazolamide produced an acid disequilibrium pH in the outer medullary collecting duct suggesting the contribution of luminal carbonic anhydrase.[69] Using a membrane-impermeant carbonic anhydrase inhibitor (F-3500; aminobenzamide coupled to a nontoxic polymer polyoxyethylene), bicarbonate absorption was reduced confirming the presence of carbonic anhydrase in the luminal membrane of the outer medullary collecting duct.[55] The K_i for inhibition of bicarbonate absorption was 5 μM, consistent with the inhibition of CAIV.

Renal Hemodynamics

Inhibition of carbonic anhydrase decreases GFR acutely. Systemic acetazolamide infusion decreased GFR by 30%. Single nephron glomerular filtration rate (SNGFR) was 23% lower during acetazolamide infusion partly because increased solute delivery to the macula densa activates the tubuloglomerular feedback (TGF) mechanism, which reduces GFR. Similar results were observed following infusion of benzolamide.[70] Nevertheless, the effects of carbonic anhydrase inhibitors to reduce GFR are not simply the result of TGF activation. Sarala^{8}- angiotensin I, an angiotensin II antagonist, prevented the decrease in SGNFR suggesting the involvement of local angiotensin II in response to benzolamide.[70] Further, infusion of benzolamide into targeted adenosine-1 receptor knockout mice (i.e., mice that lack a TGF response) reduced GFR by 21%.[71] Taken together, these results suggest complex mechanisms by which carbonic anhydrase inhibitors reduce GFR.

Pharmacokinetics

Acetazolamide is well absorbed from the gastrointestinal (GI) tract. More than 90% of the drug is plasma protein bound. The highest concentrations are found in tissues that contain large amounts of carbonic anhydrase (e.g., renal cortex, red blood cells). Renal effects are noticeable within 30 minutes and are usually maximal at 2 hours. Acetazolamide is not metabolized but is excreted rapidly by glomerular filtration and proximal tubular secretion. The half-life is approximately 5 hours and renal excretion is essentially complete in 24 hours.[16] In comparison, methazolamide is absorbed more slowly from the GI tract, and its duration of action is long, with a half-life of approximately 14 hours.

Adverse Effects

Generally, carbonic anhydrase inhibitors are well tolerated with infrequent serious adverse effects. Side effects of carbonic anhydrase inhibitors may arise from the continued excretion of electrolytes. Significant hypokalemia and metabolic acidosis may develop. In elderly patients with glaucoma treated with acetazolamide (250 to 1,000 mg per day), metabolic acidosis was a frequent finding, in comparison to a control group.[72] Acetazolamide is also associated with nephrocalcinosis and nephrolithiasis due to its effects on urine pH, facilitating stone formation. Premature infants treated with furosemide and acetazolamide are particularly susceptible to nephrocalcinosis, presumably due to the combined effect of an alkaline urine and hypercalciuria.[73] Other adverse effects include drowsiness, fatigue, central nervous system depression, and paresthesias. Bone marrow suppression has been reported.[74,75]

Clinical Use

As noted, these drugs are almost never used as first-line diuretics because of the availability of much more potent drugs. Daily use produces systemic acidemia from an increase in urinary excretion of bicarbonate. Nevertheless, acetazolamide can be administered for short-term therapy, usually in combination with other diuretics, to patients who are resistant or who do not respond adequately to other agents.[76] The rationale for using a combination of diuretic agents is based on summation of their effect at different sites along the nephron.

The major indication for the use of acetazolamide as a diuretic agent is in the treatment of patients with metabolic alkalosis accompanying edema[77,78] or the treatment of chronic respiratory acidosis in chronic obstructive lung disease.[79,80] In patients with cirrhosis, congestive heart failure, or nephrotic syndrome, aggressive diuresis with loop diuretics promotes intravascular volume depletion and secondary hyperaldosteronism, conditions that promote metabolic alkalosis. Administration of sodium chloride to correct the metabolic alkalosis simply exacerbates the edema. Acetazolamide can improve metabolic alkalosis by decreasing proximal tubule bicarbonate reabsorption thereby increasing the fractional excretion of bicarbonate. An increase in urinary pH (>7.0) indicates enhanced bicarbonaturia. However, it should be noted that potassium depletion should be corrected prior to acetazolamide use because acetazolamide will also increase potassium excretion. The time course of the acetazolamide effect is rapid. In critically ill patients on ventilators, following the correction of fluid and electrolyte disturbances, intravenous acetazolamide produced an initial effect within 2 hours and a maximum effect in 15 hours.[81]

Acetazolamide is used effectively to treat chronic open-angle glaucoma. The high bicarbonate concentration in aqueous humor is carbonic anhydrase dependent and oral carbonic anhydrase inhibition can be used to reduce aqueous humor formation. Topical formulations of carbonic anhydrase inhibitors were 82, and these drugs are now available to treat glaucoma.

Acute mountain sickness usually occurs in climbers within the 12 to 72 hours of ascending to high altitudes. Symptoms include headache, nausea, dizziness, and breathlessness. Carbonic anhydrase inhibitors improve symptoms and arterial oxygenation.[83]

The administration of acetazolamide has been used in the treatment of familial hypokalemic periodic paralysis,[84,85] a disorder characterized by intermittent episodes of muscle weakness and flaccid paralysis. Its efficacy may be related to a decrease in influx of potassium as a result of a decrease in plasma insulin and glucose[86] or to metabolic acidosis. Carbonic anhydrase inhibitors can also be used as an adjunct treatment of epilepsy,[87] pseudotumor cerebri,[88] and central sleep apnea.[89]

By increasing urinary pH, acetazolamide has been used effectively in certain clinical conditions. Acetazolamide is used to treat cystine and uric acid stones by increasing their solubility in urine, although urinary alkalinization is no longer recommended for prevention of tumor lysis syndrome.[90] Acetazolamide in combination with sodium bicarbonate infusion has been used to treat salicylate toxicity, but acetazolamide is now considered to be contraindicated in this situation. Other indications for CAIs are experimental but emerging and include possible application of CAIs in conditions as diverse as obesity, cancer, and infection.[91]

LOOP DIURETICS

The loop diuretics inhibit sodium and chloride transport along the loop of Henle and macula densa. Although these drugs also impair ion transport by proximal and distal tubules under some conditions, these effects probably contribute little to their action clinically. The loop diuretics available in the United States include furosemide, bumetanide, torsemide, and ethacrynic acid (Fig. 66.4).

Loop diuretics are organic anions. Studies that utilized radiolabeled bumetanide suggest that loop diuretics bind to one of the chloride (anion) sites on the transporter.[92] According to this model, the loop diuretic would bind because of its negative charge (and its shape) and then inhibit the transport of ions because it is not transported. Studies utilizing chimeric cloned proteins, comprising portions of different members of the cation chloride cotransporters, however, have indicated that diuretic binding and ion affinities are properties of the central hydrophobic domain of the proteins.[93] Isenring and colleagues[94,95] found that transmembrane domains 2 to 6 and 10 to 12 play roles in defining loop diuretic affinity, whereas chloride affinity is regulated by transmembrane domains 4 and 7.[95] This suggests that loop diuretics do not simply bind to one of the chloride sites on the transporter. The results of the chimeric studies, however, have been complex and it would appear that interactions between various transmembrane domains might reconcile the apparent differences in results. Recent models, based on crystallization of related proteins, may provide more definitive information about these results.[96]

Urinary Electrolyte and Water Excretion

Loop diuretics increase the excretion of water, Na, K, Cl, phosphate, magnesium, and calcium (see Table 66.1). The dose-response relationship between loop diuretic and urinary Na and Cl excretion is sigmoidal (Fig. 66.5). The steep dose response relation has led many to refer to loop diuretics as "threshold" drugs.[3] Loop diuretics have the highest natriuretic and chloruretic potency of any class of diuretics; they are sometimes called "high ceiling" diuretics for this reason. Loop diuretics can increase Na and Cl excretion up to 25% of the filtered load. If administered during water loading, solute-free water clearance (C_{H_2O}) decreases and osmolar clearance increases, although the urine always remains dilute. This effect

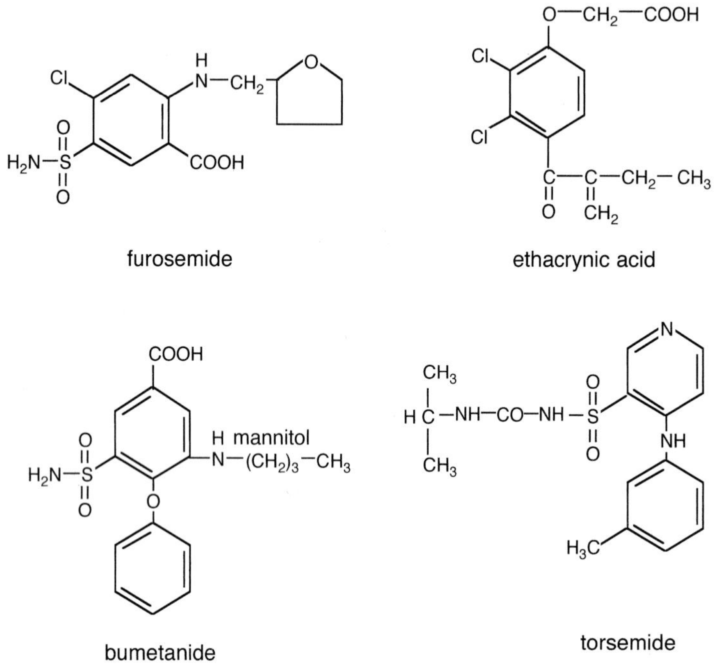

FIGURE 66.4 Structures of loop diuretics.

furosemide

ethacrynic acid

bumetanide

torsemide

contrasts with that of osmotic diuretics which increase osmolar clearance and C_{H_2O}.[97] During hydropenia, loop diuretics impair the reabsorption of solute-free water ($T^C_{H_2O}$). During maximal loop diuretic action, the urinary Na concentration is usually between 75 to 100 mM.[98] Because urinary K concentrations during furosemide-induced natriuresis remain low, this means that the clearance of electrolyte free water (C_{H_2Oe}) is increased when loop diuretics are administered during conditions of water diuresis or hydropenia.[98] This effect of loop diuretics has been exploited to treat hyponatremia, when combined with normal or hypertonic saline.[99,100]

Mechanisms of Action

Sodium and Chloride Transport

The predominant effect of loop diuretic drugs is to inhibit the electroneutral Na-K-2Cl cotransporter at the apical surface of thick ascending limb cells. The loop of Henle, defined as the region between the last surface proximal segment and the first surface distal segment, reabsorbs from 20% to 50% of the filtered Na and Cl load[101]; approximately 10% to 20% is reabsorbed by thick ascending limb cells. The model in Figure 66.6 shows key components of Na, K, and Cl transport pathways in a thick ascending limb cell. As in other nephron segments, the Na/K ATPase at the basolateral cell membrane maintains the intracellular Na concentration low (approximately 10-fold lower than interstitial) and the K concentration high (approximately 20-fold higher than interstitial). Potassium channel(s)[102] in the basolateral cell membrane permit K to diffuse out of the cell, rendering the cell membrane voltage oriented with the intracellular surface negative, relative to extracellular fluid. A chloride channel in the basolateral cell membrane permits Cl to exit the cell.[102] Together with the apical K channel, described below, this chloride channel generates a transepithelial voltage, oriented in the lumen-positive direction.

The transporter inhibited by loop diuretics is a member of the cation chloride cotransporter family.[93,103] This protein—referred to as the bumetanide-sensitive cotransporter, first isoform (BSC-1), or as the Na-K-2Cl cotransporter, second isoform (NKCC2)—is encoded by the gene *SLC12A1*. It apparently comprises 12 membrane-spanning domains, exists as a dimer,[96] and is expressed at the apical membrane of the thick ascending limb[104] and macula densa (MD) cells.[105,106] A K channel (ROMK) is also present in the same membrane, permitting potassium to recycle from the cell to the lumen.[107] Greger et al. showed that the asymmetrical orientation of channels (apical versus basolateral) and the action of the Na/K ATPase and Na-K-2Cl cotransporter combine to create a transepithelial voltage that is oriented with the lumen positive, with respect to the interstitium.[108] This lumen-positive potential drives absorption of Na^+, Ca^{2+}, and Mg^{2+} via the paracellular pathway. The paracellular component of Na reabsorption comprises 50% of the total transepithelial Na transport by thick ascending limb cells.[109] It should be noted, however, that both the transcellular and the paracellular components of Na transport are inhibited by loop diuretics, the former directly and the latter indirectly. The thick ascending limb is virtually impermeable to water. The combination of solute absorption and water impermeability determines the role of the thick ascending limb as the primary diluting segment of the kidney.

Although direct inhibition of ion transport is the most important natriuretic action of loop diuretics, other actions may contribute. Thick ascending limb cells have been shown to produce prostaglandin E_2 following stimulation with furosemide,[110]

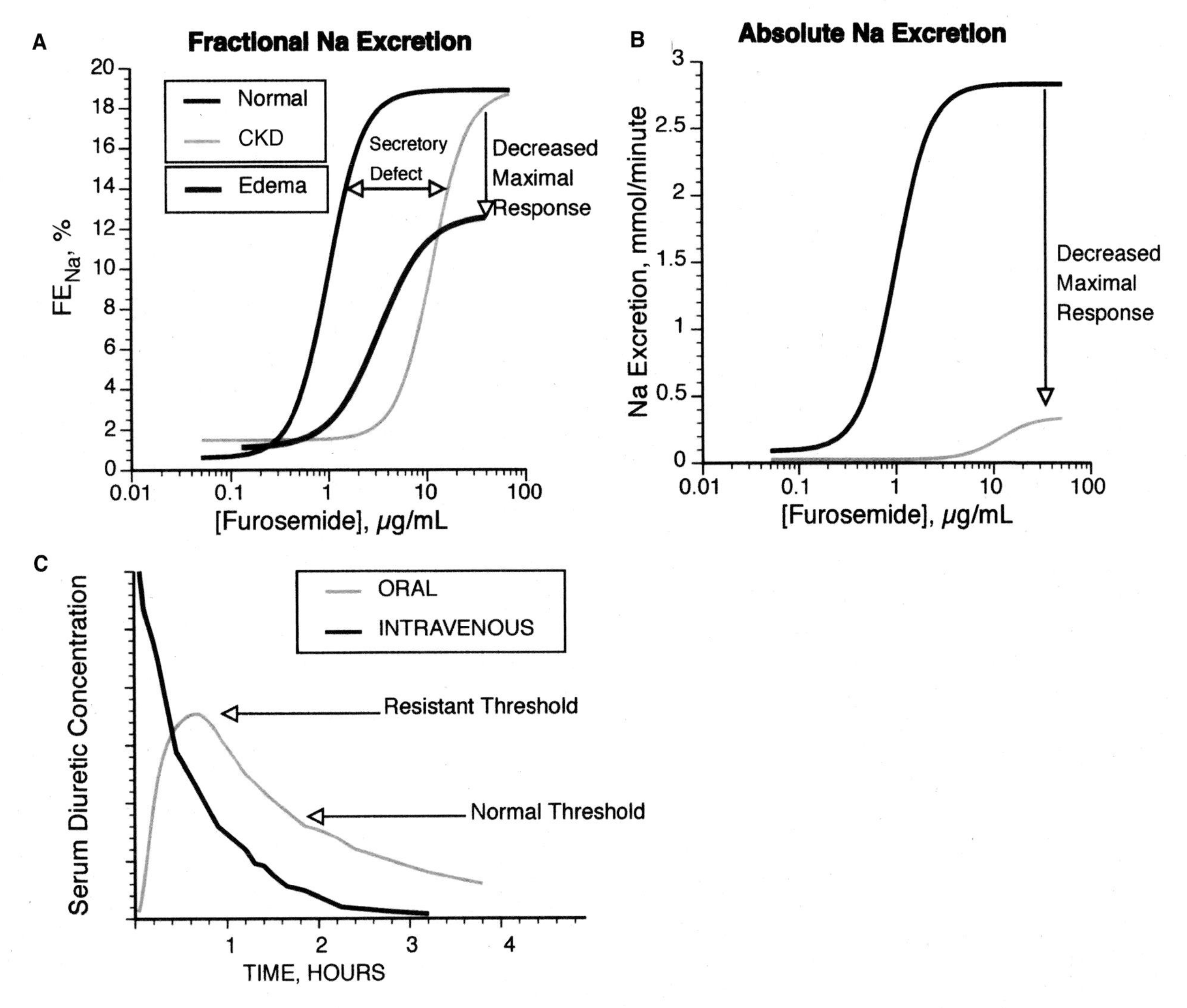

FIGURE 66.5 Dose response curve for loop diuretics. **A:** The fractional Na excretion (FE_{Na}) as a function of loop diuretic concentration. Compared with normal patients, patients with chronic renal failure (CKD) show a rightward shift in the curve, owing to impaired diuretic secretion. The maximal response is preserved when expressed as FE_{Na}, but when expressed as absolute Na excretion **(B)**, maximal natriuresis is reduced in patients with CKD. Patients with edema demonstrate a rightward and downward shift, even when expressed as FE_{Na} **(A)**. **C:** Compares the response to intravenous and oral doses of loop diuretics. In a normal individual (Normal), an oral dose may be as effective as an intravenous dose because the time above the natriuretic threshold (indicated by the *normal* line) is approximately equal. If the natriuretic threshold increases (as indicated by the *dashed line*, from an edematous patient), then the oral dose may not provide a high enough serum level to elicit natriuresis.

perhaps via inhibition of prostaglandin dehydrogenase.[111,112] Blockade of cyclooxygenase reduces the effects of furosemide to inhibit loop segment chloride transport in rats,[113,114] and this effect appears to be important clinically because nonsteroidal anti-inflammatory drugs (NSAIDs) are common causes of diuretic resistance (see below). Increases in renal prostaglandins may also contribute to the hemodynamic effects of loop diuretics, described later.

Calcium and Magnesium Transport

Loop diuretics increase the excretion of the divalent cations calcium (Ca) and magnesium (Mg). Although a component of magnesium and calcium absorption by thick ascending limbs may be active (especially when circulating parathyroid hormone levels are high[115]), a large component of their absorption is passive and paracellular, driven by the transepithelial voltage. As described above, active NaCl transport by thick ascending limb cells leads to a transepithelial voltage, oriented in the lumen positive direction. The paracellular pathway in the thick ascending limb expresses claudin-16 (paracellin-1) and claudin-19, which interact to form a tight junction that mediates both magnesium and calcium movement.[116,117] Mutations in these genes lead to the clinical syndrome familial hypomagnesemia and hypercalciuria (FHHNC), an autosomal recessive tubular disorder that is frequently associated with renal failure.[118] The positive voltage in the lumen, relative to

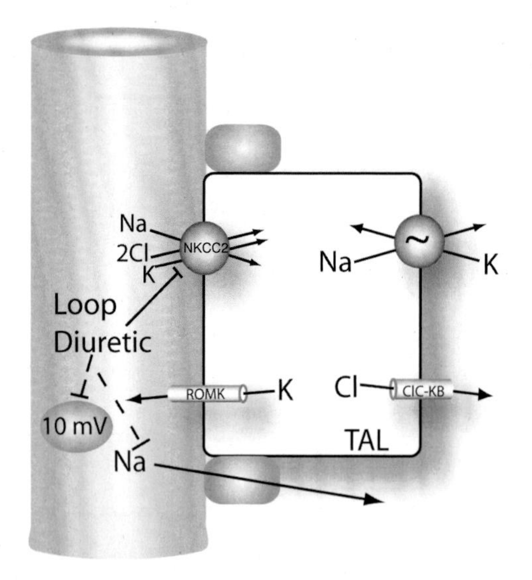

FIGURE 66.6 Mechanisms of diuretic action along the loop of Henle. Figure shows model of thick ascending limb (TAL) cells. Na and Cl are reabsorbed across the apical membrane via the loop diuretic-sensitive Na-K-2Cl cotransporter, NKCC2. Loop diuretics bind to and block this pathway directly. Note that the transepithelial voltage along the TAL is oriented with the lumen positive relative to blood (circled value, given in millivolts, mV). This transepithelial voltage drives a component of Na (and calcium and magnesium, see Fig. 66.9) reabsorption via the paracellular pathway. This component of Na absorption is also reduced by loop diuretics because they reduce the transepithelial voltage.

the interstitium, drives calcium and magnesium absorption through the paracellular pathway. Loop diuretics, by blocking the activity of the Na-K-2Cl cotransporter at the apical membrane of thick ascending limb cells, reduce the transepithelial voltage toward or to 0 mV. This stops passive paracellular calcium and magnesium absorption.

Renin Secretion

In addition to enhancing Na and Cl excretion, effects that result directly from inhibiting Na and Cl transport, loop diuretics also stimulate renin secretion. Although a component of this effect is frequently related to contraction of the extracellular fluid volume (see later), loop diuretics also stimulate renin secretion by inhibiting Na-K-2Cl cotransport directly. Macula densa cells, which control renin secretion, sense the NaCl concentration in the lumen of the thick ascending limb.[119] High luminal NaCl concentrations in the region of the macula densa lead to two distinct but related effects. First, they activate the tubuloglomerular feedback (TGF) response, which suppresses GFR. Second, they inhibit renin secretion. The relation between these two effects is complex and has been reviewed,[120] but both effects appear to result largely from NaCl movement across the apical membrane.[121] Most of the ion transport pathways of macula densa cells are expressed by thick ascending limb cells. This includes the loop diuretic-sensitive Na-K-2Cl cotransporter (NKCC2) at the apical surface.[105,106] Under normal conditions, an increase in luminal NaCl concentration in the thick ascending limb raises the NaCl concentration inside macula densa cells.[121] Because the activity of the basolateral Na/K ATPase is lower in macula densa cells than in surrounding thick ascending limb cells,[120] the cell NaCl concentration is much more dependent on luminal NaCl concentration in macula densa than in thick ascending limb cells.[122] When luminal and macula densa cell NaCl concentrations decline, production rates of nitric oxide and prostaglandin E_2 are stimulated. Although the mechanisms by which Na and Cl transport regulate nitric oxide and prostaglandin production rates are not known, both mediators appear to participate importantly in effecting renin secretion. Interestingly, loop diuretics also may stimulate renin secretion by inhibiting NKCC1, the secretory form of the three ion cotransport mechanism. Genetic deletion of NKCCC1 leads to an increase in plasma renin activity and a failure of renin exocytosis in response to furosemide,[119] suggesting a role for alternative pathways.

The constitutive (neuronal) isoform of nitric oxide synthase (nNOS) is expressed at high levels by macula densa cells, but not by other cells in the kidney.[123] Nitric oxide produced by macula densa cells has a paracrine effect to increase cellular cAMP in adjacent juxtaglomerular cells. Cyclic AMP through protein kinase A helps to stimulate renin secretion. In juxtaglomerular cells, nitric oxide may act by increasing cellular cGMP which inhibits phosphodiesterase 3,[124] leading to phosphodiesterase 3 inhibition and cAMP accumulation. Several laboratories reported that furosemide-induced stimulation of renin secretion is dependent on an intact nitric oxide system because nonspecific nitric oxide inhibition interferes with this phenomenon.[125–127] More recent studies, however, utilized knockout models to examine the role of nitric oxide in diuretic-induced renin secretion. Using this approach, it appears that neither neuronal nor endothelial nitric oxide synthases are required for loop diuretic–induced renin secretion. Instead, nitric oxide appears to play a permissive, rather than necessary, role in facilitating diuretic-induced renin secretion.[128]

Prostaglandin production also participates in regulating renin secretion. Cyclooxygenase, COX-2, is expressed by macula densa cells and by interstitial cells in the kidney.[129–132] This isoform is often found only after induction by inflammatory cytokines. Blockade of prostaglandin synthesis either by nonspecific cyclooxygenase inhibitors[133] or by specific COX-2 blockers[134,135] reduces both the natriuresis induced by loop diuretics and dramatically inhibits the renin secretory response. These results have been corroborated in humans.[136]

Renal Hemodynamics

GFR and renal blood flow (RBF) tend to be preserved during loop diuretic administration,[137] although GFR and RPF can decline if extracellular fluid volume contraction is severe. Loop diuretics reduce renal vascular resistance and increase

RBF under experimental conditions.[138,139] This effect is believed related to the diuretic-induced production of vasodilatory prostaglandins (discussed previously).

Another factor that may contribute to the tendency of loop diuretics to maintain GFR and RBF despite volume contraction is their effect on the TGF system. The sensing mechanism that activates the TGF system involves NaCl transport across the apical membrane of macula densa cells by the loop diuretic sensitive Na-K-2Cl cotransporter.[140] Under normal conditions, when the luminal concentration of NaCl reaching the macula densa rises, GFR decreases via TGF. To a large degree, the TGF-mediated decrease in GFR is believed to be due to afferent arteriole constriction. In response to changes in NaCl transport across the apical membrane of macula densa cells, ATP is released across the basolateral membranes through a NaCl sensitive ATP-permeable large-conductance (380 pS) anion channel.[141] ATP appears to be degraded to adenosine which activates A1 adenosine receptor (P1 purinergic receptor class) expressed on afferent arteriole,[142,143] as reviewed.[140] Loop diuretic drugs block TGF by blocking the sensing step of TGF.[144] In the absence of effects on the macula densa, loop diuretics would be expected to suppress GFR and RPF by increasing distal NaCl delivery and activating the TGF system. Instead, blockade of the TGF permits GFR and RPF to be maintained.

Systemic Hemodynamics

Acute intravenous administration of loop diuretics increases venous capacitance.[145] Some studies suggest that this effect results from stimulation of prostaglandin synthesis by the kidney.[146,147] Other studies suggest that loop diuretics have effects in peripheral vascular beds as well.[148] Pickkers and coworkers examined the local effects of furosemide in the human forearm. Furosemide had no effect on arterial vessels, but did cause dilation of veins, an effect that was dependent on local prostaglandin production.[149] More recently, loop diuretic-induced vasodilation was shown to depend on increased nitric oxide production.[150] Although venodilation and improvements in cardiac hemodynamics frequently result from intravenous therapy with loop diuretics, the hemodynamic response to intravenous loop diuretics may be more complex.[151] Johnston et al. reported that low dose furosemide increased venous capacitance, but that higher doses did not.[152] It was suggested that furosemide-induced renin secretion leads to angiotensin II-induced vasoconstriction. This vasoconstrictor might overwhelm the prostaglandin-mediated vasodilatory effects in some patients. In two series, 1 to 1.5 mg per kg furosemide boluses, administered to patients with chronic heart failure, resulted in transient *deteriorations* in hemodynamics (during the first hour), with declines in stroke volume index, increases in left ventricular filling pressure,[153] and exacerbation of heart failure symptoms. These changes may be related to activation of both the sympathetic nervous system and the renin/angiotensin system by the diuretic drug. Evidence for a role of the renin/angiotensin system in the furosemide-induced deterioration in systemic hemodynamics includes the temporal association between its activation and hemodynamic deterioration,[153] and the ability of angiotensin-converting enzyme (ACE) inhibitors to prevent much of the pressor effect.[154] The effects of renal denervation on sympathetic responses to furosemide were studied. These results confirm that the effects are mediated by both direct renal nerve traffic and indirectly, by activation of the renin/angiotensin axis.[155,156] Many other studies have shown that acute loop diuretic administration frequently produces a transient decline in cardiac output; whether diuretic administration increases or decreases left atrial pressure acutely may depend primarily on the state of underlying sympathetic nervous system and renin/angiotensin axis activation.

Pharmacokinetics

The three loop diuretics that are used most commonly—furosemide, bumetanide, and torsemide—are absorbed quickly after oral administration, reaching peak concentrations within 30 minutes to 2 hours. Furosemide absorption is slower than its elimination in normal subjects; thus, the time to reach peak serum level is slower for furosemide than for bumetanide and torsemide. This phenomenon is called "absorption-limited kinetics," as the rate of absorption is often slower than the rate of elimination.[3] The bioavailability of loop diuretics varies from 50% to 90% (Table 66.2); furosemide bioavailability is approximately 50%[4]; when furosemide dosing is switched from intravenous to oral, the dose may need to be increased to compensate for its poor bioavailability.[3] The half-lives of the loop diuretics available in the United States vary, but all are relatively short (ranging from approximately 1 hour for bumetanide to 3 to 4 hours for torsemide). The half-lives of muzolimine, xipamide, and ozolinone, none of which are available in the United States, are longer (6 to 15 hours).

Loop diuretics are organic anions that circulate tightly bound to albumin (>95%), thus their volume of distribution is small except during extreme hypoproteinemia.[157] Approximately 50% of an administered dose of furosemide is excreted unchanged into the urine. The remainder appears to be eliminated by glucuronidation, probably by the kidney. Torsemide and bumetanide are eliminated both by hepatic processes and through renal excretion. The differences in metabolic fate mean that the half-life of furosemide is altered by renal failure, whereas this is not true for torsemide and bumetanide. Similar to CAIs and thiazides, loop diuretics gain access to the tubular fluid almost exclusively by proximal secretion. The peritubular uptake is mediated by the organic anion transporters OAT1 and OAT3, whereas the apically located multidrug resistance–associated protein 4 (Mrp-4) mediates secretion into the tubular fluid. Mice lacking OAT1, OAT3, or Mrp-4 are remarkably resistant to both loop and thiazide diuretics, illustrating the functional importance of these proteins.[158–160] In humans, polymorphisms in the gene encoding the organic anion transporter OATP1B1 resulted in a slower elimination of torsemide.[161]

TABLE 66.2 **Pharmacokinetics of Loop Diuretics**

		Elimination Half-Life (hours)			
	Oral Bioavailability (%)	Healthy	Renal Disease	Liver Disease	Heart Failure
Furosemide	10–100	1.5–2	2.8	2.5	2.7
Bumetanide	80–100	1	1.6	2.3	1.3
Torsemide	80–100	3–4	4–5	8	6

Adapted from the data in Brater DC. Diuretic therapy. *N Engl J Med*. 1998;339:387–395.

Interestingly, the response to loop diuretics is also associated with polymorphisms in the genes encoding the more distal sodium transporters NCC and ENaC.[162]

Clinical Use

Loop diuretics are used commonly to treat the edematous conditions, congestive heart failure, cirrhosis of the liver, and nephrotic syndrome.[163] In addition, a variety of other electrolyte, fluid, and acid base disorders can respond to loop diuretic therapy. Details of loop diuretic use for the treatment of edematous conditions are beyond the scope of this chapter.

Adverse Effects

There are at least three types of adverse effects of loop diuretics. The first and most common side effects are those that result directly from the effects of these drugs on renal electrolyte and water excretion. The second class of side effects is toxic, effects that are dose-related and predictable. The third class includes idiosyncratic allergic drug reactions.

Loop diuretics are frequently administered to treat edematous expansion of the extracellular fluid volume. Edema usually results from a decrease in the "effective" arterial blood volume. Overzealous diuretic usage or intercurrent complicating illnesses can lead to excessive contraction of the intravascular volume leading to orthostatic hypotension, renal dysfunction, and sympathetic overactivity. Patients suffering from heart failure are typically treated with both diuretics and ACE inhibitors or angiotensin receptor blockers (ARBs); this combination is especially likely to worsen renal function, under certain circumstances. Functional renal failure in such patients often responds to reduced diuretic doses and liberalization of dietary NaCl intake, permitting continued administration of the ACE inhibitor/ARBs.[164,165]

Other patients at increased risk for renal dysfunction during diuretic therapy include the elderly,[166] patients with preexisting renal insufficiency,[167] patients with right-sided heart failure or pericardial disease, and patients taking NSAIDs. In a case control study of NSAID use and renal failure, diuretic users had a 2.77 relative risk of acute kidney injury, compared with nonusers.[168]

Disorders of Na and K concentration are among the most frequent adverse effects of loop diuretics. Hyponatremia is less common with loop diuretics than with distal convoluted tubule diuretics (see later), but can occur. Its pathogenesis is usually multifactorial, but involves the effect of loop diuretics to impair the clearance of solute free water. Additional factors that may contribute include the nonosmotic release of arginine vasopressin,[169] hypokalemia, and hypomagnesemia.[170] Conversely, loop diuretics have been used to treat hyponatremia when combined with hypertonic saline, in the setting of the syndrome of inappropriate ADH secretion.[100,171] The combination of loop diuretics and ACE inhibitors has been reported to ameliorate hyponatremia in the setting of congestive heart failure.[172] The value of adding a loop diuretic to treatment with a vasopressin V2 receptor antagonist for hyponatremic syndrome of inappropriate ADH secretion has been suggested.[173,174] Hypokalemia occurs commonly during therapy with loop diuretics, although the magnitude is smaller than that induced by distal convoluted tubule diuretics (loop diuretics, 0.3 mM, vs. distal convoluted tubule [DCT] diuretics, 0.5–0.9 mM).[175,176] Loop diuretics increase the delivery of potassium to the distal tubule because they block potassium reabsorption via the Na-K-2Cl cotransporter. In rats, under control conditions, approximately half the excreted potassium was delivered to the "early" distal tubule. During furosemide infusion, the delivery of potassium to the early distal tubule rose to 28% of the filtered load.[177] Thus, it appears that a large component of the effect of loop diuretics to increase potassium excretion acutely reflects their ability to block potassium reabsorption by the thick ascending limb. Nevertheless, during chronic diuretic therapy, the degree of potassium wasting correlates best with volume contraction and serum aldosterone levels.[178] These data suggest that, under chronic conditions, the predominant effect of loop diuretics to stimulate potassium excretion results from their tendency to increase mineralocorticoid hormones while simultaneously increasing distal Na and water delivery.

Metabolic alkalosis is very common during chronic treatment with loop diuretics. Loop diuretics cause metabolic alkalosis via several mechanisms. First, they increase the excretion of urine that is bicarbonate free but contains Na and Cl. This leads to contraction of the extracellular fluid around a fixed amount of bicarbonate buffer; a phenomenon known as "contraction alkalosis." This probably contributes only slightly to the metabolic alkalosis that commonly accompanies chronic loop diuretic treatment. Loop diuretics directly inhibit transport of Na and Cl into thick ascending limb cells. In some species, these cells also express an isoform of the Na/H exchanger at the apical surface. When Na entry via the Na-K-2Cl cotransporter is blocked by a loop diuretic, the decline in intracellular Na activity will stimulate H secretion via the Na/H exchanger.[179–181] Loop diuretics stimulate the renin/angiotensin/aldosterone pathway, both directly and indirectly, as discussed previously. Aldosterone stimulates Na reabsorption by principal cells of the CNT and CCT, which renders the tubule lumen more negative and increases H-ATPase activity.[182] Aldosterone also directly activates the vacuolar H^+-ATPase in the outer medullary collecting tubule.[183,184] Thus, through different mechanisms, aldosterone stimulates H^+ secretion via H^+ ATPase present at the apical membrane of α intercalated cells. Hypokalemia itself also contributes to metabolic alkalosis by increasing ammonium production,[185] stimulating bicarbonate reabsorption by proximal tubules,[186,187] and increasing the activity of the H/K ATPase in the distal nephron.[67,188] Finally, contraction of the extracellular fluid volume stimulates Na/H exchange in the proximal tubule and may reduce the filtered load of bicarbonate. All of these factors may contribute to the metabolic alkalosis observed during chronic loop diuretic treatment.

Ototoxicity is the most common toxic effect of loop diuretics that is unrelated to their effects on the kidney. Deafness, which is usually temporary but can be permanent, was reported shortly after the introduction of loop diuretics. It appears likely that all loop diuretics cause ototoxicity, because ototoxicity can occur during use of chemically dissimilar drugs such as furosemide and ethacrynic acid.[189,190] The mechanism of ototoxicity remains unclear, although the stria vascularis, which is responsible for maintaining endolymphatic potential and ion balance, appears to be a primary target for toxicity.[191] Loop diuretics reduce the striatal voltage from +80 mV to −10 to −20 mV within minutes of application.[192] A characteristic finding in loop diuretic ototoxicity is strial edema. This suggests that toxicity involves inhibition of ion fluxes.[191] Ikeda and Morizono detected functional evidence for the presence of a Na-K-2Cl cotransporter in the basolateral membrane of marginal cells in the inner ear.[193] According to the model proposed by these investigators, marginal cells resemble secretory cells in other organ systems, with a Na-K-2Cl cotransporter and Na/K ATPase at the basolateral cell membrane and channels for K and Cl at the apical surface. According to this model, loop diuretic induced shrinkage of marginal cells results from inhibition of cell Na, K, and Cl uptake across the basolateral cell membrane. This model received molecular confirmation when the secretory isoform of the Na-K-2Cl cotransporter, NKCC1, was localized in the lateral wall of the cochlea, using specific antibodies[194] and real-time polymerase chain reaction (RT-PCR).[195] Furthermore, disruption of the ubiquitous form of the Na-K-Cl cotransporter, NKCC1, leads to deafness in mice.[196–198] Loop diuretics cause loss of outer hair cells in the basal turn of the cochlea, rupture of endothelial layers, cystic formation in the stria vascularis, and marginal cell edema in the stria vascularis.[199]

Ototoxicity appears to be related to the peak serum concentration of loop diuretic and therefore tends to occur during rapid drug infusion of high doses. For this reason, this complication is most common in patients with uremia.[200] It has been recommended that furosemide infusion be no more rapid than 4 mg per minute.[201] In addition to renal failure, infants, patients with cirrhosis, and patients receiving aminoglycosides or *cis*-platinum may be at increased risk for ototoxicity.[200]

Myalgias have been reported with bolus infusion of bumetanide.[202]

DISTAL CONVOLUTED TUBULE DIURETICS

The first orally active drug to be developed that inhibited Na and Cl transport along the distal convoluted tubule (DCT) was chlorothiazide. Chlorothiazide was developed as sulfonamide-based carbonic anhydrase inhibitors were modified in pursuit of substances that increased Cl excretion rather than bicarbonate. The identification of a substance that increased Na and Cl excretion rates was immediately recognized as clinically significant, because extracellular fluid contains predominantly NaCl rather than $NaHCO_3$, and because acidosis limits the effectiveness of carbonic anhydrase inhibitors. Subsequent development led to a wide variety of benzothiadiazide (thiazide) diuretics (Fig. 66.7); all are analogs of 1,2,4-benzothiadiazine-1,1-dioxide. Other structurally related diuretics include the quinazolines (such as metolazone) and substituted benzophenone sulfonamide (such as chlorthalidone). Although the term "thiazide diuretics" is frequently used to describe this class of drugs, a more accurate descriptor is the term *distal convoluted tubule diuretics*.

Urinary Electrolyte and Water Excretion

Acute administration of these drugs increases the excretion of Na, K, Cl, HCO_3, phosphate, and urate (see Table 66.1). The increases in HCO_3, phosphate, and urate excretion are probably related primarily to carbonic anhydrase inhibition, and not to inhibition of the Na-Cl cotransporter (see later). As such, the effects of DCT diuretics to increase HCO_3, phosphate, and urate excretion may

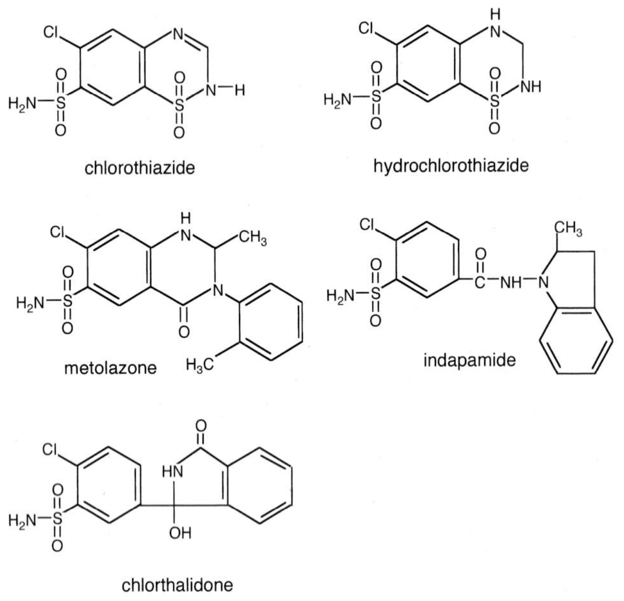

FIGURE 66.7 Structures of distal convoluted tubule diuretics.

vary, depending on the carbonic anhydrase inhibiting potency of a particular drug. Chronically, as contraction of the extracellular fluid volume occurs, uric acid excretion declines, and hyperuricemia can occur.[203] Further, bicarbonate excretion ceases, and continuing losses of chloride without bicarbonate coupled with extracellular fluid volume contraction may lead to metabolic alkalosis. In contrast to loop and proximally acting diuretics, DCT diuretics strongly reduce urinary calcium excretion.[204] Although the effects on urinary calcium excretion can be variable during acute administration,[205–207] these drugs uniformly lead to calcium retention when administered chronically.

DCT diuretics inhibit the clearance of solute free water when administered during water diuresis. This effect is similar to that of loop diuretics and originally led to the mistaken inference that they act along the thick ascending limb. In contrast to loop diuretics, however, DCT diuretics do not limit water retention during antidiuresis.

Mechanism of Action

Sodium and Water Transport in the Proximal Tubule

As discussed previously, DCT diuretics are related chemically to carbonic anhydrase inhibitors and most DCT diuretics retain some carbonic anhydrase inhibiting activity.[208] Carbonic anhydrase inhibitors interfere with the activity of the apical Na/H exchanger expressed at the luminal membrane of proximal tubule cells by indirect mechanisms described above. Although this effect of DCT diuretics may occur when these drugs are administered acutely (as during intravenous chlorothiazide administration), it probably contributes little to the overall natriuresis during chronic use.[209,210] Yet this effect may play a role in the tendency for DCT diuretics to reduce the GFR and activate the TGF mechanism.[40] The relative carbonic anhydrase inhibiting potency (shown in parentheses) of some commonly used DCT diuretics is chlorthalidone (67) > benzthiazide (50) > polythiazide (40) > chlorothiazide (14) > hydrochlorothiazide (1) > bendroflumethiazide (0.07).[211]

NaCl Absorption in the Distal Nephron

As the name indicates, the predominant site at which DCT diuretics inhibit ion transport is the DCT. This region of the nephron, between the macula densa and the confluence with another nephron to form the CCD, is cytologically heterogeneous.[212,213] It comprises a short stretch of post–macula densa thick ascending limb, the DCT, the CNT, and the initial portion of the CCD. In previous editions, the controversies surrounding the predominant sites of expression of the thiazide-sensitive transporter were described. The interested reader is referred to those editions for more details. These controversies were resolved, when the thiazide-sensitive Na-Cl cotransporter (now called NCC) was expression-cloned from the flounder bladder,[214] and later cloned from rat, mouse, rabbit, and human kidney[215–218]; the gene is *SLC12A3* and is closely related to NKCC2, and is a member of the cation chloride cotransporter gene family. In rat, human, and mouse, NCC message and protein are expressed by DCT cells. A model of NaCl transport by DCT cells is shown in Figure 66.8. In human, rat, and mouse, expression of NCC extends into a transitional segment, referred to as the DCT2, which shares properties of DCT and CNTs.[219,220] In the rabbit, the thiazide-sensitive Na-Cl cotransporter was also shown to be expressed *exclusively* by DCT cells[221]; CNT cells do not express the transporter. Thus, from a molecular standpoint, the NCC is expressed by distal convoluted tubule cells in all mammalian species examined to date.

DCT diuretics are organic anions that bind to and inhibit the transporter. Based on studies performed before NCC was identified at the molecular level, [^{3}H] metolazone binding to kidney cortical membranes was studied. DCT diuretics were shown to bind to the cotransporter at an anion site.[222] This conclusion derives from the observation that chloride inhibits the binding of [^{3}H] metolazone in a competitive manner. Unlike loop diuretic binding to the Na-K-2Cl cotransporter, [^{3}H] metolazone binding to the Na-Cl cotransporter does not require the presence of Na, suggesting either that chloride binds first to the transporter or that binding of ions to the transporter is not "ordered." Monroy and colleagues[223] studied thiazide inhibition of the cloned transporter and reported that the inhibitory activity of DCT diuretics could be inhibited by increasing concentration of *either* Cl^- or Na^+. These workers suggested a model that incorporates Na and Cl binding to the transporter in random order, with alterations in diuretic affinity occurring secondarily. Morena and colleagues used a chimeric approach to study sites of diuretic binding to NCC. They reported that

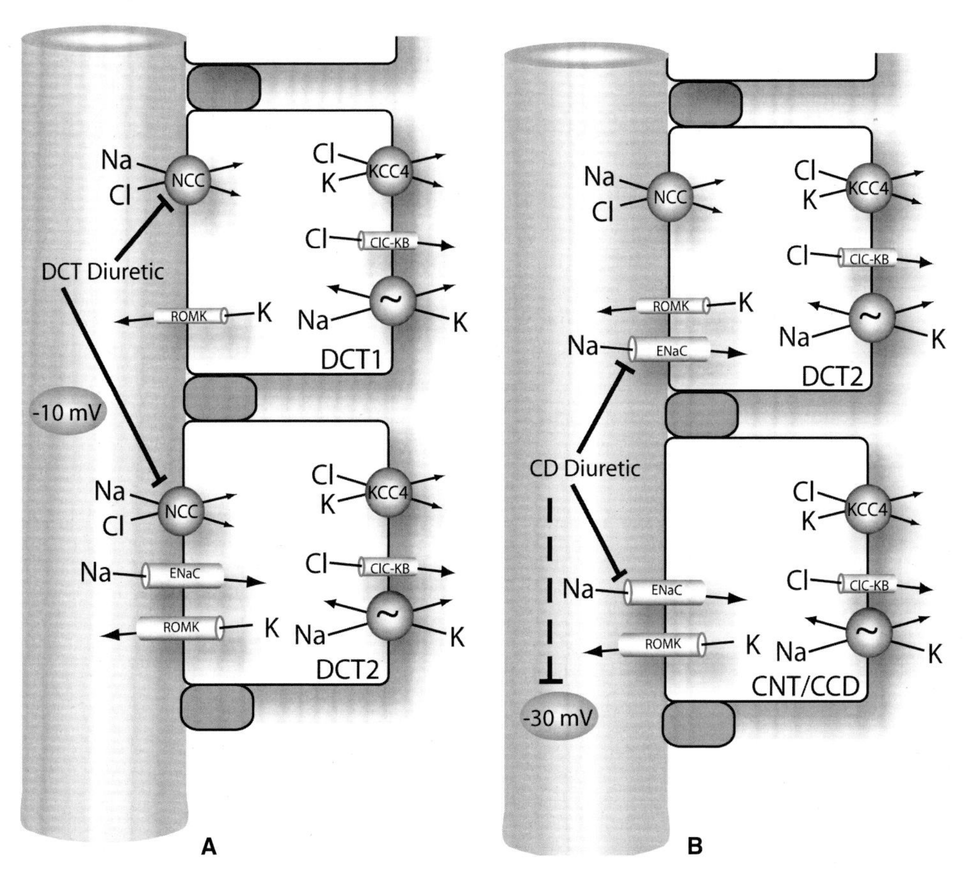

FIGURE 66.8 Mechanisms of distal convoluted tubule (DCT) and collecting duct (CD) diuretics. **A:** Mechanism of action of DCT diuretics. In rat, mouse, and human, two types of distal convoluted tubule cells have been identified, referred to here as DCT-1 and DCT-2. Na and Cl are reabsorbed across the apical membrane of DCT-1 cells only via the thiazide-sensitive Na-Cl cotransporter. This transport protein is also expressed by DCT-2 cells where Na can also cross through the epithelial Na channel, ENaC.[219,220,395] Thus, the transepithelial voltage along the DCT-1 is near to 0 mV, whereas it is finite and lumen-negative along the DCT-2. **B:** Mechanism of action of CD diuretics. The late distal convoluted tubule cells (DCT2 cells) and connecting (CNT) or CD cells are shown. Na is reabsorbed via the epithelial Na channel (ENaC), which lies in parallel with a K channel (ROMK). The transepithelial voltage is oriented with the lumen negative, relative to interstitium (shown by the *circled value*), generating a favorable gradient for transepithelial K secretion. Drugs that block the epithelial Na value reduce the voltage toward 0 mV (effect indicated by *dashed line*), thereby inhibiting K secretion.

the site determining metolazone affinity was near the last transmembrane domain, whereas the region defining chloride affinity was near the 5 to 6 transmembrane domains. Although these conclusions appear to be contradictory, it should be mentioned that in one study diuretic binding was determined, whereas in the others changes in diuretic affinity were determined. As is the case for the Na-K-2Cl cotransporter, described previously, firm conclusions about sites of diuretic binding await crystallization of the transport protein.

Evidence for thiazide action in other nephron segments has also been obtained. In vivo catheterization experiments demonstrated a component of thiazide-sensitive Na transport in medullary collecting tubules of rats.[224] Terada and Knepper detected thiazide-sensitive Na-Cl transport in rat CCDs perfused in vitro,[225] a finding recently confirmed when it was shown that thiazides can inhibit a sodium-dependent chloride-bicarbonate exchanger in the collecting duct.[226] The role of this effect in the clinical response to DCT diuretics remains to be established.

Calcium and Magnesium Transport

When administered chronically, DCT diuretics reduce calcium excretion. This effect has been utilized clinically to treat calcium nephrolithiasis (see later). Much progress in understanding mechanisms of the hypocalciuric effect of DCT diuretics has been made during the past 10 years, but the mechanisms involved remain controversial. Acute administration of DCT diuretics has a variable effect on calcium excretion, sometimes leading to increases in calcium excretion.[205,227] This probably reflects the carbonic anhydrase inhibiting capacity of these drugs, because carbonic anhydrase inhibitors increase urinary calcium excretion acutely. Calcium reabsorption by proximal tubules is coupled functionally to sodium reabsorption; drugs that inhibit proximal Na reabsorption also inhibit proximal calcium reabsorption.[228] Thus, during chronic treatment, the filtered calcium load may decrease (owing to ECF volume depletion) and proximal calcium reabsorption may increase (owing to the ECF volume contraction), which stimulates proximal Na^+ and water reabsorption.

DCT diuretics also increase renal calcium reabsorption in the distal nephron. Although rat distal nephrons reabsorb both Na and Ca, Constanzo showed[229] that thiazide diuretics dissociate the two; Na reabsorption is inhibited whereas calcium reabsorption is stimulated. Several factors are now believed to contribute to the effect of DCT diuretics to stimulate calcium reabsorption (Fig. 66.9). As in most other cells, the intracellular calcium concentration of DCT cells is low, compared with extracellular fluid calcium.[230] Calcium enters DCT cells passively, down its electrochemical gradient via specific calcium channels, primarily Trpv5.[231,232] DCT diuretics increase the intracellular calcium activity, suggesting that a primary effect is to increase apical calcium entry.[230]

Bindels and colleagues showed that a member of the transient receptor potential family, TrpV5, is expressed at the apical membranes of cells along the second part of the distal convoluted tubule (the DCT2) and along the CNT. It is regulated by vitamin D and appears to possess several characteristics suggesting that it is one of the primary apical calcium entry pathways. Lee and colleagues confirmed an acute effect of DCT diuretics on distal calcium uptake, but found that a large portion of the chronic effects of DCT diuretics results from extracellular fluid volume depletion. They speculated that acute exposure to DCT diuretics hyperpolarizes DCT cells, as suggested by Friedman and colleagues,[230] activating TRPV5 channels and also increasing their expression at the mRNA level.[233] During chronic exposure, however, ECF

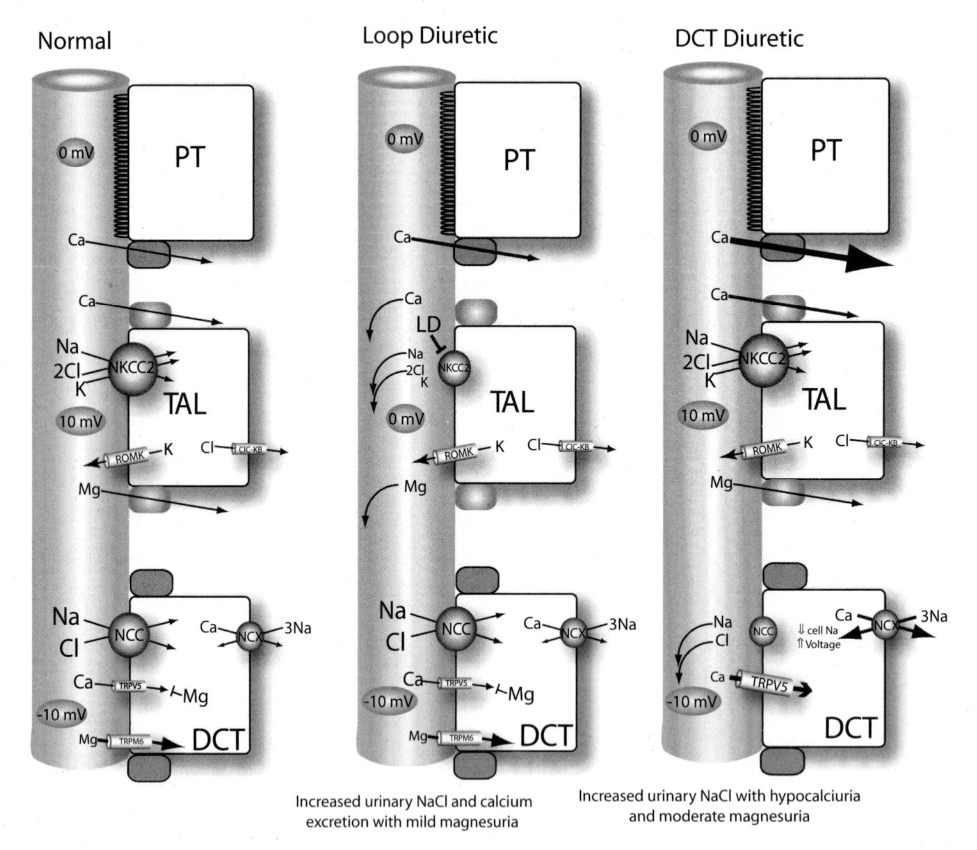

FIGURE 66.9 Possible mechanisms of diuretic effects on calcium and magnesium excretion. Typical cells from the proximal tubule (PT), thick ascending limb (TAL), distal convoluted tubule (DCT) are shown. Calcium reabsorption occurs along the DCT largely via a transient receptor potential channel (TRPV5). Magnesium reabsorption occurs along the DCT largely via a transient receptor potential channel (TRPM6). Transepithelial voltages (representative but arbitrary values, given in millivolts, mV) are shown. Net effects on electrolyte excretion are shown at the bottom. Normal conditions are at the left. Treatment with loop diuretics (LDs) is shown in the middle; treatment with DCT diuretics is shown on the right. LDs reduce the magnitude of the lumen-positive transepithelial voltage, thereby retarding passive calcium and magnesium reabsorption. Passive calcium and magnesium reabsorption appears to traverse the paracellular pathway. Chronic treatment, especially with DCT diuretics, increases proximal Na and Ca reabsorption; thus, less calcium is delivered distally. Enhanced distal calcium absorption, driven by DCT diuretics, also occurs.[204] Effects of DCT diuretics to increase magnesium excretion remain incompletely understood, but likely include decreased TRPM6 abundance.

volume contraction reduces distal NaCl delivery limiting the DCT diuretic-induced hyperpolarization.[233]

DCT diuretics not only stimulate entry of calcium across the apical membrane, but also stimulate calcium transport across the basolateral cell membrane into the interstitium. DCT cells, at least in rat, mouse, and human, express the Na/Ca exchanger and a calcium ATPase. The Na/Ca exchanger is electrogenic and is believed to carry three Na ions into the cell in exchange for one calcium ion out. When DCT diuretics block the luminal entry pathway for Na and Cl, the intracellular Na^+ concentration declines, and the cells hyperpolarize. Both the hyperpolarization and the decline in cell Na^+ concentration increase the electrochemical driving force favoring calcium movement from cell to interstitium. Although the data describing effects on apical and basolateral calcium transport were obtained in different model systems and from different species, taken together, they suggest that DCT diuretics stimulate both the apical entry pathway and the basolateral exit pathway that permit calcium reabsorption. The calcium reabsorptive pathway of the distal tubule is quite potent and the passive calcium permeability of this tubule segment is low; in stationary microperfusion experiments, the distal tubule was able to reduce the luminal calcium concentration below 0.1 mM.[229]

The net effect of DCT diuretics to reduce calcium excretion appears most likely to involve both effects along the proximal and the distal tubule. The interested reader is referred to the review by Reilly and Huang for a more detailed description of the controversy and the data supporting effects along different segments.[204]

DCT diuretics enhance magnesium excretion, but the effects are generally much less profound than their effects on calcium excretion. This is in contrast to the effects of genetic NCC deletion or inactivity, as occurs in Gitelman syndrome, where hypomagnesemia is a cardinal feature. Acute infusions have been reported to have little effect on magnesium excretion.[205,234,235] In contrast, DCT diuretics increase urinary magnesium excretion and can cause hypomagnesemia when administered chronically.[236–238] One important pathway for magnesium reabsorption across the apical membrane of DCT cells is the transient receptor potential, TRPM6.[239] This protein localizes to DCT cells (and intestinal cells) at the apical membrane and has functional characteristics suggesting it is, or is part of, the magnesium entry step along the distal nephron.[240]

The mechanisms by which chronic DCT diuretic administration lead to hypomagnesemia remain controversial. Quamme proposed that DCT diuretics, by hyperpolarizing DCT cells, enhance magnesium uptake, thereby downregulating the expression of magnesium channels, leading to magnesemia.[241] Ellison suggested that magnesium wasting consequent to DCT diuretic treatment resulted from the actions of aldosterone to increase the lumen-negative transepithelial voltage of the DCT.[242] This would be expected to increase the electrochemical gradient favoring magnesium secretion (or inhibiting its reabsorption). Loffing and colleagues suggested that magnesium wasting results from the destruction of DCT cells, resulting from apoptosis induced by DCT diuretics.[243,244] Several groups have reported that inactivation of NCC reduces the abundance of Trpm6, which would be expected to impair magnesium reabsorption.[245,246]

Renal Hemodynamics

DCT diuretics increase renal vascular resistance and decrease the GFR when given acutely. Okusa et al.[40] showed that intravenous chlorothiazide reduced the GFF by 16% when measured as whole kidney clearance or by micropuncture of a superficial distal tubule. In contrast, however, when flow to the macula densa was blocked and the single nephron GFR was measured by micropuncture of a proximal tubule, intravenous chlorothiazide had no effect on GFR. These data suggest that diuretic-induced stimulation of the TGF system mediates the effect of DCT diuretics on GFR; yet, the recent data described previously (in which carbonic anhydrase inhibition was shown to reduce the GFR of adenosine-1 receptor–deficient, TGF-deficient, animals) suggest that other mechanisms may be involved as well.[71]

During chronic treatment with DCT diuretics, mild contraction of the ECF volume develops, thereby increasing solute and water reabsorption by the proximal tubule. This effect reduces Na delivery to the macula densa. This would be expected to return GFR toward baseline values during chronic treatment with DCT diuretics.[210,247] Thus, when used chronically, DCT diuretics lead to a state of mild ECF volume contraction, increased fractional proximal reabsorption, and relatively preserved glomerular filtration.[210,247]

When administered acutely, the effect of DCT diuretics on renin secretion is variable.[248] If urinary NaCl losses are replaced, these drugs tend to suppress renin secretion,[249] probably by increasing NaCl delivery to the macula densa.[40] In contrast, during chronic administration, renin secretion increases both because solute delivery to the macula densa declines[210] and because volume depletion activates the vascular mechanism for renin secretion.

Pharmacokinetics

DCT diuretics are organic anions that circulate in a highly protein-bound state. As with loop diuretics, the amount reaching the tubule fluid by filtration across the glomerular basement membrane is small; the predominant route of entry into tubule fluid is by secretion via the organic anion secretory pathway in the proximal tubule.[3] DCT diuretics are rapidly absorbed across the gut, reaching peak concentrations within 1.5 to 4 hours.[3] The amount of administered drug that reaches the urine varies greatly,[3] as does the half-life. Short-acting DCT diuretics include bendroflumethiazide, hydrochlorothiazide, tizolemide, and trichlormethiazide. Medium-acting DCT diuretics include chlorothiazide, hydroflumethiazide, indapamide, and mefruside. Long-acting DCT diuretics include chlorthalidone, metolazone, and polythiazide.[3] The clinical effects of the differences in half-life are unclear, except in the incidence of hypokalemia, which is more common in patients taking the longer acting drugs such as chlorthalidone.[175,250] The longer half life may also contribute to their increased efficacy in essential hypertension (see following). The individual response to DCT diuretics is also associated with polymorphisms in genes encoding proteins that directly or indirectly regulate NCC, including with-no-lysine kinase 1 (WNK1)[251] and α-adducin.[252]

Clinical Use

DCT diuretics are used most commonly to treat essential hypertension.[253] Despite a great deal of debate about the potential complications of DCT diuretics, these drugs continue to be recommended as first-line therapy for hypertension because they are at least as effective as more expensive agents at reducing mortality.[254] Although hydrochlorothiazide has become most commonly used, at least to treat hypertension, there is increasing evidence that chlorthalidone and indapamide may be more effective than hydrochlorothiazide.[255]

DCT diuretics are also used occasionally to treat edematous conditions, although they may be less effective than loop diuretics. Although the maximal effect of loop diuretics to increase urinary Na, Cl, and water excretion is greater than that of DCT diuretics, Reyes and colleagues have shown that the cumulative effects of DCT diuretics on urinary Na and Cl excretion are often greater than those of once daily furosemide.[256] Although these studies were conducted in normal volunteers, they may extend to patients with mild cases of edema. In addition, DCT diuretics have proved useful to treat edematous patients who have become resistant to loop diuretics. In this case, the addition of a DCT diuretic to a regimen that includes a loop diuretic frequently increases urinary Na and Cl excretion dramatically. The interested reader is referred elsewhere for a discussion of combination diuretic therapy and diuretic synergism.[76,151]

DCT diuretics have become drugs of choice to prevent the recurrence of kidney stones in patients with idiopathic hypercalciuria. In several controlled and many uncontrolled studies, the recurrence rate for calcium stones has been reduced by up to 80%.[257–259] Relatively high doses of DCT diuretics are often employed for the treatment of nephrolithiasis.[260] Some studies suggest that the hypocalciuric effect of DCT diuretics wanes during chronic use, in the setting of absorptive hypercalciuria.[261] The observation that Gitelman syndrome, an inherited disorder of NCC inactivity, may present during adulthood with hypocalciuria suggests that compensatory mechanisms may not exist for the effects of DCT diuretics on calcium transport.[242] The ability of DCT diuretics to reduce urinary calcium excretion suggests that these drugs may prevent bone loss. Some,[262,263] but not all,[264,265] epidemiologic studies suggest that DCT diuretics reduce the risk of hip fracture and osteoporosis. A randomized controlled study confirmed that DCT diuretics reduce bone loss in women.[266] A case series suggests that DCT diuretics also provide rapid recovery of bone mass in osteoporotic men.[267] Another study confirmed an effect of DCT diuretics to reduce hip fracture, but noted that the protective effect wanes within 4 months of discontinuance.[268] Others have indicated that DCT diuretics can be effective in patients with primary hypoparathyroidism, when combined with a low salt diet.[269] Concomitant potassium bicarbonate administration may increase renal calcium retention induced by DCT diuretics.[270]

DCT diuretics are also employed to treat nephrogenic diabetes insipidus, causing a paradoxical decrease in urinary volume flow rate. This action of DCT diuretics results from the combination of mild extracellular fluid volume contraction (owing to diuretic-induced natriuresis), suppression of glomerular filtration (owing largely to diuretic-induced activation of the TGF mechanism), and impaired solute reabsorption along the DCT. The DCT, like the thick ascending limb, is nearly impermeable to water.[271] Solute reabsorption by the thiazide-sensitive Na-Cl cotransporter therefore contributes directly to urinary dilution. The central role of extracellular fluid volume contraction in the efficacy of DCT diuretics in diabetes insipidus was highlighted by the observation that dietary salt restriction is necessary to reduce urinary volume effectively.[247,272] DCT diuretics may also increase the antidiuretic hormone-independent water permeability of the medullary collecting tubule.[273] When administered to rats lacking antidiuretic hormone (similar to patients with central diabetes insipidus), DCT diuretics did not alter the abundance of the apical water channel of the collecting duct (aquaporin-2),[274] even though they reduced urine volume. In contrast, DCT diuretic treatment increased the abundance of aquaporin-2, NCC, and the alpha subunit of the epithelial Na channel[275] when administered to rats with lithium-induced nephrogenic diabetes insipidus. It was suggested that the upregulation of the abundance of the renal Na and water transporters might explain the antidiuretic effectiveness of DCT diuretics.

Adverse Effects

Electrolyte disorders, such as hypokalemia, hyponatremia, and hypomagnesemia, are common side effects of DCT diuretics. A measurable decline in serum K concentration is nearly universal in patients given DCT diuretics, but most patients do not become frankly hypokalemic. In the ALL-HAT trial, mean serum potassium concentrations declined from 4.3 to 4.0 and 4.1 mM at 2 and 4 years of treatment, respectively.[276] The clinical significance of diuretic-induced hypokalemia continues to be debated. Unlike the loop diuretics, DCT diuretics do not influence K transport directly.[277] Instead, they increase K excretion indirectly. DCT diuretics increase tubule fluid flow in the CNT and collecting duct, the predominant sites of K secretion along the nephron. Increased flow stimulates K secretion along the distal nephron, which enhances K secretion by large calcium activated K channels.[278] In addition, DCT diuretic-induced extracellular fluid volume contraction activates the renin/angiotensin/aldosterone system, further stimulating K secretion via the renal outer medullarly potassium channel (ROMK). Evidence for the central role of aldosterone in diuretic-induced hypokalemia includes the observation that hypokalemia is more common during treatment with long-acting DCT diuretics, such as chlorthalidone, than with shorter-acting DCT diuretics, such as hydrochlorothiazide, or with the very short-acting loop diuretics.[175] Another reason that DCT diuretics may produce more potassium wasting than loop diuretics is the differences in effects on calcium transport. As discussed previously, loop diuretics inhibit calcium transport by the thick ascending limb, increasing distal calcium delivery. In contrast, DCT diuretics stimulate calcium transport, reducing calcium delivery to sites of potassium secretion. Okusa and colleagues[279] showed that high luminal concentrations of calcium inhibit the functional activity of ENaC in the distal nephron, thereby inhibiting potassium secretion. DCT diuretics also increase urinary magnesium excretion and can lead to hypomagnesemia, as discussed previously. Hypomagnesemia may cause or contribute to the hypokalemia observed under these conditions.[280–282] Some studies suggest that maintenance magnesium therapy can prevent or attenuate the development of hypokalemia,[280] but this has not been supported universally.

Diuretics have been reported to contribute to more than one half of all hospitalizations for serious hyponatremia. Hyponatremia is especially common during treatment with DCT diuretics, compared with other classes of diuretics, and the disorder is potentially life-threatening.[283] A recent case control study suggested that hyponatremia during thiazide treatment is more common than generally appreciated, but that in most cases, it does not prove morbid.[284] Several factors contribute to DCT diuretic-induced hyponatremia. First, as discussed previously, DCT diuretics inhibit solute transport in the terminal portion of the "diluting segment," the DCT. This impairs the ability to excrete solute-free water. Second, DCT diuretics can reduce the GFR, primarily by activating the TGF system. This limits solute delivery to the diluting segment and impairs solute-free water clearance. Third, DCT diuretics lead to volume contraction, which increases proximal tubule solute and water reabsorption, further restricting delivery to the "diluting segment." Fourth, hyponatremia has been correlated with the development of hypokalemia in patients receiving DCT diuretics.[285] Finally, susceptible patients may be stimulated to consume water during therapy with DCT diuretics; although the mechanisms are unclear, this may contribute importantly to the sudden appearance of hyponatremia that can occur during DCT diuretic therapy. Of note, one report suggests that patients who are predisposed to develop hyponatremia during treatment with DCT diuretics will demonstrate an acute decline in serum sodium concentration in response to a single dose of the drug.[286] Other studies suggest that risk factors for DCT diuretic-induced hyponatremia include older age, lower body mass, and concomitant administration of selective serotonin reuptake inhibitors.[287,288]

DCT diuretics frequently cause mild metabolic alkalosis. The mechanisms are similar to those described above for loop diuretics, except that DCT diuretics do not stimulate Na/H exchange in the thick ascending limb.

DCT diuretics cause several disturbances of endocrine glands. Glucose intolerance has been a recognized complication of DCT diuretic use since the 1950s. This complication appears to be dose-related.[289,290] In the ALLHAT trial, patients experienced a 1.8% increase in new onset diabetes at 4 years of treatment, compared with patients treated with calcium channel blockers.[291] This difference did not translate into adverse clinical outcomes in the diuretic group, but has generated a great deal of discussion. The pathogenesis of DCT diuretic–induced glucose intolerance remains unclear, but several factors have been suggested to contribute. First, diuretic-induced hypokalemia may decrease insulin secretion by the pancreas, via effects on the membrane voltage of pancreatic β cells. When hypokalemia was prevented by oral potassium supplementation, the insulin response to hyperglycemia normalized, suggesting an important role for hypokalemia.[292] Hypokalemia may also interfere with insulin mediated glucose uptake by muscle, but most patients demonstrate relatively normal insulin sensitivity.[203] Volume depletion may stimulate catecholamine secretion, but volume depletion during therapy with DCT diuretics is usually very mild. It has also been suggested that DCT diuretics directly activate calcium-activated potassium channels that are expressed by pancreatic β cells.[293] Activation of these channels is known to inhibit insulin secretion. Inhibiting the renin/angiotensin/aldosterone axis appears to reduce the development of new diabetes.[294] Drugs that inhibit this pathway might attenuate the effects of diuretics to impair glucose homeostasis, but this has not been tested directly. Other factors may contribute to glucose intolerance as well, including drug-specific factors.[295]

DCT diuretics increase levels of total cholesterol, total triglyceride, and LDL cholesterol and reduce the HDL.[203,296] Definitive information about the mechanisms by which DCT diuretics alter lipid metabolism is not available, but many of the mechanisms that affect glucose homeostasis have been suggested to contribute. Hyperlipidemia, like hyperglycemia, is a dose-related side effect, and one that wanes with chronic diuretic use. In the ALLHAT study, treatment with chlorthalidone resulted in a total cholesterol 2.2 mg per dL higher than did treatment with ACE inhibitors.[291] In several large clinical studies, the effect of low dose DCT diuretic treatment on serum LDL was not significantly different from placebo.[297,298] Further, treatment of hypertension with DCT diuretics reduces the risk of stroke, coronary heart disease, congestive heart failure, and cardiovascular mortality.

CORTICAL COLLECTING TUBULE DIURETICS

Diuretic drugs that act primarily in the cortical collecting tubule or the CNT and CCD (potassium-sparing diuretics) comprise three pharmacologically distinct groups: aldosterone antagonists (spironolactone and eplerenone), pteridines (triamterene), and pyrazinoylguanidines (amiloride; Fig. 66.10). The site of action for all diuretics of this class

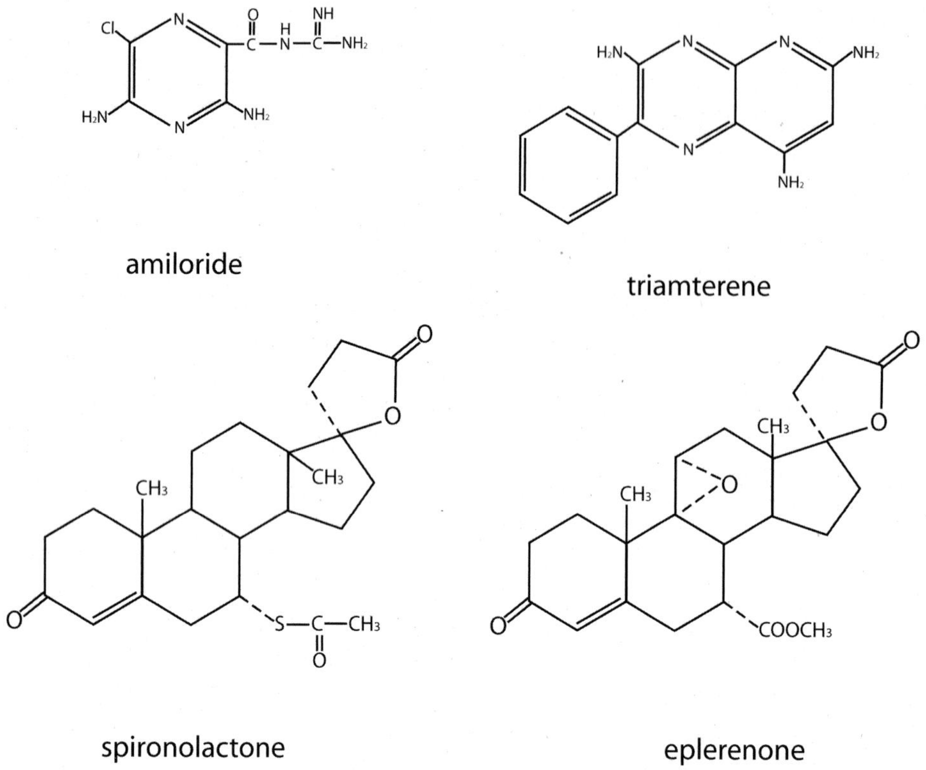

amiloride

triamterene

spironolactone

eplerenone

FIGURE 66.10 Structure of collecting duct diuretics.

is the last part of the distal convoluted tubule (the DCT2), the CNT and the CCD, where they interfere with sodium reabsorption and indirectly potassium secretion (the CNT may be especially important in this regard[299]). Because of the ability to minimize the normal tendency of diuretic drugs to increase potassium excretion, amiloride[300] and triamterene[301,302] are considered potassium sparing. The recently introduced vasopressin V2-receptor antagonists (tolvaptan, mozavaptan, and lixivaptan) also act in the collecting duct and could be categorized as diuretics.[303] These drugs selectively inhibit water reabsorption in the collecting duct and are therefore also sometimes referred to as "aquaretics." Because vasopressin-receptor antagonists are primarily used for the treatment of hyponatremia secondary to the syndrome of inappropriate antidiuretic hormone secretion, heart failure, or liver cirrhosis, these compounds are discussed in more detail in the chapter on hyponatremia.

The diuretic activity of amiloride, triamterene, and aldosterone antagonists is weak partly because fractional sodium reabsorption in the collecting tubule usually does not exceed 3% of the filtered load. Another reason, however, may relate to the tendency for these drugs to produce only partial blockade of Na channels. In support of this hypothesis, knockout or disruption of sodium channel (ENaC) function leads to profound renal salt wasting.[304] Because potassium-sparing drugs are relatively weak natriuretic agents, they are used most commonly in combination with thiazides or loop diuretics, often in a single preparation, to restrict potassium losses and sometimes augment diuretic action. However, in certain conditions potassium sparing diuretics are used as first line agents (Table 66.3). For example spironolactone is used in the treatment of edema in patients with cirrhosis[305] and amiloride or triamterene is used as a first-line treatment of Liddle syndrome.[306,307] These drugs are also used for Bartter syndrome,[308] although this indication is controversial.[309] Mineralocorticoid blocking drugs have become standard parts of the treatment of patients with systolic dysfunction heart failure. Spironolactone reduces mortality of patients with congestive heart failure.[310] Eplerenone was shown to reduce mortality in patients with left ventricular dysfunction following myocardial infarction.[311]

Urinary Electrolyte Excretion

Amiloride, triamterene, and spironolactone are weak natriuretic agents when given acutely (see Table 66.1), although some studies suggest that these drugs are as effective as furosemide in some clinical settings.[305] Additionally, these three diuretic agents decrease hydrogen ion secretion by the late distal tubule and collecting ducts. Evidence that spironolactone decreases hydrogen ion excretion comes from the finding of metabolic acidosis associated with mineralocorticoid deficiency,[312,313] and the finding that spironolactone produces metabolic acidosis in patients with cirrhosis who have mineralocorticoid excess.[314] In rats, the administration of amiloride and triamterene has been shown to inhibit urinary acidification.[300,302] A common mechanism is likely to be

TABLE 66.3 Indications for Diuretic Drugs

I. Indications for osmotic diuretics A. Acute or incipient renal failure, especially owing to heme pigment B. To reduce intraocular or intracranial pressure
II. Indications for carbonic anhydrase inhibitors A. Glaucoma (*generally outmoded) B. Acute mountain sickness C. Metabolic alkalosis D. Cystinuria E. Resistant edema (used in combination with other diuretics)
III. Indications for loop diuretics A. Edematous conditions 1. Congestive heart failure 2. Cirrhotic ascites 3. Nephrotic syndrome B. Hypercalcemia (*controversial) C. Hyperkalemia D. Hyponatremia (with hypertonic saline) E. Hyperkalemic, hyperchloremic metabolic acidosis (type 4 RTA) F. Hypermagnesemia G. Intoxications H. Hypertension I. Acute kidney injury
IV. Indications for distal convoluted tubule diuretics A. Hypertension B. Edematous conditions 1. Congestive heart failure 2. Cirrhotic ascites 3. Nephrotic syndrome C. Nephrolithiasis D. Nephrogenic diabetes insipidus E. Osteoporosis F. Hypoparathyroidism G. Diuretic resistance (used in combination with other diuretics)
V. Indications for collecting duct diuretics A. Cirrhotic ascites B. Lithium-induced diabetes insipidus C. Prevention of hypokalemia (owing to potassium-wasting diuretics) D. Prevention of hypomagnesemia (owing to potassium-wasting diuretics) E. Diuretic resistance (used in combination with other diuretics)

involved in mediating the effects of all three diuretic agents on hydrogen ion secretion. These drugs reduce the lumen-negative potential difference (voltage) and thus decrease the electrochemical gradient favoring hydrogen ion secretion.

Clearance studies in rats have demonstrated that amiloride decreases calcium excretion.[315] In these studies, amiloride produced both a decrease in the Ca clearance-to-Na clearance ratio (C_{Ca}/C_{Na}), as well as a decrease in the fractional excretion of calcium. The effect of triamterene on clearance of calcium was less clear, although it did decrease the C_{Ca}/C_{Na} ratio. In vivo microperfusion of rat distal tubules demonstrated that the effect of chlorothiazide on calcium absorption was enhanced with amiloride, but that amiloride's action was along the "late" distal tubule (probably the CNT) rather than in the true DCT.[316] Furthermore, in vitro perfusion of CNTs has shown that amiloride stimulates calcium absorption.[317] Amiloride is believed to stimulate calcium absorption through its ability to block sodium channels, thereby hyperpolarizing the apical membrane.[318] Hyperpolarization of the apical membrane stimulates calcium entry through hyperpolarization-activated calcium channels, as discussed previously. Amiloride has also been reported to reduce magnesium excretion[236,319] and to prevent the development of hypomagnesemia during therapy with a DCT diuretic.[320]

Mechanism of Action

The site of action of potassium-sparing diuretics is the DCT2, CNT, and collecting duct. Although a great deal of interest has centered on control of Na and K transport by the collecting duct, recent evidence has reemphasized the central role played by the CNT.[212,299] Molecular studies have indicated that sites of DCT diuretic action overlap with sites of CCD diuretic action. Thus, in rat, mouse and human, a transitional segment, with characteristics of both DCT and CNT, is present along the distal tubule. This segment, which may comprise the bulk of the distal tubule in humans, expresses both NCC and the amiloride-sensitive epithelial Na channel.

Although the connecting and cortical collecting tubules reabsorb only a small percentage of the filtered Na load, two characteristics render this segment important in the physiology of diuretic action. First, this nephron segment is the primary site of action of the mineralocorticoid aldosterone, a hormone that controls sodium reabsorption and potassium secretion. Second, virtually all of the potassium that is excreted is due to the secretion of potassium by the connecting and collecting tubules. Thus, this segment contributes to the hypokalemia seen as a consequence of diuretic action.

The collecting tubule is composed of two cell types that have entirely separate functions. Principal cells (collecting duct cells) are responsible for the transport of sodium, potassium, and water, whereas intercalated cells are primarily responsible for the secretion of hydrogen or bicarbonate ions. The apical membrane of principal cells expresses separate channels that permit selective conductive transport of sodium and potassium (Fig. 66.8). Connecting tubule cells also express apical Na and K channels, permitting electrogenic Na reabsorption and K secretion. The mechanism by which sodium reabsorption occurs is through conductive sodium channels. The low intracellular sodium concentration as a result of the basolateral Na, K-ATPase generates a favorable electrochemical gradient for sodium entry through sodium channels. Because sodium channels are present only in the apical membrane of principal and CNT cells, sodium conductance depolarizes the apical membrane resulting in an asymmetric voltage profile across the cell. This effect produces a lumen-negative transepithelial potential difference. The lumen-negative potential difference together with a high intracellular to lumen potassium concentration gradient provides the driving force for potassium secretion.

Amiloride-sensitive sodium conductance is a function of the epithelial sodium channel (ENaC). The functional channel comprises three homologous subunits, α, β, and γ ENaC[321]; the channel subunit structure has been debated, but the recent crystal structure of a homologous channel, and other work, suggest that it may comprise heterotrimers.[322,323] A number of factors regulate this channel, including hormones such as aldosterone, vasopressin, oxytocin; intracellular signaling elements such as G-proteins and cAMP; protein kinase C; intracellular ions sodium, hydrogen, and calcium[321]; and the cystic fibrosis transmembrane conductance regulator.[324,325] Alterations in systemic acid-base balance[326] and sodium intake[327] have also been shown to regulate ENaC function. Studies that used selective subunit antisera have demonstrated specific regulation of subunit abundance or pattern of expression. In mice adapted to a high sodium diet, the α-subunit was undetectable, and the β- and γ-subunits were expressed in the cytoplasm.[327] In contrast, mice on a low sodium diet displayed subapical or apical expression of all three subunits.[327] Administration of dDAVP to Brattleboro rats increased expression of all three subunits to varying degrees.[328] Long term acid-loading decreases and base loading increases β- and γ-subunits.[326]

The amount of sodium and potassium present in the final urine is tightly controlled by aldosterone action on connecting and collecting duct cells. Extensive studies have demonstrated that in epithelia, aldosterone produces an early increase in sodium conductance[329] followed by a sustained increase in transepithelial sodium transport. As a result, transepithelial sodium transport is increased, an effect that depolarizes the apical membrane. An increase in the lumen negative-potential in turn enhances potassium secretion through conductive potassium channels located in the apical membrane. The cellular mechanisms that are responsible for these events have been extensively studied and reviewed.[330] Aldosterone has been shown to have heterogeneous effects on ENaC subunits. In mammals, aldosterone has been shown to increase the abundance of the α subunit of ENaC,[329] to redistribute all three subunits to the apical region of principal cells,[331] and to induce a shift in the molecular weight of the γ-subunit from 85 kDa to 70 kDa. In contrast, however, a mineralocorticoid knockout mouse demonstrated essentially normal expression of ENaC subunits in the kidney, suggesting aldosterone regulation ENaC function in a posttranscriptional manner.[332] Additional nongenomic activation of ENaC function by aldosterone has been reported.[333]

Mineralocorticoid Receptor Blockers

Spironolactone (Fig. 66.10) is an analog of aldosterone that is extensively metabolized,[334,335] having the principal effect of blocking aldosterone action.[336,337] Spironolactone is converted by deacylation to 7α-thiospironolactone or by diethioacetylation to canrenone.[336] In the kidney, spironolactone and its metabolites enter target cells from the peritubular side, bind to cytosolic mineralocorticoid receptors, and act as competitive inhibitors of the endogenous hormone. In studies using radiolabelled spironolactone or aldosterone, [^{3}H]-spironolactone-receptor complexes were excluded from the nucleus. In contrast, [^{3}H]-aldosterone-receptor complexes were detected in the nucleus.[338] These results are consistent with the proposal that aldosterone antagonists block the translocation of mineralocorticoid receptors to the nucleus. The mechanism by which aldosterone antagonists block nuclear localization of antagonist-receptor complexes is not known; however, it has been suggested that they destabilize mineralocorticoid receptors facilitating proteolysis.[339] Mineralocorticoid receptors, like other steroid receptors, contain a steroid-binding unit associated with other cellular components including HSP90, in its inactive state. Steroid binding produces dissociation of HSP90 from the steroid binding unit uncapping the DNA-binding sites. Spironolactone facilitates the release of HSP90 and in combination with rapid dissociation of ligand could lead to degradation of the receptor.[339]

Spironolactone induces a mild increase in sodium excretion (1%–2%) and a decrease in potassium and hydrogen ion excretion.[340,341] Its effect depends on the presence of aldosterone. Spironolactone is ineffective in experimental adrenalectomized animals[306] and in patients with Addison disease[306] or humans on a high salt diet. In cortical collecting tubules perfused in vitro, spironolactone added to the bath solution reduced the aldosterone-induced lumen-negative transepithelial voltage.[301] By blocking sodium absorption in the collecting tubule, a decrease in lumen negative potential reduces the driving force for passive sodium and hydrogen ion secretion.[301]

Spironolactone causes troubling estrogenic side effects commonly, a fact that constrains its use (see later). Renewed interest in the utility of aldosterone blockers, especially in the setting of congestive heart failure, led to the development of antialdosterone agents that are more specific inhibitors of the mineralocorticoid receptor. Eplerenone is a second competitive aldosterone antagonist, currently in clinical use. Eplerenone (see Fig. 66.10) is Pregn-4-ene-7,21-dicarboxylic acid, 9,11-epoxy-17-hydroxy-3-oxo, γ-lactone, methyl ester (7α, 11α, 17α), and was derived from spironolactone by the introduction of a $9\alpha,11\alpha$-epoxy bridge and substitution of the 17α-thioacetal group of spironolactone with a carbomethoxy group. In vitro, eplerenone exhibits 10- to 20-fold lower affinity for the mineralocorticoid receptor than spironolactone, but in humans, it appears to be 50% to 75% as potent.[342,343] This change significantly enhances the relative affinity of the drug for mineralocorticoid receptors over other steroid receptors.

Amiloride and Triamterene

Amiloride and triamterene (see Fig. 66.10) are structurally different but are organic cations that use the same primary site of action (see Fig. 66.8). Triamterene is an aminopteridine chemically related to folic acid and amiloride is a pyrazinoylguanidine. Systemically administered amiloride results in an increase in sodium excretion and decrease in potassium excretion.[38] Their actions on sodium and potassium transport, unlike spironolactone, are not dependent on aldosterone. Systemically administered amiloride produced a small increase in sodium excretion and a much larger decrease in potassium excretion.[344,345] Sampling of tubule fluid from the distal tubule demonstrated an inhibition of the normal rise in the tubule fluid to plasma potassium ratio. These results indicated that amiloride decreased distal tubule potassium secretion. Experiments employing in vivo microperfusion of distal tubules[277,346] and in vitro perfusion of isolated cortical collecting tubules[347,348] demonstrated that luminally administered amiloride reduced sodium absorption and potassium secretion. Similar results were obtained following in vivo microperfusion with benazamil,[349] a more potent amiloride analog. Amiloride decreases potassium secretion by blocking ENaC in the apical membrane of CNT and collecting tubule cells[350,351] thereby decreasing the electrochemical gradient for potassium secretion.

In high concentrations (>100 μM), amiloride interacts with different transporters, enzymes, and receptors. At concentrations of 0.05 to 0.5 mM, however, amiloride interacts specifically with ENaC.[352,353] The molecular mechanism by which amiloride blocks ENaC remains incompletely defined. It is likely, however, that the positive charge on the guanidinium moiety plays an important role in occluding the sodium channel (see Fig. 66.8).[353,354]

Several groups, using mutational analysis[355,356] and anti-amiloride antibodies[357] have demonstrated contributions to amiloride binding by all three subunits in close proximity to the channel pore.[358] A putative amiloride binding domain, WYRFHY, of the a-subunit of ENaC has been identified.[357,359]

Clearance and free-flow micropuncture studies using triamterene demonstrated results similar to studies with amiloride[177] although the mechanism of action is not as clearly defined. In earlier studies of rabbit cortical collecting tubules perfused in vitro, triamterene produced a gradual, reversible inhibition of the potential difference after a latent period of 10 minutes. More recent studies, however, suggest that triamterene binds to the epithelial sodium channel and thus has a mechanism of action similar to amiloride.[360]

Pharmacokinetics

Spironolactone is poorly soluble in aqueous fluids. Bioavailability of an oral dose is approximately 90% in some but not all commercial preparations. The drug is rapidly metabolized in the liver into a number of metabolites. Canrenone is one metabolite of spironolactone.[334,335] This conclusion was based on fluorometric assays. Assays of spironolactone and its metabolites by the use of high performance liquid chromatography (HPLC) demonstrated that fluorometrically measured levels of canrenone overestimated true canrenone levels.[361] Using HPLC, the predominant metabolite, 7α-methylspironolactone,[362] appears to be responsible for roughly 80% of the potassium-sparing effect. Spironolactone and its metabolites are extensively bound to plasma protein (98%). In normal volunteers, taking spironolactone (100 mg per day) for 15 days, the mean half-lives for spironolactone, canrenone, 7α-thiomethylspironolactone, and 6β-hydroxy-7α-thiomethylspironolactone were 1.4, 16.5, 13.8, and 15 hours, respectively. Thus, although unmetabolized spironolactone is present in serum, it has a rapid elimination time. The onset of physiologic action is extremely slow for spironolactone, with peak response sometimes occurring 48 hours or more after the first dose; effects gradually wane over a period of 48 to 72 hours. Spironolactone is used in cirrhotic patients to induce a natriuresis. In these patients, pharmacokinetic studies indicate that the half-lives of spironolactone and its metabolites are increased. The half-lives for spironolactone, canrenone, 7α-thiomethylspironolactone, and 6β-hydroxy-7α-thiomethylspironolactone are 9, 58, 24, and 126 hours, respectively.[363]

Eplerenone is rapidly absorbed, with peak serum levels at 1.5 hours.[343] Its volume of distribution is 43 to 90 liters, with approximately 50% protein bound. It is cleared primarily via the CYP4503A4 system to inactive metabolites with an elimination half-life of 4 to 6 hours.[343] This is in contrast to spironolactone, where the half-life of the parent compound is short, but the half-life of metabolites is very long. The maximal plasma concentration and area under the curve are increased in people >65 years of age and with kidney failure; eplerenone is not removed by hemodialysis.[343]

Clinical Use

CCT diuretics can be used for the treatment of hypertension, primary aldosteronism, and secondary aldosteronism; they are also used to limit the kaliuretic effects of loop or DCT diuretics, and sometimes primarily to treat hypokalemia due to renal potassium loss of various causes.

Spironolactone (or eplerenone) plays an important role in four clinical situations. First, it is the treatment of choice in patients with primary aldosteronism (due to bilateral adrenal hyperplasia).[364,365] Second, the drug is especially appropriate for the treatment of cirrhosis with ascites, a condition invariably associated with secondary hyperaldosteronism.[305] In comparison to loop or thiazide diuretics, spironolactone is equivalent or more effective.[366] A combination of loop diuretic in addition to spironolactone can be used to boost natriuresis when the diuretic effect of spironolactone alone is inadequate, and it has been reported that a ratio of 100 mg spironolactone per 40 mg furosemide carries the best ratio of efficacy/safety.[367] A recent animal study, however, showed that amiloride may also be effective in lowering portal pressure in liver cirrhosis by inhibiting intrahepatic vasoconstriction.[368] A third use of spironolactone is in systolic heart failure, where mineralocorticoid antagonists have been shown to reduce morbidity and mortality.[369] A subsequent study showed that eplerenone reduced morbidity and mortality of patients with left ventricular dysfunction following a myocardial infarction.[370] Most recently, eplerenone, as compared with placebo, reduced both the risk of death and the risk of hospitalization among patients with systolic heart failure and even mild symptoms.[371] Finally, there is growing interest in using spironolactone to treat resistant hypertension, even when demonstrable hyperaldosteronism is not present.[372]

Triamterene or amiloride is generally used in combination with potassium-wasting diuretics (thiazide or loop diuretics), especially when maintenance of normal serum potassium concentrations is clinically important. In addition, amiloride (or triamterene) has also been used as initial therapy in potassium wasting states such as primary hyperaldosteronism,[373,374] Liddle,[307] Bartter, or Gitelman syndrome,[308] although, as noted previously, use in the latter situation has been disputed.[309] Amiloride is recommended to treat lithium-induced nephrogenic diabetes insipidus.[375] The efficacy of amiloride in this disorder relates to the ability of amiloride to block collecting duct sodium channels, a pathway which lithium uses to gain entry into cells. Recently, a small placebo-controlled cross-over trial[376] and an animal study[377] confirmed these effects.

Adverse Effects

The most serious adverse reaction encountered during therapy with spironolactone is hyperkalemia. Serum potassium should be monitored periodically even when the drug is administered with a potassium-wasting diuretic. Patients at highest risk are those with low GFRs, patients with concurrent medication predisposing to hyperkalemia, and individuals who take potassium supplements concurrently. This problem has become more important because of the wide use of aldosterone blocking drugs, together with ACE inhibitors, ARBs, and beta-blockers in patients with congestive heart failure.[378] Risk factors include kidney failure, older age, coexistent diabetes mellitus, and concomitant treatment with beta-blockers.[379] It is important to note that the original RALES study specifically excluded patients with several of these comorbidities. Renal failure appears to be another complication in this group.[379] Another group at risk for hyperkalemia are elderly patients receiving chronic treatment with spironolactone who are intermittently treated with trimethoprim-sulfamethoxazole for a urinary tract infection.[380] Surprisingly, however, another recent population-based study showed that despite a marked increase in the use of spironolactone, no increase was seen in hospital admissions for hyperkalemia and that outpatient hyperkalemia actually fell; the authors ascribed these findings to more careful monitoring.[381]

In patients with cirrhosis and ascites treated with spironolactone, hyperchloremic metabolic acidosis can develop independent of changes in renal function.[314] Gynecomastia may occur in men, especially as the dose is increased[382] but even at low doses[369]; decreased libido and impotence have also been reported. Women may develop menstrual irregularities, hirsutism, or swelling and tenderness of the breast. Spironolactone-induced agranulocytosis has also been reported.[383]

Triamterene and amiloride may also cause hyperkalemia. The risk of hyperkalemia is highest in patients with limited renal function (e.g., renal insufficiency, diabetes mellitus, and elderly patients). Additional complications included elevated serum blood urea nitrogen and uric acid, glucose intolerance, and gastrointestinal disturbances. Triamterene induces crystalluria or cylindruria[384] and may contribute to or initiate formation of renal stones[385] and acute kidney injury when combined with NSAIDs.[386,387] The drugs are contraindicated in patients with hyperkalemia, individuals taking potassium supplements in any form, and in patients with severe renal failure with progressive oliguria.

REFERENCES

1. Yang Q, Liu T, Kuklina EV, et al. Sodium and potassium intake and mortality among US adults: prospective data from the Third National Health and Nutrition Examination Survey. *Arch Intern Med.* 2011;171(13):1183–1191.

2. Okusa MD, Ellison DH. Physiology and pathophysiology of diuretic action. In: Alpern RJ, Hebert SC, eds. *The Kidney: Physiology and Pathophysiology.* 4th ed. Amsterdam: Elsevier; 2008:1051–1984.

3. Brater DC. Diuretic pharmacokinetics and pharmacodynamics. In: Seldin DW, Giebisch G, eds. *Diuretic Agents: Clinical Physiology and Pharmacology.* San Diego: Academic Press; 1997:189–208.

4. Shankar SS, Brater DC. Loop diuretics: from the Na-K-2Cl transporter to clinical use. *Am J Physiol Renal Physiol.* 2003;284(1):F11–21.

5. Better OS, Rubinstein I, Winaver JM, et al. Mannitol therapy revisited (1940–1997). *Kidney Int.* 1997;51:886–894.

6. Seely JF, Dirks JH. Micropuncture study of hypertonic mannitol diuresis in the proximal and distal tubule of the dog kidney. *J Clin Invest.* 1969;48:2330–2239.

7. Wong NLM, Quamme GA, Sutton RAL, et al. Effects of mannitol on water and electrolyte transport in dog kidney. *J Lab Clin Med.* 1979;94:683–692.

8. Gennari FJ, Kassirer JP. Osmotic diuresis. *N Engl J Med.* 1974;291(14):714–720.

9. Buerkert J, Martin D, Prasad J, et al. Role of deep nephrons and the terminal collecting duct in a mannitol-induced diuresis. *Am J Physiol.* 1981;240:F411–F422.

10. Blantz RC. Effect of mannitol on glomerular ultrafiltration in the hydropenic rat. *J Clin Invest.* 1974;54:1135–1143.

11. Johnston PA, Bernard DB, Perrin NS, et al. Prostaglandins mediate the vasodilatory effect of mannitol in the hypoperfused rat kidney. *J Clin Invest.* 1981;68:127–133.

12. Yamasaki Y, Nishiuchi T, Kojima A, et al. Effects of an oral water load and intravenous administration of isotonic glucose, hypertonic saline, mannitol and furosemide on the release of atrial natriuretic peptide in men. *Acta Endocrinol (Copenh).* 1988;119:269–278.

13. Goldberg M, Ramirez MA. Effects of saline and mannitol diuresis on the renal concentrating mechanism in dogs: alterations in renal tissue solutes and water. *Clin Sci.* 1967;32:475–493.

14. Nashat FS, Scholefield FR, Tappin JW, et al. The effect of acute changes in haematocrit in the anaesthetized dog on the volume and character of the urine. *J Physiol.* 1969;205:305–316.

15. Anderson P, Boreus L, Gordon E, et al. Use of mannitol during neurosurgery: interpatient variability in the plasma and CSF levels. *Eur J Clin Pharmacol.* 1988;35:643–649.

16. Weiner IM. Diuretics and other agents employed in the mobilization of edema fluid. In: Gilman AG, Rall TW, Nies AS, et al, eds. *The Pharmacological Basis of Therapuetics.* 8 ed. New York: Pergamon Press; 1990:713–742.

17. Lameire N, Vanholder R. Pathophysiologic features and prevention of human and experimental acute tubular necrosis. *J Am Soc Nephrol.* 2001;12 Suppl 17: S20–32.

18. Slater MS, Mullins RJ. Rhabdomyolysis and myoglobinuric renal failure in trauma and surgical patients: a review. *J Am Coll Surg.* 1998;186(6):693–716.

19. Malinoski DJ, Slater MS, Mullins RJ. Crush injury and rhabdomyolysis. *Crit Care Clin.* 2004;20(1):171–192.

20. Brown CV, Rhee P, Chan L, et al. Preventing renal failure in patients with rhabdomyolysis: do bicarbonate and mannitol make a difference? *J Trauma.* 2004;56(6):1191–1196.

21. Van Valenberg PLJ, Hoitsma AJ, Tiggeler RGWL. Mannitol as an indispensable constituent of an intraoperative hydation protocol for the prevention of acute renal failure after renal cadaveric transplantation. *Transplantation.* 1987;44:784–788.

22. Jenkins IR, Curtis AP. The combination of mannitol and albumin in the priming solution reduces positive intraoperative fluid balance during cardipulmonary bypass. *Perfusion.* 1995;10:301–305.

23. England MD, Cavaroocchi NC, O'Brien JF, et al. Influence of antioxidants (mannitol and allopurinol) on oxygen free radical generation during and after cardiopulmonary bypass. *Circulation.* 1986;74:134–137.

24. Weisberg LS, Kurnick PB, Kurnik BR. Risk of radiocontrast in patients with and without diabetes mellitus. *Kidney Int.* 1994;45:259–260.

25. Conger JD. Interventions in clinical acute renal failure: What are the data? *Am J Kid Dis.* 1995;26:565–576.

26. Solomon R, Werner C, Mann D, et al. Effects of saline, mannitol, and furosemide on acute decreases in renal function induced by radiocontrast agents. *N Engl J Med.* 1994;331:1416–1420.

27. Quon DK, Worthen DM. Dose response of intravenous mannitol on the human eye. *Ann Opthalmol.* 1981;13:1392–1393.

28. McGraw CP, Howard G. Effect of mannitol on increased intracranial pressure. *Neurosurgery.* 1983;13:269–271.

29. Kamel H, Navi BB, Nakagawa K, et al. Hypertonic saline versus mannitol for the treatment of elevated intracranial pressure: a meta-analysis of randomized clinical trials. *Crit Care Med.* 2011;39(3):554–559.

30. Gong G, Lindberg J, Abrams J, et al. Comparison of hypertonic saline solutions and dextran in dialysis-induced hypotension. *J Am Soc Nephrol.* 1993;3:1808–1812.

31. Arieff AI. Dialysis disequilibrium syndrome: Current concepts on pathogenesis and prevention. *Kidney Int.* 1994;45:629–630.

32. Makoff DL, DaSilva JA, Rosenbaum BJ. On the mechanism of hyperkalemia due to hyperosomotic expansion with saline or mannitol. *Clin Sci.* 1971;41: 383–390.

33. Hoorn EJ, Betjes MG, Weigel J, et al. Hypernatraemia in critically ill patients: too little water and too much salt. *Nephrol Dial Transplant.* 2008;23(5): 1562–1568.

34. Aiyagari V, Deibert E, Diringer MN. Hypernatremia in the neurologic intensive care unit: how high is too high? *J Crit Care.* 2006;21(2):163–172.

35. Dorman HR, Sondheimer JH, Cadnapaphornchai P. Mannitol-induced acute renal failure. *Medicine.* 1990;69:153–159.

36. Visweswaran P, Massin EK, Dubose TDJ. Mannitol-induced acute renal failure. *J Am Soc Nephrol.* 1997;8(6):1028–1033.

37. Buckalew VM, Jr., Walker BR, Puschett JB, et al. Effects of increased sodium delivery on distal tubular sodium reabsorption with and without volume expansion in man. *J Clin Invest.* 1970;49:2336–2344.

38. Puschett JB, Winaver J. Efects of diuretics on renal function. In: Windhager EE, ed. *Handbook of Physiology.* Section 8: Renal Physiology. New York: Oxford University Press; 1992:2335–2406.

39. Beck LH, Goldberg M. Effects of acetazolamide and parathyroidectomy on renal transprot of sodium, calcium and phosphate. *Am J Physiol.* 1973;224: 1136–1142.

40. Okusa MD, Erik A, Persson G, et al. Chlorothiazide effect on feedback-mediated control of glomerular filtration rate. *Am J Physiol.* 1989;257:F137–F144.

41. Malnic G, Klose RM, Giebisch G. Microperfusion study of distal tubular potassium and sodium transfer in rat kidney. *Am J Physiol.* 1966;211:548–559.

42. Good DW, Wright FS. Luminal influences on potassium secretion: sodium concentration and fluid flow rate. *Am J Physiol.* 1979;236:F192–F205.

43. Velázquez H, Wright FS, Good DW. Luminal influences on potassium secretion: chloride replacement with sulfate. *Am J Physiol.* 1982;242:F46–F55.

44. Purkerson JM, Schwartz GJ. The role of carbonic anhydrases in renal physiology. *Kidney Int.* 2007;71(2):103–115.

45. Pastorekova S, Parkkila S, Pastorek J, et al. Carbonic anhydrases: current state of the art, therapeutic applications and future prospects. *J Enzyme Inhib Med Chem.* 2004;19(3):199–229.

46. Schwartz GJ, Kittelberger AM, Barnhart DA, et al. Carbonic anhydrase IV is expressed in H(+)-secreting cells of rabbit kidney. *Am J Physiol Renal Physiol.* 2000;278(6):F894–904.

47. Alvarez BV, Loiselle FB, Supuran CT, et al. Direct extracellular interaction between carbonic anhydrase IV and the human NBC1 sodium/bicarbonate co-transporter. *Biochemistry.* 2003;42(42):12321–12329.

48. Tsuruoka S, Kittelberger AM, Schwartz GJ. Carbonic anhydrase II and IV mRNA in rabbit nephron segments: stimulation during metabolic acidosis. *Am J Physiol.* 1998;274(2 Pt 2):F259–267.

49. Purkerson JM, Schwartz GJ. Expression of membrane-associated carbonic anhydrase isoforms IV, IX, XII, and XIV in the rabbit: induction of CA IV and IX during maturation. *Am J Physiol Regul Integr Comp Physiol.* 2005;288(5): R1256–1263.

50. Tsuruoka S, Swenson ER, Petrovic S, et al. Role of basolateral carbonic anhydrase in proximal tubular fluid and bicarbonate absorption. *Am J Physiol Renal Physiol.* 2001;280(1):F146–154.

51. Schwartz GJ, Kittelberger AM, Watkins RH, et al. Carbonic anhydrase XII mRNA encodes a hydratase that is differentially expressed along the rabbit nephron. *Am J Physiol Renal Physiol.* 2003;284(2):F399–410.

52. Maren TH. Carbonic Anhydrase. *N Engl J Med.* 1985;313:179–180.

53. Boron WF. Acid-base transport by the renal proximal tubule. *J Am Soc Nephrol.* 2006;17(9):2368–2382.

54. Aronson PS. Essential roles of CFEX-mediated Cl(-)-oxalate exchange in proximal tubule NaCl transport and prevention of urolithiasis. *Kidney Int.* 2006;70(7):1207–1213.

55. Shuichi T, Schwartz GJ. HCO3– absorption in rabbit outer medullary collecting duct: role of luminal carbonic anhydrase. *Am J Physiol.* 1998;274: F139–F147.

56. DuBose TD, Lucci MS. Effect of carbonic anhydrase inhibition on superficial and deep nephron bicarbonate reabsorption inthe rat. *J Clin Invest.* 1983;71:55–65.

57. Cogan MG, Maddox DA, Warnock DG, et al. Effect of acetazolamide on bicarbonate reabsorption in the proximal tubule of the rat. *Am J Physiol.* 1979;237:F447–F454.

58. Holder LB, Hayes SL. Diffusion of sulfonamides in aqueous buffers and into red cells. *Mol Pharmacol.* 1965;1:266–279.

59. Lucci MS, Pucacco LR, DuBose TD Jr. et al. Direct evaluation of acidification by rat proximal tubule: role of carbonic anhydrase. *Am J Physiol.* 1980;238: F372–F379.

60. Tinker JP, Coulson R, Weiner IM. Dextran-bound inhibitors of carbonic anhydrase. *J Pharmacol Exp Ther.* 1981;218:600–607.

61. Lucci MS, Tinker JP, Weiner I, et al. Function of proximal tubule carbonic anhydrase defined by selective inhibition. *Am J Physiol.* 1983;245:F443–F449.

62. Alper SL. Familial renal tubular acidosis. *J Nephrol.* 2010;23 Suppl 16: S57–76.

63. Sasaki S, Marumo F. Effects of carbonic anhydrase inhibitors on basolateral base transport of rabbit proximal straight tubule. *Am J Physiol.* 1989;257: F947–F952.

64. Soleimani M, Aronson PS. Effects of acetazolamide on Na+-HCO-3 cotransport in basolateral membrane vesicles isolated from rabbit renal cortex. *J Clin Invest.* 1989;83:945–951.

65. Brown D, Hirsch S, Gluck S. An H+-ATPase in opposite plasma membrane domains in kidney epithelial cell subpopulations. *Nature.* 1988;331:622–624.

66. Wingo CS. Active proton secretion and potassium absorption in the rabbit outer medullary collecting duct: functional evidence for H-K- ATPase. *J Clin Invest.* 1990;84:361–365.

67. Okusa MD, Unwin RJ, Velázquez H, et al. Active potassium absorption by the renal distal tubule. *Am J Physiol Renal, Fluid Electrolyte Physiol.* 1992;262:F488–F493.

68. Kone BC. Renal H,K-ATPase: structure, function and regulation. *Miner Electrolyte Metab.* 1996;22:349–365.

69. Star RA, Burg MB, Knepper MA. Luminal disequilibrium pH and ammonia transport in outer medullary collecting duct. *Am J Physiol.* 1987;29984: 26980–28021.

70. Tucker BJ, Blantz RC. Studies on the mechanism of reduction in glomerular filtration rate after benzolamide. *Pflügers Arch.* 1980;388:211–216.

71. Hashimoto S, Huang YG, Castrop H, et al. Effect of carbonic anhydrase inhibition on GFR and renal hemodynamics in adenosine-1 receptor-deficient mice. *Pflugers Arch.* 2004;448(6):621–628.

72. Heller I, Halevy J, Cohen J, Theodor E. Significant metabolic acidosis induced by acetazolamide. Not a rare complication. *Arch Intern Med.* 1985;145:1815–1817.
73. Stafstrom CE, Gilmore HE, Kurtin PS. Nephrocalcinosis complicating medical treatment of posthemorrhagic hydrocephalus. *Pediatr Neurol.* 1992;8:179–182.
74. Johnson T, Kass MA. Hematologic reactions to carbonic anhydrase inhibitors. *Am J Opthal.* 1986;101:410–418.
75. Werblin TP, Pollack IP, Liss RA. Blood dyscrasias in patients using methazolamide (Neptazane) for glaucoma. *Opthalmology.* 1980;87:350–354.
76. Ellison DH. The physiologic basis of diuretic synergism: Its role in treating diuretic resistance. *Ann Intern Med.* 1991;114:886–894.
77. Rose BD. Resistance to diuretics. *Clin Investig.* 1994;72:722–724.
78. Preisig PA, Toto RD, Alpern RJ. Carbonic anhydrase inhibitors. *Renal Physiol.* 1987;10:136–159.
79. Bear R, Goldstein M, Phillipson M, et al. Effect of metabolic alkalosis on respiratory function in patients with chronic obstructive lung disease. *Can Med Assoc J.* 1977;117:900–903.
80. Miller PD, Berns AS. Acute metabolic alkalosis perpetuating hypercarbia: a role for acetazolamide in chronic obstructive pulmonary disease. *JAMA.* 1977;238:2400–2401.
81. Marik PE, Kussman BD, Lipman J, et al. Acetazolamide in the treatment of metabolic alkalosis in critically ill patients. *Heart Lung.* 1991;20:455–459.
82. Vass C, Hirn C, Sycha T, et al. Medical interventions for primary open angle glaucoma and ocular hypertension. *Cochrane Database Syst Rev.* 2007;(4):CD003167.
83. Seupaul RA, Welch JL, Malka ST, et al. Pharmacologic prophylaxis for acute mountain sickness: a systematic shortcut review. *Ann Emerg Med.* 2011 [Epub ahead of print].
84. Griggs RC, Engel WK, Resnick JS. Acetazolamide treatment of hypokalemic periodic paralysis. Prevention of attacks and improvement of persisten weakness. *Ann Intern Med.* 1970;73:39–48.
85. Resnick JS, Engle WK, Griggs RC, et al. Acetazolamide prophylaxis in hypokalemic periodic paralysis. *N Engl J Med.* 1968;278:582–586.
86. Johnsen T. Effect upon serum insulin, glucose and potassium concentrations of acetazolamide during attacks of familial periodic hypokalemic paralysis. *Acta Neurol Scand.* 1977;56:533–541.
87. Reiss WG, Oles KS. Acetazolamide in the treatment of seizures. *Ann Pharmacother.* 1996;30:514–519.
88. Shoeman JF. Childhood pseudotumor cerebri: clinical and intracranial pressure response to acetazolamide and furosemide treatment in a case series. *J Child Neurol.* 1994;9:130–134.
89. Shore ET, Millman EP. Central sleep apnea and acetazolamide therapy. *Arch Intern Med.* 1983;143:1278–1280.
90. Cairo MS, Coiffier B, Reiter A, et al. Recommendations for the evaluation of risk and prophylaxis of tumour lysis syndrome (TLS) in adults and children with malignant diseases: an expert TLS panel consensus. *Br J Haematol.* 2010;149(4):578–586.
91. Supuran CT. Carbonic anhydrases: novel therapeutic applications for inhibitors and activators. *Nat Rev Drug Discov.* 2008;7(2):168–181.
92. Haas M, McManus TJ. Bumetanide inhibits (Na + K + 2Cl) co-transport at a chloride site. *Am J Physiol.* 1983;245:C235–C240.
93. Gamba G. Molecular physiology and pathophysiology of electroneutral cation-chloride cotransporters. *Physiol Rev.* 2005;85(2):423–493.
94. Isenring P, Jacoby SC, Forbush B III. The role of transmembrane domain 2 in cation transport by the Na-K-Cl cotransporter. *Proc Natl Acad Sci U S A.* 1998;95:7179–7184.
95. Isenring P, Jacoby SC, Chang J, et al. Mutagenic mapping of the Na-K-Cl cotransporter for domains involved in ion transport and bumetanide binding. *J Gen Physiol.* 1998;112(5):549–558.
96. Monette MY, Forbush B. Regulatory activation is accompanied by movement in the C terminus of the Na-K-Cl cotransporter (NKCC1). *J Biol Chem.* 2012;287(3):2210–2220.
97. Suki WN, Eknoyan G. Physiology of diuretic action. In: Seldin DW, Giebisch G, eds. *The Kidney: Physiology and Pathophysiology.* 2nd ed. New York: Raven Press, Ltd.; 1992:3629–3670.
98. Puschett JB, Goldberg M. The acute effects of furosemide on acid and electrolyte excretion in man. *J Lab Clin Med.* 1968;71:666–677.
99. Decaux G, Waterlot Y, Genette F, et al. Treatment of the syndrome of inappropriate antidiuretic hormone with furosemide. *N Engl J Med.* 1981;304: 329–330.
100. Hantman D, Rossier B, Zohlman R, et al. Rapid correction of hyponatremia in the syndrome of inappropriate secretion of antidiuretic hormone: An alternative treatment to hypertonic saline. *Ann Intern Med.* 1973;78:870–875.
101. Khuri RN, Wiederholt M, Strieder N, et al. Effects of graded solute diuresis on renal tubular sodium transport in the rat. *Am J Physiol.* 1975;228:1262–1268.
102. di Stefano A, Greger R, Desfleurs E, et al. A Ba(2+)-insensitive K+ conductance in the basolateral cell membrane of rabbit cortical thick ascending limb cells. *Cell Physiol Biochem.* 1998;8:89–105.
103. Hebert SC, Mount DB, Gamba G. Molecular physiology of cation-coupled Cl- cotransport: the SLC12 family. *Pflugers Arch.* 2004;447(5):580–593.
104. Kaplan MR, Plotkin MD, Lee WS, et al. Apical localization of the Na-K-Cl cotransporter, rBSC1, on rat thick ascending limbs. *Kidney Int.* 1996;49:40–47.
105. Obermuller N, Kunchaparty S, Ellison DH, et al. Expression of the Na-K-2Cl cotransporter by macula densa and thick ascending limb cells of rat and rabbit nephron. *J Clin Invest.* 1996;98(3):635–640.
106. Ecelbarger CA, Terris J, Hoyer JR, et al. Localization and regulation of the rat renal Na+-K+-2Cl- cotransporter, BSC-1. *Am J Physiol Renal, Fluid Electrolyte Physiol.* 1996;271:F619–F628.
107. Xu JZ, Hall AE, Peterson LN, et al. Localization of the ROMK protein on the apical membranes of rat kidney nephron segments. *Am J Physiol.* 1997;273:F739–F748.
108. Greger R, Schlatter E. Cellular mechanism of the action of loop diuretics on the thick ascending limb of Henle's loop. *Klinische Wochenschrift.* 1983;61: 1019–1027.
109. Hebert SC, Reeves WB, Molony DA, et al. The medullary thick limb: function and modulation of the single-effect multiplier. *Kidney Int.* 1987;31:580–588.
110. Miyanoshita A, Terada M, Endou H. Furosemide directly stimulates prostaglandin E2 production in the thick ascending limb of Henle's loop. *J Pharmacol Exp Ther.* 1989;251:1155–1159.
111. Abe K, Yasuima M, Cheiba L, et al. Effect of furosemide on urinary excretion of prostaglandin E in normal volunteers and patients with essential hypertension. *Prostaglandins.* 1977;14:513–521.
112. Wright JT, Corder CN, Taylor R. Studies on rat kidney 15–hydroxyprostaglandin dehydrogenase. *Biochem Pharmacol.* 1976;25:1669–1673.
113. Kirchner KA. Prostaglandin inhibitors alter loop segment chloride uptake during furosemide diuresis. *Am J Physiol.* 1985;248:F698–F704.
114. Kirchner KA, Martin CJ, Bower JD. Prostaglandin E2 but not I2 restores furosemide response in indomethacin-treated rats. *Am J Physiol.* 1986;250: F980–F985.
115. Friedman PA. Codependence of renal calcium and sodium transport. *Annu Rev Physiol.* 1998;60:179–197.
116. Simon DB, Lu Y, Choate KA, et al. Paracellin-1, a renal tight junction protein required for paracellular Mg2+ resorption [see comments]. *Science.* 1999;285(5424):103–106.
117. Hou J, Renigunta A, Konrad M, et al. Claudin-16 and claudin-19 interact and form a cation-selective tight junction complex. *J Clin Invest.* 2008;118(2):619–628.
118. Weber S, Schneider L, Peters M, et al. Novel paracellin-1 mutations in 25 families with familial hypomagnesemia with hypercalciuria and nephrocalcinosis. *J Am Soc Nephrol.* 2001;12(9):1872–1881.
119. Schnermann J, Briggs JP. Synthesis and secretion of renin in mice with induced genetic mutations. *Kidney Int.* 2012;81(6):529–538.
120. Schnermann J. Juxtaglomerular cell complex in the regulation of renal salt excretion. *Am J Physiol.* 1998;274:R263–R279.
121. Schlatter E, Salomonsson M, Persson AEG, et al. Macula densa cells sense luminal NaCl concentration via furosemide sensitive Na+2Cl-K+ cotransport. *Pflugers Arch.* 1989;414:286–290.
122. Lapointe J-Y, Laamarti A, Hurst AM, et al. Activation of Na:2Cl:K cotransport by luminal chloride in macula densa cells. *Kidney Int.* 1995;47:752–757.
123. Mundel P, Bachmann S, Bader M, et al. Expression of nitric oxide synthase in kidney macula densa cells. *Kidney Int.* 1992;42:1017–1079.
124. Kurtz A, Gotz KH, Hamann M, et al. Stimulation of renin secretion by nitric oxide is mediated by phosphodiesterase 3. *Proc Natl Acad Sci U S A.* 1998;95:4743–4747.
125. Reid IA, Chou L. Effect of blockade of nitric oxide synthesis on the renin secretory response to frusemide in concious rabbits. *Clin Sci.* 1995;88:657–663.
126. Tharaux PL, Dussaule JC, Pauti MD, et al. Activation of renin synthesis is dependent on intact nitric oxide production. *Kidney Int.* 1997;51:1780–1787.
127. Schricker K, Hamann M, Kurtz A. Nitric oxide and prostaglandins are involved in the macula densa control of renin system. *Am J Physiol.* 1995;269: F825–F830.
128. Castrop H, Schweda F, Mizel D, et al. Permissive role of nitric oxide in macula densa control of renin secretion. *Am J Physiol Renal Physiol.* 2004;286(5): F848–857.
129. Harris RC, McKanna JA, Akai Y, et al. Cyclooxygenase-2 is associated with the macula densa of rat kidney and increases with salt restriction. *J Clin Invest.* 1994;94(6):2504–2510.

130. Guan Y, Chang M, Cho W, et al. Cloning, expression, and regulation of rabbit cyclooxygenase-2 in renal medullary interstitial cells. *Am J Physiol.* 1997;273(1 Pt 2):F18–26.
131. Komhoff M, Jeck ND, Seyberth HW, et al. Cyclooxygenase-2 expression is associated with the renal macula densa of patients with bartter-like syndrome [In Process Citation]. *Kidney Int.* 2000;58(6):2420–2424.
132. Khan KN, Venturini CM, Bunch RT, et al. Interspecies differences in renal localization of cyclooxygenase isoforms: implications in nonsteroidal antiinflammatory drug-related nephrotoxicity. *Toxicol Pathol.* 1998;26(5):612–620.
133. Frölich JC, Hollifield JW, Dormois JC, et al. Suppression of plasma renin activity by indomethacin in man. *Circ Res.* 1976;39:447–452.
134. Harding P, Sigmon DH, Alfie ME, et al. Cyclooxygenase-2 mediates increased renal renin content induced by low-sodium diet. *Hypertension.* 1997;29:297–302.
135. Kammerl MC, Nusing RM, Richthammer W, et al. Inhibition of COX-2 counteracts the effects of diuretics in rats. *Kidney Int.* 2001;60(5):1684–1691.
136. Kammerl MC, Nusing RM, Schweda F, et al. Low sodium and furosemide-induced stimulation of the renin system in man is mediated by cyclooxygenase 2. *Clin Pharmacol Ther.* 2001;70(5):468–474.
137. Hook JB, Blatt AH, Brody MJ, et al. Effects of several saluretic-diuretic agents on renal hemodynamics. *J Pharmacol Exp Ther.* 1966;154:667–673.
138. Ludens JH, Hook JB, Brody MJ, et al. Enhancement of renal blood flow by furosemide. *J Pharmacol Exp Ther.* 1968;163:456–460.
139. Dluhy RG, Wolf GL, Lauler DP. Vasodilator properties of ethacrynic acide in the perfused dog kidney. *Clin Sci.* 1970;38:347–357.
140. Schnermann J, Briggs JP. Tubuloglomerular feedback: mechanistic insights from gene-manipulated mice. *Kidney Int.* 2008;74(4):418–426.
141. Bell PD, Lapointe JY, Sabirov R, et al. Macula densa cell signaling involves ATP release through a maxi anion channel. *Proc Natl Acad Sci U S A.* 2003;100(7):4322–4327.
142. Sun D, Samuelson LC, Yang T, et al. Mediation of tubuloglomerular feedback by adenosine: evidence from mice lacking adenosine 1 receptors. *Proc Natl Acad Sci U S A.* 2001;98(17):9983–9988.
143. Castrop H, Huang Y, Hashimoto S, et al. Impairment of tubuloglomerular feedback regulation of GFR in ecto-5′-nucleotidase/CD73–deficient mice. *J Clin Invest.* 2004;114(5):634–642.
144. Wright FS, Schnermann J. Interference with feedback control of glomerular filtration rate by furosemide, triflocin, and cyanide. *J Clin Invest.* 1974;53: 1695–1708.
145. Dikshit K, Vyden JK, Forrester JS, et al. Renal and extrarenal hemodynamic effects of furosemide in congestive heart failure after acute myocardial infarction. *N Engl J Med.* 1973;288:1087–1090.
146. Bourland WA, Day DK, Williamson HE. The role of the kidney in the early nondiuretic action of furosemide to reduce elevated left atrial pressure in the hypervolemic dog. *J Pharmacol Exp Ther.* 1977;202:221–229.
147. Mukherjee SK, Katz MA, Michael UF, et al. Mechanisms of hemodynamic actions of furosemide: differentiation of vascular and renal effects on blood pressure in functionally anephric hypertensive patients. *Am Heart J.* 1981;101:313–318.
148. Schmieder RE, Messerli FH, deCarvalho JGR, et al. Immediate hemodynamic response to furosemide in patients undergoing chronic hemodialysis. *Am J Kidney Dis.* 1987;9:55–59.
149. Pickkers P, Dormans TP, Russel FG, et al. Direct vascular effects of furosemide in humans. *Circulation.* 1997;96:1847–1852.
150. Costa MA, Loria A, Elesgaray R, et al. Role of nitric oxide pathway in hypotensive and renal effects of furosemide during extracellular volume expansion. *J Hypertens.* 2004;22(8):1561–1569.
151. Ellison DH. Intensive diuretic therapy: High doses, combinations, and constant infusions. In: Seldin DW, Giebisch G, eds. *Diuretic Agents: Clinical Physiology and Pharmacology.* San Diego: Academic Press; 1997:281–300.
152. Johnston GD, Nicholls DP, Leahey WJ. The dose-response characteristics of the acute non-diuretic peripheral vascular effects of frusemide in normal subjects. *Br J Clin Pharmacol.* 1984;18:75–81.
153. Francis GS, Siegel RM, Goldsmith SR, et al. Acute vasoconstrictor response to intravenous furosemide in patients with chronic congestive heart failure. *Ann Intern Med.* 1985;103:1–6.
154. Goldsmith SR, Francis G, Cohn JN. Attenuation of the pressor response to intravenous furosemide by angiotensin converting enzyme inhibition in congestive heart failure. *Am J Cardiol.* 1989;64:1382–1385.
155. Fitch GK, Weiss ML. Activation of renal afferent pathways following furosemide treatment. II. Effect Of angiotensin blockade. *Brain Res.* 2000;861(2): 377–389.
156. Fitch GK, Patel KP, Weiss ML. Activation of renal afferent pathways following furosemide treatment. I. Effects Of survival time and renal denervation. *Brain Res.* 2000;861(2):363–376.
157. Inoue M, Okajima K, Itoh K, et al. Mechanism of furosemide resistance in analbuminemic rats and hypoalbuminemic patients. *Kidney Int.* 1987;32: 198–203.
158. Eraly SA, Vallon V, Vaughn DA, et al. Decreased renal organic anion secretion and plasma accumulation of endogenous organic anions in OAT1 knock-out mice. *J Biol Chem.* 2006;281(8):5072–5083.
159. Hasegawa M, Kusuhara H, Adachi M, et al. Multidrug resistance-associated protein 4 is involved in the urinary excretion of hydrochlorothiazide and furosemide. *J Am Soc Nephrol.* 2007;18(1):37–45.
160. Vallon V, Rieg T, Ahn SY, et al. Overlapping in vitro and in vivo specificities of the organic anion transporters OAT1 and OAT3 for loop and thiazide diuretics. *Am J Physiol Renal Physiol.* 2008;294(4):F867–873.
161. Werner U, Werner D, Heinbuchner S, et al. Gender is an important determinant of the disposition of the loop diuretic torasemide. *J Clin Pharmacol.* 2010;50(2):160–168.
162. Vormfelde SV, Sehrt D, Toliat MR, et al. Genetic variation in the renal sodium transporters NKCC2, NCC, and ENaC in relation to the effects of loop diuretic drugs. *Clin Pharmacol Ther.* 2007;82(3):300–309.
163. Schrier RW. Use of diuretics in heart failure and cirrhosis. *Semin Nephrol.* 2011;31(6):503–512.
164. Packer M, Lee WH, Medina N, et al. Functional renal insufficiencey during long-term therapy with captopril and enalapril in severe congestive heart failure. *Ann Intern Med.* 1987;106:346–354.
165. Packer M. Identification of risk factors predisposing to the development of functional renal insufficiency during treatment with converting-enzyme inhibitors in chronic heart failure. *Cardiology.* 1989;76 (Suppl. 2):50–55.
166. Smith WE, Steele TH. Avoiding diuretic related complications in older patients. *Geriatrics.* 1983;38:117–119.
167. Kaufman AM, Levitt MF. The effect of diuretics on systemic and renal hemodynamics in patients with renal insufficiency. *Am J Kidney Dis.* 1985;5: A71–A78.
168. Huerta C, Castellsague J, Varas-Lorenzo C, et al. Nonsteroidal anti-inflammatory drugs and risk of ARF in the general population. *Am J Kidney Dis.* 2005;45(3):531–539.
169. Bichet DG, Van Putten VJ, Schrier RW. Potential role of increased sympathetic activity in impaired sodium and water excretion in cirrhosis. *N Engl J Med.* 1982;307:1552–1557.
170. Dyckner T, Webster PO. Magnesium treatment of diuretic-induced hyponatremia with a preliminary report on a new aldosterone antagonist. *J Am Coll Nutr.* 1982;1:149–153.
171. Schrier RW. New treatments for hyponatremia. *N Engl J Med.* 1978;298: 214–215.
172. Dzau VJ, Hollenberg NK. Renal response to captopril in severe heart failure: role of furosemide in natriuresis and reversal of hyponatremia. *Ann Intern Med.* 1984;100:777–782.
173. Shimizu K. Combined effects of vasopressin V2 receptor antagonist and loop diuretic in humans. *Clin Nephrol.* 2003;59(3):164–173.
174. Kazama I, Hatano R, Michimata M, et al. BSC1 inhibition complements effects of vasopressin V receptor antagonist on hyponatremia in SIADH rats. *Kidney Int.* 2005;67(5):1855–1867.
175. Ram CV, Garrett BN, Kaplan NM. Moderate sodium restriction and various diuretics in the treatment of hypertension. *Arch Intern Med.* 1981;141(8): 1015–1019.
176. Palmer BF. *Potassium Disturbances Associated with the Use of Diuretics.* San Diego: Academic Press; 1997:571–583.
177. Hropot M, Fowler NB, Karlmark B, et al. Tubular action of diuretics: distal effects on electrolyte transport and acidification. *Kidney Int.* 1985;28:477–489.
178. Wilcox CS, Mitch WE, Kelly RA, et al. Factors affecting potassium balance during frusemide administration. *Clin Sci.* 1984;67:195–203.
179. Good DW, Knepper MA, Burg MB. Ammonia and bicarbonate transport by thick ascending limb of rat kidney. *Am J Physiol.* 1984;247:F35–F44.
180. Good DW. Sodium-dependent bicarbonate absorption by cortical thick ascending limb of rat kidney. *Am J Physiol.* 1985;248:F821–F829.
181. Oberleithner H, Lang F, Messner G, et al. Mechanism of hydrogen ion transport in the diluting segment of frog kidney. *Pflügers Arch.* 1984;402:272–280.
182. O'Neil RG, Helman SI. Transport characteristics of renal collecting tubules: influences of DOCA and diet. *Am J Physiol.* 1977;233:F544–F558.
183. Winter C, Schulz N, Giebisch G, et al. Nongenomic stimulation of vacuolar H+-ATPases in intercalated renal tubule cells by aldosterone. *Proc Natl Acad Sci U S A.* 2004;101(8):2636–2641.
184. Stone DK, Seldin DW, Kokko JP, et al. Mineralocorticoid modulation of rabbit medullary collecting duct acidification. *J Clin Invest.* 1983;72:77–83.
185. Tannen RL. The effect of uncomplicated potassium depletion on urine acidification. *J Clin Invest.* 1970;49:813–827.

186. Soleimani M, Grassl SM, Aronson PS. Stoichiometry of Na+-HCO3– cotransport in basolateral membrane vesicles isolated from rabbit renal cortex. *J Clin Invest.* 1987;79:1276–1280.
187. Soleimani M, Aronson PS. Ionic mechanism of Na+-HCO-3 cotransport in rabbit renal basolateral membrane vesicles. *J Biol Chem.* 1989;264: 18302–18308.
188. Wingo CS, Straub SG. Active proton secretion and potassium absorption in the rabbit outer medullary collecting duct. Functional evidence for proton-potassium-activated adenosine triphosphatase. *J Clin Invest.* 1989;84:361–365.
189. Maher JF, Schreiner GF. Studies on ethacrynic acid in patients with refractory edema. *Ann Intern Med.* 1965;62:15–29.
190. Nochy D, Callard P, Bellon B, et al. Association of overt glomerulonephritis and liver disease: A study of 34 patients. *Clin Nephrol.* 1976;6:422–427.
191. Ikeda K, Oshima T, Hidaka H, et al. Molecular and clinical implications of loop diuretic ototoxicity. *Hear Res.* 1997;107:1–8.
192. Bosher SK. The nature of ototoxicity actions of ethacrynic acid upon the mammalian endolymph system. I. Functional aspects. *Acta Otolaryngol.* 1980;89:407–418.
193. Ikeda K, Morizono T. Electrochemical profiles for monvalent ions in the stria vascularis: cellular model of ion transport mechanisms. *Hear Res.* 1989;39:279–286.
194. Mizuta K, Adachi M, Iwasa KH. Ultrastructural localization of the Na-K-Cl cotransporter in the lateral wall of the rabbit cochlear duct. *Hear Res.* 1997;106(1–2):154–162.
195. Hidaka H, Oshima T, Ikeda K, et al. The Na-K-Cl cotransporters in the rat cochlea: RT-PCR and partial sequence analysis. *Biochem Biophys Res Comm.* 1996;220:425–430.
196. Delpire E, Lu J, England R, et al. Deafness and imbalance associated with inactivation of the secretory Na-K-2Cl co-transporter. *Nat Genet.* 1999;22(2): 192–195.
197. Flagella M, Clarke LL, Miller ML, et al. Mice lacking the basolateral Na-K-2Cl cotransporter have impaired epithelial chloride secretion and are profoundly deaf. *J Biol Chem.* 1999;274(38):26946–26955.
198. Dixon MJ, Gazzard J, Chaudhry SS, et al. Mutation of the Na-K-Cl co-transporter gene Slc12a2 results in deafness in mice. *Hum Mol Genet.* 1999; 8(8):1579–1584.
199. Ryback LP. Ototoxicity of loop diuretics. *Otolaryngol Clin N America.* 1993;26:829–844.
200. Star RA. *Ototoxicity*. San Diego: Academic Press; 1997:637–642.
201. Wigand ME, Heidland A. Ototoxic side effects of high doses of furosemide in patients with uremia. *Postgrad Med J.* 1971;47:54–56.
202. Rudy DW, Voelker JR, Greene PK, et al. Loop diuretics for chronic renal insufficiency: A continuous infusion is more efficacious than bolus therapy. *Ann Intern Med.* 1991;115:360–366.
203. Toto RA. Metabolic derangements associated with diuretic use: Insulin resistance, dyslipidemia, hyperuricemia, and anti-adrenergic effects. In: Seldin DW, Giebisch G, eds. *Diuretic Agents: Clinical Physiology and Pharmacology*. San Diego: Academic Press; 1997:621–636.
204. Reilly RF, Huang CL. The mechanism of hypocalciuria with NaCl cotransporter inhibition. Nature reviews. *Nephrology*. 2011;7(11):669–674.
205. Eknoyan G, Suki WN, Martinez-Maldonado M. Effect of diuretics on urinary excretion of phosphate, calcium, and magnesium in thyroparathyroidectomized dogs. *J Lab Clin Med.* 1970;76:257–266.
206. Duarte CG, Bland JH. Calcium, phosphorous and uric acid clearances after intravenous administration of chorothiazide. *Metabolism.* 1965;14:211–219.
207. Costanzo LS, Sheehe PR, Weiner IM. Renal actions of vitamin D in D-deficient rats. *Am J Physiol.* 1974;226:1490–1495.
208. Goldfarb DS, Chan AJ, Hernandez D, et al. Effect of thiazides on colonic NaCl absorption: Role of carbonic anhydrase. *Am J Physiol Renal, Fluid Electrolyte Physiol.* 1991;261:F452–F458.
209. Kunau RT Jr, Weller DR, Webb HL. Clarification of the site of action of chlorothiazide in the rat nephron. *J Clin Invest.* 1975;56(2):401–407.
210. Walter SJ, Shirley DG. The effect of chronic hydrochlorothiazide administration on renal function in the rat. *Clin Sci (Lond).* 1986;70(4):379–387.
211. Friedman PA, Hebert SC. *Site and Mechanism of Diuretic Action.* San Diego: Academic Press; 1997:75–111.
212. Reilly RF, Ellison DH. Mammalian distal tubule: physiology, pathophysiology, and molecular anatomy. *Physiol Rev.* 2000;80(1):277–313.
213. Kriz W, Kaissling B. Structural organization of the mammalian kidney. In: Seldin DW, Giebisch G, eds. *The Kidney: Physiology and Pathophysiology*. 2nd ed. New York: Raven Press; 1992:779–802.
214. Gamba G, Saltzberg SN, Lombardi M, et al. Primary structure and functional expression of a cDNA encoding the thiazide-sensitive, electroneutral sodium-chloride cotransporter. *Proc Natl Acad Sci U S A.* 1993;90:2749–2753.
215. Miyanoshita A, Gamba G, Lytton J, et al. Primary structure and functional expression of the rat renal thiazide-sensitive Na+:Cl- cotransporter. Proceedings of the 12th International Congress of Nephrology; 1993:110.
216. Simon DB, Nelson-Williams C, Bia MJ, Ellison D, et al. Gitelman's variant of Bartter's syndrome, inherited hypokalaemic alkalosis, is caused by mutations in the thiazide-sensitive Na-Cl cotransporter. *Nat Genet.* 1996;12(1):24–30.
217. Kunchaparty S, Palcso M, Berkman J, et al. Defective processing and expression of the thiazide-sensitive Na-Cl cotransporter as a cause Gitelman's syndrome. *Am J Physiol Renal Physiol.* 1999;277:F643–F649.
218. Velázquez H, Náray-Fejes-Tóth A, Silva T, et al. The distal convoluted tubule of the rabbit coexpresses NaCl cotransporter and 11b-hydroxysteroid dehydrogenase. *Kidney Int.* 1998;54:464–472.
219. Bostanjoglo M, Reeves WB, Reilly RF, et al. 11Beta-hydroxysteroid dehydrogenase, mineralocorticoid receptor, and thiazide-sensitive Na-Cl cotransporter expression by distal tubules. *J Am Soc Nephrol.* 1998;9(8):1347–1358.
220. Obermuller N, Bernstein P, Velazquez H, et al. Expression of the thiazide-sensitive Na-Cl cotransporter in rat and human kidney. *Am J Physiol.* 1995;269 (6 Pt 2):F900–910.
221. Bachmann S, Velazquez H, Obermuller N, et al. Expression of the thiazide-sensitive Na-Cl cotransporter by rabbit distal convoluted tubule cells. *J Clin Invest.* 1995;96(5):2510–2514.
222. Tran JM, Farrell MA, Fanestil DD. Effect of ions on binding of the thiazide-type diuretic metolazone to kidney membrane. *Am J Physiol.* 1990; 258:F908–F915.
223. Monroy A, Plata C, Hebert SC, Gamba G. Characterization of the thiazide-sensitive Na(+)-Cl(-) cotransporter: a new model for ions and diuretics interaction. *Am J Physiol Renal Physiol.* 2000;279(1):F161–169.
224. Wilson DR, Honrath U, Sonnenberg H. Thiazide diuretic effect on medullary collecting duct function in the rat. *Kidney Int.* 1983;23:711–716.
225. Terada Y, Knepper MA. Thiazide-sensitive NaCl absorption in rat cortical collecting duct. *Am J Physiol Renal, Fluid Electrolyte Physiol.* 1990;259: F519–F528.
226. Leviel F, Hubner CA, Houillier P, et al. The Na+-dependent chloride-bicarbonate exchanger SLC4A8 mediates an electroneutral Na+ reabsorption process in the renal cortical collecting ducts of mice. *J Clin Invest.* 2010;120(5): 1627–1635.
227. Popovtzer MM, Subryan VL, Alfrey AC, et al. The acute effect of chlorothiazide on serum-ionized calcium. Evidence for a parathyroid hormone-dependent mechanism. *J Clin Invest.* 1975;55:1295–1302.
228. Bomsztyk K, George JP, Wright FS. Effects of luminal fluid anions on calcium transport by proximal tubule. *Am J Physiol.* 1984;246:F600–F608.
229. Costanzo LS, Windhager EE. Calcium and sodium transport by the distal convoluted tubule of the rat. *Am J Physiol.* 1978;235:F492–F506.
230. Gesek FA, Friedman PA. Mechanism of calcium transport stimulated by chlorothiazide in mouse distal convoluted tubule cells. *J Clin Invest.* 1992;90(2): 429–438.
231. Hoenderop JG, van der Kemp AW, Hartog A, et al. Molecular identification of the apical Ca2+ channel in 1, 25– dihydroxyvitamin D3–responsive epithelia. *J Biol Chem.* 1999;274(13):8375–8378.
232. Hoenderop JG, Nilius B, Bindels RJ. Calcium absorption across epithelia. *Physiol Rev.* 2005;85(1):373–422.
233. Lee CT, Shang S, Lai LW, et al. Effect of thiazide on renal gene expression of apical calcium channels and calbindins. *Am J Physiol Renal Physiol.* 2004;287(6): F1164–1170.
234. Quamme GA, Wong NL, Sutton RA, et al. Interrelationship of chlorothiazide and parathyroid hormone: a micropuncture study. *Am J Physiol.* 1975;229(1): 200–205.
235. Duarte CG. Effects of chlorothiazide and amipramizide (MK 870) on the renal excretion of calcium, phosphate and magnesium. *Metabolism.* 1968;17(5): 420–429.
236. Douban S, Brodsky MA, Whang DD. Significance of magnesium in congestive heart failure. *Am Heart J.* 1996;132:664–671.
237. Hollifield JW. Thiazide treatment of systemic hypertension: Effects on serum magnesium and ventricular ectopy. *Am J Cardiol.* 1989;63:22G-G25.
238. Quamme GA. Renal magnesium handling: New insights in undertsanding old problems. *Kidney Int.* 1997;52:1180–1195.
239. Schlingmann KP, Weber S, Peters M, et al. Hypomagnesemia with secondary hypocalcemia is caused by mutations in TRPM6, a new member of the TRPM gene family. *Nat Genet.* 2002;31(2):166–170.
240. Voets T, Nilius B, Hoefs S, et al. TRPM6 forms the Mg2+ influx channel involved in intestinal and renal Mg2+ absorption. *J Biol Chem.* 2004;279(1): 19–25.
241. Dai LJ, Ritchie G, Kerstan D, et al. Magnesium transport in the renal distal convoluted tubule. *Physiol Rev.* 2001;81(1):51–84.

242. Ellison DH. Divalent cation transport by the distal nephron: insights from Bartter's and Gitelman's syndromes. *Am J Physiol Renal Physiol.* 2000;279(4): F616–625.

243. Loffing J, Loffing-Cueni D, Hegyi I, et al. Thiazide treatment of rats provokes apoptosis in distal tubule cells. *Kidney Int.* 1996;50(4):1180–1190.

244. Loffing J, Vallon V, Loffing-Cueni D, et al. Altered renal distal tubule structure and renal Na(+) and Ca(2+) handling in a mouse model for Gitelman's syndrome. *J Am Soc Nephrol.* 2004;15(9):2276–2288.

245. Nijenhuis T, Hoenderop JG, Bindels RJ. Downregulation of Ca(2+) and Mg(2+) transport proteins in the kidney explains tacrolimus (FK506)-induced hypercalciuria and hypomagnesemia. *J Am Soc Nephrol.* 2004;15(3):549–557.

246. Nijenhuis T, Vallon V, van der Kemp AW, et al. Enhanced passive Ca2+ reabsorption and reduced Mg2+ channel abundance explains thiazide-induced hypocalciuria and hypomagnesemia. *J Clin Invest.* 2005;115(6):1651–1658.

247. Earley LE, Orloff J. The mechanism of antidiuresis associated with the administration of hydrochlorothiazide to patients with vasopressin-resistant diabetes insipidus. *J Clin Invest.* 1962;41:1988–1997.

248. McGuffin WL Jr, Gunnells JC. Intravenously administered chlorothiazide in diagnostic evaluation of hypertensive disease. *Arch Intern Med.* 1969;123:124–130.

249. Brown TC, Davis JO, Johnston CI. Acute response in plasma renin and aldosterone secretion to diuretics. *Am J Physiol.* 1966;211:437–441.

250. Siegel D, Hulley SB, Black DM, et al. Diuretics, serum and intracellular electrolyte levels, and ventricular arrhythmias in hypertensive men. *JAMA.* 1992;267:1083–1089.

251. Turner ST, Schwartz GL, Chapman AB, et al. WNK1 kinase polymorphism and blood pressure response to a thiazide diuretic. *Hypertension.* 2005;46(4):758–765.

252. Psaty BM, Smith NL, Heckbert SR, et al. Diuretic therapy, the alpha-adducin gene variant, and the risk of myocardial infarction or stroke in persons with treated hypertension. *JAMA.* 2002;287(13):1680–1689.

253. Ernst ME, Moser M. Use of diuretics in patients with hypertension. *N Engl J Med.* 2009;361(22):2153–2164.

254. Chobanian AV, Bakris GL, Black HR, et al. The Seventh Report of the Joint National Committee on Prevention, Detection, Evaluation, and Treatment of High Blood Pressure: the JNC 7 report. *JAMA.* 2003;289(19):2560–2572.

255. Messerli FH, Bangalore S. Half a century of hydrochlorothiazide: facts, fads, fiction, and follies. *Am J Med.* 2011;124(10):896–899.

256. Leary WP, Reyes AJ. Renal excretory actions of diuretics in man: Correction of various current errors and redefinition of basic concepts. In: Reyes AJ, Leary WP, eds. *Clinical Pharmacology and Therapeutic Uses of Diuretics.* 153 ed. Stuttgart: GustavFischer Verlag; 1988:153–166.

257. Ettinger B, Citron JT, Livermore B, et al. Chlorthalidone reduces calcium oxalate calculous recurrence but magnesium hydroxide does not. *J Urol.* 1988 Apr;139(4):679–684.

258. Laerum E, Larsen S. Thiazide prophylaxis of urolithiasis. A double-blind study in general practice. *Acta Med Scand.* 1984;215(4):383–389.

259. Yendt ER, Cohanim M. Prevention of calcium stones with thiazides. *Kidney Int.* 1978;13:397–409.

260. Breslau NA. Use of diuretics in disorders of calcium metabolism. In: Seldin DW, Giebisch G, eds. *Diuretic Agents: Clinical Physiology and Pharmacology.* San Diego: Academic Press; 1997:495–512.

261. Preminger GM, Pak CYC. Eventual attenuation of hypocalciuric response to hydrochlorothiazide in absorptive hypercalciuria. *J Urol.* 1987;137: 1104–1109.

262. Felson DT, Sloutskis D, Anderson JJ, et al. Thiazide diuretics and the risk of hip fracture. Results from the Framingham study. *JAMA.* 1991;265:370–373.

263. Ray WA, Griffin MR, Downey W, et al. Long-term use of thiazide diuretics and risk of hip fracture. *Lancet.* 1989;1:687–690.

264. Heidrich FE, Stergachis A, Gross KM. Diuretic drug use and the risk for hip fracture. *Ann Intern Med.* 1991;115:1–6.

265. Cauley JA, Cummings SR, Seeley DG, et al. Effects of thiazide diuretic therapy on bone mass, fractures, and falls. *Ann Intern Med.* 1993;118:666–673.

266. Reid IR, Ames RW, Orr-Walker BJ, et al. Hydrochlorothiazide reduces loss of cortical bone in normal postmenopausal women: a randomized controlled trial. *Am J Med.* 2000;109(5):362–370.

267. Adams JS, Song CF, Kantorovich V. Rapid recovery of bone mass in hypercalciuric, osteoporotic men treated with hydrochlorothiazide. *Ann Intern Med.* 1999;130(8):658–660.

268. Schoofs MW, van der Klift M, Hofman A, et al. Thiazide diuretics and the risk for hip fracture. *Ann Intern Med.* 2003;139(6):476–482.

269. Porter RH, Cox BG, Heaney D, et al. Treatment of hypoparathyroid patients with chlorthalidone. *N Engl J Med.* 1978;298:577–581.

270. Frassetto LA, Nash E, Morris RC Jr, et al. Comparative effects of potassium chloride and bicarbonate on thiazide-induced reduction in urinary calcium excretion. *Kidney Int.* 2000;58(2):748–752.

271. Coleman RA, Knepper MA, Wade JB. Rat renal connecting cells express AQP2. *J Am Soc Nephrol.* 1996;7(12):2533–2542.

272. Janjua NR, Jonassen TE, Langhoff S, et al. Role of sodium depletion in acute antidiuretic effect of bendroflumethiazide in rats with nephrogenic diabetes insipidus. *J Pharmacol Exp Ther.* 2001;299(1):307–313.

273. Cesar KR, Magaldi AJ. Thiazide induces water absorption in the inner medullary collecting duct of normal and Brattleboro rats. *Am J Physiol.* 1999; 277(5 Pt 2):F756–760.

274. Gronbeck L, Marples D, Nielsen S, et al. Mechanism of antidiuresis caused by bendroflumethiazide in conscious rats with diabetes insipidus. *Br J Pharmacol.* 1998;123(4):737–745.

275. Kim GH, Lee JW, Oh YK, et al. Antidiuretic effect of hydrochlorothiazide in lithium-induced nephrogenic diabetes insipidus is associated with upregulation of aquaporin-2, Na-Cl co-transporter, and epithelial sodium channel. *J Am Soc Nephrol.* 2004;15(11):2836–2843.

276. Major outcomes in moderately hypercholesterolemic, hypertensive patients randomized to pravastatin vs usual care: The Antihypertensive and Lipid-Lowering Treatment to Prevent Heart Attack Trial (ALLHAT-LLT). *JAMA.* 2002;288(23):2998–3007.

277. Velázquez H, Wright FS. Effects of diuretic drugs on Na, Cl, and K transport by rat renal distal tubule. *Am J Physiol.* 1986;250:F1013–F1023.

278. Sansom SC, Welling PA. Two channels for one job. *Kidney Int.* 2007;72(5): 529–530.

279. Okusa MD, Velazquez H, Ellison DH, et al. Luminal calcium regulates potassium transport by the renal distal tubule. *Am J Physiol.* 1990;258(2 Pt 2):F423–428.

280. Dorup I, Skajaa K, Thybo NK. Oral magnesium supplementation restores the concentrations of magnesium, potassium and sodium-potassium pumps in skeletal muscle of patients receiving diuretic treatment. *J Intern Med.* 1993;233:117–123.

281. Rude RK. Physiology of magnesium metabolism and the important role of magnesium in potassium deficiency. *Am J Cardiol.* 1989;63:31G-34G.

282. Huang CL, Kuo E. Mechanism of hypokalemia in magnesium deficiency. *J Am Soc Nephrol.* 2007;18(10):2649–2652.

283. Ashraf N, Locksley R, Arieff A. Thiazide-induced hyponatremia associated with death or neurologic damage in outpatients. *Am J Med.* 1981;70:1163–1168.

284. Leung AA, Wright A, Pazo V, et al. Risk of thiazide-induced hyponatremia in patients with hypertension. *Am J Med.* 2011;124(11):1064–1072.

285. Fichman MP, Vorherr H, Kleeman CR, et al. Diuretic-induced hyponatremia. *Ann Intern Med.* 1971;75:853–863.

286. Friedman E, Shadel M, Halkin H, et al. Thiazide-induced hyponatremia: Reproducibility by single dose rechallenge and an analysis of pathogenesis. *Ann Intern Med.* 1989;110:24–30.

287. Neafsey PJ. Thiazides and selective serotonin reuptake inhibitors can induce hyponatremia. *Home Healthc Nurse.* 2004;22(11):788–790.

288. Chow KM, Szeto CC, Wong TY, Leung CB, Li PK. Risk factors for thiazide-induced hyponatraemia. *QJM.* 2003;96(12):911–917.

289. Carlsen JE, Kober L, Torp-Pedersen C, et al. Relation between dose of bendrofluazide, antihypertensive effect, and adverse biochemical effects. *BMJ.* 1990;300:975–978.

290. Harper R, Ennis CN, Heaney AP, et al. A comparison of the effects of low- and conventional-dose thiazide diuretic on insulin action in hypertensive patients with NIDDM. *Diabetologia.* 1995;38:853–859.

291. Major outcomes in high-risk hypertensive patients randomized to angiotensin-converting enzyme inhibitor or calcium channel blocker vs diuretic: The Antihypertensive and Lipid-Lowering Treatment to Prevent Heart Attack Trial (ALLHAT). *JAMA.* 2002;288(23):2981–2997.

292. Helderman JH, Elahi D, Andersen DK, et al. Prevention of the glucose intolerance of thiazide diuretics by maintenance of body potassium. *Diabetes.* 1983;32(2):106–111.

293. Pickkers P, Schachter M, Hughes AD, et al. Thiazide-induced hyperglycaemia: A role for calcium-activated potassium channels? *Diabetologia.* 1996;39:861–864.

294. Scheen AJ. Renin-angiotensin system inhibition prevents type 2 diabetes mellitus. Part 2. Overview of physiological and biochemical mechanisms. *Diabetes Metab.* 2004;30(6):498–505.

295. Ellison DH, Loffing J. Thiazide effects and adverse effects: insights from molecular genetics. *Hypertension.* 2009;54(2):196–202.

296. Wilcox CS. Metabolic and adverse effects of diuretics. *Semin Nephrol.* 1999;19(6):557–568.

297. Grimm RH Jr, Flack JM, Granditis GA. Treatment of Mild Hypertension Study (TOMHS) Research Group. Long-term effects on plasma lipids of diet and drugs to treat hypertension. *JAMA.* 1996;275:1549–1556.

298. Ott SM, LaCroix AZ, Ichikawa LE, et al. Effect of low-dose thiazide diuretics on plasma lipids: results from a double-blind, randomized clinical trial in older men and women. *J Am Geriatr Soc.* 2005;51:1003–1013.

299. Meneton P, Loffing J, Warnock DG. Sodium and potassium handling by the aldosterone-sensitive distal nephron: the pivotal role of the distal and connecting tubule. *Am J Physiol Renal Physiol*. 2004;287(4):F593–601.
300. Baer J, Jones C, Spitzer S, Russo H. The potassium sparing and natriuretic activity of N-amidino-3,5 diamino-6–chloropyrazinecarboxamide hydrochloride dihydrate (amiloride hydrochloride). *J Pharmacol Exp Ther*. 1967;157:472–485.
301. Gross JB, Kokko JP. Effects of aldosterone and potassium-sparing diuretics on electrical potential differences across the distal nephron. *J Clin Invest*. 1977;59:82–89.
302. Guignard JP, Peters G. Effects of triamterene and amiloride on urinary acidification and potassium excretion in the rat. *Eur J Pharmacol*. 1970;10:255–267.
303. Decaux G, Soupart A, Vassart G. Non-peptide arginine-vasopressin antagonists: the vaptans. *Lancet*. 2008;371(9624):1624–1632.
304. McDonald FJ, Yang B, Hrstka RF, et al. Disruption of the beta subunit of the epithelial Na+ channel in mice: hyperkalemia and neonatal death associated with a pseudohypoaldosteronism phenotype. *Proc Natl Acad Sci U S A*. 1999;96(4):1727–1731.
305. Perez-Ayuso RM, Arroyo V, Planas R, et al. Randomized comparative study of efficacy of furosemide versus spironolactone in nonazotemic cirrhosis with ascites. Relationship between the diuretic response on the activity of the renin-aldosterone system. *Gastroenterology*. 1983;84:961–968.
306. Coppage WS, Liddle GW. Mode of action and clinical usefulness of aldosterone antagonists. *Ann NY Acad Sci*. 1960;88:815–820.
307. Botero-Velez M, Curtis JJ, Warnock DG. Brief Report: Liddle's syndrome revisited—a disorder of sodium reabsorption in the distal tubule. *N Engl J Med*. 1994;330(3):174–178.
308. Okusa MD, Bia MJ. Bartter's syndrome. In: Foa PP, Cohen MP, eds. *Endocrinology and Metabolism*. New York: Springer-Verlag; 1987:231–263.
309. Seyberth HW, Schlingmann KP. Bartter- and Gitelman-like syndromes: salt-losing tubulopathies with loop or DCT defects. *Pediatr Nephrol*. 2011;26(10):1789–1802.
310. Pitt B, Zannad F, Remme WJ, et al. The effect of spironolactone on morbidity and mortality in patients with severe heart failure. *N Engl J Med*. 1999;341(10):709–717.
311. Pitt B, Williams G, Remme W, et al. The EPHESUS trial: eplerenone in patients with heart failure due to systolic dysfunction complicating acute myocardial infarction. Eplerenone Post-AMI Heart Failure Efficacy and Survival Study. *Cardiovasc Drugs Ther*. 2001;15(1):79–87.
312. Kurtzman NA, White MG, Rogers PW. Aldosterone deficiency and renal bicarbonate reabsorption. *J Lab Clin Med*. 1971;77:931–940.
313. Hulter HN, Ilnicki LP, Harbottle JA, et al. Impaired renal H+ secretion and NH3 production in mineralocorticoid-deficient glucocorticoid replete dogs. *Am J Physiol*. 1977;232:F136–F146.
314. Gabow PA, Moore S, Schrier RW. Spironolactone-induced hyperchloremic acidosis in cirrhosis. *Ann Intern Med*. 1979;90:338–340.
315. Costanzo LS, Weiner IM. Relationship between clerarances of Ca and Na: effect of distal diuretics and PTH. *Am J Physiol*. 1976;230:67–73.
316. Costanzo LS. Localization of diuretic action in microperfused rat distal tubules: Ca and Na transport. *Am J Physiol*. 1985;248:F527–F535.
317. Shimizu T, Nakamura M, Yoshitomi K, et al. Interaction of trichlormethiazide or amiloride with PTH in stimulating Ca2+ absorption in rabbit CNT. *Am J Physiol*. 1991;261:F36–F43.
318. Friedman PA, Gesek FA. Stimulation of calcium transport by amiloride in mouse distal convoluted tubule cells. *Kidney Int*. 1995;48:1427–1434.
319. Bundy JT, Connito D, Mahoney MD, et al. Treatment of idiopathic renal magesium wasting with amiloride. *Am J Nephrol*. 1995;15:75–77.
320. Dyckner T, Wester P-O, Widman L. Amiloride prevents thiazide-induced intracellular potassium and magnesium losses. *Acta Med Scand*. 1988;224:25–30.
321. Schild L. The epithelial sodium channel: from molecule to disease. *Rev Physiol Biochem Pharmacol*. 2004;151:93–107.
322. Kashlan OB, Kleyman TR. ENaC structure and function in the wake of a resolved structure of a family member. *Am J Physiol Renal Physiol*. 2011;301(4):F684–696.
323. Stewart AP, Haerteis S, Diakov A, et al. Atomic force microscopy reveals the architecture of the epithelial sodium channel (ENaC). *J Biol Chem*. 2011;286(37):31944–31952.
324. Ismailov II, Awayda MS, Jovov B, et al. Regulation of epithelial sodium channels by the cystic fibrosis transmembrane conductance regulator. *J Biol Chem*. 1996;271:4725–4732.
325. Jiang Q, Li J, Dubroff R, et al. Epithelial sodium channels regulate cystic fibrosis transmembrane conductance regulator chloride channels in xenopus oocytes. *J Biol Chem*. 2000;275:13266–13274.
326. Kim GH, Martin SW, Fernandez-Llama P, et al. Long-term regulation of renal Na-dependent cotransporters and ENaC: response to altered acid-base intake. *Am J Physiol Renal Physiol*. 2000;279(3):F459–467.
327. Loffing J, Pietri L, Aregger F, et al. Differential subcellular localization of ENaC subunits in mouse kidney in response to high- and low-sodium diets. *Am J Physiol Renal Physiol*. 2000;279:F252–F258.
328. Ecelbarger CA, Kim G-H, Terris J, et al. Vasopressin-mediated regulation of epithelial sodium channel abundance in rat kidney. *Am J Physiol Renal Physiol*. 2000;279:F46–F53.
329. Verrey F. Early aldosterone action: toward filling the gap between transcription and transport. *Am J Physiol*. 1999 Sep;277(3 Pt 2):F319–327.
330. Thomas W, McEneaney V, Harvey BJ. Aldosterone-induced signalling and cation transport in the distal nephron. *Steroids*. 2008;73(9–10):979–984.
331. Masilamani S, Kim G-H, Mitchell C, et al. Aldosterone-mediated regulation of ENaCa,b and g subunits. *J Clin Invest*. 1999;104:R19–R23.
332. Berger S, Bleich M, Schmid W, et al. Mineralocorticoid receptor knockout mice: pathophysiology of Na+ metabolism. *Proc Natl Acad Sci U S A*. 1998;95(16):9424–9429.
333. Zhou ZH, Bubien JK. Nongenomic regulation of ENaC by aldosterone. *Am J Physiol Cell Physiol*. 2001;281(4):C1118–1130.
334. Karim A. Spironolactone: disposition, metabolism, pharmacodynamics and bioavailability. *Drug Metab Rev*. 1978;8:151–188.
335. Shackleton CR, Wong NLM, Sutton RA. Distal (potassium-sparing) diuretics. In: Dirks JH, Sutton RAL, eds. *Diuretics. Physiology, Pharmacology and Clinical Use*. Philadelphia: W.B. Saunders; 1986:117–134.
336. Fanestil DD. Mechanism of action of aldosterone blockers. *Sem Nephrol*. 1988;8:249–263.
337. Menard J. The 45–year story of the development of an anti-aldosterone more specific than spironolactone. *Mol Cell Endocrinol*. 2004;217(1–2):45–52.
338. Marver D, Stewart J, Funder JW, et al. Renal aldosterone receptors: Studies with [3H]aldosterone and the antimineralocorticoid [3H]spironolactone (SC26304). *Proc Natl Acad Sci*. 1974;71:1431–1435.
339. Couette B, Lombes M, Baulieu E-E, et al. Aldosterone antagonists destablilize the mineralocorticoid receptor. *Biochem J*. 1992;282:697–702.
340. Liddle GW. Aldosterone antagonists and triamterene. *Ann NY Acad Sci*. 1966;134:466–470.
341. Kagawa CM. Blocking the renal electrolyte effects of mineralocorticoids with an orally active steroidal spironolactone. *Endocrinology*. 1960;65:125–132.
342. Weinberger MH, Roniker B, Krause SL, et al. Eplerenone, a selective aldosterone blocker, in mild-to-moderate hypertension. *Am J Hypertens*. 2002;15(8):709–716.
343. Brown NJ. Eplerenone: cardiovascular protection. *Circulation*. 2003;107(19):2512–2518.
344. Duarte CG, Chomety G, Giebisch G. Effect of amiloride, ouabain, and furosemide on distal tubular function in the rat. *Am J Physiol*. 1971;221:632–639.
345. Giebisch G. Amiloride effects on distal nephron function. In: Straub RW, Bolis L, eds. *Cell Membrane Receptors for Drugs and Hormones: A Multidisciplinary Approach*. New York: Raven Press; 1978:337–342.
346. Costanzo LS. Comparison of calcium and sodium transport in early and late rat distal tubules: effect of amiloride. *Am J Physiol*. 1984;246:F937–F945.
347. Stoner LC, Burg MB, Orloff J. Ion transport in cortical collecting tubule; effect of amiloride. *Am J Physiol*. 1974;227:453–459.
348. Stokes JB. Na and K transport across the cortical and outer medullary collecting tubule of the rabbit: evidence for diffusion across the outer medullary portion. *Am J Physiol*. 1982;242:F514–F520.
349. Okusa MD, Velazquez H, Wright FS. Effect of Na-channel blockers and lumen Ca on K secretion by rat renal distal tubule. *Am J Physiol*. 1991 Mar;260(3 Pt 2):F459–465.
350. Koeppen BM, Biagi BA, Giebisch G. Intracellular microelectrode charcterization of the rabbit cortical collecting duct. *Am J Physiol*. 1983;244:F35–F47.
351. O'Neil RG, Sansom SC. Characterization of apical cell membrane Na+ and K+ conductances of cortical collecting duct using microelectrode techniques. *Am J Physiol*. 1984;247:F14–F24.
352. Garty H, Benos D. Characteristics and regulatory mechanisms of the amiloride-blockable Na+ channel. *Physiol Rev*. 1988;68:309–373.
353. Garty H. Molecular properties of epithelial, amiloride-blockable Na+ channels. *FASEB J*. 1994;8:522–528.
354. Garty H, Palmer LG. Epithelial sodium channels: function, structure, and regulation. *Physiol Rev*. 1997;77:359–396.
355. Waldmann R, Champigny G, Bassilana F, et al. Molecular cloning and functional expression of a novel amiloride-sensitive Na+ channel. *J Biol Chem*. 1995;270:27411–27414.
356. Schild L, Schneeberger E, Gautschi I, et al. Identification of amino acid residues in the a, b and g subunits of the epithelial sodium channel (ENaC) involved in amiloride block and ion permeation. *J Gen Physiol*. 1997;109:15–26.
357. Ishmailov II, Kieber-Emmons T, Lin C, et al. Identification of an amiloride binding domain within the α-subunit of the epithelial Na+ channel. *J Biol Chem*. 1997;272:21075–21083.

358. Kashlan OB, Sheng S, Kleyman TR. On the interaction between amiloride and its putative alpha-subunit epithelial Na+ channel binding site. *J Biol Chem.* 2005;280(28):26206–26215.
359. Kieber-Emmons T, Lin C, Foster MH, et al. Antiidiotypic antibody recognizes an amiloride binding domain within the a subunit of the epithelial Na+ channel. *J Biol Chem.* 1999;274:9648–9655.
360. Busch AE, Suessbrich H, Kunzelmann K, et al. Blockade of epithelial Na+ channels by triamterene-underlying mechanisms and molecular basis. *Pflügers Arch.* 1996;432:760–766.
361. Merkus FWHM, Overdiek JWPM, Cilissen J, et al. Pharmacokinetics of spironolactone after a single dose: evaluation of the true canrenone serum concentrations during 24 hours. *Clin Exp Hypertens.* 1983;[A]5:249–269.
362. Gardiner P, Schrode K, Quinlan D, et al. Spironolactone metabolism: steady-state serum levels of the sulfur-containing metabolites. *J Clin Pharmacol.* 1989;29:342–347.
363. Sungaila I, Bartle WR, Walker SE, et al. Spironolactone pharmacokinetics and pharmacodynamics in patients with cirrhotic ascites. *Gastroenterology.* 1992;102:1680–1685.
364. Ganguly A. Primary aldosteronism. *N Engl J Med.* 1998;339(25):1828–1834.
365. Brown JJ, Davies DL, Ferriss JB, et al. Comparison of surgery and prolonged spironolactone therapy in patients with hypertension, aldosterone excess, and low plasma renin. *BMJ.* 1972;2:729–730.
366. Laffi G, La Villa G, Carloni V, et al. Loop diuretic therapy in liver cirrhosis with ascites. *J Cardiovasc Pharmacol.* 1993;22 Suppl. 3:S51–S58.
367. Runyon BA. AASLD Practice Guidelines Committee. Management of adult patients with ascites due to cirrhosis. *Hepatology.* 2004;39(3):841–856.
368. Steib CJ, Hennenberg M, Beitinger F, et al. Amiloride reduces portal hypertension in rat liver cirrhosis. *Gut.* 2010;59(6):827–836.
369. Effectiveness of spironolactone added to an angiotensin-converting enzyme inhibitor and a loop diuretic for severe chronic congestive heart failure (The randomized aldactone evaluation study [RALES]). *Am J Cardiol.* 1996;78:902–907.
370. Pitt B, Remme W, Zannad F, et al. Eplerenone, a selective aldosterone blocker, in patients with left ventricular dysfunction after myocardial infarction. *N Engl J Med.* 2003;348(14):1309–1321.
371. Zannad F, McMurray JJ, Krum H, et al. Eplerenone in patients with systolic heart failure and mild symptoms. *N Engl J Med.* 2011;364(1):11–21.
372. Calhoun DA, Jones D, Textor S, et al. Resistant hypertension: diagnosis, evaluation, and treatment: a scientific statement from the American Heart Association Professional Education Committee of the Council for High Blood Pressure Research. *Circulation.* 2008;117(25):e510–526.
373. Griffing GT, Cole AG, Aurecchia SA, et al. Amiloride for primary hyperaldosteronism. *Clin Pharmacol Ther.* 1982;31:56–61.
374. Ganguly A, Weinberger MH. Triamterene-thiazide combination:alternative therapy for primary aldosteronism. *Clin Pharmacol Ther.* 1981;30:246–250.
375. Batlle DC, von Riotte AB, Gaviria M, et al. Amelioration of polyuria by amiloride in patients receiving long-term lithium therapy. *N Engl J Med.* 1985;312(7):408–414.
376. Bedford JJ, Weggery S, Ellis G, et al. Lithium-induced nephrogenic diabetes insipidus: renal effects of amiloride. *Clin J Am Soc Nephrol.* 2008;3(5): 1324–1331.
377. Kortenoeven ML, Li Y, Shaw S, et al. Amiloride blocks lithium entry through the sodium channel thereby attenuating the resultant nephrogenic diabetes insipidus. *Kidney Int.* 2009;76(1):44–53.
378. Juurlink DN, Mamdani MM, Lee DS, et al. Rates of hyperkalemia after publication of the Randomized Aldactone Evaluation Study. *N Engl J Med.* 2004;351(6):543–551.
379. Tamirisa KP, Aaronson KD, Koelling TM. Spironolactone-induced renal insufficiency and hyperkalemia in patients with heart failure. *Am Heart J.* 2004;148(6):971–978.
380. Antoniou T, Gomes T, Mamdani MM, et al. Trimethoprim-sulfamethoxazole induced hyperkalaemia in elderly patients receiving spironolactone: nested case-control study. *BMJ.* 2011;343:d5228.
381. Wei L, Struthers AD, Fahey T, et al. Spironolactone use and renal toxicity: population based longitudinal analysis. *BMJ.* 2010;340:c1768.
382. Rose LI, Underwood RH, Newmark SR, et al. Pathophysiology of spironolactone-induced gynecomastia. *Ann Intern Med.* 1977;87:398–403.
383. Whitling AM, Pergola PE, Sang JL, et al. Spironolactone-induced agranulocytosis. *Ann Pharmacother.* 1997;31:582–585.
384. Fairley KF, Woo KT, Birch DF, et al. Triamterene-induced crystalluria and cylinduria: clinical and experimental studies. *Clin Nephrol.* 1986;26:169–173.
385. Carr MC, Prien EL Jr, Babayan RK. Triamterene nephrolithiasis: Renewed attention is warranted. *J Urol.* 1990;144:1339–1340.
386. Favre L, Glasson P, Vallotton MB. Reversible acute renal failure from combined triamterene and indomethacin: a study in healthy subjects. *Ann Intern Med.* 1982;96:317–320.
387. Weinberg MS, Quigg RJ, Salant DJ, et al. Anuric renal failure precipitated by indomethacin and triamterene. *Nephron.* 1985;40:216–218.
388. Wesson LG. Magnesium, calcium and phosphate excretion during osmotic diuresis in the dog. *J Lab Clin Med.* 1967;60:422–432.
389. Benabe JE, Martinez-Maldonado M. Effects on divalent ion excretion. In: Eknoyan G, Martinez-Maldonado M, eds. *The Physiological Basis of Diuretic Therapy in Clinical Medicine.* Orlando: Grune & Stratton, Inc.; 1986:109–124.
390. Wesson LG Jr, Anslow WP. Excretion of sodium and water during osmotic diuresis in the dog. *Am J Physiol.* 1948;153:465–474.
391. Suki W, Rector FC Jr, Seldin DW. The site of action of furosemide and other sulfonamide diuretics in the dog. *J Clin Invest.* 1965;44:1458–1469.
392. Earley LE, Friedler RM. Renal tubular effects of ethacrynic acid. *J Clin Invest.* 1964;43:1495.
393. Demartini FE, Wheaton EA, Healy LA, et al. Effect of chlorothiazide on the renal excretion of uric acid. *Am J Med.* 1962;32:572–577.
394. Brater DC. Diuretic therapy. *N Engl J Med.* 1998;339:387–395.
395. Schmitt R, Ellison DH, Farman N, et al. Developmental expression of sodium entry pathways in rat nephron. *Am J Physiol.* 1999;276(3 Pt 2): F367–381.

CHAPTER

67 Cardiac Failure and the Kidney

William T. Abraham • Robert W. Schrier

The kidney plays a central role in the sodium and water retention and edema formation associated with cardiac failure. Heart failure, like liver disease and the nephrotic syndrome, represents another edematous state in which renal sodium and water retention is observed despite an excess of total body sodium and water. This finding of continued renal sodium and water retention despite total body sodium and water excess, in part, defines the clinical syndrome of heart failure. In this regard, the pathophysiology of heart failure has been described as a cardiorenal syndrome, where left ventricular systolic and/or diastolic dysfunction leads to renal sodium and water retention that in turn produces the clinical syndrome of heart failure. Manifestations of cardiac failure are almost always associated with fluid volume retention resulting in hemodynamic and clinical congestion, where the former is measured as elevated ventricular filling pressures and the latter is seen as congestive signs and symptoms. Although an abnormal cardiac output initiates renal sodium and water retention, as will be discussed later in this chapter, most of the cardinal signs and symptoms of heart failure are attributable to fluid retention rather than to an abnormal cardiac output (Table 67.1).

Moreover, worsening fluid retention is the proximate cause of heart failure hospitalization (i.e., morbidity) in nearly 90% of cases.[1,2] As will be discussed in subsequent text of this chapter, renal dysfunction as measured simply by elevated blood urea nitrogen (BUN) and/or serum creatinine portends a very poor prognosis in both acutely decompensated patients and patients with chronic heart failure.[3–6] Consequently, the kidney provides a sensitive bioassay for prognosis in patients with heart failure. This observation underscores the importance of cardiorenal interactions in the natural history of heart failure. This chapter reviews the mechanisms of edema formation and sodium and water retention associated with cardiac failure, discusses the clinical implications of cardiorenal interactions in heart failure, and reviews current and future treatment options.

THE MECHANISM OF EDEMA FORMATION

Edema is a clinical sign that indicates an increase in the volume of sodium and water in the interstitial space. This increase in interstitial-space volume is caused by an alteration of the Starling forces that govern the transfer of fluid from the vascular compartment into the surrounding tissue spaces.[7] Edema may result from local factors such as an obstruction of lymphatic or venous flow. However, the type of edema considered in this chapter reflects a generalized disturbance of sodium and water balance and is associated with a net increase in extracellular fluid (ECF) volume, a situation that is usually not present when edema results from a local disruption of normal capillary mechanisms. Generalized edema results when altered Starling forces affect all capillary beds. The development of generalized edema thus indicates a widespread disturbance in the normal balance between tissue capillary and interstitial hydrostatic and colloid osmotic pressures, which control the distribution of ECF between the vascular and extravascular (interstitial) compartments. In edematous disorders such as cardiac failure, sodium and water retention by the kidney leads to the progressive expansion of the ECF volume and alteration of the Starling forces that subsequently result in edema formation.

Transcapillary solute and fluid transport consists of two types of flow: convective and diffusive. Bulk water movement occurs via convective transport induced by the imbalance between transcapillary hydraulic pressure and colloid osmotic pressure.[7] Transcapillary hydraulic pressure is influenced by a number of factors, including systemic arterial and venous blood pressures, regional blood flow, and the resistances imposed by the precapillary and postcapillary sphincters. Cardiac output, intravascular volume, and systemic vascular resistance, in turn, determine systemic arterial blood pressure. Systemic venous pressure is determined by right atrial pressure, intravascular volume, and venous capacitance. These latter hemodynamic parameters are largely determined by sodium and water balance and by various neurohormonal factors. For

TABLE 67.1 Common Signs and Symptoms of Congestive Heart Failure

Primarily Related to Fluid Retention/Increased Ventricular Filling Pressures	Primarily Related to Abnormal Cardiac Output
Ascites	Cool extremities
Dyspnea (at rest or with exertion)	Fatigue
Hepatomegaly (RUQ fullness, pain)	Low blood pressure/ narrow pulse pressure
Jugular venous distension	Poor capillary refill
Orthopnea	
Paroxysmal nocturnal dyspnea	
Peripheral edema	
Pleural effusions	
Pulmonary rales	
Third heart sound	

RUQ, right upper quadrant.

example, right atrial pressure or right ventricular preload is modulated both by changes in the intravascular volume, which are largely determined by the kidney, and alterations in venous capacitance, which are governed in part by neuroendocrine mechanisms such as the sympathetic nervous system, the renin–angiotensin system, the nonosmotic release of arginine vasopressin (AVP), and the natriuretic peptides. As discussed in this chapter, activation of these two mechanisms (i.e., renal sodium and water retention and neurohormonal activation), which may influence transcapillary hydraulic and oncotic pressures, is observed with cardiac failure.

Several mechanisms are capable of minimizing edema formation or diminishing the transudation of solute and water across the capillary bed. In several vascular beds, the local transcapillary hydraulic pressure gradient exceeds the opposing colloid osmotic pressure gradient throughout the length of the capillary bed, so that filtration occurs across its entire length.[8] Filtered fluid consequently must return to the circulation via lymphatics. Increased lymphatic drainage and the ability of lymphatic flow to increase may thus be seen as one protective mechanism that minimizes edema formation. Other protective mechanisms that reduce interstitial fluid accumulation include precapillary vasoconstriction, increased net filtration with a resultant rise in intracapillary plasma protein concentration, and increased interstitial fluid volume with a resultant augmentation of tissue hydraulic pressure. For example, increased net filtration itself, such as that associated with hypoalbuminemia and the resultant decreased plasma oncotic pressure, leads to a dissipation of capillary hydraulic pressure, a dilution of interstitial fluid protein concentration, and a corresponding rise in intracapillary protein concentration, all of which alter the balance of the Starling forces to mitigate further interstitial fluid accumulation.

These buffering factors directed against interstitial fluid accumulation may explain why, in patients with congenital analbuminemia, positive sodium and water balance, and edema formation do not occur consistently and sodium loads are excreted.[9] Because the continued loss of intravascular fluid volume to the interstitial space without renal sodium and water retention may result in the cessation of interstitial fluid formation, the presence of generalized edema, therefore, implies concomitant renal sodium and water retention. This is unquestionably the case in cardiac failure, as well as in liver disease and the nephrotic syndrome. The disturbances in microcirculatory hemodynamics associated with edema and expansion of the ECF volume are described in Table 67.2.

THE MECHANISMS OF FLUID RETENTION IN CARDIAC FAILURE

Cardiac failure may be defined as the inability of the heart to deliver enough blood to peripheral tissues to meet metabolic demands. In the case of low-output cardiac failure, a decrease in cardiac output initiates a complex set of compensatory mechanisms in an attempt to maintain circulatory integrity. The adjustments that serve to stabilize cardiac performance and arterial perfusion in such patients include increases in plasma volume, atrial and ventricular filling pressures, peripheral vasoconstriction, and cardiac contrac-

TABLE 67.2 Disturbances in Microcirculatory Hemodynamics Associated with Edema and Expansion of Extracellular Fluid Volume

Increased venous pressure transmitted to the capillary
Adjustments in precapillary and postcapillary resistances to favor interstitial fluid accumulation
Inadequate lymphatic flow of drainage
Altered capillary permeability (K_f)

tility and heart rate. The retention of sodium and water is a major renal compensation for a failing myocardium, but it also accounts to a great extent for the familiar clinical syndrome of heart failure, which consists of pulmonary and/or peripheral edema and exercise intolerance. In fact, the inability to excrete a sodium load has been used as an index of the presence of heart failure,[10] and a defect in water excretion is regularly encountered in such patients.[11]

Classically, two theories have attempted to explain how the kidney becomes involved in renal sodium and water retention of heart failure. According to the "backward failure" hypothesis advanced by Hope[12] and Starling,[7] central venous pressure rises and then peripheral venous pressure rises as the cardiac pump fails. With this increase in peripheral venous pressure, the hydraulic pressure in the capillaries exceeds opposing forces and causes the transudation of fluid from the intravascular compartment to the interstitial space, and thus the development of edema. This loss of intravascular fluid volume then signals the kidney to retain sodium and water in an attempt to restore the circulating volume to normal. The "forward failure" theory states that as the heart fails, there is inadequate perfusion of the kidney, resulting in decreased sodium and water excretion.[13] As will become apparent from the following discussion, both an increase in central venous pressure, or "backward failure," and a decrease in cardiac output, or "forward failure," may contribute to the sodium and water retention of low-output cardiac failure via systemic and renal hemodynamic effects and through the activation of various vasoconstrictor and antinatriuretic neuroendocrine systems. According to our unifying hypothesis of body fluid–volume regulation,[14–21] neurohormonal activation plays a central role in the efferent limb of the sodium and water retention in cardiac failure, liver disease, and the nephrotic syndrome, whereas the afferent limb of this volume regulatory system is initiated by altered systemic hemodynamics. The following discussion addresses this unifying hypothesis of body fluid–volume regulation and the afferent and efferent mechanisms for sodium and water retention in edematous disorders, in particular, heart failure.

Afferent Mechanisms for Renal Sodium and Water Retention in Heart Failure

The kidney alters the amount of dietary sodium excreted in response to signals from volume receptors and chemoreceptors in the circulation. These receptors may affect kidney function by altering renal sympathetic nerve activity and changing levels of circulating hormones with vasoactive and nonvasoactive (e.g., direct sodium-retaining) effects on the kidney. Important "effector" hormones include angiotensin II (AT-II), aldosterone, AVP, endothelin, nitric oxide (NO), prostaglandins (PGs), and the natriuretic peptides, especially atrial and brain natriuretic peptides (ANP and BNP, respectively). Both high- and low-pressure baroreceptors as well as cardiac and hepatic chemoreceptors have been implicated in the activation of these neurohormonal systems.

High-Pressure Baroreceptors

In humans, evidence for the presence of volume-sensitive receptors in the arterial circulation originated from observations in patients with traumatic arterial-venous (AV) fistulae.[22] Closure of AV fistulae is associated with a decreased rate of emptying of the arterial blood into the venous circulation, as demonstrated by closure-induced increases in diastolic arterial pressure and decreases in cardiac output. This results in an immediate increase in renal sodium and water excretion without changes in either glomerular filtration rate (GFR) or renal blood flow.[22] This observation implicates the "fullness" of the arterial vascular tree as a "sensor" in modulating renal sodium and water excretion. In fact, the fullness of the arterial vascular compartment, or the so-called effective arterial blood volume (EABV),[23] has been proposed as a major determinant of renal sodium and water handling according to the unifying hypothesis of body fluid volume regulation.[14–21]

The EABV is a measure of the adequacy of arterial blood volume to "fill" the capacity of the arterial circulation. Normal EABV exists when the ratio of cardiac output to peripheral vascular resistance maintains venous return and cardiac output at normal levels. Arterial or high-pressure volume receptors, therefore, may be stimulated when either cardiac output falls or peripheral vascular resistance diminishes to such an extent that the arterial circulation is no longer effectively "full" (Fig. 67.1). Therefore, in the case of low-output cardiac failure, it is the diminution of cardiac output that is perceived by the arterial circulation as inadequate to maintain EABV. In high-output cardiac failure, decreased peripheral vascular resistance may serve as the signal for arterial underfilling.[14–21] The concept of arterial underfilling in low- and high-output cardiac failure is discussed in the following paragraphs.

Studies using one model of low-output cardiac failure—constriction of the vena cava in the dog—support the notion that a fall in cardiac output may be a primary stimulus for sodium and water retention by the kidney. Using this model, Schrier and associates[24–26] showed that constriction

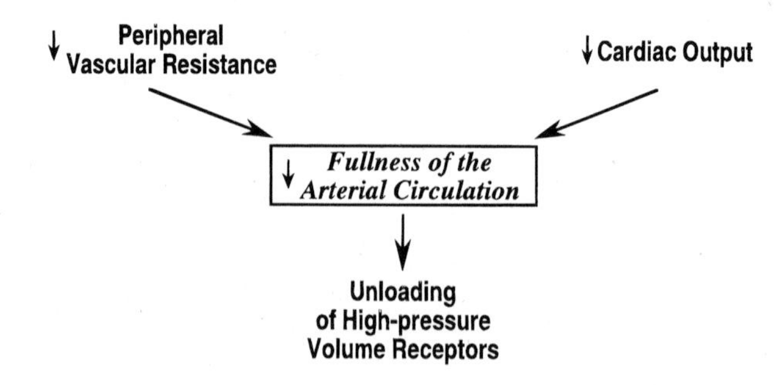

FIGURE 67.1 Peripheral vascular resistance and cardiac output as the determinants of arterial filling or the "effective arterial blood volume." Here, either a decrease in vascular resistance or diminished cardiac output results in decreased fullness of the arterial circulation with unloading of high-pressure volume receptors and activation of various neurohormonal responses (see text).

of the thoracic inferior vena cava (TIVC) is associated with a decrease in cardiac output, arterial pressure, and urinary sodium excretion, even when renal perfusion pressure and renal venous pressure were held constant. Of note, renal denervation and adrenalectomy did not abolish this antinatriuresis. Furthermore, sodium retention did not correlate with changes in GFR or renal vascular resistance. Constriction of the superior vena cava to cause a decrease in cardiac output similar to that observed in the TIVC studies resulted in a similar decrease in urinary sodium excretion despite the absence of concomitant hepatic, renal, and abdominal venous congestion. These findings support the hypothesis that the kidney decreases sodium excretion in response to a decrease in cardiac output and the associated arterial underfilling.

Migdal et al.[27] questioned this hypothesis by comparing the renal response in three different models of experimental heart failure. Specifically, they compared models of TIVC constriction, pulmonary artery occlusion (which is similar to caval constriction except that right-sided heart pressures are increased rather than decreased), and acute left ventricular infarction, another model of low-output heart failure but with increased left-sided heart pressures. This investigation demonstrated that with comparable decrements in cardiac output in all three models, only the TIVC constriction animals exhibited antinatriuresis. The authors concluded that low cardiac output per se is not the afferent signal for sodium retention in low-output heart failure. These authors[27] and others[28] suggested that in some way, decreased right-sided heart pressure mediates the antinatriuresis.

An alternative interpretation of the findings of Migdal et al.[27] is that a decrease in cardiac output is a stimulus for renal sodium and water retention, but an acute rise in atrial or ventricular end-diastolic pressures, in animals with acute pulmonary hypertension or acute left ventricular infarction, with the release of the natriuretic peptides ANP and BNP, initially obscures this effect. Support for this interpretation may be found in a report from Lee et al.,[29] who examined sodium excretion in two models of low-output heart failure in the dog, acute heart failure produced by rapid ventricular pacing, and a TIVC constriction model. Similar to the animals in the study of Migdal et al., the dogs with TIVC constriction demonstrated diminished cardiac outputs and arterial pressures without an increase in atrial pressures or plasma ANP level but with avid renal sodium retention. Of note, plasma renin activity (PRA) and plasma aldosterone concentrations were substantially elevated in these TIVC-constriction animals. In the case of pacing-induced heart failure, cardiac output and arterial pressure were similarly decreased, whereas atrial pressures and the plasma ANP concentration were significantly increased. In the animals with elevated rather than normal circulating ANP concentrations, urinary sodium excretion was maintained and PRA and plasma aldosterone concentrations were not increased. Finally, dogs with TIVC constriction were given exogenous ANP to achieve circulating concentrations comparable to that seen in the pacing-induced heart failure animals. Exogenous administration of ANP to such levels prevented sodium retention, renal vasoconstriction, and activation of the renin–angiotensin–aldosterone system. These observations support the notion that decreased cardiac output is a stimulus for renal sodium retention in heart failure and suggest an important role for the natriuretic peptides in acutely attenuating this renal response. A further discussion of the role of ANP and BNP in heart failure is presented elsewhere in this chapter.

Other experimental evidence supports a role for diminished cardiac output as a determinant of sodium and water retention in heart failure. Rats with small-to-moderate myocardial infarctions and decreased cardiac outputs exhibit decreased fractional sodium excretion despite normal right and left ventricular end-diastolic pressures.[30] Using the model of TIVC constriction, Priebe et al.[31] demonstrated that the renal retention of sodium and water was reduced markedly when cardiac output was restored to normal by autologous blood transfusions. Moreover, a reduction of pressure or stretch at the carotid sinus, like that produced by decreased cardiac output or arterial hypotension, activates the sympathetic nervous system and promotes renal sodium and water retention.[32,33] Pharmacologic or surgical interruption of sympathetic afferent neural pathways emanating from high-pressure baroreceptor sites also inhibits the natriuretic response to volume expansion.[25,26,34–38] High-pressure baroreceptors also appear to be important factors in regulating the nonosmotic release of AVP, thereby affecting renal water excretion.[39,40] Finally, the juxtaglomerular apparatus, an arterial baroreceptor located in the afferent arterioles within the kidney, has been implicated in the modulation of renal renin release[32,41,42] and thus may stimulate increases in circulating AT-II and aldosterone, both of which promote sodium retention by the kidney.

Low cardiac output cannot be the only cause of sodium and water retention in heart failure, because diminished renal sodium and water excretion is also observed in states of high-output cardiac failure. In heart failure secondary to beriberi, anemia, thyrotoxicosis, or AV fistulae, cardiac output is increased as a consequence of a decrease in peripheral vascular resistance. This decrease in vascular resistance diminishes EABV (i.e., causes arterial underfilling) and serves as the stimulus for neurohormonal activation and renal sodium and water retention in these instances of high-output heart failure.[14–21] As noted already in humans[22] and dogs,[43] closure of an AV fistula causes increased sodium excretion, whereas opening an AV fistula decreases urinary sodium excretion. These changes in renal sodium excretion correlate with changes in arterial pressure and peripheral vascular resistance rather than GFR or renal blood flow, supporting the importance of arterial circulatory "fullness" as a determinant of the renal response to heart failure.

These observations of decreased sodium and water excretion in both low- and high-output cardiac failure support the theory that arterial underfilling initiates reflex stimuli for the kidneys to retain sodium and water. In this regard, high-pressure baroreceptors in the carotid sinus, aortic arch, left ventricle, or the juxtaglomerular apparatus may comprise an important part of this reflex loop. Although these data support a role for arterial underfilling as the primary stimulus of the renal sodium and water retention of heart failure, low-pressure baroreceptors also may play an important role.

Low-Pressure Baroreceptors

In addition to the high-pressure arterial baroreceptors, the venous side of circulation seems to be a logical place for receptors sensitive to changes in blood volume to be found. In fact, 85% of blood volume may be found in the venous circulation, whereas just 15% of circulatory volume resides in the arterial circulation.[44] Although the smaller arterial blood volume may result in a higher sensitivity to detect blood volume changes, the larger amount of venous blood volume also may constitute an important component of the body fluid–volume regulatory system.

The atria of the heart are highly distensible and densely populated with nerve endings that are sensitive to small changes in passive distention.[45] Similar afferent low-pressure volume receptors may also be found in the pulmonary vasculature.[46] Increased filling of the thoracic vascular and cardiac atria would be expected to signal the kidney to increase urinary sodium excretion in order to return the blood volume to normal. As expected, maneuvers that increase this thoracic or "central" blood volume, such as weightlessness, negative-pressure breathing, head-out water immersion, recumbency, and exposure to cold, all produce a natriuresis.[47–52] Similarly, measures that decrease intrathoracic blood volume, including positive-pressure breathing, upright posture, and the application of tourniquets to the lower extremities, result in renal sodium retention.[49,53,54] Therefore, effective "central" blood volume, in addition to EABV, may serve as the afferent stimulus for the regulation of renal sodium and water excretion.

Considerable evidence implicates the left atrium as an important site of low-pressure receptors.[55–57] It is believed that changes in pressure or distention within the left atrium modulate electrical activity of the atrial receptors, which in turn may regulate renal sympathetic nerve activity. Left atrial nerves, therefore, can alter blood volume through changes in sodium excretion[57–59] as well as solute-free water excretion by influencing AVP release.[60–62] Acutely increasing left atrial volume by inflation of a balloon within the left atrium results in increased urinary volume excretion,[56] whereas hypotensive hemorrhage[63,64] and atrial tamponade[65] cause decreased atrial volume and diminish urine volume. However, in the setting of chronic heart failure, renal sodium and water retention occur despite left atrial distention and, frequently, loading of the other central baroreceptors (pulmonary veins, right atrium). Therefore, in chronic heart failure, diminished cardiac output with arterial underfilling may exert the predominant effect via the unloading of high-pressure arterial baroreceptors. Chronic studies in animals employing either experimental tricuspid insufficiency[66] or right atrial distention with an inflatable balloon[67] support this hypothesis. In these animal models, the increase in right atrial pressure was associated with avid renal sodium retention rather than the expected natriuresis. However, a concomitant fall in cardiac output could explain the sodium retention. Alternatively, alterations in cardiopulmonary baroreceptor function may occur in chronic but not acute heart failure.

Zucker et al.[68] demonstrated that the inhibition of renal sympathetic nerve activity seen during acute left atrial distention is lost during chronic heart failure in the dog. Moreover, a decrease in cardiac preload fails to produce the expected parasympathetic withdrawal and sympathetic activation in humans with heart failure.[69–71] Nishian et al.[71] described paradoxical forearm vasodilation and hemodynamic improvement during acute unloading of cardiopulmonary baroreceptors in patients with severe chronic heart failure. This paradoxical response to lower body negative pressure was associated with static plasma norepinephrine levels,[71] rather than the expected increase in plasma norepinephrine concentrations, further demonstrating this altered response to low-pressure baroreceptor unloading in heart failure. These observations confirm those made in heart failure patients during other forms of orthostatic stress.[69,70] These findings are also consistent with the observation of a strong positive correlation between left atrial pressure and coronary sinus norepinephrine, a marker of cardiac adrenergic activity, in patients with chronic heart failure.[72] Finally, Fonarow et al.[73] have shown that a reduction in left ventricular filling pressure rather than an increase in cardiac output during tailored hemodynamic management of heart failure improves survival over a 2-year period of follow-up. Taken together, these findings suggest that the normal inhibitory control of sympathetic activation accompanying increased atrial pressures is lost in heart failure patients and somehow may be converted to a stimulatory signal.

Cardiac and Pulmonary Chemoreceptors

In the heart and lungs, both vagal and sympathetic afferent nerve endings respond to a variety of exogenous and endogenous chemical substances, including capsaicin, phenyldiguanidine, bradykinin, substance P, and PGs. Baker et al.[74] demonstrated stimulation of sympathetic afferent nerve endings by bradykinin in the heart of the cat. In conscious dogs, the administration of PGE_2 and arachidonate inhibited the cardiac baroreflex.[75] Moreover, Zucker et al.[76] showed that PGI_2 attenuates the baroreflex control of renal nerve activity via an afferent vagal mechanism. Because substances such as bradykinin and PGs may circulate at increased concentrations in subjects with heart failure,[77] it is possible that altered central nervous system input from chemically sensitive cardiac or pulmonary afferents contributes to the neurohormonal activation and sodium retention of chronic heart failure. This possibility may have important implications for the treatment of heart failure, because commonly prescribed medications such as angiotensin-converting enzyme (ACE) inhibitors may alter circulating bradykinin and PG levels. At the present time, however, the exact roles of these hormones and cardiac and pulmonary chemoreceptors in heart failure are incompletely understood.

Hepatic Receptors

Theoretically, the liver should be in an ideal position to monitor dietary sodium intake and thus adjust urinary sodium excretion. Indeed, when compared with peripheral venous administration, infusion of saline solution into the portal circulation was reported to result in greater natriuresis.[78,79] Similarly, the increment in urinary sodium excretion has been claimed to be greater when the sodium load is given orally than when given intravenously.[80–82] In addition, the pathophysiologic retention of sodium in patients with severe liver disease is also consistent with an important role for the liver in the control of sodium excretion. However, some investigators[83,84] were unable to demonstrate a difference in sodium excretion between animals infused with 5% sodium chloride systemically and animals receiving the same solution via the portal vein. Moreover, Obika et al.[85] found similar sodium excretions after sodium loads given intravenously or by gastric lavage. Therefore, the experimental evidence in favor of sodium or volume hepatic receptors remains controversial.

In summary, the afferent mechanisms for sodium and water retention in chronic heart failure may be preferentially localized on the arterial or high-pressure side of the circulation where EABV may serve as the primary determinant of the renal response. However, reflexes from the low-pressure cardiopulmonary receptor system also may be altered so as to influence renal sodium and water handling in heart failure. In this regard, increases in atrial and ventricular end-diastolic pressures also stimulate the release of the natriuretic peptides and inhibit AVP release, which may be important attenuating factors in renal sodium and water retention. Finally, these afferent mechanisms for initiating sodium and water retention in chronic heart failure should not be confused with additional mechanisms that may be implicated in the setting of acute decompensated heart failure, where increased central venous pressure and renal venous congestion may also contribute to worsening renal function and sodium and water retention, as discussed later in this chapter.

Efferent Mechanisms for Renal Sodium and Water Retention in Heart Failure

The Neurohormonal Response to Cardiac Failure

As mentioned, the activation of various neurohormonal vasoconstrictor and antinatriuretic systems mediates to a large extent the renal sodium and water retention associated with the edematous disorders. Arterial underfilling secondary to a diminished cardiac output or peripheral vasodilation, perhaps in association with an alteration in low-pressure baroreceptor function, elicits these "compensatory" neuroendocrine responses in order to maintain the integrity of the arterial circulation by promoting peripheral vasoconstriction and expansion of the ECF volume through renal sodium and water retention (Fig. 67.2). The three major neurohormonal vasoconstrictor systems activated in response to arterial underfilling are the sympathetic nervous system, the renin–angiotensin–aldosterone system, and the nonosmotic release of AVP. Although other vasoconstrictor hormones may also be activated in heart failure (e.g., endothelin), their role in heart failure pathophysiology remains unclear.

The baroreceptor activation of the sympathetic nervous system appears to be the primary integrator of the hormonal vasoconstrictor systems involved in renal sodium and water retention. The nonosmotic release of AVP involves sympathetic stimulation of the supraoptic and paraventricular nuclei in the hypothalamus,[86] whereas activation of the renin–angiotensin–aldosterone system involves renal β-adrenergic stimulation.[87] However, this latter system may provide positive feedback stimulation of the sympathetic nervous system and

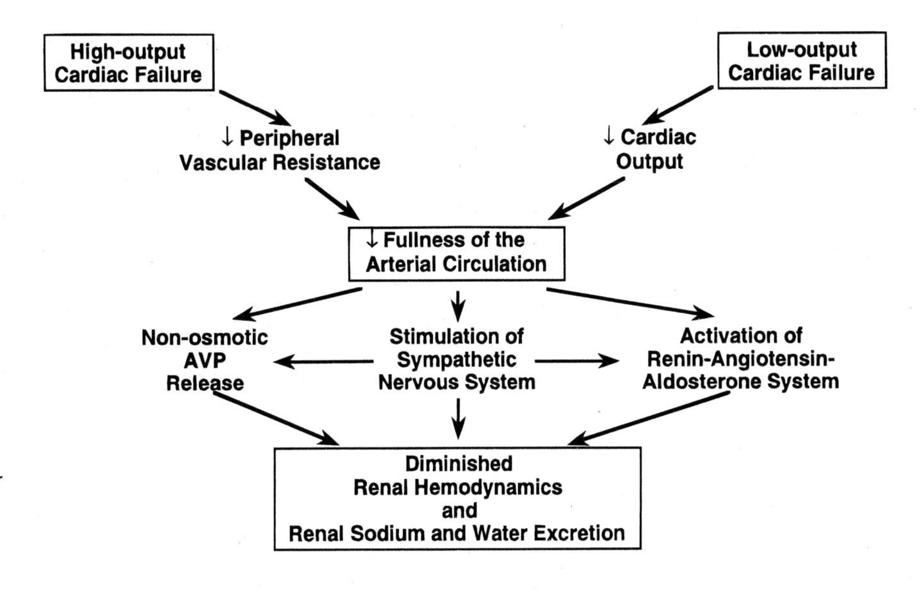

FIGURE 67.2 The mechanism explaining the defect in renal sodium and water excretion in both high- and low-output heart failure. *AVP*, arginine vasopressin.

nonosmotic AVP release. Various counterregulatory, vasodilatory, and natriuretic hormones, including the natriuretic peptides and PGs, are also activated in heart failure and the other edematous disorders, and may attenuate the renal effects of vasoconstrictor hormone activation. The effects of these neurohormonal systems, as well as the effects of alterations in systemic hemodynamics, on renal hemodynamics, and tubular sodium and water reabsorption in heart failure, are discussed in the following section.

Glomerular Filtration Rate

The GFR is usually normal in mild heart failure and is reduced only as cardiac performance becomes more severely impaired. Until 1961, it was generally accepted that the rate of glomerular filtration was a major determinant of renal sodium excretion. In 1961, de Wardener et al.[88] published their classic paper indicating that acute expansion of ECF volume by saline loading was accompanied by a brisk natriuresis even when GFR was reduced. Moreover, in sodium-retaining heart failure patients, GFR is often normal and may even be elevated in states of high-output cardiac failure. These observations argue against an important role for diminished GFR in the sodium retention of heart failure per se (i.e., in the initiation of sodium retention), although a diminished GFR may be a contributing factor in patients with advanced heart failure or comorbid disorders that directly impair this aspect of renal function. It also should be emphasized that the contribution of GFR to sodium balance is difficult to evaluate because very minute changes in GFR are difficult to measure and may account for important changes in sodium excretion. For example, under normal conditions, with a GFR of 100 mL per minute, the filtered load of sodium amounts to approximately 20,000 mEq per day. This amount of filtered sodium is enormous compared to the normal urinary sodium excretion of approximately 200 mEq per day. In view of this considerable difference, it is apparent that very small changes in GFR can result in major alterations in sodium excretion if tubular reabsorption remains unaltered. In any event, although GFR may be diminished in patients with advanced heart failure, a reduction in GFR alone is probably not an important cause of fluid retention in these patients because sodium retention can be observed in heart failure patients who have GFRs comparable to normal subjects who are capable of maintaining sodium balance.

Renal Blood Flow

Heart failure is commonly associated with an increase in renal vascular resistance and a decrease in renal blood flow.[89] In general, renal blood flow decreases in proportion to the decrease in cardiac output. Some investigators also showed a redistribution of renal blood flow from the outer cortical nephron to juxtaglomerular nephrons during experimental heart failure.[90,91] It was proposed that deeper nephrons with longer loops of Henle reabsorb sodium more avidly. Therefore, the redistribution of blood flow to these nephrons in patients with heart failure might account for or substantially contribute to the renal sodium retention observed. However, other investigators were not able to demonstrate such a redistribution of blood flow in other models of cardiac failure.[92,93] At the present time, the role of redistribution of renal blood flow in the sodium retention of cardiac failure therefore remains uncertain.

The increased renal vascular resistance in heart failure could be caused by enhanced renal sympathetic activity or increased circulating concentrations of AT-II, norepinephrine, vasopressin, or other vasoconstricting substances. Alternatively, or in addition, decreased synthesis of or the development of tachyphylaxis to known vasodilating substances such as the natriuretic peptides and PGE_2 and PGI_2 may contribute to the increased renal vascular resistance. Studies performed in rats demonstrated the ability of the adrenergic neurotransmitter norepinephrine and AT-II to promote glomerular arteriolar constriction.[94,95] In a rat model of low-output heart failure caused by myocardial infarction, the marked elevation in efferent arteriolar resistance was abolished after the infusion of an ACE inhibitor,[95] thereby implicating the renal vasoconstrictor properties of AT-II in heart failure. Clinical results from our laboratory also favor AT-II as a major renal vasoconstrictive substance in patients with heart failure.[96] In patients with advanced heart failure, GFR was improved after 1 month of treatment with the ACE inhibitor captopril. However, similar patients receiving another vasodilating agent, prazosin, with identical improvement in cardiac output and left ventricular end-diastolic pressure but without any effect on the renin–angiotensin system had no improvement in GFR.[96] Moreover, a published review of the literature on renal function alterations induced by ACE inhibition during heart failure concluded that the net effect of ACE inhibitors in patients with heart failure is to augment renal blood flow to a greater extent than cardiac output.[97] This observation also supports an important role for AT-II in the renal hemodynamic alterations of heart failure. However, the renal response to ACE inhibition in patients with heart failure is variable; as a result, it is acknowledged that volume status and the degree of neurohormonal activation may influence this response (see the following).

In heart failure, the interaction between norepinephrine or AT-II and PGs may also provide a means of preserving near constancy of renal blood flow in response to arterial underfilling. Although the inhibition of PG synthesis does not generally impair GFR in normovolemic animals[98,99] or humans,[100] in states of high plasma concentrations of endogenous AT-II induced by volume depletion, the blockade of PG synthesis may be associated with substantial declines in renal blood flow and GFR.[98,99] Recent clinical results have underscored the importance of PGs in the maintenance of renal function in patients with heart failure.[77,101] In patients with heart failure, PG activity is increased and correlates with the severity of disease as assessed by the degree of hyponatremia.[77] In these 15 patients, plasma levels of the metabolites of vasodilator PGI_2 and PGE_2 were found to be elevated 3 to 10 times above those seen in normal subjects. Of note, plasma levels of both metabolites also correlated positively with PRA and plasma AT-II concentrations. The administration of the PG synthesis inhibitor indomethacin in three of the hyponatremic heart failure patients resulted in a marked increase in peripheral vascular resistance and a fall in cardiac output. Riegger et al.[101] recently evaluated the renal effects of another PG synthesis inhibitor, acetylsalicylic acid, in patients with moderate heart failure consuming a normal sodium diet. In these patients, acetylsalicylic acid in doses that decreased the synthesis of renal PGE_2 resulted in a significant reduction in urinary sodium excretion. Moreover, the administration of a cyclooxygenase inhibitor in heart failure patients occasionally may result in acute reversible renal failure, an effect proposed to be due in part to the inhibition of vasodilating renal PGs and the resultant renal vasoconstriction.[102] It should be noted, however, that the extent to which the effects on renal function and sodium and water handling result from renal hemodynamic or the tubular actions of the PGs remains unclear.

As mentioned, norepinephrine may also contribute to the increased renal afferent arteriolar resistance in heart failure patients. In this regard, Oliver et al.[103] demonstrated that the venous to arterial norepinephrine concentration gradient across the kidney, a crude measure of renal nerve traffic, is increased in response to acute reduction of cardiac output. Moreover, Hasking et al.[104] showed that during a steady-state tritiated norepinephrine infusion, the spillover of norepinephrine to plasma from the kidney is significantly elevated in patients with heart failure. In these patients, the increased renal norepinephrine spillover substantially contributed to the increase in whole-body norepinephrine spillover. These findings demonstrate that renal adrenergic activity is increased in patients with heart failure, and thus contributes to the renal vasoconstriction. In support of this latter hypothesis, the administration of α-adrenergic receptor antagonists increased renal blood flow in edematous patients with heart failure.[105] Renal denervation studies in patients with refractory hypertension also underscore the role of renal sympathetic nerve activation in cardiovascular disease. In such patients, the catheter ablation of renal nerves reduces norepinephrine spillover from the kidneys and lowers blood pressure.[106–108] Ongoing renal denervation studies in patients with heart failure may shed further light on the role of renal sympathetic activation and the potential for catheter ablation of renal nerves in the treatment of heart failure.

Filtration Fraction, Proximal Tubular Sodium and Water Reabsorption, and Factors Acting Beyond the Proximal Tubule

Because renal blood flow falls as cardiac output decreases and GFR is usually preserved, the filtration fraction often is increased in early heart failure. An increase in the filtration fraction results in increased protein concentration and oncotic pressure in the efferent arterioles and the peritubular capillaries that surround the proximal tubule.[95] Such an increase in peritubular oncotic pressure has been proposed to increase sodium and water reabsorption in the proximal tubule.[109–113] Direct evidence for increased single-nephron filtration fraction was provided by micropuncture studies in rats with myocardial infarction induced by coronary ligation.[95] In rats with large myocardial infarctions involving approximately 40% of the left ventricular circumference, the single-nephron filtration fraction was markedly elevated (0.38 ± 0.02 versus 0.25 ± 0.02, $P < .005$) when compared with that in sham-operated control rats. The measurement of preglomerular, glomerular, and postglomerular pressures and flows revealed that these reductions in glomerular plasma flow rate and elevations in filtration fraction were associated with a profound constriction of the efferent arterioles. The effect of the latter was to sustain glomerular capillary hydraulic pressure, thereby preventing a marked fall in GFR. Significantly, fractional proximal fluid reabsorption was elevated in this model. Of interest, in these animals with myocardial infarction, the intravenous infusion of the ACE inhibitor teprotide led to the return of glomerular plasma flow rate, single-nephron filtration fraction, single-nephron GFR, efferent arteriolar resistance, and fractional proximal fluid reabsorption to or toward the levels found in the control rats.[95] Consistent with these experiments, micropuncture studies performed in other models of heart failure such as acute TIVC constriction[114] and acute cardiac tamponade[115] in dogs showed that the proximal tubule was at least one major nephron site responsible for renal sodium retention or a blunted response to saline infusion.

Despite the convincing nature of many studies, not all investigators have been able to detect an effect of peritubular oncotic pressure on proximal tubular sodium and water reabsorption. Rumrich and Ullrich,[116] Lowitz et al.,[117] Bank et al.,[118] and Holzgreve and Schrier[119] were unable to find changes in proximal reabsorption despite marked changes in peritubular oncotic pressures. Moreover, Conger et al.[120] directly perfused peritubular capillaries with either a protein-free or protein-rich solution and found that neither perfusate influences the rate of proximal reabsorption. Trying to reconcile these observations, Ott et al.[121] found that proximal reabsorption was different after changes in peritubular oncotic pressure in volume-expanded dogs compared with hydropenic animals. These authors suggested that the expansion of ECF volume resulted in an increased passive back leak that could be reversed by raising the peritubular oncotic pressure. During hydropenia, however, when passive back leak was relatively less, raising the peritubular capillary oncotic pressure did not influence proximal reabsorption.

The effects of increased filtration fraction might be expected to be exerted primarily on proximal tubular sodium reabsorption. Nevertheless, although clearance and micropuncture studies in animals with heart failure have demonstrated increased sodium reabsorption in the proximal tubule, distal sodium reabsorption also seems to be involved. In this regard, clearance and micropuncture studies performed in dogs with AV fistulae,[122] chronic pericarditis,[115] and chronic partial thoracic vena caval obstruction[123] documented enhanced distal nephron sodium reabsorption. Levy[123] also showed that the inability of dogs with chronic vena caval obstruction to excrete a sodium load is a consequence of enhanced reabsorption of sodium at the loop of Henle. This nephron segment was similarly implicated in rats with AV fistulae.[93] Physical factors also could be involved in the augmented reabsorption of sodium chloride by the loop of Henle in dogs with constriction of the vena cava.[123]

Intrarenal mechanisms, specifically decreased delivery of tubular fluid to the distal diluting segment of the nephron, may also contribute to the impaired water excretion observed in heart failure. Evidence supporting this intrarenal mechanism of water retention in heart failure has been provided by studies involving the administration of mannitol[124] or the loop diuretic furosemide[125] to patients with heart failure and hyponatremia. The administration of either of these agents converted the cardiac patient's hypertonic urine to a dilute urine.[124,125] Both mannitol and furosemide may diminish the tubular reabsorption of sodium and water in the more proximal portions of the nephron, thus increasing fluid delivery to the more distal nephron sites of urinary dilution. Other factors may, however, be implicated to explain these results: (1) the infusion of mannitol may produce volume expansion, thereby suppressing the baroreceptor-mediated release of AVP; and (2) the furosemide-induced hypotonic urine was found to not be responsive to the administration of exogenous AVP, thus suggesting antagonism of AVP by furosemide.[125] In support of this latter hypothesis, Szatalowicz et al.[126] provided further evidence that furosemide interferes with the renal action of AVP in humans.

In summary, the exact contribution of proximal versus distal nephron sites in the augmented sodium and water reabsorption seen in heart failure may depend on the severity of the heart failure and the concomitant degree of arterial underfilling. The fact that changes in the filtration fraction have been observed in patients with heart failure before changes in sodium balance occur may question the dominance of peritubular factors and proximal reabsorption in the sodium retention characteristic of heart failure.[127] This observation suggests that other factors, such as the direct tubular effects of neurohormonal activation, may play a significant role in the renal sodium and water retention of heart failure. The renal effects of these various neurohormonal systems are discussed in detail in the following section, starting with activation of the vasoconstrictor mechanisms.

Vasoconstrictor Systems

Activation of the sympathetic nervous system in heart failure. The sympathetic nervous system is activated early in patients with heart failure. Numerous studies have documented elevated peripheral venous plasma norepinephrine concentrations in heart failure patients.[104,128–131] In advanced heart failure, using tritiated norepinephrine to determine norepinephrine kinetics, Hasking et al.[104] and Davis et al.[130] demonstrated that both increased norepinephrine spillover and decreased norepinephrine clearance contribute to the elevated venous plasma norepinephrine levels seen in these patients, suggesting that increased sympathetic nerve activity is at least partially responsible for the high circulating norepinephrine levels. Our laboratory[131] has demonstrated that in earlier stages of heart failure, the rise in plasma norepinephrine in patients with heart failure was due solely to increased norepinephrine secretion (Fig. 67.3), supporting the notion that sympathetic nervous system activity is increased early in the course of heart failure. Significantly, in our heart failure patients with mild-to-moderate symptoms, plasma epinephrine, a marker of adrenal activation, was not substantially elevated, confirming the neuronal source of the increased norepinephrine.

The Studies of Left Ventricular Dysfunction (SOLVD) investigators[132] reported the presence of adrenergic activation in patients with asymptomatic left ventricular dysfunction. In this substudy of the SOLVD trials, neurohormonal activation was assessed in 56 control subjects, 151 patients with left ventricular dysfunction (ejection fractions ≤ 35%) but no overt heart failure, and 81 patients with overt heart failure, prior to randomization to receive placebo versus an ACE inhibitor. The plasma norepinephrine concentration

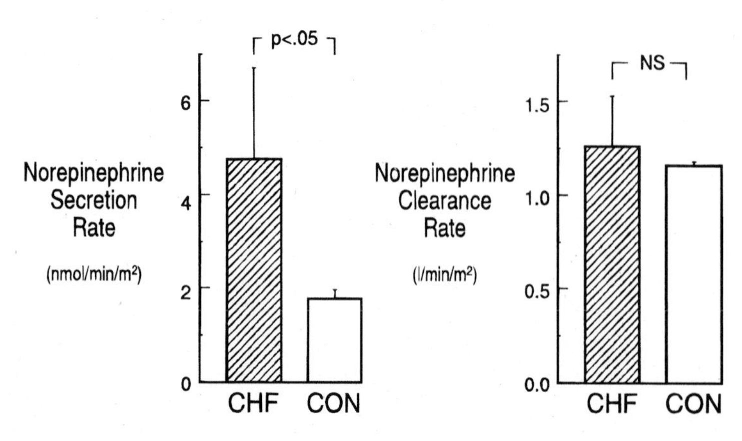

FIGURE 67.3 Plasma norepinephrine secretion and clearance rates in patients with mild-to-moderate heart failure (CHF) and in normal control subjects (CON). The findings of increased norepinephrine secretion and normal norepinephrine clearance in the CHF patients are consistent with early activation of the sympathetic nervous system in cardiac failure. *NS*, not significant. (From Abraham WT, Hensen J, Schrier RW. Elevated plasma noradrenaline concentrations in patients with low-output cardiac failure: dependence on increased noradrenaline secretion rates. *Clin Sci.* 1990;79:429, with permission.)

was significantly increased by 35% in subjects with asymptomatic left ventricular dysfunction compared to healthy control subjects, and by 65% greater than control values in the overt heart failure patients. These data also demonstrate that adrenergic activation occurs early in the course of heart failure or left ventricular dysfunction and are consistent with the observation that plasma norepinephrine concentrations or the degree of adrenergic activation are directly correlated with the degree of left ventricular dysfunction in patients with heart failure.[128,129,133,134] Finally, studies employing peroneal nerve microneurography to directly assess sympathetic nerve activity to muscle (MSNA) confirmed increased adrenergic nerve traffic in patients with heart failure.[135]

As mentioned, studies in human heart failure demonstrated the presence of renal adrenergic activation.[104] In this study of whole-body and organ-specific norepinephrine kinetics in heart failure patients, cardiac and renal norepinephrine spillovers were increased 504% and 206%, respectively, whereas norepinephrine spillover from the lungs was normal. These findings demonstrate the presence of selective cardiorenal adrenergic activation in heart failure. A discussion of the cardiac effects of this adrenergic activation is beyond the scope of this chapter. However, low heart rate variability (indicative of high cardiac sympathetic and low cardiac parasympathetic activity) assessed continuously by implantable pacemaker and/or defibrillator devices is a predictor of hospitalization for worsening heart failure.[136] Of note, in this report most hospitalizations for worsening heart failure were associated with fluid–volume overload. Therefore, measuring heart rate variability may provide insight into the systemic as well as the cardiac effects of heightened adrenergic activity. Moreover, numerous adverse effects of increased cardiac adrenergic activity have been documented in humans,[137] and positive experience with the use of β-adrenergic receptor antagonists in heart failure patients[137–143] supports the hypothesis that norepinephrine is harmful to the myocardium. In this regard, blocking the deleterious effects of norepinephrine on the heart results in the reverse of ventricular remodeling; that is, the dilated failing heart becomes smaller and stronger following chronic β-adrenergic blockade. Finally, it should be noted that a single resting venous plasma norepinephrine level provides a better guide to prognosis than do many other commonly measured indices of cardiac performance in which high plasma norepinephrine levels are associated with a poor prognosis in patients with heart failure.[144]

Renal tubular effects of adrenergic activation in heart failure. Renal nerves exert a direct influence on sodium reabsorption in the proximal tubule. Bello-Reuss et al.[58] demonstrated this direct effect of renal nerve activation to enhance proximal tubular sodium reabsorption in whole-kidney and nephron studies in the rat. In these animals, renal nerve stimulation produced an increase in the tubular fluid-to-plasma inulin concentration ratio in the late proximal tubule, a result of increased fractional sodium and water reabsorption in this segment of the nephron. On the basis of results of an elegant series of studies, DiBona et al.[145] implicated the activation of the renal nerves in the sodium and water retention observed in the various edematous disorders. Experiments were conducted in conscious, chronically instrumented rats with either heart failure (myocardial infarction), cirrhosis (common bile duct ligation), or the nephrotic syndrome (doxorubicin injection). In each experimental model, renal sodium or water excretion of an acutely administered oral or intravenous isotonic saline load was significantly less than that in control rats. Bilateral renal denervation in the experimental rats restored their renal excretory response to normal. Moreover, in response to the acute administration of a standard intravenous isotonic saline load, the decrease in efferent renal adrenergic nerve activity was significantly less in all three experimental models than in control animals. These results support an increased basal efferent renal sympathetic nerve activity in heart failure and the other edematous disorders that fail to suppress normally in response to the isotonic saline load. These findings also are consistent with the aforementioned alterations in low-pressure baroreceptor function observed in human heart failure, where adrenergic activation is seen despite chronic increased loading of these cardiopulmonary receptors.

In dogs[146] and in humans[105] with heart failure, α-adrenergic receptor blockade induces a natriuresis. Moreover, adrenergic blockade with either phenoxybenzamine or hexamethonium abolishes the sodium retention seen in acute TIVC constriction.[25] Furthermore, the comprehensive adrenergic blocking agent carvedilol, but not metoprolol, increases renal blood flow and GFR in patients with chronic heart failure.[147] Conversely, sodium retention persists in dogs with denervated transplanted kidneys and chronic vena caval constriction.[148] In addition, in dogs with pacing-induced heart failure, no differences in renal hemodynamic or electrolyte excretion between innervated or denervated kidneys in compensated or decompensated animals were observed.[149] These latter observations implicate factors in addition to renal nerves in the sodium retention of heart failure. However, in these renal denervation experiments and in human heart failure, other hormonal factors (e.g., AT-II, aldosterone, AVP) may play an important role in the sodium and water retention.

Experience with the partial β_1-adrenergic receptor agonist xamoterol in heart failure suggests a role for the renal β-receptor in modulating proximal tubular sodium reabsorption.[150] Bøtker et al.[150] examined the acute renal effects of xamoterol in 12 patients with mild-to-moderate heart failure. Each patient was given xamoterol (0.2 mg per kilogram) or placebo in random order separated by 2 weeks of a clinically stable drug washout period. Renal clearance and excretion measurements were made with the patient in the supine position at 30- to 60-minute intervals before, during, and up to 6 hours after infusion. Lithium clearance was used as a measure of proximal tubular sodium handling.[151] Blood pressure, heart rate, renal plasma flow, GFR, and urinary flow rate remained unchanged, whereas xamoterol significantly decreased renal sodium excretion by 30%. This acute decrease in sodium excretion with xamoterol was associated with an increase in proximal tubular sodium reabsorption, as indicated by decreased lithium clearance. Of note, plasma concentrations of AT-II and aldosterone were unaffected by xamoterol. These observations suggest a direct effect of acute xamoterol to enhance proximal tubular sodium reabsorption in heart failure. In patients with heart failure, the endogenous adrenergic receptor agonist and neurotransmitter norepinephrine may exert a similar effect on the proximal renal tubule.

Finally, as noted, renal nerves have been implicated as a stimulus for renin release from the kidney.[87] Therefore, with heart failure, adrenergic activation may lead to the activation of the renin–angiotensin–aldosterone system. Conversely, β-adrenergic receptor blockade may decrease renin release and improve the neurohormonal milieu in heart failure patients. In this regard, Eichhorn et al.[152] showed that the third-generation β-adrenergic receptor blocker bucindolol lowers PRA in patients with mild-to-moderate heart failure. The renal tubular effects of AT-II and aldosterone are discussed in the following paragraphs.

Activation of the renin–angiotensin–aldosterone system in heart failure. The renin–angiotensin–aldosterone system is usually activated in patients with heart failure, as assessed by PRA and plasma aldosterone.[133,153,154] In the substudy report from the SOLVD investigators,[132] PRA was increased not only in patients with established heart failure but also in subjects with asymptomatic left ventricular dysfunction. Of note, activation of the renin–angiotensin–aldosterone system is associated with hyponatremia and an unfavorable prognosis in patients with heart failure.[77,155] Dzau et al.[77] first described the association of PRA and hyponatremia in a group of 15 heart failure patients. These data showed that normal or suppressed PRA is associated with a normal serum sodium level, whereas the highest PRA is associated with the lowest serum sodium concentrations. Lee and Packer[155] subsequently confirmed this association between PRA and hyponatremia in a larger cohort of heart failure patients. Moreover, these investigators demonstrated the association of this hyponatremic, hyperreninemic state with poor survival. Finally, the proven beneficial effects of ACE inhibition or AT-II receptor blockade (ARB) on symptoms, hemodynamics, exercise capacity, and survival in heart failure patients further underscore the deleterious effects of AT-II and aldosterone in these patients.[156–161]

Recently, a positive feedback between the renin–angiotensin–aldosterone system and sympathetic activation was proposed.[162] This interaction is based in part on the ability of AT-II to augment neuronal norepinephrine release at the presynaptic level.[163] In humans, the presynaptic facilitation of norepinephrine release by AT-II may play a role in the cardiorenal adrenergic activation of heart failure. Clemson et al.[164] demonstrated AT-II–mediated increases in norepinephrine spillover in the human forearm. In heart failure patients, we demonstrated increased neuronal norepinephrine release from the heart during AT-II infusion, whereas cardiac adrenergic activity was decreased by the bolus injection of the ACE inhibitor enalaprilat.[165] In addition, Gilbert et al.[166] showed that chronic ACE inhibition with lisinopril lowers cardiac adrenergic activity in patients with chronic symptomatic heart failure. Thus, the activation of renal nerves is a stimulus for renal renin release, thereby activating the renin–angiotensin–aldosterone system, whereas activation of the renin–angiotensin–aldosterone system may further stimulate adrenergic activity at the presynaptic level.

Renal tubular effects of angiotensin II and aldosterone in heart failure. In animal models, AT-II has a direct effect on enhancing proximal tubular sodium reabsorption.[167] In these studies of the rat proximal tubule, the administration of AT-II resulted in a marked increase in the rate of sodium chloride reabsorption, whereas the infusion of the AT-II receptor antagonist saralasin significantly reduced proximal tubular sodium chloride reabsorption. Moreover, in a study from Abassi et al.,[168] the administration of the AT-II receptor antagonist losartan to decompensated sodium-retaining rats with heart failure secondary to AV fistulae produced a marked natriuresis. Although proximal tubular sodium handling was not examined in this study, the observation that losartan restored renal responsiveness to ANP is consistent with a losartan-induced increase in the delivery of sodium to the distal tubular site of ANP action. The role of distal tubular sodium delivery in the renal sodium retention of heart failure is discussed in the following paragraphs.

In humans with heart failure, the finding that urinary sodium excretion correlates inversely with PRA and urinary aldosterone excretion also supports a role for AT-II or aldosterone, or both, in renal sodium retention.[169] However, the administration of ACE inhibitors to patients with heart failure results in inconsistent effects on renal sodium excretion, despite a consistent fall in plasma aldosterone concentration.[170] A simultaneous fall in blood pressure or a decline in renal hemodynamics owing to decreased circulating AT-II concentrations, however, could obscure the beneficial renal effects of lowered AT-II and aldosterone concentrations. Support for this hypothesis may be found in a report from Motwani et al.[171] These investigators examined the hemodynamic and hormonal correlates of the initial effect of ACE inhibition with captopril on blood pressure, GFR, and natriuresis in 36 patients with moderate heart failure. In these subjects, a captopril-induced fall in GFR was predicted by a decrease in renal plasma flow, low pretreatment GFR, *and* a low absolute posttreatment serum AT-II concentration. A decrease in urinary sodium excretion was related to this fall in GFR. Conversely, Good et al.[172] showed in eight patients with chronic heart failure that long-term AT-II suppression with captopril enhances renal responsiveness to the loop diuretic furosemide. This observation also supports a role for AT-II in the renal sodium retention of heart failure.

The role of aldosterone in the renal sodium retention of heart failure has been debated for many years. In the presence of a high sodium intake, dogs with caval constriction retain sodium even after surgical removal of the adrenal source of aldosterone.[173] Moreover, patients with heart failure do not always show increased urinary sodium excretion after the administration of the aldosterone antagonist spironolactone.[174] In addition, Chonko et al.[175] showed that patients with heart failure may have edema without increased aldosterone secretion. However, a normal plasma aldosterone level in heart failure patients may be relatively high in the presence of excess total body sodium. A role for aldosterone in the renal sodium retention of human heart failure was demonstrated by our group.[176] We examined the effect of spironolactone on urinary sodium excretion in patients with mild-to-moderate heart failure who were withdrawn from all medications prior to the study. Sodium was retained in all subjects throughout the period prior to aldosterone antagonism (Fig. 67.4). With an average sodium intake of 97 ± 8 mmol per day, the average sodium excretion before spironolactone treatment was 76 ± 8 mmol per day. During therapy with spironolactone, all heart failure patients demonstrated a significant increase in urinary sodium excretion to 131 ± 13 mmol per day. Moreover, the urine sodium-to-potassium concentration ratio significantly increased during spironolactone administration, which is consistent with a decrease in aldosterone action in the distal nephron. Of note, norepinephrine concentration and PRA increased and ANP decreased during spironolactone administration, suggesting a possible explanation for the attenuation of the natriuretic effect of spironolactone in long-term studies. Therefore, the combined use of an aldosterone antagonist with other neurohormonal antagonists (e.g., ACE inhibitors, ARBs, and β-blockers) may result in an optimal long-term benefit. Several observations support this notion, including randomized controlled trials in patients with chronic heart failure or postmyocardial infarction (MI) left ventricular dysfunction.[177–180] For example, the Randomized Aldactone Evaluation Study (RALES) demonstrated that the addition of spironolactone (25 mg per day) to ACE inhibition decreased both hospitalizations and mortality by more than 30% as compared to controls in patients with advanced heart failure.[179] Another trial[180] of the selective aldosterone antagonist, eplerenone, demonstrated a 15% reduction in all-cause mortality in patients with post-MI heart failure. Although blocking aldosterone-mediated cardiac fibrosis was proposed to explain these survival benefits of aldosterone antagonism, a contribution to improved survival attributable to the renal effects of these agents cannot be excluded.

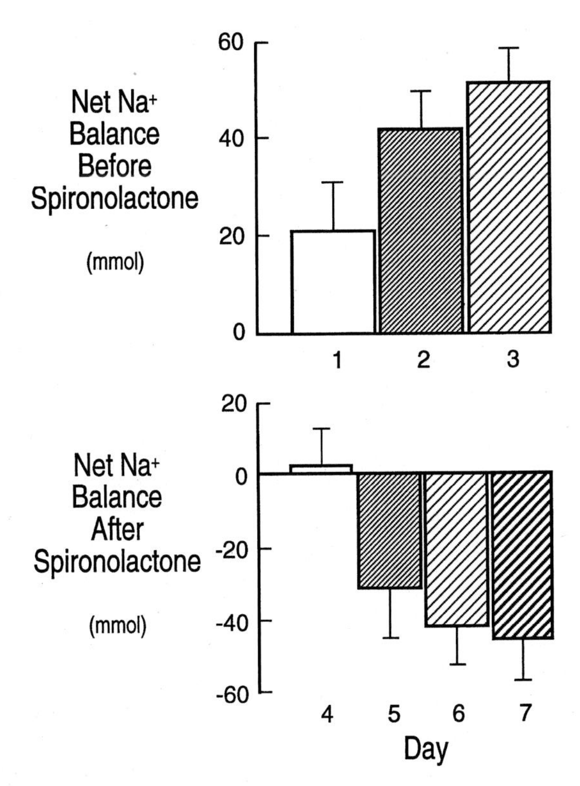

FIGURE 67.4 Reversal of sodium retention with aldosterone antagonism in patients with heart failure. The net positive cumulative sodium balance, by day, for the period before spironolactone therapy (*upper panel*) and the net negative cumulative sodium balance after the initiation of spironolactone, 400 mg per day (*lower panel*) are shown. (From Hensen J, et al. Aldosterone in congestive heart failure: analysis of determinants and role in sodium retention. *Am J Nephrol.* 1991;11:441, with permission of S. Karger AG, Basel.)

The nonosmotic release of vasopressin in heart failure. Plasma AVP is usually elevated in patients with advanced heart failure and correlates with the clinical and hemodynamic severity of disease and the serum sodium concentration.[181–186] Several clinical and experimental observations indicate that nonosmotic mechanisms are responsible for increased AVP release in heart failure. A study from our laboratory[186] found plasma AVP concentrations to be inappropriately elevated in 30 of 37 hyponatremic patients with heart failure. The 30 patients with detectable plasma AVP levels had higher levels of BUN and serum creatinine and higher ratios of BUN to serum creatinine than did the 7 patients with undetectable plasma AVP levels. This latter finding could be dissociated from diuretic use because it was also observed in 14 patients who had never received diuretics. The presence of prerenal azotemia in these patients is consistent with diminished cardiac output as a mediator of the nonosmotic AVP release. Alternatively, this observation of prerenal azotemia in association with hyponatremia also supports an intrarenal component of the impaired water excretion.

Osmotically inappropriate elevations of plasma AVP in human heart failure were also later reported by Riegger et al.,[184] Rondeau et al.,[185] and Goldsmith et al.[181] The study by Riegger et al.[184] demonstrated a decrease in the elevated plasma AVP levels after improvement in cardiac function by hemofiltration, whereas no change in plasma AVP was observed after decreasing left atrial pressure with prazosin.

Moreover, the elevated plasma AVP levels seen in patients with heart failure often,[183,187] but not always,[11] failed to suppress normally in response to acute water loading. Taken together, these observations demonstrate that there is an enhanced nonosmotic release of AVP in heart failure and support the hypothesis that diminished cardiac output, rather than alterations in atrial pressures, is responsible. As previously mentioned, the baroreceptor activation of the sympathetic nervous system in response to arterial underfilling likely mediates this nonosmotic AVP release.[86]

To shed further light on the mechanism of nonosmotic stimulation of AVP in heart failure patients and, more specifically, to determine the precise relationship between AVP release, cardiac hemodynamics, and the renin–angiotensin system, we studied 25 consecutive patients with severe heart failure (cardiac index 2.1 ± 0.1 L/minute/m^2 and pulmonary capillary wedge pressure 27.5 ± 1.5 mm Hg).[96] These patients received two water loads of 15 mL per kilogram of body weight, the first load without drugs on day 1 and the second on day 3 after receiving vasodilator therapy with either captopril or prazosin for 2 days. Baseline and hourly hemodynamic, renal, and hormonal measurements were obtained for 5 hours following the water load. Basal plasma AVP was detectable (mean 3.0 ± 0.4 pg per milliliter) in 17 of the 25 patients (group 1) despite a diminished plasma sodium concentration (P_{Na}, 133.5 mmol per liter) and low effective plasma osmolality (E_{osm}, 262 ± 3 mOsm per kilogram of H_2O). The remaining eight patients (group 2) had appropriately suppressed plasma AVP (< 0.5 pg per milliliter, undetectable) for their P_{Na} (136.5 ± 0.9 mmol per liter) and E_{osm} (268 ± 2 mOsm per kilogram of H_2O). Cardiac index (1.9 versus 2.6 L/minute/m^2, $P < .005$) and the percentage of water load excreted (31.4% versus 57.1%, $P < .005$) were lower in group 1 than in group 2 patients, but GFR was similar (55 versus 54 mL/min/1.73 m^2). The PRA and plasma aldosterone concentrations were higher in group 1 patients, suggesting arterial underfilling. In group 1 patients, vasodilators increased the cardiac index from 1.9 to 2.1 L/min/m^2 and the percentage of water load excreted from 31% to 53% (both $P < .001$). In these same patients, plasma AVP decreased from 3.0 to 1.8 pg per milliliter ($P < .01$), platelet-associated AVP decreased from 8.6 to 5.1 pg per milliliter ($P < .005$), and minimal urinary osmolality decreased from 375 to 208 mOsm per kilogram of H_2O ($P < .001$). There was no change in GFR. In group 1 patients in the control condition as well as after vasodilator therapy, plasma AVP decreased with plasma osmolality during the water load, suggesting some preservation of the osmoregulation of AVP, but with a lower osmotic threshold in these patients. Moreover, changes in the renin–angiotensin–aldosterone system were unrelated to changes in water excretion after vasodilator therapy. We consequently concluded that plasma and platelet AVP levels were the major determinants of the abnormal water excretion in many patients with heart failure. These results, therefore, favor a role of impaired cardiac function to cause arterial underfilling with resultant nonosmotic AVP release as a mediator of "resetting" the osmotic threshold for AVP in patients with heart failure. Improved cardiac function secondary to afterload reduction diminishes this resetting of the osmotic threshold. Of interest, our results are reminiscent of earlier studies that suggested that an occasional hyponatremic cardiac patient responds to a large water load by the prompt onset of a water diuresis.[11] Also, more recently, AVP secretion was found to respond in exaggerated fashion to osmotic loading in patients with heart failure undergoing radiologic procedures with radiocontrast hyperosmolar agents.[188] This latter finding also suggests a form of reset osmostat.

The renal effects of vasopressin in heart failure. Vasopressin, via the stimulation of its renal V_2 receptor,[189] induces the insertion of the aquaporin-2 (AQP2) water channel into the collecting duct apical membrane with resultant water reabsorption. Elevations in plasma vasopressin concentration and AQP2 are believed to contribute to water retention in heart failure. In animal models of heart failure, the absence of a pituitary source of AVP is associated with normal or near normal water excretion.[190,191] For example, in intact dogs with diminished cardiac outputs owing to TIVC constriction, the removal of the pituitary with glucocorticoid replacement results in the normalization of the impaired water excretion.[190] In these animals, acute constriction of the TIVC caused a significant fall in cardiac output associated with a marked increase in urinary osmolality and a decrease in solute-free water clearance. The effects of TIVC constriction were dissociated from renal hemodynamic changes and the presence or absence of renal sympathetic innervation. However, in hypophysectomized, steroid-replaced animals, both urinary osmolality and solute-free water clearance were maintained at basal levels during constriction of the TIVC. Impaired water excretion also occurs in rats with heart failure because of AV fistulae.[191] Significantly, the impairment in water excretion seen in this high-output model of heart failure was not demonstrable in Brattleboro rats with central diabetes insipidus (i.e., AVP deficiency), supporting a role for persistent AVP release in the abnormality in water excretion associated with high-output cardiac failure. Similar results were obtained by Riegger et al.[192]

Further evidence implicating a role for AVP in the water retention of heart failure comes from studies using selective peptide and nonpeptide V_2 receptor AVP antagonists in several animal models of heart failure.[193–196] Ishikawa et al.[193] assessed the antidiuretic effect of AVP in a low-output model of acute heart failure secondary to TIVC constriction in the rat. In these animals, plasma AVP concentrations were increased and a peptide antagonist of the V_2 receptor of AVP reversed the defect in solute-free water excretion. Yared et al.[194] showed a similar reversal of water retention using another peptide antagonist to the antidiuretic effect of AVP in rats with cardiac failure owing to coronary artery ligation. An orally active nonpeptide V_2 receptor AVP antagonist, OPC-31260, was described.[197] The intravenous administration of OPC-31260 during a dose-ranging study in normal human subjects increased urine output to a similar extent as 20 mg of furosemide given intravenously.[198] In these healthy volunteers, urine osmolality was significantly lower after administration of the V_2 receptor antagonist, thus indicating an increase in solute-free water clearance. Moreover, this agent reversed the impairment in renal water excretion in rats with experimental heart failure owing to myocardial infarction[195] and in dogs with pacing-induced heart failure,[196] further supporting a role for AVP in the renal water retention of heart failure. This effect of the nonosmotic release of AVP to cause water retention in cardiac failure was associated with increased transcription of messenger RNA (mRNA) for the AVP preprohormone in the rat hypothalamus.[199]

The effects of V_2 receptor antagonists on water metabolism in heart failure have now been studied at the molecular level. Kidney AQP2 expression is increased in experimental heart failure. Rats with cardiac failure due to coronary ligation demonstrate an increase in renal AQP2 expression[200,201] that was reversed with nonpeptide V_2 receptor antagonism.[186] The V_2 receptor antagonism also reversed water retention in rats with heart failure. Recent studies have been undertaken in hyponatremic heart failure patients treated with various V_2 receptor antagonists.[202–206] One investigational agent, lixivaptan, produced a dose-related increase in water excretion, a correction of hyponatremia, and a decrease in urinary AQP2 excretion.[202,205] It is known that 3% to 6% of AQP2 water channels that traffic to the luminal membrane are excreted in the urine.[207] Therefore, urine AQP2 excretion can serve as an index of AVP effect and thus V_2 receptor antagonism in vivo in humans and experimental animals. Other investigational agents, such as tolvaptan and conivaptan, have demonstrated similar effects on diuresis (aquaresis) and a correction of hyponatremia in heart failure.[203,204,206] The SALT-1 and SALT-2 studies demonstrated this effect of V_2 receptor antagonism to correct hyponatremia not only in cardiac failure but also in cirrhosis and the syndrome of inappropriate antidiuretic hormone secretion.[208] Interestingly, preliminary data suggest that AVP antagonists, like inhibitors and antagonists of the sympathetic and renin–angiotensin–aldosterone systems, may prolong survival in heart failure patients.[206] However, the large randomized Efficacy of Vasopressin Antagonism in Heart Failure Outcome Study with Tolvaptan (EVEREST) study failed to demonstrate such an effect on survival in cardiac failure patients.[209]

Endothelin in heart failure. Endothelin is a potent vasoconstrictor, and its concentration is increased in patients with heart failure.[210] Results of a study from Teerlink et al.[211] suggest that endothelin plays an important role in the maintenance of arterial pressure in experimental heart failure, as shown by a significant decrease in blood pressure following the administration of the endothelin antagonist bosentan in rats with coronary artery ligation. In the kidney, mesangial cells, endothelial cells, epithelial glomerular cells, and inner medullary collecting duct cells are capable of synthesizing endothelin.[212] In this regard, recent studies in experimental heart failure demonstrate the early activation of the cardiac and renal endothelin systems.[213] Unfortunately, the role of increased endothelin in the pathogenesis of the renal sodium and water retention of heart failure is currently unknown. However, endothelin may be a potent mediator of renal vasoconstriction via the stimulation of endothelin A (ETA) receptors and thus may influence renal sodium and water handling. In experimental cardiac failure, endothelin has been associated with an antinatriuresis.[214–217] Conversely, experimental evidence suggests that the endothelin B (ETB) receptor may play a role in renal vasodilation and/or natriuresis.[216,217] In this regard, the clinical effects of investigational nonselective endothelin antagonists in heart failure have been disappointing. The use of these agents has been associated with a greater likelihood of worsening heart failure—associated with fluid volume overload—and worse clinical outcomes.[218] Consistent with the aforementioned postulated differences between ETA and ETB receptor functions, the selective antagonism of ETA receptors may produce a more desirable effect on renal function and excretory capacity in heart failure.

In summary, the activation of the three major neurohormonal vasoconstrictor systems—the sympathetic nervous system, the renin–angiotensin–aldosterone system, and the nonosmotic release of AVP—is implicated in the renal sodium and water retention of heart failure. The role of other vasoconstrictor systems (e.g., endothelin) is less well defined. These neuroendocrine systems exert direct (tubular) and indirect (hemodynamic) effects on the kidneys to promote the retention of sodium and water. Furthermore, these observations provide the rationale for the use of neurohormonal antagonists in the treatment of heart failure (see the following paragraphs). In this regard, endogenous counterregulatory vasodilatory and natriuretic hormones may play an important attenuating role in heart failure, and the exogenous administration of these agents may be important in the treatment of heart failure.

Vasodilator Systems

Natriuretic peptides in heart failure. The natriuretic peptides, including but not limited to ANP and BNP, circulate at increased concentrations in patients with heart failure.[219–225] These peptide hormones possess natriuretic and vasorelaxant properties as well as renin, aldosterone, and possibly AVP and sympathetic-inhibiting properties.[226–231] Both of these peptide hormones appear to be released primarily from the heart in response to increased atrial or ventricular end-diastolic pressure or to increased transmural cardiac pressure.[232,233] In a study of ANP kinetics in patients with cardiac dysfunction, we demonstrated that increased ANP production rather than decreased metabolic clearance was the major factor contributing to the elevated plasma ANP concentrations in these patients.[234] This finding is consistent with the observed increase in the expression of both ANP and BNP mRNA in the cardiac ventricles of humans and animals with heart failure.[235,236] However, given the peripheral vasoconstriction and sodium retention associated with heart failure, these elevated circulating natriuretic peptide levels must be inadequate to fully block vasoconstrictor hormone activation. In this regard, volume expansion experiments performed in dogs with heart failure demonstrated a deficiency to further increase the elevated ANP levels.[237] This relative deficiency of ANP secretion may contribute to the body's limited ability to maintain hemodynamic and renal function during the advanced stages of heart failure. In a coronary ligation model of heart failure in the rat, the infusion of a monoclonal antibody shown to specifically block endogenous ANP in vivo caused a significant rise in right atrial pressure, left ventricular end-diastolic pressure, and peripheral vascular resistance.[238] Alternatively, a study by Colucci et al.[239] found that a 6-hour infusion of the recombinant human BNP, nesiritide, significantly decreased pulmonary-capillary wedge pressure and improved symptoms in patients hospitalized with symptomatic heart failure. In a pivotal trial leading to U.S. Food and Drug Administration (FDA) approval of nesiritide, infused BNP was shown to improve both hemodynamics and symptoms of decompensated heart failure.[240]

Renal effects of the natriuretic peptides in heart failure. In normal humans, ANP and BNP increase GFR and urinary sodium excretion with no change or only a slight fall in renal blood flow.[232,241] The changes in renal hemodynamics are likely mediated by afferent arteriolar vasodilation with constriction of the efferent arterioles, as indicated by micropuncture studies in rats.[242,243] In addition to increasing GFR and filtered sodium load as a mechanism of their natriuretic effect, ANP and BNP are specific inhibitors of sodium reabsorption in the collecting tubule.[244–246] An important role for endogenous ANP in the renal sodium balance of heart failure was demonstrated by the aforementioned study of Lee et al.[28] However, the administration of synthetic ANP to patients with low-output heart failure results in a much smaller increase in renal sodium excretion and less significant changes in renal hemodynamics as compared to normal subjects.[232] Like ANP, the natriuretic effect of BNP is blunted in rats with high-output heart failure produced by AV fistulae.[247] Nevertheless, in hypertensive patients with mild-to-moderate heart failure and normal renal sodium excretory capacity, the natriuretic effect of BNP appears comparable to that in control subjects.[248] Because ANP and BNP appear to share the same receptor sites,[249] it is possible that the natriuretic effect of BNP is also blunted in sodium-retaining patients with more advanced heart failure. Support for this hypothesis may be found in reports from our group[250] and from Wang et al.[251] In our study, in 16 patients with advanced decompensated New York Heart Association (NYHA) class III heart failure due to either ischemic or idiopathic dilated cardiomyopathy (left ventricular ejection fraction 18 ± 2%, cardiac index 1.84 ± 0.15 L/minute/m^2, pulmonary capillary wedge pressure 27 ± 3 mm Hg), the administration of BNP at either 0.025 or 0.050 μg/kg/min for 4 hours produced a natriuresis in only 4 patients. The effect of BNP on GFR and renal blood flow was inconsistent in these patients and did not predict the natriuretic response. It is noteworthy that the doses of BNP infused in this study were 2.5 to 5 times greater than that currently approved as an initiating dose for the treatment of heart failure. In any event, although the renal effects of BNP were blunted in some of these heart failure patients, BNP did produce a significant (50%) decrease in pulmonary capillary wedge pressure. At the higher dose, BNP also significantly lowered peripheral vascular resistance and improved cardiac performance. Wang et al.'s study[251] demonstrated essentially the same lack of beneficial renal effects of infused BNP in a similarly small group of patients with heart failure.

Concern has been raised regarding the renal effects of BNP in heart failure. A meta-analysis of five trials suggested a higher rate of worsening renal dysfunction (defined as an increase in serum creatinine of at least 0.5 mg per deciliter) in nesiritide-treated subjects compared to controls.[252] However, this analysis had several limitations including the pooling of studies using different starting doses of nesiritide. Because it is likely that the renal hemodynamic effects of BNP in heart failure relate to the relative degree of renal versus peripheral vasodilation (i.e., the distribution of regional blood flow) induced by the drug, higher doses associated with more profound reductions in peripheral vascular resistance and systemic blood pressures may be expected to produce worsening renal function, whereas lower doses may actually preserve (or perhaps improve) renal hemodynamics. Support for this hypothesis and for the renal safety of nesiritide, when used as recommended, may be found in the results of the Acute Study of Clinical Effectiveness of Nesiritide in Decompensated Heart Failure (ASCEND-HF) trial.[253] In ASCEND-HF, 7,141 patients who were hospitalized with acute heart failure were randomized to receive either nesiritide or placebo for 24 to 168 hours in addition to standard care. Using the approved dose of nesiritide, there were no significant differences in rates of death from any cause at 30 days or rates of worsening renal function, defined by more than a 25% decrease in the estimated glomerular filtration rate, between the two groups.

In contrast to the previously mentioned findings of ANP and BNP resistance in heart failure, Elsner et al.[254] recently suggested that renal responsiveness to urodilatin (ANP_{95-126}), a slightly extended form of ANP_{99-126}, is preserved in heart failure. Urodilatin appears to be produced in the kidney by different posttranslational processing of the ANP prohormone ANP_{1-126}.[255] Endogenous urodilatin appears to be confined to the kidney[256]; that is, it is not a circulating hormone like ANP and BNP. In normal humans, exogenously administered urodilatin produces hemodynamic and renal effects similar to those of ANP.[228,257] In the report from Elsner et al.,[219] 12 patients with class II or III heart failure received urodilatin, 15 ng/kg/min, or placebo ($n = 6$ in each group) for 10 hours. Although the urodilatin-treated patients did demonstrate a modest natriuresis during urodilatin infusion, it should be noted that (1) digoxin and furosemide were continued during the study, (2) the patients were maintained on an 8 g of sodium per day intake, and (3) the patients received a 500-mL water load (300 mL orally and 200 mL intravenously) during the hour preceding the study drug infusion. In the former instance, furosemide likely facilitated the delivery of sodium to the distal nephron. In the latter two cases, the high daily sodium intake and oral water load would be expected to diminish the degree of vasoconstrictor neurohormone activation. In fact, plasma vasoconstrictor hormone concentrations were, at most, mildly elevated in these patients. Therefore, these findings do not exclude the existence of renal resistance to urodilatin in patients with heart failure and more advanced degrees of neurohormonal activation. On the other hand, urodilatin is less sensitive to degradation by the neutral endopeptidase (EC 3.4.24.11) and thus, more stable in comparison to ANP.[258] Furthermore, in the kidney, ANP solely binds to cortical receptors, whereas urodilatin can also be found in medullary structures.[259] Thus, the renal effects of urodilatin in human heart failure remain uncertain. Ongoing studies of urodilatin in heart failure promise to clarify these issues.

The mechanism of the relative resistance to the natriuretic effect of ANP (and possibly BNP and urodilatin) in heart failure remains controversial. Possible mechanisms include: (1) the downregulation of renal ANP receptors,[260,261] (2) the secretion of inactive immunoreactive ANP,[262] (3) enhanced renal neutral endopeptidase activity limiting the delivery of ANP to receptor sites,[263] (4) hyperaldosteronism by an increased sodium reabsorption in the distal renal tubule,[264] and (5) diminished delivery of sodium to the distal renal tubule site of ANP action.[244–246] In sodium-retaining patients with heart failure, we found a strong positive correlation between plasma ANP and urinary cyclic guanosine monophosphate (cGMP, the second messenger for the natriuretic effect of ANP, BNP, and urodilatin in vivo).[265,266] This observation supports the active biologic responsiveness of renal ANP receptors in heart failure and thus suggests that diminished distal tubular sodium delivery may be involved in the natriuretic peptide resistance observed in patients with cardiac failure. Further support for this hypothesis is found in our experience with cirrhosis, another edematous disorder associated with renal ANP resistance, in which maneuvers that definitely increase distal tubular sodium delivery reversed the ANP resistance[267] (see the following). In addition, heart failure maneuvers that are expected to increase distal tubular sodium delivery, such as the administration of an AT-II receptor antagonist or furosemide, also improve the renal response to ANP.[170,268] Finally, studies in rats with experimental heart failure demonstrated that renal denervation reverses the ANP resistance.[269] Because proximal tubular sodium reabsorption is enhanced by adrenergic stimulation, this effect of renal denervation to enhance ANP sensitivity in experimental cardiac failure is also compatible with a role in distal sodium delivery. The proposed role of diminished distal tubular sodium delivery in natriuretic peptide resistance and impaired aldosterone escape is shown in Figure 67.5.

Summary

As the heart begins to fail, the renal tubule reabsorbs sodium and water more avidly. The afferent stimuli for this "compensatory" volume retention may involve aspects of both the forward and backward theories of heart failure. An acute fall in cardiac output may inactivate (unload) high-pressure baroreceptors located in the aortic arch, the carotid sinus, and the juxtaglomerular apparatus and thus may activate the afferent adrenergic nervous system. Diminished renal perfusion and increased renal sympathetic tone enhance the release of renin and thus activate the renin–angiotensin–aldosterone system. In acute high-output heart failure, in which the cardiac output is insufficient to meet circulatory demands, the fall in peripheral vascular resistance provides the stimulus for arterial underfilling and deactivates high-pressure receptors. Although acute loading of the low-pressure receptors of the thorax may inhibit AVP release and stimulate the release of

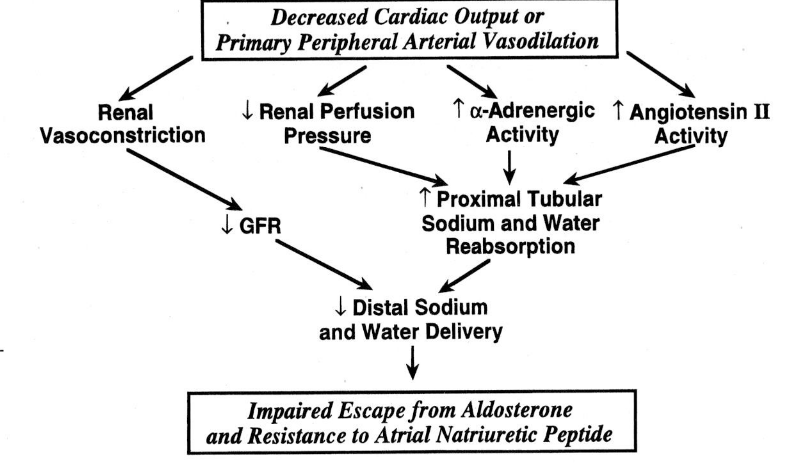

FIGURE 67.5 The proposed mechanism of natriuretic peptide resistance and impaired aldosterone escape in states of arterial underfilling. *GFR*, glomerular filtration rate. (From Schrier RW, Better OS. Pathogenesis of ascites formation. *Eur J Gastroenterol.* 1991;3:721, with permission.)

natriuretic peptides, this counterregulatory response to sodium and water retention may become ineffective because of progressive insensitivity of the cardiopulmonary receptors in the setting of chronic heart failure. Further cardiac compromise, resulting from either the progression of the primary cardiac pathology or increased cardiac demand, results in further renal sodium and water retention, expansion of the ECF volume, and overt edema formation. The development of increased cardiac filling pressures with subsequent pulmonary or peripheral edema substantially contributes to the high morbidity and mortality of heart failure.

The efferent mechanisms for renal sodium and water retention in heart failure are multifactorial. Inactivation of receptors in the high-pressure circulation and blunting of receptors in the low-pressure system initiate reflexes in which renal sympathetic tone is augmented and renal vasoconstriction results. Renal blood flow decreases to a greater extent than GFR, and therefore the filtration fraction rises. This increase alters the ultrafiltration of plasma and peritubular physical forces, which may in turn increase proximal tubular sodium reabsorption. Changes in cardiac output, ventricular filling pressures, and renal perfusion pressure also activate the renin–angiotensin–aldosterone system and the nonosmotic stimulation of AVP, and increase the secretion and/or production of PGs and the natriuretic peptides. At some point in the natural history of cardiac failure, the vasoconstrictive forces overcome the vasodilating effects of PGs, natriuretic peptides, and other vasodilating substances, and peripheral vasoconstriction and renal sodium and water retention occur. Increases in ventricular preload and afterload ensue, resulting in a further deterioration in cardiac performance and a further stimulation of neurohormonal vasoconstrictor systems.

Once initiated by arterial underfilling, sodium and water retention in heart failure leads to another vicious cycle of increasing central venous pressure, venous congestion, and worsening heart failure signs and symptoms often leading to acute decompensation, hospitalization, and worsening renal function. This cardiorenal syndrome of heart failure is associated with poor outcome (as discussed in the following section) and may be perpetuated not only by arterial underfilling but also by renal venous congestion. Support for this notion comes from a prospective cohort study of 145 patients, where an elevated central venous pressure was the most important hemodynamic factor associated with worsening renal function in patients with acute decompensated heart failure.[270] Moreover, in a retrospective analysis of 2,557 patients who underwent cardiac catheterization for hemodynamic assessment, elevated central venous pressure was the single most important prognostic factor for worsening renal function and mortality.[271] These observations are mechanistically plausible, because the transmission of venous pressure to renal veins impairs renal blood flow and glomerular filtration. Of note, diuresis in patients with right ventricular dysfunction, despite decreased cardiac output, leads to a decrease in venous congestion and a resultant improvement in renal function during the treatment of decompensated heart failure.[272] However, cardiac output remains a significant predictor of change in GFR during hospitalization in those patients without significant right ventricular dysfunction.[272] These findings speak to the importance of venous congestion and confirm the primacy of cardiac output in determining cardiorenal interactions in heart failure.

THE CLINICAL SIGNIFICANCE OF CARDIORENAL SYNDROME

As mentioned in the introduction to this chapter, the kidney represents an important marker of heart failure clinical status and a sensitive predictor of clinical outcomes in both chronic and acutely decompensated heart failure. In the PRIME II trial, an estimated GFR less than 60 mL per minute was associated with a significantly worse mortality in 1,708 chronic heart failure patients who were followed for more than 2 years.[3] Reduced GFR was a more potent predictor of mortality than many other common predictors of outcome such as the left ventricular ejection fraction, NYHA functional class ranking, hypotension, tachycardia, and the presence of comorbidity. Similarly, in 2,086 chronic heart failure patients followed in the Italian Network Project (IN-CHF), a serum creatinine level greater than 2.5 mg per deciliter was associated with a relative risk for 1-year mortality of 4.33 (95% confidence interval, 1.79 to 10.44).[4] In multivariable regression analysis, other independent clinical predictors of poor outcome included advanced NYHA class, advanced age, the presence of a third heart sound, and no ACE-inhibitor therapy. However, none of these predictors was as strong as an elevated serum creatinine. Even modest elevations of serum creatinine have been associated with an increased risk for morbidity and mortality in cardiac failure patients. A retrospective analysis of 6,797 heart failure patients enrolled in the SOLVD trial demonstrates this association.[5] The SOLVD trial excluded patients with baseline serum creatinine levels greater than 2.0 mg per deciliter. Dries et al.[5] stratified patients on the basis of serum creatinine levels into two groups, those with serum creatinine levels less than 1.5 mg per deciliter and those with serum creatinine levels between 1.5 mg per deciliter and 2.0 mg per deciliter. Those in the elevated serum creatinine group demonstrated increased risk for all-cause mortality (relative risk, 1.41; 95% confidence interval, 1.25 to 1.59), mortality due to pump failure (relative risk, 1.5; 95% confidence interval, 1.25 to 1.8), and sudden cardiac death (relative risk, 1.28; 95% confidence interval, 0.99 to 1.63). Therefore, impairment in glomerular filtration as measured by serum markers represents a potent predictor of mortality in patients with chronic heart failure.

Similarly, renal dysfunction predicts in-hospital mortality in patients with acutely decompensated heart failure. Definitive observations come from the Acute Decompensated Heart Failure National Registry (ADHERE), which has enrolled more than 150,000 patients from approximately 275 community, tertiary, and academic hospitals in the

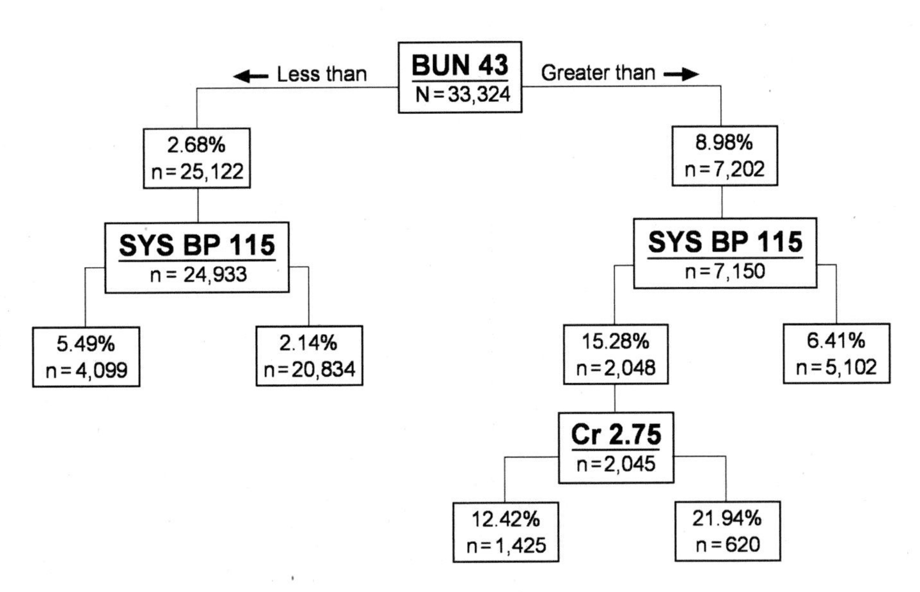

FIGURE 67.6 The ADHERE risk assessment tree from CART analysis. Numbers and percentages come from the derivation dataset and have been confirmed in a separated validation dataset (not shown). Note that two of the three predictors are measures of renal function. *BUN*, blood urea nitrogen; *SYS BP*, systolic blood pressure; *Cr*, creatinine. (From Fonarow GC, et al., for the ADHERE Scientific Advisory Committee, Study Group, and Investigators. Risk stratification for in-hospital mortality in acutely decompensated heart failure: classification and regression tree [CART] analysis. *JAMA.* 2005;293:572, with permission.)

United States.[1,6] Using classification and regression tree (CART) analysis to define covariate adjusted odds ratios of death, a practical user-friendly bedside tool for risk stratification of patients hospitalized with acute decompensated heart failure was developed.[6] Specifically, CART analysis of the ADHERE database was performed using the first 65,235 discharges enrolled. The first 33,046 hospitalizations (from October 2001 through February 2003) served as the derivation cohort and were analyzed to develop the risk-prediction model. Then, the validity of the model was prospectively tested using data from 32,229 subsequent hospitalizations (validation cohort) enrolled in ADHERE from March 2003 through July 2003. In-hospital mortality was similar in the derivation (4.2%) and validation (4.0%) cohorts. Recursive partitioning of the derivation cohort for 39 variables indicated that the best single predictor for mortality was high admission levels of BUN ($\geq$ 43 mg per deciliter), followed by low admission systolic blood pressure ($<$ 115 mm Hg), and then by high levels of serum creatinine ($\geq$ 2.75 mg per deciliter). A simple risk tree identified patient groups with mortality ranging from 2.1% to 21.9% (Fig. 67.6). The odds ratio for mortality between patients identified as high and low risk was 12.9 (95% confidence interval, 10.4 to 15.9) and similar results were seen when this risk stratification was applied prospectively to the validation cohort. These results suggest that acute decompensated heart failure patients at low, intermediate, and high risk for in-hospital mortality can be easily identified using vital sign and laboratory data obtained on hospital admission. In the context of the present chapter, it is noteworthy that two of the three most potent predictors of in-hospital mortality in ADHERE are measures of renal function. The importance of serum creatinine as a predictor of in-hospital mortality for acute decompensated heart failure was also demonstrated by the Organized Program to Initiate Lifesaving Treatment in Hospitalized Patients with Heart Failure (OPTIMIZE-HF).[273]

THE PHYSIOLOGIC BASIS FOR THE TREATMENT OF SODIUM AND WATER RETENTION IN HEART FAILURE

In heart failure, as in all of clinical medicine, effective therapy should be dictated by an understanding of the pathophysiologic process involved. Depressed ventricular function is associated with a vicious cycle of maladaptive responses, including increased neurohormonal activation, systemic vasoconstriction and renal sodium and water retention, and increased ventricular preload and afterload (Fig. 67.7). Treatment of heart failure should be directed at modifying the afferent and efferent factors responsible for the salt and water retention. Therefore, the primary goal in the treatment of cardiac failure is to improve the function of the heart as a pump. This increases the integrity of the arterial circulation and decreases the venous hypertension, thereby interrupting two of the major afferent mechanisms leading to sodium and water retention. Unfortunately, this goal of improving the contractile state of the heart is often difficult to accomplish. In certain cases of heart failure, however, left ventricular function may be improved by surgical intervention. For example, some patients with coronary artery disease and ischemic cardiomyopathy may exhibit improved cardiac function and less severe heart failure after surgical or percutaneous transluminal revascularization of the ischemic myocardium. However, a randomized controlled comparison of medical versus surgical therapies for ischemic heart failure failed to demonstrate the superiority of surgical revascularization on outcomes in a large cohort of patients.[274] Moreover, the assessment of myocardial viability did not identify patients with a differential survival benefit from bypass surgery, as compared with medical therapy alone, in this study.[275] A more classic example of surgically correctable heart failure is that seen in the setting of severe aortic stenosis. Patients with critical aortic stenosis often exhibit a severe degree of low-output heart failure with very avid

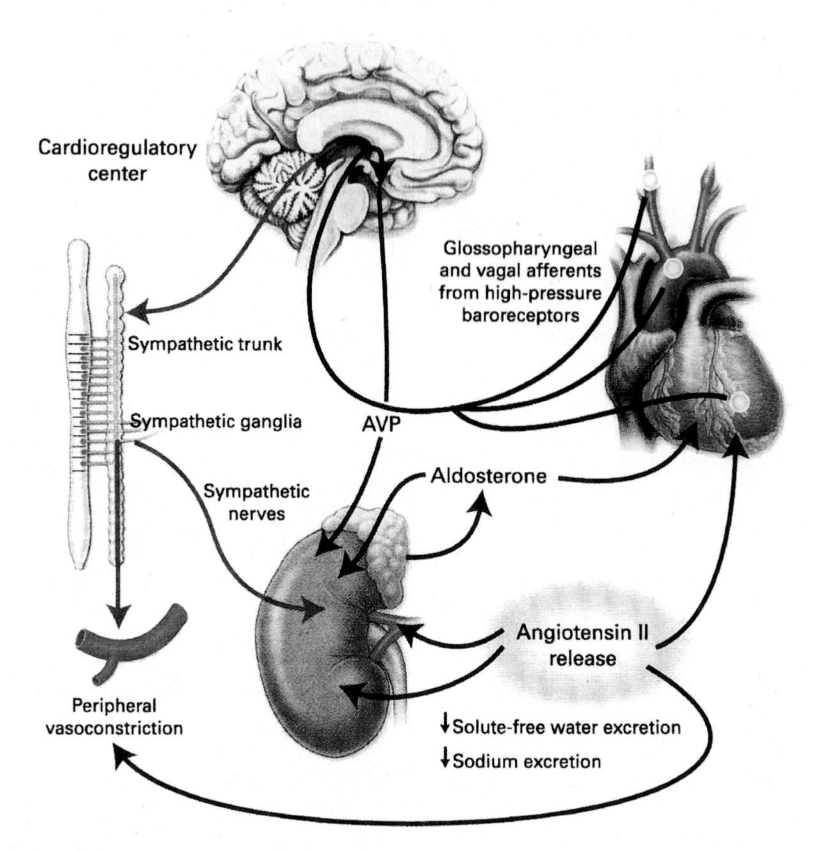

FIGURE 67.7 The pathophysiology of heart failure. Unloading of high-pressure baroreceptors (*circles*) in the left ventricle, carotid sinus, and aortic arch generates afferent signals (*black*) that stimulate cardioregulatory centers in the brain, resulting in the activation of efferent pathways in the sympathetic nervous system. The sympathetic nervous system appears to be the primary integrator of the neurohumoral vasoconstrictor response to arterial underfilling. Activation of renal sympathetic nerves stimulates the release of renin and angiotensin II, thereby activating the renin–angiotensin–aldosterone system. Concomitantly, the sympathetic stimulation of the supraoptic and paraventricular nuclei in the hypothalamus results in the nonosmotic release of arginine vasopressin (AVP). Sympathetic activation also causes peripheral and renal vasoconstriction, as does angiotensin II. Angiotensin II constricts blood vessels, stimulates the release of aldosterone from the adrenal gland, and also increases tubular sodium reabsorption and causes remodeling of cardiac myocytes. Aldosterone may have direct cardiac effects, in addition to increasing the reabsorption of sodium and the secretion of potassium and hydrogen ions in the collecting duct. The lines designate circulating hormones. (From Schrier RW, Abraham WT. Hormones and hemodynamics in heart failure. *N Engl J Med.* 1999;341:577, copyright © 2000, Massachusetts Medical Society. All rights reserved.)

renal sodium and water retention that is usually completely reversible following a replacement of the stenotic aortic valve. An emerging alternative to surgical replacement of a critically stenosed aortic valve is transcatheter aortic-valve implantation (TAVI). In patients with severe aortic stenosis who are not candidates for surgery, TAVI has been shown to significantly improve outcomes as well as cardiac symptoms, as compared with standard therapy.[276]

In other instances of heart failure, cardiac function may be augmented by the cardiac glycosides, such as digoxin, which modestly improve cardiac contractility and may favorably influence baroreceptor function.[277] However, digoxin does not improve survival in heart failure patients[278] and is thus used much less frequently than before in the treatment of chronic heart failure. Vasodilators, such as nitrates and hydralazine, and ACE inhibitors may improve cardiac function by decreasing cardiac preload and afterload.[279] The addition of a fixed dose of isosorbide dinitrate plus hydralazine to standard therapy for heart failure including neurohormonal blockers has been shown to improve survival among black patients with advanced heart failure.[280] The efficacy of ACE inhibitors in heart failure is discussed in the following paragraphs. Investigational nonglycoside inotropic agents may acutely improve cardiac output, but longer term use has been shown, thus far, to increase mortality.[281–283]. β-Adrenergic receptor antagonists, once thought to be contraindicated in patients with low-output heart failure, can exhibit a favorable effect on cardiac function and outcome in patients with chronic heart failure. In fact, these agents improve the left ventricular ejection fraction to a greater extent than do any other forms of heart failure drug therapy.[137] Carvedilol, a nonselective third-generation β-blocker/vasodilator with α_1-adrenergic receptor–blocking properties, produces a dose-related improvement in ejection fraction and a reduction in mortality in patients with class II to IV heart failure.[139] In the U.S. Carvedilol Heart Failure Trials Program, this agent reduced all-cause mortality by 65% compared to placebo in patients with mild-to-moderate heart failure.[140] Likewise, the Second Cardiac Insufficiency Bisoprolol Study demonstrated a 34% reduction in all-cause mortality versus placebo during the treatment of heart failure with this β_1 selective agent.[141] In a randomized study of metoprolol CR/XL treatment of 3,991 patients with class II to IV heart failure, treatment with metoprolol CR/XL was associated with a 34% decrease in all-cause mortality, a 38% decrease in cardiovascular mortality, a 41% decrease in sudden death, and a 49% decrease in death owing to progressive heart failure as compared to controls.[142] β-Blockers have also been shown to improve outcome in post-MI left ventricular dysfunction with or without heart failure and in severe heart failure.[133,143] However, these effects are not seen with all β-blockers.[284]

Another strategy for improving pump function and outcome in selected heart failure patients (i.e., those with ventricular dyssynchrony) is the use of cardiac resynchronization therapy. This device-based treatment for heart failure works to optimize ventricular filling and to improve the contraction pattern via atrial-synchronized biventricular pacing. Resynchronization therapy has been shown to improve hemodynamics, quality of life, functional status, and exercise capacity while reducing the risks of heart failure hospitalization and all-cause mortality.[285–291] Cardiac resynchronization has been associated with the preservation of renal function[292] and, anecdotally, a reduction in the diuretic dose in patients with chronic heart failure.

Because an improvement in pump function is a primary goal in the treatment of heart failure, agents that might further impair cardiac contractility should be avoided in this setting. Unfortunately, many medications that have been demonstrated to produce a negative effect on cardiac inotropy are commonly prescribed in cardiac disease patients. For example, most antiarrhythmic drugs and the commonly prescribed first-generation calcium channel antagonists exhibit some degree of negative inotropy in vivo.[293] Newer vascular-selective calcium channel blockers may be better tolerated in patients with heart failure but should not be used as a heart failure therapy per se.

The neuroendocrine activation in patients with heart failure provides another target for therapy. In fact, recent experience with various neurohormonal antagonists suggests that the inhibition or antagonism of neurohormonal vasoconstrictor systems may be more beneficial than nonspecific diuretic or vasodilator therapy. This is certainly the case with adrenergic blockade, as noted in the preceding text. AT-II is known to mediate myocardial hypertrophy, increase fibrosis and collagen deposition, and cause the activation of the sympathetic nervous system. Therefore, the administration of ACE inhibitors would be anticipated to decrease myocardial remodeling and hypertrophy and to decrease the activation of the sympathetic nervous system. ACE inhibition also decreases the degradation of bradykinin, which is a well-known vasodilator that can reduce cardiac afterload. The proven beneficial effects of ACE inhibition on symptoms, hemodynamics, exercise capacity, and survival in heart failure patients support this hypothesis.[147,156,282] Moreover, in the patients of the Cooperative North Scandinavian Enalapril Survival Study (CONSENSUS), all with class IV heart failure, significant reductions in mortality were consistently found in the patients treated with enalapril who had baseline hormone levels greater than median values.[156] In the group of patients treated with the ACE inhibitor, there were significant reductions from baseline to 6 weeks in levels of AT-II, aldosterone, norepinephrine, and ANP, but not epinephrine. These results suggest that the effect of enalapril on mortality was related to diminished hormonal activation in general and to the renin–angiotensin system in particular.[294] In the SOLVD studies[157] of less severe heart failure, the addition of enalapril to conventional therapy also significantly reduced mortality and hospitalization rates. Studies support the use of ACE inhibition in post-MI left ventricular dysfunction with or without clinical heart failure, as well.[158] Recent data support the noninferiority of ARBs in the treatment of post-MI ventricular dysfunction or chronic heart failure.[159–161] Such studies have led to the perceived interchangeability of ACE inhibitors and ARBs. Hospital-based quality measures from the Centers for Medicare and Medicaid Services endorse the equivalency of ACE inhibitors and ARBs in the treatment of heart failure, as do the 2005 Update to the American College of Cardiology/American Heart Association Guidelines for the Evaluation and Management of Chronic Heart Failure in the Adult.[295]

Diuretics are indicated to restore the ECF volume toward normal as heart failure becomes more advanced and when edema formation occurs. Diuretic therapy is discussed extensively elsewhere. Of note, although most patients with cardiac failure respond to a potent loop diuretic (e.g., furosemide), and this agent can increase solute-free water clearance in patients with cardiac edema,[125] cardiac output may actually decline during acute treatment due to the further activation of vasoconstrictor hormone systems.[296] Volume depletion owing to overzealous diuretic treatment must also be considered in any acute or chronic heart failure patient with worsening signs or symptoms of a low-output state. For example, diminished renal perfusion may occur in the setting of excessive diuretic treatment, resulting in elevations in BUN and serum creatinine concentrations. On the other hand, the belief that heart failure patients require elevated ventricular filling pressures to maintain an adequate cardiac output has been proved erroneous, because recent experience with heart failure management guided by implantable hemodynamic monitors demonstrates that most patients with chronic heart failure can be treated with diuretics to normalize or nearly normalize intracardiac and pulmonary artery pressures to reduce the risk of hospitalization for worsening heart failure.[297,298] One particular challenge in diuretic therapy, however, is the common circumstance of worsening renal function despite the persistence of ECF volume overload. That is, BUN and serum creatinine may rise in the face of continued fluid volume overload during diuresis. This may relate to a further reduction in cardiac output. However, in many instances, the worsening renal function appears to be due to the diuretic therapy per se. In this regard, loop diuretics have been shown to reduce GFR on average in heart failure patients.[299]

This situation of worsening renal function despite ECF volume excess during diuresis may also be associated with diuretic resistance. Diuretic resistance is not an uncommon finding in patients with advanced heart failure. Because the intraluminal delivery of loop diuretics via tubular secretion is necessary for these agents to inhibit sodium chloride reabsorption in the thick ascending limb of Henle, renal vasoconstriction may play an important role in diuretic resistance associated with heart failure (Fig. 67.8). Moreover, increased distal tubule sodium reabsorption further contributes to diuretic resistance in this condition. Therefore, the addition of a more distal acting diuretic, such as metolazone or hydrochlorothiazide, may reverse resistance to loop diuretics. In some cases, however, diuretic resistance is impossible to overcome. Such patients are often unable to be safely discharged from the hospital or are repetitively readmitted to the hospital, if discharged.

Fluid removal by intermittent or continuous ultrafiltration has been suggested to have several advantages over diuretic therapy.[300–305] In addition to the reduction of excess ECF volume in heart failure patients, it has been suggested that the ultrafiltration of cytokines, which suppress myocardial contractility, may improve cardiac function. This remains to be proven, however. As compared to diuretics, fluid/electrolyte and acid–base disturbances may be more easily corrected and avoided with ultrafiltration. Furthermore, for the same amount of fluid removal, more sodium is removed with ultrafiltration than with diuretics because the sodium concentration in the ultrafiltrate is equivalent to plasma, whereas with diuretic therapy the urinary sodium concentration is virtually always less than plasma. Recently, a simple approach to ultrafiltration using peripherally inserted catheters has been introduced for the treatment of heart failure.[304] The efficient removal of fluid has been demonstrated using this technique. Small case series support the use of ultrafiltration in hospitalized patients and intermittently in outpatients with refractory heart failure. A randomized controlled trial of ultrafiltration versus diuretics in hospitalized decompensated heart failure patients supports the benefits of this approach.[305] In the Ultrafiltration Versus IV Diuretics for Patients Hospitalized for Acute Decompensated Congestive Heart Failure (UNLOAD) trial, patients with acute decompensated heart failure randomized to early ultrafiltration compared with those assigned to standard intravenous diuretic therapy demonstrated significantly more weight and net fluid loss at 48 hours and significantly decreased rehospitalization rates at 90 days, without significant renal function differences.

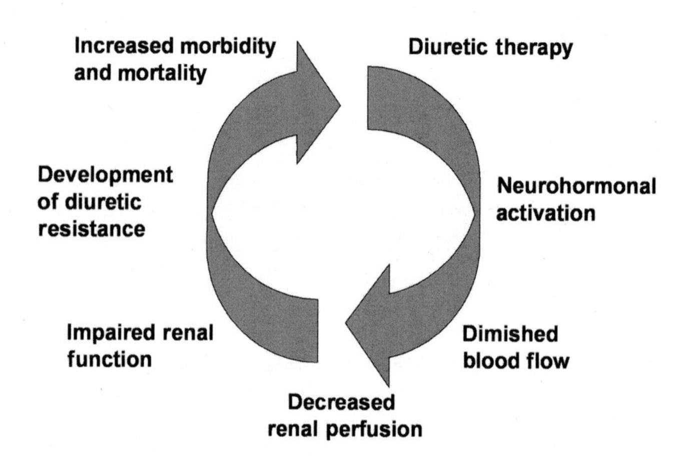

FIGURE 67.8 The "iatrogenic" cardiorenal syndrome of heart failure. A scheme by which diuretic therapy may worsen the neurohormonal and renal hemodynamic milieu of heart failure, leading to diuretic resistance and poor outcomes in heart failure patients.

Water restriction remains the mainstay of therapy in patients with heart failure who are hyponatremic. Studies also suggested that in hyponatremic patients with heart failure receiving furosemide and captopril, plasma sodium values tended to normalize, whereas they did not in patients receiving other vasodilators.[306,307] These data support the concomitant use of ACE inhibitors and loop diuretics in hyponatremic heart failure patients. Alternatively, selective V_2-receptor AVP antagonists have been shown to correct the hyponatremia of heart failure.

Finally, other measures, including sodium restriction and oxygen administration, contribute to the overall management of patients with heart failure. Special emphasis should be placed on the salutary influence of bed rest, which increases osmolar and solute-free water clearances, cardiac output, renal plasma flow, and GFR and decreases plasma catecholamines and PRA.[308] Such considerations lay the foundation for the physiologic basis of therapy in heart failure.

REFERENCES

1. Adams KF Jr, Fonarow GC, Emerman CL, et al. Characteristics and outcomes of patients hospitalized for heart failure in the United States: rationale, design, and preliminary observations from the first 100,000 cases in the Acute Decompensated Heart Failure National Registry (ADHERE). *Am Heart J.* 2005;149:209–216.

2. Friedman MM. Older adults' symptoms and their duration before hospitalization for heart failure. *Heart Lung.* 1997;26:169–176.

3. Girbes AR, Zijlstra JG. Ibopamine and survival in severe congestive heart failure: PRIME II. *Lancet.* 1997;350:147–148.

4. Maggioni AP, et al. Predictors of 1 year mortality in 2086 outpatients with congestive heart failure: data from the Italian Network on Congestive Heart Failure (abstract). *J Am Coll Cardiol.* 1998;31:218A.

5. Dries DL, Exner DV, Domanski MJ, Greenberg B, Stevenson LW. The prognostic implications of renal insufficiency in asymptomatic and symptomatic patients with left ventricular systolic dysfunction. *J Am Coll Cardiol.* 2000;35:681–689.

6. Fonarow GC, Adams KF Jr, Abraham WT, et al. Risk stratification for in-hospital mortality in acutely decompensated heart failure: classification and regression tree (CART) analysis. *JAMA.* 2005;293:572–580.

7. Starling EH. On the absorption of fluid from the connective tissue spaces. *J Physiol (Lond)*. 1896;19:312–326.

8. Intaglietta M, Zweifach BW. Microcirculatory basis of fluid exchange. *Adv Biol Med Phys*. 1974;15:111–159.

9. Bennhold H, Klaus D, Scheurlen PG. Volume regulation and renal function in analbuminemia. *Lancet*. 1960;2:1169.

10. Braunwald E, Plauth WH Jr, Morrow AG. A method for detection and quantification of impaired sodium excretion. Results of an oral sodium tolerance test in normal subjects and in patients with heart disease. *Circulation*. 1965;32:223–231.

11. Takasu T, Lasker N, Shalhoub RJ. Mechanism of hyponatremia in chronic congestive heart failure. *Ann Intern Med*. 1961;55:368–383.

12. Hope J. *A Treatise on the Diseases of the Heart and Blood Vessels*. London, England: William Kidd; 1832.

13. Mackenzie J. *Disease of the Heart*. 3rd ed. London, England: Oxford University Press; 1913.

14. Schrier RW. Pathogenesis of sodium and water retention in high-output and low-output cardiac failure, nephrotic syndrome, cirrhosis, and pregnancy. *N Engl J Med*. 1988;319:1065–1072.

15. Schrier RW. Body fluid volume regulation in health and disease: a unifying hypothesis. *Ann Intern Med*. 1990;113:155–159.

16. Schrier RW. A unifying hypothesis of body fluid volume regulation. The Lilly Lecture 1992. *J R Coll Phys (Lond)*. 1992;26:295–306.

17. Schrier RW. An odyssey into the milieu intérieur: pondering the enigmas. *J Am Soc Nephrol*. 1992;2:1549–1559.

18. Abraham WT, Schrier RW. Edematous disorders: pathophysiology of renal sodium and water retention and treatment with diuretics. *Curr Opin Nephrol Hypertens*. 1993;2:798–805.

19. Abraham WT, Schrier RW. Body fluid regulation in health and disease. In: Schrier RW, Abboud FM, Baxter JD, et al., eds. *Advances in Internal Medicine*, Vol. 39. Chicago, IL: Mosby Yearbook; 1994.

20. Schrier RW, Gurevich AK, Cadnapaphornchai MA. Pathogenesis and management of sodium and water retention in cardiac failure and cirrhosis. *Semin Nephrol*. 2001;21:157–172.

21. Schrier RW, Abraham WT. Hormones and hemodynamics in heart failure. *N Engl J Med*. 1999;341:577–585.

22. Epstein FH, Shadle OW, Ferguson TB, McDowell ME. Cardiac output and intracardiac pressure in patients with arteriovenous fistulas. *J Clin Invest*. 1953;32:543–547.

23. Papper S. The role of the kidney in Laënnec's cirrhosis of the liver. *Medicine (Baltimore)*. 1958;37:299–316.

24. Lifschitz MD, Schrier RW. Alterations in cardiac output with chronic constriction of thoracic inferior vena cava. *Am J Physiol*. 1973;225:1364–1370.

25. Schrier RW, Humphreys MH. Factors involved in the antinatriuretic effects of acute constriction of the thoracic and abdominal inferior vena cava. *Circ Res*. 1971;29:479–489.

26. Schrier RW, Humphreys MH, Ufferman RC. Role of cardiac output and autonomic nervous system in the antinatriuretic response to acute constriction of the thoracic superior vena cava. *Circ Res*. 1971;29:490–498.

27. Migdal SE, Alexander EA, Levinsky NG. Evidence that decreased cardiac output is not the stimulus to sodium retention during acute constriction of the vena cava. *J Lab Clin Med*. 1977;89:809–816.

28. Yaron M, Bennett CM. Renal sodium handling in acute right-sided heart failure in dogs. *Miner Electrolyte Metab*. 1978;1:303.

29. Lee ME, Miller WL, Edwards BS, Burnett JC Jr. Role of endogenous atrial natriuretic factor in acute congestive heart failure. *J Clin Invest*. 1989;84:1962–1966.

30. Hostetter TH, Pfeffer JM, Pfeffer MA, et al. Cardiorenal hemodynamics and sodium excretion in rats with myocardial infarction. *Am J Physiol*. 1983;245: H98–103.

31. Priebe HJ, Heimann JC, Hedley-Whyte J. Effects of renal and hepatic venous congestion on renal function in the presence of low and normal cardiac output in dogs. *Circ Res*. 1980;17:883–890.

32. Davis JO. The control of renin release. *Am J Med*. 1973;55:333–350.

33. Guyton A, Scanlon CJ, Armstrong GG. Effects of pressoreceptor reflex and Cushing's reflex on urinary output. *Fed Proc*. 1952;11:61.

34. Gilmore JP. Contribution of baroreceptors to the control of renal function. *Circ Res*. 1964;14:301–317.

35. Gilmore JP, Daggett WM. Response of chronic cardiac denervated dog to acute volume expansion. *Am J Physiol*. 1966;210:509–512.

36. Knox FG, Davis BB, Berliner RW. Effect of chronic cardiac denervation on renal response to saline infusion. *Am J Physiol*. 1967;213:174–178.

37. Pearch JW, Sonnenberg H. Effects of spinal section and renal denervation on the renal response to blood volume expansion. *Can J Physiol Pharmacol*. 1965;43:211–224.

38. Schedl HP, Bartter FC. An explanation for an experimental correction of the abnormal water diuresis in cirrhosis. *J Clin Invest*. 1960;39:248–261.

39. Anderson RJ, Cronin RE, McDonald KM, Schrier RW. Mechanism of portal hypertension induced alterations in renal hemodynamics, renal water excretion and renin secretion. *J Clin Invest*. 1976;58:964–970.

40. Schrier RW, Berl T, Anderson RJ et al. Nonosmolar control of renal water excretion. In: Andreoli T, Grantham J, Rector F, eds. *Disturbances in Body Fluid Osmolality*. Bethesda, MD: American Physiological Society; 1977.

41. Tobian L, Tomboulian A, Janecek J. The effect of high perfusion pressure on the granulation of juxtaglomerular cells in an isolated kidney. *J Clin Invest*. 1959;38:605–610.

42. Blaine EH, Davis JO, Witty RT. Renin release after hemorrhage and after suprarenal aortic constriction in dogs without sodium delivery to the macula densa. *Circ Res*. 1970;27:1081–1089.

43. Epstein FH, Post RS, McDowell M. The effects of an arteriovenous fistula on renal hemodynamics and electrolyte excretion. *J Clin Invest*. 1953;32:233–241.

44. Gauer OH, Henry JP. Neurohormonal control of plasma volume. In: Guyton AC, Cowley AW Jr, eds. *Cardiovascular Physiology II. International Review of Physiology*, Vol 9. Baltimore, MD: University Park; 1976.

45. Paintal AS. Vagal sensory receptors and their reflex effects. *Physiol Rev*. 1973;53:159–227.

46. Coleridge HM, Coleridge JC. Afferent innervation of lungs, airways, and pulmonary artery. In: Zucker IH, Gilmore JP, eds. *Reflex Control of the Circulation*. Boca Raton, FL: CRC Press; 1991.

47. Arborelius M, Ballidin UI, Lilja B, Lundgren CE. Hemodynamic changes in man during immersion with the head above water. *Aerospace Med*. 1972;43: 592–598.

48. Bichet DG, Groves BM, Schrier RW. Mechanisms of improvement of water and sodium excretion by enhancement of central hemodynamics in decompensated cirrhotic patients. *Kidney Int*. 1983;24:788–794.

49. Epstein FH. Renal excretion of sodium and the concept of a volume receptor. *Yale J Biol Med*. 1956;29:282–298.

50. Epstein M, Duncan DC, Fishman LM. Characterization of the natriuresis caused in normal man by immersion in water. *Clin Sci*. 1972;43:275–287.

51. Gauer OH, Henry JP, Sieker HO, Wendt WE. The effect of negative pressure breathing on urine flow. *J Clin Invest*. 1954;33:287–296.

52. Hulet WH, Smith HH. Postural natriuresis and urine osmotic concentration in hydropenic subjects. *Am J Med*. 1961;30:8–25.

53. Epstein FH, Goodyer AV, Lawrason FD, Relman AS. Studies of the antidiuresis of quiet standing: the importance of changes in plasma volume in glomerular filtration rate. *J Clin Invest*. 1951;30:63–72.

54. Murdaugh HV Jr, Sieker HO, Manfredi F. Effect of altered intrathoracic pressure on renal hemodynamics, electrolyte excretion and water clearance. *J Clin Invest*. 1959;38:834–842.

55. Gillespie DJ, Sandberg RL, Koike TI. Dual effect on left atrial receptors on excretion of sodium and water in the dog. *Am J Physiol*. 1973;225:706–710.

56. Henry JP, Gauer OH, Reeves JL. Evidence of the atrial location of receptors influencing urine flow. *Circ Res*. 1956;4:85–90.

57. Reinhardt HW, Kaczmarczyk G, Eisele R, et al. Left atrial pressure and sodium balance in conscious dogs on a low sodium intake. *Pflugers Arch*. 1977;370:59–66.

58. Bello-Reuss E, Trevino DL, Gottschalk CW. Effect of renal sympathetic nerve stimulation on proximal water and sodium reabsorption. *J Clin Invest*. 1976;57:1104–1107.

59. DiBona GF. Neurogenic regulation of renal tubular sodium reabsorption. *Am J Physiol*. 1977;233:F73–81.

60. de Torrente A, Robertson GL, McDonald KM, Schrier RW. Mechanism of diuretic response to increased left atrial pressure in the anesthetized dog. *Kidney Int*. 1975;8:355–361.

61. Gauer OH, Henry JP. Circulating basis of fluid volume control. *Physiol Rev*. 1963;43:423–481.

62. Share L. Effects of carotid occlusion and left atrial distension on plasma vasopressin titer. *Am J Physiol*. 1965;208:219–223.

63. Gupta PD, Henry JP, Sinclair R, Von Baumgarten R. Responses of atrial and aortic baroreceptors to nonhypotensive hemorrhage and to transfusion. *Am J Physiol*. 1966;211:1429–1437.

64. Henry JP, Gupta PD, Meehan JP, Sinclair R, Share L. The role of afferents from the low-pressure system in the release of antidiuretic hormone during nonhypotensive hemorrhage. *Can J Physiol Pharmacol*. 1968;46:287–295.

65. Goetz KL, Hermeck AS, Slick GL, Starke HS. Atrial receptors and renal function in conscious dog. *Am J Physiol*. 1970;219:1417–1423.

66. Barger AC, Yates FE, Rudolph AM. Renal hemodynamics and sodium excretion in dogs with graded valvular damage, and in congestive heart failure. *Am J Physiol*. 1961;200:601–608.

67. Stitzer SO, Malvin RL. Right atrium and renal sodium excretion. *Am J Physiol.* 1975;228:184–190.
68. Zucker IH, Gorman AJ, Cornish KG, Lang M. Impaired atrial receptor modulation of renal nerve activity in dogs with chronic volume overload. *Cardiovasc Res.* 1985;19:411–418.
69. Ferguson DW, Abboud FM, Mark AL. Selective impairment of baroreceptor-mediated vasoconstrictor responses in patients with ventricular dysfunction. *Circulation.* 1984;69:451–460.
70. Mohanty PK, Arrowood JA, Ellenbogen KA, Thames MD. Neurohormonal and hemodynamic effects of lower body negative pressure in patients with congestive heart failure. *Am Heart J.* 1989;118:78–85.
71. Nishian K, Kawashima S, Iwasaki T. Paradoxical forearm vasodilation and hemodynamic improvement during cardiopulmonary baroreceptor unloading in patients with congestive heart failure. *Clin Sci.* 1993;84:271–280.
72. Sandoval AB, et al. Hemodynamic correlates of increased cardiac adrenergic drive in the intact failing human heart. *J Am Coll Cardiol.* 1989;13:245A.
73. Fonarow GC, et al. Persistently high left ventricular filling pressure predicts mortality despite angiotensin converting enzyme inhibition in advanced heart failure (abstract). *Circulation.* 1994;90:I-488.
74. Baker DG, Coleridge HM, Coleridge JC, Nerdrum T. Search for a cardiac nociceptor: stimulation by bradykinin of sympathetic afferent nerve endings in the heart of the cat. *J Physiol.* 1980;306:519–536.
75. Panzenbeck MJ, Tan W, Hajdu MA, Cornish KG, Zucker IH. PGE_2 and arachidonate inhibit the baroreflex in conscious dogs via cardiac receptors. *Am J Physiol.* 1989;256:H999–1005.
76. Zucker IH, Panzenbeck MJ, Barker S, Tan W, Hajdu MA. PGI_2 attenuates the baroreflex control of renal nerve activity by a vagal mechanism. *Am J Physiol.* 1988;254:R424–430.
77. Dzau VJ, Packer M, Lilly LS, et al. Prostaglandins in severe congestive heart failure: relation to activation of the renin–angiotensin system and hyponatremia. *N Engl J Med.* 1984;310:347–352.
78. Daly JJ, Roe JW, Horrocks P. A comparison of sodium excretion following the infusion of saline into systemic and portal veins in the dog: evidence for a hepatic role in the control of sodium excretion. *Clin Sci.* 1967;33:481–487.
79. Passo SS, Thornborough JR, Rothballer AB. Hepatic receptors in control of sodium excretion in anesthetized cats. *Am J Physiol.* 1975;224:373–375.
80. Carey RM, Smith JR, Ortt EM. Gastrointestinal control of sodium excretion in sodium-depleted conscious rabbits. *Am J Physiol.* 1976;230:1504–1508.
81. Carey RM. Evidence for a splanchnic sodium input monitor regulating renal sodium excretion in man: lack of dependence upon aldosterone. *Circ Res.* 1978;43:19–23.
82. Lennane RJ, Peart WS, Carey RM, Shaw J. A comparison of natriuresis after oral and intravenous sodium loading in sodium-depleted rabbits: evidence for a gastrointestinal or portal monitor of sodium intake. *Clin Sci Mol Med.* 1975;49:433–436.
83. Potkay S, Gilmore JP. Renal response to vena caval and portal venous infusions of sodium chloride in unanesthetized dogs. *Clin Sci Mol Med.* 1970;39: 13–20.
84. Schneider EG, Davis JO, Robb CA, et al. Lack of evidence for a hepatic osmoreceptor in conscious dogs. *Am J Physiol.* 1970;218:42–45.
85. Obika LF, Fitzgerald EM, Gleason SD, Zucker A, Schneider EG. Lack of evidence for gastrointestinal control of sodium excretion in unanesthetized rabbits. *Am J Physiol.* 1981;240:F94–100.
86. Schrier RW Berl T, Anderson RJ. Osmotic and nonosmotic control of vasopressin release. *Am J Physiol.* 1979;236:F321–332.
87. Berl T, Henrich WL, Erickson AL, Schrier RW. Prostaglandins in the beta adrenergic and baroreceptor-mediated secretion of renin. *Am J Physiol.* 1979;235:F472–477.
88. de Wardener HE, Mills IH, Clapham WF, Hayter CJ. Studies on the efferent mechanism of the sodium diuresis which follows the intravenous administration of saline in the dog. *Clin Sci.* 1961;21:249–258.
89. Merrill AJ. Mechanism of salt and water retention in heart failure. *Am J Med.* 1949;6:357–367.
90. Kilcoyne MM, Schmidt DH, Cannon PJ. Intrarenal blood flow in congestive heart failure. *Circ Res.* 1973;47:786–797.
91. Sparks HV, Kopald HH, Carrière S, et al. Intrarenal distribution of blood flow with chronic congestive heart failure. *Am J Physiol.* 1972;223:840–846.
92. Boudreau R, Mandin H. Cardiac edema in dogs. II. Distribution of glomerular filtrate in renal blood flow. *Kidney Int.* 1976;10:578.
93. Stumpe KO, Sölle H, Klein H, Krück F. Mechanism of sodium and water retention in rats with experimental heart failure. *Kidney Int.* 1973;4:309–317.
94. Meyers BD, Deen WM, Brenner BM. Effects of norepinephrine and angiotensin II on the determinants of glomerular ultrafiltration and proximal tubule fluid reabsorption in the rat. *Circ Res.* 1975;37:101–110.
95. Ichikawa I, Pfeffer JM, Pfeffer MA, Hostetter TH, Brenner BM. Role of angiotensin II in the altered renal function in congestive heart failure. *Circ Res.* 1984;55:669–675.
96. Bichet DG, Kortas C, Mettauer B, et al. Modulation of plasma and platelet vasopressin by cardiac function in patients with heart failure. *Kidney Int.* 1986;29:1188–1196.
97. Munger MA. Renal functional alterations induced by angiotensin-converting enzyme inhibitors in heart failure. *Ann Pharmacother.* 1993;27:205–210.
98. Henrich WL, Berl T, McDonald KM, Anderson RJ, Schrier RW. Angiotensin, renal nerves and prostaglandins in renal hemodynamics during hemorrhage. *Am J Physiol.* 1978;235:F46–51.
99. Blasingham MC, Nasjletti A. Differential renal effects of cyclooxygenase inhibition in sodium-replete and sodium-deprived dog. *Am J Physiol.* 1980;239:F360–F365.
100. Dunn MJ, Zambraski EJ. Renal effect of drugs that inhibit prostaglandin synthesis. *Kidney Int.* 1980;18:609–622.
101. Riegger GA, Kahles HW, Elsner D, Kromer EP, Kochsiek K. Effects of acetylsalicylic acid on renal function in patients with chronic heart failure. *Am J Med.* 1991;90:571–575.
102. Walshe JJ, Venuto RC. Acute oliguric renal failure induced by indomethacin: possible mechanism. *Ann Intern Med.* 1979;91:47–49.
103. Oliver JA, Sciacca RR, Pinto J, Cannon PJ. Participation of the prostaglandins in the control of renal blood flow during acute reduction of cardiac output in the dog. *J Clin Invest.* 1981;67:229–237.
104. Hasking GJ, Esler MD, Jennings GL, et al. Norepinephrine spillover to plasma in patients with congestive heart failure: evidence of increased overall and cardiorenal sympathetic nervous activity. *Circulation.* 1986;73:615–621.
105. Brod J, Fejfar Z, Fejfarova MH. The role of neuro-humoral factors in the genesis of renal hemodynamic changes in heart failure. *Acta Med Scand.* 1954;148:273–290.
106. Krum H, Schlaich M, Whitbourn R, et al. Catheter-based renal sympathetic denervation for resistant hypertension: a multicentre safety and proof-of-principle cohort study. *Lancet.* 2009;373:1275–1281.
107. Esler MD, Krum H, Sobotka PA, et al. Renal sympathetic denervation in patients with treatment-resistant hypertension (The Symplicity HTN-2 Trial): a randomised controlled trial. *Lancet.* 2010;376:1903–1909.
108. Schlaich MP, Sobotka PA, Krum H, Lambert E, Esler MD. Renal sympathetic-nerve ablation for uncontrolled hypertension. *N Engl J Med.* 2009;361: 932–934.
109. Brenner BM, Falchuk KH, Keimowitz RI, Berliner RW. The relationship between peritubular capillary protein concentration and fluid reabsorption by the renal proximal tubule. *J Clin Invest.* 1969;48:1519–1531.
110. Brenner BM, Galla HH. Influence of postglomerular hematocrit and protein concentration on rat nephron fluid transfer. *Am J Physiol.* 1971;220:148–161.
111. Brenner BM, Troy JL. Postglomerular vascular protein concentration: evidence for causal role in governing fluid reabsorption in glomerulotubular balance by the renal proximal tubule. *J Clin Invest.* 1971;50:336–349.
112. Brenner BM, Troy JL, Daugharty TM, MacInnes RM. Quantitative importance of changes in postglomerular colloid osmotic pressure in mediating glomerulotubular balance in the rat. *J Clin Invest.* 1973;52:190–197.
113. Falchuk KH, Brenner BM, Tadokoro M, Berliner RW. Oncotic and hydrostatic pressure in peritubular capillaries and fluid reabsorption of proximal tubule. *Am J Physiol.* 1971;220:1427–1433.
114. Auld RB, Alexander EA, Levinsky NG. Proximal tubular function in dogs with thoracic caval constriction. *J Clin Invest.* 1971;50:2150–2158.
115. Mandin H. Cardiac edema in dogs. I. Proximal tubular and renal function. *Kidney Int.* 1976;10:185–192.
116. Rumrich G, Ullrich KJ. The minimum requirements for the maintenance of sodium chloride reabsorption in the proximal convolution of the mammalian kidney. *J Physiol.* 1968;197:69P–70P.
117. Lowitz HD, Stumpe KO, Ochwadt B. Micropuncture study of the action of angiotensin II on tubular sodium and water reabsorption in the rat. *Nephron.* 1969;6:173–187.
118. Bank N, Aynedjian HS, Wada T. Effect of peritubular capillary perfusion rate on proximal sodium reabsorption. *Kidney Int.* 1972;1:397–405.
119. Holzgreve H, Schrier RW. Effect of peritubular protein concentration on renal proximal tubular fluid reabsorption in the volume expanded rat. *Pflugers Arch.* 1972;332:R32.
120. Conger JD, Bartoli E, Earley LE. A study of in vivo peritubular oncotic pressure and proximal tubular reabsorption in the rat. *Clin Sci Mol Med.* 1976;51:379–392.
121. Ott CE, Haas JA, Cuche JL, Knox FG. Effect of increased peritubular protein concentration on proximal tubule reabsorption in the presence and absence of extracellular volume expansion. *J Clin Invest.* 1975;55:612–620.

122. Schneider EG, Dresser TP, Lynch RE, Knox FG. Sodium reabsorption by proximal tubules of dogs with experimental heart failure. *Am J Physiol.* 1971;220:952–957.
123. Levy M. Effects of acute volume expansion and altered hemodynamics on renal tubular function in chronic caval dogs. *J Clin Invest.* 1972;51:922–938.
124. Bell NH, Schedl HP, Bartter FC. An explanation for abnormal water retention and hypoosmolality in congestive heart failure. *Am J Med.* 1964;36:351–360.
125. Schrier RW, Lehman D, Zacherle B, Earley LE. Effect of furosemide on free water excretion in edematous patients with hyponatremia. *Kidney Int.* 1973;3:30–34.
126. Szatalowicz VL, Miller PD, Lacher JW, Gordon JA, Schrier RW. Comparative effect of diuretics on renal water excretion in hyponatremic edematous disorders. *Clin Sci (Lond).* 1982;62:235–238.
127. Werko L, Varnauskas E, Eliasch H, et al. Studies on the renal circulation and renal function in mitral valvular disease. I. Effect of exercise. *Circulation.* 1954;9:687–699.
128. Thomas JA, Marks BH. Plasma norepinephrine in congestive heart failure. *Am J Cardiol.* 1978;41:233–243.
129. Levine TB, Francis GS, Goldsmith SR, et al. Activity of the sympathetic nervous system and renin–angiotensin system assessed by plasma hormone levels and their relation to hemodynamic abnormalities in congestive heart failure. *Am J Cardiol.* 1982;49:1659–1666.
130. Davis D, Baily R, Zelis R. Abnormalities in systemic norepinephrine kinetics in human congestive heart failure. *Am J Physiol.* 1988;254:E760–766.
131. Abraham WT, Hensen J, Schrier RW. Elevated plasma noradrenaline concentrations in patients with low-output cardiac failure: dependence on increased noradrenaline secretion rates. *Clin Sci (Lond).* 1990;79:429–435.
132. Francis GS, Benedict C, Johnstone DE, et al. Comparison of neuroendocrine activation in patients with left ventricular dysfunction with and without congestive heart failure. A substudy of the Studies of Left Ventricular Dysfunction (SOLVD). *Circulation.* 1990;82:1724–1729.
133. Chidsey CA, Braunwald E, Morrow AG. Catecholamine excretion and cardiac stores of norepinephrine in congestive heart failure. *Am J Med.* 1965;39:442–451.
134. Cody RJ, Franklin KW, Kluger J, Laragh JH. Sympathetic responsiveness and plasma norepinephrine during therapy of congestive heart failure with captopril. *Am J Med.* 1981;72:791–797.
135. Leimbach WN Jr, Wallin BG, Victor RG, et al. Direct evidence from intraneural recordings for increased central sympathetic outflow in patients with heart failure. *Circulation.* 1986;73:913–919.
136. Adamson PB, Smith AL, Abraham WT, et al. Continuous autonomic assessment in patients with symptomatic heart failure: prognostic value of heart rate variability measured by an implanted cardiac resynchronization device. *Circulation.* 2004;110:2389–2394.
137. Lowes BD, Abraham WT, Bristow MR. Role of beta blockers in the treatment of heart failure. In: Braunwald E, ed. *Heart Disease: A Textbook of Cardiovascular Medicine—Update Summer 1994.* Philadelphia, PA: WB Saunders; 1994.
138. Dargie HJ. Effect of carvedilol on outcome after myocardial infarction in patients with left-ventricular dysfunction: the CAPRICORN randomised trial. *Lancet.* 2001;357:1385–1390.
139. Bristow MR, Gilbert E, Abraham W. Multicenter oral carvedilol assessment (MOCHA): a six-month dose-response evaluation in class II to IV patients. *Circulation.* 1995;92:I142.
140. Packer M, Bristow MR, Cohn JN, et al. The effect of carvedilol on morbidity and mortality in patients with chronic heart failure. *N Engl J Med* 1996;334:1349–1355.
141. CIBIS-II Investigators and Committees. The Cardiac Insufficiency Bisoprolol Study II (CIBIS-II): a randomized trial. *Lancet.* 1999;353:9.
142. Effect of metoprolol CR/XL in chronic heart failure: metoprolol CR/XL Randomised Intervention Trial in Congestive Heart Failure (MERIT-HF). *Lancet.* 1999;353:2001–2007.
143. Packer M, Coats AJS, Fowler MB, et al. Effect of carvedilol on survival in severe chronic heart failure. *N Engl J Med.* 2001;344:1651–1658.
144. Cohn JN, Levine TB, Olivari MT, et al. Plasma norepinephrine as a guide to prognosis in patients with chronic congestive heart failure. *N Engl J Med.* 1984;311:819–823.
145. DiBona GF, Herman PJ, Sawin LL. Neural control of renal function in edema-forming states. *Am J Physiol.* 1988;254:R1017–R1024.
146. Gill JR, Mason DT, Bartter FC. Adrenergic nervous system in sodium metabolism: effects of guanethidine and sodium-retaining steroids in normal man. *J Clin Invest.* 1964;43:177–184.
147. Abraham WT, Tsvetkova T, Lowes BD, et al. Carvedilol improves renal hemodynamics in patients with chronic heart failure. *Circulation.* 1998;98(suppl I):I-378–379.
148. Carpenter CC, Davis JO, Holman JE, Ayers CR, Bahn RC. Studies on the response of the transplanted kidney and transplanted adrenal gland to thoracic inferior vena caval constriction. *J Clin Invest.* 1961;40:196–204.
149. Mizelle HL, Hall JE, Montani JP. Role of renal nerves in control of sodium excretion in chronic congestive heart failure. *Am J Physiol.* 1989;256:F1084–1093.
150. Bøtker HE, Jensen HK, Krusell LR, Sørensen EV. Renal effects of xamoterol in patients with moderate heart failure. *Cardiovasc Drugs Ther.* 1993;7:111–116.
151. Thomsen K. Lithium clearance: a new method for determining proximal and distal tubular reabsorption of sodium and water. *Nephron.* 1984;37:217–223.
152. Eichhorn E, McGhie AL, Bedotto JB, et al. Effects of bucindolol on neurohormonal activation in congestive heart failure. *Am J Cardiol.* 1991;67:67–73.
153. Merrill AJ, Morrison JL, Brannon ES. Concentration of renin in renal venous blood in patients with chronic heart failure. *Am J Med.* 1946;1:468.
154. Watkins L Jr, Burton JA, Haber E, et al. The renin–angiotensin–aldosterone system in congestive heart failure in conscious dogs. *J Clin Invest.* 1976;57:1606–1617.
155. Lee WH, Packer M. Prognostic importance of serum sodium concentration and its modification by converting-enzyme inhibition in patients with severe chronic heart failure. *Circulation.* 1986;73:257–267.
156. Effects of enalapril on mortality in severe congestive heart failure: results of the Cooperative North Scandinavian Enalapril Survival Study (CONSENSUS). The CONSENSUS Trial Study Group. *N Engl J Med.* 1987;316:1429–1435.
157. Effect of enalapril on survival in patients with reduced left ventricular ejection fractions and congestive heart failure. The SOLVD Investigators. *N Engl J Med.* 1991;325:293–302.
158. Pfeffer MA, Braunwald E, Moyé LA, et al. Effect of captopril on mortality and morbidity in patients with left ventricular dysfunction after myocardial infarction. Results of the survival and ventricular enlargement trial. The SAVE Investigators. *N Engl J Med.* 1992;327:669–677.
159. Pfeffer MA, Swedberg K, Granger CB, et al. Effects of candesartan on mortality and morbidity in patients with chronic heart failure: the CHARM-Overall programme. *Lancet.* 2003;362:759–766.
160. Pfeffer MA, McMurray JV, Velazquez EJ, et al. Valsartan, captopril, or both in myocardial infarction complicated by heart failure, left ventricular dysfunction, or both. *N Engl J Med.* 2003;349:1893–1906.
161. Cohn JN, Tognoni G. A randomized trial of the angiotensin-receptor blocker valsartan in chronic heart failure. *N Engl J Med.* 2001;345:1667–1675.
162. Bristow MR, Abraham WT. Antiadrenergic effects of angiotensin converting enzyme inhibitors. *Eur Heart J.* 1995;16:37–41.
163. Hilgers KF, Veelken R, Rupprecht G, et al. Angiotensin II facilitates sympathetic transmission in rat hind limb circulation. *Hypertension.* 1993;21:322–328.
164. Clemson B, Gaul L, Gubin SS, et al. Prejunctional angiotensin II receptors: facilitation of norepinephrine release in the human forearm. *J Clin Invest.* 1994;93:684–691.
165. Abraham WT, Lowes BD, Rose CP, Larrabee P, Bristow MR. Angiotensin II selectively increases cardiac adrenergic activity in patients with heart failure [abstract]. *J Am Coll Cardiol.* 1994;23:215A.
166. Gilbert EM, Sandoval A, Larrabee P, et al. Lisinopril lowers cardiac adrenergic drive and increases β-receptor density in the failing human heart. *Circulation.* 1993;88:472–480.
167. Liu FY, Cogan MG. Angiotensin II: a potent regulator of acidification in the rat early proximal convoluted tubule. *J Clin Invest.* 1987;80:272–275.
168. Abassi ZA, Kelly G, Golomb E, et al. Losartan improves the natriuretic response to ANF in rats with high-output heart failure. *J Pharmacol Exper Ther.* 1994;268:224–230.
169. Cody RJ, Covit AB, Schaer GL, et al. Sodium and water balance in chronic congestive heart failure. *J Clin Invest.* 1986;77:1441–1452.
170. Pierpont GL, Francis GS, Cohn JN. Effect of captopril on renal function in patients with congestive heart failure. *Br Heart J.* 1981;46:522–527.
171. Motwani JG, Fenwick MK, Morton JJ, Struthers AD. Determinants of the initial effects of captopril on blood pressure, glomerular filtration rate, and natriuresis in mild-to-moderate chronic congestive heart failure secondary to coronary artery disease. *Am J Cardiol.* 1994;73:1191–1196.
172. Good JM, Brady AJ, Noormohamed FH, Oakley CM, Cleland JG. Effect of intense angiotensin II suppression on the diuretic response to furosemide during chronic ACE inhibition. *Circulation.* 1994;90:220–224.
173. Davis JO, Howell DS, Goodkind MJ, Hyatt RE. Accumulation of ascites during maintenance of adrenalectomized dogs with thoracic inferior vena cava constriction on a high sodium diet without hormone therapy. *Am J Physiol.* 1956;185:230–234.
174. Gill JR. Edema. *Annu Rev Med.* 1970;21:269–280.
175. Chonko AM, Bay WH, Stein JH, Ferris TF. The role of renin and aldosterone in the salt retention of edema. *Am J Med.* 1977;63:881–889.

176. Hensen J, Abraham WT, Dürr JA, Schrier RW. Aldosterone in congestive heart failure: analysis of determinants and role in sodium retention. *Am J Nephrol.* 1991;11:441–446.
177. Dahlström U, Karlsson E. Captopril and spironolactone therapy for refractory congestive heart failure. *Am J Cardiol.* 1993;71:29A–33A.
178. van Vliet AA, Donker AJ, Nauta JJ, Verheugt FW. Spironolactone in congestive heart failure refractory to high-dose loop diuretic and low-dose angiotensin-converting enzyme inhibitor. *Am J Cardiol.* 1993;71:21A–28A.
179. Pitt B, Zannad F, Remme WJ, et al. The effect of spironolactone on morbidity and mortality in patients with severe heart failure. Randomized Aldactone Evaluation Study Investigators. *N Engl J Med.* 1999;341:709–717.
180. Pitt B, Remme W, Zannad F, et al. Eplerenone, a selective aldosterone blocker, in patients with left ventricular dysfunction after myocardial infarction. *N Engl J Med.* 2003;348:1309–1321.
181. Goldsmith SR, Francis GS, Cowley AW Jr, Levine TB, Cohn JN. Increased plasma arginine vasopressin levels in patients with congestive heart failure. *J Am Coll Cardiol.* 1983;1:1385–1390.
182. Preibisz JJ, Sealey JE, Laragh JH, Cody RJ, Weksler BB. Plasma and platelet vasopressin in essential hypertension and congestive heart failure. *Hypertension.* 1983;5:129–138.
183. Pruszczynski W, Vahanian A, Ardaillou R, Acar J. Role of antidiuretic hormone in impaired water excretion of patients with congestive heart failure. *J Clin Endocrinol Metab.* 1984;58:599–605.
184. Riegger GA, Liebau G, Kochsie K. Antidiuretic hormone in congestive heart failure. *Am J Med.* 1982;72:49–52.
185. Rondeau E, de Lima J, Caillens H, et al. High plasma antidiuretic hormone in patients with cardiac failure: influence of age. *Miner Electrolyte Metab.* 1982;8:267–274.
186. Szatalowicz VL, Arnold PE, Chaimovitz C, et al. Radioimmunoassay of plasma arginine vasopressin in hyponatremic patients with congestive heart failure. *N Engl J Med.* 1981;305:263–266.
187. Goldsmith SR, Francis GS, Cowley AW Jr. Arginine vasopressin and the renal response to water loading in congestive heart failure. *Am J Cardiol.* 1986;58:295–299.
188. Uretsky BF, Verbalis JG, Generalovich T, Valdes A, Reddy PS. Plasma vasopressin response to osmotic and hemodynamic stimuli in heart failure. *Am J Physiol.* 1985;248:H396–402.
189. Guillon G, Butlen D, Cantau B, Barth T, Jard S. Kinetic and pharmacologic characterization of vasopressin membrane receptors from human kidney medulla: relation to adenylate cyclase activation. *Eur J Pharmacol.* 1982;85: 291–304.
190. Anderson RJ, Cadnapaphornchai P, Harbottle JA, McDonald KM, Schrier RW. Mechanism of effect of thoracic inferior vena cava constriction on renal water excretion. *J Clin Invest.* 1974;54:1473–1479.
191. Handelman W, Lum G, Schrier RW. Impaired water excretion in high output cardiac failure in the rat. *Clin Res.* 1979;27:173A.
192. Riegger GA, Liebau G, Bauer E, Kochsiek K. Vasopressin and renin in high output heart failure of rats: hemodynamic effects of elevated plasma hormone levels. *J Cardiovasc Pharmacol.* 1995;7:1–5.
193. Ishikawa S, Saito T, Okada K, Tsutsui K, Kuzuya T. Effect of vasopressin antagonist on renal water excretion in rats with inferior vena cava constriction. *Kidney Int.* 1986;30:49–55.
194. Yared A, Kon V, Brenner BM, et al. Role for vasopressin in rats with congestive heart failure. *Kidney Int.* 1985;27:337.
195. Fujita H, Yoshiyama M, Yamagishi H, et al. The effect of vasopressin V1 and V2 receptor antagonists on heart failure after myocardial infarction. *J Am Coll Cardiol.* 1995;25:234A.
196. Naitoh M, Suzuki H, Murakami M, et al. Effects of oral AVP receptor antagonists OPC-21268 and OPC-31260 on congestive heart failure in conscious dogs. *Am J Physiol.* 1994;267:H2245–2254.
197. Yamamura Y, Ogawa H, Yamashita H, et al. Characterization of a novel aquaretic agent, OPC-31260, as an orally effective, nonpeptide vasopressin V2 receptor antagonist. *Br J Pharmacol.* 1992;105:787–791.
198. Ohnishi A, Orita Y, Okahara R, et al. Potent aquaretic agent: a novel nonpeptide selective vasopressin 2 antagonist (OPC-31260) in men. *J Clin Invest.* 1993;92:2653–2659.
199. Kim JK, Michel JB, Soubrier F, et al. Arginine vasopressin gene expression in chronic cardiac failure in rats. *Kidney Int.* 1990;38:818–822.
200. Nielsen S, Terris J, Andersen D, et al. Congestive heart failure in rats is associated with increased expression and targeting of aquaporin-2 water channel in collecting duct. *Proc Natl Acad Sci USA.* 1997;94:5450–5455.
201. Xu DL, Martin PY, Ohara M, et al. Upregulation of aquaporin-2 water channel expression in chronic heart failure rat. *J Clin Invest.* 1997;99: 1500–1505.
202. Martin PY, Abraham WT, Lieming X, et al. Selective V2-receptor vasopressin antagonism decreases urinary aquaporin-2 excretion in patients with chronic heart failure. *J Am Soc Nephrol.* 1999;10:2165–2170.
203. Abraham WT, Suresh DP, Wagoner LE, et al. Effects of the V_{1a} and V_2 vasopressin receptor antagonist YM087 in hyponatremic patients with chronic heart failure (abstract). *J Cardiac Failure.* 1999;5(Suppl 1):51.
204. Abraham WT, Koren M, Bichet DG, et al. Treatment of hyponatremia in patients with SIADH or CHF with intravenous conivaptan (YM087), a new combined vasopressin V1a/V2 receptor antagonist [abstract]. *Eur Heart J.* 2000;21:345.
205. Abraham WT, Shamshirsaz AA, McFann K, Oren RM, Schrier RW. Aquaretic effect of lixivaptan, an oral non-peptide selective V2 receptor vasopressin antagonist, in NYHA class II and III heart failure patients. *J Am Coll Cardiol.* 2006;47:1615–1621.
206. Gheorghiade M, Gattis WA, O'Connor CM, et al. Effects of tolvaptan, a vasopressin antagonist, in patients hospitalized with worsening heart failure: a randomized controlled trial. *JAMA.* 2004;291:1963–1971.
207. Rai T, Sekine K, Kanno K, et al. Urinary excretion of aquaporin-2 water channel protein in human and rat. *J Am Soc Nephrol.* 1997;8:1357–1362.
208. Schrier RW, Gross P, Gheorghiade M, et al. Tolvaptan, a selective oral vasopressin V2-receptor antagonist, for hyponatremia. *N Engl J Med.* 2006;355: 2099–2112.
209. Konstam MA, Gheorghiade M, Burnett JC Jr, et al. Effects of oral tolvaptan in patients hospitalized for worsening heart failure: the EVEREST Outcome Trial. *JAMA.* 2007;297:1319–1331.
210. Good JM, Nihoyannopoulos P, Ghatei MA, et al. Elevated plasma endothelin concentrations in heart failure: an effect of angiotensin II? *Eur Heart J.* 1994;15:1634–1640.
211. Teerlink JR, Löffler BM, Hess P, et al. Role of endothelin in the maintenance of blood pressure in conscious rats with chronic heart failure: acute effects of the endothelin receptor antagonist Ro 470203 (bosentan). *Circulation.* 1994; 90:2510–2518.
212. Nord EP. Renal actions of endothelin. *Kidney Int.* 1993;44:451–463.
213. Motte S, van Beneden R, Mottet J, et al. Early activation of cardiac and renal endothelin systems in experimental heart failure. *Am J Physiol Heart Circ Physiol.* 2003;285:H2482–2491.
214. Schirger JA, Chen HH, Jougasaki M, et al. Endothelin A receptor antagonism in experimental congestive heart failure results in augmentation of the renin-angiotensin system and sustained sodium retention. *Circulation.* 2004; 109:249–254.
215. Bauersachs J, Braun C, Fraccarollo D, et al. Improvement of renal dysfunction in rats with chronic heart failure after myocardial infarction by treatment with the endothelin A receptor antagonist, LU 135252. *J Hypertens.* 2000; 18:1507–1514.
216. Ohnishi M, Wada A, Tsutamoto T, et al. Significant roles of endothelin-A- and -B-receptors in renal function in congestive heart failure. *J Cardiovasc Pharmacol.* 2000;36(Suppl 1):S140–143.
217. Abassi Z, Francis B, Wessale J, et al. Effects of endothelin receptors ET(A) and ET(B) blockade on renal haemodynamics in normal rats and in rats with experimental congestive heart failure. *Clin Sci (Lond).* 2002;103(Suppl 48): 245S–248S.
218. Abraham WT, et al. Effects of enrasentan, a nonselective endothelin receptor antagonist, in class II-III heart failure: results of the Enrasentan Cooperative Randomized (ENCOR) Evaluation. Presented at: Late-Breaking Clinical Trials Session, 50th Annual Scientific Session of the American College of Cardiology; March 21, 2001; Orlando, FL.
219. Bates ER, Shenker Y, Grekin RJ. The relationship between plasma levels of immunoreactive atrial natriuretic hormone and hemodynamic function in man. *Circulation.* 1986;73:1155–1161.
220. Burnett JC Jr, Kao PC, Hu DC, et al. Atrial natriuretic peptide elevation in congestive heart failure in the human. *Science.* 1986;231:1145–1147.
221. Hirata Y, Ishii M, Matsuoka H, et al. Plasma concentration of alpha-human atrial natriuretic polypeptide and cyclic GMP in patients with heart disease. *Am Heart J.* 1987;113:1463–1469.
222. Michel JB, Arnal JF, Corvol P. Atrial natriuretic factor as a marker in congestive heart failure. *Horm Res.* 1990;34:166–168.
223. Nakaoka H, Imataka K, Amano M, et al. Plasma levels of atrial natriuretic factor in patients with congestive heart failure. *N Engl J Med.* 1985;313: 892–893.
224. Raine AE, Erne P, Bürgisser E, et al. Atrial natriuretic peptide and atrial pressure in patients with congestive heart failure. *N Engl J Med.* 1986;315: 533–537.
225. Mukoyama M, Nakao K, Saito Y, et al. Increased human brain natriuretic peptide in congestive heart failure. *N Engl J Med.* 1990;323:757–758.

226. Atlas SA, Kleinert HD, Camargo MJ, et al. Purification, sequencing, and synthesis of natriuretic and vasoactive rat atrial peptide. *Nature.* 1984;309:717–719.
227. Currie MG, Geller DM, Cole BR, et al. Bioactive cardiac substances: potent vasorelaxant activity in mammalian atria. *Science.* 1983;221:71–73.
228. Molina CR, Fowler MB, McCrory S, et al. Hemodynamic, renal, and endocrine effects of atrial natriuretic peptide in severe heart failure. *J Am Coll Cardiol.* 1988;12:175–186.
229. Atarashi K, Mulrow PJ, Franco-Saenz R, Snajdar R, Rapp J. Inhibition of aldosterone production by an atrial extract. *Science.* 1984;224:992–994.
230. Samson WK. Atrial natriuretic factor inhibits dehydration and hemorrhage-induced vasopressin release. *Neuroendocrinology.* 1985;40:277–279.
231. Floras JS. Sympathoinhibitory effects of atrial natriuretic factor in normal humans. *Circulation.* 1990;81:1860–1873.
232. Cody RJ, Atlas SA, Laragh JH, et al. Atrial natriuretic factor in normal subjects and heart failure patients: plasma levels and renal, hormonal, and hemodynamic responses to peptide infusion. *J Clin Invest.* 1986;78:1362–1374.
233. Sato F, Kamoi K, Wakiya Y, et al. Relationship between plasma atrial natriuretic peptide levels and atrial pressure in man. *J Endocrinol Metab.* 1986;63:823–827.
234. Hensen J, Abraham WT, Lesnefsky EJ, et al. Atrial natriuretic peptide kinetic studies in patients with cardiac dysfunction. *Kidney Int.* 1992;42:1333–1339.
235. Saito Y, Nakao K, Arai H, et al. Atrial natriuretic polypeptide (ANP) in human ventricle: increased gene expression of ANP in dilated cardiomyopathy. *Biochem Biophys Res Commun.* 1987;148:211–217.
236. Hosoda K, Nakao K, Mukoyama M, et al. Expression of brain natriuretic peptide gene in human heart: production in the ventricle. *Hypertension.* 1991;17:1152–1155.
237. Redfield MM, Edwards BS, McGoon MD, et al. Failure of atrial natriuretic factor to increase with volume expansion in acute and chronic heart failure in the dog. *Circulation.* 1989;80:651–657.
238. Drexler H, Hirth C, Stasch HP, et al. Vasodilatory action of endogenous atrial natriuretic factor in a rat model of chronic heart failure as determined by monoclonal ANF antibody. *Circ Res.* 1990;66:1371–1380.
239. Colucci WS, Elkayam U, Horton DP, et al. Intravenous nesiritide, a natriuretic peptide, in the treatment of decompensated congestive heart failure. The nesiritide study group. *N Engl J Med.* 2000;343:246–253.
240. Publication Committee for the VMAC Investigators (Vasodilatation in the Management of Acute CHF). Intravenous nesiritide vs nitroglycerin for treatment of decompensated congestive heart failure: a randomized controlled trial. *JAMA.* 2002;287:1531–1540.
241. Biollaz J, Nussberger J, Porchet M, et al. Four-hour infusion of synthetic atrial natriuretic peptide in normal volunteers. *Hypertension.* 1986;8:II96–105.
242. Borenstein HB, Cupples WA, Sonnenberg H, Veress AT. The effect of natriuretic atrial extract on renal hemodynamics and urinary excretion in anesthetized rats. *J Physiol.* 1983;334:133–140.
243. Dunn BR, Ichikawa I, Pfeffer JM, Troy JL, Brenner BM. Renal and systemic hemodynamic effects of synthetic atrial natriuretic peptide in the anesthetized rat. *Circ Res.* 1986;58:237–246.
244. Kim JK, Summer SN, Durr J, Schrier RW. Enzymatic and binding effects of atrial natriuretic factor in glomeruli and nephrons. *Kidney Int.* 1989;35:799–805.
245. Koseki C, et al. Localization of binding sites for alpha-rat atrial natriuretic polypeptide in rat kidney. *Am J Physiol.* 1986;250:F210–216.
246. Healy DP, Fanestil DD. Localization of atrial natriuretic peptide binding sites within the rat kidney. *Am J Physiol.* 1986;250:F573–578.
247. Hoffman A, Grossman E, Keiser HR. Increased plasma levels and blunted effects of brain natriuretic peptide in rats with congestive heart failure. *Am J Hypertens.* 1991;4:597–601.
248. Yoshimura M, Yasue H, Morita E, et al. Hemodynamic, renal, and hormonal responses to brain natriuretic peptide infusion in patients with congestive heart failure. *Circulation.* 1991;84:1581–1588.
249. Gelfand RA, Frank HJ, Levin E, Pedram A. Brain and atrial natriuretic peptides bind to common receptors in brain capillary endothelial cells. *Am J Physiol.* 1991;261:E183–189.
250. Abraham WT, Lowes BD, Ferguson DA, et al. Systemic hemodynamic, neurohormonal, and renal effects of a steady-state infusion of human brain natriuretic peptide in patients with hemodynamically decompensated heart failure. *J Card Fail.* 1998;4:37–44.
251. Wang D, Dowling TC, Meadows D, et al. Nesiritide does not improve renal function in patients with chronic heart failure and worsening serum creatinine. *Circulation.* 2004;110:1620–1625.
252. Sackner-Bernstein JD, Skopicki HA, Aaronson KD. Risk of worsening renal function with nesiritide in patients with acutely decompensated heart failure. *Circulation.* 2005;111:1487–1491.
253. O'Connor CM, Starling RC, Hernandez AF, et al. Effect of nesiritide on patients with acute decompensated heart failure. *N Engl J Med.* 2011;365:32–43.
254. Elsner D, Muders F, Müntze A, et al. Efficacy of prolonged infusion of urodilatin (ANP[95–126]) in patients with congestive heart failure. *Am Heart J.* 1995;129:766–773.
255. Feller SM, Gagelmann M, Forssmann WG. Urodilatin: a newly described member of the ANP family. *Trends Pharmacol Sci.* 1989;10:93–94.
256. Drummer C, Fiedler F, König A, Gerzer R. Urodilatin, a kidney-derived natriuretic factor, is excreted with a circadian rhythm and is stimulated by saline infusion in man. *J Am Soc Nephrol.* 1991;2:1109–1113.
257. Saxenhofer H, Raselli A, Weidmann P, et al. Urodilatin, a natriuretic factor from kidneys, can modify renal and cardiovascular function in men. *Am J Physiol.* 1990;259:F832–838.
258. Gagelmann M, Hock D, Forssmann WG. Urodilatin (CDD/ANP-95–126) is not biologically inactivated by a peptidase from dog kidney cortex membranes in contrast to atrial natriuretic peptide/cardiodilatin (alpha-hANP/CDD-99–126). *FEBS Lett.* 1988;233:249–254.
259. Forssmann WG, Richter R, Meyer M. The endocrine heart and natriuretic peptides: histochemistry, cell biology, and functional aspects of the renal urodilatin system. *Histochem Cell Biol.* 1998;110:335–357.
260. Levin ER, Frank HJ, Chaudhari A, et al. Decreased atrial natriuretic factor receptors and impaired cGMP generation in glomeruli from the cardiomyopathic hamster. *Biochem Biophys Res Commun.* 1989;159:807–814.
261. Schiffrin EL. Decreased density of binding sites for atrial natriuretic peptide on platelets of patients with severe congestive heart failure. *Clin Sci (Lond).* 1988;74:213–218.
262. Gutkowska J, Genest J, Thibault G, et al. Circulating forms and radioimmunoassay of atrial natriuretic factor. *Endocrinol Metab Clin North Am.* 1987;16:183–198.
263. Wilkins MR, Settle SL, Stockmann PT, Needleman P. Maximizing the natriuretic effect of endogenous atriopeptin in a rat model of heart failure. *Proc Natl Acad Sci USA.* 1990;87:6465–6469.
264. Salerno F, Badalamenti S, Incerti P, Capozza L, Mainardi L. Renal response to atrial natriuretic peptide in patients with advanced liver cirrhosis. *Hepatology.* 1988;8:21–26.
265. Huang CL, Ives HE, Cogan MG. In vivo evidence that cGMP is the second messenger for atrial natriuretic factor. *Proc Natl Acad Sci USA.* 1986;83:8015–8018.
266. Abraham WT, Hensen J, Kim JK, et al. Atrial natriuretic peptide and urinary cyclic guanosine monophosphate in patients with chronic heart failure. *J Am Soc Nephrol.* 1992;2:1697–1703.
267. Abraham WT, Lauwaars ME, Kim JK, Peña RL, Schrier RW. Reversal of atrial natriuretic peptide resistance by increasing distal tubular sodium delivery in patients with decompensated cirrhosis. *Hepatology.* 1995;22:737–743.
268. Connelly TP, Francis GS, Williams KJ, Beltran AM, Cohn JN. Interaction of intravenous atrial natriuretic factor with furosemide in patients with heart failure. *Am Heart J.* 1994;127:392–399.
269. Koepke JP, DiBona GF. Blunted natriuresis to atrial natriuretic peptide in chronic sodium-retaining disorders. *Am J Physiol.* 1987;252:F865–871.
270. Mullens W, Abrahams Z, Francis GS, et al. Importance of venous congestion for worsening of renal function in advanced decompensated heart failure. *J Am Coll Cardiol.* 2009;53:589–596.
271. Damman K, van Deursen VM, Navis G, et al. Increased central venous pressure is associated with impaired renal function and mortality in a broad spectrum of patients with cardiovascular disease. *J Am Coll Cardiol.* 2009;53:582–588.
272. Testani JM, Khera AV, St. John Sutton MG, et al. Effect of right ventricular function and venous congestion on cardiorenal interactions during the treatment of decompensated heart failure. *Am J Cardiol.* 2010;105:511–516.
273. Abraham WT, Fonarow GC, Albert NM, et al. Predictors of in-hospital mortality in patients hospitalized for heart failure: insights from the Organized Program to Initiate Lifesaving Treatment in Hospitalized Patients with Heart Failure (OPTIMIZE-HF). *J Am Coll Cardiol.* 2008;52:347–356.
274. Velazquez EJ, Lee KL, Deja MA, et al. Coronary-artery bypass surgery in patients with left ventricular dysfunction. *N Engl J Med.* 2011;364:1607–1616.
275. Bonow RO, Maurer G, Lee KL, et al. Myocardial viability and survival in ischemic left ventricular dysfunction. *N Engl J Med.* 2011:364:1617–1625.
276. Leon MB, Smith CR, Mack M, et al. Transcatheter aortic-valve implantation for aortic stenosis in patients who cannot undergo surgery. *N Engl J Med.* 2010;363:1597–1607.
277. Arnold SB, Byrd RC, Meister W, et al. Long-term digitalis therapy improves left ventricular function in heart failure. *N Engl J Med.* 1980;303:1443–1448.

278. The effect of digoxin on mortality and morbidity in patients with heart failure. The Digitalis Investigation Group. *N Engl J Med.* 1997;336:525–533.
279. Ader R, Chatterjee K, Ports T, et al. Immediate and sustained hemodynamic and clinical improvement in chronic heart failure by an oral angiotensin-converting enzyme inhibitor. *Circulation.* 1980;61:931–937.
280. Taylor AL, Ziesche S, Yancy C, et al. Combination of isosorbide dinitrate and hydralazine in blacks with heart failure. *N Engl J Med.* 2004;351: 2049–2057.
281. Packer M, Carver JR, Rodeheffer RJ, et al. Effect of oral milrinone on mortality in severe chronic heart failure. *N Engl J Med.* 1991;325:1468–1475.
282. Feldman AM, Bristow MR, Parmley WW, et al. Effects of vesnarinone on morbidity and mortality in patients with heart failure. *N Engl J Med.* 1993;329:149–155.
283. Cohn JN, Goldstein SO, Greenberg BH, et al. A dose-dependent increase in mortality with vesnarinone among patients with severe heart failure. *N Engl J Med.* 1998;339:1810–1816.
284. Eichhorn E, Ventura H, Koch B, et al. Beta-Blocker Evaluation of Survival Trial (BEST) findings show benefit of bucindolol in moderate to severe HF patients, according to pre-specified statistical analysis plan. Poster presented at: 72nd Annual Scientific Sessions of the American Heart Association; November 7–10, 1999; Atlanta, GA.
285. Abraham WT, Fisher WG, Smith AL, et al., Cardiac resynchronization in chronic heart failure. *N Engl J Med.* 2002;346:1845–1853.
286. Young JB, Abraham WT, Smith AL, et al. Combined cardiac resynchronization and implantable cardioversion defibrillation in advanced chronic heart failure: the MIRACLE ICD Trial. *JAMA.* 2003;289:2685–2694.
287. Bristow MR, Saxon LA, Boehmer J, et al. Cardiac-resynchronization therapy with or without an implantable defibrillator in advanced chronic heart failure. *N Engl J Med.* 2004;350:2140–2150.
288. Cleland JG, Daubert JC, Erdmann E, et al. The effect of cardiac resynchronization on morbidity and mortality in heart failure. *N Engl J Med.* 2005;352: 1539–1549.
289. Linde C, Abraham WT, Gold MR, et al. Randomized trial of cardiac resynchronization in mildly symptomatic heart failure patients and in asymptomatic patients with left ventricular dysfunction and previous heart failure symptoms. *J Am Coll Cardiol.* 2008;52:1834–1843.
290. Moss AJ, Hall WJ, Cannom DS, et al. Cardiac-resynchronization therapy for the prevention of heart-failure events. *N Engl J Med.* 2009;361:1329–1338.
291. Tang AS, Wells GA, Talajic M, et al. Cardiac-resynchronization therapy for mild-to-moderate heart failure. *N Engl J Med.* 2010;363:2385–2395.
292. Boerrigter G, Costello-Boerrigter LC, Abraham WT, et al. Cardiac resynchronization therapy improves renal function in human heart failure with reduced glomerular filtration rate. *J Card Fail.* 2008;14:539–546.
293. Agostoni PG, De Cesare N, Doria E, et al. Afterload reduction: a comparison of captopril and nifedipine in dilated cardiomyopathy. *Br Heart J.* 1986;55:391–399.
294. Swedberg K, Eneroth P, Kjekshus J, Wilhelmsen L. Hormones regulating cardiovascular function in patients with severe congestive heart failure and their relation to mortality. *Circulation.* 1990;82:1730–1736.
295. Hunt SA, et al. ACC/AHA guidelines for the evaluation and management of chronic heart failure in the adult: executive summary: a report of the American College of Cardiology/American Heart Association Task Force on Practice Guidelines (Committee to revise the 2001 Guidelines for the Evaluation and Management of Heart Failure). *J Am Coll Cardiol.* 2005;46:1116.
296. Francis GS, Siegel RM, Goldsmith SR, et al. Acute vasoconstrictor response to intravenous furosemide in patients with chronic congestive heart failure. Activation of the neurohumoral axis. *Ann Intern Med.* 1985;103:1–6.
297. Ritzema J, Troughton R, Melton I, et al. Physician-directed patient self-management of left atrial pressure in advanced chronic heart failure. *Circulation.* 2010;121:1086–1095.
298. Abraham WT, Adamson PB, Bourge RC, et al. Wireless pulmonary artery haemodynamic monitoring in chronic heart failure: a randomised controlled trial. *Lancet.* 2011;377:658–666.
299. Gottlieb SS, Brater DC, Thomas I, et al. BG9719 (CVT-124), an adenosine A1 receptor antagonist, protects against the decline in renal function observed with diuretic therapy. *Circulation.* 2002;105:1348–1353.
300. DiLeo M, Pacitti A, Bergerone S, et al. Ultrafiltration in the treatment of refractory congestive heart failure. *Clin Cardiol.* 1988;11:449–452.
301. Marenzi G, Grazi S, Giraldi F, et al. Interrelation of humoral factors, hemodynamics, and fluid and salt metabolism in congestive heart failure: effects of extracorporeal ultrafiltration. *Am J Med.* 1993;94:49–56.
302. Agostoni P, Marenzi G, Lauri G, et al. Sustained improvement in functional capacity after removal of body fluid with isolated ultrafiltration in chronic cardiac insufficiency: failure of furosemide to provide the same result. *Am J Med.* 1994;96:191–199.
303. Canaud B, Leblanc M, Leray-Moragues H, et al. Slow continuous and daily ultrafiltration for refractory congestive heart failure. *Nephrol Dial Transplant.* 1998;13:51–55.
304. Jaski BE, Ha J, Denys BG, et al. Peripherally inserted veno-venous ultrafiltration for rapid treatment of volume overloaded patients. *J Card Fail.* 2003;9:227–231.
305. Costanzo MR, Guglin ME, Saltzberg MT, et al. Ultrafiltration versus intravenous diuretics for patients hospitalized for acute decompensated heart failure. *J Am Coll Cardiol.* 2007;49:675–683.
306. Dzau VJ, Hollenberg NK. Renal response to captopril in severe heart failure: role of furosemide in natriuresis and reversal of hyponatremia. *Ann Intern Med.* 1984;100:777–782.
307. Packer M, Medina M, Yushak M. Correction of dilutional hyponatremia in severe chronic heart failure by converting-enzyme inhibition. *Ann Intern Med.* 1984;100:782–789.
308. Gauer OH, Henry JP, Behn C. The regulation of extracellular fluid volume. *Annu Rev Physiol.* 1970;32:547–595.

CHAPTER

68 Liver Disease and the Kidney

Pere Ginès • Andrés Cárdenas • Elsa Solà • Robert W. Schrier

The presence of abnormalities of kidney function in patients with liver diseases has been recognized for several decades.[1] More than a century ago, Frerichs in Europe and Flint in the United States reported the association between liver diseases and kidney dysfunction.[2,3] These reports described the development of oliguria in patients with chronic liver disease in the setting of normal kidney histology and proposed the first pathophysiologic interpretation of kidney dysfunction in liver disease by linking the abnormalities in kidney function to disturbances in the systemic circulation. Since then, the relationship between the liver and kidney function has been the object of a considerable amount of research and substantial progress has been made in the last two decades with regard to the pathophysiology and management of renal dysfunction in liver diseases. Several books have been published specifically devoted to this topic.[4–13]

Most derangements of renal function in liver diseases occur in patients with cirrhosis and are pathophysiologically related to the presence of an expanded extracellular fluid volume which leads to the development of ascites and/or edema. This chapter deals with the pathophysiology, clinical features, and treatment of ascites and renal functional abnormalities in cirrhosis. The abnormalities in kidney function due to other liver diseases are not discussed.

RENAL ABNORMALITIES IN CIRRHOSIS

Most abnormalities of kidney function in cirrhosis are of functional origin (i.e., they occur in the absence of significant alterations in kidney histology).[14–18] These abnormalities are usually referred to as functional renal abnormalities, as opposed to nonfunctional renal abnormalities, which may also develop in patients with cirrhosis (i.e., glomerulonephritis).

The most common functional renal abnormalities in cirrhotic patients are an impaired ability to excrete sodium, an impaired ability to excrete solute-free water, and a reduction of the glomerular filtration rate (GFR) secondary to vasoconstriction of the renal circulation. Sodium retention is a key factor in the expansion of the extracellular fluid volume and development of ascites and edema, whereas solute-free water retention is responsible for dilutional hyponatremia. Renal vasoconstriction, when severe, leads to hepatorenal syndrome (HRS). Chronologically, sodium retention is the earliest alteration of kidney function observed in patients with cirrhosis, whereas dilutional hyponatremia and HRS are late findings. In most patients, abnormalities of kidney function usually worsen with time as the liver disease progresses. However, in some patients, a spontaneous improvement or even normalization of sodium and solute-free water excretion may occur during the course of their disease.[19–21] This improvement in renal function occurs particularly in patients with alcoholic cirrhosis after abstinence from alcohol. Spontaneous improvement of renal function after the development of type-1 HRS (see later) is extremely unusual.[22,23]

Sodium Retention and Ascites

Sodium retention is the most frequent abnormality of kidney function in patients with cirrhosis and ascites. The existence of sodium retention in cirrhosis was first documented more than 60 years ago when methods to measure electrolyte concentration in organic fluids became available.[24–26] Since then, it has been well established that sodium retention plays a key role in the pathophysiology of ascites and edema formation in cirrhosis. The amount of sodium retained within the body is dependent on the balance between the sodium ingested in the diet and the sodium excreted in the urine. As long as the amount of sodium excreted is lower than that ingested, patients accumulate ascites and/or edema. The important role of sodium retention in the pathogenesis of ascites formation is supported by the fact that ascites can disappear just by reducing the dietary sodium content in some patients or by increasing the urinary sodium excretion with the administration of diuretics in others.[26,27] Conversely, a high-sodium diet or diuretic withdrawal leads to the reaccumulation of ascites.[25,26] The achievement of a negative sodium balance (i.e., excretion higher than intake) is the essence of pharmacologic therapy of ascites. Although no studies assessing the chronologic relationship between sodium retention and the formation of ascites have been performed in patients with cirrhosis, studies in experimental animals have provided conclusive evidence indicating that sodium retention precedes ascites formation, further emphasizing the important role of this abnormality of renal function in the pathogenesis of ascites in cirrhosis.[28–32] This observation suggests that sodium retention is the cause and not the consequence of ascites formation in cirrhosis.

The severity of sodium retention in cirrhosis with ascites varies considerably from patient to patient. Some patients have relatively high urinary sodium excretion, whereas urine sodium concentrations are very low or even undetectable in others (Fig. 68.1). The proportion of patients with marked sodium retention depends on the population of cirrhotic patients considered. Most patients who require hospitalization because of severe ascites have marked sodium retention (less than 10 mEq per day). Sodium retention is particularly intense in patients with ascites refractory to diuretic treatment.[33,34] By contrast, in a population of cirrhotic patients with mild or moderate ascites, the proportion of patients with marked sodium retention is low and most patients excrete more than 10 mEq per day spontaneously (without diuretic therapy). The response to diuretic treatment is usually better in patients with moderate sodium retention than in those with marked sodium retention.[27,35,36]

Nephron Sites of Sodium Retention

In healthy subjects approximately 95% of filtered sodium is reabsorbed in the renal tubules. Approximately 60% to 70% is absorbed in the proximal tubules, another 30% to 40% gets absorbed in the thick ascending limb, and 5% to 10% of sodium is reabsorbed in the collecting ducts.[37]

In many instances, sodium retention in cirrhosis is due to increased tubular reabsorption of sodium because it occurs in the presence of normal or only moderately reduced GFR.[27,38] The exact contribution of the different segments of the nephron to this increased sodium reabsorption is not completely known. Micropuncture studies in rats with cirrhosis and ascites have demonstrated an enhanced reabsorption of sodium in the proximal tubule.[28,39] On the other hand, it has been shown that the development of a positive sodium balance and the formation of ascites in cirrhotic rats can be prevented by aldosterone antagonists, which suggests that the collecting ducts are important sites of the increased sodium reabsorption in experimental cirrhosis.[31,40,41] Studies assessing the protein abundance of renal tubular sodium transporters in rats with CCL_4– induced cirrhosis showed an increased expression of the sodium chloride cotransporters of the distal tubule (NCC/TSC) and the epithelial sodium channel of the collecting duct (ENaC), both of which are regulated by aldosterone, consistent with a major role of hyperaldosteronism in sodium retention in this animal model.[41] An increased abundance of the Na^+-K^+-$2Cl^-$ cotransporter of the thick ascending limb (NKCC/BSC1) and a decreased abundance of the proximal sodium transporters (sodium hydrogen exchanger type 3–NH-3, and sodium phosphate cotransporter isoform 2–NaPi-2) was also found, consistent with increased sodium reabsorption in the ascending limb of the loop of Henle and reduced reabsorption in the proximal tubule.[41] Other factors such as the influence of calcium on the bumetanide-sensitive $Na^+K^+2Cl^-$ cotransporter (BSC-1) located in the luminal membrane of epithelial cells lining the thick ascending limb of the loop of Henle may play a role in sodium retention.[41]

Investigations in patients with cirrhosis have also provided discrepant findings as to the most important nephron site of sodium retention. Results from earlier studies using sodium, water, or phosphate clearances to estimate the tubular handling of sodium suggest that the distal nephron is the main site of sodium retention.[42–45] Results of studies using lithium clearance, which estimates sodium reabsorption

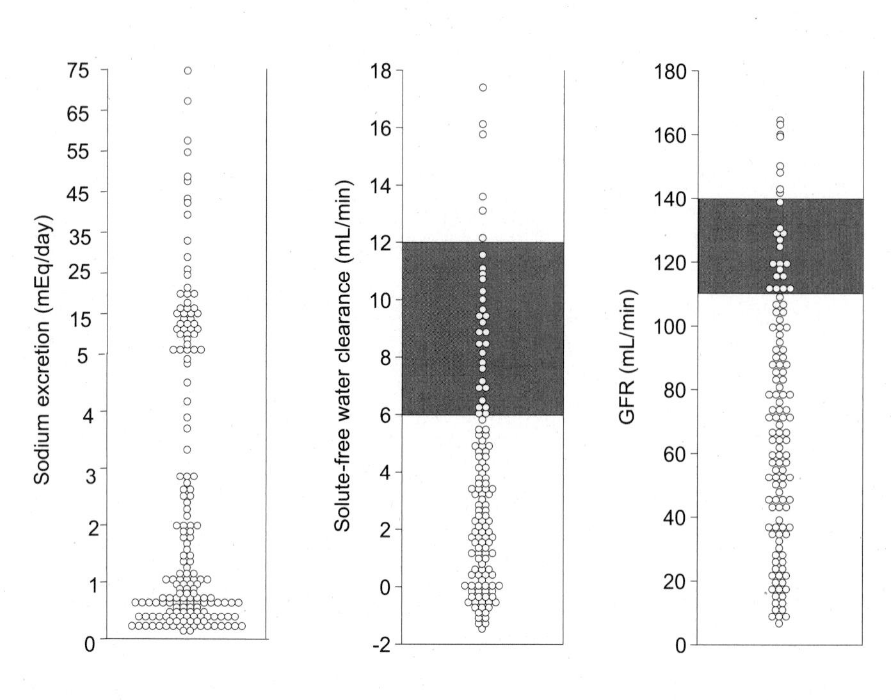

FIGURE 68.1 Individual values of sodium excretion, solute-free water clearance, and glomerular filtration rate in a large series of patients with cirrhosis and ascites without diuretic therapy and under a low-sodium diet. Lines indicate normal ranges. For urine sodium normal range is 80 to 100 mEq per day.

in the proximal tubule, suggest that cirrhotic patients with ascites show a marked increase in proximal sodium reabsorption.[46,47] Nevertheless, distal sodium reabsorption is also increased, especially in patients with more avid sodium retention.[47] Clinical studies using spironolactone to antagonize the mineralocorticoid receptor indicate that this agent induces natriuresis in a large proportion of cirrhotic patients with ascites without renal failure, which supports a major role for increased sodium reabsorption in distal sites of the nephron in these patients.[36,48–51] Taken together, these results suggest that in patients with cirrhosis without renal failure, an enhanced reabsorption of sodium in both proximal and distal tubules contributes to sodium retention. Potential mediators of this increased sodium reabsorption include changes in the hydrostatic and colloidosmotic pressures in the peritubular capillaries and increased activity of the sympathetic nervous system and the renin–angiotensin–aldosterone system (RAAS). Sodium retention is usually more marked in patients with renal failure than in those without renal failure due to both a reduction in filtered sodium load and a more marked activation of sodium-retaining mechanisms.

Clinical Consequences

Because sodium is retained together with water isoosmotically in the kidneys, sodium retention is associated with fluid retention, leading to expansion of extracellular fluid volume and increased amount of fluid in the interstitial tissue. In some patients with advanced cirrhosis, the total extracellular fluid volume may increase up to 40 L or even more (compared to the average 14 L in a 70–kg healthy adult), which represents an approximate cumulative gain of 3,400 mEq of sodium (26 L of excess extracellular fluid volume times 130 mEq per L). In most patients with advanced cirrhosis, sodium retention is manifested by the development of ascites. The most common clinical symptom of ascites is discomfort due to abdominal swelling. In cases with marked accumulation of fluid, physical activity and respiratory function may be impaired. Other clinical consequences related to the presence of ascites are the appearance of abdominal wall hernias and hydrocele and spontaneous infection of ascitic fluid (also known as spontaneous bacterial peritonitis).[52] These complications, especially infection, contribute markedly to the increased morbidity and mortality associated with the presence of ascites.

Accumulation of fluid in the subcutaneous tissue, as edema, is also common in patients with cirrhosis and sodium retention and in most cases occurs concomitantly with the existence of ascites. Edema is most commonly observed in the lower extremities, but generalized edema may occur as well. Mild or moderate pedal edema may decrease or even disappear during bed rest and reappear during the daytime, reflecting an increased natriuresis in the supine position as compared with the upright position.[53,54] Both hypoalbuminemia and increased venous pressure in the inferior vena cava due either to constriction of the vena cava within the liver or increased intra-abdominal pressure caused by ascites may contribute to the high incidence of edema in cirrhotic patients with ascites. Leg edema may occur in patients with cirrhosis treated with either surgical portacaval shunts or transjugular intrahepatic portosystemic shunts (TIPS), presumably because of the increased pressure in the inferior vena cava secondary to these procedures.

Other clinical manifestations of sodium retention in cirrhosis include pleural and/or pericardial effusions. Hepatic hydrothorax is defined as a pleural effusion in patients with cirrhosis without associated cardiac and/or pulmonary disease. This complication occurs in approximately 10% of patients with cirrhosis.[55,56] In most cases the effusion is mild or moderate, more frequent on the right side, and associated with the presence of ascites. Left-sided effusions are uncommon. Occasionally, large right pleural effusions may exist in the absence of clinically evident ascites and constitute the main manifestation of the disease.[56,57] These pleural effusions are very difficult to manage, usually recur after therapy, and are due to the existence of anatomic defects in the diaphragm which cause a communication between the peritoneal and pleural cavities. The gradient between the positive intra-abdominal pressure and the negative intrathoracic pressure explains the passage of the fluid formed in the peritoneal cavity to the pleural cavity. Although less commonly than ascitic fluid, pleural fluid may also become infected spontaneously, a condition known as spontaneous bacterial empyema.[58] Finally, between one and two thirds of cirrhotic patients with ascites also have mild or moderate pericardial effusions as demonstrated by echocardiography.[59] These disappear after the elimination of ascites and are not associated with clinical symptoms.

Assessment of Sodium Excretion in Clinical Practice

The assessment of the urinary excretion of sodium is very useful in the clinical management of patients with cirrhosis and ascites because it allows the precise quantification of sodium retention. Urine must be collected under conditions of fixed and controlled sodium intake (usually a low-sodium diet of approximately 90 mEq per day during the previous 5 to 7 days), as sodium intake may influence sodium excretion. Although the measurement of sodium concentration in a spot of urine may provide a rough estimate of sodium excretion, the assessment of sodium excretion in a 24–hour period is preferable because it is more representative of sodium excretion throughout the day and takes into account the urine output.

In clinical practice, sodium excretion should be measured without diuretic therapy when patients with ascites are first seen or when there are signs suggestive of disease progression (e.g., marked increase in ascites or edema despite compliance with the sodium-restricted diet and diuretic therapy). Baseline sodium excretion is one of the best predictors of the response to diuretic treatment and is very helpful to establish the therapeutic schedule in cirrhotic patients with ascites. Patients with marked sodium retention

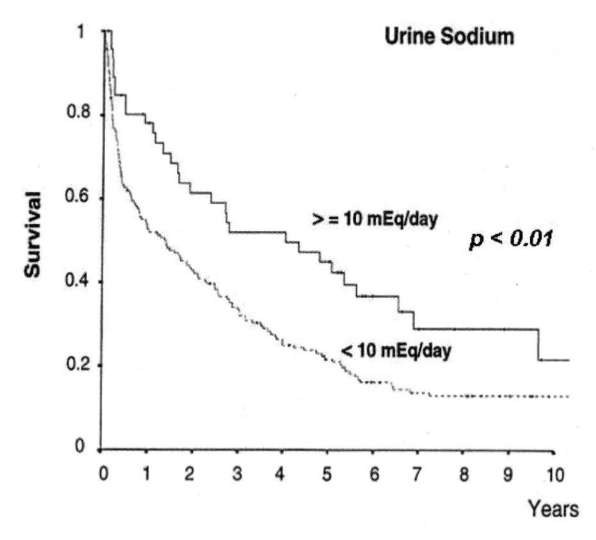

FIGURE 68.2 Long-term survival according to sodium excretion in a series of 204 patients with cirrhosis admitted to the hospital for the treatment of ascites.

(i.e., urine sodium <10 mEq per day) in whom a positive sodium balance is anticipated despite a restriction in sodium intake should be started on moderately high doses of aldosterone antagonists (e.g., spironolactone 100 to 200 mg per day) alone or in association with loop diuretics (e.g., furosemide 40 mg per day). Conversely, patients with moderate sodium retention (i.e., urine sodium >10 mEq per day) would likely respond to low doses of aldosterone antagonists (i.e., spironolactone 25 to 100 mg per day). The use of higher doses of spironolactone in these latter patients may induce overdiuresis and cause dehydration, hypovolemic hyponatremia, and prerenal renal failure. Besides its importance in helping establish the dose of diuretics, the intensity of sodium retention also provides prognostic information in patients with ascites. Patients with baseline urine sodium lower than 10 mEq per day have a median survival time of only 1.5 years compared with 4.5 years in patients with urine sodium higher than 10 mEq per day (Fig. 68.2).[60–62] Finally, the measurement of sodium excretion in patients under diuretic therapy is very useful to monitor the response to treatment.

Water Retention and Dilutional Hyponatremia

Since the pioneer studies by Papper and Saxon and Shear and colleagues,[63,64] it is well known that a derangement in the renal capacity to regulate water balance occurs in advanced cirrhosis. Cirrhotic patients without ascites usually have normal or only slightly impaired renal water handling as compared with healthy subjects. Therefore, in these patients total body water, plasma osmolality, and serum sodium concentration are normal and hyponatremia does not develop, even in conditions of excessive water intake. By contrast, an impairment in the renal capacity to excrete solute-free water is common in patients with ascites and usually it occurs late after the development of sodium retention.[63–67] In patients with ascites there is a direct correlation between urinary sodium excretion and water excretion as estimated by urine flow after a water load.[64,67] However, no correlation exists between these two parameters when only patients with marked sodium retention are considered. Therefore, sodium retention is necessary but not sufficient for the development of solute-free water retention in cirrhotic patients.

As with sodium retention, the impairment of solute-free water excretion is not uniform in all patients with ascites; rather, it varies markedly from patient to patient (Fig. 68.1). In some patients, water retention is moderate and can only be detected by measuring solute-free water excretion after a water load. These patients are able to eliminate water normally and maintain a normal serum sodium concentration as long as their fluid intake is kept within normal limits, but they may develop hyponatremia when fluid intake is increased. In other patients, the severity of the disorder is such that they retain most of their regular water intake causing hyponatremia and hypoosmolality. Therefore, hyponatremia in cirrhosis with ascites is almost always dilutional in origin since it occurs in the setting of an increased total body water. Hyponatremia is paradoxical in that it is associated with sodium retention and a marked increase in total body exchangeable sodium. The occurrence of spontaneous dilutional hyponatremia requires a profound impairment in solute-free water excretion, since it usually develops with a solute-free water clearance after a water load below 1 mL per minute.[65]

Hyponatremia in cirrhosis is currently defined as a reduction in serum sodium below 130 mEq per L.[68] The prevalence of hyponatremia using this cutoff is 22%. If the cutoff level of 135 mEq per L is used, the prevalence increases up to 49%.[69] The presence of dilutional hyponatremia in a cirrhotic patient is associated with a poor survival (Fig. 68.3).[62,65,70–79] The development of dilutional hyponatremia after a precipitating event such as hemorrhage or infection is associated with a better prognosis when compared to the spontaneous appearance of this complication.[80] This is possibly related to a higher incidence of renal dysfunction and a more advanced stage of decompensated cirrhosis associated with spontaneous dilutional hyponatremia.

Several factors may aggravate the impairment of solute-free water excretion in cirrhotic patients and precipitate the appearance of hyponatremia. These include treatment with diuretics or nonsteroidal anti-inflammatory drugs (NSAIDs), large-volume paracentesis without plasma volume expansion,[67,81–83] bacterial infections, and treatment with terlipressin for variceal bleeding.[84] Hyponatremia may also develop after the administration of hypotonic fluids in patients with ascites.

Mechanisms of Impaired Renal Water Handling

The pathogenesis of water retention in cirrhosis and dilutional hyponatremia is complex and probably involves several factors, including a reduced delivery of filtrate to the

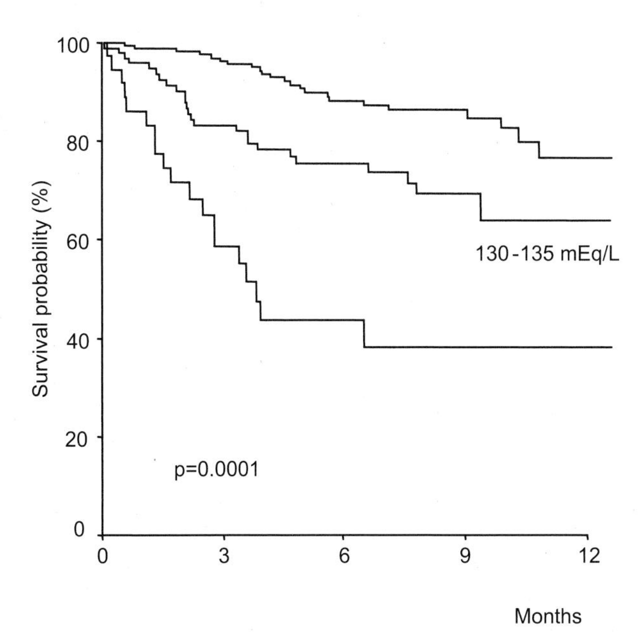

FIGURE 68.3 One-year survival before transplantation in a series of 308 patients with cirrhosis according to different values of serum sodium. (Reproduced with permission from Londoño MC, Cárdenas A, Guevara M, et al. MELD score and serum sodium in the prediction of survival of patients with cirrhosis awaiting liver transplantation. *Gut.* 2007;56:1283–1290.)

ascending limb of the loop of Henle, reduced renal synthesis of prostaglandins, and nonosmotic hypersecretion of arginine vasopressin (AVP).[68,85–87] Although definitive data about the relative importance of these factors in the pathogenesis of hyponatremia in patients with cirrhosis is lacking, it is likely that AVP hypersecretion plays a major role. This contention is supported by studies in animals and patients with cirrhosis showing that the administration of vaptans, drugs that antagonize the tubular effects of AVP (V2 receptor antagonists), improve solute-free water excretion and increase serum sodium concentration.[88–95] However, it is important to note there is a significant number of patients in whom hyponatremia does not improve despite the administration of vaptans, thus suggesting that factors other than AVP play also a role in the pathogenesis of solute-free water retention in cirrhosis. In patients with renal failure it is likely that besides AVP, a reduced distal delivery of filtrate due to decreased filtered load and increased proximal sodium and water reabsorption plays a role in solute-free water retention.

Clinical Consequences

The consequence of an impairment in solute-free water excretion is the development of dilutional hyponatremia. As indicated previously, dilutional hyponatremia in cirrhotic patients is defined as serum sodium <130 mEq per L in the presence of an expanded extracellular fluid volume, with ascites and/or edema.[68] It is associated with sodium retention and increased total body sodium and should be distinguished from hypovolemic hyponatremia that, although less common, may develop in cirrhotic patients with ascites and edema who are maintained on high doses of diuretics and sodium restriction after resolution of ascites and edema. There is limited information on the clinical consequences specifically caused by hyponatremia in cirrhosis because hyponatremia almost always occurs in the setting of advanced liver failure, which causes a wide array of clinical manifestations. Therefore, the precise identification of the clinical consequences of hyponatremia versus those of other causes has so far not been possible. This has been further hindered by the lack of an effective treatment of hyponatremia.

Hyponatremia and neurologic function. In patients without liver disease, hyponatremia is primarily associated with a broad variety of neurologic manifestations related to the existence of brain edema, such as headache, disorientation, confusion, focal neurologic deficits, seizures, and, in some cases, death due to cerebral herniation.[96] Severity of neurologic symptoms in patients with hyponatremia without liver disease correlates roughly with the levels of osmolality and sodium in the extracellular fluid. However, rather than the absolute reduction in serum sodium levels, the most important factor in determining the severity of neurologic symptoms is the rate of fall in serum sodium levels, patients with acute hyponatremia having a much higher incidence of neurologic symptoms than those with chronic hyponatremia.

Studies specifically assessing neurologic symptoms in cirrhosis with hyponatremia are lacking. However, the clinical experience indicates that significant neurologic manifestations such as headache, focal motor deficits, seizures, and cerebral herniation are very uncommon. It is likely that the relatively low incidence of neurologic manifestations in patients with cirrhosis and dilutional hyponatremia is related to the fact that in most of these patients hyponatremia is chronic rather than acute, and this gives sufficient time for the brain to adjust to hypo-osmolality of the extracellular fluid. The effects of hyponatremia on brain function have to be discussed in light of the recent hypothesis that proposes a role for a low-grade cerebral edema in the pathogenesis of hepatic encephalopathy.[97] According to this hypothesis, ammonia and other neurotoxins act synergistically to induce a low-grade cerebral edema as a result of swelling of astrocytes, which is mainly due to increased intracellular content of glutamine, secondary to ammonia metabolism. The cerebral edema would not be sufficient to cause an increase in intracranial pressure, but astrocyte swelling would result in a number of alterations of neurologic function, which would facilitate the development of hepatic encephalopathy. Evidence for such a low-grade cerebral edema derives from experimental and human studies using magnetic resonance.[98–100] In this context of low-grade cerebral edema, hyponatremia may represent a second osmotic hit to astrocytes, causing further depletion of osmotic counteractive systems (i.e., organic osmolytes). In this situation, cells

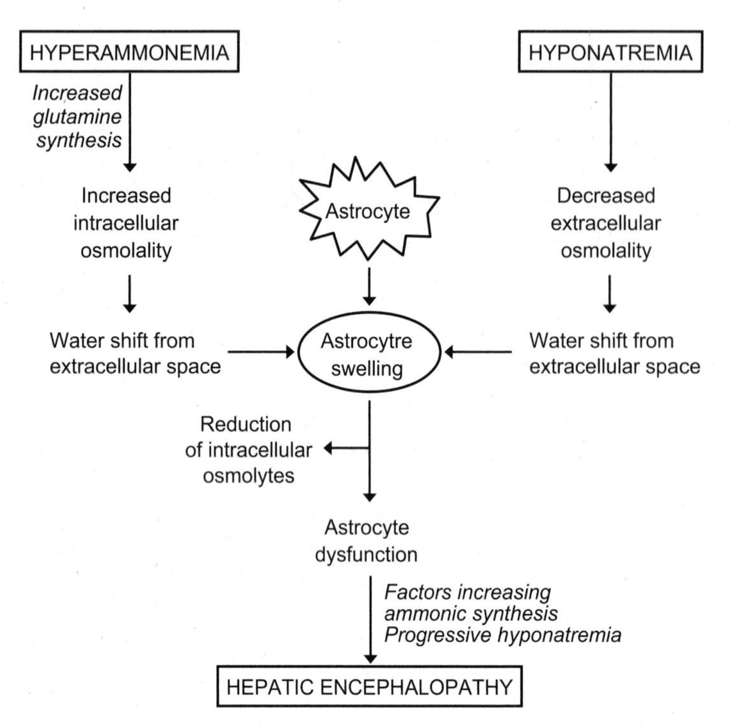

FIGURE 68.4 Proposed interaction between hyperammonemia and hyponatremia on brain astrocytes and possible pathogenic relationship with hepatic encephalopathy. (Reproduced with permission from Ginès P, Guevara M. Hyponatremia in cirrhosis: pathogenesis, clinical significance, and management. *Hepatology.* 2008;48:1002–1010.)

would probably not tolerate a further challenge to cell volume, and encephalopathy would develop due to any other osmotic stimulus, including situations associated with an increased ammonia load to the brain (gastrointestinal hemorrhage, infection) or further impairment in serum sodium concentration (Fig. 68.4). Several lines of evidence support the existence of a relationship between hepatic encephalopathy and low serum sodium concentration. First, serum sodium levels and serum ammonia levels are major factors determining electroencephalographic abnormalities in cirrhosis.[101] Second, in patients treated with transjugular intrahepatic portosystemic shunts, hyponatremia is a major risk factor for hepatic encephalopathy.[102] Third, in patients treated with diuretics (a clinical situation associated with a high incidence of hepatic encephalopathy), hyponatremia is a risk factor for hepatic encephalopathy (P. Ginès, unpublished data). Finally, serum sodium has been shown to be an independent predictive factor of hepatic encephalopathy in several series of patients with advanced cirrhosis.[103–105]

Hyponatremia and Complications of Cirrhosis. Besides hepatic encephalopathy, hyponatremia has also been reported to be associated with other complications of cirrhosis, yet information is limited. Specifically, hyponatremia is a frequent finding in patients with cirrhosis and bacterial infections.[106] In the majority of patients, hyponatremia occurs in close association with renal failure and correlates with a poor prognosis. Patients with ascites and hyponatremia constitute a unique population with a very high risk of developing HRS.[23] On the other hand, low serum sodium levels are a very common finding in patients with HRS. Information on the impact of hyponatremia on health-related quality of life in patients both with and without liver disease is very limited. In patients with cirrhosis, hyponatremia impairs quality of life because patients require a restriction of daily fluid intake to prevent further reductions in serum sodium concentration, and this is usually poorly tolerated. Moreover, in a recent study in a large population of patients with cirrhosis, hyponatremia was an independent predictive factor of the impaired health-related quality of life.[107]

Hyponatremia and Liver Transplantation. Patients with cirrhosis and hyponatremia are at increased risk of neurologic complications after transplantation, central pontine myelinolysis being the most severe, related to a rapid change in serum sodium in the early postoperative period.[108,109] The existence of hyponatremia before transplantation is associated not only with an increased risk of neurologic complications after transplantation, but also with an increased risk of renal failure and infectious complications, greater use of blood products, longer duration of hospital stay, and, more importantly, increased short-term mortality after transplantation.[110,111]

Renal Vasoconstriction and Hepatorenal Syndrome

Investigations performed by Sherlock, Schroeder, and Epstein during the late 1960s and early 1970s provided conclusive evidence indicating that the renal failure of functional origin—the so-called hepatorenal syndrome (HRS)—was due to a marked vasoconstriction of the renal circulation.[112–114] Further studies showed that, besides the striking renal vasoconstriction present in patients with HRS, mild to moderate degrees of vasoconstriction in the renal circulation are very common in patients with cirrhosis and ascites.[115–118] It has also been recognized that this vasoconstriction leading to HRS may be triggered by some precipitating factors, particularly bacterial infections.[119–121] When renal perfusion is estimated by sensitive clearance techniques, such as para-aminohippurate or inulin clearances, in a population of hospitalized patients with ascites, normal values are found in only one fifth of cases. In another 15% to 20%, renal hypoperfusion is very intense and meets the criteria of HRS. In the remaining patients, mild or moderate reductions in renal perfusion exist (Fig. 68.1). These latter patients show slightly increased serum creatinine and/or blood urea nitrogen (BUN) levels in baseline conditions (in the absence of diuretic therapy). This moderate renal vasoconstriction is clinically relevant for several reasons: first, it is often associated with marked sodium and water retention and the presence of refractory ascites[122]; second, it predisposes to the development of HRS[23,120,123]; and third, it is associated with an impaired survival.[62,73]

Definition of Hepatorenal Syndrome

The most recent definition of HRS proposed by the International Ascites Club, which is the most widely accepted, is as follows: "Hepatorenal syndrome is a potentially reversible syndrome that occurs in patients with cirrhosis, ascites and liver failure, as well as in patients with acute liver failure or alcoholic hepatitis. It is characterized by impaired renal function, marked alterations in cardiovascular function and over-activity of the sympathetic nervous system and renin-angiotensin systems. Severe renal vasoconstriction leads to a decrease of glomerular filtration rate. It appears spontaneously, but can also follow a precipitating event." This description was first proposed in 1999 and was adapted in 2007.[122,124] Although in the former definition, the existence of an ongoing bacterial infection precluded the diagnosis of HRS, with the current definition HRS can be diagnosed in the presence of an infection except in cases with septic shock.[124]

Pathogenic Mechanisms

The pathophysiologic hallmark of HRS is a vasoconstriction of the renal circulation.[114,122,125,126] Studies of renal perfusion with renal arteriography, $_{133}$Xe washout technique, para-aminohippuric acid excretion, and duplex Doppler ultrasonography have demonstrated the existence of marked vasoconstriction in the kidneys of patients with HRS, with a characteristic reduction in renal cortical perfusion.[113,126–132] The functional nature of HRS has been conclusively demonstrated by the lack of significant morphologic abnormalities in the kidney histology,[15–18,133] the normalization or improvement of renal function after liver transplantation,[134–138] and the reversibility of the syndrome by pharmacologic treatment with vasoconstrictors and albumin.[139]

The mechanism of this vasoconstriction is likely multifactorial involving changes in systemic hemodynamics, increased pressure in the portal venous system, activation of vasoconstrictor factors, and suppression of vasodilator factors acting on the renal circulation (discussed later). Contrary to the previous belief of marked vasodilation in extrarenal beds, other vascular beds besides the renal circulation are also vasoconstricted in patients with HRS, including the extremities and the cerebral circulation.[140–143] This indicates the existence of a generalized arterial vasoconstriction in nonsplanchnic vascular beds of patients with HRS and confirms that the only vascular bed responsible for arterial vasodilation and reduced total peripheral vascular resistance in cirrhosis with HRS is the splanchnic circulation.

Clinical and Laboratory Findings

HRS is a common complication of patients with cirrhosis. In patients with ascites, the probability of developing HRS during the course of the disease was reported as 18% at 1 year and 40% after 5 years of follow-up (Fig. 68.5).[23] The occurrence of HRS has been investigated in two recent studies. In one study of 129 patients, 22% of patients developed HRS during a follow-up period of 3.5 years.[144] In another study including 562 consecutive patients admitted to the hospital with renal failure, the frequency of HRS was 49% (associated with infection in 38% of cases and non-associated in 11%).[145] The clinical manifestations of patients with HRS include a combination of signs and symptoms related to renal, circulatory, and liver failure. Nonetheless, there are no specific clinical findings in HRS.

Renal failure in HRS may have a rapid or insidious onset and is associated almost constantly with intense urinary sodium retention (urine sodium <10 mEq per L), and spontaneous dilutional hyponatremia (serum sodium <130 mEq per L).[122,125,145] HRS may occur in two different clinical patterns, according to the intensity and form of onset of renal failure (Table 68.1).[122,124,146] Type 1 HRS is the classic type of HRS and represents the end of the spectrum of changes in renal perfusion in cirrhosis. The dominant clinical features of type 1 HRS are those of acutely severe renal failure

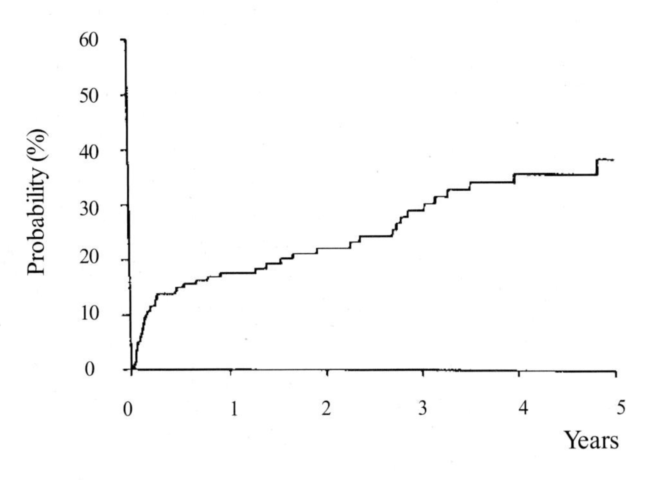

FIGURE 68.5 Probability of developing hepatorenal syndrome in a series of 234 nonazotemic cirrhotic patients with ascites. (Reproduced with permission from Ginès A, Escorsell A, Ginès P, et al. Incidence, predictive factors, and prognosis of the hepatorenal syndrome in cirrhosis with ascites. *Gastroenterology.* 1993;105:229.)

TABLE 68.1 **Clinical Types of Hepatorenal Syndrome**

Type 1	Rapid and progressive impairment of renal function as defined by a doubling of the initial serum creatinine to a level higher than 2.5 mg/dL or a 50% reduction of the initial 24-hour creatinine clearance to a level lower than 20 mL/min in less than 2 weeks.
Type 2	Impairment in renal function (serum creatinine >1.5 mg/dL) that does not meet the criteria of type 1.

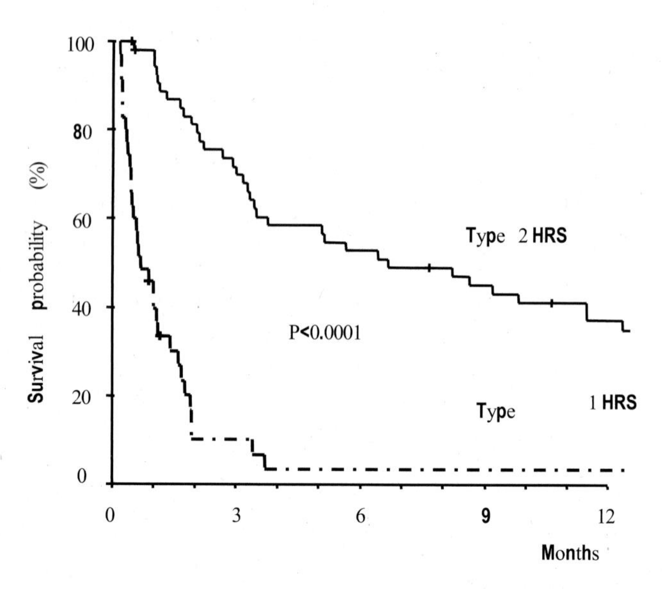

FIGURE 68.6 Survival of patients with cirrhosis according to the type of hepatorenal syndrome. (Reproduced with permission from Alessandria C, Ozdogan O, Guevara M, et al. MELD score and clinical type predict prognosis in hepatorenal syndrome: Relevance to liver transplantation. *Hepatology.* 2005;41:1282–1289.)

with rapid increase in serum levels of urea and creatinine and low urine volume in some cases, but not all of them. Type 1 HRS is characterized by a rapid and progressive impairment of renal function as defined by a doubling of the initial serum creatinine to a level higher than 2.5 mg per dL in less than 2 weeks. Despite an important reduction of GFR in these patients, serum creatinine levels are commonly lower than values observed in patients with acute renal failure of similar intensity with respect to the reduction in GFR, but without liver disease.[125,132,147,148] This is probably due to the lower endogenous production of creatinine secondary to reduced muscle mass in patients with cirrhosis compared with patients without liver disease. Type 1 HRS is associated with a very low survival expectancy, the median survival time being only 2 weeks (Fig. 68.6).[146] Type 2 HRS is characterized by a more subtle course with serum creatinine levels around 1.5 to 2.0 mg per dL. Patients are usually in a better clinical condition than those with type 1 HRS and their survival expectancy is longer, approximately 6 months (Fig. 68.6).[146] The dominant clinical feature of these patients is diuretic-resistant ascites due to the combination of intense sodium retention, reduced GFR, and marked activation of antinatriuretic systems.[122,124,146] Severe spontaneous hyperkalemia is an uncommon feature of HRS. However, marked hyperkalemia may occur if patients are treated with aldosterone antagonists, especially patients with type 1 HRS. Severe metabolic acidosis and pulmonary edema, which are frequent complications of acute renal failure of patients without liver disease, are uncommon findings in patients with HRS. Because HRS is a form of functional renal failure, the characteristics of urine are those of prerenal azotemia, with low urine sodium concentration, and increased urine osmolality and urine-to-plasma osmolality ratio.[122,149] Urine volume is not extremely reduced—in a recent series the average urine volume in 60 patients with HRS was 733 mL per day[145] and in some cases urine sodium concentration is not extremely reduced.[149,150] Table 68.2 shows the current diagnostic criteria of HRS.[124]

Circulatory failure in patients with HRS is characterized by arterial hypotension (most patients have a mean arterial pressure in the range of 70 mm Hg), and low total systemic vascular resistance, despite marked activation of the vasoconstrictor systems and the existence of severe vasoconstriction in several vascular beds, as already discussed.[122,142,143]

TABLE 68.2 **Diagnostic Criteria of Hepatorenal Syndrome**

1. Cirrhosis with ascites.
2. Serum creatinine >133 mmol/L (1.5 mg/dL).
3. No improvement of serum creatinine (decrease to a level of ≤133 mmol/L) after at least 2 days with diuretic withdrawal and volume expansion with albumin. The recommended dose of albumin is 1 g/kg of body weight per day up to a maximum of 100 g/day.
4. Absence of shock.
5. No current or recent treatment with nephrotoxic drugs.
6. Absence of parenchymal kidney disease as indicated by proteinuria >500 mg/day, microhematuria (>50 red blood cells per high power field) and/or abnormal renal ultrasonography.

Adapted from Salerno F, Gerbes A, Ginès P, et al. Diagnosis, prevention and treatment of hepatorenal syndrome in cirrhosis. *Gut.* 2007;56:1310–1318.

In addition, several studies have shown that cardiac output is low in patients with HRS, either in absolute values or relative to the reduction in total systemic vascular resistence.[151–153] This reduction in cardiac output may contribute to the reduction in the effective arterial blood volume and subsequent renal vasoconstriction.[152–154] In a longitudinal study in patients with cirrhosis it was shown that a reduction in cardiac output was associated with the occurrence of HRS.[155] Similarly, in a small series of patients with cirrhosis, those with a low cardiac output had a greater risk of HRS development.[156]

Finally, the third type of clinical manifestations of HRS is related to the existence of liver failure. The majority of patients have features of advanced liver disease with hyperbilirubinemia, elevated prothrombin time, thrombocytopenia, hepatic encephalopathy, hypoalbuminemia, poor nutritional status, and a large amount of ascites. In general, patients with type 1 HRS have more severe liver failure compared with patients with type 2 HRS.[146]

Precipitating Factors

In some patients, HRS develops without any identifiable precipitating factor, whereas in others it occurs in close chronologic relationship with bacterial infections, particularly spontaneous bacterial peritonitis.[119,122,124,157] Approximately one third of patients with spontaneous bacterial peritonitis develop renal failure during or immediately after infection, and in the absence of shock, which is currently defined as HRS[119,124] and occurs in the setting of a further decrease in effective arterial blood volume of patients with ascites, as indicated by a marked activation of vasoconstrictor systems, and increased serum and ascitic fluid levels of cytokines.[120,157] In approximately one third of patients with spontaneous bacterial peritonitis, HRS is reversible after resolution of infection. However, in the remaining patients HRS is not reversible after the resolution of the infection. Patients who develop type 1 HRS after spontaneous bacterial peritonitis have a dismal outcome, with an almost 100% hospital mortality if not treated appropriately (see below).[119,120] Similarly, large-volume paracentesis (> 5 L) without albumin expansion may precipitate type 1 HRS in up to 15% of cases.[83] This is one of the main reasons that supports the administration of intravenous albumin when large-volume paracenteses are performed.[158,159] Gastrointestinal bleeding has been classically considered as a precipitating factor of HRS.[149] However, the development of renal failure after this complication is not very common in patients with cirrhosis (approximately 10%) and occurs mainly in patients with hypovolemic shock, in most cases associated with ischemic hepatitis, which suggests that renal failure in this setting is probably related to the development of acute tubular necrosis (ATN) and not to HRS.[160] Diuretic treatment has also been classically described as a precipitating factor of HRS, but there is no clear evidence to support such a relationship.

There are several predictive factors in patients with cirrhosis and ascites associated with a greater risk of developing HRS.[23] For the most part these are related to circulatory and renal function and include severe urinary sodium retention, spontaneous dilutional hyponatremia, and low mean arterial blood pressure (<80 mm Hg). Interestingly, neither the degree of liver failure, as assessed by classic parameters of liver function (serum bilirubin, albumin, and prothrombin time) or the Child-Pugh classification, correlate with the risk of developing HRS.[23]

Diagnosis

The diagnosis of HRS is currently based on several diagnostic criteria (Table 68.2).[124] The minimum level of serum creatinine required for the diagnosis of HRS is 1.5 mg per dL (133 μmol per L). Patients with cirrhosis with a serum creatinine above 1.5 mg per dL usually have a GFR below 30 mL per minute.[125] In patients receiving diuretics, serum creatinine measurement should be repeated after diuretic withdrawal because, in some patients, serum creatinine may decrease after diuretic withdrawal.

Because no specific laboratory tests are available for the diagnosis of HRS and patients with advanced cirrhosis may develop renal failure of other etiologies (prerenal failure due to volume depletion, ATN, drug-induced nephrotoxicity, and glomerulonephritis in patients with hepatitis B or C), the most important step in the diagnosis of HRS is to rule out renal failure secondary to volume depletion or parenchymal diseases.[122,124,161] Gastrointestinal fluid losses, due to vomiting or diarrhea, or renal fluid losses, due to excessive diuresis, should be sought in all patients with cirrhosis presenting with renal failure. If renal failure is secondary to volume depletion, renal function improves rapidly after volume repletion (i.e., with intravenous saline or albumin) and treatment of the precipitating factor. Shock is another common condition in patients with cirrhosis that may lead to renal failure due to ATN. Although hypovolemic shock related with gastrointestinal bleeding is easily recognized, the presence of septic shock may be more difficult to diagnose because of the paucity of symptoms of bacterial infections in some patients with cirrhosis. Moreover, arterial hypotension due to the infection may be erroneously attributed to the underlying liver disease. In some patients with septic shock oliguria is the first sign of infection. These patients may be misdiagnosed as having HRS if signs of infection (cell blood count, examination of ascitic fluid) are not intentionally examined. On the other hand, as discussed before, patients with cirrhosis and spontaneous bacterial peritonitis may develop HRS during the course of the infection.[119,120] Renal failure in these patients may either improve with the antibiotic therapy or persist or progress, even after the resolution of the infection has been achieved. The administration of NSAIDs is another common cause of acute renal failure in patients with cirrhosis and ascites, which is clinically indistinguishable from HRS.[81,162,163] In hospitalized patients with renal failure, the administration of NSAIDs accounts for approximately 7% of all cases with renal failure.[145] Therefore, treatment with these drugs should always be ruled out before the diagnosis of HRS is made. Studies in patients with cirrhosis and ascites indicate that drugs that inhibit selectively the cyclooxygenase 2 enzyme (COX-2) do not cause renal failure, at least when administered for a short period of time.[164,165] However, studies with longer treatment duration should be performed before these drugs can be confirmed as safe for patients with cirrhosis and ascites. Patients with cirrhosis are also at high risk of developing renal failure due to ATN when treated with aminoglycosides.[162,166,167] Because of this high risk of nephrotoxicity and the existence of other effective antibiotics (e.g., third-generation cephalosporins) treatment with aminoglycosides should be avoided in patients with chronic liver disease. Finally, patients with cirrhosis due to hepatitis B and C may also develop renal failure due to glomerulonephritis.[168–170] In these cases, proteinuria and/or hematuria are almost constant and provide a clue for the diagnosis, which may be confirmed by renal biopsy in selected cases.[171]

FACTORS INVOLVED IN FUNCTIONAL RENAL ABNORMALITIES IN CIRRHOSIS

Circulatory Abnormalities

Hepatic and Splanchnic Circulation

The existence of cirrhosis causes marked structural abnormalities in the liver that result in severe disturbance of intrahepatic circulation causing increased resistance to portal flow and subsequent hypertension in the portal venous system.[172] Progressive collagen deposition and formation of nodules alter the normal vascular architecture of the liver. Moreover, selective deposition of collagen in the space of Disse, the space between sinusoidal cells and hepatocytes, may constrict the sinusoids, resulting in further mechanical obstruction to flow.[173,174] In addition to this passive resistance to portal flow there is an active component of intrahepatic resistance, which is due to the contraction of hepatic stellate cells (myofibroblastlike cells) present in sinusoids and terminal hepatic venules[175–177] and low levels of intrahepatic vasodilators. The contraction of these cells is affected by endogenous vasoconstrictors and can be modulated by vasodilators and drugs that antagonize the vasoconstrictor factors.[178–180] Moreover, there is a strong body of evidence indicating that despite the overproduction of the vasodilator nitric oxide (NO) in the splanchnic and systemic circulation in cirrhosis, there is a reduced production of NO in the intrahepatic circulation of cirrhotic livers that contributes to the increased intrahepatic resistance characteristic of portal hypertension.[181–183] There is also evidence that besides the role of fibrosis and vasoactive factors, increased hepatic neoangiogenesis and inflammation can play a role in the pathogenesis of increased intrahepatic resistance in experimental cirrhosis.[184]

Portal hypertension induces profound changes in the splanchnic circulation.[185–188] Classically, portal hypertension was considered to cause only changes in the venous side of the splanchnic circulation. However, studies in experimental animals indicate that portal hypertension also causes marked changes in the arterial side of the splanchnic vascular bed. In the venous side, the main changes consist of increased pressure and formation of portocollateral circulation, which causes the shunting of blood from the portal venous system to the systemic circulation. In the arterial side, there is marked arterial vasodilation which increases portal venous inflow.[185–189] This high portal venous inflow plays an important role in the increased pressure in the portal circulation and may explain, at least in part, why portal pressure remains increased despite the development of collateral circulation. This arteriolar vasodilation is also responsible for marked changes in splanchnic microcirculation that may predispose to increased filtration of fluid. It has been shown that chronic portal hypertension causes a much greater increase in intestinal capillary pressure and lymph flow than does an acute increase in portal pressure of the same magnitude.[190,191] This is probably due to a loss of the normal autoregulatory mechanism of the splanchnic microcirculation. The acute elevation of venous pressure in the intestine elicits a strong myogenic response, which leads to a reduction in blood flow. This phenomenon is thought to be a homeostatic response to protect the intestine against edema formation. This protective mechanism is not operative in chronic portal hypertension and arteriolar resistance is reduced and not increased.[191,192] The resultant increases in capillary pressure and filtration may be important factors in the formation of ascites in cirrhosis. The mechanism(s) by which portal hypertension induces splanchnic arteriolar vasodilation is not completely understood although a number of vasoactive mediators have been proposed (and will be discussed subsequently).[185]

Several lines of evidence indicate that portal hypertension is a major factor in the pathogenesis of ascites. First, patients with early cirrhosis without portal hypertension do not develop ascites or edema. Moreover, a certain level of portal hypertension is required for ascites formation. Ascites rarely develops in patients with portal pressure below 10 mm Hg, as assessed by the difference between wedged and free hepatic venous pressure (normal portal pressure: 5 mm Hg).[193–196] Second, cirrhotic patients treated with surgical portosystemic shunts for the management of bleeding gastroesophageal varices have lower risk of developing ascites than do patients treated with procedures that obliterate gastroesophageal varices but do not affect portal pressure (i.e., sclerotherapy, esophageal band ligation).[197] Finally, reduction of portal pressure with side-to-side or end-to-side portacaval anastomosis or TIPS (placement of a stent between a hepatic vein and the intrahepatic portion of the portal vein using a transjugular approach) is associated with an improvement of ascites, renal function, and suppression of antinatriuretic systems[198,199] in cirrhotic patients with fluid retention. The mechanism(s) by which portal hypertension contributes to renal functional abnormalities and ascites and edema formation is not completely understood, yet three pathogenic mechanisms have been proposed: (1) alterations in the splanchnic and systemic circulation which result in activation of vasoconstrictor and antinatriuretic systems and subsequent renal sodium and water retention; (2) hepatorenal reflex due to increased hepatic pressure which would cause sodium and water retention; and (3) putative antinatriuretic substances escaping from the splanchnic area through portosystemic collaterals that would have a sodium-retaining effect in the kidney. There is a large body of evidence supporting the first of these three pathogenic mechanisms.

Systemic Circulation

The development of portal hypertension is associated with marked hemodynamic changes not only in the hepatic and splanchnic circulation but also in the systemic circulation. These changes, which have been well characterized in human and experimental cirrhosis, consist of reduced systemic vascular resistance and arterial pressure, increased cardiac index, increased plasma volume, and activation of systemic vasoconstrictor and antinatriuretic factors. These changes in systemic hemodynamics appear before the formation of ascites and are more marked as the disease progresses.[40,188,200–205] The hemodynamic profile of patients with cirrhosis in different stages of the disease is summarized in Table 68.3. The factor that appears to trigger all these hemodynamic changes of cirrhosis is an arterial vasodilation located mainly in the splanchnic circulation.[185–189,205–207] The existence of a splanchnic arterial vasodilation causes an abnormal distribution of blood volume, which results in a reduction of central blood volume (heart, lungs, and aorta) that is sensed by arterial and cardiopulmonary receptors. This central underfilling triggers a neurohormonal response by activating the SNS, RAAS, and arginine vasopressin (AVP). This explains why systemic vasoconstrictor factors are activated despite an increased plasma volume that in normal conditions would suppress the activation of these systems. Investigations in patients with cirrhosis have assessed central blood volume by measuring the mean circulation time of an indicator or by magnetic resonance imaging.[205,208–211] These studies have confirmed that central blood volume is reduced in patients with cirrhosis, particularly in those with ascites and correlates directly with systemic vascular resistance and inversely with portal pressure, indicating that the greater the vasodilation and the pressure in the portal system, the lower the central blood volume. The crucial role played by the reduced central blood volume in the activation of vasoconstrictor systems has been further corroborated by studies showing that improvement of central blood volume by the combination of expansion of plasma volume or head-out water immersion and administration of pressor agents, suppresses the activation of vasoconstrictor systems.[212–215] Whether or not arterial vasodilation occurs also in nonsplanchnic territories is still controversial but most data indicate that the splanchnic circulation accounts for most, if not all, of the reduced arterial resistance in patients with cirrhosis.[185,205,216]

Despite extensive investigation, the mechanism(s) responsible for arterial vasodilation in cirrhosis is not completely understood. Several explanations have been proposed, including opening of arteriovenous fistulas, reduced sensitivity to vasoconstrictors, and increased circulating levels of vasodilator substances.[185,187,207,216–220] This latter mechanism has

TABLE 68.3 **Hemodynamic Profile of Patients with Cirrhosis in Different Stages of Disease**

	Preascitic Cirrhosis	Cirrhosis with Ascites	Hepatorenal Syndrome
Cardiac output	Normal or increased	Increased	Normal or reduced
Arterial pressure	Normal	Normal or reduced	Reduced
Systemic vascular resistance	Normal or reduced	Reduced	Markedly reduced
Plasma volume	Normal or increased	Increased	Increased
Portal pressure	Normal or increased	Increased	Increased
Vasoconstrictor systems activity	Normal	Increased[a]	Markedly increased
Renal vascular resistance	Normal	Normal or increased	Markedly increased
Brachial or femoral vascular resistance	Normal or reduced	Normal or increased	Increased
Cerebral vascular resistance	Normal	Increased	Increased

[a]May be normal in 20%–30% of patients.

been the most extensively studied. Increased production of NO, carbon monoxide, glucagon, endocannabinoids, prostaglandins, vasoactive intestinal peptide, adenosine, bile salts, platelet activating factor, substance P, calcitonin gene-related peptide, natriuretic peptides, and adrenomedullin have been proposed as possible factors of the development of splanchnic arterial vasodilation.[185,191,205,216,221–231] At present, most available data, obtained mainly from experimental cirrhosis, indicate that NO is the main mediator of arterial vasodilation in cirrhosis (Table 68.4).[232] NO synthesis from cirrhotic arterial vessels is markedly increased compared to that of normal vascular tissue. This increased NO synthesis appears to be generalized, except for the intrahepatic circulation, but predominates in the splanchnic territory. Among the different isoforms of NO synthase, the constitutive form appears to be the one responsible for the increased NO synthesis. The normalization of NO synthesis in experimental cirrhosis by the administration of inhibitors of NO synthesis is associated with a marked improvement of splanchnic and systemic hemodynamics, suppression of the increased activity of the RAAS and AVP concentration, increased sodium and water excretion, and reduction or disappearance of ascites.[233] So far, only few studies have investigated the effect of acute NO synthesis inhibition in patients with cirrhosis on systemic hemodynamia and/or renal function, with discrepant findings.[234–236] Unfortunately, no study has been reported investigating the effects of a prolonged inhibition of NO synthesis in human cirrhosis.

Neurohumoral Systems

The functional renal abnormalities that occur in cirrhosis are the result of a complex interrelationship between different systems and factors with effects on renal function. The relative contribution of a particular system in the pathogenesis of these abnormalities in cirrhosis has, therefore, been difficult to assess. This section reviews the different systems that may participate in renal dysfunction in cirrhosis. The evidence indicating their role in the pathogenesis of these abnormalities is discussed.

Renin–Angiotensin–Aldosterone System

Of all potential factors involved in pathogenesis of sodium retention in cirrhosis, aldosterone has been the most extensively studied. Plasma aldosterone levels are increased in most cirrhotic patients with ascites and marked sodium retention.[45,117,202,237–243] In ascitic patients with moderate sodium retention plasma aldosterone is either only slightly elevated or normal. It should be pointed out, however, that these "normal" concentrations occur in the presence of an increase in total body sodium of a degree that would suppress aldosterone concentration in normal subjects. Three lines of evidence indicate that aldosterone plays an important role in the pathogenesis of sodium retention in cirrhosis: (1) there is an inverse correlation between urinary sodium excretion and plasma aldosterone levels[45,117,202,237,243,244]; (2) studies in animals with experimental cirrhosis have

TABLE 68.4 Evidences for a Role of an Increased Vascular Production of Nitric Oxide (NO) in the Pathogenesis of Arterial Vasodilation and Subsequent Sodium and Water Retention in Cirrhosis

Experimental Cirrhosis

1. Reversal of the impaired pressor response to vasoconstrictors of isolated aortic rings or splanchnic vascular preparations by NO synthase inhibition.
2. Enhanced vasodilator response to NO-dependent vasodilators.
3. Increased pressor effect of systemic NO synthase inhibition.
4. Increased NO synthesis in vascular tissue.
5. Normalization of the hyperdynamic circulation, activity of antinatriuretic systems, and sodium and water retention by chronic NO synthase inhibition.
6. Increased expression of NO synthase isoenzymes in vascular tissue.

Human Cirrhosis

1. Correction of the arterial hyporesponsiveness to vasoconstrictors by NO synthase inhibition.
2. Enhanced vasodilatory response to NO-dependent vasodilators.
3. Increased plasma levels of NO and NO metabolites.
4. Increased NO in the exhaled air.
5. Increased NO synthase activity in polymorphonuclear cells and monocytes.

shown the existence of a chronologic relationship between hyperaldosteronism and sodium retention[31]; and (3) the administration of spironolactone, a specific aldosterone antagonist, is able to reverse sodium retention in the great majority of patients with ascites without renal failure.[48,49,245–248] The observation that sodium retention occurs in some cirrhotic patients in the absence of increased plasma aldosterone levels has raised the suggestion that other factors in addition to aldosterone may also contribute.[249] Nevertheless, it has also been suggested that cirrhotic patients may have an increased tubular sensitivity to aldosterone.[45,237] This may explain the natriuretic response to spironolactone in patients with normal aldosterone levels.[49,247] Thus, the possibility exists that aldosterone may participate in renal sodium retention in cirrhosis even in the presence of normal plasma concentrations of the hormone. In addition to aldosterone, increased intrarenal levels of angiotensin II may also contribute to sodium retention in patients with cirrhosis by a direct effect on tubular sodium reabsorption.[250]

The increased plasma aldosterone levels in cirrhotic patients with ascites are due to a stimulation of aldosterone secretion and not to impaired degradation, as the hepatic clearance of aldosterone is normal or only slightly reduced in these patients.[238,249,251] Among the different mechanisms that regulate aldosterone secretion an increased activity of RAAS is the most likely to be responsible for hyperaldosteronism in cirrhosis (Fig. 68.7). In fact, plasma renin activity (PRA), which estimates the activity of the RAAS, is increased in most patients with ascites and correlates closely with plasma aldosterone concentration.[117,202,239,240,252–254] Investigations using pharmacologic agents which interrupt RAAS have provided evidence suggesting that this system is activated as a result of a profound disturbance in systemic hemodynamics. The administration of angiotensin II receptor antagonists or converting-enzyme inhibitors to cirrhotic patients with ascites and increased PRA induces a marked reduction in arterial pressure and systemic vascular resistance, which suggests that the activation of RAAS is a homeostatic response to maintain arterial pressure in these patients.[255–258]

The activation of RAAS is particularly intense in patients with HRS, suggesting a role for angiotensin II in the pathogenesis of renal vasoconstriction in HRS.[259–264] This role is further supported by studies showing that the improvement of renal function in patients with HRS achieved by the administration of the vasopressin analogs ornipressin or terlipressin associated with albumin or the insertion of a TIPS is associated with a marked suppression of the activity of the RAAS.[214,215,265,266] However, because the interruption of RAAS is associated with arterial hypotension in patients with high PRA, the effects of RAAS on renal function independent of those on systemic hemodynamics have not been possible to assess. Although administration of angiotensin II blockers like losartan may induce natriuresis when given at low doses to patients with preascitic cirrhosis,[250] the use of these drugs should be avoided in patients with ascites because of a high risk of hypotension and renal failure.

Sympathetic Nervous System

Numerous studies have presented evidence indicating an increased activity of the SNS in cirrhosis. The plasma concentration of norepinephrine (NE) in the systemic circulation, an index of the activation of the SNS, is increased in most patients with ascites and normal or only slightly elevated in patients without ascites.[260,267–273] This "normal" plasma NE concentration, however, is relatively increased in the presence of plasma volume expansion, which occurs in early cirrhosis. Investigations using titrated NE, to provide a more

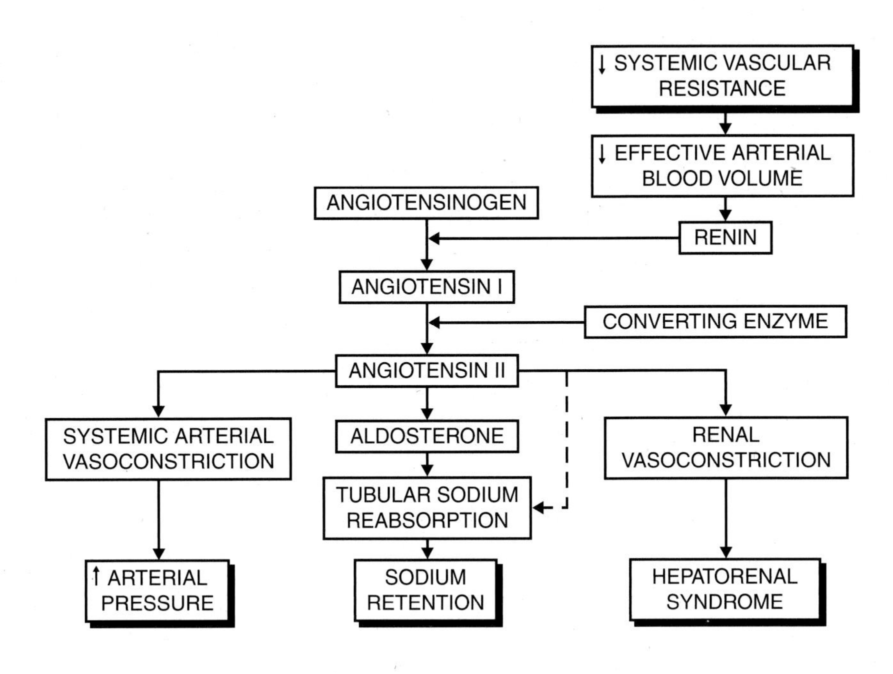

FIGURE 68.7 Proposed mechanism of activation and renal and systemic effects of renin–angiotensin–aldosterone system in cirrhosis with ascites.

accurate assessment of the SNS activity, have confirmed that the high plasma NE levels are due to an increased activity of the SNS and not to an impaired elimination of NE, as the total spillover of NE to plasma is markedly increased in cirrhotic patients with ascites whereas the plasma clearance of NE is normal.[273–278] Measurements of NE release and spillover in specific vascular beds have shown that the activity of the SNS is increased in many vascular territories, including kidneys, splanchnic organs, heart, and muscle and skin, supporting the concept of a generalized activation of the SNS.[275–279] Direct evidence of the overactivity of the SNS in cirrhosis has been provided by measuring the sympathetic nerve discharge rates from a peripheral muscular nerve. Muscular sympathetic nerve activity is markedly increased in patients with ascites and normal in patients without ascites and correlates directly with plasma NE concentration.[280]

Because the SNS has profound effects on renal function,[281] it is reasonable to presume that the increased renal sympathetic nervous activity in cirrhosis may play a role in the pathogenesis of functional renal abnormalities (Fig. 68.8). In fact, evidence suggests that the SNS is involved in sodium and water retention in cirrhosis. The activity of the SNS, either estimated by plasma NE or total NE spillover to plasma or measured from intraneural recordings, correlates inversely with sodium and water retention.[268,275,280] In addition, bilateral renal denervation increases urine volume and sodium excretion in animals with experimental cirrhosis and ascites and restores the renal capacity to eliminate a water load.[282–284] Similarly, anesthetic blockade of the lumbar SNS, a maneuver that reduces the activity of the kidney SNS, improves sodium excretion in patients with cirrhosis and ascites.[285] A study in a limited number of patients with ascites showed that administratation of diuretics together with clonidine to inhibit the sympathetic nervous activity is more effective than diuretics alone.[286] Moreover, the acute inhibition of the renal sympathetic outflow with clonidine in patients with cirrhosis is associated with a reduction in renal vascular resistance and an increase in GFR and filtration fraction, suggesting that the activation of the SNS causes renal vasoconstriction by increasing arterial tone in the afferent arteriole.[278] It has also been shown that the increased sympathetic nervous activity impairs renal blood flow autoregulation in cirrhosis.[287] On the other hand, patients with HRS have significantly higher plasma levels of NE than do patients without renal failure, and arterial and renal venous NE correlate inversely with renal blood flow (RBF), suggesting that the SNS may participate in the renal vasoconstriction observed in patients with HRS.[242,260,287,288] Moreover, the circulating levels of neuropeptide Y, a neurotransmitter with a very potent vasoconstrictor action in the renal circulation released in the setting of a marked activation of the SNS, are increased in patients with HRS but not in those with ascites without renal failure.[289] Finally, it is worth mentioning that a recent study in experimental cirrhosis suggests that the increased activity of the SNS in the splachnic circulation may contribute to bacterial infection in cirrhosis by causing increased bacterial translocation and spreading of gram negative bacteria.[290] Therefore, the SNS has important effects on the circulatory and renal function in cirrhosis.

The cause of the increased activity of the SNS in cirrhosis with ascites is not completely understood. Two major explanations have been proposed: either a baroreceptor-mediated response to a decrease in effective arterial blood volume due to arterial vasodilation[205,273,291] or a hepatorenal reflex resulting from activation of hepatic baroreceptors due to sinusoidal hypertension.[292–294] The first explanation seems more likely since the estimated central blood volume (i.e., the blood volume in the heart cavities, lungs, and central arterial tree) is reduced in cirrhotic patients and correlates inversely with SNS activity.[208,209] Furthermore, the activity of the SNS can be suppressed by maneuvers that increase effective arterial blood volume, such as the administration of vasopressin analogs and albumin, and the insertion of a peritoneovenous shunt or transjugular intrahepatic portosystemic shunt (TIPS).[214,215,265,274,295]

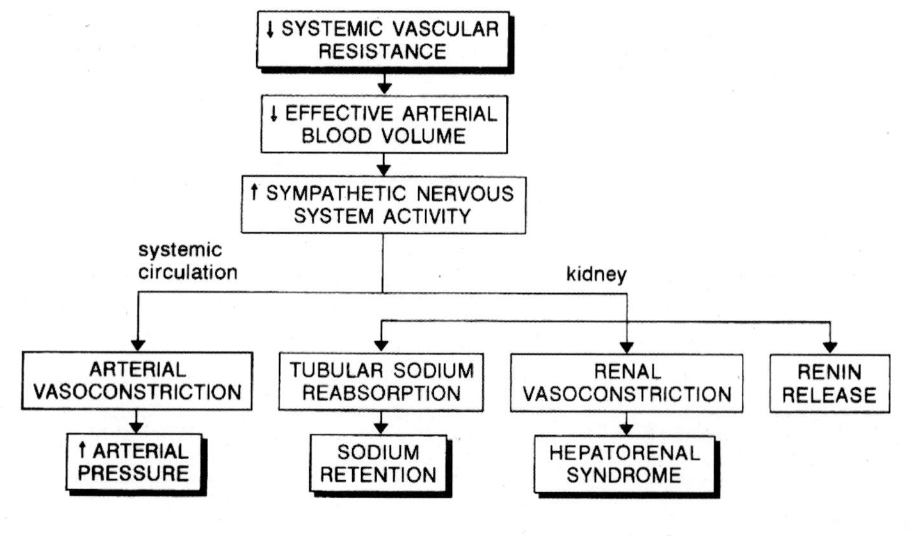

FIGURE 68.8 Proposed mechanism of activation and renal and systemic effects of sympathetic nervous system in cirrhosis with ascites.

Prostaglandins and Other Eicosanoids

Prostaglandins are known to have a protective effect on renal circulation in pathophysiologic situations associated with increased activity of renal vasoconstrictor systems.[296] According to this formulation, prostaglandins appear to play a key role in the homeostasis of renal circulation and water excretion in cirrhotic patients with ascites. The urinary excretion of prostaglandin E2 (PGE2) and 6-keto-prostaglandin F1α, which estimate the renal synthesis of PGE2 and PGI2, respectively, are increased in patients with cirrhosis and ascites without renal failure as compared to healthy subjects and patients without ascites.[118,259,260,297,298] Further evidence supporting a role for renal prostaglandins in the maintenance of RBF and GFR in cirrhosis with ascites derive from studies using NSAIDs to inhibit prostaglandin synthesis. The administration of NSAIDs, even in single doses, to cirrhotic patients with ascites causes a profound decrease in RBF and GFR in patients who have a marked activation of vasoconstrictor systems but has little or no effect in patients without activation of these systems.[81,163,260,298,299] An increased renal production of PGE2 also contributes to the maintenance of solute-free water excretion in nonazotemic cirrhotic patients with ascites as the inhibition of prostaglandin synthesis by NSAIDs in these patients impairs solute-free water excretion independently of changes in renal hemodynamics.[82]

The relationship between the renal prostaglandin system and HRS is controversial. Several studies have reported that patients with HRS have lower urinary excretion of PGE2 and 6-keto-PGF1α than do patients with ascites without renal failure, which suggests that a reduced renal synthesis of vasodilator prostaglandins may play a role in the pathogenesis of HRS.[118,259,300–302] The finding of low renal content of PGH2 synthase (medullary cyclooxygenase) in patients with HRS is also consistent with this hypothesis.[303] Other studies, however, did not find reduced urinary excretion of vasodilator prostaglandins in patients with HRS.[304,305] Nevertheless, "normal" synthesis of prostaglandins may be low relative to the increased activity of vasoconstrictor systems in cirrhosis. Because patients with HRS have the greatest activation of renal vasoconstrictor systems, an imbalance between vasoconstrictor systems and the renal production of vasodilator prostaglandins has been proposed to explain the marked reduction of RBF and GFR that occurs in this condition.[259] It has also been suggested that HRS could be the consequence of an imbalance between the renal synthesis of vasodilator and vasoconstrictor prostaglandins based on the observation of reduced urinary excretion of PGE2 and 6-keto-PGF1α and increased urinary excretion of TXB2 in patients with HRS.[302–305] These findings, however, were not confirmed by subsequent investigations.[118,301,306] Moreover, the administration of inhibitors of TXA2 synthesis does not improve renal function in these patients.[307]

Prostaglandin synthesis in cirrhosis is also increased in extrarenal organs. Patients with cirrhosis have high urinary excretion of 2-3–dinor-6-keto-PGF1α, a metabolite of PGI2 considered to be an index of systemic PGI2 production.[221,304] As prostaglandins are potent vasodilators in the systemic circulation these observations raise the possibility that an increased prostaglandin synthesis may contribute to arterial vasodilation in cirrhosis. This suggestion is consistent with the observation that the NSAID indomethacin increases systemic vascular resistance and ameliorates the hyperdynamic circulation in cirrhotic patients.[308]

Studies in rats with experimental cirrhosis and ascites have investigated the metabolic pathways leading to the increased synthesis of prostaglandins. Increased activity and expression of cytosolic phospholipase A2 (cPLA2) (the first enzyme of the metabolic cascade of eicosanoid synthesis) and cyclooxygenase-1 have been found in arterial and renal tissue of rats with cirrhosis and ascites compared with normal rats.[309–311]

The possible role of eicosanoids other than prostaglandins in the pathogenesis of functional renal abnormalities in cirrhosis is not completely understood. The urinary excretion of leukotriene E4 and *N*-acetyl-leukotriene E4, compounds with a vasoconstrictor effect in the renal circulation, is increased in cirrhotic patients with HRS as compared to healthy subjects and patients without ascites, suggesting that leukotrienes may participate in the pathogenesis of this syndrome.[312,313] Likewise, the urinary excretion of the vasoconstrictor compound 20-hydroxyeicosatetraenoic acid (20-HETE) is also increased in patients with cirrhosis as compared to healthy subjects.[314]

Arginine Vasopressin

Studies in humans and experimental animals have provided several pieces of evidence indicating that AVP plays a key role in the pathogenesis of water retention in cirrhosis with ascites. These include: (1) plasma AVP levels are often increased in cirrhotic patients and correlate closely with the reduction in solute-free water excretion, patients with higher plasma AVP levels being those with the more severe impairment in water metabolism[82,85–87,315–318]; (2) a chronologic relationship between AVP hypersecretion and impairment in water excretion can be found in rats with cirrhosis and ascites[319,320]; (3) Brattleboro rats (rats with a congenital deficiency of AVP) with cirrhosis do not develop an impairment in water excretion[321]; (4) kidneys from cirrhotic rats with ascites show increased gene expression or redistribution to plasma membrane of aquaporin-2, the AVP-regulated water channel[322,323]; (5) the administration of specific antagonists of the tubular effect of AVP (V2 antagonists) improve the renal ability to excrete solute-free water in animal as well as in human cirrhosis[88–95,324]. Nevertheless, factors other than AVP play a role in the pathogenesis of solute-free water retention because in a significant proportion of patients solute-free water excretion and serum sodium concentration do not improve despite the administration of vaptans.[93–95]

The increased plasma AVP concentrations in cirrhosis are due to an increased hypothalamic synthesis and not to a reduced systemic clearance of the peptide.[86,325–327] The hemodynamic changes occuring in cirrhosis (low arterial blood pressure, high cardiac output, and low total systemic vascular resistance) cause arterial hypotension which unloads the high pressure baroreceptors and stimulates a nonosmotic release of AVP with the subsequent increase in water reabsorption.[82,315] The mechanism of this nonosmotic hypersecretion is hemodynamic, as plasma AVP levels correlate with PRA and plasma NE concentration[82,268] and are suppressed by maneuvers that increase effective arterial blood volume, such as head-out water immersion or peritoneovenous shunting in human cirrhosis[316,328] or inhibition of NO synthesis in experimental animal cirrhosis.[233] This hemodynamic mechanism of AVP release in cirrhosis is also supported by the observation that the administration of a specific antagonist of the vascular effect of AVP (V1 antagonist) induces arterial hypotension in rats with experimental cirrhosis and ascites and water retention but not in control rats.[329] This finding suggests that AVP hypersecretion in cirrhosis contributes not only to water retention but also to the maintenance of arterial pressure (Fig. 68.9).

Natriuretic Peptides

The natriuretic hormones, represented by the atrial natriuretic peptide (ANP) and brain natriuretic peptide (BNP), are increased in patients with cirrhosis and ascites.[330–339] In patients without ascites, plasma ANP levels may be either normal or increased. In patients with ascites, the high plasma levels of ANP are due to increased cardiac secretion of the peptide and not reduced hepatic or systemic catabolism, as cardiac production of ANP is increased in cirrhotic patients with ascites but splanchnic and peripheral extraction are normal.[330,340] Consistent with these observations is the finding of increased messenger RNA expression for ANP in ventricles from cirrhotic rats with ascites.[341] In contrast to other diseases showing increased cardiac ANP secretion, in cirrhosis with ascites this increased secretion occurs in the presence of normal atrial pressure and reduced estimated central blood volume.[208,330] The mechanism(s) responsible for this increased cardiac secretion of ANP is not known. The existence of increased plasma levels of ANP in cirrhosis with ascites sufficient to have a natriuretic effect in healthy subjects, together with the presence of renal sodium retention, indicates a renal resistance to the effects of ANP. This renal resistance has been confirmed in studies in human and experimental cirrhosis in which pharmacologic doses of natriuretic peptides (ANP or BNP) were administered.[342–347] In these investigations patients with activation of antinatriuretic systems (RAAS and SNS) had a blunted or no natriuretic response after ANP infusion. This blunted response can be reversed by maneuvers that increase distal sodium delivery in human cirrhosis or by bilateral renal denervation in experimental cirrhosis, suggesting that the renal resistance to ANP in cirrhosis is related to the increased activity of antinatriuretic systems.[283,348] Limited information exists on other peptides of the natriuretic peptide family. As with ANP, the plasma concentration of BNP is increased in cirrhotic patients with ascites as compared to healthy subjects.[349] In contrast to ANP and BNP levels, the plasma levels of C-natriuretic peptide are decreased in cirrhosis, whereas the urinary excretion is increased. The plasma levels correlate inversely with arterial compliance and decreased vascular resistance, which suggests a compensatory downregulation of this peptide.[350,351] Finally, the urinary excretion of urodilatin, a member of the natriuretic peptide family exclusively synthesized in the kidney, which probably reflects the renal production of the peptide, is normal in patients with cirrhosis and ascites.[352]

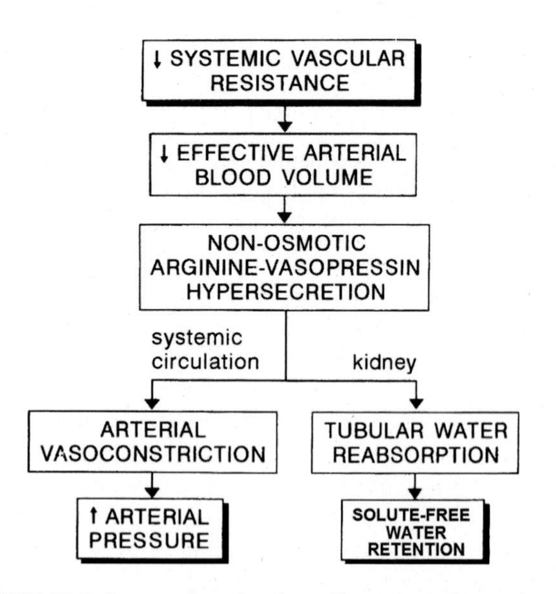

FIGURE 68.9 Proposed mechanism of hypersecretion and renal and systemic effects of arginine vasopressin in cirrhosis with ascites.

The role of natriuretic peptides in cirrhosis is not entirely clear. Because most of ANP and BNP have vasodilator properties, a role in the pathogenesis of arterial vasodilation in cirrhosis has been proposed but not proved. By contrast, data from experimental studies suggest that they play an important role in the maintenance of renal perfusion and modulation of RAAS activity, as the selective blockade of the natriuretic peptide A and B receptors causes renal vasoconstriction and increased PRA and aldosterone levels in experimental cirrhosis.[353] It could be speculated, therefore, that the cardiac synthesis of ANP and BNP is increased in an attempt to maintain renal perfusion within normal levels and limit the activation of the RAAS. Although the mechanism(s) leading to this increased synthesis of natriuretic peptides remains unknown, the hypothesis has been raised that BNP in cirrhosis may reflect the existence of a cirrhotic myocardiopathy,[339,354,355] a condition characterized by impaired myocardial function in the context of cirrhosis.[356]

Endothelins

Endothelins comprise three homologous peptides (ET-1, ET-2, and ET-3) with a very potent vasoconstrictor action.[357]

Increased plasma levels of ET-1 and ET-3 have been found in patients with cirrhosis and ascites and in patients without ascites, albeit to a lesser extent.[358–365] The increased plasma levels of ET-1 found in cirrhosis derive either from an increased production in the splanchnic circulation and/or an increased intrahepatic production. Increased levels of ET-1 and its precursor Big-ET-1 have been found in plasma samples obtained from the portal and hepatic veins of patients with cirrhosis.[366] Moreover, increased levels of ET-1 have been demonstrated in hepatic tissue in human and experimental cirrhosis.[367–370] In human cirrhosis, the increased hepatic ET-1 levels correlate with portal hypertension and the severity of ascites and liver failure.[369,370] As opposed to other vasoconstrictor factors (e.g., angiotensin II or norepinephrine), the activity of which is increased in cirrhosis, it is unlikely that hyperendothelinemia in cirrhosis is a compensatory mechanism triggered by effective arterial hypovolemia. Endothelin levels are not suppressed by maneuvers that improve circulatory function, such as plasma volume expansion with or without concomitant administration of splanchnic vasoconstrictors.[214,361,363] A role for endotoxemia in the increased endothelin levels in cirrhosis has also been proposed[358] but plasma endothelin concentration does not parallel endotoxin levels in cirrhotic patients.[363]

The role that these increased circulating ET-1 levels play in the pathogenesis of abnormalities in renal, systemic, and hepatic circulation in cirrhosis is not known. A role for ET-1 in the pathogenesis of renal vasoconstriction in HRS has been proposed on the basis of markedly increased plasma endothelin levels in patients with HRS as compared with patients with ascites without HRS[146,360] and improvement of renal function after the administration of a selective antagonist of ET_A receptors in a small group of patients.[371] Paradoxically, the administration of tezosentan, a nonselective endothelin receptor antagonist to patients with cirrhosis and type 2 HRS, was associated with a deterioration in renal function, which suggests that at least in advanced cirrhosis endothelin contributes to maintenance of renal function and not to the pathogenesis of HRS.[372] A contribution of the increased endothelin levels to the maintenance of arterial pressure in cirrhosis is unlikely because most studies in experimental models of cirrhosis and portal hypertension have found no changes in arterial pressure after chronic endothelin receptor blockade.[369,373–375] Because of the well-known vasoconstrictor effect of ET-1 in the intrahepatic circulation when infused through the portal vein, ET-1 has been postulated as a mediator of the increased intrahepatic resistance characteristic of diseases associated with portal hypertension. The results of these studies are conflicting and the role of endothelin in these abnormalities is unclear.[376] Finally, recent studies suggest an important role for ET-1 in hepatic fibrogenesis by increasing collagen synthesis from hepatic stellate cells.[368] In support of this hypothesis, a marked reduction in liver fibrosis has been demonstrated in bile duct-ligated rats chronically treated with an oral ET_A receptor antagonist.[374] Despite the great efforts aimed at elucidating the role of ET in cirrhosis its relevance in circulatory homeostasis in cirrhosis is still unclear. Further studies are needed to understand and characterize the role of ET in advanced cirrhosis.

Nitric Oxide

In addition to its effects in the regulation of systemic hemodynamics and arterial pressure, as described before NO also participates in the regulation of renal function.[377] Constitutive NO synthase has been found in several cell types in the kidney, including endothelial cells, mesangial cells, and some tubular epithelial cells. Inducible NO synthase has also been demonstrated in mesangial cells and epithelial cells. Under normal circumstances, NO participates in the regulation of glomerular microcirculation by modulating arteriolar tone and mesangial cell contractility. Moreover, NO facilitates natriuresis in response to changes in renal perfusion pressure, and regulates renin release.[377]

Three lines of evidence indicate that the renal production of NO is increased in experimental cirrhosis. First, kidneys from cirrhotic rats show enhanced endothelium-dependent vasodilator response as compared to control animals.[378] Second, infusion of L-arginine, the precursor of NO, causes a greater increase in renal perfusion in cirrhotic rats as compared to control rats.[379] Finally, increased expression of NO synthase in kidney tissue from cirrhotic rats has been found in two studies.[379,380] However, both studies showed discrepant findings with respect to the NO synthase isoform responsible for the increased NO synthesis.

The inhibition of NO synthesis in rats with cirrhosis and ascites does not result in renal hypoperfusion because of a marked rise in prostaglandin synthesis.[381] However, the simultaneous inhibition of NO and prostaglandin synthesis in experimental cirrhosis results in a marked renal vasoconstriction suggesting that NO probably interacts with prostaglandins to maintain renal hemodynamics.[382]

Endocannabinoid System

The endocannabinoid system appears to play a role in the pathogenesis of hemodynamic abnormalities (cardiovascular dysfunction and portal hypertension) in cirrhosis.[383–387] The endocannabinoid system consists of CB receptors and circulating endocannabinoids. Two G protein–coupled types of receptors (CB1 and CB2) have been identified in several tissues including the cardiovascular system and the liver.[383,384] In patients with cirrhosis, CB1 receptors in the vascular and cardiac tissue are activated by two circulating endogenous endocannabinoids; arachidonoyl ethanolamide (anandamide) and 2-arachidonoyl glycerol (2-AG).[383,384] The source of the anandamide and 2-AG are lipopolysaccharide activated macrophages.[385,386] Levels of anandamide are elevated in circulating macrophages of cirrhotic rats; in fact, injection of these macrophages into normal rats causes hypotension.[387] The role of the cannabinoid system in the hemodynamic alterations of cirrhosis is also supported by the fact that hypotension in cirrhotic rats is reversible by CB1 blockade, an effect that also reduces increased portal pressure and mesenteric blood flow.[387,388] In cirrhosis, underlying endotoxemia which activates macrophages is thought to be the principal source of endocannabinoid production by means of a lipopolysaccharide that leads to the increased levels of anandamide.[383,384] In addition, in cirrhosis there is increased expression of CB1 in vascular endothelial cells[387] and mesenteric arteries[389,390] which in turn augment the vasodilatory effects of anandamide.[388–391] In patients with cirrhosis peripheral anandamide (but not 2-AG) is increased in advanced stages; however, hepatic vein and liver tissue levels of anandamide are not increased suggesting that the liver is not the source of endogenous cannabinoids.[392,393] Experiments on isolated mesenteric resistance arteries of rats with cirrhosis and ascites demonstrate that anandamide exerts a greater vasodilatory effect when compared to control rats.[389] Interestingly, this response is not altered by L-NAME (an inhibitor of nitric oxide synthase), indicating that the effect of anadamide in resistance arteries of cirrhotic rats is perhaps independent of the functional integrity of endothelium.[389] Moreover, the effect of anandamide is selective in the mesenteric vessels because there are no changes in vascular reactivity of distal femoral arteries of cirrhotic and control rats.[389] In cirrhotic rats, rimonabant (an anandamide antagonist) caused a significant reduction in the volume and formation of ascites.[394] The antagonist also significantly improved sodium balance after 2 weeks in cirrhotic animals.[394] The role of endocannabinoids in the pathogenesis of cardiac dysfunction in cirrhosis which is mainly due to a decrease in contractility and β-adrenergic hyposensitivity is thought to be due to activation of cardiac CB1 receptors.[356,395] Studies in animals with cirrhosis have demonstrated that a decrease in baseline cardiac contractility normalizes with the administration of an endocannabinoid antagonist.[396] Although these findings suggest a potential role of endocannabinoid blockade in the treatment of complications related to portal hypertension, there are no studies evaluating the effects of rimonabant in human cirrhosis because the drug was withdrawn from the market due to significant side effects in relation to depression and anxiety.

Heme-oxygenase System

Another potential mediator in the pathogenesis of hemodynamic abnormalities in cirrhosis is the heme-oxygenase (HO) system.[397] The main byproducts of HO are carbon monoxide (CO) and biliverdin which is converted to bilirubin. There are three isoforms of HO: inducible (HO-1), constitutive (HO-2), and a secondary constitutive form with minimal activity (HO-3).[397] Several experimental and human studies indicate that CO contributes to the splanchnic vasodilation that occurs in cirrhosis and also plays a role in the regulation of hepatic vascular tone.[398–401] The mechanism by which CO causes relaxation of smooth muscle cells is by activation of soluble guanylyl cyclase which leads to an increased production of cGMP thereby opening large-conductance calcium activated channels.[397] Levels of carboxy-hemoglobin and CO in the exhaled air in patients with compensated and decompensated cirrhosis are increased and both parameters are higher in those with ascites and correlate with the Child–Pugh score but not with arterial pressure or plasma renin activity.[229] In addition, both parameters increase even more in patients with spontaneous bacterial peritonitis compared to those without infection.[229] Similar data indicate plasma-free CO is elevated in patients with cirrhosis compared with healthy controls.[229] In addition increased plasma free CO in cirrhosis without ascites correlates with plasma cGMP and is associated with impaired hemodynamics (high cardiac index and lower arterial pressure) more so than in those with ascites. Finally HO-1 activity is increased in polymorphonuclear cells of patients with cirrhosis indicating that high levels likely correlate with systemic endotoxemia. These data provide evidence that the HO pathway is activated in cirrhosis, and suggest that it may play a role in the pathogenesis of the hyperdynamic circulation of cirrhosis.[229,400] The effect of the HO system in the kidney is less studied; however, it is known that there is reduced renal expression of HO-1 in experimental cirrhosis.[402,403] One study that evaluated the renal effects of CO in cirrhotic rats indicates that impaired HO-1 expression promotes renal vasoconstriction and that chronic HO induction normalizes the sensitivity to vasoconstrictors (phenylephrine) and promotes sodium excretion.[404] Taken together, all these findings suggest that the HO system plays a role in the development of splanchnic arterial vasodilation and renal abnormalities in cirrhosis.

THE THEORIES OF ASCITES FORMATION IN CIRRHOSIS

Ascites as Primary Edema: The Overflow Theory

The existence of a primary renal sodium retention in cirrhosis with ascites was proposed in an attempt to explain the paradox of coexistence of sodium retention and increased plasma volume in patients with ascites.[405,406] According to this theory, the expansion of plasma volume would result in increased cardiac index and reduced systemic vascular resistance as adaptive circulatory mechanisms to the excess of intravascular volume. The existence of portal hypertension and circulating hypervolemia would lead to "overflow" of fluid within the peritoneal cavity. It has been proposed that the primary signal for sodium retention would arise from the liver, either as a consequence of intrahepatic portal hypertension, by means of hepatic low pressure baroreceptors, or liver failure, by means of decreased hepatic clearance of a sodium-retaining factor or reduced hepatic synthesis of a natriuretic factor.[292–294,407–411] However, the hemodynamic pattern of cirrhotic patients with ascites does not correspond with that predicted by the overflow theory because the arterial vascular compartment is not overfilled, as arterial pressure is low in most patients despite the increased plasma volume and cardiac index (Table 68.3). Moreover, there is marked overactivity of vasoconstrictor mechanisms, which would be suppressed if there were overfilling in the systemic circulation.[205,216]

Because of the increasing evidence against the existence of vascular overfilling in cirrhosis with ascites, the overflow theory has been redefined to exclusively explain changes that occur in the preascitic stage of cirrhosis. Proponents of this theory suggest that in the preascitic stage of cirrhosis subtle sodium retention leading to plasma volume expansion would have two components: one related to the circulatory changes occurring in the splanchnic circulation aimed at maintaining the effective arterial blood volume (EABV) and one related to the existence of intrahepatic portal hypertension.[412,413] Recent studies in patients with cirrhosis without ascites indicate that the existence of arterial vasodilation is of crucial importance in the development of sodium retention and ascites formation. In fact, preascitic cirrhotic patients with sinusoidal portal hypertension treated with mineralocorticoids do not show mineralocorticoid escape and develop ascites only when marked arterial vasodilation is present.[414] Moreover, pharmacologically induced vasodilation in preascitic cirrhotic patients by means of the administration of prazosin, an α-adrenergic blocker, is associated with the development of ascites and/or edema in a significant proportion of patients.[415] It is important to note that the development of sodium retention in these two studies was neither related to the degree of portal hypertension nor to the intensity of liver failure. In fact, in patients receiving prazosin, sodium retention occurred despite a reduction of portal pressure and improvement of liver perfusion.

Ascites as Secondary Edema: From the Traditional Theory to the Arterial Vasodilation Theory

The traditional concept of ascites formation in cirrhosis[416,417] considers that the key event in ascites formation is a "backward" increase in hydrostatic pressure in the hepatic and splanchnic circulation due to the increased resistance to portal flow. This would cause a disruption of the Starling equilibrium and an increased filtration of fluid into the interstitial space. Initially, this capillary hyperfiltration is compensated by an increased lymphatic flow which returns the fluid to the systemic circulation via the thoracic duct. However, as portal hypertension increases, the lymphatic system is not able to drain the excess of interstitial fluid which then accumulates in the peritoneal cavity as ascites. Loss of fluid from the intravascular compartment results in true hypovolemia which is then sensed by cardiopulmonary and arterial receptors resulting in a compensatory renal sodium retention. The retained fluid cannot adequately fill the intravascular compartment and suppress the sodium-retaining signals to the kidney because fluid is continuously leaking in the peritoneal cavity, thus creating a vicious cycle. In cases with extreme hypovolemia, renal vasoconstriction develops, leading to HRS. This hypothesis is similar to the "backward" theory of edema formation in heart failure, which suggests that sodium retention and formation of edema is secondary to the disruption of the Starling equilibrium in the microcirculation due to the backward increase in capillary hydrostatic pressure.[418] The "classic underfilling" theory of ascites formation, however, does not correspond with the systemic hemodynamic abnormalities associated with cirrhosis (Table 68.3). If this theory were correct, changes in systemic circulation would consist of reduced plasma volume and cardiac index and increased systemic vascular resistance. However, findings in patients with cirrhosis and ascites are exactly the opposite, with increased plasma volume and cardiac index and reduced systemic vascular resistance.[204,205,216]

These traditional backward theories of edema formation in cirrhosis and heart failure have been substituted by new theories that fit more precisely with the modern concepts of regulation of extracellular fluid volume, which consider that a reduction in effective arterial blood volume (EABV) is the main determinant of sodium retention in major edematous states.[419–421] Arterial vasodilation would be the triggering factor for sodium retention in cirrhosis, whereas a reduction in cardiac output would be the triggering factor in heart failure. The "arterial vasodilation" theory considers that the reduction in EABV in cirrhosis with ascites is not due to true hypovolemia, as proposed by the "traditional" theory, but rather to a disproportionate enlargement of the arterial tree secondary to arterial vasodilation (Fig. 68.10).[216,422,423] According to this theory, portal hypertension is the initial event with resultant splanchnic arteriolar vasodilation causing underfilling of the arterial circulation. The arterial receptors then sense the arterial underfilling and stimulate the SNS and the RAAS and cause nonosmotic hypersecretion of AVP. Renal sodium and water retention are the final consequence of this compensatory response to a reduction in EABV. In early stages of cirrhosis, when splanchnic arteriolar vasodilation is moderate and the lymphatic system is able to return the increased lymph production to the systemic circulation, the EABV is preserved by transient periods of sodium retention. The fluid retained by the kidneys increases plasma volume and suppresses the signals stimulating the antinatriuretic systems and sodium retention terminates. Therefore, no ascites or edema is formed at this stage and the relationship between EABV and extracellular fluid volume is maintained. As liver disease progresses, splanchnic arterial vasodilation increases, thus resulting in a more intense arterial underfilling and more marked sodium and water retention. At this time, the EABV can no longer be maintained by the increased plasma volume, probably because the retained fluid leaks from the splanchnic circulation into the peritoneal cavity as ascites and/or from the systemic circulation to the interstitial tissue as edema. A persistent stimulation of vasoconstrictor systems occurs in an attempt to maintain EABV. The activation of these systems perpetuates renal sodium and water retention, which accumulates as ascites. The correlation between EABV and extracellular fluid volume is no longer maintained as EABV remains contracted despite

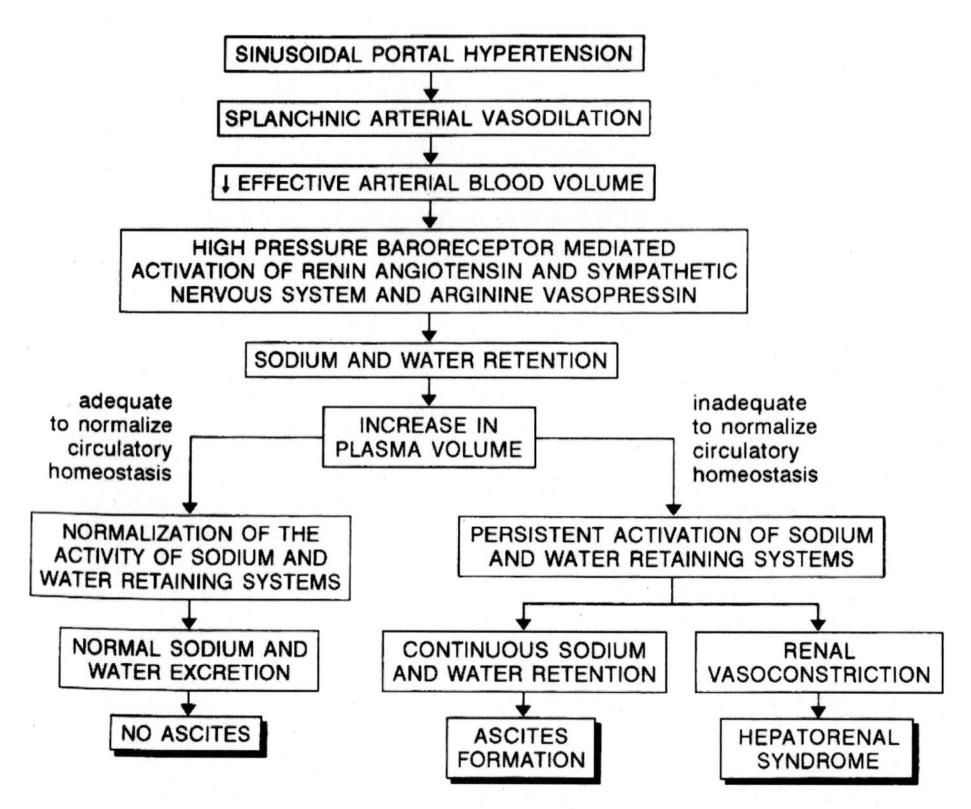

FIGURE 68.10 Pathogenesis of functional renal abnormalities and ascites formation in cirrhosis according to the arterial vasodilation hypothesis.

progressive expansion of extracellular fluid volume. HRS probably represents the most extreme manifestation of the reduction in EABV. Studies in experimental models of portal hypertension aimed at carefully investigating the chronologic relationship between abnormalities in the systemic circulation and sodium retention indicate that arterial vasodilation with reduced systemic vascular resistance precedes sodium retention and subsequent plasma volume expansion.[424]

The arterial vasodilation theory not only provides a reasonable explanation for the circulatory changes and activation of antinatriuretic systems observed in cirrhosis with ascites, but also for the preferential location of retained fluid in the peritoneal cavity. The existence of splanchnic arterial vasodilation causes a "forward" increase in splanchnic capillary pressure that enhances the effects of portal hypertension on the filtration coefficient in splanchnic capillaries, which facilitates the formation of ascites.[188,190,191]

MANAGEMENT OF COMPLICATIONS DUE TO RENAL FUNCTION ABNORMALITIES

Management of Ascites

An important step in the management of ascites is education of patients regarding a sodium-restricted diet of approximately 90 mmol per day[425,426] which may help cause a negative sodium balance and loss of ascites. A more stringent restriction is generally not well tolerated and patients become noncompliant. Additionally, fluid restriction is not necessary unless patients have associated hyponatremia. The current classification of ascites defined by the International Ascites Club divides patients in three groups.[426] Patients with grade 1 ascites are those in whom ascites is detected only by ultrasonography; these patients do not require any specific treatment, but they should be warned about avoiding foods with large amounts of salt. Patients with grade 2 ascites are those in which ascites causes moderate distension of the abdomen associated with mild/moderate discomfort. Patients with grade 3 ascites have large amounts of ascitic fluid causing marked abdominal distension and associated with significant discomfort. Patients with refractory ascites are those that do not respond to high doses of diuretics or develop side effects that preclude their use.[122]

Nonrefractory Ascites

Grade 2 ascites. These patients typically can be managed as outpatients unless other complications of cirrhosis are present. A negative sodium balance with loss of ascites is quickly and easily obtained in most cases with combination of sodium-restricted diet and diuretics.[49,159,248,427] Patients with new onset ascites respond to spironolactone 50 to 100 mg per day and the dose may be increased progressively if needed. Patients with prior episodes of ascites should receive the combination of spironolactone 100 mg per day with furosemide (20 to 40 mg per day).[49,159,248,427] If there is no response, compliance with diet and medications should be confirmed and diuretics may then be increased until there is response in a stepwise fashion every 7 days by doubling doses to a maximal dose of spironolactone of 400 mg per day and a maximal dose of furosemide of 160 mg per day. Diuretic therapy is effective in the elimination of ascites in nearly 85% to 90% of all patients.[425] Spironolactone-induced gynecomastia may cause patients to stop the drug; in these cases amiloride (5–10 mg per day) may be useful, although its potency is lower than that of spironolactone. Eplerenone, another aldosterone antagonist, has fewer endocrine adverse effects compared with spironolactone and could be a good alternative to spironolactone in patients with spironolactone-induced gynecomastia but there is limited data.[428] The goal of diuretic therapy is to achieve a maximum weight loss of 500 g per day in patients without edema and 1,000 g per day in those with peripheral edema. A greater degree of weight loss may induce volume depletion and renal failure. After minimizing ascites, the dose of diuretics should be reduced to maintain a neutral sodium balance with no more weight loss. The management of patients with grade 2 ascites is summarized in Table 68.5.

Grade 3 ascites. Patients with grade 3 ascites (large ascites) are best managed by large-volume paracentesis. Complete removal of ascites in one tap (as many liters as possible) with intravenous albumin (8 g per liter tapped) has been shown to be quick, effective, and associated with a lower number of complications than conventional diuretic therapy.[429] After a large-volume tap, postparacentesis circulatory dysfunction may develop if albumin is not given; this is a circulatory derangement with marked activation of the renin-angiotensin system that occurs 24 to 48 hours after the procedure.[430] This disorder is clinically silent, not spontaneously reversible, and associated with hyponatremia and renal impairment in up to 20% of patients.[83,429,430] In addition, it is associated with decreased survival. Postparacentesis circulatory dysfunction is prevented with the administration of albumin (8 g per L tapped).[83,431,432] Although the use of albumin after paracentesis is controversial due to the lack of data proving a survival benefit and high cost in some countries, the protective effect of albumin on the circulatory system favors its use. Thus, current guidelines recommend the use of albumin after large-volume paracentesis.[159,426,433,434] Patients with grade 3 ascites and a known history of cirrhosis and without any complications can be managed as outpatients. However, patients in whom tense ascites is the first manifestation of cirrhosis or those with associated hepatic encephalopathy, gastrointestinal bleeding, or bacterial infections require hospitalization. Most of these patients have marked sodium retention and need to be started or continued on relatively high doses of diuretics after large-volume paracentesis together with a low sodium diet (Table 68.6).

TABLE 68.5 **Therapeutic Approach to Management of Patients with Cirrhosis and Grade 2 or Moderate Ascites**

Initial Therapy

1. Start with low-sodium diet (80–120 mEq/day) and spironolactone starting at 50–100 mg/day as a single dose in patients with new onset ascites. The dose may be increased stepwise every 7 days (in 100-mg steps) to a maximum of 400 mg/day if there is no response. In patients with no response to aldosterone antagonists, low doses of loop diuretics (furosemide, 20–40 mg/day) may be used in combination with spironolactone to increase the natriuretic effect. Monitor body weight daily and urine sodium weekly. Ideal weight loss should be 300–500 g/day in patients without peripheral edema and 800–1000 g/day in patients with peripheral edema. Outpatients should be instructed to reduce the diuretic dosage in case of greater weight loss.
2. Patients with prior episodes of ascites should receive the combination of spironolactone 100 mg/day with furosemide (20–40 mg/day). If no response is seen, check compliance with treatment and low-sodium diet. Increase the dose of diuretics stepwise every 7–10 days up to 400 mg/day of spironolactone and 160 mg/day of furosemide.

Maintenance Therapy

1. Maintain sodium restriction and reduce diuretic treatment to the minimum dose necessary to prevent reaccumulation of ascites.
2. If ascites or edema does not recur, increase sodium intake progressively and maintain a low dose of diuretics.

Refractory Ascites

Nearly 10% of patients with ascites are refractory to treatment with diuretics.[122,159] In refractory ascites, a significant increase in sodium excretion cannot be achieved either because patients do not respond to high doses of diuretics (spironolactone 400 mg per day and furosemide 160 mg per day) or because they develop side effects that preclude their use.[122,435] These patients in general have features of advanced liver disease, a high recurrence rate of ascites after large-volume paracentesis, an increased risk of HRS, and a poor prognosis. Current treatment strategies include repeated large-volume paracentesis plus intravenous albumin as needed, and transjugular intrahepatic portosystemic shunts (TIPS). Large-volume paracentesis is the accepted initial therapy for refractory ascites.[159] Patients, on average, require a tap every

TABLE 68.6 **Therapeutic Approach to Management of Patients with Cirrhosis and Grade 3 or Large-volume Ascites**

Initial Therapy

1. Large-volume paracentesis plus intravenous albumin (8 g/L of ascites removed). Patients can be treated as outpatients.

Maintenance Therapy

1. Low-sodium diet (80–120 mEq/day) associated with diuretic therapy.
2. If the patient was not taking diuretics before the development of severe ascites, start with spironolactone (50–100 mg/day as a single dose) and then adjust the dose to maintain the patient with mild or no ascites or edema. Check body weight daily and urine sodium weekly. Closely monitor the patient during the first weeks of therapy. Add loop diuretics (furosemide 40 mg/day), if necessary.
3. If the patient was taking diuretics before the development of severe ascites, start with a dose slightly higher than the dose taken before paracentesis.
4. If ascites or edema increases, check compliance with treatment and the low-sodium diet. Increase the dose of diuretics stepwise every 7–10 days up to 400 mg/day of spironolactone and 160 mg/day of furosemide.
5. If ascites or edema does not recur, a balance should be maintained between sodium intake and diuretic therapy.

2 to 4 weeks and the majority may be treated as outpatients, making this option easy to perform and cost effective. TIPS, a nonsurgical method of portal decompression, reduces portal pressure and decreases ascites and diuretic requirements in these patients.[436,437] A disadvantage with TIPS is the development of side effects that include hepatic encephalopathy and impairment in liver function.[436–442] Additionally, uncovered TIPS may be complicated by stenosis of the prosthesis (18%–78%).[437] Meta-analyses of randomized controlled studies comparing TIPS versus large-volume paracentesis conclude that TIPS is better at controlling ascites but does not improve survival compared to paracentesis and increases the risk of hepatic encephalopathy.[443,444] In view of these findings, the preferred initial treatment for refractory ascites is large-volume paracentesis with albumin replacement.[159] In patients not suitable for repeated large-volume paracentesis plus albumin, TIPS placement should be evaluated on a case-by-case basis and probably reserved for patients aged <70, with preserved liver function, without hepatic encephalopathy or severe cardiopulmonary disease. The management of refractory ascites is summarized in Table 68.7.

Management of Hyponatremia

Management of dilutional hyponatremia includes water restriction of approximately 1 to 1.5 liters per day; however, this measure rarely works and although it may halt the progressive decrease in serum sodium concentration it does not correct hyponatremia. The administration of hypertonic saline solutions is not recommended because it invariably leads to further expansion of extracellular fluid volume and accumulation of ascites and edema. Several nonpeptide V2 receptor AVP antagonists including mozavaptan, lixivaptan, satavaptan, tolvaptan, and conivaptan have been evaluated in patients with cirrhosis and ascites with hyponatremia. These studies show that these drugs are effective at increasing solute-free water excretion and improve serum sodium concentration in hyponatremic patients with cirrhosis and ascites.[93–95,324,445,446] The short-term administration of vaptans is associated with an increase in serum sodium concentration that occurs within the 4 to 5 days of treatment with normalization of serum sodium concentration occurring in 30% to 55% of patients. Conivaptan is approved in the United States for short term (4 to 5 days) intravenous use (dose 20 mg per day), whereas tolvaptan is approved as an oral compound (dose starting at 15 mg per day with sequential 15 mg increments up to 60 mg per day).[324,446] The most frequent side effect of vaptans in patients with cirrhosis is thirst which can occur in up to 30% of patients. Other side effects are uncommon; however, these drugs need to be used with caution and the patient must be carefully monitored as very rapid correction of hyponatremia

TABLE 68.7 **Therapeutic Approach to Management of Patients with Cirrhosis and Refractory Ascites**

Initial Therapy

1. Repeated large-volume paracentesis plus intravenous albumin (8 g/L of ascites removed)

Maintenance Therapy

1. Maintain a low-sodium diet (80–120 mEq/day) constantly.
2. In patients taking the highest doses of diuretics, check urinary sodium. If less than 30 mEq/day, stop diuretic therapy.
3. Large-volume paracentesis plus intravenous albumin when necessary (approximately every 2–3 weeks).
4. Consider use of TIPS in patients with preserved hepatic function, no hepatic encephalopathy, either with loculated fluid, or unwilling to have repeated paracentesis.

TIPS, transjugular intrahepatic portosystemic shunt.

(e.g., >12 mEq/L/24 hours) can theoretically cause osmotic demyelination. No case of this syndrome, however, has been reported in studies so far published. The use of these agents in cirrhosis has been assessed in short-term studies; notwithstanding long-term controlled studies are needed to evaluate the safety, efficacy, and applicability of these agents in the long-term management of hyponatremia in patients with cirrhosis.

Management of Hepatorenal Syndrome

The main objective of patients with HRS, particularly those awaiting liver transplantation, is reversing renal failure in order to provide a successful bridge to transplantation. The best available therapy for HRS, other than liver transplantation, is the use of splanchnic vasoconstrictors plus albumin. Other modalities such as TIPS, renal replacement therapy, and albumin dialysis may be useful in some patients, but data on these approaches is very limited.

Vasoconstrictors

The administration of vasoconstrictors is the best medical therapy currently available for the management of HRS.[159] The rationale of this therapy is to improve circulatory function by causing vasoconstriction of the extremely dilated splanchnic arterial bed, which subsequently improves arterial underfilling, reduces the activity of the endogenous vasoconstrictor systems, and increases renal perfusion. The available vasoconstrictors used in HRS are vasopressin analogues (terlipressin) and alpha-adrenergic agonists (noradrenaline or midodrine), which act on V1 vasopressin receptors and α-1 adrenergic receptors, respectively, present in vascular smooth muscle cells (Table 68.8). In most studies, vasoconstrictors have been given in combination with intravenous albumin to further improve the arterial underfilling. Most of the published data comes from the use of intravenous terlipressin for type 1 HRS.[215,447–458] Results from randomized controlled studies and systematic reviews indicate that treatment with terlipressin together with albumin is associated with marked improvement of renal function in approximately 40% to 50% of patients.[454–458] Terlipressin is started at 1 mg per 4 to 6 hours intravenously, and the dose is increased up to a maximum of 2 mg per 4 to 6 hours after 3 days if there is no response to therapy as defined by a reduction of serum creatinine >25% of pretreatment values. Response to therapy is considered when there is marked reduction of the high serum creatinine levels, at least below 1.5 mg per dL, which is usually associated with increased urine output and improvement of hyponatremia.[454–458] The incidence of side effects (usually ischemic) requiring the discontinuation of treatment is of approximately 10%. Two randomized studies described previously[454,455] have shown that the overall population of patients treated with terlipressin and albumin do not have an improved survival compared to that of patients treated with albumin alone. However, both studies showed that responders in terms of improvement of renal function after therapy had a significant (but moderate), increase in survival compared to nonresponders. Recurrence of HRS after withdrawal of therapy occurs in less than 15% of patients and retreatment with terlipressin is generally effective. Factors associated with poor response include a bilirubin level ≥10 mg per dL, no increase in mean arterial pressure >5 mm Hg or lack of a drop in serum creatinine >0.5 mg per dL at day 3 of therapy.[459] Alpha-adrenergic agonists (noradrenaline, midodrine) represent an attractive alternative to terlipressin because of low cost, wide availability, and apparently similar efficacy compared with that of terlipressin.[266,453,460,461] However, the information on the efficacy and side effects of alpha-adrenergic agonists in patients with type 1 HRS is still very limited. Table 68.8 summarizes the treatment of HRS in patients with cirrhosis.

There are limited data on use of vasoconstrictors plus albumin for patients with type 2 HRS. However data from uncontrolled studies suggest that they are effective in decreasing serum creatinine levels in these patients. In two controlled studies, patients with type 2 HRS that received terlipressin plus albumin had a response between 67% and 88%; however, few were treated with this strategy in both studies and therefore more studies are needed in order to better define the role of vasoconstrictors plus albumin in the management of type 2 HRS.[453,455]

TABLE 68.8 **Pharmacologic Therapies for Hepatorenal Syndrome**

Vasoconstrictors
Terlipressin: 1 mg/4–6 hours intravenously; the dose is increased up to a maximum of 2 mg/4–6 hours after 3 days if there is no response to therapy as defined by a reduction of serum creatinine >25% of pretreatment values. Response to therapy is considered when there is marked reduction of the high serum creatinine levels, at least below 1.5 mg/dL (133 μmol/L). Treatment is usually given from 5–15 days.
Midodrine: 7.5 mg orally three times daily, increased to 12.5 mg three times daily if needed.
Octreotide: 100 μg subcutaneously three times daily, increased to 200 μg three times daily if needed.
Norepinephrine: 0.5–3 mg/h as continuous intravenous infusion aimed at increasing mean arterial pressure by 10 mm Hg. Treatment is maintained until serum creatinine decreases below 1.5 mg/dL.
Albumin Administration
Concomitant administration of albumin together with vasoconstrictor drugs (1g/kg body weight at day 1 followed by 20–40 g/day).

Transjugular intrahepatic portosystemic shunts. The use of TIPS for therapy of HRS has been suggested for years, but the applicability in patients with such advanced liver disease is very limited. Two small studies indicate that TIPS may improve GFR as well as reduce the activity of the RAAS and the SNS in approximately 60% of patients with type 1 HRS.[265,462] However, these studies only included patients with moderately severe liver failure and excluded those with a history of hepatic encephalopathy, Child-Pugh score ≥12 or serum bilirubin >5 mg per dL. The applicability of TIPS in patients with type 1 HRS is low because TIPS is considered contraindicated in patients with features of severe liver failure, which are common findings in the setting of type 1 HRS. The use of TIPS in type 2 HRS may improve renal function and reduce the risk of progression to type 1 HRS, but these data require confirmation in specifically designed studies.

Renal replacement therapy and other dialysis methods. Renal replacement therapy (RRT), mainly hemodialysis, has been used in the management of patients with type 1 HRS, especially in candidates for liver transplantation, in an attempt to maintain patients alive until liver transplantation is performed.[463] Unfortunately, the potential beneficial effect of this approach has not been evaluated in randomized studies comparing RRT to other forms of therapy such as vasoconstrictors. Most patients develop side effects during RRT which include severe arterial hypotension, bleeding, and infections that may contribute to death during treatment. Additionally, indications for RRT (severe fluid overload, acidosis, or hyperkalemia) are uncommon in type 1 HRS, at least in the early stages. Other methods such as the use of the molecular readsorbent recirculating system (MARS), an alternative of dialysis that clears albumin-bound substances, including vasodilators, is promising but more data are needed in order to consider it as a therapeutic device for HRS.[464–466]

Liver transplantation. Liver transplantation is the treatment of choice for candidate patients with cirrhosis and HRS. However, a major problem in liver transplantation for type 1 HRS is the high mortality rate in the waiting list due to the combination of short survival expectancy and prolonged waiting times in many transplant centers. This limitation is usually overcome by assigning these patients a high priority for transplantation. Because pretransplant renal failure is an independent risk factor of both short-term and long-term posttransplantation patient and graft survival all efforts should be made to improve renal function in order to obtain a better outcome after transplantation. The reversal of both type 1 and 2 HRS using vasoconstrictors before transplantation may help patients not only reach transplantation, but also reduce the relatively high morbidity and mortality after liver transplantation characteristic of HRS.

REFERENCES

1. Papper S. Liver–Kidney Interrelationships. A personal perspective. In: Epstein M, ed. *The Kidney in Liver Disease*, 2nd ed. New York: Elsevier Biomedical; 1983:3.
2. Frerichs T. *Tratado práctico de las enfermedades del Hígado, de los vasos hepáticos y de las vias biliares*. Madrid: Librería Extranjera y Nacional, Científica y Literaria; 1877:362.
3. Flint A. Clinical report on hydro-peritoneum, based on an analysis of forty-six cases. *Am J Med Sci.* 1863;45:306.
4. Arroyo V, Ginès P, Rodés J, Schrier RW, eds. *Ascites and Renal Dysfunction in Liver Disease. Pathogenesis, Diagnosis and Treatment*. Oxford, UK: Blackwell Science; 1999.
5. Ginès P, Arroyo V, Rodés J, Schrier RW, eds. *Ascites and Renal Dysfunction in Liver Disease. Pathogenesis, Diagnosis and Treatment*. Oxford, UK: Blackwell Publishing; 2005.
6. Ginès P, Kamath PS, Arroyo V, eds. *Chronic Liver Failure. Mechanisms and Management*. New York: Springer; 2010.
7. Bomzom A, Blendis LM. *Cardiovascular Complications of Liver Disease*. Boca Raton, FL: CRC Press; 1990.
8. Epstein M, ed. *The Kidney in Liver Disease*. 1st ed. Philadelphia: Hanley & Belfus; 1978.
9. Epstein M, ed. *The Kidney in Liver Disease*. 2nd ed. Philadelphia: Hanley & Belfus; 1983.
10. Epstein M, ed. *The Kidney in Liver Disease*. 3rd ed. Philadelphia: Hanley & Belfus; 1988.
11. Epstein M, ed. *The Kidney in Liver Disease*. 4th ed. Philadelphia: Hanley & Belfus; 1996.
12. Gerbes AL, ed. *Ascites, Hyponatremia and Hepatorenal Syndrome: Progress in Treatment. Frontiers of Gastrointestinal Research*, vol 28. Basel: Karger; 2011.
13. Terra C, Alves de Mattos A, eds. *Complicaçoes da cirrose – Ascite e Insuficiência Renal*. Rio de Janeiro: Livraria e Editora Revinter Ltda; 2009.
14. Papper S. The role of the kidney in Laënnec's cirrhosis of the liver. *Medicine (Baltimore)*. 1958;37:299.
15. Papper S, Belsky JL, Bleifer KH. Renal failure in Laënnec's cirrhosis of the liver: I. Description of clinical and laboratory features. *Ann Intern Med.* 1959;51:759.
16. Vesin P. Late functional renal failure in cirrhosis with ascites: pathophysiology, diagnosis and treatment. In: Martinin GA, Sherlock S, eds. *Aktuelle probleme der hepatologie*. Stuttgart: Georg Thieme Verlag: 1962;98.
17. Baldus WP, Feichter RN, Summerskill WHJ, et al. The kidney in cirrhosis. I. Clinical and biochemical features of azotemia in hepatic failure. *Ann Intern Med.* 1964;60:353.
18. Shear L, Kleinerman J, Gabuzda GJ. Renal failure in patients with cirrhosis of the liver: I. Clinical and pathologic characteristics. *Am J Med.* 1965;39:184.
19. Patek AJ Jr, Post J, Ratnoff OD, et al. Dietary treatment of cirrhosis of the liver. Results in one-hundred and twenty-four patients observed during a ten year period. *JAMA.* 1948;138:543.
20. Post J, Sicam L. The clinical course of Laënnec's cirrhosis under modern medical management. *Med Clin North Am.* 1960;44:639.
21. Pecikyan R, Kanzaki G, Berger EY. Electrolyte excretion during the spontaneous recovery from the ascitic phase of cirrhosis of the liver. *Am J Med.* 1967;42:359.
22. Papper S. Hepatorenal syndrome. In: Epstein M, ed. *The Kidney in Liver Disease*, 2nd ed. New York: Elsevier Biomedical; 1983;87.
23. Ginès A, Escorsell A, Ginès P, et al. Incidence, predictive factors, and prognosis of the hepatorenal syndrome in cirrhosis with ascites. *Gastroenterology.* 1993;105:229.
24. Farnsworth EB, Krakusin JS. Electrolyte partition in patients with edema of various origins. *J Lab Clin Med.* 1948;33:1545.
25. Falloon WW, Eckhardt RD, Cooper AM, et al. The effect of human serum albumin, mercurial diuretics, and a low sodium diet on sodium excretion in patients with cirrhosis of the liver. *J Clin Invest.* 1949;28:595–602.
26. Eisenmenger WJ, Blondheim SH, Bongiovanni AM, et al. Electrolyte studies on patients with cirrhosis of the liver. *J Clin Invest.* 1950;29:1491.
27. Arroyo V, Rodés J. A rational approach to the treatment of ascites. *Postgrad Med J.* 1975;51:558.
28. Levy M. Sodium retention in dogs with cirrhosis and ascites: efferent mechanisms. *Am J Physiol.* 1977;233:F586.
29. Levy M, Allotey JB. Temporal relationships between urinary salt retention and altered systemic hemodynamics in dogs with experimental cirrhosis. *J Lab Clin Med.* 1978;92:560.
30. López-Novoa JM, Rengel MA, Hernando L. Dynamics of ascites formation in rats with experimental cirrhosis. *Am J Physiol.* 1980;238:F353.
31. Jiménez W, Martínez-Pardo A, Arroyo V, et al. Temporal relationship between hyperaldosteronism, sodium retention and ascites formation in rats with experimental cirrhosis. *Hepatology.* 1985;5:245.

32. Gliedman ML, Carrol HJ, Popowitz L, et al. An experimental hepatorenal syndrome. *Surg Gynecol Obstet.* 1970;131:34.
33. Blendis LM, Greig PD, Langer B, et al. The renal and hemodynamic effects of the peritoneovenous shunt for intractable hepatic ascites. *Gastroenterology.* 1979;77:250.
34. Ginès P, Arroyo V, Vargas V, et al. Paracentesis with intravenous infusion of albumin as compared with peritoneovenous shunting in cirrhosis with refractory ascites. *N Engl J Med.* 1991;325:829.
35. Ginès P, Arroyo V, Rodés J. Complications of cirrhosis: ascites, hyponatremia, hepatorenal syndrome and spontaneous bacterial peritonitis. In: Bacon D, DiBisceglie A, eds. *Liver Disease: Diagnosis and Management.* Philadelphia: Churchill Livingstone; 2000:238.
36. Bernardi M, Laffi G, Salvagnini M, et al. Efficacy and safety of the stepped care medical treatment of ascites in liver cirrhosis: a randomized controlled clinical trial comparing two diets with different sodium content. *Liver.* 1993;13:156.
37. Fernandez-Llama P, Ginès P, Schrier RW. Pathogenesis of sodium retention in cirrhosis: the arterial vasodilation hypothesis of ascites formation. In: Ginès P, Arroyo V, Rodes J, Schrier R, eds. *Ascites and Renal Dysfunction in Liver Disease.* 2nd ed. Oxford, UK: Blackwell Publishing; 2005:201–214.
38. Cárdenas A, Bataller R, Arroyo V. Mechanisms of ascites formation. *Clin Liver Dis.* 2000;4:447.
39. López-Novoa JM, Rengel MA, Rodicio JL, at al. A micropuncture study of salt and water retention in chronic experimental cirrhosis. *Am J Physiol.* 1977;232:F315.
40. Clària J, Jiménez W. Experimental models of cirrhosis and ascites. In: Ginès P, Arroyo V, Rodes J, Schrier R, eds. *Ascites and Renal Dysfunction in Liver Disease.* 2nd ed. Oxford, UK: Blackwell Publishing; 2005:215.
41. Fernández-Llama P, Ageloff S, Fernández-Varo G, et al. Sodium retention in cirrhotic rats is associated with increased renal abundance of sodium transporter proteins. *Kidney Int.* 2005;67:622.
42. Epstein M, Ramachandran M, DeNunzio AG. Interrelationship of renal sodium and phosphate handling in cirrhosis. *Miner Electrolyte Metab.* 1982;7:305.
43. Chaimovitz C, Szylman P, Alroy G, et al. Mechanism of increased renal tubular sodium reabsorption in cirrhosis. *Am J Med.* 1972;52:198.
44. Rochman J, Chaimovitz C, Szylman P, et al. Tubular handling of sodium and phosphate in cirrhosis with salt retention. *Nephron.* 1978;20:95.
45. Wilkinson SP, Jowett TP, Slater JDH, et al. Renal sodium retention in cirrhosis: relation to aldosterone and nephron site. *Clin Sci.* 1979;56:169.
46. Angeli P, Gatta A, Caregaro L, et al. Tubular site of renal sodium retention in ascitic liver cirrhosis evaluated by lithium clearance. *Eur J Clin Invest.* 1990;20:111.
47. Diez J, Simon MA, Anton F, et al. Tubular sodium handling in cirrhotic patients with ascites analysed by the renal lithium clearance method. *Eur J Clin Invest.* 1990;20:266.
48. Eggert RC. Spironolactone diuresis in patients with cirrhosis and ascites. *Br Med J.* 1970;4:401.
49. Pérez-Ayuso RM, Arroyo V, Planas R, et al. Randomized comparative study of efficacy of furosemide versus spironolactone in nonazotemic cirrhosis with ascites. Relationship between the diuretic response and the activity of the renin-aldosterone system. *Gastroenterology.* 1983;84:961.
50. Gatta A, Angeli P, Caregaro L, et al. A pathophysiological interpretation of unresponsiveness to spironolactone in a stepped-care approach to the diuretic treatment of ascites in nonazotemic cirrhotic patients. *Hepatology.* 1991;14:231.
51. Angeli P, Gatta A. Medical treatment of ascites in cirrhosis. In: Ginès P, Arroyo V, Rodes J, Schrier R, eds. *Ascites and Renal Dysfunction in Liver Disease.* 2nd ed. Oxford, UK: Blackwell Publishing; 2005:227.
52. Ginès P, Arroyo V, Rodés J. Pathophysiology, complications and treatment of ascites. *Clin Liver Dis.* 1997;1:129.
53. Trevisani F, Bernardi M, Gasbarrini A, et al. Bed-rest-induced hypernatriuresis in cirrhotic patients without ascites: does it contribute to maintain "compensation"? *J Hepatol.* 1992;116:190.
54. Ring-Larsen H, Henriksen JH, Wilken C, et al. Diuretic treatment in decompensated cirrhosis and congestive heart failure: effect of posture. *Br Med J.* 1986;292:1351.
55. Lieberman FL, Hidemura R, Peters RL, et al. Pathogenesis and treatment of hydrothorax complicating cirrhosis with ascites. *Ann Intern Med.* 1966;64:341.
56. Strauss RM, Boyer TD. Hepatic hydrothorax. *Semin Liver Dis.* 1997;17:227.
57. Johnston RF, Loo RV. Hepatic hydrothorax. Studies to determine the source of the fluid and report of thirteen cases. *Ann Intern Med.* 1964;611:385.
58. Xiol X, Castellví JM, Guardiola J, et al. Spontaneous bacterial empyema of cirrhotic patients: a prospective study. *Hepatology.* 1996; 23:719.
59. Shah A, Variyam E. Pericardial effusion and left ventricular dysfunction associated with ascites secondary to hepatic cirrhosis. *Arch Intern Med.* 1991; 151:186.
60. Arroyo V, Bosch J, Gaya J, et al. Plasma renin activity and urinary sodium excretion as prognostic indicators in nonazotemic cirrhosis with ascites. *Ann Intern Med.* 1981;94:198.
61. Genoud E, Gonvers JJ, Schaller MD, et al. Valeur pronostique du système rènine-angiotensine dans la rèponse á la restriction sodèe et le pronostic de l'ascite cirrhotique d'origine alcoolique. *Schweiz Med Wochenschr.* 1986;116:463.
62. Llach J, Ginès P, Arroyo V, et al. Prognostic value of arterial pressure, endogenous vasoactive systems, and renal function in cirrhotic patients admitted to the hospital for the treatment of ascites. *Gastroenterology.* 1988;94:482.
63. Papper S, Saxon L. The diuretic response to administered water in patients with liver disease. II. Laënnec's cirrhosis of the liver. *Arch Intern Med.* 1959;103:750.
64. Shear L, Hall PW, Gabuzda GJ. Renal failure in patients with cirrhosis of the liver. II. Factors influencing maximal urinary flow rate. *Am J Med.* 1966;39:199.
65. Arroyo V, Rodés J, Gutièrrez-Lizárraga MA, et al. Prognostic value of spontaneous hyponatremia in cirrhosis with ascites. *Am J Dig Dis.* 1976;21:249.
66. McCullough AJ, Mullen KD, Kalhan SC. Measurements of total body and extracellular water in cirrhotic patients with and without ascites. *Hepatology.* 1991;14:1103.
67. Vaamonde CA. Renal water handling in liver disease. In: Epstein M, ed. *The Kidney in Liver Disease*, 4th ed. Philadelphia: Hanley & Belfus; 1996:33.
68. Ginès P, Berl T, Bernardi M, et al. Hyponatremia in cirrhosis: from pathogenesis to treatment. *Hepatology.* 1998;28:851.
69. Angeli P, Wong F, Watson H, Ginès P; CAPPS Investigators. Hyponatremia in cirrhosis: Results of a patient population survey. *Hepatology.* 2006;44: 1535–1542.
70. Cosby RL, Yee B, Schrier RW. New classification with prognostic value in cirrhotic patients. *Miner Electrolyte Metab.* 1989;15:261.
71. Abad-Lacruz A, Cabrè E, González-Huix F, et al. Routine tests of renal function, alcoholism, and nutrition improve the prognostic accuracy of Child-Pugh score in nonbleeding advanced cirrhosis. *Am J Gastroenterol.* 1993;88:382.
72. Salerno F, Borroni G, Moser P, et al. Survival and prognostic factors of cirrhotic patients with ascites: a study of 134 outpatients. *Am J Gastroenterol.* 1993;88:514.
73. Fernández-Esparrach G, Sánchez-Fueyo A, Ginès P, et al. A prognostic model for predicting survival in cirrhosis with ascites. *J Hepatol.* 2001;34:46.
74. Heuman DM, Abou-Assi SG, Habib A, et al. Persistent ascites and low serum sodium identify patients with cirrhosis and low MELD scores who are at high risk for early death. *Hepatology.* 2004;40:802.
75. Biggins SW, Rodriguez HJ, Bacchetti P, et al. Serum sodium predicts mortality in patients listed for liver transplantation. *Hepatology.* 2004;41:32.
76. Ruf AE, Kremers WK, Chavez LL, et al. Addition of serum sodium into the MELD score predicts waiting list mortality better than MELD alone. *Liver Transpl.* 2005;11:336.
77. Biggins SW, Rodriguez HJ, Bacchetti P, et al. Serum sodium predicts mortality in patients listed for liver transplantation. *Hepatology.* 2005;41:32–39.
78. Londoño MC, Cárdenas A, Guevara M, et al. MELD score and serum sodium in the prediction of survival of patients with cirrhosis awaiting liver transplantation. *Gut.* 2007;56:1283–1290.
79. Kim WR, Biggins SW, Kremers WK, et al. Hyponatremia and mortality among patients on the liver-transplant waiting list. *N Engl J Med.* 2008;359: 1018–1026.
80. Porcel A, Diaz F, Rendon P, et al. Dilutional hyponatremia in patients with cirrhosis and ascites. *Arch Intern Med.* 2002;162:323.
81. Boyer TD, Zia P, Reynolds TB. Effect of indomethacin and prostaglandin A1 on renal function and plasma renin activity in alcoholic liver disease. *Gastroenterology.* 1979;77:215.
82. Pèrez-Ayuso RM, Arroyo V, Camps J, et al. Evidence that renal prostaglandins are involved in renal water metabolism in cirrhosis. *Kidney Int.* 1986;26:72.
83. Ginès P, Titó Ll, Arroyo V, et al. Randomized comparative study of therapeutic paracentesis with and without intravenous albumin in cirrhosis. *Gastroenterology.* 1988;94:1493.
84. Solà E, Lens S, Guevara M, et al. Hyponatremia in patients treated with terlipressin for severe gastrointestinal bleeding due to portal hypertension. *Hepatology.* 2010;52:1783–1790.
85. Ginès P, Abraham W, Schrier RW. Vasopressin in pathophysiological states. *Semin Nephrol.* 1994;14:384.
86. Ishikawa SE, Schrier RW. Pathogenesis of hyponatremia: the role of arginine vasopressin. In: Ginès P, Arroyo V, Rodés J, Schrier RW, eds. *Ascites and Renal Dysfunction in Liver Disease.* Oxford, UK: Blackwell Publishing; 2005:305.
87. Ginès P, Guevara M. Hyponatremia in cirrhosis: pathogenesis, clinical significance, and management. *Hepatology.* 2008;48:1002–1010.
88. Tsuboi Y, Ishikawa SE, Fujisawa G, et al. Therapeutic efficacy of the nonpeptide AVP antagonist OPC-31260 in cirrhotic rats. *Kidney Int.* 1994;46:237.

89. BoschMarcè M, Poo JL, Jiménez W, et al. Comparison of two aquaretic drugs (niravoline and OPC-31260) in cirrhotic rats with ascites and water retention. *J Pharmacol Exp Ther.* 1999;289:194.
90. Inoue T, Ohnishi A, Matsuo A, et al. Therapeutic and diagnostic potential of a vasopressin-2 antagonist for impaired water handling in cirrhosis. *Clin Pharmacol Ther.* 1998;63:561.
91. Jiménez W, Serradeil-Le Gal C, Ros J, et al. Long-term aquaretic efficacy of a selective non-peptide V2–vasopressin receptor antagonist in cirrhotic rats. *J Pharm Exp Ther.* 2000;295:83.
92. Guyader D, Patat A, Ellis-Grosse EJ, et al. Pharmacodynamic effects of a nonpeptide antidiuretic hormone V2 antagonist in cirrhotic patients with ascites. *Hepatology.* 2002;36:1197.
93. Gerbes AL, Gulberg V, Ginès P, et al. Therapy of hyponatremia in cirrhosis with a vasopressin receptor antagonist: a randomized double-blind multicenter trial. *Gastroenterology.* 2003;124:933.
94. Wong F, Blei AT, Blendis LM, et al. A vasopressin receptor antagonist (VPA-985) improves serum sodium concentration in patients with hyponatremia: a multicenter, randomized, placebo-controlled trial. *Hepatology.* 2003;37:182.
95. Ginès P, Wong F, Watson H, et al. Effects of satavaptan, a selective vasopressin V(2) receptor antagonist, on ascites and serum sodium in cirrhosis with hyponatremia: a randomized trial. *Hepatology.* 2008;48:204–213.
96. Adrogué HJ, Madias NE. Hyponatremia. *N Engl J Med.*, 2000;342:1581–1589.
97. Haussinger D. Low grade cerebral edema and the pathogenesis of hepatic encephalopathy in cirrhosis. *Hepatology.* 2006;43:1187–1190.
98. Restuccia T, Gómez-Ansón B, Guevara M, et al. Effects of dilutional hyponatremia on brain organic osmolytes and water content in patients with cirrhosis. *Hepatology.* 2004;39(6):1613–1622.
99. Córdoba J, Alonso J, Rovira A, et al. The development of low-grade cerebral edema in cirrhosis is supported by the evolution of (1)H-magnetic resonance abnormalities after liver transplantation. *J Hepatol.* 2001;35:598–604.
100. Kale RA, Gupta RK, Saraswat VA, et al. Demonstration of interstitial cerebral edema with diffusion tensor MR imaging in type C hepatic encephalopathy. *Hepatology.* 2006;43:698–706.
101. Amodio P, Del Piccolo F, Petteno E, et al. Prevalence and prognostic value of quantified electroencephalogram (EEG) alterations in cirrhotic patients. *J Hepatol.* 2001;35:37–45.
102. Jalan R, Elton RA, Redhead DN, et al. Analysis of prognostic variables in the prediction of shunt failure, variceal rebleeding, early mortality and encephalopathy following the transjugular intrahepatic portosystemic stent-shunt (TIPSS). *J Hepatol.* 1995;23:123–128.
103. Guevara M, Baccaro ME, Torre A, et al. Hyponatremia is a risk factor of hepatic encephalopathy in patients with cirrhosis: a prospective study with time-dependent analysis. *Am J Gastroenterol.* 2009;104:1382–1389.
104. Guevara M, Baccaro ME, Ríos J, et al. Risk factors for hepatic encephalopathy in patients with cirrhosis and refractory ascites: relevance of serum sodium concentration. *Liver Int.* 2010;30:1137–1142.
105. Riggio O, Angeloni S, Salvatori FM, et al. Incidence, natural history, and risk factors of hepatic encephalopathy after transjugular intrahepatic portosystemic shunt with polytetrafluoroethylene-covered stent grafts. *Am J Gastroenterol.* 2008;103:2738–2746.
106. Follo A, Llovet JM, Navasa M, et al. Renal impairment after spontaneous bacterial peritonitis in cirrhosis: course, predictive factors and prognosis. *Hepatology.* 1994;20:1495–1501.
107. Ginès P, Wong F, Smajda Lew E, et al. Hyponatremia is a major determinant of impaired health-related quality of life in cirrhosis with ascites. *Hepatology.* 2007;46:567A.
108. Abbasoglu O, Goldstein RM, Vodapally MS, et al. Liver transplantation in hyponatremic patients with emphasis on central pontine myelinolysis. *Clin Transplant.* 1998;12:263–269.
109. Wszolek ZK, McComb RD, Pfeiffer RF, et al. Pontine and extrapontine myelinolysis following liver transplantation. Relationship to serum sodium. *Transplantation.* 1989;48:1006–1012.
110. Londoño MC, Guevara M, Rimola A, et al. Hyponatremia impairs early posttransplantation outcome in patients with cirrhosis undergoing liver transplantation. *Gastroenterology.* 2006;130:1135–1143.
111. Dawwas MF, Lewsey JD, Neuberger JM, et al. The impact of serum sodium concentration on mortality after liver transplantation: a cohort multicenter study. *Liver Trans.* 2007;13:1115–1124.
112. Hecker R, Sherlock S. Electrolyte and circulatory changes in terminal liver failure. *Lancet.* 1956;2:1121.
113. Schroeder ET, Shear L, Sancetta SM, et al. Renal failure in patients with cirrhosis of the liver. Evaluation of intrarenal blood flow by para-aminohippurate extraction and response to angiotensin. *Am J Med.* 1967;43:887.
114. Epstein M, Berck DP, Hollemberg NK, et al. Renal failure in the patient with cirrhosis. The role of active vasoconstriction. *Am J Med.* 1970;49:175.
115. Ginès P, Fernández-Esparrach G, Arroyo V, et al. Pathogenesis of ascites in cirrhosis. *Semin Liver Dis.* 1997;17:175.
116. Ring-Larsen H. Renal blood flow in cirrhosis: relation to systemic and portal hemodynamics and liver function. *Scand J Clin Lab Invest.* 1977;37:635.
117. Arroyo V, Bosch J, Mauri M, et al. Renin, aldosterone and renal hemodynamics in cirrhosis with ascites. *Eur J Clin Invest.* 1979;9:69.
118. Rimola A, Ginès P, Arroyo V, et al. Urinary excretion of 6–keto-prostaglandin F1*a*, thromboxane B2 and prostaglandin E2 in cirrhosis with ascites. Relationship to functional renal failure (hepatorenal syndrome). *J Hepatol.* 1986;3:111.
119. Follo A, Llovet JM, Navasa M, et al. Renal impairment after spontaneous bacterial peritonitis in cirrhosis: incidence, clinical course, predictive factors and prognosis. *Hepatology.* 1994;20:1495–1501.
120. Sort P, Navasa M, Arroyo V, et al. Effect of intravenous albumin on renal impairment and mortality in patients with cirrhosis and spontaneous bacterial peritonitis. *N Engl J Med.* 1999;341:403–409.
121. Terra C, Guevara M, Torre A, et al. Renal failure in patients with cirrhosis and sepsis unrelated to spontaneous bacterial peritonitis: value of MELD score. *Gastroenterology.* 2005;129:1944–1953.
122. Arroyo V, Ginès P, Gerbes A, et al. Definition and diagnostic criteria of refractory ascites and hepatorenal syndrome in cirrhosis. *Hepatology.* 1996; 23:164.
123. Platt JF, Ellis JH, Rubin JM, et al. Renal duplex Doppler ultrasonography: a noninvasive predictor of kidney dysfunction and hepatorenal failure in liver disease. *Hepatology.* 1994;20:362.
124. Salerno F, Gerbes A, Ginès P, et al. Diagnosis, prevention and treatment of hepatorenal syndrome in cirrhosis. *Gut.* 2007;56:1310–1318.
125. Bataller R, Ginès P, Guevara M, et al. Hepatorenal syndrome. *Semin Liver Dis.* 1997;17:233.
126. Ginès P, Rodés J. Clinical disorders of renal function in cirrhosis with ascites. In: Ginès P, Arroyo V, Rodés J, Schrier RW, eds. *Ascites and Renal Dysfunction in Liver Disease.* Malden, MA: Blackwell Publishing; 1999:36.
127. Lancestremere RG, Davidson PL, Earley LE, et al. Renal failure in Laënnec's cirrhosis. In: Ginès P, Arroyo V Rodés J, Schrier RW, eds. *Ascites and Renal Dysfunction in Liver Disease.* London, MA: Blackwell Publishing, 2005:215.
128. Epstein M. Renal sodium handling in liver disease. In: Epstein M, ed. *The kidney in Liver Disease*, 4th ed. Philadelphia: Hanley & Belfus; 1996:1.
129. Kew MC, Brunt PW, Varma RR, et al. Renal and intrarenal blood-flow in cirrhosis of the liver. *Lancet.* 1971;2:504.
130. Sacerdoti D, Merlo A, Merkel C, et al. Redistribution of renal blood flow in patients with liver cirrhosis. The role of renal PGE2. *J Hepatol.* 1986;2:253.
131. Platt JF, Marn CS, Baliga PK, et al. Renal dysfunction in hepatic disease: early identification with renal duplex Doppler US in patients who undergo liver transplantation. *Radiology.* 1992;183:801.
132. Maroto A, Ginès A, Saló J, et al. Diagnosis of functional renal failure of cirrhosis by Doppler sonography. Prognostic value of resistive index. *Hepatology.* 1994;20:839.
133. Lieberman FL. Functional renal failure in cirrhosis. *Gastroenterology.* 1970; 58:108.
134. Iwatsuki S, Popovtzer MM, Corman JL, et al. Recovery from "hepatorenal syndrome" after orthotopic liver transplantation. *N Engl J Med.* 1973;289:1155.
135. Rimola A, Gavaler J, Schade RR, et al. Effects of renal impairment on liver transplantation. *Gastroenterology.* 1987;93:148.
136. Gonwa TA, Morris CA, Goldstein RM, et al. Long-term survival and renal function following liver transplantation in patients with and without hepatorenal syndrome—experience in 300 patients. *Transplantation* 1991;51:428.
137. Gonwa TA, Wilkinson AH. Liver transplantation and renal function: results in patients with and without hepatorenal syndrome. In: Epstein M, ed. *The Kidney in Liver Disease*, 4th ed. Philadelphia: Hanley & Belfus; 1996:529.
138. Rimola A, Navasa M, Grande L. Liver transplantation in cirrhotic patients with ascites. In: Ginès P, Arroyo V, Rodés J, Schrier RW, eds. *Ascites and Renal Dysfunction in Liver Disease.* Oxford, UK: Blackwell Publishing; 2005:271.
139. Ginès P, Schrier RW. Renal failure in cirrhosis. *N Engl J Med.* 2009;361: 1279–1290.
140. Marik PE, Wood K, Starzl TE. The course of type-1 hepatorenal syndrome post-liver transplantation. *Nephrol Dial Transplant.* 2006;21:478.
141. Fernández-Seara J, Prieto J, Quiroga J, et al. Systemic and regional hemodynamics in patients with liver cirrhosis and ascites with and without functional renal failure. *Gastroenterology.* 1989;97:1304.
142. Maroto A, Ginès P, Arroyo V, et al. Brachial and femoral artery blood flow in cirrhosis: relationship to kidney dysfunction. *Hepatology.* 1993;17:788.
143. Guevara M, Bru C, Ginès P, et al. Increased cerebral vascular resistance in cirrhotic patients with ascites. *Hepatology.* 1998;28:39.
144. Montoliu S, Ballesté B, Planas R, et al. Incidence and prognosis of different types of functional renal failure in cirrhotic patients with ascites. *Clin Gastroenterol Hepatol.* 2010;8:612–622.

145. Martín-Llahí M, Guevara M, Torre A, et al. Prognostic importance of the cause of renal failure in patients with cirrhosis. *Gastroenterology.* 2011;140: 488–496.
146. Alessandria C, Ozdogan O, Guevara M, et al. MELD score and clinical type predict prognosis in hepatorenal syndrome: Relevance to liver transplantation. *Hepatology.* 2005;41:1282–1289.
147. Papadakis MA, Arieff AI. Unpredictability of clinical evaluation of renal function in cirrhosis: a prospective study. *Am J Med.* 1987;82:945.
148. Caregaro L, Menon F, Angeli P, et al. Limitations of serum creatinine level and creatinine clearance as filtration markers in cirrhosis. *Arch Intern Med.* 1994;154:201.
149. Papper S. Hepatorenal syndrome. In: Epstein M, ed. *The Kidney in Liver Disease.* New York: Elsevier Biomedical; 1978:91.
150. Dudley FJ, Kanel GC, Wood LJ, et al. Hepatorenal syndrome without sodium retention. *Hepatology.* 1986;6:248.
151. Ruíz-del-Arbol L, Urman J, Fernández J, et al. Systemic, renal, and hepatic hemodynamic derangement in cirrhotic patients with spontaneous bacterial peritonitis. *Hepatology.* 2003;38:1210.
152. Lee SS. Cardiac dysfunction in spontaneous bacterial peritonitis: a manifestation of cirrhotic cardiomyopathy?. *Hepatology.* 2003;38:1089.
153. Ginès P, Guevara M, Perez-Villa F. Management of hepatorenal syndrome: another piece of the puzzle. *Hepatology.* 2004;40:16.
154. Arroyo V, Terra C, Ginès P. Advances in the pathogenesis and treatment of type-1 and type-2 hepatorenal syndrome. *J Hepatol.* 2007;46:935–946.
155. Ruiz-del-Arbol L, Monescillo A, Arocena C, et al. Circulatory function and hepatorenal syndrome in cirrhosis. *Hepatology.* 2005;42:439–447.
156. Krag A, Bendtsen F, Henriksen JH, et al. Low cardiac output predicts development of hepatorenal syndrome and survival in patients with cirrhosis and ascites. *Gut.* 2010;59:105–110.
157. Navasa M, Follo A, Filella X, et al. Tumor necrosis factor and interleukin-6 in spontaneous bacterial peritonitis in cirrhosis: relationship with the development of renal impairment and mortality. *Hepatology.* 1998;27:1227.
158. Cárdenas A, Ginès P, Rodés J. The consequences of liver disease: Renal complications. In Schiff E, Sorrell MF, Maddrey W, eds. *Diseases of the Liver.* Philadelphia: Lippincott Willians & Wilkins; 2003:497.
159. Ginès P, Angeli P, Lenz K, et al. for the European Association for the Study of the Liver. EASL clinical practice guidelines on the management of ascites, spontaneous bacterial peritonitis, and hepatorenal syndrome in cirrhosis. *J Hepatol.* 2010;53:397–417.
160. Cárdenas A, Ginès P, Uriz J, et al. Renal failure after gastrointestinal bleeding in cirrhosis: Incidence, characteristics, predictive factors and prognosis. *Hepatology.* 2001;34:671.
161. Ginès P, Guevara M, Arroyo V, et al. Hepatorenal syndrome. *Lancet.* 2003; 362:1819–1827.
162. Salerno F, Badalamenti S. Drug-induced renal failure in cirrhosis. In: Ginès P, Arroyo V, Rodés J, Schrier RW, eds. *Ascites and Renal Dysfunction in Liver Disease.* Oxford, UK: Blackwell Publishing; 2005:372.
163. Quintero E, Ginès P, Arroyo V, et al. Sulindac reduces the urinary excretion of prostaglandins and impairs renal function in cirrhosis with ascites. *Nephron.* 1986;42:298.
164. Guevara M, Abecasis R, Terg R. Effect of celecoxib on renal function in cirrhotic patients with ascites. A pilot study. *Scand J Gastroenterol.* 2004;39:385.
165. Claria J, Kent JD, Lopez-Parra M, et al. Effects of celecoxib and naproxen on renal function in nonazotemic patients with cirrhosis and ascites. *Hepatology.* 2005;41:579.
166. Cabrera J, Arrroyo V, Ballesta AM, et al. Aminoglycoside nephrotoxicity in cirrhosis. Value of urinary beta-2 microglobulin to discriminate functional renal failure from acute tubular damage. *Gastroenterology.* 1982;82:97.
167. McCormick PA, Greensdale L, Kibbler CC, et al. A prospective randomized trial of ceftazidime versus netilmicin plus mezlocillin in the empiric therapy of presumed sepsis in cirrhosis. *Hepatology.* 1997;25:833.
168. Fabrizi F, Poordad FF, Martin P. Hepatitis C infection and the patient with end-stage renal disease. *Hepatology.* 2002;36:3–10.
169. Poole B, Schrier RW, Jani A. Glomerular disease in cirrhosis. In: Ginès P, Arroyo V, Rodés J, Schrier RW, eds. *Ascites and Renal Dysfunction in Liver Disease.* Oxford, UK: Blackwell Publishing; 2005:360.
170. Francoz C, Glotz D, Moreau R, Durand F. The evaluation of renal function and disease in patients with cirrhosis. *J Hepatol.* 2010;52:605–613.
171. Trawalé JM, Paradis V, Rautou PE, et al. The spectrum of renal lesions in patients with cirrhosis: a clinicopathological study. *Liver Int.* 2010;30:725–732.
172. Groszmann R, Loureiro-Silva M. Physiology of hepatic circulation in cirrhosis. In: Ginès P, Arroyo V Rodés J, Schrier RW, eds. *Ascites and Renal Dysfunction in Liver Disease.* London, MA: Blackwell Publishing; 2005:164.
173. Scaffner F, Popper H. Capillarization of hepatic sinusoids in man. *Gastroenterology.* 1963;44:239.
174. Orrego H, Medline A, Blendis LM, et al. Collagenisation of the Disse space in alcoholic liver disease. *Gut.* 1979;20:673.
175. Bhathal PS, Grossman HJ. Reduction of the increased portal vascular resistance of the isolated perfused cirrhotic rat liver by vasodilators. *J Hepatol.* 1985;1:325.
176. García-Pagán JC, Bosch J. The resistance of the cirrhotic liver: a new target for the treatment of portal hypertension. 1985. *J Hepatol.* 2004;40:887.
177. Gracia-Sancho J, Laviña B, Rodríguez-Vilarrupla A, et al. Enhanced vasoconstrictor prostanoid production by sinusoidal endothelial cells increases portal perfusion pressure in cirrhotic rat livers. *J Hepatol.* 2007;47(2):220–227.
178. Bataller R, Nicolás JM, Ginès P, et al. Contraction of human hepatic stellate cells activated in culture: a role for voltage-operated calcium channels. *J Hepatol.* 1998;29:398.
179. Bataller R, Ginès P, Nicolás JM, et al. Angiotensin II induces contraction and proliferation of human hepatic stellate cells *Gastroenterology.* 2000;118:1149.
180. Görbig MN, Ginès P, Bataller R, et al. Atrial natriuretic peptide antagonizes endothelin-induced calcium increase and cell contraction in cultured human hepatic stellate cells. *Hepatology.* 1999;30:501.
181. Gupta K, Toruner M, Chung MK, et al. Endothelial dysfunction and decreased production of nitric oxide in the intrahepatic microcirculation of cirrhotic rats. *Hepatology.* 1998;28:926.
182. Wiest R, Groszmann RJ. Nitric oxide and portal hypertension: its role in the regulation of intrahepatic and splanchnic vascular resistance. *Semin Liver Dis.* 1999;19:411.
183. Wiest R, Groszmann RJ. The paradox of nitric oxide in cirrhosis and portal hypertension: too much, not enough. *Hepatology.* 2002;35:478.
184. Tugues S, Fernandez-Varo G, Muñoz-Luque J, et al. Antiangiogenic treatment with sunitinib ameliorates inflammatory infiltrate, fibrosis, and portal pressure in cirrhotic rats. *Hepatology.* 2007;46:1919–1926.
185. Bosch J, García-Pagán JC. The splanchnic circulation in cirrhosis. In: Ginès P, Arroyo V Rodés J, Schrier RW, eds. *Ascites and Renal Dysfunction in Liver Disease.* Oxford, UK: Blackwell Publishing; 2005:156.
186. Abraldes JG, Iwakiri Y, Loureiro-Silva M, et al. Mild increases in portal pressure upregulate vascular endothelial growth factor and endothelial nitric oxide synthase in the intestinal microcirculatory bed, leading to a hyperdynamic state. *Am J Physiol Gastrointest Liver Physiol.* 2006;290:G980–987.
187. Iwakiri Y, Groszmann RJ. The hyperdynamic circulation of chronic liver diseases: from the patient to the molecule. *Hepatology.* 2006;43:S121–131.
188. Iwakiri Y. The systemic and splanchnic circulations. In: Ginès P, Kamath P, Arroyo V, eds. *Chronic Liver Failure. Mechanisms and Management.* New York: Springer; 2010:305.
189. Vorobioff J, Bredfeldt JE, Groszmann RJ. Increased blood flow through the portal system in cirrhotic rats. *Gastroenterology.* 1984;87:1120.
190. Korthuis RJ, Kinden DA, Brimer GE, et al. Intestinal capillary filtration in acute and chronic portal hypertension. *Am J Physiol.* 1988;254:G339.
191. Henriksen JH, Moller S. Alterations of hepatic and splanchnic microvascular exchange in cirrhosis: local factors in the formation of ascites. In: Ginès P, Arroyo V, Rodés J, Schrier RW, eds. *Ascites and Renal Dysfunction in Liver Disease.* Oxford, UK: Blackwell Publishing; 2005:174.
192. Benoit JN, Granger DN. Intestinal microvascular adaptation to chronic portal hypertension in the rat. *Gastroenterology.* 1988;94:471.
193. Casado M, Bosch J, García-Pagán JC, et al. Clinical events after transjugular intrahepatic portosystemic shunt: correlation with hemodynamic findings. *Gastroenterology.* 1998;114:1296.
194. Abraldes JG, Tarantino I, Turnes J, et al. Hemodynamic response to pharmacological treatment of portal hypertension and long-term prognosis of cirrhosis. *Hepatology.* 2003;37:902.
195. Villanueva C, López-Balaguer JM, Aracil C, et al. Maintenance of hemodynamic response to treatment for portal hypertension and influence on complications of cirrhosis. *J Hepatol.* 2004;40:757.
196. Ripoll C, Groszmann R, Garcia-Tsao G, et al. Hepatic venous pressure gradient predicts clinical decompensation in patients with compensated cirrhosis. *Gastroenterology.* 2007;133:481–488.
197. Castells A, Saló J, Planas R, et al. Impact of shunt surgery for variceal bleeding in the natural history of ascites in cirrhosis: a retrospective study. *Hepatology.* 1994;20:584.
198. Ochs A, Rössle M, Haag K, et al. The transjugular intrahepatic portosystemic stent shunt procedure for refractory ascites. *N Engl J Med.* 1995;332:1192.
199. Boyer TD, Haskal ZJ; American Association for the Study of Liver Diseases. The role of transjugular intrahepatic portosystemic shunt (TIPS) in the management of portal hypertension: update 2009. *Hepatology.* 2010;51:306.
200. Murray JF, Dawson AM, Sherlock S. Circulatory changes in chronic liver disease. *Am J Med.* 1958;32:358.
201. Kontos HA, Shapiro A, Mauck HP, et al. General and regional circulatory alterations in cirrhosis of the liver. *Am J Med.* 1964;57:526.

202. Bosch J, Arroyo V, Betriu A, et al. Hepatic hemodynamics and the renin–angiotensin–aldosterone system in cirrhosis. *Gastroenterology.* 1980;78:92.
203. Abelmann WH. Hyperdynamic circulation in cirrhosis: a historical perspective. *Hepatology.* 1994;20:1356.
204. Groszmann RJ. Hyperdynamic circulation of liver disease 40 years later: pathophysiology and clinical consequences. *Hepatology.* 1994;20:1359.
205. Moller S, Henriksen JH. The systemic circulation in cirrhosis. In: Ginès P, Arroyo V, Rodés J, Schrier RW, eds. *Ascites and Renal Dysfunction in Liver Disease.* Oxford, UK: Blackwell Publishing,; 2005:139.
206. Kotelanski B, Groszmann R, Cohn JN. Circulation times in the splanchnic and hepatic beds in alcoholic liver disease. *Gastroenterology.* 1972;63:102.
207. Sato S, Ohnishi K, Sugita S, et al. Splenic artery and superior mesenteric artery blood flow: nonsurgical Doppler US measurement in healthy subjects and patients with chronic liver disease. *Radiology.* 1987;164:347.
208. Henriksen JH, Bendtsen F, Sorensen TIA, et al. Reduced central blood volume in cirrhosis. *Gastroenterology.* 1989;97:1506.
209. Henriksen JH, Bendtsen F, Gerbes AL, et al. Estimated central blood volume in cirrhosis: relationship to sympathetic nervous activity, beta adrenergic blockade and atrial natriuretic factor. *Hepatology.* 1992;16:1163.
210. Moller S, Sondergaard L, Mogelvang J, et al. Decreased right heart blood volume determined by magnetic resonance imaging: evidence of central underfilling in cirrhosis. *Hepatology.* 1995;22:472.
211. Møller S, Hobolth L, Winkler C, et al. Determinants of the hyperdynamic circulation and central hypovolaemia in cirrhosis. *Gut.* 2011;60(9):1254–1259.
212. Shapiro MD, Nichols KM, Groves BM, et al. Interrelationship between cardiac output and vascular resistance as determinants of "effective arterial blood volume" in patients with cirrhosis. *Kidney Int.* 1985;28:206.
213. Nicholls KM, Shapiro MD, Kluge R, et al. Sodium excretion in advanced cirrhosis: effect of expansion of central volume and suppression of plasma aldosterone. *Hepatology.* 1986;6:235.
214. Guevara M, Ginès P, Fernández-Esparrach G, et al. Reversibility of hepatorenal syndrome by prolonged administration of ornipressin and plasma volume expansion. *Hepatology.* 1998;27:35.
215. Uriz J, Ginès P, Cárdenas A, et al. Terlipressin plus albumin infusion: an effective and safe therapy of hepatorenal syndrome. *J Hepatol.* 2000;33:43.
216. Ginès P, Schrier RW. The arterial vasodilation hypothesis of ascites formation in cirrhosis. In: Arroyo V, Ginès P, Rodés J, et al, eds. *Ascites and Renal Dysfunction in Liver Disease.* Malden, MA: Blackwell Science; 1999:411.
217. Schrier RW, Caramelo C. Hemodynamics and hormonal alterations in hepatic cirrhosis. In: Epstein M, ed. *The Kidney in Liver Disease.* Baltimore: Williams & Wilkins; 1988:265.
218. Norris SH, Buell JC, Kurtzman NA. The pathophysiology of cirrhotic edema: a reexamination of the "underfilling" and "overflow" hypotheses. *Semin Nephrol.* 1987;7:77.
219. Fernández-Rodríguez F, Prieto J, et al. Arteriovenous shunting, hemodynamic changes, and renal sodium retention in liver cirrhosis. *Gastroenterology.* 1993;104:1139.
220. Hennenberg M, Trebicka J, Sauerbruch T, Heller J. Mechanisms of extrahepatic vasodilation in portal hypertension. *Gut.* 2008;57:1300–1314.
221. Guarner F, Guarner C, Prieto J, et al. Increased synthesis of systemic prostacyclin in cirrhotic patients. *Gastroenterology.* 1986;90: 687.
222. Bendtsen F, Schifter S, Henriksen JH. Increased calcitonin gene-related peptide (CGRP) in cirrhosis. *J Hepatol.* 1991;12:118.
223. Gupta S, Morgan TR, Gordan GS. Calcitonin gene-related peptide in hepatorenal syndrome. *J Clin Gastroenterol.* 1992;14:122.
224. Fernández-Rodríguez CM, Prieto J, et al. Plasma levels of substance P in liver cirrhosis: relationship to the activation of vasopressor systems and urinary sodium excretion. *Hepatology.* 1995;21:35.
225. Guevara M, Ginès P, Jiménez W, et al. Increased adrenomedullin levels in cirrhosis: relationship with hemodynamic abnormalities and vasoconstrictor systems. *Gastroenterology.* 1998;114:336.
226. Henriksen JH, Moller S, Schifter S, et al. High arterial compliance in cirrhosis is related to low adrenaline and elevated circulating calcitonin gene related peptide but not to activated vasoconstrictor systems. *Gut.* 2001;49:112.
227. Batkai S, Jarai Z, Wagner JA, et al. Endocannabinoids acting at vascular CB1 receptors mediate the vasodilated state in advanced liver cirrhosis. *Nat Med.* 2001;7:827.
228. Ros J, Clària J, To-Figueras, et al. Endogenous cannabinoids: a new system involved in the homeostasis of arterial pressure in experimental cirrhosis in the rat. *Gastroenterology.* 2002;122:85.
229. De las Heras D, Fernández J, Ginès P, et al. Increased carbon monoxide production in patients with cirrhosis with and without spontaneous bacterial peritonitis. *Hepatology.* 2003;38:452.
230. Fernández-Rodriguez CM, Romero J, Petros TJ, et al. Circulating endogenous cannabinoid anandamide and portal, systemic and renal hemodynamics in cirrhosis. *Liver Int.* 2004;24:477.
231. Domenicali M, Ros J, Fernández-Varo G, et al. Increased anandamide induced relaxation in mesenteric arteries of cirrhotic rats: role of cannabinoid and vanilloid receptors. *Gut.* 2005;54:522.
232. Martin PY, Ginès P, Schrier RW. Nitric oxide as a mediator of hemodynamic abnormalities and sodium and water retention in cirrhosis. *N Engl J Med.* 1998;339:533.
233. Martin PY, Ohara M, Ginès P, et al. Nitric oxide synthase (NOS) inhibition for one week improves renal sodium and water excretion in cirrhotic rats with ascites. *J Clin Invest.* 1998;101:235.
234. La Villa G, Barletta G, Pantaleo P, et al. Hemodynamic, renal, and endocrine effects of acute inhibition of nitric oxide synthase in compensated cirrhosis. *Hepatology.* 2001;34:19.
235. Spahr L, Martin PY, Giostra E, et al. Acute effects of nitric oxide synthase inhibition on systemic, hepatic, and renal hemodynamics in patients with cirrhosis and ascites. *J Investig Med.* 2002;50:116.
236. Thiesson HC, Skott O, Jespersen B, et al. Nitric oxide synthase inhibition does not improve renal function in cirrhotic patients with ascites. *Am J Gastroenterol.* 2003;98:180.
237. Bernardi M, Trevisani F, Santini C, et al. Aldosterone related blood volume expansion in cirrhosis before and after the early phase of ascites formation. *Gut.* 1983;24:761.
238. Rosoff L Jr, Zia P, Reynolds TB. Studies on renin and aldosterone in cirrhotic patients with ascites. *Gastroenterology.* 1975;69:698.
239. Epstein M, Levinson R, Sancho J, et al. Characterization of the renin–aldosterone system in decompensated cirrhosis. *Circ Res.* 1977;41:818.
240. Chonko AM, Bay WH, Stein JH, et al. The role of renin and aldosterone in the salt retention of edema. *Am J Med.* 1977;63:881.
241. Bernardi M, De Palma R, Trevisani F, et al. Chronobiological study of factors affecting plasma aldosterone concentration in cirrhosis. *Gastroenterology.* 1986;91:683.
242. Arroyo V, Ginès P, Jiménez W, et al. Ascites, renal failure, and electrolyte disorders in cirrhosis. Pathogenesis, diagnosis, and treatment. In: McIntyre N, Benhamou JP, Bircher J, et al, eds. *Textbook of Clinical Hepatology.* Oxford: Oxford Medical Press; 1991:429.
243. Bernardi M, Domenicali M. The renin-angiotensin-aldosterone system in cirrhosis. In: Ginès P, Arroyo V, Rodés J, Schrier RW, eds. *Ascites and Renal Dysfunction in Liver Disease.* Oxford, UK: Blackwell Publishing; 2005:43.
244. Bernardi M, Santini C, Trevisani F, et al. Renal function impairment induced by change in posture in patients with cirrhosis and ascites. *Gut.* 1985;26:629.
245. Epstein M. Aldosterone in liver disease. In: Epstein M, ed. *The Kidney in Liver Disease*, 4th ed. Philadelphia: Hanley & Belfus; 1996:291.
246. Campra JL, Reynolds TB. Effectiveness of high-dose spironolactone therapy in patients with chronic liver disease and relatively refractory ascites. *Dig Dis Sci.* 1978;23:1025.
247. Bernardi M, Servadei D, Trevisani F, et al. Importance of plasma aldosterone concentration on the natriuretic effect of spironolactone in patients with liver cirrhosis and ascites. *Digestion.* 1985;31:189.
248. Angeli P, Fasolato S, Mazza E, et al. Combined versus sequential diuretic treatment of ascites in non-azotaemic patients with cirrhosis: results of an open randomised clinical trial. *Gut* 2010;59:98–104.
249. Epstein M. Aldosterone in liver disease. In: Epstein M, ed. *The Kidney in Liver Disease*, 3rd ed. Baltimore: Williams & Wilkins; 1988;356.
250. Wong F, Liu P, Allidina Y, et al. Pattern of sodium handling and its consequences in patients with preascitic cirrhosis. *Gastroenterology.* 1995;108:1820.
251. Bosch J, Arroyo V, Rodés J. Hepatic and systemic hemodynamics and the renin–angiotensin–aldosterone system in cirrhosis. In: Epstein M, ed. *The Kidney in Liver Disease.* New York, Elsevier Biomedical; 1983;286.
252. Mitch WE, Melton PK, Cooke CR, et al. Plasma levels and hepatic extraction of renin and aldosterone in alcoholic liver disease. *Am J Med.* 1979; 66:804.
253. Wernze H, Spech HJ, Muller G. Studies on the activity of the renin–angiotensin–aldosterone system (RAAS) in patients with cirrhosis of the liver. *Klin Wochenschr.* 1978;56:389.
254. Wilkinson SP, Wheeler PG, Jowett TP, et al. Factors relating to aldosterone secretion rate, the excretions of aldosterone 18–glucuronide, and the plasma aldosterone concentration in cirrhosis. *Clin Endocrinol (Oxf).* 1981;14:355.
255. Schroeder ET, Anderson GH, Goldman SH, et al. Effect of blockade of angiotensin II on blood pressure, renin and aldosterone in cirrhosis. *Kidney Int.* 1976;9:511.
256. Arroyo V, Bosch J, Mauri M, et al. Effect of angiotensin-II blockade on systemic and hepatic haemodynamics and on the renin–angiotensin–aldosterone system in cirrhosis with ascites. *Eur J Clin Invest.* 1981;11:221.
257. Pariente EA, Bataille C, Bercoff E, et al. Acute effects of captopril on systemic and renal hemodynamics and on renal function in cirrhotic patients with ascites. *Gastroenterology.* 1985;88:1255.

258. Lobden I, Shore A, Wilkinson R, et al. Captopril in the hepatorenal syndrome. *J Clin Gastroenterol.* 1985;7:354.
259. Arroyo V, Ginès P, Rimola A, et al. Renal function abnormalities, prostaglandins, and effects of nonsteroidal anti-inflammatory drugs in cirrhosis with ascites. An overview with emphasis on pathogenesis. *Am J Med.* 1986;81:104.
260. Arroyo V, Planas R, Gaya J, et al. Sympathetic nervous activity, renin–angiotensin system and renal excretion of prostaglandin E2 in cirrhosis. Relationship to functional renal failure and sodium and water excretion. *Eur J Clin Invest.* 1983;13:271.
261. Barnardo DE, Summerskill WH, Strong CG, et al. Renal function, renin activity and endogenous vasoactive substances in cirrhosis. *Am J Dig Dis.* 1970;15:419.
262. Schroeder ET, Eich RH, Smulyan H, et al. Plasma renin level in hepatic cirrhosis. Relation to functional renal failure. *Am J Med.* 1970;49:186.
263. Wong PY, Talamo RC, Williams GH. Kallikrein–kinin and renin–angiotensin systems in functional renal failure of cirrhosis of the liver. *Gastroenterology.* 1977;73:1114.
264. Wilkinson SP, Smith IK, Williams R. Changes in plasma renin activity in cirrhosis: a reappraisal based on studies in 67 patients and "low-renin" cirrhosis. *Hypertension.* 1979;1:125.
265. Guevara M, Ginès P, Bandi JC, et al. Transjugular intrahepatic portosystemic shunt in hepatorenal syndrome: effects on renal function and vasoactive systems. *Hepatology.* 1998;28:416.
266. Wong F, Pantea L, Sniderman K. Midodrine, octreotide, albumin, and TIPS in selected patients with cirrhosis and type 1 hepatorenal syndrome. *Hepatology.* 2004;40:55.
267. Henriksen JH, Christensen NJ, Ring-Larsen H. Noradrenaline and adrenaline concentrations in various vascular beds in patients with cirrhosis. Relation to haemodynamics. *Clin Physiol.* 1981;1:293.
268. Bichet DG, Van Putten VJ, Schrier RW. Potential role of increased sympathetic activity in impaired sodium and water excretion in cirrhosis. *N Engl J Med.* 1982;307:1552.
269. Burghardt W, Wernze H, Schaffrath I. Changes of circulating noradrenaline and adrenaline in hepatic cirrhosis. Relation to stage of disease, liver and renal function. *Acta Endocrinol.* 1982;99[Suppl 246]:100.
270. Bernardi M, Trevisani F, Santinin C, et al. Plasma norepinephrine, weak neurotransmitters and renin activity during active tilting in liver cirrhosis: relationship with cardiovascular hemostasis and renal function. *Hepatology.* 1983;3:56.
271. Henriksen H, Ring-Larsen H, Christensen NJ. Sympathetic nervous activity in cirrhosis. A survey of plasma catecholamine studies. *J Hepatol.* 1984;1:55.
272. Epstein M, Larios O, Johnson G. Effects of water immersion on plasma catecholamines in decompensated cirrhosis. Implications for deranged sodium and water homeostasis. *Miner Electrolyte Metab.* 1985;11:25.
273. Dudley F, Esler M. The sympathetic nervous system in cirrhosis. In: Ginès P, Arroyo V, Rodés J, Schrier RW, eds. *Ascites and Renal Dysfunction in Liver Disease.* Oxford, UK: Blackwell Publishing; 2005:54.
274. Nicholls KM, Shapiro MD, Van Putten VJ, et al. Elevated plasma norepinephrine concentrations in decompensated cirrhosis. Association with increased secretion rates, normal clearance rates, and suppressibility by central blood volume expansion. *Circ Res.* 1985;56:457.
275. Willett I, Esler M, Burke F, et al. Total and renal sympathetic nervous system activity in alcoholic cirrhosis. *J Hepatol.* 1985;1:639.
276. Henriksen JH, Ring-Larsen H, Christensen NJ. Hepatic intestinal uptake and release of catecholamines in alcoholic cirrhosis. Evidence of enhanced hepatic intestinal sympathetic nervous activity. *Gut.* 1987;28:1637.
277. MacGilchrist AJ, Howes LG, Hawksby C, et al. Plasma noradrenaline in cirrhosis: a study of kinetics and temporal relationship to ascites formation. *Eur J Clin Invest.* 1991;21:238.
278. Esler M, Dudley F, Jennings G, et al. Increased sympathetic nervous activity and the effects of its inhibition with clonidine in alcoholic cirrhosis. *Ann Intern Med.* 1992;116:446.
279. Henriksen JH, Ring-Larsen H. Renal effects of drugs used in the treatment of portal hypertension. *Hepatology.* 1993;18:688.
280. Floras JS, Legault L, Morali GA, et al. Increased sympathetic outflow in cirrhosis and ascites: direct evidence from intraneural recordings. *Ann Intern Med.* 1991;114:373.
281. DiBona GF. Neural control of the kidney: functionally specific renal sympathetic nerve fibers. *Am J Physiol.* 2000;279:R1517.
282. Zambraski E. Effects of acute renal denervation on sodium excretion in miniature swine with cirrhosis and ascites. *Physiologist.* 1985;28:268.
283. Koepke J, Jones S, DiBona G. Renal nerves mediate blunted natriuresis to atrial natriuretic peptide in cirrhotic rats. *Am J Physiol.* 1987;252:R1019.
284. Veelken R, Hilgers KF, Porst M, et al. Effects of sympathetic nerves and angiotensin II on renal sodium and water handling in rats with common bile duct ligature. *Am J Physiol Renal Physiol.* 2005;288:F1267–1275.
285. Solís-Herruzo JA, Durán A, Favela V, et al. Effects of lumbar sympathetic block on kidney function in cirrhotic patients with hepatorenal syndrome. *J Hepatol.* 1987;5:167.
286. Lenaerts A, Codden T, Meunier JC, et al. Effects of clonidine on diuretic response in ascitic patients with cirrhosis and activation of sympathetic nervous system. *Hepatology.* 2006;44:844–849.
287. Stadlbauer V, Wright GA, Banaji M, et al. Relationship between activation of the sympathetic nervous system and renal blood flow autoregulation in cirrhosis. *Gastroenterology.* 2008;134:111–119.
288. Henriksen JH, Ring-Larsen H, Christensen NJ. Autonomic nervous function in liver disease. In Bomzon A, Blendis LM, eds. *Cardiovascular Complications of Liver Disease.* Boca Raton, FL: CRC Press; 1990:63.
289. Uriz J, Ginès P, Ortega R, et al. Increased plasma levels of neuropeptide Y in hepatorenal syndrome. *J Hepatol.* 2002;36:349.
290. Worlicek M, Knebel K, Linde HJ, et al. Splanchnic sympathectomy prevents translocation and spreading of E. coli but not S. aureus in liver cirrhosis. *Gut.* 2010;59:1227–1234.
291. Better OS, Schrier RW. Disturbed volume homeostasis in patients with cirrhosis of the liver. *Kidney Int.* 1983;23:303.
292. Kostreva DR, Castaner A, Kampine JP. Reflex effects of hepatic baroreceptors on renal and cardiac sympathetic nervous activity. *Am J Physiol.* 1980;238:R390.
293. Levy M, Wexler MJ. Hepatic denervation alters first-phase urinary sodium excretion in dogs with cirrhosis. *Am J Physiol.* 1987;253: F664.
294. Levy M, Wexler MJ. Sodium excretion in dogs with low grade caval constriction: role of hepatic nerves. *Am J Physiol.* 1987;253:F672.
295. Blendis LM, Sole MJ, Campbell P, et al. The effect of peritoneovenous shunting on catecholamine metabolism in patients with hepatic ascites. *Hepatology.* 1987;7:143.
296. Conrad KP, Dunn MJ. Renal prostaglandins and other eicosanoids. In: Windhager EE, ed. *Handbook of Physiology.* New York: Oxford University Press; 1992:1707.
297. Zipser RD, Hoefs JC, Speckart PF, et al. Prostaglandins: modulators of renal function and pressor resistance in chronic liver disease. *J Clin Endocrinol Metab.* 1979;48:895.
298. Ippolito S, Moore K. Arachidonic acid metabolites and the kidney in cirrhosis. In: Ginès P, Arroyo V, Rodés J, Schrier RW, eds. *Ascites and Renal Dysfunction in Liver Disease.* Oxford, UK: Blackwell Publishing; 2005:84.
299. Planas R, Arroyo V, Rimola A, et al. Acetylsalicylic acid suppresses the renal hemodynamic effect and reduces the diuretic action of furosemide in cirrhosis with ascites. *Gastroenterology.* 1983;84:247.
300. Guarner C, Colina I, Guarner F, et al. Renal prostaglandins in cirrhosis of the liver. *Clin Sci.* 1986;70:477.
301. Uemura M, Tsujii T, Fukui H, et al. Urinary prostaglandins and renal function in chronic liver diseases. *Scand J Gastroenterol.* 1986;21:75.
302. Parelon G, Mirouze D, Michel F, et al. Prostaglandines urinaires dans le syndrome hèpatorènal du cirrhotique: rôle du thromboxane A2 et d'un dèsèquilibre des acides gras polyinsaturès prècurseurs. *Gastroenterol Clin Biol.* 1985;9:290.
303. Govindarajan S, Nast CC, Smith WL, et al. Immunohistochemical distribution of renal prostaglandin endoperoxide synthase and prostacyclin synthase: diminished endoperoxide synthase in the hepatorenal syndrome. *Hepatology.* 1987;7:654.
304. Moore K, Ward PS, Taylor GW, et al. Systemic and renal production of thromboxane A2 and prostacyclin in decompensated liver disease and hepatorenal syndrome. *Gastroenterology.* 1991;100:1069.
305. Zipser RD, Radvan GH, Kronborg I, et al. Urinary thromboxane B2 and prostaglandin E2 in the hepatorenal syndrome; evidence for increased vasoconstrictor and decreased vasodilator factors. *Gastroenterology.* 1983;84:697.
306. Laffi G, La Villa G, Pinzani M, et al. Altered renal and platelet arachidonic acid metabolism in cirrhosis. *Gastroenterology.* 1986;90:274.
307. Zipser RD, Kronberg I, Rector W, et al. Therapeutic trial of thromboxane synthesis inhibition in the hepatorenal syndrome. *Gastroenterology.* 1984; 87:1228.
308. Bruix J, Bosch J, Kravetz D, et al. Effects of prostaglandin inhibition on systemic and hepatic hemodynamics in patients with cirrhosis of the liver. *Gastroenterology.* 1985;88:430.
309. Hou MC, Cahill PA, Zhang S, et al. Enhanced cyclooxygenase-1 expression within the superior mesenteric artery of portal hypertensive rats: role in the hyperdynamic circulation. *Hepatology.* 1998;27:20.
310. Niederberger M, Ginès P, Martin PY, et al. Increased renal and vascular cytosolic phospholipase A_2 activity in rats with cirrhosis and ascites. *Hepatology.* 1998;27:42.
311. Miyazono M, Zhu D, Nemenoff R,, et al. Increased epoxyeicosatrienoic acid formation in the rat kidney during liver cirrhosis. *J Am Soc Nephrol* 2003;14:176.
312. Huber M, Kastner S, Scholmerich J, et al. Analysis of cysteinyl leukotrienes in human urine: enhanced excretion in patients with liver cirrhosis and hepatorenal syndrome. *Eur J Clin Invest.* 1989; 19:53.

313. Moore KP, Taylor GW, Maltby NH, et al. Increased production of leukotrienes in hepatorenal syndrome. *J Hepatol.* 1990;11:263.
314. Sacerdoti D, Balazy M, Angeli P, at al. Eicosanoid excretion in hepatic cirrhosis. Predominance of 20–HETE. *J Clin Invest.* 1997;100:1264.
315. Bichet D, Szatalowicz V, Chaimovitz C, et al. Role of vasopressin in abnormal water excretion in cirrhotic patients. *Ann Intern Med.* 1982;96:413.
316. Reznick RK, Langer B, Taylor BR, et al. Hyponatremia and arginine vasopressin secretion in patients with refractory hepatic ascites undergoing peritoneovenous shunting. *Gastroenterology.* 1983;84:713.
317. Castellano G, Solís-Herruzo JA, Morillas JD, et al. Antidiuretic hormone and renal function after water loading in patients with cirrhosis of the liver. *Scand J Gastroenterol.* 1991;26:49.
318. Arroyo V, Clária J, Saló J, et al. Antidiuretic hormone and the pathogenesis of water retention in cirrhosis with ascites. *Semin Liver Dis.* 1994;14:44.
319. Better OS, Aisenbrey GA, Berl T, et al. Role of antidiuretic hormone in impaired urinary dilution associated with chronic bile-duct ligation. *Clin Sci.* 1980;58:493.
320. Camps J, Solá J, Arroyo V, et al. Temporal relationship between the impairment of free water excretion and antidiuretic hormone hypersecretion in rats with experimental cirrhosis. *Gastroenterology.* 1987; 93:498.
321. Linas SL, Anderson RJ, Guggenheim SJ, et al. Role of vasopressin in impaired water excretion in conscious rats with experimental cirrhosis. *Kidney Int.* 1981;20:173.
322. Asahina Y, Izumi N, Enomoto N, et al. Increased gene expression of water channel in cirrhotic rat kidneys. *Hepatology.* 1995;21:169.
323. Fernández-Llama P, Jiménez W, Bosch-Marce M, et al. Dysregulation of renal aquaporins and Na-Cl cotransporter in CCl4–induced cirrhosis. *Kidney Int.* 2000;58:216.
324. Schrier RW, Gross P, Gheorghiade M, et al. Tolvaptan, a selective oral vasopressin V2–receptor antagonist, for hyponatremia. *N Engl J Med.* 2006;355: 2099–2112.
325. Kim JK, Summer SN, Howard RL, et al. Vasopressin gene expression in rats with experimental cirrhosis. *Hepatology.* 1993;17:143.
326. Ardaillou R, Benmansour M, Rondeau E, et al. Metabolism and secretion of antidiuretic hormone in patients with renal failure, cardiac insufficiency and renal insufficiency. *Adv Nephrol.* 1984;13:35.
327. Solís-Herruzo JA, González-Gamarra A, Castellano G, et al. Metabolic clearance rate of arginine vasopressin in patients with cirrhosis. *Hepatology.* 1992;16:974.
328. Bichet DG, Groves BM, Schrier RW. Mechanisms of improvement of water and sodium excretion by immersion in decompensated cirrhotic patients. *Kidney Int.* 1983;24:788.
329. Clária J, Jiménez W, Arroyo V, et al. Effect of V1–vasopressin receptor blockade on arterial pressure in conscious rats with cirrhosis and ascites. *Gastroenterology.* 1991;100:494.
330. Ginès P, Jiménez W, Arroyo V, et al. Atrial natriuretic factor in cirrhosis with ascites: plasma levels, cardiac release and splanchnic extraction. *Hepatology.* 1988;8:636.
331. Campbell PJ, Skorecki KL, Logan AG, et al. Acute effects of peritoneovenous shunting on plasma atrial natriuretic peptide in cirrhotic patients with massive refractory ascites. *Am J Med.* 1988;84:112.
332. Klepetko W, Muller C, Hartter E, et al. Plasma atrial natriuretic factor in cirrhotic patients with ascites. Effect of peritoneovenous shunt implantation. *Gastroenterology.* 1988;95:764.
333. Morgan TR, Imada T, Hollister AS, et al. Plasma human atrial natriuretic factor in cirrhosis and ascites with and without functional renal failure. *Gastroenterology.* 1988;95:1641.
334. Skorecki KL, Leung WM, Campbell P, et al. Role of atrial natriuretic peptide in the natriuretic response to central volume expansion induced by head-out water immersion in sodium retaining cirrhotic subjects. *Am J Med.* 1988;85:375.
335. Epstein M, Loutzenhiser R, Norsk P, et al. Relationship between plasma ANF responsiveness and renal sodium handling in cirrhotic humans. *Am J Nephrol.* 1989;9:133.
336. Salerno F, Badalamenti S, Moser P, et al. Atrial natriuretic factor in cirrhotic patients with tense ascites. Effect of large-volume paracentesis. *Gastroenterology.* 1990;98:1063.
337. Angeli P, Caregaro L, Menon F, et al. Variability of atrial natriuretic peptide plasma levels in ascitic cirrhotics: pathophysiological and clinical implications. *Hepatology.* 1992;16:1389.
338. Warner L, Skorecki K, Blendis LM, et al. Atrial natriuretic factor and liver disease. *Hepatology.* 1993;17:500.
339. Henriksen JH, Gøtze JP, Fuglsang S, et al. Increased circulating pro-brain natriuretic peptide (proBNP) and brain natriuretic peptide (BNP) in patients with cirrhosis: relation to cardiovascular dysfunction and severity of disease. *Gut.* 2003;52:1511–1517.
340. Henriksen JH, Bendtsen F, Schutten HJ, et al. Hepatic-intestinal disposal of endogenous human alpha atrial natriuretic factor 99–126 in patients with cirrhosis. *Am J Gastroenterol.* 1990;85:1155.
341. Poulos JE, Gower WR, Fontanet HL, et al. Cirrhosis with ascites: increased atrial natriuretic peptide messenger RNA expression in rat ventricle. *Gastroenterology.* 1995;108:1496.
342. Salerno F, Badalamenti S, Incerti P, et al. Renal response to atrial natriuretic peptide in patients with advanced liver cirrhosis. *Hepatology.* 1988;8:21.
343. López C, Jiménez W, Arroyo V, et al. Role of altered systemic hemodynamics in the blunted renal response to atrial natriuretic peptide in rats with cirrhosis and ascites. *J Hepatol.* 1989;9:217.
344. Beutler JJ, Koomans HA, Rabelink TJ, et al. Blunted natriuretic response and low blood pressure after atrial natriuretic factor in early cirrhosis. *Hepatology.* 1989;10:148.
345. Laffi G, Pinzani M, Meacci E, et al. Renal hemodynamic and natriuretic effects of human atrial natriuretic factor infusion in cirrhosis with ascites. *Gastroenterology.* 1989;96:167.
346. Ginès P, Tító L, Arroyo V, et al. Renal insensitivity to atrial natriuretic peptide in patients with cirrhosis and ascites. Effect of increasing systemic arterial pressure. *Gastroenterology.* 1992;102:280.
347. La Villa G, Riccardi D, Lazzeri C, et al. Blunted natriuretic response to low-dose brain natriuretic peptide infusion in nonazotemic cirrhotic patients with ascites and avid sodium retention. *Hepatology.* 1995;22:1745.
348. Abraham WT, Lauwaars M, Kim J, et al. Reversal of atrial natriuretic peptide resistance by increasing distal tubular sodium delivery in patients with decompensated cirrhosis. *Hepatology.* 1995;22:737.
349. La Villa G, Romanelli RG, Raggi VC, et al. Plasma levels of brain natriuretic peptide in patients with cirrhosis. *Hepatology.* 1992;16:156.
350. Gülberg V, Møller S, Henriksen JH, Gerbes AL. Increased renal production of C-type natriuretic peptide (CNP) in patients with cirrhosis and functional renal failure. *Gut.* 2000;47:852–857.
351. Henriksen JH, Gülberg V, Gerbes AL, et al. Increased arterial compliance in cirrhosis is related to decreased arterial C-type natriuretic peptide, but not to atrial natriuretic peptide. *Scand J Gastroenterol.* 2003;38:559–564.
352. Saló J, Jiménez W, Kuhn M, et al. Urinary excretion of urodilatin in patients with cirrhosis. *Hepatology.* 1996;24:1428.
353. Angeli P, Jiménez W, Arroyo V, et al. Renal effects of natriuretic peptide receptor blockade in cirrhotic rats with ascites. *Hepatology.* 1994;20:948.
354. Padillo J, Rioja P, Muñoz-Villanueva MC, et al. BNP as marker of heart dysfunction in patients with liver cirrhosis. *Eur J Gastroenterol Hepatol.* 2010;22:1331–1336.
355. Pimenta J, Paulo C, Gomes A, et al. B-type natriuretic peptide is related to cardiac function and prognosis in hospitalized patients with decompensated cirrhosis. *Liver Int.* 2010;30:1059–1066.
356. Alqahtani SA, Fouad TR, Lee SS. Cirrhotic cardiomyopathy. *Semin Liver Dis.* 2008;28:59–69.
357. Kusserow H, Unger T. Vasoactive peptides, their receptors and drug development. *Basic Clin Pharmacol Toxicol.* 2004;94:5.
358. Uchihara M, Izumi N, Sato C, et al. Clinical significance of elevated plasma endothelin concentration in patients with cirrhosis. *Hepatology.* 1992;16:95.
359. Uemasu J, Matsumoto H, Kawasaki H. Increased plasma endothelin levels in patients with liver cirrhosis. *Nephron.* 1992;60:380.
360. Moore K, Wendon J, Frazer M, et al. Plasma endothelin immunoreactivity in liver disease and the hepatorenal syndrome. *N Engl J Med.* 1992;327:1774.
361. Asbert M, Ginès A, Ginès P, et al. Circulating levels of endothelin in cirrhosis. *Gastroenterology.* 1993;104:1485.
362. Moller S, Emmeluth C, Henriksen JH. Elevated circulating plasma endothelin-1 concentrations in cirrhosis. *J Hepatol.* 1993;19:285.
363. Saló J, Francitorra A, Follo A, et al. Increased plasma endothelin in cirrhosis. Relationship with systemic endotoxemia and response to changes in effective blood volume. *J Hepatol.* 1995;22:389.
364. Trevisani F, Colantoni A, Gerbes A, et al. Daily profile of plasma endothelin-1 and -3 in pre-ascitic cirrhosis: relationships with the arterial pressure and renal function. *J Hepatol.* 1997;26:808.
365. Bernardi M, Gulberg V, Colantoni A, et al. Plasma endothelin-1 and -3 in cirrhosis: relationship with systemic hemodynamics, renal function and neurohumoral systems. *J Hepatol.* 1996;24:161.
366. Martinet JP, Legault L, Cernacek P, et al. Changes in plasma endothelin-1 and big endothelin-1 induced by transjugular intrahepatic portosystemic shunts in patients with cirrhosis and refractory ascites. *J Hepatol.* 1996;25:700.
367. Leivas A, Jiménez W, Lamas S, et al. Endothelin-1 does not play a major role in the homeostasis of arterial pressure in cirrhotic rats with ascites. *Gastroenterology.* 1995;108:1842.
368. Pinzani M, Milani S, DeFranco R, et al. Endothelin 1 is overexpressed in human cirrhotic liver and exerts multiple effects on activated hepatic stellate cells. *Gastroenterology.* 1996;110:534.

369. Leivas A, Jiménez W, Bruix J, et al. Gene expression of endothelin-1 and ET(A) and ET(B) receptors in human cirrhosis: relationship with hepatic hemodynamics. *J Vasc Res.* 1998;35:186.
370. Alam I, Bass NM, Bichetti P, et al. Hepatic tissue endothelin-1 levels in chronic liver disease correlate with disease severity and ascites. *Am J Gastroenterol.* 2000;95:199.
371. Soper CP, Latif AB, Bending MR. Amelioration of hepatorenal syndrome with selective endothelin-A antagonist. *Lancet.* 1996;347:1842.
372. Wong F, Moore K, Dingemanse J, Jalan R. Lack of renal improvement with nonselective endothelin antagonism with tezosentan in type 2 hepatorenal syndrome. *Hepatology.* 2008;47:160–168.
373. Poo JL, Jiménez W, Maria Muñoz R, et al. Chronic blockade of endothelin receptors in cirrhotic rats: hepatic and hemodynamic effects. *Gastroenterology.* 1999;116:161.
374. Cho JJ, Hocher B, Herbst H, et al. An oral endothelin-A receptor antagonist blocks collagen synthesis and deposition in advanced rat liver fibrosis. *Gastroenterology.* 2000;118:1169.
375. Tièche S, DeGottardi A, Kappeler A, et al. Overexpression of endothelin-1 in bile duct ligated rats: correlation with activation of hepatic stellate cells and portal pressure. *J Hepatol.* 2001;34:38.
376. Housset C. The dual play of endothelin receptors in hepatic vasoregulation. *Hepatology.* 2000;31:1025.
377. Kone BC. Nitric oxide synthesis in the kidney: isoforms, biosynthesis, and functions in health. *Semin Nephrol.* 2004;24:299.
378. García-Estañ J, Atucha N, Mario J, et al. Increased endothelium-dependent renal vasodilation in cirrhotic rats. *Am J Physiol.* 1994;267:R549.
379. Bosch-Marcè M, Morales-Ruíz M, Jiménez W, et al. Increased renal expression of nitric oxide synthase type III in cirrhotic rats with ascites. *Hepatology.* 1998;27:1191.
380. Criado M, Flores O, Ortiz MC, et al. Elevated glomerular and blood mononuclear lymphocyte nitric oxide production in rats with chronic bile duct ligation: role of inducible nitric oxide synthase activation. *Hepatology.* 1997;26:268.
381. Clária J, Jiménez W, Ros J, et al. Pathogenesis of arterial hypotension in cirrhotic rats with ascites: role of endogenous nitric oxide. *Hepatology.* 1992; 15:343.
382. Clária J, Ros J, Jiménez W, et al. Role of nitric oxide and prostacyclin in the control of renal perfusion in experimental cirrhosis. *Hepatology.* 1995;22:915.
383. Tam J, Liu J, Mukhopadhyay B, Linar R, Godlewski G, Kunos G. Endocannabinoid in liver disease. *Hepatology.* 2011;53:346–355.
384. Caraceni P, Domenicali M, Giannone F, et al.The role of the endocannabinoid system in liver diseases. *Best Pract Res Clin Endocrinol Metab.* 2009;23:65–77.
385. Varga K, Wagner JA, Bridgen DT, et al. Platelet- and macrophage-derived endogenous cannabinoids are involved in endotoxin induced hypotension. *FASEB J.* 1998;12:1035–1044.
386. Liu J, Batkai S, Pacher P, et al. Lipopolysaccharide induces anandamide synthesis in macrophages via CD14/MAPK/phosphoinositide 3–kinase/NF-kappaB independently of platelet-activating factor. *J Biol Chem.* 2003;278:45034–45039.
387. Batkai S, Jarai Z, Wagner JA, et al. Endocannabinoids acting at vascular CB1 receptors mediate the vasodilated state in advanced liver cirrhosis. *Nat Med.* 2001;7:827–832.
388. Ros J, Clària J, To-Figueras J, et al. Endogenous cannabinoids: a new system involved in the homeostasis of arterial pressure in experimental cirrhosis in the rat. *Gastroenterology.* 2002;122:85–93.
389. Domenicali M, Ros J, Fernandez-Varo G, et al. Increased anandamide induced relaxation in mesenteric arteries of cirrhotic rats: role of cannabinoid and vanilloid receptors. *Gut.* 2005;54:522–527.
390. Yang YY, Lin HC, Huang YT, et al.Role of Ca2;pq-dependent potassium channels in in vitro anandamide mediated mesenteric vasorelaxation in rats with biliary cirrhosis. *Liver Int.* 2007;27:1045–1055.
391. Orliac ML, Peroni R, Celuch SM, et al. Potentiation of anandamide effects in mesenteric beds isolated from endotoxemic rats. *J Pharmacol Exp Ther.* 2003;304:179–184.
392. Caraceni P, Viola A, Piscitelli F, et al. Circulating and hepatic endocannabinoids and endocannabinoid related molecules in patients with cirrhosis. *Liver Int.* 2010;30:816–825.
393. Fernández-Rodriguez CM, Romero J, Petros TJ, et al. Circulating endogenous cannabinoid anandamide and portal, systemic and renal hemodynamics in cirrhosis. *Liver Int.* 2004;24:477–483.
394. Domenicali M, Caraceni P, Giannone F, et al. Cannabinoid type 1 receptor antagonism delays ascites formation in rats with cirrhosis. *Gastroenterology.* 2009;137:341–349.
395. Gaskari SA, Liu H, Moezi L, et al. Role of endocannabinoids in the pathogenesis of cirrhotic cardiomyopathy in bile duct-ligated rats. *Br J Pharmacol.* 2005; 146:315–323.
396. Batkai S, Mukhopadhyay P, Harvey-White J, et al. Endocannabinoids acting at CB1 receptors mediate the cardiac contractile dysfunction in vivo in cirrhotic rats. *Am J Physiol Heart Circ Physiol,* 2007;293:H1689–H1695.
397. Ryter SW, Alam J, Choi AMK. Heme oxygenase-1/carbon monoxide: from basic science to therapeutic applications. *Physiol Rev.* 2006;86:583–650.
398. Fernandez M, Lambrecht RW, Bonkovsky HL. Increased heme oxygenase activity in splanchnic organs from portal hypertensive rats: role in modulating mesenteric vascular reactivity. *J Hepatol.* 2001;34:812–817.
399. Chen YC, Ginès P, Yang J, et al. Increased vascular heme oxygenase-1 expression contributes to arterial vasodilation in experimental cirrhosis in rats. *Hepatology.* 2004;39:1075–1087.
400. Tarquini R, Masini E, La Villa G, et al.Increased plasma carbon monoxide in patients with viral cirrhosis and hyperdynamic circulation. *Am J Gastroenterol.* 2009;104:891–897.
401. Van Landeghem L, Laleman W, Vander Elst I, et al. Carbon monoxide produced by intrasinusoidally located haem-oxygenase-1 regulates the vascular tone in cirrhotic rat liver. *Liver Int.* 2009;29:650–660.
402. Guo SB, Duan ZJ, Li Q, et al. Effect of heme oxygenase-1 on renal function in rats with liver cirrhosis. *World J Gastroenterol.* 2011;17:322–328.
403. Miyazono M, Garat C, Morris KG Jr, et al. Decreased renal heme oxygenase-1 expression contributes to decreased renal function during cirrhosis. *Am J Physiol Renal Physiol.* 2002;283(5):F1123–1131.
404. Di Pascoli M, Zampieri F, Quarta S, et al. Heme oxygenase regulates renal arterial resistance and sodium excretion in cirrhotic rats. *J Hepatol.* 2011;54: 258–264.
405. Lieberman FL, Ito S, Reynolds TB. Effective plasma volume in cirrhosis with ascites. Evidence that a decreased value does not account for renal sodium retention, a spontaneous reduction in glomerular filtration rate (GFR), and a fall in GFR during drug-induced diuresis. *J Clin Invest.* 1969;48:975.
406. Lieberman FL, Denison EK, Reynolds TB. The relationship of plasma volume, portal hypertension, ascites, and renal sodium retention in cirrhosis: the overflow theory of ascites formation. *Ann NY Acad Sci.* 1970;170:202.
407. Papper S, Rosenbaum JD. Abnormalities in the excretion of water and sodium in "compensated" cirrhosis of the liver. *J Lab Clin Med.* 1952;40:523.
408. Wensing G, Sabra R, Branch RA. The onset of sodium retention in experimental cirrhosis in rats is related to a critical threshold of liver function. *Hepatology.* 1990;11:779.
409. Rector WG Jr, Lewis F, Robertson AD, et al. Renal sodium retention complicating alcoholic liver disease: relation to portosystemic shunting and liver function. *Hepatology.* 1990;12:455.
410. Ahloulay M, Dechaux M, Hassler C, et al. Cyclic AMP is a hepatorenal link influencing natriuresis and contributing to glucagon-induced hyperfiltration in rats. *J Clin Invest.* 1996;98:2251.
411. Oliver JA, Verna EC. Afferent mechanisms of sodium retention in cirrhosis and hepatorenal syndrome. *Kidney Int.* 2010;77:669–680.
412. Levy M. The genesis of urinary sodium retention in pre-ascitic cirrhosis: the overflow theory. *Gastroenterol Int.* 1992;5:186.
413. Levy M. Pathogenesis of sodium retention in early cirrhosis of the liver: evidence for vascular overfilling. *Semin Liver Dis.* 1994;14:4.
414. La Villa G, Salmerón JM, Arroyo V, et al. Mineralocorticoid escape in patients with compensated cirrhosis and portal hypertension. *Gastroenterology.* 1992;102:2114.
415. Albillos A, Lledo JL, Rossi I, et al. Continuous prazosin administration in cirrhotic patients: effects on portal hemodynamics and liver and renal function. *Gastroenterology.* 1995;109:1257.
416. Witte MH, Witte CL, Dumont AE. Progress in liver disease: physiological factors involved in the causation of cirrhotic ascites. *Gastroenterology.* 1971; 61:742.
417. Witte CL, Witte MH, Dumont AE. Lymph imbalance in the genesis and perpetuation of the ascites syndrome in hepatic cirrhosis. *Gastroenterology.* 1980; 78:1059.
418. Braunwald E, Colucci WS, Grossman W. Clinical aspects of heart failure; high-output heart failure; pulmonary edema. In: Braunwald E, ed. *Heart Disease. A Textbook of Cardiovascular Medicine.* Philadelphia: WB Saunders; 1997:445.
419. Palmer BF, Alpern RJ, Seldin DW. Pathophysiology of edema formation. In: Seldin DW, Giebisch G, eds. *The Kidney. Physiology and Pathophysiology*, 2nd ed. New York: Raven Press; 1992:2099.
420. Schrier RW. Pathogenesis of sodium and water retention in high-output and low-output cardiac failure, nephrotic syndrome, cirrhosis and pregnancy. *N Engl J Med.* 1988;319:1065.
421. Schrier RW. Body fluid volume regulation in health and disease: a unifying hypothesis. *Ann Intern Med.* 1990;113:155.
422. Schrier RW, Arroyo V, Bernardi M, et al. Peripheral arterial vasodilation hypothesis: a proposal for the initiation of renal sodium and water retention in cirrhosis. *Hepatology.* 1988;8:1151.

423. Schrier RW, Neiderbeger M, Weigert A, et al. Peripheral arterial vasodilation: determinant of functional spectrum of cirrhosis. *Semin Liver Dis.* 1994;14:14.
424. Colombato LA, Albillos A, Groszmann RJ. Temporal relationship of peripheral vasodilatation, plasma volume expansion and the hyperdynamic circulatory state in portal-hypertensive rats. *Hepatology.* 1991;15:323.
425. Ginès P, Cárdenas A. The management of ascites and dilutional hyponatremia in cirrhosis. *Semin Liver Dis.* 2008;28:43–58.
426. Moore KP, Wong F, Ginès P, et al. The management of ascites in cirrhosis: report on the consensus conference of the International Ascites Club. *Hepatology.* 2003;38:258–266.
427. Santos J, Planas R, Pardo A, et al. Spironolactone alone or in combination with furosemide in the treatment of moderate ascites in nonazotemic cirrhosis. A randomized comparative study of efficacy and safety. *J Hepatol.* 2003; 39:187–192.
428. Mimidis K, Papadopoulos V, Kartalis G. Eplerenone relieves spironolactone-induced painful gynaecomastia in patients with decompensated hepatitis B-related cirrhosis. *Scand J Gastroenterol.* 2007;42:1516–1517.
429. Ginès P, Arroyo V, Quintero E, et al. Comparison of paracentesis and diuretics in the treatment of cirrhotics with tense ascites. Results of a randomized study. *Gastroenterology.* 1987;93:234–241.
430. Ruiz-del-Arbol L, Monescillo A, Jiménez W, et al. Paracentesis-induced circulatory dysfunction: mechanism and effect on hepatic hemodynamics in cirrhosis. *Gastroenterology.* 1997;113:579–586.
431. Cárdenas A, Ginès P, Runyon BA. Is albumin infusion necessary after large volume paracentesis? *Liver Int.* 2009;29:636–640.
432. Ginès A, Fernandez-Esparrach G, Monescillo A, et al. Randomized trial comparing albumin, dextran 70, and polygeline in cirrhotic patients with ascites treated by paracentesis. *Gastroenterology.* 1996;111:1002–1010.
433. Garcia-Tsao G, Lim JK; Members of Veterans Affairs Hepatitis C Resource Center Program. Management and treatment of patients with cirrhosis and portal hypertension: recommendations from the Department of Veterans Affairs Hepatitis C Resource Center Program and the National Hepatitis C Program. *Am J Gastroenterol.* 2009;104:1802–1829.
434. Runyon BA; AASLD Practice Guidelines Committee. Management of adult patients with ascites due to cirrhosis: an update. *Hepatology.* 2009;49:2087–2107.
435. Salerno F, Guevara M, Bernardi M, et al. Refractory ascites: pathogenesis, definition and therapy of a severe complication in patients with cirrhosis. *Liver Int.* 2010;30:937–947.
436. Casado M, Bosch J, Garcia-Pagan JC, et al. Clinical events after transjugular intrahepatic portosystemic shunt: correlation with hemodynamic findings. *Gastroenterology.* 1998;114:1296–1303.
437. Boyer TD. Transjugular intrahepatic portosystemic shunt in the management of complications of portal hypertension. *Curr Gastroenterol Rep.* 2008; 10:30–35.
438. Lebrec D, Giuily N, Hadengue A, et al. Transjugular intrahepatic portosystemic shunts: comparison with paracentesis in patients with cirrhosis and refractory ascites: a randomized trial. *J Hepatol.* 1996;25:135–144.
439. Rossle M, Ochs A, Gulberg V, et al.A comparison of paracentesis and transjugular intrahepatic portosystemic shunting in patients with ascites. *N Engl J Med.* 2000;342:1701–1707.
440. Ginès P, Uriz J, Calahorra B, et al. Transjugular intrahepatic portosystemic shunting versus paracentesis plus albumin for refractory ascites in cirrhosis. *Gastroenterology.* 2002;123:1839–1847.
441. Sanyal A, Genning C, Reddy RK, et al. The North American Study for Treatment of Refractory Ascites. *Gastroenterology.* 2003;124:634–641.
442. Salerno F, Merli M, Riggio O, et al. Randomized controlled study of TIPS versus paracentesis plus albumin in cirrhosis with severe ascites. *Hepatology.* 2004;40:629–635.
443. Albillos A, Banares R, Gonzales M, et al. A meta-analysis of transjugular intrahepatic portosystemic shunt versus paracentesis for refractory ascites. *J Hepatol.* 2005;43:990–996.
444. D'Amico G, Luca A, Morabito A, et al. Uncovered transjugular intrahepatic portosystemic shunt for refractory ascites: a meta-analysis. *Gastroenterology.* 2005;129:1282–1293.
445. Berl T, Quittnat-Pelletier F, Verbalis JG, et al. Oral tolvaptan is safe and effective in chronic hyponatremia. *J Am Soc Nephrol.* 2010;21:705–712.
446. O'Leary JG, Davis GL. Conivaptan increases serum sodium in hyponatremic patients with end-stage liver disease. *Liver Transpl.* 2009;15: 1325–1329.
447. Moreau R, Durand F, Poynard T, et al. Terlipressin in patients with cirrhosis and type 1 hepatorenal syndrome: a retrospective multicenter study. *Gastroenterology.* 2002;122:923–930.
448. Ortega R, Ginès P, Uriz J, et al. Terlipressin therapy with and without albumin for patients with hepatorenal syndrome. Efficacy and outcome. *Hepatology.* 2002;36:941–948.
449. Halimi C, Bonnard P, Bernard B. Effect of terlipressin (Glypressin) on hepatorenal syndrome in cirrhotic patients: results of a multicentre pilot study. *Eur J Gastroenterol Hepatol.* 2002;14:153–158.
450. Solanki P, Chawla A, Garg R, et al. Beneficial effects of terlipressin in hepatorenal syndrome: a prospective, randomized placebo-controlled clinical trial. *J Gastroenterol Hepatol.* 2003;18:152–156.
451. Neri S, Pulvirenti D, Malaguarnera M, et al. Terlipressin and albumin in patients with cirrhosis and type I hepatorenal syndrome. *Dig Dis Sci.* 2008;53: 830–835.
452. Triantos CK, Samonakis D, Thalheimer U, et al. Terlipressin therapy for renal failure in cirrhosis. *Eur J Gastroenterol Hepatol.* 2010;22:481–486.
453. Alessandria C, Ottobrelli A, Debernardi-Venon W, et al. Noradrenalin vs terlipressin in patients with hepatorenal syndrome: a prospective, randomized, unblinded, pilot study. *J Hepatol.* 2007;47:499–505.
454. Sanyal A, Boyer T, Garcia-Tsao G, et al. A prospective, randomized, double blind, placebo-controlled trial of terlipressin for type 1 hepatorenal syndrome (HRS). *Gastroenterology.* 2008;134:1360–1368.
455. Martin-Llahi M, Pepin MN, Guevara G, et al. Terlipressin and albumin vs albumin in patients with cirrhosis and hepatorenal syndrome: a randomized study. *Gastroenterology.* 2008;134:1352–1359.
456. Gluud LL, Christensen K, Christensen E, Krag A. Systematic review of randomized trials on vasoconstrictor drugs for hepatorenal syndrome. *Hepatology.* 2010;51:576–584.
457. Fabrizi F, Dixit V, Martin P. Meta-analysis: terlipressin therapy for the hepatorenal syndrome. *Aliment Pharmacol Ther.* 2006;24:935–944.
458. Sagi SV, Mittal S, Kasturi KS, et al. Terlipressin therapy for reversal of type 1 hepatorenal syndrome: a meta-analysis of randomized controlled trials. *J Gastroenterol Hepatol.* 2010;25:880–885.
459. Nazar A, Pereira GH, Guevara M, et al. Predictors of response to therapy with terlipressin and albumin in patients with cirrhosis and type 1 hepatorenal syndrome. *Hepatology.* 2010;51:219–226.
460. Angeli P, Volpin R, Gerunda G, et al. Reversal of type 1 hepatorenal syndrome with the administration of midodrine and octreotide. *Hepatology.* 1999; 29:1690–1697.
461. Duvoux C, Zanditenas D, Hezode C, et al. Effects of noradrenaline and albumin in patients with type 1 hepatorenal syndrome: a pilot study. *Hepatology.* 2002;36:374–380.
462. Brensing KA, Textor J, Perz J, et al. Long term outcome after transjugular intrahepatic portosystemic stent-shunt in non-transplant cirrhotics with hepatorenal syndrome: a phase II study. *Gut.* 2000;47:288–295.
463. Wong LP, Blackley MP, Andreoni KA, et al. Survival of liver transplant candidates with acute renal failure receiving renal replacement therapy. *Kidney Int.* 2005;68:362–367.
464. Bañares R, Nevens F, Larsen FS, et al Extracorporeal liver support with the molecular adsorbent recirculating system (MARS) in patients with acute-on-chronic liver failure (AOCLF). The RELIEF trial. *J Hepatol.* 2010; 52:1184A.
465. Mitzner SR, Stange J, Klammt S, et al. Improvement of hepatorenal syndrome with extracorporeal albumin dialysis MARS: results of a prospective, randomized, controlled clinical trial. *Liver Trans.* 2000;6:277–286.
466. Mitzner SR, Klammt S, Peszynski P, et al. Improvement of multiple organ functions in hepatorenal syndrome during albumin dialysis with the molecular adsorbent recirculating system. *Ther Apher.* 2001;5:417–422.

CHAPTER

69 The Nephrotic Syndrome

Jeroen K. J. Deegens • Robert W. Schrier • Jack F. M. Wetzels

The nephrotic syndrome is defined by the triad of proteinuria (>3–3.5 g per day), hypoalbuminemia (<3 g per dL), and edema. Most patients also present with hypercholesterolemia. The nephrotic syndrome is the consequence of protein loss caused by severe injury to the glomerular capillary wall, and thus a typical presentation of patients with a glomerular disorder.[1] The nephrotic syndrome should be discerned from nephrotic range proteinuria. Patients with nephrotic range proteinuria have normal or only slightly decreased serum albumin levels, and are often asymptomatic. Nephrotic range proteinuria with preserved serum albumin levels is characteristic of focal segmental glomerulosclerosis (FSGS) related to hyperfiltration.[1,2]

Complications of the nephrotic syndrome mainly result from protein loss in the urine (Table 69.1). Edema formation is the best known presenting complication of the nephrotic syndrome. Patients with the nephrotic syndrome may also have hormonal disturbances, and are at increased risk for infections, venous thromboembolism, cardiovascular events, and acute renal failure. Finally, proteinuria is the best independent predictor of progression to chronic renal failure, and patients with persistent nephrotic syndrome will almost invariably develop end-stage renal disease (ESRD).

EDEMA

Edema in the nephrotic syndrome is typically seen around the eyes in the morning, and in the lower legs and feet in the evening. Edema can be massive, resulting in weight gain of >10 kg. Edema is the consequence of an alteration in the balance of forces that govern the fluid exchange over the capillary wall as reflected in the Starling equation: $Jv = LpS\{(P_{plasma}-P_{int}) - \sigma(\pi_{plasma}-\pi_{int})\}$, where transcapillary fluid flux (Jv) is determined by the hydraulic conductivity (Lp) and the filtration surface area (S) of the capillary wall, the differences between the hydrostatic (P) and oncotic (π) pressures in plasma and interstitium (Int), and the transcapillary reflection coefficient for proteins (σ).[3] In patients with the nephrotic syndrome the hypoalbuminemia and the subsequent decrease of plasma oncotic pressure increases net capillary ultrafiltration. Initially, accumulation of interstitial fluid (and thus edema) is partly prohibited by "edema prevention forces" such as an increase in interstitial hydrostatic pressure, and increased interstitial fluid transport and lymph drainage, which transfers interstitial proteins back to the vascular compartment resulting in a decrease in interstitial oncotic pressure and unchanged $\Delta\pi$.[4] Edema develops when these opposing forces are overwhelmed.

Obviously, edema formation requires ongoing renal sodium and water retention. Two theories have been proposed to explain the sodium retention in the nephrotic syndrome. These theories and the potential afferent and efferent mechanisms of sodium and water reabsorption in the nephrotic syndrome are illustrated in Figures 69.1 and 69.2. In the underfilling theory hypoalbuminemia and the ensuing hypotonicity causes fluid loss from the intravascular space. The resultant decrease of plasma and blood volume will activate homeostatic responses which drive renal sodium retention. The overfill theory of edema formation postulates that there is primary, abnormal renal sodium retention related to intrinsic abnormalities of the kidney. In this respect patients with the nephrotic syndrome differ from patients with edema formation due to heart failure and cirrhosis of the liver, in which the kidneys are structurally normal. Indeed, in comparative studies nephrotic patients were characterized by a relatively higher arterial blood pressure, a higher glomerular filtration rate (GFR), and less impairment in sodium and water excretion.[5]

In the following paragraphs we review the evidence to support these theories, discuss new pathogenetic mechanisms, and evaluate treatment modalities. We also address other complications of the nephrotic syndrome.

RENAL SODIUM AND WATER RETENTION IN THE NEPHROTIC SYNDROME: CLINICAL OBSERVATIONS

For a long time the theory of transcapillary fluid transport, governed by the principles of the Starling equation, dominated the discussion of edema formation in the nephrotic syndrome. A reduction in the amount of circulating albumin,

TABLE 69.1 Complications of the Nephrotic Syndrome

Complication	Cause	Specific Treatment[a]
Edema	Loss of albumin	Sodium restriction Treatment with (combination of) diuretics
Hypothyroidism	Loss of thyroid hormones	Rarely supplementation with thyroid hormones necessary
Osteoporosis	Loss of vitamin D Binding protein	Treatment with vitamin D_2/D_3
Anemia	Loss of erythropoietin	No treatment Only in case of severe disabling anemia consider treatment with erythropoietin[b]
Infections	Loss of IgG	Antibiotic therapy In case of persistent nephrotic syndrome: Pneumococcal vaccination Prophylactic IgG may be useful in case of recurrent bacterial infections and hypogammaglobulinemia
Thrombosis	Loss of anticoagulant proteins	Consider prophylactic anticoagulation in patients with membranous nephropathy and serum albumin <2 g/dL *or* patients with serum albumin <2 g/dL and additional risk factor for thrombosis[c]
Cardiovascular events	Hyperlipidemia	Dietary restriction of cholesterol and saturated fat HMG CoA reductase inhibitors
Renal failure	Intrinsic renal injury Loss of transferrin with iron Proteinuria	Reduction of proteinuria and blood pressure with ACE inhibitor/ARB

[a]All patients should receive treatment aimed at the underlying disease and aimed at reduction of proteinuria preferably using ACE inhibitor/ARB.
[b]Other causes of anemia should be excluded first.
[c]Risk factors for thrombosis: previous thromboembolic event, prolonged bed rest or immobility, congestive heart failure.
ACE, angiotensin-converting enzyme; ARB, angiotensin receptor blocker; IgG, immunoglobulin G; HMG CoA, 3-hydroxy-3-methylglutaryl coenzyme A.

which is the major determinant of oncotic pressure, will promote transport of water across the capillary wall toward the interstitium. As a result plasma and blood volume will decrease. It was proposed that in patients with a nephrotic syndrome plasma and blood volume were (partly) maintained by sodium and water retention that increased the extracellular volume.[6] This increased sodium reabsorption was attributed to neurohumoral activation and renal hemodynamic changes as a consequence of the decreased blood and plasma volume.

Many studies have provided data that are in line with the sequence of events as depicted in Figure 69.1, and thus support the underfilling theory of sodium retention in the nephrotic syndrome. There is no doubt that plasma and blood volume can be severely compromised in children with a nephrotic syndrome. Van de Walle et al. reported in detail nine children with multirelapsing nephrotic syndrome due to minimal change disease.[7] These patients were studied during a severe relapse, with serum albumin concentration averaging 1.6 g per dL. The patients had symptoms of hypovolemia such as tachycardia, oliguria, peripheral vasoconstriction, and abdominal pain. These children had low GFR; elevated levels of renin, aldosterone, and vasopressin; and a markedly increased proximal tubular sodium reabsorption. Oliver studied seven children with steroid sensitive nephrotic syndrome, and observed increased urinary norepinephrine excretion in the nephrotic phase.[8] Urinary norepinephrine was positively correlated with plasma aldosterone and negatively with urinary sodium excretion. In studies that followed, these investigators showed that volume expansion with intravenous administration of albumin lowered plasma norepinephrine levels.[9] Gur et al. studied six children with lipoid nephrosis.[10] In the period of nephrosis these patients had reduced electrolyte-free water clearance, compatible with increased proximal tubular sodium reabsorption.

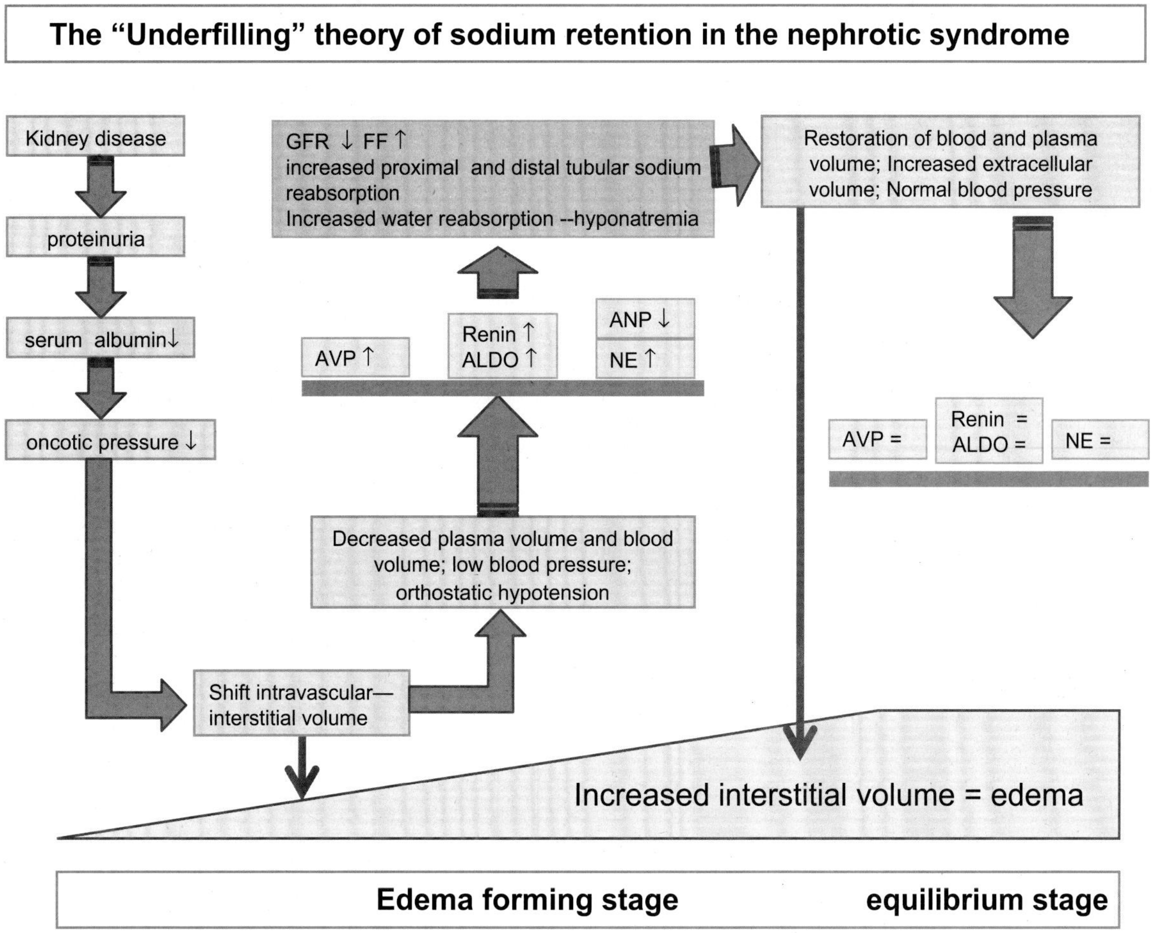

FIGURE 69.1 Pathophysiology of sodium retention in the nephrotic syndrome: the underfilling theory. Severe proteinuria and decreased serum albumin levels are the hallmark of the nephrotic syndrome. Capillary oncotic pressure decreases, resulting in increased capillary ultrafiltration. Edema will develop as soon as the edema preventing mechanisms are overwhelmed. In the edema forming phase, interstitial volume is increased and plasma volume is decreased. This will stimulate renal sodium and water reabsorption, true activation of neurohumoral mechanisms (catecholamines, renin, aldosterone, arginine vasopressin), changes in renal hemodynamics (low glomerular filtration rate, increased filtration fraction), and altered peritubular forces (increased oncotic pressure, decreased hydrostatic pressure). Ongoing water and sodium retention will normalize plasma and blood volume, at the cost of a large increase in extracellular volume, thus increasing edema. In the equilibrium phase, many parameters may be normalized. *ANP,* atrial natriuretic peptide; *AVP,* arginine vasopressin; *GFR,* glomerular filtration rate.

Support for underfilling is not limited to studies in children with steroid sensitive minimal change nephrotic syndrome. Yamauchi and Hopper described 10 adult patients who presented with hypotension and hypovolemic shock as complications of the nephrotic syndrome.[11] These patients had severe hypoalbuminemia, amounting 1.4 g per dL (range 0.4 to 2.2 g per dL). Blood volume was reduced to values ranging from 71% to 92% of the predicted values. Kunagai studied 11 patients with a nephrotic syndrome due to minimal change disease and relatively well preserved renal function.[12] These patients were studied in the stage of edema formation, during diuresis, and in remission. In the edema forming stage, the patients retained sodium and their body weight increased by >0.2 kg per day. Blood pressures were low to normal, ranging from 113/71 to 142/90 mm Hg. In the edema forming stage plasma volume (measured in supine position) was decreased, and plasma renin activity (PRA) and plasma aldosterone concentration (PAC) were increased. PRA correlated with plasma volume and PAC, and sodium excretion was lowest in patients with highest PAC. Evidence to support the role of aldosterone in sodium retention comes from clinical studies, in which spironolactone, a selective mineralocorticoid receptor antagonist, was used. Shapiro et al. studied patients with a nephrotic syndrome and a high sodium intake. Within 3 days after the start of therapy sodium excretion increased from 205 ± 20 mmol per day to 312 ± 13 mmol per day in patients on spironolactone, and remained stable in controls.[13] Other investigators evaluated the role of arginine

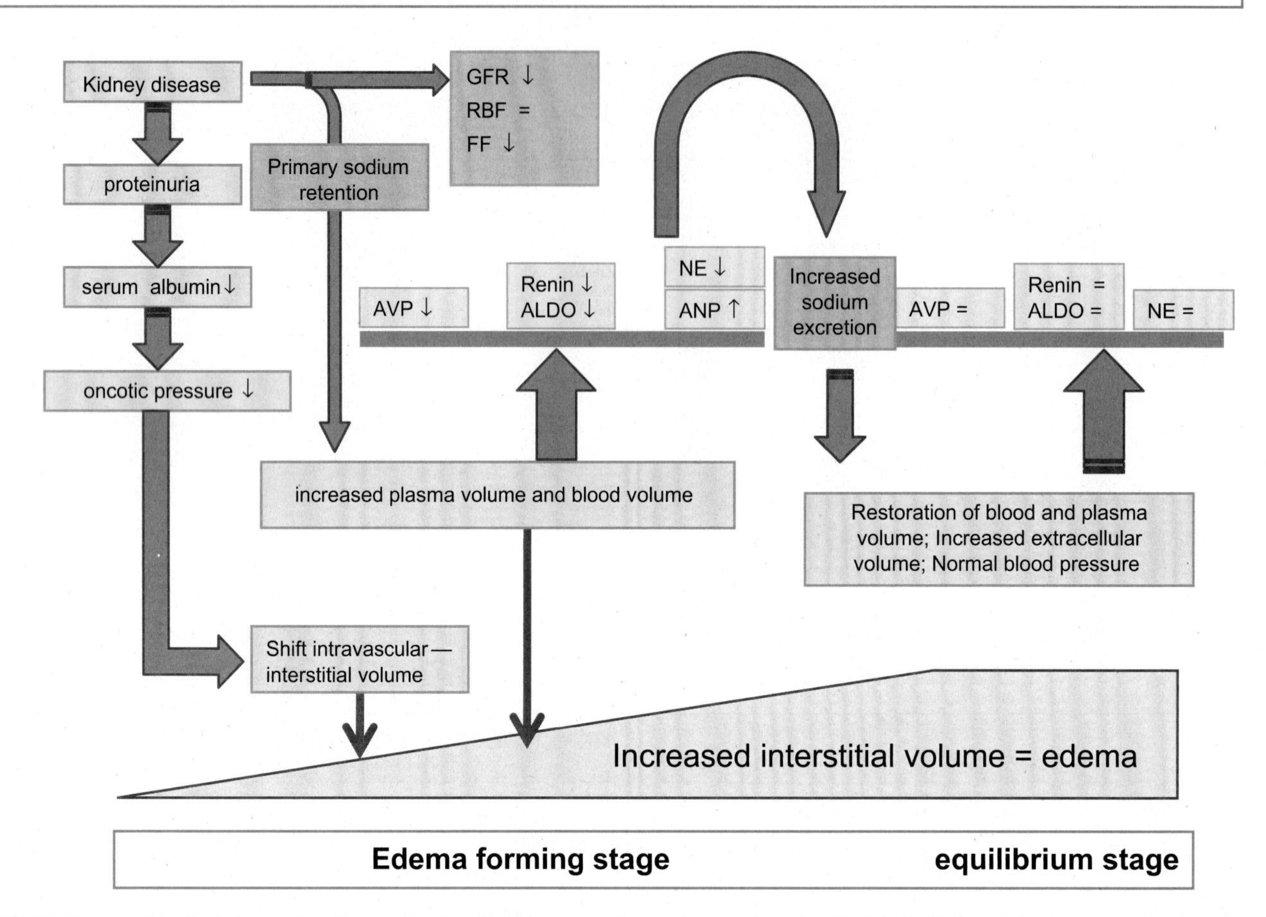

FIGURE 69.2 Pathophysiology of sodium retention in the nephrotic syndrome: the overfill theory. Kidney injury causes proteinuria and decreased serum albumin levels. Capillary oncotic pressure decreases, resulting in increased capillary ultrafiltration. Edema will develop as soon as the edema-preventing mechanisms are overwhelmed. Kidney injury also causes primary renal sodium retention. Possible mechanisms include increased activity of the epithelial sodium channel, decreased responsiveness to atrial natriuretic peptide (ANP), in addition to low glomerular filtration rate. Sodium and water retention will increase extracellular volume, with a disproportionate increase of interstitial versus plasma volume due to the altered capillary forces. Patients will present with normal or elevated plasma volume, blood pressure, and ANP, and decreased renin and aldosterone. Patients with overfilling will respond less well to volume loading, and efficacy of spironolactone may be impaired. Finally, sodium retention will cease, if equilibrium is reached. *ANP,* atrial natriuretic peptide; *AVP,* arginine vasopressin; *GFR,* glomerular filtration rate.

vasopressin (AVP). Usberti et al. studied 16 patients with a nephrotic syndrome, all with normal blood pressure and normal renal function.[14] These patients were studied while in equilibrium (no weight gain). For comparison, patients with glomerulonephritis were evaluated. The nephrotic patients had lower plasma sodium concentration and blood volume, and increased levels of plasma AVP, PRA, and urine epinephrine. Patients with the nephrotic syndrome were unable to excrete a water load: maximal urinary flow rate was 4.52 ± 1.71 mL per min (vs. 10.0 ± 2.26 mL per min in controls) and minimal urine osmolality 161 ± 50 mOsm per kg (vs. 83 ± 8 mOsm per kg). The conclusion that in the nephrotic syndrome AVP was non-osmotically stimulated was supported by subsequent experiments which showed that iso-osmotic volume expansion with human albumin decreased AVP, and increased water diuresis. Other maneuvers to increase plasma volume in patients with a nephrotic syndrome, such as water immersion and head down tilt, also increased diuresis and natriuresis.[15–17] The sympathetic nervous system has also been studied in adults with a nephrotic syndrome.[18] Sympathetic nervous system activity was assessed in six patients with a nephrotic syndrome and in six normal control subjects in the supine position. In the patients the plasma norepinephrine levels were elevated, the spillover rate of norepinephrine was markedly increased (0.30 ± 0.07 vs. 0.13 ± 0.02 μg/min/m^2, $P < .05$), whereas the norepinephrine clearance rate was comparable to that in the normal subjects (2.60 ± 0.29 vs. 2.26 ± 0.27 L per minute, not significant). Of note, PRA and plasma aldosterone, AVP, and ANP concentrations were not different in the nephrotic syndrome patients compared with control subjects.

Observations in the seventh and eighth decade of the past century provided arguments against underfilling as the only cause of renal sodium retention in the nephrotic syndrome. Dorhout-Mees et al. initially studied a group of 10 adult patients with minimal change nephrotic syndrome on 13 occasions.[19] The patients were selected for the study because of increased blood volume and blood pressure. Each patient was studied prior to and following prednisone-induced remission. After remission, blood pressure fell in 12 cases, plasma volume fell in 10 cases, and PRA increased in eight cases. Clearly, these data are most compatible with primary overfilling in the nephrotic syndrome (Fig. 69.2). Data from studies that followed supported the concept of primary renal sodium retention in the nephrotic syndrome. Geers et al. evaluated plasma and blood volume in 88 patients with nephrotic syndrome.[20] Plasma volume was 62.8 ± 9.6 mL per kg lean body mass (LBM) in nephrotic patients and 56 ± 7.1 mL per kg LBM in controls, and blood volume was 94.9 ± 15.1 mL per kg LBM in nephrotic patients versus 88.5 mL per kg LBM in controls. Blood pressures in these and other patients with a nephrotic syndrome were normal or slightly increased.[21,22] Further evidence to support overfilling comes from studies showing low PRA and PAC in many patients with a nephrotic syndrome.[21,23,24] Moreover, neither lowering aldosterone with captopril, blocking aldosterone with spironolactone, nor antagonizing angiotensin II with the analogue saralasin induced natriuresis.[23,25,26] It was also questioned if the increased levels of PRA that were observed in some patients with a nephrotic syndrome contributed to sodium retention. Brown et al. evaluated eight patients with a nephrotic syndrome and elevated PRA and PAC.[27] These patients were studied during treatment with captopril, which lowered PAC, and during treatment with intravenous (IV) albumin which decreased both PRA and PAC. Both interventions failed to restore sodium balance. The blood pressure, however, fell with captopril and could have obscured a natriuresis secondary to a decreased PAC.

Additional renal hemodynamic studies and studies of tubular function also supported the overfilling theory. Geers et al. measured GFR using Cr^{51}–EDTA clearance and ERPF using J^{131}–hippurate clearance in 41 patients with a nephrotic syndrome.[21] Mean filtration fraction was low, and averaged 14%, arguing against underfilling and a stimulated renin-angiotensin-aldosterone system (RAAS). Detailed clearance studies showed that proximal tubular sodium reabsorption was decreased rather than increased. Usberti et al. studied 21 patients with glomerulonephritis.[28] Tubular glucose reabsorption was used as a marker of proximal tubular sodium reabsorption. The threshold for glucose reabsorption was reduced in the 10 nephrotic patients with edema, suggesting diminished proximal tubular reabsorption. In studies undertaken in five nephrotic patients, a similar conclusion was reached by Grausz et al.[29] In these clearance studies, blockade of sodium reabsorption in the distal nephron with ethacrynic acid and chlorothiazide was used to assess proximal sodium reabsorption. Proximal sodium reabsorption was lower in the nephrotic patients than in normal and in cirrhotic patients.

Studies by Brown et al. and Koomans et al. also provided strong arguments against a role for hypoalbuminemia in the sodium retention of the nephrotic syndrome.[30,31] These investigators performed detailed clinical observations in patients who were treated with prednisone and developed a remission. In both studies there was a decrease of proteinuria after the start of prednisone. Immediately thereafter sodium excretion increased, well before any noticeable increase of serum albumin levels.

We must be cautious when interpreting the results of the various studies. It is important to consider the timing of the study, the characteristics of the study population, and study methodology. Studies may be done in the edema forming phase, or in the maintenance phase when patients are in equilibrium and many parameters may have normalized (Fig. 69.1). Patient characteristics include the underlying glomerular disease, the severity of renal injury, the level of GFR, and the rapidity of onset of the nephrotic syndrome. Methodology concerns include the methods used to assess plasma volume and blood volume, and the position of the patient. Measurements of plasma volume and blood volume are imprecise (coefficient of variance 10%). Studies have used different correction factors for plasma and blood volume, using body weight, dry weight, and estimated lean body mass. Plasma volume usually is calculated from the distribution of radioactive labeled albumin. Because the transcapillary escape rate of albumin is increased in patients with a nephrotic syndrome, blood samples must be taken shortly after administration of albumin. Blood volume is calculated from plasma volume or measured red cell mass and hematocrit. However, it is important to note that the ratio of peripheral hematocrit/whole body hematocrit (the so called F cell ratio) is lower in patients with a nephrotic syndrome. If this is not accounted for, calculated blood volume will be overestimated.

Another important issue is the role of body position. Most investigators have performed studies with patients in supine position. However, in patients with a nephrotic syndrome larger changes of plasma volume and blood volume occur upon change of body position. In 1960, Fawcett already studied patients with hypoalbuminemia and edema.[32] In these patients plasma and blood volume decreased to a larger extent compared to control patients as calculated from the change in hematocrit: after 60 minutes of standing hematocrit increased by 12.3 ± 3.4% in patients, and +6.6 ± 2.9% in controls. Similar findings were reported by Eisenberg and Geers.[33,34] Studies have shown that these changes are relevant, and affect natriuresis. Minutolo studied seven patients with a nephrotic syndrome and evaluated their baseline sodium excretion and the response to IV furosemide while supine and in upright position.[35] In the upright position patients had markedly higher levels of PRA and PAC, and lower sodium and water excretion. Similarly, the response to furosemide was attenuated in the upright position; 6-hour sodium excretion was 40.2 ±

7.8 mmol in the upright position and 64.1 ± 9.1 mmol while supine. Usberti also noted that fractional excretion of sodium was higher when patients were recumbent.[36]

Finally, interpretation of changes in levels of mediators of neurohumoral activation and effects of any intervention must be done with caution. Activation of PRA and sympathetic nervous system may occur as a consequence of the primary renal disease, and does not necessarily reflect underfilling. In contrast, effects of blockade of aldosterone may be masked by opposite effects of changes in blood pressure.

If we critically review the available literature, it is evident that patients with a nephrotic syndrome may present with characteristics of underfilling or overfilling. In the previously mentioned study of Van de Walle et al. only nine patients had clear signs and symptoms of hypovolemia. Ten other patients had no evidence of hypovolemia. When comparing children with and without hypovolemia, they observed higher PRA and PAC and lower blood volume in hypovolemic patients. These variations in volume status were also seen in children with a nephrotic syndrome caused by renal pathologies other than minimal change disease.[7] Similar observations have been done in adults (Table 69.2). Usberti et al. described two groups of nephrotic syndrome patients distinguished on the basis of their plasma albumin concentrations.[36] Patients in group 1 had a plasma albumin concentration of less than 1.7 g per dL associated with low blood volumes and atrial natriuretic plasma (ANP) levels, elevated plasma angiotensin II (AT-II) concentrations, and increased proximal tubular reabsorption of sodium (determined by lithium clearance). In contrast, group 2 patients with a plasma albumin concentration greater than 1.7 g per dL exhibited normal blood volumes and plasma hormone concentrations. In all patients blood volume was positively correlated with the plasma albumin concentration, and PRA was inversely correlated with both blood volume and plasma albumin concentration. Of note, GFR was not different between group 1 and group 2 patients (100 ± 25 vs. 101 ± 22 mL per minute, not significant), whereas urinary sodium excretion was substantially lower in group 1 patients (4.88 ± 5.53 vs. 29.9 ± 9.3 mEq per 4 hours, $P < .001$). Moreover, acute expansion of blood volume in group 1 patients normalized PRA, plasma AT-II and aldosterone concentrations, fractional sodium excretion, and lithium clearance, while increasing circulating ANP concentrations. Other studies have confirmed these findings, and have added relevant information. Meltzer et al. found that their hypervolemic patients tended to have more severe glomerular involvement, lower GFR, and hypertension.[37] In the study of Geers et al. this variability is also seen.[21] Patients were studied while in sodium balance, and studies were done with patients being recumbent. Overall, plasma volume, blood volume, and blood pressure were normal or above the normal range. There was a striking absence of a correlation between PRA

TABLE 69.2 **Clinical Characteristics of Patients with a Nephrotic Syndrome**

	Patients with Sodium Retention	**Patients in Sodium Balance**
Number	12	8
Age	NA	NA
Gender	NA	NA
Blood pressure (mm Hg)	NA	NA
FENa (%)	0.107 ± 0.109	0.60 ± 0.170
GFR (mL/min)	100 ± 25	101 ± 22
S albumin (g/dL)	1.4 ± 0.28	2.2 ± 0.47
Proteinuria (g/day)	9.7 (5.7–22)	6.6 (3.2–10.2)
Blood volume (mL/kg)	68 ± 6	77 ± 4
Plasma renin activity (ng/mL/hr)	5.8 ± 3.5	0.61 ± 0.43
Plasma aldosterone (pg/mL)	337 ± 228	41 ± 20

NA, not available; GFR, glomerular filtration rate; FENa, fractional excretion of sodium; data are given as means (SD) or median (range).
Adapted from Usberti M, Gazzotti RM, Poiesi C, et al. Considerations on the sodium retention in nephrotic syndrome. *Am J Nephrol.* 1995;15:38–47.

TABLE 69.3 **Factors That May Give Guidance as to Whether an Individual Patient with the Nephrotic Syndrome Has Overfill or Underfill Edema**

	Overfill	Underfill
GFR <50% of normal	+	−
GFR >75% of normal	−	+
Serum albumin >2 g/dL	+	−
Serum albumin <2 g/dL	−	+
Histology minimal change	−	+
Hypertension	+	−
Postural hypotension	−	+

GFR, glomerular filtration rate.
Reprinted from Schrier RW, Fassett RG. A critique of the overfill hypothesis of sodium and water retention in the nephrotic syndrome. *Kidney Int* 1998;53:1111, with permission.

and blood volume. However, when critically analyzing the data, it is apparent that patients with minimal change disease had lower PV, and higher PRA and PAC. Within the group of patients with minimal change disease, renal impairment was associated with higher blood pressure, PV and blood volume, and lower PRA and PAC.

Thus, patients with nephrotic syndrome can show evidence of underfilling or overfilling. The effective plasma and blood volume in a particular patient will depend on the balance between the (rapidity) of the onset of the nephrotic syndrome, the severity of hypoalbuminemia, and the magnitude of primary renal sodium retention. Thus, underfilling may be more likely in patients with minimal change disease, preserved GFR, and severe hypoalbuminemia (Table 69.3).[37,38]

With respect to the mechanisms of primary renal sodium retention, these have remained largely undisclosed in human studies. The clearance studies have pointed to an intrarenal defect at the level of the distal tubules. Koomans et al. infused albumin in patients with nephrotic syndrome.[39] Patients had increased proximal and distal sodium reabsorption. Infusion of albumin decreased proximal but not distal sodium reabsorption, compatible with a hypovolemia dependent effect on proximal and a primary renal defect of distal sodium reabsorption. In humans, resistance to ANP has been suggested as the culprit. Jespersen studied seven patients with a nephrotic syndrome and 13 age- and sex-matched controls.[40] At baseline, patients had higher blood pressures, lower levels of plasma aldosterone, and higher levels of plasma ANP levels. Both patients and controls received a bolus of 2 ug per kg ANP. Although plasma levels of ANP reached similar levels, sodium excretion was significantly lower in patients. Most importantly, these authors observed that urinary excretion of the second messenger cGMP remained lower in the patients, suggesting a defective ANP signaling. Similar studies were done by Plum et al.[22] These authors studied 31 patients and 10 controls. ANP was infused over 2 hours in 15 patients and 10 controls. At baseline ANP levels were higher in the nephrotic patients. Infusion of ANP increased absolute sodium excretion to a similar extent, in patients and controls. However, sodium excretion factored for the level of ANP was reduced in patients. Again, urinary excretion of cGMP was lower in the patients. Fractional excretion of cGMP was calculated and used as marker of tubular production of cGMP. In the controls fractional excretion of cGMP increased from 93 ± 33% to 159 ± 142%, and in the patients fractional excretion decreased (from 166 ± 77% to 130 ± 58%.), indicating that indeed the tubular production of cGMP was attenuated in the nephrotic syndrome.

RENAL SODIUM AND WATER RETENTION: ANIMAL STUDIES

Earlier work in animal models strongly suggested a pathogenetic role for aldosterone and increased sympathetic activity in the nephrotic edema: adrenalectomy prevented the sodium retention in aminonucleoside nephrosis and renal denervation restored renal excretory function in the Adriamycin model.[41–43] Micropuncture studies in the rat nephrotoxic serum nephritis model found decreased single nephron GFR and increased proximal tubular sodium reabsorption.[44] Clearly, these findings support the underfilling theory (Fig. 69.1). However, these studies and their conclusions can be questioned. Sodium retention was not overcome by saline loading,[41] sympathetic activation may be the consequence of renal injury per se and is not necessarily proof of underfilling, and in the study of Kuroda proximal tubular pressures were increased suggesting distal tubular obstruction due to protein casts.[41,44]

Different conclusions were drawn in studies that followed. Many studies have used the "puromycin aminonucleoside (PAN)" model in the rat, which is considered a model of minimal change disease. Proteinuria is induced by intravenous injection of PAN. The animals develop proteinuria and hypoalbuminemia, often associated with edema and ascites. In the PAN model a short lasting increased sodium excretion is seen at day 1, followed by sodium retention from day 2 onward. Sodium retention preceded the onset of proteinuria which occurred after day 4.[45] This time course led investigators to conclude that sodium retention could not be the consequence of the proteinuria and the ensuing hypoalbuminemia. Although plasma aldosterone levels are increased at day 6 in this model, the role of aldosterone was questioned by experiments in adrenalectomized rats that received a constant supplementation with corticosteroids. In these "corticosteroid clamped" animals injection of PAN also induced sodium retention.[46] Amiloride, but not the aldosterone receptor blocker sodium canrenoate, prevented sodium retention, thus confirming the limited role of aldosterone.[47] Additional studies indicated that sodium retention in this model was independent of systemic factors such as AVP, angiotensin II, PPARγ, nitric oxide, tumor necrosis factor alpha (TNFα), or insulin-like growth factor 1 (IGF1).[48] Deschenes and colleagues studied the activity and expression of the sodium transporters' epithelial sodium channel (ENaC) and Na-K-ATPase in the PAN model and two other models. In all models they observed an increased expression of these sodium transporters at the mRNA and protein levels in the collecting ducts. Activity of the Na-K-ATPase measured with a radioactive P^{32} labelled substrate was likewise increased and correlated with sodium excretion.[45] In similar experiments activity and expression of ENaC was increased.[46] Somewhat unexpectedly, adrenalectomy prevented the increase in expression of ENaC but not of Na-K-ATPase. Although these experiments indicate that sodium retention does occur in the absence of increased aldosterone levels, it cannot be ruled out that aldosterone plays a modulatory role. Recent studies evaluated sodium retention in mice that lacked the serum- and glucocorticoid kinase 1 (SGK1),which is induced by aldosterone and activates ENaC.[49] The nephrotic syndrome was induced by injecting doxorubicin. Sodium retention was less in the SGK1 knockout mice.

Bernard et al. performed experiments in a rat model of membranous nephropathy.[50] Micropuncture studies were done after volume expansion to limit the role of volume depletion. Urinary sodium excretion was decreased in the proteinuric rats. However, proximal tubular sodium reabsorption was not increased but decreased, and there were no differences in sodium load to the late distal tubules, suggesting that increased sodium reabsorption must have occurred beyond the late distal tubule. These findings were confirmed and extended in studies by Ichikawa et al. that virtually proved the existence of a renal defect beyond the late distal tubule as cause of the increased sodium retention in the nephrotic syndrome.[51] Ichikawa et al. selectively infused PAN in one kidney of Munich Wistar rats. They evaluated renal function, proteinuria, and single nephron function of both kidneys, which thus were exposed to the same systemic factors. Blood pressures were normal, as were serum protein levels. The data are depicted in Table 69.4. The diseased kidney was proteinuric, had slightly decreased GFR, and markedly decreased sodium excretion. Single nephron GFR and filtration fraction were decreased due to a reduction of the ultrafiltration coefficient Kf. Subsequent segmental analysis of sodium transport by micropunture showed that the amount of sodium that reached the end distal tubule was similar and amounted 0.31 nEq per minute in the perfused kidney and 0.32 nEq per minute in the nonperfused kidney. In the final urine sodium excretion was 0.08 nEq per min versus 0.24 nEq/min, indicating increased sodium reabsorption in the cortical or medullary collecting duct. Infusion of the angiotensin II blocker saralasin increased GFR but not sodium excretion, arguing against a role for the reduced GFR in the abnormal sodium excretion.[51]

TABLE 69.4 **Renal Parameters in the Unilateral Puromycin Aminonucleoside Model**

	Perfused Kidney	Control Kidney
Systolic blood pressure (mm Hg)	118	118
Protein concentration (g/dL)	5.7	5.7
Proteinuria (mg/24 hr)	101	3
GFR (mL/min)	0.82	1.35
Urinary sodium excretion (μM/24 hr)	23	76
snGFR (nL/min)	31.8	48.6
snFF	0.25	0.35
ΔP (mm Hg)	35.4	35.5
Kf (nL/s.mm Hg)	0.047	1.02
Sodium delivery at site:		
Early proximal tubule (nEq/min)	5.6	8.2
Late proximal tubule (nEq/min)	3.3	4.4
Loop of Henle (nEq/min)	0.78	0.74
Late distal tubule (nEq/min)	0.31	0.32
Urine (nEq/min)	0.08	0.24

GFR, glomerular filtration rate; snGFR, single nephron GFR; snFF, single nephron filtration fraction; ΔP: glomerular transcapillary pressure gradient; Kf, glomerular capillary ultrafiltration coefficient
Adapted from Ichikawa I, Rennke HG, Hoyer JR, et al. Role for intrarenal mechanisms in the impaired salt excretion of experimental nephrotic syndrome. *J Clin Invest.* 1983;71: 91–103.

Although the above animal studies provided direct evidence for the existence of a primary renal tubular defect as cause of the impaired sodium excretion in the nephrotic syndrome, only recently have studies clarified the mechanisms involved in this defect.

Kastner studied the relationship between proteinuria and the expression of various ion channels in a mouse model of anti-GBM glomerulonephritis.[52] To dissociate the role of glomerular protein losses from tubular dysfunction studies were done in mice that partially lacked proximal tubule megalin expression. In the diseased mice, expression of NHE3 and Na-Pi2b was decreased after injection of the antibodies, with no difference between the wild type and megalin knockout mice. Megalin knockout mice, in which reabsorption of proteins is markedly reduced, showed increased expression of fragments of αENaC and γENaC in the cortical region. In mice injected with the anti-GBM serum a further, substantial increase in the abundance of these fragments was seen, most prominent in the knockout mice. These findings were confirmed by immunohistochemistry. Similar observations by the same group were done in the rat anti-Thy-1.1 model.[53] Injection of anti-Thy1.1 antibody increased proteinuria, decreased GFR, and reduced sodium excretion. There was a major upregulation of bands of αENaC, γENAC, and Na-K-ATPase, and no change in the expression of NCC, NKCC2, and AQP2. These findings were considered compatible with increased proteolytic cleavage and thus activation of ENaC, related to the proteolytic activity of proteins in the urine. The direct role of proteinuria on renal sodium handing was substantiated in additional experiments. Svenningsen demonstrated that the nephrotic urine of patients and animals increased activity of ENaC in a cell line.[54] This effect was dependent on the presence in the urine of the serine protease plasmin. In patients with proteinuria, plasminogen is lost in the urine. Plasmin is generated by degradation of plasminogen under the influence of urokinase type plasminogen activator (uPA), which is present in the collecting ducts. In subsequent experiments it was shown that plasmin activates ENaC by cleaving and degrading an inhibitory peptide from the gamma subunit of ENaC.[55] These findings explain the efficacy of amiloride in this model; amiloride not only blocks ENaC, but also inhibits uPA.

Another potential mechanism of impaired renal sodium excretion involves ANP resistance. Perico et al. observed a blunted response to ANP in Adriamycin nephrotic rats.[56] This abnormal response preceded the water and sodium retention.[57] Valentin showed a blunted natriuretic response to infusion of saline in rats with Adriamycin nephrosis. Plasma ANP levels were higher in nephrotic rats.[58] Despite this, nephrotic rats excreted less cGMP, which was normalized by infusion of phosphodiesterase (PDE) inhibitors. There was no difference in ANP binding. These data suggested that ANP resistance was related to increased PDE activity. Similar findings were done in a Heymann nephritis model. Lower urine cGMP levels coincided with ANP resistance which was recovered by blocking PDE. Thus, these studies suggested that ANP resistance was caused by increased PDE activity.[59] Although resistance to ANP may be the consequence of volume depletion or concomitant neurohumoral activation, this is unlikely since volume loading did not alter the response to ANP, neither did renal denervation in some but not all studies. The absence of response to ANP in the isolated perfused kidney confirmed the renal defect.

A recent study pursued the potential mechanisms of ANP nonresponsiveness. Polzin studied rats made nephrotic by injection of PAN or anti-Thy-1 antibodies.[60] They observed a decreased expression of Corin in the medulla. Corin is a type 3 transmembrane serine protease that converts pro-ANP to the active ANP. Reduced Corin expression was paralleled by an increase in pro-ANP, decrease of ANP and cGMP, and an increased expression of beta-ENaC.

Although the animal studies provide convincing evidence for an intrarenal defect as cause of the altered sodium handling in the nephrotic syndrome, and the possible pathogenetic pathways are clarified in elegant in vivo and in vitro studies, a cautious note should be made: most animal models have used Adriamycin or puromycin aminonucleoside. These toxic agents not only cause glomerular injury, but may also cause direct tubular injury. As such, extrapolation of the findings in animal studies to the human situation should be done with caution. As reviewed above, the clinical observations clearly indicate that patients with the nephrotic syndrome can present with signs, symptoms, and laboratory findings of both underfilling and overfilling.

THERAPY OF SODIUM AND WATER RETENTION IN THE NEPHROTIC SYNDROME

The treatment modalities in nephrotic patients have been reviewed.[1] The first principle of treatment is to consider disease-specific treatment directed at the primary disease process, as reviewed in other chapters of this textbook. Non-disease-specific treatment is aimed at reducing proteinuria, retarding progression of renal failure, and preventing complications of the nephrotic syndrome.

Because edema formation is the consequence of renal sodium retention, restriction of dietary salt intake should be recommended to all patients. A sodium intake of between 2 and 3 g (87 and 130 mmol) per day is generally a reasonable compromise between effectiveness and palatability. However, if tolerated sodium intake can be further restricted to 1.2 g (50 mmol) per day, especially in patients with severe edema.[61] Water restriction is only needed if the patient is hyponatremic with hypo-osmolality. This is observed infrequently in patients with a nephrotic syndrome, and mostly related to too intensive diuretic therapy. Diuretic agents are needed if edema persists despite salt restriction.

In the treatment of edema of the nephrotic syndrome loop diuretics such as furosemide and bumetanide are often preferred since quantitatively most sodium is reabsorbed in the thick ascending limb of the loop of Henle.[62,63] Few controlled studies have compared the efficacy of loop diuretics in the nephrotic syndrome. Lau demonstrated that bumetanide in a dose of 2 mg was more effective than 80 mg of furosemide.[63] This was attributed to a greater effect of bumetanide on proximal tubular sodium reabsorption. Although furosemide and bumetanide are effective in the nephrotic syndrome, resistance to loop diuretics often occurs.

Diuretic resistance has been attributed to several factors, including variable gastrointestinal absorption (bioavailability), impaired renal delivery, and tubular resistance. In normal subjects bioavailability of furosemide is quite variable and ranges from 10% to 100%.[64] The effect of the nephrotic syndrome on gastrointestinal absorption is debated. Prandota reported that absorption of an oral dose of 2 mg per kg of furosemide was significantly higher in nephrotic children than in control patients with urinary tract infection and mild hypertension.[65] Bioavailability in the nephrotic children averaged 58%. In another study in children, Engle demonstrated that an intravenous dose of 1 mg per kg furosemide was twice as effective as an oral dose of 2 mg per kg.[62] Thus, a low bioavailability could explain apparent resistance to seemingly adequate doses of furosemide. This can be overcome by increasing the oral dose, administering oral bumetanide or torsemide which are absorbed more predictably (80%–100%), or by intravenous administration of the diuretic.[64]

Loop diuretics are highly bound to albumin and it has been postulated that hypoalbuminemia may result in an impaired delivery of diuretics to the kidney and reduced tubular secretion. In analbuminemic rats there indeed is insufficient delivery of loop diuretics into the tubular fluid.[66] Data from more recent studies challenge the importance of hypoalbuminemia as a cause of decreased delivery of furosemide. Fliser et al. found no significant difference in urinary furosemide excretion in patients with nephrotic syndrome (mean serum albumin 3.0 g per dL) after 60 mg furosemide IV (34.9 ± 3.7 mg) compared to furosemide 60 mg plus 40 g human albumin IV (35.1 ± 4.2 mg).[67] Moreover, only a modest increase in sodium excretion was observed after furosemide plus human albumin (312 ± 28 mmol) compared to furosemide alone (259 ± 30 mmol). The increased natriuretic action appeared to be mainly mediated by changes in renal hemodynamics but not increased delivery of furosemide. Similarly, Agarwal et al. showed that ample furosemide reached the urine in patients with nephrotic syndrome.[68]

Akcicek et al. administered a maximal dose of furosemide (bolus of 60 mg followed by 40 mg per h) to eight severely nephrotic patients (serum albumin 1.1–2.2 g per dL).[69] Neither sodium excretion (934 ± 355 μmol per min) nor volume of urine (8.49 ± 2.9 mL per min) increased with coadministration of 0.5 g per kg albumin (respectively 884 ± 453 μmol per min and 9.21 ± 4.11 mL per min).

Davison et al. treated 12 nephrotic patients, referred for a diuretic-resistant state, with furosemide in increasing doses to 500 mg per day.[70] Spironolactone up to 200 mg per day was added if diuresis did not occur with furosemide. Nine of 12 patients had a creatinine clearance rate of less than 40 mL per minute. Six (50%) patients (median serum albumin 2.2 g per dL; range 1.3–2.3 g per dL) responded satisfactorily to increased diuretic therapy. However, in the remaining six patients (median serum albumin 1.7 g per dL; range 0.9–1.8 g per dL), diuresis either was unsuccessful (two patients) or resulted in serious complications, including increasing blood urea nitrogen in three patients and hyponatremia in one patient. In the six unresponsive patients, 300 mL of a 15% solution of salt-poor albumin led to a significant diuresis and resolution of edema without worsening renal function. Thus, furosemide with albumin may be especially useful in patients with minimal change disease and severe hypoalbuminemia (<2.0 g per dL) who appear volume depleted.[71,72]

Both studies in animals and humans have shown that there is tubular resistance to the effects of loop diuretics in nephrotic syndrome.[73] Nephrotic patients show a lesser natriuretic response to equivalent excretion rates of furosemide compared to normal controls.[74,75] The resistance to furosemide has initially been attributed to its binding to albumin within the tubular fluid rendering the diuretic inactive.[76] However, blocking of albumin binding to furosemide by the administration of sulfisoxazole had no effect on diuretic reponse.[68] Although definitive conclusions cannot be drawn since patients included in the study were not diuretic resistant, the results suggest that decreased tubular responsiveness to loop diuretics and/or increased sodium reabsorption at other tubular segments are more important causes of diuretic resistance. In PAN nephrotic rats loop chloride reabsorption as a percentage of delivered load was inhibited to a lesser extent (67.9 ± 4.7%) by IV furosemide compared to normal rats (48.3 ± 3.0%), suggesting that the loop of Henle may be relatively resistant to loop diuretics.[73] Alternatively, furosemide resistance might be due mainly to the increased potency of the cortical collecting duct to reabsorb an overload of sodium. A recent study by Deschenes et al. showed normal intrinsic sensitivity of the loop of Henle in PAN nephrotic rats.[47] In contrast, in vitro perfused CCD isolated from sodium-retaining PAN nephrotic rats exhibited an extremely high transepithelial sodium reabsorption.

In view of the experimental data demonstrating enhanced sodium reabsorption in the collecting tubules, potassium-sparing diuretics that act at this level (e.g., amiloride) would also be expected to be efficacious in treating nephrotic edema. Indeed in PAN nephrotic rats administration of amiloride increased sodium excretion, normalized sodium balance, and reduced ascitic volume.[54] Preliminary data from Deschenes et al. suggest that in nephrotic patients amiloride may have similar natriuretic effects as furosemide. In six nephrotic children treatment with amiloride resulted in a negative sodium balance of -33.8 ± 48.3 mmol/m^2/day.[47] The sodium balance was comparable to a group of seven nephrotic children treated with furosemide alone (-23.4 ± 29.9 mmol/m^2/day).[77]

The response to mineralocorticoid antagonists such as spironolactone varies. Spironolactone can induce a mild but significant natriuresis in nephrotic patients with an activated RAAS,[13,23] whereas its effect is absent in nephrotic patients with a normal plasma aldosterone.[23] Currently these data are not sufficient to advise monotherapy with amiloride or spironolactone.

Based on the pathophysiologic concepts, it seems plausible that in patients with severe nephrotic syndrome who do not respond satisfactorily to treatment with a loop diuretic addition of amiloride, spironolactone or a thiazide diuretic may be considered.[70,78] Based on experimental data amiloride would be the first choice if serum potassium is normal. Deschenes administered furosemide and amiloride to seven nephrotic children which resulted in a negative sodium balance of $-73.8\pm$ 55.4 mmol/m^2/day compared to $-23.4\pm$ 29.9 mmol/m^2/day ($P < .05$) in controls using only furosemide.[77] Further evidence is certainly needed.

In daily practice, diuretic therapy for nephrotic syndrome often can be instituted in the outpatient setting.[1] Patients should be instructed to weigh themselves daily and to diminish or discontinue the diuretic if weight loss exceeds 0.5 kg per day or when edema no longer becomes a source of discomfort. Patients should also reduce or discontinue the diuretic when orthostatic lightheadedness develops. An oral thiazide diuretic is a reasonable first choice in patients with mild edema and a normal GFR (>50 mL per min).[79] Loop diuretics are indicated in case of more severe edema or renal insufficiency. Because of the previously described resistance to loop diuretic action often higher doses are required to achieve effective renal sodium excretion. The absence of a significant diuresis following ingestion of a loop diuretic usually is an indication of low tubular diuretic concentrations. Increasing the dose is indicated. Loop diuretics have a rather short half-life, and the initial natriuresis may be counterbalanced by avid sodium retention during the rest of the day. Therefore, if weight loss is insufficient in patients who respond with initially appropriate diuresis, dosing twice daily will be more effective. The total daily dose may be as high as 500 to 1,000 mg for furosemide. If natriuretic response is insufficient, amiloride, spironolactone, or a thiazide can be added. It is important to realize that the simultaneous use of diuretics from different classes increases the risk of volume contraction and potassium disturbances. Patients who do not respond to oral treatment can benefit from intravenous administration of loop diuretics. Only if these regimens fail a trial of albumin and furosemide may be indicated, especially in patients with minimal change disease and severe hypoalbuminemia (<2.0 g per dL) who appear volume depleted.[71,72] However, this form of therapy remains relatively expensive, and the diuretic effects of albumin infusion are usually short-lived.[39] Hospitalization may be required to initiate and monitor diuresis especially in the latter patients with either severe edema or marked hypoalbuminemia, especially when a significant decrease in GFR is present.

OTHER COMPLICATIONS OF THE NEPHROTIC SYNDROME

In patients with a nephrotic syndrome urinary losses of albumin are not fully compensated by the increased hepatic production, with hypoalbuminemia and edema as a consequence.[80] Many other proteins beside albumin are lost in the urine in the nephrotic syndrome. Among these are hormones and hormone-binding proteins, immunoglobulins, and proteins involved in the coagulant system. As a consequence patients with a nephrotic syndrome may present with anemia, infections, thrombosis, hypothyroidism, and vitamin D deficiency (see Table 69.1). In addition, patients with a nephrotic syndrome are at increased risk of atherosclerotic vascular disease and progression to ESRD.

Hormonal Disturbances

Many hormones are large proteins or protein bound molecules, and increased losses may occur in patients with a nephrotic syndrome. Loss of albumin and thyroid-binding globulin may reduce the binding capacity for thyroid hormones, resulting in a decrease in total triiodothyronine (T3) and thyroxin (T4) concentrations. Furthermore, loss of thyroid hormones may lead to low free thyroid hormone levels unless production is increased under the influence of thyroid stimulating hormone (TSH).[81,82] Four studies including 49 patients documented urinary loss of thyroid hormones and thyroxin-binding globulin (TBG) in patients with proteinuria.[83–86] In one study overt hypothyroidism was noted in two patients that resolved after remission of the nephrotic syndrome.[33] In a study of 159 patients with proteinuria TSH concentration was significantly higher compared to controls, and negatively correlated with serum albumin.[82] Although subclinical hypothyroidism was more frequent in the patients (11.3% vs. 1.8%), overt hypothyroidism was seen in only one patient. The relevance of subclinical hypothyroidism needs further evaluation; however, special attention is needed in pregnant women with a nephrotic syndrome.

Anemia is often observed in the nephrotic syndrome, and may be related to urinary loss of transferrin. Low serum transferrin levels can reduce serum iron concentrations and occasionally cause microcytic anemia.[87] Because transferrin transports iron to erythroid cells, severe hypotransferrinemia per se can also cause microcytic anemia in the absence of iron store depletion.[88] Supplementation of iron is often not effective. Indeed in a study in six nephrotic children treatment with oral or IV iron did not increase hemoglobin (Hb) levels.[89] Moreover, breakdown of reabsorbed transferrin can liberate iron in renal tubules, which could play a role in the nephrotoxic effects of proteinuria.[90] Thus supplemental iron may not be without risk and should not be undertaken without clear evidence of iron deficiency.

Urinary loss of erythropoietin (EPO) may also contribute to anemia in patients with a nephrotic syndrome. Erythropoietin is lost in the urine of nephrotic patients, but synthesis is not increased.[88] Administration of EPO has been successfully used in nephrotic patients, with normal renal function and repleted iron and vitamin B12 stores, resulting in a significant increase in hemoglobin levels.[89,91]

Serum levels of 25-hydroxyvitamin D, a precursor of active vitamin D (calcitriol), are reduced in the nephrotic syndrome because of urinary loss of vitamin D binding protein.[92,93] Low levels of free serum calcitriol have also been reported resulting in hypocalcemia (low ionized serum calcium or low total serum calcium corrected for albumin concentration).[94–96]

If left untreated, these metabolic disturbances can lead to secondary hyperparathyroidism and bone lesions, such as osteomalacia and osteitis fibrosa.[96] Unfortunately, there are little data available to guide treatment. In patients with nephrotic syndrome and normal renal function, daily treatment with 1,000 IU vitamin D (cholecalciferol or ergocalciferol) seems reasonable if 25-hydroxyvitamin D deficiency causes low ionized or corrected total serum calcium levels. Depending on the response, higher doses may be necessary.

Thromboembolism

Patients with a nephrotic syndrome are at increased risk for venous and arterial thrombosis. Older studies reported an overall incidence of renal vein thrombosis of 2% to 42%, of venous thrombosis 8% to 42%, of pulmonary embolism 9% to 21%, and of arterial thrombosis 4%.[97–99] Sometimes the thrombotic event is the presenting event. The increased risk of thrombosis is attributed to variable urinary losses and hepatic production of anticoagulant and procoagulant factors. In patients with a nephrotic syndrome increased concentrations of fibrinogen, factor VIII, and plasminogen activator inhibitor-1, and decreased levels of antithrombin III, plasminogen, and free protein-S have been reported.[100] This imbalance of the coagulation cascade results in a prothrombotic state. The risk of thrombosis is dependent on serum albumin levels. Two studies reported serum albumin levels of 1.5 ± .3 and 2.2 ± .6 g per dL in patients with and 2.6 ± .5 and 2.8 ± .9 g per dL in patients without thrombosis.[101,102] The majority of patients with thrombosis had serum albumin levels below 2.5 g per dL. Risk of thrombosis not only depends on serum albumin level but also on the underlying glomerular disease. Sarasin showed a two- to threefold increased risk of thrombosis in patients with idiopathic membranous nephropathy.[103] This was confirmed in a study in children.[104] The question of prophylactic anticoagulation has not been answered by prospective randomized trials. Most authors agree that patients with a membranous nephropathy and a serum albumin levels below 2.0 g per dL are at highest risk and should be considered for prophylactic anticoagulant therapy. Obviously, anticoagulation is needed in patients with risk factors for venous thromboembolism (VTE), which include a history of VTE, prolonged immobilization, congestive heart failure, morbid obesity, and abdominal, orthopedic, or gynecologic surgery.[105]

A recent retrospective study reported a high incidence rate in the first 6 months after onset of the nephrotic syndrome.[97] The incidence rate was 9.85% for VTE and 5.52% for arterial thromboembolism (ATE), a risk 140 times and 50 times higher than in the general population. In this study, neither proteinuria nor serum albumin, but rather the ratio of proteinuria to serum albumin predicted VTE. Of note, neither proteinuria nor albumin were associated with ATE, in contrast to eGFR, and known cardiovascular risk factors. This study confirmed the high risk of pulmonary embolism (PE), which exceeded the risk of deep vein thrombosis (DVT; ratio 1.3:1), whereas in the normal population the ratio PE:DVT = 1:2. The high incidence of PE is attributed to the presence of silent renal vein thrombosis in the nephrotic syndrome. The incidence of VTE and ATE decreased to values of 1% per year during follow-up. It is unclear if this reflects the true natural history, or is the mere consequence of the treatment of the nephrotic syndrome with the associated improvement in proteinuria.

Infections

Patients with a nephrotic syndrome not only develop hypoalbuminemia, but frequently also have hypogammaglobulinemia. Patients with a nephrotic syndrome are at risk for infections, notably pneumonia and peritonitis caused by encapsulated bacteria such as *Streptococcus* and *Haemophilus*. Infections were the main cause of death in children with a nephrotic syndrome before the introduction of antibiotics and prednisone. One study reported that infections in patients with proteinuria were independently associated with low serum immunoglobulin G (IgG) levels (<600 mg per dL).[106] Administration of IgG resulted in a decreased rate of bacterial infections to a level equal to that in patients with endogenous levels over 600 mg per dL.

Cardiovascular Disease and Progressive Renal Failure

An abnormal lipid metabolism is almost always present in patients with nephrotic syndrome. Both increased hepatic production of lipoproteins and decreased lipid catabolism play a role. Most prominent are an increased low-density lipoprotein (LDL) cholesterol level, hypertriglyceridemia, and an increased lipoprotein (a) [Lp(a)] level.[107,108]

The increase in Lp(a) is explained by an increased rate of synthesis.[109] The increase in LDL cholesterol appears to be partly mediated by a reduced hepatic cholesterol uptake due to an acquired LDL-receptor deficiency.[110] Studies in experimental animals point to an inefficient translation and/or increased LDL-receptor turnover as a cause for LDL-receptor deficiency.[111,112] Intracellular free cholesterol is further reduced by an increase in liver-specific acylcoenzyme A:cholesterol acyltransferase-2 (ACAT-2), the enzyme responsible for esterification of cholesterol in hepatocytes.[112,113] The reduction in hepatocellular free cholesterol can lead to upregulation of 3-hydroxy-3-methylglutaryl-coenzyme A (HMG-CoA) reductase, the rate limiting enzyme involved in synthesis of cholesterol.[114] These mechanisms all lead to increased LDL cholesterol levels. Despite the severe hypercholesterolemia in nephrotic syndrome, cholesterol 7-hydroxylase, which is the rate-limiting step in cholesterol conversion to bile acid, remains unchanged.[115]

Hypertriglyceridemia is the consequence of the inability to clear triglyceride-rich lipoproteins (VLDL, chylomicrons, and remnant particles). Several factors contribute to reduced clearance of lipoproteins in the nephrotic syndrome. Hypoalbuminemia leads to reduced amounts of endothelial bound lipoprotein lipase (LPL), resulting in decreased clearance of lipoproteins.[116] However this defect only leads to a mild increase in triglycerides.[117] More important is a deficiency in apolipoprotein (apo) E content of lipoproteins that decreases their ability to bind to LPL.[118] Shearer et al. demonstrated that binding of VLDL from nephrotic rats to endothelial cells is markedly reduced compared to controls, whereas binding of VLDL from rats with hereditary analbuminemia is increased compared to controls.[119] They also noted that HDL of nephrotic rats was deficient in apo E compared to analbuminemic and control rats. Since lipoproteins acquire apo E from HDL, the decreased clearance of lipoproteins may be caused by a reduced apo E content of nephrotic HDL.[110] Indeed, the defective binding of nephrotic VLDL was reversed by preincubation of nephrotic VLDL with HDL from either normal or analbuminemic rats but not by preincubation with nephrotic HDL.[119]

The combination of increased LDL-cholesterol, triglycerides, and Lp(a) is highly atherogenic and carries a five- to sixfold increased risk for myocardial infarction and a two- to threefold increased risk of coronary death compared to age- and sex-matched controls.[120] Lipid-lowering treatment, preferably with HMG-CoA reductase inhibitors, is indicated if proteinuria is expected to persist for at least several months or renal insufficiency is present.[121,122] In addition, reduction in protein excretion with angiotensin-converting enzyme (ACE) inhibitors or angiotensin receptor blockers (ARBs) results in a significant decline in LDL cholesterol and lipoprotein(a).[123] Although dietary restriction of cholesterol and saturated fat is advised, it is generally of limited value.

Proteinuria is an important risk factor and the best predictor of progression to ESRD in nephrotic syndrome.[124,125] Reducing proteinuria can prevent progression to renal failure and improve complications associated with nephrotic syndrome, such as hypoalbuminemia, hyperlipidemia, and edema. Strict blood pressure control is the most important measure to reduce proteinuria.[124] ACE inhibitors or, in case of side effects, ARBs are the preferred agents, as they reduce proteinuria and slow progression of kidney disease more effectively than other antihypertensive agents.[126–128] ACE inhibitors and ARBs act by reducing the intraglomerular pressure and by improving the size-selective properties of the glomerular capillary wall, both of which contribute to reducing protein excretion. ACE inhibitors and ARBs should not be started at the same time as the loop diuretic, because the combined effects of intravascular volume depletion and impairment of autoregulation increase the risk of acute renal failure. Low-dose ACE inhibitors and ARBs can be introduced once a stable dose of the loop diuretic is reached and slowly titrated upwards. Target blood pressures are $\leq$125/75 mm Hg in patients with proteinuria $\geq$1 g per day and $\leq$130/80 mm Hg if proteinuria falls below $<$1 g per day.[129] Proteinuria should be reduced to 0.5 g per day, although this target often is difficult to reach in patients with nephrotic syndrome.[130]

Dietary Protein

A high dietary protein intake should be avoided in patients with nephrotic syndrome because this can increase the rate of protein catabolism and urine protein excretion.[131] In contrast, protein restriction has been shown to slow renal function deterioration in patients with diabetic and nondiabetic renal diseases.[132] However, the optimal level of protein intake is unclear, and care must be taken to avoid malnutrition. Therefore, in patients with nephrotic syndrome a moderate protein restriction of 0.8 to 1 g per kg body weight per day plus urinary protein loss is advised while maintaining a normal caloric intake (35 kcal per kg per day).[133]

REFERENCES

1. Deegens JK, Wetzels J. Nephrotic range proteinuria. In: Daugirdas J, ed. *Handbook of Chronic Kidney Disease Management*. Philadelphia, Lippincott Williams & Wilkins; 2011.
2. Deegens JK, Dijkman HB, Borm GF, et al. Podocyte foot process effacement as a diagnostic tool in focal segmental glomerulosclerosis. *Kidney Int.* 2008;74:1568–1576.
3. Dorhout Mees EJ, Koomans HA. Understanding the nephrotic syndrome: what's new in a decade? *Nephron.* 1995;70:1–10.
4. Koomans HA, Kortlandt W, Geers AB, et al. Lowered protein content of tissue fluid in patients with the nephrotic syndrome: observations during disease and recovery. *Nephron.* 1985;40:391–395.
5. Bichet DG, Van Putten V, Schrier RW. Potential role of increased sympathetic activity in impaired sodium and water excretion in cirrhosis. *N Engl J Med.* 1982;307:1552–1557.
6. Warren JV, Merrill AJ, Stead EA. The role of the extracellular fluid in the maintenance of a normal plasma volume. *J Clin Invest.* 1943;22:635–641.
7. Van de Walle JG, Donckerwolcke RA, Greidanus TB, et al. Renal sodium handling in children with nephrotic relapse: relation to hypovolaemic symptoms. *Nephrol Dial Transplant.* 1996;11:2202–2208.
8. Oliver WJ, Owings CL. Sodium excretion in the nephrotic syndrome. Relation to serum albumin concentration, glomerular filtration rate, and aldosterone excretion rate. *Am J Dis Child.* 1967;113:352–362.
9. Kelsch RC, Light GS, Oliver WJ. The effect of albumin infusion upon plasma norepinephrine concentration in nephrotic children. *J Lab Clin Med.* 1972;79:516–525.
10. Gur A, Adefuin PY, Siegel NJ, et al. A study of the renal handling of water in lipoid nephrosis. *Pediatr Res.* 1976;10:197–201.
11. Yamauchi H, Hopper JJ. Hypovolemic shock and hypotension as a complication in the nephrotic syndrome. Report of ten cases. *Ann Intern Med.* 1964;60:242–254.
12. Kumagai H, Onoyama K, Iseki K, et al. Role of renin angiotensin aldosterone on minimal change nephrotic syndrome. *Clin Nephrol.* 1985;23: 229–235.
13. Shapiro MD, Hasbargen J, Hensen J, et al. Role of aldosterone in the sodium retention of patients with nephrotic syndrome. *Am J Nephrol.* 1990;10: 44–48.
14. Usberti M, Federico S, Meccariello S, et al. Role of plasma vasopressin in the impairment of water excretion in nephrotic syndrome. *Kidney Int.* 1984;25:422–429.
15. Berlyne GM, Sutton J, Brown C, et al. Renal salt and water handling in water immersion in the nephrotic syndrome. *Clin Sci (Lond).* 1981;61:605–610.
16. Krishna GG, Danovitch GM. Effects of water immersion on renal function in the nephrotic syndrome. *Kidney Int.* 1982;21:395–401.
17. Karnad DR, Tembulkar P, Abraham P, et al. Head-down tilt as a physiological diuretic in normal controls and in patients with fluid-retaining states. *Lancet.* 1987;2:525–528.
18. Rahman SN, Abraham WT, Van Putten V, et al. Increased norepinephrine secretion in patients with the nephrotic syndrome and normal glomerular filtration rates: evidence for primary sympathetic activation. *Am J Nephrol.* 1993;13:266–270.
19. Dorhout EJ, Roos JC, Boer P, et al. Observations on edema formation in the nephrotic syndrome in adults with minimal lesions. *Am J Med.* 1979;67: 378–384.
20. Geers AB, Koomans HA, Boer P, et al. Plasma and blood volumes in patients with the nephrotic syndrome. *Nephron.* 1984;38:170–173.
21. Geers AB, Koomans HA, Roos JC, et al. Functional relationships in the nephrotic syndrome. *Kidney Int.* 1984;26:324–330.
22. Plum J, Mirzaian Y, Grabensee B. Atrial natriuretic peptide, sodium retention, and proteinuria in nephrotic syndrome. *Nephrol Dial Transplant.* 1996;11: 1034–1042.

23. Usberti M, Gazzotti RM. Hyporeninemic hypoaldosteronism in patients with nephrotic syndrome. *Am J Nephrol.* 1998;18:251–255.

24. Brown EA, Markandu ND, Roulston JE, et al. Is the renin-angiotensin-aldosterone system involved in the sodium retention in the nephrotic syndrome? *Nephron.* 1982;32:102–107.

25. Dusing R, Vetter H, Kramer HJ. The renin-angiotensin-aldosterone system in patients with nephrotic syndrome: effects of 1–sar-8–ala-angiotensin II. *Nephron.* 1980;25:187–192.

26. Brown EA, Markandu ND, Sagnella GA, et al. Lack of effect of captopril on the sodium retention of the nephrotic syndrome. *Nephron.* 1984;37:43–48.

27. Brown EA, Markandu ND, Sagnella GA, et al. Evidence that some mechanism other than the renin system causes sodium retention in nephrotic syndrome. *Lancet.* 1982;2:1237–1240.

28. Usberti M, Federico S, Cianciaruso B, et al. Relationship between serum albumin concentration and tubular reabsorption of glucose in renal disease. *Kidney Int.* 1979;16:546–551.

29. Grausz H, Lieberman R, Earley LE. Effect of plasma albumin on sodium reabsorption in patients with nephrotic syndrome. *Kidney Int.* 1972;1:47–54.

30. Brown EA, Markandu N, Sagnella GA, et al. Sodium retention in nephrotic syndrome is due to an intrarenal defect: evidence from steroid-induced remission. *Nephron.* 1985;39:290–295.

31. Koomans HA, Boer WH, Dorhout Mees EJ. Renal function during recovery from minimal lesions nephrotic syndrome. *Nephron.* 1987;47:173–178.

32. Fawcett J, Wynn V. Effects of posture on plasma volume and some blood constituents. *J Clin Pathol.* 1960;13:304–310.

33. Eisenberg S. Postural changes in plasma volume in hypoalbuminemia. *Arch Intern Med.* 1963;112:544–549.

34. Geers AB, Koomans HA, Dorhout Mees EJ. Effect of changes in posture on circulatory homeostasis in patients with the nephrotic syndrome. *Clin Physiol.* 1986;6:63–75.

35. Minutolo R, Andreucci M, Balletta MM, et al. Effect of posture on sodium excretion and diuretic efficacy in nephrotic patients. *Am J Kidney Dis.* 2000;36:719–727.

36. Usberti M, Gazzotti RM, Poiesi C, et al. Considerations on the sodium retention in nephrotic syndrome. *Am J Nephrol.* 1995;15:38–47.

37. Meltzer JI, Keim HJ, Laragh JH, et al. Nephrotic syndrome: vasoconstriction and hypervolemic types indicated by renin-sodium profiling. *Ann Intern Med.* 1979;91:688–696.

38. Schrier RW, Fassett RG: A critique of the overfill hypothesis of sodium and water retention in the nephrotic syndrome. *Kidney Int.* 1998;53:1111–1117.

39. Koomans HA, Geers AB, Meiracker AH, et al. Effects of plasma volume expansion on renal salt handling in patients with the nephrotic syndrome. *Am J Nephrol.* 1984;4:227–234.

40. Jespersen B, Eiskjaer H, Mogensen CE, et al. Reduced natriuretic effect of atrial natriuretic peptide in nephrotic syndrome: a possible role of decreased cyclic guanosine monophosphate. *Nephron.* 1995;71:44–53.

41. Kalant N, Gupta D, Despointes R, et al. Mechanisms of edema formation in experimental nephrosis. *Am J Physiol.* 1962;202:91–96.

42. DiBona GF, Herman PJ, Sawin LL. Neural control of renal function in edema-forming states. *Am J Physiol.* 1988;254:R1017–R1024.

43. Herman PJ, Sawin LL, DiBona GF. Role of renal nerves in renal sodium retention of nephrotic syndrome. *Am J Physiol.* 1989;256:F823–F829.

44. Kuroda S, Aynedjian HS, Bank N. A micropuncture study of renal sodium retention in nephrotic syndrome in rats: evidence for increased resistance to tubular fluid flow. *Kidney Int.* 1979;16:561–571.

45. Deschenes G, Doucet A. Collecting duct (Na+/K+)-ATPase activity is correlated with urinary sodium excretion in rat nephrotic syndromes. *J Am Soc Nephrol.* 2000;11:604–615.

46. Lourdel S, Loffing J, Favre G, et al. Hyperaldosteronemia and activation of the epithelial sodium channel are not required for sodium retention in puromycin-induced nephrosis. *J Am Soc Nephrol.* 2005;16:3642–3650.

47. Deschenes G, Wittner M, Stefano A, et al. Collecting duct is a site of sodium retention in PAN nephrosis: a rationale for amiloride therapy. *J Am Soc Nephrol.* 2001;12:598–601.

48. Doucet A, Favre G, Deschenes G. Molecular mechanism of edema formation in nephrotic syndrome: therapeutic implications. *Pediatr Nephrol.* 2007;22:1983–1990.

49. Artunc F, Nasir O, Amann K, et al. Serum- and glucocorticoid-inducible kinase 1 in doxorubicin-induced nephrotic syndrome. *Am J Physiol Renal Physiol.* 2008;295:F1624–F1634.

50. Bernard DB, Alexander EA, Couser WG, et al. Renal sodium retention during volume expansion in experimental nephrotic syndrome. *Kidney Int.* 1978;14:478–485.

51. Ichikawa I, Rennke HG, Hoyer JR, et al. Role for intrarenal mechanisms in the impaired salt excretion of experimental nephrotic syndrome. *J Clin Invest.* 1983;71:91–103.

52. Kastner C, Pohl M, Sendeski M, et al. Effects of receptor-mediated endocytosis and tubular protein composition on volume retention in experimental glomerulonephritis. *Am J Physiol Renal Physiol.* 2009;296:F902–F911.

53. Gadau J, Peters H, Kastner C, et al. Mechanisms of tubular volume retention in immune-mediated glomerulonephritis. *Kidney Int.* 2009;75:699–710.

54. Svenningsen P, Bistrup C, Friis UG, et al. Plasmin in nephrotic urine activates the epithelial sodium channel. *J Am Soc Nephrol.* 2009;20:299–310.

55. Svenningsen P, Uhrenholt TR, Palarasah Y, et al. Prostasin-dependent activation of epithelial Na+ channels by low plasmin concentrations. *Am J Physiol Regul Integr Comp Physiol.* 2009;297:R1733–R1741.

56. Perico N, Delaini F, Lupini C, et al. Renal response to atrial peptides is reduced in experimental nephrosis. *Am J Physiol.* 1987;252:F654–F660.

57. Perico N, Remuzzi G: Renal handling of sodium in the nephrotic syndrome. *Am J Nephrol.* 1993;13:413–421.

58. Valentin JP, Qiu C, Muldowney WP, et al. Cellular basis for blunted volume expansion natriuresis in experimental nephrotic syndrome. *J Clin Invest.* 1992;90:1302–1312.

59. Valentin JP, Ying WZ, Sechi LA, et al. Phosphodiesterase inhibitors correct resistance to natriuretic peptides in rats with Heymann nephritis. *J Am Soc Nephrol.* 1996;7:582–593.

60. Polzin D, Kaminski HJ, Kastner C, et al. Decreased renal corin expression contributes to sodium retention in proteinuric kidney diseases. *Kidney Int.* 2010;78:650–659.

61. Orth SR, Ritz E: The nephrotic syndrome. *N Engl J Med.* 1998;338: 1202–1211.

62. Engle MA, Lewy JE, Lewy PR, et al. The use of furosemide in the treatment of edema in infants and children. *Pediatrics.* 1978;62:811–818.

63. Lau K, DeFronzo R, Morrison G, et al. Effectiveness of bumetanide in nephrotic syndrome: a double-blind crossover study with furosemide. *J Clin Pharmacol.* 1976;16:489–497.

64. Brater DC. Diuretic therapy. *N Engl J Med.* 1998;339:387–395.

65. Prandota J. Pharmacokinetics of furosemide urinary elimination by nephrotic children. *Pediatr Res.* 1983;17:141–147.

66. Inoue M, Okajima K, Itoh K, et al. Mechanism of furosemide resistance in analbuminemic rats and hypoalbuminemic patients. *Kidney Int.* 1987;32: 198–203.

67. Fliser D, Zurbruggen I, Mutschler E, et al. Coadministration of albumin and furosemide in patients with the nephrotic syndrome. *Kidney Int.* 1999;55:629–634.

68. Agarwal R, Gorski JC, Sundblad K, et al. Urinary protein binding does not affect response to furosemide in patients with nephrotic syndrome. *J Am Soc Nephrol.* 2000;11:1100–1105.

69. Akcicek F, Yalniz T, Basci A, et al. Diuretic effect of frusemide in patients with nephrotic syndrome: is it potentiated by intravenous albumin? *BMJ.* 1995;310:162–163.

70. Davison AM, Lambie AT, Verth AH, et al. Salt-poor human albumin in management of nephrotic syndrome. *Br Med J.* 1974;1:481–484.

71. Bircan Z, Kervancioglu M, Katar S, et al. Does albumin and furosemide therapy affect plasma volume in nephrotic children? *Pediatr Nephrol.* 2001;16:497–499.

72. Shankar SS, Brater DC. Loop diuretics: from the Na-K-2Cl transporter to clinical use. *Am J Physiol Renal Physiol.* 2003;284:F11–F21.

73. Kirchner KA, Voelker JR, Brater DC. Tubular resistance to furosemide contributes to the attenuated diuretic response in nephrotic rats. *J Am Soc Nephrol.* 1992;2:1201–1207.

74. Smith DE, Hyneck ML, Berardi RR, et al. Urinary protein binding, kinetics, and dynamics of furosemide in nephrotic patients. *J Pharm Sci.* 1985;74: 603–607.

75. Keller E, Hoppe-Seyler G, Schollmeyer P. Disposition and diuretic effect of furosemide in the nephrotic syndrome. *Clin Pharmacol Ther.* 1982;32: 442–449.

76. Kirchner KA, Voelker JR, Brater DC. Binding inhibitors restore furosemide potency in tubule fluid containing albumin. *Kidney Int.* 1991;40:418–424.

77. Deschenes G, Guigonis V, Doucet A. [Molecular mechanism of edema formation in nephrotic syndrome]. *Arch Pediatr.* 2004;11:1084–1094.

78. Tanaka M, Oida E, Nomura K, et al. The Na+-excreting efficacy of indapamide in combination with furosemide in massive edema. *Clin Exp Nephrol.* 2005;9:122–126.

79. Glassock RJ. Symptomatic therapy. In Ponticelli C, Glassock RJ, Eds. Treatment of primary glomerulonephritis, 2nd ed., Oxford, Oxford University Press, 2009, pp 1–46.

80. Kaysen GA, Gambertoglio J, Felts J, et al. Albumin synthesis, albuminuria and hyperlipemia in nephrotic patients. *Kidney Int.* 1987;31:1368–1376.
81. Ito S, Kano K, Ando T, et al. Thyroid function in children with nephrotic syndrome. *Pediatr Nephrol.* 1994;8:412–415.
82. Gilles R, den Heijer M., Ross AH, et al. Thyroid function in patients with proteinuria. *Neth J Med.* 2008;66:483–485.
83. Adlkofer F, Hain H, Meinhold H, et al. Thyroid function in patients with proteinuria and normal or increased serum creatinine concentration. *Acta Endocrinol(Copenh).* 1983;102:367–376.
84. Afrasiabi MA, Vaziri ND, Gwinup G, et al. Thyroid function studies in the nephrotic syndrome. *Ann Intern Med.* 1979;90:335–338.
85. Fonseca V, Thomas M, Katrak A, et al. Can urinary thyroid hormone loss cause hypothyroidism? *Lancet.* 1991;338:475–476.
86. Liappis N, Rao GS. [Behavior of the levels of free triiodothyronine, triiodothyronine, free thyroxine, thyroxine, thyrotropin and thyroxine-binding globulin in the serum of children with nephrotic syndrome]. *Klin Padiatr.* 1985;197: 423–426.
87. Hancock DE, Onstad JW, Wolf PL. Transferrin loss into the urine with hypochromic, microcytic anemia. *Am J Clin Pathol.* 1976;65:73–78.
88. Vaziri ND, Kaupke CJ, Barton CH, et al. Plasma concentration and urinary excretion of erythropoietin in adult nephrotic syndrome. *Am J Med.* 1992;92:35–40.
89. Feinstein S, Becker-Cohen R, Algur N, et al. Erythropoietin deficiency causes anemia in nephrotic children with normal kidney function. *Am J Kidney Dis.* 2001;37:736–742.
90. Cooper MA, Buddington B, Miller NL, et al. Urinary iron speciation in nephrotic syndrome. *Am J Kidney Dis.* 1995;25:314–319.
91. Gansevoort RT, Vaziri ND, de Jong PE. Treatment of anemia of nephrotic syndrome with recombinant erythropoietin. *Am J Kidney Dis.* 1996;28:274–277.
92. Haddad JG Jr, Walgate J. Radioimmunoassay of the binding protein for vitamin D and its metabolites in human serum: concentrations in normal subjects and patients with disorders of mineral homeostasis. *J Clin Invest.* 1976;58: 1217–1222.
93. Barragry JM, France MW, Carter ND, et al. Vitamin-D metabolism in nephrotic syndrome. *Lancet.* 1977;2:629–632.
94. van Hoof HJ, de Sevaux RG, van Baelen H., et al. Relationship between free and total 1,25–dihydroxyvitamin D in conditions of modified binding. *Eur J Endocrinol.* 2001;144:391–396.
95. Goldstein DA, Haldimann B, Sherman D, et al. Vitamin D metabolites and calcium metabolism in patients with nephrotic syndrome and normal renal function. *J Clin Endocrinol Metab.* 1981;52:116–121.
96. Malluche HH, Goldstein DA, Massry SG. Osteomalacia and hyperparathyroid bone disease in patients with nephrotic syndrome. *J Clin Invest.* 1979;63:494–500.
97. Mahmoodi BK, ten Kate MK, Waanders F, et al. High absolute risks and predictors of venous and arterial thromboembolic events in patients with nephrotic syndrome: results from a large retrospective cohort study. *Circulation.* 2008;117:224–230.
98. Llach F. Hypercoagulability, renal vein thrombosis, and other thrombotic complications of nephrotic syndrome. *Kidney Int.* 1985;28:429–439.
99. Rostoker G, Durand-Zaleski I, Petit-Phar M, et al. Prevention of thrombotic complications of the nephrotic syndrome by the low-molecular-weight heparin enoxaparin. *Nephron.* 1995;69:20–28.
100. Singhal R, Brimble KS. Thromboembolic complications in the nephrotic syndrome: pathophysiology and clinical management. *Thromb Res.* 2006;118: 397–407.
101. Kuhlmann U, Steurer J, Bollinger A, et al. [Incidence and clinical significance of thromboses and thrombo-embolic complications in nephrotic syndrome patients]. *Schweiz Med Wochenschr.* 1981;111:1034–1040.
102. Bellomo R, Atkins RC. Membranous nephropathy and thromboembolism: is prophylactic anticoagulation warranted? *Nephron.* 1993;63:249–254.
103. Sarasin FP, Schifferli JA. Prophylactic oral anticoagulation in nephrotic patients with idiopathic membranous nephropathy. *Kidney Int.* 1994;45:578–585.
104. Kerlin BA, Blatt NB, Fuh B, et al. Epidemiology and risk factors for thromboembolic complications of childhood nephrotic syndrome: a Midwest Pediatric Nephrology Consortium (MWPNC) study. *J Pediatr.* 2009;155:105–110.
105. Glassock RJ. Prophylactic anticoagulation in nephrotic syndrome: a clinical conundrum. *J Am Soc Nephrol.* 2007;18:2221–2225.
106. Ogi M, Yokoyama H, Tomosugi N, et al. Risk factors for infection and immunoglobulin replacement therapy in adult nephrotic syndrome. *Am J Kidney Dis.* 1994;24:427–436.
107. Joven J, Villabona C, Vilella E, et al. Abnormalities of lipoprotein metabolism in patients with the nephrotic syndrome. *N Engl J Med.* 1990;323:579–584.
108. Wanner C, Rader D, Bartens W, et al. Elevated plasma lipoprotein(a) in patients with the nephrotic syndrome. *Ann Intern Med.* 1993;119:263–269.
109. de Sain-van der Velden MG, Kaysen GA, Barrett HA, et al. Increased VLDL in nephrotic patients results from a decreased catabolism while increased LDL results from increased synthesis. *Kidney Int.* 1998;53:994–1001.
110. Vaziri ND. Molecular mechanisms of lipid disorders in nephrotic syndrome. *Kidney Int.* 2003;63:1964–1976.
111. Vaziri ND, Liang KH. Down-regulation of hepatic LDL receptor expression in experimental nephrosis. *Kidney Int.* 1996;50:887–893.
112. Vaziri ND, Sato T, Liang K. Molecular mechanisms of altered cholesterol metabolism in rats with spontaneous focal glomerulosclerosis. *Kidney Int.* 2003;63:1756–1763.
113. Vaziri ND, Liang K. Up-regulation of acyl-coenzyme A:cholesterol acyltransferase (ACAT) in nephrotic syndrome. *Kidney Int.* 2002;61:1769–1775.
114. Vaziri ND, Liang KH. Hepatic HMG-CoA reductase gene expression during the course of puromycin-induced nephrosis. *Kidney Int.* 1995;48:1979–1985.
115. Liang KH, Oveisi F, Vaziri ND. Gene expression of hepatic cholesterol 7 alpha-hydroxylase in the course of puromycin-induced nephrosis. *Kidney Int.* 1996;49:855–860.
116. Yamada M, Matsuda I. Lipoprotein lipase in clinical and experimental nephrosis. *Clin Chim Acta.* 1970; 30:787–794.
117. Davies RW, Staprans I, Hutchison FN, et al. Proteinuria, not altered albumin metabolism, affects hyperlipidemia in the nephrotic rat. *J Clin Invest.* 1990;86:600–605.
118. Shearer GC, Couser WG, Kaysen GA. Endothelial chylomicron binding is altered by interaction with high-density lipoprotein in Heymann's nephritis. *Am J Kidney Dis.* 2001;38:1385–1389.
119. Shearer GC, Stevenson FT, Atkinson DN, et al. Hypoalbuminemia and proteinuria contribute separately to reduced lipoprotein catabolism in the nephrotic syndrome. *Kidney Int.* 2001;59:179–189.
120. Ordonez JD, Hiatt RA, Killebrew EJ, et al. The increased risk of coronary heart disease associated with nephrotic syndrome. *Kidney Int.* 1993;44: 638–642.
121. Tokoo M, Oguchi H, Terashima M, et al. Effects of pravastatin on serum lipids and apolipoproteins in hyperlipidemia of the nephrotic syndrome. *Nippon Jinzo Gakkai Shi.* 1992;34:397–403.
122. Sharp Collaborative Group: Study of Heart and Renal Protection (SHARP): randomized trial to assess the effects of lowering low-density lipoprotein cholesterol among 9,438 patients with chronic kidney disease. *Am Heart J.* 2010;160:785–794.
123. Keilani T, Schlueter WA, Levin ML, et al. Improvement of lipid abnormalities associated with proteinuria using fosinopril, an angiotensin-converting enzyme inhibitor. *Ann Intern Med.* 1993;118:246–254.
124. Peterson JC, Adler S, Burkart JM, et al. Blood pressure control, proteinuria, and the progression of renal disease. The Modification of Diet in Renal Disease Study. *Ann Intern Med.* 1995;123:754–762.
125. Ruggenenti P, Perna A, Mosconi L, et al. Urinary protein excretion rate is the best independent predictor of ESRF in non-diabetic proteinuric chronic nephropathies. "Gruppo Italiano di Studi Epidemiologici in Nefrologia" (GISEN). *Kidney Int.* 1998;53:1209–1216.
126. Randomised placebo-controlled trial of effect of ramipril on decline in glomerular filtration rate and risk of terminal renal failure in proteinuric, non-diabetic nephropathy. The GISEN Group (Gruppo Italiano di Studi Epidemiologici in Nefrologia). *Lancet.* 1997;349:1857–1863.
127. Maschio G, Alberti D, Janin G, et al. Effect of the angiotensin-converting-enzyme inhibitor benazepril on the progression of chronic renal insufficiency. The Angiotensin-Converting-Enzyme Inhibition in Progressive Renal Insufficiency Study Group. *N Engl J Med.* 1996;334:939–945.
128. Kunz R, Friedrich C, Wolbers M, et al. Meta-analysis: effect of monotherapy and combination therapy with inhibitors of the renin angiotensin system on proteinuria in renal disease. *Ann Intern Med.* 2008;148:30–48.
129. Jafar T, Stark P, Schmid C, et al. Progression of chronic kidney disease: the role of blood pressure control, proteinuria, and angiotensin-converting enzyme inhibition: a patient-level meta-analysis. *Ann Intern Med.* 2003;139:244–252.
130. Praga M, Hernandez E, Montoyo C, et al. Long-term beneficial effects of angiotensin-converting enzyme inhibition in patients with nephrotic proteinuria. *Am J Kidney Dis.* 1992;20:240–248.
131. Kaysen GA, Webster S, Al-Bander H, et al. High-protein diets augment albuminuria in rats with Heymann nephritis by angiotensin II-dependent and -independent mechanisms. *Miner Electrolyte Metab.* 1998;24:238–245.
132. Kasiske BL, Lakatua JD, Ma JZ, et al. A meta-analysis of the effects of dietary protein restriction on the rate of decline in renal function. *Am J Kidney Dis.* 1998;31:954–961.
133. Maroni BJ, Staffeld C, Young VR, et al. Mechanisms permitting nephrotic patients to achieve nitrogen equilibrium with a protein-restricted diet. *J Clin Invest.* 1997;99:2479–2487.

CHAPTER

70 The Syndrome of Inappropriate Antidiuretic Hormone Secretion and Other Hypoosmolar Disorders

Joseph G. Verbalis

The syndrome of inappropriate antidiuretic hormone secretion (SIADH) is produced when plasma levels of arginine vasopressin (AVP), the only known antidiuretic hormone (ADH), are elevated at times when physiologic AVP secretion from the posterior pituitary would normally be suppressed. Because the only clinical abnormality known to result from increased secretion of AVP is a decrease in the osmotic pressure of body fluids, the hallmark of SIADH is hypoosmolality. This clinical finding led to the identification of the first well described cases of this disorder in 1957[1] and the subsequent clinical investigations that resulted in the delineation of the essential characteristics of the syndrome.[2] It is therefore appropriate to begin this chapter with a brief summary of some general issues concerning hypoosmolality and hyponatremia before discussing details that are specific to SIADH and related disorders associated with dilutional hypoosmolality of body fluids. Although much has been learned over the last five decades about the pathophysiology of SIADH and hyponatremia, it remains surprising how rudimentary our understanding is of some of the most basic aspects of this disorder.[3,4] One particularly striking example of this is the controversy concerning the most appropriate rate of correction of hyponatremic patients.[5] Nonetheless, recent and ongoing clinical and basic studies have continued to shed new light on many heretofore incompletely understood aspects of hypoosmolar disorders. In addition, we have begun an exciting new era with regard to the therapy of these disorders using antagonists of AVP receptors.[6] Although some of the specific information contained in this chapter will undoubtedly become outdated in the future, the basic concepts underlying the pathophysiology, diagnosis, and therapy of hypoosmolar disorders have withstood the tests of time and clinical utility, and likely will remain valid for some time to come.

HYPOOSMOLALITY AND HYPONATREMIA

Incidence

Hypoosmolality is one of the most common disorders of fluid and electrolyte balance encountered in hospitalized patients. The incidence and prevalence of hypoosmolar disorders depend on the nature of the patient population being studied as well as on the laboratory methods and diagnostic criteria used to ascertain hyponatremia. Most investigators have used the serum sodium concentration ([Na^+]) to determine the clinical incidence of hypoosmolality. When hyponatremia is defined as a serum [Na^+] of less than 135 mEq per L, incidences as high as 15% to 30% have been observed in studies of both acutely and chronically[7,8] hospitalized patients. These high incidences in hospitalized patients are corroborated by frequency analysis of a large population of hospitalized patients, which demonstrated that serum [Na^+] and chloride concentrations were approximately 5 mEq per L lower than those in a control group of healthy, nonhospitalized subjects.[9] However, incidences decrease to the range of 1% to 4% when only patients with serum [Na^+] less than 130 to 131 mEq per L are included,[10–12] which may represent a more appropriate level to define the occurrence of clinically significant cases of this disorder. Even when one uses these more stringent criteria to define hypoosmolality, incidences from 7% to 53% have been reported in institutionalized geriatric patients.[13,14] Perhaps most importantly, reports of all studies to date have noted a high proportion of iatrogenic or hospital-acquired hyponatremia, which has accounted for as much as 40% to 75% of all patients studied.[12,15,16] Therefore, although hyponatremia and hypoosmolality are exceedingly common, most cases are relatively mild and become manifest during the course of hospitalization.

These considerations could be interpreted to indicate that hypoosmolality is of relatively little clinical significance, but this conclusion is unwarranted for several reasons. First, severe hypoosmolality (serum [Na^+] levels <120 mEq per L), although relatively uncommon, is associated with substantial morbidity and mortality.[17,18] Second, even relatively mild hypoosmolality can quickly progress to more dangerous levels during the course of therapeutic management of other disorders. Third, overly rapid correction of hyponatremia can itself cause severe neurologic morbidity and mortality.[19] Finally, it has been observed that mortality rates are much higher, from threefold[11,20] to 60-fold,[12] in patients with even asymptomatic degrees of hypoosmolality compared to normonatremic patients. Although earlier studies associated increased mortality with serum [Na^+] levels less than130 mEq per L, more recent studies indicate an increased risk of mortality even when serum [Na^+] levels decrease below 137 mEq per L.[15] Remarkably, hyponatremia has been found to represent an independent predictor of worsened outcomes in virtually every disease ever studied, from congestive heart failure to tuberculosis to liver failure.[16] Although this is probably because hypoosmolality is more an indicator of the severity of many underlying illnesses than it is an independent contributing factor to mortality, this presumption may not be true of all cases. These considerations emphasize the importance of a careful evaluation of all hyponatremic patients, regardless of the clinical setting in which they present.

Osmolality, Tonicity, and Serum [Na^+]

As discussed in Chapter 4, the osmolality of body fluid normally is maintained within narrow limits by osmotically regulated AVP secretion and thirst. Although basal plasma osmolality can vary appreciably among individuals, the range in the general population under conditions of normal hydration lies between 275 and 295 mOsm per kg H_2O. Plasma osmolality can be determined *directly* by measuring the freezing point depression or the vapor pressure of plasma. Alternatively, it can be calculated *indirectly* from the concentrations of the three major solutes in plasma:

$$\text{Posm (mOsm/kg } H_2O) = 2 \times [Na^+] \text{ (mEq/L)} + \text{glucose (mg/dL)/18} + \text{blood urea nitrogen (mg/dL)/2.8}$$

Both methods produce comparable results under most conditions. Although either of these methods produces valid measures of total osmolality, this is not always equivalent to the effective osmolality, which is commonly referred to as the tonicity of the plasma. Only cell membrane impermeable solutes such as Na^+ and Cl^- that remain relatively compartmentalized within the extracellular fluid (ECF) space are "effective" solutes, because these solutes create osmotic gradients across cell membranes and thus generate osmotic movement of water from the intracellular fluid (ICF) compartment into the ECF compartment. By contrast, solutes that readily permeate cell membranes (e.g., urea, ethanol, and methanol) are not effective solutes, because they do not create osmotic gradients across cell membranes and thus do not generate water movement between body fluid compartments. Only the concentrations of effective solutes in plasma should be used to ascertain whether clinically significant hyperosmolality or hypoosmolality is present because these are the only solutes that directly affect body fluid distribution.[21]

Sodium and its accompanying anions represent the bulk of the major effective plasma solutes, so hyponatremia and hypoosmolality are usually synonymous. However, there are two important situations in which hyponatremia will not reflect true hypoosmolality. The first is pseudohyponatremia, which is produced by marked elevations of either lipids or proteins in plasma. In such cases the concentration of Na^+ per liter of plasma water is unchanged, but the concentration of Na^+ per liter of plasma is artifactually decreased because of the larger relative proportion of plasma volume that is occupied by the excess lipids or proteins.[22,23] However, the increased protein or lipid will not appreciably increase the total number of solute particles in solution, so the directly measured plasma osmolality will not be significantly affected under these conditions. Measurement of serum [Na^+] by ion-specific electrodes, which is now commonly employed by most clinical laboratories, is less influenced by high concentrations of lipids or proteins than is measurement of serum [Na^+] by flame photometry,[24] although recent reports have demonstrated that such errors can nonetheless still occur when using autoanalyzers that require a dilution of the plasma sample.[25–27]

The second situation in which hyponatremia does not reflect true plasma hypoosmolality occurs when high concentrations of effective solutes other than Na^+ are present in the plasma. The initial hyperosmolality produced by the additional solute causes an osmotic shift of water from the ICF to the ECF, which in turn produces a dilutional decrease in the serum [Na^+]. Once equilibrium between both fluid compartments is achieved, the total effective osmolality remains relatively unchanged. This situation most commonly occurs with hyperglycemia and represents a frequent cause of hyponatremia in hospitalized patients, accounting for up to 10% to 20% of all cases.[12] Misdiagnosis of true hypoosmolality in such cases can be avoided by measuring plasma osmolality directly, or alternatively by correcting the measured serum [Na^+] by 1.6 mEq per L for each 100 mg per dL increase in serum glucose concentration above normal levels.[28] Recent studies have shown a more complex relation between hyperglycemia and serum [Na^+], and have suggested that a more accurate correction factor may be closer to 2.4 mEq per L.[29] When the plasma contains significant amounts of unmeasured solutes, such as osmotic diuretics, radiographic contrast agents, and some toxins (e.g., ethanol, methanol, and ethylene glycol), plasma osmolality cannot be calculated accurately. In these situations, osmolality must be ascertained by direct measurement, although even this method does not yield an accurate measure of the true effective osmolality if the unmeasured solutes are noneffective solutes that permeate cell membranes (e.g., ethanol).

Because of the previously noted considerations, it should be apparent that the determination of whether true hypoosmolality is present can sometimes be difficult. Nevertheless, a straightforward and relatively simple approach will suffice in most cases:

1. The effective plasma osmolality should be calculated from the measured serum [Na^+] and glucose concentration ($2 \times [Na^+]$ + glucose/18); alternatively, the

measured serum [Na^+] can simply be corrected by 1.6 to 2.4 mEq per L for each 100 mg per dL increase in serum glucose concentration greater than normal levels (100 mg per dL).

2. If the calculated effective plasma osmolality is <275 mOsm per kg H_2O, or if the corrected serum [Na^+] is <135 mEq per L, then significant hypoosmolality exists, providing that large concentrations of unmeasured solutes or pseudohyponatremia secondary to hyperlipidemia or hyperproteinemia are not present.
3. To eliminate the latter possibilities, plasma osmolality should also be measured directly in all cases in which the hyponatremia cannot be accounted for by elevated serum glucose levels. Absence of a discrepancy between the calculated and measured total plasma osmolality (<10 mOsm per kg H_2O) will confirm the absence of significant amounts of unmeasured solutes, such as osmotic diuretics, radiocontrast agents, or ethanol; if a significant discrepancy between these measures is found (called an "osmolal gap"[30]), appropriate tests must then be conducted to rule out pseudohyponatremia or to identify possible unmeasured plasma solutes.[21,31,32] Whether significant hypoosmolality exists in the latter case will depend on the nature of the unmeasured solutes; although this determination will not always be possible, the clinician will at least be alerted to uncertainty about the diagnosis of true hypoosmolality.

Pathogenesis of Hypoosmolality

Because water moves freely between the ICF and ECF across most cell membranes, osmolality will always be equivalent in both of these fluid compartments since water distributes between them in response to osmotic gradients. Consequently, total body osmolality must always be the same as both ECF and ICF osmolality. The bulk of body solute is comprised of electrolytes, namely the exchangeable Na^+ (Na^+_E) in the ECF and the exchangeable K^+ (K^+_E) in the ICF along with their associated anions, so total body osmolality will largely be a function of these parameters[33,34]:

$$
\begin{aligned}
OSM_{ECF} &= OSM_{ICF} \\
&= \text{total body osmolality} \\
&= (\text{ECF solute} + \text{ICF solute}) / \text{body water} \\
&= (2 \times Na^+_E + 2 \times K^+_E + \text{nonelectrolyte solute}) / \text{body water}
\end{aligned}
$$

Although these calculations represent an oversimplification of complex factors that determine the relative distribution of intracellular and extracellular solutes (there is a revision of the original Edelman equation for predicting serum [Na^+] based on exchangeable body Na^+ and K^+),[35] they are sufficiently accurate for the purpose of predicting changes in serum [Na^+]. By definition, the presence of plasma hypoosmolality indicates a relative excess of water to solute in the ECF. From the preceding equations, it should be apparent that this can be produced either by an excess of body water, resulting in a dilution of remaining body solute, or alternatively by a depletion of body solute, either Na^+ or K^+, relative to the remaining body water. Table 70.1 summarizes the potential causes of hyponatremia categorized according to whether the initiating event is dilution or depletion of body solute. It should be recognized that such a classification represents an obvious oversimplification, because most clinical hypoosmolar states involve significant

TABLE 70.1 **Pathogenesis of Hypoosmolar Disorders**

Pathogenesis of Hypoosmolar Disorders
Depletion (Primary Decreases in Total Body Solute and Secondary Water Retention)
Renal Solute Loss
Diuretic use
Solute diuresis (glucose, mannitol)
Salt wasting nephropathy
Mineralocorticoid deficiency or resistance
Nonrenal Solute Loss
Gastrointestinal (diarrhea, vomiting, pancreatitis, bowel obstruction)
Cutaneous (sweating, burns)
Blood loss
Dilution (Primary Increases in Total Body Water and Secondary Solute Depletion)
Impaired Renal Free Water Excretion
Increased Proximal Reabsorption
Hypothyroidism
Impaired Distal Dilution
Syndrome of inappropriate antidiuretic hormone secretion
Glucocorticoid deficiency
Combined Increased Proximal Reabsorption and Impaired Distal Dilution
Congestive heart failure
Cirrhosis
Nephrotic syndrome
Decreased Urinary Solute Excretion
Beer potomania
Very low protein diet
Excess Water Intake
Primary polydipsia
Dilute infant formula
Fresh water drowning

components of both solute depletion and water retention. Nonetheless, it is conceptually useful as a starting point for understanding the mechanisms underlying the pathogenesis of hypoosmolality and as a framework for discussions of therapy of hypoosmolar disorders.

Solute Depletion

Depletion of body solute can result from any significant losses of ECF. Whether via renal or nonrenal routes, body fluid losses by themselves rarely cause hypoosmolality because excreted or secreted body fluids are usually isotonic or hypotonic relative to plasma and therefore tend to increase plasma osmolality. Consequently, when hypoosmolality accompanies ECF losses it is generally the result of replacement of body fluid losses by more hypotonic solutions, thereby diluting the remaining body solutes. This often occurs when patients drink water or other hypotonic fluids in response to ongoing solute and water losses, and also when hypotonic intravenous fluids are administered to hospitalized patients.[36] When the solute losses are marked, these patients can show all of the obvious signs of volume depletion (e.g., addisonian crisis). However, such patients often have a more deceptive clinical presentation because their volume deficits may be partially replaced by subsequently ingested or infused fluids. Moreover, they may not manifest signs or symptoms of cellular dehydration because osmotic gradients will draw water into the relatively hypertonic ICF. Therefore, clinical evidence of hypovolemia strongly supports solute depletion as the cause of plasma hypoosmolality, but absence of clinically evident hypovolemia never completely eliminates this as a possibility. Although ECF solute losses are responsible for most cases of depletion-induced hypoosmolality, ICF solute loss can also cause hypoosmolality as a result of osmotic water shifts from the ICF into the ECF.[33] This mechanism likely contributes to some cases of diuretic-induced hypoosmolality in which depletion of total body K^+ often occurs.[37,38]

Water Retention

Despite the obvious importance of solute depletion in some patients, most cases of clinically significant hypoosmolality are caused by increases in total body water rather than by primary loss of extracellular solute. This can occur because of either impaired renal free water excretion or excessive free water intake. However, the former accounts for most hypoosmolar disorders because normal kidneys have sufficient diluting capacity to allow excretion of up to 20 to 30 L per day of free water (see Chapter 4). Intakes of this magnitude are occasionally seen in a subset of psychiatric patients[39,40] but not in most patients, including patients with SIADH in whom fluid intakes average 2 to 3 L per day.[41] Consequently, dilutional hypoosmolality usually is the result of an abnormality of renal free water excretion. The renal mechanisms responsible for impairments in free water excretion can be subgrouped according to whether the major impairment in free water excretion occurs in proximal or distal parts of the nephron, or both (see Table 70.1).

Any disorder that leads to a decrease in glomerular filtration rate (GFR) causes increased reabsorption of both Na^+ and water in the proximal tubule. As a result, the ability to excrete free water is limited because of decreased delivery of tubular fluid to the distal nephron. Disorders causing solute depletion through nonrenal mechanisms (e.g., gastrointestinal fluid losses) also produce this effect. Disorders that cause a decreased GFR in the absence of significant ECF losses are, for the most part, edema-forming states associated with decreased effective arterial blood volume (EABV) and secondary hyperaldosteronism.[42,43] Although these conditions are typified by increased proximal reabsorption of both Na^+ and fluid, it is now clear that in most cases water retention also results from increased distal reabsorption caused by nonosmotic baroreceptor-mediated stimulated increases in plasma AVP levels,[44,45] with the possible exception of hypothyroidism.

Distal nephron impairments in free water excretion are characterized by an inability to dilute tubular fluid maximally. These disorders are usually associated with abnormalities in the secretion of AVP from the posterior pituitary. However, just as depletion-induced hypoosmolar disorders usually include an important component of secondary impairments of free water excretion, so do most dilution-induced hypoosmolar disorders involve significant degrees of secondary solute depletion. This was recognized even before the first clinical description of SIADH from studies of the effects of posterior pituitary extracts on water retention, which demonstrated that renal salt wasting was predominantly a result of the ECF volume expansion produced by the retained water.[46] Therefore, after sustained increases in total body water secondary to inappropriately elevated AVP levels, sufficient secondary solute losses, predominantly as Na^+, occur and can result in further lowering of plasma osmolality. The actual contribution of Na^+ losses to the hypoosmolality of SIADH is variable and depends in part on both the rate and volume of water retention.[47] The major factor responsible for secondary Na^+ losses appears to be renal hemodynamic effects, and specifically the phenomenon of pressure natriuresis and diuresis induced by the volume expansion.[48] However, volume-stimulated hormones such as atrial natriuretic peptide (ANP) are also elevated in response to the water retention of patients with SIADH,[49,50] and it seems likely that these factors also contribute to the secondary natriuresis, possibly via interactions with intrarenal hemodynamic effects.[51] Regardless of the actual mechanisms involved, the solute losses that occur secondary to water retention can be best understood in the context of volume regulation of the ICF and ECF compartments in response to induced hypoosmolality, which is discussed in the next section.

Some dilutional disorders do not fit particularly well into either category. Chief among these is the hyponatremia that sometimes occurs in patients who ingest large volumes of beer with little food intake for prolonged periods, called "beer potomania."[52,53] Although the volume of fluid ingested may not seem sufficiently excessive to overwhelm renal diluting mechanisms, in these cases free water excretion is limited by very low urinary solute excretion thereby causing water retention and dilutional hyponatremia. A reported case in which hyponatremia occurred in an ovolactovegetarian with a very low protein intake but no beer ingestion is consistent with this pathophysiologic mechanism.[54] However, because most such patients have very low salt intakes as well, it is likely that relative depletion of body Na^+ stores also is a contributing factor to the hypoosmolality in at least some cases.[55]

Adaptation to Hyponatremia: ICF and ECF Volume Regulation

Many studies have indicated that the combined effects of water retention plus urinary solute excretion cannot adequately explain the degree of plasma hypoosmolality observed in patients.[2,56,57] This observation originally led to the theory of cellular inactivation of solute.[2] Simply stated, this theory suggested that as ECF osmolality falls, water moves into cells along osmotic gradients, thereby causing the cells to swell. At some point during this volume expansion, the cells osmotically "inactivate" some of their intracellular solutes as a defense mechanism to prevent continued cell swelling with subsequent detrimental effects on cell function and survival. As a result of this decrease in intracellular osmolality, water then shifts back out of the ICF into the ECF, but at the expense of further worsening the dilution-induced hypoosmolality. Despite the appeal of this theory, its validity has never been demonstrated conclusively in either human or animal studies.

An appealing alternative theory has been suggested by studies of cell volume regulation, in which cell volume is maintained under hypoosmolar conditions by extrusion of potassium rather than by osmotic inactivation of cellular solute.[58,59] Whole brain volume regulation via similar types of electrolyte losses was first described by Yannet in 1940,[60] and has long been recognized as the mechanism by which the brain was able to adapt to hyponatremia and limit brain edema to sublethal levels.[61–63] Following the recognition that low molecular weight organic compounds, called organic osmolytes, also constituted a significant osmotic component of a wide variety of cell types, studies demonstrated the accumulation of these compounds in response to hyperosmolality in both kidney[64] and brain[65] tissue. Multiple groups have now shown that the brain loses organic osmolytes in addition to electrolytes during the process of volume regulation to hypoosmolar conditions in experimental animals[66–69] and human patients.[70] These losses occur relatively quickly (within 24 to 48 hours in rats) and can account for as much as one third of the brain solute losses during hyponatremia.[71] Such coordinate losses of both electrolytes and organic osmolytes from brain tissue enables very effective regulation of brain volume during chronic hyponatremia (Fig. 70.1).[72]

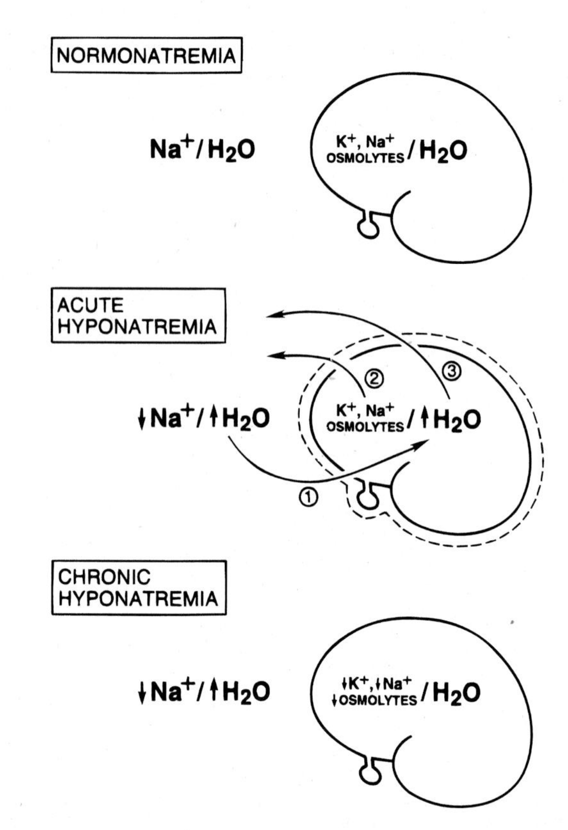

FIGURE 70.1 Schematic diagram of brain volume adaptation to hyponatremia. Under normal conditions brain osmolality and extracellular fluid (ECF) osmolality are in equilibrium (*top panel*; for simplicity the predominant intracellular solutes are depicted as K^+ and organic osmolytes, and the extracellular solute as Na^+). Following the induction of ECF hypoosmolality, water moves into the brain in response to osmotic gradients producing brain edema (*dotted line, middle panel*, #1). However, in response to the induced swelling the brain rapidly loses both extracellular and intracellular solutes (*middle panel*, #2). As water losses accompany the losses of brain solute, the expanded brain volume then decreases back toward normal (*middle panel*, #3). If hypoosmolality is sustained, brain volume eventually normalizes completely and the brain becomes fully adapted to the ECF hyponatremia (*bottom panel*).

Consequently, it is now clear that cell volume regulation in vivo in brain tissue occurs predominantly through depletion, rather than intracellular osmotic inactivation, of a variety of intracellular solutes. Ongoing experimental studies are better defining the complex cellular and molecular mechanisms that underlie this profound adaptation to hypoosmolality.

Most studies have focused on volume regulation in the brain during hyponatremia, but all cells volume regulate to varying degrees,[58] and there is little question that this process occurs throughout the body as whole organisms adapt to hypoosmolar conditions. Unexplained components of hyponatremia that led to previous speculation about cellular inactivation of solute are now better explained by cellular losses of both electrolyte and organic solutes as cells throughout the body undergo volume regulation during hypoosmolar conditions. However, volume regulatory processes are not limited to cells. Although most cases of hyponatremia clearly result from initial water retention induced by stimulated antidiuresis, it has always seemed likely that the resulting natriuresis served the purpose of regulating the volumes of the ECF and intravascular spaces. Many experimental and clinical observations are consistent with ECF volume regulation via secondary solute losses. First, dilutional decreases in concentrations of most blood constituents other than Na^+ and Cl^- do not occur in patients with SIADH,[73] suggesting that their plasma volume is not nearly as expanded as would be predicted simply by the measured decreases in serum [Na^+]. Second, an increased incidence of hypertension has never been observed in patients with SIADH,[74] again arguing against significant expansion of the arterial blood volume. Third, results of animal studies in both dogs[75] and rats[76] have clearly indicated that a significant component of chronic hyponatremia is attributable to secondary Na^+ losses rather than water retention. Furthermore, the relative contributions from water retention versus sodium loss vary with the duration and severity of the hyponatremia: water retention was found to be the major cause of decreased serum [Na^+] in the first 24 hours of induced hyponatremia in rats, but Na^+ depletion then became the predominant etiologic factor after longer periods (7–14 days) of sustained hyponatremia, particularly at very low (<115 mEq per L) serum [Na^+] levels.[76] Finally, multiple studies have attempted to measure body fluid compartment volumes in hyponatremic patients, but without consistent results that indicate either plasma or ECF volume expansion.[1,57,77,78] In particular, a report of body fluid space measurements using isotope dilution techniques in hyponatremic and normonatremic patients with small cell lung carcinoma showed no differences between the two groups with regard to exchangeable sodium space, ECF volume by $^{35}SO_4$ distribution, or total body water.[79] Such results have traditionally been explained by the relative insensitivity of isotope dilution techniques for measurement of body fluid compartment spaces, but an equally plausible possibility is that in the chronically adapted hyponatremic state body fluid compartments have regulated their volumes back toward normal via a combination of extracellular (predominantly electrolyte) and intracellular (electrolyte and organic osmolyte) solute losses.[80] Figure 70.2 schematically illustrates some of the volume regulatory processes that likely occur in response to water retention induced by inappropriate antidiuresis. The degree to which solute losses versus water retention contribute to the resulting hyponatremia will vary in association with many different factors, including the etiology of the hyponatremia, the rapidity of development of the hyponatremia, the chronicity of the hyponatremia, the volume of daily water loading and subsequent volume expansion, and undoubtedly some degree of individual variability as well. It therefore hardly seems surprising that studies of hyponatremic patients have failed to yield uniform results regarding the pathogenesis of hyponatremia in view of the marked diversity of hyponatremic patients and their presentation at different times during the process of adaptation to hypoosmolality via volume regulatory processes.

Differential Diagnosis of Hyponatremia and Hypoosmolality

Because of the multiplicity of disorders causing hypoosmolality and the fact that many involve more than one pathologic mechanism, a definitive diagnosis is not always possible at the time of initial presentation. Nonetheless, a relatively straightforward approach based on the commonly used parameters of ECF volume status and urine sodium concentration generally allows a sufficient categorization of the underlying etiology to allow appropriate decisions regarding initial therapy and further evaluation in most cases (Table 70.2).

Decreased Extracellular Fluid Volume

The presence of clinically detectable hypovolemia nearly always signifies total body solute depletion. A low urine [Na^+] indicates a nonrenal cause of solute depletion. If the urine [Na^+] is high despite hypoosmolality, renal causes of solute depletion are likely responsible. Therapy with thiazide diuretics is the most common cause of renal solute losses,[38] particularly in the elderly,[81,82] but mineralocorticoid deficiency as a result of adrenal insufficiency[83] or mineralocorticoid resistance[84] must always be considered as well. Less commonly, renal solute losses may be the result of a salt-wasting nephropathy (e.g., polycystic kidney disease,[85] interstitial nephritis,[86] or chemotherapy[87]).

Increased Extracellular Fluid Volume

The presence of clinically detectable hypervolemia usually signifies total body Na^+ excess. In these patients, hypoosmolality results from an even greater expansion of total body water caused by a marked reduction in the rate of water excretion (and sometimes an increased rate of water ingestion). The impairment in water excretion is secondary to a decreased EABV,[42,43] which increases the reabsorption of glomerular filtrate not only in the proximal nephron but also in the distal and collecting tubules by stimulating AVP secretion.[44,45] These patients generally have a low urine [Na^+] because of secondary hyperaldosteronism, which is also a product of decreased EABV. However, under certain conditions urine [Na^+] may be elevated, usually secondary to concurrent diuretic therapy but also sometimes because of a solute diuresis (e.g., glucosuria in diabetics) or after successful treatment of the underlying disease (e.g., ionotropic therapy in patients with congestive heart failure). An additional disorder that can produce hypoosmolality and hypervolemia is acute or chronic renal failure with fluid overload[12] (although in early stages of renal failure polyuria from AVP resistance is more likely[88]). Urine [Na^+] in these cases is usually elevated, but it can be variable depending on the stage of renal failure. It is important to remember that primary polydipsia will not be accompanied by signs of hypervolemia because water ingestion alone, in the absence of Na^+ retention, does not typically produce clinically apparent degrees of ECF volume expansion.

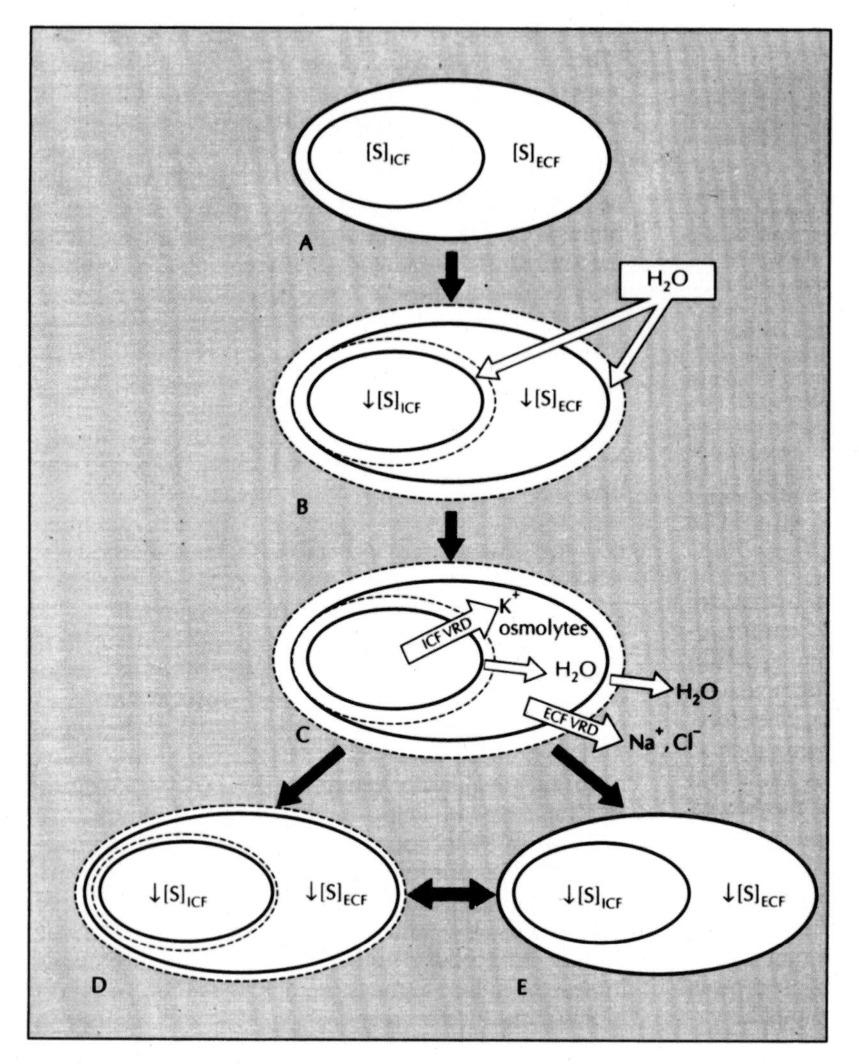

FIGURE 70.2 Schematic illustration of potential changes in whole body fluid compartment volumes at various times during adaptation to hyponatremia. Under basal conditions the concentration of effective solutes in the extracellular fluid ($[\mathbf{S}]_{ECF}$) and the intracellular fluid ($[\mathbf{S}]_{ICF}$) are in osmotic balance **(A)**. During the first phase of water retention resulting from inappropriate antidiuresis the excess water distributes across total body water, causing expansion of both ECF and ICF volumes (*dotted lines*) with equivalent dilutional decreases in $[\mathbf{S}]_{ICF}$ and $[\mathbf{S}]_{ECF}$ **(B)**. In response to the volume expansion, compensatory volume regulatory decreases (VRD) occur to reduce the effective solute content of both the ICF (via increased electrolyte and osmolyte extrusion mediated by stretch activated channels and downregulation of synthesis of osmolytes and osmolyte uptake transporters) and the ECF (via pressure diuresis and natriuretic factors) **(C)**. If both processes go to completion, such as under conditions of fluid restriction, a final steady state can be reached in which ICF and ECF volumes have returned to normal levels but $[\mathbf{S}]_{ICF}$ and $[\mathbf{S}]_{ECF}$ remain low **(E)**. In most cases this final steady state is not reached, and moderate degrees of ECF and ICF expansion persist, but significantly less than would be predicted from the decrease in body osmolality **(D)**. Consequently, the degree to which hyponatremia is due to dilution from water retention versus solute depletion from volume regulatory processes can vary markedly depending on which phase of adaptation the patient is in, and also on the relative rates at which the different compensatory processes occur (e.g., delayed ICF VRD can worsen hyponatremia due to shifts of intracellular water into the extracellular fluid as intracellular organic osmolytes are extruded and subsequently metabolized, likely accounting for some component of the hyponatremia unexplained by the combination of water retention and sodium excretion in previous clinical studies). (From Verbalis JG. Hyponatremia: epidemiology, pathophysiology, and therapy. *Curr Opin Nephrol Hyperten.* 1993;2:636–652, with permission.)

Normal Extracellular Fluid Volume

Many different hypoosmolar disorders can potentially present clinically with euvolemia, in large part because it is difficult to detect modest changes in volume status using standard methods of clinical assessment; in such cases, measurement of urine $[Na^+]$ is an especially important first step.[89] A high urine $[Na^+]$ in euvolemic patients usually implies a distally mediated, dilution-induced hypoosmolality such as SIADH. However, glucocorticoid deficiency can mimic SIADH so closely that these two disorders are often

TABLE 70.2 **Differential Diagnosis of Hyponatremia**

Extracellular Fluid Volume	Urine [Na+][a]	Presumptive Diagnosis
↓	Low	**Depletion (Nonrenal):** gastrointestinal, cutaneous, or blood ECF loss
	High	**Depletion (Renal):** diuretics, mineralocorticoid insufficiency (Addison disease), salt losing nephropathy
		Depletion (Nonrenal): any cause + hypotonic fluid replacement
→	Low	**Dilution (Proximal):** hypothyroidism, early decreased effective arterial blood volume
		Dilution (Distal): SIADH, glucocorticoid insufficiency
	High	**Dilution(Distal):** SIADH + fluid restriction
		Depletion (Renal): any cause + hypotonic fluid replacement (especially diuretic treatment)
↑	Low	**Dilution (Proximal):** decreased, effective arterial blood volume (congestive heart failure, cirrhosis, nephrosis)
	High	**Dilution (Proximal):** any cause + diuretics or improvement in underlying disease, renal failure

[a]Urine [Na+] values <30 mEq per L are generally considered to be low and values ≥30 mEq per day to be high, based on studies of responses of hyponatremic patients to infusions of isotonic saline.[89]

indistinguishable in terms of water balance.[90,91] Hyponatremia from diuretic use also can present without clinically evident hypovolemia, and the urine [Na+] will often be elevated in such cases because of the renal tubular effects of the diuretics.[38] Recent studies have suggested that the fractional excretion of uric acid may provide a better measure of ECF volume status in hyponatremic patients on diuretics.[92] A low urine [Na+] suggests a depletion-induced hypoosmolality from ECF losses with subsequent volume replacement by water or other hypotonic fluids. The solute loss often is generally nonrenal in origin, but an important exception is recent cessation of diuretic therapy, because urine [Na+] can quickly decrease to low values within 12 to 24 hours after discontinuation of the diuretic. The presence of a low serum [K+] is an important clue to diuretic use, because few of the other disorders that cause hypoosmolality are associated with significant hypokalemia. However, even in the absence of hypokalemia, any hypoosmolar, clinically euvolemic patient taking diuretics should be assumed to have solute depletion and treated accordingly; subsequent failure to correct the hypoosmolality with isotonic saline administration and persistence of an elevated urine [Na+] after discontinuation of diuretics then requires reconsideration of a diagnosis of dilutional hypoosmolality. A low urine [Na+] also can also be seen in some cases of hypothyroidism, in the early stages of decreased EABV before the development of clinically apparent sodium retention and fluid overload, or during the recovery phase from SIADH. Hence, a low urine [Na+] is less meaningful diagnostically than is a high value.

Because euvolemic causes of hypoosmolality represent the most challenging etiologies of this disease, both in terms of differential diagnosis as well as with regard to the underlying pathophysiology, the subsequent sections will discuss the major causes of euvolemic hypoosmolality and hyponatremia in greater detail.

SYNDROME OF INAPPROPRIATE ANTIDIURETIC HORMONE SECRETION

SIADH is the most common cause of euvolemic hypoosmolality. It is also the single most prevalent cause of hypoosmolality of all etiologies encountered in clinical practice, with prevalence rates ranging from 20% to 40% among all hypoosmolar patients.[12,41,93,94] The clinical criteria necessary to diagnose SIADH remain basically as set forth by Bartter and Schwartz in 1967.[2] A modified summary of these criteria is presented in Table 70.3 along with several other clinical

TABLE 70.3 Criteria for the Diagnosis of SIADH

Essential
Decreased effective osmolality of the extracellular fluid (P_{osm} <275 mOsm/kg H_2O)
Inappropriate urinary concentration (U_{osm} >100 mOsm/kg H_2O with normal renal function) at some level of hypoosmolality
Clinical euvolemia, as defined by the absence of signs of hypovolemia (orthostasis, tachycardia, decreased skin turgor, dry mucous membranes) or hypervolemia (subcutaneous edema, ascites)
Elevated urinary sodium excretion while on a normal salt and water intake
Absence of other potential causes of euvolemic hypoosmolality: hypothyroidism, hypocortisolism (Addison disease or pituitary ACTH insufficiency), and diuretic use
Supplemental
Abnormal water load test (inability to excrete at least 90% of a 20 mL/kg water load in 4 hours and/or failure to dilute U_{osm} to <100 mOsm/kg H_2O)
Plasma AVP level inappropriately elevated relative to plasma osmolality
No significant correction of serum [Na^+] with volume expansion but improvement after fluid restriction

findings that support this diagnosis. Several points about each of these criteria deserve emphasis and/or qualification:

1. True hypoosmolality must be present and hyponatremia secondary to pseudohyponatremia or hyperglycemia alone must be excluded.
2. Urinary concentration (osmolality) must be inappropriate for plasma hypoosmolality. This does not mean that urine osmolality must be greater than plasma osmolality (a common misinterpretation of this criterion), but simply that the urine must be less than maximally dilute (i.e., urine osmolality >100 mOsm per kg H_2O). It also should be remembered that urine osmolality need not be elevated inappropriately at all levels of plasma osmolality, because in the reset osmostat variant of SIADH, AVP secretion can be suppressed with resultant maximal urinary dilution and free water excretion if plasma osmolality is decreased to sufficiently low levels.[95,96] Hence, to satisfy the classical criteria for the diagnosis of SIADH, it is necessary only that urine osmolality be inadequately suppressed at some level of plasma osmolality less than 275 mOsm per kg H_2O.
3. Clinical euvolemia must be present to establish a diagnosis of SIADH, because both hypovolemia and hypervolemia strongly suggest different causes of hypoosmolality. This does not mean that patients with SIADH cannot become hypovolemic or hypervolemic for other reasons, but in such cases it is impossible to diagnose the underlying inappropriate antidiuresis until the patient is rendered euvolemic and found to have persistent hypoosmolality.
4. The criterion of renal "salt-wasting" has probably caused the most confusion regarding diagnosis of SIADH. This criterion is included because of its utility in differentiating between hypoosmolality caused by a decreased EABV, in which case renal Na^+ conservation occurs, and distal dilution-induced disorders, in which urinary Na^+ excretion is normal or increased secondary to ECF volume expansion. However, two important qualifications limit the utility of urine [Na^+] measurement in the hypoosmolar patient: urine [Na^+] also is high when solute depletion is of renal origin, as seen with diuretic use or Addison disease, and patients with SIADH can have low urine Na^+ excretion if they subsequently become hypovolemic or solute depleted, conditions that sometimes follow severe sodium and water restriction. Consequently, although a high urine Na^+ excretion is the rule in most patients with SIADH, its presence does not guarantee this diagnosis, and, conversely, its absence does not rule out the diagnosis.
5. The final criterion emphasizes that SIADH remains a diagnosis of exclusion. Thus, the presence of other potential causes of euvolemic hypoosmolality must always be excluded. This includes not only thyroid and adrenal dysfunction, but also diuretic use, because this can also sometimes present as euvolemic hypoosmolality.

Table 70.3 also lists several other criteria that support, but are not essential for a diagnosis of SIADH. The first of these, the water load test, is of value when there is uncertainty regarding the etiology of modest degrees of hypoosmolality in euvolemic patients, but it does not add useful information if the plasma osmolality is <275 mOsm per kg H_2O. Inability to excrete a standard water load normally (with normal excretion defined as a cumulative urine output of at least 90% of the administered water load within 4 hours, and suppression of urine osmolality to <100 mOsm per kg H_2O[97]) confirms the presence of an underlying defect in free water excretion. Unfortunately, water loading is abnormal in almost all disorders that cause hypoosmolality, whether dilutional or depletion-induced with secondary impairments in free water excretion. Two exceptions are primary polydipsia, in which hypoosmolality can rarely be secondary to excessive water intake alone, and the reset osmostat variant of SIADH, in which normal excretion of a water load can occur once plasma osmolality falls below the new set point for AVP secretion. The water load test may also be used to assess water excretion after treatment of an underlying disorder thought to be causing SIADH. For example, after discontinuation of a drug associated with SIADH in a patient who has already achieved a normal plasma osmolality by fluid restriction, a normal water load test can confirm the absence of persistent inappropriate antidiuresis much more quickly than can simple monitoring of the serum [Na^+] during a period of ad libitum fluid intake. Despite these limitations as a diagnostic clinical test, the water load test remains an extremely useful tool in clinical research for quantitating changes in free water excretion in response to physiologic or pharmacologic manipulations.

The second supportive criterion for a diagnosis of SIADH is an inappropriately elevated plasma AVP level in relation to plasma osmolality. At the time that SIADH was originally described, inappropriately elevated plasma levels of AVP were merely postulated because the measurement of plasma levels of AVP was limited to relatively insensitive bioassays. With the development of sensitive AVP radioimmunoassays capable of detecting the small physiologic concentrations of this peptide that circulate in plasma,[98] there was hope that measurement of plasma AVP levels might supplant the classic criteria and become the definitive test for diagnosing SIADH, as is the case for many syndromes of hormone hypersecretion. This has not occurred for several reasons. First, although plasma AVP levels are elevated in most patients with this syndrome, the elevations generally remain within the normal physiologic range and are abnormal only in relation to plasma osmolality (Fig. 70.3). Therefore, AVP levels can be interpreted only in conjunction with a simultaneous plasma osmolality and knowledge of the relation between AVP levels and plasma osmolality in normal subjects (see Chapter 4). Second, 10% to 20% of patients with SIADH do not have measurably elevated plasma AVP levels; as shown in Figure 70.3, many such patients have AVP levels that are at, or even below, the limits of detection by radioimmunoassay. Whether these cases are true examples of inappropriate antidiuresis in the absence of circulating AVP, or whether they simply represent inappropriate AVP levels that fall below the limits of detection by radioimmunoassay, is not clear. For this reason, Zerbe et al. have proposed using the term SIAD (syndrome of inappropriate antidiuresis) rather than SIADH to describe this entire group of disorders.[99] Studies of hyponatremic children have discovered two genetic mutations of the vasopressin V2 receptor (V2R) that were responsible for constitutive activation of antidiuresis in the absence of AVP-V2R ligand binding.[100] The true incidence of these, and similar V2R mutations, as well as how often they are responsible for patients with SIADH but low or unmeasurable plasma AVP levels, remains to be determined. Third, just as water loading fails to distinguish among various causes of hypoosmolality, so do plasma AVP levels. Many disorders causing solute and volume depletion are associated with elevations of plasma AVP levels secondary to hemodynamic stimuli. For similar reasons, patients with disorders that cause decreased EABV, such as congestive heart failure and cirrhosis, also have elevated AVP levels (see Chapters 67 and 68). Even glucocorticoid insufficiency has been associated with inappropriately elevated AVP levels, as is discussed in the following section.[101] Therefore, multiple different disorders cause stimulation of AVP secretion via nonosmotic mechanisms, rendering this measurement of relatively limited differential diagnostic value. Recent studies using a newly developed assay for copeptin, the glycopeptide C-terminal fragment of the AVP prohormone, have confirmed AVP secretion in most cases of dilutional hyponatremia except for primary polydipsia, where this measurement may prove to be of use diagnostically.[102]

Finally, an improvement in plasma osmolality with fluid restriction but not with volume expansion can sometimes be helpful in differentiating between disorders causing solute depletion and those associated with dilution-induced hypoosmolality. Infusion of isotonic NaCl in patients with SIADH provokes a natriuresis with little correction of osmolality, whereas fluid restriction allows such patients to achieve solute and water balance gradually through insensible free water losses.[1] In contrast, isotonic saline is the treatment of choice in disorders of solute depletion, because once volume deficits are corrected the stimulus to continued AVP secretion and free water retention is eliminated. The diagnostic value of this therapeutic response is limited somewhat by the fact that patients with proximal types of dilution-induced disorders may show a response similar to that found in patients with SIADH. However, the major drawback is that this represents a retrospective test in a situation in which

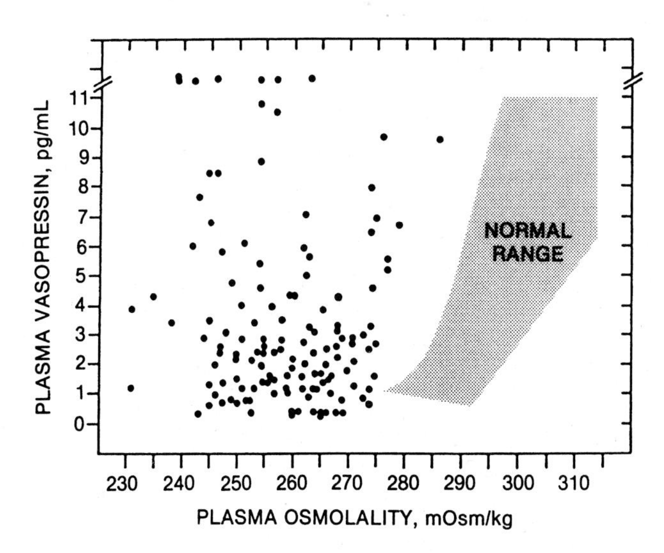

FIGURE 70.3 Plasma AVP levels in patients with SIADH as a function of plasma osmolality. Each point depicts one patient at a single point in time. The *shaded area* represents AVP levels in normal subjects over physiologic ranges of plasma osmolality. The lowest measurable plasma AVP levels using this radioimmunoassay was 0.5 pg per mL. (From Robertson GL, Aycinena P, Zerbe RL. Neurogenic disorders of osmoregulation. *Am J Med.* 1982;72:339–353, with permission.)

it would be preferable to establish a diagnosis before making a decision regarding treatment options. Nonetheless, in difficult cases of euvolemic hypoosmolality, an appropriate therapeutic response can sometimes be helpful in confirming a diagnosis of SIADH.

Etiology

Although the list of disorders associated with SIADH is long, they can be divided into four major etiologic groups (Table 70.4).

Tumors

One of the most common associations of SIADH remains with tumors. Although many different types of tumors have been associated with SIADH (Table 70.4), bronchogenic carcinoma of the lung has been uniquely associated with SIADH since the first description of this disorder in 1957.[1] In virtually all cases, the bronchogenic carcinomas causing this syndrome have been of the small cell variety; a few squamous cell types have been described, but these are rare. Incidences of hyponatremia as high as 11% of all patients with small-cell carcinoma,[103] or 33% of cases with more extensive disease,[104] have been reported. The unusually high incidence of small cell carcinoma of the lung in patients with SIADH, together with the relatively favorable therapeutic response of this type of tumor, makes it imperative that all patients presenting with an otherwise unexplained SIADH be investigated thoroughly and aggressively for a possible tumor. The evaluation should include a computed tomography (CT) or magnetic resonance imaging (MRI) scan of the thorax. In cases with a high degree of suspicion (e.g., hyponatremia in a young smoker) bronchoscopy with cytologic analysis of bronchial washings should be considered even if the results of routine chest radiography are normal, since several studies have reported hypoosmolality that predated any radiographically evident abnormality in patients who then were found to harbor bronchogenic carcinomas 3 to 12 months later.[105,106] Head and neck cancers account for another group of malignancies associated with relatively higher incidences of SIADH,[107] and some of these tumors have clearly been shown to be capable of synthesizing AVP ectopically.[108] A report from a large cancer hospital showed an incidence of hyponatremia for all malignancies combined of 3.7%, with approximately one third of these due to SIADH.[20]

Central Nervous System Disorders

The second major etiologic group of disorders causing SIADH has its origins in the central nervous system (CNS). Despite the large number of different CNS disorders associated with SIADH, there is no obvious common denominator linking them. However, this is actually not surprising when one considers the neuroanatomy of neurohypophysial innervation. The magnocellular AVP neurons receive excitatory inputs from osmoreceptor cells located in the anterior hypothalamus, but also have a major innervation from brainstem cardiovascular

TABLE 70.4 Common Etiologies of SIADH

Tumors
Pulmonary/mediastinal (bronchogenic carcinoma; mesothelioma; thymoma) Non-chest (duodenal carcinoma; pancreatic carcinoma; ureteral/prostate carcinoma; uterine carcinoma; nasopharyngeal carcinoma; leukemia)
Central Nervous System Disorders
Mass lesions (tumors; brain abscesses; subdural hematoma) Inflammatory diseases (encephalitis; meningitis; systemic lupus; acute intermittent porphyria, multiple sclerosis) Degenerative/demyelinative diseases (Guillain-Barré; spinal cord lesions) Miscellaneous (subarachnoid hemorrhage; head trauma; acute psychosis; delirium tremens; pituitary stalk section; transsphenoidal adenomectomy; hydrocephalus)
Drug Induced
Stimulated AVP release (nicotine; phenothiazines; tricyclics) Direct renal effects and/or potentiation of AVP antidiuretic effects (dDAVP; oxytocin; prostaglandin synthesis inhibitors) Mixed or uncertain actions (amiodarone; angiotensin converting enzyme inhibitors; carbamazepine and oxcarbazepine; chlorpropamide; clofibrate; clozapine; cyclophosphamide; 3,4-methylenedioxy-methamphetamine [ecstasy]; omeprazole; serotonin reuptake inhibitors; vincristine)
Pulmonary Diseases
Infections (tuberculosis; acute bacterial and viral pneumonia; aspergillosis; empyema) Mechanical/ventilatory (acute respiratory failure; COPD; positive pressure ventilation)
Other
Acquired immunodeficiency syndrome and AIDS-related complex Prolonged strenuous exercise (marathon; triathlon; ultramarathon; hot-weather hiking) Chronic inflammation (IL-6) Senile atrophy Idiopathic

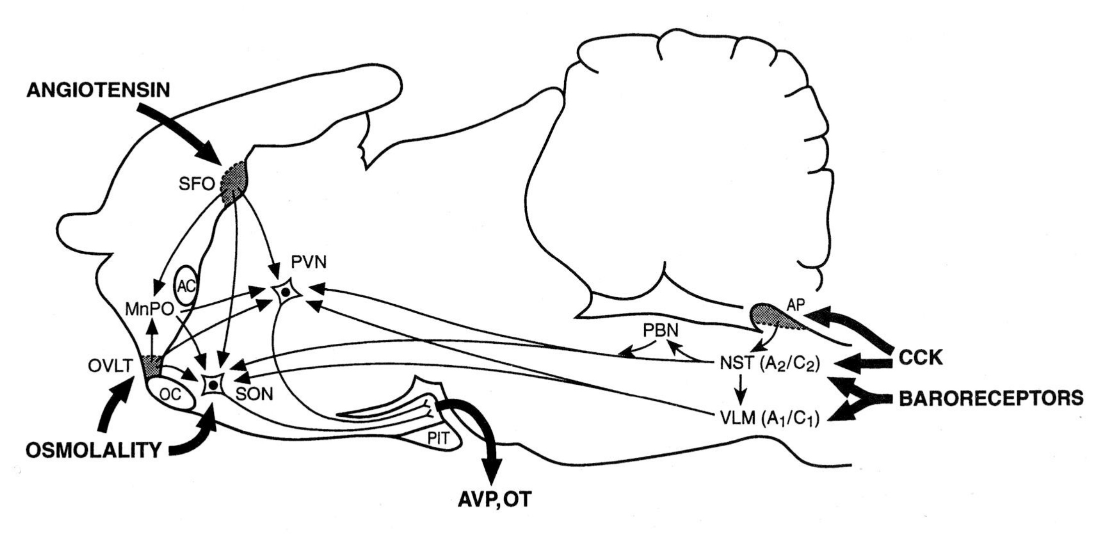

FIGURE 70.4 Diagrammatic summary of the primary brain pathways mediating AVP secretion in response to the major factors that stimulate pituitary AVP secretion. Osmolality activates neurons throughout the anterior hypothalamus, including the SFO and MnPO, but the OVLT appears to be uniquely sensitive to osmotic stimulation and is essential for osmotically stimulated AVP and OT secretion; in addition, osmotic stimulation can act directly on magnocellular neurons which themselves are intrinsically osmosensitive. Similarly, circulating angiotensin II activates cells throughout the OVLT and MnPO, but the SFO appears to be its major and essential site of action. For both of these stimuli, projections from the SFO and OVLT to the MnPO activate both excitatory and inhibitory interneurons that project to the SON and PVN and modulate the direct circumventricular inputs to these areas. Emetic stimuli act both on gastric vagal afferents which terminate in the NST and in some cases also act directly at the AP. Most of the AVP secretion appears to be a result of monosynaptic projections from catecholaminergic A2/C2 cells in the NST. Baroreceptor-mediated stimuli such as hypovolemia and hypotension are considerably more complex. Although they also arise from cranial nerves (IX and X) which terminate in the NST, most experimental data suggest that the major projection to magnocellular AVP neurons arises from catecholaminergic A1 cells of the VLM that are activated by excitatory interneurons from the NST, although some component might also arise from multisynaptic projections through other areas such as the PBN. *AC*, anterior commissure; *AP*, area postrema; *AVP*, arginine vasopressin; *MnPO*, median preoptic nucleus; *NST*, nucleus of the solitary tract; *OC*, optic chiasm; *OT*, oxytocin; *OVLT*, organum vasculosum of the lamina terminalis; *PBN*, parabrachial nucleus; *PIT*, anterior pituitary; *PVN*, paraventricular nucleus; *SFO*, subfornical organ; *SON*, supraoptic nucleus; *VLM*, ventrolateral medulla.

regulatory and emetic centers (Fig. 70.4). Although various components of these pathways have yet to be fully elucidated, many of them appear to have inhibitory as well as excitatory components.[109] Consequently, any diffuse CNS disorder can potentially cause AVP hypersecretion either by nonspecifically exciting these pathways via irritative foci, or alternatively by disrupting them and thereby decreasing the level of inhibition impinging upon the AVP neurons in the neurohypophysis. The wide variety of diverse CNS processes that can potentially cause SIADH stands in contrast to CNS causes of diabetes insipidus, which are for the most part limited to lesions localized to the hypothalamus and/or posterior pituitary that destroy the magnocellular vasopressin neurons (see Chapter 71).

Drugs

Drug-induced hyponatremia is one of the most common causes of hypoosmolality,[110] and may supplant tumors as the most common cause of SIADH. Table 70.4 lists some of the agents that have been associated with SIADH, and new drugs are being continually added to this list.[111] In general, pharmacologic agents cause this syndrome by stimulating AVP secretion, by activating AVP renal receptors to cause antidiuresis, or by potentiating the antidiuretic effect of AVP on the kidney. However, not all of the drug effects associated with inappropriate antidiuresis are fully understood; indeed, many agents may work by means of a combination of mechanisms. For example, chlorpropamide appears to have both a direct pituitary as well as a renal stimulatory effect since it has been reported to increase urine osmolality even in some patients with complete central diabetes insipidus.[112] Agents that cause AVP secretion through solute depletion, such as thiazide diuretics, are not listed here, since these are generally considered to cause depletion-induced hypoosmolality rather than true SIADH. However, some studies have suggested that in some elderly patients the precipitous hyponatremia occasionally seen after administration of thiazide diuretics is caused by polydipsia and water retention more so than by stimulated Na^+ excretion.[113] Whether this represents true SIADH independently of prior ECF volume contraction, as well as whether such cases are typical of a significant portion of patients with diuretic-induced hyponatremia, remains to be determined. A particularly interesting, and clinically important, class of agents associated with SIADH is the selective serotonin reuptake inhibitors (SSRIs). Serotonergic agents have been found to increase AVP secretion in rats in some experimental studies,[114] but most animal studies have suggested more direct effects on oxytocin rather than AVP secretion.[115] Some studies of SSRIs in humans have failed to show significant effects on AVP secretion,[116] although others support this mechanism.[117] However, hyponatremia following SSRI administration has been reported almost exclusively in the elderly, at rates as high as 22% to 28% in some studies,[118–120] although larger series have suggested an incidence closer to 1 in 200.[121] This therefore suggests the possibility that elderly patients are uniquely hypersensitive to serotonin stimulation of AVP secretion. A similar effect is likely also responsible for the recent reports of severe fatal hyponatremia caused by use of the recreational drug 3,4-methylenedioxymethamphetamine, "ecstasy,"[122,123] because this agent also possesses substantial serotonergic activity.[124] Studies of cFos expression in rats indicate that ecstasy appears to activate hypothalamic magnocellular neurons,[125] suggesting direct effects on AVP secretion as the etiology of the SIADH, and recent studies in humans support this mechanism.[126,127]

Pulmonary Disorders

Pulmonary disorders represent a relatively common but frequently misunderstood cause of SIADH. A variety of pulmonary disorders have been associated with this syndrome, but other than tuberculosis,[128] acute pneumonia,[129–131] and advanced chronic obstructive lung disease,[132] the occurrence of hypoosmolality has been noted mainly in sporadic case reports. Some bacterial infections appear to be associated with a higher incidence of hyponatremia, particularly *Legionella pneumoniae*.[133] Although one case of pulmonary tuberculosis has been reported that suggested the possibility that tuberculous lung tissue might synthesize AVP ectopically,[134] several other studies have reported that advanced pulmonary tuberculosis is associated with the reset osmostat form of SIADH,[96,128] presumably from nonosmotic stimulation of posterior pituitary AVP secretion. Most cases of pulmonary SIADH not associated with either tuberculosis or pneumonitis have occurred in the setting of respiratory failure. Although hypoxia has clearly been shown to stimulate AVP secretion in animals,[135,136] it appears to be less effective as a stimulus in humans,[137] in whom the stimulus to abnormal water retention appears to be hypercarbia more so than hypoxia.[138,139] When such patients were evaluated serially, the inappropriate AVP secretion was found to be limited to the initial days of hospitalization, when respiratory failure was most marked.[140] Even cases of tubercular SIADH generally have occurred in patients with far advanced, active, pulmonary tuberculosis, although interestingly hyponatremia was also found in 74% of a series of patients with miliary tuberculosis.[141] Therefore, SIADH in non-tumor-related pulmonary disease generally conforms to the following characteristics: (1) the pulmonary disease will always be obvious as a result of severe dyspnea or extensive radiographically evident infiltrates, and (2) the inappropriate antidiuresis will usually be limited to the period of respiratory failure—once clinical improvement has begun, free water excretion generally improves rapidly. Mechanical ventilation can cause inappropriate AVP secretion, or it can worsen any SIADH caused by other factors. This phenomenon has been associated most often with continuous positive pressure ventilation,[142] but it can also occur to a lesser degree with the use of positive end expiratory pressure.

Other Causes

One of the most recently described causes of hypoosmolality is the acquired immunodeficiency syndrome (AIDS) or AIDS-related complex (ARC), in patients with human immunodeficiency virus (HIV) infection, with incidences of hyponatremia reported as high as 30% to 38% in adults[143–145] and children.[146] Although there are many potential etiologies for hyponatremia in patients with AIDS/ARC, including dehydration, adrenal insufficiency, and pneumonitis, from 12% to 68% of AIDS patients who develop hyponatremia appear to meet criteria for a diagnosis of SIADH.[143–145] Not unexpectedly, reports have implicated some of the medications used to treat these patients as the cause of the hyponatremia, either via direct renal tubular toxicity or SIADH.[147,148]

A recent series of reports have documented a surprisingly high incidence of hyponatremia during endurance exercise events such as marathon[149] and ultramarathon[150] foot races, triathlons,[151] forced marching,[152] and hiking.[153] Occasionally, this has caused fatal outcomes associated with hyponatremic encephalopathy from acute brain edema.[154,155] Most studies support excess drinking during the exercise as the major cause of the induced hyponatremia,[156,157] but it now appears that water retention under such conditions is also contributed to by SIADH as a result of multiple potential nonosmotic stimuli (e.g., volume depletion, nausea, increased cytokine levels).[158,159]

Unexplained or idiopathic causes account for a relatively small proportion of all cases of SIADH. Although the etiology of the syndrome may not be diagnosed initially in many cases, the numbers of patients in whom an apparent cause cannot be established after consistent follow-up over time are relatively few. However, an exception to this appears to be elderly patients who sometimes develop SIADH without any apparent underlying etiology.[160–162] Coupled with the significantly increased incidence of hyponatremia in geriatric patients,[7,13,14,93,163,164] this suggests that the normal aging process may be accompanied by abnormalities of regulation of AVP secretion that predispose to SIADH. Such an effect could potentially account for the fact that virtually all causes of drug-induced hyponatremia occur much more frequently in elderly patients.[82,165,166] In several series of elderly patients meeting criteria for SIADH, 40% to 60% remained idiopathic despite rigorous evaluation,[167–169] leading some to conclude that extensive diagnostic procedures were not warranted in such elderly patients if routine history, physical examination, and laboratory evaluation failed to suggest a diagnosis.[167]

Some well-known stimuli of AVP secretion are notable primarily because of their exclusion from Table 70.4. Despite unequivocal stimulation of AVP secretion by nicotine,[170] cigarette smoking has only rarely been associated with SIADH, and primarily in psychiatric patients who have several other potential causes of inappropriate AVP secretion.[39,171,172] This is in part because of chronic adaptation to the effects of nicotine, but also because the short half-life of AVP in plasma (approximately 15 min in humans[173]) limits the duration of antidiuresis produced by relatively short-lived stimuli such as smoking. Although nausea remains the most potent stimulus to AVP secretion known in man,[174] chronic nausea is rarely associated with hypoosmolality unless accompanied by vomiting with subsequent ECF solute depletion followed by ingestion of hypotonic fluids.[175] Similar to smoking, this is probably attributable to the short half-life of AVP, but also to the fact that most such patients are not inclined to drink fluids under such circumstances. However, hyponatremia can occur when such patients are infused with high volumes of hypotonic fluids. This is likely a factor contributing to the hyponatremia that often occurs in cancer patients who are receiving chemotherapy.[103] Finally, a causal relation between stress and SIADH has often been suggested, but never conclusively established. This underscores the fact that stress, independent of associated nausea, dehydration, or hypotension, is not a major stimulus causing sustained elevations of AVP levels in humans.[176]

Pathophysiology

Sources of Arginine Vasopressin Secretion

Disorders that cause inappropriate antidiuresis secondary to elevated plasma AVP levels can be subdivided into those associated with either paraneoplastic (ectopic) or pituitary AVP hypersecretion. Most ectopic production is from tumors, and there is conclusive, cumulative evidence that tumor tissue can, in fact, synthesize AVP: (1) tumor extracts have been found to possess antidiuretic hormone bioactivity and immunologically recognizable AVP and neurophysin, which is synthesized with AVP as part of a common precursor[177–179]; (2) electron microscopy has revealed that many tumors possess secretory granules; and (3) cultured tumor tissue has been shown to synthesize not only AVP[180] but also the entire AVP prohormone (provasopressin[181,182]). Although it is therefore clear that some tumors can produce AVP, it is not certain that all tumors associated with SIADH do so, because only about half of small cell carcinomas have been found to contain AVP immunoreactivity[183] and many of the tumors listed in Table 70.4 have not been studied as extensively as have bronchogenic carcinomas. The only nonneoplastic disorder that has been reported to possibly cause SIADH by means of ectopic AVP production is tuberculosis. However, this is based on studies of a single patient in whom extracts of tuberculous lung tissue were shown by bioassay to possess antidiuretic activity.[134]

Pituitary Arginine Vasopressin Secretion: Inappropriate Versus Appropriate

In the majority of cases of SIADH the AVP secretion originates from the posterior pituitary. However, this is also true of greater than 90% of all cases of hyponatremia, including patients with hypovolemic and hypervolemic hyponatremia.[12] This raises the question of what exactly is inappropriate AVP secretion[184,185]? It is well known that AVP secretion is most sensitively stimulated by increases in osmolality, but also occurs in response to a wide variety of nonosmotic stimuli, including hypotension, hypovolemia, nausea, hypoglycemia, angiotensin, and probably other stimuli yet to be discovered[186] (see Chapter 4). Consequently, AVP secretion in response to a hypovolemic stimulus such as hemorrhage is clearly physiologically "appropriate," but when it leads to symptomatic hyponatremia from secondary water retention it could be considered to be "inappropriate" for osmotic homeostasis. Despite such semantic difficulties, it is important that the criteria for diagnosing SIADH remain as originally described, specifically excluding other clinical conditions that cause known impairments in free water excretion even when these are mediated by a secondary stimulation of AVP secretion via known physiologic mechanisms (e.g., hypovolemia, hypotension, hypocortisolism, edema-forming states, hypothyroidism, etc.). Without maintaining these distinctions, arguable as some of them may be, the definition of SIADH would become too broad to retain any degree of practical clinical usefulness.

Although measurable plasma AVP levels are found in most patients with SIADH, they are rarely elevated into pathologic ranges in most cases, even those associated with ectopic AVP production from tumors. Rather, in the majority of cases of SIADH plasma AVP levels remain in "normal" physiologic ranges, which only become abnormal under hypoosmolar conditions when plasma AVP levels should be suppressed into unmeasurable ranges (Fig. 70.3). This is important for several reasons. First, the well known vasoconstrictive effects of AVP do not come into play until much higher plasma levels are achieved (20 to 80 pg per mL[187]), whereas maximal antidiuresis is achieved with much lower levels (5 to 10 pg per mL). Consequently, it is unlikely that any of the clinical manifestations of hyponatremia can be ascribed to vasopressor effects of AVP. In this regard, it is particularly worrisome that most animal models of induced hyponatremia have employed pharmacologic doses of AVP, which generally elevate plasma AVP levels well into vasopressor ranges, raising the possibility that some results of previous studies of experimental hyponatremia were due to activation of AVP V_1 vascular and hepatic receptors. Recent results that demonstrate the absence of mortality when hyponatremia is induced in animals using the V_2–selective agonist desmopressin (dDAVP),[63] or using vasopressin infusions that maintain plasma AVP levels at lower ranges,[188] emphasize the need to take potential vasopressor effects of vasopressin into consideration in the interpretation of past and future studies. Second, the presence of "normal" plasma AVP levels, or of only mildly elevated urine osmolalities, cannot be used as arguments against SIADH as an etiology for hyponatremia. Low but nonsuppressible levels of AVP can clearly cause sufficient impairment of free water excretion to produce hypoosmolality when exogenous fluid intakes are high, as in psychiatric patients with polydipsia.[189] Recent studies of patients with SIADH and hypopituitarism have measured high nonsuppressible levels of urinary aquaporin-2 excretion that correlated with their impaired water excretion, supporting persistent activation of AVP V_2 receptors as the cause of the water retention.[190]

Patterns of Arginine Vasopressin Secretion

Studies of plasma AVP levels in patients with SIADH during graded increases in plasma osmolality produced by hypertonic saline administration have suggested four patterns of secretion (Fig. 70.5): (1) random hypersecretion of AVP; (2) a "reset osmostat" system, whereby AVP is secreted at an abnormally low threshold of plasma osmolality but otherwise displays a normal response to relative changes in osmolality; (3) inappropriate hypersecretion below the normal threshold for AVP release, but normal secretion in response to osmolar changes within normal ranges of plasma osmolality; and (4) low or undetectable plasma AVP levels despite classic clinical characteristics of SIADH.[99,191] The first pattern simply represents unregulated AVP secretion, which is often, but not always, observed in patients exhibiting ectopic AVP production. Resetting of the osmotic threshold for AVP secretion has been well described with volume depletion[192,193] and also has been shown to occur in various edema-forming states, presumably as a result of decreases in EABV.[45,194,195] However, most patients with a reset osmostat are clinically euvolemic.[95,96] It has been suggested that chronic hypoosmolality itself may reset the intracellular threshold for osmoreceptor firing, but studies in animals have not supported a major role for this mechanism since chronic hyponatremia does not appear to significantly alter the osmotic threshold for AVP secretion.[196,197] Perhaps the best-known physiologic example of a reset osmostat for AVP secretion is the hypoosmolality and hyponatremia that occurs during late pregnancy. Despite intensive studies over many years to identify potential hormonal factors that might be responsible for this resetting, a single factor has not yet been identified,[198] although some studies have indicated that the placental hormone relaxin causes a stimulation of AVP and oxytocin secretion that closely resembles the reset osmostat pattern of AVP secretion.[199,200] Perhaps the most perplexing aspect of the reset osmostat pattern is its occurrence in patients with tumors, which suggests that some of these cases represent tumor-stimulated pituitary AVP secretion rather than paraneoplastic AVP secretion.[99,191,201] The pattern of SIADH that occurs without measurable AVP secretion is not yet well understood. This form of the syndrome may be attributable to the secretion of AVP with some bioactivity but altered immunoreactivity, to the presence of other circulating antidiuretic factors, to increased renal sensitivity to very low circulating levels of AVP, or possibly to constitutively activating mutations of the AVP V_2 receptor.[100] A sufficient number of patients with this form of the disorder has not been studied to form any basis for discrimination among these possibilities, but the positive response of one such patient to a vasopressin V_2-receptor antagonist suggests that at least some of these cases may represent increased renal sensitivity to low circulating levels of AVP.[202] Despite these well-described patterns of abnormal AVP secretion in SIADH, it is surprising that no correlation has been found between any of these four patterns and the various etiologies of the syndrome.[99]

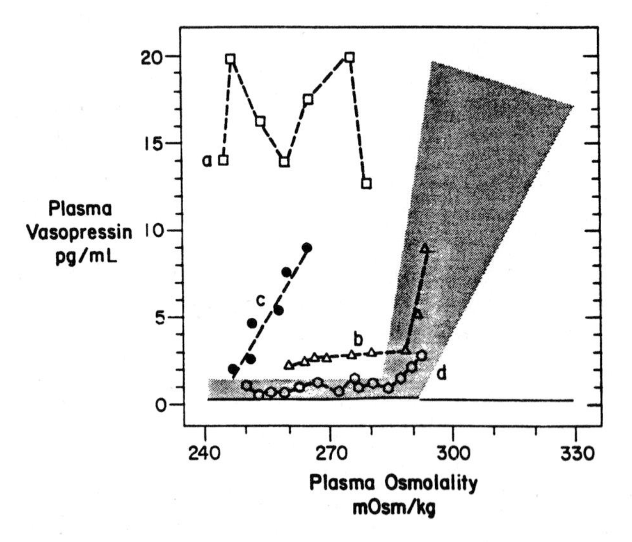

FIGURE 70.5 Schematic summary of different patterns of AVP secretion in patients with SIADH. Each line *(a–d)* represents the relation between plasma AVP and plasma osmolality of individual patients in whom osmolality was increased by infusion of hypertonic NaCl. The *shaded area* represents plasma AVP levels in normal subjects over physiologic ranges of plasma osmolality. (From Robertson GL. Thirst and vasopressin function in normal and disordered states of water balance. *J Lab Clin Med.* 1983;101:351–371, with permission.)

Stimuli to Arginine Vasopressin Secretion in Patients with SIADH

Regardless of the pattern of pituitary AVP secretion, and whether this represents an "inappropriate" or physiologically "appropriate" secretion, it is important to try to identify the cause(s) of the continued AVP secretion in patients with this disorder. Because of the variety of stimuli that can stimulate AVP secretion independent of osmolality, it seems logical to hypothesize that SIADH can be caused by continued nonosmotic stimulation of AVP secretion despite the presence of plasma hypoosmolality. The effect of hypovolemia to lower the threshold and increase the sensitivity of osmotically stimulated AVP secretion is well known, and this mechanism almost certainly accounts for the elevated plasma AVP levels in patients with edema-forming disorders in whom a decreased EABV activates baroreceptor-mediated AVP secretion.[42,43] Tumor interference with vagal pathways to brainstem baroreceptive centers could conceivably mimic or exaggerate such hypovolemic conditions, potentially accounting for the occurrence of a reset osmostat pattern of AVP secretion found in some patients with cancers. Recent reports of a 3% to 4% incidence of SIADH in patients with advanced head and neck malignancies represents a group in which some, although clearly not all,[203] of the hyponatremia might also be secondary to interference with vagal baroreceptor pathways.[204] However, not all cases of SIADH can be comfortably ascribed to nonosmotic stimuli because it is difficult to identify any such possible stimuli in many patients. Another possibility is that brain pathways conveying afferent signals that actively inhibit AVP secretion from hypothalamic magnocellular neurons may be impaired in some patients. Substantial data support the likelihood that hypoosmolality does not simply lead to decreased AVP secretion by virtue of absence of excitatory osmoreceptor inputs, but rather represents a state of active inhibition of the AVP-secreting neurons,[205] possibly via endogenous opioid[206] or gamma-amino butyric acid (GABA) pathways.[109,207] In this case, it would be easy to imagine that impairments or alterations in the activity of these inhibitory pathways might allow continued AVP secretion despite hypoosmolality. Although such abnormalities have not yet been identified, there is one clinical situation in which a decreased inhibitory tone to AVP neurons does clearly lead to enhanced AVP secretion: elderly patients have decreased AVP responses to orthostasis but exaggerated responses to osmotic stimuli.[208,209] The latter is presumably due to a diminution of inhibitory, as well as excitatory, inputs from brainstem baroreceptive centers to the hypothalamus, thereby producing an unopposed stimulation by osmotic stimuli from the anterior hypothalamus (Fig. 70.4). This phenomenon could contribute to the unusually high frequency of SIADH seen in elderly individuals.[7,13,14,163,164] Despite our lack of precise information about the mechanisms responsible for osmotically inappropriate AVP secretion, it seems certain that this will prove to be a heterogeneous group of processes rather a single dominant cause.[210]

Contribution of Natriuresis to the Hyponatremia of SIADH

Because of the original cases studied by Schwartz and Bartter, increased renal Na^+ excretion has been viewed as one of the cardinal manifestations of SIADH, indeed one which later became embedded in the requirements for its diagnosis.[2] However, next to the use of the term "inappropriate," probably no other aspect of SIADH has been so widely misinterpreted. Demonstration that the natriuresis accompanying administration of antidiuretic hormone is not due to AVP itself but rather to the volume expansion produced as a result of water retention was unequivocally shown by Leaf even before the description of the clinical occurrence of this disorder.[46] Subsequent metabolic balance studies demonstrated that excess urinary Na^+ excretion and a negative Na^+ balance occurred during the development of hyponatremia in patients with SIADH, but eventually urinary sodium excretion simply reflected daily sodium intake.[1] Patients appear to exhibit renal sodium wasting because they continue to excrete sodium despite being hyponatremic, but in reality they have simply achieved a new steady-state in which they are in neutral sodium balance, albeit at a lower serum $[Na^+]$. Although this interpretation is now supported by abundant clinical and experimental evidence, several important questions remain unanswered regarding natriuresis and hyponatremia: What physiologic and/or pathophysiologic mechanisms underlie the natriuresis? Is natriuresis in SIADH always secondary to AVP-induced water retention or is hyponatremia sometimes caused primarily by Na^+ losses? Even when natriuresis is secondary to water retention, can the natriuresis further aggravate the hyponatremia?

As described previously, studies of long-term antidiuretic-induced hyponatremia in both dogs and rats have indicated that a larger proportion of the hyponatremia is attributable to secondary Na^+ losses rather than to water retention.[75,76] However, it is important to appreciate that in these models the natriuresis actually did not worsen the hyponatremia, but rather allowed volume regulation of blood and ECF volumes to occur. Therefore, over long periods, what begins as a "purely" dilutional hyponatremia from water retention becomes a mixed hyponatremia in which urinary solute losses allow maintenance of equivalent levels of hyponatremia but with lesser degrees of volume expansion due to water retention. Much of the past difficulty in consistently demonstrating expanded plasma or ECF volumes in patients with SIADH using tracer dilution techniques[77–79] can probably be ascribed to this process. It has become clear that intrinsic renal mechanisms are capable of producing both diuresis and natriuresis in response to increases in renal perfusion pressures; this mechanism has been shown to underlie the renal escape from antidiuresis produced when AVP-infused animals are continually fluid loaded.[48] However, it has not yet been proved whether this mechanism is sufficiently sensitive to detect the relatively mild degrees of volume expansion that accompany dilutional hyponatremias. Another, not mutually exclusive, possibility is that the natriuresis is mediated via increases in circulating natriuretic peptides such as atrial natriuretic peptide (ANP) and brain natriuretic peptide (BNP). Most cases of SIADH have been shown to have elevated levels of these peptides into ranges that are capable of promoting renal sodium excretion.[49,50,211] The degree to which hyponatremia occurs primarily as a result of natriuresis has remained controversial over many years. Cerebral salt wasting (CSW) was first proposed by Peters in 1950[212] as an explanation for the natriuresis and hyponatremia that sometimes accompanies intracranial disease, particularly subarachnoid hemorrhage (SAH), in which up to one third of patients often develop hyponatremia. Following the first clinical description of SIADH in 1957, such patients were generally assumed to have hyponatremia secondary to AVP hypersecretion with a secondary natriuresis.[213] However, over the last decade, clinical and experimental data have suggested that some patients with SAH and other intracranial diseases may actually have a primary natriuresis leading to volume contraction rather than SIADH,[214–217] in which case the elevated measured plasma AVP levels may actually be physiologically appropriate for the degree of volume contraction present. The major clinical question as to the frequency of CSW as a cause of hyponatremia is dependent on the criteria used to assess the ECF volume status of these patients; opponents argue that there is insufficient evidence of true hypovolemia despite ongoing natriuresis,[218] whereas proponents argue that the combined measures that have traditionally been used to estimate ECF volume do in fact support the presence of hypovolemia in many cases.[219,220] With regard to the potential mechanisms underlying the natriuresis, both plasma and cerebrospinal fluid (CSF) ANP and BNP levels are clearly elevated in many patients with SAH,[217,221–223] and have been found to correlate variably with hyponatremia in patients with intracranial diseases.[217,223,224] However, because SIADH also is frequently associated with elevated plasma ANP and BNP levels, this finding alone does not prove causality. Ample precedent certainly exists for hyponatremia due to sodium wasting with secondary antidiuresis in Addison's disease, as well as diuretic-induced hyponatremia. Characteristic of these disorders, normalization of ECF volume with isotonic NaCl infusions restores plasma tonicity to normal ranges by virtue of shutting off secondary AVP secretion. If hyponatremia in patients with SAH occurred via a similar mechanism, it should also respond to this therapy. However, studies indicate that it does not. Nineteen patients with SAH were treated with large volumes of isotonic saline sufficient to maintain plasma volume at normal or slightly elevated levels, but despite removal of any volume stimulus to AVP secretion, 32% still developed hyponatremia in association with nonsuppressed plasma AVP levels, an incidence equivalent to that found in previous studies of SAH.[225] In contrast, other studies have demonstrated that mineralocorticoid therapy to inhibit natriuresis can reduce the incidence of hyponatremia in patients with subarachnoid hemorrhage[226]; such results are not unique to patients with intracranial diseases because a subset of elderly patients with SIADH have also been shown to respond favorably to mineralocorticoid therapy.[227] Although seemingly disparate, these types of results support the existence of disordered AVP secretion as well as a coexisting stimulus to natriuresis in many such patients. It seems most likely that SAH and other intracranial diseases represent a mixed disorder in which some patients have both exaggerated natriuresis and inappropriate AVP secretion; which effect predominates in terms of the clinical presentation will depend on their relative intensities as well as the effects of concomitant therapy. The possibility of ANP- or BNP-induced natriuresis aggravating hyponatremia is not confined to intracranial diseases, and it has been suggested that ectopic ANP production might contribute to, or even cause, the hyponatremia accompanying some small cell lung cancers.[228] In support of this, several studies have analyzed tumor cell lines from patients with hyponatremia and small cell lung carcinoma and found that many produced ANP or ANP mRNA in addition to, or in some cases instead of, AVP.[229–231] These data allow the possibility that some patients with tumors may also develop hyponatremia as a result of ectopic ANP secretion. However, in clinical studies of such patients, the hyponatremia appears to correlate more with the plasma AVP levels than the plasma ANP levels.[232] Consequently, it seems likely that such cases represent a mixture of inappropriate secretion of both hormones, analogous to patients with cerebral salt wasting, in which case the ANP and BNP could act to further exacerbate the secondary natriuresis produced primarily by AVP-induced water retention.

ADRENAL INSUFFICIENCY

The frequent occurrence of hyponatremia in patients with adrenal insufficiency was appreciated well before the discovery of the role of AVP in hypoosmolar disorders.[233] Incidences as high as 88% have been reported in patients with primary adrenal insufficiency, particularly during episodes of addisonian crisis.[234,235] This section summarizes the factors related to the development of hyponatremia in patients with adrenal insufficiency.

Etiology

The adrenal cortex produces many different types of corticosteroids, which can be broadly divided into three categories: glucocorticoids, mineralocorticoids, and androgens. Only the first two of these have been found to have significant effects on body fluid homeostasis. Disorders of impaired adrenal function can be divided into those in which the adrenal gland itself is damaged or destroyed, or primary adrenal insufficiency, and those in which the adrenal gland does not receive appropriate adrenocorticotropic hormone (ACTH) stimulation from the pituitary, or secondary adrenal insufficiency. Addison disease is the major cause of primary adrenal insufficiency and hypopituitarism is the best example of secondary adrenal insufficiency. The clinical presentation of these two types of adrenocortical insufficiency varies significantly, because adrenal destruction causes loss of both mineralocorticoids and glucocorticoids, whereas pituitary insufficiency causes only glucocorticoid insufficiency. This is because pituitary ACTH is not necessary for mineralocorticoid secretion, which is controlled primarily via the renin-angiotensin system. To understand the fluid and electrolyte abnormalities that accompany these disorders, the pathophysiology of hyponatremia due to mineralocorticoid and glucocorticoid deficiency must be considered separately.

Pathophysiology

Mineralocorticoid Deficiency

The absence of aldosterone impairs Na^+-K^+ exchange in the distal tubule. Because this defect occurs distally in the nephron, it cannot be completely compensated for by later Na^+

reabsorption, leading to the continued renal Na^+ excretion, or "salt wasting," that is the hallmark of primary adrenal insufficiency.[236] As long as sodium intake is sufficient to replace the ongoing renal losses, patients with mineralocorticoid insufficiency remain relatively stable. However, when sodium intakes are not sufficient, adrenally insufficient patients develop progressive hypovolemia, hyponatremia, and hyperkalemia, the classic fluid and electrolyte manifestations of addisonian crisis.[234,235] Proof that these effects were indeed caused primarily by the renal Na^+ losses was documented long ago by studies in animals[236,237] and addisonian patients,[238] which demonstrated that all of these abnormalities could be prevented by volume repletion with NaCl. However, the water retention of mineralocorticoid deficiency has multiple potential causes: (1) loss of aldosterone-mediated Na^+ reabsorption in the distal tubule impairs urinary dilution, similar to the use of thiazide diuretics; (2) ECF volume contraction as a result of the Na^+ losses causes increased fluid reabsorption in the proximal tubule with decreased delivery to the distal diluting segments of the nephron; and (3) ECF volume contraction also stimulates baroreceptor-mediated (i.e., nonosmotic) AVP secretion with resultant antidiuresis.

Numerous experimental studies have documented elevated plasma AVP levels despite hypoosmolality in adrenalectomized animals with mineralocorticoid insufficiency,[239–241] and the elevated AVP levels generally return to normal ranges following volume replacement with NaCl.[239] Proof that the elevations in plasma AVP levels were causally related to the water retention was provided by studies in which adrenalectomized rats replaced with only glucocorticoids were given a vasopressin V_2 receptor antagonist[242]; the antagonist significantly reduced urine osmolality in chronically, but not acutely, mineralocorticoid-deficient rats, consistent with hypovolemia-mediated stimulation of AVP secretion as a result of progressive Na^+ depletion over time. Conversely, AVP-independent effects appear to play some role in the water retention as well. Studies in adrenalectomized homozygous Brattleboro rats, which cannot synthesize AVP, have demonstrated normalization of urine dilution, free water clearance, and solute clearance following physiologic aldosterone, but not glucocorticoid, replacement.[243] These results demonstrate the contribution of multiple factors such as impaired urinary dilution due to the loss of aldosterone-mediated Na^+ reabsorption in the distal tubule, and increased proximal tubular fluid reabsorption as a result of hypovolemia, to the impaired water excretion of mineralocorticoid deficiency. The latter factor would be predicted to be reversed by volume repletion but not the former, possibly accounting for the observation that in some studies human patients with primary adrenal insufficiency still maintained higher urine osmolalities even under conditions of volume expansion,[244] although other studies in humans[238] and animals[245] have shown complete normalization of water excretion following volume expansion. Whatever the contribution of these additional factors, it nonetheless seems appropriate to conclude that the major mechanism responsible for the impaired water excretion of mineralocorticoid deficiency is hypovolemia-stimulated AVP secretion.

Glucocorticoid Deficiency

As described previously, isolated glucocorticoid deficiency generally occurs with pituitary disorders that impair normal ACTH secretion but leave other stimuli to aldosterone secretion intact. That glucocorticoid deficiency alone could also impair water excretion was recognized based on longstanding clinical observations that anterior pituitary insufficiency ameliorates, and sometimes even completely masks, the polyuria of patients with coexistent central diabetes insipidus.[246] It is not surprising, therefore, that hyponatremia occurs relatively frequently in hypopituitary patients without diabetes insipidus.[91,247,248] However, hypopituitary patients generally do not develop ECF volume contraction because they maintain adequate aldosterone secretion to prevent renal sodium wasting. Consequently, volume replacement with NaCl does not reverse the impaired water excretion of patients with secondary adrenal insufficiency as it does in primary adrenal insufficiency.[244]

Despite the lack of an apparent hypovolemia-mediated stimulus to AVP secretion, nonetheless nonosmotic AVP secretion has been strongly implicated in the impaired water excretion of glucocorticoid insufficiency. Elevated plasma AVP levels have clearly been documented in animals[249] and patients[101] with hypopituitarism (Fig. 70.6). Similarly, because primary adrenal insufficiency has components of both mineralocorticoid and glucocorticoid deficiency, adrenalectomized animals maintained only on physiologic replacement doses of mineralocorticoids also have been found to have inappropriately elevated plasma AVP levels.[250,251] That these elevated AVP levels were causally related to the impaired water excretion was again proved by studies using an AVP V_2 receptor antagonist, which demonstrated near normalization of urinary dilution in adrenalectomized mineralocorticoid-replaced rats.[242] However, as with mineralocorticoid deficiency, AVP-independent mechanisms have also been suggested to play a role in the impaired water excretion of glucocorticoid deficiency because Brattleboro rats maintained on aldosterone had somewhat decreased urine flow which increased following glucocorticoid replacement.[243] Because ECF volume depletion is generally not a manifestation of glucocorticoid deficiency, other factors must therefore be responsible for the AVP-independent aspects of the water retention. The possibility that glucocorticoids exerted direct effects on renal tubular epithelium, such that glucocorticoid insufficiency causes increased water permeability in the collecting tubules, even in the absence of AVP, has been suggested.[244] However, studies on isolated collecting tubules have failed to demonstrate any significant influence of glucocorticoids on water permeability of this tissue.[252] Consequently, the AVP-independent effects of

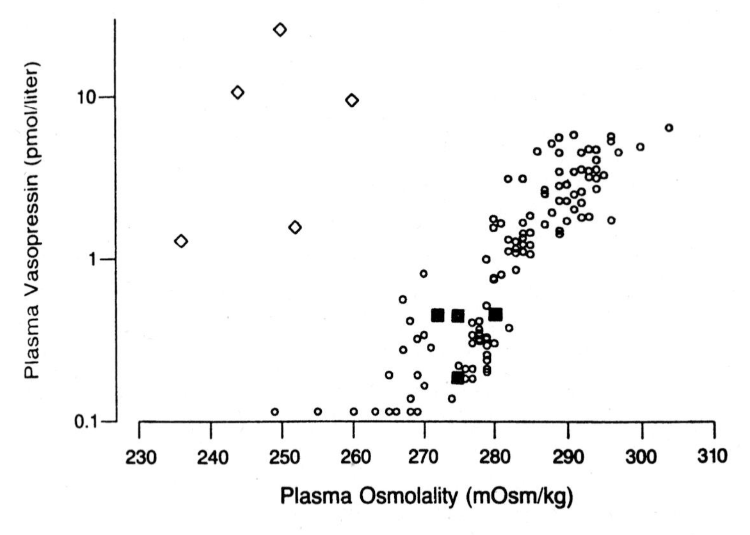

FIGURE 70.6 Plasma AVP levels as a function of plasma osmolality in patients with hypopituitarism and ACTH insufficiency. The *diamonds* show patients with untreated hypopituitarism and the *solid squares* the same patients after hydrocortisone therapy. The *open circles* depict AVP levels in normal subjects over physiologic ranges of plasma osmolality. In comparison with Figure 70.3, it is apparent that these patients would be indistinguishable from those with SIADH based on their plasma AVP-osmolality relation. (From Oelkers W. Hyponatremia and inappropriate secretion of vasopressin (antidiuretic hormone) in patients with hypopituitarism. *N Eng J Med.* 1989;321:492–496, with permission.)

glucocorticoid insufficiency remain poorly defined at the present time.

Regardless of the etiology of the AVP-independent defect in water excretion, the major mechanism responsible for the impaired water excretion of glucocorticoid deficiency appears to be nonosmotically stimulated AVP secretion. However, the stimulus to AVP secretion under these conditions also remains unclear. Studies of prolonged glucocorticoid insufficiency in dogs have shown an increased pulse pressure and decreased cardiac stroke volume,[250] and similar studies in rats have suggested decreases in cardiac index along with increased systemic vascular resistance.[251] Although these findings differ somewhat, in both cases they raise the possibility of hemodynamically mediated effects on AVP secretion. Alternatively, glucocorticoid deficiency might directly stimulate AVP secretion via two possible mechanisms. First, both clinical[253] and experimental[254] studies have shown a modest but significant effect of glucocorticoids to inhibit pituitary AVP secretion. Presumably this is mediated via glucocorticoid receptors that have been localized in magnocellular neurons[255]; interestingly, recent studies have shown that these receptors are increased during induced hypoosmolality, suggesting that glucocorticoids may play a role in the inhibition of AVP secretion under hypoosmolar conditions.[256] Second, in the absence of glucocorticoid feedback inhibition of the parvocellular AVP neurons that project to the median eminence rather than to the posterior pituitary, AVP content increases markedly in this area.[257,258] This presumably reflects increased secretion of AVP into the pituitary portal blood system in order to stimulate pituitary ACTH secretion.[259–262] Because the pituitary portal blood eventually drains into the systemic circulation, increased levels of AVP released from the median eminence could therefore increase plasma AVP levels sufficiently to produce some degree of inappropriate antidiuresis; it is important to remember that such levels need not be very high, but simply inappropriate for the plasma osmolality, as shown in Figures 70.3 and 70.6.

HYPOTHYROIDISM

Although hypothyroidism is considerably more common than adrenal insufficiency, hyponatremia secondary to hypothyroidism occurs much less frequently than hyponatremia from adrenal insufficiency. The infrequent occurrence of hyponatremia with hypothyroidism has led some to question whether hypothyroidism is in fact causally related to hyponatremia,[263] but this is likely a manifestation of the fact that impaired water excretion is only seen in more severely hypothyroid patients. Typically such patients are elderly and meet criteria for myxedema coma as a result of their altered mental status.[264,265] This section summarizes the factors related to the development of hyponatremia in patients with hypothyroidism.

Etiology

Similar to adrenal insufficiency, hypothyroidism can result from either dysfunction or damage to the thyroid gland itself, or primary hypothyroidism, or from inadequate thyroid-stimulating hormone (TSH) stimulation from the pituitary, or secondary hypothyroidism. Also similar to adrenal insufficiency, there can be significant differences in the presentation of these two disorders. However, because the only biologically active products of the thyroid gland are the hormones thyroxine (T_4) and triiodothyronine (T_3), in this case the clinical variations are due mainly to quantitative differences in the severity of the thyroid hormone deficiency rather than to qualitative differences in the nature of the hormone deficits. With moderate degrees of hypothyroidism, patients with both primary and secondary disease have similar signs and symptoms of thyroid hormone deficiency (e.g., cold intolerance, increased fatigue, dry skin, constipation, etc.), but generally only patients with primary hypothyroidism progress to more severe degrees of myxedema, including the life-threatening metabolic and neurologic abnormalities of myxedema coma. These extreme manifestations are virtually never seen with secondary hypothyroidism. This is because severe myxedema occurs only after plasma T_4 and T_3 levels have fallen to very low levels, often <1 μg per dL. This scenario can easily occur with primary hypothyroidism since in the absence of thyroid tissue there is no alternative source of thyroid hormone production. However, T_4 and T_3 levels never decrease as severely in hypopituitary patients who simply lack TSH, and frequently plasma levels remain just at or slightly below the lower limits of normal.[266] This likely reflects either some degree of constitutive thyroid hormone synthesis by the thyroid gland, or possibly low grade stimulation of TSH receptors by other circulating substances, analogous to the thyrotoxicosis produced by thyroid stimulating immunoglobulins in patients with Graves disease. Because hyponatremia is seen only in hypothyroid patients who have progressed to severe degrees of myxedema, it follows that this manifestation generally occurs in patients with primary hypothyroidism. When hyponatremia accompanies hypopituitarism it is usually a manifestation of secondary adrenal insufficiency from glucocorticoid deficiency rather than the coexisting hypothyroidism.[90,267]

Pathophysiology

Several studies have clearly confirmed abnormalities of water excretion in hypothyroid patients. However, in almost all cases, the abnormality was found to consist of a delayed excretion of water rather than major impairments in urinary dilution.[268–270] This was best shown in the studies of DeRubertis et al., in which near normal urinary dilution occurred following water loading in hypothyroid patients (Fig. 70.7), even though cumulative excretion of the water load in the hypothyroid patients lagged far behind that of euthyroid controls (39.8 ± 5.1% versus 78.7 ± 5.7%) after 2 hours.[269] Similar results have been found in studies of hypothyroid rats.[271,272] Experimental studies in hypothyroid animals have implicated decreases in renal blood flow and GFR as the primary factors responsible for the delayed water excretion. In particular, the relation between free water clearance and distal tubular Na^+ delivery was found to be identical in hypothyroid and euthyroid rats, suggesting that the observed impairments in water excretion were likely secondary to reduced delivery of glomerular filtrate to the distal nephron in the hypothyroid rats.[271] These results are consistent with findings of a decreased GFR in severely hypothyroid patients,[269,273,274] which is most likely due to decreased renal blood flow as a result of the compromised cardiac output and increased peripheral vascular resistance known to occur in severely hypothyroid patients.[275–277] Experimental studies have also supported this hypothesis because a variety of maneuvers that increase distal tubular fluid delivery (e.g., carbonic hydrase inhibition, isotonic saline infusion, and unilateral nephrectomy) all markedly increase free water clearance in hypothyroid rats.[271,278,279] Therefore, similar to patients with edema-forming states, hypothyroid patients have increased proximal Na^+ and water absorption as a result of decreased EABV with subsequent decreased delivery of tubular fluid to the distal diluting sites of the nephron, thereby accounting for much of their impaired rate of water excretion.

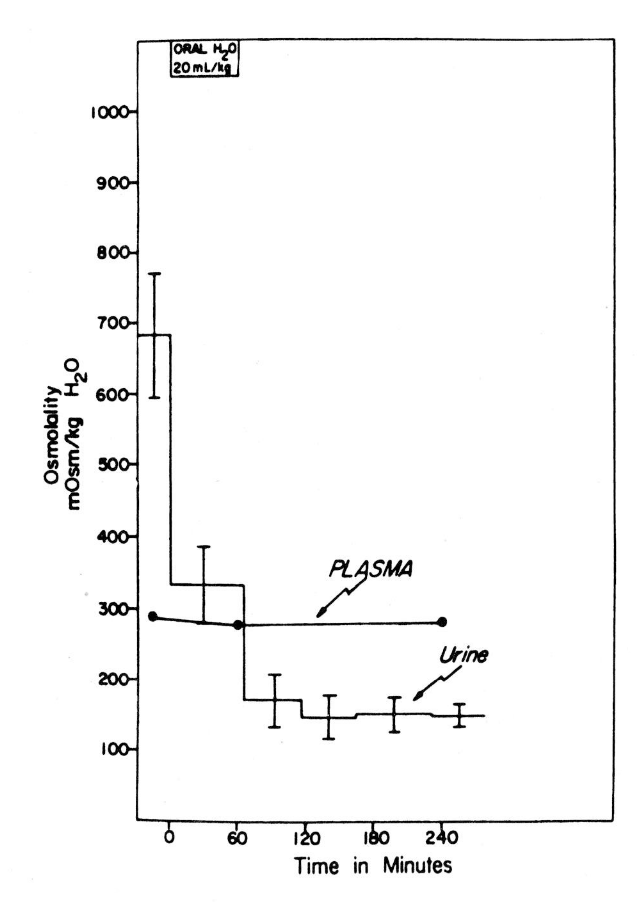

FIGURE 70.7 Mean plasma and urine osmolalities in 16 patients with untreated myxedema for 6 hours following an oral water load (20 mL per kg body weight). Urine osmolalities decreased significantly to <200 mOsm per kg H_2O by 4 hours after the water load, indicating fairly intact renal diluting mechanisms in these patients. (From Derubertis FR Jr, Michelis MF, Bloom ME, et al. Impaired water excretion in myxedema. *Am J Med.* 1971;51:41–53, with permission.)

As noted previously, patients with edema-forming states also have baroreceptor-mediated stimulation of AVP secretion that leads to further impairment of free water excretion by preventing maximal urinary dilution.[194] The results of some studies have supported a similar dual effect in hypothyroid patients as well. Fifteen of 20 patients studied by Skowsky and Kikuchi had elevated plasma AVP levels even after water loading, which then suppressed normally after the patients were made euthyroid.[270] Similarly, other investigators have found frankly elevated plasma AVP levels,[280,281] inappropriately normal levels despite plasma hypoosmolality,[281] or a decreased osmotic threshold for AVP secretion in hypothyroid patients.[282] Conversely, equal numbers of studies have failed to find evidence of inappropriately elevated plasma AVP levels, urine AVP secretion, or significantly altered osmotic thresholds for AVP secretion or urinary dilution in hypothyroid patients.[269,283–285] Consistent with these findings are several reported cases in which treatment with demeclocycline to antagonize renal AVP effects failed to increase serum [Na^+] or decrease urine osmolality in hyponatremic hypothyroid patients.[283,286] Experimental studies have also shown variable results. Hypothyroid rats have been reported to manifest higher plasma AVP levels than euthyroid rats after water loading.[272] However, hypothyroid Brattleboro rats appear to have similar defects in water excretion as rats with intact AVP secretion,[271] supporting a major role for AVP-independent mechanisms of impaired free water excretion in hypothyroid animals. Recent studies of hypothalamic AVP gene expression have failed to demonstrate upregulation of AVP synthesis in hypothyroid rats,[287] again arguing against a major stimulation of AVP secretion under these conditions, although the sensitivity of these methods for ascertaining small increases in hormone secretion and synthesis is limited. Perhaps the strongest argument against a major role for AVP-stimulated water retention in hypothyroidism has been the failure of any animal model of hypothyroidism to date to reproduce the degrees of hyponatremia commonly found in animal models of SIADH, adrenal insufficiency, and cardiac failure.

In light of the clinical and experimental observations to date, it has to be concluded that the major cause of impaired water excretion in hypothyroidism is an alteration in renal perfusion and GFR secondary to systemic effects of thyroid hormone deficiency on cardiac output and peripheral vascular resistance. Yet it must be recognized that severe hypothyroidism is a multisystem disease—just as the presentation of patients with SIADH will vary depending on the degree of volume adaptation that has occurred, it is hardly surprising that different results have been reported regarding the potential role of AVP in hypothyroidism depending on the individual characteristics of the cases studied. Therefore, in uncomplicated hypothyroidism there appears to be little elevation of plasma AVP levels, and any defects in water excretion are due primarily to effects on renal hemodynamics. As the hypothyroidism becomes more severe, EABV can decease sufficiently to stimulate AVP secretion secondarily via baroreceptor mechanisms. However, even in this case the elevated AVP levels may not be causally related to the impaired water excretion because several studies have suggested that hypothyroid animals are resistant to the effects of AVP based on decreased medullary cyclic AMP generation in response to AVP.[272,288] However, when cardiac function becomes severely compromised, as can occur with advanced myxedema, plasma AVP can become elevated sufficiently to override any renal resistance and cause an antidiuresis, which then contributes to the hemodynamic impairments of water excretion. Whether hyponatremia develops at any stage of disease progression depends on the relative balance between water intake and excretory capacity. Because maximal free water clearance decreases as these defects become more pronounced, this accounts for the increased incidence of hyponatremia as the severity of the underlying hypothyroidism worsens.

PRIMARY POLYDIPSIA

As discussed previously, excessive water intake is only rarely of sufficient magnitude to produce hyponatremia in the presence of normal renal function. However, it is often a significant factor contributing to hyponatremia in polydipsic patients, particularly those with underlying defects in free water excretion. In addition, because a positive water balance is required for the production of hyponatremia even under conditions of maximal antidiuresis in man and animals, an appreciation of the control mechanisms regulating water ingestion is important for understanding the development of hyponatremia in patients with SIADH and other hypoosmolar disorders.

Etiology

The most dramatic cases of primary polydipsia are seen in psychiatric patients, particularly in those with acute psychosis secondary to schizophrenia.[289–293] The prevalence of this disorder based on hospital admissions for acute symptomatic hyponatremia may have been underestimated, since studies of polydipsic psychiatric patients have shown a marked diurnal variation in serum [Na^+] (from 141 mEq per L at 7 AM to 130 mEq per L at 4 PM), suggesting that many such patients drink excessively during the daytime but then correct themselves via a water diuresis at night.[294] This and other considerations have led to defining this disorder as the psychosis-intermittent hyponatremia-polydipsia (PIP) syndrome. Polydipsia has been observed in up to 20% of psychiatric inpatients,[293] with incidences of intermittent hyponatremia ranging from 5% to 10%.[293,295,296] Despite the frequent occurrence of polydipsia in psychiatric patients, it is important to recognize that not all polydipsia is caused by psychiatric disease; infiltrative diseases such as CNS sarcoidosis[297] or critically placed brain tumors can also be associated with increased thirst and fluid ingestion. Consequently, polydipsic patients should be evaluated with a CT or MRI scan of the brain before concluding that excessive water intake is due to a psychiatric cause.

Pathophysiology

There is little question that excessive water intake alone can sometimes be sufficient to override renal excretory capacity and produce severe hyponatremia.[40,298] Although the water excretion rate of normal adult kidneys can exceed 20 L per day, maximum hourly rates rarely exceed 800 to 1,000 mL per hour. Recent studies of water loading in exercising athletes have indicated a similar peak urine excretion rate of 778 ± 39 mL per hour.[299] Because many psychiatric patients drink predominantly during the day or during intense drinking binges,[291,294,300,301] they can transiently achieve symptomatic levels of hyponatremia with total daily volumes of water intake less than 20 L if it is ingested sufficiently rapidly. This likely accounts for many of the cases in which such patients present with maximally dilute urine, accounting for as many as 50% of patients in some studies,[302] and correct quickly via a free water diuresis.[303] However, other cases have been found to meet the criteria for SIADH,[292,302,304–306] suggesting nonosmotically stimulated AVP secretion. As might be expected, in the face of much higher than normal water intakes, virtually any impairment of urinary dilution and water excretion can exacerbate the development of a positive water balance and thereby produce hypoosmolality. Hyponatremia has been reported in polydipsic patients taking thiazide diuretics[307,308] or drugs known to be associated with SIADH,[171,293,295,309–313] in association with smoking and presumed nicotine-stimulated AVP secretion[314–316] (although a consistent relation with smoking has not been found[172]), and adrenal insufficiency.[317] Acute psychosis itself can also cause AVP secretion,[290,318] which often appears to take the form of a reset osmostat.[189,291,305] It is therefore apparent that no single mechanism can completely explain the occurrence of hyponatremia in polydipsic psychiatric patients, but the combination of higher than normal water intakes plus even modest elevations of plasma AVP levels from a variety of potential sources appears to account for a significant portion of such cases.

Although patients with SIADH do not in general manifest the water intakes of patients with primary polydipsia, nonetheless continued water intake in the face of plasma hypoosmolality is inappropriate for maintenance of osmotic homeostasis. Analysis of daily fluid intakes of 91 hyponatremic patients showed an average fluid intake of 2.4 ± 0.2 L per 24 hours (Fig. 70.8),[41] which does not differ appreciably

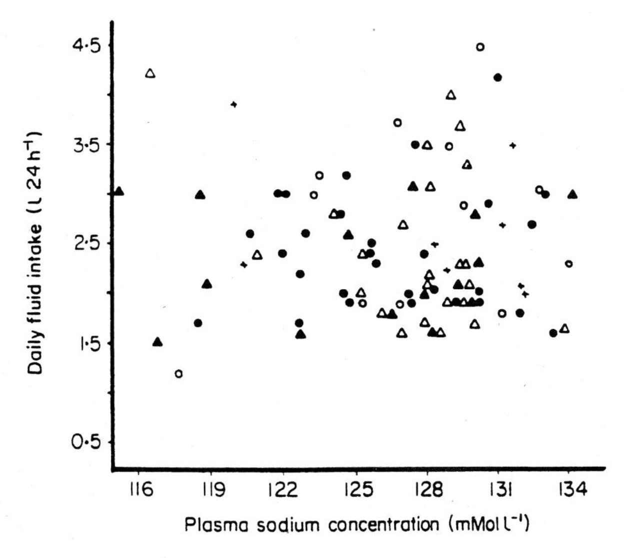

FIGURE 70.8 Daily fluid intakes of 91 hospitalized patients with hyponatremia of varying degrees and etiologies. Each point represents a single patient: *open circles*, SIADH; *open triangles*, cardiac failure; *closed circles*, volume contraction; *closed triangles*, cirrhosis; *pluses*, undiagnosed. Despite widely different etiologies for the hyponatremia, mean fluid intakes were equivalent in all groups of patients. (From Gross PA, Pehrisch H, Rascher W, et al. Pathogenesis of clinical hyponatremia: observations of vasopressin and fluid intake in 100 hyponatremic medical patients. *Eur J Clin Invest.* 1987;17:123–129, with permission.)

from earlier measured intakes of medical students or hospitalized cardiac patients (mean fluid intakes of 2.4 and 2.8 L per 24 hours, respectively[319]), or studies of middle-aged subjects (mean fluid intake of 2.1 L per 24 hours[320]). This consistent pattern of continued water intake in hyponatremic patients raises important questions as to its cause. Most, although not all, patients treated with dDAVP do not become hyponatremic because they limit their water intakes in the absence of stimulated thirst. This observation has suggested the possibility that patients with SIADH and other hypoosmolar disorders might have a coexisting defect in thirst regulation; recent studies have supported this possibility by showing a 20 mOsm per kg H_2O downward resetting of the thirst threshold in a group of patients with SIADH.[321] A potential underlying mechanism could be stimulation of thirst by central AVP hypersecretion, but to date only relatively small effects of AVP to stimulate thirst have been seen in a single species.[322] Alternatively, other animal studies have suggested that osmotic inhibition of thirst is a relatively weak phenomenon and easily overcome by a variety of nonhomeostatic stimuli causing drinking. Not only will rats increase intakes when fluids are made more palatable,[323] but rats made antidiuretic with dDAVP will continue to ingest such fluids to the point of extreme hypoosmolality and the degree of hypoosmolality achieved is proportional to the palatability of the fluid.[324] Analogous results have been obtained with schedule-induced polydipsia in rats treated with AVP.[325] In these examples drinking continued despite the production of both osmotic dilution and volume expansion, and despite drinking behavior sufficient to activate both oropharyngeal and gastrointestinal inhibitory factors that modulate fluid ingestion.[326] Obviously, drinking will not continue indefinitely in the absence of renal excretion until some factor causes inhibition of further intake, but before this happens it is possible to achieve plasma dilutions of 20% to 30%. In humans, similar to animals, there are many nonhomeostatic stimuli to drink fluids, including meal-associated drinking, oral habituation to various beverages, pleasurable sensations from palatable fluids, social interactions promoting fluid ingestion, and mouth dryness as a result of local factors, and these actually account for the major part of human fluid ingestion.[320] By themselves such stimuli are benign and simply lead to more frequent urination of dilute urine to excrete the increased fluids ingested. However, in the presence of pathologic conditions that impair renal water excretion they can lead to hyponatremia. Therefore, although direct inhibitory physiologic stimuli to thirst and fluid ingestion clearly exist, they appear to be relatively weak in comparison to excitatory stimuli and can be overridden by a variety of nonhomeostatic stimuli that cause continued fluid ingestion despite plasma hypoosmolality.[326] The extent to which such nonhomeostatic drinking versus disordered thirst regulation is responsible for the continued fluid ingestion in hypoosmolar disorders remains to be evaluated by more extensive clinical and experimental studies.

EXERCISE-ASSOCIATED HYPONATREMIA

Over the last three decades, exercise-associated hyponatremia (EAH) has emerged as an important complication of prolonged endurance physical activities. EAH is defined as the occurrence of hyponatremia in individuals engaged in prolonged physical activity who develop a serum or plasma [Na^+] below the normal reference range of the laboratory performing the test, generally less than 135 mEq per L.[327]

Etiology

The first cases of hyponatremia in association with prolonged physical activity were reported in 1985. Noakes et al. published a series of four case reports of athletes who developed hyponatremia (serum [Na^+] ranging from 115 to 125 mEq per L accompanied by fluctuating levels of consciousness, seizures, and pulmonary edema) during marathon footraces in South Africa.[150] Soon afterward, Hiller et al. reported that 27% of a prospectively studied cohort of the race finishers at the 1985 Hawaiian Ironman triathlon developed hyponatremia.[328] Since that time, well over 100 cases of EAH have been reported in the literature from physical exercise activities as diverse as forced military marches, prolonged hiking, and marathon, ultramarathon, and triathlon races, with several documented fatalities attributed to the hyponatremia.[329] Several prospective studies have been performed on subsets of runners participating in organized endurance activities and have documented incidences of hyponatremia from 13% to 29%.[151,330–332] Interestingly, for all studies in which sex differences have been examined, the incidence of hyponatremia has been found to be substantially higher in female athletes, ranging from 22% to 45%.[151,331,332] From the reported studies to date, it is clear that EAH can occur either during physical activity or within the 24-hour period after the activity, and most commonly occurs with prolonged physical activity generally lasting longer than 4 hours (although a few cases have been reported with physical activity of shorter durations[333]).

Pathophysiology

From the very first reports of EAH there has been a divergence of opinion regarding the underlying pathophysiology. Noakes has proposed that most cases of EAH represent a dilutional hyponatremia secondary to excess fluid ingestion during physical activity, similar to primary polydipsia,[156] whereas Hiller has implicated a depletional hyponatremia secondary to massive sodium losses from sweating during prolonged physical activity, especially in hot climates.[334] Multiple lines of evidence now strongly support the development of a dilutional hyponatremia from excess water retention as the primary cause of most of these cases. First, in virtually all studies where body weight has been recorded before and after exercise, there has been a consistent inverse relation between weight and serum [Na^+], indicative of fluid retention. This is best illustrated in the data from the New Zealand Ironman triathlon in 1997 (Fig. 70.9), in which the most severe hyponatremia occurred in athletes who actually gained weight during this event.[151] Second, high levels of fluid intake have been recorded in many of the athletes who develop EAH, often far in excess of the maximal renal excretory capacity of 800 to 1,000 mL per hour, and studies quantifying fluid intake have shown a significant negative correlation between ingested volumes and serum [Na^+].[331] Although fluid loses from sweating can be substantial during

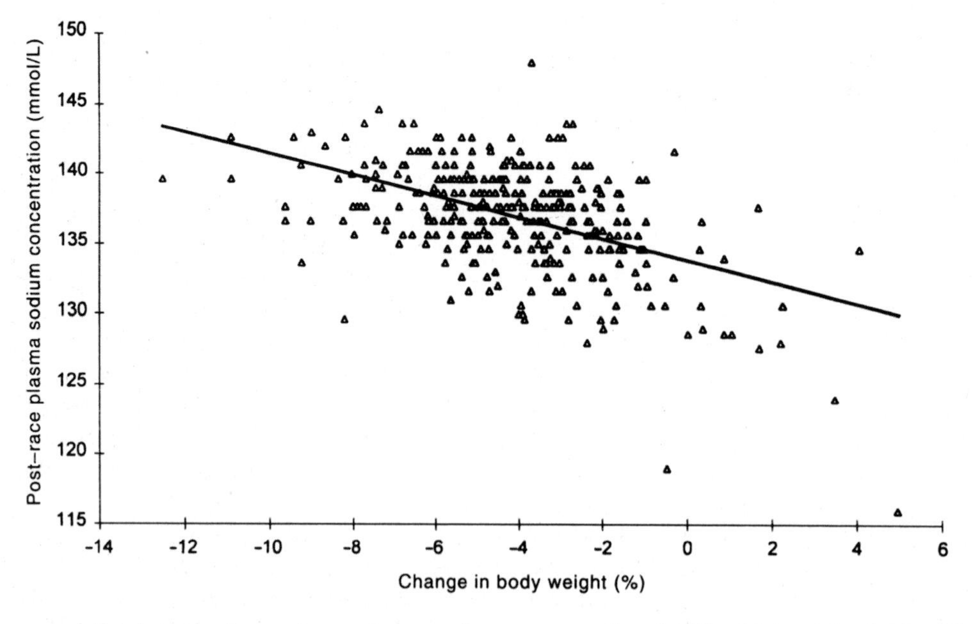

FIGURE 70.9 Inverse relation between the post-race plasma sodium concentrations in 350 athletes at the finish of the 1997 New Zealand Ironman triathlon as a function of changes in body weight during the race. (From Speedy DB, Noakes TD, Rogers IR, et al. Hyponatremia in ultradistance triathletes. *Med Sci Sports Exerc.* 1999;31(6):809–815, with permission.)

intense physical activity, this pattern of weight change suggests that fluid ingestion often exceeds the sum of fluid losses from renal excretion and sweating in EAH. Third, clinical evidence of volume depletion is not characteristic of most individuals who develop EAH (e.g., hyponatremic runners from the Houston marathon in 2000 manifested lower levels of BUN rather than developing a prerenal azotemia[331]). Fourth, two balance studies have been done on runners who developed EAH following ultramarathon races in comparison to a subset of normonatremic runners in these races.[335,336] Both of these studies showed that over a 9- to 24-hour period after the race, the hyponatremic runners corrected their serum [Na^+] via a free water diuresis of 1.3 to 3.0 L, indicating the development of water retention during the race, whereas the normonatremic runners retained 0.5 to 2.7 L, indicating the development of dehydration during the race. Both groups of runners had moderate positive sodium balances ranging from 88 to 153 mEq, indicating net sodium losses during the race, but the levels of sodium retention were not different between the hyponatremic and normonatremic runners.

Although the above data clearly implicate fluid retention as the major cause of EAH, additional data do not fully support the concept that this is solely due to excess drinking. A retrospective review of the U.S. Army inpatient data system from 1996–1997 revealed 17 cases of hyponatremia with a mean serum [Na^+] of 122 ± 5 mEq per L.[152] Virtually all of the cases occurred in the South during hot summer months, and most occurred in the first 4 weeks of military training. The majority presented with neurologic symptoms and had documented water intakes of greater than 2 quarts per hour. One recruit died from cerebral and pulmonary edema. Although these cases were all classified as due to overhydration on clinical grounds, detailed studies as to causation were not done. However, a more informative controlled study under similar conditions was performed earlier in Israel. Seventeen young males were studied during a 24-hour endurance march with ad libitum fluid ingestion. Serum [Na^+] levels decreased and were inversely related to total fluid intake, strongly suggesting a dilutional hyponatremia.[337] Despite the hyponatremia and a measured expanded plasma volume (+16%), maximal urine outputs were only 4 mL per minute with urine osmolalities of approximately 200 mOsm per kg H_2O, indicative of an inappropriate antidiuresis. Similarly instructive is a retrospective review of 44 hikers in the Grand Canyon who required medical treatment and had electrolytes measured in 1993.[153] Seven (16%) of the cases had hyponatremia, with serum [Na^+] ranging from 109 to 127 mEq per L; five of the seven had serious neurologic symptoms (three had seizures, two were disoriented) and had documented fluid intakes greater than the normonatremic patients (7.4 L versus 3.6 L), including sports drinks (4.3 L versus 0.5 L). Of particular significance, urine measurements showed osmolalities of 476 to 609 mOsm per kg H_2O and sodium levels of 36 to 120 mEq per L. A related study in Israel reported seven patients who developed hyponatremia (serum [Na^+] = 115 to 123) after moderate exercise with urine sodium levels of 74 to 122 mEq per L.[338] Most of these patients therefore met criteria for a diagnosis of SIADH, assuming the absence of thyroid and adrenal deficiencies, which are unlikely in young healthy individuals. Although SIADH had been dismissed in some reports because measured AVP levels were not "high," in this and other studies[158,159] it is clear that the plasma AVP levels were not suppressed in athletes with EAH, and consequently were inappropriate for their plasma osmolalities. It therefore seems very likely that EAH is caused by a combination of increased fluid intake in the setting of impaired renal excretory capacity during exercise. To what degree the decreased renal excretory capacity is secondary to renal hemodynamic changes, which can be marked during prolonged exercise, versus AVP-induced antidiuresis remains to be ascertained. Also unknown is the stimulus of AVP secretion during exercise. Although exercise itself is a mild stimulus of AVP secretion,[339] it is likely that hypovolemia from sweat sodium losses as well as nonhomeostatic stimuli (e.g., nausea, hypoglycemia, hypoxia, stress, increased cytokines from rhabdomyolysis) also are contributory.[158,159] The degree to which AVP secretion is stimulated, and whether it can be suppressed with sufficient fluid ingestion, will determine each individual's susceptibility to EAH as a result of fluid ingestion both before and after physical activity. Therefore, similar to the hyponatremia of schizophrenic patients, no single mechanism likely can completely explain the occurrence of hyponatremia in EAH, but the combination of higher than normal fluid intakes plus even modest elevations of plasma AVP levels from a variety of potential sources during prolonged physical activity appears to account for the majority of such cases.[340,341]

It is interesting to consider why EAH was not recognized prior to 1985. Noakes has drawn attention to the close temporal relationship between the recent reports of hyponatremia and changes in the conduct of endurance races.[156] First, these events became increasingly popular in the 1980s with large numbers of competitors, including competitors with lower fitness levels and hence longer running times. Second, multiple support stations to provide athletes with fluid at more frequent intervals during the race were introduced; prior to this time, fluid ingestion during prolonged exercise was considered unnecessary and possibly detrimental to performance. The convergence of these two developments is that athletes have more opportunity to drink during the events, and particularly the slower (i.e., novice) athletes. In support of this hypothesis, multiple studies have identified duration of time during races along with increased fluid consumption and weight gain as risk factors for the development of EAH.[331,332] Although female sex has also been frequently identified as a risk factor, a recent report from the 2002 Boston marathon has suggested that this variable might be explained by the lower body mass index (BMI) of female athletes, thus rendering them more susceptible to increased dilutional effects of excess fluid retention because of a smaller total body water volume.[332]

CLINICAL MANIFESTATIONS OF HYPOOSMOLAR DISORDERS

Regardless of the etiology of hypoosmolality, the clinical manifestations are similar. Nonneurologic symptoms are relatively uncommon, but a number of cases of rhabdomyolysis have been reported,[342,343] presumably secondary to osmotically induced swelling of muscle fibers. Hypoosmolality is primarily associated with a broad spectrum of neurologic manifestations, ranging from mild nonspecific symptoms (e.g., headache, nausea) to more significant disorders (e.g., disorientation, confusion, obtundation, focal neurologic deficits, and seizures).[344–346] This neurologic symptom complex has been termed hyponatremic encephalopathy[347] and primarily reflects brain edema resulting from osmotic water shifts into the brain because of decreased effective plasma osmolality.[348] Significant neurologic symptoms generally do not occur until the serum [Na^+] falls below 125 mEq per L, and the severity of symptoms can be roughly correlated with the degree of hypoosmolality.[344,345] However, individual variability is marked, and for any single patient, the level of serum [Na^+] at which symptoms appear cannot be predicted with great accuracy. Much of this variability can be understood within the framework provided by the process of brain volume regulation (Fig. 70.1), as discussed previously.[71,72] Although most of the neurologic symptoms associated with acute hyponatremia are caused by brain edema as a result of osmotic water movement into the CNS, a potential exception is the development of seizure activity, which may possibly be caused or aggravated by increased brain ECF concentrations of the excitatory amino acids glutamate and aspartate as a result of cellular extrusion of these osmolytes during the process of brain volume regulation to hyponatremia.[68,349]

It is also well known from animal studies that the rate of fall of serum [Na^+] is often more strongly correlated with morbidity and mortality than is the actual magnitude of the decrease.[344] This is due to the fact that the volume-adaptation process takes a finite period of time to complete; the more rapid the fall in serum [Na^+], the more brain edema will be accumulated before the brain is able to lose solute and along with it part of the increased water content. These effects are responsible for the much higher incidence of neurologic symptoms, as well as the higher mortality rates, in patients with acute hyponatremia than in those with chronic hyponatremia.[344,350] This phenomenon also likely underlies the observation that the most dramatic cases of death due to hyponatremic encephalopathy have generally been reported in postoperative patients in whom hyponatremia often develops rapidly as a result of intravenous infusion of hypotonic fluids,[18,351] or in exercise-induced hyponatremia during endurance races or forced marches as a result of excess water ingestion.[152,352,353] In such cases, nausea and vomiting are frequently overlooked as potential early signs of increased intracranial pressure in acutely hypoosmolar patients. Because hypoosmolality does not cause known direct effects on the gastrointestinal tract, the presence of unexplained nausea or vomiting in a hypoosmolar patient should be assumed to be of CNS origin and the patient treated for symptomatic hypoosmolality as described in the subsequent text. A recent study of runners in a marathon race found that vomiting was the only symptom that differentiated hyponatremia from other causes of exercise-associated collapse in this group.[331] Similarly, critically ill patients with unexplained seizures should be rapidly evaluated for possible hyponatremia, since as many as one third of such patients have been found to have serum [Na^+] less than 125 mEq per L as a contributory cause of the seizure activity.[354]

Underlying neurologic disease also affects the level of hypoosmolality at which CNS symptoms appear; moderate hypoosmolality is generally of little concern in an otherwise healthy patient, but can cause morbidity in a patient with an underlying seizure disorder. Nonneurologic metabolic disorders (e.g., hypoxia,[355] acidosis, hypercalcemia) can similarly affect the level of plasma osmolality at which CNS symptoms occur.

In the most severe cases of hyponatremic encephalopathy, death results from respiratory failure after tentorial cerebral herniation and brainstem compression. Studies of patients with severe postoperative hyponatremic encephalopathy have indicated a high incidence of hypoxia, and one fourth of these patients manifested hypercapnic respiratory failure, the expected result of brainstem compression, but three fourths had pulmonary edema as the apparent cause of the hypoxia.[356] Studies of acute hyponatremia after endurance races have similarly shown hypoxia and pulmonary edema in association with brain edema.[149,155] These results therefore suggest the possibility that hypoxia from noncardiogenic pulmonary edema may represent an early sign of developing cerebral edema even before the swelling progresses to the point of brainstem compression and tentorial herniation. Some clinical studies have also suggested that menstruating women[351] and young children[357] may be particularly susceptible to the development of neurologic morbidity and mortality during hyponatremia, especially in the acute postoperative setting.[347] However, other studies failed to corroborate these findings.[358,359] Consequently, the true clinical incidence as well as the underlying mechanisms responsible for these catastrophic cases remains to be determined.

Once the brain has volume-regulated via solute losses, thereby reducing brain edema, neurologic symptoms are not as prominent and may even be virtually absent. This accounts for the fairly common finding of relatively asymptomatic patients despite severe levels of hyponatremia.[17,345] Despite this powerful adaptation process, chronic hyponatremia is frequently associated with neurologic symptomatology, albeit milder and more subtle in nature. A recent report found a high incidence of symptoms in 223 patients with chronic hyponatremia as a result of thiazide administration: 49% had malaise or lethargy, 47% had dizzy spells, 35% had vomiting, 17% had confusion/obtundation, 17% experienced falls, 6% had headaches, and 0.9% had seizures.[360] Although dizziness can potentially be attributed to a diuretic-induced hypovolemia, symptoms such as confusion, obtundation, and seizures are more consistent with hyponatremic symptomatology. Because thiazide-induced hyponatremia can be readily corrected by stopping the thiazide and/or administering sodium, this represents an ideal situation in which to assess improvement in hyponatremia symptomatology with normalization of the serum [Na^+]; in this study, all of these symptoms improved with correction of the hyponatremia. This is one of the best examples demonstrating reversal of the symptoms associated with chronic hyponatremia by correction of the hyponatremia, because most of the patients in this study did not have underlying comorbidities that might complicate interpretation of their symptoms, as is often the case in patients with SIADH.

Even in patients adjudged to be "asymptomatic" by virtue of a normal neurologic exam, accumulating evidence suggests that there may be previously unrecognized adverse effects as a result of chronic hyponatremia. In one study, 16 patients with hyponatremia secondary to SIADH in the range of 124 to 130 mEq per L demonstrated a significant gait instability that normalized after correction of the hyponatremia to normal ranges.[361] The functional significance of the gait instability was illustrated in a study of 122 patients with a variety of levels of hyponatremia, all judged to be "asymptomatic" at the time of their visit to an emergency department (ED). These patients were compared with 244 age-, sex-, and disease-matched controls also presenting to the same ED during the same time period. Researchers found that 21% of the hyponatremic patients presented to the ED because of a recent fall, compared to only 5% of the controls; this difference was highly significant and remained so after multivariable adjustment.[361] Consequently, this study clearly documented an increased incidence of falls in so-called "asymptomatic" hyponatremic patients.

The clinical significance of the gait instability and fall data were further evaluated in a study that compared 553 patients with fractures to an equal number of age- and sex-matched controls. Hyponatremia was found in 13% of the patients presenting with fractures compared to only 4% of the controls.[362] Similar findings have been reported in a 364 elderly patients with large-bone fractures in New York,[363] and in 1,408 female patients with early chronic renal failure in Ireland.[364] More recently published studies have shown that hyponatremia is associated with increased bone loss in experimental animals and a significant increased odds ratio for osteoporosis of the femoral neck (OR, 2.87; $P < .003$) in humans over the age of 50 in the NHANES III database.[365] Thus, the major clinical significance of chronic hyponatremia may lie in the increased morbidity and mortality associated with falls and fractures in the elderly population.

THERAPY OF HYPOOSMOLAR DISORDERS

Correction of hyponatremia is associated with markedly improved neurologic outcomes in patients with severely symptomatic hyponatremia. In a retrospective review of patients who presented with severe neurologic symptoms and serum [Na^+] less than 125 mEq per L, prompt therapy with isotonic or hypertonic saline resulted in a correction in the range of 20 mEq per L over several days and neurologic recovery in almost all cases. In contrast, in patients who were treated with fluid restriction alone, there was very little correction over the study period (less than 5 mEq per L over 72 hours), and the neurologic outcomes were much worse, with most of these patients either dying or entering a persistently vegetative state.[366] Consequently, based on this and many similar retrospective analyses, prompt therapy to rapidly increase the serum [Na^+] represents the standard of care for treatment of patients presenting with severe life-threatening manifestations of hyponatremia.

As discussed previously, chronic hyponatremia is much less symptomatic as a result of the process of brain volume regulation. Because of this adaptation process, chronic hyponatremia is arguably a condition that clinicians feel they may not need to be as concerned about, which has been reinforced by the common usage of the descriptor asymptomatic hyponatremia for many such patients. However, as discussed previously, it is clear that many such patients very often do have neurologic symptoms, even if milder and more subtle in nature, including headaches, nausea, mood disturbances, depression, difficulty concentrating, slowed reaction times, unstable gait, increased falls, confusion, and disorientation.[361] Consequently, all patients with hyponatremia who manifest any neurologic symptoms that could possibly be related to the hyponatremia should be considered as potential candidates for treatment of their hyponatremia, regardless of the chronicity of the hyponatremia or the level of serum [Na^+].

Initial Evaluation

An approach to the initial evaluation and therapy of patients presenting with hyponatremia is summarized in Figure 70.10. The importance of appropriate initial evaluation and diagnosis cannot be overemphasized, as multiple studies have documented a high frequency of diagnosis- and treatment-related errors in the management of hyponatremic hospitalized patients.[367,368] Once true hypoosmolality is verified, the ECF volume status of the patient should be assessed by careful clinical examination. If fluid retention is present, the treatment of the underlying disease should take precedence over correction of plasma osmolality. Often this involves treatment with diuretics, which should simultaneously improve plasma tonicity by virtue of stimulating excretion of hypotonic urine. If hypovolemia is present, the patient must be considered to have depletion-induced hypoosmolality, in which case volume repletion with isotonic

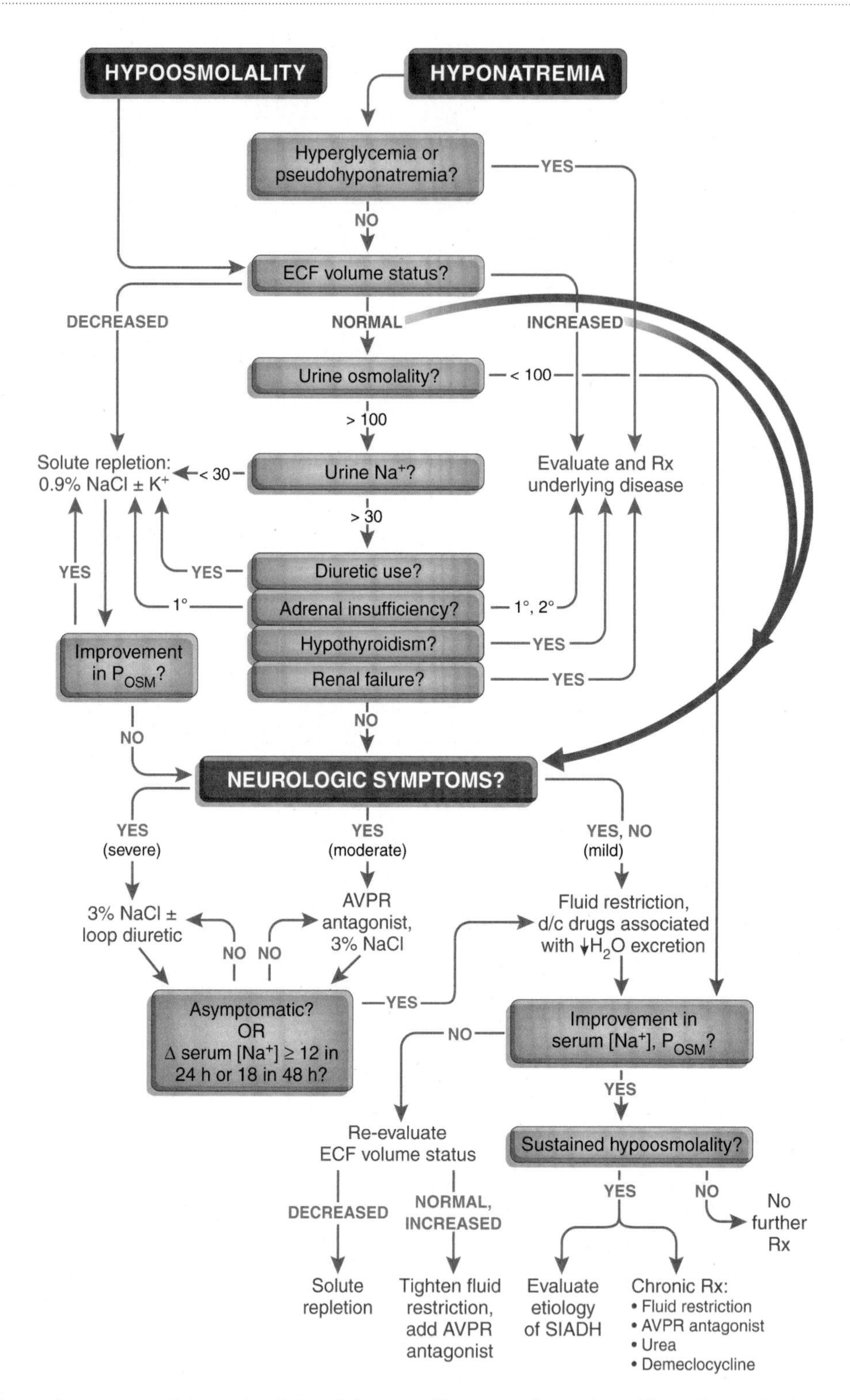

FIGURE 70.10 Schematic summary of the evaluation and therapy of hypoosmolar patients. The *red arrow* in the center emphasizes that the presence of central nervous system dysfunction due to hyponatremia should always be assessed immediately, so that appropriate therapy can be started as soon as possible in symptomatic patients while the outlined diagnostic evaluation is proceeding. (From Verbalis JG. Hyponatremia and hypo-osmolar disorders. In: Greenberg A, Cheung AK, Coffman TM, Falk RJ, Jennette JC, eds. *Primer on Kidney Diseases*. Philadelphia: Saunders Elsevier; 2009: 52–59, with permission.)

saline (0.9% NaCl) at a rate appropriate for the estimated fluid deficit should be initiated (see Chapter 66). If diuretic use is known or suspected, the isotonic saline should be supplemented with potassium (30–40 mEq per L) even if serum $[K^+]$ is not low, because of the propensity of such patients to develop total body potassium depletion. Most often, the hypoosmolar patient is clinically euvolemic, in which case the evaluation should then proceed to the measurement of urine osmolality and urine $[Na^+]$. Several situations will dictate reconsideration of solute depletion as a potential diagnosis, even in a patient without clinically apparent hypovolemia. These include: (1) a urine $[Na^+]$ less than 30 mEq per L,[89] (2) a history of recent diuretic use, and (3) any suggestion of primary adrenal insufficiency. Whenever a possibility of depletion-induced, rather than dilution-induced, hypoosmolality exists, it is most appropriate to treat the patient initially with isotonic saline, regardless of whether clinical signs of hypovolemia are present or not. An improvement in, and eventual correction of, the hyponatremia verifies solute and volume depletion. On the other hand, if the patient has SIADH rather than solute depletion, no significant harm will be done by administration of a limited volume (e.g., 1–2 L) of isotonic saline, because patients with SIADH simply excrete excess infused or ingested NaCl without significantly changing their plasma osmolality.[1] However, in the absence of an initial positive response, continued infusion of isotonic saline should be avoided because over longer periods of time sufficient free water can be retained to further lower the serum $[Na^+]$.[369]

The approach to patients with euvolemic hypoosmolality will vary according to the clinical situation (see Fig. 70.10). A patient who meets all the essential criteria for SIADH but has a low urine osmolality should be observed on a trial of modest fluid restriction. If the hypoosmolality is attributable to transient SIADH or severe polydipsia, the urine will remain dilute and the plasma osmolality will be fully corrected as free water is excreted. If, however, the patient has the reset osmostat form of the disorder, then the urine will become concentrated at some point before the plasma osmolality and serum $[Na^+]$ return to normal ranges. If either primary or secondary adrenal insufficiency is suspected, glucocorticoid replacement should be initiated immediately after the completion of a rapid ACTH stimulation test.[370,371] A prompt water diuresis after initiation of glucocorticoid treatment strongly supports a diagnosis of glucocorticoid deficiency.[372] However, absence of a quick response does not necessarily negate this diagnosis because several days of glucocorticoid replacement are sometimes required for normalization of plasma osmolality.[90] If hypothyroidism is suspected, thyroid function tests should be conducted including a plasma TSH level; usually replacement therapy is withheld pending these results unless the patient is obviously myxedematous. If renal failure is present in a patient with hypoosmolality, a more extensive evaluation of renal function will be necessary before deciding what course of treatment is most appropriate.

Currently Available Therapies for Treatment of Hyponatremia

Conventional management strategies for hyponatremia range from saline infusion and fluid restriction to pharmacologic measures to adjust fluid balance. Consideration of treatment options should always include an evaluation of the benefits as well as the potential toxicities of any therapy, and must be individualized for each patient.[373] It should always be remembered that sometimes simply stopping treatment with an agent that is associated with hyponatremia is sufficient to reverse a low serum $[Na^+]$ (see Fig. 70.10).

Isotonic Saline

The treatment of choice for depletional hyponatremia (i.e., hypovolemic hyponatremia) is isotonic saline ($[Na^+] = 154$ mEq per L) to restore ECF volume and ensure adequate organ perfusion. This initial therapy is appropriate for patients who either have clinical signs of hypovolemia, or in whom a urine Na^+ concentration is <30 mEq per L. However, this therapy is ineffective for dilutional hyponatremias such as SIADH,[1] and continued inappropriate administration of isotonic saline to a euvolemic patient may worsen their hyponatremia,[369] and/or cause fluid overload. Although isotonic saline may improve the serum $[Na^+]$ in some patients with hypervolemic hyponatremia, their volume status will generally worsen with this therapy, so isotonic saline should be avoided in such patients unless the hyponatremia is profoundly symptomatic.

Hypertonic Saline

Acute hyponatremia presenting with severe neurologic symptoms is life-threatening, and should be treated promptly with hypertonic solutions, typically 3% NaCl ($[Na^+] = 513$ mEq per L), as this represents the most reliable method to quickly raise the serum $[Na^+]$. A continuous infusion of hypertonic NaCl is usually utilized in inpatient settings. Various formulae have been suggested for calculating the initial rate of infusion of hypertonic solutions,[94] but until now there has been no consensus regarding optimal infusion rates of 3% NaCl. One of the simplest methods to estimate an initial 3% NaCl infusion rate utilizes the following relationship[373]:

Patient's weight (kg) × desired correction rate (mEq/L/h) = infusion rate of 3% NaCl (mL/h)

Depending on individual hospital policies, the administration of hypertonic solutions may require special considerations (e.g., placement in the ICU, sign-off by a consultant, etc.), which each clinician needs to be aware of in order to optimize patient care.

An alternative option for more emergent situations is administration of a 100 mL bolus of 3% NaCl, repeated once if there is no clinical improvement within 30 minutes, which has been recommended by a consensus conference organized to develop guidelines for prevention and treatment of EAH.[329] Injecting this amount of hypertonic saline intravenously raises the serum [Na^+] by an average of 2 to 4 mEq per L, which is well below the recommended maximal daily rate of change of 10 to 12 mEq per 24 hours or 18 mEq per 48 hours.[374] Because the brain can only accommodate an average increase of approximately 8% in brain volume before herniation occurs, quickly increasing the serum [Na^+] by as little as 2 to 4 mEq per L in acute hyponatremia can effectively reduce brain swelling and intracranial pressure.[375]

Many physicians are hesitant to use hypertonic saline in patients with chronic hyponatremia, because it can cause an overly rapid correction of serum sodium levels that can lead to the osmotic demyelination syndrome (ODS),[19] as discussed in the following section. Nonetheless, this remains the treatment of choice for patients with severe neurologic symptoms, even when the time course of the hyponatremia is nonacute or unknown. The administration of hypertonic saline is generally not recommended for most patients with edema-forming disorders because it acts as a volume expander and may exacerbate volume overload; consequently, as with isotonic NaCl, hypertonic saline should be avoided in such patients unless the hyponatremia is profoundly symptomatic.

Fluid Restriction

For patients with chronic hyponatremia, fluid restriction has been the most popular and most widely accepted treatment. When SIADH is present, fluids should generally be limited to 500 to 1,000 mL per 24 hours. Because fluid restriction increases the serum [Na^+] largely by underreplacing the excretion of fluid by the kidneys, some have advocated an initial restriction to 500 mL less than the 24-hour urine output.[376] When instituting a fluid restriction, it is important for the nursing staff and the patient to understand that this includes all fluids that are consumed, not just water. Generally the water content of ingested food is not included in the restriction because this is balanced by insensible water losses (perspiration, exhaled air, feces, etc.), but caution should be exercised with foods that have high fluid concentrations (such as fruits and soups). Restricting fluid intake can be effective when properly applied and managed in selected patients, but the serum [Na^+] generally increases only slowly (1–2 mEq/L/d) even with severe fluid restriction.[1] In addition, this therapy is often poorly tolerated because of an associated increase in thirst leading to poor compliance with long-term therapy. However, fluid restriction is economically favorable, and some patients do respond well to this option.

Fluid restriction should not be used with hypovolemic patients, and is particularly difficult to maintain in patients with very elevated urine osmolalities secondary to high AVP levels; in general, if the sum of urine Na^+ and K^+ exceeds the serum [Na^+], most patients will not respond to a fluid restriction since an electrolyte-free water clearance will be difficult to achieve.[377,378] In addition, fluid restriction is not practical for some patients, particularly including patients in intensive care settings who often require administration of significant volumes of fluids as part of their therapies.

Demeclocycline

Demeclocycline, a tetracycline antibiotic, inhibits adenylyl cyclase activation after AVP binds to its V_2 receptor in the kidney, and thus targets the underlying pathophysiology of SIADH. This therapy is typically used when patients find severe fluid restriction unacceptable and the underlying disorder cannot be corrected. However, demeclocycline is not approved by the U.S. Food and Drug Administration (FDA) to treat hyponatremia, and can cause nephrotoxicity in patients with heart failure and cirrhosis, although this is usually reversible if caught quickly.[379]

Mineralocorticoids

Administration of mineralocorticoids, such as fludrocortisone, has been shown to be useful in a small number of elderly patients.[227] However, the initial studies of SIADH did not show fludrocortisone to be of benefit in these patients, and it carries the risk of fluid overload and hypertension. Consequently, it is rarely used to treat hyponatremia in the United States.

Urea

Administration of urea has been successfully used to treat hyponatremia because it induces osmotic diuresis and augments free water excretion. Effective doses of urea for treatment of hyponatremia are 30 to 90 g daily, usually given in divided doses.[380] Unfortunately, its use is limited because there is no United States Pharmacopeia (USP) formulation for urea, and it is not approved by the FDA for treatment of hyponatremia. As such, urea has not been used extensively in the United States, and there are limited data to support its long-term use. In addition, urea is associated with poor palatability leading to poor patient compliance. However, patients with feeding tubes may be good candidates for urea therapy since palatability is not a concern, and the use of fluid restriction may be difficult in some patients with high obligate intake of fluids as part of their nutritional or medication therapy. Although mild azotemia can be seen with urea therapy, this rarely reaches clinically significant levels.

Furosemide and NaCl

The use of furosemide (20 to 40 mg per day) coupled with a high salt intake (200 mEq per day), which represents an extension of the treatment of acute symptomatic hyponatremia[381] to the chronic management of euvolemic hyponatremia, has also been reported to be successful in selected cases.[382] However, the long-term efficacy and safety of this approach is unknown.

Arginine Vasopressin Receptor Antagonists

Clinicians have used all of the above conventional therapies for hyponatremia over the past decades. However, conventional therapies for hyponatremia, although effective in specific circumstances, are suboptimal for many different reasons, including variable efficacy, slow responses, intolerable side effects, and serious toxicities. But perhaps the most prominent deficiency of most conventional therapies is that, with the exception of demeclocycline, these therapies do not directly target the underlying cause of almost all dilutional hyponatremias, namely inappropriately elevated plasma AVP levels. A new class of pharmacologic agents, arginine vasopressin receptor (AVPR) antagonists, that directly block AVP-mediated receptor activation have recently been approved by the FDA for treatment of euvolemic and hypervolemic hyponatremia.[383]

Conivaptan and tolvaptan are competitive receptor antagonists of the AVP V_2 (antidiuretic) receptor and have been approved by the FDA for the treatment of euvolemic and hypervolemic hyponatremia. These agents, also known as "vaptans," compete with AVP for binding at its site of action in the kidney, thereby blocking the antidiuresis caused by elevated AVP levels and directly attacking the underlying pathophysiology of dilutional hyponatremia. AVPR antagonists produce electrolyte free water excretion (called aquaresis) without significantly affecting renal sodium and potassium excretion.[384] The overall result is a reduction in body water without natriuresis, which leads to an increase in the serum [Na^+]. One of the major benefits of this class of drugs is that serum [Na^+] is significantly increased by an average of 4 to 8 mEq per L within 24 to 48 hours,[385,386] which is considerably faster than the effects of fluid restriction that can take many days. Also, compliance has not been shown to be a problem for vaptans, whereas this is a major problem with attempted long-term use of fluid restriction.

Conivaptan is FDA-approved for euvolemic and hypervolemic hyponatremia in hospitalized patients. It is available only as an intravenous preparation, and is given as a 20 mg loading dose over 30 minutes, followed by a continuous infusion of 20 or 40 mg per day.[387]Generally, the 20 mg continuous infusion is used for the first 24 hours to gauge the initial response. If the correction of serum [Na^+] is felt to be inadequate (e.g., less than 5 mEq per L), then the infusion rate can be increased to 40 mg per day. Therapy is limited to a maximum duration of 4 days because of drug-interaction effects with other agents metabolized by the CYP3A4 hepatic isoenzyme. Importantly, for conivaptan and all other vaptans, it is critical that the serum [Na^+] concentration is measured frequently during the active phase of correction of the hyponatremia (a minimum of every 6–8 hours for conivaptan, but more frequently in patients with risk factors for development of osmotic demyelination, such as severely low serum [Na^+], malnutrition, alcoholism, liver disease, and hypokalemia[373]). If the correction approaches 12 mEq per L in the first 24 hours, the infusion should be stopped and the patient monitored closely. If the correction exceeds 12 mEq per L, consideration should be given to administering sufficient water, either orally or as intravenous D_5W, to bring the overall correction below 12 mEq per L. The maximum correction limit should be reduced to 8 mEq per L over the first 24 hours in patients with risk factors for development of osmotic demyelination mentioned previously. The most common adverse effects include injection-site reactions, which are generally mild and usually do not lead to treatment discontinuation, headache, thirst, and hypokalemia.[385]

Tolvaptan, an oral AVPR antagonist, is FDA-approved for treatment of dilutional hyponatremias. In contrast to conivaptan, oral administration allows it to be used for both short- and long-term treatment of hyponatremia.[386] Similar to conivaptan, tolvaptan treatment must be initiated in the hospital so that the rate of correction can be monitored carefully. Patients with a serum [Na^+] less than 125 mEq per L are eligible for therapy with tolvaptan as primary therapy; if the serum [Na^+] is equal to or greater than 125 mEq per L, tolvaptan therapy is only indicated if the patient has symptoms that could be attributable to the hyponatremia and the patient is resistant to attempts at fluid restriction.[388] The starting dose of tolvaptan is 15 mg on the first day, and the dose can be titrated to 30 mg and 60 mg at 24-hour intervals if the serum [Na^+] remains less than 135 mEq per L or the increase in serum [Na^+] has been less than 5 mEq per L in the previous 24 hours. As with conivaptan, it is essential that the serum [Na^+] concentration is measured frequently during the active phase of correction of the hyponatremia (a minimum of every 6 to 8 hours, but more frequently in patients with risk factors for development of osmotic demyelination). Limits for safe correction of hyponatremia and methods to compensate for overly rapid corrections are the same as described previously for conivaptan. One additional factor that helps to avoid overly rapid correction with tolvaptan is the recommendation that fluid restriction not be used during the active phase of correction, thereby allowing the patient's thirst to compensate for an overly vigorous aquaresis. Common side effects include dry mouth, thirst, increased urinary frequency, dizziness, nausea, and orthostatic hypotension, which were relatively similar between placebo and tolvaptan groups in clinical trials.[386,388]

Because inducing increased renal fluid excretion via either a diuresis or an aquaresis can cause or worsen hypotension in patients with hypovolemic hyponatremia, vaptans are contraindicated in this patient population.[373] However, clinically significant hypotension was not observed in either the conivaptan or tolvaptan clinical trials in euvolemic and hypervolemic hyponatremic patients. Although vaptans are not contraindicated with decreased renal function, these agents generally will not be effective if the serum creatinine is greater than 2.5 mg per dL.

Osmotic Demyelination Syndrome

Before deciding on the therapy for any hyponatremic patient, the possibility of producing harm from correction of the hyponatremia must be carefully considered. Despite the obvious survival advantages afforded by brain volume regulation in response to hyponatremia, every adaptation made by the body in response to a perturbation of homeostasis bears within it the potential to create a new set of problems, and this is true for brain volume regulation as well. Over the last several decades it has become apparent that the demyelinating disease of central pontine myelinolysis (CPM) occurs with a significantly higher incidence in patients with hyponatremia,[389–391] and in both animal[392–396] and human studies[19,397,398] brain demyelination has clearly been shown to be associated with the correction of existing hyponatremia rather than simply to the presence of severe hyponatremia itself. Because demyelination following correction of hyponatremia has a unique etiology and frequently occurs in other white matter areas of the brain in addition to the pons, the occurrence of demyelination in hyponatremic patients has been named the osmotic demyelination syndrome (ODS).[19] Although the mechanism(s) by which correction of hyponatremia leads to brain demyelination remain under investigation, this pathologic disorder likely is precipitated by the brain dehydration that has been demonstrated to occur following correction of serum [Na^+] toward normal ranges in animal models of chronic hyponatremia. Because the degree of osmotic brain shrinkage is greater in animals that are maintained chronically hyponatremic than in normonatremic animals undergoing similar increases in plasma osmolality,[196,394,399] by analogy the brains of human patients adapted to hyponatremia are likely to be particularly susceptible to dehydration following subsequent increases in osmolality, which in turn can lead to pathologic demyelination in some patients. MRI studies have shown that chronic hypoosmolality predisposes rats to opening of the blood–brain barrier following rapid correction of hyponatremia,[400] and that the disruption of the blood–brain barrier is highly correlated with subsequent demyelination[401]; a potential mechanism by which blood–brain barrier disruption might lead to subsequent myelinolysis is via an influx of complement, which is toxic to the oligodendrocytes that manufacture and maintain myelin sheaths of neurons, into the brain.[402]

Although there has been considerable debate in the literature regarding the parameters of correction of hyponatremia associated with an increased risk of myelinolysis, studies in both patients[403–405] and experimental animals[394–396] support the notion that both the rate of correction of hyponatremia and the total magnitude of the correction over the first few days likely represent significant factors that increase the risk of demyelination. Studies in rats have shown that the initial rate of correction of hyponatremia may not be important for the development of demyelinative lesions as long as the total magnitude of the correction remains less than 20 mEq per L in 24 hours,[406] which supports clinical data indicating that magnitude of correction represents the major risk factor related to subsequent neurologic morbidity and mortality. There is still some disagreement as to the actual magnitude of correction at which patients are at risk for ODS; initial reports implicated increases in serum [Na^+] greater than 25 mEq per L over the first 24 to 48 hours of treatment,[403] whereas later studies have suggested occurrence of ODS with even lesser increases in serum [Na^+] of greater than 12 mEq per L in 24 hours or greater than 18 mEq per L in 48 hours.[374] Although overcorrection of hyponatremia to supranormal levels is also clearly a risk factor for neurologic deterioration, it is important to note that both clinical and experimental studies have found that demyelination occurred following corrections to serum [Na^+] levels still below normal ranges. Regardless of the level of increase in serum [Na^+] at which ODS occurs, the methods used to correct hyponatremia do not appear to have any significant bearing on the production of brain demyelination, since both experimental studies[396] and clinical reports[19,407–409] have demonstrated that demyelination can occur independent of the method used to correct the hyponatremia.

Other factors also can clearly influence the susceptibility to demyelination following correction of hyponatremia. Perhaps most importantly are the severity and the duration of the preexisting hyponatremia. Both of these risk factors likely relate to the degree of brain volume regulation that has occurred prior to the correction: the more severe the hyponatremia and the longer it has been maintained, the greater the degree of solute loss that will have occurred during the process of brain volume regulation. As larger amounts of solute are lost, the ability of the brain to buffer subsequent increases in plasma osmolality is impaired, resulting in greater degrees of brain dehydration as serum [Na^+] is later raised, which in turn can lead to brain demyelination via mechanisms discussed earlier. Clinical implications of this pathophysiologic mechanism are that ODS should not occur in cases of either mild or very acute hyponatremia. Both of these findings have been found to be true. ODS has only rarely been reported in patients with a starting serum [Na^+] greater than 120 mEq per L,[19,374,410] and also does not appear to occur in most patients with psychogenic polydipsia who are well known to develop hyponatremia acutely from episodes of massive water ingestion followed by rapid correction as they diurese the excess fluid.[303] There are also some independent risk factors for the occurrence of CPM, particularly chronic alcoholism and malnutrition, which led to the original description of this disorder in 1959.[411] Although no studies to date have clearly documented interactive effects between these risk factors and ODS, it seems likely that the threshold for increases in serum [Na^+] that increase the risk for ODS will be lower in alcoholic and malnourished patients, and reports of myelinolysis in patients with chronic alcoholism in whom the rate of correction stayed within the recommended guidelines supports this likelihood.[412,413] Interestingly, one factor that appears to protect hyponatremic patients from myelinolysis following rapid correction of hyponatremia is uremia. Although uremic patients on dialysis frequently have large swings of serum [Na^+], only rare cases of osmotically induced demyelination have been reported in this group.[414] A study in rats showed that azotemic rats were able to sustain large increases in serum [Na^+] without brain damage, purportedly because the urea acts as an intracellular osmolyte to stabilize intracellular volume and thereby reduces the degree of brain dehydration produced following rapid correction of hyponatremia.[415]

Several other aspects of this unique disease deserve emphasis. First, apropos the widespread nature of the neuropathologic lesions, a much broader range of neurologic disorders is now being reported in patients following correction of hyponatremia, including cognitive, behavioral, and neuropsychiatric disorders, presumably as a result of demyelination in subcortical, corpus callosal, and hippocampal white matter,[416,417] and movement disorders, as a result of demyelination in the basal ganglia.[418–420] Second, MRI scans often fail to demonstrate the characteristic demyelinative lesions in many cases because scans are usually negative until sufficient time has passed (generally 3–4 weeks) after the correction of hyponatremia and the onset of neurologic symptoms.[421–423] Consequently, the presence of positive MRI findings strongly (though not unequivocally[424]) supports a diagnosis of ODS, but the absence of radiologic findings can never eliminate the possibility of this disorder. Third, although most cases of ODS have been associated with rapid correction of hyponatremia, the disorder has also been reported with severe hypernatremia in both animal models[425] and patients.[426] This is consistent with the hypothesis that brain dehydration with subsequent disruption of the blood–brain barrier is related to the pathogenesis of the demyelinative process.[401,402] Finally, it is clear that given our present knowledge, we cannot predict with any degree of certainty which patients will develop demyelination regardless of the parameters used to correct hyponatremia. Many patients undergo very rapid and large corrections of their serum [Na^+] without subsequent neurologic complications,[427] as is true of experimental animals as well.[396,406] Consequently, overly rapid correction of hyponatremia should be viewed as a factor that puts patients at risk for ODS, but does not inevitably precipitate this disorder.

Hyponatremia Treatment Guidelines

Based on the previous discussions of hyponatremic encephalopathy and the osmotic demyelination syndrome, it follows that optimal treatment of hyponatremic patients must entail balancing the risks of hyponatremia against the risks of correction for each patient individually. Although individual variability in response is great, and consequently one cannot always accurately predict which patients will develop neurologic complications from either hyponatremia or its correction, consensus guidelines for treating hypoosmolar patients allow a rational approach to minimizing the risks of both these complications. Implicit in these guidelines is the realization that treatment must be individualized and tailored to each patient's clinical presentation: appropriate therapy for one hyponatremic patient may be inappropriate for another despite equivalent degrees of hypoosmolality.[5,428] To accomplish this, three factors should be taken into consideration when making a treatment decision in a hypoosmolar patient: (1) the severity of the hyponatremia, (2) the duration of the hyponatremia, and (3) the patient's neurologic symptomatology. The importance of duration and symptomatology both relate to how well the brain has adapted to the hyponatremia and consequently its degree of risk for subsequent demyelination with rapid correction. However, of these factors, the severity of the hypoosmolality is the single most important consideration. The red arrow in Figure 70.10 emphasizes that hypoosmolar patients should always be evaluated quickly for the presence of neurologic symptoms so that appropriate therapy can be initiated, if indicated, even whereas other results of the diagnostic evaluation are still pending.

Although various authors have published recommendations on the treatment of hyponatremia,[94,348,373,429,430] no standardized treatment algorithms have yet been widely accepted. A synthesis of existing expert recommendations for treatment of hyponatremia is illustrated in Figure 70.11.

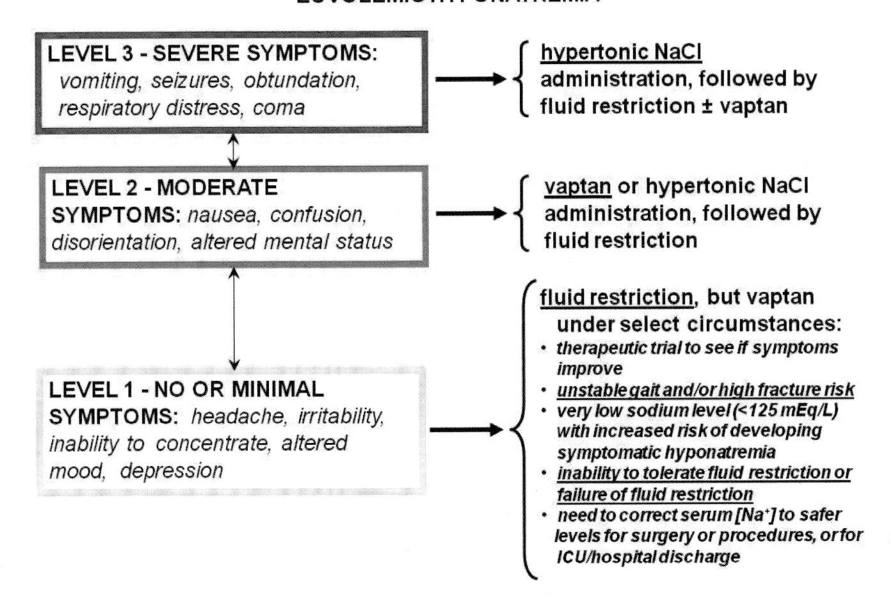

FIGURE 70.11 Algorithm for treatment of patients with euvolemic hyponatremia based on their presenting symptoms. The *arrows* between the symptom boxes indicate movement of patients between different symptom levels. (Modified from Verbalis JG. Managing hyponatremia in patients with syndrome of inappropriate antidiuretic hormone secretion. *Endocrinol Nutr.* 2010;57 Suppl 2:30–40, with permission.)

This treatment algorithm is based primarily on the symptomatology of hyponatremic patients, rather than the serum [Na^+] or on the chronicity of the hyponatremia, which is often difficult to ascertain. A careful neurologic history and assessment should always be done to identify potential causes for the patient's symptoms other than hyponatremia, although it will not always be possible to exclude an additive contribution from the hyponatremia to an underlying neurologic condition. In this algorithm, patients are divided into three groups based on their presenting symptoms.

Level 1 (Severe) Symptoms

The presence of seizures, coma, respiratory arrest, obtundation, and vomiting usually indicate a more acute onset or worsening of hyponatremia requiring immediate active treatment. Therapies that will quickly raise serum sodium levels are required to reduce cerebral edema and decrease the risk of potentially fatal herniation.

Level 2 (Moderate) Symptoms

Nausea, confusion, disorientation, and altered mental status are more moderate hyponatremic symptoms. These symptoms may be either a manifestation of chronic or acute hyponatremia, but allow time to elaborate a more deliberate approach to treatment.

Level 3 (Mild) Symptoms

This group consists of minimal symptoms such as a headache, irritability, inability to concentrate, altered mood, and depression, to a virtual absence of discernible symptoms, and indicate that the patient may have chronic or slowly evolving hyponatremia. These symptoms necessitate a more cautious and deliberate approach, especially when patients have underlying co-morbidities.

Patients with severe symptoms (level 1) should be treated with hypertonic saline as first-line therapy, followed by fluid restriction with or without AVPR antagonist therapy. Patients with moderate symptoms will benefit from a regimen of vaptan therapy or limited hypertonic saline administration, followed by fluid restriction or long-term vaptan therapy. Although moderate neurologic symptoms can indicate that a patient is in an early stage of acute hyponatremia, they more often indicate a chronically hyponatremic state with sufficient brain volume adaptation to prevent marked symptomatology from cerebral edema. Regardless, close monitoring of these patients in a hospital setting is warranted until the symptoms improve or stabilize. Patients with no or minimal symptoms should be managed initially with fluid restriction, although subsequent treatment with vaptans may be appropriate for a wide range of specific clinical conditions, foremost of which is the failure to improve the serum [Na^+] despite reasonable attempts at fluid restriction (see Fig. 70.11).

A special case is when rapid correction of hyponatremia occurs at an undesirably rapid rate as a result of the onset of a spontaneous aquaresis. This can occur following cessation of desmopressin therapy in a patient who has become hyponatremic, replacement of glucocorticoids in a patient with adrenal insufficiency, replacement of solutes in a patient with diuretic-induced hyponatremia, or spontaneous resolution of transient SIADH. Brain damage from ODS can clearly ensue in this setting if the preceding period of hyponatremia has been of sufficient duration (usually greater than 48 hours) to allow brain volume regulation to occur. If the previously discussed correction parameters have been exceeded and the correction is proceeding more rapidly than planned (usually because of continued excretion of hypotonic urine), the pathologic events leading to demyelination can be reversed by readministration of hypotonic fluids and desmopressin. Efficacy of this approach is suggested both from animal studies[431] as well as reports in humans,[429,432] even when patients are overtly symptomatic.[433]

Although this classification is based on presenting symptoms at the time of initial evaluation, it should be remembered that in some cases patients initially exhibit more moderate symptoms because they are in the early stages of hyponatremia. In addition, some patients with minimal symptoms are prone to develop more symptomatic hyponatremia during periods of increased fluid ingestion. In support of this, approximately 70% of 31 patients presenting to a university hospital with symptomatic hyponatremia and a mean serum [Na^+] of 119 mEq per L had preexisting asymptomatic hyponatremia as their most common risk factor identified.[434] Consequently, therapy of hyponatremia should also be considered to prevent progression from lower to higher levels of symptomatic hyponatremia, particularly in patients with a past history of repeated presentations for symptomatic hyponatremia.

Monitoring the Serum [Na^+] in Hyponatremic Patients

Regardless of the initial rate of correction chosen, acute treatment should be interrupted once any of three endpoints is reached: (1) the patient's symptoms are abolished, (2) a safe serum [Na^+] (generally greater than 120 mEq per L) is achieved, or (3) a total magnitude of correction of 12 mEq per L in 24 h or 18 mEq per L in 48 h is achieved (see Fig. 70.10). Once any of these endpoints is reached, the active correction should be stopped and the patient treated with slower acting therapies, such as oral rehydration or fluid restriction, depending on the etiology of the hypoosmolality. It follows from these recommendations that serum [Na^+] levels must be carefully monitored at frequent intervals during the active phases of treatment to adjust therapy to keep the correction within these maximum limits.

The frequency of serum [Na^+] monitoring is dependent on both the severity of the hyponatremia and the therapy chosen. In all hyponatremic patients neurologic symptomatology should be carefully assessed very early in the diagnostic evaluation to evaluate the symptomatic severity of the hyponatremia and to determine whether the patient requires more urgent therapy. All patients undergoing active treatment with hypertonic saline for level 1 or level 2 symptomatic hyponatremia should have frequent monitoring of serum [Na$^+$] and ECF volume status (every 2–4 hours) to ensure that the serum [Na$^+$] does not exceeded the recommended levels during the active phase of correction,[373] since overly rapid correction of serum sodium can cause ODS.[19] Patients treated with vaptans for level 2 or level 3 symptoms should have serum [Na$^+$] monitored every 6 to 8 hours during the active phase of correction, which will generally be the first 24 to 48 hours of therapy. Importantly, ODS has not yet been reported either in clinical trials or with therapeutic use of any vaptan to date. In patients with a stable level of serum [Na$^+$] treated with fluid restriction or therapies other than hypertonic saline, measurement of serum [Na$^+$] daily is generally sufficient, because levels will not change that quickly in the absence of active therapy or large changes in fluid intake or administration.

Management of Overly Rapid Correction of Hyponatremia

Despite the best attempts at treating hyponatremia, occasional patients will exceed the recommended maximal limits of correction of 12 mEq per L in 24 hours or 18 mEq per L in 48 hours. As discussed previously, this is common with rapid corrections as a result of spontaneous aquaresis. However, overly rapid correction also has been found to accompany corrections of thiazide-induced hyponatremia and use of hypertonic saline.[435] Regardless of how it occurs, the occurrence of an overly rapid correction requires active intervention to decrease the risk of ODS.[436]The only exceptions to this are cases in which the hyponatremia is known to be acute (i.e., less than 48 hours duration), in which case complete brain volume regulation has not occurred and patients do not appear to be at risk of ODS with rapid correction of their serum [Na$^+$] to normal levels.[303] For any patient with chronic hyponatremia who is found to be correcting overly rapidly, attempts should be made to prevent further correction and to bring the correction back to safe limits for that patient. In most patients this will be the recommended maximal limits of correction of 12 mEq per L in 24 hours or 18 mEq per L in 48 hours,[374] but in patients at high risk of ODS (severely low serum [Na$^+$] less than 105 mEq per L, malnutrition, alcoholism, liver disease, or hypokalemia), the maximal correction should not exceed 8 mEq per L in 24 hours.[373]

In order to prevent further correction, all active therapies should be stopped, including saline infusions and pharmacologic therapies such as vaptans. However this will not be sufficient if the patient is undergoing a spontaneous aquaresis because the ongoing water excretion will cause continued increases in the serum [Na$^+$]. One option in such cases is to give water, orally or intravenously as 5% dextrose solution, at a volume that equals the hourly urine output. However, this can be difficult to do, since urine output can reach 800 to 1,000 mL per hour in the setting of suppressed AVP levels. An alternative is to give dDAVP (1 to 2 μg subcutaneously) in order to stop the aquaresis, an approach that has been successfully employed.[437] As each dose of dDAVP wears off (generally in 6–12 hours) and urine output increases, a decision will need to be made regarding re-dosing based on the desired further correction of the serum [Na$^+$]. With the combined use of dDAVP and water administration, it is possible to control corrections of hyponatremia to within acceptable limits in virtually all patients.

In cases in which an overcorrection has already occurred, consideration should be given to lowering the serum [Na$^+$] back to the maximally desired correction in that patient, again using water administration and/or dDAVP. Animal models have suggested that lowering the serum [Na$^+$] after overcorrection can prevent subsequent brain damage from occurring,[431,438] and this would be consistent with the occurrence of a delayed immunologic demyelination as a result of complement influx into the brain following a sustained blood–brain barrier disruption.[402] A case report in which delayed lowering of serum [Na$^+$] was associated with a reversal of symptoms suggestive of early myelinolysis also supports this as a potential therapy in similar cases.[439] Experimental studies in animals have shown that administration of high-dose glucocorticoids can prevent the development of osmotic demyelination after rapid correction of hyponatremia in rats,[440] again likely via stabilization of the blood–brain barrier to prevent or minimize disruption. Although controlled clinical studies with glucocorticoids have not yet been done in humans, it would seem prudent to employ this relatively benign intervention in cases where a correction of hyponatremia in excess of current guidelines has already occurred, or prior to correction in cases at high risk for development of ODS. More recent promising experimental studies suggest that the drug minocycline may be able to prevent or reduce demyelination following rapid correction of hyponatremia by inhibiting brain microglial activation[441,442]; controlled clinical studies will be necessary to determine the dosing, efficacy, and safety of this drug in humans.

Long-term Treatment of Chronic Hyponatremia

Some patients will benefit from continued treatment of hyponatremia following discharge from the hospital. In many cases, this will consist of a continued fluid restriction. However, as discussed previously, long-term compliance with this therapy is poor due to the increased thirst that occurs with more severe degrees of fluid restriction. For selected patients who have responded to tolvaptan in the hospital, consideration should be given to continuing the treatment as an outpatient after discharge. In patients with established chronic hyponatremia, tolvaptan has been shown to be effective at maintaining a normal [Na$^+$] for as long as 4 years of continued daily therapy.[443] However, many patients with inpatient hyponatremia will have a transient form of SIADH without any need for long-term therapy. In the conivaptan open-label study, approximately 70% of patients treated as an inpatient for 4 days had normal serum [Na+] concentrations 7 and 30 days after cessation of the vaptan therapy in the absence of chronic therapy for hyponatremia. Selection of which patients with inpatient hyponatremia are candidates for long-term therapy should be based on the etiology of the SIADH. Figure 70.12 shows estimates of the relative probability that patients with different causes of SIADH will have persistent hyponatremia that may benefit from long-term treatment with tolvaptan following discharge from the hospital. Nonetheless, for any individual patient this simply represents an estimate of the likelihood of requiring long-term therapy. In all cases, consideration should be given to a trial of stopping the drug at 2 to 4 weeks following discharge to determine if hyponatremia is still present.

A reasonable period of tolvaptan cessation to evaluate the presence of continued SIADH is 7 days, since this period was sufficient for demonstration of a recurrence of hyponatremia in the tolvaptan clinical trials.[386,443] Serum [Na+] should be monitored every 2 to 3 days following cessation of tolvaptan so that the drug can be resumed as quickly as possible in those patients with recurrent hyponatremia because the longer the patient is hyponatremic the greater the risk of subsequent osmotic demyelination with overly rapid correction of the low serum [Na+].

Future of Hyponatremia Treatment

Guidelines for the appropriate treatment of hyponatremia, and particularly the role of vaptans, are still evolving, and will undoubtedly change substantially over the next several years. Of special interest will be studies to assess whether more effective treatment of hyponatremia can reduce the incidence of falls and fractures in elderly patients, whether more effective treatment of hyponatremia can reduce utilization of healthcare resources for both inpatients and outpatients with hyponatremia, and whether more effective treatment of hyponatremia can reduce the markedly increased morbidity and mortality of patients with hyponatremia across multiple disease states. A potential role for vaptans in the treatment of heart failure has already been studied. A large trial in patients with heart failure (EVEREST) demonstrated short-term improvement in dyspnea, but no long-term survival benefit.[444] However, this trial was not powered to evaluate the outcomes of hyponatremic patients with heart failure. Consequently, the potential therapeutic role of AVPR antagonists in the treatment of water-retaining disorders must await further studies specifically designed to assess specific clinical outcomes of hyponatremic patients treated with vaptans,

Etiology of SIADH	Likely duration of SIADH*	Relative risk of chronic SIADH
Tumors producing vasopressin ectopically (small-cell lung carcinoma, head and neck carcinoma)	Indefinite	High
Drug-induced, with continuation of offending agent (carbamazepine, SSRI)	Duration of drug therapy	
Brain tumors	Indefinite	
Idiopathic (senile)	Indefinite	
Subarachnoid hemorrhage	1–4 weeks	
Stroke	1–2 weeks	
Inflammatory brain lesions	Dependent on response to therapy	Medium
Respiratory failure (chronic obstructive lung disease)	Dependent on response to therapy	
HIV infection	Dependent on response to therapy	
Traumatic brain injury	2–7 days to indefinite	
Drug-induced, with cessation of offending agent	Duration of drug therapy	
Pneumonia	2–5 days	
Nausea, pain, prolonged exercise	Variable depending on cause	
Postoperative hyponatremia	2–3 days postoperatively	Low

*Time frames are based on clinical experience.

FIGURE 70.12 Estimated probability of the need for long-term treatment of SIADH depending on the underlying etiology of hyponatremia. The time frames of likely duration of SIADH are estimates based on clinical experience with these etiologies. (Modified from Verbalis JG. Managing hyponatremia in patients with syndrome of inappropriate antidiuretic hormone secretion. *Endocrinol Nutr.* 2010;57 Suppl 2:30–40, with permission.)

as well as increased clinical experience to better delineate efficacies as well as potential toxicities of all treatments for hyponatremia. Nonetheless, it is abundantly clear that the vaptans clearly have ushered in a new era in the evaluation and treatment of hyponatremic disorders.

REFERENCES

1. Schwartz WB, Bennett S, Curelop S, et al. A syndrome of renal sodium loss and hyponatremia probably resulting from inappropriate secretion of antidiuretic hormone. *Am J Med.* 1957;23:529–542.
2. Bartter FC, Schwartz WB. The syndrome of inappropriate secretion of antidiuretic hormone. *Am J Med.* 1967;42:790–806.
3. Verbalis JG. Hyponatremia: answered and unanswered questions. *Am J Kidney Dis.* 1991;18:546–552.
4. Verbalis JG. Escape from antidiuresis: a good story. *Kidney Int.* 2001;60(4):1608–1610.
5. Berl T. Treating hyponatremia: damned if we do and damned if we don't. *Kidney Int.* 1990;37:1006–1018.
6. Verbalis JG. Vasopressin V2 receptor antagonists. *J Mol Endocrinol.* 2002;29(1):1–9.
7. Hawkins RC. Age and gender as risk factors for hyponatremia and hypernatremia. *Clin Chim Acta.* 2003;337(1–2):169–172.
8. Upadhyay A, Jaber BL, Madias NE. Epidemiology of hyponatremia. *Semin Nephrol.* 2009;29(3):227–238.
9. Owen JA, Campbell DG. A comparison of plasma electrolyte and urea values in healthy persons and in hospital patients. *Clin Chim Acta.* 1968;22:611–618.
10. Flear CT, Gill GV, Burn J. Hyponatraemia: mechanisms and management. *Lancet.* 1981;2:26–31.
11. Brunsvig PF, Os I, Frederichsen P. Hyponatremia. A retrospective study of occurrence, etiology and mortality. *Tidsskrift for Den Norske Laegeforening.* 1990;110:2367–2369.
12. Anderson RJ, Chung HM, Kluge R, et al. Hyponatremia: a prospective analysis of its epidemiology and the pathogenetic role of vasopressin. *Ann Intern Med.* 1985;102:164–168.
13. Sorensen IJ, Matzen LE. Serum electrolytes and drug therapy of patients admitted to a geriatric department. *Ugeskrift for Laeger.* 1993;155:3921–3924.
14. Miller M, Morley JE, Rubenstein LZ. Hyponatremia in a nursing home population. *J Am Geriatr Soc.* 1995;43(12):1410–1413.
15. Wald R, Jaber BL, Price LL, et al. Impact of hospital-associated hyponatremia on selected outcomes. *Arch Intern Med.* 2010;170(3):294–302.
16. Upadhyay A, Jaber BL, Madias NE. Incidence and prevalence of hyponatremia. *Am J Med.* 2006;119(7 Suppl 1):S30–S35.
17. Sterns RH. Severe symptomatic hyponatremia: treatment and outcome. A study of 64 cases. *Ann Intern Med.* 1987;107:656–664.
18. Arieff AI. Hyponatremia, convulsions, respiratory arrest, and permanent brain damage after elective surgery in healthy women. *N Eng J Med.* 1986;314:1529–1535.
19. Sterns RH, Riggs JE, Schochet SS Jr. Osmotic demyelination syndrome following correction of hyponatremia. *N Engl J Med.* 1986;314:1535–1542.
20. Berghmans T, Paesmans M, Body JJ. A prospective study on hyponatraemia in medical cancer patients: epidemiology, aetiology and differential diagnosis. *Support Care Cancer.* 2000;8(3):192–197.
21. Oster JR, Singer I. Hyponatremia, hyposmolality, and hypotonicity: tables and fables [see comments]. *Arch Intern Med.* 1999;159(4):333–336.
22. Albrink MJ, Hald PM, Man EBPJP. The displacement of serum water by the lipids of hyperlipemic serum: a new method for the rapid determination of serum water. *J Clin Invest.* 1955;34:1483–1488.
23. Weisberg LS. Pseudohyponatremia: a reappraisal. [Review]. *Am J Med.* 1989;86:315–318.
24. Ladenson JH, Apple FS, Koch DD. Misleading hyponatremia due to hyperlipemia: a method-dependent error. *Ann Intern Med.* 1981;95:707–708.
25. Turchin A, Wiebe DA, Seely EW, et al. Severe hypercholesterolemia mediated by lipoprotein X in patients with chronic graft-versus-host disease of the liver. *Bone Marrow Transplant.* 2005;35(1):85–89.
26. Lawn N, Wijdicks EF, Burritt MF. Intravenous immune globulin and pseudohyponatremia. *N Engl J Med.* 1998;339(9):632.
27. Steinberger BA, Ford SM, Coleman TA. Intravenous immunoglobulin therapy results in post-infusional hyperproteinemia, increased serum viscosity, and pseudohyponatremia. *Am J Hematol.* 2003;73(2):97–100.
28. Katz MA. Hyperglycemia-induced hyponatremia—calculation of expected serum sodium depression. *N Engl J Med.* 1973;289:843–844.
29. Hillier TA, Abbott RD, Barrett EJ. Hyponatremia: evaluating the correction factor for hyperglycemia. *Am J Med.* 1999;106(4):399–403.
30. Dorwart WV, Chalmers L. Comparison of methods for calculating serum osmolality from chemical concentrations, and the prognostic value of such calculations. *Clin Chem.* 1975;21(2):190–194.
31. Gennari FJ. Current concepts. Serum osmolality. Uses and limitations. *N Engl J Med.* 1984;310:102–105.
32. Jacobsen D, Bredesen JE, Eide I, et al. Anion and osmolal gaps in the diagnosis of methanol and ethylene glycol poisining. *Acta Med Scand.* 1982;212:17–20.
33. Rose BD. New approach to disturbances in the plasma sodium concentration. *Am J Med.* 1986;81:1033–1040.
34. Edelman IS, Leibman J. Anatomy of body water and electrolytes. *Am J Med.* 1959;27:256.
35. Nguyen MK, Kurtz I. New insights into the pathophysiology of the dysnatremias: a quantitative analysis. *Am J Physiol. Renal Physiol.* 2004;287(2):F172–F180.
36. Moritz ML, Ayus JC. Prevention of hospital-acquired hyponatremia: a case for using isotonic saline. *Pediatrics.* 2003;111(2):227–230.
37. Fichman MP, Vorherr H, Kleeman CR, et al. Diuretic-induced hyponatremia. *Ann Intern Med.* 1971;75:853–863.
38. Spital A. Diuretic-induced hyponatremia. *Am J Nephrol.* 1999;19(4):447–452.
39. Vieweg WV, Karp BI. Severe hyponatremia in the polydipsia-hyponatremia syndrome. *J Clin Psych.* 1994;55:355–361.
40. Gillum DM, Linas SL. Water intoxication in a psychotic patient with normal renal water excretion. *Am J Med.* 1984;77:773–774.
41. Gross PA, Pehrisch H, Rascher W, et al. Pathogenesis of clinical hyponatremia: observations of vasopressin and fluid intake in 100 hyponatremic medical patients. *Eur J Clin Invest.* 1987;17:123–129.
42. Schrier RW. Pathogenesis of sodium and water retention in high-output and low-output cardiac failure, nephrotic syndrome, cirrhosis, and pregnancy (1). *N Engl J Med.* 1988;319:1065–1072.
43. Schrier RW. Pathogenesis of sodium and water retention in high-output and low-output cardiac failure, nephrotic syndrome, cirrhosis, and pregnancy (2). *N Engl J Med.* 1988;319:1127–1134.
44. Szatalowicz VL, Arnold PE, Chaimovitz C, et al. Radioimmunoassay of plasma arginine vasopressin in hyponatremic patients with congestive heart failure. *N Engl J Med.* 1981;305:263–266.
45. Bichet D, Szatalowicz V, Chaimovitz C, et al. Role of vasopressin in abnormal water excretion in cirrhotic patients. *Ann Intern Med.* 1982;96:413–417.
46. Leaf A, Bartter FC, Santos RF, et al. Evidence in man that urinary electrolyte loss induced by pitressin is a function of water retention. *J Clin Invest.* 1953;32:868–878.
47. Nolph KD, Schrier RW. Sodium, potassium and water metabolism in the syndrome of inappropriate antidiuretic hormone secretion. *Am J Med.* 1970;49:534–545.
48. Hall JE, Montani JP, Woods LL, et al. Renal escape from vasopressin: role of pressure diuresis. *Am J Physiol.* 1986;250:F907–F916.
49. Kamoi K, Ebe T, Kobayashi O, et al. Atrial natriuretic peptide in patients with the syndrome of inappropriate antidiuretic hormone secretion and with diabetes insipidus. *J Clin Endocrinol Metab.* 1990;70:1385–1390.
50. Cogan E, Debieve MF, Pepersack T, et al. Natriuresis and atrial natriuretic factor secretion during inappropriate antidiuresis. *Am J Med.* 1988;84:409–418.
51. Mizelle HL, Hall JE, Hildebrandt DA. Atrial natriuretic peptide and pressure natriuresis: interactions with the renin-angiotensin system. *Am J Physiol.* 1989;257:R1169–R1174.
52. Demanet JC, Bonnyns M, Bleiberg H, et al. Coma due to water intoxication in beer drinkers. *Lancet.* 1971;2:1115–1117.
53. Hilden T, Svendsen TL. Electrolyte disturbances in beer drinkers. A specific "hypo- osmolality syndrome". *Lancet.* 1975;2:245–246.
54. Thaler SM, Teitelbaum I, Berl T. "Beer potomania" in non-beer drinkers: effect of low dietary solute intake. *Am J Kidney Dis.* 1998;31(6):1028–1031.
55. Musch W, Xhaet O, Decaux G. Solute loss plays a major role in polydipsia-related hyponatraemia of both water drinkers and beer drinkers. *QJM.* 2003;96(6):421–426.
56. Cooke CR, Turin MD, Walker WG. The syndrome of inappropriate antidiuretic hormone secretion (SIADH): pathophysiologic mechanisms in solute and volume regulation. *Medicine.* 1979;58:240–251.
57. Stormont JM, Waterhouse C. The genesis of hyponatremia associated with marked overhydration and water intoxication. *Circulation.* 1961;24:191–203.
58. Grantham JJ. Pathophysiology of hyposmolar conditions: a cellular perspective. In: Andreoli TE, Grantham JJ, Rector FC, eds. *Disturbances in Body Fluid Osmolality.* Bethesda: American Physiological Society, 1977:217–225.
59. Grantham J, Linshaw M. The effect of hyponatremia on the regulation of intracellular volume and solute composition. *Circ Res.* 1984;54:483–491.

60. Yannet H. Changes in the brain resulting from depletion of extracellular electrolytes. *Am J Physiol.* 1940;128:683–689.

61. Holliday MA, Kalayci MN, Harrah J. Factors that limit brain volume changes in response to acute and sustained hyper- and hyponatremia. *J Clin Invest.* 1968;47:1916–1928.

62. Melton JE, Patlak CS, Pettigrew KD, et al. Volume regulatory loss of Na, Cl, and K from rat brain during acute hyponatremia. *Am J Physiol.* 1987;252: F661–F669.

63. Verbalis JG, Drutarosky MD. Adaptation to chronic hypoosmolality in rats. *Kidney Int.* 1988;34:351–360.

64. Garcia-Perez A, Burg MB. Renal medullary organic osmolytes. *Phys Rev.* 1991;71:1081–1115.

65. Heilig CW, Stromski ME, Blumenfeld JD. Characterization of the major brain osmolytes that accumulate in salt-loaded rats. *Am J Physiol.* 1989;257: F1108–F1116.

66. Thurston JH, Hauhart RE, Nelson JS. Adaptive decreases in amino acids (taurine in particular), creatine, and electrolytes prevent cerebral edema in chronically hyponatremic mice: rapid correction (experimental model of central pontine myelinolysis) causes dehydration and shrinkage of brain. *Metabol Brain Dis.* 1987;2:223–241.

67. Lien YH, Shapiro JI, Chan L. Study of brain electrolytes and organic osmolytes during correction of chronic hyponatremia. Implications for the pathogenesis of central pontine myelinolysis. *J Clin Invest.* 1991;88:303–309.

68. Verbalis JG, Gullans SR. Hyponatremia causes large sustained reductions in brain content of multiple organic osmolytes in rats. *Brain Res.* 1991;567:274–282.

69. Sterns RH, Baer J, Ebersol S, et al. Organic osmolytes in acute hyponatremia. *Am J Physiol.* 1993;264:F833–F836.

70. Videen JS, Michaelis T, Pinto P, et al. Human cerebral osmolytes during chronic hyponatremia. *J Clin Invest.* 1995;95:788–793.

71. Gullans SR, Verbalis JG. Control of brain volume during hyperosmolar and hypoosmolar conditions. *Annu Rev Med.* 1993;44:289–301.

72. Verbalis JG. Brain volume regulation in response to changes in osmolality. *Neuroscience.* 2010;168(4):862–870.

73. Graber M, Corish D. The electrolytes in hyponatremia. *Am J Kidney Dis.* 1991;18:527–545.

74. Padfield PL, Brown JJ, Lever AF, et al. Blood pressure in acute and chronic vasopressin excess: studies of malignant hypertension and the syndrome of inappropriate antidiuretic hormone secretion. *N Engl J Med.* 1981;304:1067–1070.

75. Smith MJ Jr, Cowley AW Jr, Guyton AC, et al. Acute and chronic effects of vasopressin on blood pressure, electrolytes, and fluid volumes. *Am J Physiol.* 1979;237:F232–F240.

76. Verbalis JG. Pathogenesis of hyponatremia in an experimental model of the syndrome of inappropriate antidiuresis. *Am J Physiol.* 1994;267:R1617–R1625.

77. Jaenike JR, Waterhouse C. The renal response to sustained administration of vasopressin and water in man. *J Clin Endocrinol Metab.* 1961;21:231–242.

78. Kaye M. An investigation into the cause of hyponatremia in the syndrome of inappropriate secretion of antidiuretic hormone. *Am J Med.* 1966;41:910–926.

79. Southgate HJ, Burke BJ, Walters G. Body space measurements in the hyponatraemia of carcinoma of the bronchus: evidence for the chronic 'sick cell' syndrome? *Ann Clin Biochem.* 1992;29:90–95.

80. Verbalis JG. Whole-body volume regulation and escape from antidiuresis. *Am J Med.* 2006;119(7 Suppl 1):S21–S29.

81. Clark BA, Shannon RP, Rosa RM, et al. Increased susceptibility to thiazide-induced hyponatremia in the elderly. *J Am Soc Nephrol.* 1994;5(4):1106–1111.

82. Sharabi Y, Illan R, Kamari Y, et al. Diuretic induced hyponatraemia in elderly hypertensive women. *J Hum Hypertens.* 2002;16(9):631–635.

83. Werbel SS, Ober KP. Acute adrenal insufficiency. *Endocrinol Metab Clin North Am.* 1993;22(2):303–328.

84. Zennaro MC. Mineralocorticoid resistance. *Steroids.* 1996;61(4):189–192.

85. D'Angelo A, Mioni G, Ossi E, et al. Alterations in renal tubular sodium and water transport in polycystic kidney disease. *Clin Nephrol.* 1975;3(3):99–105.

86. Nzerue C, Schlanger L, Jena M, et al. Granulomatous interstitial nephritis and uveitis presenting as salt-losing nephropathy. *Am J Nephrol.* 1997;17(5): 462–465.

87. Hutchison FN, Perez EA, Gandara DR, et al. Renal salt wasting in patients treated with cisplatin. *Ann Intern Med.* 1988;108(1):21–25.

88. Teitelbaum I, McGuinness S. Vasopressin resistance in chronic renal failure. Evidence for the role of decreased v2 receptor mrna. *J Clin Invest.* 1995;96(1): 378–385.

89. Chung HM, Kluge R, Schrier RW, et al. Clinical assessment of extracellular fluid volume in hyponatremia. *Am J Med.* 1987;83:905–908.

90. Carroll PB, McHenry L, Verbalis JG. Isolated adrenocorticotrophic hormone deficiency presenting as chronic hyponatremia. *N Y State J Med.* 1990;90:210–213.

91. Diederich S, Franzen NF, Bahr V, et al. Severe hyponatremia due to hypopituitarism with adrenal insufficiency: report on 28 cases. *Eur J Endocrinol.* 2003;148(6):609–617.

92. Fenske W, Stork S, Koschker AC, et al. Value of fractional uric acid excretion in differential diagnosis of hyponatremic patients on diuretics. *J Clin Endocrinol Metab.* 2008;93(8):2991–2997.

93. Misra SC, Mansharamani GG. Hyponatremia in elderly hospital in-patients. *Brit J Clin Prac.* 1989;43:295–296.

94. Ellison DH, Berl T. Clinical practice. The syndrome of inappropriate antidiuresis. *N Engl J Med.* 2007;356(20):2064–2072.

95. Michelis MF, Fusco RD, Bragdon RW, et al. Reset of osmoreceptors in association with normovolemic hyponatremia. *Am J Med.* Sci 1974;267:267–273.

96. DeFronzo RA, Goldberg M, Agus ZS. Normal diluting capacity in hyponatremic patients. Reset osmostat or a variant of the syndrome of inappropriate antidiuretic hormone secretion. *Ann Intern Med.* 1976;84:538–542.

97. Robertson GL. Posterior pituitary. In: Felig P, Baxter J, Broadus A, Frohman L, eds. *Endocrinology and Metabolism.* New York: McGraw-Hill; 1986:338–385.

98. Robertson GL, Mahr EA, Athar S, et al. Development and clinical application of a new method for the radioimmunoassay of arginine vasopressin in human plasma. *J Clin Invest.* 1973;52:2340–2352.

99. Zerbe R, Stropes L, Robertson G. Vasopressin function in the syndrome of inappropriate antidiuresis. *Annu Rev Med.* 1980;31:315–327.

100. Feldman BJ, Rosenthal SM, Vargas GA, et al. Nephrogenic syndrome of inappropriate antidiuresis. *N Engl J Med.* 2005;352(18):1884–1890.

101. Oelkers W. Hyponatremia and inappropriate secretion of vasopressin (antidiuretic hormone) in patients with hypopituitarism. *N Engl J Med.* 1989; 321:492–496.

102. Fenske W, Stork S, Blechschmidt A, et al. Copeptin in the differential diagnosis of hyponatremia. *J Clin Endocrinol Metab.* 2009;94(1):123–129.

103. List AF, Hainsworth JD, Davis BW, et al. The syndrome of inappropriate secretion of antidiuretic hormone (SIADH) in small-cell lung cancer. *J Clin Oncol.* 1986;4:1191–1198.

104. Maurer LH, O'Donnell JF, Kennedy S, et al. Human neurophysins in carcinoma of the lung: relation to histology, disease stage, response rate, survival, and syndrome of inappropriate antidiuretic hormone secretion. *Cancer Treat Rep.* 1983;67:971–976.

105. Gschwantler M, Weiss W. Hyponatremic coma as the first symptom of a small cell bronchial carcinoma. *Deutsche Medizinische Wochenschrift.* 1994;119:261–264.

106. Kamoi K, Kurokawa I, Kasai H, et al. Asymptomatic hyponatremia due to inappropriate secretion of antidiuretic hormone as the first sign of a small cell lung cancer in an elderly man [see comments]. *Intern Med.* 1998;37(11): 950–954.

107. Ferlito A, Rinaldo A, Devaney KO. Syndrome of inappropriate antidiuretic hormone secretion associated with head neck cancers: review of the literature. *Ann Otol Rhinol Laryngol.* 1997;106(10 Pt 1):878–883.

108. Kavanagh BD, Halperin EC, Rosenbaum LC, et al. Syndrome of inappropriate secretion of antidiuretic hormone in a patient with carcinoma of the nasopharynx. *Cancer.* 1992;69:1315–1319.

109. Renaud L. Hypothalamic magnocellular neurosecretory neurons: intrinsic membrane properties and synaptic connections. *Prog Brain Res.* 1994;100: 133–137.

110. Moses AM, Miller M. Drug-induced dilutional hyponatremia. *N Engl J Med.* 1974;291:1234–1239.

111. Liamis G, Milionis H, Elisaf M. A review of drug-induced hyponatremia. *Am J Kidney Dis.* 2008;52(1):144–153.

112. Robertson GL. Posterior pituitary. In: Felig P, Baxter J, Frohman L, eds. *Endocrinology and Metabolism.* New York: McGraw-Hill, 1995:385–432.

113. Friedman E, Shadel M, Halkin H, et al. Thiazide-induced hyponatremia. Reproducibility by single dose rechallenge and an analysis of pathogenesis. *Ann Intern Med.* 1989;110:24–30.

114. Gibbs DM, Vale W. Effect of the serotonin reuptake inhibitor fluoxetine on corticotropin- releasing factor and vasopressin secretion into hypophysial portal blood. *Brain Res.* 1983;280(1):176–179.

115. Mikkelsen JD, Jensen JB, Engelbrecht T, et al. D-fenfluramine activates rat oxytocinergic and vasopressinergic neurons through different mechanisms. *Brain Res.* 1999;851(1–2):247–251.

116. Faull CM, Rooke P, Baylis PH. The effect of a highly specific serotonin agonist on osmoregulated vasopressin secretion in healthy man. *Clin Endocrinol (Oxf).* 1991;35(5):423–430.

117. Fabian TJ, Amico JA, Kroboth PD, et al. Paroxetine-induced hyponatremia in older adults: a 12–week prospective study. *Arch Intern Med.* 2004;164(3):327–332.

118. Strachan J, Shepherd J. Hyponatraemia associated with the use of selective serotonin reuptake inhibitors. *Aust N Z J Psychiatry.* 1998;32(2):295–298.

119. Bouman WP, Pinner G, Johnson H. Incidence of selective serotonin reuptake inhibitor (ssri) induced hyponatraemia due to the syndrome of inappropriate antidiuretic hormone (siadh) secretion in the elderly. *Int J Geriatr Psychiatry.* 1998;13(1):12–15.
120. Odeh M, Seligmann H, Oliven A. Severe life-threatening hyponatremia during paroxetine therapy. *J Clin Pharmacol.* 1999;39(12):1290–1291.
121. Wilkinson TJ, Begg EJ, Winter AC, et al. Incidence and risk factors for hyponatraemia following treatment with fluoxetine or paroxetine in elderly people. *Br J Clin Pharmacol.* 1999;47(2):211–217.
122. Maxwell DL, Polkey MI, Henry JA. Hyponatraemia and catatonic stupor after taking "ecstasy" [see comments]. *BMJ.* 1993;307:1399.
123. Parr MJ, Low HM, Botterill P. Hyponatraemia and death after "ecstasy" ingestion. *Med J Aust.* 1997;166(3):136–137.
124. Burgess C, O'Donohoe A, Gill M. Agony and ecstasy: a review of MDMA effects and toxicity. *Eur Psychiatry.* 2000;15(5):287–294.
125. Stephenson CP, Hunt GE, Topple AN, et al. The distribution of 3,4-methylenedioxymethamphetamine "Ecstasy"-induced c-fos expression in rat brain. *Neuroscience.* 1999;92(3):1011–1023.
126. Fallon JK, Shah D, Kicman AT, et al. Action of MDMA (ecstasy) and its metabolites on arginine vasopressin release. *Ann N Y Acad Sci.* 2002;965: 399–409.
127. Simmler LD, Hysek CM, Liechti ME. Sex differences in the effects of MDMA (Ecstasy) on plasma copeptin in healthy subjects. *J Clin Endocrinol Metab.* 2011;96(9):2844–2850.
128. Hill AR, Uribarri J, Mann J, et al. Altered water metabolism in tuberculosis: role of vasopressin. *Am J Med.* 1990;88:357–364.
129. Breuer R, Rubinow A. Inappropriate secretion of antidiuretic hormone and mycoplasma pneumonia infection. *Respiration.* 1981;42:217–219.
130. Pollard RB. Inappropriate secretion of antidiuretic hormone associated with adenovirus pneumonia. *Chest.* 1975;68:589–591.
131. Rosenow EC, Segar WE, Zehr JE. Inappropriate antidiuretic hormone secretion in pneumonia. *Mayo Clin Proc.* 1972;47:169–174.
132. Farber MO, Roberts LR, Weinberger MH, et al. Abnormalities of sodium and H_2O handling in chronic obstructive lung disease. *Arch Intern Med.* 1982;142:1326–1330.
133. Sabria M, Campins M. Legionnaires' disease: update on epidemiology and management options. *Am J Respir Med.* 2003;2(3):235–243.
134. Vorherr H, Massry SG, Fallet R, et al. Antidiuretic principle in tuberculous lung tissue of a patient with pulmonary tuberculosis and hyponatremia. *Ann Intern Med.* 1970;72:383–387.
135. Raff H, Shinsako J, Keil LC, et al. Vasopressin, ACTH, and blood pressure during hypoxia induced at different rates. *Am J Physiol.* 1983;245(5 Pt 1): E489–E493.
136. Kelestimur H, Leach RM, Ward JP, et al. Vasopressin and oxytocin release during prolonged environmental hypoxia in the rat. *Thorax.* 1997;52(1):84–88.
137. Baylis PH, Stockley RA, Heath DA. Effect of acute hypoxaemia on plasma arginine vasopressin in conscious man. *Clin Sci Mol Med.* 1977;53(4):401–404.
138. Farber MO, Bright TP, Strawbridge RA, et al. Impaired water handling in chronic obstructive lung disease. *J Lab Clin Med.* 1975;85:41–49.
139. Leach RM, Forsling ML. The effect of changes in arterial PCO2 on neuroendocrine function in man. *Exp Physiol.* 2004;89(3):287–292.
140. Dhawan A, Narang A, Singhi S. Hyponatraemia and the inappropriate ADH syndrome in pneumonia. *Ann Trop Ped.* 1992;12:455–462.
141. Hussain SF, Irfan M, Abbasi M, et al. Clinical characteristics of 110 miliary tuberculosis patients from a low HIV prevalence country. *Int J Tuberc Lung Dis.* 2004;8(4):493–499.
142. Baratz RA, Ingraham RC. Renal hemodynamics and antidiuretic hormone release associated with volume regulation. *Am J Physiol.* 1960;198:565.
143. Agarwal A, Soni A, Ciechanowsky M, et al. Hyponatremia in patients with the acquired immunodeficiency syndrome. *Nephron.* 1989;53:317–321.
144. Cusano AJ, Thies HL, Siegal FP, et al. Hyponatremia in patients with acquired immune deficiency syndrome. *J Acq Immune Def Syn.* 1990;3:949–953.
145. Tang WW, Kaptein EM, Feinstein EI, et al. Hyponatremia in hospitalized patients with the acquired immunodeficiency syndrome (AIDS) and the AIDS-related complex. *Am J Med.* 1993;94:169–174.
146. Tolaymat A, al-Mousily F, Sleasman J, et al. Hyponatremia in pediatric patients with HIV-1 infection. *South Med J.* 1995;88(10):1039–1042.
147. Noto H, Kaneko Y, Takano T, et al. Severe hyponatremia and hyperkalemia induced by trimethoprim-sulfamethoxazole in patients with pneumocystis carinii pneumonia. *Intern Med.* 1995;34(2):96–99.
148. Yeung KT, Chan M, Chan CK. The safety of i.v. pentamidine administered in an ambulatory setting. *Chest.* 1996;110(1):136–140.
149. Young M, Sciurba F, Rinaldo J. Delirium and pulmonary edema after completing a marathon. *Am Rev Respir Dis.* 1987;136:737–739.
150. Noakes TD, Goodwin N, Rayner BL, et al. Water intoxication: a possible complication during endurance exercise. *Med Sci Sports Exerc.* 1985;17(3): 370–375.
151. Speedy DB, Noakes TD, Rogers IR, et al. Hyponatremia in ultradistance triathletes. *Med Sci Sports Exerc.* 1999;31(6):809–815.
152. O'Brien KK, Montain SJ, Corr WP, et al. Hyponatremia associated with overhydration in U.S. Army trainees. *Mil Med.* 2001;166(5):405–410.
153. Backer HD, Shopes E, Collins SL, et al. Exertional heat illness and hyponatremia in hikers. *Am J Emerg Med..* 1999;17(6):532–539.
154. Garigan TP, Ristedt DE. Death from hyponatremia as a result of acute water intoxication in an Army basic trainee. *Mil Med.* 1999;164(3):234–238.
155. Ayus JC, Varon J, Arieff AI. Hyponatremia, cerebral edema, and noncardiogenic pulmonary edema in marathon runners. *Ann Intern Med.* 2000;132(9): 711–714.
156. Noakes TD. The hyponatremia of exercise. [Review]. *Int J Sport Nutr.* 1992;2: 205–228.
157. Speedy DB, Noakes TD, Schneider C. Exercise-associated hyponatremia: a review. *Emerg Med (Fremantle).* 2001;13(1):17–27.
158. Siegel A, Verbalis JG, Clement SC. Exertional hyponatremia is associated with inappropriate secretion of arginine vasopressin. *Am J Med.* 2007; 120(5):461.
159. Hew-Butler T. Arginine vasopressin, fluid balance and exercise: is exercise-associated hyponatraemia a disorder of arginine vasopressin secretion? *Sports Med.* 2010;40(6):459–479.
160. Goldstein CS, Braunstein S, Goldfarb S. Idiopathic syndrome of inappropriate antidiuretic hormone secretion possibly related to advanced age. *Ann Intern Med.* 1983;99:185–188.
161. Hamilton DV. Inappropriate secretion of antidiuretic hormone associated with cerebellar and cerebral atrophy. *Postgrad Med J.* 1978;54:427–428.
162. Miller M. Hyponatremia: age-related risk factors and therapy decisions. *Geriatrics.* 1998;53(7):32–33, 37–38, 41–42:assim.
163. Kleinfeld M, Casimir M, Borra S. Hyponatremia as observed in a chronic disease facility. *J Am Geriatrics Soc.* 1979;27:156–161.
164. Miller M, Hecker MS, Friedlander DA, et al. Apparent idiopathic hyponatremia in an ambulatory geriatric population. *J Am Geriatr Soc.* 1996;44(4): 404–408.
165. Pillans PI, Coulter DM. Fluoxetine and hyponatraemia—a potential hazard in the elderly. *N Zealand Med J.* 1994;107:85–86.
166. Rault RM. Case report: hyponatremia associated with nonsteroidal antiinflammatory drugs. *Am J Med Sci.* 1993;305:318–320.
167. Hirshberg B, Ben-Yehuda A. The syndrome of inappropriate antidiuretic hormone secretion in the elderly. *Am J Med.* 1997;103(4):270–273.
168. Arinzon Z, Feldman J, Jarchowsky J, et al. A comparative study of the syndrome of inappropriate antidiuretic hormone secretion in community-dwelling patients and nursing home residents. *Aging Clin Exp Res.* 2003;15(1):6–11.
169. Anpalahan M. Chronic idiopathic hyponatremia in older people due to syndrome of inappropriate antidiuretic hormone secretion (SIADH) possibly related to aging. *J Am Geriatr Soc.* 2001;49(6):788–792.
170. Rowe JW, Kilgore A, Robertson GL. Evidence in man that cigarette smoking induces vasopressin release via an airway-specific mechanism. *J Clin Endocrinol Metab.* 1980;51:170–172.
171. Ellinas PA, Rosner F, Jaume JC. Symptomatic hyponatremia associated with psychosis, medications, and smoking. *J Natl Med Assoc.* 1993;85:135–141.
172. Vieweg WV, David JJ, Rowe WT, et al. Correlation of cigarette-induced increase in serum nicotine levels with arginine vasopressin concentrations in the syndrome of self-induced water intoxication and psychosis (SIWIP). *Can J Psych -Rev Can Psych.* 1986;31:108–111.
173. Lausen HD. Metabolism of the neurohypophyseal hormones. In: Greep RO, Astwood EB, Knobil E, Sawyer WH, Geiger SR, eds. *Handbook of Physiology.* Washington: American Physiological Society; 1974: 287–393.
174. Rowe JW, Shelton RL, Helderman JH, et al. Influence of the emetic reflex on vasopressin release in man. *Kidney Int.* 1979;16:729–735.
175. Coslovsky R, Bruck R, Estrov Z. Hypo-osmolal syndrome due to prolonged nausea. *Arch Intern Med.* 1984;144:191–192.
176. Edelson JT, Robertson GL. The effect of the cold pressor test on vasopressin secretion in man. *Psychoneuroendocrinology.* 1986;11:307–316.
177. North WG, Friedmann AS, Yu X. Tumor biosynthesis of vasopressin and oxytocin. *Ann N Y Acad Sci.* 1993;689:107–121.
178. Legros JJ, Geenen V, Carvelli T, et al. Neurophysins as markers of vasopressin and oxytocin release. A study in carcinoma of the lung. *Hormone Res.* 1990;34:151–155.
179. Ishikawa S, Kuratomi Y, Saito T. A case of oat cell carcinoma of the lung associated with ectopic production of ADH, neurophysin and ACTH. *Endocrinol Jpn.* 1980;27:257–263.

180. George JM, Capen CC, Phillips AS. Biosynthesis of vasopressin in vitro and ultrastructure of a bronchogenic carcinoma. Patient with the syndrome of inappropriate secretion of antidiuretic hormone. *J Clin Invest.* 1972;51:141–148.
181. Rosenbaum LC, Neuwelt EA, Van Tol HH, et al. Expression of neurophysin-related precursor in cell membranes of a small-cell lung carcinoma. *Proc Natl Acad Sci U S A.* 1990;87:9928–9932.
182. Yamaji T, Ishibashi M, Yamada N, et al. Biosynthesis of the common precursor to vasopressin and neurophysin in vitro in transplantable human oat cell carcinoma of the lung with ectopic vasopressin production. *Endocrinol Jpn.* 1983;30:451–461.
183. Vorherr H, Massry SG, Utiger RD, et al. Antidiuretic principle in malignant tumor extracts from patients with inappropriate ADH syndrome. *J Clin Endocrinol Metab.* 1968;28(2):162–168.
184. Verbalis JG. Hyponatremia: epidemiology, pathophysiology, and therapy. *Curr Opin Nephrol Hyperten.* 1993;2:636–652.
185. Schrier RW. Editorial: "Inappropriate" versus "appropriate" antidiuretic hormone secretion. *West Med J.* 1974;121:62–64.
186. Schrier RW, Berl T, Anderson RJ. Osmotic and nonosmotic control of vasopressin release. *Am J Physiol.* 1979;236:F321–F332.
187. Cowley AW Jr. Vasopressin and cardiovascular regulation. *Int Rev Physiol.* 1982;26:189–242.
188. Verbalis JG. Hyponatremia induced by vasopressin or desmopressin in female and male rats. *J Am Soc Nephrol.* 1993;3:1600–1606.
189. Goldman MB, Luchins DJ, Robertson GL. Mechanisms of altered water metabolism in psychotic patients with polydipsia and hyponatremia. *N Engl J Med.* 1988;318:397–403.
190. Saito T, Ishikawa SE, Ando F, et al. Exaggerated urinary excretion of aquaporin-2 in the pathological state of impaired water excretion dependent upon arginine vasopressin. *J Clin Endocrinol Metab.* 1998;83(11):4034–4040.
191. Robertson GL, Aycinena P, Zerbe RL. Neurogenic disorders of osmoregulation. *Am J Med.* 1982;72:339–353.
192. Robertson GL, Athar S. The interaction of blood osmolality and blood volume in regulating plasma vasopressin in man. *J Clin Endocrinol Metab.* 1976;42:613–620.
193. Robertson GL. The regulation of vasopressin function in health and disease. *Rec Prog Horm Res.* 1976;33:333–385.
194. Schrier RW. Body fluid volume regulation in health and disease: a unifying hypothesis. *Ann Intern Med.* 1990;113:155–159.
195. Kortas C, Bichet DG, Rouleau JL, et al. Vasopressin in congestive heart failure. *J Cardiovas Pharm.* 1986;8 Suppl 7:S107–S110.
196. Verbalis JG, Baldwin EF, Robinson AG. Osmotic regulation of plasma vasopressin and oxytocin after sustained hyponatremia. *Am J Physiol.* 1986;250: R444–R451.
197. Verbalis JG, Dohanics J. Vasopressin and oxytocin secretion in chronically hypoosmolar rats. *Am J Physiol.* 1991;261:R1028–R1038.
198. Lindheimer MD, Davison JM. Osmoregulation, the secretion of arginine vasopressin and its metabolism during pregnancy. *Eur J Endocrinol.* 1995;132(2): 133–143.
199. Weisinger RS, Burns P, Eddie LW, et al. Relaxin alters the plasma osmolality-arginine vasopressin relationship in the rat. *J Endocrinol.* 1993;137(3):505–510.
200. Wilson BC, Summerlee AJ. Effects of exogenous relaxin on oxytocin and vasopressin release and the intramammary pressure response to central hyperosmotic challenge. *J Endocrinol.* 1994;141(1):75–80.
201. Wall BM, Crofton JT, Share L, et al. Chronic hyponatremia due to resetting of the osmostat in a patient with gastric carcinoma. *Am J Med.* 1992;93: 223–228.
202. Kamoi K. Syndrome of inappropriate antidiuresis without involving inappropriate secretion of vasopressin in an elderly woman: effect of intravenous administration of the nonpeptide vasopressin v2 receptor antagonist opc-31260. *Nephron.* 1997;76(1):111–115.
203. Kavanaugh BD, Halperin EC, Rosenbaum LC, et al. Syndrome of inappropriate secretion of antidiuretic hormone in a patient with carcinoma of the nasopharynx. *Cancer.* 1992;69:1315–1319.
204. Talmi YP, Hoffman HT, McCabe BF. Syndrome of inappropriate secretion of arginine vasopressin in patients with cancer of the head and neck. *Ann Otol Rhinol Laryngol.* 1992;101:946–949.
205. Verbalis JG. Osmotic inhibition of neurohypophysial secretion. *Ann N Y Acad Sci.* 1993;689:146–160.
206. Dohanics J, Verbalis JG. Naloxone disinhibits magnocellular responses to osmotic and volemic stimuli in chronically hypoosmolar rats. *J Neuroendocrinol.* 1995;7:57–62.
207. Nissen R, Renaud LP. GABA receptor mediation of median preoptic nucleus-evoked inhibition of supraoptic neurosecretory neurons in the rat. *J Physiol.* 1994;479.2:207–216.
208. Helderman JH, Vestal RE, Rowe JW, et al. The response of arginine vasopressin to intravenous ethanol and hypertonic saline in man: the impact of aging. *J Gerontol.* 1978;33:39–47.
209. Rowe JW, Minaker KL, Sparrow D, et al. Age-related failure of volume-pressure-mediated vasopressin release. *J Clin Endocrinol Metab.* 1982;54:661–664.
210. Hodak SP, Verbalis JG. Abnormalities of water homeostasis in aging. *Endocrin Metab Clinics North Am.* 2005;34(4):1031–1046.
211. Manoogian C, Pandian M, Ehrlich L, et al. Plasma atrial natriuretic hormone levels in patients with the syndrome of inappropriate antidiuretic hormone secretion. *J Clin Endocrinol Metab.* 1988;67:571–575.
212. Peters JP, Welt KG, Sims EAH, et al. A salt-wasting syndrome associated with cerebral disease. *Trans Ass Am Physiol.* 1950;63:57–64.
213. Doczi T, Tarjanyi J, Huszka E, et al. Syndrome of inappropriate secretion of antidiuretic hormone (SIADH) after head injury. *Neurosurgery.* 1982;10:685–688.
214. Nelson PB, Seif S, Gutai J, et al. Hyponatremia and natriuresis following subarachnoid hemorrhage in a monkey model. *J Neurosurg.* 1984;60:233–237.
215. Wijdicks EF, Vermeulen M, Hijdra A, et al. Hyponatremia and cerebral infarction in patients with ruptured intracranial aneurysms: is fluid restriction harmful? *Ann Neurol.* 1985;17:137–140.
216. Wijdicks EF, Ropper AH, Hunnicutt EJ, et al. Atrial natriuretic factor and salt wasting after aneurysmal subarachnoid hemorrhage. *Stroke.* 1991;22:1519–1524.
217. Diringer MN, Lim JS, Kirsch JR, et al. Suprasellar and intraventricular blood predict elevated plasma atrial natriuretic factor in subarachnoid hemorrhage. *Stroke.* 1991;22:577–581.
218. Oh MS, Carroll HJ. Cerebral salt-wasting syndrome. We need better proof of its existence. *Nephron.* 1999;82(2):110–114.
219. Maesaka JK, Gupta S, Fishbane S. Cerebral salt-wasting syndrome: does it exist? *Nephron.* 1999;82(2):100–109.
220. Palmer BF. Hyponatremia in patients with central nervous system disease: SIADH versus CSW. *Trends Endocrinol Metab.* 2003;14(4):182–187.
221. Sviri GE, Shik V, Raz B, et al. Role of brain natriuretic peptide in cerebral vasospasm. *Acta Neurochir (Wien).* 2003;145(10):851–860.
222. Espiner EA, Leikis R, Ferch RD, et al. The neuro-cardio-endocrine response to acute subarachnoid haemorrhage. *Clin Endocrinol (Oxf).* 2002;56(5):629–635.
223. McGirt MJ, Blessing R, Nimjee SM, et al. Correlation of serum brain natriuretic peptide with hyponatremia and delayed ischemic neurological deficits after subarachnoid hemorrhage. *Neurosurgery.* 2004;54(6):1369–1373.
224. Weinand ME, O'Boynick PL, Goetz KL. A study of serum antidiuretic hormone and atrial natriuretic peptide levels in a series of patients with intracranial disease and hyponatremia. *Neurosurgery.* 1989;25:781–785.
225. Diringer MN, Wu KC, Verbalis JG, et al. Hypervolemic therapy prevents volume contraction but not hyponatremia following subarachnoid hemorrhage. *Ann Neurol.* 1992;31:543–550.
226. Mori T, Katayama Y, Kawamata T, et al. Improved efficiency of hypervolemic therapy with inhibition of natriuresis by fludrocortisone in patients with aneurysmal subarachnoid hemorrhage. *J Neurosurg.* 1999;91(6):947–952.
227. Ishikawa S, Fujita N, Fujisawa G, et al. Involvement of arginine vasopressin and renal sodium handling in pathogenesis of hyponatremia in elderly patients. *Endocr J.* 1996;43(1):101–108.
228. Kamoi K, Ebe T, Hasegawa A, et al. Hyponatremia in small cell lung cancer. Mechanisms not involving inappropriate ADH secretion. *Cancer.* 1987;60: 1089–1093.
229. Gross AJ, Steinberg SM, Reilly JG, et al. Atrial natriuretic factor and arginine vasopressin production in tumor cell lines from patients with lung cancer and their relationship to serum sodium. *Cancer Res.* 1993;53:67–74.
230. Shimizu K, Nakano S, Nakano Y, et al. Ectopic atrial natriuretic peptide production in small cell lung cancer with the syndrome of inappropriate antidiuretic hormone secretion. *Cancer.* 1991;68:2284–2288.
231. Bliss DP Jr, Battey JF, Linnoila RI, et al. Expression of the atrial natriuretic factor gene in small cell lung cancer tumors and tumor cell lines. *J Natl Cancer Inst.* 1990;82:305–310.
232. Johnson BE, Chute JP, Rushin J, et al. A prospective study of patients with lung cancer and hyponatremia of malignancy. *Am J Respir Crit Care Med.* 1997;156(5):1669–1678.
233. Thorn GW. *The Diagnosis and Treatment of Adrenal Insufficiency.* Springfield, IL: Charles C Thomas; 1951.
234. Knowlton AI. Addison's disease: a review of its clinical course and management. In: Christy NP, editor. *The Human Adrenal Cortex.* New York: Harper & Row; 1971: 329–358.
235. Nerup J. Addison's disease - clinical studies. *Acta Endocrinol.* 1974;76: 127–141.
236. Loeb RF, Atchley DW, Benedict EM. Electrolyte balance studies in adrenalectomized dogs with particular reference to excretion of sodium. *J Exp Med.* 1933;57:775.

237. Harrop GA, Soffer LJ, Ellsworth R. Studies on the suprarenal cortex. III. Plasma electrolytes and electrolyte excretion during suprarenal insufficiency in the dog. *J Exp Med.* 1933;58:17.
238. Gill JR Jr, Gann DS, Bartter FC. Restoration of water diuresis in Addisonian patients by expansion of the volume of the extracellular fluid. *J Clin Invest.* 1962;41:1078–1085.
239. Share L, Travis RH. Plasma vasopressin concentration in the adrenally insufficient dog. *Endocrinology.* 1970;86:196–201.
240. Seif SM, Robinson AG, Zimmerman EA, et al. Plasma neurophysin and vasopressin in the rat: response to adrenalectomy and steroid replacement. *Endocrinology.* 1978;103:1009–1015.
241. Boykin J, DeTorrente A, Robertson GL, et al. Persistent plasma vasopressin levels in the hypoosmolar state associated with mineralocorticoid deficiency. *Miner Electrolyte Metab.* 1979;2:310–315.
242. Ishikawa S, Schrier RW. Effect of arginine vasopressin antagonist on renal water excretion in glucocorticoid and mineralocorticoid deficient rats. *Kidney Int.* 1982;22:587–593.
243. Green HH, Harrington AR, Valtin H. On the role of antidiuretic hormone in the inhibition of acute water diuresis in adrenal insufficiency and the effects of gluco- and mineralocorticoids in reversing the inhibition. *J Clin Invest.* 1970;49:1724–1736.
244. Cutler RE, Kleeman CR, Koplowitz J, et al. Mechanisms of impaired water excretion in adrenal and pituitary insufficiency. III. The effect of extracellular or plasma volume expansion, or both, on the impaired diuresis. *J Clin Invest.* 1962;41:1524–1530.
245. Ufferman RC, Schrier RW. Importance of sodium intake and mineralocorticoid hormone in the impaired water excretion in adrenal insufficiency. *J Clin Invest.* 1972;51:1639–1646.
246. Ikkos D, Luft R, Olivecrona H. Hypophysectomy in man: effect on water excretion during the first two postoperative months. *J Clin Endocrinol Metab.* 1955;15:553–567.
247. Bethune JE, Nelson DH. Hyponatremia in hypopituitarism. *N Engl J Med.* 1965;272:771.
248. Stacpoole PW, Interlandi JW, Nicholson WE. Isolated ACTH deficiency: a heterogeneous disorder. *Medicine.* 1982;61:13–24.
249. Mandell IN, DeFronzo RA, Robertson GL, et al. Role of plasma arginine vasopressin in the impaired water diuresis of isolated glucocorticoid deficiency in the rat. *Kidney Int.* 1980;17:170–195.
250. Boykin J, DeTorrente A, Erickson A, et al. Role of plasma vasopressin in impaired water excretion of glucocorticoid deficiency. *J Clin Invest.* 1978;62:738–744.
251. Linas SL, Berl T, Robertson GL, et al. Role of vasopressin in the impaired water excretion of glucocorticoid deficiency. *Kidney Int.* 1980;18:58–67.
252. Schwartz MJ, Kokko JP. Urinary concentrating defect of adrenal insufficiency: permissive role of adrenal steroids on the hydroosmotic response across the rabbit cortical collecting tubule. *J Clin Invest.* 1980;66:234–242.
253. Aubry RH, Nankin HR, Moses AM, et al. Measurement of the osmotic threshold for vasopressin release in human subjects, and its modification by cortisol. *J Clin Endocrinol Metab.* 1965;25:1481–1492.
254. Raff H. Interactions between neurohypophysial hormones and the ACTH-adrenocortical axis. *Ann N Y Acad Sci.* 1993;689:411–425.
255. Kiss JZ, Van Eckelen AM, Reul JMHM. Glucocorticoid receptor in magnocellular neurosecretory neurons. *Endocrinology.* 1988;122:444–449.
256. Berghorn KA, Knapp LT, Hoffman GE, et al. Induction of glucocorticoid receptor expression in hypothalamic neurons during chronic hypoosmolality. *Endocrinology.* 1995;136:804–807.
257. Stillman MA, Recht LD, Rosario SL, et al. The effects of adrenalectomy and glucocorticoid replacement on vasopressin and vasopressin-neurophysin in the zona externa of the rat. *Endocrinology.* 1977;101:42–49.
258. Robinson AG, Seif SM, Verbalis JG, et al. Quantitation of changes in the content of neurohypophyseal peptides in hypothalamic nuclei after adrenalectomy. *Neuroendocrinology.* 1983;36:347–350.
259. Recht LD, Hoffman DL, Haldar J, et al. Vasopressin concentrations in hypophysial portal plasma; insignificant reduction following removal of the posterior pituitary. *Neuroendocrinology.* 1981;33:88–90.
260. Rivier C, Vale W. Modulation of stress-induced ACTH release by corticotropin-releasing factor, catecholamines and vasopressin. *Nature.* 1983;305:325–327.
261. Antoni FA. Hypothalamic control of adrenocorticotropin secretion: advances since the discovery of 41–residue corticotropin-releasing factor. *Endocrine Rev.* 1986;7:351–378.
262. Verbalis JG, Baldwin EF, Ronnekleiv OK, et al. In vitro release of vasopressin and oxytocin from rat median eminence tissue. *Neuroendocrinology.* 1986;42:481–488.
263. Hanna FW, Scanlon MF. Hyponatraemia, hypothyroidism, and role of arginine-vasopressin. *Lancet.* 1997;350(9080):755–756.
264. Curtis RH. Hyponatremia in primary myxedema. *Ann Intern Med.* 1956;44:376.
265. Chinitz A, Turner FL. The association of primary hypothyroidism and inappropriate secretion of the antidiuretic hormone. *Arch Intern Med.* 1965;116:871–874.
266. Larsen PR, Ingbar SH. The thyroid gland. In: Wilson JD, Foster DW, editors. *Williams Textbook of Endocrinology*. Philadelphia: W.B. Saunders; 1992:357–487.
267. LeRoith D, Broitman D, Sukenik S, et al. Isolated ACTH deficiency and primary hypothyroidism: volume-dependent elevation of antidiuretic hormone secretion in the presence of hyponatremia. *Israel J Med Sci.* 1980;16:440–443.
268. Crispell KR, Parson W, Sprinkle PA. A cortisone-resistant abnormality in the diuretic response to ingested water in primary myxedema. *J Clin Endocrinol Metab.* 1954;14:640.
269. Derubertis FR Jr, Michelis MF, Bloom ME, et al. Impaired water excretion in myxedema. *Am J Med.* 1971;51:41–53.
270. Skowsky WR, Kikuchi TA. The role of vasopressin in the impaired water excretion of myxedema. *Am J Med.* 1978;64:613–621.
271. Emmanouel DS, Lindheimer MD, Karz AI. Mechanism of impaired water excretion in the hypothyroid rat. *J Clin Invest.* 1974;54:926–934.
272. Seif SM, Robinson AG, Zenser TV, et al. Neurohypophyseal peptides in hypothyroid rats: Plasma levels and kidney response. *Metabolism.* 1979;28:137–143.
273. Hlad CJ, Bricker NS. Renal function and I^{125} clearance in hyperthyroidism and myxedema. *J Clin Endocrinol Metab.* 1954;14:1539.
274. Ford RV, Owens JC, Curd GW. Kidney function in various thyroid states. *J Clin Endocrinol Metab.* 1961;21:548.
275. Davies CE, Mackinnon J, Platts MM. Renal circulation and cardiac output in low-output heart failure and in myxedema. *BMJ.* 1952;2:595.
276. Graettinger JS, Muenster JJ, Checchia CS, et al. A correlation of clinical and hemodynamic studies in patients with hypothyroidism. *J Clin Invest.* 1958;37:502–510.
277. Amidi M, Leon DF, DeGroot WJ. Effect of the thyroid state on myocardial contractility and ventricular ejection rate in man. *Circulation.* 1968;38:229–239.
278. Holmes EW, DiScala VA. Studies on the exaggerated natriuretic response to a saline infusion in the hypothyroid rat. *J Clin Invest.* 1970;49:1224–1236.
279. Michael UF, Kelley J, Alpert H, et al. Role of distal delivery of filtrate in impaired renal dilution of the hypothyroid rat. *Am J Physiol.* 1976;230:699–705.
280. Archambeaud-Mouveroux F, Dejax C, Jadaud JM, et al. Myxedema coma with hypervasopressinism. 2 cases. *Ann Intern Med.* 1987;138:114–118.
281. Salomez-Granier F, Lefebvre J, Racadot A, et al. Antidiuretic hormone levels (arginine-vasopressin) in cases of peripheral hypothyroidism. 26 cases. *Presse Medicale - Paris* 1983;12:1001–1004.
282. Laczi F, Janaky T, Ivanyi T, et al. Osmoregulation of arginine-8–vasopressin secretion in primary hypothyroidism and in Addison's disease. *Acta Endocrinol.* 1987;114:389–395.
283. Macaron C, Famuyiwa O. Hyponatremia of hypothyroidism. Appropriate suppression of antidiuretic hormone levels. *Arch Intern Med.* 1978;138:820–822.
284. Iwasaki Y, Oiso Y, Yamauchi K, et al. Osmoregulation of plasma vasopressin in myxedema. *J Clin Endocrinol Metab.* 1990;70:534–539.
285. Hochberg Z, Benderly A. Normal osmotic threshold for vasopressin release in the hyponatremia of hypothyroidism. *Hormone Res.* 1983;17:128–133.
286. Caron C, Plante GE, Belanger R, et al. Hypothyroid hyponatremia: dilution defect non-correctable with demeclocycline. *Can Med Assoc J.* 1980;123:1019–1021.
287. Howard RL, Summer S, Rossi N, et al. Short-term hypothyroidism and vasopressin gene expression in the rat. *Am J Kidney Dis.* 1992;19:573–577.
288. Kim JK, Summer SN, Schrier RW. Cellular action of arginine vasopressin in the isolated renal tubules of hypothyroid rats. *Am J Physiol.* 1987;253:F104–F110.
289. Barlow ED, DeWardner HE. Compulsive water drinking. *Q J Med.* 1959;28:235.
290. Dubovsky SL, Grabon S, Berl T, et al. Syndrome of inappropriate secretion of antidiuretic hormone with exacerbated psychosis. *Ann Intern Med.* 1973;79:551–554.
291. Hariprasad MK, Eisinger RP, Nadler IM, et al. Hyponatremia in psychogenic polydipsia. *Arch Intern Med.* 1980;140:1639–1642.
292. Kramer DS, Drake ME Jr. Acute psychosis, polydipsia, and inappropriate secretion of antidiuretic hormone. *Am J Med.* 1983;75:712–714.
293. de Leon J, Verghese C, Tracy JI, et al. Polydipsia and water intoxication in psychiatric patients: a review of the epidemiological literature. *Bio Psych.* 1994;35:408–419.
294. Vieweg WV, Robertson GL, Godleski LS, et al. Diurnal variation in water homeostasis among schizophrenic patients subject to water intoxication. *Schizophrenia Res.* 1988;1:351–357.

295. Gleadhill IC, Smith TA, Yium JJ. Hyponatremia in patients with schizophrenia. *South Med J.* 1982;75:426–428.
296. Ohsawa H, Kishimoto T, Hirai M, et al. An epidemiological study on hyponatremia in psychiatric patients in mental hospitals in Nara Prefecture. *Jpn J Psych Neurol.* 1992;46:883–889.
297. Stuart CA, Neelon FA, Lebovitz HE. Disordered control of thirst in hypothalamic-pituitary sarcoidosis. *N Engl J Med.* 1980;303:1078–1082.
298. Kushnir M, Schattner A, Ezri T, et al. Schizophrenia and fatal self-induced water intoxication with appropriately-diluted urine. *Am J Med.* Sci 1990;300:385–387.
299. Noakes TD, Wilson G, Gray DA, et al. Peak rates of diuresis in healthy humans during oral fluid overload. *S Afr Med J.* 2001;91(10):852–857.
300. Mendelson WB, Deza PC. Polydipsia, hyponatremia, and seizures in psychotic patients. *J Nerv Ment Dis.* 1976;162:140–143.
301. Vieweg WV, Carey RM, Godleski LS, et al. The syndrome of psychosis, intermittent hyponatremia, and polydipsia: evidence for diurnal volume expansion. *Psych Med.* 1990;8:135–144.
302. Bouget J, Thomas R, Camus C, et al. Water intoxication in psychiatric patients. 13 cases of severe hyponatremia. *Rev Med Interne.* 1989;10:515–520.
303. Cheng JC, Zikos D, Skopicki HA, et al. Long-term neurologic outcome in psychogenic water drinkers with severe symptomatic hyponatremia: the effect of rapid correction. *Am J Med.* 1990;88:561–566.
304. Rosenbaum JF, Rothman JS, Murray GB. Psychosis and water intoxication. *J Clin Psych.* 1979;40:287–291.
305. Delva NJ, Crammer JL, Lawson JS, et al. Vasopressin in chronic psychiatric patients with primary polydipsia. *Brit J Psych.* 1990;157:703–712.
306. Emsley R, Potgieter A, Taljaard F, et al. Water excretion and plasma vasopressin in psychotic disorders. *Am J Psych.* 1989;146:250–253.
307. Levine S, McManus BM, Blackbourne BD, et al. Fatal water intoxication, schizophrenia and diuretic therapy for systemic hypertension. *Am J Med.* 1987;82:153–155.
308. Shah PJ, Greenberg WM. Water intoxication precipitated by thiazide diuretics in polydipsic psychiatric patients. *Am J Psych.* 1991;148:1424–1425.
309. Kimelman N, Albert SG. Phenothiazine-induced hyponatremia in the elderly. *Gerontology.* 1984;30:132–136.
310. Gossain VV, Hagen GA, Sugawara M. Drug-induced hyponatraemia in psychogenic polydipsia. *Postgrad Med J.* 1976;52:720–722.
311. Tildesley HD, Toth E, Crockford PM. Syndrome of inappropriate secretion of antidiuretic hormone in association with chlorpromazine ingestion. *Can J Psych -Rev Can Psych.* 1983;28:487–488.
312. Kastner T, Friedman DL, Pond WS. Carbamazepine-induced hyponatremia in patients with mental retardation. *Am J Ment Retard.* 1992;96:536–540.
313. Madhusoodanan S, Bogunovic OJ, Moise D, et al. Hyponatraemia associated with psychotropic medications. A review of the literature and spontaneous reports. *Adverse Drug React Toxicol Rev.* 2002;21(1–2):17–29.
314. Blum A. The possible role of tobacco cigarette smoking in hyponatremia of long-term psychiatric patients. *JAMA.* 1984;252:2864–2865.
315. Allon M, Allen HM, Deck LV, et al. Role of cigarette use in hyponatremia in schizophrenic patients. *Am J Psych.* 1990;147:1075–1077.
316. Finch CK, Andrus MR, Curry WA. Nicotine replacement therapy-associated syndrome of inappropriate antidiuretic hormone. *South Med J.* 2004;97(3):322–324.
317. Lever EG, Stansfeld SA. Addison's disease, psychosis, and the syndrome of inappropriate secretion of antidiuretic hormone. *Brit J Psych.* 1983;143:406–410.
318. Goldman MB, Robertson GL, Luchins DJ, et al. Psychotic exacerbations and enhanced vasopressin secretion in schizophrenic patients with hyponatremia and polydipsia. *Arch Gen Psychiatry.* 1997;54(5):443–449.
319. Holmes JH. Thirst and fluid intake problems in clinical medicine. In: Wayner MJ, ed. *Thirst.* Oxford: Pergamon Press; 1964: 57–75.
320. de Castro J. A microregulatory analysis of spontaneous fluid intake in humans: evidence that the amount of liquid ingested and its timing is mainly governed by feeding. *Physiol Behav.* 1988;3:705–714.
321. Smith D, Moore K, Tormey W, et al. Downward resetting of the osmotic threshold for thirst in patients with SIADH. *Am J Physiol Endocrinol Metab.* 2004;287(5):E1019–E1023.
322. Szczepanska-Sadowska E, Sobocinska J, Sadowski B. Central dipsogenic effect of vasopressin. *Am J Physiol.* 1982;242:R372–R379.
323. Ernits T, Corbit JD. Taste as a dipsogenic stimulus. *J Comp Physiol Psychol.* 1973;83:27–31.
324. Verbalis JG. An experimental model of syndrome of inappropriate antidiuretic hormone secretion in the rat. *Am J Physiol.* 1984;247:E540–E553.
325. Stricker EM, Adair ER. Body fluid balance, taste, and postprandial factors in schedule-induced polydipsia. *J Comp Physiol Psychol.* 1966;62:449–454.
326. Verbalis JG. Inhibitory controls of drinking. In: Ramsay DJ, Booth DA, eds. *Thirst: Physiological and Psychological Aspects.* Springer-Verlag: London; 1991: 313–334.
327. Hew-Butler T, Almond C, Ayus JC, et al. Consensus statement of the 1st International Exercise-Associated Hyponatremia Consensus Development Conference, Cape Town, South Africa 2005. *Clin J Sport Med.* 2005;15(4):208–213.
328. Hiller WD, O'Toole ML, Fortess EE, et al. Medical and physiological considerations in triathlons. Am *J Sports Med.* 1987;15(2):164–167.
329. Hew-Butler T, Ayus JC, Kipps C, et al. Statement of the Second International Exercise-Associated Hyponatremia Consensus Development Conference, New Zealand, 2007. *Clin J Sport Med.* 2008;18(2):111–121.
330. Hiller WD. Dehydration and hyponatremia during triathlons. *Med Sci Sports Exerc.* 1989;21(5 Suppl):S219–S221.
331. Hew TD, Chorley JN, Cianca JC, et al. The incidence, risk factors, and clinical manifestations of hyponatremia in marathon runners. *Clin J Sport Med.* 2003;13(1):41–47.
332. Almond CS, Shin AY, Fortescue EB, et al. Hyponatremia among runners in the Boston Marathon. *N Engl J Med.* 2005;352(15):1550–1556.
333. Speedy DB, Rogers I, Safih S, et al. Hyponatremia and seizures in an ultradistance triathlete. *J Emerg Med.* 2000;18(1):41–44.
334. Hiller WD. Dehydration and hyponatremia during triathlons. [Review]. *Med Sci Sports Exerc.* 1989;21:S219–S221.
335. Irving RA, Noakes TD, Buck R, et al. Evaluation of renal function and fluid homeostasis during recovery from exercise-induced hyponatremia. *J Appl Physiol.* 1991;70:342–348.
336. Speedy DB, Rogers IR, Noakes TD, et al. Exercise-induced hyponatremia in ultradistance triathletes is caused by inappropriate fluid retention. *Clin J Sport Med.* 2000;10(4):272–278.
337. Galun E, Tur-Kaspa I, Assia E, et al. Hyponatremia induced by exercise: a 24–hour endurance march study. *Miner Electrolyte Metab.* 1991;17:315–320.
338. Zelingher J, Putterman C, Ilan Y, et al. Case series: hyponatremia associated with moderate exercise. *Am J Med.* Sci 1996;311(2):86–91.
339. Wade CE. Response, regulation, and actions of vasopressin during exercise: a review. *Med Sci Sports Exerc.* 1984;16(5):506–511.
340. Hew-Butler T. Arginine vasopressin, fluid balance and exercise: is exercise-associated hyponatraemia a disorder of arginine vasopressin secretion? *Sports Med.* 2010;40(6):459–479.
341. Rosner MH, Kirven J. Exercise-associated hyponatremia. *Clin J Am Soc Nephrol.* 2007;2(1):151–161.
342. Tomiyama J, Kametani H, Kumagai Y, et al. Water intoxication and rhabdomyolysis. *Jpn J Med.* 1990;29:52–55.
343. Trimarchi H, Gonzalez J, Olivero J. Hyponatremia-associated rhabdomyolysis. *Nephron.* 1999;82(3):274–277.
344. Arieff AI, Llach F, Massry SG. Neurological manifestations and morbidity of hyponatremia: correlation with brain water and electrolytes. *Medicine.* 1976;55:121–129.
345. Daggett P, Deanfield J, Moss F. Neurological aspects of hyponatraemia. *Postgrad Med J.* 1982;58:737–740.
346. Arieff AI. Central nervous system manifestations of disordered sodium metabolism. *Clin Endocrinol Metab.* 1984;13:269–294.
347. Fraser CL, Arieff AI. Epidemiology, pathophysiology, and management of hyponatremic encephalopathy. *Am J Med.* 1997;102:67–77.
348. Adrogue HJ, Madias NE. Hyponatremia. *N Engl J Med.* 2000;342(21): 1581–1589.
349. Pasantes-Morales H, Lezama RA, Ramos-Mandujano G, et alL. Mechanisms of cell volume regulation in hypo-osmolality. *Am J Med.* 2006;119(7 Suppl 1): S4–11.
350. Kleeman CR. The kidney in health and disease: X. CNS manifestations of disordered salt and water balance. *Hosp Pract.* 1979;14(5):59–68, 73.
351. Ayus JC, Wheeler JM, Arieff AI. Postoperative hyponatremic encephalopathy in menstruant women. *Ann Intern Med.* 1992;117:891–897.
352. Noakes TD, Sharwood K, Collins M, et al. The dipsomania of great distance: water intoxication in an Ironman triathlete. *Br J Sports Med.* 2004;38(4):E16.
353. Gardner JW. Death by water intoxication. *Mil Med.* 2002;167(5):432–434.
354. Wijdicks EF, Sharbrough FW. New-onset seizures in critically ill patients. *Neurology.* 1993;43:1042–1044.
355. Vexler ZS, Ayus JC, Roberts TP, et al. Hypoxic and ischemic hypoxia exacerbate brain injury associated with metabolic encephalopathy in laboratory animals. *J Clin Invest.* 1994;93:256–264.
356. Ayus JC, Arieff AI. Pulmonary complications of hyponatremic encephalopathy. noncardiogenic pulmonary edema and hypercapnic respiratory failure [see comments]. *Chest.* 1995;107(2):517–521.
357. Arieff AI, Ayus JC, Fraser CL. Hyponatraemia and death or permanent brain damage in healthy children. *BMJ.* 1992;304:1218–1222.

358. Wattad A, Chiang ML, Hill LL. Hyponatremia in hospitalized children. *Clin Ped.* 1992;31:153–157.
359. Wijdicks EF, Larson TS. Absence of postoperative hyponatremia syndrome in young, healthy females. *Ann Neurol.* 1994;35:626–628.
360. Chow KM, Kwan BC, Szeto CC. Clinical studies of thiazide-induced hyponatremia. *J Natl Med Assoc.* 2004;96(10):1305–1308.
361. Renneboog B, Musch W, Vandemergel X, et al. Mild chronic hyponatremia is associated with falls, unsteadiness, and attention deficits. *Am J Med.* 2006;119(1):71.
362. Gankam KF, Andres C, Sattar L, et al. Mild hyponatremia and risk of fracture in the ambulatory elderly. *QJM.* 2008;101(7):583–588.
363. Sandhu HS, Gilles E, DeVita MV, et al. Hyponatremia associated with large-bone fracture in elderly patients. *Int Urol Nephrol.* 2009;41(3):733–737.
364. Kinsella S, Moran S, Sullivan MO, et al. Hyponatremia independent of osteoporosis is associated with fracture occurrence. *Clin J Am Soc Nephrol.* 2010;5(2):275–280.
365. Verbalis JG, Barsony J, Sugimura Y, et al. Hyponatremia-induced osteoporosis. *J Bone Miner Res.* 2010;25(3):554–563.
366. Ayus JC. Diuretic-induced hyponatremia [editorial]. *Arch Intern Med.* 1986;146(7):1295–1296.
367. Hoorn EJ, Lindemans J, Zietse R. Development of severe hyponatraemia in hospitalized patients: treatment-related risk factors and inadequate management. *Nephrol Dial Transplant.* 2006;21(1):70–76.
368. Gill G, Huda B, Boyd A, et al. Characteristics and mortality of severe hyponatraemia—a hospital-based study. *Clin Endocrinol (Oxf).* 2006;65(2):246–249.
369. Steele A, Gowrishankar M, Abrahamson S, et al. Postoperative hyponatremia despite near-isotonic saline infusion: a phenomenon of desalination [see comments]. *Ann Intern Med.* 1997;126(1):20–25.
370. Lindholm J, Kehlet H, Blichert-Toft M, et al. Reliability of the 30-minute ACTH test in assessing hypothalamic-pituitary-adrenal function. *J Clin Endocrinol Metab.* 1978;47:272–274.
371. May ME, Carey RM. Rapid adrenocorticotropic hormone test in practice. *Am J Med.* 1985;79:679–684.
372. Davis BB, Bloom ME, Field JB, et al. Hyponatremia in pituitary insufficiency. *Metabolism.* 1969;18:821–832.
373. Verbalis JG, Goldsmith SR, Greenberg A, et al. Hyponatremia treatment guidelines 2007: expert panel recommendations. *Am J Med.* 2007;120(11 Suppl 1): S1–21.
374. Sterns RH, Cappuccio JD, Silver SM, et al. Neurologic sequelae after treatment of severe hyponatremia: a multicenter perspective. *J Am Soc Nephrol.* 1994;4:1522–1530.
375. Battison C, Andrews PJ, Graham C, et al. Randomized, controlled trial on the effect of a 20% mannitol solution and a 7.5% saline/6% dextran solution on increased intracranial pressure after brain injury. *Crit Care Med.* 2005;33(1): 196–202.
376. Robertson GL. Regulation of arginine vasopressin in the syndrome of inappropriate antidiuresis. *Am J Med.* 2006;119(7 Suppl 1):S36–S42.
377. Furst H, Hallows KR, Post J, et al. The urine/plasma electrolyte ratio: a predictive guide to water restriction. *Am J Med Sci.* 2000;319(4):240–244.
378. Berl T. Impact of solute intake on urine flow and water excretion. *J Am Soc Nephrol.* 2008;19(6):1076–1078.
379. Singer I, Rotenberg D. Demeclocycline-induced nephrogenic diabetes insipidus. In-vivo and in- vitro studies. *Ann Intern Med.* 1973;79(5):679–683.
380. Decaux G, Genette F. Urea for long-term treatment of syndrome of inappropriate secretion of antidiuretic hormone. *BMJ Clin Res.* 1981;283:1081–1083.
381. Hantman D, Rossier B, Zohlman R, et al. Rapid correction of hyponatremia in the syndrome of inappropriate secretion of antidiuretic hormone. An alternative treatment to hypertonic saline. *Ann Intern Med.* 1973;78:870–875.
382. Decaux G, Waterlot Y, Genette F, et al. Treatment of the syndrome of inappropriate secretion of antidiuretic hormone with furosemide. *N Engl J Med.* 1981;304:329–330.
383. Greenberg A, Verbalis JG. Vasopressin receptor antagonists. *Kidney Int.* 2006;69(12):2124–2130.
384. Ohnishi A, Orita Y, Okahara R, et al. Potent aquaretic agent. A novel nonpeptide selective vasopressin 2 antagonist (OPC-31260) in men. *J Clin Invest.* 1993;92(6):2653–2659.
385. Zeltser D, Rosansky S, van Rensburg H, et al. Assessment of the efficacy and safety of intravenous conivaptan in euvolemic and hypervolemic hyponatremia. *Am J Nephrol.* 2007;27(5):447–457.
386. Schrier RW, Gross P, Gheorghiade M, et al. Tolvaptan, a selective oral vasopressin V2–receptor antagonist, for hyponatremia. *N Engl J Med.* 2006; 355(20):2099–2112.
387. Vaprisol (conivaptan hydrochloride injection) prescribing information. Deerfield, IL: Astellas Pharma US, Inc., 2006.
388. Otsuka Pharmaceutical Co L, Tokyo J. Samsca (tolvaptan) prescribing information. 2009.
389. Tomlinson BE, Pierides AM, Bradley WG. Central pontine myelinolysis. Two cases with associated electrolyte disturbance. *Q J Med.* 1976;45:373–386.
390. Burcar PJ, Norenberg MD, Yarnell PR. Hyponatremia and central pontine myelinolysis. *Neurology.* 1977;27:223–226.
391. Wright DG, Laureno R, Victor M. Pontine and extrapontine myelinolysis. *Brain.* 1979;102:361–385.
392. Kleinschmidt-DeMasters BK, Norenberg MD. Rapid correction of hyponatremia causes demyelination: relation to central pontine myelinolysis. *Science.* 1981;211:1068–1070.
393. Laureno R. Central pontine myelinolysis following rapid correction of hyponatremia. *Ann Neurol.* 1983;13:232–242.
394. Sterns RH, Thomas DJ, Herndon RM. Brain dehydration and neurologic deterioration after rapid correction of hyponatremia. *Kidney Int.* 1989;35:69–75.
395. Ayus JC, Krothapalli RK, Armstrong DL, et al. Symptomatic hyponatremia in rats: effect of treatment on mortality and brain lesions. *Am J Physiol.* 1989;257:F18–F22.
396. Verbalis JG, Martinez AJ. Neurological and neuropathological sequelae of correction of chronic hyponatremia. *Kidney Int.* 1991;39:1274–1282.
397. Karp BI, Laureno R. Pontine and extrapontine myelinolysis: a neurologic disorder following rapid correction of hyponatremia. *Medicine.* 1993;72: 359–373.
398. Norenberg MD, Leslie KO, Robertson AS. Association between rise in serum sodium and central pontine myelinolysis. *Ann Neurol.* 1982;11: 128–135.
399. Cserr H, DePasquale M, Patlak CS. Regulation of brain water and electrolytes during acute hyperosmolality. *Am J Physiol.* 1987;253:F522–F529.
400. Adler S, Verbalis JG, Williams D. Effect of rapid correction of hyponatremia on the blood brain barrier of rats. *Brain Res.* 1995;679:135–143.
401. Adler S, Martinez J, Williams DS, et al. Positive association between blood brain barrier disruption and osmotically-induced demyelination. *Mult Scler.* 2000;6(1):24–31.
402. Baker EA, Tian Y, Adler S, et al. Blood-brain barrier disruption and complement activation in the brain following rapid correction of chronic hyponatremia. *Exp Neurol.* 2000;165(2):221–230.
403. Ayus JC, Krothapalli RK, Arieff AI. Treatment of symptomatic hyponatremia and its relation to brain damage. A prospective study. *N Engl J Med.* 1987;317:1190–1195.
404. Kumar S, Berl T. Sodium. *Lancet.* 1998;352(9123):220–228.
405. Sterns RH, Silver S, Kleinschmidt-DeMasters BK, et al. Current perspectives in the management of hyponatremia: prevention of CPM. *Expert Rev Neurother.* 2007;7(12):1791–1797.
406. Soupart A, Penninckx R, Stenuit A, et al. Treatment of chronic hyponatremia in rats by intravenous saline: comparison of rate versus magnitude of correction. *Kidney Int.* 1992;41:1662–1667.
407. Verbalis JG. Hyponatremia. Endocrinologic causes and consequences of therapy. *Trends Endocrinol Metab.* 1992;3:1–7.
408. Ellis SJ. Extrapontine myelinolysis after correction of chronic hyponatraemia with isotonic saline. *Br J Clin Pract.* 1995;49(1):49–50.
409. Lin SH, Chau T, Wu CC, et al. Osmotic demyelination syndrome after correction of chronic hyponatremia with normal saline. *Am J Med Sci.* 2002; 323(5):259–262.
410. Lohr JW. Osmotic demyelination syndrome following correction of hyponatremia: association with hypokalemia. *Am J Med.* 1994;96:408–413.
411. Adams RD, Victor M, Mancall EL. Central pontine myelinolysis: A hitherto undescribed disease occurring in alcoholic and malnourished patients. *Arch Neurol Psych.* 1959;81:154–172.
412. Kelly J, Wassif W, Mitchard J, et al. Severe hyponatraemia secondary to beer potomania complicated by central pontine myelinolysis. *Int J Clin Pract.* 1998;52(8):585–587.
413. Leens C, Mukendi R, Foret F, et al. Central and extrapontine myelinolysis in a patient in spite of a careful correction of hyponatremia. *Clin Nephrol.* 2001;55(3):248–253.
414. Loo CS, Lim TO, Fan KS, et al. Pontine myelinolysis following correction of hyponatraemia. *Med J Malaysia.* 1995;50(2):180–182.
415. Soupart A, Penninckx R, Stenuit A, et al. Azotemia (48 h) decreases the risk of brain damage in rats after correction of chronic hyponatremia. *Brain Res.* 2000;852(1):167–172.
416. Price BH, Mesulam MM. Behavioral manifestations of central pontine myelinolysis. *Arch Neurol.* 1987;44:671–673.
417. Vermetten E, Rutten SJ, Boon PJ, et al. Neuropsychiatric and neuropsychological manifestations of central pontine myelinolysis. *Gen Hosp Psychiatry.* 1999;21(4):296–302.

418. Maraganore DM, Folger WN, Swanson JW, et al. Movement disorders as sequelae of central pontine myelinolysis: report of three cases. *Mov Disord.* 1992;7:142–148.

419. Sullivan AA, Chervin RD, Albin RL. Parkinsonism after correction of hyponatremia with radiological central pontine myelinolysis and changes in the basal ganglia. *J Clin Neurosci.* 2000;7(3):256–259.

420. Koussa S, Nasnas R. Catatonia and Parkinsonism due to extrapontine myelinolysis following rapid correction of hyponatremia: a case report. *J Neurol.* 2003;250(1):103–105.

421. Brunner JE, Redmond JM, Haggar AM, et al. Central pontine myelinolysis after rapid correction of hyponatremia: a magnetic resonance imaging study. *Ann Neurol.* 1988;23:389–391.

422. Brunner JE, Redmond JM, Haggar AM, et al. Central pontine myelinolysis and pontine lesions after rapid correction of hyponatremia: a prospective magnetic resonance imaging study. *Ann Neurol.* 1990;27:61–66.

423. Kumar SR, Mone AP, Gray LC, et al. Central pontine myelinolysis: delayed changes on neuroimaging. *J Neuroimaging.* 2000;10(3):169–172.

424. Miller GM, Baker HL Jr, Okazaki H, et al. Central pontine myelinolysis and its imitators: MR findings. *Radiology.* 1988;168:795–802.

425. Soupart A, Penninckx R, Namias B, et al. Brain myelinolysis following hypernatremia in rats. *J Neuropathol Exp Neurol.* 1997;55:106–113.

426. McComb RD, Pfeiffer RF, Casey JH, et al. Lateral pontine and extrapontine myelinolysis associated with hypernatremia and hyperglycemia. *Clin Neuropathol.* 1989;8(6):284–288.

427. Ayus JC, Olivero JJ, Frommer JP. Rapid correction of severe hyponatremia with intravenous hypertonic saline solution. *Am J Med.* 1982;72:43–48.

428. Verbalis JG. Adaptation to acute and chronic hyponatremia: implications for symptomatology, diagnosis, and therapy. *Semin Nephrol.* 1998;18(1):3–19.

429. Sterns RH, Nigwekar SU, Hix JK. The treatment of hyponatremia. *Semin Nephrol.* 2009;29(3):282–299.

430. Verbalis JG. Hyponatremia and hypo-osmolar disorders. In: Greenberg A, Cheung AK, Coffman TM, Falk RJ, Jennette JC, eds. *Primer on Kidney Diseases.* Philadelphia. PA: Saunders Elsevier; 2009: 52–59.

431. Soupart A, Penninckx R, Crenier L, et al. Prevention of brain demyelination in rats after excessive correction of chronic hyponatremia by serum sodium lowering. *Kidney Int.* 1994;45:193–200.

432. Goldszmidt MA, Iliescu EA. DDAVP to prevent rapid correction in hyponatremia. *Clin Nephrol.* 2000;53(3):226–229.

433. Oya S, Tsutsumi K, Ueki K, et al. Reinduction of hyponatremia to treat central pontine myelinolysis. *Neurology.* 2001;57(10):1931–1932.

434. Bissram M, Scott FD, Liu L, et al. Risk factors for symptomatic hyponatraemia: the role of pre-existing asymptomatic hyponatraemia. *Intern Med J.* 2007;37(3):149–155.

435. Mohmand HK, Issa D, Ahmad Z, et al. Hypertonic saline for hyponatremia: risk of inadvertent overcorrection. *Clin J Am Soc Nephrol.* 2007;2(6): 1110–1117.

436. Sterns RH, Hix JK. Overcorrection of hyponatremia is a medical emergency. *Kidney Int.* 2009;76(6):587–589.

437. Perianayagam A, Sterns RH, Silver SM, et al. DDAVP is effective in preventing and reversing inadvertent overcorrection of hyponatremia. *Clin J Am Soc Nephrol.* 2008;3(2):331–336.

438. Soupart A, Penninckx R, Stenuit A, et al. Reinduction of hyponatremia improves survival in rats with myelinolysis-related neurologic symptoms. *J Neuropathol Exp Neurol.* 1996;55(5):594–601.

439. Soupart A, Ngassa M, Decaux G. Therapeutic relowering of the serum sodium in a patient after excessive correction of hyponatremia. *Clin Nephrol.* 1999;51(6):383–386.

440. Sugimura Y, Murase T, Takefuji S, et al. Protective effect of dexamethasone on osmotic-induced demyelination in rats. *Exp Neurol.* 2005;192(1): 178–183.

441. Suzuki H, Sugimura Y, Iwama S, et al. Minocycline prevents osmotic demyelination syndrome by inhibiting the activation of microglia. *J Am Soc Nephrol.* 2010;21(12):2090–2098.

442. Gankam-Kengne F, Soupart A, Pochet R, et al. Minocycline protects against neurologic complications of rapid correction of hyponatremia. *J Am Soc Nephrol.* 2010;21(12):2099–2108.

443. Berl T, Quittnat-Pelletier F, Verbalis JG, et al. Oral tolvaptan is safe and effective in chronic hyponatremia. *J Am Soc Nephrol.* 2010;21(4): 705–712.

444. Konstam MA, Gheorghiade M, Burnett JC Jr, et al. Effects of oral tolvaptan in patients hospitalized for worsening heart failure: the EVEREST Outcome Trial. *JAMA.* 2007;297(12):1319–1331.

CHAPTER

71 Nephrogenic and Central Diabetes Insipidus

Daniel G. Bichet

Diabetes insipidus is a disorder characterized by the excretion of abnormally large volumes (greater than 30 mL per kilogram of body weight per day for an adult patient) of dilute urine (less than 250 mmol per kilogram). This definition excludes osmotic diuresis, which occurs when excess solute is being excreted (e.g., glucose in the polyuria of diabetes mellitus). Other agents that produce osmotic diuresis are mannitol, urea, glycerol, contrast media, and loop diuretics. Osmotic diuresis should be considered when solute excretion exceeds 60 mmol per hour. Four basic defects can be involved. The most common, a deficient secretion of the antidiuretic hormone (ADH) arginine vasopressin (AVP), is referred to as neurogenic (or central, neurohypophyseal, cranial, or hypothalamic) diabetes insipidus. Diabetes insipidus can also result from renal insensitivity to the antidiuretic effect of AVP, which is referred to as nephrogenic diabetes insipidus. Excessive water intake can result in polyuria, which is referred to as primary polydipsia; it can be due to an abnormality in the thirst mechanism, referred to as dipsogenic diabetes insipidus, or it can be associated with a severe emotional cognitive dysfunction, referred to as psychogenic polydipsia. Finally, the increased metabolism of vasopressin during pregnancy is referred to as gestational diabetes insipidus.

ARGININE VASOPRESSIN

Synthesis

The regulation of the release of AVP from the posterior pituitary is primarily dependent, under normal circumstances, on tonicity information relayed by central osmoreceptor neurons expressing transient receptor potential channel 1 (TRPV1) (Fig. 71.1)[1] and peripheral osmoreceptor neurons expressing TRPV4.[2] AVP and its corresponding carrier, neurophysin II, are synthesized as a composite precursor by the magnocellular neurons of the supraoptic and paraventricular nuclei of the hypothalamus.[3] The precursor is packaged into neurosecretory granules and transported axonally in the stalk of the posterior pituitary. En route to the neurohypophysis, the precursor is processed into the active hormone. Preprovasopressin has 164 amino acids and is encoded by the 2.5 kb *AVP* gene located in chromosome region 20p13.[4,5] The *AVP* gene (coding for AVP and neurophysin II) and the *OXT* gene (coding for oxytocin and neurophysin I) are located in the same chromosome region, at a very short distance from each other (12 kb in humans) in a head-to-head orientation. Data from transgenic mouse studies indicate that the intergenic region between the *OXT* and the *AVP* genes contains the critical enhancer sites for cell-specific expression in the magnocellular neurons.[3] It is phylogenetically interesting to note that *cis* and *trans* components of this specific cellular expression have been conserved between the *Fugu* isotocin (the homolog of mammalian oxytocin) and rat oxytocin genes.[6] Exon 1 of the *AVP* gene encodes the signal peptide, AVP, and the NH_2-terminal region of neurophysin II. Exon 2 encodes the central region of neurophysin II, and exon 3 encodes the COOH-terminal region of neurophysin II and the glycopeptide. Provasopressin is generated by the removal of the signal peptide from preprovasopressin and from the addition of a carbohydrate chain to the glycopeptide (Fig. 71.2). Additional posttranslation processing occurs within neurosecretory vesicles during the transport of the precursor protein to axon terminals in the posterior pituitary, yielding AVP, neurophysin II, and the glycopeptide. The AVP-neurophysin II complex (Fig. 71.3) forms tetramers that can self-associate to form higher oligomers.[7] Neurophysins should be seen as chaperonelike molecules facilitating intracellular transport in magnocellular cells. In the posterior pituitary, AVP is stored in vesicles. Exocytotic release is stimulated by minute increases in serum osmolality (hypernatremia, osmotic regulation) and by more pronounced decreases in extracellular fluid (hypovolemia, nonosmotic regulation). Oxytocin and neurophysin I are released from the posterior pituitary by the suckling response in lactating females.

Immunocytochemical and radioimmunologic studies have demonstrated that oxytocin and vasopressin are synthesized in separate populations of the supraoptic nuclei and the paraventricular nuclei neurons,[8,9] the central and vascular projections of which have been described in great detail.[10]

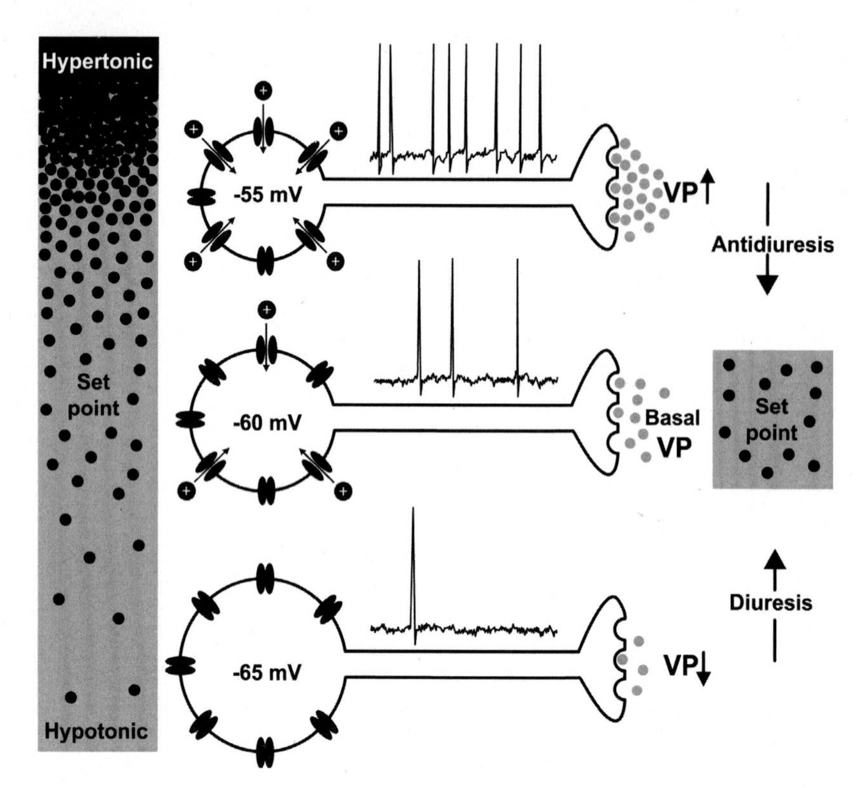

FIGURE 71.1 Osmoreception in vasopressin neurons. Changes in osmolality cause inversely proportional changes in soma volume. Shrinkage activates nonselective cation channels (NSCCs) and the ensuing depolarization increases the action potential firing rate and vasopressin (VP) release from axon terminals in the neurohypophysis. Increased VP levels in blood enhance water reabsorption by the kidney (antidiuresis) to restore extracellular fluid osmolality toward the set point. Hypotonic stimuli inhibit NSCCs. The resulting hyperpolarization and the inhibition of firing reduces VP release and promotes diuresis. (Modified from Prager-Khoutorsky and Bourque.[15])

Some cells express the *AVP* gene and other cells express the *OXT* gene. Immunohistochemical studies have revealed a second vasopressin neurosecretory pathway that transports high concentrations of the hormone to the anterior pituitary gland from parvocellular neurons to the hypophyseal portal system. In the portal system, the high concentration of AVP acts synergistically with corticotropin-releasing hormone (CRH) to stimulate adrenocorticotropic hormone (ACTH) release from the anterior pituitary. More than half of parvocellular neurons coexpress both *CRH* and *AVP*. In addition, while passing through the median eminence and the hypophyseal stalk, magnocellular axons can also release AVP into the long portal system. Furthermore, a number of neuroanatomic studies have shown the existence of short

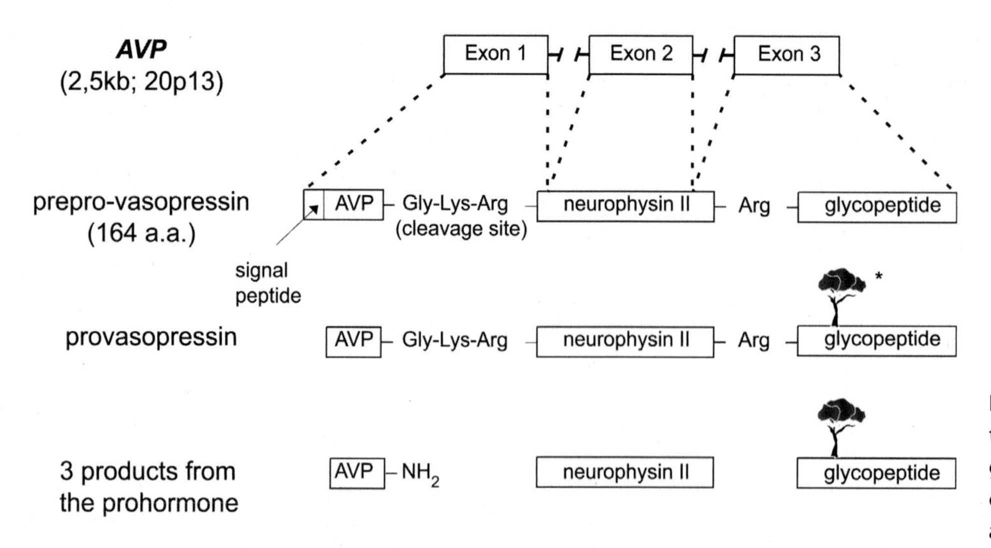

FIGURE 71.2 The structure of the human vasopressin (AVP) gene and prohormone. The cascade of vasopressin biosynthesis and signal peptide; AVP and arginine-vasopressin; neurophysin; and glycoprotein.

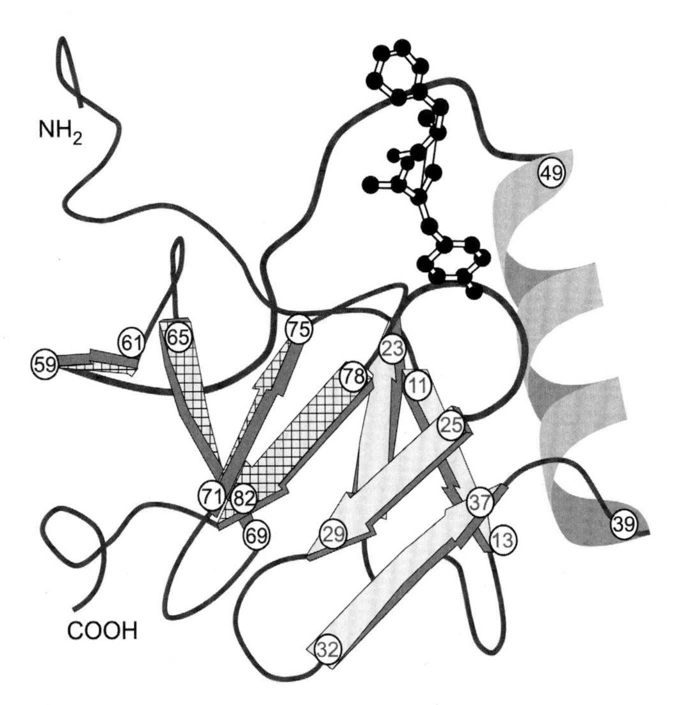

FIGURE 71.3 A three-dimensional structure of a bovine peptide-neurophysin monomer complex. The structure of each chain is 12% helix and 40% β-sheet. The chain is folded into two domains as predicted by disulfide-pairing studies. The amino-terminal domain begins in a long loop (residues 1–10), then enters a four-stranded (residues 11–13, 19–23, 25–29, and 32–37) antiparallel β-sheet (sheet I; *four solid arrows*), followed by a three-turn 3_{10}-helix (residues 39–49) and another loop (residues 50–58). The carboxyl-terminal domain is shorter, consisting of only a four-stranded (residues 59–61, 65–69, 71–75, and 78–82) antiparallel β-sheet (sheet II; *four cross-hatched arrows*).[7] The arginine vasopressin molecule (balls and sticks model) is shown in the peptide-binding pocket of the neurophysin monomer. The strongest interactions in this binding pocket are salt-bridge interactions between the $\alpha NH3^+$ group of the peptide, the γ-COO^- group of Glu^{NP47} (residue number 47 of the neurophysin molecule), and the side chain of Arg^{NP8}. The γ-COO^- group of Glu^{NP47} plays a bifunctional role in the peptide-binding pocket: (1) it directly interacts with the hormone, and (2) it interacts with other neurophysin residues to establish the correct, local structure of the peptide-neurophysin complex. Arg^{NP8} and Glu^{NP47} are conserved in all neurophysin sequences from mammals to invertebrates.

portal vessels that allow communication between the posterior and anterior pituitary. Therefore, in addition to parvocellular vasopressin, magnocellular vasopressin is able to influence ACTH secretion.[11,12]

OSMOTIC AND NONOSMOTIC STIMULATION

The regulation of ADH release from the posterior pituitary is dependent primarily on two mechanisms involving the osmotic and nonosmotic pathways (Fig. 71.4).[13] Although magnocellular neurons are themselves osmosensitive, they require input from the lamina terminalis to respond fully to osmotic challenges (Fig. 71.5). Neurons in the lamina terminalis are also osmosensitive and because the subfornical organ (SFO) and the organum vasculosum of the lamina terminalis (OVLT) lie outside the blood–brain barrier, they can integrate this information with endocrine signals borne of circulating hormones, such as angiotensin II (AT-II), relaxin, and atrial natriuretic peptide (ANP). Although circulating AT-II and relaxin excite both oxytocin and vasopressin magnocellular neurons, ANP inhibits vasopressin neurons.[14]

The nonosmotic pathways are more physiologically described now as "osmoregulatory gain."[15] A stable and approximately linear relation is normally observed between vasopressin concentration and plasma osmolality under resting conditions (Fig. 71.4A).[16] The slope of this relation reflects the overall sensitivity of this homeostatic mechanism and the term "osmoregulatory gain" refers to this parameter. Osmoregulatory gain is increased during hypovolemia to help maintain arterial pressure and restore blood volume.[17] Conversely, osmoregulatory gain is attenuated during hypervolemia to promote homeostasis by favoring diuresis (Fig. 71.6). The enhancement of osmosensory gain is mediated by circulating AT-II: neurons in the SFO (Fig. 71.5) contain AT-II and the release of this peptide during hypovolemia or hypotension can lead to an increase in the osmotic activation of magnocellular cells producing vasopressin. Good et al.[18] and Zhang and Bourque[19] found that AT-II enhances osmosensory gain by amplifying mechanosensory transduction, an F actin–dependent phenomenon probably part of a scaffolding complex.

In addition to an angiotensinergic path from the SFO, the OVLT and the median preoptic nucleus provide direct glutaminergic and GABAergic projections to the hypothalamoneurohypophyseal system. Nitric oxide may also modulate neurohormone release.[3] The neuropeptide apelin is colocalized with AVP in supraoptic nucleus (SON) magnocellular neurons, and physiologic experiments indicate that AVP and apelin are conversely regulated to facilitate systemic AVP release and to suppress antidiuresis.[20]

The cellular basis for osmoreceptor potentials has been characterized using patch-clamp recordings and morphometric analysis in magnocellular cells isolated from the supraoptic nucleus of the adult rat. In these cells, stretch-inactivating cationic channels transduce osmotically evoked changes in cell volume into functionally relevant changes in membrane potential. In addition, magnocellular neurons also operate as intrinsic Na^+ detectors. The N-terminal variant of the TRPV1 is an osmotically activated channel expressed in the magnocellular cells producing vasopressin[21] and in the circumventricular organs, the OVLT, and the SFO.[22] Because osmoregulation still operates in $Trpv1^{-/-}$ mice, other osmosensitive neurons or pathways must compensate for the loss of central osmoreceptor function.[21–23] Afferent neurons expressing the osmotically activated ion channel TRPV4 in the thoracic dorsal root ganglia that innervate hepatic blood

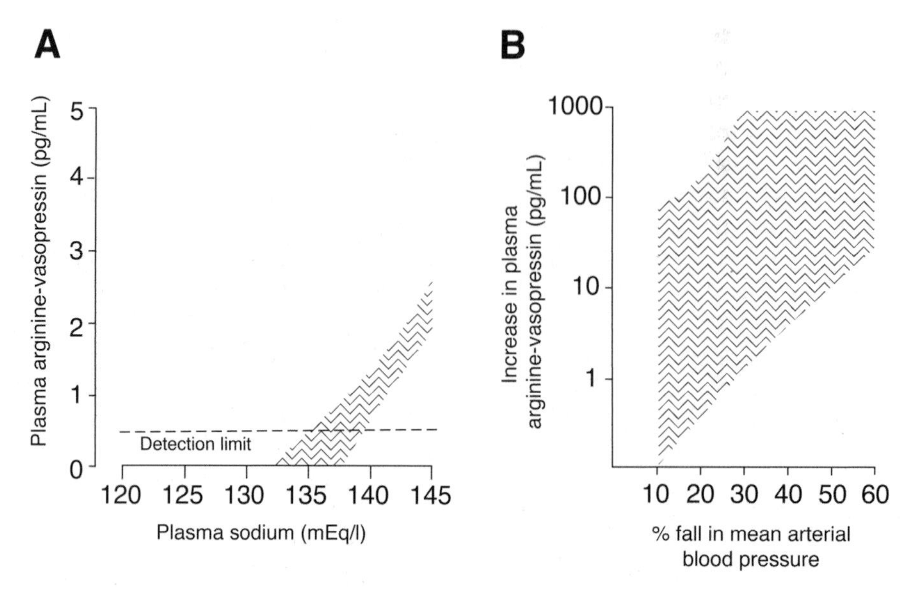

FIGURE 71.4 A: The osmotic and nonosmotic stimulation of arginine vasopressin (AVP). The relationship between plasma AVP (P_{AVP}) and plasma sodium (P_{Na}) in 19 normal subjects is described by the area with *vertical lines*, which includes the 99% confidence limits of the regression line P_{Na}/P_{AVP}. The osmotic threshold for AVP release is approximately 280 to 285 mmol per kilogram or 136 mEq of Na per liter. AVP secretion should be abolished when plasma sodium is less than 135 mEq per liter.[214] **B:** The increase in plasma AVP during hypotension (*vertical lines*). Note that a large diminution in blood pressure in normal humans induces large increments in AVP. (From Zerbe RL, Henry DP, Robertson GL. Vasopressin response to orthostatic hypotension: etiological and clinical implications. *Am J Med.* 1983;74:265, with permission.)

vessels and detect physiologic hypo-osmotic shifts in blood osmolality have recently been identified.[2]

In mice lacking the osmotically activated ion channel TRPV4, hepatic sensory neurons no longer exhibit osmosensitive inward currents and the activation of peripheral

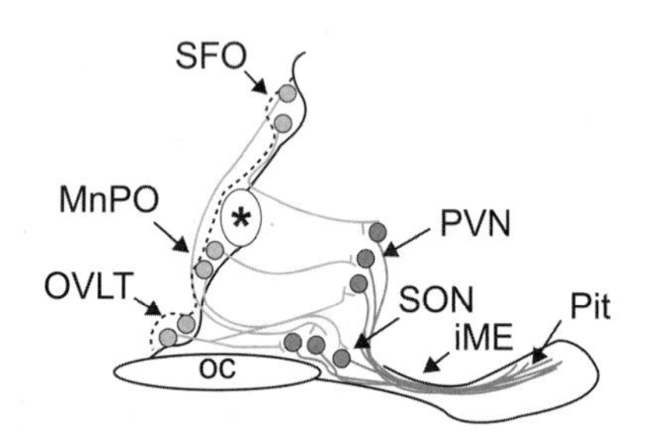

FIGURE 71.5 A schematic representation of the osmoregulatory pathway of the hypothalamus (sagittal section of midline of ventral brain around the third ventricle in mice). Neurons (*lightly filled circles*) in the lamina terminalis (OVLT), median preoptic nucleus (MnPO), and subfornical organ (SFO), which are responsive to plasma hypertonicity, send efferent axonal projections (*grey lines*) to magnocellular neurons of the paraventricular (PVN) and supraoptic nuclei (SON). The OVLT is one of the brain circumventricular organs and is a key osmosensing site in the mammalian brain (vide infra). The processes (*dark lines*) of these magnocellular neurons form the hypothalamoneurohypophyseal pathway that courses in the median eminence to reach the posterior pituitary, where neurosecretion of vasopressin and oxytocin occurs. (Modified from Wilson et al., 2002 with permission, Copyright (2002), National Academy of Sciences USA.)

osmoreceptors in vivo is abolished. In a large cohort of human liver transplantees, who presumably have denervated livers, plasma osmolality is significantly elevated compared to healthy controls, suggesting the presence of an inhibitory vasopressin effect of hyponatremia perceived in the portal vein from hepatic afferents.[2] TRPV1 (expressed in central neurons) and TRPV4 (expressed in peripheral neurons) thus appear to play entirely complementary roles in osmoreception. McHugh et al.[24] have therefore identified the primary afferent neurons that constitute the afferent arc of a well-characterized reflex in man, which was recently identified in rodents. This reflex engages the sympathetic nervous system to raise blood pressure and stimulate metabolism.[25,26] Of clinical interest, it has already been demonstrated that orthostatic hypotension and postprandial hypotension respond to water drinking.[27–29] Moreover, water drinking in man can prevent neutrally mediated syncope during blood donation or after prolonged standing.[30] Finally, water drinking is also associated with weight loss in overweight individuals.[31] Other peripheral sensory neurons expressing other mechanosensitive proteins may also be involved in osmosensitivity.[32]

The osmotic stimulation of AVP release by dehydration, hypertonic saline infusion, or both, is regularly used to determine the vasopressin secretory capacity of the posterior pituitary. This secretory capacity can be assessed *directly* by comparing the plasma AVP concentrations measured sequentially during the dehydration procedure with the normal values[33] and then correlating the plasma AVP values with the urine osmolality measurements obtained simultaneously (Fig. 71.7).

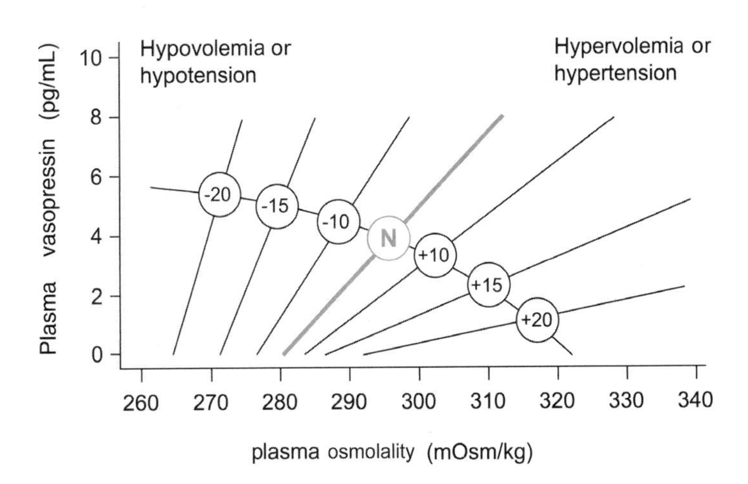

FIGURE 71.6 A schematic representation of the relationship between plasma vasopressin and plasma osmolality in the presence of differing states of blood volume and/or pressure. The line labeled *N* represents normovolemic normotensive conditions. Minus numbers to the left indicate a percent fall, and positive numbers to the right represent a percent rise in blood volume or pressure. Data from Vokes and Robertson.[230]

The AVP release can also be assessed *indirectly* by measuring plasma and urine osmolalities at regular intervals during the dehydration test.[34] The maximal urine osmolality obtained during dehydration is compared with the maximal urine osmolality obtained after the administration of vasopressin (Pitressin, 5 U subcutaneously in adults, 1 U subcutaneously in children) or 1-desamino-8-D-arginine vasopressin (desmopressin [dDAVP], 1 to 4 μg s.c. or intravenously [IV], over 5 to 10 minutes).

The nonosmotic stimulation of AVP release can be used to assess the vasopressin secretory capacity of the posterior pituitary in a rare group of patients with the essential hyponatremia and hypodipsia syndrome.[35] Although some of these patients may have partial central diabetes insipidus, they respond normally to nonosmolar AVP release signals such as hypotension, emesis, and hypoglycemia.[35] In all other cases of suspected central diabetes insipidus, these nonosmotic stimulation tests will not give additional clinical information.[36]

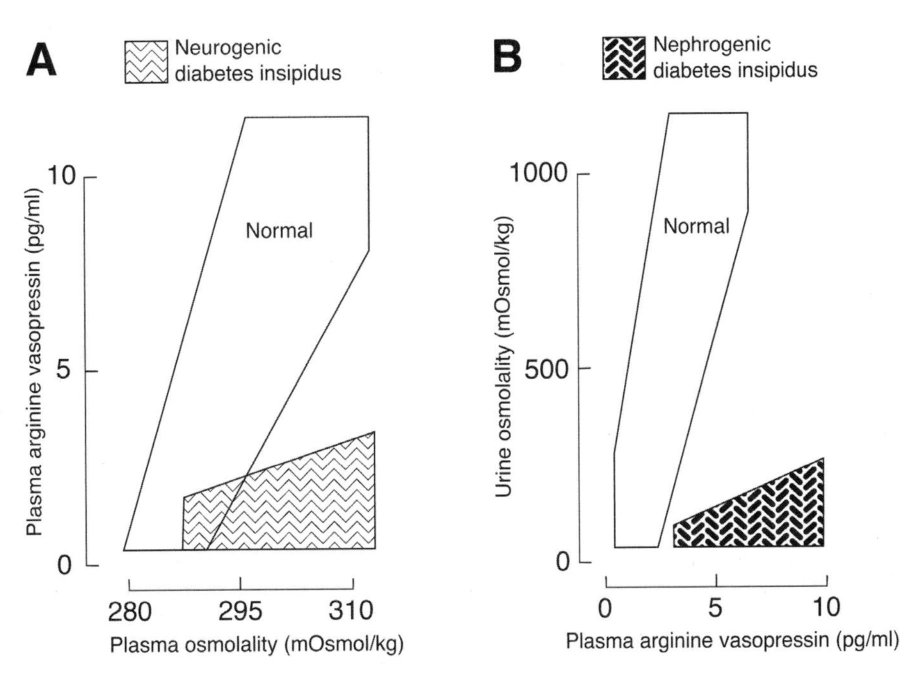

FIGURE 71.7 A: The relationship between plasma arginine vasopressin (AVP) and plasma osmolality during the infusion of a hypertonic saline solution. Patients with primary polydipsia and nephrogenic diabetes insipidus have values within the normal range (*open area*) in contrast to patients with neurogenic diabetes insipidus, who show subnormal plasma antidiuretic hormone (ADH) responses (*cross-hatched area*). **B:** The relationship between urine osmolality and plasma ADH during dehydration and water loading. Patients with neurogenic diabetes insipidus and primary polydipsia have values within the normal range (*open area*) in contrast to patients with nephrogenic diabetes insipidus, who have hypotonic urine despite high plasma ADH (*stippled area*). (Modified from Zerbe RL, Robertson GL. Disorders of ADH. *Med North Am.* 1984;13:1570.[231])

CLINICALLY IMPORTANT HORMONAL INFLUENCES ON THE SECRETION OF VASOPRESSIN

Angiotensin is a well-known dipsogen and has been shown to increase thirst in all the species tested.[37] However, knockout models for angiotensinogen[38] or for angiotensin-1A (AT-IA) receptor[39,40] did not alter thirst or water balance. Disruption of the AT-II receptor induced only mild abnormalities of thirst postdehydration.[41,42] However, as described earlier, AT-II enhances osmosensory gain. Earlier reports suggested that the intravenous administration of atrial peptides inhibits the release of vasopressin,[43] but this was not confirmed by Goetz et al.[44] Furthermore, Ogawa et al.[45] found no evidence that ANP, administered centrally or peripherally, was important in the physiologic regulation of plasma AVP release in conscious rats. A very rapid and robust release of AVP is seen in humans after a cholecystokinin (CCK) injection.[46] Nitric oxide is an inhibitory modulator of the hypothalamoneurohypophyseal system in response to osmotic stimuli.[47–50] Vasopressin secretion is under the influence of a glucocorticoid-negative feedback system,[51] and the vasopressin responses to a variety of stimuli (hemorrhage, hypoxia, hypertonic saline) in normal humans and animals appear to be attenuated or eliminated by pretreatment with glucocorticoids. Finally, nausea and emesis are potent stimuli of AVP release in humans and seem to involve dopaminergic neurotransmission.[52]

CELLULAR ACTIONS OF VASOPRESSIN

The neurohypophyseal hormone AVP has multiple actions, including the inhibition of diuresis, the contraction of smooth muscle, the aggregation of platelets, the stimulation of liver glycogenolysis, the modulation of adrenocorticotropic hormone release from the pituitary, and the central regulation of somatic functions (thermoregulation and blood pressure) and the modulation of social and reproductive behavior.[53] These multiple actions of AVP can be explained by the interaction of AVP with at least three types of G protein–coupled receptors: the V_{1a} (vascular, hepatic, and brain) and V_{1b} (anterior pituitary) receptors act through phosphatidylinositol hydrolysis to mobilize calcium, and the V_2 (kidney) receptor is coupled to adenylate cyclase.[54–56]

The transfer of water across the principal cells of the collecting ducts is now known at such a detailed level that billions of molecules of water traversing the membrane can be represented; see useful teaching tools at http://www.mpibpc.gwdg.de/abteilungen/073/gallery.html and http://www.ks.uiuc.edu/research/aquaporins. The 2003 Nobel Prize in Chemistry was awarded to Peter Agre and Roderick MacKinnon, who solved two complementary problems presented by the cell membrane: How does a cell let one type of ion through the lipid membrane to the exclusion of other ions? And, how does it permeate water without ions? See Figure 71.8. This contributed to a momentum and renewed interest in basic discoveries related to the transport of water and indirectly to diabetes insipidus.[57,58] The first step in the action of AVP on water excretion is its binding to arginine vasopressin type 2 receptors (hereafter referred to as V_2 receptors) on the basolateral membrane of the collecting duct cells (Fig. 71.9). The human *AVPR2* gene that codes for the V_2 receptor is located in chromosome region Xq28 and has three exons and two small introns.[59,60] The sequence of the cDNA predicts a polypeptide of 371 amino acids with seven transmembrane, four extracellular, and four cytoplasmic domains (Fig. 71.10). The activation of the V_2 receptor on renal collecting tubules stimulates adenylyl cyclase via the stimulatory G protein (Gs) and

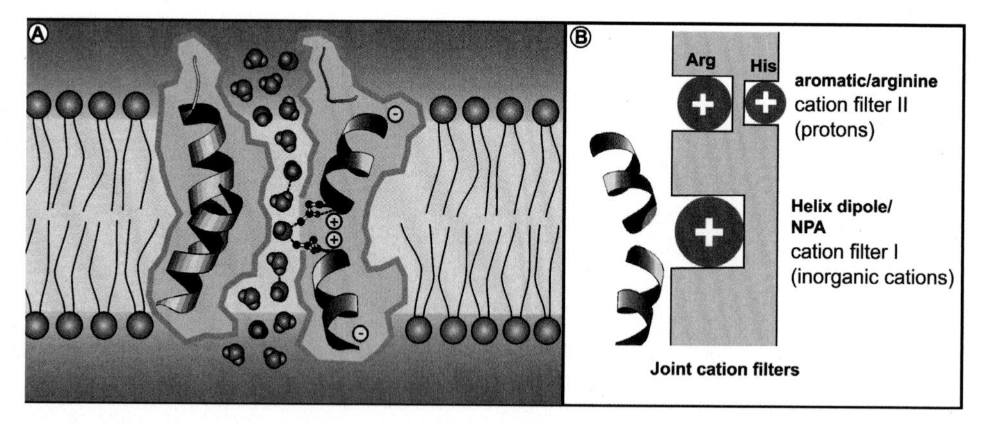

FIGURE 71.8 Schematic representations explaining the mechanism for blocking proton permeation of aquaporin 1 (AQP1). **A:** A diagram illustrating how partial charges from the helix dipoles restrict the orientation of the water molecules passing through the constriction of the pore. (From Murata K, Mitsuoka K, Hirai T, et al. Structural determinants of water permeation through aquaporin-1. *Nature.* 2000;407:599.) **B:** A diagram illustrating how primordial AQPs selected against inorganic cations, such as Na+ and K+, because of a positive electrostatic field from the helix dipoles and the lack of cation coordination sites in the NPA region (filter I); yet, protons leaked through. Later, a second cation filter evolved in the ar/R region, which fully excluded protons (filter II) and provided individual selectivity properties for water, glycerol, urea, and ammonia.[232]

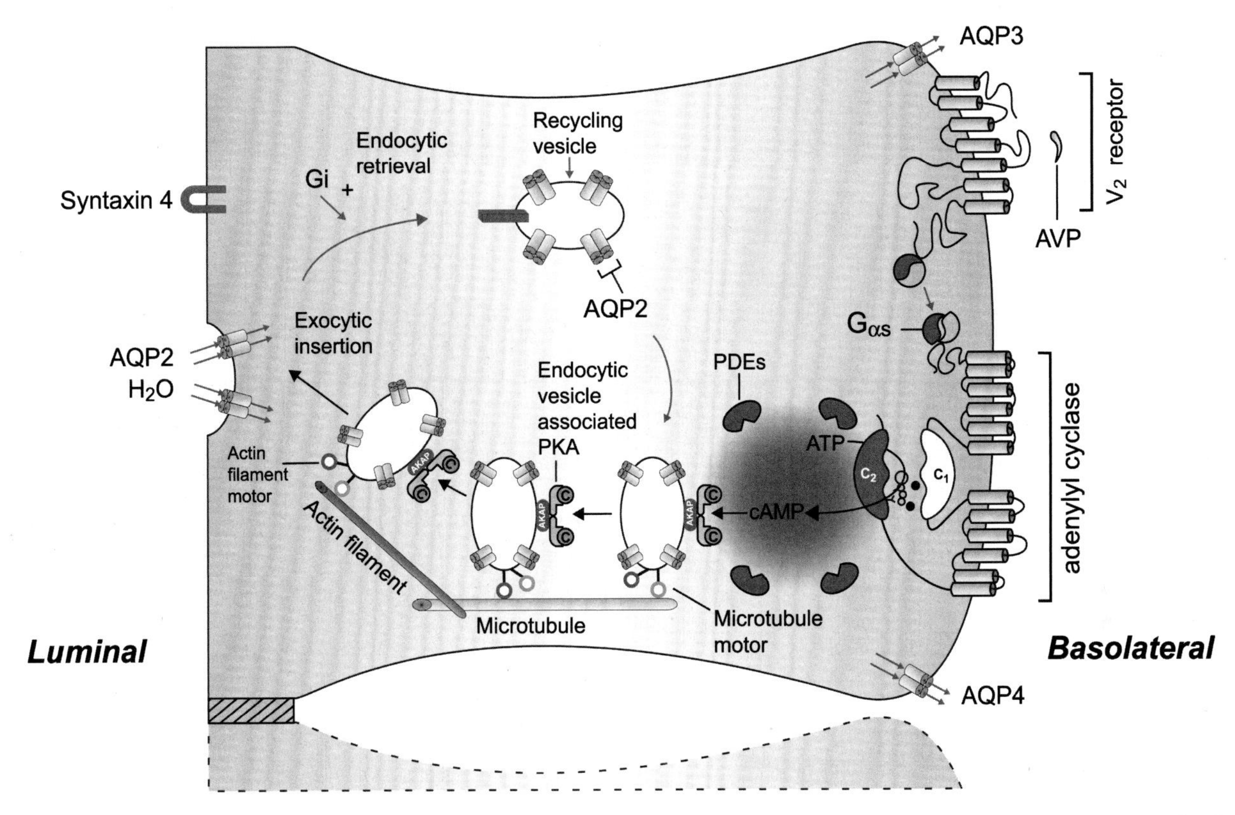

FIGURE 71.9 A schematic representation of the effect of vasopressin (AVP) to increase water permeability in the principal cells of the collecting duct. AVP is bound to the V_2 receptor (a G-protein–linked receptor) on the basolateral membrane. The basic process of G-protein–coupled receptor signaling consists of three steps: a heptahelical receptor that detects a ligand (in this case, AVP) in the extracellular milieu, a G-protein ($G_{\alpha s}$) that dissociates into subunits bound to GTP and bg subunits after interaction with the ligand-bound receptor, and an effector (in this case, adenylyl cyclase) that interacts with dissociated G-protein subunits to generate small-molecule second messengers. AVP activates adenylyl cyclase, increasing the intracellular concentration of cAMP. The topology of adenylyl cyclase is characterized by two tandem repeats of six hydrophobic transmembrane domains separated by a large cytoplasmic loop and terminates in a large intracellular tail. The dimeric structure (C_1 and C_2) of the catalytic domains is represented. Conversion of ATP to cAMP takes place at the dimer interface. Two aspartate residues (in C_1) coordinate two metal cofactors (Mg^{2+} or Mn^{2+} represented here as two *small black circles*), which enable the catalytic function of the enzyme.[233] Adenosine is shown as an *open circle* and the three phosphate groups (ATP) are shown as *smaller open circles*. Protein kinase A (PKA) is the target of the generated cAMP. The binding of cAMP to the regulatory subunits of PKA induces a conformational change, causing these subunits to dissociate from the catalytic subunits. These activated subunits (C), as shown here, are anchored to an aquaporin-2 (AQP2)-containing endocytic vesicle via an A-kinase anchoring protein. The local concentration and distribution of the cAMP gradient is limited by phosphodiesterases (PDEs). Cytoplasmic vesicles carrying the water channels (represented as homotetrameric complexes) are fused to the luminal membrane in response to AVP, thereby increasing the water permeability of this membrane. The dissociation of the A-kinase anchoring protein from the endocytic vesicle is not represented. Microtubules and actin filaments are necessary for vesicle movement toward the membrane. When AVP is not available, AQP2 water channels are retrieved by an endocytic process, and water permeability returns to its original low rate. Aquaporin-3 (AQP3) and aquaporin-4 (AQP4) water channels are expressed constitutively at the basolateral membrane.

promotes the cyclic adenosine monophosphate (cAMP)-mediated incorporation of water channels into the luminal surface of these cells. There are two ubiquitously expressed intracellular cAMP receptors: (1) the classical protein kinase A (PKA) that is a cAMP-dependent protein kinase, and (2) the recently discovered exchange protein directly activated by cAMP that is a cAMP-regulated guanine nucleotide exchange factor. Both of these receptors contain an evolutionally conserved cAMP-binding domain that acts as a molecular switch for sensing intracellular cAMP levels to control diverse biologic functions.[61] Several proteins participating in the control of cAMP-dependent aquaporin-2 AQP2 trafficking have been identifieD (e.g., A-kinase anchoring proteins tethering PKA to cellular compartments; phosphodiesterases regulating the local cAMP

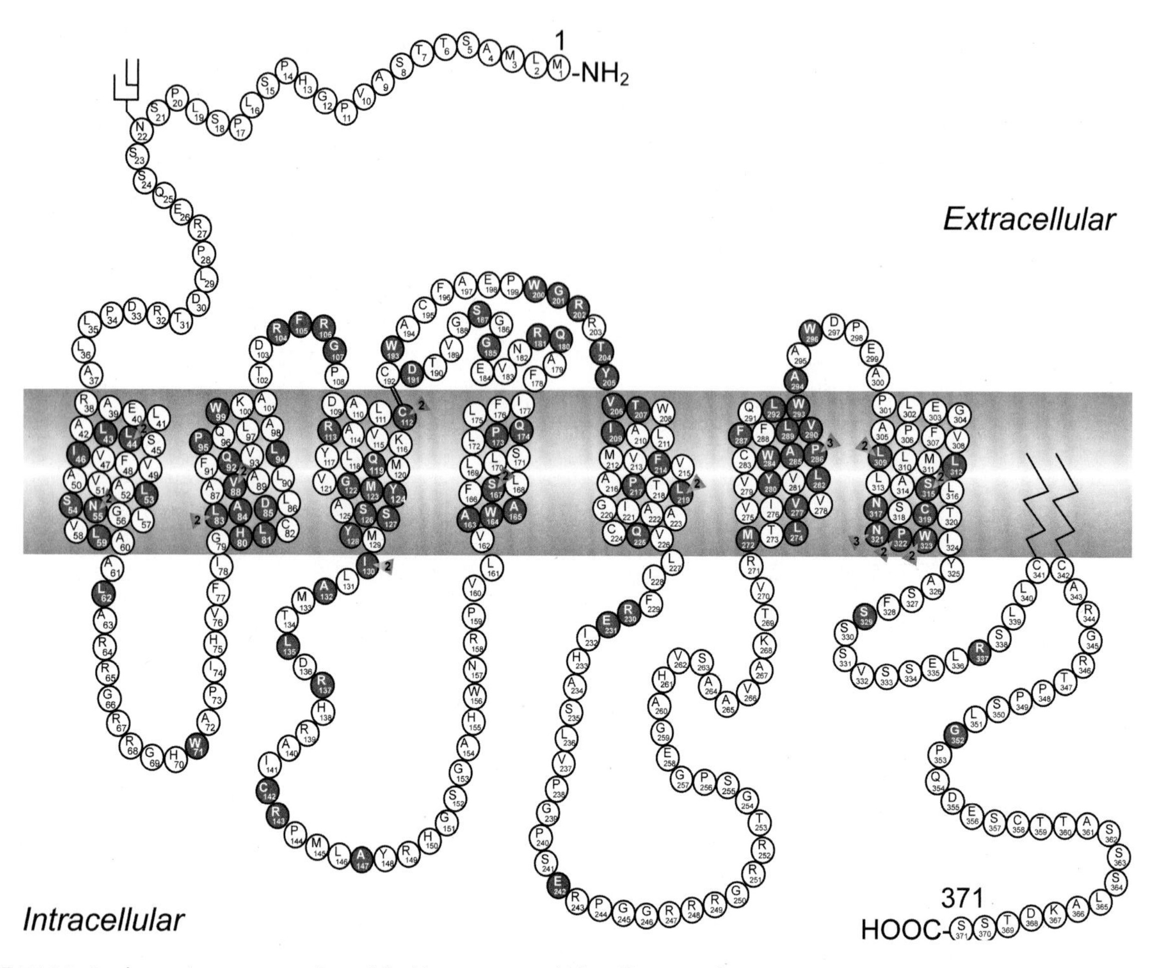

FIGURE 71.10 A schematic representation of the V_2 receptor and identification of 193 putative disease-causing AVPR2 mutations. Predicted amino acids are shown as the one-letter amino acid code. A *solid symbol* indicates a codon with a missense or nonsense mutation; a *number* indicates more than one mutation in the same codon; other types of mutations are not indicated on the figure. There are 95 missense, 18 nonsense, 46 frameshift deletion or insertion, 7 in-frame deletion or insertion, 4 splice site, 22 large deletion mutations, and 1 complex mutation.

level; cytoskeletal components such as F-actin and microtubules; small GTPases of the Rho family controlling cytoskeletal dynamics; motor proteins transporting AQP2-bearing vesicles to and from the plasma membrane for exocytic insertion and endocytic retrieval; soluble N-ethylmaleimide-sensitive fusion protein attachment protein receptors (SNAREs) inducing membrane fusions, hsc70, a chaperone important for endocytic retrieval). These processes are the molecular basis of the vasopressin-induced increase in the osmotic water permeability of the apical membrane of the collecting tubule.[62–64]

AVP also increases the water reabsorptive capacity of the kidney by regulating the urea transporter UT-A1 that is present in the inner medullary collecting duct, predominantly in its terminal part.[65,66] AVP also increases the permeability of principal collecting duct cells to sodium.[67] Finally, the vasopressin V_2 receptor has been located in the primary cilium and Bardet-Biedl syndrome–derived unciliated renal epithelial cells were unable to respond to luminal AVP and to activate luminal AQP2.[68]

In summary, in the absence of AVP stimulation, collecting duct epithelia exhibit very low permeabilities to sodium urea and water. These specialized permeability properties permit the excretion of large volumes of hypotonic urine formed during intervals of water diuresis. By contrast, AVP stimulation of the principal cells of the collecting ducts leads to selective increases in the permeability of the apical membrane to water, urea, and sodium.

These actions of vasopressin in the distal nephron are possibly modulated by prostaglandin E2 (PGE2), nitric oxide,[69] and by luminal calcium concentration. High levels of E-prostanoid-3 receptors are expressed in the kidney.[70] However, mice lacking E-prostanoid-3 receptors for PGE2 were found to have quasinormal regulation of urine volume and osmolality in response to various physiologic stimuli.[70] PGE2 is synthesized and released in the collecting duct, which expresses all E-prostanoid receptors.[71–73] An apical calcium/polycation receptor protein expressed in the terminal portion of the inner medullary collecting duct of the rat has been shown to reduce AVP-elicited osmotic water permeability when luminal calcium concentration rises.[74] This possible link between calcium and water metabolism may play a role in the pathogenesis of renal stone formation.[74]

KNOCKOUT MICE WITH URINARY CONCENTRATION DEFECTS

A useful strategy to establish the physiologic function of a protein is to determine the phenotype produced by pharmacologic inhibition of protein function or by gene disruption. Transgenic knockout mice deficient in AQP1, AQP2, AQP3, AQP4, AQP3, and AQP4; CLCNK1; NKCC2; AVPR2; AGT; or adenylyl cyclase 6 (AC6) have been engineered.[75–84] Angiotensinogen (AGT)-deficient mice are characterized by both concentrating and diluting defects secondary to a defective renal papillary architecture.[76]

As reviewed by Rao and Verkman,[85] the extrapolation of data in mice to humans must be made with caution. For example, the maximum osmolality of mice (greater than 3,000 mOsmol per kilogram of H_2O) is much greater than that of human urine (1,000 mOsmol per kilogram of H_2O), and normal serum osmolality in mice is 330 to 345 mOsmol per kilogram of H_2O, substantially greater than that in humans (280 to 290 mOsmol per kilogram of H_2O). These differences are related to renal anatomy and metabolic rate: (1) the mouse kidney exhibits much larger loops of Henle in the inner medulla and papillae and (2) because of the large difference in body size (30 g to 70 kg) the mouse metabolic rate (and thus the food intake) per gram of body mass is 20 times greater than that of humans. The amount of osmoles that need to be excreted by the kidney is also disproportionately larger when expressed per gram of body mass or kidney mass. These two features account for the much higher urine concentrating ability of the mouse as compared to humans. Protein expression patterns, and thus the interpretation of phenotype studies, may also be species dependent. For example, AQP4 is expressed in both the proximal tubule and the collecting duct in mice but only in the collecting duct in rats and humans.[85]

The *Aqp3*, *Aqp4*, *Clcnk-1*, and *Agt* knockout mice have no identified human counterparts. Of interest, *AQP1*-null individuals have no obvious symptoms.[86] Yang et al.[87] have generated an AQP2-T126M conditional knockin model of nephrogenic diabetes insipidus (NDI), to recapitulate the clinical features of the naturally occurring human AQP2 mutation T126M.[88] The conditional knockin adult mice showed polyuria, urinary hypo-osmolality, and endoplasmic reticulum (ER) retention of AQP2-T126M in the collecting duct. The screening of candidate protein folding correctors in AQP2-T126M–transfected kidney cells showed increased AQP2-T126M plasma membrane expression with the Hsp90 inhibitor 17-allylamino-17-demethoxygeldanamycin (17-AAG), a compound currently in clinical trials for tumor therapy. 17-AAG increased urine osmolality in the AQP2-T126M mice (without effect in AQP2 null mice) and partially rescued defective AQP2-T126M cellular processing. These proof-of-concept findings suggest the possibility of using existing drugs for therapy of some forms of NDI. Ethylnitrosourea-mutagenized mice heterozygous for the *F204V* mutation in the *Aqp2* gene have been described.[89] The homozygous mice are viable because of a moderate phenotype with a possibility to concentrate urine from 161 to 470 mOsmol per kilogram of H_2O in response to dDAVP. Cell biology experiments performed on renal tissue from *Aqp2*$F^{204V/+}$ animals suggest that the mutant protein is being rescued by the wild-type protein.

Mice lacking the AVPR2 receptor failed to thrive and died within the first week after birth due to hypernatremic dehydration.[78] Li et al.[90] generated mice in which the *Avpr2* gene could be conditionally deleted during adulthood by the administration of 4-OH-tamoxifen. Adult mice displayed all characteristic symptoms of X-linked NDI (XNDI), including polyuria, polydipsia, and resistance to the antidiuretic actions of vasopressin. Gene expression analysis suggested that the activation of renal EP4 PGE_2 receptors might compensate for the lack of renal V2R activity in X-linked NDI mice, and both acute and chronic treatment of the mutant mice with a selective EP4 receptor agonist greatly reduced all major manifestations of XNDI. This beneficial effect is likely secondary to the intracellular generation of cAMP at the principal cell level by EP4 PGE_2 receptors.

The absence of the gene coding for the NaK2Cl cotransport (NKCC2) in the luminal membrane of the thick ascending loop of Henle in the mouse also caused polyuria that was not compensated elsewhere in the nephron and recapitulated many features of the human classical Bartter syndrome.[79] The absence of transcellular NaCl transport via NKCC2 probably abolished the lumen-positive transepithelial voltage that enables paracellular reabsorption of Na and K across the wall of the thick ascending tubule. The combined absence of transcellular and paracellular transport of salt across the thick ascending limb cells prevents the establishment of the normal osmotic gradient necessary for urine concentration.

EXPRESSION OF THE VASOPRESSIN GENE IN DIABETES INSIPIDUS RATS (BRATTLEBORO RATS)

The animal model of diabetes insipidus that has been most extensively studied is the Brattleboro rat. Discovered in 1961, the rat lacks vasopressin and its neurophysin, whereas the synthesis of the structurally related hormone oxytocin is not affected by the mutation.[91] Its inability to synthesize vasopressin is inherited as an autosomal recessive trait. Schmale and Richter[92] isolated and sequenced the vasopressin gene from homozygous Brattleboro rats, and found that the defect is due to a single nucleotide deletion of a G residue within the second exon encoding the carrier protein neurophysin (Fig. 71.11). The shift in the reading frame caused by this deletion predicts a precursor with an deleted in Brattleboro rat

```
GGA AGC GGA GGC CGC TGC GCT GCC    Rat
Gly Ser Gly Gly Arg Cys Ala Ala

GGG AGC GGG GGC CGC TGC GCC GCC    Human
Gly Ser Gly Gly Arg Cys Ala Ala
 62  63  64  65  66  67  68  69
```

FIGURE 71.11 A neurophysin II genomic and amino acid sequence showing the 1 bp (G) deleted in the Brattleboro rat. The human sequence (GenBank entry M11166) is also shown. It is almost identical to the rat prepro sequence. In the Brattleboro rat, G1880 is deleted with a resultant frameshift after 63 amino acids (amino acid 1 is the first amino acid of neurophysin II).

entirely different C terminus. The messenger RNA (mRNA) produced by the mutated gene encodes a normal AVP but an abnormal NPII moiety,[92] which impairs transport and processing of the AVP-NPII precursor and its retention in the endoplasmic reticulum of the magnocellular neurons where it is produced.[93,94] Homozygous Brattleboro rats may still demonstrate some V2 (vide infra) antidiuretic effects since the administration of a selective nonpeptide V2 antagonist (SR 121463A, 10 mg per kilogram i.p.) induced a further increase in urine flow rate (200 to 354 ± 42 mL per 24 hours) and a decline in urinary osmolality (170 to 92 ± 8 mmol per kilogram).[95] This decline in urine osmolality following the administration of a nonpeptide V2r antagonist could also be secondary to the "inverse agonist" properties of SR121463A: the intrinsic activity, or tone, of the V2R would be deactivated by the SR121463A compound (for the inverse agonist properties of SR121463A (see reference 96). There is also an alternative explanation to this relatively high urine osmolality of 170 because, in Brattleboro rats, low levels of hormonally active AVP are produced from alternate forms of AVP preprohormone. Due to a process called molecular misreading, one transcript contains a 2-bp deletion downstream from the single nucleotide deletion that restores the reading frame and produces a variant AVP preprohormone that is smaller in length by one amino acid and differs from the normal product by only 13 amino acids in the neurophysin II moiety.[97] Oxytocin, which is present at enhanced plasma concentrations in Brattleboro rats, may be responsible for the antidiuretic activity observed.[98,99] Oxytocin is not stimulated by increased plasma osmolality in humans.

CLINICAL CHARACTERISTICS OF DIABETES INSIPIDUS DISORDERS

Central Diabetes Insipidus

Common Forms

Failure to synthesize or secrete vasopressin normally limits maximal urinary concentration and, depending on the severity of the disease, causes varying degrees of polyuria and polydipsia. Experimental destruction of the vasopressin-synthesizing areas of the hypothalamus (the supraoptic and paraventricular nuclei) causes a permanent form of the disease. Similar results are obtained by sectioning the hypophyseal-hypothalamic tract above the median eminence. Sections below the median eminence, however, produce only transient diabetes insipidus. Lesions to the hypothalamic-pituitary tract are often associated with a three-stage response both in experimental animals and in humans,[100] which consists of:

1. An initial diuretic phase lasting from a few hours to 5 to 6 days.
2. A period of antidiuresis unresponsive to fluid administration. This antidiuresis is probably due to vasopressin release from injured axons and may last from a few hours to several days. Because urinary dilution is impaired during this phase, continued water administration can cause severe hyponatremia.
3. A final period of diabetes insipidus. The extent of the injury determines the completeness of the diabetes insipidus and, as already discussed, the site of the lesion determines whether the disease will or will not be permanent.

A detailed assessment of water balance following transsphenoidal surgery has been reported.[101] There were 101 patients who underwent transsphenoidal pituitary surgery at the National Institutes of Health Clinical Center and were studied. Of the patients, 25% developed spontaneous isolated hyponatremia, 20% developed diabetes insipidus, and 46% remained normonatremic. Normonatremia, hyponatremia, and diabetes insipidus were associated with increasing degrees of surgical manipulation of the posterior lobe and pituitary stalk during surgery.

The etiologies of central diabetes insipidus in adults and in children are listed in Table 71.1.[102–104] Rare causes of central diabetes insipidus include leukemia, thrombotic thrombocytopenic purpura, pituitary apoplexy, sarcoidosis, and Wegener granulomatosis.[105] A distinctive syndrome characterized by early diabetes insipidus with subsequent progressive spastic cerebellar ataxia has also been described.[106] Five patients who all presented with central diabetes insipidus and hypogonadism as first manifestations of neurosarcoidosis have been reported.[107] Finally, circulating antibodies to vasopressin do not play a role in the development of diabetes insipidus.[108] Antibodies to vasopressin occasionally develop during treatment with ADH and, when they do, almost always result in secondary resistance to its antidiuretic effect.[108,109] Maghnie et al.[102] studied 79 patients with central diabetes insipidus who were seen at four pediatric endocrinology units between 1970 and 1996. There were 37 male and 42 female patients whose median age at diagnosis was 7 years (range, 0.1 to 24.8 years). In 11 patients, central diabetes insipidus developed during an infectious illness or less than 2 months afterward (varicella in 5 patients,

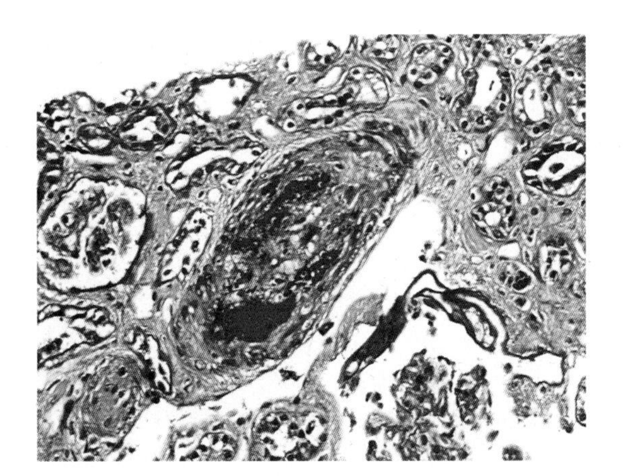

FIGURE 53.31

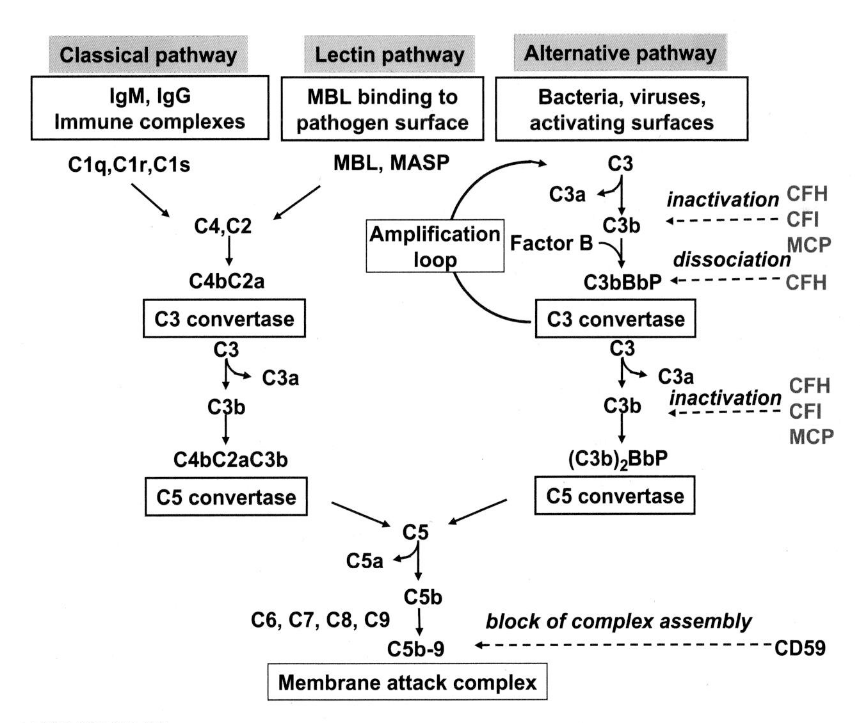

FIGURE 55.12

Erythropoietin (green) Fibroblasts (blue) Combined staining

FIGURE 57.1

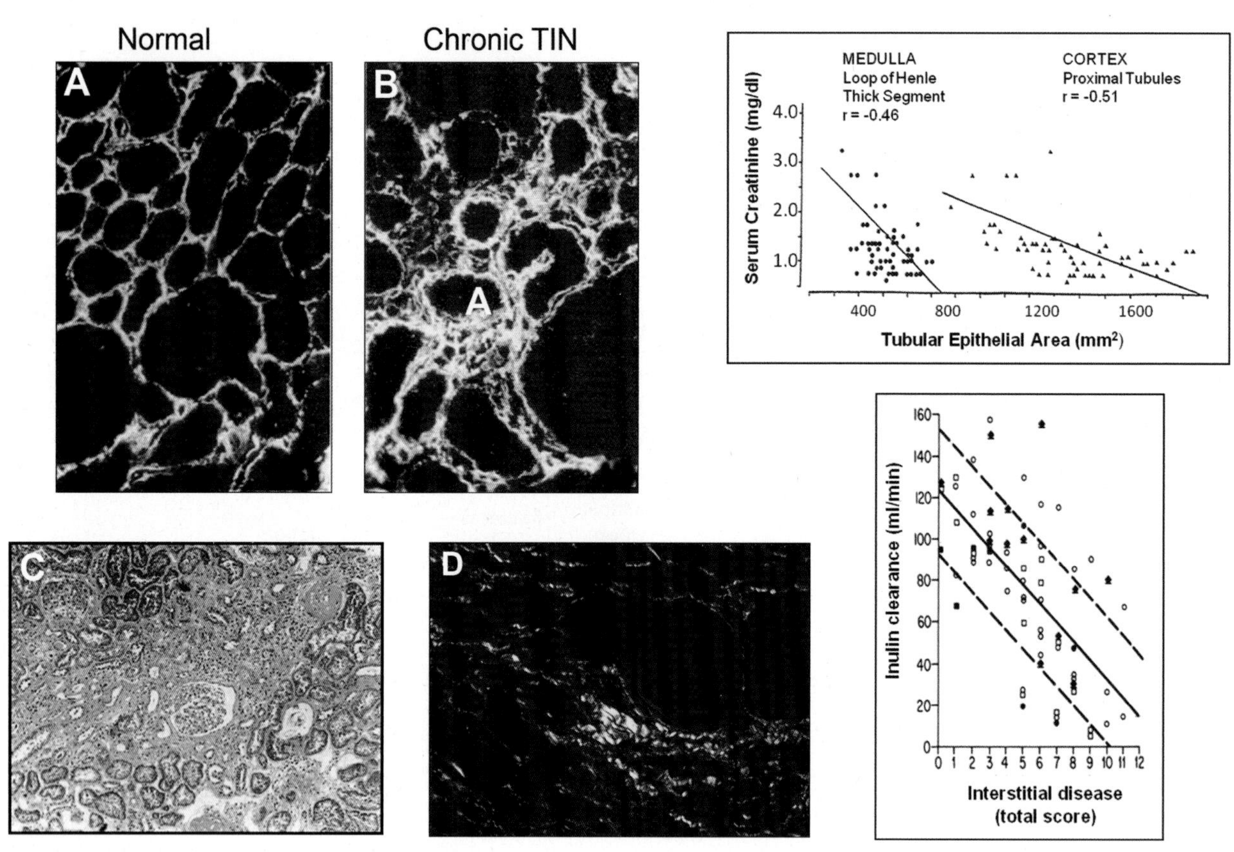

FIGURE 57.2

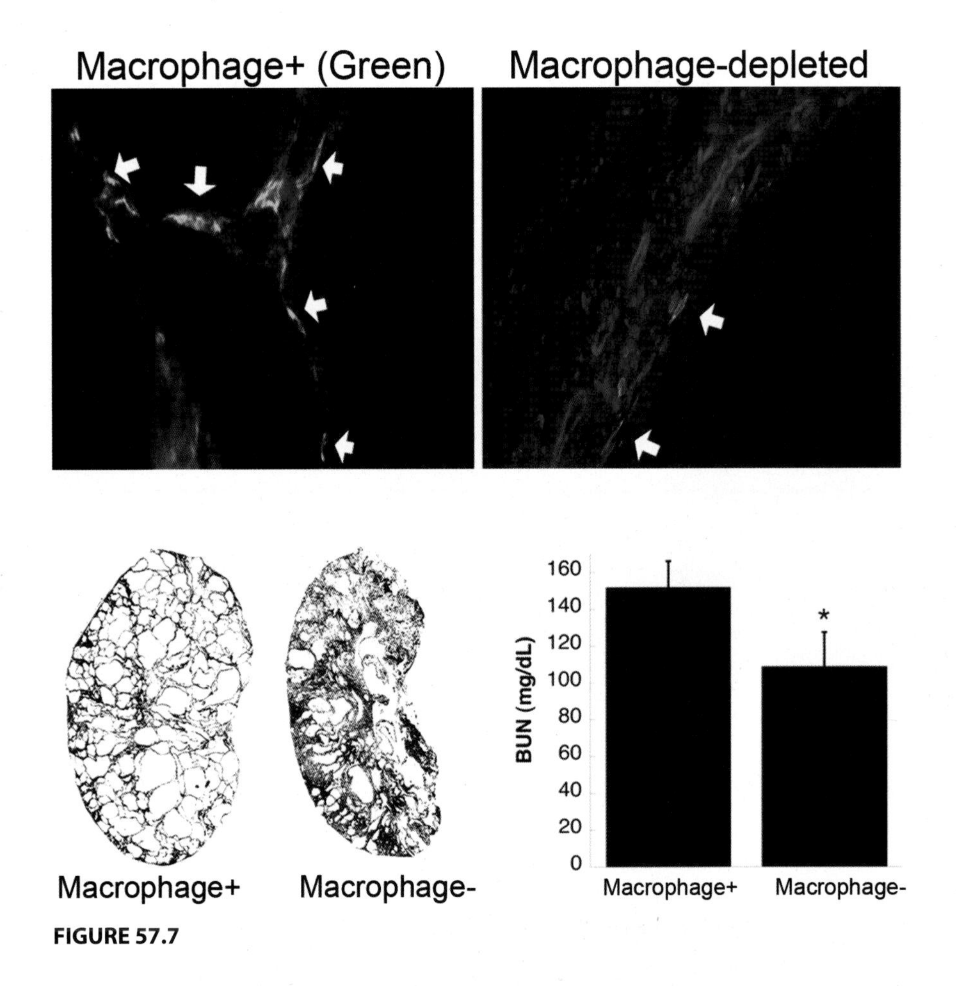
Macrophage+ (Green)
Macrophage-depleted
160
140
120
100
80
60
40
20
0
BUN (mg/dL)
*
Macrophage+
Macrophage-
Macrophage+
Macrophage-

FIGURE 57.7

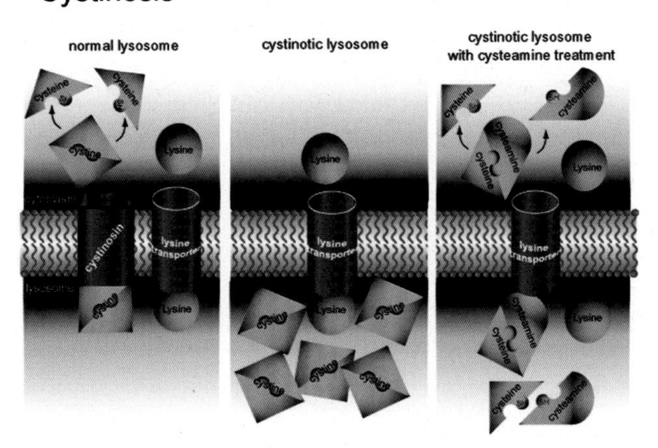
Cystinosis
normal lysosome
cystinotic lysosome
cystinotic lysosome
with cysteamine treatment
cysteine
cystine
Lysine
cystinosin
lysine transporter
cysteamine

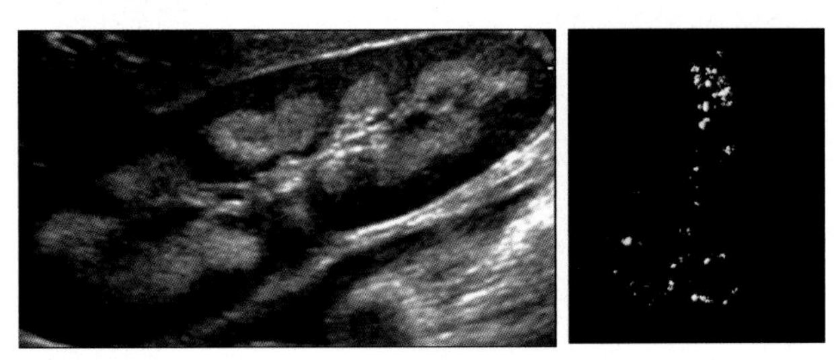
Oxalosis

FIGURE 57.8

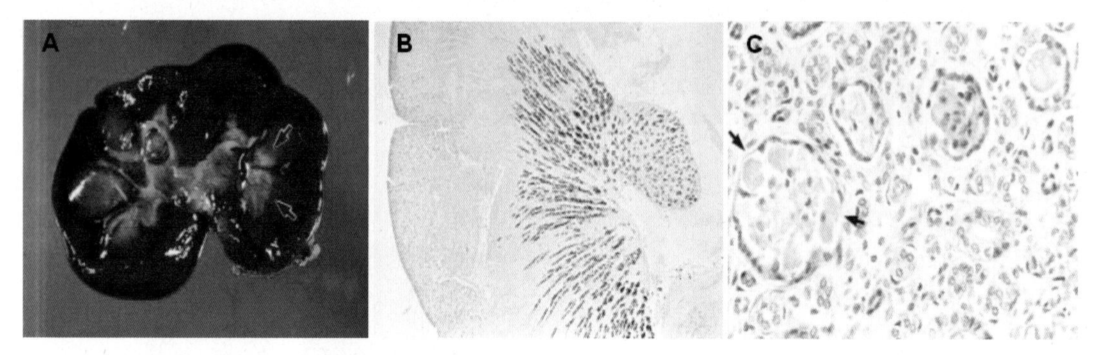

FIGURE 61.3

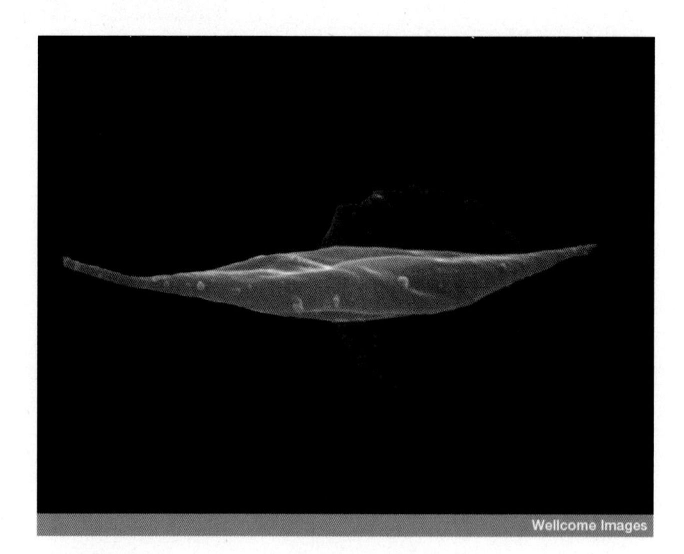

FIGURE 62.1

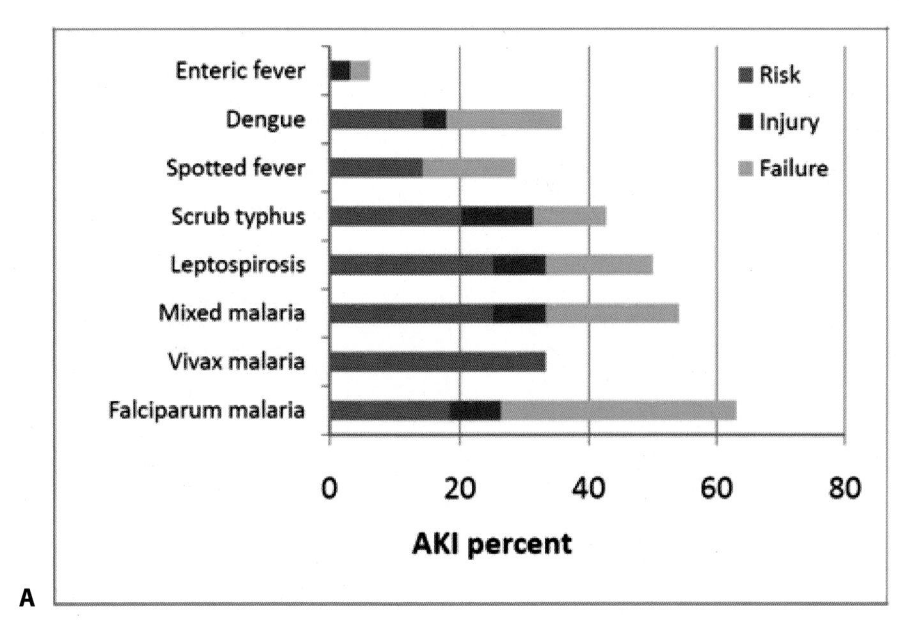

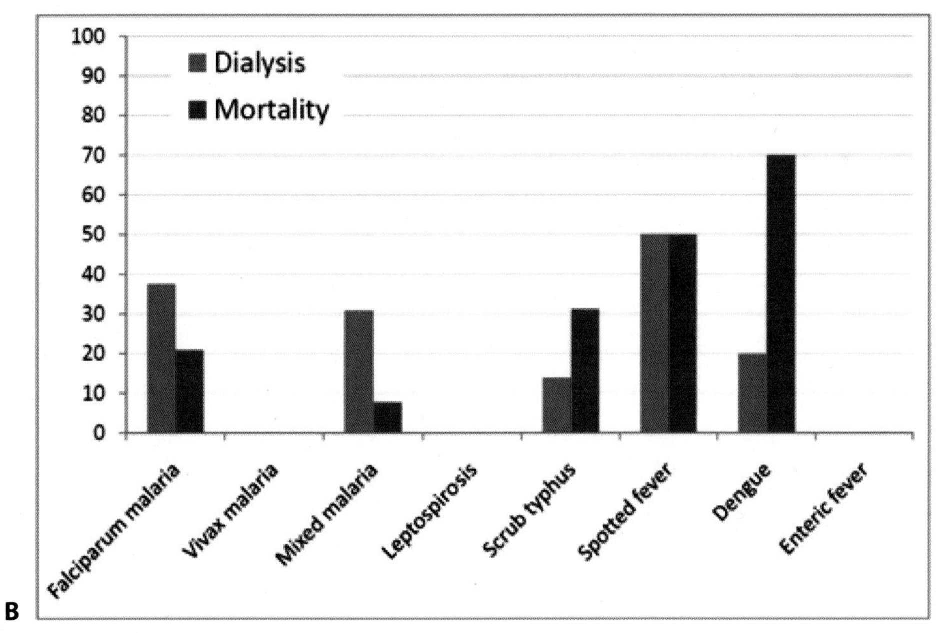

FIGURE 63.3A,B

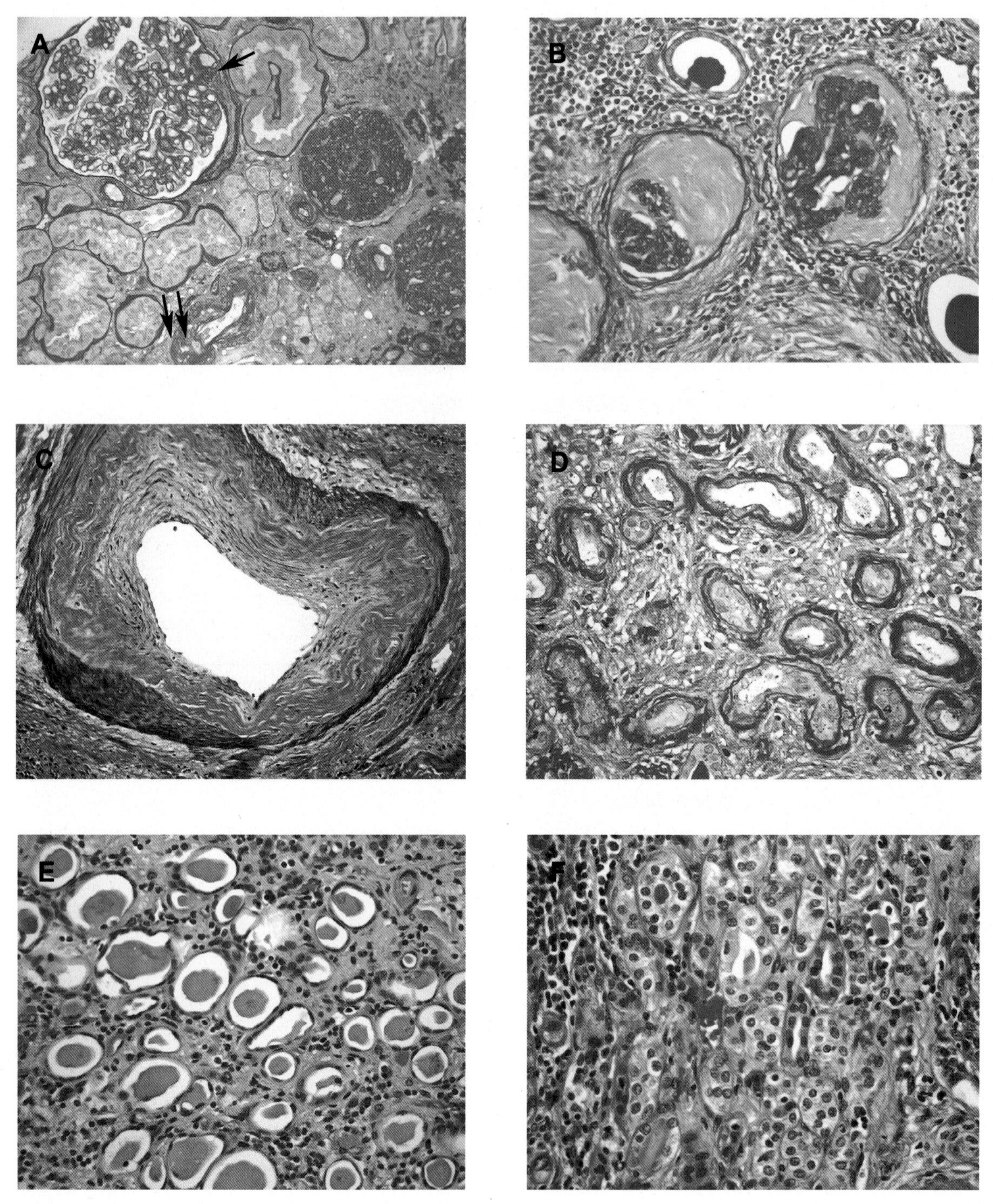

FIGURE 65.1

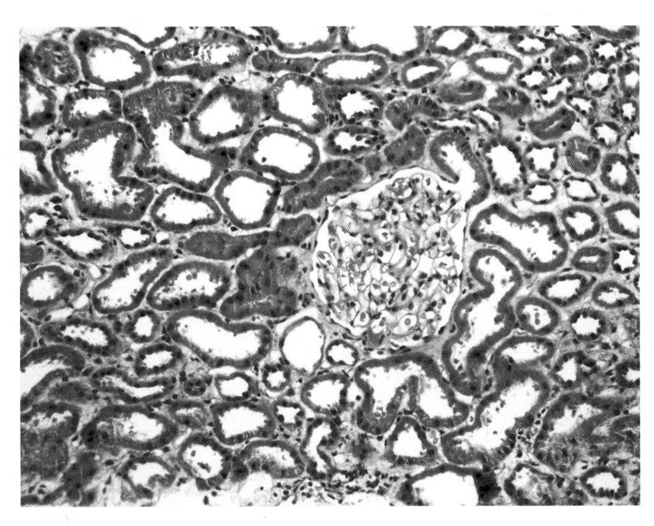

FIGURE 65.3

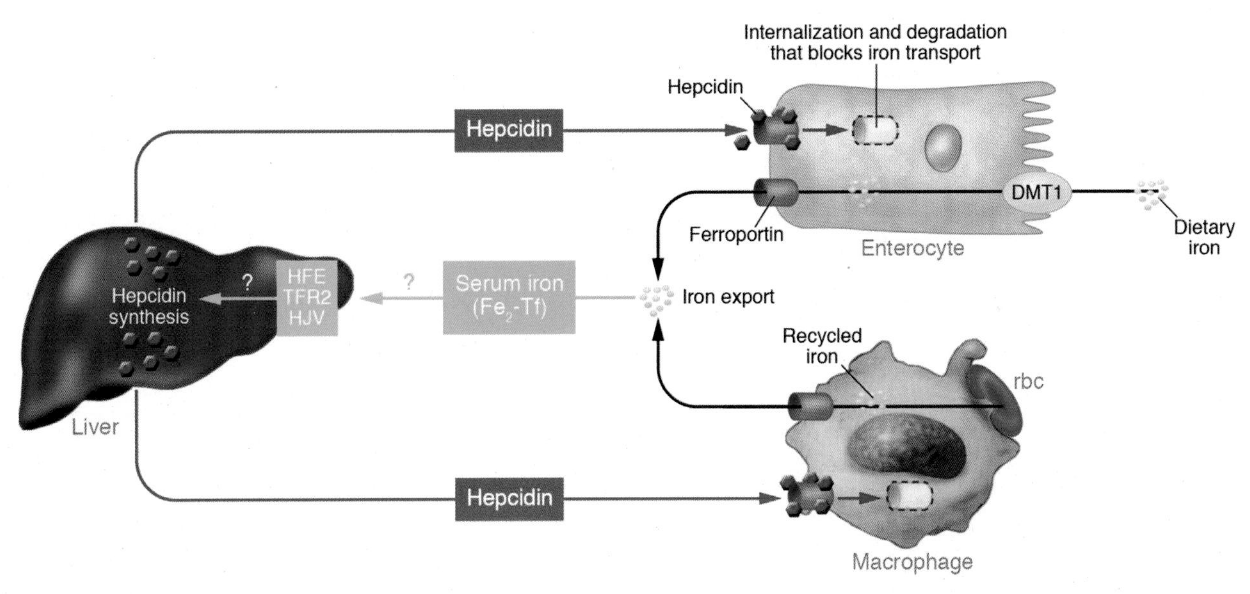

FIGURE 76.3

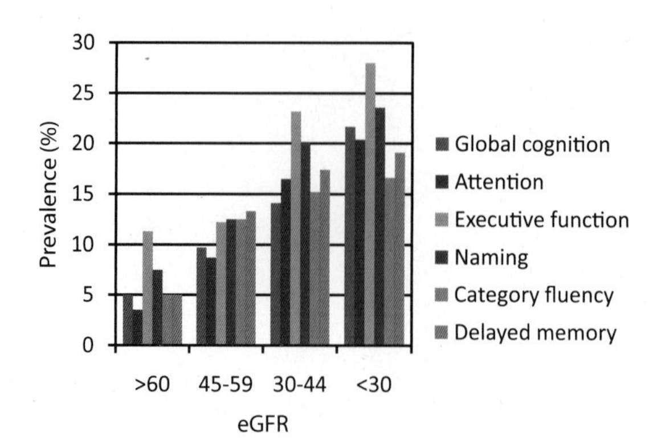

FIGURE 78.2

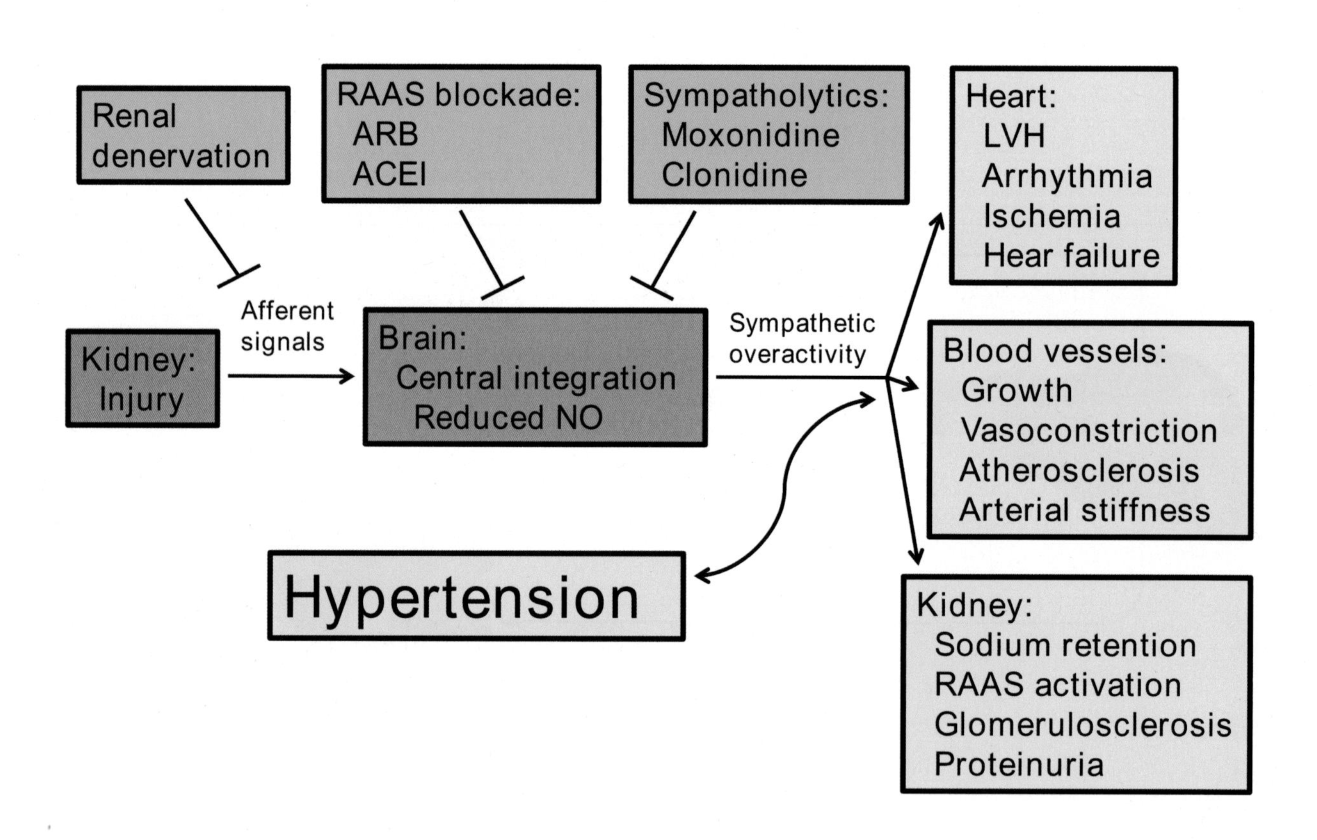

FIGURE 78.7

TABLE 71.1 Etiology of Hypothalamic Diabetes Insipidus in Children and Adults[102–105]

	Children (%)	Children and Young Adults (%)	Adults (%)
Primary brain tumor[a]	49.5	22	30
Before surgery	33.5		13
After surgery	16		17
Idiopathic (isolated or familial)	29	58	25
Histiocytosis	16	12	—
Metastatic cancer[b]	—		8
Trauma[c]	2.2	2.0	17
Postinfectious disease	2.2	6.0	—

[a]Primary malignancy: Craniopharyngioma, dysgerminoma, meningioma, adenoma, glioma, astrocytoma.
[b]Secondary: Metastatic from lung or breast, lymphoma, leukemia, dysplastic pancytopenia.
[c]Trauma could be severe or mild.

mumps in 3 patients, and measles, toxoplasmosis, and hepatitis B in 1 patient each). Deficits in anterior pituitary hormones were documented in 48 patients (61%) a median of 0.6 year (range, 0.1 to 18.0 years) after the onset of diabetes insipidus. The most frequent abnormality was growth hormone deficiency (59%), followed by hypothyroidism (28%), hypogonadism (24%), and adrenal insufficiency (22%). Of the patients with histiocytosis of the Langerhans cells, 75% had an anterior pituitary hormone deficiency that was first detected at a median of 3.5 years after the onset of diabetes insipidus. The frequency and progression of histiocytosis of the Langerhans cells related to anterior pituitary and other nonendocrine hypothalamic dysfunction and their response to treatment in 12 adult patients has also been reviewed.[110] None of the patients with central diabetes insipidus secondary to *AVP* mutations developed anterior pituitary hormone deficiencies.

Rare Forms

Inherited neurohypophyseal diabetes insipidus (OMIM 125700)[111] is due to mutations in the *AVP* gene (OMIM 192340)[111] and Wolfram syndrome 1 (OMIM 222300)[111] is due to mutations in the *WFS1* gene. Historically, Lacombe[112] and Weil[113] described a familial non–X-linked form of diabetes insipidus without any associated mental retardation. The descendants of the family described by Weil were later found to have autosomal dominant neurogenic diabetes insipidus.[114–116]

Patients with autosomal dominant neurohypophyseal diabetes insipidus retain some limited capacity to secrete AVP during severe dehydration, and the polyuria–polydipsic symptoms usually appear after the first year of life,[117] when the infant's demand for water is more likely to be understood by adults. In neurohypophyseal diabetes insipidus, termed familial neurohypophyseal diabetes insipidus (FNDI), levels of AVP are insufficient and patients show a positive response to treatment with dDAVP. Growth retardation might be observed in untreated children with autosomal dominant FNDI.[118] Over 50 mutations in the prepro-arginine-vasopressin-neurophysin II *AVP* gene located on chromosome 20p13 have been reported in dominant FNDI (adFNDI). Knockin mice heterozygous for a nonsense mutation in the AVP carrier protein neurophysin II showed progressive loss of AVP-producing neurons over several months correlated with increased water intake, increased urine output, and decreased urine osmolality. The data suggest that vasopressin mutants accumulate as fibrillar aggregates in the endoplasmic reticulum and cause cumulative toxicity to magnocellular neurons explaining the later age of onset.[119,120] To date, recessive FNDI has only been described in two studies.[121,122] A study by Christensen et al.[123] examined the differences in cellular trafficking between dominant and recessive AVP mutants and found that dominant forms were concentrated in the cytoplasm whereas recessive forms were localized to the tips of neurites. The expression of regulated secretory proteins such as granins and prohormones, including provasopressin, generates granulelike structures in a variety of neuroendocrine cell lines due to aggregation in the trans-Golgi.[124] Costaining experiments unambiguously distinguished between these granulelike structures and the accumulations by pathogenic dominant mutants formed in the ER, because the latter, but not the trans-Golgi granules, colocalized with specific ER markers.[119] As studies concerning both dominant and recessive FNDI accumulate, it is becoming evident that

FNDI exhibits a variable age of onset and this may be related to the cellular handling of the mutant AVP. This progressive toxicity, sometimes called a toxic gain of function, shares mechanistic pathways with other neurodegenerative diseases such as Huntington disease and Parkinson disease.

WOLFRAM SYNDROME

Wolfram syndrome, also known as DIDMOAD, is an autosomal recessive neurodegenerative disorder accompanied by insulin-dependent diabetes mellitus and progressive optic atrophy. The acronym DIDMOAD describes the following clinical features of the syndrome: diabetes insipidus, diabetes mellitus, optic atrophy, and sensorineural deafness. An unusual incidence of psychiatric symptoms has also been described in patients with this syndrome. These included paranoid delusions, auditory or visual hallucinations, psychotic behavior, violent behavior, organic brain syndrome typically in the late or preterminal stages of their illness, progressive dementia, and severe learning disabilities or mental retardation or both. Wolfram syndrome patients develop diabetes mellitus and bilateral optical atrophy mainly in the first decade of life, the diabetes insipidus is usually partial and of gradual onset, and the polyuria can be wrongly attributed to poor glycemic control. Furthermore, a severe hyperosmolar state can occur if untreated diabetes mellitus is associated with an unrecognized posterior pituitary deficiency. The dilatation of the urinary tract observed in DIDMOAD syndrome may be secondary to chronic high urine flow rates and, perhaps, to some degenerative aspects of the innervation of the urinary tract. The gene responsible for Wolfram syndrome, located in chromosome region 4p16.1, encodes a putative 890 amino acid transmembrane protein referred to as wolframin. Wolframin is an endoglycosidase H-sensitive glycoprotein, which localizes primarily in the endoplasmic reticulum of a variety of neurons, including neurons in the supraoptic nucleus and neurons in the lateral magnocellular division of the paraventricular nucleus.[125,126] Disruption of the *Wfs1* gene in mice cause progressive beta cell loss and impaired stimulus-secretion coupling in insulin secretion but central diabetes insipidus is not observed in $Wfs^{-/-}$ mice.[127] Miner1, another endoplasmic reticulum protein, is causative in Wolfram syndrome 2,[128] and WFS1 negatively regulates a key transcription factor involved in ER stress signaling.[129]

THE SYNDROME OF HYPERNATREMIA AND HYPODIPSIA

Some patients with the hypernatremia and hypodipsia syndrome may have partial central diabetes insipidus. These patients also have persistent hypernatremia that is not due to any apparent extracellular volume loss, absence or attenuation of thirst, and a normal renal response to AVP. In almost all the patients studied to date, the hypodipsia has been associated with cerebral lesions in the vicinity of the hypothalamus. It has been proposed that in these patients there is a "resetting" of the osmoreceptor because their urine tends to become concentrated or diluted at inappropriately high levels of plasma osmolality. However, using the regression analysis of plasma AVP concentration versus plasma osmolality, it has been shown that in some of these patients the tendency to concentrate and dilute urine at inappropriately high levels of plasma osmolality is due solely to a marked reduction in sensitivity or a gain in the osmoregulatory mechanism.[130,131] This finding is compatible with the diagnosis of partial central diabetes insipidus. In other patients, however, plasma AVP concentrations fluctuate in a random manner, bearing no apparent relationship to changes in plasma osmolality. Such patients frequently display large swings in serum sodium concentration and frequently exhibit hypodipsia. It appears that most patients with essential hypernatremia fit one of these two patterns (Fig. 71.12). Both of these groups of patients consistently respond normally to nonosmolar AVP release signals, such as hypotension, emesis, or hypoglycemia, or all three. These observations suggest that (1) the osmoreceptor may be anatomically as well as functionally separate from the nonosmotic efferent pathways, and neurosecretory neurons for vasopressin and a hypothalamic lesion may impair the osmotic release of AVP while the nonosmotic release of AVP remains intact; and (2) the osmoreceptor neurons that regulate vasopressin secretion are not totally synonymous with those that regulate thirst, although they appear to be anatomically close if not overlapping.

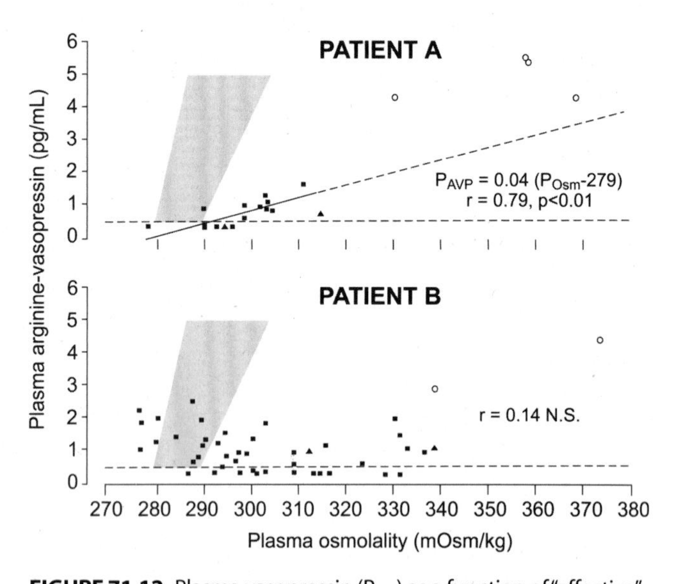

FIGURE 71.12 Plasma vasopressin (P_{AVP}) as a function of "effective" plasma osmolality (P_{OSM}) in two patients with adipsic hypernatremia. *Open circles* indicate values obtained on admission; *filled squares* indicate those obtained during forced hydration; *filled triangles* indicate those obtained after 1 to 2 weeks of ad libitum water intake; *shaded areas* indicate a range of normal values. (From: Robertson GL. The physiopathology of ADH secretion. In: Tolis G, Labrie F, Martin JB, et al., eds. *Clinical Neuroendocrinology: A Pathophysiological Approach*. New York, NY: Raven Press; 1979: 247, with permission from Wolters Kluwer/Lippincott Williams & Wilkins.[234])

NEPHROGENIC DIABETES INSIPIDUS

In NDI, AVP levels are normal or elevated but the kidney is unable to concentrate urine. The clinical manifestations of polyuria and polydipsia can be present at birth and must be immediately recognized to avoid severe episodes of dehydration. Most (> 90%) of the congenital patients with NDI have X-linked mutations in the *AVPR2* gene, the Xq28 gene coding for the vasopressin V_2 (antidiuretic) receptor. In less than 10% of the families studied, congenital NDI has an autosomal recessive inheritance, and approximately 46 mutations have been identified in the AQP2 gene (*AQP2*) located in chromosome region 12q13; that is, the vasopressin-sensitive water channel (Fig. 71.13).[132] For the *AVPR2* gene, 211 putative disease-causing mutations have now been published in 326 unrelated families with XNDI (Fig. 71.10). When studied in vitro, most *AVPR2* mutations lead to receptors that are trapped intracellularly and are unable to reach the plasma membrane.[133] A minority of the mutant receptors reach the cell surface but are unable to bind AVP or to trigger an intracellular cAMP signal. Similarly, *AQP2* mutant proteins are trapped intracellularly and cannot be expressed at the luminal membrane. This AQP2-trafficking defect is correctable, at least in vitro, by chemical chaperones. Other inherited disorders with mild, moderate, or severe inability to concentrate urine include Bartter syndrome (MIM601678),[134] cystinosis, and autosomal dominant hypocalcemia,[135,136] nephronophthisis, and apparent mineralocorticoid excess.[137]

Clinical Presentation and History of X-Linked Nephrogenic Diabetes Insipidus

XNDI (OMIM 304800) is secondary to *AVPR2* mutations, which result in a loss of function or dysregulation of the V_2 receptor.[138] Males who have an *AVPR2* mutation have a phenotype characterized by early dehydration episodes, hypernatremia, and hyperthermia as early as the first week of life. Dehydration episodes can be so severe that they lower arterial blood pressure to a degree that is not sufficient to sustain adequate oxygenation to the brain, kidneys, and other organs. Mental and physical retardation and renal failure are the classical "historical" consequences of a late diagnosis and lack of treatment. Heterozygous females may exhibit variable degrees of polyuria and polydipsia because of skewed X chromosome inactivation.[139]

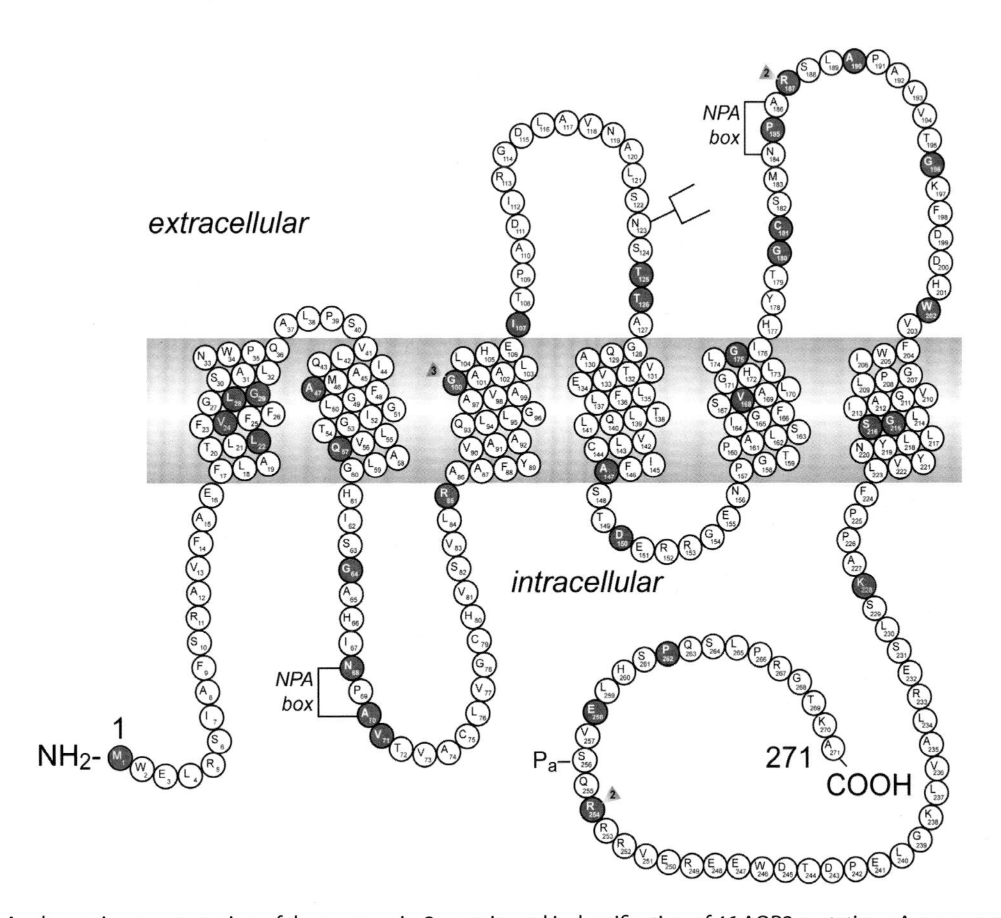

FIGURE 71.13 A schematic representation of the aquaporin-2 protein and indentification of 46 AQP2 mutations. A monomer is represented with six stetches of hydrophobic sequences that are suggestive of six transmembrane helices. The MIP proteins share an NPA (Asn-Pro-Ala) motiff in each of the two prominent loops. AQP1 (and, by analogy, AQP2) is homotetramer containing four independent aqueous channels. The location of the protein kinase A phosphorylation site is indicated. This site is possibly involved in the vasopressin-induced trafficking of AQP2 from intracellular vesicles to the plasma membrane and in the subsequent stimulation of endocytosis.

The "historical" clinical characteristics include hypernatremia, hyperthermia, mental retardation, and repeated episodes of dehydration in early infancy.[140] Mental retardation, a consequence of repeated episodes of dehydration, was prevalent in the Crawford and Bode study,[140] in which only 9 of 82 patients (11%) had normal intelligence. Early recognition and treatment of XNDI with an abundant intake of water allows a normal life span with normal physical and mental development.[141] Two characteristics suggestive of XNDI are the familial occurrence and the confinement of mental retardation to male patients. It is then tempting to assume that the family described in 1892 by McIlraith[142] and discussed by Reeves and Andreoli[143] was an XNDI family. Lacombe[112] and Weil[113] described a familial form of diabetes insipidus with autosomal transmission and without any associated mental retardation. The descendants of the family originally described by Weil were later found to have neurohypophyseal adFNDI (OMIM 192340).[144] Patients with adFNDI retain some limited capacity to secrete AVP during severe dehydration, and the polyuro-polydipsic symptoms usually appear after the first year of life when the infant's demand for water is more likely to be understood by adults.

The severity in infancy of NDI was clearly described by Crawford and Bode.[140] The first manifestations of the disease can be recognized during the first week of life. The infants are irritable, cry almost constantly, and although eager to suck, will vomit milk soon after ingestion unless prefed with water. The history given by the mothers often includes persistent constipation, erratic unexplained fever, and failure to gain weight. Even though the patients characteristically show no visible evidence of perspiration, increased water loss during fever or in warm weather exaggerates the symptoms. Unless the condition is recognized early, children will experience frequent bouts of hypertonic dehydration, sometimes complicated by convulsions or death; mental retardation is a frequent consequence of these episodes. The intake of large quantities of water, combined with the patient's voluntary restriction of dietary salt and protein intake, leads to hypocaloric dwarfism beginning in infancy. Affected children frequently develop lower urinary tract dilatation and obstruction, probably secondary to the large volume of urine produced. Dilatation of the lower urinary tract is also seen in primary polydipsic patients and in patients with neurogenic diabetes insipidus.[145,146] Chronic renal insufficiency may occur by the end of the first decade of life and could be the result of episodes of dehydration with thrombosis of the glomerular tufts.[140] More than 20 years ago our group observed that the administration of dDAVP, a V_2 receptor agonist, increased plasma cAMP concentrations in normal subjects but had no effect in 14 male patients with XNDI.[147] Intermediate responses were observed in obligate carriers of the disease, possibly corresponding to half of the normal receptor response. Based on these results, we predicted that the defective gene in these patients with XNDI was likely to code for a defective V_2 receptor (see Fig. 71.10).[147]

XNDI is a rare disease with an estimated prevalence of approximately 8.8 per million male live births in the Province of Quebec (Canada).[139] In defined regions of North America, however, the prevalence is much higher: we estimated the incidence in Nova Scotia and New Brunswick (Canada) to be 58 per million,[139] and is due to common ancestors. An early example is the Mormon pedigree, with its members residing in Utah (Utah families); this pedigree was originally described by Cannon.[148] The "Utah mutation" is a nonsense mutation (L312X) predictive of a receptor that lacks transmembrane domain 7 and the intracellular COOH-terminus.[149] The largest known kindred with XNDI is the Hopewell family, named after the Irish ship *Hopewell,* which arrived in Halifax, Nova Scotia, in 1761.[150] Aboard the ship were members of the Ulster Scot clan, descendants of Scottish Presbyterians who migrated to Ulster, Ireland in the 17th century and left Ireland for the New World in the 18th century. Whereas families arriving with the first emigration wave settled in northern Massachusetts in 1718, the members of a second emigration wave, passengers of the *Hopewell,* settled in Colchester County, Nova Scotia. According to the Hopewell hypothesis,[150] most patients with NDI in North America are progeny of female carriers of the second emigration wave. This assumption is mainly based on the high prevalence of NDI among descendants of the Ulster Scots residing in Nova Scotia. In two villages with a total of 2500 inhabitants, 30 patients have been diagnosed, and the carrier frequency has been estimated at 6%. Given the numerous mutations found in North American XNDI families, the Hopewell hypothesis cannot be upheld in its originally proposed form. However, among XNDI patients in North America, the W71X (the Hopewell mutation) mutation is more common than another *AVPR2* mutation. It is a null mutation (W71X),[149,151] predictive of an extremely truncated receptor consisting of the extracellular NH_2-terminus, the first transmembrane domain, and the NH_2-terminal half of the first intracellular loop. Because the original carrier cannot be identified, it is not clear whether the Hopewell mutation was brought to North America by *Hopewell* passengers or by other Ulster Scot immigrants. The diversity of *AVPR2* mutations found in many ethnic groups (Caucasians, Japanese, African Americans, Africans) and the rareness of the disease is consistent with an X-linked recessive disease that in the past was lethal for male patients and was balanced by recurrent mutations. In XNDI, loss of mutant alleles from the population occurs because of the higher mortality of affected males compared with healthy males, whereas a gain of mutant alleles occurs by mutation. If affected males with a rare X-linked recessive disease do not reproduce and if mutation rates are equal in mothers and fathers, then, at genetic equilibrium, one third of new cases of affected males will be due to new mutations. We and others have described ancestral mutations, de novo mutations, and potential mechanisms of mutagenesis.[139] These data are reminiscent of those obtained from patients with late-onset autosomal-dominant retinitis pigmentosa. In one fourth of patients, the disease is caused by mutations in the light receptor rhodopsin. Here too, many different mutations (approximately 100) spread throughout the coding region of the rhodopsin gene have been found.[152]

The basis of loss of function or dysregulation of 28 different mutant V_2 receptors (including nonsense, frameshift, deletion, or missense mutations) has been studied using in vitro expression systems. Most of the mutant V_2 receptors tested were not transported to the cell membrane and were thus retained within the intracellular compartment. Our group and others also demonstrated that misfolded *AVPR2* mutants could be rescued in vitro[153,154] and in vivo[155] by nonpeptide vasopressin antagonists acting as pharmacologic chaperones. This new therapeutic approach could be applied to the treatment of several hereditary diseases resulting from errors in proteins folding and kinesis.[156]

Only four *AVPR2* mutations (D85N, V88M, G201D, P322S) have been associated with a mild phenotype.[157–159] In general, the male infants bearing these mutations are identified later in life and the classic episodes of dehydration are less severe. This mild phenotype is also found in expression studies: the mutant proteins are expressed on the plasma membrane of cells transfected with these mutants and demonstrate a stimulation of cAMP for higher concentrations of agonists.[157,159,160]

Gain of Function of the Vasopressin V_2 Receptor: Nephrogenic Syndrome of Inappropriate Antidiuresis

The clinical phenotype here is opposite to NDI. Rare cases of infants or adults with hyponatremia, concentrated urine, and suppressed AVP plasma concentrations have been described bearing the mutations R137C or R137L in their *AVPR2* gene.[161–164] It is interesting to note that another mutation in the same codon (R137H) is a relatively frequent mutation causing classical NDI; however, the phenotype may be milder in some patients.[165] With cell-based assays, both R137C and R137L were found to have elevated basal signaling through the cAMP pathway and to interact with beta-arrestins in an agonist independent manner.[166] It is my opinion that *AVPR2* mutations with gain of function are extremely rare. We have sequenced the *AVPR2* gene in many patients with hyponatremia and never found a mutation. By contrast, we continue to identify new and recurrent loss-of-function *AVPR2* mutations in patients with classical NDI.

Loss-of-Function Mutations of AQP2 (OMIM 107777)

The AQP2 gene is located on chromosome region 12q12-q13. Approximately 10% of NDI cases are due to autosomal mutations in AQP2, of which 40 mutations have been reported, which can be autosomal recessive (32 mutations reported) or autosomal dominant (8 mutations reported).[167] Males and females affected with congenital NDI have been described who are homozygous for a mutation in the AQP2 gene or carry two different mutations (Fig. 71.13).[158,168] Autosomal recessive mutations give rise to misfolded proteins that are retained in the ER and eventually degraded.[132] Autosomal dominant mutations are believed to be restricted to the C-terminal end of the AQP2 protein and operate through a dominant-negative effect where the mutant protein associates with functional AQP2 proteins within intracellular stores, thus preventing normal targeting and function.[167,169] To study the behavior of various AQP2 mutants on membrane water permeability, oocytes of the African clawed frog (*Xenopus laevis*) have provided a useful system. Functional expression studies showed that Xenopus oocytes injected with mutant cRNA had abnormal coefficient of water permeability, whereas Xenopus oocytes injected with both normal and mutant cRNA had coefficient of water permeability similar to that of normal constructs alone. These findings provide conclusive evidence that NDI can be caused by homozygosity for mutations in the AQP2 gene. A patient with a partial phenotype has also been described to be a compound heterozygote for the L22V and C181W mutations.[170] Immunolocalization of AQP2-transfected CHO cells showed that the C181W mutant had an endoplasmic reticulumlike intracellular distribution, whereas L22V and wild-type AQP2 showed endosome and plasma membrane staining. The authors suggested that the L22V mutation was key to the patient's unique response to desmopressin. The leucine 22 residue might be necessary for proper conformation or for the binding of another protein important for normal targeting and trafficking of the molecule. More recently, we obtained evidence to suggest that both autosomal dominant and autosomal recessive NDI phenotypes could be secondary to novel mutations in the AQP2 gene.[169,171–175] Reminiscent of expression studies done with AVPR2 proteins, studies also demonstrated that the major cause underlying autosomal recessive NDI is the misrouting of AQP2 mutant proteins.[88,171,173,176–179] To determine if the severe AQP2-trafficking defect observed with the naturally occurring mutations T126M, R187C, and A147T is correctable, cells were incubated with the chemical chaperone glycerol for 48 hours. Redistribution of AQP2 from the ER to the membrane-endosome fractions was observed by immunofluorescence. This redistribution was correlated to improved water permeability measurements.[177] We recently studied the ability of myo-inositol to stimulate water permeability in oocytes expressing six different mutant AQP2s. Only two mutants (D150E and S256L) were sensitive to the effect of myo-inositol, whereas no changes were seen with mutants A70D, V71M, and G196D.[180]

POLYURIA, POLYDIPSIA, ELECTROLYTE IMBALANCE, AND DEHYDRATION IN CYSTINOSIS, NEPHRONOPHTHISIS, AND APPARENT MINERALOCORTICOID EXCESS

Polyuria may be as mild as persistent enuresis and as severe to contribute to death from dehydration and electrolyte abnormalities in infants with cystinosis who have acute gastroenteritis.[136] Nephronophthisis and apparent mineralocorticoid excess are also associated with low urine osmolality that is unresponsive to vasopressin.[137]

Polyuria in Hereditary Hypokalemic Salt-Losing Tubulopathies

Patients with polyhydramnios, hypercalciuria, and hypo- or isosthenuria have been found to bear *KCNJ1* (ROMK) and *SLC12A1* (NKCC2) mutations.[134,181] Patients with polyhydramnios, profound polyuria, hyponatremia, hypochloremia, metabolic alkalosis, and sensorineural deafness were found to bear *BSND* mutations.[182–185] These studies demonstrate the critical importance of the proteins ROMK, NKCC2, and Barttin to transfer NaCl in the medullary interstitium and, together with urea, to thereby generate a hypertonic milieu (Fig. 71.14).

Acquired Nephrogenic Diabetes Insipidus

Acquired NDI is much more common than congenital NDI, but it is rarely as severe. The ability to produce hypertonic urine is usually preserved even though there is inadequate

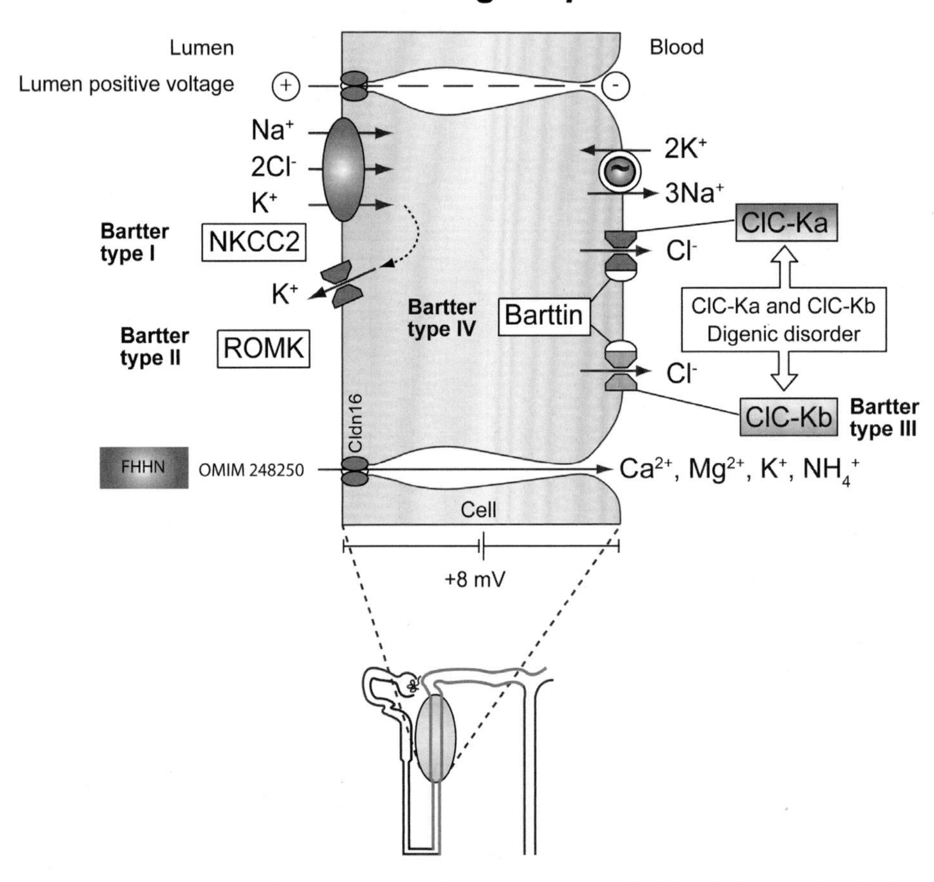

FIGURE 71.14 A schematic representation of transepithelial salt resorption in a cell of the thick ascending limb (TAL) of the loop of Henle. Of the filtered sodium chloride, 30% is reabsorbed in the TAL and most of the energy for concentration and dilution of the urine derives from active NaCl transport in the TAL. Filtered NaCl is reabsorbed through NKCC2, which uses the sodium gradient across the membrane to transport chloride and potassium into the cell. The potassium ions are recycled (100%) through the apical membrane by the potassium channel ROMK. Sodium leaves the cell actively through the basolateral Na-K-ATPase. Chloride diffuses passively through two basolateral channels, ClC-Ka and ClC-Kb. Both of these chloride channels must bind to the b subunit of barttin to be transported to the cell surface. Four types of Bartter syndrome (types I, II, III, and IV) are attributable to recessive mutations in the genes that encode the NKCC2 cotransporter, the potassium channel (ROMK), one of the chloride channels (ClC-Kb), and barttin, respectively. A fifth type of Bartter syndrome has also been shown to be a digenic disorder that is attributable to loss-of-function mutations in the genes that encode the chloride channels ClC-Ka and ClC-Kb.[223] As a result of these different molecular alterations, sodium chloride is lost into the urine, positive lumen voltage is abolished, and calcium (Ca^{2+}), magnesium (Mg^{2+}), potassium (K^{+}), and ammonium (NH_4^{+}) cannot be reabsorbed in the paracellular space. In the absence of mutations, the recycling of potassium maintains a lumen-positive gradient (+8 mV). Claudin 16 (CLDN16) is necessary for the paracellular transport of calcium and magnesium. (Modified from Bichet DG, Fujiwara TM: Reabsorption of sodium chloride—lessons from the chloride channels. *N Engl J Med.* 2004 350:1281–1283.[235])

concentrating ability of the nephron. Polyuria and polydipsia are therefore moderate (3 to 4 L per day).

Among the more common causes of acquired NDI, lithium administration has become the most frequent cause; 54% of 1105 unselected patients on chronic lithium therapy developed NDI.[186] Of the patients, 19% had polyuria, as defined by a 24-hour urine output exceeding 3 L. The dysregulation of aquaporin-2 expression is the result of cytotoxic accumulation of lithium, which enters via the epithelial sodium channel (ENaC) on the apical membrane and leads to the inhibition of signaling pathways that involve glycogen synthase kinase type 3 beta.[187] The concentration of lithium in urine of patients on well-controlled lithium therapy (i.e., 10 to 40 mOsmol per liter) is sufficient to exert this effect. For patients on long-term lithium therapy, amiloride has been proposed to prevent the uptake of lithium in the collecting ducts, thus preventing the inhibitory effect of intracellular lithium on water transport.[188]

Primary Polydipsia

Primary polydipsia is a state of hypotonic polyuria secondary to excessive fluid intake. Primary polydipsia was extensively studied by Barlow and de Wardener in 1959[189]; however, the understanding of the pathophysiology of this disease has made little progress. Barlow and de Wardener[189] described seven women and two men who were compulsive water drinkers; their ages ranged from 48 to 59 years except for one patient who was 24. Eight of these patients had histories of previous psychological disorders, which ranged from delusions, depression, and agitation, to frank hysterical behavior. The other patient appeared normal. The consumption of water fluctuated irregularly from hour to hour or from day to day; in some patients, there were remissions and relapses lasting several months or longer. In eight of the patients, the mean plasma osmolality was significantly lower than normal. Vasopressin tannate in oil made most of these patients feel ill; in one, it caused overhydration. In four patients, the fluid intake returned to normal after electroconvulsive therapy or a period of continuous narcosis; the improvement in three was transient, but in the fourth it lasted 2 years. Polyuric female subjects might be heterozygous for de novo or previously unrecognized *AVPR2* mutations or autosomal dominant *AQP2* mutations[169] and may be classified as compulsive water drinkers.[190] Therefore, the diagnosis of compulsive water drinking must be made with care and may represent our ignorance of yet undescribed pathophysiologic mechanisms. Robertson[190] has described under the term *dipsogenic diabetes insipidus* a selective defect in the osmoregulation of thirst. Three studied patients had, under basal conditions of ad libitum water intake, thirst, polydipsia, polyuria, and high-normal plasma osmolality. They had a normal secretion of AVP, but their osmotic threshold for thirst was abnormally low. Such cases of dipsogenic diabetes insipidus might represent up to 10% of all patients with diabetes insipidus.[190] Primary polydipsic rats had low serum sodium, suppressed AVP, low urine osmolality, and decreased AQP2 protein abundance in their inner medulla.[191]

DIABETES INSIPIDUS AND PREGNANCY

Pregnancy in a Patient Known to Have Diabetes Insipidus

An isolated deficiency of vasopressin without a concomitant loss of hormones in the anterior pituitary does not result in altered fertility and, with the exception of polyuria and polydipsia, gestation, delivery, and lactation are uncomplicated.[192] Patients may require increasing dosages of dDAVP. The increased thirst may be due to a resetting of the thirst osmostat.[193]

Increased polyuria also occurs during pregnancy in patients with partial NDI.[194] These patients may be obligatory carriers of the NDI gene[195] or may be homozygotes, compound heterozygotes, or may have dominant AQP2 mutations.

Syndromes of Diabetes Insipidus that Begin During Gestation and Remit After Delivery

Barron et al.[196] described three pregnant women in whom transient diabetes insipidus developed late in gestation and subsequently remitted postpartum. In one of these patients, dilute urine was present despite high plasma concentrations of AVP. Hyposthenuria in all three patients was resistant to administered aqueous vasopressin. Because excessive vasopressinase activity was not excluded as a cause of this disorder, Barron et al. labeled the disease vasopressin resistant rather than NDI.

A well-documented case of enhanced activity of vasopressinase has been described in a woman in the third trimester of a previously uncomplicated pregnancy.[197] She had massive polyuria and markedly elevated plasma vasopressinase activity. The polyuria did not respond to large intravenous doses of AVP but responded promptly to dDAVP, a vasopressinase-resistant analog of AVP. The polyuria disappeared with the disappearance of the vasopressinase. It is suggested that pregnancy may be associated with several different forms of diabetes insipidus, including central, nephrogenic, and vasopressinase mediated.[194,198–200]

DIFFERENTIAL DIAGNOSIS OF POLYURIC STATES

Plasma sodium and osmolality are maintained within normal limits (136 to 143 mmol per liter for plasma sodium, 275 to 290 mmol per kilogram for plasma osmolality) by a thirst-ADH-renal axis. Thirst and ADH, both stimulated by increased osmolality, have been termed a double-negative feedback system.[201] Therefore, even when the ADH limb of this double-negative regulatory feedback system is lost, the thirst mechanism still preserves the plasma sodium and osmolality within the normal range but at the expense of pronounced polydipsia and polyuria. Consequently, the plasma sodium concentration or osmolality of an untreated patient with diabetes insipidus may be slightly higher than the mean normal value, but because the values usually remain within the normal range, these small increases have no diagnostic significance.

Theoretically, it should be relatively easy to differentiate between central diabetes insipidus, NDI, and primary polydipsia. A comparison of the osmolality of urine obtained during dehydration from patients with central diabetes insipidus or NDI with that of urine obtained after the administration of AVP should reveal a rapid increase in osmolality only in patients with central diabetes insipidus. Urine osmolality should increase normally in response to moderate dehydration in primary polydipsia patients.

However, these distinctions may not be as clear as one might expect because of several factors.[202] First, chronic polyuria of any etiology interferes with the maintenance of the medullary concentration gradient, and this washout effect diminishes the maximum concentrating ability of the kidney. The extent of the blunting varies in direct proportion to the severity of the polyuria and is independent of its cause. Hence, for any given level of basal urine output, the maximum urine osmolality achieved in the presence of saturating concentrations of AVP is depressed to the same extent in patients with primary polydipsia, central diabetes insipidus, and NDI (Fig. 71.15). Second, most patients with central diabetes insipidus maintain a small, but detectable, capacity to secrete AVP during severe dehydration, and urine osmolality may then rise above plasma osmolality. Third, many patients with acquired NDI have an incomplete deficit in AVP action, and concentrated urine could again be obtained during dehydration testing. Finally, all polyuric states (whether central, nephrogenic, or psychogenic) can

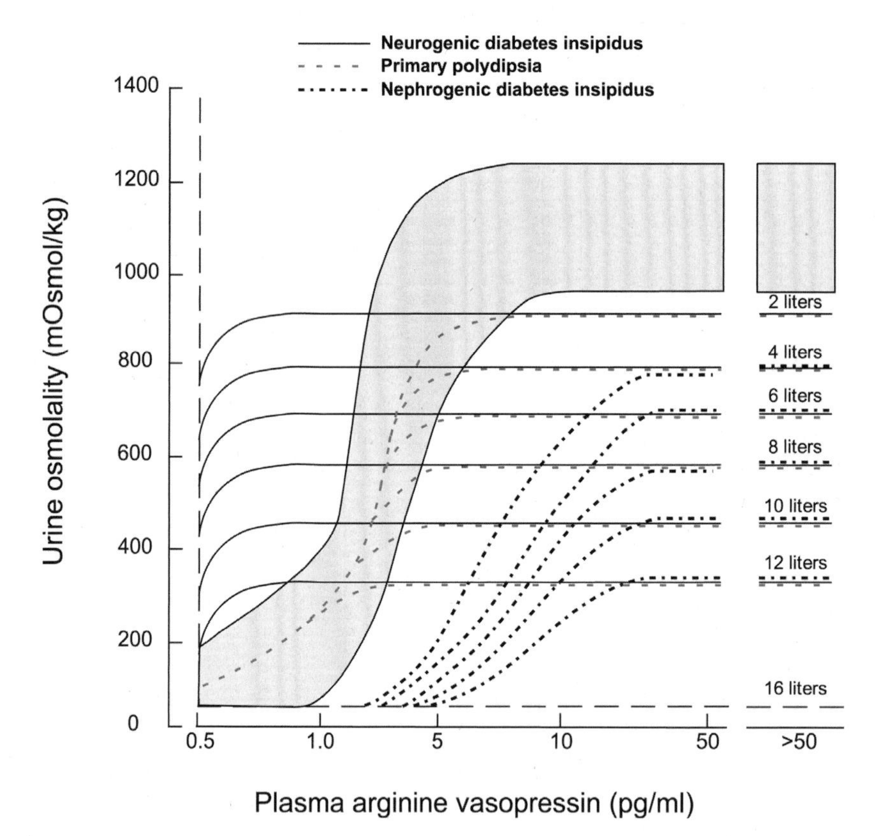

FIGURE 71.15 The relationship between urine osmolality and plasma vasopressin in patients with polyuria of diverse etiology and severity. Note that for each of the three categories of polyuria (neurogenic diabetes insipidus, nephrogenic diabetes insipidus, and primary polydipsia), the relationship is described by a family of sigmoid curves that differ in height. These differences in height reflect differences in maximum concentrating capacity due to "washout" of the medullary concentration gradient. They are proportional to the severity of the underlying polyuria (indicated in liters per day at the right end of each plateau) and are largely independent of the etiology. Therefore, the three categories of diabetes insipidus differ principally in the submaximal or ascending portion of the dose-response curve. In patients with partial neurogenic diabetes insipidus, this part of the curve lies to the left of normal, reflecting increased sensitivity to the antidiuretic effects of very low concentrations of plasma AVP. In contrast, in patients with partial nephrogenic diabetes insipidus, this part of the curve lies to the right of normal, reflecting decreased sensitivity to the antidiuretic effects of normal concentrations of plasma arginine vasopressin. In primary polydipsia, this relationship is relatively normal. (From Robertson GL. Diagnosis of diabetes insipidus. In: Czernichow P, Robinson AG, eds. *Frontiers of Hormone Research,* Vol. 13. Basel, Germany: S. Karger; 1985: 176, with permission.)

TABLE 71.2 **Urinary Responses to Fluid Deprivation and Exogenous Vasopressin in Recognition of Partial Defects in Antidiuretic Hormone Secretion**[34]

	No. of Cases	Maximum U_{osm} with Dehydration (mmol/kg)	U_{osm} after Vasopressin (mmol/kg)	% Change (U_{osm})	U_{osm} Increase after Vasopressin (%)
Normal subjects	9	1068 ± 69	979 ± 79	9 ± 3	< 9
Complete central diabetes insipidus	18	168 ± 13	445 ± 52	183 ± 41	> 50
Partial central diabetes insipidus	11	438 ± 34	549 ± 28	28 ± 5	> 9 < 50
Nephrogenic diabetes insipidus	2	123.5	174.5	42	< 50
Compulsive water drinking	7	738 ± 53	780 ± 73	5.0 ± 2.2	< 9

induce large dilations of the urinary tract and bladder.[203–205] As a consequence, the urinary bladder of these patients may contain an increased residual capacity, and changes in urine osmolalities induced by diagnostic maneuvers might be difficult to demonstrate.

The Indirect Test

The measurements of urine osmolality after dehydration followed by vasopressin administration are usually referred to as indirect testing because vasopressin secretion is indirectly assessed through changes in urine osmolalities.

The patient is maintained on a complete fluid restriction regimen until urine osmolality reaches a plateau, as indicated by an hourly increase of less than 30 mmol per kilogram for at least 3 successive hours. After the plasma osmolality is measured, 5 U of aqueous vasopressin or 4 μg of dDAVP is administered subcutaneously. Urine osmolality is measured 30 and 60 minutes later. The last urine osmolality value obtained before the vasopressin injection and the highest value obtained after the injection are compared. The patients are then separated into five categories according to previously published criteria (Table 71.2).[34]

The Direct Test

The two approaches of Zerbe and Robertson[33] are used. First, during the dehydration test, plasma is collected and assayed for vasopressin. The results are plotted on a nomogram depicting the normal relationship between plasma sodium or osmolality and plasma AVP in normal subjects (Fig. 71.7). If the relationship between plasma vasopressin and osmolality falls below the normal range, the disorder is diagnosed as central diabetes insipidus.

Second, partial NDI and primary polydipsia can be differentiated by analyzing the relationship between plasma AVP and urine osmolality at the end of the dehydration period (Figs. 71.7 and 71.15). However, a definitive differentiation between these two disorders might be impossible because a normal or even supranormal AVP response to increased plasma osmolality occurs in polydipsic patients. None of the patients with psychogenic or other forms of severe polydipsia studied by Robertson[202] have ever shown any evidence of pituitary suppression. Zerbe and Robertson[33] found that in the differential diagnosis of polyuria, all seven of the cases of severe neurogenic diabetes insipidus diagnosed by the standard indirect test were confirmed when diagnosed by the plasma vasopressin assay. However, two of six patients diagnosed by the indirect test as having partial neurogenic diabetes insipidus had normal vasopressin secretion as measured by the direct assay; one was found to have primary polydipsia and the other, NDI. Moreover, 3 of 10 patients diagnosed as having primary polydipsia by the indirect test had clear evidence of partial vasopressin deficiency by the direct assay.[33] These patients were thus wrongly diagnosed as primary polydipsic! A *combined* direct and indirect testing of the AVP function is described in Table 71.3. Urinary vasopressin measurements and copeptin plasma levels might also be useful.[206,207]

The Therapeutic Trial

In selected patients with an uncertain diagnosis, a closely monitored therapeutic trial of desmopressin (10 μg intranasally twice a day) may be used to distinguish partial NDI from partial neurogenic diabetes insipidus and primary polydipsia. If desmopressin at this dosage causes a significant antidiuretic

TABLE 71.3 **Direct and Indirect Tests of Arginine Vasopressin Function in Patients with Polyuria[236]**

Measurements of AVP cannot be used in isolation but must be interpreted in light of four other factors:
Clinical history
Concurrent measurements of plasma osmolality, urine osmolality, and maximal urinary response to exogenous vasopressin in reference to the basal urine flow

AVP, arginine vasopressin.

effect, NDI is effectively excluded. If polydipsia as well as polyuria is abolished and plasma sodium does not fall below the normal range, the patient probably has central diabetes insipidus. Conversely, if desmopressin causes a reduction in urine output without a reduction in water intake and hyponatremia appears, the patient probably has primary polydipsia. Because fatal water intoxication is a remote possibility, the desmopressin trial should be carried out with closed monitoring.

Recommendations

Table 71.4 lists recommendations for obtaining a differential diagnosis of diabetes insipidus.[208]

RADIOIMMUNOASSAY OF AVP AND OTHER LABORATORY DETERMINATIONS

Radioimmunoassay of Arginine Vasopressin

Three developments were basic to the elaboration of a clinically useful radioimmunoassay for plasma AVP[209,210]: (1) the extraction of AVP from plasma with petrol-ether and acetone and the subsequent elimination of nonspecific immunoreactivity, (2) the use of highly specific and sensitive rabbit antiserum, and (3) the use of a tracer (^{125}I-AVP) with high specific activity. More than 25 years later, the same extraction procedures are widely used,[211–214] and commercial tracers (^{125}I-AVP) and antibodies are available. AVP can also be extracted from plasma by using Sep-Pak C18 cartridges.[215–217]

Blood samples collected in chilled 7-mL lavender-stoppered tubes containing ethylenediaminetetraacetic acid (EDTA) are centrifuged at 4°C, 1000 g (3000 rpm in a usual lab centrifuge), for 20 minutes. This 20-minute centrifugation is mandatory for obtaining platelet-poor plasma samples because a large fraction of the circulating vasopressin is associated with the platelets in humans.[213,218] The tubes may be kept for 2 hours on slushed ice prior to centrifugation. Plasma is then separated, frozen at −20°C, and extracted within 6 weeks of sampling. Details for sample preparation (Table 71.5) and the assay procedure (Table 71.6) can be found in writings by Bichet et al.[213,214] An AVP radioimmunoassay should be validated by demonstrating (1) a good

TABLE 71.4 **Differential Diagnosis of Diabetes Insipidus[208]**

1.	Measure plasma osmolality and/or sodium concentration under conditions of ad libitum fluid intake. If they are greater than 295 mmol per kilogram and 143 mmol per liter, the diagnosis of primary polydipsia is excluded, and the workup should proceed directly to step 5 and/or 6 to distinguish between neurogenic and nephrogenic diabetes insipidus. Otherwise,
2.	Perform a dehydration test. If urinary concentration does not occur before plasma osmolality and/or sodium reaches 295 mmol per kilogram or 143 mmol per liter, the diagnosis of primary polydipsia is again excluded, and the workup should proceed to step 5 and/or 6. Otherwise,
3.	Determine the ratio of urine to plasma osmolality at the end of the dehydration test. If it is < 1.5, the diagnosis of primary polydipsia is again excluded, and the workup should proceed to step 5 and/or 6. Otherwise,
4.	Perform a hypertonic saline infusion with measurements of plasma vasopressin and osmolality at intervals during the procedure. If the relationship between these two variables is subnormal, the diagnosis of diabetes insipidus is established. Otherwise,
5.	Perform a vasopressin infusion test. If urine osmolality rises by more than 150 mOsmol per kilogram greater than the value obtained at the end of the dehydration test, nephrogenic diabetes insipidus is excluded. Alternately,
6.	Measure urine osmolality and plasma vasopressin at the end of the dehydration test. If the relationship is normal, the diagnosis of nephrogenic diabetes insipidus is excluded.

TABLE 71.5 **Arginine Vasopressin Measurements: Sample Preparation**

4°C—blood in EDTA tubes
Centrifugation 1000 g × 20 minutes
Plasma frozen −20°C
Extraction: 2 mL acetone + 1 mL plasma 1000 g × 30 minutes 4°C Supernatant + 5 mL of petrol-ether 1000 g × 20 minutes 4°C Freeze −80°C Throw nonfrozen upper phase Evaporate lower phase to dryness Store desiccated samples at −20°C

AVP, arginine vasopressin; EDTA, ethylenediaminetetraacetic acid.

correlation between plasma sodium or osmolality and plasma AVP during dehydration and infusion of hypertonic saline solution (Fig. 71.15) and (2) the inability to obtain detectable values of AVP in patients with severe central diabetes insipidus. Plasma AVP immunoreactivity may be elevated in patients with diabetes insipidus following hypothalamic surgery.[219]

In pregnant patients, the blood contains high concentrations of cystine aminopeptidase, which can (in vitro) inactivate enormous quantities (ng × mL^{-1} × min^{-1}) of AVP. However, phenanthroline effectively inhibits these cystine aminopeptidases (Table 71.7).

TABLE 71.6 **Arginine Vasopressin Measurements: Assay Procedure**

Day 1: Assay Setup
400 μL/tube (200 μL sample or standard + 200 μL of antiserum or buffer) Incubation 80 hours, 4°C
Day 4: ^{125}I-AVP 100 μL/tube
1000 cpm/tube Incubation 72 hours, 4°C
Day 7: Separation dextran + Charcoal

AVP, arginine vasopressin.

TABLE 71.7 **Measurements of Arginine Vasopressin Levels in Pregnant Patients[212]**

1,10-Phenanthrolene monohydrate (Sigma)
60 mg/mL—solubilized with several drops of glacial acetic acid
0.1 mL/10 mL of blood

AVP, arginine vasopressin.

Aquaporin-2 Measurements

Urinary AQP2 excretion could be measured by radioimmunoassay[220] or by quantitative Western analysis[221] and could provide an additional indication of the responsiveness of the collecting duct to AVP.[221,222]

Plasma Sodium and Plasma and Urine Osmolality Measurements

Measurements of plasma sodium and plasma and urine osmolality should be immediately available at various intervals during dehydration procedures. Plasma sodium is easily measured by flame photometry or with a sodium-specific electrode.[223] Plasma and urine osmolalities are also reliably measured by freezing point depression instruments with a coefficient of variation at 290 mmol per kilogram of less than 1%.

In our clinical research unit, plasma sodium and plasma and urine osmolalities are measured at the beginning of each dehydration procedure and at regular intervals (usually hourly) thereafter, depending on the severity of the polyuric syndrome explored.

In one case, an 8-year-old patient (31 kg body weight) with a clinical diagnosis of congenital NDI (later found to bear the de novo AVPR2 mutant 274insG)[224] continued to excrete large volumes of urine (300 mL per hour) during a short 4-hour dehydration test. During this time, the patient had severe thirst, his plasma sodium was 155 mEq per liter, his plasma osmolality was 310 mmol per kilogram, and his urine osmolality was 85 mmol per kilogram. The patient received 1 μg of desmopressin intravenously and was allowed to drink water. Repeated urine osmolality measurements demonstrated a complete urinary resistance to desmopressin.

It would have been dangerous and unnecessary to prolong the dehydration further in this young patient. Therefore, the usual prescription of overnight dehydration should not be used in patients, especially children, with severe polyuria and polydipsia (more than 4 L per day). Great care should be taken to avoid any severe hypertonic state arbitrarily defined as a plasma sodium greater than 155 mEq per liter.

At variance with published data,[33,213] we have found that plasma and serum osmolalities are equivalent (i.e., similar values are obtained). Blood taken in heparinized tubes is easier to handle because the plasma can be more readily removed after centrifugation. The tube used (green-stoppered tube) contains a minuscule concentration of lithium and sodium, which does not interfere with plasma sodium or osmolality measurements. Frozen plasma or urine samples can be kept for a further analysis of their osmolalities because the results obtained are similar to those obtained immediately after blood sampling, except in patients with severe renal failure. In the latter patients, plasma osmolality measurements are increased after freezing and thawing, but the plasma sodium values remain unchanged.

Plasma osmolality measurements can be used to demonstrate the absence of unusual osmotically active substances (e.g., glucose and urea in high concentrations, mannitol, and ethanol).[225] With this information, plasma or serum sodium measurements are sufficient to assess the degree of dehydration and its relationship to plasma AVP. Nomograms describing the normal plasma sodium–plasma AVP relationship (Fig. 71.4) are equally as valuable as classical nomograms describing the relationship between plasma osmolality and effective osmolality (i.e., plasma osmolality minus the contribution of "ineffective" solutes: glucose and urea).

Magnetic Resonance Imaging in Patients with Diabetes Insipidus

Magnetic resonance imaging (MRI) permits the visualization of the anterior and posterior pituitary glands and the pituitary stalk. The pituitary stalk is permeated by numerous capillary loops of the hypophyseal-portal blood system. This vascular structure also provides the principal blood supply to the anterior pituitary lobe, because there is no direct arterial supply to this organ. In contrast, the posterior pituitary lobe has a direct vascular supply. Therefore, the posterior lobe can be more rapidly visualized in a dynamic mode after the administration of gadolinium (gadopentetate dimeglumine) as a contrast material during MRI. The posterior pituitary lobe is easily distinguished by a round, high-intensity signal (the posterior pituitary "bright spot") in the posterior part of the sella turcica on T1-weighted images. Loss of the pituitary hyperintense spot or bright spot on a T1-weighted MRI image reflects a loss of functional integrity of the neurohypophysis and is a nonspecific indicator of neurohypophyseal diabetes insipidus regardless of the underlying cause.[102,226] It is now reasoned that the bright spot represents normal AVP storage in the posterior lobe of the pituitary, that the intensity is correlated with the amount of AVP, and that, after 60 years of age, the signal is often less intense with irregularities in the normally smooth convex edge.[227,228] An MRI is reported to be the best technique with which to evaluate the pituitary stalk and infundibulum in patients with idiopathic polyuria. A thickening or enlargement of the pituitary stalk may suggest an infiltrative process destroying the neurohypophyseal tract.[229]

Treatment

In most patients with complete hypothalamic diabetes insipidus, the thirst mechanism remains intact. Thus, hypernatremia does not develop in these patients and they suffer only from the inconvenience associated with marked polyuria and polydipsia. If hypodipsia develops or access to water is limited, then severe hypernatremia can supervene. The treatment of choice for patients with severe hypothalamic diabetes insipidus is dDAVP, a synthetic, long-acting vasopressin analog with minimal vasopressor activity but a large antidiuretic potency. The usual intranasal daily dose is between 5 and 20 μg. To avoid the potential complication of dilutional hyponatremia, which is exceptional in these patients as a result of an intact thirst mechanism, dDAVP can be withdrawn at regular intervals to allow the patients to become polyuric. Aqueous vasopressin (Pitressin) or dDAVP (4.0 mg per 1-mL ampule) can be used intravenously in acute situations such as after hypophysectomy or for the treatment of diabetes insipidus in the brain-dead organ donor. Pitressin tannate in oil and nonhormonal antidiuretic drugs are somewhat obsolete and are now rarely used. For example, chlorpropamide (250 to 500 mg daily) appears to potentiate the antidiuretic action of circulating AVP, but the troublesome side effects of hypoglycemia and hyponatremia do occur.

In the treatment of congenital NDI, an abundant unrestricted water intake should always be provided, and affected patients should be carefully followed during their first years of life. Water should be offered every 2 hours day and night, and temperature, appetite, and growth should be monitored. The parents of these children easily accept setting their alarm clock every 2 hours during the night. Hospital admission may be necessary to allow for continuous gastric feeding. A low-osmolar and low-sodium diet, hydrochlorothiazide (1 to 2 mg per kilogram per day) alone or with amiloride, and indomethacin (0.75 to 1.5 mg per kilogram) substantially reduce water excretion and are helpful in the treatment of children. Many adult patients receive no treatment.

ACKNOWLEDGMENTS

I thank Ellen Buschman and Danielle Binette for editorial and computer graphics expertise.

REFERENCES

1. Bourque CW. Central mechanisms of osmosensation and systemic osmoregulation. *Nat Rev Neurosci.* 2008;9:519–531.

2. Lechner SG, Markworth S, Poole K, et al. The molecular and cellular identity of peripheral osmoreceptors. *Neuron.* 2011;69:332–344.

3. Burbach JP, Luckman SM, Murphy D, Gainer H. Gene regulation in the magnocellular hypothalamo-neurohypophyseal system. *Physiol Rev.* 2001;81: 1197–1267.

4. Rao VV, Loffler C, Battey J, Hansmann I. The human gene for oxytocin-neurophysin I (OXT) is physically mapped to chromosome 20p13 by in situ hybridization. *Cell Genet.* 1992;61:271–273.

5. Sausville E, Carney D, Battey J. The human vasopressin gene is linked to the oxytocin gene and is selectively expressed in a cultured lung cancer cell line. *J Biol Chem.* 1985;260:10236–10241.

6. Venkatesh B, Si-Hoe SL, Murphy D, Brenner S. Transgenic rats reveal functional conservation of regulatory controls between the Fugu isotocin and rat oxytocin genes. *Proc Natl Acad Sci USA.* 1997;94:12462–12466.

7. Chen L, Rose JP, Breslow E, et al. Crystal structure of a bovine neurophysin II dipeptide complex at 2.8 Angström determined from the single-wave length anomalous scattering signal of an incorporated iodine atom. *Proc Natl Acad Sci USA.* 1991;88:4240–4244.

8. Vandesande F, Dierickx K. Identification of the vasopressin producing and of the oxytocin producing neurons in the hypothalamic magnocellular neurosecretroy system of the rat. *Cell Tissue Res.* 1975;164:153–162.

9. Swaab D, Pool WC, Novelty F. Immunofluorescence of vasopressin and oxytocin in the rat hypothalamo-neurohypophyseal system. *J Neural Transm.* 1975;36:195–215.

10. Sofroniew M. *Morphology of Vasopressin and Oxytocin Neurons and Their Central and Vascular Projections.* New York, NY: Elsevier; 1883.

11. Yanovski JA, Friedman TC, Nieman LK, et al. Inferior petrosal sinus AVP in patients with Cushing's syndrome. *Clin Endocrinol (Oxf).* 1997;47:199–206.

12. Kalogeras KT, Nieman LN, Friedman TC, et al. Inferior petrosal sinus sampling in healthy human subjects reveals a unilateral corticotropin-releasing hormone-induced arginine vasopressin release associated with ipsilateral adrenocorticotropin secretion. *J Clin Invest.* 1996;97:2045–2050.

13. Robertson G, Berl T, eds. *Pathophysiology of Water Metabolism.* Philadelphia, PA: WB Saunders Co.; 1996.

14. Wilson Y, Nag N, Davern P, et al. Visualization of functionally activated circuitry in the brain. *Proc Natl Acad Sci USA.* 2002;99:3252–3257.

15. Prager-Khoutorsky M, Bourque CW. Osmosensation in vasopressin neurons: changing actin density to optimize function. *Trends Neurosci.* 2010;33:76–83.

16. Zerbe RL, Henry DP, Robertson GL. Vasopressin response to orthostatic hypotension. Etiologic and clinical implications. *Am J Med.* 1983;74:265–271.

17. Robertson GL, Athar S. The interaction of blood osmolality and blood volume in regulating plasma vasopressin in man. *J Clin Endocrinol Metab.* 1976;42:613–620.

18. Good MC, Zalatan JG, Lim WA. Scaffold proteins: hubs for controlling the flow of cellular information. *Science.* 2011;332:680–686.

19. Zhang Z, Bourque CW. Amplification of transducer gain by angiotensin II-mediated enhancement of cortical actin density in osmosensory neurons. *J Neurosci.* 2008;28:9536–9544.

20. De Mota N, Reaux-Le Goazigo A, El Messari S, et al. Apelin, a potent diuretic neuropeptide counteracting vasopressin actions through inhibition of vasopressin neuron activity and vasopressin release. *Proc Natl Acad Sci USA.* 2004;101:10464–10469.

21. Sharif Naeini R, Witty MF, Seguela P, Bourque CW. An N-terminal variant of Trpv1 channel is required for osmosensory transduction. *Nat Neurosci.* 2006;9:93–98.

22. Ciura S, Bourque CW. Transient receptor potential vanilloid 1 is required for intrinsic osmoreception in organum vasculosum lamina terminalis neurons and for normal thirst responses to systemic hyperosmolality. *J Neurosci.* 2006;26:9069–9075.

23. Taylor AC, McCarthy JJ, Stocker SD. Mice lacking the transient receptor vanilloid potential 1 channel display normal thirst responses and central Fos activation to hypernatremia. *Am J Physiol Regul Integr Comp Physiol.* 2008;294:R1285–1293.

24. McHugh J, Keller NR, Appalsamy M, et al. Portal osmopressor mechanism linked to transient receptor potential vanilloid 4 and blood pressure control. *Hypertension.* 2010;55:1438–1443.

25. Tank J, Schroeder C, Stoffels M, et al. Pressor effect of water drinking in tetraplegic patients may be a spinal reflex. *Hypertension.* 2003;41:1234–1239.

26. Boschmann M, Steiniger J, Franke G, et al. Water drinking induces thermogenesis through osmosensitive mechanisms. *J Clin Endocrinol Metab.* 2007;92:3334–3337.

27. Shannon JR, Diedrich A, Biaggioni I, et al. Water drinking as a treatment for orthostatic syndromes. *Am J Med.* 2002;112:355–360.

28. Schroeder C, Bush VE, Norcliffe LJ, et al. Water drinking acutely improves orthostatic tolerance in healthy subjects. *Circulation.* 2002;106:2806–2811.

29. Jordan J, Shannon JR, Black BK, et al. The pressor response to water drinking in humans: a sympathetic reflex? *Circulation.* 2000;101:504–509.

30. Claydon VE, Schroeder C, Norcliffe LJ, Jordan J, Hainsworth R. Water drinking improves orthostatic tolerance in patients with posturally related syncope. *Clin Sci (Lond).* 2006;110:343–352.

31. Stookey JD, Constant F, Popkin BM, Gardner CD. Drinking water is associated with weight loss in overweight dieting women independent of diet and activity. *Obesity (Silver Spring).* 2008;16:2481–2488.

32. Coste B, Mathur J, Schmidt M, et al. Piezo1 and Piezo2 are essential components of distinct mechanically activated cation channels. *Science.* 2010; 330:55–60.

33. Zerbe RL, Robertson GL. A comparison of plasma vasopressin measurements with a standard indirect test in the differential diagnosis of polyuria. *N Engl J Med.* 1981;305:1539–1546.

34. Miller M, Dalakos T, Moses AM, Fellerman H, Streeten DH. Recognition of partial defects in antidiuretic hormone secretion. *Ann Intern Med.* 1970;73: 721–729.

35. Bichet DG, Kluge R, Howard RL, Schrier RW. Hyponatremic states. In: Seldin DW, Giebisch G, eds. *The Kidney: Physiology and Pathophysiology.* New York, NY: Raven Press; 1992: 1727–1751.

36. Baylis PH, Gaskill MB, Robertson GL. Vasopressin secretion in primary polydipsia and cranial diabetes insipidus. *Q J Med.* 1981;50:345–358.

37. Rolls B, Rolls E. *Thirst (Problems in the Behavioural Sciences).* Cambridge, UK: Cambridge University Press; 1982:194.

38. Nimura F, Labosky P, Kakuchi J, et al. Gene targeting in mice reveals a requirement for angiotensin in the development and maintenance of kidney morphology and growth factor regulation. *J Clin Invest.* 1995;96:2947–2954.

39. Sugaya T, Nishimatsu S, Tanimoto K, et al. Angiotensin II type 1a receptor-deficient mice with hypotension and hyperreninemia. *J Biol Chem.* 1995;270:18719–18722.

40. Ito M, Oliverio MI, Mannon PJ, et al. Regulation of blood pressure by the type 1A angiotensin II receptor gene. *Proc Natl Acad Sci USA.* 1995;92: 3521–3525.

41. Hein L, Barsh G, Pratt R, Dzau V, Kobilka B. Behavioural and cardiovascular effects of disrupting the angiotensin II type-2 receptor gene in mice. *Nature.* 1995;377:744–747.

42. Morris M, Li P, Callahan MF, et al. Neuroendocrine effects of dehydration in mice lacking the angiotensin AT1a receptor. *Hypertension.* 1999;33:482–486.

43. Samson WK. Atrial natriuretic factor inhibits dehydration and hemorrhage-induced vasopressin release. *Neuroendocrinology.* 1985;40:277–279.

44. Goetz KL, Wang BC, Geer PG, Sundet WD, Needleman P. Effects of atriopeptin infusion versus effects of left atrial stretch in awake dogs. *Am J Physiol.* 1986;250:R221–226.

45. Ogawa K, Arnolda LF, Woodcock EA, Hiwatari M, Johnston CI. Lack of effect of atrial natriuretic peptide on vasopressin release. *Clin Sci (Lond).* 1987;72:525–530.

46. Abelson JL, Le Melledo J, Bichet DG. Dose response of arginine vasopressin to the CCK-B agonist pentagastrin. *Neuropsychopharmacology.* 2001;24:161–169.

47. Wang H, Morris JF. Constitutive nitric oxide synthase in hypothalami of normal and hereditary diabetes insipidus rats and mice: role of nitric oxide in osmotic regulation and its mechanism. *Endocrinology.* 1996;137:1745–1751.

48. Kadowaki K, Kishimoto J, Leng G, Emson PC. Up-regulation of nitric oxide synthase (NOS) gene expression together with NOS activity in the rat hypothalamo-hypophyseal system after chronic salt loading: evidence of a neuromodulatory role of nitric oxide in arginine vasopressin and oxytocin secretion. *Endocrinology.* 1994;134:1011–1017.

49. Yasin S, Costa A, Trainer P, et al. Nitric oxide modulates the release of vasopressin from rat hypothalamic explants. *Endocrinology.* 1993;133:1466–1469.

50. Ota M, Crofton JT, Festavan GT, Share L. Evidence that nitric oxide can act centrally to stimulate vasopressin release. *Neuroendocrinology.* 1993;57:955–959.

51. Raff H. Glucocorticoid inhibition of neurohypophyseal vasopressin secretion. *Am J Physiol.* 1987;252:R635–644.

52. Rowe JW, Shelton RL, Helderman JH, Vestal RE, Robertson GL. Influence of the emetic reflex on vasopressin release in man. *Kidney Int.* 1979;16:729–735.

53. Donaldson ZR, Young LJ. Oxytocin, vasopressin, and the neurogenetics of sociality. *Science.* 2008;322:900–904.

54. Walum H, Westberg L, Henningsson S, et al. Genetic variation in the vasopressin receptor 1a gene (AVPR1A) associates with pair-bonding behavior in humans. *Proc Natl Acad Sci USA.* 2008;105:14153–14156.

55. Serradeil-Le Gal C, Wagnon J, Simiand J, et al. Characterization of (2S,4R)-1-[5-chloro-1-[(2,4-dimethoxyphenyl)sulfonyl]-3-(2-methoxy-phenyl)-2-oxo-2,3-dihydro-1H-indol-3-yl]-4-hydroxy-N,N-dimethyl-2-pyrrolidine carboxamide (SSR149415), a selective and orally active vasopressin V1b receptor antagonist. *J Pharmacol Exp Ther.* 2002;300:1122–1130.

56. Thibonnier M, Coles P, Thibonnier A, Shoham M. The basic and clinical pharmacology of nonpeptide vasopressin receptor antagonists. *Annu Rev Pharmacol Toxicol.* 2001;41:175–202.

57. Murata K, Mitsuoka K, Hirai T, et al. Structural determinants of water permeation through aquaporin-1. *Nature.* 2000;407:599–605.

58. Tajkhorshid E, Nollert P, Jensen MO, et al. Control of the selectivity of the aquaporin water channel family by global orientational tuning. *Science.* 2002;296:525–530.

59. Seibold A, Brabet P, Rosenthal W, Birnbaumer M. Structure and chromosomal localization of the human antidiuretic hormone receptor gene. *Am J Hum Genet.* 1992;51:1078–1083.

60. Birnbaumer M, Seibold A, Gilbert S, et al. Molecular cloning of the receptor for human antidiuretic hormone. *Nature.* 1992;357:333–335.

61. Rehmann H, Wittinghofer A, Bos JL. Capturing cyclic nucleotides in action: snapshots from crystallographic studies. *Nat Rev Mol Cell Biol.* 2007;8:63–73.

62. Nedvetsky PI, Tamma G, Beulshausen S, et al. Regulation of aquaporin-2 trafficking. *Handb Exp Pharmacol.* 2009;(190):133–157.

63. Boone M, Deen PM. Physiology and pathophysiology of the vasopressin-regulated renal water reabsorption. *Pflugers Arch.* 2008;456:1005–1024.

64. Nielsen S, Frokiaer J, Marples D, Kwon TH, Agre P, Knepper MA. Aquaporins in the kidney: from molecules to medicine. *Physiol Rev.* 2002;82: 205–244.

65. Smith CP. Mammalian urea transporters. *Exp Physiol.* 2009;94:180–185.

66. Yang B, Bankir L, Gillespie A, Epstein CJ, Verkman AS. Urea-selective concentrating defect in transgenic mice lacking urea transporter UT-B. *J Biol Chem.* 2002;277:10633–10637.

67. Bankir L, Fernandes S, Bardoux P, Bouby N, Bichet DG. Vasopressin-V2 receptor stimulation reduces sodium excretion in healthy humans. *J Am Soc Nephrol.* 2005;16:1920–1928.

68. Marion V, Schlicht D, Mockel A, et al. Bardet-Biedl syndrome highlights the major role of the primary cilium in efficient water reabsorption. *Kidney Int.* 2011;79:1013–1025.

69. Morishita T, Tsutsui M, Shimokawa H, et al. Nephrogenic diabetes insipidus in mice lacking all nitric oxide synthase isoforms. *Proc Natl Acad Sci USA.* 2005;102:10616–10621.

70. Fleming EF, Athirakul K, Oliverio MI, et al. Urinary concentrating function in mice lacking EP3 receptors for prostaglandin E2. *Am J Physiol.* 1998; 275:F955–961.

71. Breyer MD, Jacobson HR, Davis LS, Breyer RM. In situ hybridization and localization of mRNA for the rabbit prostaglandin EP3 receptor. *Kidney Int.* 1993;44:1372–1378.

72. Guan Y, Zhang Y, Breyer RM, et al. Prostaglandin E2 inhibits renal collecting duct Na^+ absorption by activating the EP1 receptor. *J Clin Invest.* 1998;102:194–201.

73. Jensen BL, Stubbe J, Hansen PB, Andreasen D, Skott O. Localization of prostaglandin E(2) EP2 and EP4 receptors in the rat kidney. *Am J Physiol Renal Physiol.* 2001;280:F1001–1009.

74. Sands JM, Naruse M, Baum M, et al. Apical extracellular calcium/polyvalent cation-sensing receptor regulates vasopressin-elicited water permeability in rat kidney inner medullary collecting duct. *J Clin Invest.* 1997;99:1399–1405.

75. Rieg T, Tang T, Murray F, et al. Adenylate cyclase 6 determines cAMP formation and aquaporin-2 phosphorylation and trafficking in inner medulla. *J Am Soc Nephrol.* 2010;21:2059–2068.

76. Okubo S, Niimura F, Matsusaka T, et al. Angiotensinogen gene null-mutant mice lack homeostatic regulation of glomerular filtration and tubular reabsorption. *Kidney Int.* 1998;53:617–625.

77. Yang B, Gillespie A, Carlson EJ, Epstein CJ, Verkman AS. Neonatal mortality in an aquaporin-2 knock-in mouse model of recessive nephrogenic diabetes insipidus. *J Biol Chem.* 2001;276:2775–2779.

78. Yun J, Schoneberg T, Liu J, Schulz A, et al. Generation and phenotype of mice harboring a nonsense mutation in the V2 vasopressin receptor gene. *J Clin Invest.* 2000;106:1361–1371.

79. Takahashi N, Chernavvsky DR, Gomez RA, et al. Uncompensated polyuria in a mouse model of Bartter's syndrome. *Proc Natl Acad Sci USA.* 2000;97: 5434–5439.

80. Ma T, Song Y, Yang B, et al. Nephrogenic diabetes insipidus in mice lacking aquaporin-3 water channels. *Proc Natl Acad Sci USA.* 2000;97:4386–4391.

81. Chou CL, Knepper MA, Hoek AN, et al. Reduced water permeability and altered ultrastructure in thin descending limb of Henle in aquaporin-1 null mice. *J Clin Invest.* 1999;103:491–496.

82. Matsumura Y, Uchida S, Kondo Y, et al. Overt nephrogenic diabetes insipidus in mice lacking the CLC-K1 chloride channel. *Nat Genet.* 1999;21:95–98.

83. Ma T, Yang B, Gillespie A, et al. Severely impaired urinary concentrating ability in transgenic mice lacking aquaporin-1 water channels. *J Biol Chem.* 1998;273:4296–4299.

84. Ma T, Yang B, Gillespie A, et al. Generation and phenotype of a transgenic knockout mouse lacking the mercurial-insensitive water channel aquaporin-4. *J Clin Invest.* 1997;100:957–962.

85. Rao S, Verkman AS. Analysis of organ physiology in transgenic mice. *Am J Physiol Cell Physiol.* 2000;279:C1–C18.

86. Preston GM, Smith BL, Zeidel ML, Moulds JJ, Agre P. Mutations in aquaporin-1 in phenotypically normal humans without functional CHIP water channels. *Science.* 1994;265:1585–1587.

87. Yang B, Zhao D, Qian L, Verkman AS. Mouse model of inducible nephrogenic diabetes insipidus produced by floxed aquaporin-2 gene deletion. *Am J Physiol Renal Physiol.* 2006;291:F465–472.

88. Mulders SM, Knoers NV, van Lieburg AF, et al. New mutations in the AQP2 gene in nephrogenic diabetes insipidus resulting in functional but misrouted water channels. *J Am Soc Nephrol.* 1997;8:242–248.

89. Lloyd DJ, Hall FW, Tarantino LM, Gekakis N. Diabetes insipidus in mice with a mutation in aquaporin-2. *PLoS Genet.* 2005;1:e20.

90. Li JH, Chou CL, Li B, et al. A selective EP4 PGE2 receptor agonist alleviates disease in a new mouse model of X-linked nephrogenic diabetes insipidus. *J Clin Invest.* 2009;119:3115–3126.

91. Valtin H, North WG, Edwards BR, Gellai M. Animal models of diabetes insipidus. *Front Horm Res.* 1885;13:105–126.

92. Schmale H, Richter D. Single base deletion in the vasopressin gene is the cause of diabetes insipidus in Brattleboro rats. *Nature.* 1984;308:705–709.

93. Schmale H, Bahnsen U, Fehr S, Nahke D, Richter D, eds. *Hereditary Diabetes Insipidus in Man and Rat.* Paris, France: John Libbey Eurotext; 1991: 57–62.

94. Richter D, ed. *Reflections on Central Diabetes Insipidus: Retrospective and Perspectives.* Paris: John Libbey Eurotext; 1993: 3–14.

95. Serradeil-Le Gal C, Lacour C, Valette G, et al. Characterization of SR 121463A, a highly potent and selective, orally active vasopressin V2 receptor antagonist. *J Clin Invest.* 1996;98:2729–2738.

96. Jean-Alphonse F, Perkovska S, Frantz MC, et al. Biased agonist pharmacochaperones of the AVP V2 receptor may treat congenital nephrogenic diabetes insipidus. *J Am Soc Nephrol.* 2009;20:2190–2203.

97. Evans DA, De Bree FM, Nijenhuis M, et al. Processing of frameshifted vasopressin precursors. *J Neuroendocrinol.* 2000;12:685–693.

98. Chou CL, DiGiovanni SR, Luther A, Lolait SJ, Knepper MA. Oxytocin as an antidiuretic hormone II. Role of V2 vasopressin receptor. *Am J Physiol.* 1995;269 (1 Pt 2):F78–F85.

99. Balment RJ, Brimble MJ, Forsling ML. Oxytocin release and renal actions in normal and Brattleboro rats. *Ann N Y Acad Sci.* USA 1982;394:241–253.

100. Verbalis JG, Robinson AG, Moses AM, eds. *Postoperative and post-traumatic diabetes insipidus.* Basel, Germany: S. Karger; 1985.

101. Olson BR, Gumowski J, Rubino D, Oldfield EH. Pathophysiology of hyponatremia after transsphenoidal pituitary surgery. *J Neurosurg.* 1997;87: 499–507.

102. Maghnie M, Cosi G, Genovese E, et al. Central diabetes insipidus in children and young adults. *N Engl J Med.* 2000;343:998–1007.

103. Greger NG, Kirkland RT, Clayton GW, Kirkland JL. Central diabetes insipidus. 22 years' experience. *Am J Dis Child.* 1986;140:551–554.

104. Czernichow P, Pomarede R, Brauner R, eds. *Neurogenic Diabetes Insipidus in Children.* Basel, Germany: S. Karger; 1985.

105. Moses AM, Blumenthal SA, Streeten DH, eds. *Acid-Base and Electrolyte Disorders Associated with Endocrine Disease: Pituitary and Thyroid.* New York, NY: Churchill Livingstone; 1985.

106. Birnbaum DC, Shields D, Lippe B, Perlman S, Phillipart M. Idiopathic central diabetes insipidus followed by progressive spastic cerebral ataxia. Report of four cases. *Arch Neurol.* 1989;46:1001–1003.

107. Bullmann C, Faust M, Hoffmann A, et al. Five cases with central diabetes insipidus and hypogonadism as first presentation of neurosarcoidosis. *Eur J Endocrinol.* 2000;142:365–372.

108. Vokes TJ, Gaskill MB, Robertson GL. Antibodies to vasopressin in patients with diabetes insipidus. Implications for diagnosis and therapy. *Ann Intern Med.* 1988;108:190–195.

109. Bichet DG, Kortas C, Manzini C, Barjon JN. A specific antibody to vasopressin in a man with concomitant resistance to treatment with Pitressin. *Clin Chem.* 1986;32:211–212.

110. Kaltsas GA, Powles TB, Evanson J, et al. Hypothalamo-pituitary abnormalities in adult patients with Langerhans cell histiocytosis: clinical, endocrinological, and radiological features and response to treatment. *J Clin Endocrinol Metab.* 2000;85:1370–1376.

111. McKusick VA. Online Mendelian Inheritance in Man (OMIM). http://www.ncbi.nlm.nih.gov/omim/ Accessed April 26, 2012.

112. Lacombe UL. *De la Polydipsie.* Paris, France: Imprimerie et Fonderie de Rignoux; 1841: 87.

113. Weil A. Ueber die hereditäre form des diabetes insipidus. *Arch Klin Med (Virchow's Arch).* 1884;95:70–95.

114. Camerer JW. Eine ergänzung des Weilschen diabetes-insipidus-stammbaumes. *Archiv Rassen-und Gesellschaftshygiene Biologic.* 1935;28:382–385.

115. Dölle W. Eine weitere ergänzung des Weilschen diabetes-insipidus-stammbaumes. *Zschr Menschl Vererb.* 1951;30:372–374.

116. Weil A. Ueber die hereditäre form des diabetes insipidus. *Deutch Arch Klin Med.* 1908;93:180–290.

117. Rittig R, Robertson GL, Siggaard C, et al. Identification of 13 new mutations in the vasopressin-neurophysin II gene in 17 kindreds with familial autosomal dominant neurohypophyseal diabetes insipidus. *Am J Hum Genet.* 1996;58:107–117.

118. Brachet C, Birk J, Christophe C, et al. Growth retardation in untreated autosomal dominant familial neurohypophyseal diabetes insipidus caused by one recurring and two novel mutations in the vasopressin-neurophysin II gene. *Eur J Endocrinol.* 2011;164:179–187.

119. Birk J, Friberg MA, Prescianotto-Baschong C, Spiess M, Rutishauser J. Dominant pro-vasopressin mutants that cause diabetes insipidus form disulfide-linked fibrillar aggregates in the endoplasmic reticulum. *J Cell Sci.* 2009; 122:3994–4002.
120. Castino R, Davies J, Beaucourt S, Isidoro C, Murphy D. Autophagy is a prosurvival mechanism in cells expressing an autosomal dominant familial neurohypophyseal diabetes insipidus mutant vasopressin transgene. *FASEB J.* 2005; 19:1021–1023.
121. Abu Libdeh A, Levy-Khademi F, Abdulhadi-Atwan M, et al. Autosomal recessive familial neurohypophyseal diabetes insipidus: onset in early infancy. *Eur J Endocrinol.* 2009;162:221–226.
122. Willcutts MD, Felner E, White PC. Autosomal recessive familial neurohypophyseal diabetes insipidus with continued secretion of mutant weakly active vasopressin. *Hum Mol Genet.* 1999;8:1303–1307.
123. Christensen JH, Siggaard C, Corydon TJ, et al. Differential cellular handling of defective arginine vasopressin (AVP) prohormones in cells expressing mutations of the AVP gene associated with autosomal dominant and recessive familial neurohypophyseal diabetes insipidus. *J Clin Endocrinol Metab.* 2004; 89:4521–4531.
124. Beuret N, Stettler H, Renold A, Rutishauser J, Spiess M. Expression of regulated secretory proteins is sufficient to generate granule-like structures in constitutively secreting cells. *J Biol Chem.* 2004;279:20242–20249.
125. Takeda K, Inoue H, Tanizawa Y, et al. WFS1 (Wolfram syndrome 1) gene product: predominant subcellular localization to endoplasmic reticulum in cultured cells and neuronal expression in rat brain. *Hum Mol Genet.* 2001;10:477–484.
126. Domenech E, Gomez-Zaera M, Nunes V. Study of the WFS1 gene and mitochondrial DNA in Spanish Wolfram syndrome families. *Clin Genet.* 2004; 65:463–469.
127. Ishihara H, Takeda S, Tamura A, et al. Disruption of the WFS1 gene in mice causes progressive beta-cell loss and impaired stimulus-secretion coupling in insulin secretion. *Hum Mol Genet.* 2004;13:1159–1170.
128. Conlan AR, Axelrod HL, Cohen AE, et al. Crystal structure of Miner1: The redox-active 2Fe-2S protein causative in Wolfram syndrome 2. *J Mol Biol.* 2009;392:143–153.
129. Fonseca SG, Ishigaki S, Oslowski CM, et al. Wolfram syndrome 1 gene negatively regulates ER stress signaling in rodent and human cells. *J Clin Invest.* 2010;120:744–755.
130. Crowley RK, Sherlock M, Agha A, Smith D, Thompson CJ. Clinical insights into adipsic diabetes insipidus: a large case series. *Clin Endocrinol (Oxf).* 2007;66:475–482.
131. Howard RL, Bichet DG, Schrier RW. Hypernatremic and polyuric states. In: Seldin DW, Giebisch, eds. *The Kidney: Physiology and Pathophysiology*. New York, NY: Raven Press, Ltd.; 1992: 1753–1778.
132. Robben JH, Knoers NV, Deen PM. Cell biological aspects of the vasopressin type-2 receptor and aquaporin 2 water channel in nephrogenic diabetes insipidus. *Am J Physiol Renal Physiol.* 2006;291:F257–270.
133. Spanakis E, Milord E, Gragnoli C. AVPR2 variants and mutations in nephrogenic diabetes insipidus: review and missense mutation significance. *J Cell Physiol.* 2008;217:605–617.
134. Peters M, Jeck N, Reinalter S, et al. Clinical presentation of genetically defined patients with hypokalemic salt-losing tubulopathies. *Am J Med.* 2002;112:183–190.
135. Konrad M, Weber S. Recent advances in molecular genetics of hereditary magnesium-losing disorders. *J Am Soc Nephrol.* 2003;14:249–260.
136. Gahl WA, Thoene JG, Schneider JA. Cystinosis. *N Engl J Med.* 2002;347: 111–121.
137. Bockenhauer D, van't Hoff W, Dattani M, et al. Secondary nephrogenic diabetes insipidus as a complication of inherited renal diseases. *Nephron Physiol.* 2010;116:23–29.
138. Fujiwara TM, Bichet DG. Molecular biology of hereditary diabetes insipidus. *J Am Soc Nephrol.* 2005;16:2836–2846.
139. Arthus M-F, Lonergan M, Crumley MJ, et al. Report of 33 novel *AVPR2* mutations and analysis of 117 families with X-linked nephrogenic diabetes insipidus. *J Am Soc Nephrol.* 2000;11:1044–1054.
140. Crawford JD, Bode HH. Disorders of the posterior pituitary in children. In: Gardner LI, ed. *Endocrine and Genetic Diseases of Childhood and Adolescence*. Philadelphia, PA: W.B. Saunders; 1975: 126–158.
141. Niaudet P, Dechaux M, Trivin C, Loirat C, Broyer M. Nephrogenic diabetes insipidus: Clinical and pathophysiological aspects. *Adv Nephrol Necker Hosp.* 1984;13:247–260.
142. McIlraith CH. Notes on some cases of diabetes insipidus with marked family and hereditary tendencies. *Lancet.* 1892;2:767–768.
143. Reeves WB, Andreoli TE. Nephrogenic diabetes insipidus. In: Scriver CR, Beaudet AL, Sly WS, Valle D, eds. *The Metabolic Basis of Inherited Disease*. New York, NY: McGraw-Hill; 1995: 3045–3071.
144. Christensen JH, Rittig S. Familial neurohypophyseal diabetes insipidus—an update. *Semin Nephrol.* 2006; 26:209–223.
145. Ulinski T, Grapin C, Forin V, et al. Severe bladder dysfunction in a family with ADH receptor gene mutation responsible for X-linked nephrogenic diabetes insipidus. *Nephrol Dial Transplant.* 2004;19:2928–2929.
146. Shalev H, Romanovsky I, Knoers NV, Lupa S, Landau D. Bladder function impairment in aquaporin-2 defective nephrogenic diabetes insipidus. *Nephrol Dial Transplant.* 2004;19:608–613.
147. Bichet DG, Razi M, Arthus M-F, et al. Epinephrine and dDAVP administration in patients with congenital nephrogenic diabetes insipidus. Evidence for a pre-cyclic AMP V2 receptor defective mechanism. *Kidney Int.* 1989;36:859–866.
148. Cannon JF. Diabetes insipidus clinical and experimental studies with consideration of genetic relationships. *Arch Intern Med.* 1955;96:215–272.
149. Bichet DG, Arthus M-F, Lonergan M, et al. X-linked nephrogenic diabetes insipidus mutations in North America and the Hopewell hypothesis. *J Clin Invest.* 1993;92:1262–1268.
150. Bode HH, Crawford JD. Nephrogenic diabetes insipidus in North America: The Hopewell hypothesis. *N Engl J Med.* 1969;280:750–754.
151. Holtzman EJ, Kolakowski LF, O'Brien D, Crawford JD, Ausiello DA. A null mutation in the vasopressin V2 receptor gene (AVPR2) associated with nephrogenic diabetes insipidus in the Hopewell kindred. *Hum Mol Genet.* 1993;2:1201–1204.
152. Vaithinathan R, Berson EL, Dryja TP. Further screening of the rhodopsin gene in patients with autosomal dominant retinitis pigmentosa. *Genomics.* 1994;21:461–463.
153. Robben JH, Kortenoeven ML, Sze M, et al. Intracellular activation of vasopressin V2 receptor mutants in nephrogenic diabetes insipidus by nonpeptide agonists. *Proc Natl Acad Sci USA.* 2009;106:12195–12200.
154. Morello JP, Salahpour A, Laperrière A, et al. Pharmacological chaperones rescue cell-surface expression and function of misfolded V2 vasopressin receptor mutants. *J Clin Invest.* 2000;105:887–895.
155. Bernier V, Morello JP, Zarruk A, et al. Pharmacologic chaperones as a potential treatment for X-linked nephrogenic diabetes insipidus. *J Am Soc Nephrol.* 2006;17:232–243.
156. Ulloa-Aguirre A, Janovick JA, Brothers SP, Conn PM. Pharmacologic rescue of conformationally-defective proteins: implications for the treatment of human disease. *Traffic.* 2004;5:821–837.
157. Bockenhauer D, Carpentier E, Rochdi D, et al. Vasopressin type 2 receptor V88M mutation: molecular basis of partial and complete nephrogenic diabetes insipidus. *Nephron Physiol.* 2009;114:1–10.
158. Vargas-Poussou R, Forestier L, Dautzenberg MD, et al. Mutations in the vasopressin V2 receptor and aquaporin-2 genes in 12 families with congenital nephrogenic diabetes insipidus. *J Am Soc Nephrol.* 1997;8:1855–1862.
159. Sadeghi H, Robertson GL, Bichet DG, Innamorati G, Birnbaumer M. Biochemical basis of partial NDI phenotypes. *Mol Endocrinol.* 1997;11:1806–1813.
160. Ala Y, Morin D, Mouillac B, et al. Functional studies of twelve mutant V2 vasopressin receptors related to nephrogenic diabetes insipidus: molecular basis of a mild clinical phenotype. *J Am Soc Nephrol.* 1998;9:1861–1872.
161. Marcialis MA, Faa V, Fanos V, et al. Neonatal onset of nephrogenic syndrome of inappropriate antidiuresis. *Pediatr Nephrol.* 2008;23:2267–2271.
162. Soule S, Florkowski C, Potter H, et al. Intermittent severe, symptomatic hyponatraemia due to the nephrogenic syndrome of inappropriate antidiuresis. *Ann Clin Biochem.* 2008;45:520–523.
163. Decaux G, Vandergheynst F, Bouko Y, et al. Nephrogenic syndrome of inappropriate antidiuresis in adults: high phenotypic variability in men and women from a large pedigree. *J Am Soc Nephrol.* 2007;18:606–612.
164. Feldman BJ, Rosenthal SM, Vargas GA, et al. Nephrogenic syndrome of inappropriate antidiuresis. *N Engl J Med.* 2005;352:1884–1890.
165. Kalenga K, Persu A, Goffin E, et al. Intrafamilial phenotype variability in nephrogenic diabetes insipidus. *Am J Kidney Dis.* 2002;39:737–743.
166. Kocan M, See HB, Sampaio NG, et al. Agonist-independent interactions between beta-arrestins and mutant vasopressin type II receptors associated with nephrogenic syndrome of inappropriate antidiuresis. *Mol Endocrinol.* 2009;23:559–571.
167. Noda Y, Sohara E, Ohta E, Sasaki S. Aquaporins in kidney pathophysiology. *Nat Rev Nephrol.* 2010;6:168–178.
168. Deen PM, Verdijk MA, Knoers NV. Requirement of human renal water channel aquaporin-2 for vasopressin-dependent concentration of urine. *Science.* 1994;264:92–95.
169. Mulders SM, Bichet DG, Rijss JP, et al. An aquaporin-2 water channel mutant which causes autosomal dominant nephrogenic diabetes insipidus is retained in the Golgi complex. *J Clin Invest.* 1998;102:57–66.
170. Canfield MC, Tamarappoo BK, Moses AM, Verkman AS, Holtzman EJ. Identification and characterization of aquaporin-2 water channel mutations causing nephrogenic diabetes insipidus with partial vasopressin response. *Hum Mol Genet.* 1997;6:1865–1871.

171. Leduc-Nadeau A, Lussier Y, Arthus MF, et al. New autosomal recessive mutations in aquaporin-2 causing nephrogenic diabetes insipidus through deficient targeting display normal expression in Xenopus oocytes. *J Physiol.* 2010; 588:2205–2218.
172. Kuwahara M, Iwai K, Ooeda T, et al. Three families with autosomal dominant nephrogenic diabetes insipidus caused by aquaporin-2 mutations in the C-terminus. *Am J Hum Genet.* 2001;69:738–748.
173. Marr N, Bichet DG, Hoefs S, et al. Cell-biologic and functional analyses of five new aquaporin-2 missense mutations that cause recessive nephrogenic diabetes inspidus. *J Am Soc Nephrol.* 2002;13:2267–2277.
174. Kamsteeg EJ, Bichet DG, Konings IB, et al. Reversed polarized delivery of an aquaporin-2 mutant causes dominant nephrogenic diabetes insipidus. *J Cell Biol.* 2003;163:1099–1109.
175. de Mattia F, Savelkoul PJ, Bichet DG, et al. A novel mechanism in recessive nephrogenic diabetes insipidus: wild-type aquaporin-2 rescues the apical membrane expression of intracellularly retained AQP2-P262L. *Hum Mol Genet.* 2004;13:3045–3056.
176. Deen PM, Croes H, van Aubel RA, Ginsel LA, van Os CH. Water channels encoded by mutant aquaporin-2 genes in nephrogenic diabetes insipidus are impaired in their cellular routing. *J Clin Invest.* 1995;95:2291–2296.
177. Tamarappoo BK, Verkman AS. Defective aquaporin-2 trafficking in nephrogenic diabetes insipidus and correction by chemical chaperones. *J Clin Invest.* 1998;101:2257–2267.
178. Levin MH, Haggie PM, Vetrivel L, Verkman AS. Diffusion in the endoplasmic reticulum of an aquaporin-2 mutant causing human nephrogenic diabetes insipidus. *J Biol Chem.* 2001;276:21331–21336.
179. Lin SH, Bichet DG, Sasaki S, et al. Two novel aquaporin-2 mutations responsible for congenital nephrogenic diabetes insipidus in Chinese families. *J Clin Endocrinol Metab.* 2002;87:2694–2700.
180. Lussier Y, Bissonnette P, Bichet DG, Lapointe JY. Stimulating effect of external Myo-inositol on the expression of mutant forms of aquaporin 2. *J Membr Biol.* 2010;236:225–232.
181. Bettinelli A, Bianchetti MG, Girardin E, et al. Use of calcium excretion values to distinguish two forms of primary renal tubular hypokalemic alkalosis: Bartter and Gitelman syndromes. *J Pediatr.* 1992;120:38–43.
182. Estevez R, Boettger T, Stein V, et al. Barttin is a Cl- channel beta-subunit crucial for renal Cl- reabsorption and inner ear K+ secretion. *Nature.* 2001;414:558–561.
183. Waldegger S, Jeck N, Barth P, et al. Barttin increases surface expression and changes current properties of ClC-K channels. *Pflugers Arch.* 2002;444:411–418.
184. Jeck N, Reinalter SC, Henne T, et al. Hypokalemic salt-losing tubulopathy with chronic renal failure and sensorineural deafness. *Pediatrics.* 2001;108:E5.
185. Birkenhager R, Otto E, Schurmann MJ, et al. Mutation of BSND causes Bartter syndrome with sensorineural deafness and kidney failure. *Nat Genet.* 2001;29:310–314.
186. Scherling B, Verder H, Nielsen MD, Christensen P, Giese J. Captopril treatment in Bartter's syndrome. *Scand J Urol Nephrol.* 1990;24:123–125.
187. Winterborn MH, Hewitt GJ, Mitchell MD. The role of prostaglandins in Bartter's syndrome. *Int J Pediatr Nephrol.* 1984;5:31–38.
188. Mackie FE, Hodson EM, Roy LP, Knight JF. Neonatal Bartter syndrome—use of indomethacin in the newborn period and prevention of growth failure. *Pediatr Nephrol.* 1996;10:756–758.
189. Barlow ED, de Wardener HE. Compulsive water drinking. *Q J Med.* 1959; 28:235–258.
190. Robertson GL. Dipsogenic diabetes insipidus: a newly recognized syndrome caused by a selective defect in the osmoregulation of thirst. *Trans Assoc Am Physicians.* 1987;100:241–249.
191. Cadnapaphornchai MA, Summer SN, Falk S, et al. Effect of primary polydipsia on aquaporin and sodium transporter abundance. *Am J Physiol Renal Physiol.* 2003;285:F965–971.
192. Amico JA. Diabetes insipidus and pregnancy. In: Czernichow P, ed. *Frontiers of Hormone Research.* Basel, Germany: S. Karger; 1985: 266–277.
193. Davison JM, Shiells EA, Philips PR, Lindheimer MD. Serial evaluation of vasopressin release and thirst in human pregnancy. Role of human chorionic gonadotrophin in the osmoregulatory changes of gestation. *J Clin Invest.*;1988;81:798–806.
194. Iwasaki Y, Oiso Y, Kondo K, et al. Aggravation of subclinical diabetes insipidus during pregnancy. *N Engl J Med.* 1991;324:522–526.
195. Forssman J. On hereditary diabetes insipidus, with special regard to a sex-linked form. *Acta Med Scand.* 1945;159:1–196.
196. Barron WM, Cohen LH, Ulland LA, et al. Transient vasopressin-resistant diabetes insipidus of pregnancy. *N Engl J Med.* 1984;310:442–444.
197. Durr JA, Hoggard JG, Hunt JM, Schrier RW. Diabetes insipidus in pregnancy associated with abnormally high circulating vasopressinase activity. *N Engl J Med.* 1987;316:1070–1074.
198. Lindheimer MD. Polyuria and pregnancy: its cause, its danger. *Obstet Gynecol.* 2005;105:1171–1172.
199. Hiett AK, Barton JR. Diabetes insipidus associated with craniopharyngioma in pregnancy. *Obstet Gynecol.* 1990;76:982–984.
200. Brewster UC, Hayslett JP. Diabetes insipidus in the third trimester of pregnancy. *Obstet Gynecol.* 2005;105:1173–1176.
201. Leaf A. Nephrology forum: neurogenic diabetes insipidus. *Kidney Int.* 1979; 15:572–580.
202. Robertson GL. Diagnosis of diabetes insipidus. In: Czernichow P, ed. *Frontiers of Hormone Research.* Basel: S. Karger; 1985: 176.
203. van Lieburg AF, Knoers NV, Monnens LA. Clinical presentation and follow-up of 30 patients with congenital nephrogenic diabetes insipidus. *J Am Soc Nephrol.* 1999;10:1958–1964.
204. Gautier B, Thieblot P, Steg A. Mégauretère, mégavessie et diabète insipide familial. *Sem Hop.* 1981;57:60–61.
205. Boyd SD, Raz S, Ehrlich RM. Diabetes insipidus and nonobstructive dilatation of urinary tract. *Urology.* 1980;16:266–269.
206. Fenske W, Quinkler M, Lorenz D, et al. Copeptin in the differential diagnosis of the polydipsia-polyuria syndrome—revisiting the direct and indirect water deprivation tests. *J Clin Endocrinol Metab.* 2011;96:1506–1515.
207. Diederich S, Eckmanns T, Exner P, et al. Differential diagnosis of polyuric/polydipsic syndromes with the aid of urinary vasopressin measurement in adults. *Clin Endocrinol (Oxf).* 2001;54:665–671.
208. Robertson GL. Diseases of the posterior pituitary. In: Felig D, Baxter JD, Broadus AE, eds. *Endocrinology and Metabolism.* New York, NY: McGraw-Hill; 1981: 251.
209. Robertson GL, Mahr EA, Athar S, Sinha T. Development and clinical application of a new method for the radioimmunoassay of arginine vasopressin in human plasma. *J Clin Invest.* 1973;52:2340–2352.
210. Robertson GL, Klein LA, Roth J, Gorden P. Immunoassay of plasma vasopressin in man. *Proc Natl Acad Sci USA.* 1970;66:1298–1305.
211. Vokes TP, Aycinena PR, Robertson GL. Effect of insulin on osmoregulation of vasopressin. *Am J Physiol.* 1987;252:E538–548.
212. Davison JM, Gilmore EA, Durr J, Robertson GL, Lindheimer MD. Altered osmotic thresholds for vasopressin secretion and thirst in human pregnancy. *Am J Physiol.* 1984;246:F105–109.
213. Bichet DG, Arthus MF, Barjon JN, Lonergan M, Kortas C. Human platelet fraction arginine-vasopressin. Potential physiological role. *J Clin Invest.* 1987; 79:881–887.
214. Bichet DG, Kortas C, Mettauer B, et al. Modulation of plasma and platelet vasopressin by cardiac function in patients with heart failure. *Kidney Int.* 1986; 29:1188–1196.
215. Ysewijn-Van Brussel KA, De Leenheer AP. Development and evaluation of a radioimmunoassay for Arg8-vasopressin, after extraction with Sep-Pak C18. *Clin Chem.* 1985;31:861–863.
216. LaRochelle FT Jr, North WG, Stern P. A new extraction of arginine vasopressin from blood: the use of octadecasilyl-silica. *Pflugers Arch.* 1980;387:79–81.
217. Hartter E, Woloszczuk W. Radioimmunological determination of arginine vasopressin and human atrial natriuretic peptide after simultaneous extraction from plasma. *J Clin Chem Clin Biochem.* 1986;24:559–563.
218. Preibisz JJ, Sealey JE, Laragh JH, Cody RJ, Weksler BB. Plasma and platelet vasopressin in essential hypertension and congestive heart failure. *Hypertension.* 1983;5:I129–I138.
219. Seckl JR, Dunger DB, Bevan JS, et al. Vasopressin antagonist in early postoperative diabetes insipidus. *Lancet.* 1990;335:1353–1356.
220. Kanno K, Sasaki S, Hirata Y, et al. Urinary excretion of aquaporin-2 in patients with diabetes insipidus. *N Engl J Med.* 1995;332:1540–1545.
221. Elliot S, Goldsmith P, Knepper M, Haughey M, Olson B. Urinary excretion of aquaporin-2 in humans: a potential marker of collecting duct responsiveness to vasopressin. *J Am Soc Nephrol.* 1996;7:403–409.
222. Saito T, Ishikawa SE, Sasaki S, et al. Urinary excretion of aquaporin-2 in the diagnosis of central diabetes insipidus. *J Clin Endocrinol Metab.* 1997;82:1823–1827.
223. Maas AH, Siggaard-Andersen O, Weisberg HF, Zijlstra WG. Ion-selective electrodes for sodium and potassium: a new problem of what is measured and what should be reported. *Clin Chem.* 1985;31:482–485.
224. Bichet DG, Birnbaumer M, Lonergan M, et al. Nature and recurrence of AVPR2 mutations in X-linked nephrogenic diabetes insipidus. *Am J Hum Genet.* 1994;55:278–286.
225. Gennari FJ. Current concepts. Serum osmolality. Uses and limitations. *N Engl J Med.* 1984;310:102–105.
226. De Buyst J, Massa G, Christophe C, Tenoutasse S, Heinrichs C. Clinical, hormonal and imaging findings in 27 children with central diabetes insipidus. *Eur J Pediatr.* 2007;166:43–49.
227. Cattin F, Bonneville F, Chayep C. Imagerie par resonance magnetique du diabete insipide. *Feuillets de Radiologie.* 2005;45:425–434.

228. Fujisawa I. Magnetic resonance imaging of the hypothalamic-neurohypophyseal system. *J Neuroendocrinol.* 2004;16:297–302.
229. Rappaport R. Magnetic resonance imaging in pituitary disease. *Growth Genet Hor.* 1995;11:1–5.
230. Vokes TP, Robertson GL, eds. *Physiology of Secretion of Vasopressin*. Basel: S. Karger; 1985: 127–155.
231. Zerbe RL, Robertson GL. Disorders of ADH. *Med North Am.* 1984;13:1570.
232. Wu B, Steinbronn C, Alsterfjord M, Zeuthen T, Beitz E. Concerted action of two cation filters in the aquaporin water channel. *EMBO J.* 2009;28:2188–2194.
233. Gainer H, Chin H. Molecular diversity in neurosecretion: reflections on the hypothalamo-neurohypophyseal system. *Cell Mol Neurobiol.* 1998;18: 211–230.
234. Robertson G. The pathophysiology of ADH secretion. In: Tolis G, Labrie F, Martin JB, eds. *Clinical Neuroendocrinology: A Pathophysiological Approach*. New York, NY: Raven Press; 1979.
235. Bichet DG, Fujiwara TM. Reabsorption of sodium chloride—lessons from the chloride channels. *N Engl J Med.* 2004;350:1281–1283.
236. Stern P, Valtin H. Verney was right, but. *N Engl J Med.* 1981;305:1581–1582.

CHAPTER

72 Disorders of Potassium and Acid–Base Metabolism in Association with Renal Disease

Mark A. Perazella • Asghar Rastegar

In this chapter, we review disturbances in potassium and acid–base homeostasis seen in patients with renal disease. Our discussion is, however, limited to disorders of potassium and acid–base homeostasis seen in (1) patients with progressive chronic kidney disease (CKD) and (2) patients with renal insufficiency and defects in the renin–aldosterone axis or in the tubular response to aldosterone. We briefly review potassium and acid–base homeostasis in healthy humans before focusing on patients with underlying renal disease. We do not, however, discuss normal renal handling of potassium and only briefly review renal handling of hydrogen ion. These two topics are extensively reviewed in Chapter 6: Tubular Potassium Transport, and Chapter 7: Renal Acid–Base Transport, respectively.

POTASSIUM HOMEOSTASIS

Potassium is the most abundant cation in the body. The distribution of potassium is such that 98% of total body potassium is intracellular, whereas only 2% is extracellular. Serum potassium is normally between 3.8 and 5.0 mEq per liter, whereas the intracellular potassium concentration is 120 to 140 mEq per liter. The high intracellular to extracellular potassium ratio (K_i/K_o) is crucial to normal cell function, because it is the major determinant of the resting membrane potential. The body is able to maintain this distribution in a highly regulated and efficient fashion through the hormonal modulation of Na-K-ATPase pump activity.[1,2] Humans, as carnivorous intermittent eaters, are continuously challenged by large potassium loads. On a long-term basis, this challenge is met primarily by the renal excretion of potassium load; however, on a short-term basis, a significant amount of potassium is shifted intracellularly.[3] This shift temporarily buffers the expected change in the K_i/K_o ratio until potassium intake is balanced by a comparable output. Therefore, potassium homeostasis is regulated through both extrarenal as well as renal mechanisms (Fig. 72.1).[4]

Extrarenal Potassium Homeostasis

The kidney is able to excrete only about 50% of the administered potassium during the first 4 hours after intravenous or oral intake of potassium. Approximately 80% of the retained potassium is shifted intracellularly, and only 20% (or 10% of the total intake) remains in the extracellular space.[5–7] The retained potassium will be excreted completely over the next 24 hours.[8] The major regulators of this internal redistribution are: (1) insulin, (2) catecholamines, and (3) mineralocorticoids. In addition to these physiologic regulators, serum potassium is also regulated by acid–base status as well as plasma osmolality. Factors that increase or decrease plasma potassium concentration are noted in Figure 72.2.

Insulin

The ability of insulin to shift potassium intracellularly has been known for over 70 years[9] and has been used therapeutically for the treatment of hyperkalemia. Pancreatectomized dogs tolerate exogenous potassium loads poorly.[10] This is reversed by the exogenous replacement of insulin.[11,12] The partial inhibition of endogenous insulin in dogs by somatostatin infusion results in a twofold rise in serum potassium compared to controls.[6] If physiologic doses of insulin were added to the somatostatin infusion, potassium tolerance returned to normal. In healthy volunteers, somatostatin infusion in the postabsorptive state led to a 50% decline in the plasma insulin concentration and a 0.5 to 0.7 mEq per liter rise in serum potassium that was reversed by a physiologic infusion of exogenous insulin.[6] A similar phenomenon was observed in maturity-onset diabetic patients who have normal or increased fasting plasma insulin levels, but not in insulin-deficient juvenile diabetic patients.[13]

The primary sites of insulin-mediated potassium uptake include muscle and the liver, and to a lesser degree, adipose tissue.[14,15] In normal volunteers on variable insulin doses, the liver is the primary site of potassium uptake during the first hour.[15] However, during the second hour, despite a continued decrease in serum potassium, there is net release of potassium from the portal and splanchnic bed, indicating a shift of potassium uptake to the peripheral tissue, especially muscle.[15]

At the cellular level, insulin interacts with specific receptors on the plasma membrane,[16] increasing the activity

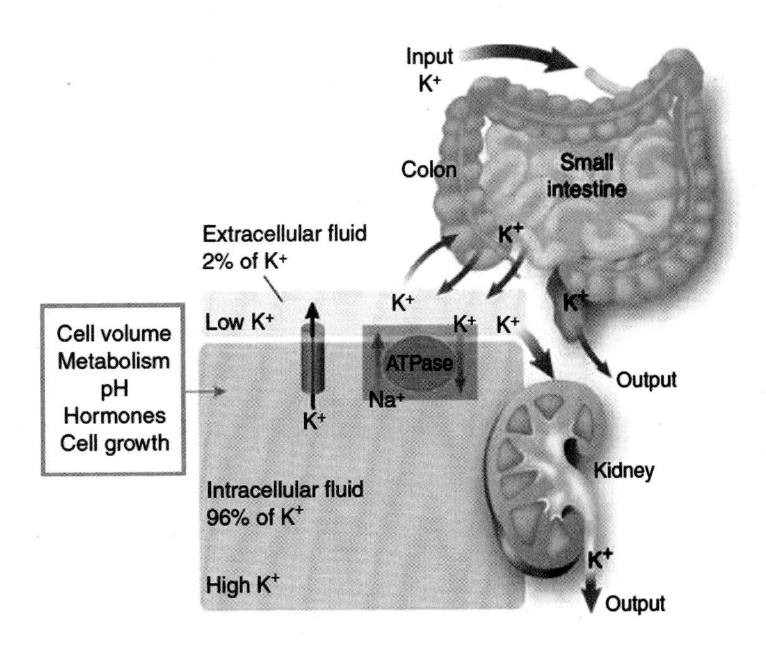

FIGURE 72.1 The distribution of potassium (K) in the body. Potassium is primarily located in cells (96%), with distribution controlled by a pump-leak mechanism involving both Na-K-ATPase and membrane potassium channels. The kidneys excrete more than 90% of the daily potassium load, and the intestines excrete the rest. (From Giebisch G, Krapf R, Wagner C. Renal and extrarenal regulation of potassium. *Kidney Int.* 2007;397, with permission.)

of the Na-K-ATPase pump in the skeletal and heart muscle, epithelial cells of the kidney and bladder, as well as liver and fat cells.[17] This results in a series of intracellular events leading to hyperpolarization of cell membranes.[17] The time course for this interaction is consistent with both an increase in enzyme activity as well as the rapid recruitment of Na-K-ATPase pumps to the cellular membrane. In contrast, chronic stimulation by insulin probably increases the total number of available pump sites. This occurs through the regulation of the Na-K-ATPase pump at the transcriptional and posttranscriptional levels by inducing the synthesis of new α and β subunits.[1] McDonough and Youn,[18] using a potassium clamp, have recently shown that after 10 days of potassium deprivation in rats Na-K-ATPase activity decreased by more than 50% and insulin-mediated potassium shift decreased by 94%, whereas in rats deprived of potassium for only 2 days the number of pumps did not decrease, but insulin-mediated potassium shift decreased by 80%. This would indicate that insulin resistance precedes a decrease in the number of pump expression during hypokalemia. The molecular mechanism underlying this response, however, remains poorly understood.[19] Several in vitro studies, including one study in humans, have shown that insulin-driven potassium uptake by both muscle and the liver is independent of glucose uptake.[15,20]

Catecholamines

D'Silva,[21] beginning in 1934, first observed a biphasic response of plasma potassium to epinephrine injection. Plasma potassium rose during the first 1 to 3 minutes, but

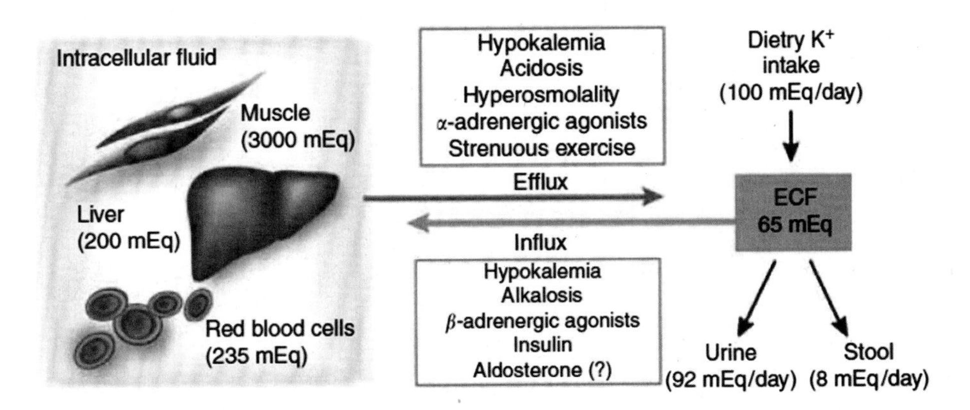

FIGURE 72.2 The distribution of potassium (K) between the intracellular and extracellular fluid compartments. Potassium distribution between the intra- and extracellular fluid is controlled by a pump-leak mechanism involving both Na-K-ATPase and membrane potassium channels. The factors noted in the figure drive potassium into or out of cells. (From Giebisch G, Krapf R, Wagner C. Renal and extrarenal regulation of potassium. *Kidney Int.* 2007;397, with permission.)

with continued infusion, fell and remained lower than baseline. Other investigators have shown increased potassium tolerance in animals infused with pharmacologic doses of epinephrine[22,23] despite a pancreatectomy or nephrectomy.[24] Brown and coworkers[25] have shown that the infusion of stress-level doses of epinephrine resulted in a decrease in serum potassium by 0.4 to 0.6 mEq per liter. Because epinephrine inhibits the renal excretion of potassium,[26,27] the decline in potassium concentration is entirely accounted for by enhanced cellular potassium uptake.

Specific receptors are involved in the cellular disposal of potassium by catecholamines. Alpha stimulation in humans by phenylephrine[28] significantly impairs cellular potassium tolerance, which is reversed by the α-antagonist phentolamine. This phenomenon may explain the initial rise in serum potassium after the infusion of catecholamine.[26,27] β_2-blockade impairs the catecholamine-induced shift of potassium into extrarenal tissues[29,30] and causes hyperkalemia despite an increase in renal excretion of this ion. In normal volunteers who exercise while taking β-adrenergic blocking agents, the serum potassium level is raised 2- to 2.5-fold higher than during similar exercise performed without a β blockade.[3,31] The effect of nonspecific β-blockers such as propranolol on serum potassium is mimicked by specific β_2-blockers[32] but not β_1-blockers. Although an important role for catecholamine-stimulated uptake of potassium by muscle has been demonstrated, the role of the liver remains controversial. The effect of potassium on catecholamine levels is less clear.

At the cellular level, epinephrine binds to the β_2-receptor resulting in the stimulation of adenyl cyclase and the conversion of adenosine triphosphate to cyclic 3′,5′-adenosine mono- phosphate (cAMP). It is postulated that cAMP then activates protein kinase A, which then phosphorylates the Na-K-ATPase pump, increasing its activity and promoting potassium influx into the cell and Na^+ efflux.[31] Binding catecholamines to the α receptor decreases cellular potassium uptake by inhibiting adenylate cyclase activity and decreasing Na-K-ATPase pump activity.[32] In addition, activation of the α-1 receptor alters cytoplasmic calcium, thereby increasing intracellular calcium concentration and opening calcium-activated potassium channels, which allow potassium to exit the cell.[32] Interestingly, the effect of insulin and epinephrine on plasma potassium is additive, which confirms a separate mechanisms of action.[31] In insulin-induced hypoglycemia, hypokalemia is therefore due to the combined effect of both insulin and the hypoglycemia-induced rise in catecholamines.[31]

Mineralocorticoids

Mineralocorticoids play a major role in external potassium homeostasis by increasing its excretion by the kidney,[33] colon,[34] salivary,[35] and sweat glands.[36] However, aldosterone's role in internal potassium homeostasis is less clear.[37,38] Anephric rats adapted to high potassium intake handle an acute potassium load more efficiently than do nonadapted rats. This adaptation is lost by prior adrenalectomy and restored by exogenous mineralocorticoid replacement.[39] However, Spital and Sterns[40,41] observed that during the 20 hours of fasting before a nephrectomy and acute potassium loading, these rats became potassium depleted owing to marked kaliuresis resulting from high serum potassium coupled with a high aldosterone level. In adrenalectomized dogs, Young and Jackson[42] have shown that plasma potassium concentration at any exchangeable potassium level was a function of aldosterone replacement dose. High-dose aldosterone in anephric rabbits delays death due to hyperkalemia.[43] Similarly, baseline potassium was significantly higher in hormonally deficient adrenalectomized rats despite negative potassium balance compared to exogenously replaced controls, thus supporting a defect in the cellular uptake of potassium.[5,44] This impairment was corrected by either aldosterone or epinephrine replacement. In rats, aldosterone has been shown to increase Na-K-ATPase pump activity by inducing the synthesis of new α- and β-subunits in heart and vascular smooth muscle.[1] This effect presumably represents the action of aldosterone on Na-K-ATPase pump gene expression and supports a role for aldosterone in cellular potassium homeostasis. In anephric humans treated with deoxycorticosterone acetate (DOCA), spironolactone, or placebo for 3 days, the baseline potassium was similar; however, the DOCA-treated subjects showed greater tolerance to acute potassium load than did the other two groups.[45] In a study of 15 patients on hemodialysis that were treated with 0.05 to 2.0 mg per day of fludrocortisone acetate, the serum K^+ decreased significantly.[46] Interestingly, the effect of exogenous mineralocorticoid was more pronounced in patients with a low compared to a high plasma aldosterone concentration. Low dose spironolactone (25 mg per day) was associated with an increase in a mean serum K^+ concentration of 0.3 mEq per liter over 4 weeks of therapy in 15 chronic hemodialysis patients.[47] In the largest study to date, serum potassium in 50 hemodialysis patients treated with 25 mg per day of spironolactone increased from baseline 4.96 to 5.16 in 2 weeks and remained stable for 6 months.[48] Very low dose spironolactone (25 mg thrice weekly), however, did not increase serum K^+ in hemodialysis patients,[49] whereas a very high dose (300 mg per day) induced a significant rise in plasma potassium (0.5 mEq per liter) and caused hyperkalemia after 3 weeks of therapy in nine chronically hemodialyzed end-stage renal disease (ESRD) patients (three were anephric).[50] In summary, these studies support a small but significant role for aldosterone in internal potassium homeostasis in anephric animals and ESRD patients.

Acid–Base Balance

The role of acid–base balance on the internal distribution of potassium[51] is based on the concept that during the development of acute acidemia, the hydrogen ion enters the cell in exchange for potassium and that the reverse occurs during the development of alkalemia.[51–53] This dynamic interrelationship has been simplified clinically to a general rule that for each 0.1 U change in serum pH, the serum potassium changes in the opposite direction by 0.6 mEq per liter. However, the relationship between serum potassium and serum pH is much more complex and depends on the type and severity of the acid–base disorder, the anion accompanying hydrogen, the duration of acidosis, changes in plasma bicarbonate concentration independent of changes in pH and the extent of intracellular buffering, and renal adaptation as well as hormonal changes in response to the disorder.[54] In addition, in clinical settings, there are often other physiologic and pathophysiologic processes that may be present, which would affect both transcellular as well as the renal and extrarenal handling of potassium. The following generalizations should therefore be used with caution.

1. On the whole, acidosis is accompanied by a greater change in serum potassium than is alkalosis.[55]
2. Mineral acidosis (Fig. 72.3) causes the greatest shift (0.24 to 1.7 mEq per liter for each 0.1 U in pH change), whereas organic acidosis has a much smaller effect.[53,56,57] Mild mineral acidosis (a decrease in serum bicarbonate by 5 mEq per liter and an increase in hydrogen ion concentration by 0.45 nmol per liter), however, does not result in a significant change in serum potassium.[58]
3. Acute respiratory alkalosis paradoxically results in a small but significant rise in serum potassium (+0.30 mEq per liter with a drop in pCO_2 of 16 to 22.5 mm Hg). The rise was primarily due to stimulation of α-adrenergic receptors by catecholamine.[59] Chronic respiratory alkalosis, however, results in sustained hypokalemia due to a renal loss of potassium.[60]
4. The amounts of potassium shifted into the cell in metabolic and chronic respiratory alkalosis are approximately similar (0.1 to 0.4 mEq per liter for each 0.1 U of pH change).
5. Acute respiratory acidosis resulting in a decrease in pH to 7.24 had no effect on serum K^+.[61]
6. Changes in serum bicarbonate, independent of serum pH, have an inverse effect on the serum potassium concentration.
7. In chronic acidosis and alkalosis, the final serum K^+ is a function of the effect of acid–base disturbance on the renal handling of potassium, as well as on the transcellular distribution of this ion. In dogs with ammonium chloride–induced acidosis, Magner and associates[62] noted a fall in serum potassium below baseline by days 3 to 5, owing to severe kaliuresis.

Osmolality

The acute hyperkalemic effect of a sudden rise in plasma osmolality is probably caused by the shift of potassium-rich intracellular fluid by solvent drag.[63] Clinically, this phenomenon is most commonly observed in hyperosmolar diabetic patients (Fig. 72.4), with or without ketoacidosis[64–67] when insulin deficiency augments the rise in potassium. Although chronic hyperkalemia in diabetic patients is multifactorial, a sudden rise in plasma osmolality seems to play a contributory role. The infusion of hypertonic mannitol in healthy humans[68] or hypertonic saline[69] or hypertonic contrast media[70] in patients with chronic kidney disease results in a modest rise in serum potassium (0.4 to 0.6 mEq per liter). Hyperkalemia can be severe, especially in diabetic patients with little or no

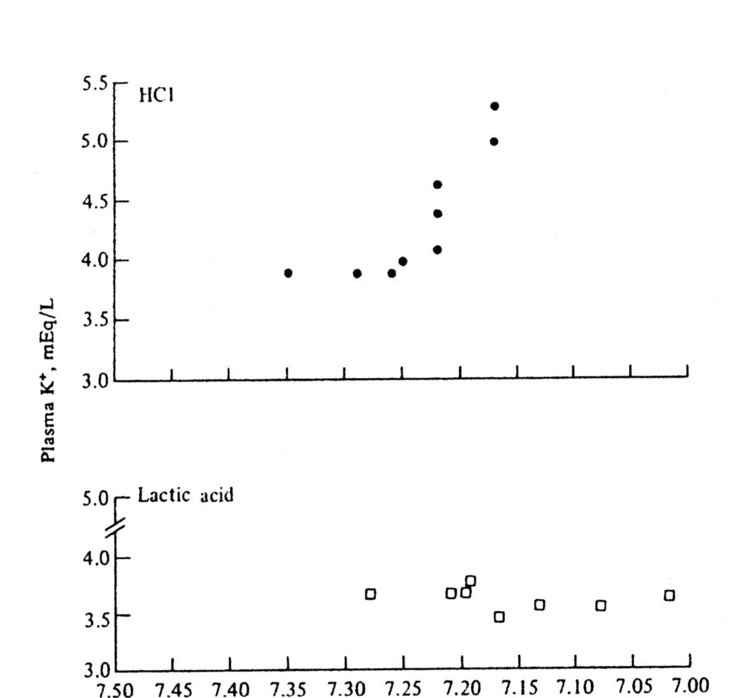

FIGURE 72.3 The effect of arterial pH on plasma potassium concentration in experimentally induced mineral acidosis (hydrochloric acid-HCl) and lactic acidosis in dogs. (From Perez GO, Oster JR, Vaamonde CA. Serum potassium concentration in acidemic states. *Nephron.* 1981;27:233, with permission.)

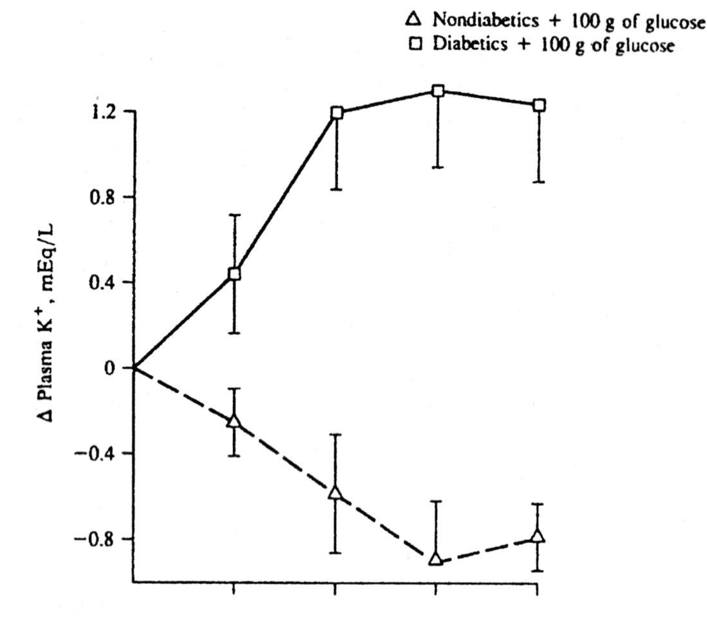

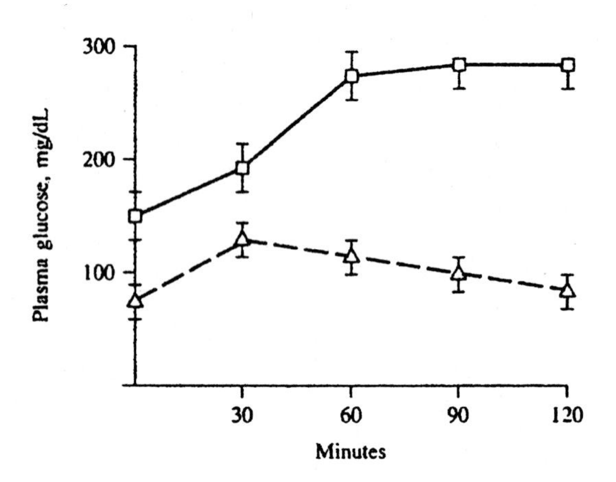

FIGURE 72.4 The effect of glucose infusion on plasma potassium and glucose concentrations in diabetics *(squares)* and normal subjects *(triangles)*. The plasma potassium rises in diabetics owing to the development of hyperosmolality (hyperglycemia) but falls in normal subjects as a result of the glucose-induced release of endogenous insulin. (From Nicolis GL, Kahn T, Sanchez A, et al. Glucose-induced hyperkalemia in diabetic subjects. *Arch Intern Med.* 1981;141:49, with permission.)

renal function facing sudden hyperglycemia.[71] These clinical observations support an independent role of sudden osmolar shifts in the regulation of serum potassium.

Feedback or Feedforward Control of Potassium Homeostasis. It is well known that an increase in potassium concentration directly stimulates renal potassium excretion through an increase in potassium secretion in the collecting duct. This is accomplished by the direct stimulation of Na-K-ATPase, an increased tubular flow, and an increase in aldosterone. However, as Rabinowitz et al.[72] first noted an increase in renal potassium excretion after meals in sheep was independent of change in serum potassium and aldosterone. In normal human subjects, urinary potassium excretion increased significantly 20 minutes after the ingestion of potassium salts before any change in serum potassium. Kaliuresis was more robust if potassium is ingested with meals rather than without meals or given intravenously. These and other observations support a role for a direct gut–kidney axis in potassium homeostasis favoring a feedforward rather than a feedback homeostatic mechanism (Fig. 72.5). The specific gut sensor and the gut–kidney loop remains speculative at this point. For a more detailed discussion, readers are referred to two recent reviews of this topic.[73,74]

POTASSIUM HOMEOSTASIS IN RENAL FAILURE

Patients with renal failure are able to maintain a near normal serum potassium concentration despite a marked decrease in glomerular filtration rate (GFR).[75–78] Although hyperkalemia could be due to increased potassium intake and/or rapid shifts of potassium from the cell, renal failure is the most important cause of hyperkalemia, accounting for 77% of the cases reported by Acker and coworkers.[79] In a random sample of 300 CKD patients (serum creatinine [Cr] levels

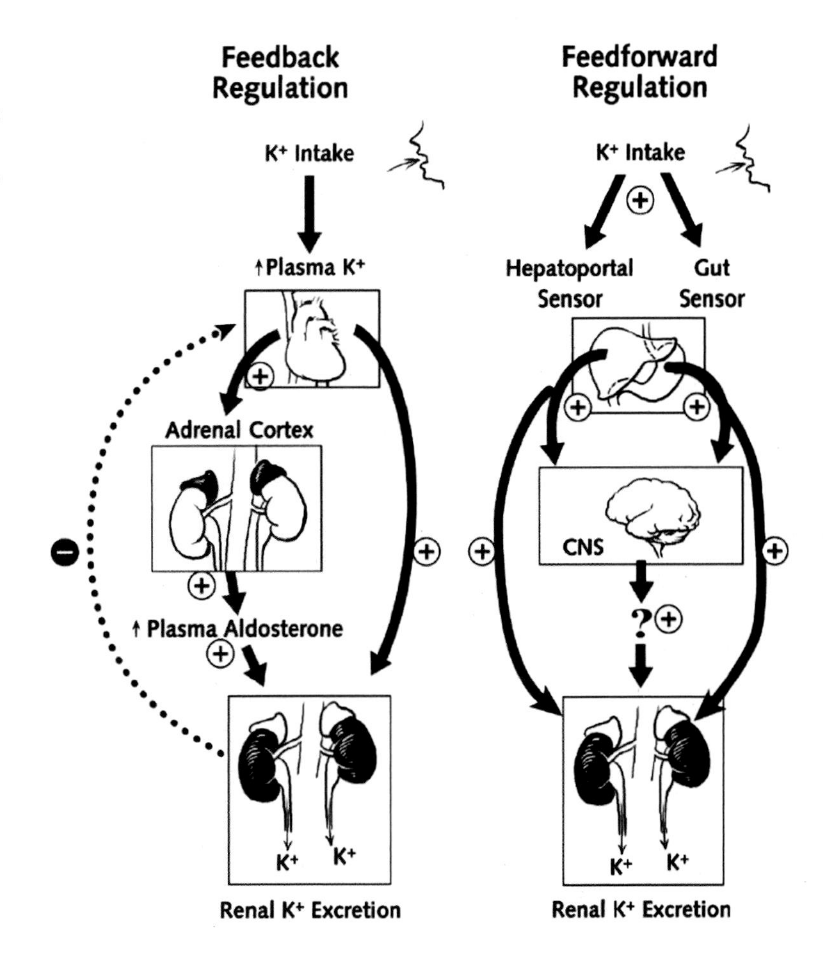

FIGURE 72.5 The integrated model of the regulation of body potassium balance: feedback and feedforward regulation. Renal potassium excretion is controlled by both feedback signals (plasma potassium concentration) and feedforward signals (liver and gut). CNS, central nervous system. (From Greenlee M, Wingo CS, McDonough AA, et al. Narrative review: evolving concepts in potassium homeostasis and hypokalemia. *Ann Intern Med.* 2009;150:619, with permission.)

1.5 to 6.0 mg per deciliter) not receiving drugs that interfered with potassium homeostasis, 55% were noted to have hyperkalemia ($K^+ \geq 5.0$ mEq per liter).[80] Treatment with drugs that interfere with potassium handling would be expected to further increase the development of hyperkalemia (see the following). Serum potassium rises with decreasing GFR; however, it often remains within normal range with GFR above 40 mL per minute.[75] In this study, the rate of hyperkalemia ($[K^+] > 5.0$) was 17% and was primarily limited to patients with CKD stage 4 and 5. However, under certain conditions, hyperkalemia may occur in patients with mild-to-moderate renal failure (Table 72.1). In a longitudinal study of patients with CKD, hyperkalemia ($[K] > 5.5$) was reported in only 8% of patients and, surprisingly, hypokalemia ($[K] < 4.0$) was more frequently seen in 15% of patients. Hypokalemia was not related to nutrition and was most likely secondary to the use of diuretics.[78] This observation would indicate that electrolyte disturbances in patients with CKD are partly related to the underlying disease and partly to medications used in the management of concomitant comorbidities such as fluid overload and hypertension. However, it should be emphasized that the risk of hyperkalemia in patients with CKD, including those treated with renin–angiotensin–aldosterone system (RAAS) blockers, is relatively small.[81]

In this section, we initially discuss total body potassium content in patients with renal failure before treatment with dialysis and then review internal and external potassium homeostasis in these patients. In the subsequent section, we discuss hyperkalemia seen in patients with renal insufficiency with a defect in the renin–angiotensin–aldosterone axis or in the tubular responsiveness to aldosterone.

TABLE 72.1 Etiologies of Hyperkalemia in Patients with Renal Insufficiency

GFR < 20 mL/min
Defects in the renin–angiotensin–aldosterone axis
Tubular defects in potassium secretion
Potassium input (e.g., rhabdomyolysis, hemolysis, severe catabolic states, gastrointestinal bleeding, exogenous potassium administration)
Shift of potassium from intracellular compartment
Drugs that interfere with renal and extrarenal potassium homeostasis

GFR, glomerular filtration rate.

Total Body and Cellular Potassium Content in Renal Failure

Total body potassium content is a reflection of the balance between potassium intake and potassium output, whereas the cellular content reflects the distribution of potassium between the intracellular and the extracellular compartments. Exchangeable potassium (K_e) in pre-ESRD patients has been generally reported as lower than normal.[82] However, Berlyne and associates,[83] after excluding patients with intercurrent problems (such as vomiting, diarrhea, or malnutrition), reported a normal value. It should also be noted that malnutrition is common in patients with CKD and many serum and anthropomorphic measurements of protein-energy nutritional status show progressive decline with the progression of CKD.[84] As Patrick[85] has pointed out, the normal range for K_e is not well defined and depends on age, sex, and the reference points used (e.g., total body weight, lean body weight, intracellular water). These reference points may be distorted in patients with CKD. The measurement of total body potassium by the use of a naturally occurring isotope (^{40}K) also has given normal values.[86]

Cellular potassium content has been estimated by the use of muscle biopsy.[87–92] Bergstrom and colleagues[87] studied 102 patients with serum creatinine levels ranging from 4.8 to 25.0 mg per deciliter before therapy. In this and other studies, the intracellular potassium concentration was low owing to an increase in intracellular water despite normal intracellular potassium content.[87,90] However, Bilbrey and coworkers[93] and Montanari and coworkers[92] have reported normal intracellular potassium concentrations. Importantly, the intracellular potassium content was either low or normal (but not increased) in all four studies.[87,90–93] The low intracellular potassium (and high intracellular sodium content) has also been reported in erythrocytes[92,94,95] and leukocytes[82,96] from these patients. This bespeaks of a decrease in the number and/or the activity of the Na-K-ATPase pumps in the cell membrane. In chronic dialysis patients, the pump transport rate is higher immediately after fluid removal,[97,98] and the abnormal levels of intracellular sodium and potassium in uremic patients return to normal following several weeks of dialysis.[95] Because the number of pump sites inversely correlates with intracellular sodium, and a change in their number requires the production of new cells with lower intracellular sodium, the acute effect of fluid removal by dialysis may result from the removal of a volume-sensitive pump inhibitor.[99] In contrast, the long-term effect of dialysis reflects the production of new cells with lower intracellular sodium and a higher number of pump sites. For a detailed discussion, refer to the article by Kaji and Kahn.[99]

Internal Potassium Homeostasis in Chronic Kidney Disease

The role of cellular uptake of potassium in renal failure has been studied in both humans[76,77,100] and animals.[101–103] Schon and associates[103] have shown that the cellular uptake of potassium in rats with a remnant kidney is similar to that in normal rats maintained on a comparable diet but is lower than normal when both groups consume a high potassium diet. In contrast, in two different models of renal failure in rats, Bia and DeFronzo[101] showed impairment in the cellular disposal of an acute potassium load. Bourgoignie and associates[102] challenged chronically uremic dogs (remnant kidney model) that were adapted to different potassium intakes with an acute potassium load. Whereas the percentage of retained potassium that was shifted into the intracellular compartment was greater in normal dogs (90%), the absolute amount was significantly less than that in dogs with a remnant kidney (9.0 versus 20.5 mEq, respectively). They concluded that extrarenal cellular uptake was normal in the dogs with renal failure. Gonick and colleagues[76] challenged patients with moderate renal failure with an oral potassium load. Whereas serum potassium 5 hours postchallenge was slightly higher in patients than in controls (5.2 versus 4.7 mEq per liter), this result was entirely because of a lower urinary excretion. In a study of patients with tubulointerstitial disease, the absolute amount of potassium shifted into the cell was greater in patients compared with controls, but the relative amount (expressed as a percentage of total potassium retained) was similar.[100] In contrast, Kahn and colleagues[77] observed a significantly greater rise in serum potassium in patients compared with controls when dietary potassium was increased by 50 mEq per day. This study[77] cannot be strictly compared with others because they relied on 24-hour urinary potassium measurements, and their study reflected a long-term adaptation to a high potassium diet in patients with CKD. In hemodialysis patients, serum potassium rose significantly more in patients than in controls challenged with acute potassium load (1.06 versus 0.39 mEq per liter). However, the baseline potassium was significantly higher in patients than in controls (5.17 versus 3.59 mEq per liter), making the interpretation of this study difficult.[104] More recently, Allon and colleagues[105] noted a similar response in these patients with lower baseline potassium. Finally, the effect of vigorous exercise on serum potassium in hemodialysis patients was similar to the control group.[106] It is reasonable to conclude that the extrarenal cellular uptake of an acute potassium load in CKD patients is near normal.

As discussed previously, internal potassium homeostasis is regulated by insulin, catecholamines, and, to a lesser extent, aldosterone. Although the serum insulin level is increased in renal failure,[106–108] several studies provide strong support for normal insulin-stimulated potassium uptake[106,108,109] by the splanchnic as well as by the peripheral tissues.[109] Alvestrand and coworkers,[109] using the euglycemic insulin clamp technique, demonstrated a similar uptake of potassium by both splanchnic and leg tissues in patients with CKD. The inhibition of endogenous insulin by somatostatin results in a significantly greater rise in serum potassium in uremic rats than in controls (1.0 versus 0.2 mEq per liter at 60 minutes).[110] The administration of glucose with potassium stimulates insulin secretion and attenuates the rise in potassium in patients on dialysis as well as normal controls.[105]

Elevated serum catecholamine levels have been reported in CKD.[106,111,112] Yang and coworkers[113] noted higher mean potassium in patients on propranolol. Infusion of epinephrine resulted in two different responses: In 4 of 10 patients, serum potassium did not fall; in the remaining 6, an exaggerated response was noted. The authors felt that the latter group of patients is those who have a propensity to develop hyperkalemia while on propranolol. Gifford and associates,[114] using a much lower epinephrine dose, could not show a hypokalemic response in patients with ESRD. Plasma aldosterone is normal or high in most CKD patients.[115–119] As noted, patients with ESRD who are taking DOCA, spironolactone, or placebo have similar baseline potassium levels; however, patients on DOCA can dispose an acute potassium load more promptly than the other groups.[45] In addition, ESRD patients on spironolactone have a small but significant rise in serum potassium levels.[48] These studies would support a minor role for aldosterone in internal potassium homeostasis in ESRD patients. In summary, extrarenal potassium homeostasis is near normal in patients with severe renal failure, although a cellular defect in potassium disposal due to abnormal response to catecholamines has been reported in a subgroup of patients on dialysis.

External Potassium Homeostasis in Severe Renal Failure

Renal Adaptation

Patients with a marked decrease in GFR are able to excrete the ingested dietary potassium load and maintain near normal potassium balance. This adaptive process is reflected by an increase in the fractional excretion of potassium (FE_K) modulated by an increase in secretory rate per functioning nephron. However, this adaptive response is limited and a sudden increase in potassium intake may result in life-threatening hyperkalemia. The quantitative aspects as well as the anatomic and functional characteristics of this adaptive response are briefly reviewed herein.

In conscious dogs with a 10% remnant kidney, Schultze and coworkers[119] showed that potassium excretion by the remnant kidney increased fourfold by 18 hours and approached 85% of the control value by the 7th day. Kunau and Whinnery[120] and Wilson and Sonnenberg[103] reported similar data in rats. In experiments by Schultze and associates,[119] animals with a remnant kidney manifested an exaggerated kaliuresis following a potassium load. In contrast to these data and independent of previous potassium intake, dogs with 25% remnant kidney were only able to excrete 30% to 37% of the load in 5 hours compared with 70% to 90% in the control animals.[102] There is no easy resolution to the differences in these two studies.[102,119]

Gonick and colleagues[76] documented that human subjects with CKD were able to excrete only 20% of an oral potassium load in 6 hours compared with 46% in normal controls. Similar data were reported by Perez and colleagues[100] in patients with tubulointerstitial disease. Kahn and colleagues[77] demonstrated in 10 patients with stable chronic kidney disease renal adaptation to increased dietary potassium. In summary, it can be concluded that residual renal tissue is able to maintain external potassium homeostasis in the postabsorptive state. However, the initial phase of this adaptation is impaired when an acute potassium load is administered.

The nephron sites involved in this adaptation have been studied using a variety of techniques in both rats and rabbits and appear to include both the distal convoluted tubule and the collecting duct.[103,119–123] The discrepancies reported in the literature most likely owe to interspecies and intraspecies differences as well as the anatomic definition of different distal tubular segments.

The mechanisms involved in this renal adaptation have been partially defined. In both humans[115] and rodents,[124] aldosterone has been shown to play an important role in the adaptive ability of the diseased kidney to maintain a normal rate of potassium excretion. This renal adaptation has been shown to be independent of dietary sodium intake.[125] Schultze and coworkers[119] argued that aldosterone is not important in the renal potassium adaptation that occurs following a reduction in renal mass, because uremic dogs maintained on constant aldosterone replacement maintained normal rates of potassium excretion. However, the replacement dose of aldosterone in this study was in the high pharmacologic range. Serum potassium concentration itself plays an important role in augmenting urinary potassium excretion.[81] Bourgoignie and colleagues[102] found a direct relationship between serum potassium and both the absolute and fractional potassium excretion (EE_k). The slope of the curve relating serum potassium to the absolute rate of urinary potassium excretion was much steeper in normal dogs than in dogs with a remnant kidney. However, the slope of the curve relating serum potassium to the FE_K was similar in the control and uremic dogs.

Microperfusion studies by Fine and associates[122] indicate that adaptation is an inherent characteristic of the renal tubular cells of uremic animals and, once learned, it can be retained in vitro, at least for short periods of time. Schon and associates[103] showed that augmented potassium excretion is associated with an increase in Na-K-ATPase in the outer medulla in animals subjected to a three-quarter nephrectomy. This increase is quite specific to this enzyme and occurs only in the kidney[103] and the colon.[126] Muto and colleagues[127] demonstrated that an increase in peritubular [K^+] increased renal potassium excretion by also enhancing K^+ conductance (ROMK) and Na^+ conductance (ENaC) in principal cells (Fig. 72.6). Other mechanisms may include a higher rate of potassium delivery and an increase in tubular flow rate in the distal nephron.[120]

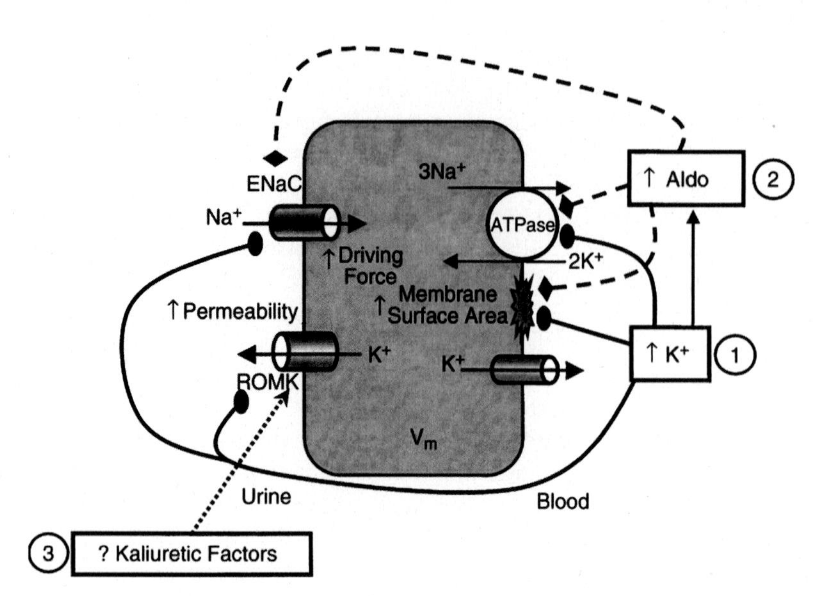

FIGURE 72.6 The major factors that regulate potassium secretion in principal cells. Sodium is reabsorbed across the luminal membrane through ENaC (epithelial sodium channels) with resultant cellular depolarization increasing the electrical driving force for potassium secretion through ROMK (potassium channels). The effects of aldosterone (Aldo) and hyperkalemia (↑K^+) on potassium secretion are noted. (From Gennari FJ, Segal AS. Hyperkalemia: an adaptive response in chronic renal insufficiency. *Kidney Int.* 2002;62:1, with permission.)

Intestinal Potassium Excretion in Renal Failure

Patients with renal failure secrete more potassium in the stool than do normal controls.[115,128,129] Net colonic secretion of potassium is increased significantly above control levels in rats with renal insufficiency.[128] This increase is associated with an increase in Na-K-ATPase activity in colonic mucosa and is functionally similar to the increase seen with the administration of DOCA, glucocorticoids, or high dietary potassium.[130] Although the rise in fecal potassium concentration is significant, the absolute amount of K^+ lost through this route in patients with mild-to-moderate CKD is small and contributes only minimally to the external K^+ homeostasis. In patients with advanced renal insufficiency (GFR < 5 to 10 mL per minute), however, up to 30% to 40% of the ingested potassium load may be excreted in the stool.[129]

Acid–Base Homeostasis in Renal Failure

The ability of the kidney to excrete a hydrogen ion is progressively diminished with the diminution of GFR. A significant decrease in serum bicarbonate does not usually occur until GFR falls below 25 to 30 mL per minute.[75,131] Widmer and colleagues,[132] in 41 ambulatory patients with CKD who had multiple electrolyte measurements over time, noted a serum bicarbonate reduction from 28 to 22 mEq per liter in patients with a moderate renal failure defined as a creatinine level of 2 to 4 mg per deciliter and a further reduction to 19 mEq per liter in patients with a creatinine level of 4 to 14 mg per deciliter. The anion gap remained unchanged in the first group and rose significantly with a further decrease in GFR. This study is criticized for the use of serum creatinine to define severity of renal failure rather than the use of a more accurate measurement of renal function. The concept of orderly progression of metabolic acidosis of renal failure from hyperchloremic to anion gap acidosis, however, occurs in the minority of patients. Wallia and colleagues[133] studied the electrolyte pattern in 70 patients with ESRD just before dialytic therapy was begun. Five patterns were found: 14 patients with normal electrolytes; 14 with anion gap metabolic acidosis; 21 with hyperchloremic acidosis; 11 with mixed hyperchloremic and anion gap acidosis; and 10 with normal serum chloride, low serum bicarbonate, and normal anion gap. This last group, however, had the lowest serum sodium and therefore were relatively hyperchloremic. Therefore, among these 70 patients with ESRD, 31 (44%) had hyperchloremic acidosis, only 14 (20%) had classic anion gap acidosis, and interestingly, another 14 (20%) had normal electrolytes. Patients with an increased anion gap, however, had a slight but significantly higher serum creatinine than patients with pure hyperchloremic acidosis or with normal electrolytes (13.2 versus 10.0 versus 9.0 mg per deciliter, respectively). In addition, these two studies did not support the common impression that hyperchloremic acidosis occurs more often in patients with tubulointerstitial rather than glomerular disease.[132,133] Interestingly, diabetic patients with moderately severe renal failure (GFR < 30 mL per minute) have recently been reported to have milder metabolic acidosis than nondiabetic patients with similar renal function.[134]

Renal tubular acidosis (RTA) defines a group of disorders characterized by the presence of metabolic acidosis out of proportion to the decrease in GFR. The hallmark of these disorders is the presence of significant metabolic acidosis with hyperchloremia and a normal anion gap. Renal tubular acidosis in patients with mild-to-moderate renal insufficiency is often associated with significant hyperkalemia and is discussed later in this chapter.

The Pathophysiology of Metabolic Acidosis in Chronic Kidney Disease

Many studies have shown that acid production in renal failure is normal, and therefore, uremic acidosis reflects a decrease in net acid excretion, defined as the difference between proton excretion in the form of titratable acid and ammonium ion (NH_4^+) and bicarbonate excretion.[135–137] Careful metabolic studies by Goodman and colleagues[137] documented that patients with chronic renal failure have a daily bicarbonate deficit of approximately 13 to 19 mEq. It is notable that despite this persistent deficit, serum bicarbonate in patients with CKD after an initial drop remains stable over long periods of time.[138,139] This is due chiefly to the buffering of excess hydrogen ions by bone buffers, including calcium carbonate.[138]

Renal Excretion of Bicarbonate

Several studies demonstrate that some patients with severe kidney disease have significant bicarbonate wasting.[135,140–144] In an early study by Schwartz and coworkers,[135] three out of four patients with renal failure had significant bicarbonaturia, which disappeared only after the fall of serum bicarbonate to below 20 mEq per liter. In a more detailed study in 17 uremic patients (serum creatinine of 5.6 to 18.9 mg per deciliter), the majority had significant bicarbonate wasting (fractional excretion of HCO_3 of 0% to 17.56%) despite the presence of metabolic acidosis (serum HCO_3 of 16 to 23 mEq per liter). After NH_4Cl loading, serum bicarbonate decreased to below 14 mEq per liter, and bicarbonaturia disappeared in all but four patients.[144] Interestingly, the bicarbonate wasting in these four patients also disappeared with the institution of a low-sodium diet.[144] These two studies support the presence of a diminished maximal tubular reabsorption (T_m) for bicarbonate in the majority of patients with renal failure. Further, they demonstrate that the low T_m is partly responsive to volume status.

Arruda and colleagues[143] and Wong and associates,[145] working with a remnant kidney model in dogs with variable levels of volume expansion and serum bicarbonate, noted that the ratio of absolute bicarbonate to sodium reabsorption was increased in CKD. In addition, Wong and associates,[145] using a micropuncture method, showed that this ratio was also higher at the beginning of the distal tubule, indicating avid bicarbonate absorption by the proximal tubule of the remnant kidney. Although absolute absorption was higher, the absolute amount of bicarbonate delivered to the distal tubule was also higher, reflecting the marked increase in filtered load per nephron owing to an increase in single nephron GFR.[145] In summary, the whole kidney T_m for bicarbonate is, in general, diminished in CKD despite an absolute increase in bicarbonate resorption at the single nephron. The discrepancy in these findings may reflect the variation in the experimental designs and the role of nonvolume regulators in bicarbonate handling by the kidney.

Renal Excretion of Titratable Acid

The excretion of titratable acids chiefly reflects the amount of urinary phosphate and the urinary pH. Most CKD patients are able to maximally acidify their urine,[135,146] and urine-serum PCO_2, as a measure of hydrogen pump activity in the distal tubule, is normal.[147] The amount of titratable acids in these patients is normal.[137,138–150] This is primarily owing to an increase in the fractional excretion of phosphate initiated by secondary hyperparathyroidism. It should be noted, however, that urinary phosphate does decrease with severe renal failure. This reflects both a decrease in dietary phosphate as well as the effect of phosphate binders commonly used in these patients.

Renal Excretion of Ammonium

Although bicarbonaturia may contribute to metabolic acidosis, the major abnormality is a decrease in renal excretion of ammonium. Ammonium is primarily produced by the deamination of amino acids, chiefly glutamine, in the proximal tubule and, to a much lesser extent, in the loop of Henle and the distal convoluted tubule.[130,131] This is reviewed in detail in Chapter 7, Renal Acid–Base Transport and will not be reviewed here. In CKD, fractional renal ammonium excretion initially increases by severalfold, thereby resulting in the maintenance of a normal absolute excretion rate.[151] However, as the GFR decreases below 20 mL per minute, despite a maximal increase in fractional excretion of ammonium, the absolute excretory rate decreases significantly. Thus, progressive metabolic acidosis results. This decrease in the rate of ammonium excretion also reflects a decreased ability of the kidney to trap ammonia in the collecting duct.[146] Warnock[139] has suggested that the decrease in ammonia trapping in the remnant kidney model may be secondary to excess delivery of bicarbonate to the collecting duct, thereby resulting in an unfavorable environment for the diffusion and trapping of ammonia.

The role of aldosterone in ammonium excretion is complex. Aldosterone increases the rate of Na^+-dependent and Na^+-independent H^+ secretion in the cortical and medullary collecting duct.[152,153] Hypoaldosteronism is associated with a decrease in the rate of H^+ secretion, whereas the ability to maintain a steep H^+ gradient between urine and plasma, as measured by urinary pH and urine minus blood PCO_2 in alkaline urine, is not affected.[154,155] The decrease in the rate of H^+ secretion is associated with a decrease in the availability of ammonium buffer in the urine that is not augmented appropriately in response to sodium sulfate infusion.[156,157] Hypoaldosteronism is universally associated with a decreased potassium excretion and hyperkalemia. Hyperkalemia decreases renal ammonium excretion significantly. A decrease in accumulation of ammonium in the renal interstitium despite normal production by the proximal tubule underlies this effect.[158] In the syndrome of hyperkalemic renal tubular acidosis, this mechanism probably plays the major role in the production of hyperchloremic acidosis seen early in the course of renal failure (Fig. 72.7).[159] Reversal of hyperkalemia with sodium binding resin,[160] mineralocorticoids,[161] or low-potassium diet[162] ameliorates the metabolic acidosis by increasing ammonium secretion.

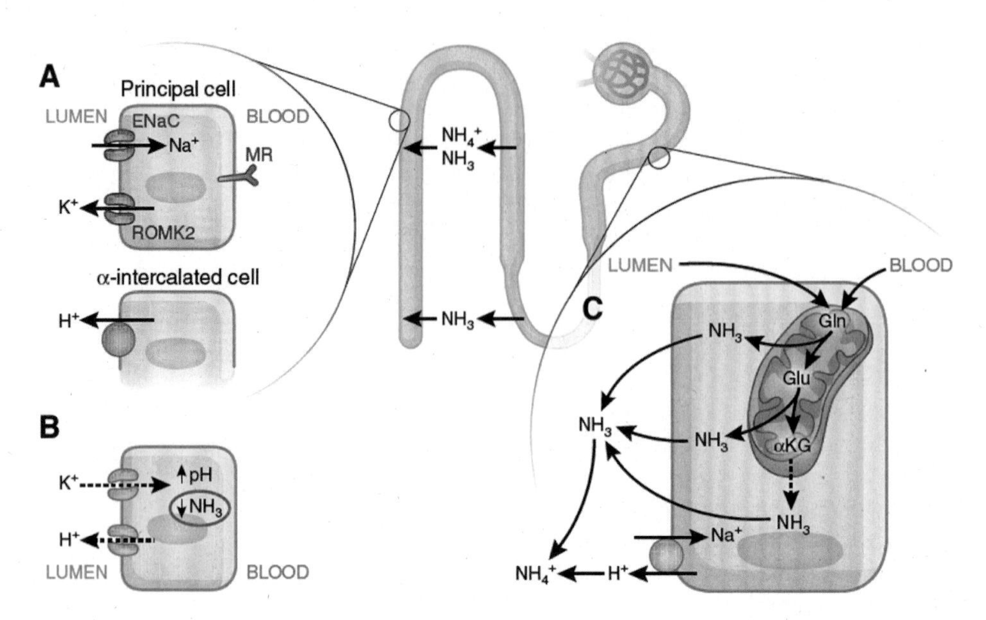

FIGURE 72.7 The factors involved in hyperkalemic acidosis. **A:** ENaC function at the apical surface of principal cells allows potassium secretion by ROMK (potassium channels) and the hydrogen ion by adjacent intercalated cells. **B:** Hyperkalemia increases intracellular pH by proton exchange, impairing the enzyme involved in ammoniagenesis. **C:** The process of ammoniagenesis involves deamination of glutamine, which allows ammonia to buffer the hydrogen ion in the urine. Ammonia and ammonium are reabsorbed in the medullary loop and are then excreted in the urine in the distal nephron. (From Karet FE. Mechanisms in hyperkalemic renal tubular acidosis. *J Am Soc Nephrol.* 2009;20:251, with permission.)

In summary, the metabolic acidosis develops universally in all patients with CKD as GFR decreases to below 20 mL per minute. The pathogenesis of this disorder is complex and reflects renal defect in both resorption as well as the generation of bicarbonate. The major mechanism, however, is in a decrease in absolute ammonia excretion despite the presence of acidosis.

HYPERKALEMIC RENAL TUBULAR ACIDOSIS OWING TO A DEFECT IN RENIN–ANGIOTENSIN–ALDOSTERONE AXIS OR TUBULAR UNRESPONSIVENESS TO ALDOSTERONE

Although a decrease in GFR may be associated with the development of significant hyperkalemia and hyperchloremic (HCA) or anion gap metabolic acidosis, this usually occurs only with severe reductions in GFR, below 15 to 20 mL per minute. However, some patients with underlying renal disease and mild-to-moderate azotemia present with striking hyperkalemia with or without HCA. The elevated serum potassium in these patients is primarily owing to a disturbance in the renin–angiotensin–aldosterone axis or to renal tubular responsiveness to aldosterone (see Fig. 72.6 and Table 72.2). Since the report by Hudson and associates,[163] numerous cases have been described in which hyperkalemia with or without HCA developed in the presence of only mild-to-moderate renal insufficiency.[164] The majority of these cases are diabetic or hypertensive nephropathy or chronic interstitial nephritis.[165] In 1972, Schambelan and colleagues[166] presented evidence linking hypoaldosteronism with hyporreninism in six patients with this syndrome. This association was verified in subsequent reports,[167–170] and the entity became known as hyporeninemic hypoaldosteronism (HHA). However, it quickly became clear that a significant minority of these patients had normal renin levels. DeFronzo,[171] in 1980, after reviewing 81 published cases, came to the conclusion that in 20% of cases the low plasma aldosterone levels could not be explained by renin deficiency, and therefore a primary abnormality in aldosterone synthesis had to be postulated. At the same time, some patients with sickle cell disease,[172,173] systemic lupus erythematosus,[174–177] and renal transplantation[178–180] have a renal tubular secretory defect resulting in hyperkalemia despite a normal renin–aldosterone axis. Therefore, at the present time, these patients can be divided into two large categories: (1) hyperkalemia resulting from hypoaldosteronism with or without hyporreninism; and (2) hyperkalemia resulting from a primary renal tubular potassium secretory defect. One could consider this entity as a spectrum ranging from pure aldosterone deficiency with normal tubular responsiveness to severe tubular resistance with normal aldosterone secretion. Between these two extremes there are many overlapping presentations in which either the defect in the hormonal axis or the tubular responsiveness dominates. Although Table 72.2 summarizes all the hormonal or tubular defects that can lead to hyperkalemia,

TABLE 72.2 **Etiology of Chronic Hyperkalemia Due to Disturbances in Renal Potassium Excretion**

I. Decrease in GFR
  A. Acute renal failure
  B. Chronic kidney disease (GFR $<$ 15–20 mL/min)
II. Defect in renal tubular secretion of potassium
  A. Disturbance in the renin–angiotensin–aldosterone axis
    1. Hyporeninism: associated with renal insufficiency (diabetes mellitus, interstitial nephritis)
    2. Disturbance in angiotensin II activation or function (captopril, saralasin)
    3. Hypoaldosteronism
      a. With glucocorticoid deficiency (Addison disease, enzyme deficiency)
      b. Block in aldosterone synthesis (heparin, 18-methyloxidase deficiency)
      c. Primary hypoaldosteronism
  B. Tubular resistance to the action of aldosterone (renal tubular hyperkalemia)
    1. Pseudohypoaldosteronism
    2. Hyperkalemia, hypertension, and normal renal function
    3. Hyperkalemia with mild-to-moderate renal insufficiency and variable plasma aldosterone levels (sickle cell disease, systemic lupus erythematosus, renal transplant, obstructive uropathy, miscellaneous)
    4. Pharmacologic inhibition of the tubular action of aldosterone (spironolactone, eplerenone, triamterene, amiloride, pentamidine, trimethoprim) in distal nephron

GFR, glomerular filtration rate.

often with HCA, our discussion is limited to the disturbances associated with renal insufficiency.

Hyperkalemic Renal Tubular Acidosis Owing to a Defect in Renin–Angiotensin–Aldosterone Axis

This group comprises approximately 80% of the patients with renal insufficiency and hyperkalemia.[171,181–183] The hallmark of this group is a low plasma aldosterone concentration. The majority (80%) of this group also has low plasma renin activity (PRA) and therefore represents the classic syndrome of HHA. However, 20% have a normal PRA. Clinically and physiologically, these patients present with fairly uniform features. Several large series[166,184] have defined the characteristics of these patients first summarized in a review by DeFronzo.[171] These include: (1) a mean age of about 60 years, (2) the presence of diabetes mellitus in about 50%, (3) the presence of mild-to-moderate renal failure in the majority, and (4) a lack of symptoms referable to hyperkalemia in 75%. Physiologic features include: (1) low or low-normal baseline and/or stimulated aldosterone levels, (2) normal plasma cortisol, (3) low baseline and/or stimulated renin values in 80%, (4) normal aldosterone response to angiotensin or adrenocorticotropic hormone (ACTH) stimulation in the minority, (5) presence of hyperchloremic acidosis in well over 50%, and (6) a lack of significant salt wasting.

To gain an understanding of the physiologic basis of this syndrome, we initially review the defect in renin secretion and then summarize our present understanding of aldosterone deficiency in this syndrome.

Hyporreninism

At present, no single abnormality can explain the low PRA seen in 80% of these patients.[171,182,183] Evidence has been presented in support of a defect in one or more physiologic regulators of renin secretion including volume, autonomic nervous system, serum potassium concentration, and prostaglandins.

Oh and colleagues,[169] Perez and colleagues,[185] and others[186,187] have demonstrated that long-term sodium and volume depletion in these patients is associated with a significant increase in the PRA. However, comparable data in normal controls with the same degree of volume depletion were not provided. In the report of Oh and colleagues,[169] after 3 to 6 weeks of salt depletion, the PRA rose into the normal range, but plasma aldosterone remained subnormal. In the study by Chan and coworkers, 8 of the 12 patients with hyporreninism responded to 2 weeks of furosemide with an increase in PRA without a similar response in plasma aldosterone.[187] In a study of four patients with acute postinfectious glomerulonephritis,[155] plasma renin and aldosterone concentrations were low during the acute phase, but returned to normal following recovery from acute nephritis. Interestingly, in two patients, the renin and aldosterone levels remained low during the acute phase despite an excellent response to diuretics. These two patients, however, responded appropriately to physiologic doses of fludrocortisone. This study,[155] coupled with previous studies of acute glomerulonephritis,[188,189] supports the concept that although physiologic suppression of the renin–aldosterone axis by volume expansion may play a significant role in certain patients with glomerular disease, hypertension, and edema, other factors such as decreased GFR and damage to the juxtaglomerular apparatus play an important contributory role. Gordon and colleagues[190] have described a patient with hypertension, acidosis, hyperkalemia, and normal renal function associated with HHA. Prolonged sodium restriction resulted in a correction of these abnormalities. A similar pathophysiologic mechanism has been postulated in hypertensive patients with hyperkalemia and renal insufficiency.[191]

The autonomic nervous system plays an important physiologic role in the regulation of renin secretion. Sympathetic nerve terminals are known to innervate the juxtaglomerular apparatus, and renin secretion is stimulated by epinephrine.[192,193] Therefore, autonomic insufficiency could result in a state of hyporreninemia. This hypothesis has been investigated primarily in diabetic patients, in whom autonomic neuropathy is common and circulating catecholamine levels are often low.[194] In five diabetic patients with autonomic neuropathy, Tuck and colleagues[195] reported low basal PRA as well as diminished plasma aldosterone and norepinephrine concentrations. In addition, the infusion of isoproterenol, a β-adrenergic agonist, did not increase PRA, indicating a possible block at or beyond the receptor level. In contrast, normal circulating catecholamine levels have previously been reported in diabetic patients with the syndrome of hypoaldosteronism.[154,167,196,197] Fernandez-Cruz and coworkers[198] compared stimulated PRA in 16 normotensive diabetic patients without overt nephropathy and 9 age-matched controls. The stimulated PRA was significantly lower in these patients and correlated directly with the degree of autonomic dysfunction as measured by the velocity of esophageal peristalsis. de Chatel and colleagues,[199] however, were unable to demonstrate in a large group of diabetic individuals any correlation between the plasma epinephrine concentration and abnormalities in the renin–aldosterone axis. Therefore, although autonomic neuropathy may play a role in the development of hypoaldosteronism in some diabetic patients, it is not a uniform finding and certainly cannot explain the occurrence of this syndrome in nondiabetic patients.

Hyperkalemia is known to inhibit PRA[200]; consequently, one could hypothesize that hyporreninemia is not a primary defect but is secondary to hyperkalemia. In two studies,[166,170] short-term normalization of serum potassium did not increase PRA significantly; however, long-term studies have not been undertaken to examine this very important question.

Prostaglandins E_2, I_2, and D_2 are known stimulators of renin release,[201,202] whereas prostaglandins E_1 and E_2 directly increase aldosterone biosynthesis in vitro.[203] Furthermore, hyperkalemia has been reported following treatment with indomethacin, a potent prostaglandin inhibitor[204] as well as selective cyclooxygenase-2 (COX-2) inhibitors,[205] suggesting that a defect in prostaglandin synthesis may play a role in the development of HHA in some hyperkalemic patients. Consistent with this possibility, Tan and colleagues[206] found a strong correlation between urinary PGE_2 levels and the ratio of active to inactive renin in normal controls and in patients with the syndrome of hypoaldosteronism. In four of the nine patients, low urinary PGE_2 was associated with a low ratio of active to inactive renin. In normal controls, the inhibition of prostaglandin synthesis with indomethacin resulted in a similar decrease in this ratio. These authors postulated that prostaglandins may play a critical role in the activation of renin, and therefore hypoaldosteronism in these patients may be secondary to a prostaglandin deficiency. In two patients with diabetes mellitus and hypoaldosteronism, the total renin concentration was normal, whereas PRA was low.[207] The fractionation of the plasma yielded an inactive renin precursor (prorenin or "big renin"); unfortunately, prostaglandin levels were not measured in these diabetic patients. It should be noted, however, that other investigators have failed to find an association between prostaglandin deficiency and the development of HHA.[208]

Another hypothesis that links CKD with hyporreninism is fibrosis of the juxtaglomerular apparatus owing to intrinsic renal disease. Although occasional reports of juxtaglomerular apparatus fibrosis have appeared,[187] this is a rare finding. Besides, the presence of juxtaglomerular apparatus damage alone does not explain the development of hypoaldosteronism.

Hyperfiltration hypothesis has been linked to the development of HHA in both diabetic and nondiabetic CKD patients.[209] According to this hypothesis, as the number of nephrons is reduced, there is an adaptive increase in the renal plasma flow and GFR by the remaining functioning glomeruli. These alterations in renal hemodynamics serve to inhibit renin synthesis and release, leading secondarily to the development of hypoaldosteronism.

Hypoaldosteronism

The hallmark of the syndrome of HHA is a low basal or low stimulated plasma aldosterone level in spite of normal levels of glucocorticoids and other ACTH-dependent steroids such as DOCA or corticosterone. Aldosterone secretion is primarily stimulated by the renin–angiotensin system. However, ACTH and serum potassium, as well as other regulators, play independent roles.

As stated previously, hyporreninemia is present in 80% of patients with hypoaldosteronism,[171,179,183] and therefore it is logical to consider that the primary defect in these patients lies in renin synthesis or release. Schambelan and colleagues[183] showed that the stimulation of renin by volume contraction resulted in a rise in plasma aldosterone that was appropriate for the increase in PRA. The slope of the curve relating plasma renin and aldosterone was similar in patients with HHA and normal controls. Surprisingly, for any given level of PRA, the plasma aldosterone concentration was disproportionately elevated, probably because of the independent stimulatory effect of plasma potassium on aldosterone secretion. Nevertheless, the highest levels of renin and aldosterone achieved in these patients were comparable only to the basal levels in control subjects. In contrast, as indicated, other investigators have found a clear disconnect between renin and aldosterone level after stimulation with volume depletion[185–187] and captopril.[187] In all studies, however, the response of aldosterone was significantly blunted despite increased renin and persistent hyperkalemia. In addition, most investigators have reported a marked impairment in the ability of angiotensin II (AT-II) to stimulate aldosterone secretion.[171,183] This finding, coupled with a subnormal aldosterone response to ACTH stimulation, and the failure of hyperkalemia to stimulate aldosterone secretion, has strengthened the possibility of a primary adrenal defect in some patients with hypoaldosteronism. This is further supported by the observation that 20% of patients with hypoaldosteronism have normal PRA.[171,179,183] It is possible that the poor response of aldosterone to ACTH, AT-II, and hyperkalemia may be secondary to long-term atrophy of the zona glomerulosa of the adrenal gland rather than to a specific enzymatic defect in aldosterone production. Consistent with this possibility, Fredlund and colleagues[210] provided evidence in isolated adrenal glomerulosa cells that the aldosterone response to hyperkalemia is dependent on the circulating angiotensin level. However, no study so far has evaluated the response of the adrenal gland to prolonged stimulation by AT-II in patients.

The serum potassium concentration is an important regulator of the plasma aldosterone level.[211–213] In nephrectomized patients, a significant correlation between serum potassium and plasma aldosterone exists,[214] and this relationship is independent of renin or ACTH. Therefore, in interpreting a given plasma aldosterone level, the effect of serum potassium must be considered. Schambelan and colleagues[183] categorized 31 patients into two groups based on the ratio of urinary aldosterone excretion to serum potassium concentration. Group A (23 patients) had a low ratio and was considered to have hypoaldosteronism. Group B (8 patients) had a normal ratio and was considered to have a primary tubular defect in potassium secretion. In group A, 20% had a normal PRA. Therefore, hypoaldosteronism in this group, in spite of normal PRA and high plasma potassium, is probably owing to a defect in aldosterone synthesis.

Another regulator of aldosterone secretion and plasma volume is atrial natriuretic factor (ANF). ANF has been shown to be a strong inhibitor of baseline as well as stimulated aldosterone in humans.[215,216] In normal humans, ANF also prevents a potassium-stimulated rise in the aldosterone level.[217] In addition, the ANF level is markedly elevated 10- to 50-fold in patients with hypoaldosteronism.[217] Although the rise in ANF (and the suppression of aldosterone) could be secondary to volume expansion, ANF also suppresses potassium, angiotensin, and ACTH-stimulated aldosterone secretion, supporting the presence of a common cellular mechanism for its action possibly through the stimulation of cyclic guanosine monophosphate (cGMP).[218]

Several investigators have explored the possibility of an enzymatic defect in aldosterone biosynthesis,[185,197,200] and an enzymatic block involving the conversion of 18-hydroxycorticosterone to aldosterone has been postulated, but these findings have not been supported by other studies.[219,220]

As indicated, diabetic patients constitute a large percentage of patients with HHA. To explain this high incidence, two other postulates have been presented. Insulin is an important regulator of potassium uptake by a variety of tissues, and chronic hypoinsulinemia (absolute or relative) might be expected to result in a state of intracellular potassium deficiency. Furthermore, intracellular potassium concentration is an important regulator of aldosterone synthesis.[171] Potassium-deficient cultured zona glomerulosa cells have a blunted aldosterone response to AT-II and ACTH.[210,221] Insulinopenia, by decreasing intracellular potassium, may lead to a defect in aldosterone synthesis and the syndrome of hypoaldosteronism. A second hypothesis is offered by Smith and DeFronzo[222] and involves the concept of tubuloglomerular feedback. Normal tubuloglomerular balance is disrupted in the presence of osmotic agents in the renal tubule,[223,224] including glucose.[225–227] It is postulated that, in diabetic patients with a high filtered glucose load, sodium chloride delivery out of the proximal tubule is enhanced, leading to an increased delivery of solute to the loop of Henle. Enhanced chloride reabsorption by the thick ascending limb of Henle (TALH) may inhibit renin secretion,[228] which secondarily leads to the development of hypoaldosteronism.

In summary, at present, a unified etiologic hypothesis cannot explain the occurrence of the syndrome of HHA in different patients. It is likely that this syndrome is quite heterogeneous and can be explained only by multiple etiologic abnormalities. In a given patient, the role of different regulatory systems (i.e., volume status, prostaglandins, ANF, autonomic nervous system, structural damage to the juxtaglomerular apparatus, enzymatic defects in aldosterone and renin biosynthesis, and intracellular adrenal potassium deficiency) should be considered and evaluated.

Hyperkalemic Renal Tubular Acidosis Owing to a Renal Tubular Secretory Defect

This group of disorders (see Table 72.2 and Fig. 72.8) includes patients who have hyperkalemia out of proportion to the degree of renal failure or hypoaldosteronism. The primary defect is a partial resistance to the physiologic effect of aldosterone to promote potassium secretion. Perez and coworkers[229] named this syndrome renal tubular hyperkalemia and divided it into three groups: group I, patients with pseudohypoaldosteronism; group II, patients with hyperkalemia, hypertension, and normal renal function; and group III, patients with hyperkalemia, mild-to-moderate renal insufficiency, and normal-plasma aldosterone (group IIIa), low-plasma aldosterone (group IIIb), or high-plasma aldosterone (IIIc) (Table 72.2).

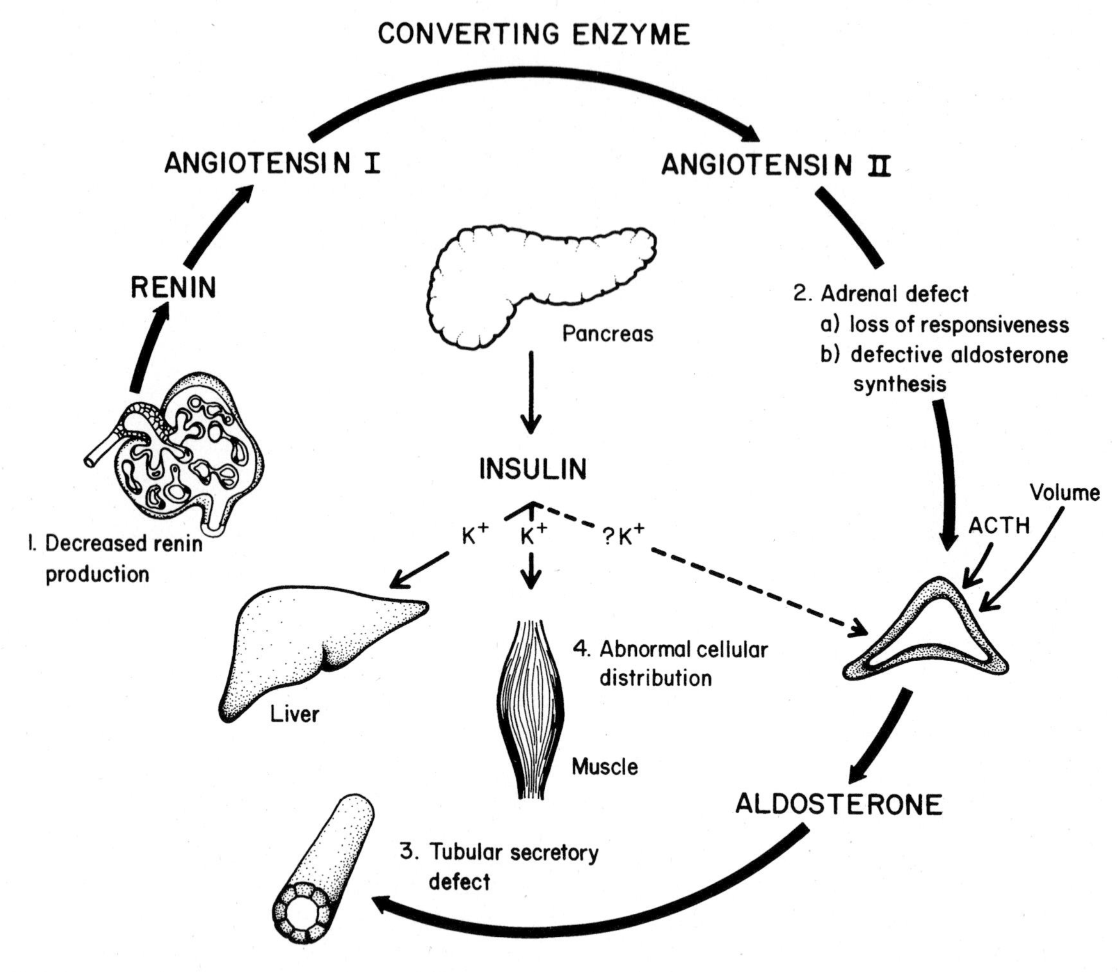

FIGURE 72.8 A schematic representation of potential hormonal, renal, and extrarenal defects resulting in hyperkalemia. Hyperkalemia may result from one of the following conditions: (**1**) decreased renin production, (**2**) decreased aldosterone production despite normal renin secretion (adrenal defect), (**3**) a renal tubular secretory defect, or (**4**) an abnormal distribution of potassium between intracellular and extracellular fluid compartments. ACTH, adrenocorticotropic hormone. (From DeFronzo RA, et al. Nonuremic hypokalemia: a possible role for insulin deficiency. *Arch Intern Med.* 1979;137:842, with permission.)

Groups I and II represent examples of a pure tubular secretory defect without renal insufficiency and are not discussed here. In this section we deal only with group III patients, who present with mild-to-moderate renal insufficiency, hyperkalemia, hyperchloremic acidosis, variable plasma renin and aldosterone levels, and resistance to physiologic doses of mineralocorticoids. This clinical entity has been described in patients with sickle cell disease, systemic lupus erythematosus, renal transplant, obstructive uropathy, AIDS, and a group of miscellaneous diseases including lead nephropathy and chronic interstitial nephritis.

Sickle Cell Disease

A renal tubular potassium secretory defect in sickle cell disease was first reported in patients with normal renal function and normal serum electrolyte concentrations[7] and, later, in patients with sickle cell nephropathy,[171,230] sickle cell trait,[172] and sickle cell disease.[173] Although basal and stimulated aldosterone levels were normal in all subjects, these patients were unable to excrete a potassium load normally. The infusion of potassium chloride, sodium sulfate, and furosemide failed to augment potassium secretion normally. This defect is thought to result from ischemic damage to the collecting tubules and medullary area by sickle cells. An immunologic reaction against a renal tubular antigen also has been suggested. It should be noted that the syndrome of HHA also occurs in sickle cell disease.[171,230]

Systemic Lupus Erythematosus

Patients with systemic lupus erythematosus (SLE) may have multiple tubular defects, including type I and IV RTA.[176,177] In the largest study of 30 patients with active SLE, 18 patients had defects in the handling of potassium, sodium, and/or hydrogen ions. Eight patients had distal renal tubular acidosis (dRTA) due to an isolated proton secretory defect. Five had dRTA of the gradient or acid back leak type.

Three had voltage-dependent dRTA. One individual had hyporeninemic hypoaldosteronism and one had dRTA plus hypoaldosteronism. Clinically, patients with the abnormal tubular study results more often presented with nephritis or nephrotic sediment, peripheral edema, or anemia.[176] A defect in potassium secretion, similar to the defect in sickle cell disease, has also been reported in several patients with SLE.[174,175] The defect is often accompanied by a defect in hydrogen ion secretion.[174,175,231] In a study of two patients with SLE and hyperkalemic RTA, Bastani and associates[232] showed the presence of autoantibodies to collecting duct cells in one patient. The serum from the patient with autoantibodies labeled the intercalated cell in rat kidney section. However, the serum from both patients did not react with the affinity-purified bovine H^+ATPase or human H^+ATPase beta subunit. This is in contrast to the finding in a single patient with Sjögren syndrome who had an absence of vacuolar H^+ATPase in intercalated cells.[233] These findings support the concept that cellular and molecular mechanisms in these patients probably are heterogeneous in nature.

Obstructive Uropathy

Hyperkalemic RTA, as a complication of obstructive uropathy, is common and best described in a report of 13 patients by Batlle and associates.[181] Two patterns were noted: (1) Five patients had normal plasma aldosterone levels but failed to increase urinary potassium excretion after the administration of acetazolamide, fludrocortisone, and sodium sulfate. The primary defect in this group is renal tubular unresponsiveness to aldosterone. (2) Eight patients had low plasma aldosterone levels but failed to augment renal potassium excretion with mineralocorticoid administration. As noted, this reflects a combined defect in this group. Furthermore, urinary acidification in response to systemic acidosis and sodium sulfate infusion was abnormal in 8 of 13 patients. In a rat model of acute ureteral obstruction, no change in the number or tubular distribution of vacuolar H^+ATPase was noted; however, the intracellular distribution was changed with a significant decrease in plasma membrane bound pumps in intercalated cells.[234] This finding may explain hyperchloremic metabolic acidosis (HMA), which is commonly noted in these patients.

Renal Transplantation

In the precyclosporine era, hyperkalemia was a relatively unusual phenomenon following a successful renal transplantation.[179,180,235] However, two series from Australia and the United States[179,180] and a series from Israel[236] have reported the occurrence of renal tubular hyperkalemia in this group. In the largest series, 23 of 75 patients with a successful kidney transplant had hyperkalemia unrelated to rejection episodes, renal failure, oliguria, or acidosis.[180] The renin–angiotensin–aldosterone axis was normal in these patients, and hyperkalemia did not respond to furosemide. The hyperkalemia was transient, disappearing spontaneously, and did not correlate with clinical or laboratory evidence of rejection. In contrast, in two patients studied by Batlle and coworkers,[235] hyperkalemia was associated with very low levels of aldosterone, which did not respond to volume contraction. Urinary potassium was low and did not respond to the infusion of sodium sulfate or acetazolamide. The etiology of this disorder is not clear, but immunologic damage to the renal tubular cells is postulated.[180] In the cyclosporine era, hyperkalemia is more common in kidney transplant recipients.[180,237,238]

In a study of 12 transplant patients on cyclosporine, Kamel et al.[238] noted low renin and aldosterone levels associated with a poor response to fludrocortisone. Transtubular potassium gradients (TTKGs), however, rose significantly with bicarbonaturia initiated with acetazolamide, supporting the hypothesis that a tubular defect was due to an inability to generate a favorable electrical and chemical gradient in the cortical collecting duct.[238] In a recent series of 567 transplant patients for more than 12 months and GFR $>$ 40 mL per minute, RTA was diagnosed in 76 (13%). Using standard tools including urine pH, urine anion gap, as well as bicarbonate loading, the authors divided the group as follows: 28 (37%) with classical RTA, 11 (14%) with classical RTA but with elevated potassium, and 37 (49%) with type IV RTA (some with normal potassium). In multivariate analysis, the presence of RTA correlated with lower GFR, higher parathyroid hormone (PTH) level, the use of tacrolimus, and renin–angiotensin blockers. It was estimated that the use of renin–angiotensin blockers accounted for 25% of patients with RTA.[180]

Hyperkalemic Renal Tubular Acidosis Associated with AIDS

Acid–base and electrolyte disturbances, with or without renal failure, are common in patients with AIDS. As reviewed by Perazella and Brown,[239] the incidence varies from 5% to 53% and is owing to a variety of causes including adrenal insufficiency, renal failure, type IV RTA, and finally as a complication of drugs used in these patients.[240] The syndrome of hyporenin–hypoaldosteronism is relatively uncommon and usually is associated with HIV-related nephropathy. Patients with AIDS are exposed to a variety of drugs that could result in hyperkalemia, which is often associated with HCA and/or renal insufficiency.

Miscellaneous Conditions

Renal tubular hyperkalemia has been reported in a variety of other renal diseases. These include chronic interstitial nephritis of unknown etiology,[241] nephrosclerosis,[184] diabetes mellitus,[183] postinfectious glomerulonephritis,[188,189] lead nephropathy,[242] and drug-induced acute interstitial nephritis.[243] Although in our experience this entity seems to be relatively common in nonspecific interstitial nephritis, no incidence or prevalence data are available.

Drugs Associated with Hyperkalemia in Patients with Kidney Disease

In patients with underlying kidney disease, prescribed drugs or over-the-counter medications and supplements play an increasingly dominant role in the development of hyperkalemia. It is therefore important to recognize that a variety of products are capable of elevating serum potassium concentration through multiple mechanisms (Table 72.3). Hyperkalemia, depending on the criteria used, has been reported to develop in anywhere from 1.3% to 10% of patients and is often multifactorial. Of the many factors involved, culprit medications, either alone or in association with other disturbances in potassium homeostasis, were a contributing cause of hyperkalemia in 35% to 75% of hospitalized patients.[244–248] Of note, kidney disease and older age (> 60 years) were important predisposing risk factors in many studies.[244–246]

Increased Potassium Input

Enteral and parenteral inputs of potassium are very common causes of hyperkalemia in hospitalized patients. Nonetheless, chronic hyperkalemia does not occur with these products unless an underlying defect in potassium homeostasis also is present. Deliberate potassium intake often lies at the root of hyperkalemia, although unsuspected potassium delivery also occurs. A 3.6% incidence of hyperkalemia among 4,921 patients taking physician-prescribed potassium supplements was documented in the Boston Collaborative Drug

TABLE 72.3 Common Drugs That Cause Hyperkalemia and the Mechanism of Action

Medication	Mechanism of Action
Potassium supplement	Increase intake
Salt substitutes	Increase intake
Nutritional/herbal supplements	Increase intake
β_2-blocking agents	Decrease potassium movement into cells, decrease renin/aldosterone
Digoxin intoxication	Decrease Na^+-K^+-ATPase activity
Lysine, arginine, and ε-aminocaproic acid	Shift of potassium out of cells
Succinylcholine	Shift of potassium out of cells
Potassium-sparing diuretics	
Spironolactone, eplerenone, drospirenone	Aldosterone antagonism
Triamterene	Block Na^+ channels in principal cells
Amiloride	Block Na^+ channels in principal cells
NSAIDs, COX-2 selective inhibitors	Decrease renin/aldosterone Decrease RBF and GFR
ACE inhibitors and AT-II	Decrease aldosterone synthesis
receptor antagonists	Decrease RBF and GFR
Heparin	Decrease aldosterone synthesis
Trimethoprim and pentamidine	Block Na^+ channels in principal cells
Cyclosporine and tacrolimus	Decrease aldosterone synthesis Decrease Na^+-K^+-ATPase activity Decrease K^+ channel activity

NSAIDs, nonsteroidal anti-inflammatory drugs; COX-2, cyclooxygenase-2; GFR, glomerular filtration rate; ACE, angiotensin-converting enzyme; AT-II, angiotensin II.

Surveillance Program.[244] The mean peak K^+ concentration in these patients was 6.0 mEq per liter, whereas a level greater than 7.5 mEq per liter was noted in 13 of the 179 patients (7.3%). Azotemia and older age were more frequent among those with hyperkalemia. In addition, several other studies reveal that potassium supplements cause or contribute to hyperkalemia in 15% to 40% of hospitalized patients.[245–248]

The new *Dietary Guidelines for Americans* stresses the importance of reducing sodium intake and increasing dietary potassium. As a result, food manufacturers have focused on meeting these guidelines by replacing sodium in their products with potassium-based alternatives. Potassium salt substitutes and alternatives, which provide a rich source of potassium, are not new but are recently receiving a second look from food processors.[249] Pressure exerted by the government and public health advocates to reduce dietary sodium has led the food industry to experiment with salt substitutes. Manufacturers also assert that improved product formulas significantly reduce the metallic aftertaste often noted with potassium chloride, thereby making it more palatable. Some potassium salt substitutes contain 10 to 13 mEq of potassium per gram.[250]

A number of nutritional supplements contain as much as 49 to 54 mEq of potassium per liter, whereas foods prepared as low sodium contain greater amounts of potassium (because potassium replaces sodium in these foods). As a result, enteral feeds employing these products and some herbal remedies, such as noni juice (K^+, 56.3 mEq per liter) can deliver excessive amounts of potassium to patients with impaired potassium homeostasis.[251] An emerging source of potassium in foods is so-called "enhanced" fresh meat, which is injected with a solution of water with sodium and potassium salts. Food companies claim that this salt-based injection ensures that meat will be tender and tasty despite how it is cooked by the consumer. In an analysis of the potassium content of 36 fresh meat products purchased from local grocery stores, enhanced products often contained 2 to 3 times more potassium than comparable cuts of nonenhanced meat.[252] Most concerning was the absence of potassium content on most labels.

Another unsuspected source of potassium excess in the hospital includes the antibiotic penicillin G potassium (1.7 mEq of K^+ per 1 million units), which can cause hyperkalemia if administered in sufficiently high doses.[254] The urinary alkalinizing agent potassium citrate (2 mEq of potassium per 1 mL), and packed red blood cells transfused after 10 or more days of storage (7.5 to 13 mEq of K^+ per liter) can precipitate hyperkalemia in at risk patients.[255,256] A potassium-containing cardioplegia solution employed during cardiac surgery may also cause hyperkalemia in patients with a defect in potassium handling.

Impaired Cellular Potassium Homeostasis

As discussed previously, the cellular uptake of a potassium load is the primary mechanism by which the body acutely prevents the development of hyperkalemia. Several commonly prescribed drugs can impair this protective cellular response. β-Adrenergic–blocking drugs through the inhibition of renin secretion as well as cellular uptake of potassium have been associated with the development of mild and, on rare occasions, life-threatening hyperkalemia.[257,258] Hyperkalemia often develops rapidly, as one would expect with the disruption of cellular potassium homeostasis, but rarely develops in the absence of heavy exercise or other risk factors for hyperkalemia.[3,258] As an example, three renal transplant recipients developed severe hyperkalemia (K^+ range 6.0 to 8.3 mEq per liter) within hours of treatment with intravenous labetalol.[259] Most studies evaluating hyperkalemia in hospitalized patients have shown that β-adrenergic blockers have caused or at least contributed to hyperkalemia in anywhere from 4% to 17% of patients.[248,260–262] Not unexpectedly, the hyperkalemic potential of β-adrenergic blockers is increased by underlying renal insufficiency, the coexistence of diabetes mellitus or hypoaldosteronism, and concurrent therapy with other medications that reduce renal potassium excretion.[256,257]

Digoxin, by blocking the Na-K-ATPase pump function, has also been demonstrated to disrupt potassium homeostasis.[263] As a result of this effect, the impaired cellular uptake of potassium as well as reduced renal potassium excretion occurs. In general, therapeutic digoxin levels do not lead to hyperkalemia but, in rare circumstances, can be a contributing factor.[263] Nonetheless, digoxin intoxication will result in hyperkalemia, which at times is fatal.[263,264]

Both natural (lysine, arginine) and synthetic (ε-aminocaproic acid) amino acids have been associated with hyperkalemia.[265–269] This is owing to the shift of potassium out of cells.[265–269] Levinsky and colleagues[265] demonstrated lysine uptake into isolated rat muscle within 1 hour in an amount equivalent to the potassium lost from the muscle tissue. In intact animals, the infusion of lysine was associated with hyperkalemia, with a 1.0 to 1.5 mEq per liter rise in plasma K^+ concentration noted for every 10 mEq per liter increase in plasma lysine concentration.[266] Hyperkalemia has also been described with intravenous arginine administration.[267–269] In normal humans, serum potassium increased by approximately 1 mEq per liter following the infusion of 30 to 60 g of arginine, whereas patients with ESRD developed a mean increase in serum K^+ of 1.5 mEq per liter at 2 hours after 30 g of intravenous arginine.[268] In two patients with mild renal insufficiency and liver disease, K^+ concentrations were 7.5 and 7.1 mmol per liter, respectively, after the infusion of arginine.[269] Serum potassium concentrations increased as early as 45 minutes after arginine infusion and peaked between 2 to 6 hours following injection, bespeaking a disturbance in cellular potassium homeostasis.[268,269] Hyperkalemia can also develop in subjects treated with the synthetic amino acid, ε-aminocaproic acid, which is structurally similar to both lysine and arginine.[270] A study in nephrectomized dogs demonstrated a significant rise in serum K^+ in animals administered intravenous ε-aminocaproic acid as either a constant infusion (2 or 4 g per hour) or a bolus injection of 2.5 g.[270] Clinical relevance in humans was demonstrated in a case report where hyperkalemia (potassium, 6.7 mEq per liter) developed acutely in a patient with chronic renal insufficiency treated with ε-aminocaproic acid (three boluses of 10 g) to reduce perioperative blood loss during cardiac surgery.[271] The rapid onset of hyperkalemia following ε-aminocaproic acid therapy in this patient suggested that a cellular release of potassium was the cause of this electrolyte disturbance. In addition, Perazella and coworkers[272] in a retrospective study in patients undergoing cardiac surgery noted higher intraoperative serum potassium concentrations (K^+, 5.9 mEq per liter) in 232 patients treated with intravenous ε-aminocaproic acid as compared with 371 well-matched controls (K^+, 5.5 mEq per liter) who did not receive this medication. Other possible confounding factors did not explain the rapid development of hyperkalemia in these patients. It is therefore likely that intravenous ε-aminocaproic acid causes hyperkalemia through the cellular release of potassium in exchange for this synthetic amino acid.

The anesthetic agent succinylcholine, by the depolarization of the cell membrane, can cause hyperkalemia.[273–275] A rapid cellular potassium leak induced by these agents, resulting in the abrupt onset of hyperkalemia, has been demonstrated in muscle preparations in intact animals and humans. Plasma K^+ increased by 0.5 mEq per liter within 3 to 5 minutes in patients with normal muscle, whereas increases as high as 3.0 mEq per liter occurred in patients afflicted by trauma or nervous system disease.[4,300] In 12 patients with renal insufficiency, plasma K^+ concentration rose by 1.2 mEq per liter in one patient and up to 0.7 mEq per liter in the rest.[275]

An interesting study that examined the effect of the dual inhibition of the RAAS with 4 weeks of spironolactone and lisinopril as compared with placebo (randomized, crossover in 18 participants) noted a higher serum potassium concentration with drug therapy (4.87 mEq per liter versus 4.37 mEq per liter). However, using an hourly measurement of renal potassium excretion following a 35 mEq oral potassium challenge, the reduction in renal excretion (0.44 mEq per liter) did not entirely explain the increase in serum potassium (0.67 mEq per liter), suggesting an effect to reduce cellular potassium disposition.[276]

Impaired Renal Potassium Excretion

Although an increase in K^+ intake can contribute to hyperkalemia, impaired renal excretion almost always plays the dominant role in this process. Potassium-sparing diuretics are used to enhance renal sodium losses and diminish potassium excretion in patients with hypertension and edematous states.[277,278] Two basic mechanisms underlie the pharmacologic actions of these diuretics, which act to modulate principal cells residing in the collecting duct.[279] The aldosterone antagonists, spironolactone and eplerenone, compete with aldosterone binding to cytoplasmic aldosterone receptors, thereby preventing the nuclear uptake of the receptor and blunting aldosterone's effects on the principal cell.[280,281] Amiloride and triamterene directly block sodium channel activity in the luminal membrane of the principal cell, effectively inhibiting sodium reabsorption through the epithelium and decreasing the driving force for potassium secretion.[282,283] Moderate-to-severe hyperkalemia has been reported in 4% to 19% of patients treated with these medications.[261,280–292] In one small study, treatment with the combination of triamterene and hydrochlorothiazide resulted in hyperkalemia in 26% of the patients.[283] In a retrospective chart review, five patients were noted to develop severe hyperkalemia (K^+ concentrations in the 9.4 to 11 mEq per liter range) within 8 to 18 days of combination therapy with amiloride/hydrochlorothiazide and an angiotensin-converting enzyme (ACE) inhibitor.[286] All of these patients had diabetes and three had underlying CKD.

The combination of spironolactone and losartan increased plasma K^+ by 0.8 mEq per liter (up to 5.0 mEq per liter) and decreased urinary potassium excretion (from 108 to 87 mEq per liter) in eight normal subjects studied.[288] Hyperkalemia occurred most frequently in patients with preexisting renal insufficiency or diabetes mellitus, and those taking K^+ supplements or another medication that also impairs potassium excretion.[285,286,289–292] Several studies have demonstrated a brisk increase in the incidence of hyperkalemia from the use of either spironolactone or eplerenone in patients with heart failure following the publication of the Randomized Aldactone Evaluation Study (RALES) and Eplerenone Post-Acute Myocardial Infarction Heart Failure Efficacy and Survival Study (EPHESUS) trials.[293,294] For example, the spironolactone prescription rate increased from 34 per 1,000 patients in 1994 to 149 per 1,000 patients in 2001 following the publication of RALES.[294] This was associated with an increase in the rate of hospitalization for hyperkalemia (2.4 per 1,000 patients in 1994; 11.0 per 1,000 patients in 2001) (Fig. 72.9) and mortality (0.3 per 1,000 patients in 1994; 2.0 per 1,000 patients in 2001) in heart failure patients treated with ACE inhibitors.[294] In the EPHESUS trial, significant hyperkalemia ($K^+ >$ 6.0 mEq per liter) developed in 5.5% of treated patients versus 3.9% in placebo-treated patients.[295] Hyperkalemia (K^+ $>$ 6.0 mEq per liter) was most prevalent in patients with impaired kidney function (creatinine clearance $<$ 50 mL per minute) as 10.1% of eplerenone-treated patients developed this complication as compared with 5.9% of placebo-treated patients.[295] However, these data are refuted by a population-based longitudinal analysis of patients in Scotland who were treated with spironolactone for heart failure, cirrhosis, and resistant hypertension before and after the publication of RALES.[296] Using the record linkage database, the number of spironolactone prescriptions, hospital admissions for hyperkalemia, and hyperkalemia and kidney function without admission were analyzed. The authors found that despite a significant increase in spironolactone prescriptions (2,847 in the first half of 1999; 6,582 in the second half of 2001; and 8,619 by 2007), there was not an increase in the number of admissions for hyperkalemia in 1995 before the publication

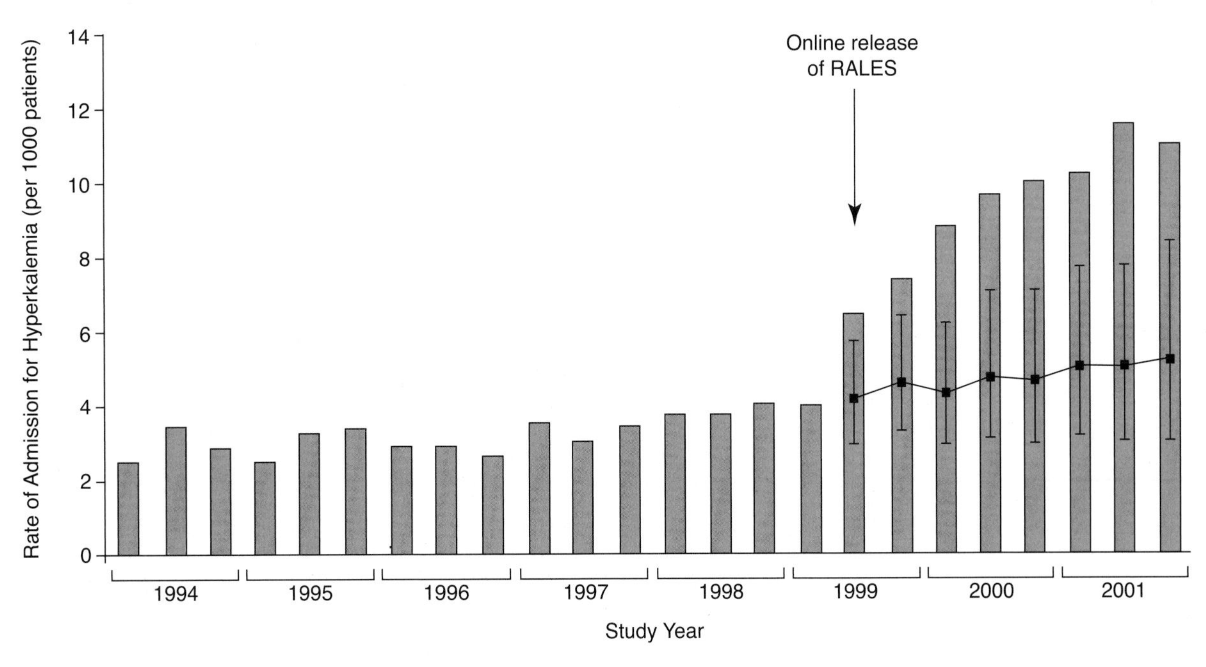

FIGURE 72.9 The rate of hospital admissions for hyperkalemia among patients recently hospitalized for heart failure who were receiving angiotensin-converting enzyme (ACE) inhibitors. Each bar demonstrates the rate of hospital admission for hyperkalemia per 1,000 patients during one 4-month interval. *RALES,* Randomized Aldactone Evaluation Study. (From Juurlink DN, et al. Rates of hyperkalemia after publication of the Randomized Aldactone Evaluation Study. *New Engl J Med.* 2004;351:543, with permission.)

of RALES and in 2001 and 2007 after the publication of RALES. A separate analysis of heart failure patients also prescribed ACE inhibitors demonstrated a significant increase in spironolactone prescriptions but no increase in outpatient hyperkalemia. Thus, it appears that spironolactone can be used safely with an appropriate monitoring in this group of patients. Another drug with the potential to induce hyperkalemia is drospirenone, which is combined with ethinyl estradiol, and is used for contraception, premenstrual syndrome, and postmenopausal osteoporosis. Drospirenone is a novel progestin and mineralocorticoid antagonist, which has the capacity to reduce renal potassium excretion and potentially cause hyperkalemia in patients with advanced kidney failure and/or in those who are receiving other medications that impair renal potassium excretion. Currently, no cases of serious hyperkalemia have been reported; however, plasma potassium does increase during therapy with this medication. A study in postmenopausal women aged 44 to 70 years (~one third diabetes mellitus) all on either an ACE-inhibitor or AT-II receptor blockers (ARB) were randomized to 28 days of drospirenone/ethinyl estradiol or placebo.[297] Baseline creatinine clearance was greater than 100 mL per minute in both groups. Serum potassium was higher in the drug arm, with hyperkalemia ($K^+ > 5.5$ mEq per liter) developing in 7.3% of drug-treated versus 2.6% in placebo-treated patients ($P = .13$).

Nonsteroidal anti-inflammatory drugs (NSAIDs) are widely prescribed for a variety of inflammatory diseases and pain syndromes. Hyperkalemia is one of the many renal complications associated with NSAID therapy, and over-the-counter availability of these agents further increases the risk of drug toxicity.[298] NSAIDs disturb potassium homeostasis via the inhibition of renal prostaglandin synthesis, especially prostaglandin E2 (PGE2) and prostaglandin I2 (PGI2).[299] The inhibition of prostaglandin synthesis decreases potassium secretion through (1) a lack of activation of the renin–angiotensin system, (2) the direct inhibition of potassium channels in principal cells, and (3) the decreased renal blood flow and diminished delivery of sodium to the distal nephron.[204,298–301] Several reports have confirmed the hyperkalemic complication of NSAIDs prescribed to normal subjects, diabetic patients, and patients with underlying renal insufficiency.[250,300–305] This is especially problematic in patients with reduced effective renal perfusion such as those with intravascular fluid depletion, congestive heart failure (CHF), and third-spacing of intravascular fluid.[297–300] Predictably, NSAID-induced hyperkalemia occurs more often in patients with preexisting hyporeninemic hypoaldosteronism, renal insufficiency, and concomitant therapy with potassium-sparing diuretics and ACE inhibitors.[298–304] As with the traditional NSAIDs, selective COX-2 inhibitors (celecoxib) cause hyperkalemia in at risk patients.[305] The induction of hyporeninemic hypoaldosteronism, reduced sodium delivery to the cortical collecting duct, and renal insufficiency are the mechanisms by which these drugs promote hyperkalemia.[305]

A retrospective analysis of a large national cohort of patients cared for at the Veterans Health Administration (VHA) demonstrated an increased rate of hyperkalemia in CKD patients treated with RAAS antagonists (versus non-CKD patients). Most concerning was the increased odds ratio of death within 1 day of the hyperkalemic event in patients with moderate (≥ 5.5 mEq per liter and < 6.0 mEq per liter) and severe hyperkalemia (≥ 6.0 mEq per liter) for all stages of CKD, suggesting that use of RAAS blockers in CKD patients should be monitored closely.[306]

ACE inhibitors indirectly reduce renal potassium excretion by inducing a state of hypoaldosteronism.[250,307,308] These drugs may additionally impair renal potassium excretion by reducing the effective GFR in patients with volume depletion, renal artery stenosis, and/or moderate-to-severe chronic renal insufficiency. In these conditions, ACE inhibitors interfere with AT-II production and blunt the postglomerular arteriolar constriction induced by this hormone, thereby lowering the effective filtration pressure and GFR. Ultimately, a reduction in the distal nephron delivery of sodium and water, together with decreased aldosterone production, may precipitate hyperkalemia.[307] In hospitalized patients, ACE inhibitors have been noted to be the culprit drug in 9% to 38% of patients who developed hyperkalemia.[261,262,309] In outpatients treated with an ACE inhibitor for 1 year, 10% developed a serum potassium concentration greater than 6.0 mEq per liter.[310] In this study, patients with renal impairment who were over the age of 70 years were at highest risk. Most studies suggest that the risk of ACE inhibitor–induced hyperkalemia is directly proportional to the existing degree of renal insufficiency.[261,262,307–309] However, serum potassium concentrations can rise significantly in patients with only modest renal insufficiency.[307,308,311] For example, a rise in serum K^+ concentration, a positive cumulative potassium balance, and a reduction in both plasma and urinary aldosterone were demonstrated in 22 of 23 patients treated with high-dose captopril for 10 days despite a creatinine clearance greater than 50 mL per minute.[308] In addition, another study noted a fall in aldosterone excretion and a rise in serum K^+ concentration (mean rise 0.8 mEq per liter) in 23 of 33 hypertensive patients after 1 week of captopril therapy.[307] In this study, all but 3 of the patients had a creatinine clearance above 60 mL per minute and the peak serum K^+ concentration was not predicted by the pretherapy serum creatinine concentration. In contrast, Memon and colleagues[309] demonstrated a significant positive correlation of hyperkalemia with serum creatinine and a negative correlation with creatinine clearance, emphasizing the importance of the underlying level of renal function. In patients with renal impairment, reducing the dose of an ACE inhibitor and initiating a low-potassium diet has been shown to decrease the development of hyperkalemia in a significant percentage of patients.[309,311] Unfortunately, as many as one-third of patients still require the discontinuation of this medication because of ongoing hyperkalemia.[309] Predictably, combination therapy with an ACE inhibitor and other medications capable of altering potassium homeostasis can increase plasma potassium and precipitate hyperkalemia in patients with only modest renal impairment.[250,307,308,312–317] As an example, elderly patients on an ACE inhibitor who were hospitalized for hyperkalemia were 27 times more likely to have been prescribed a potassium-sparing diuretic in the week prior to hospital admission.[318] Other notable risk factors include hypoaldosteronism and states of effective arterial volume depletion, such as CHF and cirrhosis.[250,307,308,319,320] Using patients with hypertensive CKD (GFR, 20 to 65 mL/min/1.73 m^2) from the AASK trial, Weinberg et al.[321] noted that ACE-I therapy was associated with an increased hazard ratio for hyperkalemia than either calcium channel blockers or β-receptor blockers. However, this effect was only present in patients with GFR 31 to 40 mL/min/1.73 m^2 (heart rate [HR], 3.61) and GFR < 30 mL/min/1.73 m^2 (HR, 6.81), because risk was not increased in those with GFR 41 to 50 mL/min/1.73 m^2. In addition, diuretic use reduced hyperkalemia risk by 59%.[321] Johnson et al.[322] analyzed a retrospective cohort of CKD patients in the Kaiser Health Maintenance Organization who were initiated on lisinopril and who developed hyperkalemia (potassium ≥ 5.5 mEq per liter or diagnosis code). They then used Cox regression to synthesize a risk score from a priori predictors in the medical record. They noted a 90-day hyperkalemia risk of 2.8% in the population and found seven predictors: age, estimated GFR, diabetes mellitus, heart failure, potassium supplements, potassium sparing diuretics, and high lisinopril dose. The risk score was able to separate high-risk from low-risk patients with excellent accuracy (predicted and observed risks agreed within 1% for each quintile). Although the risk score must be validated in other populations, it has the potential to help guide clinician practice in avoiding potentially lethal hyperkalemia.[322]

ARBs are a relatively new class of drugs marketed for the treatment of hypertension. Their action to block binding of AT-II to its receptor ultimately decreases AT-II–driven adrenal synthesis of aldosterone, causing hyperkalemia through the induction of hypoaldosteronism in a manner similar to ACE inhibitors. Data are conflicting with regard to the effect of this class of drugs on the development of hyperkalemia. In healthy patients with essential hypertension, the ARB, losartan (100 mg), and the ACE inhibitor, enalapril (20 mg), similarly depressed plasma aldosterone levels (50% decrease) and 24-hour urinary aldosterone excretion.[323] The effect of these two drugs on the RAAS did not include the evaluation of serum K^+ concentrations in these patients.[323] Data pooled from 16 double-blind clinical trials evaluating the safety of therapy with losartan as compared with ACE inhibitors in healthy patients with hypertension demonstrated no significant difference in the development of hyperkalemia (K^+ > 5.5 mEq per liter) between the two drug classes (1.3% versus 1.5%).[324] It is important to remember that the patients evaluated in these studies were healthy and at very low risk of developing hyperkalemia.[324] The evaluation of the effect of losartan in elderly patients demonstrated a significant rise in serum potassium (> 0.5 mEq per liter) in 19% of patients, whereas hyperkalemia actually developed in 7% of patients.[325] A clinical history of diabetic nephropathy and a serum creatinine greater than 1.3 mg per deciliter were predictors of a significant increase in serum potassium. Bakris and colleagues[326] compared the effects of the ACE inhibitor, lisinopril, to the ARB, valsartan, on serum potassium concentration, urinary potassium excretion, and plasma aldosterone in 35 subjects with a mean GFR of approximately 71 mL/min/1.73 m^2.[326] After 4 weeks of therapy with lisinopril, serum K^+ increased (0.2 mEq per liter), whereas plasma aldosterone and urinary potassium excretion decreased. In contrast, serum potassium, plasma aldosterone, and urinary potassium excretion were essentially unchanged in the valsartan group.[326]

Combination therapy with ACE inhibitors and ARBs raises concerns that patients may experience an increase in the development of hyperkalemia from a more complete blockade of the RAS. The combined decline in GFR and the more pronounced suppression of aldosterone synthesis may promote serious hyperkalemia. A multicenter randomized active-controlled parallel group trial studied patients with renal insufficiency (average creatinine clearance 20 to 45 mL per minute).[327] Patients were randomized to either valsartan alone or in combination with benazepril. Dual therapy, however, was associated with a very low risk of hyperkalemia. Serum K^+ concentration rose in each group ranging from 0.28 mEq per liter to 0.48 mEq per liter. An identical percentage (4.5%) of patients on monotherapy and dual blockade developed a serum K^+ concentration greater than 6.0 mEq per liter. Other studies note similar rates of hyperkalemia, although small numbers of patients developed serum K^+ levels greater than 6.0 mEq per liter.[328] Weir and Rolfe[329] reviewed 39 studies that used RAAS inhibitors in the treatment of patients with hypertension, heart failure, or CKD and the rate of hyperkalemia. In patients without other risk factors for hyperkalemia, the incidence of hyperkalemia with drug monotherapy was $\leq$ 2%, whereas it increased to 5% with dual drug therapy. In patients with CKD or heart failure, hyperkalemia incidence increased to 5% to 10%, with serum potassium increases of 0.1 to 0.3 mEq per liter, but a low rate of drug withdrawal (1% to 5%). Thus, although RAAS inhibitor use in high-risk patients is fraught with more hyperkalemia, the actual increases are generally small and serious hyperkalemia is relatively rare.[329] Despite these generally reassuring data, a risk remains for the development of hyperkalemia when these drugs are used alone or in combination. Clinicians should therefore monitor follow-up serum K^+ levels within 1 to 2 weeks once therapy has been initiated.

Trimethoprim and pentamidine are antimicrobial agents employed to treat infections in both HIV-infected patients as well as other hosts. Hyperkalemia evolves through a reduction in renal potassium secretion, the result of competitive inhibition of sodium transport channels in the luminal membranes of the distal nephron by these drugs.[330] The blockade of epithelial sodium channel transport indirectly inhibits potassium secretion (Fig. 72.10),[349] because potassium movement into the distal nephron lumen is electrogenically linked to the movement of sodium out of the lumen.[278,279,330] This action is identical to that exhibited by amiloride, which has a molecular structure very similar to both trimethoprim and pentamidine.[330] Hyperkalemia was first described in a patient treated with "high-dose" trimethoprim (20 mg/kg/day) for *Pneumocystis carinii* pneumonia.[331] Subsequently, a 50% incidence of mild hyperkalemia ($K^+ > 5.0$ mEq per liter) and a 10% to 12% incidence of severe hyperkalemia ($K^+ > 6.0$ mEq per liter) were observed in HIV-infected patients receiving high-dose trimethoprim.[330] Shortly thereafter, 21% of hospitalized non-HIV patients treated with standard dose trimethoprim (360 mg per day) developed hyperkalemia ($K^+ > 5.5$ mEq per liter).[332] Mild renal impairment (serum creatinine $\leq$ 1.2 mg per deciliter) was significantly associated with the development of a higher serum potassium concentration.[332] A prospective, randomized controlled study in healthy outpatients treated with standard-dose trimethoprim revealed that 18% (9/51) and 6% (3/51) of trimethoprim-treated patients developed serum K^+ concentrations greater than 5.0 and 5.5 mEq per liter, respectively.[333] Older age, diabetes mellitus, and a higher serum creatinine level appeared to predispose a patient to more severe hyperkalemia. Additionally, therapy with pentamidine also has been complicated by hyperkalemia.[334] A retrospective study in 32 patients with AIDS noted a significant increase in mean serum K^+ from 4.2 to 4.7 mEq per liter, with 24% of the patients developing severe hyperkalemia.[335] All cases of hyperkalemia were associated with renal insufficiency, providing an underlying risk factor in these patients. A sevenfold risk for hyperkalemia-associated hospitalization was noted within 14 days of concurrent trimethoprim-sulfamethoxazole and RAAS inhibitor therapy in a cohort of elderly patients. This population-

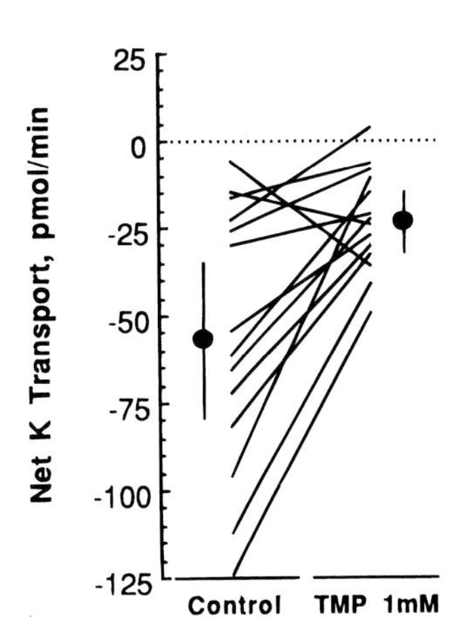

FIGURE 72.10 The net potassium transport during perfusion of 14 distal tubules with control and trimethoprim (TMP) solutions. Lines connect measurements in the same tubules. *Black circles* and *vertical lines* indicate means and confidence intervals. Positive values indicate absorption; negative values indicate secretion. (From Velazquez H, Perazella MA, Wright F, et al. Renal mechanism of trimethoprim-induced hyperkalemia. *Ann Intern Med.* 1993;119:296, with permission.)

based, nested case-control study in Canadian residents did not note such a risk with other antibiotics (amoxicillin, ciprofloxacin, norfloxacin, or nitrofurantoin), suggesting that the potassium-sparing effects of trimethoprim combined with RAAS blockade should be avoided or used cautiously in the elderly.[335] However, in a study using the same population of patients, a further increased risk of trimethoprim-sulfamethoxazole–associated hospitalization for hyperkalemia with concurrent β-blocker use was not noted.[336]

Heparin and its congeners have been shown to inhibit adrenal aldosterone production and precipitate hyperkalemia in approximately 8% of patients treated with at least 10,000 U per day.[337] This drug reduces both the number and affinity of AT-II receptors in the adrenal zona glomerulosa, thus decreasing the principal stimulus for aldosterone synthesis.[337] Heparin also directly inhibits the final enzymatic steps of aldosterone formation (18-hydroxylation) and promotes atrophy of the zona glomerulosa in rats following prolonged administration, further reducing aldosterone production.[337] Finally, excess anticoagulation with heparin may rarely precipitate adrenal hemorrhage and induce frank adrenal insufficiency. Although heparin-associated hyperkalemia has been reported in normal subjects, patients with preexisting hypoaldosteronism, kidney disease, or diabetes mellitus and patients treated with other medications that disrupt K^+ homeostasis more commonly develop hyperkalemia.[337]

Cyclosporine and tacrolimus have been associated with the development of hyperkalemia in organ transplant recipients. In the precyclosporine era, 31% (23/75) of renal transplant patients were noted to develop transient hyperkalemia because of an underlying disturbance in potassium excretion.[235] Not unexpectedly, therapy with cyclosporine and tacrolimus increases the risk of this disorder in these patients.[180] Heering and Grabensee[237] documented the presence of incomplete RTA in 8 of 35 recipients on cyclosporine compared with none of the 15 on azathioprine. Four of the former group also had HHA syndrome. In a detailed study of 12 cadaveric recipients with hyperkalemia on cyclosporine, Kamel and colleagues[238] documented the presence of low urinary potassium excretion that did not respond to 0.2 mg of fludrocortisone. Renal K^+ excretion, however, responded to bicarbonaturia initiated by acetazolamide, suggesting a defect in generating a favorable electrochemical gradient in the distal tubule, leading to hyperkalemia and varying degrees of hyperchloremic acidosis. Recently, Yu and coworkers[338] demonstrated higher serum potassium concentrations and lower TTKGs in 35 renal transplant recipients receiving cyclosporine as compared with matched normal controls, thus supporting a disturbance in renal potassium excretion. Tacrolimus has similarly caused hyperkalemia in solid organ transplant patients. Hyperkalemia was noted in 26 of 49 (53%) pediatric heart transplant recipients treated with tacrolimus.[339] Of note, the majority of subjects who developed hyperkalemia had impaired renal function. The reduction in renal potassium excretion that occurs with these two drugs is likely owing to a dose-dependent decrease in the activity of the basolateral Na-K-ATPase pumps in principal cells in the distal nephron.[340,341] Calcineurin, which modulates sodium pump function through its regulation of phosphatase activity, is inhibited by both cyclosporine and tacrolimus.[341] In vitro inhibition of calcineurin by these two drugs has been shown to decrease Na-K-ATPase pump activity and probably explains the observed reduction in renal potassium excretion. Ling and Eaton[342] have also demonstrated the inhibition of apical secretory potassium channels by cyclosporine, providing yet another possible mechanism of decreased renal potassium excretion and hyperkalemia. Cyclosporine also impairs cellular potassium homeostasis and causes transient hyperkalemia by acutely increasing potassium efflux from cells.[343] Although the mechanism is currently unknown, cyclosporine may cause hyperkalemia through the impairment of Na-K-ATPase pumps in muscle and liver cell membranes.

Acute Treatment of Serious Hyperkalemia

Severe hyperkalemia is a potentially life-threatening disorder because of its toxic effect on cardiac and other excitable neuromuscular tissues. Importantly, patients with underlying renal disease and disturbances in potassium homeostasis can develop serious hyperkalemia. It is therefore imperative that this electrolyte disturbance is rapidly recognized and aggressively treated. Symptoms of hyperkalemia are sometimes impressive and quite obvious; however, serious hyperkalemia also may present with only very subtle symptoms or signs. Rarely, patients may have absolutely no clinical evidence of this disorder, the presence of renal impairment or other disturbances in potassium homeostasis providing the only clues to hyperkalemia. Nonspecific muscle weakness and generalized malaise are common, but severe muscle weakness, paresthesias, and ascending paralysis may rarely be seen in these patients with extreme elevations in serum potassium levels.[344] The cardiac toxicity of hyperkalemia may manifest as weakness or dizziness from arrhythmias that induce hypotension and cerebral hypoperfusion.[344] Cardiac monitoring or a 12-lead electrocardiogram (ECG) may reveal a rhythm suspicious of hyperkalemia. These include tenting of the T waves (K^+, 5.5 to 6.0 mEq per liter), lengthening of the P-R interval and widening of the QRS complex (K^+, 6.0 to 7.0 mEq per liter), disappearance of the P waves (K^+, 7.0 to 7.5 mEq per liter), and finally the sine wave pattern (K^+, 8.0 mEq per liter or greater). These ECG changes may occur at different concentrations (higher or lower) of potassium, depending on underlying heart disease and acuity of hyperkalemia.[344] The presence of hypocalcemia, hypomagnesemia, and hyponatremia potentiate the toxic effects of hyperkalemia on the cardiac conduction system and potassium concentrations in the 6.0 to 6.5 mEq per liter range can precipitate life-threatening arrhythmias.[344] Additionally, patients with underlying cardiac disease may deteriorate directly to a ventricular arrhythmia in the absence of other ECG changes.

Once the clinician judges that hyperkalemia warrants treatment (plasma $K^+ > 6.0$ to 6.5 mEq per liter, clinical manifestations, or ECG changes), immediate therapy should be commenced. The stabilization of excitable cell membranes—in particular, cardiac tissue—is the most urgent priority in the treatment of hyperkalemia. Intravenous calcium, as either calcium gluconate (10% solution, calcium ion at 3 mEq per milliliter) or calcium chloride (10% solution, calcium ion at 13 mEq per milliliter), is the treatment of first choice and should be administered in a monitored setting (Table 72.4). Calcium acts within 1 to 3 minutes, and the effect persists for approximately a half hour.[344] If no effect is noted within 5 minutes following the first dose, repeated administration may provide benefit. Patients who have been treated with digoxin should receive a slower infusion of calcium (calcium mixed in 100 mL of 5% dextrose) over 10 to 20 minutes.[344]

Intravenous administration of regular insulin as a 10-U bolus followed by 50 mL of intravenous 50% dextrose (Table 72.4) should be the next therapeutic choice.[345,346] Twenty units of intravenous insulin may promote an even greater reduction in plasma K^+.[347] The beneficial effect of insulin is observed within 15 minutes and lasts approximately 3 to 6 hours.[345–347] Dextrose is given to prevent hypoglycemia in nondiabetic patients. However, because a high incidence of hypoglycemia occurs even with this regimen, it is prudent to monitor blood glucose levels and redose dextrose based on levels.[345–347] Dextrose should not be infused before insulin because an acute worsening of hyperkalemia can occur with hyperglycemia through a shift of potassium out of cells. Glucose levels should be checked prior to the administration of dextrose to diabetic patients.[345–347]

High-dose nebulized albuterol (10 to 20 mg), which is fourfold to eightfold higher than used to treat asthma, also effectively lowers potassium concentrations in patients with hyperkalemia (Table 72.4).[348] However, the potassium-lowering effect of albuterol is less reliable in ESRD patients, and as many as 40% of these patients are resistant to the potassium-lowering effect of this β-agonist.[348] In general, the plasma potassium concentration declines significantly at 30 minutes following albuterol inhalation and remains depressed for approximately 2 hours.[348] To date, no adverse cardiovascular effects from albuterol have been documented in ESRD patients.[348] Therefore, nebulized albuterol is useful to acutely lower plasma potassium concentration in most hyperkalemic patients; however, it should not replace insulin as the most important therapy to move potassium into cells. Subcutaneous terbutaline (7 μg per kilogram) was shown in a study of 14 CKD patients to significantly lower serum potassium (mean reduction, 1.31 +/− 0.5 mEq per liter), with reasonably good safety because the major adverse effect was asymptomatic tachycardia.[349]

Combined therapy with intravenous insulin and nebulized albuterol has been shown to be additive in the reduction of plasma K^+ concentrations.[348] Plasma K^+ decreases approximately 0.6 mEq per liter with 10 U of insulin, whereas 20 mg of nebulized albuterol lowers plasma K^+ to a similar degree[347]; however, the combination of these agents lowers plasma K^+ by approximately 1.2 mEq per L.[274] As a result, it is worthwhile to combine these two agents to treat severe hyperkalemia (Table 72.4). Combined therapy with sodium bicarbonate and insulin reduced plasma K^+ more effectively, whereas sodium bicarbonate plus nebulized albuterol was no better than monotherapy.[348]

Although sodium bicarbonate is listed as a useful treatment for hyperkalemia, the critical evaluation of the

TABLE 72.4 **Acute Treatment of Serious Hyperkalemia**

Stabilize Excitable Tissues (Cardiac and Neuromuscular) Calcium gluconate (10% solution), given as a 10- to 20-mL intravenous bolus. Calcium chloride (10% solution), given as a 5-mL intravenous bolus. Each may be repeated every 5 min, if ECG appearance does not improve. Calcium gluconate should be mixed in 100 mL of 5% and infused over 10–20 min if the patient has been treated with digoxin.
Shift Potassium into Cells Regular insulin, 10 to 20 U plus 50% dextrose (50 mL), given as an intravenous bolus, followed by 10% dextrose at 50 mL/min until definitive therapy. Check glucose levels at 1- to 2-hr intervals. Albuterol (5 mg/mL), 10–20 mg, nebulized over approximately 10 min. Terbutaline, 7 mcg/kg, subcutaneous injection. Combination therapy of insulin/dextrose and nebulized albuterol.
Remove Potassium from the Body Acute hemodialysis (low potassium dialysate) to remove potassium in patients with severe renal insufficiency. Sodium polystyrene sulfonate (15–30 g) plus sorbitol (15–30 mL), oral ingestion (avoid in postsurgical patients and those with gastrointestinal disease).

ECG, electrocardiogram.

literature suggests that this agent is ineffective as an isolated therapy to acutely lower plasma potassium.[350,351] In studies where bicarbonate infusion successfully lowered plasma potassium concentrations in ESRD patients, the effect was not observed until at least 4 hours after treatment. Similarly, other studies have confirmed the use of sodium bicarbonate therapy in the chronic (not acute) lowering of plasma K^+ concentrations.[350,351] In contrast, patients with severe metabolic acidosis and concurrent hyperkalemia should receive bicarbonate to correct pH and stabilize cardiac tissue. In this setting, sodium bicarbonate (50 mEq) may be given intravenously to correct pH and serum bicarbonate levels in patients who are normokalemic and can tolerate the sodium load.[350,351]

THE WORKUP AND MANAGEMENT OF CHRONIC HYPERKALEMIC RENAL TUBULAR ACIDOSIS

Although acute hyperkalemia with or without significant HCA requiring immediate treatment occurs in patients with impaired potassium handling, the major challenge is the workup and treatment of chronic hyperkalemia seen in this setting. Given the frequency of this syndrome and the lack of individualized treatment for specific subgroups, most patients can be adequately managed without complex workups. However, in certain patients, it may be important to make a more specific pathophysiologic diagnosis. Although HCA is the dominant finding in some patients, hyperkalemia is the prominent presentation requiring workup and treatment.

Figure 72.11 summarizes a simple pathophysiologic approach to chronic hyperkalemia in these patients. The first question to be answered is, "Is the hyperkalemia owing to an increase in intake or a decrease in output?" Although dietary history and pertinent clinical data may be helpful, a specific laboratory test that would answer this question could simplify the workup. Urinary potassium concentration and the urinary to serum potassium ratio do not account for the variability in the urinary potassium concentration as a function of water reabsorption in the collecting duct. The fractional excretion of potassium (FE_K^+) normalizes potassium excretion for GFR; however, because potassium is primarily secreted (and therefore, less dependent on filtration), its clinical use is questionable.

Halperin and colleagues[58,352–354] have suggested correcting the urinary (U_K) to serum potassium (S_K) concentration by the ratio of urine (U_{Osm}) to serum osmolality (S_{Osm}) to normalize the data for water reabsorption. This ratio ($U_K^+/S_K^+ X\ S_{Osm}U_{Osm}$), called the TTKG, attempts to approximate the gradient across potassium-secreting cells in the distal nephron. Despite several pitfalls (urine more diluted than the plasma or very low urinary sodium), a value less than 6 in patients with hyperkalemia suggests a lack of aldosterone or response to aldosterone; a value above 6 is in favor of an increase in potassium intake, with or without renal abnormality in potassium handling. It should, however, be noted that the published clinical experience with the use of TTKG is still very limited and often is limited to case reports. Therefore, the values given here should be used with caution and evaluated in light of other data.[355] If the TTKG is normal, one should search for excessive potassium intake, either externally (e.g., potassium supplements, salt substitutes) or internally (e.g., severe hemolysis, rhabdomyolysis, acidosis). In general, given the renal ability to handle a large oral potassium load (e.g., serum potassium rising by less than 1.0 mEq per liter on a 400-mEq diet), a significant increase in serum potassium is indicative of either a major internal shift of potassium or a decrease in urinary excretion output. If the TTKG is low in the face of hyperkalemia, the aldosterone level should be measured to separate the group with tubular unresponsiveness from that with low aldosterone. Patients also can be challenged with exogenous mineralocorticoids (0.05 to 1.0 mg of fludrocortisone). If the TTKG increases to 7 or above, hypoaldosteronism is probably the major factor in the development of hyperkalemia.[354,355] The role of renin–angiotensin in patients with hypoaldosteronism can be evaluated by measuring the renin level. A low renin associated with low aldosterone is the hallmark of the most common subgroup (i.e., hyporenin-hypoaldosteronism). If the renin level is normal, then either the generation of

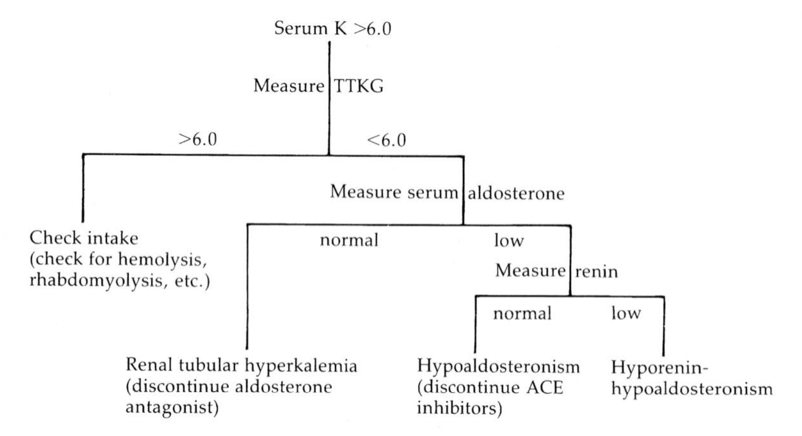

FIGURE 72.11 The pathophysiologic approach to chronic hyperkalemia. *ACE*, angiotensin-converting enzyme; *TTKG*, transtubular potassium gradient.

AT-II is abnormal (e.g., in patients on ACE inhibitors) or the synthesis and secretion of aldosterone are abnormal. The adrenal response to AT-II infusion would provide appropriate answers to this question.

In practice, this type of workup should be reserved for unusual patients who do not represent the commonly recognized groups with this syndrome (e.g., diabetic, hypertensive patients), or as part of a research protocol. In addition, it should be noted that this approach does not lead to an etiologic diagnosis, but only a pathophysiologic one. The etiologic diagnosis (as discussed elsewhere in this chapter) should depend on other diagnostic evaluations.

Some patients with type IV RTA present primarily with HCA. In these patients, the diagnostic workup should focus on the pathogenesis and etiology of this abnormality. The major defect leading to HCA is either a loss of bicarbonate, often through the gastrointestinal tract, or a decrease in the regeneration of bicarbonate by the kidney through the stimulation of ammoniagenesis. Urinary ammonium should be high in the former and low in the latter group. However, urinary ammonium is not commonly measured in clinical laboratories. Clinicians are forced to rely on measurements of surrogates for urinary ammonium excretion. The most commonly used surrogate is the urinary anion gap, which is the difference between major urinary cations (Na + K) and urinary anions ($Cl + HCO_3$). As the amount of bicarbonate is very small in acid urine (urine pH < 6.5), the difference between urinary Na^+, K^+, and Cl^- reflects the major missing ion (i.e., ammonium). Using this formula, one can demonstrate an inverse relationship between the urinary anion gap and the amount of ammonium in the urine (Fig. 72.12).[356,357] In the presence of extrarenal acidosis, the urinary ammonium excretion should increase severalfold, resulting in a very negative anion gap value. In contrast, in distal RTA, the urinary ammonium will remain low, resulting in a positive anion gap. The amount of ammonium in the urine also can be deduced from a modified urinary osmolar gap using the following formula:

$$\text{Urinary Ammonium} = 1/2\ (\text{Urine Osmolality} - 2(\text{Na} + \text{K}) + \text{Urea Nitrogen}/2.8 + \text{Glucose}/18) \quad (1)$$

This is based on the concept that NH_4^+, with its accompanying anion, is the major missing osmole accounting for the osmolar gap.[358] It should be noted that neither calculation predicts the exact amount of ammonium in the urine but rather provides a qualitative estimate of it. This is still helpful if used to answer the appropriate question in a patient with HCA.

The major use of urinary anion or osmolar gap is to differentiate renal from extrarenal causes of hyperchloremic acidosis such as diarrhea or the ingestion of hydrochloric acid or its equivalent where the gap is negative. However, a low or negative anion gap in itself does not establish the diagnosis of type IV RTA, because this is also seen in classic RTA as well as uremic acidosis. Batlle and colleagues[357]

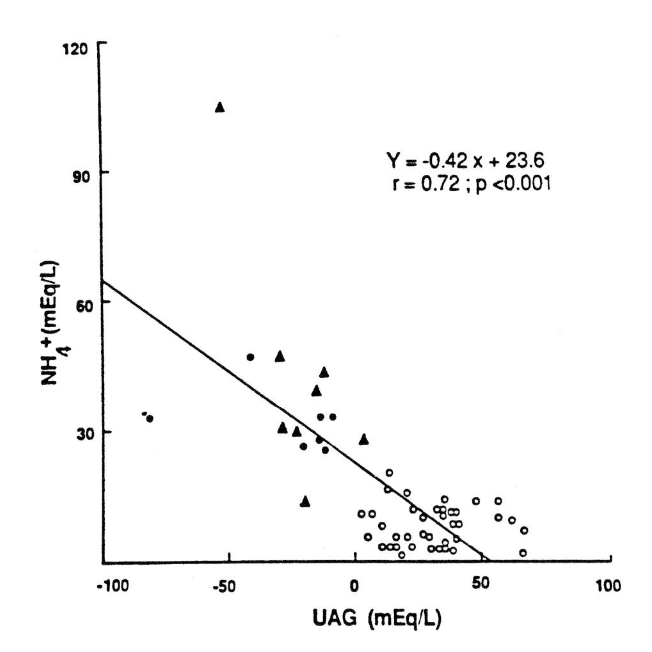

FIGURE 72.12 Urinary ammonium (NH_4^+) in relation to the urinary anion gap (UAG). The 38 patients with altered distal urinary acidification are represented by *open circles*; the 7 normal subjects receiving ammonium chloride are represented by *closed circles*; and the 8 patients with hyperchloremic metabolic acidosis associated with diarrhea are represented by *triangles*. (From Batlle DC, et al. The use of urinary anion gap in the diagnosis of hyperchloremic metabolic acidosis. *N Engl J Med.* 1988;318:594, with permission.)

studied a group of patients with classic RTA, hyperkalemic RTA, and selective aldosterone deficiency and compared the results to controls with a serum pH 7.30 to 7.35. These investigators noted a urinary anion gap of -20 ± 5.7 in controls and $+23 \pm 4.1$, $+30 \pm 4.2$, and $+39 \pm 4.2$ mEq per liter in patients, respectively. The major pitfall in using urinary anion gap is the presence of a significant amount of bicarbonate or an unexpected charged molecule, such as penicillin or ketoacids, in the urine. In summary, urinary anion gap is a physiologic concept that indirectly assesses the amount of urinary ammonium. This measurement, in conjunction with other data, is helpful in establishing the pathogenesis of HCA in selected patients.[359]

In patients with hyperkalemic RTA, the treatment of chronic hyperkalemia should be instituted only when absolutely necessary (i.e., when clinical signs of hyperkalemia are present or plasma K^+ is over 6.0 mEq per liter). If therapy is deemed necessary, simple modalities should be tried first before more complex therapies with their associated side effects are instituted.

Discontinuation of Drugs That Cause Hyperkalemia

As these patients have an intrinsic difficulty in the excretion of potassium, any drugs that can cause hyperkalemia should be immediately discontinued. The list of drugs that should be stopped includes those discussed in the previous section.

Dietary Intervention

The next step in patients with mild-to-moderate hyperkalemia is to decrease K^+ intake to less than 60 mEq per day. This can be done by the elimination of potassium-rich foods. This may be difficult if the patient is on a low-sodium diet because such a diet, by definition, contains foods that are high in potassium content. Also, an increased replacement of sodium with potassium by the food industry as well as "meat enhancing" will make potassium-containing foods more prevalent.

Treatment of Acidemia

Because HCA is commonly associated with hyperkalemia, the correction of the acidosis by sodium bicarbonate decreases the serum potassium concentration. The effect of bicarbonate is partly related to a change in H^+ concentration and is partly independent of pH change. As acidemia is corrected, H^+ moves out of cells in exchange for potassium. The inhibitory effect of acidemia on renal K^+ secretion also is removed. In addition, sodium bicarbonate, through volume expansion and the delivery of both sodium and bicarbonate to the distal potassium exchange site, may also increase renal excretion of potassium.

In some patients with significant metabolic acidosis (HCO_3 < 16 mEq per liter and/or pH < 7.30), it is important to treat acidosis with base replacement to prevent mobilization of bone calcium and protein catabolism. Bone provides a buffer sink for the hydrogen ion, resulting in a release of calcium and its loss in the urine.[137,360] This phenomenon is independent of vitamin D, the parathyroid hormone, and calcitonin.[361,362] In addition, there is increasing evidence for a catabolic role for metabolic acidosis independent of uremia in patients with chronic renal failure.[363] This is thought to result in muscle wasting secondary to the stimulation of muscle protein degradation through the ubiquitin-proteasome system.[364] Both effects can be reversed by alkali therapy. More recently, the relationship between serum bicarbonate and the rate of decline in renal function has been explored in several studies. Low serum bicarbonate in patients with CKD is associated with higher mortality.[365,366] In one study, the relationship between serum bicarbonate and mortality was U shaped, indicating that both low and high bicarbonate was associated with increased mortality.[366] Two studies have also shown that the treatment of metabolic acidosis with alkali improves both the nutritional state as well as decreases the rate of decline in kidney function[367,368] and the need for dialysis.[368] The mechanism of acidosis-induced injury is unclear and may involve complement activation and/or the induction of endothelin production resulting in tubulointerstitial injury.[368,369] Although these provocative findings will require further substantiation with randomized prospective studies, it is recommended that alkali therapy be used to raise serum bicarbonate to > 22mEq per liter. The bicarbonate needed in these patients is close to 0.5 to 0.75 mEq/kg/day and can be easily supplied as citric acid-sodium citrate (Shohl) solution, which contains 1 mEq of bicarbonate equivalent per milliliter. Interestingly, such therapy is well tolerated and has not resulted in volume overload or worsening of hypertension.

Volume Expansion

Volume expansion may enhance potassium excretion by increasing distal fluid and sodium delivery. This therapy is especially effective in patients with chronic volume depletion owing to mild sodium wastage.

Diuretic Therapy

Use of most diuretics, especially loop blockers and thiazides, results in hypokalemic, hypochloremic metabolic alkalosis. In patients with hyperkalemia, the previously mentioned side effects may ameliorate hyperkalemia and, when present, metabolic acidosis. To prevent volume depletion with its resultant decrease in distal tubular sodium and fluid delivery, a high salt intake can be added to the diuretic regimen. Thiazide diuretics have proved effective in some patients with renal tubular hyperkalemia despite the failure of loop blockers such as furosemide.

Mineralocorticoids

Mineralocorticoid replacement represents the most logical approach to therapy in these patients. DeFronzo[171] reported an 84% success rate with this therapy; however, the effective dose of fludrocortisone (up to 0.4 to 1.0 mg per day) was much higher than the true physiologic dose. This observation suggests that most of these patients possess some degree of tubular resistance to the potassium stimulatory effect of mineralocorticoids. Surprisingly, although such high doses were needed to augment renal potassium excretion and normalize serum potassium levels, the sodium-retaining effects of aldosterone remained intact in some patients, resulting in marked edema formation, hypertension, and CHF. In general, if the dose of fludrocortisone required to maintain normokalemia exceeds 0.2 mg per day, side effects are common, and these drugs probably should be combined with diuretics or not employed at all. Use of mineralocorticoids should be limited to patients who have not responded to other maneuvers and continue to have clinically significant hyperkalemia.

Sodium-Potassium Exchange Resins

Sodium polystyrene sulfonate (SPS) resin was first used as a therapy to treat hyperkalemia in 1958 and a study in 1961 documented its efficacy in significantly lowering serum potassium (1.8 mEq per liter at the end of study) in 22 hyperkalemic patients.[370] Studies demonstrated a reliable lowering of serum potassium in hyperkalemic patients using oral SPS mixed either with water or the cathartic sorbitol, which was added to reduce SPS retention and prevent obstipation.[371] In general, a decline in serum potassium requires at least 2 hours, peaks at 4 to 6 hours, and may take 10 hours or longer following oral administration. SPS retention enemas in water were found to be less efficacious. On average, SPS resin efficiency is approximately 33%; that is, 10 mEq of potassium is bound by 30 g of resin (compared with 1 mEq per gram of resin in vitro).[372] As a result, SPS mixed in sorbitol (33% or 70% sorbitol) became a standard therapy for hyperkalemia in both the acute and chronic setting. However, in 2009, the U.S. Food and Drug Administration (FDA) recommended against the "concomitant use of sorbitol" with SPS powder because of associated complications such as colonic necrosis, gastrointestinal injury (bleeding, ischemic colitis, perforation), and rectal stenosis. A close examination of the cases where complications developed reveals the following: (1) SPS enemas with 70% sorbitol were primarily associated with gastrointestinal injury, and (2) postsurgical patients and those with compromised gastrointestinal function were the group most often developing these complications. Although the incidence of complications is difficult to estimate, a study of 752 hospitalized patients treated with SPS resin mixed with sorbitol provides insight.[373] Only two cases of colonic necrosis developed and these patients were given the mixture within 1 week of surgery. This was an incidence of 1.8% in postsurgical patients. If the entire SPS-treated hospital group is examined, the incidence declines to 0.3%. Thus, it is reasonable to continue to use oral SPS mixed in 33% sorbitol in hyperkalemic patients who do not have gastrointestinal dysfunction or who are not in the immediate postsurgical period. Also, SPS enemas should never be employed as therapy for hyperkalemia.

REFERENCES

1. Ewart HS, Klip A. Hormonal regulation of the Na+-K+-ATPase: mechanisms underlying rapid and sustained changes in pump activity. *Am J Physiol.* 1995;269:C295.
2. Yang S, Curtis B, Thompson J, et al. Extrarenal regulation of potassium homeostasis: muscle Na, K-ATPase and NKCCl subcellular distribution. *J Am Soc Nephrol.* 1999;10:49A.
3. Bia MJ, DeFronzo RA. Extrarenal potassium homeostasis. *Am J Physiol.* 1981;240:F257.
4. Giebisch G, Krapf R, Wagner C. Renal and extrarenal regulation of potassium. *Kidney Int.* 2007;397.
5. DeFronzo RA, Lee R, Jones A, Bia M. Effect of insulinopenia and adrenal hormone deficiency on acute potassium tolerance. *Kidney Int.* 1980;17:586.
6. DeFronzo RA, Sherwin RS, Dillingham M, et al. Influence of basal insulin and glucagon secretion on potassium and sodium metabolism. *J Clin Invest.* 1978;61:472.
7. DeFronzo RA, Taufield PA, Black H, et al. Impaired renal tubular potassium secretion in sickle cell disease. *Ann Intern Med.* 1979;90:310.
8. Brown RS. Extrarenal potassium homeostasis. *Kidney Int.* 1986;30:116.
9. Briggs AP, Koechig I, Doisy EA, et al. Some changes in the composition of blood due to the injection of insulin. *J Biol Chem.* 1924;58:721.
10. Hiatt N, Yamakawa T, Davidson MB. Necessity for insulin in transfer of excess infused K to intracellular fluid. *Metabolism.* 1974;23:43.
11. Pettit GW, Vick RL. Contribution of pancreatic insulin to extrarenal potassium homeostasis: a two compartmental model. *Am J Physiol.* 1974;226:319.
12. Santeusanio F, Faloona GR, Knochel JP, et al. Evidence for a role of endogenous insulin and glucagon in the regulation of potassium homeostasis. *J Lab Clin Med.* 1973;81:809.
13. DeFronzo RA, Sherwin RS, Felig P, et al. Nonuremic diabetic hyperkalemia: a possible role of insulin deficiency. *Arch Intern Med.* 1977;137:842.
14. Clausen T, Hansen O. Active Na-K transport and the rate of ouabain binding. The effect of insulin and other stimuli on skeletal muscle and adipocytes. *J Physiol.* 1977;270:415.
15. DeFronzo RA, Felig P, Ferrannini E, et al. Effect of graded doses of insulin on splanchnic and peripheral potassium metabolism in man. *Am J Physiol.* 1980;238:E421.
16. Kahn CR. The molecular mechanism of insulin action. *Ann Rev Med.* 1985;36:429.
17. Moore RD. Effects of insulin upon ion transport. *Biochim Biophys Acta.* 1983;737:1.
18. McDonough AA, Youn JH. Role of muscle in regulating extracellular [K+]. *Semin Nephrol.* 2005;25:335.
19. Benziane B, Chibalin AV. Frontiers: skeletal muscle sodium pump regulation: a translocation paradigm. *Am J Physiol Endocrinol Metab.* 2008 Sep;295(3): E553.
20. Cohen P, Barzilai N, Lerman A, et al. Insulin effects on glucose and potassium metabolism in vivo: evidence for selective insulin resistance in humans. *J Clin Endocrinol Metab.* 1991;73:564.
21. D'Silva JH. The action of adrenaline on serum potassium. *J Physiol (Lond).* 1935;86:219.
22. Lockwood RH, Lum BK. Effects of adrenergic agonists and antagonists on potassium metabolism. *J Pharmacol Exp Ther.* 1974;189:119.
23. Lockwood RH, Lum BK. Effects of adrenalectomy and adrenergic antagonists on potassium metabolism. *J Pharmacol Exp Ther.* 1977;203:103.
24. Hiatt N, Chapman LW, Davidson MB. Influence of epinephrine and propranolol on transmembrane K transfer in anuric dogs with hyperkalemia. *J Pharmacol Exp Ther.* 1979;209:282.
25. Brown MJ, Brown DC, Murphy MB. Hypokalemia from β 2 receptor stimulation by circulating epinephrine. *N Engl J Med.* 1983;309:1414.
26. DeFronzo RA, Stanton B, Klein-Robbenhaar G, et al. Inhibitory effect of epinephrine on renal potassium secretion: a micropuncture study. *Am J Physiol.* 1983;245:F303.
27. Katz L, D'Avella J, DeFronzo RA. Effect of epinephrine on renal potassium excretion in the isolated perfused rat kidney. *Am J Physiol.* 1984;247:F331.
28. Berend N, Marlin GE. Characterization of β-adrenoreceptor subtype mediating the metabolic actions of salbutamol. *Br J Clin Pharmacol.* 1978;5:207.
29. Bia MJ, Lu D, Tyler K, et al. β adrenergic control of extrarenal potassium disposal. A β-2 mediated phenomenon. *Nephron.* 1986;43:117.
30. DeFronzo RA, Bia M, Birkhead G. Epinephrine and potassium homeostasis. *Kidney Int.* 1981;20:83.
31. Flatman JA, Clausen T. Combined effects of adrenaline and insulin on active electrogenic Na^+-K^+ transport in rat soleus muscle. *Nature.* 1979;281:580.
32. Peterson KG, Shuter KJ, Kemp L. Regulation of serum potassium during insulin-induced hypoglycemia. *Diabetes.* 1982;31:615.
33. Wright FS. Potassium transport by successive segments of the mammalian nephron. *Fed Proc.* 1981;40:2398.
34. Hayslett JP, Halevy J, Pace PE, et al. Demonstration of net potassium absorption in mammalian colon. *Am J Physiol.* 1982;242:G209.
35. Simpson SAS, Tait JF. Recent progress on methods of isolation, chemistry, and physiology of aldosterone. *Recent Prog Horm Res.* 1955;11:183.
36. Conn JW. Aldosteronism in man. Some clinical and climatological aspects. *JAMA.* 1963;183:775.
37. Adler S. An extrarenal action of aldosterone on mammalian skeletal muscle. *Am J Physiol.* 1970;218:616.
38. Lim VS, Webster GD. The effect of aldosterone on water and electrolyte composition of incubated rat diaphragms. *Clin Sci.* 1967;33:261.
39. Alexander EA, Levinsky NG. An extrarenal mechanism of potassium adaptation. *J Clin Invest.* 1968;47:740.
40. Spital A, Sterns RH. Extrarenal potassium adaptation: the role of aldosterone. *Clin Sci.* 1989;76:213.
41. Spital A, Sterns RH. Paradoxical potassium depletion: a renal mechanism for extrarenal potassium adaptation. *Kidney Int.* 1986;30:532.
42. Young DB, Jackson TE. Effects of aldosterone on potassium distribution. *Am J Physiol.* 1982;243:R526.
43. Ross EJ. *Aldosterone and Aldosteronism.* London, England: The Whitefriars; 1975.
44. Bia MJ, Tyler KA, DeFronzo RA. Regulation of extrarenal potassium homeostasis by adrenal hormones in rats. *Am J Physiol.* 1982;242:F641.
45. Sugarman A, Brown RS. The role of aldosterone in potassium tolerance: studies in anephric humans. *Kidney Int.* 1988;34:397.
46. Furuya R, Kumagai H, Sakao T, et al. Potassium-lowering effect of mineralocorticoid therapy in patients undergoing hemodialysis. *Nephron.* 2002;92:576.

47. Hussain S, Dreyfus DE, Marcus RJ, et al. Is spironolactone safe for dialysis patients? *Nephrol Dial Transplant.* 2003;18:2365.
48. Matsumotoa Y, Kageyamab S, Yakushigawac T, et al. Long-term low-dose spironolactone therapy is safe in oligoanuric hemodialysis patients. *Cardiology.* 2009;114:32–38.
49. Saudan P, Mach F, Perneger T, et al. Safety of low-dose spironolactone administration in chronic haemodialysis patients. *Nephrol Dial Transplant.* 2003;18:2359.
50. Papadimitriou M, Vyzantiadis A, Milionis A, et al. The effect of spironolactone in hypertensive patients on regular haemodialysis and after renal allotransplantation. *Life Support Systems.* 1983;1:197.
51. Simmons DH, Avedon M. Acid base alterations and plasma potassium concentrations. *Am J Physiol.* 1959;197:319.
52. Adler S, Fraley DS. Potassium and intracellular pH. *Kidney Int.* 1977;11:433.
53. Perez GO, Oster JR, Vaamonde CA. Serum potassium concentration in acidemic states. *Nephron.* 1981;27:233.
54. Krapf R. Acid-base and potassium homeostasis. *Nephrol Dial Transplant.* 1995;10:1537.
55. Adrogue HJ, Madias NE. Changes in plasma potassium concentration during acute acid–base disturbances. *Am J Med.* 1981;71:456.
56. Fulop M. Serum potassium in lactic acidosis and ketoacidosis. *N Engl J Med.* 1979;300:1087.
57. Oster JR, Perez GO, Castro A, et al. Plasma potassium response to metabolic acidosis induced by mineral and nonmineral acids. *Miner Electrolyte Metab.* 1980;4:28.
58. Wiederseiner J-M, Muser J, Lutz T, et al. Acute metabolic acidosis: Characterization and diagnosis of the disorder and the plasma potassium response. *J Am Soc Nephrol.* 2004;15:1589.
59. Krapf R, Caduff P, Wagdi P, et al. Plasma potassium response to acute respiratory alkalosis. *Kidney Int.* 1995;47:217.
60. Krapf R, Beeler I, Hertne D, et al. Chronic respiratory alkalosis—the effect of sustained hyperventilation on renal regulation of acid–base equilibrium. *N Engl J Med.* 1991;324:1394.
61. Natalini G, Seramondi D, Fassini P, et al. Acute respiratory acidosis does not increase plasma potassium in normokalemic anaesthetized patients. A controlled randomized trial. *Eur J Anaesthesiol.* 2001;18:394.
62. Magner PO, Robinson L, Halperin RM, et al. The plasma potassium concentration in metabolic acidosis: a re-evaluation. *Am J Kidney Dis.* 1988;11:220.
63. Moreno M, Murphy C, Goldsmith C. Increase in serum potassium resulting from the administration of hypertonic mannitol and other solutions. *J Lab Clin Med.* 1969;73:291.
64. Goldfarb S, Cox M, Singer I. Acute hyperkalemia induced by hyperglycemia: hormonal mechanisms. *Ann Intern Med.* 1976;84:426.
65. Goldfarb S, Strunk B, Singer I, Goldberg M. Paradoxical glucose-induced hyperkalemia. Combined aldosterone-insulin deficiencies. *Am J Med.* 1975;59:744.
66. Nicolis GL, Kahn T, Sanchez A. Glucose-induced hyperkalemia in diabetic subjects. *Arch Intern Med.* 1981;141:49.
67. Rado JP. Glucose-induced paradoxical hyperkalemia in patients with suppression of the renin–aldosterone system: prevention by sodium depletion. *J Endocrinol Invest.* 1979;2:401.
68. Bratusch-Marrain PR, DeFronzo RA. Impairment of insulin-mediated glucose metabolism by hyperosmolality in man. *Diabetes.* 1983;32:1028.
69. Conte G, Dal Canton A, Imperatore P, et al. Acute increase in plasma osmolality as a cause of hyperkalemia in patients with renal failure. *Kidney Int.* 1990;38:301.
70. Sirken G. Raja R, Garces J, et al. Contrast-induced translocational hyponatremia and hyperkalemia in advanced kidney disease. *Am J Kidney Dis.* 2004; 24:1127.
71. Rohrscheib M, Tzamaloukas AH, Ing TS, et al. Serum potassium concentration in hyperglycemia of chronic dialysis. *Adv Perit Dial.* 2005;21:102.
72. Rabinowitz L. Aldosterone and potassium homeostasis. *Kidney Int.* 1996,49: 1738.
73. Greenlee M, Wingo CS, McDonough AA, et al. Narrative review: evolving concepts in potassium homeostasis and hypokalemia. *Ann Intern Med.* 2009;150:619.
74. Youn JH, McDonough AA. Recent advances in understanding integrative control of potassium homeostasis. *Annu Rev Physiol.* 2009;71:381.
75. Moranne O, Froissart M, Rossert J. Timing of onset of CKD-related metabolic complications. *J Am Soc Nephrol.* 2009;20:164.
76. Gonick HC, Kleeman CR, Rubini ME, et al. Functional impairment in chronic renal disease. 3. Studies of potassium excretion. *Am J Med Sci.* 1971;261:281.
77. Kahn T, Kaji DM, Nicolis G, et al. Factors related to potassium transport in chronic stable renal disease in man. *Clin Sci Mol Med.* 1978;54:661.
78. Korgaonkar S, Tilea A, Gillespie BW, et al. Serum potassium and outcomes in CKD: insights from the RRI-CKD Cohort Study. *Clin J Am Soc Nephrol.* 2010;5:762.
79. Acker CG, Johnson JP, Palevsky M, et al. Hyperkalemia in the hospital. *J Am Soc Nephrol.* 1996;7:1346.
80. Gennari FJ, Segel AS. Hyperkalemia: an adaptive response in chronic renal insufficiency. *Kidney Int.* 2002;62:1.
81. Weinberg JM, Appel LJ, Bakris G, et al. Risk of hyperkalemia in nondiabetic patients with chronic kidney disease receiving antihypertensive therapy. *Arch Intern Med.* 2009;169(17):1587.
82. Adesman J, Goldberg M, Castelman L, et al. Simultaneous measurement of body sodium and potassium using Na^{22} and K^{42}. *Metabolism.* 1960;9:561.
83. Berlyne GM, Van Laethem L, Ben Ari J. Exchangeable potassium and renal potassium handling in advanced chronic renal failure in man. *Nephron.* 1971;8:264.
84. Kopple JD. Relationship between nutritional status and the glomerular filtration rate: results from the MDRD Study. *Kidney Int.* 2000;57:1688.
85. Patrick J. The assessment of body potassium stores. *Kidney Int.* 1977;11: 476.
86. Boddy K, King PC, Lindsay RM, et al. Exchangeable and total body potassium in patients with chronic renal failure. *Br Med J.* 1972;1:140.
87. Bergstrom J, Alvestrand A, Fürst P, et al. Muscle intracellular electrolytes in patients with chronic uremia. *Kidney Int Suppl.* 1983;16:S153.
88. Bergstrom J, Hultman E. Water, electrolyte and glycogen content of muscle tissue in patients undergoing regular dialysis therapy. *Clin Nephrol.* 1974;2:24.
89. Ericsson F, Carlmark B. Potassium in whole body, skeletal muscle and erythrocytes in chronic renal failure. *Nephron.* 1983;33:173.
90. Graham JA, Lawson DH, Linton AL. Muscle biopsy water and electrolyte contents in chronic renal failure. *Clin Sci.* 1970;38:583.
91. Montanari A, Montanari A, Borghi L, et al. Studies on cell water and electrolytes in chronic renal failure. *Clin Nephrol.* 1978;9:200.
92. Montanari A, Montanari A, Graziani G, et al. Skeletal muscle water and electrolytes in chronic renal failure. Effects of long-term regular dialysis treatment. *Nephron.* 1985;39:316.
93. Bilbrey GL, Carter NW, White MG, et al. Potassium deficiency in chronic renal failure. *Kidney Int.* 1973;4:423.
94. Cole CH. Decreased ouabain-sensitive adenosine triphosphatase activity in the erythrocyte membrane of patients with chronic renal disease. *Clin Sci.* 1973;45:775.
95. Welt LG, Sachs JR, McManus TJ. An ion transport defect in erythrocytes from uremic patients. *Trans Assoc Am Phys.* 1964;77:169.
96. Patrick J, Jones NF. Cell sodium, potassium and water in uraemia and the effects of regular dialysis as studied in the leucocyte. *Clin Sci.* 1974;46:583.
97. Cole CH, Balfe JW, Welt LG. Induction of an ouabain-sensitive ATPase defect by uremic plasma. *Trans Assoc Am Phys.* 1968;81:213.
98. Edmondson RP, Hilton PJ, Jones NF, et al. Leucocyte sodium transport in uraemia. *Clin Sci Mol Med.* 1975;49:213.
99. Kaji D, Kahn T. Na^+-K^+ pump in chronic renal failure. *Am J Physiol.* 1987;252:F785.
100. Perez GO, Pelleya R, Oster JR, et al. Blunted kaliuresis after an acute potassium load in patients with chronic renal failure. *Kidney Int.* 1983;24:656.
101. Bia MJ, DeFronzo RA. The medullary collecting duct (MCD) does not play a primary role in potassium (K) adaptation following decreased GFR. *Clin Res.* 1978;26:457A.
102. Bourgoignie JJ, Kaplan M, Pincus J, et al. Renal handling of potassium in dogs with chronic renal insufficiency. *Kidney Int.* 1981;20:482.
103. Schon DA, Silva P, Hayslett JP. Mechanism of potassium excretion in renal insufficiency. *Am J Physiol.* 1974;227:1323.
104. Fernandez J, Oster JR, Perez GO. Impaired extrarenal disposal of an acute oral potassium load in patients with end stage renal disease on chronic hemodialysis. *Miner Electrolyte Metab.* 1986;12:125.
105. Allon M, Dansby L, Shanklin N. Glucose modulation of the disposal of an acute potassium load in patients with end-stage renal disease. *Am J Med.* 1993;94:475.
106. Clark BA, Shannon C, Brown RS, et al. Extrarenal potassium homeostasis with maximal exercise in end-stage renal disease. *Am Soc Nephrol.* 1996;7:1223.
107. DeFronzo RA, Cooke CR, Andres R, et al. The effect of insulin on renal handling of sodium, potassium, calcium, and phosphate in man. *J Clin Invest.* 1975;55:845.
108. Westervelt FB. Insulin effect in uremia. *J Lab Clin Med.* 1969;74:79.
109. Alvestrand A, Wahren J, Smith D, et al. Insulin-mediated potassium uptake is normal in uremic and healthy subjects. *Am J Physiol.* 1984;246:E174.

110. Goecke IA, Bonilla S, Marusic ET, et al. Enhanced insulin sensitivity in extrarenal potassium handling in uremic rats. *Kidney Int.* 1991;39:39.
111. Atuk NO, Westervelt FB, Peach M. Altered catecholamine metabolism, plasma renin activity and hypertension in renal failure. *Int Cong Nephrol.* 1975;475A.
112. Henrich WL, Katz FH, Molinoff PB, et al. Competitive effects of hypokalemia and volume depletion on plasma renin activity, aldosterone and catecholamine concentrations in hemodialysis patients. *Kidney Int.* 1977;12:279.
113. Yang WC, Huang TP, Ho LT, et al. β-adrenergic-mediated extrarenal potassium disposal in patients with end-stage renal disease: effect of propranolol. *Miner Electrolyte Metab.* 1986;12:186.
114. Gifford JD, Rutsky EA, Kirk KA, et al. Control of serum potassium during fasting in patients with end-stage renal disease. *Kidney Int.* 1989;35:90.
115. Schrier RW, Regal EM. Influence of aldosterone on sodium, water and potassium metabolism in chronic renal disease. *Kidney Int.* 1972;1:156.
116. Weidmann P, Maxwell MH, De Lima J, et al. Control of aldosterone responsiveness in terminal renal failure. *Kidney Int.* 1975;7:351.
117. Weidmann P, Maxwell MH, Rowe P, et al. Role of the renin–angiotensin–aldosterone system in the regulation of plasma potassium in chronic renal disease. *Nephron.* 1975;15:35.
118. Williams GH, Bailey GL, Hampers CL, et al. Studies on the metabolism of aldosterone in chronic renal failure and anephric man. *Kidney Int.* 1973;4:280.
119. Schultze RG, Taggart DD, Shapiro H, et al. On the adaptation of potassium excretion associated with nephron reduction in the dog. *J Clin Invest.* 1971;50:1061.
120. Kunau RT, Whinnery MA. Potassium transfer in distal tubule of normal and remnant kidneys. *Am J Physiol.* 1978;235:F186.
121. Bank N, Aynedjian HS. A micropuncture study of potassium excretion by the remnant kidney. *J Clin Invest.* 1973;52:1480.
122. Fine LG, Yanagawa N, Schultze RG, et al. Functional profile of the isolated uremic nephron: potassium adaptation in the rabbit cortical collective tubule. *J Clin Invest.* 1979;64:1033.
123. Rocha A, Marcondes M, Malnic G. Micropuncture study in rats with experimental glomerulonephritis. *Kidney Int.* 1973;3:14.
124. Bia MJ, Tyler K, DeFronzo RA. Role of glucocorticoids and mineralocorticoids in potassium adaptation after decreased GFR. *Kidney Int.* 1983;23:211A.
125. Espinel CH. Effect of proportional reduction of sodium intake on the adaptive increase in glomerular filtration rate/nephron and potassium and phosphate excretion in chronic renal failure in the rat. *Clin Sci Mol Med.* 1975;49:193.
126. Charney AN, Kinsey MD, Myers L, et al. Na+-K+-activated adenosine triphosphatase and intestinal electrolyte transport. Effect of adrenal steroids. *J Clin Invest.* 1975;56:653.
127. Muto S, Asano Y, Seldin D, et al. Basolateral Na+ pump modulates apical Na+ and K+ conductances in rabbit cortical collecting ducts. *Am J Physiol.* 1999;276:F143.
128. Bastl C, Hayslett JP, Binder HJ. Increased large intestinal secretion of potassium in renal insufficiency. *Kidney Int.* 1977;12:9.
129. Hayes CP, MacLeod ME, Robinson RR. An extrarenal mechanism for the maintenance of potassium balance in severe chronic renal failure. *Trans Assoc Am Phys.* 1964;80:207.
130. Pitts RF. Symposium on acid–base homeostasis. Control of renal production of ammonia. *Kidney Int.* 1972;1:297.
131. Hsu CY, Chertow GM. Elevations of serum phosphorus and potassium in mild to moderate chronic renal insufficiency. *Nephrol Dial Transplant.* 2002;17:1419.
132. Widmer B, Gerhardt RE, Harrington IT, et al. Serum electrolyte and acid–base composition. The influence of graded degrees of chronic renal failure. *Arch Intern Med.* 1979;139:1099.
133. Wallia R, Greenberg A, Piraino B, et al. Serum electrolyte patterns in end-stage renal disease. *Am J Kidney Dis.* 1986;8:98.
134. Caravaca F, Arrobas M, Pizarro JL, et al. Metabolic acidosis in advanced renal failure: differences between diabetic and nondiabetic patients. *Am J Kidney Dis.* 1999;33:892.
135. Schwartz WB, Hall PW 3rd, Hays RM, Relman AS. On the mechanism of acidosis in chronic renal disease. *J Clin Invest.* 1959;38:39.
136. Relman AS, Lennon EJ, Lemann J Jr. Endogenous production of fixed acid and measurement of the net balance acid in normal subject. *J Clin Invest.* 1961;40:1621.
137. Goodman AD, Lemann J, Lennon EJ, et al. Production, excretion, and net balance of fixed acid in patient with renal acidosis. *J Clin Invest.* 1965;44:495.
138. Litzow JR, Lemann J Jr, Lennon EJ. The effect of treatment of acidosis on calcium balance in patients with chronic azotemic renal disease. *J Clin Invest.* 1967;46:280.
139. Warnock DG. Uremic acidosis. *Kidney Int.* 1988;34:278.
140. Wrong O, Davies HEF. The excretion of acid in renal disease. *Q J Med.* 1959;28:259.
141. Slatopolsky E, Hoffsten P, Purkerson M, et al. On the influence of extracellular fluid volume expansion and uremia of bicarbonate reabsorption in man. *J Clin Invest.* 1970;49:988.
142. Muldowney F, Donohoe JF, Carroll DV, et al. Parathyroid acidosis in uremia. *Q J Med.* 1972;41:321.
143. Arruda JA, Carrasquillo T, Cubria A, et al. Bicarbonate reabsorption in chronic renal failure. *Kidney Int.* 1976;9:481.
144. Lameire N, Matthys E. Influence of progressive salt restriction on urinary bicarbonate wasting in uremic acidosis. *Am J Kidney Dis.* 1986;8:151.
145. Wong NL, Quamme GA, Dirks JH. Tubular handling of bicarbonate in dogs with experimental renal failure. *Kidney Int.* 1984;25:912.
146. Buerkert J, Martin D, Trigg D, et al. Effect of reduced renal mass on ammonium handling and net acid formation by the superficial and juxtamedullary nephron of the rat. *J Clin Invest.* 1983;71:1661.
147. Oster JR. Renal acidification in patients with chronic renal insufficiency. PCO_2 of alkaline urine and response to ammonium chloride. *Miner Electrolyte Metab.* 1978;1:253.
148. Brigg AP, Waugh WH, Harms WS, et al. Pathophysiology of uremic acidosis as indicated by urinary acidification on a controlled diet. *Metabolism.* 1961;10:749.
149. Gonick HC, Maxwell MH, Rubini ME, et al. Functional impairment in chronic renal disease. II. Studies of acid excretion. *Nephron.* 1969;6:28.
150. Simpson DP. Control of hydrogen ion homeostasis and renal acidosis. *Medicine.* 1971;50:503.
151. MacClean AJ, Hayslett JP. Adaptive change in ammonia excretion in renal insufficiency. *Kidney Int.* 1980;17:595.
152. Stone DK, Seldin DW, Kokko JP, et al. Mineralocorticoid modulation of rabbit medullary collecting duct acidification. A sodium-independent effect. *J Clin Invest.* 1983;72:77.
153. Koeppen BM, Helmann SI. Acidification of luminal fluid by the rabbit cortical collecting tubule perfused in vitro. *Am J Physiol.* 1982;242:F521.
154. Al-Awqati Q, Norby LH, Mueller A, et al. Characteristics of stimulation of H^+ transport by aldosterone in turtle urinary bladder. *J Clin Invest.* 1976;58:351.
155. Kurtzman NA. Acquired distal renal tubular acidosis. *Kidney Int.* 1983;24:807.
156. DiTella PJ, Sodhi B, McCreary J, et al. Mechanism of the metabolic acidosis of selective mineralocorticoid deficiency. *Kidney Int.* 1978;14:466.
157. Hulter HN, Ilnicki LP, Harbottle JA, et al. Impaired renal H^+ secretion and NH^3 production in mineralocorticoid-deficient glucocorticoid-replete dogs. *Am J Physiol.* 1977;232:F136.
158. Good DW. Active absorption of NH_4^+ by rat medullary thick ascending limb: inhibition by potassium. *Am J Physiol.* 1988;255:F78.
159. Karet FE. J Mechanisms in hyperkalemic renal tubular acidosis. *Am Soc Nephrol.* 2009;20:251.
160. Szylman P, Better OS, Chaimowitz C, et al. Role of hyperkalemia in the metabolic acidosis of isolated hypoaldosteronism. *N Engl J Med.* 1976;294:361.
161. Sebastian A, Schambelan M, Lindenfeld S, et al. Amelioration of metabolic acidosis with fludrocortisone therapy in hyporeninemic hypoaldosteronism. *N Engl J Med.* 1977;297:576.
162. Matsuda O, Nonoguchi H, Tomita K, et al. Primary role of hyperkalemia in the acidosis of hyporeninemic hypoaldosteronism. *Nephron.* 1988;49:203.
163. Hudson J, Chobanian A, Relman A. Hypoaldosteronism. A clinical study of a patient with an isolated adrenal mineralocorticoid deficiency, resulting in hyperkalemia and Stokes-Adams attacks. *N Engl J Med.* 1957;257:529.
164. Christlieb AR, Hickler RB, Lauler DP, et al. Hypertension with inappropriate aldosterone stimulation. *N Engl J Med.* 1969;281:128.
165. Don BR, Schambelan M. Hyperkalemia in acute glomerulonephritis due to transient hyporeninemic hypoaldosteronism. *Kidney Int.* 1990;38:1159.
166. Schambelan M, Stockigt JR, Biglieri EG. Isolated hypoaldosteronism in adults. A renin-deficiency syndrome. *N Engl J Med.* 1972;287:573.
167. Brown J, Chinn RH, Fraser F, et al. Recurrent hyperkalemia due to selective aldosterone deficiency: correction by angiotensin infusion. *Br Med J.* 1973;1:650.
168. Perez G, Siegel L, Schreiner G. Selective hypoaldosteronism with hyperkalemia. *Ann Intern Med.* 1972;76:757.
169. Oh MS, Carroll HJ, Clemmons JE, et al. A mechanism for hyporeninemic hypoaldosteronism in chronic renal disease. *Metabolism.* 1974;23:1157.
170. Weidmann P, Reinhart R, Maxwell MH, et al. Syndrome of hyporeninemic hypoaldosteronism and hyperkalemia in renal disease. *J Clin Endocrinol Metab.* 1973;36:965.
171. DeFronzo RA. Hyperkalemia and hyporeninemic hypoaldosteronism. *Kidney Int.* 1980;17:118.

172. Rosansky SJ, Kennedy M. Sickle cell trait with episodic acute renal failure and type IV renal tubular acidosis. *Ann Intern Med.* 1980;93:643.
173. Roseman MK, Sehy JT, Arruda JAL, et al. Studies on the mechanism of hyperkalemic distal renal tubular acidosis (dRTA): gradient type dRTA in SC hemoglobinopathy. *Kidney Int.* 1977;12:473.
174. DeFronzo RA, Cooke CR, Goldberg M, et al. Impaired renal tubular potassium secretion in systemic lupus erythematosus. *Ann Intern Med.* 1977;86:268.
175. Hadler NM, Gill JR, Gardner JD. Impaired renal tubular secretion of potassium, elevated sweat sodium chloride concentration and plasma inhibition of erythrocyte sodium outflux as complications of systemic lupus erythematosus. *Arthritis Rheum.* 1972;15:515.
176. Kozeny GA, Barr W, Bansal VK, et al. Occurrence of renal tubular dysfunction in lupus nephritis. *Arch Intern Med.* 1987;147:891.
177. Li SL, Liu LB, Fang JT, et al. Symptomatic renal tubular acidosis (RTA) in patients with systemic lupus erythematosus: an analysis of six cases with new association of type 4 RTA. *Rheumatology.* 2005;44:1176.
178. DeFronzo RA, Goldberg M, Cooke CR, et al. Investigations into the mechanisms of hyperkalemia following renal transplantation. *Kidney Int.* 1977;11:357.
179. Gyory AZ, Stewart JH, George CRP, et al. Renal tubular acidosis, acidosis due to hyperkalemia, hypercalcemia, disordered citrate metabolism and other tubular dysfunctions following human renal transplantation. *Q J Med.* 1969;38:231.
180. Schwartz C, Benesch T, Kodras K, et al. Complete renal tubular acidosis late after kidney transplantation. *Nephrol Dial Transplant.* 2006;21:2615.
181. Batlle DC, Arruda JA, Kurtzman NA. Hyperkalemic distal renal tubular acidosis associated with obstructive uropathy. *N Engl J Med.* 1981;304:373.
182. Glassock RJ, Goldstein DA, Goldstone R, et al. Diabetes mellitus, moderate renal insufficiency and hyperkalemia. *Am J Nephrol.* 1983;3:233.
183. Schambelan M, Sebastian A, Biglieri EG. Prevalence, pathogenesis, and functional significance of aldosterone deficiency in hyperkalemic patients with chronic renal insufficiency. *Kidney Int.* 1980;17:89.
184. Arruda JA, Batlle DC, Sehy JT, et al. Hyperkalemia and renal insufficiency: role of selective aldosterone deficiency and tubular unresponsiveness to aldosterone. *Am J Nephrol.* 1981;1:160.
185. Perez GO, Lespier LE, Oster JR, et al. Effect of alterations of sodium intake in patients with hyporeninemic hypoaldosteronism. *Nephron.* 1977;18:259.
186. Phelps KR, Lieberman RL, Oh MS, et al. Pathophysiology of the syndrome of hyporeninemic hypoaldosteronism. *Metabolism.* 1980;29:186.
187. Chan R, Sealey JE, Michelis MF, et al. Renin–aldosterone system can respond to furosemide in patients with hyperkalemic hyporeninism. *J Lab Clin Med.* 1998;132:229.
188. Birkenhager WH. Interrelations between arterial pressure, fluid-volumes, and plasma-renin concentration in the course of acute glomerulonephritis. *Lancet.* 1970;1:1086.
189. Powell HR, Rotenberg E, Williams AL, et al. Plasma renin activity in acute post streptococcal glomerulonephritis and the haemolytic-uraemic syndrome. *Arch Dis Child.* 1974;49:802.
190. Gordon RD, Geddes RA, Pawsey CG, et al. Hypertension and severe hyperkalemia associated with suppression of renin and aldosterone and completely reversed by dietary sodium restriction. *Aust Ann Med.* 1970;4:287.
191. Rado JP, Boer P, Dorhout Mees EJ, et al. Outpatient hyperkalemia syndrome in renal and hypertensive patients with suppressed aldosterone production. *J Med.* 1979;10:145.
192. DeChamplain J, Genest J, Veyratt R, et al. Factors controlling renin in man. *Arch Intern Med.* 1966;117:355.
193. Wagermark J, Ungerstedt U, Ljungqvist A. Sympathetic innervation of the juxtaglomerular cells of the kidney. *Circ Res.* 1968;22:149.
194. Christensen NJ. Plasma catecholamines in long-term diabetes with and without neuropathy and in hypophysectomized subjects. *J Clin Invest.* 1972;51:779.
195. Tuck ML, Sambhi MP, Levin L. Hyporeninemic hypoaldosteronism in diabetes mellitus. Studies of the autonomic nervous system's control of renin release. *Diabetes.* 1979;28:237.
196. Gossain VV, Ferrara EV, Werk EE, et al. Impaired renin responsiveness with secondary hypoaldosteronism. *Arch Intern Med.* 1973;132:885.
197. Vagnucci AH. Selective aldosterone deficiency. *J Clin Endocrinol Metab.* 1969;29:279.
198. Fernandez-Cruz A, Noth RH, Lassman MN, et al. Low plasma renin activity in normotensive patients with diabetes mellitus: relationship to neuropathy. *Hypertension.* 1981;3:87.
199. de Chatel R, Weidmann P, Flammer J, et al. Sodium, renin, aldosterone, catecholamines, and blood pressure in diabetes mellitus. *Kidney Int.* 1977;12:412.
200. Tuck ML, Mayes DM. Mineralocorticoid biosynthesis in patients with hyporeninemic hypoaldosteronism. *J Clin Endocrinol Metab.* 1980;50:341.
201. Dunn MJ, Zambraski EJ. Renal effects of drugs that inhibit prostaglandin synthesis. *Kidney Int.* 1980;18:609.
202. Yun J, Kelly G, Bartter FC, et al. Role of prostaglandins in the control of renin secretion in the dog. *Circ Res.* 1977;40:459.
203. Saruta T, Kaplan NM. Adrenocortical steroidogenesis: the effects of prostaglandins. *J Clin Invest.* 1972;51:2246.
204. Tan SY, Shapiro RS, Franco R, et al. Indomethacin-induced prostaglandin inhibition with hyperkalemia. A reversible cause of hyporeninemic hypoaldosteronism. *Ann Intern Med.* 1979;90:783.
205. Aljadhey H Tu W, Hansen RA, et al. Risk of hyperkalemia associated with selective COX-2 inhibitors. *Pharmacoepidemiol Drug Saf.* 2010;19:1194.
206. Tan SY, Antonipillai I, Mulrow PJ. Inactive renin and prostaglandin production in hyporeninemic hypoaldosteronism. *J Clin Endocrinol Metab.* 1980;51:849.
207. deLeiva A, Christlieb AR, Melby JC, et al. Big renin and biosynthetic defect of aldosterone in diabetes mellitus. *N Engl J Med.* 1976;295:639.
208. Farese RV, Rodriguez-Colome M, O'Malley BC. Urinary prostaglandins following furosemide treatment and salt depletion in normal subjects with diabetic hyporeninemic hypoaldosteronism. *Clin Endocrinol.* 1980;13:447.
209. Brenner BM, Meyer TW, Hostetter TH. Dietary protein intake and the progressive nature of kidney disease. (The role of hemodynamically mediated glomerular injury in the pathogenesis of progressive glomerular sclerosis in aging, renal ablation, and intrinsic renal disease.) *N Engl J Med.* 1982;307:652.
210. Fredlund P, Saltman S, Catt KJ, et al. Aldosterone production by isolated glomerulosa cells: modulation of sensitivity to angiotensin II and ACTH by extracellular potassium concentration. *Endocrinology.* 1977;100:481.
211. Dluhy RG, Axelrod L, Underwood RH, et al. Studies of the control of plasma aldosterone concentration in normal man. II. Effect of dietary potassium and acute potassium infusion. *J Clin Invest.* 1972;51:1950.
212. Himathongkam T, Dluhy RG, Williams GH. Potassium-aldosterone-renin interrelationships. *J Clin Endocrinol Metab.* 1975;41:153.
213. Walker WG, Cooke CR. Plasma aldosterone regulation in anephric man. *Kidney Int.* 1973;3:1.
214. Bayard F, Cooke CR, Tiller DJ, et al. The regulation of aldosterone secretion in anephric man. *J Clin Invest.* 1971;50:1585.
215. Williams TDM, Walsh KP, Lightman SI, et al. Atrial natriuretic peptide inhibits postural release of renin and vasopressin in humans. *Am J Physiol.* 1988;255:R368.
216. Tuchelt H, Eschenhagen G, Bahr V, et al. Role of atrial natriuretic factor in changes in the responsiveness of aldosterone to angiotensin II secondary to sodium loading and depletion in man. *Clin Sci.* 1990;79:57.
217. Clark BA, Brown RS, Epstein FH. Effect of atrial natriuretic peptide on potassium-stimulated aldosterone secretion: potential relevance to hypoaldosteronism in man. *J Clin Endocrinol Metab.* 1992;75:399.
218. Barret PQ, Isales CM. The role of cyclic nucleotides in atrial natriuretic peptide-mediated inhibition of aldosterone secretion. *Endocrinology.* 1988;122:799.
219. McGiff JC, Muzzarelli RE, Duffy PA, et al. Interrelationships of renin and aldosterone in a patient with hypoaldosteronism. *Am J Med.* 1970;48:247.
220. Mellinger RC, Petermann FL, Jurgenson JC. Hyponatremia with low urinary aldosterone occurring in an old woman. *J Clin Endocrinol Metab.* 1972;34:85.
221. Tait JF, Tait SA. The effect of changes in potassium concentration on the maximal steroidogenic response of purified zona glomerulosa cells to angiotensin II. *J Steroid Biochem.* 1976;7:687.
222. Smith JD, DeFronzo RA. *Clinical Disorders of Potassium Metabolism, Fluid, Electrolyte and Acid–Base Disorders.* New York, NY: Churchill Livingstone; 1985.
223. Schnermann J, Persson AE, Agerup B. Tubuloglomerular feedback. Nonlinear relation between glomerular hydrostatic pressure and loop of Henle perfusion rate. *J Clin Invest.* 1973;52:862.
224. Schnermann J, Wright FS, Davis JM, et al. Regulation of superficial nephron filtration rate by tubuloglomerular feedback. *Pflugers Arch.* 1970;318:147.
225. Blantz RC, Konnen KS. Relation of distal tubular delivery and reabsorptive rate to nephron filtration. *Am J Physiol.* 1977;233: F315.
226. Blantz RC, Peterson OW, Gushwa L, et al. Effect of modest hyperglycemia on tubulo-glomerular feedback activity. *Kidney Int.* 1982;22:S206.
227. Tucker BJ, Tucker BJ, Gushwa L, et al. Mechanism of diuresis with modest hyperglycemia. *Clin Res.* 1981;29:478A.
228. Wright FS, Briggs JP. Feedback control of glomerular blood flow, pressure, and filtration rate. *Physiol Rev.* 1979;59:958.
229. Perez GO, Pelleya R, Oster JR. Renal tubular hyperkalemia. *Am J Nephrol.* 1982;2:109.
230. Battle DC, Itsarayoungyuen K, Arruda JAL, et al. Hyperkalemic hyperchloremic metabolic acidosis in sickle cell hemoglobinopathies. *Am J Med.* 1982;72:188.
231. Morris RC, McSherry E. Symposium on acid–base homeostasis. Renal acidosis. *Kidney Int.* 1972;1:322.

232. Bastani B, Underhill D, Chu N, et al. Preservation of intercalated cell H(+)-ATPase in two patients with lupus nephritis and hyperkalemic distal renal tubular acidosis. *J Am Soc Nephrol.* 1997;8:1109.
233. Cohen EP, Bastani B, Cohen MR, et al. Absence of H(+)-ATPase in cortical collecting tubules of a patient with Sjögren's syndrome and distal renal tubular acidosis. *J Am Soc Nephrol.* 1992;3:264.
234. Purcell H, Bastani B, Harris KP, et al. Cellular distribution of H(+)-ATPase following acute unilateral ureteral obstruction in rats. *Am J Physiol.* 1991;261:F365.
235. Batlle DC, Mozes MF, Manaligod J, et al. The pathogenesis of hyperchloremic metabolic acidosis associated with kidney transplantation. *Am J Med.* 1981;70:786.
236. Roll D, Licht A, Rösler A, et al. Transient hypoaldosteronism after renal allotransplantation. *Isr J Med Sci.* 1979;15:29.
237. Heering P, Grabensee B. Influence of cyclosporine A on renal tubular function after kidney transplantation. *Nephron.* 1991;59:66.
238. Kamel SK, Ethier JH, Quaggin S, et al. Studies to determine the basis of hyperkalemia in recipients of a renal transplant who are treated with cyclosporine. *J Am Soc Nephrol.* 1992;2:1279.
239. Perazella MA, Brown E. Electrolyte and acid–base disorders associated with AIDS: an etiologic review. *J Gen Int Med.* 1994;9:232.
240. Peter SA. Electrolyte disorders and renal dysfunction in acquired immunodeficiency syndrome patients. *J Natl Med Assoc.* 1991;83:889.
241. Popovtzer MM, Katz FH, Pinggera WF, et al. Hyperkalemia in salt-wasting nephropathy. Study of the mechanisms. *Arch Intern Med.* 1973;132:203.
242. Morgan JM. Hyperkalemia and acidosis in lead nephropathy. *South Med J.* 1976;69:881.
243. Cogan MC, Arieff AI. Sodium-wasting, acidosis and hyperkalemia induced by methicillin interstitial nephritis. Evidence for selective distal tubular dysfunction. *Am J Med.* 1978;64:500.
244. Lawson DH. Adverse reactions to potassium chloride. *Q J Med.* 1974;43:433.
245. Lawson DH, O'Connor PC, Jick H, et al. Drug attributed alterations in potassium handling in congestive cardiac failure. *Eur J Clin Pharmacol.* 1982;23:21.
246. Paice B, Gray JM, McBride D, et al. Hyperkalemia in patients in hospital. *Br Med J.* 1983;286:1189.
247. Shapiro S, Slone D, Lewis GP, et al. Fatal drug reactions among medical inpatients. *J Am Med Assoc.* 1971;216:467.
248. Shemer J, Ezra D, Modan M, et al. Incidence of hyperkalemia in hospitalized patients. *Isr J Med Sci.* 1983;19:659.
249. Tarver T. Desalting the food grid. *Food Technology.* 2010; 64(8).
250. Ponce SP, Jennings AE, Madias NE, et al. Drug-induced hyperkalemia. *Medicine.* 1985;64:357.
251. Mueller BA, Scott MK, Sowinski KM, et al. Noni juice (*Morinda citrifolia*): hidden potential for hyperkalemia? *Am J Kidney Dis.* 2000;35:310.
252. Sherman RA, Mehta O. Phosphorus and potassium content of enhanced meat and poultry products: implications for patients who receive dialysis. *Clin J Am Soc Nephrol.* 2009;4:1370.
253. Mercer CW, Logic JR. Cardiac arrest due to hyperkalemia following intravenous penicillin administration. *Chest.* 1973;64:358.
254. Browning JJ, Channer KS. Hyperkalaemic cardiac arrhythmia caused by potassium citrate mixture. *Br Med J.* 1981;283:1366.
255. Michael JM, Dorner I, Bruns D, et al. Potassium load in CPD-preserved whole blood and two types of packed red blood cells. *Transfusion.* 1975;15:144.
256. Bethune DW, McKay R. Paradoxical changes in serum potassium during cardiopulmonary bypass in association with non-cardioselective β-blockade. *Lancet.* 1978;2:380.
257. Lundborg P. The effect of adrenergic blockade on potassium concentrations in different conditions. *Acta Med Scand.* 1983;672:121.
258. Traub YM, Rabinov M, Rosenfeld JB, et al. Elevation of serum potassium during β blockade: absence of relationship to the renin–aldosterone system. *Clin Pharmacol Ther.* 1980;28:765.
259. Arthur S, Greenberg A. Hyperkalemia associated with intravenous labetalol therapy for acute hypertension in renal transplant recipients. *Clin Nephrol.* 1990;33:269.
260. Borra S, Shaker R, Kleinfeld M. Hyperkalemia in an adult hospitalized population. *Mt Sinai J Med.* 1988;55:226.
261. Rimmer JM, Horn JF. Hyperkalemia as a complication of drug therapy. *Arch Intern Med.* 1987;147:867.
262. Ahmed EU, Mohammed BN, Matute R, et al. Etiology of hyperkalemia in hospitalized patients: an answer to Harrinton's question. *J Am Soc Nephrol.* 1999;10:103A.
263. Smith TW, Willerson JT. Suicidal and accidental digoxin ingestion. Report of five cases with serum digoxin level correlations. *Circulation.* 1971;44:29.
264. Reza MJ, Kovick RB, Shine KI, et al. Massive intravenous digoxin overdosage. *N Engl J Med.* 1974;291:777.
265. Levinsky NG, Tyson I, Miller RB, et al. The relationship between amino acids and potassium in isolated rat muscle. *J Clin Invest.* 1962;41:480.
266. Dickerman HW, Walker WG. Effect of cationic amino acid infusion on potassium metabolism *in vivo*. *Am J Physiol.* 1964;206:403.
267. Alberti KGM, Johnston HH, Lauler DP, et al. Effect of arginine on electrolyte metabolism in man. *Clin Res.* 1967;15:476A.
268. Hertz P, Richardson JA. Arginine-induced hyperkalemia in renal failure patients. *Arch Intern Med.* 1972;130:778.
269. Bushinsky DA, Gennari FJ. Life-threatening hyperkalemia induced by arginine. *Ann Intern Med.* 1978;89:632.
270. Carroll HJ, Tice DA. The effects of epsilon amino-caproic acid upon potassium metabolism in the dog. *Metabolism.* 1966;15:449.
271. Perazella MA, Biswas P. Acute hyperkalemia associated with intravenous epsilon-aminocaproic acid therapy. *Am J Kidney Dis.* 1999;33:782.
272. Perazella MA, Garwood S, Matthew J, et al. Hyperkalemia associated with IV epsilon-aminocaproic acid. *J Am Soc Nephrol.* 1999;10:123A.
273. Weintraub HD, Heisterkamp DV, Cooperman LH. Changes in plasma potassium concentration after depolarizing blockers in anaesthetized man. *Br J Anaesth.* 1969;41:1048.
274. Yentis SM. Suxamethonium and hyperkalaemia. *Anaesth Intens Care.* 1990;18:92.
275. Gronert GA, Theye RA. Pathophysiology of hyperkalemia induced by succinylcholine. *Anesthesiology.* 1975;43:89.
276. Preston RA, Afshartous D, Garg D, et al. Mechanisms of impaired potassium handling with dual rennin-angiotensin-aldosterone blockade in chronic kidney disease. *Hypertension.* 2009;53:754.
277. Laragh JH. Amiloride, a potassium-conserving agent new to the USA: mechanisms and clinical relevance. *Curr Ther Res.* 1982;32:173.
278. Ramsay LE, Hettiarachchi J, Fraser R, et al. Amiloride, spironolactone, and potassium chloride in thiazide-treated hypertensive patients. *Clin Pharmacol.* 1980;4:533.
279. Good DW, Wright FS. Luminal influences on potassium secretion: sodium concentration and fluid flow rate. *Am J Physiol.* 1979;236:F192.
280. Udezue FU, Harrold BP. Hyperkalaemic paralysis due to spironolactone. *Postgrad Med.* 1980;56:254.
281. Greenblatt DJ, Koch-Weser J. Adverse reactions to spironolactone. A report from Boston Collaborative Drug Surveillance Program. *JAMA.* 1973;225:40.
282. Whiting GF, McLaran CJ, Bochner F. Severe hyperkalaemia with moduretic. *Med J Aust.* 1979;1:409.
283. Petersen AG. Letter: dyazide and hyperkalemia. *Ann Intern Med.* 1976;84:612.
284. Feinfeld DA, Carvounis CP. Fatal hyperkalemia and hyperchloremic acidosis. Association with spironolactone in the absence of renal impairment. *J Am Med Assoc.* 1978;240:1516.
285. Jaffey L, Martin A. Malignant hyperkalemia after amiloride/hydrochlorothiazide treatment. *Lancet.* 1981;1:1272.
286. Chiu TF, Bullard MJ, Chen JC, et al. Rapid life-threatening hyperkalemia after addition of amiloride HCl/hydrochlorothiazide to angiotensin-converting enzyme inhibitor therapy. *Ann Emerg Med.* 1997;30:612.
287. Maddox RW, Arnold WS, Dewell WM Jr . Extreme hyperkalemia associated with amiloride. *South Med J.* 1985;78:365.
288. Henger A, Tutt P, Riesen WF, Hulter HN, Krapf R. Acid–base effects of inhibition of aldosterone and angiotensin II action in chronic metabolic acidosis in humans. *J Am Soc Nephrol.* 1999;10:121A.
289. McNay JL, Oran E. Possible predisposition of diabetic patients to hyperkalemia following administration of potassium-retaining diuretic, amiloride (MK-870). *Metabolism.* 1970;19:58.
290. Mor R, Pitlik S, Rosenfeld JB, et al. Indomethacin- and moduretic-induced hyperkalemia. *Isr J Med Sci.* 1983;19:535.
291. Walker BR, Capuzzi DM, Alexander F, et al. Hyperkalemia after triamterene in diabetic patients. *Clin Pharmacol Ther.* 1972;13:643.
292. Wan HH, Lye MDW. Moduretic-induced metabolic acidosis and hyperkalemia. *Postgrad Med J.* 1980;56:348.
293. Pitt B, Zannad F, Remm WJ, et al. The effect of spironolactone on morbidity and mortality in patients with severe heart failure. *New Engl J Med.* 1999;341:709.
294. Juurlink DN, Mamdani MM, Lee DS, et al. Rates of hyperkalemia after publication of the Randomized Aldactone Evaluation Study. *N Engl J Med.* 2004;351:543.
295. Pitt B, Remme W, Zannad F, et al. Eplerenone, a selective aldosterone blocker, in patients with left ventricular dysfunction after myocardial infarction. *N Engl J Med.* 2003;348:1309.
296. Wei L, Struthers AD, Fahey T, Watson AD, MacDonald TM. Spironolactone use and renal toxicity: population based longitudinal analysis. *Br Med J.* 2010; 18;340:c1768.

297. Preston RA, White WB, Pitt B, et al. Effects of drospirenone/17-beta estradiol on blood pressure and potassium balance in hypertensive postmenopausal women. *Am J Hypertens.* 2005;18:797.
298. Schlondorff D. Renal complications of nonsteroidal anti-inflammatory drugs. *Kidney Int.* 1993;44:643.
299. Garella S, Matarese RA. Renal effects of prostaglandins and clinical adverse effects of nonsteroidal anti-inflammatory agents. *Medicine.* 1984;63:165.
300. Mactier RA, Khanna R. Hyperkalemia induced by indomethacin and naproxen and reversed by fludrocortisone. *South Med J.* 1988;81:799.
301. Kimberly RP, Bowden RE, Keiser HR, et al. Reduction of renal function by newer non-steroidal anti-inflammatory drugs. *Am J Med.* 1978;64:799.
302. Corwin HL, Bonventre JV. Renal insufficiency associated with nonsteroidal anti-inflammatory agents. *Am J Kidney Dis.* 1984;4:147.
303. Frais MA, Burgess ED, Mitchell LB. Piroxicam-induced renal failure and hyperkalemia. *Ann Intern Med.* 1983;99:129.
304. Galler M, Volkert VW, Schlondorff D, et al. Reversible acute renal insufficiency and hyperkalemia following indomethacin therapy. *J Am Med Assoc.* 1981;246:154.
305. Perazella MA. COX-2 selective inhibitors: Analysis of the renal effects. *Expert Opin Drug Saf.* 2002;1:53.
306. Einhorn LM, Zhan M, Hsu VD, et al. The frequency of hyperkalemia and its significance in chronic kidney disease. *Arch Intern Med.* 2009;169:1156.
307. Textor SC, Bravo EL, Fouad FM, et al. Hyperkalemia in azotemic patients during angiotensin-converting enzyme inhibition and aldosterone reduction with captopril. *Am J Med.* 1982;73:719.
308. Atlas SA, Case DB, Sealey JE, et al. Interruption of the renin–angiotensin system in hypertensive patients by captopril induces sustained reduction in aldosterone secretion, potassium retention and natriuresis. *Hypertension.* 1979;1:274.
309. Memon A, et al. Incidence and predictors of hyperkalemia in patients with chronic renal failure on angiotensin converting enzyme inhibitors. *J Am Soc Nephrol.* 1999;10:294A.
310. Reardon LC, Macpherson DS. Hyperkalemia in outpatients using angiotensin-converting enzyme inhibitors. How much should we worry? *Arch Intern Med.* 1998;158:26.
311. Keilani T, Danesh FR, Schlueter WA, et al. A subdepressor low dose of ramipril lowers urinary protein excretion without increasing plasma potassium. *Am J Kidney Dis.* 1999;33:450.
312. Russo D, Pisani A, Balletta MM. Additive antiproteinuric effect of converting enzyme inhibitor and losartan in normotensive patients with IgA nephropathy. *Am J Kidney Dis.* 1999;33:851.
313. Heeg JE, de Jong PE, Vriesendorp R, et al. Additive antiproteinuric effect of the NSAID indomethacin and the ACE inhibitor lisinopril. *Am J Nephrol.* 1990;10:94.
314. White WB, Aydelotte ME. Clinical experience with labetalol and enalapril in combination in patients with severe essential and renovascular hypertension. *Am J Med Sci.* 1988;296:187.
315. Dahlstrom U, Karlsson E. Captopril and spironolactone therapy for refractory congestive heart failure. *Am J Cardiol.* 1993;71:29A.
316. Hannedouche T, Landais P, Goldfarb B, et al. Randomised controlled trial of enalapril and β blockers in non-diabetic chronic renal failure. *Br Med J.* 1994;309:833.
317. Apperloo AJ, De Zeeuw D, Sluiter HE, et al. Differential effects of enalapril and atenolol on proteinuria and renal haemodynamics in non-diabetic renal disease. *Br Med J.* 1991;303:821.
318. Juurlink DN, Mamdani M, Kopp A, et al. Drug-drug interactions among elderly patients hospitalized for drug toxicity. *JAMA.* 2003;289:1652.
319. Ferder L, Daccordi H, Martello M, et al. Angiotensin converting enzyme inhibitors versus calcium antagonists in the treatment of diabetic hypertensive patients. *Hypertension.* 1992;19:II237.
320. Kjekshus J, Swedberg K. Tolerability of enalapril in congestive heart failure. *Am J Cardiol.* 1988;62:67A.
321. Weinberg JM, Appel LJ, Bakris G, et al. Risk of hyperkalemia in nondiabetic patients with chronic kidney disease receiving antihypertensive therapy. *Arch Intern Med.* 2009;169:1587.
322. Johnson ES, Weinstein JR, Thorp ML, et al. Predicting the risk of hyperkalemia in patients with chronic kidney disease starting lisinopril. *Pharmacoepidemiol Drug Saf.* 2010;19:266.
323. Goldberg MR, Bradstreet TE, McWilliams EJ, et al. Biochemical effects of losartan, a nonpeptide angiotensin II receptor antagonist, on the renin–angiotensin–aldosterone system in hypertensive patients. *Hypertension.* 1995;25:37.
324. Goldberg AI, Dunlay MC. Safety and tolerability of losartan potassium, an angiotensin II receptor antagonist, compared with hydrochlorothiazide, atenolol, felodipine ER, and angiotensin-converting enzyme inhibitors for the treatment of systemic hypertension. *Am J Cardiol.* 1995;75:793.
325. Savoy A, Palant CE, Patchin G, et al. Losartan effects on serum potassium in an elderly population. *J Am Soc Nephrol.* 1998;9:111A.
326. Bakris GL, Siomos M, Bolton WK, et al. Differential effects of valsartan and lisinopril on potassium homeostasis in hypertensive patients with nephropathy. *J Am Soc Nephrol.* 1999;10:68A.
327. Ruilope LM, Aldigier JC, Ponticelli C, et al. Safety of combination of valsartan and benazepril in patients with chronic kidney disease. European Group for the Investigation of Valsartan in Chronic Renal Disease. *J Hypertens.* 2000; 18:89.
328. Luno J, Barrio V, Goicoechea MA, et al. Effects of dual blockade of the renin-angiotensin system in primary proteinuric nephropathies. *Kidney Int.* 2002;62:S47.
329. Weir MR, Rolfe M. Potassium homeostasis and renin-angiotensin-aldosterone system inhibitors. *Clin J Am Soc Nephrol.* 2010;5:531.
330. Velázquez H, Perazella MA, Wright FS, et al. Renal mechanism of trimethoprim-induced hyperkalemia. *Ann Intern Med.* 1993;119:296.
331. Kaufman AM, Hellman G, Abramson RG, et al. Renal salt wasting and metabolic acidosis with trimethoprim-sulfamethoxazole therapy. *Mt Sinai J Med.* 1983;50:238.
332. Alappan R, Perazella MA, Buller GK. Hyperkalemia in hospitalized patients treated with trimethoprim-sulfamethoxazole. *Ann Intern Med.* 1996;124:316.
333. Alappan R, Buller GK, Perazella MA. Trimethoprim-sulfamethoxazole therapy in outpatients: is hyperkalemia a significant problem? *Am J Nephrol.* 1999;19:389.
334. Briceland LL, Bailie GR. Pentamidine-associated nephrotoxicity and hyperkalemia in patients with AIDS. *DICP.* 1991;25:1171.
335. Antoniou T, Gomes T, Juurlink DN, et al. Trimethoprim-sulfamethoxazole-induced hyperkalemia in patients receiving inhibitors of the renin-angiotensin system: a population-based study. *Arch Intern Med.* 2010;170:1045.
336. Weir MA, Juurlink DN, Gomes T, et al. Beta-blockers, trimethoprim-sulfamethoxazole, and the risk of hyperkalemia requiring hospitalization in the elderly: a nested case-control study. *CJASN.* 2010;5:1544.
337. Oster JR, Singer I, Fishman LM. Heparin-induced aldosterone suppression and hyperkalemia. *Am J Med.* 1995;98:575.
338. Yu HS, Chang HS, Han DJ, et al. Change of transtubular potassium gradient (TTKG) in renal transplant recipients. *J Am Soc Nephrol.* 1999;10:14A.
339. Asante-Korang A, Boyle GJ, Webber SA, et al. Experience of FK506 immune suppression in pediatric heart transplantation: a study of long term adverse effects. *J Heart Lung Transplant.* 1996;15:415.
340. Tumlin JA, Sands JM. Nephron segment-specific inhibition of Na+/K(+)-ATPase activity by cyclosporin A. *Kidney Int.* 1993;43:246.
341. Lea JP, Sands JM, McMahon SJ, et al. Evidence that the inhibition of Na+/K(+)-ATPase activity by FK506 involves calcineurin. *Kidney Int.* 1994;46:647.
342. Ling BN, Eaton DC. Cyclosporin A inhibits apical secretory K+ channels in rabbit cortical collecting tubule principal cells. *Kidney Int.* 1993;44:974.
343. Pei Y, Richardson R, Greenwood C, et al. Extrarenal effect of cyclosporine A on potassium homeostasis in renal transplant recipients. *Am J Kidney Dis.* 1993;22:314.
344. DeFronzo RA, Smith JD. Disorders of potassium metabolism-hyperkalemia. In: Arieff AI, DeFronzo RA, eds. *Fluid, Electrolyte and Acid–Base Disorders.* New York, NY: Churchill-Livingstone; 1995:319.
345. Moore RD. Stimulation of Na:H exchange by insulin. *Biophys J.* 1981;33: 203.
346. Gourley DRH. Effect of insulin on potassium exchange in normal and ouabain-treated skeletal muscle. *J Pharmacol Exp Ther.* 1965;148:339.
347. Kamel K, Wei C. Controversial issues in the treatment of hyperkalemia. *Nephrol Dial Transplant.* 2003;18:2215.
348. Allon M, Copkney C. Albuterol and insulin for treatment of hyperkalemia in hemodialysis patients. *Kidney Int.* 1990;38:869.
349. Sowinski KM, Cronin D, Mueller BA, et al. Subcutaneous terbutaline use in CKD to reduce potassium concentrations. *Am J Kidney Dis.* 2005;45:1040.
350. Ngugi N, McLigeyo SO, Kayima JK, et al. Treatment of hyperkalemia by altering the transcellular gradient in patients with renal failure: efficacy of various therapeutic approaches. *East Afr Med J.* 1997;74:503.
351. Blumberg A, Weidmann P, Shaw S, et al. Effect of various therapeutic approaches on plasma potassium and major regulating factors in terminal renal failure. *Am J Med.* 1988;85:507.
352. Ethier JH, Kamel KS, Magner PO, et al. The transtubular potassium concentration in patients with hypokalemia and hyperkalemia. *Am J Kidney Dis.* 1990;15:309.
353. Kamel KS, Ethier JH, Richardson RM, et al. Urine electrolytes and osmolality: when and how to use them. *Am J Nephrol.* 1990;10:89.
354. Zettle RM, West ML, Josse RG, et al. Renal potassium handling during states of low aldosterone bio-activity: a method to differentiate renal from non-renal causes. *Am J Nephrol.* 1987;7:360.

355. Choi MJ, Ziyadeh FN. The utility of the transtubular potassium gradient in the evaluation of hyperkalemia. *J Am Soc Nephrol.* 2008;19:424.
356. Goldstein MB, Bear R, Richardson RM, et al. The urine anion gap: a clinically useful index of ammonium excretion. *Am J Med Sci.* 1986;292:198.
357. Batlle DC, Hizon M, Cohen E, et al. The use of urinary anion gap in the diagnosis of hyperchloremic metabolic acidosis. *N Engl J Med.* 1988;318:594.
358. Dyck RF, Asthana S, Kalra J, et al. A modification of the urine osmolal gap: an improved method for estimating urine ammonium. *Am J Nephrol.* 1990;10:359.
359. Halperin ML, Richardson RM, Bear RA, et al. Urine ammonium: the key to the diagnosis of distal renal tubular acidosis. *Nephron.* 1988;50:1.
360. Dominguez JH, Raisz LG. Effects of changing hydrogen ion, carbonic acid, and bicarbonate concentrations on bone resorption in vitro. *Calcif Tissue Int.* 1979;29:7.
361. Adams ND, Gray RW, Lemann J Jr. The calciuria of increased fixed acid production: evidence against a role for parathyroid hormone and 1, 25(OH)2-vitamin D. *Calcif Tiss Int.* 1979;28:233.
362. Kraut JA, Mishler DR, Kurokawa K. Effect of colchicine and calcitonin on calcemic response to metabolic acidosis. *Kidney Int.* 1984;25:608.
363. Greiber S, Mitch WE. Catabolism in uremia: metabolic acidosis and activation of specific pathways. *Contrib Nephrol.* 1992;98:20.
364. Workeneh BT, Mitch WE. Review of muscle wasting associated with chronic kidney disease. *Am J Clin Nutr.* 2010;91(suppl):1128S.
365. Kovesdy CP, Anderson JE, Kalantar-Zadeh K. Association of serum bicarbonate levels with mortality in patients with non-dialysis-dependent CKD. *Nephrol Dial Transplant.* 2009;24:1232.
366. Menon V, Tighiouart H, Vaughn NS, et al. Serum bicarbonate and long-term outcomes in CKD. *Am J Kidney Dis.* 56:907.
367. de Brito-Ashurst I, Varagunam M, Raftery MJ, et al. Bicarbonate supplementation slows progression of CKD and improves nutritional status. *Am Soc Nephrol.* 2009;20:2075.
368. Phisitkul S, Khanna A, Simoni J, et al. Amelioration of metabolic acidosis in patients with low GFR reduced kidney endothelin production and kidney injury, and better preserved GFR. *Kidney Int.* 2010;77:617.
369. Nath KA, Hostetter MK, Hostetter TH. Pathophysiology of chronic tubulo-interstitial disease in rats. Interactions of dietary acid load, ammonia, and complement component C3. *J Clin Invest.* 1985;76:667.
370. Scherr L, Ogden DA, Mead AW, et al. Management of hyperkalemia with a cation-exchange resin. *N Engl J Med.* 1961;19;264:115.
371. Flinn RB, Merrill JP, Welzant WR. Treatment of the oliguric patient with a new sodium-exchange resin and sorbitol; a preliminary report. *N Engl J Med.* 1961;19;264:111.
372. Watson M, Abbott KC, Yuan CM. Damned if you do, damned if you don't: potassium binding resins in hyperkalemia. *Clin J Am Soc Nephrol.* 2010;5:1723.
373. Gerstman BB, Kirkman R, Platt R. Intestinal necrosis associated with postoperative orally administered sodium polystyrene sulfonate in sorbitol. *Am J Kidney Dis.* 1992;20:159.

CHAPTER

73 Disorders of Phosphorus, Calcium, and Magnesium Metabolism

Keith A. Hruska • Moshe Levi • Eduardo Slatopolsky

PHOSPHORUS

Phosphorus is a common anion ubiquitously distributed throughout the body. Approximately 80% to 85% of the phosphorus is present in the skeleton. The rest is widely distributed in the form of organic phosphate compounds that play fundamental roles in several aspects of cellular metabolism. The energy required for many cellular reactions including biosynthesis derives from hydrolysis of adenosine triphosphate (ATP). Organic phosphates are important components of cell membrane phospholipids. In the extracellular fluid (ECF), phosphorus is present predominantly in the inorganic form (Pi). The physiologic concentration of serum phosphorus ranges from 2.5 to 4.5 mg/dL (0.9 to 1.45 mmol/L) in adults.[373] In serum, phosphorus exists mainly as the free ion, and only a small fraction (less than 15%) is protein bound.[274,683] There is a diurnal variation in serum phosphorus of 0.6 to 1.0 mg/dL, with the nadir occurring between 8 AM and 11 AM.

Phosphorus Balance and Gastrointestinal Absorption

Approximately 1 g of phosphorus is ingested daily in an average diet in the United States. About 300 mg is excreted in the stool, and 700 mg is absorbed (Fig. 73.1). Most of the phosphorus is absorbed in the duodenum and jejunum with minimal absorption occurring in the ileum.[204] Phosphorus transport in proximal segments of the small intestine appears to involve both passive and active components and to be under the influence of vitamin D. The movement of phosphorus from the intestinal lumen to the blood requires (1) transport across the luminal brush-border membrane of the intestine; (2) transport through the cytoplasm; and (3) transport across the basolateral plasma membrane of the epithelium. The rate-limiting step and the main driving force of absorption is the luminal membrane step.[373]

Intestinal Epithelial Luminal Membrane Transport

The mechanism of transport across the intestinal brush border epithelial membrane involves a sodium–phosphate (NaPi) cotransport system, NaPi-IIb.[265] The NaPi cotransporters are a secondary active form of ion transport using the energy of the Na gradient from outside to inside the cell to move phosphate ion uphill against an electrochemical gradient (Fig. 73.2).

The intestinal NaPi-IIb transporter is upregulated by a low phosphate diet and 1,25-dihydroxyvitamin D3.[258,314] Although low phosphate diets upregulate1,25-dihydroxyvitamin D3, studies in vitamin D–receptor (VDR) null mice indicate that the intestinal NaPi cotransport adaptation to a low phosphate diet occurs independent of vitamin D.[585]

Intestinal NaPi cotransport activity and NaPi-IIb protein is also regulated by several other factors—including the aging process,[722] glucocorticoids,[26] epidermal growth factor (EGF),[723] and liver X receptor (LXR)[106]—that decrease intestinal NaPi transport, and estrogen[724] and metabolic acidosis[638] that increase intestinal NaPi transport.

Studies of phosphorus accumulation by rat intestinal brush-border vesicles have demonstrated that it is affected by the transmembrane potential, indicating that like the renal type IIa cotransporter, NaPi-IIa, the intestinal type IIb cotransporter, NaPi-IIb, is electrogenic.[265] The $K_m(P_i)$ of NaPi-IIb is approximately 50 μm, similar to the renal transport protein. In contrast to the renal NaPi-IIa isoform, the intestinal NaPi-IIb cotransporter is less dependent on the pH level.

Transcellular Movement of Phosphorus

The second component of transcellular intestinal phosphorus transport involves the movement of phosphorus from the luminal to the basolateral membrane. Although little is known about the cellular events that mediate this transcellular process, evidence suggests a role for the microtubular microfilament system of intestinal cells.[204] Microfilaments in the cell may be important in conveying phosphorus from the brush-border membrane to the basolateral membrane and may be involved in the extrusion of phosphorus at the basolateral membrane from the epithelial cell.

Phosphate Exit at Basolateral Membrane

Little is known about the mechanisms of phosphorus extrusion at the basolateral membrane of intestinal epithelial cells.

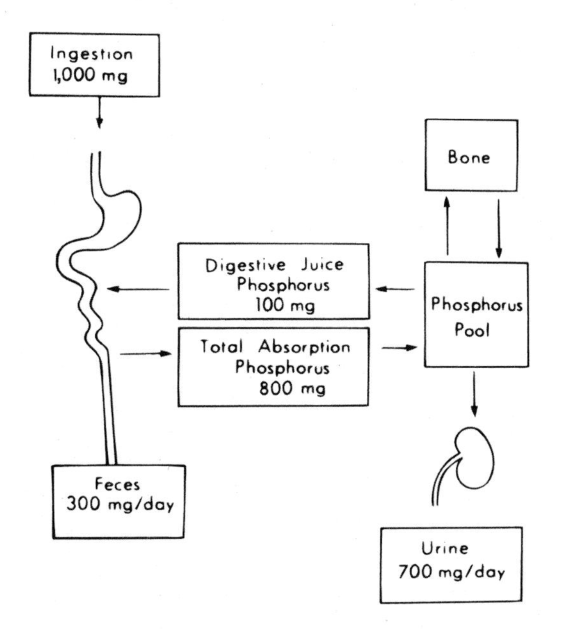

FIGURE 73.1 Summary of phosphorus metabolism in humans. Approximately 1 g of phosphorus is ingested daily, of which 300 mg is excreted in the stool and 700 mg in the urine. The gastrointestinal tract, bone, and kidney are the major organs involved in phosphorus homeostasis.

The electrochemical gradient for phosphorus favors movement from the intracellular to the extracellular compartment because the interior of the cell is electrically negative compared with the basolateral external surface. Therefore, the presumption has been that the exit of phosphorus across the basolateral membrane represents a mode of passive transport.[321]

Renal Excretion of Phosphorus, Reabsorption

Most of the inorganic phosphorus in serum (90% to 95%) is ultrafiltrable at the level of the glomerulus. At physiologic levels of serum phosphorus, approximately 7 g of phosphorus is filtered daily by the kidney, of which 80% to 90% is reabsorbed by the renal tubules and the remainder is excreted in the urine (approximately 700 mg on a 1-g phosphorus diet)

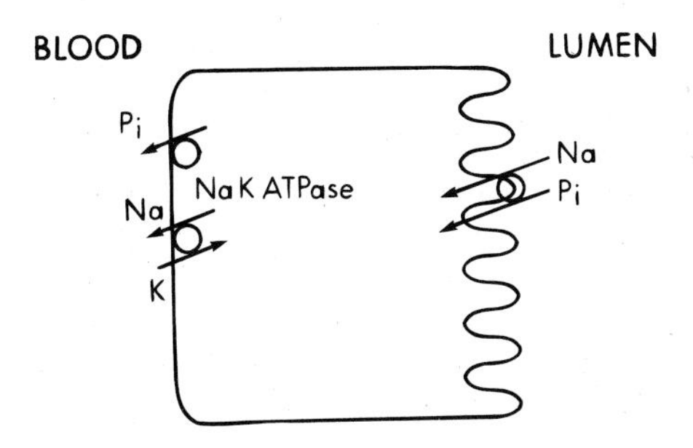

FIGURE 73.2 The apical membrane sodium–inorganic phosphate (Pi) cotransport proteins utilize the electrochemical driving force for sodium to move Pi into the cell. The electrochemical sodium gradient is maintained by active sodium extrusion across the basolateral membrane through the action of Na^+-K^+-ATPase.

equal to intestinal absorption.[332] As a result, adults are generally in balance between phosphorus intake and excretion (Fig. 73.1). Micropuncture studies have demonstrated that 60% to 70% of the filtered phosphorus is reabsorbed in the proximal tubule. However, there is also evidence that a significant amount of filtered phosphorus is reabsorbed in distal segments of the nephron.[502] When serum phosphorus levels increase and the filtered load of phosphorus increases, the capacity to reabsorb phosphorus also increases. However, a maximum rate of transport (Tm) for phosphorus reabsorption is obtained usually at serum phosphorus concentrations of 6 mg per dL. There is a direct correlation between Tm phosphorus values and glomerular filtration rate (GFR) even when the GFR is varied over a broad range. Micropuncture studies suggest two different mechanisms responsible for phosphorus reabsorption in the proximal tubule. In the first third of the proximal tubule, in which only 10% to 15% of the filtered sodium and fluid is reabsorbed, the ratio of tubular fluid (TF) phosphorus to plasma ultrafiltrable (UF) phosphorus falls to values of approximately 0.6. This indicates that the first third of the proximal tubule accounts for approximately 50% of the total amount of phosphorus reabsorbed in this segment of the nephron. In the last two thirds of the proximal tubule, the reabsorption of phosphorus parallels the movement of salt and water. In the remaining 70% of the pars convoluta, the TF:UF phosphorous ratio remains at a value of 0.6 to 0.7, whereas fluid reabsorption increases to approximately 60% to 70% of the filtered load. Thus, in the last two thirds of proximal tubule, the TF:UF phosphorus reabsorption ratio is directly proportional to sodium and fluid reabsorption. A significant amount of phosphorus, perhaps on the order of 20% to 30%, is reabsorbed beyond the portion of the proximal tubule that is accessible to micropuncture. There is little phosphorus transport within the loop of Henle, with most transport distal to micropuncture accessibility occurring in the distal convoluted tubule. In this location, Pastoriza-Munoz et al.[502] found that approximately 15% of filtered phosphorus is reabsorbed under baseline conditions in animals subjected to parathyroidectomy, but that the value falls to about 6% after administration of large doses of parathyroid hormone (PTH). The collecting duct is a potential site for distal nephron reabsorption of phosphorus.[115,508,592] Transport in this nephron segment may explain the discrepancy between the amount of phosphorus delivered to the late distal tubule in micropuncture studies and the considerably smaller amount of phosphorus that appears in the final urine of the same kidney. Phosphorus transport in the cortical collecting tubule is independent of regulation by PTH. This is in agreement with the absence of PTH-dependent adenylate cyclase in the cortical collecting tubule.[115]

Comparison of Superficial and Deep Nephron Transport

The contribution of superficial nephrons and deep nephrons of the kidney to phosphorus homeostasis differs.

Nephron heterogeneity in phosphorus handling has been evaluated under a number of conditions by puncture of the papillary tip and the superficial early distal tubule, with the recorded fractional delivery representing deep and superficial nephron function, respectively. Microinjection of phosphorus tracer into thin ascending and descending limbs of loops of Henle reveals that only 80% of phosphorus was recovered in the urine, whereas 88% to 100% of phosphorus was recovered when the tracer was injected into the late superficial distal tubule. It was concluded that a significant amount of phosphorus must be reabsorbed by juxtamedullary distal tubules or by segments connecting the juxtamedullary distal tubules to the collecting ducts to account for the discrepancy between the results of superficial nephron injection and juxtamedullary nephron injections. These data support an increased reabsorptive capacity for phosphorus in deep as opposed to superficial nephrons and increased responsiveness to body Pi requirements.[253,254]

In summary, phosphorus transport occurs in the distal nephron, particularly in the distal convoluted tubule and cortical collecting tubular system. This transport may be considerable under certain experimental conditions, but the importance of the terminal nephron system in day-to-day phosphorus homeostasis remains to be defined. It is also evident from data obtained from various micropuncture and microinjection studies that juxtamedullary and superficial nephrons have different capacities for phosphorus transport. The increased responsiveness of the deep nephrons to phosphorus intake suggests a key regulatory role for this system in phosphorus homeostasis.

Cellular Mechanisms of Phosphate Reabsorption in the Kidney

The apical membrane of renal tubular cells is the initial barrier across which phosphorus and other solutes present in the tubular fluid must pass to be transported into the peritubular capillary network. Because the electrical charge of the cell interior is negative to the exterior, and phosphorus concentrations are higher in the cytosol, phosphorus must move against an electrochemical gradient into the cell interior, whereas at the antiluminal membrane, the transport of phosphorus into the peritubular capillary is favored by the high intracellular phosphorus concentration and the electronegativity of the cell interior. Studies with apical membrane vesicles have demonstrated cotransport of Na^+ with phosphate across the brush-border membrane, whereas the transport of phosphorus across the basolateral membrane is independent of that of Na^+.[272] The apical membrane Na^+-phosphate cotransport protein (NaPi-IIa) energizes the uphill transport of phosphate across the brush-border membrane (BBM) by the movement of Na^+ down its electrochemical gradient. The latter gradient is established and maintained by active extrusion of Na^+ across the basolateral cell membrane into the peritubular capillary through the action of Na^+-K^+-ATPase (Fig. 73.2).[571]

Three families of NaPi cotransport proteins of the proximal tubule (types I, II, and III) have been cloned.[414,472,473,636,661,709] The DNA clones encode 80- to 95-kd proteins that reconstitute Na^+-dependent concentrative, or "uphill," transport of phosphate.[203,414,636] The type I cotransporter, Npt1/SLC17, is expressed predominantly in the renal proximal tubule, and it accounts for about 13% of the known NaPi cotransporter mRNA in the mouse kidney.[662] Npt1 is not regulated by dietary Pi, and studies in Npt1-cRNA–injected oocytes revealed that it may function not only as a NaPi cotransporter but also as a chloride and organic anion channel.[103]

The type II cotransporter NaPi-II/SLC34 proteins are similar between several species including humans.[472,473,661] In addition to NaPi-IIa, the predominant isoform in the renal proximal tubule, another isoform, NaPi-IIc, has been discovered.[486,584,586,660] Nephron localization of NaPi-II proteins has been limited to the proximal tubule of superficial and deep nephrons (greatest in the latter, concordant with physiologic studies).[472,473,661] Immunolocalization studies in renal epithelial cells demonstrated apical membrane and subapical membrane vesicle staining,[472,473,661] suggesting that a functional pool of transporters is available for insertion into or retrieval from the BBM itself. This has been postulated to be a major mechanism of Pi transport regulation in response to acute changes in phosphorus, PTH, MEPE, and fibroblast growth factor 23 (FGF23) levels.[33,472,473,609,661] The NaPi-II family is upregulated at message and protein levels by chronic feeding of low-Pi diets[368,403] and downregulated at message and protein levels by PTH[136,368,403] and dietary potassium deficiency.[92]

The type III NaPi cotransporters SLC20 were originally identified as retroviral receptors for gibbon ape leukemia virus (Glvr1) and rat amphotropic virus (Ram1).[317] They are ubiquitously expressed, and they comprise about 1% of the known NaPi cotransporter mRNAs in the mouse kidney.[662] Pit-2 protein is expressed in the apical membrane of the renal proximal tubule and the levels are regulated by dietary Pi,[678] dietary potassium,[92] and LXR.[106]

Studies of phosphorus exit across the basolateral membrane suggest that it is accompanied by the net transfer of a negative charge and occurs down a favorable electrochemical gradient via sodium-independent mechanisms.[582]

Proteins that Interact with the Type IIa and Type IIc Na/Pi Cotransporter Proteins

Several proteins with PDZ domains have been identified that interact with the NaPi-IIa and NaPi-IIc protein and are localized in the BBM or the subapical compartment (Fig. 73.3). PDZ domains are modular protein interaction domains that often occur in scaffolding proteins and bind in a sequence-specific fashion to the C-terminal peptide sequence or at times the internal peptide sequences of target proteins. These domains of approximately 90 amino acids are known by an acronym of the first three PDZ-containing proteins identified including the postsynaptic protein PSD-95/SAP90, the

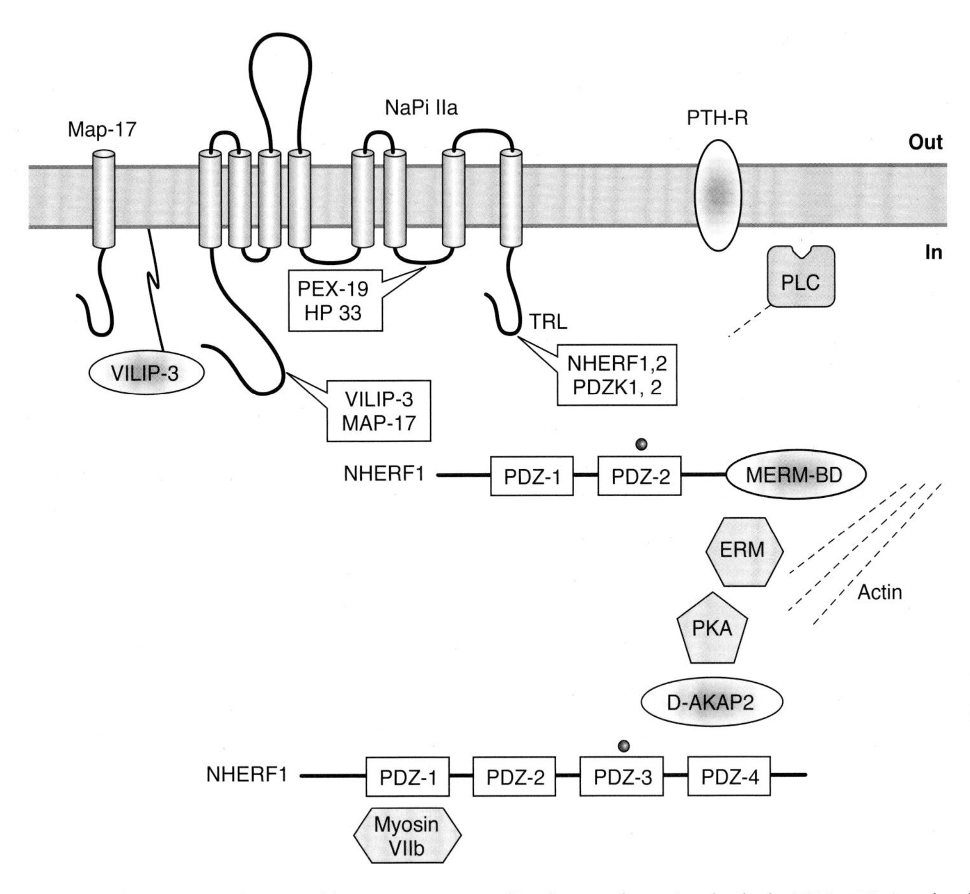

FIGURE 73.3 Interactions of NaPi-IIa with several proteins expressed in the renal proximal tubule. MAP-17 is involved in the apical location of PDZK1 (via PDZ-4) in OK cells. (From Biber J, Gisler SM, Hernando N, et al. PDZ interaction and proximal tubular phosphate reabsorption. *Am J Physiol Renal Physiol.* 2004;287:F871.)

Drosophila septate junction protein Discs-large, and the tight junction protein ZO-1.[255,288,367,596]

PDZ domain containing proteins including NHERF-1, NHERF-2, PDZK1, CAL, and ZO-1 play an important role in: (1) the regulation of the expression and activity of renal proximal tubular BBM transport proteins including NHE-3,[596,697–700] NaPi IIa,[33,359] and NaPi-IIc[219,677] and basolateral membrane transport proteins including Na-K-ATPase[359] and Na-HCO_3 cotransporter (NBC)[696]; (2) the regulation of the expression and activity of cystic fibrosis transmembrane conductance regulator (CFTR), a cAMP-regulated chloride channel and channel regulator[389,477,540,653,686]; (3) parathyroid hormone 1 receptor signaling[417] and endocytic sorting of the β2-adrenergic receptor[107] and platelet-derived growth factor receptor (PDGFR)[313,436]; (4) epithelial cell polarity and formation of tight junctions[64,289]; and (5) maintaining the integrity of the glomerular barrier to proteins through interactions with podocalyxin, negatively charged sialoprotein expressed on the surface of podocytes, the glomerular visceral epithelial cells.[284,285,490,503,504,655]

In addition to their interaction with membrane proteins and receptors, the PDZ domain-containing proteins also interact with the F-actin cytoskeleton through their interactions with the ezrin-radixin-moesin (ERM) proteins (Fig. 73.3).[91,524,633] ERM proteins are typically located peripherally in the membrane and link the cytoplasmic tails of membrane proteins and receptors to the cortical actin cytoskeleton. The ERM proteins play an important role in the formation of microvilli, cell-cell junctions, and membrane ruffles and also participate in signal transduction pathways. The ERM proteins contain an F-actin binding site within their carboxy-terminal 30 residues. In addition, the ERM proteins have FERM (**f**our-point one, **e**zrin, **r**adixin, **m**oesin) domains, which are generally located at or near the amino terminal, and act as multifunctional protein and lipid binding sites. The FERM domain of ezrin interacts strongly with NHERF-1 and NHERF-2. NHERF-1 and NHERF-2 have 2 PDZ domains and have a carboxy-terminal sequence of 30 amino acids that bind ezrin.

Using the molecular approach (yeast two-hybrid) several proteins with PDZ domains that interact with the C terminus of NaPi-IIa have been identified including: (1) NHERF-1/EBP50, (2) NHERF-2/E3KARP, (3) PDZK1/NaPi-Cap1, (4) PDZK2/NaPi-Cap2, and (5) CAL, a CFTR-associated ligand.[60,68,220–222,263,456,516,594]

Different studies suggest that apical expression of NaPi-IIa depends on the presence of NHERF-1. Expression of NaPi-IIa was reduced upon introduction of dominant-negative form of NHERF-1 in OK cells.[220–222,263] The in vivo importance of the

NaPi-IIa interaction with NHERF-1 was also shown in a study where targeted disruption of the mouse NHERF-1 gene was associated with decreased BBM expression and increased intracellular localization of NaPi-IIa resulting in decreased renal phosphate reabsorption and renal phosphate wasting.[595] On the other hand targeted disruption of NHERF-1 did not modulate the BBM expression and localization of NHE3; however, there was impaired regulation of NHE3 in response to PKA.[595]

In contrast to NHERF-1, targeted disruption of the PDZK1 gene failed to modulate the BBM expression of NaPi-IIa.[108,334] NHERF-1, therefore, plays a critical and unique role in the renal proximal tubular apical membrane targeting of NaPi-IIa protein and maintenance of phosphate homeostasis. However targeted disruption of PDZK1modulates the BBM expression of NaPi-IIc, as compared to NaPi-IIa PDZK1, which has preferential interactions with NaPi-IIc.[219,677]

Recent studies have identified at least three additional proteins that may be important in the regulation of NaPi-IIa targeting and trafficking: (1) the peroxisomal protein PEX 19, a farnesylated protein that confers PTH responsiveness to NaPi-IIa[297]; (2) the calcium binding protein Vilip-3, a myristoleated protein that may be important in calcium dependent regulation of NaPi-IIa[517]; and (3) MAP 17 which may be important for apical expression of PDZK1 (Fig. 73.3).[516]

Factors that Affect the Urinary Excretion of Phosphorus

Of the multiplicity of factors that regulate phosphate transport in the kidney, the most important are dietary phosphate, PTH, and FG23.

Alterations in Dietary Phosphorus Intake

The mechanism by which the kidney modulates phosphorus excretion when dietary phosphorus is reduced or increased continues to be intriguing. Earlier micropuncture studies suggested that the most striking adaptive increase in phosphorus transport occurs in the proximal tubule. Later studies[707] suggested that the entire nephron participates in the reduction of phosphorus excretion during dietary phosphorus deprivation. It has been shown that isolated perfused tubules obtained from rabbits that were fed a normal or low-phosphorus diet differ in their capacity to reabsorb phosphate. In normal animals, the proximal convoluted tubule (PCT) is capable of reabsorbing 7.2 $\pm$ 0.8 pmol/mL/min, whereas tubules obtained from phosphorus-deprived animals reabsorb 11.1 $\pm$ 1.3 pmol/mL/min. Conversely, animals that are fed a high phosphorus diet show reduced phosphorus reabsorption when the proximal tubules are perfused in vitro (2.7 $\pm$ 2.6 pmol/mL/min).

The effect of reduced dietary phosphorus to stimulate renal phosphorus transport is intrinsic to the renal tubular epithelium and occurs at the BBM Na^+-phosphate cotransporter. The adaptation to phosphate supply by the sodium–phosphate cotransporter is biphasic.[61,85,113] Incubation of cells in a low-phosphate medium result in a twofold increase in Na^+-independent phosphate cotransport. The first phase of adaptation is observed rapidly (within 10 minutes) and is characterized by an increase in the V_{max} of the transporter. This initial phase is independent of new protein synthesis.[368,369,403] A slower phase resulting in a doubling of the phosphate transport rate, also through an increase in V_{max}, occurs over several hours and is inhibited by blocking new protein synthesis.[708] The adaptation to acute Pi deprivation occurs independent of de novo transcription and protein synthesis and is mediated by apical insertion of cytoplasmic NaPi-II a transporters by a microtubule dependent mechanism (Fig. 73.4).[402] Secondly, through gene transcription and increased NaPi protein synthesis, additional units are produced and inserted into the brush border. Dietary Pi deprivation also induces the upregulation of NaPi-IIc and Pit-2 in the apical brush border membrane; however, the response of these two transporters is delayed and unlike NaPi-IIa may be dependent on de novo protein synthesis.[677]

Effects of Parathyroid Hormone on Phosphorus Reabsorption by the Kidney

Parathyroidectomy decreases urinary phosphorus excretion, whereas PTH administration increases phosphorus excretion.[57,525] Micropuncture studies indicate that PTH inhibits phosphorus transport in the proximal tubule[9] and in segments of the nephron located beyond the proximal tubule.[502] TF:UF phosphorus ratio reaches a value of 0.6 by the S_2 segment of the proximal tubule and, once achieved, this equilibrium ratio is maintained along the accessible portion of the proximal tubule. Within 6 to 24 hours after parathyroidectomy, the proximal TF:UF phosphorus ratio falls to a value of 0.2 to 0.4, indicating an increase in phosphorus reabsorption.[41,43,707] TF phosphorus falls progressively with continuous fluid absorption along the length of the tubule, so by the end of the proximal tubule, the reabsorption of phosphorus is 70% to 85% of the filtered load, resulting in decreased phosphorus delivery to distal segments of the nephron. In the nonphosphorus-loaded, acutely parathyroidectomized animal, virtually all the distal load of phosphorus is reabsorbed by the distal nephron, reducing urinary phosphorus excretion to very low levels.[333,358] In the phosphorus-loaded animal, the distal reabsorption of phosphorus increases until saturation is approached and urinary phosphorus excretion begins to rise. Acute administration of PTH to phosphorus-loaded parathyroidectomized dogs sharply lowers the distal reabsorption.

Administration of PTH in vivo results in decreased rates of Na^+-dependent phosphorus transport in brush-border membrane vesicles isolated from the kidneys of treated rats.[184,252] Intravenous infusion of dibutyryl cyclic adenosine monophosphate (cAMP) also decreased Na^+-dependent phosphorus uptake in isolated brush-border vesicles, but neither PTH nor dibutyryl cAMP decreased phosphate transport when added directly to membrane vesicles.[184] PTH stimulates two signaling pathways in proximal tubule cells: adenylate cyclase and phospholipase C (PLC), resulting in activation of protein

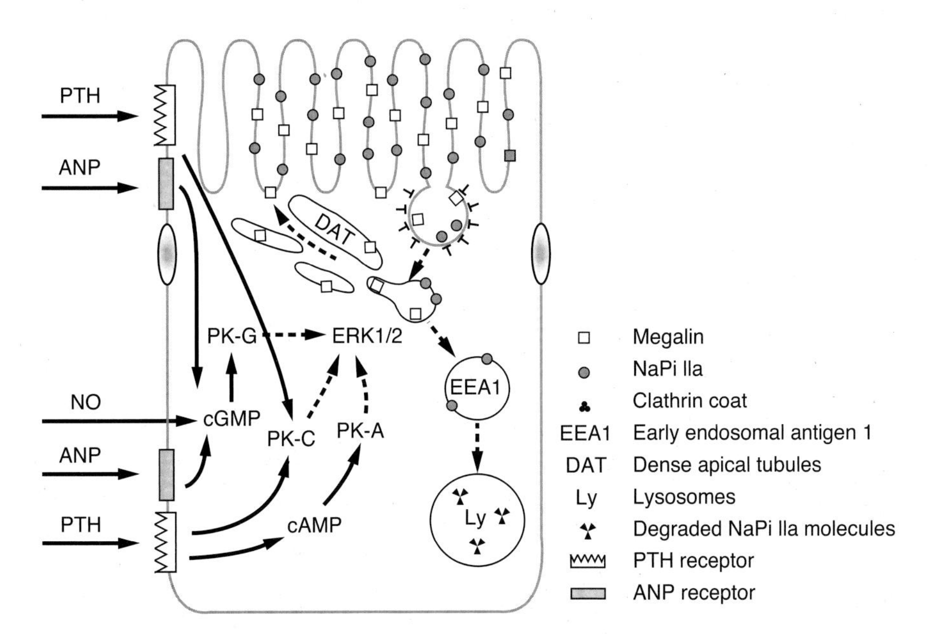

FIGURE 73.4 Mechanisms of NaPi-IIa traffic in the apical membranes of proximal tubular cells. Microvillar NaPi-IIa is retrieved in megalin containing clathrin coated vesicles. NaPi-IIa moves from the vesicles into an endosomal pool marked by EEA-1, whereas megalin is recycled through dense apical tubules back to the microvilli. The endosomal NaPi-IIa is targeted for lysosomal degradation. The process of NaPi-IIa retrieval and lysosomal degradation is stimulated by several factors (parathyroid hormone, atrial natriuretic peptide, nitric oxide) whose mechanisms of signal transduction (PK-A, PK-C, PK-G) merge in activation of ERK1/2 that modulates the process. (From Bacic D, Wagner CA, Hernando N, et al. Novel aspects in regulated expression of the renal type IIa Na/Pi-cotransporter. *Kidney Int.* 2004;66:S5, with permission.)

kinase A (PKA), and protein kinase C (PKC).[174] The first pathway, activation of the adenylate cyclase, differs from that of PKC. Studies in OK cells show that PKA activation by PTH decreases the expression of NaPi-IIa cotransporter likely due to internalization and degradation of the transporter. Binding of PTH to its receptor leads to activation of PLC with the subsequent hydrolysis of phosphatidylinositol 4,5-bisphosphate to inositol 1,4,5-trisphosphate (IP_3) and 1,2-diacylglycerol (DAG). IP_3 generation leads to the release of intracellular calcium stores. DAG activates PKC.[174] In addition to its direct effect on NaPi-IIa, PTH inhibits NaPi transport indirectly by inhibiting the Na^+-K^+-ATPase by decreasing the favorable Na^+ gradient for Pi entry into the cell.[546] Recent studies indicate that the activation of PKA and PKC signaling pathways by PTH also activates mitogen activated protein (MAP) kinase (MAPK) or extracellular receptor kinase (ERK1/2) which also induces inhibition of NaPi transport.[32,360]

Measurement studies of in vivo renal reabsorption of phosphorus and calculations of kinetic parameters of Na^+-dependent phosphorus transport in membrane vesicles isolated from the renal brush-border membranes of normal dogs, parathyroidectomized dogs, dogs fed a low-phosphorus diet, and dogs receiving human growth hormone were performed.[252,281] The latter three groups of dogs had greater baseline values for absolute tubular reabsorption of phosphorus compared with normal dogs. Na^+-dependent phosphate transport in BBM vesicles isolated from kidneys of these dogs was significantly increased compared with transport in brush-border vesicles from kidneys of normal dogs. Administration of PTH decreased significantly the apparent V_{max} for Na^+-dependent phosphorus transport in BBM vesicles isolated from kidneys of each of the four groups of dogs. The apparent K_m (intrinsic binding affinity) for Na^+-dependent phosphorus transport was not significantly changed by experimental maneuvers. Absolute tubular reabsorption of phosphorus measured in vivo was decreased by administration of PTH in each group of dogs with the exception of the dogs fed a low-phosphorus diet.[252,281] Thus, alterations in phosphorus reabsorption measured in vivo were paralleled by alterations in Na^+-dependent phosphorus transport in isolated membrane vesicles, and the administration of PTH in vivo resulted in altered transport characteristics of the isolated BBMs.

The cloning of the NaPi-IIa cotransport proteins did not completely elucidate the mechanisms of PTH action on phosphate transport. Because the phosphaturic effect of PTH can be reproduced by analogs of cAMP, the intracellular mechanism of phosphate transport regulation is thought to involve the cAMP/PKA signal pathway. However, the NaPi-IIa transport proteins are not characterized by a PKA–mediated phosphorylation site.[259] Phosphorylation of BBM proteins in vitro occurs in parallel with inhibition with NaPi-IIa cotransport.[252] Parathyroidectomy of rats causes a twofold to threefold increase in the NaPi-IIa protein content of BBM vesicles.[319] Immunocytochemistry reveals the increase in protein exclusively in apical BBMs of proximal tubules. PTH treatment of parathyroidectomized rats for 2 hours decreased protein levels and decreased the abundance of NaPi-IIa-specific messenger RNA (mRNA) by 31%.[319] Parathyroidectomy did not affect NaPi-IIa mRNA levels. The effects of PTH were apparent within 2 hours of administration and indicate that PTH regulation of NaPi-IIa is determined by changes in the expression of NaPi-IIa protein in the renal BBMs.[319]

PTH decreases the NaPi-IIa protein content of the apical membrane by a endocytic retrieval pathway which is megalin and myosin VI dependent (Fig. 73.4).[31,67] In megalin intact mice or rats, following treatment with PTH NaPi-IIa is internalized via clathrin-coated pits, and NaPi-IIa is then delivered to early endosomes and eventually to the lysosomes where the protein is degraded. At the present time unlike some of the other proximal tubular transport proteins or receptors, there is no evidence that the NaPi-IIa protein is present at the recycling endosomes.

PTH also regulates the NaPi-IIc protein content of the apical membrane by an endocytic retrieval pathway that is myosin VI–dependent, but the time course is delayed compared to NaPi-IIa.[351]

Fibroblast Growth Factor 23

Through studies of familial hypophosphatemia and tumor induced osteomalacia, a new hormone operating in a systems biology network regulating phosphate homeostasis between the skeleton and the kidney has been discovered (Fig. 73.5).[307,600] The hormone is FGF23, secreted by skeletal osteocytes in response to changes in bone formation and serum phosphorus.[487] The physiology is that the osteocyte monitors deposition of phosphorus into the skeletal reservoir and the saturation of the exchangeable phosphorus pool. When Pi levels increase within the pool due to decreased exit into the skeleton (bone formation) or due to increased plasma phosphorus, osteocytes secrete FGF23, which acts on the renal proximal tubule to decrease reabsorption and increase phosphorus excretion.[279,604]

FGF23 actions at the proximal tubule (PCT) have not been studied as extensively as the actions of PTH, which were described above. Studies indicate that FGF23 acts to decrease expression of NaPi-IIa and NaPi-IIc in the PCT.[209,604] The actions of FGF23 on the PCT are mediated through binding to a FGF receptor—predominantly FGFR1(IIIc) and a coreceptor, Klotho.[673] Signal transduction is stimulated through phosphorylation of extracellular signal-regulated kinase (ERK) and the immediate early response gene, early growth response-1 (Erg-1), a zinc finger transcription factor.[212,673] A matter of current uncertainty is related to KLOTHO expression which is mainly in the renal distal tubule whereas its signaling function is in the PCT. Recent studies have shown that it is expressed in the PCT which would resolve this issue (M. Kuro-o, personal communication).

Besides inhibiting PCT renal Pi transport, FGF23 signaling inhibits PCT CYP27B1, the 25-OH cholecalciferol 1α hydroxylase, and activates 24-OH hydroxylase (CYP24R1) resulting in decreased production and increased catabolism of calcitriol.[600] In addition, activation of 24-OH hydroxylase results in the high prevalence of vitamin D deficiency associated with elevations of FGF23 levels, especially in chronic kidney disease (CKD). Calcitriol increases FGF23, closing the feedback loop in the system (Fig. 73.5).

Vitamin D

Controversy still surrounds the regulatory role of vitamin D in renal phosphorus handling. Several studies have demonstrated that the chronic administration of vitamin D to parathyroidectomized animals is phosphaturic.[75,467,647] Conversely, other investigators reported that vitamin D acutely stimulates proximal tubular phosphorus transport in both

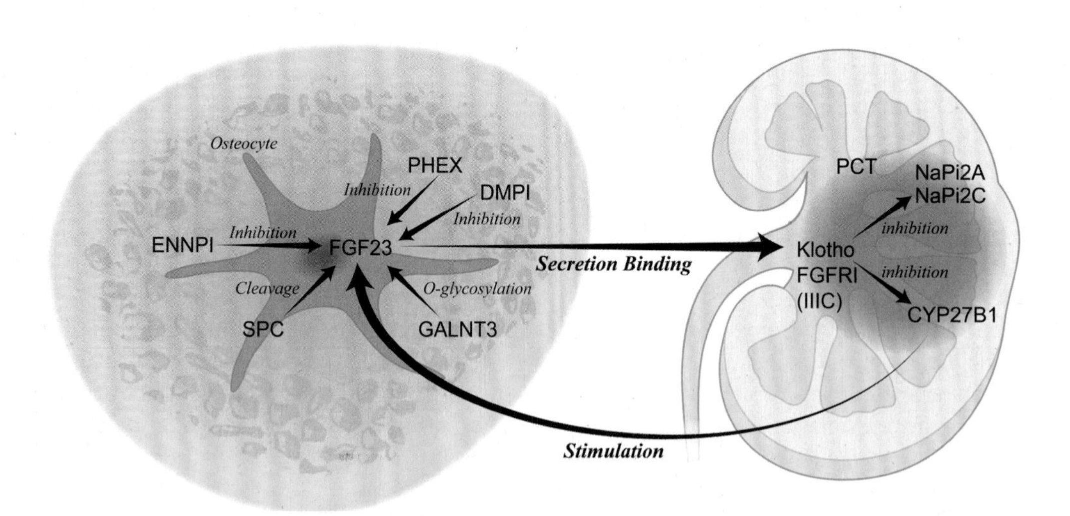

FIGURE 73.5 The skeletal–kidney endocrine axis: regulation of Pi in the exchangeable pool. FGF23 is a hormone secreted by the osteocyte to regulate proximal tubular cell Pi transport and calcitriol production. Multiple mechanisms of increased FGF23 levels cause hypophosphatemic rickets. Calcitriol stimulates FGF23 to maintain Pi levels in response to stimulation of intestinal absorption. Function of various proteins in the endocrine axis and the genetic diseases they cause are listed in Table 73.2.

parathyroidectomized and vitamin D–depleted rats.[211] A unifying interpretation of these studies was hampered by the fact that the dosages of vitamin D administered and the status of the serum calcium, phosphorus, and PTH varied considerably from study to study.

Liang et al.[384] administered 1,25-dihydroxycholecalciferol to vitamin D–deficient chicks and subsequently examined the transport characteristics of isolated renal tubule cells. Three hours after the in vivo administration of vitamin D, phosphorus uptake by the cells was significantly increased, whereas 17 hours after the administration of vitamin D, phosphorus uptake was reduced. The serum phosphorus concentration, however, was significantly increased at 17 hours after administration, and administration of phosphorus to vitamin D–depleted animals so their serum phosphorus levels were comparable to those of the 17-hour vitamin D–replenished group resulted in a similar decrease in phosphorus uptake.[384] In response to in vitro preincubation with as little as 0.01 pm of 1,25-dihydroxycholecalciferol, renal cells isolated from vitamin D–deficient chicks demonstrated a specific increase in sodium-dependent phosphorus uptake, which was blocked by pretreatment with actinomycin D. The stimulatory effect was relatively specific for 1,25-dihydroxycholecalciferol, and kinetic analysis indicated that the V_{max} of the phosphorus transport system was increased, whereas the affinity of the system for phosphorus was unaffected.[384]

Kurnik and Hruska[346] also examined the relationship between vitamin D and renal phosphorus excretion in a normocalcemic, normophosphatemic weanling rat model fed a vitamin D–deficient diet. The animals were mildly vitamin D deficient (92 pg per mL of 1,25-dihydroxycholecalciferol versus 169 pg per mL in controls) but had no evidence of secondary hyperparathyroidism. Clearance studies performed in the basal partially vitamin D–deficient state showed an increase in both absolute and fractional phosphorus excretion compared with controls. Animals that were replenished with 1,25-dihydroxycholecalciferol and maintained on diets designed to protect against the development of hyperphosphatemia demonstrated a significant decrease in urinary phosphorus excretion. Other animals were similarly replenished with vitamin D but did not receive dietary adjustment; and in this group, both the serum phosphorus and the urinary phosphorus excretion level increased significantly. A third group was fed a normal diet and received smaller doses of 1,25-dihydroxycholecalciferol (15 pmol per g of body weight) for shorter periods, and although this dose had no effect on the serum phosphorus concentration, the phosphaturia was completely resolved.

Studies on BBM vesicles prepared from these animals revealed that in the partially vitamin D–deficient state, sodium-dependent phosphorus uptake was significantly reduced compared with control animals. Animals that were replenished with vitamin D and fed a controlled diet had a greater sodium-dependent phosphorus uptake than both vitamin D–depleted and vitamin D–replenished animals not maintained on controlled diets.

The results of this series of studies suggest that the primary action of 1,25-dihydroxycholecalciferol is to increase tubular phosphorus reabsorption. Long-term administration of vitamin D, however, represents a more complex situation, where phosphaturia may occur secondary to changes in the filtered load of phosphorus, in the body distribution of phosphorus, or in intracellular phosphorus activity.

Effects of Changes in Acid–Base Balance on Phosphate Excretion

The effect of acid–base status on the renal excretion and transport of phosphate is complex. Acute respiratory acidosis increases and acute respiratory alkalosis decreases phosphate excretion.[275] These effects occur independently of PTH and plasma or luminal bicarbonate levels.[275] However, other studies suggest that the effects of respiratory acid–base changes may be mediated by changes in plasma phosphate.[275]

Acute metabolic acidosis has minimal effects on phosphate excretion; however, the phosphaturic effect of PTH is blunted.[43] Acute metabolic alkalosis causes an increase in phosphate excretion independently of PTH.[206,345,448,526,530] This effect is due, in part, to volume expansion produced by the infusion of bicarbonate.[448,530]

Chronic acidosis increases phosphate excretion, again independent of PTH or changes in ionized Ca^{2+}.[144,234,345,509] The effect appears to be directly on the sodium-dependent phosphate transport mechanism.[674] Chronic alkalosis decreases phosphate excretion, probably by the same mechanism as acidosis, operating in the opposite direction.[206,535]

Acute and chronic acidosis in rats decreases the proximal tubule cell luminal membrane expression of the NaPi-IIa cotransporter.[18] In acute acidosis, there is rapid internalization of the transporter and the total cortical homogenate cotransporter expression is unchanged. In chronic acidosis, there are parallel changes in NaPi-IIa protein and mRNA abundance. The effects of acid–base perturbations are complex and depend on antecedent dietary intake, the chronicity of the change, and whether the change affects luminal or intracellular pH, or both.

Adrenal Hormones

Administration of pharmacologic amounts of cortisol leads to phosphaturia. Acute adrenalectomy reduces the GFR and increases the reabsorption of phosphorus in the proximal tubule. Frick and Durasene[195] concluded that glucocorticoid hormones could play an important role in the regulation of fractional reabsorption of phosphorus. Indeed administration of glucocorticoids to animals has been shown to decrease proximal tubular NaPi cotransport activity and induce phosphaturia by causing parallel decreases in NaPi-IIa protein and mRNA levels.[370] The inhibitory effects of glucocorticoids in NaPi transport is in part mediated by the concomitant alterations in renal proximal tubular apical BBM glycosphingolipid composition, as inhibition of glycosphingolipid synthesis prevents in part the decrease in renal NaPi cotransport activity. In contrast to glucocorticoid administration, adrenalectomy with mineralocorticoid administration, resulting in selective glucocorticoid deficiency, is associated with increased renal proximal tubular NaPi-IIa protein expression.[396]

Growth Hormone

An increase in serum phosphorus and a rise in renal phosphorus transport are characteristics of growth hormone (GH) excess during the period of rapid growth in the child, during acromegaly, or during exogenous GH administration to experimental animals. Hammerman et al. reexamined this phenomenon in the BBM vesicle preparation in the dog[252] and demonstrated that GH treatment resulted in an increased sodium-dependent phosphorus transport. These data reassert the importance of BBM phosphorus uptake in regulating overall renal phosphorus reabsorptive capacity. The action of growth hormone is likely mediated by insulin-like growth factor-1.[114]

Studies have further identified the nephron sites and mechanisms by which GH regulates renal Pi uptake.[716] Micropuncture experiments were performed after acute thyroparathyroidectomy in the presence and absence of PTH in adult (14- to 17-week-old), juvenile (4-week-old), and GH-suppressed juvenile male rats. Although the phosphaturic effect of PTH was blunted in the juvenile rat compared with the adult, suppression of GH in the juvenile restored fractional Pi excretion to adult levels. In the presence or absence of PTH, GH suppression in the juvenile rat caused a significant increase in the fractional Pi delivery to the late proximal convoluted (PCT) and early distal tubule, so that delivery was not different from that in adults. These data were confirmed by Pi uptake studies into BBM vesicles. Immunofluorescence studies indicate increased BBM type IIa NaPi cotransporter (NaPi-II) expression in the juvenile compared with adult rat, and GH suppression reduced NaPi-II expression to levels observed in the adult. GH replacement in the [N-acetyl-Tyr(1)-d-Arg(2)]-GRF-(1-29)-NH(2)-treated juveniles restored high NaPi-II expression and Pi uptake. Together, these novel results demonstrate that the presence of GH in the juvenile animal is crucial for the early developmental upregulation of BBM NaPi-II and, most importantly, describe the enhanced Pi reabsorption along the PCT and proximal straight nephron segments in the juvenile rat.[716]

Thyroid Hormone

Because Pi is intensively used in general metabolism, Pi homeostasis should be regulated by factors controlling the rate of metabolism itself. One such factor is thyroid hormone, and its role in Pi reabsorption regulation has been extensively analyzed.[45,637,729] Pharmacologic doses of T_3 have been shown to increase Na/Pi cotransport in BBM vesicles from rat proximal tubules.[54,729] In addition, T_3 concentrations approximating the association constant (K_m) of the thyroid hormone nuclear receptor also elicited a similar increase in P_i transport in opossum kidney (OK) cells.[637] In both cases, the increase in transport rate was caused by an increase in the capacity of the transport system, whereas the affinity was not modified. Euzet et al.[182,183] have shown an important role for T_3 in the maturation of the renal Na/Pi cotransporter, which was associated with changes in both K_m and V_{max}, as well as in the type II Na/Pi cotransporter (NaPi-II) protein and mRNA abundance.

Sorribas et al. have determined the role of physiologic concentrations of thyroid hormone in renal phosphate transport in vivo. In addition, they also determined the potential role of thyroid hormone in impairment of phosphate reabsorption that accompanies the aging kidney.[16] Their results show that chronically treated hypothyroid rats, using a physiologic dose of T_3, exhibit increases in serum Pi levels, NaPi-II mRNA and protein content, and Na/Pi cotransport activity in superficial and juxtamedullary renal cortex, all these effects by means of enhanced transcription of the corresponding NaPi-II gene. The stimulatory effect of the hormone was less evident in the aging kidney, which shows a lower level of basal phosphate reabsorption. In this study, only pharmacologic hyperthyroidism was able to restore partially the level of serum Pi observed in young animals.

Epidermal Growth Factor

Epidermal growth factor (EGF) is a 53-amino acid polypeptide. The kidney is a major site of synthesis of the EGF precursor, prepro-EGF. In renal epithelial cells grown in culture, EGF has been shown to modulate sodium gradient-dependent phosphate transport (Na-Pi cotransport) activity, but the directionality of the modulation in cell culture has been controversial.[22,232,510] A study also determined whether EGF regulates Na-Pi cotransport activity in vivo and whether the effect of EGF to regulate Na-Pi cotransport is dependent on the developmental stage of the animal (i.e., suckling [12-day-old] vs. weaned [24-day-old] rats). This study demonstrated that proximal tubule BBMV Na-Pi cotransport activity, NaPi-II protein abundance, and NaPi-II mRNA abundance are higher in weaned than in suckling rats and that EGF inhibits Na-Pi cotransport activity in BBMV isolated from suckling and weaned rats by a decrease in NaPi-II protein abundance, in the absence of a change in NaPi-II mRNA.[23]

Aging

The aging process is associated with impairment in renal tubular reabsorption of Pi and renal tubular adaptation to a low Pi diet. In experiments using 3- to 4-month-old young adult rats and 12- to 16-month-old aged rats, it was found that there was an age-related twofold decrease in proximal tubular apical BBM Na-Pi cotransport activity, which was associated with similar decreases in BBM NaPi-II protein abundance and renal cortical NaPi-II mRNA level. Immunohistochemistry showed lower NaPi-II protein expression in the BBM of proximal tubules of superficial, midcortical, and juxtamedullary nephrons. This study also found that in response to chronic (7 days) and/or acute (4 hour) feeding of a low Pi diet, there were similar adaptive increases in BBM Na-Pi cotransport activity and BBM NaPi-II protein abundance in both young and aged rats. However, BBM Na-Pi cotransport activity and BBM NaPi-II protein abundance were still significantly lower in aged rats, in spite of a significantly lower serum Pi concentration in aged rats. Thus, impaired expression of the type II renal Na-Pi cotransporter protein at the level of the apical BBM plays an important role in the age-related impairment in renal tubular reabsorption of Pi and renal tubular adaptation to a low Pi diet.[635]

Stanniocalcin

Stanniocalcin is a calcium and phosphate regulating hormone found in serum and the kidney. In teleost fish, it is produced in the corpuscles of Stannius, specialized endocrine organs closely associated with the kidneys. Stanniocalcin plays a major role in the calcium and phosphate homeostasis of fish. It inhibits calcium uptake by the gills and gut and stimulates phosphate reabsorption by the kidney.[151,157,294,406,413,489,680,733]

Two mammalian homologues of Stanniocalcin have been identified. Stanniocalcin 1 and Stanniocalcin 2, with seemingly opposing effects on renal phosphate transport. Stanniocalcin I induces increased gastrointestinal (GI) and renal Pi transport.[295] Stanniocalcin 2 on the other hand causes inhibition of renal Pi transport by transcriptional mechanisms.[295]

Diuretics

Acetazolamide inhibits phosphate reabsorption by its effects on proximal tubule decreases in Na^+-dependent bicarbonate transport, essential for the maintenance of the Na^+ gradient. Furosemide inhibits carbonic anhydrase activity and thus decreases phosphate transport. Similar effects have been demonstrated with the administration of large doses of thiazide diuretics.[246]

Hypophosphatemia

Hypophosphatemia refers to serum phosphorus concentrations of less than 2.5 mg per dL. Hypophosphatemia usually results from one or a combination of the following factors (Fig. 6)[328,340]: (1) increased excretion of phosphorus in the urine; (2) decreased GI absorption of phosphorus; or (3) translocation of phosphorus from the extracellular to the intracellular space. The major causes of hypophosphatemia are shown in Table 73.1.

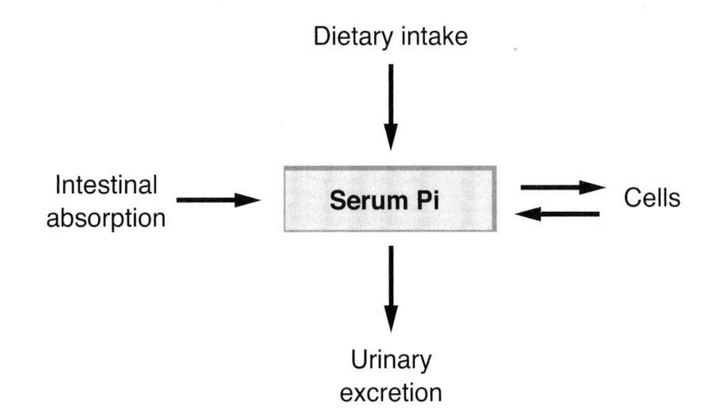

FIGURE 73.6 The major determinants of serum inorganic phosphate (Pi) concentration.

TABLE 73.1 Causes of Hypophosphatemia

I. Increased excretion of phosphorus in the urine
  A. Familial
  B. Primary hyperparathyroidism
  C. Secondary hyperparathyroidism
  D. Renal tubular defects (Fanconi syndrome)
  E. Diuretic phase of acute tubular necrosis
  F. Postobstructive diuresis
  G. Extracellular fluid volume expansion
    1. X-linked hypophosphatemia
    2. Autosomal dominant hypophosphatemic rickets
    3. Autosomal recessive hypophosphatemic rickets 1; autosomal recessive hypophosphatemic rickets 2
    4. Oncogenic hypophosphatemic osteomalacia (TIO) - Phos
    5. McCune-Albright syndrome/Fibrous dysplasia
    6. Mutations in NaPi-IIa
    7. Hereditary hypophosphatemic rickets with hypercalciuria
  H. Posttransplant hypophosphatemia
II. Decrease in gastrointestinal absorption of phosphorus
  A. Abnormalities of vitamin D metabolism
    1. Vitamin D–deficient rickets
    2. Familial
      a. Vitamin D–dependent rickets
      b. X-linked hypophosphatemia
  B. Malabsorption
  C. Malnutrition-starvation
III. Miscellaneous causes/translocation of phosphorus
  A. Leukemia, lymphoma
  B. Diabetes mellitus: during treatment for ketoacidosis
  C. Severe respiratory alkalosis
  D. Recovery phase of malnutrition
  E. Alcohol withdrawal
  F. Toxic shock syndrome
  G. Severe burns

Increased Excretion of Phosphorus in the Urine

Several pathophysiologic conditions increase excretion of phosphorus in the urine. Some of these are characterized by elevated levels of circulating PTH or FGF23. Because PTH and FGF23 decrease phosphorus reabsorption by the kidney, elevations of the hormones increase urinary excretion (Table 73.1). Decreased tubular reabsorption of phosphorus may also occur without increased levels of PTH and may be due to changes in the reabsorption of salt and water or to renal tubular defects specific for the reabsorption of certain solutes or phosphorus. Hypophosphatemia may also occur in the diuretic phase of acute tubular necrosis or in postobstructive diuresis, presumably due to a combination of high levels of PTH and decreased tubular reabsorption of salt and water.

Primary Hyperparathyroidism

Primary hyperparathyroidism is a common entity in clinical medicine.[27] PTH is secreted in excess of the physiologic needs for mineral homeostasis due to either adenomas or hyperplasia of the parathyroid glands.[54] This results in decreased phosphorus reabsorption by the kidney. The losses of phosphorus in the urine result in hypophosphatemia. The degree of hypophosphatemia may vary considerably among patients, because mobilization of phosphorus from bone will in part mitigate the hypophosphatemia. Moreover, if the patient ingests large amounts of dietary phosphorus, the degree of hypophosphatemia observed may be mild. Because these patients also have elevated levels of serum calcium, the diagnosis is made relatively easy in most cases by the finding of elevated levels of immunoreactive PTH.

Secondary Hyperparathyroidism

Although secondary hyperparathyroidism is present in most patients with chronic renal disease, hyperphosphatemia rather than hypophosphatemia occurs in such patients because of decreased phosphorus excretion in the urine resulting from the fall in GFR. However, certain conditions characterized by malabsorption of calcium from the GI tract may produce hypocalcemia, leading to development of secondary hyperparathyroidism.[224] The elevated levels of PTH will decrease phosphorus reabsorption by the kidney, resulting in hypophosphatemia. Thus, patients with GI tract abnormalities resulting in calcium malabsorption and secondary hyperparathyroidism will have low levels of serum calcium and phosphorus. In these patients, the hypocalcemia is responsible for the increased release of PTH. In addition, decreased intestinal absorption of phosphorus as a result of the primary GI tract disease may also contribute to the decrement in the levels of serum phosphorus. In general, these patients have

TABLE 73.2 **Inherited Disorders of Phosphate Homeostasis Cause Hypophosphatemic Rickets or Hyperphosphatemia and Are Components of a Bone Kidney Endocrine Axis**

Protein/Gene	Function	Disease
FGF23	Hormone regulating phosphate excretion and calcitriol production	ADHR: excess tumoral calcinosis: deficiency
PHEX	Unclear, inhibits FGF23 secretion/production	XLH
DMPI	Matrix protein, inhibits FGF23 secretion/production	ARHR1
ENNPI	Produces pyrophosphate in osteocyte/osteoblast extracellular fluid/inhibits FGF23 secretion/production	ARHR2: homozygous infantile calcific arteriopathy: homozygous
GALNT3	O-glycosylation of FGF23, deficiency increases SPC mediated FGF23 cleavage	Tumoral calcinosis
KLOTHO	FGF23 co-receptor	Tumoral calcinosis Hyperphosphatemia Early senescence
NaPi2c/SLC34A3	Proximal tubule phosphate transport protein	HHRC
CYP27BI	Produces calcitriol which stimulates FGF23 production	Vitamin D dependent rickets
NaPi2a/SLCH34A1	Proximal tubule phosphate transport protein	Nephrolithiasis

FGF23, fibroblast growth factor 23; ADHR, autosomal dominant hypophosphatemic rickets; PHEX, phosphate regulating gene with homologies to endopeptidases on the X chromosome; XLH, x-linked hypophosphatemia; DMPI, dentin matrix protein 1; ARHR1, autosomal recessive hypophosphatemic rickets 1; ENNPI, ectonucleotide pyrophosphatase 1; ARHR2, autosomal recessive hypophosphatemic rickets 2; GALNT3, N- acetylglucosaminyltransferase 3; SLC34A3, solute carrier family 34A3; HHRC, hereditary hypophosphatemic rickets with calciuria; CYP27BI, cytochrome P450 family 27 subfamily B polypeptide I.

urinary losses of phosphorus that are out of proportion to the hypophosphatemia in contrast to patients with predominant phosphorus malabsorption and no secondary hyperparathyroidism in whom urinary excretion of phosphorus is low.

Familial Hypophosphatemia

Studies of hereditary (Table 73.2), and acquired (oncogenic hypophosphatemic osteomalacia [OHO] and McCune-Albright syndrome) renal phosphate wasting disorders have led to the identification of novel genes involved in the regulation of renal Pi transport and calcitriol synthesis.[70,87,536,537,561,579,659] The discovery of these genes has established a bone-kidney axis responsible for maintaining phosphate homeostasis (Fig. 73.5).

X-linked Hypophosphatemia

X-linked hypophosphatemia (XLH) is a common cause of rickets with a prevalence of approximately 1 in 20,000. It is inherited in an X-linked dominant manner. Manifestations of XLH include short stature, bone pain, tooth abscesses, calcification of tendon insertions, ligaments, joint capsules, and lower extremity deformities. However, with genetic sequencing causing reclassification of some presumed XLH patients into autosomal dominant hypophosphatemic rickets (ADHR) or autosomal recessive hypophosphatemic rickets (ARHR) categories, the clinical manifestations may change. For example, posterior longitudinal ligament ossification may be a manifestation mainly of ARHR2.[379] XLH is characterized by hypophosphatemia, decreased reabsorption of phosphorus by the renal tubule, decreased absorption of calcium and phosphorus from the GI tract, and varying degrees of rickets or osteomalacia. Patients with this disorder exhibit normal to reduced levels of 1,25-dihydroxycholecalciferol despite hypophosphatemia and reduced Na-phosphate transport in the proximal tubule. The message levels of NaPi-IIa are reduced by 50% in the PCT of *Hyp* mice similar to the reduction in apical membrane vesicle NaPi-IIa protein levels.[663]

The gene responsible for XLH was designated **PHEX** for **PH**osphate regulating gene with homology to **E**ndopeptidases on the **X** chromosome.[3] PHEX is a member of the M13 family of type II cell surface zinc-dependent metallopeptidases which includes neprilysin, endothelin-converting enzymes 1 and 2, KELL, and DINE/X-converting enzyme. The mouse PHEX DNA sequence is highly homologous to that of humans and the inactivating mutations of PHEX have been identified in the mouse homologues of XLH, *Hyp* and *Gy* mice. More than 180 mutations in the PHEX gene have been shown to result in XLH. PHEX is expressed predominantly in osteoblasts, osteocytes, and odontoblasts, but not in the kidney. The hypophosphatemia and rickets of XLH is produced by excess FGF23 in the circulation.[307,726] How PHEX inactivation variably increases FGF23 secretion is currently unknown (Fig. 73.5). However, the finding that homozygous ablation of FGF23 in the *Hyp* background produced the phenotype of FGF23 deficiency (hyperphosphatemia, elevated calcitriol, and vascular calcification) and loss of the *Hyp* phenotype demonstrates that FGF23 is causative of hypophosphatemia in *Hyp* and XLH.[619] The initial thought that FGF23 was a PHEX substrate[84] proved untrue.[47,244,392,393] In fact, FGF23 has recently been shown to be cleaved by subtilisin-like protein convertases (SPC) (Fig. 73.5). SPCs are a seven-member family of calcium-dependent serine proteases responsible for the processing of peptide hormones, neuropeptides, adhesion molecules, receptors, growth factors, cell surface glycoproteins, and enzymes. Instead PHEX, most likely through the actions of unidentified PHEX substrates or other downstream effectors, regulates FGF23 secretion as part of a hormonal axis between bone and kidneys that controls systemic phosphate homeostasis and mineralization.[47]

From a therapeutic point of view, the combination of neutral phosphate and 1,25-dihydroxycholecalciferol has led to an improvement in the bone disease of patients with XLH and in the Hyp mice.[225,676] The administration of phosphorus in X-linked hypophosphatemia is usually divided into four doses, with the total amount ranging between 1 to 4 g per day. Pharmacologic doses of 1,25-dihydroxycholecalciferol on the order of 1 to 3 μg per day may be necessary to correct the skeletal alterations. 1,25-dihydroxycholecalciferol does not correct the increased fractional excretion of phosphate. The enthusiasm for this regimen is tempered by a high incidence of nephrocalcinosis and occasional renal failure.[196,225,676]

Autosomal Dominant Hypophosphatemic Rickets

The clinical presentation of ADHR is similar to XLH. However, ADHR exhibits male to male transmission, consistent with autosomal dominant inheritance, and is characterized by incomplete penetrance and variable age of onset. Adults typically complain of bone pain, fatigue, and/or weakness, and can present with stress fractures or pseudofractures. Renal phosphate wasting and inappropriately normal serum calcitriol levels are the most typical laboratory findings.

The gene responsible for ADHR is a member of the FGF family, FGF23.[4] FGF23 is a 251 amino acid peptide secreted by osteocytes and processed to amino- and carboxy-terminal peptides at a consensus pro-protein convertase (furin) site. In four unrelated ADHR families missense mutations have been identified in FGF23 in the proteolytic cleavage site (R176Q, R179W, and R179Q) that interfere with peptide processing and result in gain of function of FGF23.[603,712,713]

Administration of wild-type FGF23 or FGF23 expressing the ADHR mutations in the furin cleavage site (R176Q, R179W, or R179Q) to rats and mice has been shown to induce hypophosphatemia, increased urinary phosphate excretion via inhibition of the type IIa NaPi cotransport protein, and decreased 1,25 $(OH)_2D_3$ levels.[36,572,586,600] Chronic administration of FGF23 and increased expression of FGF23 (FGF23 transgenic mice) has also been shown to induce osteomalacia and decreased 1,25 $(OH)_2D_3$ levels via decrease in 25-hydroxyvitamin D 1α-hydroxylase mRNA.[35,353,604]

In vitro studies in OK cells have demonstrated that FGF23 inhibits Na/Pi cotransport activity and type IIa NaPi cotransport protein abundance by the MAPK signaling dependent pathway.[725]

In contrast, targeted ablation of FGF23 in mice results in significantly increased serum Pi levels with increased renal Pi absorption. These mice also have increased serum 1,25 $(OH)_2D_3$ levels that is due to increased expression of renal 25-hydroxyvitamin D 1α-hydroxylase (1α-OHase).[601] Another study with homozygous ablation of FGF23 in mice revealed that these mice have marked hyperphosphatemia, increased serum 1,25 $(OH)_2D_3$ levels, growth retardation, increased total body bone mineral content but decreased bone mineral density of the limbs, and excessive mineralization in soft tissues, including in the heart, vasculature, and kidneys.[619]

Autosomal Recessive Hypophosphatemic Rickets

Genetic studies have led to the discovery of autosomal recessive inheritance familial hypophosphatemic rickets. The genes involved are dentin matrix protein 1 (DMP1) in ARHR1, and ectonucleotide pyrophosphatase/phosphodiesterase 1 (ENPP1) in ARHR2 (Fig. 73.5).[188,400,401] Circulating levels of FGF23 are elevated in ARHR1 and 2, and FGF23 is thought to be the basis of the hypophosphatemia and rickets. The clinical picture of ARHR resembles that of ADHR and XLH. Therefore, genetic studies may be needed in the future to establish molecular etiology of hypophosphatemic rickets.

Oncogenic Hypophosphatemic Osteomalacia or Tumor-Induced Osteomalacia

Tumor-induced osteomalacia (TIO) is an acquired disorder of renal phosphate wasting with clinical and biochemical features similar to XLH and ADHR. This disorder is characterized by hypophosphatemia associated with tumors. It was described initially in association with benign mesenchymal tumors; however, other reports have emphasized the association of this syndrome with malignant tumors.[501,565] The other characteristics of this syndrome are increased phosphate excretion, low plasma 1,25-dihydroxycholecalciferol concentrations, and osteomalacia. All of the biochemical and pathologic abnormalities disappear when the tumor is resected.

The tumors associated with this syndrome have been found to secrete substances that inhibit the renal tubular reabsorption of phosphate and suppress 25-hydroxycholecalciferol 1α-hydroxylase activity. The TIO substances include FGF23, MEPE, sFRP4, and others.[53] FGF23 has been cloned from the tumors of patients who have presented with TIO and FGF23 is the most prevalent factor causing both the impaired renal Pi reabsorption resulting in hypophosphatemia and also the decreased serum 1,25 $(OH)_2D_3$ levels.[150,602,648] Several studies have shown increased serum levels of FGF23 and/or immunohistochemical detection of FGF23 in patients who present with TIO and the serum levels to normalize after the resection of the tumors.[193,354,479,656,688] sFRP-4 has been detected in patients with TIO and it has been shown to inhibit Pi transport in OK cells and also in normal rats by PTH-independent mechanisms.[53] sFRP-4 antagonizes Wnt signaling but at this time the role of the Wnt pathway in regulation of renal Pi transport or 25-hydroxyvitamin D 1α-hydroxylase has not been established.

MEPE is exclusively expressed in osteoblasts, osteocytes, and odontoblasts and is markedly upregulated in murine XLH (*Hyp*) osteoblasts and TIO tumors (Fig. 73.5).[24,90,300,561,562] The recombinant human-MEPE has been shown to result in dose-dependent inhibition of renal Pi reabsorption, phosphaturia, and hypophosphatemia.[564] In addition, human-MEPE dose dependently inhibited BMP-2 mediated mineralization of a murine osteoblast cell line (2T3) in vitro.[563]

A protease-resistant carboxy-terminal MEPE peptide containing the acidic serine-aspartate rich motif (ASARM) peptide has been shown to play a role in the inhibition of the mineralization (minhibin). PHEX prevents proteolysis of MEPE and release of ASARM. In XLH mutated PHEX may, therefore, contribute to the increased ASARM peptide seen in that disorder.[563] Recent studies using surface plasmon resonance (SPR) indicates that MEPE binds to PHEX via the MEPE-ASARM motif which can provide a molecular basis for the inhibition of bone mineralization in XLH subjects and *Hyp* mice.[563] The potential role of ASARM in regulation of renal Pi transport or 25-hydroxyvitamin D 1α-hydroxylase, however, remains to be determined.

In contrast to the potential role of MEPE and ASARM to inhibit bone mineralization, disruption of MEPE gene in mice results in increased bone mass, resistance to age-associated trabecular bone loss, increased mineralization apposition rate, and accelerated mineralization in ex vivo osteoblast cultures.[233] These mice, however, have normal serum Pi levels, perhaps due to normal FGF23 and PHEX expression.

McCune-Albright Syndrome and Fibrous Dysplasia

McCune-Albright syndrome (MAS) is characterized by the clinical triad of polyostotic fibrous dysplasia (FD), café au lait skin pigmentation, and endocrine/metabolic disorders. The endocrine disorders include autonomous secretion of various hormones such as GH, thyroid hormone, cortisol, estradiol, and testosterone. Rickets and osteomalacia due to hyperphosphaturic hypophosphatemia are prominent components of the syndrome.[14,58,59,134,140,146,386,387,443,551,569,704]

The disorders of the syndrome share in common excessive function of cells whose actions are normally regulated by hormones that induce cAMP generation. The molecular basis for the phenotype is an activating mutation of GNAS1 which encodes the $G_S\alpha$ protein (α component of the stimulatory heterotrimeric guanosine triphosphate binding protein, G_S) in cells from affected tissues from patients with the syndrome.[14,58,59,134,140,146,386,387,443,551,569,704] Kidney tissue, presumably proximal tubule, from patients has been reported to contain cells with the mutation.

A study using a combination of real-time polymerase chain reaction (RT-PCR), in situ hybridization, enzyme-linked immunosorbent assay (ELISA) of media conditioned by normal and FD stromal cells and trabecular bone cells, and measurements of FGF23 in the serum has determined that FGF23 is expressed in FD tissues and osteogenic cells and that high levels of circulating FGF23 correlate with renal Pi wasting in FD/MAS patients.[550]

Mutations in the Type IIa NaPi Cotransporter (SLC34A1)

Epidemiologic studies suggest that genetic factors confer a predisposition to the formation of renal calcium stones or bone demineralization. Low serum phosphate concentrations due to a decrease in renal phosphate reabsorption have been reported in some patients with these conditions, suggesting that genetic factors leading to a decrease in renal phosphate reabsorption may contribute to them. Prie and colleagues investigated if mutations in the gene coding for the main renal sodium-phosphate cotransporter (NaPi-IIa) may be present in patients with these disorders. Twenty patients with urolithiasis or bone demineralization and persistent idiopathic hypophosphatemia associated with a decrease in maximal renal phosphate reabsorption were studied. The coding region of the gene for NaPi-IIa was sequenced in all patients. The functional consequences of the mutations identified were analyzed by expressing the mutated RNA in Xenopus laevis oocytes. Two patients, one with recurrent urolithiasis and one with bone demineralization, were found to be heterozygous for two distinct mutations. One mutation resulted in the substitution of phenylalanine for alanine at position 48, and the other in a substitution of methionine for valine at position 147. Phosphate-induced current and sodium-dependent phosphate uptake were impaired in oocytes expressing the mutant NaPi-IIa. Coinjection of oocytes with wild-type and mutant RNA indicated that the mutant protein had altered function. This study, therefore, concluded that heterozygous mutations in the NaPi-IIa gene may be responsible for hypophosphatemia and urinary phosphate loss in persons with urolithiasis or bone demineralization.[520]

A follow-up study by Virkki and colleagues recreated the two mutants, expressed them in Xenopus oocytes, and analyzed their kinetic behavior by two-electrode voltage clamp. They also performed coexpression experiments where they injected mRNA for wild-type (WT) and mutants containing an additional S462C mutation, enabling complete inhibition of cotransport function with cysteine-modifying reagents. Finally, WT and mutant NaPi-IIa as C-terminal fusions to green fluorescent protein (GFP) in opossum kidney (OK) cells was expressed They found in oocyte expression experiments that Pi-induced currents were reduced in both mutants, whereas Pi and Na affinities and other transport characteristics were not affected. The amount of cotransport activity remaining after cysteine modification, corresponding to WT activity, was not affected by coexpression of either mutant. Finally, GFP-tagged WT and mutants were expressed at the apical membrane in OK cells, showing that both mutants are correctly targeted in a mammalian cell.[679] This, therefore, suggests that the heterozygous A48F and V147M mutations cannot explain the pathologic phenotype observed by Prie and colleagues. In this regard Prie and colleagues reported mutations in NaPi-IIa interacting PDZ domain containing protein NHERF1 that result in renal phosphaturia.[312,372,518,519] In addition Magen and Skorecki and colleagues have also reported a loss of function mutation in NaPi-IIa in ARHR with renal Fanconi syndrome.[415]

Mutations in the Type IIc NaPi Cotransporter (SLC34A3)

Hereditary hypophosphatemic rickets with hypercalciuria (HHRH) is an autosomal form of hypophosphatemic rickets.[666] The gene involved in HHRH is NaPi-IIc (SLC34A3). The disease is characterized, and differs from other forms of hereditary hypophosphatemic rickets and/or osteomalacia, by increased serum levels of 1,25-dihydroxyvitamin D, increased GI calcium absorption, and hypercalciuria. Some of the NaPi-IIc mutations cause mistargeting of NaPi-IIc protein and uncoupling of NaPi cotransport activity.[50,301,371,658]

Renal Tubular Defects

Several conditions characterized by single or multiple tubular defects have been described in which phosphorus reabsorption is decreased. In the Fanconi syndrome,[559] patients excrete not only increased amounts of phosphorus in the urine but also increased quantities of amino acids, uric acid, and glucose, resulting in hypouricemia and hypophosphatemia. Rare familial forms of hypercalciuria are often associated with one or more of the components of the Fanconi syndrome including hypophosphatemia or hyperphosphaturia.[210,394,665] Interestingly, these familial syndromes, Dent disease, and its variants have been found to be caused by a mutation in the CLCN5 chloride channel,[394,578] which is an intracellular vesicular channel, perhaps related to the vesicles that harbor the NaPi cotransport proteins.[242,304,305,331] There are other conditions in which an isolated defect in the renal tubular transport of phosphorus has been found, for example, fructose intolerance, which is an autosomal-recessive disorder.[278] After renal transplantation, an acquired renal tubular defect may be responsible for the persistence of hypophosphatemia in some patients.[366,556]

Diuretic Phase of Acute Tubular Necrosis

Most patients with acute renal failure develop secondary hyperparathyroidism and hyperphosphatemia during the oliguric phase. During the recovery phase of acute renal failure, the combined occurrence of a profound diuresis, secondary hyperparathyroidism, and continued use of phosphate binders may lead to severe hypophosphatemia. This hypophosphatemia is usually short lived, and serum phosphorus levels return to within the normal range as the diuretic phase of acute tubular necrosis subsides.

Postobstructive Diuresis

A marked phosphaturia may develop in some patients after relief of urinary tract obstruction. This phosphaturia may be severe enough in a few patients to lead to hypophosphatemia.[185]

Extracellular Fluid Volume Expansion

Expansion of the ECF volume by the administration of solutions containing sodium increases the urinary excretion of phosphorus. An important mechanism by which ECF volume expansion produces phosphaturia consists of a fall in ionized calcium and subsequent release of PTH.[42] This condition is probably of minor importance in clinical medicine, and restoration of the ECF volume to within the normal range results in the return of phosphorus reabsorption to physiologic levels.

Posttransplant Hypophosphatemia

Posttransplant hypophosphatemia, a common disorder, is well described in the literature. Although described mainly in patients following renal transplantation,[56,208,234,245,458,488,492,500,555,574,643,687] posttransplant hypophosphatemia also occurs in patients undergoing bone marrow transplantation.[143,538] In all reports, the decrease in serum Pi concentration was associated with an increase in urinary phosphate excretion and a significant decrease in the measured or derived ratio of maximal rate of renal tubular transport of phosphate to glomerular filtration rate (TmPi/GFR).[684] In addition to the impairment in renal tubular phosphate reabsorption, evidence indicates that intestinal phosphate absorption is impaired in transplant patients.[186,366,429,557]

The mechanism for posttransplant hypophosphatemia has not been fully elucidated, but it is linked to disordered regulation of renal tubular reabsorption of Pi. As discussed earlier, PTH leads to a reduction in the expression of type II Na/Pi cotransport at the BBMs, which accounts for the phosphaturic action of PTH. Given this property of PTH, it has been postulated that increased PTH activity during chronic renal failure (CRF) may be the major mechanism responsible for maintaining Pi balance during CRF. According to this hypothesis, posttransplant hypophosphatemia has been attributed to persistent hyperparathyroidism (HPT), that is, incomplete involution of hyperplastic glands produced by renal failure prior to transplantation would cause hypophosphatemia and increased phosphaturia during the early posttransplant period.[262] Several studies, however, have documented that protracted HPT cannot account for the phenomenon of posttransplant hypophosphatemia since it can be seen in transplant patients with normal PTH levels. Moreover, transplant recipients failed to decrease Pi excretion in the urine even when PTH was suppressed by calcium infusion.[555] In addition, the phosphaturia following kidney transplantation could not be ascribed to the effects of nephrectomy or to the influence of immunosuppressive drugs.[555]

A study by Green et al. determined that a non-PTH humoral mechanism accounted for the entity of posttransplant hypophosphatemia.[237] The factor, however, had characteristics different from FGF-23, sFRP-4, and MEPE, phosphatonins discussed earlier.[237] However, recent studies continue to focus on PTH and FGF23 as the causes of posttransplant hypophosphatemia in the early posttransplant period.

Decrease in Gastrointestinal Absorption of Phosphorus

Abnormalities of Vitamin D Metabolism

Vitamin D and its metabolites play an important role in phosphorus homeostasis.[236] Vitamin D promotes the intestinal absorption of calcium and phosphorus and is necessary to maintain the normal mineralization of bone. Dietary deficiencies of vitamin D increase the amount of osteoid tissue in the skeleton and decrease normal mineralization. Bone mineralization is a complex process that is not completely understood. Normally, the osteoblast is responsible for laying down normal collagen that is well organized and distributed in a lamellar fashion. Between the recently deposited collagen and the old bone, there is an area called the mineralization front. Initially, amorphous calcium phosphate is deposited in the mineralization front and eventually matures into hydroxyapatite $[Ca_{10}(PO_4)_6(OH)_2]$. Thus, the osteoid tissue changes into bone. Optimal mineralization requires the following: (1) normal bone cell activity; (2) normal supply of minerals; (3) the appropriate pH level (7.4 to 7.6); (4) normal synthesis and composition of the matrix; and (5) control of inhibitors of calcification.

The appositional growth rate in normal bone is about 1 μm per day and complete mineralization of the osteoid requires 13 to 21 days. Thus, the thickness of the osteoid usually does not exceed 20 μm. Less than 20% of the surface of the bone is normally covered by osteoid. When a biopsy is performed in a healthy subject who has previously ingested two doses of tetracycline separately and 3 weeks apart, one usually detects two fluorescent rings or bands, indicating the locations of the mineralization front. In a patient with osteomalacia, usually a single band, no band, or an irregular and spotty uptake of tetracycline is seen. In rickets or osteomalacia, there is a quantitative and qualitative defect in bone mineralization.

Vitamin D–Deficient Rickets

Diets deficient in vitamin D lead to the metabolic disorder known as rickets when it occurs in children or osteomalacia when it appears in adults.[480] Vitamin D deficiency in childhood results in severe deformities of bone because of rapid growth. These deformities are characterized by soft loose areas in the skull known as craniotabes and costochondral swelling or bending (known as rachitic rosary). The chest usually becomes flattened, and the sternum may be pushed forward to form the so-called pigeon chest. Thoracic expansion may be greatly reduced with impairment of respiratory function. Kyphosis is a common finding. There is remarkable swelling of the joints, particularly the wrists and ankles, with characteristic anterior bowing of the legs, and fractures of the "greenstick" variety may also be seen. In adults, the symptoms are not as striking and are usually characterized by bone pain, weakness, radiolucent areas, and pseudofractures. Pseudofractures represent stretch fractures in which the normal process of healing is impaired because of a mineralization defect. Mild hypocalcemia may be present; however, hypophosphatemia is the most frequent biochemical alteration. This metabolic abnormality responds well to administration of small amounts of vitamin D.

Vitamin D–Dependent Rickets

These are recessively inherited forms of vitamin D–refractory rickets. The conditions are characterized by hypophosphatemia, hypocalcemia, elevated levels of serum alkaline phosphatase, and, sometimes, generalized aminoaciduria and severe bone lesions. Currently, two main forms of vitamin D–dependent rickets have been characterized. The serum concentrations of 1,25-dihydroxycholecalciferol serves to differentiate the two types of vitamin D–dependent rickets.

Type I vitamin D–dependent rickets is associated with reduced calcitriol levels. It is caused by a mutation in the gene converting 25(OH)D to 1,25-dihydroxycholecalciferol, the renal 1α-hydroxylase enzyme.[178,202] This condition responds to very large doses of vitamin D_2 and D_3 (100 to 300 times the normal requirement of physiologic doses), or to 0.5 to 1.0 μg per day of 1,25-dihydroxycholecalciferol.

Type II vitamin D–dependent rickets is characterized by end-organ resistance to 1,25-dihydroxycholecalciferol. Plasma levels of 1,25-dihydroxycholecalciferol are elevated. This finding, in association with radiographic and biochemical signs of rickets, implies resistance to 1,25-dihydroxycholecalciferol in the target tissues. Cellular defects found in patients with vitamin D–resistant rickets type II are heterogeneous, providing in part an explanation for the different clinical manifestations of this disorder. Among the cellular defects are (1) decreased number of cytosolic receptors, (2) deficient maximal hormonal binding, (3) deficient hormone binding affinity, (4) normal hormonal binding but undetectable nuclear localization, and (5) abnormal DNA binding domain for the 1,25-dihydroxycholecalciferol receptor.[385]

Numerous studies[119,187,264,266,419,445,544,632] have demonstrated that hereditary type II vitamin D–resistant rickets is a genetic disease affecting the vitamin D receptor (VDR). Defects in the hormone binding domain[119,187] and the DNA binding domain[266,419] have been defined. In addition, several cases of human vitamin D–resistant rickets have been studied and no abnormality in the coding region of the VDR has been found,[264] suggesting a defect elsewhere in the hormone action pathway. An unexplained feature of this disease in adolescents is the tendency for calcium levels to normalize and for the radiographic abnormalities of rickets to improve, thus giving the appearance that they outgrow the disease. Human vitamin D–resistant rickets as a genetic defect in the VDR varies significantly from other genetic diseases of steroid hormone receptors caused by resistance to thyroid hormone, androgens, and estrogens.[445,544,632] For example, individuals heterozygous for VDR mutations are apparently completely healthy. Secondly, no dominant negative mutations, which are prominent in thyroid hormone resistance, have been identified as a cause of human vitamin D–resistant rickets. Thus, much remains to be learned from the genetic analysis of this disease. The treatment of this condition requires large pharmacologic doses of calcium, which overcome the receptor defects and maintain bone remodeling.[266] Studies in mice with targeted disruption of the *VDR* gene, an animal model of vitamin D–dependent rickets type II, confirm that many aspects of the clinical phenotype are due to decreased intestinal ion transport and can be overcome by adjustments of dietary intake.[382]

Malabsorption

Because most of the absorption of phosphorus from the GI tract occurs in the duodenum and jejunum, gastrointestinal tract disorders such as celiac disease, tropical and nontropical sprue, and regional enteritis may decrease the absorption of phosphorus.[224] Phosphorus malabsorption has also been described in patients who have undergone surgical bypass procedures for morbid obesity. The degree of hypophosphatemia varies among patients with intestinal malabsorption, being extremely mild in some and severe in others.

Malnutrition

Most of the phosphorus ingested in the diet is present in protein, particularly meat, cheese, milk, and eggs. In many parts of the world where protein consumption is extremely low, hypophosphatemia occurs predominantly in children. Overall growth is retarded and a series of metabolic abnormalities are present.[324]

Administration of Phosphate Binders

Certain compounds, mainly aluminum salts (aluminum hydroxide, aluminum carbonate gel) and calcium carbonate, are used in the treatment of hyperphosphatemia.[598] However, when these compounds are given in excess, they may produce profound hypophosphatemia. These gels trap phosphorus in the small intestine and increase the amount of phosphorus in the stool. Patients ingesting large amounts of phosphate binders and not followed closely may develop phosphate depletion. With time, such individuals may develop severe weakness, bone pain, and osteomalacia.

Miscellaneous Causes of Hypophosphatemia

Major reviews of the causes of hypophosphatemia in hospitalized patients[309,352] attributed most instances to intravenous administration of carbohydrate. However, many other causes were found, including diuretic usage, hyperalimentation, alcoholism, respiratory alkalosis, and use of phosphate binders.[55] A 31% incidence of hypophosphatemia was seen in patients admitted to a general medical ward, and a further fall in serum concentrations occurred in all patients with acute alcoholism between the second and fifth day after admission to a medical ward.[570] Hypophosphatemia is also seen frequently during treatment of diabetic ketoacidosis.[587] When diabetic patients develop ketoacidosis, they usually have an increase in phosphate excretion in the urine; however, the serum phosphate level may be slightly elevated due to acidosis. During the administration of insulin, there is a rapid decrease in the level of glucose with translocation of phosphate from the extracellular to the intracellular space, resulting in hypophosphatemia.

Acute respiratory alkalosis decreases urinary phosphate excretion but produces marked hypophosphatemia.[465] In contrast, patients who receive sodium bicarbonate excrete large amounts of phosphate in the urine; however, the hypophosphatemia that may develop is only moderate in nature. It has been postulated that in respiratory alkalosis, there is an increase in the intracellular pH level with activation of glycolysis and increased formation of phosphate-containing sugars, leading to a precipitous fall in the concentration of serum phosphorus. The mild hypophosphatemia that may be seen during administration of sodium bicarbonate is probably secondary to increased renal phosphate excretion due to a decrease in ionized calcium and release of PTH, as well as to the consequences of ECF volume expansion.

In addition, new clinical disorders have been identified in which hypophosphatemia is an important aspect of the pathologic condition. Marked hypophosphatemia has been associated with acute leukemia or with lymphomas in the leukemic phase.[8,435,730] These individuals typically present with hypophosphatemia, normocalcemia, and no evidence of excess PTH activity. Urinary phosphate concentration is typically extremely low. Although kinetic studies have not been performed in this setting, the facts that serum phosphate concentration correlates with a growth phase of the tumors and that hyperphosphatemia is seen when cells are destroyed by chemotherapy or radiotherapy strongly suggest that serum phosphorus was initially used in the rapid growth of new cells. Because these patients are often severely ill and under treatment with glucose infusions, as well as antacids and other drugs known to induce hypophosphatemia, they may be at great risk of developing severe acute phosphorus depletion.

Another clinical condition in which hypophosphatemia has been a prominent feature is the toxic shock syndrome. Chesney et al.[124] described 22 women with this disorder who showed hypocalcemia and hypophosphatemia as prominent manifestations. Whether respiratory alkalosis or staphylococcal sepsis–induced release of substances were responsible for acute phosphorus shifts into cells is unknown. Lindquist et al.[363] studied in a prospective fashion the importance of hypophosphatemia in patients with severe burns. In 33 patients studied for 2 weeks after injury, transient hypophosphatemia was seen in the second to tenth day in all these individuals. Five of seven patients who died from complications of the terminal injury had severe hypophosphatemia. Because urinary phosphorus excretion was not increased, tissue uptake seems to be the predominant mechanism responsible for the hypophosphatemia. Levy[378] reported the occurrence of severe hypophosphatemia during the rewarming phase in a profoundly hypothermic patient. In this individual, urinary excretion of phosphorus was minimal, suggesting that a shift of phosphate into the cells occurred as a result of rewarming. Finally, the development of hypophosphatemia resulting from refeeding clinically starved patients has been emphasized. Silvis et al.[612] showed that the classic phosphorus-depletion syndrome, consisting of paresthesias, weakness, seizures, and hypophosphatemia, can occur in individuals who receive oral caloric supplements after a prolonged period of starvation. To further evaluate this issue, they performed studies in normal dogs that had been starved or had received normal diets and found that the infusion of calories through an intragastric catheter to previously starved animals resulted in a fall in serum phosphorus concentration from an average of 4.8 mg per dL to 1.6 mg per dL. Nearly 50% of starved animals developed clinical signs of phosphate depletion after oral refeeding. Weinsier and Krumdiek reported two patients who developed the phosphorus-depletion syndrome in association with cardiopulmonary decompensation following overzealous hyperalimentation after prolonged caloric deprivation.[701]

Clinical and Biochemical Manifestations of Hypophosphatemia

The manifestations of hypophosphatemia are presented in Table 73.3. It has been suggested that the clinical manifestations of hypophosphatemia and severe phosphorus depletion are related to disturbances in cellular energy and metabolism. Studies have examined the effects of phosphate depletion on cellular energetics and other components of cell function. A study of glycolytic intermediates and adenine nucleotides during insulin treatment of patients with diabetic ketoacidosis emphasized the important effects of insulin-induced cellular phosphate depletion on cell metabolism.[337] These results demonstrated that the reduced level of 2,3-diphosphoglycerate (2,3-DPG) seen during insulin treatment of diabetes is due to intracellular phosphorus depletion, producing a decrease in glyceraldehyde 3-phosphate dehydrogenase activity rather than inhibition of the phosphofructokinase enzyme system. Ditzel[163] has suggested that repeated transient decreases in red cell oxygen delivery due to reduced 2,3-DPG with insulin-induced hypophosphatemia could contribute over many years to the microvascular

TABLE 73.3 **Clinical and Biochemical Manifestations of Marked Hypophosphatemia**

I. Cardiovascular and skeletal muscle
  A. Decreased cardiac output
  B. Muscle weakness
  C. Decreased transmembrane resting potential
  D. Rhabdomyolysis
II. Carbohydrate metabolism
  A. Hyperinsulinemia
  B. Decreased glucose metabolism
III. Hematologic alterations
  A. Red blood cells
    1. Decreased adenosine triphosphate (ATP) content
    2. Decreased 2,3-DPG
    3. Decreased P_{50}
    4. Increased oxygen affinity
    5. Decreased lifespan
    6. Hemolysis
    7. Spherocytosis
  B. Leukocytes
    1. Decreased phagocytosis
    2. Decreased chemotaxis
    3. Decreased bactericidal activity
  C. Platelets
    1. Impaired clot retraction
    2. Thrombocytopenia
    3. Decreased ATP content
    4. Megakaryocytosis
    5. Decreased lifespan
IV. Neurologic manifestations
  A. Anorexia
  B. Irritability
  C. Confusion
  D. Paresthesias
  E. Dysarthria
  F. Ataxia
  G. Seizures
  H. Coma
V. Skeletal abnormalities
  A. Bone pain
  B. Radiolucent areas (X-ray)
  C. Pseudofractures
  D. Rickets or osteomalacia
VI. Biochemical and renal manifestations
  A. Low parathyroid hormone levels
  B. Increased $1,25(OH)_2D_3$
  C. Hypercalciuria
  D. Hypomagnesemia
  E. Hypermagnesuria
  F. Hypophosphaturia
  G. Decreased glomerular filtration rate
  H. Decreased T_m for bicarbonate
  I. Decreased renal gluconeogenesis
  J. Decreased titratable acid excretion
  K. Increased creatinine phosphokinase
  L. Increased aldolase

From Slatopolsky E. Pathophysiology of calcium, magnesium, and phosphorus. In: Klahr S, ed. *The Kidney and Body Fluids in Health and Disease.* New York: Plenum Press; 1983:269, with permission.

disease seen in diabetic patients. Patients with mild degrees of hypophosphatemia are usually asymptomatic. However, if hypophosphatemia is severe—that is, if serum phosphorus levels are less than 1.5 mg per dL—a series of hematologic, neurologic, and metabolic disorders may develop. In general, the patients become anorectic and weak, and mild bone pain may be present if the hypophosphatemia persists for several months (Table 73.3).

Cardiovascular and Skeletal Muscle Manifestations

Severe cardiomyopathy with decreased cardiac output has been described in patients and animals with severe hypophosphatemia.[484,731] Studies revealed that the resting muscle membrane potential fell, sodium chloride and water content of the tissue increased, and potassium content decreased in severe hypophosphatemia.[205] These values returned to within the normal range after phosphate was administered. Skeletal muscle weakness and electromyographic abnormalities are associated with chronic hypophosphatemia and phosphate depletion. Dogs that were fed low-phosphate diets for several months developed changes in muscle, rhabdomyolysis, and characteristic increases in their levels of creatinine kinase and aldolase in blood.[329] Rhabdomyolysis has been observed in alcoholic patients with hypophosphatemia.[330] Knochel et al.[329] showed that myopathy associated with phosphate depletion in dogs did lead to changes in cell water content, sodium concentration, and transmembrane potential difference. Kretz et al.[341] examined the possibility that changes in calcium transport in the sarcoplasmic reticulum of muscle were responsible for the clinical myopathy seen in acute phosphate depletion. Despite significant hypophosphatemia and a reduction in muscle phosphorus concentration, they found no significant changes in the rate of calcium uptake of calcium-concentrating ability in vesicles prepared from muscle sarcoplasmic reticulum of phosphate-depleted rats. Thus, the role of altered transcellular calcium movements in phosphate-depleted tissues is yet to be completely resolved.

Effects on Carbohydrate Metabolism

Hyperinsulinemia and abnormal glucose metabolism suggesting insulin resistance have been described in phosphate depletion. DeFronzo and Lange[155] have used the glucose and insulin clamp technique to study the kinetics of glucose metabolism in patients with various chronic hypophosphatemic conditions including vitamin D–resistant rickets. When glucose was infused to maintain constant glycemia at 125 mg per dL, hypophosphatemic individuals required 36% less glucose to maintain these glycemic levels than controls. Also when euglycemia was achieved by combined insulin and glucose infusion, the hypophosphatemic individuals required 40% less glucose to maintain euglycemia than controls. Insulin catabolism was apparently unaffected in these hypophosphatemic individuals. These data indicate that hypophosphatemia is associated with impaired glucose metabolism in both hyperglycemic and euglycemic patients.

Hematologic Manifestations

Hematologic abnormalities of hypophosphatemia are a major manifestation of this syndrome.[388,668] In addition to defects in affinity of oxyhemoglobin leading to generalized tissue hypoxia, there may be increased hemolysis.[298,327] Quantitative and functional defects have also been described in platelets and leukocytes.[142] These defects lead to diminished platelet aggregation and abnormalities in chemotaxis and phagocytosis of white blood cells. The latter may contribute to the increased risk of gram-negative sepsis reported in hypophosphatemic patients.[549] This is of particular concern in immunosuppressed patients receiving phosphate-poor alimentation through a central venous line.

Neurologic Manifestations

Manifestations at the level of the central nervous system, resulting in generalized anorexia and malaise or more severe disturbances such as ataxia, seizures, and coma, have been described in hypophosphatemia.[404,405,522] Neuromuscular abnormalities include paresthesias and weakness, the result of both myopathic changes and diminished nerve conduction.[72]

Skeletal Abnormalities

The skeletal abnormalities associated with hypophosphatemia, particularly in vitamin D–resistant rickets, may be quite marked. In addition, bony abnormalities, including osteomalacia and pathologic fractures, have been described in antacid-induced phosphate depletion,[37,139] as well as in hypophosphatemic patients undergoing hemodialysis who did not receive phosphate binding gels.[11] A rheumatic syndrome resembling ankylosing spondylitis also has been reported in hypophosphatemic patients.[464]

Gastrointestinal Disturbances

These manifestations include anorexia, nausea, and vomiting.[405] It has been speculated that hypophosphatemia in the alcoholic patient may further impair hepatic function through hypoxic insult.

Renal Manifestations

There is decreased phosphorus excretion and decreased tubular reabsorption of calcium, magnesium, bicarbonate, and glucose.[130,165,181,227,228,230] The renal conservation of phosphorus occurs early in the syndrome and is the result of a primary increase in the tubular reabsorption of the anion and a decrease in the GFR and consequently in the filtered load of phosphorus.[230,468] This mechanism results in complete renal conservation of phosphorus, with net losses representing only a small fraction of total body phosphorus stores.[405] The increase in phosphorus reabsorption seen with phosphorus depletion is independent of several hormones known to influence phosphorus transport under other circumstances, including PTH, vitamin D, calcitonin, and thyroxine.[640] The possibility that serum phosphorus concentration per se (or intracellular phosphorus) may in some manner regulate its absorption along the nephron seems plausible. Hypercalciuria of enough magnitude to produce a negative calcium balance is seen commonly in hypophosphatemic patients. Several factors contribute to this increase in calcium excretion including increased calcium mobilization from bone, enhanced GI tract calcium absorption, and inhibition of renal tubular calcium reabsorption.[130,165,181,227,228,230] These effects appear to be independent of PTH activity and may be the result of a direct effect of phosphate on these transport processes.

Acid–Base Disturbances

Renal bicarbonate wasting, diminished titratable acid excretion, and decreased ammoniagenesis have been reported in hypophosphatemia.[165,485] However, these defects are counterbalanced to some extent by the mobilization of alkali from bone. Thus, steady-state pH may be near normal at the expense of skeletal buffers.[181]

Differential Diagnosis of Hypophosphatemia

In general, the cause of hypophosphatemia can be determined either from the medical history or from the clinical setting in which it occurs. When the cause is in doubt, measurement of the urinary phosphorus excretion level may be helpful. If the urinary phosphorus concentration is less than 4 mg per dL when the serum phosphorus level is less than 2 mg per dL, renal losses may be excluded.[256] Of the three major extrarenal causes including diminished phosphorus intake, increased extrarenal losses (GI tract), and translocation into the intracellular space, the last is the most common, particularly in the hospitalized patient.[309,364]

When the urinary phosphorus excretion level is high, the differential diagnosis includes hyperparathyroidism, a primary renal tubular abnormality, or vitamin D–dependent or –resistant renal rickets. Measurements of serum calcium, PTH, and vitamin D and its metabolites, as well as urinary excretion of other solutes (glucose, amino acids, and bicarbonate), will usually elucidate the underlying disturbance that is responsible for the hypophosphatemia.

Treatment of Hypophosphatemia

There are several general principles that apply to the treatment of hypophosphatemic patients. As with any predominantly intracellular ion (e.g., potassium), the state of total body phosphorus stores, as well as the magnitude of phosphorus losses, cannot be readily assessed by measurement of the concentrations in serum. In fact, under conditions in which a rapid shift of phosphorus has resulted from glucose infusion or hyperalimentation, total body stores of phosphorus may be normal, although with diminished intake and renal losses, there may be severe phosphorus depletion. Furthermore, the volume of distribution of phosphorus may vary widely, reflecting in part the intensity and duration of the underlying cause.[364]

In clinical situations in which hypophosphatemia is to be expected (e.g., glucose infusion or hyperalimentation in the alcoholic or nutritionally compromised patient during treatment of diabetic ketoacidosis), careful monitoring of the concentration of serum phosphorus is crucial. In these situations, addition of phosphorus supplementation to prevent the development of severe hypophosphatemia may prove very helpful. Certainly, other contributing causes of hypophosphatemia in this setting should be identified and treated. This is particularly true of the use of phosphate binding antacids (aluminum and magnesium hydroxide) for peptic ulcer disease, which may be replaced by aluminum phosphate antacids (Phosphagel) or cimetidine (Tagamet). It is now generally recommended that hyperalimentation solutions contain a phosphorus concentration of 12 to 15 mmol per L or 37 to 46.5 mg per dL, in order to provide an appropriate amount of phosphorus in the patient in whom renal impairment is absent.[364] Phosphorus supplementation during glucose infusion or during the treatment of ketoacidosis is usually withheld until the serum phosphorus levels decrease to less than 1 mg per dL. Phosphorus may be given orally to these patients and others with mild asymptomatic hypophosphatemia in the form of skim milk, which contains 0.9 mg per mL, Neutra-phos (3.3 mg per mL), or phosphorus soda (129 mg per mL). However, intestinal absorption is quite variable, and diarrhea often complicates the oral administration of phosphate-containing compounds. For these reasons, parenteral administration is usually recommended in the hospitalized patient. If oral therapy is permissible, Fleet Phospho-Soda may be given at a dosage of 60 mmol daily in three doses (21 mmoL per 5 mL or 643 mg per 5 mL). A convenient method is to provide the phosphorus together with potassium replacement in these patients. Addition of 5 mL of potassium phosphate (K phosphate) into 1 L of intravenous fluid provides 22 mEq of potassium and 15 mmol (466 mg) of phosphorus.[364] However, because potassium losses may greatly exceed the phosphorus deficit, the repletion of potassium should not be totally linked to phosphorus therapy. In patients with severe phosphate depletion, it is difficult to determine the magnitude of the total deficit of phosphorus and to calculate a precise initial dose. It is usually prudent to proceed with caution and repair the deficit slowly. The most frequently recommended regimen is 0.08 mmol per kg of body weight (2.5 mg per kg body weight) given over 6 hours for severe but uncomplicated hypophosphatemia and 0.016 mmol per kg of body weight (5 mg per kg of body weight) in symptomatic patients.[364] Parenteral administration should be discontinued when the serum phosphorus concentration is greater than 2 mg per dL.

Calcium administration may be needed during phosphate repletion to prevent severe hypocalcemia. Calcium must not be added to bicarbonate- or phosphate-containing solutions because of the potential precipitation of calcium salts. Intravenous infusion of calcium gluconate or calcium chloride may be given until tetany abates. In addition to hypocalcemia, metastatic calcification, hypotension, hyperkalemia, and hypernatremia are potential side effects of parenteral infusion of phosphorus. These problems can be prevented by judicious use of therapy and frequent monitoring of serum electrolyte concentrations.

Hyperphosphatemia

Hyperphosphatemia is said to occur when the serum phosphorus concentration exceeds 4.6 mg per dL in adults. In children, serum levels of phosphorus of up to 6 mg per dL may be physiologic. The most frequent cause of hyperphosphatemia is decreased excretion of phosphorus in the urine as a result of a fall in the GFR. However, increases in serum phosphorus concentration can also occur as a result of increased entry into the ECF due to excessive intake of phosphorus, increased release of phosphorus from tissue breakdown, and release of phosphorus from the skeletal reservoir through bone resorption. The major causes of hyperphosphatemia are listed in Table 73.4.

Decreased Excretion of Phosphorus in Urine

Decreased Renal Function

In progressive kidney failure, phosphorus homeostasis is maintained by a progressive increase in phosphorus excretion per nephron.[624,625] As a result of increased phosphorus excretion per nephron, it is unusual to see marked hyperphosphatemia until GFRs decrease to less than 25 mL per minute.[624,625] Under physiologic conditions with a GFR of 120 mL per minute, a fractional excretion of 5% to 15% of the filtered load of phosphorus is adequate to maintain phosphorus homeostasis. However, as renal insufficiency progresses and the number of nephrons decreases, fractional excretion of phosphorus may increase to as high as 60% to

TABLE 73.4 **Causes of Hyperphosphatemia**

I. Decreased renal excretion of phosphate
   A. Renal insufficiency
      1. Chronic
      2. Acute
   B. Hypoparathyroidism
   C. Pseudohypoparathyroidism
      1. Type I
      2. Type II
   D. Abnormal circulating parathyroid hormone
   E. Acromegaly
   F. Tumoral calcinosis
   G. Administration of bisphosphonates
II. Increased entrance of phosphorus into the extracellular fluid
   A. Neoplastic diseases
      1. Leukemia
      2. Lymphoma
   B. Increased catabolism
   C. Respiratory acidosis
III. Increased intake and gastrointestinal absorption of phosphorus
   A. Pharmacologic administration of vitamin D metabolites
   B. Ingestion and/or administration of phosphate salts
IV. Miscellaneous
   A. Cortical hyperostosis
   B. Intermittent hyperphosphatemia
   C. Artifacts

From Slatopolsky E. Pathophysiology of calcium, magnesium, and phosphorus. In: Klahr S, ed. *The Kidney and Body Fluids in Health and Disease.* New York: Plenum Press; 1983:269, with permission.

80% of the filtered load. This progressive phosphaturia per nephron serves to maintain the concentration of phosphorus within normal limits in plasma as renal disease progresses. The decrease in phosphate reabsorption per nephron is stimulated by increased PTH and FGF23 levels. However, when the number of nephrons is greatly diminished, if the dietary intake of phosphorus remains constant, phosphorus homeostasis can no longer be maintained and hyperphosphatemia develops. This usually occurs when the GFR falls to less than 25 mL per minute. As hyperphosphatemia develops the filtered load of phosphorus per nephron increases, phosphorus excretion rises, and phosphorus balance is reestablished but at higher concentrations of serum phosphorus, PTH, and FGF23. Hyperphosphatemia is a usual finding in patients with far-advanced renal insufficiency unless phosphorus intake in the diet has decreased through dietary manipulations or the patient is receiving phosphate binders such as calcium carbonate, sevelamer, or lanthanum carbonate that decrease the absorption of phosphate from the GI tract.[568] In patients with acute kidney injury (AKI), hyperphosphatemia is a common finding.[430] The degree of hyperphosphatemia in patients with acute renal failure varies considerably. It is quite marked in patients with renal insufficiency secondary to severe trauma or nontraumatic rhabdomyolysis.[335] Hyperphosphatemia in CKD and AKI directly stimulates osteocyte, osteoblast, odontoblast, and vascular smooth muscle cell signaling that results in gene transcription of *RUNX2* and *osterix*.[434] In vascular smooth muscle cells of neointimal atherosclerotic plaques and cardiac valves, stimulation of *RUNX2* and *osterix* produce matrix calcification akin to bone formation.[590] In mineralizing vascular smooth muscle cells, Pi is a signal stimulating molecule, and the sodium-dependent Pi transport protein PIT1 may be the phosphorus sensing receptor.[381] Thus, hyperphosphatemia is related to vascular calcification and both of these are cardiovascular risk factors in CKD.[69,398] Cardiovascular mortality is extremely high in CKD and hyperphosphatemia and vascular calcification account for much of this.[192,630]

Decreased or Absent Levels of Circulating Parathyroid Hormone

Hypoparathyroidism is characterized by low or absent levels of PTH, low levels of serum calcium, and hyperphosphatemia.[498] The most common causes of hypoparathyroidism result from injury to the parathyroid glands, or their blood supply during thyroid, parathyroid, or radical neck surgery. Idiopathic hypoparathyroidism is a rare disease. Because PTH normally inhibits the renal reabsorption of phosphorus, its absence leads to an elevation in the Tm for phosphorus and a decrease in the excretion of the anion in the urine. Balance is reestablished when the serum phosphorus concentration rises to 6 to 8 mg per dL. At this concentration of serum phosphorus, the filtered load of phosphate is increased, exceeding the Tm for phosphorus reabsorption, and a new steady-state is reestablished. Patients with hypoparathyroidism are easily diagnosed by the findings of a low level of serum calcium, hyperphosphatemia, and undetectable levels of circulating immunoreactive PTH. After several years of hypoparathyroidism, other signs may become manifest such as cataracts and bilateral symmetrical calcification of the basal ganglia on X-ray films of the skull. The most striking symptoms in patients presenting with hypoparathyroidism are related to an increase in neuromuscular excitability resulting from a decrease in the levels of ionized calcium in serum. Some patients may not develop hypocalcemia and severe tetany, but increased neuromuscular excitability may be demonstrated by contraction of facial muscles in response to stimulus over the facial nerve (Chvostek's sign) or by carpal spasm (Trousseau's sign) occurring 2 or 3 minutes after inflating a blood pressure cuff around the arm above systolic blood pressure. In other patients, psychiatric disturbances, paresthesias, numbness, muscle cramps, and dysphagia may be presenting symptoms.

Pseudohypoparathyroidism

This is a relatively rare condition characterized by end-organ resistance to the action of PTH.[13] Characteristically, the kidney and skeleton do not respond appropriately to the action of PTH. Some patients with pseudohypoparathyroidism (PHP) may have specific somatic characteristics such as short stature, round face, short metacarpal bones and phalanges, and some degree of mental retardation. Biochemically, these patients, like those with hypoparathyroidism, have low concentrations of serum calcium and hyperphosphatemia. However, there are two important points in the differential diagnosis. First, in most patients with PHP, the circulating levels of immunoreactive PTH are elevated, whereas in patients with true hypoparathyroidism PTH levels are low or absent. Second, patients with PHP do not respond to the administration of exogenous PTH with phosphaturia. Patients with true hypoparathyroidism demonstrate a heightened phosphaturic response to administration of exogenous PTH. Two major types of PHP have been described. In type I, patients fail to increase the excretion of cAMP or phosphate in the urine in response to the administration of exogenous PTH. PHP type Ia is due to defects in the guanosine triphosphate (GTP) binding protein, $G_{S\alpha}$(the alpha subunit of the heterotrimeric stimulatory G protein), which is a product of the *GNAS* gene locus, whereas PHP type Ib is due to methylation defects in the imprinted *GNAS* cluster.[425] In other patients, there is an increase in cAMP in response to the administration of exogenous PTH but no phosphaturic response. This condition has been termed PHP type II.[169]

Abnormal Circulating Parathyroid Hormone

This syndrome is characterized by hyperphosphatemia, hypocalcemia, chronic tetany, and cataracts. These manifestations, as described previously, are those observed in patients with hypoparathyroidism, but these patients have normal or high serum levels of PTH. However, in contrast to patients with pseudohypoparathyroidism, they do respond to the exogenous administration of PTH, with an increase in the excretion of cAMP and phosphaturia. It has been postulated that the defect in these patients relates to an abnormal form of endogenous PTH that is devoid of physiologic effects.[137] However, this postulate has not been substantiated by characterization and analysis of the circulating PTH in these patients.

Acromegaly

GH decreases the urinary excretion of phosphorus and increases the Tm for phosphorus.[350] Hypersecretion of GH may lead to development of gigantism if the increased secretion occurs before the closure of the epiphysis or to acromegaly if the excessive secretion occurs after puberty. Hyperphosphatemia has been described in patients with acromegaly. It is known that serum phosphorus concentrations are higher in children (5 to 8 mg per dL) than in adults. This may be related in part to increased levels of circulating GH in children.

Tumoral Calcinosis

This condition, which is seen more frequently in young African Americans, is characterized by hyperphosphatemia, ectopic calcification around large joints, normal levels of circulating immunoreactive PTH, and a normal response to administration of exogenous PTH.[408,732] The extensive calcification of soft tissues observed in patients with this condition is most likely due to an elevated phosphorus–calcium product in blood. Despite the development of hyperphosphatemia, patients with tumoral calcinosis do not develop secondary hyperparathyroidism. This may be due to the fact that circulating levels of 1,25-dihydroxycholecalciferol remain within the normal range in these patients despite hyperphosphatemia. These normal levels of 1,25-dihydroxycholecalciferol maintain a normal GI tract absorption of calcium. This, combined with the decreased urinary calcium observed in these patients, may serve to maintain normal serum calcium values and prevent the development of secondary hyperparathyroidism.

The pathogenesis of this disease has been clarified by genetic studies of rare familial forms, see below. Mutations in three genes, *FGF23*, *KLOTHO*, and *GALNT3*, all related to FGF23 function, have been found to cause tumoral calcinosis.[48,291,667] Because acquired tumoral calcinosis is most often observed in association with kidney disease, which is characterized by reduced *KLOTHO* and FGF23 signaling, tumoral calcinosis is probably related to decreased phosphorus excretion by the kidney.[454]

Familial Tumoral Calcinosis

Familial tumoral calcinosis (FTC) is inherited in both autosomal recessive and autosomal dominant patterns.[407,409,410,455,495,521,629] The disease most commonly appears before the second decade of life, presenting as periarticular calcified masses of the hip, elbow, or shoulder. This disorder is associated with hyperphosphatemia and increased renal tubular Pi reabsorption, but with normal serum levels of calcium and parathyroid hormone. Serum levels of 1,25-dihydroxyvitamin D may be normal or elevated.

Biallelic mutations in the UDP-*N*-acetyl-alpha-D-galactosamine:polypeptide N-acetylglucosaminyltransferase 3 (*GALNT3*) gene have been identified in two large families as a cause of FTC.[290] *GALNT3* encodes a glycosyltransferase responsible for initiating mucin-type O-glycosylation. FGF23 is O-glycosylated which blocks the recognition sequence for SPC and processing of FGF23. Thus, lack of *GALNT3* function leads to reduced FGF23 levels. Furthermore, inactivating mutations of FGF23 have been shown to cause tumoral calcinosis.[48] Recently, mutations in the *KLOTHO* gene have also been shown to cause familial tumoral calcinosis.[291] Thus, familial tumoral calcinosis is a disease of decreased FGF23 signaling.

Administration of Bisphosphonates

Administration of bisphosphonates, which are used in the treatment of Paget disease and osteoporosis, may result in the development of hyperphosphatemia.[685] The mechanisms by which bisphosphonates increase serum phosphorus are not completely clear but may involve an alteration in phosphate distribution between different cellular compartments and a decrease in renal phosphorus excretion. It appears that the levels of both circulating PTH and the urinary excretion of cAMP after administration of exogenous PTH are within the normal range in patients receiving bisphosphonates.

Redistribution of Phosphorus between Intracellular and Extracellular Pools

Tumor Lysis Syndrome

Various syndromes of tissue breakdown may result in the development of hyperphosphatemia and subsequent hypocalcemia. Hyperphosphatemia has been described in patients with several types of lymphomas. Patients receiving treatment for lymphoblastic leukemia may develop hyperphosphatemia with a concomitant decrease in serum calcium concentration.[734] The phosphorus load originates primarily from the destruction of lymphoblasts, which have about four times the concentration of organic and inorganic phosphorus present in mature lymphocytes.

Similar findings have been described during treatment of Burkitt lymphoma. Cohen et al.[133] reviewed the acute tumor lysis syndrome associated with the treatment of Burkitt lymphoma. In 37 patients with American Burkitt lymphoma, azotemia occurred in 14 patients and preceded chemotherapy in eight. Pretreatment of azotemia was associated with elevated levels of lactate dehydrogenase (LDH) and uric acid and sometimes extrinsic ureteral obstruction by the tumor. After chemotherapy, major metabolic complications related to tumor lysis were associated with large tumors and high LDH levels and were manifested by hyperkalemia, hyperphosphatemia, and hyperuricemia. Elevated phosphorus levels were seen in 31% of nonazotemic patients and in all azotemic patients. Hemodialysis was required in three patients for control of azotemia, hyperuricemia, hyperphosphatemia, or hyperkalemia.

Tsokos et al.[669] studied the renal metabolic complications of other undifferentiated lymphomas and lymphoblastic lymphomas. These workers found that serum LDH concentration before chemotherapy correlated well with the stage of disease and predicted the serum levels of creatinine, uric acid, and phosphorus in the posttreatment period. Patients with LDH values of more than 2,000 IU were likely to develop severe hyperphosphatemia. When azotemia developed in the post-chemotherapy period, it was attributed to hyperuricemia or hyperphosphatemia. Some of these patients had elevated serum phosphorus levels in the range of 20 to 30 mg per dL, which may contribute to the development of renal insufficiency due to calcium deposition in the kidney and other tissues.

Thus, there is a great risk of hyperphosphatemia in patients undergoing chemotherapy for rapidly growing malignant lymphomas. The best method of prevention of this complication, as well as the best therapeutic intervention, has not been well defined. Initially, it appears useful to attempt to increase the renal excretion of phosphate during the induction of remission by chemotherapy in these patients. This requires infusion of large amounts of saline and possibly bicarbonate, which has been shown to increase renal phosphorus excretion above and beyond the mere effects of volume expansion. Acetazolamide, a potent phosphaturic agent, might also be beneficial in these individuals. The general recommendation of hemodialysis as the prime therapeutic modality for hyperphosphatemia and acute renal insufficiency resulting from tumor lysis is not based on experimental data. Although hemodialysis no doubt rapidly lowers serum phosphorus levels, the mass of phosphorus continually presented to the extracellular space from ongoing tissue breakdown is not continuously treated by this modality. Thus, it is possible that combined hemodialysis and peritoneal dialysis, or even peritoneal dialysis alone, might be as, if not more, beneficial and safer in individuals with tumor lysis syndrome.

Increased Catabolism

Conditions characterized by increased protein breakdown (e.g., severe tissue muscle damage and severe infections) may sometimes be accompanied by hyperphosphatemia. Although the hyperphosphatemia may be related simply to translocation of phosphorus into the extracellular space, other factors seem to play a role. Hyperphosphatemia has been described in patients with ketoacidosis before treatment. After administration of intravenous fluids and insulin therapy, the entrance of glucose into the cells is usually followed by movement of phosphorus back into the intracellular space, and some patients now may develop hypophosphatemia. Thus, the combination of dehydration, acidosis, and tissue breakdown in different catabolic states may lead to hyperphosphatemia.

Respiratory Acidosis

Acute respiratory acidosis may lead to a marked increase in serum phosphorus concentration.[217] By contrast, chronic respiratory acidosis is usually not manifested by sustained elevated levels of serum phosphorus. Acute rises in P_{CO_2} in experimental animals have been shown to lead to increased serum phosphorus levels. The modest degree of hyperphosphatemia seen in chronic respiratory acidosis is probably related to renal compensation and increased phosphorus excretion via the kidney to maintain phosphorus homeostasis.

Increased Intake and Gastrointestinal Absorption of Phosphorus

Administration of Phosphate Salts or Vitamin D or Its Metabolites

Administration of vitamin D_3 or its metabolites, particularly 1,25-dihydroxycholecalciferol, may result in increases in serum phosphorus, particularly in uremic patients. These compounds very likely may result in hyperphosphatemia in uremic individuals by increasing phosphorus absorption from the gut and perhaps by potentiating the effect of PTH on the skeleton with increased release of phosphorus from bone. Decreased renal function limits the compensatory mechanism of the kidney to excrete the increased load of phosphate entering the extracellular space. In addition to elevating serum phosphorus levels, vitamin D metabolites may result in hypercalcemia. An increase in the phosphorus–calcium product may result in tissue deposition of calcium, particularly in the kidney, leading to further renal functional deterioration.

Ingestion or Administration of Salts Containing Phosphate

Hyperphosphatemia has been observed in adults ingesting laxative-containing phosphate salts or after administration of enemas containing large amounts of phosphate.[273,441] Intravenous phosphate administration has been used in the treatment of hypercalcemia of malignancy. The administration of 1 to 2 g of phosphate intravenously decreases the concentration of serum calcium. Unfortunately, the severe hyperphosphatemia induced by administration of large amounts of phosphorus intravenously may lead to calcium-phosphate precipitation in important organs such as the heart and kidney, and several deaths resulting from this form of therapy have been reported. Hyperphosphatemia may develop in newborn infants who are fed cow's milk, which is higher in phosphorus content than human milk. This may be an important factor in the genesis of neonatal tetany.

Clinical Manifestations of Hyperphosphatemia

Acute hyperphosphatemia following administration of phosphate enemas or oral sodium phosphate solution has been associated with acute and chronic renal failure or acute phosphate nephropathy.[5,426] Otherwise, most of the clinical effects of hyperphosphatemia are related to secondary changes of calcium metabolism. Hyperphosphatemia produces hypocalcemia by several mechanisms (Fig. 73.7), including decreased production of 1,25-dihydroxycholecalciferol, precipitation of calcium, and decreased absorption of calcium from the gastrointestinal tract, presumably due to a direct effect of phosphorus on calcium absorption.[462] In addition to the manifestations by hypocalcemia, which are described elsewhere in this chapter, ectopic calcification is one of the important manifestations of hyperphosphatemia. The association of hyperphosphatemia and ectopic calcification has been observed in several clinical settings including in patients with chronic renal failure, hypoparathyroidism, and tumoral calcinosis. It appears that when the calcium–phosphorus product exceeds 70, the likelihood for calcium precipitation is greatly increased. In addition to the calcium–phosphorus product, local tissue factors may play an important role in calcium deposition. For example, regional changes in pH (local alkalosis) may favor

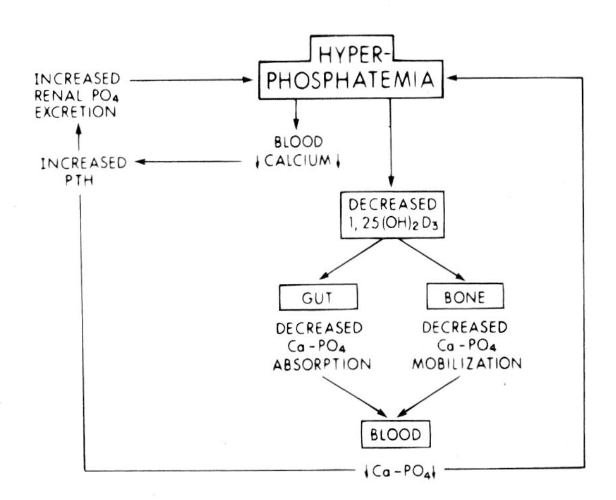

FIGURE 73.7 Pathophysiologic changes occurring during the development of hyperphosphatemia. These changes tend to increase the urinary excretion of phosphorus and to correct the hyperphosphatemia.

calcification in tissue such as cornea and lungs. In patients with severe calcification (calciphylaxis), it appears that high levels of circulating PTH may also aggravate this condition. Hyperphosphatemia plays a key role in the development of secondary hyperparathyroidism in patients with renal insufficiency. It has been observed that when phosphate ingestion is decreased and hyperphosphatemia is prevented in experimental animals with induced renal insufficiency, hyperparathyroidism can be prevented.[622] The mechanisms presumably relate to maintenance of serum calcium levels with prevention of hyperphosphatemia and, at the same time, continued synthesis of 1,25-dihydroxycholecalciferol, the circulating levels of which may directly influence the secretion of PTH.[229,628] Several investigators[156,499,611,623] have demonstrated that dietary phosphate markedly influences the rate of parathyroid cell proliferation and PTH synthesis and secretion independent of changes in ionized calcium or 1,25-dihydroxycholecalciferol. It seems that the mechanism by which phosphorus increases PTH synthesis and secretion is posttranscriptional. Moreover, in experimental uremic rats, it has been shown that phosphate restriction suppresses parathyroid cell growth by inducing p21, a repressor of the cell cycle. On the other hand, a high phosphate intake rapidly (3 to 5 days) induces significant parathyroid cell hyperplasia by inducing an increase in transforming growth factor α (TGFα).[344] TGFα, which is known to promote growth not only in malignant transformation but also in normal tissues,[170,176] is enhanced in hyperplastic and adenomatous human parathyroid glands.[226] In patients on chronic hemodialysis, the degree of hyperparathyroidism correlates well with the concentration of serum phosphorus. Patients who do not adhere to their therapeutic prescriptions requiring ingestion of phosphate binders seem to develop more severe and persistent hyperphosphatemia with marked secondary hyperparathyroidism and bone disease than patients who adhere carefully to dietary and therapeutic prescriptions.

Vascular calcification has been observed in some patients with chronic renal insufficiency and severe calcification, hyperphosphatemia, and hyperparathyroidism, leading to necrosis and gangrene of extremities. Slit-lamp examination may show ocular calcification, and some patients may develop acute conjunctivitis, the so-called red eye syndrome of uremia. Precipitation of calcium in the skin may be in part responsible for pruritus, a symptom that is usually seen in patients with far-advanced uremia. It has been reported that parathyroidectomy in such patients may alleviate the symptoms. From the therapeutic point of view, the most efficacious way of controlling hyperphosphatemia is through the use of phosphate binders that decrease the absorption of phosphorus from the GI tract. In patients with adequate renal function, expansion of the ECF with saline will greatly increase phosphorus excretion in the urine and contribute to correction of the hyperphosphatemia.

Treatment of Hyperphosphatemia

Decreased absorption of phosphate from the GI tract is a cornerstone of treatment of hyperphosphatemia. Phosphate absorption from the GI tract can be markedly decreased by decreasing the amount of phosphorus in the diet, by administering phosphate binding agents capable of decreasing absorption of phosphorus, or both. Because protein requirements limit the amount of phosphorus restriction that can be achieved through dietary manipulation, from a practical point of view, administration of agents capable of decreasing phosphorus absorption from the GI tract is the mainstay of treatment. Administration of calcium salts has replaced aluminum salts as the traditional treatment to control hyperphosphatemia. Most of these preparations require the administration of two to four tablets or capsules three or four times daily. If the patient develops constipation, one of the complications of such medications, magnesium salts may be incorporated into these preparations. However, if the patient has hyperphosphatemia secondary to severe renal insufficiency, magnesium should not be given because of the likelihood of producing severe hypermagnesemia, which may lead to magnesium intoxication, muscle paralysis, and death.

The elucidation of aluminum toxicity, which results from prolonged administration of aluminum-containing salts, as phosphate binders to patients with chronic renal insufficiency, has led to diminished use of these agents or their elimination.[52,689] Several studies indicate that calcium carbonate[463,626,627] is an effective agent for control of hyperphosphatemia in chronic renal failure. However, numerous investigators have demonstrated an increase in the number of aortic and mitral valve calcifications in patients on dialysis when compared with the general population. Cardiovascular events are responsible for a 40% to 60% mortality rate of patients on dialysis.[240,397,547,558] Morbidity and mortality rates increase as the Ca–PO_4 product raises to more than 60. Braun et al.,[88] with the use of electron beam computed tomography (CT), demonstrated a significant deposition of calcium in the coronary arteries of patients on dialysis. Although coronary artery calcifications worsen with age, this abnormality has been demonstrated in young patients.[231] In fact, postmortem examination of children with renal failure demonstrated that 60% to 70% had calcification of the heart, lungs, and blood vessels.[452] Positive calcium balances of 500 to 900 mg daily were demonstrated in uremic patients receiving large doses of calcium carbonate.[627] Thus, it is critical not only to reduce the Ca–PO_4 product to less than 60, but also to significantly decrease the calcium load that patients receive to control serum phosphorus.

To avoid these deleterious side effects, well-tolerated calcium albumin–free phosphate binders have been developed—sevelamer hydrochloride or carbonate and lanthanum carbonate that are not absorbed from the GI tract that interact with phosphate ions. Several short-term clinical studies in patients with end-stage renal disease (ESRD) have established that they are effective phosphate binders without increasing the calcium load to the patients.[121,621] In addition, sevelamer hydrochloride decreases low-density lipoprotein cholesterol by 30% to 40%, and in long-term studies increases high-density lipoprotein cholesterol by 20% to 30%; it does not affect triglycerides.[122]

Studies have shown that nicotinamide may also be an effective agent to decrease serum phosphorus levels. Because nicotinamide is an inhibitor of sodium-dependent phosphate cotransport in rat renal tubule and small intestine,[315,719] studies have examined whether nicotinamide reduces serum levels of phosphorus and intact parathyroid hormone (iPTH) in patients undergoing hemodialysis. Sixty-five hemodialysis patients with a serum phosphorus level of more than 6.0 mg per dL after a 2-week washout of calcium carbonate were enrolled in this study. Nicotinamide was administered for 12 weeks. The starting dose was 500 mg per day, and the dose was increased by 250 mg per day every 2 weeks until serum phosphorus levels were well controlled at less than 6.0 mg per dL. A 2-week posttreatment washout period followed the cessation of nicotinamide. Blood samples were collected every week for measurement of serum calcium, phosphorus, lipids, iPTH, and blood nicotinamide adenine dinucleotide (NAD). The mean dose of nicotinamide was 1080 mg per day. The mean blood NAD concentration increased from 9.3 ± 1.9 nmol per 105 erythrocytes before treatment to 13.2 ± 5.3 nmol per 105 erythrocytes after treatment. The serum phosphorus concentration increased from 5.4 ± 1.5 mg per dL to 6.9 ± 1.5 mg per dL with the pretreatment washout, then decreased to 5.4 ± 1.3 mg per dL after the 12-week nicotinamide treatment, and rose again to 6.7 ± 1.6 mg per dL after the posttreatment washout. Serum calcium levels decreased during the pretreatment washout from 9.1 ± 0.8 mg per dL to 8.7 ± 0.7 mg per dL with the cessation of calcium carbonate. No significant changes in serum calcium levels were observed during nicotinamide treatment. Median serum iPTH levels increased with pretreatment washout from 130.0 (32.8 to 394.0) pg per mL to 200.0 (92.5 to 535.0) pg per mL and then decreased from the maximum 230.0

(90.8 to 582.0) pg per mL to 150.0 (57.6 to 518.0) pg per mL after the 12-week nicotinamide treatment. With nicotinamide, serum high-density lipoprotein (HDL) cholesterol concentrations increased from 47.4 ± 14.9 mg per dL to 67.2 ± 22.3 mg per dL and serum low-density lipoprotein (LDL) cholesterol concentrations decreased from 78.9 ± 18.8 mg per dL to 70.1 ± 25.3 mg per dL; serum triglyceride levels did not change significantly.[654] This study demonstrated that nicotinamide may provide an alternative for controlling hyperphosphatemia and hyperparathyroidism without inducing hypercalcemia in hemodialysis patients.

Although decreased GI absorption of phosphorus is an effective way to control hyperphosphatemia in patients with renal insufficiency, excretion of phosphorus through the kidney is also an important mechanism. Thus expansion of the ECF volume may markedly increase phosphorus excretion by the kidney. This result is presumably related both to direct effects of volume expansion on the kidney, which decreases salt and water reabsorption and hence phosphorus reabsorption, and to increased PTH release, particularly as a consequence of decreased ionized calcium during volume expansion. In patients with marked renal insufficiency or with marked degrees of hyperphosphatemia due to tumor lysis or chemotherapy, peritoneal dialysis or hemodialysis may be used to remove large quantities of phosphorus from the extracellular space. Redistribution of phosphorus from the intracellular to the extracellular space can sometimes be rapidly corrected by the administration of glucose and insulin. In general, mild degrees of hyperphosphatemia can be tolerated, particularly if calcium levels are not markedly elevated. The goal in patients with chronic renal insufficiency is to keep phosphorus levels at less than 4.5 mg per dL to avoid falls in serum ionized calcium and marked development of severe hyperparathyroidism.

CALCIUM

Calcium, the most abundant cation of the body and the principal mineral of the human skeleton, is essential to the integrity and function of cell membranes, neuromuscular excitability, transmission of nerve impulses, multiple enzymatic reactions, and regulation of hormones such as PTH, calcitonin, and 1,25-dihydroxycholecalciferol. A complex homeostatic system involving the interplay of the bones, the kidneys, and the intestine has evolved to maintain calcium concentrations within a narrow range.

Distribution of Calcium

The total amount of calcium in the human body ranges from 1,000 to 1,200 g or 20 to 25 g per kg of fat-free body tissue. Approximately 99% of body calcium resides in the skeleton; the other 1% is present in the extracellular and intracellular spaces. About 1% of the calcium in the skeleton is freely exchangeable with calcium in the ECF. Together, these two fractions are known as the exchangeable pool of calcium and account for 2% of total body calcium. Calcium in bone is primarily crystalline hydroxyapatite, although some calcium exists as amorphous crystals in combination with phosphate. The normal calcium:phosphate ratio in bone is 1.5:1.

Extracellular Calcium

In humans, the serum calcium concentration is kept remarkably constant, between 9.0 and 10.4 mg per dL, or 4.5 to 5.2 mEq per L, or 2.25 to 2.6 mmol per L. About 50% of serum calcium is ionized and 10% is complexed with citrate, phosphate, bicarbonate, and lactate. These two fractions, ionized plus complexed calcium (*ultrafiltrable calcium*), make up approximately 60% of the total serum calcium. The rest, 40%, is protein bound, mainly to albumin. In hypoproteinemic states, such as the nephrotic syndrome or cirrhosis, although total serum calcium may be low, the ionized fraction may be within the normal range. Five to 10% of the calcium is bound to globulins. It is unusual for total serum calcium concentrations to change because of alterations in the levels of serum globulins. However, in severe hyperglobulinemia, such as may occur in patients with multiple myeloma or other dysproteinemias, elevations of total serum calcium concentrations may be observed.

Intracellular Calcium

Calcium is the major intracellular ionic messenger for the activation of many biologic processes.[286] The intracellular concentration of calcium is approximately 0.15 μM (Table 73.5 and Fig. 73.8). Cells extrude calcium via pumps or exchangers, sequester it in intracellular organelles, or use low-affinity binding sites with large capacities to maintain free calcium, Ca^{2+}, at the 0.15 μM level.[109,303] Intracellular calcium is complexed with ions such as orthophosphate or pyrophosphate and is bound to organic molecules such as ATP and proteins. Three major cellular calcium pools exist: (1) bound to multiple diverse sites, (2) sequestered in intracellular organelles, and (3) bound or free within the cytosol.[286]

Extrusion of Ca^{2+} from the cell and sequestration in intracellular organelles are transport functions generally carried out by two mechanisms, Na^+-Ca^{2+} exchange and Ca-ATPase (Table 73.5 and Fig. 73.8).[109,166,303,416,481,577,714] In cardiac muscle, nerve, brain, and kidney, calcium extrusion is directly coupled to sodium transport.[481,545] The Na^+-Ca^{2+} transport system depends on the asymmetric distribution of Na^+ across the plasma membrane. The Na-K-ATPase of the plasma membrane maintains the Na^+ gradient. Thus, the movement of Na^+ into the cell is coupled to the flux of Ca^{2+} out of the cell. This Na^+-Ca^{2+} antiport system is electrogenic with a stoichiometry of three Na^+ per Ca^{2+}.[111,545] A second and more ubiquitous mechanism of calcium efflux energizes uphill transport of calcium by the hydrolysis of high-energy–yielding phosphate bonds of ATP.[416,577,639]

The cytosolic calcium concentration is also maintained by an active transport into mitochondria and the endoplasmic reticulum (Fig. 73.8). It has been shown that mitochondria accumulate Ca^{2+} through a Ca-uniporter, with Ca^{2+} moving down an electrochemical gradient. The K_m for

TABLE 73.5 **Epithelial Calcium Transporters**

Plasma membrane
A. Calcium channels
1. TRPV5
2. TRPV6
B. Calcium buffer proteins
1. Calbindin −9K
2. Calbindin −28K
C. Calcium/Na exchangers
1. NCX1
2. NCX2
3. NCX3
D. Calcium ATPases
1. PCA1
2. PMCA2
3. PMCA3
4. PMCA4
Endoplasmic reticulum/Golgi
A. Calcium ATPase
1. SERCA: IP_3 sensitive Ca release channel
Mitochondria
A. Calcium channel (uniporter)

Ca^{2+} of the uniporter is about 1 μmmol per L. Mitochondria also contain an Na^+-Ca^{2+} exchange mechanism. In the mitochondria, calcium and phosphate ions form insoluble amorphous tricalcium phosphate, a reaction that releases hydrogen ions into the cytosol. Cell injury may lead to a rise in intracellular calcium sufficient for Ca^{2+} to be sequestered in the mitochondria.[168] Ca^{2+} is sequestered in the endoplasmic reticulum by the action of a Ca-ATPase, which differs in properties from that found on the plasma membrane and Golgi apparatus.[343,466] During the early response of cells to certain stimuli, production of IP_3 and cyclic adenosine diphosphate ribose stimulates the opening of Ca^{2+} channels in the endoplasmic reticulum, serving to transiently increase cytosolic Ca^{2+} and allow the ion to act as an intracellular signal. Recently, polycystin-2 has been identified as an IP_3 sensitive ER Ca release channel.[339] Polycystin-2 is the product of the gene mutated in type 2 autosomal dominant polycystic kidney disease (ADPKD).[339] This identifies polycystin-2 as a critical regulator of renal tubular epithelial cell Ca signaling, and suggests that disordered Ca signaling during development leads to polycystic kidney disease.

Skeletal Calcium

More than 99% of the total body calcium is found in the skeleton. Bone consists of approximately 40% mineral, 30% organic matrix, and 30% water. Bone mineral exists

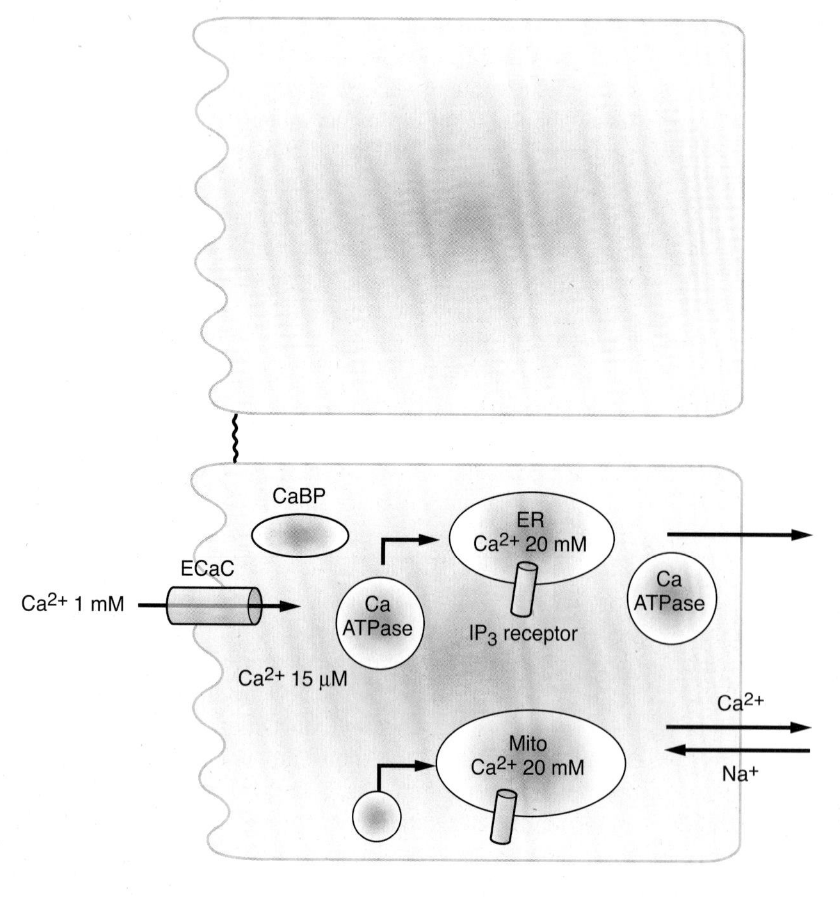

FIGURE 73.8 Control of intracellular calcium. The distal tubule epithelial cell is portrayed as an example of cellular control of cytosolic Ca^{2+} concentrations. Cells extrude Ca by energy (ATP) dependent pumps to maintain cytosolic levels at the 0.15 μM range. Intracellular stores in the endoplasmic reticulum (ER) and the mitochondria (Mito) have pumps to load in Ca and release channels, the IP_3 receptor, and the ryanodine receptor for the ER. Entry of calcium is controlled by entry channels, TRPV5 (which was originally called ECaC) in the case of the distal tubule epithelium and Na/Ca exchange transporters. Ca entering the cell is sequestered by vesicles enriched in calbindin 8K (CaBP) or 25K in the kidney and intestine, respectively.

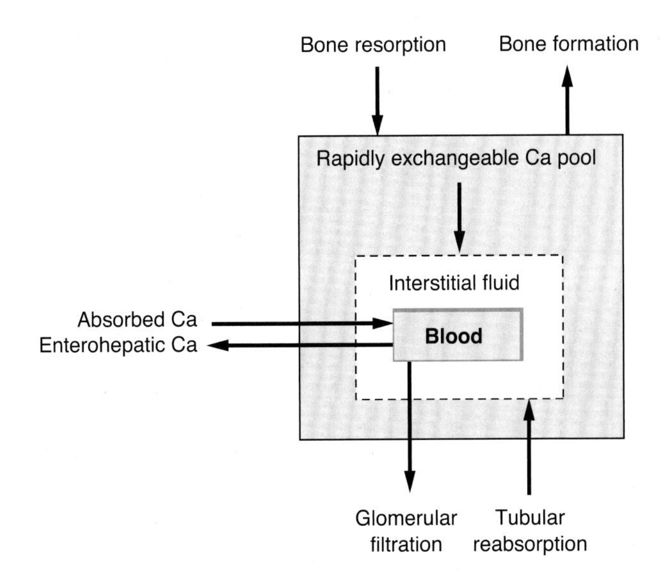

FIGURE 73.9 The exchangeable Ca pool. Absorbed Ca from the intestine enters the interstitial fluid and blood compartments. These compartments are in equilibrium with a larger complexed Ca compartment located in the mineralization fronts at sites of skeletal remodeling and bone formation. Ca leaves the exchangeable pool by the enterohepatic circulation, glomerular filtration, and bone formation. Besides intestinal absorption, Ca enters the exchangeable pool by bone resorption and tubular reabsorption.

in two physical forms, the amorphous and the crystalline. The amorphous form consists mainly of brushite and tricalcium phosphate; the crystalline form is composed mainly of hydroxyapatite. More than 90% of the organic material of the bone matrix is in the form of collagen fibers that are arranged in bundles with specific interaction with hydroxyapatite. Crystalline skeletal Ca is the huge Ca depot that is slowly exchangeable with blood and interstitial fluid pools of extracellular Ca. A large rapidly exchangeable Ca pool is also found in the skeleton (Fig. 73.9). The nature of the freely exchangeable calcium pool in bone is unknown, but it is unlikely to be collagen-associated hydroxyapatite. The Ca pool is likely amorphous and found associated with areas of active bone formation (mineralization fronts) where Ca is being deposited into the crystalline (poorly exchangeable) pool of bone.

A coupled process of bone resorption and formation (remodeling) is responsible for exit of calcium from the exchangeable pool (bone formation) and release of skeletal calcium (bone resorption) into the exchangeable pool. Remodeling imbalance contributes to serum calcium in certain disease states, especially CKD. Pathologic states in which bone resorption is increased (i.e., when bone resorption is greater than bone formation) produce profound changes in calcium homeostasis. In states wherein bone formation is decreased and bone resorption continues in excess (i.e., the renal adynamic bone disorder), hypercalcemia is often observed.[347] Bone remodeling is a coupled process because the activation of a remodeling unit sets two cell differentiation programs into operation—that of the osteoblast and that of the osteoclast. Bone marrow stromal cells, the osteoprogenitors that will become osteoblasts, harbor the receptors that are recognized by the factors capable of activating bone remodeling. Their stimulation results in the synthesis of a cell-attached ligand for RANK (receptor for activation of nuclear factor kappa B) on osteoclast progenitors, known as RANK ligand (RANKL).[102,336,349] RANKL and macrophage colony-stimulating factor (MCSF-1) are the critical osteoclast differentiation factors, and these local bone marrow factors are sufficient to direct osteoclast formation. Thus, stimulation of osteoblastic cells leads to stimulation of osteoclasts, and the process of skeletal remodeling represents bone formation and bone resorption.

The osteoclasts responsible for bone resorption are multinucleated giant cells lying in irregular indentations of the bone surface known as Howship's lacunae. Bone resorption depends on the number and activity of osteoclasts. The process of bone resorption performed by the osteoclasts includes the production of an acidic environment by proton secretion and matrix degradation by cathepsin K. The osteoblasts, on the other hand, are the cells responsible for the repair process after bone resorption (bone formation). Differentiation of the cells in the osteoblast lineage begins with specification of mesenchymal stem cells to the lineage by expression of osteoblast-specific transcription factors—RUNX2[172] and Osterix.[476] RUNX2 expression is stimulated by the bone morphogenetic protein subfamily of the TGFβ superfamily responsible for the direction of osteoblast differentiation and bone formation. Cells early in the process of osteoblast differentiation initiate bone matrix production by the biosynthesis of collagen. Thereafter, the matrix is mineralized by the deposition of calcium and phosphate, with formation of amorphous material initially and then development of hydroxyapatite. The deposition of mineral occurs along a well-defined front ("mineralization front"), outside of which there is an osteoid border or seam. The osteoid begins to calcify about 10 days after deposition. From the architectural point of view, the skeleton is composed of two types of bone: (1) compact cortical bone, which surrounds the marrow cavity and forms the shaft of the long bones, and (2) cancellous or trabecular bone, which is the main component of flat bones, such as ribs, and vertebra.

A differentiation between two other general types of bone is critical in the diagnosis of metabolic bone disease. The first, called woven bone (immature bone)[1] is a loosely organized, highly mineralized bone in which the collagen fibers are coarsely arranged and the osteocytes are large and irregular in size and shape. Woven bone is formed by simultaneous and unorganized actions of many cells. The calcification of the tissue is patchy, occurring in a speckled pattern and independent of the presence of vitamin D activity. Woven bone is present in the fetus, but after age 14 is no longer found in the human skeleton, except with pathologic conditions such as chronic kidney disease, Paget disease, hyperparathyroidism and during rapid bone turnover, as in the presence of healing fractures.[1,2,670] The second general type of bone is lamellar bone (mature bone), which is the major component of the normal adult skeleton. It is a highly organized tissue in which the collagen bundles are arranged in successive layers, between which are cells called osteocytes. Lamellar bone is the product of synchronized activity by the osteoblast depositing collagen materials at a specific cell surface.

Another difference between woven bone and lamellar bone relates to the relation of mineral to collagen. In lamellar bone, the relative amounts of collagen and minerals are closely related, making hypermineralization in these bones difficult. Mineralization of woven bone is disorderly, and the degree of mineralization varies enormously; thus, hypermineralization (osteosclerosis) may occur in this type of bone.[1,2,86]

PTH, in conjunction with PTH-related peptide (PTHrP), other locally produced cytokines, and vitamin D, play key roles in bone turnover. At physiologic doses, PTH has an anabolic effect, increasing bone formation. Thus, PTH, by increasing calcium reabsorption by the kidney and gut and through stimulation of the osteoblast, affects the rate of bone formation. However, in pathologic conditions (e.g., hyperparathyroidism), the concentration of PTH in serum may be increased 10- to 50-fold. At this high concentration, PTH increases the activity and number of osteoclasts; thus, bone resorption predominates over bone formation, and minerals and organic matrix are removed from bone and enter the ECF. Not only PTH but also other hormones such as PTH-related proteins, thyroxine, interleukin-1 (IL-1), and tumor necrosis factor can produce severe hypercalcemia by increasing the activity of osteoclasts. The bone remodeling in these conditions, such as renal failure, is characterized by increased woven bone.[86,280,421]

Calcium Balance

Approximately 700 to 2,000 mg of Ca is ingested daily in the diet. However, this amount may vary depending on the amount of milk consumed. Milk and cheese are the major sources of Ca, contributing 50% to 70% of the total amount ingested in the diet. In the United States, 1 L of milk contains approximately 800 to 900 mg of Ca. About 10 to 15 mg of Ca per kilogram of body weight is the recommended daily intake. Ca needs may vary widely; for instance during the last trimester of pregnancy, there is an increased requirement for Ca because approximately 20 to 30 g of Ca enters the fetus. Transfer of Ca from the mother to milk during lactation is another instance of increased Ca demand.[675] In these states, intestinal absorption may not be sufficient and regulation of extracellular Ca by the calcium sensor, PTH and PTHrP, regulate the intestine and the skeleton to supply the needed Ca. With age, active intestinal Ca absorption declines; thus, an increase in Ca intake may be necessary to maintain Ca homeostasis. When 1 g of Ca is ingested in the

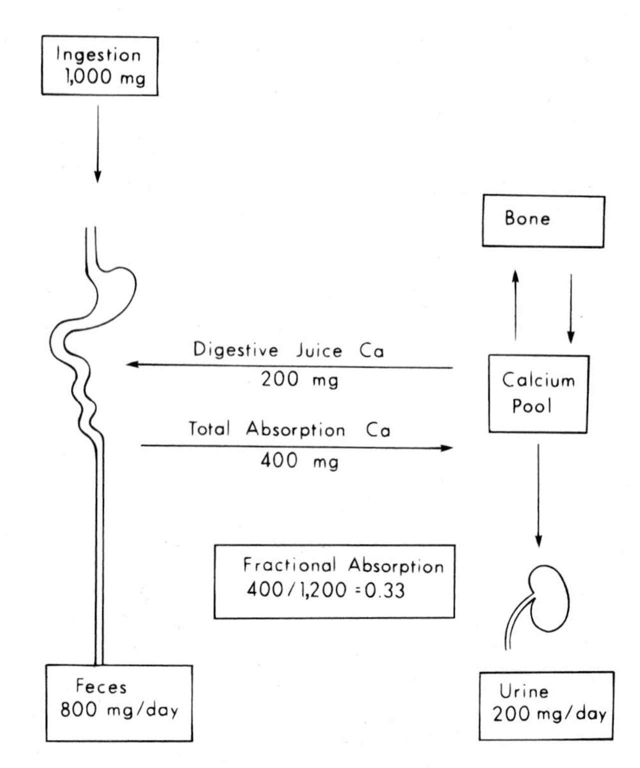

FIGURE 73.10 Diagrammatic representation of Ca metabolism in humans showing the contribution of the gastrointestinal tract, the kidney, and bone to the maintenance of the Ca pool.

diet, approximately 800 mg is excreted in the feces and 200 mg in the urine (Fig. 73.10). With a normal Ca intake (700 to 1,000 mg per day), approximately 30% to 40% of ingested Ca is absorbed in the intestine. However, on lower Ca diets, the percentage of Ca absorbed increases, and the percentage of Ca absorbed decreases when the diet has a high Ca content (more than 1,500 mg per day). The mechanisms responsible for this adaptation have been partially characterized and require the participation of PTH, vitamin D, and perhaps calcitonin. With low-Ca diet feeding, mild hypocalcemia activates the parathyroid gland chief cell Ca sensor and the release of PTH, which increases the conversion of 25-hydroxycholecalciferol to 1,25-dihydroxycholecalciferol in the renal cortex. 1,25-Dihydroxycholecalciferol is the hormonal metabolite of vitamin D, and it increases the intestinal absorption of Ca and mobilizes Ca from bone, synergistically with PTH. Thus, serum Ca levels return to normal. On the other hand, if the patient is fed a high-Ca diet, the mild hypercalcemia inhibits the chief cell Ca sensor, suppressing PTH, and stimulates the release of calcitonin from the C cells of the thyroid. In the absence of PTH, the activity of the 1α-hydroxylase is diminished and the 24-hydroxylase is activated; thus, the kidney makes preferentially 24,25-dihydroxycholecalciferol [24,25$(OH)_2D_3$], which is less efficient than 1,25-dihydroxycholecalciferol in promoting Ca absorption from the GI tract and mobilizing calcium from the skeleton. Fecal calcium consists of the fraction of ingested Ca that is not absorbed plus 100 to 200 mg of Ca secreted by the intestine daily. The secreted digestive juice Ca is known as endogenous fecal calcium. The amount of Ca secreted by the intestine is fairly constant and is not greatly influenced by hypercalcemia.

Intestinal Calcium Absorption

The mechanisms of Ca transport across the intestinal mucosa are complex, but our understanding of the physiology is rapidly improving. Intestinal Ca absorption occurs by two general mechanisms: active and passive transport (Fig. 73.11).[690,691] The passive process involves paracellular movement of Ca in some intestinal segments, and active transport involves movement through mucosal epithelial cells. When the intestine is perfused in vitro with increasing Ca concentrations, the rate of movement of Ca from the mucosa to the serosa increases without evidence of saturation or a maximum transport rate. An active transport process would be expected to be saturable. It has been estimated that at luminal Ca concentrations of more than 7.0 mmol per L, Ca is transported primarily by a diffusional process.[95]. This suggests that in regions of the intestine such as the ileum, where the Ca concentration is high, the passive transport process predominates. In the duodenum and jejunum, where the luminal Ca concentration is lower than 6.0 mmol per L, the active transport process assumes a predominant role.[442]

Active intestinal calcium transport involves three steps: (1) the transport of Ca from the lumen into the cell; (2) the movement of Ca within the cell; and (3) the movement of Ca from the cell into the interstitial fluid (Fig. 73.11). Insulation of the cell interior from the millimolar Ca concentrations of plasma suggests that a brush-border component is instrumental in the transfer of Ca into the epithelial cell. The transfer of Ca across the intestinal brush-border surface is modulated by vitamin D.[19,190,383] The early effects of 1,25-dihydroxycholecalciferol on Ca transport are mediated by changes in the structure of the luminal membrane of the intestine.[543] Administration of 1,25-dihydroxycholecalciferol leads to an increase in de novo synthesis and total content of phosphatidylcholine of the BBM. These changes in lipid structure precede or occur simultaneously with the change in calcium transport rate.[543] However, the major mechanism of Ca entry across the intestinal enterocyte brush border of the duodenum, proximal jejunum, and cecum is through a channel, TRPV6,[267,270] which shares high

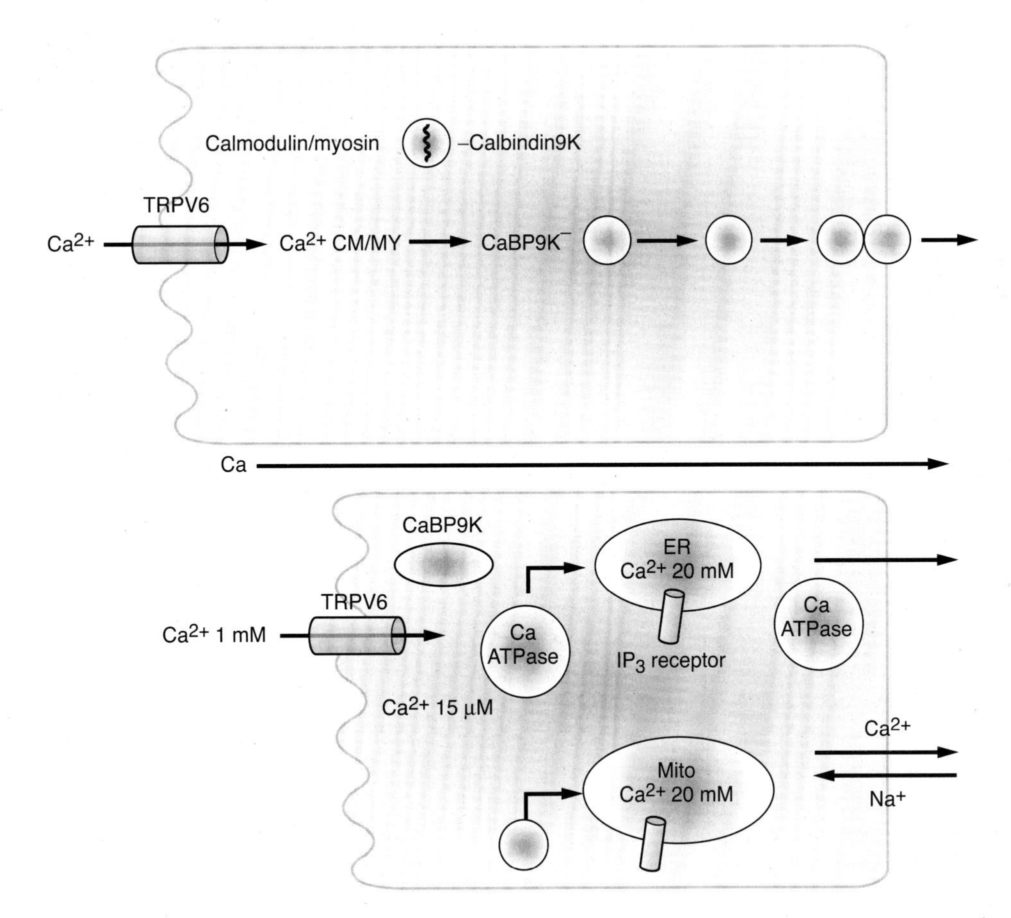

FIGURE 73.11 Intestinal Ca transport in jejunal enterocytes. Ca transport may be through the paracellular space or by an active process through the cell. Transport of Ca from the jejunal lumen through the microvillar membrane is through the TRPV6 channel. Ca is shuttled down the microvillar stalk by calmodulin/myosin (CM/MY) to the glycocalyx where it is bound to calbindin 9K and vesicle sequestered, Ca vesicles deliver Ca to the endoplasmic reticulum and to the efflux pathway, a Ca ATPase in the basolateral membrane.

homology (75%) with the renal tubular epithelial calcium channel (TRPV5).[283,482] The TRPV acronym stands for the Transient Release Potential (TRP), family of Ca channels of the Vanilloid (V) receptor type, TRPV.[283] TRPV6 is voltage-dependent and permeant to Sr and Ba but not Mg. It is inhibited by the trivalent cations Gd and La, and the divalent Cd and Co.[267,270,271]

Less is known about the movement of Ca within the intestinal cell. When Ca enters the cell, it either diffuses or is carried across the cell to the basolateral membrane, where it is pumped out into the serosal medium. Studies suggest that Ca entering through the apical membrane is accumulated in subcellular organelles within the terminal web of the microvillus. This process is stimulated by 1,25-dihydroxycholecalciferol through nongenomic mechanisms.[322] Calmodulin is the major Ca binding protein in the microvillus.[62,63] Its concentration in the microvillus is increased by 1,25-dihydroxycholecalciferol by redistribution from the cytosol. No new calmodulin synthesis is required or observed after 1,25-dihydroxycholecalciferol administration.[62] Calmodulin is thought to play a major role in Ca transport within the microvillus, whereas calbindin is thought to be the dominant Ca binding protein in the cytoplasm. The hypothesis put forth by Bikle et al.[62,63] is that calmodulin and myosin 1 regulate Ca movement within the microvillus to where Ca accumulates within intracellular organelles through the action of calbindin. Movement in the intracellular organelle provides Ca access to the efflux mechanisms. Thus, Ca is transported across the cell without affecting cytoplasmic Ca levels. Specific Ca binding proteins have been demonstrated in the mucosal cells of the intestine of many species.[657,692–694] Their molecular weights are 8,000 to 25,000 and they are referred to as calbindins. Calbindins are transcriptionally regulated by vitamin D, and calbindin-$_{9K}$ is present in intestinal mucosal cells, whereas calbindin-$_{25K}$ is present in distal renal tubular cells involved in active transepithelial Ca^{2+} transport and the brain, but not in bone or other cells. The time course of the calbindins' appearance after vitamin D treatment is similar to the time course of changes in Ca transport, and they are localized in the glycocalyx surface of the brush border of the mucosal intestinal cells. The exact role of these proteins in Ca transport by mucosal cells is still unknown, but it appears to be related to movement of Ca from the entry channel to a shuttle mechanism delivering it to the cell exit mechanism (Fig. 73.11). Increased intestinal Ca absorption is accompanied by an increase in calbindin levels without changes in their intrinsic binding affinity (K_m) for Ca.

Calcium movement from the mucosa to the serosal surface of the intestinal epithelia occurs against a concentration gradient. The intestinal cells contain a "pump" capable of moving calcium against an electrochemical gradient,[109] a Ca-dependent ATPase that is increased by vitamin D.[639] The increase in Ca ATPase parallels the change in Ca transport after vitamin D repletion. Delivery of intracellular Ca to the exit pump is a process largely unknown but appears to involve calbindins.

Many factors regulate intestinal Ca absorption including (1) dietary Ca intake; (2) vitamin D intake; (3) age of the patient; (4) the general state of Ca balance; and (5) circulating levels of PTH, which all affect active transport. In addition to PTH and vitamin D, other factors such as phosphate influence Ca absorption. High-phosphate diets decrease Ca absorption, possibly due to the formation of relatively insoluble calcium–phosphate complexes that decrease the availability of Ca for transepithelial uptake and to decreased 1,25-dihydroxycholecalciferol synthesis secondary to hyperphosphatemia. Experimentally, large concentrations of lactose or other sugars (mannose, xylose) or certain amino acids (lysine, arginine) inhibit intestinal Ca absorption. The physiologic significance of these observations is unknown. The decreased Ca absorption produced by glucocorticoids has therapeutic implications in the management of hypercalcemic disorders associated with excessive intake or increased sensitivity to vitamin D.

Renal Handling of Calcium

In humans who have a GFR of 170 L per 24 hours and serum ultrafiltrable Ca concentrations of 6 mg per dL, roughly 10 g of Ca is filtered per day. The amount of Ca excreted in the urine usually ranges from 100 to 200 mg per 24 hours; hence, 98% to 99% of the filtered load of Ca is reabsorbed by the renal tubular epithelium (Fig. 73.12). There are remarkable similarities in the handling of Ca and Na by the kidney. Less than 2% of their filtered load is excreted normally, and there is no evidence of tubular secretion of either Ca or Na in the mammalian nephron. Urinary excretion of either Na or Ca is controlled by adjustments in tubular reabsorption. Approximately 60% of the filtered Ca is reabsorbed in the PCT (Fig. 73.12), 20% to 30% in the loop of Henle, 10% by the distal convoluted tubule, and 1% by the collecting system. The terminal nephron (connecting segment, distal tubule, and collecting duct), although responsible for the reabsorption of only 10% of the filtered Ca load, is the major site for regulation of Ca excretion.

Calcium in the Glomerular Filtrate

Micropuncture studies of the kidney in the Munich-Wistar rat with surface glomeruli have demonstrated that the ratio of Ca in fluid of Bowman's space to plasma (TF/P calcium) is 0.6, indicating that only the serum Ca not bound to protein is filterable.[256] Thus, approximately 60% of the total Ca, which is the ultrafiltrable Ca, is filtered across the glomerulus.

Proximal Convoluted Tubule

Potential factors regulating Ca reabsorption in the PCT include convection (solvent drag), concentration (increased Ca concentration in tubular fluid due to absorption of Na and water), and transepithelial potential difference. Microperfusion studies of the rabbit PCT in vitro[73,474] and micropuncture of the rat in vivo[672] indicate that fluid absorption and

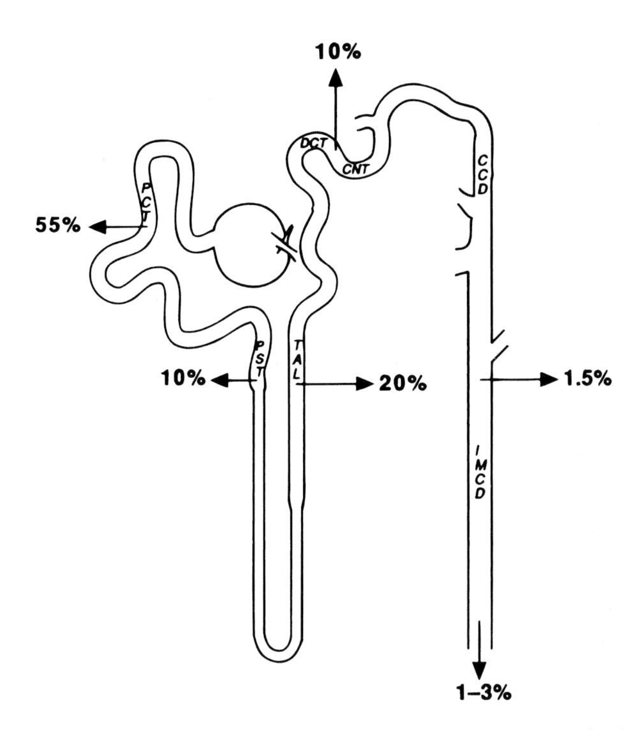

FIGURE 73.12 Schematic illustration of the reabsorption of calcium by different segments of the nephron. *CCD*, cortical collecting duct; *CNT*, connecting tubule; *DCT*, distal convoluted tubule; *IMCD*, intramedullary collecting duct; *PCT*, proximal convoluted tubule; *PST*, proximal straight tubule; *TAL*, thick ascending limb. (From Friedman P, Gesek F. Calcium transport in renal epithelial cells. *Am J Physiol.* 1993;264:F181, with permission.)

solvent drag, as well as diffusion along an electrochemical gradient, contribute to net Ca flux. The reabsorption of Ca in the PCT parallels that of Na and water: The ratio of tubular fluid to plasma ultrafiltrable calcium in the earliest portion of the PCT rises to 1.1 and remains at this value along the rest of the PCT. This is compatible with passive Ca reabsorption secondary to Na and water reabsorption along most of the PCT. The transepithelial movement occurs through the paracellular pathway across the tight junction. Although the passive movement of Ca through a paracellular pathway accounts for most of the Ca transport across the proximal tubule, there is evidence of an active transport component in this segment of the nephron (Fig. 73.13).[73,171,201,356,672] During stop-flow microperfusion experiments measuring net PCT efflux, Ullrich et al. demonstrated that the tubular fluid Ca concentration was lower than that in the capillary.[672] They calculated the active transport rate as 3.4×10^{-13} mol/cm/second, which is in the range of 20% to 30% of the total reabsorptive rate for this segment.

The reabsorption of Ca transcellularly rather than through intercellular channels is a multistep process in which Ca enters the cell across apical membranes and exits across basolateral plasma membranes. Calcium-permeable channels in PCT cells have been described.[189,438–440] However, these are activated by membrane stretch and, therefore, are thought to participate in cell volume regulation.[439] Basolateral efflux of calcium PCTs may be mediated in whole or in part by Na^+-Ca^{2+} exchange.[167,199,583,672,727]

Proximal Straight Tubule (Pars Recta)

Calcium is transported in the pars recta by a process that is not inhibited by ouabain.[560] Because ouabain abolishes water and sodium transport, this suggests that the sodium–calcium exchange is not the major mechanism for Ca extrusion across the basolateral membrane in this segment of the nephron. Approximately one third of the Ca transported can be attributed to sodium and water, and thus, it would seem that an active transport component plays an important role in the reabsorption of Ca in the proximal straight tubule.

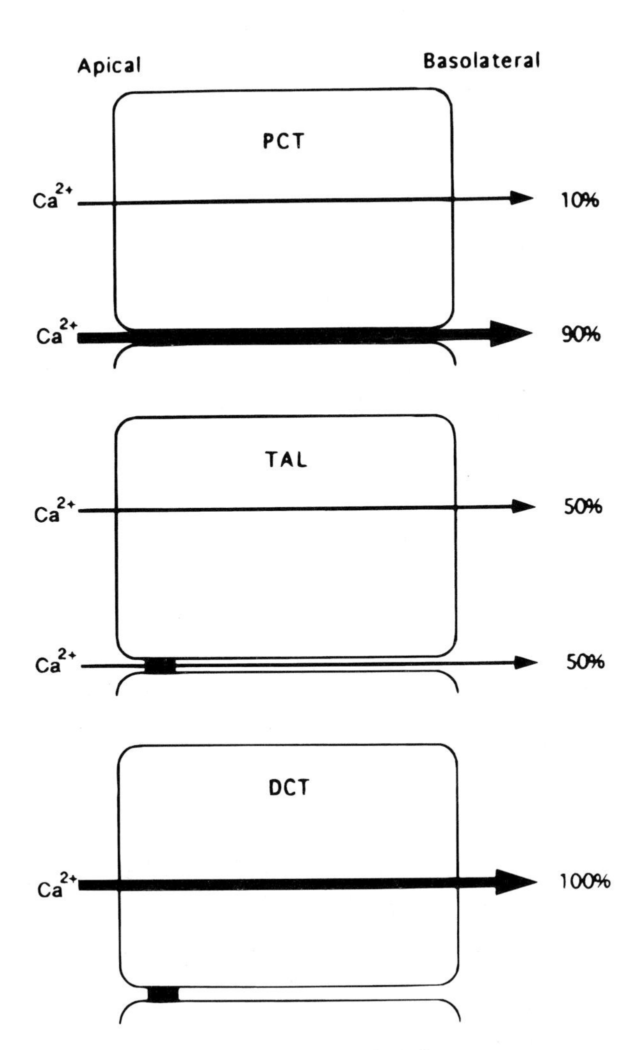

FIGURE 73.13 Cellular and paracellular calcium transport pathways along the nephron. Relative percentage of calcium absorbed by cellular or paracellular pathways in the proximal convoluted tubule (*PCT*), thick ascending limb (*TAL*), and distal convoluted tubule (*DCT*). (From Friedman P, Gesek F. Calcium transport in renal epithelial cells. *Am J Physiol.* 1993;264:F181, with permission.)

Loop of Henle

Neither the thin descending limb nor the thin ascending limb (TAL) of the loop of Henle plays an important role in calcium reabsorption.[560] In contrast, in vitro studies have shown that the TAL of the loop of Henle reabsorbs Ca from lumen to both in the absence of water movement. About 20% of the filtered Ca is reabsorbed in this segment of the nephron. The transepithelial flux of Ca is proportional to the positive transepithelial potential gradient generated by sodium chloride transport mechanisms.[81,591,593] Much of this flux is probably paracellular (Fig. 73.13). Studies of the TAL suggest that the flux ratio for Ca may be greater than can be accounted for by the positive intraluminal potential; thus, an additional active transport process for Ca is present in this segment,[292,552,651] and it accounts for up to 50% of the total Ca transported (Fig. 73.13). This transcellular component is regulated by PTH[201,552] and calcitonin in the cortical and medullary TALs, respectively.[201,651]

Under resting conditions, Ca^{2+} transport is passive in the TAL. Changes in the electrochemical drive for Ca^{2+} determine the magnitude of passive, paracellular absorption. Under these circumstances, the transepithelial voltage is the primary determinant of the driving force, and the magnitude of the voltage, oriented electropositive in the lumen, is set by the rate of Na^+ absorption. As Na^+ absorption increases, transepithelial voltage increases[198,261] and Ca^{2+} flux increases. Peptide hormones that enhance Na^+ transport and thereby increase the transepithelial voltage in medullary TALs would be expected to stimulate passive Ca^{2+} absorption. Extensive evidence consistent with this model has been provided.[158,162,180] Inhibition of Na^+ absorption reduces the transepithelial voltage and would be expected to decrease passive Ca absorption. Furosemide, bumetanide, and ethacrynic acid, which block sodium transport in the TAL of the loop of Henle, also block Ca transport. The tight junction of the TAL has a specific permeability for Ca that participates in the voltage-dependent paracellular flux of the cation. This was proven by the discovery that mutations in the gene *PCLN1* which encodes for the protein Paracellin-1 (PCLN1), a member of the claudin family of epithelial tight junction proteins,[207] cause a syndrome of renal magnesium wasting, hypercalciuria, and nephrocalcinosis.[613]

Distal Convoluted Tubule, Connecting Tubule, and Collecting Tubule

Calcium transport in the distal convoluted tubule, connecting tubule, and collecting ducts is an active process. It occurs against an electrochemical gradient. The epithelium is considered "tight," meaning there is very little fluid or electrolyte flux through the paracellular route (Fig. 13).[395] Free flow micropuncture studies in the rat demonstrate that TF_{Ca2+}/UF_{Ca2+} falls from a value of 0.6 in the early PCT to 0.3 by the early portion of the cortical collecting duct. This is consistent with active transcellular calcium movement.

Active transcellular Ca^{2+} absorption in the distal convoluted tubule and connecting tubule is a three-step process. Ca^{2+} enters the cell across apical plasma membranes, diffuses across the cytosol bound to calcium binding proteins, and is actively extruded from the cell across basolateral membranes (Fig. 73.14). The mechanism of Ca^{2+} entry into the cells was defined with the expression cloning of the ECaC (now TRPV5) (Fig. 73.14).[270] Apical influx is considered the rate-limiting step in transcellular Ca transport and, therefore, the regulatory target of stimulatory and inhibitory hormones (Fig. 73.15).[201,634] Evidence suggests that hormonal stimuli of Ca^{2+} transport produce an insertion of Ca channels into the apical membrane (Fig. 73.15).[34,482,634] Furthermore, thiazide diuretics stimulate Ca^{2+} transport in this segment.[605,664] Thiazides produce their diuretic action by inhibiting a Na^+-Cl^- cotransport protein of the apical membrane.[138,605,664] How this is translated into a stimulation of Ca^{2+} transport was elucidated by Shimizu et al.[605] and Bordeau and Lau[83] (Fig. 73.16). In the presence of inhibited apical Na^+ entry, there is increased Na^+ flux into the cell across the basolateral membranes, which is coupled to Ca^{2+} extrusion, in other words actuation of a basolateral Na^+-Ca^{2+} exchanger. This nephron segment is also characterized by a hormonally regulated isoform of the Ca-ATPase, PMCA1b, found only in epithelia involved in active Ca^{2+} transport (Fig. 73.14).[79] In addition, the vitamin D–regulated calcium binding protein, calbindin-$_{28K}$, associated with Ca^{2+} transport is also localized in the distal tubule (Fig. 73.14).[78,395]

The apical Na-Cl cotransport, which is thiazide sensitive, appears mainly in the distal tubule (Figs. 73.16 and 73.17). In the connecting tubule and the collecting duct, Na^+ entry occurs through an apical, amiloride-sensitive Na^+ channel.[395,494,664] Amiloride also stimulates Ca^{2+} reabsorption in these segments. The mechanism appears to be, as for thiazides, a limitation of apical Na^+ entry stimulating basolateral Na^+ entry through a Na^+-Ca^{2+} exchange, activating Ca^{2+} efflux (Figs. 73.16 and 73.17).

Factors that Regulate Calcium Transport

Maneuvers such as administration of parathyroid hormone (PTH),[30,115,197,459,460] cAMP,[593] and calcitonin,[116,524] ECF volume expansion,[10,525] insulin administration,[153,154,526,527] and phosphate depletion[204,357,717] have all been shown to inhibit proximal tubular reabsorption of Ca and increase the delivery of Ca to the more distal nephron segments. The relationship of these maneuvers on urinary Ca excretion, however, may be a decrease, no change, or an increase in Ca excretion, emphasizing again the critical role of the distal tubule in the final regulation of Ca excretion. Both metabolic acidosis[652] and phosphate depletion[41,357,717] are accompanied by increased Ca excretion in the urine. Experimental studies in animals suggest that the "defect" in Ca reabsorption in metabolic acidosis[652] and phosphate depletion[717] is located in the distal tubule and probably through an effect on the TRPV5,[271] although phosphate depletion may also affect Ca transport in the proximal tubule. The administration of sodium bicarbonate, which rapidly corrects acidosis, increases Ca reabsorption in the late distal tubule. Similar

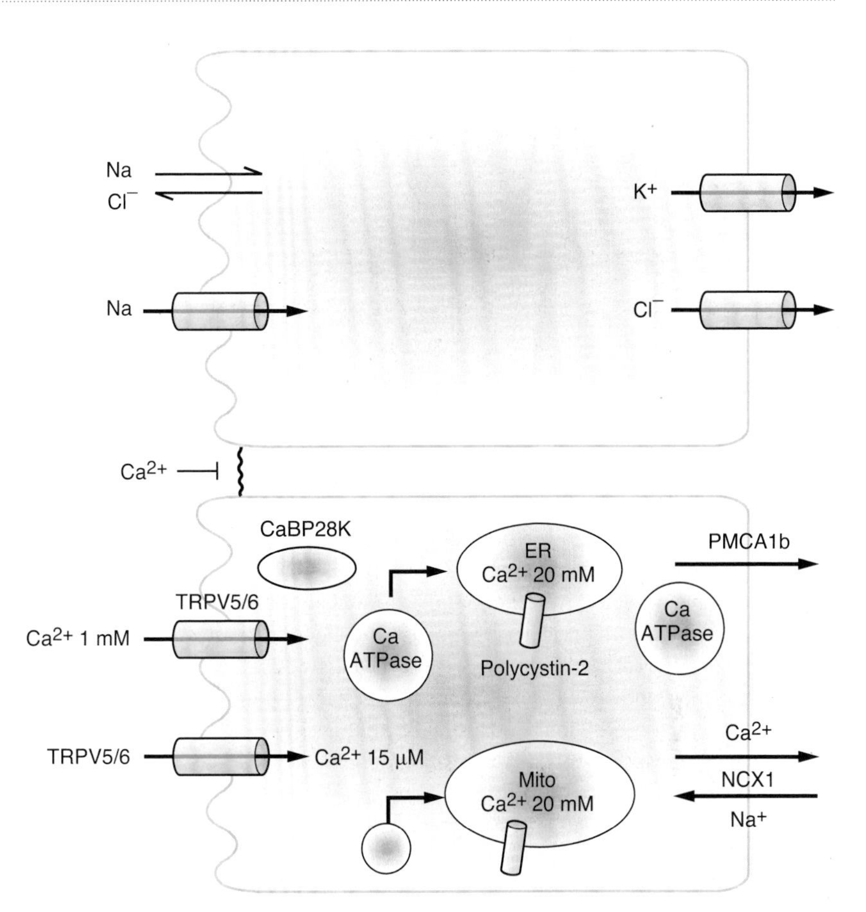

FIGURE 73.14 Calcium transport in distal convoluted tubule and connecting tubule. Transport mechanisms involved in transcellular Ca flux are depicted in the lower cell, whereas other transport proteins whose actions impinge on Ca absorption (apical NaCl cotransport, Na channels, basolateral chloride channels, and basolateral potassium channels) are shown in the top cell. There is no paracellular flux. The apical NaCl cotransport is inhibited by thiazide diuretics whose action in Ca transport is thought to be a limitation of Na availability leading to increased activity in the basolateral Na/Ca exchange, NCX1, causing increased Ca efflux. Likewise, the epithelial Na channel is inhibited by amiloride diuretics whose action also stimulates Ca transport similar to thiazide diuretics. Ca entry is facilitated by the apical epithelial Ca channel TRPV6/5 which assembles as homo- or heterotetramers. Subsequently, the ion binds to CABP28K and may be delivered to the endoplasmic reticulum. The ER may come into close association with PMCA1b resulting in delivery of Ca to the efflux pathways.

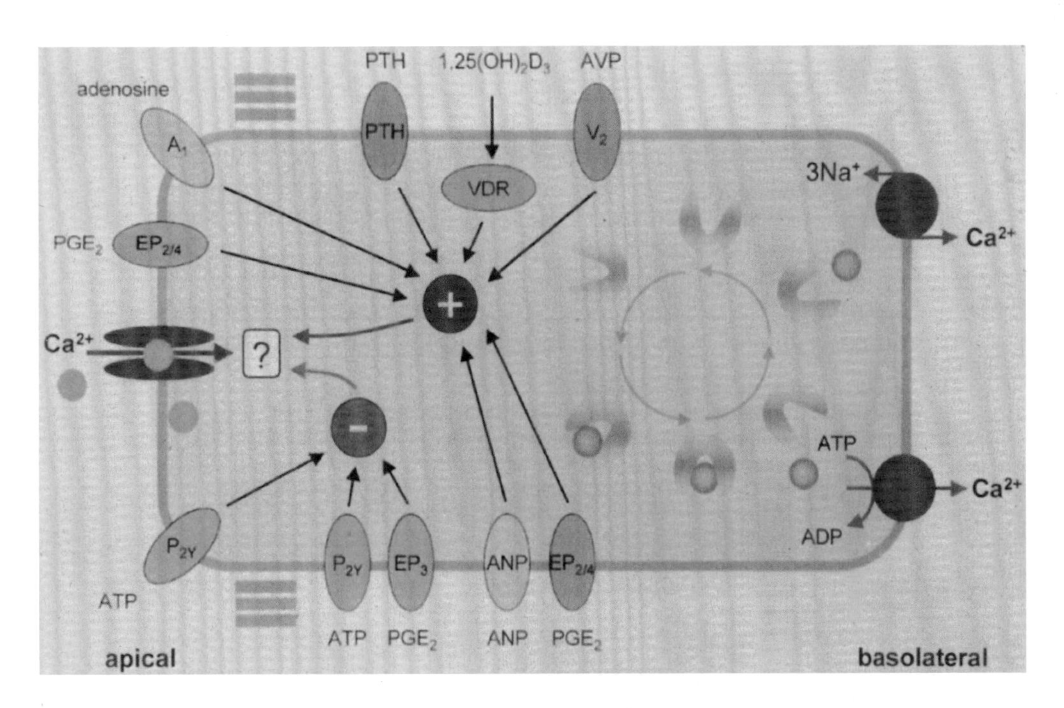

FIGURE 73.15 Schematic model for hormonal regulation of transcellular Ca^{2+} transport in distal nephron. Parathyroid hormone (PTH), V_2, atrial natriuretic peptide (ANP), and EP_3 receptors are localized in the basolateral membrane, whereas A_1 is present in the apical membrane. $EP_{2/4}$ and P_{2Y} are present in both membranes. 1,25-dihydroxycholecalciferol passes plasma membranes and binds to the intracellular vitamin D receptor (VDR). Hormones can be divided into stimulatory hormones, including PTH, arginine vasopressin, ANP, prostaglandin E_2 (PGE_2) (via $EP_{2/4}$), and adenosine, and inhibitory hormones such as adenosine triphosphate and PGE_2 (via EP_3). (From Hoenderop JG, Willems PH, Bindels RJ. Toward a comprehensive molecular model of active calcium reabsorption. *Am J Physiol Renal.* 2000;278:F352, with permission.)

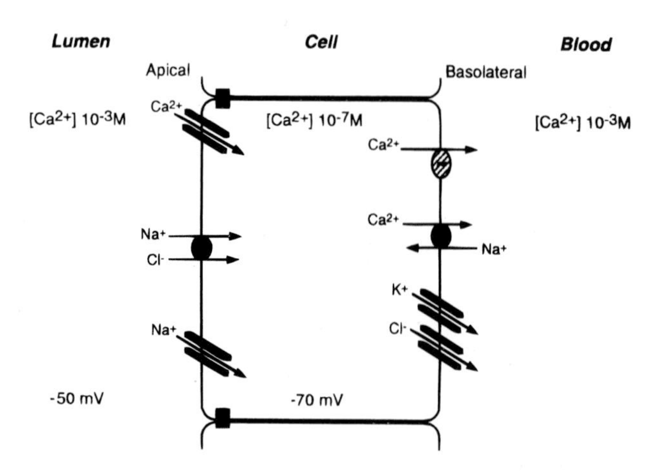

FIGURE 73.16 Model of Ca^{2+} transport in distal convoluted tubule, connecting tubule, and cortical collecting duct cells. Transport mechanisms involved in apical Ca^{2+} entry (channels) and basolateral efflux (Ca^{2+}-ATPase and Na^{+}-Ca^{2+} exchange) are depicted. Other transport proteins whose action impinges on Ca^{2+} absorption (apical Na^{+}-Cl cotransport, Na^{+} channels, basolateral Cl channels, and basolateral K^{+} channels) are shown. The apical Na^{+}-Cl cotransport is inhibited by thiazide diuretics whose action on Ca^{2+} transport is thought to be a limitation of Na^{+} availability leading to increased activity of the basolateral Na^{+}-Ca^{2+} exchange causing increased Ca^{2+} efflux. This would assume basal activity of Ca^{2+} channel activity. The dependency of the thiazide effect on the presence of parathyroid hormone (PTH) would be expected because PTH stimulates insertion of Ca^{2+} channels into the apical membrane. (From Friedman P, Gesek F. Calcium transport in renal epithelial cells. *Am J Physiol.* 1993;264:F181.)

results are found when phosphate is given to an animal that has been previously phosphate depleted.

PTH plays an important role in the regulation of Ca transport and reduces urinary Ca excretion (Fig. 73.15). In humans, the status of the parathyroid gland greatly influences the amount of Ca excreted in the urine. At equal filtered loads of Ca, patients with high levels of circulating PTH have less Ca in the urine than those in whom the levels of PTH in serum are low. Experimental evidence indicates the main effect of PTH is in the distal tubule and connecting tubule[30,197,605–607] and is mediated through the adenylate cyclase system. Although PTH inhibits proximal tubular reabsorption of Na and Ca, the main action of PTH is localized in more distal segments of the nephron.

Studies in rabbits have shown a PTH-sensitive Ca transport mechanism in the cortical TAL.[459,460] Little is known about how PTH affects the paracellular pathway for Na^{+} and Ca^{2+} reabsorption of the PCT. Studies in isolated renal cortical BBM vesicles indicate that PTH mimics the effect of membrane phosphorylation on Ca binding and translocation.[320,634] Phosphorylation of BBM vesicles produces an increase in membrane-bound Ca due to production of negatively charged phospholipids.[282] Aminoglycosides compete for the binding of Ca to phospholipids. In the presence of a chemical potential for Ca, PTH also stimulates Ca binding that is aminoglycoside inhibitable, as well as an increase in the BBM content of the acidic phospholipids produced by phosphorylation.[282] The control of Ca efflux across the basolateral membrane of the PCT by PTH involves the Na^{+}-Ca^{2+}

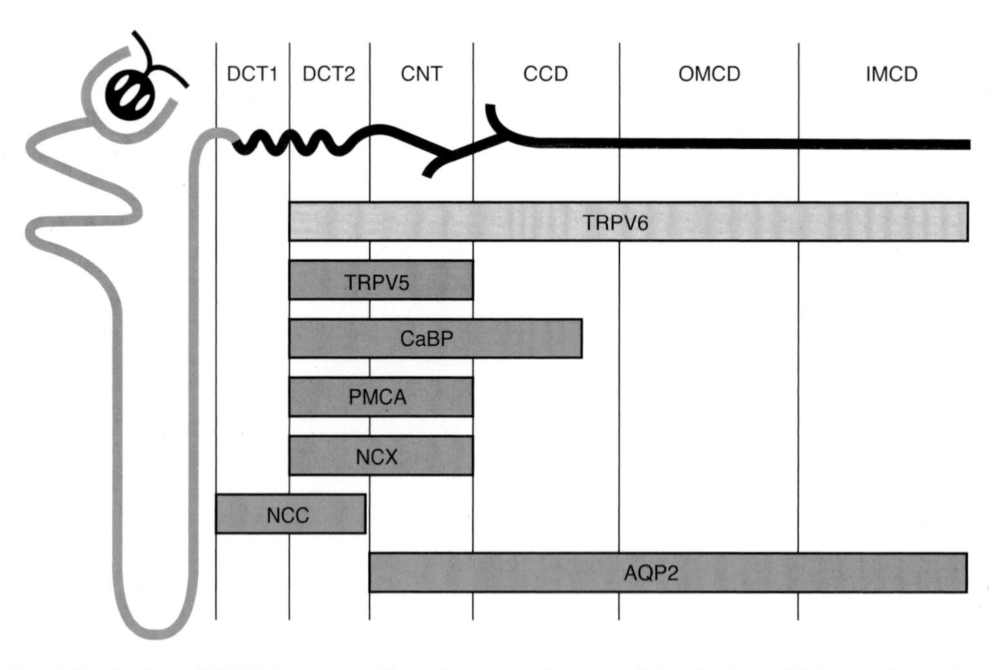

FIGURE 73.17 Renal distribution of TRPV6 in mouse kidney. Summary of the renal distribution of TRPV6 as determined by immunohistochemistry. *DCT*, distal convoluted tubule; *CNT*, connecting tubule; *CCD*, cortical collecting duct; *OMCD*, outer medullary collecting duct; *IMCD*, inner medullary collecting duct; *PMCA*, plasma membrane Ca^{2+}-ATPase; *NCX*, Na^{+}/Ca^{2+} exchanger; *NCC*, Na^{+}-Cl^{-} cotransporter; *AQP2*, aquaporin-2. (From Nijenhuis T, Hoenderop JG, vander Kamp AW, et al. Localization and regulation of the epithelial Ca^{2+} channel TRPV6 in the kidney. *J Am Soc Nephrol.* 2003;14:2731, with permission.)

exchange. Scoble et al.[583] and Jayakumar et al.[302] demonstrated sodium gradient (outside > inside) dependent on Ca efflux stimulated by PTH in basolateral membrane vesicles from dog and rat renal cortex. These studies were thought to use membranes from the proximal tubule. However, more recent studies suggested that the Na^+-Ca^{2+} exchange activity is the highest in the distal tubule and the earlier studies may have been affected by contaminants from these segments.[541]

PTH stimulation of Ca^{2+} transport in the TAL of the loop of Henle is localized to the cortical portion, whereas the calcitonin effect is exerted in the medullary portion. Because PTH does not stimulate Na^+ or Cl^- transport, it is unlikely that it works to increase the lumen-positive transepithelial electrical driving force. Rather, its main action has been suggested to be at the level of the permeability to Ca^{2+} of the paracellular pathway[80,82] and to be related to the function of paracellin-1 (PCLN1), also referred to as claudin-16, the tight junction Ca/Mg permeability factor. Recent thought indicates that an effect on transcellular transport may be involved.[197,200]

Significant progress has been made in the understanding of PTH actions on Ca^{2+} transport in the connecting tubule and the cortical collecting duct. Here, Ca^{2+} reabsorption is transcellular and an active energy consuming process. Studies[30,197,200,214] suggest that PTH hyperpolarizes the epithelium and produces insertion of voltage-operated Ca^{2+} channels in the apical membrane.[34,200] Patch clamp studies of PTH-stimulated distal convoluted tubule cells[200,215,538,540] demonstrated an increase in open time of apical membrane channels with increasing membrane voltage.[652] However, these findings remain controversial,[200,214,215] and the mechanism of anomalous function of the apical Ca entry channel remains to be elucidated. Voltage-operated epithelial Ca channels are complex heterotetramers consisting of TRPV5 and TRPV6 subunits (Fig. 73.16).[269] Identification of the distal nephron Ca entry channel, TRPV5 (Fig. 73.14),[268,270,271] which is insensitive to membrane potential, failed to shed light on the mechanism of Ca entry associated with hyperpolarization,[728] and although the discovery of heterotetramers may explain the divergent electrophysiologic results,[269] other Ca entry mechanisms probably await discovery.

Hypocalcemia

Hypocalcemia decreases the renal excretion of Ca, secondary to a decrease in the filtered load of Ca and enhanced tubular reabsorption of Ca. Hypocalcemia triggers the release of PTH, which increases Ca reabsorption in the TAL and distal tubule. The effects on the TAL could also be observed in the TPTX setting.[529] Recent studies have indicated that the Ca sensor receptor (CaSR) inactivation plays an important role in the enhancement of Ca transport in the TAL during hypocalcemia.[30,97,260]

Hypercalcemia

In general, patients with hypercalcemia have increased amounts of v in the urine, partly due to an increase in the filtered load of Ca and partly to suppression of PTH secretion. Activation of the CaSR also may increase the excretion of Ca by decreasing the activity of the apical K^+ channel and decreasing the positive potential difference (PD). Thus, less Ca and Mg are reabsorbed via the paracellular pathway in the TAL.[30,97]

Volume Status

Volume contraction decreases and volume expansion increases the renal excretion of Na and Ca. Volume expansion decreases tubular reabsorption of both Na and Ca even if the filtered load is reduced,[431] clearly demonstrating that the regulation of these ions is primarily by changes in tubular reabsorption.

Diuretics

Furosemide produces a significant increase in Na^+ and Ca^{2+} excretion by inhibiting the reabsorption of both ions in the TAL.[179] Furosemide decreases the PD in the TAL. Because the reabsorption of Ca in this segment of the nephron is passive, a decrease in the positive voltage of the lumen diminishes the movement of Ca through the paracellular pathway. Thiazide, on the other hand, produces dissociation between Na and Ca excretion. A mild natriuresis is usually accompanied by a decrease in Ca excretion. Micropuncture studies have shown that this mechanism occurs in the distal portion of the nephron. Thiazide stimulates Ca entry through the apical Ca^{2+} channel by activating Cl channels (Fig. 73.13).[213] These effects are independent of PTH, although PTH is important for the presence of TRPV5 in the apical membrane of the connecting tubule. The chronic administration of thiazide produces significant decrease in Ca excretion secondary to volume contraction, because this effect can be reversed by the administration of NaCl.

Vitamin D

The acute administration of 1,25-dihydroxycholecalciferol increases renal transepithelial Ca transport by its effects on the distal, connecting, and collecting duct system. In these segments of the nephron, the transport of Ca is mainly active. 1,25-Dihydroxycholecalciferol has a positive transcriptional effect on TRPV5 gene transcription. In addition, an increase in calbindin-28K and on the Ca ATPase in the basolateral side of the cell is also transcriptionally regulated by 1,25-dihydroxycholecalciferol (Fig. 73.15).[271]

The chronic administration of 1,25-dihydroxycholecalciferol increases the excretion of Ca secondary to an increase in the filtered load of Ca. This is due to an increase in Ca absorption in the gut and Ca resorption in the skeleton.

Clinical Effects of Plasma Calcium Concentrations

Hypocalcemia

The clinical manifestations of hypocalcemia vary greatly among patients.[581] Patients who suddenly become hypocalcemic, such as those with postsurgical hypoparathyroidism, may develop profound symptomatology, including tetany, even after a moderate decrease in serum Ca levels. On the other hand, patients with chronic renal insufficiency adjust well to low levels of serum Ca and seldom become symptomatic. Before the pathophysiologic mechanisms responsible for the hypocalcemia can be correlated with the clinical symptomatology, it is critical to determine whether both total and ionized Ca levels are low. In conditions such as the nephrotic syndrome and cirrhosis with severe hypoalbuminemia, total serum Ca may be decreased, but ionized Ca levels may be within the normal range or only slightly decreased, and the patient remains asymptomatic.

Clinical Symptoms

Patients with significant hypocalcemia have increased neuromuscular irritability.[411] The hallmark of hypocalcemia is tetany. Latent tetany may be detected by tapping over the facial nerves, which results in contraction of the facial muscles (Chvostek's sign), or by occluding the arterial blood supply to the forearm, which produces carpal spasm (Trousseau's sign). The symptomatology depends on the rapidity of onset of hypocalcemia. Patients with chronic renal failure occasionally have marked hypocalcemia; however, tetany is extremely rare. This may be due in part to the presence of metabolic acidosis. However, the changes in ionized Ca produced by metabolic acidosis in the majority of patients with profound hypocalcemia are not sufficient to bring the ionized Ca level back to normal. On the other hand, respiratory alkalosis due to hyperventilation can precipitate tetany. Clinically, the patient may complain of tingling in the tips of the fingers, stiff muscles, and cramps and may develop convulsions or impaired mental function. Children may develop mental retardation, and dementia may occur in adults. Extrapyramidal disorders also have been found in some patients. Psychiatric manifestations are characterized by confusion and hallucinations. Proximal muscle weakness is more frequently seen when the hypocalcemia is secondary to vitamin D deficiency.

Severe complications of hypocalcemia include development of cataracts,[293] papilledema, and rarely, optic neuritis. In general, the skin may be dry and puffy, and the patient may develop dermatitis. Hypocalcemia may produce hypotension and a delay in ventricular repolarization, thus increasing the QT interval and ST segment. Ventricular arrhythmias and atrial fibrillation refractory to digoxin[126] have been seen in patients with hypocalcemia. Because Ca, as mentioned previously, has an inotropic effect, hypocalcemia may be responsible in part for a decrease in cardiac output.[100,135,216]

The pathogenetic mechanisms responsible for the development of hypocalcemia are described in Table 73.6 and include: (1) absence of PTH; (2) decreased Ca mobilization from bone; (3) reduced Ca absorption in the gastrointestinal tract; (4) translocation of Ca between different compartments of the body; and (5) miscellaneous conditions.

TABLE 73.6 Causes of Hypocalcemia

I. Hypocalcemia secondary to low or absent levels of parathyroid hormone in blood
   A. Hypoparathyroidism
      1. Congenital
      2. Idiopathic
      3. DiGeorge syndrome
      4. Postsurgical
      5. Infiltration of parathyroid glands by malignancy or amyloidosis
   B. Transient hypoparathyroidism
      1. Neonatal
      2. Postsurgical (for parathyroid adenoma)
II. Hypocalcemia secondary to a decrease in calcium mobilization from bone
   A. Vitamin D deficiency
      1. Decreased ingestion
      2. Decreased absorption (gastrointestinal disorders)
         a. Partial gastrectomy
         b. Intestinal bypass
         c. Sprue
         d. Pancreatic insufficiency
   B. $25(OH)D_3$ deficiency
      1. Severe liver disease
         a. Biliary cirrhosis
         b. Amyloidosis
      2. Ingestion of anticonvulsant medication
      3. Nephrotic syndrome
   C. $1,25(OH)_2D_3$ deficiency
      1. Advanced renal failure
      2. Severe hyperphosphatemia
      3. Hypoparathyroidism
   D. Pseudohypoparathyroidism types I and II
   E. Magnesium deficiency
III. Hypocalcemia secondary to reduced calcium absorption in the gastrointestinal tract
   A. Deficiency of vitamin D or its metabolites
IV. Hypocalcemia secondary to translocation of calcium into different compartments
   A. Hyperphosphatemia
   B. Administration of citrate
   C. Administration of ethylenediaminetetraacetic acid
   D. Urinary excretion
V. Miscellaneous conditions
   A. Ca receptor gene mutations
   B. Pancreatitis
   C. Colchicine intoxication
   D. Pharmacologic dose of calcitonin
   E. Administration of mithramycin
   F. "Hungry bone" syndrome

From Slatopolsky E. Pathophysiology of calcium, magnesium, and phosphorus. In: Klahr S, ed. *The Kidney and Body Fluids in Health and Disease.* New York: Plenum Press; 1983:269, with permission.

Hypocalcemia Secondary to Low or Absent Levels of Parathyroid Hormone in Blood

A decrease or absence of PTH will have significant effects on Ca metabolism.[373,475,597] Because PTH plays a key role in the regulation of osteoclasts, which are the cells responsible for bone resorption, through the production of RANKL, a decrease in the activity or in the number of osteoclasts will eventually reduce the efflux of Ca from bone. In the absence of PTH, the capacity of the ascending portion of the loop of Henle and distal nephron to transport Ca is decreased; thus, at any filtered load of Ca, a greater amount of Ca will be excreted in the urine. Moreover, the absence of PTH decreases the activity of 1α-hydroxylase in the kidney and leads to decreased formation of 1,25-dihydroxycholecalciferol and a reduction in Ca absorption from the GI tract. Thus, decreased mobilization of Ca from bone, excretion of larger amounts of Ca in the urine, and decreased absorption of Ca from the gut lead to profound hypocalcemia. The most common cause of hypoparathyroidism is excision or damage to the parathyroid glands at surgery. This may be secondary to thyroid or parathyroid surgery or to radical neck dissection performed for the treatment of cancer.[149,575] Some patients might develop transient hypocalcemia. This phenomenon is observed in patients who have one adenoma of the parathyroid gland. The hypercalcemia produced by the excessive secretion of PTH by the adenoma usually suppresses secretion from the other glands, and the removal of the adenoma may produce a transient period of hypoparathyroidism and hypocalcemia. However, the remaining glands, if they are intact, will respond to the hypocalcemia, and this abnormality will be reversible in a relatively short period of time.

Idiopathic hypoparathyroidism is a rare disease, and tetany may occur soon after birth. Idiopathic hypoparathyroidism may be associated with congenital absence of the thymus (DiGeorge syndrome).[161,323,451] These patients have depressed cell immunity and many other malformations; they frequently have mucosal candidiasis and usually die in early childhood of severe hypocalcemia or severe infections.[323] The parathyroid gland may be transiently suppressed at birth as a result of maternal hypercalcemia; thus, neonatal tetany should be looked for in the presence of hypercalcemia of any cause in the mother. The fetal parathyroid glands are suppressed by maternal hypercalcemia and when the hypocalcemic infant is stressed—for example, with a phosphate load (cow's milk)—tetany may result. Another factor that plays a key role in the secretion of PTH is magnesium.[21,118,365,566,649] As will be discussed in a subsequent section, profound hypomagnesemia may decrease the release of PTH. In this syndrome, administration of magnesium to correct the hypomagnesemia increases the release of PTH within minutes.

Hypocalcemia Secondary to Decreased Calcium Mobilization from Bone

Vitamin D has a synergistic effect with PTH that increases the mobilization of calcium from bone. The mechanism by which vitamin D and its metabolites increase bone resorption is not fully understood. Both hormones are key factors in the differentiation of osteoclasts,[642,695] and both factors regulate the osteoblast through differentiation of osteoblast precursors and direct regulation of bone matrix protein gene transcription.[642,695] Many disorders can alter the metabolism of vitamin D, and different vitamin D metabolites could be responsible for decreased mobilization of Ca from bone. In vitamin D–deficient rickets, a nutritional condition observed in children, the lack of vitamin D is responsible for hypocalcemia, hypophosphatemia, and mild secondary hyperparathyroidism.[112,496] Disorders of the GI tract such as partial gastrectomy, intestinal bypass, tropical and nontropical sprue, and Crohn disease may impair the absorption of vitamin D from the diet. Pathologic processes that involve the liver, such as hepatobiliary cirrhosis, may decrease the production of 25-hydroxycholecalciferol.[77] The lack of this metabolite greatly diminishes the mineralization front, and adults with low levels of 25-hydroxycholecalciferol may develop osteomalacia. Although there may be an increase in the level of PTH, osteoclasts are unable to remove Ca because the osteoid material lacks minerals; therefore, there is decreased mobilization of Ca from bone. Administration of anticonvulsant medication may also result in low serum levels of 25-hydroxycholecalciferol, possibly due to the enhanced microsomal activity in the liver with increased catabolism of 25-hydroxycholecalciferol.[129,249,610]

Chronic Renal Failure/1,25(OH)$_2$D$_3$ Deficiency

Chronic renal failure is characterized by moderate hypocalcemia. Serum calcium seldom falls to less than 7.0 mg per dL. The pathogenesis of hypocalcemia in chronic renal failure is multifactorial. However, phosphate retention and low levels of 1,25-dihydroxycholecalciferol play a key role in its genesis.[128] In patients with profound hypomagnesemia, the skeleton becomes resistant to the action of PTH, and there is decreased Ca mobilization from bone.[365,566]

Pseudohypoparathyroidism

Another important condition causing hypocalcemia is PHP, which is a genetic disorder characterized by skeletal and somatic defects including short stature, rounded face, brachydactyly, subcutaneous calcification, and subnormal intelligence.[15,152,391,423] The secretion of PTH is increased as assessed by elevated levels of immunoreactive PTH; thus, the hypocalcemia in PHP is felt to represent a bone resistance to the effects of PTH.[355,703] This syndrome is collectively referred to as Albright hereditary osteodystrophy (AHO).[376,424] Many patients also have renal resistance to the action of the hormone because administration of exogenous PTH does not lead to increased urinary excretion of cAMP and phosphate. The syndrome has been subclassified as PHP type Ia (PHP-Ia), in which there is neither a cAMP nor a phosphaturic response to exogenous PTH. Maternally inherited mutations in one of the 13 GNAS exons encoding $G_{S\alpha}$ cause PHP-Ia.[355,375,505] The mRNA for G_S is also reduced about 50% in these patients.[505] Heterozygous mutations of the $G_{S\alpha}$ gene have been identified in families of subjects with AHO, providing molecular confirmation that transmission of the $G_{S\alpha}$ gene defects accounts for the autosomal-dominant inheritance of AHO.[453,702] When the same $G_{S\alpha}$ mutations are inherited paternally, affected individuals develop AHO in the absence of hormone resistance, and this condition is referred to as pseudopseudohypoparathyroidism (PPH).[355] Thus, the development of hormone resistance in a patient with a $G_{S\alpha}$ mutation is subject to paternal imprinting; that is, it develops only after maternal transmission.[355,573,703] Genomic imprinting is a process by which specific genes undergo allele-specific epigenetic changes that lead to allele-specific differences in gene expression. One or more of the epigenetic changes is established in the male or female germline during gametogenesis. Often, imprinting is associated with allele-specific differences in DNA methylation at CpG dinucleotides during gametogenesis and maintained throughout development. Imprinting may be incomplete, as in tissue specific, as is the case for GNAS. $G_{S\alpha}$ is biallelically expressed in most tissues, but in the renal proximal tubule and some endocrine organs, it is expressed primarily from the maternal allele. As a result of this tissue-specific imprinting, patients who inherit $G_{S\alpha}$ null mutations from their mother develop multihormone resistance of PHP-1a.[573]

Some subjects with PHP type I lack features of AHO. Patients with this subtype, termed PHP type Ib (PHP-Ib), typically show hormone resistance that is limited to PTH target organs and have normal $G_{S\alpha}$ activity.[374] This variant has been genetically linked to the GNAS locus on chromosome 20q13-3, and the pattern of inheritance indicates paternal imprinting (maternal transmission). Furthermore, affected individuals with autosomal dominant PHP-Ib show loss of GNAS exon A/B methylation and a heterozygous ~3 kb microdeletion located within STX1b approximately 220kb centromeric of GNAS exon A/B.[355] Hormone resistance in PHP-Ib is limited to the PTH dependent actions in the renal proximal tubule and a few other tissues in which $G_{S\alpha}$ is paternally imprinted such as the thyroid.[355]

PHP type II, in which there is no phosphaturia despite a normal cAMP excretion rate in response to PTH,[117,169,274,325,483,553] is a heterogeneous disorder. Some of these patients have low levels of 1,25-dihydroxycholecalciferol, perhaps representing renal resistance to PTH-stimulated 1α-hydroxylase activity. Thus, the high levels of PTH and the lack of response to the exogenous administration of PTH differentiate this syndrome from true hypoparathyroidism. The hyperphosphatemia that is present in this syndrome also may be partly responsible for the low levels of 1,25-dihydroxycholecalciferol. Thus, PHP is a heterogeneous disorder; some patients have resistance to PTH at the renal level only, others at the skeletal level, and still others in both organs.

Hypocalcemia Secondary to Reduced Intestinal Calcium Absorption

A healthy individual who ingests a low calcium diet usually does not develop hypocalcemia or develops it to a minimal degree because compensatory secondary hyperparathyroidism will correct mild hypocalcemia. Hypocalcemia is usually associated with pathologic processes of the GI tract that affect the absorption of vitamin D. Under these circumstances, the low absorption of calcium, plus abnormalities in vitamin D metabolism, greatly affects calcium homeostasis, and the patient may develop profound hypocalcemia. Growing animals fed a low calcium diet develop severe hypocalcemia.

Hypocalcemia Secondary to Translocation of Calcium into Different Compartments

Precipitation of ionized Ca is seen in disorders in which there is retention of phosphorus. Patients with advanced renal insufficiency, malignancies,[730] or severe rhabdomyolysis and hyperphosphatemia[335] may precipitate Ca rapidly and may develop symptoms characterized by tremors, muscular irritability, and tetany. In the neonate, administration of cow's milk, which is high in phosphorus content compared with human milk, may produce severe hyperphosphatemia and hypocalcemia. Neonatal parathyroid function is not adequate to cope with this challenge, and the neonate may develop severe symptoms secondary to hypocalcemia. When large amounts of blood containing citrate are given to patients (open heart surgery, exchange transfusions for neonatal hyperbilirubinemia), the ionized calcium is complexed by citrate and hypocalcemia leading to tetany may develop.

Hypocalcemia secondary to increased urinary excretion of Ca is rare and self-limited. The expansion of the ECF compartment produces a remarkable decrease in the reabsorption of Na and Ca, and large amounts of these cations may be excreted in the urine. However, these are transitory mechanisms that are rapidly corrected by the release of PTH. Thus, if the PTH, vitamin D, and skeletal axis are intact, an increase in urinary Ca excretion should not result in significant hypocalcemia. Diuretics such as furosemide or ethacrynic acid, which block the reabsorption of Ca in the thick ascending portion of the loop of Henle, are effective drugs in the treatment of hypercalcemia. However, very seldom do patients ingesting these drugs develop hypocalcemia.

Miscellaneous Conditions

Defects in the human CaSRs have been shown to cause familial hypocalciuria, hypercalcemia, and neonatal severe hyperparathyroidism.[127,507,511] Recently, Pollak et al.[513] demonstrated that a missense mutation (GLU128 Ala) in this gene causes familial hypocalcemia in affected membranes of one family. In this syndrome, an alteration in the CaSR shifts the "set point" for calcium to the left, and the parathyroid glands are hyperresponsive to extracellular Ca.

Approximately 10% to 20% of patients with acute pancreatitis develop some degree of hypocalcemia. The hypocalcemia is related to deposition of calcium salts in areas of lipolysis and tissue necrosis.[250] Some investigators have postulated that proteolytic digestion of PTH may explain the lack of elevated levels of PTH in the serum of patients with acute pancreatitis.

Some drugs such as calcitonin, mithramycin (used for testicular carcinoma), and colchicine (used in gout) can produce profound hypocalcemia by decreasing bone resorption. A series of disorders are characterized by increased bone formation in which the uptake of Ca by the skeleton is greatly increased. Such patients may develop profound hypocalcemia. A disorder known as "hungry bone syndrome" is seen in patients with chronic renal insufficiency and severe secondary hyperparathyroidism. The removal of the parathyroid glands in these uremic patients produces profound hypocalcemia, which sometimes is difficult to correct even with pharmacologic doses of 1,25-dihydroxycholecalciferol. Under these conditions, when the factors producing bone resorption have been removed and the osteoblastic activity is greatly increased, there is a remarkable flux of Ca into bone due to bone formation. The great uptake of minerals by the skeleton may produce profound hypocalcemia.

Hypercalcemia

Hypercalcemia is an elevation of total serum Ca levels to more than 10.5 mg per dL (when serum protein values are within the normal range). The manifestations of hypercalcemia differ among patients.[94] Mild hypercalcemia may be totally asymptomatic and may be detected during routine blood chemistry tests; however, hypercalcemia may be severe enough to produce lethargy, disorientation, coma, and death.

Clinical Symptoms of Hypercalcemia

Patients with mild hypercalcemia may be totally asymptomatic[66]; however, as serum Ca increases, usually to more than 11.5 mg per dL, numerous symptoms may be present and practically every organ of the body is affected. The most common symptoms are nausea, vomiting, polyuria, polydipsia, lack of concentration, fatigue, somnolence, mental confusion, and even death (Table 73.7).

TABLE 73.7 Clinical Manifestations of Hypercalcemia

I. General: apathy, lethargy, weakness
II. Cardiovascular: cardiac arrhythmias, hypertension, vascular calcification
III. Renal: polyuria, hypercalciuria, stones, nephrocalcinosis-impaired concentration of urine renal insufficiency
IV. Gastrointestinal: anorexia, nausea, vomiting, polydipsia, constipation, abdominal pain, gastric ulcer, pancreatitis
V. Neuropsychiatric and muscular: headache, impaired concentration, loss of memory, confusion, hallucination, coma, myalgia, muscle weakness, arthralgia
VI. Heterotopic calcification: band keratopathy, conjunctival irritation, vascular calcification, periarticular calcification

From Slatopolsky E. Pathophysiology of calcium, magnesium, and phosphorus. In: Klahr S, ed. *The Kidney and Body Fluids in Health and Disease*. New York: Plenum Press; 1983:269, with permission.

Renal Effects

Hypercalcemia may cause either an acute and reversible decrement in the GFR or a chronic nephropathy. There are numerous mechanisms by which hypercalcemia decreases the GFR.[287,377,515] Hypercalcemia may lead to vasoconstriction of the afferent arterioles and decreased renal blood flow. It can decrease ultrafiltration across glomerular capillaries. In addition, acute hypercalcemia may produce natriuresis and ECF volume contraction. In chronic hypercalcemic nephropathy, there is a fall in the GFR and a decrease in the maximum urinary concentrating capacity, and the urine is free of cells or casts, although mild proteinuria may be observed. The findings are similar to those seen in patients with interstitial nephritis. The characteristic abnormality of hypercalcemic nephropathy is an inability to concentrate the urine.[40,110,218] This abnormality persists even after the administration of antidiuretic hormone (ADH).[44] The mechanisms by which hypercalcemia impairs concentration of the urine are multiple.[241,422,650] The osmotic gradient of the medulla is decreased, partly because of decreased sodium transport in the thick ascending portion of the loop of Henle. Moreover, hypercalcemia decreases the permeability of the collecting duct to water by inhibiting the adenylate cyclase activity and generation of cAMP in response to ADH. There is some evidence to suggest that increased prostaglandin synthesis may mediate part of this effect. Prostaglandin E_2 (PGE_2) enhances medullary blood flow, inhibits sodium chloride transport in the loop of Henle, and antagonizes the effect of ADH on the collecting duct.[390] It is possible that several of the effects of hypercalcemia on the concentrating mechanism are related to increased prostaglandin synthesis in the medulla. Thus, a salt-wasting nephropathy and the inability to concentrate the urine may explain some of the symptoms such as polyuria and polydipsia seen in patients with hypercalcemia. Chronic persistent hypercalcemia eventually leads to the development of nephrocalcinosis, most commonly localized to the medulla of the kidney.

Gastrointestinal Manifestations

Anorexia, nausea, and vomiting are frequently seen in patients with hypercalcemia. Occasionally, abdominal pain, distention, and ileus may be present.[478] There is an increased incidence of peptic ulcer in patients with primary hyperparathyroidism, and it has been shown that Ca increases the release of gastrin and hydrochloric acid in the stomach. Moreover, the incidence of pancreatitis is also greatly increased. Several mechanisms have been implicated in the development of pancreatitis. Usually, hypercalcemia increases pancreatic enzyme secretion, and intraductal proteins may cause obstruction of the pancreatic duct. Enhanced conversion of trypsinogen to trypsin due to elevated Ca levels may contribute to the inflammatory process.

Cardiovascular Effects

Calcium has an inotropic effect on the cardiovascular system. Calcium increases peripheral resistance, and hypertension occurs in 20% to 30% of patients with chronic hypercalcemia.[51,131,418] Renal parenchymal damage with elevated levels of renin, increased cardiac output, and severe vasoconstriction may participate in the development of hypertension. The most significant change in the electrocardiogram is a shortening of the QT interval. Because the positive inotropic effect of digitalis is enhanced by Ca, digitalis toxicity may be aggravated by hypercalcemia.

Neurologic and Psychiatric Effects of Hypercalcemia

Patients with hypercalcemia are frequently admitted to psychiatric wards because of nonspecific complaints characterized by lethargy, apathy, depression, and decreased memory. Patients with hypercalcemia secondary to increased PTH levels have electroencephalographic changes that are reversible after removal of the parathyroid adenoma. Moreover, the administration of large doses of PTH to dogs results in increased brain Ca and changes in the electroencephalogram.[25]

Heterotopic Calcification

Patients with hypercalcemia may develop band keratopathy, which is the appearance of corneal calcification. The changes in the cornea are usually permanent. However, conjunctival irritation disappears after correction of the hypercalcemia. Arterial and periarticular calcifications are observed more frequently in patients who have some degree of renal insufficiency,[399] especially those who also have hyperphosphatemia. Vascular calcification has become a critical complication of chronic kidney disease.[120,123,141,398,539] Vascular calcification in CKD associated with the adynamic bone disorder is often associated with hypercalcemia.[147,148,399]

Hypercalcemia

Pathologically, three general mechanisms may lead to the development of hypercalcemia (Table 73.8): (1) increased mobilization of Ca from bone, by far the most common and important mechanism; (2) increased absorption of Ca from the GI tract; and (3) decreased urinary excretion of Ca (of minor importance). In some clinical disorders, although one

TABLE 73.8 **Causes Of Hypercalcemia**

I. Hypercalcemia secondary to increased calcium mobilization from bone
   A. Malignancy
      1. Metastatic
      2. Nonmetastatic
         a. Osteoclastic-activating factor
         b. Prostaglandin E_2
         c. Ectopic hyperparathyroidism
   B. Hyperparathyroidism
      1. Primary
         a. Adenoma
         b. Hyperplasia
         c. Neoplastic
      2. Secondary
      3. Multiple endocrine neoplasias
         a. Type I with pituitary and pancreatic tumors
         b. Type II with medullary carcinoma of thyroid and pheochromocytoma
   C. Immobilization
   D. Hyperthyroidism
   E. Vitamin D intoxication
   F. Renal disease
      1. Chronic renal failure
      2. After renal transplantation
      3. Diuretic phase of acute renal failure
   G. Vitamin A intoxication
II. Hypercalcemia secondary to an increase in calcium absorption from the gastrointestinal tract
   A. Sarcoidosis
   B. Vitamin D intoxication
   C. Milk-alkali syndrome
III. Hypercalcemia secondary to a decrease in urinary calcium excretion
   A. Thiazide diuretics
   B. Familial hypocalciuric hypercalcemia
IV. Miscellaneous
   A. Adrenal insufficiency
   B. Tuberculosis
   C. Berylliosis
   D. Dysproteinemias
   E. Hemoconcentration
   F. Hyperalimentation regimens

From Slatopolsky E. Pathophysiology of calcium, magnesium, and phosphorus. In: Klahr S. *The Kidney and Body Fluids in Health and Disease.* New York: Plenum Press; 1983:269, with permission.

or more of these mechanisms may be operative, compensatory adaptations develop and hypercalcemia may not occur. For example, in idiopathic hypercalciuria due to increased Ca absorption from the GI tract, increased urinary excretion of Ca may prevent the development of hypercalcemia. On the other hand, in hyperparathyroidism, all three mechanisms (increased bone resorption, augmented GI absorption of Ca, and decreased urinary calcium excretion) lead to the development of hypercalcemia.

Hypercalcemia Secondary to Increased Calcium Mobilization from Bone

Hypercalcemia Secondary to Malignancies/Humoral Hypercalcemia of Malignancy

Malignancy is the most common cause of hypercalcemia. Multiple mechanisms underlie the development of hypercalcemia of malignancy, but in general, it is due to a combined disorder of increased mobilization of Ca from the skeleton secondary to increased bone resorption by osteoclasts and variable decreases in the renal excretion of calcium.[74,644] This increased resorption could be due to the action of malignant cells that have metastasized to bone from tumors of such organs as the breast, prostate, kidney, lung, and thyroid.[644] The tumor cells in the bone metastasis produce RANKL and macrophage colony stimulating factor (MCSF) that stimulate production of active osteoclasts and local osteolysis. However, on some occasions, hypercalcemia occurs with no evidence of bone metastasis, and generally, the removal of the tumor results in correction of the hypercalcemia. In these cases, humoral agents are involved. The major humoral osteoclast-stimulating factor is PTH-related peptide (PTHrP).[238,644,720] This factor, which is a endochondral bone morphogen and an endogenous paracrine of the adult mammary glands, oviduct, fibroblasts, and vascular smooth muscle, has sufficient homology with PTH in its amino terminal region to act through PTH receptors on PTH target cells such as the osteoblast and the distal connecting tubule.[277,675,721] Thus, its production by tumors mimics the action of high PTH levels in stimulating bone resorption and renal Ca retention. PTHrP accounts for about 80% of the hypercalcemia associated with malignancies. Other mechanisms of hypercalcemia due to tumors include secretion of PGE_2,[29,145,299,326] especially by solid tumors, the production of TNFα, as in patients with multiple myeloma and lymphosarcoma,[470] and the secretion of IL-1 and TGFβ. The latter factors are often produced in association with PTHrP. TGFα works through epidermal growth factor receptors and stimulates bone resorption. Its production is highly prevalent (40%) in tumors associated with hypercalcemia, and it may play a secondary role in association with many cases in which PTHrP is being produced. In metastatic bone disease, there are usually two effects: (1) an increase in bone resorption and (2) an increase in woven bone formation. If the osteoblastic process (bone formation) predominates, hypercalcemia may not develop. However, if the osteolytic process predominates, the patient develops severe hypercalciuria and hypercalcemia. In contrast to tumors that produce a "parathyroid-like material," the serum phosphorus level or the tubular reabsorption of phosphate usually is not decreased in metastatic bone disease. However, the patient may develop hypophosphatemia when the disease progresses and malnutrition becomes evident. Although many tumors may secrete PTHrP (59 of 72 cases with hypercalcemia)[682] the two most important ones are the epidermoid squamous cell carcinoma of the lung and renal cell carcinoma. Rarely, patients with hypercalcemia of malignancy have elevated levels of circulating immunoreactive PTH.[644,682] Most often this is due to coexistent parathyroid disease and malignancy.[644,682]

Primary Hyperparathyroidism

Primary hyperparathyroidism is the most common endocrine disorder causing hypercalcemia.[65] It is probably the major cause of asymptomatic hypercalcemia in young people and older women. A single adenoma of the parathyroid gland is the most common cause of primary hyperparathyroidism. In contrast, chief cell hyperplasia is commonly observed in patients with secondary hyperparathyroidism caused by renal insufficiency. The incidence of primary hyperparathyroidism increases substantially in both men and women older than 50 years but is two to four times more common in women.[65] The mechanism of hypercalcemia is due to the action of PTH in the skeleton and kidney. The levels of PTH measurable by radioimmunoassay are elevated in primary hyperparathyroidism. The percentage of positive results to confirm the diagnosis depends on the type of antibody used and the sensitivity of each particular radioimmunoassay for PTH. Sensitive assays, using a carboxyterminal antibody, demonstrate elevated levels of PTH in 90% to 95% of patients with primary hyperparathyroidism, but these assays were sensitive to retention of fragments in kidney failure and have been replaced by assays measuring the intact hormone without loss of sensitivity.[65,671] As PTH increases the activity and number of osteoclasts, bone resorption is seen on bone histology. X-ray films of the phalanges show subperiosteal bone resorption. The increased Ca mobilization from bone raises the filtered load of Ca and leads to the development of hypercalciuria despite the effect of PTH in increasing the reabsorption of Ca in the distal nephron. Moreover, the hypercalcemia is aggravated by increased Ca absorption from the gut secondary to high levels of 1,25-dihydroxycholecalciferol in response to high levels of PTH in blood. PTH decreases the renal reabsorption of phosphorus in the proximal and distal tubules, resulting in hypophosphatemia. Patients with primary hyperparathyroidism have a high incidence of peptic ulcer, renal stones, soft tissue calcification, neuromuscular disease, and psychiatric disorders. Because hypercalcemia interferes with the renal countercurrent mechanism responsible for the concentration of the urine, the patient develops polyuria and polydipsia. The treatment of this condition is surgery (parathyroidectomy), except in mild cases of asymptomatic hypercalcemia (plasma calcium concentration of less than 11 mg per dL), especially in older adults.[66,506,645,705]

Immobilization

Patients who are immobilized for several days develop some degree of hypercalciuria. However, some of these patients may develop hypercalcemia.[51,631] This occurs in diseases involving increased bone turnover such as Paget disease. Hypercalcemia is seen frequently in immobilized patients with multiple fractures. It seems that prolonged periods of immobilization disrupt the balance between bone resorption and formation. The resorptive process predominates because of the depression of osteoblastic activity, and calcium mobilization occurs.

Hyperthyroidism

Serum Ca concentration may increase in thyrotoxicosis. Usually the increment is mild and does not produce severe symptoms. Bone histology reveals an increase in osteoclastic bone resorption and fibroblastic proliferation resembling osteitis fibrosa cystica. Moreover, patients with thyrotoxicosis who present with hypercalcemia usually have low or undetectable levels of PTH in blood.

Vitamin D Intoxication

Vitamin D increases both Ca absorption from the GI tract and bone resorption. Metabolites of vitamin D have been shown to increase the efflux of Ca from bone in vitro. Moreover, administration of 1,25-dihydroxycholecalciferol to dogs fed low Ca diets leads to hypercalcemia, suggesting that the effect on bone was responsible for the rise in extracellular Ca. The manifestations of vitamin D intoxication include high levels of 25-hydroxycholecalciferol in blood, whereas the circulating levels of 1,25-dihydroxycholecalciferol may remain within the normal range. Of course, if a patient receives pharmacologic doses of 1,25-dihydroxycholecalciferol, the hormonal derivative of vitamin D produces toxic effects and the characteristic hypercalcemia.

Renal Disease

Hypercalcemia is rare in patients with chronic kidney failure[620] prior to dialysis. Most patients with renal disease have hypocalcemia, which leads to the development of secondary hyperparathyroidism. Hypercalcemia in patients with end-stage kidney failure receiving treatment is commonly associated with the administration of vitamin D analogs and the adynamic bone disorder.[347] The mechanism of hypercalcemia is both intestinal resorption and excess bone resorption over formation.[280] Extreme hyperplasia of the parathyroid glands may also develop in these patients, and progress to a point at which they no longer respond to normal feedback mechanisms due to the development of clonal adenomatous change.[28] Thus, a greater degree of hypercalcemia may be necessary to suppress PTH secretion by such enlarged glands. In some patients, hypercalcemia may be seen after significant reductions of serum phosphorus levels or after ingestion of large amounts of Ca carbonate usually associated with vitamin D analog treatment.

A mineralization defect described in a substantial number of patients maintained on chronic hemodialysis[620,683] has been shown to be due to aluminum deposition in the interface between osteoid and mineralized bone is responsible for this defect. Many of these patients have mild hypercalcemia and relatively low levels of PTH. This finding has led to the elimination of aluminum from the chronic dialysis environment.

Hypercalcemia occurs more frequently after a successful renal transplantation than in patients with chronic renal insufficiency.[620] Because patients receiving kidney transplants usually have severe secondary hyperparathyroidism, the amount of 1,25-dihydroxycholecalciferol produced by the new kidney, if the graft is successful, is greatly increased due to both high levels of PTH and decreased serum phosphate levels due to the marked phosphaturia after the transplantation. Synergistically, 1,25-dihydroxycholecalciferol and PTH would increase calcium mobilization from bone, leading to hypercalcemia. Obviously, 1,25-dihydroxycholecalciferol also increases Ca absorption from the GI tract. In most patients, the hypercalcemia does not require specific treatment and subsides after 3 to 4 weeks. However, in some patients, specific measures should be taken to prevent nephrocalcinosis, and if the hypercalcemia is severe and persists for several months or years, the patient may require surgical parathyroidectomy.

Vitamin A Intoxication

This is a very rare cause of hypercalcemia and is seen more frequently in children than adults.[132,308,316]

Hypercalcemia Secondary to Increased Calcium Absorption from the Gastrointestinal Tract

There are several clinical entities such as sarcoidosis, vitamin D intoxication, and milk alkali syndrome that are characterized by increased Ca absorption from the gut and positive Ca balance. Some patients also have widespread soft tissue calcification and nephrocalcinosis. Most of these patients have low or undetectable levels of PTH.

Sarcoidosis

About 10% to 20% of patients with sarcoidosis have mild hypercalcemia.[437] This abnormality is secondary to an increase in Ca absorption, and the mechanism responsible for the increased Ca absorption is unregulated production of calcitriol in macrophages of the sarcoid lesions. Serum levels of 1,25-dihydroxycholecalciferol may be elevated in sarcoidosis, but this is not uniform.[38,46] Recent studies in an anephric patient with sarcoidosis with high levels of 1,25-dihydroxycholecalciferol[38] clearly indicate an extrarenal production of 1,25-dihydroxycholecalciferol in sarcoidosis. Adams et al.[7] first demonstrated that alveolar macrophages obtained by bronchial lavage from a patient with sarcoidosis and hypercalcemia converted 25-hydroxycholecalciferol to 1,25-dihydroxycholecalciferol. In general, patients with sarcoidosis are sensitive to small doses of vitamin D and exposure to ultraviolet radiation of the skin. The administration of corticosteroids in these patients decreases intestinal calcium absorption and corrects the hypercalcemia. Hypercalcemia also has been demonstrated in patients with histoplasmosis,[681] tuberculosis,[6] disseminated coccidioidomycosis,[361] and berylliosis,[646] all due to unregulated calcitriol production by macrophages associated with disease lesions.

Vitamin D Intoxication

Vitamin D and its metabolites, especially 1,25-dihydroxycholecalciferol, increase intestinal Ca absorption. Thus, high concentrations of vitamin D metabolites (mainly 25-hydroxycholecalciferol) in blood are responsible for the hypercalcemia observed in vitamin D intoxication. As described already, vitamin D metabolites may also have a direct effect on bone resorption, which contributes to the development of hypercalcemia.

Milk Alkali Syndrome

This syndrome was seen frequently in patients with peptic ulcer disease who ingested large amounts of Na and Ca bicarbonate.[444,491] Calcium carbonate contains 40% of elemental Ca. Some patients who ingested up to 20 g of Ca carbonate in 24 hours developed severe hypercalcemia. Moreover, alkalosis increases renal Ca reabsorption in the distal tubule and reduces bone turnover, thus decreasing Ca uptake by bone.

Hypercalcemia Secondary to Decreased Urinary Calcium Excretion

The decrease in urinary excretion of Ca may be secondary to a fall in the filtered load of Ca or to an increase in the tubular reabsorption of Ca. The fall in the filtered load of Ca may be secondary to a decrease in serum Ca level or the GFR. By definition, if the patient has a disorder that produces hypocalcemia with a decrease in urinary Ca excretion, he or she cannot be at the same time hypercalcemic; thus, such disorders can be excluded. A fall in the GFR may decrease Ca delivery to the distal tubule, and less Ca may be excreted in the urine. This situation, which may occur in profound dehydration, is self-limited and the hypercalcemia does not persist for a prolonged time. Moreover, dehydration or other conditions that decrease GFR may also modify the transport of Na and water and affect the reabsorption of Ca by the nephron.

Thiazide Diuretics

Patients taking thiazide diuretics may develop moderate hypercalcemia.[93,420,497,514] The mechanisms for the hypercalcemia are not fully understood, and a number of factors are involved. Thiazides decrease urinary excretion of Ca by increasing Ca resorption in the distal tubule. This reduction in urinary Ca seems to require some degree of ECF volume contraction and the presence of PTH, because patients with hypoparathyroidism do not greatly reduce the amount of Ca in the urine after the administration of thiazides. Thus, in patients with increased Ca mobilization from bone, the administration of thiazides may blunt the expected hypercalciuria and potentially raise serum Ca. However, thiazides also have a direct effect on the skeleton.[420] Administration of thiazides intravenously produces a mild change in ionized Ca. This effect is apparently potentiated by PTH because the effect is greater in patients with hyperparathyroidism than in healthy subjects.[514] Finally, there is controversy about whether thiazides per se increase the release of PTH. Most of the evidence indicates that this is not the case.

Familial Hypocalciuric Hypercalcemia and Neonatal Severe Hyperparathyroidism

Marx et al.[427,428] describe a syndrome characterized by hypocalciuria and mild hypercalcemia. Usually several members of the same family are affected. Familial hypocalciuric hypercalcemia is characterized by autosomal dominant transmission and generally follows a benign course. Some patients may have a mild degree of hyperparathyroidism; however, the hypercalcemia persists after subtotal parathyroidectomy. The main characteristic of this syndrome is a decrease in urinary Ca. Thus, the calcium:creatinine ratio provides an important diagnostic tool to differentiate familial hypocalciuric hypercalcemia from primary hyperparathyroidism. The development of hypercalcemia in young members of the family also favors this diagnosis. The pathogenesis of this syndrome is due to mutations in the Ca sensor of the parathyroid gland chief cells and the TAL/distal nephron epithelia or to autoantibodies.[96,493,548] As a result, these cells do not downregulate PTH secretion and Ca transport with the correct sensitivity to the plasma calcium. Mutations in the Ca sensor are also responsible for neonatal primary hyperparathyroidism. Two abnormal alleles for calcium sensor mutations produce the primary hyperparathyroidism, whereas single abnormal alleles produce familial hypocalciuric hypercalcemia.[512]

Treatment of Disorders of Calcium Metabolism

Hypocalcemia

The treatment of severe hypocalcemia and tetany is a medical emergency. Administration of Ca intravenously is mandatory to prevent severe complications and even death in these patients. If the patient has severe hypocalcemia and tetany in the absence of hypomagnesemia, the symptoms can be easily relieved by administration of 1 or 2 ampules of Ca gluconate given intravenously over 10 minutes (1 ampule of Ca gluconate has approximately 100 mg of elemental Ca). This initial treatment can be followed by administration of 1.0 g of elemental Ca dissolved in 500 mL of dextrose in water and given intravenously over 4 to 6 hours. If the condition responsible for the hypocalcemia cannot be corrected (e.g., hypoparathyroidism), a program for the chronic treatment of hypocalcemia should be instituted. The amount of Ca in the diet should be supplemented by 1 to 3 g of elemental Ca. Calcium carbonate has roughly 40% of elemental Ca; commercial preparations such as 3M Titralac or Os-Cal can be used in this situation. However, in many circumstances, administration of large amounts of Ca may not be sufficient to increase absorption by the intestine; therefore, different metabolites of vitamin D should be used. In chronic situations, 1,25-dihydroxycholecalciferol could be used. The dosage used ranges from 0.5 to 2 μg per 24 hours. Most patients eventually require 0.5 μg per day. If this metabolite of vitamin D is not available, vitamin D_2 or D_3, about 50,000 U three times a week, could be used instead. The dosage can be gradually increased up to 50,000 to 100,000 units daily. The serum Ca should be carefully monitored to prevent severe hypercalcemia, nephrocalcinosis, and potentially irreversible renal disease.

Hypercalcemia

A useful maneuver to correct hypercalcemia is to increase urinary Ca excretion (Table 73.9).[469] As discussed previously, only 1% to 2% of the filtered load of Ca is excreted by the kidney. This percentage can be greatly increased, and the kidney may thus become an excellent excretory organ for Ca. Because most patients with hypercalcemia develop dehydration and volume contraction with a consequent decrease in GFR, one of the first therapeutic maneuvers is the expansion of the ECF space. Expansion with saline requires several liters per day; therefore, it is mandatory that strict records be kept to maintain accurate determination of the intake and output of fluids. In most patients, it is convenient to determine the central venous pressure (CVP), which will allow volume expansion and prevent the potential risk of overexpansion and heart failure. Thus, after a CVP line is inserted, volume expansion with saline should be instituted until the venous pressure increases to 10 to 14 mm Hg. This maneuver alone will increase the GFR and decrease the reabsorption of Ca in the proximal tubule and in the ascending portion of the loop of Henle. Thus, fractional excretion of Ca will be greatly increased. This effect can be enhanced by administration of diuretics such as furosemide, bumetanide, or ethacrynic acid. The administration of 40 to 120 mg of furosemide every 4 hours is recommended in most patients. Using these maneuvers, fractional excretion of Ca can be increased to 10% of the filtered load. Thus, 1 g of Ca can be easily excreted in the urine in 24 hours. The administration of large amounts of saline and diuretics usually increases the excretion of potassium. To prevent arrhythmias, serum potassium should be maintained between 3.5 and 5.0 mEq per L. This can be achieved by adding 10 to 30 mEq of potassium to each liter of saline.

Although expansion of the ECF may control the hypercalcemia, this effect is temporary, and because in most circumstances, hypercalcemia is secondary to increased mobilization of Ca from bone, the physician may be forced to add a second line of medications to decrease the efflux of Ca from bone. In addition, many patients with hypercalcemia have renal failure and are not responsive to diuretics.

Bisphosphonates

A derivative of the bisphosphonates, disodium dichloroethylene diphosphonate,[618] was originally used with success on an experimental basis in patients with tumors and bone metastases and severe hypercalcemia.[616] Pamidronate, ibandronate, and zoledronic acid, second- and third-generation bisphosphonates, respectively, have become the standard of therapy for hypercalcemia of malignancy[39,49,71,239,576] and other causes of hypercalcemia requiring inhibition of bone resorption. One or two doses of 30 to 60 mg of pamidronate or a single dose of zoledronic acid intravenously are usually effective.[24] Potent bisphosphonates, including alendronate and risedronate, have become available and are effective as oral agents for hypercalcemia. Renal toxicity has to be considered when using these agents.[554]

Cinacalcet

Cinacalcet maintains long-term normocalcemia in patients with mild or asymptomatic primary hyperparathyroidism.[506] Cinacalcet is an orally bioavailable calcimimetic that increases the sensitivity of Ca sensing receptors to extracellular calcium. Cinacalcet in doses of 30 to 50 mg twice daily is sufficient to normalize serum Ca in hyperparathyroidism. Cinacalcet is also used in the treatment of secondary hyperparathyroidism seen in CKD.[457]

Calcitonin produces hypocalcemia by decreasing the activity of osteoclasts. The dose commonly used ranges from 2 to 5 MRC U per kg of body weight every 6 to 12 hours. The degree of hypocalcemia produced by this drug is mild, and the decrease is usually 1 to 3 mg per dL.[311] Calcitonin can be given either intramuscularly or intravenously in a concentration of 5 MRC U per kg dissolved in 500 mL of 5% dextrose in water to be given over 6 hours. Calcitonin is also available as a nasal spray. Unfortunately, in most patients, there is an escape from the hypocalcemic effect of calcitonin after 6 to 10 days of administration.

Miscellaneous Approaches

Mithramycin is an antibiotic originally introduced for the treatment of testicular tumors. Mithramycin blocks the activity of osteoclasts and may result in severe hypocalcemia.[615,617] It is usually given intravenously over 3 to 4 hours in a dose of 25 μg per kg of body weight dissolved in 500 mL of 5% dextrose in water or saline. Mithramycin is an effective drug. However, the effects may be seen only after 48 to 72 hours. One of the toxic effects of the drug is severe thrombocytopenia and bleeding. In general, the drug should not be given more than once every 4 or 5 days, and its use has been almost eliminated by development of effective, less toxic agents such as the bisphosphonates.[616]

TABLE 73.9 **Treatment of Hypercalcemia**

Agent	Dosage	Route of Administration	Effect	Mechanism of Action	Side Effects
I. Measures directed to enhance renal excretion of calcium					
Saline	1 to 3 L	IV	4 to 8 hours	GFR; tubular reabsorption of Ca	Heart failure, electrolyte imbalance
Furosemide	40 to 20 mg every 2 to 4 hours	IV	2 to 4 hours	Tubular reabsorption of Ca	Hypokalemia
II. Measures directed at decreasing bone resorption					
Bisphosphonates					
Paminodrate	60 to 90 mg	IV	24 to 72 hours	DBR effect on osteoclasts	Hypocalcemia, mandibular osteonecrosis
Alendronate	5 to 10 mg daily	PO	2 to 3 days	DBR effect on osteoclasts	Gastrointestinal disorders
Risedronate	30 mg daily	PO	2 to 3 days	DBR effect on osteoclasts	Gastrointestinal disorders
Zoledronic Acid	4 mg once/year	IV	24 to 72 hours	DBR effect on osteoclasts	Renal failure
Cinacalcet	15 to 30 mg daily	PO	24 to 72 hours	Decreases PTH levels	Hypocalcemia
Calcitonin	2 to 5 MRC/kg every 4 to 8 hours	IM	4 to 12 hours	DBR effect on osteoclasts	Allergic reaction, nausea, flushing
Mithramycin	25 μg/kg in 500 mL saline	IV	24 to 72 hours	DBR (marked)	Thrombocytopenia, bleeding
Indomethacin	75 mg q12h	PO	2 to 4 days	DBR secondary to prostaglandins	Gastrointestinal disorders
Aspirin	1 g q6h	PO	2 to 4 days	DBR secondary to prostaglandins	Gastrointestinal disorders, allergic
III. Measures directed to decrease calcium absorption in gastrointestinal tract					
Prednisone	20 to 30 mg q12h	PO	2 to 4 days	Decreased gastrointestinal absorption	Acute toxic steroid effects
IV. Measures directed to decrease serum calcium					
Hemodialysis	Low dialysate calcium		30 minutes	Direct removal from serum	

IV, intravenous; IM, intramuscular; PO, by mouth; MRC, Medical Research Council; DBR, decreased bone resorption; GFR, glomerular filtration rate; q, every.

There are rare tumors that produce prostaglandins that have resulted in the development of hypercalcemia. The use of aspirin in a dosage of 1 g four times daily or indomethacin 75 mg twice daily has ameliorated the hypercalcemia.[89,296,589]

If hypercalcemia is mainly due to increased absorption of Ca from the GI tract, such as in sarcoidosis, it is obviously important to decrease the amount of Ca in the diet and to administer corticosteroids, which will result in decreased absorption.[471,715] Usually prednisone (20 mg twice daily) has been effective in conditions such as sarcoidosis, which is characterized by increased 1,25-dihydroxycholecalciferol production by macrophages in the granulomas. The dose of corticosteroid should be titrated down to the lowest dose required to maintain normocalcemia.

Phosphate has been used in the treatment of hypercalcemia.[433] However, the presence of a normal or slightly elevated serum phosphorus level or decreased renal function precludes the use of this medication. Phosphorus should be given only when the serum phosphorus level is low, and its use is generally discouraged. If an elevation of the serum phosphorus level is achieved and the serum Ca level decreases, the patient may deposit Ca phosphate in soft tissues.

There are some general measures that are important in the treatment of hypercalcemia. Immobilization should be avoided as much as possible, especially in patients with rapid bone turnover such as those with Paget disease. Because most patients with hypercalcemia have an underlying tumor that is causing the hypercalcemia, physicians should be aware of this pathogenetic mechanism and join efforts with oncologists in the diagnosis and treatment of the malignancy. Finally, when the hypercalcemia is very severe and the patient has advanced renal insufficiency, acute hemodialysis is an effective method of correcting the hypercalcemia (Table 73.9).

MAGNESIUM

General Considerations

Magnesium is the second most abundant intracellular cation (after potassium) and the fourth most abundant cation of the body (after Ca, K, Na). Magnesium (Mg^{2+}) is divalent and has an atomic weight of 24. Mg^{2+} has an essential role as a cofactor for various enzymes, most of which use ATP. Mg^{2+} increases the stimulus threshold in nerve fibers and in pharmacologic doses has a curare-like action on neuromuscular function, probably inhibiting the release of acetylcholine at the neuromuscular junction. Mg^{2+} decreases peripheral resistance and lowers blood pressure. Like Ca^{2+}, Mg^{2+} plays a role in the regulation of PTH secretion. Hypermagnesemia suppresses the release of PTH. Acute hypomagnesemia has the opposite effect; however, profound magnesium depletion decreases the release of PTH. In vitro, magnesium increases the solubility of both calcium and phosphorus.

Body Stores of Magnesium

The total body magnesium concentration is approximately 2,000 mEq, or 25 g. As with calcium, only a small fraction (about 1%) of the body magnesium is present in the ECF compartment. Approximately 60% of the total body magnesium is found in bone. Most of the magnesium in bone is associated with apatite crystals, and a significant amount is present as a surface-limited ion on the bone crystal and is freely exchangeable. Approximately 20% of the total body magnesium is localized in the muscle. The remaining 20% is localized in other tissues of the body; the liver has a high magnesium content. The concentration of magnesium in blood is maintained within narrow limits, ranging between 1.5 and 1.9 mEq per L. Approximately 75% to 80% of the magnesium in serum is ultrafiltrable, and the rest is protein bound.[99,432] Most of the ultrafiltrable magnesium is present in the ionized form. Red cell magnesium concentration is approximately 5 mEq per L.

Intracellular free Mg^{2+} levels in renal tubular cells are in the range of 500 μmol per L.[380] High-performance liquid chromatography and fluorescent methods have been used to ascertain intracellular Mg^{2+} levels. Mitochondrial inhibitors that deplete intracellular ATP produce modest increases in intracellular Mg^{2+} and Ca^{2+}. The effects of these inhibitors are due to the changes in ATP levels.[380] Another agent, antimycin, diminishes ATP levels and decreases intracellular Mg^{2+} to 430 μmol per L but increases cytosolic Ca^{2+}, indicating that Mg^{2+} movements can be distinguished from those of Ca^{2+} by fluorescent techniques. Also, these studies indicate that intracellular regulation of Mg^{2+} is distinctive from that of Ca^{2+}. The role of intracellular Mg^{2+} in the control of cell function remains poorly understood.[160] However, intracellular Mg^{2+} levels are rapidly changed through a number of different influences that have important effects on cell function.

Magnesium Balance

Approximately 300 mg, or 25 mEq, of magnesium is ingested daily in the diet (1 mEq = 12 mg). A large portion of dietary magnesium is provided by the ingestion of green vegetables. A minimal magnesium intake of 0.3 mEq per kg of body weight is apparently necessary to maintain magnesium balance in the average person. Of the total amount of magnesium ingested in the diet, about one third is eliminated in urine and the rest in feces (Fig. 73.18). Thus, on a normal diet containing approximately 300 mg of magnesium, 30% to 40% of the ingested magnesium is absorbed (Fig. 73.18). Small amounts of magnesium, on the order of 15 to 30 mg per day, are secreted by the GI tract. Many studies have shown that animals fed low-magnesium diets can excrete urine that is very low in magnesium.[99,160,173] However, the GI tract continues to secrete small amounts of magnesium, and the animal becomes magnesium depleted. Most of the magnesium is absorbed in the upper GI tract. Magnesium shares with calcium similar pathways for absorption in

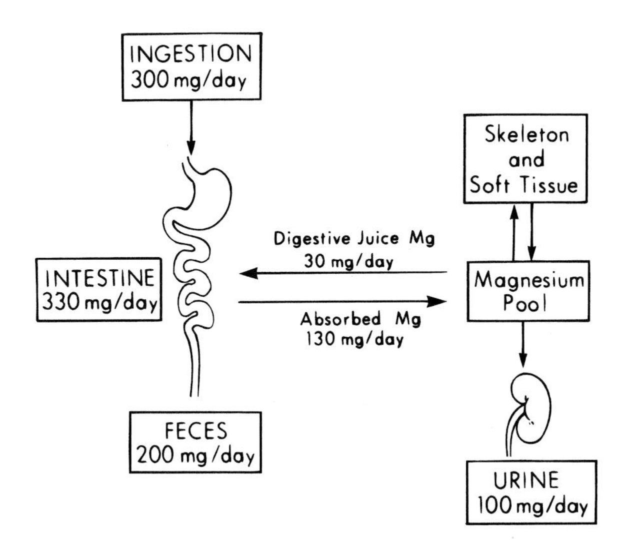

FIGURE 73.18 Diagrammatic representation of magnesium metabolism in humans showing the contribution of the gastrointestinal tract, the kidney, bone, and soft tissues to the magnesium pool. (From Slatopolsky E, Rosenbaum R, Mennes P, et al. The hypocalcemia of magnesium depletion. In: Massry S, Ritz E, Rapado A, eds. *Homeostasis of Phosphate and Other Minerals*. New York: Plenum; 1978:263.)

the intestine, but whereas most of the evidence suggests that calcium is actively absorbed from the GI tract, magnesium is absorbed mainly by ionic diffusion and "solvent drag" resulting from the bulk flow of water. A carrier mechanism also may be involved in this process.[12,235] Intestinal magnesium absorption occurs via two different pathways: a nonsaturable paracellular passive transport and a saturable active transport. At low intraluminal concentrations, magnesium is absorbed primarily via the active cellular route, and with increasing concentrations, via the paracellular pathway. In hypomagnesemia with secondary hypocalcemia, all magnesium is absorbed via the paracellular pathway. This is evidenced by mutations in TRPM6 which leads to disruption of transcellular magnesium absorption in the intestine and kidney.[338] The factors controlling the absorption of magnesium from the bowel are not fully understood. Although there is some evidence to suggest that vitamin D may influence the absorption of magnesium, this role seems to be less important for magnesium than for the absorption of calcium.[446,449] It is known that patients with severe renal insufficiency and low levels of 1,25-dihydroxycholecalciferol may develop profound hypermagnesemia by slightly increasing the amount of magnesium in the diet without modifying the metabolites of vitamin D in serum. The sigmoid colon has the capability of absorbing magnesium, and there are several reports in the literature of patients who developed magnesium toxicity after receiving enemas containing magnesium; most of these patients also had renal insufficiency. Experimental evidence in different species suggests an interrelationship between magnesium and calcium absorption from the GI tract. Diets high in calcium decrease the absorption of magnesium, and diets low in magnesium increase the absorption of calcium.

Renal Handling of Magnesium

Approximately 2 g of magnesium is filtered daily by the kidney, and about 100 mg appears in the urine. Thus, 95% to 97% of the filtered load of magnesium is reabsorbed, and 1% to 3% is excreted in the urine (Fig. 73.19).[159,160] In states of magnesium deficiency, the kidney can reduce the amount of magnesium excreted in the urine to less than 0.5% of the filtered load. On the other hand, during magnesium infusion or in patients with far-advanced renal insufficiency, as is commonly seen, the kidney can excrete 40% to 80% of the filtered load of magnesium.[641] The proximal tubule is poorly permeable to magnesium,[98,99,159,257,641,718] and probably no more than 15% to 20% is reabsorbed in this segment (Fig. 73.19). This is in contrast to the amount of sodium and calcium (60%) reabsorbed in this segment of the nephron. The tubular fluid magnesium is usually 1.5-fold greater than the plasma magnesium,[12] and it increases along perfused tubules in a linear manner, with net water reabsorption. Further studies indicated a low level of backflux from peritubular membrane into the lumen.[528,608] In the descending limb of the loop of Henle, the magnesium concentration is raised severalfold over the ultrafiltrable serum concentration due to water removal. The TAL of the loop of Henle seems to play a critical role in the reabsorption of magnesium. Early studies by LeGrimellec et al.[362] and by Morel et al.[461] demonstrated that the loop of Henle was the major site for magnesium reabsorption. Approximately 60% to 70% of the filtered magnesium was reabsorbed between the last accessible portion of the proximal tubule and the early distal tubule (Fig. 73.19).[534] In the presence of a normal plasma magnesium concentration, magnesium absorption increases with intraluminal magnesium concentration, without indication of a T_{max} for magnesium. On the other hand, an increase in plasma magnesium concentration (i.e., on the basolateral membrane) resulted in a significant depression of magnesium absorption, suggesting that hypermagnesemia decreases magnesium absorption in the loop of Henle by inhibiting magnesium transport at the basolateral membrane. Thus, the permeability of the TAL to magnesium is quite different from that of the proximal tubule. Two mechanisms have been proposed to explain magnesium transport in the TAL of the loop of Henle: (1) passive,[81] secondary to the potential difference generated by the active transport of sodium chloride, which facilitates paracellular movement of Mg^{2+}; and (2) active,[292,552,593] because the chemical concentration of magnesium in the cells is higher than that in the lumen, and the potential gradient may not be great enough to explain the entry of magnesium into cells. Diets deficient in magnesium or the administration of PTH enhances the reabsorption of magnesium in the TAL of the loop of Henle. On the other hand, diets containing large amounts of magnesium or factors that decrease the reabsorption of sodium chloride in this portion of the nephron (ECF volume

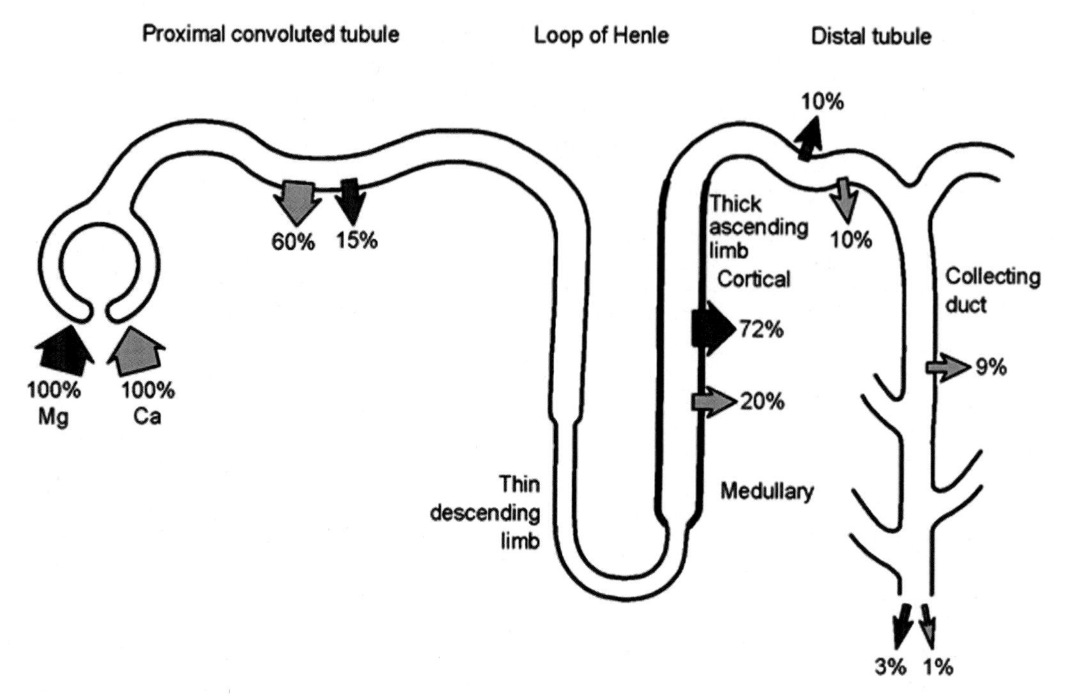

FIGURE 73.19 Summary of segmental magnesium absorption along the nephron relative to sodium and calcium reabsorption. (From Quamme GA, De Rouffignac C. Renal magnesium handling. In Selding D, Giebisch G, eds. *The Kidney*. New York: Lippincott Williams & Wilkins; 2004:1711.)

expansion, administration of diuretics such as furosemide, bumetanide, or ethacrynic acid) also decrease the reabsorption of magnesium.

Hypomagnesemia with Hypercalciuria and Nephrocalcinosis

Recently a protein, paracellin 1 (PCLN1), was detected in the TAL and in the distal tubule.[613] PCLN1 or claudin16 is a member of the claudin family of high-junction proteins. PCLN1 is a highly negative-charged protein, with 10 negatively charged residues and a net charge of −5 (Fig. 73.20).[613] Mutations in the protein induce renal Mg^{2+} wasting, hypercalciuria, nephrocalcinosis, and renal failure. PCLN1 plays an important role in the conductance of the TAL. The negative charges may contribute to the cationic selectivity of the paracellular pathway for the reabsorption of calcium and magnesium.[613]

The terminal segment of the nephron (late distal tubule and collecting duct) appears to play a minor role in the reabsorption of magnesium under normal conditions.[527,532,534] However, more recent studies by the same investigators indicate that the distal tubule also plays an important role in magnesium conservation.[531] The distal tubule normally reabsorbs about 10% of the filtered load of magnesium. Because there is little reabsorption of magnesium in the collecting duct, the distal tubule plays a key role in determining the final urinary excretion of magnesium.

Recent studies with immortalized DCT cell lines have shown that magnesium uptake is specific and regulated by factors shown to influence distal magnesium reabsorption. Quamme and DeRouffignac[533] speculated that Mg^{2+} entry is through a channel, and transport is dependent on the transmembrane voltage. The active step is at the basolateral membrane where Mg^{2+} leaves the cell against both electrical and concentration gradient. Na^{+}–Mg^{2+} exchange may occur, with Na^{+} moving back into the cell, coupled with Mg^{++} exiting from the cell into the interstitium. A large number

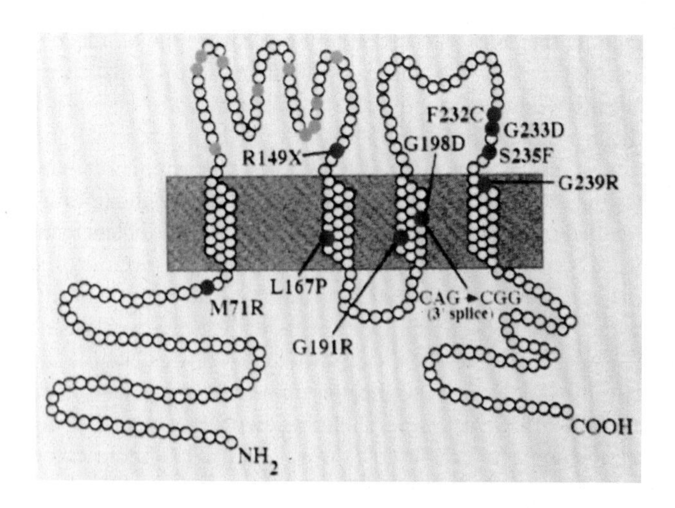

FIGURE 73.20 Structure of the *PCLN-1* human gene. The red dots indicate mutations in *PCLN-1* in patients with recessive renal hypomagnesemia. (From Simon DB, Lu Y, Cahote KA, et al. Paracellin-1, a renal tight junction protein required for paracellular Mg^{2+} resorption. *Science*. 1999;285:103.)

of hormones, such as PTH, calcitonin, glucagon, and vasopressin, stimulate Mg^{2+} reabsorption in the thick ascending loop and distal tubule; however, they have no effect in the proximal tubule.

Chronic administration of mineralocorticoids increases magnesium excretion. Several interrelationships between calcium and magnesium reabsorption have been demonstrated. The administration of one of these two elements decreases the reabsorption of the other. When large amounts of magnesium are given intravenously, there is a remarkable decrease in the renal reabsorption of calcium and vice versa. Alcohol also affects the handling of magnesium by the kidney. A remarkable short-lived hypermagnesuria is seen after alcohol is given to experimental animals or humans. The intravenous administration of glucose has a similar effect.

In summary, in contrast to calcium, the thick ascending portion of the loop of Henle is the most important portion of the nephron in the regulation of magnesium reabsorption. Magnesium reabsorption in the loop occurs within the cortical TAL primarily by passive means driven by the transepithelial voltage through the paracellular pathway. On the other hand, magnesium reabsorption in the distal tubule is transcellular and active in nature. Moreover, the reabsorption of magnesium in the proximal tubule, in contrast to that of sodium, calcium, and phosphate, is rather limited.

Hypermagnesemia

By far the most common cause of hypermagnesemia is chronic renal insufficiency.[542] The kidney can excrete large amounts of magnesium in the urine. Thus, hypermagnesemia is seldom seen in patients with normal renal function, even if the patient ingests large amounts of magnesium such as antacids containing magnesium or laxatives such as milk of magnesia. Mild hypermagnesemia may be seen in patients with GFRs of approximately 10 mL per minute. However, moderate hypermagnesemia is usually seen in patients with GFRs of less than 5 mL per minute. As renal insufficiency progresses, the fractional excretion of magnesium in the urine significantly increases. Patients with a GFR of 120 mL per minute excrete approximately 5% of the filtered load of magnesium. However, patients with far-advanced renal failure (GFR of less than 10 mL per minute) may excrete up to 40% to 80% of the filtered load of magnesium.[542] Thus, patients with chronic renal failure may not be able to increase magnesium excretion further after ingestion of large amounts of magnesium. Therefore, if magnesium ingestion is increased (after administration of laxatives or antacids containing magnesium) in patients with advanced renal failure, profound hypermagnesemia and death may occur. In obstetric wards, magnesium is still used for the treatment of eclampsia.[523] In some of these patients, the GFR is decreased, and the administration of large amounts of magnesium sulfate may result in hypermagnesemia. Although most of the magnesium is absorbed in the small intestine, the sigmoid colon can also absorb magnesium. Healthy subjects receiving large amounts of magnesium sulfate per rectum have been found to have serum magnesium levels of more than 10 mEq per L.[164]

Symptoms and Signs of Hypermagnesemia

Profound hypermagnesemia blocks neuromuscular transmission and depresses the conduction system of the heart. The neuromuscular effects of magnesium are antagonized by the administration of calcium. Mild hypermagnesemia is well tolerated. However, if serum magnesium levels increase to 5 to 6 mg per dL, there may be a decrease in tendon reflexes[706] and some degree of mental confusion. If the serum magnesium level increases to 7 to 9 mg per dL, the respiratory rate slows and the blood pressure falls. If serum magnesium levels increase to about 10 to 13 mg per dL, there is usually profound hypotension and severe mental depression. When the levels increase further to about 15 mg per dL, death may occur.[17,164,706] In uremic patients, the adverse effect of hypermagnesemia may be worsened by the presence of hypocalcemia. Acute hypermagnesemia may also produce mild hypocalcemia. This may be due to (1) suppression of the release of PTH and (2) competition for tubular reabsorption between calcium and magnesium, leading to decreased calcium reabsorption and hypercalciuria, which aggravates the hypocalcemia produced by decreased release of PTH. In chronic renal insufficiency, there is probably an increase in red cell magnesium and muscle magnesium, but the results are controversial. The amount of magnesium in bone is apparently increased in cortical and trabecular bone.[17]

Hypomagnesemia

Hypomagnesemia is defined as a decrease in serum magnesium to levels less than 1.5 mg per dL. Diseases involving the small intestine may decrease magnesium absorption and are the most common cause of hypomagnesemia (Table 73.10). It is difficult to predict the degree of total body magnesium deficiency by determining only serum magnesium concentration. Because only 1% of magnesium is present in the ECF compartment, changes in intracellular magnesium and skeletal magnesium can modify the concentration of serum magnesium, and it may not be possible to assess precisely the degree of magnesium deficiency by determining serum magnesium level. Probably the determination of skeletal or muscle magnesium may provide a better index of magnesium deficiency. However, these determinations are not practical in clinical medicine. In patients with magnesium deficiency, the administration of 50 to 100 mEq of magnesium per day usually corrects the hypomagnesemia after a short time. Magnesium depletion can also produce changes in other electrolytes. Usually there is an increase in potassium excretion in the urine, and patients may develop hypokalemia.[710] In several experimental studies, it has been shown in humans[599] and animals[711] that magnesium depletion is accompanied by urinary potassium losses. Potassium alone did not increase muscle potassium unless

TABLE 73.10 **Causes of Hypomagnesemia**

I. Decreased intestinal absorption
  A. Severe diarrhea
  B. Intestinal bypass
  C. Surgical resection
  D. Tropical and nontropical sprue
  E. Celiac disease
  F. Invasive and infiltrative process; lymphomas
  G. Prolonged gastrointestinal suction
II. Decreased intake
  A. Starvation
  B. Protein energy malnutrition
  C. Chronic alcoholism
  D. Prolonged therapy with intravenous fluids lacking magnesium
III. Excessive urinary losses
  A. Diuretic phase of acute tubular necrosis
  B. Postobstructive diuresis
  C. Diuretic therapy
  D. Diabetic ketoacidosis (during treatment)
  E. Chronic alcoholism
  F. Hypercalcemic states
  G. Primary aldosteronism
  H. Inappropriate antidiuretic hormone secretion
  I. Aminoglycoside toxicity
  J. Idiopathic renal magnesium wasting
  K. Cisplatinum
  L. Cyclosporine
  M. Gitelman syndrome

From Slatopolsky E. Pathophysiology of calcium, magnesium, and phosphorus. In: Klahr S, ed. *The Kidney and Body Fluids in Health and Disease.* New York: Plenum Press; 1983:269, with permission.

magnesium replacement was given as well to patients receiving diuretics.[177] It has been suggested that the effect of magnesium on intracellular potassium is a result of magnesium stimulating Na-K-ATPase activity, allowing the cell to maintain a potassium gradient.[588] However, the most important manifestation of hypomagnesemia is the development of hypocalcemia and tetany. Experimental animals fed a low-magnesium diet develop hypocalcemia.[125,175,348,450] However, the rat becomes hypercalcemic. The pathogenesis of hypocalcemia in magnesium depletion is multifactorial. Hypomagnesemia has profound effects on PTH metabolism and bone physiology. It is known that mild hypomagnesemia increases acutely the levels of PTH in vivo[101] or in vitro[247]; on the other hand, profound hypomagnesemia decreases the levels of PTH in blood.[21] It seems that neither the biosynthesis nor the conversion of pro-PTH to PTH is greatly affected by the concentration of magnesium.[248,251] However, the release of PTH is influenced by the serum magnesium concentration.[20] Several investigators have demonstrated that the administration of magnesium to patients with severe hypomagnesemia who have low levels of immunoreactive PTH in serum increases the release of PTH a few minutes after magnesium administration. Also, there is evidence to indicate that during hypomagnesemia, the skeleton is resistant to the action of PTH,[136,567] and in general, the administration of mildly pharmacologic doses of PTH does not elicit a normal calcemic response in patients with magnesium depletion. Studies by Freitag et al.[194] have further clarified this abnormality. The uptake of PTH by bones obtained from dogs with experimental magnesium depletion was greatly diminished, and the release of cAMP by bone was also blunted in hypomagnesemia. In addition to a decrease in the release of PTH and skeletal resistance to this hormone, in magnesium depletion there is evidence that the ionic exchange from the hydration shell of bone between calcium and magnesium also is decreased[412]; thus, on a physicochemical basis, less calcium is mobilized from bone in hypomagnesemia. Thus, the decrease in the release of PTH, the low uptake of PTH by bone, and the decreased heteroionic exchange of calcium for magnesium in bone are all pathogenetic factors responsible for the hypocalcemia observed in patients with profound magnesium depletion.

Clinical Manifestations of Hypomagnesemia

Patients with severe hypomagnesemia usually develop some degree of anorexia, mental confusion, and vomiting. In general, there is increased neuromuscular irritability, and tremors and seizures are usually observed in these patients. Muscle fasciculation and positive Trousseau's and Chvostek's signs can be observed. Nodal or sinus tachycardia and premature atrial or ventricular contractions may occur. The electrocardiogram may show prolongation of the QT interval and broadening and flattening or even inversion of the T waves. Magnesium deficiency potentiates the action of digitalis, and there is an enhanced sensitivity to the toxic effects of digitalis. Because magnesium plays a key role in regulating the activity of Na-K-ATPase, which is the enzyme responsible for the maintenance of intracellular potassium concentration, severe alterations in skeletal muscle and myocardial function are observed. Sometimes it is difficult to decide whether the changes in the electrocardiogram are related to magnesium or potassium depletion. Most of these patients also have profound hypocalcemia, and sometimes it is difficult to determine whether the symptoms are due to magnesium deficiency or to the concomitant hypocalcemia. Other neurologic manifestations may include vertigo, ataxia, nystagmus, and dysarthria. Changes in personality, depression, and sometimes hallucinations and psychosis have been observed. Patients also may show some degree of hypophosphatemia. In the rat, it has been shown that magnesium deficiency promotes renal phosphate excretion.[342]

Mechanisms Responsible for the Development of Hypomagnesemia

From the pathogenetic point of view, three main mechanisms are responsible for the development of hypomagnesemia: (1) decreased intestinal absorption, (2) decreased intake, and (3) excessive urinary losses.

Hypomagnesemia Secondary to Decreased Intestinal Absorption of Magnesium

By far the most common causes responsible for the development of hypomagnesemia are pathologic entities affecting the small bowel. In these conditions, the kidney adapts to the hypomagnesemia and decreases the urinary excretion of magnesium. However, the amount of magnesium in the stool does not decrease appropriately (probably the secretion of magnesium is not greatly reduced), and the patient develops hypomagnesemia. Severe magnesium depletion is associated with steatorrheic syndromes.[76] Pathologic processes such as celiac disease, tropical and nontropical sprue, malignancies (characteristically lymphoma), surgical resection, intestinal bypass, and profound diarrhea have all been considered responsible for the development of hypomagnesemia. From 1960 to 1975, when the number of surgical bypass procedures for the treatment of obesity increased greatly, it was noted that many of these patients developed profound hypomagnesemia and tetany. Hypomagnesemia is especially prominent in patients with idiopathic steatorrhea and diseases affecting the terminal ileum.

As described before, the characterization of TRPM6 mutations demonstrated a key role in hypomagnesemia and hypocalcemia secondary to a decrease in intestinal absorption and renal reabsorption of magnesium.

Hypomagnesemia Secondary to Decreased Magnesium Intake

Magnesium depletion has been described in children with protein-calorie malnutrition.[105] The hypomagnesemia results from a combination of decreased intake and GI losses due to diarrhea or severe vomiting. In a hospital setting, perhaps the most common cause of hypomagnesemia is prolonged therapy with intravenous fluids lacking magnesium. Often, when surgical patients require intestinal suction, they are given intravenous fluid, sometimes for several weeks, and seldom is magnesium added to the intravenous fluids. Alcoholism is probably the most common cause of hypomagnesemia in the United States.[191,306,447] The chronic ingestion of alcohol produces hypomagnesemia. The mechanisms are multifactorial. Usually patients with chronic alcoholism ingest diets poor in magnesium. Alcohol increases the urinary excretion of magnesium.[310] From the point of view of differential diagnosis, the clinical history, evidence of malnutrition, the presence of diarrhea and vomiting, or a history of surgery may help to differentiate individuals with decreased absorption of magnesium due either to a primary GI disease or to decreased intake from individuals with increased urinary excretion of magnesium. As mentioned previously, when there is decreased intake or absorption of magnesium from the GI tract, the amount of magnesium excreted in the urine is greatly reduced, on the order of 10 to 15 mg per day.

Hypomagnesemia Secondary to Increased Urinary Losses of Magnesium

Because 60% to 70% of magnesium is absorbed in the TAL of the loop of Henle, any factor that blocks the reabsorption of sodium chloride in this part of the nephron will also promote the urinary excretion of magnesium. In conditions in which the ECF volume is increased and in entities characterized by profound diuresis (diuretic phase of acute tubular necrosis, postobstructive diuresis), the patient may excrete 20% to 30% of the filtered load of magnesium and may develop profound hypomagnesemia. Administration of large amounts of diuretics such as ethacrynic acid, bumetanide, or furosemide has a significant effect on renal magnesium excretion. Patients with ketoacidosis may develop hypomagnesemia. Serum magnesium, phosphorus, and potassium concentrations may be elevated during periods of ketoacidosis; however, the levels usually fall after the administration of insulin and fluid replacement. Increased excretion of magnesium has been seen after the treatment of diabetic ketoacidosis[104] and in metabolic conditions characterized by an excess of mineralocorticoids[276] such as primary aldosteronism. A specific defect has been described in patients receiving aminoglycosides[318] or cisplatin (an antitumoral agent).[580] The usual lesions produced by aminoglycosides are acute tubular necrosis, renal insufficiency, and hypermagnesemia; however, several patients have developed a specific tubular defect characterized by profound hypermagnesuria and hypomagnesemia that may persist for several weeks after the drug is discontinued. Some of these patients also developed hypokalemia.

Gitelman Syndrome

Patients with chronic hypokalemia and a phenotype other than that of Bartter syndrome, who have hypomagnesemia and excess urinary magnesium, are described as having Gitelman syndrome.[223] Gitelman syndrome is actually more common than Bartter syndrome and is characterized as follows. The patients may be children or adults with primary renal tubular hypokalemic metabolic alkalosis with magnesium deficiency, hypocalciuria, and skin lesions. Hyperreninemic hyperaldosteronism is present, as are the other features of Bartter syndrome. The inheritance is autosomal recessive, and linkage analysis to the locus encoding the renal thiazide–sensitive Na-Cl cotransporter is uniform.[614] Thus, reduced sodium chloride reabsorption in the diluting segment is the pathogenesis of the disease, and it further leads to abnormalities in magnesium transport.

Treatment of Alterations in Magnesium Metabolism

Hypermagnesemia

Hypermagnesemia is seen very seldom in clinical medicine. In general, it is observed in patients with far-advanced renal insufficiency, usually with a GFR of less than 10 mL per minute. The treatment is similar to that for hypercalcemia (i.e., volume expansion with saline and administration of furosemide). However, care is required because this therapeutic regimen will also increase the excretion of calcium in the urine and potentiate the toxic effects of hypermagnesemia. Thus, if expansion with saline and furosemide is used, calcium should be added to the solutions, approximately 1 to 3 ampules of calcium gluconate per liter of saline, to prevent hypocalcemia. If the patient's GFR is extremely low, and volume expansion with saline and diuretics is not effective, dialysis with a low or zero magnesium dialysate should be instituted. Hypermagnesemia is also seen clinically when large amounts of magnesium are given intravenously to patients. A decrease in the dose administered will rapidly correct the condition.

Hypomagnesemia

Profound magnesium depletion may be accompanied by hypocalcemia and tetany. Thus, the treatment of severe hypomagnesemia may constitute a medical emergency. Profound hypomagnesemia can be easily corrected by administration of magnesium intravenously, provided that the patient has fairly normal renal function. In patients with compromised renal function, magnesium should be given cautiously, and serum magnesium should be closely monitored. Fifty to 75 mEq of magnesium sulfate or magnesium chloride should be mixed in 500 mL of dextrose in water and given intravenously over 6 to 8 hours. The next morning, serum magnesium should be measured and, if hypomagnesemia persists, the amount of magnesium should be increased to 100 mEq dissolved in the same type of solution and given over 8 hours. In some circumstances, this procedure should be repeated two or three times until the serum magnesium level increases to 2.5 mg per dL. If the patient requires magnesium orally over a prolonged period, magnesium salts can be given to these patients. One gram of magnesium oxide has roughly 50 mEq, or 600 mg, of magnesium. Thus, magnesium oxide in a dose of 250 to 500 mg can be given to patients two to four times daily. Larger doses are not well tolerated, and most patients will develop diarrhea. It is important to emphasize that a normal diet provides approximately 25 mEq, or 300 mg, of magnesium.

ACKNOWLEDGMENTS

This work was supported by grants NIH R01-DK070790, NIH R01 DK066029, and NIH R01 DK062209 by the National Institutes of Health.

REFERENCES

1. *The Physiological and Cellular Basis of Metabolic Bone Disease*. Baltimore: Williams & Wilkins Co.; 1974.
2. *Bone Histomorphometry*. New York: Raven Press; 1994.
3. A gene (PEX) with homologies to endopeptidases is mutated in patients with X-linked hypophosphatemic rickets. The HYP Consortium. *Nat Genet.* 1995;11:130.
4. Autosomal dominant hypophosphatasemic rickets is associated with mutations in FGF23. *Nat Genet.* 2000;26:345.
5. Aasebø W, Scott H, Ganss R. Kidney biopsies taken before and after oral sodium phosphate bowel cleansing. *Nephrol Dial Transplant.* 2007;22:920.
6. Abassi AA, Chemplavil JK, Farah S. Hypercalcemia in active tuberculosis. *Ann Intern Med.* 1979;90:324.
7. Adams JS, Sharma OP, Singer FR. Metabolism of 25-hyperoxyvitamin D_3 by alveolar macrophages in sarcoidosis. *Clin Res.* 1983;31:499A.
8. Aderka D, Shoenfeld Y, Santo M, et al. Life-threatening hypophosphatemia in a patient with acute myelogenous leukemia. *Acta Haematol.* 1980;64:117.
9. Agus ZS, Gardner LB, Beck LH, et al. Effects of parathyroid hormone on renal tubular reabsorption of calcium, sodium and phosphate. *Am J Physiol.* 1973;224:1143.
10. Agus ZS, Goldfarb S, Wasserstein A. eds. Disorders of Calcium and Phosphate Balance. In: Brenner BM, Rector FCJ, eds. *The Kidney*. Philadelphia: Saunders, 1981; 940.
11. Ahmed KY, Varghese Z, Willis MR, et al. Persistent hypophosphatemia and osteomalacia in dialysis patients not on oral phosphate-binders: Response to dihydrotachysterol therapy. *Lancet.* 1976;1:439.
12. Aikawa JK, Rhoades EL, Gordon GS. Urinary and fecal excretion of orally administered Mg^{2+}. *Proc Soc Exp Biol Med.* 1958;98:29.
13. Albright F, Burnett CH, Smith PH, Parson W. Pseudohypoparathyroidism—an example of "Seabright-Bantam syndrome". *Endocrinology.* 1942;30:922.
14. Albright F, Butler AM, Hampton AO, Smith P. Syndrome characterized by osteitis fibrosa disseminata, areas of pigmentation and endocrine dysfunction with precocious puberty in females. *N Eng J Med.* 1937;216:727.
15. Albright F, Forbes AP, Hinneman PH. Pseudopseudohypoparathyroidism. *Trans Assoc Am Physicians.* 1952;65:337.
16. Alcalde AI, Sarasa M, Raldua D, et al. Role of thyroid hormone in regulation of renal phosphate transport in young and aged rats. *Endocrinology.* 1999;140:1544.
17. Alfrey AC, Miller NL. Bone magnesium pools in uremia. *J Clin Invest.* 1973;52:3019.
18. Ambuhl PM, Zajicek HK, Wang H, et al. Regulation of renal phosphate transport by acute and chronic metabolic acidosis in the rat. *Kidney Int.* 1998;53:1288.
19. Amling M, Priemel M, Holzmann T, et al. Rescue of the skeletal phenotype of vitamin D receptor-ablated mice in the setting of normal mineral ion homeostasis: Formal histomorphometric and biomechanical analyses. *Endocrinology.* 1999;140:4982.
20. Anast CA, Winnocker JL, Forte LR. Impaired release of parathyroid hormone in magnesium deficiency. *J Clin Endocrinol. Metab.* 1976;42:707.
21. Anast CW, Mohs JM, Kaplan SL. Evidence for parathyroid failure in magnesium deficiency. *Science.* 1972;177:606.
22. Arar M, Baum M, Biber J, Murer H, Levi M. Epidermal growth factor inhibits Na-Pi cotransport and mRNA in OK cells. *Am J Physiol.* 1995;268:309.
23. Arar M, Zajicek HK, Elshihabi I, Levi M. Epidermal growth factor inhibits Na-Pi cotransport in weaned and suckling rats. *Am J Physiol.* 1999;276:72.
24. Argiro L, Desbarats M, Glorieux FH, Ecarot B. Mepe, the gene encoding a tumor-secreted protein in oncogenic hypophosphatemic osteomalacia, is expressed in bone. *Genomics.* 2001;74:342.
25. Arieff AI, Massry SG. Calcium metabolism of brain in acute renal failure. *J Clin Invest.* 1974;53:387.
26. Arima K, Hines ER, Kiela PR, Drees JB, Collins JF, Ghishan FK. Glucocorticoid regulation and glycosylation of mouse intestinal type IIb Na-P(i) cotransporter during ontogeny. *Am J Physiol. Gastrointest Liver Physiol.* 2002;283:426.
27. Arnaud CD, Clar OH. eds. Primary Hyperparathyroidism. In: Krieger DT, Bardin CW, eds. *Current Therapy in Endocrinology 1983–1984*. Philadelphia and St. Louis: Decker and Mosby, 1983; 270.
28. Arnold A, Brown MF, Urena P, Gaz RD, Sarfati E, Drueke TB. Monoclonality of parathyroid tumors in chronic renal failure and in primary parathyroid hyperplasia. *J Clin Invest.* 1995;95:2047.
29. Atkins D, Ibbotson KJ, Hillier K. Secretion of prostaglandins as bone resorbing agents by renal cortical carcinoma in culture. *Br J Cancer.* 1971;36:601.
30. Ba J, Friedman PA. Calcium-sensing receptor regulation of renal mineral ion transport. *Cell Calcium.* 2004;35:229.

31. Bachmann S, Schlichting U, Geist B, et al. Kidney-specific inactivation of the megalin gene impairs trafficking of renal inorganic sodium phosphate cotransporter (NaPi-IIa). *J Am Soc Nephrol.* 2004;15:892.

32. Bacic D, Schulz N, Biber J, et al. Involvement of the MAPK-kinase pathway in the PTH-mediated regulation of the proximal tubule type IIa Na+/Pi cotransporter in mouse kidney 88. *Pflugers Arch.* 2003;446:52.

33. Bacic D, Wagner CA, Hernando N, Kaissling B, Biber J, Murer H. Novel aspects in regulated expression of the renal type IIa Na/Pi-cotransporter. *Kidney Int. Suppl.* 2004;66:S5–S12.

34. Bacskai BJ, Friedman PA. Activation of latent Ca^{2+} channels in renal epithelial cells by parathyroid hormone. *Nature.* 1990;347:388.

35. Bai X, Miao D, Li J, Goltzman D, Karaplis AC. Transgenic mice overexpressing human fibroblast growth factor 23 (R176Q) delineate a putative role for parathyroid hormone in renal phosphate wasting disorders. *Endocrinology.* 2004; 145:5269.

36. Bai XY, Miao D, Goltzman D, Karaplis AC. The autosomal dominant hypophosphatemic rickets R176Q mutation in fibroblast growth factor 23 resists proteolytic cleavage and enhances in vivo biological potency. *J Biol Chem.* 2003;278:9843.

37. Baker LRI, Ackrill P, Cattell WR, Stamp TC, Watson L. Latrogenic osteomalacia and myopathy due to phosphate depletion. *Br Med J.* 1974;3:150.

38. Barbour GL, Coburn JW, Slatopolsky E. Hypercalcemia in an anephric patient with sarcoidosis: Evidence for extra-renal generation of 1,25-dihydroxyvitamin D. *N Engl J Med.* 1982;305:440.

39. Beall DP, Scofield RH. Milk-alkali syndrome associated with calcium carbonate consumption. *Medicine.* 1995;74:89.

40. Beck D, Levitin H, Epstein FH. The effect of intravenous infusion of calcium on renal concentrating ability. *Am J Physiol.* 1959;197:1118.

41. Beck LH, Goldberg M. Effects of acetazolamide and parathyroidectomy on renal transport of sodium, calcium and phosphate. *Am J Physiol.* 1973;224:1136.

42. Beck LH, Goldberg M. Mechanism of the blunted phosphaturia in saline-loaded thyroparathyroidectomized dogs. *Kidney Int.* 1974;6:18.

43. Beck N. Effect of metabolic acidosis on renal response to parathyroid hormone in phosphorus-deprived rats. *Am J Physiol.* 1981;241:F23–F27.

44. Beck N, Singh H, Reed SW. Pathogenic role of cyclic AMP in the impairment of urinary concentrating ability in acute hypercalcemia. *J Clin Invest.* 1974;54:1049.

45. Beers KW, Dousa TP. Thyroid hormone stimulates the Na(+)-PO4 symporter but not the Na(+)-SO4 symporter in renal brush border. *Am J Physiol.* 1993;265:323.

46. Bell HH, Stern PH, Pantzer E, Sinha TK, DeLuca HF. Evidence that increased circulating 1α,25-dihydroxyvitamin D is the probable cause for abnormal calcium metabolism in sarcoidosis. *J Clin Invest.* 1979;64:218.

47. Benet-Pages A, Lorenz-Depiereux B, Zischka H, et al. FGF23 is processed by proprotein convertases but not by PHEX. *Bone.* 2004;35:455.

48. Benet-Pages A, Orlik P, Strom TM, et al. An FGF23 missense mutation causes familial tumoral calcinosis with hyperphosphatemia. *Hum Mol Genet.* 2005;14:385–390.

49. Berenson J, Hirschberg R. Safety and convenience of a 15-minute infusion of zoledronic acid. *Oncologist.* 2004;9:319.

50. Bergwitz C, Roslin NM, Tieder M, et al. SLC34A3 mutations in patients with hereditary hypophosphatemic rickets with hypercalciuria predict a key tole for the sodium-phosphate cotransporter NaPi-IIc in maintaining phosphate homeostasis. *Am J Hum Genet.*. 2006;78:179.

51. Berliner BC, Shenker IR, Weinstock MS. Hypercalcemia associated with hypertension due to prolonged immobilization (an unusual complication of extensive burns). *Pediatrics.* 1972;49:92.

52. Berlyne GM, Ben-Ari J, Pest D, Weinberger J, et al. Hyperaluminaemia from aluminum resins in renal failure. *Lancet.* 1970;2:494.

53. Berndt T, Craig TA, Bowe AE, et al. Secreted frizzled-related protein 4 is a potent tumor-derived phosphaturic agent. *J Clin Invest.* 2003;112:785.

54. Berson SA, Yalow RS. Parathyroid hormone in plasma in adenomatous hyperparathyroidism, uremia and bronchogenic carcinoma. *Science.* 1966;154:907.

55. Betro MG, Pain RW. Hypophosphatemia and hyperphosphatemia in a hospital population. *Br Med J.* 1972;1:273.

56. Better OS. Tubular dysfunction following kidney transplantation. *Nephron.* 1980;25:209.

57. Beutner EH, Munson PL. Time course of urinary excretion of inorganic phosphate by rats after parathyroidectomy and after injection of parathyroid extract. *Endocrinology.* 1960;66:610.

58. Bianco P, Riminucci M, Majolagbe A, et al. Mutations of the GNAS1 gene, stromal cell dysfunction, and osteomalacic changes in non-McCune-Albright fibrous dysplasia of bone. *J Bone Miner Res.* 2000;15:120.

59. Bianco P, Robey PG, Wientroub S. eds. Fibrous dysplasia of bone. In: Glorieux FH, Pettifor J, Juppner H., eds. *Pediatric Bone Biology and Disease.* New York: Academic Press, 2003; 509.

60. Biber J, Gisler SM, Hernando N, et al. PDZ interactions and proximal tubular phosphate reabsorption. *Am J Physiol. Renal Physiol.* 2004;287:871.

61. Biber J, Murer H. Na-P_i cotransport in LLC-PK_1 cells: fast adaptive response to P_i deprivation. *Am J Physiol.* 1985;249:C430–C434.

62. Bikle DD, Munson S. 1,25-dihydroxyvitamin D increases calmodulin binding to specific proteins in the chick duodenal brush border membrane. *J Clin Invest.* 1985;76:2312.

63. Bikle DD, Munson S, Chafouleas J. Calmodulin may mediate 1,25-dihydroxyvitamin D-stimulated calcium transport. *FEBS Lett.* 1984;174:30.

64. Bilder D, Schober M, Perrimon N. Integrated activity of PDZ protein complexes regulates epithelial polarity. *Nat Cell Biol.* 2003;5:53.

65. Bilezikian JP, Brandi ML, Rubin M, et al. Primary hyperparathyroidism: new concepts in clinical, densitometric and biochemical features. *J Intern Med.* 2005;257:6.

66. Bilezikian JP, Silverberg SJ. Asymptomatic primary hyperparathyroidism. *N Engl J Med.* 2004;350:1746.

67. Blaine J, Okamura K, Giral H, et al. PTH-induced internalization of apical membrane NaPi2a: role of actin and myosin VI. *Am J Physiol. Cell Physiol.* 2009;297:C1339–C1346.

68. Blasco T, Aramayona JJ, Alcalde AI, et al. Rat kidney MAP17 induces cotransport of Na-mannose and Na-glucose in Xenopus laevis oocytes. *Am J Physiol. Renal Physiol.* 2003;285:799.

69. Block GA, Hulbert-Shearon TE, Levin NW, et al. Association of serum phosphorus and calcium X phosphate product with mortality risk in chronic hemodialysis patients: a national study. *Am J Kidney Dis.* 1998;31:607–617.

70. Blumsohn A. What have we learnt about the regulation of phosphate metabolism? *Curr Opin Nephrol Hypertens.* 2004;13:397.

71. Body JJ, Dumon JC. Treatment of tumor-induced hypercalcemia with the bisphosphonate pamidronate: dose-response relationship and influence of tumor type. *Ann Oncol.* 1994;5:359.

72. Boelens PA, Norwood W, Kjellstrand C, et al. Hypophosphatemia with muscle weakness due to antacids and hemodialysis. *Am J Dis Child.* 1970;120:350.

73. Bomsztyk K, Wright FS. Effects of transepithelial fluid flux on transepithelial voltage and transport of calcium, sodium, chloride and potassium by renal proximal tubule. *Kidney Int.* 1982;21:269.

74. Bonjour J-P, Philippe J, Guelpa G, et al. Bone and renal components in hypercalcemia of malignancy and response to a single infusion of clodronate. *Bone.* 1998;9:123.

75. Bonjour JP, Preston C, Fleisch H. Effect of 1,25 dihydroxyvitamin D_3 on renal handling of P_i in thyroparathyroidectomized rats. *J Clin Invest.* 1977;60:1419.

76. Booth CC, Babouris N, Hanna S. Incidence of hypomagnesemia in intestinal malabsorption. *Med J.* 1963;2:141.

77. Bordier P, Rasmussen H, Marie P. Vitamin D metabolites and bone mineralization in man. *Clin Endocrinol Metab.* 1978;46:284.

78. Borke JL, Caride A, Verma AK. Plasma membrane calcium pump and 28-kDa calcium protein in cells of rat kidney distal tubules. *Am J Physiol.* 1989;257:F842.

79. Borke JL, Minami J, Verma A, et.al. Monoclonal antibodies to human erythrocyte membrane Ca^{++}-Mg^{++} adenosine trisphosphatase pump recognize an epitope in the basolateral membrane of human kidney distal tubule cells. *J Clin Invest.* 1987;80:1225.

80. Bourdeau JE. Calcium transport across the cortical thick ascending limb of Henle's loop. In: Bronner F, Peterlik M, eds. *Calcium and Phosphate Transport Across Biomembranes.* New York: Academic Press; 1981:199.

81. Bourdeau JE, Burg MB. Voltage dependence of calcium transort in the thick ascending limb of Henle's loop. *Am J Physiol.* 1979;236:F357.

82. Bourdeau JE, Burg MB. Effect of PTH on calcium transport across the thick ascending limb of Henle's loop. *Am J Physiol.* 1980;239:F121.

83. Bourdeau JE, Lau K. Basolateral cell membrane Ca-Na exchange in single rabbit connecting tubules. *Am J Physiol.* 1990;258:F1497–F1503.

84. Bowe AE, Finnegan R, Jan de Beur SM, et al. FGF-23 inhibits renal tubular phosphate transport and is a PHEX substrate. *Biochem Biophys Res Commun.* 2001;284:977.

85. Boyce BF, Yoneda T, Lowe C, et al. Requirement of pp60c-src expression for osteoclasts to form ruffled borders and resorb bone in mice. *J Clin Invest.* 1992;90:1622.

86. Boyce TM, Bloebaum RD. Cortical aging differences and fracture implications for the human femoral neck. *Bone.* 1993;14:769.

87. Brame LA, White KE, Econs MJ. Renal phosphate wasting disorders: clinical features and pathogenesis. *Semin Nephrol.* 2004;24:39.

88. Braun J, Oldendorf M, Moshage W, et al. Electron beam computed tomography in the evaluation of cardiac calcification in chronic dialysis patients. *AJKD.* 1996;27:394.

89. Brereton HD, Halushka PV, Alexander RW. Indomethacin-responsive hypercalcemia in a patient with renal cell adenocarcinoma. *N Engl J Med.* 1974; 291:83.

90. Bresler D, Bruder J, Mohnike K, et al. Serum MEPE-ASARM-peptides are elevated in X-linked rickets (HYP): implications for phosphaturia and rickets. *J Endocrinol.* 2004;183:1.
91. Bretscher A, Edwards K, Fehon RG. ERM proteins and merlin: integrators at the cell cortex. *Nat Rev Mol Cell Biol.* 2002;3:586.
92. Breusegem SY, Takahashi H, Giral-Arnal H, et al. Differential regulation of the renal sodium-phosphate cotransporters NaPi-IIa, NaPi-IIc, and PiT-2 in dietary potassium deficiency. *Am J Physiol. Renal Physiol.* 2009;297:F350–F361.
93. Brickman AS, Massry SG, Coburn JW. Changes in serum and urinary calcilum during treatment of hydrochlorothiazide studies on mechanisms. *J Clin Invest.* 1972;51:945.
94. Bringhurst FR, Demay MB, Kronenberg HM. eds. Hormones and disorders of mineral metabolism. In: Larsen PR, Kronenberg HM, Melmed S, Polonsky KS, eds. *Williams Textbook of Endocrinology*. Philadelphia: W.B. Saunders; 2003:1303.
95. Bronner F, Siepchenko B, Wood RJ, et al. The role of passive transport in calcium absorption [letter]. *J Nutr.* 2003;133:1426.
96. Brown EM, Gamba G, Riccardi D, et al. Cloning and characterization of an extracellular Ca2+-sensing receptor from bovine parathyroid. *Nature.* 1993;366:575–580.
97. Brown EM, Hebert SC. A cloned Ca^{2+}-sensing receptor; a mediator of direct effects of extracellular Ca^{2+} on renal function? *J Am Soc Nephrol.* 1995;6:1530.
98. Brunette MG, Vigneault N, Carriere S. Micropuncture study of magnesium transport along the nephron in the young rat. *Am J Physiol.* 1974;227:891.
99. Brunette MG, Vigneault N, Carriere S. Micropouncture study of renal magnesium transport in magnesium-loaded rats. *Am J Physiol.* 1975;229:1695.
100. Brunvand L, Haga P, Tangsrud SE, et al. Congestive heart failure caused by vitamin D deficiency? *Acta Paediatr.* 1995;84:106.
101. Buckle RH, Care AD, Cooper CW. The influence of plasma magnesium concentration on parathyroid hormone secretion. *J Endocrinol.* 1968;42:529.
102. Burgess TL, Qian Y-X, Kaufman S, Ring BD, et al. The ligand for osteoprotegrin (OPGL) directly activates mature osteoclasts. *J Cell Biol.* 1999;145:527.
103. Busch AE, Schuster A, Waldegger S. Expression of a renal type I sodium/phosphate transporter (NaPi-1) induces a conductance in Xenopus oocytes permeable for organic and inorganic anions. *Proc Natl Acad Sci U S A.* 1996;93:5347.
104. Butler AM, Talbot NB, Burnett CH. Metabolic studies in diabetic coma. *Trans Assoc Am Physicians.* 1947;60:102.
105. Caddell JL, Goddard DR. Studies in protein-calorie malnutrition 1. Chemical evidence for magnesium deficiency. *N Engl J Med.* 1967;275:533.
106. Caldas YA, Giral H, Cortazar MA, et al. Liver X receptor-activating ligands modulate renal and intestinal sodium-phosphate transporters. *Kidney Int.* 2011;80:535.
107. Cao TT, Deacon HW, Reczek D, et al. A kinase-regulated PDZ-domain interaction controls endocytic sorting of the beta2-adrenergic receptor. *Nature.* 1999;401:286.
108. Capuano P, Bacic D, Stange G, et al. Expression and regulation of the renal Na/phosphate cotransporter NaPi-IIa in a mouse model deficient for the PDZ protein PDZK1. *Pfluegers Arch.* 2004;449:392.
109. Carafoli E. Calcium pump of the plasma membrane. *Phys Rev.* 1991;71:129.
110. Carone FA. The effects upon the kidney of transient hypercalcemia induced by parathyroid extract. *Am J Pathol.* 1960;36:77.
111. Caroni P, Reinlib L, Carafoli E. Charge movements during the Na^{+}-Ca^{++} exchange in heart sarcolemmal vesicles. *Proc Natl Acad Sci U S A.* 1980;77:6354.
112. Carpenter TO, Insogna KL. eds. The hypocalcemic disorders: Differential diagnosis and therapeutic use of vitamin D. In: Feldman D, Glorieux FH, Pike JW, eds. *Vitamin D.* San Diego: Academic Press, 1997; 923.
113. Caverzasio J, Brown CD, Biber J, et al. Adaptation of phosphate transport in phosphate-deprived LLC-PK_1 cells. *Am J Physiol.* 1985;248:F122–F127.
114. Caverzasio J, Montessuit C, Bonjour J-P. Stimulatory effect of insulin-like growth factor-1 on renal Pi transport and plasma 1,25-dihydroxyvitamin D_3. *Endocrinol.* 1990;127:453.
115. Chabardes D, Imbert M, Clique A, Montegut M, Morel F. PTH sensitive adenyl cyclase activity in different segments of the rabbit nephron. *Pflugers Arch (Euro J Physiol).* 1975;354:229.
116. Chabardes D, Imbert-TeBoule M, Clique A. Distribution of calcitonin-sensitive adenylate cyclase along the rabbit kidney tubule. *Proc Natl Acad Sci U S A.* 1976;73:3608.
117. Chase LR, Melson GL, Aurbach GD. Pseudohypoparathyroidism: Defective excretion of 3′-5′-AMP in response to parathyroid hormone. *J Clin Invest.* 1969;48:1832.
118. Chase LR, Slatopolsky E. Secretion and metabolic efficacy of parathyroid hormone in patients with severe hypomagnesemia. *J Clin Endocrinol Metab.* 1974;38:363.
119. Chen TL, Hirst MA, Cone CM, Hochberg Z, Tietze H-U, Feldman D. 1,25-dihydroxyvitamin D resistance, rickets and alopecia: Analysis of receptors and bioresponse in cultured fibroblasts from patients and parents. *J Clin Endocrinol Metab.* 1984;59:383.
120. Chertow GM. Slowing the progression of vascular calcification in hemodialysis. *J Am Soc Neph.* 2003;14:S310–S314.
121. Chertow GM, Burke SK, Lazarus JM, et al. Poly[allylamine hydrochloride] (RenaGel): a noncalcemic phosphate binder for the tratment of hyperphosphatemia in chronic renal failure. *AJKD.* 1997;29:66.
122. Chertow GM, Burke SK, Dillon MA, et al. Long-term effects of sevelamer hydrochloride on the calcium × phosphate product and lipid profile of haemodialysis patients. *Nephrol Dial Transplant.* 1999;14:2907.
123. Chertow GM, Burke SK, Raggi P. Sevelamer attenuates the progression of coronary and aortic calcification in hemodialysis patients. *Kidney Int.* 2002;62:245.
124. Chesney PJ, Davis JP, Purdy WK, Wand PJ, Chesney RW. Clinical manifestations of toxic shock syndrome. *JAMA.* 1981;246:741.
125. Chiemchaisri H, Phillips PH. Certain factors including fluoride which affect magnesium calcinosis in the dog and rat. *J Nutrition.* 1965;86:23.
126. Chopra D, Janson P, Sawin CT. Insensitivity to digoxin associated with hypocalcemia. *N Engl J Med.* 1977;296:917.
127. Chou YH, Pollak MR, Brandi ML, et al. Mutations in the human Ca2+-sensing-receptor gene that cause familial hypocalciuric hypercalcemia. *Am J Hum Genet.* 1995;56:1075.
128. Coburn J, Slatopolsky E. eds. Vitamin D, PTH and renal osteodystrophy. In: Brenner B, Rector F, eds. *The Kidney*. Philadelphia: Saunders, 1981; 2213.
129. Coburn JW, Brautbar N. eds. Disease states and related to Vitamin D. In: Norman AW, Decker M, eds. *Vitamin D, Clinical and nutritional aspects*. New York: 1986.
130. Coburn JW, Massry SG. Changes in serum and urinary calcium during phosphate depletion: Studies on mechanisms. *J Clin Invest.* 1970;49:1073.
131. Coburn JW, Massry SG, DePalma JR. Rapid appearance of hypercalcemia with initiation of hemodialysis. *J Am Med Assoc.* 1969;210:2276.
132. Cohen EP, Trivedi C. Hypercalcemia from non-prescription vitamin A. *Nephrol Dial Transplant.* 2004;19:2929.
133. Cohen LF, Balow JE, Magrath IT, et al. Acute tumor lysis syndrome. A review of 37 patients with Burkitt's lymphoma. *Am J Med.* 1980;68:486.
134. Collins MT, Chebli C, Jones J, et al. Renal phosphate wasting in fibrous dysplasia of bone is part of a generalized renal tubular dysfunction similar to that seen in tumor-induced osteomalacia, *J Bone Miner Res.* 2001;16:806.
135. Connor TB, Rosen BL, Blaustein MP. Hypocalcemia precipitating congestive heart failure. *N Engl J Med.* 1982;307:869.
136. Connor TBP, Toskes J, Mahaffey LG. Parathyroid functon during chronic magnesium deficiency. *Johns Hopkins Med J.* 1972;131:100.
137. Connors MH, Irias JJ, Golabi M. Hypo-hyperparathyroidism: evidence for a defective parathyroid hormone. *Pediatrics.* 1977;60:343.
138. Constanzo LS. Localization of diuretic action in microperfused rat distal tubules; Ca and Na transport. *Nature.* 1990;347:388.
139. Cooke N, Teitelbaum S, Avioli LV. Antacid-induced osteomalacia and nephrolithiasis. *Arch Intern Med.* 1978;138:1007.
140. Corsi A, Collins MT, Riminucci M, et al. Osteomalacic and hyperparathyroid changes in fibrous dysplasia of bone: core biopsy studies and clinical correlations. *J Bone Miner Res.* 2003;18:1235.
141. Coulter-Mackie MB, Tung A, Henderson HE, et al. The AGT gene in Africa: a distinctive minor allele haplotype, a polymorphism (V326I), and a novel PH1 mutation (A112D) in black Africans. *Mol Genet Metab.* 2003;78:44.
142. Craddock PR, Yawata Y, Van Santen L, et ak. Acquired phagocyte dysfunction: A complication of the hypophosphatemia of parental hyperalimentation. *N Engl J Med.* 1974;290:1403.
143. Crook M, Swaminathan R, Schey S. Hypophosphataemia in patients undergoing bone marrow transplantation. *Leuk Lymphoma.* 1996;22:335.
144. Cuche JL, Ott CE, Marchand GR, Diaz-Buxo JA, Knox FG. Intrarenal calcium in phosphate handling. *Am J Physiol.* 1976;230:790.
145. Cummings KB, Robertson RP. Prostaglandin: Increased production by renal cell carcinoma. *J Urol.* 1977;118:720.
146. Dachille RD, Goldberg JS, Wexler ID, Shons AR. Fibrous dysplasia-induced hypocalcemia/rickets. *J Oral Maxillofac Surg.* 1990;48:1319.
147. Davies MR, Lund RJ, Hruska KA. BMP-7 is an efficacious treatment of vascular calcification in a murine model of atherosclerosis and chronic renal failure. *J Am Soc Nephrol.* 2003;14:1559.
148. Davies MR, Lund RJ, Mathew S, et al. Low turnover osteodystrophy and vascular calcification are amenable to skeletal anabolism in an animal model of chronic kidney disease and the metabolic syndrome. *J Am Soc Nephrol.* 2005;16:917–928.
149. Davis RH, Fourman P, Smith JWG. Prevalence of parathyroid insufficiency after thyroidectomy. *Lancet.* 1961;2:1432.
150. De Beur SM, Finnegan RB, Vassiliadis J, et al. Tumors associated with oncogenic osteomalacia express genes important in bone and mineral metabolism. *J Bone Miner Res.* 2002;17:1102.

151. De Niu P, Olsen HS, Gentz R, et al. Immunolocalization of stanniocalcin in human kidney. *Mol Cell Endocrinol.* 1998;137:155.

152. de Sanctis L, Vai S, Andreo MR, et al. Brachydactyly in 14 genetically characterized pseudohypoparathyroidism type Ia patients. *J Clin Endocrinol. Metab.* 2004;1989:1650.

153. DeFronzo RA, Cooke CR, Andres R. The effect of insulin on renal handling of sodium, potassium, calcium and phosphate in man. *J Clin Invest.* 1975;55:845.

154. DeFronzo RA, Goldberg M, Agus ZS. The effects of glucose and insulin on renal electrolyte transport. *J Clin Invest.* 1976;58:83.

155. DeFronzo RA, Lang R. Hypophosphatemia and glucose intolerance: evidence for tissue insensitivity to insulin. *N Engl J Med.* 1980;303:1259.

156. Denda M, Finch J, Slatopolsky E. Phosphorus accelerates the development of parathyroid hyperplasia and secondary hyperparathyroidism in rats with renal failure. *AJKD.* 1996;28:596.

157. Deol H, Stasko SE, De Niu P, et al. Post-natal ontogeny of stanniocalcin gene expression in rodent kidney and regulation by dietary calcium and phosphate. *Kidney Int.* 2001;60:2142.

158. DeRouffignac C, DiStefano A, Wittner M, et al. Consequences of different effects of ADH and other peptide hormones on thick ascending limb of mammalian kidney. *Am J Physiol.* 1991;260:R1023.

159. DeRouffignac C, Mandon B, Wittner M, et al. Hormonal control of renal magnesium handling. *Min Elec Metab.* 1993;19:226.

160. DeRouffignac C, Quamme G. Renal magnesium handling and its hormonal control. *Phys Rev.* 1994;74:305.

161. DiGeorge AM. Congenital absence of the thymus and its immunologic consequence: Concurrence with congenital hypoparathyroidism. *Birth Defects.* 1968; 4:16.

162. DiStefano A, Wittner M, Nitschke R, et al. Effects of glucagon on Na^+, Cl^-,K^+, Mg^{2+}, and Ca^{2+} transports in cortical medullary thick ascending limbs of mouse kidney. *Pflugers Arch.* 1989;414:640.

163. Ditzel J. Changes in red cell oxygen release capacity in diabetes mellitus. *Fed Proc.* 1979;38:2484.

164. Ditzler JW. Epsom salts poisoning and a review of magnesium-ion physiology. *Anesthesiology.* 1970;32:378.

165. Dominguez JH, Gray RW, Lemann JJ. Dietary phosphate deprivation in women and men: Effects on mineral and acid balances, parathyroid hormone and the metabolism of 25-OH-vitamin D. *J Clin Endocrinol Metab.* 1976;43:1056.

166. Dominguez JH, Juhaszova M, Feister HA. The renal sodium-calcium exchanger. *J Lab Clin Med..* 1992;119:640.

167. Dominguez JH, Mann C, Rothrock JK, et al. Na^+-Ca^{2+} exchange and Ca^{2+} depletion in proximal tubules. *Am J Physiol.* 1991;261:F328.

168. Dong Z, Saikumar P, Griess GA, et al. Intracellular Ca2+ thresholds that determine survival or death of energy-deprived cells. *Am J Pathol.* 1998;152;231.

169. Drezner M, Neelon FA, Lebovitz HE. Pseudohypoparathyroidism type II: A possible defect in the reception of the cyclic AMP signal. *N Engl J Med.* 1973;289:1056.

170. Driman DK, Kobrin MS, Kudlow JE, et al. Transforming growth factor-alpha in normal and neoplastic human endocrinal tissues. *Hum Pathol.* 1992;23:1360.

171. Duarte CG, Watson JG. Calcium reabsorption in proximal tubule of the dog nephron. *Am J Physiol.* 1967;212:1355.

172. Ducy P, Zhang R, Geoffroy V, et al. Osf2/Cbfa1: A transcriptional activator of osteoblast differentiation. *Cell* 1997;89:747.

173. Dudley HR, Ritchie AC, Schilling A. Pathological changes associated with the use of sodium ethylene diamine tetra-acetate in the treatment of hypercalcemia. *N Engl J Med.* 1955;252:331.

174. Dunlay R, Hruska KA. Parathyroid hormone receptor coupling to phospholipase C is an alternate pathway of signal transduction in the bone and kidney. *Am J Physiol.* 1990;258:F223–F231.

175. Dunn MJ. Magnesium depeletion in the rhesus monkey: Induction of magnesium-dependent hypocalcaemia. *Clin Sci Mol Med.* 1971;41:333.

176. Dusso AS, Lu Y, Pavlopoulos T, et al. A role of enhanced expression of transforming growth factor alpha (TGF-alpha) in the mitogenic effect of high dietary phosphorus on parathyroid cell growth in uremia. *J Am Soc Neph.* 1999;10;617.

177. Dyckner T, Webster PO. Ventricular extrasystoles and intracellular electrolytes before and after potassium and magnesium infusions in patients on diuretic therapy. *Am Heart J.* 1979;97:12.

178. Eberle M, Traynor-Kaplan AE, Sklar LA, et al. Is there a relationship between phosphatidylinositol trisphosphate and F-actin polymerization in human neutrophils? *J Biol Chem.* 1990;265:16725.

179. Edwards BR, Baer PG, Sutton RA, et al. Micropuncture study of diuretic effects on sodium and calcium reabsorption in the dog nephron. *J Clin Invest.* 1973;52:2418.

180. Elalouf JM, Roinel N, DeRouffignac C. ADH-like effects of calcitonin on electrolyte transport by Henle's loop of rat kidney. *Am J Physiol.* 1984;246: F213–F220.

181. Emmett M, Goldfarb S, Agus ZS, et al. The pathophysiology of acid-base changes in chronically phosphate-depleted rats: bone-kidney interactions. *J Clin Invest.* 1977;59:291.

182. Euzet S, Lelievre-Pegorier M, Merlet-Benichou C. Maturation of rat renal phosphate transport: effect of triiodothyronine. *J Physiol.* 1995;488 (Pt 2):449.

183. Euzet S, Lelievre-Pegorier M, Merlet-Benichou C. Effect of 3,5,3′-triiodothyronine on maturation of rat renal phosphate transport: kinetic characteristics and phosphate transporter messenger ribonucleic acid and protein abundance. *Endocrinology.* 1996;137:3522.

184. Evers C, Murer H, Kinne R. Effect of parathyrin on the transport properties of isolated renal brush-border vesicles. *Biochem J.* 1978;172:49.

185. Falls WFJ, Stacey WK. Postobstructive diuresis. Studies in a dialyzed patient with a solitary kidney. *Am J Med.* 1973;54:404.

186. Farrington K, Varghese Z, Newman SP, et al. Dissociation of absorptions of calcium and phosphate after successful cadaveric renal transplantation. *Br Med J.* 1979;1:712.

187. Feldman D, Chen T, Cone C, et al. Vitamin D resistant rickets with alopecia: cultured skin fibroblasts exhibit defective cytoplasmic receptors and unresponsiveness to $1,25(OH)_2D_3$. *J Clin Endocrinol Metab.* 1982;55:1020.

188. Feng JQ, Ward LM, Liu S, et al. Loss of DMP1 causes rickets and osteomalacia and identifies a role for osteocytes in mineral metabolism. *Nat Genet.* 2006;38:1310.

189. Filipovic D, Sackin H. A calcium-permeable stretch-activated cation channel in renal proximal tubule. *Am J Physiol.* 1991;260:F119.

190. Fleet JC, Wood RJ. Specific $1,25(OH)_2D_3$-mediated regulation of transcellular calcium transport in Caco-2 cells. *Am Physiol Soc.* 1999;276:G958–G964.

191. Flilnk EB, Stutzman FL, Anderson AR. Magnesium deficiency after prolonged parenteral fluid administration and after chronic alcoholism, complicated by delirium tremens. *J Lab Clin Med.* 1954;43:169.

192. Foley RN. Phosphorus comes of age as a cardiovascular risk factor. *Arch Intern Med.* 2007;167:873.

193. Folpe AL, Fanburg-Smith JC, Billings SD, et al. Most osteomalacia-associated mesenchymal tumors are a single histopathologic entity: an analysis of 32 cases and a comprehensive review of the literature. *Am J Surg Pathol.* 2004;28:1.

194. Freitag J, Martin K, Conrades M. Evidence for skeletal resistance to parathyroid hormone magnesium depletion. *J Clin Invest.* 1979;64:1238.

195. Frick A, Durasin I. Proximal tubular reabsorption of inorganic phosphate in adrenalectomized rats. *Pflugers Arch (Euro J Physiol).* 1980;385:189.

196. Friedman NE, Lobaugh B, Drezner MK. Effects of calcitriol and phosphorus therapy on the growth of patients with X-linked hypophosphatemia. *J Clin Endocrinol Metab.* 1993;76:839.

197. Friedman PA. Mechanisms of renal calcium transport. *Exp Nephrol.* 2000; 8:343.

198. Friedman PA, Andreoli TE. CO2-stimulated NaCl absorption in the mouse renal cortical thick ascending limb of Henle. Evidence for synchronous Na+/H+ and Cl/HCO3-exchange in apical plasma membranes. *J Gen Physiol.* 1982;80:683.

199. Friedman PA, Figueiredo JF, Maack T, et al. Sodium-calcium interactions in renal proximal convoluted tubule of the rabbit. *Am J Physiol.* 1981;240:F558.

200. Friedman PA, Gesek FA. Calcium transport in renal epithelial cells. *Am J Physiol.* 1993;264:F181.

201. Friedman PA, Gesek FA. Cellular calcium transport in renal epithelia: measurement, mechanisms, and regulation. *Physiol Rev* 1995;75:429.

202. Fu GK, Lin D, Zhang MY, et al. Cloning of human 25-hydroxyvitamin D-1 alpha-hydroxylase and mutations causing vitamin D-dependent rickets type 1. *Mol Endocrinol.* 1997;11:1961.

203. Fucentese M, Murer H, Biber J. Expression of rat renal Na/cotransport of phosphate and sulfate in Sf9 insect cells. *J Am Soc Nephrol.* 1994;5:860.

204. Fuchs R, Peterlik M. eds. Intestinal phosphate transport. In: Massry SG, Ritz E, Jahn H, eds. *Phosphate and Minerals in Health and Disease.* New York: Plenum Press; 1980:381.

205. Fuller TJ, Nichols WW, Brenner BJ, et al. Reversible depression in myocardial performance in dogs with experimental phosphorus deficiency. *J Clin Invest.* 1978;62:1194.

206. Fulop M, Brazeau P. The phosphaturic effect of sodium bicarbonate and acetazolamide in dogs. *J Clin Invest.* 1968;47:983.

207. Furuse M, Fujita K, Hiiragi T, et al. Claudin-1 and -2: Novel integral membrane proteins localizing at tight junctions with no sequence similarity to occludin*g. J Cell Biol.* 1998;141:1539.

208. Garabedian M, Silve C, Levy D, et al. Chronic hypophosphatemia in kidney transplanted children and young adults. *Adv Exp Med Biol.* 1980;128:249.

209. Gattineni J, Bates C, Twombley K, et al. FGF23 decreases renal NaPi-2a and NaPi-2c expression and induces hypophosphatemia in vivo predominantly via FGF receptor 1. *Am J Physiol Renal Physiol.* 2009;297:F282–F291.
210. Gazit D, Tieder M, Liberman UA, et al. Osteomalacia in hereditary hypophosphatemic rickets with hypercalciuria: a correlative clinical-histomorphometric study. *J Clin Endocrin Metab.* 1991;72:229.
211. Gekle DJ, Stroder J, Rostock D. The effect of vitamin D on renal inorganic phosphate reabsorption on normal rats, parathyroidectomized rats, and rats with rickets. *Pediatr Res.* 1971;5:40.
212. Genovese G, Friedman DJ, Ross MD, et al. Association of trypanolytic apoL1 variants with kidney disease in African Americans. *Science.* 2010;329:841.
213. Gesek FA, Friedman PA. Mechanism of calcium transport stimulated by chlorothiazide in mouse distal convoluted tubule cells. *J Clin Invest.* 1992;90:429.
214. Gesek FA, Friedman PA. On the mechanism of parathyroid hormone stimulation of calcium uptake by mouse distal convoluted tubule cells. *J Clin Invest.* 1992;90:749.
215. Gesek FA, Friedman PA. Calclitonin stimulates calcium transport in distal convoluted tubule cells. *Am J Physiol.* 1993;264:F744.
216. Ghent S, Judson MA, Rosansky SJ. Refractory hypotension associated with hypocalcemia and renal disease. *Am J Kidney Dis.* 1994;23:430.
217. Giebisch G, Berger L, Pitts RF. The extra-renal response to acute acid-base disturbances of respiratory origin. *J Clin Invest.* 1955;34:231.
218. Gill JR, Bartter FC. On the impairment of renal concentrating ability in prolonged hypercalcemia and hypercalciuria in man. *J Clin Invest.* 1961;49:16.
219. Giral H, Lanzano L, Caldas Y, et al. Role of PDZK1 protein in apical membrane expression of renal sodium-coupled phosphate transporters. *J Biol Chem.* 2011;286:15032.
220. Gisler SM, Madjdpour C, Bacic D, et al. PDZK1: II. An anchoring site for the PKA-binding protein D-AKAP2 in renal proximal tubular cells. *Kidney Int.* 2003;64:1746.
221. Gisler SM, Pribanic S, Bacic D, et al. PDZK1: I. A major scaffolder in brush borders of proximal tubular cells. *Kidney Int.* 2003;64:1733.
222. Gisler SM, Stagljar I, Traebert M, et al. Interaction of the type IIa Na/Pi cotransporter with PDZ proteins. *J Biol Chem.* 2001;276:9206.
223. Gitelman HJ, Graham JB, Welt LG. A new familial disorder characterized by hypokalemia and hypomagnesemia. *Trans Assoc Am Physicians.* 1966;79:221.
224. Glikman RM. Malabsorption: pathophysiology and diagnosis. In: Wyngaarden JB, Smith LHJ, eds. *Cecil's Textbook of Medicine.* Philadelphia: Saunders; 1985:710.
225. Glorieux FH, Marie PJ, Pettifor JM, et al. Bone response to phosphate salts, ergocalciferol, and calcitriol in hypophosphatemic vitamin D-resistant rickets. *N Engl J Med.* 1980;303:1023.
226. Gogusev J, Duchambon P, Stoermann-Chopard C, et al. De novo expression of transforming growth factor-alpha in parathyroid gland tissue of patients with primary or secondary uraemic hyperparathyroidism. *Nephrol Dial Transplant.*1996;11:2155.
227. Gold LW, Massry SG, Arieff AI, et al. Renal bicarbonate wasting during phosphate depletion: A possible cause of altered acid-base homeostasis in hyperparathyroidism. *J Clin Invest.* 1973;52:2556.
228. Gold LW, Massry SG, Friedler RM. Effect of phosphate depletion on renal tubular reabsorption of glucose. *J Lab Clin Med.* 1977;89:554.
229. Golden P, Mazey R, Greenwalt A, et al. Vitamin D: A direct effect on the parathyroid gland. *Miner Electrolyte Metab.* 1979;2:1.
230. Goldfarb S, Westby GR, Goldberg M, et al. Renal tubular effects of chronic phosphate depletion. *J Clin Invest.* 1977;59:770.
231. Goodman WG, Goldin J, Kuizon BD, et al. Coronary-artery calcification in young adults with end-stage renal disease who are undergoing dialysis. *N Engl J Med.* 2000;342:1478.
232. Goodyer PR, Kachra Z, Bell C, et al. Renal tubular cells are potential targets for epidermal growth factor. *Am J Physiol.* 1988;255:1191.
233. Gowen LC, Petersen DN, Mansolf AL, et al. Targeted disruption of the osteoblast/osteocyte factor 45 gene (OF45) results in increased bone formation and bone mass. *J Biol Chem.* 2003;278:1998.
234. Graf H, Kovarik J, Stummvoll HK, et al. Handling of phosphate by the transplanted kidney. *Proc Eur Dial Transplant Assoc.* 1979;16:624.
235. Granam LACJJ, Burger ASV. Gastrointestinal absorption and excretion of Mg^{28} in man. *Metabolism.* 1960;9:646.
236. Gray RW, Wilz DR, Caldas AE, et al. The importance of phosphate in regulating plasma $1,25(OH)_2$ vitamin D levels in humans: Studies in healthy subjects, in calcium-stone formers and in patients with primary hyperparathyroidism. *J Clin Endocrinol Metab.* 1977;45:299.
237. Green J, Debby H, Lederer E, et al. Evidence for a PTH-independent humoral mechanism in post-transplant hypophosphatemia and phosphaturia. *Kidney Int.* 2001;60:1182.
238. Grill V, Martin TJ. eds. Parathyroid hormone-related protein as a cause of hypercalcemia in malignancy. In: Bilezikian JP, Marcus R, Levine MA, eds. *The Parathyroids: Basic and Clinical Concepts.* New York: Raven Press; 1994:295.
239. Gucalp R, Theriault R, Gill I, et al. Treatment of cancer-associated hypercalcemia: Double-blind comparison of rapid and slow intravenous infusion regimens of pamidronate disodium and saline alone. *Arch Intern Med.* 1994;154:1935.
240. Guerin AP, London GM, Marchais SJ, et al. Arterial stiffening and vascular calcifications in end-stage renal disease. *Nephrol Dial Transplant.* 2000;15:1014.
241. Guignard JP, Jones NF, Barraclough MA. Effect of brief hypercalcemia on free water reabsorption during solute diuresis: Evidence for impairment of sodium transport in Henle's loop. *Clin Sci.* 1970;39:337.
242. Gunther W, Luchow A, Cluzeaud F, et al. ClC-5, the chloride channel mutated in Dent's disease, colocalizes with the proton pump in endocytotically active kidney cells. *Proc Natl Acad Sci U S A.* 1998;95:8075.
243. Guntupalli J, Eby B, Lau K. Mechanism for the phosphaturia of NH_4Cl: Dependence on acidemia but not on diet PO_4 or PTH. *Am J Physiol.* 1982;242: F552–F560.
244. Guo R, Liu S, Spurney RF, et al. Analysis of recombinant Phex: an endopeptidase in search of a substrate. *Am J Physiol Endocrinol Metab* 2001;281:837.
245. Gyory AZ, Stewart JH, George CR, et al. Renal tubular acidosis, due to hyperkalemia, hypercalcemia, disordered citrate metabolism and other tubular dysfunction following human renal transplantation. *Q J Med.* 1969;38:231.
246. Haas JA, Larson MV, Marchand GR, et al. Phosphaturic effect of furosemide: role of TH and carbonic anhydrase. *Am J Physiol.* 1977;232:F105–F110.
247. Habener JF, Potts JT Jr. Regulation of parathyroid hormone secretion in vitro. Quantitative aspects of calcium and magnesium ion control. *Endocrinology.* 1971;88:1477.
248. Habener JF, Potts JT Jr. Relative effectiveness of magnesium and calcium on the secretion and biosynthesis of parathyroid hormone *in vitro. Endocrinology.* 1976;98:197.
249. Habener JL, Mahaffey JE. Osteomalacia and disorders of vitamin D metabolism. *Ann Rev Med.* 1978;29:327.
250. Haldiman B, Goldstein DA, Akmal M. Renal function and blood levels of divalent ions in acute pancreatitis: A prospective study in 99 patients. *Miner Electrolyte Metab.* 1980;3:190.
251. Hamilton JW, Spierto FW, MacGregor RR. Studies on the biosynthesis in vitro of parathyroid hormone. II. The effect of calcium and magnesium on synthesis of parathyroid hormone isolated from bovine parathyroid tissue and incubation medium. *J Biol Chem.* 1971;246:3224.
252. Hammerman MR, Hruska KA. Cyclic AMP-dependent protein phosphorylation in canine renal brush-border membrane vesicles is associated with decreased Pi transport. *J Biol Chem.* 1982;257:992.
253. Haramati A, Haas JA, Knox FG. Adaptation of deep and superficial nephrons to changes in dietary phosphate intake. *Am J Physiol.* 1983;244:F265–F269.
254. Haramati A, Haas JA, Knox FG. Nephron heterogeneity of phosphate reabsorption: Effect of parathyroid hormone. *Am J Physiol.* 1984;246:F155–F158.
255. Harris BZ, Lim WA. Mechanism and role of PDZ domains in signaling complex assembly. *J Cell Sci.* 2001;114:3219.
256. Harris CA, Bauer PG, Chirito E, Dirks JH. Composition of mammalian glomerular filtrate. *Am J Physiol.* 1974;227:972.
257. Harris CA, Burnatowska MA, Seely JF. Effects of parathyroid hormone on electrolyte transport in the hampster nephron. *Am J Physiol.* 1979;236:342.
258. Hattenhauer O, Traebert M, Murer H, et al. Regulation of small intestinal Na-P(i) type IIb cotransporter by dietary phosphate intake. *Am J Physiol.* 1999;277:756.
259. Hayes G, Busch AE, Lang F, et al. Protein kinase C consensus sites and the regulation of renal Na/Pi-cotransport (NaPi-2) expressed in XENOPUS laevis oocytes. *Pflugers Arch (Euro J Physiol).* 1995;430:819.
260. Hebert SC, Brown EM. The scent of an ion: calcium-sensing and its roles in health and disease. *Curr Opin Nephrol Hypertens.* 1996;5:45.
261. Hebert SC, Culpepper RM, Andreoli TE. NaCl transport in mouse medullary thick ascending limbs: I. Functional nephron heterogeneity and ADH-stimulated NaCl co-transport. *Am J Physiol.* 1981;241:F412.
262. Herdman RC, Michael AF, Vernier RL, et al. Renal function and phosphorus excretion after human renal homotransplantation. *Lancet.* 1966;1:121.
263. Hernando N, Deliot N, Gisler SM, et al. PDZ-domain interactions and apical expression of type IIa Na/P(i) cotransporters. *Proc Natl Acad Sci U S A.* 2002;99:11957.
264. Hewison M, Rut AR, Kristjansson K, et al. Tissue resistance to 1,25-dihydroxyvitamin D without a mutation of the vitamin D receptor gene. *Clin Endocrinol.* 1993;39:663.
265. Hilfiker H, Hattenhauer O, Traebert M, et al. Characterization of a murine type II sodium-phosphate cotransporter expressed in mammalian small intestine. *Proc Natl Acad Sci U S A.* 1998;95:14564.

266. Hochberg Z, Weisman Y. Calcitriol-resistant rickets due to vitamin D receptor defects. *Trends Endocrinol Metab* 1995;6:216.
267. Hoenderop JG, Hartog A, Stuiver M, et al. Localization of the epithelial Ca^{2+} channel in rabbit kidney and intestine. *J Am Soc Nephrol.* 2000;11:1171.
268. Hoenderop JG, Nilius B, Bindels RJ. Molecular mechanisms of active Ca^{2+} reabsorption in the distal nephron. *Ann Rev Physiol.* 2002;64:529.
269. Hoenderop JG, Voets T, Hoefs S, et al. Homo- and heterotetrameric architecture of the epithelial Ca2+ channels, TRPV5 and TRPV6. *EMBO J.* 2003;22:776.
270. Hoenderop JGJ, vanderKemp AWCM, Hartog A, et al. Molecular identification of the apical Ca^{2+} channel in 1,25-dihydroxyvitamin D_3-responsive epithelia. *J Biol Chem.* 1999;274:8375.
271. Hoenderop JGJ, Willems PHGM, Bindels RJM. Toward a comprehensive molecular model of active calcium reabsorption. *Am J Physiol Renal.* 2000;278: F352–F360.
272. Hoffmann N, Thees M, Kinne R. Phosphate transport by isolated renal brush border vesicles. *Pflugers Arch (Euro J Physiol).* 1976;362:147.
273. Honig PJ, Holtzapple PG. Hypocalcemic tetany following hypertonic phosphate enemas. *Clin Pediatr.* 1975;14:678.
274. Hopkins T, Howard JE, Eisenberg H. Ultrafiltration studies on calcium and phosphorus in human serum. *Bull Johns Hopkins Hospital.* 1952;91:1.
275. Hoppe A, Metler M, Berndt TJ, et al. Effect of respiratory alkalosis on renal phosphate excretion. *Am J Physiol.* 1982;243:F471–F475.
276. Horton R, Biglieri EG. Effect of aldosterone on the metabolism of magnesium. *J Clin Endocrinol. Metab.* 1962;22:1187.
277. Horwitz MJ, Tedesco MB, Sereika SM, et al. Direct comparison of sustained infusion of human parathyroid hormone-related protein-(1-36) [hPTHrP-(1-36)] versus hPTH-(1-34) on serum calcium, plasma 1,25-dihydroxyvitamin D concentrations, and fractional calcium excretion in healthy human volunteers. *J Clin Endo Metab.* 2003;88:1603.
278. Howell RR. Essential fructosuria and hereditary fructose intolerance. In: Wyngaarden JB, Smith LHJ, eds. *Cecil's Textbook of Medicine*. Philadelphia: Saunders; 1985:1100.
279. Hruska KA, Mathew S. eds. The chronic kidney disease mineral bone disorder (CKD-MBD). *Primer on the Metabolic Bone Diseases and Disorders of Mineral Metabolism*, Philadelphia: Lippincott Williams & Wilkins, 2008.
280. Hruska KA. Pathophysiology of renal osteodystrophy. *Pediatr Nephrol.* 2000;14:636.
281. Hruska KA, Hammerman MR. Parathyroid hormone inhibition of phosphate transport in renal brush border vesicles from phosphate-depleted dogs. *Biochim Biophys Acta.* 1981;645:351.
282. Hruska KA, Mills SC, Khalifa S. Phosphorylation of renal brush border membrane vesicles of calcium uptake and membrane content of polyphosphoinositides. *J Biol Chem.* 1983;258:2501.
283. Huang CL. The transient receptor potential superfamily of ion channels. *J Am Soc Nephrol.* 2004;15:1690.
284. Huber TB, Schmidts M, Gerke P, et al. The carboxyl terminus of Neph family members binds to the PDZ domain protein zonula occludens-1. *J Biol Chem.* 2003;278:13417.
285. Hugo C, Nangaku M, Shankland SJ, et al. The plasma membrane-actin linking protein, ezrin, is a glomerular epithelial cell marker in glomerulogenesis, in the adult kidney and in glomerular injury. *Kidney Int.* 1998;54:1934.
286. Humes HD. Regulation of intracellular calcium. *Semin Nephrol.* 1984; 4(2):117.
287. Humes HD, Ichikawa I, Troy JL. Influence of calcium on the determinants of glomerular ultrafiltration. *Trans Assoc Am Physicians.* 1977;90:228.
288. Hung AY, Sheng M. PDZ domains: structural modules for protein complex assembly. *J Biol Chem.* 2002;277:5699.
289. Hurd TW, Gao L, Roh MH, et al. Direct interaction of two polarity complexes implicated in epithelial tight junction assembly. *Nat Cell Biol.* 2003;5:137.
290. Ichikawa S, Lyles KW, Econs MJ. A novel GALNT3 mutation in a pseudoautosomal dominant form of tumoral calcinosis: Evidence that the disorder is autosomal recessive. *J Clin Endocrinol Metab.* 2005;90:2420–2423.
291. Ichikawa S, Imel EA, Kreiter ML, et al. A homozygous missense mutation in human KLOTHO causes severe tumoral calcinosis. *J Clin Invest.* 2007;117:2684–2691.
292. Imai M. Calcium transport across the rabbit thick ascending limb of Henle's loop perfused in vitro. *Pflugers Arch.* 1978;374:255.
293. Ireland AW, Hornbrook HW, Neale FC. The crystalline lens in chronic surgical hypoparathyroidism. *Arc Intern Med.* 1968;122:408.
294. Ishibashi K, Imai M. Prospect of a stanniocalcin endocrine/paracrine system in mammals. *Am J Physiol Renal Physiol.* 2002;282:367.
295. Ishibashi K, Miyamoto K, Taketani Y, et al. Molecular cloning of a second human stanniocalcin homologue (STC2). *Biochem Biophys Res Commun.* 1998;250:252.
296. Ito H, Sanada T, Katayama T. Indomethacin-responsive hypercalcemia. *N Engl J Med.* 1975;293:558.
297. Ito M, Iidawa S, Izuka M, et al. Interaction of a farnesylated protein with renal type IIa Na/Pi co-transporter in response to parathyroid hormone and dietary phosphate. *Biochem J.* 2004;377:607.
298. Jacob HS, Amsden T. Acute hemolytic anemia and rigid red cells in hypophosphatemia. *N Engl J Med.* 1971;285:1446.
299. Jaffe BM, Parker CW, Philpott GW. Immunochemical measurement of prostaglandin or prostaglandin-like activity from normal and neoplastic cultured tissue. *Surg Forum.* 1971;22:90.
300. Jain A, Fedarko NS, Collins MT, et al. Serum levels of matrix extracellular phosphoglycoprotein (MEPE) in normal humans correlate with serum phosphorus, parathyroid hormone and bone mineral density. *J Clin Endocrinol Metab.* 2004;89:4158.
301. Jaureguiberry G, Carpenter TO, Forman S, et al. A novel missense mutation in SLC34A3 that causes hereditary hypophosphatemic rickets with hypercalciuria in humans identifies threonine 137 as an important determinant of sodium-phosphate cotransport in NaPi-IIc. *Am J Physiol Renal Physiol.* 2008;295:F371–F379.
302. Jayakumar A, Liang CT, Sacktor B. Na^{+} gradient-dependent Ca^{2+} transport in rat.
303. Jencks WP. How does a calcium pump pump calcium? *J Biol Chem.* 1989;264:18855.
304. Jentsch TJ, Gunther W. Chloride channels: an emerging molecular picture. *BioEssays.* 1997;19:117.
305. Jentsch TJ, Poet M, Fuhrmann JC, et al. Physiological functions of CLC Cl^{-} channels gleaned from human genetic disease and mouse models. *Annu Rev Physiol.* 2005;67:779.
306. Jones JE, Shane SR, Jacobs WH. Magnesium balance studies in chronic alcoholism. *N Y Acad Sci.* 1969;162:934.
307. Jonsson KB, Zahradnik R, Larsson T, et al. Fibroblast growth factor 23 in oncogenic osteomalacia and X-linked hypophosphatemia. *N Engl J Med.* 2003;348:1656.
308. Jowsey J, Riggs BL. Bone changes in a patient with hypervitaminosis. *J Clin Endocrinol. Metab.* 1968;28:1833.
309. Juan D, Elrazak MA. Hypophosphatemia in hospitalized patients. *JAMA.* 1979;242:163.
310. Kalbfleish JM, Lindeman RD, Ginn HE. Effects of ethanol administration on urinary excretion of magnesium and other electrolytes in alcoholic and normal subjects. *J Clin Invest.* 1963;42:1471.
311. Kammerman S, Canfield RE. Effect of porcine calcitonin on hypercalcemia in man. *J Clin Endocrinol.* 1970;31:70.
312. Karim Z, Gerard B, Bakouh N, et al. NHERF1 mutations and responsiveness of renal parathyroid hormone. *NEJM.* 2008;359:1128.
313. Karthikeyan S, Leung T, Ladias JA. Structural determinants of the Na+/H+ exchanger regulatory factor interaction with the beta 2 adrenergic and platelet-derived growth factor receptors. *J Biol Chem.* 2002;277:18973.
314. Katai K, Miyamoto K, Kishida S, et al. Regulation of intestinal Na+-dependent phosphate co-transporters by a low-phosphate diet and 1,25-dihydroxyvitamin D3. *Biochem J.* 1999;343 Pt 3:705.
315. Katai K, Tanaka H, Tatsumi S, et al. Nicotinamide inhibits sodium-dependent phosphate cotransport activity in rat small intestine. *Nephrol Dial Transplant.* 1999;14:1195.
316. Katz CM, Tzagournis M. Chronic adult hypervitaminosis A with hypercalcemia. *Metabolism.* 1972;21:1171.
317. Kavanaugh MP, Miller DG, Zhang W, et al. Cell-surface receptors for gibbon ape leukemia virus and amphotropic murine retroviruses are inducible sodium-dependent phosphate symporters. *Proc Natl Acad Sci U S A.* 1994;91:7071.
318. Keating MJ, Sethi MR, Bodey GP. Hypocalcemia with hypoparathyroidism and renal tubular dysfunction associated with aminoglycoside therapy. *Cancer.* 1977;39:1410.
319. Kempson SA, Lotscher M, Kaissling B, et al. Parathyroid hormone action on phosphate transporter mRNA and protein in rat renal proximal tubules. *Am J Physiol.* 1995;268:F784–F791.
320. Khalifa S, Mills SC, Hruska K. Stimulation of calcium uptake by parathyroid hormone in renal border membrane vesicles. *J Biol Chem.* 1983;258:400.
321. Kikuchi K, Ghishan FK. Phosphate transport by basolateral plasma membranes of human small intestine. *Gastroenterology.* 1987;93:106.
322. Kim YS, McDonald PN, Dedhar S, et al. Association of 1α,25-dihydroxyvitamin D3-occupied vitamin D receptors with cellular membrane acceptance sites. *Endocrinology.* 1996;137:3649.
323. Kitsiou-Tzeli S, Kolialexi A, Fryssira H, et al. Detection of 22q11.2 deletion among 139 pateints with Di George/Velo cardiofacial syndrome features. *In Vivo.* 2004;18:603.
324. Klahr S, Davis TA. Changes in renal function with chronic protein-calorie malnutrition. In: Mitch WE, Klahr S, eds. *Nutrition and the Kidney*. Boston: Little, Brown and Co; 1988:59.

325. Klahr S, Slatopolsky E. eds. Urinary phosphate and cyclic AMP in pseudohypoparathyroidism. In: Massry SG, Ritz E, Rapado A, eds. *Homeostasis of Phosphate and Other Minerals*. New York: Plenum; 1977:173.

326. Klein DC, Raisz LA. Prostaglandin stimulation of bone resorption in tissue culture. *Endocrinology.* 1970;86:1436.

327. Klock JC, Williams HE, Mentzer WC. Hemolytic anemia and somatic cell dysfunction in severe hypophosphatemia. *Arch Intern Med.* 1974;134:360.

328. Knochel JP. The pathophysiology and clinical characteristics of severe hyperphosphatemia. *Arch Intern Med.* 1977;137:203.

329. Knochel JP, Barcenas C, Cotton JR, et al. Hypophosphatemia and rhabdomyolysis. *J Clin Invest.* 1978;62:1240.

330. Knochel JP, Bilbrey GL, Fuller TJ. The muscle cell in chronic alcoholism: the possible role of phosphate depletion in alcoholic myopathy. *Ann N Y Acad Sci.* 1975;252:274.

331. Knohl SJ, Scheinman SJ. Inherited hypercalciuric syndromes: Dent's disease (CLC-5) and familial hypomagnesemia with hypercalciuria (paracellin-1). *Semin Nephrol.* 2004;24:55.

332. Knox FG, Osswald H, Marchand GR, et al. Phosphate transport along the nephron. *Am J Physiol.* 1977;233:F261–F268.

333. Knox FG, Preiss J, Kim JK, et al. Mechanism of resistance to the phosphaturic effect of the parathyroid hormone in the hamster. *J Clin Invest.* 1977;59:675.

334. Kocher O, Yesilaltay A, Cirovic C, et al. Targeted disruption of the PDZK1 gene in mice causes tissue-specific depletion of the high density lipoprotein receptor scavenger receptor class B type I and altered lipoprotein metabolism. *J Biol Chem.* 2003;278:52820.

335. Koffler A, Friedler RM, Massry SG. Acute renal failure due to nontraumatic rhabdomyolysis. *Ann Intern Med.* 1976;85:23.

336. Kong Y-Y, Yoshida H, Sarosi I, et al. OPGL is a key regulator of osteoclastogenesis, lymphocyte development and lymph-node organogenesis. *Nature.* 1999;397:315.

337. Kono N, Kuwajima M, Tarui S. Alteration of glycolytic intermediary metabolism in erythrocytes during diabetic ketoacidosis and its recovery phase. *Diabetes.* 1981;30:346.

338. Konrad M, Schlingmann KP, Gudermann T. Insights into the molecular nature of magnesium homeostasis. *Am J Physiol. Renal Physiol.* 2003;286:F599–F605.

339. Koulen P, Cai Y, Geng L, et al. Polycystin-2 is an intracellular calcium release channel. *Nature Cell Biol.* 2002;4:191.

340. Kreisberg RA. Phosphorus deficiency and hypophosphatemia. *Hosp Pract.* 1977;12:121.

341. Kretz J, Sommer G, Boland R, et al. Lack of involvement of sarcoplasmic reticulum in myopathy of acute phosphorus depletion. *Klin Wochenschr.* 1980;58:833.

342. Kreusser WJ, Kurokawa K, Aznar E. Effect of phosphate depletion on magnesium homeostasis in rats. *J Clin Invest.* 1978;61:573.

343. Kulkarni RN, Roper MG, Dahlgren G, et al. Islet secretory defect in insulin receptor substrate 1 null mice is linked with reduced calcium signaling and expression of sarco(endo)plasmic reticulum Ca2+-ATPase (SERCA)-2b and -3. *Diabetes.* 2004;1953:1517.

344. Kumar V, Bustin SA, McKay IA. Transforming growth factor alpha. *Cell Biol Int.* 1995;19:373.

345. Kuntziger HE, Amiel C, Couette S, et al. Localization of parathyroid-hormone-independent sodium bicarbonate inhibition of tubular phosphate reabsorption. *Kidney Int.* 1980;17:749.

346. Kurnik BR, Hruska KA. Effects of 1,25-dihydroxycholecalciferol on phosphate transport in vitamin D-deprived rats. *Am J Physiol.* 1984;247:F177–F184.

347. Kurz P, Monier-Faugere M-C, Bognar B, et al. Evidence for abnormal calcium homeostasis in patients with adynamic bone disease. *Kidney Int.* 1994;46:855–861.

348. L'Estrange JL, Axford RFE. A study of magnesium and calcium metabolism in lactating ewes semi-purified diet low in magnesium. *J Agric Sci.* 1964;62:353.

349. Lacey DL, Timms E, Tan H-L, et al. Osteoprotegrin ligand is a cytokine that regulates osteoclast differentiation and activation. *Cell.* 1998;93:165.

350. Lambert PP, Corvilan J. eds. Site of action of parathyroid hormone and role of growth hormone in phosphate excretion. In: Williams PC, eds. *Hormones and the Kidney (Memoirs of the Society of Endocrinology, No. 13)*. New York: Academic Press; 1963:130.

351. Lanzano L, Lei T, Okamura K, et al. Differential modulation of the molecular dynamics of the type IIa and IIc sodium phosphate cotransporters by parathyroid hormone. *Am J Physiol Cell Physiol.* 2011;301:C850–C861.

352. Larsson L, Rebel K, Sorbo B. Severe hypophosphatemia—a hospital survey. *Acta Med Scand.* 1983;214:221.

353. Larsson T, Marsell R, Schipani E, et al. Transgenic mice expressing fibroblast growth factor 23 under the control of the alpha1(I) collagen promoter exhibit growth retardation, osteomalacia, and disturbed phosphate homeostasis. *Endocrinology.* 2004;145:3087.

354. Larsson T, Zahradnik R, Lavigne J, et al. Immunohistochemical detection of FGF-23 protein in tumors that cause oncogenic osteomalacia. *Eur J Endocrinol.* 2003;148:269.

355. Laspa E, Bastepe M, Juppner H, et al. Phenotypic and molecular genetic aspects of pseudohypoparathyroidism type Ib in a Greek kindred: evidence for enhanced uric acid excretion due to parathyroid hormone resistance. *J Clin Endocrinol Metab.* 2004;1989;5942.

356. Lassiter WE, Gottschalk CW, Mylle M. Micropuncture study of tubular reabsorption of calcium in normal rodents. *Am J Physiol.* 1963;204:771.

357. Lau YK, Goldfarb S, Goldberg M. Effects of phosphate administration on tubular calcium transport. *J Lab Clin Med.* 1982;99:317.

358. Le Grimellec C, Roinel N, Morel F. Simultaneous Mg, Ca, P, K and Cl analysis in rat tubular fluid. IV. During acute phosphate plasma loading. *Pflugers Arch (Euro J Physiol).* 1974;346:189.

359. Lederer ED, Khundmiri SJ, Weinman EJ. Role of NHERF-1 in regulation of the activity of Na-K ATPase and sodium-phosphate co-transport in epithelial cells. *J Am Soc Nephrol.* 2003;14:1711.

360. Lederer ED, Sohi SS, McLeish KR. Parathyroid hormone stimulates extracellular signal-regulated kinase (ERK) activity through two independent signal transduction pathways: role of ERK in sodium-phosphate cotransport. *J Am Soc Nephrol.* 2000;11:222.

361. Lee JC, Catanzaro A, Parthemore JG. Hypercalcemia in disseminated coccidioidomycosis. *N Engl J Med.* 1977;297:431.

362. LeGrimellec C, Roinel N, Morel F. Simultaneous Mg, Ca, P, K, Na, and Cl analysis in rat tubular fluid: I. During perfusion of either insulin or ferrocyanide. *Pflugers Arch.* 1973;340:181.

363. Lennquist S, Lindell B, Nordstrom H, et al. Hypophosphatemia in severe burns: A prospective study. *Acta Chir Scand.* 1979;145:1.

364. Lentz RD, Brown DM, Kjellstrand CM. Treatment of severe hypophosphatemia. *Ann Intern Med.* 1978;89:941.

365. Levi J, Massry SG, Coburn JW. Hypocalcemia in magnesium depleted dogs: Evidence for reduced responsiveness to parathyoid hormone and relative failure of parathyroid gland function. *Metabolism.* 1974;23:323.

366. Levi M. Post-transplant hypophosphatemia. *Kidney Int.* 2001;59:2377.

367. Levi M. Role of PDZ domain-containing proteins and ERM proteins in regulation of renal function and dysfunction. *J Am Soc Nephrol.* 2003;14:1949.

368. Levi M, Kempson SA, Lotscher M, et al. Molecular regulation of renal phosphate transport. *J Membrane Biology.* 1996;154:1.

369. Levi M, Lotscher M, Sorribas V, et al. Cellular mechanisms of acute and chronic adaptation of rat renal P(i) transporter to alterations in dietary P(i). *Am J Physiol.* 1994;267:F900–F908.

370. Levi M, Shayman JA, Abe A, et al. Dexamethasone modulates rat renal brush border membrane phosphate transporter mRNA and protein abundance and glycosphingolipid composition. *J Clin Invest.* 1995;96:207.

371. Levi M. Novel NaPi-2c mutations that cause mistargeting of NaPi-2c protein and uncoupling of Na-Pi cotransport cause HHRH. *Am J Physiol Renal Physiol.* 2008;295:F369–F370.

372. Levi M, Breusegem S. Renal phosphate–transporter regulatory proteins and nephrolithiasis. *N Engl J Med.* 2008;359:1171.

373. Levine BS, Kleeman CR. Hypophosphatemia and hyperphosphatemia: clinical and pathophysiologic aspects. In: Maxwell MH, Kleeman CR, eds. *Clinical Disorders of Fluid and Electrolyte Metabolism*. New York: McGraw-Hill; 1994:1040.

374. Levine MA. Resistance to multiple hormones in patients with pseudohypoparathyroidism: Association with deficient activity of guanine nucleotide regulatory protein. *Am J Med.* 1983;74:545.

375. Levine MA, Jap TS, Mauseth RS, et al. Activity of the stimulatory guanine nucleotide-binding protein is reduced in erythrocytes from patients with pseudohypoparathyroidism and pseudopseudohypoparathyroidism: Biochemical, endocrine, and genetic analysis of Albright's hereditary osteodystrophy in six kindreds. *J Clin Endocrinol. Metab.* 1986;62:497.

376. Levine MA, Schwindinger WF, Downs RW Jr, Moses AM. Pseudohypoparathyroidism: Clinical, biochemical, and molecular features. In: Bilezikian JP, Marcus R, Levine MA, eds. *The Parathyroids: Basic and Clinical Concepts*. New York: Raven Press; 1994:781.

377. Levitt MF, Halpern MH, Polimeros DP. The effect of abrupt changes in plasma calcium concentrations on renal function and electrolyte excretion in man and monkey. *J Clin Invest.* 1958;37:294.

378. Levy LA. Severe hypophosphatemia as a complication of the treatment of hypothermia. *Arch Intern Med.* 1980;140:128.

379. Levy-Litan V, Hershkovitz E, Avizov L, et al. Autosomal-recessive hypophosphatemic rickets is associated with an inactivation mutation in the ENPP1 gene. *Am J Hum Genet.* 2010;86:273.

380. Li HY, Dai LJ, Quamme GA. Effect of chemical hypoxia on intracellular ATP and cytosolic levels. *J Lab Clin Med.* 1993;122:232.

381. Li X, Yang HY, Giachelli CM. Role of the sodium-dependent phosphate cotransporter, Pit-1, in vascular smooth muscle cell calcification. *Circ Res.* 2006;98:905–912.
382. Li YC, Amling M, Pirro AE, et al. Normalization of mineral ion homeostasis by dietary means prevents hyperparathyroidism, rickets, and osteomalacia, but not alopecia in vitamin D receptor-ablated mice. *Endocrinology.* 1998;139:4391.
383. Li YC, Pirro AE, Amling M, et al. Targeted ablation of the vitamin D receptor: An animal model of vitamin D-dependent rickets type II with alopecia. *Proc Natl Acad Sci U S A.* 1997;94:9831.
384. Liang CT, Barnes J, Cheng L, et al. Effects of 1,25(OH)$_2$D$_3$ administered in vivo on phosphate uptake by isolated chick renal cells. *Am J Physiol.* 1982;242:C312–C318.
385. Liberman UA, Eil C, Marx SJ. Resistance of 1,25 dihydroxyvitamin D. Associated with heterogeneous defects in cultured skin fibroblasts. *J Clin Invest.* 1983;71:192.
386. Lichtenstein L. Polyostotic fibrous dysplasia. *Arch Surg.* 1938;36:874.
387. Lichtenstein L, Jaffe HL. Fibrous dysplasia of bone: a condition affecting one, several or many bones, the graver case of which may present abnormal pigmentation of skin, premature sexual development, hyperthyroidism and still other extraskeletal abnormalities. *Arch Pathol.* 1942;33:777.
388. Lichtman MA, Miller DR, Cohen J, Waterhouse C. Reduced red cell glycolysis, 2,3-diphosphoglycerate and adenosine triphosphate concentration and increased hemoglobin-oxygen affinity caused by hypophosphatemia. *Ann Intern Med.* 1971;74:562.
389. Liedtke CM, Yun CH, Kyle N, et al. Protein kinase C epsilon-dependent regulation of cystic fibrosis transmembrane regulator involves binding to a receptor for activated C kinase (RACK1) and RACK1 binding to Na+/H+ exchange regulatory factor. *J Biol Chem.* 2002;277:22925.
390. Lipschitz MD, Stein JH. Renal vasoactive homrones. In: Brenner B, Rector F, eds. *The Kidney*. Philadelphia: Saunders; 1981:650.
391. Liu J, Nealon JG, Weinstein LS. Distinct patterns of abnormal GNAS imprinting in familial and sporadic pseudohypoparathyroidism type IB. *Hum Mol Genet.* 2005;1914:95.
392. Liu S, Guo R, Simpson LG, et al. Regulation of fibroblastic growth factor 23 expression but not degradation by PHEX. *J Biol Chem.* 2003;278:37419.
393. Liu S, Guo R, Tu Q, et al. Overexpression of Phex in osteoblasts fails to rescue the Hyp mouse phenotype. *J Biol Chem.* 2002;277:3686.
394. Lloyd SE, Pearce SHS, Fisher SE, et al. A common molecular basis for three inherited kidney stone diseases. *Nature.* 1996;379:445.
395. Loffing J, Loffing-Cueni D, Valderrabano V, et al. Distribution of transcellular calcium and sodium transport pathways along mouse distal nephron. *Am J Phys (Renal).* 2001;291:F1021–F1027.
396. Loffing J, Lotscher M, Kaissling B, et al. Renal Na/H exchanger NHE-3 and Na-PO4 cotransporter NaPi-2 protein expression in glucocorticoid excess and deficient states. *J Am Soc Nephrol.* 1998;9:1560.
397. London GM, Dannier B, Marchais SJ, et al. Calcification of the aortic valve in the dialyzed patient. *J Am Soc Nephrol.* 2000;11:778.
398. London GM, Guerin AP, Marchais SJ, et al. Arterial media calcification in end-stage renal diseases: impact on all-cause and cardiovascular mortality. *Nephrol Dial Transplant.* 2003;18:1731.
399. London GM, Marty C, Marchais SJ, et al. Arterial calcifications and bone histomorphometry in end-stage renal disease. *J Am Soc Neph.* 2004;15:1943.
400. Lorenz-Depiereux B, Bastepe M, et-Pages A, et al. DMP1 mutations in autosomal recessive hypophosphatemia implicate a bone matrix protein in the regulation of phosphate homeostasis. *Nat Genet.* 2006;38:1248.
401. Lorenz-Depiereux B, Schnabel D, Tiosano D, et al. Loss-of-function ENPP1 mutations cause both generalized arterial calcification of infancy and autosomal-recessive hypophosphatemic rickets. *Am J Hum Genet.* 2010;86:267.
402. Lotscher M, Kaissling B, Biber J, et al. Role of microtubules in the rapid regulation of renal phosphate transport in response to acute alterations in dietary phosphate content. *J Clin Invest.* 1997;99:1302.
403. Lotscher M, Wilson P, Nguyen S, et al. New aspects of adaptation of rat renal Na-Pi cotransporter to alterations in dietary phosphate. *Kidney Int.* 1996;49:1012.
404. Lotz M, Ney R, Bartter FC. Osteomalacia and debility resulting from phosphorus depletion. *Trans Ass Amer Physicians.* 1964;77:281.
405. Lotz M, Zisman E, Bartter FC. Evidence for a phosphorus-depletion syndrome in man. *N Engl J Med.* 1968;278:409.
406. Lu M, Wagner GF, Renfro JL. Stanniocalcin stimulates phosphate reabsorption by flounder renal proximal tubule in primary culture. *Am J Physiol.* 1994;267:1356.
407. Lufkin EG, Kumar R, Heath H III. Hyperphosphatemic tumoral calcinosis: effects of phosphate depletion on vitamin D metabolism, and of acute hypocalcemia on parathyroid hormone secretion and action. *J Clin Endocrinol Metab.* 1983;56:1319.
408. Lufkin EG, Wilson DM, Smith LH, et al. Phosphorus excretion in tumoral calcinosis: Response to parathyroid hormone and acetazolamide. *J Clin Endocrinol Metab.* 1980;50:648.
409. Lufkin EG, Wilson DM, Smith LH, et al. Phosphorus excretion in tumoral calcinosis: response to parathyroid hormone and acetazolamide. *J Clin Endocrinol Metab.* 1980;50:648.
410. Lyles KW, Burkes EJ, Ellis GJ, et al. Genetic transmission of tumoral calcinosis: autosomal dominant with variable clinical expressivity. *J Clin Endocrinol Metab.* 1985;60:1093.
411. Macefield G, Burke D. Parasthesiae and tetany induced by voluntary hyperventilation: Increased excitability of human cutaneous and motor axons. *Brain.* 1991;114:527.
412. MacManus J, Heaton FW. The influence of magnesium in calcium release from bone in vitro. *Biochim Biophys Acta.* 1970;215:360.
413. Madsen KL, Tavernini MM, Yachimec C, et al. Stanniocalcin: a novel protein regulating calcium and phosphate transport across mammalian intestine. *Am J Physiol.* 1998;274:96.
414. Magagnin S, Werner A, Markovich D, et al. Expression cloning of human and rat renal cortex Na/Pi cotransport. *Proc Natl Acad Sci U S A.* 1993;90:5979.
415. Magen D, Berger L, Coady MJ, et al. A loss-of-function mutation in NaPi-IIa and renal fanconi's syndrome. *N Engl J Med.* 2010;362:1102.
416. Magyar CE, White KE, Rojas R, et al. Plasma membrane Ca2+-ATPase and NCX1 Na+/Ca2+ exchanger expression in distal convoluted tubule cells. *Am J Phys (Renal).* 2002;283:F29–F40.
417. Mahon MJ, Donowitz M, Yun CC, et al. Na(+)/H(+) exchanger regulatory factor 2 directs parathyroid hormone 1 receptor signalling. *Nature.* 2002;417:858.
418. Mallette LE, Bilezikian JP, Heath DA. Primary hyperparathyroidism: Clinical and biochemical features. *Medicine.* 1974;83:127.
419. Malloy PJ, Hochberg Z, Pike JW, et al. Abnormal binding of vitamin D receptors to deoxyribonucleic acid in a kindred with vitamin D-dependent rickets, type II. *J Clin Endocrinol Metab.* 1989;68:263.
420. Malluche HH, Meyer-Sabellek WA, Singer FR. Evidence for a direct effect of thiazides on bone. *Miner Electrolyte Metab.* 1980;4:89.
421. Malluche HH, Ritz E, Lange HP. Bone histology in incipient and advanced renal failure. *Kidney Int.* 1976;9:355–362.
422. Manitius A, Levitin H, Beck D. On the mechanism of impairment of renal concentrating ability in hypercalcemia. *J Clin Invest.* 1960;39:693.
423. Mann JB, Alterman S, Hills AG. Albright's hereditary osteodystrophy comprising pseudohypoparathyroidism. *Ann Intern Med.* 1962;36:315.
424. Mantovani G, Bondioni S, Locatelli M, et al. Biallelic expression of the Gs{alpha} gene in human bone and adipose tissue. *J Clin Endocrinol Metab.* 2004;1989;6316.
425. Mantovani G, de Sanctis L, Barbieri AM, et al. Pseudohypoparathyroidism and GNAS epigenetic defects: clinical evaluation of Albright hereditary osteodystrophy and molecular analysis in 40 patients. *J Clin Endocrinol Metab.* 2010;95:651.
426. Markowitz GS, Stokes MB, Radhakrishnan J, et al. Acute phosphate nephropathy following oral sodium phosphate bowel purgative: an underrecognized cause of chronic renal failure. *J Am Soc Nephrol.* 2005;16:3389.
427. Marx SJ, Spiegel AM, Brown EM. Divalent cation metabolism: Familial hypocalciuric hypercalcemia versus typical primary hyperparathyroidism. *Am J Med.* 1978;65:235.
428. Marx SJ, Stock JL, Attie MF. Familial hypocalciuric hypercalcemia: Recognition among patients referred after unsuccessful parathyroid exploration. *Ann Intern Med.* 1980;92:351.
429. Massari PU. Disorders of bone and mineral metabolism after renal transplantation. *Kidney Int.* 1997;52:1412.
430. Massry SG, Arieff AI, Coburn JW, et al. Divalent ion metabolism in patients with acute renal failure: studies on the mechanism of hypocalcemia. *Kidney Int.* 1974;5:437.
431. Massry SG, Coburn JW, Chapman LW, et al. Effect of NaCl infusion on urinary Ca^{++} and Mg^{++} during reduction in their filtered loads. *Am J Physiol.* 1967;213:1218.
432. Massry SG, Coburn JW, Kleeman CR. Renal handling of magnesium in the dog. *Am J Physiol.* 1969;216:1460.
433. Massry SG, Mueller E, Silverman AG. Inorganic phosphate treatment of hypercalcemia. *Intern Med* 1968;12:307.
434. Mathew S, Tustison KS, Sugatani T, et al. The mechanism of phosphorus as a cardiovascular risk factor in chronic kidney disease. *J Am Soc Nephrol.* 2008;19:1092–1105.
435. Matzner Y, Procócimer M, Polliack A, et al. Hypophosphatemia in a patient with lymphoma in leukemic phase. *Arch Intern Med.* 1981;141:805.
436. Maudsley S, Zamah AM, Rahman N, et al. Platelet-derived growth factor receptor association with Na(+)/H(+) exchanger regulatory factor potentiates receptor activity. *Mol Cell Biol.* 2000;20:8352.

437. Mayock RL, Bertrand P, Morrison CE. Manifestations of sarcoidosis: Analysis of 145 patients, with review of nine selected from the literature. *Am J Med.* 1963;35:67.

438. McCarty NA, O'Neil RG. Dihydropyridine-sensitive cell volume regulation in proximal tubule: the calcium window. *Am J Physiol.* 1990;259:950.

439. McCarty NA, O'Neil RG. Calcium-dependent control of volume regulation in renal proximal cells. II. Roles of dihydropyridine-sensitive and insensitive Ca^{2+} entry pathways. *J Membr Biol.* 1991;123:161.

440. McCarty NA, O'Neil RG. Calcium-dependent control of volume regulation in renal proximal cells. I. Swelling-activated Ca^{2+} entry and release. *J Membr Biol.* 1991;123:149.

441. McConnell TH. Fatal hypocalcemia from phosphate absorption from laxative preparation. *JAMA.* 1971;216:147.

442. McCormick CC. Passive diffusion does not play a major role in the absorption of dietary calcium in normal adults. *J Nutr.* 2002;132:3428.

443. McCune DJ, Bruch H. Progress in pediatrics: osteodystrophia fibrosa. *Am J Dis Child.* 1937;54:806.

444. McMillan DE, Freeman RB. The milk alkali syndrome: A study of the acute disorder with comments on the development of the chronic condition. *Medicine.* 1965;44:485.

445. McPhaul MJ, Marcelli M, Zoppi S, et al. Genetic basis of endocrine disease. 4. The spectrum of mutations in the androgen receptor gene that causes androgen resistance. *J Clin Endocrinol Metab.* 1993;76:17.

446. Meintzer RB, Steenbock H. Vitamin D and magnesium absorption. *J Nutr.* 1955;56:285.

447. Mendelsoh JH, Barnes B, Mayman C. The determination of exchangeable magnesium in alcoholic patients. *Metabolism.* 1965;14:88.

448. Mercado A, Slatopolsky E, Klahr S. On the mechanisms responsible for the phosphaturia of bicarbonate administration. *J Clin Invest.* 1975;56:1386.

449. Miller ER, Ullrey DE, Zutaut CL. Effect of dietary vitamin D2 levels upon calcium, phosphorus and magnesium balance. *J Nutr.* 1965;85:255.

450. Miller ER, Ullrey DE, Zutaut CL. Magnesium requirement of the baby pig. *J Nutr.* 1965;85:13.

451. Miller MJ, Frame B, Poyanski A. Branchial anomalies in idiopathic hypoparathyroidism: Branchial dysembryogenesis. *Henry Ford Hosp Med J.* 1972;20:3.

452. Milliner DS, Zinsmeister AR, Lieberman L, et al. Soft tissue calcification in pediatric patients with end-stage renal disease. *Kidney Int.* 1990;38:931.

453. Miric A, Vechio JD, Levine MA. Heterogeneous mutations in the gene encoding the alpha subunit of the stimulatory G protein of adenylyl cyclase in Albright hereditary osteodystrophy. *J Clin Endocrinol Metab.* 1993;76:1560.

454. Mitnick PD, Goldbarb S, Slatopolsky E, et al. Calcium and phosphate metabolism in tumoral calcinosis. *Ann Intern Med.* 1980;92:482.

455. Mitnick PD, Goldfarb S, Slatopolsky E, et al. Calcium and phosphate metabolism in tumoral calcinosis. *Ann Intern Med.* 1980;92:482.

456. Moe OW. Scaffolds: Orchestrating proteins to achieve concerted function. *Kidney Int.* 2003;64:1916.

457. Moe SM, Chertow GM, Coburn JW, et al. Achieving NKF-K/DOQI™ bone metabolism and disease treatment goals with cinacalcet HCl. *Kidney Int.* 2005;67:760.

458. Moorhead JF, Wills MR, Ahmed KY, et al. Hypophosphataemic osteomalacia after cadaveric renal transplantation. *Lancet.* 1974;1:694.

459. Morel F. Sites of hormone action in the mammalian nephron. *Am J Physiol.* 1981;240:F159.

460. Morel F, Chabardes D, Imbert M. Functional segmentation of the rabbit distal tubule by microdetermination of hormone dependent adenylate cyclase activity. *Kidney Int.* 1976;9:264.

461. Morel F, Roinel N, LeGrimellec C. Electron probe analysis of tubular fluid composition. *Nephron.* 1969;6:350.

462. Morgan DB. eds. Calcium and phosphorus transport across the intestine. In: Girdwood RM, Smith AW, eds. *Malabsorption*. Baltimore: Williams & Wilkins; 1969.

463. Moriniere PH, Roussel A, Tahira Y, et al. Substitution of aluminum hydroxide by high doses of calcium carbonate in patients on chronic hemodialysis: disappearance of hyperalbuminemia and equal control of hyperparathyroidism. *Proc Eur Dial Transplant Assoc.* 1982;19:784.

464. Moser CR, Fessel WJ. Rheumatic manifestations of hypophosphatemia. *Arch Intern Med.* 1974;134:674.

465. Mostellar ME, Tuttle EPJ. Effects of alkalosis on plasma concentration and urinary excretion of urinary phosphate in man. *J Clin Invest.* 1964;43:138.

466. Mueller B, Zhao M, Negrashov IV, et al. SERCA structural dynamics induced by ATP and calcium. *Biochemistry.* 2004;43:12846.

467. Muhlbauer RC, Bonjour J-P, Fleisch H. Tubular handling of Pi: localization of effects of $1,25(OH)_2D_3$ and dietary Pi in TPTX rats. *Am J Physiol.* 1981; 241:F123–F128.

468. Mühlbauer RC, Bonjour JP, Fleisch H. Tubular localization to dietary phosphate in rats. *Am J Physiol.* 1978;234:F342–F348.

469. Mulder JE, Bilezikian JP. eds. Acute management of hypercalcemia. In: Bilezikian JP, Marcus R, Levine MA, eds. *The Parathyroids: Basic and Clinical Concepts*. San Diego: Academic Press; 2001:729.

470. Mundy GR. Evaluation and treatment of hypercalcemia. *Hosp Prac.* 1994; 29:79.

471. Mundy GR, Luben RA, Raisz LG. Evidence for the secretion of an osteoclast stimulating factor in myeloma. *N Engl J Med.* 1974;291:1041.

472. Murer H, Forster I, Biber J. The sodium phosphate cotransporter family SLC34. *Pflugers Arch.* 2004;447:763.

473. Murer H, Hernando N, Forster I, et al. Regulation of Na/Pi transporter in the proximal tubule. *Annu Rev Physiol.* 2003;65:531.

474. Murphy E, Mandel JL. Cytosolic free calcium levels in rabbit proximal kidney tubules. *Am J Physiol.* 1982;242:6124.

475. Nagant de Deuxchaisnes C, Krane SM. eds. Hypoparathyroidism. In: Avioli LV, Krane SM, eds. *Metabolic Bone Disease*. New York: Academic Press; 1978:217.

476. Nakashima K, Zhou X, Kunkel G, et al. The novel zinc finger-containing transcription factor osterix is required for osteoblast differentiation and bone formation. *Cell.* 2002;108:17.

477. Naren AP, Cobb B, Li C, et al. A macromolecular complex of beta 2 adrenergic receptor, CFTR, and ezrin/radixin/moesin-binding phosphoprotein 50 is regulated by PKA. *Proc Natl Acad Sci U S A.* 2003;100:342.

478. Neer RM, Potts JT Jr. Medical management of hypercalcemia and hyperparathyroidism. In: DeGroot LJCGF, Martini L, eds. *Endocrinology*. New York: Grune & Stratton; 1979:725.

479. Nelson AE, Bligh RC, Mirams M, et al. Clinical case seminar: Fibroblast growth factor 23: a new clinical marker for oncogenic osteomalacia. *J Clin Endocrinol Metab.* 2003;88:4088.

480. Nemere I, Norman AW. The rapid, hormonally stimulated transport of calcium (transcaltachia). *J Bone Miner Res.* 1987;2:167.

481. Nicoll DA, Longoni S, Philipson KD. Molecular cloning and functional expression of the cardiac sarcolemmal Na^+-Ca^{2+} exchanger. *Science.* 1990;250:562.

482. Nijenhuis T, Hoenderop JGJ, Van Der Kemp AWCM, et al. Localization and regulation of the epithelial Ca^{2+} channel TRPV6 in the kidney. *J Am Soc Neph.* 2003;14:2731.

483. Nusynowitz ML, Frame B, Kolb FO. The spectrum of the hypoparathyroid states: A classification based on physiologic principles. *Medicine.* 1976;55:105.

484. Nutter DO, Glenn JR. Reversible severe congestive cardiomyopathy in three cases of hypophoisphatemia. *Ann Intern Med.* 1983;99:275.

485. O'Donovan DJ, Lotspeich WD. Activation of kidney mitochondrial glutaminase by inorganic phosphate and organic acids. *Nature.* 1966;212:930.

486. Ohkido I, Segawa H, Yanagida R, et al. Cloning, gene structure and dietary regulation of the type-IIc Na/Pi cotransporter in the mouse kidney. *Pflugers Arch.* 2003;446:106.

487. Ohkido I, Yokoyama K, Kagami S, et al. The hypothesis that bone turnover influences FGF23 secretion. *Kidney Int.* 2010;77:743.

488. Olgaard K, Madsen S, Lund B, et al. Pathogenesis of hypophosphatemia in kidney necrograft recipients: a controlled trial. *Adv Exp Med Biol.* 1980;128:255.

489. Olsen HS, Cepeda MA, Zhang QQ, et al. Human stanniocalcin: a possible hormonal regulator of mineral metabolism. *Proc Natl Acad Sci U S A.* 1996; 93:1792.

490. Orlando RA, Takeda T, Zak B, et al. The glomerular epithelial cell anti-adhesin podocalyxin associates with the actin cytoskeleton through interactions with ezrin. *J Am Soc Nephrol.* 2001;12:1589.

491. Orwoll ES. The milk-alkali syndrome: Current concepts. *Ann Intern Med.* 1982;97:242.

492. Pabico RC, McKenna BA. Metabolic problems in renal transplant patients. Persistent hyperparathyroidism and hypophosphatemia: effects of intravenous calcium infusion. *Transplant Proc.* 1988;20:438.

493. Pallais JC, Kifor O, Chen YB, et al. Acquired hypocalciuric hypercalcemia due to autoantibodies against the calcium-sensing receptor. *N Engl J Med.* 2004;351:362.

494. Palmer LG, Frindt G. Amiloride-sensitive Na channels from the apical membrane of the rat cortical collecting tubule. *Proc Natl Acad Sci U S A.* 1986; 83:2767.

495. Palmer PE. Tumoural calcinosis. *Br J Radiol.* 1966;39:518.

496. Panda DK, Miao D, Bolivar I, et al. Inactivation of the 25-hydroxyvitamin D 1α-hydroxylase and vitamin D receptor demonstrates independent and interdependent effects of calcium and vitamin D on skeletal and mineral homeostasis. *J Biol Chem.* 2004;279:16754.

497. Parfitt AM. The interactions of thiazide diuretics with parathyroid hormone and vitamin D: Studies in patients with hypoparathyroidism. *J Clin Invest.* 1972;51:1879.

498. Parfitt AM. The spectrum of hypoparathyroidism. *J Clin Endocrinol Metab.* 1972;34:152.
499. Parfitt AM. The hyperparathyroidism of chronic renal failure: a disorder of growth. *Kidney Int.* 1997;52:3.
500. Parfitt AM, Kleerekoper M, Cruz C. Reduced phosphate reabsorption unrelated to parathyroid hormone after renal transplantation: implications for the pathogenesis of hyperparathyroidism in chronic renal failure. *Miner Electrolyte Metab.* 1986;12:356.
501. Parker MS, Klein I, Haussler MR, et al. Tumor-induced osteomalacia: Evidence of a surgically correctable alteration in vitamin D metabolism. *JAMA.* 1981;245:492.
502. Pastoriza-Munoz E, Colindres RE, Lassiter WE, et al. Effect of parathyroid hormone on phosphate reabsorption in rat distal convolution. *Am J Physiol.* 1978;235:F321–F330.
503. Patrie KM, Drescher AJ, Goyal M, et al. The membrane-associated guanylate kinase protein MAGI-1 binds megalin and is present in glomerular podocytes. *J Am Soc Nephrol.* 2001;12:667.
504. Patrie KM, Drescher AJ, Welihinda A, et al. Interaction of two actin-binding proteins, synaptopodin and alpha-actinin-4, with the tight junction protein MAGI-1. *J Biol Chem.* 2002;277:30183.
505. Patten JL, Levine MA. Immunochemical analysis of the α-subunit of the stimulatory G-protein of adenylyl cyclase in patients with Albright's hereditary osteodystrophy. *J Clin Endocrinol Metab.* 1990;71:1208.
506. Peacock M, Bilezikian JP, Klassen PS, et al. Cinacalcet hydrochloride maintains long-term normocalcemia in patients with primary hyperparathyroidism. *J Clin Endo Metab.* 2005;90:135.
507. Pearce SHS, Brown EM. Calcium-sensing receptor mutations: insights into a structurally and functionally novel receptor. *J Clin Endo Metab.* 1996;81:1309.
508. Peraino RA, Suki WN. Phosphate transport by isolated rabbit cortical collecting tubule. *Am J Physiol.* 1980;238:F358–F362.
509. Pitts RF, Alexander RS. The renal reabsorptive mechanism for inorganic phosphate in normal and acidotic dogs. *Am J Physiol.* 1944;142:648.
510. Pizurki L, Rizzoli R, Caverzasio J, et al. Effect of transforming growth factor-alpha and parathyroid hormone-related protein on phosphate transport in renal cells. *Am J Physiol.* 1990;259:929.
511. Pollak MR, Brown EM, Chou YH, et al. Mutations in the human Ca2+-sensing receptor gene cause familial hypocalciuric hypercalcemia and neonatal severe hyperparathyroidism. *Cell.* 1993;75:1297.
512. Pollak MR, Brown EM, Chou YH, et al. Mutations in the human Ca^{2+}-sensing receptor gene cause familial hypocalciuric hypercalcemia and neonatal severe hyperparathyroidism. *Cell.* 1993;75:1297.
513. Pollak MR, Brown EM, Estep HL, et al. Autosomal dominant hypocalcaemia caused by a Ca^{2+}-sensing receptor gene mutation. *Nat Genet.* 1994;8:303.
514. Popovtzer MM, Subryan VL, Alfrey AC. The acute effect of chlorothiazide on serum ionized calcium: Evidence for a parathyroid hormone-dependent mechanism. *J Clin Invest.* 1975;55:1295.
515. Poulos PP. The renal tubular reabsorption and urinary excretion of calcium by the dog. *J Lab Clin Med.* 1957;49:253.
516. Pribanic S, Gisler SM, Bacic D, et al. Interactions of MAP17 with the NaPi-IIa/PDZK1 protein complex in renal proximal tubular cells. *Am J Physiol Renal Physiol.* 2003;285:784.
517. Pribanic S, Loffing J, Madjdpour C, et al. Expression of visinin-like protein-3 in mouse kidney. *Nephron Physiol.* 2003;95:76.
518. Prie D, Beck L, Friedlander G, et al. Sodium-phosphate cotransporters, nephrolithiasis and bone demineralization. *Curr Opin Nephrol Hypertens.* 2004;13:675.
519. Prie D, Beck L, Silve C, et al. Hypophosphatemia and calcium nephrolithiasis. *Nephron Exper Nephrol.* 2004;98:50.
520. Prie D, Huart V, Bakouh N, et al. Nephrolithiasis and osteoporosis associated with hypophosphatemia caused by mutations in the type 2a sodium-phosphate cotransporter. *N Engl J Med.* 2002;347:983.
521. Prince MJ, Schaeffer PC, Goldsmith RS, et al. Hyperphosphatemic tumoral calcinosis: association with elevation of serum 1,25-dihydroxycholecalciferol concentrations. *Ann Intern Med.* 1982;96:586.
522. Prins JG, Schrijver H, Staghouwer JM. Hyperalimentation, hypophosphatemia and coma. *Lancet.* 1973;1:1253.
523. Pritchard JA. The use of magnesium ion in the management of eclamptogenic toxemias. *Surg Gynecol Obstet.* 1955;100:131.
524. Pruyne D, Evangelista M, Yang C, et al. Role of formins in actin assembly: nucleation and barbed-end association. *Science.* 2002;297:612.
525. Pullman TN, Lavender AR, Aho I, et al. Direct renal action of a purified parathyroid extract. *Endocrinology.* 1960;67:570.
526. Puschett JB, Goldberg M. The relationship between the renal handling of phosphate and bicarbonate in man. *J Lab Clin Med.* 1969;73:956.
527. Quamme GA. Effect of calcitonin and magnesium transport in the rat nephron. *Am J Physiol.* 1980;238:573.
528. Quamme GA. Influence of volume expansion on Mg influx into the superficial proximal tubule. *Kidney Int.* 1980;17:721A.
529. Quamme GA. Effect of hypercalcemia on renal tubular handling of calcium and magnesium. *Canadian J Physiol Pharmacol.* 1982;60:1275.
530. Quamme GA. Urinary alkalinization may not result in an increase in urinary phosphate excretion. *Kidney Int.* 1984;25:150.
531. Quamme GA. Renal magnesium handling: new insights in understanding old problems. *Kidney Int.* 1997;52:1180.
532. Quamme GA, Carney SC, Wong NLM. Effect of parathyroid hormone on renal calcium and magnesium reabsorption in magnesium deficient rats. *Pflugers Arch.* 1980;58:1.
533. Quamme GA, De Rouffignac C. Renal magnesium handling. In: Selding D, Giebisch G, eds. *The Kidney.* Lippincott Williams and Williams; 2004:1711.
534. Quamme GA, Dirks JH. Intraluminal and contraluminal magnesium on magnesium and calcium transfer in the rat nephron. *Am J Physiol.* 1980;238:F187–F198.
535. Quamme GA, Mizgala CL, Wong NLM, et al. Effects of intraluminal pH and dietary phosphate on phosphate transport in the proximal convoluted tubule. *Am J Physiol.* 1985;249:F759–F768.
536. Quarles LD. Evidence for a bone-kidney axis regulating phosphate homeostasis. *J Clin Invest.* 2003;112:642.
537. Quarles LD. FGF23, PHEX, and MEPE regulation of phosphate homeostasis and skeletal mineralization. *Am J Physiol Endocrinol Metab.* 2003;285:1.
538. Raanani P, Berkowicz M, Harden I, et al. Severe hypophosphataemia in autograft recipients during accelerated leucocyte recovery. *Br J Haematol.* 1995;91:1031.
539. Raggi P, Boulay A, Chasan-Taber S, et al. Cardiac calcification in adult hemodialysis patients. A link between end-stage renal disease and cardiovascular disease? *J Am Coll Cardiol.* 2002;39:695.
540. Raghuram V, Mak DD, Foskett JK. Regulation of cystic fibrosis transmembrane conductance regulator single-channel gating by bivalent PDZ-domain-mediated interaction. *Proc Natl Acad Sci U S A.* 2001;98:1300.
541. Ramachandran C, Brunette MG. Renal Na/Ca^{2+} exchange system is located exclusively in the distal tubule. *Biochem J.* 1989;257:259.
542. Randall RE Jr, Chen MD, Spray CC. Hypermagnesemia in renal failure. *Ann Intern Med.* 1949;61:73.
543. Rasmussen H, Fontaine O, Max EE, et al. Effect of 1alpha-hydroxy-vitamin D_3 administration on calcium transport in chick intestine brush border membrane vesicles. *J Biol Chem.* 1979;254:2993.
544. Refetoff S, Weiss RE, Usala SJ. The syndromes of resistance to thyroid hormone. *Endocrine Rev.* 1993;14:348.
545. Reilly RF, Shugrue CA. cDNA cloning of a renal Na^+/Ca^{2+} exchanger. *Am J Physiol.* 1992;262:F1105–F1109.
546. Ribeiro CP, Mandel LJ. Parathyroid hormone inhibits proximal tubule. *Am J Physiol.* 1992;262:F209–F216.
547. Ribeiro S, Ramos A, Brandao A, et al. Cardiac valve calcification in haemodialysis patients: role of calcium-phosphate metabolism. *Nephrol Dial Transplant.* 1998;13:2037.
548. Riccardi D, Park J, Lee WS, et al. Cloning and functional expression of a rat kidney extracellular calcium/polyvalent cation-sensing receptor. *Proc Natl Acad Sci U S A.* 1995;92:131.
549. Riedler GF, Scheitlin WA. Hypophosphatemia in septicemia: Higher incidence in gram-negative than in gram-positive infections. *Br Med J.* 1969;1:753.
550. Riminucci M, Collins MT, Fedarko NS, et al. FGF-23 in fibrous dysplasia of bone and its relationship to renal phosphate wasting. *J Clin Invest.* 2003;112:683.
551. Riminucci M, Fisher LW, Shenker A, et al. Fibrous dysplasia of bone in the McCune-Albright syndrome: abnormalities in bone formation. *Am J Pathol.* 1997;151:1587.
552. Rocha AS, Magaldi JB, Kokko JP. Calcium and phosphate transport in isolated segments of rabbit Henle's loop. *J Clin Invest.* 1977;59:975.
553. Rodriguez HJ, Villareal H, Klahr S. Pseudohypoparathyroidism type II: Restoration of normal renal responsiveness to parathyroid hormone by calcium administration. *J Clin Endocrinol Metab.* 1974;39:693.
554. Rosen LS, Gordon D, Kaminski M, et al. Zoledronic acid versus pamidronate in the treatment of skeletal metastases in patients with breast cancer or osteolytic lesions of multiple myeloma: a phase III, double-blind comparative trial. *Cancer J.* 2001;7:377.
555. Rosenbaum RW, Hruska KA, Korkor A, et al. Decreased phosphate reabsorption after renal transplantation: Evidence for a mechanism independent of calcium and parathyroid hormone. *Kidney Int.* 1981;19:568.
556. Rosenbaum RW, Hruska KA, Korkor A, et al. Decreased phosphate reabsorption after renal transplantation: Evidence for a mechanism independent of calcium and parathyroid hormone. *Kidney Int.* 1981;19:568.

557. Rosental R, Babarykin D, Fomina O, et al. Hypophosphatemia after successful transplantation of the kidney. Clinico-experimental study. *Z Urol Nephrol.* 1982;75:393.
558. Rostand SG, Sanders C, Kirk KA, et al. Myocardial calcification and cardiac dysfunction in chronic renal failure. *Am J Med.* 1988;85:651.
559. Roth KS, Foreman JW, Segal S. The Fanconi syndrome and mechanisms of tubular dysfunction. *Kidney Int.* 1981;20:705.
560. Rouse D, Ng RCK, Suki WN. Calcium transport in the pars recta and thin descending limb of Henle of the rabbit, perfused in vitro. *J Clin Invest.* 1980;65:37.
561. Rowe PS. The wrickkened pathways of FGF23, MEPE and PHEX. *Crit Rev Oral Biol Med.* 2004;15:264.
562. Rowe PS, de Zoysa PA, Dong R, et al. MEPE, a new gene expressed in bone marrow and tumors causing osteomalacia. *Genomics.* 2000;67:54.
563. Rowe PS, Garrett IR, Schwarz PM, et al. Surface plasmon resonance (SPR) confirms that MEPE binds to PHEX via the MEPE-ASARM motif: a model for impaired mineralization in X-linked rickets (HYP). *Bone.* 2005;36:33.
564. Rowe PS, Kumagai Y, Gutierrez G, et al. MEPE has the properties of an osteoblastic phosphatonin and minhibin. *Bone.* 2004;34:303.
565. Rowe PSN, Ong ACM, Cockerill FJ, et al. Candidate 56 and 58 kDa protein(s) responsible for mediating the renal defects in oncogenic hypophosphatemic osteomalacia. *Bone.* 1996;18:159.
566. Rude RK. Magnesium deficiency in parathyroid function. In: Bilezikian JP, Marcus R, Levine MA, eds. *The Parathyroids: Basic and Clinical Concepts.* San Diego: Academic Press; 2001:763.
567. Rude RK, Oldham SB, Singer FR. Functional hypoparathyroidism and parathyroid hormone organ resistance in human magnesium deficiency. *Clin Endocrinol.* 1976;5:209.
568. Rutherford E, Mercado A, Hruska K, et al. An evaluation of a new and effective phosphate binding agent. *Trans Am Soc Artif Intern Organs.* 1973;19:446.
569. Ryan WG, Nibbe AF, Schwartz TB, et al. Fibrous dysplasia of bone with vitamin D resistant rickets: a case study. *Metabolism.* 1968;17:988.
570. Ryback RS, Eckardt MJ, Pautler CP. Clinical relationships between serum phosphorus and other blood chemistry values in alcoholics. *Arch Intern Med.* 1980;140:673.
571. Sacktor B. Transport in membrane vesicles isolated from the Mammalian kidney and intestine. In: Sanadi R, ed. *Current Topics in Bioenergetics.* New York: Academic Press; 1977:30.
572. Saito H, Kusano K, Kinosaki M, et al. Human fibroblast growth factor-23 mutants suppress Na+-dependent phosphate co-transport activity and 1alpha,25-dihydroxyvitamin D3 production. *J Biol Chem.* 2003;278:2206.
573. Sakamoto A, Liu J, Greene A, et al. Tissue-specific imprinting of the G protein Gs{alpha} is associated with tissue-specific differences in histone methylation. *Hum Mol Genet.* 2004;1913:819.
574. Sakhaee K, Brinker K, Helderman JH, et al. Disturbances in mineral metabolism after successful renal transplantation. *Miner Electrolyte Metab.* 1985;11:167.
575. Salander H, Tisell LE. Incidence of hypoparathyroidism after radical surgery for thyroid carcinoma and autotransplantation of parathyroid glands. *Am J Surg.* 1977;134:358.
576. Saunders Y, Ross JR, Broadley KE, et al. Systematic review of bisphosphonates for hypercalcaemia of malignancy. *Palliat Med.* 2004;18:418.
577. Schatzmann HJ. The red cell calcium pump. *Ann Rev Physiol.* 1983;45:303.
578. Scheinman SJ. X-linked hypercalciuric nephrolithiasis: Clinical syndromes and chloride channel mutations. *Kidney Int.* 1998;53:3.
579. Schiavi SC, Kumar R. The phosphatonin pathway: New insights in phosphate homeostasis. *Kidney Int.* 2004;65:1.
580. Schilsky RL, Anderson T. Hypomagnesemia and renal magnesium wasting in patients receiving cisplatin. *Ann Intern Med.* 1979;90:926.
581. Schneider AB, Sherwood LM. Pathogenesis and management of hypoparathyroidism and hypocalcemic disorders. *Metabolism.* 1975;24:871.
582. Schwab SJ, Hammerman MR. Mechanisms of phosphate exit across the basolateral membrane of the renal proximal tubule cell. *Clin Res.* 1984;32:530.
583. Scoble J, Mills S, Hruska KA. Calcium transport (Ca^{2+}) in renal basolateral vesicles (BLMV): Effects of parathyroid hormone (PTH). *J Clin Invest.* 1985;75:1096.
584. Segawa H, Kaneko I, Takahashi A, et al. Growth-related renal type II Na/Pi cotransporter. *J Biol Chem.* 2002;277:19665.
585. Segawa H, Kaneko I, Yamanaka S, et al. Intestinal Na-P(i) cotransporter adaptation to dietary P(i) content in vitamin D receptor null mice. *Am J Physiol Renal Physiol.* 2004;287:39.
586. Segawa H, Kawakami E, Kaneko I, et al. Effect of hydrolysis-resistant FGF23-R179Q on dietary phosphate regulation of the renal type-II Na/Pi transporter. *Pflugers Arch.* 2003;446:585.
587. Seldin DW, Tarail R. The metabolism of glucose and electrolytes in diabetic acidosis. *J Clin Invest.* 1950;29:552.
588. Seller RH, Cangiano J, Kim EE. Digitalis toxicity and hypomagnesemia. *Am Heart J.* 1970;79:57.
589. Seyberth HW, Segre GV, Hamet P. Characterization of the group of patients with hypercalcemia of cancer who respond to treatment with prostaglandin synthesis inhibitors. *Trans Assoc Am Physicians.* 1976;89:92.
590. Shanahan CM, Cary NRB, Metcalfe JC, et al. High expression of genes for calcification-regulating proteins in human atherosclerotic plaques. *J Clin Invest.* 1994;93:2393.
591. Shareghi GR, Agus ZS. Magnesium transport in the cortical thick ascending limb of Henle's loop of the rabbit. *J Clin Invest.* 1982;69:759.
592. Shareghi GR, Agus ZS. Phosphate transport in the light segment of the rabbit cortical collecting tubule. *Am J Physiol.* 1982;242:F379–F384.
593. Shareghi GR, Stoner LC. Calcium transport across segments of the rabbit distal nephron in vitro. *Am J Physiol.* 1978;235:F367.
594. Shenolikar S, Voltz JW, Cunningham R, et al. Regulation of ion transport by the NHERF family of PDZ proteins. *Physiology (Bethesda).* 2004;19:362.
595. Shenolikar S, Voltz JW, Minkoff CM, et al. Targeted disruption of the mouse NHERF-1 gene promotes internalization of proximal tubule sodium-phosphate cotransporter type IIa and renal phosphate wasting. *Proc Natl Acad Sci U S A.* 2002; 99:11470.
596. Shenolikar S, Weinman EJ. NHERF: targeting and trafficking membrane proteins. *Am J Physiol Renal Physiol.* 2001;280:389.
597. Sherwood LM, Santora AC. Hypoparathyroid states in the differential diagnosis of hypocalcemia. In: Bilezikian JP, Marcus R, Levine MA, eds. *The Parathyroids: Basic and Clinical Concepts.* New York: Raven Press; 1994:747.
598. Shields HM. Rapid fall of serum phosphorus secondary to antacid therapy. *Gastroenterology.* 1978;75:1137.
599. Shils ME. Experimental human magnesium depletion. *Medicine.* 1969;48:61.
600. Shimada T, Hasegawa H, Yamazaki Y, et al. FGF-23 is a potent regulator of vitamin D metabolism and phosphate homeostasis. *J Bone Miner Res.* 2004; 19:429.
601. Shimada T, Kakjitani M, Hasegawa H, et al. Targeted ablation of FGF-23 causes hyperphosphatemia. Increased 1,25-dihydroxyvitamin D level and severe growth retardation. *J Bone Min Res.* 2002;17(1):S168.
602. Shimada T, Mizutani S, Muto T, et al. Cloning and characterization of FGF23 as a causative factor of tumor-induced osteomalacia. *Proc Natl Acad Sci U S A.* 2001;98:6500.
603. Shimada T, Muto T, Urakawa I, et al. Mutant FGF-23 responsible for autosomal dominant hypophosphatemic rickets is resistant to proteolytic cleavage and causes hypophosphatemia in vivo. *Endocrinology.* 2002;143:3179.
604. Shimada T, Urakawa I, Yamazaki Y, et al. FGF-23 transgenic mice demonstrate hypophosphatemic rickets with reduced expression of sodium phosphate cotransporter type IIa. *Biochem Biophys Res Commun.* 2004;314:409.
605. Shimizu T, Nakamura M, Yoshitomi K. Interaction of trichlormethiazide or amiloride with PTH in stimulating calcium absorption in the rabbit connecting tubule. *Am J Physiol.* 1991;261:F36.
606. Shimizu T, Yoshitomi K, Nakamura M. Effect of parathyroid hormone on the connecting tubule from the rabbit kidney: Biphasic response of transmural voltage. *Pflugers Arch.* 1990;416:257.
607. Shimizu T, Yoshitomi K, Nakamura M, et.al. Effects of PTH, calcitonin, and cAMP on calcium transport in rabbit distal nephron segments. *Am J Physiol.* 1990;259:F408–F414.
608. Shirley DG, Poujeol P, LeGrimellec C. Phosphate, calcium and magnesium fluxes into the lumen of the rat proximal convoluted tubule. *Pflugers Arch.* 1976;362:247.
609. Shirley DG, Faria NJR, Unwin RJ, et al. Direct micropuncture evidence that matrix extracellular phosphoglycoprotein inhibits proximal tubular phosphate reabsorption. *Nephrol Dial Transplant.* 2010;25:3191.
610. Silver J, Neale G, Thompson GR. Effect of phenobarbitone treatment on vitamin D metabolism in mammals. *Clin Sci Mol Med.* 1974;46:433.
611. Silver J, Sela SB, Naveh-Man T. Regulation of parathyroid cell proliferation. *Curr Opin Nephrol Hypertens.*1997;6:321.
612. Silvis SE, DiBartolomeo AG, Aaker HM. Hypophosphatemia and neurologic changes secondary to oral caloric intake: A variant of hyperalimentation syndrome. *Am J Gastroenterol.* 1980;73:215.
613. Simon DB, Lu Y, Chaote KA, et al. Paracellin-I, a renal tight junction protein required for paracellular Mg^{2+} resorption. *Science.* 1999;285:103.
614. Simon DB, Nelson-Williams C, Bia MJ, et al. Gitelman's variant of Bartter's syndrome, inherited hypokalaemic alkalosis, is caused by mutations in the thiazide-sensitive Na-Cl cotransporter. *Nat Genet.* 1996;12:24.
615. Singer FR, Neer RM, Murray JM. Mithramycin treatment of intractable hypercalcemia due to parathyroid adenomas. *N Engl J Med.* 1970;283:634.

616. Singer FR, Ritch PS, Lad TE. Treatment of hypercalcemia of malignancy with intravenous etidronate. *Arch Intern Med.* 1991;151:471.

617. Singer FR, Sharp CF, Rude RK. Pathogenesis of hypercalcemia in malignancy. *Miner Electrolyte Metab.* 1979;2:161.

618. Siris ES, Sherman WH, Baguiran DC. Effects of dichloromethylene-diphosphonate on skeletal mobilization of calcium in multiple myeloma. *N Engl J Med.* 1980;302:310.

619. Sitara D, Razzaque MS, Hesse M, et al. Homozygous ablation of fibroblast growth factor-23 results in hyperphosphatemia and impaired skeletogenesis, and reverses hypophosphatemia in Phex-deficient mice. *Matrix Biol.* 2004; 23:421.

620. Slatopolsky E. Pathophysiology of calcium, magnesium and phosphorus. In: Klahr S, ed. *The Kidney and Body Fluids in Health and Disease*. New York: Plenum Press; 1984:269.

621. Slatopolsky E, Burke SK, Dillon MA. RenaGel, a nonabsorbed calcium and aluminum-free phosphate-binder, lowers serum phosphorus and parathyroid hormone. *Kidney Int.* 1999;55:299.

622. Slatopolsky E, Caglar S, Gradowska L, et al. On the prevention of secondary hyperparathyroidism in experimental chronic renal disease using "proportional reduction" of dietary phosphorus intake. *Kidney Int.* 1972;2:147.

623. Slatopolsky E, Finch J, Denda M, et al. Phosphorus restriction prevents parathyroid gland growth. High phosphorus directly stimulates PTH secretion in vitro. *J Clin Invest.* 1996;97:2534.

624. Slatopolsky E, Gradowska L, Kashemsant C. The control of phosphate excretion in uremia. *J Clin Invest.* 1966;45:672.

625. Slatopolsky E, Robson AM, Elkan I, et al. Control of phosphate excretion in uremic man. *J Clin Invest.* 1968;47:1865–1874.

626. Slatopolsky E, Weerts C, Lopez-Hilker S, et al. Calcium carbonate as a phosphate binder in patients with chronic renal failure undergoing dialysis. *N Engl J Med.* 1986;315:157.

627. Slatopolsky E, Weerts C, Norwood K, et al. Long-term effects of calcium carbonate and 2.5 mEq/liter calcium dialysate on mineral metabolism. *Kidney Int.* 1989;36:897.

628. Slatopolsky E, Weerts C, Thielan J. Marked suppression of secondary hyperparathyroidism by intravenous administration of 1,25-dihydroxycholecalciferol in uremic patients. *J Clin Invest.* 1984;74:2136.

629. Slavin RE, Wen J, Kumar D, et al. Familial tumoral calcinosis. A clinical, histopathologic, and ultrastructural study with an analysis of its calcifying process and pathogenesis. *Am J Surg Pathol.* 1993;17:788.

630. Slinin Y, Foley RN, Collins AJ. Calcium, phosphorus, parathyroid hormone, and cardiovascular disease in hemodialysis patients: The USRDS waves 1, 3, and 4 Study. *J Am Soc Nephrol.* 2005;16:1788–1793.

631. Smith EL, Gilligan C. Exercise and bone mass. In: DeLuca HF, Mazess R, eds. *Osteoporosis: Physiological Basis, Assessment and Treatment*. New York: Elsevier Science Publishing; 1990:285.

632. Smith EP, Boyd J, Frank GR, et al. Estrogen resistance caused by a mutation in the estrogen receptor gene in a man. *N Engl J Med.* 1994;331:1088.

633. Smith WJ, Nassar N, Bretscher A, et al. Structure of the active N-terminal domain of Ezrin. Conformational and mobility changes identify keystone interactions. *J Biol Chem.* 2003;278:4949.

634. Sneddon WB, Magyar CE, Willick GE, et al. Ligand-selective dissociation of activation and internalization of the parathyroid hormone (PTH) receptor: conditional efficacy of PTH peptide fragments. *Endocrinology.* 2004;145:2815.

635. Sorribas V, Lotscher M, Loffing J, et al. Cellular mechanisms of the age-related decrease in renal phosphate reabsorption. *Kidney Int.* 1996;50:855.

636. Sorribas V, Markovich D, Hayes G, et al. Cloning of a Na/Pi cotransporter from opossum kidney cells. *J Biol Chem.* 1994;269:6615.

637. Sorribas V, Markovich D, Verri T, et al. Thyroid hormone stimulation of Na/Pi-cotransport in opossum kidney cells. *Pflugers Arch.* 1995;431:266.

638. Stauber A, Radanovic T, Stange G, et al. Regulation of intestinal phosphate transport. II. Metabolic acidosis stimulates Na(+)-dependent phosphate absorption and expression of the Na(+)-P(i) cotransporter NaPi-IIb in small intestine. *Am J Physiol. Gastrointest Liver Physiol.* 2005;288:501.

639. Stauffer TP, Guerini D, Carafoli E. Tissue distribution of the four gene products of the plasma membrane Ca^{2+} pump - a study using specific antibodies. *J Biol Chem.* 1995;270:12184.

640. Steele TH, Stromberg BA, Larmore CA. Renal resistance to parathyroid hormone during phosphorus deprivation. *J Clin Invest.* 1976;58:1461.

641. Steele TH, Weng SF, Evenson MA. The contributions of the chronically diseased kidney to magnesium homeostasis in man. *J Lab Clin Med.* 1968; 71:455.

642. Stein GS, Lian JB. Molecular mechanisms mediating proliferation/differentiation interrelationships during progressive development of the osteoblast phenotype. *Endocrine Rev* 1993;14:424.

643. Steiner RW, Ziegler M, Halasz NA, et al. Effect of daily oral vitamin D and calcium therapy, hypophosphatemia, and endogenous 1-25 dihydroxycholecalciferol on parathyroid hormone and phosphate wasting in renal transplant recipients. *Transplantation.* 1993;56:843.

644. Stewart AF. Hypercalcemia associated with cancer. *N Eng J Med.* 2005; 352:373.

645. Stock JL, Marcus R. eds. Medical management of primary hyperparathyroidism. In: Bilezik JP, Marcus R, Levine MA, eds. *The Parathyroids: Basic and Clinical Concepts*. New York: Raven Press; 1994:519.

646. Stoeckle JD, Hardy HL, Weber AL. Chronic beryllium disease: Long-term follow up of sixty cases and selective review of the literature. *Am J Med.* 1969;46:545.

647. Stoll R, Kinne R, Murer H, et al. Phosphate transport by rat renal brush border membrane vesicles: Influence of dietary phosphate, thyroparathyroidectomy, and 1,25-dihydroxyvitamin D_3. *Pflugers Arch.* 1979;380:47.

648. Strewler GJ. FGF23, hypophosphatemia, and rickets: has phosphatonin been found? *Proc Natl Acad Sci U S A.* 2001;98:5945.

649. Suh SM, Tashjian AH, Matsuo N. Pathogenesis of hypocalcemia in primary hypomagnesemia: Normal end-organ responsiveness to parathyroid hormone, impaired parathyroid gland function. *J Clin Invest.* 1973;52:153.

650. Suki WN, Eknoyan G, Rector FC. The renal diluting and concentrating mechanisms in hypercalcemia. *Nephron.* 1969;6:50.

651. Suki WN, Rouse D, Ng RCK, et al. Calcium transport in the thick ascending limb of Henle: Heterogeneity of function in the medullary and cortical segments. *J Clin Invest.* 1980;68:1004.

652. Sutton RAL, Wong NLM, Dirks JH. Effects of metabolic acidosis and alkalosis on sodium transport in the dog kidney. *Kidney Int.* 1979;15:520.

653. Swiatecka-Urban A, Duhaime M, Coutermarsh B, et al. PDZ domain interaction controls the endocytic recycling of the cystic fibrosis transmembrane conductance regulator. *J Biol Chem.* 2002;277:40099.

654. Takahashi Y, Tanaka A, Nakamura T, et al. Nicotinamide suppresses hyperphosphatemia in hemodialysis patients. *Kidney Int.* 2004;65:1099.

655. Takeda T, McQuistan T, Orlando RA, et al. Loss of glomerular foot processes is associated with uncoupling of podocalyxin from the actin cytoskeleton. *J Clin Invest.* 2001;108:289.

656. Takeuchi Y, Suzuki H, Ogura S, et al. Venous sampling for fibroblast growth factor-23 confirms preoperative diagnosis of tumor-induced osteomalacia. *J Clin Endocrinol Metab.* 2004;89:3979.

657. Taylor AN, Wasserman RH. Immunofluorescent localization of vitamin D-dependent calcium-binding proteins. *J Histochem Cytochem.* 1970;18:107.

658. Tencza AL, Ichikawa S, Dang A, et al. Hypophosphatemic rickets with hypercalciuria due to mutation in SLC34A3/type IIc sodium-phosphate cotransporter: presentation as hypercalciuria and nephrolithiasis. *J Clin Endocrinol Metab.* 2009;94:4433.

659. Tenenhouse HS. Regulation of phosphorus homeostasis by the type IIa Na/phosphate cotransporter. *Annu Rev Nutr.* 2005;25:10.1–10.18.

660. Tenenhouse HS, Martel J, Gauthier C, et al. Differential effects of Npt2a gene ablation and X-linked Hyp mutation on renal expression of Npt2c. *Am J Physiol Renal Physiol.* 2003;285:1271.

661. Tenenhouse HS, Murer H. Disorders of renal tubular phosphate transport. *J Am Soc Nephrol.* 2003;14:240.

662. Tenenhouse HS, Roy S, Martel J, et al. Differential expression, abundance, and regulation of Na+-phosphate cotransporter genes in murine kidney. *Am J Physiol.* 1998;275:F527–F534.

663. Tenenhouse HS, Werner A, Biber J, et al. Renal Na^+-phosphate cotransport in murine X-linked hypophosphatemic rickets: molecular characterization. *J Clin Invest.* 1994;93:671.

664. Terada Y, Knepper MA. Thiazide-sensitive NaCl absorption in rat cortical collecting duct. *Am J Physiol.* 1990;259:F519.

665. Tieder M. Hereditary hypophosphatemic rickets with hypercalciuria. *N Engl J Med.* 1985;312:611.

666. Tieder M, Arie R, Bab I, et al. A new kindred with hereditary hypophosphatemic rickets with hypercalciuria: implications for correct diagnosis and treatment. *Nephron.* 1992;62:176.

667. Topaz O, Shurman DL, Bergman R, et al. Mutations in GALNT3, encoding a protein involved in O-linked glycosylation, cause familial tumoral calcinosis. *Nat Genet.* 2004;36:579.

668. Travis SF, Sugarman HJ, Ruberg RL, et al. Alterations of red-cell glycolytic intermediates and oxygen transport as a consequence of hypophosphatemia in patients receiving intravenous hyperalimentation. *N Engl J Med.* 1971;285:763.

669. Tsokos GC, Balow JE, Spiegel RJ, et al. Renal and metabolic complications of undifferentiated and lymphoblastic lymphomas. *Medicine* 1981;60:218.

670. Turner CH, Forwood MR. What role does the osteocyte network play in bone adaptation? *Bone.* 1995;16:283.

671. Turner JJO, Stacey JM, Harding B, et al. UROMODULIN mutations cause familial juvenile hyperuricemic nephropathy. *J Clin Endocrinol Metab.* 2003; 88:1398.
672. Ullrich KJ, Rumrich G, Kloss S. Active Ca^{2+} reabsorption in the proximal tubule of the rat kidney. Dependence on sodium and buffer transport. *Pflugers Arch (Euro J Physiol).* 1976;364:223.
673. Urakawa I, Yamazaki Y, Shimada T, et al. Klotho converts canonical FGF receptor into a specific receptor for FGF23. *Nature.* 2006;444:770.
674. van den Heuvel L, Op de Koul K, Knots E, et al. Autosomal recessive hypophosphatasemic rickets with hypercalciuria is not caused by mutations in the type II renal sodium/phosphate cotransporter gene. *Nephrol Dial Transplant.* 2001;16:48.
675. VanHouten J, Dann P, McGeoch G, et al. The calcium-sensing receptor regulates mammary gland parathyroid hormone-related protein production and calcium transport. *J Clin Invest.* 2005;113:598.
676. Verge CF, Lam A, Simpson JM, et al. Effect of therapy in X-linked hypophosphatemic rickets. *N Engl J Med.* 1991;325:1875.
677. Villa-Bellosta R, Barac-Nieto M, Breusegem SY, et al. Interactions of the growth-related, type IIc renal sodium/phosphate cotransporter with PDZ proteins. *Kidney Int.* 2007;73:456.
678. Villa-Bellosta R, Ravera S, Sorribas V, et al. The Na+-Pi cotransporter PiT-2 (SLC20A2) is expressed in the apical membrane of rat renal proximal tubules and regulated by dietary Pi. *Am J Physiol Renal Physiol.* 2009;296: F691–F699.
679. Virkki LV, Forster IC, Hernando N, et al. Functional characterization of two naturally occurring mutations in the human sodium-phosphate cotransporter type IIa. *J Bone Miner Res.* 2003;18:2135.
680. Wagner GF, Vozzolo BL, Jaworski E, et al. Human stanniocalcin inhibits renal phosphate excretion in the rat. *J Bone Miner Res.* 1997;12:165.
681. Walker JV, Baran D, Yakub DN. Histoplasmosis with hypercalcemia, renal failure, and papillary necrosis: confusion with sarcoidosis. *JAMA.* 1977;237:1350.
682. Walls J, Ratcliffe WA, Howell A, et al. Parathyroid hormone and parathyroid-hormone related protein in the investigation of hypercalcemia in two hospital populations. *Clin Endocrinol.* 1994;41:407.
683. Walser M. Ion association. VI. Interactions between calcium, magnesium, inorganic phosphate, citrate and protein in normal human plasma. *J Clin Invest.* 1961;40:723.
684. Walton RJ, Bijvoet OL. Nomogram for derivation of renal threshold phosphate concentration. *Lancet.* 1975;2:309.
685. Walton RJ, Russell RG, Smith R. Changes in the renal and extrarenal handling of phosphate induced by disodium etidronate (EHDP) in man. *Clin Sci Mol Med.* 1975;49:45.
686. Wang S, Yue H, Derin RB, et al. Accessory protein facilitated CFTR-CFTR interaction, a molecular mechanism to potentiate the chloride channel activity. *Cell.* 2000;103:169.
687. Ward HN, Pabico RC, McKenna BA, et al. The renal handling of phosphate by renal transplant patients: correlation with serum parathyroid hormone (SPTH), cyclic 3′,5′-adenosine monophosphate (cAMP) urinary excretion, and allograft function. *Adv Exp Med Biol.* 1977;81:173.
688. Ward LM, Rauch F, White KE, et al. Resolution of severe, adolescent-onset hypophosphatemic rickets following resection of an FGF-23-producing tumour of the distal ulna. *Bone.* 2004;34:905.
689. Ward MK, Feest TG, Ellis HA. Osteomalacic dialysis osteodystrophy: Evidence for a water-borne aetiological agent, probably aluminum. *Lancet.* 1978;1:841.
690. Wasserman RH. Intestinal absorption of calcium and phosphorus. *Fed Proc.* 1981;40:68.
691. Wasserman RH. Vitamin D and the dual processes of intestinal calcium absorption. *J Nutrition.* 2004;134:3137.
692. Wasserman RH, Corradino RA, Taylor AN. Vitamin D-dependent calcium binding protein: purification and some properties. *J Biol Chem.* 1968;243:3970.
693. Wasserman RH, Taylor AN. Vitamin D_3-induced calcium binding protein in chick intestinal mucosa. *Science* 1966;152:791.
694. Wasserman RH, Taylor AN. Evidence for a vitamin D_3-induced calcium-binding protein in new world primates. *Proc Soc Exp Biol Med.* 1970;136:25.
695. Watson P, Lazowski D, Han V, et al. Parathyoid hormone restores bone mass and enhances osteoblast insulin-like growth factor I gene expression in ovariectomized rats. *Bone.* 1995;16:357.
696. Weinman EJ, Evangelista CM, Steplock D, et al. Essential role for NHERF in cAMP-mediated inhibition of the Na+-HCO3- co-transporter in BSC-1 cells. *J Biol Chem.* 2001;276:42339.
697. Weinman EJ, Minkoff C, Shenolikar S. Signal complex regulation of renal transport proteins: NHERF and regulation of NHE3 by PKA. *Am J Physiol Renal Physiol.* 2000;279:393.
698. Weinman EJ, Steplock D, Donowitz M, et al. NHERF associations with sodium-hydrogen exchanger isoform 3 (NHE3) and ezrin are essential for cAMP-mediated phosphorylation and inhibition of NHE3. *Biochemistry.* 2000;39:6123.
699. Weinman EJ, Steplock D, Shenolikar S. NHERF-1 uniquely transduces the cAMP signals that inhibit sodium-hydrogen exchange in mouse renal apical membranes. *FEBS Lett.* 2003;536:141.
700. Weinman EJ, Steplock D, Wade JB, et al. Ezrin binding domain-deficient NHERF attenuates cAMP-mediated inhibition of Na(+)/H(+) exchange in OK cells. *Am J Physiol Renal Physiol.* 2001;281:374.
701. Weinsier RL, Krumdiek CL. Death resulting from overzealous total parenteral nutrition: the refeeding syndrome revisited. *Am J Clin Nutr.* 1981;34:393.
702. Weinstein LS. Mutations of the Gs alpha-subunit gene in Albright hereditary osteodystrophy detected by denaturing gradient gel electrophoresis. *Proc Natl Acad Sci U S A.* 1990;87:8287.
703. Weinstein LS, Liu J, Sakamoto A, et al. Minireview: GNAS: normal and abnormal functions. *Endocrinology.* 2004;145:5459.
704. Weinstein LS, Shenker A, Gejman PV, et al. Activating mutations of the stimulatory G protein in the McCune-Albright syndrome. *N Engl J Med.* 1991;325:1688.
705. Wells SA Jr, Doherty GM. The surgical management of hyperparathyroidism. In: Bilezikian JP, Marcus R, Levine MA, eds. *The Parathyroids: Basic and Clinical Concepts.* San Diego: Academic Press; 2001:487.
706. Welt LG, Gitelman H. Disorders of magnesium metabolism. *Dis Mon.* 1965;1:1.
707. Wen SF. Micropuncture studies of phosphate transport in the proximal tubule of the dog. The relationship of sodium reabsorption. *J Clin Invest.* 1974; 53:143.
708. Werner A, Kempson SA, Biber J, et al. Increase of Na/P_i-cotransport encoding mRNA in response to low P_i diet in rat kidney cortex. *J Biol Chem.* 1994; 269:6637.
709. Werner A, Moore ML, Mantei N, et al. Cloning and expression of cDNA for a Na/Pi cotransport system of kidney cortex. *Proc Natl Acad Sci.* USA 1991;88:9608.
710. Whang R, Oei TO, Hamiter T. Frequency of hypomagnesemia associated with hypokalemia in hospitalized patients. *Am J Clin Pathol.* 1979;71:610.
711. Whang R, Welt LG. Observations in experimental magnesium depletion. *J Clin Invest.* 1963;42:305.
712. White KE, Carn G, Lorenz-Depiereux B, et al. Autosomal-dominant hypophosphatemic rickets (ADHR) mutations stabilize FGF-23. *Kidney Int.* 2001; 60:2079.
713. White KE, Jonsson KB, Carn G, et al. The autosomal dominant hypophosphatemic rickets (ADHR) gene is a secreted polypeptide overexpressed by tumors that cause phosphate wasting. *J Clin Endocrinol Metab.* 2001;86:497.
714. Windhager EE, Frindt G, Milovanovic S. The role of Na-Ca exchange in renal epithelia: an overview. *Ann N Y Acad Sci.* 1991;639:577.
715. Winnacker JL, Becker KL, Katz S. Endocrine aspects of sarcoidosis. *N Engl J Med.* 1968;278:427.
716. Woda CB, Halaihel N, Wilson PV, et al. Regulation of renal NaPi-2 expression and tubular phosphate reabsorption by growth hormone in the juvenile rat. *Am J Physiol Renal Physiol.* 2004;287:117.
717. Wong NL, Quamme GA, O'Callaghan TJ. Renal tubular transport and phosphate depletion: A micropuncture study. *Can J Physiol Pharmacol.* 1980;58:1063.
718. Wong NLM, Quamme GA, Dirks JH. Tubular reabsorptive capacity for magnesium in the dog kidney. *Am J Physiol.* 1983;224:62.
719. Wu KI, Bacon RA, Al-Mahrouq HA, et al. Nicotinamide as a rapid-acting inhibitor of renal brush-border phosphate transport. *Am J Physiol.* 1988;255:15.
720. Wysolmerski JJ, Broadus AE. Hypercalcemia of malignancy: the central role of parathyroid hormone-related protein. *Ann Rev Med.* 1994;45:189.
721. Wysolmerski JJ, Stewart AF. The physiology of parathyroid hormone-related protein: An emerging role as a developmental factor. *Annu Rev Physiol.* 1998;60:431.
722. Xu H, Bai L, Collins JF, et al. Age-dependent regulation of rat intestinal type IIb sodium-phosphate cotransporter by 1,25-(OH)(2) vitamin D(3). *Am J Physiol Cell Physiol.* 2002;282:487.
723. Xu H, Inouye M, Hines ER, et al. Transcriptional regulation of the human NaPi-IIb cotransporter by EGF in Caco-2 cells involves c-myb. *Am J Physiol Cell Physiol.* 2003;284:1262.
724. Xu H, Uno JK, Inouye M, et al. Regulation of intestinal NaPi-IIb cotransporter gene expression by estrogen. *Am J Physiol Gastrointest Liver Physiol.* 2003;285:1317.
725. Yamashita T, Konishi M, Miyake A, et al. Fibroblast growth factor (FGF)-23 inhibits renal phosphate reabsorption by activation of the mitogen-activated protein kinase pathway. *J Biol Chem.* 2002;277:28265.
726. Yamazaki Y, Okazaki R, Shibata M, et al. Increased circulatory level of biologically active full-length FGF-23 in patients with hypophosphatemic rickets/ osteomalacia. *J Clin Endocrinol Metab.* 2002;87:4957.

727. Yang JM, Lee CO, Windhager EE. Regulation of cytosolic free calcium in isolated perfused proximal tubules of *Necturus*. *Am J Physiol*. 1988;255: F787.
728. Yu ASL, Hebert SC, Brenner BM, et al. Molecular characterization and nephron distribution of a family of transcripts encoding the pore-forming subunit of Ca^{2+} channels in the kidney. *Proc Natl Acad Sci U S A*. 1992;89:10494.
729. Yusufi AN, Murayama N, Keller MJ, et al. Modulatory effect of thyroid hormones on uptake of phosphate and other solutes across luminal brush border membrane of kidney cortex. *Endocrinology*. 1985;116:2438.
730. Zamkoff KW, Kirshner JJ. Marked hypophosphatemia associated with acute myelomonocytic leukemia: Indirect evidence of phosphorus uptake by leukemic cells. *Arch Intern Med*. 1980;140:1523.
731. Zazzo J-F, Troche G, Ruel P, et al. High incidence of hypophosphatemia in surgical intensive care patients: efficacy of phosphorus therapy on myocardial function. *Intensive Care Med*. 1995;21:826.
732. Zerwekh JE, Sanders LA, Townsend J, et al. Tumoral calcinosis: evidence for concurrent defects in renal tubular phosphorus transport and in 1alpha,25-dihydroxycholecalciferol synthesis. *Calcif Tissue Int*. 1980;32:1.
733. Zlot C, Ingle G, Hongo J, et al. Stanniocalcin 1 is an autocrine modulator of endothelial angiogenic responses to hepatocyte growth factor. *J Biol Chem*. 2003;278:47654.
734. Zusman J, Brown DM, Nesbit ME. Hyperphosphatemia, hyperphosphaturia and hypocalcemia in acute lymphoblastic leukemia. *N Engl J Med*. 1973;289:1335.

CHAPTER 74

Fluid–Electrolyte and Acid–Base Disorders Complicating Diabetes Mellitus

Horacio J. Adrogué • Nicolaos E. Madias

Diabetes mellitus, the most prevalent endocrine disorder, is a very challenging condition responsible for the development of severe abnormalities in whole body composition and damage of critical functions. The deranged metabolic pathways lead to defects in the normal fluid–electrolyte and acid–base homeostasis, which are reviewed in this chapter. We examine the basic defects of diabetes mellitus, and describe each of the various disturbances of water, electrolyte, and acid–base composition observed in association with this disease.

KETOSIS AND KETOACIDOSIS

Ketosis is an abnormal state of nutrient metabolism that develops when the rate of production of ketones exceeds their removal; as a result, ketones accumulate in body fluids as reflected by high blood and urine levels.[1–4] Because ketones are largely organic acids (β-hydroxybutyric and acetoacetic acid) that dissociate almost completely at the pH of the body fluids, their production generates H^+ ions, which consume HCO_3^- and lead to metabolic acidosis (ketoacidosis). The term ketosis is used to describe a mild form of the disturbance, reserving the term ketoacidosis for the full-blown condition that features substantial metabolic acidosis.[5]

The mechanisms underlying ketoacidosis are essentially the same whether it develops as an acute complication of diabetes mellitus or in nondiabetic subjects (e.g., starvation ketosis, alchoholic ketoacidosis). Abnormal levels or action of insulin and glucagon are required for the development of ketosis.[5–10] Insulin deficiency or resistance impairs glucose utilization in skeletal muscle and increases adipose tissue and muscle breakdown, thereby augmenting delivery of glycerol and alanine (gluconeogenic substrates) to the liver. Hepatic gluconeogenesis, in turn, is stimulated by insulin deficiency and, more importantly, by glucagon excess. The fatty acids released from the enhanced lipolysis are converted to ketones by the hepatocytes under the influence of glucagon excess. Pancreatic β cell destruction is largely responsible for the hormonal imbalance observed in most cases of diabetic ketoacidosis. Conversely, insulin deficiency in the presence of normal β cells plays a major role in ketosis associated with fasting, starvation, ethanol ingestion, and some liver diseases.

Diabetic ketoacidosis (DKA) is a disease state characterized by the presence of hyperglycemia and hyperosmolality, metabolic acidosis due to ketoacid accumulation, extracellular and intracellular fluid depletion, and varying degrees of electrolyte deficiency, particularly of potassium and phosphate.[9–11]

ROLES OF INSULIN AND GLUCAGON

In normal fasting individuals, the major source of glucose (approximately 90%) is from the liver, through glycogenolysis and gluconeogenesis. The kidney contributes the remaining 10% through synthesis of glucose from three-carbon precursors (gluconeogenesis). After a meal, glucose absorption increases the plasma glucose level. The resultant hyperglycemia-induced stimulation of insulin secretion suppresses hepatic glucose production, largely through inhibition of glycogenolysis, and stimulates glucose uptake by the liver, the gut, and peripheral tissues, including skeletal muscle.

The abnormal metabolism of carbohydrates and lipids observed in DKA is largely caused by a rise in the molar ratio of glucagon/insulin in plasma. The two hormones are metabolic antagonists with respect to fuel production and utilization but their primary effects occur on different tissues. Insulin acts on muscle and adipose tissue augmenting glucose transport and inhibiting lipolysis. Conversely, glucagon primarily acts on the liver increasing glycogenolysis, gluconeogenesis, and ketogenesis. Insulin's action on the hepatocyte is essentially that of an antiglucagon hormone, as it has minimal hepatic effects in the absence of glucagon-induced metabolic changes. Insulin decreases glucagon release from α cells in the pancreatic islets and inhibits a glucagon-activated, cAMP-dependent protein kinase in the hepatocyte.[5] Beyond the critical role of glucagon in ketone body production, other hormones, including catecholamines, cortisol, growth hormones, and thyroid hormones, increase hepatic ketogenesis and may participate in the pathogenesis of diabetic ketoacidosis (Fig. 74.1).[12]

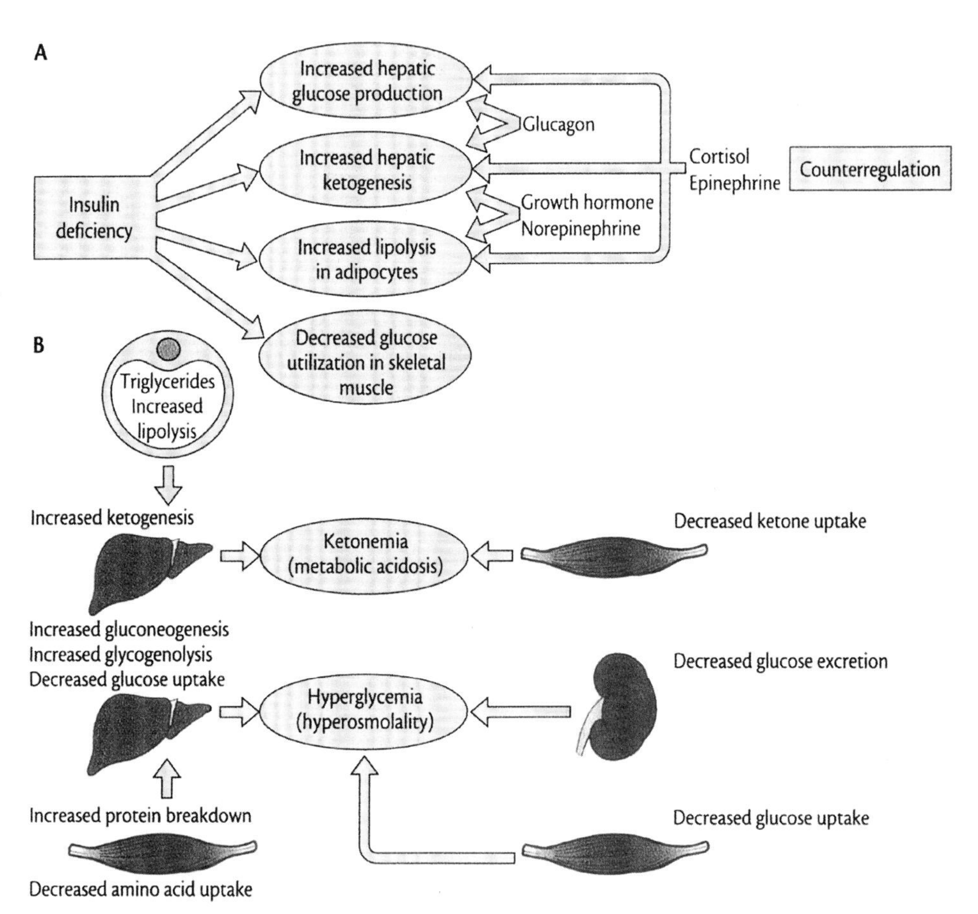

FIGURE 74.1 Role of insulin deficiency, counterregulatory hormones, and various tissues and organs in the pathogenesis of hyperglycemia and ketosis in diabetic ketoacidosis (DKA). **A:** Metabolic processes affected by insulin deficiency, on the one hand, and excess of glucagon, cortisol, epinephrine, norepinephrine, and growth hormone, on the other. **B:** The roles of the adipose tissue, liver, skeletal muscle, and kidney in the pathogenesis of hyperglycemia and ketonemia. Excessive hepatic production of glucose and impairment of glucose utilization are the main determinants of hyperglycemia. Increased hepatic production of ketones and their reduced utilization by peripheral tissues account for the ketonemia. (From Adrogué HJ, Madias NE. Disorders of acid–base balance. In: Berl T, Bonventre JV, eds. *Atlas of Diseases of the Kidney*. Boston: Blackwell Scientific; 1999.)

DISTURBANCES IN BODY COMPOSITION

The major fluid–electrolyte and acid–base disorders complicating diabetes mellitus are conveniently classified as single disturbances and combinations of multiple disturbances (Table 74.1). Each of the single disturbances, including defects in homeostasis of glucose, lipids, water, sodium, potassium, phosphate, and acid–base balance, is characterized by unique features that are reviewed in this section. Combinations of multiple disturbances comprising the simultaneous presence of defects in the homeostasis of glucose, fluid, electrolyte, and acid–base balance are responsible for the development of the full-blown clinical pictures of diabetic ketoacidosis, nonketotic hyperglycemia (NKH), and renal failure complicating diabetes mellitus. These combined disturbances are examined thereafter, with the exception of renal failure, which is discussed elsewhere.

Single Disturbances

Defect in Glucose Homeostasis

In uncontrolled diabetes, hyperglycemia is caused by increased hepatic and renal glucose production and decreased glucose utilization in muscle and adipose tissue. Decreased glucose utilization, once considered the major contributor to hyperglycemia in uncontrolled diabetes, is currently believed to play a smaller role than excessive glucose production. Figure 74.2 depicts the hepatic and renal contribution to endogenous glucose production in conscious normal and diabetic dogs.[13] The rise in the glucagon/insulin ratio in plasma characteristic of uncontrolled diabetes activates key enzymes that accelerate the rates of both glycogenolysis and gluconeogenesis. The increased ratio also promotes glucose overproduction by modulating the effects of other hormones, availability of substrate, and rates of fatty acid oxidation (Fig. 74.1). Volume depletion secondary to hyperglycemia-induced osmotic diuresis reduces the urinary loss of glucose, thereby worsening hyperglycemia.

An important contributor to the development of hyperglycemia in uncontrolled diabetes may be the prevailing acidemia.[14–18] In animals with hypercapnia-induced acidemia, for example, a substantially smaller glucose infusion rate maintains euglycemia as compared to dogs without respiratory acidosis during constant insulin infusion, reflecting less glucose entry into cells for a given insulin level (Fig. 74.3).[19] Although the sympathetic surge characteristic of acidemia undoubtedly contributes to glucose intolerance, adrenergic blockade during acute respiratory acidosis does not prevent the disturbed glucoregulation. Nor do plasma levels of insulin fall during acute respiratory acidosis. In fact, acidemia reduces tissue extraction of insulin and, more specifically,

TABLE 74.1 **Major Fluid–Electrolyte and Acid–Base Disorders Complicating Diabetes Mellitus**

Condition	Defect in Homeostasis of	Specific Entity
Single disturbance	Glucose	Hyponatremia (hypertonic or translocational)
		Hypernatremia
	Lipids	Pseudohyponatremia
	Water	Hyponatremia (hypotonic)
		Hypernatremia
	Sodium	Volume depletion
		Volume expansion
	Potassium	Hypokalemia, K^+ depletion
		Hyperkalemia
	Acid–base balance	Ketoacidosis
		Hyperchloremic acidosis
		Renal tubular acidosis
		Lactic acidosis
Combination of multiple disturbances	Glucose, fluid, and acid–base balance	Diabetic ketoacidosis
		Hyperosmolar nonketotic syndrome
		Renal failure

insulin uptake by the liver.[19] Although plasma glucagon levels also increase during metabolic or respiratory acidosis, the glucagon/insulin ratio in the portal circulation remains unchanged, thereby reducing the possible role of glucagon in the hyperglycemia of acidemic states. The weight of the evidence suggests that the hyperglycemia of acidemia is mediated by reduction of insulin binding to its receptor and decreased tissue sensitivity to the hormone.[19–22]

The defect in glucose homeostasis observed in uncontrolled diabetes might lead to either hyponatremia or hypernatremia.[23–25] The hyperglycemia-induced increase in effective osmotic pressure of the extracellular fluid (ECF) triggers a shift of water out of cells, most prominently skeletal muscle, which reduces serum $[Na^+]$. An increase of 100 mg per dL (5.6 mmol per L) in the glucose concentration decreases serum $[Na^+]$ by approximately 1.7 mEq per L, the end result being a rise in serum osmolality by approximately 2.0 mOsm per kg H_2O.[25,26] The resulting ECF expansion is, however, brief due to simultaneous renal and extrarenal loss of fluids. The hyperglycemia-induced increase in the filtered load of glucose exceeds the renal tubular reabsorptive capacity resulting in substantial glucosuria—one of the hallmarks of DKA. In turn, glucosuria causes osmotic diuresis that results in urinary losses of 75 to 150 mL per kg of water and 7 to 10 mEq per kg of Na^+ and Cl^- over an entire episode of DKA.

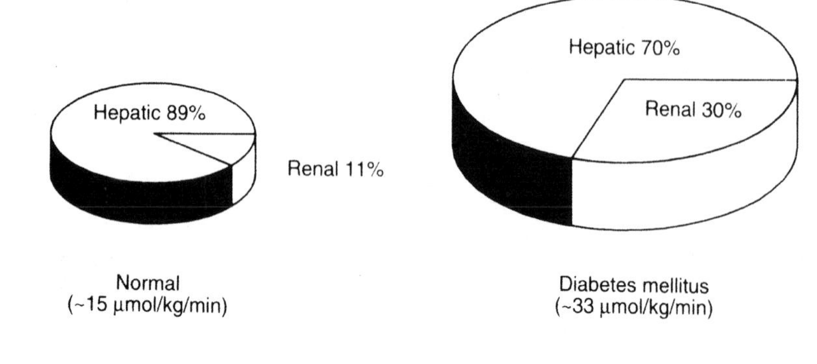

FIGURE 74.2 Contributions of the liver and the kidney to endogenous glucose production in conscious normal and diabetic dogs. Total glucose production is indicated in parentheses. (From Adrogué HJ. Glucose homeostasis and the kidney. *Kidney Int.* 1992;42:266.)

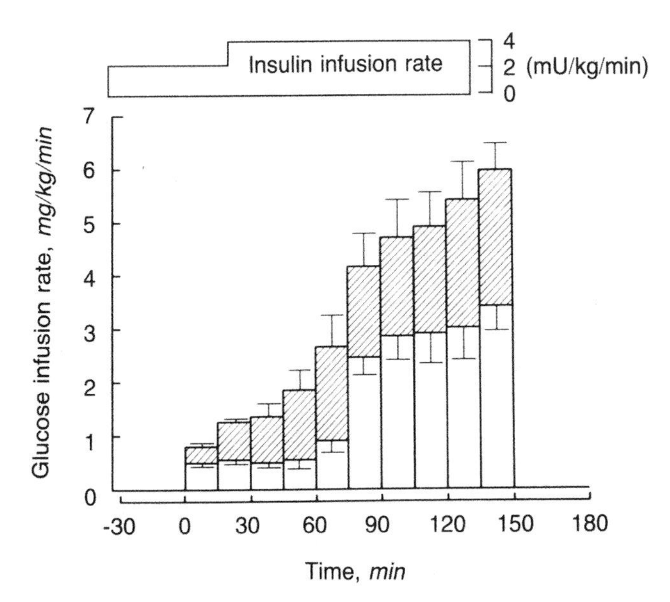

FIGURE 74.3 Rate of glucose infusion required to maintain euglycemia during insulin infusion studies in normal and acidemic dogs (respiratory acidosis, arterial pH = 7.18). Open area in each column represents the value in acidemic dogs; the entire column is the value in normal dogs. (From Adrogué HJ. Glucose homeostasis and the kidney. *Kidney Int.* 1992;42:1266.)

Because the total of the Na^+ and K^+ concentrations in the urine falls short of that in serum, osmotic diuresis elevates serum [Na^+] and [Cl^-]; moderation of hyponatremia or frank hypernatremia can ensue.[23,27] However, other factors also act to modify the serum [Na^+] and [Cl^-].[27] Some Na^+ enters cells replacing cellular K^+ losses, thereby decreasing serum [Na^+]. Urinary losses of Na^+ as ketone salts tend to increase serum [Cl^-], whereas selective Cl^- depletion during vomiting tends to cause hypochloremia. Further, the intake of fluid and electrolytes (sodium, potassium, and chloride) influences serum [Na^+] and [Cl^-]. Differences in the magnitude of these phenomena from one patient to another account for the variability in serum electrolyte composition observed at presentation. Table 74.2 reviews the admitting laboratory values of patients with DKA.[8] Note that serum [Na^+] is usually depressed; the rare presence of hypernatremia is indicative of a profound water depletion, usually seen in the most critically ill patients.

Prerenal azotemia due to volume depletion is almost always present in uncontrolled diabetes and is usually reversible, but occasionally it can progress to acute tubular necrosis.[28,29] The levels of plasma urea nitrogen, creatinine, total protein, uric acid, hematocrit, and hemoglobin can all be elevated on admission for DKA, a reflection of ECF contraction, and/or renal dysfunction, but they normalize swiftly after volume repletion.

Hyperlipidemia

Diabetes mellitus is commonly associated with hyperlipidemia, which in turn may reduce measured serum sodium concentration, causing the so-called pseudohyponatremia or false hyponatremia. This electrolyte disorder is characterized by a normal [Na^+] in plasma water despite a diminished [Na^+] in a plasma or serum sample. The decreased [Na^+] arises from an increased solid phase of plasma owing to severe hyperlipidemia or hyperproteinemia (e.g., myeloma). If [Na^+] is measured directly (without dilution of the sample) with ion-sensitive electrodes instead of flame photometry (the latter being the classic method), a normal value will be found; thus, this type of hyponatremia is false because: (1) the [Na^+] in plasma water is normal, and (2) its detection is dependent on the method used for measurement of [Na^+]. Pseudohyponatremia does not produce, of course, any of the symptoms associated with hypotonic hyponatremia. Furthermore, measured plasma osmolality is normal in pseudohyponatremia, because the solute concentration in plasma water is not altered.[23]

Let us compare the hyponatremia owing to hyperglycemia or hypertonic infusions (e.g., mannitol) with that caused by hyperlipidemia. The decreased [Na^+] owing to hyperglycemia or hypertonic infusions is not a form of pseudohyponatremia because [Na^+] in plasma water also is diminished. The ECF accumulation of solutes of relatively small molecular size, observed with hyperglycemia or hypertonic infusions, increases extracellular tonicity, which in turn osmotically pulls water from the intracellular fluid (ICF), diluting the [Na^+] in ECF. By contrast, high plasma levels of large-molecular-size solutes (e.g., hypertriglyceridemia) fail to alter extracellular tonicity and, therefore, do not cause a shift of water from the ICF to the ECF. Thus, pseudohyponatremia is a spurious form of isoosmolar and isotonic hyponatremia identified when severe hyperlipidemia or paraproteinemia increases substantially the solid phase of plasma and the [Na^+] is measured by means of flame photometry. The increasing availability of direct measurement of serum sodium with ion-specific electrodes has all but eliminated this laboratory artifact.[23]

Defect in Water Homeostasis

Examination of the defect in water homeostasis that accompanies diabetes mellitus requires a brief overview of this topic.[23–25] The disorders of salt and water balance may be classified into three major categories: (1) abnormalities in the size of body fluid compartments, (2) disturbances in the tonicity of body fluids, and (3) a selective deficit or excess of chloride with respect to sodium.[25] The first group of disorders comprises an enlargement ("volume expansion") and a reduction ("volume depletion or contraction") in the size of the ECF compartment, which are produced by a combined salt and water excess and a combined salt and water deficit, respectively. Disturbances in the tonicity of body fluids include increases (e.g., hypernatremia) and decreases (e.g., hypotonic hyponatremia) in the effective osmolality of body fluids. In contrast to the first group in which salt and water excess or deficit develops with normal proportionality, a discordant abnormality in salt and water balance occurs in disorders of body fluid tonicity. The third group of salt and

TABLE 74.2 **Salient Laboratory Abnormalities on Admission for Diabetic Ketoacidosis**

Parameter	Value			Comments
Glucose	250 to 750 mg/dL			Values below 200 mg/dL ("euglycemic DKA") can be seen, especially in alcoholics or pregnant insulin-dependent diabetics; also, values above 1,000 mg/dL can be seen, especially in severe volume contraction leading to renal failure and interruption of glucosuria; glucose concentration not related to severity of DKA
Serum ketones	Positive in plasma diluted 1:1 or greater			Nitroprusside reagent (Ketostix, Acetest) does not react with β-hydroxybutyrate; color reaction is mostly (>80%) due to acetoacetate
Bicarbonate	<18 mmol/L			Always reduced in DKA unless complicated by coexisting metabolic alkalosis
pH	<7.30			Always reduced in DKA unless complicated by coexisting metabolic alkalosis or respiratory alkalosis
	Plasma Concentration			
	Low	**Normal**	**High**[a]	
Sodium	67	26	7	Body stores depleted (7–10 mEq/kg)
Chloride	33	45	22	
Potassium	18	43	39	Body stores depleted (3–5 mEq/kg)
Magnesium	7	25	68	
Phosphate	11	18	71	Body stores depleted (5–7 mEq/kg)
Calcium	28	68	4	
BUN, creatinine	High			Because creatinine can be spuriously elevated (cross-reaction with acetoacetate), BUN can better reflect renal function
White blood cell count	Usually high			Not necessarily indicative of infection; associated with lymphopenia and eosinopenia
Hemoglobin, hemacri, total protein	Frequently increased			Due to intravascular volume depletion
SGOT, SGPT, LDH, CPK	High, 20% to 65%			Partially due to interference of acetoacetate with colorimetric assays; elevated CPK might be related to phosphate depletion and possible associated rhabdomyolysis
Amylase	Often increased			Isoenzyme evaluation reveals that site of origin is pancreas (50%), salivary (36%), or mixed (14%)

[a]Modified from Kreisberg RA. Diabetic ketoacidosis: new concepts and trends in pathogenesis and treatment. *Ann Intern Med.* 1978;88:681.
DKA, diabetic ketacidosis; BUN, blood urea nitrogen; SGOT, serum glutamic-oxaloacetic transaminase; SGPT, serum glutamic-pyruvic transaminase; LDH, lactate dehydrogenase; CPK, creatine phosphokinase.

water disorders is characterized by an abnormal relationship between the $[Na^+]_p$ and $[Cl^-]_p$ (plasma concentration). Although the $[Na^+]_p$ is generally maintained within normal limits in these disorders because it is dependent on overall water homeostasis, the $[Cl^-]_p$ is either abnormally low or high. The major representatives of a selective deficit or excess of chloride with respect to sodium are hypochloremic metabolic alkalosis and hyperchloremic metabolic acidosis, respectively. These acid–base disorders are reviewed in the section dealing with such abnormalities.

Disturbances in salt balance are the primary causes of volume excess and depletion, whereas disorders in water balance are responsible for the development of the tonicity disorders, hypertonicity (hypernatremia), and hypotonicity (hyponatremia). Because sodium chloride (NaCl) excess only transiently increases tonicity, leading to augmented antidiuretic hormone (ADH) (i.e., arginine vasopressin) secretion and secondary water retention, hypernatremia is not clinically observed. Expansion of the ECF volume, instead, is the hallmark of a primary NaCl excess. In a comparable fashion, NaCl deficit only transiently decreases tonicity, inhibiting ADH secretion with secondary increase in water excretion, so that hyponatremia is not observed, whereas volume depletion becomes the major manifestation of this electrolyte imbalance. A primary and exclusive disturbance in water balance, deficit and excess, causes hypertonicity (hypernatremia) and hypotonicity (hyponatremia), respectively, but does not produce a major alteration in the size of the fluid compartments because the latter is primarily determined by the osmolar content in each compartment, and the change in water content is distributed throughout the body fluids.[25]

Dysnatremias in Diabetes Mellitus. A defect in water homeostasis in patients with diabetes mellitus might lead to either hypotonic hyponatremia or hypernatremia in response to positive or negative water balance, respectively.[25] Water and electrolyte losses caused by vomiting or diarrhea are commonly encountered in uncontrolled diabetes as well as patients with diabetes experiencing target organ damage in the alimentary tract (e.g., gastroparesis, nocturnal diarrhea). In addition, excessive urinary fluid losses may develop as a result of osmotic diuresis, use of diuretics, adrenal insufficiency, or other causes. Whether hypotonic hyponatremia or hypernatremia develops is dependent on the concomitant water intake. Hypernatremia might be observed if water intake is insufficient, whereas a large salt-free fluid intake might lead to hyponatremia. Long-standing diabetes mellitus commonly predisposes or leads to heart failure, renal failure, or both, thereby impairing renal water excretion that may lead to hypotonic hyponatremia. Concomitant medication, including diuretics, might also play a role in the development of hyponatremia.

Abnormal $[Na^+]_p$ can produce signs and symptoms owing to central nervous system dysfunction and the clinical manifestations elicited by opposite changes in tonicity are remarkably similar, except for seizures that are mostly caused by cerebral edema secondary to dilutional (hypotonic) hyponatremia. When the patient's osmoregulating mechanisms (thirst, changes in water intake and ADH levels, renal water retention or excretion) fail, an increase or decrease in plasma tonicity and $[Na^+]_p$ develops. Plasma hypertonicity induces brain water loss, whereas hypotonicity produces water gain in this organ, accompanied in both cases by parallel volume changes. As a defense mechanism to correct brain volume changes, the intracellular osmolytes of this organ increase in hypernatremia and decrease in hypotonic hyponatremia. The adaptive increase in brain osmolytes reflects a modest increase in cellular K^+ and accumulation of organic solutes (e.g., glutamine, glutamate, and other organic metabolites), which are referred to as idiogenic osmoles. Conversely, the adaptive decrease in brain osmolytes reflects a decrease in cellular K^+ accompanied by a diminished concentration of idiogenic osmoles. These secondary responses of the brain to altered extracellular tonicity can be demonstrated within a few hours of the initiation of abnormal tonicity and are complete within a few days.

Hypotonic or Dilutional Hyponatremia. It represents an excess of water in relation to existing sodium stores, which can be decreased, essentially normal, or increased. Retention of water most commonly reflects the presence of conditions that impair renal excretion of water; in a minority of cases, however, it is caused by excessive water intake, with a normal or nearly normal excretory capacity.

Conditions of impaired renal excretion of water are categorized according to the characteristics of the ECF volume, as determined by clinical assessment. Decreased ECF volume can result from renal sodium loss (e.g., glucosuria-induced osmotic diuresis) or extrarenal sodium loss (e.g., vomiting). Conditions with essentially normal ECF volume include thiazide diuretics, syndrome of inappropriate secretion of antidiuretic hormone, decreased intake of solutes, hypothyroidism, and glucocorticoid insufficiency. Increased ECF volume with hyponatremia can be observed in pregnancy, renal failure, congestive heart failure, cirrhosis, and nephrotic syndrome. With the exception of renal failure, these conditions are characterized by high plasma concentrations of ADH despite the presence of hypotonicity; arterial underfilling induces baroreceptor-mediated nonosmotic release of ADH that overrides the osmotic regulation of the hormone, thereby impairing urinary dilution and causing hyponatremia. Depletion of potassium accompanies many of these disorders and contributes to hyponatremia because the sodium concentration is determined by the ratio of the "exchangeable" (i.e., osmotically active) portions of the body's sodium and potassium content to total body water. Patients with hyponatremia induced by thiazides can present with variable hypovolemia or apparent euvolemia, depending on the magnitude of the sodium loss and water retention.

Excessive water intake can cause hyponatremia by overwhelming normal water excretory capacity (e.g., 15 to 20 L per day). Frequently, however, psychiatric patients with excessive water intake have plasma arginine vasopressin concentrations that are not fully suppressed and urine that is not maximally dilute, thus contributing to water retention.

The optimal treatment of hypotonic hyponatremia requires balancing the risks of hypotonicity against those of therapy.[23] The presence of symptoms and their severity largely determine the pace of correction. Patients with symptomatic hyponatremia and dilute urine (osmolality, <200 mOsm per kg water) but with less serious symptoms usually require only water restriction and close observation. Severe symptoms (e.g., seizures or coma) call for infusion of hypertonic saline. On the other hand, patients who have symptomatic hyponatremia with concentrated urine (osmolality ≥200 mOsm per kg water) in association with a hypovolemic state are best treated with isotonic saline; those having clinical euvolemia or hypervolemia require infusion of hypertonic saline.

There is no consensus about the optimal treatment of symptomatic hyponatremia.[23] Nevertheless, correction should be of a sufficient pace and magnitude to reverse the manifestations of hypotonicity but not be so rapid and large as to pose a risk of the development of central pontine myelinolysis. Osmotic demyelination is a serious disorder and can develop one to several days after aggressive treatment of hyponatremia by any method, including water restriction alone. Shrinkage of the brain triggers demyelination of pontine and extrapontine neurons that can cause neurologic dysfunction, including quadriplegia, pseudobulbar palsy, seizures, coma, and even death. Hepatic failure, potassium depletion, and malnutrition increase the risk of the complication. Physiologic considerations indicate that a relatively small increase in the serum $[Na^+]$, on the order of 5%, should substantially reduce cerebral edema in patients with symptomatic hypotonic hyponatremia. Even seizures induced by hyponatremia can be stopped by rapid increases in the serum $[Na^+]$ that average only 3 to 7 mEq per L. Most reported cases of osmotic demyelination occurred after rates of correction that exceeded 12 mEq per L per day were used, but isolated cases occurred after corrections of only 9 to 10 mEq per L in 24 hours or 19 mEq per L in 48 hours. After weighing the available evidence and the all-too-real risk of overshooting the mark, we recommend a targeted rate of correction that does not exceed 8 mEq per L on any day of treatment. Remaining within this target, the initial rate of correction can still be 1 to 2 mEq per L per hour for several hours in patients with severe symptoms.

The rate of infusion of the selected solution can be derived expediently by applying the following equations:

$$\Delta[Na^+]_s = \frac{[Na^+]_{inf} - [Na^+]_s}{TBW + 1} \tag{74.1}$$

Equation 74.1 projects the impact of 1 L of any infusate on the patient's $[Na^+]_s$

$$\Delta[Na^+]_s = \frac{[Na^+ + K^+]_{inf} - [Na^+]_s}{TBW + 1} \tag{74.2}$$

Equation 74.2 is a simple derivative of equation 74.1 and projects the impact of 1 L of any infusate containing sodium and potassium on the patient's $[Na^+]_s$

The preceding equations project the change in serum $[Na^+]$ elicited by the retention of 1 L of any infusate.[30] Dividing the change in serum sodium targeted for a given treatment period by the output of this equation determines the volume of infusate required, and hence the rate of infusion. Although water restriction ameliorates all forms of hyponatremia, as explained, it is not the optimal therapy in all cases.

Corrective measures for nonhypotonic hyponatremia are directed at the underlying disorder rather than at the hyponatremia itself. Administration of insulin is the basis of treatment for uncontrolled diabetes, but deficits of water, sodium, and potassium also should be corrected.

Hypernatremia. Defined as a rise in the $[Na^+]_p$ to a value exceeding 145 mEq per L, it represents a deficit of water in relation to the body's sodium stores, which can result from a net water loss or a hypertonic sodium gain.[24] Net water loss accounts for the majority of cases of hypernatremia. It can occur in the absence of a sodium deficit (pure water loss) or in its presence (hypotonic fluid loss). Net water loss can result from pure water (e.g., hypodipsia, diabetes insipidus) or hypotonic fluid loss, the latter secondary to renal, gastrointestinal, or cutaneous causes.

An equation[31] that allows projection of the expected $\Delta[Na^+]_s$ in response to losing 1 L of fluid (fl) of variable electrolyte content from the renal or extrarenal route is as follows:

$$\Delta[Na^+]_s = \frac{[Na^+]_s - [Na^+ + K^+]_{fl}}{TBW - 1} \tag{74.3}$$

Multiplying the output of the equation by the volume of the fluid loss in liters provides a quantitative estimate of the impact of the fluid loss on $[Na^+]_s$. Obviously, application of this equation has greater practical value in the presence of large fluid losses (e.g., large gastrointestinal drainage, polyuria).

Hypertonic sodium gain usually results from clinical interventions (e.g., sodium bicarbonate infusion, hypertonic enemas) or accidental sodium loading. Signs and symptoms of hypernatremia largely reflect central nervous system dysfunction and are prominent when the increase in the serum $[Na^+]$ is large or occurs rapidly (i.e., over a period of hours). Most outpatients with hypernatremia are either very young or very old. Common symptoms in infants include hyperpnea, muscle weakness, restlessness, a characteristic high-pitched cry, insomnia, lethargy, and even coma. Convulsions are typically absent except in cases of inadvertent sodium loading or aggressive rehydration. Brain shrinkage induced by hypernatremia can cause vascular rupture, with cerebral bleeding, subarachnoid hemorrhage, and permanent neurologic damage or death. Brain shrinkage is countered by an adaptive response that is initiated promptly and consists of solute gain by the brain that tends to restore lost water.

Proper treatment of hypernatremia requires a two-pronged approach: addressing the underlying cause and correcting the prevailing hypertonicity.[24] Managing the underlying cause may mean stopping gastrointestinal fluid losses; controlling pyrexia, hyperglycemia, and glucosuria; withholding lactulose and diuretics; treating hypercalcemia and hypokalemia; moderating lithium-induced polyuria; or correcting the feeding preparation. In patients with hypernatremia that has developed over a period of hours (e.g., those with accidental sodium loading) rapid correction improves the prognosis without increasing the risk of cerebral edema, because accumulated electrolytes are rapidly extruded from brain cells. In such patients reducing the $[Na^+]_p$ by 1 mEq/L/hour is appropriate. A slower pace of correction is prudent in patients with hypernatremia of longer or unknown duration, because the full dissipation of accumulated brain solutes occurs over a period of several days. In such patients, reducing the $[Na^+]_p$ at a maximal rate of 0.5 mEq/L/hour prevents cerebral edema and convulsions. Consequently, we recommend a targeted fall in the $[Na^+]_p$ of 10 mEq/L/day for all patients with hypernatremia except those in whom the disorder has developed over a period of hours. The goal of treatment is to reduce the $[Na^+]_p$ to 145 mEq per L. Because ongoing losses of hypotonic fluids, whether obligatory or incidental, aggravate the hypernatremia, allowance for these losses must also be made.

The preferred route for administering fluids is the oral route or a feeding tube; if neither is feasible, fluids should be given intravenously. Only hypotonic fluids are appropriate, including pure water, 5% dextrose, 0.2% NaCl (referred to as one quarter isotonic saline), and 0.45% NaCl (one half isotonic saline). The more hypotonic the infusate, the lower the infusion rate required. The volume should be restricted to that required to correct hypertonicity because the risk of cerebral edema increases with the volume of the infusate. Except in cases of frank circulatory compromise, 0.9% NaCl (isotonic saline) is unsuitable for managing hypernatremia.

After selecting the appropriate infusate, the physician must determine the rate of infusion. This can be easily calculated with the use of equations 74.1 and 74.2 which estimate the change in the serum sodium concentration caused by the retention of 1 L of any infusate. The sole indication for administering isotonic saline to a patient with hypernatremia is a depletion of ECF volume sufficient to cause substantial hemodynamic compromise. Even in this case, after a limited amount of isotonic saline has been administered to stabilize the patient's circulatory status, a hypotonic fluid (i.e., 0.2% or 0.45% NaCl) should be substituted in order to restore normal hemodynamic values while correcting the hypernatremia. If a hypotonic fluid is not substituted for isotonic saline, the ECF volume may become seriously overloaded.

Defect in Sodium Homeostasis

The quantity of solutes in each of the main fluid compartments determines its size, so that deficit or excess of solutes in a particular space will shrink or swell that space in comparison with the other compartments.[25] The partition of water is determined by the osmotic activity of the solutes confined to each body compartment. One major solute is responsible for the size of each fluid compartment. These solutes are potassium, sodium, and proteins, for the intracellular, extracellular, and intravascular spaces, respectively. Because the hydraulic permeability of most cell membranes is very high, solute-free water freely and rapidly moves across all body compartments.

Body stores of NaCl are determined by the balance of its intake and excretion. Under normal circumstances, NaCl intake is derived from the diet and its excretion occurs by urinary loss. A positive NaCl balance (intake exceeds excretion) increases salt stores, whereas a negative one (excretion exceeds intake) decreases salt stores. The effect of increased NaCl stores is expansion of ECF volume, whereas decreased NaCl stores lead to a reduced ECF volume. Thus, an NaCl deficit in body fluids (e.g., vomiting, diarrhea) reduces ECF volume, including the intravascular compartment. By contrast, NaCl excess (e.g., congestive heart failure) expands ECF volume and can produce overt peripheral edema and accumulation of fluid in major body cavities (pleural effusion, ascites). A major decrease in serum protein concentration (mostly albumin) diminishes intravascular volume and promotes expansion of the interstitial compartment (e.g., nephrotic syndrome, hepatic cirrhosis). Diabetes mellitus is a common cause of both volume depletion and volume expansion. The former disturbance is characteristically observed in the course of severe metabolic complications of this disease, namely, DKA and NKH. Conversely, volume expansion is observed in patients having chronic diabetic complications, including congestive heart failure, nephrotic syndrome, and renal failure.

Volume Depletion. Volume depletion in diabetic patients can result from fluid loss (e.g., renal and/or extrarenal) or from fluid sequestered into a "third space" (e.g., acute pancreatitis). Renal losses may occur in the presence of normal intrinsic renal function (e.g., osmotic diuresis caused by glucosuria or urea diuresis, adrenal insufficiency, diuretics) or in acute and chronic renal disease (e.g., acute tubular necrosis, diabetic glomerulosclerosis). Osmotic diuresis owing to renal excretion of glucose can produce a large natriuresis, leading to volume depletion. Patients with significant hyperglycemia, including those with DKA or nonketotic coma, may have a fluid deficit of 10% or more of body weight. Extrarenal losses include those from the gastrointestinal tract (e.g., vomiting, diarrhea, gastrointestinal suction, fistulas) and those from the skin (sweat, burns, extensive skin lesions). Fluid sequestration into a third space occurs with abdominal accumulation (e.g., intestinal obstruction, pancreatitis, peritonitis), bleeding, skeletal fractures, and obstruction of a major venous system.

The patient's history, physical examination, and laboratory data are critical elements in the evaluation of volume depletion, allowing the physician to (1) assess the severity of the deficit, and (2) establish its cause. Immediate recognition of hypovolemic shock is of utmost importance, because rapid intravascular volume expansion might prevent tissue injury and death. Evaluation of its severity allows establishment of the rate of infusion and the total fluid requirements. Recognition of the factors responsible for fluid loss permits initiation of specific therapeutic measures to correct the volume depletion.[25]

Patients with volume depletion have signs and symptoms related to (1) the process responsible for volume depletion, and (2) the hemodynamic consequences of fluid loss. Through the first group of manifestations it is possible to recognize the cause of volume depletion, such as loss or sequestration of fluid. The second group of signs and symptoms includes hypotension, decreased cardiac output, and tachycardia owing to intravascular volume depletion. In addition, diminished tissue perfusion produces altered mental status, generalized weakness, and occasionally severe organ damage (e.g., acute tubular necrosis, cerebral ischemia, myocardial infarction).

The severity of volume deficit may be estimated through evaluation of blood pressure, heart rate, neck veins and venous pressure, skin turgor, moistness of mucous membranes, changes in body weight, and blood and urine indices. If volume depletion results from mechanisms other than hemorrhage, the fluid loss produces hemoconcentration with increased hematocrit (Hct). The ECF volume deficit can be estimated in states of a primary extravascular fluid loss from the rise in Hct as follows:

$$\text{ECV volume deficit} = 0.25 \times \text{body weight (kg)} \times (\text{actual Hct/normal Hct} - 1) \quad (74.4)$$

where 0.25 represents the fraction of ECF per kg of body weight (250 mL per kg). Because the normal range of Hct is relatively wide (38% to 45%), the patient's baseline Hct usually is unknown, and blood loss may have occurred, the reliability of changes in Hct is only modest. Therefore, a precise estimation of volume deficit is difficult. The loss of body weight from its baseline level (body weight prior to the episode of volume depletion) is a clinically useful index to estimate volume deficit, as follows:

$$\Delta \text{ body weight (kg)} = \text{fluid deficit (L)} \quad (74.5)$$

The change in body weight is unreliable for the estimation of fluid deficit in patients with "third space" sequestration. If $[Na^+]_p$ remains within normal limits, the weight loss in kilogram truly represents loss of isotonic fluid. Volume deficit accompanied by hypernatremia or hyponatremia indicates the existence of a disproportionate water loss compared to Na^+ loss.

Pertinent blood indices that are most useful in the diagnosis and management of volume depletion include: (1) blood urea nitrogen (BUN) and serum creatinine levels; (2) Hct, total plasma protein, and/or albumin values; and (3) levels of serum electrolytes, including Na^+, K^+, Cl^-, and total carbon dioxide (almost identical to plasma $[HCO_3^-]$). In volume depletion, BUN and plasma creatinine increase because of an overall depression of renal function, manifested by oliguria, and reduced glomerular filtration rate (GFR) and renal plasma flow. Increased plasma creatinine is caused by a reduced GFR (when muscle necrosis, which could release this substance into the circulation, is absent). Conversely, an elevated BUN, not accompanied by increased plasma creatinine and reduced GFR, reflects enhanced renal reabsorption of urea accompanied by increased salt and water reabsorption. Consequently, the ratio of BUN over plasma creatinine increases from its normal value of 10:1 to 15:1 or more. Hematocrit and concentration of plasma proteins also can increase in volume depletion, a process referred to as hemoconcentration. Alterations in serum electrolytes are commonly observed and they depend on the composition of the fluid lost (e.g., vomiting produces hypokalemia and metabolic alkalosis) as well as the concomitant water and electrolyte intake.

With respect to fluid therapy in volume depletion, considering that oral intake is the physiologic pathway for the entry of fluids, this route should be always considered. Oral replacement therapy is effective, relatively inexpensive, and noninvasive; does not require hospitalization; and saves several million patients (mostly children in developing nations) each year from death. Nevertheless, the presence of vomiting, ileus, or altered mental status precludes its use, mandating intravenous administration of fluid. Most frequently, however, volume repletion in hospitalized patients is performed by the parenteral (intravenous) route.

Volume repletion should be promptly secured because severe volume depletion frequently produces a major reduction in intravascular volume and hypovolemic shock. The type of fluid to be used depends on the cause of volume depletion. Hypovolemia caused by bleeding (e.g., peptic ulcer, rupture of aortic aneurysm) must be treated with blood products or plasma volume expanders (e.g., packed red cells, albumin, or dextran solutions), whereas that resulting from renal or extrarenal losses and fluid sequestration in body cavities (e.g., ileus, ascites) must be treated with saline, dextrose in saline, or Ringer's solution. Plasma volume expanders can be used in the initial phase of treatment to secure a more rapid restoration of hemodynamic status in all patients with shock.

Various intravenous solutions can be selected in fluid therapy.[25] The most commonly used intravenous fluids consist of a NaCl-containing solution (NaCl 0.23%, 0.45%, and 0.9%, known as ¼ normal saline, ½ normal saline, and normal saline, respectively) with or without 5% dextrose. The term normal used in reference to intravenous solutions does not imply "normality" (chemical notation) but simply refers to the isotonicity of intravenous solutions with respect to body fluids. It is more proper to refer to these solutions as ¼ isotonic saline, ½ isotonic saline, and isotonic saline. Although 5% dextrose in water is isotonic with body fluids, the glucose is metabolized so that this solution provides solute-free water without effective long-lasting osmoles (yet providing some caloric intake). The NaCl added to intravenous solutions provides effective osmoles that are preferentially retained in ECF. The efficacy of the various solutions with respect to volume deficit correction is a function of their NaCl concentration, with normal saline as the most effective one and dextrose in water without NaCl the least effective. The selection of intravenous solution is also determined by the patient's $[Na^+]_p$; hypernatremic patients are most frequently treated with NaCl-free solutions (e.g., 5% dextrose in water), whereas those with hyponatremia are usually given isotonic saline or hypertonic (e.g., NaCl 3.0%) saline solutions. It is important to realize the expected changes in the volume of ECF and ICF in response to various solutions. The infusion of normal saline expands the ECF exclusively (ECF volume increment is identical to the volume infused); thus, ICF volume remains unaltered. The infusion of ½ isotonic saline expands both the ECF and ICF, with the former receiving 73% and the latter 27% of the volume load. Finally, a salt-free water infusion (e.g., 5% dextrose in water) will also expand both the ECF and ICF, but in this case, the latter receives 60% of the volume load. In summary, a pure water infusion expands all body compartments but predominantly the ICF, whereas isotonic saline expands the ECF exclusively.[23]

Because patients in hypovolemic shock are at immediate risk of death or ischemic tissue injury, the initial fluid infusion should be at the maximal flow allowed by the intravenous catheter ("wide open"); once blood pressure and tissue perfusion return to acceptable levels, the rate must be diminished to approximately 100 mL per hour to minimize the risk of pulmonary edema, owing to rapid intravascular expansion. Patients with acceptable hemodynamic parameters should receive fluid at initial rates of 100 to 200 mL per hour, with subsequent reduction after 6 to 12 hours to rates of about 100 mL per hour, to secure gradual repletion of all fluid compartments without imposing undue stress on the circulation. Exceptions to these rules are patients with extreme volume depletion (e.g., DKA, NKH) or large ongoing fluid losses (e.g., continuous drainage of large volume of gastrointestinal secretions, postobstructive diuresis, and diabetes insipidus) who might require fluids at a higher rate of infusion as described in the corresponding section of this chapter.

Proper monitoring of fluid replacement therapy is accomplished by evaluation of arterial blood pressure, presence of collapsed or distended neck veins, and urine output to establish the optimum rate of fluid replacement. Additional information might be necessary in critically ill patients, including monitoring of left- and right-sided heart filling pressures, blood pressure measurement through an intra-arterial line, arterial and/or venous blood gas analysis, and sequential chest X-ray films to detect pulmonary venous congestion and interstitial edema.

Volume Expansion. A syndrome of volume expansion caused by overt salt and water retention is commonly observed in long-standing diabetes mellitus.[32,33] Both forms of generalized edema, the so-called primary as well as the secondary types, are encountered. In primary edema, renal retention of salt and water is the initial event that leads to expansion of ECF volume (e.g., diabetic glomerulosclerosis with reduced GFR and avid tubular reabsorption of salt and water). In secondary edema, also called underfill edema, the presence of renal hypoperfusion, owing to decreased "effective arterial circulating blood volume," initiates salt and water retention by the kidney (e.g., diabetes mellitus with congestive heart failure). Thus, the kidney is always involved in the development of positive salt and water balance that leads to generalized edema.[25] It must be recognized that salt and water retention, owing to primary renal disease and congestive heart failure, is the main cause of generalized edema and normal or near-normal serum albumin. Absence of proteinuria argues against renal disease as the primary cause of fluid retention. Patients with heart failure usually have either minimal or mild urinary protein excretion (1+ or 2+ on dipstick determination), whereas those with nephrotic syndrome have, as a rule, severe proteinuria (4+ dipstick). The fluid retention observed in nephrotic syndrome appears to occur as a combination of primary and secondary edema.

The management of localized and generalized edema must be directed, if possible, at the primary cause of fluid accumulation. Effective treatment of the primary cause leads to resolution of the edema. Therapy of the primary process in congestive heart failure can involve the use of afterload-reducing agents, digoxin, and diuretics. Patients with generalized edema most frequently require treatment of the fluid overload in addition to that directed at the primary disease. Correction of fluid overload involves restriction of dietary NaCl, and if this is unsuccessful, the use of diuretic therapy. In addition, both localized and generalized edema are ameliorated by bed rest and elevation of the edematous body area. The management of generalized edema caused by congestive heart failure, nephrotic syndrome, and diabetic glomerulosclerosis is examined in detail in other chapters.

Defect in Potassium Homeostasis

The levels of total body K^+ stores are established by the external K^+ balance, which in turn is determined by the difference between K^+ intake and excretion. The internal K^+ balance refers to the control mechanisms for the distribution of total body K^+ stores between the ICF and the ECF. The major factors that alter internal K^+ balance include hormones (insulin, catecholamines), the acidity of body fluids, the levels of other electrolytes, the tonicity of body fluids, and drugs.[34]

Insulin is a major modulator of extrarenal K^+ homeostasis and promotes K^+ uptake in many cell types, including those from skeletal muscle and liver. The hypokalemic action occurs at very low concentrations of insulin and is independent of the effect of insulin on glucose uptake. The precise mechanism of this action remains to be fully defined but appears to involve the activation of several transport proteins, including stimulation of the Na^+-K^+-ATPase, stimulation of the Na^+-H^+ exchanger, and changes in ionic conductance of certain K^+ channels.[35] Direct stimulation of the Na^+-K^+ pump by insulin induces the translocation of K^+ into the cell interior (entry of two K^+ and exit of three Na^+). This action results in hyperpolarization of the membrane potential (a more negative cell interior). Such hyperpolarization of the cell membrane establishes a new electrical gradient, which favors cellular K^+ entry, and deactivates K^+ channels, which inhibits cellular K^+ exit. Thus, the secondary effects of insulin on the membrane potential increase the hypokalemic action of this hormone.

By stimulating the Na^+-H^+ exchanger, insulin promotes the cellular entry of Na^+ and the cellular exit of H^+. The entry of Na^+ increases the intracellular $[Na^+]$, which further stimulates the Na^+-K^+-ATPase. The cellular exit of H^+ results in cytosolic alkalinization, which in turn increases the K^+-binding capacity for intracellular anions and stimulates the Na^+-K^+ pump, therefore favoring cellular K^+ loading.

A third mechanism for the hypokalemic effect of insulin is mediated from its action on K^+ channels. Insulin controls gating of the inward rectifier K^+ channel of skeletal muscle. This channel is responsible for most of the K^+ conductance of the skeletal muscle in the resting state. It allows K^+ to flow into cells much more easily than it exits from them. Consequently, when the cell membrane is hyperpolarized, the high inward conductance facilitates cellular K^+ entry, whereas when the cell membrane is depolarized, the low outward conductance reduces K^+ exit from cells. Insulin exaggerates the inward rectifying properties of this class of K^+ channel by a dual effect of stimulation of K^+ entry and depression of K^+ exit.

Glucagon also has significant effects on internal K^+ balance and plasma potassium levels.[36] Glucagon induces glycogen breakdown in the hepatocytes, releasing glucose and K^+; therefore, high glucagon levels can elicit a transient increase in $[K^+]_P$. An increase in plasma glucagon in acute metabolic acidosis has been described and this hormonal response might play a role in acidosis-induced hyperkalemia.[35]

K^+ Depletion with Hyperkalemia. The development of uncontrolled diabetes, including DKA, is usually accompanied by varying degrees of total body potassium depletion, which results from multiple causes, including massive kaliuresis secondary to glucosuria, decreased intake, and frequent vomiting. However, plasma potassium levels are rarely low at the time of hospitalization, ranging in most instances from normal to high levels and occasionally attaining dangerously elevated values. This paradoxical relationship has been classically attributed to the concomitant changes in blood acidity that would affect a shift of potassium out of the cells in exchange for hydrogen ions moving intracellularly.[37] However, several of the metabolic derangements observed in patients presenting with DKA are known to alter potassium metabolism and may contribute to the development of hyperkalemia. Endogenous ketoacidemia and hyperglycemia correlate with increased plasma potassium concentration on admission in patients with DKA.[36] However, exogenous ketoacidemia and hyperglycemia in the otherwise normal experimental animal fails to increase plasma potassium levels,[38,39] suggesting that the insulin deficit per se is the major cause of the hyperkalemia that develops in DKA.[36]

Serum pH and bicarbonate levels are known to alter plasma potassium levels. Whereas some studies indicated that the changes in plasma potassium concentration observed during acute acid–base disorders are consequent to the attendant changes in plasma pH, others showed that a low plasma bicarbonate concentration, under isohydric conditions, may induce hyperkalemia.[40,41] Increased effective serum osmolality is another abnormality characteristic of DKA that may affect serum potassium; extracellular hypertonicity resulting from the infusion of saline, mannitol, or glucose results in the translocation of potassium-rich cell water to the extracellular compartment.[42] Hyperglycemia of either endogenous or exogenous origin unaccompanied by ketoacidosis results in hyperkalemia in insulin-deficient diabetics, especially when hypoaldosteronism also is present.[39]

As previously described, glucagon may also play a role in the hyperkalemia of DKA. This hormone may cause an increased potassium output from the liver, an effect that is usually transient because of the counterregulatory enhancement of insulin secretion. However, in the presence of an impaired insulin secretion, as in patients with DKA, increments in plasma glucagon levels may result in uncontrolled hyperkalemia.[43]

An additional mechanism that may be involved in the deranged potassium homeostasis observed in diabetes mellitus is the sympathetic nervous system. Potassium tolerance has been found to be markedly impaired in chemically sympathectomized animals, but is improved in animals given a simultaneous infusion of epinephrine.[44] The effects of the adrenergic agents on the internal potassium balance are mediated by their effect on the plasma levels of insulin and glucagon, and a direct cellular effect on K^+ transport. Therefore, any physiologic condition or pharmacologic maneuver that blocks the β-adrenergic system could result in hyperkalemia, particularly during states of increased potassium load. Diabetic patients may have a suboptimal epinephrine response or altered peripheral sympathetic activity, resulting in potassium movement from the intracellular to the extracellular space as well as an impairment in cellular entry of potassium.

K^+ Depletion with Hypokalemia. Hypokalemia can result from the redistribution or depletion of K^+ stores. The hypokalemia that results from redistribution is caused by cellular uptake of K^+ from the ECF; K^+ redistribution can occur simultaneously with K^+ depletion so that the two processes leading to hypokalemia can have additive effects. The hypokalemia observed with K^+ depletion is characterized by a reduction in the K^+ content of all body fluids.[34]

Potassium depletion can occur with diabetes mellitus when dietary K^+ intake is very low and therefore fails to counterbalance the obligatory urinary K^+ losses associated with glucosuria. However, if K^+ losses are abnormally high, potassium depletion might develop in association with a normal dietary K^+ intake. Potassium losses may be renal or extrarenal, but a combination of losses is commonly encountered. Total body K^+ deficit results in a greater absolute reduction of K^+ content in ICF than in ECF. Nevertheless, the percent deviation in K^+ content is considerably smaller in ICF than in ECF. In a similar fashion, the decrease in intracellular $[K^+]$ with K^+ depletion is significantly smaller than the decrease in $[K^+]_p$. With respect to the relationship between $[K^+]_p$ and the degree of K^+ deficit, a linear relationship with a slope of 0.3 mEq/L per 100 mEq of K^+ deficit $[\Delta[K^+]_p/\Delta K^+$ stores$]$ has been described for patients with K^+ depletion in the absence of redistribution of K^+ stores. According to this relationship, a K^+ depletion of 10% of total body K^+ stores (350 mEq) produces a decrease in $[K^+]_p$ of approximately 1 mEq per L.

Diabetic gastroparesis is a common cause of vomiting leading to fluid and electrolyte losses. Protracted vomiting leads to hypokalemia that is largely caused by increased renal K^+ excretion. The increased kaliuresis is owing to HCO_3^- excretion consequent to HCl depletion (metabolic alkalosis) and to secondary hyperaldosteronism resulting from ECF volume depletion. The direct loss of K^+ as a result of vomiting is relatively small, considering that $[K^+]$ in gastric juice averages 15 mEq per L. Diuretic therapy for the management of accompanying hypertension and congestive heart failure is a common additional cause of potassium depletion. Within a week from the start of diuretic therapy, a mild decrease (0.3 to 0.6 mEq per L) in $[K^+]_p$ occurs, and this level remains constant thereafter unless an intercurrent illness that decreases K^+ intake (vomiting) or increases K^+ loss (diarrhea) develops. Hypokalemia is most commonly observed with thiazides (5% of patients) than with loop diuretics (1% of patients). The decrease in $[K^+]_p$ is directly proportional to the daily dosage and duration of action of the diuretic; thus, daily administration and high-dosage regimens of chlorthalidone, a long-acting thiazide, are more likely to produce severe K^+ depletion and hypokalemia. The antihypertensive effect of thiazides is achieved with small dosages (6.25 to 25.0 mg daily), which have a small effect on K^+ balance; consequently, high dosages of thiazides are not warranted because they will result in K^+ depletion without better blood pressure control. Insulin administration in the course of treating DKA, a condition in which K^+ depletion is usually present, can result in profound and symptomatic hypokalemia.

K^+ Overload with Hyperkalemia. Potassium overload leading to hyperkalemia can occur because of increased K^+ intake or decreased renal K^+ excretion. The former occurs when the adaptive increase in renal K^+ excretion is insufficient to match the larger-than-normal K^+ intake. Salt substitutes are K^+ salts (KCl) that mimic the taste of NaCl and their use may lead to hyperkalemia. As these products are available over the counter, patients frequently use them whether they are recommended by physicians or not. A low NaCl intake reduces the ability of the kidney to excrete K^+; simultaneous ingestion of salt substitutes (K^+ salts) can lead to hyperkalemia owing to the combination of increased K^+ intake and reduced renal K^+ excretion. In fact, a low NaCl intake is the single most commonly observed contributing factor in the development of hyperkalemia in clinical practice. Removing the salt restriction promotes increased kaliuresis, which might partially or fully correct the hyperkalemia.

Diabetes mellitus commonly damages the renal mechanisms of potassium excretion.[34] Such abnormality might result from decreased GFR, decreased tubular secretion of K^+, hypoaldosteronism or pseudohypoaldosteronism, or drugs. In the absence of generalized renal failure, a diminished renal K^+ excretion reflects either a defect in the renin–angiotensin–aldosterone axis or renal resistance to aldosterone.

Renin deficiency leads to a low plasma aldosterone level that might reduce renal K^+ excretion. It occurs in certain physiologic states (advanced age, expansion of ECF volume), with the use of various drugs (β-adrenergic blockers, inhibitors of prostaglandin synthesis, methyldopa), with certain toxins (lead), in some systemic diseases (diabetes mellitus), and in some renal diseases (obstructive uropathy, interstitial nephritis). A common cause of renin deficiency is the so-called type 4 renal tubular acidosis, which is characterized by impaired excretion of both K^+ and H^+. Perhaps its most common presentation is in elderly diabetic patients. Angiotensin-converting enzyme (ACE) inhibitors lead to hypoaldosteronism, which reduces renal K^+ excretion and can increase $[K^+]_p$.

One or more of the various syndromes of diminished aldosterone activity may be observed in diabetes mellitus. A diminished aldosterone activity can occur as a result of:

1. A primary defect in the adrenal synthesis of aldosterone owing to a disease or defect in the adrenal cortex.
2. A secondary defect in the adrenal synthesis of aldosterone owing to failure in the production, release, or action of the various components of the renin-angiotensin-aldosterone axis (e.g., renin deficiency).
3. End-organ resistance to aldosterone, owing to either drugs acting on the kidney (e.g., spironolactone) or renal disease.

Drug-induced mechanisms of hypoaldosteronism leading to hyperkalemia are commonly encountered in diabetic patients. Prostaglandin synthetase inhibitors, such as the nonsteroidal anti-inflammatory drugs (NSAIDs), and cyclosporine inhibit renin secretion, producing hyporeninemic hypoaldosteronism. These drugs can also cause hemodynamically induced decreases in GFR as well as direct nephrotoxicity, thereby impairing further K^+ excretion. ACE inhibitors decrease plasma levels of angiotensin II resulting in decreased levels of aldosterone. Heparin acts directly on the adrenal gland, inhibiting aldosterone secretion. Increased $[K^+]_p$ can occur with heparin administration in approximately 5% of hospitalized patients.

Diabetes mellitus is also associated with end-organ resistance to aldosterone, leading to hyperkalemia, a syndrome known as pseudohypoaldosteronism. This entity can develop as a result of drug administration or renal diseases. Hyperkalemia caused by spironolactone, eplerenone, triamterene, and amiloride, collectively known as K^+-sparing diuretics, exemplifies drug-induced pseudohypoaldosteronism. Renal diseases that primarily damage the renal tubules (with minor decreases in GFR), collectively known as tubulointerstitial renal diseases, elicit this hyperkalemic syndrome (e.g, obstructive uropathy).

Diabetes mellitus is the single major cause of end-stage renal disease (ESRD), and therefore commonly leads to hyperkalemia because of decreased renal function (diminished GFR). In the presence of renal insufficiency, potassium balance might be maintained within normal limits until the GFR decreases to less than 25% of normal. The ability of the kidney with decreased GFR to maintain K^+ balance depends on the development of compensatory mechanisms, collectively known as K^+ adaptation, that increase the fractional K^+ excretion (FE_K) by the kidney.[34] Because $[K^+]_p$ might remain within normal limits in patients with only 25% of overall renal function (GFR), whereas K^+ intake remains unchanged, a fourfold increase in $FE_K{}^+$ must be present. As the calculated FE_K in normal individuals amounts to approximately 10%, the estimated FE_K in a patient with this degree of renal insufficiency is about 40%.

Management of Hyperkalemia. The management of K^+ retention should be initiated even in the presence of a mild degree of hyperkalemia.[34] Several measures should be undertaken at once in patients who have high-normal $[K^+]_p$ (i.e., 5.0 mEq per L) and a disease that predisposes to hyperkalemia, such as diabetes mellitus with renal dysfunction. Severe restriction of dietary NaCl intake should be avoided because it impairs renal K^+ excretion; dietary NaCl intake should be at least 4 g per day. Restriction of dietary K^+ must be enforced. Medications that impair the renal excretion of K^+, such as K^+-sparing diuretics, should be discontinued. Metabolic acidosis, if present, should be treated with alkali therapy.

Proper management of simultaneous retention of Na^+ and K^+ in patients with diabetes mellitus and a salt-retaining disease (hypertension, congestive heart failure, nephrotic syndrome, renal insufficiency), who have an elevated $[K^+]_p$ or even a high-normal $[K^+]_p$ (i.e., 5.0 mEq per L), is effectively achieved by avoiding severe restriction of dietary NaCl intake while concomitantly administering diuretics (e.g., furosemide, thiazides). This recommendation with respect to the dietary NaCl intake should be instituted once a large ECF volume excess is no longer present. A moderate dietary NaCl intake of about 4 g per day will not result in ECF volume expansion if increased urine excretion of NaCl is achieved with the use of diuretics. This strategy secures adequate kaliuresis. Diuretics should not be administered to patients with ESRD because a meaningful kaliuretic response is not expected. A negative external K^+ balance is achieved in all patients with ESRD by: (1) the utilization of cation exchange resins (such as Kayexalate, a sodium polystyrene sulfonate) that promote the excretion of K^+ in the stools, and (2) dialysis (hemodialysis or peritoneal dialysis).

Hyperkalemia is the major threat to life in patients with type 4 renal tubular acidosis; therefore, the main focus of attention should be placed on correcting this electrolyte abnormality. That is the reason why dietary K^+ restriction, diuretics (furosemide, thiazides), and K^+-binding resins are so valuable in these patients. The intake of NaCl should be encouraged, because the availability of Na^+ in the collecting tubules is a major determinant of renal K^+ excretion. The administration of fludrocortisone (Florinef) in daily doses of 0.1 to 0.3 mg helps in the correction of hyperkalemia and acidosis (enhances distal acidification), yet the associated volume expansion may induce hypertension or increase its severity. Alkali therapy (1 to 2 mEq/kg/day) is useful to ensure correction of hyperkalemia and acidosis.

The following three strategies must be considered whenever severe hyperkalemia is present in any patient[34]:

1. To counterbalance the effect of hyperkalemia on the excitability of myocardial and skeletal muscle. This modality is not aimed at reducing the increased $[K^+]_p$.
2. To modify internal K^+ balance, promoting the translocation of K^+ from ECF to ICF. This modality will not alter the total body K^+ stores.
3. To modify external K^+ balance, inducing a net K^+ loss from the body.

The treatment of hyperkalemia with agents that ameliorate the effects of hyperkalemia on myocardial and skeletal muscle excitability involves the administration of Ca^{2+} salts (chloride or gluconate). These agents diminish tissue excitability by widening the difference between resting and threshold potentials. Calcium gluconate (20 mL of a 10% solution) can be infused intravenously over a 10-minute period. The intravenous administration of Ca^{2+} salts is definitely indicated when $[K^+]_p$ reaches 7.0 mEq per L or when significant electrocardiographic abnormalities (absence of P waves, prolongation of QRS complexes, etc.) are present. The effects of Ca^{2+} infusion are short lasting, with peak effect noted about 5 minutes after infusion.

The most important therapeutic agent that promotes cellular K^+ entry is insulin. Insulin leads to tissue uptake of K^+ as well as glucose; therefore, the latter must be infused to prevent hypoglycemia in patients presenting without hyperglycemia. Considering that hyperglycemia of endogenous and exogenous origin can result in hyperkalemia (especially in diabetics), caution should be exercised as to the rate of glucose infusion. Consequently, a situation that mimics a euglycemic insulin clamp (providing enough exogenous glucose to maintain normal plasma glucose level during insulin administration) must be instituted. Additional but less important strategies that might translocate K^+ from ECF to ICF are administration of β_2 agonists and infusion of sodium bicarbonate.

The first two modalities in the therapy of hyperkalemia are only temporary measures that remove the immediate threat to life resulting from hyperkalemia. Achievement of a net K^+ loss is the most effective therapeutic modality to reduce and sustain a normal $[K^+]_p$ in patients with severe and persistent hyperkalemia. Consequently, treatment of severe and persistent hyperkalemia must combine all three modalities.

The presence of associated clinical and laboratory abnormalities can prevent use of one or more treatment modalities of hyperkalemia. The use of K^+ exchange resins by oral or rectal routes is contraindicated in patients with significant gastrointestinal symptoms. Calcium infusions are contraindicated in patients with hypercalcemia. Sodium bicarbonate infusions are contraindicated in patients with alkalemia, patients with high $[HCO_3^-]_p$, those with hypernatremia, or in patients at a significant risk of developing pulmonary edema or with significant ECF volume expansion. Severe hyperkalemia accompanied by preserved renal function usually can be corrected without dialysis. Potassium removal can be achieved in these patients by inducing an enhanced kaliuresis with the administration of fluids containing NaCl or $NaHCO_3$, or both, and with the use of diuretics. The majority of patients who develop severe hyperkalemia, however, have renal failure, and dialysis is the treatment of choice.

Defect in Phosphate Homeostasis

The osmotic diuresis of hyperglycemia leads to decreased renal reabsorption of phosphate accounting for phosphate depletion in DKA.[45] Nonetheless, serum phosphate levels are usually normal or increased at presentation (Table 74.2). The initial serum phosphate correlates positively with serum osmolality, glucose, and anion gap. Insulin deficiency and metabolic acidosis induce a shift of phosphate from cells to the extracellular compartment thereby masking phosphate depletion. Insulin therapy shifts phosphate back into cells, rapidly lowering the serum levels.[46–48]

Defect in Acid–Base Balance

Ketoacidosis and Hyperchloremic Metabolic Acidosis. Although the metabolic acidosis of DKA is mostly caused by the overproduction of β-hydroxybutyric and acetoacetic acids, additional acids, including lactic acid, free fatty acids, and other organic acids, can contribute to the fall in plasma $[HCO_3^-]$.[5] Insulin deficiency, coupled with counterregulatory hormone excess (largely glucagon), activates cAMP, which in turn leads to phosphorylation and activation of lipase in adipocytes, thereby promoting lipolysis.[49–52] Lipolysis of triglyceride stores in the adipocyte provides long-chain fatty acids, which are the principal substrate for hepatic ketogenesis.[53,54] However, hepatic triglycerides might also serve as a source of fatty acids in the presence of fatty liver, a not uncommon condition in patients with diabetes.[5]

Role of Fatty Acid Oxidation. In addition to augmented substrate in the form of long-chain fatty acids, development of substantial ketogenesis by the hepatocyte mitochondria requires a major increase in fatty acid oxidation. A transport system, the carnitine shuttle, is needed for long-chain fatty acids to enter the mitochondrial matrix. This carrier system consists of two carnitine palmitoyl-transferases (CPT)—an outer CPT I and an inner CPT II—and carnitine/acylcarnitine translocase. The key regulatory step for fatty acid oxidation takes place in a transesterification reaction catalyzed by CPT I.[53,55] This enzyme controls the entry of acyl-coenzyme A (CoA) esters, which are derived from the long-chain fatty acids, from the cytosol into the mitochondria (Fig. 74.4).[5] In the normal fed state and in well-controlled diabetes, CPT I is inhibited such that fatty acids cannot enter the mitochondria for oxidation and ketoacid formation, but are re-esterified to triglycerides and transported out of the cytosol as very-low-density plasma lipoproteins. Inhibition of CPT I is provided by malonyl-CoA, a metabolite whose level is dependent on adequate glycolysis and activity of acetyl-CoA carboxylase.[56–59] The concentration of malonyl-CoA is maximal in the fed state, but it sharply decreases with fasting and uncontrolled diabetes. In these conditions, an increase in the glucagon/insulin ratio blocks glycolysis and inhibits acetyl-CoA carboxylase, two processes that lead to a major drop in malonyl-CoA levels. Consequently, CPT I activity is enhanced, allowing conversion of the acyl-CoA esters of long-chain fatty acids to acylcarnitines that can be transported toward the interior of mitochondria.[60] The transesterification to acylcarnitine is then reversed by CPT II, which works in conjuction with the translocase, allowing the release of fatty acyl-CoA in the mitochondrial matrix. The capacity of the hepatocytes for fatty acid oxidation is large and most of the fatty acyl-CoA molecules entering the mitochondria are oxidized to ketone bodies.

The Anion Gap. During the development of DKA, ketoacids released into the body fluids are titrated by HCO_3^- and other body buffers.[61–65] As a result of this buffering process, HCO_3^- ions are replaced by ketoanions in the extracellular fluid producing the characteristic increase in plasma unmeasured anions (the so-called "anion gap"). In uncomplicated DKA, the increment in the anion gap (AG) above its normal value should be approximately equal to the decrement in plasma $[HCO_3^-]$.[61,64] Thus, the ratio of excess AG

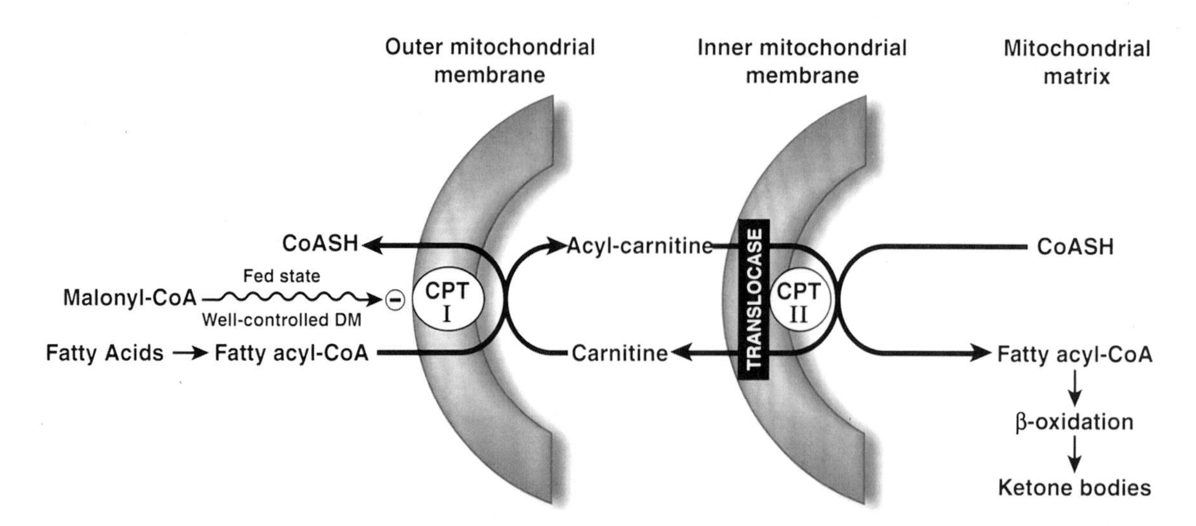

FIGURE 74.4 Regulation of hepatic ketogenesis. Synthesis of ketones in the liver depends on transfer of fatty acyl-CoA into the mitochondria by carnitine palmitoyl-transferase I (CPT I). In the fed state and in well-controlled diabetes, CPT I activity is inhibited by cytoplasmic malonyl CoA. During fasting and in patients with uncontrolled diabetes, the increase in the glucagon/insulin molar ratio suppresses malonyl CoA synthesis, allowing for increased transfer of fatty acyl-CoA into the mitochondria and increased ketogenesis. (From Foster DW, McGarry JD. Acute complications of diabetes mellitus: ketoacidosis, hyperosmolar coma, and lactic acidosis. In: DeGroot LJ, Jameson JL. *Endocrinology*. 4th ed.; 2001.)

(i.e., measured AG minus normal AG) in mEq/L to the decrement in $[HCO_3^-]$ (i.e., normal plasma $[HCO_3^-]$ minus measured plasma $[HCO_3^-]$) should be approximately 1.0. In fact, this pattern is seen in most patients with DKA.[64,66–72] Table 74.3 presents admission data obtained or calculated from several published reports of patients with DKA. Note that the mean decrement in plasma $[HCO_3^-]$ was essentially equal to the mean excess AG in most of these studies (in two studies, ΔAG actually exceeds $\Delta[HCO_3^-]$ by 6 to 8 mEq per L, most likely due to a preexisting metabolic alkalosis).

TABLE 74.3 **Comparison of Admission Data in Diabetic Ketoacidosis**

	Danowski et al.[66] (*n* = 8)	**Seldin et al.[67] (*n* = 10)**	**Nabarro et al.[68] (*n* = 7)**	**Shaw et al.[69] (*n* = 30)**	**Assal et al.[70] (*n* = 9)**	**Oh et al.[71] (*n* = 35)**	**Adrogué et al.[64] (*n* = 150)[a]**
Blood pH					7.06 ± 0.03	7.07 ± 0	7.06 ± 0.0
$[Na]_p$, mEq/L	130 ± 3.2	129 ± 3.7	136 ± 0.5	131 ± 1.4	146 ± 3.0	136 ± 1.6	132 ± 0.6
$[K]_p$, mEq/L	4.9 ± 0.5	4.7 ± 0.2	5.7 ± 0.2	5.8 ± 0.3	5.6 ± 0.3		5.7 ± 0.1
$[Cl]_p$, mEq/L	94 ± 2.8	94 ± 3.5	93 ± 1.0	96 ± 1.3	106 ± 3.0	101 ± 1.4	98 ± 0.6
$[HCO_3]_p$, mEq/L	7.0 ± 0.8	7.4 ± 1.0	7.5 ± 1.1	5.0 ± 0.6[a]	5.6 ± 1.0	9.6 ± 0.3	6.2 ± 0.2[a]
Anion gap, mEq/L	34.3 ± 1.3	32.1 ± 1.5	40.8 ± 2.1	36.7 ± 1.7	40.0	25.0 ± 1.2[b]	33.5 ± 0.6
$\Delta[HCO_3]_p$, mEq/L[c]	17.0 ± 0.8	16.6 ± 1.0	16.5 ± 1.1	22.0 ± 0.6[a]	18.4	14.4 ± 0.3	20.8 ± 0.2
ΔAnion gap, mEq/L[d]	18.3 ± 1.3	16.1 ± 1.5	24.8 ± 2.1	20.7 ± 1.7	24.0	13.0 ± 0.9	17.5 ± 0.6

[a] TCO_2 was measured.
[b] The value was calculated with $[K]_p$.
[c] The values were derived using a baseline value of either 24 mEq/L or 27 mmol/L depending on whether $[HCO_3]_p$ or TCO_2 were measured, respectively.
[d] The values were derived using a baseline value of 16 mEq/L.

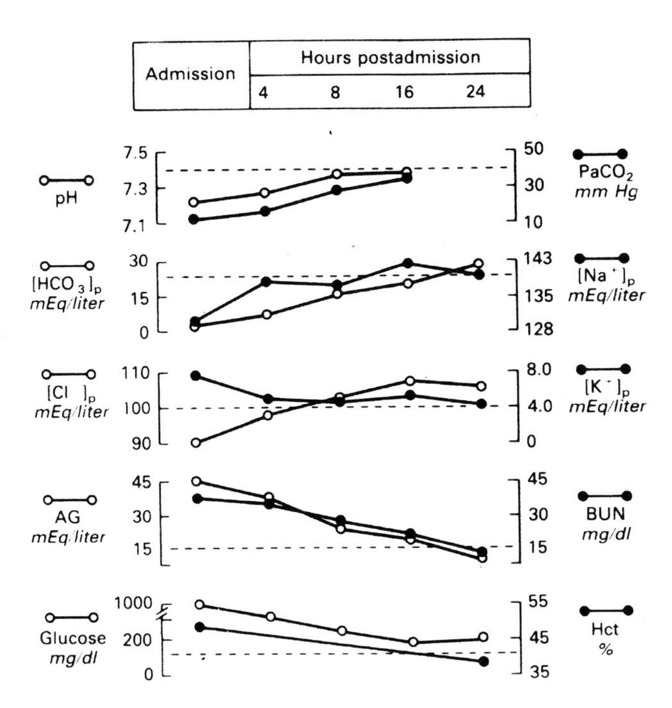

FIGURE 74.5 Laboratory data on admission and follow-up values in a patient admitted for diabetic ketoacidosis and featuring pure anion gap acidosis. Each symbol represents a single measurement. (From Adrogué HJ, Eknoyan G, Suki WN. Diabetic ketoacidosis: role of the kidney in the acid–base homeostasis re-evaluated. *Kidney Int.* 1984;25:591.)

Figure 74.5 charts the course of treatment in a patient with DKA presenting with a typical high AG acidosis.[72] In this patient, the decrement in plasma $[HCO_3^-]$ was essentially equal to the increase in AG before treatment was begun. During the course of therapy, plasma $[HCO_3^-]$ increased as the AG fell, and serum $[Cl^-]$ rose concomitantly. By 16 hours after admission, serum $[HCO_3^-]$ was 16 mEq per L, and blood pH was almost normal. Of note, the BUN was increased on admission, reflecting a prerenal fall in renal function, which was corrected by treatment (see later text).

Although most patients with DKA have an increased AG, one occasionally encounters a patient with pure hyperchloremic metabolic acidosis.[32,73] The presenting data and course of treatment in one such patient are depicted in Figure 74.6.[72] Severe metabolic acidosis, accompanied by the appropriate respiratory response, was present on admission, but the decrement in plasma $[HCO_3^-]$ was not associated with an increase in the AG (AG = 16 ± 4 mEq per L in this example, which includes $[K^+]$ in the calculation). A notable additional feature is that the BUN concentration is within normal limits. Despite standard treatment, 60 hours elapsed before the serum $[HCO_3^-]$ rose to 17 mEq per L. Serum $[Cl^-]$, although elevated on admission, increased further during treatment, and was associated with a reciprocal decrement in the AG. The fall in the AG was due, at least in part, to a major reduction in the serum protein concentration. Thus, two differences are noteworthy in patients with DKA and a normal AG. The first is that there is less evidence of impairment of renal function, and the second is a slower recovery from metabolic acidosis compared with patients presenting with an increased AG. Considering that the DKA patient is unable to properly metabolize ketoacids, whether ketoanions are retained in the ECF or are wasted in the urine should have no major effect on the severity of the acid–base disorder.

The representative cases depicted in Figures 74.5 and 74.6 portray the extremes of the acid–base patterns observed on admission for uncomplicated DKA.[72] In fact, most patients have elements of both increased AG and hyperchloremic acidosis with one element being dominant (Table 74.4). Although various factors could potentially alter the stoichiometric relationship between the increment in AG and the decrement in plasma bicarbonate, the overall level of renal function appears to be the major determinant of the type of metabolic acidosis encountered on admission for DKA.

Additional conditions might alter the ratio of excess AG/bicarbonate deficit in patients with DKA, including hyperproteinemia, vomiting, exogenous bicarbonate therapy, and hypocapnia. Differences in the apparent distribution volume of bicarbonate and ketone anions have also been proposed to explain the hyperchloremic acidosis of DKA; this hypothesis, however, has not been verified experimentally.[64]

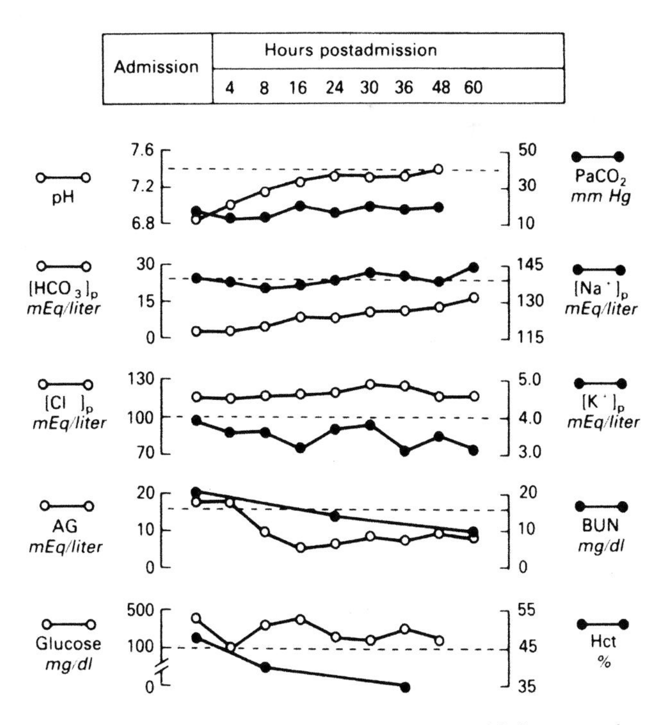

FIGURE 74.6 Laboratory data on admission and follow-up values in a patient admitted for diabetic ketoacidosis and featuring pure hyperchloremic acidosis. Each symbol represents a single measurement. (From Adrogué HJ, Eknoyan G, Suki WN. Diabetic ketoacidosis: role of the kidney in the acid–base homeostasis re-evaluated. *Kidney Int.* 1984;25:591.)

TABLE 74.4 **Acid–Base Patterns of Patients with Diabetic Ketoacidosis**

	Pure High Anion Gap Acidosis	Mixed Forms	Pure Hyperchloremic Acidosis
Associated clinical features before start of therapy			
Fluid intake	Poor	⇔	Adequate
Extrarenal fluid loss	Present	⇔	Absent
ECF volume deficit	Severe	⇔	Mild
Impairment of renal function	Severe	⇔	Mild
Associated laboratory features before start of therapy			
Hematocrit, hemoglobin, serum proteins	Higher	⇔	Lower
BUN, creatinine, uric acid	Higher	⇔	Lower
Cause of changes in $\Delta AG/\Delta HCO_3$ after initiation of therapy[a]	Bicarbonate administration	⇔	Infusion of chloride-rich solutions

[a]AG, anion gap; AG, $[Na^+]_p - ([Cl^-]_p + [HCO_3^-]_p)$. Excess AG (mEq/L) equals measured AG minus normal AG, and bicarbonate deficit (mEq/L) equals normal plasma bicarbonate minus measured plasma bicarbonate. Expected value of $\Delta AG/\Delta HCO_3^-$ is 1.0 as the bicarbonate deficit is the result of its titration by ketoacids.
ECF, extracellular fluid; BUN, blood urea nitrogen.

Role of the Kidney in Modulating the Anion Gap. Because renal reabsorption of filtered plasma ketoanions is limited and the production of ketoacids can reach levels as high as 1,000 to 2,000 mEq per day, the urinary excretion of the sodium and potassium salts of the ketoacid anions can be enormous.[67,68,74–76] The renal "wasting" of ketone salts in association with glucosuria-induced osmotic diuresis, poor fluid intake, and vomiting result in ECF volume depletion and a resultant reduction in renal function. Renal blood flow and GFR both fall during DKA, with recovery to normal values following the episode.[77,78] Increased urea production from enhanced catabolism of amino acids in patients with DKA also contributes to the elevation of blood urea nitrogen levels.

Patients with DKA who develop substantial volume depletion will tend to present with an increased AG metabolic acidosis because of their limited ability to excrete ketone salts. Conversely, patients with DKA who are able to maintain sodium and water intake, thereby minimizing ECF volume depletion, will tend to present with variable degrees of hyperchloremic acidosis, due to urinary excretion of ketone salts and retention of chloride.[64,72]

Effect of Treatment on Anion Gap. Volume replacement with saline infusions during treatment of DKA causes dilution of both ketones and bicarbonate; thus, the AG decreases due to replacement of an unmeasured anion (ketones) with a measured anion (Cl^-). Additionally, correction of K^+ depletion with the chloride salt results in the cellular uptake of K^+ in exchange for H^+, whereas most of the chloride remains in the ECF. Because the H^+ extruded is titrated by HCO_3^-, the net effect is the development of hyperchloremic acidosis.

Renal Response to Ketoacidosis. Diabetic ketoacidosis stimulates renal acid excretion, leading to a several-fold increase in net acid excretion. It should be recalled that a voltage-dependent stimulus for H^+ secretion exists in the distal nephron whenever sodium is absorbed without an accompanying anion. A substantial electrical gradient favoring distal H^+ secretion is present in DKA as a result of increased distal sodium delivery (ketonuria and osmotic diuresis), avid sodium reabsorption (ECF volume contraction), and the presence of poorly reabsorbable anions (ketones). As a result, daily renal net acid excretion, as ammonium and titratable acid, can attain levels as high as 250 and 500 mEq, respectively.[75] Although this vigorous response suggests that the kidney very effectively defends acid–base homeostasis in the course of DKA, such a conclusion is untenable. Maximal stimulation of renal acidification in DKA does not suffice to compensate for the large urinary loss of HCO_3^- precursors in the form of salts of ketoacids. In fact, experimental studies have shown that despite maximal stimulation of urinary acidification, for each mmol of β-hydroxybutyrate excreted, the kidney could salvage only about 0.5 mEq of potential base.[79] Although ketones have been shown to inhibit the rate of renal ammoniagenesis in the experimental animal, this effect most probably plays only a minor role in humans, as a large increment in urinary ammonium excretion is present in DKA.[80]

Effect of Treatment on Renal Response. Balance studies carried out in the early period after admission for DKA revealed that correction of volume depletion resulted in massive urinary loss of bicarbonate precursors (salts of ketoacids) that exceeded the elevated levels of urinary ammonium and titratable acidity (Table 74.5).[72] Thus, in the initial period after admission, the kidneys behave in a maladaptive fashion relevant to the systemic acid–base composition.[72] Only when the plasma ketones have fallen substantially is stimulation of urinary excretion of ammonium and titratable acidity capable of generating sufficient new HCO_3^- to begin to correct the ketoacidosis.

Lactic Acidosis. Patients with diabetes mellitus may develop lactic acidosis, which represents a potentially serious condition.[81] Its diagnosis is warranted in the presence of a high anion gap metabolic acidosis associated with blood lactate levels equal to or higher than 4 mEq per L. This acid–base disorder results from the imbalance between production and utilization of lactate; thus, lactic acidosis might result from increased production, decreased utilization, or both. The skeletal muscle and gut are the organs involved in the development of lactic acidosis because of overproduction. The liver and, to a lesser degree, the kidney are the organs playing the major role in lactate removal. Diabetes mellitus has been shown to be associated with type A as well as type B lactic acidosis. However, this classification has lost its appeal in clinical practice because patients frequently display features of type A as well as type B lactic acidosis simultaneously.[82] Type A includes clinical conditions associated with impaired tissue oxygenation. Examples of type A lactic acidosis are clinical states with either reduced oxygen delivery (shock, cardiac arrest, severe hypoxemia, and sepsis) or those with increased oxygen demand (vigorous exercise, shivering, and generalized seizures). Type B includes clinical conditions in which there is no apparent oxygenation defect to explain the hyperlactatemia. Although patients with type A acidosis develop clinical signs of tissue hypoxia or underperfusion, patients with type B lactic acidosis lack these manifestations. Examples of type B acidosis include congenital defects in glucose or lactate metabolism and many

TABLE 74.5 **Role of the Kidney in the Acid–Base Defense in Normal Subjects and During Recovery from Diabetic Ketoacidosis**

	Normal Subjects[a] $TA + NH_4^+ - HCO_3^-$		Diabetic Ketoacidosis[b] $TA + NH_4^+ - HCO_3^{-c}$	
	Balance	Cum. balance	Balance	Cum. balance
Post admission	mEq		mEq	
0 to 4 hours	12.7	12.7	−45.0 ± 8.2	−45.0 ± 8.2
4 to 8 hours	12.7	25.4	−10.3 ± 13.5	−55.3 ± 20.8
8 to 12 hours	12.7	38.1	1.8 ± 6.8	−53.5 ± 27.1
12 to 16 hours	12.7	50.8	−16.5 ± 2.0	−37.0 ± 28.3
16 to 20 hours	12.7	63.5	−14.3 ± 2.3	−22.7 ± 28.9
20 to 24 hours	12.7	76.2	−21.2 ± 4.8	−1.5 ± 31.2

[a]Estimate based on net acid excretion equal to 1.25 mEq/kg body weight/day and a body weight equal to that of the diabetic patients (61 kg).
[b]The values presented are means ± 1 SE of four studies.
[c]Actual plus potential bicarbonate is shown; ketone salts other than ammonium represent potential bicarbonate.
From Adrogué HJ, Eknoyan G, Suki WN. Diabetic ketoacidosis: role of the kidney in the acid–base homeostasis re-evaluated. *Kidney Int.* 1984;25:591–598.

acquired conditions (e.g., diabetes mellitus, malignancies, toxins, and liver disease). Lactic acidosis caused by metabolic defects comprises: (1) disorders of glucoregulation, including hypoglycemia and diabetes mellitus; (2) major organ failure, involving hepatic, renal, or multiple organ failure; and (3) neoplasias, especially lymphomas, leukemias, sarcomas, and lung carcinomas.

Several drugs and toxins might cause lactic acidosis in diabetic and nondiabetic patients. Ethanol abuse is probably the most common cause within this group. The oral hypoglycemic agents of the biguanides group (phenformin and metformin) used to be a major cause of lactic acidosis, particularly in patients with impaired renal function; the limited worldwide use of these drugs, at the present time, explains their diminishing importance in the etiology of lactic acidosis. Many other drugs, including salicylates, methanol, ethylene glycol, propylene glycol, nitroprusside, and isoniazid, might cause this condition.

Correction of the underlying cause of lactic acidosis is the cornerstone of treatment of this condition. The high mortality associated with lactic acidosis can be reduced by securing adequate support of vital functions. The hemodynamic status and tissue perfusion might improve by correcting volume deficit, enhancing cardiac output, and avoiding vasoconstricting drugs (e.g., norepinephrine). Tissue oxygenation must be optimized by correcting anemia or providing a higher inspired oxygen mixture with or without mechanical ventilation. Energy stores must be replenished to prevent the development of hypoglycemia. If drugs or toxins are responsible for the lactic acidosis, it is mandatory to remove these agents promptly from the patient's tissues by whatever means available (i.e., hemodialysis or hemoperfusion, if necessary). Sepsis must be treated aggressively. Other measures in the management of lactic acidosis might include alkali therapy as well as the use of dichloroacetate (DCA), which enhances the oxidation of pyruvate, as described later.

The utilization of alkali therapy in the treatment of lactic acidosis is controversial because the rising pH associated with this treatment tends to further increase hyperlactatemia. It has been known for years that acidosis inhibits glycolysis, whereas alkalosis stimulates it and consequently results in elevated plasma lactate levels; this effect, however, is generally mild and usually results in an increase in plasma lactate of only 1 to 3 mEq per L. This pH feedback system is not unique to lactic acid but also occurs with other organic acids, including ketoacids, whose production is inhibited by acidosis and stimulated by alkalosis. Additionally, HCO_3^- therapy neither alters the natural course of the deranged metabolism leading to lactic acidosis nor diminishes the mortality of this condition. Yet, most experts advise HCO_3^- therapy in lactic acidosis in the presence of severe acidemia (blood pH <7.20) or $[HCO_3^-]_p$ lower than 10 to 12 mEq per L. Bicarbonate administration, however, has several potential adverse effects that are described elsewhere in this chapter.

Other therapeutic measures include the administration of Carbicarb (0.33 mol per L sodium carbonate and 0.33 mol per L sodium bicarbonate) and DCA. The alkalinizing capacity of Carbicarb is identical to that of $NaHCO_3$, but Carbicarb produces less carbon dioxide.[82] Thus, the potential risk of tissue acidosis owing to H_2CO_3 accumulation appears to be lower when Carbicarb is used instead of pure $NaHCO_3$. However, the use of Carbicarb in clinical practice is not universally accepted. DCA limits lactate production by stimulating pyruvate dehydrogenase activity, resulting in oxidation of pyruvate to acetyl CoA. The usual dose in adults with lactic acidosis is 50 mg per kg of body weight, diluted in 50 mL of isotonic saline for intravenous infusion over a 30-minute period. This dose might be repeated if plasma lactate levels remain substantially elevated. Limited experience with DCA indicates that this therapy can be beneficial in some cases of lactic acidosis.

Renal Tubular Acidosis. A normal anion gap acidosis, also known as hyperchloremic acidosis, might develop either from a primary loss of HCO_3^- or a failure to replenish HCO_3^- stores depleted by the daily production of fixed acids. These two defects are commonly encountered in patients with diabetes mellitus.[61] A primary loss of HCO_3^- might result from intestinal (e.g., diarrhea) or urinary losses of alkali or its precursors (e.g., ketone salts of sodium and potassium). Hyperchloremic metabolic acidosis that results from failure to replace HCO_3^- stores that have been depleted by the daily production of fixed acids is observed in diabetics with distal tubular acidosis. In this condition, the daily net acid excretion by the kidney falls short of the daily acid production, leading to metabolic acidosis owing to depletion of HCO_3^- stores. The major causes of distal renal tubular acidosis accompanied by hyperkalemia (type 4 renal tubular acidosis) include diabetic renal disease, hypoaldosteronism, obstructive uropathy, sickle cell nephropathy, and renal transplant rejection.[83]

Combination of Multiple Disturbances

The full-blown forms of DKA and NKH represent the most frequently observed acute metabolic complications of uncontrolled diabetes mellitus.[84,85] Clinicians generally consider that each of these two entities represents a distinct condition that develops in isolation from the other in the course of diabetes mellitus. In addition, major textbooks commonly describe DKA and NKH as different processes having little in common, thereby perpetuating such a notion. In fact, these conditions are closely interrelated and represent different expressions of a remarkably similar pathophysiologic process.[84–87] Mixed forms having features of DKA and NKH are observed at least as frequently as the pure forms (Tables 74.6 and 74.7). As depicted in Figure 74.7, insulin deficiency or resistance and excessive counterregulation are present in both DKA and NKH, yet the severity of these abnormalities differs in the two clinical conditions. The profound ketosis characteristic of DKA is caused by severe insulin deficiency or resistance in association with a mild degree of excessive counterregulation.

TABLE 74.6 **Contrasting Clinical Features of Pure Forms of Diabetic Ketoacidosis and Nonketotic Hyperglycemia**[a]

Feature	Pure DKA	Mixed forms	Pure NKH
Incidence	5 to 10 times higher	⇔	5 to 10 times lower
Mortality	5% to 10%	⇔	10% to 60%
Onset	Rapid (<2 days)	⇔	Slow (>5 days)
Age of patient	Usually <40 years	⇔	Usually >40 years
Type 1 diabetes	Common	⇔	Rare
Type 2 diabetes	Rare	⇔	Common
First indication of diabetes	Often	⇔	Rare
Volume depletion	Mild/moderate	⇔	Severe
Renal failure (most commonly of prerenal nature)	Mild	⇔	Severe
Subsequent therapy with insulin	Always	⇔	Occasional

[a]Mixed forms of DKA–NKH have intermediate features denoted by the symbol ⇔.
DKA, diabetic ketoacidosis; NKH, nonketotic hyperglycemia.

Conversely, the profound hyperglycemia observed in NKH results from mild insulin deficiency or resistance in association with severe activation of counterregulatory hormones as well as superimposed renal failure.

The pathogenesis of ketosis and hyperglycemia in diabetes mellitus always involves the presence of either absolute or relative insulin deficiency. Such insulin deficit might occur because of augmented insulin requirements relative to a fixed insulin dosage, withdrawal of insulin therapy, or failure of the pancreatic β-cells. Resistance to insulin action also participates in the ketosis and hyperglycemia. Factors that contribute to insulin resistance include counterregulatory

TABLE 74.7 **Contrasting Biochemical Features of Pure Diabetic Ketoacidosis and Nonketotic Hyperglycemia**[a]

Plasma Levels	Pure DKA	Mixed Forms	Pure NKH
Glucose	<600 mg/dL	⇔	>600 mg/dL
Ketone bodies	4+ in 1:1 dilution	⇔	Not 4+ in 1:1 dilution
Effective osmolality	<340 mOsm/kg	⇔	>340 mOsm/kg
pH	Decreased	⇔	Normal
$[HCO_3^-]$	Decreased	⇔	Normal
$[Na^+]$	Normal or low	⇔	Normal or high
$[K^+]$	Variable	⇔	Variable

[a]Mixed forms of DKA–NKH have intermediate features denoted by the symbol ⇔.
DKA, diabetic ketoacidosis; NKH, nonketotic hyperglycemia.

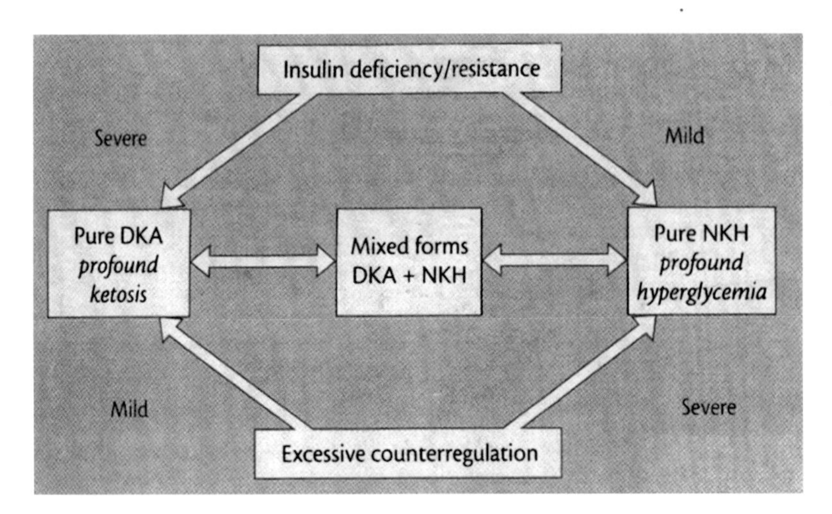

FIGURE 74.7 Diabetic ketoacidosis (DKA) and nonketotic hyperglycemia (NKH) are different forms of the same disease process.

hormones, deficiency of electrolytes (mostly potassium), increased tonicity of body fluids, and acidemia. Counterregulatory hormones play a major role in the development of hyperglycemia. Elevated levels of cortisol, growth hormone, and epinephrine depress insulin-mediated glucose uptake in peripheral tissues (e.g., skeletal muscle) and promote the release of gluconeogenic precursors from myocytes and adipocytes. The latter effect combined with augmented glucagon levels contributes to enhanced gluconeogenesis by the liver and kidney (less important role).

Figure 74.1 depicts the dominant derangements observed in the liver and peripheral tissues that are responsible for the ketonemia and hyperglycemia in decompensated diabetes. Triglycerides stored in adipocytes are decomposed into free fatty acids and glycerol by activation of a "hormone-sensitive" lipase within these cells. Whereas insulin inhibits this lipase, growth hormone, glucagon, and epinephrine stimulate its activity. Consequently, the hormonal disarray of uncontrolled diabetes augments the release of ketone precursors. The increased plasma levels of free fatty acids promote their uptake by hepatocytes where fatty acids are converted to their fatty acyl CoA derivatives. The long-chain fatty acyl CoA may be consumed in the cytosol for the synthesis of fatty acids (including malonyl CoA), triglycerides, and phospholipids (dominant pathway in the normal state) or transported by the carnitine shuttle into the mitochondria where it undergoes β-oxidation producing acetyl CoA (dominant pathway in uncontrolled diabetes mellitus). Within the mitochondria of healthy individuals, the acetyl CoA condenses mostly with oxaloacetate for oxidation in Krebs tricarboxylic acid cycle forming carbon dioxide. The alternative pathway of acetyl CoA within the mitochondria is that two molecules of this compound combine with each other to form the "ketone bodies," acetoacetate and β-hydroxybutyrate (ketoacids). The latter route is greatly stimulated in uncontrolled diabetes mellitus because oxaloacetate is in short supply (being removed from the mitochondria for the augmented gluconeogenesis) and excessive acetyl CoA cannot be accommodated through the Krebs cycle so that it overflows in the ketogenic pathway.[88] The carnitine shuttle is inhibited by cytosolic malonyl CoA, which is produced during fatty acid synthesis, ensuring that newly formed fatty acids are not immediately transported into the mitochondria and broken down. Because insulin augments, whereas glucagon and catecholamines diminish, the concentration of malonyl CoA, the hormonal imbalance of uncontrolled diabetes produces low cytosolic levels of malonyl CoA, enhancing fatty acid transport toward the mitochondria and thereby stimulating ketogenesis. In summary, synthesis of ketones in the liver largely depends on transfer of fatty acyl CoA into the mitochondria by CPT I. In the fed state of normal individuals, CPT activity is inhibited by cytoplasmic malonyl CoA. During fasting and in patients with ketoacidosis, malonyl CoA synthesis is suppressed, allowing for increased transfer of fatty acyl CoA into the mitochondria and increased ketogenesis. Decreased consumption of ketone bodies by peripheral tissues also contributes to the high levels of plasma ketones in DKA.

Clinical Manifestations and Diagnosis of Diabetic Ketoacidosis

Diabetic ketoacidosis is a medical emergency most often observed in type 1 diabetes. Less frequently, DKA is the presenting condition in obese patients with newly diagnosed type 2 diabetes. In patients with uncontrolled type 2 diabetes, DKA can be observed in combination with nonketotic hyperglycemia. The risk of developing DKA in type 1 diabetics is approximately 1% to 2% each year.[90,91] The morbidity associated with DKA is dependent on the severity of the acid–base and electrolyte disturbances present. Despite advances in treatment, mortality of DKA remains approximately 7% in the United States.[91]

Precipitating Events. Omission of insulin administration or noncompliance with treatment, various forms of stress, and dietary indiscretions (especially a large alcohol intake) represent common precipitating events of DKA and NKH

TABLE 74.8 Precipitating Factors for Diabetic Ketoacidosis and Nonketotic Hyperglycemia

1.	Infection (urinary tract infection, pneumonia, sepsis) ~40%	
2.	Inadequate insulin regimen or noncompliance with treatment ~25%	
3.	New-onset diabetes (~15% for DKA) and previously undiagnosed disease (for NKH)	
4.	Acute illness and other conditions	
	Myocardial infarction	Cerebrovascular accident
	Acute pancreatitis	Alcohol abuse
	Intestinal obstruction	Complicated pregnancy
	Renal failure	Endocrine disorders (thyrotoxicosis, Cushing syndrome, acromegaly)
	Peritoneal dialysis (NKH)	Trauma
	Stress	Surgery
	Dental abscess	Drugs (e.g., cocaine, corticosteroids, thiazides)
	Heavy use of concentrated carbohydrate beverages	Idiopathic (20% to 30%)
	Total parenteral nutrition	

DKA, diabetic ketoacidosis; NKH, nonketotic hyperglycemia.

(Table 74.8).[92–94] In young individuals with type 1 diabetes, emotional stress can trigger repeated episodes of DKA over short intervals. Infectious illnesses often precipitate DKA and must be aggressively treated if the ketoacidosis is to be controlled. Such common etiologies include seemingly trivial viral infections as well as pneumonia, pyelonephritis, and septicemia.[73] Pregnancy, myocardial infarction, cerebrovascular accident, intra-abdominal catastrophes (including pancreatitis), K^+ depletion, and drugs such as corticosteroids can also precipitate DKA.[84]

Symptoms and Signs. Weakness, malaise, air hunger, thirst, polyuria, vomiting, and altered sensorium are commonly observed.[1–3] Severe abdominal pain secondary to ketosis (possibly a hypertriglyceridemia-induced pancreatitis) can be observed, and these patients sometimes are mistakenly triaged to surgery.[92] However, the abdominal pain can represent an independent process, such as acute appendicitis (that requires surgery) or pyelonephritis, which in turn may have precipitated DKA. Increased rate and depth of respirations, the so-called Kussmaul breathing, is an almost constant finding. Signs of volume depletion, including orthostatic hypotension, tachycardia, decreased skin turgor, and soft eyeballs, can be evident on physical examination.[95,96] Although DKA is sometimes referred to as diabetic coma, only 10% of patients are unconscious at presentation and about 20% are alert.[92] The majority of patients present, however, with a clouded sensorium. Severe obtundation, coma, or convulsions, rarely seen in pure DKA, are prominent manifestations of severe nonketotic hyperglycemia. The patient's temperature is often decreased but the presence of hypothermia does not rule out an infectious process.[95] Conversely, if fever is present, the likelihood of infection is high. A search for tooth or skin infection, perirectal abscess, or other infectious precipitating event is most important. Patients might describe experiencing the distinct taste and smell of ketones, and the examiner might notice a fruity odor in the subject's breath.

Serum Ketones. The clinical diagnosis of DKA depends on semiquantitative assessment of serum ketones with reagent sticks or tablets; reagent tablets should be powdered before use (Table 74.9). A "large" reading (4+ reaction) for ketones in plasma diluted 1:1 or greater is diagnostic of DKA—such a reading in a urine sample is not diagnostic of DKA, however, as it can be observed in other conditions, including ordinary fasting, fasting induced by an illness that has precipitated lactic acidosis or nonketotic hyperglycemia, or nonketotic hyperglycemia itself.[5] The low renal threshold for ketones accounts for the possible development of a sufficiently high urine ketone concentration in all ketotic states to be detected as a "large" test response (4+ reaction).

The semiquantitive test for ketones measures only acetoacetate and acetone (a product derived from nonenzymatic decarboxylation of acetoacetate); it does not detect β-hydroxybutyrate. The latter ketoacid is formed from the reduction of acetoacetate in a reaction utilizing nicotinamide adenine dinucleotide (NADH). Because the β-hydroxybutyrate concentration in all ketotic states is at least two to three times higher than that of acetoacetate, a relatively high plasma ketone level of at least 6 mmol per L is required to achieve a "large" test reading in an undiluted sample. Therefore, a "large" test reading in plasma diluted 1:1 or greater indicates that at least 12 mmol per L of ketones are present, a level found in DKA but rarely present in other ketotic states.[97,98] Exceptions

TABLE 74.9 Diagnostic Criteria for Diabetic Ketoacidosis and Nonketotic Hyperglycemia

	DKA: Mild	DKA: Moderate	DKA: Severe	NKH
Plasma glucose (mg/dL)	>250	>250	>250	>600
Arterial pH	7.25–7.30	7.00–7.24	<7.00	>7.30
Serum bicarbonate (mEq/L)	15–18	10 to <15	<10	>18
Urine ketones[a]	Positive	Positive	Positive	Small
Serum ketones[a]	Positive	Positive	Positive	Small
Effective serum osmolality (mOsm/kg)[b]	Variable	Variable	Variable	>320
Anion gap[c]	>10	>12	>12	Variable
Alteration in sensorium or mental obtundation	Alert	Alert/drowsy	Stupor	Stupor/coma

[a]Nitroprusside reaction method
[b]2 [measured Na^+ (mEq/L) + glucose (mg/dL divided 18)]
[c]$Na^+ - (Cl^- + HCO_3^-)$
DKA, diabetic ketoacidosis; NKH, nonketotic hyperglycemia.
From Kitabchi AE, Umpierrez GE, Miles JM, et al. Hyperglycemic crises in adult patients with diabetes: a consensus statement from the American Diabetic Association. *Diabetes Care*. 2009;32:1335.

include a short-term fast in late pregnancy, lactating women, and some alcoholic patients.[99–102]

The altered redox state of hepatocytes observed in tissue hypoxia, ethanol ingestion, or with high rates of fatty acid oxidation increases further the ratio of β-hydroxybutyrate to acetoacetate making the semiquantitative assay less reliable for detection of ketosis. Sulfhydryl drugs, including captopril, can produce a false positive ketone test.[103] An interaction of the colorimetric assay for creatinine with acetoacetate (chromogen) results in higher measured serum creatinine levels on admission for DKA, followed by large decreases after insulin's lowering effects on ketone levels. Table 74.2 presents a summary of salient abnormalities of blood measurements in patients presenting with DKA.

Diagnosis. The diagnosis is made by recognition of characteristic symptoms and signs, coupled with biochemical features that include hyperglycemia and ketosis.[84] A commonly used but more restrictive diagnostic criterion of DKA includes a triad of hyperglycemia (plasma glucose >250 mg per dL), ketosis (serum ketones 4+ positive by the nitroprusside reaction in a dilution 1:1 or greater), and metabolic acidosis (plasma bicarbonate <18 mEq per L, blood pH <7.30). However, the hypobicarbonatemia and acidemia might be absent in DKA because of the coexistence of additional acid–base disorders.[104]

Differential Diagnosis. The differential diagnosis of DKA includes conditions with symptoms and signs related to the neurologic, gastrointestinal, or respiratory systems. Neurologic disorders include metabolic diseases (e.g., hypoglycemia, uremia, nonketotic hyperglycemia, lactic acidosis), toxic encephalopathies (e.g., ethanol, methanol, ethylene glycol, opium derivatives, other narcotics), head trauma, cerebrovascular accident, meningitis, and encephalitis. Gastroenteritis (abdominal pain, nausea, vomiting) and pneumonia (dyspnea) can also resemble DKA.

Nonketotic Hyperglycemia. Nonketotic hyperglycemia (NKH) is a syndrome characterized by the presence of severe hyperglycemia (usually >600 mg per dL) and the absence of clinically significant ketosis (Tables 74.7 and 74.9).[84,85] DKA and NKH share the same general pathogenesis—insulin deficiency/resistance and excessive counterregulation (the most important element being high glucagon levels), but the importance of each of these endocrine abnormalities appears to differ.[86,87] Pure DKA, which features profound ketosis, might emanate from severe insulin deficiency/resistance, with milder abnormalities in counterregulation (Fig. 74.7). By contrast, NKH, which features marked hyperglycemia without ketosis, appears to reflect relatively mild insulin deficiency/resistance but more intense counterregulation. The most important clinical distinction, however, is that the

TABLE 74.10 **Fluid Deficit and Glucose Load as Precipitating Factors of Nonketotic Hyperglycemia in Diabetes Mellitus**

Condition	Physiologic Derangement	Clinical Entity
Fluid deficit	Poor water intake	
	Relatively preserved CNS function	Elderly/nursing home patients
	Major CNS abnormality	Cerebrovascular accident, subdural hemorrhage
	Increased urinary fluid loss	Large osmotic diuresis, diuretics
	Extrarenal fluid loss	
	Gastrointestinal	Gastroenteritis, peptic ulcer disease, gastrointestinal bleeding, pancreatitis
	Skin	Heat stroke, burns
Glucose load	Increased glucose intake	Highly sweetened drinks, enteral or tube-feeding; hyperalimentation, peritoneal dialysis
	Increased endogenous glucose production	
	Stress	Psychological/physical trauma
	Infection	Pneumonia, pyelonephritis, sepsis
	Major illness	Myocardial infarction
	Medication	Corticosteroids, phenytoin, calcium channel blockers[a]

[a]Phenytoin and calcium channel blockers may decrease insulin release and precipitate the nonketotic hyperglycemia.
CNS, central nervous system.

severity of the fluid deficit and secondary renal dysfunction is greater in NKH than in DKA. This finding in NKH plays a critical pathogenetic role in the profound hypertonicity observed (Table 74.9).[105–108] In some instances, a large exogenous source of glucose can be of great importance in the development of this condition (Table 74.10).[13]

Hypertonicity and Renal Dysfunction. Renal dysfunction, most commonly caused by volume depletion, must be present to generate and sustain the extreme hyperglycemia observed in most patients with NKH.[13] Fluid deficit can be caused by poor fluid intake (e.g., in patients who are frail and unable to perceive or respond to thirst because of sedation, stroke, or other causes) and/or abnormal fluid losses due to osmotic diuresis, vomiting, diarrhea, fever, or diuretics. A simple calculation demonstrates the virtual impossibility of maintaining plasma glucose levels substantially higher than 400 mg per dL in the presence of normal renal function, because of the magnitude of obligatory glucosuria.[13] In a patient with a plasma glucose of 400 mg per dL and a normal GFR, for example, the amount of glucose that escapes reabsorption (difference between plasma glucose and the "renal threshold concentration," 180 mg per dL) is approximately 400 g per day. Glucose is also removed by cellular metabolism; whole-body glucose utilization is approximately 200 g per day under euglycemic conditions, and increases in proportion to the glucose concentration even in the absence of insulin. In patients with severe hyperglycemia and adequate renal function, therefore, substantial glucose removal, on the order of 600 to 1,000 g per day, would result both from glucosuria and internal disposal. An equal amount of new glucose must enter the circulation to satisfy these demands in steady-state, severe hyperglycemia. Thus, unless the patient has an exceptionally high level of endogenous glucose production (in excess of three times the normal value observed in the fasting state) or an extremely large exogenous source of glucose is present, severe hyperglycemia cannot be sustained in the absence of renal failure. Exogenous sources of glucose include tube-feeding solutions, parenteral hyperalimentation, or peritoneal dialysis with a high glucose concentration in the dialysate. Table 74.10 summarizes the role of fluid deficit and glucose load as precipitating factors of NKH.[13]

Absence of Ketosis

There are several theories to account for the absence of substantial ketosis in NKH.[109–111] It has been proposed that in NKH there is sufficient insulin to inhibit lipolysis but not enough to stimulate peripheral glucose uptake. This theory is based on the presumed less severe insulin deficit of patients with NKH, and the known inhibition of ketosis by relatively low insulin levels. Because hypertonicity has been shown to inhibit lipolysis in vitro, it may also be partly responsible for the absence of substantial ketoacidosis in NKH.[112] A more recent explanation offered for the absence of ketosis is hepatic resistance to glucagon, such that malonyl-CoA levels do not decrease as much as in DKA.[113–115]

Diagnosis

Typically, patients with this disorder are elderly with type 2 diabetes, and present with depressed sensorium, progressing to obtundation and finally coma (Table 74.9). They may be oliguric or anuric. Patients with "pure" NKH have no acid–base abnormalities, no clinically significant ketonemia, a markedly elevated blood glucose concentration, and elevated BUN and creatinine concentrations. The diagnosis is based on the presence of severe hyperglycemia (glucose levels >600 mg per dL), hypertonicity (>320 mOsm per kg), absence of significant ketosis, and profound volume depletion.[84] A comparison of the most salient clinical and biochemical features that distinguish pure forms of DKA from NKH are displayed in Tables 74.6 and 74.7. Notably, many patients exhibit a mixed pattern with clinical and biochemical features of both DKA and NKH. These patients should be diagnosed as having DKA-NKH.[81]

Clinical Manifestations

Depression of the sensorium, somnolence, obtundation, and coma are prominent manifestations of NKH, and the degree of CNS depression correlates with the severity of serum hypertonicity.[105] Water loss from the central nervous system with brain shrinkage has been documented within 1 hour of severe hyperglycemia in experimental animals, but brain volume recovers at 4 to 6 hours. Neither ketosis nor metabolic acidosis, features that are consistently present in DKA but usually absent in NKH, produce extreme depression of the sensorium.[105] In fact, a serum tonicity (i.e., effective osmolality) of 340 mOsm per kg H_2O or higher appears to be necessary for the development of coma, and such levels are commonly observed in NKH but not in DKA.[84,105] Circulatory collapse secondary to profound volume depletion can be observed in NKH. All other symptoms and signs previously described for patients in DKA (except for dyspnea and Kussmaul respiration that arise from metabolic acidosis) may also be observed in NKH.

Assessment of Effective Osmolality

To estimate serum tonicity (effective osmolality), one should use only the sodium and glucose concentrations (effective osmolality = 2 × $[Na^+]$ + glucose/18). Not infrequently, a comatose diabetic patient is found to have, for example, a measured osmolality of 350 mOsm per kg H_2O but the calculated effective osmolality is only 310 mOsm per kg H_2O; in this case, the patient's coma is more likely to be due to conditions other than NKH (e.g., alcohol, uremia, cerebrovascular accident). Conversely, a comatose diabetic patient who is admitted with a calculated effective osmolality of 350 mOsm per kg H_2O most likely has NKH encephalopathy. Nonetheless, one should always exclude other causes of coma. Sometimes it is difficult to establish whether a neurologic finding is a cause or effect. For example, stroke can lead to NKH, and conversely NKH can cause a cerebrovascular accident.[116–118] Rapid reversal of the neurologic syndrome with therapy for NKH indicates that the neurologic event was not the cause but the effect of this metabolic disorder.

Therapy of Diabetic Ketoacidosis and Nonketotic Hyperglycemia

The main therapeutic goals of the successful management of DKA and NKH include repletion of fluid deficit and securing an adequate circulation, reversal of the altered intermediary metabolism, correction of the electrolyte and acid–base imbalance, and treatment of the initiating event.[119–125] To accomplish these objectives, a number of requirements must be fulfilled: continuous physician availability; 24-hour access to laboratory facilities; equipment and drugs for handling medical emergencies; and maintenance of a flowchart documenting evaluations of vital signs, mental condition, serum chemistries, urine tests, insulin intake, fluid administration (intravenous and oral), urine output, electrolyte intake, and other medications. A synopsis of the bedside and laboratory procedures for the diagnosis, management, and monitoring of DKA and NKH is presented in Table 74.11.

Fluids

Intravenous saline infusion should be started at once to correct the impaired hemodynamic status and the renal dysfunction; in addition, it lowers plasma glucose levels by enchancing glucosuria and decreasing counterregulatory hormone release (catecholamines).[126,127] Isotonic saline (i.e., 0.9%, NaCl) should be infused at the fastest rate possible in patients in circulatory shock (Table 74.12). Patients who do not have an extreme volume deficit should receive about 500 mL per hour for the first four hours followed by 250 mL per hour for the next 4 hours. More rapid administration is not recommended, as it can delay correction of acidemia (see earlier) and increase the risk of cerebral edema.[127] Some experts prefer lactated Ringer's solution to minimize the increase in serum $[Cl^-]$, but there is no evidence that such a practice is of benefit[5]; further, it has the potential of inducing rebound metabolic alkalosis, as it loads the patient with the HCO_3^- precursor, lactate. Once the patient is hemodynamically stable, the use of half-isotonic saline with the addition of 20 to 40 mEq of potassium per each L of infusate is appropriate to also secure potassium repletion.

Patients presenting with extreme volume depletion can require a fluid infusion of as much as 5 to 10 L within the first 24 hours.[128–131] Fluid challenges of this magnitude demand that the patient receive careful monitoring for signs of pulmonary edema. Central venous or pulmonary artery catheterization may be required in some patients to accurately monitor intravascular volume.

It is unwise to allow oral fluid intake in the early phase of DKA and NKH because vomiting is common, especially if acute gastric distention is present. Although efforts should be made to avoid routine bladder catheterization in patients with uncontrolled diabetes to prevent the development or exacerbation of a urinary tract infection, a catheter might be required if the patient is stuporous or urine output cannot be monitored reliably.

TABLE 74.11 **Procedures/Studies for Diagnosis, Management, and Monitoring of Diabetic Ketoacidosis and Nonketotic Hyperglycemia[a]**

Bedside	Laboratory Procedures/Studies
	Blood
1. Assess vital signs and cardiorespiratory status (every 30 minutes for 4 hours, hourly for next 4 hours, then every 2 to 4 hours) until stable	1. Glucose (hourly by test strip until <250 mg/dL, then every 2 hours; confirm in laboratory every 2 to 4 hours) until stable
2. Assess volume status, body weight, and skin turgor	2. Serum electrolytes (every 2 to 4 hours) and monitoring of serum anion gap until stable
3. Assess mental status (hourly) (consider head CT scan, lumbar puncture)	3. Venous pH, PCO_2, HCO_3^- (every 2 to 4 hours) until stable
4. Blood glucose (test strips)	4. Urea nitrogen, creatinine
5. Blood and urine ketones (test strips or tablets)	5. Osmolality
6. Urine output (hourly for 6 hours and every 4 hours thereafter) until stable	6. Hb, WBC, and differential
7. Fluid intake and output (hourly monitoring)	7. Cardiac enzymes
8. Complete flow chart	8. Amylase (spuriously elevated ?)
9. Electrocardiogram	9. Cultures
10. Chest X-ray	**Urine**
	1. Microscopy and cultures
	2. Glucose, ketones

[a]The frequency of repeat tests indicated above represents general guidelines that might require adjustments depending on the patient's presentation and response to treatment.
CT, computed tomography; Hb, hemoblobin; WBC, white blood cell.

TABLE 74.12 **Synopsis of Intravenous Fluids and Insulin Therapy in the Management of Diabetic Ketoacidosis and Nonketotic Hyperglycemia**

1. IV fluids
   Shock: fluid resuscitation with 0.9% NaCl (isotonic saline), as needed
   Moderate to severe volume depletion: 500–1,000 mL/hr isotonic saline for 4 hours, and half the initial rate for the next 4 hours
   Mild volume depletion and
      Normal or high $[Na^+]_s$ (corrected): 0.45% NaCl at 250–500 mL/hr
      Low $[Na^+]_s$ (corrected): isotonic saline at 250–500 mL/hr
   Add dextrose (i.e., 5% dextrose in 0.45% NaCl) when serum glucose is ≤200 mg/dL
2. Insulin
   Replete K^+ first if $[K^+]_s$ <3.5 mEq/L while holding insulin
   SC route (uncomplicated DKA): regular insulin 0.3 units/kg followed by 0.2 units/kg every 2 hrs
   IV route: regular insulin as IV bolus (0.1 unit/kg) followed by continuous infusion (0.1 unit/kg/hr)
   Double insulin dose if initial glucose fall <50–70 mg/dL
   Reduce insulin dose when glucose ≤200 mg/dL or change to SC
   Keep glucose 150–200 mg/dL until resolution

DKA, diabetic ketoacidosis; NKH, nonketotic hyperglycemia; IV, intravenous; SC, subcutaneous.

Insulin

All patients with uncontrolled diabetes require insulin to reverse the ketoacidosis and correct hyperglycemia.[132–134] These actions of insulin largely reflect suppression of ketone and glucose production in the liver because of insulin's antiglucagon effect. Of lesser importance is the insulin-induced enhancement of glucose utilization in muscle and adipose tissue as well as inhibition of lipolysis. Regular insulin should be given, if possible, intravenously.[5,85]

Mild insulin resistance is virtually a constant finding, although occasionally it may be extreme.[135,136] Consequently, insulin requirements in DKA are always several-fold higher than in normal persons. A loading dose of 15 to 30 units given as a bolus on arrival is recommended to secure binding of insulin to anti-insulin antibodies that might be present in patients who have been previously treated with animal insulin, and to assure saturation of insulin receptors.[137] In patients who are markedly volume depleted, insulin therapy should be withheld for the initial 30 to 60 minutes to allow some repletion of the ECF volume with isotonic saline. In the absence of saline, insulin can exacerbate ECF volume depletion by translocating glucose into cells, thereby causing a fall in ECF tonicity and a shift of water to the ICF compartment. In fact, fluid repletion alone in the absence of insulin administration reduces plasma glucose concentration by 35 to 70 m per dL per hour.[138]

Table 74.12 presents a synopsis of insulin therapy for the management of DKA and NKH.[139–144] Although continuous intravenous insulin infusion is most commonly used, intramuscular or subcutaneous administration appears to be as effective in correcting hyperglycemia and ketoacidosis.[46] Plasma glucose should fall at approximately 5% to 10% per hour. As the glucose level approaches 300 mg per dL, 5% dextrose in water at 50 mL per hour should be included in the intravenous fluids and the plasma glucose concentration should be followed closely.

A solution containing 100 units of insulin in 100 mL of isotonic saline is commonly used, adjusting the infusion rate to secure the insulin dosage desired. Because some patients are very resistant to insulin, much larger doses might be required. In all cases, the hourly dose should be doubled if the expected reduction in the plasma glucose is not observed within a few hours. Monitoring serum ketones during therapy is unnecessary since it does not help in the adjustment of insulin dosage.[144]

Alkali

Bicarbonate administration should theoretically be unnecessary in DKA (at least in patients with predominantly increased AG acidosis) because ketones, when finally metabolized to CO_2 and H_2O, regenerate HCO_3^-.[1–3] Indeed, several studies have shown that HCO_3^- administration did nothing to improve the recovery of patients with DKA who presented with very severe acidemia (arterial pH of 6.90 to 7.10).[145,146] The administration of HCO_3^- in DKA may also have some potentially deleterious effects because it can augment hepatic ketogenesis and lead to worsening of the CNS acidosis, hypokalemia, and rebound metabolic alkalosis.[145–147]

Nonetheless, there are proponents of alkali administration. The controversy regarding its utility is based on variable assessment of the associated risks and benefits by different workers.[84,147–151] The potential advantages and disadvantages of HCO_3^- administration are summarized in Table 74.13.

Table 74.14 summarizes our recommendations in terms of indications, goals, and dose estimation for HCO_3^- administration in DKA.[151,152] After weighing the arguments, it appears that judicious administration of HCO_3^- to severely acidemic patients, especially those with predominant hyperchloremic metabolic acidosis, confers net benefit; the goal is to support the arterial pH at 7.10 to 7.20 and serum $[HCO_3^-]$ at approximately 10 mEq per L. Bicarbonate should be added to an IV infusion, if possible, instead of administering by intravenous bolus (unless hyperkalemia is present), because of the risk of severe hypokalemia.

Potassium

The typical patient with DKA has a potassium deficit of 4 to 8 mEq per kg at the time of admission, yet the initial serum $[K^+]$ will usually be normal or elevated (see earlier and Table 74.2). Serum $[K^+]$ decreases with therapy because of insulin-mediated uptake by cells, dilution due to volume repletion by intravenous fluids, correction of metabolic acidosis, and urinary K^+ losses. Thus, K^+ supplementation is required.[1–3] Specifically, after the initial fluid challenge has restored the urinary output and assuming that serum $[K^+]$ is below 5.0 mEq per L, an intravenous infusion of 10 to 20 mEq per hour should be started and continued until the DKA is controlled and serum $[K^+]$ is 4.0 to 5.0 mEq per L. Serum $[K^+]$ should be monitored periodically and the K^+ infusion rate adjusted, as needed. Details about K^+ supplementation are provided in Table 74.15.

Phosphate

Because phosphate administration is of unproven clinical significance and potentially dangerous (i.e., it might result in hypocalcemia and hypomagnesemia), it should not be infused unless the serum phosphate is below 0.5 mg per dL; in those circumstances, 10 to 30 mmol of potassium phosphate might be added to the intravenous infusion and repeated if necessary to correct persistent hypophosphatemia. The hypophosphatemia of DKA may have serious consequences (e.g., impaired myocardial and/or skeletal muscle contractility) if it occurs in undernourished patients, such as chronic alcoholics. In this population, parenteral phosphate replacement of 60 to 120 mmol administered over a 24-hour period is recommended.

Cerebral Edema and Other Complications of Therapy

Patients with DKA may be admitted with a relatively normal mental status and subsequently become unconscious within the first 12 hours of therapy, in spite of a partial or complete correction of the hyperglycemia and ketoacidosis.[153] These

TABLE

74.13 Potential Advantages and Disadvantages of Bicarbonate Administration in the Management of Diabetic Ketoacidosis

Advantages

1. Improves hemodynamic status if shock persists after volume repletion and severe metabolic acidosis is present
2. Increases myocardial contractility and enhances cardiac and vascular responsiveness to catecholamines
3. Aids correction of hyperkalemia, especially in patients with prerenal azotemia
4. Prevents a rapid fall in CSF osmolality and therefore might decrease risk of cerebral edema
5. Aids correction of cell metabolism and function (including CNS), impaired by severe acidosis
6. Improves acidosis-induced glucose intolerance and insulin resistance

Disadvantages

1. Induces or worsens hypokalemia, leading to cardiac arrhythmias (especially in digitalized patients) and/or dysfunction of respiratory muscles (respiratory failure)
2. Produces ECF volume expansion that can cause pulmonary edema
3. Reduces cerebral blood flow (pH effect) and O_2 delivery to the brain
4. Worsens hypophosphatemia due to cellular uptake of phosphate and depresses O_2 delivery to tissues (increased affinity of Hb for O_2)
5. Produces hypernatremia and increased serum osmolality
6. Decreases further CSF pH, leading to worsening of CNS function
7. Induces overshoot (rebound) alkalosis once conversion of ketone salts to bicarbonate takes place
8. Aggravates ketogenesis and lactic acidosis
9. Predisposes to tetany resulting from hypocalcemia and alkalemia

CSF, cerebrospinal fluid; CNS, central nervous system; ECF, extracellular fluid.

TABLE

74.14 Indications, Goals, and Dose Estimation for Bicarbonate Administration in the Management of Diabetic Ketoacidosis

INDICATION

1. Extreme metabolic acidosis (pH <7.00, TCO_2 <5 mmol/L), independent of prevailing hemodynamic status
2. Severe metabolic acidosis (pH <7.15, TCO_2 <10 mmol/L) in association with one or more of the following:
   - Shock unresponsive to volume repletion
   - Persistence or worsening of acidemia after several hours of therapy
   - Predominant hyperchloremic acidosis instead of the usual high anion gap acidosis
   - Worsening of mental status and CNS depression
3. Severe hyperkalemia ($[K^+]_p$ >7 mEq/L)

GOALS AND DOSE ESTIMATION

1. If TCO_2 <5 mmol/L (indication 1), it should be increased to no more than 8 to 10 mmol/L
2. If TCO_2 is 5 to 10 mmol/L (indication 2), it should be increased to no more than 13 to 15 mmol/L
3. Dose estimation: (desired plasma TCO_2 − current plasma TCO_2) × b.wt (kg) × 0.5^a
4. Calculated bicarbonate dose can be added to IV infusion (1 to 2 ampules or 44 to 88 mEq $NaHCO_3$ per L) or given by IV bolus (50% of estimated dose immediately, and the rest within 2 to 4 hours provided that hypokalemia is not present or is simultaneously treated and that evidence of pulmonary edema is not found)
5. Monitor blood acid–base status every 30 to 60 min (for 2 to 4 hours) after initiation of bicarbonate therapy to adjust dose to patient's needs

[a]Derives from the "apparent space of distribution" of bicarbonate (retained HCO_3^- in mEq/kg divided by the $\Delta[HCO_3^-]_p$ from preinfusion) that is approximately 50% of body weight in normal subjects but higher in hypobicarbonatemic states. Thus, this formula purposefully underestimates bicarbonate requirements to avoid the risk of overcorrection.
CNS, central nervous system; IV, intravenous.

TABLE 74.15 **Potassium Supplementation in the Management of Diabetic Ketoacidosis and Nonketotic Hyperglycemia**

KCl should *not be* added to the initial 2 L of IV infusion to avoid hyperkalemia because
- Urinary output is initially unknown
- Initial $[K^+]_p$ is usually normal or high

Exception to the above rule on K^+ supplementation: add K^+ to the initial 2 L of IV fluids if
- Initial $[K^+]_p$ <4.0 mEq/L and
- Adequate diuresis is secured

KCl should *be* added to the third L of IV infusion and subsequently if
- Urinary output is adequate (should be at least 30 to 60 mL/hr) and
- $[K^+]_p$ <5.0 mEq/L

Rate of IV K^+ supplementation:
 20 to 30 mEq/hour if $[K^+]_p$ <4.0 mEq/L
 10 to 20 mEq/hour if $[K^+]_p$ >4.0 mEq/L

Concentration of K^+ in IV infusions:
 20 mEq/L when IV supplementation is started and subsequently if $[K^+]_p$ <4.0 mEq/L, and IV infusion rate is = 1 L/hour
 40 mEq/L (maximum) if $[K^+]_p$ <4.0 mEq/L and IV infusion rate is <1 L/hour

Monitoring of K^+ supplementation is accomplished by
 $[K^+]_P$ every 2 to 4 hours during the initial 12 to 24 hours of therapy
 ECG every 30 to 60 minutes during the initial 4 to 6 hours (i.e., only lead II)

IV, intravenous.

patients are typically, but not exclusively, children or young adults, and their morbidity and mortality is relatively high.[154] Often, the fatal outcome is unexpected, as these patients do not have the underlying vascular, cardiac, and renal abnormalities found in older diabetics. At autopsy, cerebral edema is consistently present.[154] Although cerebral edema leading to death or chronic sequelae (e.g., isolated growth hormone deficiency) is fortunately rare, milder forms can be regularly found in the course of standard treatment of DKA.[5,155,156]

The pathogenesis of this condition remains poorly understood.[116,157–159] Osmotic disequilibrium between brain cells and the cerebrospinal fluid (CSF) is often cited as the principal determinant of cerebral edema. In response to hyperglycemia, brain cells increase their osmolar content within hours to defend themselves against shrinkage. Once this cellular adaptation to hypertonicity has occurred, a sudden decrease in CSF osmolality, due to hypotonic fluid infusions or a fall in plasma glucose, may cause swelling of these adapted cells and produce cerebral edema. Insulin administration also activates the plasma membrane Na^+/H^+ exchanger (NHE–1), which promotes sodium entry in brain cells, facilitating development of cerebral edema. The effects of rapid crystalloid volume loading in diabetic patients with DKA and the resulting dilutional hypoalbuminemia have been studied and some degree of brain swelling or increase in CSF pressure was found.[160–165] Alterations in CSF pH and oxygen tension following HCO_3^- administration may also contribute to the development of cerebral edema.

These mechanisms are only hypotheses, however, and the pathogenesis of cerebral edema in DKA remains uncertain. Still, it seems prudent in the course of therapy of DKA (and that

TABLE 74.16 **Complications Of Diabetic Ketoacidosis and Nonketotic Hyperglycemia**

1. Cardiogenic shock
2. Septic shock
3. Cerebral thrombosis
4. Hypoglycemia
5. Hypokalemia and hyperkalemia
6. Fluid overload (pulmonary edema)
7. Cerebral edema (with possible neurologic sequelae or death)
8. Acute gastric dilatation, erosive gastritis
9. Infection: urinary tract, pneumonia, mucormycosis
10. Venous and arterial thrombosis
11. Acute tubular necrosis (renal failure)

of nonketotic hyperglycemia) to avoid excessively aggressive volume replacement, sudden changes in the patient's serum glucose and [Na^+], and excessive use of HCO_3^-.

A number of life-threatening complications may develop in the course of DKA and NKH in spite of adequate medical care (Table 74.16). Shock of cardiac origin or resulting from sepsis or volume depletion, as well as cerebral thrombosis and edema, are among the most prominent complications.[92,166] Cerebral edema leading to death or responsible for chronic sequelae[118,155] fortunately is rare, yet milder forms may be regularly found with the standard treatment of DKA[160] and NKH.[167] Mortality from DKA has declined from more than 40% in the 1930s to less than 5% in some institutions, as the result of improvements in medical technology and appreciation of the seriousness of the disease. Yet, the prognosis of patients with NKH is substantially worse, as evidenced by the higher mortality associated with this metabolic complication (10% to 60%).[85]

Acknowledgments

The authors are indebted to Geri Tasby for skillful assistance in preparing the manuscript.

REFERENCES

1. Felig P. Diabetic ketoacidosis. *N Engl J Med.* 1974;290:1360.
2. Kreisberg RA. Diabetic ketoacidosis: new concepts and trends in pathogenesis and treatment. *Ann Intern Med.* 1978;88:681.
3. Adrogué HJ, Maliha G. Diabetic ketoacidosis. In: Adrogué HJ, ed. *Acid–base and Electrolyte Disorders. Contemporary Management in Critical Care.* New York: Churchill Livingstone; 1991:21.
4. Karam JH, Salber PR, Forsham PH. Pancreatic hormones and diabetes mellitus. In: Greenspan FS, Forsham PH, eds. *Basic and Clinical Endocrinology.* East Norwalk: Lange Medical Publications; 1986.
5. Foster, DW, McGarry JD. Acute complications of diabetes mellitus: ketoacidosis, hyperosmolar coma, and lactic acidosis. In: DeGroot LJ, Jameson JL, eds. *Endocrinology.* 4th ed. Philadelphia: WB Saunders; 2001:908.
6. Halperin ML, Goguen JM, Cheema-Dhadli S, et al. Diabetic emergencies. In: Arieff A, DeFronzo RA, eds. *Fluid, Electrolyte, and Acid–base Disorders.* New York: Churchill Livingstone; 1995:741.
7. Skillman TG. Diabetes mellitus. In: Mazzaferri EL, ed. *Endocrinology.* New York: Medical Examination Publishing; 1986:595.
8. Kreisberg RA. Diabetic ketoacidosis, alcoholic ketosis, lactic acidosis, and hyporeninemic hypoaldosteronism. In: Ellenberg M, Rifkin H, eds. *Diabetes Mellitus.* New York: Medical Examination Publishing; 1983: 621.
9. Felts PW. Ketoacidosis. *Med Clin North Am.* 1983;67:831.
10. Fleckman AM. Diabetic ketoacidosis. *Endocr Metab Clin North Am.* 1993;22:181.
11. Foster DW, McGarry JD. The metabolic derangements and treatment of diabetic ketoacidosis. *N Engl J Med.* 1983;309:159.
12. Adrogué HJ, Madias NE. Disorders of acid–base balance. In: Berl T, Bonventre JV, eds. *Atlas of Diseases of the Kidney.* Boston: Blackwell Science 1999;6:20.
13. Adrogué HJ. Glucose homeostasis and the kidney. *Kidney Int.* 1992;42:1266.
14. Alberti KG, Cuthbert C. The hydrogen ion normal metabolism: a review. In: Porter R, Lawrenson G. *Metabolic Acidosis.* London: Pitman; 1982:1.
15. Cuthbert C, Alberti KG. Acidemia and insulin resistance in the diabetic ketoacidotic rat. *Metabolism.* 1978;27:1903.
16. Guest GM, Mackler B, Knoles HC. Effects of acidosis on insulin action and on carbohydrate and mineral metabolism. *Diabetes.* 1952;1:276.
17. Walker BG, Phear DN, Martin FI, et al. Inhibition of insulin by acidosis. *Lancet.* 1963;2:964.
18. Misbin Rl, Pulkkinen AJ, Loften SA, et al. Ketoacids and the insulin receptor. *Diabetes.* 1978;27:539.
19. Adrogué HJ, Chap Z, Okuda Y, et al. Acidosis-induced glucose intolerance is not prevented by adrenergic blockade. *Am J Physiol.* 1988;255:E812.
20. Van Putten JP, Wieringa T, Krans HM. Low pH and ketoacids induce insulin receptor binding and postbinding alterations in cultured 3T3 adipocytes. *Diabetes.* 1985;34:744.
21. Waelbroeck M. The dependence of insulin binding. A quantitative study. *J Biol Chem.* 1982;257:8284.
22. Whittaker JC, Cuthbert C, Hammond VA, et al. The effects of metabolic acidosis on insulin binding to isolated rat adipocytes. *Metabolism.* 1982;31:553.
23. Adrogué HJ, Madias NE. Hyponatremia. *N Engl J Med.* 2000;342:1581.
24. Adrogué HJ, Madias NE. Hypernatremia. *N Engl J Med.* 2000;342:1493.
25. Adrogué HJ, Wesson DE. *Salt & Water. Blackwell's Basics of Medicine Series.* Boston: Blackwell Scientific; 1994.
26. Gennari FJ. Hypo-hypernatraemia: disorders of water balance. In: *Oxford Textbook of Clinical Nephrology.* 2nd ed. Oxford: Oxford University Press; 1998:175.
27. Roscoe JM, Halperin ML, Rolleston FS, et al. Hyperglycemia-induced hyponatremia: metabolic considerations in calculation of serum sodium depression. *Can Med Assoc J.* 1975;112:452.
28. Trever RW, Cluff LE. The problem of increasing azotemia during management of diabetic acidosis. *Am J Med.* 1958;24:368.
29. Linton AL, Kennedy AC. Diabetic ketosis complicated by acute renal failure. *Postgrad Med J.* 1963;39:364.
30. Adrogué HJ, Madias NE. Aiding fluid prescription for the dysnatremias. *Intensive Care Med.* 1997;23:309.
31. Adrogué HJ, Madias NE. Quantitative projection of the impact of measured water and electrolyte losses on serum sodium concentration for managing hyponatremia and hypernatremia. *J Am Soc Nephrol.* 2004;15:781A.
32. Adrogué HJ, Barrero J, Dolson GM. Diabetic ketoacidosis. In: Suki WN, Massry SG, eds. *Therapy of Renal Diseases and Related Disorders.* 2nd ed. Boston: Martinus Nijhoff; 1991:193.
33. Narins RG, Krisna GG, Kopyt NP. Fluid-electrolyte and acid–base disorders complicating diabetes mellitus. In: Schrier RW, Gottschalk CW, eds. *Diseases of the Kidney.* 5th ed. Boston: Little, Brown; 1993.
34. Adrogué HJ, Wesson DE. *Potassium. Blackwell's Basics of Medicine Series.* Boston: Blackwell Scientific; 1994.
35. Adrogué HJ. Mechanisms of transcellular potassium shifts in acid–base disorders. In: Hatano M, ed. *Proceedings of the XIth International Congress on Nephrology, Tokyo, Japan.* Tokyo: Springer; 1991.
36. Adrogué HJ, Lederer ED, Suki WN, et al. Determinants of plasma potassium levels in diabetic ketoacidosis. *Medicine.* 1986;65:163.
37. Adrogué HJ, Madias NE. Changes in plasma potassium concentration during acute acid–base disturbances. *Am J Med.* 1981;71:456.
38. Adrogué HJ, Chap Z, Ishida T, et al. Role of the endocrine pancreas in the kalemic response to acute metabolic acidosis in conscious dogs. *J Clin Invest.* 1985;75:798.
39. Goldfarb S, Cox M, Singer I, et al. Acute hyperkalemia induced by hyperglycemia: hormonal mechanisms. *Ann Intern Med.* 1976;84:426.
40. Fraley DS, Adler S. Isohydric regulation of plasma potassium by bicarbonate in the rat. *Kidney Int.* 1976;9:333.
41. Fraley DS, Adler S. Correction of hyperkalemia by bicarbonate despite constant blood pH. *Kidney Int.* 1977;12:354.
42. Makoff DL, da Silva JA, Rosenbaum BJ, et al. Hypertonic expansion: acid–base and electrolyte changes. *Am J Physiol.* 1970;218:1201.
43. Massara F, Martelli S, Cagliero E, et al. Influence of glucagon on plasma levels of potassium in man. *Diabetologia.* 1980;19:414.
44. Silva P, Spokes K. Sympathetic system in potassium homeostasis. *Am J Physiol.* 1981;241:F151.
45. Kebler R, McDonald FD, Cadnapaphornchai P. Dynamic changes in serum phosphorus levels in diabetic ketoacidosis. *Am J Med.* 1985;79:571.
46. Fisher JN, Shahshahani MN, Kitabchi AE. Diabetic ketoacidosis: low-dose insulin therapy by various routes. *N Engl J Med.* 1977;297:238.
47. Pfeifer MA, Samols E, Wolter CF, et al. Low-dose versus high-dose insulin therapy for diabetic ketoacidosis. *Southern Med J.* 1979;72:149.
48. Carroll P, Matz R. Uncontrolled diabetes mellitus in adults: experience in treating diabetic ketoacidosis and hyperosmolar nonketotic coma with low-dose insulin and a uniform treatment regimen. *Diabetes Care.* 1983;6:579.
49. Gerich JE, Lorenzi M, Bier DM, et al. Prevention of human diabetic ketoacidosis by somatostatin: evidence for an essential role of glucagon. *N Engl J Med.* 1975;292:985.
50. Dobbs R, Sakurai H, Sasaki H, et al. Role in the hyperglycemia of diabetes mellitus. *Science.* 1975;187:544.
51. Unger RH. Role of glucagon in the pathogenesis of diabetes. The status of the controversy. *Metabolism.* 1978;27:1691.
52. Unger RH, Orci L. Glucagon and the A cell: physiology and pathophysiology. *N Engl J Med.* 1981;304:1518.

53. McGarry JD, Foster DW. Regulation of hepatic fatty acid oxidation and ketone body production. *Annu Rev Biochem*. 1980;49:395.

54. Foster DW. From glycogen to ketones—and back. *Diabetes*. 1984;33:1188.

55. McGarry JD, Woeltje KF, Kuwajima M, et al. Regulation of ketogenesis and the renaissance of carnitine palmitoyltransferase. *Diabetes Metab Rev*. 1989;5:271.

56. McGarry JD, Leatherman GF, Foster DW. Carnitine palmitoyltransferase I: the site of inhibition of hepatic fatty acid oxidation by malonyl-CoA. *J Biol Chem*. 1978;253:4128.

57. DiMarco JP, Hoppel C. Hepatic mitochondrial function in ketogenic states: diabetes, starvation and after growth hormone administration. *J Clin Invest*. 1975;55:1237.

58. McGarry JD, Brown NF. The mitochondrial carnitine palmitoyltransferase system—from concept to molecular analysis. *Eur J Biochem*. 1997;244:1.

59. McGarry JD, Takabayashi Y, Foster DW. The role of malonyl-CoA in the coordination of fatty acid synthesis and oxidation in isolated rat hepatocytes. *J Biol Chem*. 1978;253:8294.

60. Murphy MS, Pande SV. Mechanism of carnitine acylcarnitine translocase-catalyzed import of acylcarnitines into mitochondria. *J Biol Chem*. 1984; 259:9082.

61. Adrogué HJ, Wesson DE. *Acid–Base Blackwell's Basics of Medicine*. Boston: Blackwell Scientific; 1994.

62. Oster JR, Epstein M. Acid–base aspects of ketoacidosis. *Am J Nephrol*. 1984;4:137.

63. Keller U. Diabetic ketoacidosis: current views on pathogenesis and treatment. *Diabetologia*. 1986;29:71.

64. Adrogué HJ, Wilson H, Boyd AE, et al. Plasma acid–base patterns in diabetic ketoacidosis. *N Engl J Med*. 1982;307:1603.

65. Kleeman CR, Narins RG. Diabetic acidosis and coma. In: Maxwell MH, Kleeman CR, eds. *Clinical Disorders of Fluid and Electrolyte Metabolism*. New York: McGraw-Hill; 1980;1339.

66. Danowski TS, Peters JH, Rathbun JC, et al. Studies in diabetic acidosis and coma, with particular emphasis on the retention of administered potassium. *J Clin Invest*. 1949;28:1.

67. Seldin DW, Tarail R. The metabolism of glucose and electrolytes in diabetic acidosis. *J Clin Invest*. 1950;29:552.

68. Nabarro JD, Spencer AG, Stowers JM. Metabolic studies in severe diabetic ketosis. *Q J Med*. 1952;21:225.

69. Shaw CE, Hurwitz GE, Schmukler M, et al. A clinical and laboratory study of insulin dosage in diabetic acidosis: comparison with small and large doses. *Diabetes*. 1962;11:23.

70. Assal JP, Aoki TT, Manzano FM, et al. Metabolic effects of sodium bicarbonate in management of diabetic ketoacidosis. *Diabetes*. 1974;23:405.

71. Oh MS, Carroll HJ, Goldstein DA, et al. Hyperchloremic acidosis during the recovery phrase of diabetic ketoacidosis. *Ann Intern Med*. 1978;89:925.

72. Adrogué HJ, Eknoyan G, Suki WN. Diabetic ketoacidosis: role of the kidney in the acid–base homeostasis reevaluated. *Kidney Int*. 1984;25:591.

73. Adrogué HJ, Barrero J, Ryan JE, et al. Diabetic ketoacidosis: a practical approach. *Hospital Practice*. 1989;24:83.

74. Pitts RF. The renal regulation of acid base balance with special reference to the mechanism for acidifying the urine. *Science*. 1945;102:49.

75. Pitts RF. Acid–base regulation by the kidneys. *Am J Med*. 1950;9:356.

76. Daughaday WH. Hydrogen ion metabolism in diabetic acidosis. *Arch Intern Med*. 1961;107:63.

77. Bernstein LM, Foley EF, Hoffman WS. Renal function during and after diabetic coma. *J Clin Invest*. 1952;31:711.

78. Reubi FC. Glomerular filtration rate, renal blood flow and blood viscosity during and after diabetic coma. *Circ Res*. 1953;1:410.

79. Guest GM, Rapoport S. Electrolytes of blood plasma and cells in diabetic acidosis and during recovery. *Proc Am Diabetes Assn*. 1947;7:97.

80. Pitts RF. *Renal regulation of acid–base balance. Physiology of the kidney and body fluids*. Chicago: Year Book; 1974:198.

81. Adrogué HJ, Tannen RL. Ketoacidosis, hyperosmolar states, and lactic acidosis. In: Tannen RL, Kokko JP, eds. *Fluids and Electrolytes*. 3rd ed. Philadelphia: WB Saunders; 1995.

82. Adrogué HJ, Madias NE: Management of life-threatening acid–base disorders. (First of two parts). *N Engl J Med*. 1998;338:26.

83. Adrogué HJ, Madias NE. Renal tubular acidosis. In: Davison AM, Cameron JS, Grünfeld J-P, et al., eds. *Oxford Textbook of Clinical Nephrology*. 3rd ed. Oxford: Oxford University Press; 2005.

84. Alberti KG. Diabetic acidosis, hyperosmolar coma, and lactic acidosis. In: Becker KL, ed. *Principles and Practice of Endocrinology and Metabolism*. Philadelphia: JB Lippincott; 1990.

85. Marshall SM, Walker M, Alberti KG. Diabetic ketoacidosis and hyperglycaemic non-ketotic coma. In: Alberti KG, et al., eds. *International Textbook of Diabetes Mellitus*. Chichester: Wiley; 1992.

86. Davidson MB. Diabetic ketoacidosis and hyperosmolar nonketotic syndrome. In: Davidson MB, ed. *Diabetes Mellitus, Diagnosis and Treatment*. New York: Churchill Livingstone; 1991.

87. Genuth SM. Diabetic ketoacidosis and hyperglycemic hyperosmolar coma. In: Bardin CW, ed. *Current Therapy in Endocrinology and Metabolism*. Philadelphia: BC Decker; 1991;348.

88. Salway JG. *Metabolism at a Glance*. Oxford: Blackwell Scientific; 1994.

89. Johnson DD, Palumbo PJ, Chu CP. Diabetic ketoacidosis in a community-based population. *Mayo Clin Proc*. 1980;55:83.

90. Wetterhall SF, Olson DR, DeStafano F, et al. Trends in diabetes and diabetic complications. *Diabetes Care*. 1992;15:960.

91. Clements RS, Vourganti B. Fatal diabetic ketoacidosis: major causes and approaches to their prevention. *Diabetes Care*. 1978;1:314.

92. Alberti KG, Hockaday TD. Diabetic coma: a reappraisal after five years. *Clin Endocrinol Metab*. 1977;6:421.

93. Morris AD, Boyle DI, McMahon AD, et al. Adherence to insulin treatment, glycaemic control, and ketoacidosis in insulin-dependent diabetes mellitus. *Lancet*. 1997;350:1505.

94. Tattersall R. Brittle diabetes. *Clin Endocrinol Metab*. 1977;6:403.

95. Cohen AS, Vance VK, Runyan JW, et al. Diabetic acidosis: an evaluation of the cause, course and therapy of 73 cases. *Ann Intern Med*. 1960;52:55.

96. Beigelman PM. Severe diabetic ketoacidosis (diabetic "coma"): 482 episodes in 257 patients; experience of three years. *Diabetes*. 1971;20:490.

97. Cahill GF, Herrera MG, Morgan AP, et al. Hormone-fuel interrelationships during fasting. *J Clin Invest*. 1966;45:1751.

98. Owen OE, Morgan AP, Kemp HG, et al. Brain metabolism during fasting. *J Clin Invest*. 1967;46:1589.

99. Mahoney CA. Extreme gestational starvation ketoacidosis: case report and review of pathophysiology. *Am J Kidney Dis*. 1992;20:276.

100. Chernow B, Finton C, Rainey TG, et al. "Bovine ketosis" in a nondiabetic postpartum woman. *Diabetes Care*. 1982;5:47.

101. Levy LJ, Duga J, Girgis M, et al. Ketoacidosis associated with alcoholism in nondiabetic subjects. *Ann Intern Med*. 1973;78:213.

102. Wren KD, Slovis CM, Minion GE, et al. The syndrome of alcoholic ketoacidosis. *Am J Med*. 1991;91:119.

103. Csako G, Elin RJ. Unrecognized false-positive ketones from drugs containing free-sulfhydryl groups (letter). *JAMA*. 1993;269:1634.

104. Cronin JW, Kroop SF, Diamond J, et al. Alkalemia in diabetic ketoacidosis. *Am J Med*. 1984;77:192.

105. Fulop M, Rosenblatt A, Kreitzer SM, et al. Hyperosmolar nature of diabetic coma. *Diabetes*. 1975;24:594.

106. Gerich JE, Martin MM, Recant L. Clinical and metabolic characteristics of hyperosmolar nonketotic coma. *Diabetes*. 1971;20:228.

107. Matz R. Coma in the nonketotic diabetic. In: Ellenberg M, Rifkin H, eds. New York: Diabetes Mellitus Medical Examination Publishing; 1983: 655.

108. Matz R. Uncontrolled diabetes mellitus: diabetic ketoacidosis and hyperosmolar coma. In: Bergman M, ed. *Principles of Diabetes Management*. New York: Medical Examination Publishing; 1987:109.

109. Schade DS, Eaton RP. Dose response to insulin in man: differential effects on glucose and ketone body regulation. *J Clin Endocrinol Metab*. 1977;44:1038.

110. Joffe BI, Goldberg RB, Krut LH, et al. Pathogenesis of nonketotic hyperosmolar diabetic coma. *Lancet*. 1975;1:1069.

111. Lindsey CA, Faloona GR, Unger RH. Plasma glucagon in nonketotic hyperosmolar coma. *JAMA*. 1974;229:1171.

112. Gerich J, Panhaus JC, Gutman RA, et al. Effect of dehydration and hyperosmolarity on glucose, free fatty acid and ketone body metabolism in the rat. *Diabetes*. 1973;22:264.

113. Yen TT, Stamm NB, Fuller RW, et al. Hepatic insensitivity to glucagon in ob/ob mice. *Res Commun Chem Pathol Pharmacol*. 1980;30:29.

114. Azain MJ, Fukuda N, Chao FF, et al. Contributions of fatty acid and sterol synthesis to triglyceride and cholesterol secretion by the perfused rat liver in genetic hyperlipemia and obesity. *J Biol Chem*. 1985;260:174.

115. Begin-Heick N. Absence of the inhibitory effect of guanine nucleotides on adenylate cyclase activity in white adipocyte membranes of the ob/ob mouse: effect of the ob gene. *J Biol Chem*. 1985;260:6187.

116. Guisado R, Arieff AI. Neurologic manifestations of diabetic comas: correlation with biochemical alterations in the brain. *Metabolism*. 1975;24:665.

117. Maccario M, Messis CP, Vastola EF. Focal seizures as a manifestation of hyperglycemia without ketoacidosis: a report of seven cases with review of the literature. *Neurology*. 1965;15:195.

118. Maccario M. Neurological dysfunction associated with nonketotic hyperglycemia. *Arch Neurol*. 1968;19:525.

119. Beigelman PM, Martin HE, Miller LV, et al. Severe diabetic ketoacidosis. *JAMA*. 1969;210:1082.

120. Taylor AL. Diabetic ketoacidosis. *Postgrad Med.* 1980;68:161.
121. Davidson MB. Diabetic ketoacidosis and hyperosmolar nonketotic coma. In: Davidson MB, ed. *Diabetes Mellitus: Diagnosis and Treatment*. New York: Wiley Medical; 1981:193.
122. Kitabchi AE, Matteri R, Murphy MB. Optimal insulin delivery in diabetic ketoacidosis (DKA) and hyperglycemic hyperosmolar nonketotic coma (HHNC). *Diabetes Care.* 1982;5(Suppl 1):78.
123. Beigelman PM. Severe diabetic ketoacidosis. In: Beigelman PM, Kumar D, eds. *Diabetes Mellitus for the Houseofficer*. Baltimore: Williams & Wilkins; 1986:23.
124. Ellemann K, Soerensen JN, Pedersen L, et al. Epidemiology and treatment of diabetic ketoacidosis in a community population. *Diabetes Care.* 1984;7:528.
125. Johnson DG. Diabetic ketoacidosis. In: Bressler R, Johnson DG, eds. *Management of Diabetes Mellitus*. Boston: John Wright PSG; 1982:153.
126. Waldhaüsl W, Klienberger G, Korn A, et al. Severe hyperglycemia: effects of rehydration on endocrine derangements and blood glucose concentration. *Diabetes.* 1979;28:577.
127. Adrogué HJ, Barrero J, Eknoyan G. Salutary effects of modest fluid replacement in the treatment of adults with diabetic ketoacidosis. *JAMA.* 1989; 262:2108.
128. Kandel G, Aberman A. Selected developments in the understanding of diabetic ketoacidosis. *Can Med Assoc J.* 1983;128:392.
129. Brown RH, Rossini AA, Callaway CW, et al. Caveat on fluid replacement in hyperglycemic, hyperosmolar, nonketotic coma. *Diabetes Care.* 1978;1:305.
130. Fulop M. The treatment of severely uncontrolled diabetes mellitus. *Adv Int Med.* 1984;29:327.
131. Khardori R, Soler NG. Hyperosmolar hyperglycemic nonketotic syndrome. *Am J Med.* 1984;77:899.
132. Kitabchi AE, Young R, Sacks H, et al. Diabetic ketoacidosis. Reappraisal of therapeutic approach. *Ann Rev Med.* 1979;30:339.
133. Kozak GP, Rolla AR. Diabetic comas. In: Kozak GP, ed. *Clinical Diabetes Mellitus*. Philadelphia: WB Saunders; 1982;109.
134. Unger RH, Foster DW. Diabetes mellitus. In: Wilson JD, Foster DW, Kronenberg HM, et al., eds. *Williams' Textbook of Endocrinology*. 9th ed. Philadelphia: WB Saunders; 1998:973.
135. Barrett EJ, DeFronzo RA, Bevilacqua S, et al. Insulin resistance in diabetic ketoacidosis. *Diabetes.* 1982;31:923.
136. Pedersen O, Beck-Nielsen H. Insulin resistance and insulin-dependent diabetes mellitus. *Diabetes Care.* 1987;10:516.
137. Flier JS. Lilly lecture: syndromes of insulin resistance. From patient to gene and back again. *Diabetes.* 1992;41:1207.
138. Luzi L, Barrett EJ, Groop LC, et al. Metabolic effects of low-dose insulin therapy on glucose metabolism in diabetic ketoacidosis. *Diabetes.* 1988;37:1470.
139. Barrett EJ, DeFronzo RA. Diabetic ketoacidosis: diagnosis and treatment. *Hosp Pract.* 1984;19(4):89,99.
140. Brown PM, Tompkins CV, Juul S, et al. Mechanism of action of insulin in diabetic patients: a dose-related effect on glucose production and utilization. *Br Med J.* 1978;1:1239.
141. Rosenthal NR, Barrett EJ. An assessment of insulin action in hyperosmolar hyperglycemic nonketotic diabetic patients. *J Clin Endocrinol Metab.* 1985;60:607.
142. Page MM, Alberti KG, Greenwood R, et al. Treatment of diabetic coma with continuous low-dose insulin infusion. *Br Med J.* 1974;2:687.
143. Padilla AJ, Loeb JN. "Low dose" versus "high dose" insulin regimens in the management of uncontrolled diabetes. A survey. *Am J Med.* 1977;63:843.
144. Fulop M, Murthy V, Michilli A, et al. Serum betahydroxybutyrate measurement in patients with uncontrolled diabetes mellitus. *Arch Intern Med.* 1999;159:381.
145. Bureau MA, Begin R, Berthiaume Y, et al. Cerebral hypoxia from bicarbonate infusion in diabetic acidosis. *J Pediatrics.* 1980;96:968.
146. Lever E, Jaspan JB. Sodium bicarbonate therapy in severe diabetic ketoacidosis. *Am J Med.* 1983;75:263.
147. Okuda Y, Adrogué HJ, Field JB, et al. Counterproductive effects of sodium bicarbonate in diabetic ketoacidosis. *J Clin Endocrinol Metab.* 1996;81:314.
148. Morris LR, Murphy MB, Kitabchi AE. Bicarbonate therapy in severe diabetic ketoacidosis. *Ann Intern Med.* 1986;105:836.
149. Levine SN, Loewenstein JE. Treatment of diabetic ketoacidosis. *Arch Intern Med.* 1981;141:713.
150. Narins RG, Arieff AI. Alkali therapy of metabolic acidosis due to organic acids. *AKF Nephrol Lett.* 1985;2:13.
151. Narins RG, Cohen JJ. Bicarbonate therapy for organic acidosis: the case for the continued use. *Ann Intern Med.* 1987;106:615.
152. Adrogué HJ, Brensilver J, Cohen JJ, et al. Influence of steady-state alterations in acid–base equilibrium on the fate of administered bicarbonate in the dog. *J Clin Invest.* 1983;71:867.
153. Clements RS, Morrison AD, Blumenthal SA, et al. Increased cerebrospinal-fluid pressure during treatment of diabetic ketosis. *Lancet.* 1971;2:671.
154. Young E, Bradley RF. Cererbral edema with irreversible coma in severe diabetic ketoacidosis. *N Engl J Med.* 1967;276:665.
155. Keller RJ, Wolfsdorf JI. Isolated growth hormone deficiency after cerebral edema complicating diabetic ketoacidosis. *N Engl J Med.* 1987;316:857.
156. Krane EJ, Rockoff MA, Wallman JK, et al. Subclinical brain swelling in children during treatment of diabetic ketoacidosis. *N Engl J Med.* 1985; 312:1147.
157. Arieff AI, Kleeman CR. Studies on mechanisms of cerebral edema in diabetic comas. *J Clin Invest.* 1973;52:571.
158. Arieff AI, Kleeman CR. Cerebral edema in diabetic comas. II. Effects of hyperosmolality, hyperglycemia and insulin in diabetic rabbits. *J Clin Endocrinol Metab.* 1974;38:1057.
159. Winegrad AI, Kern EF, Simmons DA. Cerebral edema in diabetic ketoacidosis. *N Engl J Med.* 1985;312:1184.
160. Ohman JL, Marliss EB, Aoki TT, et al. The cerebrospinal fluid in diabetic ketoacidosis. *N Engl J Med.* 1971;284:283.
161. Fein IA, Rackow EC, Sprung CL, et al. Relation of colloid osmotic pressure to arterial hypoxemia and cerebral edema during crystalloid volume loading of patients with diabetic ketoacidosis. *Ann Intern Med.* 1982;96:570.
162. Rosenbloom AL. Intracerebral crisis during treatment of diabetic ketoacidosis. *Diabetes Care.* 1990;13:22.
163. Durr JA, Hoffman WH, Sklar AH, et al. Correlates of brain edema in uncontrolled IDDM. *Diabetes.* 1992;41:627.
164. Harris GD, Fiordalisi I, Harris WL, et al. Minimizing the risk of brain herniation during treatment of diabetic ketoacidosis: a retrospective and prospective study. *J Pediatr.* 1990;117:22.
165. Silver SM, Clark EC, Schroeder BM, et al. Pathogenesis of cerebral edema after treatment of diabetic ketoacidosis. *Kidney Int.* 1997;51:1237.
166. Bryan CS, Reynolds KL, Metzger WT. Bacteremia in diabetic patients: comparison of incidence and mortality with nondiabetic patients. *Diabetes Care.* 1985;8:244.
167. Maccario M, Messis CP. Cerebral edema complicating treated non-ketotic hyperglycemia. *Lancet.* 1969;2:352.

CHAPTER 75

Pathophysiology and Nephron Adaptation in Chronic Kidney Disease

Radko Komers • Timothy W. Meyer • Sharon Anderson

That we are endowed with a surfeit of nephrons above that needed to maintain normal homeostasis is shown by the ability of a single kidney to carry out the functions previously performed by two, after a uninephrectomy. The surplus is even more apparent in progressive chronic kidney disease (CKD), where solute and water balance are well maintained until late in the course. This chapter first reviews the compensatory changes in function and structure that occur when nephron number is reduced and that enable maintenance of homeostasis. Alterations in handling of individual solutes and water are then described. We then describe the mechanisms that underlie adaptation, and then the transition stage in which these compensatory changes can prove maladaptive and accelerate remaining nephron loss.

PRINCIPLES AND PATTERNS OF NEPHRON ADAPTATION: INTACT NEPHRONS AND GLOMERULOTUBULAR BALANCE

As nephrons fail during the course of CKD, each remaining nephron must increase its single nephron excretion of the filtered load of water and solutes. In 1952, Robert Platt[1] reasoned that the work of each remaining unit is increased, making an analogy with the remaining workers in a factory putting in overtime when their numbers are reduced by illness. Bricker and colleagues[2,3] later noted that the functional capacity of the residual nephrons determines the degree to which homeostasis is preserved, and that maintenance of homeostasis implies preservation (or even enhancement) of normal glomerular and tubular function in the remaining nephrons. Reasoning that globally hypofunctioning nephrons could not maintain homeostasis, these investigators coined the intact nephron hypothesis to explain the preserved ability of the remnant nephrons to excrete the required load of water and solutes.[2,3] Each remnant nephron presumably transports water and solutes in proportion to its individual glomerular filtration rate (GFR), whether it is reduced by disease or increased by compensatory hyperfiltration and hypertrophy.

Another essential component of adaptation is maintenance of glomerulotubular balance. For example, in experimental glomerulonephritis, despite a wide range of single nephron (SN)GFR values, proximal fluid reabsorption correlates closely with SNGFR in individual nephrons, so that fractional reabsorption is the same in hypofiltering and hyperfiltering nephrons.[4] Presumably, structural changes in the proximal tubule (PT) and the peritubular capillary network act together with alterations in Starling forces to perpetuate glomerulotubular balance.

FUNCTIONAL ADAPTATIONS TO NEPHRON LOSS

Surgical ablation of renal tissue has long been used to mimic the more gradual nephron loss that occurs in CKD. In this experimental model, the reduction of renal mass leads to structural and functional hypertrophy of the remaining nephrons. Remnant nephron hyperfiltration is beneficial in the short term, because it minimizes the decrease in total GFR that would otherwise ensue. However, as will be described, sustained activity of these compensatory forces contributes to a loss of GFR and structural injury in the long term. Most commonly, functional adaptations precede changes in structure, though functional and structural adaptations are closely interrelated, often sharing common pathophysiologic mediators. Adaptive and maladaptive mechanisms will be discussed in parallel, with an emphasis on putative mechanisms or factors underlying transition from adaptation to maladaptation.

FUNCTIONAL ADAPTATIONS

Renal Hemodynamic Adaptations and Maladaptations: Compensatory Hyperfiltration

Remaining nephrons compensate for nephron loss by increased perfusion and filtration rates. Studies in renal transplant donors indicate that within weeks after a nephrectomy,

GFR and the renal plasma flow (RPF) rate in the remaining kidney increase by about 40%, so that GFR is about 70% of the prenephrectomy value.[5] In rat models,[6,7] vascular resistance is reduced in the afferent and efferent arterioles, allowing an increase in the glomerular capillary plasma flow rate (Q_A). Because the decrease in afferent arteriolar resistance (R_A) is proportionally greater than that in efferent arteriolar resistance (R_E), the hydraulic pressure in the glomerular capillary (P_{GC}) increases. Together, glomerular capillary hyperperfusion and hypertension account for the compensatory single nephron hyperfiltration. The magnitude of increase in SNGFR is proportional to the degree of renal mass reduction.[8,9] With a uninephrectomy, the increase in SNGFR is largely due to an increase in Q_A. However, in more extensive renal ablation, substantial increases in P_{GC} occur. The magnitude of the adaptive increase in SNGFR is similar in superficial and juxtamedullary nephrons,[10] and the tubuloglomerular feedback mechanism remains intact, with its set point altered in a way that permits hyperfiltration.[11]

Of the glomerular hemodynamic determinants of adaptive hyperfiltration, glomerular capillary hypertension appears to be the crucial cause of eventual structural injury. In a study by Hostetter et al.,[8] untreated rats subjected to 85% nephrectomy exhibited elevated SNGFR, due to elevations in P_{GC} and Q_A. These hemodynamic adaptations were associated with the development of proteinuria and extensive focal and segmental glomerular sclerosis (FSGS).[12] When dietary protein restriction was used to blunt the adaptive hyperfiltration, values for SNGFR, Q_A, and P_{GC} were nearly normalized, and structural injury was limited. Studies with angiotensin converting enzyme inhibitors (ACEIs) helped to clarify the role of specific determinants of hyperfiltration in causing subsequent injury. ACEIs reduce R_E and P_{GC} without affecting Q_A or SNGFR. In rats with renal ablation, selective control of glomerular hypertension is protective, even with persistent hyperfiltration and hyperperfusion. Conversely, antihypertensive therapy that lowers systemic but not intraglomerular pressure may not protect the kidney at risk.[9]

Loss of renal mass is often accompanied by substantial systemic hypertension[8,9] and studies in hypertensive renal disease models have demonstrated the hemodynamic mechanisms of hypertensive injury. Afferent arteriolar vasodilation and an impaired ability to autoregulate in response to changes in perfusion pressure result in enhanced transmission of systemic pressure into the glomerular capillary network and thereby in glomerular capillary hypertension.[13]

Alterations in Glomerular Permeability

Another index of glomerular function is the ability to restrict passage of macromolecules into the urinary space.[14] Permselectivity is characterized by examining the extent to which the glomerular capillary wall discriminates among molecules of different size, charge, and configuration. A uninephrectomy is associated with modest, late development of proteinuria in the rat,[15] and in some cases, humans.[16] With more extensive renal ablation, proteinuria results from defects in both size selectivity and charge selectivity,[12,17] with increased flux through the shunt pathway. As is discussed in the following section, this adaptation is associated with a lesser capability of podocytes to adapt to the loss of nephron mass.

Functional Adaptations: Tubular

Adaptive changes in SNGFR and in proximal tubular reabsorptive capacity are accompanied by mechanisms that enable the excretion of a constant solute load in the face of a dwindling number of functioning nephrons. When this capability is exceeded, the complications of CKD ensue.

As elucidated by Bricker and Fine,[3] there are three major patterns of adaptation to advancing CKD (Fig. 75.1), which are reflected by the change in the serum concentration of specific solutes with the fall in GFR. If there is no regulation or adaptation, the plasma concentration increases (curve A of Fig. 75.1). Examples include urea and creatinine, in which the rate of excretion depends on the filtered load, and tubular reabsorption and secretion mechanisms fail to adapt sufficiently to prevent a rise in the serum concentration. Curve B represents regulation with limitation (i.e., maintenance of normal plasma concentration until late stages of CKD); when GFR falls below a critical level, excretion can no longer keep up with intake, and plasma concentration rises. Solutes in this class, such as phosphate and urate, are excreted by filtration and tubular reabsorption, secretion, or both. The third pattern (curve C) is termed complete regulation. Serum concentration is maintained in the normal range until terminal CKD stages; examples include sodium, potassium, and magnesium. For normal serum levels to be maintained, increased single nephron excretion results from altered tubular transport patterns, as discussed in the following. Changes in individual solute handling in CKD have been reviewed extensively elsewhere[18] and are briefly summarized here.

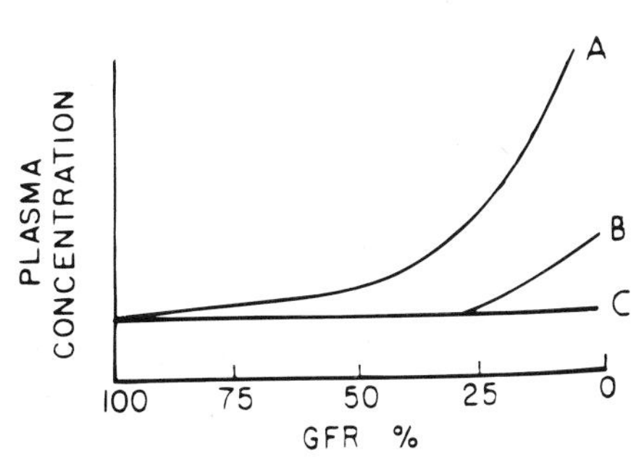

FIGURE 75.1 Patterns of adaptation for different solutes in chronic progressive renal disease. **A:** No regulation or adaptation. **B:** Regulation with limitation. **C:** Complete regulation. See text for discussion. *GFR,* glomerular filtration rate. (Reprinted from Bricker NS, Fine LG. The renal response to progressive nephron loss. In: Brenner BM, Rector FC Jr, eds. *The Kidney.* Philadelphia: WB Saunders, 1981:1058, with permission.)

Sodium Excretion and the Regulation of Extracellular Fluid Volume

Extracellular fluid (ECF) volume is maintained remarkably close to normal until the very late stages of CKD. Although absolute sodium (Na) reabsorption in the PT increases in parallel with the rise in SNGFR, fractional excretion of Na and water increase.[19] These changes result in increased Na delivery to the thick ascending limb of Henle and the distal nephron.[10]

Chronic adaptations enable the maintenance of normal Na balance until the late stages, though the natriuretic response to a large Na challenge is impaired.[20] Natriuresis after Na loading is reduced less than is GFR, so acute volume expansion causes a greater increase in fractional Na excretion in uremic animals than in normal controls, a "magnification" phenomenon.[20,21] In advanced CKD, the ability to conserve Na is also compromised, such that most patients are unable to lower Na excretion below 20 to 30 mEq per day (a "salt floor").[3,22] With high Na intakes, the smaller number of functioning nephrons may be unable to increase Na excretion enough to maintain Na balance, and thus may be termed as having a low salt ceiling. As CKD progresses, the distance between floor and ceiling increases, and the maintenance of Na balance becomes more difficult,[3] though slowly reducing Na intake may lead to more efficient reductions in Na excretion.[23]

Early investigators postulated that decreased aldosterone formation or effect might be involved in the adaptive changes in Na handling. However, observations that serum aldosterone levels are normal or high, that responsiveness to aldosterone antagonist therapy is present,[24] and that exogenous mineralocorticoid therapy does not cause Na retention in CKD patients[19,25] have cast doubt on a major role for this mechanism. Later, the discovery of atrial natriuretic peptide (ANP) turned attention toward that hormone as a mediator of Na excretion in CKD. Rats with renal ablation exhibit increased ANP levels, which are related to dietary Na intake and fractional Na excretion.[26] Increased ANP levels in CKD patients have been related to increased blood volume and to increased blood pressure.[27] Interpretation of these studies is complicated by the presence of heart failure and errors in the plasma ANP assay caused by related peptides that are retained in CKD. However, studies with an ANP antagonist confirm that increased ANP levels contribute to increased fractional Na excretion in experimental CKD[28] and giving a monoclonal anti-ANP antibody prevents the postnephrectomy diuresis in rats by blunting both proximal and distal tubular Na reabsorption.[29]

Hypertension may contribute to increased fractional Na excretion in CKD, as suggested by Guyton's group.[30] According to this view, the maintenance of constant Na intake in the setting of fewer nephrons leads to Na retention and expansion of ECF and blood volumes; the consequent higher blood pressure in turn causes a higher fractional Na excretion. However, blood pressure is higher in CKD patients than in normal subjects whose blood volumes have been increased by salt loading, and reducing dietary salt intake does not consistently prevent hypertension in rats with renal ablation.[31] Thus, blood pressure alone is not the sole factor of regulating Na excretion in CKD.

The molecular basis for Na transport after a reduction in nephron number has been explored. Using microdissected tubule segments of 5/6 nephrectomized rats, Terzi et al.[32] found increased Na-K-ATPase activity along the nephron when expressed per unit of nephron length. Enzymatic activity correlated with the degree of tubular hypertrophy. However, when expressed per tubule surface unit, no changes were found, suggesting that the density of pumps remained stable during compensatory tubular hypertrophy. Kwon et al.[33] found a decrease in total kidney Na/H exchanger, Na-phosphate cotransporter, and basolateral Na-K-ATPase in remnant kidneys as compared to controls. Densities of these transporters did not increase proportionally to the nephron hypertrophy and GFR. These findings reflected mainly changes in the PT and were associated with increased remnant nephron Na excretion. In contrast, expression of bumetanide-sensitive channels in thick ascending limb and thiazide-sensitive channels in distal tubules was increased, and Na-K-ATPase expression was maintained in these segments. These changes indicate compensatory increases in distal segments in CKD, partly because of elevated vasopressin and aldosterone levels. In contrast to rats with extensive renal ablation, studies in uninephrectomized rats have shown upregulation and activation of NHE-3 (Na/H exchanger). Moreover, the inhibition of NHE-3 was associated with the inhibition of compensatory growth in the remnant kidney.[34]

Potassium Homeostasis

The kidney retains the ability to maintain potassium (K) homeostasis and normal serum K levels until very late stages of CKD. K secretion per nephron increases, and experimentally, the fractional excretion of K may exceed 100% of the filtered load. Similar to Na handling, there is a significant inverse correlation between the fractional excretion of K and GFR. The major factors responsible for increased K excretion per nephron appear to be the elevation of plasma and intracellular K concentrations following K ingestion, particularly early in the course; later, an adaptive tubule process also augments K secretion.[35] In uninephrectomized rats, K secretion occurs within hours after a nephrectomy and is mediated by amiloride-sensitive channels.[36] In addition, reduced K reabsorption by the loop of Henle may facilitate the excretion of acute potassium loads in CKD.[37]

Following the ingestion of a K load, serum K increases by about the same increment in CKD patients and in normal subjects, inducing an increase in distal K secretion. When factored for GFR, the kaliuresis in patients with moderate CKD is the same as in normal subjects.[38] However, because the CKD patient excretes K more slowly than in the normal subject, there is prolonged elevation of serum K following an oral load.

Later in the course, distal tubular adaptations—specifically, increased activity of Na-K-ATPase and basolateral surface area in principal cells of the cortical collecting duct—promote K excretion.[39] In addition, as CKD progresses, intestinal K excretion also increases in concert with increased colonic Na-K-ATPase activity[40,41] and potassium permeability.[42] The administration of spironolactone to patients with CKD may result in dangerous hyperkalemia. Thus, it appears that adequate aldosterone levels are required to facilitate increased K secretion per nephron, and that hyperkalemia may occur earlier in CKD patients with low plasma aldosterone levels.[43]

Water Homeostasis

The capacity to generate solute-free water is remarkably well maintained in moderate CKD.[3,44,45] However, water excretory capacity is impaired, as reflected in a reduction in the minimum attainable urine osmolality. In contrast to the somewhat preserved diluting mechanisms, concentrating ability starts to fail relatively early in CKD, resulting in decreased fractional reabsorption of solute-free water. In CKD, severe dehydration is usually avoided because intact thirst mechanisms allow the patient to compensate for the urinary water losses. Accordingly, nocturia is the predominant symptom.

Urinary concentration requires the maintenance of hypertonicity of the medullary interstitium and normal water transport across distal nephron segments in response to antidiuretic hormone (ADH). The maintenance of medullary interstitial hypertonicity in turn requires structural preservation of the countercurrent system. Part of the urinary concentrating defect in CKD may be attributed to the high solute load imposed on each nephron. However, disruption of medullary architecture in tubulointerstitial diseases may cause disproportionate impairment of concentrating ability.[46] The presence of a concentration defect despite elevated plasma ADH levels in CKD suggests a distal tubular defect. Limited ADH responsiveness may be due to two factors. First, ADH-stimulated adenylate cyclase activity and water permeability in the distal nephron may be impaired.[47,48] Also, increased tubular flow rates may limit the fraction of water that can be reabsorbed by the distal nephron in response to ADH. Teitelbaum and McGuinness[49] described the absence of ADH V2 receptor mRNA in the inner medulla of rats with CKD. Kwon et al.[50] studied protein expression of aquaporins (AQP) in rat remnant kidneys. AQP1 is found mainly in the proximal tubule and in the descending limb of the loop of Henle, whereas AQP2 and 3 localize in the apical and basolateral membranes of the collecting ducts, respectively. All three channels were markedly reduced in remnant kidneys. Furthermore, decreased AQP expression was resistant to treatment with ADH.[50] Downregulation of the Na cotransporter rat bumetanide-sensitive cotransporter (rBSCl) has also been reported.[51] Several molecular mechanisms involving AQP in CKD have been suggested (reviewed in Holmes[52]).

Acid–Base Homeostasis

Metabolic acidosis is characteristic of CKD, due to reduced renal ability to excrete acid.[53,54] Early in the course, hydrogen balance is maintained by increased ammonium excretion per functioning nephron.[53–55] Later, this adaptation proves insufficient and acidosis is maintained due to reduced ammonia synthetic capacity. Ammonium excretion per total GFR rises to three to four times normal,[56] but the increase is insufficient to counteract the reduced nephron number. Impaired ammonia excretion was originally attributed to the impairment of countercurrent mechanisms, which were thought to increase ammonium concentration in the medulla and facilitate "trapping" of ammonia by acidified luminal fluid in the collecting duct. However, it is now recognized that ammonia enters tubule fluid by active secretion as well as by trapping.

Renal acid excretion also requires the reabsorption of filtered bicarbonate and the generation of a large hydrogen ion gradient in the distal nephron. Following a uninephrectomy, the stimulation of PT bicarbonate reabsorption occurs, as a result of a doubled transport rate. An increase in Na/H exchange contributes to this phenomenon.[57] There may be slight increases in the fractional reabsorption of bicarbonate[58] and studies of proximal tubule brush-border vesicles from rats with renal ablation have shown increases in V_{max} of the Na-H antiporter.[59] However, clinically, a decrease in bicarbonate reabsorptive ability develops,[60] corresponding to findings of reduced NHE-3 in the proximal tubules of rat remnant kidneys.[33] In severe CKD, the threshold for bicarbonate reabsorption may also be reduced.[61]

Distal acidification is generally better maintained than proximal bicarbonate reabsorption in CKD, except in patients with distal renal tubular acidosis. However, CKD patients are unable to lower urinary pH as well as normal subjects with experimental acidemia,[53] and so a relative decrease in distal hydrogen ion pump capacity may also contribute to acidosis. Failure to attain normal minimal urinary pH prevents optimal titration of nonammonia buffers and thus reduces the excretion of the titratable acid. Dietary phosphate restriction may further contribute to the reduced excretion of titratable acid in CKD.

Phosphate Homeostasis

Abnormalities of phosphate and calcium metabolism and their contributions to metabolic bone disease are discussed elsewhere in this book. Intrarenal adaptations that contribute to calcium and phosphate homeostasis in CKD are discussed here. A progressive increase in fractional phosphate excretion maintains phosphate balance in early CKD.[62] Later in the course, phosphate excretion is maintained by a further increase in the fractional excretion, along with increased serum phosphate levels. Slatopolsky et al.[62–64] suggested that increased parathyroid hormone (PTH) caused the increase in fractional phosphate excretion. In dogs with renal ablation, the fractional excretion of phosphorus increased and the magnitude of the increased fractional excretion correlated with the magnitude of the increase in circulating PTH levels. Restricting phosphate intake prevented increases in both PTH levels and fractional phosphate excretion. These observations formed the basis for Bricker's "trade-off hypothesis,"[65] postulating that some of the major stigmata of uremia may occur as indirect consequences of the adaptations in the nephron function.[3] According to this hypothesis, hyperparathyroidism is the biologic price paid to maintain the excretion of a constant dietary phosphate load when the nephron number is reduced. With each decrement in GFR, a transient period of phosphate retention and decreased plasma calcium would stimulate PTH synthesis and secretion, and the increased PTH activity would act to partially restore phosphate balance by augmented phosphate excretion.[66] This adverse trade-off could be avoided by reducing phosphate intake as renal function declined.

However, some studies indicate that the increased fractional phosphate excretion does not depend on an increase in PTH levels or tubule responsiveness to PTH.[67] These data suggest that the increased fractional excretion is achieved via decreased phosphate reabsorption in the proximal nephron, as occurs in intact animals fed a high phosphate diet.[68] Phosphate uptake per unit tubule mass is reduced in the proximal nephron segments isolated from uremic rabbits, and sodium-phosphate cotransport activity is reduced in brush-border membrane vesicles from uremic dogs[69] and rats[33], but these reductions do not fully account for the reduction in proximal phosphate reabsorption observed in vivo. Although reduced proximal reabsorption accounts for most of the increased fractional phosphate excretion, there is also evidence of altered distal phosphate transport (or reabsorption).[68] Nevertheless, the principal tenets of the intact nephron hypothesis continue to inform studies of adaptation in CKD.[70]

Calcium Homeostasis

As CKD advances, the production of active vitamin D [$1,25(OH_2)D_3$] is impaired, leading to reduced intestinal calcium reabsorption and renal calcium excretion; the fractional calcium excretion then increases.[71] The mechanism responsible for the increased fractional calcium excretion in advanced CKD is unclear. Possible factors include acidosis, the suppression of vitamin D production, increased distal nephron flow rates, and ECF volume expansion. Animal studies suggest that the increase in remnant nephron calcium excretion associated with ECF expansion may be mediated by ANP.[72]

STRUCTURAL ADAPTATIONS

Renal hypertrophy is an early development in the adaptive response to loss of renal mass.[73–75] Enlargement is due primarily to growth of the proximal convoluted tubules,[76] resulting in the disproportionate enlargement of the cortex in comparison to the medulla. In 1917, Addis[77] reasoned that the excretion of urea required energy, and that renal enlargement was a reflection of the need for added renal "work." Although he subsequently disproved his own hypothesis with regard to urea, the notion that the kidney grows in response to the added workload remains. Despite ingenious experimentation over the years, the question of whether hyperfiltration drives hypertrophy, or vice versa, remains incompletely answered. However, new understandings of the mechanisms and consequences of mechanotransduction are helping to elucidate this question.

Compensatory Renal Hypertrophy

Structural Changes in Individual Renal Compartments

Glomerular Hypertrophy Glomeruli also undergo progressive enlargement. A uninephrectomy in the rat increases glomerular tuft volume (V_G) by up to 75%.[78] In more exuberant hypertrophic states, as occur with extensive ablation or mineralocorticoid-salt hypertension, the degree of V_G enlargement is even greater.[78–80] Increased V_G does not necessarily parallel increased whole kidney size; V_G may continue to increase after renal growth slows. Serial structure–function studies in the rat have shown that V_G and SNGFR increase in parallel after uninephrectomy.[79,80] Morphometric studies demonstrate an increase in the total volume occupied by cellular constituents in the remnant glomeruli of nephrectomized rats.[79–86] Overall, the glomerular fractions occupied by different structural components remain constant as V_G enlarges, at least in the early phases of adaptation. However, long-term adaptation may follow a different pattern, with the mesangial volume fraction increasing only later in the course.[81]

An early study found a prominent increase in the number of glomerular endothelial, mesangial, and epithelial cells following a uninephrectomy in very young rats.[84] Later studies confirmed increased mesangial cellularity.[86] A proliferative response involving glomerular endothelial cells is apparent,[87–89] as is an increase in endothelial cell volume.[87]

Increases in glomerular capillary length and radius occur, such that capillary surface area increases.[81,86] Afferent and efferent arteriolar diameters also increase.[86] Morphometric measurements have been used to estimate the filtering capacity of the enlarged remnant glomeruli. The glomerular capillary ultrafiltration coefficient (K_f) is the product of the surface area available for filtration (S) and the hydraulic permeability of the glomerular capillary wall (k). It is not clear which anatomic boundary constitutes the surface corresponding to S. As estimated by measuring the glomerular capillary area in direct apposition to epithelial foot processes, S increases following a nephrectomy, albeit to a slightly lesser degree than total glomerular volume.[79] However, most functional studies have not found an increase in K_f of remnant glomeruli after extensive renal ablation.[8,9]

It is conceivable that k is reduced, because a decrease in S cannot be involved to explain the fall in K_f. In theory, an increase in average foot-process width would cause a decrease in the length of filtration slit overlying each unit area of peripheral capillary surface and thereby could decrease k in remnant glomeruli. In fact, morphometric studies have revealed an increase in the average width of epithelial cell foot processes in rats subjected to extensive renal ablation.[80] Alternatively, it may be that the filtering surface estimated by morphologic techniques in remnant glomeruli does not represent effective area available for filtration in vivo. Theoretical studies suggest that much of the glomerular capillary network is relatively underperfused in rats with extensive renal ablation.[90] No increase in S was found following a uninephrectomy in rats when the infusion of glomerular basement membrane antibody was used to estimate capillary surface area in vivo.[91] Alternatively, it may be that the decrease in K_f in remnant glomeruli is more functional than structural, at least early on, because ACEI therapy raises K_f to supranormal levels.[9]

Compensatory glomerular hypertrophy has been proposed as a trigger of FSGS as well. Many models show a strong association between increased V_G and the development of proteinuria and FSGS.[31,78,79,92] Conversely, there may be a protective effect of low V_G.[93] Miller et al.[94] compared the rate of development of proteinuria and FSGS in normal and uninephrectomized rats treated with a pressor dose of angiotensin (Ang) II, which increases P_{GC}. Despite the fact that the Ang II dose was halved in uninephrectomized rats, these rats demonstrated a markedly faster development of renal injury. There were no differences in P_{GC} between those groups; however, V_G was increased in the uninephrectomized animals.

The combination of increases in both glomerular capillary intraluminal pressure and capillary radius exerts increased tension on the glomerular capillary wall (following Laplace law), thus contributing to disruption of capillary wall integrity, the induction of mechanical stress-induced signaling, the activation of local humoral systems, and the podocyte changes discussed in the following. Normalizing P_{GC} may limit, but does not prevent, glomerular hypertrophy following renal ablation. Studies comparing two models of renal ablation showed differences in systemic and glomerular blood pressure, the expression of prosclerotic factors, and the rate of development of renal injury, but similar degrees of glomerular hypertrophy.[95] These studies indicate that the protective effect of reducing P_{GC} cannot be solely attributed to reduction in V_G.

Podocyte Biology after Nephron Loss. The potential additive deleterious effects of glomerular capillary hypertension and glomerular enlargement also suggest that injury may be mediated by effects on the glomerular visceral epithelial cells[79,92] and their lower ability to adapt. Adult podocytes possess diminished ability to divide in response to stressful stimuli.[96,97] Podocytes undergo exaggerated stress as glomeruli enlarge, resulting in their dysfunction and possibly destruction, in the pathogenesis of FSGS.[79,82]

Though unable to replicate, podocytes are able to undergo hypertrophy in response to a loss of renal mass and glomerular enlargement.[82,83] As reviewed by Kriz and LeHir,[97] glomerular enlargement without podocyte replication leads to structural changes including foot-process effacement, cell-body attenuation, pseudocyst formation, accumulation of absorption droplets, and finally, detachment. The loss of podocytes then triggers the onset of FSGS, as is further discussed.

Mechanisms of Renal Hypertrophy

General Principles: Hypertrophy Versus Hyperplasia

The term compensatory hypertrophy has been used to describe the aggregate changes in nephron structure, including both cellular hypertrophy and hyperplasia, which follow a loss of renal mass (reviewed in Fine and Norman,[98] Wolf,[99] Terzi et al.[100]). Renal cells react to physical, biochemical, and humoral stimuli imposed by reduced nephron number with coordinate activation of a variety of signaling pathways and changes in expression of their molecular components, with a resultant induction of genes encoding proteins involved in structural adaptive and maladaptive responses.

Hyperplasia is a result of an increase in cell number associated with DNA replication and cell division, whereas hypertrophy is defined as cell enlargement due to increases in protein and RNA content without DNA replication.[75] Both processes are involved in renal compensatory growth. During hyperplasia, cells progress through the whole cell cycle; hypertrophy occurs when the cells are engaged in the cycle but cannot progress to later stages. An interaction of the cell with growth factors that modulate the activity of cell cycle regulators then determines whether the cell will engage in hyperplasia or hypertrophy.

The Role of Physical Forces

Cortes and coworkers[101,102] showed that glomeruli can enlarge as perfusion pressure rises. In the remnant kidney, the transmission of pressure fluctuations into the glomerular capillary tuft is not prevented by myogenic autoregulatory control. This results in glomerular distension and increased V_G. Glomerular compliance is determined by capillary wall tension, size of the glomerulus, and glomerular stiffness, and is increased in remnant kidneys. This process is independent of humoral or biochemical factors, at least initially. Indeed, an increase in glomerular capillary radius is the earliest morphologic finding after a uninephrectomy.[82,83]

Increased glomerular capillary pressures and/or plasma flow rates alter the growth and activity of glomerular component cells, inducing the expression of cytokines and other mediators, which then stimulate mesangial matrix production and promote structural injury. Hemodynamic physical forces, such as shear stress or changes in blood flow, are well recognized to influence activity of endothelial and vascular smooth muscle cells (VSMC). Mechanical stress imposed on renal cells by enhanced capillary and tubular flows and pressures triggers a variety of physiologic and pathophysiologic responses. A key component of these responses, representing the actual link between mechanical stresses and growth in glomeruli and tubules, is stress-induced signaling or mechanotransduction. Intrarenal mechanotransduction has been demonstrated using in vitro systems capable of simulating stretch or pulsatile stresses imposed upon endothelial, mesangial, and tubular cells, or podocytes.

Principles of Mechanotransduction

Physical stimuli are sensed by cells and transmitted through intracellular signal transduction pathways to cytosolic effectors or to the nucleus, resulting in the induction of inappropriate genes.[103–105] The responses to mechanical stress lead to both adaptive and maladaptive processes following the nephron loss.

A spectrum of molecules has been implicated in mechanosensing; mechanical stress may directly perturb the cell surface and alter conformation of receptors and their immediate downstream effectors such as G proteins, guanine nucleotide exchange factors, and small GTPases of the Rho family, thereby initiating signaling pathways. The role of integrins, cadherin junctional complexes, and the cytoskeleton in mechanosensing has also been suggested by multiple lines of evidence.[103–107] The extracellular matrix (ECM) protein organization is sensed by integrins, transmembrane receptors that mediate cell attachment to ECM proteins. Integrins act as mediators of cell adhesion, but can also transmit extracellular stimuli into intracellular signaling events. In the vascular system, the transient receptor potential (TRP) ion channel superfamily has also been implicated in mechanosensing, as well as in stress-induced Ca^{2+} influx and vascular functional alterations,[108] but their role in renal responses to nephron loss remains unknown. Also, new caveolae are formed in endothelial cells in response to shear stress, and act as mechanosensors resulting in ras-raf-extracellular signal-related kinase (ERK) and Akt kinase activation.[109]

Mechanosensing molecules transduce signals to downstream kinases and other signaling mediators. In vascular and renal cells, mechanotransduction involves the activation of the mitogen-activated protein kinase (MAPK) family.[110] These serine/threonine kinases transduce signals in response to multiple agonists acting through GFRs with intrinsic tyrosine kinases, G protein–coupled receptors, via nonreceptor tyrosine kinases, and cellular stresses. ERKs have been implicated in mitogenic cellular responses, whereas c-Jun N-terminal kinase (JNK) and p38 activation is associated with inflammatory cytokine action, oxidative stress, prosclerotic actions, production of ECM, and apoptosis.[111,112] Activated MAPKs can translocate to the nucleus and can lead to phosphorylation and activation of transcriptional factors (which follow) or phosphorylate their cytosolic substrates.[113]

Protein kinase C (PKC) is another major family of serine/threonine kinases that are active in mechanotransduction. PKC are typically activated by lipid-derived second messengers, such as diacylglycerol or phospholipids. PKC has a number of downstream targets involved in hypertrophic signaling and the production of vasoactive factors.[114] PKC has also been shown to contribute to shear stress-induced MAPK activation.

Phosphatidylinositol-3 kinase (PI-3K), another multifactional kinase activated by upstream G proteins, is stimulated by shear stress[111] and contributes to shear stress-induced JNK activation in endothelial cells. PI3K is also involved in endothelial mechanotransduction sensed by integrins.[112] Akt kinase (protein kinase B) is a major downstream target of PI-3K. Akt is a potent survival kinase, transducing signals leading to the inhibition of apoptosis promoting cell proliferation and cell cycle regulation. Akt kinase may also transduce potentially protective signals, such as shear stress–induced generation of nitric oxide.[115]

Rho associated kinases, the effectors of the Rho family of small G proteins that act as possible mechanosensors, have been implicated in mediating cell contraction, adhesion, migration, cytoskeleton organization, and proliferation, and have been identified as major players in the pathophysiology of CKD.[116,117]

Activation of growth promoting systems leads to the upregulation of transcription factors such as activator-protein 1 (AP-1), a transcription factor formed by the heterodimerization of fos and jun proteins, or nuclear factor-κB (NF-κB), and early response genes or proto-oncogenes, the protein products of which regulate the transcriptional control of large numbers of other genes, which are early steps in cell proliferation and differentiation evoked by stress signaling, mitogens, and growth factors.

The Impact of Mechanical Stress

Expansion of the glomerular capillaries and stretching of the mesangium in response to hypertension might be a force that translates high P_{GC} into increased mesangial matrix formation. In microperfused rat glomeruli, increased P_{GC} is associated with increased V_G; in cultured mesangial cells, cyclic stretching results in the enhanced synthesis of protein, total collagen, collagen IV, collagen I, laminin, fibronectin, and transforming growth factor (TGF)-β.[101] Additionally, growing mesangial cells under pulsatile conditions stimulates the Ang II receptor; angiotensinogen mRNA levels[118] and protein kinase C, calcium influx, and proto-oncogene expression[119]; as well as altered extracellular matrix protein processing enzymes.[120,121] In vivo, Shankland et al.[122] observed that the increased P_{GC} induced by uninephrectomy in spontaneously hypertensive rats (SHR) was associated with the glomerular expression of TGF-β and platelet-derived growth factor (PDGF). Normalization of P_{GC} with an ACEI decreased glomerular TGF-β and PDGF. Similarly, Griffin et al.[95] compared P_{GC} in relation to glomerular TGF-β and PDGF expression between the excision and infarction models of renal ablation. The rats subjected to renal infarction demonstrated higher systemic and glomerular pressures, and a markedly higher expression of TGF-β and PDGF mRNA in glomeruli.

Ingram and coworkers[110,114] found stretch-induced activation of p42/44, JNK, and p38 in mesangial cells. These changes resulted in the activation of the AP-1 family, and were in part Ca^{2+} and PKC dependent. Stretch-induced activation of p38 MAPK in mesangial cells leads to increased production of TGF-β.[111] Of note, Ohashi et al.[112] found that the inhibition of enhanced renal p38 MAPK activity in rats with renal ablation leads to the acceleration of renal injury, with more proteinuria, FSGS, and interstitial fibrosis, but less tubular cell apoptosis. p38 Inhibition was associated with ERK 1/2 activation, a possible factor explaining the worsening FSGS. Thus, activation of p38 in remnant kidneys might play a protective role associated with inhibitory actions on ERKs signaling.

AP-1 and NF-κB are increased in remnant kidneys and downregulated by nephroprotective treatment.[123,124] Mirza et al.[125] reported an important function of NF-κB in regulating of the enzyme transglutaminase, which is an activator of latent TGF-β. Transglutaminase also cross-links matrix proteins, possibly contributing to interstitial fibrosis in the remnant kidney model.[126] The activation of NF-κB may have an important role in mediating cortical interstitial monocyte infiltration and tubular injury in proteinuric tubulointerstitial inflammation.[127,128] Studies of expression of early response genes in the remnant kidney following a uninephrectomy have been inconsistent. For example, the renal activity of c-fos, c-myc, c-egr1, c-jun, and c-H-ras following a uninephrectomy has been found to increase in some studies, but not in others.[129–132] Importantly, however, these studies suggest that proto-oncogene activation after uninephrectomy is modest or absent, consistent with the low risk of deterioration of GFR in this modest degree of nephron loss.

Cell Cycle Regulation as an Important Determinant of Structural Response to Nephron Loss

Genes induced by nephron loss include those coding for cell cycle regulatory proteins.[133] Positive regulation (the stimulation of transition from quiescent cell phase to ultimate cell division by mitosis) is carried out by cyclins and their partner molecules, cyclin-dependent kinases (CDK). Although CDK are constitutively expressed, cyclins are transcriptionally regulated and their levels are increased by specific mitogens such as growth factors. Negative regulation of the cell cycle is accomplished by CDK inhibitors, which bind to cyclin-CDK complexes and inhibit their activity. In addition to the preceding processes, the cells also engage in apoptosis. The total number of cells in a particular organ reflects the balance between proliferation and apoptosis. Apoptotic cells exit from the cell cycle. The initiation of apoptosis also is regulated by cyclin-CDK complexes, and the progression of the cell into mitosis or apoptosis seems to be determined by the level of CDK inhibitor p27.[133]

Liu and Preisig[134] studied renal tubular cell cycle regulation after a uninephrectomy and the resulting compensatory hypertrophy. In both rats and mice, compensatory PT growth after the uninephrectomy was hypertrophic and was associated with a cell cycle-dependent mechanism. The development of hypertrophy required that the cells enter the G1 phase and initiate the events of this phase, such as increased protein synthesis, increased cdk4/cyclin D kinase activity, and maintaining retinoblastoma protein in the hypophosphorylated state. However, the cells did not progress to the S phase, where DNA synthesis occurs. Unlike the cdk4/cyclin D activation, there was insufficient or absent activation of cdk2/cyclin E, preventing the progression of cell cycle into the S phase, resulting in hypertrophy instead of hyperplasia. This pattern of differential activation of cdk4/cyclin D and cdk2/cyclin E may reflect the previously mentioned differences in the expression and activities of p21 and p27. Compensatory hypertrophy after renal ablation is associated with cyclin E and CDK2 expression coinciding with the early proliferative response.[135]

CDK inhibitors also play a key role. These molecules are regulated by factors that have been implicated in ablation nephropathy, including Ang II and TGF-β.[136,137] p21 knockout mice subjected to renal ablation are resistant to the development of FSGS, as compared to wild-type animals.[138] In the absence of the p21 gene, the growth response in the remnant kidney is relatively more hyperplastic than hypertrophic. The authors alluded to a proposal, made by Goss[139] 45 years ago, suggesting that when an organ accommodates increased work by hypertrophy rather than hyperplasia, it is at a serious physiologic disadvantage and is more likely to undergo regression of structure and function.

Mechanotransduction in Podocytes and Its Consequences for Glomerular Injury. The additive deleterious effects of glomerular capillary hypertension and glomerular enlargement have also prompted speculation that injury may be mediated by detrimental effects on the glomerular visceral epithelial cells.[79,83,92] Podocytes undergo exaggerated stress as glomeruli enlarge, resulting in their dysfunction and possibly destruction.[79,82] Adult podocytes possess a diminished ability to divide in response to stressful stimuli[96,97]; though unable to replicate, they are able to undergo hypertrophy. As reviewed by Kriz and LeHir,[97] glomerular enlargement without podocyte replication leads to structural changes including foot-process effacement, cell-body attenuation, pseudocyst formation, accumulation of absorption droplets, and finally, detachment. The loss of podocytes then triggers the onset of FSGS, as is discussed below.

Mechanical stress induces a unique reorganization of the actin cytoskeleton in podocytes.[115] The F-actin reorganization in response to mechanical stress depends on Ca^{2+} influx and Rho kinase. A dynamic cytoskeleton allows podocytes to withstand significant mechanical stress with elevation of P_{GC}. Podocytes respond to fluid shear stress with a changed expression of focal contact markers and downregulation of ZO-1 followed by a loss of cell–cell contacts.[140] That process leads to an intermediate adhesive state, which may be a promoter of podocyte detachment. That study also demonstrated that the activation of specific tyrosine kinases is required for the podocytes to withstand increased fluid shear stress.[140]

Stretch-induced p38 in podocytes is associated with an enhanced prostanoid production via cyclooxygenase-2 (COX-2), an increased expression of the EP4 prostanoid receptor, and consequent alterations in podocyte cytoskeletal dynamics that could compromise filtration barrier function under conditions of increased P_{GC}.[141] In CKD, inhibitors have been implicated in mechanical stretch-induced podocyte hypertrophy.[142] Stretch reduces cell-cycle progression in wild-type and p27 knockout mice and induces hypertrophy, whereas hypertrophy is not induced in single p21 and double p21/p27 knockout podocytes. Stretch-induced hypertrophy is inhibited by blocking ERK 1/2 or Akt, but not p38.

Integrins are essential for podocyte adhesion to the glomerular basement membrane and therefore to the integrity of glomerular filter. Every integrin binds to a restricted number of ECM ligands. The laminin binding integrin $\alpha3\beta$ is the most highly expressed integrin on podocytes, and the key integrin mediating podocyte adhesion to the GBM.[143] Podocyte adhesion to the GBM via integrin $\alpha3\beta1$ is enhanced by its interaction with the tetraspanin protein CD151,[144,145] which regulates the tightness of integrin-dependent adhesion, cell morphology, and cell migration. The role of mechanical stress in podocyte injury and the consequent development of FSGS is further supported by evidence in CD151 knockout mice.[144] These observations have suggested that podocyte adhesion to the GBM promoted by CD151 is required to prevent the development of FSGS under conditions of high P_{GC}, and that ACEIs induce their therapeutic effects, at least in part by limiting podocyte detachment from the GBM.

Tubular Structural Adaptations

Quantitatively, the proximal convoluted tubule enlarges by approximately 15% in luminal and outside diameter and by 35% in length after the uninephrectomy in the rat,[76] and PT enlargement is proportional to the extent of the nephron number reduction.[146] The increased tubule size follows the increase in fluid reabsorption by segments of the isolated proximal straight tubule.[147] Later in the course, the increased reabsorptive rate approximates the increase in PT size and protein content.[148] The distal convoluted tubule enlarges by approximately 10% in the luminal and outside diameter by 17% in length in the rat.[76] In the distal convoluted tubules and collecting ducts, the cross-sectional area of both lumen and epithelium is increased, but to a lesser degree.[76] Tubular cells do not enlarge symmetrically; enlargement of basolateral portions of cells is more prominent as compared to the luminal surface.[149]

Tubular changes are accompanied by a transient increase in the proliferation of peritubular endothelial cells after a uninephrectomy.[88,89] This increase is followed by decreased peritubular capillary proliferation with consequences for progression, as discussed in the following. Similar to the role of hemodynamic responses in the development of glomerular hypertrophy, increased solute burden and luminal flow contribute to tubular hypertrophy after renal ablation.

Tubular Mechanotransduction

Compensatory hyperfiltration exposes tubular cells to increased flow and pressures of tubular fluid, and studies have linked tubular flow and growth. Sigmon et al.[150] showed that preventing nitric oxide (NO)-dependent hyperperfusion in uninephrectomized rats is associated with lack of compensatory renal hypertrophy, further suggesting a link between the tubular growth and hemodynamics. In another study, PT expression of angiotensinogen after a uninephrectomy in mice correlated with hyperfiltration, suggesting a role for tubular flow in the local regulation of renin-angiotensin system (RAS) activity.[151] Signaling events associated with stress-induced tubular hypertrophy are starting to be understood. Alexander et al.[152] found that cyclic stretch applied on rabbit PT cells triggered intensity-dependent ERK activation. Phospholipase A2 was identified as a part of the upstream mechanosensing process; a requirement for extracellular Ca^{2+} and stretch-activated Ca^{2+} channels was also noted. Cyclic stretch also caused rapid phosphorylation of the EGF receptor kinase and c-Src. Furthermore, arachidonic acid itself induced time- and dose-dependent phosphorylation of c-Src. As recently reviewed,[153] tubular stretch induces robust expression of a variety of mediators, which contribute to the inflammatory and ultimately fibrotic milieu.

Epithelial-Mesenchymal Transition (EMT)

Much recent attention has focused on the potential role of epithelial-mesenchymal transition (EMT) in the pathogenesis of renal fibrosis.[154–157] According to this hypothesis, the accumulation of the ECM in the tubulointerstitial space is mediated primarily by myofibroblasts, which are derived from resident interstitial fibroblasts, tubular epithelial cells, periadventitial cells, and possibly also mesenchymal stem cells and endothelial cells.[154] There are a number of proposed stimuli for this process, including proteinuria. However, although there is ample confirmatory evidence in vitro, the role of EMT in vivo remains controversial.[156,157]

Mediators of Functional and Structural Adaptations

In addition to changes induced by mechanical stress, nephron loss leads to altered levels and/or activity of many endogenous mediators that contribute to the adaptive changes after nephron loss. Many of the factors involved in hemodynamic adaptations are, in parallel, important determinants of renal growth responses.

Renin–Angiotensin–Aldosterone System

Ang II, the major effector peptide of the renin–angiotensin–aldosterone system (RAAS), causes vasoconstriction of afferent and efferent arterioles, mesangial cell contraction, and elevation in P_{GC}.[158,159] By increasing R_E, Ang II helps to sustain glomerular capillary hypertension.[9] Ang II may further elevate

P_{GC} by promoting sodium retention and causing systemic hypertension.[160] After a uninephrectomy, renin mRNA increases in proximal tubules and glomeruli of the remnant kidney.[161] In rats with ablation by partial renal infarction, renin activity is concentrated in areas adjacent to the infarcted tissue.[162] Renin production by hypoperfused nephrons adjacent to the infarcted tissue could explain why blood pressure is not increased when nephron number is halved by a uninephrectomy[79] and tends to be higher when ablation is accomplished by infarction as compared with surgical removal.[163,164] The generalized renin overexpression in tubular cells[165] and the expression of interstitial Ang II[166] are found in rat remnant kidneys, further supporting the notion of the indirect effect of Ang II in mediating increased P_{GC}. Ang II AT_1 receptor mRNA is decreased in remnant kidneys, likely as a result of increased tissue levels of Ang II,[167] whereas there is a counterregulatory increase in expression of the AT_2 receptor.[168]

Another effector molecule of the RAAS, aldosterone, has been implicated in the changes that occur after renal ablation. Plasma aldosterone levels are high in this model,[169] and sometimes in CKD patients.[24] Adrenalectomy[170] ameliorates CKD in experimental renal ablation, and the nephroprotective effects of RAAS blockers are offset by the concomitant infusion of aldosterone.[169] Arima et al.[171] reported direct, nongenomic actions of aldosterone in the glomerular microcirculation, with dose-dependent increases in R_A and predominantly in R_E, which would raise P_{GC}. The fact that P_{GC} is increased in mineralocorticoid salt models of hypertension[78] provides further evidence for a contribution of aldosterone to the progression of CKD. Aldosterone receptor antagonists reduce proteinuria clinically, though evidence for the slowing of CKD in experimental models is variable. Additional mechanisms by which aldosterone may contribute to injury include the upregulation of plasminogen-activator inhibitor-1 (PAI-1) via the mineralocorticoid receptor and TGF-β, the activation of MAPK, and the stimulation of reactive oxygen species via the upregulation of nicotinamide adenine dinucleotide phosphate (NADPH) oxidase (see reviews in Ponda and Hostetter,[172] Brem et al.,[173] Bertoccio et al.,[174] and Briet and Schiffrin[175]).

Ang II exerts a number of other actions that influence renal morphology.[176–178] Among these effects are the stimulation of proto-oncogenes, the stimulation of a plethora of growth factors (e.g., TGF-β, PDGF), the activation of NF-κB, the stimulation of monocyte chemotactic protein-1 (MCP-1), and increasing ECM accumulation by increased synthesis (fibronectin, collagen, laminin, osteopontin) or diminished degradation (metalloproteinases, PAI-1) of profibrosis cytokines.[176–178] RAS components can be activated by shear stress and altered physical forces in mesangial cells[118] and in podocytes in vitro and in vivo.[179]

Nitric Oxide, Oxidative Stress, and Endothelial Dysfunction

NO would be a good candidate for mediating hyperfiltration associated with reduced nephron mass in view of its renal hemodynamic actions[180] and evidence of shear-stress induced activation of NO generation.[181] There are, however, striking differences between studies exploring renal NO activity in uninephrectomized models, and models with a more radical nephron reduction. Uninephrectomized rats demonstrate greater renal vasoconstrictor responses to NO synthase (NOS) inhibition, and increased inducible NOS protein expression, as compared with sham-operated controls.[182] In contrast, in rats with 5/6 nephrectomy, there is decreased renal expression and enzymatic activity of all three NOS isoforms.[183,184] Furthermore, treatment with L-arginine, a NO precursor, or the NO donor molsidomine, ameliorated increases in P_{GC} or renal injury in the same model.[185,186] A blunted response to nonspecific NOS inhibition has also been shown in 5/6 nephrectomized rats.[187] Because chronic inhibition of NO production with L-arginine analogs causes severe glomerular injury associated with an increase in P_{GC},[188,189] suppression of NO synthesis in remnant glomeruli and vasculature could contribute to the development of FSGS. As discussed in the following, the NO-deficient state of reduced renal mass may be associated with enhanced oxidative stress in remnant nephrons.[190] Furthermore, the development of oxidative stress in conjunction with a shift from enhanced to reduced NO bioavailability may be a demarcation point characterizing the transition from adaptive to maladaptive responses after renal mass reduction.

In a related area, the role of oxidative stress in remnant nephron pathophysiology has been well recognized.[191] Reactive oxygen species (ROS) generated during this process not only alter the integrity of a large spectrum of proteins and lipids, but also act as signaling molecules.[192] Expression and, in particular, activities of antioxidant enzymes, such as catalase, copper/zinc superoxide dismutase, and glutathione peroxidase, increase during the course of CKD in the remnant kidney.[193] Corresponding to clinical evidence suggesting endothelial dysfunction in CKD patients,[194] impaired endothelium-dependent vasodilation of resistance arteries occurs in partially nephrectomized rats.[195] Treatment with the membrane-permeable superoxide dismutase (SOD)-mimetic tempol prevents the development of hypertension and restores vascular responsiveness to acetylcholine in vitro. Experimentally, antioxidant therapy with alpha-tocopherol attenuates the development of FSGS and interstitial fibrosis.[196] However, there is as yet no persuasive clinical evidence that antioxidant treatment per se will significantly alter the progression of clinical CKD.

Enhanced ROS production is closely linked to reduced NO bioavailability in a given vascular bed or tissue. As demonstrated by Vaziri et al.[197] in rats with renal ablation, renal and vascular oxidative stress, which promote the enhanced production of reactive carbonyl compounds and lipoperoxides and the accumulation of advanced glycation and lipoxidation end products, also leads to NO quenching, producing cytotoxic reactive nitrogen species capable of nitrating proteins and damaging other molecules. Renal and vascular expression of nitrotyrosine, a marker of tissue NO and ROS interaction, is markedly increased in rats with renal ablation.

Furthermore, these abnormalities are ameliorated by antioxidant treatment. In this context, the evidence suggests a protective role of NO in the development of injury in the remnant kidney. The chronic inhibition of NO accelerates the progression of renal injury in the remnant kidney, in association with more rapid loss of peritubular capillaries and altered tubular vascular endothelial growth factor (VEGF) expression.[198] Furthermore, treatment with L-arginine, a NO precursor, or the NO donor molsidomine, ameliorates increases in P_{GC} and renal injury in the same model,[185,186] although the protective effects of L-arginine may be observed even in the absence of changes in P_{GC}.[185] Nephroprotective effects in rats with renal ablation have also been reported with the administration of tetrahydrobiopterin, a key cofactor for appropriate eNOS enzymatic activity.[199]

NO is also an important modulator of stress-induced signaling in renal cells. In vitro, the stretch-induced activation of p42/44, JNK, and p38 MAPK, their nuclear translocation, and the stimulation of downstream transcription factors, such as AP-1 and NF-κB, in mesangial cells can be inhibited by the nitric oxide-cyclic guanosine monophosphate (NO-cGMP) pathway.[200,201] These inhibitory effects are associated with NO-induced destabilization of the actin cytoskeleton[202] and are mediated via the inhibition of RhoA-Rho kinase signaling.[203] These mechanisms may be responsible, at least in part, for the protective effect of NO in animal models with glomerular hypertension. In addition to endothelial nitric oxide synthase (eNOS)-derived NO, evidence suggests a protective role of neuronal nitric oxide synthase (nNOS)-derived NO in the remnant kidney.[204]

Recent attention has focused on the contributions of asymmetric dimethylarginine (ADMA), which inhibits NOS, and its isomer symmetric dimethylarginine (SDMA), which does not inhibit NOS, in the pathogenesis of CKD.[205–207] ADMA accumulates in the plasma in CKD and is believed to be an independent predictor of progressive CKD and cardiovascular disease. Experimentally, ADMA impairs the glomerular filtration barrier[208] and induces hypertension, oxidative stress, and glomerular and vascular fibrosis, along with increasing the expression of collagen I mRNA and TGF-β1.[209] Inducing the overexpression of dimethylarginine dimethylaminohydrolase (DDAH), an enzyme which degrades ADMA, is associated with the preservation of glomerular capillaries and reduced glomerular sclerosis in the remnant kidney model.[210]

Prostaglandins

Increased susceptibility to acute kidney injury with nonsteroidal anti-inflammatory drugs (NSAIDs) suggests a strong dependence of hemodynamics on prostaglandins (PGs) in CKD. The synthesis of PGE2, PGI2, and thromboxane A2 are increased in glomeruli isolated from subtotally nephrectomized rats, and the per nephron excretion of PGE2 and thromboxane A2 is increased.[211,212] Acute PG synthesis inhibition reduces Q_A and SNGFR but not P_{GC} in remnant kidney rats, whereas chronic thromboxane synthesis inhibition decreases vascular resistance and increases Q_A and SNGFR.[213,214] PG synthesis inhibition reduces RPF and GFR experimentally[215] and clinically.[216] Goncalves et al.[166] and Fujihara et al.[217] found a mild reduction of P_{GC} and significant nephroprotection in remnant kidney rats after treatment with nitroflurbiprofen, a compound combining nonselective cyclooxygenase (COX) inhibition and an NO-donating moiety, preventing the critical depression of renal function. Additional studies confirm a nephroprotective effect of COX-2 inhibition alone, at least experimentally.[218,219]

COX is a key enzyme in the synthesis of PG and thromboxanes from arachidonic acid. COX-2–derived PGs play a role in the physiologic regulation in the normal kidney, being involved in modulation of afferent arteriolar vasoconstriction and myogenic afferent responses to increases in renal perfusion pressure[220] and stimulation of renin release.[219] The expression of COX-2 is increased in the macula densa of remnant kidneys,[166,221] and increased activity of COX-2 is involved in the altered renal function and progression of CKD.[218,219]

The nephroprotective effect of specific COX-2 inhibition may also be mediated via the suppression of TGF-β.[218] Because thromboxane A2 is a product of the COX pathway, the authors hypothesized that thromboxanes contribute to the development of injury by stimulating TGF-β. However, vasoactive hormones, such as prostaglandin E2 (PGE2), may challenge the integrity of the actin cytoskeleton, alter podocyte morphology, and compromise glomerular permeability. PGE2 synthesis correlates with the onset of proteinuria and increased P_{GC} following reduced nephron mass.[221]

Endothelin

Endothelin (ET) infusion increases P_{GC} in the normal kidney,[222] and the ET receptor blockade is associated with the preservation of renal function and structure in remnant kidney rats.[223] In the absence of micropuncture data, it is difficult to determine whether the nephroprotective effects of ET receptor blockers are due to the inhibition of hemodynamic actions or growth actions, or both. However, in other models of CKD, the ET receptor blockade reduces P_{GC}.[224]

ET-1 is a potent mitogen and fibrogenic molecule that can contribute to interstitial fibrosis by causing ischemia due to its vasoconstrictor effects. ET-1 also has direct in vitro effects on matrix production, tubular cell proliferation, and upregulation of TGF-β (see reviews in Kohan,[225] Gagliardini et al.,[226] and Fligny et al.[227]). It appears that the ETA receptor mediates the damage, whereas the ETB receptor is more likely protective.[228] However, clinical studies have raised concerns. A recent trial,[229] in which the ET blocker avosentan was tested in patients with diabetic nephropathy, was terminated prematurely due to excess cardiovascular events in the avosentan treatment group.

Atrial Natriuretic Peptide

Another mediator of hyperfiltration is ANP, which is a potent vasodilator of the glomerular afferent arteriole. Plasma ANP levels[26] and ANP mRNA expression[230] are increased following renal ablation, and hyperfiltration is reversed with the administration of an ANP receptor antagonist.[28]

Uric Acid

Hyperuricemia has been postulated as a novel risk factor for the progression of cardiovascular and renal disease.[231–233] In addition to the stimulation of vascular smooth muscle cell proliferation, the induction of endothelial dysfunction, and growth effects, uric acid may contribute to progression via hemodynamic mechanisms. In rat models, mild hyperuricemia has been reported to induce glomerular capillary hypertension in normal[234] and remnant kidney[235] rats.

Growth Factors

The role of growth factors in initiating compensatory renal growth has been suspected since at least 1896, when Sacerdotti[236] infused blood from bilaterally nephrectomized dogs into normal dogs and induced renal growth in the recipients. In the 1950s, Braun Menéndez[237] postulated the existence of a humoral renal growth factor, termed renotropin. Fractions of urine, serum, and liver from uninephrectomized animals, and urine and serum from humans, stimulate biochemical changes (such as the incorporation of radiolabeled nucleotides into DNA) in isolated renal tissue preparations, and stimulate growth in cultures of kidney-derived cells. Such studies have been proposed as further evidence for the existence of renotropin.[238] These data do not establish that these fractions induce whole kidney growth, however, and no true renotropic hormone has been isolated.

Early evidence for the role of growth factors in the structural adaptation to nephron loss was based on in vitro observations in cultured renal cells. In general, however, these factors promote growth in many cell types, and are thus likely to participate in compensatory renal hypertrophy in a nonspecific manner. Moreover, factors that cause growth of kidney cells in vitro may not necessarily contribute importantly in vivo. For example, Ang II induces the growth of PT and mesangial cells in culture, but Ang II blockade does not prevent compensatory hypertrophy in vivo. Here we focus on those growth factors that have been implicated in hemodynamic and/or structural adaptation using several experimental approaches, including in vivo studies.

Insulinlike Growth Factor (IGF-1)

Insulinlike growth factor (IGF-1) increases renal perfusion and filtration in normal rats,[239] and levels of IGF-1 increase in the remnant kidney.[240] IGF-1 inhibition ameliorates hyperfiltration after a uninephrectomy.[241] The administration of IGF-1 increases GFR and kidney weight in intact rats, although it is not clear whether the kidneys grow disproportionately to body weight.[242,243] Following renal ablation, renal IGF-1 levels increase, whereas IGF-1 receptor levels remain constant.[242,244] Whether IGF-1 mRNA increases is also controversial. Overall, the data suggest that IGF-1 participates in, but does not initiate, compensatory renal growth, although the amelioration of compensatory hypertrophy with the early initiation of an IGF-1 receptor antagonist has been reported.[245] In rats with renal ablation, IGF-1 antagonism inhibited compensatory renal hypertrophy, but did not attenuate the development of renal fibrosis.[246]

Some studies suggest that IGF may even be protective. IGF-1 transgenic mice do not develop FSGS despite similar glomerular hypertrophy.[247] Furthermore, IGFBP-1 transgenic mice, with a decreased availability of IGF-1, develop FSGS without glomerular hypertrophy.[248]

Epidermal Growth Factor (EGF)

Epidermal growth factor (EGF) has both growth promoting and hemodynamic actions, in that it has been shown to affect arteriolar resistances and to increase P_{GC}.[249] Increased EGF content and reduced EGF receptor levels occur only after compensatory renal hypertrophy is established,[250] so it is possible that EGF plays a pathophysiologic role later in the course of the hypertrophic response to nephron loss. Of note, the functional inactivation of the EGF receptor (EGFR) by the targeted expression of a dominant-negative EGFR in renal PT cells reduces tubulointerstitial lesions in mice with 75% renal mass reduction,[251] and inhibiting the EGFR with a specific tyrosine kinase inhibitor slows progression experimentally.[252]

Hepatocyte Growth Factor (HGF)

Hepatocyte growth factor (HGF) is a potentially protective factor. Liu et al.[253] found increased renal and systemic HGF production in rats with renal ablation. With the administration of an anti-HGF antibody, rats experienced a rapid decrease in GFR and increased renal fibrosis, in association with increased ECM accumulation. Parallel in vitro data suggest that HGF preserves kidney structure by activating matrix degradation pathways via increased collagenase and matrix metalloproteinase-9 (MMP-9) expression and suppression of tissue inhibitors of metalloproteinase (TIMP), which are endogenous MMP inhibitors.[253]

The link between HGF and renal matrix degradation via the modulation of MMPs and TIMP has been confirmed in studies using treatment with recombinant HGF.[254,255] For example, in rats with renal ablation, HGF infusion halted proteinuria and decreased renal collagen accumulation. The treatment also attenuated renal inflammation in vivo and in vitro in PT cells. In contrast, HGF neutralization had the opposite effect, worsening renal fibrosis.[255]

HGF is functionally linked to the action of TGF-β. TGF-β1 induces the expression of c-met, a protoncogene encoding HGF, in renal tubular epithelial cells,[256] suggesting that HGF may act as a natural TGF-β antagonist. In TGF-β1 transgenic mice with renal ablation, HGF suppressed the expression of connective tissue growth factor (CTGF), a downstream effector of TGF-β in the remnant kidney, thus attenuating the renal fibrosis and improving the survival rate.[257] Recently, it was reported that the activation of HGF, via peroxisome proliferator-activated receptor-γ (PPAR-γ), may be a renoprotective mechanism of the RAAS blockade.[258]

Vascular Endothelial Growth Factor

There may also be a role for VEGF, a pluripotent angiogenic factor essential for kidney development. The administration of a neutralizing antibody to VEGF partially attenuates renal hypertrophy and fully prevents glomerular hypertrophy after a uninephrectomy in mice.[259] However, other evidence suggests a protective role for VEGF, particularly with respect to the tubulointerstitial changes in CKD. Kang et al.[88,260] found that a loss of peritubular capillaries and impaired angiogenesis in renal microvasculature coincides with the progressive course of CKD in remnant kidneys and is associated with a decreased expression of VEGF. This decrease in VEGF expression may be a consequence of progressive macrophage infiltration, the production of macrophage-associated cytokines, and the antiangiogenic factor thrombospondin-1. Thus, the VEGF-induced preservation and neoformation of glomerular and peritubular capillaries may limit structural injury after severe nephron loss. In addition, differences in VEGF expression after nephron loss may underlie differences in susceptibility to the progression of renal injury between male and female genders.[260]

Platelet-Derived Growth Factor

PDGF is a potent mitogen acting on glomerular cells.[261] Similar to TGF-β, PDGF is stimulated by Ang II.[262] TGF-β can be stimulated by PDGF, resulting in a transition from cell proliferation to hypertrophy and fibroproduction.[263] PDGF is upregulated in kidneys after experimental ablation[264] and in clinical CKD.[265] A pathophysiologic role in the development of FSGS is further supported by studies with PDGF in transgenic rats.[266]

Fibroblast Growth Factor 23

Fibroblast growth factor (FGF-23) is a newly discovered regulator of phosphate and mineral metabolism[267] that has recently been demonstrated to play a potential role in the progression of CKD.[268,269] FGF-23 levels rise and the responsiveness to the hormone declines as GFR falls. Progressively, FGF-23 is unable to contribute to maintain normal phosphate homeostasis.[267] Recent epidemiologic studies indicate that elevated FGF-23 is a strong independent risk factor for the progression of CKD, including diabetic nephropathy.[270,271]

Transforming Growth Factor β

TGF-β, a multifunctional prosclerotic growth cytokine, is involved in a wide array of physiologic and pathophysiologic processes and in many of the signaling and growth pathways that eventuate in CKD (see reviews in Bottinger and Bitzer[272] and Schnaper et al.[273]). The trophic effects of Ang II are, at least in part, mediated by TGF-β, and renoprotection by the RAAS blockade is associated with a reduction of renal TGF-β expression.[274]

The Smad proteins, including Smad2, Smad3, and Smad7, are essential components of downstream TGF-β signaling, which either positively (via activation of Smad2/3) or negatively (through the negative feedback mechanism of Smad7) regulate biologic activities of TGF-β1.[275] Treatment with Smad7 substantially inhibits Smad2/3 activation and preserves renal function and structure in rats with renal ablation, without affecting blood pressure.[276]

TGF-β is under the control of several miRNA families,[277] and TGF-β–induced changes in miRNA expression contribute to its effects on gene targets.[278] Sun et al.[279] reported that the beneficial structural effects and the suppression of TGF-β signaling by paclitaxel in remnant kidney rats was associated with amelioration of disbalance in the expression of several miRNA families. Although this field remains controversial, sometimes with conflicting findings, miRNA-targeted therapies may prove useful as a future treatment of CKD.[280]

Connective Tissue Growth Factor

CTGF is another strong profibrotic cytokine acting as one of the effectors of TGF-β via Smad-dependent mechanisms, as well as in a Smad-independent manner in response to stimulation by Ang II or metabolic factors.[281] Evidence also suggests that CTGF is a target of mechanosensing machinery.[282] It is expressed in PT epithelial cells that have been engulfed by interstitial fibrosis in the remnant kidneys of TGF-β transgenic mice.[257] In subtotally nephrectomized TGF-β1 transgenic mice, treatment with CTGF antisense oligodeoxynucleotide significantly blocked CTGF expression in the PT cells despite the sustained level of TGF-β1 mRNA. This reduction in CTGF mRNA level paralleled a reduction in mRNA levels of matrix molecules as well as proteinase inhibitors PAI-1 and TIMP-1,[283] suppressing renal interstitial fibrogenesis and suggesting a nephroprotective potential for this new treatment.

ECM accumulation is a hallmark of FSGS and interstitial fibrosis, and there is a delicate balance between ECM production and degradation. ECM proteins are being constantly degraded by connective tissue proteases, such as cathepsins or MMPs, and activity is further controlled by their tissue inhibitors.[284] The balance between proteinases and their tissue inhibitors is regulated by growth factors such as Ang II, TGF-β, PDGF, and others.[285] Evidence suggests a role for PAI-1 in CKD.[286,287] The amelioration of FSGS in remnant kidney rats treated with RAAS blockade is associated with inhibition of PAI-1.[286]

Modulators of Structural Adaptations after Nephron Loss

Hypertension

The most widely accepted risk factor for the progression of CKD is hypertension, which is covered elsewhere in this book. As discussed earlier, one major mechanism of hypertensive renal injury is the associated transmission of high pressure into the glomerular capillary network, with induction and maintenance of glomerular capillary hypertension.

This higher force is transmitted via mechanotransduction to the component cells of the glomerulus, with subsequent predisposition to the development of FSGS. Hypertensive vascular disease may further promote glomerular obsolescence by reducing renal and glomerular capillary blood flow.

The Role of Gender

Male gender is a risk factor for the progression of CKD.[288] It was originally suggested that the magnitude of compensatory hypertrophy is not influenced by androgens or gender. However, some clinical studies reported an increased risk in uninephrectomized males as compared to females.[16] After a uninephrectomy, the initial hypertrophy is comparable between the sexes, but later, kidney growth is greater in males.[289] Accelerated growth in males is accompanied by glomerular hypertrophy and glomerular and tubular lesions, and is associated with the presence of testosterone. Furthermore, females show more hyperplastic responses than males.[290] Thus, a uninephrectomy in the female rat theoretically can be viewed as a model of true adaptation with a minimal risk for the development of renal injury.

Many mechanisms contribute to gender differences in the progression of CKD. In vivo, female gender and/or estrogen therapy are renoprotective in a number of CKD models, and in vitro, estradiol modulates cellular activities via mechanisms consistent with a protective effect.[291,292] Exposure of mesangial cells to mechanical strain increases 44/42 mitogen-activated protein kinase (MAPK) and JNK activities, as well as the nuclear translocation of p44/42 MAPK and stress-activated protein kinase (SAPK) and nuclear protein binding to AP-1; these changes are inhibited by pretreatment with 17β-estradiol.[293] Similar findings were noted in endothelial cells exposed to cyclical strain.[294] Gender-related differences in NO appear to contribute to the relative protection observed in females.[295] Another mechanism relates to the preservation of peritubular capillary architecture. Kang et al.[260] found that male gender is associated with the downregulation of renal VEGF and the loss of peritubular capillaries, thus leading to tubulointerstitial fibrosis in remnant kidney rats, as compared with a more benign course in females. Podocytes express estrogen receptor alpha, and the presence of the receptor is protective against apoptosis,[296] whereas testosterone induces podocyte apoptosis.[297]

Dietary Factors

Feeding a low-protein diet to rats with renal ablation limits hyperfiltration and hypertrophy, whereas feeding a high-protein diet augments hypertrophy.[15] These observations suggest that the stimuli to hyperfiltration and hypertrophy associated with a nephrectomy and protein feeding are additive. After a nephrectomy, kidney weights are lower in nephrectomized rats ingesting diets that are restricted in sodium,[31] phosphate,[298] total calories,[299] or carbohydrates,[300] or are high in water.[301] Though mechanisms are not yet fully understood, the oral administration of a novel dietary adsorbent, AST-120, has also been shown to limit the progression of CKD in rats with renal ablation[124]; clinical studies are in progress to determine whether this drug can slow the progression of CKD.

Age

Age at the nephrectomy affects the magnitude of compensatory renal growth, with greater responses being seen in the younger kidneys.[302] The increased magnitude of compensatory renal hypertrophy in youth may reflect generally greater responsiveness of young tissue to stimuli responsible for organ growth, as similar increases occur in compensatory growth of other organs.

Hyperlipidemia and Lipid Nephrotoxicity

In 1982, Moorhead and coworkers[303] put forth the lipid nephrotoxicity hypothesis, suggesting that hyperlipidemia could precipitate glomerular and tubulointerstitial injury. Experimentally, feeding a high-cholesterol diet accelerates injury, whereas hypolipidemic therapy slows progression.[304] Mechanisms of lipid-induced injury include the stimulation of renal cellular proliferation by low-density lipoproteins (LDL); synergistic interactions among LDL and various growth factors; and interactions among dyslipidemia, atherosclerosis, inflammation, and oxidative stress.[304,305] As in atherosclerosis, hyperlipidemia may act synergistically with other risk factors, such as hypertension, in promoting glomerular injury. However, clinical evidence proving a beneficial effect of hypolipidemic therapy in reducing proteinuria and slowing CKD remains inconclusive.[306]

Glomerular Capillary Thrombosis

It has been suggested that early endothelial cell injury precipitates capillary thrombosis in the remnant glomeruli, contributing to FSGS by the direct occlusion of capillary lumina and the release of platelet-derived factors that aggravate glomerular injury.[73,307] Some evidence supports this experimentally; for example, heparin is protective in the remnant kidney model.[308] Heparin may also protect remnant glomeruli by other mechanisms, including the reduction of blood pressure,[308] the suppression of ET-1[309] and mesangial ECM accumulation,[310] and the inhibition of mesangial cell expression of basic FGF and PDGF, and of extracellular matrix proteins.[311] However, safety concerns have precluded clinical trials, and studies of anticoagulants in specific forms of CKD have not yet yielded practical interventions.

Altered Phosphate Metabolism and Renal Calcium Deposition

Alfrey and coworkers[312] provided the first evidence that intrarenal calcium deposition contributes to the progressive loss of renal function in experimental CKD. These studies showed that restricting phosphate intake reduced renal calcium content, preserved renal function, and prolonged life span in rats with renal ablation or nephrotoxic serum nephritis. Phosphorus restriction may also protect remnant nephrons by lowering circulating lipid levels, reducing tubule energy consumption, altering glomerular hemodynamic function, or reducing glomerular volume.[313–315] Calcium citrate, which is used clinically to bind dietary phosphate, slows the progression of CKD in rats with renal ablation, in association with improved metabolic acidosis, and the reduction in proliferative activity of glomerular and tubular cells.[316] However, despite widespread clinical usage, there remains no convincing data that oral phosphate binders slow the progression of clinical CKD, and data available thus far are not promising.[317]

Tubule-Specific Mechanisms: Proteinuria of Glomerular Origin

Proteins of glomerular origin may trigger tubular maladaptive processes by several mechanisms. First, tubular and interstitial cells can be activated by a number of growth-promoting factors generated by glomerular cells. These factors can be reabsorbed from the tubular fluid and further transported into the interstitium,[318] or they can reach the tubulointerstitial compartment via the postglomerular vasculature. Second, Remuzzi et al.[319] have suggested that glomerular proteinuria per se can exert deleterious effects on the tubulointerstitial compartment. According to this hypothesis, as protein traffic across the glomerular barrier increases, the protein concentration in the Bowman capsule and tubules also increase. PT cells actively reabsorb filtered proteins by phagocytosis. Increasing protein loads in PT cells cause organelle congestion, lysosomal swelling, and rupture, exposing the tubular cells and interstitium to lysosomal enzymes. Furthermore, protein may upregulate genes involved in tubulointerstitial infiltration and injury. For example, PT cells exposed to higher loads of proteins such as albumin or immunoglobulin may respond with an increase in ET-1 production. The release is primarily basolateral, suggesting a link with the development of interstitial injury.[320] In addition to these injurious effects of glomerular protein leakage, primary tubulointerstitial processes may contribute to remnant nephron destruction following renal ablation. The applicability of this mechanism to the progression of CKD remains controversial. Clinically, interventions that reduce proteinuria and slow the loss of GFR, showing an association, but not a tight cause-and-effect relationship. A detailed discussion of this controversy can be found in the review of Kriz and LeHir.[97]

Hypoxia Theory

Fine and coworkers[321] introduced the theory that hypoxia of tubular and interstitial cells may be a major trigger of events resulting in tubulointerstitial injury. Blood flow and oxygen delivery to the interstitial and peritubular capillary network is compromised by glomerular injury, and the tubulointerstitial capillary network may suffer the same hemodynamic injury as glomeruli. Peritubular capillaries may be compressed by hypertrophic tubules.[322] In addition, increased metabolic demands caused by enhanced reabsorptive work may contribute to tubular hypoxia.[191,323,324] Hypoxia stimulates the expression of growth factors, vasoactive molecules, cytokines, adhesion molecules, and other mediators of injury. At the level of gene transcription, hypoxia response elements (HREs) have been identified in a number of genes forming a binding site for the hypoxia-inducible transcription factor (HIF-1α).[325] HIF-1α acts in concert with other transcription factors, such as NF-κB and the fos and jun families, to induce gene expression.[325] It is now recognized that HIFs induce the expression of many genes involved in hematopoiesis, angiogenesis, resistance to oxidative stress, cell proliferation, survival and apoptosis, and extracellular matrix homeostasis, among others,[326] and that these factors contribute to tubulointerstitial injury.[327–329]

Changes in Interstitial Osmolarity

Bouby and associates[301] found a nephroprotective effect of high water intake in rats with subtotal nephrectomy, and ascribed those effects to the inhibition of the process of urinary concentration. In vitro, hypertonicity activates latent TGF-β into the biologically active form.[330] In vivo, the reduction of interstitial osmolality by high water intake in remnant kidney rats results in a decrease in TGF-β and fibronectin mRNA expression, and the amelioration of not only predominantly tubulointerstitial, but also glomerular, injury.[331]

Increased Ammoniagenesis

Increased ammonia production by remnant nephrons has been associated with intrarenal complement activation and interstitial inflammation. The administration of sodium bicarbonate reduces remnant nephron ammonia production, limits tubulointerstitial injury in rats with renal ablation,[332] and has shown promise in preliminary clinical studies.[333]

THE PRICE OF ADAPTATION: PROGRESSIVE CHRONIC KIDNEY DISEASE

Whatever the initial cause, after enough nephrons are lost, the kidney will fail. These observations suggest that, after a certain point, a reduction in the functioning nephron number leads to failure of the remaining units, because adaptive mechanisms turn maladaptive.[334] The following sections will briefly describe the glomerular and tubulointerstitial sequelae of the loss of functioning nephrons. More detail can be found in several excellent reviews.[73,97,334–336]

Glomerulosclerosis

Rennke[73] summarized the glomerular morphologic changes associated with the transition from glomerular hypertrophy to obsolescence (FSGS). The expansion of mesangial elements is a typical feature in conditions associated with sustained hyperfiltration. Both mesangial hypercellularity and increased synthesis of ECM contribute to the expansion.

In advanced stages, mesangial expansion leads to the obliteration of capillaries and glomerular obsolescence. The process is linked to the filtration of molecules into the mesangium due to increased P_{GC}, and the local generation of growth factors by intrinsic renal (endothelial and mesangial) and blood-borne (platelets and leukocytes) cells. Subendothelial hyaline deposition occurs in association with increased P_{GC} and podocyte changes. A greatly hypertrophied or stretched podocyte may no longer maintain an efficient attachment to the underlying basement membrane and capillary loop, resulting in the formation of areas with high hydraulic conductivity. Large macromolecules are filtered into these areas, forming aggregates that may ultimately occlude the capillary lumen. The formation of microthrombi is another feature often associated with hyperfiltering states. This process is most likely a consequence of glomerular endothelial injury and the local production of proclotting factors. Finally, capillary microaneurysms may occur, in particular in conditions characterized by a rapid rise in P_{GC}.[73]

The essential role of the podocyte was reiterated in an elegant description presented by Kriz and LeHir.[97] In this formulation, the pattern of injury following nephron loss is considered to be degenerative. When podocytes are exposed to chronic stress (e.g., glomerular hypertension, and abnormal activity of growth factors or vasoactive compounds), the consequences are twofold. Functionally, the size selectivity of the glomerular barrier is lost. Structurally, podocytes undergo a pattern of foot-process effacement, followed by cell-body attenuation, pseudocyst formation, the accumulation of absorption droplets, sometimes microvillus transformation, and then detachment. The decreased density of these terminally differentiated cells leads to hypertrophy, but eventually the podocytes are unable to cover the tuft, parietal cells adhere to naked glomerular basement membrane (GBM), and adhesion of the tuft to the Bowman capsule results. The adherent tuft portion allows capillaries to leak protein-rich filtrate into the interstitium instead of the Bowman space. In response, interstitial fibroblasts move in, forming a crescent-shaped space that eventually leads to the formation of synechia and FSGS.[97]

The role of those events, and the contributions of other intrinsic glomerular cells, was summarized by El Nahas and Bello.[336] There is evidence that endothelial cells may initiate this process.[337] According to this formulation, systemic factors such as hypertension, dyslipidemia, and smoking lead to endothelial damage and dysfunction, with the proliferation of mesangial cells and injury to podocytes (Fig. 75.2). Hypertension-induced shear stress leads to injury and then activation and dysfunction of glomerular endothelial cells, which in turn initiates glomerular microinflammation leading to interactions between inflammatory cells (macrophages) and mesangial cells, with the activation, proliferation, and dysfunction of the latter. Under the influence of growth factors, particularly TGF-β1, mesangial cells regress to an embryonic mesenchymal phenotype (mesangioblasts) capable of producing ECM, leading to mesangial expansion. Simultaneously, podocytes are undergoing the effacement described earlier. The outcome of this glomerular remodeling depends on the balance of healing and scarring influences.[336]

After injury, the glomerulus may either enter a phase in which its cellular constituents dedifferentiate into their mesenchymal embryonic precursors (reverse embryogenesis), or it may attract hematopoietic embryonic stem cells to recapitulate embryogenesis.[338] The outcome will depend in part on the activity of the environmental (modulating) forces at hand, as well as the potential influx of bone marrow–derived mesangial progenitor cells.[339] Another aspect of the process is the degree of apoptosis. In the process of renal scarring, renal cells undergo enhanced apoptosis. Successful interventions, such as control of hypertension, have been associated with marked decreases in apoptotic markers.[340]

Tubulointerstitial Injury

A critical reduction of the nephron number often leads to profound tubulointerstitial expansion and fibrosis.[284,335] Indeed, the degree of tubulointerstitial involvement has been suggested to be the strongest morphologic predictor of progression of CKD.[341] As ECM production increases, tubules and peritubular capillaries disappear. Loss of the linkage between glomeruli and tubules leads to atubular glomeruli, with open capillary loops but no attached tubules,[335,342,343] thus helping to explain the decline in GFR. As summarized by Eddy,[284] the interstitial scar is composed of normal interstitial ECM proteins (collagens, fibronectin, tenascin), basement membrane proteins (collagen IV, laminin), proteoglycans, and glycoproteins (hyaluronan, thrombospondin, and secreted protein acidic and rich in cysteine [SPARC]). α-Integrins[344] may be involved in binding fibronectin in the insoluble matrix. The matrix proteins that accumulate in the interstitium are assembled into a complex three-dimensional scaffold supported by cross-linking of protein chains. Studies exploring the cellular origin of proteins involved in interstitial scarring identified tubular epithelial cells and interstitial fibroblasts. Whether these cells are capable of EMT is controversial, as mentioned previously. In addition to resident renal cells, interstitial macrophages and infiltrating monocytes represent an important source of growth factors involved in fibroproduction, vasoactive molecules, and matrix proteins. Indeed, FSGS in remnant kidney rats is ameliorated by immunosuppressive agents such as mycophenolate mofetil.[345]

PATHOPHYSIOLOGY OF PROGRESSIVE CHRONIC KIDNEY DISEASE AFTER NEPHRON LOSS: UNIFYING SCENARIO

The different mechanisms proposed to account for CKD are not mutually exclusive; indeed, there are most likely extensive interactions among them.[73,74,97] Given the close apposition and functional interdependency of glomerular cell types, such interaction among injury mechanisms should be expected. The foregoing studies suggest that the progression

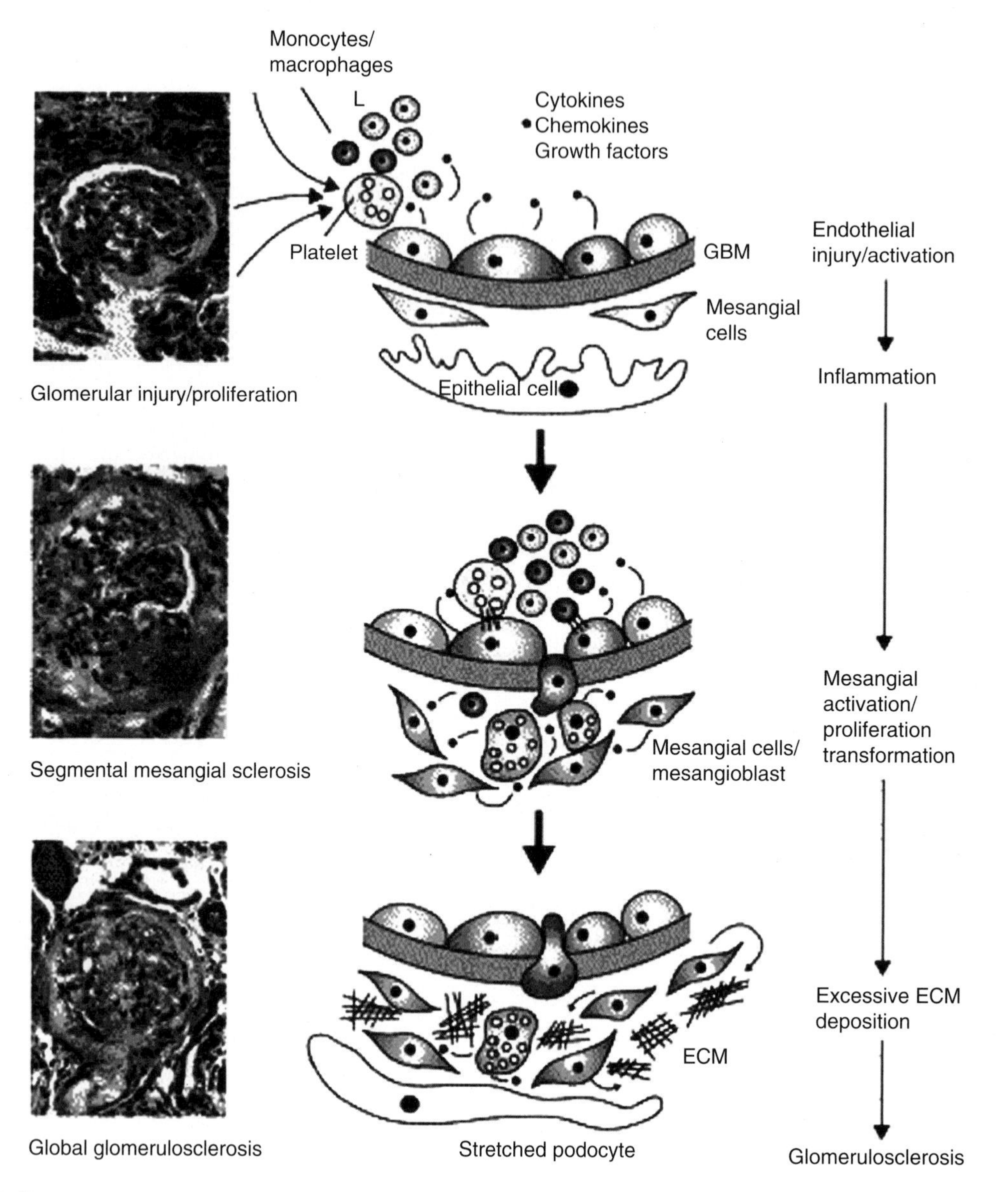

FIGURE 75.2 A diagrammatic representation of the stages of focal and segmental glomerular sclerosis (FSGS). *GBM,* glomerular basement membrane; *ECM,* extracellular matrix. (Reprinted from El Nahas AM, Bello AK. Chronic kidney disease: the global challenge. *Lancet* 2005;365:331, with permission.)

of CKD associated with systemic hypertension is mediated by the resultant adaptive increase in P_{GC}, which then contributes to structural injury. The sequence of events whereby alterations in hemodynamics, oxygen delivery, and glomerular permeability initiate growth factor overexpression and subsequent cellular injury is schematized in Figure 75.3.[100] All glomerular cell types participate. Glomerular hypertension and hypertrophy also may cause FSGS by promoting the movement of circulating macromolecules through the glomerular capillary wall. These permselective defects are associated with changes in podocyte structure and activity, as described earlier. The subendothelial deposition of large macromolecules in areas where macromolecule passage through the capillary wall is increased may result in hyalinosis, eventually proceeding to the occlusion of capillary lumina. Together, damage to these cellular elements results in FSGS.

Meanwhile, tubulointerstitial injury develops due to a primary interstitial process, or secondary to glomerular events. The cells in the tubulointerstitial compartment are injured by hypoxia, resulting from high metabolic demands imposed by the increased burden of molecules they process, impaired blood flow from obstruction in diseased glomeruli, and/or vascular injury of the interstitial capillary network. Increased protein trafficking secondary to leakage from affected glomeruli causes direct tubular toxicity, and includes humoral mediators of tubulointerstitial injury. Under these pathophysiologic stimuli, tubulointerstitial cells generate an array of prosclerotic and profibrotic mediators and transdifferentiate to

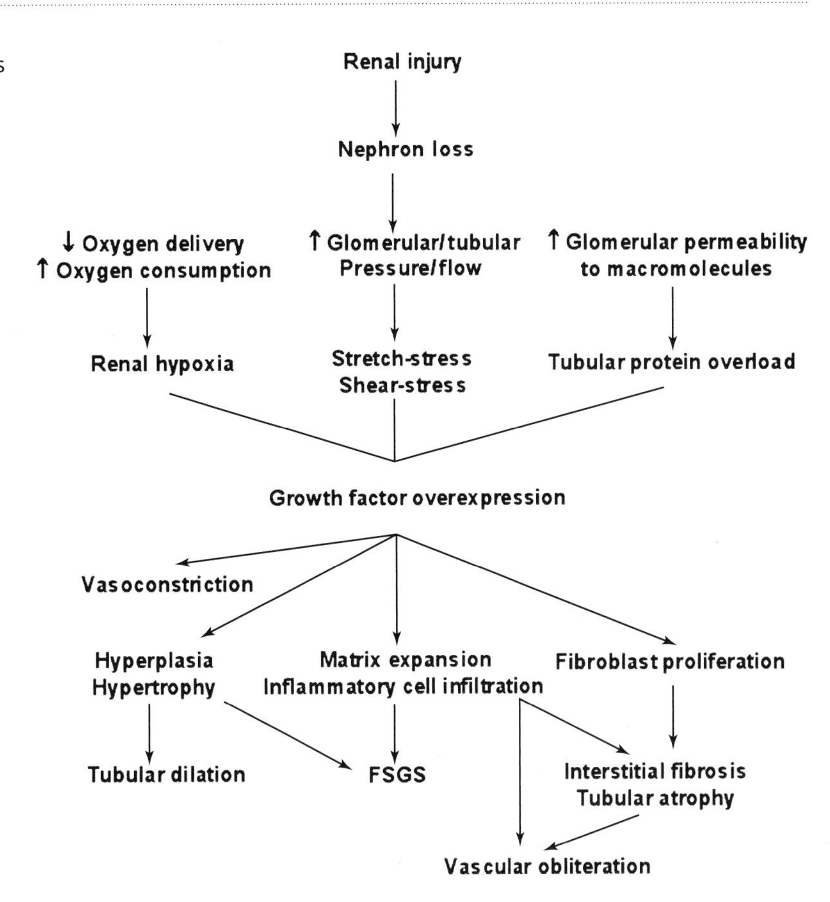

FIGURE 75.3 A hypothetical schema of pathways that link nephron reduction to the development of renal lesions via hemodynamic forces and growth factor overexpression. FSGS, focal and segmental glomerular sclerosis. (Reprinted from Terzi F, Burtin M, Friedlander G. Early molecular mechanisms in the progression of renal failure: role of growth factors and protooncogenes. *Kidney Int.* 1998;53:S68, with permission.)

more primitive cell types that further contribute to progressive injury. Tubulointerstitial injury then perpetuates nephron loss by creating atubular glomeruli.[335,343] Progressive nephron destruction in turn contributes to systemic and glomerular hypertension, thus perpetuating the cycle.

THE PROGRESSION OF HUMAN CHRONIC KIDNEY DISEASE: THERAPEUTIC IMPLICATIONS

Understanding the pathways leading to nephron destruction has prompted clinical trials exploring the potential of slowing the progression of clinical CKD. The wide spectrum of pathophysiologic mechanisms suggests that the problem can be approached from many different directions.[346,347] Experimental and, in some cases, clinical observations indicate a number of risk factors and markers for the initiation and progression of CKD, and help to point out future areas for investigation.

Systemic and glomerular hypertension remain the most practical targets for intervention. Moreover, the same interventions can also ameliorate renal growth abnormalities, resulting in beneficial effects in the tubulointerstitial as well as glomerular compartments. The inhibition of the RAAS still represents the major pharmacologic therapy of progressive CKD, with beneficial effects on hemodynamics and growth factor abnormalities. These agents are most protective in the setting of proteinuria and/or diabetes. However, control of hypertension per se affords some protection in most nephropathies, regardless of the class of agent used. In general, therapies that afford cardiovascular protection are also likely to slow the development of CKD associated with aging and probably other forms of CKD,[346] although clinical proof remains inconclusive.

Finally, the efficacy of specific pharmaceutical blockers, such as those that limit the action of endothelin, TGF-β, PPAR-γ agonists,[348] receptors for advanced glycation end products (RAGE) antagonists,[349] and other mediators, is likely to undergo clinical testing in the coming years. Several novel interventions are currently in clinical testing. Bardoxolone, an oral antioxidant inflammation modulator, has shown promise in phase II testing in diabetic nephropathy,[350] and is currently in phase III trials. Pirfenidone, an antifibrotic and anti-inflammatory investigational agent,[351] has shown promise in early clinical trials.[352] Recently, vitamin D has been proposed as having renoprotective properties,[353] and clinical trials are beginning. On the horizon are newer strategies involving the application of proteomics,[354] and stem cell therapies.[355,356] As our understanding of the disease process matures, novel treatments will come forward.

REFERENCES

1. Platt R. Structural and functional adaptation in renal failure. *Br Med J.* 1952;52:1313.

2. Bricker NS, Morrin PA, Kime SW Jr. The pathologic physiology of chronic Bright's disease: an exposition of the "intact nephron hypothesis". *Am J Med.* 1960;28:77.

3. Bricker NS, Fine LG. The renal response to progressive nephron loss. In: Brenner BM, Rector FO Jr, eds. *The Kidney*. 2nd ed. Philadelphia: Saunders; 1981:1056.

4. Ichikawa I, Hoyer JR, Seiler MW, Brenner BM. Mechanism of glomerulotubular balance in the setting of heterogeneous glomerular injury: preservation of a close functional linkage between individual nephrons and surrounding microvasculature. *J Clin Invest.* 1982;69:185.

5. Krohn AG, Ogden DA, Holmes JH. Renal function in 29 healthy adults before and after nephrectomy. *JAMA.* 1966;196:322.

6. Meyer TW, Rennke HG. Progressive glomerular injury after limited renal infarction in the rat. *Am J Physiol.* 1988;254:F856.

7. Deen WM, Maddox DA, Robertson CR, Brenner BM. Dynamics of glomerular ultrafiltration in the rat: VII. Response to reduced renal mass. *Am J Physiol.* 1974;227:F556.

8. Hostetter TH, Olson JL, Rennke HG, Venkatachalam MA, Brenner BM. Hyperfiltration in remnant nephrons: a potentially adverse response to renal ablation. *Am J Physiol.* 1981;241:F85.

9. Anderson S, Rennke HG, Brenner BM. Therapeutic advantage of converting enzyme inhibitors in arresting progressive renal disease associated with systemic hypertension in the rat. *J Clin Invest.* 1986;77:1993.

10. Buerkert J, Martin D, Prasad J, Chambless S, Klahr S. Response of deep nephrons and the terminal collecting duct to a reduction in renal mass. *Am J Physiol.* 1979;236:F454.

11. Salmond R, Seney FD Jr. Reset tubuloglomerular feedback permits and sustains glomerular hyperfunction after extensive renal ablation. *Am J Physiol.* 1991;260:F395.

12. Olson JL, Hostetter TH, Renneke HG, Brenner BM, Venkatachalam MA. Altered glomerular permselectivity and progressive sclerosis following extreme ablation of renal mass. *Kidney Int.* 1982;22:112.

13. Bidani AK, Schwartz MM, Lewis EJ. Renal autoregulation and vulnerability to hypertensive injury in remnant kidneys. *Am J Physiol.* 1987;252:F1003.

14. Anderson S, Komers R, Brenner BM. Systemic and renal manifestations of glomerular disease. In: Brenner BM, ed. *The Kidney*. 7th ed. Philadelphia: Saunders; 2004:1927.

15. Hostetter TH, Meyer TW, Rennke HG, Brenner BM. Chronic effects of dietary protein on renal structure and function in the rat with intact and reduced renal mass. *Kidney Int.* 1986;30:509.

16. Hakim RM, Goldszer RC, Brenner BM. Hypertension and proteinuria: long-term sequelae of uninephrectomy in humans. *Kidney Int.* 1984;25:930.

17. Yoshioka T, Shiraga H, Yoshida Y, et al. "Intact nephrons" as the primary origin of proteinuria in chronic renal disease: study in the rat model of subtotal nephrectomy. *J Clin Invest.* 1988;82:1614.

18. Komers R, Meyer TW, Anderson S. Pathophysiology and nephron adaptation in chronic kidney disease. In: Schrier RW, ed. *Diseases of the Kidney & Urinary Tract*. 8th ed. Philadelphia: Lippincott Williams & Wilkins; 2007:2380.

19. Slatopolsky E, Elkan IO, Weerts C, Bricker NS. Studies on the characteristics of the control system governing sodium excretion in uremic man. *J Clin Invest.* 1968;47:521.

20. Bourgoignie JJ, Kaplan M, Gavellas G, Jaffe D. Sodium homeostasis in dogs with chronic renal insufficiency. *Kidney Int.* 1982;21:820.

21. Gutmann FD, Rieselbach RE. Disproportionate inhibition of sodium reabsorption in the unilaterally diseased kidney of dog and man after an acute saline load. *J Clin Invest.* 1971;50:422.

22. Coleman AJ, Arias M, Carter NW, Rector FC, Seldin DW. The mechanism of salt wastage in chronic renal disease. *J Clin Invest.* 1966;45:116.

23. Danovitch GM, Bourgoignie JJ, Bricker NS. Reversibility of the "salt-losing" tendency of chronic renal failure. *N Engl J Med.* 1977;296:14.

24. Hené RJ, Boer P, Koomans HA, Mees EJ. Plasma aldosterone concentrations in chronic renal disease. *Kidney Int.* 1982;21:98.

25. Schrier RW, Regal EM. Influence of aldosterone on sodium, water and potassium metabolism in chronic renal disease. *Kidney Int.* 1972;1:156.

26. Smith S, Anderson S, Ballermann BJ, Brenner BM. Role of atrial natriuretic peptide in the adaptation of sodium excretion with reduced renal mass. *J Clin Invest.* 1986;77:1395.

27. Yamamoto Y, Higa T, Kitamura K, et al. Plasma concentration of human atrial natriuretic polypeptide in patients with impaired renal function. *Clin Nephrol.* 1987;27:84.

28. Zhang PL, Mackenzie HS, Troy JL, Brenner BM. Effects of natriuretic peptide receptor inhibition on remnant kidney function in rats. *Kidney Int.* 1994;46:414.

29. Valentin JP, Ribstein J, Neuser D, Nüssberger J, Mimran A. Effect of monoclonal anti-ANP antibodies on the acute functional adaptation to unilateral nephrectomy. *Kidney Int.* 1993;43:1260.

30. Guyton AC, Coleman TG, Young DB, Lohmeier TE, DeClue JW. Salt balance and long-term blood pressure control. *Annu Rev Med.* 1980;31:15.

31. Daniels BS, Hostetter TH. Adverse effects of growth in the glomerular microcirculation. *Am J Physiol.* 1990;258:F1409.

32. Terzi F, Cheval L, Barlet-Bas C, et al. Na-K-ATPase along rat nephron after subtotal nephrectomy: effect of enalapril. *Am J Physiol.* 1996;270:F997.

33. Kwon TH, Frøkiaer J, Fernández-Llama P, et al. Altered expression of Na transporters NHE-3, NaPi-II, Na-K-ATPase, BSC-1, and TSC in CRF rat kidneys. *Am J Physiol.* 1999;277:F257.

34. Girardi AC, Rocha RO, Britto LR, Rebouças NA. Upregulation of NHE3 is associated with compensatory cell growth response in young uninephrectomized rats. *Am J Physiol Renal Physiol.* 2002;283:F1296.

35. Bengele HH, Evan A, McNamara ER, Alexander EA. Tubular sites of potassium regulation in the normal and uninephrectomized rat. *Am J Physiol.* 1978;234:F146.

36. Aizman RI, Rabinowitz L, Mayer-Harnisch C. Early effects of uninephrectomy on K homeostasis in unanesthetized rats. *Am J Physiol.* 1996;270:R434.

37. Milanes CL, Jamison RL. Effect of acute potassium load on reabsorption in Henle's loop in chronic renal failure in the rat. *Kidney Int.* 1985;27:919.

38. Gonick HC, Kleeman CR, Rubini ME, Maxwell MH. Functional impairment in chronic renal disease: 3. Studies of potassium excretion. *Am J Med Sci.* 1971;261:281.

39. Stanton BA, Biemesderfer D, Wade JB, Giebisch G. Structural and functional study of the rat distal nephron: effects of potassium adaptation and depletion. *Kidney Int.* 1981;19:36.

40. Schon DA, Silva P, Hayslett JP. Mechanism of potassium excretion in renal insufficiency. *Am J Physiol.* 1974;227:F1323.

41. Finkelstein FO, Hayslett JP. Role of medullary Na-K-ATPase in renal potassium adaptation. *Am J Physiol.* 1975;229:F524.

42. Mathialahan T, Maclennan KA, Sandle LN, Verbeke C, Sandle GI. Enhanced large intestinal potassium permeability in end-stage renal disease. *J Pathol.* 2005;206:46.

43. Schambelan M, Sebastian A, Biglieri EG. Prevalence, pathogenesis, and functional significance of aldosterone deficiency in hyperkalemic patients with chronic renal insufficiency. *Kidney Int.* 1980;17:89.

44. Bricker NS, Dewey RR, Lubowitz H, Stokes J, Kirkensgaard T. Observations on the concentrating and diluting mechanisms of the diseased kidney. *J Clin Invest.* 1959;38:516.

45. Kleeman CR, Adams DA, Maxwell MH. An evaluation of maximal water diuresis in chronic renal disease. 1. Normal solute intake. *J Lab Clin Med.* 1961;58:169.

46. Finkelstein FO, Hayslett JP. Role of medullary structures in the functional adaptation of renal insufficiency. *Kidney Int.* 1974;6:419.

47. Pennell JP, Bourgoignie JJ. Water reabsorption by papillary collecting ducts in the remnant kidney. *Am J Physiol.* 1982;242:F657.

48. Pedersen EB, Thomsen EM, Lauridsen TG. Abnormal function of the vasopressin-cyclic-AMP-aquaporin2 axis during urine concentrating and diluting in patients with reduced renal function. A case control study. *BMC Nephrol.* 2010 Oct 5;11:28.

49. Teitelbaum I, McGuinness S. Vasopressin resistance in chronic renal failure. Evidence for the role of decreased V2 receptor mRNA. *J Clin Invest.* 1995;96:378.

50. Kwon TH, Frøkiaer J, Knepper MA, Nielsen S. Reduced AQP1, -2, and -3 levels in kidneys of rats with CRF induced by surgical reduction in renal mass. *Am J Physiol.* 1998; 275:F724.

51. Michimata M, Kazama I, Mizukami K, et al. Urinary concentration defect and limited expression of sodium cotransporter, rBSC1, in a rat model of chronic renal failure. *Nephron Physiol.* 2003;93:34.

52. Holmes RP. The role of renal water channels in health and disease. *Mol Aspects Med.* 2012.

53. Wrong O, Davies HE. Excretion of acid in renal disease. *Q J Med.* 1959; 28:259.

54. Widmer B, Gerhardt RE, Harrington JT, Cohen JJ. Serum electrolyte and acid base composition: the influence of graded degrees of chronic renal failure. *Arch Intern Med.* 1979;139:1099.

55. Dourhout-Mees EJ, Machado M, Slatopolsky E, Klahr S, Bricker NS. The functional adaptation of the diseased kidney. III. Ammonium excretion. *J Clin Invest.* 1966;45:289.

56. Schoolwerth AC, Sandler RS, Hoffman PM, Klahr S. Effects of nephron reduction and dietary protein content on renal ammoniagenesis in the rat. *Kidney Int.* 1975;7:397.

57. Ohno A, Beck FX, Pfaller W, Giebisch G, Wang T. Effects of chronic hyperfiltration on proximal tubule bicarbonate transport and cell electrolytes. *Kidney Int.* 1995;48:712.

58. Maddox DA, Horn JF, Famiano FC, Gennari FJ. Load dependence of proximal tubule fluid and bicarbonate reabsorption in the remnant kidney of the Munich-Wistar rat. *J Clin Invest.* 1986;77:1639.

59. Lubowitz H, Purkerson ML, Rolf DB, Weisser F, Bricker NS. Effect of nephron loss on proximal tubular bicarbonate reabsorption in the rat. *Am J Physiol.* 1971;220:457.
60. Schwartz WB, Hall PW III, Hays RM, Relman AS. On the mechanism of acidosis in chronic renal failure. *J Clin Invest.* 1959;38:39.
61. Arruda JA, Nascimento L, Arevelo G, et al. Bicarbonate reabsorption in chronic renal failure: studies in man and the rat. *Pflugers Arch.* 1978; 376:193.
62. Slatopolsky E, Robson AM, Elkan I, et al. Control of phosphate excretion in uremic man. *J Clin Invest.* 1968;47:1865.
63. Slatopolsky E, Gradowska L, Kashemsant C, et al. The control of phosphate excretion in uremia. *J Clin Invest.* 1966;45:672.
64. Slatopolsky E, Caglar S, Gradowska L, et al. On the prevention of secondary hyperparathyroidism in experimental chronic renal disease using "proportional reduction" of dietary phosphorous intake. *Kidney Int.* 1972;2:147.
65. Bricker NS. On the pathogenesis of the uremic state: an exposition of the "trade off hypothesis." *N Engl J Med.* 1972;286:1093.
66. Bricker NS, Slatopolsky E, Reiss E, Avioli LV. Calcium, phosphorus, and bone in renal disease and transplantation. *Arch Intern Med.* 1969;123:543.
67. Milanes CL, Pernalete N, Starosta R, et al. Altered response of adenylate cyclase to parathyroid hormone during compensatory renal growth. *Kidney Int.* 1989;36:802.
68. Bank N, Su WS, Aynedjian HS. A micropuncture study of renal phosphate transport in rats with chronic renal failure and secondary hyperparathyroidism. *J Clin Invest.* 1978;61:884.
69. Hruska KA, Klahr S, Hammerman MR. Decreased luminal membrane transport of phosphate in chronic renal failure. *Am J Physiol.* 1982;242:F17.
70. Slatopolsky E. The intact nephron hypothesis: the concept and its implications for phosphate management in CKD-related mineral and bone disorder. *Kidney Int.* 2011;79(Suppl 121):S3.
71. Coburn JW, Popovtzer MM, Massry SG, Kleeman CR. The physicochemical state and renal handling of divalent ions in chronic renal failure. *Arch Intern Med.* 1969;124:302.
72. Ortola FV, Ballermann BJ, Brenner BM. Endogenous ANP augments fractional excretion of Pi, Ca, and Na in rats with reduced renal mass. *Am J Physiol.* 1988;255:F1091.
73. Rennke HG. Pathology of glomerular hyperfiltration. In: Mitch WE, Brenner BM, Stein JH, eds. *The Progressive Nature of Renal Disease.* New York: Churchill Livingstone; 1986:111.
74. Rennke HG, Anderson S, Brenner BM. Structural and functional correlations in the progression of renal disease. In: Tisher CC, Brenner BM, eds. *Renal Pathology.* 2nd ed. Philadelphia: JB Lippincott; 1994:116.
75. Fine LG. The biology of renal hypertrophy. *Kidney Int.* 1986;29:619.
76. Hayslett JP, Kashgarian M, Epstein FH. Functional correlates of compensatory renal hypertrophy. *J Clin Invest.* 1968;47:774.
77. Addis T. The ratio between the urea content of the urine and of the blood after the administration of large quantities of urea: an approximate index of the quantity of actively functioning kidney tissue. *J Urol.* 1917;1:263.
78. Dworkin LD, Hostetter TH, Rennke HG, Brenner BM. Hemodynamic basis for glomerular injury in rats with desoxycorticosterone-salt hypertension. *J Clin Invest.* 1984;73:1448.
79. Fries JW, Sanstrom DJ, Meyer TW, Rennke HG. Glomerular hypertrophy and epithelial cell injury modulate progressive glomerulosclerosis in the rat. *Lab Invest.* 1989;60:205.
80. Shea SM, Raskova J, Morrison AB. A stereologic study of glomerular hypertrophy in the subtotally nephrectomized rat. *Am J Pathol.* 1978;90:201.
81. Schwartz MM, Evans J, Bidani AK. The mesangium in the long-term remnant kidney model. *J Lab Clin Med.* 1994;124:644.
82. Nagata M, Kriz W. Glomerular damage after uninephrectomy in young rats. I. Hypertrophy and distortion of capillary architecture. *Kidney Int.* 1992;42:136.
83. Nagata M, Schörer K, Kriz W. Glomerular damage after uninephrectomy in young rats. II. Mechanical stress on podocytes as a pathway to sclerosis. *Kidney Int.* 1992;42:148.
84. Olivetti G, Anversa P, Melissari M, et al. Morphometry of the renal corpuscle during postnatal growth and compensatory hypertrophy. *Kidney Int.* 1980;17:438.
85. Schwartz MM, Bidani AK. Mesangial structure and function in the remnant kidney. *Kidney Int.* 1991;40:226.
86. Nyengaard JR. Number and dimensions of rat glomerular capillaries in normal development and after nephrectomy. *Kidney Int.* 1993;43:1049.
87. Adamczak M, Gross ML, Krtil J, Koch A, et al. Reversal of glomerulosclerosis after high-dose enalapril treatment in subtotally nephrectomized rats. *J Am Soc Nephrol.* 2003: 2833.
88. Kang DH, Joly AH, Oh SW, et al. Impaired angiogenesis in the remnant kidney model: I. Potential role of vascular endothelial growth factor and thrombospondin-1. *J Am Soc Nephrol.* 2001;12:1434.
89. Kanda S, Hisamatsu H, Igawa T, et al. Peritubular endothelial cell proliferation in mice during compensatory renal growth after unilateral nephrectomy. *Am J Physiol.* 1993;265:F712.
90. Shea SM, Raskova J. Glomerular hemodynamics and vascular structure in uremia: a network analysis of glomerular path lengths and maximal blood transit times computed for a microvascular model reconstructed from serial ultrathin sections. *Microvasc Res.* 1984;28:37.
91. Knutson DW, Chieu F, Bennett CM, Glassock RJ. Estimation of relative glomerular capillary surface area in normal and hypertrophic rat kidneys. *Kidney Int.* 1978;14:437.
92. Miller PL, Scholey JW, Rennke HG, Meyer TW. Glomerular hypertrophy aggravates epithelial cell injury in nephrotic rats. *J Clin Invest.* 1990;85:1119.
93. Grond J, Beukers JY, Schilthuis MS, Weening JJ, Elema JD. Analysis of renal structural and functional features in two rat strains with a different susceptibility to glomerular sclerosis. *Lab Invest.* 1986;54:77.
94. Miller PL, Rennke HG, Meyer TW. Glomerular hypertrophy accelerates hypertensive glomerular injury in rats. *Am J Physiol.* 1991;261:F459.
95. Griffin KA, Picken MM, Churchill M, Churchill P, Bidani AK. Functional and structural correlates of glomerulosclerosis after renal mass reduction in the rat. *J Am Soc Nephrol.* 2000;11:497.
96. Kriz W. Progressive renal failure–inability of podocytes to replicate and the consequences for development of glomerulosclerosis. *Nephrol Dial Transplant.* 1996;11:1738.
97. Kriz W, LeHir M. Pathways to nephron loss starting from glomerular diseases: insights from animal models. *Kidney Int.* 2005;67:404
98. Fine LG, Norman J. Cellular events in renal hypertrophy. *Annu Rev Physiol.* 1989;51:19.
99. Wolf G. Cellular mechanisms of tubule hypertrophy and hyperplasia in renal injury. *Miner Electrolyte Metab.* 1995;21:303.
100. Terzi F, Burtin M, Friedlander G. Early molecular mechanisms in the progression of renal failure: role of growth factors and protooncogenes. *Kidney Int.* 1998;53:S68.
101. Riser BL, Cortes P, Zhao X, et al. Intraglomerular pressure and mesangial stretching stimulate extracellular matrix formation in the rat. *J Clin Invest.* 1992;90:1932.
102. Cortes P, Zhao X, Riser BL, Narins RG. Regulation of glomerular volume in normal and partially nephrectomized rats. *Am J Physiol.* 1996;270:F356.
103. Chen CS, Tan J, Tien J. Mechanotransduction at cell-matrix and cell-cell contacts. *Annu Rev Biomed Eng.* 2004;6:275.
104. Katsumi A, Orr AW, Tzima E, Schwartz MA. Integrins in mechanotransduction. *J Biol Chem.* 2004:279:12001.
105. Ingber DE. Mechanobiology and diseases of mechanotransduction. *Ann Med.* 2003:35:564.
106. Shyy JY, Chien S. Role of integrins in endothelial mechanosensing of shear stress. *Circ Res.* 2002;91:769.
107. Tzima E, Irani-Tehrani M, Kiosses WB, et al. A mechanosensory complex that mediates the endothelial cell response to fluid shear stress. *Nature.* 2005;437:426.
108. Yin J, Kuebler WM. Mechanotransduction by TRP channels: General concepts and specific role in the vasculature. *Cell Biochem Biophys.* 2010;56:1.
109. Boyd NL, Park H, Boo YC, et al. Chronic shear induces caveolae formation and alters ERK and Akt responses in endothelial cells. *Am J Physiol.* 2003;285:H1113.
110. Ingram AJ, Ly H, Thai K, et al. Activation of mesangial cell signaling cascades in response to mechanical strain. *Kidney Int.* 1999;55:476.
111. Gruden G, Zonca S, Hayward A, et al. Mechanical stretch-induced fibronectin and transforming growth factor-beta1 production in human mesangial cells is p38 mitogen-activated protein kinase-dependent. *Diabetes.* 2000,49:655.
112. Ohashi R, Nakagawa T, Watanabe S, et al. Inhibition of p38 mitogen-activated protein kinase augments progression of remnant kidney model by activating the ERK pathway. *Am J Pathol.* 2004;164:477.
113. Tian W, Zhang Z, Cohen DM. MAPK signaling in the kidney. *Am J Physiol.* 2000;279:F593.
114. Ingram AJ, James L, Ly H, Thai K, Scholey JW. Stretch activation of jun N-terminal kinase/stress-activated protein kinase in mesangial cells. *Kidney Int.* 2000;58:1431.
115. Endlich N, Kress KR, Reiser J, et al. Podocytes respond to mechanical stress in vitro. *J Am Soc Nephrol.* 2001;12:413.
116. Kanda T, Wakino S, Hayashi K, et al. Effect of fasudil on Rho-kinase and nephropathy in subtotally nephrectomized spontaneously hypertensive rats. *Kidney Int.* 2003;64:2009.
117. Komers R, Oyama TT, Beard DR, et al. Rho kinase inhibition protects kidneys from diabetic nephropathy without reducing blood pressure. *Kidney Int.* 2011;79:432.

118. Becker BN, Yasuda T, Kondo S, et al. Mechanical stretch/relaxation stimulates a cellular renin-angiotensin system in cultured rat mesangial cells. *Exp Nephrol.* 1998;6:57.
119. Harris RC, Haralson MA, Badr KF. Continuous stretch-relaxation in culture alters rat mesangial cell morphology, growth characteristics, and metabolic activity. *Lab Invest.* 1992;66:548.
120. Yasuda T, Kondo S, Homma T, Harris RC. Regulation of extracellular matrix by mechanical stress in rat glomerular mesangial cells. *J Clin Invest.* 1996;98:1991.
121. Harris RC, Akai Y, Yasuda T, Homma T. The role of physical forces in alterations of mesangial cell function. *Kidney Int.* 1995;45:S17.
122. Shankland SJ, Ly H, Thai K, Scholey JW. Increased glomerular capillary pressure alters glomerular cytokine expression. *Circ Res.* 1994;75:844.
123. Terzi F, Burtin M, Hekmati M, et al. Sodium restriction decreases AP-1 activation after nephron reduction in the rat: role in the progression of renal lesions. *Exp Nephrol.* 2000;8:104.
124. Komiya T, Miura K, Tsukamoto J, et al. Possible involvement of nuclear factor-kB inhibition in the renal protective effect of oral adsorbent AST-120 in a rat model of chronic renal failure. *Int J Mol Med.* 2004;13:133.
125. Mirza A, Liu SL, Frizell E, et al. A role for tissue transglutaminase in hepatic injury and fibrogenesis, and its regulation by NF-kappaB. *Am J Physiol.* 1997;272:G281.
126. Johnson TS, Griffin M, Thomas GL, et al. The role of transglutaminase in the rat subtotal nephrectomy model of renal fibrosis. *J Clin Invest.* 1997;99:2950.
127. Morrissey J, Klahr S. Transcription factor NF-kappaB regulation of renal fibrosis during ureteral obstruction. *Semin Nephrol.* 1998;18:603.
128. Rangan GK, et al. Inhibition of nuclear factor-kappaB activation reduces cortical tubulointerstitial injury in proteinuric rats. *Kidney Int.* 1999;56:118.
129. Sawczuk IS, Olsson CA, Hoke G, Buttyan R. Immediate induction of c-fos and c-myc transcripts following unilateral nephrectomy. *Nephron.* 1990;55:193.
130. Nakamura T, Ebihara I, Tomino Y, et al. Gene expression of growth-related proteins and ECM constituents in response to unilateral nephrectomy. *Am J Physiol.* 1992;262:F389.
131. Kujubu DA, Norman JT, Herschman HR, Fine LG. Primary response gene expression in renal hypertrophy and hyperplasia: evidence for different growth initiation processes. *Am J Physiol.* 1991;260:F823.
132. Terzi F, Ticozzi C, Burtin M, et al. Subtotal but not unilateral nephrectomy induces hyperplasia and protooncogene expression. *Am J Physiol.* 1995;268:F793.
133. Shankland SJ, Wolf G. Cell cycle regulatory proteins in renal disease: role in hypertrophy, proliferation, and apoptosis. *Am J Physiol.* 2000;278:F515.
134. Liu B, Preisig PA. Compensatory renal hypertrophy is mediated by a cell cycle-dependent mechanism. *Kidney Int.* 2002;62:1650.
135. Shankland SJ, Hamel P, Scholey JW. Cyclin and cyclin-dependent kinase expression in the remnant glomerulus. *J Am Soc Nephrol.* 1997;8:368.
136. Wolf G, Mueller E, Stahl RA, Ziyadeh FN. Angiotensin II-induced hypertrophy of cultured murine proximal tubular cells is mediated by endogenous transforming growth factor-beta. *J Clin Invest.* 1993;92:1366.
137. Wolf G, Stahl RA. Angiotensin II-stimulated hypertrophy of LLC-PK1 cells depends on the induction of the cyclin-dependent kinase inhibitor p27Kip1. *Kidney Int.* 1996;50:2112.
138. Megyesi J, Price PM, Tamayo E, Safirstein RL. The lack of a functional p21(WAF1/CIP1) gene ameliorates progression to chronic renal failure. *Proc Natl Acad Sci USA.* 1999;96:10830.
139. Goss RJ. Hypertrophy versus hyperplasia. *Science.* 1966;153:1615.
140. Friedrich C, Endlich N, Kriz W, et al. Podocytes are sensitive to fluid shear stress in vitro. *Am J Physiol Renal Physiol.* 2006; 291: F856.
141. Martineau LC, McVeigh LI, Jasmin BJ, Kennedy CR. p38 MAP kinase mediates mechanically induced COX-2 and PG EP4 receptor expression in podocytes: implications for the actin cytoskeleton. *Am J Physiol.* 2004;286:F693.
142. Petermann AT, Pippin J, Durvasula R, et al. Mechanical stretch induces podocyte hypertrophy in vitro. *Kidney Int.* 2005;67:157.
143. Pozzi A, Jarad G, Moeckel GW, et al. Beta1 integrin expression by podocytes is required to maintain glomerular structural integrity. *Dev Biol.* 2008;316:288.
144. Sachs N, Claessen N, Aten J, et al. Blood pressure influences end-stage renal disease of CD151 knockout mice. *J Clin Invest.* 2012;122:348.
145. Sachs N, Kreft M, van den Bergh Weerman MA, et al. Kidney failure in mice lacking the tetraspanin CD151. *J Cell Biol.* 2006;175:33.
146. Oliver J. New direction in renal morphology: a method, its results and its future. *Harvey Lecture Series.* 1945;XL:102.
147. Tabei K, Levenson DJ, Brenner BM. Early enhancement of fluid transport in rabbit proximal straight tubules after loss of contralateral renal excretory function. *J Clin Invest.* 1983;72:871.
148. Johnston JR, Brenner BM, Hebert SC. Uninephrectomy and dietary protein affect fluid absorption in rabbit proximal straight tubules. *Am J Physiol.* 1987;253:F222.
149. Salehmoghaddam S, Bradley T, Mikhail N, et al. Hypertrophy of basolateral Na-K pump activity in the proximal tubule of the remnant kidney. *Lab Invest.* 1985;53:443.
150. Sigmon DH, Gonzalez-Feldman E, Cavasin MA, et al. Role of nitric oxide in the renal hemodynamic response to unilateral nephrectomy. *J Am Soc Nephrol.* 2004;15:1413.
151. Gociman B, Rohrwasser A, Lantelme P, et al. Expression of angiotensinogen in proximal tubule as a function of glomerular filtration rate. *Kidney Int.* 2004;65:2153.
152. Alexander LD, Alagarsamy S, Douglas JG. Cyclic stretch-induced cPLA2 mediates ERK 1/2 signaling in rabbit proximal tubule cells. *Kidney Int.* 2004; 65:551.
153. Rohatgi R, Flores D. Intratubular hydrodynamic forces influence tubulointerstitial fibrosis in the kidney. *Curr Opin Nephrol Hypertens.* 2010;19:65.
154. Strutz FM. EMT and proteinuria as progression factors. *Kidney Int.* 2009;75:475.
155. Burns WC, Thomas MC. The molecular mediators of type 2 epithelial to mesenchymal transition (EMT) and their role in renal pathophysiology. *Expert Rev Mol Med.* 2010;12:e17.
156. Quaggin SE, Kapus A. Scar wars: mapping the fate of epithelial-mesenchymal-myofibroblast transition. *Kidney Int.* 2011;80:41.
157. Kriz W, Kaissling B, Le Hir M. Epithelial-mesenchymal transition (EMT) in kidney fibrosis: fact or fantasy? *J Clin Invest.* 2011;121:468.
158. Blantz RC, Konnen KS, Tucker BJ. Angiotensin II effects upon the glomerular microcirculation and ultrafiltration coefficient of the rat. *J Clin Invest.* 1976;57:419.
159. Myers BD, Deen WM, Brenner BM. Effects of norepinephrine and angiotensin II on the determinants of glomerular ultrafiltration and proximal tubule fluid reabsorption in the rat. *Circ Res.* 1975;37:101.
160. Baboolal K, Meyer TW. The effect of acute angiotensin II blockade on renal function in rats with reduced renal mass. *Kidney Int.* 1994;46:980.
161. Tank JE, Moe OW, Star RA, Henrich WL. Differential regulation of rat glomerular and proximal tubular renin mRNA following uninephrectomy. *Am J Physiol.* 1996;270:F776.
162. Rosenberg ME, Correa-Rotter R, Inagami T, Kren SM, Hostetter TH. Glomerular renin synthesis and storage in the remnant kidney in the rat. *Kidney Int.* 1991;40:677.
163. Terzi F, Beaufils H, Laouari D, et al. Renal effect of anti-hypertensive drugs depends on sodium diet in the excision remnant kidney model. *Kidney Int.* 1992;42:354.
164. Griffin KA, Picken M, Bidani AK. Method of renal mass reduction is a critical modulator of subsequent hypertension and glomerular injury. *J Am Soc Nephrol.* 1994;4:2023.
165. Gilbert RE, Wu LL, Kelly DJ, et al. Pathological expression of renin and angiotensin II in the renal tubule after subtotal nephrectomy. Implications for the pathogenesis of tubulointerstitial fibrosis. *Am J Pathol.* 1999;155:429.
166. Goncalves AR, Fujihara CK, Mattar AL, et al. Renal expression of COX-2, ANG II, and AT1 receptor in remnant kidney: strong renoprotection by therapy with losartan and a nonsteroidal anti-inflammatory. *Am J Physiol.* 2003;286:F945.
167. Wang DH, Yao A, Zhao H, DiPette DJ. Regulation of ANG II receptor in hypertension: role of ANG II. *Am J Physiol.* 1996;271:H120.
168. Vazquez E, et al. Angiotensin II-dependent induction of AT(2) receptor expression after renal ablation. *Am J Physiol* 2005;288:F207.
169. Greene EL, Kren S, Hostetter TH. Role of aldosterone in the remnant kidney model in the rat. *J Clin Invest.* 1996;98:1063.
170. Quan ZY, Walser M, Hill GS. Adrenalectomy ameliorates ablative nephropathy in the rat independently of corticosterone maintenance level. *Kidney Int.* 1992;41:326.
171. Arima S. Rapid non-genomic vasoconstrictor actions of aldosterone in the renal microcirculation. *J Steroid Biochem Mol Biol.* 2006;102:170.
172. Ponda MP, Hostetter TH. Aldosterone antagonism in chronic kidney disease. *Clin J Am Soc Nephrol.* 2006;1:668.
173. Brem AS, Morris DJ, Gong R. Aldosterone-induced fibrosis in the kidney: questions and controversies. *Am J Kidney Dis.* 2011;58:471.
174. Bertoccio JP, Warnock DG, Jaisser F. Mineralocorticoid receptor activation and blockade: an emerging paradigm in chronic kidney disease. *Kidney Int.* 2011:79:1051.
175. Briet M, Schiffrin EL. Aldosterone: effects on the kidney and cardiovascular system. *Nat Rev Nephrol.* 2010;6:261.
176. Ichikawa I, Harris RC. Angiotensin actions in the kidney: renewed insight into the old hormone. *Kidney Int.* 1991;40:583.
177. Siragy HM, Carey RM. Role of the intrarenal renin-angiotensin-aldosterone system in chronic kidney disease. *Am J Nephrol.* 2010;31:541.
178. Taal MW, Brenner BM. Renoprotective benefits of RAS inhibition: from ACEI to angiotensin II antagonists. *Kidney Int.* 2000;57:1803.

179. Durvasula RV, Petermann AT, Hiromura K, et al. Activation of a local tissue angiotensin system in podocytes by mechanical strain. *Kidney Int.* 2004;65:333.
180. Deng A, Baylis C. Locally produced EDRF controls preglomerular resistance and ultrafiltration coefficient. *Am J Physiol.* 1993;264:F212.
181. Buga GM, Gold ME, Fukuto JM, Ignarro LJ. Shear stress-induced release of nitric oxide from endothelial cells grown on beads. *Hypertension.* 1991;17:187.
182. Valdivielso JM, Pérez-Barriocanal F, Garcia-Estan J, López-Novoa JM. Role of nitric oxide in the early renal hemodynamic response after unilateral nephrectomy. *Am J Physiol.* 1999;276:R1718.
183. Vaziri ND, Ni Z, Wang XQ, Oveisi F, Zhou XJ. Downregulation of nitric oxide synthase in chronic renal insufficiency: role of excess PTH. *Am J Physiol.* 1998;274:F642.
184. Roczniak A, Fryer JN, Levine DZ, Burns KD. Downregulation of neuronal nitric oxide synthase in the rat remnant kidney. *J Am Soc Nephrol.* 1999;10:704.
185. Katoh T, Takahashi K, Klahr S, et al. Dietary supplementation with L-arginine ameliorates glomerular hypertension in rats with subtotal nephrectomy. *J Am Soc Nephrol.* 1994;4:1690.
186. Benigni A, Zoja C, Noris M, et al. Renoprotection by nitric oxide donor and lisinopril in the remnant kidney model. *Am J Kidney Dis.* 1999;33:746.
187. Tapia E, et al. Role of nitric oxide on glomerular dynamics in arterial hypertension with renal ablation. *J Am Soc Nephrol.* 1991;2:484A.
188. Baylis C, Mitruka B, Deng A. Chronic blockade of nitric oxide synthesis in the rat produces systemic hypertension and glomerular damage. *J Clin Invest.* 1992;90:278.
189. Ribeiro MO, Antunes E, de Nucci G, et al. Chronic inhibition of nitric oxide synthesis. A new model of arterial hypertension. *Hypertension.* 1992;20:298.
190. Modlinger PS, Wilcox CS, Aslam S. Nitric oxide, oxidative stress, and progression of chronic renal failure. *Semin Nephrol.* 2004;24:354
191. Okamura DM, Himmelfarb J. Tipping the redox balance of oxidative stress in fibrogenic pathways in chronic kidney disease. *Pediatr Nephrol.* 2009;24:2309.
192. Lassègue B, Griendling KK. NADPH oxidases: functions and pathologies in the vasculature. *Arterioscler Thromb Vasc Biol.* 2010;30:653.
193. Van Den Branden C, Ceyssens B, De Craemer D, et al. Antioxidant enzyme gene expression in rats with remnant kidney induced chronic renal failure. *Exp Nephrol.* 2000;8:91.
194. London GM, Pannier B, Agharazii M, et al. Forearm reactive hyperemia and mortality in end-stage renal disease. *Kidney Int.* 2004;65:700.
195. Hasdan G, Benchetrit S, Rashid G, et al. Endothelial dysfunction and hypertension in 5/6 nephrectomized rats are mediated by vascular superoxide. *Kidney Int.* 2002;61:586.
196. Hahn S, Kuemmerle NB, Chan W, et al. Glomerulosclerosis in the remnant kidney rat is modulated by dietary alpha-tocopherol. *J Am Soc Nephrol.* 1998;9:2089.
197. Vaziri ND, Ni Z, Oveisi F, Liang K, Pandian R. Enhanced nitric oxide inactivation and protein nitration by reactive oxygen species in renal insufficiency. *Hypertension.* 2002;39:135.
198. Kang DH, Nakagawa T, Feng L, Johnson RJ. Nitric oxide modulates vascular disease in the remnant kidney model. *Am J Pathol.* 2002;161:239.
199. Podjarny E, Hasdan G, Bernheim J, et al. Effect of chronic tetrahydrobiopterin supplementation on blood pressure and proteinuria in 5/6 nephrectomized rats. *Nephrol Dial Transplant.* 2004;19:2223.
200. Ingram AJ, James L, Ly H, et al. Nitric oxide modulates stretch activation of mitogen-activated protein kinases in mesangial cells. *Kidney Int.* 2000;58:1067.
201. Ingram AJ, James L, Thai K, et al. Nitric oxide modulates mechanical strain-induced activation of p38 MAPK in mesangial cells. *Am J Physiol.* 2000;279:F243.
202. Ingram AJ, James L, Cai L, et al. NO inhibits stretch-induced MAPK activity by cytoskeletal disruption. *J Biol Chem.* 2000;275:40301.
203. Krepinsky JC, Ingram AJ, Tang D, et al. Nitric oxide inhibits stretch-induced MAPK activation in mesangial cells through RhoA inactivation. *J Am Soc Nephrol.* 2003;14:2790.
204. Szabo AJ, Wagner L, Erdley A, Lau K, Baylis C. Renal neuronal nitric oxide synthase protein expression as a marker of renal injury. *Kidney Int.* 2003;64:1765.
205. Ueda S, Yamagishi S, Okuda S. New pathways to renal damage: role of ADMA in retarding renal disease progression. *J Nephrol.* 2010:23:377.
206. Schwedhelm E, Böger RH. The role of asymmetric and symmetric dimethylarginines in renal disease. *Nat Rev Nephrol.* 2011;7:275.
207. Baylis C. Nitric oxide synthase derangements and hypertension in kidney disease. *Curr Opin Nephrol Hypertens.* 2012;21:1.
208. Sharma A, Zhou Z, Miura H, et al. ADMA injures the glomerular filtration barrier: role of nitric oxide and superoxide. *Am J Physiol Renal Physiol.* 2009;296:F1386.
209. Mihout F, Shweke N, Bigé N, et al. Asymmetric dimethylarginine (ADMA) induces chronic kidney disease through a mechanism involving collagen and TGF-β1 synthesis. *J Pathol.* 2011;223:37.
210. Ueda S, Yamagishi S, Matsumoto Y, et al. Involvement of asymmetric dimethylarginine (ADMA) in glomerular capillary loss and sclerosis in a rat model of chronic kidney disease (CKD). *Life Sci.* 2009;84:853.
211. Nath KA, Chmielewski DH, Hostetter TH. Regulatory role of prostanoids in glomerular microcirculation of remnant nephrons. *Am J Physiol.* 1987; 252:F829.
212. Stahl RA, Kudelka S, Paravicini M, Schollmeyer P. Prostaglandin and thromboxane formation in glomeruli from rats with reduced renal mass. *Nephron.* 1986;42:252.
213. Griffin KA, Bidani AK, PIcken M, et al. Prostaglandins do not mediate impaired autoregulation or increased renin secretion in remnant rat kidneys. *Am J Physiol.* 1992;263:F1057.
214. Purkerson ML, Joist JH, Yates J, et al. Inhibition of thromboxane synthesis ameliorates the progressive kidney disease of rats with subtotal ablation. *Proc Natl Acad Sci USA.* 1985;82:193.
215. Kirschenbaum MA, Serros ER. Effect of prostaglandin inhibition on glomerular filtration rate in normal and uremic rabbits. *Prostaglandins.* 1981;22:245.
216. Ciabattoni G, Cinotti GA, Pierucci A, et al. Effects of sulindac and ibuprofen in patients with chronic glomerular disease: evidence for the dependence of renal function on prostacyclin. *N Engl J Med.* 1984;310:279.
217. Fujihara CK, Malheiros DM, Donato JL, et al. Nitroflurbiprofen, a new nonsteroidal anti-inflammatory, ameliorates structural injury in the remnant kidney. *Am J Physiol.* 1998;274:F573.
218. Wang JL, Cheng HF, Shappell S, Harris RC. A selective cyclooxygenase-2 inhibitor decreases proteinuria and retards progressive renal injury in rats. *Kidney Int.* 2000;57:2334.
219. Sanchez PL, Salgado LM, Ferreri NR, Escalante B. Effect of cyclooxygenase-2 inhibition on renal function after renal ablation. *Hypertension.* 1999;34:848.
220. Ichihara A, Imig JD, Navar LG. Cyclooxygenase-2 modulates afferent arteriolar responses to increases in pressure. *Hypertension.* 1999;34:843.
221. Wang JL, Cheng HF, Zhang MZ, et al. Selective increase of cyclooxygenase-2 expression in a model of renal ablation. *Am J Physiol.* 1998;275:F613.
222. King AJ, Brenner BM, Anderson S. Endothelin: a potent renal and systemic vasoconstrictor peptide. *Am J Physiol.* 1989;256:F1051.
223. Benigni A, Zoja C, Corna D, et al. A specific endothelin subtype A receptor antagonist protects against injury in renal disease progression. *Kidney Int.* 1993;44:440.
224. Qiu C, Baylis C. Endothelin and angiotensin mediate most glomerular responses to nitric oxide inhibition. *Kidney Int.* 1999;55:2390.
225. Kohan DM. Endothelin, hypertension, and chronic kidney disease: new insights. *Curr Opin Nephrol Hypertens.* 2010;19:134.
226. Gagliardini E, Buelli S, Benigni A. Endothelin in chronic proteinuric kidney disease. *Contrib Nephrol.* 2011;172:171.
227. Fligny C, Barton M, Tharaux PL. Endothelin and podocyte injury in chronic kidney disease. *Contrib Nephrol.* 2011;172:120.
228. Okada Y, Nakata M, Izumoto H, et al. Role of endothelin ETB receptor in partial ablation-induced chronic renal failure in rats. *Eur J Pharmacol.* 2004;494:63.
229. Mann JF, Green D, Jamerson K, et al. Avosentan for overt diabetic nephropathy. *J Am Soc Nephrol.* 2010;21:527.
230. Totsune K, Mackenzie HS, Totsune H, et al. Upregulation of atrial natriuretic peptide gene expression in remnant kidney of rats with reduced renal mass. *J Am Soc Nephrol.* 1998;9:1613.
231. Johnson RJ, Kang DH, Feig D, et al. Is there a pathogenetic role for uric acid in hypertension and cardiovascular and renal disease? *Hypertension.* 2003;41:1183.
232. Feig DI. Uric acid – a novel mediator and marker of risk in chronic kidney disease? *Curr Opin Nephrol Hypertens.* 2009;18:526.
233. Feig DI, Kang DH, Johnson RJ. Uric acid and cardiovascular risk. *N Engl J Med.* 2008;359:1811.
234. Sánchez-Lozada LG, Tapia E, Avila-Casado C, et al. Mild hyperuricemia induces glomerular hypertension in normal rats. *Am J Physiol Renal Physiol.* 2002;283:F1105.
235. Sánchez-Lozada LG, Tapia E, Santamaria J, et al. Mild hyperuricemia induces vasoconstriction and maintains glomerular hypertension in normal and remnant kidney rats. *Kidney Int.* 2005;67:237.
236. Sacerdotti C. Uber die compensatorische hypertrophie der nieren. *Virchows Arch Pathol Anat.* 1896;146:267.
237. Braun Menéndez E. Hypertension and relation between kidney weight and body weight. *Stanford Med Bull.* 1952:10:65.
238. Preuss HG. Does renotropin have a role in the pathogenesis of hypertension? *Am J Hypertens.* 1989;2:65.
239. Hirschberg R, Kopple JD. The growth hormone insulin-like growth factor I axis and renal glomerular function. *J Am Soc Nephrol.* 1992;2:1417.
240. Rogers SA, Miller SB, Hammerman MR. Enhanced renal IGF-I expression following partial kidney infarction. *Am J Physiol.* 1993;264:F963.

241. Haylor JL, McKillop IH, Oldroyd SD, El Nahas MA. IGF-I inhibitors reduce compensatory hyperfiltration in the isolated rat kidney following unilateral nephrectomy. *Nephrol Dial Transplant.* 2000;15:87.
242. Lajara R, Rotwein P, Bortz JD, et al. Dual regulation of insulin-like growth factor I expression during renal hypertrophy. *Am J Physiol.* 1989;257:F252.
243. Miller SB, Hansen VA, Hammerman MR. Effects of growth hormone and IGF-I on renal function in rats with normal and reduced renal mass. *Am J Physiol.* 1990;259:F747.
244. Hise MK, Lahn JS, Shao ZM, et al. Insulin-like growth factor-I receptor and binding proteins in rat kidney after nephron loss. *J Am Soc Nephrol.* 1993;4:62.
245. Haylor J, Hickling H, El Eter E, et al. JB3, an IGF-1 receptor antagonist, inhibits early renal growth in diabetic and uninephrectomized rats. *J Am Soc Nephrol.* 2000;11:2027.
246. Oldroyd SD, Miyamoto Y, Moir A, et al. An IGF-I antagonist does not inhibit renal fibrosis in the rat following subtotal nephrectomy. *Am J Physiol Renal Physiol.* 2006;290:F695.
247. Doi T, Striker LJ, Quaife C, et al. Progressive glomerulosclerosis develops in transgenic mice chronically expressing growth hormone and growth hormone releasing factor but not in those expressing insulinlike growth factor-1. *Am J Pathol.* 1988;131:398.
248. Doublier S, Seurin D, Fouqueray B, et al. Glomerulosclerosis in mice transgenic for human insulin-like growth factor-binding protein-1. *Kidney Int.* 2000;57:2299.
249. Harris RC, et al. Evidence for glomerular actions of epidermal growth factor in the rat. *J Clin Invest* 1988;82:1028.
250. Sack EM, Arruda JA. Epidermal growth factor binding to cortical basolateral membranes in compensatory renal hypertrophy. *Regul Peptides.* 1991;33:339.
251. Terzi F, Burtin M, Hekmati M, et al. Targeted expression of a dominant-negative EGF-R in the kidney reduces tubulo-interstitial lesions after renal injury. *J Clin Invest.* 2000;106:225.
252. Lautrette A, Li S, Alili R, et al. Angiotensin II and EGF receptor cross-talk in chronic kidney diseases: a new therapeutic approach. *Nat Med.* 2005;11:867.
253. Liu Y, Rajur K, Tolbert E, Dworkin LD. Endogenous hepatocyte growth factor ameliorates chronic renal injury by activating matrix degradation pathways. *Kidney Int.* 2000;58:2028.
254. Dworkin LD, Gong R, Tolbert E, et al. Hepatocyte growth factor ameliorates progression of interstitial fibrosis in rats with established renal injury. *Kidney Int.* 2004;65:409.
255. Gong R, Rifai A, Tolbert EM, et al. Hepatocyte growth factor ameliorates renal interstitial inflammation in rat remnant kidney by modulating tubular expression of macrophage chemoattractant protein-1 and RANTES. *J Am Soc Nephrol.* 2004;15:2868.
256. Zhang X, Yang J, Li Y, Liu Y. Both Sp1 and Smad participate in mediating TGF-{beta}1-induced HGF receptor expression in renal epithelial cells. *Am J Physiol.* 2005;288:F16.
257. Inoue T, Okada H, Kobayashi T, et al. Hepatocyte growth factor counteracts transforming growth factor-beta1, through attenuation of connective tissue growth factor induction, and prevents renal fibrogenesis in 5/6 nephrectomized mice. *FASEB J.* 2003;17:268.
258. Kusunoki H, Taniyama Y, Azuma J, et al. Telmisartan exerts renoprotective actions via peroxisome proliferator-activated receptor-γ/hepatocyte growth factor pathway independent of angiotensin II type 1 receptor blockade. *Hypertension.* 2012:59:308.
259. Flyvbjerg A, Schrijvers BF, De Vriese AS, Tilton RG, Rasch R. Compensatory glomerular growth after unilateral nephrectomy is VEGF dependent. *Am J Physiol.* 2002;283:E362.
260. Kang DH, Yu ES, Yoon KI, Johnson R. The impact of gender on progression of renal disease: potential role of estrogen-mediated vascular endothelial growth factor regulation and vascular protection. *Am J Pathol.* 2004;164:679.
261. Huwiler A, Stabel S, Fabbro D, Pfeilschifter J. Platelet-derived growth factor and angiotensin II stimulate the mitogen-activated protein kinase cascade in renal mesangial cells: comparison of hypertrophic and hyperplastic agonists. *Biochem J.* 1995;305:777.
262. Johnson RJ, Alpers CE, Yoshimura A, et al. Renal injury from angiotensin II-mediated hypertension. *Hypertension.* 1992;19:464.
263. Throckmorton DC, Brogden AP, Min B, et al. PDGF and TGF-beta mediate collagen production by mesangial cells exposed to advanced glycosylation end products. *Kidney Int.* 1995;48:111.
264. Kliem V, Johnson RH, Alpers CE, et al. Mechanisms involved in the pathogenesis of tubulointerstitial fibrosis in 5/6-nephrectomized rats. *Kidney Int.* 1996;49:666.
265. Gesualdo L, Di Paolo S, Milani S, et al. Expression of platelet-derived growth factor receptors in normal and diseased human kidney. An immunohistochemistry and in situ hybridization study. *J Clin Invest.* 1994;94:50.
266. Isaka Y, Fujiwara Y, Ueda N, et al. Glomerulosclerosis induced by in vivo transfection of transforming growth factor-beta or platelet-derived growth factor gene into the rat kidney. *J Clin Invest.* 1993;92:2597.
267. Juppner H. Phosphate and FGF-23. *Kidney Int.* 2011:79(Suppl 121):S24.
268. Bernheim J, Benchetrit S. The potential roles of FGF23 and Klotho in the prognosis of renal and cardiovascular diseases. *Nephrol Dial Transplant.* 2011:26:2433.
269. de Borst MH, Vervloet MG, ter Wee PM, Navis G. Cross talk between the renin-angiotensin-aldosterone system and vitamin d-FGF-23-klotho in chronic kidney disease. *J Am Soc Nephrol.* 2011;22:1603.
270. Isakova T, Xie H, Yang W, et al. Fibroblast growth factor 23 and risks of mortality and end-stage renal disease in patients with chronic kidney disease. *JAMA.* 2011; 305:2432.
271. Titan SM, Zatz R, Graciolli FG, dos Reis LM, et al. FGF-23 as a predictor of renal outcome in diabetic nephropathy. *Clin J Am Soc Nephrol.* 2011;6:241.
272. Bottinger EP, Bitzer M. TGF-beta signaling in renal disease. *J Am Soc Nephrol.* 2002;13:2600.
273. Schnaper HW, Hayashida T, Hubchak SC, Poncelet AC. TGF-beta signal transduction and mesangial cell fibrogenesis. *Am J Physiol.* 2003;284:F243.
274. Junaid A, Hostetter TH, Rosenberg ME. Interaction of angiotensin II and TGF-β1 in the rat remnant kidney. *J Am Soc Nephrol.* 1997;8:1732.
275. Kretzschmar M, Massague J. Smads: mediators and regulators of TGF-β signaling. *Curr Opin Genet Dev.* 1998;8:103.
276. Hou CC, Wang W, Huang XR, et al. Ultrasound-microbubble-mediated gene transfer of inducible Smad7 blocks transforming growth factor-beta signaling and fibrosis in rat remnant kidney. *Am J Pathol.* 2005;166:761.
277. Kato M, Arce L, Natarajan R. MicroRNAs and their role in progressive kidney diseases. *Clin J Am Soc Nephrol.* 2009;4:1255.
278. Wang B, Komers R, Carew R, et al. Suppression of microRNA-29 expression by TGF-β1 promotes collagen expression and renal fibrosis. *J Am Soc Nephrol.* 2012;23:252.
279. Sun L, Zhang D, Liu F, et al. Low-dose paclitaxel ameliorates fibrosis in the remnant kidney model by down-regulating miR-192. *J Pathol.* 2011;225:364.
280. Lorenzen JM, Haller H, Thum T. MicroRNAs as mediators and therapeutic targets in chronic kidney disease. *Nat Rev Nephrol.* 2011:7:286.
281. Yang F, Chung AC, Huang XR, Lan HY. Angiotensin II induces connective tissue growth factor and collagen I expression via transforming growth factor-beta-dependent and -independent Smad pathways: the role of Smad3. *Hypertension.* 2009;54:877.
282. Feng Y, Yang JH, Huang H, et al. Transcriptional profile of mechanically induced genes in human vascular smooth muscle cells. *Circ Res.* 1999;85:1118.
283. Okada H, Kikuta T, Kobayashi T, et al. Connective tissue growth factor expressed in tubular epithelium plays a pivotal role in renal fibrogenesis. *J Am Soc Nephrol.* 2005;16:133.
284. Eddy AA. Molecular basis of renal fibrosis. *Pediatr Nephrol.* 2000;15:290.
285. Gomez DE, Alonso DF, Yoshiji H, Thorgeirsson UP. Tissue inhibitors of metalloproteinases: structure, regulation and biological functions. *Eur J Cell Biol.* 1997;74:111.
286. Ma LJ, Fogo AB. PAI-1 and kidney fibrosis. *Front Biosci.* 2009;14:2028.
287. Eddy AA, Fogo AB. Plasminogen activator inhibitor-1 in chronic kidney disease: evidence and mechanisms of action. *J Am Soc Nephrol.* 2006;17:2999.
288. Silbiger S, Neugarten J. Gender and human chronic renal disease. *Gend Med.* 2008; 5 Suppl A:S3.
289. Mulroney SE, Woda C, Johnson M, Pesce C. Gender differences in renal growth and function after uninephrectomy in adult rats. *Kidney Int.* 1999;56:944.
290. Mulroney SE, Pesce C. Early hyperplastic renal growth after uninephrectomy in adult female rats. *Endocrinology.* 2000;141:932.
291. Dubey RK, Jackson EK. Estrogen-induced cardiorenal protection: potential cellular, biochemical, and molecular mechanisms. *Am J Physiol.* 2001;280:F365.
292. Doublier S, Lupia E, Catanuto P, Elliot SJ. Estrogens and progression of diabetic kidney damage. *Curr Diabetes Rev.* 2011;7:28.
293. Krepinsky J, Ingram AJ, James L, et al. 17beta-estradiol modulates mechanical strain-induced MAPK activation in mesangial cells. *J Biol Chem.* 2002;277:9387.
294. Juan SH, Chen JJ, Chen CH, et al. 17beta-estradiol inhibits cyclic strain-induced endothelin-1 gene expression within vascular endothelial cells. *Am J Physiol.* 2004;187:H1254.
295. Baylis C. Sexual dimorphism in the aging kidney: differences in the nitric oxide system. *Nat Rev Nephrol.* 2009;5:384.
296. Kummer S, Jeruschke S, Wegerich LV, et al. Estrogen receptor alpha expression in podocytes mediates protection against apoptosis in-vitro and in-vivo. *PLoS One.* 2011;6:e27457.
297. Doublier S, Lupia E, Catanuto P, et al. Testosterone and 17β-estradiol have opposite effects on podocyte apoptosis that precedes glomerulosclerosis in female estrogen receptor knockout mice. *Kidney Int.* 2011;79:404.

298. Klahr S, Buerkert J, Purkerson ML. Role of dietary factors in the progression of chronic renal disease. *Kidney Int.* 1983;24:579.

299. Kobayashi S, Venkatachalam MA. Differential effects of caloric restriction on glomeruli and tubules of the remnant kidney. *Kidney Int.* 1992;42:710.

300. Kleinknecht C, Laouari D, Hinglais N, et al. Role of amount and nature of carbohydrates in the course of experimental renal failure. *Kidney Int.* 1986;30:687.

301. Bouby N, Bachmann S, Bichet D, Bankir L. Effect of water intake on the progression of chronic renal failure in the 5/6 nephrectomized rat. *Am J Physiol.* 1990;258:F973.

302. Hayslett JP. Effect of age on compensatory renal growth. *Kidney Int.* 1983; 23:599.

303. Moorhead JF, Chan MK, El-Nahas M, Varghese Z. Lipid nephrotoxicity in chronic progressive glomerular and tubule-interstitial disease. *Lancet.* 1982:2:1309.

304. Keane WF. Lipids and the kidney. *Kidney Int.* 1994;46:910.

305. Ruan XZ, Varghese Z, Moorhead JF. An update on the lipid nephrotoxicity hypothesis. *Nat Rev Nephrol.* 2009;5:713.

306. Krane V, Wanner C. Statins, inflammation and kidney disease. *Nat Rev Nephrol.* 2011;7:385.

307. Floege J, Burns MW, Alpers CE, et al. Glomerular cell proliferation and PDGF expression precede glomerulosclerosis in the remnant kidney model. *Kidney Int.* 1992;41:297.

308. Olson JL. Role of heparin as a protective agent following reduction of renal mass. *Kidney Int.* 1984;25:376.

309. Kohno M, Yokokawa K, Horio T, et al. Heparin inhibits endothelin-1 production in cultured rat mesangial cells. *Kidney Int.* 1994;45:137.

310. Tang WW, Wilson CB. Heparin decreases mesangial matrix accumulation after selective antibody-induced mesangial cell injury. *J Am Soc Nephrol.* 1992;3:921.

311. Floege J, Eng E, Young BA, et al. Heparin suppresses mesangial cell proliferation and matrix expansion in experimental mesangioproliferative glomerulonephritis. *Kidney Int.* 1993;43:369.

312. Ibels LS, Alfrey AC, Haut L, Huffer WE. Preservation of function in experimental renal disease by dietary restriction of phosphate. *N Engl J Med.* 1978;298:122.

313. Lumlertgul D, Burke TJ, Gillum DM, et al. Phosphate depletion arrests progression of chronic renal failure independent of protein intake. *Kidney Int.* 1986;29:658.

314. Lau K. Phosphate excess and progressive renal failure: the precipitation-calcification hypothesis. *Kidney Int.* 1989;36:918.

315. Harris DC, Chan L, Schrier RW. Remnant kidney hypermetabolism and progression of chronic renal failure. *Am J Physiol.* 1988;254:F267.

316. Gadola L, Noboa O, Márquez MN, et al. Calcium citrate ameliorates the progression of chronic renal injury. *Kidney Int.* 2004;65:1224.

317. Kovesdy CP, Kuchmak O, Lu JL, Kalantar-Zadeh K. Outcomes associated with phosphorus binders in men with non-dialysis-dependent CKD. *Am J Kidney Dis.* 2010;56:842.

318. Wang SN, Hirschberg R. Growth factor ultrafiltration in experimental diabetic nephropathy contributes to interstitial fibrosis. *Am J Physiol.* 2000;278:F554.

319. Remuzzi G, Ruggenenti P, Benigni A. Understanding the nature of renal disease progression. *Kidney Int.* 1997;51:2.

320. Zoja C, Moigi M, Figliuzzi M, et al. Proximal tubular cell synthesis and secretion of endothelin-1 on challenge with albumin and other proteins. *Am J Kidney Dis.* 1995;26:934.

321. Fine LG, Orphanides C, Norman JT. Progressive renal disease: the chronic hypoxia hypothesis. *Kidney Int.* 1998;65:S74.

322. Bohle A, Wehrmann M, Bogenschütz I, et al. The long-term prognosis of the primary glomerulonephritides. A morphological and clinical analysis of 1747 cases. *Pathol Res Pract.* 1992;88:908.

323. Harris DC, Chan L, Schrier RW. Remnant kidney hypermetabolism and progression of chronic renal failure. *Am J Physiol.* 1988;254:F267.

324. Schrier RW, Harris DC, Chan L, Shapiro JI, Caramelo C. Tubular hypermetabolism as a factor in the progression of chronic renal failure. *Am J Kidney Dis.* 1988;12:243.

325. Bunn HF, Poyton RO. Oxygen sensing and molecular adaptation to hypoxia. *Physiol Rev.* 1996;76:839.

326. Myllyharju J, Schipani E. Extracellular matrix genes as hypoxia-inducible targets. *Cell Tissue Res.* 2010;339:19.

327. Nangaku M. Chronic hypoxia and tubulointerstitial injury: a final common pathway to end-stage renal failure. *J Am Soc Nephrol.* 2006;17:17-25.

328. Mayer G. Capillary rarefaction, hypoxia, VEGF and angiogenesis in chronic renal disease. *Nephrol Dial Transplant.* 2011:26:1132.

329. Higgins DF, Kimura K, Iwano M, Haase VH. Hypoxia-inducible factor signaling in the development of tissue fibrosis. *Cell Cycle.* 2008; 7:1128.

330. Sugiura T, Yamauchi A, Kitamura H, et al. Effects of hypertonic stress on transforming growth factor-beta activity in normal rat kidney cells. *Kidney Int.* 1998;53:1654.

331. Sugiura T, Yamauchi A, Kitamura H, et al. High water intake ameliorates tubulointerstitial injury in rats with subtotal nephrectomy: possible role of TGF-beta. *Kidney Int.* 1999;55:1800.

332. Nath KA, Hostetter MK, Hostetter TH. Pathophysiology of chronic tubulo-interstitial disease in rats: interactions of dietary acid load, ammonia, and complement component C3. *J Clin Invest.* 1985;76:667.

333. de Brito-Ashurst I, Varagunam M, Raftery MJ, Yaqoob MM. Bicarbonate supplementation slows progression of CKD and improves nutritional status. *J Am Soc Nephrol.* 2009;20:2075.

334. Brenner BM, Meyer TW, Hostetter TH. Dietary protein intake and the progressive nature of kidney disease. *N Engl J Med.* 1982;307:652.

335. Meyer TW. Tubular injury in glomerular disease. *Kidney Int.* 2003;63:774.

336. El Nahas AM, Bello AK. Chronic kidney disease: the global challenge. *Lancet.* 2005;365:331.

337. Lee LK, Meyer TW, Pollock AS, Lovett DH. Endothelial cell injury initiates glomerular sclerosis in the rat remnant kidney. *J Clin Invest.* 1995;96:953.

338. El Nahas AM. Plasticity of kidney cells: role in kidney remodeling and scarring. *Kidney Int.* 2003;64:1553.

339. Ito T, Suzuki A, Imai E, Okabe M, Hori M. Bone marrow is a reservoir of repopulating mesangial cells during glomerular remodeling. *J Am Soc Nephrol.* 2001;12:2625.

340. Soto K, Gómez-Garre D, Largo R, et al. Tight blood pressure control decreases apoptosis during renal damage. *Kidney Int.* 2004;65:811.

341. Bohle A, Strutz F, Muller GA. On the pathogenesis of chronic renal failure in primary glomerulopathies: a view from the interstitium. *Exp Nephrol.* 1994;2:205.

342. Marcussen N. Atubular glomeruli and the structural basis for chronic renal failure. *Lab Invest.* 1992;66:265.

343. Gandhi M, Olson JL, Meyer TW. Contribution of tubular injury to loss of remnant kidney function. *Kidney Int.* 1998;54:1157.

344. Roy-Chaudhury P, HIllis G, McDonald S, Simpson JG, Power DA. Importance of the tubulointerstitium in human glomerulonephritis. II. Distribution of integrin chains beta 1, alpha 1 to 6 and alpha V. *Kidney Int.* 1997;52:103.

345. Fujihara CK, Malheiros DM, Zatz R, Noronha IL. Mycophenolate mofetil attenuates renal injury in the rat remnant kidney. *Kidney Int.* 1998;54:1510.

346. El Nahas M. Cardio-kidney-damage: a unifying concept. *Kidney Int.* 2010:78:14.

347. Kronenberg F. Emerging risk factors and markers of chronic kidney disease progression. *Nat Rev Nephrol.* 2009;5:677.

348. Fogo AB. PPARγ and chronic kidney disease. *Pediatr Nephrol.* 2011;26:347.

349. D'Agati V, Schmidt AM. RAGE and the pathogenesis of chronic kidney disease. *Nat Rev Nephrol.* 2010:6:352.

350. Pergola PE, Raskin P, Toto RD, et al. Bardoxolone methyl and kidney function in CKD with type 2 diabetes. *New Engl J Med.* 2011;365:327.

351. Cho ME, Kopp JB. Pirfenidone: an anti-fibrotic therapy for progressive kidney disease. *Expert Opin Invest Drugs.* 2010;19:275.

352. Sharma K, Ix JH, Mathew AV, et al. Pirfenidone for diabetic nephropathy. *J Am Soc Nephrol.* 2011;22:1144.

353. Agarwal R. Vitamin D, proteinuria, diabetic nephropathy, and progression of CKD. *Clin J Am Soc Nephrol.* 2009:4:1523.

354. Klein J, Kavvadas P, Prakoura N, et al. Renal fibrosis: insight from proteomics in animal models and human disease. *Proteomics.* 2011;11:805.

355. Imai N, Kaur T, Rosenberg ME, Gupta S. Cellular therapy of kidney diseases. *Semin Dial.* 2009;22:629.

356. Yeagy BA, Cherqui S. Kidney repair and stem cells: a complex and controversial process. *Pediatr Nephrol.* 2011;26:1427.

CHAPTER

76

Anemia in Chronic Kidney Disease

James E. Novak • Jerry Yee

INTRODUCTION

Anemia in patients with chronic kidney disease (CKD), including end-stage renal disease (ESRD) and kidney transplantation, is a complex condition with important prognostic and therapeutic implications. Anemia is defined by the World Health Organization (WHO) as hemoglobin (Hb) < 13 g per deciliter in men and < 12 g per deciliter in women, and the National Kidney Foundation (NKF) recommends an evaluation when Hb is < 13.5 g per deciliter in men and < 12 g per deciliter in women.[1] Nonetheless, a more precise characterization of anemia in CKD is problematic, and involves consideration of numerous hematologic, gastrointestinal, and hormonal abnormalities. In this chapter, we review the most recent evidence concerning the epidemiology, pathophysiology, diagnosis, and treatment of anemia in kidney disease. When applicable, we distinguish among CKD, ESRD, and transplant populations.

EPIDEMIOLOGY

The prevalence of stages 1 through 4 CKD in the United States has been estimated at 13.1%, or about 40 million people.[2] Anemia is common in CKD, and its prevalence increases as kidney function decreases. Claims data from the 2010 United States Renal Data System (USRDS) include a diagnosis of anemia in 43% of patients with stages 1 to 2 and 57% of those with stages 3 to 5 CKD.[3] African Americans have correspondingly higher rates of 48% and 64% for stages 1 to 2 and 3 to 5 CKD, respectively. In contrast, anemia is present in 12% to 14% of subjects at risk for kidney disease (Kidney Early Evaluation Program [KEEP]) and only 5% to 6% of the general population (National Health and Nutrition Examination Survey [NHANES] 1999 to 2004).[4]

As of December 31, 2008, the combined hemodialysis (HD) and peritoneal dialysis (PD) population in the United States was approximately 381,000 persons.[3] Because the use of erythropoiesis-stimulating agents (ESAs) has decreased (see the following), the mean Hb of incident ESRD patients has fallen from approximately 10.5 g per deciliter in 2006 to 9.9 g per deciliter in 2008. The Kidney Disease Outcomes Quality Initiative (KDOQI) target Hb of 11 to 12 g per deciliter, established in 2007, was achieved by only 37% to 38% of prevalent dialysis patients in 2008.[3] Even considering 6-month rolling averages, this target was consistently achieved by < 50% of HD patients.[5]

Hb variability, defined as the spontaneous change in Hb concentration above or below the desired range with time, is common in CKD and ESRD patients.[6] In the HD population, the standard deviation (SD) of Hb levels around the mean is 1.1 to 1.3 g per deciliter, and only 8% to 18% of patients maintain stable Hb over 6 to 12 months.[7] In contrast, in the general population, the SD of Hb levels is < 0.6 g per deciliter. This variability may[8–10] or may not[11] have important implications for morbidity and mortality in CKD and ESRD patients (see the following). Hb also varies normally with age, sex, and race, as well as under the influence of infection, inflammation, other comorbidities, and HD parameters such as adequacy and water quality.[6,12]

In patients with CKD, anemia is associated with increased all-cause and cardiovascular mortality and higher rates of left ventricular hypertrophy (LVH), congestive heart failure (CHF), major adverse cardiovascular events (MACE), and progression to ESRD.[13] In a cohort of > 1300 men without clinical history of CHF, the presence of both Hb < 13 g per deciliter and glomerular filtration rate (GFR) < 60 mL/min/1.73 m^2, compared to either anemia or CKD alone, was associated with a significantly higher rate of previously unrecognized LV dysfunction (ejection fraction [EF] < 40%).[14] Rates of CHF hospitalization and death were 3 to 5 times higher in the group with anemia and CKD compared to the group with neither anemia nor CKD. Among European HD patients (Dialysis Outcomes and Practice Patterns Study [DOPPS]), the relative risk (RR) for hospitalization and death increased by 4% and 5%, respectively, with each 1 g per deciliter decrease in Hb within the 10 to 13 g per deciliter range.[15] Consistent with these data, in a recent study of HD patients from the United Kingdom Renal Registry, the relative hazard for death increased by nearly threefold with each 1 g per deciliter decrease in Hb within the 9 to 13 g per deciliter range.[16] Among U.S. PD patients, the hazard ratio

(HR) for hospitalization and death increased similarly with decreased Hb within the same range.[17]

Anemia is increasingly recognized as a major cause of signs and symptoms previously attributed to uremia, including fatigue, weakness, dizziness, cold intolerance, shortness of breath, decreased exercise tolerance, and decreased muscle strength.[6,18,19] Anemia in CKD is also associated with functional and mobility impairment, increased risk of falls, and decreased health-related quality of life (QOL).

PATHOPHYSIOLOGY

Anemia: Historical Overview

The Bible and ancient medicine portrayed blood as a symbol of life, and most physical and mental disease was attributed to disorders of the blood.[20] The first xenogeneic (animal-to-human) blood transfusion was reported in Paris in 1667. Physician-in-Ordinary to Louis XIV, Jean-Baptiste Denis, and surgeon Paul Emmerez transfused whole lamb blood into a patient who had previously been bled 20 times for fever, whose symptoms of anemia improved markedly following the procedure. The first successful allogeneic (human-to-human) blood transfusion was reported in London in 1825, when James Blundell transfused a man's blood into his wife to treat postpartum hemorrhage.[20]

The idea that the bone marrow is the site of erythropoiesis in response to hypoxia was first proposed in 1823 and gradually expanded during the following century.[20–22] In 1863, Jourdanet observed that blood viscosity was higher in Mexicans living at high altitudes than in those living at sea level.[23] In 1891, Viault extended this observation to red blood cell (RBC) counts in Peruvians.[24] Carnot and DeFlandre[25] reported in 1906 that serum from bled rabbits, when injected into normal rabbits, stimulated RBC production. They tentatively coined the term "hemopoietine" to identify the presumed erythropoietic substance transferred by the serum. Similar experiments, in which serum or plasma from anemic or hypoxemic rabbits caused a reticulocytosis in recipient rabbits, were conducted from 1932 to 1953.[22] Brown and Roth[26] determined in 1922 that the anemia of chronic nephritis resulted from hypoactive bone marrow. In 1950, Reissmann[27] used parabiotic rats to show that, although only one animal was exposed to low O_2 tension, both partners exhibited bone marrow erythroid hyperplasia, reticulocytosis, and polycythemia, again strongly suggesting the presence of a humoral erythropoietic factor acting on the bone marrow. In 1948, Bonsdorff and Jalavisto[27a] named this factor erythropoietin (EPO).

In subsequent years, the tissue origin of EPO was elucidated. In 1957, it was shown that a bilateral nephrectomy prevented the rise in plasma EPO levels in bled rats.[28] Experiments from 1961 to 1974 showed that perfusates from hypoxic rabbit and dog kidneys could stimulate presynthesized EPO release and subsequent reticulocytosis.[21,22] In 1983, *EPO* mRNA from hypoxic rat kidneys, injected into frog oocytes, was translated into EPO, and experiments from 1988 to 1996 demonstrated *EPO* transcripts and biologically active EPO in the peritubular interstitial cells of kidneys from a number of species.[29]

More recent discoveries have included the description of EPO physiology and molecular biology, especially pertaining to kidney disease. Erythropoietic activity was quantified from 1955 to 1961 by the measurement of increased ^{59}Fe uptake by RBCs in polycythemic rats and in normal rats that had been injected with plasma from anemic rats.[30,31] The inverse relationship between EPO concentration and hematocrit was reported in 1968.[32] EPO itself was ultimately purified in 1977 by concentrating 2550 L of urine from patients with aplastic anemia.[33] Isolation of the purified protein facilitated the development of an EPO radioimmunoassay in 1979,[34] followed by the cloning and expression of the *EPO* gene in 1985.[34,35] Clinical trials of recombinant human erythropoietin (rHuEPO), which showed improved Hb in ESRD patients, were conducted from 1986 to 1987, thereby ushering in the era of ESA therapy for the anemia of CKD.[36,37]

Normal Erythropoiesis

Tissue hypoxia, primarily in the kidney, provides the major physiologic stimulus for RBC production. Importantly, a fall in renal blood flow (RBF) is coupled with a decrease in GFR, which leads to reduced oxygen use by tubule transport proteins. Thus, tissue oxygenation is relatively independent of RBF across a wide range.[38,39]

Hypoxia-inducible factors (HIFs) are helix-loop-helix heterodimeric transcription factors that consist of O_2-regulated α subunits and constitutively expressed β subunits.[39] In normoxic cells, O_2, Fe^{2+}, and ascorbic acid activate prolyl-4-hydroxylase domain (PHD) proteins, which catalyze the hydroxylation of key proline residues in HIF-α subunits.[40,41] HIF-α then binds the von Hippel-Lindau protein, is polyubiquitinated by E3 ubiquitin ligase, and then is swiftly degraded by the proteasome.[20,42] Conversely, in hypoxic cells, low O_2 tension and high concentrations of tricarboxylic acid cycle intermediates inhibit PHD proteins, allowing HIF-α to translocate to the nucleus, heterodimerize, and activate hypoxia response elements (HREs) that regulate gene transcription for numerous cellular processes, including erythropoiesis, angiogenesis, and anaerobic metabolism (Fig. 76.1).

Of the three HIF proteins currently known, HIF-2 is the most strongly implicated in the hypoxic induction of EPO.[39,42] HIF-2α knockout mice are pancytopenic with bone marrow hypocellularity and attenuated EPO levels; RBC production normalizes with the addition of recombinant EPO.[43] In addition, the postnatal deletion of HIF-2 abolishes EPO production by the kidney and liver, and overexpression of HIF-2 causes erythrocytosis.[44] HIF-2–mediated *EPO* transcription may require the cooperative binding of other transcription factors, such as hepatocyte nuclear factor 4, to the HREs.[45] HIF-1, on the other hand, is more important in regulating glycolysis, whereas some HIF-3 splice

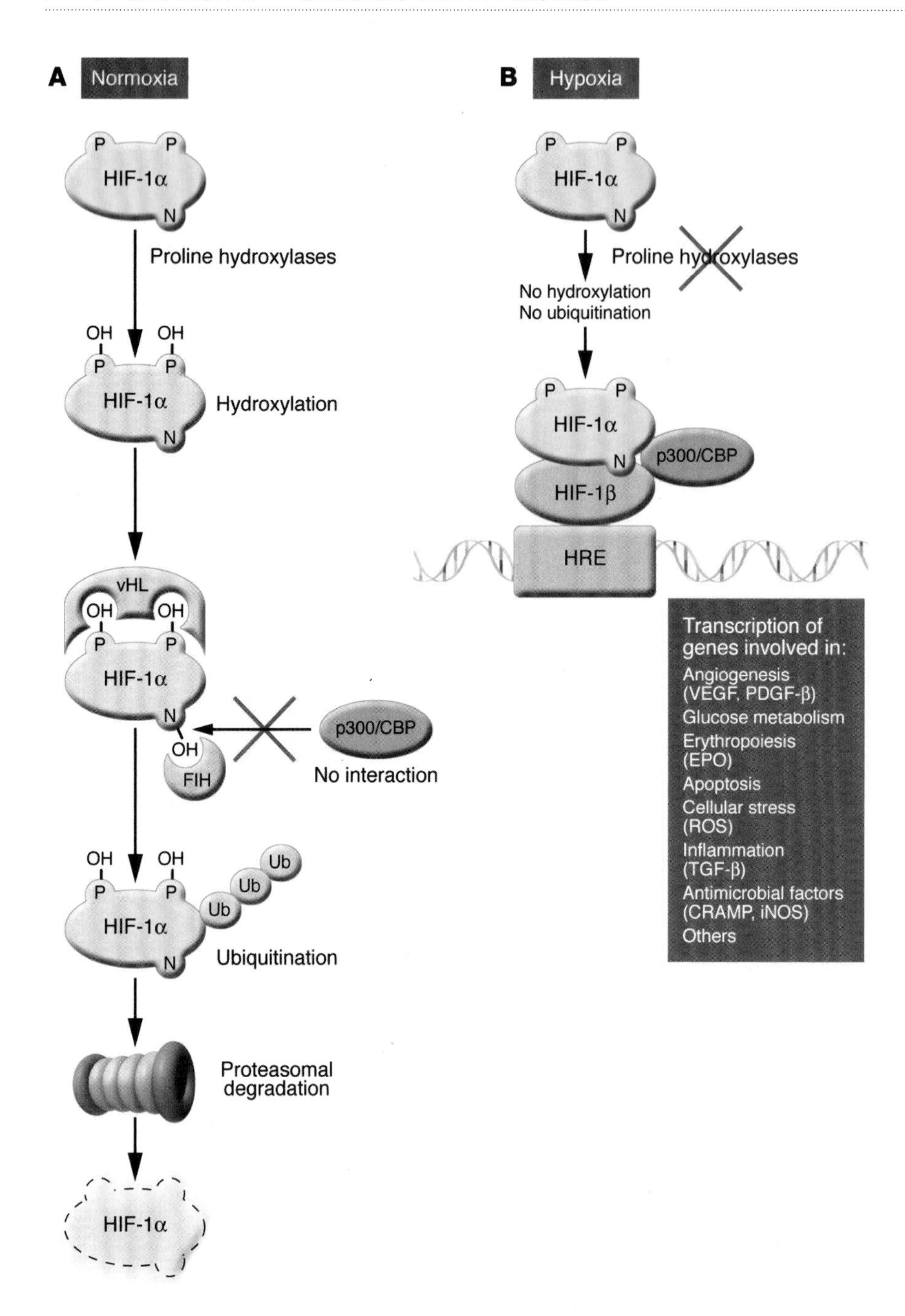

FIGURE 76.1 The regulation of hypoxia-inducible factor (HIF) expression. Under normoxic conditions **(A)**, proline hydroxylases (prolyl-4-hydroxylase domain proteins) target HIF for von Hippel-Lindau (vHL) protein binding, ubiquitination, and degradation. Under hypoxic conditions **(B)**, proline hydroxylases are inhibited, facilitating HIF-α heterodimerization and nuclear translocation, with consequent gene transcription. CBP, cAMP response element-binding protein; HRE, hypoxia response elements; VEGF, vascular endothelial growth factor; PDGF-β, platelet-derived growth factor-beta; ROS, reactive oxygen species; TGF-beta, transforming growth factor-beta; CRAMP, cathelin-related antimicrobial peptide; iNOS, inducible nitric oxide synthase. (Reproduced with permission from Zarember KA, Malech HL. HIF-1α: a master regulator of innate host defenses? *J Clin Invest.* 2005;115:1702.)

variants may actually inhibit transcription.[39] Interestingly, the HIF proteins activate the transcription of *PHD-2* and *PHD-3*, thereby creating a negative feedback loop resulting in their own degradation.

EPO is a 165-amino acid (AA) glycoprotein hormone with a molecular weight of 30 kDa.[39] In adults, 90% of the EPO produced in response to anemia originates from the kidney, specifically from a population of cortical peritubular fibroblasts with neuronlike morphology in the inner cortex and the outer medulla, regions that tend to be especially susceptible to hypoxia.[46] *EPO* expression in other cell types is normally suppressed by transcription factors that bind to the tetranucleotide sequence, G-A-T-A, in the core promoter region of the gene (GATA transcription factors). Mild hypoxia, rather than increasing the transcription of *EPO* messenger RNA (mRNA), actually stimulates the brisk recruitment of previously quiescent clusters of cells within the kidney, each of which then generates EPO at a fixed rate. Moderate hypoxia, however, fuels additional EPO production by the liver, mainly from hepatocytes near the central veins and, to a lesser extent, from stellate or Ito cells.[39,46] *EPO* transcripts have also been isolated from bone marrow, the spleen, the brain, the lungs, hair follicles, and the reproductive tract, but are unlikely to contribute significantly to plasma EPO levels, because protein expression by these tissues has not been demonstrated.[20]

The erythropoietin receptor (EPO-R) is a 484-AA glycoprotein with a single membrane-spanning domain that homodimerizes during synthesis in the endoplasmic reticulum.[20,47] Each EPO-R binds to the tyrosine kinase, Janus kinase-2 (JAK-2), and the entire complex associates with the type 2 transferrin receptor (TfR-2) for trafficking to the cell membrane. TfR-2, a disulfide-bonded homodimer, is required to optimize the sensitivity of the EPO-R complex to circulating EPO and to efficiently synthesize growth differentiation factor (GDF)-15 (see the following).[47] Parenthetically, the Friend spleen focus-forming virus glycoprotein (gp55), a very different disulfide-bonded homodimer, can substitute for TfR-2 in facilitating EPO-R homodimerization and trafficking from the endoplasmic reticulum, resulting in EPO-independent EPO-R activation, autonomous erythroid proliferation, and leukemia in mice. Under normal conditions, the EPO-R:TfR-2 complex, upon binding EPO, undergoes a conformational change that allows its cytoplasmic domains to be tyrosine phosphorylated by JAK-2, stimulating signal transduction and activator of transcription (STAT)-5, mitogen-activated protein kinase (MAPK), phosphatidylinositol-3-kinase (PI-3K), and protein kinase C (PKC).[39,48] The acute effects of EPO last only 30 to 60 minutes, after which JAK-2 and the EPO-R are dephosphorylated and the EPO:EPO-R complex may be internalized and degraded by the proteasome.[49] In addition, EPO also activates the phosphotyrosine phosphatase SHP-1, which binds to the EPO-R, dephosphorylates JAK-2, and terminates the propagation of the other intracellular signals. However, the primary signaling cascade set in motion by EPO-R activation is critical for the synthesis of erythrocytes.

Erythropoiesis takes place in the bone marrow, which is unquestionably the principal target of EPO activity. RBC production begins with the EPO-independent differentiation of the multipotent hematopoietic stem cell into the colony-forming unit granulocyte, erythrocyte, monocyte, megakaryocyte (CFU-GEMM), which in turn develops into the burst-forming unit erythroid (BFU-E).[50] The BFU-E is the first cell type in the erythroid lineage to express the EPO-R, and EPO is required for its survival and subsequent proliferation into several colony-forming units erythroid (CFU-E), a process that requires 10 to 13 days (Fig. 76.2). Of all the

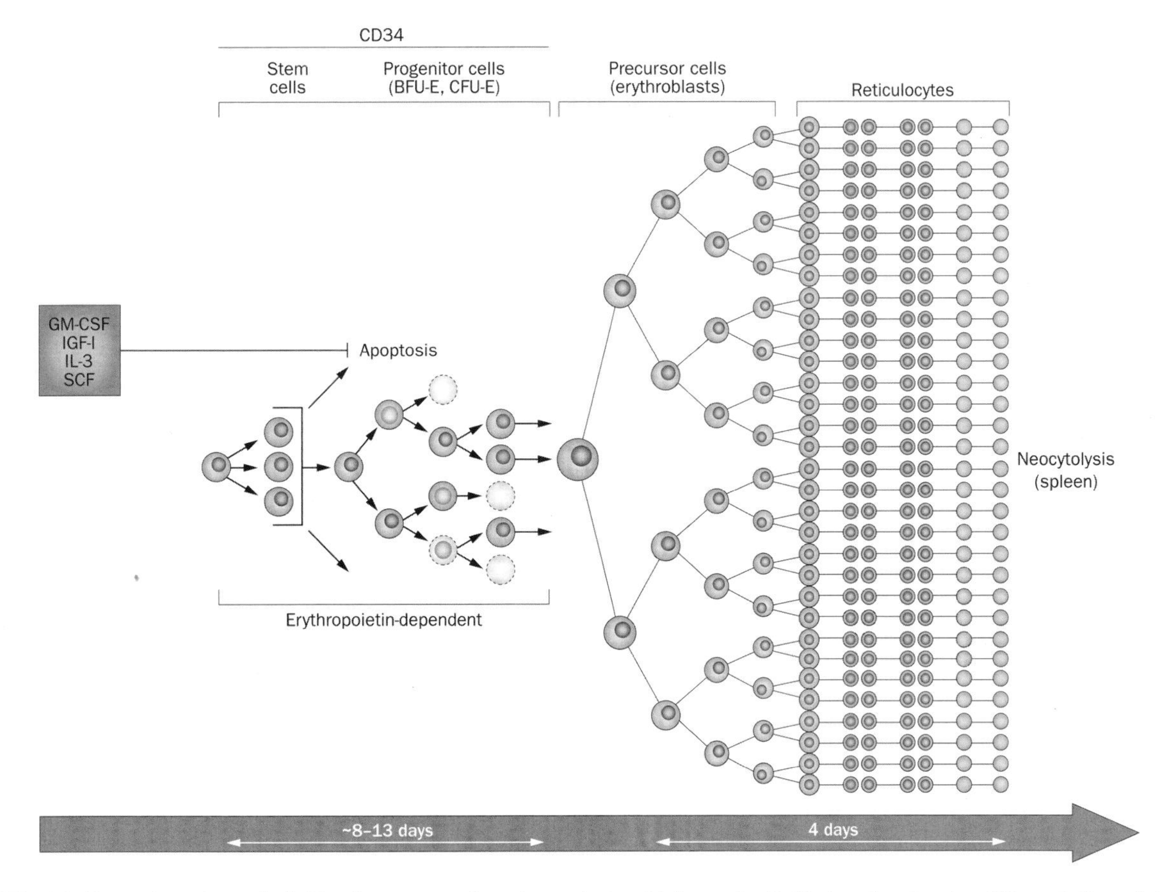

FIGURE 76.2 Normal erythropoiesis. The first stages of erythropoiesis, which require 8–13 days, involve the differentiation of the multipotent stem cell into the burst forming unit-erythroid (BFU-E) and colony forming unit-erythroid (CFU-E). These precursors require erythropoietin (EPO) and other growth factors to prevent apoptosis. The second stages of erythropoiesis, which require 4 days, involve the differentiation of erythroblasts to reticulocytes. Reticulocytes require EPO to avoid neocytolysis (premature destruction in the spleen). (Reproduced with permission from Besarab A, Coyne DW. Iron supplementation to treat anemia in patients with chronic kidney disease. *Nat Rev Nephrol.* 2010;6:699.)

erythroid precursors, the CFU-E has the highest membrane density of EPO-Rs, albeit < 1000 per cell, and additionally expresses TfR and GATA-1.[51] In the presence of EPO, GATA-1 promotes transcription of the antiapoptotic protein bcl-x_L, which allows the CFU-E to multiply. Conversely, in the absence of EPO, proapoptotic caspases are activated, and the CFU-E dies. A host of other growth factors, such as interleukin (IL)-3 and IL-9; granulocyte-colony stimulating factors and granulocyte, monocyte-colony stimulating factors (G-CSF and GM-CSF); and stem cell factors (SCFs) are also required for CFU-E proliferation.[50]

Subsequent phases of erythroid differentiation take place within erythroblastic islands.[51] Each erythroblastic island is a distinct, erythropoietic unit that consists of one central macrophage closely apposed to several maturing erythroblasts. Cell-specific molecular interactions, such as the binding between β1 integrins and vascular cell adhesion molecule (VCAM)-1, are critical to maintain the structure of these islands.[52] The CFU-E first differentiates into the proerythroblast, which again requires exposure to EPO to escape apoptosis. The proerythroblast has a large nucleus and expresses numerous membrane adhesion molecules such as CD44, intercellular adhesion molecule (ICAM)-1, and α4β1 and α5β1 integrins.[53] During maturation, the nucleus condenses and adhesion molecule expression is greatly diminished. Of note, CD44, the expression of which decreases by 30-fold during the progression from the proerythroblast to the orthochromatic normoblast, may be a more reliable marker of erythroid differentiation than the commonly used TfR, the expression of which remains relatively constant.

Terminal erythroid differentiation occurs as the erythroblast progresses through the basophilic, polychromatic, and orthochromatic normoblast stages. During this sequence, the cell acquires Hb, Rh factor, and the Duffy antigen, as well as skeletal proteins such as α- and β-spectrin, ankyrin, proteins 4.1R and 4.2, and the band 3 glycoprotein, which promotes membrane elasticity and stability.[53] The orthochromatic normoblast extrudes its pyknotic nucleus, which is ingested by the central macrophage and digested by deoxyribonuclease II, and becomes a reticulocyte.[51] This enucleated, multilobed reticulocyte is transformed into a biconcave erythrocyte during the next 2 to 3 days, initially in the bone marrow and then in the circulation, a process that involves membrane vesiculation, stabilization, and reorganization, as well as decreased cell volume. During erythrocyte maturation, cell membrane concentrations of aquaporin-1 (AQP-1), the glucose transporter (GLUT-4), the Na^+/H^+ exchanger (NHE-1), and the Na^+/K^+ pump are decreased, whereas the membrane skeletal proteins are retained.[54]

The Importance of Iron

Iron is essential for normal erythropoiesis. Total body iron is 50 mg per kilogram of body weight, or approximately 3500 mg for a 70-kg man.[55] This iron is distributed as about 65% in Hb; 10% in myoglobin (Mb), cytochromes, and enzymes; and the remainder in the reticuloendothelial system (RES), liver, and bone marrow. To meet the daily requirement of 300 billion fresh erythrocytes, differentiating erythroblasts need approximately 20 to 30 mg per day of iron, most of which is obtained from the recycling of senescent RBCs by phagocytic macrophages of the RES.[56] Heme from these cells is metabolized by heme oxygenase, and the Fe^{2+} released is sequestered by ferritin, which itself may undergo lysosomal degradation to hemosiderin.[55] The central macrophage of the erythroblastic island, acting as a "nurse cell," releases ferritin to its satellite erythroblasts, thus facilitating Hb synthesis and uninterrupted differentiation.[54]

Ferritin is indispensable for concentrating iron to the levels required for iron/oxygen chemistry, including aerobic metabolism, while avoiding the generation of insoluble ferric oxide and toxic oxygen radicals.[57] Ferritin is a hollow sphere with an external diameter of 12 nm and molecular weight of 480 kDa, consisting of 24 heavy and light polypeptide chains folded into four-helix bundles.[58] The center of the molecule's cavity has an internal diameter of ~7 to 8 nm, accessible via eight protein pores, which can accumulate up to 4000 atoms of iron. Iron must be reduced to Fe^{2+} to travel through the pores to the interior of the ferritin molecule, where it undergoes ferroxidase-catalyzed conversion to Fe^{3+} for storage.[57] Sequestration by ferritin increases the effective solubility of iron by 15 orders of magnitude.

Although only 1 to 2 mg per day of iron is obtained from the diet, gastrointestinal (GI) absorption of iron is required to offset minor losses from epithelial desquamation and microscopic bleeding.[56] The typical dietary intake of iron is 15 to 20 mg per day. Only 10% of dietary iron is present as relatively bioavailable heme compounds, which are readily absorbed into enterocytes and degraded by heme oxygenase to release Fe^{2+}. The remaining nonheme iron exists in the relatively unavailable Fe^{3+} state and must be reduced to Fe^{2+} by ferrireductase in conjunction with ascorbic acid; iron is then transported into the enterocyte by divalent metal transporter (DMT)-1.[55,59]

Cytosolic iron, whether present in duodenal enterocytes, macrophages, or hepatocytes, is delivered to the circulation via ferroportin (FP)-1, oxidized to Fe^{3+}, and bound to plasma transferrin.[60] In order to provide sufficient iron for reticulocyte production, transferrin-bound iron must be recycled 6 to 7 times daily.[7] Iron enters the erythroblast when two transferrin molecules bind TfR-1, which then undergoes endocytosis into a clathrin-coated siderosome.[55] The siderosome is acidified, releasing Fe^{3+} that is again reduced to Fe^{2+} by ferrireductase and exported to the cytoplasm via DMT-1. The apotransferrin:TfR-1 complex is recycled to the cell membrane and released into the circulation.[60] Meanwhile, cytosolic iron enters the mitochondrion, where ferrochelatase catalyzes its insertion into protoporphyrin IX to form heme, the critical component of Hb.[55,61]

Iron homeostasis is largely regulated at the level of GI absorption. One regulatory model postulates that plasma iron is sensed by duodenal crypt enterocytes via the TfR.[55] When iron is scarce, low cytosolic iron induces the transcription of

TfR-1, DMT-1, and FP-1 mRNA, all of which stimulate iron absorption. A second, compatible model proposes that iron absorption is downregulated by hepcidin, a 25-AA polypeptide produced by hepatocytes when iron is abundant. Hepcidin binds to FP-1 in enterocytes, macrophages, and hepatocytes themselves, promoting the JAK-2–mediated tyrosine phosphorylation, internalization, and degradation of FP-1; thus, hepcidin inhibits both the efflux of iron from the duodenum into the plasma as well as the mobilization of iron from the RES.[62] Hepcidin expression is itself regulated at critical points in the homeostatic loop. Specifically, hepcidin transcription is inhibited by HIF during tissue hypoxia, by soluble hemojuvelin during iron deficiency, and by EPO, GDF-15, and twisted gastrulation (TWSG-1) during erythroblast maturation. Conversely, hepcidin transcription is stimulated by iron-mediated production of bone morphogenetic proteins (BMPs), lipopolysaccharide, and IL-6 in states of systemic inflammation.[55,56,63,64] The biology of hepcidin is summarized in Figure 76.3.

A third model of iron regulation involves host defense pathways. Under conditions of infection or inflammation, macrophages generate DMT-1 and neutrophils release apolactoferrin and neutrophil gelatinase–associated lipocalin (NGAL), all of which remove iron from the circulation and decrease its availability to iron-dependent microorganisms.[60] NGAL is a 25-kDa protein, which similarly to hepcidin, sequesters iron during the acute phase response.[65] NGAL binds siderophores, high-affinity iron chelators produced by bacteria, and also functions as a nontransferrin pool of circulating iron.[66] During the acute phase response, cytokines such as IL-1β and tumor necrosis factor (TNF)-α also stimulate the translation of presynthesized ferritin subunit transcripts.[58] Presumably, this ferritin-mediated iron trapping is protective in states of acute inflammation, such as bacterial infection, but maladaptive in states of chronic inflammation, such as CKD.

Lastly, iron availability may regulate its own use via iron-regulatory elements (IREs). When cytosolic iron is abundant, transcription factors known as iron-regulatory proteins (IRPs) are rendered unable to bind their IRE; specifically, IRP-1 is converted into an aconitase and IRP-2 is degraded by the proteasome.[39,67] On the other hand, when iron is absent, IRPs bind to 3′- or 5′-regions of specific coding sequences, stimulating or inhibiting transcription, respectively. The IRP/IRE complex increases the transcription and translation of TfR-1 and DMT-1, promoting iron uptake into cells. Conversely, IRP/IRE decreases the expression of ferritin, which prevents iron sequestration; HIF-2α, which prevents EPO synthesis; and δ-aminolevulinic acid synthase 2, which prevents heme synthesis. Thus, scarcity of cytosolic iron blocks erythropoiesis and further iron consumption.[68]

Mechanisms of Anemia in Kidney Disease

The anemia of CKD and ESRD is the result of a confluence of many pathophysiologic processes. The most well-known of these is a deficiency of EPO relative to the degree of anemia. In subjects with normal Hb and kidney function, the EPO concentration is roughly 3 to 30 mU per milliliter,

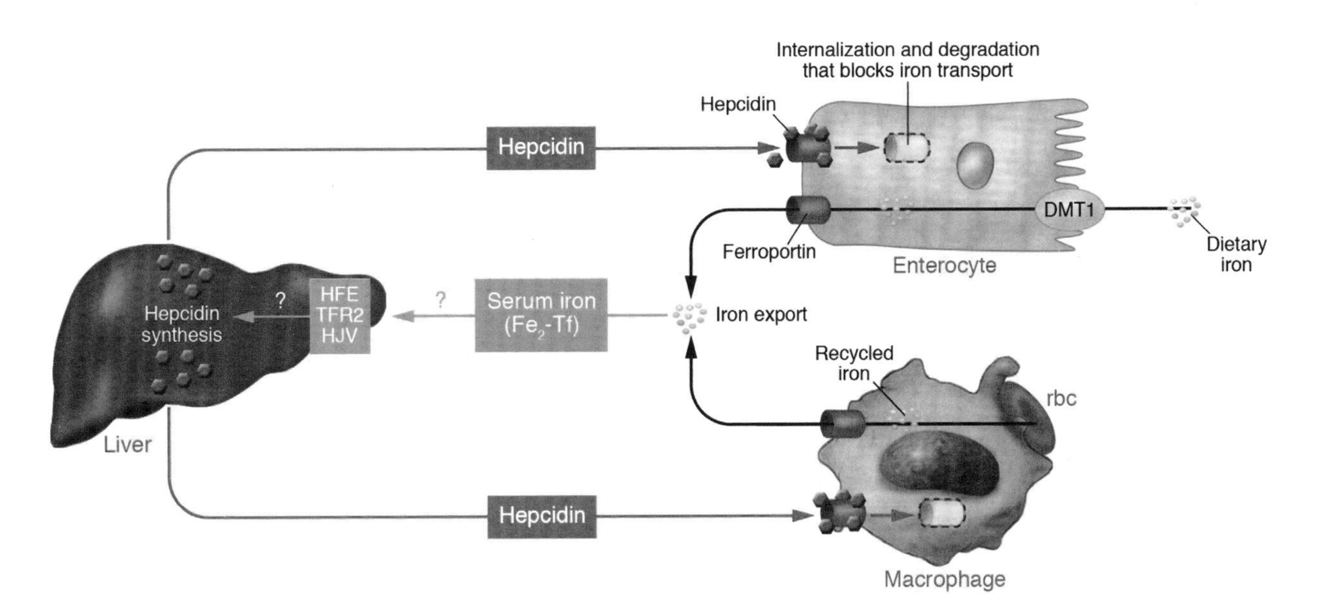

FIGURE 76.3 Hepcidin and iron homeostasis. Dietary iron uptake into the enterocyte involves transit via the divalent metal transporter 1 (DMT1). Iron recycled from senescent red blood cells (rbc) is stored in macrophages. Under conditions of iron sufficiency, increased diferric transferrin (Fe_2-Tf) is sensed by the human hemochromatosis (HFE) protein, type 2 transferrin receptor (TFR2), and the hemojuvelin (HJV) protein, and stimulates hepcidin production. Hepcidin binds to its ligand, ferroportin, and internalizes it back into the cytoplasm of enterocytes and macrophages, thereby sequestering iron and inhibiting its export from these cells. (Reproduced with permission from Vaulont S, Lou D-Q, Viatte L, et al. Of mice and men: the iron age. *J Clin Invest.* 2005;115:2079.) (See Color Plate.)

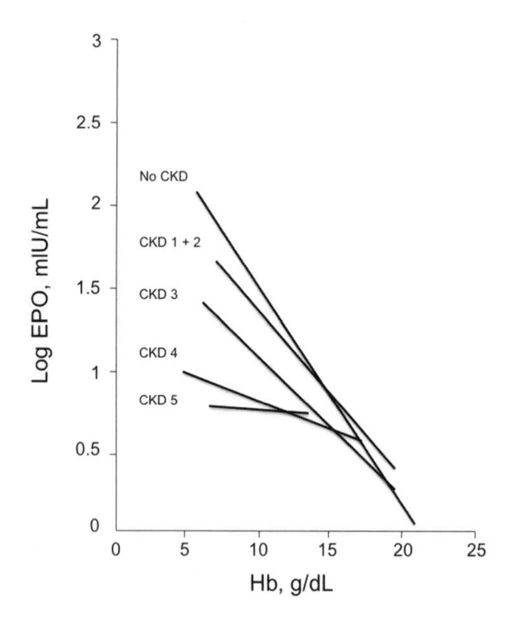

FIGURE 76.4 The relationship between hemoglobin (Hb) and log erythropoietin (EPO) concentrations. Each line represents the relationship for a specific stage of chronic kidney disease (CKD). (Reproduced with permission from Artunc F, Risler T. Serum erythropoietin concentrations and responses to anaemia in patients with or without chronic kidney disease. *Nephrol Dial Transplant.* 2007;22:2900.)

which increases by 100-fold as Hb falls.[69] In patients with kidney disease, the inverse relationship between EPO and Hb evaporates as kidney function declines, with little correlation at GFR or creatinine clearance (CrCl) $<$ 30 to 40 mL per minute (Fig. 76.4).[69,70] In stages 4 through 5 CKD, this sluggish EPO response produces a normochromic, normocytic anemia.

Several mechanisms have been proposed to account for relative EPO deficiency in advanced CKD. (1) The diseased kidney adapts to an increased single-nephron sodium load by attenuating tubular sodium absorption. This change decreases O_2 consumption, improves oxygenation in the outer medulla, and reduces the stimulus for EPO production.[69] (2) EPO secreted into the circulation may be neutralized by soluble EPO-R, a 27-kDa splice variant identified in dialysis patients, the transcription of which is induced by inflammatory mediators, such as IL-6 and TNF-α.[71] (3) EPO may be inactivated by desialylation, a process mediated by proteases, the activity of which is increased in uremic patients.[72] (4) Even if EPO does reach the bone marrow intact and in sufficient quantity to stimulate erythropoiesis, its action may be blunted by the absence of permissive factors, such as IL-3, calcitriol, and CD4 cells, as well as by the presence of inhibitory factors, such as polyamines, ribonuclease, and parathyroid hormone (PTH).[72,73]

Iron deficiency, both absolute and relative, contributes significantly to anemia in kidney disease. Absolute iron deficiency is caused by blood loss, such as from repeated phlebotomy, colonic angiodysplasias, and occasionally, uremic bleeding. HD patients can also lose blood in the dialysis circuit, with cumulative iron losses averaging 1 to 3 g per year.[64] In addition, oral (PO) iron is poorly absorbed in advanced CKD, both because of hepcidin (see the following) as well as because of concomitantly prescribed medications such as proton pump inhibitors and calcium-, aluminum-, and lanthanum-containing compounds.[74]

Relative, or functional, iron deficiency occurs when the body is unable to mobilize otherwise adequate iron stores for erythropoiesis, a condition chiefly attributed to hepcidin. Hepcidin accumulates with progressive CKD; from 73 ng per milliliter in controls to 270 ng per milliliter in stages 2 through 4 CKD to 652 ng per mL in stage 5 CKD.[75] This increase probably results from a combination of persistent inflammation, frequent iron administration, and decreased renal clearance of hepcidin.[61,64] Interestingly, although anemia, hypoxia, the use of ESAs, and clearance by HD would be expected to decrease hepcidin levels, factors that induce hepcidin transcription clearly predominate. As previously mentioned, hepcidin binds to FP-1 and inhibits both the absorption of iron from the duodenum as well as the mobilization of iron from ferritin in the RES. NGAL, as well as hepcidin, is increased in HD patients and may contribute to functional iron deficiency.[76]

Iron deficiency is associated with reactive thrombocytosis in CKD and ESRD.[7] One mechanism to explain this effect involves the sequence homology between thrombopoietin and EPO.[77] As iron becomes scarce, EPO levels rise to compensate; in addition, patients may be given ESAs therapeutically. These high concentrations of either endogenous or exogenous hormone may accordingly stimulate platelet production. Thrombocytosis in response to iron deficiency, occasionally $>$ 1,000,000 platelets per microliter, can be complicated by thromboembolic events, such as ischemic stroke, venous thromboembolism, central retinal vein occlusion, and cerebral venous sinus thrombosis.[78,79]

In patients with advanced CKD and ESRD, erythrocytes undergo accelerated destruction, a process that involves both young (neocytolysis) and old (senescence) RBC. Iron-poor, hypochromic cells are broken down during nadirs in EPO levels and undergo early phagocytosis because of abnormally high expression of phosphatidylserine.[80] The RBC cell membrane in HD patients is poorly deformable and lipid peroxidated, with unusual proportions of spectrin, ankyrin, protein 4.1, and band 3.[80,81] Many other changes in the composition of RBC membranes and intracellular machinery have been described in ESRD patients, involving AQP-1, the Na^+-K^+ pump, hexokinase, lactate dehydrogenase, and adenosine triphosphate (ATP), but the clinical significance of these abnormalities or their correction during dialysis is unknown.[82–84] Intravascular hemolysis can occur as a side effect of oxidizing medications, such as dapsone, primaquine, and nitrofurantoin. Hemolysis can also occur during HD because of mechanical lysis and exposure to water contaminants such as chloramines, nitrates, fluorine, arsenic, copper, and zinc.[85]

Nutritional deficiencies are easily overlooked causes of anemia in kidney disease. B-complex vitamins, specifically B_6 (pyridoxine), B_9 (folic acid), and B_{12} (cobalamin), are all essential cofactors in erythropoiesis. Deficiency of L-carnitine, a constituent of mitochondrial shuttle proteins involved in β-oxidation of fatty acids, occurs with the loss of kidney mass and via hemodialytic clearance. L-Carnitine supplementation induces heme oxygenase-1, activates the antiapoptotic protein Bcl-2, and increases CFU-E in animal cell cultures.[86,87] Hypophosphatemia, presumably via ATP depletion, impairs erythrocyte membrane deformability, leading to early senescence or even acute hemolytic anemia.[88] Moreover, scarcity of phosphorus decreases the availability of 2,3-bisphosphoglycerate for unloading O_2 from Hb, leading to tissue hypoxia.

DIAGNOSIS

As previously mentioned, the 2006 KDOQI guidelines advise an evaluation when Hb is < 13.5 g per deciliter in men and is < 12 g per deciliter in women, which are the mean Hb levels of the lowest 5th percentiles of the sex-specific adult population.[1] Hb is preferred over hematocrit (Hct) measurement, because the latter varies with glucose concentration, storage conditions, and analysis technique. Nonetheless, Hb measurements may vary by up to 0.5 g per deciliter within the same blood sample.[6] In CKD and PD patients, the timing of the Hb assessment is flexible. Conversely, in HD patients, Hb levels vary substantially during both the interdialytic and intradialytic periods, such that each 1 L of ultrafiltration increases Hb by 0.4 g per deciliter. Hb in these patients should be measured at the start of dialysis following a short (2-day) interdialytic interval (i.e., the midweek dialysis session). Hb measured at this time most closely approximates the mean weekly time-averaged Hb.[89]

The preliminary evaluation of anemia consists of a complete blood count (CBC), absolute reticulocyte count, ferritin, and either transferrin saturation (TSAT) or reticulocyte Hb content (CHr).[1] The CBC is useful for excluding aplastic anemia, myelodysplasia, or other bone marrow disorders (leukopenia, thrombocytopenia), folate or vitamin B_{12} deficiency (macrocytosis), and iron deficiency (microcytosis, hypochromia). The reticulocyte count, reticulocyte index, and reticulocyte production index estimate the erythropoietic response to anemia. The anemia of CKD and ESRD is nearly always hypoproliferative, especially at CrCl < 40 mL per minute. Even in this setting, EPO levels in most patients are within the normal range. For these reasons, the determination of EPO concentration in CKD and ESRD is of limited value.[69]

Iron status is a fundamental determinant of anemia, and iron deficiency can actually exist in the absence of anemia.[90] Fatigue, regardless of the Hb concentration, may be a prominent presenting symptom of iron deficiency because of the involvement of iron in enzymatic oxidative metabolism. The best parameter for assessing iron status remains elusive. RBC indices, such as low mean corpuscular Hb (MCH) or mean corpuscular volume (MCV) and a high red cell distribution width (RDW) often suggest iron deficiency but are nonspecific. A low RDW may be the earliest index of iron deficiency, but a low MCH may be more reliable.[90]

One commonly used test for iron deficiency is serum ferritin. Under normal conditions, 1 ng per milliliter of ferritin corresponds to approximately 8 mg of stored iron, but in states of chronic inflammation, serum ferritin is a poor marker of tissue ferritin, which is physiologically more significant but less easily measurable.[90] Serum ferritin can often reflect a leakage from tissue sources, is more highly glycosylated than the tissue form, and because it corresponds to molecular apoferritin, may contain little to no actual iron.[58,91] In CKD patients, a serum ferritin level < 10 to 30 ng per milliliter is associated with a fall in Hb, but levels of ferritin also correlate poorly with bone marrow iron (ferritin < 175 ng per milliliter, sensitivity and specificity to diagnose iron deficiency both 71%).[92,93] In HD patients, the relationship between ferritin and Hb is unclear, although ferritin levels < 500 ng per milliliter may more accurately reflect marrow iron scarcity.[94] Conversely, iron overload syndromes such as hemosiderosis are uncommon unless ferritin levels are > 2000 ng per milliliter.[58]

TSAT is calculated as serum iron divided by total iron binding capacity (TIBC) and represents the circulating iron available for erythropoiesis, specifically, iron-bound transferrin. Transferrin is a negative acute phase reactant, and in chronically inflamed CKD patients, TIBC is decreased from the normal mean of 330 to about 220 μg per deciliter.[7] TSAT varies diurnally, with maximal values occurring between 12:00 A.M. and 8:00 A.M. and minimal values (up to 58% less) occurring in the late afternoon and early evening.[95] This variability may confound an interpretation of TSAT unless the time of collection is standardized.[96] In the CKD population, Hb declines linearly with TSAT without a specific threshold, although action levels of 16% to 20% have been proposed.[1,92]

Because of these limitations, other assays have been advocated for the determination of iron status in patients with kidney disease. CHr measures the amount of Hb in reticulocytes, and provides a "snapshot" of iron available for erythropoiesis within the preceding 1 to 2 days.[96] CHr correlates reasonably well with TSAT, and threshold values of 29 to 32 pg per cell have been proposed to diagnose iron deficiency in HD patients. The reticulocyte Hb equivalent (RET-Hb), a related assay, facilitates the determination of CHr using commonly available blood analyzers.[97] In contrast, the percentage of hypochromic red blood cells (PHRC) measures the amount of Hb in the entire population of RBC, but suffers from inconsistency because RBC may sometimes expand during specimen storage.[96] Another test includes the measurement of soluble TfR, which is secreted by iron-hungry erythroblasts in states of iron deficiency in the presence of sufficient EPO or ESA. Increased TfR may be one of the first

TABLE 76.1 A Comparison of Markers to Diagnose Iron Deficiency in Chronic Kidney Disease and End-Stage Renal Disease[7,58]

Marker	Diagnostic Threshold	Advantages	Disadvantages
Ferritin	< 100–200 ng/mL	Widely available	High variability, nonspecific if ↑
TSAT	< 20–25%	Widely available, ↑ sensitivity vs. ferritin	High variability
CHr	< 29–32 pg/cell	Accurate, inexpensive	Limited availability, ? diagnostic threshold
PHRC	< 6–10%	Accurate, inexpensive	Impractical with sample storage
sTfR	> 2.4 μg/mL	Accurate	Limited availability, ? diagnostic threshold
ZnPP	> 40–80 μmol/mol	Limited confounding by inflammation	Affected by lead concentration
Hepcidin	Unknown	Reflects functional iron deficiency	No reliable assay available
Bone marrow/ liver Bx	Unknown	Gold standard	Invasive, semiquantitative

TSAT, transferrin saturation; CHr, reticulocyte hemoglobin content; PHRC, percentage of hypochromic red blood cells; sTfR, soluble transferrin receptor; ZnPP, erythrocyte zinc protoporphyrin; Bx, biopsy.

signals of iron deficiency and is unaffected by inflammation.[98] In a recent study of HD patients, the soluble TfR-ferritin index had a higher predictive value for iron deficiency than either ferritin or TSAT alone.[99] Nonetheless, the diagnostic cut-off values of ferritin < 100 ng per milliliter, TSAT < 20%, and soluble TfR > 2.4 μg per milliliter appear to be poorly correlated.[98] High erythrocyte protoporphyrin and serum hepcidin concentrations have also been investigated as markers of iron deficiency, although an accurate measurement of the latter currently requires mass spectrometry and is thus impractical.[75,100] Table 76.1 lists some of the parameters that have been proposed to diagnose iron deficiency in CKD and ESRD.

TREATMENT

Therapy for the anemia of kidney disease has undergone a transformation during the past 5 to 10 years. ESAs remain a cornerstone of treatment, but successive randomized, controlled trials (RCTs) have demonstrated evidence of harm from using these agents to target higher Hb levels, leaving the nephrology community scrambling for alternate therapeutic agents. One such alternative is intravenous (IV) iron, various formulations of which improve Hb while concomitantly reducing doses of ESA. Moreover, there are several novel agents in active development that hold great promise for the treatment of anemia.

Erythropoiesis-Stimulating Agents

The U.S. Food and Drug Administration (FDA) first approved rHuEPO in 1989.[101,102] The first-generation ESAs include epoetin alfa (Epogen, Procrit, Eprex, Erypo, Espo) and beta (Neo-Recormon, Epogen), which are produced in Chinese hamster ovary cells, and epoetin omega (Epomax, Repotin), which is produced in baby hamster kidney cells. These compounds have the identical amino acid sequence as human EPO but differ in the degree of *N*- and *O*-linked glycosylation (Fig. 76.5). Conversely, epoetin delta derives from a human fibrosarcoma cell line, lacks the foreign *N*-glycolylneuraminic acid residues found in other rHuEPO congeners, and therefore more closely approximates the structure of endogenous EPO.[103] The second-generation ESAs, darbepoetin alfa (DPO, Aranesp) and methoxy polyethylene glycol-epoetin beta or continuous erythropoietin receptor activator (CERA, Mircera), are glycosylated in order to increase biologic half-life ($t_{1/2}$) and to decrease frequency of administration (see the following).[101,104] Although neither epoetin delta nor CERA are currently available because of financial and legal considerations, respectively, the development of newer, biosimilar ESAs continues in many countries worldwide.

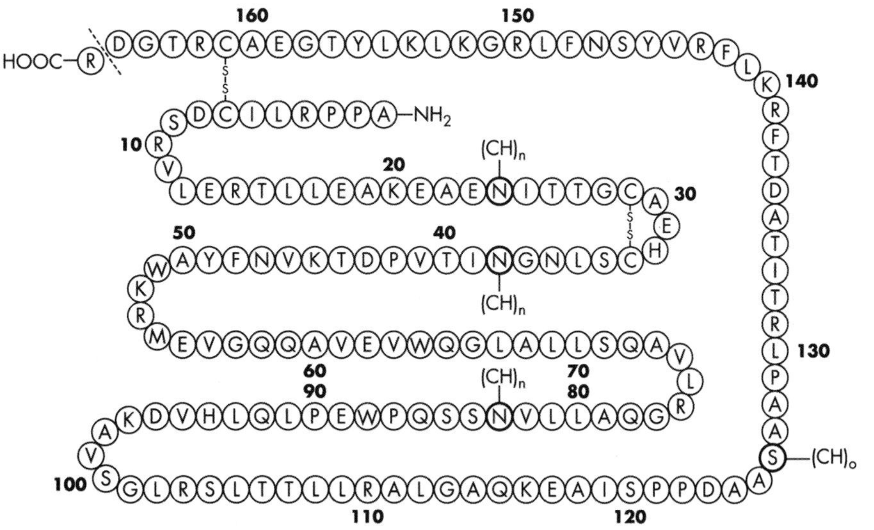

FIGURE 76.5 The amino acid sequence and structure of erythropoietin. $(CH)_n$ indicates *N*-linked glycosylation at asparagine residues 24, 38, and 83; $(CH)_o$ indicates *O*-linked glycosylation at serine residue 126. The C-terminal arginine at position 166 is cleaved prior to erythropoietin secretion. (Reproduced with permission from Ng T, Marx G, Littlewood T, et al. Recombinant erythropoietin in clinical practice. *Postgrad Med J.* 2003;79:367.)

The ESAs were approved on the basis of improved Hb and the avoidance of transfusions in small clinical trials, and observational studies suggested that ESA use was beneficial. In an adjusted analysis of nearly 90,000 Medicare ESRD patients, those who received ESAs most consistently 2 years before dialysis, as compared to those who received ESAs least consistently, had a 68% RR of 1-year mortality.[105,106] Furthermore, in a retrospective review of > 3000 patients undergoing maintenance dialysis, those who received epoetin beta had a 20% RR of 1-year mortality.[107] Recent systematic reviews and meta-analyses of studies in CKD and ESRD populations, prospective but of variable quality, have concluded that correcting anemia with ESAs is associated with improvements in left ventricular mass index (LVMI), a frequently cited surrogate for mortality, as well as both subjective and objective assessments of physical functioning and exercise tolerance.[18,108,109] A small trial, again in CKD and ESRD patients, has also demonstrated that the treatment of anemia with ESAs improves electrophysiologic markers of cognitive function.[110]

Notwithstanding the apparent benefits of ESA suggested by such studies, numerous large-scale RCTs have now compelled a belated reassessment of the hazards of aggressive ESA titration. Two landmark RCTs, the Correction of Hemoglobin and Outcomes in Renal Insufficiency (CHOIR) and the Cardiovascular Risk Reduction by Early Anemia Treatment with Epoetin Beta (CREATE), were published in late 2006.[111–113] In CHOIR, 1432 patients with CKD stages 3 through 4 were treated with epoetin alfa to achieve Hb 11.3 or 13.5 g per deciliter. The trial was discontinued early because of a higher rate of a composite of death, stroke, myocardial infarction (MI), and hospitalization for CHF in the arm randomized to the higher Hb target. In CREATE, 603 patients with CKD stages 3 through 4 were treated with epoetin beta to achieve Hb 10.5 to 11.5 or 13 to 15 g per deciliter. This trial was completed and demonstrated a higher rate of dialysis initiation and hypertension (HTN) in the arm randomized to the higher Hb target. Most importantly, the Trial to Reduce Cardiovascular Events with Aranesp Therapy (TREAT), which gained notoriety as the first placebo-controlled RCT of ESAs, was reported in 2009.[114] In TREAT, 4038 patients with type 2 diabetes and CKD stages 3 through 4 were treated either with DPO titrated to target Hb 13 g per deciliter, or with placebo, with rescue DPO given if Hb fell to < 9 g per deciliter. This study showed a higher rate of stroke, arterial and venous thromboembolic events, and cancer deaths in those with preexisting malignancy in the arm randomized to DPO. However, there were also improved measures of QOL and fewer transfusions in those assigned to active treatment.[114] The Normal Hematocrit trial, originally published in 1998 but recently updated with the release of supplemental data, previously reported comparable outcomes in HD patients. In the final analysis, 1265 patients on maintenance HD with CHF or ischemic heart disease were treated with epoetin alfa to achieve Hct 30% or 42%.[115] Again, the study was discontinued because of a trend toward a higher rate of death and nonfatal MI in the arm randomized to the higher Hct target.

Meta-analyses and systematic reviews of clinical trials involving ESA therapy in CKD and ESRD patients have yielded the same conclusions. One meta-analysis of nine RCTs, which included > 5000 patients with CKD, showed a higher risk of all-cause mortality with rHuEPO-targeted Hb of 12 to 16 g per deciliter (Fig. 76.6; RR 1.17, 95% confidence interval 1.01 to 1.35).[116] Also reported in this analysis and the accompanying editorial were a higher risk of HD access thrombosis, uncontrolled HTN, and MACE with more aggressive anemia correction.[117] A recent meta-analysis and a systematic review analyzed health-related QOL outcomes in 11 RCTs and showed no clinically meaningful differences in Short Form (SF)-36 scores, regardless of Hb levels achieved by ESA treatment.[118]

The route of administration of ESA has several important implications. Subcutaneous (SC) dosing of rHuEPO, compared to IV dosing, yields lower bioavailability (48.8%

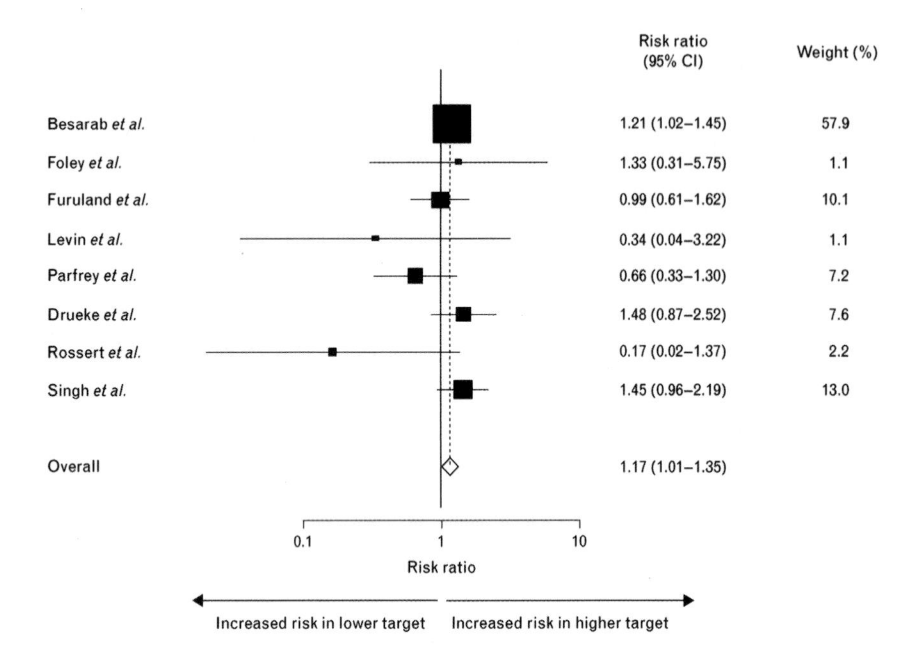

FIGURE 76.6 The risk of all-cause mortality in higher versus lower hemoglobin target groups in recent clinical trials (fixed effects analysis). (Reproduced with permission from Phrommintikul A, Haas SJ, Elsik M, et al. Mortality and target haemoglobin concentrations in anaemic patients with chronic kidney disease treated with erythropoietin: a meta-analysis. *Lancet.* 2007;369:381.)

and 100%, respectively) but higher and more sustained concentrations of the drug ($t_{1/2}$ = 19 to 25 hours and 5 to 11 hours, respectively).[119] Sustained levels of rHuEPO, within a critical range of 40 to 200 IU per kilogram, are required to trigger erythroid differentiation and to avoid neocytolysis, the process by which nascent RBCs undergo premature phagocytosis in the absence of circulating EPO. The SC administration of ESA, compared to the IV administration, thus may be more physiologic, and indeed causes less frequent dose-associated HTN. Because of the aforementioned pharmacokinetic differences, SC treatment, compared to IV treatment, also translates into a 14% to 32% decrease in dose and therefore cost. Hb levels may[120,121] or may not[122] be as stable with rHuEPO given SC dosing versus IV dosing. Because of logistical and patient compliance considerations, CKD and PD patients are often given DPO SC during clinic visits, whereas HD patients are currently given rHuEPO IV during dialysis.

Erythropoiesis-Stimulating Agent Hyporesponsiveness

Some patients with CKD and ESRD are unable to reach or maintain Hb levels of 11 to 12 g per deciliter, the range currently recommended by KDOQI, irrespective of ESA dose titration. This phenomenon is termed hyporesponsiveness, and has been defined as a continued need for rHuEPO at doses of > 300 IU/kg/week SC or > 400 to 450 IU/kg/week IV, or DPO at a dose of > 1.5 μg/kg/week SC (Table 76.2).[1,123] Inflammation, which is associated with a variety of clinical circumstances, is one of the main causes of ESA hyporesponsiveness.[124] The most familiar example of inflammation is the malnutrition, inflammation, atherosclerosis (MIA) or malnutrition-inflammation complex syndrome (MICS), which is found in 35% to 65% of HD patients. This syndrome is characterized by the presence of decreased Hb, transferrin, cholesterol, homocysteine, creatinine, and albumin and increased ferritin, IL-6, TNF-α, C-reactive protein (CRP), serum amyloid A, haptoglobin, and fibrinogen.[125] MICS is associated with lower QOL and higher rates of hospitalization and death, but its causes remain ambiguous. Potential etiologies include oxidative and carbonyl stress, loss of nutrients and antioxidants during dialysis, the accumulation of uremic toxins and inflammatory cytokines, and volume overload. In patients with MICS, the profusion of cytokines, particularly IL-1, IL-6, and TNF-α, inhibits endogenous EPO production and blocks the effect of rHuEPO on erythroid differentiation.[124]

Many clinical scenarios are associated with inflammatory ESA hyporesponsiveness. CKD patients with active malignancy, systemic lupus erythematosus (SLE), human immunodeficiency virus (HIV), or diabetic foot infections may have anemia that responds poorly to ESAs. CKD patients with chronic or acute decompensated CHF have increased levels of IL-1, IL-6, IL-18, TNF-α, endotoxins, aldosterone, angiotensin II, soluble adhesion molecules, and the soluble receptors TNFR-1, TNFR-2, IL-6R, and gp130, as well as volume overload, all of which may contribute to inflammation and anemia.[124,126] HD patients with periodontal disease often have an abnormal Hb, CRP, and erythrocyte sedimentation rate (ESR), the parameters of which improve with the treatment of disease.[127] HD patients who are underdialyzed (Kt/V < 1.33) show an association between dialysis adequacy and Hb, a finding that suggests that the elimination of uremic toxins is required to sustain adequate erythropoiesis.[128] Furthermore, HD patients who are exposed to endotoxin, impure dialysate, and bioincompatible membranes may have refractory anemia.[129] Patients who undergo HD via a tunneled, cuffed catheter (TCC) or an arteriovenous graft (AVG), compared to those who use an arteriovenous fistula

TABLE 76.2 **Causes of Erythropoiesis-Stimulating Agent Hyporesponsiveness**

Causes	Examples
Inflammation	MICS, SLE, CHF, malignancy, failed kidney allograft Chronic infection: HIV, osteomyelitis, periodontal disease Hemodialysis-associated: impure dialysate, bioincompatible membranes, TCC/AVG use, inadequate dialysis
Iron restriction	Relative iron deficiency: inflammation Absolute iron deficiency: bleeding
Bone marrow disorders	Myelofibrosis, myelodysplastic syndrome Hemoglobinopathies: sickle cell anemia, thalassemia
Hemolysis	Oxidizing medications: dapsone, primaquine, nitrofurantoin Hemodialysis-associated: impure dialysate (e.g., chloramines, copper), mechanical destruction
Nutritional deficiencies	Pyridoxine, folic acid, cobalamin, L-carnitine, phosphorus
Miscellaneous	Pure red cell aplasia, severe SHPT, aluminum, ACEI/ARB

MICS, malnutrition-inflammation complex syndrome; SLE, systemic lupus erythematosus; CHF, congestive heart failure; HIV, human immunodeficiency virus; TCC, tunneled, cuffed catheter; AVG, arteriovenous graft; SHPT, secondary hyperparathyroidism; ACEI, angiotensin-converting enzyme inhibitor; ARB, angiotensin receptor blocker.

(AVF), are also more likely to show ESA hyporesponsiveness, presumably because of inflammation associated with a subclinical infection or the presence of foreign material in the vasculature.[130,131] Inflammatory ESA hyporesponsiveness has been treated with statins, vitamins C and E, oxpentifylline (also referred to as pentoxifylline), ultrapure water and biocompatible membranes in HD patients, and transplant nephrectomy in patients with failed allografts.[123]

Iron-restricted erythropoiesis is a common cause of ESA hyporesponsiveness. Functional iron deficiency, as previously discussed, occurs in patients with chronic inflammation, and is characterized by high ferritin and low TSAT, corresponding to the role of these biomarkers as acute phase and negative acute phase reactants, respectively. In 2005, 60% of HD patients had serum ferritins > 500 ng per milliliter, and 22% of HD patients had serum ferritins > 800 ng per milliliter.[124,132] Absolute iron deficiency, in contrast, occurs in patients with total body iron depletion, such as from GI bleeding, and is characterized by low ferritin and low TSAT. Iron supplementation may be beneficial in the treatment of both types of iron deficiency (see the following).

A rare but noteworthy cause of ESA hyporesponsiveness is pure red cell aplasia (PRCA), which occurs when patients previously exposed to ESAs develop anti-EPO antibodies.[133,134] Patients may be sensitized by treatment with any of the commercially available ESAs, although most cases have been reported in conjunction with a 2002 formulation of epoetin alfa (Eprex), in which albumin had been replaced by polysorbate-80. The neutralizing antibodies formed cross-react with rHuEPO as well as endogenous EPO, thus blocking activation of the EPO-R and subsequent erythropoiesis. Patients present with rapidly progressive anemia (Hb decreases by 0.1 g/dL/day), severe reticulocytopenia (< 10,000 cells per microliter), and an absence of erythroid precursors on bone marrow biopsy. In addition, the failure of erythropoiesis results in a surfeit of iron (ferritin > 1000 ng per milliliter and TSAT > 70%). The detection of anti-EPO antibodies is necessary but not sufficient for a diagnosis of PRCA, because some patients with measurable antibody titers may not exhibit clinical symptomatology. PRCA is treated by withdrawing the ESA and prescribing corticosteroids with or without cyclosporine or cyclophosphamide.

Other causes of ESA hyporesponsiveness are also uncommon but may be valuable diagnostic considerations. Primary bone marrow disorders, such as myelofibrosis and myelodysplasia, as well as hemoglobinopathies, such as sickle cell anemia and thalassemia, are associated with a poor response to ESAs.[123] Secondary hyperparathyroidism is also linked to ESA-resistant anemia, possibly by causing increased fragility of RBCs, the inhibition of EPO synthesis and erythropoiesis, and the stimulation of bone marrow fibrosis. Small clinical trials show higher achieved Hb levels in response to a lower ESA dose after a parathyroidectomy.[135] Aluminum, by interfering with heme synthesis or iron bioavailability, and angiotensin-converting enzyme inhibitors (ACEIs) and angiotensin receptor blockers (ARBs), by blocking angiotensin II-mediated EPO release or hematopoietic stem cell maturation, are rarely reported causes of ESA hyporesponsiveness.[123,124,136] Hemolysis and nutrient deficiencies, as previously discussed, also contribute to ESA-refractory anemia.

Novel and Experimental Erythropoiesis-Stimulating Agents

New ESAs under development may have advantages over currently used agents, including a longer $t_{½}$, an absence of sequence homology with endogenous EPO, and in some cases, diverse mechanisms of action. CERA is synthesized by the integration of EPO with a 30-kDa methoxy polyethylene glycol polymer. This modification increases the $t_{½}$ from 8.5 hours with endogenous EPO to 130 hours with CERA.[103] CERA is administered either IV or SC every 2 to 4 weeks, compared to DPO, which is optimally given every 1 to 2 weeks, and rHuEPO, which is given every 2 to 3 days. Clinical trials have shown that CERA maintains stable Hb levels in both CKD and ESRD patients.[137,138] Other EPO-like molecules and derivatives, including synthetic erythropoiesis protein-polymers and fusion proteins in which EPO molecules are linked to flexible polypeptides, the Fc region of human IgG, or albumin have also been developed as means to enhance $t_{½}$.[103] Some of these compounds can be administered by ingestion, transdermal absorption, or aerosol inhalation.

Peginesatide (Hematide) is a pegylated, synthetic, dimeric peptide that activates the EPO-R but shares no sequence homology with endogenous EPO.[139] In vitro, peginesatide stimulates the proliferation and differentiation of erythroid progenitors, and in rodent and monkey models, the drug causes a dose-dependent rise in Hb levels. Because of its unique molecular structure, peginesatide should be unrecognizable to anti-EPO antibodies, and therefore could be used to treat PRCA. In an open-label trial involving 14 CKD patients with anti-EPO antibody-mediated PRCA, 28 months of peginesatide administration led to > 10-fold increase in reticulocyte counts, the suppression of anti-EPO antibody titers, a rise in Hb from median levels of 9 to 11.4 g per deciliter, and the elimination of transfusion requirements in most patients.[140] This molecule also has a $t_{½}$ of 14 to 60 hours, allowing monthly dosing in the same manner as CERA. Data from phase III clinical trials of peginesatide have been recently reported.[141,142] In PEARL 1 and 2,[141] a total of 983 CKD patients were randomized to either peginesatide or DPO to achieve Hb levels of 11 to 12 g per deciliter. These trials demonstrated the noninferiority of peginesatide to reach Hb targets, but a pooled analysis identified a higher risk of death, arrhythmia, and unstable angina in patients given peginesatide versus those given DPO (22% and 17%, respectively).[143] In EMERALD 1 and 2,[142] a total of 1626 HD patients were randomized to either peginesatide or rHuEPO to achieve Hb levels of 10 to 12 g per deciliter. These trials also demonstrated the noninferiority of peginesatide, but in this case showed no worrying safety signals. The discordance between the PEARL and EMERALD findings is currently unexplained.

HIF prolyl-hydroxylase inhibitors (PHIs) act in a manner mechanistically distinct from ESAs. The PHIs are orally active oxoglutarate analogs that inhibit PHD proteins, which are responsible for the hydroxylation, the ubiquitination, and the degradation of HIF-α, as discussed previously. These compounds mimic a hypoxic stimulus and lead to the stabilization of HIF-α, followed by heterodimerization, nuclear translocation, and HRE-mediated transcription of a multitude of genes. In fact, more than 100 genes are upregulated by PHIs, and the consequences of this pleiotropic activation are not yet fully understood.[103,144] Salutary effects include the stimulation of EPO release, the inhibition of hepcidin transcription, the amelioration of diabetic kidney disease, and protection from ischemia–reperfusion injury. Potentially deleterious effects include enhanced glycolysis, impaired mitochondrial respiration, aggravated tubulointerstitial injury, and increased vascular endothelial growth factor (VEGF)-mediated angiogenesis. In a small study, the administration of FG-2216, a first-generation PHI, increased EPO levels in six anephric ESRD patients from 7.8 to 240.6 mU per milliliter and in healthy controls from 6.4 to 81.2 mU per milliliter.[145] Although clinical trials of FG-2216 were halted following a case of fatal hepatic necrosis, studies with the related agent FG-4592 are ongoing and appear promising.

Additional therapeutic approaches to the anemia of CKD are the subject of active preclinical research. As discussed previously, some of the GATA transcription factors block *EPO* gene transcription, and GATA-2 inhibitors enhance HIF-1 activity, EPO levels, CFU-E and reticulocyte counts, and Hb concentration in a mouse model of anemia.[103,146] Separately, the phosphotyrosine phosphatase SHP-1, also known as hematopoietic cell phosphatase (HCP), binds to the *src*-homology 2 domain of the EPO-R, dephosphorylates JAK-2, and terminates the propagation of EPO-mediated signaling. HCP antisense oligonucleotide increases STAT-5 expression and BFU-E recovery in cells cultured from ESA-hyporesponsive HD patients.[147]

Iron Supplementation

Iron-restricted erythropoiesis, as previously mentioned, is common in CKD and ESRD patients. Correction of the iron deficiency should thus address one of the root causes of anemia and thereby reduce the dose of ESA required to maintain adequate Hb levels. In addition, iron supplementation may have nonhematologic benefits, such as improved cognition, thermoregulation, immune function, and exercise adaptation, as well as decreased restless legs syndrome and aluminum absorption.[148] The 2006 KDOQI guidelines recommend iron administration to maintain TSAT > 20% and ferritin 100 to 500 ng per milliliter in CKD and PD patients, and TSAT > 20% or CHr > 29 pg per cell and ferritin 200 to 500 ng per milliliter in HD patients.[1]

Recent evidence suggests that iron supplementation is beneficial in treating both absolute (ferritin < 100 to 200 ng per milliliter) and functional (ferritin > 100 to 200 ng per milliliter) iron deficiency. Specifically, the efficacy of IV iron in treating functional iron deficiency was evaluated in the Dialysis Patients' Response to IV Iron with Elevated Ferritin (DRIVE) trial.[112,149] In DRIVE, 134 HD patients with Hb levels < 11 g per deciliter, TSAT < 25%, and ferritin levels of 500 to 1,200 ng per milliliter were randomized to receive either ferric gluconate 125 mg IV during eight consecutive HD sessions (total dose, 1 g) or no iron. Patients with a malignancy or an active infection requiring systemic antibiotics were excluded. The EPO dose was ≥ 225 IU/kg/week or ≥ 22,500 IU per week at baseline and was increased by 25% at randomization. At 6 weeks, Hb increased by 1.6 ± 1.3 g per deciliter in the treatment group compared to 1.1 ± 1.4 g per deciliter in the control group ($P = .028$), with no difference in the rate of adverse events. TSAT and ferritin also increased in the patients given IV iron. DRIVE-II, a 6-week cohort follow-up of the original trial, showed that the rHuEPO dose fell by 7527 ± 18,021 IU per week in the treatment group compared to 649 ± 19,987 IU per week in the control group ($P = .017$).[150]

The choice between PO and IV iron therapy, especially in CKD patients, is somewhat controversial. PO iron includes the nonheme compounds, ferrous sulfate, chloride, fumarate, and gluconate, as well as the relatively new heme iron polypeptide (HIP).[74,151] Overdosing with PO iron is less likely than with IV iron, because hepcidin prevents GI absorption of excess iron in states of sufficiency (see previous). In advanced CKD, however, the unregulated excess of hepcidin and other acute phase and host defense molecules is precisely the cause of iron deficiency and iron-restricted erythropoiesis. Furthermore, the absorption of PO iron may be impaired by the concomitant ingestion of specific medications, and compliance with the increased pill burden is problematic. In four recent RCTs involving CKD patients, PO iron produced a lesser Hb response than IV iron.[152] Notwithstanding these limitations, PO iron is generally cost-effective, easily administered, and worth a trial of therapy before proceeding to IV infusion in CKD patients.

In contrast, PO iron is usually ineffective in HD and PD patients.[153] This poor response has been attributed to (1) dialysis-associated losses that exceed the amount of elemental iron absorbed orally, (2) increased time to maximal incorporation of PO iron into RBCs (33 days PO versus 8.6 days IV), and (3) high levels of hepcidin that block the duodenal uptake of PO iron.[74,154] A possible exception is HIP, which is absorbed from the GI tract 10 times more effectively than nonheme iron. A 6-month trial of HIP in maintenance HD patients concluded that PO heme iron successfully replaced IV iron and was associated with increased rHuEPO efficiency.[151] The oral HEMe iron polypeptide Against Treatment with Oral Controlled Release Iron Tablets (HEMATOCRIT) trial, a 6-month study of HIP in PD patients, is currently under way.[155]

A common clinical conundrum in ESRD patients is whether to prescribe iron in low doses at regular intervals (maintenance dosing) or in high doses after iron deficiency develops (repletion dosing). Repletion dosing, which consists of ≥ 1 g of iron administered during 1 to 8 infusions, is given when TSAT is < 20% to 25% or ferritin levels are < 100 to 200 ng per milliliter. This dose is considered an adequate test of iron responsiveness, which is assessed by the serial measurement of iron indices and Hb.[74] Maintenance dosing, which consists of 22 to 65 mg of iron administered weekly, may be advantageous in minimizing Hb variability, maximizing ESA sensitivity, and overcoming ESA hyporesponsiveness.[156,157] This approach is recommended by the most current KDOQI guidelines.[1]

Intravenous Iron: Options and Toxicity

Many formulations of IV iron are available, and are useful in both CKD and ESRD patients (Table 76.3). The iron dextrans are formulated as high molecular weight ([HMW] 265 kDa; Imferon, DexFerrum) and low molecular weight ([LMW] 165 kDa; INFeD) compounds. Because of the association of the HMW agents with anaphylactoid reactions, Imferon has been withdrawn from the market, and DexFerrum is increasingly avoided. The risk of adverse events, including life-threatening episodes, is much less with LMW (< 1 in 200,000 doses) than with HMW iron dextran.[148,158,159] Iron dextran has been given in doses of 2 to 3 g within 4 to 10 minutes, although in clinical practice, doses of 1 to 3 g are infused during the course of a 4-hour HD session. Advantages of LMW iron dextran include providing ≥ 1 g of iron in a single infusion and saving an estimated $250 million yearly when used instead of more expensive preparations. Conversely, the preferential use of proprietary IV iron formulations to avoid the rare adverse events associated with LMW iron dextran would cost $7.8 million USD to prevent a single life-threatening event and $33 million USD to prevent a single death.[148,159]

IV iron is also manufactured as iron sucrose (Venofer) and ferric gluconate (Ferrlecit), which is available as a generic equivalent (Watson Pharmaceuticals, Corona, CA). Iron sucrose is delivered at doses ≤ 200 to 300 mg during a 2-hour infusion, because single doses of 400 to 500 mg have been linked to infusion-associated hypotension and coronary vasospasm.[160,161] Ferric gluconate is delivered at doses of 125 to 250 mg during a 1- to 4-hour infusion; again, doses exceeding this range have been linked to hypotension. Both agents thus require four to eight sequential infusions to achieve a cumulative dose of 1 g of elemental iron. Ferric gluconate, compared to iron sucrose and iron dextran, donates iron most readily to apotransferrin, a property that should theoretically increase the efficiency of erythropoiesis and should decrease the oxidative stress provoked by free iron, although the clinical relevance of these observations is unknown.[154,162] On a separate note, small studies in CKD patients have shown consistently that albuminuria, enzymuria, and the excretion of N-acetyl-β-glucosaminidase (NAG) increase following the

TABLE 76.3 **Currently Available and Investigational Intravenous Iron Formulations**[148,175,177]

Generic Name	Trade Name	Standard Dose	Infusion Rate	WAC (USD)
LMW iron dextran	INFeD	1–3 g	2–4 hours	$24.10 (100 mg/vial)
HMW iron dextran	DexFerrum	1–3 g	2–4 hours	$36.00 (100 mg/vial)
Iron sucrose	Venofer	200–300 mg	2–3 hours	$55.00 (100 mg/vial)
Ferric gluconate	Ferrlecit	125–250 mg	1–4 hours	$31.80 (62.5 mg/ampule)
Ferumoxytol	Feraheme	510 mg	17 seconds	$396.78 (510 mg/vial)
Ferric carboxymaltose	Ferinject	750–1,000 mg	15 minutes	N/A
Iron isomaltoside 1000	Monofer	1.5–1.7 g	1 hour	N/A

WAC, wholesale acquisition cost (as of March 28, 2011); USD, United States dollars; LMW, low molecular weight; HMW, high molecular weight; N/A, not available.

administration of iron sucrose but not ferric gluconate.[163–165] Iron sucrose, compared to ferric gluconate and iron dextran, causes the most severe injury to proximal tubule and endothelial cells in vitro, although all three agents induce significant lipid peroxidation.[166] This result has been recapitulated in HD patients, in whom the infusion of iron sucrose caused increased peroxidation of polyunsaturated fatty acids as measured by the generation of malondialdehyde.[167]

Additional concerns have surfaced about the use of IV iron, regardless of the formulation. The possibility of iron overload and hemosiderosis has caused considerable anxiety. Before the ESA era, repeated blood transfusions led to more frequent parenchymal iron deposition, but serum ferritin levels in these cases were often $>$ 5000 ng per milliliter.[74] The risk of iron overload, which begins when total body iron is $>$ 5 g (the capacity of the RES), is low as long as ferritin levels are $<$ 2000 ng per milliliter. A hypothetical risk of IV iron is the acceleration of systemic infection by the suppression of phagocytosis and the provenance of iron to microorganisms.[148] Clinical data underpinning this fear are limited, and both prospective and retrospective clinical studies have failed to link bacteremia to the use of IV iron.[168,169]

Novel and Experimental Iron Agents

The newer PO iron compounds have been designed to have better bioavailability than their older congeners. HIP was discussed previously. Soluble ferric pyrophosphate (SFP) has been found, in vitro, to increase ferritin production compared to ferric sulfate and chloride, with less sensitivity to inhibition by divalent cations.[170] Furthermore, an emulsification of ferric pyrophosphate within albumin microspheres is superior to SFP, as assessed by total absorption from the GI tract in a rat model.[171] Low doses of sodium feredetate, a different formulation, have proven more effective than high doses of ferric fumarate in pregnant, anemic women.[172] Conversely, the efficacy of iron hydroxide polymaltose in treating iron-deficiency anemia has been repeatedly questioned.[173] The value of any of these medications in treating CKD and ESRD patients is unknown.

One of the newest formulations of IV iron is ferumoxytol (Feraheme), a carbohydrate-coated, superparamagnetic iron oxide nanoparticle.[174] The chief advantage of ferumoxytol is the ability to give a 510-mg dose by IV push in as little as 17 seconds without adverse effects. This speedy delivery is possible because of the absence of free iron in the formulation, and is clearly an attractive alternative to prolonged IV infusions in ambulatory CKD and PD patients. In RCTs involving CKD and HD patients, two doses of ferumoxytol 510 mg IV were more effective than 3 weeks of ferrous fumarate 200 mg per day PO, with the rare occurrence of anaphylactoid and hypersensitivity reactions and hypotension. Ferumoxytol may also affect magnetic resonance imaging (MRI) studies for up to 3 months after administration.

Ferric carboxymaltose (Ferinject) is a carbohydrate shell–stabilized ferric hydroxide core.[175] Ferric carboxymaltose also contains little free iron and can be given as a 1-g dose in $\leq$ 15 minutes. In RCTs involving CKD and ESRD patients, ferric carboxymaltose 1 g IV was more effective than ferric sulfate 65 mg three times per day PO and as effective as equivalent doses of iron sucrose, as assessed by improvements in TSAT, ferritin, Hb, and health-related QOL. Adverse events with ferric carboxymaltose were rare and less frequent than with iron sucrose. The Randomized Evaluation of Efficacy and Safety of Ferric Carboxymaltose in Patients with Iron Deficiency Anemia and Impaired Renal Function (REPAIR-IDA) trial will randomize CKD patients to two 750-mg doses of ferric carboxymaltose versus five 200-mg doses of iron sucrose.[176]

Iron isomaltoside 1000 (Monofer) is the latest addition to the IV iron armamentarium and may possess some unique advantages. Iron isomaltoside 1000 can be given in doses of up to 20 mg per kilogram of body weight and is relatively pure. In contrast, ferric carboxymaltose is limited to doses of 15 mg per kilogram of body weight and contains up to 75 μg per milliliter of aluminum and 5.5 mg per milliliter of sodium, the impurities of which may be problematic for patients with kidney disease.[177] In an open-label trial involving 182 CKD and ESRD patients, iron isomaltoside 1000, administered as either bolus injections of 100 to 200 mg or as a fast high-dose infusion, resulted in increased TSAT, ferritin, and Hb, with no immediate or delayed allergic reactions.[178]

CONCLUSION

Anemia is common in the CKD population and is associated with increased morbidity and mortality. The anemia of CKD has its origins within a confluence of pathobiologic circumstances that include relative EPO and iron deficiencies. Unraveling its etiologic and diagnostic characteristics remains challenging. During the course of modern history, the management of anemia in patients with kidney disease has progressed from the archaic, involving whole blood transfusions, to the contemporary, encompassing evidence-based and Hb-targeted ESA and iron administration, and continues to evolve with the discovery of new mechanisms and therapeutic agents. As scientific inquiry proceeds, we anticipate significant advances in the treatment of this complex condition, the anemia of chronic kidney disease.

REFERENCES

1. KDOQI Clinical Practice Guidelines and Clinical Practice Recommendations for Anemia in Chronic Kidney Disease. *Am J Kidney Dis.* 2006;47:S11.

2. Coresh J, Selvin E, Stevens LA, et al. Prevalence of chronic kidney disease in the United States. *JAMA.* 2007;298:2038.

3. Collins AJ, Foley RN, Herzog C, et al. US Renal Data System 2010 Annual Data Report. *Am J Kidney Dis.* 2011;57:A8.

4. McFarlane SI, Chen SC, Whaley-Connell AT, et al. Prevalence and associations of anemia of CKD: Kidney Early Evaluation Program (KEEP) and National Health and Nutrition Examination Survey (NHANES) 1999-2004. *Am J Kidney Dis.* 2008;51:S46.

5. Berns JS, Elzein H, Lynn RI, et al. Hemoglobin variability in epoetin-treated hemodialysis patients. *Kidney Int.* 2003;64:1514.

6. Kalantar-Zadeh K, Aronoff GR. Hemoglobin variability in anemia of chronic kidney disease. *J Am Soc Nephrol.* 2009;20:479.

7. Besarab A, Hörl WH, Silverberg D. Iron metabolism, iron deficiency, thrombocytosis, and the cardiorenal anemia syndrome. *Oncologist.* 2009;14 (Suppl 1):22.

8. Boudville NC, Djurdjev O, Macdougall IC, et al. Hemoglobin variability in nondialysis chronic kidney disease: examining the association with mortality. *Clin J Am Soc Nephrol.* 2009;4:1176.

9. Gilbertson DT, Ebben JP, Foley RN, et al. Hemoglobin level variability: associations with mortality. *Clin J Am Soc Nephrol.* 2008;3:133.

10. Yang W, Israni RK, Brunelli SM, et al. Hemoglobin variability and mortality in ESRD. *J Am Soc Nephrol.* 2007;18:3164.

11. Eckardt KU, Kim J, Kronenberg F, et al. Hemoglobin variability does not predict mortality in European hemodialysis patients. *J Am Soc Nephrol.* 2010;21:1765.

12. Ebben JP, Gilbertson DT, Foley RN, et al. Hemoglobin level variability: associations with comorbidity, intercurrent events, and hospitalizations. *Clin J Am Soc Nephrol.* 2006;1:1205.

13. Astor BC, Coresh J, Heiss G, et al. Kidney function and anemia as risk factors for coronary heart disease and mortality: the Atherosclerosis Risk in Communities (ARIC) Study. *Am Heart J.* 2006;151:492.

14. Bhatti S, Hakeem A, Dillie KS, et al. Prevalence, prognosis, and therapeutic implications of unrecognized left ventricular systolic dysfunction in patients with anemia and chronic kidney disease. *Congest Heart Fail.* 2010;16:271.

15. Locatelli F, Pisoni RL, Combe C, et al. Anaemia in haemodialysis patients of five European countries: association with morbidity and mortality in the Dialysis Outcomes and Practice Patterns Study (DOPPS). *Nephrol Dial Transplant.* 2004;19:121.

16. Macdougall IC, Tomson CR, Steenkamp M, et al. Relative risk of death in UK haemodialysis patients in relation to achieved haemoglobin from 1999 to 2005: an observational study using UK Renal Registry data incorporating 30,040 patient-years of follow-up. *Nephrol Dial Transplant.* 2010;25:914.

17. Li S, Foley RN, Collins AJ. Anemia, hospitalization, and mortality in patients receiving peritoneal dialysis in the United States. *Kidney Int.* 2004; 65:1864.

18. Gandra SR, Finkelstein FO, Bennett AV, et al. Impact of erythropoiesis-stimulating agents on energy and physical function in nondialysis CKD patients with anemia: a systematic review. *Am J Kidney Dis.* 2010;55:519.

19. Cesari M, Penninx BW, Lauretani F, et al. Hemoglobin levels and skeletal muscle: results from the InCHIANTI study. *J Gerontol A Biol Sci Med Sci.* 2004;59:249.

20. Jelkmann W. Erythropoietin after a century of research: younger than ever. *Eur J Haematol.* 2007;78:183.

21. Besarab A, Ayyoub F. Anemia in renal disease. In: Schrier RW, ed. *Diseases of the Kidney and Urinary Tract*, 8th ed. Philadelphia, PA: Lippincott Williams & Wilkins; 2007: 2405.

22. Fisher JW. Landmark advances in the development of erythropoietin. *Exp Biol Med (Maywood).* 2010;235:1398.

23. Jourdanet D. *De l'Anemie des Altitudes et de l'Anemie in General dans ses Raports avec la Pression del l'Atmosphere.* Paris, France: Balliere; 1863.

24. Viault F. Sur la quantite d'oxygene continue dans le sang des animaux des hauts plateaux l'Amerique du Sud. *CR Acad Sci (Paris).* 1891;112:295.

25. Carnot P, DeFlandre C. Sur l'activite hematopoietique de serum au cours de la regeneration di sang. *CR Acad Sci (Paris).* 1906;143:384.

26. Brown GE, Roth GM. The anemia of chronic nephritis. *Arch Intern Med.* 1922;30:817.

27. Reissmann KR. Studies on the mechanism of erythropoietin stimulation in parabiotic rats during hypoxia. *Blood.* 1950;5:372.

27a. Bonsdorff E, Jalavisto E. *Acta Physiol Scand* 1948;16:150.

28. Jacobson LO, Goldwasser E, Fried W, et al. Role of the kidney in erythropoiesis. *Nature.* 1957;179:633.

29. Mach B, Ucla C, Fisher J, et al. Translation of mRNA from kidneys of hypoxic rats into biologically active erythropoietin following microinjection into frog oocytes. *Clin Res.* 1983;31:484A.

30. Plzak LF, Fried W, Jacobson LO, et al. Demonstration of stimulation of erythropoiesis by plasma from anemic rats, using Fe59. *J Lab Clin Med.* 1955;46:671.

31. Cotes PM, Baugham DR. Bioassay of erythropoietin in mice made plethoric by exposure to air at reduced pressure. *Nature.* 1961;191:1065.

32. Adamson JW. The erythropoietin/hematocrit relationship in normal and polycythemic man: implications of marrow regulation. *Blood.* 1968;32:597.

33. Miyake T, Kung CKH, Goldwasser E. Purification of human erythropoietin. *J Biol Chem.* 1977;252:5558.

34. Garcia JF, Sherwood J, Goldwasser E. Radioimmunoassay of erythropoietin. *Blood Cells.* 1979;5:405.

35. Lin FK, Suggs S, Lin CH, et al. Cloning and expression of the erythropoietin gene. *Proc Natl Acad Sci.* USA 1985;92:7850.

36. Eschbach JW, Egrie JC, Downing MR, et al. Correction of the anemia of end-stage renal disease with recombinant human erythropoietin. Results of a combined phase I and II clinical trial. *N Engl J Med.* 1987;316:73.

37. Winearls GC, Oliver DO, Pippard MJ, et al. Effect of human erythropoietin derived from recombinant DNA on the anemia of patients maintained by chronic hemodialysis. *Lancet.* 1986;2:1175.

38. Evans RG, Gardiner BS, Smith DW, et al. Intrarenal oxygenation: unique challenges and the biophysical basis of homeostasis. *Am J Physiol Renal Physiol.* 2008;295:F1259.

39. Haase VH. Hypoxic regulation of erythropoiesis and iron metabolism. *Am J Physiol Renal Physiol.* 2010;299:F1.

40. Masson N, Willam C, Maxwell PH, et al. Independent function of two destruction domains in hypoxia-inducible factor-alpha chains activated by prolyl hydroxylation. *EMBO J.* 2001;20:5197.

41. Schofield CJ, Ratcliffe PJ. Oxygen sensing by HIF hydroxylases. *Nat Rev Mol Cell Biol.* 2004;5:343.

42. Semenza GL. Hypoxia-inducible factor 1 (HIF-1) pathway. *Sci STKE.* 2007;2007:cm8.

43. Scortegagna M, Ding K, Zhang Q, et al. HIF-2alpha regulates murine hematopoietic development in an erythropoietin-dependent manner. *Blood.* 2005;105:3133.

44. Kim WY, Safran M, Buckley MR, et al. Failure to prolyl hydroxylate hypoxia-inducible factor alpha phenocopies VHL inactivation in vivo. *EMBO J.* 2006;25:4650.

45. Warnecke C, Zaborowska Z, Kurreck J, et al. Differentiating the functional role of hypoxia-inducible factor (HIF)-1alpha and HIF-2alpha (EPAS-1) by the use of RNA interference: erythropoietin is a HIF-2alpha target gene in Hep3B and Kelly cells. *FASEB J.* 2004;18:1462.

46. Obara N, Suzuki N, Kim K, et al. Repression via the GATA box is essential for tissue-specific erythropoietin gene expression. *Blood.* 2008;111:5223.

47. Forejtnikova H, Vieillevoye M, Zermati Y, et al. Transferrin receptor 2 is a component of the erythropoietin receptor complex and is required for efficient erythropoiesis. *Blood.* 2010;116:5357.

48. Jelkmann W, Bohlius J, Hallek M, et al. The erythropoietin receptor in normal and cancer tissues. *Crit Rev Oncol Hematol.* 2008;67:39.

49. Verdier F, Walrafen P, Hubert N, et al. Proteasomes regulate the duration of erythropoietin receptor activation by controlling down-regulation of cell surface receptors. *J Biol Chem.* 2000;275:18375.

50. Elliott S, Pham E, Macdougall IC. Erythropoietins: a common mechanism of action. *Exp Hematol.* 2008;36:1573.

51. Jelkmann W. Molecular biology of erythropoietin. *Intern Med.* 2004; 43:649.

52. Soni S, Bala S, Gwynn B, et al. Absence of erythroblast macrophage protein (Emp) leads to failure of erythroblast nuclear extrusion. *J Biol Chem.* 2006;281:20181.

53. Chen K, Liu J, Heck S, et al. Resolving the distinct stages in erythroid differentiation based on dynamic changes in membrane protein expression during erythropoiesis. *Proc Natl Acad Sci USA.* 2009;106:17413.

54. An X, Mohandas N. Erythroblastic islands, terminal erythroid differentiation and reticulocyte maturation. *Int J Hematol.* 2011;93:139.

55. Munoz M, Garcia-Erce JA, Remacha AF. Disorders of iron metabolism. Part 1: molecular basis of iron homoeostasis. *J Clin Pathol.* 2011;64:281.

56. Nemeth E. Iron regulation and erythropoiesis. *Curr Opin Hematol.* 2008;15:169.

57. Theil EC. Ferritin: at the crossroads of iron and oxygen metabolism. *J Nutr.* 2003;133:1549S.

58. Kalantar-Zadeh K, Kalantar-Zadeh K, Lee GH. The fascinating but deceptive ferritin: to measure it or not to measure it in chronic kidney disease? *Clin J Am Soc Nephrol.* 2006;1(Suppl 1):S9.

59. Fleming RE, Bacon BR. Orchestration of iron homeostasis. *N Engl J Med.* 2005;352:1741.

60. Malyszko J, Tesar V, Macdougall IC. Neutrophil gelatinase-associated lipocalin and hepcidin: what do they have in common and is there a potential interaction? *Kidney Blood Press Res.* 2010;33:157.

61. Andrews NC. Forging a field: the golden age of iron biology. *Blood.* 2008; 112:219.

62. Ramey G, Deschemin JC, Durel B, et al. Hepcidin targets ferroportin for degradation in hepatocytes. *Haematologica.* 2010;95:501.

63. Choi SO, Cho YS, Kim HL, et al. ROS mediate the hypoxic repression of the hepcidin gene by inhibiting C/EBPalpha and STAT-3. *Biochem Biophys Res Commun.* 2007;356:312.

64. Babitt JL, Lin HY. Molecular mechanisms of hepcidin regulation: implications for the anemia of CKD. *Am J Kidney Dis.* 2010;55:726.

65. Tong Z, Wu X, Ovcharenko D, et al. Neutrophil gelatinase-associated lipocalin as a survival factor. *Biochem J.* 2005;391:441.

66. Goetz DH, Holmes MA, Borregaard N, et al. The neutrophil lipocalin NGAL is a bacteriostatic agent that interferes with siderophore-mediated iron acquisition. *Mol Cell.* 2002;10:1033.

67. Muckenthaler MU, Galy B, Hentze MW. Systemic iron homeostasis and the iron-responsive element/iron-regulatory protein (IRE/IRP) regulatory network. *Annu Rev Nutr.* 2008;28:197.

68. Sanchez M, Galy B, Muckenthaler MU, et al. Iron-regulatory proteins limit hypoxia-inducible factor-2alpha expression in iron deficiency. *Nat Struct Mol Biol.* 2007;14:420.

69. Fehr T, Ammann P, Garzoni D, et al. Interpretation of erythropoietin levels in patients with various degrees of renal insufficiency and anemia. *Kidney Int.* 2004;66:1206.

70. Artunc F, Risler T. Serum erythropoietin concentrations and responses to anaemia in patients with or without chronic kidney disease. *Nephrol Dial Transplant.* 2007;22:2900.

71. Khankin EV, Mutter WP, Tamez H, et al. Soluble erythropoietin receptor contributes to erythropoietin resistance in end-stage renal disease. *PLoS One.* 2010;5:e9246.

72. Glaser M. Growth characteristics of circulating hematopoietic progenitors in terminal renal failure. *Med Sci Monit.* 2006;12:CR113.

73. Aucella F, Scalzulli RP, Gatta G, et al. Calcitriol increases burst-forming unit-erythroid proliferation in chronic renal failure. A synergistic effect with r-HuEpo. *Nephron Clin Pract.* 2003;95:c121–c127.

74. Besarab A, Coyne DW. Iron supplementation to treat anemia in patients with chronic kidney disease. *Nat Rev Nephrol.* 2010;6:699.

75. Zaritsky J, Young B, Wang HJ, et al. Hepcidin—a potential novel biomarker for iron status in chronic kidney disease. *Clin J Am Soc Nephrol.* 2009;4:1051.

76. Malyszko J, Malyszko JS, Kozminski P, et al. Possible relationship between neutrophil gelatinase-associated lipocalin, hepcidin, and inflammation in haemodialysed patients. *Nephron Clin Pract.* 2010;115:c268–c275.

77. Bilic E, Bilic E. Amino acid sequence homology of thrombopoietin and erythropoietin may explain thrombocytosis in children with iron deficiency anemia. *J Pediatr Hematol Oncol.* 2003;25:675.

78. Kinoshita Y, Taniura S, Shishido H, et al. Cerebral venous sinus thrombosis associated with iron deficiency: two case reports. *Neurol Med Chir (Tokyo).* 2006;46:589.

79. Nagai T, Komatsu N, Sakata Y, et al. Iron deficiency anemia with marked thrombocytosis complicated by central retinal vein occlusion. *Intern Med.* 2005;44:1090.

80. Handelman GJ, Levin NW. Red cell survival: relevance and mechanism involved. *J Ren Nutr.* 2010;20:S84.

81. Costa E, Rocha S, Rocha-Pereira P, et al. Altered erythrocyte membrane protein composition in chronic kidney disease stage 5 patients under haemodialysis and recombinant human erythropoietin therapy. *Blood Purif.* 2008;26:267.

82. Buemi M, Floccari F, Di Pasquale G, et al. AQP1 in red blood cells of uremic patients during hemodialytic treatment. *Nephron.* 2002;92:846.

83. Debska-Slizien A, Owczarzak A, Lysiak-Szydlowska W, et al. Erythrocyte metabolism during renal anemia treatment with recombinant human erythropoietin. *Int J Artif Organs.* 2004;27:935.

84. Gambhir KK, Parui R, Agarwal V, et al. The effect of hemodialysis on the transport of sodium in erythrocytes from chronic renal failure patients maintained on hemodialysis. *Life Sci.* 2002;71:1615.

85. Junglee NA, Rahman SU, Wild M, et al. When pure is not so pure: chloramine-related hemolytic anemia in home hemodialysis patients. *Hemodial Int.* 2010;14:327.

86. Calo LA, Davis PA, Pagnin E, et al. Carnitine-mediated improved response to erythropoietin involves induction of haem oxygenase-1: studies in humans and in an animal model. *Nephrol Dial Transplant.* 2008;23:890.

87. Hedayati SS. Dialysis-related carnitine disorder. *Semin Dial.* 2006;19:323.

88. Brunelli SM, Goldfarb S. Hypophosphatemia: clinical consequences and management. *J Am Soc Nephrol.* 2007;18:1999.

89. Bellizzi V, Minutolo R, Terracciano V, et al. Influence of the cyclic variation of hydration status on hemoglobin levels in hemodialysis patients. *Am J Kidney Dis.* 2002;40:549.

90. Muñoz M, García-Erce JA, Remacha AF. Disorders of iron metabolism. Part II: iron deficiency and iron overload. *J Clin Pathol.* 2011;64:287.

91. Yamanishi H, Iyama S, Yamaguchi Y, et al. Relation between iron content of serum ferritin and clinical status factors extracted by factor analysis in patients with hyperferritinemia. *Clin Biochem.* 2002;35:523.

92. Hsu CY, McCulloch CE, Curhan GC. Iron status and hemoglobin level in chronic renal insufficiency. *J Am Soc Nephrol.* 2002;13:2783.

93. Stancu S, Stanciu A, Zugravu A, et al. Bone marrow iron, iron indices, and the response to intravenous iron in patients with non-dialysis-dependent CKD. *Am J Kidney Dis.* 2010;55:639.

94. Rocha LA, Barreto DV, Barreto FC, et al. Serum ferritin level remains a reliable marker of bone marrow iron stores evaluated by histomorphometry in hemodialysis patients. *Clin J Am Soc Nephrol.* 2009;4:105.

95. Guillygomarc'h A, Christian J, Romain M, et al. Circadian variations of transferrin saturation levels in iron-overloaded patients: implications for the screening of C282Y-linked haemochromatosis. *Br J Haematol.* 2003;120:359.

96. Wish JB. Assessing iron status: beyond serum ferritin and transferrin saturation. *Clin J Am Soc Nephrol.* 2006;1(Suppl 1):S4.

97. Miwa N, Akiba T, Kimata N, et al. Usefulness of measuring reticulocyte hemoglobin equivalent in the management of haemodialysis patients with iron deficiency. *Int J Lab Hematol.* 2010;32:248.

98. Beerenhout C, Bekers O, Kooman JP, et al. A comparison between the soluble transferrin receptor, transferrin saturation and serum ferritin as markers of iron state in hemodialysis patients. *Nephron.* 2002;92:32.

99. Chen YC, Hung SC, Tarng DC. Association between transferrin receptor-ferritin index and conventional measures of iron responsiveness in hemodialysis patients. *Am J Kidney Dis.* 2006;47:1036.
100. Macdougall IC, Malyszko J, Hider RC, et al. Current status of the measurement of blood hepcidin levels in chronic kidney disease. *Clin J Am Soc Nephrol.* 2010;5:1681.
101. Goldsmith D. 2009: a requiem for rHuEPOs—but should we nail down the coffin in 2010? *Clin J Am Soc Nephrol.* 2010;5:929.
102. Jelkmann W. Biosimilar epoetins and other "follow-on" biologics: update on the European experiences. *Am J Hematol.* 2010;85:771.
103. Macdougall IC. Novel erythropoiesis-stimulating agents: a new era in anemia management. *Clin J Am Soc Nephrol.* 2008;3:200.
104. Curran MP, McCormack PL. Methoxy polyethylene glycol-epoetin beta: a review of its use in the management of anaemia associated with chronic kidney disease. *Drugs.* 2008;68:1139.
105. Novak JE, Inrig JK, Patel UD, et al. Negative trials in nephrology: what can we learn? *Kidney Int.* 2008;74:1121.
106. Xue JL, St Peter WL, Ebben JP, et al. Anemia treatment in the pre-ESRD period and associated mortality in elderly patients. *Am J Kidney Dis.* 2002;40:1153.
107. Mocks J. Cardiovascular mortality in haemodialysis patients treated with epoetin beta - a retrospective study. *Nephron.* 2000;86:455.
108. Johansen KL, Finkelstein FO, Revicki DA, et al. Systematic review and meta-analysis of exercise tolerance and physical functioning in dialysis patients treated with erythropoiesis-stimulating agents. *Am J Kidney Dis.* 2010;55:535.
109. Parfrey PS, Lauve M, Latremouille-Viau D, et al. Erythropoietin therapy and left ventricular mass index in CKD and ESRD patients: a meta-analysis. *Clin J Am Soc Nephrol.* 2009;4:755.
110. Singh NP, Sahni V, Wadhwa A, et al. Effect of improvement in anemia on electroneurophysiological markers (P300) of cognitive dysfunction in chronic kidney disease. *Hemodial Int.* 2006;10:267.
111. Drueke TB, Locatelli F, Clyne N, et al. Normalization of hemoglobin level in patients with chronic kidney disease and anemia. *N Engl J Med.* 2006;355:2071.
112. Novak JE, Szczech LA. Triumph and tragedy: anemia management in chronic kidney disease. *Curr Opin Nephrol Hypertens.* 2008;17:580.
113. Singh AK, Szczech L, Tang KL, et al. Correction of anemia with epoetin alfa in chronic kidney disease. *N Engl J Med.* 2006;355:2085.
114. Pfeffer MA, Burdmann EA, Chen CY, et al. A trial of darbepoetin alfa in type 2 diabetes and chronic kidney disease. *N Engl J Med.* 2009;361:2019.
115. Besarab A, Goodkin DA, Nissenson AR. The normal hematocrit study—follow-up. *N Engl J Med.* 2008;358:433.
116. Phrommintikul A, Haas SJ, Elsik M, et al. Mortality and target haemoglobin concentrations in anaemic patients with chronic kidney disease treated with erythropoietin: a meta-analysis. *Lancet.* 2007;369:381.
117. Strippoli GF, Tognoni G, Navaneethan SD, et al. Haemoglobin targets: we were wrong, time to move on. *Lancet.* 2007;369:346.
118. Clement FM, Klarenbach S, Tonelli M, et al. The impact of selecting a high hemoglobin target level on health-related quality of life for patients with chronic kidney disease: a systematic review and meta-analysis. *Arch Intern Med.* 2009;169:1104.
119. Besarab A. Optimizing anaemia management with subcutaneous administration of epoetin. *Nephrol Dial Transplant.* 2005;20(Suppl 6):vi10–vi15.
120. Grzeszczak W, Sulowicz W, Rutkowski B, et al. The efficacy and safety of once-weekly and once-fortnightly subcutaneous epoetin beta in peritoneal dialysis patients with chronic renal anaemia. *Nephrol Dial Transplant.* 2005;20:936.
121. Weiss LG, Clyne N, Divino Fihlho J, et al. The efficacy of once weekly compared with two or three times weekly subcutaneous epoetin beta: results from a randomized controlled multicentre trial. Swedish Study Group. *Nephrol Dial Transplant.* 2000;15:2014.
122. Patel T, Hirter A, Kaufman J, et al. Route of epoetin administration influences hemoglobin variability in hemodialysis patients. *Am J Nephrol.* 2009;29:532.
123. Johnson DW, Pollock CA, Macdougall IC. Erythropoiesis-stimulating agent hyporesponsiveness. *Nephrology (Carlton).* 2007;12:321.
124. Elliott J, Mishler D, Agarwal R. Hyporesponsiveness to erythropoietin: causes and management. *Adv Chronic Kidney Dis.* 2009;16:94.
125. Kalantar-Zadeh K, Ikizler TA, Block G, et al. Malnutrition-inflammation complex syndrome in dialysis patients: causes and consequences. *Am J Kidney Dis.* 2003;42:864.
126. von Haehling S, Schefold JC, Lainscak M, et al. Inflammatory biomarkers in heart failure revisited: much more than innocent bystanders. *Heart Fail Clin.* 2009;5:549.
127. Kadiroglu AK, Kadiroglu ET, Sit D, et al. Periodontitis is an important and occult source of inflammation in hemodialysis patients. *Blood Purif.* 2006;24:400.
128. Movilli E, Cancarini GC, Vizzardi V, et al. Epoetin requirement does not depend on dialysis dose when Kt/N > 1.33 in patients on regular dialysis treatment with cellulosic membranes and adequate iron stores. *J Nephrol.* 2003;16:546.
129. Sitter T, Bergner A, Schiffl H. Dialysate related cytokine induction and response to recombinant human erythropoietin in haemodialysis patients. *Nephrol Dial Transplant.* 2000;15:1207.
130. Goicoechea M, Caramelo C, Rodriguez P, et al. Role of type of vascular access in erythropoietin and intravenous iron requirements in haemodialysis. *Nephrol Dial Transplant.* 2001;16:2188.
131. Roberts TL, Obrador GT, St Peter WL, et al. Relationship among catheter insertions, vascular access infections, and anemia management in hemodialysis patients. *Kidney Int.* 2004;66:2429.
132. Kinney R. 2005 Annual Report: ESRD Clinical Performance Measures Project. *Am J Kidney Dis.* 2006;48:S1.
133. Pollock C, Johnson DW, Horl WH, et al. Pure red cell aplasia induced by erythropoiesis-stimulating agents. *Clin J Am Soc Nephrol.* 2008;3:193.
134. Casadevall N, Nataf J, Viron B, et al. Pure red-cell aplasia and antierythropoietin antibodies in patients treated with recombinant erythropoietin. *N Engl J Med.* 2002;346:469.
135. Lee CT, Chou FF, Chang HW, et al. Effects of parathyroidectomy on iron homeostasis and erythropoiesis in hemodialysis patients with severe hyperparathyroidism. *Blood Purif.* 2003;21:369.
136. Rossert J, Gassmann-Mayer C, Frei D, et al. Prevalence and predictors of epoetin hyporesponsiveness in chronic kidney disease patients. *Nephrol Dial Transplant.* 2007;22:794.-
137. Provenzano R, Besarab A, Macdougall IC, et al. The continuous erythropoietin receptor activator (C.E.R.A.) corrects anemia at extended administration intervals in patients with chronic kidney disease not on dialysis: results of a phase II study. *Clin Nephrol.* 2007;67:306.
138. Sulowicz W, Locatelli F, Ryckelynck JP, et al. Once-monthly subcutaneous C.E.R.A. maintains stable hemoglobin control in patients with chronic kidney disease on dialysis and converted directly from epoetin one to three times weekly. *Clin J Am Soc Nephrol.* 2007;2:637.
139. Fan Q, Leuther KK, Holmes CP, et al. Preclinical evaluation of Hematide, a novel erythropoiesis stimulating agent, for the treatment of anemia. *Exp Hematol.* 2006;34:1303.
140. Macdougall IC, Rossert J, Casadevall N, et al. A peptide-based erythropoietin-receptor agonist for pure red-cell aplasia. *N Engl J Med.* 2009;361:1848.
141. Macdougall IC, Provenzano R, Pergola PE, et al. Primary results from two phase 3 randomized, active-controlled, open-label studies (PEARL 1 and PEARL 2) of the safety and efficacy of Hematide/peginesatide for the correction of anemia in patients with chronic renal failure not on dialysis and not receiving treatment with erythropoiesis-stimulating agents. *J Am Soc Nephrol Abstr.* 2010;21:2B.
142. Schiller B, Locatelli F, Covic AC, et al. Primary results from two phase 3 randomized, active-controlled, open-label studies (EMERALD 1 and EMERALD 2) of the safety and efficacy of Hematide/peginesatide for the maintenance treatment of anemia in patients with chronic renal failure who were receiving hemodialysis and were previously treated with epoetin alfa or epoetin beta. *J Am Soc Nephrol Abstr.* 2010;21:2B.
143. Fishbane S, Besarab A, Schiller B, et al. Results from a composite safety endpoint used to evaluate the cardiovascular safety of Hematide/peginesatide in patients with anemia due to chronic renal failure. *J Am Soc Nephrol Abstr.* 2010;21:1B.
144. Tanaka T, Nangaku M. The role of hypoxia, increased oxygen consumption, and hypoxia-inducible factor-1 alpha in progression of chronic kidney disease. *Curr Opin Nephrol Hypertens.* 2010;19:43.
145. Bernhardt WM, Wiesener MS, Scigalla P, et al. Inhibition of prolyl hydroxylases increases erythropoietin production in ESRD. *J Am Soc Nephrol.* 2010;21:2151.
146. Nakano Y, Imagawa S, Matsumoto K, et al. Oral administration of K-11706 inhibits GATA binding activity, enhances hypoxia-inducible factor 1 binding activity, and restores indicators in an in vivo mouse model of anemia of chronic disease. *Blood.* 2004;104:4300.
147. Akagi S, Ichikawa H, Okada T, et al. The critical role of SRC homology domain 2-containing tyrosine phosphatase-1 in recombinant human erythropoietin hyporesponsive anemia in chronic hemodialysis patients. *J Am Soc Nephrol.* 2004;15:3215.
148. Hayat A. Safety issues with intravenous iron products in the management of anemia in chronic kidney disease. *Clin Med Res.* 2008;6:93.
149. Coyne DW, Kapoian T, Suki W, et al. Ferric gluconate is highly efficacious in anemic hemodialysis patients with high serum ferritin and low transferrin saturation: results of the Dialysis Patients' Response to IV Iron with Elevated Ferritin (DRIVE) Study. *J Am Soc Nephrol.* 2007;18:975.
150. Kapoian T, O'Mara NB, Singh AK, et al. Ferric gluconate reduces epoetin requirements in hemodialysis patients with elevated ferritin. *J Am Soc Nephrol.* 2008;19:372.

151. Nissenson AR, Berns JS, Sakiewicz P, et al. Clinical evaluation of heme iron polypeptide: sustaining a response to rHuEPO in hemodialysis patients. *Am J Kidney Dis.* 2003;42:325.
152. Macdougall IC. Iron supplementation in the non-dialysis chronic kidney disease (ND-CKD) patient: oral or intravenous? *Curr Med Res Opin.* 2010;26:473.
153. Johnson DW. Intravenous versus oral iron supplementation in peritoneal dialysis patients. *Perit Dial Int.* 2007;27(Suppl 2):S255.
154. Yee J, Besarab A. Iron sucrose: the oldest iron therapy becomes new. *Am J Kidney Dis.* 2002;40:1111.
155. Barraclough KA, Noble E, Leary D, et al. Rationale and design of the oral HEMe iron polypeptide Against Treatment with Oral Controlled Release Iron Tablets trial for the correction of anaemia in peritoneal dialysis patients (HEMATOCRIT trial). *BMC Nephrol.* 2009;10:20.
156. Singh A. Hemoglobin control, ESA resistance, and regular low-dose IV iron therapy: a review of the evidence. *Semin Dial.* 2009;22:64.
157. Besarab A. Resolving the paradigm crisis in intravenous iron and erythropoietin management. *Kidney Int Suppl.* 2006;69:S13.
158. Auerbach M, Al Talib K. Low-molecular weight iron dextran and iron sucrose have similar comparative safety profiles in chronic kidney disease. *Kidney Int.* 2008;73:528.
159. Chertow GM, Mason PD, Vaage-Nilsen O, et al. Update on adverse drug events associated with parenteral iron. *Nephrol Dial Transplant.* 2006;21:378.
160. Chandler G, Harchowal J, Macdougall IC. Intravenous iron sucrose: establishing a safe dose. *Am J Kidney Dis.* 2001;38:988.
161. George P, Das J, Pawar B, et al. Coronary artery vasospasm with iron sucrose. *Nephrol Dial Transplant.* 2007;22:1795.
162. Bishu K, Agarwal R. Acute injury with intravenous iron and concerns regarding long-term safety. *Clin J Am Soc Nephrol.* 2006;1(Suppl 1):S19.
163. Agarwal R, Rizkala AR, Kaskas MO, et al. Iron sucrose causes greater proteinuria than ferric gluconate in non-dialysis chronic kidney disease. *Kidney Int.* 2007;72:638.
164. Agarwal R, Vasavada N, Sachs NG, et al. Oxidative stress and renal injury with intravenous iron in patients with chronic kidney disease. *Kidney Int.* 2004;65:2279.
165. Leehey DJ, Palubiak DJ, Chebrolu S, et al. Sodium ferric gluconate causes oxidative stress but not acute renal injury in patients with chronic kidney disease: a pilot study. *Nephrol Dial Transplant.* 2005;20:135.
166. Zager RA, Johnson AC, Hanson SY, et al. Parenteral iron formulations: a comparative toxicologic analysis and mechanisms of cell injury. *Am J Kidney Dis.* 2002;40:90.
167. Roob JM, Khoschsorur G, Tiran A, et al. Vitamin E attenuates oxidative stress induced by intravenous iron in patients on hemodialysis. *J Am Soc Nephrol.* 2000;11:539.
168. Aronoff GR, Bennett WM, Blumenthal S, et al. Iron sucrose in hemodialysis patients: safety of replacement and maintenance regimens. *Kidney Int.* 2004;66:1193.
169. Furuland H, Linde T, Ahlmen J, et al. A randomized controlled trial of haemoglobin normalization with epoetin alfa in pre-dialysis and dialysis patients. *Nephrol Dial Transplant.* 2003;18:353.
170. Zhu L, Glahn RP, Nelson D, et al. Comparing soluble ferric pyrophosphate to common iron salts and chelates as sources of bioavailable iron in a Caco-2 cell culture model. *J Agric Food Chem.* 2009;57:5014.
171. Shivakumar HN, Vaka SR, Murthy SN. Albumin microspheres for oral delivery of iron. *J Drug Target.* 2010;18:36.
172. Sarkate P, Patil A, Parulekar S, et al. A randomised double-blind study comparing sodium feredetate with ferrous fumarate in anaemia in pregnancy. *J Indian Med Assoc.* 2007;105:278.
173. Ruiz-Arguelles GJ, Diaz-Hernandez A, Manzano C, et al. Ineffectiveness of oral iron hydroxide polymaltose in iron-deficiency anemia. *Hematology.* 2007;12:255.
174. Schwenk MH. Ferumoxytol: a new intravenous iron preparation for the treatment of iron deficiency anemia in patients with chronic kidney disease. *Pharmacotherapy.* 2010;30:70.
175. Lyseng-Williamson KA, Keating GM. Ferric carboxymaltose: a review of its use in iron-deficiency anaemia. *Drugs.* 2009;69:739.
176. Szczech LA, Bregman DB, Harrington RA, et al. Randomized evaluation of efficacy and safety of ferric carboxymaltose in patients with iron deficiency anaemia and impaired renal function (REPAIR-IDA): rationale and study design. *Nephrol Dial Transplant.* 2010;25:2368.
177. Gozzard D. When is high-dose intravenous iron repletion needed? Assessing new treatment options. *Drug Des Devel Ther.* 2011;5:51.
178. Wikström B, Bhandari S, Barany P, et al. Iron isomaltoside 1000: a new intravenous iron for treating iron deficiency in chronic kidney disease. *J Nephrol.* 2011;24:589.

CHAPTER 77

Mineral and Bone Disorder in Chronic Kidney Disease

Elvira O. Gosmanova • Darryl L. Quarles

Historically, renal osteodystrophy (ROD) was a term used to describe the metabolic bone disease caused by abnormalities in mineral homeostasis resulting from kidney failure.[1] In recent years, the recognition of a complex endocrine regulation of mineral and bone metabolism, the prominent extra skeletal manifestations of chronic kidney disease (CKD), and the association between abnormalities in mineral metabolism and increased morbidity and mortality in patients with kidney failure led to formulation of a new term—chronic kidney disease–mineral and bone disorder (CKD-MBD) (Table 77.1)[1]—which describes a broader clinical syndrome, including metabolic/endocrine abnormalities, parathyroid gland dysfunction, bone disease, and unique CKD-associated cardiovascular risk factors as well as other adverse clinical outcomes, such as fractures and vascular and soft tissue calcifications (Fig. 77.1). In this chapter we review separate components of CKD-MBD, clinical manifestations, and general principles of CKD-MBD treatment.

Four organ systems, including the *gut* (absorption of calcium [Ca] and inorganic phosphate [Pi]), *kidneys* (reabsorption and excretion of Ca, Pi, and calcitriol synthesis), *bones* (interchange of Ca and Pi with extracellular pool, and FGF23 secretion), and *parathyroid gland* (parathyroid hormone [PTH] secretion) are involved in regulating mineral homeostasis[2] and each play a role in the pathogenesis of CKD-MBD (Fig. 77.2).

BIOCHEMICAL ABNORMALITIES IN CKD-MBD

Calcium

There are three Ca pools in our body. The majority of Ca (99%) is found in bone. The remaining Ca is either intracellular (mostly protein bound), and extracellular (45% protein bound and 55% free calcium). PTH is a key regulator of serum calcium levels. The extracellular Ca concentration is tightly regulated by changes in PTH through sensing of calcium by the calcium-sensing receptor (CaSR)[3] and through actions of PTH on bone and kidney. In turn, Ca controls PTH secretion, synthesis, and degradation as well as parathyroid cell hypertrophy and hyperplasia.[4,5] PTH directly regulates the excretion of Ca by the kidney and also influences the exchange between bone and extracellular pools. PTH stimulates gut calcium absorption indirectly through the stimulation of $1,25(OH)_2D_3$ production by the kidney, which in turn activates calcium absorption through vitamin D receptor (VDR)-dependent mechanisms. Decrements in $1,25(OH)_2 D_3$ levels occur prior to elevations of PTH during the progressive loss of glomerular filtration rate (GFR). The increments in PTH maintain serum calcium concentrations in the normal range until late in the course of CKD (Fig. 77.3A,B).[6]

Phosphorus

Pi is required for cellular function and skeletal mineralization and excess phosphate is associated with soft tissue and vascular calcifications. Serum Pi level is less tightly regulated than Ca, but is maintained in normal range through a complex interplay between intestinal absorption, exchange with intracellular and bone storage pools, and renal tubular reabsorption. Pi is abundant in the diet, and intestinal absorption of Pi is stimulated by $1,25(OH)_2D$. The kidney is a major regulator of Pi homeostasis, where increases or decreases in its Pi reabsorptive capacity under the control of various hormones determine serum Pi levels. The crucial regulated step in Pi homeostasis is the transport of Pi across the renal proximal tubule via the type II sodium-dependent phosphate (Na/Pi) cotransporter 2a (NPT2a) and 2c (NPT2c). PTH and FGF23 are the two principal hormones that regulate NPT2 translocation to the proximal tubular brush border membrane. PTH inhibits renal phosphate reabsorption due to reductions in membrane expression of NPT2. FGF23, a bone-derived hormone originally identified as the causative factor in inherited and acquired hypophosphatemic disorders also inhibits proximal tubular phosphate transport through mechanisms that remain to be defined. Increments in FGF23 appear to precede elevations of PTH in CKD, but both work in concert to prevent elevations in serum Pi by increasing renal phosphate excretion.[6–14] Like Ca, serum Pi levels remain in the normal range until late in the course of

TABLE 77.1 Classification of Chronic Kidney Disease: Mineral and Bone Disorder

CKD-MBD is either one or combination of the following:
- Abnormalities of calcium, phosphorus, PTH, or vitamin D metabolism, as measured by laboratory values
- Abnormalities in bone turnover, mineralization, volume, linear growth, or strength, as measured mainly by bone histology
- Vascular or other soft tissue calcifications

CKD-MBD, chronic kidney disease–mineral and bone disorder; PTH, parathyroid hormone.
Adopted from KDIGO clinical practice guideline for the diagnosis, evaluation, prevention, and treatment of Chronic Kidney Disease-Mineral and Bone Disorder (CKD-MBD). *Kidney Int Suppl.* 2009;(113):S1–130.

CKD, typically when glomerular filtration rate (GFR) is <30 to 40 mL/min/m^2.[6,8,11,15]

Vitamin D

Decrements in both 25(OH)D and 1,25$(OH)_2$D occur early in the course of CKD-MBD. Low levels of vitamin D are associated with increased mortality in CKD and treatment with vitamin D analogues are believed to have a survival benefit.[16] The mechanism for decreased circulating 25(OH)D levels in CKD are not well understood, but may result from poor nutritional status caused by chronic illness. Patients with CKD, however, may also be refractory to nutritional vitamin D supplementation, suggesting other mechanisms for decreased 25(OH)D levels.

1,25$(OH)_2D_3$, the active form of vitamin D, is synthesized from 25 (OH)D by 1α-hydroxylase- cytochrome P450, family 27, subfamily B, polypeptide 1(CYP27B1) located in the kidney proximal tubule. CYP27B1 is stimulated by PTH and inhibited by FGF23. Both 25(OH)D and 1,25$(OH)_2$D are catabolized by 25-hydroxyvitamin $D_3$24-hydroxylase (CYP24), which is also present in the proximal tubule. CYP24 is stimulated by FGF23 and inhibited by PTH. Decrements in 1,25$(OH)_2$D occur early in CKD. Diminished 1,25$(OH)_2$D levels are seen with early GFR decline to less than 60 to 70 mL/min/m^2 and are inversely related to elevation in FGF23.[8] The reductions in 1,25$(OH)_2$D in CKD were thought to be the result of reduced production of this hormone caused by the diseased kidney, but more recently it has been recognized that the suppression of 1,25$(OH)_2$D production is a regulated process due to the effects of FGF23 on CYP27B1-mediated production and/or CYP24–mediated degradation of 1,25$(OH)_2$D.[17–19] Reduced GFR can additionally contribute to 1,25$(OH)_2$D deficiency via decrease in renal uptake of 25-hydroxyvitamin D by proximal tubular cells for its activation to 1,25$(OH)_2$D through decrease in amount of filtered 25-hydroxyvitamin D bound to vitamin D-binding protein available for uptake. Moreover, CKD leads to a decrease in kidney megalin content that is essential for the internalization of 25-hydroxyvitamin D into proximal tubular cells.[20]

The principal functions of 1,25$(OH)_2$D are to promote active intestinal absorption of Ca and Pi, suppress PTH gene transcription in the parathyroid gland, stimulate bone formation and resorption in bone, as well as regulate the innate immune response in other tissues. Alterations in 1,25$(OH)_2$D directly suppresses PTH gene expression through a genomic action[21] via VDR on parathyroid cells. 1,25$(OH)_2$D also indirectly regulates parathyroid gland function through elevations in serum calcium and stimulation of CaSR. Mouse genetic studies suggest that CaSR is dominant to VDR in regulation of parathyroid gland function, because calcium exerts PTH and VDR regulation in absence of any vitamin D source,[22] whereas ablation of VDR in the parathyroid gland results in hyperparathyroidism that can be rescued by raising serum calcium levels.[23,24] Several additional factors lead to impaired action of 1,25$(OH)_2$D on parathyroid gland in uremia, such as diminished activation of VDR with reduced 1,25$(OH)_2$D levels in CKD, and decrease in parathyroid VDR content, especially when nodular parathyroid hyperplasia is present.

FGF23

Elevations in circulating FGF23 levels are one of the earliest abnormalities in CKD-MBD and are strongly associated with increased all-cause mortality.[25,26] Elevations of FGF23

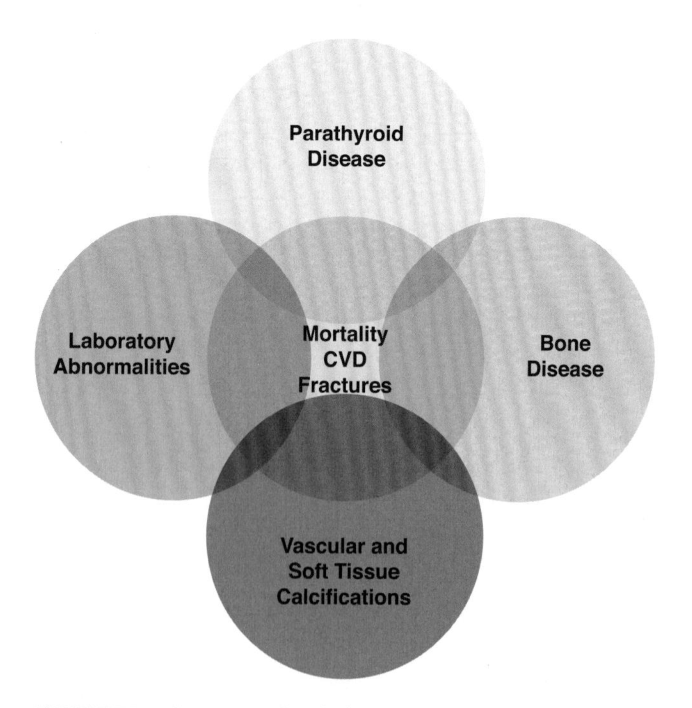

FIGURE 77.1 Spectrum of pathology in chronic kidney disease–mineral and bone disorder. (Modified from KDIGO clinical practice guideline for the diagnosis, evaluation, prevention, and treatment of Chronic Kidney Disease-Mineral and Bone Disorder (CKD-MBD). *Kidney Int Suppl.* 2009;(113):S1–130.)

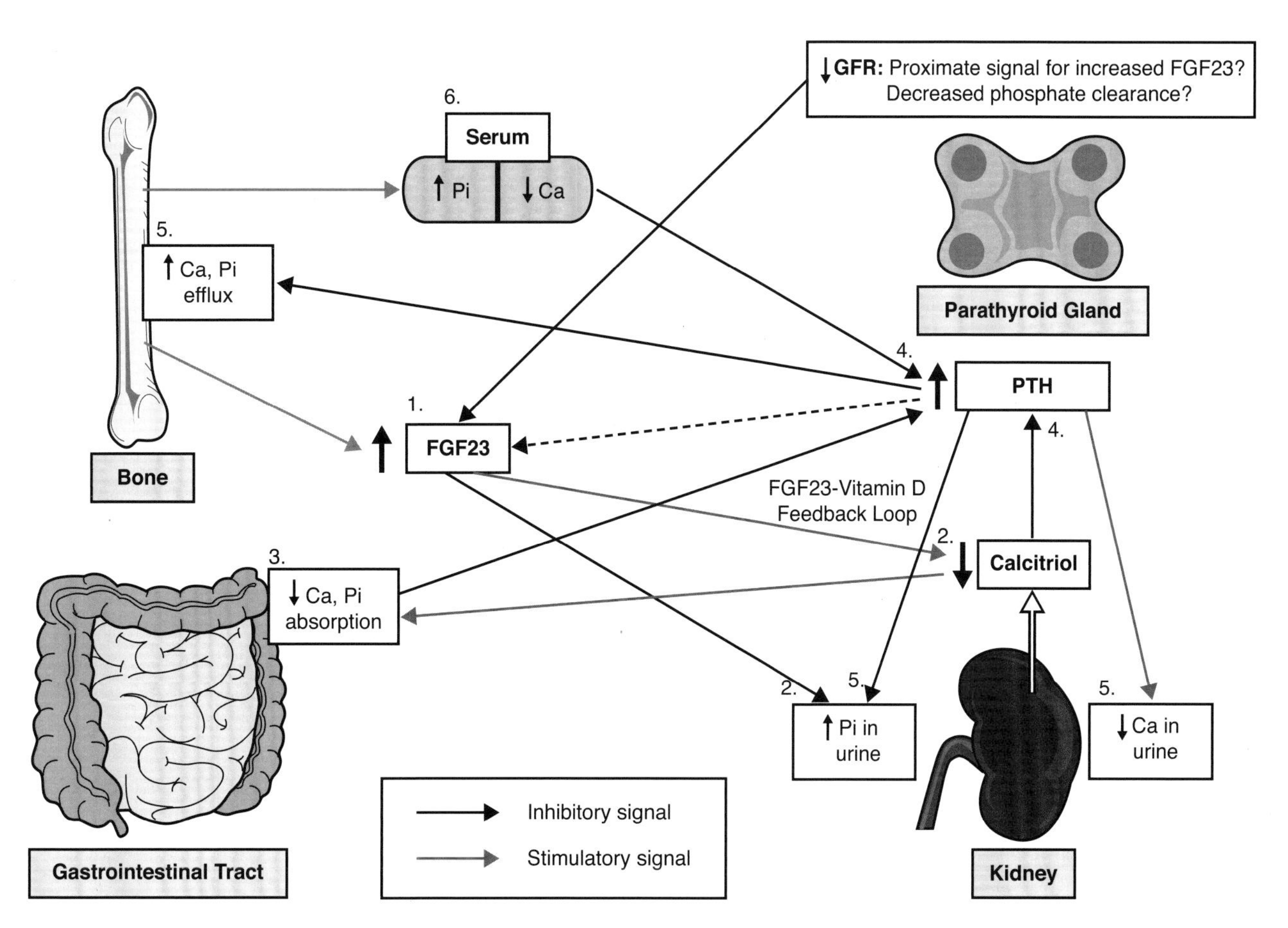

FIGURE 77.2 The schematic representation of chronic kidney disease–mineral and bone disorder pathogenesis. *Ca,* calcium; *Pi,* phosphorus. 1, Increase in FGF23; 2, suppression of calcitriol and increased urinary phosphate; 3, decreased gastrointestinal calcium and phosphorus absorption; 4, increased parathyroid hormone; 5, increased bone resorption/calcium and phosphorus bone efflux; increased phosphorus and decreased calcium in urine; 6, maintenance of serum phosphorus and calcium in normal range until stage V chronic kidney disease.

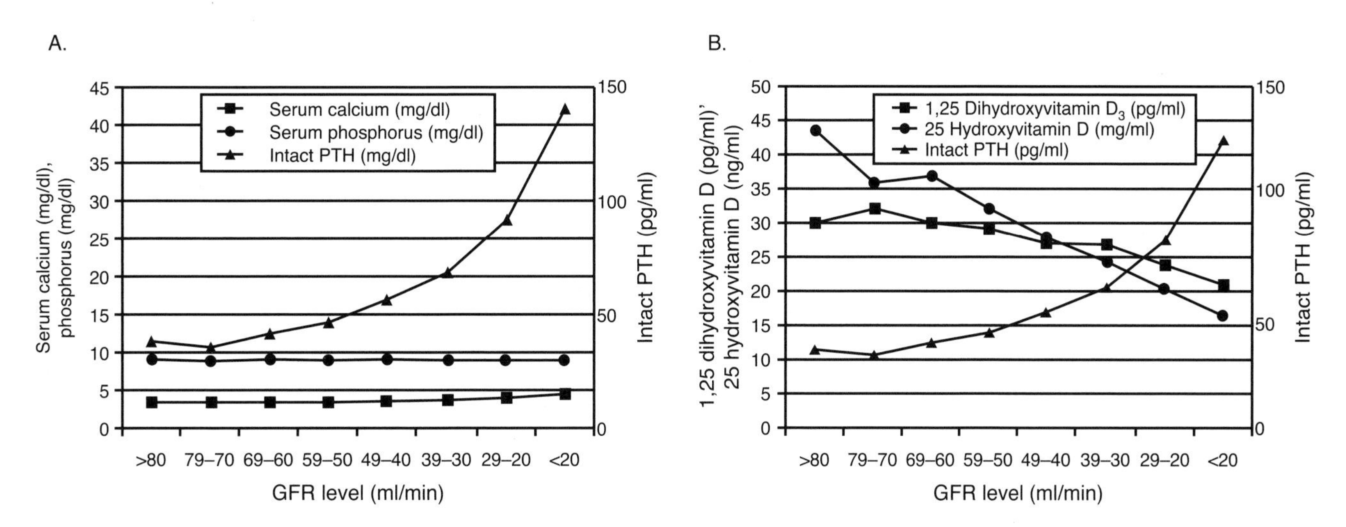

FIGURE 77.3 Relationship between glomerular filtration rate (GFR) and parathyroid hormone (PTH), calcium, phosphorus, and calcitriol levels in patients with chronic kidney disease. **A:** Median values of serum calcium, phosphorus, and intact PTH by GFR levels. **B:** Median values of 1,25-dihydroxyvitamin D, 25-hydroxyvitamin D, and intact PTH by GFR levels. (Adopted from Levin A, Bakris GL, Molitch M, et al. Prevalence of abnormal serum vitamin D, PTH, calcium, and phosphorus in patients with chronic kidney disease: results of the study to evaluate early kidney disease. *Kidney Int.* 2007;71(1):31–38.)

inversely correlate with GFR.[8,27–29] Patients with end-stage renal disease (ESRD) have markedly elevated levels of FGF23 that parallels with degree of hyperphosphatemia[30] and secondary hyperparathyroidism (SHPT).[31]

FGF23 is a 32-kDa protein with an N-terminal region containing the FGF-homology domain and a novel 71-amino acid C terminus[32,33] that interacts with FGF receptor (FGFR) in the presence of the members of Klotho family of proteins.[34,35] In vitro studies indicate that Klotho is an essential cofactor for FGF23 to activate FGFR.[34,36,37] Circulating FGF23 is mainly produced and secreted by osteoblasts and osteocytes in bone.[38] The target organs for FGF23 are defined by the coexpression of the membrane form of Klotho and FGFR.[37,39] Klotho is expressed in high levels in parathyroid gland, kidney, and several other organs; however, the kidney is the principal physiologically defined target for FGF23, where it inhibits phosphate reabsorption and $1,25(OH)_2D$ synthesis. The parathyroid gland is also a target for FGF23 action, but it is not clear if FGF23 stimulates or inhibits PTH secretion. Elevated levels of FGF23 in human disease and mouse models are associated with hyperparathyroidism (HPT),[40,41] likely due to the effect of FGF23 to suppress $1,25(OH)_2D$ leading to the secondary development of HPT. In contrast, in vitro studies demonstrated that FGF23 activates extracellular regulated kinases 1/2 - *Egr-1* pathway leading to inhibition of PTH mRNA expression and PTH secretion from parathyroid cells.[42,43] Additionally, FGF23 suppresses parathyroid cell proliferation and increases CaSR and VDR expression in normal parathyroid gland.[44] In individuals with normal kidney function, FGF23 exerts negative feedback on the parathyroid gland; however, the fact that in CKD patients PTH remains high despite elevated FGF23 suggests the presence of resistance to FGF23 action. This possibility was reinforced by a finding of a reduced Klotho and FGFR expression in surgically removed parathyroid glands from uremic patients.[42]

The mechanism of increased FGF23 in CKD is poorly understood. The increase in serum FGF23 is not explained by reduced FGF23 clearance; and the proximate stimulus in early CKD that leads to increments in FGF23 are not clear. Nevertheless, FGF23 production is likely increased to counteract Pi retention due to reduced nephron mass by promoting urinary Pi excretion.[45] Elevations in FGF23 precede increments in PTH in CKD[46] and animal studies show that blockade of FGF23 by neutralizing antibodies lead to normalization of $1,25(OH)_2D$ and PTH levels in models of CKD.[47] On the other hand, there is also strong evidence supporting the ability of PTH to stimulate FGF23 expression in bone in patients with CKD. In this regard, parathyroidectomy reduces FGF23 in humans with ESRD and animal models of kidney failure.[48,49] Recent studies also demonstrate the ability of PTH to directly stimulate FGF23 expression in osteoblast cultures and overexpression of a constitutively active PTH stimulates FGF23 expression in bone of transgenic mice. Regardless, the discovery and elucidation of FGF23 functions as phosphaturic[50,51] and $1,25(OH)_2D$ counter-regulatory hormone[8,10,51] provided new insight for the understanding of SHPT. Primary decrease in Pi excretion due to loss of functioning renal mass when GFR falls below ~70 mL/min/m^2 somehow leads to increase in FGF23 secretion from bone, which in turn inhibits renal Pi reabsorption and suppresses production of $1,25(OH)_2D$.[52] Reduction in $1,25(OH)_2D$, leads to increase in PTH production.[12] Both PTH and elevated FGF23 work in concert to increase Pi excretion and to maintain normal serum Pi. Further loss of renal function and elevations of PTH further stimulate FGF23 in an abnormal positive feed forward loop.

Parathyroid Hormone

As noted previously, elevations in PTH occur early in the course of CKD, just after increments in FGF23 and decrements in $1,25(OH)_2D$ and before demonstrable alterations in serum calcium and phosphate levels.

PTH actions are mediated through PTH receptor (PTH1R) in the kidney—which inhibits renal Pi reabsorption, increases renal tubular calcium excretion, and increases $1,25(OH)_2D$ production—and in osteoblasts in bone, which stimulates bone formation and osteoclastic bone resorption.[53] Chronic elevation of PTH in SHPT leads to increased bone remodeling which plays a crucial role in mineral homeostasis by providing access to the stores in bones' Ca and Pi. PTH orchestrates a coordinated process of increased bone resorption by osteoclasts followed by new bone formation by osteoblasts. PTH stimulates osteoclast formation indirectly by binding to its receptor (PTH1R) on osteoblastic cells. This in turn triggers production of receptor activator of NFkB ligand (RANKL) and suppresses the RANKL decoy receptor osteoprotegerin (OPG), thereby stimulating maturation of osteocytes by RANKL.[54] PTH also increases osteoblast number and activity, possibly through release of growth factors from bone matrix during its resorption, although the mechanism is not entirely understood.[55] However, the net result of these changes by continuous PTH stimulation in SHPT is the loss of cortical bone and increased bone fragility. Additionally, PTH was implicated in reduced red cell production by causing marked bone marrow fibrosis.[56] Interestingly, PTH can exert anabolic or catabolic action on the bone depending on whether it acts on the bone in continuous or pulsatile fashion. Intermittent administration of PTH inhibits osteoblast apoptosis and increases osteoblast number, whereas chronic administration of PTH increases mostly osteoclast number.[57] The PTH1R is also found in nonclassical PTH target tissues such as breast, skin, heart, blood vessels, liver, and other tissues.

PTH is secreted as linear protein consisting of 84 amino acids also called intact PTH (iPTH). Interaction of the 1–34 amino acid N-terminal portion of PTH is required for activation of PTH1R. In addition to full length PTH, other PTH fragment are produced from 1–84 PTH in parathyroid gland and the liver, such as bioactive N-terminal fragment (1–34), as well as various C-terminal fragments that are found in blood.

There is increase in half-life of circulating PTH and especially C-terminal fragments observed in serum of patients with uremia, possibly due to reduced clearance as the kidney is one of the principal sites for the degradation of PTH and its fragments. Patients with advanced CKD also exhibit abnormal ratio in serum between circulating 1–84 PTH and its fragments as compared with healthy controls.[58] Conventional two-site immunoassays for intact (1–84) PTH can register long N-truncated C terminal PTH fragments that lack full N terminal region (1–34) necessary for PTH1R activation. These long N-truncated C terminal fragments accumulate disproportionally to 1–84 PTH in kidney failure and may constitute up to 50% or more to total PTH immunoreactivity, as compared to 15% to 20% in normal subjects. Some of these fragments have been identified as 7–84 PTH and studies in animal models demonstrated that 7–84 PTH can antagonize effects of 1–84 PTH on increased bone turnover and serum Ca levels.[59] It has been documented that patients with CKD have impaired serum Ca response to PTH and higher PTH levels are required to maintain eucalcemia. Several possible explanations of bone PTH resistance include presence of inhibitors, such as 7–84 PTH and elevated osteoprotegerin, as well as downregulation of *PTH1R mRNA* in animal models and patients with CKD.[60,61]

As noted previously, CaSR is the major regulator of PTH secretion and production as well as parathyroid gland hyperplasia. VDR plays an important modulating role on PTH gene transcription. Hyperphosphatemia may stimulate PTH secretion independently from low Ca or $1,25(OH)_2D$[62, 63] through poorly defined posttranslational mechanisms.[21,64,65]

Clinical Significance of Abnormal Biochemistries in Chronic Kidney Disease

The growing body of evidence links disordered values of all CKD-MBD laboratory markers and all-cause and cardiovascular mortality in patients with CKD. In the international study of ESRD patients, lowest mortality was observed for Ca at 8.6 to 10.0 mg per dL, corrected to albumin Ca of 7.6 to 9.5 mg per dL, phosphorus at 3.6 to 5.0 mg/dL, and PTH between 101 and 300 pg per mL, with the highest mortality for Ca or corrected to albumin Ca levels greater than 10.0 mg per dL, Pi levels greater than 7.0 mg per dL, and PTH levels greater than 600 pg per mL.[66] However, recent meta-analysis challenged the association between levels of Ca and PTH and all-cause or cardiovascular mortality, whereas still strongly supporting the association between rising levels of Pi and these outcomes.[67] There is also an evidence of possible nonlinear U-shape or J-shape association between levels of Ca, Pi, PTH, and mortality with both very low and high levels predicting poor outcomes.[68,69] FGF23 has also been strongly linked in several large observational studies to all-cause mortality in CKD patients both with earlier stages not requiring renal replacement therapy (RRT) as well as hemodialysis.[25,26,70] Additionally, higher FGF23 levels are associated with the faster progression of CKD to need of RRT.[70–72] The strong adverse association between disordered markers of CKD-MBD and mortality and risk of ESRD progression necessitates the need of clinical control studies aiming to improve these outcomes in CKD patients.

BONE ABNORMALITIES

Bone is central to the pathogenesis of CKD-MBD because it is: (1) a reservoir for calcium and phosphate; (2) a target for PTH, which activates PTH receptors located in osteoblasts to increase osteoblast-mediated bone resorption and to stimulate osteoclast mediated bone resorption through the release of Rank ligand; (3) a target for 1,25(OH)2D, which binds to VDR:RXR complexes to activate gene transcription in both osteoblasts and osteoclasts; and (4) the principal source of the phosphaturic and VDR hormone FGF23, which is made by osteoblasts and osteocytes.

Renal osteodystrophy (ROD) is a general term to describe the variety of skeletal histologic abnormalities that result from the changes in hormones and calcium/phosphate homeostasis in CKD.[73] The classification of ROD is based on quantitative bone histomorphometric analysis of bone biopsy that measures bone turnover (i.e., bone formation rates and resorption), mineralization of extracellular matrix, and trabecular bone volume and cortical porosity) (Tables 77.2 and 77.3). Based on the degree of bone remodeling and mineralization abnormalities, bone biopsy diagnoses typically include osteitis fibrosa cystica (characterized by excessive PTH-mediated increases in bone formation and resorption accompanied by peritrabecular fibrosis, woven osteoid, and increased cortical porosity), osteomalacia (characterized by excess unmineralized osteoid and prolonged mineralization lag time), and adynamic bone (characterized by severely diminished bone formation and resorption). Milder forms of these abnormalities can occur and combinations of abnormal bone turnover and mineralization can occur (referred to as mixed uremic osteodystrophy). Additionally, cortical osteopenia due to excess PTH and osteoporosis due to loss of trabecular bone volume can be found in CKD and lead to increased fracture risks. Other systemic abnormalities leading to skeletal abnormalities such as β_2–microglobulin amyloidosis and acidosis induced demineralization can also occur in patients with CKD.

The majority of epidemiologic data on ROD were obtained from cross-sectional analysis of bone biopsies in predialysis patients or patients on RRT; therefore, accurate data on patients with earlier stages of CKD are uncertain. The reported prevalence of ROD in CKD stage 4 and 5 ranges from 62% to 100%[5]; however, given the importance of bone remodeling as a target for PTH and 1,25(OH)2D in the maintenance of calcium metabolism, virtually all patients in the late stages of CKD would be expected to have high turnover ROD, either osteitis fibrosa (OF) or mixed uremic osteodystrophy (MUO).[74]

TABLE 77.2 Classification of Bone Disease in Chronic Kidney Disease Patients

Renal Osteodystrophy
High-turnover bone disease (represented by increased bone formation rate, increased osteoblastic/osteoclastic activity and number, reduced osteoid volume, and high peritrabecular fibrosis surface area) ■ Osteitis fibrosa (associated with severe hyperparathyroidism) ■ Mild disease (associated with mild to moderate hyperparathyroidism)
Low-turnover bone disease (low bone formation rate is characterized as being equal to or below the lower value observed in normal individuals) ■ Osteomalacia (defined as markedly increased osteoid volume and thickness with decreased fibrosis and defective bone mineralization) ■ Adynamic bone disease (characterized by paucity of bone cells with severely reduced osteoid seams and absence of fibrosis)
Mixed uremic osteodystrophy (includes findings of increased osteoid volume and fibrosis surfaces and may present with different degrees of bone formation rate that vary from high to normal and low)
Osteopenia and Osteoporosis
Other Causes of Bone Pathology in CKD
■ Acidosis ■ β_2–microglobulin amyloidosis

CKD, chronic kidney disease.
Adopted from Sprague SM. The role of the bone biopsy in the diagnosis of renal osteodystrophy. *Semin Dial*. 2000;13(3):152–155.

TABLE 77.3 TMV Classification System for Renal Osteodystrophy

Turnover	Mineralization	Volume
Low	Normal	Low
Normal	Abnormal	Normal
High		High

TMV, bone turnover, mineralization, and volume.
Adopted from Moe S, Drueke T, Cunningham J, et al. Definition, evaluation, and classification of renal osteodystrophy: a position statement from Kidney Disease: Improving Global Outcomes (KDIGO). *Kidney Int*. 2006;69(11):1945–1953.

Although data are incomplete, the epidemiology of ROD appears to have changed in the last three decades, with a decline of OF and a higher prevalence of low bone remodeling states of uncertain clinical significance and etiology. Types of ROD also vary depending whether or not the patient already started RRT and on modality of RRT, with low turnover bone remodeling being the most common lesion in predialysis patients (27%–48%) and patients on peritoneal dialysis (48%–62%), whereas OF (32%–37%) and low turnover bone remodeling (32%–36%) occur with similar frequency in hemodialysis patients. Mixed disease represents about 10% to 13% of cases of ROD, and low turnover osteomalacia is present in 3% to 8% of patients. We lack diagnostic tools to accurately assess bone remodeling and mineralization, other than bone biopsy, making it difficult to determine the type and magnitude of bone abnormalities in an individual patient with CKD.

When GFR declines below 60 mL/min/m^2,[75] excess PTH and decrements in 1,25$(OH)_2$D are the major factors leading to abnormalities of high bone remodeling and abnormal mineralization in CKD that characterize OF and MUO. The pathogenesis of PTH and 1,25$(OH)_2$D alterations in CKD were discussed earlier in this chapter.

Low turnover bone disease is at the opposite end of the bone remodeling spectrum and is characterized by a diminished bone formation rate, a paucity of bone cells, an absence of fibrosis, and an abnormal bone mineralization. Adynamic bone disease (ABD) and osteomalacia are variants of low turnover bone disease in CKD. A reduction in the osteoid accumulation and number of bone remodeling sites are predominant features of ABD, which represent a primary defect in osteoblast-mediated bone formation or osteoclast-mediated bone resorption, whereas increased relative osteoid defines the presence of osteomalacia, which is a primary defect in the mineralization of extracellular matrix.

The cause of low turnover bone disease in CKD is poorly understood and it is likely to be a multifactorial condition. First reports of low turnover bone disease were osteomalacic lesions associated with aluminum toxicity; however, it was quickly recognized that low turnover bone disease can occur without aluminum accumulation in the bone. Presently, the emphasis on pathogenesis of ABD in CKD is placed on oversuppression of circulating PTH levels and concomitant skeletal resistance to PTH actions due to downregulation of PTH1R. Exposure to high Ca through the use of Ca-containing phosphate binders and dialysate with high Ca is a risk factor for ABD. Metabolic acidosis and uremia-induced oxidative stress are additional CKD-related risk factors that can induce low turnover bone disease via suppression of active vitamin D and collagen synthesis and reduction of osteoblast life span, respectively.[76] An advanced age, presence of diabetes,

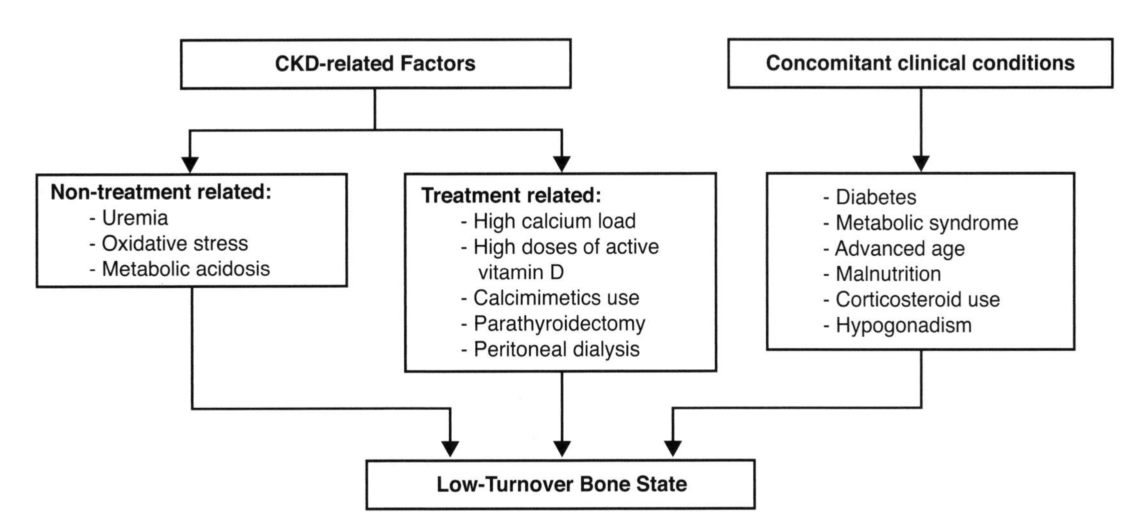

FIGURE 77.4 Low-turnover bone state risk factors.

hypogonadism, and a treatment with corticosteroids are also important clinical conditions associated with low turnover bone disease.[77] There is growing evidence linking ABD to the malnutrition-inflammation complex syndrome. Higher rates of ABD are reported in peritoneal dialysis patients with low albumin levels.[78] Additionally, several proinflammatory cytokines such as interleukin-1β and interleukin-6 were shown to inhibit PTH secretion in vitro.[79,80] Therefore, the development of ABD is influenced by patient characteristics, as well as treatment options for CKD-MBD (Fig. 77.4).

PTH is the most widely used surrogate marker of bone turnover (Table 77.4). Although relatively low to normal iPTH levels (<50–100 pg per mL) in ESRD patients are associated with biopsy proven ABD, higher iPTH levels (>300 pg per mL) can be also be seen in patients with biopsy-proven ABD,[81] especially in African Americans.[82,83] There are several proposed explanations of this variability of iPTH levels and ABD. First, iPTH assays and their ability to discriminate between whole PTH and its fragments differ across the studies. Some PTH fragments, such as 7–84PTH, can be actually inhibitory on bone formation and these fragments tend to accumulate in ESRD; therefore, higher PTH may not be equivalent of presence of high biointact PTH. Additionally, treatment modalities

TABLE 77.4 Factors Regulating Parathyroid Hormone Secretion

Factor	Mechanism
Decreased PTH secretion	
Calcium	Direct activation of CaSR leading to posttranslational decrease in PTH secretion
Calcitriol	Direct inhibition of *preproPTH* gene transcription via VDR
	Indirect inhibition via increase in CaSR in parathyroid gland
FGF23	Direct inhibition of *PTH mRNA* expression
Increased PTH secretion	
High phosphorus	Posttranslational increase in PTH via stabilization of *PTH mRNA*
Low calcium	Indirectly via increase in unbound to calcium calreticulin that inhibits calcitriol action on PTH secretion
	Direct decrease in activation of CaSR
FGF23	Indirect increase in PTH secretion through decrease in calcitriol synthesis

PTH, parathyroid hormone; CaSR, calcium-sensing receptor; VDR, vitamin D receptor.

may influence bone formation rate independently from PTH levels. Lastly, PTH is not a bone-derived marker and therefore may never be a fully accurate indicator of bone turnover. At present, it is unknown what levels of PTH are associated with ABD in patients with less severe CKD not yet on renal replacement therapy. Bone-specific alkaline phosphatase (BSAP) may be an additional useful marker of ABD. Low levels of BSAP predict ABD and BSAP correlates with bone turnover in ESRD patients treated with hemodialysis.[82]

Fracture Risks in Chronic Kidney Disease

Patients with ESRD have fourfold increased risk of fractures; and the highest risk (10- to 100-fold increase) of fractures is observed in ESRD patients below age 65 as compared with age-matched individuals from the general population.[84] The risk of fractures is also augmented in early CKD.[85,86] Vertebral and hip fractures are shown to independently increase all-cause mortality in CKD patients.[87,88] The fracture risk in patients with low turnover bone disease remains controversial as no biopsy-proven studies are available investigating the association between adynamic bone disease and fractures in CKD patients. Because ABD is linked to PTH oversuppression, several studies demonstrated the association between relatively low to normal PTH levels and the risk of vertebral and hip fractures.[89,90] However, in a case-control study, dialysis patients who underwent parathyroidectomy were found to have 32% lower risk for hip fractures, and 31% lower risk for any fractures as compared with matched controls.[91]

Bone Disease and Vascular Calcifications

Vascular calcifications, and especially arterial calcifications, are very common in patients with CKD and correlate with cardiovascular complications.[92] The prevalence of vascular calcifications is the highest among patients with ESRD[93,94]; however, patients with CKD stages 2 to 4 are also found to have increased vascular calcifications on imaging studies as compared with the general population.[95] There are two types of arterial calcifications with different clinical consequences: one affects intimal layer of arteries and is associated with atherosclerotic plaque, and the second type involves medial wall or arteries (Mönckeberg sclerosis). The atherosclerotic plaques are usually patchy in distribution and lead to chronic and acute end-organ ischemia from vessel lumen obstruction from the plaque itself or acute thrombosis following plaque rupture, respectively. On the other hand, medial arterial calcifications are more diffuse and increase vessel stiffness and reduce vascular compliance. As the result of the latter, blood pressure rises with the development of left ventricular hypertrophy that compromises myocardial perfusion during diastole and is associated with high mortality rates in patients with ESRD.[96,97] The mechanism of vascular calcification is not completely understood and is likely multifactorial, involving factors promoting transformation of vascular smooth muscle cell into "bone-like" cells, elevation of calcium and phosphorus due to altered bone and mineral metabolism, low levels of circulating and locally produced inhibitors, impaired renal excretion, and current therapies such as the use of calcium-containing phosphate binders and active vitamin D.[98] There is well documented association between increased vascular[99,100] and soft tissue calcifications[101] and the biopsy-proven ABD in ESRD patients. ABD is characterized by a reduced bone ability to incorporate extracellular calcium and, therefore, diminished ability to buffer calcium load leading to more frequent hypercalcemia.[102,103] Cardiovascular mortality is shown to be increased in dialysis patients with higher burden of vascular calcifications and some observational studies also revealed increased mortality in patients with relatively low to normal PTH supporting ABD as a strong risk factor for cardiovascular death.[104] Interestingly, parathyroidectomy in ESRD patients was shown to improve long term survival by 15% in observational study; although postoperative PTH levels were not provided.[105]

PARATHYROID GLAND ABNORMALITIES

Parathyroid cells are generally quiescent and rarely divide under normal physiologic conditions. In addition to increased PTH secretion, stimulation of parathyroid gland (PTG) during the course of CKD leads initially to diffuse polyclonal proliferation (hyperplasia) followed by monoclonal nodular hyperplasia, which can be diffuse or have a predominant nodule.[106] Factors associated with PTG hyperplasia are listed in Table 77.5. Low Ca is involved in activation of parathyroid gland growth. In animal models, a diet low in Ca was shown to increase parathyroid cell proliferation 10-fold,[107] and in rats with kidney failure, the administration of a calcimimetic compound that binds to CaSR attenuated the parathyroid cell proliferation.[108] In addition to low serum Ca, high serum Pi is the major factor leading to parathyroid cell proliferation[107] and low Pi diet reduces parathyroid cell proliferation and PTH mRNA levels. In severe hyperparathyroidism, there is also a reduction in the number of CaSR, effectively shifting the calcium-PTH set point toward greater PTH secretion for any given serum Ca concentration and a loss of inhibitory Ca role on PTG growth.[109,110] Decrease in CaSR and VDR expression is observed during parathyroid proliferation and is especially pronounced in nodular hyperplasia.[44,58,111,112] Density of VDR was reported to be negatively correlated with both the weight and proliferative activity of the glands.[113] Administration of calcitriol and calcimimetics was shown to result in decrease of parathyroid cell proliferation and was associated with elevation of CaSR and VDR.[114,115] Moreover, low serum Ca may interfere with $1,25(OH)_2D$ action by inducing resistance to vitamin D via reduction of VDR[116] and upregulation of calreticulin.

TABLE 77.5 **Factors Regulating Parathyroid Gland Proliferation**

Factor	Mechanism
Inhibitors of polyclonal PTG proliferation	
$1,25(OH)_2D$	Decreased *c-myc* expression that modulates cell cycle progression via VDR
	Activation of *p21* gene expression that inhibits cell cycle
	Downregulation of EGFR signaling
	Indirect effect via upregulation of CaSR
Calcium	Direct effect via activation of CaSR
Stimulator of polyclonal PTG proliferation	
High phosphorus	Inhibits *p21* gene expression and promotes cell cycle
Stimulators of monoclonal transformation	
Decreased CaSR gene expression	Decreased activation of CaSR
Decreased VDR gene expression	Decreased activation of VDR
Increased expression of EGFR	Decreased VDR gene expression

$1,25(OH)_2D$, active vitamin D; VDR, vitamin D receptor; EGFR, epidermal growth factor receptor; CaSR, calcium-sensing receptor, PTG, parathyroid gland.

Calreticulin is a calcium-binding intracellular protein, and when is unbound can inhibit $1,25(OH)_2D$ action on PTH gene transcription.[117] Enhanced expression of two receptors for potent growth promoters such as transforming growth factor alpha (TGFα) and epidermal growth factor (EGF) was also described to contribute to PTG hyperplasia in patients with CKD.[118,119] In nodular hyperplasia, activation of EGFR by TGFα was shown to be associated with 80% reduction of VDR mRNA levels leading to $1,25(OH)_2D$ resistance.[118] It is uncertain, at present, if impaired apoptosis contributes to PTG hyperplasia.

The reversibility of PTG hyperplasia is a subject of debate.[120,121] Size of PTG as determined by ultrasound has been shown to be a sensitive indicator of therapeutic responsiveness to pharmacologic treatment of SHPT. Histologic studies demonstrated that PTG heavier than 0.5 to 1.0 g were composed in the majority of cases of nodular hyperplasia[122] and were refractory to therapy with calcitriol or its analogs.[123,124]

CLINICAL MANIFESTATIONS OF CKD-MBD

Patients with SHPT frequently remain asymptomatic even with advanced disease and presence of biochemical and imagining abnormalities. In general, signs and symptoms are nonspecific (Table 77.6) and related to osteitis fibrosa or electrolyte changes such as hypercalcemia and/or hyperphosphatemia. The severity of symptoms also varies from moderate bone or joint pains and bone deformities and fractures to life threatening calciphylaxis and cardiovascular disease as a result of calcium deposition in vasculature and other organs. Fracture risk, vascular calcifications, and mortality associated with CKD-MBD were discussed earlier in this chapter.

DIAGNOSIS OF CKD-MBD

Diagnostic tests for CKD-MBD are divided into biochemical, imaging, and bone biopsy and will be briefly discussed in the following sections.

Serum Markers of CKD-MBD

Parathyroid Hormone

The biochemical diagnosis of SHPT relies on finding of elevated serum iPTH. The most commonly used assays for PTH determination represent second generation two-site immunometric assays that recognize full length intact 1–84 PTH; however, this assay also cross reacts with large PTH fragments, such as 7–84 PTH which antagonizes PTH action on elevation of serum Ca levels and osteoblasts.[59]

TABLE 77.6 **Signs and Symptoms of Secondary Hyperparathyroidism**

Skeletal	Extraskeletal
Osteoporosis	Vascular calcification leading to cardiovascular disease
Bone fractures	Calciphylaxis (calcific uremic arteriopathy)
Bone and joint pain	Pruritus
Bone deformities	Anemia
Growth retardation in children	Red eye syndrome

1–84 PTH usually represents only 50% to 60% of whole PTH determined by these assays. There has been developed a new third generation assay that measures only the full length 1–84 PTH (biointact PTH) and not amino-terminally truncated fragments.[125] Additionally, the measurement of a ratio of 1–84 PTH to large C-terminal fragments has been proposed[126] for evaluation of high turnover bone disease; however, the usefulness of these new methods remains to be elucidated.

Calcium and Phosphate

Ca and Pi usually remain normal until GFR reaches below 30 to 40 mL/min/m^2 and then Ca tends to fall while Pi rises.[6] Nonetheless, hypercalcemia can also be observed in setting of large doses of vitamin D administration, especially while using calcium-containing phosphate binders, or with the development of severe hyperparathyroid bone disease. Pi is almost uniformly high in untreated patients with ESRD; however, normal and even low Pi may be present with concomitant malnutrition.

Vitamin D Metabolites

25-hydroxyvitamin D deficiency is common in CKD patients.[6,127] 25-Hydroxyvitamin D is shown to correlate with PTH levels and the rate of bone turnover[128] and is considered as the best index of vitamin D status in CKD patients because of its long half-life (about 3 weeks) and ability to access both endogenous and exogenous sources of vitamin D. Additionally, levels of 25-hydroxyvitamin D positively correlate with serum 1,25(OH)$_2$D in CKD patients but not in healthy individuals,[129,130] suggesting that 1,25(OH)$_2$D production is more dependent on substrate availability in CKD. 1,25(OH)$_2$D is not routinely measured in patients with CKD because its levels do not differentiate between different histologic variants of renal osteodystrophy nor predict any other clinical outcomes.

Markers of Bone Formation and Resorption

Bone formation markers such as total alkaline phosphatase (TALP) and bone-specific alkaline phosphatase (BSALP) are useful markers of bone turnover in CKD. Importantly, metabolism of TALP and BSALP is not impaired by the presence of reduced GFR and higher levels of BSALP correlate with high rates of bone turnover and PTH.[131,132] Usefulness of BSALP in the predicting of high and low turnover bone disease is further increased if BSALP is combined with simultaneous measurements of iPTH.[133,134] Osteocalcin (OC) and tartrate-resistant acid phosphatase (TRACP) are two markers of bone resorption that also have been shown in small studies to correlate with histomorphometric parameters of bone turnover.[132] OC accumulates with CKD and its low levels are sensitive in predicting low turnover bone disease,[135] whereas TRACP levels are not affected by CKD and high levels predict osteoclastic activity and high turnover bone disease.[136] Nevertheless, the role of OC and TRACP is still under investigation.

FGF23

Elevated FGF23 predicts all-cause mortality and faster evelopment of ESRD as discussed previously. Therefore, FGF23 level may be a useful prognostic marker; however, its determination is available only in experimental research.

Imagining Studies

X-rays

Although routine radiography is not used in diagnosis of ROD, plane X-rays can help in differential workup by revealing several skeletal abnormalities of CKD-MBD.[137,138] Subperiosteal bone resorption is a feature of advanced SPHPT and in adults most commonly affects the phalangeal tufts, the radial aspect of the proximal and middle phalanges of the fingers, the metatarsals, the rib margins, the lamina dura, and the medial margins of the proximal humerus, femur, and tibia. Subchondral resorption can occur at several sites, including the sternoclavicular and acromioclavicular joints, the symphysis pubis, the sacroiliac joints, and the diskovertebral joints. Additionally, an erosive type arthropathy is reported with secondary hyperparathyroidism. Brown tumors are a manifestation of advanced SHPT and are seen rarely with modern therapy of CKD-MBD. Brown tumors radiographically can look similar to lytic lesions and can occur essentially in any bone. Plain X-ray also detects extra-osseous calcifications developing with SHPT such as vascular calcifications, calcified pulmonary nodules, chondrocalcinosis, and calcifications of various organs (breast, heart, liver, and kidney).

Computer Tomography

Computed tomography (CT) is not routinely used for diagnosis of ROD, as CT scan is not sensitive in detecting changes related to SHPT. However, several CT techniques have been successfully applied for the diagnosis of vascular calcifications.[139]

Bone Biopsy

Bone biopsy with quantitative histomorphometric analysis is a gold standard in diagnosis of renal osteodystrophy. Yet, bone biopsy is not routinely performed because of its invasive nature and the ability of iPTH to predict type of bone disease in CKD patients due to reasonably reliable correlation between levels of iPTH and bone histology. Nevertheless, bone biopsy remains an important tool in differentiation of low and normal bone turnover disease, or when aluminum-related bone disease is suspected. General indications for bone biopsy are listed in Table 77.7. We will conclude this chapter by discussing general therapeutic approaches for the treatment of CKD-MBD.

TREATMENT OF CKD-MBD

General Strategy Overview

Treatment strategies differ for the various stages of CKD. The abnormalities in mineral metabolism begin from stages 2 to 4 of CKD; therefore, the prevention and treatment of CKD-MBD should be started early in the course of kidney disease before elevations in serum phosphate or reductions in serum calcium. At present serum PTH and FGF23 levels are not routinely measured in patients with mild degrees of renal dysfunction. Serum 25(OH)D levels are commonly measured in the general population and efforts to normalize 25(OH)D levels in CKD seem to be a reasonable therapeutic goal as low levels of 25(OH)D are known to cause secondary HPT even in patients with normal kidney function.[140] Treatment with phosphate binders in early CKD is theoretically attractive when there is evidence for increased fractional excretion of phosphate, but at present the use of phosphate binders in CKD patients with normal serum phosphate levels is not approved and their effects have not been studied in clinical trials. Once secondary hyperparathyroidism has developed, as evidenced by elevated serum PTH levels, treatment with calcium supplementation and use of active vitamin D sterols can be considered. Calcimimetics are not approved for use in early stages of CKD stages 3 to 5 and their use in this setting suppresses PTH but increases serum phosphate levels. In contrast, active vitamin D analogues suppress PTH in CKD stages 3 and 4 without increasing serum phosphate levels, possibly due to their effect to also stimulate FGF23. The asymptomatic nature of CKD-MBD contributes to the challenge of treating this disorder. In CKD stage 5D, combinations of treatments are needed to reduce serum phosphate levels while suppressing PTH concentrations that include the use of calcium and noncalcium phosphate binders (for phosphate control) and the use of active vitamin D analogues and calcimimetics (alone or in combination) to suppress circulating PTH levels and to prevent the progression of parathyroid gland diseases, while optimizing bone health. Different treatment strategies include: (1) use of increasing doses of active vitamin D analogues and increasing does of phosphate binders versus (2) use of increasing doses of cinacalcet, fixed physiologic replacement doses of active vitamin D analogues, and phosphate binders to suppress PTH and treat hyperphosphatemia.

TABLE 77.7 Indications for Bone Biopsy in Patients with Chronic Kidney Disease

Discrepancy between biochemical parameters leading to no conclusion
Fracture or unexplained bone pain
Severe progressing vascular calcifications
Unexplained hypercalcemia
Suspicion of aluminum intoxication
If considering treating a patient for fractures

Treatment Target Guidelines

There are several clinical practice guidelines such as Kidney Disease Outcomes Quality Initiative (KDOQI),[141] Kidney Disease: Improving Global Outcomes (KDIGO),[1] and Japanese Society of Dialysis Therapy (JSDT)[142] that developed recommendations for the target levels of serum Ca, Pi, and PTH at different stages of CKD (Table 77.8). All these guidelines regarded CKD-MBD as systemic disorder and uniformly agreed on the paramount importance of maintaining Ca and Pi homeostasis as close to normal as possible irrespective of degree of renal impairment in order to avoid the development of vascular calcifications. However, KDOQI, KDIGO, and JSTA have different target ranges for PTH. KDOQI PTH targets between 150 and 300 pg per mL is based on the estimated levels of PTH to maintain normal bone remodeling, with the higher than normal range reflecting the resistance to PTH actions and assessment of circulating inactive PTH fragments in dialysis patients.[143] The emphasis of changes in PTH and higher (i.e., $<$600 pg per mL) threshold PTH concentrations in the KDIGO recommendations reflects the variability in existing PTH assays in measuring bioactive PTH and the recognitions that high PTH values are associated with increased mortality. In contrast, for the patients with ESRD JSTA advocates PTH concentrations closer to the normal range for the general population, which emphasizes the prevention of progressive parathyroid gland hyperplasia.[144]

TABLE 77.8 Target Levels for Calcium, Phosphorus, and Parathyroid Hormone

	KDOQI	KDIGO	JSDT
Calcium			
CKD stage 3–5	Normal range	Normal range	N/A
CKD stage 5D	Normal range	Normal range: 8.4–10 mg/dL	Preferably 8.4–9.5 mg/dL
Phosphorus			
CKD stage 3–4	2.7–4.6 mg/dL	Normal range	N/A
CKD stage 5	3.5–5.5 mg/dL	Normal range	N/A
CKD stage 5D	3.5–5.5 mg/dL	Toward normal range	3.5–6 mg/dL
Intact PTH			
CKD stage 3	35–70 pg/mL	Optimal level is unknown	N/A
CKD stage 4	70–110 pg/mL	Optimal level is unknown	N/A
CKD stage 5	200–300 pg/mL	Optimal level is unknown	N/A
CKD stage 5D	200–300 pg/mL	2–9 times above upper limit of normal	60–180 pg/mL

KDOQI, Kidney Disease Outcomes Quality Initiative; KDIGO, Kidney Disease: Improving Global Outcomes; JSDT, Japanese Society of Dialysis Therapy; PTH, parathyroid hormone; CKD stage 3: glomerular filtration rate (GFR) 30–59 mL/min/m^2; CKD stage 4, GFR 15–29 mLmin/m^2; CKD stage 5, GFR ≤15 mL/min/m^2 but not on dialysis; CKD stage 5D, GFR ≤15 mL/min/m^2 on dialysis.

Specific Treatments

Maintenance of Neutral Phosphorus Balance

The maintenance of normal Pi level is the goal. The rationale to maintain normal Pi level in CKD comes from human observational studies linking Pi levels above the normal range with the increased mortality, presence of soft tissue and vascular calcifications, and from the experimental data strongly supporting the role of Pi in the development of SHPT, calcitriol deficiency, and extraskeletal calcifications. Recommended level of Pi depends on stage of CKD with the goal to maintain normal serum Pi in mild to moderate CKD (stages 3 to 4) or 2.7 to 4.6 mg per dL, and toward normal levels for ESRD, 3.5 to 5.5 mg per dL.[141] Adequate Pi level can be achieved by the restriction of amount of Pi absorbed in gastrointestinal (GI) tract by limiting dietary Pi intake and the use of Pi binders. Dietary Pi absorption is dependent on active vitamin D; therefore limiting dose of vitamin D analogs administered for the control of elevated PTH may also reduce the amount of absorbed Pi in the intestine. In patients with ESRD, hemodialysis and peritoneal dialysis also contribute to normal Pi balance by elimination of Pi from the body.

Diet. Pi retention due to reduced nephron mass from CKD plays a critical role in the development of CKD-MBD. Therefore, it is logical to implement primary prevention of CKD-MBD by introducing moderate Pi restriction by means of mild protein restriction from earliest stages of CKD, even before any abnormalities in Pi level or PTH are detected.[141] KDOQI[141] specifically recognized the limitations of the above conclusion as it is based on: (1) studies that primarily restricted protein intake and therefore, only indirectly restricted Pi intake; (2) it is possible to restrict protein intake without restricting Pi intake; (3) most of the reports provided analysis for "prescribed diet" rather than "consumed diet"; and (4) in many studies, the patients had concomitant therapy with vitamin D and/or phosphate binders making interpretation of the results difficult. In order to accomplish the Pi restriction, it is critical to gain the knowledge on the best but yet minimally invasive and less costly way to educate patients on low Pi diet. It is essentially unknown what intervention is needed for patients to reduce their Pi intake. Additionally, it is unknown if low Pi diet could actually achieve its goal of reducing CKD-MBD. The data about beneficial effects of low Pi diet on improving parameters of CKD-MBD are scarce and controversial at present, with some studies showing no benefit in PTH or FGF23,[145] whereas others showing improvement in PTH levels.[146,147]

Dietary Pi consumption parallels intake of protein and it is not uncommon to observe normal and even low levels of Pi in uremic patients who have inadequate protein intake. It is important to avoid malnutrition while minimizing Pi intake and this potentially could be achieved by choosing protein from plant sources. Pi in meats is stored in organic form which is easily hydrolyzed and absorbed in gastrointestinal tract. Three fourths of Pi in plant proteins is in inorganic form and humans lack the enzyme phytase that is necessary

TABLE 77.9 **Classification of Phosphate Binders: Advantages and Disadvantages**

Drug	Advantages	Disadvantages
Calcium-containing	Effective, inexpensive	May cause hypercalcemia and/or promote vascular calcifications
Sevelamer	Effective, may reduce GI side effects (nausea, vomiting, vascular calcifications, diarrhea, bloating, abdominal pain) due to less hypercalcemia	Expensive, higher pill burden as compared with Ca-based binders
Lanthanum	Effective, less hypercalcemia	Expensive, long-term safety unknown, various GI side effects
Magnesium-containing	Effective, inexpensive	GI side effects (diarrhea), rare respiratory depression
Aluminium-containing[a]	Effective, inexpensive	Encephalopathy, anemia, osteomalacia

[a]Aluminum-based binder use should be limited to 4 weeks.[1]
GI, gastrointestinal; Ca, calcium.

for its hydrolysis and subsequent absorption. Therefore, bioavailability of Pi from plant sources is significantly less than from animal origin.

Phosphate Binders. With the progression of CKD, dietary Pi restriction alone is not sufficient to maintain normal Pi levels. Therefore, specific treatment is usually needed in the form of oral Pi binders aimed to prevent systemic Pi absorption from the gut. Nevertheless, the use of Pi binders should always be combined with dietary Pi restriction in order to reduce pill burden from Pi binders and their potential side effects. Many compounds have been found to be effective Pi binders such as aluminum, magnesium, iron, calcium, and lanthanum salts, and nonabsorbable polymers. Their efficacy and side effects vary widely and are summarized in Table 77.9. Calcium-containing phosphorus binders and sevelamer have become most commonly used contemporary Pi binders. Ca-containing binders are cheap, effective, and well tolerated by patients. Their popularity has been decreasing in recent years due to accumulating evidence that Ca binders may contribute to progression of vascular calcifications and low turnover bone disease in patients with CKD, and therefore, higher CV mortality as compared with sevelamer-containing binders, although no data from randomized controlled trials exists to support this theory. Most common side effects of Ca-containing Pi-binders is hypercalcemia and KDOQI recommends limiting daily Ca intake to 2,000 mg of elemental Ca including Ca from Ca-based agents.[141] Nonabsorbabale polymer sevelamer, which acts as an anion-exchange resin, has many potential advantages over Ca-based binders as its use is not associated with Ca load and also can lower LDL cholesterol; therefore, having potential advantageous effect on cardiovascular disease. However, there is a controversy as to whether sevelamer use is associated with reduced risk of vascular calcifications, and there is no data to support its superior role in reducing cardiovascular mortality on CKD patients. Additionally, it is expensive and requires significantly higher pill count to achieve adequate Pi control as compared with Ca-based binders. Lanthanum is a newest and highly potent Pi binder. It is expensive and its long-term safety is still unknown.

Removal of Phosphate with Hemodialysis and Peritoneal Dialysis. Once a patient with CKD reaches ESRD, RRT in a form of hemodialysis (HD) or peritoneal dialysis (PD) becomes an additional means of Pi elimination. HD is more efficient in removing Pi with a single 4-hour HD session eliminating about 800 mg of Pi. About 300 mg of Pi is removed during daily PD but weekly removal of Pi is comparable in both modalities, as PD is a daily treatment, as opposed to thrice weekly conventional HD. It is important to recognize that neither conventional HD nor PD can substitute for normal kidneys for the elimination of all absorbed dietary Pi. Even with moderate Pi restriction to 800 mg per day, assuming that 40% to 80% of dietary Pi absorbed, up to 5,600 mg of Pi is gained per week in patients with ESRD, whereas only about 2,400 mg of Pi can be removed with RRT, leading to a positive Pi balance. Therefore, patients with ESRD must continue to follow dietary Pi restriction and use Pi binders on daily basis. The limitation of Pi removal with hemodialysis is due to majority of body Pi being distributed intracellularly. When dialysis is started, the plasma concentration of Pi falls rapidly during first 60 to 90 minutes.[148] After this initial phase, the removal of Pi is limited by Pi transfer from intracellular to intravascular space which is rate-limited step in Pi clearance. Different approaches tested, such as use of low and high flux dialyzer membranes,[149,150] delayed correction of metabolic acidosis,[151] or lengthening the hemodialysis session were not found to increase Pi removal with hemodialysis. However, increasing frequency of HD sessions to six or seven times per week as with short daily HD or nocturnal HD can lead to improved Pi control with lesser dose of Pi binders and even discontinuation of Pi binders.[152,153]

Other Approaches for Reduction of Dietary Phosphate Absorption

Reduction of Dose of Active Vitamin D and Its Analogs. Because the administration of active vitamin D analogs increases GI Ca and Pi absorption, their use is associated with both hypercalcemia and hyperphosphatemia. Therefore, the prescription of lower doses of active vitamin D analogs and alternative strategies to suppress PTH may lead to lower Pi absorption by the GI tract, and lower serum Pi.

Niacin. Niacin is converted into niacinamide during its metabolism and reduces intestinal transport of Pi via inhibition of Na-Pi cotransporter 2b which is responsible for up to 50% of absorbed Pi. Both niacin and niacinamide are available pharmacologically. As oppose to niacin, niacinamide does not cause vasodilatation or flushing because it does not activate G-protein coupled receptors for niacin. However, niacinamide has no lipid-lowering properties of niacin. Niacinamide has been shown in small clinical trials to effectively reduce serum Pi levels in hemodialysis patients,[154,155] as well as peritoneal dialysis patients.[156] Niacin was also found to successfully lower Pi while additionally elevating high density lipoprotein cholesterol in a prospective observational study.[157]

Maintenance of Normal Calcium Level

Maintenance of Ca in normal range is the goal in CKD, and both hypocalcemia stimulating PTH release and hypercalcemia that can lead to vascular and soft tissue calcifications should be avoided. Ca intake in patients with CKD requires individualization to account for the use of Ca-based Pi binders, presence of vascular calcifications, and low turnover bone disease. It is recommended that most CKD patient consume no more than 2 g of elemental Ca per day to avoid hypercalcemia. However, patients after parathyroidectomy may be an exclusion from this rule and require substantial amounts of Ca to maintain eucalcemia. Because Ca absorption in GI tract is vitamin D dependent, CKD patients should be screened for vitamin D deficiency and treated to maintain 25-hydroxyvitamin D levels above 30 ng per mL.[141]

Administration of Vitamin D

There are three forms of vitamin D (Fig. 77.5): (1) provitamin D (or simply vitamin D) includes ergocalciferol of plant source (vitamin D_2) and cholecalciferol (vitamin D_3) which could be of animal source or produced from skin 7-dehydrocholesterol under exposure to ultraviolet B solar radiation; (2) 25-hydroxyvitamin D (25(OH)D), precursor of active form of vitamin D that is produced in the liver after vitamins D_2

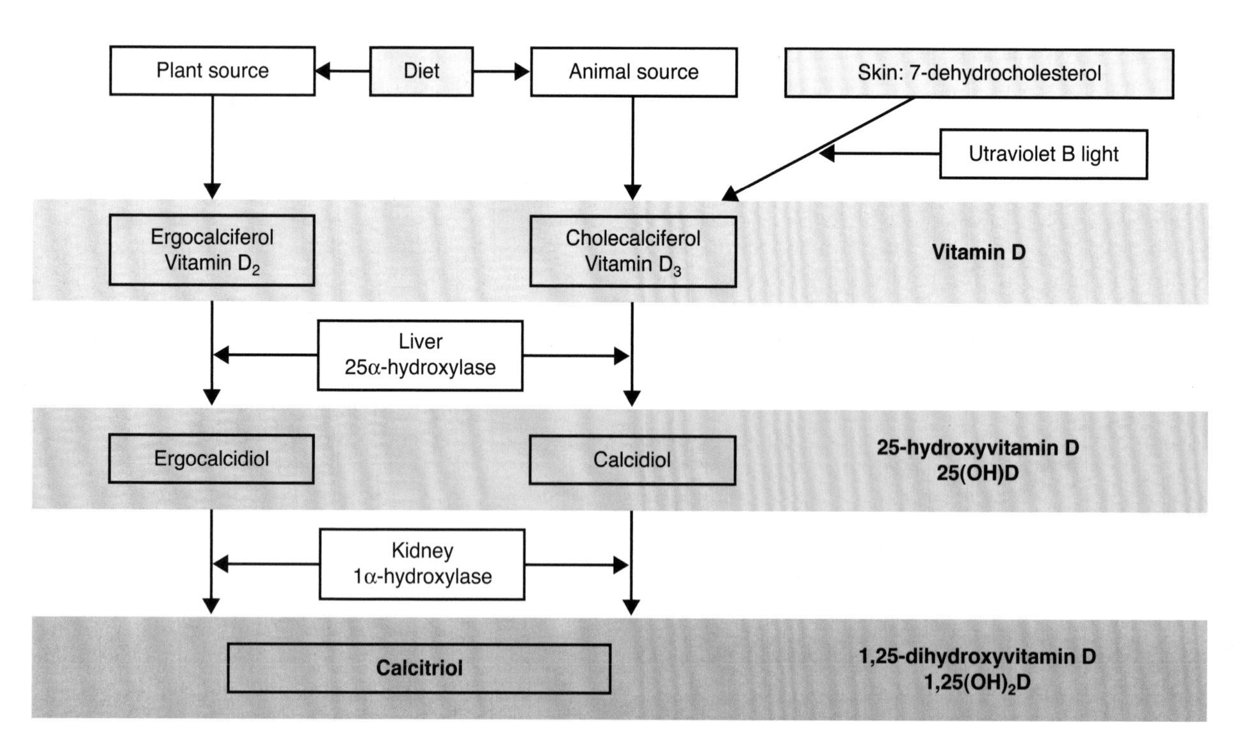

FIGURE 77.5 Sources, pathways of conversion, and classification of vitamin D.

and D_3 undergo hydroxylation by 25α-hydroxylase; and (3) active vitamin D or 1,25-dihydroxyvitamin D or calcitriol ($1,25(OH)_2D$) is produced in the kidneys after additional hydroxylation of 25(OH)D by 1alpha-hydroxylase. The therapeutically available forms of vitamin D include naturally occurring ergocalciferol, cholecalciferol, calcidiol, calcitriol, and synthetic forms such as vitamin D_2 analogs (doxercalciferol, paricalcitol), and vitamin D_3 analogs (alfacalcidol, falecalcitriol, maxacalcitol). Vitamin D analogs do not require 1alpha-hydroxylation for their activity.

Vitamin D deficiency in CKD patients is common and the administration of 25(OH)D to achieve its serum levels above 30 mg per mL (75 nmol/L) has been shown to positively impact elevated levels of PTH in patients with CKD stages 3 to 4.[158,159] Nutritional vitamin D therapy is less effective in reducing PTH[160] and restoring bone histology to normal[161] in hemodialysis patients. Nevertheless, in addition to the role of active vitamin D in bone health and regulation of mineral homeostasis, the local extrarenal tissue conversion of 25(OH)D into $1,25(OH)_2D$ is important for the regulation of immune responses, oxidative stress, cell differentiation, and blood pressure regulation.[162,163] A study of hemodialysis patients demonstrated that cholecalciferol administration was associated with the reduction in production of inflammatory cytokines by circulating monocytes.[164] The recommended by KDOQI ergocalciferol dose is 50,000 units and its frequency ranges from once a week to once a month for a total course of 6 months depending on the severity of vitamin D deficiency.[141]

If despite adequate 25(OH)D level PTH remains elevated, then active vitamin therapy in the form of calcitriol or vitamin D analogs can be successfully used for the treatment of elevated PTH in CKD.[1,141] Calcitriol and vitamin D analogs effectively lower PTH levels in stages 2 to 5 of CKD including patients on RRT, and all can cause hypercalcemia and hyperphosphatemia in a dose-dependent manner.[1] There are no comparative trials on the superiority among different active vitamin D regimens in reducing PTH of CKD patients not yet on RRT; and only two studies that compared calcitriol to maxacalcitol[165] and calcitriol to paricalcitol[166] in hemodialysis patients. These trials revealed similar efficacy of these agents in reducing PTH and comparable adverse profiles, including the incidence of developing elevated Ca and Pi levels and oversuppression of PTH. Therefore, Ca, Pi, and PTH levels need to be closely monitored during vitamin D therapy. In addition to PTH-lowering effect, calcitriol and vitamin D analogs have been shown to improve bone histology,[167] and offered survival benefit for CKD patients in observational studies; however, this hypothesis needs to be confirmed in randomized trials.[168]

Use of Calcimimetics to Suppress Parathyroid Hormone

It is a unique group of drugs that allosterically regulate CaSR and inhibit PTH secretion by sensitizing the parathyroid calcium receptor to extracellular calcium, and hence, "mimic" effects of increased extracellular calcium.[112,169] Cinacalcet is the only drug of this class that is available in clinical practice for the treatment of SHPT in patients with stage 5 CKD on dialysis since its U.S. Food and Drug Administration (FDA) approval in 2004; cinacalcet effectively lowers PTH in ESRD patients (treated with both hemodialysis and peritoneal dialysis).[170,171] In the OPTIMA study, the addition of cinacalcet was shown to increase the proportion of patients achieving serum PTH, Ca, and Pi within KDOQI target levels as compared to conventional therapy (active vitamin D therapy and phosphorus binders) alone.[172] Moreover, cinacalcet is useful for PTH control in patients with elevated calcium and Pi[173]: in hemodialysis patients with PTH controlled by high dose of vitamin D therapy but elevated serum Ca and Pi, addition of cinacalcet to a usual treatment (active vitamin D and phosphorus binders) allowed patients to maintain PTH within KDOQI targets while lowering serum Ca and Pi as compared with the usual treatment alone. The ability of cinacalcet to lower serum Pi in dialysis patients is likely related to PTH reduction and, therefore, reduced Pi translocation from the bone while having no effect on intestinal Pi reabsorption that defer cinacalcet from active vitamin D therapy. In contrast to CKD5D, cinacalcet is not recommended in the treatment of SHPT in patients with earlier CKD stages (3–4)[1] because its use was associated with documented hypocalcemia and paradoxical increase in serum Pi levels and need for Pi-binders.[174] However, the latter phenomenon in that study was likely related to the more frequent vitamin D use in the cinacalcet group.

The data on the effects of calcimimetics on bone histomorphology in patients with CKD are limited. As expected from its ability to suppress PTH, cinacalcet use is associated with higher incidence of development of low turnover bone disease as compared with the placebo.[175] On the other hand, there is a theoretical advantage of using cinacalcet for the prevention of ABD development while treating secondary hyperparathyroidism in patients at high risk for ABD, such as elderly diabetic patients: cinacalcet is able to maintain pulsatile PTH secretion pattern which is anabolic for the bone. In animal CKD models, cinacalcet restored low bone formation[176] and in phase 3 clinical trials use of cinacalcet in combination with active vitamin D analogues reduced fracture risk.[177] Unlike active vitamin D analogues, cinacalcet treatment does not lead to further elevations of circulating FGF23.[178] Current trials are under way that investigate the effects of cinacalcet on mortality in patients with ESRD.

Parathyroidectomy

The surgical correction remains the final therapy of the most severe forms of SHPT which cannot be controlled by medical management. Failure of medical treatment could result from ineffectiveness of medical therapy (combination of low Pi diet, Pi binders, active vitamin D, and cinacalcet)

TABLE 77.10 **Indications for Parathyroidectomy**

ESRD patients and severe HPT (generally PTH> 800 pg/mL and elevated AP) **and additional:** Persistent hypercalcemia Persistent hyperphosphatemia Persistently elevated PTH despite adequate treatment Progressive extraskeletal calcifications, including calciphylaxis Persistent pruritus
Kidney transplant candidates with Persistently elevated PTH and parathyroid hyperplasia[a]
Kidney transplant recipients with Persistently elevated PTH with hypercalcemia Persistently elevated PTH with unexplained worsening of allograft function

[a]Specific level of PTH is not established.
ESRD, end-stage renal disease; HPT, hyperparathyroidism; PTH, parathyroid hormone; AP, alkaline phosphatase.

leading to the complications of SHPT, or patient intolerance of medical treatment due to its side effects. There is a paucity of data available on effects of parathyroidectomy on cardiovascular, bone histology, biochemical, or other outcomes as discussed previously in clinical manifestation section. General indications for parathyroidectomy are listed in Table 77.10. Most commonly, two types of parathyroidectomy are performed: subtotal parathyroidectomy or total parathyroidectomy with autotransplantation. The presence of severe form of SHPT is ascertained by clinical, biochemical, and radiologic evidence. Clinical symptoms such as pruritus and periarticular pain are nonspecific and cannot be used in isolation as indication for parathyroidectomy. Similarly, hypercalcemia even in presence of soft tissue calcifications is not sufficient to warrant parathyroidectomy, because low turnover bone disease can also be associated with hypercalcemia and elevated Pi. In general, patients requiring parathyroidectomy have PTH levels exceeding 800 pg per mL and with elevation of alkaline phosphatase. Parathyroidectomy is recommended for kidney transplant recipients with persistent PTH elevation associated with hypercalcemia and worsening of kidney function. Additionally, parathyroidectomy can be considered in kidney transplant candidates even without severe symptoms if they have continuously high levels of PTH and parathyroid hyperplasia that is unlikely to regress after kidney transplantation—although no specific level of PTH at which parathyroidectomy would be warranted is established.

Special Consideration for the Treatment of Adynamic Bone Disease

Despite growing prevalence of ABD, its treatment is poorly investigated. The general approach for the treatment of ABD consists of restoration of PTH activity via limiting Ca load by reduction of calcium-containing phosphate-binders and lowering dialysate Ca, and decreasing or discontinuing active vitamin D or cinacalcet therapies. The use of synthetic PTH (1–34) teriparatide as an anabolic agent to restore bone formation in ABD has not been studied in patients with CKD.

Limiting Calcium Load

Ca is the most potent suppressor of PTH release. Several small studies demonstrated that patients treated with Ca-containing phosphate binders exhibited higher rates of development of ABD and were less likely to have an improvement in bone formation during follow-up as compared to non-calcium-containing binders.[179,180] Therefore, sevelamer and lanthanum may be preferable Pi binders for the patients at risk or with already developed ABD. Exposure of ESRD patients to high-calcium dialysate during RRT (both PD and HD) can also contribute to PTH oversuppression. In agreement with this observation, it has been demonstrated that lowering Ca concentration in dialysate for PD or HD improves bone histomorphology and markers of bone turnover.[181–183] Patients treated with PD exhibit higher rates of ABD as compared with HD treated patients. One possible explanation is that PD patients have continuous exposure to high-calcium dialysate versus thrice weekly exposure in HD patients.

Limiting Active Vitamin D Treatment

The use of active vitamin D leads to effective lowering of PTH and improving bone histology in OF via a reduction in bone formation, which, if excessive, can cause ABD. The oversuppression of bone turnover with calcitriol can occur even in presence of relatively normal to high PTH levels suggestive of its possible direct bone suppressive effect.[184,185] However, a recent report that compared effects of calcitriol and doxercalciferol (active vitamin D analog) on changes in bone histomorphology in pediatric ESRD patients treated with peritoneal dialysis did not find any increase in the development of ABD with the careful monitoring of Ca levels.[186] Additionally, there is accumulating evidence from animal models that active vitamin D exerts anabolic effects on the bone by modulating osteoblast and osteoclast activity.[187,188] It is possible that low doses of active vitamin D are beneficial for hyperparathyroid bone disease, whereas in higher doses, vitamin D is more likely to oversuppress bone formation; however, this point of view requires further exploration.

REFERENCES

1. KDIGO clinical practice guideline for the diagnosis, evaluation, prevention, and treatment of chronic kidney disease-mineral and bone disorder (CKD-MBD). *Kidney Int Suppl.* 2009;(113):S1–130.

2. Quarles LD. Endocrine functions of bone in mineral metabolism regulation. *J Clin Invest.* 2008;118(12):3820–3828.

3. Brown EM, Pollak M, Seidman CE, et al. Calcium-ion-sensing cell-surface receptors. *N Engl J Med.* 1995;333(4):234–240.

4. Silver J, Levi R. Cellular and molecular mechanisms of secondary hyperparathyroidism. *Clin Nephrol.* 2005;63(2):119–126.

5. D'Amour P, Rakel A, Brossard JH, et al. Acute regulation of circulating parathyroid hormone (PTH) molecular forms by calcium: utility of PTH fragments/PTH(1–84) ratios derived from three generations of PTH assays. *J Clin Endocrinol Metab.* 2006;91(1):283–289.

6. Levin A, Bakris GL, Molitch M, et al. Prevalence of abnormal serum vitamin D, PTH, calcium, and phosphorus in patients with chronic kidney disease: results of the study to evaluate early kidney disease. *Kidney Int.* 2007;71(1):31–38.

7. Craver L, Marco MP, Martinez I, et al. Mineral metabolism parameters throughout chronic kidney disease stages 1–5--achievement of K/DOQI target ranges. *Nephrol Dial Transplant.* 2007;22(4):1171–1176.

8. Gutierrez O, Isakova T, Rhee E, et al. Fibroblast growth factor-23 mitigates hyperphosphatemia but accentuates calcitriol deficiency in chronic kidney disease. *J Am Soc Nephrol.* 2005;16(7):2205–2215.

9. Berndt T, Kumar R. Phosphatonins and the regulation of phosphate homeostasis. *Annu Rev Physiol.* 2007;69:341–359.

10. Liu S, Quarles LD. How fibroblast growth factor 23 works. *J Am Soc Nephrol.* 2007;18(6):1637–1647.

11. Shigematsu T, Kazama JJ, Yamashita T, et al. Possible involvement of circulating fibroblast growth factor 23 in the development of secondary hyperparathyroidism associated with renal insufficiency. *Am J Kidney Dis.* 2004;44(2): 250–256.

12. Evenepoel P, Meijers B, Viaene L, et al. Fibroblast growth factor-23 in early chronic kidney disease: additional support in favor of a phosphate-centric paradigm for the pathogenesis of secondary hyperparathyroidism. *Clin J Am Soc Nephrol.* 2010;5(7):1268–1276.

13. Rostand SG, Drueke TB. Parathyroid hormone, vitamin D, and cardiovascular disease in chronic renal failure. *Kidney Int.* 1999;56(2):383–392.

14. Slinin Y, Foley RN, Collins AJ. Calcium, phosphorus, parathyroid hormone, and cardiovascular disease in hemodialysis patients: the USRDS waves 1, 3, and 4 study. *J Am Soc Nephrol.* 2005;16(6):1788–1793.

15. Ramos AM, Albalate M, Vazquez S, et al. Hyperphosphatemia and hyperparathyroidism in incident chronic kidney disease patients. *Kidney Int Suppl.* 2008;(111):S88–93.

16. Wolf M, Shah A, Gutierrez O, et al. Vitamin D levels and early mortality among incident hemodialysis patients. *Kidney Int.* 2007;72(8):1004–1013.

17. Inouye K, Sakaki T. Enzymatic studies on the key enzymes of vitamin D metabolism; 1 alpha-hydroxylase (CYP27B1) and 24-hydroxylase (CYP24). *Biotechnol Annu Rev.* 2001;7:179–194.

18. Sakaki T, Sawada N, Komai K, et al. Dual metabolic pathway of 25-hydroxyvitamin D3 catalyzed by human CYP24. *Eur J Biochem.* 2000;267(20): 6158–6165.

19. Zierold C, Mings JA, DeLuca HF. Regulation of 25-hydroxyvitamin D3-24-hydroxylase mRNA by 1,25-dihydroxyvitamin D3 and parathyroid hormone. *J Cell Biochem.* 2003;88(2):234–237.

20. Takemoto F, Shinki T, Yokoyama K, et al. Gene expression of vitamin D hydroxylase and megalin in the remnant kidney of nephrectomized rats. *Kidney Int.* 2003;64(2):414–420.

21. Silver J, Kilav R, Naveh-Many T. Mechanisms of secondary hyperparathyroidism. *Am J Physiol Renal Physiol.* 2002;283(3):F367–376.

22. Russell J, Bar A, Sherwood LM, et al. Interaction between calcium and 1,25-dihydroxyvitamin D3 in the regulation of preproparathyroid hormone and vitamin D receptor messenger ribonucleic acid in avian parathyroids. *Endocrinology.* 1993;132(6):2639–2644.

23. Li YC, Amling M, Pirro AE, et al. Normalization of mineral ion homeostasis by dietary means prevents hyperparathyroidism, rickets, and osteomalacia, but not alopecia in vitamin D receptor-ablated mice. *Endocrinology.* 1998;139(10): 4391–4396.

24. Meir T, Levi R, Lieben L, et al. Deletion of the vitamin D receptor specifically in the parathyroid demonstrates a limited role for the receptor in parathyroid physiology. *Am J Physiol Renal Physiol.* 2009;297(5):F1192–1198.

25. Gutierrez OM, Mannstadt M, Isakova T, et al. Fibroblast growth factor 23 and mortality among patients undergoing hemodialysis. *N Engl J Med.* 2008;359(6):584–592.

26. Jean G, Terrat JC, Vanel T, et al. High levels of serum fibroblast growth factor (FGF)-23 are associated with increased mortality in long haemodialysis patients. *Nephrol Dial Transplant.* 2009;24(9):2792–2796.

27. Larsson T, Nisbeth U, Ljunggren O, et al. Circulating concentration of FGF-23 increases as renal function declines in patients with chronic kidney disease, but does not change in response to variation in phosphate intake in healthy volunteers. *Kidney Int.* 2003;64(6):2272–2279.

28. Westerberg PA, Linde T, Wikstrom B, et al. Regulation of fibroblast growth factor-23 in chronic kidney disease. *Nephrol Dial Transplant.* 2007;22(11): 3202–3207.

29. Ix JH, Shlipak MG, Wassel CL, et al. Fibroblast growth factor-23 and early decrements in kidney function: the Heart and Soul Study. *Nephrol Dial Transplant.* 2010;25(3):993–997.

30. Weber TJ, Liu S, Indridason OS, et al. Serum FGF23 levels in normal and disordered phosphorus homeostasis. *J Bone Miner Res.* 2003;18(7):1227–1234.

31. Komaba H, Goto S, Fuji H, et al. Depressed expression of Klotho and FGF receptor 1 in hyperplastic parathyroid glands from uremic patients. *Kidney Int.* 2010;77(3):232–238.

32. Shimada T, Mizutani S, Muto T, et al. Cloning and characterization of FGF23 as a causative factor of tumor-induced osteomalacia. *Proc Natl Acad Sci U S A.* 2001;98(11):6500–6505.

33. Yamashita T, Yoshioka M, Itoh N. Identification of a novel fibroblast growth factor, FGF-23, preferentially expressed in the ventrolateral thalamic nucleus of the brain. *Biochem Biophys Res Commun.* 2000;277(2):494–498.

34. Kurosu H, Yamamoto M, Clark JD, et al. Suppression of aging in mice by the hormone Klotho. *Science.* 2005;309(5742):1829–1833.

35. Tsujikawa H, Kurotaki Y, Fujimori T, et al. Klotho, a gene related to a syndrome resembling human premature aging, functions in a negative regulatory circuit of vitamin D endocrine system. *Mol Endocrinol.* 2003;17(12):2393–2403.

36. Kuro-o M, Matsumura Y, Aizawa H, et al. Mutation of the mouse klotho gene leads to a syndrome resembling ageing. *Nature.* 1997;390(6655):45–51.

37. Urakawa I, Yamazaki Y, Shimada T, et al. Klotho converts canonical FGF receptor into a specific receptor for FGF23. *Nature.* 2006;444(7120):770–774.

38. Liu S, Zhou J, Tang W, et al. Pathogenic role of Fgf23 in Hyp mice. *Am J Physiol Endocrinol Metab.* 2006;291(1):E38–49.

39. Kurosu H, Ogawa Y, Miyoshi M, et al. Regulation of fibroblast growth factor-23 signaling by klotho. *J Biol Chem.* 2006;281(10):6120–6123.

40. Bai X, Miao D, Li J, et al. Transgenic mice overexpressing human fibroblast growth factor 23 (R176Q) delineate a putative role for parathyroid hormone in renal phosphate wasting disorders. *Endocrinology.* 2004;145(11):5269–5279.

41. Kazama JJ, Geivyo F, Shigematsu T, et al. Role of circulating fibroblast growth factor 23 in the development of secondary hyperparathyroidism. *Ther Apher Dial.* 2005;9(4):328–330.

42. Ben-Dov IZ, Galitzer H, Lavi-Moshayoff V, et al. The parathyroid is a target organ for FGF23 in rats. *J Clin Invest.* 2007;117(12):4003–4008.

43. Krajisnik T, Bjorklund P, Marsell R, et al. Fibroblast growth factor-23 regulates parathyroid hormone and 1-hydroxylase expression in cultured bovine parathyroid cells. *J Endocrinol.* 2007;195(1):125–131.

44. Canalejo R, Canalejo A, Martinez-Moreno JM, et al. FGF23 fails to inhibit uremic parathyroid glands. *J Am Soc Nephrol.* 2010;21(7):1125–1135.

45. Quarles LD. The bone and beyond: 'Dem bones' are made for more than walking. *Nat Med.* 2011;17(4):428–430.

46. Isakova T, Guiterrez O, Shah A, et al. Postprandial mineral metabolism and secondary hyperparathyroidism in early CKD. *J Am Soc Nephrol.* 2008;19(3): 615–623.

47. Hasegawa H, Nagano N, Urakawa I, et al. Direct evidence for a causative role of FGF23 in the abnormal renal phosphate handling and vitamin D metabolism in rats with early-stage chronic kidney disease. *Kidney Int.* 2010;78(10):975–980.

48. Lavi-Moshayoff V, Wasserman G, Meir T, et al. PTH increases FGF23 gene expression and mediates the high-FGF23 levels of experimental kidney failure: a bone parathyroid feedback loop. *Am J Physiol Renal Physiol.* 2010;299(4): F882–889.

49. Sato T, Tominaga Y, Ueki T, et al. Total parathyroidectomy reduces elevated circulating fibroblast growth factor 23 in advanced secondary hyperparathyroidism. *Am J Kidney Dis.* 2004;44(3):481–487.

50. Mirza MA, Larrson A, Lind L, et al. Circulating fibroblast growth factor-23 is associated with vascular dysfunction in the community. *Atherosclerosis.* 2009; 205(2):385–390.

51. Shimada T, Hasegawa H, Yamazaki Y, et al. FGF-23 is a potent regulator of vitamin D metabolism and phosphate homeostasis. *J Bone Miner Res.* 2004;19(3):429–435.

52. Wetmore JB, Quarles LD. Calcimimetics or vitamin D analogs for suppressing parathyroid hormone in end-stage renal disease: time for a paradigm shift? *Nat Clin Pract Nephrol.* 2009;5(1):24–33.

53. Murray TM, Rao LG, Divieti P, et al. Parathyroid hormone secretion and action: evidence for discrete receptors for the carboxyl-terminal region and related biological actions of carboxyl- terminal ligands. *Endocr Rev.* 2005;26(1):78–113.

54. Lee SK, Lorenzo JA. Parathyroid hormone stimulates TRANCE and inhibits osteoprotegerin messenger ribonucleic acid expression in murine bone marrow cultures: correlation with osteoclast-like cell formation. *Endocrinology.* 1999;140(8):3552–3561.

55. Pfeilschifter J, Mundy GR. Modulation of type beta transforming growth factor activity in bone cultures by osteotropic hormones. *Proc Natl Acad Sci U S A.* 1987;84(7):2024–2028.

56. Drueke TB, Eckardt KU. Role of secondary hyperparathyroidism in erythropoietin resistance of chronic renal failure patients. *Nephrol Dial Transplant.* 2002;17 Suppl 5:28–31.

57. McSheehy PM, Chambers TJ. Osteoblastic cells mediate osteoclastic responsiveness to parathyroid hormone. *Endocrinology.* 1986;118(2):824–828.

58. Lewin E, Garfia B, Reico FL, et al. Persistent downregulation of calcium-sensing receptor mRNA in rat parathyroids when severe secondary hyperparathyroidism is reversed by an isogenic kidney transplantation. *J Am Soc Nephrol.* 2002;13(8):2110–2116.

59. Langub MC, Monier-Fauqere MC, Wang G, et al. Administration of PTH-(7–84) antagonizes the effects of PTH-(1–84) on bone in rats with moderate renal failure. *Endocrinology.* 2003;144(4):1135–1138.

60. Picton ML, Moore PR, Mawer EB, et al. Down-regulation of human osteoblast PTH/PTHrP receptor mRNA in end-stage renal failure. *Kidney Int.* 2000;58(4):1440–1449.

61. Smogorzewski M, Tian J, Massry SG. Down-regulation of PTH-PTHrP receptor of heart in CRF: role of [Ca2+]i. *Kidney Int.* 1995;47(4):1182–1186.

62. Hernandez A, Concepcion MT, Rodruquez M, et al. High phosphorus diet increases preproPTH mRNA independent of calcium and calcitriol in normal rats. *Kidney Int.* 1996;50(6):1872–1878.

63. Kilav R, Silver J, Naveh-Many T. Parathyroid hormone gene expression in hypophosphatemic rats. *J Clin Invest.* 1995;96(1):327–333.

64. Almaden Y, Canalejo A, Hernandez A, et al. Direct effect of phosphorus on PTH secretion from whole rat parathyroid glands in vitro. *J Bone Miner Res.* 1996;11(7):970–976.

65. Spasovski GB, Bervoets AB, Behets G, et al. Spectrum of renal bone disease in end-stage renal failure patients not yet on dialysis. *Nephrol Dial Transplant.* 2003;18(6):1159–1166.

66. Tentori F, Blayney MJ, Albert JM, et al. Mortality risk for dialysis patients with different levels of serum calcium, phosphorus, and PTH: the Dialysis Outcomes and Practice Patterns Study (DOPPS). *Am J Kidney Dis.* 2008;52(3):519–530.

67. Palmer SC, Hayen A, Macaskill P, et al. Serum levels of phosphorus, parathyroid hormone, and calcium and risks of death and cardiovascular disease in individuals with chronic kidney disease: a systematic review and meta-analysis. *JAMA.* 2011;305(11):1119–1127.

68. Floege J, Kim J, Ireland E, et al. Serum iPTH, calcium and phosphate, and the risk of mortality in a European haemodialysis population. *Nephrol Dial Transplant.* 2011;26(6):1948–1955.

69. Block GA, Klassen PS, Lazarus JM, et al. Mineral metabolism, mortality, and morbidity in maintenance hemodialysis. *J Am Soc Nephrol.* 2004;15(8): 2208–2218.

70. Isakova T, Xie H, Yang W, et al. Fibroblast growth factor 23 and risks of mortality and end-stage renal disease in patients with chronic kidney disease. *JAMA.* 2011;305(23):2432–2439.

71. Fliser D, Kollerits B, Neyer U, et al. Fibroblast growth factor 23 (FGF23) predicts progression of chronic kidney disease: the Mild to Moderate Kidney Disease (MMKD) Study. *J Am Soc Nephrol.* 2007;18(9):2600–2608.

72. Titan SM, Zatz R, Graciolli FG, et al. FGF-23 as a predictor of renal outcome in diabetic nephropathy. *Clin J Am Soc Nephrol.* 2011;6(2):241–247.

73. Moe S, Drueke T, Cunningham J, et al. Definition, evaluation, and classification of renal osteodystrophy: a position statement from Kidney Disease: Improving Global Outcomes (KDIGO). *Kidney Int.* 2006;69(11):1945–1953.

74. Gal-Moscovici A, Sprague SM. Role of bone biopsy in stages 3 to 4 chronic kidney disease. *Clin J Am Soc Nephrol.* 2008;3(Supplement 3):S170–S174.

75. Malluche HH, Ritz E, Lange HP, et al. Bone histology in incipient and advanced renal failure. *Kidney Int.* 1976;9(4):355–362.

76. Andress DL. Adynamic bone in patients with chronic kidney disease. *Kidney Int.* 2008;73(12):1345–1354.

77. Goodman WG. Perspectives on renal bone disease. *Kidney Int.* 2006;70: S59–S63.

78. Sanchez-Gonzalez MC, Lopez-Barea F, Bajo M, et al. Serum albumin levels, an additional factor implicated in hyperparathyroidism outcome in peritoneal dialysis: a prospective study with paired bone biopsies. *Adv Perit Dial.* 2006;22: 198–202.

79. Carlstedt E, Ridefelt P, Lind L, et al. Interleukin-6 induced suppression of bovine parathyroid hormone secretion. *Biosci Rep.* 1999;19(1):35–42.

80. Nielsen PK, Rasmussen AK, Butters R, et al. Inhibition of PTH secretion by interleukin-1 beta in bovine parathyroid glands in vitro is associated with an up-regulation of the calcium-sensing receptor mRNA. *Biochem Biophys Res Commun.* 1997;238(3):880–885.

81. Barreto FC, Barreto DV, Moyses RM, et al. K/DOQI-recommended intact PTH levels do not prevent low-turnover bone disease in hemodialysis patients. *Kidney Int.* 2008;73(6):771–777.

82. Moore C, Yee J, Malluche H, et al. Relationship between bone histology and markers of bone and mineral metabolism in African-American hemodialysis patients. *Clin J Am Soc Nephrol.* 2009;4(9):1484–1493.

83. Sawaya BP, Butros R, Naqvi S, et al. Differences in bone turnover and intact PTH levels between African American and Caucasian patients with end-stage renal disease. *Kidney Int.* 2003;64(2):737–742.

84. Alem AM, Sherrard DJ, Gillen DL, et al. Increased risk of hip fracture among patients with end-stage renal disease. *Kidney Int.* 2000;58(1):396–399.

85. Dukas L, Schacht E, Stahelin HB. In elderly men and women treated for osteoporosis a low creatinine clearance of <65 ml/min is a risk factor for falls and fractures. *Osteoporos Int.* 2005;16(12):1683–1690.

86. Ensrud KE, Lui LY, Taylor BC, et al. Renal function and risk of hip and vertebral fractures in older women. *Arch Intern Med.* 2007;167(2):133–139.

87. Nitsch D, Mylne A, Roderick PJ, et al. Chronic kidney disease and hip fracture-related mortality in older people in the UK. *Nephrol Dial Transplant.* 2009;24(5):1539–1544.

88. Rodriguez-Garcia M, Gomez-Alonso C, Naves-Diaz M, et al. Vascular calcifications, vertebral fractures and mortality in haemodialysis patients. *Nephrol Dial Transplant.* 2009;24(1):239–246.

89. Atsumi K, Kushida K, Yamazaki K, et al. Risk factors for vertebral fractures in renal osteodystrophy. *Am J Kidney Dis.* 1999;33(2):287–293.

90. Danese MD, Kim J, Doan QV, et al. PTH and the risks for hip, vertebral, and pelvic fractures among patients on dialysis. *Am J Kidney Dis.* 2006;47(1):149–156.

91. Rudser KD, de Boer IH, Dooley A, et al. Fracture risk after parathyroidectomy among chronic hemodialysis patients. *J Am Soc Nephrol.* 2007;18(8): 2401–2407.

92. Goodman WG, Goldin J, Kuizon BD, et al. Coronary-artery calcification in young adults with end-stage renal disease who are undergoing dialysis. *N Engl J Med.* 2000;342(20):1478–1483.

93. Damjanovic T, Djuric S, Schlieper G, et al. Clinical features of hemodialysis patients with intimal versus medial vascular calcifications. *J Nephrol.* 2009;22(3):358–366.

94. Gelev S, Spasovski G, Dzikova S, et al. Vascular calcification and atherosclerosis in hemodialysis patients: what can we learn from the routine clinical practice? *Int Urol Nephrol.* 2008;40(3):763–770.

95. Russo D, Palmiero G, De Blasio AP, et al. Coronary artery calcification in patients with CRF not undergoing dialysis. *Am J Kidney Dis.* 2004;44(6):1024–1030.

96. Blacher J, Guerin AP, Pannier B, et al. Arterial calcifications, arterial stiffness, and cardiovascular risk in end-stage renal disease. *Hypertension.* 2001;38(4): 938–942.

97. Klassen PS, Lowrie EG, Reddan DN, et al. Association between pulse pressure and mortality in patients undergoing maintenance hemodialysis. *JAMA.* 2002;287(12):1548–1555.

98. Moe SM, Chen NX. Mechanisms of vascular calcification in chronic kidney disease. *J Am Soc Nephrol.* 2008;19(2):213–216.

99. Barreto DV, Barreto FC, Carvalho AB, et al. Coronary calcification in hemodialysis patients: the contribution of traditional and uremia-related risk factors. *Kidney Int.* 2005;67(4):1576–1582.

100. London GM, Marty C, Marchais SJ, et al. Arterial calcifications and bone histomorphometry in end-stage renal disease. *J Am Soc Nephrol.* 2004;15(7): 1943–1951.

101. Mawad HW, Sawaya BP, Sarin R, et al. Calcific uremic arteriolopathy in association with low turnover uremic bone disease. *Clin Nephrol.* 1999;52(3): 160–166.

102. Kurz P, Monier-Faugere MC, Bognar B, et al. Evidence for abnormal calcium homeostasis in patients with adynamic bone disease. *Kidney Int.* 1994; 46(3):855–861.

103. Meric F, Yap P, Bia MJ. Etiology of hypercalcemia in hemodialysis patients on calcium carbonate therapy. *Am J Kidney Dis.* 1990;16(5):459–464.

104. Jean G, Lataillade D, Genet L, et al. Association between very low PTH levels and poor survival rates in haemodialysis patients: results from the French ARNOS Cohort. *Nephron Clin Pract.* 2011;118(2):c211–216.

105. Kestenbaum B, Andress DL, Schwartz SM, et al. Survival following parathyroidectomy among United States dialysis patients. *Kidney Int.* 2004;66(5): 2010–2016.

106. Arnold A, Brown MF, Urena P, et al. Monoclonality of parathyroid tumors in chronic renal failure and in primary parathyroid hyperplasia. *J Clin Invest.* 1995;95(5):2047–2053.
107. Naveh-Many T, Rahamimov R, Livni N, et al. Parathyroid cell proliferation in normal and chronic renal failure rats. The effects of calcium, phosphate, and vitamin D. *J Clin Invest.* 1995;96(4):1786–1793.
108. Wada M, Furuya Y, Sakiyama J, et al. The calcimimetic compound NPS R-568 suppresses parathyroid cell proliferation in rats with renal insufficiency. Control of parathyroid cell growth via a calcium receptor. *J Clin Invest.* 1997;100(12):2977–2983.
109. Gogusev J, Duchambon P, Hory B, et al. Depressed expression of calcium receptor in parathyroid gland tissue of patients with hyperparathyroidism. *Kidney Int.* 1997;51(1):328–336.
110. Kifor O, Moore FD Jr, Wang P, et al. Reduced immunostaining for the extracellular Ca2+-sensing receptor in primary and uremic secondary hyperparathyroidism. *J Clin Endocrinol Metab.* 1996;81(4):1598–1606.
111. Canalejo A, Canalejo R, Rodriguez ME, et al. Development of parathyroid gland hyperplasia without uremia: role of dietary calcium and phosphate. *Nephrol Dial Transplant.* 2010;25(4):1087–1097.
112. Mizobuchi M, Hatamura I, Ogata H, et al. Calcimimetic compound upregulates decreased calcium-sensing receptor expression level in parathyroid glands of rats with chronic renal insufficiency. *J Am Soc Nephrol.* 2004;15(10): 2579–2587.
113. Tokumoto M, Tsuruya K, Fukuda K, et al. Reduced p21, p27 and vitamin D receptor in the nodular hyperplasia in patients with advanced secondary hyperparathyroidism. *Kidney Int.* 2002;62(4):1196–1207.
114. Lopez I, Mendoza FJ, Aguilero-Tejero E, et al. The effect of calcitriol, paricalcitol, and a calcimimetic on extraosseous calcifications in uremic rats. *Kidney Int.* 2008;73(3):300–307.
115. Rodriguez ME, Almaden Y, Canadillas A, et al. The calcimimetic R-568 increases vitamin D receptor expression in rat parathyroid glands. *Am J Physiol Renal Physiol.* 2007;292(5):F1390–1395.
116. Garfia B, Canadillas S, Canalejo A, et al. Regulation of parathyroid vitamin D receptor expression by extracellular calcium. *J Am Soc Nephrol.* 2002;13(12):2945–2952.
117. Sela-Brown A, Russell J, Koszewski NJ, et al. Calreticulin inhibits vitamin D's action on the PTH gene in vitro and may prevent vitamin D's effect in vivo in hypocalcemic rats. *Mol Endocrinol.* 1998;12(8):1193–1200.
118. Arcidiacono MV, Sato T, Alvarez-Hernandez D, et al. EGFR activation increases parathyroid hyperplasia and calcitriol resistance in kidney disease. *J Am Soc Nephrol.* 2008;19(2):310–320.
119. Dusso AS, Pavlopoulous T, Naumovich L, et al. p21(WAF1) and transforming growth factor-alpha mediate dietary phosphate regulation of parathyroid cell growth. *Kidney Int.* 2001;59(3):855–865.
120. Fukagawa M, Okazaki R, Takano K, et al. Regression of parathyroid hyperplasia by calcitriol-pulse therapy in patients on long-term dialysis. *N Engl J Med.* 1990;323(6):421–422.
121. Quarles LD, Yohay DA, Carroll BA, et al. Prospective trial of pulse oral versus intravenous calcitriol treatment of hyperparathyroidism in ESRD. *Kidney Int.* 1994;45(6):1710–1721.
122. Tominaga Y, Tanaka Y, Sato K, et al. Histopathology, pathophysiology, and indications for surgical treatment of renal hyperparathyroidism. *Semin Surg Oncol.* 1997;13(2):78–86.
123. Okuno S, Ishimura E, Kitatani K, et al. Relationship between parathyroid gland size and responsiveness to maxacalcitol therapy in patients with secondary hyperparathyroidism. *Nephrol Dial Transplant.* 2003;18(12):2613–2621.
124. Tominaga Y, Inaguma D, Matsuoka S, et al. Is the volume of the parathyroid gland a predictor of Maxacalcitol response in advanced secondary hyperparathyroidism? *Ther Apher Dial.* 2006;10(2):198–204.
125. John MR, Goodman WG, Gao P, et al. A novel immunoradiometric assay detects full-length human PTH but not amino-terminally truncated fragments: implications for PTH measurements in renal failure. *J Clin Endocrinol Metab.* 1999;84(11):4287–4290.
126. Monier-Faugere MC, Geng Z, Mawad H, et al. Improved assessment of bone turnover by the PTH-(1–84)/large C-PTH fragments ratio in ESRD patients. *Kidney Int.* 2001;60(4):1460–1468.
127. Jean G, Charra B, Chazot C. Vitamin D deficiency and associated factors in hemodialysis patients. *J Ren Nutr.* 2008;18(5):395–399.
128. Coen G, Mantella D, Manni M, et al. 25–hydroxyvitamin D levels and bone histomorphometry in hemodialysis renal osteodystrophy. *Kidney Int.* 2005;68(4):1840–1848.
129. Ishimura E, Nishizawa Y, Inaba M, et al. Serum levels of 1,25–dihydroxyvitamin D, 24,25–dihydroxyvitamin D, and 25–hydroxyvitamin D in nondialyzed patients with chronic renal failure. *Kidney Int.* 1999;55(3):1019–1027.
130. Papapoulos SE, Clemens TL, Fraher LJ, et al. Metabolites of vitamin D in human vitamin-D deficiency: effect of vitamin D3 or 1,25–dihydroxycholecalciferol. *Lancet.* 1980;2(8195 pt 1):612–615.
131. Coen G, Ballanti P, Fischer MS, et al. Bone markers in the diagnosis of low turnover osteodystrophy in haemodialysis patients. *Nephrol Dial Transplant.* 1998;13(9):2294–2302.
132. Urena P, De Vernejoul MC. Circulating biochemical markers of bone remodeling in uremic patients. *Kidney Int.* 1999;55(6):2141–2156.
133. Ferreira A, Drueke TB. Biological markers in the diagnosis of the different forms of renal osteodystrophy. *Am J Med Sci.* 2000;320(2):85–89.
134. Urena P, Hruby M, Ferreira A, et al. Plasma total versus bone alkaline phosphatase as markers of bone turnover in hemodialysis patients. *J Am Soc Nephrol.* 1996;7(3):506–512.
135. Couttenye MM, D'Haese PC, Van Hoof VO, et al. Low serum levels of alkaline phosphatase of bone origin: a good marker of adynamic bone disease in haemodialysis patients. *Nephrol Dial Transplant.* 1996;11(6):1065–1072.
136. Chu P, Chao TY, Lin YF, et al. Correlation between histomorphometric parameters of bone resorption and serum type 5b tartrate-resistant acid phosphatase in uremic patients on maintenance hemodialysis. *Am J Kidney Dis.* 2003; 41(5):1052–1059.
137. Ambrosoni P, Olaizola I, Heuquerot C, et al. The role of imaging techniques in the study of renal osteodystrophy. *Am J Med Sci.* 2000;320(2):90–95.
138. Tigges S, Nance EP, Carpenter WA, et al. Renal osteodystrophy: imaging findings that mimic those of other diseases. *AJR Am J Roentgenol.* 1995;165(1): 143–148.
139. McIntyre CW. Is it practical to screen dialysis patients for vascular calcification? *Nephrol Dial Transplant.* 2006;21(2):251–254.
140. Khaw KT, Sneyd MJ, Compston J. Bone density parathyroid hormone and 25–hydroxyvitamin D concentrations in middle aged women. *BMJ.* 1992; 305(6848):273–277.
141. K/DOQI clinical practice guidelines for bone metabolism and disease in chronic kidney disease. *Am J Kidney Dis.* 2003;42(4 Suppl 3):S1–201.
142. Kazama JJ. Japanese Society of Dialysis Therapy treatment guidelines for secondary hyperparathyroidism. *Ther Apher Dial.* 2007;11 Suppl 1:S44–47.
143. Quarles LD, Lobaugh B, Murphy G. Intact parathyroid hormone overestimates the presence and severity of parathyroid-mediated osseous abnormalities in uremia. *J Clin Endocrinol Metab.* 1992;75(1):145–150.
144. Nakai S, Akiba T, Kazama J, et al. Effects of serum calcium, phosphorous, and intact parathyroid hormone levels on survival in chronic hemodialysis patients in Japan. *Ther Apher Dial.* 2008;12(1):49–54.
145. Isakova T, Gutierrez OM, Smith K, et al. Pilot study of dietary phosphorus restriction and phosphorus binders to target fibroblast growth factor 23 in patients with chronic kidney disease. *Nephrol Dial Transplant.* 2011;26(2):584–591.
146. Llach F, Massry SG. On the mechanism of secondary hyperparathyroidism in moderate renal insufficiency. *J Clin Endocrinol Metab.* 1985;61(4):601–606.
147. Portale AA, Booth BE, Halloran BP, et al. Effect of dietary phosphorus on circulating concentrations of 1,25–dihydroxyvitamin D and immunoreactive parathyroid hormone in children with moderate renal insufficiency. *J Clin Invest.* 1984;73(6):1580–1589.
148. Pohlmeier R, Vienken J. Phosphate removal and hemodialysis conditions. *Kidney Int Suppl.* 2001;78:S190–194.
149. Chauveau P, Poignet JL, Kuno T, et al. Phosphate removal rate: a comparative study of five high-flux dialysers. *Nephrol Dial Transplant.* 1991;6 Suppl 2:114–115.
150. Kerr PG, Lo A, Chin M, et al. Dialyzer performance in the clinic: comparison of six low-flux membranes. *Artif Organs.* 1999;23(9):817–821.
151. Harris DC, Yuill E, Chesher DW. Correcting acidosis in hemodialysis: effect on phosphate clearance and calcification risk. *J Am Soc Nephrol.* 1995; 6(6):1607–1612.
152. Ayus JC, Mizani MR, Achinger SG, et al. Effects of short daily versus conventional hemodialysis on left ventricular hypertrophy and inflammatory markers: a prospective, controlled study. *J Am Soc Nephrol.* 2005;16(9):2778–2788.
153. Kooienga L. Phosphorus balance with daily dialysis. *Semin Dial.* 2007;20(4): 342–345.
154. Cheng SC, Young DO, Huang Y, et al. A randomized, double-blind, placebo-controlled trial of niacinamide for reduction of phosphorus in hemodialysis patients. *Clin J Am Soc Nephrol.* 2008;3(4):1131–1138.
155. Takahashi Y, Tanaka A, Nakamura T, et al. Nicotinamide suppresses hyperphosphatemia in hemodialysis patients. *Kidney Int.* 2004;65(3):1099–1104.
156. Young DO, Cheng SC, Delmez JA, et al. The effect of oral niacinamide on plasma phosphorus levels in peritoneal dialysis patients. *Perit Dial Int.* 2009;29(5): 562–567.
157. Muller D, Mehling H, Otto B, et al. Niacin lowers serum phosphate and increases HDL cholesterol in dialysis patients. *Clin J Am Soc Nephrol.* 2007;2(6): 1249–1254.

158. Al-Aly Z, Qazi RA, Gonzalez EA, et al. Changes in serum 25–hydroxy-vitamin D and plasma intact PTH levels following treatment with ergocalciferol in patients with CKD. *Am J Kidney Dis.* 2007;50(1):59–68.
159. Zisman AL, Hristova M, Ho LT, et al. Impact of ergocalciferol treatment of vitamin D deficiency on serum parathyroid hormone concentrations in chronic kidney disease. Am *J Nephrol.* 2007;27(1):36–43.
160. Berl T, Berns AS, Hufer WE, et al. 1,25 dihydroxycholecalciferol effects in chronic dialysis. A double-blind controlled study. *Ann Intern Med.* 1978;88(6):774–780.
161. Malluche HH, Ritz E, Werner E, et al. Long-term administration of vitamin D steroles in incipient and advanced renal failure: effect on bone histology. *Clin Nephrol.* 1978;10(6):219–228.
162. Panichi V, Migliori M, Taccola D, et al. Effects of calcitriol on the immune system: new possibilities in the treatment of glomerulonephritis. *Clin Exp Pharmacol Physiol.* 2003;30(11):807–811.
163. Richart T, Li Y, Staessen JA. Renal versus extrarenal activation of vitamin D in relation to atherosclerosis, arterial stiffening, and hypertension. *Am J Hypertens.* 2007;20(9):1007–1015.
164. Stubbs JR, Idiculla A, Slusser J, et al. Cholecalciferol supplementation alters calcitriol-responsive monocyte proteins and decreases inflammatory cytokines in ESRD. *J Am Soc Nephrol.* 2010;21(2):353–361.
165. Hayashi M, Tsuchiya Y, Itaya Y, et al. Comparison of the effects of calcitriol and maxacalcitol on secondary hyperparathyroidism in patients on chronic haemodialysis: a randomized prospective multicentre trial. *Nephrol Dial Transplant.* 2004;19(8):2067–2073.
166. Sprague SM, Llach F, Amdahl M, et al. Paricalcitol versus calcitriol in the treatment of secondary hyperparathyroidism. *Kidney Int.* 2003;63(4): 1483–1490.
167. Malluche HH, Mawad H, Monier-Faugere MC. Effects of treatment of renal osteodystrophy on bone histology. *Clin J Am Soc Nephrol.* 2008;3 Suppl 3: S157–163.
168. Shoben AB, et al. Association of oral calcitriol with improved survival in nondialyzed CKD. *J Am Soc Nephrol.* 2008;19(8):1613–1649.
169. Goodman WG, Frazao JM, Goodkin DA, et al. A calcimimetic agent lowers plasma parathyroid hormone levels in patients with secondary hyperparathyroidism. *Kidney Int.* 2000;58(1):436–445.
170. Lindberg JS, Culleton B, Wong G, et al. Cinacalcet HCl, an oral calcimimetic agent for the treatment of secondary hyperparathyroidism in hemodialysis and peritoneal dialysis: a randomized, double-blind, multicenter study. *J Am Soc Nephrol.* 2005;16(3):800–807.
171. Block GA, Zaun D, Smits G, et al. Cinacalcet for secondary hyperparathyroidism in patients receiving hemodialysis. *N Engl J Med.* 2004;350(15): 1516–1525.
172. Messa P, Macario F, Yagoob M, et al. The OPTIMA study: assessing a new cinacalcet (Sensipar/Mimpara) treatment algorithm for secondary hyperparathyroidism. *Clin J Am Soc Nephrol.* 2008;3(1):36–45.
173. Chertow GM, Blumenthal S, Turner S, et al. Cinacalcet hydrochloride (Sensipar) in hemodialysis patients on active vitamin D derivatives with controlled PTH and elevated calcium × phosphate. *Clin J Am Soc Nephrol.* 2006;1(2):305–312.
174. Chonchol M, Locatelli F, Abboud HE, et al. A randomized, double-blind, placebo-controlled study to assess the efficacy and safety of cinacalcet HCl in participants with CKD not receiving dialysis. *Am J Kidney Dis.* 2009;53(2): 197–207.
175. Malluche HH, Monier-Faugere MC, Wang G, et al. An assessment of cinacalcet HCl effects on bone histology in dialysis patients with secondary hyperparathyroidism. *Clin Nephrol.* 2008;69(4):269–278.
176. Ishii H, Wada M, Furuya Y, et al. Daily intermittent decreases in serum levels of parathyroid hormone have an anabolic-like action on the bones of uremic rats with low-turnover bone and osteomalacia. *Bone.* 2000;26(2): 175–182.
177. Cunningham J, Danese M, Olson K, et al. Effects of the calcimimetic cinacalcet HCl on cardiovascular disease, fracture, and health-related quality of life in secondary hyperparathyroidism. *Kidney Int.* 2005;68(4):1793–1800.
178. Wetmore JB, Liu S, Krebill R, et al. Effects of cinacalcet and concurrent low-dose vitamin D on FGF23 levels in ESRD. *Clin J Am Soc Nephrol.* 2010;5(1): 110–116.
179. D'Haese PC, Spasovski GB, Sikole A, et al. A multicenter study on the effects of lanthanum carbonate (Fosrenol) and calcium carbonate on renal bone disease in dialysis patients. *Kidney Int Suppl.* 2003;(85):S73–78.
180. Ferreira A, Frazao JM, Monier-Faugere MC, et al. Effects of sevelamer hydrochloride and calcium carbonate on renal osteodystrophy in hemodialysis patients. *J Am Soc Nephrol.* 2008;19(2):405–412.
181. Haris A, Sherrard DJ, Hercz G. Reversal of adynamic bone disease by lowering of dialysate calcium. *Kidney Int.* 2006;70(5):931–937.
182. Spasovski G, Geleve S, Masin-Spasovska J, et al. Improvement of bone and mineral parameters related to adynamic bone disease by diminishing dialysate calcium. *Bone.* 2007;41(4):698–703.
183. Lezaic V, Pejanovic S, Kostic S, et al. Effects of lowering dialysate calcium concentration on mineral metabolism and parathyroid hormone secretion: a multicentric study. *Ther Apher Dial.* 2007;11(2):121–130.
184. Goodman WG, Ramirez JA, Belin TR, et al. Development of adynamic bone in patients with secondary hyperparathyroidism after intermittent calcitriol therapy. *Kidney Int.* 1994;46(4):1160–1166.
185. Salusky IB, Kuizon BD, Belin TR, et al. Intermittent calcitriol therapy in secondary hyperparathyroidism: a comparison between oral and intraperitoneal administration. *Kidney Int.* 1998;54(3):907–914.
186. Wesseling-Perry K, Pereira RC, Sahney S, et al. Calcitriol and doxercalciferol are equivalent in controlling bone turnover, suppressing parathyroid hormone, and increasing fibroblast growth factor-23 in secondary hyperparathyroidism. *Kidney Int.* 2011;79(1):112–119.
187. Baldock PA, Thomas GP, Hodge JM, et al. Vitamin D action and regulation of bone remodeling: suppression of osteoclastogenesis by the mature osteoblast. *J Bone Miner Res.* 2006;21(10):1618–1626.
188. Okuda N, Takeda S, Shinomiya K, et al. ED-71, a novel vitamin D analog, promotes bone formation and angiogenesis and inhibits bone resorption after bone marrow ablation. *Bone.* 2007;40(2):281–292.
189. Sprague SM. The role of the bone biopsy in the diagnosis of renal osteodystrophy. *Semin Dial.* 2000;13(3):152–155.

CHAPTER 78

Nervous System Manifestations of Renal Disease

Yeong-Hau Howard Lien

Patients with chronic kidney disease (CKD) manifest a variety of neurologic disorders involving central, peripheral, and autonomic nervous systems. The severity of these nervous system manifestations increases in parallel to the advance of CKD. Without dialysis, patients with end-stage renal disease (ESRD) will develop uremic encephalopathy, uremic neuropathy, and uremic autonomic neuropathy. Some of these symptoms are partially or completely reversed by renal replacement therapy (i.e., dialysis or kidney transplantation). On the other hand, neurologic complications may occur due to improper hemodialysis, such as dialysis disequilibrium syndrome (DDS) and dialysis dementia, or due to complications of arteriovenous fistula (AVF) placement, such as ischemic monomelic neuropathy and vascular steal syndrome. In this chapter, CKD-associated neurologic disorders are reviewed in three sections: the central nervous system (CNS), the peripheral nervous system (PNS), and the autonomic nervous system (ANS).

CENTRAL NERVOUS SYSTEM

Several distinct CNS syndromes have been recognized in patients with ESRD: uremic encephalopathy,[1] DDS,[2] and dialysis dementia.[3] In addition, dementia and cognition impairment, common in elderly populations, are significantly worsened by renal impairment, but poorly recognized in ESRD patients.[4] These disorders are multifactorial and associated with prolonged hospitalization and an increased risk of mortality. Lastly, restless leg syndrome (RLS), a poorly understood syndrome, probably related to dopaminergic dysfunction in the subcortical system, affects 10% to 20% of ESRD patients[5] and is discussed under the CNS section.

Uremic Encephalopathy

Manifestations

Uremic encephalopathy is an acute or subacute organic brain syndrome that occurs in patients with advanced renal failure and is frequently associated with GFR less than 10 mL/min/1.73 m^2. The term *uremic encephalopathy* is used to describe the early appearance and dialysis responsiveness of the nonspecific neurologic symptoms of uremia. Patients with uremic encephalopathy display variable disorders of consciousness, psychomotor behavior, thinking, memory, speech, perception, and emotion.[6,7] The symptoms may include sluggishness and easy fatigue; daytime drowsiness and insomnia with a tendency toward sleep inversion; inability to focus or sustain attention or to perform mental (cognitive) tasks and manipulation; inability to manage ideas and abstractions; slurring of speech; anorexia, nausea, and vomiting probably of central origin; imprecise memory; volatile emotionality and withdrawal; myoclonus and asterixis; paranoid thought content; disorientation and confusion with bizarre behavior; hallucinosis; transient pareses and aphasic episodes; coma; and convulsions.[6,8]

With an early recognition of CKD and the timely initiation of renal replacement therapy, severe uremic encephalopathy has been rare and is mainly related to acute kidney injury or unattended CKD due to a lack of health care. The severe neurologic symptoms of uremic encephalopathy such as seizure, confusion, myoclonus, and asterixis, are usually improved after a few runs of dialysis, and rarely recur if dialysis clearance is adequate. However, uremic encephalopathy may occur in patients on maintenance dialysis if they are not compliant with dialysis treatment, or if their dialysis prescriptions are not adequate. It should be mentioned that even with adequate dialysis, patients on maintenance dialysis may still have mild CNS symptoms, such as cognitive dysfunction as part of a "residual syndrome" because dialysis only replaces a fraction of total renal function.[9]

Pathogenesis

The mechanisms of uremic encephalopathy are multifactorial and largely unknown.[1] It has been proposed that uremic encephalopathy is due to an accumulation of uremic toxins. Although many uremic toxins have been identified, exact toxins responsible for uremic encephalopathy are still unclear.[10] Table 78.1 lists selected examples of uremic toxins grouped according to their structure. The source and characteristics of these toxins are provided.[8]

TABLE 78.1 **Uremic Toxins**[8]

Solute Group	Example	Source	Characteristics
Peptides and small proteins	β2-microglobulin	Shed from MHC	Poorly dialyzed because of large size
Guanidines	Guanidine, creatinine, guanidinosuccinic acid, methylguanidine	Arginine	Increased production in uremia
Phenols	p-Cresol sulfate	Phenylalanine, tyrosine	Protein bound, produced by gut bacteria
Indoles	Indican	Tryptophan	Protein bound, produced by gut bacteria
Aliphatic amines	Dimethylamine, trimethylamine	Choline	Large volume of distribution, produced by gut bacteria
Furans	CMPF	Unknown	Tightly protein bound
Polyols	Myoinositol	Dietary intake, cell synthesis from glucose	Normally degraded by the kidney rather than excreted
Nucleosides	Pseudouridine	tRNA	Most prominent of several altered RNA species
Dicarboxylic acids	Oxalate	Ascorbic acid	Formation of crystal deposits
Carbonyls	Glyoxal	Glycolytic intermediates	Reaction with proteins to form advanced glycation end products

MHC, major histocompatibility complex; CMPF, 3-carboxy-4-methyl-5-propyl-2-furanpropionic acid.
Modified from Meyer TW, Hostetter TH. Uremia. *N Engl J Med.* 2007;357:1316–1325.

Among them, uremic guanidino compounds, including creatinine, guanidine, guanidinosuccinic acid (GSA), and methylguanidine, are highly elevated in both the serum and cerebrospinal fluid (CSF) of uremic patients. GSA is a potential candidate as a uremic neurotoxin because it induces convulsion in animals at a dosage that produces a brain GSA level comparable to that of uremic patients.[11] In vitro, GSA blocks both γ-aminobutyric acid (GABA) A receptors and glycine receptors. However, GSA-induced convulsions only respond to N-methyl-D-aspartate (NMDA) receptor antagonists. Further studies revealed that GSA causes neurotoxicity via activation of the NMDA receptor and by increasing Ca^{2+} influx.[11] Whether these in vitro and in vivo findings have pathophysiologic significance in uremic encephalopathy is still controversial.

Parathyroid hormone (PTH) is another neurotoxin in a uremic state.[1] PTH causes neurotoxicity by increasing intracellular Ca^{2+} concentration in brain cells. The total brain Ca^{2+} content is elevated in uremic patients and animals.[1] The electroencephalogram (EEG) findings in uremic dogs are similar to those in patients with uremic encephalopathy. Both increased brain calcium content and EEG abnormalities in the uremic dog can be prevented by a parathyroidectomy.[12] Furthermore, the intracellular Ca^{2+} level in brain synaptosomes is increased in uremic animals, which can be prevented by parathyroidectomy or reduced by verapamil, a calcium channel blocker.[13] The increased intracellular Ca in uremic synaptosomes can be explained by an increased Ca^{2+} uptake and a decreased Ca^{2+} extrusion, both of which are mediated by PTH.[13–15] Because calcium is an essential mediator of neurotransmitter release and a regulator of intracellular metabolic and enzymatic processes, alterations in brain calcium are likely to affect cerebral function.

Abnormal neurotransmitter content or release in the brain has been reported in uremic animals. Decreased brain norepinephrine content, uptake and release,[16] and increased acetylcholine content and release[17] are found in uremic rats. In addition, the basal outflow of GABA and glutamate, but not the K^+-stimulated outflow in the hypothalamus, which is measured by microdialysis, is increased in uremic rats. However, the K^+-stimulated release of GABA is less sensitive to Ca depletion.[18] Whether these changes in neurotransmitters in uremic rats are related to uremic encephalopathy in humans is not clear at present.

Diagnosis

Clinically, the diagnosis of uremic encephalopathy is suspected in patients with advanced CKD who present with a constellation of neurologic clinical signs and symptoms, as described earlier. The diagnosis can be confirmed with the resolution of signs and symptoms after a series of dialysis. Electroencephalographic findings in uremic encephalopathy are nonspecific. Typical findings are generalized slowing with an excess of delta and theta waves and sometimes bilateral spike–wave complexes.[19] EEG is rarely needed for diagnosing uremic encephalopathy.

Similarly, brain images are rarely performed for patients with uremic encephalopathy. In one study, a diffusion-weighted magnetic resonance imaging (MRI) was performed prior to the initiation of hemodialysis in eight ESRD patients. The average blood urea nitrogen (BUN) level was 161 mg per deciliter. None of these patients had prior neurologic disorders. MRI revealed diffuse interstitial brain edema with a increased apparent diffusion coefficient.[20] However, reversible diffuse cytotoxic brain edema was reported in a patient with left facial palsy, aphasia and confusion, and a BUN level of 220 mg per deciliter.[21] It appears that uremic encephalopathy is associated with brain edema, which may advance from interstitial form to cytotoxic form if left untreated.

In patients on maintenance dialysis, the diagnosis of uremic encephalopathy can be difficult. The neurologic symptoms and signs are similar between uremic encephalopathy and other brain pathologies such as strokes, hepatic encephalopathy, hypertensive encephalopathy, Wernicke encephalopathy, and others (Table 78.2). Other differential diagnoses include electrolyte and endocrine abnormalities, drug and food effects, dementia, and depression (Table 78.2). In ESRD patients, an altered mental status may occur due to electrolyte and endocrine abnormalities such as hyponatremia, hypernatremia, hypocalcemia, hypercalcemia, and hypoglycemia. The drugs listed in Table 78.2 are commonly associated with neurotoxicity in patients with ESRD. They cause confusion or seizure probably due to changes in drug metabolism or clearance of the drugs, or their potentially toxic metabolites. Starfruit (Fig. 78.1), a popular fruit in Southeast Asia and Central and South America, can cause neurologic symptoms in patients with advanced CKD within hours. Symptoms include hiccups, vomiting, confusion, seizure, and even death.[22] In one series from Taiwan, the mortality was as high as 40%.[23]

TABLE 78.2 Differential Diagnosis for Altered Mental Status in Patients with Advanced Chronic Kidney Disease[19,22,23,48]

Uremic encephalopathy
Hepatic encephalopathy
Hypertensive encephalopathy
Wernicke encephalopathy
Dialysis disequilibrium syndrome
Strokes and transient ischemic attack
Subdural hematoma
Electrolyte and metabolic abnormalities: Hyponatremia, hypernatremia, hypocalcemia, hypercalcemia, hypoglycemia
Drugs: Opioid analgesics, antibiotics (cephalosporin), antiviral agents (acyclovir), gabapentin, cimetidine, metoclopramide, isoniazid, encainide, cinacalcet, and others
Food: Starfruit (Averrhoa carambola)
Dementia: Vascular dementia and Alzheimer dementia
Depression

If BUN and serum creatinine (Cr) levels are elevated, uremic encephalopathy due to inadequate dialysis can be diagnosed without difficulties. Frequently, BUN and serum Cr levels may not be elevated due to malnutrition and sarcopenia, which are frequently associated with inadequate dialysis. A careful evaluation of dialysis records and physical and laboratory findings are needed to eliminate possibilities of other encephalopathies because the management could be quite different for each disease. For example, Wernicke encephalopathy (ophthalmoplegia, ataxia, and disturbance of consciousness) is due to the depletion of thiamine from dialysis removal of this water-soluble vitamin, and can be treated with supplementation of thiamine along with other water soluble vitamins.[24] If uremic encephalopathy is highly suspected, a therapeutic trial with renal replacement frequently ameliorates CNS symptoms and confirms the diagnosis.

Of note, there are a few case reports of posterior reversible encephalopathy syndrome (PRES) in patients with ESRD and neurologic symptoms.[25–27] These patients had bilateral

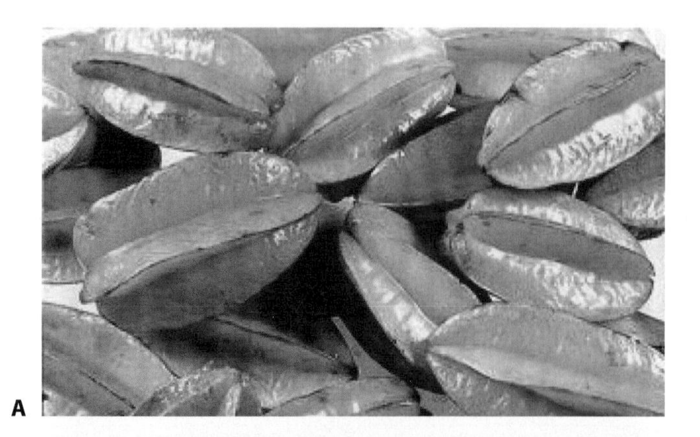

A

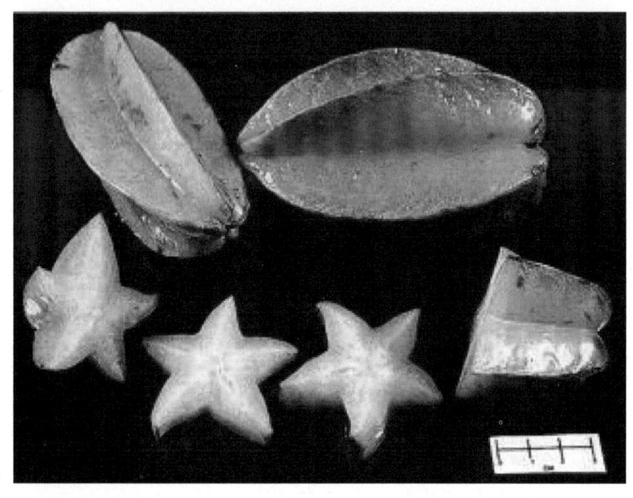

B

FIGURE 78.1 Starfruit (*Averrhoa carambola*), a lethal fruit for the ESRD patient. (From Neto MM, da Costa JA, Garcia-Cairasco N, et al. Intoxication by star fruit (Averrhoa carambola) in 32 uraemic patients: treatment and outcome. *Nephrol Dial Transplant.* 2003;18:120–125.)

symmetric hypodense lesions in the territories of the posterior circulation, which were reversible after hypertension was controlled. Almost all of them presented with uncontrolled hypertension (frequently > 200 mm Hg systolically). The brain edema is due to the leakage of fluid from hypertension-damaged blood vessels, so called "vasogenic edema." The edema occurs preferentially in the posterior of the brain, whereas brain edema associated with uremic encephalopathy is diffuse. Because the pathogenesis and treatment of these two diseases are different, it is critical to distinguish them as separate disease entities.

Prevention and Treatment

Uremic encephalopathy can be largely eliminated with the early referral of CKD patients to nephrologists and the timely initiation of dialysis. For patients on maintenance dialysis, the routine evaluation of dialysis adequacy and increased dialysis clearance for those who fall behind are effective in preventing uremic encephalopathy. As for treatment, intensive dialysis therapy—frequently, daily dialysis—should improve neurologic symptoms and signs within a week or two. A lack of response should prompt physicians to look for other etiologies. Although secondary hyperparathyroidism has been implicated in the pathogenesis of uremic encephalopathy, reducing the PTH level is rarely needed to improve neurologic symptoms. It is possible that repeated hemodialysis may reduce brain Ca^{21} content, thus reducing neurologic symptoms.[1]

Dialysis Disequilibrium Syndrome

Manifestations

DDS occurs rarely in current nephrology practice because of the early initiation of renal replacement therapy and routine orders of slow blood flow rate and short dialysis duration during the initial dialysis sessions. The cardinal symptoms of DDS are the symptoms caused by elevated intracranial pressure such as headache, nausea, and vomiting. These symptoms may progress into confusion, seizure, and even death if unrecognized and left untreated. The onset of DDS is usually during or immediately after aggressive hemodialysis, frequently in the setting of the first hemodialysis session.

Pathogenesis

The hallmark of DDS is brain edema that is induced by dialysis. Evidence accumulated that the "reverse urea effect" is the cause of DDS.[2] Hemodialysis rapidly removes urea from the blood, but does not remove urea from the brain as efficiently. As a consequence, the urea concentration is higher in the brain than in the blood. This brain–blood urea gradient drives water to enter into brain tissue and causes brain edema and raises intracranial pressure. Elevated brain urea concentration and increased brain water content have been demonstrated in animals undergoing aggressive hemodialysis.[28] When urea was added to the dialysate to keep the blood urea concentration equal to that in the brain, brain edema did not occur after hemodialysis. Using MRI, Galons et al.[29] reported that the apparent diffusion coefficient of brain water increased in nephrectomized rats after hemodialysis. These results strongly suggest that the brain edema induced by hemodialysis in uremic rats is due to interstitial edema rather than cytotoxic edema, further supporting the reverse urea effect as the pathogenetic mechanism of brain edema in DDS. The increased diffusion coefficient of brain water after fast hemodialysis has been confirmed in patients with ESRD.[20]

More recently, a potential molecular basis for the reverse urea effect has been identified. In uremic rats, the brain expression of urea transporter 1 (UTB1) is reduced by 50%, whereas water channels aquaporin 4 (AQP4) and AQP9 were upregulated. Because of low UTB abundance, urea exit from the brain is likely delayed during the rapid removal of extracellular urea through fast dialysis. This creates an osmotic driving force that promotes water entry into the brain and subsequent brain swelling.[30]

There are other hypotheses for the pathogenesis of DDS, such as the creation of idiogenic osmoles, or paradoxical intracellular acidosis by hemodialysis.[31,32] However,

Silva et al.[28] measured most known organic osmoles in the brain after hemodialysis and did not find any significant changes in their concentrations. As for the acidosis hypothesis, it is not clear how intracellular acidosis causes interstitial edema. Although frequently quoted as the pathogenesis of DDS, one may wonder if cerebral acidosis is the consequence, rather than the cause, of brain edema in DDS.

Diagnosis

The diagnosis of DDS is mainly based on the onset of symptoms, the history of prolonged and untreated renal failure, markedly elevated BUN levels, and the association with hemodialysis. Unfortunately, up to now there are no clinical criteria for the diagnosis of DDS. As a result, DDS has become a wastebasket for any neurologic symptoms that occur after hemodialysis. Although DDS is rarely encountered in current nephrology practice, there have been several cases reported in recent literature, including two lethal cases.[33–37] These cases are summarized in Table 78.3. Most of them are young, with a predialysis BUN level in the range of 109 to 241 mg per deciliter and a decrease in the BUN level of 60 to 92 mg per deciliter. The blood flow rate and dialysis time in some cases are excessive. The onset of symptoms is closely related to hemodialysis. Most of them had documented brain edema with imaging studies. Two out of 5 patients died, and the others recovered without sequelae. From these case reports, it appears that a predialysis BUN level greater than 100 mg per deciliter with a decrease in BUN level greater than 60 mg per deciliter are reasonable criteria for the diagnosis of clinically significant DDS (i.e., altered mental status, seizure, and neurologic defects). The onset of symptoms occurs immediately after hemodialysis and brain edema, which are demonstrated by imaging studies that may further confirm the diagnosis. It should be mentioned that uremic patients with a head injury, subdural hematoma, stroke, malignant hypertension, and other conditions associated with brain edema are at a higher risk of DDS due to existing conditions that predispose them to cerebral edema.[36]

Prevention and Treatment

It has been well established that limiting dialysis efficiency at the initiation of hemodialysis is the best way to prevent DDS (i.e., performing hemodialysis with a low blood flow rate, short dialysis time, and a small dialysis filter). This gentle dialysis treatment does not remove blood urea rapidly, thus preventing the formation of the brain–blood urea gradient.[36] It is helpful to estimate the urea reduction rate from the dialysis prescription and target urea reduction to less than 60 mg per deciliter. Another common practice for preventing DDS is infusing mannitol during hemodialysis to raise serum osmolarity in order to reduce the brain–blood osmolarity gradient. The infusion of mannitol during hemodialysis is recommended for preventing DDS only in high-risk patients with marked azotemia (BUN level $>$ 150 mg per deciliter) or in those with preexisting risk factors, as mentioned earlier. Mannitol infusion can cause acute volume expansion and congestive heart failure, and thus should not be used routinely for the initiation of hemodialysis.

TABLE 78.3 **Clinical Parameters of Cases with Dialysis Disequilibrium Syndrome**

Reference	Age (years)	Sex	Pre-HD BUN	Post-HD BUN	ΔBUN	BFR (mL/min)	HD Time (hour)	Onset (hour after HD)	Brain Edema	Outcome
Harris et al., 1989 (33)	22	F	109	47	62	NA	1.5	0	Yes	Death
DiFresco et al., 2000 (35)	22	F	199	110	89	150	1.5	0	Yes[a]	Recovery
Bagshaw et al., 2004 (34)	22	M	130	38	92	250–350	4	0	Yes	Death
Patel et al., 2008 (36)	54	M	131	71	60	250–300	4	1	No	Recovery
Attur et al., 2008 (37)	15	M	241	160	81	150	4	0	Yes	Recovery

[a]Dialysis disequilibrium syndrome with brain edema recurred during the second hemodialysis session (pre- and post-HD BUN levels were not available for the second hemodialysis session).
Pre-HD, prehemodialysis; post-HD, posthemodialysis; ΔBUN, change in BUN after hemodialysis; BFR, blood flow rate; F, female, M, male; NA, not available.

Dialysis Dementia

Manifestation

This mysterious syndrome haunted dialysis patients in the 1970s, but it has now nearly vanished completely. Dialysis dementia, also named dialysis encephalopathy, is a progressive, frequently fatal neurologic disease almost appearing exclusively in patients being treated with chronic hemodialysis for more than 2 years. Early manifestations consist of a mixed dysarthria–apraxia of speech with slurring, stuttering, and hesitancy. Patients subsequently develop personality changes, including psychoses, paranoid thinking, or delirium, and global dementia, myoclonus, and seizures. In most cases, the disease progressed to death within 6 to 12 months.[3] Observation studies revealed that dialysis dementia is a part of a multisystem disease that may include encephalopathy, osteomalacic bone disease, proximal myopathy, and anemia.[3,38]

Pathogenesis

Aluminum intoxication was first implicated in this disorder by Alfrey et al.[39] Aluminum content of the brain's gray matter, of bone, and of other soft tissue is markedly elevated in patients with dialysis dementia. Strong epidemiologic evidence links dialysis dementia to aluminum intoxication from the dialysate water and/or from oral phosphate binders containing aluminum.[3] Furthermore, citrate was frequently used to correct metabolic acidosis in patients with advanced CKD. The gastrointestinal (GI) absorption of aluminum is markedly enhanced by the concomitant use of citrate.[40] After a routine deionization of dialysate with reverse osmosis for removing contaminated aluminum in dialysis facilities and the limited use of aluminum containing phosphate binders, dialysis dementia has been nearly eliminated.

Diagnosis

Dialysis dementia is suspected in patients on maintenance dialysis who develop speech disorders, personality changes, and dementia. EEGs are diagnostic for dialysis dementia. The characteristic EEG changes are a mild slowing of the dominant rhythm with increased low voltage theta and bursts of anteriorly predominant high voltage delta. Occasionally, the paroxysmal activity may take the form of a 1.3 to 3.0 c per second spike and wave, mainly in the frontocentral region.[3] Blood aluminum levels may not be elevated, but should be increased after the infusion of the chelating agent, deferoxamine (DFO).[41] The concurrence of osteomalacia and microcytic anemia also prompts physicians to look for aluminum toxicity.

Prevention and Treatment

As mentioned earlier, dialysis dementia is nearly eliminated due to the use of reverse osmosis and the replacement of aluminum-containing phosphate binders with calcium-based binders or sevelamer. As mentioned earlier, citrate-containing alkylating agents enhance aluminum absorption and should not be used in conjunction with aluminum-based binders. As for treatment, DFO has been used for chelating aluminum. DFO is usually given at the end of hemodialysis. During the following dialysis session, the DFO-Al complex can be removed effectively by a polysulfone dialyzer.[42] Aggravation of dialysis dementia by DFO may occur due to the release of aluminum from tissue.[43]

Dementia and Cognitive Impairment

Manifestations

With the marked reduction in the occurrence of uremic encephalopathy, DDS, and dialysis dementia, cognitive impairment and dementia have become the major CNS disorders in patients with ESRD. Dementia is characterized by a loss of function in multiple cognitive domains such as a decline in memory from previously higher levels of functioning, together with at least one of the following: aphasia, apraxia, agnosia, or disturbances in executive functioning. Cognitive impairment indicates that a patient's ability to function in their work, personal, or social environment is affected.[4] Both dementia and cognitive impairment are highly prevalent in patients with ESRD. Murray et al.[44] reported that in 338 prevalent hemodialysis patients, 37% had severe cognitive impairment, qualified as dementia, 36% had moderate impairment, and 13% had mild impairment. In addition, the prevalence of cognitive impairment in ESRD patients increases with aging. It is 20% to 30% in patients 55 to 84 years of age, and increased to 50% to 60% in those 85 years or older.[4]

Cognitive impairment may already be present in patients with CKD stages 3 and 4. In the Heart Estrogen/Progestin Replacement (HERS) study, which involves 1,015 menopausal women with coronary artery disease, there is a fivefold risk of cognitive impairment if the estimated glomerular filtration rate (eGFR) is < 30 (stages 4 and 5) and patients with cognitive impairment tend to have a rapid progression of CKD.[45] In the Reasons for Geographic and Racial Differences in Stroke (REGARDS) study[46] involving over 23,000 adults > 45 years of age, it was found that eGFR < 60 is associated with a 23% increase in the prevalence of cognitive impairment after adjustment for demographic characteristics, prevalent cardiovascular disease, and cardiovascular (CV) risk factors.[46] The prevalence of cognitive impairment increases in multiple areas with the decline of eGFR, as shown in Figure 78.2.[47] For example, the prevalence of global cognition increases by 5% for each reduction of eGFR by 15 mL/min/1.73 m^2. Other studies also confirm the association of CKD and cognitive impairment.[46,48] In addition, the decline in cognitive function is faster in patients with CKD compared with non-CKD patients.[49]

Pathogenesis

There is strong evidence that indicates CKD-associated cognitive impairment is predominantly vascular in nature.

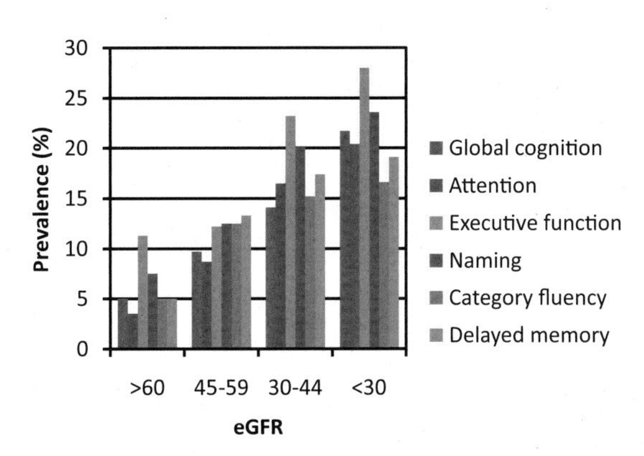

FIGURE 78.2 The unadjusted prevalence of cognitive impairment among 825 older adults (55 years or older) with mild-to-moderate renal insufficiency, according to estimated glomerular filtration rate (eGFR). Data taken from Yaffe K, Ackerson L, Kurella Tamura M, et al. Chronic Renal Insufficiency Cohort Investigators. Chronic kidney disease and cognitive function in older adults: findings from the chronic renal insufficiency cohort cognitive study. *J Am Geriatr Soc.* 2010;58:338–345. (See Color Plate.)

In the Cardiovascular Health Cognition (CVHS) study, it was found that moderate renal impairment in elderly adults (65 years or older) is associated with a 58% increase in the incidence of vascular dementia, but with no increase in the incidence of pure Alzheimer dementia. The overall incidence of vascular dementia and pure Alzheimer dementia in this cohort is 1.5% and 1.7% per year, respectively.[50] In the Northern Manhattan Study (NOMAS), a prospective, community-based cohort of which a subset of stroke-free participants underwent MRIs, CKD stages 3 and 4 are associated with an increase in white matter hyperintensity volume, which is a marker for stroke, cognitive decline, and dementia.[51] The increase of white matter lesions in CKD patients is confirmed by Ikram et al.[52] More recently, Kobayashi et al.[53] demonstrated that CKD also increases silent brain infarcts, and both the prevalence and the number of silent brain infarct increase with declining GFR.[53] Furthermore, CKD is also associated with a rapid progression of carotid intima-media thickness in a community study.[54]

The incidence of vascular dementia in ESRD patients is even higher than in those with moderate renal impairment. Fukunishi et al.[55] reported that the 1-year incidence rate of vascular dementia and Alzheimer dementia is 3.7% and 0.5%, respectively, in aged Japanese hemodialysis patients. The incidence of vascular dementia was 7.4 times of that in the general elderly population. Furthermore, although in patients with moderate renal impairment the incidence of vascular and Alzheimer dementia is about the same, vascular dementia outgrows the Alzheimer dementia by sevenfold in ESRD patients.[50,55]

Therefore, it is likely that patients with CKD are at risk of vascular dementia and the progression of CKD is parallel to the progression of cerebrovascular disease—primarily, atherosclerotic disease. The pathogenesis of dementia and cognitive impairment in patients with ESRD is multifactorial, as illustrated in Figure 78.3. There are shared mechanisms for both CKD and neurovascular disorders, but nephrogenic and dialysis-associated mechanisms also play important roles in the development of dementia. The shared risk factors for CKD and cerebrovascular disease are aging, nonwhite race, low socioeconomic status/low education, diabetes, hypertension, hyperlipidemia.[4] In addition, with declining renal function, several nephrogenic risk factors are likely to facilitate cerebrovascular disease, such as sympathetic overactivity, inflammation, oxidative stress, anemia, uremic toxins, and vascular calcification.[4] Lastly, complications of hemodialysis such as intradialytic hypotension, hyperviscosity, thrombotic events, and hemorrhage due to heparin use will further worsen cerebrovascular disease.[4,48]

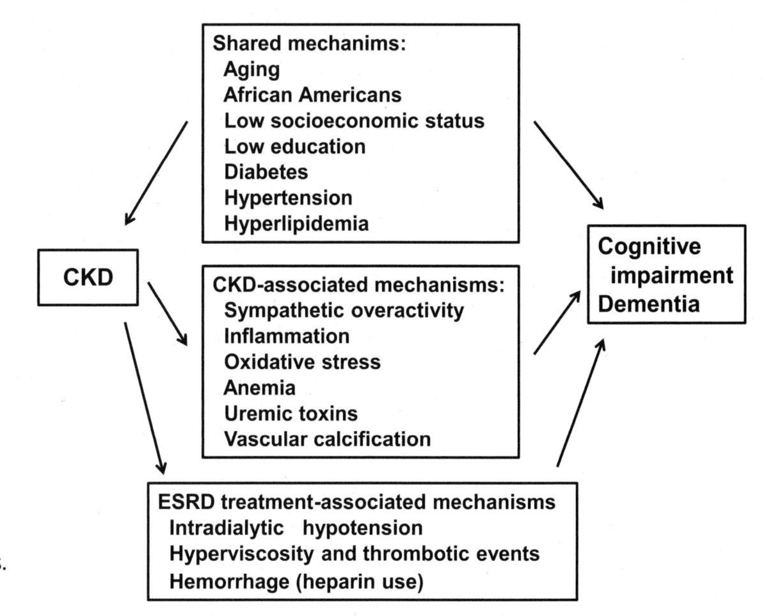

FIGURE 78.3 The proposed mechanisms of cognitive impairment and dementia in end-stage renal disease (ESRD). *CKD,* chronic kidney disease. (Modified from Kurella Tamura M, Yaffe K. Dementia and cognitive impairment in ESRD: diagnostic and therapeutic strategies. *Kidney Int.* 2010;79:14–22.)

Diagnosis

Cognitive impairment and dementia in CKD patients are frequently ignored. As a result, they tend to progress rapidly to an irreversible state. The prevalence of dementia in ESRD patients has been reported to be as high as 37%[44]; however, in a cohort of 16,694 patients in the Dialysis Outcomes and Practice Patterns Study, dementia was documented in the medical records as a comorbid condition in 4% of the entire study population.[56] It is recommended that screening for cognitive impairment should start from the onset of ESRD. There are many screening tests available. The Mini-Mental State Exam (MMSE) is perhaps the most studied cognitive test for dementia. There are other tests such as Mini-Cog and the Kidney Disease Quality of Life test, which can be used annually to assess the progression of cognitive impairment.[4,48] The most critical part of the evaluation of dementia is the search for reversible causes of altered mental status, including electrolyte abnormalities, drug effects, infections, depression, uremia, hepatic or cardiac failure, and others (Table 78.2). The laboratory evaluation should include HIV serologies, vitamin B12 levels, and thyroid function tests.[4]

Brain imaging studies are valuable for diagnosing cognitive impairment and dementia in CKD patients, particularly for identifying vascular dementia. Two major MRI findings are related to cerebral small vessel disease: lacunar infarct and white matter lesions. Both of them are increased in patients with CKD.[51–53] However, these findings are common in CKD patients; thus, the presence of these findings does not exclude other causes of cognitive impairment.

Prevention and Treatment

Because cognitive impairment and dementia associated with CKD are vascular in nature, reducing all cardiovascular risks before progressing to ESRD is critical for preventing these CNS disorders. Treatments targeted at controlling blood pressure, blood sugar, lipid profiles, proteinuria, and mineral metabolism may slow down the progression of both CKD and neurodegenerative diseases. Whether increasing dialysis clearance has a benefit on cognitive function has been controversial. Higher dialyzer urea clearance × time/urea volume of distribution (Kt/V) values have been associated with poorer cognitive function in patients on maintenance hemodialysis.[44,57] However, in a small study with 12 patients, switching from conventional hemodialysis to nocturnal daily hemodialysis for 6 months resulted in a 22% reduction in cognitive symptoms, a 7% improvement in psychomotor efficiency and processing speed, and a 32% improvement in attention and working memory.[58] Further studies are needed to substantiate these benefits from nocturnal hemodialysis.

Once dementia is diagnosed, the prognosis is poor in general because current drugs for treating dementia can only provide modest clinical benefit and none of them have been tested in patients with ESRD.[4] The management of dementia associated with ESRD requires a multidisciplinary approach involving the primary care physician, caregiver, nephrologist, and staff at the dialysis facility and nursing facility to define the goals of care and to facilitate end-of-life care planning.

Restless Leg Syndrome

Manifestations

RLS is a common neurologic condition in patients with ESRD. The prevalence is 10% to 20% based on clinical diagnosis,[5,59,60] but increases to 58% if diagnosed with a polysomnogram.[61] RLS is characterized by an imperative need to move the leg because of uncomfortable and unpleasant sensations in the legs. It occurs primarily at rest, which is usually worse in the evening and alleviated by movement.

Pathogenesis

RLS is predominantly a disorder of the central rather than the peripheral nervous system. Dopaminergic dysfunction in the subcortical system appears to play a central role in idiopathic RLS. Reduced iron stores in the brain have been demonstrated, suggesting that the homeostatic control of iron is altered.[62] Because iron is necessary for the activity of tyrosine hydroxylase, the rate-limiting step in dopamine synthesis, it is possible that a link exists between CNS iron deficiency and dopaminergic dysfunction. Compared with idiopathic RLS, RLS associated with ERSD progresses faster and responds poorly to a dopaminergic agent.[63] Interestingly, iron deficiency seems to be linked to RLS in CKD patients with[5] or without dialysis.[64] Further studies are needed to define the role of disturbed iron homeostasis in the development of RLS in CKD patients. In addition, RLS tends to be exacerbated by caffeine, alcohol, and medications including dopamine antagonists, lithium, selective serotonin reuptake inhibitors, and tricyclic antidepressants.[65]

Diagnosis

The diagnosis is mainly based on symptomatology and the effects of resting and movement on restless legs. The neurologic examination is typically normal in RLS. Polysomnography is useful for diagnosing RLS, and 90% of patients with RLS manifest an increased rate of periodic limb movements.[61]

Prevention and Treatment

Based on the association between iron deficiency and RLS in CKD patients, it is possible that the early detection and treatment of iron deficiency may prevent RLS; however, this hypothesis has not been proven. As for treatment, many drugs have been tried with variable success including dopaminergic agonists, gabapentin, and benzodiazepines.[65] Fortunately, successful kidney transplantation leads to the resolution of RLS symptoms within 1 to 21 days, which may remain in remission for several years. However, RLS tends to recur when transplants fail.[66]

THE PERIPHERAL NERVOUS SYSTEM

There are several unique PNS abnormalities that are caused by ESRD or due to an AVF created for hemodialysis. Uremic neuropathy is a common neurologic complication caused by unknown uremic toxins.[19] Carpel tunnel syndrome (CTS) in patients with prolonged hemodialysis treatment is the early symptom of dialysis-related amyloidosis caused by β2-microglobulin.[67] AVF may also cause CTS and other syndromes such as vascular steal syndrome and ischemic monomelic neuropathy.[68]

Uremic Neuropathy

Manifestations

Uremic neuropathy typically presents as a slowly progressive symmetrical peripheral neuropathy, initially affecting the distal regions of the limbs, and later progressing proximally. The earliest symptoms reflect sensory loss, resulting in symptoms of paresthesia, pain, and numbness in lower extremities. With disease progression, motor involvement develops, which is characterized by weakness and muscle atrophy, again most prominent distally.[69] Finally, the proximal regions of lower extremities as well as the upper extremities are affected. Uremic neuropathy usually occurs after GFR is less than 10 mL/min/1.73 m^2. Unlike uremic encephalopathy, which improves with renal replacement therapy and remains stable, uremic neuropathy may improve initially, but progresses slowly in spite of adequate dialysis treatment.[70] As a result, the prevalence of uremic neuropathy in ESRD patients is 60% to 90%, which is increased with the vintage of dialysis.[19,69] Laaksonen et al.[71] evaluated 21 patients on maintenance hemodialysis for a mean of 2 years with a battery of neurophysiologic parameters. None of those patients had other causes of peripheral neuropathy such as diabetes, alcoholism, or amyloidosis. They found that only 4 patients had no detectable sign of neuropathy, 4 had asymptomatic neuropathy, 10 had nondisabling symptomatic neuropathy with two or more positive neurologic tests, and 3 had disabling neuropathy. They also found that positive sensory symptoms correlated well with both motor and sensory neurologic tests.[71] Overall, uremic neuropathy affects the majority of ESRD patients and may cause significant morbidity in 10% to 20% of these patients. The increased severity appears to correlate with the vintage of dialysis treatment.[70]

Pathogenesis

Uremic neuropathy presents as a length-dependent polyneuropathy involving large, myelinated sensory and motor fibers. Although small fibers may be involved in some cases, isolated small fiber involvement has not been reported in association with uremic neuropathy.[72] Axon degeneration occurs in uremic neuropathy and is different from demyelination, or a loss of the myelin sheath, as seen in chronic inflammatory demyelinating neuropathy (Fig 78.4).[72] Clinically significant

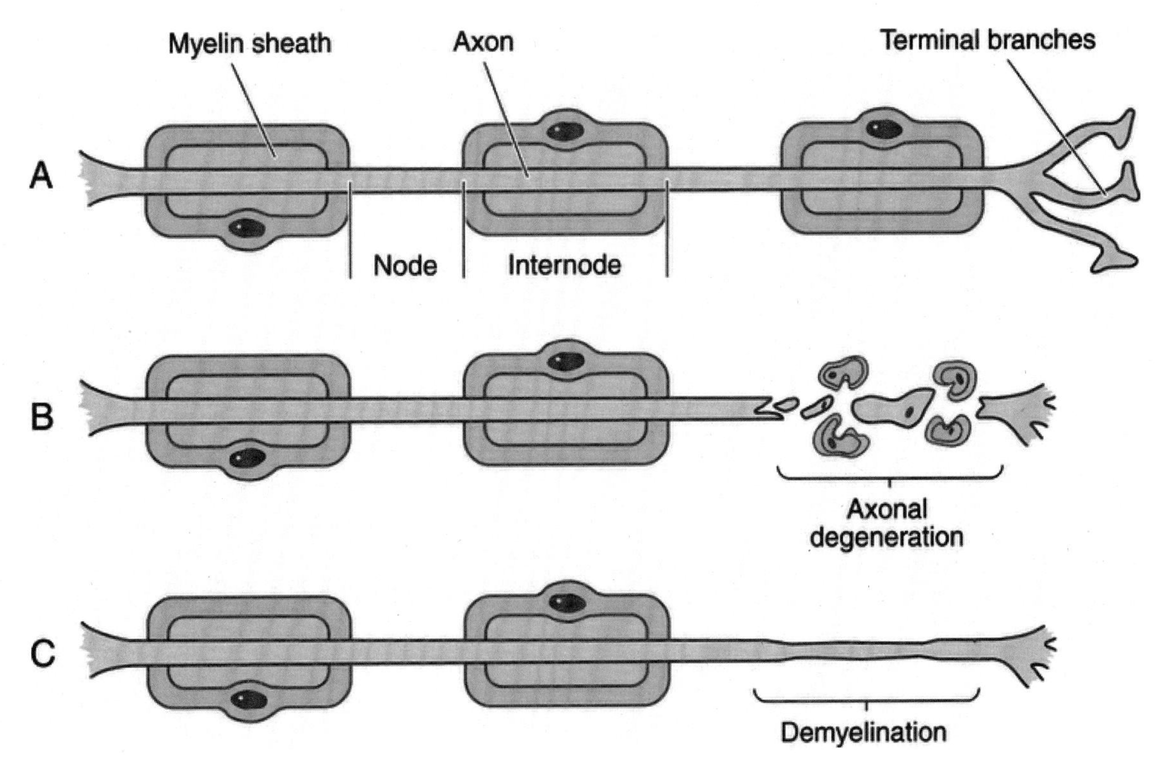

FIGURE 78.4 Differences between axonal degeneration and demyelinating disease of the peripheral nerve fibers. **A:** The normal axon, surrounded by myelin, laid down by Schwann cells and arranged in a multilamellar spiral fashion, which provides an insulating sheath, which is essential for rapid saltatory conduction of action potentials. **B:** Axonal degeneration ("dying-back" phenomenon), as occurs in length-dependent uremic neuropathy. **C:** Demyelination, with loss of the myelin sheath, occurs in chronic inflammatory demyelinating polyneuropathy. (From Krishnan AV, Pussell BA, Kiernan MC. Neuromuscular disease in the dialysis patient: an update for the nephrologist. *Semin Dial.* 2009;22:267–278.)

uremic neuropathy does not occur until patients reach ESRD. Although symptoms of uremic neuropathy, particularly paresthesia, improve after the initiation of dialysis, long-term dialysis does not reduce the prevalence of uremic neuropathy. These observations suggest that uremic toxins, particularly middle molecules, may be involved in axon degeneration; however, such molecules have not been identified.

More recently, a new hypothesis suggests that hyperkalemia, even a mild form with serum K at 5.0 mEq per liter, is associated with significant abnormalities in nerve excitability.[72,73] These abnormalities are corrected after hemodialysis, which normalizes serum K levels. Most ESRD patients have persistent hyperkalemia, which would lead to chronic membrane depolarization and subsequent reverse activation of the Na^+/Ca^{2+} exchanger, leading to an influx of Ca^{2+} and, eventually, axonal degeneration.[69,72] Further studies are needed to validate this provocative hypothesis because until now, predialysis hyperkalemia has not been identified as an independent risk factor for uremic neuropathy. Furthermore, hyperkalemia rarely occurs in patients on peritoneal dialysis, yet the progression of uremic neuropathy is not significantly different between patients receiving peritoneal dialysis versus hemodialysis.[74]

Diagnosis

Nerve conduction studies remain the mainstay in the diagnosis of uremic neuropathy. In order to make a correct diagnosis of uremic neuropathy, nerve conduction studies should not be performed on the limb with AVF because AVF itself may affect peripheral nerve function.[71] In uremic neuropathy, nerve conduction studies demonstrate features of axonal degeneration with a reduction in sensory amplitudes and, to a lesser extent, motor amplitudes. However, the delayed latency of the F-wave on lower limb nerves is the most sensitive test. Sensory and motor nerve conduction velocities are relatively reserved.[71,75] In uremic neuropathy, denervation of a portion of muscle fibers is readily compensated for by collateral reinnervation from surviving motor units. Therefore, the motor amplitude remains normal in mild-to-moderate neuropathy. Because there is no compensatory mechanism for the sensory nerve, reduced sensory amplitude is more sensitive for detecting uremic neuropathy.[71] In addition, vibration detection thresholds on the foot are also a sensitive test for detecting uremic neuropathy.[71,74] Because diabetic nephropathy is also a length-dependent neuropathy, nerve conduction studies cannot distinguish between uremic neuropathy and diabetic neuropathy.[72]

The progression of uremic neuropathy is typically a slow process. When patients present with a rapidly progressive course with significant weakness, demyelinating neuropathy should be ruled out. Nerve conduction studies in these disorders demonstrate a significant reduction in nerve conduction velocities and relatively reserved sensory and motor amplitudes in the early stage. Serology tests, including inflammatory markers, antinuclear antibodies, rheumatoid factors, antineutrophil cytoplasmic antibodies, hepatitis antibodies (B and C), and cryoglobulins, should be performed. Combined nerve and muscle biopsies are likely needed for confirming the diagnosis if immunosuppressive therapy is indicated.[72]

Prevention and Treatment

Uremic neuropathy is one of indications for the initiation of dialysis treatment. Symptoms are usually improved after the initial dialysis treatment, but may recur if dialysis clearance is inadequate. Thus, adequate dialysis clearance is important for preventing uremic neuropathy.[76] However, even with adequate dialysis treatment, uremic neuropathy may progress slowly. Bazzi et al.[70] reported that about 50% of patients on hemodialysis for less than 10 years have mild uremic neuropathy, but for patients on hemodialysis more than 10 years, the prevalence of mild, moderate, and severe neuropathy is 81%, 11%, and 3%, respectively.[70] The only treatment for uremic neuropathy in patients on maintenance dialysis treatment is a kidney transplant, and the recovery may not be complete for those with advanced disease.[77,78]

For patients with neuropathic pain, antidepressants such as amitriptyline and anticonvulsants such as gabapentin, may be useful for symptomatic management.[72] Vitamin supplementation with pyridoxine[79] and methylcobalamin[80] has been shown to improve uremic neuropathy, probably through the stimulation of nerve metabolism and the enhancement of regeneration. However, these preliminary results need to be confirmed.

Carpal Tunnel Syndrome

Manifestations

The initial symptoms of CTS are paresthesia, numbness, and pain confined to the median nerve territory or diffusely in the hand, with a characteristic nocturnal exacerbation. In some patients, these symptoms are localized to more proximal regions of the affected arm. Symptoms are usually bilateral, but more severe in the dominant hand. As CTS progresses, it affects motor function, leading to weakness and muscle atrophy. The prevalence of CTS in ESRD patients ranges from 10% to 30%, but increases sharply to 50% in patients who have been on hemodialysis for more than 20 years.[67,81] In some patients, particularly those without prolonged dialysis vintage, CTS appears to be related to AVF.[82]

Pathogenesis

The carpal tunnel is narrow and bounded by the transverse carpal ligament superiorly and the carpal bones inferiorly. Given this narrow passageway, the median nerve is susceptible to injury. In the general population, the causes of CTS include chronic trauma, arthritis, amyloidosis, and myxedema. In patients with ESRD, there are two unique pathogenetic mechanisms accounting for most of the reported cases of dialysis-related CTS: deposition of β2-microglobulin

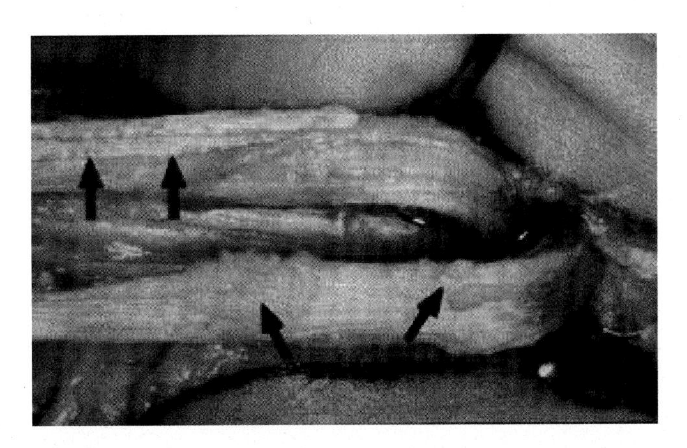

FIGURE 78.5 The dialysis-related amyloid (*arrows*) deposited in the peritenons and the synovial membranes of the carpal tunnel. From Yamamoto S, Gejyo F. Historical background and clinical treatment of dialysis-related amyloidosis. *Biochim Biophys Acta*. 2005;1753:4–10.

(Fig. 78.5)[67] and AVF.[82] The deposition of β2-microglobulin causes dialysis-related amyloidosis, which is characterized by CTS, arthropathy, and bone cysts. The pathologic specimens are positive for Congo red staining and for immunochemistry staining for β2-microglobulin. The accumulation of β2-microglobulin is related to the duration of ESRD and dialysis membrane.[67,83] Because of the switch to a high flux dialysis membrane, dialysis-related amyloidosis has been reported mainly in patients with prolonged dialysis, usually more than 10 to 20 years.[67] In Japan, where the survival of ESRD patients with prolonged dialysis is common, nearly all reported cases of CTS are due to β2-microglobulin.[81] This is not the case in other countries. In one series from France, β2-microglobulin accounts for 60% of dialysis-related CTS.[84] In a study from the United States, about one half of specimens from the transverse carpal ligament were positive for amyloid staining.[82] The presence of AVF does cause significant abnormalities in nerve conduction velocities and latencies in both median and ulnar nerves.[85] It is possible that nerve ischemia due to steal syndrome and venous congestion due to increased downstream pressure may contribute to the development of CTS.[85]

Diagnosis

Two bedside tests are useful for a diagnosis of CTS in patients who have typical symptoms of paresthesia, numbness, and pain in the median nerve territory: the Phalen test and the Tinel sign. The Phalen test involves placing the wrist into an end-of-range palmar flexion for 1 minute to increase intratunnel pressure. The test is positive if symptoms in the median nerve territory are reproduced.[86] The Tinel sign refers to a tingling sensation over the territory of the median nerve when it is tapped. The positive rate of the Phalen test and the Tinel sign in patients with CTS is 70% and 50%, respectively.[86] In advanced CTS, sensory loss in the median nerve territory and weakness and atrophy in distal median-innervated muscles, particularly the abductor pollicis brevis, are detected. Nerve conduction studies demonstrate a slowing of the distal median nerve conduction in sensory and motor fibers at the level of the wrist. Sensory and motor amplitudes are normal in the early stages, but may be reduced in the later stages, which is indicative of axonal loss.[72] The interpretation of nerve conduction studies may be complicated by coexisting uremic or diabetic neuropathy. The diagnosis of CTS is supported by significantly worse nerve parameters in the median nerve when compared with other nerves.

Because the management of β2-microglobulin-induced and AVF-induced CTS is different, it is important to distinguish between these two causes. Patients with CTS should be evaluated for bone cysts and arthropathy.[84] If patients undergo surgical treatment, biopsy samples should be submitted for a microscopic examination of β2-microglobulin. Of note, the predialysis serum β2-microglobulin levels are not helpful for diagnosing dialysis-related amyloidosis because the commonly used high flux membrane has effectively removed β2-microglobulin.[81] As for AVF-related CTS, signs of ischemia distal to AVF and limb swelling should prompt a thorough vascular examination to rule out vascular steal syndrome and venous hypertension. In addition, AVF-related CTS may involve nerves other than the median nerve.

Prevention and Treatment

The incidence of CTS has been reduced after the widespread use of high flux membrane for hemodialysis therapy.[83] Hemodiafiltration[87] and β2-microglobulin adsorption column[88] have been shown to remove β2-microglobulin even more efficiently. They can be used in patients at a high risk of dialysis-related amyloidosis; however, neither of them have been approved by the U.S. Food and Drug Administration (FDA) in the United States. For preventing AVF-related CTS, monitoring ischemic changes, arm swelling, and AVF function, and the early management of vascular steal syndrome and venous hypertension may be important for the prevention of AVF-related CTS.

As for treatment, conservative treatment such as nocturnal splinting is appropriate for dialysis-related CTS with mild symptoms and mild conduction slowing with normal sensory and motor amplitudes. A corticosteroid injection may induce median nerve injury and should be avoided. In patients with severe CTS symptoms with marked reductions in median nerve compound amplitudes, surgical decompression is indicated.[67] Most patients have symptom relief after surgery, but the outcome is not as good as for nondialysis patients and CTS may recur if the primary cause is not eliminated.[82]

Arteriovenous Fistula-Related Neuropathy

Manifestation

AVF has been associated with a variety of peripheral neuropathies due to acute or chronic ischemia. Ischemic monomelic neuropathy refers to neurologic symptoms in the ipsilateral limb, which occurs immediately following the

TABLE 78.4 **Differential Diagnosis Between Steal Syndrome and Ischemic Monomelic Neuropathy[68]**

	Vascular Steal Syndrome	Ischemic Monomelic Neuropathy
Onset	Usually insidious	Acute
Predilection for diabetes	Strong	Almost all
Access location	Wrist, forearm, upper arm	Forearm, upper arm
Degree of ischemia	Severe, diffuse	Mild–moderate
Radial pulse presence	No	Yes/No
Digital pressures	Very low	Mildly reduced or normal
Tissue affected	Skin > muscle > nerve	Nerve
Reversibility	Variable	Very poor with late intervention

Modified from Miles AM. Vascular steal syndrome and ischaemic monomelic neuropathy: two variants of upper limb ischaemia after haemodialysis vascular access surgery. *Nephrol Dial Transplant*. 1999;14:297–300.

creation of AVF. It is due to acute nerve ischemia induced by the shunting of arterial blood away from the distal parts of the limb. Patients manifest distal sensory loss and weakness in the muscles of the forearm and hand without soft tissue changes.[68] Vascular steal syndrome occurs insidiously usually days or weeks after the fistula creation. Neurologic symptoms include numbness and pain, which are worse during a dialysis session.[68] The comparison between ischemic monomelic neuropathy and vascular steal syndrome is summarized in Table 78.4. CTS and ulnar neuropathy with pain and numbness in the domain of the median and ulnar nerves, respectively, also have been reported to be associated with AVF.[85]

Pathogenesis

Ischemic monomelic neuropathy has been largely reported in patients with diabetes, particularly those with preexisting peripheral vascular disease or neuropathy.[89] It is likely that preexisting chronic nerve ischemia is the underlying mechanism of the catastrophic event after an AVF creation.[90] As for vascular steal syndrome, chronic ischemia is caused by retrograde flow from the distal and palmar arch arteries through the fistula, which acts as a low-pressure system.[91]

Diagnosis

Ischemic monomelic neuropathy is diagnosed by the immediate onset of severe pain and weakness in the ipsilateral limb after an AVF creation and frequently involves multiple nerves. Electromyogram (EMG), and nerve conduction studies, are useful to demonstrate axon loss in multiple nerves distal to the AVF.[68,90]

Vascular steal syndrome is characterized by cyanosis, coldness, reduced sensation, and the presence of ischemic ulcers. Vascular Doppler studies or a digital pressure measurement may demonstrate the steal phenomenon and nerve conduction studies reveal slow conduction and low amplitudes in multiple nerves distal to the AVF.[68,91]

Prevention and Treatment

Ischemic monomelic neuropathy occurs mainly in patients with diabetes; however, it is difficult to predict with preoperative evaluation. Early diagnosis is essential to preserve neurologic functions of the hand. Early ligation or revision of the fistula may cause significant clinical and electrophysiologic improvement,[72] whereas the outcome of delayed surgery is frequently poor.[89]

For vascular steal syndrome, vigilant monitoring of AVF functions and signs of ischemia may prevent the development of vascular steal syndrome. Several surgical treatments have been used for steal syndrome: access ligation, banding, elongation, distal arterial ligation, and distal revascularization–interval ligation.[91]

THE AUTONOMIC NERVOUS SYSTEM

Abnormalities in the autonomic nerve system are common in patients with CKD. Both sympathetic and parasympathetic nerve systems are involved. The severity of autonomic dysfunction increases as renal function declines. As a result, multiple organ systems are affected in patients with ESRD. All these abnormalities are discussed under uremic autonomic neuropathy.

Uremic Autonomic Neuropathy

Manifestations

Uremic autonomic neuropathy refers to renal failure-induced autonomic dysfunction, which is observed in patients with uremia. Unlike uremic encephalopathy or uremic neuropathy, which occurs when GFR is less than 10 mL per minute, autonomic dysfunction occurs early in patients with CKD. In those patients, autonomic dysfunction, mainly sympathetic overactivity, contributes to the increased risk of hypertension, heart failure, coronary artery diseases and strokes, as well as the progression of CKD.[92] For CKD patients with mild-to-moderate renal insufficiency, perhaps "nephrogenic" autonomic neuropathy is a better term because they do not have any uremic symptoms.

In ESRD patients, symptoms suggestive of autonomic dysfunction such as male impotency, dyspepsia, constipation, diarrhea, bladder dysfunction, postural dizziness, and intradialytic hypotension are reported from 40% to 70% of nondiabetic patients maintained on hemodialysis.[69,93] However, only male impotency correlates well with autonomic dysfunction diagnosed with traditional tests for cardiovascular autonomic functions.[93] The prevalence of autonomic dysfunction is much increased when diabetic patients are included.[94] Additional cardiac manifestations related to autonomic dysfunction include resting tachycardia with a fixed heart rate, exercise intolerance, silent myocardial infarction, arrhythmia, and sudden cardiac arrest or death.[94–99] Many of these symptoms and signs of autonomic dysfunction are nonspecific; therefore, autonomic function tests are required to confirm the diagnosis of uremic autonomic neuropathy.

Pathogenesis

The key elements of uremic autonomic neuropathy are sympathetic overactivity and parasympathetic hypoactivity. Sympathetic overactivity is primarily due to increased renal afferent signaling, which occurs at the beginning of renal injury.[92,100] The kidneys are subserved with abundant sympathetic innervation of the renal vasculature, renal tubules, and the juxtaglomerular apparatus. Renal injury stimulates afferent signaling via sensory renal nerves.[101] The increased sympathetic activity can be detected by recording muscular sympathetic nerve activity (MSNA) in patients with ESRD.[102] The role of renal injury on sympathetic overactivity in ESRD is confirmed by reducing MSNA with a bilateral nephrectomy.[102] Furthermore, even in the presence of a functioning renal graft, MSNA is still hyperactive until the removal of both native kidneys, as shown in Figure 78.6.[103]

The increased afferent signaling is independent of GFR because it occurs in patients with early stage polycystic kidney disease[104] or in animals with localized renal injury,[100] both of which have normal GFR. The generation, integration, and consequences of renal afferent signaling from renal injury are shown in Figure 78.7. These afferent signals from the injured kidney are centrally integrated and result in sympathetic outflow to the kidney, heart, and vasculature in order to restore renal perfusion. The suppression of brain nitric oxide synthase activity in CKD removes the tonic inhibition on the sympathetic outflow from the brainstem. With constant renal signaling and suppression of brainstem inhibition, organs receiving chronically elevated sympathetic outflow start to deteriorate resulting in left ventricular hypertrophy, arrhythmias, vasoconstriction, sodium retention, and renin-angiotensin-aldosterone system activation. These changes aggravate hypertension, which in return worsens cardiac and renal functions, atherosclerosis, and glomerulosclerosis.[92]

There are other mechanisms that may contribute to increased sympathetic activity in CKD patients. Tonic arterial chemoreceptor activation may be involved in sympathetic activation associated with renal impairment. The deactivation of arterial chemoreceptors by the inhalation of

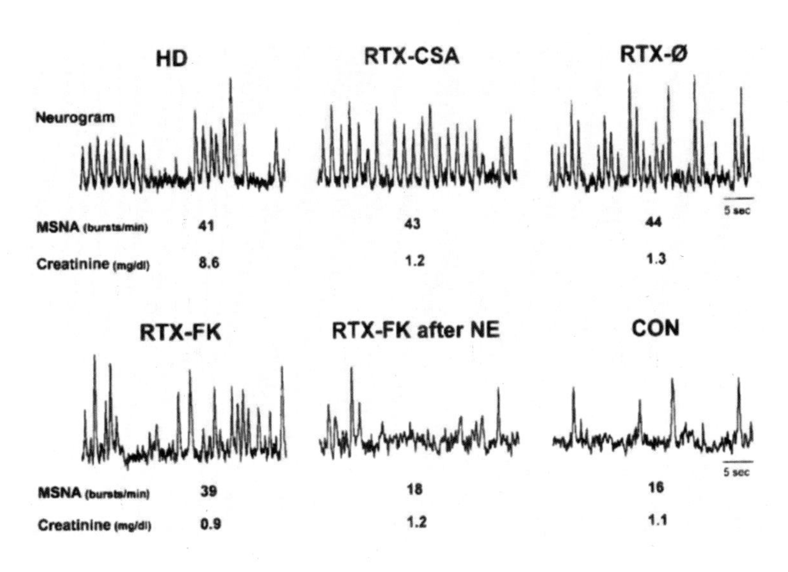

FIGURE 78.6 Representative tracings of sympathetic neurograms from a hemodialysis patient (*HD*), the same patient after a successful kidney transplantation receiving cyclosporine (*RTX-CSA*), a renal transplantation patient without calcineurin inhibitor treatment (*RTX-Ø*), a renal transplantation patient receiving tacrolimus before (*RTX-FK*) and after native kidney nephrectomy (*RTX-FK after NE*), and a healthy volunteer (*CON*). The renal transplant recipients had serum creatinine concentrations similar to that of the healthy volunteer; however, muscle sympathetic nerve activity (MSNA) declined not with transplantation but with native kidney nephrectomy. (From Hausberg M, Kosch M, Harmelink P, et al. Sympathetic nerve activity in end-stage renal disease. *Circulation.* 2002;106:1974–1979.)

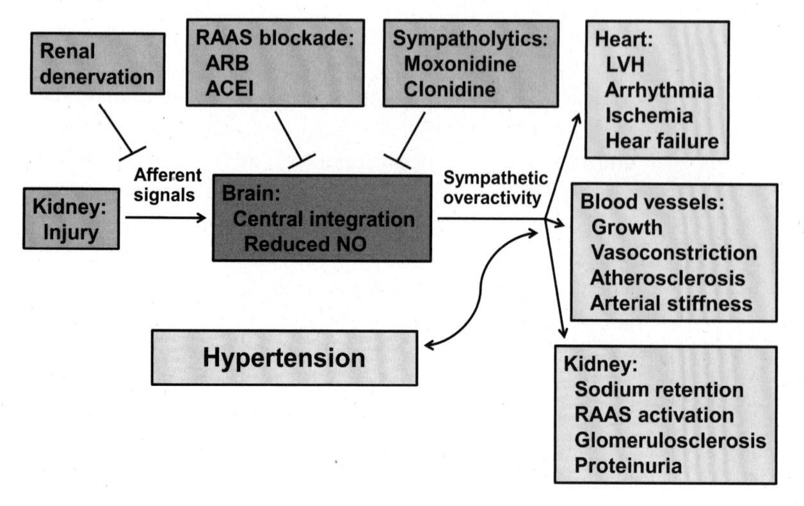

FIGURE 78.7 Causes and consequences of sympathetic activation in chronic kidney disease and the potential treatment. See text for explanation. Color codes: red: cause; blue: integration; yellow: consequences; and green: treatment. RAAS, renin-angiotensin-aldosterone system; ARB, angiosten receptor blocker; ACEI, angiotensinogen converting enzyme inhibitor; LVH, left ventricular hypertrophy; NO, nitric oxide. (Modified from Schlaich MP, Socratous F, Hennebry S, et al. Sympathetic activation in chronic renal failure. *J Am Soc Nephrol.* 2009 May;20(5):933–939.) (See Color Plate.)

100% oxygen substantially decreased MSNA in patients with chronic renal disease, but not in healthy control subjects.[105] Another novel mechanism for sympathetic overactivity is mediated by reduced renalase release. Renalase is a novel soluble monoamine oxidase that metabolizes catecholamines such as dopamine and norepinephrine.[106] Renalase is released from the kidney into the blood in an inactive form (prorenalase). Catecholamines not only activate prorenalase, but also induce its release from the kidney; as a consequence, active renalase metabolizes circulating catecholamines as an important regulatory mechanism for hemodynamic homeostasis.[107] In rats with 5/6 nephrectomy, blood levels of renalase are markedly reduced, which lead to increased plasma catecholamine levels and subsequent sympathetic overactivity.[107]

As for parasympathetic hypoactivity, it is likely to be mediated by impaired baroreceptor sensitivity (BRS). The baroreflexes are neurocardiovascular reflexes that maintain circulatory homeostasis. When systemic blood pressure (BP) rises, the arterial stretch triggers the firing of the baroreceptors in the carotid artery and aorta. The afferent impulses are transmitted to the CNS, signals are integrated, and the efferent arm of the reflex projects neural signals systemically via the sympathetic and parasympathetic branches of the ANS. By inhibiting the efferent sympathetic outflow, vascular tone, cardiac chronotropy, and inotropy are reduced, whereas the increase in parasympathetic outflow reduces cardiac chronotropy.[108]

CKD promotes carotid artery intimal thickening and increases arterial stiffness. The arterial stiffness becomes worse in patients with advanced CKD because of vascular calcification. Chesterton et al.[109] have demonstrated that decreased BRS in patients on hemodialysis correlates with arterial stiffness measured with central pulse wave analysis and vascular calcification measured with a computed tomography (CT) scan. Additionally, parasympathetic hypoactivity is associated with heart failure, which is common in ESRD patients.[110]

The cardiac parasympathetic function in experimental CKD animals has been studied.[111] Using a 5/6 nephrectomy model in rats, Kuncova et al.[111] reported diminished cardiac parasympathetic tone in CKD rats. These rats have resting tachycardia and a blunted response to atropine injection. However, there are no differences in negative chronotropic responses to the stimulation of the vagus nerves, nor in chronotropic and inotropic responses to carbachol. Furthermore, the relative expression of muscarinic (M2) receptors, the high affinity choline transporter, the vesicular acetylcholine transporter, and the choline acetyltransferase in cardiac tissues is also unchanged.[111] These studies indicate that in 5/6 nephrectomy rats, parasympathetic hypoactivity is mainly due to suppression of the afferent limb while the efferent parasympathetic limb remains intact. Similar mechanisms are likely to occur in patients with CKD or early stage ESRD. However, whether the efferent parasympathetic limb remains intact after a prolonged duration of dialysis treatment is unknown.

Although sympathetic overactivity may explain hypertension associated with CKD, particularly in those patients with adult-onset polycystic kidney disease,[104] it seems to be at odds with the fact that some ESRD patients develop baseline hypotension, orthostatic hypotension, or intradialytic hypotension, and that the prevalence of hypotension increases with dialysis vintage.[112,113] The majority of these hypotensive patients have relatively preserved cardiac function. Because ESRD patients without a nephrectomy have increased sympathetic afferent signaling from injured kidneys, how do they develop hypotension, which is associated with reduced peripheral resistance from decreased sympathetic activity? It is likely that in spite of a hyperactive afferent limb, these patients may develop end organ unresponsiveness. Reduced adrenoreceptor responsiveness has been reported in ESRD with hypotension before or during dialysis. Daul et al.[112] reported reduced platelet α2 adrenoreceptor, blunted blood pressure responses to phenylephrine injection, and elevated plasma norepinephrine levels in these patients. They found that these abnormalities correlated well with duration of dialysis. They proposed that elevated catecholamine may downregulate adrenoreceptors in platelets and, possibly, in blood vessels.[112] These results are confirmed by another study comparing ESRD patients with or without hypotension. The mean duration of dialysis treatment was 10 and 3 years, for hypotensive and normotensive patients, respectively. Hypotensive patients had lower platelet $\alpha 2$ adrenoreceptor and lymphocyte $\beta 2$ adrenoreceptor densities and elevated plasma epinephrine levels.[113] In animal studies, a reduced $\alpha 1$ adrenoreceptor in mesentery arteries and elevated plasma epinephrine levels are observed in rats with 5/6 nephrectomy. Interestingly, a parathyroidectomy did not affect adrenoreceptor or epinephrine levels in these animals.[114] In addition to adrenergic receptor downregulation, sympathetic denervation is another plausible possibility for reduced sympathetic activity in spite of increased sympathetic signaling. Recently, Chao et al.[115] reported that in patients with advanced CKD, mostly ESRD, there is a high percentage of skin denervation (67.5%), which correlates with the presence of autonomic dysfunction as measured by heart rate variability and sympathetic skin response. The skin denervation also correlates well with the duration of CKD and dialysis, suggesting that unknown uremic toxins may be responsible for the damage of small nerve fibers in the skin. Because these skin nerves are small myelinated or unmyelinated nerves that are similar to postganglionic autonomic nerves,[116] it is possible that a similar denervation may occur in sympathetic and parasympathetic nerve systems and results in reduced efferent sympathetic and parasympathetic flow in patients with prolonged ESRD. More studies are needed to test this hypothesis.

Autonomic dysfunction has been implicated in the pathogenesis of intradialytic hypotension. Converse et al.[117] elegantly demonstrated that patients with intradialytic hypotension did have increased sympathetic activities consisting of hypertension and tachycardia right before a hypotensive episode, but then developed a paradoxical withdrawal of sympathetic vasoconstrictor drive that is consistent with a vasodepressor syncope. An ECG (echocardiograph) right before hypotension showed a near collapse of the left ventricle at the end of systole, which may activate cardiac afferents and may trigger the reflex inhibition of sympathetic outflow (Bezold-Jarisch reflex).[117,118] Similarly, Chesterton et al.[119] reported that patients with reduced BRS, but who were resistant to intradialytic hypotension, were able to raise total peripheral resistance to maintain BP probably via increased sympathetic activity, whereas patients with reduced BRS who are prone to intradialytic hypotension were not able to do so, which is consistent with sympathetic withdrawal. The decrease in their cardiac output is closely related to the volume of fluid removal. Therefore, although autonomic dysfunction predisposes ESRD patients to intradialytic hypotension, the intrinsic cardiac disease and fluid removal are still the major factors for intradialytic hypotension.

Uremic autonomic neuropathy also contributes to increasing GI symptoms in patients with ESRD, including dyspepsia (nausea, vomiting, abdominal distension, early satiety, and anorexia), constipation, and diarrhea. The prevalence of GI symptoms in patients with ESRD is in the range of 70% to 80%.[120] However, the correlation between GI symptoms and autonomic dysfunction is poor.[93] Gastroparesis has been implicated in dyspeptic symptoms in patients with ESRD. Delayed gastric emptying is associated with autonomic dysfunction in ESRD patients,[121] but it does not consistently correlate with dyspeptic symptoms.[122,123] An electrogastrogram was also abnormal and consistent with gastric emptying delay.[124] Overall, it appears that uremic autonomic neuropathy may incur delayed gastric emptying that may or may not cause dyspeptic symptoms.

Erectile dysfunction is another common symptom of autonomic dysfunction in patients with ESRD. About 65% of male dialysis patients report a difficulty in achieving and maintaining an erection, and 40% report a difficulty in achieving orgasm.[125] Vita et al.[93] reported that erectile dysfunction is the only symptom that correlates well with abnormal autonomic tests. The correlation between erectile dysfunction and abnormal responses to the Valsalva maneuver has been demonstrated.[126] However, there are other factors that contribute to erectile dysfunction in patients with ESRD, such as hypothalamic-pituitary-gonadal axis imbalance, accelerated vascular disease, and medications such as antihypertensives, antidepressants, diuretics, and histamine receptor blockers.[125]

The erectile activity is completely dependent on autonomic innervation from the spinal cord.[127] Norepinephrine and neuropeptide Y (NPY) are released in the penis by the terminals of the sympathetic fibers. Norepinephrine is the major contractile agent of the smooth muscles of the penis and penile arteries, and NPY augments its effects. Norepinephrine plays a role in flaccidity and detumescence; thus, the sympathetic activity is antierectile. The terminals of the parasympathetic fibers release acetylcholine, vasoactive intestinal polypeptide (VIP), and nitric oxide. Acetylcholine activates endothelial cells that in turn release nitric oxide. Nitric oxide increases the production of cyclic guanosine 3′5′-monophosphate (cGMP) in smooth muscle fibers and is recognized as the most important activator of the local relaxation of the penis smooth muscle. VIP is also a smooth muscle relaxant. Therefore, parasympathetic activity is proerectile.[127] Most ESRD patients with erectile dysfunction have autonomic dysfunction and reduced HRV in high frequency (HF) and low frequency (LF), indicating that they have increased sympathetic activity and reduced parasympathetic activity, a combination affecting erectile activity negatively.[93]

Diagnosis

Patients with ESRD frequently report symptoms of autonomic dysfunction, such as impotence, GI symptoms, and postural dizziness. In addition to uremic autonomic neuropathy, autonomic dysfunction may be secondary to other etiologies. Diseases such as diabetes, amyloidosis, and Fabry disease may cause ESRD and autonomic dysfunction independently.[116] Autoimmune diseases such as systemic lupus erythematosus (SLE), scleroderma, mixed connective tissue diseases, and Sjögren disease may also develop various forms of autonomic

TABLE 78.5 **Cardiovascular Autonomic Dysfunction Detected with Various Autonomic Function Tests in Patients with End-Stage Renal Disease**

Tests	Measurement	ESRD pre-HD	ESRD on HD	Kidney TX
Valsalva maneuver	Ratio of longest R-R interval during release phase to the shortest R-R during strain phase	Reduced (parasympathetic hypoactivity)[102]	Improved[102,153]	Normalized[153]
Orthostasis	Changes in BP and HR during orthostasis	Abnormal fall in BP, but normal increase in HR due to NE resistance[102]	Improved[102,153]	Normalized[153]
Handgrip exercise	Changes in BP and HR during handgrip exercise	Reduced increment in BP (NE resistance) and HR (parasympathetic hypoactivity)[102]	BP but not heart rate improved[102]	Normalized[153]
Muscle sympathetic nerve activity	Microneurography of muscle sympathetic nerve	Increased (increased renal efferent signaling)[130]	Unchanged[103]	Unchanged[103]
Heart rate variability	Time domains	Reduced (parasympathetic hypoactivity and sympathetic overactivity)[131]	Improved[132]	Improved[135]
	Frequency domains	Reduced in LF (mainly sympathetic overactivity) Reduced in HF (parasympathetic hypoactivity)[131]	Not improved[132] Improved[134]	Improved[135]
Baroreceptor sensitivity	Regression slope between R-R intervals and beat-to-beat BP changes	Reduced[137]	Improved[137]	Improved/ normalized[137,138]

BP, blood pressure; HR, heart rate; HD, hemodialysis; TX, transplantation; NE, norepinephrine; LF, low frequency.

dysfunction, frequently before the development of ESRD.[116] These nonuremic causes of autonomic dysfunction should be recognized in patients with ESRD, which is likely to worsen uremic autonomic neuropathy.

Many tests have been used clinically or for research purposes to diagnose uremic autonomic neuropathy. Clinically, autonomic dysfunction has an important impact as an independent predictor for cardiovascular mortality and morbidity.[96,98] Most studies of autonomic activity in patients with ESRD used cardiovascular parameters to assess autonomic dysfunction. Table 78.5 lists the tests used for CKD-associated autonomic dysfunction in the cardiovascular system, results in patients with ESRD, and the effects of dialysis and successful kidney transplantation.

The key components of autonomic dysfunction associated with CKD are sympathetic overactivity and parasympathetic hypoactivity. Tests for sympathetic activities include measurements of blood pressure responses to orthostasis change and handgrip exercises. Tests for parasympathetic activities include measurements of heart rate responses to blood pressure change (baroreceptor sensitivity), respiration, the Valsalva maneuver, and orthostasis.[128] More recently, noninvasive techniques have been developed to assess BRS and heart rate variability (HRV). Using power spectrum analysis, these convenient bedside tests provide high volumes of quality data for determining autonomic functions and predicting outcomes of patients with ESRD.

The classic studies on autonomic dysfunction by Campese et al.[102] provide excellent insight of uremic autonomic neuropathy. Using classic physiologic methods, including the Valsalva maneuver, handgrip exercise, and orthostasis, they characterized uremic autonomic neuropathy prior to initiation of hemodialysis. These patients failed to reduce the heart rate at the release phase of the Valsalva maneuver and had fewer blood pressure and heart rate responses to handgrip exercise. When changing from a supine to a standing position, their blood pressure dropped in spite of a normal tachycardic response. Uremic patients had higher baseline plasma norepinephrine (NE) levels and a larger increment in plasma NE levels after ambulating for 60 minutes. When NE was injected intravenously, the increment in blood pressure and the reduction in the heart rate were significantly less in uremic patients when compared to normal individuals. This classic study demonstrates that uremic patients have markedly reduced parasympathetic activity, increased sympathetic activity, but resistance to NE. Dialysis treatment reduces NE resistance and improves orthostatic hypotension and parasympathetic hypoactivity.[102]

Increased sympathetic activity can be demonstrated using microneurography by inserting electrodes into muscle sympathetic nerves. MSNA is markedly increased in ESRD patients with or without hemodialysis.[129,130] Hemodialysis fails to correct sympathetic overactivity. In fact, even successful kidney transplantation fails to suppress MSNA. However, native kidney nephrectomy completely normalized MSNA in both hemodialysis[117] and transplant patients.[103]

HRV has been increasingly used for evaluating autonomic dysfunction. It refers to beat-to-beat alterations in heart rate as measured by periodic variation in the R-R interval. HRV provides a noninvasive method for investigating autonomic input into the heart. Normal individuals have a high degree of HRV, which can be analyzed in either time or frequency domains. The time domain analysis measures normal R-R intervals over a period of time and is expressed in many different ways, such as standard deviation of all normal R-R intervals during a 24-hour period (SDNN), a standard deviation of a 5-minute average of normal R-R intervals (SDANN), an average of a 5-minute SDNN (ASDNN), the root-mean square of the difference of successive R-R intervals (rMSSD), and the number of instances per hour in which two consecutive R-R intervals differ by more than 50 ms over 24 hours (pNN50). The SDNN and its variables may represent the sympathetic limb of the autonomic nervous system, whereas rMSSD, NN50, and pNN50, in the presence of a normal sinus rhythm and atrioventricular-nodal function, represent the parasympathetic limb.[99] The frequency domain analysis splits the heart rate signal into constituent frequency components using the fast Fourier transformation. The clinically important frequencies are low frequency (LF), 0.04 to 0.15 Hz, and high frequency (HF), 0.15 to 0.40 Hz. The former is affected by the baroreceptor reflex and is thought to reflect sympathetic and parasympathetic tone, whereas the latter is influenced by respiratory frequency and is thought to reflect parasympathetic tone. The LF/HF ratio is an index of sympathovagal balance.[99,128] Reduced HRV is common (about 50%) in patients with advanced CKD with or without dialysis.[131] The reduction of HRV in HF is consistent with parasympathetic hypoactivity, whereas reduced LF or time domain may be related to sympathetic overactivity or the combination of these two abnormalities. Short-term hemodialysis improved time domain HRV, but not frequency domain HRV in one study.[132] On the other hand, dialysis vintage is an independent predictor for reduced HRV.[133] Preliminary studies have shown that nocturnal hemodialysis has improved both HF power and LF/HF ratio in nine ESRD patients after switching from a conventional hemodialysis.[134] A reduction in both time- and frequency-domain HRV can be improved or normalized after successful kidney transplantation.[135]

BRS is another test for evaluating autonomic dysfunction. BRS measures regression slope between R-R intervals and beat-to-beat BP changes. Reduced BRS accounts for parasympathetic hypoactivity, which is common in patients with advanced CKD[136] and patients on dialysis.[137] Interestingly, successful kidney transplantation is capable of normalizing BRS.[137,138]

Prevention and Treatment

Autonomic dysfunction is an independent predictor for cardiovascular events in patients with CKD.[98,128,139] Recent epidemiology studies have shown that reduced HRV in patients with CKD predicts ESRD and CKD-related hospitalization.[140] However, treatment options for CKD-induced autonomic dysfunction are limited (Fig. 78.7). Angiotensin-converting enzyme inhibitors and angiotensin-receptor blockers reduce sympathetic activity by 20% to 25%.[141–143] The addition of moxonidine, a centrally acting imidazoline-I1 receptor agonist and sympatholytic agent, to angiotensin receptor blocker (ARB) normalized sympathetic overactivity in patients with advanced CKD.[144] Moxonidine also reduced MSNA in patients with ESRD.[145] Notably, moxonidine is excreted by the kidney and dose adjustment is required for patients with reduced renal function. In the CKD and ESRD studies mentioned earlier, 0.2 mg and 0.3 mg per day was used, respectively, and was well tolerated.[144,145] Moxonidine reduces both blood pressure and MSNA in patients with CKD, but reduces MSNA only without affecting blood pressure in ESRD patients. Volume overload in patients with ESRD may account for this difference. Lastly, the modulation of sympathetic activity by angiotensin converting enzyme (ACE) inhibitors, ARB, or moxonidine in CKD patients does not affect the BRS.[141,144] Moxonidine has not been approved by the FDA in the United States. It has been shown to increase cardiac mortality and hospitalization rates in a clinical trial for heart failure, which may be related to the designed target dose, 3 mg per day, a dose 10 times higher than that in the studies for renal patients.[146] Clonidine, an imidazoline and an α2-receptor agonist, has been shown to reduce sympathetic activity in heart failure patients.[147] Whether clonidine has similar effects as moxonidine in CKD patients has not been studied. In patients who tolerate clonidine, it may be an alternative drug for lowering sympathetic activities.

Renal denervation ideally is the treatment of choice for CKD-associated sympathetic overactivity because it specifically targets the pathogenetic mechanism without adverse effects from the suppression of a sympathetic reflex induced by sympatholytic agents. A novel catheter-based method using radiofrequency ablation of the renal sympathetic nerve has been developed and is effective for treating resistant hypertension.[148] Whether this procedure is cost-effective at reducing cardiovascular complications and the progression of renal disease in CKD patients remains to be tested.

As for parasympathetic hypoactivity, the main goal is to prevent arterial stiffness, vascular calcification, and heart failure in order to preserve BRS and improve parasympathetic activity.[128] The treatment plan should include controlling volume status, blood pressure, blood sugar, hemoglobin, lipid profiles, and mineral metabolism parameters (calcium, phosphorus, and parathyroid hormone).

Obviously, renal transplantation is the best option for treating uremic autonomic neuropathy. Successful kidney transplantation normalizes multiple parameters of both sympathetic and parasympathetic systems, except MSNA (Table 78.5).[103,138,149]

As for the symptomatic treatment for uremic autonomic neuropathy, sildenafil has been shown to be effective and well tolerated for erectile dysfunction.[150] Gastroprokinetic medications such as metoclopramide or erythromycin given before each meal and at bedtime have been shown to improve the nutritional status in ESRD patients probably through the improvement of gastroparesis.[151] For intradialytic hypotension, midodrine, an oral α1-adrenoceptor agonist, given 15 to 30 minutes before the hemodialysis session appears to be effective and safe.[152]

REFERENCES

1. Smogorzewski MJ. Central nervous dysfunction in uremia. *Am J Kidney Dis.* 2001;38(4 Suppl 1):S122–S128.

2. Silver SM, Sterns RH, Halperin ML. Brain swelling after dialysis: old urea or new osmoles? *Am J Kidney Dis.* 1996 Jul;28(1):1–13.

3. Alfrey AC. Dialysis encephalopathy syndrome. *Annu Rev Med.* 1978;29:93–98.

4. Kurella Tamura M, Yaffe K. Dementia and cognitive impairment in ESRD: diagnostic and therapeutic strategies. *Kidney Int.* 2011;79(1):14–22.

5. Winkelman JW, Chertow GM, Lazarus JM. Restless legs syndrome in end-stage renal disease. *Am J Kidney Dis.* 1996;28(3):372–378.

6. Mahoney CA, Arieff AI. Uremic encephalopathies: clinical, biochemical, and experimental features. *Am J Kidney Dis.* 1982 Nov;2(3):324–336.

7. Teschan PE, Bourne JR, Reed RB, Ward JW. Electrophysiological and neurobehavioral responses to therapy: the National Cooperative Dialysis Study. *Kidney Int Suppl.* 1983;(13):S58–S65.

8. Meyer TW, Hostetter TH. Uremia. *N Engl J Med.* 2007;357(13):1316–1325.

9. Depner TA. Uremic toxicity: urea and beyond. *Semin Dial.* 2001;14(4):246–251.

10. Vanholder R, Baurmeister U, Brunet P, et al. A bench to bedside view of uremic toxins. *J Am Soc Nephrol.* 2008;19(5):863–870.

11. De Deyn PP, Vanholder R, Eloot S, Glorieux G. Guanidino compounds as uremic (neuro)toxins. *Semin Dial.* 2009;22(4):340–345.

12. Arieff AI, Massry SG. Calcium metabolism of brain in acute renal failure. Effects of uremia, hemodialysis, and parathyroid hormone. *J Clin Invest.* 1974;53(2):387–392.

13. Hajjar SM, Smogorzewski M, Zayed MA, Fadda GZ, Massry SG. Effect of chronic renal failure on $Ca2^+$ ATPase of brain synaptosomes. *J Am Soc Nephrol.* 1991;2(6):1115–1121.

14. Fraser CL, Sarnacki P, Arieff AI. Calcium transport abnormality in uremic rat brain synaptosomes. *J Clin Invest.* 1985;76(5):1789–1795.

15. Fraser CL, Sarnacki P. Parathyroid hormone mediates changes in calcium transport in uremic rat brain synaptosomes. *Am J Physiol.* 1988;254(6 Pt 2):F837–844.

16. Smogorzewski M, Campese VM, Massry SG. Abnormal norepinephrine uptake and release in brain synaptosomes in chronic renal failure. *Kidney Int.* 1989;36(3):458–465.

17. Ni Z, Smogorzewski M, Massry SG. Derangements in acetylcholine metabolism in brain synaptosomes in chronic renal failure. *Kidney Int.* 1993;44(3):630–637.

18. Schaefer F, Vogel M, Kerkhoff G, et al. Experimental uremia affects hypothalamic amino acid neurotransmitter milieu. *J Am Soc Nephrol.* 2001;12(6):1218–1227.

19. Brouns R, De Deyn PP. Neurological complications in renal failure: a review. *Clin Neurol Neurosurg.* 2004;107(1):1–16.

20. Chen CL, Lai PH, Chou KJ, et al. A preliminary report of brain edema in patients with uremia at first hemodialysis: evaluation by diffusion-weighted MR imaging. *AJNR Am J Neuroradiol.* 2007;28(1):68–71.

21. Pruss H, Siebert E, Masuhr F. Reversible cytotoxic brain edema and facial weakness in uremic encephalopathy. *J Neurol.* 2009;256(8):1372–1373.

22. Neto MM, da Costa JA, Garcia-Cairasco N, et al. Intoxication by star fruit (Averrhoa carambola) in 32 uraemic patients: treatment and outcome. *Nephrol Dial Transplant.* 2003;18(1):120–125.

23. Chang JM, Hwang SJ, Kuo HT, et al. Fatal outcome after ingestion of star fruit (Averrhoa carambola) in uremic patients. *Am J Kidney Dis.* 2000;35(2):189–193.

24. Hung SC, Hung SH, Tarng DC, et al. Thiamine deficiency and unexplained encephalopathy in hemodialysis and peritoneal dialysis patients. *Am J Kidney Dis.* 2001;38(5):941–947.

25. Port JD, Beauchamp NJ Jr. Reversible intracerebral pathologic entities mediated by vascular autoregulatory dysfunction. *Radiographics.* 1998;18(2):353–367.

26. Schmidt M, Sitter T, Lederer SR, Held E, Schiffl H. Reversible MRI changes in a patient with uremic encephalopathy. *J Nephrol.* 2001;14(5):424–427.

27. Lee VH, Wijdicks EF, Manno EM, Rabinstein AA. Clinical spectrum of reversible posterior leukoencephalopathy syndrome. *Arch Neurol.* 2008;65(2):205–210.

28. Silver SM. Cerebral edema after rapid dialysis is not caused by an increase in brain organic osmolytes. *J Am Soc Nephrol.* 1995;6(6):1600–1606.

29. Galons JP, Trouard T, Gmitro AF, Lien YH. Hemodialysis increases apparent diffusion coefficient of brain water in nephrectomized rats measured by isotropic diffusion-weighted magnetic resonance imaging. *J Clin Invest.* 1996;98(3):750–755.

30. Trinh-Trang-Tan MM, Cartron JP, Bankir L. Molecular basis for the dialysis disequilibrium syndrome: altered aquaporin and urea transporter expression in the brain. *Nephrol Dial Transplant.* 2005;20(9):1984–1988.

31. Arieff AI, Kerian A, Massry SG, DeLima J. Intracellular pH of brain: alterations in acute respiratory acidosis and alkalosis. *Am J Physiol.* 1976;230(3):804–812.

32. Arieff AI. Dialysis disequilibrium syndrome: current concepts on pathogenesis and prevention. *Kidney Int.* 1994;45(3):629–635.

33. Harris CP, Townsend JJ. Dialysis disequilibrium syndrome. *West J Med.* 1989;151(1):52–55.

34. Bagshaw SM, Peets AD, Hameed M, et al. Dialysis disequilibrium syndrome: brain death following hemodialysis for metabolic acidosis and acute renal failure—a case report. *BMC Nephrol.* 2004;5:9.

35. DiFresco V, Landman M, Jaber BL, White AC. Dialysis disequilibrium syndrome: an unusual cause of respiratory failure in the medical intensive care unit. *Intensive Care Med.* 2000;26(5):628–630.

36. Patel N, Dalal P, Panesar M. Dialysis disequilibrium syndrome: a narrative review. *Semin Dial.* 2008;21(5):493–498.

37. Attur RP, Kandavar R, Kadavigere R, Baig WW. Dialysis disequilibrium syndrome presenting as a focal neurological deficit. *Hemodial Int.* 2008;12(3):313–315.

38. Pierides AM, Edwards WG Jr, Cullum UX Jr, McCall JT, Ellis HA. Hemodialysis encephalopathy with osteomalacic fractures and muscle weakness. *Kidney Int.* 1980;18(1):115–124.

39. Alfrey AC, LeGendre GR, Kaehny WD. The dialysis encephalopathy syndrome. Possible aluminum intoxication. *N Engl J Med.* 1976;294(4):184–188.

40. Molitoris BA, Froment DH, Mackenzie TA, Huffer WH, Alfrey AC. Citrate: a major factor in the toxicity of orally administered aluminum compounds. *Kidney Int.* 1989;36(6):949–953.

41. Milliner DS, Nebeker HG, Ott SM, et al. Use of the deferoxamine infusion test in the diagnosis of aluminum-related osteodystrophy. *Ann Intern Med.* 1984;101(6):775–779.

42. Molitoris BA, Alfrey AC, Alfrey PS, Miller NL. Rapid removal of DFO-chelated aluminum during hemodialysis using polysulfone dialyzers. *Kidney Int.* 1988;34(1):98–101.

43. Sherrard DJ, Walker JV, Boykin JL. Precipitation of dialysis dementia by deferoxamine treatment of aluminum-related bone disease. *Am J Kidney Dis.* 1988;12(2):126–130.

44. Murray AM, Tupper DE, Knopman DS, et al. Cognitive impairment in hemodialysis patients is common. *Neurology*. 2006;67(2):216–223.

45. Kurella M, Yaffe K, Shlipak MG, Wenger NK, Chertow GM. Chronic kidney disease and cognitive impairment in menopausal women. *Am J Kidney Dis.* 2005;45(1):66–76.

46. Kurella Tamura M, Wadley V, Yaffe K, et al. Kidney function and cognitive impairment in US adults: the Reasons for Geographic and Racial Differences in Stroke (REGARDS) Study. *Am J Kidney Dis*. 2008;52(2):227–234.

47. Yaffe K, Ackerson L, Kurella Tamura M, et al. Chronic kidney disease and cognitive function in older adults: findings from the chronic renal insufficiency cohort cognitive study. *J Am Geriatr Soc.* 2010;58(2):338–345.

48. McQuillan R, Jassal SV. Neuropsychiatric complications of chronic kidney disease. *Nat Rev Nephrol*. 2010;6(8):471–479.

49. Buchman AS, Tanne D, Boyle PA, et al. Kidney function is associated with the rate of cognitive decline in the elderly. *Neurology*. 2009;73(12):920–927.

50. Seliger SL, Siscovick DS, Stehman-Breen CO, et al. Moderate renal impairment and risk of dementia among older adults: the Cardiovascular Health Cognition Study. *J Am Soc Nephrol*. 2004;15(7):1904–1911.

51. Khatri M, Wright CB, Nickolas TL, et al. Chronic kidney disease is associated with white matter hyperintensity volume: the Northern Manhattan Study (NOMAS). *Stroke*. 2007;38(12):3121–3126.

52. Ikram MA, Vernooij MW, Hofman A, et al. Kidney function is related to cerebral small vessel disease. *Stroke*. 2008;39(1):55–61.

53. Kobayashi M, Hirawa N, Yatsu K, et al. Relationship between silent brain infarction and chronic kidney disease. *Nephrol Dial Transplant*. 2009;24(1): 201–207.

54. Desbien AM, Chonchol M, Gnahn H, Sander D. Kidney function and progression of carotid intima-media thickness in a community study. *Am J Kidney Dis*. 2008;51(4):584–593.

55. Fukunishi I, Kitaoka T, Shirai T, et al. Psychiatric disorders among patients undergoing hemodialysis therapy. *Nephron*. 2002;91(2):344–347.

56. Kurella M, Mapes DL, Port FK, Chertow GM. Correlates and outcomes of dementia among dialysis patients: the Dialysis Outcomes and Practice Patterns Study. *Nephrol Dial Transplant*. 2006;21(9):2543–2548.

57. Kurella Tamura M, Larive B, Unruh ML, et al. Prevalence and correlates of cognitive impairment in hemodialysis patients: the Frequent Hemodialysis Network trials. *Clin J Am Soc Nephrol*. 2010;5(8):1429–1438.

58. Jassal SV, Devins GM, Chan CT, Bozanovic R, Rourke S. Improvements in cognition in patients converting from thrice weekly hemodialysis to nocturnal hemodialysis: a longitudinal pilot study. *Kidney Int*. 2006;70(5):956–962.

59. Takaki J, Nishi T, Nangaku M, et al. Clinical and psychological aspects of restless legs syndrome in uremic patients on hemodialysis. *Am J Kidney Dis*. 2003;41(4):833–839.

60. Mucsi I, Molnar MZ, Ambrus C, et al. Restless legs syndrome, insomnia and quality of life in patients on maintenance dialysis. *Nephrol Dial Transplant*. 2005;20(3):571–577.

61. Rijsman RM, de Weerd AW, Stam CJ, Kerkhof GA, Rosman JB. Periodic limb movement disorder and restless legs syndrome in dialysis patients. *Nephrology (Carlton)*. 2004;9(6):353–361.

62. Satija P, Ondo WG. Restless legs syndrome: pathophysiology, diagnosis and treatment. *CNS Drugs*. 2008;22(6):497–518.

63. Enomoto M, Inoue Y, Namba K, Munezawa T, Matsuura M. Clinical characteristics of restless legs syndrome in end-stage renal failure and idiopathic RLS patients. *Mov Disord*. 2008;23(6):811–816.

64. Merlino G, Lorenzut S, Gigli GL, et al. A case-control study on restless legs syndrome in nondialyzed patients with chronic renal failure. *Mov Disord*. 2010;25(8):1019–1025.

65. Novak M, Mendelssohn D, Shapiro CM, Mucsi I. Diagnosis and management of sleep apnea syndrome and restless legs syndrome in dialysis patients. *Semin Dial*. 2006;19(3):210–216.

66. Winkelmann J, Stautner A, Samtleben W, Trenkwalder C. Long-term course of restless legs syndrome in dialysis patients after kidney transplantation. *Mov Disord*. 2002;17(5):1072–1076.

67. Yamamoto S, Gejyo F. Historical background and clinical treatment of dialysis-related amyloidosis. *Biochim Biophys Acta*. 2005;1753(1):4–10.

68. Miles AM. Vascular steal syndrome and ischaemic monomelic neuropathy: two variants of upper limb ischaemia after haemodialysis vascular access surgery. *Nephrol Dial Transplant*. 1999;14(2):297–300.

69. Krishnan AV, Kiernan MC. Neurological complications of chronic kidney disease. *Nat Rev Neurol*. 2009;5(10):542–551.

70. Bazzi C, Pagani C, Sorgato G, et al. Uremic polyneuropathy: a clinical and electrophysiological study in 135 short- and long-term hemodialyzed patients. *Clin Nephrol*. 1991;35(4):176–181.

71. Laaksonen S, Metsarinne K, Voipio-Pulkki LM, Falck B. Neurophysiologic parameters and symptoms in chronic renal failure. *Muscle Nerve*. 2002;25(6):884–890.

72. Krishnan AV, Pussell BA, Kiernan MC. Neuromuscular disease in the dialysis patient: an update for the nephrologist. *Semin Dial*. 2009;22(3):267–278.

73. Krishnan AV, Phoon RK, Pussell BA, et al. Altered motor nerve excitability in end-stage kidney disease. *Brain*. 2005;128(Pt 9):2164–2174.

74. Tegner R, Lindholm B. Uremic polyneuropathy: different effects of hemodialysis and continuous ambulatory peritoneal dialysis. *Acta Med Scand*. 1985;218(4):409–416.

75. Jovanovic DB, Matanovic DD, Simic-Ogrizovic SP, et al. Polyneuropathy in diabetic and nondiabetic patients on CAPD: is there an association with HRQOL? *Perit Dial Int*. 2009;29(1):102–107.

76. Laaksonen S, Voipio-Pulkki L, Erkinjuntti M, Asola M, Falck B. Does dialysis therapy improve autonomic and peripheral nervous system abnormalities in chronic uraemia? *J Intern Med*. 2000;248(1):21–26.

77. Oh SJ, Clements RS Jr, Lee YW, Diethelm AG. Rapid improvement in nerve conduction velocity following renal transplantation. *Ann Neurol*. 1978;4(4):369–373.

78. Hupperts RM, Leunissen KM, van Hooff JP, Lodder J. Recovery of uremic neuropathy after renal transplantation. *Clin Neurol Neurosurg*. 1990;92(1):87–89.

79. Okada H, Moriwaki K, Kanno Y, et al. Vitamin B6 supplementation can improve peripheral polyneuropathy in patients with chronic renal failure on high-flux haemodialysis and human recombinant erythropoietin. *Nephrol Dial Transplant*. 2000;15(9):1410–1413.

80. Kuwabara S, Nakazawa R, Azuma N, et al. Intravenous methylcobalamin treatment for uremic and diabetic neuropathy in chronic hemodialysis patients. *Intern Med*. 1999;38(6):472–475.

81. Shin J, Nishioka M, Shinko S, et al. Carpal tunnel syndrome and plasma beta2-microglobulin concentration in hemodialysis patients. *Ther Apher Dial*. 2008;12(1):62–66.

82. Gilbert MS, Robinson A, Baez A, et al. Carpal tunnel syndrome in patients who are receiving long-term renal hemodialysis. *J Bone Joint Surg Am*. 1988;70(8):1145–1153.

83. Jaradat MI, Moe SM. Effect of hemodialysis membranes on beta 2-microglobulin amyloidosis. *Semin Dial*. 2001;14(2):107–112.

84. Chary-Valckenaere I, Kessler M, Mainard D, et al. Amyloid and non-amyloid carpal tunnel syndrome in patients receiving chronic renal dialysis. *J Rheumatol*. 1998;25(6):1164–1170.

85. Knezevic W, Mastaglia FL. Neuropathy associated with Brescia-Cimino arteriovenous fistulas. *Arch Neurol*. 1984;41(11):1184–1186.

86. MacDermid JC, Wessel J. Clinical diagnosis of carpal tunnel syndrome: a systematic review. *J Hand Ther*. 2004;17(2):309–319.

87. Lornoy W, Becaus I, Billiouw JM, et al. On-line haemodiafiltration. Remarkable removal of beta2-microglobulin. Long-term clinical observations. *Nephrol Dial Transplant*. 2000;15 Suppl 1:49–54.

88. Koda Y, Nishi S, Miyazaki S, et al. Switch from conventional to high-flux membrane reduces the risk of carpal tunnel syndrome and mortality of hemodialysis patients. *Kidney Int*. 1997;52(4):1096–1101.

89. Hye RJ, Wolf YG. Ischemic monomelic neuropathy: an under-recognized complication of hemodialysis access. *Ann Vasc Surg*. 1994;8(6):578–582.

90. Riggs JE, Moss AH, Labosky DA, et al. Upper extremity ischemic monomelic neuropathy: a complication of vascular access procedures in uremic diabetic patients. *Neurology*. 1989;39(7):997–998.

91. Schanzer H, Eisenberg D. Management of steal syndrome resulting from dialysis access. *Semin Vasc Surg*. 2004;17(1):45–49.

92. Schlaich MP, Socratous F, Hennebry S, et al. Sympathetic activation in chronic renal failure. *J Am Soc Nephrol*. 2009;20(5):933–939.

93. Vita G, Bellinghieri G, Trusso A, et al. Uremic autonomic neuropathy studied by spectral analysis of heart rate. *Kidney Int*. 1999;56(1):232–237.

94. Pop-Busui R, Roberts L, Pennathur S, et al. The management of diabetic neuropathy in CKD. *Am J Kidney Dis*. 2010;55(2):365–385.

95. Thomson BJ, McAreavey D, Neilson JM, Winney RJ, Ewing DJ. Heart rate variability and cardiac arrhythmias in patients with chronic renal failure. *Clin Auton Res*. 1991;1(2):131–133.

96. Jassal SV, Coulshed SJ, Douglas JF, Stout RW. Autonomic neuropathy predisposing to arrhythmias in hemodialysis patients. *Am J Kidney Dis*. 1997;30(2):219–223.

97. Zoccali C, Mallamaci F, Parlongo S, et al. Plasma norepinephrine predicts survival and incident cardiovascular events in patients with end-stage renal disease. *Circulation*. 2002;105(11):1354–1359.

98. Fukuta H, Hayano J, Ishihara S, et al. Prognostic value of heart rate variability in patients with end-stage renal disease on chronic haemodialysis. *Nephrol Dial Transplant*. 2003;18(2):318–325.
99. Ranpuria R, Hall M, Chan CT, Unruh M. Heart rate variability (HRV) in kidney failure: measurement and consequences of reduced HRV. *Nephrol Dial Transplant*. 2008;23(2):444–449.
100. Ye S, Zhong H, Yanamadala S, Campese VM. Oxidative stress mediates the stimulation of sympathetic nerve activity in the phenol renal injury model of hypertension. *Hypertension*. 2006;48(2):309–315.
101. DiBona GF, Esler M. Translational medicine: the antihypertensive effect of renal denervation. *Am J Physiol Regul Integr Comp Physiol*. 2010;298(2):R245–253.
102. Campese VM, Romoff MS, Levitan D, Lane K, Massry SG. Mechanisms of autonomic nervous system dysfunction in uremia. *Kidney Int*. 1981;20(2):246–253.
103. Hausberg M, Kosch M, Harmelink P, et al. Sympathetic nerve activity in end-stage renal disease. *Circulation*. 2002;106(15):1974–1979.
104. Klein IH, Ligtenberg G, Oey PL, Koomans HA, Blankestijn PJ. Sympathetic activity is increased in polycystic kidney disease and is associated with hypertension. *J Am Soc Nephrol*. 2001;12(11):2427–2433.
105. Hering D, Zdrojewski Z, Krol E, et al. Tonic chemoreflex activation contributes to the elevated muscle sympathetic nerve activity in patients with chronic renal failure. *J Hypertens*. 2007;25(1):157–161.
106. Xu J, Li G, Wang P, et al. Renalase is a novel, soluble monoamine oxidase that regulates cardiac function and blood pressure. *J Clin Invest*. 2005;115(5):1275–1280.
107. Li G, Xu J, Wang P, et al. Catecholamines regulate the activity, secretion, and synthesis of renalase. *Circulation*. 2008;117(10):1277–1282.
108. Monahan KD. Effect of aging on baroreflex function in humans. *Am J Physiol Regul Integr Comp Physiol*. 2007;293(1):R3–R12.
109. Chesterton LJ, Sigrist MK, Bennett T, Taal MW, McIntyre CW. Reduced baroreflex sensitivity is associated with increased vascular calcification and arterial stiffness. *Nephrol Dial Transplant*. 2005;20(6):1140–1147.
110. Nishimura M, Hashimoto T, Kobayashi H, et al. Association between cardiovascular autonomic neuropathy and left ventricular hypertrophy in diabetic haemodialysis patients. *Nephrol Dial Transplant*. 2004;19(10):2532–2538.
111. Kuncova J, Sviglerova J, Kummer W, et al. Parasympathetic regulation of heart rate in rats after 5/6 nephrectomy is impaired despite functionally intact cardiac vagal innervation. *Nephrol Dial Transplant*. 2009;24(8):2362–2370.
112. Daul AE, Wang XL, Michel MC, Brodde OE. Arterial hypotension in chronic hemodialyzed patients. *Kidney Int*. 1987;32(5):728–735.
113. Esforzado Armengol N, Cases Amenos A, Bono Illa M, et al. Autonomic nervous system and adrenergic receptors in chronic hypotensive haemodialysis patients. *Nephrol Dial Transplant*. 1997;12(5):939–944.
114. Fadda GZ, Massry SG, el-Refai M, Campese VM. Alpha 1 adrenergic receptors in mesenteric arteries of rats with chronic renal failure. *Kidney Int*. 1988;34(4):463–466.
115. Chao CC, Wu VC, Tan CH, et al. Skin denervation and its clinical significance in late-stage chronic kidney disease. *Arch Neurol*. 2011;68(2):200–206.
116. Freeman R. Autonomic peripheral neuropathy. *Lancet*. 2005;365(9466):1259–1270.
117. Converse RL Jr, Jacobsen TN, Jost CM, et al. Paradoxical withdrawal of reflex vasoconstriction as a cause of hemodialysis-induced hypotension. *J Clin Invest*. 1992;90(5):1657–1665.
118. Daugirdas JT. Pathophysiology of dialysis hypotension: an update. *Am J Kidney Dis*. 2001;38(4 Suppl 4):S11–17.
119. Chesterton LJ, Selby NM, Burton JO, et al. Categorization of the hemodynamic response to hemodialysis: the importance of baroreflex sensitivity. *Hemodial Int*. 2010;14(1):18–28.
120. Shirazian S, Radhakrishnan J. Gastrointestinal disorders and renal failure: exploring the connection. *Nat Rev Nephrol*. 2010;6(8):480–492.
121. Dumitrascu DL, Barnert J, Kirschner T, Wienbeck M. Antral emptying of semisolid meal measured by real-time ultrasonography in chronic renal failure. *Dig Dis Sci*. 1995;40(3):636–644.
122. Van Vlem B, Schoonjans R, Vanholder R, et al. Delayed gastric emptying in dyspeptic chronic hemodialysis patients. *Am J Kidney Dis*. 2000;36(5):962–968.
123. Strid H, Norstrom M, Sjoberg J, et al. Impact of sex and psychological factors on the water loading test in functional dyspepsia. *Scand J Gastroenterol*. 2001;36(7):725–730.
124. Chen JD, Lin Z, Pan J, McCallum RW. Abnormal gastric myoelectrical activity and delayed gastric emptying in patients with symptoms suggestive of gastroparesis. *Dig Dis Sci*. 1996;41(8):1538–1545.
125. Finkelstein FO, Shirani S, Wuerth D, Finkelstein SH. Therapy insight: sexual dysfunction in patients with chronic kidney disease. *Nat Clin Pract Nephrol*. 2007;3(4):200–207.
126. Campese VM. Autonomic nervous system dysfunction in uraemia. *Nephrol Dial Transplant*. 1990;5(Suppl 1):98–101.
127. Giuliano F, Rampin O. Neural control of erection. *Physiol Behav*. 2004;83(2):189–201.
128. Robinson TG, Carr SJ. Cardiovascular autonomic dysfunction in uremia. *Kidney Int*. 2002;62(6):1921–1932.
129. Converse RL Jr, Jacobsen TN, Toto RD, et al. Sympathetic overactivity in patients with chronic renal failure. *N Engl J Med*. 1992;327(27):1912–1918.
130. Klein IH, Ligtenberg G, Neumann J, et al. Sympathetic nerve activity is inappropriately increased in chronic renal disease. *J Am Soc Nephrol*. 2003;14(12):3239–3244.
131. Hathaway DK, Cashion AK, Milstead EJ, et al. Autonomic dysregulation in patients awaiting kidney transplantation. *Am J Kidney Dis*. 1998;32(2):221–229.
132. Mylonopoulou M, Tentolouris N, Antonopoulos S, et al. Heart rate variability in advanced chronic kidney disease with or without diabetes: midterm effects of the initiation of chronic haemodialysis therapy. *Nephrol Dial Transplant*. 2010;25(11):3749–3754.
133. Tamura K, Tsuji H, Nishiue T, et al. Determinants of heart rate variability in chronic hemodialysis patients. *Am J Kidney Dis*. 1998;31(4):602–606.
134. Chan CT, Hanly P, Gabor J, et al. Impact of nocturnal hemodialysis on the variability of heart rate and duration of hypoxemia during sleep. *Kidney Int*. 2004;65(2):661–665.
135. Rubinger D, Sapoznikov D, Pollak A, Popovtzer MM, Luria MH. Heart rate variability during chronic hemodialysis and after renal transplantation: studies in patients without and with systemic amyloidosis. *J Am Soc Nephrol*. 1999;10(9):1972–1981.
136. Bavanandan S, Ajayi S, Fentum B, et al. Cardiac baroreceptor sensitivity: a prognostic marker in predialysis chronic kidney disease patients? *Kidney Int*. 2005;67(3):1019–1027.
137. Agarwal A, Anand IS, Sakhuja V, Chugh KS. Effect of dialysis and renal transplantation on autonomic dysfunction in chronic renal failure. *Kidney Int*. 1991;40(3):489–495.
138. Rubinger D, Backenroth R, Sapoznikov D. Restoration of baroreflex function in patients with end-stage renal disease after renal transplantation. *Nephrol Dial Transplant*. 2009;24(4):1305–1313.
139. Penne EL, Neumann J, Klein IH, et al. Sympathetic hyperactivity and clinical outcome in chronic kidney disease patients during standard treatment. *J Nephrol*. 2009;22(2):208–215.
140. Brotman DJ, Bash LD, Qayyum R, et al. Heart rate variability predicts ESRD and CKD-related hospitalization. *J Am Soc Nephrol*. 2010;21(9):1560–1570.
141. Ligtenberg G, Blankestijn PJ, Oey PL, et al. Reduction of sympathetic hyperactivity by enalapril in patients with chronic renal failure. *N Engl J Med*. 1999;340(17):1321–1328.
142. Klein IH, Ligtenberg G, Oey PL, Koomans HA, Blankestijn PJ. Enalapril and losartan reduce sympathetic hyperactivity in patients with chronic renal failure. *J Am Soc Nephrol*. 2003;14(2):425–430.
143. Neumann J, Ligtenberg G, Klein IH, et al. Sympathetic hyperactivity in hypertensive chronic kidney disease patients is reduced during standard treatment. *Hypertension*. 2007;49(3):506–510.
144. Neumann J, Ligtenberg G, Oey L, Koomans HA, Blankestijn PJ. Moxonidine normalizes sympathetic hyperactivity in patients with eprosartan-treated chronic renal failure. *J Am Soc Nephrol*. 2004;15(11):2902–2907.
145. Hausberg M, Tokmak F, Pavenstädt H, Kramer BK, Rump LC. Effects of moxonidine on sympathetic nerve activity in patients with end-stage renal disease. *J Hypertens*. 2010;28(9):1920–1927.
146. Cohn JN, Pfeffer MA, Rouleau J, et al. Adverse mortality effect of central sympathetic inhibition with sustained-release moxonidine in patients with heart failure (MOXCON). *Eur J Heart Fail*. 2003;5(5):659–667.
147. Grassi G, Turri C, Seravalle G, et al. Effects of chronic clonidine administration on sympathetic nerve traffic and baroreflex function in heart failure. *Hypertension*. 2001;38(2):286–291.
148. Krum H, Schlaich M, Whitbourn R, et al. Catheter-based renal sympathetic denervation for resistant hypertension: a multicentre safety and proof-of-principle cohort study. *Lancet*. 2009;373(9671):1275–1281.
149. Heidbreder E, Schafferhans K, Heidland A. Disturbances of peripheral and autonomic nervous system in chronic renal failure: effects of hemodialysis and transplantation. *Clin Nephrol*. 1985;23(5):222–228.
150. Rosas SE, Wasserstein A, Kobrin S, Feldman HI. Preliminary observations of sildenafil treatment for erectile dysfunction in dialysis patients. *Am J Kidney Dis*. 2001;37(1):134–137.
151. Ross EA, Koo LC. Improved nutrition after the detection and treatment of occult gastroparesis in nondiabetic dialysis patients. *Am J Kidney Dis*. 1998;31(1):62–66.
152. Prakash S, Garg AX, Heidenheim AP, House AA. Midodrine appears to be safe and effective for dialysis-induced hypotension: a systematic review. *Nephrol Dial Transplant*. 2004;19(10):2553–2558.
153. Heidbreder E, Schafferhans K, Heidland A. Autonomic neuropathy in chronic renal insufficiency. Comparative analysis of diabetic and nondiabetic patients. *Nephron*. 1985;41(1):50–56.

CHAPTER

79 Cardiac Disease in Chronic Kidney Disease

Patrick S. Parfrey • Sean W. Murphy

INTRODUCTION

Acute or chronic dysfunction in the heart or kidneys can cause dysfunction in the other organ, producing cardiorenal syndromes that were classified in 2008 by Ronco and colleagues[1] into five different types. In type I, or acute cardiorenal syndrome, an abrupt worsening of cardiac function leads to acute kidney injury. In type II, or chronic cardiorenal syndrome, chronic cardiac dysfunction causes progressive and potentially permanent chronic kidney function impairment. In type III, or acute renocardiac syndrome, an abrupt worsening of kidney function causes acute cardiac dysfunction. In type IV, or chronic renocardiac syndrome, chronic kidney dysfunction contributes to cardiac dysfunction. In type V, or secondary cardiorenal syndrome, a systemic condition such as diabetes mellitus or sepsis causes both cardiac and renal dysfunction. This chapter will focus on type IV, chronic renocardiac syndrome.

Both estimated glomerular filtration rate (eGFR) and albuminuria are independent predictors of cardiovascular (CV) events.[2] In over a million enrollers in the California Kaiser Permanente health maintenance organization (HMO), the degree of kidney function impairment independently and incrementally predicted subsequent cardiac events, hospitalization, and all-cause mortality.[3] Among 11,640 patients with type 2 diabetes, a tenfold increment in urinary albumin to creatinine ratio independently increased the risk of CV events by 2.5-fold and that of CV death by 3.9-fold.[4] Every halving of baseline eGFR was associated with a 2.2-fold increase in a risk of CV events and a 3.6-fold increase in risk of CV death.[4] In a recent meta-analysis, mortality risk was doubled at eGFR levels of 30 to 45 mL/min/1.73 m^2 or urine albumin to creatinine ratio > 11.3 mg per millimole as compared with their normal ranges.[5] Furthermore, patients with higher levels of proteinuria within a given level of eGFR had an increased risk of adverse outcomes.[6]

Not only is the baseline eGFR predictive of CV events, but so is the rate of decline of eGFR. The Cardiovascular Health Study demonstrated that those that had a more rapid decline in eGFR over a 7-year period had increased risk of CV events during the subsequent 8-year period: an increased risk of heart failure of about 30% and an increased risk of myocardial infarction (MI) of about 40%.[7] In the U.S. Atherosclerosis Risk in Communities (ARIC) study, individuals with greatest annual declines in eGFR had higher risk of incident coronary heart disease and of all-cause mortality at 3 and 9 years than those with stable eGFRs.[8]

In the Cardiovascular Health Study, the 3-year probability of CV events increased as the GFR declined below 70 mL per minute.[9] However, the probability decreased substantially after adjustment for traditional risk factors. Below a eGFR level of 30 mL per minute, the CV event rate is very high and likely influenced by uremia-related risk factors. After starting dialysis therapy, atheromatous event rates are much higher than before dialysis. In the United States, the incidence of de novo coronary events, stroke, and peripheral vascular disease of hemodialysis patients, after 2.2 years follow-up from the start of dialysis, were 10.2%, 2.2%, and 14%, respectively.[10] In addition, the uremic state is certainly cardiomyopathic and predisposes the patient to heart failure. This is supported by numerous studies: a high incidence of heart failure in CKD,[11] a high prevalence of cardiac failure on starting dialysis,[12] a higher rate of de novo symptomatic heart failure in renal transplant recipients than in the general population,[13] and a high incidence of de novo cardiac failure in hemodialysis patients (13.6% over a 2.2-year mean follow-up in the United States and 17% over a 3.4-year follow-up in Canada).[14,15]

The rate of CV death in patients on dialysis is substantially higher than that of the general population in all age groups, particularly in the younger group (Fig. 79.1).[16] This enormous burden of cardiac disease is related to the high prevalence of different cardiac/vascular diseases, the high rate of traditional cardiac risk factors, and the cardiopathic and vasculopathic hemodynamic and metabolic milieu associated with chronic kidney disease (CKD).

The Pathogenesis of Cardiac Disease

The CV disorders associated with CKD are multiple and often present in the same patient (Fig. 79.2). Atherosclerotic events occur frequently among patients with CKD[11]

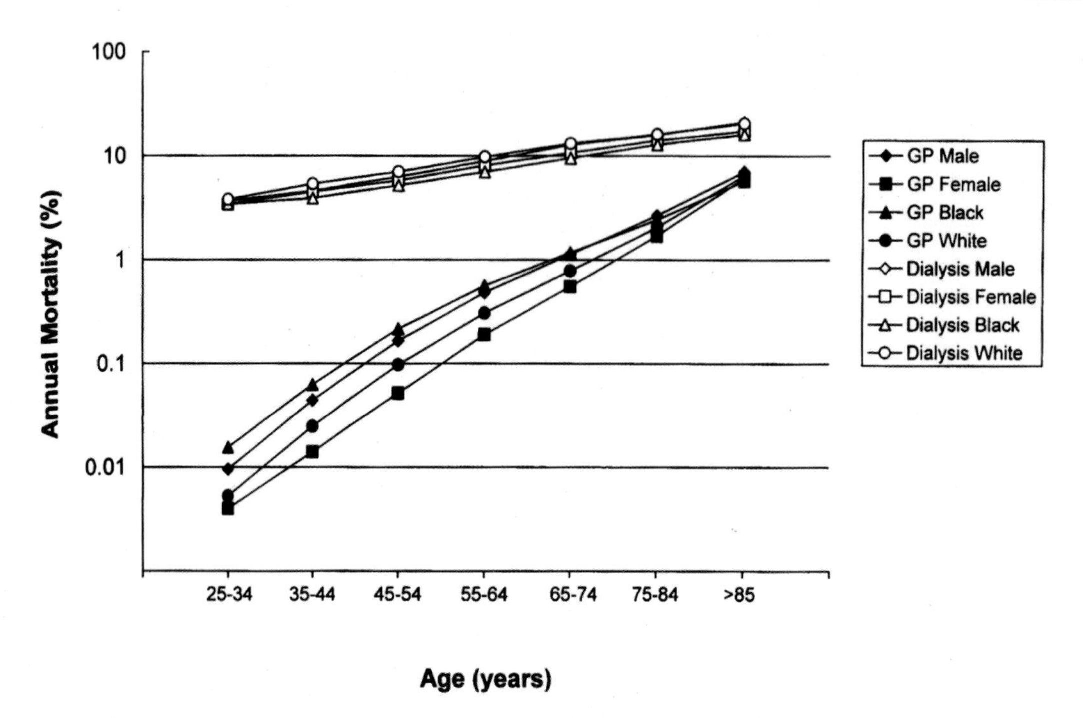

FIGURE 79.1 Annual cardiovascular mortality by age group in the general population (GP) and in patients on dialysis. (From Foley RN, Parfrey PS, Sarnak MJ. Epidemiology of cardiovascular disease in chronic renal disease. *J Am Soc Nephrol.* 1998;9:S16, with permission.)

because of the high prevalence of diabetes, hypertension, dyslipidemia, and the likelihood that uremia-related factors increase atherosclerotic risk, particularly when eGFR falls below 30mL/min/1.73 m^2. Arteriosclerosis, a diffuse disorder of large conduit arteries, is characterized by dilated, ectatic, noncompliant vessels. Such noncompliance can be exacerbated by metastatic vascular calcification.[17]

Concentric left ventricular hypertrophy (LVH) also occurs frequently because of LV pressure overload caused by hypertension, arteriosclerosis, and sometimes aortic stenosis.[18] Eccentric LVH results from LV volume overload associated with hypervolemia, arteriovenous fistula, and anemia. During years on dialysis LV growth occurs,[19] although it regresses following renal transplantation.[20] LVH can progress

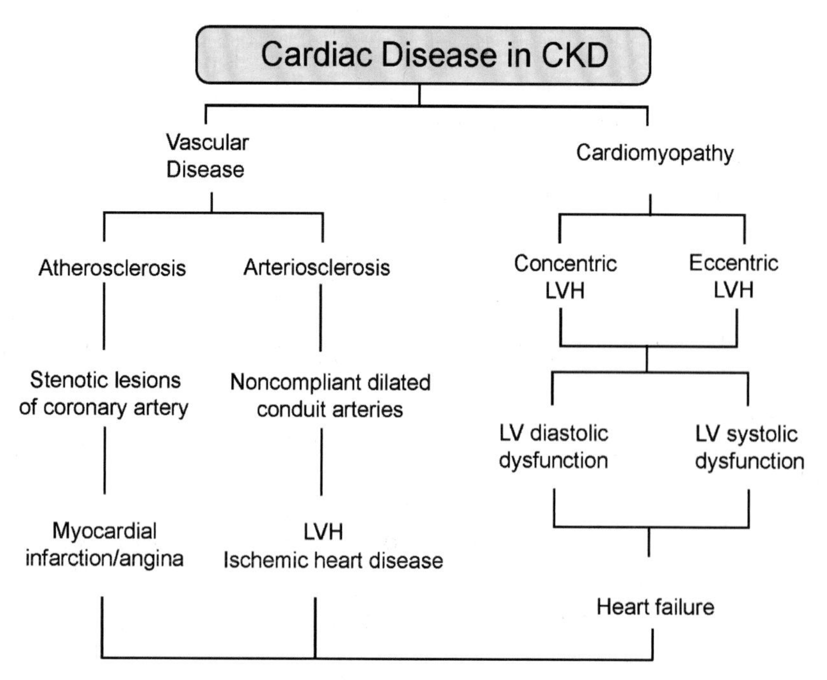

FIGURE 79.2 The pathogenesis of cardiovascular disease in chronic kidney disease (CKD). *LV,* left ventricular; *LVH,* left ventricular hypertrophy.

to LV systolic dysfunction through progressive myocyte loss, but LV diastolic dysfunction also frequently results in symptomatic pulmonary edema.[21]

Ischemic Heart Disease

Coronary artery disease. Symptomatic myocardial ischemia usually results from flow-limiting critical coronary atherosclerotic disease, but may be present in the absence of significant angiographic disease in approximately 25% of patients (Fig. 79.3).[22] In the latter case, small-vessel disease or a decrease in myocardial capillary density consequent to LVH or fibrosis may contribute to the ischemic symptoms.[23–25] LVH itself may predispose the patient to ischemia, and it may be associated with increased diastolic coronary blood flow caused by arteriosclerosis.

In non-CKD populations, the initiating event of atherosclerosis appears to be endothelial injury caused by mechanical stress (e.g., hypertension) or endothelial toxins (nicotine, oxidative stress, hyperlipidemia, and inflammation) that alter the endothelial phenotype to a more permeable, procoagulant state.[26] Endothelial denudation or, more commonly, alterations in cell surface receptor expression, permits the access of lipoproteins and macrophages into the subintimal space.[26,27] The oxidative modification of lipoproteins, particularly of low-density lipoprotein (LDL), is chemotactic for macrophages and facilitates the uptake of oxidized lipids by macrophages, resulting in the formation of foam cells.[28] Oxidized LDL stimulates the elaboration of growth factors that are mitogenic for smooth muscle and are profibrotic.[29] These processes result in the accumulation of oxidatively modified lipids and inflammatory cells at the center of a fibrous "cap" of variable thickness. This cap may rupture, causing subocclusive thromboses that may be minimally symptomatic or associated with acute coronary syndromes (e.g., unstable angina, myocardial infarction). These thrombi eventually become organized in the wall of the vessel. Calcific deposits may develop. The mature atheroma thus may contain, in addition to lipids, inflammatory cells, collagen, an organized thrombus, and calcium.[30] The propensity for rupture varies with the composition of the atheroma. Lipid and inflammatory cell–rich atheromas with thin fibrous caps are thought to be more

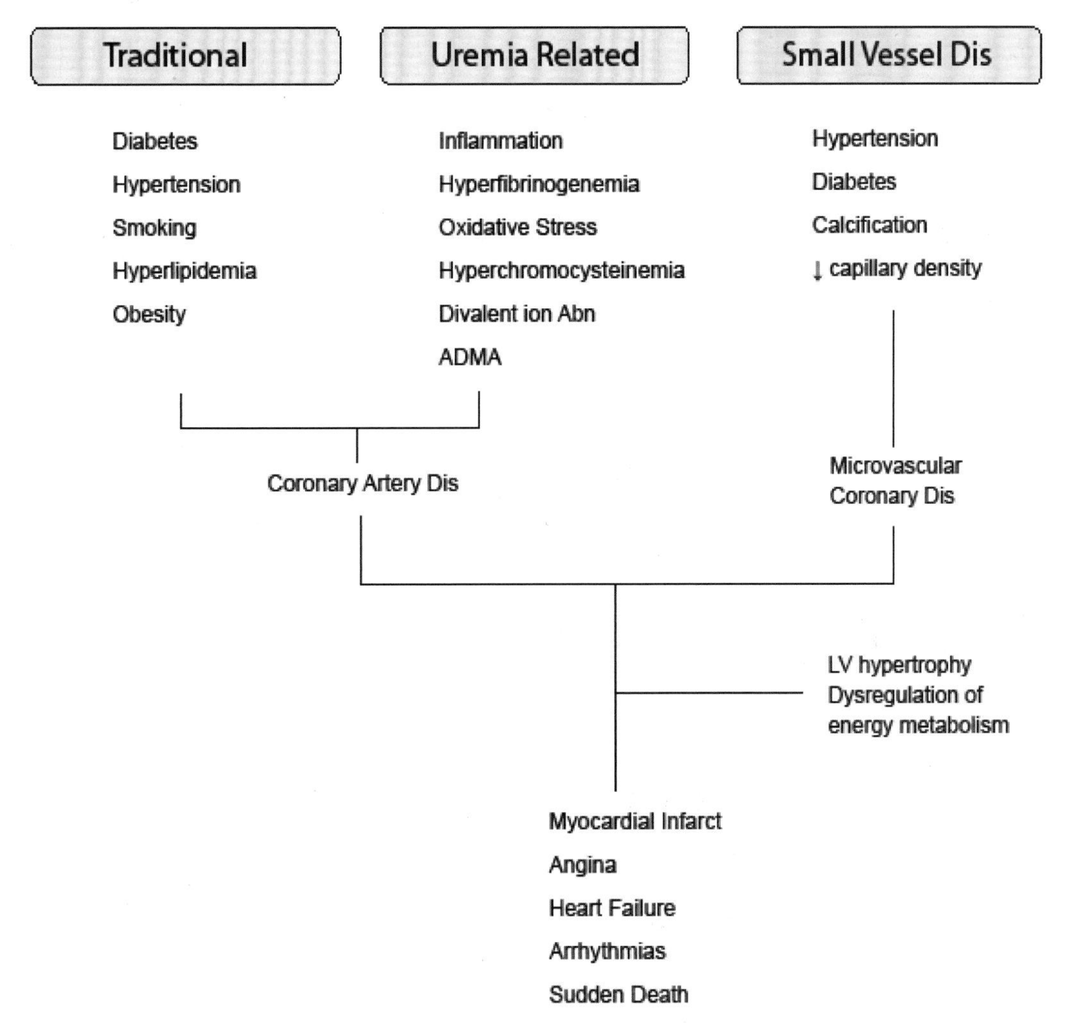

FIGURE 79.3 The etiology of ischemic heart disease in chronic kidney disease. *Dis,* disease; *ADMA,* asymmetric dimethyl arginine; *LV,* left ventricular

unstable than those with a greater degree of fibrosis and those that are less lipid.[31]

The histologic classification of coronary artery disease (CAD) lesions is outlined in Figure 79.4.[32] Initial lesions, type I through III, are small and silent, whereas types IV to VI may produce clinical events or may remain silent. The riskiest lesion is type VI, where surface defects and hematoma and a thrombus occur. The anatomic study of carotid plaque composition in 46 CKD patients with critical stenosis was compared to plaques in 56 CAD patients with normal renal function.[33] In CKD patients compared to controls, plaques were more frequently unstable (83% versus 52%), ruptured (59% versus 36%), and calcified (17% versus 7%), and the fibrous component was reduced (40% versus 57%).

Postmortem data from patients with CKD show increased vascular medial thickness and a smaller lumen area relative to control subjects matched for age and gender.[31] Although carotid artery intima-media thickness is a marker of atherosclerotic plaques in the general population, in CKD it may be increased by factors unrelated to atherosclerosis. In 406 patients with CKD and without overt CV disease (CVD), intima-media thickness was inversely correlated with eGFR, but had no association with traditional CV risk factors.[34] Furthermore, following a renal transplantation, intima-medial thickness normalized within 90 days. It is possible that shear stress associated with fluid overload, endothelial dysfunction, or other factors induce the increase in intima-media thickness seen in CKD.

Theoretically, renal failure can modify the atherogenic process at multiple levels. Hypertension and flow overload may increase stresses on the vascular wall at bifurcations. In many patients on dialysis, a prooxidant and chronic inflammatory state pertains, and both may contribute to endothelial dysfunction.[35] Hyperhomocysteinemia may promote endothelial activation and thrombosis by mechanisms that are yet unclear.[36] Hyperparathyroidism and divalent ion abnormalities may promote vascular calcification and medial hypertrophy.[17] The presence of calcium identified by electron beam tomography correlates with advanced atherosclerosis and appears to be more prevalent in patients with end-stage renal disease (ESRD).[37–38]

Asymmetric dimethyl arginine (ADMA) is an endogenous competitive inhibitor of nitric oxide synthase (NOS) and reduces nitric oxide generation, thus inhibiting the beneficial affect of nitric oxide on vasodilation, arterial stiffness, and endothelial function. The accumulation of ADMA inhibits NOS in endothelial cells and induces endothelial dysfunction, vasoconstriction, and atherosclerosis. ADMA levels are inversely related to GFR in patients with mild-to-moderate CKD. In renal transplant recipients, ADMA levels were an independent and a significant risk factor for major cardiac events and all-cause mortality.[39] A similar association was previously reported for dialysis patients.[40]

Matrix metalloproteinases and their specific tissue inhibitors regulate the proteolysis of the vascular extracellular matrix, and their balance is important in atherosclerosis and plaque destabilization. A cross-sectional study of 111 patients with stage 1 through 4 CKD, 217 dialysis patients, and 50 healthy controls demonstrated elevated levels of circulating metalloproteinase-10 associated with a severity of CKD.[41] A composite atherosclerosis score was highest in dialysis patients, and the severity of atherosclerosis was associated with the elevated levels of circulating metalloproteinase-10. It is possible that the riskier plaques seen in CKD may be caused, at least in part, by the high levels of metalloproteinases.

Microvascular disease. In the absence of flow-limiting CAD, ischemic symptoms may result from a reduction in coronary vasodilator reserve and altered myocardial oxygen delivery. Intracoronary ultrasonography has shown that angiographically normal vessel segments may contain areas of nonencroaching atheroma. Endothelial function is impaired in these vessels and may reduce coronary vasodilator reserve (i.e., the ability of the vessel to dilate above baseline in response to increased myocardial oxygen demand).[42] Vasodilator reserve is clearly impaired in vessels with lumen-encroaching disease.[43] The resulting mismatch of supply and demand may give rise to symptomatic ischemia.

Small vessel disease may occur in LVH and diabetes, and because of uremia per se. In LVH, small vessel smooth muscle hypertrophy and endothelial abnormalities can diminish coronary reserve. Diabetes may be associated with microvascular disease characterized by endothelial proliferation, subendothelial fibrosis, and exudative deposits of hyaline in the intima.[44] In uremic rats, LVH is associated with a severe reduction in myocardial capillary density compared with hypertensive rats that were matched for weight and blood pressure (BP).[25] Small vessel calcification may also impair coronary reserve.

Dysregulation of energy metabolism. An impairment in energy supply in the myocyte may increase cellular susceptibility to ischemia. A reduced myocardial phosphocreatine-adenosine triphosphate ratio under stress has been observed in uremic animals.[45] Hyperparathyroidism may play a critical role in the dysregulation of cellular energetics, and may thus exacerbate ischemic damage to the myocardium.[46]

Impaired myocardial fatty acid metabolism and insulin resistance, both of which reduce the synthesis of myocardial adenosine triphosphate, cause a deficiency in the myocardial energy supply. Visualization of impaired fatty acid metabolism is possible using single-photon emission computed tomography (SPECT) with the iodinated fatty acid analog iodine, 123-B-methyliodophenyl pentadecanoic acid (BMIPP). Uptake of this analog on SPECT images has been graded in 17 segments using a 5-point scale, and provides a measure of recurrent myocardial ischemia.[47] Among 155 prevalent hemodialysis patients without obstructive coronary artery disease on angiography, subsequent cardiac death was associated with both BMIPP score > 12 and also with increased insulin resistance scores, suggesting an important role for impairment in

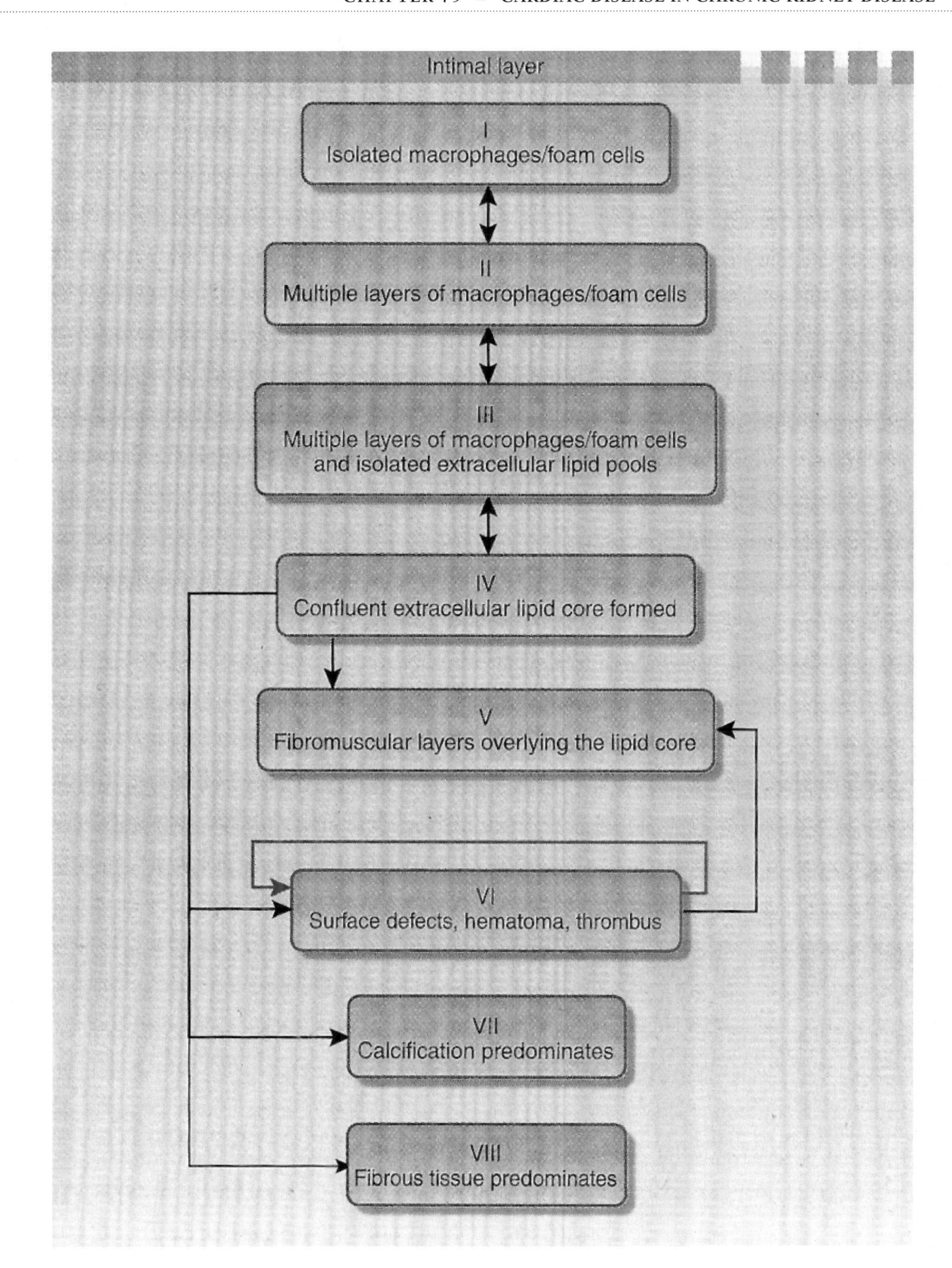

FIGURE 79.4 The histologic classification of atherosclerotic lesions. Thick lines identify preferential pathways of lesion evolution. Box VI highlights type VI plaques, which are the riskiest lesions. The line above it identifies a vicious cycle that may rapidly lead to vessel occlusion. (From Zoccali C, Secks S. What makes plaques vulnerable in CKD?: a fresh look at metalloproteinases. *Kidney Int.* 2010;78:1207, with permission.)

myocardial energy supply in the occurrence of cardiac death in these patients.[47] In a prospective study of a larger group (N = 318) of asymptomatic hemodialysis patients without a clinical history of MI or coronary revascularization who were followed for 3.6 ± 1 year, a BMIPP score > 12 was again strongly associated with cardiac death (hazard ratio [HR]: 22; 95% confidence interval [CI] = 8.5 to 56.1).[48]

Arteriosclerosis

Increased CV morbidity and mortality have been correlated, either directly or indirectly, with various estimates of elevated LV afterload in patients with CKD.[49–51] Postulated etiologic factors include increased arterial wall stiffness,[49] raised sympathetic tone mediated by elevated noradrenaline levels,[52,53] cardiac natriuretic peptides,[54] nocturnal hypoxemia,[55] and autonomic dysregulation.[56] These factors are associated with two established components of LV afterload: hypertension and reduced arterial wall compliance. Before examining these, however, it is important first to recognize the pathophysiologic similarities and differences by which they are characterized.

Hypertension has usually been attributed to a reduction in the caliber or number of muscular arteries (150 to 400 μm diameter), resulting in an increase in peripheral resistance. This approach, however, does not take into account the fact that BP fluctuates during the cardiac cycle, and that systolic and diastolic levels represent only the limits of this fluctuation. A Fourier analysis of the BP curve can determine both its steady state (mean BP) and oscillatory (fluctuation about the mean) components. The former is determined exclusively by cardiac output and peripheral resistance (pressure and flow considered constant over time). The oscillatory component is determined by the pattern of LV ejection, the viscoelastic properties of large conduit arteries, and the reflection of pulse waves.[57] A faster pulse wave velocity (PWV) is primarily associated with arterial stiffness, which, in CKD, is an acceleration of the normal aging process with vessel dilatation and a diffuse, nonocclusive medial and intimal wall hypertrophy (arteriosclerosis). It has been correlated with shortened stature, male gender, smoking, BP, diabetes, volume overload, humoral imbalance, and age.[58–60]

The clinical characteristics of hypertension therefore will depend on the predominant abnormality. Increased peripheral resistance is characterized principally by an increased diastolic and mean BP, whereas increased arterial stiffness and early wave reflections are indicated by an increased systolic and widened pulse pressure. Because the peripheral resistance of most dialysis patients is within the normal range, it is likely that effects from an accelerated PWV contribute more significantly to CV morbidity than an elevation in mean BP. Increased systolic BP and pulse pressure are observed in dialysis patients and are closely correlated with LV hypertrophy.[61,62]

Vascular calcification. An increased calcium X phosphate product, elevated levels of promoters of calcification, and reduced levels of inhibitors of calcification, in addition to hyperparathyroidism, insulin resistance, oxidant stresses, and dyslipidemia, promote metastatic vascular calcification and heart fibrosis in patients with ESRD.[63] Multiple inhibitors of vascular calcification have been identified, the transcription and synthesis of which are downregulated during inflammation. A study in a mouse model revealed that fetuin-A, an inhibitor of vascular calcification, protects against vascular calcification in CKD, suggesting that the patients who develop calcification might be those with inflammation and low levels of circulating inhibitors of vascular calcification.[64]

Vascular smooth muscle cells have the ability to transform into cells with chondrocytelike or osteoblastlike phenotypes, the consequences of which include the local production of collagen and noncollagenous proteins in intimal and medial layers, the incorporation of calcium and phosphorus into matrix vesicles, and vascular mineralization. This active process is associated with CKD, aging, diabetes, and inflammation.[63]

The cellular origin of medial vascular calcifications is suggested by ultrastructural analysis of the iliac arteries in 30 dialysis patients, obtained before renal transplantation, which demonstrated that arterial microcalcifications seem to originate from nanocrystals, and they often exhibit a core-shell structure.[65]

Two types of vascular calcification occur: patchy calcification of the intima associated with atherosclerotic plaques and diffuse calcification of the media, in the absence of cholesterol deposits, associated with arteriosclerosis. Metastatic vascular calcification decreases compliance of large conduit vessels and thus increases PWV. An early rebound of pressure waves from the distal vessels increases systolic pressure and predisposes the patient to LVH, and low diastolic pressure predisposes the patient to diminished coronary flow during diastole.

Controversy exists as to whether these are two distinct entities in CKD or rather are a continuum of advanced vascular pathology consistent with accelerated atherosclerotic calcification.[66,67] Coronary artery calcification scoring by computed tomography is used to estimate the likelihood of coronary artery disease in the general population and is a predictor of all-cause mortality. In 225 diabetic patients with proteinuria, coronary artery calcification was diagnosed in 86% of the patients, and it was not associated with eGFR, serum calcium, phosphate, parathyroid hormone, or 25-hydroxy vitamin D.[69] This suggests that the coronary calcification was associated with atherosclerotic disease rather than medial calcification induced by CKD. The severity of coronary artery calcification early in the course of CKD was an independent predictor of all-cause mortality.[68]

A recent autopsy study[69] of patients at different stages of CKD reported the occurrence of coronary intimal sclerosis in all CKD stages, but medial sclerosis in patients with stage 4 and 5 CKD (18%). Moreover, medial calcification was generally associated with intimal sclerosis, which is supportive of the belief that medial calcification is an amplification of preexisting atherosclerosis.

Cardiomyopathy

Left ventricular hypertrophy. Ventricular growth occurs in response to mechanical stresses, primarily volume or pressure overload (Fig. 79.5). LV volume overload results in the addition of new sarcomeres in series, leading to an increased cavity diameter.[70] A larger diameter results in increased wall tension, a direct consequence of the Laplace law, which states that all wall tension (T) is proportional to the product of intraventricular pressure (P) multiplied by the ventricular diameter (D), divided by the wall thickness (M), or T = PD/M. An increase in wall tension secondarily stimulates the addition of new sarcomeres in parallel. This remodeling thickens the ventricular wall, distributing the tension over a larger cross-sectional area of muscle and returning the tension in each individual fiber back to normal, thereby alleviating the stimulus to further hypertrophy. This combination of cavity enlargement and wall thickening is called eccentric hypertrophy. Pressure overload increases wall tension by increasing the intraventricular pressure, resulting directly in the parallel addition of new sarcomeres and their functional consequences, as described. Because sarcomeres are not added in series, isolated pressure overload does not lead to cavity enlargement (concentric hypertrophy).

Both eccentric and concentric hypertrophies are initially beneficial. Dilation permits an increase in stroke volume without an increase in the inotropic state of the myocardium and, as such, is an efficient adaptation to volume overload.[70] It also permits the maintenance of normal stroke volume and cardiac output in the presence of decreased contractility. Muscular hypertrophy returns the tension per unit muscle fiber back to normal, thereby decreasing ventricular stress.

The uremic milieu of chronic renal disease can potentiate many of these processes. Anemia, salt and water excess, and arteriovenous fistulae in patients on dialysis are prevalent causes of volume overload, whereas hypertension is a major cause of pressure overload. These disturbances are probably the primary stimuli to ventricular remodeling in uremia. These same stimuli promote arterial remodeling in the large

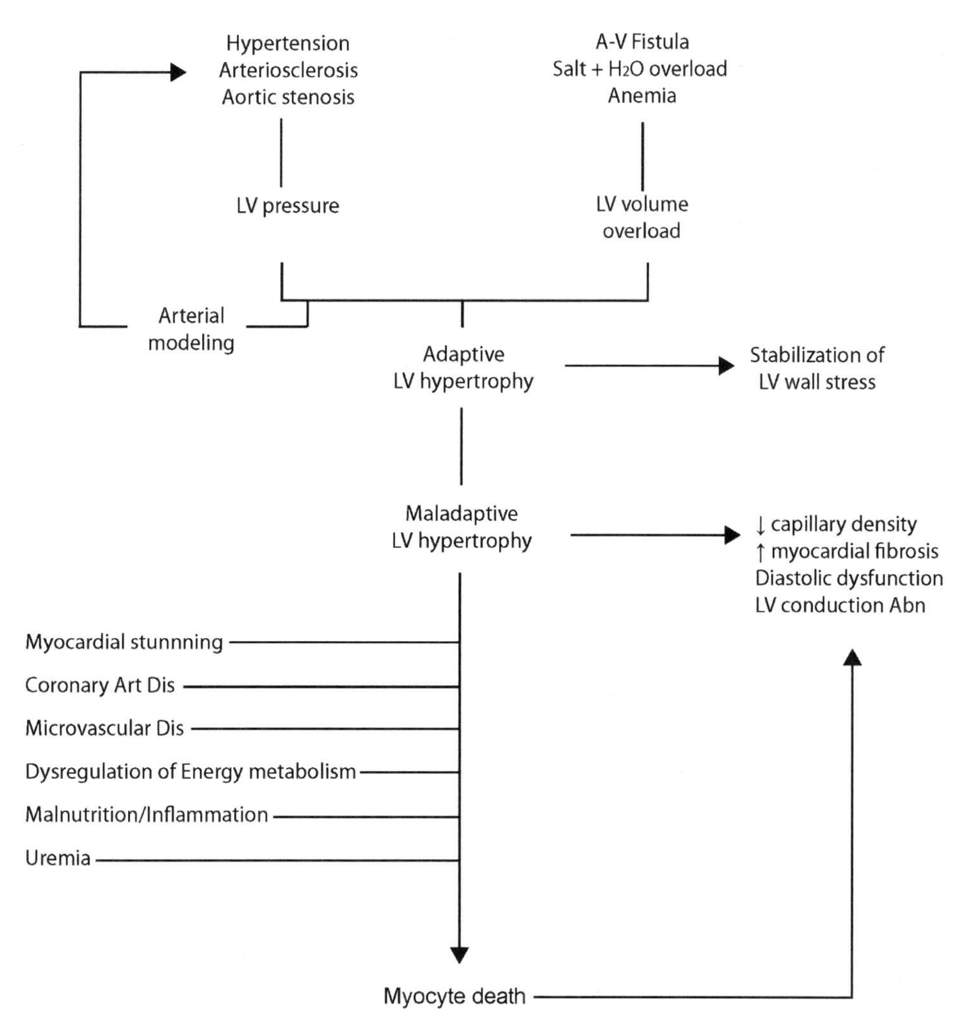

FIGURE 79.5 The evolution of cardiomyopathy in chronic kidney disease. *A-V,* atrioventricular; *LV,* left ventricular; *Art Dis,* artery disease; *Dis,* disease.

and resistance arteries, which is characterized by diffuse arterial thickening and stiffening (arteriosclerosis), which can increase the effective load on the left ventricle independently of mean arterial pressure.[71,72] Secondary hyperparathyroidism and raised calcium phosphate product may be associated with aortic valve calcification and, in some cases, stenosis, which is a less frequent cause of pressure overload.[73]

Progressive concentric LVH and hyperkinesis occur in hemodialysis patients, which is partly explained by hypertension but not by a wide array of potential risk factors, including moderate anemia.[19] Another explanation may be that primary stimuli independent of LV load might initiate or contribute to LVH and fibrosis in patients with CKD. Several signaling pathways could have a role in this process, including defects in insulin signaling through the protein kinase, Akt, and downstream, the mammalian target of rapamycin (mTOR) pathway.[74] Siedlecki et al.[75] created normotensive CKD using a mouse model in which kidney parenchyma was resected so as to avoid excessive renin-angiotensin system (RAS) activation. Progressive LVH and fibrosis developed, which was associated with de novo protein synthesis and activation of the mTOR pathway. The administration of rapamycin, which inhibits the mTOR pathway, prevented cardiac hypertrophy.

Myocyte death. Ultimately, in persistent LV overload, LVH becomes maladaptive (Fig. 79.5). Muscular hypertrophy is associated with several progressive, deleterious changes in cell function and tissue architecture. Early in the evolution of LV hypertrophy, slow reuptake of calcium by the sarcoplasmic reticulum leads to abnormal ventricular relaxation. Combined with decreased passive compliance of a thickened ventricular wall, these changes may precipitate diastolic dysfunction.[76] More advanced sarcoplasmic reticulum dysfunction is associated with calcium overload and cell death. Decreased capillary density, impaired coronary reserve, and abnormal relaxation may decrease subendocardial perfusion, promoting ischemia.[25,77] The frequent coexistence of CAD may exacerbate ischemia and myocyte attrition. Fibrosis of the cardiac interstitium also occurs and appears to be more marked in pressure than in volume overload.[77] Myocyte apoptosis, ischemia, and neurohormonal activation (e.g., increased catecholamines, angiotensin II, and aldosterone) are thought to contribute to myocardial dysfunction.[78,79] In the late phases of chronic and sustained overload, oxidative stress may contribute to cellular dysfunction and demise.[35] Together, these various processes lead to progressive cellular attrition, fibrosis, pump failure, and, ultimately, death.

The attrition of myocytes in chronic uremia may be exacerbated by several factors. An underlying coronary artery disease promotes ischemia and infarction. Hyperparathyroidism increases susceptibility to ischemia through dysregulation of the cellular energy metabolism,[46] and appears to promote myocardial fibrosis directly.[80] Malnutrition, oxidative stress, and inadequate dialysis may additionally promote myocyte death. Such cell death in the presence of LVH and continuing pressure and volume overload may be catastrophic, leading to a severe overload cardiomyopathy and, ultimately, death.[81]

Pathologic studies support this etiologic pathway. Cardiac pathology in patients who had diabetes, heart failure, and no evidence of coronary artery disease on angiography revealed cell loss as a result of apoptosis and necrosis of cardiac myocytes and endothelial cells, with the extent of fibrosis, apoptosis, and hypertrophy all greater in hypertensive patients than in those without hypertension.[82] Myocardial biopsies of dialysis patients with dilated cardiomyopathy revealed abnormal cardiac myocyte anatomy and interposition of dense fibrosis.[83] The extent of myocardial fibrosis in patients with ESRD was more marked than in patients with diabetes mellitus or essential hypertension with similar LV mass.[84]

Myocardial stunning. Another cardiopathic mechanism that may predispose to a patient arrhythmia or to heart failure is recurrent reperfusion injury. The coronary arteries of dialysis patients are often narrowed, the microcirculation is often underdeveloped, and the LV may be hypertrophied. In this scenario, transient hypoperfusion could produce severe ischemia, followed by reperfusion necrosis.[85] The frequent, although minor elevations in troponin observed in ESRD patients may reflect this myocardial damage. A phenomenon called myocardial stunning supports this hypothesis.

Myocardial stunning has been defined as a 20% reduction in regional wall motion in two or more segments and hyperkinesis as either a $> 20\%$ or a $> 50\%$ increase in shortening fraction. This was measured using echocardiography before hemodialysis, during hemodialysis, and 15 minutes after hemodialysis in 12 children without structural cardiac disease. Eleven of the 12 developed myocardial stunning with varying degrees of compensatory hyperkinesis in unaffected segments, thus maintaining LV ejection fraction throughout dialysis.[86] This regional hypokinesis is associated with reduced myocardial blood flow. Four patients without coronary artery disease had myocardial blood measured during dialysis using serial intradialytic $H_2{}^{15}O$ positron emission tomography scanning and had their regional wall motion assessed using serial concurrent echocardiography.[87] Segmental myocardial blood flow was reduced to a significantly greater extent in areas that developed regional wall motion abnormalities compared with those that did not.

Valvular Disease

Most valvular lesions observed in patients with CKD are acquired and develop from dystrophic calcification of the valvular annulus and leaflets, particularly the aortic and mitral valves.[88] The prevalence of aortic valve calcification in dialysis patients is up to 55%, similar to that in the elderly general population, although it occurs 10 to 20 years earlier.[88,89] Aortic valve orifice stenosis in CKD evolves from valve sclerosis, which itself is now generally recognized to be associated with an increased cardiovascular mortality.[90] In dialysis patients, the prevalence of aortic stenosis is 3% to 13%.[45] It may sometimes evolve rapidly (within 6 months) to hemodynamically significant stenosis, with a worsening of LVH and rapidly evolving symptoms. Age, duration of dialysis, a raised phosphate level, and an elevated calcium phosphate product appear to be the most important risk factors for the development of aortic stenosis.[88]

Mitral valve calcification is not as common as aortic valve disease in CKD and may have a somewhat different pathophysiology. In one study[88] evaluated by echocardiography, mitral annulus calcification was present in 45% of 92 hemodialysis patients (compared to 10% of age-and gender-matched controls). In a study[91] of 135 peritoneal dialysis patients with low parathyroid hormone levels, a constant involvement of the posterior cusp, together with left atrial enlargement, was observed. Valve calcification has also been associated with rhythm and cardiac conduction defects, valvular insufficiency, and peripheral vascular calcification. Although most studies have identified abnormalities in calcium phosphate metabolism as the predominant underlying risk factor, additional factors include the duration of dialysis and the duration of predialysis systolic hypertension. Factors associated with decreased survival include the severity of calcification, mitral regurgitation, and reduced LV function.[92]

Diagnosis

Coronary Artery Disease

Symptoms of myocardial ischemia in patients with CKD are, in general, similar to those in the nonuremic population. However, the prevalence of silent myocardial ischemia in this group of patients is very high.[93,94] This has been best demonstrated in diabetic patients with ESRD because they often are subjected to a screening coronary angiography before renal transplantation. In one series[95] of 100 diabetic patients with ESRD, for example, 75% of the patients with angiographically demonstrated CAD had no typical angina symptoms. The prevalence of asymptomatic CAD in nondiabetic patients with ESRD is not as well studied. Exertional dyspnea is also less specific for cardiac disease in patients with CKD than in the general population. Such symptoms may be attributable to anemia, acidosis, heart failure, or fluid overload; therefore, a careful interpretation within the clinical context is required.

Patients with CKD and symptomatic ischemic heart disease (IHD) should be investigated in a manner similar to patients with normal renal function, provided that revascularization will be considered should critical coronary artery disease (CAD) be identified. Routine screening for CAD in asymptomatic patients with CKD therefore is not recommended.[96] It is appropriate to apply clinical practice guidelines for a CAD screening of patients before noncardiac surgery to the CKD population as well.[97] Generally, CAD screening is recommended before surgery when the combination of risk factors and the nature of the operation place the patient at moderate or higher risk of a cardiovascular event. Patients being evaluated for renal transplantation are an exception to the aforementioned recommendations. The adverse prognostic implications of CAD, the desire to avoid allograft injury from posttransplantation invasive cardiac testing, and the need to ration transplantable organs are justification for screening all but the lower risk patients. The American Society of Transplant Physicians has published guidelines for the evaluation of renal transplantation candidates that include recommendations for the investigation of CAD.[98]

Biomarkers for ischemic heart disease. Cardiac troponin T and troponin I are currently the standard biomarkers of myocardial injury. These tests are more specific for myocardial damage than creatinine kinase-myocardial band but still are not always indicative of an ischemic mechanism of injury.[99] First-generation troponin T levels in ESRD patients are often high, whereas troponin I levels are high less frequently.[100] Although there is no difference between the diagnostic and prognostic accuracy of troponin T versus troponin I in the general population in suspected acute coronary syndrome,[101] the lower incidence of increased troponin I in the renal failure population suggests that this is the preferred test in this clinical setting.[100]

Despite concerns about falsely positive tests, troponins are clearly very useful in the evaluation of suspected ACS. In one retrospective analysis,[102] troponin I was shown to be the best performing marker in suspected acute coronary syndrome (ACS) in patients with CKD or ESRD when compared to alternatives such as creatine kinase or myoglobin. Although troponin T is more likely to be elevated at baseline in patients with renal impairment, a normal level has useful negative predictive value. A sequential rise in either of the serum troponins is consistent with new myocardial damage regardless of symptoms.[103]

Noninvasive testing for coronary artery disease. Exercise electrocardiography (ECG) has been the traditional method of a noninvasive diagnosis of CAD. The sensitivity of this test is only 50% to 60% for single vessel disease but is greater than 85% for triple vessel CAD in the general population.[104] These figures are based on the assumption that the patient reaches an adequate exercise level (i.e., 85% of the age-adjusted predicted maximal heart rate). A large proportion of patients with ESRD are unable to achieve this target because of poor exercise tolerance, anemia, poorly controlled hypertension, or the use of cardiac medications. One study[105] of 85 diabetic uremic patients showed that only 6 achieved an adequate exercise level. Pharmacologic agents, therefore, often are used for noninvasive testing for CAD in these patients. The diagnostic utility of dipyridamole-thallium testing in patients with ESRD is poor,[106] whereas that of dobutamine stress echocardiography is better,[107] and therefore may be the method of choice where it is available.

Nuclear scintigraphic scanning. Nuclear scintigraphy can be used both for the assessment of myocardial systolic function and for ischemia. The former method examines the ejection fraction of the left and/or right ventricles and relies upon gated analysis techniques. Care must be taken with regard to associated valve regurgitation, which when present, can substantially confound functional estimates. If valve function is intact, accurate estimates of systolic function at rest and with exercise can be achieved.

The predominant role for nuclear scanning techniques, however, is in the assessment of myocardial ischemia, both as a screening tool in the work-up for transplantation and in cases of diagnostic uncertainty. Exercise-based studies as well as the use of dipyridamole to enhance vasodilation are commonly used, together with one or other of technetium-99m (^{99m}Tc)-labeled thallium, methoxyisobutylisonitrile (MIBI), or metaiodobenzylguanidine (MIBG). Inherent problems with scintigraphy must be taken into consideration. BP may be too high or too low to permit the safe administration of a vasodilatory agent; high endogenous circulating levels of adenosine may blunt the efficacy of dipyridamole; coronary flow reserve may be reduced due to LV hypertrophy and small vessel disease; and symmetrical coronary disease and/or a blunted tachycardic response due to autonomic neuropathy can mask significant pathology.[108,109]

Dahan and colleagues[110] found a positive and negative predictive value of 47% and 91%, respectively, for dipyridamole-thallium combined imaging in the diagnosis of coronary disease by coronary angiography in a study of 60 asymptomatic hemodialysis patients. It is likely that both on-site expertise and the recognized testing limitations in patients with CKD influence the utility of nuclear scanning and therefore dictate the interpretation and screening strategy for a particular center.

Computed tomography. Electron-beam ultrafast computed tomography–derived coronary artery calcification assessment relies upon the principle that coronary artery calcification is a reliable surrogate for significant coronary atherosclerosis, but this is far from certain in patients with CKD.[66,67] It has been used recently to demonstrate a reduction in coronary artery calcification after treatment with the non–calcium-containing medication sevelamer and with cinacalcet.[111,112] The role of this technique in evaluating risk or disease in transplant patients is unknown. Severe coronary artery calcification measured by electron beam–computed tomography in stage 3 through 5 CKD occurs much more frequently in diabetics (56%) than in nondiabetics (4%). In CKD stages 1 and 2, the prevalence was 10% in diabetics and 1% in nondiabetics.[113]

In the Multi-Ethnic Study of Atherosclerosis, 562 adults with eGFR < 60 mL per minute had assessments of coronary artery calcification.[114] The prevalence of coronary artery calcification at baseline was 66%, and the incidence was 6.1% per year in women and 14.8% in men. Progression occurred in 17% of subjects per year across all subgroups, and diabetes was associated with a 65% adjusted risk of progression.

The accuracy and clinical utility of noninvasive testing for coronary artery disease was evaluated in 517 Dutch patients referred for an evaluation of chest pain symptoms, using coronary arteriography as the gold standard.[115] Stress testing was sufficient as a diagnostic test for patients with a low pretest probability of coronary disease based on their Duke classification clinical score. Computed tomography coronary angiography was useful in patients with intermediate pretest probability, because it could distinguish which patients required invasive angiography. In patients with high pretest probability, proceeding directly to invasive angiography, without a noninvasive test evaluation, was recommended.

Coronary angiography. Cardiac catheterization and coronary angiography remain the gold standard for the diagnosis of CAD. A major disadvantage associated with this mode of investigation is the potential for renal toxicity from radiocontrast agents. CKD, especially in diabetic patients, is a major risk factor for contrast-induced acute renal failure.[116] The risk of clinical nephrotoxicity is related to the severity of prior renal impairment. Although most patients who develop nephropathy eventually recover renal function, there is a risk that contrast administration may precipitate ESRD in patients with severe impairment in renal function at baseline. The risk of contrast nephropathy in high-risk patients may be reduced by using nonionic contrast media and a saline infusion. Many interventions to reduce the risk of nephropathy have been studied, but none have been shown to be consistently effective.[116] A number of trials using N-acetylcysteine in CKD patients have demonstrated a reduction in the incidence of contrast nephropathy, whereas others have not. A meta-analysis of this topic indicated that the relative risk of nephropathy is reduced by N-acetylcysteine (relative risk 0.65; 95% CI, 0.43 to 1.00), but there has been significant heterogeneity in studies to date.[117] Given its low cost and lack of adverse effects, it is reasonable to use N-acetylcysteine in high-risk patients prior to angiography. A large trial with clinically meaningful outcomes is still required before it can be universally recommended.

Arteriosclerosis

Aortic PWV is the best available measure of aortic stiffness and correlates well with a subsequent risk for CVD.[118]

Cardiomyopathy

Because echocardiography is widely available, simple, and reproducible, it has become the method of choice for the assessment of LVH. Systolic dysfunction is defined as an ejection fraction of less than 40%, which indicates impaired myocardial contractility. It often is associated with LV dilation (LV end-diastolic diameter ≥ 5.6 cm), which is defined echocardiographically as an LV cavity volume index greater than 90 mL per square meter.[119] Concentric LVH is characterized by a thickened LV wall (≥ 1.2 cm during diastole) with normal cavity volume. LV mass index is a calculated parameter that reflects the degree of muscular hypertrophy in the LV. Epidemiologic studies in nonrenal patients have established that the upper limits of LV mass index are 130 g per square meter for adult men and 102 g per square meter for adult women.[120] Values above these limits indicate hypertrophy. The calculation of LV mass and volume are not independent of volume status. As a result, patients should be euvolemic when the echocardiogram is performed. In patients on hemodialysis, it is important to standardize the time and conditions of the study in relation to the dialysis session and to have patients at their dry weight.

Cardiac magnetic resonance is a volume-independent technique to assess cardiac structure and LV mass. This technique is now used as a surrogate outcome measure in randomized controlled trials (RCTs).[121] Of 246 Scottish hemodialysis patients, 64% had LV hypertrophy using this technique, and the principal associations of LV mass were end-diastolic volume, predialysis BP, and calcium X phosphate product.[122]

In the Cardiovascular Risk Reduction by Early Anemia Treatment with Epoetin Beta (CREATE) trial,[123] in patients with stage 3 and 4 CKD, the prevalence of LV hypertrophy using echocardiography at baseline was 47%, with eccentric hypertrophy more prevalent than concentric. During the study, LVH prevalence and mean LV mass index did not increase significantly, but LV geometry fluctuated considerably within 2 years in both groups.

Levin et al.[124] have reported a prevalence of LVH in 27% of patients with a creatinine clearance rate greater than 50 mL per minute, in 31% of those with clearances of 25 to 49 L per minute, and in 45% of those with clearances less than 25 mL per minute. In the prospective arm of this study, an association between rising LV mass index and falling GFR was observed. The overall prevalence of LVH among patients beginning dialysis was 75%.[125] In a large prospective cohort study, only 16% had normal echocardiograms at inception. Fifteen percent (15%) had systolic dysfunction, 28% had dilation with preserved contractility, and 41% had concentric LVH.[126] In a subset of these patients on dialysis who underwent yearly consecutive echocardiograms, LV mass index and LV cavity volume progressively increased, and the biggest increase occurred between baseline and 1 year.[127] This progressive LV growth was confirmed in a recent prospective study.[19]

In patients about to undergo transplantation, the distribution of echocardiographic abnormalities is similar to those in patients on dialysis: normal, 17%; concentric LVH, 41%; dilation, 32%; and systolic dysfunction, 12%.[128] In this longitudinal study, the proportion of patients with normal studies doubled (36%) and systolic function normalized in all patients with fractional shortening of less than 25% at 1 year posttransplantation.[128]

Clinical Manifestations

Myocardial Infarction or Angina

The most frequent manifestations of ischemic heart disease are MI and angina. The incidence rate of atherosclerotic events (MI, CV events, peripheral vascular disease) in predialysis CKD is very high. In a Medicare population of nondiabetic CKD patients, it was 36 per 100 patient years, and in diabetic CKD, it was 49 per 100 patient years.[11]

In Canada, a prospective study[12] demonstrated that by the time patients reach ESRD, the prevalence of angina was 21% and of patients who had had a MI, it was 18%. The annual incidence of angina or MI among Canadian patients on hemodialysis is 10%.[129] Among renal transplant recipients, the annual incidence of MI, revascularization, or death from MI was 1.5%.[130] In another study, the rate of de novo angina or MI was 1.22 per 100 patient years.[13]

Both traditional and nontraditional risk factors predict coronary heart disease in CKD. Results from the atherosclerosis risk in communities (ARIC) study[131] identified that independent of age, gender, and diabetes the following are risk factors: smoking, hypertension, hyperglycemia, and hypercholesterolemia. In addition to these traditional risk factors, nontraditional risk factors identified were increased waist circumference, hyperlipoproteinemia B, anemia, hypoalbuminemia, and hyperfibrinogenemia (Table 79.1).[131]

TABLE 79.1 **Traditional and Nontraditional Risk Factors as Predictors of Coronary Artery Disease in Chronic Kidney Disease (Results from the ARIC study)[131]**

Traditional	Adjusted RR	95% CI
Age, 5 years	1.33	1.1–1.6
Male	3.96	2.25–6.2
Smoking	1.91	1.2–3.2
Hypertension	1.79	1.1–2.9
Systolic BP, 20 mm Hg	1.26	1.05–1.5
Glucose, 40 mg/dL	1.26	1.15–1.4
Diabetes	2.88	1.9–4.5
Total chol, 43 mg/dL	1.46	1.3–1.7
Nontraditional		
Waist circum, 13 cm	1.24	1.0–1.6
Apolipoprotein B, 29 mg/dL	1.28	1.1–1.5
Anemia	2.01	1.2–3.4
S. Albumin, 0.33 mg/dL	0.76	0.6–0.9
Fibrinogen, 69 mg/dL	1.23	1.1–1.4

ARIC, atherosclerosis risk in communities; RR, relative risk; CI, confidence interval; BP, blood pressure; chol, cholesterol; circum, circumference.

In an incident cohort of dialysis patients, independent predictors of de novo ischemic heart disease events were diabetes, hypertension, and hypoalbuminemia.[132] In an incident cohort of renal transplant recipients,[13] the major predictors were diabetes and hypertension, and in a more recent cohort study,[133] hypercholesterolemia was identified as a predictor of cardiac events.

Congestive Heart Failure

Congestive heart failure (CHF) may result from systolic dysfunction or diastolic dysfunction,[21] the latter occurring because of concentric or eccentric hypertrophy (Fig. 79.2). IHD is an additional independent predictor. Among patients with diastolic dysfunction, CHF results from impaired ventricular relaxation; this leads to an exaggerated increase in LV end-diastolic pressure for a given increase in end-diastolic volume. As a result, a small excess of salt and water can rapidly lead to a large increase in LV end-diastolic pressure, culminating in pulmonary edema. The development of CHF, even in the presence of salt and water overload, suggests an underlying cardiac abnormality. Because the management of diastolic dysfunction differs from that of systolic dysfunction, an echocardiogram of the left ventricle is useful in planning management.

Approximately half of patients with CHF have CKD, as defined by a GFR ≤ 60 mL per minute.[134] Differentiating type II chronic cardiorenal syndrome from type IV chronic cardiorenal syndrome may be difficult, because chronic heart failure may cause CKD, and CKD predisposes a patient to heart failure. In predialysis, CKD heart failure events occur as frequently as atherosclerotic events, particularly in patients with diabetic nephropathy; in nondiabetic CKD patients, the event rate was 31 per 100 patient years and in diabetic CKD patients it was 52 per 100 patient years.[11]

On starting dialysis, 35% of patients have had a previous episode of CHF.[12] A baseline history of CHF carries a twofold risk of death independent of age, diabetes, and heart disease.[125] The risk for the development of pulmonary edema requiring hospitalization or ultrafiltration after starting maintenance hemodialysis is 10% annually.[129] Among patients free of CHF at the initiation of dialysis, de novo CHF developed in 25% over 41 months of observation.[15] In a cohort of 244 CKD patients, 20% developed new or worsening cardiac symptoms, including a change in their CHF symptoms.[134] Renal transplant recipients who were free of cardiac disease 1 year after transplantation developed de novo CHF as frequently as de novo IHD (1.26 versus 1.22 events per 100 patient years, respectively).[13]

In an incident cohort of dialysis patients without a previous history of CHF, the significant predictors of the de novo development of CHF, independent of age, diabetes, and systolic dysfunction at baseline, were hypertension, anemia, hypoalbuminemia, and hypocalcemia.[15] It appears that factors that predispose a patient to volume or flow overload (e.g., anemia), pressure overload (e.g., hypertension), and cell death (e.g., malnutrition, hypocalcemia/hyperparathyroidism, and IHD) are associated with CHF in dialysis.

The presence of concentric LV hypertrophy, LV dilation, or systolic dysfunction at the time of ESRD therapy has been associated with progressively higher risks of congestive heart failure independent of age, sex, diabetes, and ischemic heart disease.[126] Furthermore, changes in echocardiographic measurements following the initiation of dialysis also predicted the development of heart failure.[135]

In a large cohort of renal transplant recipients (RTRs) without cardiac disease 1 year after transplantation, age, diabetes, gender, high BP, and anemia were identified as independent risk factors for de novo CHF.[13]

Arrhythmias

In patients without renal failure, LVH and CAD appear to be associated with an increased risk of arrhythmias. As outlined earlier, these cardiac diseases occur frequently in patients with CKD. In addition, serum electrolyte levels that can affect cardiac conduction, including potassium, calcium, magnesium, and hydrogen, are often abnormal or undergo rapid fluctuations during hemodialysis.

In cross-sectional studies, the prevalence of arrhythmias is high: between 68% and 88% for atrial arrhythmias, 56% to 76% for ventricular arrhythmias, and premature ventricular complexes were found in 14% to 21%.[136,137] Older age, preexisting heart disease, LVH, and digoxin therapy were associated with a higher prevalence and a greater severity of cardiac arrhythmias. However, because of the considerable variation in the frequency and severity of arrhythmias during and after dialysis, the clinical significance in a given patient is unclear.

Most atrial arrhythmias are of low clinical significance. However, a sustained, rate-related (fast or slow) impairment of LV filling can certainly produce hemodynamic consequences. The majority of the premature ventricular contractions are unifocal and number less than 30 per hour. The finding of high-grade ventricular arrhythmias in the presence of CAD has been associated with an increased risk of cardiac mortality and sudden death.[138] Dialysis-associated hypotension may precipitate high-grade ventricular arrhythmias.

Arrhythmias in peritoneal dialysis patients appear different from those in hemodialysis patients. Severe cardiac arrhythmias occurred in only 4% of 27 peritoneal dialysis patients compared to 33% of 27 hemodialysis patients.[139] Patients in both groups were matched for age, sex, duration of treatment, and etiology of chronic renal failure. The lower frequency of LVH, the maintenance of a relatively stable BP, the absence of sudden hypotensive events, and the significantly lower incidence of hyperkalemia in patients on peritoneal dialysis may explain the lower incidence of severe arrhythmias.

Atrial Fibrillation

The prevalence of atrial fibrillation in ESRD is extremely high, and it is associated with increased mortality in hemodialysis patients.[140] Of 17,513 randomly sampled patients in the

Dialysis Outcomes and Practice Patterns Study (DOPPS),[141] 2,188 (12.5%) had preexisting atrial fibrillation and the incidence of de novo atrial fibrillation during follow-up was 1 per 100 patient years. Advanced age, non-black race, higher facility mean dialysate calcium, prosthetic heart valves, and valvular heart disease were associated with a higher risk of de novo atrial fibrillation. The risk of ischemic stroke in the general population is best estimated with the CHADS2 score (1 point each for congestive heart failure, hypertension, age ≥ 75 years, and diabetes; 2 points for prior stroke or transient ischemic attack). The CHADS2 score identified approximately equal-sized groups of hemodialysis patients at low (< 2) and high risk (> 4) for subsequent strokes.

The prevalence of atrial fibrillation in predialysis CKD is also high and likely related to comorbidity rather than severity of CKD. Of 2010 nondialysis patients with CKD in two community hospitals in Chicago, 21% had atrial fibrillations.[142] This was associated with older age, white race, increasing left atrial diameter, lower systolic BP, and congestive heart failure, but was not associated with eGFR.

Registry data in the United States revealed that the cumulative incidence of new onset atrial fibrillation was 3.6% at 12 months and 7.3% at 36 months after renal transplantation, and declined below the demographics adjusted cumulative incidence on the waiting list by about 17 months.[143] Baseline independent predictors of atrial fibrillation included older recipient age, male gender, white race, renal failure from hypertension, and coronary artery disease. Transplant factors included donor age, delayed graft function, posttransplantation hypertension, anemia, new onset diabetes, MI, and graft failure.

Sudden Death

The proportion of deaths designed as sudden is similar in both patients with CKD and the general population. In a British community-based study,[144] approximately 70% of deaths were the result of cardiac disease, and roughly half of those cardiovascular deaths were sudden. Among diabetic hemodialysis patients in the Die Deutsche Diabetes Dialysis (4D) study in 178 German dialysis centers,[145] 26% of adjudicated cardiac deaths were sudden, whereas coronary artery disease, heart failure, and other cardiac etiologies were the cause of 9%, 6%, and 3% of the adjudicated deaths, respectively. A study of 4,120 deaths in the United States during a 2-year follow-up of 12,833 prevalent hemodialysis patients showed that the greatest percentage of all deaths (27%) was caused by sudden cardiac arrest, whereas other cardiovascular conditions (including CAD, vascular heart disease, cardiomyopathy, arrhythmia, pericarditis/cardiac tamponade, and pulmonary edema) accounted for 20% of all deaths.[146]

A high rate of sudden cardiac death in 5,830 dialysis patients who underwent coronary artery bypass (CABG) surgery in the United States was reported by Herzog et al.[147] All-cause and arrhythmias-related mortality were 290 and 76 deaths per 1,000 patient years, respectively. Deaths from sudden cardiac arrest or arrhythmia accounted for approximately 25% of all-cause deaths.

The rate of sudden cardiac death was also examined in 19,440 U.S. patients with CKD who had undergone cardiac catheterization at a single institution[148]: 522 sudden cardiac deaths occurred and 25% of cases had an eGFR < 60 mL/min/1.73 m^2. The sudden cardiac death rate increased with increasing severity of CKD; the hazard ratio (HR) for each 10 mL/min/1.73 m^2 decline in eGFR was 1.11 (95% CI = 1.06 to 1.7).

Among patients undergoing dialysis, the frequency of sudden cardiac death increased both with the duration of time that the patient had been undergoing dialysis and with the duration of time since their previous dialysis session, and was highest among individuals with diabetes.[149,150] Furthermore, the ratio of observed to expected deaths was higher than expected in the first 12 hours after the initiation of the hemodialysis session, and increased as the time from start of the dialysis session exceeded 36 hours.[150] The number of observed deaths was three times higher than expected in the period 60 to 72 hours after the start of the dialysis session. Other risk factors for sudden death included hospitalization within the past 30 days and a decrease in systolic BP of 30 mm Hg during hemodialysis.[150] Patients with ESRD and diabetes have a higher risk of sudden death than nondiabetic ESRD patients, with an incidence of 20% within the first 2 years after the dialysis is initiated.[151]

Cardiac arrest. Four hundred cardiac arrests occurred in a total of 5,744,708 hemodialysis sessions, which is equivalent to a rate of 7 arrests per 100,000 hemodialysis sessions.[149] In another cohort study of 295,913 incident dialysis patients surviving at least 1 year on dialysis, the rate of cardiac arrest was 93 events per 1,000 patient years at year 1, and 164 events per 1,000 patient years at year 4.[152] Among patients with diabetes who were undergoing dialysis, the rate of cardiac arrest at year 1 was 110 events per 1,000 patient years, rising to 208 events per 1,000 patient years at year 4.[152]

The survival rates following cardiac arrest reported by Herzog[152] were 32% at 30 days and 17% at 1 year after arrest, respectively, and dropped to 13% at year 1 in patients with diabetes. On the other hand, 60% of patients with ESRD who experienced cardiac arrest in the dialysis unit died within 48 hours of cardiac arrest; 13% of these deaths occurred while in dialysis units.[149]

Mechanisms of sudden death. Clearly, the adverse cardiomyopathic and vasculopathic milieu predisposes individuals with CKD to arrhythmias and conduction abnormalities, which are manifestations of cardiac disease associated with sudden cardiac death. This predisposition is likely exacerbated by electrolyte shifts, increased ultrafiltration volumes, divalent ion abnormalities, diabetes, and sympathetic overactivity, in addition to inflammation and possibly iron deposition (Fig. 79.6). Impaired baroreflex effectiveness and sensitivity, as well as obstructive sleep apnea, might also

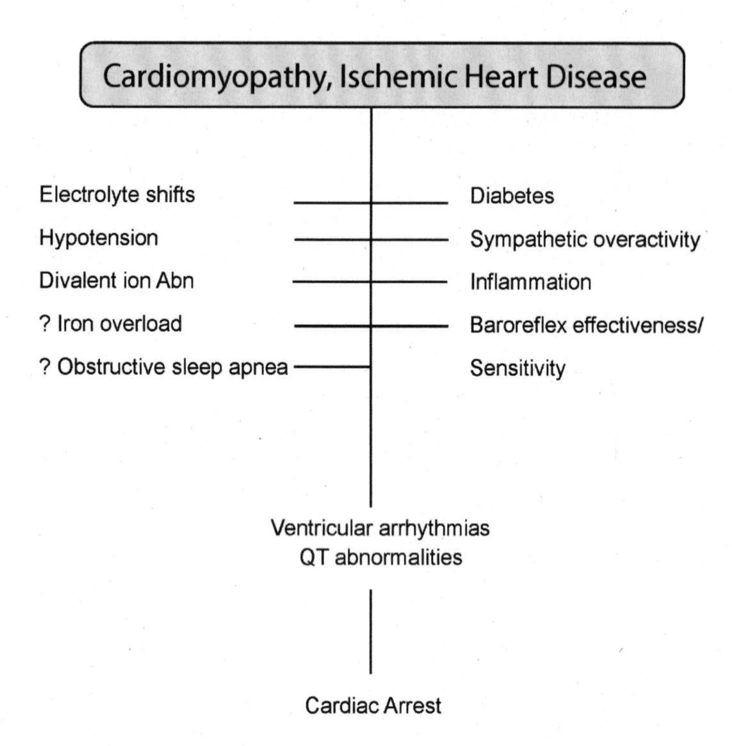

FIGURE 79.6 The mechanisms of sudden cardiac death in chronic kidney disease.

contribute to the risk of sudden death. Each of these risk factors is discussed in greater detail in the following.

Prolonged corrected QT (QTc) intervals in patients with CKD and ESRD usually result from inhomogeneity of both myocardial depolarization and repolarization that occurs secondary to LVH and intercardiomyocytic fibrosis. Measures of the temporal variability in myocardial repolarization include QT dispersion and QT variability index. The former is defined as the difference between the maximal and minimal QT intervals on a standard ECG (QTmax – QTmin) and is associated with an increased risk of ventricular arrhythmias and mortality in patients with congestive heart failure and in the general population.[153] The latter is calculated as the logarithm of the ratio between the variances of the normalized QT and RR intervals. It can predict the subsequent risk of sudden cardiac death or ventricular arrhythmia in patients who present for electrophysiologic investigation.[154]

Left ventricular hypertrophy. LVH could predispose individuals to sudden death through the prolongation of the QTc interval or by increasing arrhythmogenesis. The QTc interval is substantially longer in hemodialysis patients than in those who have near normal kidney function, and is associated with several manifestations of uremic cardiomyopathy, including increased LV mass index and end-diastolic volume, and a reduced LV ejection fraction.[155] In addition, more premature ventricular complexes (PVCs) occur during hemodialysis in patients with LVH compared with those without LVH.[138]

Ischemic heart disease. In the general population, coronary heart disease is an important cause of sudden death. In patients undergoing hemodialysis, CAD probably causes arrhythmogenesis because severe coronary stenosis is associated with the induction and lengthy persistence of ventricular arrhythmias during and after hemodialysis.[156] Furthermore, the number of PVCs during and after hemodialysis is higher in patients with ischemic heart disease than in those without it.[138,156]

Novel markers of coronary ischemia can identify patients who are at a high risk of cardiac death. Ischemia modified albumin (IMA) is a novel biomarker of acute ischemia that has high sensitivity and moderate specificity.[157,158] In 114 patients with ESRD, an IMA level of 95 KU per liter predicted all-cause mortality with a sensitivity and specificity of 76% and 74%, respectively, whereas an elevated cardiac troponin level $\geq$ 0.06 μg per liter predicted mortality with a sensitivity of 75% and a specificity of 72%.[159] Cardiac mortality risk was increased sevenfold in patients with combined elevated IMA and cardiac troponin levels (odds ratio [OR] = 7.12; 95% CI, 4.14 to 10.12).

QT dispersion and variability. Elevated QT dispersion was evident in 20 hemodialysis patients and 20 patients treated with continuous ambulatory peritoneal dialysis, and was significantly higher than in healthy controls.[160] The difference in QT dispersion rates between patients undergoing hemodialysis and those on chronic ambulatory peritonial dialysis (CAPD) was not statistically significant. In a retrospective cohort study of 147 adult patients undergoing dialysis, a QTc interval dispersion that occurred for longer than 74 ms was an independent predictor of all-cause mortality (relative risk [RR], 1.5; 95% CI, 1.2 to 2.0), and of cardiovascular mortality (RR, 1.6; 95% CI, 1.2 to 2.4).[161]

The QT variability index was increased by 47% in 163 patients with advanced CKD (43 individuals with stage

4 CKD, 67 patients undergoing hemodialysis, and 43 patients on CAPD) during a 30-minute rest period compared with 39 age-matched healthy controls.[162] The variability index was similar in patients with stage 4 CKD and in those on dialysis, whereas it was higher in patients with diabetes compared with nondiabetic patients with renal failure. Furthermore, in a multiple linear regression analysis, a history of diabetes or CAD were the only independent predictors of the QT variability index in patients with advanced CKD. The elevated index in patients with advanced CKD was the result of both reduced RR interval variance (secondary to reduced autonomic control of heart rate) and increased QT interval variance.[162]

It should be noted that several drugs (such as typical and atypical antipsychotics, sotalol, and antiarrhythmic agents) could prolong cardiac repolarization (QT interval) and trigger torsades de pointes, and could increase the risk of sudden cardiac death in patients with CKD.[163]

Baroreflex effectiveness and sensitivity. Impaired arterial baroreflex function is associated with an increased risk of ventricular arrhythmia and sudden cardiac death.[164] In healthy individuals, an appropriate baroreflex response is usually obtained in 25% of all systolic BP ramps during the day and in 15% of ramps during the night.[165] The ability of the arterial baroreflex to preserve short-term BP homeostasis—defined as arterial baroreflex sensitivity—has been identified as a prognostic marker of cardiovascular mortality in patients with MI.[166] The baroreflex effectiveness index is defined as the ratio between the number of systolic BP ramps, followed by baroreflex-mediated changes in heart rate, and the total number of systolic BP ramps during the recording period.[167]

In 216 patients with hypertension and stage 4 or 5 CKD, the baroreflex sensitivity was reduced by 51% and the baroreflex effectiveness index was reduced by 49% compared with age-matched healthy controls ($n = 43$).[164] Although the treatment modality for renal failure had no effect on baroreflex sensitivity or effectiveness, patients with CKD and diabetes had a greater reduction in both baroreflex sensitivity and effectiveness than patients with CKD who did not have diabetes. During the 41-month follow-up period, 69 patients with hypertension died.[167] Sudden cardiac death occurred in 15 of these patients (22% of all deaths). The reduced baroreflex effectiveness index was an independent predictor of all-cause mortality, whereas reduced baroreflex sensitivity was an independent predictor of sudden cardiac death.[167]

Inflammation. Inflammation has been associated with sudden cardiac death independently of traditional cardiovascular risk factors.[168] After adjusting for demographic characteristics, comorbidities, and laboratory factors, the highest tertiles of the inflammatory markers C-reactive protein (CRP) and interleukin 6 (IL-6) were associated with a doubled risk of sudden cardiac death compared with the lowest tertiles, whereas a decrease in serum albumin level was associated with a 1.35-fold increased risk of sudden cardiac death in the highest tertile compared with the lowest tertile.[169] Inflammation could trigger sudden cardiac death through premature atherosclerosis and cytokine-induced plaque instability or by a direct effect on the myocardium and the electrical conduction system.

Impact of the hemodialysis prescription. A rapid change in the extracellular concentration of electrolytes during a dialysis session leads to a secondary shift of electrolytes between the intracellular and extracellular milieu, which depends on the electrochemical gradient. As a result, cellular membrane polarization and stability may be affected. Data from patients treated at Fresenius Medical Care North America–affiliated centers showed that dialysis with a potassium dialysate concentration of zero or 1 mmol per liter was a significant risk factor for cardiac arrest.[149] This prescription had been used in 17.1% of patients who experienced a cardiac arrest compared with 8.8% of controls ($P < .0001$).[149] Cardiac arrests were more frequent during dialysis sessions carried out on a Monday as compared to Wednesday ($P = .001$) and Friday ($P = .004$). Although the mechanism for this observation was not studied, it may be due to increased fluctuations in potassium concentrations or perhaps increased ultrafiltration volumes.

Further evidence to support modifiable risk factors associated with the hemodialysis prescription causing sudden cardiac arrest has been reported recently. From the DaVita/Gambro Healthcare database of 43,200 outpatient dialysis patients, 502 patients who experienced a sudden cardiac arrest were compared to 1,632 age-and dialysis vintage–matched controls.[169] Independent factors associated with sudden cardiac arrest included low potassium dialysate < 2 mEq per liter, increased ultrafiltration volume, exposure to low calcium dialysate, and low serum creatinine levels. This study suggests that modification of the hemodialysis prescription may reduce the risk of sudden cardiac arrest, although the case-control research design is of low evidentiary power.

Evidence to support increased ultrafiltration volume as a CV risk factor was reported in a cohort of 1,846 patients. Rates over 13 mL/hr/kg, compared to ultrafiltration rates up to 10 mL/hr/kg, were significantly associated with all-cause and CV-related mortality (adjusted hazard ratio = 1.59 and 1.71, respectively).[170] In the subset of patients with congestive heart failure, ultrafiltration rates between 10 and 13 mL/hr/kg were also significantly associated with all-cause mortality.

In addition to low potassium dialysate, a decreasing potassium profile during hemodialysis may be harmful; complex arrhythmias were observed more frequently during and after hemodialysis in those with a decreasing potassium profile compared with individuals whose potassium levels were kept constant (2.5 mmol per liter).[171]

Abnormalities in calcium homeostasis may also be cardiotoxic. In 68 nondiabetic patients with ESRD who were undergoing hemodialysis with a normal maximal ECG stress test and no evidence of LVH on ECG, hemodialysis increased QTc intervals from 421 ± 26 ms before hemodialysis to 434 ± 29 ms after hemodialysis ($P = .005$).[172] Abnormally prolonged QTc intervals (> 440 ms) after hemodialysis were recorded 1.5 to 2.3 times more often than in the high-risk diabetic population. In addition, patients with greater increases in QTc intervals after hemodialysis had higher baseline plasma calcium levels ($r = 0.47$; $P < .001$), and lower calcium levels after hemodialysis ($r = 0.33$; $P < .05$). These data suggest that abnormalities in calcium hemostasis may induce the prolongation of QTc, and thus may predispose a patient to sudden death.

Drugs. In a large, retrospective study of 43,200 patients undergoing hemodialysis, 729 patients experienced a cardiac arrest.[173] β-Blockers were prescribed more frequently among those who survived than among those who died from a sudden cardiac arrest (53% versus 40%; OR, 0.59; 95% CI, 0.43 to 0.80). Among those who survived, β-blockers were associated with a significantly lower risk of death at 24 hours and 6 months after cardiac arrest. In addition, a positive correlation was observed between increasing β-blocker dose and survival. The use of angiotensin-converting enzyme (ACE) inhibitors and angiotensin-receptor blockers (ARBs) was associated with a significantly reduced risk of sudden cardiac death after 6 months of treatment (adjusted OR, 0.51; 95% CI, 0.28 to 0.95; $P = .03$) in survivors of a cardiac arrest.[173] A positive correlation was observed between the dose of ACE inhibitor and/or ARB and survival. Selection bias in the treatment group could, however, potentiate the positive effect of β-blockers on survival, because patients with very poor cardiac function, low BP, and/or intradialytic hypotension might not be prescribed these drugs.

All Cause Mortality

Incident cardiac events. The severity of CKD portends a worse prognosis if a cardiac event occurs. A study of 3,106 patients with MI reported an in-hospital mortality of 2% for patients with normal renal function, 6% for mild CKD, 14% for moderate CKD, 21% for severe CKD, and 30% for patients dependent on dialysis.[174] A meta-analysis of trials of thrombosis for MI indicated an inverse correlation between GFR and mortality at 1 month.[175]

In a large prospective register of nearly 50,000 cases of ST-segment elevation MI and non–ST-segment elevation infarction, the prevalence of CKD was high: 30% in the former group and over 40% in the latter.[176] Cases with CKD had a greater prevalence of diabetes, hypertension, and prior CVD than those without CKD. Even in patients with early stage 3 CKD, the risk of short-term mortality after acute coronary syndrome was twofold higher than in those without CKD. Patients with CKD were less likely to undergo invasive therapies, and had lower rates of β-blocker and statin use.

CKD is an important predictor of mortality risk in patients with CHF.[177,178] In a secondary analysis of the Digoxin Intervention Group trial, Shlipak et al.[179] found that patients with stable CHF and an ejection fraction less than 45% had a higher risk of death with a GFR ≤ 50 mL per minute (HR, 2.6; 95% CI, 1.69 to 2.51). Patients with a GFR of 50 to 60 mL per minute had no increase in mortality relative to the patients with better renal function.

Baseline cardiomyopathy. The presence of concentric LVH, LV dilation with normal contractility, and systolic dysfunction at the time of ESRD therapy initiation has been associated with progressively worse survival, independent of age, sex, diabetes, and IHD.[126] In a study of CKD stage 3/4 patients CV event-free survival was significantly worse in the presence of concentric and eccentric LVH compared with the absence of LVH.[123]

Excessive hypertrophy in concentric LVH (high LV mass to volume ratio) and inadequate hypertrophy in LV dilation (low LV mass to volume ratio) were independently associated with late mortality in a Canadian dialysis cohort.[18] However, in 596 incident hemodialysis patients, an adjusted association between baseline LV mass index and subsequent CV events or death was eliminated by adjusting for age, diabetes, systolic BP, and N-terminal pro-B type natriuretic peptide.[19]

Among renal transplant recipients, LVH at the time of transplantation was an independent risk factor for death (RR, 1.9; 95% CI, 1.22 to 3.22) and CHF (RR, 2.27; 95% CI, 1.08 to 4.81) in the subsequent 5 years.[180]

In a Japanese study of 1,254 consecutive incident hemodialysis patients, 8.5% had an LV ejection fraction of 40% to 50%, 3.3% had an ejection fraction of 30% to 40%, and 1.4% had an ejection fraction < 30%. Seven year event-free survival for the respective groups was 57%, 46%, and 23%, respectively, as compared to about 67% in the group with an ejection fraction above 50%. After adjusting for other risk factors, a decreasing ejection fraction was a strong independent predictor for CV death.[181]

Sixty-four percent of 70 prevalent HD patients had significant myocardial stunning during hemodialysis.[182] A significantly increased hazard of death occurred in those with myocardial stunning and elevated cardiac troponin T than in those with elevated levels alone. The LV ejection fraction at rest fell from 62% at baseline to 55% after 12 months in those with regional wall motion abnormalities compared to a fall from 60% to 56% in those without regional wall motion abnormalities.

Baseline calcification. In a prospective study of 117 nondialyzed Brazilian patients with CKD, the presence of coronary artery calcification was significantly associated with the subsequent occurrence of CV events independent of age and diabetes.[183]

Recently, 1,084 prevalent dialysis patients had scoring of abdominal aortic calcification using plain lateral abdominal X-rays and measurements of carotid femoral PWVs, and were followed for 2 years.[184] Compared with the lowest tertile of aortic calcification, the risk of a CV event was increased by a factor of 3.7 in patients with a score in the middle tertile, and by a factor of 8.6 in the highest tertile. The risk associated with an increased PWV was less pronounced at higher levels of calcification. After accounting for age, diabetes, and serum albumin, both aortic calcification and PWV were independent predictors of outcome.

Among 140 patients with ESRD who underwent ECG and coronary angiography, 56 (40%) had mitral annular calcifications, which was associated with a significant increase in all-cause mortality (P = .04).[92] Mitral annular calcification was also independently associated with substantial CAD, defined as luminal stenosis > 70% by visual estimation in at least one coronary artery (OR, 12; 95% CI, 3.3 to 26.1).

Baseline symptomatic cardiac disease. In a Canadian prospective cohort study, patients with clinical IHD at the start of dialysis were more likely to have an admission for CHF (RR, 1.7) or to die (RR, 1.5) than patients free of IHD at baseline, after adjusting for age and diabetes.[132] In these patients, most of the excess mortality associated with IHD seemed to be through the development of CHF. In diabetic renal transplants, the presence of IHD was associated with a fourfold risk of future events and death.[185]

For dialysis patients, CHF has a poor prognosis; the median survival of patients who had heart failure at or before the initiation of ESRD therapy was 36 months, compared with 62 months in subjects without baseline CHF.[15] This adverse prognosis was independent of age, diabetes, and IHD. Among patients who had heart failure at baseline, recurrent heart failure developed in 56% and the remaining 44% were failure free during follow-up. Median survival in those with recurrent CHF was 29 months, which was significantly less than in those without recurrence (45 months). For RTRs, the development of new onset CHF carries a prognosis similar to that for new IHD (RR for death, 1.78; 95% CI, 1.21 to 2.61 for CHF versus RR for death, 1.50; 95% CI, 1.05 to 2.13 for IHD).[13]

Risk Factors

Although experimental studies in animal models and cross-sectional or case-control studies in small groups of patients can lend insights into the mechanisms of disease in renal failure, only large, rigorous, prospective studies in relevant clinical populations (free of cardiac disease at baseline), can identify widely generalizable risk factors for CVD. The Framingham Study is the archetypal population-based cohort study in the field of CVD, and the risk factors identified by it have been widely vindicated in subsequent intervention trials on BP control and cholesterol reduction. Unfortunately, few large, adequately designed prospective cohort studies on CV outcomes have been performed in renal failure populations. We await with interest the results of the large Chronic Renal Insufficiency Cohort (CRIC) study ongoing in the United States, which should be powered enough to identify the most important independent risk factors for CV events.[186]

Table 79.2 outlines independent predictors of cardiac events identified by studies such as ARIC in CKD,[8,131,187] the Canadian cohort of incident dialysis patients all of whom had echocardiography at baseline,[15,125–128,132,188–191] the U.S. incident cohort of dialysis patients enrolled in CHOICE,[192–194] the 4D study of prevalent diabetic hemodialysis patients,[195–201] the Canadian incident renal transplant cohort,[13,180] and others. Whether these predictors of CV risk can be modified by risk factor intervention is also summarized in Table 79.2.

Nonmodifiable Risk Factors

Age. Older age has been independently associated with the occurrence of coronary events[131] and with the development or worsening of CVD in the CKD population.[202,203] Among dialysis patients, older age is predictive of the de novo occurrence of angina pectoris, MI, or coronary revascularization[132] and of de novo heart failure.[15] Among renal transplant recipients, age is an independent risk factor for MI or coronary revascularization or death from MI[130] and the development of de novo heart failure.[13]

Gender. Gender is an inconsistent predictor of CV events in CKD, although male gender was associated with coronary events in CKD,[131] and female gender with ischemic heart disease events in renal transplant recipients.[13]

Diabetes mellitus. Almost half the cases of ESRD are caused by diabetes mellitus, particularly type 2.[151] Diabetes confers a substantially increased risk of coronary events in CKD patients (Table 79.1).[131] On starting dialysis, diabetics had more concentric LVH, IHD, and cardiac failure than nondiabetic patients.[191] Among patients on dialysis, diabetes is independently associated with the development of de novo IHD but not with de novo heart failure (Table 79.3A).[191] In renal transplant recipients, diabetes was associated with de novo ischemic heart disease and heart failure events (Table 79.3B).[13] In another study of renal transplant recipients, diabetes was strongly associated with multiple atherosclerotic outcomes (RR of 2.09 for MI, revascularization, or death from MI; RR of 2.98 for ischemic stroke; and RR of 25.7 for development of peripheral vascular disease).[130]

The impact of diabetes in all renal populations may well be underestimated. Angiographic studies in asymptomatic diabetic patients on dialysis show that approximately one-third have at least one coronary artery stenosis of 50% or greater.[93] Among asymptomatic diabetic patients referred for renal transplantation, 88% of those older than 45 years had significant coronary stenosis.[185]

There is evidence for a specific diabetic cardiomyopathy in diabetic patients without ESRD.[204,205] Furthermore, LVH, along with cardiac fibrosis, is a more frequent finding in hypertensive diabetic patients than in hypertensive nondiabetic patients.[84]

Modifiable Traditional Risk Factors

Hypertension

Predictor of CV events. The primary cause of ESRD in the United States is hypertension (27% of cases).[151] Furthermore, CKD, whatever its cause, is usually associated with hypertension. In the Modification of Diet in Renal Disease (MDRD) Study, although 91% of CKD patients were treated

TABLE 79.2 **Traditional and Nontraditional Modifiable High-risk Factors for Cardiovascular Disease in Chronic Kidney Disease: Evidence from Cohort Studies and Randomized Controlled Trials**

	Cohort		RCT	
	CKD	Dialysis	CKD	Dialysis
Traditional				
Hypertension	+	+	+	?
Smoking	+	+	NA	NA
Hyperlipidemia	+	+	+	−/+
Hyperglycemia	+	+	ND	ND
Obesity	+	+	ND	ND
Nontraditional				
Moderate anemia	+	+	−	−
Hypoalbuminemia	+	+	ND	ND
Inflammation	+	+	ND	ND
Hyperfibrinogenemia	+	+	+	+
Troponin	?	+	ND	ND
Oxidant stress	ND	ND	−	+
Hyperhomocysteinemia	+	+	−	IP
Hyperphosphatemia	+	+	ND	ND
Hyperparathyroidism	ND	+	ND	IP
Degree of renal impairment	+	NA	+	NA
Mode of dialysis	NA	+	NA	+
Salt + H_2O overload	+	+	ND	?
A-V fistula/graft	NA	−	NA	+

CKD, chronic kidney disease; RCT, randomized controlled trial; +, positive; –, negative; ND, not done; NA, not applicable; IP, in progress; A-V, arterio-venous.

with antihypertensive agents, only 54% had BPs of 140/90 mm Hg or less.[206] Hypertension is present in 86% of U.S. dialysis patients, yet it is adequately controlled in only 30% of cases.[207] In the ARIC Study, hypertension substantially increased the risk of coronary heart disease (Table 79.1).[131] Hypertension has been shown to promote LV growth in a large cohort of patients with CKD[124] and its control may prevent or regress LVH.[208,209]

In patients on dialysis, each 10 mm Hg increment in BP is associated with a 48% higher risk for the development of LVH.[188] Furthermore, higher systolic BP over time was an independent predictor for progressive LVH.[19] Hypertension is an independent predictor of de novo heart failure and of de novo IHD events in incident dialysis patients (Table 79.3A).[188]

After transplantation, hypertension was associated with the progression to LVH in patients with normal hearts

TABLE 79.3 **Predictors of De Novo Cardiovascular Events in Incident Dialysis Patients[15,132] and in Incident Transplant Recipients[13]**

A. Dialysis Patients	**Heart Failure**		**MI/Angina**	
(n = 432)	HR	P	HR	P
Diabetes		NS	3.2	0.0002
Hypertension per 10 mm Hg rise in SBP	1.44	0.007	1.39	0.05
Anemia per 1 g/dL decrease	1.28	0.02		NS
Hypoalbuminemia per 10 g/L fall	1.30	0.007	1.49	< 0.001
B. Transplant Recipients[a]	**Heart Failure**		**MI/Angina**	
(n = 638)	HR	95% CI	HR	95% CI
Diabetes	2.30	1.4–3.7	2.4	1.5–3.9
Hypertension per 10 mm Hg rise in SBP	1.29	1.1–1.5	1.41	1.0–1.9
Anemia per 10 g/L decrease	1.24	1.1–4.1		NS
Hypoalbuminemia per 10 g/L fall	2.10	1.1–4.1		NS

[a]Alive and free of clinical heart disease at 1 year.
HR, hazard ratio; MI, myocardial infarction; CI, confidence interval; SBP, systolic blood pressure; NS, not stated.

at transplantation.[210] A prospective cohort study demonstrated that diastolic BP was an independent risk factor for increasing LV mass between the first and fifth years after transplantation, but systolic BP was the only predictor of de novo LVH at 5 years.[180] Hypertension was also an independent risk factor for cardiac events in renal transplant recipients (Table 79.3B).[13]

Despite these strong data substantiating hypertension as a predictor of CV events in CKD, there is a U-shaped curve association of BP and mortality in hemodialysis patients,[211,212] with lower BP predicting higher mortality. However, the high prevalence of cardiac disease at the start of ESRD therapy is a confounding issue even for well-executed, prospective cohort studies. Because cardiac dysfunction can cause low BP and is independently associated with death, even prospective studies cannot exclude the possibility that low BP is simply a surrogate marker for poor pump function, unless patients with cardiac abnormalities at baseline are excluded from analysis. This is difficult to do in practice because most patients (75% to 80%) have ECG abnormalities at the start of maintenance dialysis.[125] In one prospective cohort study[188] of 433 patients on dialysis, high BP was positively associated with the development of de novo heart failure, which in turn was associated with both a drop in mean arterial pressure and subsequent death. These observations suggest, but do not prove, the following causal sequence:

Hypertension → IHD and LVH → Pump failure → hypotension and death

This chain of events is supported by the changing relationship of BP with mortality over time in 16,959 incident dialysis patients.[213] For those with systolic BP < 120 mm Hg, increased mortality was observed in the first 2 years after the initiation of dialysis, whereas in those with systolic BP ≥ 150 mm Hg, increased mortality was observed after year 2. Using time-varying analyses, mild-to-moderate hypertension was relatively well tolerated. Furthermore, in an incident cohort of hemodialysis patients without symptomatic cardiac disease at baseline, hypertension was an independent predictor of CV events during 2 years of follow-up.[19]

Treatment in CKD patients. Control of BP in predialysis CKD is probably best undertaken by the normalization of blood volume and the use of inhibitors/blockers of the renin-angiotensin system. The use of ACE inhibitors or ARBs are considered the agents of first choice in most patients due to their documented benefit in delaying the progression of CKD in both diabetic and nondiabetic disease, particularly with associated proteinuria.[214] Ramipril has improved CVD outcomes in patients with decreased GFR and at least one CVD risk factor, in addition to either diabetes or manifest vascular disease.[2] The ARB, losartan, has reduced hospitalization for heart failure in diabetics with overt nephropathy.[215] In 1,715 adults with diabetic nephropathy, irbesartan (another ARB) significantly reduced the incidence of CHF compared to placebo (HR = 0.72; 95% CI, 0.52 to 1.0).[216] It appears that the beneficial impact of blockade of the renin-angiotensin system is more than can be accounted for by lowering of BP.

An analysis of the achieved BP in the Irbesartan Diabetic Nephropathy Trial (N = 17.5) demonstrated that the progressive lowering of systolic BP to 120 mm Hg was associated with renal protection and decrement in mortality and CV events.[217] However, with systolic BP < 120 mm Hg, renal protection was observed but there was an increase in all-cause mortality, CV mortality, and CHF in patients who have a more severe underlying cardiac disease. Assignment to irbesartan lowered the risk for heart failure by 29%, lowering the systolic BP by 20 mm Hg did so by 25%, and the combination of both lowered the risk by 53%.

Management of hypertension should generally aim for levels less than 130/80 mm Hg for CKD, particularly in those with ≥ 1 g per day of proteinuria.[218] In some patients, particularly diabetics with moderate-to-advanced renal dysfunction, BP can be highly resistant to intervention, requiring extensive combination treatment. However, this Kidney Disease Outcomes Quality Initiative (KDOQI) target BP was driven by observational data or secondary analyses from RCTs.[218] Results of RCTs establishing the benefits or harm in meeting a goal BP < 130/80 mm Hg in CKD patients are necessary because no primary analysis of any RCT supports lower BP goals.[219] In the interim, individualization of therapy is recommended.

In renal transplant recipients, calcium channel blockers (CCBs) are widely used because they are well tolerated and because of their effects in counteracting calcineurin-mediated vasoconstriction. The use of ACE inhibitors or ARBs is probably justified in most patients, particularly because the regression of LVH has been reported in renal transplant recipients with ARBs. However, issues relating to hyperkalemia, anemia, and a reduction in eGFR warrant consideration, particularly in the first 12 months posttransplantation.

Treatment in dialysis patients. The mainstay of therapy in dialysis patients is the maintenance of normal extracellular fluid volume, as suggested by the results of a dialysis regimen of long, slow ultrafiltration, which was associated with normotension, regression of LV hypertrophy, and improved survival.[220] In a RCT of hypertensive patients on hemodialysis, 100 patients were assigned to receive ultrafiltration, prescribed as an additional weight loss of 0.1 kg per 10 kg of body weight per dialysis above that which is required to remove interdialytic fluid gain. There were 50 patients assigned to the control group.[221] At 4 weeks, a mean reduction in postdialysis weight of 0.9 kg was achieved, which resulted in significant improvements in BP (7 mm Hg in systolic and 3 mm Hg in diastolic). This demonstrates that extracellular volume expansion, even in the absence of clinical signs of volume overload, mediates, at least in part, hypertension in hemodialysis patients.

RCTs of the CV effects of ACE inhibitors or ARBs in hemodialysis are few in number, consist of few patients, and are of variable quality.

London and colleagues[222] compared the effects of an ACE inhibitor (perindopril) with a CCB (nitrendipine) in a double-blinded, randomized trial involving 24 hemodialysis patients with LVH over a period of 12 months. At baseline, each group displayed LVH due predominantly to an increased LV end-diastolic diameter. Similar and significant changes were found in BP, total peripheral resistance, aortic and arterial PWVs, and arterial wave reflections. After treatment, there was a significant decrease in LV mass in the perindopril-treated group only. It was also found that LV mass reductions were related not to changes in LV wall thickness but rather to a reduction in LV end-diastolic diameter.

The FOSIDIAL study,[223] a placebo-controlled randomized trial of prevalent hemodialysis patients with established LVH, did not show a substantial adjusted effect of the ACE inhibitor fosinopril on the primary end point (the combined fatal and nonfatal first cardiovascular events) in the intention to treat analysis (RR, 0.93; 95% CI, 0.68 to 1.26) or in the per protocol analysis (adjusted RR, 0.79; 95% CI, 0.59 to 1.10). However, this study was underpowered for the primary event rate. Furthermore, patients assigned to the treatment group had a higher baseline risk (such as LVH, CAD, diabetes, and duration on hemodialysis) than the control group.

In a small randomized controlled trial of 80 patients undergoing hemodialysis, who had no clinical evidence of cardiac disease, use of the angiotensin II type I–receptor blocker, candesartan, was associated with a reduced incidence of CV events and mortality compared with placebo: 46.3% versus 53.8%.[224]

A meta-analysis (5 RCTs) of ACE inhibitor and ARB use resulted in a statistically significant reduction in LV mass, with a weighted mean difference compared to controls of 15.4 g per square meter (95% CI, 7.4 to 23.3).[225] In 3 RCTs, the relative risk of CV events associated with ACE inhibitor or ARB use was 0.66, but the 95% CIs were 0.35 to 1.25.

A cohort of patients was examined for the effects of BP changes on 150 dialysis patients over a mean of 51 months.[49] Independent predictors of CV mortality included no reduction in PWV in response to a BP decrease (RR, 2.59; 95% CI, 1.51 to 4.43), an increased LV mass (RR, 1.11 per 10 g increase in LV mass index, 95% CI, 1.03 to 1.19), age (RR, 1.69; 95% CI, 1.32 to 2.17), preexisting CVD, and lack of ACE inhibitor treatment (RR, 0.19; 95% CI, 0.14 to 0.43). These findings were consistent with earlier descriptive studies, but for the first time suggested that there might be a survival advantage in reducing PWV. Importantly, ACE inhibitors appeared also to have a favorable effect on survival in this patient group, which was independent of BP change.

A reasonable target BP for antihypertensive treatment is a predialysis BP < 140/90 mm Hg, unless the patient develops symptomatic hypotension or low BP during or after dialysis. Patients with a BP > 140/90 mm Hg after achievement of their base day weight should have antihypertensive drugs prescribed.

The selection of antihypertensive agents is best guided by the presence of associated comorbidities. There are not, however, large randomized trials to support one agent over another. Hence, patients with reduced LV systolic function are likely to benefit from ACE inhibitors or ARBs, and patients with relatively intact LV function postmyocardial infarction should be treated with a β-receptor antagonist. Practical difficulties in this patient group in particular include associated cerebrovascular or coronary disease, advanced age, and CV instability in relation to ultrafiltration. In such situations, BP will require individual targeting and some compromise on the optimal target will be necessary.

Smoking

Predictor of cardiovascular events. Although 25% of patients with CKD were current or former smokers as of 2001,[226] the prevalence of current smokers is probably decreasing. In a recent RCT[227] only 5% were current smokers, although 40% were previous smokers.

The Cardiovascular Health Study[228] investigated 5,808 people who had CKD and were ≥ 65 years, and observed 20 extra deaths per 1,000 patient years in current smokers. In the ARIC population-based study of CKD patients,[131] the relative risk for coronary disease was 1.91 in current smokers (Table 79.1). Smoking has been independently associated with subsequent de novo heart failure, peripheral vascular disease, and death at the start of dialysis.[14] Among renal transplant recipients, a smoking exposure has been independently associated with ischemic stroke, peripheral vascular disease, and death.[229]

Intervention. RCTs are not necessary to demonstrate that cessation of smoking is beneficial. However, in renal transplant patients, most continued to smoke after transplantation despite admonitions to quit.[230]

Obesity. Obesity is an independent predictor of coronary events in CKD (Table 79.1),[131] but there is no evidence to suggest it is an independent risk factor in patients on any type of dialysis.

Hyperlipidemia

Predictor of cardiovascular events. An atherogenic lipid profile is highly prevalent in patients with renal disease, particularly in patients with nephrotic syndrome.[231] In CKD, hypercholesterolemia and hyperapolipoproteinuria B are independent predictors of coronary disease (Table 79.1).[131] The prevalence of dyslipidemias in renal transplant recipients is high. Hypercholesterolemia has been linked to ischemic events in this population.[130,133]

In dialysis patients, the highest mortality risk appears to be associated with low, not high serum cholesterol.[232] This may be because low total cholesterol is strongly correlated with poor nutritional status, inflammation, and low albumin levels, which are themselves associated with increased mortality risk. In CHOICE,[193] a prospective study of patients starting dialysis, high serum cholesterol was associated with low all-cause mortality risk in the presence of inflammation, but with increased risk in individuals without inflammation (HR, 1.32 per 1.0 mmol per liter increment in total cholesterol; 95% CI, 1.07 to 1.63). This supports the hypothesis that the inverse association of total cholesterol level with mortality in dialysis patients is likely due to the cholesterol-lowering effect of systemic inflammation and malnutrition, not to a protective effect of high cholesterol concentrations.

In stage 3 and 4 CKD, the presence of malnutrition/inflammation also modified the relationship of serum cholesterol with CVD. African Americans with hypertensive CKD were stratified using body mass index (BMI) < 23 kg per square meter or C-reactive protein > 10 mg per deciliter. In the group without evidence of malnutrition/inflammation, the adjusted cholesterol HR increased progressively across cholesterol level, but in those with malnutrition/inflammation, the HRs did not vary significantly by cholesterol level.[233]

Although lipoprotein (a) is elevated in patients on dialysis and is independently associated with IHD and death,[234] its clinical utility as a test is limited.

Intervention. The data on the efficacy of statin (HMG coenzyme A [CoA] inhibitor) therapy in CKD arises from RCTs in patients with or at high risk of coronary disease, and CKD patients are clearly at the highest risk of atherosclerotic events. Tonelli et al.[235] performed a secondary analysis of a subset of patients with a GFR of 30 to 60 mL per minute from three randomized trials of pravastatin versus placebo. Among the 4,491 subjects identified, pravastatin significantly reduced the incidence of MI, coronary death, or coronary revascularization (HR, 0.77; 95% CI, 0.68 to 0.86), which is similar to the effect of pravastatin on the primary outcome in subjects with normal function (HR, 0.78; 95% CI, 0.65 to 0.94).[235] A pooled analysis of 30 completed RCTs investigating the effect of fluvastatin in patients with creatinine clearance < 50 mL per minute demonstrated a 41% reduction in combined cardiac death and MI compared to placebo.[236]

These results were not replicated in three RCTs in ESRD populations. An RCT in renal transplant recipients of fluvastatin (40 to 80 mg per day) in 2,102 RTRs failed to find a benefit with respect to primary composite cardiac end points (MI, cardiac death, and cardiac intervention). Post hoc analysis using alternative outcomes suggested that fluvastatin reduced the incidence of cardiac death or definite MI from 104 to 70 events (RR, 0.65; 95% CI, 0.48 to 0.88).[237] The 4D Study, a randomized trial of atorvastatin versus placebo in type 2 diabetics who had been on hemodialysis for no more than 2 years, demonstrated no reduction in the rate of CV mortality and of nonfatal MI compared to placebo.[195] The AURORA study,[238] an RCT of rosuvastatin in hemodialysis patients who had low-density lipoprotein (LDL) cholesterol of 2.6 mmol per liter at baseline, revealed no difference in primary event rate (cardiovascular death, nonfatal MI, or stroke) in the rosuvastatin-treated group compared to placebo. This trial was probably underpowered to answer the research question, patients already on statins were excluded (which probably amounted to 40% of the hemodialysis population), and discontinuation of the assigned treatment occurred in about half of the enrolled patients, all of which limit the conclusions that can be made.

The disappointing results of 4D and AURORA have been recently countered by the results from the Study of Heart and Renal Protection (SHARP)[239] where 9,438 CKD patients (3,191 on dialysis and 6,247 not on dialysis) with no history of MI or coronary revascularization were randomly allocated to lipid lowering agents ezetimibe/simvastatin or placebo. During median follow-up of 4.9 years, major atherosclerotic events occurred significantly less frequently in the ezetimibe/simvastatin group compared to placebo (RR, 0.83; 95% CI, 0.74 to 0.94), with similar reductions observed in both dialysis and nondialysis patients.

Because of the benefit of statins that were demonstrated in predialysis CKD and in SHARP, together with the clear benefit observed in the general population, it seems reasonable to treat CKD patients in a similar manner, provided their life expectancy is such as to benefit from these drugs. The KDOQI guidelines for managing dyslipidemia in CKD recommend that patients with CKD should be considered in the highest risk group for CV events.[240] Thus LDL cholesterol levels of 100 mg per deciliter (2.56 mmol per liter) or more and 130 mg per deciliter (3.33 mmol per liter) or more are treatment thresholds for diet and drug therapy, respectively. Drug therapy is recommended if LDL cholesterol levels remain in the range of 100 to 129 mg per deciliter despite 3 months of lifestyle changes. The target LDL level is 100 mg per deciliter (2.56 mmol per liter) or less. A cholesterol-lowering diet should be part of the treatment program, but most patients require pharmacologic therapy. For patients with high LDL levels, statins are recommended as first-line therapy. These agents are safe and effective in uremic patients, but screening for myositis should be undertaken. Fibrates are also effective in CKD patients, but dose reduction appropriate to the level of renal failure is important. The combination of a statin and a fibrate is associated with a high risk of muscle toxicity and in general should be avoided. The KDOQI guidelines suggest that fibrates may be used either for patients with triglyceride levels greater than 500 mg per deciliter or statin-intolerant patients who have triglycerides greater than 200 mg per deciliter with non-high-density lipoprotein (HDL) cholesterol > 130 mg per deciliter. Similar guidelines have been published for the renal transplant population.[241]

Hyperglycemia

In addition to the presence of diabetes mellitus, hyperglycemia is an independent risk factor for the development of CAD in CKD (Table 79.1).[131] In the 4D study of prevalent diabetic hemodialysis patients, poor glycemic control was strongly associated with sudden cardiac death, which accounted for increased CV events and mortality.[196] In contrast, the rate of MI was not affected. However, in another study, higher glucose and HbA1C levels were not associated with mortality in 1,484 incident hemodialysis patients with and without diabetes.[242] Whether interventions to achieve tighter glycemic control will improve cardiac outcomes in CKD is unknown.

Uremia-Related Risk Factors

Anemia

Predictor of cardiovascular events. Anemia is a predictor of CAD in CKD (Table 79.1),[131] of the development of de novo cardiac failure in dialysis (Table 79.3A),[15] and of de novo heart failure in renal transplant recipients (Table 79.3B).[13] As hemoglobin levels fell below normal, there was a linear increase in the incidence of de novo heart failure,[13] suggesting that moderate anemia was a potential risk factor for heart failure.

Intervention. Partial correction of severe anemia with erythropoietin-stimulating agents was associated with regression of hypertrophy in cohort studies (i.e., without a control group),[243] but in an RCT of full correction of anemia, compared to partial correction, changes in LV mass index and LV volume index were similar in both groups.[244] In addition, CV event rates were similar in diabetic CKD patients with moderate anemia treated with darbepoetin alpha compared to placebo.[227] This suggests that moderate anemia is not a cause of cardiac disease in CKD but a marker for some other unidentified cardiomyopathic factors associated with CKD.

The partial correction of severe anemia with erythropoietin-stimulating agents in dialysis patients has had a substantial impact on blood transfusion rates and has improved patients' quality of life,[245] although the safety of this intervention is unknown. Normalization of hemoglobin with erythropoiesis-stimulating agents was associated with harm, such as strokes,[227,244] vascular access clotting,[246] and hypertension.[247] It seems reasonable to prevent hemoglobin levels from falling below 9 g per deciliter using erythropoietin-stimulating agents to prevent transfusions and to maintain it in the 10 to 11.5 g per deciliter range to improve quality of life.

Hypoalbuminemia. Several studies have shown that hypoalbuminemia is a powerful predictor of poor outcome in the different groups of patients with CKD. It has been associated with CAD events in CKD (Table 79.1),[131] with de novo heart failure and ischemic heart disease events in dialysis patients (Table 79.3A),[189] and with de novo heart failure in renal transplant recipients (Table 79.3B).[13] The mechanisms underlying this association are unknown. Hypoalbuminemia may be a marker of a chronic inflammatory state, a hypercoagulable state, malnutrition, inadequate dialysis, or vitamin deficiency, all of which hypothetically could accelerate myocyte death and the development of cardiomyopathy, as discussed previously.

Inflammation

Predictor of cardiovascular events. Markers of inflammation have been associated with CV events in dialysis patients. CRP is an acute phase reactant, which is elevated in inflammation and is a predictor of CV death and of sudden cardiac death in incident dialysis patients.[248] In the 4D study of prevalent diabetic hemodialysis patients, CRP was strongly associated with CV events and mortality, and was a much better predictor of these events than LDL cholesterol.[198]

Endotoxemia may be a cause of inflammation because CKD patients are exposed to endotoxemia from the gut, which is induced by systemic circulatory stress and recurrent regional ischemia. Endotoxemia is associated with systemic inflammation, malnutrition markers, cardiac injury, and reduced survival.[249] Soluble endotoxin receptor CD14 may result from subclinical endotoxemia, and was an independent predictor of mortality among prevalent patients on hemodialysis.[250]

Circulating plasma advanced glycation end products (AGE) accumulate in CKD. AGEs bind to their receptor for advanced glycation end products (RAGE) and induce an inflammatory response. Soluble RAGE (SRAGE) is shed from the cell-surface RAGE and binds circulating ligands, thus antagonizing downstream RAGE signaling. S100A12 is an extracellular newly identified RAGE binding protein (EN-RAGE), which is a ligand for RAGE. Circulating S100A12 and SRAGE are both elevated in hemodialysis patients. However, in prevalent patients, only S100A12 is associated with mortality, which is partly explained by its link with inflammation.[251]

Intervention. Statins may reduce inflammation in CKD. In the 4D study of 1,255 diabetic hemodialysis patients, CRP levels remained stable at 6 months on atorvastatin but increased in the placebo group.[197] Although CRP levels were highly predictive of outcome, atorvastatin treatment was not associated with reduced relative risks in the composite vascular end point or mortality. Aspirin may also reduce inflammation (see the following).

Hyperfibrinogenemia. Hyperfibrinogenemia is an independent predictor of CAD in CKD (Table 79.1).[131] Aspirin exerts its beneficial effect on the CV system by improving the procoagulant milieu that predisposes one to atherosclerotic events. In one large meta-analysis of non-CKD patients examining primary prevention of CAD, the absolute benefit of aspirin was a 0.15% reduction per year in MI compared with an increased risk of 0.04% per year for major noncerebral hemorrhage (noncerebral bleeds causing death, transfusion, or surgery) and 0.18% per year for minor hemorrhage.[252] Among hemodialysis patients ($n = 2{,}632$) in 14 RCTs, antiplatelet therapy resulted in a 41% reduction in CV events.[252]

Aspirin therapy probably worsens the platelet defects in CKD and increases the risk of bleeding. Despite these risks, patients with overt CVD should probably be prescribed low-dose aspirin to reduce the risk of subsequent CV events.[253] However, individual treatment decisions must be based on the considerations of patients' individual risks, likely benefits, and preferences.

Troponin levels. Troponin T and I are markers of myocardial injury. In ESRD patients not suspected of having acute coronary syndrome, elevated levels of troponin T (> 0.1 ng per milliliter) identified a subgroup who had poor survival and a high risk of cardiac death.[254] Troponin T may be a potential risk stratification tool, and the myocardial injury for which it is a marker may eventually be modifiable.

Oxidative Stress

Predictor of cardiovascular events. Oxidative stress occurs when there is an imbalance between the formation of reactive oxygen species (ROS) and antioxidant defense mechanisms. A number of enzymatic and nonenzymatic defense mechanisms have evolved to "detoxify" ROS. The predominant nonenzymatic agents include vitamin E, vitamin C, selenium, and zinc. Superoxide dismutase and glutathione peroxidase are the main antioxidant enzymes. Enhanced oxidative stress may be identified by an increase in the products of lipid peroxidation (e.g., malondialdehyde), a decrease in substances that enhance oxidative resistance (e.g., plasmalogen), or a decrease in reducing substances (e.g., glutathione). It is thought that oxidative stress is important in the formation of atheroma, but the ability of oxidative stress biomarkers to predict CVD has yet to be established.[255,256]

In CKD, markers of oxidative stress are increased. In fact, inflammation and oxidative stress are evident early in autosomal dominant polycystic kidney disease, even with normal renal function.[257] Dialysis may also further contribute to oxidative stress through the removal of antioxidants or through the stimulation of ROS by the use of incompatible dialysis components. However, the role of oxidative stress as a predictor of subsequent CV events has not been evaluated in large longitudinal studies.[258]

Two small RCTs in ESRD have reported good outcomes with antioxidants. In 196 hemodialysis patients, 800 U of vitamin E was compared to placebo in the secondary prevention of CVD, and a significantly lower incidence of ischemic events was reported.[259] In the other RCT, acetylcysteine (600 mg BID) was compared to placebo in 134 hemodialysis patients and also reported a significantly lower incidence of composite ischemic events.[260]

However, the Heart Outcomes Prevention Evaluation (HOPE) study[261] found no significant difference in the composite primary outcomes (MI, stroke, or CV death) using vitamin E in patients with moderate CKD (serum creatinine, 1.4 to 2.3 mg per deciliter). Furthermore, in HOPE – TOO,[262] where 3,994 enrolled patients continued to take study medication (ramipril, vitamin E, or placebo), there were no differences in CV events with vitamin E therapy on longer follow-up, but there were higher rates of heart failure. These dissonant results do not permit recommendations in favor of antioxidant therapy at present.

Homocysteine

Predictor of cardiovascular events. Homocysteine is a byproduct of methionine metabolism, a sulfhydryl-containing essential amino acid, and lies at the junction of two metabolic pathways, transsulfuration and remethylation. The rate of homocysteine elimination is facilitated by cofactors, particularly B_{12} and folate. Progressive renal failure is associated with increasing homocysteine levels: 83% of patients have levels above the 90th percentile for the general population by the time they reach ESRD,[263] and prospective studies suggest an association between homocysteine and combined CV end points in hemodialysis patients and renal transplant recipients.[264,265]

Intervention. High-dose folate supplementation (15 mg per day) can reduce but does not normalize homocysteine levels in ESRD.[266] An improvement in clinical outcomes for dialysis patients with high-dose folic acid relative to low-dose supplementation (i.e., 1 mg per day) was not observed.[267] In CKD patients and in renal transplant recipients, therapy with supraphysiologic doses of vitamins B_6, B_{12}, and folic acid may reduce homocysteine to normal levels.[266] However, a RCT of vitamin B therapy versus placebo in 283 patients with diabetic nephropathy demonstrated that, rather than lowering vascular events, the intervention was associated with an increase in these events and a greater decrease in GFR.[268]

In an RCT of 650 hemodialysis patients randomized to a high dose of combined B vitamins and compared to a low-dose total mortality did not differ between the two arms of the study, but there was a nonsignificant 20% reduction in the risk of CV events in the high-dose arm (HR, 0.8; 95% CI, 0.60 to 1.07).[269]

A definitive answer may be likely when the Folic Acid for Vascular Outcome Reduction in Transplantation (FAVORIT) Trial is completed.[270] This study has enrolled 4,110 renal transplant recipients to assess the impact of high doses of folic acid, B_6, and B_{12} on CV events.

Increased extracellular volume. Salt and water overload is a persistent problem in patients on dialysis and is also problematic in patients with CKD and in renal transplant recipients. LV diameter changes with changes in blood volume in hemodialysis patients.[271] Observational studies suggest that greater interdialytic weight gain and noncompliance with the prescribed dialysis regimen are independently associated with higher blood pressure.[272,273] In a prospective study of peritoneal dialysis patients, sodium and fluid removal as well as hypertension were predictive of death within 3 years of starting dialysis.[273] LVH is possibly more severe in long-term peritoneal dialysis patients, a finding that is associated with pronounced volume expansion, hypertension, and hypoalbuminemia.[274]

High natriuretic peptide levels can result from volume expansion and/or myocardial dysfunction. Levels of B-type natriuretic peptide (BNP) are highest in patients who are on dialysis and have CV comorbidities.[275] In patients with CKD, serum BNP can be elevated and high BNP levels are a predictor of progressive renal disease and mortality.[276,277] In incident hemodialysis, patients' N-terminal pro-BNP (NT pro-BNP) was an independent predictor of future CV events.[19]

In the 4D study of prevalent diabetic hemodialysis patients, high baseline and increasing levels over time in N-terminal pro-BNP were predictive for sudden cardiac death, CV events, and mortality.[201] In 965 peritoneal dialysis patients enrolled in a trial[278] of increased quantity of dialysis using peritoneal dialysis, baseline values of natriuretic peptides were elevated and were inversely correlated with levels of residual renal function. The relative risk of NT pro-BNP for the bottom two quintiles compared to the remainder was 0.63, which was significant and independent of multiple other predictors. Whether the high BNP levels were associated with increased blood volume, and thus potentially modifiable by interventions to normalize blood volume, is unknown, but this seems likely. Trials to assess the clinical impact of interventions that maintain normal blood volume should be undertaken.

Arteriovenous Fistulae

Blood flow in arteriovenous fistulae and grafts predisposes a patient to LV volume overload. In one study, 20 renal transplant recipients with a mean fistula flow of 1790 ± 648 mL per minute were assessed.[279] Three to 4 months after fistula closure, LV end-diastolic diameter decreased from 51.5 to 49.3 minutes ($P < .01$) and the LV mass index fell from 135 to 120 g per square meter ($P < .01$). These findings were confirmed in another similar study.[280]

Abnormalities in Divalent Ion Metabolism

Predictor of cardiovascular events. An attractive hypothesis that is gaining traction is that disturbed divalent ion metabolism promotes vascular calcification, which produces noncompliant large conduit vessels. This in turn predisposes the patient to LVH, cardiac failure, and subsequent death.

Hyperphosphatemia usually develops as kidney function deteriorates and is a common problem among patients with ESRD. Phosphate combines with calcium in the blood and the resultant hypocalcemia induces secondary hyperparathyroidism. The persistent overstimulation of the parathyroid glands engenders autonomous growth, and this tertiary hyperparathyroidism may be associated with hyperphosphatemia, increased calcium X phosphate product, and elevated parathyroid hormone (PTH) levels.

In a study of 12,833 patients undergoing hemodialysis,[281] a 0.3 mmol per liter incremental increase in serum PO_4 levels was associated with a 9% increase in the risk of death related to CAD and a 6% increase in the risk of sudden cardiac death. Deaths related to CAD and sudden cardiac death correlated with elevated levels of Ca × PO_4 product in a linear manner. Sudden cardiac deaths were also related to log parathyroid hormone in a nonlinear fashion (U-shaped relationship), but were strongly associated with serum parathyroid hormone > 52.1 ng per liter (RR, 1.25; $P < .05$).[281] An analysis of 40,538 prevalent hemodialysis patients from the U.S. Renal Data System (USRDS) registry also demonstrated that high serum phosphate, serum calcium, and serum parathyroid hormone concentrations were associated with increased all-cause and CV mortality.[282] These two studies included only survivors of dialysis, thus limiting the conclusions that can be made. The CHOICE study[194] enrolled incident hemodialysis patients, and confirmed the adverse impact of divalent ion abnormalities. This prospective study of 776 hemodialysis and 259 peritoneal dialysis patients had a median follow-up of 2.5 years, during which time 460 deaths occurred. The adjusted RR of death for time-dependent serum phosphate levels > 6.0 mg per deciliter was 1.6 (95% CI, 1.1 to 2.3); for time-dependent serum calcium levels > 9.7 mg per deciliter, it was 1.5 (95% CI, 1.0 to 2.3); and for time-dependent PTH levels > 308 pg per milliliter, it was 1.7 (95% CI, 1.0 to 2.8). The association between high PTH levels and mortality was confirmed in the 4D study, but this impact was nullified in those who had wasting, which was defined by serum albumin levels < 3.8 g per deciliter and a BMI < 23.[199]

The adverse outcomes associated with hyperphosphatemia in dialysis patients have been extended to patients with predialysis CKD and to community-based cohorts. In patients with CKD, data from the Veterans' Affairs Consumer Health Information and Performance Sets (CHIPS) of 6,730 patients with CKD revealed that a serum phosphate level > 3.5 mg per deciliter was associated with mortality independent of other risk factors and eGFR.[283] In 1,036 stage 3 and 4 CKD patients from a single United Kingdom center, the highest quartile of serum phosphate compared to that in the lowest quartile was a predictor of all-cause and CV mortality, independent of age, gender, proteinuria, eGFR, diabetes, hemoglobin (Hb), systolic BP, current smoking, CVD, renal replacement therapy, vitamin D analog use, and phosphate binder use.[284] However, it is possible that serum phosphate colocalizes with some other factor(s) associated with CKD that actually causes CVD.

Five community-based prospective cohort studies examined the relationship between serum phosphate and CVD. Graded associations with cardiac calcification, LVH, CV events were observed, and CV risk seemed to accelerate with serum phosphate 3.5 to 4 mg per deciliter.[285]

In CKD, fibroblast growth factor 23 levels are increased to maintain normal concentrations of serum phosphate. Increased levels are associated with increased LV mass and an increased risk of LVH in predialysis CKD patients.[286]

In 1,094 participants in the African American Study of Kidney Disease Hypertension (AASK), following an adjustment for demographics, drug and BP groups, comorbidity, liver function, serum calcium, and phosphorus, each doubling of serum alkaline phosphatase was associated with a HR of 1.55 (95% CI, 1.03 to 2.33).[287] It is possible that raised serum alkaline phosphatase reflects more severe hyperparathyroidism or vitamin D deficiency.

Levels of 25-hydroxyvitamin D were measured in 1,108 diabetic hemodialysis patients in the 4D study and followed for a median time of 4 years.[200] Severe vitamin D deficiency was strongly associated with higher rate of sudden cardiac death and CV results. However, whether vitamin D supplementation will decrease these adverse outcomes is unknown.

Evidence to support the link between divalent on abnormalities and metastatic calcification has also evolved. An increased prevalence and the extent of coronary artery calcification, particularly in young dialysis patients, has been significantly associated with higher serum phosphate, calcium–phosphate product, and calcium intake.[17] Whether this calcification represents specific changes within atherosclerotic plaques or is a stage associated with arteriosclerosis is not clear. The presence of vascular calcification in hemodialysis patients was associated in one study with increased stiffness of large capacity, elastic-type arteries such as the aorta and the common carotid artery. The extent of arterial calcifications increased with the use of calcium-based phosphate binders.[17] As discussed earlier, aortic calcification is predictive of death in dialysis patients.[184]

Treatment. Patients with CKD are in substantial positive calcium balance from an early stage of the disease. Attempts to minimize the calcium X phosphate product by treating hyperparathyroidism and by phosphate control have a sound teleologic base, as does the appropriate use of vitamin D analogs. However, evidence of better CV event outcomes with these therapies compared to placebo have not been reported. The relative benefits of sevelamer hydrochloride (a noncalcium, noncarbonate binder) was compared to calcium carbonate in 114 hemodialysis patients. It showed that at 52 weeks, patients treated with calcium carbonate had significant increases in coronary artery (34%, $P < .01$) and aortic (32%, $P < .01$) calcification compared to the sevelamer-treated patients.[111]

Cinacalcet is a calcimimetic, which reduces parathyroid hormone levels. In 360 hemodialysis patients with moderate-to-severe secondary hyperparathyroidism, an RCT of cinacalcet plus low-dose vitamin D sterols compared to flexible doses of vitamin D sterols alone was recently reported.[112] Increases in calcification scores were consistently less in the aorta, in the aortic valve, and in the mitral valve among the cinacalcet group and the differences were significant at the aortic valve. Whether these observations translate into improvement in CV outcomes is unknown.

An observational study of 19,186 hemodialysis patients, 5,976 of whom received cinacalcet, reported a significant lower all-cause mortality among cinacalcet-treated patients compared with nontreated patients (adjusted HR, 0.74; 95% CI, 0.67 to 0.83).[288] Like all observational studies, adjustment for multiple different potential confounding factors does not remove the bias caused by selecting particular patients for cinacalcet therapy. Consequently, one should await the results of the Evaluation of Cinacalcet Therapy to Lower Cardiovascular Events (EVOLVE) study before adopting cinacalcet as a strategy to reduce CV events in patients with secondary hyperparathyroidism. This is an RCT that has enrolled around 4,000 hemodialysis patients comparing cinacalcet to placebo, and has as its primary end point a composite of major CV events.[289]

Iron Overload

The role of iron in the pathogenesis of CVD in patients with ESRD is not well defined; iron overload has, however, been associated with elevated rates of hospitalization and mortality in patients with ESRD.[290] Iron can promote the production of ROS and free radicals resulting in intercardiomyocytic fibrosis. In a study of 102 nondiabetic patients undergoing peritoneal dialysis who were matched with 102 healthy patients with a serum creatinine level < 133 μmol per liter (1.5 mg per deciliter), the mean QTc dispersion among the patients was significantly longer than in control participants (69.8 ± 40.0 versus 55.2 ± 33.6 ms; $P < .01$).[291] High iron saturation > 35.2% was an independent factor for QTc dispersion longer than 74 ms (sensitivity, 71.4%; specificity, 55.3%; r = 0.432; $P < .001$).

Sympathetic Overactivity

Sympathetic overactivity is an early event in the pathophysiology of acute and chronic kidney injury of various etiologies. Augmented sympathetic drive is seen even during hemodialysis sessions, suggesting that this event is volume independent. Such events usually subside following a bilateral nephrectomy.[292] Sympathetic overactivity may aggravate hypertension, ventricular hypertrophy, and heart failure and may result in an increased risk of sudden cardiac death.[52]

Autonomic imbalance may result from high sympathetic tone and/or low parasympathetic tone, and can be assessed using heart rate variability measurements. In the ARIC study, a higher resting heart rate and lower heart rate variability were significantly associated with incident ESRD and CKD-related hospitalizations.[293]

In 239 subjects enrolled in the Frequent Hemodialysis Network Trial Holter monitor findings were characterized by sympathetic overactivity and vagal withdrawal, and were associated with a higher LV mass.[56] As discussed earlier, β-blockers, which diminish sympathetic activity, have been shown to improve some CV outcomes in CKD.

Obstructive Sleep Apnea

Obstructive sleep apnea causes episodes of nocturnal arterial oxygen desaturation, and this syndrome occurs more frequently in patients undergoing dialysis compared with the general population. In 30 clinically stable hemodialysis patients, 25 (83%) had sleep disordered breathing, with an apnea–hypopnea index > 5 episodes per hour. The percent of sleeping time with saturated arterial 0_2 < 90% was 4.2%.[294] In the 4D study, 40% of people who died as a result of sudden cardiac arrest were found dead in bed in the morning.[145] The investigators postulated that this outcome might be related to obstructive sleep apnea. This suggestion was supported by a recent study. Of 93 prevalent peritoneal dialysis patients, 51 were diagnosed with sleep apnea syndrome, which was a predictor of mortality independent of age, gender, and diabetes.[295] The absolute increase in the apnea–hypopnea index was associated with incremental risk of CV events. In addition, nocturnal hypoxemia and night–day arterial pressure changes have been linked to LV geometry in dialysis patients.[55] Sleep apnea is improved by daily dialysis[56] but whether this translates into better CV outcomes is unknown.

Mode of Dialysis Therapy

Although RCTs in hemodialysis patients[296] and in peritoneal dialysis patients[297] failed to show that an increased quantity of dialysis improved clinical outcomes, suggestive evidence has recently been reported that nocturnal/daily dialysis may have a beneficial effect on the heart. Culleton et al.[298] have demonstrated an improvement in LV mass index measured by magnetic resonance imaging (MRI) in those randomly allocated to daily hemodialysis compared to conventional dialysis. In the Frequent Hemodialysis Network Trial, 125 patients were randomly allocated to hemodialysis six times per week and were compared to 120 patients allocated three times per week.[121] Frequent hemodialysis was associated with a significant benefit for the coprimary outcome, death or increase in LV mass measured using MRI (HR, 0.61; 95% CI, 0.46 to 0.82); improved control of hypertension; and improved control of hyperphosphatemia. It is possible that these beneficial effects on the cardiac structure are mediated by better blood volume control, and daily dialysis certainly has the potential to prevent CV events.

A cohort study of 94 patients who were treated with nocturnal hemodialysis was compared to 10 propensity score–matched controls treated with conventional hemodialysis for each patient.[299] Nocturnal hemodialysis was associated with significant reductions in mortality risk (HR, 0.36; 95% CI, 0.22 to 0.61) and in risk for death, acute MI, or stroke (HR, 0.56; 95% CI, 0.35 to 0.89).

It has been postulated that more atherogenic lipid profiles in peritoneal dialysis patients could predispose them to more atherosclerotic events and that the intermittent blood volume increases seen in hemodialysis patients could predispose them to more heart failure events. Evidence to support the former hypothesis was reported from outcomes in 24,587 patients who commenced dialysis in Australia and New Zealand between 1997 and 2008.[300] Peritoneal dialysis was consistently associated with an increased hazard of CV death compared to hemodialysis after 1 year of treatment. This increased risk in peritoneal patients was largely associated with an increased risk of death due to MIs. Surprisingly, in an analysis of registry data from more than 100,000 incident dialysis patients, patients with CHF treated with peritoneal dialysis had higher levels of mortality over 2 years compared to hemodialysis patients (RR, 1.24; 95% CI, 1.14 to 1.35).[301]

Multiple Risk Factor Intervention

The objective of enhancing the appropriate use of interventions to slow the progression of renal disease and to prevent CVD requires a multifaceted, multidisciplinary approach, which may not be feasible with current primary care–provided models. Furthermore, the poor outcomes of CVD in ESRD suggest that a preventive strategy at an earlier phase of CKD may be more fruitful than a secondary prevention strategy after cardiac events have occurred. This strategy would require risk intervention in multiple factors simultaneously. The excellent results achieved in an RCT[302] of diabetic patients receiving intensive therapy, and of heart failure patients treated in multidisciplinary clinics, suggest that a similar approach in patients with CKD could produce better outcomes than conventional health care delivery models.

Recently, a RCT of 474 stage 3/4 CKD patients identified in the community was reported examining a nurse-coordinated model of care for multiple risk factor interventions versus usual care determined by the family doctor.[303] The important conclusions were (1) patients with CKD identified through community laboratories largely had nonprogressive kidney disease but had quite a high rate of cardiovascular events, (2) the nurse-coordinated model during the 2-year study provided similar control of most risk factors compared to conventional management and was associated with more use of appropriate drugs in eligible patients, and (3) it was less costly.[303,304] Whether this model of care can improve renal and CV outcomes in patients with progressive kidney disease requires investigation.

Interventions for Symptomatic Cardiac Disease

Ischemic Heart Disease

There are no randomized trials concerning the treatment of either the acute coronary syndrome (unstable angina and acute MI) or the nonacute presentations of CAD (stable angina and CHF) in patients with CKD. In the absence of such data, the treatment should be the same as in the nonuremic population. Unfortunately, observational data suggest that dialysis patients with an acute MI are far less likely to receive standard therapy (i.e., aspirin, β-blockers, and ACE inhibitors) compared to other patients.[305] Control of extracellular fluid volume and partial correction of severe anemia with erythropoietin-stimulating agents is a therapeutic adjunct specific to CKD patients, particularly those on dialysis.

Medical Management

As in the general population, patients with CKD and stable angina pectoris who have not had an MI should be treated with antianginal agents for the relief of symptoms. Coronary arteriography is recommended for patients with symptoms at rest or after minimal exertion, LV dysfunction, or signs of severe ischemia at low level of exercise during a stress test. For patients who have had an MI, β-adrenergic blockers are recommended indefinitely, as is an ACE inhibitor for patients with LV dysfunction.[306] In the general population, aspirin therapy is of proven benefit in the treatment of acute MI and after acute MI, as well as for long-term use in patients with a wide range of prior manifestations of CVD.[307] Although far fewer data are available for the CKD population, a study of 1,724 patients with an acute MI categorized patients into quartiles based on their renal function. In the group with the lower GFR (< 46.3 mL per minute), aspirin and β-blocker use was the lowest among all groups of patients, yet the observed risk reduction was similar among all ranges of GFR. This suggests that aspirin and β-blockers are at least as effective in CKD and in dialysis patients as in the nonrenal-failure populations.[308] This, combined with the substantial improvement in CVD outcomes in nonuremic patients with preexisting CVD, is sufficient to recommend that patients with CKD or ESRD with ACS or established CAD should be treated with aspirin and β-blockers in a manner similar to patients with normal renal function.

Although the general population appears to benefit from newer antiplatelet therapies such as aspirin plus clopidogrel,[309,310] the relative safety and efficacy of such a treatment in patients with CKD or ESRD is not yet known.

There is overwhelming evidence that the treatment of dyslipidemia in the general population for the secondary prevention of atherosclerotic events provides substantial survival benefit. In view of the data presented earlier, it seems reasonable to treat CKD patients in a similar manner, provided that life expectancy is such as to benefit from these drugs.

Revascularization

Coronary artery bypass graft surgery. The potential risks and benefits of coronary revascularization procedures in patients with CKD or ESRD are different from those in the general population. The reported perioperative mortality rate of CABG surgery in patients on dialysis has ranged from 0% to 20%, which is significantly higher than in the general population, but the studies on which these figures are based are mostly small and retrospective, and do not make adjustment for comorbid factors. When the results of these studies are combined, the perioperative mortality rate is approximately 8% to 9%, roughly three times the expected rate for patients without ESRD.[311–313] The perioperative morbidity rate of CABG surgery is also greater, both in patients on dialysis and nondialysis-dependent patients with CKD than in matched control patients.[314–316] The 5-year cumulative survival rate of patients on dialysis after CABG is approximately 50%.[311,312] These survival rates are comparable with those seen in the overall ESRD population, but are considerably lower then the overall 5-year survival rate of 85% after CABG, as observed in the Coronary Artery Surgery Study.[317] There are few data as to the outcome of revascularization procedures in patients who have had renal transplantation. Transplanted patients with near normal renal function have a perioperative mortality rate and long-term survival rate close to those observed in the non-ESRD population.[318,319]

The only randomized trial of revascularization versus medical therapy in patients with ESRD to date enrolled 26 asymptomatic diabetic patients who were found to have CAD on screening coronary angiography before renal transplantation.[320] Ten of 13 medically managed and 2 of

13 revascularized patients had a CV end point (unstable angina, MI, or cardiac death), and the trial was stopped early by an external review committee. This provides some evidence that revascularization may improve the prognosis of asymptomatic CAD in this select population, but medical therapy in this instance consisted only of a calcium channel–blocking drug and aspirin. Regardless of any survival benefit, CABG usually offers good relief from angina.[314]

Coronary artery stenting. The role of percutaneous transluminal angioplasty (PTCA) in the CKD or ESRD patients is controversial. Despite a high rate of initial technical success in patients with ESRD, PTCA seems to be associated with frequent recurrence of symptoms, usually resulting from restenosis.[312,321,322] PTCA with stenting of dilated vessels in the dialysis population is certainly feasible, but patients treated with PTCA compared to CABG do have a significantly higher long-term risk of MI or a recurrence of ischemic symptoms.[311] CABG appears to have better outcomes in dialysis patients than PTCA with or without stenting.[323,324] However, it is important to remember that all comparisons between vascularization procedures in CKD patients are from registries or observational studies, and thus are prone to selection bias and confounding by indication. Herzog et al.[324] analyzed USRDS data from dialysis patients undergoing their first revascularization procedure. After comorbidity adjustment, the RR for CABG (versus PTCA) patients was 0.80 (95% CI, 0.76 to 0.84), for all-cause death, and 0.72 (95% CI, 0.67 to 0.77) for cardiac death. For stent (versus PTCA) patients, the RR was 0.94 (95% CI, 0.88 to 0.99) for all-cause death, and 0.92 (95% CI, 0.85 to 0.99) for cardiac death.[324] To date, there have been no studies comparing PTCA with medical management of patients with ESRD or CKD and CAD.

The recent advent of drug-eluting stents may be a step forward in the management of CAD. In a large registry of all comers for percutaneous coronary intervention, CKD was an independent predictor of adverse late outcomes.[325] In patients with ESRD requiring hemodialysis frequencies of restenosis and 2-year major adverse cardiac event rates after sirolimus-eluting stent implantation were markedly higher than in nonhemodialysis CKD patients.[326] However, the selective use of drug-eluting stents in patients with CKD was safe and effective in the long term, with a lower risk of all-cause death, target vessel revascularization, and major adverse cardiac events, and a similar risk of MI and stent thrombosis as compared with bare metal stents.[327] In another registry study,[328] the results in patients with severely decreased GFR were not as impressive. In patients with nondialysis CKD and multivessel CAD, CABG was associated with better survival than angioplasty and placement of drug-eluting stents, but CABG patients had a greater short-term risk of requiring permanent hemodialysis.[329]

In summary, the indications for coronary revascularization in patients with CKD or ESRD are, in general, the same as those in the nonuremic population. Revascularization appears to be beneficial in high-risk patients. Those with persistent symptoms of myocardial ischemia, despite maximal medical therapy, should have a coronary arteriography to identify critical coronary stenosis, provided that their life expectancy is otherwise reasonable. Based on the existing evidence, CABG appears to be the revascularization procedure of choice. PTCA with a drug-eluting stent seems to be a reasonable alternative in single-vessel disease or multiple-vessel disease with culprit lesions.

Congestive Heart Failure

For all patients with symptoms of heart failure, potentially reversible precipitating and aggravating factors (e.g., ischemia, tachycardia, dysrhythmias, or hypertension) should be sought and appropriately managed. The treatment of heart failure differs for those with systolic and diastolic dysfunction in that inotropic agents such as digoxin and vasodilators should be avoided in those with diastolic dysfunction.

β-Adrenergic receptor blockers. A large amount of data from recent, well-designed trials supports the use of β-adrenergic receptor antagonists in the management of LV systolic dysfunction. Improvement in mortality or hospitalization rates have been shown in patients with mild-to-moderate symptomatic heart failure treated with carvedilol, bisoprolol, or controlled-release metoprolol.[330] The use of β-receptor antagonists with intrinsic sympathomimetic activity appears to be detrimental, and these agents should not be used in patients with heart failure. Current guidelines for the general population suggest the routine use of β-receptor antagonists in clinically stable patients with an LV ejection fraction < 40% and mild-to-moderate heart failure symptoms who are on standard therapy (e.g., diuretics, ACE inhibitors, and digoxin).[330] Such therapy also should be considered for asymptomatic patients with an LV ejection fraction < 40%, but the evidence supporting its use in this setting is not as strong. In one of the few randomized trials performed in dialysis patients, Cice et al.[331] have demonstrated that carvedilol treatment in patients with dilated cardiomyopathy reduced 2-year mortality (51.7% in the carvedilol group, compared with 73.2% in the placebo group [$P < .01$]). There were fewer cardiovascular deaths (29.3%) and hospital admissions (34.5%) among patients receiving carvedilol than among those receiving a placebo (67.9% and 58.9%, respectively; $P < .00001$). This supports the notion that β-receptor antagonists may be safely used in the CKD and ESRD population in the same manner recommended for the general heart failure population. As in the nonrenal-failure population, however, the agents should be started in low doses with careful clinical reevaluations during the titration phase.

Angiotensin-converting enzyme inhibitors/blockers. The use of this class of drugs for the management of heart failure has been well demonstrated in the general population. ACE inhibitors have been found to improve symptoms, reduce morbidity, and improve survival, thus making them an important component of CHF therapy.[330] Although trials in the CKD or ESRD population have not been conducted, the high degree of benefit shown in other patients makes it very reasonable to treat these patients in a similar manner. Therefore, ACE inhibitor therapy is recommended for patients with symptomatic heart failure, for post-MI patients with an LV ejection fraction < 40%, and for asymptomatic patients with an LV ejection fraction less than 35%.[330] Angiotensin II–receptor blockers are good alternatives to ACE inhibitors in the treatment of heart failure for those who cannot tolerate ACE inhibitors.

In the absence of large, double-blinded randomized controlled trials in patients undergoing dialysis, the use of ACE inhibitors, ARBs, or both should follow indications derived from trials in patients without renal disease.

Digoxin. In the nonrenal population, digoxin may be beneficial in the treatment of heart failure and atrial fibrillation. However, in hemodialysis patients, digoxin use has been associated with excess mortality.[332] It should be noted that the research design in the study was observational and thus limited by selection bias. However, digoxin levels > 1.0 ng per milliliter were associated with excess mortality, which is consistent with the belief that the narrow therapeutic window, the long half-life, and the potential for lethal arrhythmias, especially in the presence of hypokalemia, make digoxin a poor choice for use in ESRD patients.

Diuretics. These drugs remain an essential component of the symptomatic treatment for heart failure in nondialysis-dependent patients with CKD, although multiple agents at high doses may be required in patients with more advanced renal impairment. Loop diuretics are widely used to maintain euvolemia in most patients with CHF, but their effect may be negligible in patients requiring dialysis. Thiazide diuretics usually become ineffective with a GFR < 30 mL per minute and are therefore not useful in patients with severe renal impairment. Aldosterone antagonists are similarly ineffective in patients with ESRD, but hyperkalemia can result when these drugs are combined with renin angiotensin system blockade and β-receptor antagonists. They should be avoided in such patients.

Warfarin in atrial fibrillation. An observational study (DOPPS)[141] identified an increased risk of stroke associated with warfarin use in dialysis patients with atrial fibrillation, a risk also identified in another study.[333] For patients with CKD, atrial fibrillation and a CHADS2 score ≥ 2 anticoagulation with warfarin has been recommended, provided there is access to high quality monitoring of coagulation.[334]

Cardiac Arrest

Automated external defibrillators. A total of 110 cardiac arrests in two hemodialysis facilities in King County, Seattle, Washington, were identified over 14 years; 65% of these events occurred during hemodialysis sessions and were secondary to ventricular fibrillation.[35] The risk of ventricular fibrillation was much higher after the dialysis session compared with the period during dialysis. Thirty-four cardiac arrests occurred after an automated external defibrillator was made available within the dialysis units. However, these devices were only used in 50% of these arrests. A shock was delivered on 83% of the occasions when the defibrillator was used. Survival to hospital discharge was not notably different between patients who arrested before or after an external defibrillator was provided at the dialysis unit.[335] Although data do not exist to support a survival benefit of external defibrillator placement in dialysis centers, it seems reasonable to provide them for use in patients who want resuscitation if they arrest.

Implantable cardioverter-defibrillators. Implantable cardioverter-defibrillators (ICDs) decrease the risk of sudden cardiac death, but the majority of trials using these devices have excluded patients with advanced renal insufficiency. Dasgupta et al.[336] reported complication rates for cardiac rhythm management devices (permanent pacemakers or ICDs) in 41 patients with ESRD and in 123 control participants without ESRD. Major complications (such as pneumothorax requiring a chest tube, a pocket infection requiring device extraction, or thrombosis) occurred in 29% of ESRD patients versus 5% of controls ($P < .03$). No fatal complications occurred in either group. Furthermore, patients with advanced renal insufficiency could be less responsive to ICD therapy, probably owing to higher defibrillation thresholds.

In a retrospective study[337] of 230 patients who received an ICD for primary or secondary indications, renal insufficiency was a strong predictor of an arrhythmia eliciting appropriate ICD shocks. Patients with higher degrees of renal dysfunction were more likely to have shorter times to ICD therapy (defined as shock and antitachycardia pacing). Patients were divided into three groups according to their serum creatinine levels (< 88.4 μmol per liter, 88.4 to 123.8 μmol per liter, and > 123.8 μmol per liter). The 1-year incidence of appropriate ICD shock was 3.8%, 10.8%, and 22.7% in these groups, respectively ($P = .003$). The 1-year incidence of any appropriate ICD therapy was 8.8%, 20.8%, and 26.3% ($P = .02$). Serum creatinine was an independent predictor of the time to first appropriate ICD shock (HR, 6.0 for the third group compared with the first group; $P = .001$) or the first appropriate ICD therapy (HR, 3.0 for the third compared with the first group; $P = .015$). Seven patients (3%) were on hemodialysis at the time of device implantation. These patients experienced more appropriate ICD shocks for documented ventricular tachyarrhythmias than those not undergoing dialysis (57% versus 11%; $P = .006$). The 1-year incidence of appropriate ICD shock was 37.5% for patients on dialysis and 10.7% for those not on dialysis ($P < .0001$), and the 1-year incidence of any appropriate ICD therapy for patients on dialysis versus those not on dialysis was 33.3% versus 16.5% ($P = .0005$).

Patients who received an ICD for the primary prevention of sudden cardiac death ($n = 222$) were stratified by CKD, defined as serum creatinine levels ≥ 176.8 μmol per liter, or on dialysis.[338] The 1-year survival for patients with ($n = 35$) and without ($n = 194$) CKD was 61.2% and 96.3%, respectively. CKD was the most significant independent predictor of mortality (HR, 10.5; 95% CI, 4.8 to 23.1). Furthermore, each 10 mL per minute drop in creatinine clearance was associated with a 55% rise in the HR of death ($P < .001$). It was concluded that in patients receiving an ICD for the primary prevention of sudden cardiac death, CKD significantly reduced long-term survival, which may limit the impact of ICD therapy in this patient population.

A decision analysis and Markov modeling of whether to implant a cardioverter-defibrillator for the primary prevention of sudden cardiac death in patients with CKD[339] found that the benefit of ICD use depends primarily on the patient's age and secondarily on the stage of kidney disease. ICDs reduce mortality in patients with stage 1 and 2 CKD, whereas the benefit is less notable in patients with stage 3 through 5 CKD, and the effect is age dependent. These findings could be attributed to a higher procedural risk and complications in addition to decreased life expectancy in patients with advanced CKD compared with control individuals.[340] With a standard procedural mortality of 0.5% per procedure, cardioverter-defibrillator implantation is preferential in patients < 80 years of age for stage 3 CKD (GFR, 30 to 59 mL/min/1.73 m^2), in patients < 75 years of age for stage 4 CKD (GFR, 15 to 29 mL/min/1.73 m^2), and in patients < 65 years of age for stage 5 CKD (GFR < 15 mL/min/1.73 m^2).[339] Thus, advanced stages of CKD and older age favor the no ICD strategy. No health technology assessment of ICD use in patients with CKD is available. However, a study published in 2005 showed that prophylactic ICD use in patients with heart failure has a cost-effectiveness ratio below US$100,000 per quality-adjusted life year gained, provided that the ICD reduced mortality by 7 years or more.[340]

CONCLUSIONS

CKD is a state of high cardiomyopathic, atherosclerotic, and arteriosclerotic disease. The high prevalence of traditional CV risk factors is partly responsible, including the modifiable factors of hypertension, smoking, hyperlipidemia, hyperglycemia, and obesity. Furthermore, uremia-related predictors of CV disease have been identified, including inflammation, hyperfibrinogenemia, high troponin levels, hyperhomocysteinemia, hypophosphatemia, hyperparathyroidism, and blood volume expansion caused by severe anemia, atrioventricular fistula/graft, and salt and water retention. Whether modification of these predictors will result in fewer CV events is unknown. Although the outcomes of the CV events in stage 4/5 CKD are worse than those in the general population, efficacious therapies are available. The greatest opportunity for improvement in CV outcomes lies in the prevention of CVD in the earlier phases of CKD, and in the development of interventions to modify uremia-related CV risk factors, particularly reducing inflammation, treating divalent ion abnormalities, and normalizing blood volume.

REFERENCES

1. Ronco C, House AA, Haapio M. Cardiorenal syndrome: refining the definition of a complex symbiosis gone wrong. *Intensive Care Med.* 2008;34:957–962.
2. Mann JF, Gerstein HC, Pogue J, Bosch J, Yusuf S. Renal insufficiency as a predictor of cardiovascular outcome and the impact of Ramipril. The HOPE randomized trial. *Ann Intern Med.* 2001;134: 629–636.
3. Go AS, Chertow GM, Fau D, et al. Chronic kidney disease and the risks of death, cardiovascular events and hospitalization. *N Engl J Med.* 2004;351: 1296–1305.
4. Ninomiya T, Perkovic V, de Galan BE, et al. Albuminuria and kidney function independently predict cardiovascular and renal outcomes in diabetes. *J Am Soc Nephrol.* 2009;20:1813–1821.
5. Chronic Kidney Disease Prognosis Consortium. Association of estimated glomerular filtration rate and albuminuria with all-cause and cardiovascular mortality in general population cohorts: a collaborative meta-analysis. *Lancet.* 2010;375:2073–2081.
6. Hemmelgarn BR, Manns BJ, Lloyd A, et al. Relation between kidney function, proteinuria and adverse outcomes. *JAMA.* 2010;303:423–429.
7. Shlipak MG, Katz R, Kestenbaum B, et al. Rapid decline of kidney function increases cardiovascular risk in the elderly. *J Am Soc Nephrol.* 2009;20:2625–2630.
8. Matsushita K, Selvin E, Bash LD, et al. Change in estimated GFR associates with coronary heart disease and mortality. *J Am Soc Nephrol.* 2009;20: 2617–2624.
9. Manjunath G, Tighiouart H, Coresh J, et al. Level of kidney function as a risk factor for cardiovascular outcomes in the elderly. *Kidney Int.* 2003;63: 1121–1129.
10. Reddan DN, Marcus RJ, Owen WWF Jr, et al. Long-term outcomes of revascularization for peripheral vascular disease in end-stage renal patients. *Am J Kidney Dis.* 2001;38:57–63.
11. Foley RN, Murray AM, Li S, et al. Chronic kidney disease and the risk for cardiovascular disease, renal replacement, and death in the United States Medicare population, 1998 to 1999. *J Am Soc Nephrol.* 2005;16:489–495.
12. Barrett BJ, Parfrey PS, Morgan J, et al. Prediction of early death in end-stage renal disease patients starting dialysis. *Am J Kidney Dis.* 1997;29(2):214–222.
13. Rigatto C, Parfrey P, Foley R, et al. Congestive heart failure in renal transplant recipients: Risk factors, outcomes, and relationship with ischemic heart disease. *J Am Soc Nephrol.* 2002;13:1084–1090.
14. Foley RN, Herzog CA, Collins AJ. Smoking and cardiovascular outcomes in dialysis patients: The United States Renal Data System Wave 2 study. *Kidney Int.* 2003;63(4):1462–1467.
15. Harnett JD, Foley RN, Kent GM, et al. Congestive heart failure in dialysis patients: Prevalence, incidence, prognosis, and risk factors. *Kidney Int.* 1995;47:884–890.
16. Foley RN, Parfrey PS, Sarnak MJ. Clinical epidemiology of cardiovascular disease in chronic renal disease. *Am J Kidney Dis.* 1998;32(5 Suppl 3):S112–0S119.
17. London GM, Marchais SJ, Guérin AP, et al. Associations of bone activity, calcium load, aortic stiffness and calcifications in ESRD. *J Am Soc Nephrol.* 2008;19:1827–1835.
18. Foley RN, Parfrey PS, Harnett JD, et al. The prognostic importance of left ventricular geometry in uremic cardiomyopathy. *J Am Soc Nephrol.* 1995;5: 805–813.
19. Foley RN, Curtis BM, Randell EW, Parfrey PS. Left ventricular hypertrophy in new hemodialysis patients without symptomatic cardiac disease. *Clin J Am Soc Nephrol.* 2010;5:805–813.
20. Rigatto C, Foley RN, Kent GM, Guttmann R, Parfrey PS. Long-term changes in left ventricular hypertrophy after renal transplantation. *Transplantation.* 2002;70:570–575.
21. Parfrey PS, Harnett JD, Griffiths S, Gault MH, Barre PE. Congestive heart failure in dialysis patients. *Arch Intern Med.* 1988;148:1519–1525.
22. Rostand SG, Kirk KA, Rutsky EA. Dialysis-associated ischemic heart disease: insights from coronary angiography. *Kidney Int.* 1984;25:653.
23. Mosseri M, Yarom R, Gotsman MS, et al. Histologic evidence for small-vessel coronary artery disease in patients with angina pectoris and patent large coronary arteries. *Circulation.* 1986;74:964.
24. James TN. Morphologic characteristics and functional significance of focal fibromuscular dysplasia of small coronary arteries. *Am J Cardiol.* 1990;65:12G.
25. Amann K, Wiest G, Zimmer G, et al. Reduced capillary density in the myocardium of uremic rats – a stereological study. *Kidney Int.* 1992;42:1079.

26. Diaz MN, Frei B, Vita JA, et al. Antioxidants and arteriosclerotic heart disease. *N Engl J Med.* 1997;337:408.
27. Cominacini L, Garbin U, Pasini AF, et al. Antioxidants inhibit the expression of intercellular cell adhesion molecule-1 and vascular cell adhesion molecule-1 induced by oxidized LDL on human umbilical vein endothelial cells. *Free Radic Biol Med.* 1997;22:117.
28. Westhuyzen J. The oxidation hypothesis of atherosclerosis: an update. *Ann Clin Lab Sci.* 1997;27:1.
29. Ananyeva NM, Tjurmin AV, Berliner JA, et al. Oxidized LDL mediates the release of fibroblast growth factor-1. *Arterioscler Thromb Vasc Biol.* 1997;17:445.
30. Stary HC. Composition and classification of human atherosclerotic lesions. *Virchows Arch A Pathol Anat Histopathol.* 1992;421–477.
31. Schwarz U, Buzello M, Ritz E, et al. Morphology of coronary atherosclerotic lesions in patients with end-stage renal failure. *Nephrol Dial Transplant.* 2000;15:218.
32. Zoccali C, Beck S, What makes plaques vulnerable in CKD: a fresh look at metalloproteinases. *Kidney Int.* 2010;78:1206–1208.
33. Pelisek J, Assadian A, Sarkar O, Eckstein HH, Frank H. Carotid plaque composition in chronic kidney disease: a retrospective analysis of patients undergoing carotid endarterectomy. *Eur J Vasc Endovasc Surg.* 2010;39:11–16.
34. Yilmaz MI, Qureshi AR, Carrero JJ, et al. Predictors of carotid artery intima – media thickness in chronic kidney disease and kidney transplant patients without overt cardiovascular disease. *Am J Nephrol.* 2010;31:214–221.
35. Rigatto C, Singal P. Oxidative stress in uremia: impact on cardiac disease in dialysis patients. *Semin Dial.* 1999;12:91.
36. Boston AG, Culleton BF. Hyperhomocysteinemia in chronic renal disease. *J Am Soc Nephrol.* 1999;10:891.
37. Goodman WG, Goldin J, Kuizon BD, et al. Coronary artery calcification in young adults with end-stage renal disease who are undergoing dialysis. *N Engl J Med.* 2000;342:1478.
38. Oh J, Wunsch R, Turzer M, et al. Advanced coronary and carotid arteriopathy in young adults with childhood-onset chronic renal failure. *Circulation.* 2002;106:100.
39. Abedini S, Meinitzer A, Holme I, et al. Asymmetrical dimethylarginine is associated with renal and cardiovascular outcomes and all-cause mortality in renal transplant recipients. *Kidney Int.* 2010;77:44–50.
40. Zoccali C, Bode-Boger S, Mallamaci F, et al. Plasma concentration of asymmetrical dimethylarginine and mortality in patients with end-stage renal disease: a prospective study. *Lancet.* 2001;358(9299):2113–2117.
41. Coll B, Rodriguez JA, Craver L, et al. Serum levels of metalloproteinase −10 are associated with the severity of atherosclerosis in patients with chronic kidney disease. *Kidney Int.* 2010;78:1275–1280.
42. Erbel R, Ge J, Bockisch A, et al. Value of intracoronary ultrasound and Doppler in the differentiation of angiographically normal coronary arteries: a prospective study in patients with angina pectoris. *Eur Heart J.* 1996;17:880.
43. Uren NG, Melin JA, De Bruyne B, et al. Relation between myocardial blood flow and the severity of coronary-artery stenosis. *N Engl J Med.* 1994;330:1782.
44. Zoneraich S. Unravelling the conundrums of the diabetic heart diagnosed in 1876: prelude to genetics. *Can J Cardiol.* 1994;10:945.
45. Raine AE, Seymour AM, Roberts AF, et al. Impairment of cardiac function and energetics in experimental renal failure. *J Clin Invest.* 1993;92:2934.
46. Massry SG, Smogorzewski M. Mechanisms through which parathyroid hormone mediates its deleterious effects on organ function in uremia. *Semin Nephrol.* 1994;14;219.
47. Nishimura M, Tsukamoto K, Tamaki N, et al. Risk stratification for cardiac death in hemodialysis patients without obstructive coronary artery disease. *Kidney Int.* 2011;79:363–371.
48. Nishimura M, Tsukamoto K, Hasebe N, et al. Prediction of cardiac death in hemodialysis patients by myocardial fatty acid imaging. *J Am Coll Cardiol.* 2008;51:146–148.
49. Guerin AP, Blacher J, Pannier B, et al. Impact of aortic stiffness attenuation on survival of patients in end-stage renal failure. *Circulation.* 2001;103(7):987–992.
50. Benedetto FA, Mallamaci F, Tripepi G, Zoccali C. Prognostic value of ultrasonographic measurement of carotid intima media thickness in dialysis patients. *J Am Soc Nephrol.* 2001;12:2458–2464.
51. Tozawa M, Iseki K, Iseki C, Takishita S. Pulse pressure and risk of total mortality and cardiovascular events in patients on chronic hemodialysis. *Kidney Int.* 2002;61:717–726.
52. Zoccali C, Mallamaci F, Tripepi G, et al. CREED investigators. Norepinephrine and concentric hypertrophy in patients with end-stage renal disease. *Hypertension.* 2002;40:41–46.
53. Zoccali C, Mallamaci F, Parlongo S, et al. Plasma norepinephrine predicts survival and incident cardiovascular events in patients with end-stage renal disease. *Circulation.* 2002;105:1354–1359.
54. Zoccali C, Mallamaci F, Benedetto FA, et al. Cardiac natriuretic peptides are related to left ventricular mass and function and predict mortality in dialysis patients. *J Am Soc Nephrol.* 2001;12:1508–1515.
55. Zoccali C, Benedetto FA, Tripepi G, et al. Nocturnal hypoxemia, night-day arterial pressure changes and left ventricular geometry in dialysis patients. *Kidney Int.* 1998;53:1078–1084.
56. Chan CT, Levin NW, Chertow GM, et al. Determinants of cardiac autonomic dysfunction in ESRD. *Clin J Am Soc Nephrol.* 2010;5:1821–1827.
57. London GM, Marchais SJ, Guerin AP, et al. Cardiac hypertrophy and arterial alterations in end-stage renal disease: Hemodynamic factors. *Kidney Int Suppl.* 1993;41:S42–S49.
58. Marchais SJ, Guerin AP, Pannier BM, et al. Wave reflections and cardiac hypertrophy in chronic uremia. Influence of body size. *Hypertension.* 1993;22(6):876–883.
59. Savage T, Giles M, Tomson CV, et al. Gender differences in mediators of left ventricular hypertrophy in dialysis patients. *Clin Nephrol.* 1998;49(2);107–112.
60. Greaves SC, Gamble GD, Collins JF, et al. Determinants of left ventricular hypertrophy and systolic dysfunction in chronic renal failure. *Am J Kidney Dis.* 1995;24(5):768–776.
61. de Lima JJ, Abensur H, Krieger EM, et al. Arterial blood pressure and left ventricular hypertrophy in haemodialysis patients. *J Hypertens.* 1996;14: 1019–1024.
62. Blacher J, Guerin AP, Pannier B, et al. Impact of aortic stiffness on survival in end-stage renal disease. *Circulation.* 1999;99(18):2434–2439.
63. Moe SM, Chen NX. Mechanisms of vascular calcification in chronic kidney disease. *J Am Soc Nephrol.* 2008;19:213–216.
64. Westenfeld R, Schäfer C, Krüger T, et al. Fetuin-A protects against atherosclerotic calcification in CKD. *J Am Soc Nephrol.* 2009;20:1264–1274.
65. Schlieper G, Aretz A, Verberckmoes SC, et al. Ultrastructural analysis of vascular calcifications in uremia. *J Am Soc Nephrol.* 2010;21:689–696.
66. Amann K. Media calcification and intima calcification are distinct entities in chronic kidney disease. *Clin J Am Soc Nephrol.* 2008;3:1599–1605.
67. McCullough PA, Agrawal V, Danielewicz E, Abela GS. Accelerated atherosclerotic calcification and Monckeberg's sclerosis: a continuum of advanced vascular pathology in chronic kidney disease. *Clin J Am Soc Nephrol.* 2008;3:1585–1598.
68. Chiu YW, Adler SG, Budoff MJ, et al. Coronary artery calcification and mortality in diabetic patients with proteinuria. *Kidney Int.* 2010;77:1107–1114.
69. Nakamura S, Ishibashi-Ueda H, Zizuma S, et al. Coronary artery calcification in patients with chronic kidney disease and coronary artery disease. *Clin J Am Soc Nephrol.* 2009;4:1892–1900.
70. Grossman W. Cardiac hypertrophy: useful adaptation or pathologic process? *Am J Med.* 1980;69:576.
71. London GM, Guerin AP, Marchais SJ, et al. Cardiac and arterial interactions in end-stage renal disease. *Kidney Int.* 1996;50:600.
72. London GM, Drueke TB. Atherosclerosis and arteriosclerosis in chronic renal failure. *Kidney Int.* 1997;51:1678.
73. Raine AE. Acquired aortic stenosis in dialysis patients. *Nephron.* 1994; 68:159.
74. Semple D, Smith K, Bhandari S, et al. Uremic cardiomyopathy and insulin resistance: a critical role for Akt? *J Am Soc Nephrol.* 2011;22:207–215.
75. Siedlecki AM, Jin X, Muslin AJ. Uremic cardiac hypertrophy is reversed by rapamycin but not by lowering of blood pressure. *Kidney Int.* 2009;75:800–808.
76. Rozich JD, Smith B, Thomas JD, et al. Dialysis-induced alternations in left ventricular filling: mechanisms and clinical significance. *Am J Kidney Dis.* 1991;17:277.
77. Hoffman JI. Transmural myocardial perfusion. *Prog Cardiovasc Dis.* 1987; 29:429.
78. Cheng W, Li B, Kajstura J, et al. Stretch-induced programmed myocyte cell death. *J Clin Invest.* 1995;96:2247.
79. Suzuki H, Schaefer L, Ling H, et al. Prevention of cardiac hypertrophy in experimental chronic renal failure by long-term ACE inhibitor administration: potential role of lysosomal proteinases. *Am J Nephrol.* 1995;15:129.
80. Amann K, Ritz E, Wiest G, et al. A role of parathyroid hormone for the activation of cardiac fibroblasts in uremia. *J Am Soc Nephrol.* 1994;4:1814.
81. Katz AM. The cardiomyopathy of overload: an unnatural growth response in the hypertrophied heart. *Ann Intern Med.* 1994;121:363.
82. Frustaci A, Kajstura J, Chimenti C, et al. Myocardial cell death in human diabetes. *Circ Res.* 2000;87:1123–1132.
83. Aoki J, Nakajima H, Mori M. Clinical and pathologic characteristics of dilated cardiomyopathy in hemodialysis patients. *Kidney Int.* 2005;67:333–341.
84. van Hoeven KH, Factor SM. A comparison of the pathological spectrum of hypertensive, diabetic, and hypertensive-diabetic heart disease. *Circulation.* 1990;82:848–855.

85. Sniderman AD, Solhpour A, Alam A, Williams K, Sloand JA. Cardiovascular death in dialysis patients: lessons we can learn from AURORA. *Clin J Am Soc Nephrol.* 2010;5:335–340.
86. Hothi DK, Rees L, Marek J, Buron J, McIntyre CW. Pediatric myocardial stunning underscores the cardiac toxicity of conventional hemodialysis treatments. *Clin J Am Soc Nephrol.* 2009;4:790–797.
87. McIntyre CW, Burton JO, Selby NM, et al. Hemodialysis-induced cardiac dysfunction is associated with an acute reduction in global and segmental myocardial blood flow. *Clin J Am Soc Nephrol.* 2008;3:19–26.
88. Ribeiro S, Ramos A, Brandao A, et al. Cardiac valve calcification in haemodialysis patients: Role of calcium-phosphate metabolism. *Nephrol Dial Transplant.* 1998;13(8):2037–2040.
89. London GM, Pannier B, Marchais SJ, Guerin AP. Calcification of the aortic valve in the dialyzed patient. *J Am Soc Nephrol.* 2000;11(4):778–783.
90. Otto CM, Lind BK, Kitzman DW, et al. Association of aortic-valve sclerosis with cardiovascular mortality and morbidity in the elderly. *N Engl J Med.* 1999;341(3):142–147.
91. Fernandez-Reyes MJ, Auxiliadora Bajo M, Robles P, et al. Mitral annular calcification in CAPD patients with a low degree of hyperparathyroidism. An analysis of other possible risk factors. *Nephrol Dial Transplant.* 1995;10:2090–2095.
92. Rufino M, García S, Jiménez A, et al. Heart valve calcification and calcium × phosphorus product in hemodialysis patients: analysis of optimum values for its prevention. *Kidney Int Suppl.* 2003;85:S115–S118.
93. Weinrauch L, D'Elia JA, Healy RW, et al. Asymptomatic coronary artery disease: angiographic assessment of diabetics evaluated for renal transplantation. *Circulation.* 1978;58:1184.
94. Lorber MI, Van Buren CT, Flechner SM, et al. Pretransplant coronary arteriography for diabetic renal transplant recipients. *Transplant Proc.* 1987;19:1539.
95. Braun WE, Phillips DF, Vidt DG, et al. Coronary artery disease in 100 diabetics with end-stage renal failure. *Transplant Proc.* 1984;16:603.
96. Murphy SW, Foley RN, Parfrey PS. Screening and treatment for cardiovascular disease in patients with chronic renal disease. *Transplant Proc.* 1984;16:603.
97. Eagle KA, Berger PB, Calkins H, et al. ACC/AHA guideline update for perioperative cardiovascular evaluation for noncardiac surgery: executive summary. A report of the American College of Cardiology/American Heart Association Task Force on Practice Guidelines (Committee to Update the 1996 Guidelines on Perioperative Cardiovascular Evaluation for Noncardiac Surgery). *Circulation.* 2002;105:1257.
98. Kasiske BL, Cangro CB, Hariharan S, et al. The evaluation of renal transplantation candidates: clinical practice guidelines. *Am J Transplant.* 2001;1(Suppl 2):3.
99. Herzog CA, Apple FS. Cardiac biomarkers in the new millennium. *Semin Dial.* 2001;14:322.
100. Li D, Jialal I, Keffer J. Greater frequency of increased cardiac troponin T than increased cardiac troponin I in patients with chronic renal failure. *Clin Chem.* 1996;42:114.
101. Fleming SM, Daly KM. Cardiac troponins in suspected acute coronary syndrome: a meta-analysis of published trials. *Cardiology.* 2001;95:66.
102. McCullough PA, Nowak RM, Foreback C, et al. Performance of multiple cardiac biomarkers measured in the emergency department in patients with chronic kidney disease and chest pain. *Acad Emerg Med.* 2002;9:1389.
103. Freda BJ, Tang WH, Van Lente F, et al. Cardiac troponins in renal insufficiency: review and clinical implications. *J Am Coll Cardiol.* 2002;40:2065.
104. Coley CM, Eagle KA. Preoperative assessment and perioperative management of cardiac ischemic risk in noncardiac surgery. *Curr Probl Cardiol.* 1996;21:289.
105. Morrow CE, Schwartz JS, Sutherland DE, et al. Predictive value of thallium stress testing for coronary and cardiovascular events in uremic diabetic patients before renal transplantation. *Am J Surg.* 1983;146:331.
106. Schmidt A, Stefenelli T, Schuster E, et al. Informational contribution of noninvasive screening tests for coronary artery disease in patients on chronic renal replacement therapy. *Am J Kidney Dis.* 2001;37:56.
107. Herzog CA, Marwick TH, Pheley AM, et al. Dobutamine stress echocardiography for the detection of significant coronary artery disease in renal transplant candidates. *Am J Kidney Dis.* 1999;33:1080.
108. Reis G, Marcovitz PA, Leichtman AB, et al. Usefulness of dobutamine stress echocardiography in detecting coronary artery disease in end-stage renal disease. *Am J Cardiol.* 1995;75:707–710.
109. Le A, Wilson R, Douek K, et al. Prospective risk stratification in renal transplant candidates for cardiac death. *Am J Kidney Dis.* 1994;24:65–71.
110. Dahan M, Viron BM, Faraggi M, et al. Diagnostic accuracy and prognostic value of combined dipyridamole-exercise thallium imaging in hemodialysis patients. *Kidney Int.* 1998;54:255–262.
111. Chertow GM, Burke SK, Raggi P. Treat to Goal Working Group. Sevelamer attenuates the progression of coronary and aortic calcification in hemodialysis patients. *Kidney Int.* 2002;62:245–252.
112. Raggi P, Chertow GM, Torres PU, et al. The ADVANCE study: a randomized study to evaluate the effects of cinacalcet plus low-dose vitamin D on vascular calcification in patients on hemodialysis. *Nephrol Dial Transplant.* 2011;26(4):1327–1339.
113. Kramer H, Toto R, Peshock R, Cooper R, Victor R. Association between chronic kidney disease and coronary artery calcification: The Dallas Heart Study. *J Am Soc Nephrol.* 2005;16:507–513.
114. Kestenbaum BR, Adeney KL, de Boer IH, et al. Incidence and progression of coronary calcification in chronic kidney disease: The Multi-Ethnic Study of Atherosclerosis. *Kidney Int.* 2009;76:991–998.
115. Weustink AC, Mollet NR, Neefjes LA, et al. Diagnostic accuracy and clinical utility of noninvasive testing for coronary artery disease. *Ann Intern Med.* 2010;152:630–639.
116. Barrett BJ, Parfrey PS. Clinical practice: preventing nephrotoxicity induced by contrast medium. *N Engl J Med.* 2006;354:379–386.
117. Pannu N, Manns B, Lee H, et al. Systematic review of the impact of N-acetylcyteine on contrast nephropathy. *Kidney Int.* 2004;65:1366.
118. DeLoach SS, Townsend RR. Vascular stiffness: its management and significance for epidemiologic and outcome studies. *Clin J Am Soc Nephrol.* 2008;3:184–192.
119. Pombo JF, Troy BL, Russell RO Jr. Left ventricular volumes and ejection fraction by echocardiography. *Circulation.* 1971;43:480.
120. Levy D, Savage DD, Garrison RJ, et al. Echocardiographic criteria for left ventricular hypertrophy: the Framingham Heart Study. *Am J Cardiol.* 1987;59:956.
121. FHN Trial Group, Chertow GM, Levin NW, et al. In-centre hemodialysis six times per week versus three times per week. *N Engl J Med.* 2010;363:2287–2300.
122. Patel RK, Oliver S, Mark PB, et al. Determinants of left ventricular mass and hypertrophy in hemodialysis patients assessed by cardiac magnetic resonance imaging. *Clin J Am Soc Nephrol.* 2009;4:1477–1483.
123. Eckardt KU, Scherhag A, Macdougall IC, et al. Left ventricular geometry predicts cardiovascular outcomes associated with anemia correction in CKD. *J Am Soc Nephrol.* 2009;20:2651–2660.
124. Levin A, Singer J, Thompson CR, et al. Prevalent left ventricular hypertrophy in the predialysis population: identifying opportunities for intervention. *Am J Kidney Dis.* 1996;327–347.
125. Foley RN, Parfrey PS, Harnett JD, et al. Clinical and echocardiographic disease in patients starting end-stage renal disease. *Kidney Int.* 1995;47:186.
126. Parfrey PS, Foley RN, Harnet JD, et al. Outcome and risk factors for left ventricular disorders in chronic uremia. *Nephrol Dial Transplant.* 1996;11: 1277–1285.
127. Foley RN, Parfrey PS, Kent GM, et al. Long-term evolution of cardiomyopathy in dialysis patients. *Kidney Int.* 1998;54:1720.
128. Parfrey PS, Harnett JD, Foley RN, et al. Impact of renal transplantation on uremic cardiomyopathy. *Transplantation.* 1995;60:908–914.
129. Churchill DN, Taylor DW, Cook RJ, et al. Canadian hemodialysis morbidity study. *Am J Kidney Dis.* 1992;19:214.
130. Kasiske BL, Guijarro C, Massy ZA, et al. Cardiovascular disease after renal transplantation. *J Am Soc Nephrol.* 1996;7:158.
131. Muntner P, He J, Astor BC, et al. Traditional and nontraditional risk factors predict coronary heart disease in chronic kidney disease: results from the Atherosclerosis Risk in Communities Study. *J Am Soc Nephrol.* 2005;16;529.
132. Parfrey PS, Foley RN, Harnett JD, et al. Outcome and risk factors of ischemic heart disease in chronic uremia. *Kidney Int.* 1996;49:1428–1434.
133. Jardine AG, Fellstrom B, Logan JO, et al. Cardiovascular risk and renal transplantation: post hoc analyses of the Assessment of Lescol in Renal Transplantation (ALERT) Study. *Am J Kid Dis.* 2005;46:529–536.
134. Hillege HL, Girbes AR, de Kam PJ, et al. Renal function, neurohormonal activation, and survival in patients with chronic heart failure. *Circulation.* 2000;102:203.
135. Foley RN, Parfrey PS, Kent GM, et al. Serial change in echocardiographic parameters and cardiac failure in end-stage renal disease. *J Am Soc Nephrol.* 2000;11:912–916.
136. Kimura K, Tabei K, Asano J, Hosoda S. Cardiac arrhythmias in hemodialysis patients. A study of incidence and contributory factors. *Nephron.* 1989;53:201–207.
137. Multicentre cross-sectional study of ventricular arrhythmias in chronically hemodialysed patients. Gruppo Emodialist e Pathologia Cardiovasculari. *Lancet.* 1988;6:305–309.
138. Sforzini S, Latini R, Mingadi G, et al. Ventricular arrhythmias and four-year mortality in hemodialysis patients. *Lancet.* 1992;339:212–213.
139. Canziani ME, Cendoroglo Neto M, Saragoça MA, et al. Hemodialysis versus continuous ambulatory peritoneal dialysis: Effects on the heart. *Artif Organs.* 1995;19:241–244.

140. Genovesi S, Vincenti A, Rossi E, et al. Atrial fibrillation and morbidity and mortality in a cohort of long-term hemodialysis patients. *Am J Kid Dis*. 2008;51: 2550–2562.

141. Wizemann V, Tong L, Stayathum S, et al. Atrial fibrillation in hemodialysis patients: clinical features and associations with anti-coagulant therapy. *Kidney Int*. 2010;77:1098–1106.

142. Ananthapanyasut W, Napan S, Rudolph EH, et al. Prevalence of atrial fibrillation and its predictors in nondialysis patients with chronic kidney disease. *Clin J Am Soc Nephrol*. 2010;5:173–181.

143. Lentine KL, Schnitzler MA, Abbott KC, et al. Incidence, predictors, and associated outcomes of atrial fibrillation after kidney transplantation. *Clin J Am Soc Nephrol*. 2006;1:288–296.

144. Thomas AC, Knapman, PA, Krikler DM, David MJ. Community study of the causes of "natural" sudden death. *BMJ*. 1988;297:1453–1456.

145. Ritz E, Wanner C. The challenge of sudden death in dialysis patients. *Clin J Am Soc Nephrol*. 2008;3:920–929.

146. Ganesh SK, Stack AG, Levin NW, Hulbert-Shearon T, Port FK. Association of elevated serum PO_4, Ca × PO_4 product, and parathyroid hormone with cardiac mortality risk in chronic hemodialysis patients. *J Am Soc Nephrol*. 2001;12:2131–2138.

147. Herzog CA, Strief JW, Collins AJ, Gilbertson DT. Cause-specific mortality of dialysis patients after coronary revascularization: why don't dialysis patients have better survival after coronary intervention? *Nephrol Dial Transplant*. 2008;23:2629–2633.

148. Pun PH, Smarz TR, Honeycutt ER, et al. Chronic kidney disease is associated with increased risk of sudden cardiac death among patients with coronary artery disease. *Kidney Int*. 2009;76:652–658.

149. Karnik JA, Young BS, Lew NL, et al. Cardiac arrest and sudden death in dialysis units. *Kidney Int*. 2001;60:350–357.

150. Bleyer AJ, Hartman J, Brannon PC, et al. Characteristics of sudden death in hemodialysis patients. *Kidney Int*. 2006;69:2268–2273.

151. US Renal Data System. USRDS 2008 Annual Data Report. National Institutes of Health, National Institutes of Diabetes and Digestive and Kidney Diseases.

152. Herzog CA. Cardiac arrest in dialysis patients: approaches to alter an abysmal outcome. *Kidney Int*. 2003;63(Suppl. 84):197–200.

153. de Bruyne MC, Hoes AW, Kors JA, et al. QTc dispersion predicts cardiac mortality in the elderly: the Rotterdam Study. *Circulation*. 1998;97:467–472.

154. Atiga WL, Calkins H, Lawrence JH, et al. Beat-to-beat repolarization lability identifies patients at risk for sudden cardiac death. *J Cardiovasc Electrophysiol*. 1998;9:899–908.

155. Stewart GA, Gansevoort RT, Mark PB, et al. Electrocardiographic abnormalities in uremic cardiomyopathy. *Kidney Int*. 2005;67:217–226.

156. Kitano Y, Kasuga H, Watanabe M, et al. Severe coronary stenosis is an important factor for induction and lengthy persistence of ventricular arrhythmias during and after hemodialysis. *Am J Kidney Dis*. 2004;44:328–336.

157. Sinha MK, Gaze DC, Tippins JR, Collinson, PO, Kaski JC. Ischemia modified albumin is a sensitive marker of myocardial ischemia after percutaneous coronary intervention. *Circulation*. 2003;107:2403–2405.

158. Pollack C, Peacock WF, Summers RW, Morris DL. Ischemic modified albumin is useful in risk stratification of emergency department chest pain patients. *Acad Emerg Med*. 2003;10:555–556.

159. Sharma R, Gaze DC, Pellerin D, et al. Ischemia-modified albumin predicts mortality in ESRD. *Am J Kidney Dis*. 2006;47:493–502.

160. Kantarci G, Ozener C, Tokay S, Bihorac A, Akoglu E. QT dispersion in hemodialysis and CAPD patients. *Nephron*. 2002;91:739–741.

161. Beaubien ER, Pylypchuk GB, Akhtar J, Biem HJ. Value of corrected QT interval dispersion in identifying patients initiating dialysis at increased risk of total and cardiovascular mortality. *Am J Kidney Dis*. 2002;39:834–842.

162. Johansson M, Gao SA, Friberg P, et al. Elevated temporal QT variability index in patients with chronic renal failure. *Clin Sci (Lond)*. 2004;107: 583–588.

163. Patanè S, Marte F, Di Bella G, Currò A, Coglitore S. QT interval prolongation, torsade de pointes and renal disease. *Int J Cardiol*. 2008;130:371–373.

164. Johansson M, Gao SA, Friberg P, et al. Reduced baroreflex effectiveness index in hypertensive patients with chronic renal failure. *Am J Hypertens*. 2005;18:995–1000.

165. Di Rienzo M, Parati G, Castiglioni P. et al. Baroreflex effectiveness index: an additional measure of baroreflex control of heart rate in daily life. *Am J Physiol Regul Integr Camp Physiol*. 2001;280:744–751.

166. La Rovere MT, Bigger JT Jr, Marcus FI, Mortara A, Schwartz PJ. Baroreflex sensitivity and heat-rate variability in prediction of total cardiac mortality after myocardial infarction ATRAMI (Autonomic Tone and Reflexes After Myocardial Infarction) Investigators. *Lancet*. 1998;351:478–484.

167. Johansson M, Gao SA, Friberg P, et al. Baroreflex effectiveness index and baroreflex sensitivity predict all-cause mortality and sudden death in hypertensive patients with chronic renal failure. *J Hypertens*. 2007;25:163–168.

168. Parekh RS, Plantinga LC, Kao WH, et al. The association of sudden cardiac death with inflammation and other traditional risk factors. *Kidney Int*. 2008;74:1335–1342.

169. Pun PH, Lehrich RQ, Honeycutt EF, Herzog CA, Middleton JP. Modifiable risk factors associated with sudden cardiac arrest within hemodialysis clinics. *Kidney Int*. 2011;79:218–227.

170. Flythe JE, Kimmel SE, Brunelli SM. Rapid fluid removal during dialysis is associated with cardiovascular morbidity and mortality. *Kidney Int*. 2011; 790:250–257.

171. Santoro A, Mancini E, London G, et al. Patients with complex arrhythmias during and after hemodialysis suffer from different regimens of potassium removal. *Nephrol Dial Transplant*. 2008;23:1415–1421.

172. Covic A, Diaconita M, Gusbeth-Tatomir P, et al. Hemodialysis increases QT(c) interval but not QT(c) dispersion in ESRD patients without manifest cardiac disease. *Nephrol Dial Transplant*. 2002;17:2170–2177.

173. Pun PH, Lehrich RW, Smith SR, Middleton JP. Predictors of survival after cardiac arrest in outpatient hemodialysis clinics. *Clin J Am Soc Nephrol*. 2007;2: 491–500.

174. Wright RS, Reeder GS, Herzog CA, et al. Acute myocardial infarction and renal dysfunction: a high-risk combination. *Ann Intern Med*. 2002;137:563.

175. Gibson CM, Pinto DS, Murphy SA, et al. Association of creatinine and creatinine clearance on presentation in acute myocardial infarction with subsequent mortality. *J Am Coll Cardiol*. 2003;42:1535.

176. Fox CS, Muntner P, Chen AY, et al. Use of evidence based therapies in short-term outcomes of ST-segment elevation myocardial infarction and non-ST-segment elevation myocardial infarction in patients with chronic kidney disease: a report from National Cardiovascular Data Acute Coronary Treatment and Intervention Outcomes Network Registry. *Circulation*. 2010;121:357–365.

177. Al-Ahmad A, Rand WM, Manjunath G, et al. Reduced kidney function and anemia as risk factors for mortality in patients with left ventricular dysfunction. *J Am Coll Cardiol*. 2001;38:955.

178. Kearney MT, Fox KA, Lee AJ, et al. Predicting death due to progressive heart failure in patients with mild-to-moderate chronic heart failure. *J Am Coll Cardiol*. 2002;40:1801.

179. Shlipak MG, Smith GL, Rathore SS, et al. Renal function, digoxin therapy, and heart failure outcomes: evidence from the digoxin intervention group trial. *J Am Soc Nephrol*. 2004;15:2195.

180. Rigatto C, Foley R, Jeffrey J, et al. Electrocardiographic left ventricular hypertrophy in renal transplant recipients: prognostic value and impact of blood pressure and anemia. *J Am Soc Nephrol*. 2003;14:462–468.

181. Yamada S, Ishii H, Takahashi H, et al. Prognostic value of reduced left ventricular ejection fraction at start of hemodialysis therapy on cardiovascular and all-cause mortality in end-stage renal disease patients. *Clin J Am Soc Nephrol*. 2010;5:1793–1798.

182. Burton JO, Jefferies HJ, Selby NM, McIntryre CW. Hemodialysis-induced cardiac injury: determinants and associated outcomes. *Clin J Am Soc Nephrol*. 2009;4:914–920.

183. Watanabe R, Lemos MM, Manfredi SR, Draibe SA, Canziani ME. Impact of cardiovascular calcifications in nondialyzed patients after 24 months of follow-up. *Clin J Am Soc Nephrol*. 2010;5:189–194.

184. Verbeke F, Van Biesen W, Honkanen E, et al. Prognostic value of aortic stiffness and calcification for cardiovascular events and mortality in dialysis patients: outcome of the Calcification Outcome in Renal Disease (CORD) study. *Clin J Am Soc Nephrol*. 2011;6:153–159.

185. Manske CL, Thomas W, Wang Y, et al. Screening diabetic transplant candidates for coronary artery disease: identification of a low risk subgroup. *Kidney Int*. 1993;44:617.

186. Kurella Tamura M, Xie D, Yaffe K, et al. Vascular risk factors and cognitive impairment in chronic kidney disease: The Chronic Renal Insufficiency Cohort (CRIC) Study. *Clin J Am Soc Nephrol*. 2011;6:248–256.

187. Abramson JL, Jurkovitz CT, Vaccarino V, et al. Chronic kidney disease, anemia, and incident stroke in a middle-aged, community-based population: The ARIC Study. *Kidney Int*. 2003;64610–64615.

188. Foley RN, Parfrey PS, Harnett JD, et al. Impact of hypertension on cardiomyopathy, morbidity and mortality in end-stage renal disease. *Kidney Int*. 1996;49:1379–1385.

189. Foley RN, Parfrey PS, Harnett JD, et al. Hypoalbuminemia, cardiac morbidity, and mortality in end-stage renal disease. *J Am Soc Nephrol*. 1996;7:728–736.

190. Foley RN, Parfrey PS, Harnett JD, et al. The impact of anemia on cardiomyopathy, morbidity, and mortality in end-stage renal disease. *Am J Kidney Dis*. 1996;28:53–61.

191. Foley RN, Culleton BF, Parfrey PS, et al. Cardiac disease in diabetic end-stage renal disease. *Diabetologia*. 1997;40:1307–1312.
192. Plantinga LC, Fink NE, Levin NW, et al. Early, intermediate, and long-term risk factors for mortality in incident dialysis patients: the Choices for Healthy Outcomes in Caring for ESRD (CHOICE) Study. *Am J Kidney Dis*. 2007;49:831–840.
193. Liu Y, Coresh J, Eustace JA, et al. Association between cholesterol level and mortality in dialysis patients: Role of inflammation and malnutrition. *JAMA*. 2004;291:451–459.
194. Melamed ML, Eustace JA, Plantinga L, et al. Changes in serum calcium, phosphate, and PTH and the risk of death in incident dialysis patients: a longitudinal study. *Kidney Int*. 2006;70:351–357.
195. Wanner C, Krane V, März W, et al. Atorvastatin in patients with type 2 diabetes mellitus undergoing hemodialysis. *N Engl J Med*. 2005; 353:238–348.
196. Drechsler C, Krane V, Ritz E, März W, Wanner C. Glycemic control and cardiovascular events in diabetic hemodialysis patients. *Circulation*. 2009;120: 2421–2428.
197. Krane V, Winkler K, Drechsler C, et al. Effect of atorvastatin on inflammation and outcome in patients with type 2 diabetes mellitus on hemodialysis. *Kidney Int*. 2008;74:1461–1467.
198. Krane V, Winkler K, Drechsler C, Lilienthal J, et al. Association of LDL cholesterol and inflammation with cardiovascular events and mortality in hemodialysis patients with type 2 diabetes mellitus. *Am J Kidney Dis*. 2009;54:902–911.
199. Drechsler C, Krane V, Grootendorst DC, et al. The association between parathyroid hormone and mortality in dialysis patients is modified by wasting. *Nephrol Dial Transplant*. 2009;24:3151–3157.
200. Drechsler C, Pilz S, Obermayer-Pietsch B, et al. Vitamin D deficiency is associated with sudden cardiac death, combined cardiovascular events, and mortality in haemodialysis patients. *Eur Heart J*. 2010;31:2253–2261.
201. Winkler K, Wanner C, Drechsler C, et al. Change in N-terminal-pro-B-type-natriuretic-peptide and the risk of sudden death, stroke, myocardial infarction, and all-cause mortality in diabetic dialysis patients. *Eur Heart J*. 2008;29:2092–2099.
202. Levin A, Djurdjev O, Barrett B, et al. Cardiovascular disease in patients with chronic kidney disease: getting to the heart of the matter. *Am J Kidney Dis*. 2001;38:1398.
203. Goicoechea M, de Vinuesa SG, Gomez-Campdera F, et al. Predictive cardiovascular risk factors in patients with chronic kidney disease (CKD). *Kidney Int Suppl*. 2005;S35.
204. Galderisi M, Anderson KM, Wilson PW, et al. Echocardiographic evidence for the existence of a distinct diabetic cardiomyopathy: the Framingham Heart Study. *Am J Cardiol*. 1991;68–85.
205. Grossman E, Messerli FH. Diabetic and hypertensive heart disease. *Ann Intern Med*. 1996;125:304.
206. Buckalew VM Jr, Berg RL, Wang SR, et al. Prevalence of hypertension in 1,795 subjects with chronic renal disease: the modification of diet in renal disease study baseline cohort. Modification of Diet in Renal Disease Study Group. *Am J Kidney Dis*. 1996;28:811.
207. Agarwal R, Nissenson AR, Batle D, et al. Prevalence, treatment, and control of hypertension in chronic hemodialysis patients in the United States. *Am J Med*. 2003;115:291.
208. Cannella G, Paoletti E, Delfino R, et al. Regression of left ventricular hypertrophy in hypertensive dialyzed uremic patients on long-term antihypertensive therapy. *Kidney Int*. 1993;44:881.
209. Cruickshank JM, Lewis J, Moore V, et al. Reversibility of left ventricular hypertrophy by differing types of antihypertensive therapy. *J Hum Hypertens*. 1992;6:85.
210. Rigatto C, Foley RN, Kent GM, et al. Long-term changes in left ventricular hypertrophy after renal transplantation. *Transplantation*. 2000;70:570.
211. Zager PG, Nikolic J, Brown RH, et al. "U" curve association of blood pressure and mortality in hemodialysis patients. Medical Directors of Dialysis Clinic, Inc. *Kidney Int*. 1998;54:561.
212. Goodkin DA, Bragg-Gresham JL, Koenig KG, et al. Association of comorbid conditions and mortality in hemodialysis patients in Europe, Japan, and the United States: the Dialysis Outcomes and Practice Patterns Study (DOPPS). *J Am Soc Nephrol*. 2003;14:3270.
213. Stidley CA, Hunt WC, Tentori F, et al. Changing relationship of blood pressure with mortality over time among hemodialysis patients. *J Am Soc Nephrol*. 2006;16:513–520.
214. Jafar TH, Schmid CH, Landa M, et al. Angiotensin-converting enzyme inhibitors and progression of nondiabetic renal disease. A meta-analysis of patient-level data. *Ann Intern Med*. 2001;135(2):73–87.
215. Brenner BM, Cooper ME, de Zeeuw D, et al. Effects of losartan on renal and cardiovascular outcomes in patients with type 2 diabetes and nephropathy. *N Engl J Med*. 2001;345:861–869.
216. Berl T, Hunsicker LG, Lewis JB, et al. Cardiovascular outcomes in the Irbesartan Diabetic Nephropathy Trial of patients with type 2 diabetes and overt nephropathy. *Ann Intern Med*. 2003;138:542–549.
217. Berl T, Hunsickers LG, Lewis JB, et al. Impact of achieved blood pressure on cardiovascular outcomes in the irbesartan diabetic nephropathy trial. *J Am Soc Nephrol*. 2005;16:2170–2179.
218. National Kidney Foundation. K/DOQI clinical practice guidelines or hypertension and antihypertensive agents in chronic kidney disease. *Am J Kid Dis*. 2004;43(Suppl 1):S1–S290.
219. Lewis JB. Blood pressure control in chronic kidney disease: is less really more. *J Am Soc Nephrol*. 2010;21:1086–1092.
220. Charra B, Calemard E, Ruffet M, et al. Survival as an index of adequacy of dialysis. *Kidney Int*. 1992;41:1286–1291.
221. Agarwal R, Alborzi P, Setyan A, Light RP. Dry-weight reduction in hypertensive hemodialysis patients (DRIP): a randomized controlled trial. *Hypertension*. 2009;53:500–507.
222. London GM, Pannier B, Guerin AP, et al. Cardiac hypertrophy, aortic compliance, peripheral resistance, and wave reflection in end-stage renal disease. Comparative effects of ACE inhibition and calcium channel blockade. *Circulation*. 1994;90:2786–2796.
223. Zannad R, Kessler M, Lehert P, et al. Prevention of cardiovascular events in end-stage renal disease: results of a randomized trial of fosinopril and implications for future studies. *Kidney Int*. 2006;70:1318–1324.
224. Takahashi A, Takase H, Toriyama T, et al. Candesartan, an angiotensin II type-1 receptor blocker, reduces cardiovascular events in patients on chronic hemodialysis—a randomized study. *Nephrol Dial Transplant*. 2006;21:2507–2512.
225. Tai DJ, Lim TW, James MT, et al. Cardiovascular effects of angiotensin converting enzyme inhibitor or angiotensin receptor blockage in hemodialysis: a meta-analysis. *Clin J Am Soc Nephrol*. 2010;5:623–630.
226. Tonelli M, Bohm C, Pandeya S, et al. Cardiac risk factors and the use of cardioprotective medications in patients with chronic renal insufficiency. *Am J Kidney Dis*. 2001;37;484.
227. Pfeffer MA, Burdmann EA, Chen CY, et al. A trial of darbepoetin alfa in type 2 diabetes and chronic kidney disease. *N Engl J Med*. 2009;361:2019–2032.
228. Shlipak MG, Fried LF, Cushman M, et al. Cardiovascular mortality risk in chronic kidney disease: comparison of traditional and novel risk factors. *JAMA*. 2005;293:1737–1745.
229. Kasiske BL, Chakkera HA, Roel J. Explained and unexplained ischemic heart disease risk after renal transplantation. *J Am Soc Nephrol*. 2000;11:1735–1743.
230. Kasiske BL, Klinger D. Cigarette smoking in renal transplant recipients. *J Am Soc Nephrol*. 2000;11:753.
231. Kasiske BL. Hyperlipidemia in patients with chronic renal disease. *Am J Kidney Dis*. 1998;32:S142.
232. Lowrie EG, Lew NL. Commonly measured laboratory variables in hemodialysis patients: relationships among them and to death risk. *Semin Nephrol*. 1992;12:276.
233. Contreres G, Hu B, Astor BC, et al. Malnutrition-inflammation modifies the relationship of cholesterol with cardiovascular disease. *J Am Soc Nephrol*. 2010;21:2131–2141.
234. Cressman MD, Heyka RJ, Paganini EP, et al. Lipoprotein (a) is an independent risk factor for cardiovascular disease in hemodialysis patients. *Circulation*. 1992;86:475.
235. Tonelli M, Isles C, Curhan GC, et al. Effect of pravastatin on cardiovascular events in people with chronic kidney disease. *Circulation*. 2004;110:1557.
236. Holdaas H, Wanner C, Abletshauser C, et al. The effect of fluvastatin on cardiac outcomes in patients with moderate to severe renal insufficiency: a pooled analysis of double-blind, randomized trials. *Int J Cardiol*. 2007;117:64–74.
237. Jardine AG, Holdaas H, Fellstrom B, et al. Fluvastatin prevents cardiac death and myocardial infarction in renal transplant recipients: post-hoc subgroup analyses of the ALERT study. *Am J Transplant*. 2004;4:988.
238. Fellström BC, Jardine AG, Schmieder RE, et al. Statin therapy offered no cardiovascular benefit to patients undergoing hemodialysis. *N Engl J Med*. 2009;360:1395–1407.
239. Baigent C, Landray M, and SHARP investigators. The effects of lowering LDL cholesterol with simvastatin plus ezetimide in patients with chronic kidney disease (Study of Heart and Renal Protection): a randomized placebo-controlled trial. *Lancet* 2011;377:2181–2192.
240. Kidney Disease Outcomes Quality Initiative (K/DOQI) Group. K/DOQI clinical practice guidelines for management of dyslipidemias in patients with kidney disease. *Am J Kidney Dis*. 2003;41:S1.
241. Kasiske B, Cosio EG, Beto J, et al. Clinical practice guidelines for managing dyslipidemias in kidney transplant patients: a report from the Managing Dyslipidemias in Chronic Kidney Disease Work Group of the National Kidney Foundation Disease Outcomes Quality Initiatives. *Am J Transplant*. 2004;4(Suppl 7):13.

242. Shurraw S, Majumdar SR, Thadhani R, et al. Glycemic control and the risk of death in 1484 patients receiving hemodialysis. *Am J Kidney Dis.* 2010;55:875–884.

243. Parfrey PS, Lauve M, Latremouille-Viau D, Lefebvre P. Erythropoietin therapy and left ventricular mass index in CKD and ESRD patients: a meta-analysis. *Clin J Am Soc Nephrol.* 2009;4:455–462.

244. Parfrey PS, Foley RN, Wittreich BH, et al. Double-blind comparison of full and partial anemia correction in incident hemodialysis patients without symptomatic heart disease. *J Am Soc Nephrol.* 2005;16:2180–2189.

245. CESG Canadian Erythropoietin Study Group. Association between recombinant human erythropoietin and quality of life and exercise capacity of patients receiving haemodialysis. *Br Med J.* 1990;300:573–578.

246. Besarab A, Bolton WK, Browne JK, et al. The effects of normal as compared to low hematocrit values in patients with cardiac disease who are receiving hemodialysis and epoetin. *N Engl J Med.* 1998;339:584–590.

247. Palmer SC, Navaneethan SD, Craig JC, et al. Meta-analysis: Erythropoiesis-stimulating agents in patients with chronic kidney disease. *Ann Intern Med.* 2010; 153:23–33.

248. Parekh RS, Plantinga LC, Kao WH, et al. The association of sudden cardiac death with inflammation and other traditional risk factors. *Kidney Int.* 2008;74: 1335–1342.

249. McIntyre CW, Harrison LE, Eldehni MT, et al. Circulating endotoxemia: a novel factor is systemic inflammation and cardiovascular disease in chronic kidney disease. *Clin J Am Soc Nephrol.* 2011;5:133–141.

250. Raj DS, Shah VO, Rambod M, et al. Association of soluble endotoxin receptor CD14 and mortality among patients undergoing hemodialysis. *Am J Kid Dis.* 2009;54:1062–1071.

251. Nakashima A, Carrero JJ, Qureshi AR, et al. Effect of circulating soluble receptor for advanced glycation end products (SRAGE) and the proinflammatory RAGE ligand (EN-RAGE, SIOOAIZ) on mortality in hemodialysis patients. *Clin J Am Soc Nephrol.* 2010;5:2213–2219.

252. Sanmuganathan PS, Ghahramani P, Jackson RR, et al. Aspirin for primary prevention of coronary heart disease: Safety and absolute benefit related to coronary risk derived from meta-analysis of randomized trials. *Heart.* 2001;85: 265–271.

253. Antithrombotic Trialists' Collaboration. Collaborative meta-analysis of randomized trials of antiplatelet therapy for prevention of death, myocardial infarction and stroke in high risk patients. *BMJ.* 2002;324:71–86.

254. Khan NA, Hemmelgarn BR, Tonelli M, Thompson CR, Levin A. Prognostic value of troponin T and I among asymptomatic patients with end-stage renal disease: a meta-analysis. *Circulation.* 2005;112:3088–3096.

255. Strobel NA, Fassett RG, Marsh SA, Coombs JS. Oxidative stress biomarkers as predictors of cardiovascular disease. *Int J Cardiol.* 2011;147:191–201.

256. Himmelfarb J, Stenvinkel P, Ikizler TA, Hakim RM. The elephant in uremia: oxidant stress as a unifying concept of cardiovascular disease in uremia. *Kidney Int.* 2002;62:1524–1538.

257. Menon V, Rudym D, Chandra P, et al. Inflammation, oxidative stress and insulin resistance in polycystic kidney disease. *Clin J Am Soc Nephrol.* 2011;6:7–13.

258. Del Vecchio L, Locatelli F, Carini M. What we know about oxidative stress in patients with chronic kidney disease on dialysis—clinical effects, potential treatment, and prevention. *Semin Dial.* 2011;24:56–64.

259. Boaz M, Smetana S, Weinstein T, et al. Secondary prevention with antioxidants of cardiovascular disease in end-stage renal disease (SPACE): Randomised placebo-controlled trial. *Lancet.* 2000;356:1213–1218.

260. Tepel M, van der Giet M, Statz M, et al. The antioxidant acetylcysteine reduces cardiovascular events in patients with end-stage renal failure: A randomized, controlled trial. *Circulation.* 2003;107:992–995.

261. Mann JF, Lonn EM, Yi Q, et al. Effects of vitamin E on cardiovascular outcomes in people with mild-to-moderate renal insufficiency: Results of the HOPE Study. *Kidney Int.* 2004;65(4):1375–1380.

262. Lonn EM, Bosch J, Yusuf S, et al. Effects of long-term vitamin E supplementation on cardiovascular outcomes and cancer: a randomized controlled trial. *JAMA.* 2005;293;1338–1347.

263. Bostom AG, Lathrop L. Hyperhomocysteinemia in end-stage renal disease: prevalence, etiology, and potential relationship to arteriosclerosis outcomes. *Kidney Int.* 1997;52:10.

264. Mallamaci F, Zoccali C, Tripepi G, et al. Hyperhomocysteinemia predicts cardiovascular outcomes in hemodialysis patients. *Kidney Int.* 2002;61;609.

265. Wald D, Law M, Morris JK. Homocysteine and cardiovascular disease: evidence on causality from a meta-analysis. *BMJ.* 2022;325:1202.

266. Shemin D, Bostom AG, Selhub J. Treatment of hyperchomocysteinemia in end-stage renal disease. *Am J Kidney Dis.* 2001;38:S91.

267. Wrone EM, Hornberger JM, Zehnder JL, et al. Randomized trial of folic acid for prevention of cardiovascular events in end-stage renal disease. *J Am Soc Nephrol.* 2004;14:420.

268. House AA, Eliasziw M, Cattran DC, et al. Effect of B-vitamin therapy on progression of diabetic nephropathy: a randomized controlled trial. *JAMA.* 2010;303:1603–1609.

269. Heinz J, Kropf S, Domröse U, et al. B vitamins and the risk of total mortality and cardiovascular disease in end-stage renal disease: results of a randomized controlled trial. *Circulation.* 2010;121:1432–1438.

270. Bostom AG, Carpenter MA, Hunsicker L, et al. Baseline characteristics of participants in the Folic Acid for Vascular Outcome Reduction in Transplantation (FAVORIT) Trial. *Am J Kidney Dis.* 2009;53:121–128.

271. Harnett JD, Murphy B, Collingwood P, et al. The reliability and validity of echocardiographic measurement of left ventricular mass index in hemodialysis patients. *Nephron.* 1993;65:212.

272. Rahman M, Fu P, Sehgal AR, et al. Interdialytic weight gain, compliance with dialysis regimen, and age are independent predictors of blood pressure in hemodialysis patients. *Am J Kidney Dis.* 2000;35:257.

273. Ates K, Nergizoglu G, Keven K, et al. Effect of fluid and sodium removal on mortality in peritoneal dialysis patients. *Kidney Int.* 2001;60:767.

274. Enia G, Mallamaci F, Benederro FA, et al. Long-term CAPD patients are volume expanded and display more severe left ventricular hypertrophy than hemodialysis patients. *Nephrol Dial Transplant.* 2001;16:1459.

275. Parfrey PS. BNP in hemodialysis patients. *Clin J Am Soc Nephrol.* 2010;5:954–955.

276. Roberts MA, Srivastava PM, Macmillan N, et al. B-type natriuretic peptides strongly predict mortality in patients who are treated with long-term dialysis. *Clin J Am Soc Nephrol.* 2008;3:1057–1065.

277. Spanaus KS, Kronenberg F, Ritz E, et al. B-type natriuretic peptide concentrations predict the progression of nondiabetic chronic kidney disease: the Mild-to-Moderate Kidney Disease Study. *Clin Chem.* 2007;53:1264–1272.

278. Paniagua R, Amato D, Mugais S, et al. Predictive value of brain natriuretic peptides in patients on peritoneal dialysis: results from the ADEMEX Trial. *Clin J Am Soc Nephrol.* 2008;3:407–415.

279. van Duijnhoven ED, Cheriex EC, Tordoir JH, et al. Effect of closure of the arteriovenous fistula on left ventricular dimensions in renal transplant patients. *Nephrol Dial Transplant.* 2001;16:368–372.

280. Unger P, Velez-Roa S, Wissing KM, et al. Regression of left ventricular hypertrophy after arteriovenous fistula closure in renal transplant recipients: A long-term follow-up. *J Transplant.* 2004;4(12):2038–2044.

281. Ganesh SK, Stack AG, Levin NW, Hulbert-Shearon T, Port FK. Association of elevated serum PO_4 Ca × PO_4 product, and parathyroid hormone with cardiac mortality risk in chronic hemodialysis patients. *J Am Soc Nephrol.* 2001;12: 2131–2138.

282. Block GA, Klassen PS, Lazarus JM, et al. Mineral metabolism, mortality, and morbidity in maintenance hemodialysis. *J Am Soc Nephrol.* 2004;15(8): 2208–2218.

283. Kestenbaum B, Sampson JN, Rudser KD, et al. Serum phosphate levels and mortality risk among people with chronic kidney disease. *J Am Soc Nephrol.* 2005;16(2):520–528.

284. Eddington H, Hoefield R, Sinha S, et al. Serum phosphate and mortality in patients with chronic kidney disease. *Clin J Am Soc Nephrol.* 2010;5: 2251–2257.

285. Foley RN. Phosphate levels and cardiovascular disease in the general population. *Clin J Am Soc Nephrol.* 2009;4:1136–1139.

286. Gutiérrez OM, Januzzi JL, Isakova T, et al. Fibroblast growth factor 23 and left ventricular hypertrophy in chronic kidney disease. *Circulation.* 2009;119: 2545–2552.

287. Beddhu S, Ma X, Baird B, Cheung AK, Greene T. Serum alkaline phosphatase and mortality in African Americans with chronic kidney disease. *Clin J Am Soc Nephrol.* 2009;4:1805–1810.

288. Block GA, Zaun D, Smits G, et al. Cinacalcet hydrochloride treatment significantly improves all-cause and cardiovascular survival in a large cohort of hemodialysis patients. *Kidney Int.* 2010;78:578–589.

289. Chertow GM, Pupim LB, Block GA, et al. Evaluation of cinacalcet therapy to lower cardiovascular events (EVOLVE): rational and design overview. *Clin J Am Soc Nephrol.* 2007;2:898–905.

290. Besarab A. Iron and cardiac disease in the end-stage renal disease setting. *Am J Kidney Dis.* 1999;34:S18–S24.

291. Wu VC, Huang JW, Wi MS, et al. The effect of iron stores on corrected QT dispersion in patients undergoing peritoneal dialysis. *Am J Kidney Dis.* 2004;44:720–728.

292. Rump LC, Amann K, Orth S, Ritz E. Sympathetic overactivity in renal disease: a window to understand progression and cardiovascular complications of uremia? *Nephrol Dial Transplant.* 2000;15:1735–1738.

293. Brotman DJ, Bash LD, Qayyum R, et al. Heart rate variability predicts ESRD and CKD-related hospitalization. *J Am Soc Nephrol.* 2010;21:1560–1570.

294. Jung HH, Lee JH, Baek HJ, Kim SJ, Lee JJ. Nocturnal hypoxemia and periodic limb movement predict mortality in patients on maintenance hemodialysis. *Clin J Am Soc Nephrol*. 2010;5:1607–1613.
295. Tang SC, Lam B, Yao TJ, et al. Sleep apnea is a novel risk predictor of cardiovascular morbidity and death in patients receiving peritoneal dialysis. *Kidney Int*. 2010;77:1031–1038.
296. Eknoyan G, Beck GJ, Cheung AK, et al. Effect of dialysis dose and membrane flux in maintenance hemodialysis. *New Engl J Med*. 2002;347:2010–2019.
297. Paniagua R, Amato D, Vouesh E, et al. Effects of increased peritoneal clearances on mortality rates in peritoneal dialysis: ADEMEX, a prospective randomized controlled trial. *J Am Soc Nephrol*. 2002;13:1307–1320.
298. Culleton BF, Walsh M, Klarenbach SW, et al. Effect of frequent nocturnal hemodialysis vs conventional hemodialysis on left ventricular mass and quality of life. *JAMA*. 2007;298:1291–1299.
299. Johansen KL, Zhang R, Huang Y, et al. Survival and hospitalization among patients using nocturnal and short daily compared to conventional hemodialysis: a USRDS study. *Kidney Int*. 2009;76:984–990.
300. Johnson DW, Dent H, Hawley CM, et al. Association of dialysis modality and cardiovascular mortality in incident dialysis patients. *Clin J Am Soc Nephrol*. 2009;4:1620–1628.
301. Stack AG, Molony DA, Rahman NS, et al. Impact of dialysis modality on survival of new ESRD patients with congestive heart failure in the United States. *Kidney Int*. 2003;64:1071–1079.
302. Gaede P, Vedel P, Parving HH, Pedersen O. Intensified multifactorial intervention in patients with type 2 diabetes mellitus and microalbuminuria: The Steno type 2 randomised study. *Lancet*. 1999;353:617–622.
303. Barrett BJ, Garg AX, Goeree R, et al. A nurse co-ordinated model of care versus usual care for stage 3/4 chronic kidney disease in the community: a randomized controlled trial. *Clin J Am Soc Nephrol*. 2011;6(6):1241–1247.
304. Hopkins R, Garg AX, Levin A, et al. Cost-effectiveness analysis of a randomized trial comparing care models for chronic kidney disease. *Clin J Am Soc Nephrol*. 2011;6(6):1248–1257.
305. Berger AK, Duval S, Krumholz HM. Aspirin, beta-blocker, and angiotensin-converting enzyme inhibitor therapy in patients with end-stage renal disease and acute myocardial infarction. *J Am Coll Cardiol*. 2003;42:201.
306. Solomon AJ, Gersh BJ. Management of chronic stable angina: medical therapy, percutaneous transluminal coronary angioplasty, and coronary artery bypass graft surgery. Lessons from the randomized trials. *Ann Intern Med*. 1998;128:216.
307. Hennekens CH, Dyken ML, Fuster V. Aspirin as a therapeutic agent in cardiovascular disease: a statement for healthcare professionals from the American Heart Association. *Circulation*. 1997;96:2751.
308. McCullough PA, Sandberg KR, Borzak S, et al. Benefits of aspirin and beta-blockade after myocardial infarction in patients with chronic kidney disease. *Am Heart J*. 2002;144:226.
309. Yusuf S, Zhao F, Mehta SR, et al. Effects of clopidogrel in addition to aspirin in patients with acute coronary syndromes without ST-segment elevation. *N Engl J Med*. 2001:345:494.
310. Peters RJ, Mehta SR, Fox KA, et al. Effects of aspirin dose when used along or in combination with clopidogrel in patients with acute coronary syndromes: observations from the Clopidogrel in Unstable Angina to Prevent Recurrent Events (CURE) Study. *Circulation*. 2003;108:1682.
311. Koyanagi T, Nishida H, Kitamura M, et al. Comparison of clinical outcomes of coronary artery bypass grafting and percutaneous transluminal coronary angioplasty in renal dialysis patients. *Ann Thorac Surg*. 1996;61:1793.
312. Rinehart AL, Herzog CA, Collins AJ, et al. A comparison of coronary angioplasty and coronary artery bypass grafting outcomes in chronic dialysis patients. *Am J Kidney Dis*. 1995;25:281.
313. Samuels LE, Sharma S, Morris RJ, et al. Coronary artery bypass grafting in patients with chronic renal failure: a reappraisal. *J Card Surg*. 1996;11:128.
314. Owen CH, Cummings RG, Sell TL, et al. Coronary artery bypass grafting in patients with dialysis-dependent renal failure. *Ann Thorac Surg*. 1994;58:1729.
315. Rao V, Weisel RD, Buth KJ, et al. Coronary artery bypass grafting in patients with non-dialysis-dependent renal insufficiency. *Circulation*. 1997;96:38.
316. Zanardo G, Michielon P, Paccagnella A, et al. Acute renal failure in the patient undergoing cardiac operation: prevalence, mortality rate, and main risk factors. *J Thorac Cardiovasc Surg*. 1994;107:1489.
317. Coronary Artery Surgery Study (CASS): a randomized trial of coronary artery bypass surgery. Survival data. *Circulation*. 1983;68:939.
318. Bolman RM, Anderson RW, Molina JE, et al. Cardiac operations in patients with functioning renal allografts. *J Thorac Cardiovasc Surg*. 1984;88:537.
319. Hueb WA, Oliveira SA, Bittencourt D, et al. Coronary bypass surgery for patients with renal transplantation. *Cardiology*. 1986;73:151.
320. Manske Cl, Wang Y, Rector T, et al. Coronary revascularization in insulin-dependent diabetic patients with chronic renal failure. *Lancet*. 1992;340:998.
321. Ahmed WH, Shubrooks SJ, Gibson CM, et al. Complications and long-term outcomes after percutaneous coronary angioplasty in chronic hemodialysis patients. *Am Heart J*. 1994;128:252.
322. Schoebel FC, Gradaus F, Ivens K, et al. Restenosis after elective coronary balloon angioplasty in patients with end stage renal disease: a case-control study using quantitative coronary angiography. *Heart*. 1997;78:337.
323. Szczech LA, Reddan DN, Owen WF, et al. Differential survival after coronary revascularization procedures among patients with renal insufficiency. *Kidney Int*. 2001;60:292.
324. Herzog CA, Ma JZ, Collins AJ. Comparative survival of dialysis patients in the United States after coronary angioplasty, coronary artery stenting, and coronary artery bypass surgery and impact of diabetes. *Circulation*. 2002;106:2207–2211.
325. Appleby CE, Ivanov J, Lavi S, et al. The adverse long-term impact of renal impairment in patients undergoing percutaneous coronary intervention in the drug-eluting stent era. *Circ Cardiovasc Interv*. 2009;2:309–316.
326. Ota T, Umeda H, Yokota S, et al. Relationship between severity of renal impairment and 2 year outcomes after sirolimus-eluting stent implantation. *Am Heart J*. 2009;158:92–98.
327. Shenoy C, Boura J, Orshaw P, Harjai KJ. Drug-eluting stents in patients with chronic kidney disease: a prospective registry study. *PLoS One*. 2010;5:e15070.
328. Charytan DM, Varma MR, Silbaugh TS, et al. Long-term clinical outcomes following drug-eluting or bare-metal stent placement in patients with severely reduced GFR: results of the Massachusetts Data Analysis Centre (Mass-DAC) State Registry. *Am J Kidney Dis*. 2011;57:202–211.
329. Ashrith G, Lee VV, Elayda MA, Reul RM, Wilson JM. Short and long-term outcomes of coronary artery bypass grafting or drug-eluting stent implantation for multivessel coronary artery disease in patients with chronic kidney disease. *Am J Cardiol*. 2010;106:348–353.
330. Hunt SA, Baker DW, Chin MH, et al. ACC/AHA guidelines for the evaluation and management of chronic heart failure in the adult: executive summary. A report of the American College of Cardiology/American Heart Association Task Force on Practice Guidelines (Committee to Revise the 1995 Guidelines for the Evaluation and Management of Heart Failure): Developed in collaboration with the International Society for Heart and Lung Transplantation; endorsed by the Heart Failure Society of America. *Circulation*. 2001;104:2996.
331. Cice G, Ferrara L, D'Andrea A, et al. Carvedilol increases two-year survival in dialysis patients with dilated cardiomyopathy: a prospective, placebo-controlled trial. *J Am Coll Cardiol*. 2003;41:1438.
332. Chan KE, Lazarus JM, Hakim RM. Digoxin associated with mortality in ESRD. *J Am Soc Nephrol*. 2010;21:1550–1559.
333. Chan KE, Lazarus JM, Thadhani R, Hakim RM. Warfarin use associates with increased risk for stroke in hemodialysis patients with atrial fibrillation. *J Am Soc Nephrol*. 2009;20:2223–2232.
334. Reinecke H, Brand E, Mesters R, et al. Dilemmas in the management of atrial fibrillation in chronic kidney disease. *J Am Soc Nephrol*. 2009;20:705–711.
335. Davis TR, Young BA, Eisenberg MS, et al. Outcome of cardiac arrests attended by emergency medical services staff at community outpatient dialysis centers. *Kidney Int*. 2008;73:933–939.
336. Dasgupta A, Montalvo J, Medendorp S, et al. Increased complication rates of cardiac rhythm management devices in ESRD patients. *Am J Kidney Dis*. 2007;49: 656–663.
337. Hreybe H, Ezzeddine R, Bedi M, et al. Renal insufficiency predicts the time to first appropriate defibrillator shock. *Am Heart J*. 2006;151:852–856.
338. Cuculich PS, Sánchez JM, Kerzner R, et al. Poor prognosis for patients with chronic kidney disease despite ICD therapy for the primary prevention of sudden death. *Pacing Clin Electrophysiol*. 2007;30:207–213.
339. Amin MS, Fox AD, Kalahasty G, et al. Benefit of primary prevention implantable cardioverter-defibrillators in the setting of chronic kidney disease: a decision model analysis. *J Cardiovasc Electrophysiol*. 2008;19:1275–1280.
340. Sanders GD, Hlatky MA, Owens DK. Cost-effectiveness of implantable cardioverter defibrillators. *N Engl J Med*. 2005;353:1471–1480.

CHAPTER

80

Metabolic and Endocrine Dysfunctions in Uremia

Eberhard Ritz • Marcin Adamczak • Andrzej Wiecek

PATHOMECHANISMS UNDERLYING ENDOCRINE DISORDERS IN PATIENTS WITH CHRONIC KIDNEY DISEASE

Disturbances of endocrine function in patients with chronic kidney disease may arise from a number of different causes, which are summarized in Table 80.1.

The clinician has at his or her disposal measurements of hormone concentration, which may or may not be abnormal. However, endocrinologic assessment is more than looking at plasma hormone concentrations. Hormone concentrations per se fail to provide a proper assessment of the adequacy of the hormonal state (e.g., hormone concentrations may be inappropriate to the stimulating or suppressing signal, the test may detect inactive hormone isoforms, or the response of the target organ may be abnormal). It is, therefore, indispensable to interpret hormone levels in the appropriate context (e.g., insulin concentration relative to glucose concentration, parathyroid hormone [PTH] in relation to serum ionized calcium concentration, and plasma 1,25-dihydroxycholecalciferol [$1,25(OH)_2D_3$] concentration).

DISORDERS OF CARBOHYDRATE METABOLISM IN PATIENTS WITH CHRONIC KIDNEY DISEASE

In patients with chronic kidney disease (CKD) abnormalities in carbohydrate metabolism are encountered at different levels of the insulin-glucose cascade (Table 80.2). Patients with chronic kidney disease almost always display resistance to the peripheral action of insulin, although the half-life of insulin is prolonged, because insulin removal by the damaged kidney and by the extrarenal organs is impaired so that plasma insulin concentrations tend to be higher.[1,2] The normal response of the β cell to insulin resistance is to increase the secretion of insulin and, therefore, hyperglycemia as a pointer to glucose intolerance is seen only when this adaptive response of β cells fails. In CKD patients, glucose intolerance is seen only in patients who have both insulin resistance and impaired insulin secretion.[3]

Peripheral Resistance to Insulin Action

Peripheral glucose uptake is reduced in uremic patients as shown by the euglycemic insulin clamp technique.[1,2] Peripheral resistance to insulin is seen even in patients with early stages of CKD. It is clinically important, because of its tight correlation to the enhanced cardiovascular risk[4] and to the rate of progression of CKD.[5]

Liver and skeletal muscles are the major sites of peripheral glucose uptake. The liver and, more recently appreciated, the kidney are the major sites of glucose production in the fasting state.[6] Glucose metabolism by the liver is usually not impaired in CKD: hepatic glucose production[2] as well as its suppression by insulin.[2]

The skeletal muscles are the primary sites of decreased insulin sensitivity. The defect is not at the level of the insulin receptor.[7] The defect is presumably at the postreceptor level. As a result, higher levels of insulin will be required to increase glucose uptake.[7]

The insulin-regulated glucose transporter (GLUT-4) in muscle and adipose tissue is unchanged in CKD.[8] In the heart of uremic rats, however, we observed (in unpublished studies) diminished insulin-dependent glucose uptake and unchanged total GLUT-4, but reduced GLUT-4 incorporation into the plasma membrane.

Peripheral resistance to insulin action is often found early in the course of renal disease and is present in the majority of patients with advanced CKD[9] and is markedly improved after several weeks of hemodialysis[10] and of peritoneal dialysis. Sera of uremic patients contain a compound that inhibits glucose metabolism by normal rat adipocytes.[11]

Insulin Secretion and Pancreatic Islet Metabolism

Glucose-induced insulin secretion starts with the uptake of glucose by the β cells, followed by its metabolism and production of adenine triphosphate (ATP), which facilitates closure of ATP-dependent K^+ channels, followed by cell depolarization, and subsequent activation of voltage-sensitive Ca^{++} channels. As a consequence, calcium enters the islets,

TABLE 80.1 **Different Pathomechanisms Underlying Endocrine Disorders in Chronic Kidney Disease**

	Example
Abnormalities of Hormone Production/Catabolism	
Reduced production of hormone in the kidney	Diminished or inappropriate concentrations of $1,25(OH)_2D_3$ and erythropoietin
Reduced production of hormone in extrarenal production sites (testes, ovary)	Diminished concentrations of testosterone and estrogen(s)
Abnormal secretion pattern (pulsatility; circadian rhythm)	PTH, GH, LH
Reactive hypersecretion of hormone to reestablish homeostasis	PTH, FGF 23
Inappropriate hypersecretion due to disturbed feedback	LH, prolactin, corticotropin
Decreased metabolic clearance	Particularly peptide hormones (e.g., PTH, insulin, gastrin, MSH, ghrelin, leptin, adiponectin)
Abnormalities of Hormone Action	
Disturbed activation of prohormones	Proinsulin/insulin, proinsulinlike growth factor 1A, thyroxine (T_4)
Increased isoforms with potentially less bioactivity (from glycosylation, sialylation)	LH
Increased hormone binding proteins reducing availability of free hormone	IGF
Decreased hormone binding proteins increasing availability of free hormone	Leptin
Abnormal target organ response	
Inhibitory factors	$PTH_{1,84}$ versus $PTH_{7,84}$
Changed receptor number, structure, modification	Low parathyroid vitamin D receptor
Disturbed postreceptor steps	Insulin, GH

PTH, parathyroid hormone; GH, growth hormone; LH, luteinizing hormone; FGF 23, fibroblast growth factor 23; MSH, melanocyte stimulating hormone; IGF, insulinlike growth factor.

TABLE 80.2 **Glucose and Insulin Metabolism in Patients with Chronic Kidney Disease**

- Usually normal fasting blood glucose, but tendency for spontaneous hypoglycemia
- Fasting hyperinsulinemia with prolonged insulin half-life and elevated blood levels of proinsulin and C peptide
- Decreased requirement for insulin by diabetic patients
- Usually decreased early, but exaggerated late-insulin response to hyperglycemia induced by oral or intravenous glucose administration
- Elevated plasma immunoreactive glucagon concentration
- Impaired glucose tolerance (decreased peripheral sensitivity to insulin action, but normal suppression of hepatic glucose production by insulin)

causing an acute rise in cytosolic Ca^{++} concentration and secretion of insulin.

PTH impairs insulin secretion in CKD and it is improved when PTH secretion is suppressed.[12] Glucose-induced insulin secretion by pancreatic islets is impaired in parathyroid intact but is normal in PTX uremic rats. Conversely, glucose-induced insulin secretion is impaired in rats with normal renal function treated with PTH.[13]

Islet cells express the vitamin D receptor.[14] Insulin secretion is impaired in vitamin D–deficient rats with normal renal function reversibly with the administration of vitamin D. An acute intravenous administration of $1,25(OH)_2D_3$ to dialysis patients improved early and late phases of insulin secretion.[15]

Insulin Clearance

Insulin is filtered by the glomeruli and reabsorbed in the proximal tubule.[16] Renal insulin clearance (200 mL per minute) exceeds glomerular filtration rate (GFR), indicating additional peritubular uptake.[17] Insulin removal by the kidney accounts for 25% to 40% of total removal.

A decreased metabolic clearance rate of insulin is seen at GFR < 40 mL per minute, and a significant prolongation of insulin half-life is observed at GFR < 20 mL per minute.[18] When dialysis is started, insulin clearance increases.

In CKD patients, diminished renal and extrarenal (liver and muscles) insulin clearance accounts for fasting hyperinsulinemia and higher insulin concentrations, fasting after administration of glucose, and decreased insulin requirements in diabetic patients with impaired renal function.[19]

Hypoglycemia

Episodes of spontaneous hypoglycemia may be seen in diabetic and even in nondiabetic CKD patients.[20] In diabetic patients, decreased degradation of administered insulin may cause excessive blood insulin levels; in diabetics, repeated episodes of hypoglycemia may be the first clinical sign of impaired renal function. Many sulfonylurea compounds or their active metabolites are cleared via the kidney.[21] Appropriate dose adjustment is again necessary, but it is even better to switch the patients to insulin. The sulfonylurea gliquidone is eliminated predominantly by the liver and does not accumulate.

Spontaneous hypoglycemia is also occasionally seen in nondiabetic CKD patients.[20,22] The underlying mechanism is not clear. Poor nutritional status, diminished gluconeogenesis, impaired glycogenolysis, and impaired degradation in insulin may all contribute.[22]

Hypoglycemia may exacerbate the cardiovascular risk via increased adrenergic activity, coronary ischemia, and arrhythmia.[20]

Clinical Consequences

Hyperglycemia and insulin resistance may contribute to accelerated atherogenesis in renal failure. Shinohara et al.[4] followed 183 nondiabetic hemodialysis patients for more than 5 years. Cumulative cardiovascular deaths were significantly more frequent in subjects in the top tertile of insulin resistance assessed by the homeostasis model assessment of insulin resistance (HOMA) technique. The adverse effect of insulin resistance on mortality was independent on body mass, hypertension, and dyslipidemia. Hyperinsulinemia and insulin-resistance contribute to hypertension[23] and lipid abnormalities.

Insulin is also an important regulator of lipoprotein lipase activity and its activity is reduced by insulin deficiency as well as insulin resistance.[24] Lipoprotein lipase plays a major role in triglyceride removal. In patients with CKD, lipoprotein lipase activity is impaired and this is the major cause of hypertriglyceridemia in these patients.

Insulin resistance may also contribute to malnutrition, commonly found in CKD[25] by inflammatory mechanisms.[26,27] Insulin deficiency stimulates muscle breakdown and activates the ubiquitin–proteasome system.[28] Insulin resistance increases salt sensitivity via increased tubular sodium reabsorption and contributes to hypertension.[29]

An interesting link between insulin resistance, metabolic syndrome, and kidney disease as a result of excessive fructose ingestion has recently been proposed by Johnson et al.[30]

DISORDERS OF LIPID METABOLISM IN CHRONIC KIDNEY DISEASE

In the 19th century, Richard Bright[31] commented on the milky aspect of the serum of patients suffering from kidney diseases. After this early observation, dyslipidemia and hyperlipidemia of renal patients had become well known, but only in the recent decades did it attract more general interest after it had been recognized that atherosclerotic complications are extremely frequent in patients with impaired renal function, at least partially as the result of dyslipidemia.

It had long been underappreciated how severe dyslipidemia actually is because measurements were usually restricted to the determination of total cholesterol and triglycerides in plasma. Only today's more sophisticated analyses of lipid subfractions, postprandial lipid changes, apolipoprotein (apo) concentrations, and modification by oxidation, glycation, and carbamylation have fully disclosed the profound and highly atherogenic character of the lipid changes in uremia (Fig. 80.1).

Dyslipoproteinemia was initially attributed to reduced renal function, but it has increasingly been recognized that concomitant pathologies (diabetes, metabolic syndrome, proteinuria, steroid treatment, and genetic background) play an important ancillary role.

Lipid Abnormalities in Kidney Disease

The Spectrum of Dyslipidemia in Uremia

Dyslipidemia in uremia is mainly characterized by:

- Hypertriglyceridemia
- Higher remnant lipoproteins (chylomicron remnants, intermediate density lipoproteins [IDLs])
- Lower high density lipoprotein (HDL) cholesterol
- Higher small dense low density lipoproteins [sd(LDL)], lipoprotein (a) [Lp(a)], apolipoprotein A-IV (apo A-IV)
- Normal plasma LDL cholesterol (except in nephrotic syndrome and in peritoneal dialysis)

(For details, see Table 80.3.)

Exogenous and Endogenous Pathways

The plasma–lipid spectrum is influenced through two different pathways. In the exogenous pathway, dietary lipids transported from the intestine into the systemic circulation yield triglyceride-rich chylomicrons, which are quickly metabolized by endothelium-associated lipoprotein lipase. Chylomicron remnants are taken up by the liver. Chylomicrons, that is, large triglyceride-rich particles of intestinal origin, are only transiently present in plasma in the postprandial state under physiologic conditions. In CKD patients, the

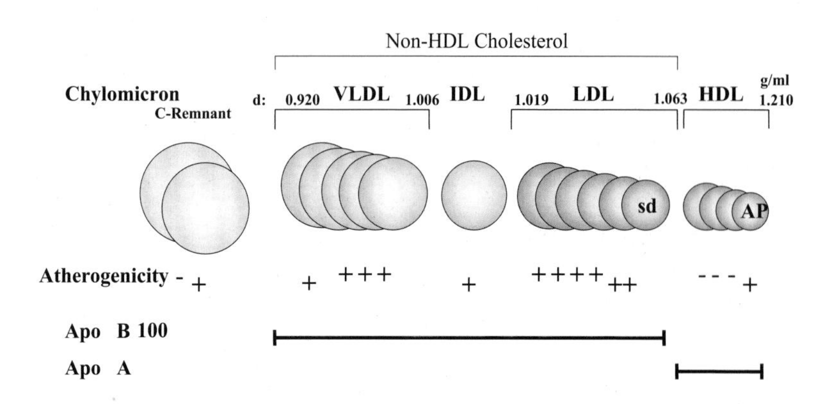

FIGURE 80.1 The atherogenicity of major lipoprotein classes. *HDL,* high density lipoprotein; *Apo,* apolipoprotein; *VLDL,* very low density lipoprotein; *IDL,* intermediate density lipoprotein; *LDL,* low density lipoprotein. (From Otvos J. Measurement of triglyceride-rich lipoproteins by nuclear magnetic resonance spectroscopy. *Clin Cardiol.* 1999;22:21, with permission.)

clearance of chylomicrons is severely impaired.[32] This abnormality contributes to the hypertriglyceridemia in CKD.

In the endogenous pathway, the liver synthesizes and secretes triglyceride-rich very low density lipoproteins (VLDLs) for export from the liver to peripheral tissues. Chylomicrons are metabolized stepwise to yield IDLs, which are either further converted into LDL particles or taken up by the liver (Fig. 80.2). This pathway is severely disturbed in CKD and end-stage renal disease (ESRD).

TABLE 80.3 **Abnormalities of Lipid Metabolism in Patients with Chronic Kidney Disease**

Quantitative Changes in Plasma Lipid Profile
Moderate elevation of plasma triglyceride concentrations
Low plasma HDL cholesterol concentration
High plasma VLDL and IDL cholesterol
Normal plasma LDL cholesterol
High ratio total cholesterol/HDL cholesterol
High ratio LDL cholesterol/HDL cholesterol
Quantitative Changes in Plasma Lipoproteins
Decreased plasma concentrations of apo A-I and A-II
Normal or elevated plasma concentration of apo B
High plasma concentrations of apo C-I, C-II, and C-III
Postprandial Changes in Plasma Lipoproteins
Prolonged persistence of chylomicrons in the circulation postprandially
Qualitative Lipoprotein Changes
Postribosomal modification of apolipoproteins by oxidation, glycation, and carbamylation
Alteration in HDL component (changed it from antioxidant to pro-oxidant lipoprotein)
Accumulation of small dense LDL
Atherogenic apo A phenotype (low molecular weight)

LDL, low density lipoprotein; VLDL, very low density lipoprotein; IDL, intermediate density lipoprotein; HDL, high density lipoprotein; apo, apolipoprotein.

Lipid Spectrum

The lipid spectrum in kidney disease is characterized by quantitative and qualitative changes.

Triglycerides. Triglycerides start to increase in early stages of CKD.[33] They are more strikingly increased in advanced CKD and dialysis, specifically in peritoneal dialysis, and are highest in the nephrotic syndrome. Chylomicrons and VLDL are enriched in triglycerides. This reflects both abnormalities in particle production and in the low fractional catabolic rate of particles. Their reduced fractional catabolic rate is caused by the lower activity of lipoprotein lipase (LPL) and of the hepatic triglyceride lipase. In part, this is the result of the increased apo C-III/apo C-II ratio; apo C-III inhibits and apo C-II activates LPL. The result is an accumulation of intermediate particles, (e.g., chylomicron remnants and IDLs).

High density lipoprotein. In patients with CKD, HDL cholesterol concentrations are commonly reduced and this is accompanied by an abnormal spectrum of HDL subfractions resulting from low apo A-I levels and decreased lecithin:cholesterol acyltransferase (LCAT) activity with consecutive diminishing of esterification of free cholesterol and conversion of HDL_3 to HDL_2. In uremia, HDLs are modified by paraoxonase, inhibiting the oxidation of LDLs, and by inflammation, converting HDLs from antioxidant in pro-oxidant particles. HDL particles are involved in reverse cholesterol transport from the periphery (e.g., cell membranes) to the liver. The apo A lipoprotein in HDL activates LCAT, which esterifies cholesterol and facilitates transport.

Apo lipoprotein A-IV. Apo A-IV is synthesized in the small intestine and protects against atherosclerosis by promoting reverse cholesterol transport from the periphery to the liver. It is an activator of LCAT. The beneficial effect of high plasma apo A-IV levels is illustrated by the inverse relationship between apo A-IV and coronary artery disease in healthy individuals and in uremia.[34] Low apo A-IV also correlates to progression in CKD.[35]

Low density lipoprotein. Elevated LDL is not a typical feature in CKD and ESRD (except in patients with nephrotic syndrome). Behind normal LDL concentrations are hidden

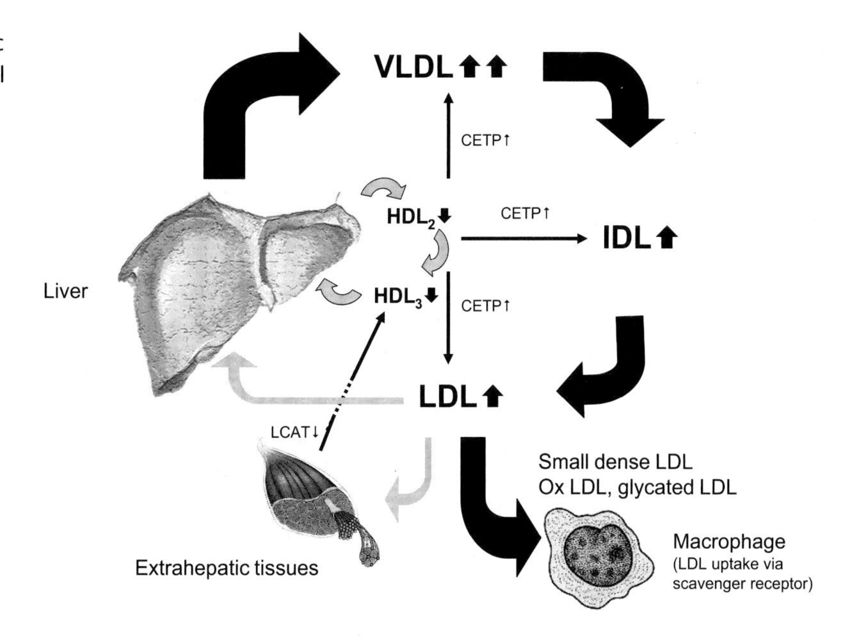

FIGURE 80.2 Lipoprotein metabolism in chronic kidney disease patients. *LCAT*, lecithin-cholesterol acyltransferase; *CETP*, cholesterol ester transfer protein; *LPL*, lipoprotein lipase; *VLDL*, very low density lipoproteins; *IDL*, intermediate density lipoprotein; *LDL*, low density lipoproteins.

qualitative changes, particularly an increased proportion of atherogenic sdLDL and IDL. Not only the activity of lipoprotein lipase, however, but also the activity of hepatic triglyceride lipase is decreased in animal models and patients with CKD.[36,37] The decreased activities of both lipases cause a major defect in the catabolism of triglyceride-rich lipoproteins. Reduced lipoprotein lipase activity explains the disturbed first step in the breakdown of both chylomicrons (circulating after the absorption of fat from the gut) and of VLDL (synthesized and secreted by the liver). Because of the reduced activity of the hepatic triglyceride lipase, the second step (i.e., the clearance of partially metabolized lipoproteins and chylomicrons) is disturbed as well. The VLDL receptor is expressed in skeletal muscle, the heart, the brain, and adipose tissue, which use fatty acids for energy production or storage. The expression of the VLDL receptor was reduced in experimental uremia.[38] In addition to quantitative changes in lipoprotein particles, several qualitative lipoprotein changes have been demonstrated to occur in CKD. These include postribosomal modification of apos by oxidation, glycation, and carbamylation. Modified lipoproteins are not recognized by their respective receptors.[39] Their half-life in the circulation is increased. The prolonged residence time in the circulation permits their uptake by the nonsaturable scavenger receptor pathway. Oxidation does not reduce the affinity of oxidized LDL to the scavenger receptor, and oxidized LDL uptake by the macrophage scavenger receptor is increased, thus favoring the formation of foam cells. In addition to its pivotal role in foam cell formation, oxidized LDL exhibits additional atherogenic properties, including cytotoxicity and stimulation of thrombotic as well as inflammatory events.[40] LDL oxidation is currently considered as an early key event in the pathogenesis of atherosclerosis. HDL protects against oxidation of LDL. In hemodialysis patients, the capacity of HDL to prevent LDL oxidation is reduced, however.

Lipoprotein (a). Lipoprotein (Lp)(a) is an LDL-like lipoprotein consisting of apo A covalently bound to an LDL particle. The plasma Lp(a) concentrations are strongly determined by genetic factors: individuals with the high molecular weight isoform have lower plasma Lp(a) concentrations and plasma Lp(a) levels begin to start to rise early in CKD. The increase is more delayed in individuals with low molecular weight isoforms. The level of Lp(a) is determined by the degree of proteinuria.[41,42] Furthermore, the turnover of Lp(a) is reduced, causing increasing residence time.[43] In prospective studies, Kronenberg et al.[44] and Longenecker et al.[45] found in hemodialysis patients that the small apo A genotype predicted coronary events and total mortality.

Predictive Parameters

Disorders of lipid metabolism in chronic kidney disease are not adequately reflected by the simple conventionally measured parameters (i.e., plasma concentrations of total cholesterol, LDL-cholesterol, and triglycerides). The previous parameters do not provide information on further lipid abnormalities, which almost certainly impact on the atherogenic risk: (1) abnormal concentrations of apolipoproteins (low apo A-I and apo A-II; and high apo B, apo C-II, and apo E serum concentrations); (2) postribosomal modification of apolipoproteins by oxidation, glycation, and carbamylation; (3) inflammation-induced alterations of HDL (transforming HDL from an antioxidant to a prooxidant lipoprotein); (4) accumulation of IDL and small, dense LDLs; (5) prolonged postprandial persistence of chylomicrons in the circulation; and (6) atherogenic apo A genotypes (Table 80.3).

Shoji et al.[46] demonstrated that the plasma IDL concentration is an independent risk factor for aortic atherosclerosis as determined by pulse-wave Doppler sonography and proposed non-HDL cholesterol (i.e., the sum of LDL and VLDL cholesterol, as a predictor [target < 130 mg per deciliter]).

Epidemiology

The constellation of (1) high plasma LDL cholesterol, (2) low HDL cholesterol, and (3) high triglycerides increase the risk of cardiovascular atherosclerosis.[47] The correlation between lipid concentrations and cardiovascular (CV) events is not very strong, however, possibly because apos may be more important than the lipid parts of the particles or because prolonged residence time permits the modification of the particles.

The recently proposed index of non-HDL cholesterol reflects the sum of LDL and VLDL particles and appears to be more sensitive. It is a superior predictor of cardiovascular risk (Table 80.3).[48,49]

Dialysis modalities and lipid profile. In hemodialyzed patients, the improvement of dyslipidemia has also been documented in patients with the studies addressing alternative dialysis treatment modalities (e.g., comparing of conventional hemodialysis against hemodialysis using high-flux membranes)[50] and also nocturnal hemodialysis.[51] A randomized crossover study showed that treatment with high-flux polysulfone and modified cellulose membranes significantly lowered serum triglyceride concentration when compared with low-flux dialysis with polysulfone membrane.

In patients treated with continuous ambulatory peritoneal dialysis (CAPD), the concentrations of total plasma cholesterol, LDL cholesterol, and triglycerides are even higher than in hemodialysis patients.[52,53] Such aggravation is most likely due to two additional factors: a loss of protein (7 to 14 g per day) with peritoneal dialysate and the absorption of glucose (150 to 200 mg per day) from the dialysis fluid. The protein loss may concern not only albumin, but also apolipoproteins, and possibly further lipoprotein-regulating substances, as occurs in the nephrotic syndrome. The glucose load increases the availability of free fatty acids and stimulates the synthesis of triglycerides and lipoproteins by the liver. This hypothesis is supported by the observation that conversion of patients from conventional glucose-containing dialysis fluids to icodextrin-containing dialysis fluids in the overnight dwell reduced plasma cholesterol concentrations.[54]

Dyslipidemia and Outcome—An Example of Reverse Epidemiology

Following the seminal report of Degoulet et al.,[55] numerous investigators found a paradoxical inverse relationship between plasma cholesterol concentration and overall mortality, as well as cardiovascular mortality.[56,57] Usually a U- or J-shaped relationship was noted between plasma cholesterol concentration and cardiovascular mortality (i.e., a higher mortality at low as well as high plasma cholesterol concentrations).[56] The most plausible explanation for this paradox is that this represents an example of reverse epidemiology[58] (i.e., a relationship that is reversed by a confounding factor). The work of Liu et al.[59] is important in this respect.[59] They identified microinflammation as a major confounding factor. In dialysis patients with low high sensitivity C-reactive protein (hs) CRP concentrations, a direct positive relation was noted between LDL cholesterol and cardiovascular mortality as in individuals with no renal disease. In contrast, in patients with high hsCRP concentrations, the mortality was higher at low LDL cholesterol concentrations.[59] This finding is important because in such circumstances, serum cholesterol and LDL cholesterol concentrations may no longer be a valid guide to establish the indication for lipid-lowering therapy.

Treatment of Dyslipidemia in Renal Failure

In the treatment of dyslipidemia in patients with CKD and ESRD, the best documented intervention of high current interest is the administration of statins. Because of the negative outcome of past intervention trials in dialysis patients (4D and AURORA), the indication for lipid lowering had not been evidence based until recently. There is no doubt that in early stages of renal dysfunction, lipid lowering by statins provides a benefit by significantly lowering cardiovascular events and possibly even the progression of CKD.[60,61,62] In dialysis patients, however, the overall outcome (cardiovascular mortality) in two underpowered studies on the use of statins (i.e., atorvastatin in the 4D study[63] and rosuvastatin in the AURORA study[64]) was negative. But, after approximately 3 years, there was a delayed nonsignificant tendency for fewer coronary events. A major drawback was that coronary events (the primary treatment target) accounted only for approximately 10% of mortality, whereas the contribution of sudden death and other noncoronary causes of cardiac death was approximately 30%.

Today, the results of the sufficiently powered Study of Heart and Renal Protection (SHARP) have clarified the dilemma. The SHARP study recruited about 8,000 patients (i.e., CKD patients or dialysis patients).[65] A significant overall survival benefit was found in patients treated with atorvastatin (± ezetimibe) and this will be reported soon.

Which other intervention strategies do we have? There is no doubt that dyslipidemia in patients with advanced CKD can be modified by dietary interventions. A reduced intake of saturated fatty acids and carbohydrates reverses VLDL overproduction by the liver and thus lowers plasma triglyceride levels.[66] Caloric restriction will also achieve weight loss and improve lipid levels in obese patients with advanced CKD. Both interventions have not gained universal acceptance,[67] however, because of their obvious side effects, particularly catabolism. Another nonpharmacologic approach is physical exercise, which has been shown to reduce insulin resistance and improve the lipid pattern in CKD patients, just as it does in nonrenal patients.[68] In our experience, however, adherence to this intervention is less than optimal.

What is the role of alternative pharmacologic treatments?

The spectrum of dyslipidemia of renal patients is mainly characterized by low HDL and high triglycerides. This constellation would require an a priori call for medications that increase HDL and decrease triglyceride concentrations.

Current efforts in cardiology target cholesteryl ester transfer protein (CETP) to raise HDL cholesterol levels in order to overcome residual dyslipidemia despite statin therapy.[69] Although the outcome of the effect of torcetrapib on glucose, insulin, and hemoglobin A1c in subjects in the ILLUMINATE study was negative,[70] presumably resulting from "off target" side effects of torcetrapib, novel agents also targeting CETP (e.g., dalcetrapib, anacetrapib) are currently under investigation.[69]

There are further interesting approaches (e.g., maturation of HDL with the orally absorbable amphipathic apo A-I mimetic peptide 4F).[71]

The pattern of hypertriglyceridemia associated with low-plasma HDL cholesterol concentration appears, at first sight, as an ideal indication for peroxisome proliferator-activated receptor alpha (PPAR-α) agonists (i.e., fibrates). Fibrates mimic the structure of free fatty acids and increase the HDL cholesterol concentration up to 20%, in part by reducing plasma CETP activity as a result of modulating CETP gene expression through the activation of PPAR-α.[69] Fibrates reduce inflammation markers independently of effects on lipid and glucose metabolism.[72] The problem is that fibrates accumulate in renal insufficiency. Therefore, except for gemfibrozil, the dose must be reduced in CKD patients depending on the level of GFR.[73] Fibrates may cause massive rhabdomyolysis with acute renal failure[74,75] and deterioration of kidney function even in the absence of rhabdomyolysis.[76] Therefore, fibrates are no longer recommended for treatment in CKD patients.

Nicotinic acid (niacin) lowers elevated concentrations of triglyceride-rich lipoproteins, (i.e., IDL, LDL, and Lp[a]); in addition, it raises HDL dose dependently by up to 30%.[77] Upregulation of apo A-I at HDL-C is the result of (1) the upregulation of apo A-I production, (2) the inhibition of hormone-sensitive triglyceride lipase in adipose tissue, and (3) the reduction of plasma CETP activity. Unfortunately, nicotinic acid frequently causes side effects, particularly flushing and occasionally worsening glucose tolerance and hepatotoxicity. Studies investigating the effect of nicotinic acid in hemodialysis patients are sparse.[78,79,80] Currently, nicotinic acid analogs with fewer side effects are under investigation.

DISORDERS OF PROTEIN AND AMINO ACID METABOLISM IN CHRONIC KIDNEY DISEASE

Nutrients can be divided into six general classes: proteins, lipids, carbohydrates, minerals, vitamins, and water. The first three classes serve as sources of energy required for carrying out the biochemical and functional activities of organs and cells. In addition to being an energy source, proteins in the diet provide the amino acids that are used to synthesize body proteins. Proteins and their constituent amino acids are essential to life.

The protein requirement of an individual is defined as the lowest level of dietary protein intake that will balance the losses of nitrogen from the body and maintain energy balance at modest levels of physical activity. The need for dietary protein largely arises because turnover of tissue and organ proteins is accompanied by an inefficient capture of their constituent amino acids to form new body proteins. The amino acids are lost via oxidative metabolism. Most estimates of protein and amino acid requirements in humans have been obtained directly or indirectly from measurements of nitrogen balance. In the course of carrying out their functional roles, proteins and amino acids turn over, and part of their nitrogen and carbon is lost via excretory pathways. This includes carbon dioxide in expired air and urea and ammonium in urine. Thus, to maintain an adequate protein and amino acid balance, these losses must be replaced by an appropriate dietary supply of a usable source of nitrogen and by indispensable and conditionally indispensable amino acids. These are required to replace amino acids that are lost during the course of metabolic processes or those that are deposited during growth and tissue replacement. Adults in stable conditions synthesize and degrade approximately 3.5 to 4.5 g of protein per kilogram of body weight (i.e., 245 to 315 g of protein in a 70-kg adult person) each day.[81] The protein content of muscle is about 20%. Therefore, the daily protein turnover is the equivalent of 1.2 to 2 kg of muscle. Because protein turnover is so large, even a small increase in protein degradation or a decrease in the protein synthesis rate, persisting for longer periods, can cause a marked loss of lean body mass.

The essential amino acids are valine, leucine, isoleucine, threonine, methionine, phenylalanine, lysine, tryptophan, and histidine. The nonessential amino acids are glycine, alanine, serine, cystine, aspartic acid, glutamic acid, and hydroxyproline. A third category, conditionally indispensable, is based on the observation that under specific dietary conditions, function is best maintained when these amino acids are part of nutrient intake. These conditionally indispensable amino acids are glycine, cystine, tyrosine, proline, arginine, citrulline, glutamine, and taurine.[82]

Recently, the concept of protein-energy wasting (PEW) has been introduced by The International Society Of Clinical Nutrition and Metabolism.[83] PEW is characterized by the loss of adequate nutrient intake, decreased body protein, and reduced body energy reserves as a cause of malnutrition and/or inflammation. PEW is estimated to be present in 6% to 8% of ESRD patients. The diagnostic criteria for PEW are given in Table 80.4.

In catabolic conditions, Du et al.[84] identified activation of caspase 3 as the initial step triggering accelerated muscle proteolysis in catabolic conditions of different causes (including fasting, cancer cachexia, streptozotocin diabetes,

TABLE 80.4 **Indices of Protein–Energy Wasting in Patients with Chronic Kidney Disease**

Biochemical Parameters
Plasma albumin concentration < 3.8 g/dL
Plasma transthyretin concentration < 30 mg/dL
Plasma cholesterol concentration < 100 mg/dL
Body Mass
Body mass index < 22 kg/m^2 (for ≤ 65 years) or < 23 kg/m^2 (for > 65 years)
Unintentional weight loss over time; ≥ 5% in 3 months or ≥ 10% in 6 months
Total body fat percentage < 10%
Muscle Mass
Muscle wasting; reduced muscle mass ≥ 5% in 3 months or ≥ 10% in 6 months
Reduced midarm muscle circumference area; > 10 % reduction in relation to 50th percentile of reference population
Dietary Intake
Unintentional low dietary protein intake < 0.80 g/kg/d for at least 2 months for maintenance dialysis patients or < 0.60 g/kg/d for patients with CKD stages 2 to 5 with ≤ 5g/d of urinary protein loss
Unintentional low dietary energy intake < 25 kcal/kg/d for at least 2 months

CKD, chronic kidney disease.

and uremia induced by subtotal nephrectomy).[85] A common set of genes (atrogenes) was affected in these catabolic states, including polyubiquitins, ubiquitin ligases, and others, suggesting that different types of muscle atrophies shared a common transcription program.[86]

Abnormalities in Plasma and Intracellular Amino Acid Concentrations in Chronic Kidney Disease

Some disturbances in the amino acids' plasma concentrations are observed in chronic kidney disease even before renal replacement therapy is started.[87] The severity of amino acid abnormalities is related to the degree of chronic kidney disease and the presence of uremic symptoms.[88]

Plasma concentrations of tryptophan, tyrosine, and the branched-chain amino acids, particularly valine, are low in chronic renal failure[87] and plasma concentrations of citrulline, methylhistidine, and the sulfur-containing amino acids, cystine, and methionine, are high.[87,89,90] In summary, plasma concentrations of essential amino acids, with some exceptions, tend to be decreased, whereas plasma concentrations of the nonessential amino acids tend to be increased. The pattern of the plasma amino acid concentrations does not accurately reflect the intracellular pattern.[91] The intracellular concentrations of valine, threonine, tyrosine, and taurine in muscle are decreased[92] as a result of acidosis. The concentrations of phenylalanine, alanine, arginine, and citrulline are increased.[92] The molecular pathways of muscle wasting with CKD have been reviewed by Workeneh and Mitch.[93]

In CKD patients, low plasma amino acid concentrations and low intracellular amino acid concentrations may be due to: (1) anorexia, (2) decreased amino acid synthesis, (3) increased catabolism, (4) loss during the dialysis procedure, and (5) impaired binding to serum albumin caused by substances that accumulate in the blood in uremia.

As in nonuremic individuals, in CKD patients, poor dietary intake of protein and nutrients leads also to decreased concentrations of such amino acids as histidine, isoleucine, leucine, valine, and tyrosine.[94] In CKD patients, the plasma concentrations of several amino acids are inversely correlated with protein intake.[95]

In rats with experimental chronic renal disease, the principal cause of low plasma concentrations of branched-chain amino acids (valine, leucine, isoleucine) is increased catabolism.[92] This is stimulated by acidosis and is caused by increased activity of branched-chain keto acid dehydrogenase, a key enzyme in the amino acid degradation pathway.[92] The correction of metabolic acidosis increases the concentration of the previous three amino acids in muscle.[96] Reduced binding by albumin probably accounts for the low total plasma tryptophan concentration.[97] Also, low intracellular levels of taurine with normal or slightly elevated concentrations of this amino acid in plasma are found in CKD patients. Because the plasma concentration of precursors of taurine, such as cystine, methionine, and cystine sulfonic acid are elevated, a selective metabolic block at the level of cystine sulfonic acid decarboxylase has been proposed to explain the decrease in intracellular taurine.[98] In addition, low intracellular levels of threonine and lysine and low ratios of essential to nonessential amino acids (valine–glycine and phenylalanine–tyrosine) have been found in patients with CKD.[99]

Protein Metabolism in Chronic Kidney Disease

The detailed observations of renal patients by Richard Bright[100] pointed to an important role of inanition in kidney disease. More recently, a high prevalence of protein malnutrition has been reported in hemodialysis patients as well. Mild-to-moderate protein malnutrition occurs in approximately 33% of hemodialysis patients and severe malnutrition occurs in an additional 6% to 8% of these individuals.[101] The interpretation, however, of what constitutes malnutrition and how it relates to patient outcome remains controversial.[102] Pure-energy protein malnutrition (kwashiorkor) is not associated with accelerated atherogenesis and cardiovascular events. These events, however, are commonly found in wasted dialysis patients and are associated with markers of microinflammation, such as high hsCRP, low plasma concentrations of albumin and fetuin, as well as high plasma concentrations of interleukin (IL)-6, IL-18, and tumor necrosis factor (TNF)-α.[103] This constellation has been rephrased as the malnutrition, inflammation, and atherosclerosis (MIA) syndrome.[104] It has remained uncertain, however, whether low muscle and body mass per se[105] or rather the process of active wasting have negative effects on outcome.[104] The paradoxical finding that survival is best in dialysis patients with a high body mass index (BMI), even in the range of frank obesity, may indicate that obesity increases tolerance toward episodes of catabolism. Energy expenditure is increased in uremia.[105] In addition, some factors common in uremic patients may trigger catabolism, such as fasting resulting from a loss of appetite. Acidosis or insulin resistance activates the ubiquitin proteasome system as the final common pathway of protein breakdown.[86] It is important that proteolytic mechanisms, not malnutrition caused by loss of muscle mass in chronic renal failure[106] with insulin resistance, triggered the activation of the ubiquitin proteasome pathway as an upstream component.[107] There is also evidence that the dialysis procedure per se is a catabolic stimulus.[108] A study by Pupim at al.[109] confirmed that dialysis causes whole body and muscle proteolysis, which can be overcome, at least acutely, by an intravenous infusion of amino acids, glucose, and lipids.

The rates of synthesis and degradation of proteins can be quantitated by the infusion of either radiolabeled or stable isotopes bearing amino acids. This allows the calculation of total body protein synthesis and total average proteolysis, as well as amino acid oxidation.[110] Patients with stable CKD have been studied using this methodology when ingesting either of two different levels of dietary protein: 0.6 g per kilogram of body weight or 1.0 g per kilogram of body weight. Studies were performed both after overnight fasting and in the fed state. No differences were found in either the rate of protein turnover or the amino acid oxidation as compared to control subjects. Thus, the dynamics of amino acid metabolism are apparently normal at the whole body level in stable, nonacidotic patients with chronic kidney disease.[111]

In contrast to nondialyzed, stable CKD patients, nitrogen balance studies indicate that hemodialysis patients are unable to conserve nitrogen normally and have increased dietary requirements.[112] The increased protein needs are higher than accounted for by a loss of amino acids, peptides, and proteins into the dialysate. These findings are consistent with the existence of a chronic, low-grade catabolic state in hemodialysis patients. Such a catabolic state may be due to the presence of chronic inflammation, acidosis, insulin resistance, or a combination of these conditions.[113]

When protein intake is restricted, supplemental calories may improve nitrogen balance.[114] If calorie intake is inadequate in patients eating a low protein diet, the risk of catabolizing body protein is increased.[114]

Caloric Requirements in Patients with Chronic Kidney Disease

Inadequate caloric intake may be present when energy requirements are increased, when caloric intake is decreased, or when a combination of both is present.

In a study on 10 hemodialysis patients, Ikizler et al.[108] found 7% higher than expected energy expenditure during both dialysis and nondialysis days, suggesting that uremia per se increases energy expenditure. This conclusion is controversial, however. Monteon et al.[115] measured energy expenditure of CKD patients during rest and exercise; CKD patients did not differ from control subjects. This issue may be clinically important, because a prospective study showed a correlation between high resting energy expenditure and increased mortality or cardiovascular death in patients on continuous ambulatory peritoneal dialysis.[116]

In CKD patients, caloric intake tends to be decreased.[117] CKD patients do not ingest a prescribed amount of calories despite dietary counseling: in the Modification of Diet in Renal Disease (MDRD) study, initial energy intake was below the recommended limit (30 to 35 kcal per kilogram of body weight per day) and, during the study, energy intake declined further despite intensive dietary counseling.[118]

Nutrition in Hemodialysis Patients

Hypercatabolism is common in dialysis patients and is presumably related to an intradialytic loss of amino acids, as well as cytokine activation, particularly IL-6. There is an interesting dichotomy: muscle protein breakdown increases during hemodialysis, whereas whole-body proteolysis is not increased.[119] It has been suggested that avoiding a negative protein balance requires both the provision of nutrients and the inhibition of inflammatory signals.[119] Hypoalbuminemia, negative nitrogen balance, loss of muscle mass, and wasting are commonly seen in long-term dialysis patients.[119] Several tests have been used to diagnose PEW, but they do not exactly measure the same abnormality.[102] The procedures range from the well-known anthropometric measurements, such as skinfold thickness and midarm muscle circumference, BMI, waist-to-hip ratio, to a subjective global assessment. Low plasma albumin concentrations are closely related to mortality,[120] whereas BMI and urine creatinine excretion as an index of muscle mass are not. Even small decrements in plasma albumin concentration (in the range of 3.5 to 3.9 g per deciliter) have been associated with increased mortality in hemodialysis patients. The plasma albumin concentration appears to be a late index of malnutrition. Because of its relatively long half-life (21 days) and the vast capacity of the liver to synthesize albumin, a decrease in serum albumin concentration lags behind the onset of malnutrition by several months.[121] Other indicators of PEW include prealbumin levels, plasma cholesterol concentrations (< 150 mg per deciliter), decreased plasma transferrin, and a decrease in body weight.[102] Indices of PEW in CKD patients undergoing renal replacement therapy are shown in Table 80.4.

TABLE 80.5 Factors That Affect the Nutritional Status of Patients with Chronic Kidney Disease

Gastrointestinal Disturbances
Anorexia
Gastroparesis and delayed gastric emptying
Malabsorption
Esophagitis, gastritis
Intestinal bacterial colonization
Subjective feeling of fullness from dialysate in the abdomen (in peritoneal dialysis patients)
Biochemical Derangements
Metabolic acidosis
Low grade inflammation
Insulin resistance
Iatrogenic Factors
Dialysate amino acids, protein and glucose losses
Bioincompatibility of dialysis membranes
Multiple medications, particularly sedatives
Other Factors
Long-term, low protein intake
Low socioeconomic status
Depression
Underlying illness
Frequent hospitalizations

Factors That Affect Nutritional Status in Chronic Kidney Disease

Several factors contribute to the high prevalence of PEW in CKD patients (Table 80.5). The catabolic factors that may participate in the pathogenesis of PEW in CKD are (1) metabolic acidosis, (2) inflammation, (3) insulin resistance, (4) dialysate loss of amino acids and glucose losses, and (5) bioincompatibility of dialysis membrane.

Metabolic acidosis is one of the most important factors causing excessive catabolism of amino acids and proteins in CKD patients. Metabolic acidosis activates the specific pathways involved in the degradation of branched-chain amino acids catalyzed by branched-chain keto acid dehydrogenase.[92] It also activates the ubiquitin–proteasome system, the final common pathway of muscle protein degradation.[122] Profound acidemia following the ingestion of ammonium chloride causes cachexia in humans without CKD.[123] Conversely, in CKD patients, correction of metabolic acidosis decreases protein degradation considerably.[124] Long-term therapy with a higher concentration of lactate buffer in peritoneal dialysate caused decreased expression of mRNA encoding ubiquitin in muscle.[125] Correction of metabolic acidosis by oral sodium bicarbonate supplementation in dialysis patients increases plasma albumin concentration and muscle mass,[126] and may even slow down progression in CKD.[127,128]

In a sizable proportion of hemodialyzed patients, high plasma concentration of proinflammatory cytokines are found[129] (e.g., high TNF-α, which are known to stimulate protein degradation in muscle). Another factor is insulin resistance. Absence of, and potentially resistance to, insulin stimulates the ubiquitin–proteasome system, that is, the common proteolytic pathway, in muscle.[28]

The hemodialysis procedure may also be catabolic. Protein breakdown is acutely stimulated during a dialysis session.[105] This effect may be mediated, at least in part, via complement activation by contact between blood and bioincompatible membranes.[130] The use of more biocompatible dialysis membranes may prevent PEW by reducing complement activation. Unfortunately, two long-term, prospective studies on this issue yielded conflicting results,[131,132] and the issue of the relation between bioincompatibility and malnutrition remains a matter of debate.

A further important factor contributing to malnutrition in CKD patients is a loss of appetite. Changes in the motility and function of the gastrointestinal tract, including gastroparesis, malabsorption, intestinal bacterial colonization, and constipation, are further contributory factors.

Dietary and Energy Intake Recommended in Patients Undergoing Dialysis Replacement Therapy

The recommended nutrient intake for patients undergoing maintenance hemodialysis or peritoneal dialysis is summarized in Table 80.6.[133]

ENDOCRINE DISORDERS IN CHRONIC KIDNEY DISEASE

Abnormalities in the Hormones of the Hypothalamic–Pituitary–Gonadal Axis

Both female and male CKD patients present a variety of derangements of the hypothalamic–pituitary–gonadal axis (Table 80.7). In males, these abnormalities are involved in the pathogenesis of impotence and gynecomastia. In females, these abnormalities account for anovulatory menstrual cycles and infertility.

The Hypothalamic–Pituitary–Gonadal Axis in Male Chronic Kidney Disease Patients

Luteinizing Hormone

In CKD, the lack of appropriate cyclic release of gonadotropin-releasing hormone (GnRH) by the hypothalamus leads to a loss of normal pulsatile luteinizing hormone (LH) release by the pituitary, which results in impaired ovulation in women and reduced testosterone and sperm production in men.[134] The cause of impaired cyclic release of GnRH is unclear, but

TABLE 80.6 **Recommended Dietary Protein and Energy Intake for Patients Undergoing Maintenance Hemodialysis or Peritoneal Dialysis**

	Maintenance Hemodialysis	Continuous Ambulatory or Cyclic Peritoneal Dialysis
Protein	1.2 g/kg/d ≥50% high biologic-value protein	1.2–1.3 g/kg/d ≥50% high biologic-value protein Unless a patient has demonstrated adequate protein nutritional status on 1.2 g/kg/d diet, 1.3 g/kg/d should be prescribed
Energy	≥ 35 kcal/kg/d 30 to 35 kcal/kg/d for patients 60 years or older	

Based on Kidney diseases outcomes quality initiative clinical practice guidelines for nutrition in chronic renal failure. *Am J Kidney Dis.* 2000;35[suppl 2].

hyperprolactinemia, elevated endorphins, and high levels of GnRH and LH caused mainly by reduced clearance may contribute.[134]

In the majority of CKD patients, basal plasma LH concentrations are higher by a factor of approximately 1.5 to 2 compared with healthy controls. Such concentrations approach the concentrations in patients with primary hypogonadism. High plasma LH concentrations in CKD are mainly due to a decreased rate of catabolism of LH[135] and, conversely, its half-life of LH in CKD is increased by a factor of 2 to 4 compared to normal subjects.[135] Apart from an abnormal basal LH concentration, there is also an abnormality of pulsatile LH secretion. Schaefer et al.[136] found decreased amplitudes of the secretory bursts of bioactive and immunoreactive LH, but no change in the number of bursts.

LH stimulates the production of testosterone by the Leydig cells of the testes. Testosterone, in turn, exerts negative feedback control on the secretion of GnRH and, secondarily, on LH. Low plasma testosterone concentration in CKD[137] may, therefore, contribute to the elevation of LH concentration.

TABLE 80.7 **Abnormalities of the Hypothalamic–Pituitary–Gonadal Axis in Patients with Chronic Kidney Disease**

	Male	Female
Basal prolactin	↑	↑
Prolactin response to TRH	↓	↓ and delayed
Prolactin suppression test	Impaired	Impaired
Basal FSH	↑	N
FSH response to GnRH	N but delayed	N
Basal LH	↑	↑
LH response to GnRH	N	N
Testosterone	↓	—
Estradiol	N	↓
Progesterone	—	↓

TRH, thyrotropin-releasing hormone; FSH, follicle-stimulating hormone; GnRH, gonadotropin-releasing hormone; LH, luteinizing hormone; N, normal.

Follicle-Stimulating Hormone

In CKD patients, the basal plasma concentrations of follicle-stimulating hormone (FSH) are in the upper normal range or elevated.[134] FSH is important for spermatogenesis. It stimulates testicular growth and increases the production of testosterone-binding protein by Sertoli cells. In testicular tubules, FSH accounts for the high local concentrations of testosterone required for sperm maturation. In CKD patients, spermatogenesis is impaired despite elevated blood levels of FSH,[134] a finding that is consistent with the following explanations: (1) resistance of the testis to the action of FSH causes testicular damage with a consequent increase in FSH concentrations, and/or (2) testicular damage is the primary abnormality and the elevated FSH concentrations represent the normal response of the hypothalamic–pituitary axis. In either case, the negative feedback between testes and the hypothalamic–pituitary axis appears to be normal in CKD.

Prolactin

Plasma prolactin concentrations are elevated in the majority (40% to 70%) of male hemodialysis patients.[138] As CKD progresses, elevated plasma prolactin concentrations correlate with plasma creatinine concentration.[139] Apart from elevated basal prolactin concentrations, the circadian rhythm of prolactin secretion is also disturbed. Finally, the characteristic sleep-induced secretory bursts are not observed, although episodic secretion occurs during the daytime.[139]

It seems that both diminished prolactin clearance[140] and increased autonomous production rate contribute to hyperprolactinemia in CKD. The response to the stimulation or suppression of prolactin is diminished in CKD. This observation is consistent with the notion of increased autonomous production.[138,140] The underlying mechanism is presumably an inadequate dopaminergic inhibition of prolactin release from pituitary lactrotrophs.[141]

It is of interest that in some patients, correction of the hyperprolactinemia by bromocriptine also caused improvement of sexual dysfunction.[142]

Testicular Hormones

In most male hemodialysis patients, plasma testosterone concentrations are low.[143,144] In a recent paper, Carrero et al.[137] found that testosterone deficiency was present in 44% of the hemodialysis patients, whereas 33% showed testosterone insufficiency (10 to 14 nmol per liter), and only 23% had normal testosterone values (>14 nmol per liter). The normal circadian rhythm of plasma testosterone concentrations, with a peak at 4 to 8 AM and nadir at 8 to 12 PM is maintained in CKD patients.[145] It is unknown whether the decreased plasma testosterone concentrations are due to reduced synthesis, increased catabolism, or a combination of both. LH stimulates testosterone secretion; however, despite numerous studies, it is not clear whether the deranged LH metabolism accounts for the reduced testosterone concentrations. The reduced amplitude of pulsatile secretory LH bursts, found in CKD, may be more critical for testosterone secretion than the sustained elevation of LH concentration. Alternatively, LH resistance of testosterone-producing cells may lead to impaired testosterone production and/or secretion. A circulating LH-receptor inhibitor was found in CKD patients, which suggested that it might contribute to Leydig cell resistance and an impaired feedback mechanism at the hypothalamic–pituitary level.[146] In this context, it is also possible that elevated prolactin concentrations interfere with the action of LH on the testes and contribute to LH resistance.[147] The response to 4 days of administration of human gonadotropin is sluggish and delayed; no increase of testosterone concentration was seen after 8 hours, but a two- to threefold increase was seen after 4 days.[148] Malnutrition is also likely to participate in the reduction of plasma testosterone concentration in CKD male patients. In CKD patients on a low-protein diet, essential amino acids and keto analog supplementation raised low testosterone plasma concentration.[149]

With respect to the other androgens, increased plasma dihydrotestosterone and androstanediol concentrations[150] as well as decreased plasma concentration of androstenedione and dehydroepiandrosterone sulfate have been reported.[151]

Androgen deficit in CKD males may cause changes in body composition. Body fat increases while lean body mass is reduced. An androgen deficit may be associated with reduced muscle mass, osteoporosis, and a higher incidence of bone fractures.[147] In addition to its negative effects on body composition, the androgen deficit also may impair libido and sexual function and might lead to depression.[147] Moreover, testosterone was strongly and inversely correlated to inflammatory markers (CRP, IL-6, and fibrinogen).[137] Finally, it was recently shown that low testosterone concentrations were associated with worse outcomes in male hemodialysis patients.[143,144]

Abnormalities in the Hormones of the Hypothalamic–Pituitary–Gonadal Axis in Female Chronic Kidney Disease Patients

Luteinizing Hormone

Pulsatile secretion of GnRH at 90-minute intervals during the follicular phase of the cycle is essential for effective hypophyseal gonadotropin secretion. In healthy premenopausal females, the secretion of LH is pulsatile. In female CKD patients, the spontaneous pulsatile LH secretion is disturbed.[152] Plasma LH concentration is elevated in most premenopausal CKD patients. The response to stimulation with GnRH is delayed.[153] Diurnal pulsatile LH secretion and high preovulatory peaks of GnRH and LH plasma concentrations are absent in most female CKD patients. In healthy females, estradiol lowers the amplitude of LH pulses. In females with CKD, estradiol fails to influence the LH surge, suggesting impaired positive feedback.[153]

Follicle-Stimulating Hormone

In contrast to the abnormal plasma LH concentration, the plasma FSH concentration is normal in most premenopausal CKD patients[154] and the FSH/LH ratio is decreased. The decreased FSH/LH ratio argues against primary ovarian failure and suggests hypothalamic–hypophyseal dysregulation in CKD females.

Prolactin

Plasma prolactin concentrations are often elevated in female hemodialysis patients,[154] but the increase of plasma prolactin after the administration of thyrotropin-releasing hormone (TRH) is blunted.[154] In CKD females, amenorrhea is frequent in patients with high plasma prolactin concentrations, and conversely, in females with regular menstruation plasma prolactin, concentrations are lower.[155]

Estrogens

In female CKD patients, the plasma estradiol concentrations are normal or low[152,156] and are consistently lower in CKD females with hyperprolactinemia.[157] In the second half of the menstrual cycle, plasma progesterone concentrations are low because of defective luteinization of the follicles.[156] The hormonal derangements of females with CKD are clearly the consequence of abnormal regulation at the level of the hypothalamus.

A major consequence of the low plasma estrogen concentration concerns bone disease. Weisinger et al.[158] studied young female hemodialysis patients. Amenorrheic patients had not only significantly lower plasma estrogen concentrations, but also significantly lower bone mineral density compared to normally menstruating female dialysis patients. Furthermore, in amenorrheic patients, a significant positive correlation was found between bone mineral density and both plasma estradiol concentration[158] and free estrogen index.[159] A causal role is suggested by the observation of Matuszkiewicz-Rowinska et al.[160] In a small group of postmenopausal women on dialysis, they showed that treatment with transdermal estradiol and cyclic addition of norethisterone acetate for 1 year increased lumbar spine bone mineral density significantly. Similarly, in a placebo-controlled randomized trial, 1 year of treatment with raloxifene, a selective estrogen receptor modulator (SERM), significantly increased bone mineral density of the lumbar spine in hemodialyzed postmenopausal females.[161] In view of concern about the potential adverse cardiovascular effects of hormonal replacement therapy, it must be emphasized that currently long-term studies on the effectiveness and safety of hormone replacement or SERM therapy in CKD female are not available.

TABLE 80.8 **Abnormalities in the Growth Hormone–Insulinlike Growth Factor (Somatotropic) Axis in Patients with Chronic Kidney Disease**

Growth Hormone (GH)
Increased plasma GH concentration
Decreased plasma concentrations of high-affinity GH-binding protein
Peripheral resistance to GH due to defect in GH intracellular signal transduction
Insulinlike Growth Factor (IGF)
Slightly decreased IGF-1 and increased IGF-2 plasma concentration
Reduced free IGF-1 plasma concentration
Increased IGFBPs (IGFBP-1, -2, -3, -4, and -6) plasma concentration
Presence of low molecular weight (1,000 Da) inhibitor of IGF-1 in plasma
Peripheral resistance to IGF-1 probably due to postreceptor defect in IGF-1 action

IGFBP, IGF-binding protein.

Abnormalities in the Growth Hormone–Insulinlike Growth Factor (Somatotropic) Axis

The somatotropic axis comprises growth hormone (GH), insulinlike growth factor 1 and 2 (IGF-1 and -2), six IGF-binding proteins (IGFBP-1 to -6), and the IGFBP proteases (BP-Pr). All are involved in the modulation of somatic growth, cellular proliferation, metabolism, and numerous other processes. Poor growth and reduced final height are well-known complications of children with CKD. Data from the North American Pediatric Renal Trials and Collaborative Studies (NAPRTCS) 2005 database revealed that 36.9% of children with CKD had growth impairment.[162] It is not surprising that several abnormalities (Table 80.8) in the somatotropic axis have been reported in children and adults with CKD.

Growth Hormone

GH is produced and secreted by the somatotrophs of the pituitary glands. The secretion of GH is pulsatile. A diurnal rhythm also exists; the secretion is high before awakening and decreases toward the end of the day. The secretion of GH is mainly controlled by two opposing hypothalamic factors; growth hormone-releasing hormone (GHRH), which stimulates GH secretion, and somatostatin, which inhibits GH secretion. The kidney is the main site of GH degradation.[163]

In children and adult patients with CKD, the plasma concentration of GH is usually elevated.[164] The increase in plasma GH concentration is correlated negatively to GFR.[164] The increase in plasma GH concentration is caused by a reduction of the metabolic clearance rate and by an increase of GH secretion. In CKD, the metabolic clearance rate of GH is reduced[165] and the GH secretion rate is elevated, as documented in adult hemodialysis patients.[166] The latter finding is not consistent, however, and in pubertal patients with advanced CKD, the GH secretion rate was decreased.[167] Plasma GH concentrations are higher in CAPD than in hemodialysis patients.[168]

The dysregulation of GH secretion is explained by several abnormalities of the central neuroendocrine control mechanisms. This issue has been investigated by suppressing and stimulating maneuvers testing the hypothalamic–pituitary function in CKD patients. Hyperglycemia by glucose infusion suppresses GH secretion in normal individuals, but fails to do so in CKD patients.[169] Conversely, in CKD patients, the response of GH secretion to the administration of GHRH[169] or L-3,4-dihydroxyphenylalanine (L-DOPA)[170] is exaggerated. Exogenous TRH does not affect GH release in normal subjects, but stimulates GH secretion in CKD[170] and a sustained exaggerated increase of GH secretion is also seen after stimulatory maneuvers, such as arginine infusion and insulin-induced hypoglycemia.[170,171]

Approximately 45% of plasma GH is bound to plasma proteins. Decreased plasma concentrations of the high affinity GH-binding protein have been found in CKD.[172] The constellation of increased concentrations of plasma GH and decreased concentrations of the high-affinity GH-binding protein implies that the fraction of free hormone is increased to which target tissues are exposed. When chondrocytes are isolated from bones of uremic rats and exposed to growth hormone or IGF-1, the response was blunted, however,[173] suggesting that in CKD the high concentrations of free GH are counteracted by peripheral resistance to GH.

The resistance appears to be both at the receptor and the postreceptor level. Determination of the concentration of serum growth hormone binding protein (GHBP), which is a cleaved product of the GH receptor, may be used to assess GH receptor density in tissues. GHBP plasma concentration is low in children and adults with CKD and proportionate to the degree of renal dysfunction.[162] Experiments of Rabkin et al.[174] suggest that resistance to GH is due to defective intracellular signal transduction. The authors found impaired phosphorylation and nuclear translocation of GH-activated signal transducer and activator of transcription (STAT) protein.[174]

Insulinlike Growth Factors

GH promotes linear growth partially by stimulating systemic and local concentrations of IGFs. The two most important IGFs are IGF-1 and IGF-2. These peptide growth factors are produced locally by most tissues, including the growth plate, but the liver is the main source of circulating hormones. The synthesis of IGFs is stimulated by GH. Conversely, as part of a negative feedback loop, IGF-1 inhibits GH presumably through stimulation of somatostatin secretion by the hypothalamus. Plasma IGF-1 forms complexes with six IGF-binding proteins (IGFBP-1 to -6). IGFBP-3 is the predominant IGFBP isoform in human plasma. Its main production site is the liver. IGFBP-3 binds IGF-1 and binding prolongs the half-life of IGF and serves as a reservoir of IGF-1.

In advanced CKD, the plasma concentration of total IGF-1 is slightly decreased and that of IGF-2 is increased.[175] The plasma concentration of free IGF-1 is lower by 50%.[176] Moreover, the so-called somatomedin bioactivity in blood, an index of IGF activity measured by sulfate incorporation into porcine costal cartilage, is reduced in uremia.[177]

The discrepancy between normal or elevated total IGF plasma concentration and low bioactivity in CKD may be explained by one or a combination of the following: (1) increased plasma concentration of IGFBPs, (2) circulating IGF inhibitor, and (3) receptor or postreceptor defect. There is some evidence for all three possibilities.

Plasma concentrations of five of the six IGF-binding proteins (IGFBP-1, -2, -3, -4, and -6) are markedly higher in CKD patients.[178] The increased binding capacity of IGF-1 decreases the concentration of free IGF-1.[179] This imbalance between plasma IGF-1 and plasma IGFBP concentrations seems to be relevant in the pathogenesis of growth failure in CKD. A significant negative correlation is found between plasma concentrations of IGFBP-1, -2, and -4, on the one hand, and standardized height in CKD children, on the other hand.[175,179]

A low molecular weight (1,000 Da) inhibitor of IGF-1 has been identified in the plasma of CKD patients,[180] but molecular details have not yet been characterized.

Finally, Ding et al.[181] characterized a postreceptor defect to the action of IGF-1 in the epitrochlearis muscle of uremic rats (i.e., both autophosphorylation of the IGF-1R tyrosine kinase and activity of the IGF-1R tyrosine kinase to the exogenous insulin receptor substrate 1 [IRS-1], a natural substrate for IGF-1 receptor tyrosine kinase, are diminished). These are in line with observations of Fouque et al.,[182] who found resistance to the metabolic effects of recombinant human IGF-1 in patients with advanced CKD.

Clinical Consequences

It was shown that growth failure in CKD is associated with increased morbidity and mortality. Furth et al.[183] demonstrated from the U.S. Renal Data System (USRDS) database that patients with severe-to-moderate growth failure had increased hospitalization rates and increased risk of death.[183]

Elevation of plasma GH concentration and low IGF bioactivity is compatible with the notion that growth failure in CKD is mainly due to end-organ hyporesponsiveness to growth hormone. The demonstration of the resistance to the action of GH and IGF-1 in CKD provides the rationale for the use of GH in the treatment of CKD children with retarded growth despite normal or elevated hormone concentrations. In a multicenter randomized double-blind placebo-controlled study, 2 years of administration of recombinant human GH in 125 prepubertal children with CKD caused an increase in growth rate and in standardized height without undue advancement of bone age or significant side effects.[184] Haffner et al.[185] studied the effect of GH treatment on the final adult height of children with CKD that, in contrast to the controls, had persistent growth failure; children treated with rhGH demonstrated sustained catch-up growth.[185]

Abnormalities in the Adrenocorticotropin–Cortisol Axis

The adrenocorticotropin–cortisol axis is only mildly affected in CKD. In CKD patients, plasma adrenocorticotropin (ACTH) concentrations are normal or elevated.[186,187] In CKD patients, ACTH secretion following the administration of corticotropin-releasing hormone (CRH) occurs earlier, but the magnitude of the response is blunted.[188,189]

In CKD patients, the basal blood levels of cortisol are normal[188] or modestly elevated.[189,190] No significant correlation was found between free cortisol concentrations and GFR.[191] The circadian rhythm of cortisol secretion is not disturbed. The cortisol half-life is prolonged in CKD patients,[190] and decreased catabolism may contribute to the mildly elevated basal levels of cortisol.

A reduced stimulated cortisol secretion to CRH despite prolonged elevation of ACTH has been observed in hemodialysis patients,[192] but the results are not uniform.

Zager et al.[186] found a normal cortisol response to exogenous ACTH.

In CKD patients, ACTH secretion cannot be suppressed by standard oral doses of dexamethasone.[190] This is probably due to reduced dexamethasone absorption in the gut, because higher doses of dexamethasone suppress ACTH secretion. Therefore, when Cushing syndrome is suspected in CKD patients, a 2-day dexamethasone test is recommended. Overall, the adrenocorticotropin–cortisol axis is either normal or only mildly altered in CKD; the clinical significance of this finding is unknown.

Abnormalities in Vasopressin

In CKD patients, the plasma vasopressin concentration is elevated.[193,194] The major cause is a decreased metabolic clearance rate.[195]

The main physiologic stimuli for vasopressin secretion are increased plasma osmolality and decreased cardiac output or arterial vasodilation. Most studies found an intact osmotic regulation of vasopressin secretion in CKD.[193] The vasopressin response to nonosmotic stimuli is apparently also normal. In hemodialyzed patients, the plasma vasopressin concentration increases during ultrafiltration[196] and plasma volume contraction.[197] Conversely, it decreases during central hypervolemia induced by water immersion.[194] It was shown that in hemodialysis patients, the hierarchy of stimuli-regulating vasopressin secretion is osmotic followed by nonosmotic factors.[197]

The clinical significance of the elevated blood levels of vasopressin in CKD is still uncertain. Experimental studies suggest that vasopressin (AVP) may participate in the genesis and exacerbation of renal damage and CKD. It was shown that a sustained stimulation of vasopressin receptors induces intrarenal renin–angiotensin system activation, podocyte alterations, glomerular hyperfiltration, and hypertrophy eventuating in proteinuria and kidney damage. Furthermore, AVP directly stimulates the contraction and proliferation of mesangial cells and the accumulation of extracellular matrix and glomerulo-sclerosis.[198]

Copeptin (or C-terminal proarginine vasopressin; CT-proAVP) is the C-terminal part of the vasopressin prohormone, which is secreted stoichiometrically with AVP and easier to estimate its plasma concentration than AVP itself. It was shown that in patients with diabetic nephropathy, CT-proAVP is directly associated with serum creatinine and predicts cardiovascular mortality.[199] Moreover Meijer et al.[200] found in a recent cohort study in 548 renal transplant patients that high CT-proAVP entails a negative renal prognosis. In this study, the plasma concentrations of this peptide predicted renal function loss over 3.2 years.[200] Selective and nonselective AVP type 2 antagonists, also denominated aquaretic agents, have already been tested in various hyponatremia-related disorders such as chronic heart failure. However, no clinical trial has been done to investigate the potential nephroprotective effect of this class of drugs.

Abnormalities in the Thyroid Gland and Hypothalamic-Pituitary–Thyroid Axis

Abnormalities in the structure and function of the thyroid gland and in the metabolism and plasma concentrations of thyroid hormones are common in patients with CKD.[201] These derangements may be due to the uremic state per se, to nonthyroid disorders (chronic disease), or to concomitant disorders of the thyroid, the pituitary, or the hypothalamus. A detailed profile of the prevalent indices of thyroid status in CKD as compared to primary hypothyroidism and chronic nonthyroid illness is presented in Table 80.9.

Goiters, Thyroid Nodules, and Thyroid Carcinoma

Available data indicate that the prevalence of goiters is increased in CKD patients.[202,203] Ultrasound scanning shows an increase of thyroid volume in about 50% of hemodialysis patients.[203] Kaptein et al.[202] studied 306 CKD patients and compared them to 139 hospitalized control patients without renal disease. A goiter was present in 40% of the CKD patients and in 43% of those treated with dialysis, compared to 6.5% in the control group. The frequency of goiters was higher in patients treated for more than 1 year with hemodialysis (50%) than in those treated for a shorter time (39%).

TABLE 80.9 **Abnormalities of the Hypothalamic–Pituitary–Thyroid Axis in Patients with Chronic Kidney Disease, Chronic Nonthyroidal Nonkidney Illness, and Primary Hypothyroidism**

	Free T_4	Free T_3	rT_3	TSH
Chronic kidney disease	N, ↓	↓	N	N
Chronic nonthyroidal nonkidney illness	N, ↓	↓	↑	N
Primary hypothyroidism	↓	↓	N	↑

N, normal; TSH, thyroid-stimulating hormone; T_4, thyroxine; T_3, triiodothyronine; rT_3, reverse triiodothyronine.

It has been suggested that in CKD, goiter formation is the result of increased plasma iodide concentrations.[201,204]

Thyroid nodules are more common in CKD patients than in the general population and were found in 55% of female hemodialysis patients compared with 21% of normal females.[205] We emphasize that it is necessary to exclude malignancy in CKD patients with solitary nodules.

The prevalence of thyroid carcinoma is increased in CKD patients. In a large sample of patients in the United States, the relative risk of thyroid malignancy was increased 2.9 times in females but not in males (1.2 times).[206] In Europe (the European Dialysis and Transplantation Association-European Renal Association [EDTA-ERA] registry), the frequency of thyroid cancer was increased by a factor of 4 to 8 in young female dialysis patients and by a factor of 2 in older dialysis patients.[207]

Thyroid Hormones

The plasma concentrations of both thyroxine (T_4) and triiodothyronine (T_3) are normal or reduced in CKD patients.[201,202,204] Plasma T_3 is more often and more markedly decreased than T_4.[201]

The reduced plasma T_3 concentration in CKD patients is the result of decreased peripheral conversion of T_4 to T_3 in several tissues. In contrast, the production of T_3 in the thyroid gland is normal. T_3 clearance rates are normal or decreased.[208] The impaired conversion of T_4 to T_3 may also be the result of malnutrition, because in CKD patients, a significant positive correlation was found between total plasma T_3 concentration and plasma albumin, as well as transferrin concentrations.[202] Chronic metabolic acidosis associated with CKD may contribute to this effect.[209]

In contrast to the other chronic nonthyroid diseases, reverse T_3 (rT_3) plasma concentration is normal in CKD patients.[210]

Although T_3 is the most active thyroid hormone, CKD patients with low plasma T_3 concentrations appear clinically euthyroid.[211] The expression of messenger RNA of T_3 receptors by mononuclear cells is increased in CKD patients compared with normal subjects.[212] This response of the receptor may help to maintain a euthyroid state despite low free T_3 concentrations.

In CKD, abnormal thyroid hormone indices do not indicate a state of hypothyroidism, but are a reflection of the state of chronic illness and/or malnutrition. Therefore, abnormal thyroid hormone indices (low T_3 and T_4 plasma concentrations) do not require therapy, which even carries a hazard. In CKD patients with low plasma T_3 concentration, it has been shown that triiodothyronine supplementation causes a negative protein balance.[213] The low T_3 state of CKD can be viewed as being protective, promoting the conservation of protein.

The Hypothalamic-Pituitary–Thyroid Axis

Despite a tendency to low plasma concentrations of T_4 and T_3, the plasma concentration of thyroid-stimulating hormone (TSH) is usually normal in CKD patients.[214] The normal plasma TSH concentration despite a low plasma concentration of the thyroid hormones suggests an abnormal regulation of the hypothalamic-pituitary–thyroid axis. The TSH response to TRH is usually blunted.[202,215] In CKD patients, the normal diurnal rhythm of TSH with a peak in the late evening or early morning is blunted,[216,217] and the nocturnal TSH surge is reduced.[216] The pattern of pulsatile TSH secretion is altered by the appearance of low-amplitude, high-frequency pulses.[217]

Primary Hypothyroidism and Hyperthyroidism

Primary hypothyroidism is two to three times more frequent in CKD patients than in the general population.[202] Risk factors are female sex, age greater than 50 years,[202] and increased iodine intake.[218] A recent study has shown a prevalence of subclinical hypothyroidism in 7% of patients with estimated GFR $\geq$ 90 mL/min/1.73 m^2 that increased to 17.9% in subjects with GFR < 60 mL/min/1.73 m^2.[219]

It is very difficult to make the clinical diagnosis of hypothyroidism in CKD patients. The signs and symptoms of hypothyroidism, such as pallor, hypothermia, and asthenia, are also found in patients with advanced CKD and no hypothyroidism.[201] The only reliable procedure to diagnose hypothyroidism in renal failure is the finding of an elevated plasma concentration of TSH associated with clearly low plasma concentrations of T_4. Because heparin competes with T_4 at the binding site of the hormone-binding protein, causing an increase of plasma T_4 concentrations for at least 24 hours, blood for the determination of thyroid hormones should be sampled before heparin administration at the beginning of a dialysis session.[220]

The prevalence of hyperthyroidism in CKD is similar to that found in the general population, in areas with an inadequate intake of iodine.[221]

Abnormalities in the Vitamin D Metabolites

Vitamin D is first hydroxylated in the liver to 25-hydroxyvitamin D_3 ($25[OH]D_3$). The prevalence of 25-vitamin D_3 deficiency increases with the progression of CKD and approaches 80% in CKD stage 5 patients.[222] Moreover, in patients with nephrotic syndrome, the $25(OH)D_3$ and vitamin D-binding protein is lost in the urine.[223] Similarly, 25(OH) D_3 is lost in the peritoneal fluid in CKD patients treated with peritoneal dialysis.[224] Therefore, both patients with nephrotic syndrome and CKD patients treated with peritoneal dialysis have a low $25(OH)D_3$ plasma concentration. Although repletion with high-dose ergocalciferol (20,000 U per week during 9 months) is considered safe, it achieves the desired level in only about 50% of hemodialysis patients.[225] A small randomized trial found that 50,000 U of cholecalciferol weekly for 12 weeks was safe and effective in satisfying $25(OH)D_3$ levels in stage 3 and 4 CKD patients.[226] In the general population, vitamin D deficiency has been linked to increased prevalence of hypertension, metabolic syndrome, insulin resistance, obesity, cardiovascular diseases (CVD), and albuminuria.[227]

$25(OH)D_3$ is transported to the kidneys for further hydroxylation, resulting in the production of the active metabolite 1,25$(OH)_2D_3$. It is known that with worsening renal function, there is progressive decline in the activity of 1α-hydroxylase, the enzyme critical in converting 25(OH) D_3 to 1,25-dihydroxyvitamin D_3 (calcitriol).[228] As a consequence, in anephric patients and in those in CKD stage 5, the blood levels of 1,25$(OH)_2D_3$ are usually very low.[228] Moreover, patients with CKD display end-organ resistance to the action of 1,25$(OH)_2D_3$. There is a decrease in the concentration of 1,25$(OH)_2D_3$ receptors (VDR) in these patients.[229]

1,25$(OH)_2D_3$ exerts its action by binding to an intracellular VDR, which is located predominantly in the nucleus. The hormone–receptor complex interacts with DNA-responsive elements in target genes with the synthesis of proteins. The deficiency of 1,25$(OH)_2D_3$ plays a paramount role in the genesis of many of the disturbances of divalent ions observed in patients with CKD. These abnormalities include secondary hyperparathyroidism, defective intestinal absorption of calcium, skeletal resistance to the calcemic action of PTH, defective mineralization of bone, growth retardation in children, and proximal myopathy.

The number of recent clinical studies suggest that 1,25$(OH)_2D_3$ deficiency leads to increased mortality in CKD patients. The results of the small interventional studies suggest that treatment with calcitriol or other VDR agonists reduce the mortality among these patients. Kovesdy et al.[230] found in a single-center, nonrandomized, observational study of 520 males with CKD an association between calcitriol treatment and reduced mortality. Shoji et al. showed in a small observational study that patients taking alfacalcidol had a reduced risk of CVD death compared to patients who were not on vitamin D. Tentori et al.[231] published similar findings in a larger cohort treated with a VDR agonist. However, these studies are small, and more large studies are needed in this area.

The number of recent clinical studies suggest that 1,25$(OH)_2D_3$ deficiency increases proteinuria in CKD patients. Recently, it was shown that low 25$(OH)D_3$ and 1,25$(OH)_2D_3$ were independently associated with increased albuminuria in CKD patients.[233] Moreover, Agarwal et al.[234] found an antiproteinuric effect of oral paricalcitol in CKD patients.[235] However, again, these studies are small, and more large studies are needed in this area.

The other abnormalities in the endocrine regulation of calcium and phosphate metabolism (among others, PTH and fibroblast growth factor-23) in CKD were discussed in other chapters of this text.

Alterations of the Renin–Angiotensin–Aldosterone System in Chronic Kidney Disease

The renin–angiotensin–aldosterone system (RAAS) is both an endocrine and a paracrine system, which plays a major role under physiologic and pathophysiologic conditions. The RAAS is involved in the regulation of blood pressure, control of volume, and sodium balance, as well as growth and remodeling of cardiovascular and renal tissues under pathologic conditions, to name only a few. Space does not permit giving an exhaustive overview, and we restrict the discussion to problems where measurement of the components of the system provides guidance to the clinician.

Plasma Renin Activity

In CKD patients suffering from primary renal disease, the activity of the renin-angiotensin system is inappropriately high. Weidmann et al.[236] documented that in hemodialysis patients, plasma renin activity (PRA) is higher at any given level of exchangeable body sodium than in normal subjects. These observations demonstrate that sodium retention and hypervolemia do not adequately suppress renin secretion, indicating disruption of the negative feedback between volume state and renin secretion. In renal disease, an important mechanism that accounts for increased and unregulated renin secretion is luminal narrowing of preglomerular vessels because of vascular sclerosis. Consequently, the "baroreceptor" in the juxtaglomerular apparatus will measure falsely low perfusion pressures, which is analogous to the kidney with a Goldblatt clip of the renal artery. Renin will, therefore, be secreted even when blood pressure is high and exchangeable sodium is increased. Normally, PRA decreases asymptotically with increasing blood pressure. In contrast, in patients with renal disease, renin secretion is not adequately suppressed by high blood pressure values, and PRA remains inappropriately high.

In CKD patients, the basal values of PRA, as measured in peripheral blood, vary. These variations are most likely due to variable degrees of renal ischemia in different renal diseases, to variable disruption of the negative feedback-control system between body fluid volume and renin secretion, and to nonstandardized conditions of examination. Weidmann and Maxwell[237] reported that PRA is highest in patients with nephrotic syndrome. On the other hand, in some patients with renal disease, particularly diabetic nephropathy, obstructive uropathy, or interstitial nephritis, hyporeninemic hypoaldosteronism with low PRA values is seen rather frequently.[238] It should also be mentioned that hypertensive CKD patients are treated with medications that may affect renin secretion, thus contributing to the variability of PRA. After hemodialysis, PRA may increase dramatically as a result of ultrafiltration and hypovolemia.[239]

It should be mentioned that PRA in the circulation does not adequately reflect the activity of local tissue RAAS systems. The paradox that drugs, which block the RAAS, are highly effective and renoprotective (e.g., in patients with diabetic nephropathy as documented by the Lewis trial[240] and the IDNT[241] or RENAAL trials[242]) is explained by the activation of local renin systems in proximal tubular epithelial cells, in podocytes, in mesangial cells, among others, despite low PRA in the circulation.[243]

The importance of the RAAS in CKD is illustrated by the fact that in CKD patients, blockade of the system reduces progression,[240–242] lowers elevated blood pressure,[244] and induces partial regression of cardiovascular structural abnormalities, such as left ventricular hypertrophy (LVH).[245]

In CKD patients, a treatment blockade of the RAAS carries an increased risk of hyperkalemia.[246]

Aldosterone

In early experimental studies, it was shown in subtotally nephrectomized rats that after adrenalectomy, less proteinuria and structural lesions were seen.[247] Conversely, DOCA salt administration caused malignant nephrosclerosis.[248] The pathogenetic role of aldosterone in CKD was shown in the model of subtotal nephrectomy: despite a RAAS blockade with the administration of an angiotensin converting enzyme inhibitor (ACEI) and the ARB administration of aldosterone, increased proteinuria as well as glomerular lesions and also increased heart weight occurred, thus documenting the adverse effects of aldosterone on the kidney and the heart.[249] More remarkably, the administration of spironolactone even caused a regression of the established glomerulosclerosis in the subtotal nephrectomy model.[250] Xue et al.[251] documented local synthase and aldosterone production in the cortex of adrenalectomized diabetic rats. In a model of diabetic nephropathy, spironolactone ameliorated signs of inflammation,[252] thus underlining the importance of the anti-inflammatory effect of mineralocorticoid receptor blockade. It is important that aldosterone induces target organ damage in the kidney and the heart only in a high salt environment,[253] thus identifying salt as a permissive factor.

The important role of aldosterone in CKD is also supported by numerous clinical observations. Plasma aldosterone concentrations were elevated in patients when GFR was < 70 mL per minute,[254] and a correlation between plasma aldosterone concentration and the rate of progression was noted by Walker[255] and Ruggenenti et al.[256]

The first proposal to use spironolactone to reduce proteinuria despite a RAAS blockade in CKD patients was made by Chrysostomou and Becker.[257] Eight patients with proteinuria > 1 g per 24 hours despite ACEI treatment were given 25 mg spironolactone. Proteinuria decreased from an average of 3.81 to 1.75 g per 24 hours without a significant change in blood pressure or creatinine clearance. Meanwhile, this finding has been confirmed in numerous studies. In a meta-analysis, Bomback et al.[258] found that proteinuria was decreased by 15% to 54% in proteinuric patients on an RAAS blockade, which was accompanied by a decrease in GFR. A meta-analysis by Navaneethan et al.[259] also showed a significant reduction of proteinuria, but this did not translate into a reduction in GFR. Whether this reflects reversal of hyperfiltration or whether observation times were not sufficient is currently unclear.

Abnormalities in the Cardiac Natriuretic Peptides

Cardiomyocytes produce and secrete a pulsatile family of related peptide hormones named cardiac natriuretic hormones, which have potent diuretic, natriuretic, and vascular smooth muscle relaxing effects.[260] Cardiac natriuretic hormones include the atrial natriuretic peptide (ANP), the brain natriuretic peptide (BNP), and their related peptides. ANP is released by atrial myocytes in response to stretches associated with increased atrial pressure, whereas the ventricular production and release of this peptide are triggered only in the presence of ventricular hypertrophy. BNP is produced by ventricular myocytes and its generation rate is increased in heart failure and left ventricular hypertrophy. Therefore, the plasma concentration of cardiac natriuretic hormones is increased in diseases characterized by expanded fluid volume, including renal failure, liver cirrhosis, and heart failure.[261]

In CKD patients, plasma concentrations of ANP and BNP are elevated.[262–264] Moreover, in these patients, the pulsatile secretion of ANP and BNP is preserved with abnormally high amplitude.[265] In the predialysis phase of CKD, there is a significant correlation between plasma ANP and serum creatinine concentrations.[264] The causes of high plasma concentrations of ANP and BNP in advanced CKD are multifactorial and depend on: (1) an increase in intravascular filling and atrial distension,[263] (2) concomitant heart failure, and (3) diminished renal clearance.[266,267] Indeed, the removal of fluid by ultrafiltration during dialysis therapy is associated with a decrease in the plasma ANP and BNP concentrations.[268]

The measurement of ANP and BNP plasma concentration was used as a biochemical marker of volume overload in the CKD patient for the improved identification of "dry weight."[269] The use of ANP and BNP to improve the definition of dry weight has yielded variable results, however.[269] The weight of evidence indicates that measurements of ANP and BNP plasma concentration add little to the clinical examination.[269] This is because of (1) a wide variability in results, (2) a lack of correlation with measures of extracellular volume, (3) an inability to detect volume depletion (no differences between normovolemia and hypovolemia), and (4) often, the presence of cardiac dysfunction as a confounder.

Results of recent studies suggest that, in general, the estimation of plasma concentrations of cardiac natriuretic hormones (BNP and N-terminal proBNP) could be useful for a differential diagnosis of heart failure.[270] Moreover, a number of studies in heart failure showed a prognostic relevance of plasma concentrations of cardiac natriuretic hormones.[270] In CKD patients, most studies indicate that the upward adjustment of diagnostic cut points preserves the usefulness of BNP and N-terminal proBNP for the differential diagnosis of heart failure.[271]

Left ventricular hypertrophy and left ventricular dysfunction are considered predictors of cardiovascular and total mortality in dialysis patients. Mallamaci et al.[272] found that measuring the plasma concentrations of cardiac natriuretic hormones, particularly BNP, may be useful in identifying dialysis patients with left ventricular hypertrophy or for excluding systolic dysfunction.

In CKD stage 5d patients, it was found that both BNP and ANP plasma concentrations are strongly related to left atrial volume (LAV) and predict LAV changes over time.[273] Moreover, in a prospective study of a cohort of dialysis patients without overt heart failure, Zoccali et al.[274] found that high plasma concentrations of cardiac natriuretic peptides, particularly BNP, were strong predictors of cardiovascular mortality. The prognostic value of concentrations of cardiac natriuretic peptides in hemodialysis patients was confirmed by several recent studies.[275–277]

Abnormalities in Gastrointestinal Hormones

Elevated plasma gastrin concentrations have been reported in CKD patients.[278–280] Hypergastrinemia in CKD is due predominantly to "big" gastrin (G34). Plasma concentrations of "little" gastrin (G17) are normal in CKD patients.[279] G34 is biologically 6 to 8 times less active than G17. Postprandial gastrin release in CKD patients in the first 30 minutes was similar to that in normal subjects, but the peak values were attained later and the response was more prolonged.[280] Because the kidney is the main site of gastrin biodegradation,[281] hypergastrinemia in uremic patients is regarded mainly as the consequence of reduced renal degradation of this hormone.

Ghrelin is a gut peptide that stimulates the production of GH from the pituitary gland.[282] Ghrelin and synthetic ghrelin analogs increase food intake by an action exerted at the level of the hypothalamus. They activate cells in the arcuate nucleus that include the orexigenic NPY neurons.[282] The two major forms of circulating ghrelin are acylated ($<$ 10%) and des-acyl ghrelin.[282] Acylated ghrelin promotes food intake, whereas des-acyl ghrelin induces negative energy balance.[282] Elevated plasma ghrelin levels were observed in CKD stage 5d patients.[283] However, only plasma des-acyl ghrelin levels were elevated in CKD. It is suggested that in elevated des-acyl ghrelin levels, plasma concentration is involved in anorexia in CKD patients.[284] Increased total ghrelin levels in CKD are due to the decreased degradation of ghrelin in the kidney.[284] The results of two small interventional clinical studies suggest that ghrelin treatment in uremia results in an improved nutritional status. A single subcutaneous injection of ghrelin enhanced short-term (3 days) food intake.[285] A subsequent report from the same group indicated that the daily administration of synthetic ghrelin stimulated food intake over a period of 7 days.[286] Importantly, energy expenditure was unchanged and there was no subsequent compensatory reduction in energy intake in these patients. Results of these two preliminary studies on ghrelin have renewed hope for the successful treatment of uremic PEW.

The plasma concentrations of other gastrointestinal hormones, such as cholecystokinin,[287] gastric inhibitory peptide,[288] pancreatic polypeptide,[289] secretin,[290] gastrin releasing peptide,[290] and motilin,[278] are elevated in CKD patients. Both normal[279] and markedly elevated[291] plasma concentrations of vasoactive intestinal polypeptide (VIP) were found in CKD patients. The pathophysiologic importance of these findings remains to be elucidated.

Abnormalities in the Hormones of Adipose Tissue

The adipose tissue is an important endocrine organ producing biologically active substances with local and/or systemic action. An incomplete list comprises plasminogen activator inhibitor type-1 (PAI-1), transforming growth factor β (TGF-β), tissue factor (TF), complement factors (e.g., adipsin), adipocyte complement–related protein, TNF-α, acylation stimulating protein (ASP), angiotensinogen (Ang), prostaglandin (PGI–2α), IGF-1, macrophage inhibitory factor (MIF), sex hormones, glucocorticoids, Ang II, visfatin, omentin, leptin, adiponectin, and resistin.[292]

Leptin

Leptin is a protein that is predominantly produced by adipocytes. It is encoded by the *ob* gene. It is presumed that leptin is involved in the regulation of appetite, food intake and energy expenditure, sexual maturation and fertility, hematopoiesis, and activity of the hypothalamic-pituitary-gonadal axis. Obese individuals have high plasma leptin concentrations.

Patients with advanced CKD have elevated plasma leptin concentrations compared to body mass index (BMI) and sex-matched healthy individuals.[293] Leptin concentrations are normalized by a successful kidney transplantation.[294] Interestingly, the influence of impaired kidney function on the plasma leptin concentration is less pronounced in noninflammatory acute renal failure than in CKD, suggesting the participation of the other factors influencing leptin secretion in this state.[295]

It was shown that the decreased leptin clearance by insufficient kidneys leads to its accumulation in the circulation.[296,297] Results of kinetic studies suggest that the renal metabolism of leptin involves an active uptake of leptin by the renal tissue.[298] Cumin et al.[299] studied changes of plasma leptin concentration in Zucker obese rats subjected to a bilateral nephrectomy or a bilateral ureteral ligation. A bilateral ureteral ligation reduced glomerular filtration by increasing tubular pressure. Following the bilateral nephrectomy in these experiments, plasma leptin concentrations increased by 300%, a value much higher than only the 50% increase after a bilateral ureteral ligation. Results of this elegant experimental study suggest that leptin elimination is only partly dependent on glomerular filtration.[299] Therefore, renal elimination is not necessarily affected by the disease in direct proportion to changes in glomerular filtration.

The increased plasma leptin concentration in CKD is not due to oversecretion of this protein. It was shown that leptin gene expression in adipocytes in CKD patients is lower than in healthy individuals.[300] Leptin plasma concentrations are not reduced by low-flux dialysis membranes, whereas high-flux dialysis membranes decrease leptin levels.[301] CAPD patients are characterized by higher plasma leptin concentrations than hemodialysis patients.[302]

There is growing evidence that leptin, originally considered exclusively as an anorexigenic hormone, exerts actions in the periphery outside of the central nervous system.

Indeed, leptin receptors are found in many tissues. It was initially thought that hyperleptinemia was an adequate explanation for anorexia in CKD patients.[303] However, subsequent studies addressing the relation between nutritional status and plasma leptin concentration in CKD yielded conflicting results.[304,305] Therefore, the role of high plasma leptin concentration in anorexia and malnutrition in CKD patients is not proved. Leptin stimulates the proliferation and the differentiation of hematopoietic stem cells.[306] It is likely that the effects of leptin and erythropoietin are synergistic. It deserves consideration whether high plasma leptin concentrations in CKD patients counteract the development of anemia when a plasma erythropoietin concentration is relatively decreased.

Leptin may also participate in CKD progression. It was shown in rats that leptin infusion led to the increase of glomerular TGF-β and collagen intravenous (IV) expression and to the enhancement of proteinuria.[307]

Apart from this, leptin likely plays a pathophysiologic role in hypertension, cardiovascular diseases, and endothelial dysfunction.[308] Leptin receptors are highly expressed in carotid plaques while they correlate with macrophage density. Leptin may contribute to the development of hypertension mainly through increased sympathetic nervous activation both centrally and at the kidney; endothelial dysfunction through the regulation of blood vessel tonus and imbalance between endothelial nitric oxide synthase (eNOS) expression and intracellular L-arginine; and atherogenesis through the stimulation of platelet aggregation, inflammation, endothelial dysfunction, neointimal hyperplasia, and vascular smooth muscle cell (VSMC) proliferation and migration.[308] Whether the hyperleptinemia seen in CKD contributes to the uremic cardiovascular risk is unexplored.

Adiponectin

Adiponectin is one of the protein hormones secreted by adipocytes, which circulate in the bloodstream in relatively high concentrations (almost 0.01% of total plasma protein) with presumed antiatherogenic and insulin-sensitizing properties. Within the circulation, adiponectin is present as a wide range of multimers: from trimers (low molecular weight [LMW]), hexamers (medium molecular weight [MMW]), to dodecamers or 18-mers (high molecular weight [HMW]). It was demonstrated that HMW is the most active form of adiponectin to improve insulin sensitivity. In hemodialysis and peritoneal dialysis CKD patients, plasma adiponectin concentrations are approximately 3 times higher than in healthy subjects.[309] Impaired kidney function does not affect the relative proportion of plasma fractions of adiponectin (i.e., HMW, MMW, or LMW adiponectin).[309] Also, the expression of receptors for adiponectin in CKD patients is preserved and similar to those observed in healthy subjects.[310] The increased plasma adiponectin concentration in CKD patients is due to the disturbances of its renal biodegradation and elimination. The kidney is the main organ participating in the biodegradation and elimination of adiponectin from circulation. Thus, as expected, successful kidney transplantation is accompanied by a prompt reduction of plasma adiponectin concentration.[311] Another piece of evidence is provided by the inverse relationship between plasma adiponectin concentration and GFR in apparently healthy individuals,[312] mild or moderate CKD,[313] and kidney transplant patients.[314] Iwashima et al.[309] showed a gradual increase of plasma adiponectin concentration in parallel to the stages of CKD. An additional argument supporting renal elimination of adiponectin is the lower concentration of this protein in plasma samples from renal veins than in samples from the aorta.[315] The increased plasma adiponectin concentration in CKD patients cannot be explained by its oversecretion by adipose tissue. The expression of adiponectin gene (ApM1) in adipocytes is even decreased in patients with advanced CKD.[316] A possible cause of lower adiponectin gene expression in CKD patients is the frequently coexisting microinflammation, increased oxidative stress in these subjects, and increased sympathetic nervous activity.[317]

It has been shown that in hemodialyzed patients, similarly to subjects with normal kidney function, lower plasma adiponectin concentrations are associated with cardiovascular complications, such as coronary artery disease or peripheral arterial occlusive disease.[318,319] Similarly, plasma adiponectin concentrations in peritoneal dialysis patients with carotid artery plaque were lower than in those without.[320] Moreover, in hemodialyzed patients, an inverse relationship was found between plasma adiponectin concentrations and intima-media thickness of the common carotid artery, which is an early marker of atherosclerotic changes.[321] Even in interlobular kidney arteries, the presence and complexity of arteriosclerotic lesions was negatively related to plasma adiponectin concentration as demonstrated by Iwasa et al.[322] in kidney biopsies of patients with immunoglobulin A (IgA) nephropathy.

Zoccali et al.[323] showed that low plasma adiponectin concentrations are a new risk factor for cardiovascular morbidity in hemodialysis patients. This observation was confirmed in peritoneal dialysis patients[324] and in mild-to-moderate CKD.[313] However, more recent studies[325–327] show contradictory results.

Animal experiments suggest that adiponectin normalizes albuminuria and improves podocyte foot process effacement. Therefore, it could be hypothesized that a high plasma adiponectin concentration slows CKD progression. However, current clinical evidence suggests that high, not low, adiponectin is associated with CKD progression at least in patients with diabetic kidney disease.[325,328]

Trying to reconcile the previously described contradictions, it has been proposed that increased adiponectin may be a reflection of a reparatory response to the microvascular insults in CKD.[308]

REFERENCES

1. De Fronzo RA, Andres R, Edgar P, et al. Carbohydrate metabolism in uremia: a review. *Medicine (Baltimore)*. 1973;52:469.

2. De Fronzo RA, Alvestrand A, Smith D, et al. Insulin resistance in uremia. *J Clin Invest*. 1981;67:563.

3. De Fronzo RA. Pathogenesis of glucose intolerance in uremia. *Metabolism.* 1978;27:1866.

4. Shinohara K, Shoji T, Emoto M, et al. Insulin resistance as an independent predictor of cardiovascular mortality in patients with end-stage renal disease. *J Am Soc Nephrol.* 2002;13:1894.

5. Becker B, Kronenberg F, Kielstein JT, et al. Renal insulin resistance syndrome, adiponectin and cardiovascular events in patients with kidney disease: the mild and moderate kidney disease study. *J Am Soc Nephrol.* 2005;16:1091.

6. Stumvoll M, Meyer C, Perriello G, et al. Human kidney and liver gluconeogenesis: evidence for organ substrate selectivity. *Am J Physiol.* 1998;274:E817.

7. Smith D, De Fronzo RA. Insulin resistance in uremia mediated by postbinding defects. *Kidney Int.* 1982;22:54.

8. Friedman JE, Dohm GL, Elton CW, et al. Muscle insulin resistance in uremic humans: glucose transport, glucose transporters, and insulin receptors. *Am J Physiol.* 1991;261:E87.

9. De Fronzo RA, Tobin JD, Rowe JW, et al. Glucose intolerance in uremia: quantification of pancreatic beta cell sensitivity to glucose and tissue sensitivity to insulin. *J Clin Invest.* 1978;62:425.

10. Kobayashi S, Maejima S, Ikeda T, et al. Impact of dialysis therapy on insulin resistance in end-stage renal disease: comparison of haemodialysis and continuous ambulatory peritoneal dialysis. *Nephrol Dial Transplant.* 2000;15:65.

11. McCaleb ML, Wish JB, Lockwood DH. Insulin resistance in chronic renal failure. *Endocrinol Res.* 1985;11:113.

12. Mak RH, Bettinelli A, Turner C, et al. The influence of hyperparathyroidism on glucose metabolism in uremia. *J Clin Endocrinol Metab.* 1985;60:229.

13. Perna AF, Fadda GZ, Zhou XJ, et al. Mechanisms of impaired insulin secretion after chronic excess of parathyroid hormone. *Am J Physiol.* 1990;259:F210.

14. Christakos S, Norman AW. Studies on the mode of action of calciferol: biochemical characterization of 1,25-dihydroxyvitamin D_3 receptors in chick pancreas and kidney cytosol. *Endocrinology.* 1981;108:140.

15. Mak RH. Intravenous 1,25-dihydroxycholecalciferol corrects glucose intolerance in hemodialysis patients. *Kidney Int.* 1992;41:1049.

16. Rabkin R, Rubenstein AH, Colwell JA. Glomerular filtration and maximal tubular absorption of insulin (^{125}I). *Am J Physiol.* 1972;223:1093.

17. Rabkin R, Jones J, Kitabchi AE. Insulin extraction from the renal peritubular circulation in the chicken. *Endocrinology.* 1977;101:1828.

18. Rabkin R, Simon NM, Steiner S, et al. Effect of renal disease on renal uptake and excretion of insulin in man. *N Engl J Med.* 1970;282:182.

19. Rabkin R, Unterhalter SA, Duckworth WC. Effect of prolonged uremia on insulin metabolism by isolated liver and muscle. *Kidney Int.* 1979;16:433.

20. Moen MF, Zhan M, Hsu VD, et al. Frequency of hypoglycemia and its significance in chronic kidney disease. *Clin J Am Soc Nephrol.* 2009;4:1121.

21. Krepinsky J, Ingram AJ, Clase CM. Prolonged sulfonylurea-induced hypoglycemia in diabetic patients with end-stage renal disease. *Am J Kidney Dis.* 2000;35:500.

22. Arem R. Hypoglycemia associated with renal failure. *Endocrinol Metab Clin North Am.* 1989;18:103.

23. Ferrannini E, Buzzigoli G, Bonadonna R, et al. Insulin resistance in essential hypertension. *N Engl J Med.* 1987;317:350.

24. Eckel RH, Yost TJ, Jensen DR. Alterations in lipoprotein lipase in insulin resistance. *Int J Obes Relat Metab Disord.* 1995;19:S16.

25. Noori N, Kopple JD. Effect of diabetes mellitus on protein-energy wasting and protein wasting in end-stage renal disease. *Semin Dial.* 2010;23:178.

26. da Costa JA, Ikizler TA. Inflammation and insulin resistance as novel mechanisms of wasting in chronic dialysis patients. *Semin Dial.* 2009;22:652.

27. Siew ED, Ikizler TA. Insulin resistance and protein energy metabolism in patients with advanced chronic kidney disease. *Semin Dial.* 2010;23:378.

28. Mitch WE. Insights into the abnormalities of chronic renal disease attributed to malnutrition. *J Am Soc Nephrol.* 2002;13:S22.

29. Ritz E. Metabolic syndrome and kidney disease. *Blood Purif.* 2008;26:59.

30. Johnson RJ, Sanchez-Lozada LG, Nakagawa T. The effect of fructose on renal biology and disease. *J Am Soc Nephrol.* 2010;21:2036.

31. Bright R. *Reports of Medical Cases Selected with a View of Illustrating the Symptoms and Cure of Diseases by Reference to Morbid Anatomy*. London, England: Longman, Rees, Orme, Brown & Green; 1827.

32. Weintraub M, Burstein A, Rassin T, et al. Severe defect in clearing postprandial chylomicron remnants in dialysis patients. *Kidney Int.* 1992;42:1247.

33. Kwan BC, Kronenberg F, Beddhu S, et al. Lipoprotein metabolism and lipid management in chronic kidney disease. *J Am Soc Nephrol.* 2007;18:1246.

34. Kronenberg F, Kuen E, Ritz E, et al. Apolipoprotein A-IV serum concentrations are elevated in patients with mild and moderate renal failure. *J Am Soc Nephrol.* 2002;13:461.

35. Boes E, Fliser D, Ritz E, et al. Apolipoprotein A-IV predicts progression of chronic kidney disease: The mild to moderate kidney disease study. *J Am Soc Nephrol.* 2006;17:528.

36. Oi K, Hirano T, Sakai S, et al. Role of hepatic lipase in intermediate-density lipoprotein and small, dense low-density lipoprotein formation in hemodialysis patients. *Kidney Int.* 1999;71:S227.

37. Gonzalez AI, Schreier L, Elbert A, et al. Lipoprotein alterations in hemodialysis: differences between diabetic and nondiabetic patients. *Metabolism.* 2003;52:116.

38. Vaziri ND, Liang K. Down-regulation of VLDL receptor expression in chronic experimental renal failure. *Kidney Int.* 1997;51:913.

39. Kramer-Guth A, Quaschning T, Galle J, et al. Structural and compositional modifications of diabetic low-density lipoproteins influence their receptor-mediated uptake by hepatocytes. *Eur J Clin Invest.* 1997;27:460.

40. Itabe H. Oxidized low-density lipoproteins: what is understood and what remains to be clarified. *Biol Pharm Bull.* 2003;26:1.

41. Kronenberg F, Kuen E, Ritz E, et al. Lipoprotein(a) serum concentrations and apolipoprotein(a) phenotypes in mild and moderate renal failure. *J Am Soc Nephrol.* 2000;11:105.

42. Kronenberg F, Lingenhel A, Lhotta K, et al. The apolipoprotein(a) size polymorphism is associated with nephrotic syndrome. *Kidney Int.* 2004;65:606.

43. Frischmann KE, Kronenberg F, Trenkwalder E, et al. In vivo turnover study demonstrates diminished clearance of lipoprotein(a) in hemodialysis patients. *Kidney Int.* 2007;71:1036.

44. Kronenberg F, Neyer U, Lhotta K, et al. The low molecular weight apo(a) phenotype is an independent predictor for coronary artery disease in hemodialysis patients: a prospective follow-up. *J Am Soc Nephrol.* 1999;10:1027.

45. Longenecker JC, Klag MJ, Marcovina SM, et al. Small apolipoprotein(a) size predicts mortality in end-stage renal disease: the CHOICE Study. *Circulation.* 2002;106:2812.

46. Shoji T, Nishizawa Y, Kawagishi T, et al. Intermediate-density lipoprotein as an independent risk factor for aortic atherosclerosis in hemodialysis patients. *J Am Soc Nephrol.* 1998;9:1277.

47. Wilson PW, D'Agostino RB, Levy D, et al. Prediction of coronary heart disease using risk factor categories. *Circulation.* 1998;97:1837.

48. Nishizawa Y, Shoji T, Kakiya R, et al. Non-high-density lipoprotein cholesterol (non-HDL-C) as a predictor of cardiovascular mortality in patients with end-stage renal disease. *Kidney Int.* 2003;63:S117.

49. Belani SS, Goldberg AC, Coyne DW. Ability of non-high-density lipoprotein cholesterol and calculated intermediate-density lipoprotein to identify nontraditional lipoprotein subclass risk factors in dialysis patients. *Am J Kidney Dis.* 2004;43:320.

50. House AA, Wells GA, Donnelly JG, et al. Randomized trial of high-flux vs low-flux hemodialysis: effects on homocysteine and lipids. *Nephrol Dial Transplant.* 2000;15:1029.

51. Bugeja AL, Chan CT. Improvement in lipid profile by nocturnal hemodialysis in patients with end-stage renal disease. *ASAIO J.* 2004;50:328.

52. Attman PO, Samuelsson O, Johansson AC, et al. Dialysis modalities and dyslipidemia. *Kidney Int.* 2003;63:110.

53. Dieplinger H, Schoenfeld PY, Fielding CJ. Plasma cholesterol metabolism in end-stage renal disease: difference between treatment by hemodialysis or peritoneal dialysis. *J Clin Invest.* 1986;77:1071.

54. Bredie SJ, Bosch FH, Demacker PN, et al. Effects of peritoneal dialysis with an overnight icodextrin dwell on parameters of glucose and lipid metabolism. *Perit Dial Int.* 2001;21:275.

55. Degoulet P, Legrain M, Reach I, et al. Mortality risk factors in patients treated by chronic hemodialysis. Report of the Diaphane collaborative study. *Nephron.* 1982;31:103.

56. Lowrie EG, Lew NL. Death risk in hemodialysis patients: the predictive value of commonly measured variables and an evaluation of death rate differences between facilities. *Am J Kidney Dis.* 1990;15:458.

57. Iseki K, Yamazato M, Tozawa M, et al. Hypocholesterolemia is a significant predictor of death in a cohort of chronic hemodialysis patients. *Kidney Int.* 2002;61:1887.

58. Kalantar-Zadeh K, Block G, Humphreys MH, et al. Reverse epidemiology of cardiovascular risk factors in maintenance dialysis patients. *Kidney Int.* 2003;63:793.

59. Liu Y, Coresh J, Eustace JA, et al. Association between cholesterol level and mortality in dialysis patients: role of inflammation and malnutrition. *JAMA.* 2004;291:451.

60. Tonelli M, Isles C, Curhan GC, et al. Effect of pravastatin on cardiovascular events in people with chronic kidney disease. *Circulation.* 2004;110:1557.

61. Navaneethan SD, Pansini F, Perkovic V, et al. HMG CoA reductase inhibitors (statins) for people with chronic kidney disease not requiring dialysis. *Cochrane Database Syst Rev.* 2009;CD007784.

62. Colhoun HM, Betteridge DJ, Durrington PN, et al. Effects of atorvastatin on kidney outcomes and cardiovascular disease in patients with diabetes: an analysis from the Collaborative Atorvastatin Diabetes Study (CARDS). *Am J Kidney Dis.* 2009;54:810.

63. Wanner C, Krane V, März W, et al. Atorvastatin in patients with type 2 diabetes mellitus undergoing hemodialysis. *N Engl J Med.* 2005;353:238.

64. Fellström BC, Jardine AG, Schmieder RE, et al. Rosuvastatin and cardiovascular events in patients undergoing hemodialysis. *N Engl J Med.* 2009;360:1395.
65. Baigent C, Landry M. Study of Heart and Renal Protection (SHARP). *Kidney Int Suppl.* 2003;84:S207.
66. Sanfelippo ML, Swenson RS, Reaven GM. Response of plasma triglycerides to dietary change in patients on hemodialysis. *Kidney Int.* 1978;14:180.
67. Axelsson TG, Irving GF, Axelsson J. To eat or not to eat: dietary fat in uremia is the question. *Semin Dial.* 2010;23:383.
68. Goldberg AP, Hagberg JM, Delmez JA, Metabolic effects of exercise training in hemodialysis patients. *Kidney Int.* 1980;18:754.
69. Chapman MJ, Le Goff W, Guerin M, et al. Cholesteryl ester transfer protein: at the heart of the action of lipid-modulating therapy with statins, fibrates, niacin, and cholesteryl ester transfer protein inhibitors. *Eur Heart J.* 2010; 31:149.
70. Barter PJ, Caulfield M, Eriksson M, et al. Effects of torcetrapib in patients at high risk for coronary events. *N Engl J Med.* 2007;357:2109.
71. Kaysen GA. Potential restoration of HDL function with apolipoprotein A-I mimetic peptide in end-stage renal disease. *Kidney Int.* 2009;76:359.
72. Belfort R, Berria R, Cornell J, et al. Fenofibrate reduces systemic inflammation markers independent of its effects on lipid and glucose metabolism in patients with the metabolic syndrome. *J Clin Endocrinol Metab.* 2010; 95:829.
73. Pasternack A, Vanttinen T, Solakivi T, et al. Normalization of lipoprotein lipase and hepatic lipase by gemfibrozil results in correction of lipoprotein abnormalities in chronic renal failure. *Clin Nephrol.* 1987;27:163.
74. Tahmaz M, Kumbasar B, Ergen K, et al. Acute renal failure secondary to fenofibrate monotherapy-induced rhabdomyolysis. *Ren Fail.* 2007;29:927.
75. Unal A, Torun E, Sipahioglu MH, et al. Fenofibrate-induced acute renal failure due to massive rhabdomyolysis after coadministration of statin in two patients. *Intern Med.* 2008;47:1017.
76. Polanco N, Hernández E, González E, et al. Fibrate-induced deterioration of renal function. *Nefrologia.* 2009;29:208.
77. Taylor AJ, Villines TC, Stanek EJ, et al. Extended-release niacin or ezetimibe and carotid intima-media thickness. *N Engl J Med.* 2009;361:2113.
78. Shoji T, Nishizawa Y, Kawasaki K, et al. Effects of the nicotinic acid analogue niceritrol on lipoprotein Lp(a) and coagulation-fibrinolysis status in patients with chronic renal failure on hemodialysis. *Nephron.* 1997;77:112.
79. Nakahama H, Nakanishi T, Uyama O, et al. Niceritrol reduces plasma lipoprotein(a) levels in patients undergoing maintenance hemodialysis. *Ren Failure.* 1993;15:189.
80. Nishizawa Y, Shoji T, Tabata T, et al. Effects of lipid-lowering drugs on intermediate-density lipoprotein in uremic patients. *Kidney Int Suppl.* 1999;71:S134.
81. Mitch WE, Goldberg AL. Mechanisms of muscle wasting. The role of the ubiquitin-proteasome pathway. *N Engl J Med.* 1996;335:1897.
82. Young VR, Krauss RM. Nutritional requirements of normal adults. In: Mitch WE, Klahr S, eds. *Nutrition and the Kidney*. 4th ed. Philadelphia, PA: Lippincott–Raven Press; 2002: 1.
83. Dukkipati R, Kopple JD. Causes and prevention of protein-energy wasting in chronic kidney failure. *Semin Nephrol.* 2009;29:39.
84. Du J, Wang X, Miereles C, et al. Activation of caspase-3 is an initial step triggering accelerated muscle proteolysis in catabolic conditions. *J Clin Invest.* 2004;113:115.
85. Lecker SH, Jagoe RT, Gilbert A, et al. Multiple types of skeletal muscle atrophy involve a common program of changes in gene expression. *FASEB J.* 2004;18:39.
86. Du J, Mitch WE. Identification of pathways controlling muscle protein metabolism in uremia and other catabolic conditions. *Curr Opin Nephrol Hypertens.* 2005;14:378.
87. Broyer M, Jean G, Dartois AM, et al. Plasma and muscle free amino acids in children at the early stages of renal failure. *Am J Clin Nutr.* 1980;33:1396.
88. Dalton RN, Chantler C. The relationship between branched-chain amino acids and alpha-keto acids in blood in uremia. *Kidney Int.* 1983;16:S61.
89. Bergström J, Alvestrand A, Fürst P. Plasma and muscle free amino acids in maintenance hemodialysis patients without protein malnutrition. *Kidney Int.* 1990;38:108.
90. Suliman ME, Anderstam B, Lindholm B, et al. Total, free and protein-bound sulphur amino acids in uremic patients. *Nephrol Dial Transplant.* 1997;12:2332.
91. Bergström J, Furst P, Noree LO, et al. Intracellular free amino acids in muscle tissue of patients with chronic uraemia: effect of peritoneal dialysis and infusion of essential amino acids. *Clin Sci Mol Med.* 1978;54:51.
92. Hara Y, May RC, Kelly RA, et al. Acidosis, not azotemia, stimulates branched-chain, amino acid catabolism in uremic rats. *Kidney Int.* 1987;32:808.
93. Workeneh BT, Mitch WE. Review of muscle wasting associated with chronic kidney disease. *Am J Clin Nutr.* 2010;91:1128S.
94. Edozien JC. The free amino acids of plasma and urine in kwashiorkor. *Clin Sci.* 1966;31:153.
95. Hara Y, May RC, Kelly RA, et al. Acidosis, not azotemia, stimulates branched-chain, amino acid catabolism in uremic rats. *Kidney Int.* 1987;32:808.
96. Lofberg E, Wernerman J, Anderstam B, et al. Correction of metabolic acidosis in dialysis patients increases branched-chain and total essential amino acid levels in muscle. *Clin Nephrol.* 1997;48:230.
97. Cernacek P, Becvarova H, Gerova Z, et al. Plasma tryptophan level in chronic renal failure. *Clin Nephrol.* 1980;14:246.
98. Suliman ME, Anderstam B, Lindholm B, et al. Evidence of taurine depletion and accumulation of cysteinesulfinic acid in chronic dialysis patients. *Kidney Int.* 1996;50:1713.
99. Canepa A, Divino Filho JC, Forsberg AM, et al. Nutritional status and muscle amino acids in children with end-stage renal failure. *Kidney Int.* 1992;41:1016.
100. Bright R. *Reports of Medical Cases Selected with a View of Illustrating the Symptoms and Cure of Diseases by Reference to Morbid Anatomy.* Vol 2. London, England: Longman, Rees, Orme, Brown & Green; 1830.
101. Kopple JD. Amino acid and protein metabolism in chronic renal failure. In: Massry SG, Glassock RJ, eds. *Massry and Glassock's Textbook of Nephrology*. 4th ed. Philadelphia, PA: Lippincott Williams & Wilkins; 2001:1356.
102. Stenvinkel P, Heimburger O, Lindholm B. Wasting, but not malnutrition, predicts cardiovascular mortality in end-stage renal disease. *Nephrol Dial Transplant.* 2004;19:2181.
103. Pecoits-Filho R, Lindholm B, Stenvinkel P. The malnutrition, inflammation, and atherosclerosis (MIA) syndrome—the heart of the matter. *Nephrol Dial Transplant.* 2002;17:28.
104. Stenvinkel P, Heimburger O, Lindholm B, et al. Are there two types of malnutrition in chronic renal failure? Evidence for relationships between malnutrition, inflammation and atherosclerosis (MIA syndrome). *Nephrol Dial Transplant.* 2000;15:953.
105. Ikizler TA, Wingard RL, Sun M, et al. Increased energy expenditure in hemodialysis patients. *J Am Soc Nephrol.* 1996;7:2646.
106. Mitch WE. Proteolytic mechanisms, not malnutrition, cause loss of muscle mass in kidney failure. *J Ren Nutr.* 2006;16:208–211.
107. Wang X, Hu Z, Hu J, Du J, et al. Insulin resistance accelerates muscle protein degradation: Activation of the ubiquitin-proteasome pathway by defects in muscle cell signaling. *Endocrinology.* 2006;147:4160.
108. Ikizler TA, Pupim LB, Brouillette JR, et al. Hemodialysis stimulates muscle and whole body protein loss and alters substrate oxidation. *Am J Physiol Endocrinol Metab.* 2002;282:E107.
109. Pupim LB, Flakoll PJ, Brouillette JR, et al. Intradialytic parenteral nutrition improves protein and energy homeostasis in chronic hemodialysis patients. *J Clin Invest.* 2002;110:483.
110. Bier DM. Intrinsically difficult problems: the kinetics of body proteins and amino acids in man. *Diabetes Metab Rev.* 1989;5:111.
111. Goodship TH, Mitch WE, Hoerr RA. Adaptation to low-protein diets in renal failure: leucine turnover and nitrogen balance. *J Am Soc Nephrol.* 1990;1:66.
112. Pupim LB, Flakoll PJ, Ikizler TA. Protein homeostasis in chronic hemodialysis patients. *Curr Opin Clin Nutr Metab Care.* 2004;7:89.
113. Mitch WE. Insights into abnormalities of chronic renal disease attributed to malnutrition. *J Am Soc Nephrol.* 2002;13:S22.
114. Kopple JD, Monteon FJ, Shaib JK. Effect of energy intake on nitrogen metabolism in nondialyzed patients with chronic renal failure. *Kidney Int.* 1986;29:734.
115. Monteon FJ, Laidlaw SA, Shaib JK, et al. Energy expenditure in patients with chronic renal failure. *Kidney Int.* 1986;30:741.
116. Wang AY, Sea MM, Tang N, et al. Resting energy expenditure and subsequent mortality risk in peritoneal dialysis patients. *J Am Soc Nephrol.* 2004;15:3134.
117. Ikizler TA, Greene JH, Wingard RL, et al. Spontaneous dietary protein intake during progression of chronic renal failure. *J Am Soc Nephrol.* 1995;6:1386.
118. Kopple JD, Levey AS, Greene T, et al. Effect of dietary protein restriction on nutritional status in Modification of Diet in Renal Disease (MDRD) Study. *Kidney Int.* 1997;52:778.
119. Raj DS, Sun Y, Tzamaloukas AH. Hypercatabolism in dialysis patients. *Curr Opin Nephrol Hypertens.* 2008;17:589.
120. Pupim LB, Caglar K, Hakim RM, et al. Uremic malnutrition is a predictor of death independent of inflammatory status. *Kidney Int.* 2004;66:2054.
121. Hakim RM, Levin N. Malnutrition in hemodialysis patients. *Am J Kidney Dis.* 1993;21:125.
122. Rajan V, Mitch WE. Ubiquitin, proteasomes and proteolytic mechanisms activated by kidney disease. *Biochim Biophys Acta.* 2008;1782:795.
123. Relman AS, Shelburne PF, Talman A. Profound acidosis resulting from excessive ammonium chloride in previously healthy subjects. A study of two cases. *N Engl J Med.* 1961;264:848.

124. Graham KA, Reaich D, Channon SM, et al. Correction of acidosis in hemodialysis decreases whole-body protein degradation. *J Am Soc Nephrol.* 1997;8:632.
125. Pickering WP, Price SR, Bircher G, et al. Nutrition in CAPD: serum bicarbonate and the ubiquitin-proteasome system in muscle. *Kidney Int.* 2002; 61:1286.
126. Szeto CC, Wong TY, Chow KM, et al. Oral sodium bicarbonate for the treatment of metabolic acidosis in peritoneal dialysis patients: a randomized placebo-control trial. *J Am Soc Nephrol* 2003;14:2119.
127. de Brito-Ashurst I, Varagunam M, Raftery MJ, et al. Bicarbonate supplementation slows progression of CKD and improves nutritional status. *J Am Soc Nephrol.* 2009;20:2075.
128. Kraut JA, Madias NE. Consequences and therapy of the metabolic acidosis of chronic kidney disease. *Pediatr Nephrol.* 2011;26:19.
129. Bergstrom J, Lindholm B, Lacson E Jr, et al. What are the causes and consequences of the chronic inflammatory state in chronic dialysis patients? *Semin Dial.* 2000;13:163.
130. Stein A, Moorhouse J, Iles-Smith H, Baker F, et al. Role of an improvement in acid-base status and nutrition in CAPD patients. *Kidney Int.* 1997;52:1089.
131. Parker TF, Wingard RL, Husni L, et al. Effect of the membrane biocompatibility on nutritional parameters in chronic hemodialysis patients. *Kidney Int.* 1996;49:551.
132. Locatelli F, Mastangelo F, Redacelli B, et al. Effects of different membranes and dialysis technologies on patients' treatment tolerance and nutritional parameters. The Italian Cooperative Dialysis Study Group. *Kidney Int.* 1996;49:1293.
133. Kidney diseases outcomes quality initiative clinical practice guidelines for nutrition in chronic renal failure. *Am J Kidney Dis.* 2000;35(suppl 2):1.
134. Holley JL. The hypothalamic-pituitary axis in men and women with chronic kidney disease. *Adv Chronic Kidney Dis.* 2004;11:337.
135. de Kretser DM, Atkins RC, Paulsen CA. Role of the kidney in the metabolism of luteinizing hormone. *J Endocrinol.* 1973;58:425.
136. Schaefer F, Veldhuis JD, Robertson WR, et al. Immunoreactive and bioactive luteinizing hormone in pubertal patients with chronic renal failure: Cooperative Study Group in Pubertal Development in Chronic Renal Failure. *Kidney Int.* 1994;45:1465.
137. Carrero JJ, Qureshi AR, Nakashima A, et al. Prevalence and clinical implications of testosterone deficiency in men with end-stage renal disease. *Nephrol Dial Transplant.* 2011;26:184.
138. Lim VS, Kathpalia SC, Frohman LA. Hyperprolactinemia and impaired pituitary response to suppression and stimulation in chronic renal failure: reversal after transplantation. *J Clin Endocrinol Metab.* 1979;48:101.
139. Biasioli S, Mazzali A, Foroni R, et al. Chronobiological variations of prolactin (PRL) in chronic renal failure (CRF). *Clin Nephrol.* 1988;30:86.
140. Emmanouel DS, Fang VS, Katz AI. Prolactin metabolism in the rat: role of the kidney in degradation of the hormone. *Am J Physiol.* 1981;240:F437.
141. Adachi N, Lei B, Deshpande G, et al. Uremia suppresses central dopaminergic metabolism and impairs motor activity in rats. *Intensive Care Med.* 2001; 27:1655.
142. Ramirez G, Butcher DE, Newton JL, et al. Bromocriptine and the hypothalamic hypophyseal function in patients with chronic renal failure on chronic hemodialysis. *Am J Kidney Dis.* 1985;6:111.
143. Gungor O, Kircelli F, Carrero JJ, et al. Endogenous testosterone and mortality in male hemodialysis patients: is it the result of aging? *Clin J Am Soc Nephrol.* 2010;5:2018.
144. Carrero JJ, Qureshi AR, Parini P, et al. Low serum testosterone increases mortality risk among male dialysis patients. *J Am Soc Nephrol.* 2009;20:613.
145. Zadeh JA, Koutsaimanis KG, Roberts AP, et al. The effect of maintenance haemodialysis and renal transplantation on the plasma testosterone levels of male patients in chronic renal failure. *Acta Endocrinol (Copenhagen).* 1975;80:577.
146. Dunkel L, Raivio T, Laine J, et al. Circulating luteinizing hormone receptor inhibitor(s) in boys with chronic renal failure. *Kidney Int.* 1997;51:777.
147. Schmidt A, Luger A, Hörl WH. Sexual hormone abnormalities in male patients with renal failure. *Nephrol Dial Transplant.* 2002;17:368.
148. de Kretser DM, Atkins RC, Hudson B, et al. Disordered spermatogenesis in patients with chronic renal failure and undergoing maintenance hemodialysis. *Aust NZ J Med.* 1974;4:178.
149. Fioretti P, Melis GB, Ciardella F, et al. Parathyroid function and pituitary-gonadal axis in male uremics: effects of dietary treatment and of maintenance hemodialysis. *Clin Nephrol.* 1986;25:155.
150. Van Kammen E, Thijssen JH, Schwarz F. Sex hormones in male patients with chronic renal failure. I. The production of testosterone and of androstenedione. *Clin Endocrinol (Oxf).* 1978;8:7.
151. van Coevorden A, Stolear JC, Dhaene M, et al. Effect of chronic oral testosterone undecanoate administration on the pituitary-testicular axes of hemodialyzed male patients. *Clin Nephrol.* 1986;26:48.
152. Lim VS, Henriquez C, Sievertsen G, et al. Ovarian function in chronic renal failure: evidence suggesting hypothalamic anovulation. *Ann Intern Med.* 1980;93:21.
153. Swamy AP, Woolf PD, Cestero RV. Hypothalamic-pituitary-ovarian axis in uremic women. *J Lab Clin Med.* 1979;93:1066.
154. Rudolf K, Rudolf H, Ruting M, et al. Behavior of basal and stimulated serum levels of prolactin, growth hormone and gonadotropins in females with chronic uremia. *Z Gesamte Inn Med.* 1988;43:542.
155. Michaelides N, Humke W. Erfahrunegen bei der gynäkologischen Betrteuung von patientinnen mit chronischer Nireninsuffizienz. *Nieren und Hochdruckkrankheiten.* 1993;22:187.
156. Zingraff J, Jungers P, Pelissier C, et al. Pituitary and ovarian dysfunctions in women on haemodialysis. *Nephron.* 1982;30:149.
157. Gomez F, de la Cueva R, Wauters JP, et al. Endocrine abnormalities in patients undergoing long-term hemodialysis. The role of prolactin. *Am J Med.* 1980;68:522.
158. Weisinger JR, Gonzalez L, Alvarez H, et al. Role of persistent amenorrhea in bone mineral metabolism of young hemodialyzed women. *Kidney Int.* 2000;58:331.
159. Sugiya N, Nakashima A, Takasugi N, et al. Endogenous estrogen may prevent bone loss in postmenopausal hemodialysis patients throughout life. *Osteoporos Int.* 2011;22:1573.
160. Matuszkiewicz-Rowinska J, Skorzewska K, Radowicki S, et al. The benefits of hormone replacement therapy in pre-menopausal women with oestrogen deficiency on haemodialysis. *Nephrol Dial Transplant.* 1999;14:1238.
161. Hernandez E, Valera R, Alonzo E, et al. Effects of raloxifene on bone metabolism and serum lipids in postmenopausal women on chronic hemodialysis. *Kidney Int.* 2003;63:2269.
162. Mahesh S, Kaskel F. Growth hormone axis in chronic kidney disease. *Pediatr Nephrol.* 2008;23:41.
163. Johnson V, Maack T. Renal extraction, filtration, absorption, and catabolism of growth hormone. *Am J Physiol.* 1977;233:F185.
164. Ramírez G, Bittle PA, Sanders H, et al. The effects of corticotropin and growth hormone releasing hormones on their respective secretory axes in chronic hemodialysis patients before and after correction of anemia with recombinant human erythropoietin. *J Clin Endocrinol Metab.* 1994;78:63.
165. Schaefer F, Baumann G, Haffner D, et al. Multifactorial control of the elimination kinetics of unbound (free) growth hormone (GH) in the human: regulation by age, adiposity, renal function, and steady state concentrations of GH in plasma. *J Clin Endocrinol Metab.* 1996;81:22.
166. Veldhuis JD, Iranmanesh A, Wilkowski MJ, et al. Neuroendocrine alterations in the somatotropic and lactotropic axes in uremic men. *Eur J Endocrinol.* 1994;131:489.
167. Schaefer F, Veldhuis JD, Stanhope R, et al. Alterations in growth hormone secretion and clearance in peripubertal boys with chronic renal failure and after renal transplantation. Cooperative Study Group of Pubertal Development in Chronic Renal Failure. *J Clin Endocrinol Metab.* 1994;78:1298.
168. Iglesias P, Díez JJ, Fernández-Reyes MJ, et al. Growth hormone, IGF-1 and its binding proteins (IGFBP-1 and -3) in adult uraemic patients undergoing peritoneal dialysis and haemodialysis. *Clin Endocrinol.* 2004;60:741.
169. Ramirez G, O'Neill WA, Bloomer HA, et al. Abnormalities in the regulation of growth hormone in chronic renal failure. *Arch Intern Med.* 1978;138:267.
170. Ramirez G, Bercu BB, Bittle PA, et al. Response to growth hormone-releasing hormone in adult renal failure patients on hemodialysis. *Metabolism.* 1990;39:764.
171. Marumo F, Sakai T, Sato S. Response of insulin, glucagon and growth hormone to arginine infusion in patients with chronic renal failure. *Nephron.* 1979;24:81.
172. Postel-Vinay MC, Tar A, Crosnier H, et al. Plasma growth hormone-binding activity is low in uraemic children. *Pediatr Nephrol.* 1991;5:545.
173. Mak RH, Pak YK. End-organ resistance to growth hormone and IGF-1 in epiphyseal chondrocytes of rats with chronic renal failure. *Kidney Int.* 1996;50:400.
174. Rabkin R, Sun DF, Chen Y, et al. Growth hormone resistance in uremia, a role for impaired JAK/STAT signaling. *Pediatr Nephrol.* 2005;20:313.
175. Tönshoff B, Blum WF, Wingen AM, et al, Serum insulin-like growth factors (IGFs) and IGF binding proteins 1, 2, and 3 in children with chronic renal failure: relationship to height and glomerular filtration rate. *J Clinical Endocrinol Metab.* 1995;80:2684.
176. Frystyk J, Ivarsen P, Skjaerbaek C, et al. Serum-free insulin-like growth factor I correlates with clearance in patients with chronic renal failure. *Kidney Int.* 1999;56:2076.
177. Phillips LS, Kopple JD. Circulating somatomedin activity and sulfate levels in adults with normal and impaired kidney function. *Metabolism.* 1981;30:1091.

178. Nanba K, Nagake Y, Miyatake N, et al. Relationships of serum levels of insulin like growth factors with indices of bone metabolism and nutritional conditions in hemodialysis patients. *Nephron.* 2001;89:145.
179. Powell DR, Liu F, Baker BK, et al. Insulin-like growth factor-binding protein-6 levels are elevated in serum of children with chronic renal failure. *J Clin Endocrinol Metab.* 1997;82:2978.
180. Phillips LS, Fusco AC, Unterman TG, et al. Somatomedin inhibitor in uremia. *J Clin Endocrinol Metab.* 1984;59:764.
181. Ding H, Gao XL, Hirschberg R, et al. Impaired actions of insulin-like growth factor 1 on protein synthesis and degradation in skeletal muscle of rats with chronic renal failure: evidence for a postreceptor defect. *J Clin Invest.* 1996;97:1064.
182. Fouque D, Peng SC, Kopple JD. Impaired metabolic response to recombinant insulin-like growth factor I in dialysis patients. *Kidney Int.* 1995;47:876.
183. Furth SL, Hwang W, Yang C, et al. Growth failure, risk of hospitalization and death for children with end-stage renal disease. *Pediatr Nephrol.* 2002;17:450.
184. Fine RN, Kohaut EC, Brown D, et al. Growth after recombinant human growth hormone treatment in children with chronic renal failure: report of a multicenter randomized double-blind placebo-controlled study. *J Pediatr.* 1994;124:374.
185. Haffner D, Schaefer F, Nissel R, et al. Effect of growth hormone treatment on the adult height of children with chronic renal failure. German Study Group for Growth Hormone Treatment in Chronic Renal Failure. *N Engl J Med.* 2000;343:923.
186. Zager PG, Spalding CT, Frey HJ, et al. Low dose adrenocorticotropin infusion in continuous ambulatory peritoneal dialysis patients. *J Clin Endocrinol Metab.* 1985;61:1205.
187. Luger A, Lang I, Kovarik J, et al. Abnormalities in the hypothalamic–pituitary–adrenocortical axis in patients with chronic renal failure. *Am J Kidney Dis.* 1987;9:51.
188. Siamopoulos KC, Dardamanis M, Kyriaki D, et al. Pituitary adrenal responsiveness to corticotropin releasing hormone in chronic uremic patients. *Peritoneal Dial Int.* 1990;10:153.
189. Ramirez G, Brueggemeyer C, Ganguly A. Counterregulatory hormonal response to insulin-induced hypoglycemia in patients on chronic hemodialysis. *Nephron.* 1988;49:231.
190. McDonald WJ, Golper TA, Mass RD, et al. Adrenocorticotropin–cortisol axis abnormalities in hemodialysis patients. *J Clin Endocrinol Metab.* 1979;48:92.
191. Betts PR, Howse PM, Morris R, et al. Serum cortisol concentrations in children with chronic renal insufficiency. *Arch Dis Child.* 1975;50:3.
192. Grant AC, Rodger RS, Mitchell R, et al. Hypothalamo-pituitary-adrenal axis in uraemia: evidence for primary adrenal dysfunction? *Nephrol Dial Transplant.* 1993;8:307.
193. Fasanella d'Amore T, Wauters JP, Waeber B, et al. Response of plasma vasopressin to change in extracellular volume and/or plasma osmolality in patients on maintenance hemodialysis. *Clin Nephrol.* 1985;23:299.
194. Kokot F, Grzeszczak W, Zukowska-Szczechowska E, et al. Water immersion induced alterations of plasma atrial natriuretic peptide level and its relationship to the renin–angiotensin–aldosterone system and vasopressin secretion in acute and chronic renal failure. *Clin Nephrol.* 1989;31:247.
195. Benmansour M, Rainfray M, Paillard F, et al. Metabolic clearance rate of immunoreactive vasopressin in man. *Eur J Clin Invest.* 1982;12:475.
196. Pruszczynski W, Viron B, Mignon F, et al. Massive plasma arginine vasopressin (AVP) removal during hemofiltration stimulates AVP secretion in humans. *J Clin Endocrinol Metab.* 1987;64:383.
197. Odar-Cedelof I, Eriksson CG, Theodorsson E, et al. Antidiuretic hormone regulation in hemodialysis. *ASAIO Trans.* 1991;37:M227.
198. Bolignano D, Zoccali C. Vasopressin beyond water: implications for renal diseases. *Curr Opin Nephrol Hypertens.* 2010,19:499.
199. Maier C, Clodi M, Neuhold S, et al. Endothelial markers may link kidney function to cardiovascular events in type 2 diabetes. *Diabetes Care.* 2009;32:1890.
200. Meijer E, Bakker SJ, de Jong PE, et al. Copeptin, a surrogate marker of vasopressin, is associated with accelerated renal function decline in renal transplant recipients. *Transplantation.* 2009; 88:561.
201. Iglesias P, Diez JJ. Thyroid dysfunction and kidney disease. *Eur J Endocrinol.* 2009;160:503.
202. Kaptein EM, Quiion-Verde H, Chooljian CJ, et al. The thyroid in end-stage renal disease. *Medicine.* 1988;67:187.
203. Hegedus L, Andersen JR, Poulsen LR, et al. Thyroid gland volume and serum concentrations of thyroid hormones in chronic renal failure. *Nephron.* 1985;40:171.
204. Kaptein EM. Thyroid hormone metabolism and thyroid diseases in chronic renal failure. *Endocrin Rev.* 1996;17:45.
205. Miki H, Oshimo K, Inoue H, et al. Thyroid nodules in female uremic patients on maintenance hemodialysis. *J Surg Oncol.* 1993;54:216.
206. Kantor AF, Hoover RN, Kinlen LJ, et al. Cancer in patients receiving long-term dialysis treatment. *Am J Epidemiol.* 1987;126:370.
207. Brunner FP, Landais P, Selwood NH. Malignancies after renal transplantation: the EDTA-ERA registry experience. European Dialysis and Transplantation Association-European Renal Association. *Nephrol Dial Transplant.* 1995;10:74.
208. Faber J, Heaf J, Kirkegaard C, et al. Simultaneous turnover studies of thyroxine, 3,5,3′ and 3,3′,5′-triiodothyronine, 3,5-, 3,3′-, and 3′,5′-diiodothyronine, and 3′-monoiodothyronine in chronic renal failure. *J Clin Endocrinol Metab.* 1983;56:211.
209. Wiederkehr MR, Kalogiros J, Krapf R. Correction of metabolic acidosis improves thyroid and growth hormone axes in haemodialysis patients. *Nephrol Dial Transplant.* 2004;19:1190.
210. Kaptein EM, Feinstein EI, Nicoloff JT, et al. Serum reverse triiodothyronine and thyroxine kinetics in patients with chronic renal failure. *J Clin Endocrinol Metab.* 1983;57:181.457.
211. Spector DA, Davis PJ, Helderman JH, et al. Thyroid function and metabolic state in chronic renal failure. *Ann Intern Med.* 1976;85:724.
212. Williams GR, Franklyn JA, Newberger JM, et al. Thyroid hormone receptor expression in the sick euthyroid syndrome. *Lancet.* 1989;2:1477.
213. Lim VS, Tsalikian E, Flanigan MJ. Augmentation of protein degradation by L-triiodothyronine in uremia. *Metabolism.* 1989;38:1210.
214. Davis FB, Spector DA, Davis PJ, et al. Comparison of pituitary-thyroid function in patients with endstage renal disease and in age- and sex-matched controls. *Kidney Int.* 1982;21:362.
215. Gonzalez-Barcena D, Kastin AJ, Schalch DS, et al. Response to thyrotropin releasing hormone in patients with renal failure and after infusion in normal man. *J Clin Endocrinol Metab.* 1973;36:117.
216. Bartalena L, Pacchiarotti A, Palla R, et al. Lack of nocturnal serum thyrotropin (TSH) surge in patients with chronic renal failure undergoing regular maintenance hemofiltration: a case of central hypothyroidism. *Clin Nephrol.* 1990; 34:30.
217. Wheatley T, Clark PM, Clark JD, et al. Abnormalities of thyrotrophin (TSH) evening rise and pulsatile release in haemodialysis patients: evidence for hypothalamic-pituitary changes in chronic renal failure. *Clin Endocrinol (Oxf).* 1989;31:39.
218. Takeda S, Michigishi T, Takazakura E. Iodine-induced hypothyroidism in patients on regular dialysis treatment. *Nephron.* 1993;65:51.
219. Chonchol M, Lippi G, Salvagno G, et al. Prevalence of subclinical hypothyroidism in patients with chronic kidney disease. *Clin J Am Soc Nephrol.* 2008;3:1296.
220. van Leusen R, Meinders AE. Cyclical changes in serum thyroid hormone concentrations related to hemodialysis: movement of hormone into and out of the extravascular space as a possible mechanism. *Clin Nephrol.* 1982;18:193.
221. Ramirez G, O'Neill W Jr, Jubiz W et al. Thyroid dysfunction in uremia: evidence for thyroid and hypophyseal abnormalities. *Ann Intern Med.* 1976;84:672.
222. Blair D, Byham-Gray L, Lewis E, et al. Prevalence of vitamin D [25(OH) D] deficiency and effects of supplementation with ergocalciferol (vitamin D2) in stage 5 chronic kidney disease patients. *J Ren Nutr.* 2008;18:375.
223. Rojas-Rivera J, de la Piedra C, Ramos A, et al. The expanding spectrum of biological actions of vitamin D. *Nephrol Dial Transplant* 2010;25:2850.
224. Delmez JA, Slatopolsky E, Martin KJ, et al. Mineral, vitamin D and parathyroid hormone in continuous ambulatory peritoneal dialysis. *Kidney Int.* 1982;21:862.
225. Tokmak F, Quack I, Schieren G, et al. High-dose cholecalciferol to correct vitamin D deficiency in haemodialysis patients. *Nephrol Dial Transplant.* 2008;23:4016.
226. Chandra P, Binongo JN, Ziegler TR, et al. Cholecalciferol (vitamin D3) therapy and vitamin D insufficiency in patients with chronic kidney disease: a randomized controlled pilot study. *Endocr Pract.* 2008;14:10.
227. Wang TJ, Pencina MJ, Booth SL, et al. Vitamin D deficiency and risk of cardiovascular disease. *Circulation.* 2008;117:503.
228. Patel T, Singh AK. Role of vitamin D in chronic kidney disease. *Semin Nephrol.* 2009; 29:113.
229. Korkor AB. Reduced binding of (H) 1,25-dihydroxyvitamin D3 in the parathyroid glands of patients with renal failure. *N Engl J Med.* 1987;316:1573.
230. Kovesdy CP, Ahmadzadeh S, Anderson JE, et al. Association of activated vitamin D treatment and mortality in chronic kidney disease. *Arch Intern Med.* 2008;168:397.
231. Tentori F, Hunt WC, Stidley CA, et al. Mortality risk among hemodialysis patients receiving different vitamin D analogs. *Kidney Int.* 2006;70:1858.
232. Teng M, Wolf M, Lowrie E, et al. Survival of patients undergoing hemodialysis with paricalcitol or calcitriol therapy. *N Engl J Med.* 2003;349:446.

233. Isakova T, Gutiérrez OM, Patel NM, et al. Vitamin D deficiency, inflammation, and albuminuria in chronic kidney disease: complex interactions. *J Ren Nutr.* 2010;21:295–302.
234. Agarwal R, Acharya M, Tian J, et al. Antiproteinuric effect of oral paricalcitol in chronic kidney disease. *Kidney Int.* 2005;68:2823.
235. Alborzi P, Patel NA, Peterson C, et al. Paricalcitol reduces albuminuria and inflammation in chronic kidney disease: a randomized double-blind pilot trial. *Hypertension.* 2008;52:249.
236. Weidmann P, Beretta-Piccoli C, Steffen F, et al. Hypertension in terminal renal failure. *Kidney Int.* 1976;9:294.
237. Weidmann P, Maxwell MH. The renin-angiotensin system in terminal renal failure. *Kidney Int.* 1975;8:S219.
238. DeFronzo RA. Hyperkalemia and hyporeninemic hypoaldosteronism. *Kidney Int.* 1980;17:118.
239. Iitake K, Kimura T, Matsui K, et al. Effect of haemodialysis in plasma ADH levels, plasma renin activity and plasma aldosterone levels in patients with end-stage renal disease. *Acta Endocrinol (Copenhagen).* 1985;110:207.
240. Lewis EJ, Hunsicker LG, Bain RP, et al. The effect of angiotensin-converting-enzyme inhibition on diabetic nephropathy. *N Engl J Med.* 1993;329:1456.
241. Lewis EJ, Hunsicker LG, Clarke WR, et al. Collaborative Study Group. Renoprotective effect of the angiotensin-receptor antagonist irbesartan in patients with nephropathy due to type 2 diabetes. *N Engl J Med.* 2001;345:851.
242. Brenner BM, Cooper MK, de Zeeuw D, et al. RENAAL Study Investigators. Effects of losartan on renal and cardiovascular outcomes in patients with type 2 diabetes and nephropathy. *N Engl J Med.* 2001;345:861.
243. Price DA, Porter LE, Gordon M, et al. The paradox of the low-renin state in diabetic nephropathy. *J Am Soc Nephrol.* 1999;10:2382.
244. Maschio G, Marcantoni C, Bernich P. Lessons from large interventional trials on antihypertensive therapy in chronic renal disease. *Nephrol Dial Transplant.* 2002;17 Suppl 11:47.
245. Shibasaki Y, Masaki H, Nishiue T, et al. Angiotensin II type 1 receptor antagonist, losartan, causes regression of left ventricular hypertrophy in end-stage renal disease. *Nephron.* 2002;90:256.
246. Knoll GA, Sahgal A, Nair RC, et al. Renin-angiotensin system blockade and the risk of hyperkalemia in chronic hemodialysis patients. *Am J Med.* 2002;112:110.
247. Quan ZY, Walser M, Hill GS. Adrenalectomy ameliorates ablative nephropathy in the rat independently of corticosterone maintenance level. *Kidney Int.* 1992;41:326.
248. Gavras H, Brunner HR, Laragh JH, et al. Malignant hypertension resulting from deoxycorticosterone acetate and salt excess: role of renin and sodium in vascular changes. *Circ Res.* 1975;36:300.
249. Greene EL, Kren S, Hostetter TH. Role of aldosterone in the remnant kidney model in the rat. *J Clin Invest.* 1996; 98:1063.
250. Aldigier JC, Kanjanbuch T, Ma LJ, et al. Regression of existing glomerulosclerosis by inhibition of aldosterone. *J Am Soc Nephrol.* 2005;16:3306.
251. Xue C, Siragy HM. Local renal aldosterone system and its regulation by salt, diabetes, and angiotensin II type 1 receptor. *Hypertension.* 2005;46:584.
252. Han SY, Kim CH, Kim HS, et al. Spironolactone prevents diabetic nephropathy through an anti-inflammatory mechanism in type 2 diabetic rats. *J Am Soc Nephrol.* 2006;17:1362.
253. Rocha R, Funder JW. The pathophysiology of aldosterone in the cardiovascular system. *Ann NY Acad Sci.* 2002;970:89.
254. Hené RJ, Boer P, Koomans HA, et al. Plasma aldosterone concentrations in chronic renal disease. *Kidney Int.* 1982;21:98.
255. Walker WG. Hypertension-related renal injury: a major contributor to end-stage renal disease. *Am J Kidney Dis.* 1993;22:164.
256. Ruggenenti P, Perna A, Gherardi G, et al. Renal function and requirement for dialysis in chronic nephropathy patients on long-term ramipril: REIN follow-up trial. Gruppo Italiano di Studi Epidemiologici in Nefrologia (GISEN). Ramipril efficacy in nephropathy. *Lancet.* 1998;352:1252.
257. Chrysostomou A, Becker G. Spironolactone in addition to ACE inhibition to reduce proteinuria in patients with chronic renal disease. *N Engl J Med.* 2001;345:925.
258. Bomback AS, Kshirsagar AV, Amamoo MA, et al. Change in proteinuria after adding aldosterone blockers to ACE inhibitors or angiotensin receptor blockers in CKD: a systematic review. *Am J Kidney Dis.* 2008;51:199.
259. Navaneethan SD, Nigwekar SU, Sehgal AR, et al. Aldosterone antagonists for preventing the progression of chronic kidney disease. *Cochr Data System Rev.* 2009;4:542–551.
260. Vanderheyden M, Bartunek J, Goethals M. Brain and other natriuretic peptides: molecular aspects. *Eur J Heart Fail.* 2004;6:261.
261. Clerico A, Iervasi G, Mariani G. Pathophysiologic relevance of measuring the plasma levels of cardiac natriuretic peptide hormones in humans. *Horm Metab Res.* 1999;31:487.
262. Ishizaka Y, Yamamoto Y, Fukunaga T, et al. Plasma concentration of human brain natriuretic peptide in patients on hemodialysis. *Am J Kidney Dis.* 1994;24:461.
263. Deray G, Maistre G, Basset JY, et al. Plasma levels of atrial natriuretic peptide in chronically dialyzed patients. *Kidney Int.* 1988;25(Suppl):S86.
264. Predel HG, Kipnowski J, Meyer-Lehnert H, et al. Human atrial natriuretic peptide in non-dialyzed patients with chronic renal failure. *Clin Nephrol.* 1989;31:150.
265. Pedersen EB, Bacevicus E, Bech J, et al. Abnormal rhythmic oscillations of atrial natriuretic peptide and brain natriuretic peptide in chronic renal failure. *J Clin Sci.* 2006;110:491.
266. Tonolo G, McMillan M, Polonia J, et al. Plasma clearance and effects of alpha-hANP infused in patients with end-stage renal failure. *Am J Physiol.* 1988;254:F895.
267. Buckley MG, Sethi D, Markandu ND, et al. Plasma concentrations and comparisons of brain natriuretic peptide and atrial natriuretic peptide in normal subjects, cardiac transplant recipients and patients with dialysis-independent or dialysis-dependent chronic renal failure. *Clin Sci (London).* 1992;83:437.
268. Corboy JC, Walker RJ, Simmonds MB, et al. Plasma natriuretic peptides and cardiac volume during acute changes in intravascular volume in haemodialysis patients. *Clin Sci (London).* 1994;87:679.
269. Ishibe S, Peixoto AJ. Methods of assessment of volume status and intercompartmental fluid shifts in hemodialysis patients: implications in clinical practice. *Semin Dial.* 2004;17:37.
270. Clerico A, Emdin M. Diagnostic accuracy and prognostic relevance of the measurement of cardiac natriuretic peptides: a review. *Clin Chem.* 2004; 50:33.
271. Dhar S, Pressman GS, Subramanian S, et al. Natriuretic peptides and heart failure in the patient with chronic kidney disease: a review of current evidence. *Postgrad Med J.* 2009;85:299–302.
272. Mallamaci F, Zoccali C, Tripepi G, et al. Diagnostic potential of cardiac natriuretic peptides in dialysis patients. The Cardiovascular Risk Extended Evaluation. *Kidney Int.* 2001;59:1559.
273. Tripepi G, Mattace-Raso F, Mallamaci F, et al. Biomarkers of left atrial volume: a longitudinal study in patients with end stage renal disease. *Hypertension.* 2009;54:818.
274. Zoccali C, Mallamaci F, Benedetto FA, et al. Cardiac natriuretic peptides are related to left ventricular mass and function and predict mortality in dialysis patients. *J Am Soc Nephrol.* 2001;12:1508.
275. Nakatani T, Naganuma T, Masuda C, et al. The prognostic role of atrial natriuretic peptides in hemodialysis patients. *Blood Purif.* 2003;21:395.
276. Goto T, Takase H, Toriyama T, et al. Increased circulating levels of natriuretic peptides predict future cardiac event in patients with chronic hemodialysis. *Nephron.* 2002;92:610.
277. Naganuma T, Sugimura K, Wada S, et al. The prognostic role of brain natriuretic peptides in hemodialysis patients. *Am J Nephrol.* 2002;22:437.
278. Sirinek KR, O'Dorisio TM, Gaskill HV, et al. Chronic renal failure: effect of hemodialysis on gastrointestinal hormones. *Am J Surg.* 1984;148:732.
279. El Ghonaimy E, Barsoum R, Soliman M, et al. Serum gastrin in chronic renal failure: morphological and physiological correlations. *Nephron.* 1985;39:86.
280. Muto S, Murayama N, Asano Y, et al. Hypergastrinaemia and achlorhydria in chronic renal failure. *Nephron.* 1985;40:143.
281. Grace SG, Davidson WD, State D. Renal mechanism for removal of gastrin from the circulation. *Surg Forum.* 1974;25:323.
282. Cheung WW, Mak RK. Ghrelin in chronic kidney disease. *Int J Pept.* 2010; 2010 pii:567343.
283. Pèrez-Fontan M, Cordido F, Rodrıguez-Carmona A, et al. Plasma ghrelin levels in patients undergoing haemodialysis and peritoneal dialysis. *Nephrol Dial Transplant.* 2004;19:2095.
284. Yoshimoto A, Mori K, Sugawara A, et al. Associations between plasma ghrelin levels and body composition in endstage renal disease: a longitudinal study. Plasma ghrelin and desacyl ghrelin concentrations in renal failure. *J Am Soc Nephrol.* 2002;13:2748.
285. Wynne K, Giannitsopoulou K, Small CJ, et al. Subcutaneous ghrelin enhances acute food intake in malnourished patients who receive maintenance peritoneal dialysis: a randomized, placebo-controlled trial. *J Am Soc Nephrol.* 2005;16:2111.
286. Ashby DR, Ford HE, Wynne KJ, et al. Sustained appetite improvement in malnourished dialysis patients by daily ghrelin treatment. *Kidney Int* 2009;76:199.
287. Wright M, Woodrow G, O'Brien S, et al. Cholecystokinin and leptin: their influence upon the eating behaviour and nutrient intake of dialysis patients. *Nephrol Dial Transplant.* 2004;19:133.
288. Owyang C, Miller LJ, DiMagno EP, et al. Gastrointestinal hormone profile in renal insufficiency. *Mayo Clin Proc.* 1979;54:769.

289. Grekas DM, Raptis S, Tourkantonis AA. Plasma secretin, pancreozymin and somatostatin-like hormone in chronic renal failure patients. *Uremia Invest.* 1984;8:117.

290. Hegbrant J, Thysell H, Ekman R. Plasma levels of gastrointestinal regulatory peptides in patients receiving maintenance hemodialysis. *Scand J Gastroenterol.* 1991;26:599.

291. Henriksen JH, Staun-Olsen P, Borg Mogensen N, et al. Circulating endogenous vasoactive intestinal polypeptide (VIP) in patients with uraemia and liver cirrhosis. *Eur J Clin Invest.* 1986;16:211.

292. Wiecek A, Kokot F, Chudek J, et al. The adipose tissue—a novel endocrine organ of interest to the nephrologist. *Nephrol Dial Transplant.* 2002;17:191.

293. Heimbürger O, Lönnqvist F, Danielsson A, et al. Serum immunoreactive leptin concentration and its relation to the body fat content in chronic renal failure. *J Am Soc Nephrol.* 1997;8:1423.

294. Kokot F, Adamczak M, Wiecek A. Plasma leptin concentration in kidney transplant patients during the early post-transplant period. *Nephrol Dial Transplant.* 1998;13:2276.

295. Ficek R, Kokot F, Chudek J, et al. Plasma leptin concentration in patients with acute renal failure. *Clin Nephrol.* 2004;62:84.

296. Cumin F, Baum HP, Levens N. Mechanism of leptin removal from the circulation by the kidney. *J Endocrinol.* 1997;155:577.

297. Meyer C, Robson D, Rackovsky N, et al. Role of the kidney in human leptin metabolism. *Am J Physiol.* 1997;273:E903.

298. Zeng J, Patterson BW, Klein S, et al. Whole body leptin kinetics and renal metabolism in vivo. *Am J Physiol.* 1997;273:E1102.

299. Cumin F, Baum HP, de Gasparo M, et al. Removal of endogenous leptin from the circulation by the kidney. *Int J Obesity Relat Metab Disord.* 1997;21:495.

300. Nordfors L, Lönnqvist F, Heimbürger O, et al. Low leptin gene expression and hyperleptinemia in chronic renal failure. *Kidney Int.* 1998;54:1267.

301. van Tellingen A, Grooteman MP, Schoorl M, et al. Enhanced long-term reduction of plasma leptin concentrations by super-flux polysulfone dialysers. *Nephrol Dial Transplant.* 2004;19:1198.

302. Fontan MP, Rodriguez-Carmona A, Cordido F, et al. Hyperleptinemia in uremic patients undergoing conservative management, peritoneal dialysis, and hemodialysis: a comparative analysis. *Am J Kidney Dis.* 1999;34:824.

303. Young GA, Woodrow G, Kendall S, et al. Increased plasma leptin/fat ratio in patients with chronic renal failure: a cause of malnutrition? *Nephrol Dial Transplant.* 1997;12:2318.

304. Johansen KL, Mulligan K, Tai V, et al. Leptin, body composition, and indices of malnutrition in patients on dialysis. *J Am Soc Nephrol.* 1998;9:1080.

305. Chudek J, Adamczak M, Kania M, et al. Does plasma leptin concentration predict the nutritional status of hemodialyzed patients with chronic renal failure? *Med Sci Monit.* 2003;9:CR377.

306. Stenvinkel P, Heimburger O, Lonnqvist F, et al. Does the ob gene product leptin stimulate erythropoiesis in patients with chronic renal failure? *Kidney Int.* 1998;53:1430.

307. Wolf G, Hamann A, Han DC, et al. Leptin stimulates proliferation and TGF-beta expression in renal glomerular endothelial cells: potential role in glomerulosclerosis. *Kidney Int.* 1999;56:860.

308. Carrero JJ, Cordeiro AC, Lindholm B, et al. The emerging pleiotrophic role of adipokines in the uremic phenotype. *Curr Opin Nephrol Hypertens.* 2010;19:37–42.

309. Iwashima Y, Horio T, Kumada M, et al. Adiponectin and renal function and implication as a risk of cardiovascular disease. *Am J Cardiol.* 2006; 98:1603.

310. Shen YY, Charlesworth JA, Kelly JJ, et al. The effect of renal transplantation on adiponectin and its isoforms and receptors. *Metabolism.* 2007;56:1201.

311. Chudek J, Adamczak M, Karkoszka H, et al. Plasma adiponectin concentration before and after successful kidney transplantation. *Transplant Proc.* 2003;35:2186.

312. Adamczak M, Rzepka E, Chudek J, et al. Ageing and plasma adiponectin concentration in apparently healthy males and females. *Clin Endocrinol.* 2005;62:114.

313. Becker B, Kronenberg F, Kielstein JT, et al. Renal insulin resistance syndrome, adiponectin and cardiovascular events in patients with kidney disease: the mild and moderate kidney disease study. *J Am Soc Nephrol.* 2005;16:1091.

314. Adamczak M, Szotowska M, Chudek J, et al. Plasma adiponectin concentration in patients after successful kidney transplantation—a single centre, observational study. *Clin Nephrol.* 2007;67:381.

315. Adamczak M, Czerwieńska B, Chudek J, et al. Renal extraction of circulating adiponectin in patients with renovascular hypertension. *Acta Physiol Hung.* 2007;94:143.

316. Marchlewska A, Stenvinkel P, Lindholm B, et al. Reduced gene expression of adiponectin in fat tissue from patients with end-stage renal disease. *Kidney Int.* 2004;66:46.

317. Adamczak M, Chudek J, Wiecek A. Adiponectin in patients with chronic kidney disease. *Seminar Dial.* 2009;22:391.

318. Rao M, Li L, Tighiouart H, et al. Plasma adiponectin levels and clinical outcomes among haemodialysis patients. *Nephrol Dial Transplant.* 2008; 23:2619.

319. Saito O, Saito T, Okuda K, et al. Serum adiponectin and markers of endothelial injury in hemodialysis patients with arteriosclerosis obliterans. *Clin Exp Nephrol.* 2008;12:58.

320. Malyszko J, Wolczynski S, Mysliwiec M. Adiponectin, leptin and thyroid hormones in patients with chronic renal failure and on renal replacement therapy: are they related? *Nephrol Dial Transplant.* 2006;21:145.

321. Karabinis A, Kyriazis J, Vardas P, et al. Adiponectin and cardiovascular remodeling in end-stage renal disease and co-morbid diabetes mellitus. *Am J Nephrol.* 2006;26:340.

322. Iwasa Y, Otsubo S, Ishizuka T, et al. Influence of serum high-molecular-weight and total adiponectin on arteriosclerosis in IgA nephropathy patients. *Nephron Clin Pract.* 2008;108:c226.

323. Zoccali C, Mallamaci F, Tripepi G, et al. Adiponectin, metabolic risk factors, and cardiovascular events among patients with end-stage renal disease. *J Am Soc Nephrol.* 2002;13:134.

324. Yu ZZ, Ni ZH, Gu LY, et al. Adiponectin is related to carotid artery plaque and a predictor of cardiovascular outcome in a cohort of non-diabetic peritoneal dialysis patients. *Blood Purif.* 2008;26:386.

325. Jorsal A, Tarnow L, Frystyk J, et al. Serum adiponectin predicts all-cause mortality and end stage renal disease in patients with type I diabetes and diabetic nephropathy. *Kidney Int.* 2008;74:649.

326. Menon V, Li L, Wang X, et al. Adiponectin and mortality in patients with chronic kidney disease. *J Am Soc Nephrol.* 2006;17:2599.

327. Drechsler C, Krane V, Winkler K, et al. Changes in adiponectin and the risk of sudden death, stroke, myocardial infarction, and mortality in hemodialysis patients. *Kidney Int.* 2009;76:567.

328. Saraheimo M, Forsblom C, Thorn L, et al. Serum adiponectin and progression of diabetic nephropathy in patients with type 1 diabetes. *Diabetes Care.* 2008;31:1165.

CHAPTER 81

Immunobiology and Immunopharmacology of Renal Allograft Rejection

Choli Hartono • Terry B. Strom • Manikkam Suthanthiran

Renal transplantation is the treatment of choice for patients with irreversible renal failure and has moved from a high risk, experimental procedure to a safe, clinical procedure in the relatively short time of five decades.[1] The substantive gains in patient and graft survival owe much to an improved understanding of the antiallograft repertoire, better preservation of donor kidneys, judicious usage of immunosuppressive drugs and monoclonal/polyclonal antibodies, and the clinical application of infection prophylaxis protocols.

IMMUNOBIOLOGY OF RENAL TRANSPLANTATION

The Antiallograft Response

Allograft rejection is contingent on the coordinated activation of alloreactive T cells and antigen-presenting cells (APCs). Through the intermediacy of cytokines and cell-to-cell interactions, a heterogeneous contingent of lymphocytes, including CD4+ helper T cells, CD8+ cytotoxic T cells, antibody-forming B cells, and other proinflammatory leukocytes are recruited into the antiallograft response (Fig. 81.1 and Table 81.1).

T Cell Activation and the Immunologic Synapse: Signal One

The immunologic synapse consists of a multiplicity of T cell-surface protein forms and clusters, thereby creating a platform for antigen recognition and generation of crucial T cell activation-related signals.[2] The synapse begins to form when the initial adhesions between certain T cell (e.g., CD2, LFA-1) and APC surface proteins (e.g., CD58, ICAM-1) are formed (Table 81.2). These physical contacts between T cells and APCs provide an opportunity for the antigen reactive T cells to recognize cognate antigen. Antigen-driven T cell activation, a highly coordinated, preprogrammed process, begins when T cells recognize intracellularly processed fragments of foreign proteins (approximately 8 to 16 amino acids) embedded within the groove of the major histocompatibility complex (MHC) proteins expressed on the surface of APCs.[3–5] Some of the recipient's T cells directly recognize the allograft (i.e., donor antigen[s] presented on the surface of donor APCs) and this process is termed direct recognition whereas other T cells recognize the donor antigen after it is processed and presented by self-APCs[6] (Fig. 81.1) and this process is designated indirect recognition.

The T cell antigen receptor (TCR)–CD3 complex is composed of clonally distinct TCR α and β peptide chains that recognize the antigenic peptide in the context of MHC proteins and clonally invariant CD3 chains that propagate intracellular signals originating from antigenic recognition (Fig. 81.2).[2,7,8] The TCR variable, diversity, junction, and constant region genes (i.e., genes for regions of the clone-specific antigen receptors) are spliced together in a cassette-like fashion during T cell maturation.[7] A small population of T cells expresses TCR γ and δ chains instead of the TCR α and β chains.

CD4 and CD8 proteins, expressed on reciprocal T cell subsets, bind to nonpolymorphic domains of human leukocyte antigen (HLA) class II (DR, DP, DQ) and class I (A, B, C) molecules, respectively (Fig. 81.1 and Table 81.2).[2,7] A threshold of TCR to MHC-peptide engagements is necessary to stabilize the immunologic synapse stimulating a redistribution of cell-surface proteins and coclustering of the TCR/CD3 complex with the T cell-surface proteins.[8–10] Additional T cell surface proteins such as CD5 proteins join the synapse.[9,10] The TCR cluster already includes integrins (e.g., LFA-1) and nonintegrins (e.g., CD2)[2,8,9] that have created T cell–APC adhesions. Hence, antigen recognition stimulates a redistribution of cell-surface proteins and coclustering of the TCR/CD3 complex with the T cell-surface proteins[2,7–9] and signaling molecules. This multimeric complex functions as a unit in initiating T cell activation.

Following activation by antigen, the TCR–CD3 complex and coclustered CD4 and CD8 proteins are physically associated with intracellular protein–tyrosine kinases (PTKs)

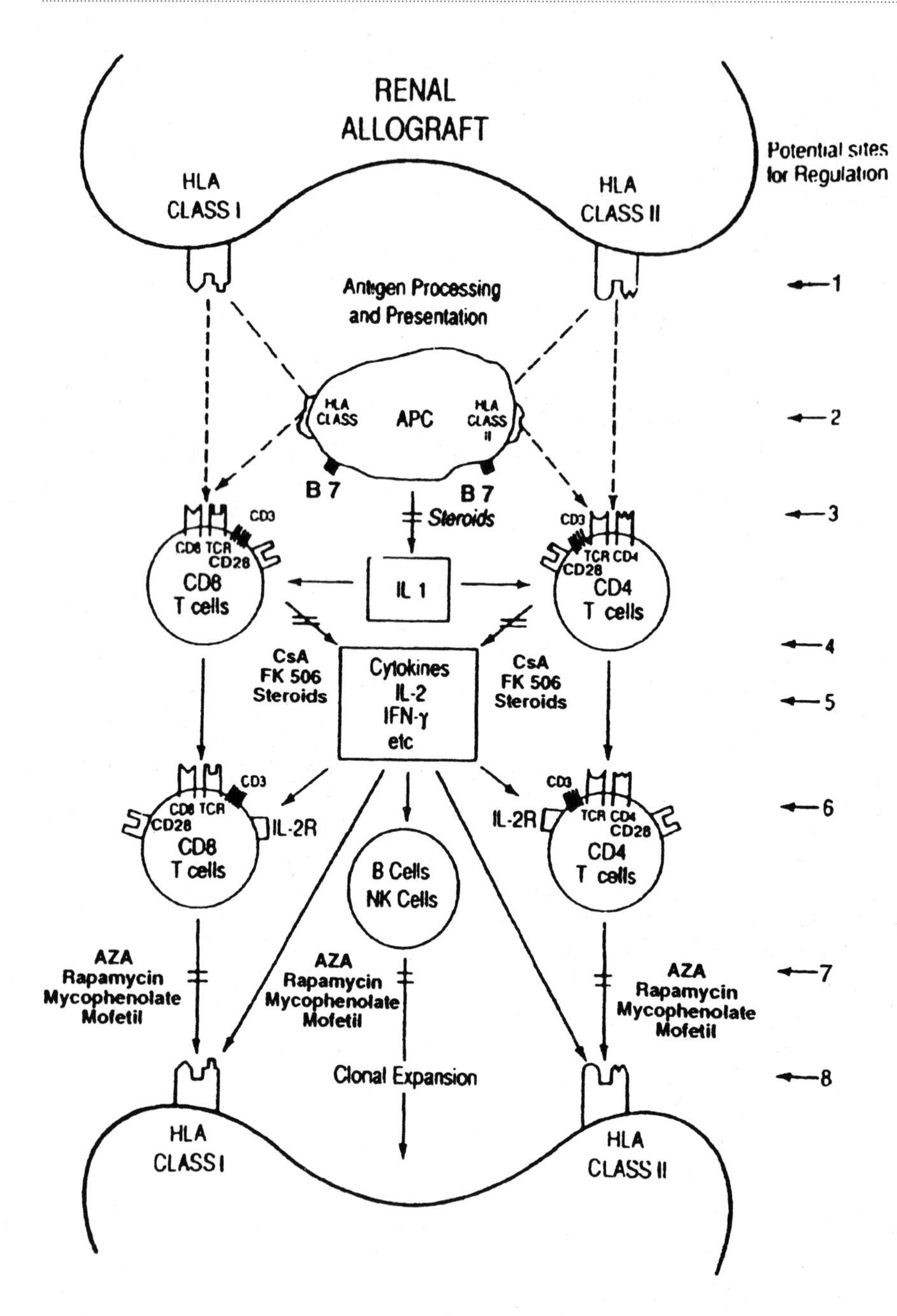

FIGURE 81.1 The antiallograft response. Schematic representation of human leukocyte antigens (HLA), the primary stimuli for the initiation of the antiallograft response, cell-surface proteins participating in antigenic recognition and signal transduction, contribution of the cytokines and multiple cell types to the immune response, and the potential sites for the regulation of the antiallograft response. *Site 1*: Minimizing histoincompatibility between the recipients and the donor (e.g., HLA matching). *Site 2*: Prevention of monokine production by antigen-presenting cells (e.g., corticosteroids). *Site 3*: Blockade of antigen recognition (e.g., OKT3 mAbs). *Site 4*: Inhibition of T cell cytokine production (e.g., cyclosporin A [CsA]). *Site 5*: Inhibition of cytokine activity (e.g., anti-interleukin-2 [IL-2] antibody). *Site 6*: Inhibition of cell cycle progression (e.g., anti-IL-2 receptor antibody). *Site 7*: Inhibition of clonal expansion (e.g., azathioprine [AZA]). *Site 8*: Prevention of allograft damage by masking target antigen molecules (e.g., antibodies directed at adhesion molecules). HLA class I: HLA-A, B, and C antigens; HLA class II: HLA-DR, DP, and DQ antigens. *IFN-γ*, interferon-γ; *NK cells*, natural killer cells.

of two different families, the src (including $p59^{fyn}$ and $p56^{lck}$) and ZAP 70 families.[2] The CD45 protein, a tyrosine phosphatase, contributes to the activation process by dephosphorylating an autoinhibitory site on the $p56^{lck}$ PTK. Intracellular domains of several TCR/CD3 proteins contain activation motifs that are crucial for antigen-stimulated signaling. Certain tyrosine residues within these motifs serve as targets for the catalytic activity of src family PTKs. Subsequently, these phosphorylated tyrosines serve as docking stations for the SH2 domains (recognition structures for select phosphotyrosine-containing motifs) of the ZAP-70 PTK. Following antigenic engagement of the TCR/CD3 complex, select serine residues of the TCR and CD3 chains are also phosphorylated.[2,5]

The waves of tyrosine phosphorylation triggered by antigen recognition encompass other intracellular proteins and are a cardinal event in initiating T cell activation. Tyrosine phosphorylation of the phospholipase $C\gamma_1$ activates this coenzyme and triggers a cascade of events that leads to full expression of T cell programs: hydrolysis of phosphatidylinositol 4,5-biphosphate (PIP_2) and generation of two intracellular messengers, inositol 1,4,5-triphosphate (IP_3) and diacylglycerol (Fig. 81.2).[11] IP_3, in turn, mobilizes ionized calcium from intracellular stores, while diacylglycerol, in the presence of increased cytosolic free Ca^{2+}, binds to and translocates protein kinase C (PKC)—a phospholipid/Ca^{2+}-sensitive protein serine/threonine kinase—to the membrane in its enzymatically active form.[5,11] Sustained activation of PKC is dependent on diacylglycerol generation from hydrolysis of additional lipids, such as phosphatidylcholine.

The increase in intracellular free Ca^{2+} and sustained PKC activation promote the expression of several nuclear regulatory proteins (e.g., nuclear factor of activated T cells

TABLE 81.1 **Cellular Elements Contributing to the Antiallograft Response**

Cell Type	Functional Attributes
T cells	The CD4+ T cells and the CD8+ T cells participate in the antiallograft response. CD4+ T cells recognize antigens presented by HLA class II proteins; CD8+ T cells recognize antigens presented by HLA class I proteins. The CD3/TCR complex is responsible for recognition of antigen and generates and transduces the antigenic signal.
CD4+ T cells	CD4+ T cells function mostly as helper T cells and secrete cytokines such as IL-2, a T cell growth/death factor, and IFN-γ, a proinflammatory polypeptide that can upregulate the expression of HLA proteins as well as augment cytotoxic activity of T cells and NK cells. Recently, three main types of CD4+ T cells have been recognized: CD4+ TH1, CD4+ TH2, and CD4 TH17. IL-2 and IFN-γ are produced by CD4+ TH1 type cells, IL-4 and IL-5 are secreted by CD4+ TH2 type cells, and IL-17 family of cytokines CD4+CD17 cells. Each cell type can regulate the secretion of the other and the regulated secretion is important in the expression of host immunity.
CD8+ T cells	CD8+ T cells function mainly as cytotoxic T cells. A subset of CD8+ T cells expresses suppressor cell function. CD8+ T cells can secrete cytokines such as IL-2 and IFN-γ and can express molecules, such as perforin, granzymes that function as effectors of cytotoxicity.
APCs	Monocytes/macrophages and dendritic cells function as potent APCs. Donor's APCs can process and present donor antigens to recipient's T cells (direct recognition) or recipient's APCs can process and present donor antigens to recipient's T cells (indirect recognition). The relative contribution of direct recognition and indirect recognition to the antiallograft response has not been resolved. Direct recognition and indirect recognition might also have differential susceptibility to inhibition by immunosuppressive drugs.
B cells	B cells require T cell help for the differentiation and production of antibodies directed at donor antigens. The alloantibodies can damage the graft by binding and activating complement components (complement-dependent cytotoxicity) and/or binding the Fc receptor of cells capable of mediating cytotoxicity (antibody-dependent, cell-mediated cytotoxicity).
NK cells	The precise role of NK cells in the antiallograft response is not known. Increased NK cell activity has been correlated with rejection. NK cell function might also be important in immune surveillance mechanisms pertinent to the prevention of infection and malignancy.

APCs, antigen presenting cells; IFN, interferon; IL, interleukin; HLA, human leukocyte antigen; NK, natural killer; TCR, T cell antigen receptor.
Reproduced from Suthanthiran M, Morris RE, Strom TB. Transplantation immunobiology.
In: Walsh PC, Retik AB, Vaughn ED Jr, et al., eds. *Campbell's Urology,* 7th ed. Philadelphia, PA: Saunders; 1997:491, with permission.

[NF-AT], nuclear factor kappa B [NF-κB], activator protein 1 [AP-1]) and the transcriptional activation and expression of genes central to T cell growth (e.g., interleukin-2 [IL-2] and receptors for IL-2 and IL-15).[2,5,12]

Calcineurin, a Ca^{2+}- and calmodulin-dependent serine/threonine phosphatase, is crucial to Ca^{2+}-dependent, TCR-initiated signal transduction.[13,14] Inhibition by cyclosporine and tacrolimus (FK-506) of the phosphatase activity of calcineurin is considered central to their immunosuppressive activity.[15]

Costimulatory Signals: Signal Two

Signaling of T cells via the TCR/CD3 complex (signal one) is necessary, but insufficient, to induce T cell proliferation; full activation of T cells is dependent on both the antigenic signals and the costimulatory signals (signal two) engendered by the contactual interactions between cell-surface proteins expressed on antigen-specific T cells and APCs (Fig. 81.3 and Table 81.2).[16,17] The interaction of the CD2 protein on the T cell surface with the CD58 (leukocyte function-associated antigen 3 [LFA-3]) protein on the surface of APCs, and that of the CD11a/CD18 (LFA-1) proteins with the CD54 (intercellular adhesion molecule 1 [ICAM-1]) proteins,[18] and/or the interaction of the CD5 with the CD72 proteins[10] aids in imparting such a costimulatory signal.

Recognition of the B7-1 (CD80) and B7-2 (CD86) proteins expressed upon CD4+ T cells generates a very

TABLE 81.2 Cell-Surface Proteins Important for T Cell Activation[a]

T Cell Surface	APC Surface	Functional Response	Potential Consequence of Blockade
LFA-1 (CD11a, CD18)	ICAM (CD54)	Adhesion	Immunosuppression
ICAM1 (CD54)	LFA-1 (CD11a, CD18)	Adhesion	Immunosuppression
CD8, TCR, CD3	MHCI	Antigen recognition	Immunosuppression
CD4, TCR, CD3	MHCII	Antigen recognition	Immunosuppression
CD2	LFA3 (CD58)	Costimulation	Immunosuppression
CD40L (CD154)	CD40	Costimulation	Immunosuppression
CD5	CD72	Adhesion	Immunosuppression
CD28	B7-1 (CD80)	Costimulation	Anergy
CD28	B7-2 (CD86)	Costimuation	Anergy
CTLA4 (CD152)	B7-1 (CD80)	Inhibition	Immunostimulation
CTLA4 (CD152)	B7-2 (CD86)	Inhibition	Immunostimuation

[a]Receptor/counterreceptor pairs that mediate interactions between T cells and APCs are shown in this table. Inhibition of each protein-to-protein interaction, except the CTLA4–B7.1/B7.2 interaction, results in an abortive in vitro immune response. Initial contact between T cells and APCs requires an antigen-independent adhesive interaction. Next, the T cell antigen-receptor complex engages processed antigen presented within the antigen-presenting groove of MHC molecules. Finally, costimulatory signals are required for full T cell activation. An especially important signal is generated by B7-mediated activation of CD28 on T cells. Activation of CD28 by B7.2 may provide a more potent signal than activation by B7.1. CTLA4, present on activated but not resting T cells, imparts a negative signal. Monoclonal antibodies directed at the T cell CD2 protein, used as component of a preconditioning regimen, has been associated with tolerance to histoincompatble human renal allografts.[23]

APC, antigen-presenting cell; ICAM, intercellular adhesion molecule; LFA, leukocyte function-associated; MHC, major histocompatibility complex.

Reproduced from Suthanthiran M, Morris RE, Strom TB. Transplantation immunobiology. In: Walsh PC, Retik AB, Vaughn ED Jr, et al., eds. *Campbell's Urology,* 7th ed. Philadelphia: WB Saunders, 1997:491, with permission.

powerful T cell costimulus.[19] A subset of monocytes and dendritic cells constitutively express CD80 and CD86 at low levels and cytokines (e.g., granulocyte–macrophage colony-stimulating factor [GMCSF] or interferon-γ [IFN-γ]) stimulate heightened expression of CD80 and CD86 on monocytes, B cells, and dendritic cells.[19] Many T cells express B7-binding proteins (i.e., CD28 proteins that are constitutively expressed on the surface of CD4+ T cells and CTLA-4 [CD152]), a protein whose ectodomain is closely related to that of CD28, and is expressed upon activated CD4+ and CD8+ T cells. CD28 binding of B7 molecules stimulates a Ca^{2+}-independent activation pathway that leads to stable transcription of the IL-2, IL-2 receptors, and other activation genes resulting in vigorous T cell proliferation.[19] For some time, the terms CD28 and the costimulatory receptor were considered synonymous by some, but the demonstration that robust T cell activation occurs in CD28-deficient mice indicated that other receptor ligand systems contribute to signal two.[20] In particular, the interaction between CD40 expressed upon APCs and CD40 ligand (CD154) expressed by antigen-activated CD4+ T cells has received great attention as a potent second signal.[21]

The delivery of the antigenic first signal and the costimulatory second signal leads to stable transcription of the IL-2, several T cell growth-factor receptors, and other pivotal T cell activation genes (Table 81.2). The Ca^{2+}-independent costimulatory CD28 pathway is relatively more resistant to inhibition by cyclosporine or FK-506 as compared to the calcium-dependent pathway of T cell activation. Whereas the interactions between B7 proteins and its counter receptor CD28 result in positive costimulation, the interactions between B7 proteins by CTLA-4, a protein primarily expressed on activated T cells, result in the generation of a negative signal to T cells. This coinhibitory signal is a prerequisite for peripheral T cell tolerance.[22]

The formulation that full T cell activation is dependent on the costimulatory signal, as well as the antigenic signal, is most significant, as T cell molecules responsible for costimulation and their cognate receptors on the surface

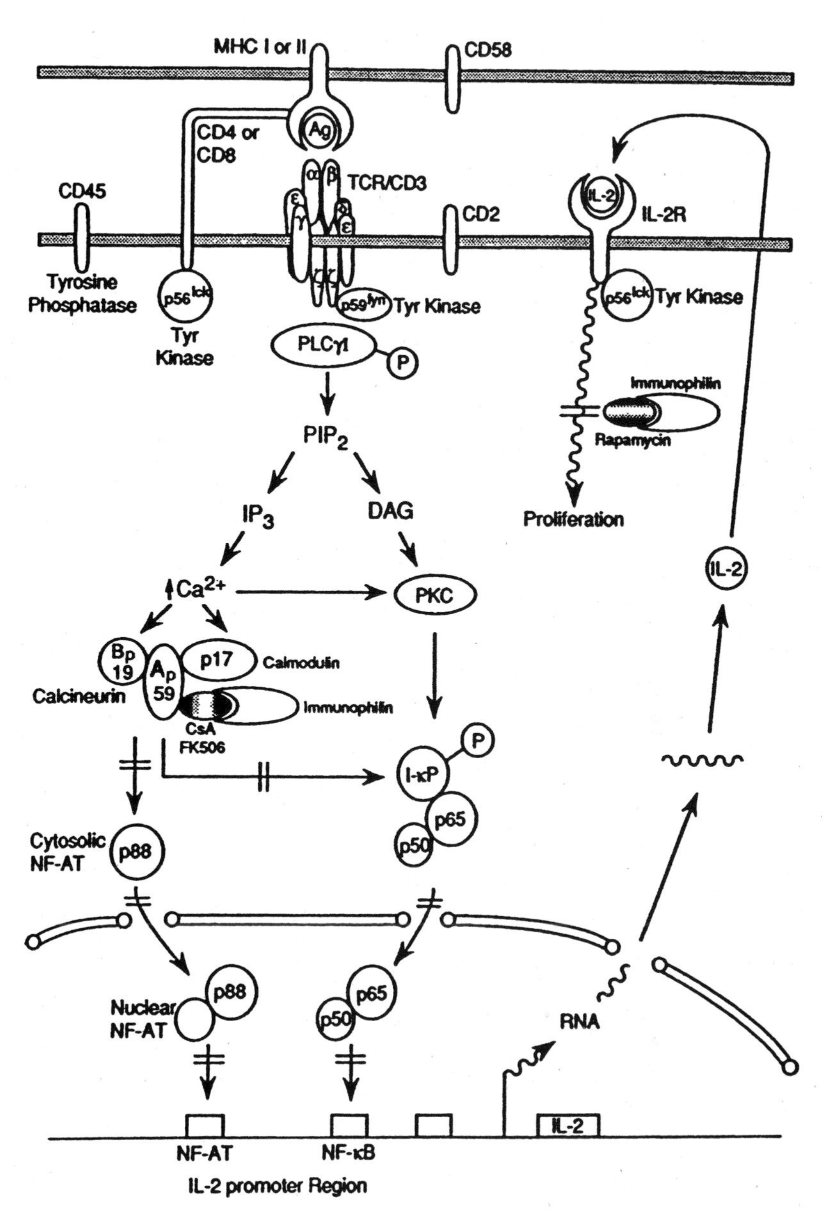

FIGURE 81.2 Signal transduction in T cells and mechanisms of action of cyclosporin A (CsA), FK-506, or rapamycin. Signaling molecules and transmembrane signaling events participating in the transduction of antigenic signals from the plasma membrane of the T cells to the nucleus are schematically shown. The sites of action of the drug (CsA/FK-506/rapamycin)–immunophilin complex are also shown. *Ag,* antigen; *Ap59* and *Bp19,* subunits of calcineurin; *DAG,* diacylglycerol; *I-κB,* inhibitory factor kappa B; *IL-2,* interleukin-2; *immunophilin,* cyclophilin or FK-binding protein; *IP$_3$,* inositol 1,4,5-triphosphate; *MHC,* major histocompatibility complex; *NF-AT,* nuclear factor of activated T cells; *NF-κB,* nuclear factor kappa B; *P,* phosphotyrosine; *PIP$_2$,* phosphatidylinositol 4,5-biphosphate; *PKC,* protein kinase C; *PLCγ1,* phospholipase C gamma-1; *Tyr kinase,* tyrosine kinase. (Adapted from Schreier MH, Baumann G, Zenke G, et al. Inhibition of T-cell signaling pathways by immunophilin drug complexes: Are side effects inherent to immunosuppressive properties? *Transplant Proc* 1993;25:502.)

of APCs then represent target molecules for the regulation of the antiallograft response. Indeed, transplantation tolerance has been induced in experimental models by targeting a variety of cell-surface molecules that contribute to the generation of costimulatory signals, and tolerance to histoincompatible human kidney allografts has been accomplished with a conditioning regimen that includes monoclonal antibodies directed at the CD2 protein.[23]

Interleukin-2/Interleukin-15 Stimulated T Cell Proliferation

Autocrine type of T cell proliferation occurs as a consequence of the T cell activation-dependent production of IL-2 and the expression of multimeric high affinity IL-2 receptors on T cells (Fig. 81.2) formed by the noncovalent association of three IL-2-binding peptides (α, β, γ).[12,24–26] IL-15 is a paracrine-type T cell-growth factor family member with very similar overall structural and identical T cell stimulatory qualities to IL-2.[12] The IL-2 and IL-15 receptor complexes share β and γ chains that are expressed in low abundance upon resting T cells; expression of these genes is amplified in activated T cells. The α-chain receptor components of the IL-2 and IL-15 receptor complexes are distinct and expressed upon activated, but not resting, T cells. The intracytoplasmic domains of the IL-2 receptor β and γ chains are required for intracellular signal transduction. The ligand-activated, but not resting, IL-2/IL-15 receptors are associated with intracellular PTKs.[12,27–29] Raf-1, a protein serine/threonine kinase associates with the intracellular domain of the shared β chain,[30] and this association and the kinase activity are prerequisites to IL-2/IL-15-triggered cell proliferation. Translocation of IL-2 receptor-bound Raf-1 serine/threonine kinase into the cytosol requires IL-2/IL-15-stimulated

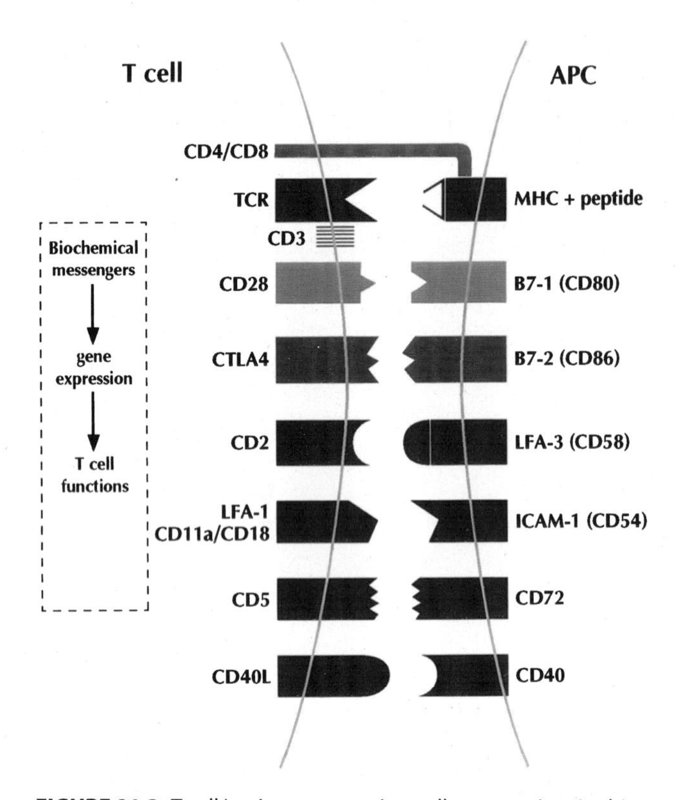

FIGURE 81.3 T cell/antigen-presenting cell contact sites. In this schema of T cell activation, the antigenic signal is initiated by the physical interaction between the clonally variant T cell antigen receptor (TCR) α-, β-heterodimer, and the antigenic peptide displayed by MHC on antigen-presenting cells (APCs). The antigenic signal is transduced into the cell by the CD3 proteins. The CD4 and the CD8 antigens function as associative recognition structures, and restrict TCR recognition to class II and class I antigens of MHC, respectively. Additional T cell- surface receptors generate the obligatory costimulatory signals by interacting with their counterreceptors expressed on the surface of the APCs. The simultaneous delivery to the T cells of the antigenic signal and the costimulatory signal results in the optimum generation of second messengers (such as calcium), expression of transcription factors (such as nuclear factor of activated T cells), and T cell growth-promoting genes (such as IL-2). The CD28 antigen as well as the CTLA4 antigen can interact with both the B7-1 and B7-2 antigens. The CD28 antigen generates a stimulatory signal, and CTLA4, unlike CD28, generates a negative signal. *CD,* cluster designation; *ICAM-1,* intercellular adhesion molecule-1; *LFA-1,* leukocyte function-associated antigen-1; *MHC,* major histocompatibility complex. (From Suthanthiran M. Transplantation tolerance: fooling mother nature. *Proc Natl Acad Sci U S A.* 1996;93:12072.)

PTK activity. The ligand-activated common γ chain recruits a member of the Janus kinase family, Jak 3, to the receptor complex that leads to activation of a member of the STAT family. Activation of this particular Jak–STAT pathway is essential for the proliferation of antigen-activated T cells. The subsequent events leading to IL-2/IL-15-dependent proliferation are not fully resolved; however, IL-2/IL-15–stimulated expression of several DNA binding proteins including Bcl-2, c-jun, c-fos, and c-myc contributes to cell cycle progression.[31,32] It is interesting and probably significant that IL-2, but not IL-15, triggers apoptosis of many antigen-activation T cells. In this way, IL-15–triggered events may be more detrimental to the antiallograft response than those initiated by IL-2. As IL-15 is not produced by T cells, IL-15 expression is not regulated by cyclosporine or tacrolimus.

Humoral Rejection

Antibody-mediated rejection (AMR) is a form of humoral rejection wherein antibodies directed at the donor HLA antigens (DSAs) serve as the main effector for the immune response directed at the allograft. Antibodies directed at non-HLA antigens such as endothelial cell associated antigens and MHC class I-related chain A antigens (MICA) have also been implicated in the pathogenesis of AMR. Whereas most acute T cell mediated rejections (TMRs) are responsive to steroid therapy, AMR is typically steroid-resistant and requires additional treatment such as plasmapheresis, anti-B cell, and intravenous immunoglobulin (IVIG) therapy. The incidence of AMR has been estimated at less than 10% but appears to be on the rise due to multiple reasons including acute TMR being effectively prevented by current immunosuppressive regimens, better definition of AMR, and transplantation of individuals with humoral presenitization and repeat transplants. Patients with AMR invariably harbor anti-HLA DSA although, in certain cases, histopathologic evidence of AMR may be apparent without any anti-HLA DSA. Acute AMR may occur within 1 week after engraftment even in the setting of antithymocyte globulin induction therapy. The diagnosis of AMR requires the presence of C4d complement staining in the peritubular capillaries in addition to peritubular capillary inflammation with polymorphonuclear and mononuclear leukocytes or the presence of fibrinoid changes/transumural arterial inflammation or acute tubular necrosis (ATN)-like tissue injury.[33] In the current Banff classification schema, those who present with histolgic features consistent with AMR but without concurrent intragraft C4d deposition or circulating DSA are classified as supicious for AMR—it is possible that the offending antibodies may be of the noncomplement fixing IgG subtypes and/or non-HLA antibodies (because most screening assays for DSA utilize HLA as target antigens).

A novel form of humoral rejection has also been documented. Antibodies directed against two epitopes of the angiotensin II type I (AT_1) receptor have been associated with refractory vascular allograft rejection in a series of 16 patients and these patients did not have anti-HLA antibodies at the time of incident humoral rejection.[34]

Immunobiology and Molecular Diagnosis of Rejection

The net consequence of cytokine production and acquisition of cell-surface receptors for these transcellular molecules is the emergence of antigen-specific and graft-destructive T cells and antibody producing B cells/plasma cells (Fig. 81.1). Cytokines facilitate not only the T cell effector arm and TCR but also the B cell/plasma cell arm by promoting the production of cytopathic antibodies. Moreover, cytokines such as IFN-γ and tumor necrosis factor-α (TNF-α) can amplify the ongoing immune response by upregulating the expression of HLA molecules as well as costimulatory molecules (e.g., B7) on graft parenchymal cells and APCs (Fig. 81.1). We and others have demonstrated the presence of antigen-specific cytotoxic T lymphocytes (CTL) and anti-HLA antibodies during or preceding a clinical rejection episode.[35,36] We have detected messenger RNA (mRNA) encoding the CTL-selective serine protease (granzyme B), perforin, Fas-ligand attack molecules, and immunoregulatory cytokines, such as IL-10 and IL-15, in human renal allografts undergoing acute rejection.[37] Indeed, these gene expression events may anticipate clinically apparent rejection. More recent efforts to develop a noninvasive method for the molecular diagnosis of rejection have proved rewarding. Using either peripheral blood[38] or urinary leukocytes[39] rejection-related, gene expression events evident in renal biopsy specimens are robustly detected in peripheral blood or urinary sediment specimens. Initial results from large-scale multicenter trials (e.g., Clinical Trials in Organ Transplantation, CTOT-04) support the hypothesis that noninvasive diagnosis of acute TMR is feasible by measurement of genes encoding cytotoxic attack molecules in urine, and the urinary cell mRNA profiles may anticipate the future development of acute TMR.[40] We speculate as well that a noninvasive, molecular diagnostic approach to rejection would be of value toward the detection of insidious, clinically silent rejection episodes that, although rarely detected through standard measures, are steroid-sensitive but usually lead to chronic rejection.[41]

Immunopharmacology of Allograft Rejection

Glucocorticosteroids

Glucocorticosteroids inhibit T cell proliferation, T cell-dependent immunity, and cytokine gene transcription (including IL-1, IL-2, IL-6, IFN-γ, and TNF-α gene).[42–44] Although no single cytokine can reverse the inhibitory effects of corticosteroids on mitogen-stimulated T cell proliferation, a combination of cytokines is effective.[45] The glucocorticoid and glucocorticoid–receptor bimolecular complex block IL-2 gene transcription via impairment of the cooperative effect of several DNA-binding proteins.[46] Corticosteroids also inhibit formation of free NF-κB, a DNA-binding protein required for cytokine and other T cell-activation gene expression events (Fig. 81.1 and Table 81.3).[47]

Azathioprine

Azathioprine (AZA), a thioguanine derivative of 6-mercaptopurine,[48] is a purine analog, acts as a nonspecific inhibitor of purine biosynthesis, and is an effective antiproliferative agent (Fig. 81.1 and Table 81.3).[48,49] In a randomized conversion trial from mycophenolate mofetil (MMF) to AZA in 48 stable kidney transplant recipients at 6 months following engraftment, it was observed that acute rejection rates

TABLE 81.3 Mechanisms of Action of Small Molecule Immunosuppressants[a]

Immunosuppressant	Subcellular Site(s) of Action
Azathioprine	Inhibits purine synthesis
Corticosteroids	Blocks cytokine gene expression
CsA/tacrolimus	Blocks Ca^{2+}-dependent T cell activation pathway via binding to calcineurin
Mycophenolate mofetil	Inhibits inosine monophosphate dehydrogenase and prevents de novo guanosine and deoxyguanosine synthesis in lymphocytes
Sirolimus/everolimus	Blocks IL-2 and other growth factor signal transduction; blocks CD28-mediated costimulatory signals
Leflunomide/FK778	Inhibits dihydroorotate dehydrogenase—a key enzyme for de novo pyramidine biosynthesis
FTY720	Phosphorylated FTY720 binds sphingolipid 1-phosphate receptor and prevents S1P signaling of cells; sequestration of lymphocytes within the lymph nodes and prevention of cell egress into the peripheral circulation

CsA, cyclosporin A; IL, interleukin.

were comparable (4.5% vs. 3.8%) after a 6-month observation period in the MMF (n = 22) or AZA (n = 26) arm. The trial participants received cyclosporine and prednisone as maintenance immunosuppressive therapy and antithymocyte globulin induction was used in 27% of the recipients maintained on MMF and 46% in the AZA conversion group. It is worth noting that high-risk patients including retransplant recipients, highly sensitized, and those with a history of steroid-resistant rejection were all excluded from the trial.[50]

The Calcineurin Inhibitors: Cyclosporine and Tacrolimus (FK-506)

Cyclosporine, a small cyclic fungal peptide, and FK-506, a macrolide antibiotic, block the Ca^{2+}-dependent antigen triggered T cell activation (signal one) (Fig. 81.2).[51] The immunosuppressive effects of cyclosporine and FK-506 are dependent on the formation of a heterodimeric complex that consists of the drug cyclosporine or FK-506 and its respective cytoplasmic receptor "immunophilin" proteins, cyclophilin and FK-binding protein (FKBP), respectively. The heterodimeric cyclosporine–cyclophilin complex and the FK-506–FKBP complex target and bind calcineurin and inhibit its phosphatase activity (Table 81.3). The inhibition of the enzymatic activity of calcineurin is considered central to the immunosuppressive effects of cyclosporine and FK-506.

One of the well-documented consequences of calcium/calmodulin dependent activation of calcineurin is dephosphorylation of cytoplasmic NF-AT in T cells, import of NF-AT into the nucleus, binding of NF-AT with its nuclear partmer, and transcription of the IL-2 gene. The cyclosporine–FK-506 mediated inhibition of phosphatase activity of calcineurin results in the lack of dephosphorylation of cytoplasmic NF-AT and retention of the phosphorylated NF-AT in the cytoplasm. In addition to inhibiting the expression of NF-AT, cyclosporine also inhibits other DNA-binding proteins, such as NF-κB and AP-1.[52]

The phosphorylation status of transcription factors can also affect their DNA binding ability and interaction with the rest of the transcriptional machinery. For example, the DNA binding activities of c-jun increase upon dephosphorylation.

Blockade of cytokine gene activation does not totally account for the antiproliferative effect of cyclosporine and FK-506. It is significant that cyclosporine as well as FK-506, in striking contrast to their inhibitory activity on the induced expression of IL-2, enhance the expression of transforming growth factor-β (TGF-β).[53,54] Because TGF-β is a potent inhibitor of T cell proliferation and generation of antigen-specific CTL,[55] heightened expression of TGF-β must contribute to the antiproliferative/immunosuppressive activity of cyclosporine/tacrolimus. This TGF-β inducing effect of cyclosporine/tacrolimus also suggests a mechanism for some of the complications (e.g., renal fibrosis and tumor metastasis) of therapy with calcineurin inhibitors, because TGF-β is a fibrogenic and proangiogenic cytokine.

Mycophenolate Mofetil and Enteric-Coated Mycophenolate Sodium

MMF is a semisynthetic derivative of mycophenolic acid (MPA). MMF inhibits allograft rejection in rodents, diminishes proliferation of T and B cells, decreases generation of cytotoxic T cells, and suppresses antibody formation.[56–58] MMF inhibits inosine monophosphate dehydrogenase (IMPDH), an enzyme in the de novo pathway of purine synthesis. Lymphocytes are dependent on this biosynthetic pathway to satisfy their guanosine requirements (Table 81.3).[58] Early clinical trials have utilized MMF to replace azathioprine in the cyclosporine- and steroid-based immunosuppressive regimen. These controlled, prospective trials have shown a diminished incidence of early acute rejection episodes.[58–60] Although follow-up studies over a 3-year period have indicated an advantage for MMF over azathioprine,[60] a recent randomized trial comparing MMF with azathioprine in recipients of a first kidney transplant from a deceased donor found similar levels of acute rejection in the first 6 months of transplantation.[61]

Enteric-coated mycophenolate sodium (EC-MPS) was developed to improve the gastrointestinal tolerability of MPA. An international phase III, randomized, double-blinded, parallel group trial demonstrated the therapeutic equivalence of MMF and EC-MPS.[62] The two parallel groups received equivalent concomitant antibody induction, corticosteroids, and calcineurin inhibitor (CNI) therapy. At 12 months, the incidence of acute rejection, graft loss, and death was comparable for both treatment groups. Interestingly, in the phase III pivotal trial gastrointestinal complications were not significantly different between MMF and EC-MPS. Within 12 months of enrollment, dose changes were required for gastrointestinal adverse events in 19.5% versus 15% of subjects (P = not significant [NS]) in the MMF and EC-MPS groups, respectively.[62]

Sirolimus (Rapamycin)

Rapamycin[63–65] is a macrocyclic lactone isolated from *Streptomyces hygroscopicus* that, like FK-506, binds to FKBP. However, rapamycin and FK-506 affect different and distinctive sites in the signal transduction pathway (Fig. 81.2 and Table 81.3). Whereas rapamycin blocks IL-2 and other growth factor-mediated signal transduction, FK-506 (or cyclosporine) has no such capacity. Also, the rapamycin–FKBP complex, unlike the FK-506–FKBP complex, does not bind calcineurin. The antiproliferative activity of the rapamycin–FKBP complex is linked to blockade of the activation of the 70-kDa S6 protein kinases and blockade of expression of the bcl-2 proto-oncogene. Rapamycin also blocks the Ca^{2+}-independent CD28-induced costimulatory pathway. Substitution of rapamycin for azathioprine in a triple-therapy regimen reduced the frequency and severity of acute rejection.[66] The CONVERT trial, an international randomized, prospective, open-label study tested the efficacy and safety of converting CNI-based maintenance therapy for renal transplant recipients to a sirolimus-based CNI-free immunosuppressive regimen.[67] The mean Nankivell glomerular filtration rates (GFRs) at 12 months were 63.6 mL per min vs. 61.1 mL per min ($P = .006$) and at 24 months were 62.6 mL per min vs. 59.9 mL per min ($P = .009$) in the converted CNI-free group. The rejection, graft survival, and patient survival rates were similar in both CNI and sirolimus groups. The malignancy rates were significantly lower after conversion to sirolimus (3.8% vs. 11.0%, $P < .001$). The mean urinary protein/creatinine ratios or calculated daily proteinuria at 24 months was higher after sirolimus conversion when compared to baseline (mean ± standard deviation [SD], 0.72 ± 1.50 vs. 0.04 ± 0.04, $P < .001$). In the Spare-the-Nephron trial, 299 patients were randomized to MMF/CNI or MMF/sirolimus.[68] Iothalamate estimation of GFR at 1 year showed the mean percentage improvement from baseline of GFR was higher in the MMF/sirolimus group when compared to the MMF/CNI group (24.4% vs. 5.2%, $P = .012$). The percentage change in GFR from baseline at 2 years remained higher in the CNI-free group but was not statistically significant (8.6% vs. 3.4%, $P = .54$).

Everolimus (RAD)

Everolimus is a derivative of rapamycin. The use of everolimus in phase II clinical trials involving cyclosporine, steroids, and basiliximab induction resulted in excellent graft survival at 36 months.[69] In a short-term phase III trial, everolimus was comparable to MMF with cyclosporine and steroids in preventing acute rejection.[70] The U.S. Food and Drug Administration (FDA) approved everolimus in 2010 for the prevention of kidney transplant rejection following its approval in 2009 for the treatment of advanced renal cell carcinoma in patients who have failed sunitinib or sofrafenib therapy.

Leflunomide

Leflunomide is a synthetic isoxazole derivative that inhibits dihydroorotate dehydrogenase—a key enzyme for de novo pyrimidine synthesis. It belongs to the family of drugs known as malonitrilamides and is currently approved for the treatment of rheumatoid arthritis. Leflunomide has antiviral effects against cytomegalovirus, herpes simplex virus type 1, and polyomavirus (BK virus).[71–73] A short-term, open-label, prospective crossover trial of leflunomide comprised of 22 patients with chronic renal allograft dysfunction found 100% patient survival and 91% graft survival at 6 months posttransplantation, and was well tolerated, with anemia being the most common adverse effect.[74]

FK778

FK778 is an analog of the active metabolite (A771726) of leflunomide. A phase II European multicenter randomized, double-blind, and FK778 dose-controlled trial was performed in 149 renal transplant recipients divided into three groups: group 1, high-level FK778/tacrolimus/steroids; group 2, low- level FK778/tacrolimus/steroids; and group 3, placebo/tacrolimus/steroids.[75] The incidence of acute rejection in groups 1, 2, and 3 were 28.6%, 25.9%, and 34.8%, respectively, and patients who reached target levels had a lower incidence of acute rejection. Anemia was a commonly reported complication and was observed in 43% in group 1, 31% in group 2, and 20% in group 3. A phase II randomized, open-label, two-arm, parallel-group, multicenter trial tested the efficacy of FK778 against BK nephropathy in comparison to standard of care (reduction of immunosuppression). The treatment group had a statistically significant reduction in BK viremia but without significant improvement in renal function or histology based on the Drachenberg criteria. When compared to the standard of care, the FK778 treated group also experienced multiple rejection epidoses and had a higher incidence of biopsy-proven acute rejection.[76]

Muromonab–CD3 (OKT3)

OKT3 is a murine monoclonal antibody directed against the CD3 component of the T cell receptor complex. It was initially tested for its efficacy as an antirejection agent and was found to be superior to corticosteroids in the treatment of acute rejection of renal allografts. Later, OKT3 was utilized as an induction agent in renal transplantation and for the treatment of steroid-resistant acute rejection. The OKT3 associated first dose reaction as a result of cytokine release may be severe and include fever, chills, respiratory symptoms, and headaches. Currently, OKT3 has lost favor with the transplant community primarily because of the first dose reaction and because of the availability of other induction agents. A humanized preparation (HuM291) that potentially reduces cytokine release reaction is being investigated[77] and may restore CD3–directed therapy in organ transplanttion.

Antithymocyte Globulin

Immunizing either rabbits or equines with human thymocytes produces antithymocyte globulin preparations. The antibodies generated are polyclonal in nature and are directed against several cell-surface antigens including: CD2, CD3, CD4, CD8, CD11a, CD18, CD25, CD44, CD45, HLA-DR, and HLA class I heavy chain.[78] Antithymocyte globulin (ATG) preparations are used both as an induction agent, especially in high-risk renal transplant recipients, and for the treatment of acute rejection. In a steroid rapid-withdrawal protocol using calcineurin inhibitor and MMF or sirolimus, rabbit ATG was selected as the induction agent for low-risk, mostly Caucasian, renal transplant recipients and the actuarial acute rejection-free graft survival was 92% at 3 years.[79] The surviving peripheral T cell subsets were analyzed in five patients following antibody-mediated T cell depletion therapy with ATG.[80] The study found a significant reduction in the absolute lymphocyte population but heterogeneity in the degree of depletion of T cell subsets. Whereas both CD8+ naïve T cells and CD4+ naïve T cells were depleted by over 98%, both CD4+CD25+ T cell subset and CD4+CD45RA-CD62L-T cell subset were only depleted by 90% (P = .001). The CD4+CD45RA-CD62L-effector memory T cells represented 88 ± 3% of the postdepletion resistant T cell subset in contrast to their usual prevalence of 10% to 20% in normal volunteers. These memory T cells may potentially serve as the progenitor cells for mounting an immune response against the allograft even in the setting of lymphopenia. The CD4+CD25+ may include regulatory T cells and their relative sparing may be of significance for counter-regulating the anti-allograft response. Clearly more data with a larger cohort are needed but the initial implication of the study is that T cell depletion therapy with ATG has differential effects on T cell subsets with some beneficial (a sparing of regulatory T cells) and some detrimental (lack of full depletion of memory T cells).

Interleukin-2 Receptor Antagonists: Basiliximab and Daclizumab

IL-2 receptor antagonists (IL-2Ra) inhibit allograft rejection by competitively binding CD25 antigen (IL-2 receptor α chain or Tac subunit) on activated T lymphocytes. Both basiliximab (chimeric human/murine monoclonal $IgG_{1\kappa}$) and daclizumab (humanized monoclonal IgG1) are commonly utilized as induction agents for renal transplantation. A meta-analysis of clinical trials involving monoclonal antibodies directed at CD25 showed that, when combined with standard double or triple immunosuppressive regimens, the use of these antibodies reduced the incidence of acute rejection by 34% and by 49% the incidence of steroid-resistant rejection.[81] The meta-analysis also showed that the efficacy of anti-CD25 monoclonal antibodies in preventing acute rejection was similar to that of OKT3 and that of polyclonal antibody preparations and, importantly, with fewer side effects. A large prospective randomized international trial tested the efficacy of a 5-day course of ATG versus two doses of basiliximab induction therapy in 278 deceased-donor renal transplants at risk for acute rejection or delayed graft function.[82] Participants in the ATG group (n = 141) had lower incidence of acute rejection at 12 months when compared to the basiliximab group (n = 137) (15.6% vs. 25.5%). However, the incidence of delayed graft function (40.4% vs. 44.5%), death (4.3% vs. 4.4%), as well as graft loss (9.2% vs. 10.2%), were similar in the two groups.

Alemtuzumab

Alemtuzumab is a humanized monoclonal $IgG_{1\kappa}$ directed against CD52, which is a glycoprotein expressed on B and T cells, natural killer (NK) cells, monocytes, and macrophages. It is approved by the FDA for the treatment of B cell chronic lymphocytic leukemia. In a pilot study of 29 primary renal transplant recipients treated with alemtuzumab and sirolimus monotherapy, profound and sustained depletion of lymphocytes was observed; however, 8 of 29 patients developed acute rejection with 7 requiring conversion to standard triple therapy.[83] In an investigation of 44 renal allograft recipients treated with alemtuzumab, tacrolimus (trough levels of 5 to 7 ng per mL), and MMF (500 mg twice a day), and with a median follow-up of 9 months, four patients developed acute rejection and four developed infection and the patient and graft survival rates were 100%.[84] The use of alemtuzumab induction was associated with an elevated serum B-cell activating factor (BAFF) level in kidney transplantation and may increase the risk of humoral rejection in the absence of concomitant CNI maintenance therapy.[85]

The INTAC study group tested alemtuzumab against conventional induction agents in a randomized prospective multicenter trial.[86] High risk participants received rabbit ATG whereas low risk participants in the trial received basiliximab conventional induction therapy. All participants received tacrolimus and MMF maintenance immunosuppression with rapid steroid discontinuation after 5 days of therapy. When compared to basiliximab, alemtuzumab induction in the low risk group resulted in a significantly lower rate of biopsy-proven acute rejection at 6 months (2% vs. 18%, $P < .001$), 12 months (3% vs. 20%, $P < .001$), and 36 months (10% vs. 22%, $P \leq .003$). When compared to rabbit ATG, alemtuzumab induction in the high-risk group resulted in equivalent rates of biopsy-proven acute rejection at 6 months (6% vs. 9%; P = .49), 12 months (10% vs. 13%; P = .53), and 36 months (18% vs. 15%; P = .63). Patient survival at 3 years was similar between alemtuzumab and basiliximab or ATG in the low risk (95% vs. 98%; P = .19) or high risk (99% vs. 91%; P = .07) groups. After censoring for deaths, graft survival at 3 years was similar between alemtuzumab and basiliximab or ATG in the low-risk (97% vs. 94%; P = .17) or high-risk (91% vs. 84%; P = .32) groups. However, the rates of late biopsy-proven acute rejection (between 12 and 36 months) were higher in the alemtuzumab cohort when compared to participants in the conventional induction cohorts (8% vs. 3%, P = .03) thus suggesting that surveillance for late rejection is important when using alemtuzumab as an induction agent.

Rituximab

Rituximab is a chimeric murine/human monoclonal $IgG_{1\kappa}$ directed against the CD20 antigen expressed on the surface of B cells. It was FDA approved for the treatment of CD20-positive, B cell non-Hodgkin lymphoma. Initial experience with rituximab has shown promising results in the treatment of steroid-resistant acute renal allograft rejection.[87] Rituximab has also been used as a component of a preconditioning regimen to prepare patients for renal transplantation from ABO incompatibile donors.[88] In an open-label, controlled trial randomizing rituximab against daclizumab induction, the study was closed after excessive acute rejection episodes in the rituximab arm (first five of six patients) in the initial 3 months after transplant (83% vs. 14%). Both arms received steroid-free maintenance with tacrolimus and MMF. All episodes of rejection responded to intravenous methylprednisolone and the GFR was similar at 1 year in the 2 arms (44.4 ± 8.1 vs.

48.9 ± 10.6 mL/min/1.73 m^2). The authors hypothesized that rituximab therapy, by disrupting regulatory B cells and transiently increasing the release of inflammatory cytokines, contributed to an anti-allograft immune response.[89]

Intravenous Immune Globulins

IVIG is used to treat a variety of autoimmune diseases based on its immodulatory effects.[90] In the renal transplantation arena, IVIG is being utilized to reduce humoral immunity in two distinct settings: (1) to reduce the level of preexisting anti-HLA antibodies and convert a positive crossmatch recipient to a negative crossmatch recipient,[91] and (2) to treat humoral rejection.[92] It has been reported that a combination desensitizing regimen of IVIG and rituximab facilitated, in a safe manner, rapid transplantation of 16 of 20 highly sensitized patients.[93]

FTY720

FTY720 is a synthetic analog derived from the ascomycete *Isaria sinclairii*. The phosphorylated metabolite, FTY720-phosphate, is the biologically active compound. FTY720 affects the normal trafficking of lymphocytes and prevents their transmigration from lymph nodes to the allograft by binding lymphocytic sphingolipid 1-phosphate $(S1P)_1$ receptors. This process prevents the signaling of lymphocytes by serum S1P and the egress into the periphery in response to systemic inflammation.[94] In the first human trial of FTY720 in stable renal allograft recipients, transient but asymptomatic bradycardia was noted following 10 of 24 doses examined.[95] In a randomized, multicenter, double-blind, and placebo-controlled, phase I study of stable renal allograft recipients, a dose-dependent decrease in peripheral blood lymphocytes was observed.[96] A phase IIA trial comparing FTY720 to MMF in combination with cyclosporine and steroids in de novo renal transplant recipients showed equivalent efficacy and safety with regard to prevention of acute rejection.[97] A 12-month phase III international randomized trial compared three groups of patients: group 1, reduced dose cyclosporine and FTY720 (5 mg); group 2, full dose cyclosporine and FTY720 (2.5 mg); and group 3, MMF and full dose cyclosporine.[98] All study patients received corticosteroids as part of the maintenance regimen. Participants in group 1 had a prohibitively higher risk of acute rejection and the group was discontinued from the trial on the recommendation by the study Data Safety Monitoring Board (DSMB). Participants in groups 2 and 3 had similar rates of acute rejection at 22%. Analysis of a composite efficacy endpoint showed that group 2 did not achieve statistical noninferiority compared to group 3. The rate of discontinuation of study drugs was also higher in group 2 versus group 3 with patients receiving FTY720 having an increased incidence of macular edema. A second phase III trial failed to demonstrate any benefit of combining FTY720 and reduced dose cyclosporine when compared to the MMF-based standard of care regimen for de novo kidney transplant recipients.[99]

Belatacept

Belatacept (BMS-224818) is a fusion protein of cytotoxic T lymphocyte-associated antigen 4 and Fc piece of immunoglobulin (CTLA4Ig) and was designed to block the B7/CD28 costimulatory pathway. A phase II trial comparing belatacept to cyclosporine (in a regimen consisting of basiliximab, MMF, and corticosteroids) yielded promising results in preventing acute rejection of renal allografts.[100] Phase III trials, BENEFIT and BENEFIT-EXT, were conducted to test the effectiveness of belatacept as part of a CNI-free regimen.[101,102] The BENEFIT study was a 3-year randomized, parallel group designed trial conducted at 100 transplant sites worldwide. Following basiliximab induction, participants were randomized to one of three groups consisting of a more intensive belatacept regimen, a less intensive belatacept regimen, or cyclosporine with the addition of maintenance MMF and corticosteroids. The incidence of acute rejection at 12 months was higher in the belatacept groups (22% and 17%) compared to the cyclosporine group (7%). More participants also developed type IIa and IIb rejections in the belatacept cohorts but without an increase in donor-specific antibody production when compared to the cyclosporine-treated group. The mean GFR was superior at 12 months for the belatacept groups compared to the cyclosporine group. The BENEFIT-EXT trial was a 3-year randomized, multicenter trial performed at 79 transplant sites worldwide to test the benefit of a CNI-free regimen containing belatacept in patients undergoing high risk transplant from expanded criteria donors. Following basiliximab induction, participants were randomized to one of three groups consisting of a more intensive belatacept regimen, a less intensive belatacept regimen, or cyclosporine with the addition of maintenance MMF and corticosteroids. The incidence of acute rejection was not different among the three groups but CNI-free belatacept regimens resulted in more type IIb rejections. The mean GFR was significantly higher at 12 months for the more intensive belatacept group (52.1 mL/min/1.73 m^2) but not significant for the less intensive belatacept group (49.5 mL/min/1.73 m^2) compared to the cyclosporine group (45.2 mL/min/1.73 m^2). Both the BENEFIT and BENEFIT-EXT trials showed that neither the more intensive nor less intensive belatacept regimens were noninferior to cyclosporine on patient and graft survival. In the 2-year follow-up report, the salutary effects on GFR remained apparent for both the BENEFIT and BENEFIT-EXT trials with 16 to 17 mL per min and 8 to 10 mL per min higher GFR observed in the belatacept cohort of both trials when compared to the CNI group.[103] Belatacept was approved by the FDA in 2011 for the prophylaxis of organ rejection in kidney transplant recipients.

Alefacept

Alefacept, LFA3-Ig, is a dimeric fusion protein made by linking the CD2 binding portion of the human lymphocyte function-associated antigen-3 (LFA-3) to the Fc portion of human IgG1. In addition to pretransplant whole blood donor-specific transfusion (DST), costimulatory blockade using CTLA4-Ig for 8 weeks and sirolimus for 90 days, alefacept given weekly for 8 weeks was able to significantly prolong renal allograft survival in rhesus monkeys when compared to control animals.[104] LFA3-Ig and CTLA4-Ig combination therapy given to the animals prevented the development of alloantibodies and five of eight treated monkeys had greater than 90 days of rejection-free period.[104] A phase II randomized, open-label, parallel group, multicenter trial has recently been completed to test alefacept in de novo kidney transplant using tacrolimus, MMF, and steroids.[105] The primary endpoint was incidence of biopsy proven acute rejection (BPAR) at 6 months. The trial enrolled 309 subjects randomized to the following four arms: control (basilixmab induction with full dose tacrolimus, MMF, and steroids), alefacept/low dose tacrolimus/MMF/steroids (A), alefacept/full dose tacrolimus/steroids (B), and every other week alefacept/low dose tacrolimus/MMF/steroids (C). The authors found that the incidence of BPAR was significantly higher in group A when compared to the control arm (26.3% vs. 12.7%; $P < .05$) whereas the MMF replacement arm (B) and group C had similar rates of BPAR when compared to the control arm (18.8% and 16.7%, respectively). At six months, patient and graft survival as well as renal function were similar in all groups.[105]

Janus Kinase (JAK)3 inhibitor

JAK3 inhibitor (CP-690,550) inhibits the tyrosine kinase required for signal transduction downstream of cytokine receptors and is important for the activation and function of T-cells as well as NK cells. A phase IIA randomized, open-label, multicenter trial was conducted in de novo kidney transplant recipients.[106] Following induction with monoclonal antibodies directed at the IL-2Ra, participants were randomized to lower dose JAK3 inhibitor (CP15), higher dose JAK3 inhibitor (CP30), and tacrolimus along with maintenance MMF and corticosteroids. The trial was converted into an exploratory study without sufficient power to address its primary and secondary objectives due to four cases of BK nepropathy (BKN) that occurred in the CP30 group. The CP15 group had a similar rejection rate when compared to the tacrolimus control group. Paradoxically, the CP30 group had a higher rejection rate than the tacrolimus control group. In this trial, combination JAK3 inhibition with MMF therapy yielded excessive viral opportunistic infections such as BKN and CMV disease.

Efalizumab

Efalizumab is a humanized IgG1 anti-CD11a monoclonal antibody approved by the FDA for treatment of psoriasis. LFA-1, a member of the heterodimeric B2 integrin family and adhesion molecule on T cell, interacts with ICAM-1 (CD54) on APC to facilitate T-cell activation. CD11a and CD18 constitute the alpha and beta chains of LFA-1. Although an early phase II study in kidney transplants was promising, a voluntary phased withdrawal of the product in the U.S. market was instituted in 2009 due to increased risk of progressive multifocal leukoencephalopathy.[107]

Eculizumab

Eculizumab is a humanized monoclonal antibody against complement 5a molecule and is approved by the FDA for the treatment of paroxysmal nocturnal hematuria. Several case reports described the use of eculizumab in renal transplant recipients with atypical hemolytic-uremic syndrome, as salvage therapy for antibody-mediated rejection, and renal transplant patients with catastrophic antiphospholipid antibody syndrome.[108-110]

Bortezomib

Bortezomib is a proteasome inhibitor and is approved by the FDA for the treatment of multiple myeloma and mantle cell lymphoma. Proteasomes are large cytosolic protease complexes and with ubiquitin they perform basic housekeeping protein degradation in all eukaryotic cells. The ubiquitin-proteasome pathway is essential for numerous important physiologic functions such as oncogenesis, inflammation, apoptosis, cell cycle progression, and immune activation. Plasma cells are professional antibody secreting cells and in the process of producing antibodies they are subjected to tremendous intracellular stress leading to proteasomal insufficiency and cell death if accumulation of polyubiquitinated proteins are left unchecked.[111] Even nonmalignant plasma cells are susceptible to proteasome inhibition. Preliminary studies have been completed testing bortezomib in antibody-mediated kidney rejection and appear promising.[112] Clearly further studies with larger cohorts are needed to fully define the usefulness of bortezomib.

Immunosuppressive Regimens

Immunologic considerations, including antirejection therapy, are organized around a few general principles. The first consideration is careful patient preparation and, in the circumstance of living donor renal transplantation, selection of the best available ABO-compatible HLA match in the event that several potential living related donors are available for organ donation. Second is a multitiered approach to immunosuppressive therapy similar, in principle, to that used in chemotherapy; several agents are used simultaneously, each of which is directed at a different molecular target within the allograft response (Fig. 81.1 and Table 81.3). Additive/synergistic effects are achieved through application of each agent at a relatively low dose, thereby limiting the toxicity of each individual agent while increasing the total immunosuppressive effect. Third is the principle that higher immunosuppressive drug doses and/or more individual immunosuppressive drugs are required to gain early engraftment and to treat established rejection than are needed to maintain immunosuppression in the long term. Hence, intensive induction and lower dose maintenance drug protocols are used. Fourth is careful investigation of each episode of posttransplant graft dysfunction, with the realization that most of the common causes of graft dysfunction, including rejection, can (and often do) coexist. Successful therapy, therefore, often involves several simultaneous therapeutic maneuvers. Fifth is the appropriate reduction or withdrawal of an immunosuppressive drug when that drug's toxicity exceeds its therapeutic benefit.

The basic immunosuppressive protocol used in most transplant centers involves the use of at least two and often three drugs, each directed at a discrete site in the T cell activation cascade (Fig. 81.1) and each with distinct side effects. Although a calcineurin inhibitor plus MMF plus glucocorticoids is the most widely used regimen, there are concerns regarding nephrotoxicity associated with long-term use of calcineurin inhibitors[113] and several popular variations of the "triple" drug protocol are being explored in the clinic. A calcineurin-free regimen consisting of sirolimus, MMF, and glucocorticosteroids has been reported to result in better renal function.[114] In a randomized controlled trial of cyclosporine withdrawal in recipients of first deceased donor renal grafts, a 3-month course of cyclosporine followed by azathioprine and steroid maintenance therapy was superior to continuous cyclosporine-alone protocol.[115] Early cyclosporine withdrawal from a regimen of cyclosporine, sirolimus, and steroids has been associated with a better renal function and renal allograft histology compared to patients maintained on the three-drug regimen.[116]

Many centers employ induction therapy with antilymphocyte preparations. Monoclonal anti–CD25 antibodies or polyclonal antithymocyte antibodies are used as induction therapy in the immediate posttransplant period, thereby establishing an immunosuppressive umbrella that enables early engraftment without immediate use of calcineurin inhibitors during the early posttransplant period. During this critical period, the graft may be particularly vulnerable to CsA–tacrolimus-induced nephrotoxic effects. The incidence of early rejection episodes is reduced by the prophylactic use of anti-CD25 or antithymocyte antibodies. This protocol is particularly beneficial for patients at high risk for immunologic graft failure (e.g., broadly presensitized or retransplant patients). The efficacy of the polyclonal antilymphocyte antibody preparation (e.g., thymoglobulin) or mAbs (e.g., CAMPATH-1H) in preventing rejection is impressive, but profound lymphopenia and an increase in the incidence of opportunistic infections and lymphoma results. Because of selective targeting of IL-2R+ T cells, anti-CD25 mAb treatment appears to be safer than treatment with thymoglobulin or anti-T cell mAbs.[81] Insofar as activated but not resting T cells express the IL-2 receptor α chain, anti-CD25 mAbs are employed as humanized[117,118] or chimeric[119,120] mAbs to selectively target and destroy alloreactive T cells. These efforts are based on successful exploration and application of IL-2–receptor targeted therapy in preclinical models.[121] Low-dose tacrolimus and sirolimus protocol[122] may prove to rival the current sequential immune therapy regimens for use in patients at high risk to reject an allograft. Induction therapy protocols using either basiliximab or daclizumab have also been utilized to enable successful early steroid withdrawal in the first week of renal transplantation.[123,124]

HLA and Renal Transplantation

The genes that code for the HLA antigens are located within the short arm of chromosome 6.[125,126] The class I proteins, HLA-A, B, and C antigens, are composed of a 41-kDa polymorphic chain linked noncovalently to a 12-kDa β_2-microglobulin chain that is encoded in chromosome 15. The class I molecules are expressed by all nucleated cells and platelets. The class II molecules, HLA-DR, DP, and DQ, are composed of a chain of 34 kDa and a β chain of 29 kDa. MHC class II molecules are constitutively expressed on the surface of B cells, monocytes/macrophages, and dendritic cells. Additional lymphoid cells, such as T cells and many nonlymphoid cells, such as renal tubular epithelial cells, express class II proteins only on stimulation with cytokines.

The clinical benefits of HLA matching are readily appreciable in the recipients of renal grafts from living related donors. An analysis of the United Network for Organ Sharing (UNOS) scientific renal transplant registry data has revealed that the 1-year graft survival rate is 94% in recipients of two haplotype-matched, HLA-identical kidneys. It is 89% and 90%, respectively, when a one haplotype-matched parent or sibling is the donor (Fig. 81.4A).[127] The Collaborative Transplant Study, an international study that draws on 305 transplant centers located in 47 countries for data, has also demonstrated that the survival rate of HLA-identical transplants is superior to that of one-haplotype-matched grafts, even in the cyclosporin era.[128]

The advantage of HLA-matching is maintained beyond the first year of transplantation. UNOS registry data[127] show estimated half-lives (the time needed for 50% of the grafts functioning at 1 year posttransplantation to fail) of 26.9 years for HLA-identical grafts and 12.2 years and 10.8 years for one-haplotype-matched sibling grafts and parental grafts, respectively. Data from the Collaborative Transplant Study, comprising 22,414 living related grafts, have also revealed a substantial long-term benefit[128] of HLA matching in recipients of living related grafts.

The effect of matching for HLA in deceased donor graft recipients has been examined in a prospective U.S. study[129] in which kidneys were shared nationally on the basis of matching for HLA-A, B, and DR antigens. All transplantation centers in the United States participated in this study. The 1-year graft survival rate was 88% for HLA-matched kidneys and 79% for HLA-mismatched kidneys (Fig. 81.4B). Moreover, the benefit of HLA matching persisted beyond the first year posttransplantation; the estimated half-life of the HLA-matched renal graft was 17.3 years and that of HLA-mismatched renal allografts was 7.8 years.

Since the inception of the U.S. national kidney-sharing program in 1987, more than 7,500 deceased donor kidneys have been distributed to transplantation centers located in 48 states, and a recent analysis confirmed and extended the

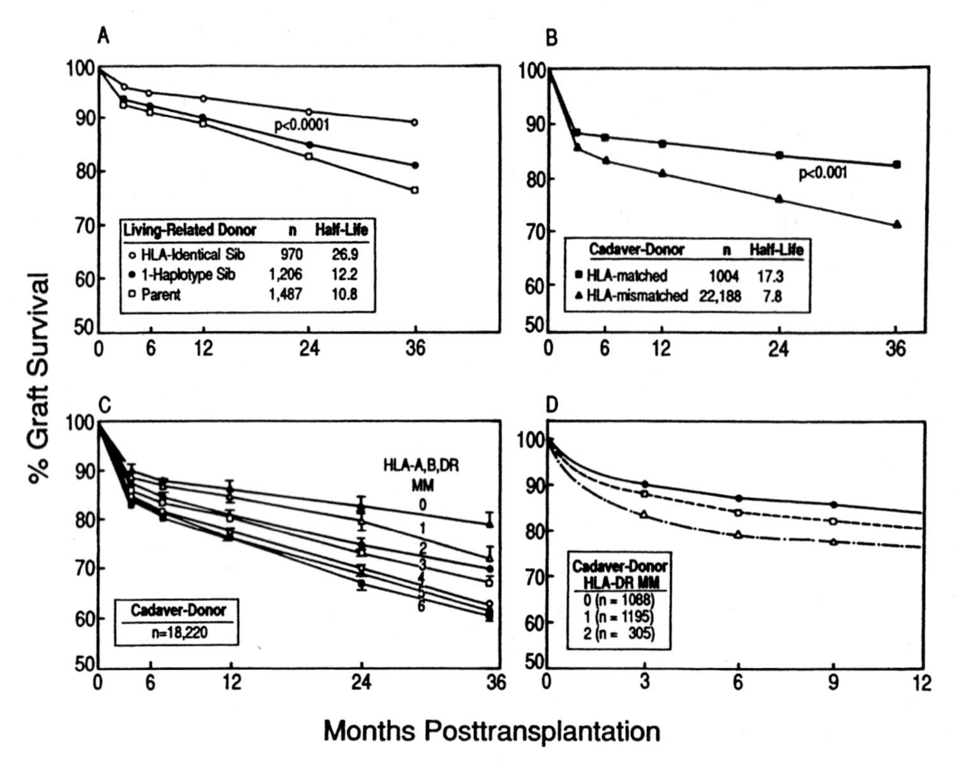

FIGURE 81.4 Impact of human leukocyte antigen (HLA) matching on renal allograft survival rates. **A:** The effect of haplotype matching in living related renal transplantation.[68] **B:** The superior results found with HLA-matched (A, B, and DR antigens) deceased donor renal grafts compared with HLA-mismatched deceased donor renal grafts.[70] **C:** The impact of different levels of HLA-A, B, and DR mismatching on the survival of deceased donor renal grafts.[72] **D:** The stepwise improvement in the survival of deceased donor grafts following matching for the HLA-DR antigens identified by DNA typing (number of DR mismatches: •—•, 0;—, 1; •—Δ—•, 2 .[75]

observation that HLA-matched transplants have a superior outcome compared to HLA-mismatched transplants.[130] The estimated 10-year rate of deceased donor graft survival was 52% for HLA-matched transplants and was 37% for HLA-mismatched transplants. Furthermore, the incidence of rejection was lower in HLA-matched transplants compared to mismatched ones. Interestingly, the mean duration of cold-ischemia time of nationally shared kidneys was not that different from locally transplanted kidneys; it was 23 hours compared to 22 hours for nonshared kidneys.[130]

A stepwise increase in the survival rate of deceased donor renal allografts has also been documented with increasing levels of HLA-A, B, and DR antigen matching (Fig. 81.4C). The improvement in the graft survival rate following HLA matching is more apparent when matching is based on better resolved HLA antigens (HLA split antigens) than when based on broad HLA antigens; the improvement in the graft survival rate between the best-matched and the worst-matched grafts increases with time.[131] In the UNOS registry data, the difference in the graft survival rate between the best-matched and worst-matched recipient was 10% at 1-year posttransplantation and this difference increased to 18% by 3 years posttransplantation. The Collaborative Transplant Study of more than 67,000 primary cadaver grafts has also demonstrated a significant correlation between the number of HLA mismatches and graft loss.[128]

A threshold level of HLA matching might exist: Allografts that are matched for four or more HLA antigens (or two or less HLA mismatches) have a superior short- as well as long-term outcome compared to less than four HLA antigen matches (or greater than two antigen mismatches).[131] It is noteworthy that the beneficial effect of different degrees of matching/mismatching for the HLA-A, B, and DR antigens,[132] with the exception of phenotypically identical HLA transplants, is more evident in white recipients as compared to black recipients of deceased donor renal allografts.[127,131]

The impact of each of the HLA loci—HLA-A locus, HLA-B locus, and HAL-DR locus—on renal allograft outcome has been investigated. Each locus impacts graft outcome. In the Collaborative Transplant Study, the influence of HLA-DR mismatches was greater than that of HLA-A or HLA-B mismatches in the first year following transplantation; with increased posttransplantation time, mismatches at any of the three loci impacted adversely on graft survival rates.[128]

Molecular techniques are currently used for the typing of HLA and for finer resolution of the HLA system.[133] The clinical advantage of molecular matching was suggested originally by the observation that the 1-year deceased donor renal graft survival rate is 87% in patients who receive kidneys that are HLA-DR identical, not only by the serologic methods but also by molecular methods (DNA-RFLP method). This figure drops to 69% for patients who receive kidneys that are not HLA-DR identical by the molecular methodology.[134] Application of molecular techniques for the identification of HLA-DR antigens has also resulted in the appreciation of a stepwise increase in the survival of deceased donor renal allografts matched for zero, one, or two HLA-DR antigens (Fig. 81.4D).[128,133] Molecular typing has also been used to detect mismatches at the HLA-A or HLA-B locus. Mismatches that were missed by conventional serologic techniques, but identified by molecular techniques, were found to adversely impact graft survival.[128]

Previous data has suggested minimal impact of matching for HLA-C locus antigens. Matching for the HLA-DP antigen, on the other hand, appears to be important in repeat but not primary grafts.[128] Emerging data support the importance of matching for HLA-C antigens. Using the polymerase chain reaction-sequence specific primer method, a cohort of 2,260 deceased-donor renal transplant recipients was typed for the HLA-C locus as well as assessed for presensitization using lymphocytotoxicity testing. Mismatching at the HLA-C locus had a significantly negative impact on graft survival in presensitized but not in non-presensitized recipients.[135]

Crossmatch

Crossmatches, testing of the recipient's serum for antibodies reacting with the donor's HLA antigens, must be performed prior to renal transplantation. The standard crossmatch test (CDC) consists of incubating the serum from the recipient with the donor's lymphocytes in the presence of rabbit serum as a source of complement.

The presence in the recipient's serum of cytotoxic antibodies directed at the donor's class I antigen (positive T cell crossmatch) is an absolute contraindication to transplantation because 80% to 90% of transplants performed in the presence of a positive crossmatch are subject to hyperacute rejection.[136] The sensitivity of the standard crossmatch test has been increased by the addition of sublytic concentrations of antihuman globulin (AHG) to the test system. The graft survival rate is about 5% lower in recipients with a positive AHG test compared to recipients with a negative AHG test.[137]

The significance of antibodies reacting with the donor's class II antigens (positive B cell crossmatch) is not fully resolved. A survival disadvantage, 7% in primary transplants and 15% in repeat transplants, however, has been noted in recipients with a positive B cell crossmatch.[137]

A number of centers are currently using flow cytometry-based methodology to detect donor-specific antibodies. Flow cytometry crossmatches permit detection of low, sublytic concentrations of complement fixing as well as noncomplement-fixing antibodies. In the UNOS kidney transplant registry data,[138] a positive flow cytometry crossmatch was associated with an increased incidence of early graft dysfunction requiring dialytic support, primary nonfunction of the allograft, prolonged hospitalization, and a greater incidence of allograft rejection. The negative impact of a positive flow cytometry crossmatch was greater in repeat transplants compared to primary transplants. Whereas a positive flow crossmatch was associated with a 5% decrease in the 3-year survival rate of primary grafts, a 19% decrease was observed in the 3-year survival of repeat grafts. In primary transplants, a T+B+ flow cytometry crossmatch and a T–B+ crossmatch had a similar outcome (76% vs. 74% at 3 years posttransplantation), and in repeat transplants a T+B+ flow cytometry crossmatch has a much inferior outcome compared to a T–B+ crossmatch (60% vs. 73% at 3 years posttransplantation).

The presence of posttransplant donor-specific anti-HLA antibodies has been shown in an international cooperative study from 36 centers to be detrimental to the survival of the kidney allograft.[139] From the study, the overall frequency of HLA antibodies found among kidney transplant recipients was 20.9%. The frequency of antibodies detected remained relatively constant in patients who were transplanted from 1 year (17.8%) to greater than 10 years (26.9%). In a separate study, data also support the negative impact of posttransplant de novo donor HLA-specific antibodies on graft outcome. In addition, they appear to predict rejection in kidney transplant recipients.[140]

Solid phase assays were introduced to enhance anti-HLA antibody detection either via enzyme-linked immunosorbent assay (ELISA)-based methods or Luminex technology (Austen, TX).[141] The ELISA technique detects anti-HLA antibodies from test serum via their binding with individual or groups of HLA molecules on the surface of the ELISA well with the appropriate specificity. A positive read is indicated by a change in color following the addition of a second enzyme-linked anti-human IgG antibody and a suitable substrate for the reaction. The Luminex platform-based method has greater sensitivity than the ELISA technique and is now widely used by transplant programs to screen for HLA-specific antibodies.

The Luminex single antigen fluorescent bead technology is based on a series of polysytrene beads with embedded fluorochromes of varying intensity that display predetermined HLA molecules on their surfaces. A test serum containing primary anti-HLA antibodies will interact with the appropriate HLA molecules, which are attached to the beads. Phycoerythrin-labelled anti-human IgG antibodies are then added to bind the primary anti-HLA antibodies. Lasers excite both the fluorochromes in the beads and the phycoerythrin bound to the primary anti-HLA antibodies. The unique combination of signals detected by the sensor determines the specificity of the anti-HLA antibody in question.

The solid-phase assays and Luminex in particular screen only for anti-HLA antibodies whereas the CDC method may detect non-HLA antibodies such as autoantibodies, antibodies directed at non-HLA molecules, and even immune complexes. The CDC assay may also pick up IgM anti-HLA antibodies whereas the Luminex method requires the addition of anti-IgM antibodies to detect anti-HLA IgM antibodies. On the other hand, the Luminex assay will detect all classes of IgG antibodies irrespective of their complement fixing abilities, which is required for detection by the CDC method. Luminex technology also permits the testing of sera following the administration of rituximab given during desensitization procedures whereas the CDC assay may yield a false positive reaction due to the interaction of the monoclonal antibodies and CD20 molecules on the B cells. A calculated panel reactive antibody (PRA) may be obtained with Luminex single antigen fluorescent bead technology by determining the frequencies of the HLA antigens in a given population. Finally, the Luminex platform assay allows a pretransplant virtual crossmatch to be performed in order to predict the success of high-risk presensitized live or deceased donor transplants.

TRANSPLANTATION TOLERANCE

Transplantation tolerance can be defined as an inability of the organ graft recipient to express a graft destructive immune response. Although this statement does not restrict either the mechanistic basis or the quantitative aspects of immune unresponsiveness of the host, true tolerance is antigen-specific, induced as a consequence of prior exposure to the specific antigen, and is not dependent on the continuous administration of exogenous nonspecific immunosuppressants.

A classification of tolerance on the basis of the mechanisms involved, site of induction, extent of tolerance, and the cell primarily tolerized is provided in Table 81.4. Induction strategies for the creation of peripheral tolerance are listed in Table 81.5.

Several hypotheses, not necessarily mutually exclusive and, at times, even complementary, have been proposed for the cellular basis of tolerance. Data from several laboratories support the following mechanistic possibilities for the creation of a tolerant state: clonal deletion, clonal anergy, and immunoregulation.

Clonal Deletion

Clonal deletion is a process by which self–antigen-reactive cells (especially those with high affinity for the self-antigens), are eliminated from the organism's immune repertoire. This process is called central tolerance. In the case of T cells, this process takes place in the thymus, and the death of immature T cells is considered to be the ultimate result of high-affinity interactions between a T cell with productively rearranged TCR and the thymic nonlymphoid cells, including dendritic cells that express the self-MHC antigen. This purging of the immune repertoire of self-reactive T cells is termed negative selection and is distinguished from the positive selection process responsible for the generation of the T cell repertoire involved in the recognition of foreign antigens in the context of self-MHC molecules. Clonal deletion or at least marked depletion of mature T cells as a consequence of apoptosis can also occur in the periphery.[142] The form of graft tolerance, occurring as a consequence of mixed hematopoietic chimerism, entails massive deletion of alloreactive clones.[143] Tolerance to renal allografts has been achieved in patients who have accepted a bone marrow graft from the same donor.[144,145] It is interesting that IL-2, the only T cell-growth factor that triggers T cell proliferation as well as apoptosis, is an absolute prerequisite for the acquisition of organ graft tolerance through use of nonlymphoablative treatment regimens.[146,147] Tolerance achieved under these circumstances also involves additional mechanisms, including clonal anergy and suppressor mechanisms.[148-150]

TABLE 81.5 Potential Approaches for the Creation of Tolerance

A. Cell Depletion Protocols
   1. Whole body irradiation
   2. Total lymphoid irradiation
   3. Panel of monoclonal antibodies
B. Reconstitution Protocols
   1. Allogeneic bone marrow cells with or without T cell depletion
   2. Syngeneic bone marrow cells
C. Combination of Strategies A and B
D. Cell-Surface Molecule Targeted Therapy
   1. Anti-CD4 mAbs
   2. Anti-ICAM-1 + anti-LFA-1 mAbs
   3. Anti-CD3 mAbs
   4. Anti-CD2 mAbs
   5. Anti-IL-2 receptor α (CD25) mAbs
   6. CTLA4Ig fusion protein
   7. Anti-CD40L mAbs
E. Drugs
   1. Azathioprine
   2. Cyclosporine
   3. Rapamycin
F. Additional Approaches
   1. Donor-specific blood transfusions with concomitant mAb or drug therapy
   2. Intrathymic inoculation of cells/antigens
   3. Oral administration of cells/antigens

TABLE 81.4 Classification of Tolerance

A. Based on the Major Mechanism Involved
   1. Clonal deletion
   2. Clonal anergy
   3. Suppression
B. Based on the Period of Induction
   1. Fetal
   2. Neonatal
   3. Adult
C. Based on the Cell Tolerized
   1. T cell
   2. B cell
D. Based on the Extent of Tolerance
   1. Complete
   2. Partial, including split
E. Based on the Main Site of Induction
   1. Central
   2. Peripheral

Clonal Anergy

Clonal anergy refers to a process in which the antigen-reactive cells are functionally silenced. The cellular basis for the hyporesponsiveness resides in the anergic cell itself and the current data suggest that the anergic T cells fail to express the T cell-growth factor, IL-2, and other crucial T cell activation genes because of defects in the antigen-stimulated signaling pathway.

T cell clonal anergy can result from suboptimal antigen-driven signaling of T cells, as mentioned earlier. The full activation of T cells requires at least two signals, one signal generated via the TCR–CD3 complex, and the second (costimulatory) signal initiated/delivered by the APCs. Stimulation of T cells via the TCR–CD3 complex alone—provision of signal 1 without signal 2—can result in T cell anergy/paralysis (Fig. 81.5 and Table 81.2).

B cell activation, in a fashion analogous to T cell activation, requires at least two signals. The first signal is initiated via the B cell antigen receptor immunoglobulin and the second costimulatory signal is provided by cytokines or cell-surface proteins of T cell origin. Thus, delivery of the antigenic signal alone to the B cells without the instructive cytokines or T cell help can lead to B cell anergy and tolerance.

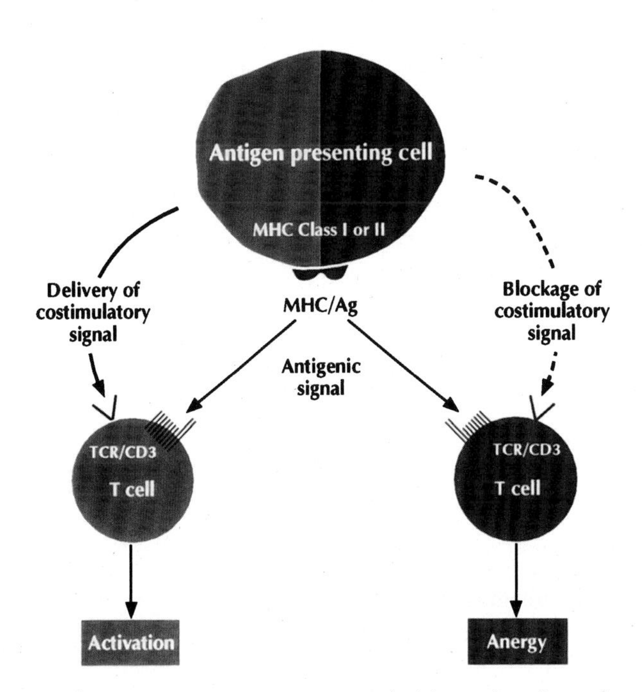

FIGURE 81.5 T cell activation/anergy decision points. Several potential sites for the regulation of T cell signaling are shown. The antigenic peptide displayed by major histocompatibility complex (MHC) (*site 1*), costimulatory signals (*site 2*), T cell antigen receptor (TCR) (*site 3*), and cytokine signaling (*site 4*) can influence the eventual outcome. Altered peptide ligands, blockade of costimulatory signals, downregulation of TCR, and interleukin (IL)-10 favor anergy induction, whereas fully immunogenic peptides, delivery of costimulatory signals, appropriate number of TCRs, and IL-12 prevent anergy induction and facilitate full activation of T cells. (From Suthanthiran M. Transplantation tolerance: fooling mother nature. *Proc Natl Acad Sci U S A.* 1996;93:12072.)

Immunoregulatory (Suppressor) Mechanisms

Antigen-specific T or B cells are physically present and are functionally competent in tolerant states resulting from suppressor mechanisms. The cytopathic and antigen-specific cells are restrained by the suppressor cells or factors or express noncytopathic cellular programs. Each of the major subsets of T cells, the CD4 T cells and the CD8 T cells, has been implicated in mediating suppression. Indeed, a cascade involving MHC antigen-restricted T cells, MHC antigen-unrestricted T cells, and their secretory products have been reported to collaborate to mediate suppression. Recently, a subset of CD4+ T cells, the CD4+ CD25+ cells that express FOXP3 (Tregs), has been identified to mediate potent suppressive activity.[151,152] There are two major types of CD4+CD25+ T regs: naturally occurring CD4+CD25+Foxp3+ T-regs (nTregs) that arise from the thymus and induced CD4+CD25+Foxp3+ T-regs (iTregs) that originate in the periphery. IL-2 and TGF-β, a prototypic anti-inflammatory cytokine, are important for the maintenance of nTregs and TGF-β can differentiate CD4+CD25-Foxp3–T cells into CD4+CD25+Foxp3+ T cells. IL-6, a pro-inflammatory cytokine, inhibits the generation of Tregs and in the presence of TGF-β induces naïve T cells to differentiate into Th17 cells. Th 17 cells are a newly discovered effector T helper cell subset that produce IL-17, a proinflammatory cytokine, which activates the NF-κB and mitogen-activated protein kinases pathways.[153] Although not completely proven, Th 17 cells may contribute to acute allograft rejection that is resistant to suppression by Tregs.[154]

At least four distinct mechanisms have been advanced to explain the cellular basis for suppression:

1. An anti-idiotypic regulatory mechanism in which the idiotype of the TCR of the original antigen-responsive T cells functions as an immunogen and elicits an anti-idiotypic response. The elicited anti-idiotypic regulatory cells, in turn, prevent the further responses of the idiotype-bearing cells to the original sensitizing stimulus.
2. The veto process by which recognition by alloreactive T cells of alloantigen-expressing veto cells results in the targeted killing (veto process) of the original alloreactive T cells by the veto cells.
3. Immune deviation, a shift in CD4+ T cell programs away from Th1-type (IL-2, IFN-γ expressing) toward the Th2-type (IL-4, IL-10 expressing) program.
4. The production of suppressor factors or cytokines (e.g., the production of TGF-β by myelin basic protein-specific CD8 T cells or other cytokines with antiproliferative properties[155]). The process leading to full tolerance is infectious. Tolerant T cells recruit nontolerant T cells into the tolerant state.[149] The tolerant state also establishes a condition in which foreign tissues housed in the same microenvironment as the specific antigen to which the host has been tolerized are protected from rejection.[149] Tolerance is clearly a multistep process.[148-150]

It is very likely that more than one mechanism is operative in the induction of tolerance (Fig. 81.5). The tolerant state is not an all-or-nothing phenomenon, but is one that has several gradations. Of the mechanisms proposed for tolerance, clonal deletion might be of greater importance in the creation of self-tolerance and clonal anergy and immunoregulatory mechanisms might be more applicable to transplantation tolerance. More recent data suggest both clonal depletion and immunoregulatory mechanisms are needed to create and sustain central or peripheral tolerance. From a practical viewpoint, a nonimmunogenic allograft (e.g., located in an immunologically privileged site or physically isolated from the immune system) might also be "tolerated" by an immunocompetent organ-graft recipient.

Authentic tolerance has been difficult to identify in human renal allograft recipients. Nevertheless, the clinical examples, albeit infrequent, of grafts functioning without any exogenous immunosuppressive drugs (either due to noncompliance of the patient or due to discontinuation of drugs for other medical reasons) does suggest that some long-term recipients of allografts develop tolerance to the transplanted organ and accept the allografts.[156] The recent progress in our understanding of the immunobiology of graft rejection and tolerance and the potential to apply molecular approaches to the bedside hold significant promise for the creation of a clinically relevant tolerant state and transplantation without exogenous immunosuppressants—the ultimate goal of the transplant physician.

Clinical Trials in Transplant Tolerance

Small and large animal studies have successfully demonstrated the concept of "mixed chimerism" in achieving allograft tolerance. In these models, transplanting the donor's hematopoietic stem cells in tandem with the allograft create a bone marrow lymphohematopoietic chimera in which the donor and recipient hematopoiesis coexist thereby allowing the acceptance of the allograft. In a landmark trial, following a pretransplant nonmyeloablative-conditioning regimen, a total of five patients underwent combined bone marrow and kidney transplants from HLA single-haplotype mismatched living-related donors.[23] All five patients developed transient chimerism with one allograft failure due to irreversible humoral rejection and four patients achieving tolerance after discontinuation of all immunosuppressive regimens at 240, 244, 272, and 422 days after transplantation. Analysis of kidney allograft biopsy specimens from tolerant patients revealed the presence of high levels of the regulatory T-cell signature, FOXP3 mRNA, and the absence of the cellular rejection biomarker, granzyme B mRNA.

In a study of 25 tolerant kidney transplant patients who were off immunosuppressive medications for at least a year, unique B cell signatures were identified from peripheral whole blood specimens using gene microarrays and urinary cell sediments using real-time quantitative polymerase chain reaction (PCR) assays.[156] The predictive genes for tolerance (IGKV4-1, IGLLA, IGKV1D-13) were important for B cell differentiation and activation. They encode lambda and kappa light chains, which were increased during transition from pre- to mature B cells and during class switching and receptor editing. The study also showed that in tolerant patients, there was an increase in transitional B cells (CD38+CD24+) producing IL-10 cytokine.

Tolerance-inducing protocols and transplant tolerance trials are very likely to be tested in the clinic as novel conditioning immunosuppressive regimens become available to the transplant community.

CONCLUSION

Successful organ transplantation represents the fruition of the dedicated efforts of basic scientists, clinicians, and allied personnel. An excellent paradigm for the effective application of knowledge gained by basic research to the alleviation of life-threatening illness, renal transplantation also affords marvelous opportunities for the investigation of the systemic basis for renal disease independent of organ-specific mechanisms. Synergistic therapeutic protocols that target discrete steps in antigen recognition, signal transduction, and effector immunity are being explored in the clinic. The ultimate prize of transplantation would be that the basic principles learned would facilitate the prevention of the disease that necessitated transplantation in the first place.

Acknowledgments

The authors are grateful to our colleagues for the stimulating discussions and very importantly to our patients who have always inspired us by their courage and tolerance as we strive to improve knowledge in our chosen field.

REFERENCES

1. Suthanthiran M, Strom TB. Renal transplantation. *N Engl J Med.* 1994;334:365.
2. Dustin ML, Cooper JA. The immunological synapse and the actin cytoskeleton: molecular hardware for T cell signaling. *Nature Immunol.* 2000;1:23.
3. Unanue ER, Cerottini JC. Antigen presentation. *FASEB J.* 1989;3:2496.
4. Germain RN. MHC-dependent antigen processing and peptide presentation: providing ligands for T lymphocyte activation. *Cell.* 1994;76:287.
5. Acuto O, Cantrell D. T cell activation and the cytoskeleton. *Annu Rev Immunol.* 2000;18:165.
6. Shoskes DA, Wood KJ. Indirect presentation of MHC antigens in transplantation. *Immunol Today.* 1994;15:32.
7. Jorgensen JL, Reay PA, Ehrich EW, et al. Molecular components of T cell recognition. *Annu Rev Immunol.* 1992;10:835.
8. Suthanthiran M. A novel model for the antigen-dependent activation of normal human T cells: transmembrane signaling by crosslinkage of the CD3/T cell receptor-alpha/beta complex with the cluster determinant 2 antigen. *J Exp Med.* 1990;171:1965.
9. Brown MH, et al. The CD2 antigen associates with the T-cell antigen receptor CD3 antigen complex on the surface of human T lymphocytes. *Nature (London).* 1989;339:551.
10. Beyers AD, Spruyt LL, Williams AF. Molecular associations between the T-lymphocyte antigen receptor complex and the surface antigens CD2, CD4, or CD8 and CD5. *Proc Natl Acad Sci U S A.* 1992;89:2945.
11. Nishizuka Y. Intracellular signaling by hydrolysis of phospholipids and activation of protein kinase C. *Science.* 1992;258:607.

12. Waldmann T, Tagaya Y, Bamford R. Interleukin-2, interleukin-15, and their receptors. *Int Rev Immunol.* 1998;16:205.

13. O'Keefe SJ, et al. FK506- and CsA-sensitive activation of the IL-2 promoter by calcineurin. *Nature (London).* 1992;357:692.

14. Clipstone NA, Crabtree GR. Identification of calcineurin as a key signalling enzyme in T-lymphocyte activation. *Nature (London).* 1992;357:695.

15. Liu J, et al. Calcineurin is a common target of cyclophilin-cyclosporin A and FKBP-FK506 complexes. *Cell.* 1991;66:807.

16. Schwartz RH. T cell anergy. *Sci Am.* 1993;269:62.

17. Suthanthiran M. Signaling features of T cells: implication for the regulation of the anti-allograft response. *Kidney Int Suppl.* 1993;43:S3.

18. Dustin ML, Springer TA. T-cell receptor cross-linking transiently stimulates adhesiveness through LFA-1. *Nature (London).* 1989;341:619.

19. Lenschow DJ, Walunas TL, Bluestone JA. CD28/B7 system of T cell costimulation. *Annu Rev Immunol.* 1996;14:233.

20. Shahinian A, Pfeffer K, Lee KP, et al. Differential T cell costimulatory requirements in CD28-deficient mice. *Science.* 1993;261:609.

21. Noelle RJ. CD40 and its ligand in host defense. *Immunity.* 1996;4:415.

22. Oosterwegel MA, Greenwald RJ, Mandelbrot DA, et al. CTLA-4 and T cell activation. *Curr Opin Immunol.* 1999;11:294.

23. Kawai T, Cosimi AB, Spitzer TR, et al. HLA-mismatched renal transplantation without maintenance immunosuppression. *N Engl J Med.* 2008;358:353.

24. Smith KA. Interleukin-2: inception, impact, and implications. *Science.* 1988;240:1169.

25. Waldman TA. The interleukin-2 receptor. *J Biol Chem.* 1991;266:2681.

26. Takeshita T, Asao H, Ohtani K. Cloning of the gamma chain of the human IL-2 receptor. *Science.* 1992;257:379.

27. Hatakeyama M, et al. Interaction of the IL-2 receptor with the src-family kinase $p56^{lck}$: identification of novel intermolecular association. *Science.* 1991;252:1523.

28. Fung MR, et al. A tyrosine kinase physically associates with the alpha-subunit of the human IL-2 receptor. *J Immunol.* 1991;147:1253.

29. Remillard B, et al. Interleukin-2 receptor regulates activation of phosphatidylinositol 3-kinase. *J Biol Chem.* 1991;266:14167.

30. Maslinski W, Remillard B, Tsudo M, et al. Interleukin-2 (IL-2) induces tyrosine kinase-dependent translocation of active Raf-1 from the IL-2 receptor into the cytosol. *J Biol Chem.* 1992;267:15281.

31. Shibuya H, et al. IL-2 and EGF receptors stimulate the hematopoietic cell cycle via different signaling pathways: demonstration of a novel role for c-myc. *Cell.* 1992;70:57.

32. Taniguchi T. Cytokine signalling through non-receptor protein tyrosine kinases. *Science.* 1995;260:251.

33. Racusen LC, Colvin RB, Solez K, et al. Antibody-mediated rejection criteria – an addition to the Banff '97 classification of renal allograft rejection. *Am J Transplant.* 2003;3:709.

34. Dragun D, Muller DN, Brasen JH, et al. Angiotensin II type 1-receptor activating antibodies in renal-allograft rejection. *N Engl J Med.* 2005;352:558.

35. Strom TB, Tilney NL, Carpenter CB, et al. Identity and cytotoxic capacity of cells infiltrating renal allografts. *N Engl J Med.* 1975;292:1257.

36. Suthanthiran M, Garovoy MR. Immunologic monitoring of the renal transplant recipient. *Urol Clin North Am.* 1983;10:315.

37. Strom TB, Suthanthiran M. Prospects and applicability of molecular diagnosis of allograft rejection. *Semin Nephrol.* 2000;20:103.

38. Vasconcellos LM, Schachter AD, Zheng XX, et al. Cytotoxic lymphocyte gene expression in peripheral blood leukocytes correlates with rejecting renal allografts. *Transplantation.* 1998;66:562.

39. Li B, Hartono C, Ding R, et al. Noninvasive diagnosis of renal-allograft rejection by measurement of messenger RNA for perforin and granzyme B in urine. *N Engl J Med.* 2001;344:947.

40. Suthanthiran M, Ding R, Sharma V, et al. Urinary cell messenger RNA expression signatures anticipate acute cellular rejection: A report from CTOT-04. Abstract [1] presented at the American Transplant Congress 2011.

41. Rush D, Nickerson P, Gough J, et al. Beneficial effects of treatment of early subclinical rejection: a randomized study. *J Am Soc Nephrol.* 1998;9:2129.

42. Knudsen PJ, Dinarello CA, Strom TB. Glucocorticoids inhibit transcriptional and post-transcriptional expression of interleukin-1 in U937 cells. *J Immunol.* 1987;139:4129.

43. Zanker B, Walz G, Wieder KJ, et al. Evidence that glucocorticosteroids block expression of the human interleukin-6 gene by accessory cells. *Transplantation.* 1990;49:183.

44. Arya SK, Won-Staal J, Gallo RC. Dexamethasone-mediated inhibition of human T cell growth factor and gamma-interferon messenger RNA. *J Immunol.* 1984;133:273.

45. Almawi WY, et al. Abrogation of glucocorticosteroid-mediated inhibition of T cell proliferation by the synergistic action of IL-1, IL-6 and IFN-gamma. *J Immunol.* 1991;146:3523.

46. Vacca A, et al. Glucocorticoid receptor-mediated suppression of the interleukin-2 gene expression through impairment of the cooperativity between nuclear factor of activated T cells and AP-1 enhancer elements. *J Exp Med.* 1992;175:637.

47. Auphan N, DiDonato J, Rosette C, et al. Immunosuppression by glucocorticoids: inhibition of NF-$_{\kappa}$B activity through induction of I$_{\kappa}$B synthesis. *Science.* 1995;270:286.

48. Elion GB. Biochemistry and pharmacology of purine analogues. *Fed Proc.* 1967;26:898.

49. Bach JF, Strom TB. The mode of action of immunosuppressive agents. In: Bach JF, Strom TB, eds. *Research Monographs in Immunology.* Amsterdam: Elsevier; 1986:105.

50. Wuthrich RP, Cicvara S, Ambuhl PM, et al. Randomized trial of conversion from mycophenolate mofetil to azathioprine 6 months after renal allograft transplantation. *Neph Dial Transplant.* 2000;15:1228.

51. Schreiber SL. Immunophilin-sensitive protein phosphatase action in cell signaling pathways. *Cell.* 1992;70:365.

52. Li B, Sehajpal PK, Khanna A, et al. Differential regulation of transforming growth factor beta and interleukin-2 genes in human T cells: demonstration by usage of novel competitor DNA constructs in the quantitative polymerase chain reaction. *J Exp Med.* 1991;174:1259.

53. Sehajpal PK, Sharma VK, Ingulli E, et al. Synergism between the CD3 antigen- and CD2 antigen-derived signals: exploration at the level of induction of DNA-binding proteins and characterization of the inhibitory activity of cyclosporine. *Transplantation.* 1993;55:1118.

54. Khanna A, Cairns V, Hosenpud JD. Tacrolimus induces increased expression of transforming growth factor-beta1 in mammalian lymphoid as well as nonlymphoid cells. *Transplantation.* 1999;67:614.

55. Kehrl JH, Wakefield LM, Roberts AB, et al. Production of transforming growth factor beta by human T lymphocytes and its potential role in the regulation of T cell growth. *J Exp Med.* 1986;163:1037.

56. Morris RE, Wang J. Comparison of the immunosuppressive effects of mycophenolic acid and the morpholinoethyl ester of mycophenolic acid (RS-61433) in recipients of heart allografts. *Transplant Proc.* 1999;23:493.

57. Sweeney MJ. Metabolism and biochemistry of mycophenolic acid. *Cancer Res.* 1972;32:1803.

58. Lui SL, Halloran PF. Mycophenolate mofetil in kidney transplantation. *Curr Opin Nephrol Hypertens.* 1996;5:508.

59. Sollinger HW and U.S. Renal Transplant Mycophenolate Mofetil Study Group. Mycophenolate mofetil for the prevention of acute rejection in primary cadaveric renal allograft recipients. *Transplantation.* 1995;60:225.

60. European Mycophenolate Mofetil Cooperative Study Group. Mycophenolate mofetil in renal transplantation: 3-year results from the placebo-controlled trial. *Transplantation.* 1999;68:391.

61. Remuzzi G, Lesti M, Gotti E, et al. Mycophenolate mofelil versus azathioprine for prevention of acute rejection in renal transplantation (MYSS): a randomised trial. *Lancet.* 2004;364:503.

62. Salvadori M, Holzer H, de Mattos A, et al. Enteric-coated mycophenolate sodium is therapeutically equivalent to mycophenolate mofetil in *de novo* renal transplant patients. *Am J Transplant* 2003;4:231.

63. Morris RE. Rapamycins: antifungal, antitumor, antiproliferative, and immunosuppressive macrolides. *Transplant Rev.* 1992;6:39.

64. Chung J, Kuo CJ, Crabtree GR, et al. Rapamycin-FKBP specifically blocks growth-dependent activation of and signaling by the 70-kd 56 protein kinases. *Cell.* 1992;69:1227.

65. Kuo CJ, et al. Rapamycin selectively inhibits interleukin-2 activation of p70 56 kinase. *Nature (London).* 1992;358:70.

66. Kahan BD. Efficacy of sirolimus compared with azathioprine for reduction of acute allograft rejection: a randomized multicentre study. *Lancet.* 2000;356:194.

67. Schena FP, Pascoe MD, Alberu J, et al. Conversion from calcineurin inhibitors to sirolimus maintenance therapy in renal allograft recipients: 24-month efficacy and safety results from the CONVERT trial. *Transplantation.* 2009;87:233.

68. Weir MR, Mulgaonkar S, Chan L, et al. Mycophenolate mofetil-based immunosuppression with sirolimus in renal transplantation: a randomized, controlled Spare-the-Nephron trial. *Kidney Int.* 2011;79:897.

69. Nashan B, Curtis J, Ponticelli C, et al. Everolimus and reduced-exposure cyclosporine in de novo renal-transplant recipients: a three-year phase II, randomized, multicenter, open-label study. *Transplantation.* 2004;78:1332.

70. Vitko S, Margreiter R, Weimar W, et al. Everolimus (certican) 12-month safety and efficacy versus mycophenolate mofetil in de novo renal transplant recipients. *Transplantation.* 2004;78:1532.

71. Waldman WJ, Knight DA, Lurain NS, et al. Novel mechanism of inhibition of cytomegalovirus by the experimental immunosuppressive agent leflunomide. *Transplantation.* 1999;68:814.

72. Knight DA, Hejmanowski AQ, Dierksheide JE, et al. Inhibition of herpes simplex virus type 1 by the experimental immunosuppressive agent leflunomide. *Transplantation.* 2001;71:170.

73. Farasati NA, Shapiro R, Vats A, et al. Effect of leflunomide and cidofovir on replication of BK virus in an in vitro culture system. *Transplantation.* 2005; 79:116.65.

74. Hardinger KL, Wang CD, Schnitzler MA, et al. Prospective, pilot, open-label, short-term study of conversion to leflunomide reverses chronic renal allograft dysfunction. *Am J Transplant.* 2002;2:867.

75. Vanrenterghem Y, van Hooff JP, Klinger M, et al. The effects of FK778 in combination with tacrolimus and steroids: a phase II multicenter study in renal transplant patients. *Transplantation.* 2004;78:9.

76. Guasch A, Roy-Chaudhury P, Woodle ES, et al. Assessment of efficacy and safety of FK778 in comparison with standard care in renal transplant recipients with untreated BK nephropathy. *Transplantation.* 2010;90:897.

77. Norman DJ, Vincenti F, De Mattos AM, et al. Phase I trial of HuM291, a humanized anti-CD3 antibody, in patients receiving renal allografts from living donors. *Transplantation.* 2000;70:1707.

78. Prescribing information for Thymoglobulin® Genzyme Corporation. 2008.

79. Khwaja K, Asolati M, Harmon J, et al. Outcome at 3 years with a prednisone-free maintenance regimen: a single-center experience with 349 kidney transplant recipients. *Am J Transplant.* 2004;4:980.

80. Pearl JP, Parris J, Hale DA, et al. Immunocompetent T-cells with a memory-like phenotype are the dominant cell type following antibody-mediated T-cell depletion. *Am J Transplant.* 2005;5:465.

81. Webster AC, Playford EG, Higgins G, et al. Interleukin 2 receptor antagonists for renal transplant recipients: a meta-analysis of randomized trials. *Transplantation.* 2004;77:166.

82. Brennan DC, Daller JA, Lake KD, et al. Rabbit antithymocyte globulin versus basiliximab in renal transplantation. *N Engl J Med.* 2006;355:1967.

83. Knechtle SJ, Pirsch JD, Fechner JH Jr, et al. Campath-1H induction plus rapamycin monotherapy for renal transplantation: results of a pilot study. *Am J Transplant.* 2003;3:722.

84. Ciancio G, Burke GW, Gaynor JJ, et al. The use of Campath-1H as induction therapy in renal transplantation: preliminary results. *Transplantation.* 2004;78:426.

85. Bloom D, Chang Z, Pauly K, et al. BAFF is increased in renal transplant patients following treatment with alemtuzumab. *Am J Transplant.* 2009;9:1835.

86. Hanaway MJ, Woodle ES, Mulgaonkar S, et al. Alemtuzumab induction in renal transplant. *N Engl J Med.* 2011;364:1909.

87. Becker YT, Becker BN, Pirsch JD, et al. Rituximab as treatment for refractory kidney transplant rejection. *Am J Transplant.* 2004;4:996.

88. Tyden G, Kumlien G, Genberg H, et al. ABO incompatible kidney transplantations without splenectomy, using antigen-specific immunoadsorption and rituximab. *Am J Transplant.* 2005;5:145.

89. Clatworthy MR, Watson CJE, Plotnek G, et al. B-cell-depleting induction therapy and acute cellular rejection. *N Engl J Med.* 2009;360:2683.

90. Kazatchkine MD, Kaveri SV. Immunomodulation of autoimmune and inflammatory diseases with intravenous immune globulin. *N Engl J Med.* 2001;345:747.

91. Jordan SC, Tyan D, Stablein D, et al. Evaluation of intravenous immunoglobulin as an agent to lower allosensitization and improve transplantation in highly sensitized adult patients with end-stage renal disease: report of the NIH IG02 Trial. *J Am Soc Nephrol.* 2004;15:3256.

92. White NB, Greenstein SM, Cantafio AW, et al. Successful rescue therapy with plasmapheresis and intravenous immunoglobulin for acute humoral renal transplant rejection. *Transplantation.* 2004;78:772.

93. Vo AA, Lukovsky M, Toyoda M, et al. Rituximab and intravenous immune globulin for desensitization during renal transplantation. *N Engl J Med.* 2008;359:242.

94. Brinkmann V, Cyster JG, Hla T. FTY720: sphingosine 1-phosphate receptor 1 in the control of lymphocyte egress and endothelial barrier function. *Am J Transplant.* 2004;4:1019.

95. Budde K, Schmouder RL, Brunkhorst R, et al. First human trial of FTY720, a novel immunomodulator, in stable renal transplant patients. *J Am Soc Nephrol.* 2002;13:1073.

96. Kahan BD, Karlix JL, Ferguson RM, et al. Pharmacodynamics, pharmacokinetics, and safety of multiple doses of FTY720 in stable renal transplant patients: a multicenter, randomized, placebo-controlled, phase 1 study. *Transplantation.* 2003;76:1079.

97. Tedesco-Silva H, Mourad G, Kahan BD, et al. FTY720, a novel immunomodulator: efficacy and safety results from the first phase 2A study in de novo renal transplantation. *Transplantation.* 2004;77:1826.

98. Salvadori M, Budde K, Charpentier B, et al. FTY720 versus MMF with cyclosporine in *de novo* renal transplantation: a 1-year, randomized controlled trial in Europe and Australasia. *Am J Transplant.* 2006;6:2912.

99. Tedesco-Silva H, Pescovitz MD, Cibrik D, et al. Randomized controlled trial of FTY720 versus MMF in *de novo* renal transplantation. *Transplantation.* 2006;82:1689.

100. Vincenti F, Muehlbacher F, Nashan B, et al. Co-stimulation blockade with LEA29Y in a calcineurin inhibitor free maintenance regimen in renal transplant: 6-month efficacy and safety. Abstract [1037] presented at the American Transplant Congress 2004.

101. Vincenti F, Charpentier B, Vanrenterghem Y, et al. A phase III study of belatacept-based immunosuppression regimens versus cyclosporine in renal transplant recipients (BENEFIT Study). *Am J Transplant.* 2010;10:535.

102. Durrbach A, Pestana JM, Pearson T, et al. A phase III study of belatacept versus cyclosporine in kidney transplants from extended criteria donors (BENEFIT-EXT Study). *Am J Transplant.* 2010;10:547.

103. Larsen CP, Grinyo J, Medina-Pestana J, et al. Belatacept-based regimens versus a cyclosporine A-based regimen in kidney transplant recipients: 2-year results from the BENEFIT and BENEFIT-EXT studies. *Transplantation.* 2010; 90:1528.

104. Weaver TA, Charafeddine AH, Agarwal A, et al. Alefacept promotes co-stimulation blockade based allograft survival in primates. *Nat Med.* 2009;15:746.

105. Bromberg J, Cibrik D, Steinberg S, et al. A phase 2 study to assess the safety and efficacy of alefacept (ALEF) in de novo kidney transplant recipients. Abstract [533] presented at the American Transplant Congress 2011.

106. Busque S, Leventhal J, Brennan DC, et al. Calcineurin-inhibitor-free immunosuppression based on the JAK inhibitor CP-690,550: a pilot study in *de novo* kidney allograft recipients. *Am J Transplant.* 2009;9:1936.

107. Vincenti F, Mendez R, Pescovitz M, et al. A phase I/II randomized open-label multicenter trial of efalizumab, a humanized anti-CD11a, anti-LFA-1 in renal transplantation. *Am J Transplant.* 2007;7:1770.

108. Lonze BE, Singer AL, Montgomery RA. Eculizumab and renal transplantation in a patient with CAPS. *N Engl J Med.* 2010;362:1744.

109. Locke JE, Magro CM, Singer AL, et al. The use of antibody to complement protein C5 for salvage treatment of severe antibody-mediated rejection. *Am J Transplant.* 2009;9:231.

110 . Zimmerhackl LB, Hofer J, Cortina G, et al. Prophylactic eculizumab after renal transplantation in atypical hemolytic-uremic syndrome. *N Engl J Med.* 2010;362:1746.

111. Perry DK, Burns JM, Pollinger HS, et al. Proteasome inhibition causes apoptosis of normal human plasma cells preventing alloantibody production. *Am J Transplant.* 2008;8:1.

112. Everly MJ, Everly, JJ, Susskind B, et al. Bortezomib provides effective therapy for antibody- and cell-mediated acute rejection. *Transplantation.* 2008; 86:1754.

113. Nankivell BJ, Borrows RJ, Fung CLS, et al. Calcineurin inhibitor nephrotoxicity: longitudinal assessment by protocol histology. *Transplantation.* 2004; 78:557.

114. Kreis H, Cisterne JM, Land W, et al. Sirolimus in association with mycophenolate mofetil induction for the prevention of acute graft rejection in renal allograft recipients. *Transplantation.* 2000;69:1252.

115. Gallagher MP, Hall B, Craig J, et al. A randomized controlled trial of cyclosporine withdrawal in renal-transplant recipients: 15-year results. *Transplantation.* 2004;78:1653.

116. Ruiz JC, Campistol JM, Grinyo JM, et al. Early cyclosporine A withdrawal in kidney-transplant recipients receiving sirolimus prevents progression of chronic pathologic allograft lesions. *Transplantation.* 2004;78:1312.

117. Vincenti F, Kirkman R, Light S, et al. Interleukin-2 receptor blockade with daclizumab to prevent acute rejection in renal transplantation. Daclizumab Triple Therapy Study Group. *N Engl J Med.* 1998;338:161.

118. Ekbergh H, Backman L, Tufveson G, et al. Daclizumab prevents acute rejection and improves patient survival post transplantation: 1 year pooled analysis. *Transplant Int.* 2000;13:151.

119. Kahan BD, Rajagopalan PR, Hall M. Reduction of the occurrence of acute cellular rejection among renal allograft recipients treated with basiliximab, a chimeric anti-interleukin-2-receptor monoclonal antibody. United States Simulect Renal Study Group. *Transplantation.* 1999;67:276.

120. Hong JC, Kahan BD. Use of anti-CD25 monoclonal antibody in combination with rapamycin to eliminate cyclosporine treatment during the induction phase of immunosuppression. *Transplantation.* 1999;68:701.

121. Strom TB, et al. Interleukin-2 receptor-directed therapies: antibody- or cytokine-based targeting molecules. *Annu Rev Med.* 1993;44:343.

122. McAlister VC, Gao Z, Peltekian K, et al. Sirolimus tacrolimus combination immunosuppression. *Lancet.* 2000;355:376.

123. Woodle ES, Vincenti F, Lorber MI, et al. A multicenter pilot study of early (4-day) steroid cessation in renal transplant recipients under Simulect, Tacrolimus and Sirolimus. *Am J Transplant.* 2005;5:157.
124. ter Meulen CG, van Riemsdijk I, Hene RJ, et al. Steroid-withdrawal at 3 days after renal transplantation with anti-IL-2 receptor α therapy: a prospective, randomized, multicenter study. *Am J Transplant.* 2004;4:803.
125. Klein J, Sato A. The HLA system. First of two parts. *N Engl J Med.* 2000; 343:702.
126. Klein J, Sato A. The HLA system. Second of two parts. *N Engl J Med.* 2000; 343:782.
127. Cecka JM, Terasaki PI. The UNOS Scientific Renal Transplant Registry—1991. In: Terasaki PI, Cecka JM, eds. *Clinical Transplants 1991.* Los Angeles: UCLA Tissue Typing Laboratory; 1992:1.
128. Opelz G, Wujciak T, Dohler B, et al. HLA compatibility and organ transplant survival. *Rev Immunogen.* 1999;1:334.
129. Takemoto S, Terasaki PI, Cecka JM, et al. Survival of nationally shared, HLA-matched kidney transplants from cadaveric donors. *N Engl J Med.* 1992; 327:834.
130. Takemoto SK, Terasaki PI, Gjertson DW, et al. Twelve years' experience with national sharing of HLA-matched cadaveric kidneys for transplantation. *N Engl J Med.* 2000;343:1078.
131. Cicciarelli J, Cho Y. HLA matching: univariate and multivariate analyses of UNOS Registry data. In: Terasaki PI, Cecka JM, eds. *Clinical Transplants 1991.* Los Angeles: UCLA Tissue Typing Laboratory; 1992:325.
132. Terasaki PI, et al. UCLA and UNOS Registries: overview. In: Terasaki PI, Cecka JM, eds. *Clinical Transplants 1992.* Los Angeles: UCLA Tissue Typing Laboratory; 1992:409.
133. Opelz G, Wujciak T, Mytilineos J, et al. Revisiting HLA matching for kidney transplants. *Transplant Proc.* 1993;25:173.
134. Opelz G, et al. Survival of DNA HLA-DR typed and matched cadaver kidney transplants. *Lancet.* 1991;338:461.
135. Tran TH, Dohler B, Heinold A, et al. Deleterious impact of mismatching for human leukocyte antigen-C in presensitized recipients of kidney transplants. *Transplantation.* 2011;92:419.
136. Williams GM, et al. "Hyperacute" renal-homograft rejection in man. *N Engl J Med.* 1968;279:611.
137. Ogura, K. Clinical transplants 1992. In: Terasaki PI, Cecka JM, eds. *Clinical Transplants 1992.* Los Angeles: UCLA Tissue Typing Laboratory; 1993:357.
138. Cook DJ, El Fettouh HIA, Gjertson DW, et al. Flow cytometry crossmatching (FXCM) in the UNOS kidney transplant registry. In: Terasaki PI, Cecka JM, eds. *Clinical Transplants 1998.* Los Angeles: UCLA Tissue Typing Laboratory; 1999:413.
139. Terasaki PI, Ozawa M. Predicting kidney graft failure by HLA antibodies: a prospective trial. *Am J Transplant.* 2004;4:438.
140. Worthington JE, Martin S, Al-Husseini DM, et al. Posttransplantation production of donor HLA-specific antibodies as a predictor of renal transplant outcome. *Transplantation.* 2003;75:1034.
141. Tait BD, Hudson F, Cantwell L, et al. Review article: Luminex technology for HLA antibody detection in organ transplantation. *Nephrology.* 2009;14:247.
142. Van Parijs L, Abbas AK. Homeostasis and self-tolerance in the immune system: turning lymphocytes off. *Science.* 1998;280:243.
143. Wekerle T, Sayegh MH, Hill J, et al. Extrathymic T cell deletion and allogeneic stem cell engraftment induced with costimulatory blockade is followed by central T cell tolerance. *J Exp Med.* 1998;187:2037.
144. Sayegh MH, Fine NA, Smith JL, et al. Immunologic tolerance to renal allografts after bone marrow transplants from the same donors. *Ann Intern Med.* 1991;114:954.
145. Spitzer TR, Delmonico F, Tolkoff-Rubin N, et al. Combined histocompatibility leukocyte antigen-matched donor bone marrow and renal transplantation for multiple myeloma with end stage renal disease: the induction of allograft tolerance through mixed lymphohematopoietic chimerism. *Transplantation.* 1999;68:480.
146. Dai Z, Konieczny BT, Baddoura FK, et al. Impaired alloantigen-mediated T cell apoptosis and failure to induce long-term allograft survival in IL-2-deficient mice. *J Immunol.* 1998;161:1659.
147. Li Y, Li XC, Zheng XX, et al. Blocking both signal 1 and signal 2 of T-cell activation prevents apoptosis of alloreactive T cells and induction of peripheral allograft tolerance. *Nature Med.* 1999;5:1298.
148. Li SC, Wells AD, Strom TB, et al. The role of T cell apoptosis in transplantation tolerance. *Curr Opin Immunol.* 2000;12:522.
149. Waldmann H. Transplantation tolerance—where do we stand? *Nature Med.* 1999;5:1245.
150. Suthanthiran M. Transplantation tolerance: fooling mother nature. *Proc Natl Acad Sci U S A.* 1996;93:12072.
151. Sakaguchi S, Sakaguchi N, Shimizu J, et al. Immunologic tolerance maintained by CD25+CD4+ regulatory T cells: their common role in controlling autoimmunity, tumor immunity, and transplantation tolerance. *Immunol Rev.* 2001;182:18.
152. Maloy KJ, Powrie F. Regulatory T cells in the control of immune pathology. *Nat Immunol.* 2001;2:816.
153. Awasthi A, Murugaiyan G, Kuchroo VK. Interplay between effector Th17 and regulatory T cells. *J Clin Immunol.* 2008;28:660.
154. Burrell BE, Bishop DK. Th17 cells and transplant acceptance. *Transplantation.* 2010;90:945.
155. Miller A, Lider O, Roberts AB, et al. Suppressor T cells generated by oral tolerization to myelin basic protein suppress both in vitro and in vivo immune responses by the release of transforming growth factor β after antigen-specific triggering. *Proc Natl Acad Sci U S A.* 1992;89:421.
156. Newell KA, Asare A, Kirk AD, et al. Identification of a B cell signature associated with renal transplant tolerance in humans. *J Clin Invest.* 2010;120:1836.

CHAPTER

82 Clinical Aspects of Renal Transplantation

Alexander C. Wiseman • James E. Cooper • Laurence Chan

INTRODUCTION

Since the first successful renal transplant over 50 years ago,[1] more than 500,000 patients with renal failure have had their lives prolonged with renal allografts. Renal transplantation is associated with improved longevity compared to dialysis[2] with increased quality of life,[3] and currently is the preferred treatment modality for eligible patients with chronic kidney disease (glomerular filtration rate [GFR] <20 mL per minute).

The progressive increase in the incidence and prevalence of severe chronic kidney disease (CKD) has led to a parallel increase in the number of patients waiting for a transplant. This increase substantially outpaces the supply of available organs (Fig. 82.1). The reported average waiting time for a deceased donor kidney transplant (DDKT) is more than 3.5 years (2009 Scientific Registry of Transplant Recipients [SRTR] Annual Report Table 5.2). For this reason, efforts have been made to increase living kidney donor transplantation. Unfortunately, living donation rates in the Unites States have not increased in recent years, and modest growth in kidney transplantation has occurred as a result of increased deceased donor use.[4,5] Worldwide, rates of kidney transplantation and use of living donors for kidney transplant vary widely due to societal differences in the perception of transplantation and of organ donation following brain death or cardiac death (Fig. 82.2).

Patient and graft survival after kidney transplant are affected by a large number of variables (Table 82.1). Primary factors include: age, sex, and race of the recipient and donor; type of donor (living versus deceased, expanded criteria versus standard criteria); tissue compatibility; prior sensitization to human leukocyte antigens (HLA); original renal disease, pretransplant health status, and concomitant extrarenal disease of the recipient; adherence of the recipient; donor factors, such as age, cold ischemia time, and nephron dosing effect; and choice of immunosuppressive agents (Figs. 82.3 and 82.4). Short-term outcomes have improved substantially over the past 15 years, with 1-year graft survival averaging 90% to 94% and patient survival averaging 94% to 97%; however, improvements in long-term graft survival have been more difficult to achieve. An analysis by Hariharan et al.[6] of graft survival for all 93,934 renal transplantations performed in the United States between 1988 and 1996, suggested that the estimated half-life for grafts from living donors increased steadily from 12.7 to 21.6 years, and that for deceased donor grafts increased from 7.9 to 13.8 years. However, in this analysis graft survival was calculated upon projected, not actual, graft survival. A later analysis of graft outcomes from 1988 to 1995 demonstrated that actual graft survival demonstrated far less improvement in graft half-life of 6.0 to 8.0 years for deceased donor grafts.[7] A recent analysis of transplants from 1989 to 2009 suggests slow improvements in graft survival over time, primarily in higher risk transplants (the expanded criteria donor, described later) (Table 82.2). For living donor kidney transplants, the estimated graft half-life did not change appreciably for transplants performed from 1989 to 2005 (11.4 years to 11.9 years).[8] With greater understanding of the causes of graft loss, it is hoped that this will translate into better outcomes in renal transplantation with improved long-term graft and patient survival. In the subsequent sections of this chapter, we will discuss each of the factors influencing outcomes of renal transplantation, the recipient and donor evaluation prior to transplantation, immunosuppressive drugs, posttransplantation management, and complications.

PATIENT SELECTION AND PRETRANSPLANT EVALUATION

General Philosophy in Recipient Selection

In general, patients with CKD stage IV through V (GFR <30 mL per minute) should be presented with information regarding dialysis modalities and transplantation. Patients who express an interest in undergoing kidney transplantation should be fully evaluated by the transplant team. This is typically as an outpatient during a clinic visit; however, some centers may provide this on an inpatient basis. Early referral prior to the onset of dialysis should be encouraged, because

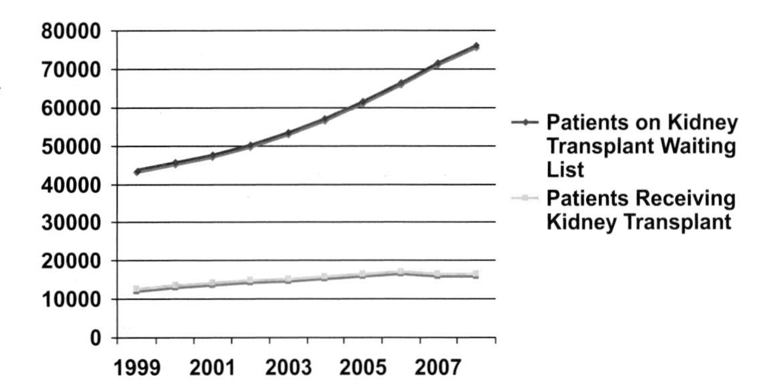

FIGURE 82.1 Counts of patients on the renal transplant waiting list and counts of renal transplants by year in the United States from 1999 to 2008. (From Scientific Registry of Transplant Recipients 2009 Annual Data Report, Ann Arbor MI, Tables 5.1a, 5.1b, 5.4, 5.4d, with permission.)

the degree of dialysis time prior to transplant has been associated with poorer graft survival following transplant.[9]

There are few absolute contraindications to kidney transplantation, and many of these contraindications are relative (Table 82.3). The current protocols for a transplant evaluation focus on ensuring the safety of undergoing surgery and the ability to assume the risks of immunosuppressive therapy in order to optimize successful kidney transplant outcomes. This evaluation is tailored to the individual candidate's risk for complications, and includes consideration of the patient's age, diabetes, and heart disease status. These factors are also associated with a higher risk of death in the general population and in patients with end-stage renal disease (ESRD) treated by dialysis.

Age

The adolescent patient (age 12 to 17) and the elderly recipient (age >65) have poorer graft survival than other age groups (SRTR Annual Report Table 5.8c). In the former, this is due primarily to difficulties in medication adherence, whereas in the latter, this is due to complications of immunosuppressive therapy leading to death or to nontransplant-related complications, in particular, cardiovascular disease in the elderly leading to death.[10,11]

In the United States, national kidney allocation policy prioritizes pediatric candidates to ensure a minimum of waiting time to promote the beneficial effects of transplantation, including growth and development. The challenge of ensuring appropriate medical support for young people with solid organ transplants as they move into adult-centered services has become a topic of significant interest in the field of organ transplantation. Proceedings from a consensus conference of the major transplant societies has outlined the need for collaborative transitional care between pediatric and adult providers and the need for research in this area.[12]

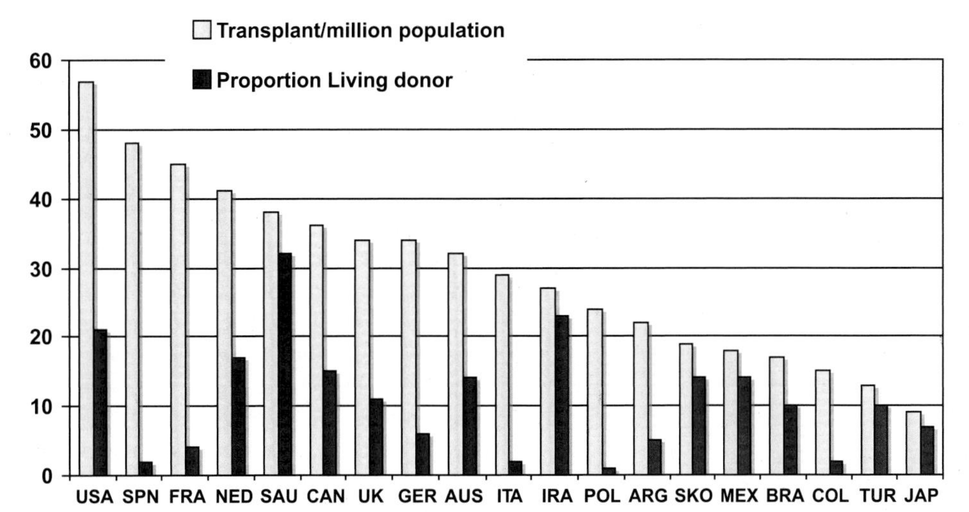

FIGURE 82.2 Transplantation rates for countries reporting more than 500 kidney transplants in 2006 (count of new renal transplants per million total population) and number of transplants arising from living donors. *SPN,* Spain; *FRA,* France; *NED,* Netherlands; *SAU,* Saudi Arabia; *CAN,* Canada; *UK,* United Kingdom; *GER,* Germany; *AUS,* Australia; *ITA,* Italy; *IRA,* Iran; *POL,* Poland; *ARG,* Argentina; *SKO,* South Korea; *MEX,* Mexico; *BRA,* Brazil; *COL,* Columbia; *TUR,* Turkey; *JAP,* Japan. (Data from Horvat LD, Shariff SZ, Garg AX. Global trends in the rates of living kidney donation. *Kidney International* 2009; 75:1088–1098.)

TABLE 82.1 **Factors Influencing the Outcome of Renal Transplantation**

Immunologic	Nonimmunologic
Immunosuppressive protocol	Delayed graft function/ ischemic time
Matching for HLA	Medication adherence
Sensitization	Cardiovascular disease
Rejection	Recipient age
	Nephron dose/donor and recipient gender

HLA, human leukocyte antigens.

With the improvements in perioperative management and immunosuppressive strategies, advanced age itself is no longer a contraindication to renal transplantation. Based on a retrospective analysis of wait-listed patients >70 years old from the SRTR, 1990 to 2004, elderly transplant recipients had a 41% lower overall risk of death compared with wait-listed candidates.[13] These benefits also extend to selected patients over age 80.[14] Older patients may have better immunologic survival despite the higher mortality from cardiovascular disease. One explanation may be an age-related change in immunologic function that confers less alloreactivity with aging, as suggested by a registry analysis that demonstrated that acute rejection rates significantly fell with advancing recipient age.[15] Recipients older than 65 years demonstrated significantly elevated numbers of memory T cells, whereas counts for naive T cells were significantly reduced.[16] For this reason, many centers advocate the use of lower immunosuppression in elderly patients. In summary, kidney transplantation can now be safely and successfully performed in selected elderly patients but requires comprehensive screening of underlying cardiovascular disease and occult malignancy.

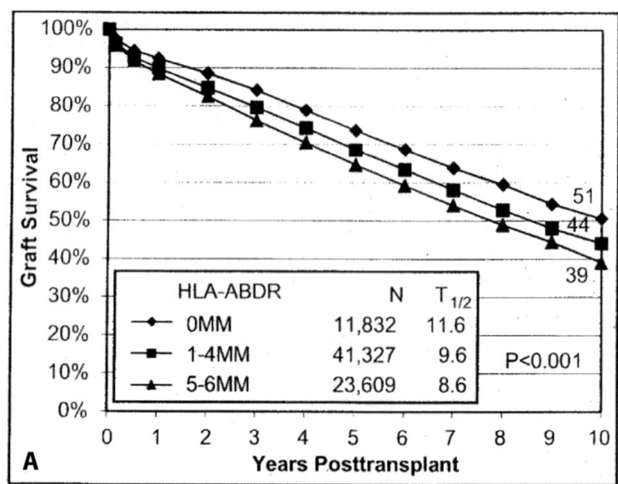

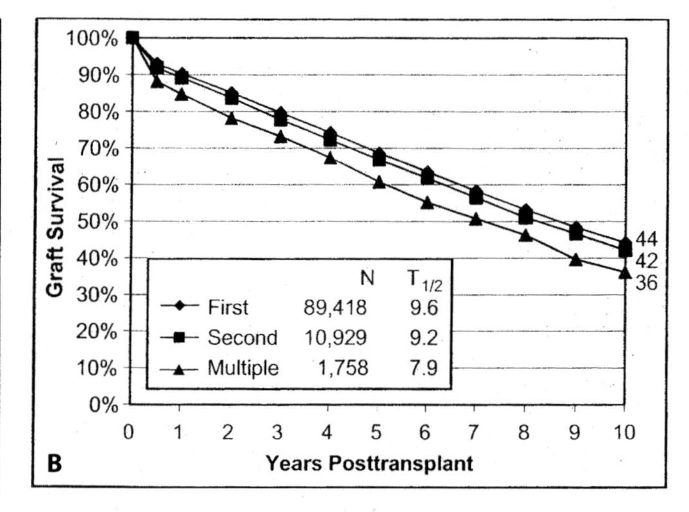

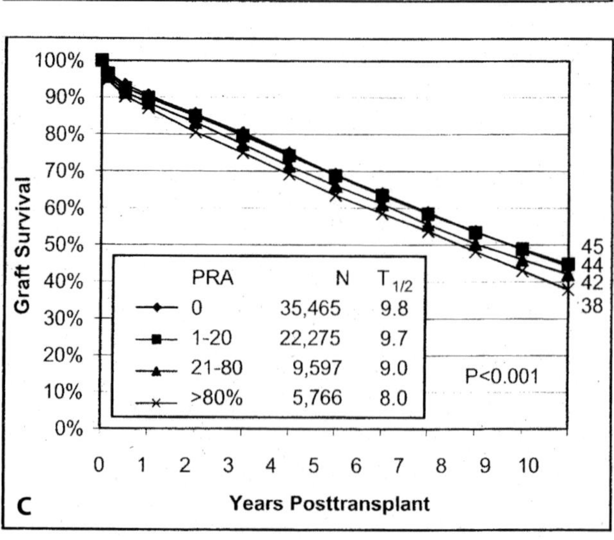

FIGURE 82.3 Graft survival related to immunologic factors. **A.** Effects of human leukocyte antigen (HLA) mismatches (MM) on the survival of first diseased donor transplants. Graft survival rates declined as the number of HLA-A, HLA-B, and HLA-DR MMs increased. The difference in graft half-life between the best and the worst matched grafts was 3 years (11.6 years vs. 8.6 years). **B.** Graft survival among first and repeat deceased donor transplant recipients. The differences between first and subsequent transplants have diminished, with no significant differences in graft survival. **C.** Graft survival related to HLA sensitization. HLA sensitization remains a significant risk factor for graft loss. Highly sensitized recipients (panel reactive antibody [PRA] >80%) have a lower long-term graft survival than patients with PRA <20%. Data are from the United Network for Organ Sharing Scientific Renal Transplant Registry, 1996–2005. (From: Cecka J, Terasaki P, eds. *Clinical Transplants 2008*. Los Angeles, CA: UCLA Tissue Typing Laboratory; 2008:1–18, with permission.)

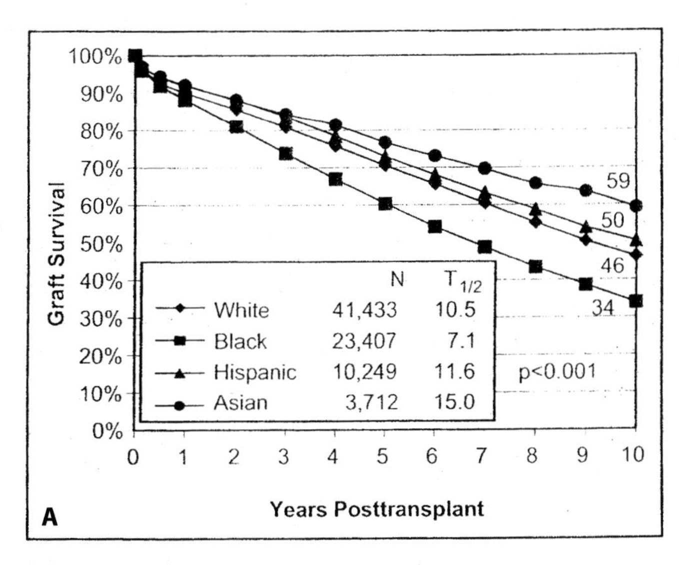

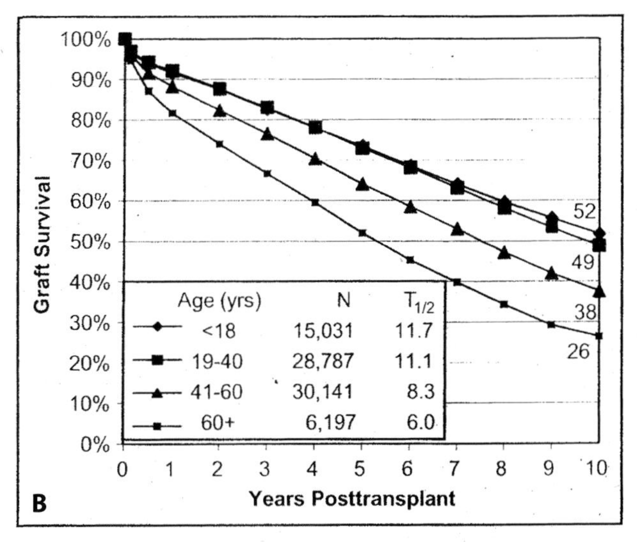

FIGURE 82.4 Graft survival rates of deceased donor kidney transplants are related to donor and recipient factors. **A.** The effect of recipient race on graft survival. The race of the recipients was a significant factor in the outcome of the first deceased donor transplants. Asian patients had the highest graft survival rates—59% at 10 years, respectively—whereas blacks had the poorest survival rates—34% at 10 years. **B.** The effect of donor age on graft survival. Donor age remains one of the most important factors in deceased donor kidney transplant graft survival. Data are from the United Network for Organ Sharing Scientific Renal Transplant Registry, 1996–2005. (From: Cecka J, Terasaki P, eds. *Clinical Transplants 2008.* Los Angeles, CA: UCLA Tissue Typing Laboratory; 2008:1–18, with permission.)

Obesity

Obesity alone is rarely an absolute contraindication to transplantation, yet it is a well-defined risk factor. Lower graft survival rates, higher postoperative mortalities, and complications have been demonstrated in patients with a body mass index (BMI) greater than 35 kg per square meter.[17,18] The large body size is also a risk factor for progression and subsequent premature failure due to the physiologic changes that have been linked to nephron hyperfiltration.[18] Although weight reduction is important for obese dialysis patients before proceeding to transplantation, often patients will regain weight following transplantation and mandatory weight loss pretransplant may not substantially improve longer term outcomes.[19]

TABLE 82.2 Actual Transplant Half-Life for Transplants Performed in 1997, and Projected Transplant Half-Life for Transplants Performed in 2004[9]

Transplant Subgroup	Actual Graft Half-Life, 1997 Transplants	Actual Graft Half-Life, 1997 Transplants	Projected Graft Half-Life, 2004 Transplants	Projected Graft Half-Life, 2004 Transplants
	All recipients	African American recipients	All recipients	African American recipients
All deceased donor transplants	8.2 yr	6.3 yr	8.8 yr	7.1 yr
SCD	8.9 yr	6.8 yr	9.7 yr	7.7 yr
ECD (first transplant)	5.1 yr	4.4 yr	5.9 yr	5.4 yr
Living donor	12.0 yr	8.7 yr	14.2 yr	10.8 yr

SCD, Standard criteria donor; ECD, Expanded criteria donor.

TABLE 82.3 Contraindications to Transplantation

Absolute	Relative
Active infection	Renal disease with high recurrence rate
Disseminated malignancy	Urologic abnormalities
Extensive vascular disease	Active systemic illness
High risk for perioperative mortality	Ongoing substance abuse
Persistent coagulation abnormality	Uncontrolled psychosis
Informed patient refusal of consent	Refractory nonadherence

Prior Kidney Transplantation

Renal allograft failure is now one of the most common causes of ESRD, accounting for about 30% of patients awaiting renal transplantation. Graft survival of a second transplant is decreased compared to that of the first, but outcomes have improved over time (Fig. 82.3).[7] Evaluation of a potential recipient for a repeat allograft requires careful attention to the reason for the graft failure, such as nonadherence with immunosuppressive medications, recurrent renal disease, or high alloreactivity with high panel reactive antibody (PRA) titers. These patients may also manifest complications of prior immunosuppressive therapy and, as such, should be screened for complications associated with these medications, such as infection and malignancy.[20] No controlled, prospective studies have been performed to determine the best method for tapering or withdrawal of immunosuppression following renal allograft failure, with some suggestion that nephrectomy after graft loss may improve patient survival and rates of retransplantation.[21] Most centers have adopted a policy of immediate withdrawal of immunosuppression combined with preemptive nephrectomy for patients with early allograft failure. However, this practice is less common for patients with late graft failure. A longer taper of immunosuppression may permit the maintenance of some residual renal function while on dialysis. Further studies are needed to determine the optimal means of immunosuppression withdrawal or nephrectomy in patients who return to dialysis.

Underlying Renal Diseases

It is most important to assess the cause of the potential recipient's renal failure. The primary pathologies leading to renal failure are expected to influence outcome depending on the etiologic mechanisms, propensity for recurrence, and status of the immune system.

Diabetes Mellitus

Although patients with diabetes are at a higher risk for posttransplant complications primarily related to their pretransplant comorbidities, kidney transplantation is the treatment of choice for otherwise eligible patients due to their high mortality rate while on dialysis.[22] In particular, patients with type 1 diabetes (T1DM) enjoy the highest net mortality benefit of transplantation compared to dialysis following receipt of a simultaneous pancreas kidney transplant (SPK) when compared to other kidney transplant recipients.[23] Patient survival and pancreas graft survival rates continue to improve, with data from U.S. centers demonstrating 95% and 86% 1-year patient and pancreas graft survival, and 85% and 70% 5-year patient and pancreas graft survival, respectively.[4]

With the increase in use of living donors for kidney transplantation, solitary pancreas transplant after kidney transplant (PAK) is often considered for patients with T1DM. Although this offers the benefit of timely kidney transplant, ideally prior to the need for hemodialysis, this strategy requires two separate survival procedures, two different HLA-mismatched organs, and the risks inherent to surgery. Pancreas allograft survival is worse as a PAK than SPK likely due to the additional immunologic factors of a second organ and the lack of use of renal function changes as a surrogate marker of pancreas function changes. Recommendations for patients with T1DM approaching kidney failure should be tailored to the individual's circumstance, and should include an assessment of the following: (1) can a living donor be identified; (2) is the patient (and transplant program) willing to accept a higher risk of early death and possibility of pancreas graft loss (~2% and ~15% in the first year, respectively) when considering SPK versus living donor kidney transplant; (3) how debilitating are the patient's diabetes-related quality-of-life issues and achieved level of glycemic control; and (4) what is the expected waiting time for an SPK in the patient's geographic region.[24] In general, SPK appears to offer advantages over kidney transplantation alone with respect to long-term survival if the waiting time for a deceased donor is not excessive and dialysis time can be minimized (perhaps to less than 6 months). For those patients who are unable to wait for SPK, a living donor kidney transplant followed by a later pancreas transplant appears to be associated with better kidney graft function with a risk of mortality that is similar to living donor kidney transplant alone.[25] One suggested algorithm for patients with T1DM and CKD considering their transplant options is provided in Figure 82.5.

Another treatment option in development for the patient with T1DM is pancreatic islet cell transplantation (ICT). In experienced centers, ICT can achieve insulin independence in 80% to 90% of recipients at 1 year; however, <30% have remained insulin free after 5 years.[26] At present, this therapy should still be considered experimental, because

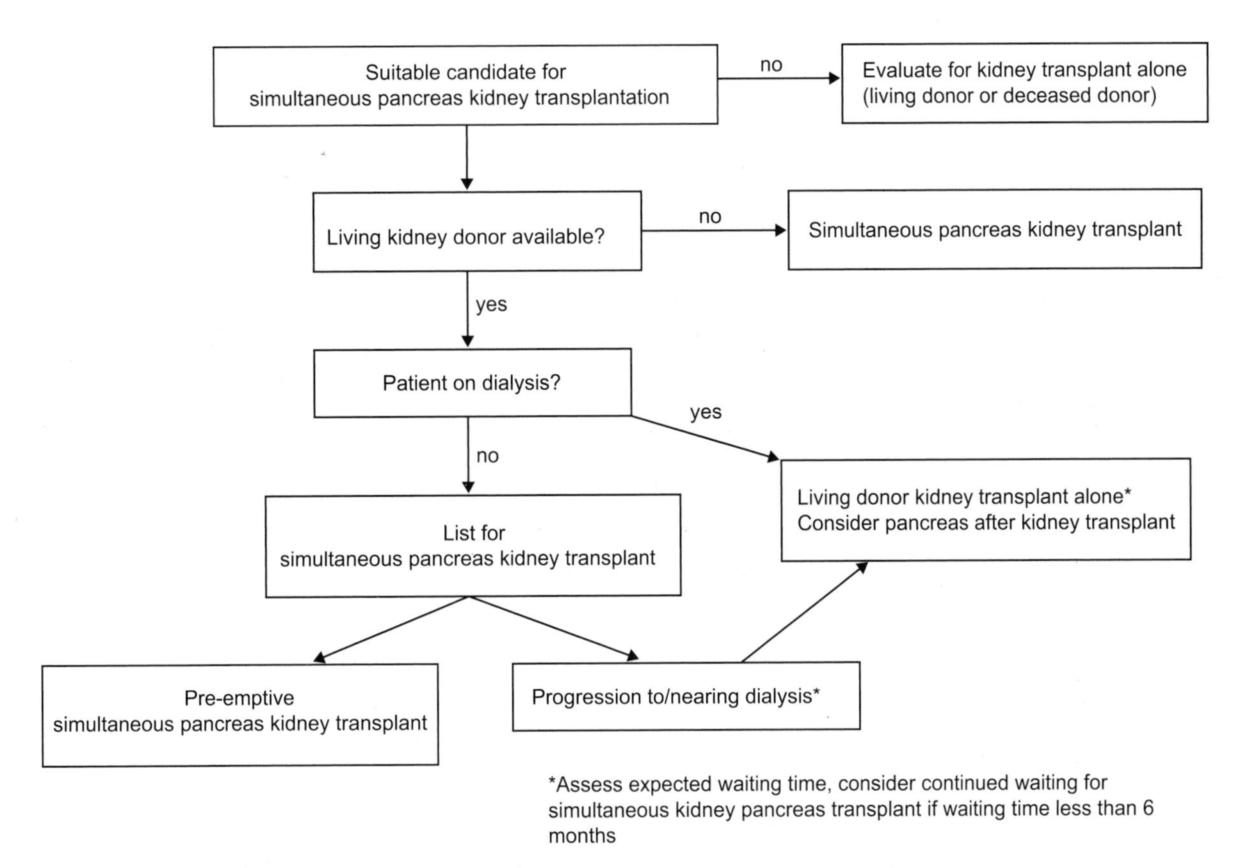

FIGURE 82.5 Proposed algorithm for type 1 diabetic patients requiring transplant. (Adapted from Wiseman AC. Simultaneous pancreas kidney transplantation: a critical appraisal of the risks and benefits compared with other treatment alternatives. *Adv Chronic Kidney Dis.* 2009;16(4):278–287, with permission.)

the long-term graft survival is unknown and the risks of immunosuppression and HLA sensitization must be weighed against the benefits of normalization of blood glucose.

Recurrence of the diabetic nephropathy in T1DM recipients is a late and slowly developing complication. An examination of biopsy specimens early after transplantation indicates that there are few glomerular pathologic abnormalities other than frequent afferent and efferent arteriosclerosis. Glomerular basement immunoglobulin G (IgG) deposition is seen <2 years after transplantation, but the onset and progression of glomerular basement membrane thickening and mesangial expansion only occurs after 2 years, and the typical nodular glomerular hyalinosis is rarely seen in these patients. Long-term follow-up has shown that recurrent nephropathy progresses to ESRD with the same time course as primary type I diabetic nephropathy. The mean time to recurrent ESRD is estimated to be 15 to 20 years. Therefore, recurrence of the lesion is not a barrier to long-term renal graft survival in diabetic recipients. The frequency and natural history of recurrence in type II diabetic recipients remain to be elucidated.

Metabolic and Congenital Disorders

Results of renal transplantation in the metabolic and congenital disorders causing end-stage renal failure such as Alport syndrome, amyloidosis, cystinosis, familial nephritis, gout, and cystic disease are similar to those of the more common causes of end-stage renal failure with the exception of primary hyperoxaluria, sickle cell, and Fabry disease, as discussed in detail in the following paragraphs.

Primary Hyperoxaluria

Although often presenting in childhood, inherited deficiencies in alanine:glyoxalate aminotransferase (AGT) levels or function may present in the young adult as calcium oxalate nephrolithiasis, nephrocalcinosis, renal failure, and systemic oxalate deposition. Registry analyses generally favor combined liver-kidney transplantation (to correct the AGT defect and promote long-term kidney graft survival), but occasionally, patients may have a functional AGT deficiency that is pyridoxine sensitive, and 5 to 10 mg/kg/day of pyridoxine may decrease oxalate levels to a level that is acceptable to consider kidney transplantation alone.[27,28] To reduce the chance of oxalate accumulation, dialysis treatment or kidney transplantation should be considered when the GFR approaches 20 mL per minute. Aggressive dialysis schedules should be implemented before transplantation to deplete the oxalate metabolic pool. Medical therapy with pyridoxine, neutral phosphate, and magnesium should be given after transplantation to reduce oxalate deposition and recurrence (Fig. 82.6).

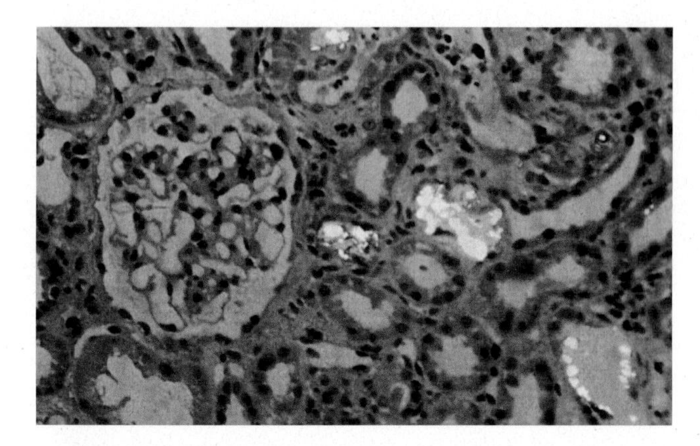

FIGURE 82.6 A renal biopsy specimen from a transplanted kidney showing calcium oxalate deposition in a patient with primary hyperoxaluria and a recurrence of oxalosis.

Unlike primary hyperoxaluria, secondary oxalosis is due to excessive intake or absorption of oxalates from the diet. Secondary oxalosis is seen primarily in fat malabsorption, short bowel syndromes after gastrointestinal surgery, and high-oxalate diets. For these patients, consideration should be given to reanastomosis of gastric bypass, hydration, and dietary restriction of oxalates. Good allograft function can be achieved when attention is paid to reduce the oxalate excretion load.[29]

Cystinosis

Cystine stones recur after transplantation, but have little effect on graft function.[30] Renal transplantation has been recommended as a preferred therapy in children with ESRD due to cystinosis. The systemic effects of cystine accumulation, including corneal crystallization and retinal degeneration, leading to blindness, progress after renal transplantation but can be reduced with chronic cysteamine therapy.[31]

Sickle Cell Disease

The autosomal recessive conditions of sickle cell disease and sickle cell trait may be complicated by a variety of renal abnormalities, which may eventually lead to ESRD.[32] The North American Pediatric Renal Transplant Cooperative Study (NAPRTCS) reports favorable outcomes in pediatric patients with patient survival of 89%, and graft survival at 12 and 24 months posttransplant of 89% and 71%, respectively.[33] A second registry analysis demonstrates comparable short-term but diminished long-term outcomes compared to other causes of ESRD.[34] The importance of recurrence after transplantation is difficult to determine because of the relatively nonspecific nature of sickle cell nephropathy.

Fabry Disease

Fabry disease is an X-linked disorder of glycosphingolipid metabolism due to a ceramide trihexosidase. Fabry nephropathy does not recur in the allograft, and transplantation provides superior outcomes to Fabry patients on dialysis.[35] Graft survival at 5 years is comparable to patients with other causes of ESRD, but with a higher risk of death.[36] Enzyme replacement therapy with agalsidase alfa is well tolerated in patients with Fabry disease following renal transplantation, but data regarding an impact on survival has yet to be determined.[37] Transplantation is considered the optimal mode of renal replacement therapy for otherwise eligible patients with Fabry disease.

Amyloidosis

Recurrent nephrotic syndrome and graft failure can occur in primary and secondary amyloidosis. Although transplantation is uncommonly performed for patients with primary amyloid light chain (AL) amyloidosis, in selected patients kidney transplantation has been shown to be successful.[38] Often, the treatment for this disorder requires chemotherapy and autologous stem cell transplantation. The decision to perform stem cell transplant before or after kidney transplant has been debated; reports of living donor kidney transplant followed by stem cell transplant have demonstrated favorable results.[39] Without definitive treatment, the recurrence of renal AL amyloidosis is common following kidney transplant.[40] Familial Mediterranean fever (FMF), rheumatoid arthritis, and osteomyelitis are the most common causes of secondary amyloidosis. FMF is an autosomal recessive disorder that occurs in Sephardic Jews, Armenians, Turks, and Arabs of the Levant. In Israel, amyloidosis constitutes 6% of all patients on dialysis, compared to 0.6% in Europe. Although there has been a higher early mortality rate in the transplanted patients in the past, the incidence of rejection episodes is lower than in patients without amyloidosis. Reduced immunosuppression has decreased postoperative mortality and morbidity. Colchicine at 1 to 2 mg per day dramatically relieves the symptoms and reduces the incidence of attacks in FMF, and interleukin (IL)-1 receptor antagonism is an increasingly attractive treatment alternative.[41]

Alport Syndrome

Dialysis and transplantation pose no particular problems for patients with Alport syndrome. Recurrent disease has not been well documented. Improvement or stabilization of deafness after renal transplantation has occasionally been reported. There is a 3% to 5% risk of developing de novo antiglomerular basement membrane (anti-GBM) nephritis after transplantation, typically occurring within the first year and resulting in graft loss.[42]

Polycystic Kidney Disease

Autosomal dominant polycystic kidney disease is responsible for approximately 4% to 12% of ESRD cases in the United States and Europe. Native kidney removal is only required if the kidneys are massive due to polycystic disease or there is associated persistent infection or severe hypertension. Embolization of native kidneys prior to transplant may be a less invasive treatment strategy in the future.[43] Occasionally, patients with severe liver cysts will require combined liver-kidney transplantation, primarily due to symptoms related to cyst volume and the impact on nutritional status.[44] Screening for cerebral aneurysms prior to transplant is generally directed toward those with a family history or with new onset headaches.[45]

Glomerulonephritis

Almost all types of glomerulonephritis have been reported to recur after transplantation. There is, however, much variation between the various types of glomerulonephritis with regard to the frequency of recurrence, the clinical course, and the prognosis. The overall incidence of recurrence is less than 10% to 20% and recurrent disease accounts for less than 2% to 4% of all graft failures (Table 82.4).[46]

Focal Segmental Glomerulosclerosis

Recurrent focal sclerosis may be seen early after transplantation, presenting with nephrotic-range proteinuria and a rapid decline in renal function. Histologically, the features on light microscopy that permit categorization are focal and segmental sclerosis, affecting a small number of glomeruli, often those in the deep juxtamedullary cortex. The development of foot-process fusion can be immediate after transplantation and precede glomerular segmental sclerosis by weeks to months (Fig. 82.7). The frequency of recurrence is about 20% in adults and may be as high as 40% in children. When stringent definitions of primary focal segmental glomerulosclerosis (FSGS) are applied (i.e., the nonfamilial inheritance pattern from patient history and documented biopsy-proven disease), the recurrence rate approaches 50%.[47] Patients presenting with rapid progression of renal disease from the time of diagnosis of nephrotic syndrome to ESRD have higher risk for recurrence. If a transplant patient suffers graft loss because of recurrent FSGS, there is ~50% risk of subsequent allograft failure within 5 years of a second transplantation. With increasing understanding of the genetic causes of FSGS (e.g., podocin and nephrin mutations) a more tailored approach to FSGS may be possible in the future, with avoidance of living donors with similar genetic risk.[48]

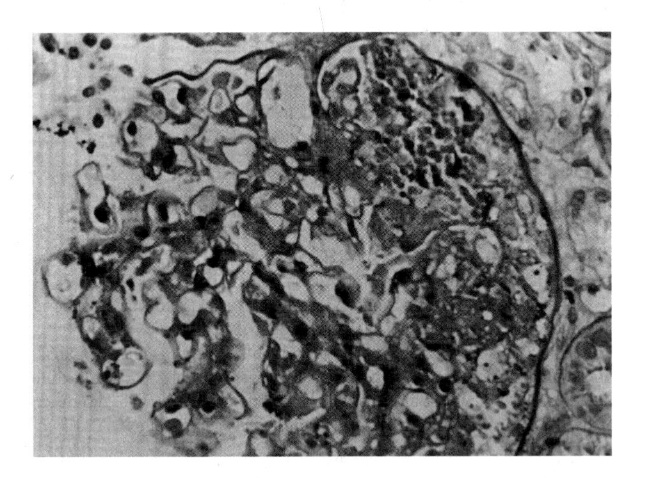

FIGURE 82.7 A renal biopsy specimen of a transplanted kidney showing recurrence of focal segmental glomerulosclerosis. (Periodic acid–Schiff stain, magnification ×250.)

TABLE 82.4 Recurrent Disease in Renal Allografts

Disease	Approximate Recurrence Rate (%)	Graft Loss Due to Recurrence
Primary Glomerulonephritis		
Membranous	10%–30%	Uncommon
FSGS	30%–60%	Common
HUS	20%–50%	Common
Type I MPGN	20%–30%	Common
Type II MPGN	80%–100%	Common
HSP	15%–50%	Uncommon
IgA nephropathy	30%–50%	Uncommon
Anti-GBM	Rare	Uncommon
ANCA associated	20%	Common
Systemic Disease		
Hyperoxaluria	80%–100%	Common
Cystinosis	50%–100%	Uncommon
Fabry disease	Rare	Common
Sickle cell disease	Rare	Common
Diabetes type I	100%	Uncommon
SLE	<10%	Uncommon

FSGS, focal segmental glomerulosclerosis; HUS, hemolytic uremic syndrome; MPGN, membranoproliferative glomerulonephritis; HSP, Henoch-Schonlein Purpura; IgA, IgA nephropathy; GBM, anti-glomerular basement membrane disease; ANCA, antineutrophil cytoplasmic antibody associated vasculitis; SLE, systemic lupus erythematosis.

Treatment for recurrent FSG remains disappointing. Heavy proteinuria and nephrotic syndrome are usually resistant to steroids.[49] Cyclosporine (CsA) or other immunosuppressants do not seem to prevent recurrence. In many cases, the rapidity of recurrence immediately post-transplant strongly suggests the presence of a circulating factor in primary FSGS that is toxic to the glomerular epithelial cell/podocyte interface. It has been shown that sera from some patients with FSGS increases the permeability of isolated glomeruli to albumin.[50] Recently, this circulating factor has been suggested to be urokinase receptor (uPAR) potentially derived from circulating neutrophils.[51] Use of a regenerating protein adsorption column or plasma exchange can reduce protein excretion in patients with recurrent FSGS in the transplant. More prolonged remissions have been achieved using plasma exchange that is initiated promptly after the onset of proteinuria or the combination of plasma exchange and cyclophosphamide. These prolonged beneficial results have also been reported in children treated with plasma exchange and cyclophosphamide.[52]

Antiglomerular Basement Membrane Disease

Based on histology and fluorescence studies, anti-GBM disease is associated with >50% recurrence rate in the allograft. However, only 25% of patients with biopsy-proved IgG staining along the capillary wall have evidence for clinical disease activity. Furthermore, graft failure due to recurrent disease is less common, estimated at <5%.[53] Although engraftment during the presence of anti-GBM antibodies has been reported to be successful, many transplant centers still prefer serologic quiescence of anti-GBM antibody production for 6 to 12 months before proceeding with transplantation to reduce the risk for recurrent anti-GBM disease. Despite delaying transplantation to allow anti-GBM antibody to fall, recurrence has been reported.[54]

Hemolytic Uremic Syndrome (HUS)

Typical (diarrhea-associated) hemolytic uremic syndrome (HUS) does not recur in the transplant, although atypical (nondiarrheal) aHUS has a high recurrence rate that usually leads to graft loss.[55] aHUS is the clinical manifestation of complement dysregulation, either via complement deficiencies or autoantibodies. Recurrence rates of 80% to 100% have been reported for factor H or I deficiencies, whereas membrane cofactor protein (MCP) deficiency does not usually recur. The recurrence rate may be higher in recipients of living-related transplants, those of an older age at the onset of HUS, those with a short duration between disease onset and ESRD or transplantation, who use living related donors, and, to a lesser degree, in those who had been administered calcineurin inhibitors (CsA or tacrolimus).[56] There is no treatment for recurrent HUS that has been proven to be consistently successful. Salicylates, dipyridamole, plasma infusion, and plasma exchange have been shown to be of limited benefit. However, case reports of successful treatment and prevention of recurrent HUS in kidney transplant with the anti-C5a antibody eculizumab have generated encouraging results.[57,58] In preparation for transplant, patients with suspected aHUS should be screened at a minimum for factor H, I, and MCP deficiencies to aid in prognosis and in potential peritransplant treatment with plasma exchange and/or eculizumab. CsA and tacrolimus have both been associated with altered coagulation mechanisms and the development of de novo HUS in renal transplant recipients, particularly in combination with sirolimus.[59] These agents should, therefore, be used with caution in patients whose original kidney disease was due to HUS.

IgA Nephropathy/Henoch-Schönlein Purpura

In many parts of the world, IgA nephropathy (IgAN) is the most common type of glomerulonephritis. Although histologic recurrence of IgAN is common (up to 75%), its presentation is often clinically mild, and graft loss specifically due to IgAN is uncommon (<5%).[46] Patients with IgAN have at least comparable if not better graft survival rates than those with other diseases.[60]

The closely related Henoch-Schönlein purpura (HSP) has been reported to recur with similar frequency and outcomes as IgAN.[61] Clinically, recurrent HSP or IgAN can be severe with crescentic glomerulonephritis, nephrotic syndrome, graft failure, and variable recurrence of purpura.[62] To reduce recurrence, the delay of engraftment is recommended for at least 6 to 12 months after the skin lesions of HSP have resolved.

Membranoproliferative Glomerulonephritis Type I and Type II

Type I and type II membranoproliferative glomerulonephritis (MPGN) can recur posttransplant and can negatively impact long-term graft survival.[63] Type II MPGN may recur at a higher frequency (60% to 100%) than type I MPGN (15% to 30%).[64,65] The early development of nephrotic syndrome and persistent microscopic hematuria from the time of transplantation are clinical markers suggesting recurrence rather than rejection. Levels of serum C3 do not accurately predict recurrences. Specific disease-targeted therapy is not well defined, except in the case of MPGN type II with known complement factor deficiency (factor H or I) in which plasma exchange is warranted.[66]

Membranous Nephropathy (MN)

Graft survival for patients with membranous nephropathy (MN) is similar to the general transplant population despite a recurrence rate of up to 40%.[67,68] MN can also present as a primary de novo condition in allograft recipients.[69] Recurrent MN with nephrotic syndrome generally occurs earlier, at an average of 10 months compared with de novo MN, which is usually seen about 18 to 20 months after transplantation (Fig. 82.8). Rituximab has been shown in initial reports to be of benefit in proteinuria regression and renal function stabilization.[68,70]

Systemic Lupus Erythematosus (SLE)

Recurrence of clinically significant systemic lupus erythematosus (SLE) is relatively rare following transplant.[71] Similarly, the reactivation of other nonrenal manifestations of SLE after transplantation is extremely infrequent and is often controlled by the immunosuppressive medications when it occurs.[72] Recurrence is not predictable with serologic monitoring. However, there should be no systemic disease activity prior to transplantation.[73] Recurrences can be successfully treated with steroids, mycophenolate mofetil, or chlorambucil.

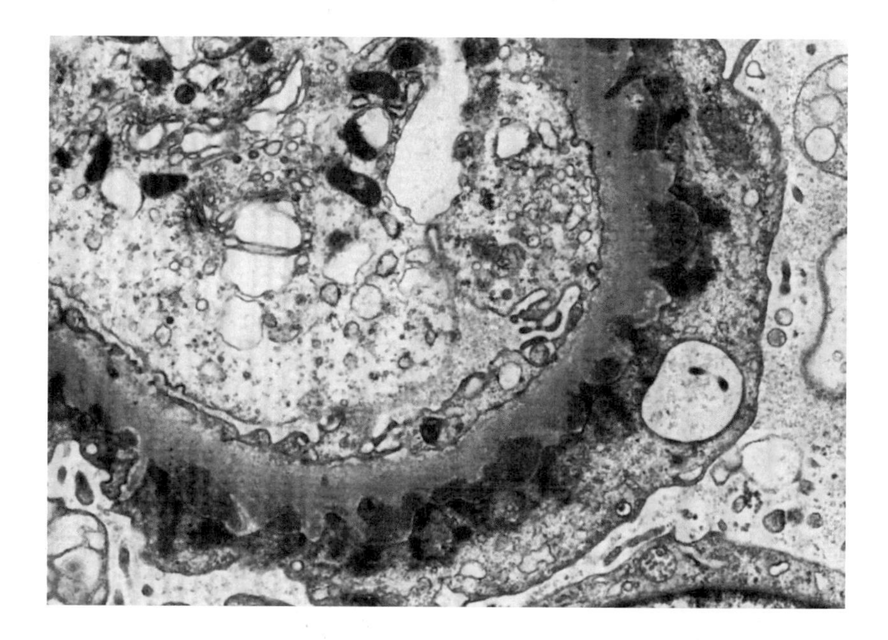

FIGURE 82.8 An electron micrograph of de novo membranous glomerulonephritis.

Antineutrophil Cytoplasmic Antibody–Associated Small Vessel Vasculitis

Patients with antineutrophil cytoplasmic antibody (ANCA)-related vasculitis have graft survival rates comparable to nondiabetic transplant populations.[74] As a relapsing and remitting disease, its recurrence rate following transplant is ~20%, which is slightly less than those remaining on dialysis.[75] ANCA titers do not appear to be predictive of recurrence posttransplant, thus transplantation can be reasonably pursued once clinical remission is achieved.[76] Recurrences are not prevented by baseline transplant immunosuppression, but can be treated successfully by adding cyclophosphamide and by increasing the steroid dose, together with decreasing or discontinuing some transplant medications.

Progressive Systemic Sclerosis (Scleroderma)

Transplant outcomes for patients with scleroderma are worse than in other diseases but are better than their wait-listed counterparts on dialysis.[77] Recurrence in the graft can occur within the first few months after transplantation. Recurrent scleroderma renal crisis in the allograft may be preceded by systemic features of scleroderma, such as the progression of diffuse skin thickening, new onset anemia, and cardiac complications.[78] The current recommendation for transplantation is that the patient should be clinically stable with an absence of visceral progressive systemic sclerosis activity prior to transplantation. Patients with early diffuse scleroderma should be closely monitored for new onset hypertension and should be treated continuously with angiotensin-converting enzyme (ACE) inhibitors. The majority of patients with scleroderma will improve generally after transplantation with a loss of Raynaud syndrome and improvement of the skin condition.[77] Therefore, transplantation is justified if the patient has not been severely debilitated by the systemic effects of scleroderma.

Interstitial Disease

Chronic Pyelonephritis

Chronic pyelonephritis is a diagnosis that has been frequently used for nonspecific interstitial nephritis, not necessarily caused by bacterial infection. The presence or history of significant urinary infection is important to identify. Because of the risk of residual foci of infection that may predispose a patient to bacteremia or may seed the urinary tract and transplant kidney, pretransplant nephrectomy may be indicated in these patients.

Analgesic Nephropathy

Patients with analgesic nephropathy need to be identified because cessation of the use of nephrotoxic analgesics is essential for these patients. Kidney function may improve after cessation of the use of analgesics, and damage to the allograft is a significant risk if this use persists. There is an increase in the incidence of transitional cell carcinoma of the urinary tract in patients with analgesic nephropathy.

GENERAL EVALUATION

This assessment should include not only a complete medical evaluation and a determination where possible of the underlying disease causing renal failure, but also a careful surveillance for problems that might arise following transplantation (Table 82.5).[79]

A careful physical examination should be performed to identify coexisting cardiovascular disease, infection, and malignancy. Additional examinations should assess pulmonary reserve, gastrointestinal (GI) disease, and genitourinary (GU) disease, as indicated by the patient's history. A psychosocial assessment should be performed to screen for potential barriers to successful transplantation.

TABLE 82.5 **Pretransplantation Recipient Medical Evaluation**

1. History and physical examination
2. Social and psychiatric evaluation
3. Determine primary kidney disease activity and residual kidney function
4. Dental evaluation
5. Laboratory studies
   Complete blood cell count and blood chemistry
   HBsAg
   HIV
   Antibodies to cytomegalovirus and Epstein–Barr virus
   HLA typing and antibodies screening
   Urine analysis and urine culture
6. Chest X-ray
7. Electrocardiogram
8. Special procedures for selected patients
   Abdominal ultrasound of gallbladder
   Upper gastrointestinal study or endoscopy
   Barium enema or colonoscopy
   Purified protein derivative (PPD) skin test for tuberculosis
   Cardiac stress testing
   Angiogram: coronary
   Cystourethrography
9. Consults (optional)
   Psychiatric
   Gynecology evaluation and mammography (for female >40 yr)
   Urologic assessment (voiding cystourethrography, cystoscopy, or urodynamic studies in patients with vesicoureteric reflux, neurogenic bladder, bladder neck obstruction, or strictures)

HBsAg, hepatitis B surface antigen; HLA, human leukocyte antigen; PPD, purified protein derivative.

The laboratory evaluation should include routine hematologic tests to detect leukopenia or thrombocytopenia, liver function tests to identify patients in whom the metabolism of immunosuppressive agents may be abnormal, complete hepatitis and HIV profiles, viral titers, and urinalysis when possible.

In general, there are few absolute contraindications to transplantation (Table 82.2). Conditions excluding a patient from renal transplantation may include the presence of severe ischemic heart disease, the presence of persistent infection, or untreated cancer. When a patient has had previous curative therapy for cancer, it is generally thought appropriate to wait at least 2 years with proven freedom from recurrence before proceeding with transplantation, although individual tumor types and patient circumstances may shorten this waiting time.[80]

Cardiovascular Evaluation

Cardiovascular disease is a major cause of morbidity and mortality for the patient with CKD and ESRD, whether the patient remains on dialysis or chooses to have a kidney transplant.[81,82] Risk factor assessment and modification should be pursued. Patients considered at high risk for heart disease (for patients with CKD, men >45 years and women >55, those with an abnormal ECG, history of DM or of prior ischemic heart disease) should undergo further investigation with a stress test and/or coronary angiography.[83] Up to 50% of asymptomatic diabetic transplant candidates have significant coronary artery disease, which may be missed on stress testing.[84] Thus, some centers consider angiography as the initial screening test for this subgroup. Although most centers will intervene on identified asymptomatic coronary lesions either with stenting or coronary artery bypass grafting, no randomized trial has clarified the value of this preemptive strategy, and in the nontransplant scenario (major vascular surgery), intervention has not been shown to be of benefit.[85,86] Additional assessment of peripheral arterial disease should be considered in those with known atherosclerotic disease, diabetes, and poor femoral or peripheral pulses on exam.

Hepatitis Screening

Hepatitis B Virus

Patients should undergo routine screening for the hepatitis B surface antigen (HBsAg), surface antibody, and core antibody pretransplant. Because of the poor conversion rate in patients with ESRD, a hepatitis B vaccination of patients should be given early in the course of progressive renal failure.[87] Previously vaccinated patients who are HBsAg-negative should be tested annually for antihepatitis B virus (HBV) antibodies and should receive booster vaccinations when the titer decreases to <10 mIU per milliliter. No known loss of graft function has occurred as a result of active vaccination with the hepatitis B vaccine.[88] Given the success of antiviral therapy (lamivudine, entecavir, tenofovir, and adefovir) against hepatitis B, chronic HBV infection is not a contraindication to transplantation.[89] Pretransplant management should include a liver biopsy to determine the degree of underlying liver disease and risk of progressive liver failure after transplantation. Patients with decompensated cirrhosis and ESRD should be evaluated for a combined liver–kidney transplant rather than kidney or liver transplant alone because of the high mortality risk associated with cirrhosis in this population.[90] To minimize the risk of viral replication and progressive liver disease, HBsAg-seropositive kidney transplant recipients should be treated with antiviral therapy at the time of transplantation, irrespective of their HBV–DNA level.

Hepatitis C Virus (HCV)

The prevalence of antihepatitis C virus (HCV) antibody positivity in kidney transplant recipients is estimated to be between 6% and 46% depending on the transplant center and/or country.[91] Although HCV-related liver disease can worsen after transplantation in the setting of chronic immunosuppression, the survival benefit of transplantation over dialysis outweighs this risk. Transplant candidates who are HCV+ with detectable RNA and no clinical stigmata of cirrhosis should undergo liver biopsy to determine histologically the degree of underlying liver disease. In those with cirrhosis, combined liver–kidney transplantation should be considered (Fig. 82.9). In those without cirrhosis, antiviral therapy should be considered to minimize the risk of developing posttransplant complications.[92] Goals of therapy are not only to avoid progressive liver disease, but also to avoid the extrahepatic complications such as the development of new onset diabetes after transplantation (NODAT) or glomerulonephritis that may occur in HCV infected renal transplant recipients.[93] A 48-week course of pegylated interferon (IFN)-α and ribavirin is often used in non-CKD populations. Unfortunately, in the setting of CKD, rapid accumulation of ribavirin can occur, which can lead to significant hemolysis. In the setting of CKD, pegylated IFN-α is associated with a high rate of adverse effects that lead to discontinuation of this therapy with no demonstrable benefit in sustained viral response (SVR) over nonpegylated IFN-α. Therefore, in patients on dialysis, monotherapy with nonpegylated IFN-α for 24 to 48 weeks is suggested as first-line therapy, with viral response rates as high as 70% to 80%, with the average SVR of 30% to 40%.

HIV Screening

All patients should be screened for HIV prior to transplantation. Successful transplantation in HIV individuals is now common.[94] Current disease-specific inclusion criteria for transplantation include an undetectable viral load, CD4 T-cell count >200 cells per milliliter, in addition to other features from the medical history including absence of multidrug-resistant fungal infection, history of malignancy, or progressive multifocal leukoencephalopathy. Unique considerations in the management of the patient with HIV following transplant include the potential for significant drug interactions between protease inhibitors, nonnucleoside reverse transcriptase inhibitors and calcineurin inhibitors and mammalian target of rapamycin (mTOR) inhibitors, and the surprisingly high rate of acute rejection encountered in HIV+ transplant recipients.[95] For these reasons, management is often coordinated with infectious disease consultation at experienced transplant centers.

Malignancy Screening

Patients with no history of malignancy should be screened using age-appropriate guidelines developed for the general population. Additionally, screening for renal cell carcinoma via ultrasound is gaining attention given its increased prevalence in patients with end-stage kidney disease and following a transplant.[96,97] Patients with a history of malignancy should be disease free prior to transplantation. Generally, it is recommended that patients should have a disease-free interval of 2 to 5 years prior to transplantation, due to the increase in malignancy risk ascribed to immunosuppressive medications following the transplant. However, with advances in treatment options for patients with various forms of malignancy, it is often difficult to ascribe a specific waiting period following successful treatment. The Canadian Society of Transplantation

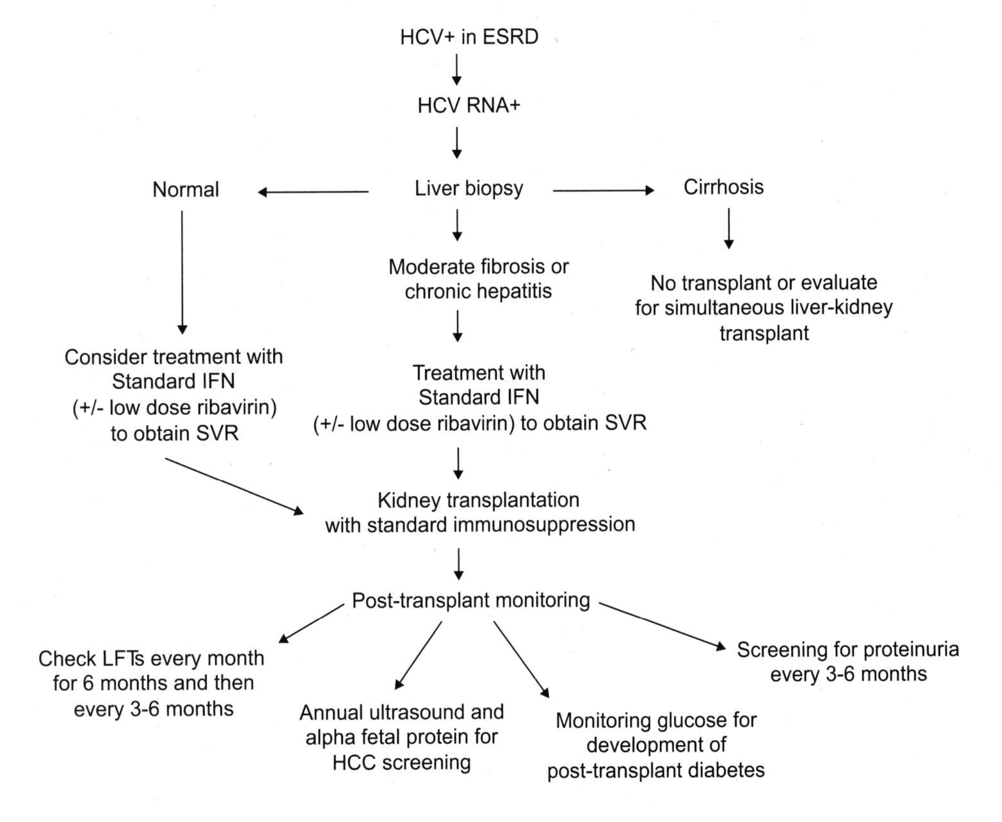

FIGURE 82.9 An algorithm for pre- and posttransplant management of HCV+ patients. *ESRD,* end-stage renal disease; *IFN,* interferon; *SVR,* sustained viral response; *HCC,* hepatocellular carcinoma. (Adapted from Huskey J, Wiseman AC. Chronic viral hepatitis in kidney transplantation. *Nat Rev Nephrol.* 7(3):156–165, with permission.)

has published consensus guidelines that attempt to take into consideration a number of more common clinical circumstances, but these must continue to be reviewed in the context of emerging data.[80] Oncology referral and discussion of expected disease-free survival is an important part of the evaluation process for those with a history of malignancy.

Infection

Patients should be free of active infection prior to transplantation. Appropriate immunizations against influenza, pneumococcus, hepatitis B, and, when appropriate, varicella, should be performed prior to transplant. Patients in areas with high prevalence rates of tuberculosis and those with an abnormal chest X-ray suggesting granulomatous disease should undergo purified protein derivative (PPD) testing. If the PPD is nonreactive (as is common in patients with renal failure) or if the patient has a history of BCG vaccination, IFN-γ release assay testing may be of benefit in the diagnosis of latent tuberculosis.[98]

Additional Pretransplant Evaluation Considerations

Gastrointestinal Evaluation

In patients with symptomatic cholelithiasis, a cholecystectomy should be performed to eliminate the risk of possible sepsis after transplantation. Patients with diabetes and asymptomatic gallstones seen with ultrasonography (~20% to 30% prevalence) may also benefit from pretransplant elective cholecystectomy.[99] A colonoscopy should be performed for patients >50 years of age to screen for colon cancer. Those with known colonic disease, especially those with diverticulitis, should be evaluated with a barium enema and a colonoscopy and, if appropriate, should be treated with surgical resection prior to transplantation.

Genitourinary Evaluation

An accurate evaluation of the lower urinary tract function prior to transplantation is important to minimize postoperative urologic complications. The original renal disease must be clearly defined. Any history of prior bladder surgery, repeated urinary infections, and current reports of urine cultures should be obtained. A voiding cystourethrogram should be performed if there is clinical or historical evidence of a bladder or ureteric abnormality. Cystoscopy and urodynamic studies should be performed in patients with evidence of bladder dysfunction. Urologic operations are necessary either to correct or improve obstructive lesions or sometimes to provide a conduit in the presence of a neurogenic bladder or a previous cystectomy.

Immunologic Evaluation

The human HLA system—encoded on the short arm of chromosome 6—encodes antigens that play a major role in host immune responses. The importance of these antigens in the practice of organ transplantation became evident when immunologic mechanisms were found to be responsible for immediate allograft destruction in early attempts at kidney transplant between non-HLA identical pairs.[100] Antibodies against HLA antigens are formed as a result of pregnancy, transfusions, and prior organ transplantation and have the potential to cause hyperacute, acute, or chronic antibody-mediated allograft rejection (AMR).[101] A landmark study by Drs. Patel and Terasaki in 1969 described a complement-dependent cytotoxicity assay (CDC) for anti-HLA antibodies that was highly predictive of hyperacute graft rejection.[102] The CDC assay screens for donor-directed complement fixing antibodies in the sera of recipients via in vitro mixing studies with donor lymphocytes, and became the first routinely used cross-match technique in organ transplantation.

Although CDC cross-matching revolutionized the pretransplant immunologic evaluation and has remained in use for 5 decades, it is associated with limited sensitivity and requires a subjective visual assessment of cell lysis. Flow cytometry (FCXM) was introduced in the 1980s as a method for screening recipient sera for donor-directed HLA antibodies with up to a threefold higher sensitivity compared to CDC. FCXM involves the incubation of donor T and B lymphocytes with recipient sera, allowing for the binding of any donor-directed HLA antibodies that may be present. After the addition of a fluorochrome-conjugated secondary (anti-IgG) antibody, anti-HLA antibody strength is measured by mean fluorescence intensity (MFI) or channel shift. Positive FCXM has been shown to be predictive of rejection and graft loss.[103] In addition to a more sensitive antibody detection, FCXM involves independent testing of B and T lymphocytes and thus allows for further characterization of HLA antibodies as specific to antigens belonging to either class I (present on all nucleated cells) or class II (present only on antigen-presenting cells such as B cells).

More recently, the practice of pretransplant antibody screening was again revolutionized by the introduction of solid phase testing using antigen-coated microbeads (SAB).[104] This assay, unlike the cell-based CDC and FCXM, uses microparticle "beads" coated with a single HLA antigen peptide incubated with recipient sera and a fluorochrome-conjugated secondary antibody. The strength of antibody binding is again determined by MFI; however, the identification of exact antigen specificities is now possible with anti-HLA antibodies further characterized as donor specific (DSA) or not. The presence of pretransplant DSA detected by single antigen beads (SAB) has been associated with an increased risk of antibody-mediated rejection (AMR) in multiple reports, however the antibody strength (MFI) that correlates with poor graft outcomes remains a matter of debate.

In addition to HLA and blood group ABO typing, most patients undergo a final cross-match prior to the kidney transplant in order to minimize the risk of hyperacute and acute AMR. There is considerable center-to-center variation in the cross-match technique and it includes CDC, FCXM, SAB, or any combination of the three. In general, contraindications to transplant include a positive CDC cross-match or T-cell FCXM.[105] A number of transplant centers in the United States have forgone the CDC method in favor of FCXM and SAB analysis, tests that offer improved sensitivity at the likely expense of decreased specificity. For example, although a positive CDC cross-match has remained an absolute contraindication to transplant, the clinical implications of a weak FCXM or low level antibodies detected by SAB are less clear and are currently a matter of intense clinical research. Thus, the evolution of cross-match techniques has resulted in increasing protection against early AMR at the expense of potentially withholding the transplant in patients with clinically irrelevant antibodies detected by sensitive assays.

Although pretransplant cross-matching serves to minimize the risk of early AMR between a recipient and a particular donor, the overall level patient sensitization helps to estimate the likelihood of positive cross-match with the general population. Patients with high levels of circulating anti-HLA antibodies are regarded as sensitized and of higher immunologic risk. Sensitization is quantified by the degree of PRA, or more recently by calculated PRA (cPRA). Historically, PRA has been determined by complement-dependent cytotoxicity mixing studies of recipient sera with a panel of lymphocytes derived from the general population, where positive reactions in 50% of samples would correspond to a PRA of 50%. It should be noted that the degree of sensitization has no bearing on the outcome of a cross-match between recipient and an individual donor, serving instead to estimate the probability of a positive cross-match between recipient and any given potential donor in the general population. As increasing levels of PRA correspond to decreasing numbers of donors to which the recipient will have a negative cross-match, sensitized patients wait much longer for transplants and are transplanted at a lower rate per year. Strategies aimed at desensitizing patients with either high PRA or positive cross-matches to potential living donors using plasmapheresis, intravenous immunoglobulin (IVIG), and anti-B cell agents bortezomib and rituximab have been met with variable success and are associated with high rates of posttransplant AMR.[106,107]

In October 2009, the United Network for Organ Sharing (UNOS) implemented a strategy replacing conventional PRA measurements with cPRA, a measure of sensitization based on unacceptable antibody levels as determined by SAB analysis.[108] Potential transplant patients are screened for antibodies against HLA antigens by SAB assays at various intervals while on the waiting list, with antigens to which the patient has significant levels of antibody listed as "unacceptable" by the transplant center. The cPRA is determined by entering the patient's unacceptable antigens into a formula that calculates the relative frequency of these antigens in the general population. Using this strategy, patients are able to undergo a "virtual" cross-match with prospective donors, taking into account both the donor HLA profile and the previously listed unacceptable antigens for the recipient. Final cross-matching is then performed only if the virtual cross-match is negative. An initial analysis of virtual cross-matching shows improved organ allocation efficiency and improved access to transplantation for sensitized patients on the waiting list compared to prior eras.[109]

DONOR SELECTION

Live Kidney Donation

Living donor transplants comprise about 35% of all transplants performed in the United States (Fig. 82.2), whereas their proportion is much less (10% to 15%) in Europe and Australia, and much higher in the Middle East.[110] Outcomes of related versus unrelated donor kidney transplants are comparable, with the exception of the 2-haplotype HLA matched living related donor transplant, and are superior compared to kidney transplants from a deceased donor.[4] This is due to a number of factors that include the minimization of cold ischemia time and the risk of delayed graft function, as well as the benefits imparted by the opportunity to perform a detailed history and medical assessment of the donor.

The initial series of tests for a potential living donor include ABO blood group and HLA tissue typing, which can be completed at a brief outpatient visit. The living donor not only needs a thorough medical evaluation, with particular attention to renal function and the urinary tract, but also a renal angiography or magnetic resonance angiography to identify vascular or anatomic variation of the kidneys or the collecting systems (Table 82.6). It is important to ascertain that both kidneys are of normal size and configuration and that a donor kidney with a single renal artery can be obtained. Several long-term follow-up studies have not revealed any adverse problems for the living donor with a single kidney and support the judicious use of the live kidney donor.[111,112] The donor surgical mortality risk is 3.1 per 10,000 donors, and life expectancy in the donor remains unaffected.[112] Although compensatory hyperfiltration occurs in the remaining kidney, the achieved glomerular filtration rate is typically 70% of baseline after 2 to 4 weeks. Blood pressure appears to increase by ~5 mm 5 to 10 years from donation over pretransplant values, adjusted for blood pressure increases with aging.[113] Black donors appear to have a greater risk of hypertension than white donors, thus it may be reasonable to have more stringent blood pressure thresholds for the black potential kidney donor.[114] Women who may desire pregnancy following kidney donation should be counseled that current observational data suggest a similar rate of fetal loss, preeclampsia, gestational diabetes, and gestational hypertension compared to the general population, but higher rates of each of these parameters compared to pregnancies that had occurred in donors prior to donation.[115,116]

Efforts to increase transplantation rates have led to the consideration of living donors with mild medical conditions and from extended social relationships from the potential recipient (Table 82.7). The nondirected kidney donor, an individual who contacts transplant centers wishing to

TABLE 82.6 Suggested Evaluation Process for Potential Living Donors

Donor screening
Educate patient regarding deceased and live donation
Take family and social history and screen for potential donors
Review ABO compatibilities of potential donors
Tissue type and cross-match ABO-compatible potential donors
Choose primary potential donor with patient and family
Educate donor regarding process of evaluation and donation
Donor evaluation
Complete history and physical examination
Comprehensive laboratory screening to include complete blood count, chemistry panel, HIV, very low-density lipoprotein, hepatitis B and C serology, cytomegalovirus, glucose tolerance test (for diabetic families)
Urinalysis, urine culture, pregnancy test
Protein, 24-hr urine collection
Creatinine, 24-hr urine collection
Chest radiograph, cardiac stress test for patients >50 years of age
Helical computed tomography urogram
Psychosocial evaluation
Repeat cross-match before transplantation

TABLE 82.7 Exclusion Criteria for Living Kidney Donors

Age <18 or >65–70 yr
Significant medical illness (e.g., cardiovascular/pulmonary diseases, recent malignancy)
History of recurrent kidney stones
History of thrombosis or thromboembolism
Psychiatric contraindications
Obesity
Hypertension (>140/90 mm Hg or necessity for medication)
Proteinuria (>250 mg/24 hr)
Microscopic hematuria
Abnormal glomerular filtration rate (<80 mL/min)
Diabetes (abnormal glucose tolerance test or hemoglobulin A_{1c})
Urologic/vascular abnormalities in donor kidneys

donate a kidney for purely altruistic reasons, provides an opportunity to benefit individuals who may have an incompatible donor or individuals without a living donor option.[117] Paired exchange programs have been developed to identify two potential donors who wish to donate to a family or friend but are unable to due to blood group incompatibility or a positive cross-match. Two such donors and their prospective recipients are then paired, with donor A donating to recipient B and donor B donating to recipient A. When an altruistic donor is introduced to paired exchange programs, it may result in significant opportunity for transplantation of a number of incompatible pairs.[118,119] Another circumstance is the matched donor in which a prospective recipient pays a monthly fee to a coordinating site, which presumably has access to a list of potential parties interested in donating their kidney. In the United States, assurances required from these donor/recipient circumstances must include the lack of monetary benefit for the donor (altruism). The U.S. Organ Transplantation Act of 1984 (HR5580, Title II) makes it a federal crime to engage in organ sale and commerce. Other countries have eliminated the waiting list with the use of monetary incentives for living unrelated donation, a topic that continues to be debated worldwide.[120,121]

Deceased Kidney Donation

Deceased kidney donors can be classified as those donors who are deceased by brain death (DBD) or those who are deceased by cardiac death (DCD). The criteria for the diagnosis of brain death have been well defined in most Western countries, although the requirements vary little from country to country (Table 82.8). Protocols exist that vary from country to country regarding DCD donation, but generally involve a waiting period of 5 minutes following the declaration of death prior to organ procurement.

DBD donors have been subcategorized as standard criteria donors (SCD) or expanded criteria donors (ECD). ECD donors are defined based on the presence of variables

TABLE 82.8 Medical Evaluation of the Potential Deceased Donor

I. Diagnosis of death
  A. Preconditions
    1. Positive diagnosis of brain death (irremediable structural brain damage)
    2. Planned withdrawal of cardiopulmonary support for irreversible conditions
  B. Exclusions
    1. Primary hypothermia (<33°C)
    2. Drugs
    3. Severe metabolic or endocrine disturbances
  C. Tests
    1. Absent brainstem reflexes
    2. Apnea (strictly define)
II. No preexisting renal disease
III. No active infection tests:
  A. HBsAg; five antibodies to cytomegalovirus and hepatitis C virus
  B. HIV antibodies
  C. HIV antigen in high-risk patients

HBsAg, hepatitis B surface antigen.

that increased the risk for graft failure by 70% compared with an SCD kidney and include donors over the age of 60, or donors between the ages of 50 to 59 with two of three additional criteria: (1) cerebrovascular accident as a cause of death, (2) prior diagnosis of hypertension, or (3) terminal serum creatinine greater than 1.5 mg per day. The rationale for making the distinction between SCD and ECD was to allocate kidneys efficiently to those in greatest need (those at greatest risk for mortality while on dialysis).[122] The survival benefit of ECD transplant over dialysis is present across all candidates, but in particular is of benefit to those with diabetes over the age of 40 or who are in regions with waiting times for a transplant of >1,350 days.[5]

DCD donors can be controlled (with a planned withdrawal of cardiopulmonary support following a consent for donation) or uncontrolled (a cardiopulmonary death in a medical setting with rapid perfusion of organs, prior to consent). The latter is practiced in countries in which there are national policies of presumed consent.[123] The additional warm ischemia time that occurs during the DCD procurement process results in higher rates of delayed graft function and primary nonfunction, but with comparable long-term graft survival to SCD kidney transplants.[124] Figure 82.10 summarizes the most recent graft survival data from the United States by type of organ.

For all organ donors, there should be no evidence of primary renal disease and no generalized viral or bacterial infection. Biopsies are often performed to determine glomerulosclerosis in cases in which there is a question of suitability for transplant, but this has not consistently demonstrated a predictive value for graft function or longevity.[125] Screening for hepatitis B, C, and HIV infection is performed to exclude donors, although in the case of hepatitis C reactivity, these donors may be used for selected recipients with chronic hepatitis C infection with good results.[126] Epstein–Barr virus (EBV) and cytomegalovirus (CMV) testing is performed to assess the risk of transmission and posttransplant complications for the recipient.

THE TRANSPLANT OPERATION–DONOR PROCUREMENT

Living Donor Nephrectomy

A living donor nephrectomy can be performed via either an open or a laparoscopic approach. The open approach entails a flank incision by an open nephrectomy. The approach to the kidney, typically the left kidney because this has the longer renal vein, may be either below or through the bed of the 12th rib using a retroperitoneal approach, or rarely via an anterior transperitoneal approach using a midline incision. Care

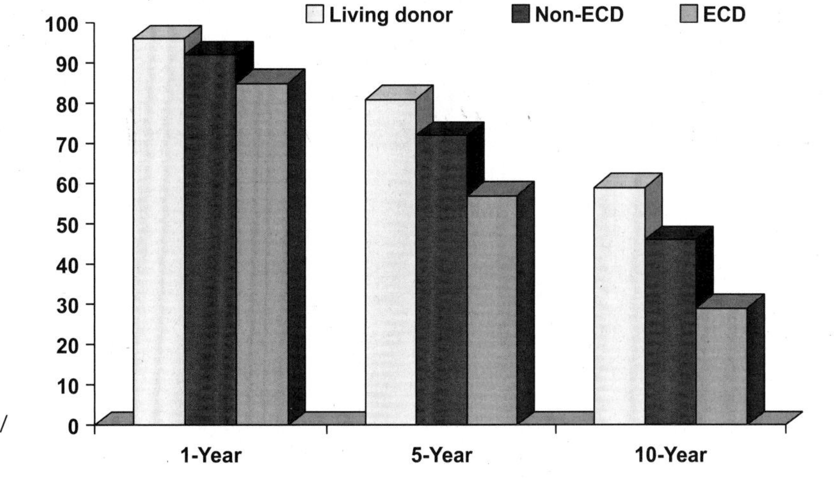

FIGURE 82.10 One, 5-, and 10-year kidney graft survival from living donors (LD), standard criteria donors (non-SCD), and expanded criteria donors (ECD). (Adapted with permission from 2009 OPTN/UNOS Annual Report, Tables 5.10a, b, d.)

TABLE 82.9 **Advantages and Disadvantages of Laparoscopic Nephrectomy**

Advantages
Less postoperative pain
Minimal surgical scarring
Rapid return to fill activities and work (approx. 4 weeks)
Shorter hospital stay
Magnified view of renal vessels
Disadvantages
Longer operative time, impaired early graft function, graft loss or damage during "learning curve"
Pneumoperitoneum may compromise renal blood flow
Tendency to have shorter renal vessels and multiple arteries
Added expense of specialized instrumentation

must be given to retraction of the kidney during its removal to avoid traction injury of the renal artery and dissection in the hilum of the kidney, particularly between the ureter and the renal artery, which should be avoided to prevent damage to the ureteric blood supply. Furthermore, in removing the ureter down to the brim of the pelvis, care should be taken to leave an adequate amount of periureteric tissue. A living donor nephrectomy for transplantation can also be performed by laparoscopic approach.[127] This approach results in less postoperative surgical pain, a shorter hospital stay, and a quicker recovery than the standard open donor nephrectomy (Table 82.9). The laparoscopic techniques have been rapidly adopted worldwide; an analysis from Australia/New Zealand transplant centers upon the introduction of the laparoscopic technique in 1997 through 2004 demonstrates comparable rates of technical failure, delayed graft function, and graft survival to an open nephrectomy, with a conversion rate to open procedures of 6%.[128] This conversion rate is much higher than that reported for experienced centers of 1%.[129]

Deceased Donor Nephrectomy

Currently, most kidneys will be removed as part of a multiple-organ procurement procedure in which not only the kidneys are removed, but also the liver and heart and, occasionally, the lungs and pancreas. There are two basic approaches to a deceased donor nephrectomy. In one, each kidney is removed individually with a patch of aorta via an anterior approach, whereas in the other, which is the more satisfactory technique, both kidneys are removed en bloc with the appropriate segment of the aorta and vena cava. The dissection of the vessels and the kidneys can then be completed after hypothermic perfusion and storage. In situ perfusion may be performed in both cases before and during removal.

Renal Preservation

The effective preservation of the kidney is an integral part of a kidney transplantation program and has evolved on the basis of known principles of preservation because of a need for longer storage of kidneys.[130] The ability to preserve kidneys provides time for tissue typing and cross-matching and the selection of the most appropriate recipients for a particular donor on the basis of matching, as well as the preparation of the patients selected, who often may need dialysis before transplantation, and, finally, the transport of the kidneys to a center where an appropriately matched recipient may be awaiting a transplant.

There are two methods of preservation: simple cold storage in ice after flushing with a hypothermic solution to give a renal core temperature of 0°C and a more complicated approach of continuous perfusion of the kidney with an oxygenated colloid solution. The simple cold storage approach is most commonly used, and provides adequate preservation for at least 24 to 30 hours. The kidneys are initially flushed free of blood with a cold solution via the aorta and renal artery while the kidney is in situ. Many different flushing solutions have been used; currently the most common preservation solutions in use in the United States are Viaspan (University of Wisconsin [UW] solution or Belzer solution) and Custodiol (histidine-tryptophan-ketoglutarate [HTK]) (Table 82.10).[131] Drugs, metabolites, and other agents have been used to enhance the effects of cold preservation. The aim of these maneuvers is to reduce the incidence of posttransplant acute tubular necrosis.

In the absence of any warm ischemia, which is generally the case with a brain-dead donor on a ventilator, the immediate function can be obtained in most kidneys with up to 24 hours of preservation and even after 48 hours of preservation in some patients. However, from 24 hours onward, most kidneys will have a significant period of delayed function ranging from 1 day to several weeks and there will be a significant incidence of primary nonfunction. Because 18 to 36 hours is an adequate time for most units and also allows time for transport of kidneys within a region or country, there has been widespread adoption of the simple cold storage (CS) technique for preservation.

Compared to the more traditional CS technique, machine perfusion (MP) involves placing kidneys from a deceased donor on a perfusion device that provides either continuous or pulsatile flow of a hypothermic solution through the renal vasculature.[132] In theory, by eliminating toxic metabolic byproducts and providing nutrients and oxygen, MP may protect deceased-donor kidneys from peritransplant ischemia/reperfusion injury that is responsible for the majority of clinically significant delayed graft function (DGF), an event independently associated with acute rejection and poor graft survival.[133] In recent years, the use

TABLE 82.10 **Contents of Commonly Used Cold Preservation Solutions**

	Custodiol (HTK)	UW
Sodium (mM)	15	30
Potassium (mM)	10	120
Magnesium (mM)	4	5
Histidine (mM)	198	—
Tryptophan (mM)	2	—
Alpha-ketoglutarate	n/a	
Mannitol (mM)	30	—
Sulfate (mM)	—	5
Phosphate (mM)	—	25
Lactobionate (mM)	—	100
Raffinose (mM)	—	30
Adenosine (mM)	—	5
Allopurinol (mM)	—	1
Glutathione (mM)	—	3
Insulin (units/L)	—	100
Dexamethasone (mg/L)	—	8
Hydroxyethyl starch (g/L)	—	50

HTK, histidine-tryptophan-ketoglutarate; UW, University of Wisconsin.

of kidneys from less traditional donors has been on the rise, including ECD and DCD, both of which are associated with significantly higher rates of DGF.[134,135] As a result, a number of recent clinical trials have studied preservation methods in an attempt to demonstrate improved rates of DGF in deceased donor kidney transplants.

Most recent clinical trials have shown improved DGF rates with the use of MP compared to CS. For example, in the largest prospective randomized controlled trial to date, Moers et al.[136] studied the outcomes of 336 kidney pairs, where 1 kidney per pair underwent MP and the other CS, and reported both lower rates of DGF and improved 1-year allograft survival in the MP group. Subsequent prospective extensions of this trial demonstrate lower DGF rates for both ECD and DCD, improved 1-year graft survival for ECD, but comparable 1-year graft survival for DCD kidneys with MP versus CS transplants.[137,138] In contrast, a UK-based paired kidney analysis of DCD kidneys undergoing either MP or CS failed to show any difference in terms of DGF rates or 1-year graft survival.[139] Despite these mixed results, MP likely results in modestly less DGF for deceased donor kidney transplants of any type compared to CS. Whether the increased cost associated with MP can be offset by improved long-term graft outcomes has yet to be clarified.

THE TRANSPLANT OPERATION–RECIPIENT SURGERY

The surgical technique of renal transplantation is standardized.[140] In cadaver transplantation, the kidney must first be inspected to ensure that it is suitable for transplantation before undertaking the operation. This procedure should be carried out in the operating room on a sterile back table. The procedure is to remove the unnecessary fatty tissue and to prepare the donor vessels. In small pediatric donors, both kidneys can be used en bloc for transplantation in adults.

The transplanted kidney is implanted in the retroperitoneal space in either the right or left iliac fossa through an oblique incision extending from the suprapubic area to a point just above and medial to the anterior superior iliac crest. For transplantation, after failed transplants in both iliac fossae, a lower midline intraperitoneal approach should be used.

The iliac vessels should be carefully dissected[141] and the lymphatics ligated to prevent lymphocele formation. The donor renal vein is anastomosed end to side to the external iliac vein. The renal artery is anastomosed to the external or common iliac artery end to side using a cuff of aorta as a patch for the anastomosis, or it is anastomosed end to end to the internal iliac artery, which has been previously ligated and divided. The end-to-side anastomosis using a cuff of aorta is the simpler anastomosis; it is the most appropriate one to use in cadaver transplantation when the renal artery is provided with a cuff of aorta. The end-to-end anastomosis to the internal iliac artery is technically more demanding and should only be used in living donor kidney transplantation.

Implantation of the ureter in the bladder is performed in one of two ways.[142] The first is to anastomose the spatulated end of the ureter mucosa to the dome of the bladder drawing muscle over the anastomosis to provide a tunnel. The second technique is to bring the ureter through the lateral wall of the bladder and down through a 2- to 3-cm submucosal tunnel and out in the vicinity of the patient's own ureteric orifices at the trigone, where it is anastomosed mucosa to mucosa. The success of the first technique is greater than the second. Preventive antibiotics with appropriate broad-spectrum activity should be given with the premedication, in particular to protect against the possibility of infection being transmitted with the transplanted kidney.

General Postoperative Management and Follow-up

Routine postoperative observations should include the monitoring of vital signs, fluid intake, and urine output. A postoperative hematuria is usually transient. The Foley catheter is generally left in these patients for 3 to 4 days because of high urine outflow rates that occur during this time in order to prevent overdistension of the bladder. This is particularly important in diabetic patients who frequently have neurogenic bladders and can have extremely large bladder volumes before they develop an urge to micturate. Catheters should also be carefully monitored for obstruction and irrigated under sterile conditions if occluded by a clot.

Immediate function of the transplanted kidney makes postoperative management of the patient in the first few days much simpler than if the kidney is not functioning. The patient, particularly in the case of a living related transplant, may have a massive diuresis in the first 48 hours, and, for this reason, hourly monitoring of the urine output and a central venous line are essential to balance the fluid requirements appropriately. A very basic regimen, at least for the first few hours, is to replace fluid at the rate of the last hour's output plus 50 mL per hour of IV fluid. This can then be modified according to the kidney function and the central venous pressure.

Within 48 hours, particularly with a functioning kidney, the patient's restored sense of well-being is quite remarkable and most patients can get out of bed on the second postoperative day. Provided that no complications ensue and that any early rejection episode can be dealt with satisfactorily with appropriate treatment, these patients are ready to leave the hospital by the 3rd to 5th or 6th postoperative day.

After discharge from the hospital, the follow-up interval will depend on the patient's general condition and the development of additional problems. Routine biochemistry, hematology, and urine analysis should be obtained at each clinic visit. General guidelines for the frequency and type of posttransplant monitoring have been proposed by the Kidney Disease Improving Global Outcomes (KDIGO) workgroup,[143] which for the stable patient, include suggestions for monitoring laboratory parameters and clinic visits as frequently as every 2 to 3 times per week in the immediate posttransplant period tapering to a weekly, biweekly, and monthly schedule over the first 6 months.

IMMUNOSUPPRESSIVE THERAPY

Immunosuppressive therapy in renal transplant recipient consists of: (1) continuous baseline therapy (maintenance immunosuppression) to prevent the development of rejection and (2) short courses of intensive therapy peritransplant (termed induction therapy), or in the setting of acute rejection (antirejection therapy) to more completely abrogate the immunologic antidonor rejection response. The agents used for induction and antirejection therapy are similar and include high-dose methylprednisolone, monoclonal antibodies or polyclonal antisera, such as antilymphocyte globulin (ALG) and antithymocyte globulin (ATG), and B-cell directed therapies when the antidonor antibody is identified. The use of induction therapy in the United States now approaches 80% of all transplants and is employed for varying goals, including (1) the minimization of maintenance immunosuppresion such as corticosteroid withdrawal or calcineurin inhibitor minimization, avoidance or withdrawal (see later sections), (2) the minimization of risk for acute rejection in patients considered at increased immunologic risk, and (3) the delayed introduction of maintenance immunosuppression such as calcineurin inhibitors in settings of increased risk of delayed graft function/acute tubular necrosis, to avoid the vasoconstrictive effects and the potential for prolongation or potentiation of graft injury. Baseline immunosuppression traditionally involves the use of multiple drugs, each directed at a discrete site in the T-cell activation cascade and each with distinct side effects. The use of multiple agents at lower doses may provide greater protection from immunologic injury with fewer side effects than single agent therapy, thus two- and three-drug immunosuppression regimens are commonly employed. The maintenance immunosuppressive agents can be classified on the basis of their primary site of action as inhibitors of transcription (the calcineurin inhibitors cyclosporine and tacrolimus), inhibitors of nucleotide synthesis (azathioprine and mycophenolate), inhibitors of growth factor signal transduction (the mTOR inhibitors sirolimus and everolimus), and an oral corticosteroid, a broad immunosuppressant with inhibitory activity against lymphocytes, macrophages, and neutrophils. Current standard practice for chronic immunosuppression includes a calcineurin inhibitor (CsA or tacrolimus), an antiproliferative agent (mycophenolate, mTORi or azathioprine), and steroids. Many corticosteroid tapering schedules have been employed and are typically based on the immunologic risk of the recipient as well as the induction and baseline immunosuppression used. A conservative corticosteroid taper would be prednisone starting with a 20 to 30 mg daily dose for the first month and tapered by 2.5 to 5 mg every 2 weeks to a maintenance dose of 5 to 10 mg per day. Most centers do not routinely discontinue or switch to alternate-day steroids unless the patient is having problems with side effects (including worsening glucose control, hypercholesterolemia, or difficulties in blood pressure control) and has had stable renal allograft function with no episodes of acute rejection within the preceding 6 to 12 months. However, steroid-withdrawal strategies continue to be of significant interest to both transplant centers and potential transplant recipients. Overall, cumulative high-dose immunosuppression leads to a myriad of complications, increased infections, malignancy, and cardiovascular morbidity and mortality. The goal of transplant immunosuppression is to reduce immunosuppression to a level that will prevent or suppress rejection, but minimize the risk of life-threatening infections and other problems related to the treatment.

Induction Agents

Common induction agents currently in use can be defined as T-cell depleting or non–T-cell depleting agents. Although historically, equine antithymocyte serum (ATGAM) and murine monoclonal anti-CD3 (OKT3, now no longer in production) had been prominently used as T-cell depleting agents, these have largely been replaced in clinical use by rabbit antithymocyte globulin (rATG, Thymoglobulin) and monoclonal humanized anti-CD52 (alemtuzumab, Campath 1-H), which also acts as a B-cell–depleting agent. These agents primarily function to eliminate the T-cell alloimmune response, with T-cell depletion lasting weeks (for rATG) to months (for anti-CD52). Although ATGAM and rATG have similar general mechanisms of action (both are pooled polyclonal antibodies developed from the administration of T cells to animals (the horse in the case of ATGAM, and the rabbit in the case of rATG), the relative efficacy of the two have been compared in one clinical trial,[144] suggesting a therapeutic advantage to rATG. The nondepleting induction agents include the IL-2 receptor antagonists daclizumab (currently not in production) and basiliximab. These agents function to inhibit the proliferation of activated T cells.

Many centers use induction agents in the immediate posttransplant period. In 2008, the use of rATG, anti-CD52, and IL-2ra for induction in the United States was 45%, 11%, and 29%, respectively (SRTR Annual Report 2009). For higher risk patients such as those with prior sensitization (elevated PRA), prior transplant, or African American ethnicity, induction therapy is usually combined with standard doses of immunosuppression to prevent rejection. For those with a lower risk (living donor kidney recipients, primary kidney transplants), induction therapy is often employed in an effort to minimize exposure to maintenance immunosuppression.

In low-risk patients, the need for induction therapy remains controversial when using a standard three-drug maintenance immunosuppression. A meta-analysis of 24 studies examining IL-2ra versus placebo reported a reduction in risk of both graft loss of 25% and acute rejection within the first year of 28%.[145] However, only three studies were included in the analysis that used tacrolimus/mycophenolate (TAC/MMF) as maintenance immunosuppression, and the rejection rate in the placebo/no induction arm was 38%. This rate is much higher than present day reports with TAC/MMF-based immunosuppression. A recent analysis of 28,000 patients treated between 2000 and 2008 with tacrolimus, mycophenolate, prednisone, and either IL-2ra or no induction suggests a minimal reduction in acute rejection rates and no impact on graft survival.[146]

For patients at a higher risk of acute rejection, two trials have compared nondepleting agents (IL-2ra) versus the T-cell depleting agent rATG in the prevention of rejection. Although the trials differed in inclusion criteria, the dosing regimen of rATG, and the baseline calcineurin inhibitor, they demonstrated similar findings of reduced rates of acute rejection in the rATG group (15% to 16%) versus the IL-2ra group (26% to 27%).[147,148] On the basis of these experiences, depleting agents generally are favored in the transplant recipient at elevated risk for rejection. A comparison of alemtuzumab and rATG has not been performed in the setting of triple agent maintenance immunosuppression, thus statements of efficacy differences between these agents cannot be accurately made.

With regard to safety, all depleting agents carry concerns regarding long-term risk of infection and malignancy.[149] Registry analyses suggest that there is an increased risk of a future development of lymphoma with depleting agents compared to nondepleting agents or no induction therapy, an association that appears to be dose dependent.[150, 151] For this reason, repeated or prolonged courses of depleting antibody therapy must be considered with this risk balanced by the potential for graft recovery or prolongation. A review of the mechanisms of action, administration, and side effects of commonly used induction agents is provided in the following paragraphs.

T-Cell Depleting Agents

Polyclonal Antisera to Human T Cells: Thymoglobulin and Equine Antithymocyte Serum

As described previously, antithymocyte globulins (rATG-Thymoglobulin, and equine ATG-ATGAM) are polyclonal antisera derived from immunization of lymphocytes, lymphoblasts, or thymocytes into rabbits or horses. The immunosuppressive product contains cytotoxic antibodies directed against a variety of T-cell–surface markers including the major histocompatibility complex (MHC) antigens. The administration leads to the depletion of peripheral blood lymphocytes. The lymphocytes are either lysed or cleared by the reticuloendothelial system, and their surface antigen may be masked by the antibody.

Dosing of either agent has not been defined, with a number of reports of efficacy using rATG given as 1 to 2 mg per kilogram intravenously for 3 to 14 days, whereas alternate day dosing and T-cell count-monitored dosing has demonstrated efficacy. Equine ATG is typically given 15 mg/kg/day for 7 to 14 days. Data suggest that rATG is superior to equine ATG for the prevention and/or reversal of rejection.[144]

Potential side effects of rATG and equine ATG include fever, chills, erythema, thrombocytopenia, local phlebitis, serum sickness due to cytokine release, and anaphylaxis. The potential for development of host anti-antithymocyte antibodies has not been a significant problem because of the use of less immunogenic preparations and additionally because rATG and equine ATG suppress the immune response to the foreign protein itself. To avoid allergic reactions and symptoms related to cytokine release, the patients receive intravenous medications consisting of methylprednisolone (30 mg) and diphenhydramine hydrochloride (50 mg) 30 minutes before injection. Acetaminophen should be given before and 4 hours after the commencement of infusion for fever control. Thrombocytopenia and leukopenia may necessitate reduction or curtailment of drug dosage.

Muromonab-CD3 (OKT3) Monoclonal Antibodies

OKT3 is a mouse monoclonal antibody directed against the CD3 molecule, which is a subunit of the T-cell receptor of the T lymphocyte. Administration leads to the depletion of peripheral blood lymphocytes. As mentioned previously,

OKT3 is currently not produced, primarily due a decrease in use over the last decade due to side effects related to cytokine release, but is presented briefly within this chapter as a number of analogs remain in clinical development.

OKT3 was commonly given 5 mg per day once daily for 7 to 14 days and administered as an IV push over <1 minute at a final concentration of 1 mg per milliliter. Premedication with Solu-Medrol at 15 mg per kilogram IV is administered prior to the first dose to decrease the incidence of reactions, which include fever, rigors, diarrhea, myalgia, arthralgia, aseptic meningitis, dyspnea, and wheezing. The release of tumor necrosis factor (TNF), IL-2, and IFN-γ in the serum are found after an OKT3 injection. The acute pulmonary compromise due to a capillary-leak syndrome is more common in patients who are > 3% of dry weight before the initiation of OKT3 treatment.

The development of host anti-OKT3 antibodies complicates the reuse of this drug in previously treated patients. Approximately 33% to 100% of patients develop anti–mouse antibodies after the first exposure to OKT3, depending on concomitant immunosuppression.[152] Anti-OKT3 titers of 1:10,000 or more usually correlate with a lack of clinical response. If anti-OKT3 antibodies are of low titer, retreatment with OKT3 is typically successful. If retreatment is attempted with anti–mouse titers of 1:100 or more, the peripheral lymphocyte count, CD3 T cells, and trough-free circulating OKT3 should be monitored. If the absolute CD3 T-lymphocyte count is greater than 10/μL or the free-circulating trough OKT3 level is not detected, it may be indicative of an inadequate dose of OKT3. Under these circumstances, increasing the dose of OKT3 from 5 to 10 mg per day can overcome the anti–mouse antibody response.

Nondepleting T-Cell Agents

IL-2 Receptor Antagonists: Basiliximab and Daclizumab

Basiliximab (Simulect) is a chimeric (murine/human) immunosuppressant monoclonal antibody that binds and blocks the alpha chain of the IL-2 receptor complex expressed on activated T cells, leading to a reduction in T-cell proliferation. Daclizumab similarly is a chimeric (90% human, 10% murine) monoclonal IgG antibody produced by recombinant DNA technology with the same binding site and mechanism of action.

Both were approved for use in kidney transplantation as induction agents but, as mentioned previously, daclizumab is currently not produced due to planned discontinuation by the manufacturer. Basiliximab is given 20 mg intravenously as a bolus or infusion over 20 to 30 minutes on days 0 and day 4, whereas daclizumab is given 1 mg per kilogram within 24 hours before transplantation (day 0), then every 14 days for 4 additional doses (total of 5 doses).

Notably, and in direct contrast to the depleting agents, the administration of basiliximab or daclizumab did not increase the incidence or severity of adverse effects over placebo in clinical trials.

B- and T-Cell Depleting Agents

Anti-CD52 (Alemtuzumab, Campath 1-H)

Alemtuzumab is a humanized recombinant DNA-derived monoclonal antibody directed against the cell surface molecule CD52 present on both B and T cells. As described previously, it has been used as an efficient T-cell depleting agent but also leads to the depletion of B cells. This effect occurs within hours of infusion and its effects may last beyond 6 months. This prolonged lymphopenia raises concerns regarding the potential for delayed acute rejection episodes, because T- and B-cell reconstitution occurs much later in the posttransplant course during which time monitoring may not be as frequent. Concerns have been expressed regarding an increased risk of unusual infections, reports have noted a comparable safety profile to other depleting induction agents, and reduced incidence of posttransplant lymphoproliferative disease.

Although no formal dosing strategy has been extensively evaluated, experiences with 30 mg intravenously given perioperatively and followed by a second 30 mg dose on day 1 or 2 is frequently reported, with few infusion-related side effects reported.

B-Cell–Targeted Therapy

Greater attention has been focused in recent years on the role of B cells and donor-specific antibody production (HLA and non-HLA) and graft injury. At the outset of transplantation, B-cell/antibody reduction strategies (referred to as "desensitization") may permit transplantation under circumstances that would previously result in rapid rejection (often referred to as hyperacute rejection, or delayed hyperacute rejection, see the following). Acute antibody-mediated rejection can occur at any time following a transplant, either with or without a T-cell component, and these agents have been used in this setting as well. Finally, the pathologic entity of chronic antibody-mediated rejection has been increasingly described, with small case series reports of B-cell therapies in this setting. Although the presentation, pathology, and management of antibody-mediated rejection is provided in a later section, a review of the agents used for B-cell/antibody–directed therapy is provided in the following sections. These interventions include bortezomib, rituximab, intravenous immunoglobulin, and plasma exchange.

Bortezomib. Bortezomib is a proteasome inhibitor that causes apoptosis of plasma cells among other effects. It has been approved for use in the United States for patients with multiple myeloma to control B-cell production of immunoglobulins. It has been used in small studies to inhibit HLA antibody production in the setting of acute antibody-mediated rejection, and may prove to be of value in desensitization protocols perioperatively.

For the treatment of multiple myeloma, a treatment cycle of 1.3 mg per square meter intravenously twice weekly for 2 weeks is usually repeated for a total of six to nine cycles.

Modeling this experience, transplant centers have adopted the four-dose, 2-week cycle as initial therapy with additional cycles depending on clinical response and reduction in donor-specific antibody titer.

In patients with multiple myeloma treated with repeated cycles, the incidence of peripheral neuropathy increases (up to 28% to 64% in those receiving up to 8 biweekly cycles) but resolved in 85% within a median of 98 days.[153]

Rituximab. Rituximab (Rituxan) is a humanized anti-CD20 antibody that binds to CD20 on mature B cells, resulting in B-cell depletion. Unlike bortezomib, it is not effective against plasma cells, because plasma cells do not express CD20 on the cell surface. It is approved for use in the United States for the treatment of certain non-Hodgkin lymphomas, and has been used experimentally to reduce donor-specific antibodies pretransplant as well as for treatment of acute humoral rejection and forms of posttransplant lymphoproliferative disease (PTLD) following transplant.

A common dosing strategy is 375 to 500 mg per square meter intravenously for one to four doses.[154] Fifty percent of patients will experience infusion-related side effects within the first 2 hours of the first rituximab infusion, 90% of which are mild and may include nausea, skin rash and pruritus, headache, fever, chills, dyspnea, and angioedema. These symptoms generally resolve within 3 hours. Subsequent infusions are associated with a lower risk of reactions. More severe reactions including bronchospasm and severe hypotension/anaphylaxis are rare (5% to 10%) but have been reported. Although the risk of infections appears low when used as monotherapy, there may be an increased risk of later opportunistic infections when used in conjunction with other B-cell modulating therapies and in the background of intensified maintenance immunosuppression.

Intravenous Immunoglobulin

Infusion of IVIG may provide blocking or anti-idiotypic antibodies that can reduce the production of anti-HLA antibodies in the pretransplant period and also has a number of additional effects that may modulate the immune response, including the blockade of Fc receptors, the decrease of inflammation, and the regulation of T cells.[155] There is also limited experience in the use of IVIG in the treatment of allograft rejection. Successful prevention and the treatment of acute humoral rejection were reported in a series of kidney transplant patients with steroid and antilymphocyte-resistant rejection.[156]

When used in desensitization protocols in the absence of plasma exchange, a dose of 1 to 2 g per kilogram is commonly used for up to six doses.[107,157] When used with plasma exchange, 100 to 200 mg per kilogram IV after each exchange has been reported.[158] When used as a treatment for acute rejection, a similar dosing strategy is typically employed.[158]

Infusion-related side effects may include flushing, chills, and myalgia, and arthralgia may occur in ~5% of patients. Aseptic meningitis has been reported in up to 11%, and typically lasts for up to 72 hours after infusion. An increased risk for venous thrombotic events has been suggested; currently, a U.S. Food and Drug Administration (FDA) warning exists for this potential adverse event.

Maintenance Immunosuppressive Agents

Maintenance immunosuppression has evolved from an era in which azathioprine and oral corticosteroids were the sole agents used for kidney transplant immunosuppresion to the cyclosporine era in which acute rejection rates within the first year fell from ~70% to ~50%, to an era in which newer calcineurin inhibitors and antiproliferative agents were introduced. Together with induction agents, acute rejection rates are commonly less than 20% in the first year and are often nearer to 10% in lower risk patient populations. With the improvement in prevention of acute rejection come greater considerations for the safety profiles of these agents, not only in terms of graft outcomes but in terms of patient risk factors such as cardiovascular, infectious, and malignancy risks. Within this context, the agents used for maintenance immunosuppression will be reviewed with a discussion of clinical trials that support (or fail to support) one strategy over another.

Corticosteroids

Corticosteroids have been known for more than 40 years to have a suppressive effect on the immune system. Their first use in renal transplantation was in 1960, when cortisone was used to reverse a rejection episode in a living related donor transplant recipient who had been immunosuppressed by total-body irradiation. Since then, steroids have been used for the treatment of rejection episodes and as part of the standard immunosuppressive regimen for the prevention of rejection. The complications of steroid therapy are numerous and involve many organ systems. Acute side effects include fluid and salt retention, which may exacerbate hypertension; steroid-induced diabetes, which may result from impaired glucose tolerance; or preexisting diabetes, and rarely, central nervous system (CNS) changes, such as steroid psychosis or pseudotumor cerebri. These changes occur when high doses of prednisone or methylprednisolone are given during the initial posttransplant period or in the treatment of a rejection episode. Generally, these short-term effects lessen or disappear when the doses of steroids are tapered. The long-term side effects are more insidious in onset and are associated with Cushingnoid changes, poor wound healing, and increased frequency of infections. Other side effects include cataracts, proximal myopathy, osteoporosis, and osteonecrosis.

In an effort to reduce the incidence of metabolic and infectious complications, the current trend is to use lower doses of steroids for maintenance and IV pulses of methylprednisolone for the treatment of rejection. Because of the growth-suppressive effects of corticosteroids, alternate day steroid therapy is often used in children. However, this regimen has not been evaluated in randomized controlled trials in adults.

Steroid Withdrawal. Given the number of cosmetic, metabolic, and cardiovascular side effects attributable to chronic prednisone use, the elimination of corticosteroids from maintenance immunosuppression regimens have been an active area of study. Early corticosteroid cessation (within 7 days following a transplant) has become increasingly popular in the United States. In 2006, over 30% of all patients were discharged following transplant without maintenance prednisone therapy. Typically, patients at lower immunologic risk (low panel reactive antibodies, first transplants) are selected, and immunosuppression includes induction therapy, a calcineurin inhibitor (CNI), and an antiproliferative agent. Acute rejection rates in single center studies range from 10% to 15%.[159] In the only prospective, double-blind, multicenter study of corticosteroid cessation to date, a rapid elimination of steroids at 7 days posttransplant was compared to a standard steroid taper to 5 mg at 6 months versus a background of induction therapy plus a TAC/MMF-based immunosuppression.[160] Corticosteroid withdrawal was associated with less bone disease, less cataract formation, and lower triglyceride levels with similar graft function at 5 years. However, other cardiovascular risk factors and weight gain were equivalent, and rejection rates were higher in the corticosteroid withdrawal arm (18% versus 11%, $P = .04$). Post hoc analysis suggested a higher rate of chronic allograft nephropathy in the corticosteroid withdrawal arm. Outcomes using a strategy of steroid avoidance have recently been reported in an open-label study in comparison with a steroid withdrawal strategy after 7 days, or standard chronic steroid use (all in the setting of induction with basiliximab and chronic immunosuppression with CsA and MMF).[161] Both the steroid avoidance cohort and the steroid withdrawal cohort experienced a significantly higher amount of biopsy-proven acute rejection (31.5% and 26.4%, respectively) compared to the chronic steroid arm (14.7%).

Similar to the early steroid withdrawal experience, single center studies and uncontrolled analyses demonstrate the potential for benefit in the withdrawal of steroids later after transplant (3 to 12 months).[162] When studied in a randomized controlled fashion, steroid withdrawal at 3 months following transplant has been shown to result in unacceptably high acute rejection rates, particularly in African Americans.[163] Thus, an element of caution is required before recommending the routine use of steroid withdrawal. Clinicians must weigh the increased risk of acute rejection and the potential for chronic allograft injury versus the patient's interest in avoiding the side effects of chronic steroid use when determining if steroid withdrawal is appropriate.

Calcineurin Inhibitors: Cyclosporine and Tacrolimus

The calcineurin inhibitor CsA was first introduced in renal transplantation by Calne and his colleagues[164] in 1978 and resulted in a dramatic reduction in acute rejection rates, quickly becoming the standard immunosuppressive agent in transplantation. Tacrolimus (FK506 or Prograf) is a macrolide immunosuppressant introduced in clinical trials in the mid-1990s and is similar to CsA in its mode of action. Although cyclosporine is a fungal peptide that binds to cyclophilin, TAC binds to an immunophilin, FKBP (FK506 binding protein). Both the block of calcineurin-mediated T-cell receptor signal transduction leading to the inhibition of several T-cell growth-promoting genes such as IL-2, and the inhibition of T-cell–dependent B-cell activation. The original formulation of cyclosporine (Sandimmune) has been replaced by microemulsion formulations (Neoral and the generic formulations, Gengraf and cyclosporine USP). These are available as 25 and 100 mg capsules. TAC is available in branded (Prograf) and generic formulations in 0.5-, 1-, and 5-mg capsules. A long-acting formulation of TAC given once daily (Advagraf) is available in Europe but not in the United States.

CsA and TAC are administered orally as two 12-hourly doses. The starting oral dosage for CsA is 4 to 6 mg/kg/day and for TAC is 0.1 to 0.2 mg/kg/day, and adjusted according to graft function and trough (C0) levels. Both TAC and CsA are available in intravenous forms but are rarely used due to excellent bioavailability. When necessary (patients with ileus or other gastrointestinal dysfunction) the IV dosage is one-third of the oral dose. CsA should be given in a slow infusion with 0.9% sodium chloride or 5% dextrose over 2 to 6 hours, whereas TAC should be given as a continuous infusion. African American patients often require a higher dose of TAC (mean 37% higher dose than Caucasian patients) to achieve comparable blood concentrations.

Therapeutic Drug Monitoring of Calcineurin Inhibitor. Therapeutic monitoring is important due to the inter- and intra-patient variation in metabolism. Similar goals should be applied for generic formulations, as no adverse events have yet been reported regarding their use. Some consider the 2-hour peak as more predictive of CsA toxicity than C0 levels, but this has not been widely implemented. Typical C0 goals for TAC and CsA as compared in a recent pivotal head-to-head trial are listed in Table 82.11. Although the results of this trial compared trough level goals that are currently in clinical practice and thus form the basis of current recommendations, dosing may require modification in the individual patient. For example, for those who may not be able to tolerate an antiproliferative agent, higher calcineurin inhibitor exposure and a higher trough level goal may be required, whereas for those who suffer complications of overimmunosuppression, such as posttransplant lymphoproliferative disorder or polyomavirus nephropathy, a lower calcineurin inhibitor exposure and lower trough level goal is required.

Side Effects. A number of side effects have been observed in patients receiving calcineurin inhibitors. CNI nephrotoxicity

TABLE 82.11 **Acute Rejection and Graft Survival Rates from a Clinical Trial Comparing CNI-based Immunosuppression to MTOR-based Immunosuppression**

Regimen	Acute Rejection (%)	Graft Survival (%)	GFR (mL/min)
Cyclosporine "standard": C0 goal CsA150–300 ng/mL × 3 months, then 100–200 ng/mL	25.8	89.3	57.1
Cyclosporine "low dose": Daclizumab induction, C0 goal CSA 50–100 ng/mL	24.0	93.1	59.4
Tacrolimus "low dose": Daclizumab induction, C0 goal TAC 3–7 ng/mL	12.3*	94.2*	65.4*
Sirolimus "low dose": Daclizumab induction, C0 goal sirolimus 4–8 ng/mL	37.2	89.3	56.7
*$P < .05$			

* $P < .05$. CNI, calcineurin inhibitor; MTOR, mammalian target of rapamycin; GFR, glomerular filtration rate.

is a concern particularly at higher dosing and C0 concentrations, and is discussed in a later section addressing the long-term management of the transplant recipient. Other side effects include hypertension, fluid retention, hyperkalemia, hypomagnesemia, hyperuricemia, and rarely, a microangiopathic hemolytic anemia in association with hemolytic uremic syndrome. Other side effects that are more common to CsA than TAC include hypertrichosis, gingival hypertrophy, hyperuricemia, and hyperlipidemia, whereas those that are more common to TAC include more prominent neurologic side effects such as tremor, headache, insomnia, and more prominent metabolic side effects such as posttransplant diabetes, more frequent alopecia, an increased incidence of polyoma virus infection, and a higher rate of posttransplant diabetes.[165] Hypertrophic cardiomyopathy has also been reported in children treated with TAC.

Drug Interactions. Cyclosporine is metabolized almost entirely in the liver through the cytochrome P450 system. Most of the drug is excreted in the bile and liver dysfunction causes it to accumulate and serum levels to rise. TAC is absorbed primarily by the small intestine and its oral bioavailability is about 25%. Impaired renal function does not affect plasma or whole blood levels because only about 0.1% of the native drug is detected in the urine and only 10% of the metabolites of the parent compound are excreted in the urine. Like CsA, it is primarily metabolized by hepatic cytochrome P450. Therefore, the calcineurin inhibitor exposure level will be influenced by the concomitant administration of medications that affect cytochrome P450. The well-known interactions are listed in Table 82.12. Drugs that induce hepatic enzymes, such as rifampicin, phenytoin, phenobarbital, norfloxacin, and nafcillin, will increase the rate of metabolism of the calcineurin inhibitor and lower blood levels of the parent compound. Drugs that increase calcineurin inhibitor levels include calcium channel blockers, such as diltiazem, verapamil and nicardipine, erythromycin, and ketoconazole. It is important to consider the possibility of drug–drug interactions with any medication that is added to the transplant recipient's regimen given the potential influence on calcineurin inhibitor exposure (both inhibitors and inducers of the P450 system). A number of drugs can enhance CNI nephrotoxicity irrespective of drug–drug interactions.

TABLE 82.12 **Cyclosporine or Tacrolimus Drug Interactions**

Increase Level	Decrease Level	Additive Nephrotoxicity
Erythromycin	Barbiturate	Aminoglycosides
Diltiazem	Carbamazepine	Amphotericin B
Ketoconazole	Isoniazid	Cotrimoxazole
Metoclopramide	Phenytoin	Trimethoprim
Oral contraceptives	Rifampicin	Acyclovir
Nicardipine		

These include aminoglycosides, amphotericin B, trimethoprim, and cotrimoxazole.

Cyclosporine Versus Tacrolimus: Efficacy and Side Effects

Most randomized trials comparing TAC to CsA demonstrate lower rejection rates with TAC. In a large multicenter randomized controlled trial using lower doses of tacrolimus (3 to 7 ng per milliliter) and CsA (50 to 100 ng per milliliter) in conjunction with IL-2ra, MMF, and steroids, the acute rejection rate in the TAC arm was 12% at 1 year, whereas in the CsA arm the acute rejection rate was statistically and clinically significantly higher (24%).[166] However, accompanying these benefits come an increased risk of diabetes and neurologic and GI side effects. The relative differences in efficacy may be overcome with more potent induction therapy.[167] A meta-analysis of randomized controlled trials generally favors TAC over CsA for the prevention of acute rejection. Treating 100 patients with TAC instead of cyclosporine would prevent 12 patients from experiencing acute rejection, and would form graft loss in 2, but would cause an additional 5 patients to develop insulin-requiring diabetes.[168]

Mycophenolate Mofetil and Enteric-Coated Mycophenolate Sodium

MMF and enteric-coated mycophenolate sodium (EC-MPS) are converted in vivo to mycophenolic acid (MPA), a noncompetitive and reversible inhibitor of inosine monophosphate dehydrogenase (Fig. 82.11). This enzyme is responsible for the conversion of inosine monophosphate to guanosine monophosphate (GMP), which is required for the production of nucleic acids and other critical steps in cellular activation. Lymphocytes require the de novo synthesis of GMP, so that MPA causes a profound inhibition of T- and B-cell function. Most other cells possess a salvage pathway that permits a resynthesis of guanine derivatives and are relatively resistant to MPA. EC-MPS is an enteric-coated formulation of mycophenolate sodium that releases the active moiety MPA in the small intestine instead of the stomach with the aim of improving MPA-related upper GI adverse events.

The recommended initial dosing of MMF is 1 g administered twice daily, whereas the recommended dose of EC-MPS is 720 mg administered twice daily 1 hour before or 2 hours after food intake. For African Americans, a higher dose (the equivalent of 1.5 g twice daily) is preferable when given with

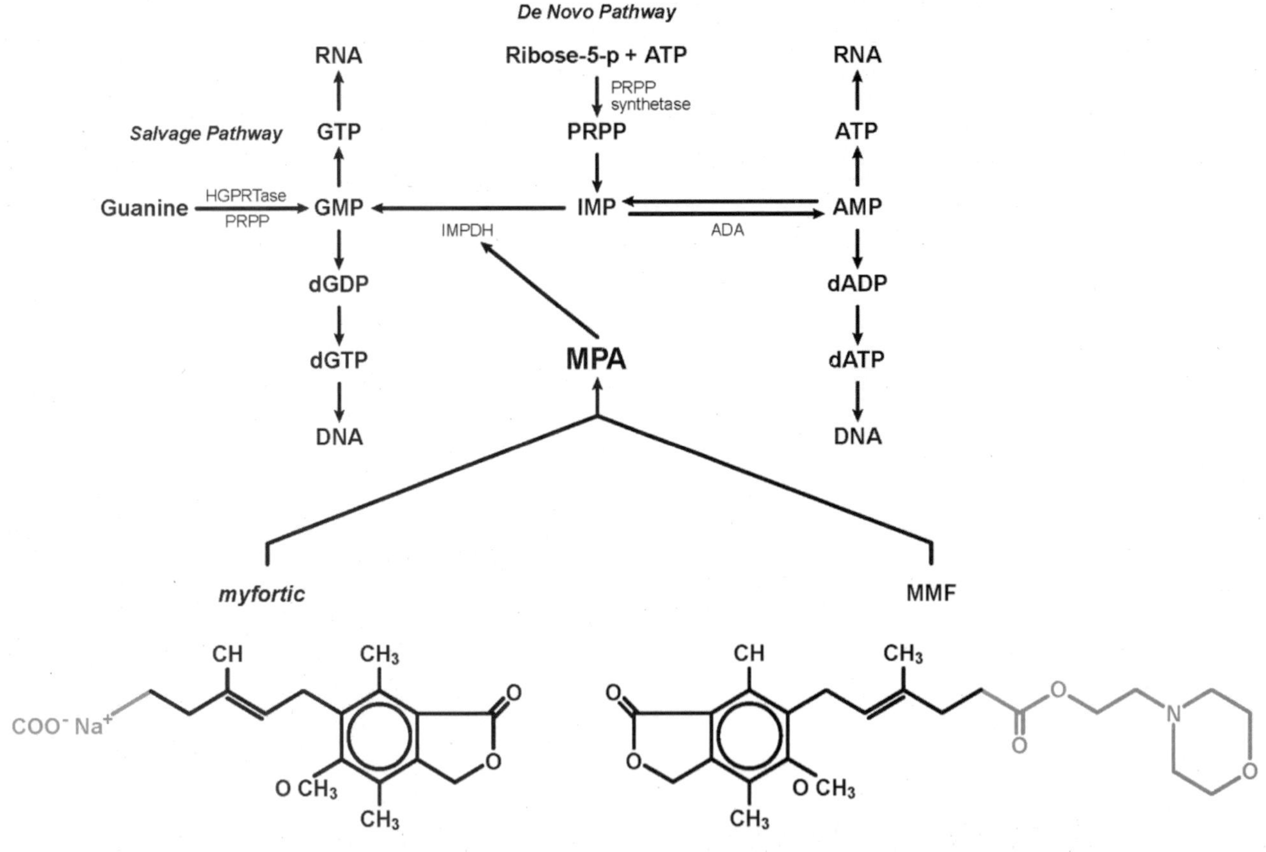

FIGURE 82.11 The site of inhibition by mycophenolic acid (MPA). MPA is the active moiety of myfortic (MMF). It is a potent, selective, and reversible inhibitor of inosine monophosphate dehydrogenase (*IMPDH*). The de novo pathway for the generation of guanosine monophosphate (*GMP*) is dependent on the conversion of inosine monophosphate (IMP) by IMPDH. *GTP*, guanasine triphosphate; *PRPP*, phosphoribosyl pyrophosphate; *AMP*, adenosine monophosphate; *dGDP*, deoxyguanosine diphosphate; *dGTP*, deoxyguanosine triphosphate. (From Allison AC, Eugui EM, Sollinger HW. Mycophenolate mofetil (RS-61443): mechanisms of action and effects in transplantation. *Transplantation Reviews* 1993;7:129–139.)

CsA. Efficacy is similar between EC-MPS and MMF in both de novo and maintenance patients. In the de novo setting, the incidence of GI adverse events was comparable between the two treatment groups throughout the 12-month study period, but the incidence of dose changes due to GI side effects was lower in the EC-MPS group, suggesting potentially less severe GI adverse events.[169]

Therapeutic drug monitoring of mycophenolate has not consistently correlated with outcomes, and in particular has not been formally tested in the case of EC-MPS.[170] high performance liquid chromatography (HPLC) methods have been established for the measurement of MMF, MPA, and mycophenolic acid glucuronide (MPAG), the principal metabolite that is pharmacologically inactive. Orally administered MMF is rapidly absorbed and hydrolyzed to MPA in the liver and is then glucuronidated to an inactive form of MPAG. The bioavailability of MMF is 90% with a half-life of 12 hours. There is no accumulation of MPA in hepatic or renal impairment. The maximum concentration of MPA and the area under the curve (AUC) value determined immediately after transplantation were only 30% to 50% of those measured for patients 3 months after transplantation, suggesting a need to increase dosing in the immediate posttransplant period. There is evidence of pharmacologic interaction between MMF and TAC, in that MPA exposure increases when MMF is used with TAC compared to cyclosporine.

The major side effects of MMF and EC-MPA include mild neutropenia and GI intolerance, such as diarrhea, esophagitis, and gastritis at high doses. The reason for leukopenia in transplant patients treated with MMF remains to be determined, because leukopenia was not predicted based on the mechanism of action of MMF and was not noted in patients with psoriasis or rheumatoid arthritis who were treated with this drug. The incidence of infection is not increased overall, although there may be a slight increase in tissue-invasive cytomegalovirus infection of the GI tract and liver.[171]

The mTOR Inhibitors: Sirolimus and Everolimus

mTOR is a regulatory kinase in the process of cell division. The term mTOR inhibitor refers to two similar immunosuppressant drugs, the mode of action of which is closely linked to the inhibition of this kinase. Sirolimus (SRL), also known as rapamycin, is a macrolide antibiotic compound that is structurally related to TAC and was approved in 1999 in the United States for the prophylaxis of organ rejection in patients receiving renal transplants. Everolimus (EVL, Zortress or Certican) is a structural analog of sirolimus with greater bioavailability (18% versus 10%) and a shorter half-life (18 to 35 hours versus 62 hours) than sirolimus. Everolimus was approved for use in kidney transplant recipients in Europe in 2005 and in the United States for low-to-moderate risk recipients in 2010.

The immunosuppressive function of the mTORi SRL and EVL ultimately results from the inhibition of cytokine and growth-factor activity upon T, B, and nonimmune cells. mTORi bind to the immunophilin FK506-binding protein 12 (FKBP12), a property shared with TAC. However, instead of inhibiting calcineurin like the TAC-FKBP12 complex, the EVL-FKBP12 complex inhibits the protein kinase mTOR, which causes an arrest in the G1 cell cycle.[172] mTOR belongs to the phosphoinositide 3-kinase (PI3K)-related protein kinases (PIKK) family and its signaling pathway couples energy and nutrient abundance to the execution of cell growth and division. mTOR complex 1 (mTORC1) and mTORC2 exert their actions by regulating other important kinases, such as S6 kinase (S6K) and Akt. At therapeutically relevant concentrations, the mTORi-FKBP12 complex mainly inhibits mTORC1 and thus inactivates the p70 S6 kinase in lymphocytes, resulting in the selective inhibition of the synthesis of ribosomal proteins and thus immunosuppression.

SRL is given at a dose of 2 to 6 mg orally once daily 4 hours after the morning dose of either CsA or concomitantly with TAC. A loading dose of 6 to 12 mg is often given on the first day of treatment due to its long half-life. The concomitant administration of SRL and Neoral formulation of CsA increased the AUC for SRL by 230% compared with the administration of SRL alone, whereas the administration 4 hours after the CsA dose increased the AUC by 80%. For this reason, it is recommended that SRL be administered 4 hours after the morning CsA dose. The pharmacologic interaction between SRL and TAC has not been rigorously explored. The recommended target trough levels vary between 5 to 15 ng per deciliter. Blood levels of SRL can be determined by HPLC with ultraviolet (UV) light detection or HPLC–mass spectrometry.

EVL can be started at 0.75 to 1.5 mg orally twice daily without a loading dose and can be given concomitantly with either CsA or TAC. The recommended therapeutic range for trough blood concentrations is 3 to 8 ng per milliliter in combination with CNIs. Potential benefits of the shorter half-life of EVL include the lack of necessity for a loading dose, the fact that the steady state is reached more quickly, and the fact that the drug is eliminated more quickly, which may permit a more rapid clinical response to changes in dose (e.g., in response to a drug–drug interaction or side effect).

The primary systemic side effects of mTORi are dyslipidemia, thrombocytopenia, and delayed wound healing. Side effects specific to kidney transplantation include increased lymphocele formation, proteinuria, the potential for prolongation of delayed graft function, and an enhancement of CNI-related nephrotoxicity. Although the drug is minimally nephrotoxic when used alone, the combination of SRL and CsA has caused synergistic toxicity in animals.[173] The mechanisms for the increased association of proteinuria with mTORi may include a loss of tubular reabsorption of protein, an inhibitory action of SRL on vascular endothelial growth factor, and a loss of nephrin in glomeruli.[174,175]

Azathioprine

Azathioprine (AZA) is an antimetabolite, a purine analog that incorporates into cellular DNA and inhibits the synthesis and metabolism of RNA. AZA was first used as an immunosuppressive agent for kidney transplantation in 1962,[176] and for many years AZA at a dose of 1.75 to 2.5 mg/kg/day was used with high-dose steroids. Prior to the introduction of CsA in the 1980s, AZA and steroids were the mainstays of maintenance immunosuppression. Although largely replaced by mycophenolate and mTORi, due to better antirejection efficacy with the latter agents, its use is still of value in reducing medication costs and as a safe alternative in pregnancy.

When used as a secondary agent in combination with a CNI or mTORi, 1 to 2 mg/kg/day in a single oral dose is recommended. When used as the primary immunosuppressant, the dose should be increased to 2 to 3 mg/kg/day.

AZA can cause bone marrow depression with granulocytopenia, hepatic dysfunction, pancreatitis, and an increased risk of infection and neoplasia. Macrocytic anemia with megaloblastic erythrocytosis, pure red cell aplasia, thrombocytopenia, and suppression of all marrow cell lines have been reported. Trimethoprim–sulfamethoxazole, when administered with AZA, may lead to neutropenia and thrombocytopenia, possibly because of the antibiotic's antifolate effect, resulting in enhanced 6-MP marrow toxicity. Similarly, allopurinol inhibits the breakdown of AZA and thus acts to enhance drug exposure; concomitant allopurinol and AZA use is therefore discouraged. If necessary, AZA should be reduced by 25% to 50% when starting allopurinol, with frequent white blood cell and platelet count monitoring.

Selection of Antimetabolite

Clinical decision making as to whether a mycophenolate agent, an mTORi, or AZA should be used for a given patient is usually determined by efficacy (the prevention of acute rejection) and the side effect profile. When used in conjunction with CNI (without depleting induction therapy), AZA is considered to be inferior to MPA in preventing acute rejection based on MMF registration trials, and mTORi is considered to be at least equally effective in preventing acute rejection.[177–179] The Tricontinental Mycophenolate Mofetil Renal Transplantation Study Group compared the effectiveness of MMF at two doses: 3 g per day (164 patients) and 2 g per day (173 patients), to AZA (100 to 150 mg per day, 166 patients). Patients were treated with equivalent doses of corticosteroids and CsA. The MMF groups have a lower incidence of rejection—16% and 20% versus 36% with AZA; decreased use of antilymphocyte antibody for severe or steroid-resistant rejection episodes (4.9% and 8.8% versus 15.4%); and a nonsignificant trend toward improved graft survival at 1 year. At 3 years, both MMF groups continued to show a nonsignificant trend toward better graft survival and a lower rate of graft loss from rejection as compared to the AZA group.

When comparing acute rejection rates and short-term graft outcomes with MPA versus mTORi-containing, CNI-based regimens, acute rejection rates generally are comparable.[180] However, GFR on >1 year follow-up in most studies tends to be lower with mTORi, and registry analyses suggest a slight decrease in 5-year graft survival using TORi versus MPA as the antiproliferative agent.[181,182] This is likely due to enhanced CNI toxicity, which is noted with mTORi versus MPA. A reduction in CNI exposure with mTORi use may lead to similar kidney function without increasing acute rejection rates.[179]

With regard to differences in side effect profiles between antiproliferative agents, AZA is associated with the fewest side effects necessitating discontinuation, whereas mTORi tends to have the highest rates of discontinuation. Common side effects that prompt a transition from one agent to another include skin cancer/other malignancy (transition from AZA or MPA to mTORi), GI side effects (MPA to AZA or mTORi), and proteinuria (mTORi to MPA or AZA).

Calcineurin Inhibitor Avoidance and Minimization Strategies

Given the nephrotoxicity as well as metabolic and cosmetic side effects common with CNI use, the elimination or withdrawal of CNI from maintenance immunosuppression has been an area of active study. CNI minimization strategies can be segregated to (1) CNI avoidance, and (2) CNI withdrawal/conversion at time points following early CNI use (either "early" withdrawal/conversion, typically 3 to 6 months posttransplant, or "late" withdrawal/conversion, following the identification of graft dysfunction).

Calcineurin Inhibitor Avoidance. Most trials suggest that MMF/prednisone is inadequate for initial immunosuppression due to unacceptably high acute rejection rates of 50% to 70%. De novo SRL/MMF/prednisone maintenance immunosuppression has met with mixed results, with most randomized trials suggesting an increased acute rejection rate compared to CNI/MMF/prednisone-based control groups. A retrospective analysis from registry data also supports the findings of inferior graft survival and higher discontinuation rates in patients maintained on SRL/MMF compared to CNI/MMF combinations. In the largest comparison of SRL-based immunosuppression versus TAC or CsA-based immunosuppression (the ELITE-Symphony study), acute rejection rate at 1 year within the SRL cohort (goal trough 4 to 8 ng per milliliter) was 37% with 1-year graft survival of 89%, whereas in the low dose CsA cohort (trough 50 to 100 ng per milliliter) acute rejection at 1 year was 24%, and in the low dose tacrolimus (trough 3 to 7 ng per milliliter) cohort, acute rejection rate was 12%.[166] These findings have generally dampened enthusiasm for de novo CNI avoidance with medications currently available for use in transplantation.

Calcineurin Inhibitor Withdrawal (Early: 1 to 6 Months Posttransplant). Given the acute rejection rates noted previously with CNI avoidance and the perioperative complications that may result from mTORi such as an increased rate of lymphocele formation and delayed wound healing, an alternative strategy to de novo CNI avoidance is a brief period of CNI followed by CNI withdrawal, with or without addition of another agent. In the large, prospective, multicenter CEASAR study, 536 patients on CsA, MMF, and prednisone maintenance were randomized to either undergo CsA withdrawal at 4 months, continue standard dose CsA (trough 150 to 300 ng per milliliter), or taper to low dose CsA (trough 50 to 100 ng per milliliter).[183] Although no difference was seen in the primary end point of GFR at 12 months, significantly higher rejection rates were noted in the CsA withdrawal group (38%) compared to either of the CsA continuation groups (25% to 27%). With SRL as the antiproliferative agent, 430 patients in the multicenter Rapamune Maintenance Regimen Trial on CsA, SRL, and prednisone were randomized to CsA withdrawal and increased SRL target trough levels 3 months after transplant, or remained on triple therapy. At 1 and 4 years, GFR was significantly better in the CsA withdrawal arm, despite a nominally higher acute rejection rate.[184] Although SRL may be more effective than MMF in CNI withdrawal strategies in combination with prednisone, issues of tolerability may limit this approach. To address this, the Spare the Nephron trial studied the efficacy and tolerability of the combination of both lower dose SRL and MMF in patients who undergo CNI discontinuation 1 to 6 months posttransplantation. Although this regimen was better tolerated and did not lead to an increase in acute rejection rates, differences in GFR using the CNI withdrawal strategy were small and not statistically significant after 24 months.[185]

Later Calcineurin Inhibitor Withdrawal/Conversion. When GFR is noted to steadily deteriorate or when biopsy findings suggest chronic nephrotoxicity and/or fibrosis, it is unclear if CNI withdrawal is safe or beneficial in slowing the rate of graft loss. A suggestion of benefit was noted in the Creeping Creatinine study,[186] in which the effect of removing CsA with MMF maintenance was compared to CsA maintenance (either alone or in combination with AZA or steroids). GFR stabilized without episodes of acute rejection in patients who underwent CsA discontinuation.[186] Another common CNI withdrawal strategy is conversion from CNI to SRL in patients on a CNI/MMF/prednisone regimen. Data from the multicenter randomized CONVERT trial, in which 830 patients 6 to 60 months post–kidney transplant were randomized 2:1 to SRL conversion versus CNI maintenance, suggests that subjects with GFR >40 mL per minute and minimal proteinuria (urine protein/creatinine ratio <0.11) at baseline experienced improved renal function at 24 months following CNI conversion to SRL without increased acute rejection rates, whereas those with proteinuria or GFR <40 mL per minute did not derive benefit from the transition.[187] As with single center experiences, improvements in renal function are noted, but issues of increased proteinuria and high rates of discontinuation of SRL due to adverse events remain common themes.[188] Taken together, CNI withdrawal appears most promising after a period of stability but prior to significant graft dysfunction. Novel agents currently are under investigation and may prove to be more effective than our current immunosuppressive agents in achieving CNI-free immunosuppression.

New Immunosuppressive Agents

New agents such as janus kinase (JAK) inhibitors, costimulatory blockade (primarily cytotoxic T-lymphocyte-associated protein 4-immunoglobulin [CTLA4-Ig] and anti-CD154 mAb), and PKC inhibitors are currently under experimental and clinical studies for maintenance immunosuppression as well as for the treatment of acute rejection.[189] Of these, the CTLA4-Ig Belatacept has completed phase II/III clinical trials.[190] In a CNI-free regimen, belatacept in combination with MMF and prednisone demonstrated improved GFR, less findings of interstitial fibrosis on biopsy, and less formation of donor-specific antibodies at 1 year compared to CsA-based immunosuppresion, but was also paradoxically associated with higher acute rejection rates and a higher incidence of posttransplant lymphoproliferative disease.[191] Longer-term follow-up of these findings will determine whether this agent becomes available for use in kidney transplantation.

COMMON POSTTRANSPLANT COMPLICATIONS

Surgical Complications of Renal Transplantation

The surgical technique of renal transplantation is reasonably standardized and overall direct surgical complication rates are low, accounting for only a small percentage of graft losses. Nevertheless, the transplant physician must be familiar with the diagnosis and treatment of surgically related complications to minimize recipient morbidity and mortality. The allograft is placed extraperitoneally into the iliac fossa in most cases. Thus, intraperitoneal bleeding, or bowel obstruction from adhesions or internal herniation, should not occur as a direct result of the surgery. In small children or in some recipients with a supravesical urinary diversion, the transplant is placed intraperitoneally and the potential surgical complications listed previously must be considered.

Wound Complications

The most important causes of wound infections stem from the operative complications of hematomas, urine leaks, and lymphoceles. Transplant recipients are vulnerable to wound infections because of postoperative immunosuppressive medications and poorly controlled uremia. Wound infections following transplantation are extremely bothersome, because if they are deep-seated infections around the arterial anastomosis, a secondary hemorrhage may occur. On presentation of a wound infection, adequate drainage should be provided immediately and appropriate antibiotic therapy should be introduced. However, the prevention of contamination during a donor nephrectomy and the use of preventive antibiotics before transplantation should ensure that the incidence of wound infection after transplantation is no more than 3% or 4%.

Patients with high fever but benign-appearing incision sites can harbor large purulent abscesses, emphasizing the effect of steroids on masking signs of inflammation. If unexplained fevers persist, ultrasonography or computed tomography (CT) scanning of the wound may localize a fluid collection; needle aspiration of a fluid collection is indicated. Prophylaxis with the administration of intraoperative intravenous antibiotics has reduced both wound infections and sepsis.

Bleeding

A secondary hemorrhage following a renal transplant is, fortunately, an unusual event and is always secondary to infection, which usually has been introduced at the time of operation. During a fulminant rejection episode, acute swelling of the kidney may lead to rupture through its cortex, often originating at a previous biopsy site. Urgent surgical exploration is necessary in most cases of hemorrhage. The kidney and its surroundings should be examined, the source of bleeding should be identified if possible, and the wound should be evacuated to eliminate a potential nidus of infection. If a small cortical rupture is present without a venous obstruction, it may be repaired by packing it with autologous muscle or microfibrillar collagen. If the rupture is large or venous compromise is present, transplant nephrectomy is almost invariably indicated.

Vascular Complications

Arterial Thrombosis. A thrombosis of the renal artery is a rare complication in the early days after transplantation, probably due both to the high flow through the kidney and also to the associated anemia and coagulation defects present in most patients with end-stage renal failure. It occurs in less than 1% of renal transplants. Factors that may predispose one to thrombosis include a preexisting hypercoagulable state, technical difficulties with the anastomosis, heavy arteriosclerotic involvement of recipient or donor vessels, kidneys with multiple renal arteries, and hypotension. Thrombosis may also occur owing to CsA-associated arteriopathy or because of hyperacute humoral rejection. CsA has been associated with increased thromboembolic complications, possibly because of the enhancement of platelet aggregation. Thrombosis due to an error in suture technique may occur in any case, but would be extraordinarily rare in an end-to-side anastomosis performed between a patch of donor aorta to an arteriotomy in the common or external iliac artery. In the later weeks after transplantation, renal artery thrombosis may be seen secondarily to arteriolar thrombosis in an acutely rejecting kidney, but the major vessel thrombosis is not the primary event. A renogram will quickly establish the presence of an arterial blood supply to the kidney if this is in doubt.

A sudden cessation of urine flow in the setting of a previously working allograft and a patent urinary catheter should suggest the possibility of renal artery thrombosis. An emergency renal ultrasound study or radionuclide renal scan will confirm the presence or absence of parenchymal blood flow. A digital subtraction angiogram is reserved for the very few cases with a no flow renal scan. Attempts to remove the thrombus are usually unsuccessful because of extensive intrarenal clotting beyond the main arterial branches.

Venous Thrombosis. Thrombosis of the renal vein as an acute event in the transplanted kidney is unusual and is usually due to a technical mishap at the time of operation. Thrombosis of the renal vein at some later period after transplantation is probably more common than is realized. It may occur secondarily to thrombosis of the common iliac vein or may occur occasionally as the primary event. Venous thrombosis may be related to CsA use, but it may also occur after placement of the allograft into a tight scarred, retroperitoneal pocket after removal of a previous graft.

In the absence of the clinical features of thrombosis of the common iliac vein, thrombosis of the renal vein itself may present with proteinuria and a marked increase in the size of the kidney, but may also occur without any notable features. A partial obstruction of the iliac vein by the pressure of the allograft can produce unilateral leg swelling on the side of the graft and rarely may lead to deep venous thrombosis. If the diagnosis of deep venous thrombosis is confirmed by Doppler plethysmography or venography, anticoagulation therapy should be initiated unless there are absolute contraindications. A venography is the best test to confirm the diagnosis.

Treatment for a well-localized thrombosis involves a thrombectomy and revascularization. Alternatively, it can be treated with systemic anticoagulation. Treatment often is successful if the condition was due to a transient hypercoagulable state, but rarely succeeds if the process was one manifestation of severe rejection and high renal vascular resistance with low flow. In practical terms, however, by the time the diagnosis is confirmed by angiography or radionuclide scanning, salvage of the kidney is unlikely and transplant nephrectomy is the usual outcome. Deep vein thrombosis occurs with a frequency of around 10% of transplant patients. Anticoagulation of these patients for several months is required because a pulmonary embolism is not an uncommon cause of death in renal transplant patients.

Other Vascular Problems. In kidneys with multiple renal arteries, the thrombosis of a polar branch can lead to ureteral necrosis or segmental parenchymal infarction with the potential development of a calyceal cutaneous fistula. Careful attention to these tenuous, small-caliber polar branches has decreased the incidence of these complications. In cadaveric kidneys harvested en bloc, a small aortic cuff (Carrel patch) can be made surrounding the orifices of the renal arteries. The cuff can then be anastomosed end to side to the external iliac artery, thus preventing any possibility of anastomotic compromise. If no cuff is available, the polar branches can be anastomosed end to side to the main renal artery, followed by anastomosis of the main artery to the recipient.

Many male patients with ESRD have erectile dysfunction because of decreased penile arterial flow, neuropathy, or both. Repeat transplant recipients should have an end-to-side reno-iliac arterial anastomosis if the contralateral hypogastric artery was used in the first transplant.

Urologic Complications

An accurate evaluation of lower urinary tract function prior to transplantation is important to minimize postoperative urologic complications. There are many approaches to the correction of these urologic complications, but, as a general rule, the approach should be early and aggressive rather than conservative. Many of the complications are preventable with careful attention to the technique of donor nephrectomy.

Urine Leak. Urine leak is an infrequent but serious problem and occurs in approximately 2% of renal transplant patients. It is seen early after transplantation and is usually secondary to necrosis of the entire or distal portion of the ureter or to infarction of the renal pelvis. This usually is due to the interruption or thrombosis of the ureteral artery, which is the main arterial supply to the donor ureter.

The source of the leak may be from the ureter, calyces, or the bladder. Upper urinary tract leakage is due to ischemia resulting from the loss of vascular supply during organ procurement. The preservation of hilar vessels and periurethral fat and adventitia is the key to prevention of this problem. A bladder urine leak may occur at the site of the ureteral reimplant or along the cystotomy closure.

The clinical presentation of a urine leak may be subtle unless a wound drain is in place. The leakage of urine from the lower end of the ureter is not usually evident until at least 1 week after transplantation and often much later. It may be associated with a decrease in urine output, fever, local tenderness, and swelling due to the localized collection of urine known as urinoma. Other clinical signs include unexplained fever and edema of the scrotum, labia, or thigh ipsilateral to the graft.

An ultrasonography is the preferred study for diagnosis of a suspected urine leak. Aspiration of the fluid mass and comparison of the fluid creatinine or urea content to serum values confirms the diagnosis of a urine leak. The dynamic phase of a renal scan also may demonstrate urinary extravasation. A cystography with oblique and drainage films will confirm whether the leak is from the bladder. Confirmation of an upper urinary tract leakage is more difficult, because attempts at retrograde pyelography in the early postoperative period often are unsuccessful.

Urine is a strong chemical irritant to tissues and predisposes the fresh vascular anastomoses to infection. Prolonged catheter drainage may be adequate treatment for a small bladder leak. Insertion of a percutaneous nephrostomy or ureteral stent can also be used to provide initial urinary drainage and stabilization of the patient. After function returns to baseline, surgical reexploration and repair is usually attempted. If the distal ureter is necrotic or stenotic, the necrotic portion can be removed and the vascularized proximal ureter can be reimplanted into the bladder. If the ureter is too short or the renal pelvis is necrotic, the ipsilateral native ureter can be detached from the native kidney near the pelvis and connected to the renal transplant by means of a ureteropyeloplasty. The anastomosis is protected by a temporary nephrostomy and ureteral stent. If a native ureter is not available or adequate, then the bladder can be mobilized and a Boari flap ureteronephrostomy can be constructed, or the bladder is anastomosed directly to the kidney pelvis, and a nephrostomy tube is left in place for several weeks.

Ureteral Obstruction. Acute ureteral obstruction in the early postoperative period may be due to distal ischemia, infarction, or rejection. Transient obstruction by a clot in the ureter or bladder immediately postoperatively may cause erratic urine output and can usually be taken care of by bladder catheter irrigation. Technical error as an early cause of obstruction of the ureterovesical junction is rare. Oliguria or anuria in the immediate posttransplant period should make one suspect the diagnosis. A cystogram is usually performed first to rule out a bladder leak. The diagnosis is confirmed by the presence of hydronephrosis by ultrasonography (Fig. 82.12) or by decreased flow from ureter to bladder or evidence of extravasation on percutaneous nephrostogram (Fig. 82.13). The site of obstruction can be identified by an antegrade pyelogram. Occasionally, obstruction of the ureter may be secondary to a hydrocele or hematoma, which can occur after a percutaneous needle biopsy.

Obstruction of the ureter may occur at some time remote from transplantation, often due to the development of a stricture, presumably as a result of previous ischemia. Progressive stenosis of the distal transplant ureter secondary

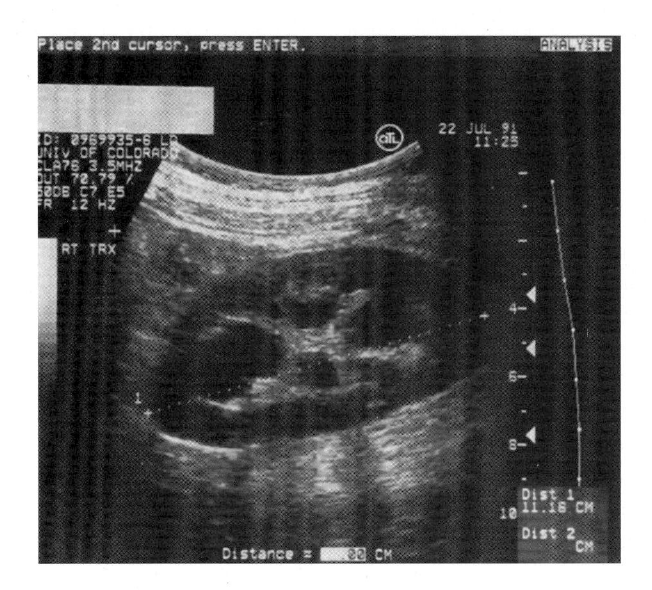

FIGURE 82.12 An ultrasound scan of a renal transplant showing hydronephrosis due to ureteric obstruction.

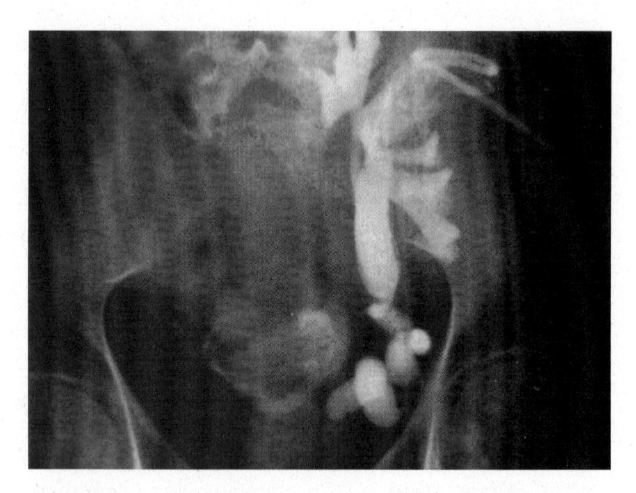

FIGURE 82.13 A percutaneous nephrostogram of a renal transplant. A nephrostomy tube placement with antegrade pyelogram to identify the site of obstruction.

to fibrosis or chronic ischemia may present as progressive azotemia over several months. An ultrasonography and an intravenous pyelogram or an antegrade pyelogram should confirm the diagnoses. A ureteric obstruction should always be considered in the patient with a gradual deterioration of renal function. Options for treatment include cystoscopic or percutaneous radiologic placement of an indwelling double-J ureteral stent, use of percutaneous nephrostomy, balloon dilatation, and surgical repair.

Reflux. Vesicoureteral reflux into the transplanted ureter has a reported incidence of 4% to 65%, depending on the technique of ureteral anastomosis; the creation of a distinct submucosal tunnel through the bladder wall has resulted in a lower incidence. The presence of vesicoureteral reflux in the transplanted allograft has not been found to increase the rate of urinary tract infections compared with nonrefluxing grafts.[192] Mathew and coworkers[193] found an increased incidence of proteinuria, microhematuria, hypertension, and graft failure in the refluxing group, a finding that has not been confirmed in additional studies.

Lymphocele. The major complication associated with lymphatics is the occurrence of a lymphocele, which usually presents in the first 2 or 3 months after transplantation as a large cystic mass in the vicinity of the kidney.[194] It is usually asymptomatic. Its presenting features are due to pressure on surrounding structures; it may cause deterioration in renal function due to pressure on the ureter, swelling of the leg due to pressure on the iliac vein, urgency due to pressure on the bladder, and diarrhea and tenesmus due to pressure on the rectum. An ultrasonography can confirm the presence of a perinephric (lymph) collection. Studies with radiolabeled lymph reveal that the major source of fluid in lymphoceles is from the lymphatics along the recipient iliac vessels and not from the renal hilum. Therefore, the meticulous ligation of the lymphatics during exposure of the vessels is the best prevention. Aspiration of the mass and measurement of fluid creatinine and potassium levels compared with the values in serum establishes the diagnosis of lymphocele and excludes urine leak, hematoma, or abscess. Sometimes, the lymphocele will not recur after two or three aspirations. However, if the lymphocele continues to recur, then it should be marsupialized into the peritoneal cavity after checking the aspirate for urine products and bacterial growth.

Assessing Renal Dysfunction in the Transplanted Kidney

An assessment of the cause of renal dysfunction is warranted in any patient with a sustained increase in serum creatinine >0.3 mg per deciliter or decrease in renal function of >20%. The differential diagnosis immediately following transplant (Table 82.13) and its assessment (Table 82.14) typically involves ruling out structural abnormalities with noninvasive testing, verifying drug level monitoring, and assessing for acute rejection. Noninvasive imaging of the transplanted kidney can be quite useful in differentiating the different causes of acute allograft dysfunction, particularly in the early posttransplant period.

Radionuclide Imaging. Renal perfusion can be assessed by technetium diethylene triamine pentaacetic acid (DTPA) or technetium-99m mercaptoacetyltriglycine (MAG3) and tubular function by iodohippurate (Hippuran) I^{131} uptake. A decline in initial renal blood flow and a decrease in tubular function often occur during acute rejection. Occasionally, scans can help diagnose uncommon posttransplant complications, such as venous thrombosis or urinary leak.

Ultrasound. Real-time and duplex Doppler sonography of the renal allograft is useful for evaluating recipients

TABLE 82.13 **Causes of Acute Renal Failure Associated with Renal Transplantation**

Prerenal	Hypovolemia Arterial stenosis or thrombosis Venous thrombosis
Renal	Acute tubular necrosis Hyperacute/accelerated rejection Acute rejection Nephrotoxicity
Postrenal	Ureteral obstruction Urinary leak Lymphocele Hematoma

TABLE 82.14 **Approach to the Patient with Acute Renal Failure Following Transplantation**

Immediate Acute Renal Failure (48 hr)
Rule out catheter obstruction
Rule out hypovolemia
Radioisotope scan to rule out vascular catastrophe
Ultrasound to rule out urinary extravasation or obstruction
Radiocontrast studies (if indicated by previous)
Early or Late Acute Renal Failure (After 48 hr)
History and physical examination to detect oliguria, tender swelling graft, fever
Urine sodium, FENa (especially if baseline available)
CsA or tacrolimus levels
Radioisotope scan
Ultrasound
Therapeutic trial of steroids/lowering cyclosporine dose
Renal biopsy

FENa, fractional excretion of sodium; CsA, cyclosporine.

with surgical complications, including perinephric fluid collections, hydronephrosis, and vascular complications (Fig. 82.14). The sonography reveals variable findings in acute rejection, such as graft enlargement, enhanced echogenicity of the parenchyma, and increased resistive index (>70%) of the vessels. The studies will not confirm the diagnosis of rejection, but will serve to exclude allograft thrombosis and urinary obstruction, and will indicate that a percutaneous transplant kidney biopsy with pathologic examination should be performed.

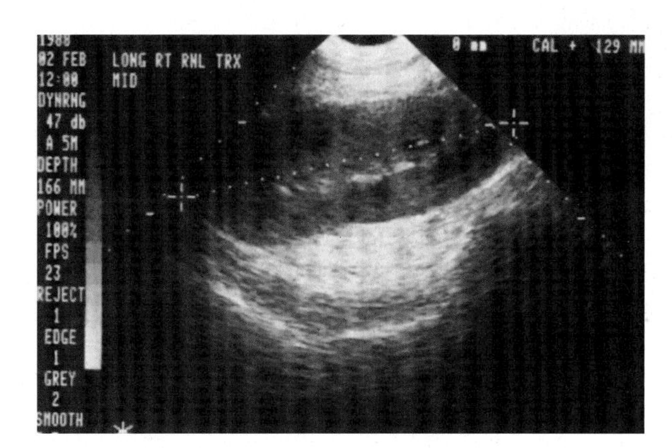

FIGURE 82.14 A normal renal ultrasound of a transplanted kidney.

Renal Transplant Biopsy. A biopsy will help to confirm the diagnosis of acute tubular necrosis (ATN) by the exclusion of a histologic picture of severe rejection (Table 82.15). A needle biopsy of the donor kidney just prior to or after implantation is helpful to detect renal disease or preservation injury that might confound the interpretation of delayed renal allograft function. However, a poor understanding of the natural history of transplant histology makes it an imperfect gold standard.

Technique of Renal Transplant Kidney Biopsy. The use of a percutaneous biopsy of the transplant kidney to diagnose rejection was first performed in 1967.[195] Since then, the technique has been well established as a useful tool in the differential diagnosis of allograft dysfunction. The position and alignment of the transplant kidney can vary from patient to patient (Fig. 82.15). In most instances, the transplant kidney is palpable and the orientation of the kidney can be estimated by reviewing an isotope scan of the transplant kidney (Fig. 82.16).

A biopsy can be obtained with a Vim–Silverman needle, a 14G to 16G disposable Tru-Cut biopsy needle, or an 18G

TABLE 82.15 **Histopathology of Renal Allograft Using Needle Biopsy**

Changes Associated with Rejection
Glomerular
Swelling of endothelium
Endothelial/mesangial proliferation
Exudation of polymorphs, mononuclear cells
Interstitial
Edema
Infiltration of mononuclear cells
Macrophages
Eosinophils
Vascular
Endothelial edema
Mural infiltration
Necrosis, hemorrhage
Severe vasculitis (especially interstitial hemorrhage) predicts eventual graft failure
Changes Associated with Cyclosporine
Tubular changes
Giant mitochondria
Vacuolization
Microcalcification
Interstitium
Mononuclear infiltration
Vascular changes
Arteriolar necrosis

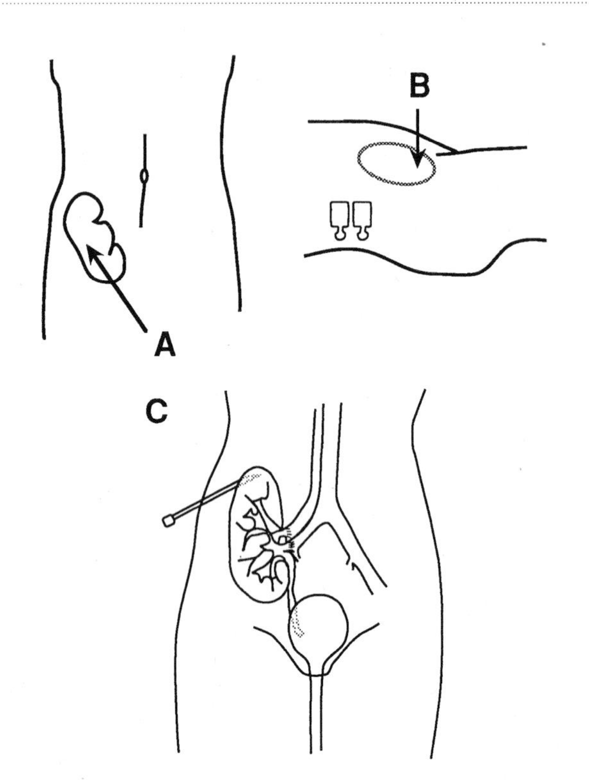

FIGURE 82.15 The site of biopsy for the transplanted kidney. The orientation of the transplanted kidney is localized by palpation and a review of the operative record and renal scan. The kidney is approached either tangentially or vertically **(A),** in a plane tangential to the lateral curvature of the allograft or **(B)** in a plane perpendicular to the kidney directed to the lower pole. **C:** Tangential across the upper pole of the transplanted kidney.

automatic Biopty or Monopty needle (Fig. 82.17). It is best performed under sonographic guidance. Relative contraindications to biopsy include abnormal coagulation studies or a low platelet count, an active urinary tract infection, and significant renal allograft hydronephrosis. Hydronephrosis, indicative of a urinary tract obstruction, should be further investigated. In patients with prolonged bleeding time due to uremia, intravenous desamino-D-arginine vasopressin (dDAVP) (0.3 μg per kilogram) can be used to correct the coagulation defect prior to a biopsy procedure. If the kidney has been transplanted via an intra-abdominal approach or is difficult to localize, then consideration should be given to a CT-guided direction, or occasionally, via a limited open surgical approach in the operating room. A biopsy considered adequate for analysis involves a sampling of at least 10 glomeruli and two small arteries, stained for hematoxylin and eosin (H&E), periodic acid-Schiff (PAS) or silver, and trichrome stains, whereas a biopsy with 7 to 9 glomeruli and one artery is considered of marginal adequacy. When performed for clinical indications (renal dysfunction), two separate cores should be obtained because the findings of rejection are often patchy in distribution.[196]

Novel Diagnostic Techniques. Although a percutaneous needle biopsy is currently the gold standard for the diagnosis of renal allograft dysfunction, it is a time- and resource-intensive invasive procedure that is subject to sampling error as well as potential procedure-related complications. The noninvasive diagnosis of allograft dysfunction using biomarker profiles is an attractive alternative to invasive methods, and numerous reports have described targets identified in either blood or urine samples that are predictive and/or diagnostic of events such as acute rejection (AR) and DGF.

Because cytotoxic T lymphocytes play a dominant role in cell-mediated rejection, their effector molecules perforin, granzyme B, and FasL have been assessed noninvasively in transplant recipients for correlation with clinical sequelae. These effector molecules have been shown to be upregulated in both the blood and urine of patients with AR in some[197] but not all[198] reports. Moreover, elevated levels of urine perforin, granzyme B, and FasL mRNA have been described in conditions of nonimmune-mediated graft injury, including

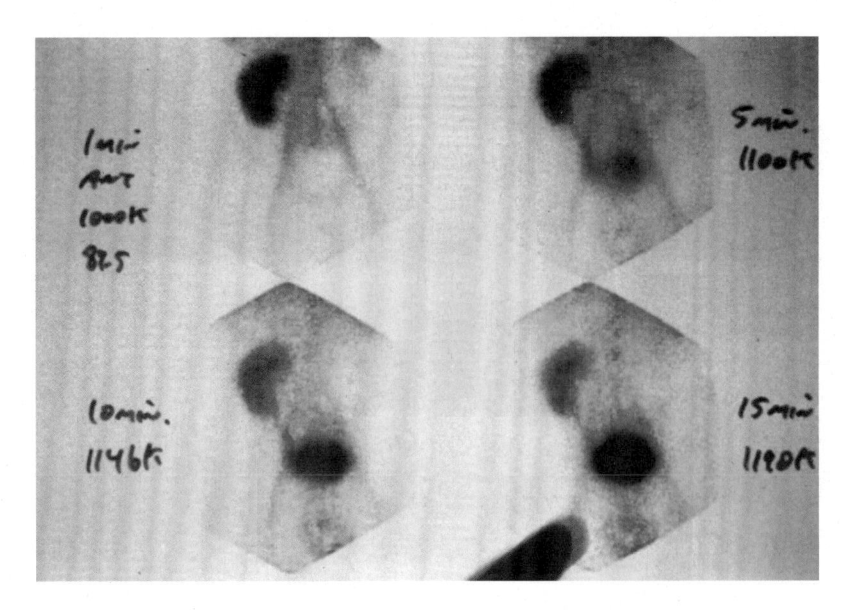

FIGURE 82.16 A diethylenetriamine pentaacetic acid scan showing good renal perfusion in a transplanted kidney.

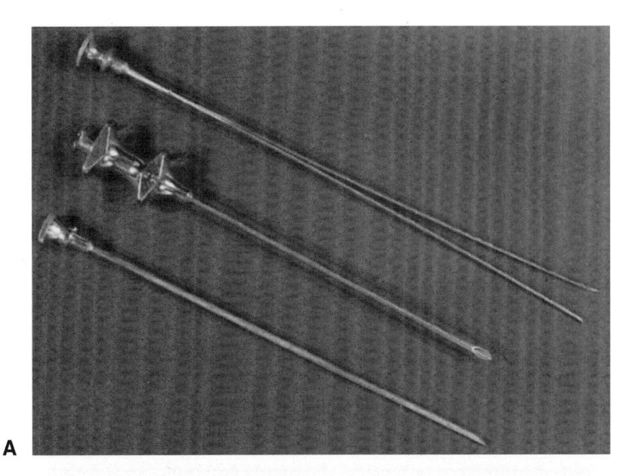

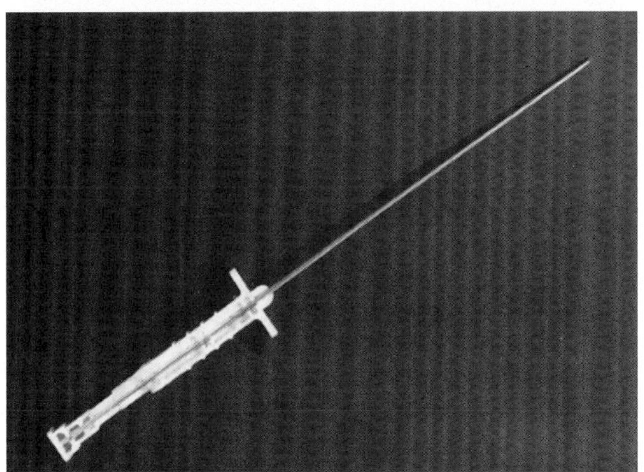

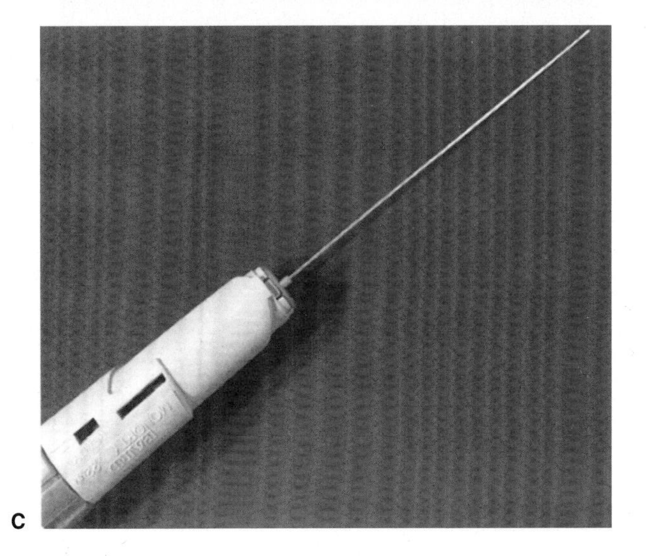

FIGURE 82.17 Different types of biopsy needles. **A:** Vim-Silverman. **B:** Tru-Cut 14 G (disposable needle). **C:** Biopty gun 18 G (disposable needle).

bacterial urinary tract infection, CMV infection, and DGF, potentially limiting their diagnostic use. Urinary levels of FOXP3 mRNA from T-regulatory cells has been shown to be increased in episodes of AR, and mRNA levels correlate with serum creatinine at the time of allograft biopsy.[199] TIM-3, a protein expressed on the surface of T-helper 1 cells, was also shown to be helpful in differentiating ATN from AR in 50 patients with DGF, where blood and urine mRNA levels were significantly higher in patients with AR with a sensitivity and specificity of 100%.[200] Finally, of interest in the setting of AMR is the Affymetrix microarray assay (Affymetrix Inc., Santa Clara, CA), which has shown higher intragraft expression of endothelial-associated transcripts in patients with AR compared to those without, and even higher levels in those with AMR versus cell-mediated rejection.[201] Despite the appeal of noninvasive diagnostic techniques and the encouraging data described previously, large clinical trials validating biomarkers as reliable alternatives to percutaneous biopsy have yet to be performed and their use remains experimental.

Medical Causes of Acute Allograft Injury

The transplanted kidney is susceptible to postsurgical, infectious, and immunologic insults, which are exacerbated by the lack of autoregulation that exists as a result of denervation following a kidney transplantation. In the immediate posttransplant period, there may be DGF or cessation of function after the initial good function. The most likely cause of renal failure during this period is ischemic tubular damage, but a vascular accident, ureteric obstruction, a urine leak, acute CNI nephrotoxicity, or rejection are all possible etiologies, and more than one cause of dysfunction can occur together (Table 82.13). Knowledge of the natural history of several clinical entities is extremely helpful in limiting the differential diagnosis.

Acute Tubular Necrosis

The pathogenesis of acute tubular necrosis (ATN) may arise from ischemic damage secondary to hypovolemia and hypotension in the donor and prolonged warm ischemia and cold ischemia during preservation. In the transplant setting, ATN is often interchangeable with DGF, although a complete diagnostic assessment should rule out all other causes prior to reaching this diagnosis. The most common definition of DGF is the need for dialysis within the first week following transplant. Using this definition, DGF is strongly associated with 1-year graft loss.[202]

Allograft Rejection

Rejection is a major cause of graft failure. It is important to diagnose acute rejection as soon as possible in order to promptly institute antirejection therapy. The classification can be made based on pathologic criteria with therapy directed at the specific pathogenic process (Table 82.16).

Hyperacute Antibody-Mediated Rejection. This form of rejection is caused by preformed antibodies against alloantigens that are present in response to previous exposure to antigens through prior transplantations, blood transfusions, or multiple pregnancies. When present at the time of surgery, alloantibody leads to the clinical manifestation of hyperacute rejection, a failure of the kidney to perfuse properly on

TABLE 82.16 **Banff 2007 Diagnostic Categories for Renal Allograft Biopsies**

1. Normal
   The presence of patchy mononuclear cell infiltrates without tubulitis is not uncommon in normally functioning renal allografts and, when considered alone, does not warrant the diagnosis of acute rejection.
2. Antibody-mediated rejection (Rejection demonstrated to be due, at least in part, to antidonor antibody)
   Acute:
   I. ATN-like: C4d+, minimal inflammation
   II. Capillary: margination and/or thromboses, C4d+
   III. Arterial: v3, C4d+
   Chronic: active antibody-mediated rejection (Glomerular double contours and/or peritubular capillary basement membrane multilayering and/or interstitial fibrosis/tubular atrophy and/or fibrous intimal thickening in arteries, C4d+)
3. Borderline changes: "Suspicious" for acute rejection, foci of tubulitis and no arteritis, not reaching threshold of IA that follows
   This category is used when no intimal arteritis is present, but there are foci of mild tubulitis (1 to 4 mononuclear cells/tubular cross-section)
4. T-cell–mediated rejection

Acute T-Cell–Mediated Rejection

Type (Grade)	Histopathologic Findings
IA	Cases with significant interstitial infiltration (>25% of parenchyma affected) and foci of moderate tubulitis (>4 mononuclear cells/tubular cross-section or group of 10 tubular cells)
IB	Cases with significant interstitial infiltration (>25% of parenchyma affected) and foci of severe tubulitis (>10 mononuclear cells/tubular cross-section or group of 10 tubular cells)
IIA	Cases with mild-to-moderate intimal arteritis
IIB	Cases with severe intimal arteritis comprising >25% of luminal area
III	Cases with "transmural" arteritis and/or arterial fibrinoid change and necrosis of medial smooth muscle cells

Chronic active T-cell–mediated rejection
(Chronic allograft arteriopathy: arterial intimal fibrosis with mononuclear cell infiltration in fibrosis, formation of neo-intima)

5. Interstitial fibrosis and tubular atrophy, no evidence of any specific etiology

Grade	Histopathologic Findings
I (mild)	Mild interstitial fibrosis and tubular atrophy (<25% of cortical area)
II (moderate)	Moderate interstitial fibrosis and tubular atrophy (26-50% of cortical area)
III (severe)	Severe interstitial fibrosis and tubular atrophy (>50% of cortical area)

6. Other changes not considered to be due to rejection
   Posttransplant lymphoproliferative disorder
   Polyomavirus-associated interstitial nephritis
   Acute tubular necrosis
   Acute interstitial nephritis
   Cyclosporine or FK506-associated change

release of the vascular clamps just after vascular anastomosis is completed. The kidney initially becomes firm and then rapidly becomes blue, spotted, and flabby. The presence of neutrophils in the glomeruli and peritubular capillaries in the kidney biopsy confirms the diagnosis, and is supported by the finding of markers of complement deposition (C4d) in peritubular capillaries.[203] It can be prevented by careful testing of recipients for the presence of the preformed cytotoxic antibodies. Although hyperacute rejection is rare due to effective pretransplant HLA typing and cross-matching, delayed

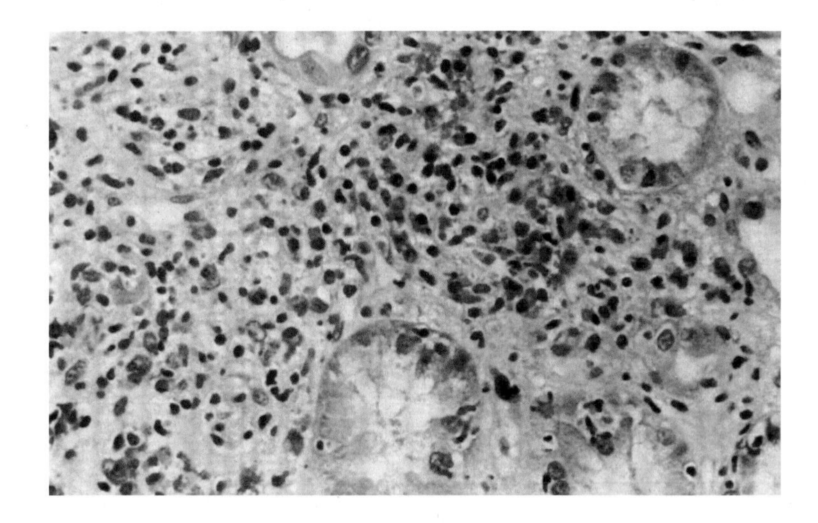

FIGURE 82.18 Acute cellular rejection, Banff 1b. A percutaneous renal transplant biopsy specimen showing tubulitis with tubular epithelial infiltrates of lymphocytes and plasma cells.

hyperacute rejection has become more common as centers attempt to transplant across incompatible HLA and ABO types with desensitization strategies. In the previously sensitized patient in whom preformed anti-HLA antibodies are present, the memory B-cell response is upregulated in the week following transplant and donor-specific antibodies are formed, which lead to rapid decline in renal function and a similar clinical picture to that mentioned for hyperacute rejection.

Acute antibody-mediated rejection can occur at any time following transplantation either in combination with a T-cell–mediated process, or in isolation with the development of donor specific antibodies (Table 82.16). Diagnosis is made by a triad of findings comprised of tissue injury (classically, peritubular capillaritis composed primarily of neutrophils), the presence of circulating antidonor antibodies (donor-specific antibodies), and evidence of complement activation via staining for C4d. Although the presence of all three findings is specific for acute antibody-mediated rejection, all three findings are not required to make this diagnosis and initiate therapy in the setting of rapid graft dysfunction.

Acute T-Cell–Mediated (Cellular) Rejection (ACR). Acute T-cell–mediated rejection (ACR) episodes may occur as early as 5 to 7 days, but are generally seen between 1 and 4 weeks after transplantation. The classic acute rejection episode of the earlier era in a patient treated with AZA/prednisone was accompanied by swelling and tenderness of the kidney and the onset of oliguria with an associated rise in serum creatinine, and was usually accompanied by a significant fever. However, in patients who have been treated with higher degrees of immunosuppression, the clinical features of an acute rejection can be minimal in that there is perhaps some swelling of the kidney, usually no tenderness, and there commonly is an absence of fever. Because such an acute rejection may occur at a time when there is a distinct possibility of acute CsA or TAC toxicity, the differentiation between the two entities may be extremely difficult and requires a biopsy for an accurate diagnosis.

Pathologic changes of acute cellular rejection include interstitial infiltration with mononuclear cells and disruption of the tubular basement membranes (tubulitis) by the infiltrating cells (Fig. 82.18).[196] The presence of patchy mononuclear cell infiltrates without tubulitis is not uncommon in normal functioning renal allografts and is not sufficient to make the diagnosis of acute rejection. The finding of interstitial infiltrates and tubulitis in a kidney transplant biopsy is not specific to acute cellular rejection and other etiologies such as viral nephropathy (BK virus, less commonly cytomegalovirus [CMV]), pyelonephritis, or posttransplant lymphoproliferative disease should be considered based on the clinical presentation. In contrast, the histologic finding of endothelialitis is pathognomonic of acute cellular rejection. The intrarenal arteries and arterioles show characteristic changes of intimal thickening and the presence of inflammatory cells within and adherent to the endothelium (Fig. 82.19). The glomerular changes are usually unremarkable in rejection. However, glomerular capillary and vascular intimal infiltrates can occur in the setting of mixed humoral and cellular rejection (Fig. 82.20). A periodic examination of histologic features in the absence of changes in renal function (protocol biopsies) may reveal silent allograft rejection (subclinical rejection). Although potentially predictive of chronic graft dysfunction, treatment of subclinical rejection is of unclear benefit.[204]

Treatment of acute rejection. Treatment of T-cell–mediated acute rejection is often directed by the findings on biopsy and the clinical response to pulse corticosteroids. For the patient with graft dysfunction and biopsy-proven rejection, treatment with intravenous methylprednisolone 3 to 5 mg per kilogram (250 to 500 mg per day) for 3 to 5 days is often effective if the histologic injury is tubulointerstitial (Banff class IA or IB) (see Fig. 82.18). If there is an inadequate response following corticosteroid pulse therapy or if there is vascular involvement (Banff class IIA, IIB) (Fig. 82.19), corticosteroids often must be supplemented with T-cell–depleting antibody therapies in a similar dosing strategy, but a longer treatment course when compared to their use for induction. Most studies have

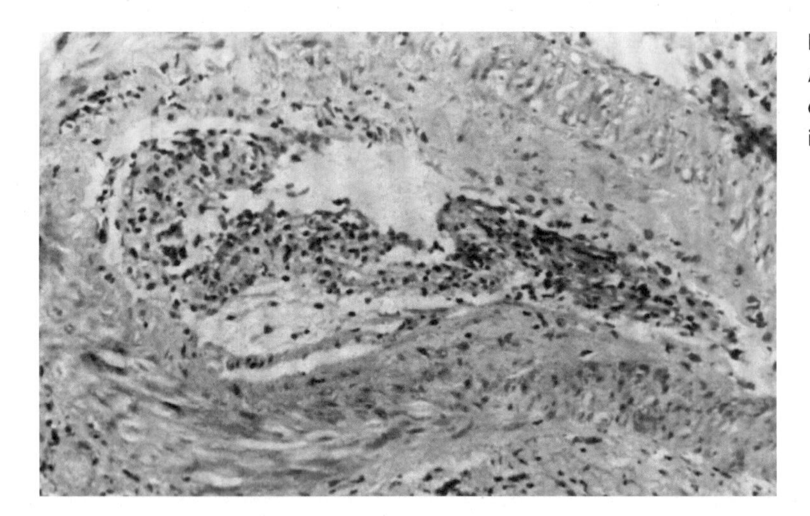

FIGURE 82.19 Acute cellular rejection, Banff IIb. A renal transplant biopsy specimen showing marked endovasculitis and acute inflammatory endothelial infiltrates.

used these agents in 7- to 14-day treatment courses, with no clinical trials investigating the efficacy of shorter courses versus longer courses. For patients who are on a maintenance regimen that is not TAC based, TAC conversion may also be considered in the setting of rejection with an inadequate response to corticosteroids. For patients on a corticosteroid-free regimen, the reinstitution of maintenance prednisone may be warranted. The treatment of acute antibody-mediated rejection is indicated when the triad of graft injury, C4d+ staining in peritubular capillaries on biopsy, and circulating donor-specific antibody is present, but should also be considered in high-risk circumstances (prior desensitization or known donor-specific antibody) even if all three criteria are not met. Treatment entails the removal of the pathogenic immunoglobulin(s) with plasma exchange and inhibition/suppression of antibody production with IVIG. In general at least 5 plasma exchange treatments should be administered with 1 to 2 g per kilogram total dose IVIG. Because IVIG is removed by plasma exchange, a common strategy employed is to administer IVIG 100 to 200 mg per kilogram after each exchange. For refractory acute humoral rejection, rituximab or bortezomib may be considered. Finally, there are case reports of splenectomy for refractory acute antibody-mediated rejection.[205] These therapies are typically coupled with targeted T-cell therapy such as high dose steroids and/or depleting antibody therapy, because helper T-cell function may contribute to an enhanced B-cell response.

Acute Calcineurin Inhibitor Nephrotoxicity. Nephrotoxicity is the most frequently encountered and the most important side effect of CNI therapy. Acute CNI nephrotoxicity can occur within days or weeks after renal transplantation. The pathogenesis of acute nephrotoxicity is due to a dose-dependent CNI-induced renal arteriolar vasoconstriction leading to a decline in renal blood flow with a consequent fall in GFR.[206] A small increment in serum creatinine occurs, which is frequently correlated with high serum CNI trough levels. Serum creatinine returns to baseline within 24 hours of reduction of CNI dosage. In the early posttransplant period, functional CNI nephrotoxicity has clinical features similar to those of acute renal allograft rejection, and an allograft biopsy specimen should be obtained if the diagnosis is uncertain. Histologically, acute CNI nephrotoxicity can be distinguished from acute rejection chiefly by the absence

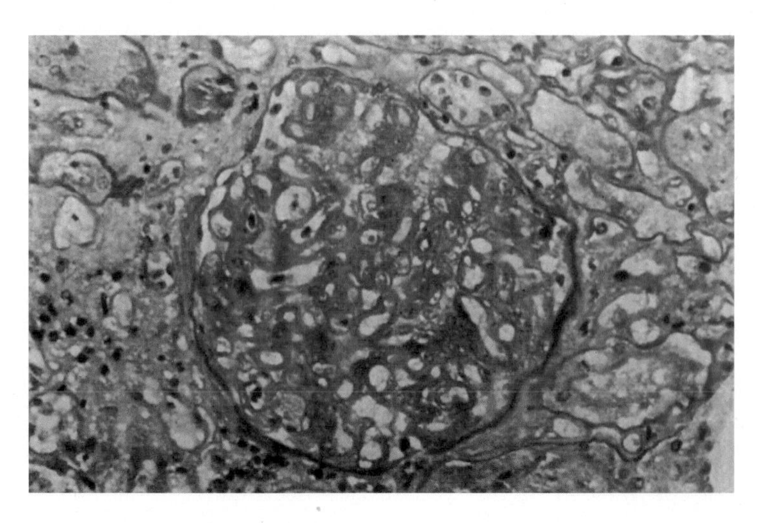

FIGURE 82.20 Acute cellular and humoral rejection. Glomerular and vascular endothelial infiltrates and swelling.

of an extensive inflammatory infiltrate. Rarely, a thrombotic microangiopathic vascular lesion can be seen, presumably due to endothelial injury. This appears to be more common with CsA than TAC and is more prevalent when mTORi is used rather than MPA as concurrent therapy.[59]

Causes of Subacute/Chronic Allograft Injury

Although early after transplant the differential diagnosis of graft dysfunction primarily involves surgical complications and acute rejection, after a period of stability, the progressive loss of graft function is common and is often due to both immunologic and nonimmunologic factors. Recently, a series of 1,317 patients who were on standard CNI-based immunosuppression were assessed by biopsy for etiologies for graft loss.[207] They reported that following the acute transplant period, the most common causes of graft loss were glomerular disease (37%), interstitial fibrosis/tubular atrophy (IF/TA) (31%), followed by acute rejection (12%) and other medical/surgical etiologies (16%). Graft losses due to glomerular injury were equally divided into recurrent glomerulonephritis, de novo glomerulonephritis, and glomerular disease associated with anti-HLA antibodies, whereas those due to IF/TA were comprised primarily of patients with prior acute rejection episodes, BK virus infections, and recurrent pyelonephritis episodes, which could explain the IF/TA lesion. Thus, the differential of subacute and chronic graft dysfunction must focus on glomerular etiologies and a determination of potential clinical clues that may lead to IF/TA.

Polyomavirus. Both the BK virus (*Polyomavirus hominis*) and the JC virus (*Polyomavirus hominis*) belong to the human Papovavirus family. About 60% to 80% of adults are seropositive for the BK virus. In immunocompetent individuals, the virus has little clinical significance, residing in a latent state in the kidney. However, in immunocompromised/suppressed patients, the BK virus can undergo replication, which leads to an immune response that causes an interstitial nephritis. In addition, renal allograft recipients were reported to have BK virus associated with ureteral stenosis and bone marrow transplant recipients from hemorrhagic cystitis. Histologically, it can be difficult to distinguish from the tubulitis and interstitial inflammation of acute cellular rejection. The presence of BKV-associated interstitial nephritis is suggested by the finding of large basophilic intranuclear viral inclusion bodies in tubular epithelial cells along the entire nephron and also the transitional cell layer and confirmed by special staining with SV40 (simian virus, related to BKV) immunohistochemical staining. Graft loss is common when identified late in its presentation, thus screening protocols have been recommended to detect early BKV reactivation in order to intervene at an earlier stage.[208] Screening can be from urine (via Papanicolaou staining for decoy cells or urine polymerase chain reaction [PCR]) or blood by PCR (Fig. 82.21). The primary risk factor for BK virus disease is high-dose immunosuppression. No established therapy for a polyomavirus infection is available and the reduction of immunosuppression offers the best therapeutic option. Leflunomide, cidofovir, IVIG, and corticosteroids have been used as potential therapeutic options but have not been studied in controlled trials.

Chronic Calcineurin Inhibitor Nephrotoxicity. The debate about long-term nephrotoxicity of CNI remains unresolved. Prospective biopsy series using CsA report a high incidence of lesions consistent with chronic CNI nephrotoxicity increasing to near universal presence over 10 years but without functional consequence, whereas a more recent series using TAC suggest that CNI-related fibrosis is uncommon and not uniformly progressive.[209,210] CNI-based immunosuppression can provide stable, long-term allograft function.[211] Support for the role of CNI in CKD derives primarily from nonrenal transplants in whom the cumulative incidence of CKD <30 mL per minute at 5 years ranged from 7% (recipients of heart–lung transplants) to 21% (recipients of intestine transplants).[212] While the classic renal biopsy findings of obliterative arteriopathy (suggesting primary endothelial damage), ischemic collapse or scarring of the glomeruli, vacuolization of the tubules, global and focal segmental glomerulosclerosis, and focal areas of tubular atrophy and interstitial fibrosis (producing a picture of striped fibrosis) may be present, unfortunately many of these lesions may overlap with lesions due to hypertension, vascular disease, or chronic T-cell–mediated rejection. Therefore, the diagnosis of isolated CNI nephrotoxicity may be an unusual occurrence.[207]

The treatment of chronic CNI nephrotoxicity is nonspecific, with immunosuppression manipulation (CNI dose reduction, withdrawal, or substitution with another agent) all meeting with modest and sporadic improvements, likely due to the significant overlap with other etiologies of renal injury that occur.

Chronic T-Cell–Mediated Rejection and Chronic Antibody-Mediated Rejection. Chronic antibody-mediated rejection is likely the result of an indolent alloimmune response that results in transplant glomerulopathy and arteriopathy. Although transplant glomerulopathy is often associated with circulating donor-specific antibodies and with C4d deposition, 30% to 50% of cases will be identified in the absence of these diagnostic markers.[213] This suggests that these lesions are not solely due to a humoral immune response, or that the lack of a temporal relationship of donor-specific antibodies or C4d deposition to biopsy findings is related to the waxing/waning nature of the humoral immune response. The diagnosis of chronic antibody-mediated rejection is suggested by (1) evidence of donor-specific antibodies, (2) C4d deposition in peritubular capillaries, and (3) evidence of chronic tissue injury. The forms of chronic tissue injury may include duplication of the glomerular basement membrane, multilamination of the peritubular capillary basement membrane, arterial intimal fibrosis without elastosis, and/or interstitial fibrosis with tubular atrophy.

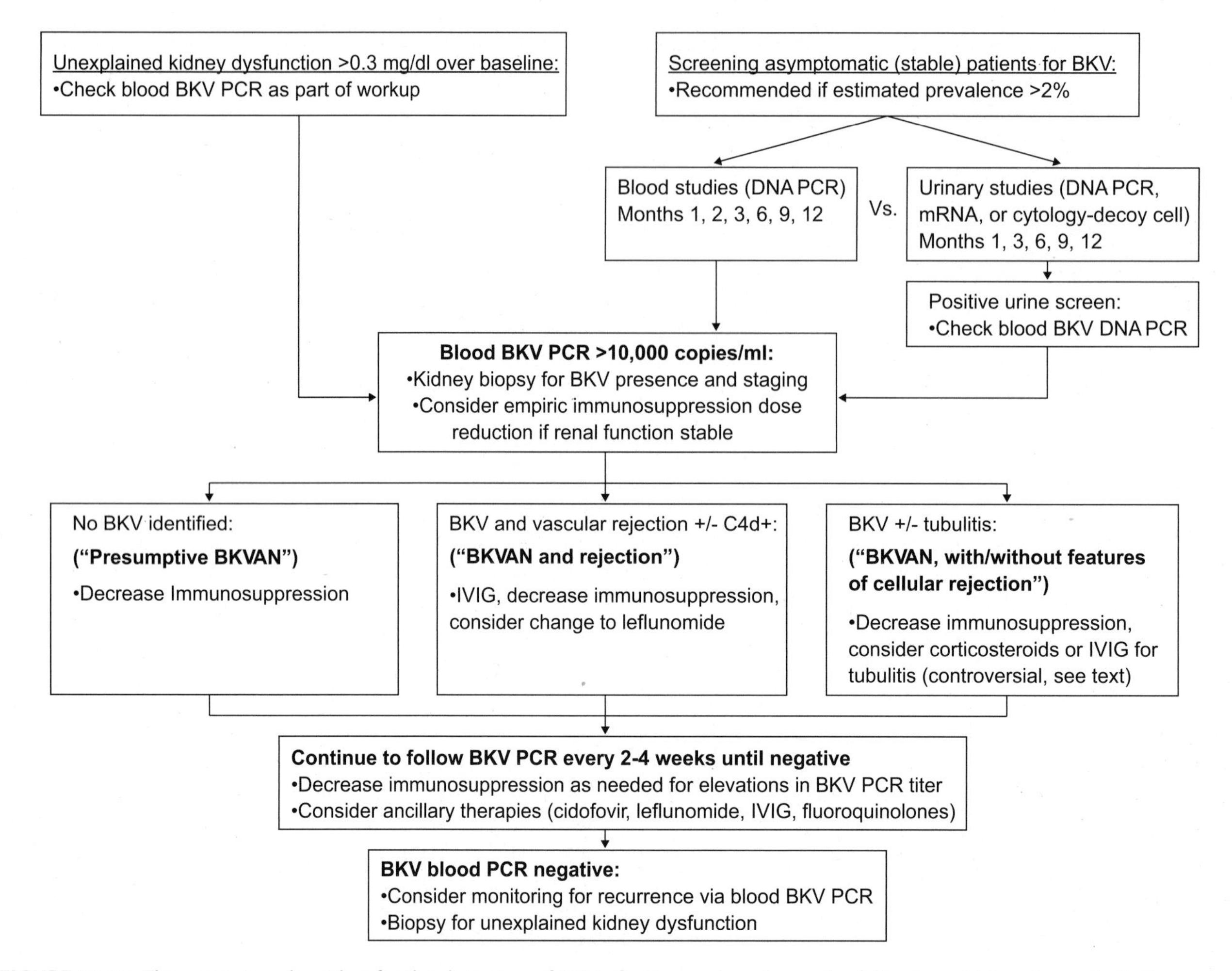

FIGURE 82.21 The screening algorithm for the detection of BKV infection and nephropathy following a kidney transplantation. *PCR,* polymerase chain reaction; *BKVAN,* BKV associated nephropathy; *IVIG,* intravenous immunoglobulin. (From Wiseman AC. Polyomavirus nephropathy: a current perspective and clinical considerations. *Am J Kidney Dis.* 2009;54(1):131–142, with permission.)

Chronic active T-cell–mediated rejection is a histologic diagnosis that refers to arterial intimal fibrosis, specifically with evidence of mononuclear cell infiltration and the formation of neointima. This is distinguished from chronic antibody-mediated rejection by the location of vascular injury and a lack of evidence of the pathogenic antibody, and is distinguished from other nonimmunologic processes that may lead to vascular and interstitial fibrosis (such as CNI nephrotoxicity) by the presence of persistent infiltrating cells within vessels (Fig. 82.22).

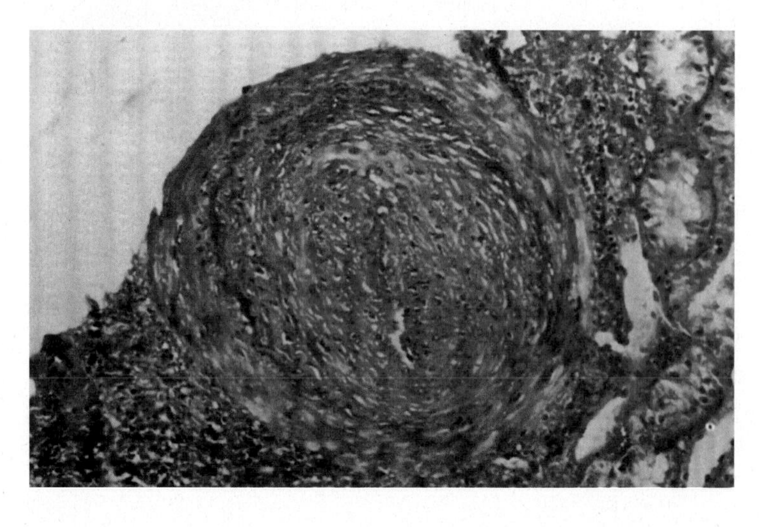

FIGURE 82.22 Chronic T-cell mediated rejection. A renal transplant biopsy specimen showing obliterative arteriopathy and fibrointimal vascular narrowing.

Glomerular Injury in Allografts

Four main etiologies of glomerular injury may occur in allografts: (1) the donor kidney may be the seat of glomerular disease before grafting; (2) recurrent glomerular disease may develop due to the persistence of the original stimulus and recurrence of the original disease in the recipient; (3) transplant glomerulopathy may occur as a result of host response to the graft; and (4) de novo glomerulopathies may arise in a previously normal allograft.

Nephritis of Donor Origin. Diseased donor kidneys may have unsuspected glomerulonephritis. Interestingly, donor glomerulonephritis may resolve following transplant.[214] When possible, pretransplant donor biopsies can provide a good understanding of the nature of preexisting glomerulopathies. Proteinuria immediately posttransplant cannot be used as a guide for recipients versus a donor-related source of glomerular disease, because proteinuria posttransplant may still arise from the recipient's native renal residual function for the first 2 to 6 weeks.[215]

Recurrence of Primary Renal Disease. Essentially all glomerulopathies have been described to recur in renal allografts (see Patient Selection, previously).[216] However, there is much variation between the various types of glomerulonephritis with regard to the frequency of recurrence, the clinical pattern, and the prognosis (Table 82.4). The clinical manifestations of recurrent glomerulonephritis include microscopic hematuria and proteinuria, which may progress to nephrotic syndrome. Recurrent glomerulonephritis is the most common cause of nephrotic syndrome following transplantation. Proteinuria may also be a manifestation of de novo glomerular disease or chronic rejection. Although the documented overall incidence of graft failure from recurrent disease is less than 2%, this is an underestimate due to difficulty in firmly establishing this diagnosis and in defining the cause of primary ESRD and graft dysfunction or whether loss occurred because of the same pathologic process.

Transplant Glomerulopathy. Transplant glomerulopathy is an entity that may be considered a special form of chronic alloimmune injury. It is believed to be related to alloantibody because the frequency of glomerular lesions was found to be inversely related to HLA compatibility and is often found in conjunction with circulating donor-specific HLA antibodies (see Chronic T-Cell–Mediated Rejection and Chronic Antibody-Mediated Rejection, previously). Histologically, it may resemble membrano-proliferative glomerulonephritis (type I MPGN) with mesangial proliferation and thickening or reduplication of the glomerular basement membrane. It is the most common cause of nephrotic syndrome in renal transplant patients. Along with proteinuria, the clinical presentations include microscopic hematuria and progressive graft dysfunction.

De Novo Glomerulopathy. The development of glomerular lesions in patients with no history of glomerulonephritis suggests the presence of a de novo process in the allograft. For example, de novo membranous nephropathy (Fig. 82.8) is reported to occur with an incidence of less than 1%. Nephrotic range proteinuria occurred at a mean time of 1 to 2 years after transplantation. In contrast to the indolent course of idiopathic membranous glomerulonephritis in nontransplant patients, de novo membranous nephropathy can lead to graft loss. This may be due to superimposed glomerular and interstitial lesions associated with chronic rejection.

Focal segmental glomerulosclerosis is not uncommon among transplant recipients whose original disease was not FSGS. The mechanisms underlying de novo glomerulosclerosis are not clear. It may represent a nonspecific response to chronic rejection, glomerular ischemia, vesicoureteral reflux, or infections such as hepatitis B and HIV. Circulating anti-GBM antibodies and anti-GBM disease can develop in some patients with Alport disease after renal transplantation. Patients with Alport disease lack a component of the GBM and do not bind anti-GBM antibodies isolated from patients with Goodpasture syndrome. When the allograft, which contains these GBM proteins, is transplanted, the recipient may mount a humoral response against these proteins, which may lead to anti-GBM disease.

Other Causes of Chronic Graft Injury. Nonimmunologic causes can also contribute to the decline in renal function. Atheromatous renovascular disease of the transplant kidney can be responsible for a significant number of cases of progressive graft failure (Fig. 82.23). The reduction in nephron mass as a result of earlier immunologic injury, donor-recipient size mismatching, or donor renal disease (in the case of expanded criteria or older donors), likely contributes to a further decline in function. Retrospective analyses suggest that control of hypertension preserves graft function, but a specific agent has not been shown to be superior to another.[217,218]

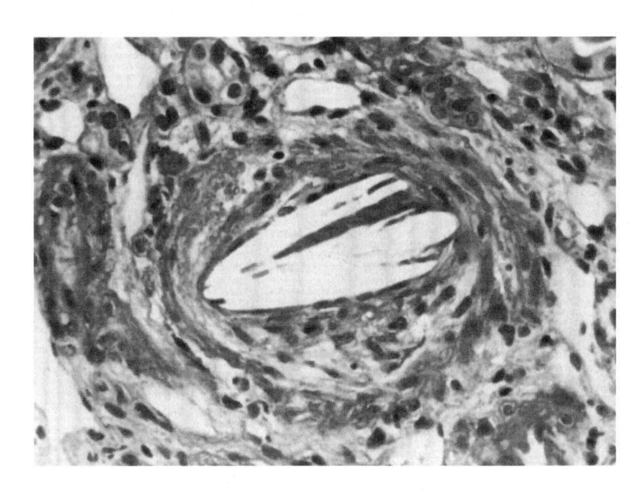

FIGURE 82.23 A percutaneous needle biopsy of a kidney 20 years posttransplantation showing an atheroembolus in a small artery. (Trichrome stain, magnification ×400.)

SYSTEMIC COMPLICATIONS

Infectious complications of immunosuppressive therapy, cardiovascular diseases, and malignancy are the most important causes of death following a kidney transplantation.[11,219,220] Additional concerns following transplantation include but are not limited to bone disease, nutritional status, growth and development in children, and pregnancy in women.

Infection

The occurrence of infection is due primarily to the interplay between two factors: the degree of immunosuppression in the patient and the epidemiologic exposures that the patient encounters. The most common presentation of an infection in a transplant patient is fever; some guidelines to the approach to the patient with fever are given in Table 82.17. The prevalence of particular infections vary according to the degree of immunosuppression; thus, it is helpful to consider the time posttransplant in the diagnostic approach to a patient with a possible infection. During the first posttransplantation month, opportunistic infections are rare and the major infectious disease hazards are similar to those for patients undergoing major urologic surgery. The period between 1 and 6 months after transplantation is when most serious infections occur. This is because of the maximal effect of the immunosuppressive drugs on the host's defense system, as well as it coinciding with the period when attempts are made to reverse rejection episodes with potent antirejection therapy. As in other states of immune deficiencies, opportunistic infections derived from endogenous flora including *Cryptococcus*, *Candida*, *Aspergillus*, *Pneumocystis carinii*, CMV, and herpes zoster are seen after transplantation. *Candida albicans*, a normal inhabitant in healthy individuals of the oropharynx, intestine, and vagina, may cause severe pharyngitis, esophagitis, vaginitis, and systemic infections in immunosuppressed patients. Wound infections and urinary infections are commonly due to bacterial infections. Septicemia is not uncommon after transplantation and is usually due to a gram-negative organism with the primary focus in the urinary tract. However, *Staphylococcus aureus*, *Listeria*, and *Candida* may also cause septicemia. Although awaiting the results of blood culture, appropriate broad-spectrum antimicrobial treatment should be commenced. A vigorous search for the focus of infection must be made and dealt with as appropriate.

TABLE 82.17 The Diagnostic Approach to the Transplant Patient with an Unexplained Fever

Possible sites of infection
Chest: pulmonary infection, pericarditis, endocarditis
Mouth: *Candida*
Lower limb: deep venous thrombosis
Soft tissues: skin (e.g., fungi, *Nocardia*, mycobacteria), joints
Transplant wound: rejection, abscess, urine leak, hematoma
Peritoneal cavity: pancreas, colon, dialysis catheter
Urinary tract: bladder, prostate, native kidneys
Central nervous system (CNS): *Listeria*, *Cryptococcus*, *Aspergillus*, tuberculosis, *Nocardia*
Systemic: viral infection, tuberculosis
Investigations
Chest X-rays
Ultrasound of transplanted kidney
Cultures: mouth, sputum, urine, blood, stool, access sites
Serology: viral antibodies, especially cytomegalovirus
Lumbar puncture and computed tomography of head if CNS infection suspected

Viral Infections

Cytomegalovirus. CMV is one of the most important viral infections that occur in transplant recipients. The incidence and severity of CMV infection depend on the presence of latent infection in the donor, the immune status of the recipient, and the degree of immunosuppression.[221] CMV infection (defined as evidence of CMV viremia either via culture techniques, or more commonly, detection by blood PCR) occurs in 20% to 70% of patients depending on the serostatus of donor and recipient. CMV infection takes two forms: namely, that of a primary infection, which occurs in patients who are seronegative at the time of transplantation and received a kidney from a seropositive donor, and that of a secondary (or reactivated) infection. Use of DNA-restriction enzyme analytic methods to detect different CMV serotypes indicates that many of the clinical CMV infections in individuals seropositive for CMV before transplantation are due to superinfection with the donor virus strain. Patients with a secondary infection or reactivation of latent CMV often are not symptomatic, whereas those with superinfection of a new viral strain may demonstrate the acute symptoms of active CMV. CMV infection has been associated with decreased survival and decreased allograft survival rates.[221,222]

CMV infection can progress to clinical symptoms and tissue invasion, which is referred to as CMV disease. A common presentation is that of a fever that may be spiking or constant and usually occurs between 4 and 10 weeks after transplantation or after discontinuation of antiviral prophylaxis. It may be associated with neutropenia, liver function abnormalities, or GI symptoms, and atypical lymphocytes may be identified in the blood smear. CMV pneumonia is a serious complication of CMV infection and should be ruled out in any seronegative transplant recipient who received a kidney from a seropositive donor and presents with a fever

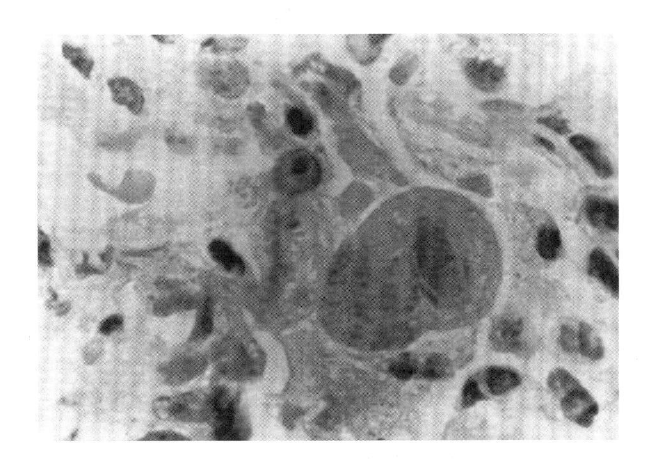

FIGURE 82.24 A typical cytomegalovirus-infected lung cell showing cytomegaly, large intracellular inclusions with peripheral chromatin clumping, and abundant intracytoplasmic inclusions. (Hematoxylin and eosin stain, magnification ×1,000.)

and radiologic pulmonary infiltrates (Fig. 82.24). Less commonly, hepatitis, arthralgia, splenomegaly, myalgia, and GI ulceration may be presenting features. In rare instances, chorioretinitis can occur, occasionally without prior evidence of CMV activity. CMV encephalitis, transverse myelitis, and cutaneous vasculitis also have been reported.[223]

The impact of CMV on graft function has been debated. A deterioration in renal transplant function may be seen during the early stages of CMV infection, and a frank glomerulopathy has been reported to occur.[224] It has been proposed that CMV infection, through the elaboration of lymphokines and IFNs, may cause upregulation of histocompatibility antigens on the allograft. This change results in the induction of immune responses that histologically lead to glomerular endothelial changes and possibly increase the risk for acute rejection[225] and contribute to allograft dysfunction.

Management of CMV after transplant should take into account a patient's risk for CMV infection and disease, with consideration of monitoring and/or prophylactic therapy and aggressive treatment in established disease. The prophylactic administration of oral ganciclovir (ganciclovir or valganciclovir) and valacyclovir to renal allograft recipients for 12 weeks after transplantation has been shown to reduce symptomatic active CMV infections. Valganciclovir is the L-valine ester of ganciclovir and is administered orally at 450 to 900 mg per day for CMV prophylaxis. This dose produces similar AUC values to IV ganciclovir (5 mg/kg/day) and much higher values than oral ganciclovir (3 g per day). The major side effects of ganciclovir and valganciclovir are bone marrow suppression, sterility, and potential nephrotoxicity. Dose adjustment is necessary for patients with renal impairment (Table 82.18).

Trials investigating two approaches to the management of CMV prevention following transplant, a prophylaxis approach (prophylaxis) versus a monitoring and preemptive therapeutic approach (preemptive), have generally been found to be similarly effective in preventing CMV disease. For high-risk recipients (seronegative recipients of kidneys from seropositive donors), late CMV disease that occurs after stopping prophylaxis has been problematic. In this patient population, extending the time of prophylactic therapy from 3 to 6 months after transplant may be considered.[226]

Treatment of overt CMV disease requires high-dose ganciclovir therapy (either IV ganciclovir 5 mg/kg/day or oral valganciclovir 900 mg twice per day (bid), adjusted for renal function) and reduction in immunosuppressive therapy. High-dose therapy should be given for 21 days or until clinical CMV disease is absent and CMV viremia is no longer present. Prophylaxis should be reinitiated and continued until stable on reduced dose immunosuppression for 3 to 6 months.

TABLE 82.18 **Dosage Adjustment for Intravenous Ganciclovir and Valganciclovir in the Initial Treatment of CMV Infection**

Estimated GFR	Ganciclovir (IV)	Valganciclovir (PO)
>60 mL/min	5 mg/kg q12hr	900 mg q12hr
40–59 mL/min	2.5 mg/kg q12hr	450 mg q12hr
25–39 mL/min	2.5 mg/kg q24hr	450 mg q24h
10–24 mL/min	1.25 mg/kg q24hr	450 mg q48h
Dialysis	1.25 mg/kg 3×/week after dialysis	Not recommended

GFR, glomerular filtration rate; IV, intravenous; PO, by mouth.

Herpes Simplex Virus. Reactivation of latent herpes simplex virus (HSV) infections is extremely common in transplant patients. The most common lesion is the orolabial HSV type 1 infection. Occasionally, an anogenital lesion due to an HSV type 2 infection may occur. Rarely, a Kaposi varicelliform eruption, due to a disseminated HSV infection in the skin, may develop in transplant patients. Therapy of acute HSV infection with acyclovir or valacyclovir will lead to clinical improvement.

Varicella Zoster. Varicella zoster is frequently seen in transplant patients and can occur at any time after transplantation. It is commonly presented as a localized zoster due to the reactivation of the latent virus present in the dorsal root ganglion since childhood chickenpox. For localized dermatomes, oral acyclovir can be used, but with multidermatomal involvement or optic nerve involvement, intravenous acyclovir is the treatment of choice. Chickenpox is a rare but often extremely virulent infection. Should a patient without humoral immunity to varicella zoster be exposed to chickenpox, varicella zoster immune globulin should be given within 72 hours of the exposure. If chickenpox develops, intravenous acyclovir needs to be instituted without delay.

Epstein–Barr Virus. In general, EBV is not a common problem in transplant patients, although occasionally EBV may be the cause of a glandular febrile illness. However, infection or reactivation of latent EBV can cause an acute lymphoproliferative syndrome or even a polyclonal lymphoma. Using the DNA hybridization technique, EBV has been identified in lymphoma and lymphoproliferative lesions of renal transplant patients, described under "Cancer in Transplant Patients," which follows.

HIV. The impact of HIV infection and AIDS on recipients of organ transplantation has not yet been fully realized. In patients who have clinically quiescent disease and are on stable antiretroviral therapy, there does not seem to be an increase in the progression of HIV or deterioration in CD4 counts with standard immunosuppression, although depleting antibody induction therapy may indeed lead to prolonged depression of CD4 counts.[94] Close monitoring of CD4 count and viral load is appropriate following transplant.

Hepatitis

Chronic liver function impairment is not rare after renal transplantation. Viral hepatitis and drug-related hepatitis are the most common causes. Drugs that may cause hepatic dysfunction include CsA, AZA, antihypertensives, and lipid-lowering agents. CsA- and AZA-induced liver enzyme elevation usually resolves on dosage reduction. For the patient with elevated liver enzymes following transplant, a careful review of medications should be followed by retesting for hepatitis viral infections.

Hepatitis B Virus. HBV is a relatively uncommon viral infection after transplantation, but the main cause for concern is the outcome of transplantation in a patient who is a carrier of the hepatitis B antigen. There is considerable concern about the possible progression of liver disease leading to liver failure. Additionally, the incidence of hepatoma in those chronic carriers of hepatitis B is 15%, much higher than in the general population who contract hepatitis. Immunosuppression enables persistent viral replication, leading to a greater frequency of hepatitis e-antigen, viral DNA, and viral DNA polymerase in the sera of transplanted individuals.

The natural history of liver disease due to chronic hepatitis B in transplant patients differs from that in both the general population and hemodialysis patients. Transplant recipients who have hepatitis B typically remain surface antigen–positive for longer than 6 months and do not revert to seronegativity. Most episodes of hepatitis in the early posttransplantation period are relatively mild, but an unusually high rate of transformation from chronic persistent to chronic active hepatitis occurs in this patient population. Patients who have persistent hepatitis e-antigenemia or concomitant delta virus infection are at higher risk for chronic active hepatitis and more rapid deterioration.

For kidney transplant recipients with chronic HBV infection, the use of antiviral therapy has provided a major advancement in pretransplant and posttransplant management and patient outcome. Lamivudine is an oral nucleoside analog that effectively inhibits viral replication. However, the development of antiviral resistance is common, which increases progressively with treatment duration and has been reported to be >70% after 8 years of continuous treatment. Other treatment alternatives include initial prophylactic treatment with tenofovir or entecavir. Therapy should be continued indefinitely.[92]

Hepatitis C Virus. The prevalence of anti-HCV positivity in renal transplant recipients is estimated to be between 6% to 46% depending on the center and/or country.[91] Patients with hepatitis C are at increased risk of liver disease, cardiovascular disease, infection, sepsis, proteinuria, and a significantly higher rate of NODAT. In the setting of posttransplant immunosuppression, HCV loads can increase, but these do not reliably predict progressive liver disease.[227] Antiviral therapy posttransplant is less effective than pretransplant treatment and is associated with an increased risk of acute rejection. Because posttransplant noninvasive monitoring is unreliable and pretransplant cirrhosis is associated with increased posttransplant mortality, liver ultrasound should be performed every 1 to 2 years in patients with active hepatitis C following a transplant to monitor for hepatoma, and attention to the biochemical and the clinical stigmata of ongoing liver injury should be continuously monitored.

Pneumocystis carinii Pneumonia. This is a relatively common pathogen that can cause pulmonary infection in states of significant immunosuppression. In the transplant setting, this risk is highest in the first 1 to 6 months following transplant, thus antibiotic prophylaxis is often used during this period. The preferred therapy is trimethoprim/sulfamethoxazole (TMP/SMZ), but in the case of sulfa allergy, aerosolized pentamidine or oral dapsone therapy may be considered. Patients with suspected pneumocystis pneumonia typically present with a fever and are often associated with some dyspnea, but with very few physical signs on examination. A chest X-ray shows diffuse shadowing that tends to be linear in distribution but can be normal. TMP/SMZ in high doses is the antimicrobial of choice.

Mycobacterial Infections

The incidence of tuberculosis in transplant recipients varies from region to region, but certainly is more common in transplant recipients than in the general population.[228] The symptoms are frequently nonspecific and the site of infection is often in organs other than the lungs. Treatment of the established case should be the routine antituberculous therapy (e.g., rifampicin and isoniazid). It should be remembered that these drugs are metabolized in the liver. Rifampicin induces hepatic enzymes; therefore, CNI or mTOR levels must be closely monitored. Chemoprophylaxis should be considered in patients with calcification on a chest roentgenogram and in the presence of a positive tuberculin skin test. Therapy for 6 to 9 months with isoniazid should be given to patients who have never received adequate treatment and who are PPD positive.[229]

Fungal Infections

Fungal infections are relatively common in transplant patients and must always be considered as a possible cause of fever and pneumonia, especially in the presence of excessive immunosuppressive therapy. Pulmonary infiltrates due to fungal infection include *Aspergillus*, *Cryptococcus*, *Coccidioides*, *Candida,* and *Histoplasma capsulatum*. *Aspergillus* is a hyphal saprophytic fungus in which infection is started by the inhalation of spores; the lungs are, therefore, the primary site of infection. In the lung, *Aspergillus* causes a patchy infiltration followed by a consolidation and abscess formation (Fig. 82.25). Histoplasmosis is another fungal pneumonia, caused by *H. capsulatum*, which can occur in renal transplant recipients. This may also be acquired or result from reactivation and usually presents with fever, pulmonary infiltrates, and skin lesions at any time after transplantation. These infections require aggressive therapy with conventional amphotericin B, a lipid-based amphotericin B preparation (Abelcet, AmBisome, or Amphotec), or an appropriate azole antifungal agent. Ketoconazole, fluconazole, and itraconazole are useful for treating mucocutaneous fungal infections and infections of the GU tract and GI system, lungs, and under specific conditions, the central nervous system. All of the triazole antifungals impair calcineurin inhibitor metabolism and increase blood levels of CsA and TAC. CsA or TAC dose reduction, therefore, may be necessary while patients are on triazole treatment.[230]

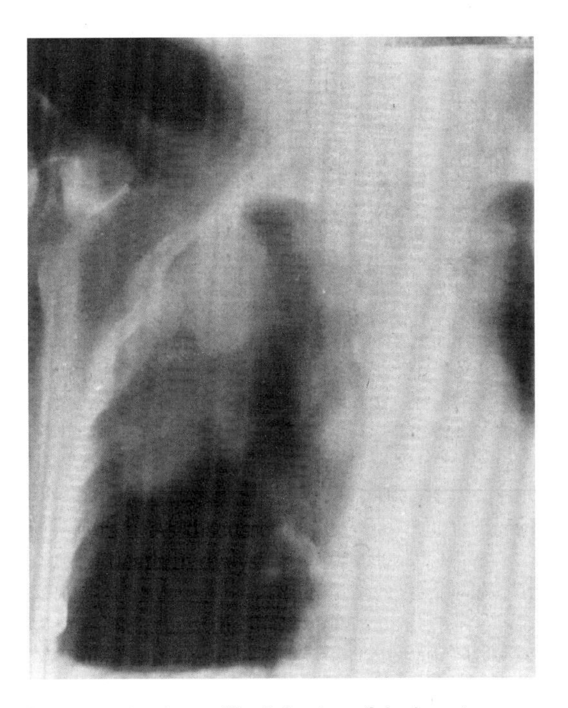

FIGURE 82.25 An *Aspergillus* infection of the lung in a patient who underwent renal transplantation after several courses of antirejection therapy with high-dose intravenous methylprednisolone. (From Morris PJ. *Kidney Transplantation: Principles and Practice*. 2nd ed. New York: Grune & Stratton; 1984, with permission.)

Central Nervous System Infection

Infections of the CNS after renal transplantation typically present between 1 and 12 months posttransplant and are characterized by a subacute onset and the frequent lack of systemic signs. Organisms commonly associated with a CNS infection in renal transplant recipients include *Listeria*, *Cryptococcus*, *Mycobacterium*, *Nocardia*, *Aspergillus*, fungi of the Mucorales order, *Toxoplasma*, *Candida*, and *Strongyloides*. *Listeria* may cause an acute or focal brain infection. *Cryptococcus* and, less often, *Mycobacterium* and *Coccidioides* are important causes of subacute meningitis. Focal lesions are most common with *Aspergillus*, *Toxoplasma*, and *Nocardia*. HIV can cause a variety of CNS syndromes, most predominantly, a global-dementing illness. JC virus infection can also cause dementia with progressive multifocal leukoencephalopathy.

In acute meningoencephalitis, nuchal rigidity may be absent. The development of fever and mild headache should be sufficient to alert the physician to the possibility of CNS infection. The aseptic meningitis that occurs during OKT3 or IVIG administration is self-limited, but if severe or persistent, may require diagnostic workup to rule out infection. Focal findings on neurologic examination are not common except with well-developed focal brain infections. Because the early findings in these infections are often nonspecific, lumbar puncture and cranial CT scanning or magnetic resonance imaging (MRI) should not be delayed.

Aspergillus. *Aspergillus* may cause pneumonia in the immunocompromised host and may disseminate to the brain, skin, kidney, and gut. *Aspergillus*, which infiltrates the vasculature, is not found free in the cerebrospinal fluid (CSF) and is often impossible to diagnose before death. The organism may be suspected in patients with clinical evidence for meningitis and CSF cytology and chemistry determinations consistent with meningitis, especially in the absence of a positive culture, inflammatory foci, and culture or serologic findings consistent with cryptococcal infection. The treatment of choice is amphotericin B.

Cryptococcus. Although rare, *Cryptococcus* is another cause of meningitis in the transplant patient. It tends to be seen relatively late in the transplantation course and has a rather nonspecific presentation, and hence, the diagnosis is often delayed. Lung involvement is also common when this infection is present. Amphotericin B is again the indicated treatment.

Coccidioides. *Coccidioides* is quite rare in Europe but does occur commonly in parts of the United States. It may cause destructive lesions of the lungs, liver, brain, and spleen and is sometimes due to reactivation of an existing latent infection. Amphotericin B is the appropriate treatment.

Listeria monocytogenes. *Listeria monocytogenes* may present as meningitis, brain abscess, or as meningoencephalitis. It may occur at any time after transplantation, but is usually associated with increased or excessive immunosuppressive therapy for rejection. *Listeria* should be the primary suspect in a patient with meningoencephalitis because other causes of meningitis are rare in transplant recipients. CSF findings may not be striking. Treatment with ampicillin should be commenced as soon as CSF and other specimens for culture have been taken.

Nocardia. *Nocardia* usually presents as respiratory illness with an unproductive cough, fever, malaise, and a nodular infiltrate on the chest X-ray. Occasionally, the infection may spread to the brain, presenting as a space-occupying lesion, but it may also be seen as skin abscesses or joint infections. The treatment of choice is probably sulfonamide, which is given for at least 2 months, although some would advocate treatment for 12 months.

Urinary Tract Infection

A urinary tract infection is the most common bacterial infection following transplantation. Urinary tract infections appearing within the first 3 or 4 months after transplantation are often associated with transplant pyelonephritis, septicemia, and relapse after standard antibiotic therapy. Patients with an anatomic abnormality requiring urinary diversion or stent placement and those with pyelonephritis should receive chronic suppressive antibiotics in addition to the 4- to 6-week course of primary treatment. Uncomplicated urinary tract infections that occur later after transplantation can be treated with a standard 1- or 2-week course of oral antibiotics.

Cancer in Transplant Patients

The incidence of cancer in transplant recipients varies considerably from region to region, ranging from a low incidence of 1.6% of patients developing cancer after transplantation in Europe to as high as 24% of patients in Australia.[231,232] Much of this variation is due to the high incidence of skin cancer in those areas at risk for these cancers. In regions with limited exposure to the risk, there is a four- to sevenfold increase, but in areas with copious sunshine there is an almost 29-fold increase in incidence as compared with the control population. There is also a well-recognized and highly significant increase in the risk of developing a malignant (non-Hodgkin) lymphoma. Even with skin cancers and malignant lymphomas excluded from the analysis, there is an increased incidence in all forms of cancer in patients after transplantation (Table 82.19).

TABLE 82.19 **Common Malignancies Encountered in Renal Transplant Recipients**

Cancer	Increased Risk Compared to General Population
Cancers of the Skin and Lips	>20×
Squamous cell carcinomas	
Basal cell carcinomas	
Malignant melanoma	
Malignant Lymphomas	>20×
Non-Hodgkin lymphoma	
Reticulum cell sarcoma	
B-cell lymphoproliferative syndrome (Epstein–Barr virus)	
Kaposi Sarcoma	>20×
Cutaneous form	
Visceral and cutaneous form	
Genitourinary Cancer	>15×
Carcinoma of native kidney (acquired cystic disease)	
Carcinoma of transplanted kidney (hypernephroma)	
Carcinoma of the urinary bladder (cyclophosphamide associated)	
Uroepithelial tumors (associated with analgesic nephropathy)	
Gynecologic Cancer	5×
Carcinoma of cervix	
Ovarian cancer	

Careful physical examination to detect the common malignancies is essential in the long-term follow-up of renal transplant patients. The increased incidence of cervical cancer in females after transplantation implies that all female transplant patients should have an annual cervical smear, and although the cost-effectiveness of screening for breast, colorectal, and prostate disease remains an unresolved issue, it appears that the benefits of screening may outweigh harm.[233]

A number of factors contribute to the increased risk of cancers in immunosuppressed recipients of a kidney transplant. These include depression of immune surveillance, chronic antigenic stimulation in the presence of immunosuppression, a directly neoplastic action of the immunosuppressive drugs themselves, and increased susceptibility to oncogenic viral infection. First, alterations in the immune surveillance due to immunosuppressive therapy may allow potentially malignant cell mutants to become established in the host because they cannot be detected and killed in the usual fashion. The allograft with its foreign HLA may also stimulate the host lymphoreticular system, resulting in the development of lymphoid malignancies. Depleting T-cell induction therapy has been associated with an increased risk of lymphomas.[151] Finally, latent oncogenic viruses may be activated in immunosuppressed hosts who are simultaneously experiencing stimulation immunologically by an antigen. An association exists between the papilloma virus and the development of squamous skin cancer, as well as condyloma acuminatum with cervical carcinoma. EBV has also been implicated in polyclonal B cell lymphoproliferative disease. In addition to primary cancer developed de novo in patients after transplantation, cancer may be transferred in the transplanted kidney from a donor with cancer undetected at the time of donor nephrectomy.

Skin cancer is the most common neoplasia in transplant patients, with an incidence 4 to 21 times the population average.[234] Squamous cell carcinoma predominates over basal cell skin cancer. Patients who live in warm climates should be carefully advised after transplantation to use sun-blocking creams and to wear appropriate clothing while in the sun. The appearance of neoplasia can be atypical, and an early biopsy of any suspicious lesion is indicated. The prognosis after the resection of skin cancer is excellent, provided strict avoidance of sun exposure is followed. A reduction in immunosuppression may be considered if the malignancy is extensive or rapidly progressive.

Lymphoma occurs earlier than other tumors and accounts for 20% to 30% of posttransplant neoplasms. The incidence of this neoplasm is relatively higher in the last decade, which is probably related to the use of monoclonal or polyclonal globulin and other immunosuppression. Two types of lymphoproliferative disease are seen in patients after transplantation.[235] The first presents with an infectious mononucleosislike illness within the first year of transplantation with fever, sore throat, and lymphadenopathy. The clinical course is often short and can be fatal. Cessation of the immunosuppression will lead to regression in some patients. This type of lymphoproliferative disease is due to infection with EBV. With acyclovir treatment, remission can occasionally be achieved without the cessation of immunosuppression. The second group of lymphoproliferative diseases presents as localized solid tumor masses and can be localized to the graft or to the CNS in a high percentage of patients. Lymphoma, therefore, should be considered in the differential diagnosis of any CNS abnormality. These lymphomas are often more rapidly progressive than those seen in the normal population and, although responsive to conventional therapy for non-Hodgkin lymphoma, carry a high mortality rate. In addition to the standard established treatment for each malignancy, consideration must be given to reduce or cease immunosuppressive medications. Many of the therapeutic agents are cytotoxic and additive suppression of the bone marrow can occur. An initial course of rituximab can be considered, with or without additional cytotoxic therapy.[236] In most cases, regression does not appear to occur with the cessation of immunosuppression, and the patients do not respond to acyclovir.

The incidence of Kaposi sarcoma is 300 to 400 times that of the normal population and accounts for 5% to 10% of posttransplant neoplasms. Those with Kaposi sarcoma involving only the skin do better than those with visceral disease, with complete remission in 50% compared with 14%, respectively, after chemotherapy or the cessation of immunosuppression. Remissions in Kaposi sarcoma confined to the skin may occur with the discontinuation of immunosuppression as the sole therapy. mTOR inhibitors have been shown to be effective in achieving remission while preserving graft function.[237]

Cardiovascular Complications

Cardiovascular Disease

Cardiovascular disease is a major cause of morbidity and death after renal transplantation. This risk can be attributed to the cause of the underlying disease for renal failure (e.g., diabetes), and to chronic kidney disease as an independent cardiovascular risk factor.[238] Independent predictors of cardiovascular disease include tobacco use, diabetes, obesity, hypertension, and dyslipidemia. Once the patient has been transplanted, it is essential that rigorous advice be given to the management of these risk factors.

Hyperlipidemia

It has been known for some time that uremic patients frequently have type IV hyperlipidemia with marked hypertriglyceridemia. Total cholesterol is usually normal or low. In particular, high-density lipoprotein (HDL) levels are abnormally low. After transplantation, the hypertriglyceridemia of uremia shifts toward hypercholesterolemia. Very low-density lipoprotein and low-density lipoprotein cholesterol levels are elevated in transplant patients. Hypertriglyceridemia may persist, but triglyceride levels often decrease. Overall, the incidence of hyperlipidemia following transplantation is about 50%.

Immunosuppressive agents contribute to hyperlipidemia following transplant, in particular mTOR inhibitors and corticosteroids. Hypertriglyceridemia is a common side effect of mTOR inhibitor therapy.[239] High dose prednisone contributes to the development of mixed hyperlipidemia, but improves after the reduction of the initial steroid dose, HDL levels increase and become normal, with normal proportions of HDL3 and HDL2, but hypertriglyceridemia may persist.[160] Dietary therapy should be initiated during the first 6 months after transplantation when hypercholesterolemia is most often marked. Patients should be advised to avoid high-calorie, high-carbohydrate, and high-fat diets. Supplementation of the diet with omega-3 fatty acids may reduce triglyceride and cholesterol levels, and may increase HDL levels. If hypercholesterolemia persists beyond 6 months on diet therapy and on maintenance steroid dose, drug therapy should be considered. Potential pharmacologic agents include niacin, bile-binding resins, fibrates, and statins. Niacin lowers triglyceride and cholesterol levels. A slow-release preparation of niacin may reduce the side effects of flushing and GI distress. Bile-binding resins are rarely used because they may interfere with immunosuppressive drug absorption. Fibrates (gemfibrozil) primarily reduce triglyceride levels, but they can lower cholesterol when triglyceride levels are normal. Statins inhibit 3-hydroxy-3-methylglutaryl-coenzyme A (HMG-CoA) reductase, the rate-limiting enzyme in cholesterol biosynthesis, and are effective at reducing cholesterol levels. Liver enzymes should be monitored in all patients receiving niacin, gemfibrozil, and statins because hepatitis is a major adverse effect. Reports have been made of myositis and myalgia occurring at low frequency secondary to gemfibrozil and statins. An increased risk of myositis has been described in those patients receiving CsA who also were treated with lovastatin.

The cardiovascular benefits of LDL reduction with statin therapy are well known in the general population. In the kidney transplant setting, one randomized, double-blind controlled trial of fluvastatin (n = 1,050) or placebo (n = 1,052) lowered LDL cholesterol concentrations by 32% and was associated with a 35% reduction in risk for cardiac deaths or non-fatal myocardial infarction.[240] In a 2-year extension study, patients randomized to fluvastatin had a 29% reduction in cardiac death or non-fatal MI, supporting the use of aggressive LDL cholesterol management to LDL $<$100 mg per deciliter.[241]

Hypertension

Hypertension is extremely common after renal transplantation. Hypertension after transplant is associated with reduced graft function and patient survival after transplant.[217] Hypertension in the transplant recipient may be due to the native kidney disease, chronic allograft injury/CKD of the transplanted kidney, renal artery stenosis in the transplanted kidney, and medication side effects of corticosteroids, and calcineurin inhibitors. The relationship between hypertension and activity of the renin–angiotensin system in patients with a renal transplant is unclear. It is apparent that the patient's native kidneys may contribute to hyperreninemia, but conflicting reports exist concerning the role of the renin–angiotensin system in the transplanted kidney as a cause of hypertension.

Although steroid therapy certainly contributes to hypertension, this is less common now that low-dose steroid protocols are used by most centers. The incidence of hypertension in patients treated with CNIs, either with or without steroids, is greater than that seen in patients treated with CNI-free regimens.[184] The degree to which CsA might increase blood pressure is dose dependent, as demonstrated by the fact that there is a general decrease in blood pressure following the reduction of the CsA dose to a maintenance therapy level of 4 mg/kg/day.

The initial management of hypertension in patients with stable graft function includes salt restriction, weight reduction, elimination or reduction of medications that may contribute to hypertension, and the use of antihypertensive agents.

Most standard therapies have been demonstrated to be safe and effective after renal transplantation. There are, however, a number of management issues that are unique to transplant recipients. Transplant patients may be more prone to decreased renal function resulting from diuretic use than are hypertensive patients in the general population. Patients may occasionally develop decreased renal function after ACE inhibitor therapy, especially if patients exhibit renal artery stenosis or chronic allograft nephropathy. Anemia and hyperkalemia may also be associated with the use of ACE inhibitors and angiotensin II (Ang II) receptor antagonists. Several studies have shown, however, that these drugs are generally safe, effective, and well tolerated. They may reduce proteinuria and may stabilize the deterioration in renal function in chronic allograft failure, possibly by reducing TGF-β. They may also have additional benefits in reducing the incidence of cardiovascular events in high-risk patients.

ACE inhibitors are useful in treating posttransplantation hypertension in patients who do not have transplant artery stenosis. Calcium channel blockers are often used in the treatment of hypertension, because there is evidence that these agents may counteract the decreased effective renal plasma flow and increased renovascular resistance of calcineurin inhibitors. Patients with hypertension associated with renal dysfunction should be evaluated to determine the cause of the dysfunction. Possibilities might include chronic immunologic injury, CNI nephrotoxicity, or a recurrence of the original disease. A renal biopsy may be appropriate to rule out rejection. If hypertension is severe or associated with worsening renal function, with no evidence for rejection, transplant artery stenosis may be pursued by arteriography.

Renal Artery Stenosis

When hypertension cannot be controlled, particularly if attempts to reduce blood pressure results in decreased renal function, the possibility of renal allograft artery stenosis should be considered. Transplant renal artery stenosis (RAS) currently is diagnosed in <2% of cases. Occasionally, RAS may occur in the early months after transplantation; at this time it is always due to a technical defect at the anastomosis. For deceased donor kidney transplants, the use of end-to-side anastomosis of an aortic patch containing the renal artery origin onto the recipient external iliac artery has resulted in much lower rates of transplant RAS. RAS may present 1 to several years after transplantation with poorly controlled hypertension and a deterioration of renal function. Other causes of arterial stenosis include arteriosclerosis, the development of a fibrous plaque in the artery at the anastomotic site or constriction beyond it, technical narrowing of the anastomosis, perfusion injury, kinking of the vessels, and chronic microvascular rejection. A sudden occurrence or increase in severity of hypertension, the presence of a new bruit over the allograft, or a decline in renal function in the absence of rejection all suggest the possibility of RAS. A rise in the serum creatinine level after treatment with an ACE inhibitor for hypertension is very suggestive of renal allograft arterial stenosis. On occasion, renal vein and peripheral renin levels may be of value. Angiographic evidence of RAS is relatively common in the transplanted kidney, but this does not necessarily mean that it is the cause of hypertension. Making the diagnosis of a functional RAS is difficult. In the presence of poorly controlled hypertension and deteriorating renal function, a magnetic resonance angiography of the kidney or renal arteriography as well as a renal biopsy should be considered. If the biopsy shows evidence of moderate-to-severe chronic allograft injury with intimal fibrosis of the arteries and arterioles, correction of the RAS is unlikely to be very successful. Another more diagnostic sign of a functional stenosis is a loss of renal function following treatment with an ACE inhibitor, such as captopril or enalapril. This does imply a prominent role for the renin–angiotensin system in the etiology of the hypertension. A radionuclide scan may show a delay and a decrease in allograft blood flow but is a relatively insensitive tool for the diagnosis of RAS. Doppler ultrasonography is a moderately sensitive and noninvasive means of establishing the diagnosis; however, many false negative studies occur. If a significant chronic allograft injury can be excluded, surgical correction of the stenosis can be considered, but because of the difficulty of the surgery, a percutaneous transluminal angioplasty is considered the treatment of choice for renal artery stenoses.[242]

Erythrocytosis

Erythrocytosis, defined as a hematocrit value greater than 52%, occurs with a frequency of up to 15% in kidney transplant recipients, typically within the first year after transplantation. It can present in settings of good allograft function, chronic allograft injury, transplant RAS, and hydronephrosis, and may be caused by native kidney and hepatic erythropoietin production and the use of androgenic steroids. In patients with good allograft function, it is postulated that correction of the uremic milieu allows overzealous red blood cell production because of a reset marrow response to erythropoietin (EPO).[243] In patients with RAS or hydronephrosis, intrarenal hypoxemia may stimulate EPO production. In most cases, the precise etiology is uncertain, but studies of EPO levels after transplantation indicate that graft function restores the hematopoietic response to normal. The phenomenon usually is self-limited, lasting 3 to 12 months. Low-dose ACE inhibition can be used to reduce the hematocrit because Ang II appears to promote EPO in bone marrow precursors, and ACE inhibitors can induce anemia in some renal transplant recipients without erythrocytosis. The effect begins within 6 weeks and is complete in 3 to 6 months. Compatible with the role of an EPO-independent mechanism is the observation that withdrawal of the ACE inhibitor results in a gradual rise in hematocrit without a concurrent elevation in EPO levels. An alternative to ACE inhibition is theophylline. Theophylline appears to act as an adenosine antagonist in this setting, suggesting that adenosine facilitates both the release and perhaps the bone marrow response to EPO. In severe cases (hematocrit >52%), a phlebotomy should be considered to prevent thromboembolic complications.

Bone Complications

The main types of renal osteodystrophy are secondary hyperparathyroidism and osteomalacia. After a successful transplantation, the metabolic milieu of bone changes, with correction of acidosis, cessation of aluminum hydroxide gel therapy, and improved vitamin D metabolism, whereas immunosuppressive agents such as corticosteroids and CNIs contribute to osteoporosis. This leads to varying degrees of resolution of preexisting renal osteodystrophy and osteomalacia. A progressive resolution of hyperparathyroidism occurs as early as 3 months after transplantation, but many patients have sustained hyperparathyroidism lasting more than 1 year. Indications for a parathyroidectomy include the progressive elevation of parathyroid hormone (PTH) and alkaline phosphatase levels, progressive or new metabolic bone disease, osteonecrosis, metastatic calcification, and severe symptoms of pruritus and proximal myopathy. Osteoporosis is primarily related to steroid therapy. Vertebral bone loss occurs at a more rapid rate in the first 6 months posttransplant, and decreases at a slower rate as corticosteroids are tapered.[244] The development of osteopenia places the patient at increased risk for pathologic fractures. The prevalence of atraumatic fractures in the renal transplant recipient may be as high as 22%; these fractures occur primarily at sites of high cancellous bone, such as the vertebrae and ribs. Glucocorticoid suppression of bone formation is the most important factor in the genesis of early bone loss. Steroids are directly toxic to osteoblasts and lead to increased osteoclast activity. They also have other effects that promote calcium loss and the development of osteopenia. These include decreased calcium absorption, reduced gonadal hormone production, diminished insulin-like growth factor-1 production, and decreased sensitivity to PTH. Cyclosporine, which induces a high turnover osteopenia in rodents, also may contribute to bone loss, especially in long-term survivors and in subjects treated only with cyclosporine. A higher rate of bone disease-related complications is reported with doses of prednisone as low as 5 mg per day compared to corticosteroid-free regimens.[160]

The main bone disorder that can be directly attributed to high-dose corticosteroids is avascular necrosis or osteonecrosis, which most commonly affects the hips (Fig. 82.26) and tends to be bilateral, but may affect other joints, including the wrists, elbows, knees, ankles, and shoulders. Pain may be severe and is the most common presenting symptom, usually occurring between 1 and 3 years after transplantation. The mean time to onset was 12 months after transplantation (range, 6 to 21 months). The incidence of avascular necrosis is ~2% using current immunosuppressive protocols.[160,166] Pain usually precedes any radiologic changes by several months. In well-established cases, the diagnosis can be made on plain radiographs, whereas CT scanning, MRI, and nuclear bone scanning may detect earlier changes. If performed early, core decompression to relieve the intramedullary venous outflow obstruction can prevent osteonecrosis. With more severe disease, prosthetic total hip replacement has been used with excellent functional recovery. In general, surgery should be performed early in order to facilitate rehabilitation.

The management of bone disease posttransplant is challenging, given the many different factors that contribute to bone disease in the renal transplant recipient. It is important to monitor bone mineral density in the renal transplant recipient using dual-energy X-ray absorptiometry (DEXA). It is recommended that lumbar spine and hip-bone mineral densities should be measured at the time of transplant, after 6 months, and then every 12 months if results are abnormal. Those subjects displaying rapid bone loss and/or a low initial bone density should be considered for treatment. Calcium supplementation (1 g per day) should be considered in nonhypercalcemic patients. The administration of vitamin D analogs (such as calcitriol) can further improve calcium absorption. Vitamin D levels should be measured and corrected. If bone loss is severe and/or rapid, consideration should be given to the administration of calcitonin or other antiresorptive agents, such as the bisphosphonates. Although not approved for use in kidney transplant recipients, cinacalcet may be considered in the patient with persistently elevated PTH after transplant provided hypocalcemia is not a concern.

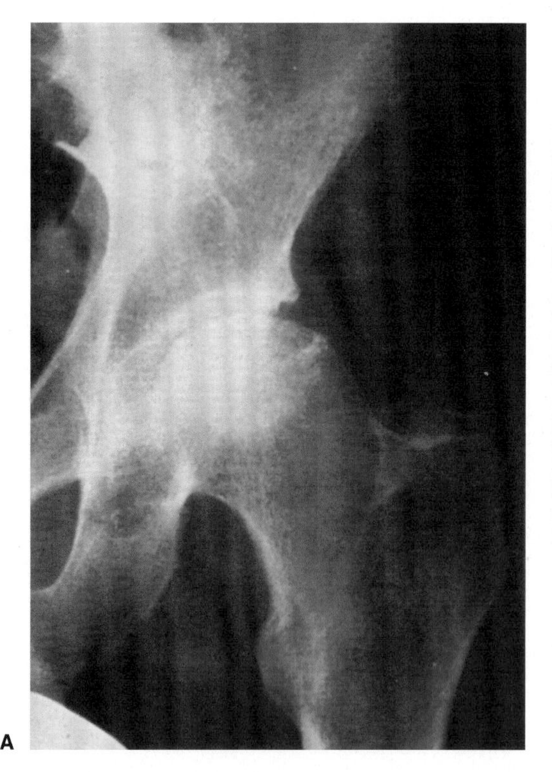

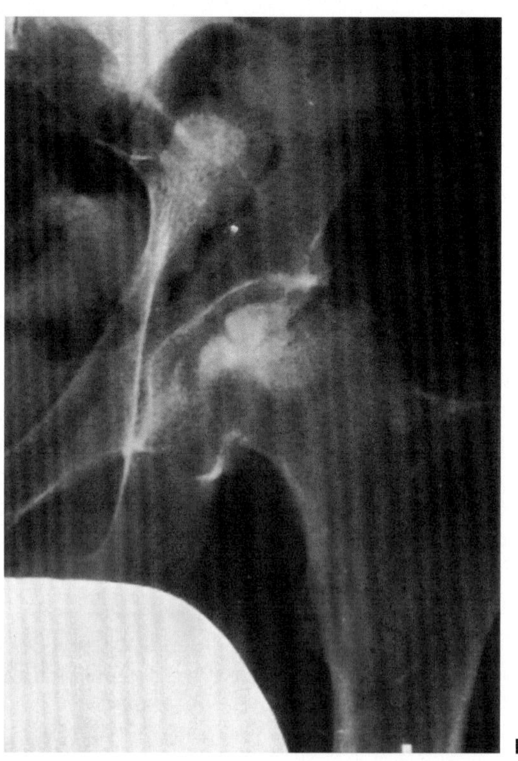

FIGURE 82.26 An avascular necrosis of the head of the femur after transplantation. **A.** A normal radiograph of the hip 10 months after transplantation, at which time the patient was complaining of pain. **B.** The same hip 8 months later. This patient had received azathioprine and high-dose steroids and subsequently had a successful hip replacement. (From Morris PJ. *Kidney Transplantation: Principles and Practice*. 2nd ed. New York: Grune & Stratton; 1984, with permission.)

Gastrointestinal Complications

GI complications include peptic ulceration, esophagitis, intestinal or colonic perforation and hemorrhage, pseudomembranous colitis, necrotizing enterocolitis, and diverticulitis.

Complications of a peptic ulcer, either hemorrhage or perforation, are associated with a high mortality in transplant patients. Whereas about 8% of patients with negative peptic ulcer histories before engraftment later develop gastroduodenal complications, 19% of those with previous episodes of uremic gastritis develop further complications after transplantation. Most transplant centers now prescribe proton pump inhibitors or histamine antagonists prophylactically during the first few months after transplantation to prevent these complications. Both hemorrhage and perforation from a peptic ulcer after transplantation should be treated promptly and aggressively by surgery.

Infection of the gastrointestinal tract presents commonly as *Candida* stomatitis or esophagitis. This is particularly common in transplant patients who are debilitated from other complications or infections or who have the presence of leukopenia or excess immunosuppressive therapy. Esophageal candidiasis is probably the most severe form of local infection due to this pathogen, but occasionally a septicemia may ensue. The epiglottitis and esophagitis respond to local nystatin, but more severe infections should be treated with amphotericin B or fluconazole. Classic enteric pathogens are not notably common after transplantation.

Spontaneous perforation of the small intestine is rare and the etiology is often not understood, although CMV infection, obstruction, intestinal ischemia, and the use of steroids have been implicated. Hemorrhage of the large bowel with ulceration and perforation occurs in 0.9% of such patients. Possible causes include uremia, the effects of immunosuppressive therapy, the use of antibiotics, atherosclerosis, and the sequelae of irradiation. The administration of sodium polystyrene resin in sorbitol to treat patients with hyperkalemia can also be complicated by colonic perforation.

Pseudomembranous colitis is an antibiotic-associated diarrhea and thus may occur in transplant patients who are receiving broad-spectrum antibiotic therapy for a concomitant bacterial infection. However, it may also occur in transplant units where *Clostridium difficile* infection is endemic. This condition is highly infectious and should be treated as such to avoid spread within a transplant unit. Occasionally, a necrotizing enterocolitis with gangrene of part or all of the colon, and even occasionally involving only the small bowel, is seen. This is inevitably fatal and the cause is uncertain, although it has been associated with CMV infection. Solitary ulcers, which may bleed or perforate, may also be encountered, especially in the cecum. A colonoscopy is a useful diagnostic tool in some of these colonic complications.

Diverticulitis is no more common in the transplant patient than the normal population except perhaps in patients with polycystic kidneys, but again, complicated diverticulitis does present a very serious problem with a high mortality. For this reason, some surgeons believe that the presence of diverticulosis in patients before transplantation is an indication for colectomy in order to avoid complications arising after transplantation.

Pancreatitis

Although mild hyperamylasemia without pancreatitis is common in patients with poor graft function, due to decreased clearance of the enzyme, high serum amylase and lipase levels suggest active pancreatitis. Acute pancreatitis has been reported to occur in 2% to 12% of transplant recipients. Several causes have been considered. Inflammatory changes, possibly due to secondary hyperparathyroidism, may be seen in the glands of uremic patients. Microscopic examinations occasionally have revealed changes consistent with the presence of CMV, but the role of this organism is unknown. Corticosteroids may produce pancreatitis both experimentally and clinically, and AZA and CsA can be rare causes of pancreatitis. Acute pancreatitis in renal transplant patients often follows a fulminating course with an acute abdomen, electrolyte disturbances, tetany, jaundice, and hypotension.

Renal Electrolyte and Tubular Disorders

Proximal bicarbonate wasting occurs most often in the early transplantation course and resolves gradually. Proximal renal tubular acidosis may be related to ischemic preservation injury, secondary hyperparathyroidism, malnutrition, acute tubular necrosis, and acute rejection. Distal renal tubular acidosis sometimes occurs either as a consequence of acute rejection or as a result of the interstitial nephropathy caused by chronic allograft injury. Hyperkalemia is common in patients on CNIs and is readily reversible by lowering of the dose. The mechanism is unclear but the decreased potassium excretion may be due to diminished serum aldosterone levels or to a primary tubular defect.

Hypercalcemia

Acute hypercalcemia usually occurs in the setting of severe secondary hyperparathyroidism. Because of the improved management of secondary hyperparathyroidism preoperatively, this is less frequently seen with oral phosphate binders, calcium supplementation, and vitamin D administration. Most hypercalcemic patients have transient elevations in serum calcium levels, in the range of 11 to 12 mg per deciliter. The treatment of hypercalcemia includes a dietary reduction of calcium and the cessation of thiazide diuretics and vitamin D supplements, which may exacerbate hypercalcemia. Persistent mild hypercalcemia is generally managed conservatively with serial serum calcium determinations, unless there are indications for a more aggressive intervention with a parathyroidectomy. Serum-intact PTH should be measured at 6 and 12 months and then annually posttransplantation.[143]

Indications for a parathyroidectomy in these patients include severe symptomatic hypercalcemia and persistent hypercalcemia in association with elevated PTH for longer than 6 to 12 months. Approximately 4% to 10% of patients remain hypercalcemic after 1 year. An elective parathyroidectomy should be considered if the plasma calcium concentration remains above 12.5 mg per deciliter (3.1 mmol per liter) for more than 1 year, particularly if associated with a radiologic evidence of increased bone resorption.

Hypophosphatemia

Hypophosphatemia (serum phosphorus levels <2.6 mg per deciliter) is very common in the early weeks after transplantation. The newly transplanted kidney may waste phosphate due to PTH-dependent and -independent mechanisms.[245] Hypophosphatemia is usually not symptomatic and typically resolves over 6 to 12 months. Hypophosphatemia is observed in 60% to 70% of patients within 1 year after transplantation. Hypophosphatemia may persist for more than 1 year in 20% to 25% of cases, even in the absence of hyperparathyroidism, a phenomenon that may be related to persistent elevations of the phosphaturic hormone FGF-23.[246] Plasma phosphate levels below 1.0 to 1.5 mg per deciliter (0.32 to 0.48 mmol per liter) can cause muscle weakness. Severe and prolonged hypophosphatemia can lead to osteomalacia and fractures. Oral phosphate replacements are required if hypophosphatemia persists. One important exception is the patient with significant persistent hyperparathyroidism, as detected by elevated plasma-intact PTH levels. In this setting, the administration of phosphate can exacerbate the hyperparathyroidism in part by complexing with calcium and lowering intestinal calcium absorption.

Hypomagnesemia

Hypomagnesemia (serum total magnesium levels <1.5 mg per deciliter) is common in the early weeks after transplantation. It can result from CsA- or tacrolimus-induced renal magnesium wasting via the downregulation of calcium and magnesium transport proteins,[247] and may be present in up to 25% of long-term CNI-treated patients. The prevalence decreases with time after transplantation, possibly because of decreasing CNI blood levels. Muscle weakness, hypokalemia, hypocalcemia, and rarely, seizures may result from severe hypomagnesemia. Treatment for asymptomatic hypomagnesemia with oral agents such as magnesium oxide are effective, but if symptoms potentially related to hypomagnesemia are present, consideration for the intravenous administration of magnesium sulfate is warranted.

Hyperuricemia

Renal handling of uric acid is reduced by the use of CNI agents, particularly CsA, and leads to an increase in gout attacks following transplantation.[248] Asymptomatic hyperuricemia occurs in 55% of patients receiving CsA and in 25% of those taking AZA. There is no report of graft failure due to urate nephropathy in the transplanted kidney. Crystal-induced erosive arthritis can occur in these patients. The optimal therapy for acute attacks remains colchicine with or without a brief corticosteroid pulse (20 to 30 mg for 2 to 3 days) and tapering. Nonsteroidal anti-inflammatory agents should be avoided because of the potential negative influence on renal hemodynamics and the development of interstitial nephritis. For patients with hyperuricemia and recurrent gout attacks, allopurinol, a xanthine oxidase inhibitor, can be used with attention to renal-adjusted dosing. However, allopurinol should be avoided in patients taking AZA because the concomitant administration of allopurinol and AZA results in marrow suppression and a fourfold increase in immunosuppression.

New Onset Diabetes after Transplant

Rates of NODAT have been reported at a rate of 4% to 18%, depending on the clinical trial and the immunosuppressive agents used. Both mTOR inhibitors and CNIs may cause pancreatic toxicity, with hyperglycemia occurring in a dose-dependent fashion and exacerbated by prednisone administration.[160,166] TAC appears to have a greater diabetogenic effect than CsA, and patients treated with TAC and sirolimus have the highest rate of NODAT, compared to CsA and MMF.[249] Older individuals, patients with hepatitis C, and African American and Hispanic patients are most susceptible. Transplant recipients who develop diabetes are at a greater risk of death, and support the concept of individualized immunosuppressive agent selection based on the risk for rejection versus risk for NODAT.[250]

Obesity

Lower graft survival rates, higher postoperative mortalities, and complications have been demonstrated in patients with a body mass index (BMI) >35 kg per square meter.[17,18] However, approximately 40% of renal transplant recipients are obese, defined as a BMI >30 kg per square meter or more than 130% of the ideal body weight, 1 year after transplantation. Increased calorie intake may occur after transplantation primarily because of enhanced appetite associated with corticosteroid use. If obesity ensues, it may contribute to the development or exacerbation of hypertension, hyperlipidemia, cardiovascular disease, and steroid-induced diabetes. Weight loss is recommended to improve the lipid profile, to lower blood pressure, and to improve glycemic control for patients with T2DM. In addition to limiting calorie intake, the management of posttransplantation obesity includes behavior modification, an exercise program, and early nutritional counseling. Although corticosteroid use is often implicated in posttransplant weight gain, 5 mg per day did not result in a greater weight gain compared to a steroid withdrawal strategy.[160]

Cataracts

Posterior lenticular cataracts appear in up to 10% of transplant patients receiving high-dose steroids. Usually the cataracts are small and do not present a severe handicap to the patient, although in some instances, cataracts are large and require the removal of the lens.

TABLE 82.20 **Criteria for Renal Transplantation Desiring Pregnancy**

1. Preferably 1 yr after transplantation
2. Stable graft function with minimal immunosuppression, serum creatinine <1.5–2.0 mg/dL
3. No evidence of graft rejection
4. No significant proteinuria
5. Good blood pressure control
6. No evidence of pelvicalyceal distortion

Parenthood after Renal Transplant

Chronic renal failure is associated with a loss of libido, amenorrhea in women, and impotence in men. After a successful transplantation, menstruation returns in young women, and men usually redevelop their libido and potency. Women have had successful pregnancies and men have fathered children. Spontaneous abortions and ectopic pregnancies do not appear to be more frequent in posttransplant pregnancies compared to the general population, but there is a higher rate of preeclampsia, hypertension, proteinuria, preterm delivery, and intrauterine growth retardation.[251] Given these potential complications, it is generally recommended that women have stable graft function (creatinine [Cr] <2.0 mg per deciliter, ideally <1.5 mg per deciliter and < 1 g proteinuria) for 1 year prior to conception (Table 82.20).[143] Medications should be reviewed for potential teratogenicity. Mycophenolate has been associated with congenital fetal abnormalities and should be discontinued in patients considering pregnancy.[252] Little data exist for the use of mTOR inhibitors during pregnancy; however, in men there has been an association with impaired spermatogenesis.[253]

There are no reported adverse effects of CsA or TAC on human fetuses. Although rare, steroids may cause adrenal insufficiency in the neonate. Steroids and low concentrations of AZA and CsA are found in breast milk. Because there are few data on the effect of continued exposure to low doses of immunosuppressive agents to the infant, no definitive recommendations can be offered regarding the safety of breastfeeding. With the established safety of TAC, cyclosporine, AZA, and prednisone in pregnancy, a common strategy is to use these agents whenever possible.

CURRENT SUCCESSES AND FUTURE CHALLENGES

Dramatic improvements have occurred in the outcome of renal transplantation over the past 50 years. Immunosuppressive drug regimens have become more sophisticated with better graft survival and less morbidity and mortality. Currently, the 1-year graft and patient survival rates are over 90% and 95% in most transplant centers, despite the fact that an increasing number of high risk patients are undergoing transplantation as a replacement therapy for ESRD. The long-term issues confronting the patient and physician are both the relentless decline in allograft function resulting in poor graft survival beyond 5 years and the medical complications, particularly those resulting from the use of chronic immunosuppression. Renal allograft failure is now one of the most common causes of ESRD, accounting for 20% to 30% of patients awaiting renal transplantation. Future efforts will continue to be directed toward increasing the supply of donor organs and increasing the safety of the immunosuppressive regimen.

REFERENCES

1. Hume DM, Merrill JP, Miller BF, Thron GW. Experiences with renal homotransplantation in the human: report of nine cases. *J Clin Invest*. 1955;34(2):327–382.
2. Wolfe RA, Ashby VB, Milford EL, et al. Comparison of mortality in all patients on dialysis, patients on dialysis awaiting transplantation, and recipients of a first cadaveric transplant. *N Engl J Med*. 1999;341(23):1725–1730.
3. Laupacis A, Keown P, Pus N, et al. A study of the quality of life and cost-utility of renal transplantation. *Kidney Int*. 1996;50(1):235–242.
4. Axelrod DA, McCullough KP, Brewer ED, et al. Kidney and pancreas transplantation in the United States, 1999-2008: the changing face of living donation. *Am J Transplant*. 2010;10(4 Pt 2):987–1002.
5. Merion RM, Ashby VB, Wolfe RA, et al. Deceased-donor characteristics and the survival benefit of kidney transplantation. *JAMA*. 2005;294(21):2726–2733.
6. Hariharan S, Johnson CP, Bresnahan BA, et al. Improved graft survival after renal transplantation in the United States, 1988 to 1996. *N Engl J Med*. 2000;342(9):605–612.
7. Meier-Kriesche HU, Schold JD, Kaplan B. Long-term renal allograft survival: have we made significant progress or is it time to rethink our analytic and therapeutic strategies? *Am J Transplant*. 2004;4(8):1289–1295.
8. Lamb KE, Lodhi S, Meier-Kriesche HU. Long-term renal allograft survival in the United States: a critical reappraisal. *Am J Transplant*. 2011;11(3):450–462.
9. Schold JD, Sehgal AR, Srinivas TR, et al. Marked variation of the association of ESRD duration before and after wait listing on kidney transplant outcomes. *Am J Transplant*. 2010;10(9):2008–2016.
10. Dobbels F, Ruppar T, De Geest S, et al. Adherence to the immunosuppressive regimen in pediatric kidney transplant recipients: a systematic review. *Pediatr Transplant*. 2010;14(5):603–613.
11. Ojo AO. Cardiovascular complications after renal transplantation and their prevention. *Transplantation*. 2006;82(5):603–611.
12. Bell LE, Bartosh SM, Davis CL, et al. Adolescent Transition to Adult Care in Solid Organ Transplantation: a consensus conference report. *Am J Transplant*. 2008;8(11):2230–2242.
13. Rao PS, Merion RM, Ashby VB, et al. Renal transplantation in elderly patients older than 70 years of age: results from the Scientific Registry of Transplant Recipients. *Transplantation*. 2007;83(8):1069–1074.
14. Huang E, Poommipanit N, Sampaio MS, et al., Intermediate-term outcomes associated with kidney transplantation in recipients 80 years and older: an analysis of the OPTN/UNOS database. *Transplantation*. 2010;90(9):974–979.
15. Tullius SG, Tran H, Guleria I, et al. The combination of donor and recipient age is critical in determining host immunoresponsiveness and renal transplant outcome. *Ann Surg*. 2010;252(4):662–674.
16. Pratschke J, Merk V, Reutzel-Selke A, et al. Potent early immune response after kidney transplantation in patients of the European senior transplant program. *Transplantation*. 2009;87(7):992–1000.
17. Gore JL, Pham PT, Danovitch GM, et al. Obesity and outcome following renal transplantation. *Am J Transplant*. 2006;6(2):357–363.
18. Armstrong KA, Campbell SB, Hawley CM, et al. Obesity is associated with worsening cardiovascular risk factor profiles and proteinuria progression in renal transplant recipients. *Am J Transplant*. 2005;5(11):2710–2718.
19. Schold JD, Srinivas TR, Guerra G, et al. A "weight-listing" paradox for candidates of renal transplantation? *Am J Transplant*. 2007;7(3):550–559.
20. Kendrick EA, Davis CL. Managing the failing allograft. *Semin Dial*. 2005;18(6):529–539.

21. Ayus JC, Achinger SG, Lee S, Syegh MH, Go AS. Transplant nephrectomy improves survival following a failed renal allograft. *J Am Soc Nephrol.* 2010; 21(2):374–380.

22. Gruessner RW, Sutherland DE, Gruessner AC. Mortality assessment for pancreas transplants. *Am J Transplant.* 2004;4(12):2018–2026.

23. Wolfe RA, McCullough KP, Schaubel DE, et al. Calculating life years from transplant (LYFT): methods for kidney and kidney-pancreas candidates. *Am J Transplant.* 2008;8(4 Pt 2):997–1011.

24. Wiseman AC. Simultaneous pancreas kidney transplantation: a critical appraisal of the risks and benefits compared with other treatment alternatives. *Adv Chronic Kidney Dis.* 2009;16(4):278–287.

25. Sampaio MS, Poommipanit N, Cho YW, Shah T, Bunnapradist S. Transplantation with pancreas after living donor kidney vs. living donor kidney alone in type 1 diabetes mellitus recipients. *Clin Transplant.* 2010;24(6):812–820.

26. Shapiro AM, Ricordi C, Hering BJ, et al. International trial of the Edmonton protocol for islet transplantation. *N Engl J Med.* 2006;355(13): 1318–1330.

27. Bergstralh EJ, Monico CG, Lieske JC, et al. Transplantation outcomes in primary hyperoxaluria. *Am J Transplant.* 2010;10(11):2493–2501.

28. Cibrik DM, Kaplan B, Arndorfer JA, Meier-Kriesche HU. Renal allograft survival in patients with oxalosis. *Transplantation.* 2002;74(5):707–710.

29. Roberts RA, Sketris IS, MacDonald AS, Belitsky P. Renal transplantation in secondary oxalosis. *Transplantation.* 1988;45(5):985–986.

30. Langlois V, Geary D, Murray L, et al. Polyuria and proteinuria in cystinosis have no impact on renal transplantation. A report of the North American Pediatric Renal Transplant Cooperative Study. *Pediatr Nephrol.* 2000;15(1–2):7–10.

31. Nesterova G, Gahl W. Nephropathic cystinosis: late complications of a multisystemic disease. *Pediatr Nephrol.* 2008;23(6):863–878.

32. Scheinman JI. Sickle cell disease and the kidney. *Nat Clin Pract Nephrol.* 2009;5(2):78–88.

33. Warady BA, Sullivan EK. Renal transplantation in children with sickle cell disease: a report of the North American Pediatric Renal Transplant Cooperative Study (NAPRTCS). *Pediatr Transplant.* 1998;2(2):130–133.

34. Ojo AO, Govaerts TC, Schmouder RL, et al. Renal transplantation in end-stage sickle cell nephropathy. *Transplantation.* 1999;67(2):291–295.

35. Mignani R, Feriozzi S, Schaefer RM, et al. Dialysis and transplantation in Fabry disease: indications for enzyme replacement therapy. *Clin J Am Soc Nephrol.* 2010;5(2):379–385.

36. Shah T, Gill J, Malhotra N, Takemoto SK, Bunnapradist S. Kidney transplant outcomes in patients with Fabry disease. *Transplantation.* 2009;87(2): 280–285.

37. Cybulla M, Walter KN, Schwarting A, et al. Kidney transplantation in patients with Fabry disease. *Transpl Int,* 2009;22(4):475–481.

38. Sattianayagam PT, Gibbs SD, Pinney JH, et al. Solid organ transplantation in AL amyloidosis. *Am J Transplant.* 2010;10(9):2124–2131.

39. Leung N, Griffin MD, Dispenzieri A, et al. Living donor kidney and autologous stem cell transplantation for primary systemic amyloidosis (AL) with predominant renal involvement. *Am J Transplant.* 2005;5(7):1660–1670.

40. Sethi S, Fervenza FC, Miller D, Norby S, Leung N. Recurrence of amyloidosis in a kidney transplant. *Am J Kidney Dis.* 2010;56(2):394–398.

41. Ozen S, Bilginer Y, Aktay Ayaz N, Calguneri M. Anti-interleukin 1 treatment for patients with familial Mediterranean fever resistant to colchicine. *J Rheumatol.* 2011;38(3):516–518.

42. Gobel J, Olbricht CJ, Offner G, et al. Kidney transplantation in Alport's syndrome: long-term outcome and allograft anti-GBM nephritis. *Clin Nephrol.* 1992;38(6):299–304.

43. Cornelis F, Couzi L, Le Bras Y, et al. Embolization of polycystic kidneys as an alternative to nephrectomy before renal transplantation: a pilot study. *Am J Transplant.* 2010;10(10):2363–2369.

44. Ueno T, Barri YM, Netto GJ, et al. Liver and kidney transplantation for polycystic liver and kidney-renal function and outcome. *Transplantation.* 2006; 82(4):501–507.

45. Schrier RW, Belz MM, Johnson AM, et al. Repeat imaging for intracranial aneurysms in patients with autosomal dominant polycystic kidney disease with initially negative studies: a prospective ten-year follow-up. *J Am Soc Nephrol.* 2004;15(4):1023–1028.

46. Ivanyi B. A primer on recurrent and de novo glomerulonephritis in renal allografts. *Nat Clin Pract Nephrol.* 2008;4(8):446–457.

47. Hickson LJ, Gera M, Amer H, et al. Kidney transplantation for primary focal segmental glomerulosclerosis: outcomes and response to therapy for recurrence. *Transplantation.* 2009;87(8):1232–1239.

48. Löwik MM, Groenen PJ, Levtchenko EN, et al. Molecular genetic analysis of podocyte genes in focal segmental glomerulosclerosis—a review. *Eur J Pediatr.* 2009;168(11):1291–1304.

49. Tejani A, Stablein DH. Recurrence of focal segmental glomerulosclerosis posttransplantation: a special report of the North American Pediatric Renal Transplant Cooperative Study. *J Am Soc Nephrol.* 1992;2(12 Suppl):S258–263.

50. Savin VJ, Sharma R, Sharma M, et al. Circulating factor associated with increased glomerular permeability to albumin in recurrent focal segmental glomerulosclerosis. *N Engl J Med.* 1996;334(14):878–883.

51. Wei C, Möller CC, Altintas MM, et al. Modification of kidney barrier function by the urokinase receptor. *Nat Med.* 2008;14(1):55–63.

52. Ulinski T. Recurrence of focal segmental glomerulosclerosis after kidney transplantation: strategies and outcome. *Curr Opin Organ Transplant.* 2010; 15(5):628–632.

53. Levy JB, Turner AN, Rees AJ, Pusey CD. Long-term outcome of anti-glomerular basement membrane antibody disease treated with plasma exchange and immunosuppression. *Ann Intern Med.* 2001;134(11):1033–1042.

54. Khandelwal M, McCormick BB, Lajoie G, et al. Recurrence of anti-GBM disease 8 years after renal transplantation. *Nephrol Dial Transplant.* 2004;19(2): 491–494.

55. Noris M, Remuzzi G. Thrombotic microangiopathy after kidney transplantation. *Am J Transplant.* 2010;10(7):1517–1523.

56. Ducloux D, Rebibou JM, Semhoun-Ducloux S, et al. Recurrence of hemolytic-uremic syndrome in renal transplant recipients: a meta-analysis. *Transplantation.* 1998;65(10):1405–1407.

57. Zimmerhackl LB, Hofer J, Cortina G, et al. Prophylactic eculizumab after renal transplantation in atypical hemolytic-uremic syndrome. *N Engl J Med.* 2010;362(18):1746–1748.

58. Larrea CF, Cofan F, Oppenheimer F, et al. Efficacy of eculizumab in the treatment of recurrent atypical hemolytic-uremic syndrome after renal transplantation. *Transplantation.* 89(7):903–904.

59. Fortin MC, Raymond MA, Madore F, et al. Increased risk of thrombotic microangiopathy in patients receiving a cyclosporin-sirolimus combination. *Am J Transplant.* 2004;4(6):946–952.

60. Han SS, Huh W, Park SK, et al. Impact of recurrent disease and chronic allograft nephropathy on the long-term allograft outcome in patients with IgA nephropathy. *Transpl Int.* 2010;23(2):169–175.

61. Han SS, Sun HK, Lee JP, et al. Outcome of renal allograft in patients with Henoch-Schönlein nephritis: single-center experience and systematic review. *Transplantation.* 2010;89(6):721–726.

62. Moroni G, Gallelli B, Diana A, et al. Renal transplantation in adults with Henoch-Schonlein purpura: long-term outcome. *Nephrol Dial Transplant.* 2008;23(9):3010–3016.

63. Angelo JR, Bell CS, Braun MC. Allograft failure in kidney transplant recipients with membranoproliferative glomerulonephritis. *Am J Kidney Dis.* 2011;57(2):291–299.

64. Braun MC, Stablein DM, Hamiwka LA, et al. Recurrence of membranoproliferative glomerulonephritis type II in renal allografts: The North American Pediatric Renal Transplant Cooperative Study experience. *J Am Soc Nephrol.* 2005;16(7):2225–2233.

65. Lorenz EC, Sethi S, Leung N, et al. Recurrent membranoproliferative glomerulonephritis after kidney transplantation. *Kidney Int.* 2010;77(8):721–728.

66. Noris M, Remuzzi G. Translational mini-review series on complement factor H: therapies of renal diseases associated with complement factor H abnormalities: atypical haemolytic uraemic syndrome and membranoproliferative glomerulonephritis. *Clin Exp Immunol.* 2008;151(2):199–209.

67. Moroni G, Gallelli B, Quaglini S, et al. Long-term outcome of renal transplantation in patients with idiopathic membranous glomerulonephritis (MN). *Nephrol Dial Transplant.* 2010;25(10):3408–3415.

68. El-Zoghby ZM, Grande JP, Fraile MG, et al. Recurrent idiopathic membranous nephropathy: early diagnosis by protocol biopsies and treatment with anti-CD20 monoclonal antibodies. *Am J Transplant.* 2009;9(12):2800–2807.

69. Dabade TS, Grande JP, Norby SM, Fervenza FC, Cosio FG. Recurrent idiopathic membranous nephropathy after kidney transplantation: a surveillance biopsy study. *Am J Transplant.* 2008;8(6):1318–1322.

70. Sprangers B, Lefkowitz GI, Cohen SD, et al. Beneficial effect of rituximab in the treatment of recurrent idiopathic membranous nephropathy after kidney transplantation. *Clin J Am Soc Nephrol.* 2010;5(5):790–797.

71. Contreras G, Mattiazzi A, Guerra G, et al. Recurrence of lupus nephritis after kidney transplantation. *J Am Soc Nephrol.* 2010;21(7):1200–1207.

72. Dong G, Panaro F, Bogetti D, et al. Standard chronic immunosuppression after kidney transplantation for systemic lupus erythematosus eliminates recurrence of disease. *Clin Transplant.* 2005;19(1):56–60.

73. Grimbert P, Frappier J, Bedrossian J, et al. Long-term outcome of kidney transplantation in patients with systemic lupus erythematosus: a multicenter study. Groupe Cooperatif de Transplantation d'ile de France. *Transplantation.* 1998;66(8):1000–1003.

74. Geetha D, Seo P. Renal transplantation in the ANCA-associated vasculitides. *Am J Transplant.* 2007;7(12):2657–2662.
75. Allen A, Pusey C, Gaskin G. Outcome of renal replacement therapy in antineutrophil cytoplasmic antibody-associated systemic vasculitis. *J Am Soc Nephrol.* 1998;9(7):1258–1263.
76. Nachman PH, Segelmark M, Westman K, et al. Recurrent ANCA-associated small vessel vasculitis after transplantation: A pooled analysis. *Kidney Int.* 1999;56(4):1544–1550.
77. Gibney EM, Parikh CR, Jani A, et al. Kidney transplantation for systemic sclerosis improves survival and may modulate disease activity. *Am J Transplant.* 2004;4(12):2027–2031.
78. Pham PT, Pham PC, Danovitch GM, et al. Predictors and risk factors for recurrent scleroderma renal crisis in the kidney allograft: case report and review of the literature. *Am J Transplant.* 2005;5(10):2565–2569.
79. Kasiske BL, Cangro CB, Hariharan S, et al. The evaluation of renal transplantation candidates: clinical practice guidelines. *Am J Transplant.* 2001;1 Suppl 2:3–95.
80. Knoll G, Cockfield S, Blydt-Hansen T, et al. Canadian Society of Transplantation: consensus guidelines on eligibility for kidney transplantation. *CMAJ.* 2005;173(10):S1–25.
81. Lentine KL, Hurst FP, Jindal RM, et al. Cardiovascular risk assessment among potential kidney transplant candidates: approaches and controversies. *Am J Kidney Dis.* 55(1):152–167.
82. Jones DG, Taylor AM, Enkiri SA, et al. Extent and severity of coronary disease and mortality in patients with end-stage renal failure evaluated for renal transplantation. *Am J Transplant.* 2009;9(8):1846–1852.
83. Pilmore H. Cardiac assessment for renal transplantation. *Am J Transplant.* 2006;6(4):659–665.
84. Ramanathan V, Goral S, Tanriover B, et al. Screening asymptomatic diabetic patients for coronary artery disease prior to renal transplantation. *Transplantation.* 2005;79(10):1453–1458.
85. McFalls EO, Ward HB, Moritz TE, et al. Coronary-artery revascularization before elective major vascular surgery. *N Engl J Med.* 2004;351(27):2795–2804.
86. Boden WE, O'Rourke RA, Teo KK, et al. Optimal medical therapy with or without PCI for stable coronary disease. *N Engl J Med.* 2007;356(15):1503–1516.
87. Stevens CE, Alter HJ, Taylor PE, et al. Hepatitis B vaccine in patients receiving hemodialysis. Immunogenicity and efficacy. *N Engl J Med.* 1984;311(8):496–501.
88. Feuerhake A, Muller R, Lauchart W, Pichlmayr R, Schmidt FW. HBV-vaccination in recipients of kidney allografts. *Vaccine.* 1984;2(4):255–256.
89. Ghany MG, Doo EC. Antiviral resistance and hepatitis B therapy. *Hepatology.* 2009;49(5 Suppl):S174–184.
90. Mathurin P, et al. Impact of hepatitis B and C virus on kidney transplantation outcome. *Hepatology.* 1999;29(1):257–263.
91. Fabrizi F, Martin P, Ponticelli C. Hepatitis C virus infection and renal transplantation. *Am J Kidney Dis.* 2001;38(5):919–934.
92. Huskey J, Wiseman AC. Chronic viral hepatitis in kidney transplantation. *Nat Rev Nephrol.* 2011;7(3):156–165.
93. Fabrizi F, Messa P, Basile C, Martin P. Hepatic disorders in chronic kidney disease. *Nat Rev Nephrol.* 2010;6(7):395–403.
94. Frassetto LA, Tan-Tam C, Stock PG. Renal transplantation in patients with HIV. *Nat Rev Nephrol.* 2009;5(10):582–589.
95. Stock PG, Barin B, Murphy B, et al. Outcomes of kidney transplantation in HIV-infected recipients. *N Engl J Med.* 363(21):2004–2014.
96. Hurst FP, Jindal RM, Graham LJ, et al. Incidence, predictors, costs, and outcome of renal cell carcinoma after kidney transplantation: USRDS experience. *Transplantation.* 2010;90(8):898–904.
97. Goh A, Vathsala A. Native renal cysts and dialysis duration are risk factors for renal cell carcinoma in renal transplant recipients. *Am J Transplant.* 2011;11(1):86–92.
98. Pai M, Zwerling A, Menzies D. Systematic review: T-cell-based assays for the diagnosis of latent tuberculosis infection: an update. *Ann Intern Med.* 2008;149(3):177–184.
99. Lowell JA, Stratta RJ, Taylor RJ, et al. Cholelithiasis in pancreas and kidney transplant recipients with diabetes. *Surgery.* 1993;114(4):858–863; discussion 863–864.
100. Doyle AM, Lechler RI, Turka LA. Organ transplantation: halfway through the first century. *J Am Soc Nephrol.* 2004;15(12):2965–2971.
101. Colvin RB. Antibody-mediated renal allograft rejection: diagnosis and pathogenesis. *J Am Soc Nephrol.* 2007;18(4):1046–1056.
102. Patel R, Terasaki PI. Significance of the positive crossmatch test in kidney transplantation. *N Engl J Med.* 1969;280(14):735–739.
103. Mahoney RJ, Ault KA, Given SR, et al. The flow cytometric crossmatch and early renal transplant loss. *Transplantation.* 1990;49(3):527–535.
104. Pei R, Lee JH, Shih NJ, Chen M, Terasaki PI. Single human leukocyte antigen flow cytometry beads for accurate identification of human leukocyte antigen antibody specificities. *Transplantation.* 2003;75(1):43–49.
105. Gebel HM, Bray RA, Nickerson P. Pre-transplant assessment of donor-reactive, HLA-specific antibodies in renal transplantation: contraindication vs. risk. *Am J Transplant.* 2003;3(12):1488–1500.
106. Gloor J, Stegall MD. Sensitized renal transplant recipients: current protocols and future directions. *Nat Rev Nephrol.* 2010;6(5):297–306.
107. Vo AA, Lukovsky M, Toyoda M, et al. Rituximab and intravenous immune globulin for desensitization during renal transplantation. *N Engl J Med.* 2008;359(3):242–251.
108. Cecka JM. Calculated PRA (CPRA): the new measure of sensitization for transplant candidates. *Am J Transplant.* 2010;10(1):26–29.
109. Cecka JM, Kucheryavaya AY, Reinsmoen NL, Leffell MS. Calculated PRA: initial results show benefits for sensitized patients and a reduction in positive crossmatches. *Am J Transplant.* 2011;11(4):719–724.
110. Horvat LD, Shariff SZ, Garg AX. Global trends in the rates of living kidney donation. *Kidney Int.* 2009;75(10):1088–1098.
111. Ibrahim HN, Foley R, Tan L, et al. Long-term consequences of kidney donation. *N Engl J Med.* 2009;360(5):459–469.
112. Segev DL, Muzaale AD, Caffo BS, et al. Perioperative mortality and long-term survival following live kidney donation. *JAMA.* 2010;303(10):959–966.
113. Boudville N, Prasad GV, Knoll G, et al. Meta-analysis: risk for hypertension in living kidney donors. *Ann Intern Med.* 2006;145(3):185–196.
114. Lentine KL, Schnitzler MA, Xiao H, et al. Racial variation in medical outcomes among living kidney donors. *N Engl J Med.* 2010;363(8):724–732.
115. Reisaeter AV, Røislien J, Henriksen T, Irgens LM, Hartmann A. Pregnancy and birth after kidney donation: the Norwegian experience. *Am J Transplant.* 2009;9(4):820–824.
116. Ibrahim HN, Akkina SK, Leister E, et al. Pregnancy outcomes after kidney donation. *Am J Transplant.* 2009;9(4):825–834.
117. Matas AJ, Garvey CA, Jacobs CL, Kahn JP. Nondirected donation of kidneys from living donors. *N Engl J Med.* 2000;343(6):433–436.
118. Roodnat JI, Zuidema W, van de Wetering J, et al. Altruistic donor triggered domino-paired kidney donation for unsuccessful couples from the kidney-exchange program. *Am J Transplant.* 2010;10(4):821–827.
119. Rees MA, Kopke JE, Pelletier RP, et al. A nonsimultaneous, extended, altruistic-donor chain. *N Engl J Med.* 2009;360(11):1096–1101.
120. Rizvi AH, Naqvi AS, Zafar NM, Ahmed E. Regulated compensated donation in Pakistan and Iran. *Curr Opin Organ Transplant.* 2009;14(2):124–128.
121. The Declaration of Istanbul on Organ Trafficking and Transplant Tourism. *Clin J Am Soc Nephrol.* 2008;3(5):1227–1231.
122. Metzger RA, Delmonico FL, Feng S, et al. Expanded criteria donors for kidney transplantation. *Am J Transplant.* 2003;3 Suppl 4:114–125.
123. Rao PS, Ojo A. The alphabet soup of kidney transplantation: SCD, DCD, ECD—fundamentals for the practicing nephrologist. *Clin J Am Soc Nephrol.* 2009;4(11):1827–1831.
124. Doshi MD, Hunsicker LG. Short- and long-term outcomes with the use of kidneys and livers donated after cardiac death. *Am J Transplant.* 2007;7(1):122–129.
125. Cockfield SM, Moore RB, Todd G, Solez K, Gourishankar S. The prognostic utility of deceased donor implantation biopsy in determining function and graft survival after kidney transplantation. *Transplantation.* 2010;89(5):559–566.
126. Kucirka LM, Singer AL, Ros RL, et al. Underutilization of hepatitis C-positive kidneys for hepatitis C-positive recipients. *Am J Transplant.* 2010;10(5):1238–1246.
127. Sener A, Cooper M. Live donor nephrectomy for kidney transplantation. *Nat Clin Pract Urol.* 2008;5(4):203–210.
128. Brook NR, Gibbons N, Nicol DL, McDonald SP. Open and laparoscopic donor nephrectomy: activity and outcomes from all Australasian transplant centers. *Transplantation.* 2010;89(12):1482–1488.
129. Leventhal JR, Paunescu S, Baker TB, et al. A decade of minimally invasive donation: experience with more than 1200 laparoscopic donor nephrectomies at a single institution. *Clin Transplant.* 2010;24(2):169–174.
130. Belzer FO, Southard JH. Principles of solid-organ preservation by cold storage. *Transplantation.* 1988;45(4):673–676.
131. Sung RS, Galloway J, Tuttle-Newhall JE, et al. Organ donation and utilization in the United States, 1997–2006. *Am J Transplant.* 2008;8(4 Pt 2):922–934.
132. St Peter SD, Imber CJ, Friend PJ. Liver and kidney preservation by perfusion. *Lancet.* 2002;359(9306):604–613.
133. Perico N, Cattaneo D, Sayegh MH, Remuzzi G. Delayed graft function in kidney transplantation. *Lancet.* 2004;364(9447):1814–1827.
134. Pascual J, Zamora J, Pirsch JD. A systematic review of kidney transplantation from expanded criteria donors. *Am J Kidney Dis.* 2008;52(3):553–586.

135. Kokkinos C, Antcliffe D, Nanidis T, et al. Outcome of kidney transplantation from nonheart-beating versus heart-beating cadaveric donors. *Transplantation.* 2007;83(9):1193–1199.
136. Moers C, Smits JM, Maathuis MH, et al. Machine perfusion or cold storage in deceased-donor kidney transplantation. *N Engl J Med.* 2009;360(1):7–19.
137. Treckmann J, Moers C, Smits JM, et al. Machine perfusion versus cold storage for preservation of kidneys from expanded criteria donors after brain death. *Transpl Int.* 2011;24(6):548–554.
138. Jochmans I, Moers C, Smits JM, et al. Machine perfusion versus cold storage for the preservation of kidneys donated after cardiac death: a multicenter, randomized, controlled trial. *Ann Surg.* 2010;252(5):756–764.
139. Watson CJ, Wells AC, Roberts RJ, et al. Cold machine perfusion versus static cold storage of kidneys donated after cardiac death: a UK multicenter randomized controlled trial. *Am J Transplant.* 2010;10(9):1991–1999.
140. Murray JE, Harrison JH. Surgical management of fifty patients with kidney transplants including eighteen pairs of twins. *Am J Surg.* 1963;105:205–218.
141. Gorey TF, Bulkley GB, Spees EK Jr, Sterioff S. Iliac artery ligation: the relative paucity of ischemic sequelae in renal transplant patients. *Ann Surg.* 1979;190(6):753–757.
142. Weil R III, Simmons RL, Tallent MB, et al. Prevention of urological complications after kidney transplantation. *Ann Surg.* 1971;174(1):154–160.
143. KDIGO clinical practice guideline for the care of kidney transplant recipients. *Am J Transplant.* 2009;9 Suppl 3: S1–155.
144. Gaber AO, First MR, Tesi RJ, et al. Results of the double-blind, randomized, multicenter, phase III clinical trial of Thymoglobulin versus Atgam in the treatment of acute graft rejection episodes after renal transplantation. *Transplantation.* 1998;66(1):29–37.
145. Webster AC, et al. Interleukin 2 receptor antagonists for kidney transplant recipients. *Cochrane Database Syst Rev.* (1):CD003897.
146. Gralla J, Wiseman AC. The impact of IL2ra induction therapy in kidney transplantation using tacrolimus- and mycophenolate-based immunosuppression. *Transplantation.* 2010;90(6):639–644.
147. Noël C, Abramowicz D, Durand D, et al. Daclizumab versus antithymocyte globulin in high-immunological-risk renal transplant recipients. *J Am Soc Nephrol.* 2009;20(6):1385–1392.
148. Brennan DC, Daller JA, Lake KD, et al. Rabbit antithymocyte globulin versus basiliximab in renal transplantation. *N Engl J Med.* 2006;355(19):1967–1977.
149. Clatworthy MR, Friend PJ, Calne RY, et al. Alemtuzumab (CAMPATH-1H) for the treatment of acute rejection in kidney transplant recipients: long-term follow-up. *Transplantation.* 2009;87(7):1092–1095.
150. Caillard S, Dharnidharka V, Agodoa L, Bohen E, Abbott K. Posttransplant lymphoproliferative disorders after renal transplantation in the United States in era of modern immunosuppression. *Transplantation.* 2005;80(9):1233–1243.
151. Kirk AD, Cherikh WS, Ring M, et al. Dissociation of depletional induction and posttransplant lymphoproliferative disease in kidney recipients treated with alemtuzumab. *Am J Transplant.* 2007;7(11):2619–2625.
152. Carey G, Lisi PJ, Schroeder TJ. The incidence of antibody formation to OKT3 consequent to its use in organ transplantation. *Transplantation.* 1995; 60(2):151–158.
153. Richardson PG, Briemberg H, Jagannath S, et al. Frequency, characteristics, and reversibility of peripheral neuropathy during treatment of advanced multiple myeloma with bortezomib. *J Clin Oncol.* 2006;24(19):3113–3120.
154. Becker YT, Becker BN, Pirsch JD, Sollinger HW. Rituximab as treatment for refractory kidney transplant rejection. *Am J Transplant.* 2004;4(6):996–1001.
155. Kazatchkine MD, Kaveri SV. Immunomodulation of autoimmune and inflammatory diseases with intravenous immune globulin. *N Engl J Med.* 2001; 345(10):747–755.
156. Luke PP, Scantlebury VP, Jordon ML, et al. Reversal of steroid- and anti-lymphocyte antibody-resistant rejection using intravenous immunoglobulin (IVIG) in renal transplant recipients. *Transplantation.* 2001;72(3):419–422.
157. Jordan SC, Tyan D, Stablein D, et al. Evaluation of intravenous immunoglobulin as an agent to lower allosensitization and improve transplantation in highly sensitized adult patients with end-stage renal disease: report of the NIH IG02 trial. *J Am Soc Nephrol.* 2004;15(12):3256–3262.
158. Montgomery RA, Zachary AA, Racusen LC, et al. Plasmapheresis and intravenous immune globulin provides effective rescue therapy for refractory humoral rejection and allows kidneys to be successfully transplanted into cross-match-positive recipients. *Transplantation.* 2000;70(6):887–895.
159. Matas AJ, Kandaswamy R, Gillingham KJ, et al. Prednisone-free maintenance immunosuppression—a 5-year experience. *Am J Transplant.* 2005;5(10):2473–2478.
160. Woodle ES, First MR, Pirsch J, et al. A prospective, randomized, double-blind, placebo-controlled multicenter trial comparing early (7 day) corticosteroid cessation versus long-term, low-dose corticosteroid therapy. *Ann Surg.* 2008;248(4):564–577.
161. Vincenti F, Schena FP, Paraskevas S, et al. A randomized, multicenter study of steroid avoidance, early steroid withdrawal or standard steroid therapy in kidney transplant recipients. *Am J Transplant.* 2008;8(2):307–316.
162. Opelz G, Dohler B, Laux G. Long-term prospective study of steroid withdrawal in kidney and heart transplant recipients. *Am J Transplant.* 2005; 5(4 Pt 1):720–728.
163. Ahsan N, et al. Prednisone withdrawal in kidney transplant recipients on cyclosporine and mycophenolate mofetil—a prospective randomized study. Steroid Withdrawal Study Group. *Transplantation.* 1999;68(12):1865–1874.
164. Calne RY, White DJ, Thiru S, et al. Cyclosporin A in patients receiving renal allografts from cadaver donors. *Lancet.* 1978;2(8104–5):1323–1327.
165. Pirsch JD, Miller J, Deierhoi MH, Vincenti F, Filo RS. A comparison of tacrolimus (FK506) and cyclosporine for immunosuppression after cadaveric renal transplantation. FK506 Kidney Transplant Study Group. *Transplantation.* 1997;63(7):977–983.
166. Ekberg H, Tedesco-Silva H, Demirbas A, et al. Reduced exposure to calcineurin inhibitors in renal transplantation. *N Engl J Med.* 2007;357(25): 2562–2575.
167. Hardinger KL, Bohl DL, Schnitzler MA, et al. A randomized, prospective, pharmacoeconomic trial of tacrolimus versus cyclosporine in combination with thymoglobulin in renal transplant recipients. *Transplantation.* 2005; 80(1):41–46.
168. Webster A, Woodroffe RC, Taylor RS, Chapman JR, Craig JC. Tacrolimus versus cyclosporin as primary immunosuppression for kidney transplant recipients. *Cochrane Database Syst Rev.* 2005;(4):CD003961.
169. Salvadori M, Holzer H, de Mattos A, et al. Enteric-coated mycophenolate sodium is therapeutically equivalent to mycophenolate mofetil in de novo renal transplant patients. *Am J Transplant.* 2004;4(2):231–236.
170. de Winter BC, Mathot RA, Sombogaard F, Vilto AG, van Gelder T. Nonlinear relationship between mycophenolate mofetil dose and mycophenolic acid exposure: implications for therapeutic drug monitoring. *Clin J Am Soc Nephrol.* 2011;6(3):656–663.
171. Halloran P, Mathew T, Tomlanovich S, et al., Mycophenolate mofetil in renal allograft recipients: a pooled efficacy analysis of three randomized, double-blind, clinical studies in prevention of rejection. The International Mycophenolate Mofetil Renal Transplant Study Groups. *Transplantation.* 1997;63(1):39–47.
172. Zoncu R, Efeyan A, Sabatini DM. mTOR: from growth signal integration to cancer, diabetes and ageing. *Nat Rev Mol Cell Biol.* 2011;12(1):21–35.
173. Andoh TF, Burdmann EA, Fransechini N, Houghton DC, Bennett WM. Comparison of acute rapamycin nephrotoxicity with cyclosporine and FK506. *Kidney Int.* 1996;50(4):1110–1117.
174. Straathof-Galema L, Wetzels JF, Dijkman HB, et al. Sirolimus-associated heavy proteinuria in a renal transplant recipient: evidence for a tubular mechanism. *Am J Transplant.* 2006;6(2):429–433.
175. Biancone L, Bussolati B, Mazzucco G, et al. Loss of nephrin expression in glomeruli of kidney-transplanted patients under m-TOR inhibitor therapy. *Am J Transplant.* 2010;10(10):2270–2278.
176. Hitchings GH, Elion GB. Chemical suppression of the immune response. *Pharmacol Rev.* 1963;15:365–405.
177. A blinded, randomized clinical trial of mycophenolate mofetil for the prevention of acute rejection in cadaveric renal transplantation. The Tricontinental Mycophenolate Mofetil Renal Transplantation Study Group. *Transplantation.* 1996;61(7):1029–1037.
178. Sollinger HW. Mycophenolate mofetil for the prevention of acute rejection in primary cadaveric renal allograft recipients. U.S. Renal Transplant Mycophenolate Mofetil Study Group. *Transplantation.* 1995;60(3):225–232.
179. Tedesco Silva H Jr, Cibrik D, Johnston T, et al. Everolimus plus reduced-exposure CsA versus mycophenolic acid plus standard-exposure CsA in renal-transplant recipients. *Am J Transplant.* 2010;10(6):1401–1413.
180. Ciancio G, Burke GW, Gaynor JJ, et al. A randomized long-term trial of tacrolimus/sirolimus versus tacrolimus/mycophenolate versus cyclosporine/sirolimus in renal transplantation: three-year analysis. *Transplantation.* 2006; 81(6):845–852.
181. Gralla J, Wiseman AC. Tacrolimus/sirolimus versus tacrolimus/mycophenolate in kidney transplantation: improved 3-year graft and patient survival in recent era. *Transplantation.* 2009;87(11):1712–1719.
182. Meier-Kriesche HU, Schold JD, Srinivas TR, et al. Sirolimus in combination with tacrolimus is associated with worse renal allograft survival compared to mycophenolate mofetil combined with tacrolimus. *Am J Transplant.* 2005;5 (9):2273–2280.
183. Ekberg H, Grinyó J, Nashan B, et al. Cyclosporine sparing with mycophenolate mofetil, daclizumab and corticosteroids in renal allograft recipients: the CAESAR Study. *Am J Transplant.* 2007; 7(3):560–570.

184. Oberbauer R, Segoloni G, Campistol JM, et al. Early cyclosporine withdrawal from a sirolimus-based regimen results in better renal allograft survival and renal function at 48 months after transplantation. *Transpl Int*. 2005;18(1):22–28.
185. Weir MR, Mulgaonkar S, Chan L, et al. Mycophenolate mofetil-based immunosuppression with sirolimus in renal transplantation: a randomized, controlled Spare-the-Nephron trial. *Kidney Int*. 2011;79(8):897–907.
186. Dudley C, Pohanka E, Riad H, et al. Mycophenolate mofetil substitution for cyclosporine in renal transplant recipients with chronic progressive allograft dysfunction: the "creeping creatinine" study. *Transplantation*. 2005;79(4):466–475.
187. Schena FP, Pascoe MD, Alberu J, et al. Conversion from calcineurin inhibitors to sirolimus maintenance therapy in renal allograft recipients: 24-month efficacy and safety results from the CONVERT trial. *Transplantation*. 2009;87(2):233–242.
188. Mulay AV, Cockfield S, Stryker R, Fergusson D, Knoll GA. Conversion from calcineurin inhibitors to sirolimus for chronic renal allograft dysfunction: a systematic review of the evidence. *Transplantation*. 2006;82(9):1153–1162.
189. Vincenti F, Kirk AD. What's next in the pipeline. *Am J Transplant*. 2008;8(10):1972–1981.
190. Larsen CP, Pearson TC, Adams AB, et al. Rational development of LEA29Y (belatacept), a high-affinity variant of CTLA4-Ig with potent immunosuppressive properties. *Am J Transplant*. 2005;5(3):443–453.
191. Vincenti F, Charpentier B, Vanrenterghem Y, et al. A phase III study of belatacept-based immunosuppression regimens versus cyclosporine in renal transplant recipients (BENEFIT study). *Am J Transplant*. 2010;10(3):535–546.
192. Yadav RV, Johnson W, Morris PJ, et al. Vesico-ureteric reflux following renal transplantation. *Br J Surg*. 1972; 59(1):33–35.
193. Mathew TH, Kincaid-Smith P, Vikraman P. Risks of vesicoureteric reflux in the transplanted kidney. *N Engl J Med*. 1977;297(8):414–418.
194. Schweizer RT, Cho S, Koutz SL, Belzer FO. Lymphoceles following renal transplantation. *Arch Surg*. 1972;104(1):42–45.
195. Mathew TH, Kincaid-Smith P, Eremin J, Marshall VC. Percutaneous needle biopsy of renal homografts. *Med J Aust*. 1968;1(1):6–7.
196. Racusen LC, Solez K, Colvin RB, et al. The Banff 97 working classification of renal allograft pathology. *Kidney Int*. 1999;55(2):713–723.
197. Li B, Hartono C, Ding R, et al. Noninvasive diagnosis of renal-allograft rejection by measurement of messenger RNA for perforin and granzyme B in urine. *N Engl J Med*. 2001;344(13):947–954.
198. Graziotto R, Del Prete D, Rigotti P, et al. Perforin, Granzyme B, and fas ligand for molecular diagnosis of acute renal-allograft rejection: analyses on serial biopsies suggest methodological issues. *Transplantation*. 2006;81(8):1125–1132.
199. Muthukumar T, Dadhania D, Ding R, et al. Messenger RNA for FOXP3 in the urine of renal-allograft recipients. *N Engl J Med*. 2005;353(22):2342–2351.
200. Manfro RC, Aquino-Dias EC, Joelsons G, et al. Noninvasive Tim-3 messenger RNA evaluation in renal transplant recipients with graft dysfunction. *Transplantation*. 2008;86(12):1869–1874.
201. Sis B, Jhangri GS, Bunnag S, et al. Endothelial gene expression in kidney transplants with alloantibody indicates antibody-mediated damage despite lack of C4d staining. *Am J Transplant*. 2009;9(10):2312–2323.
202. Quiroga I, McShane P, Koo DD, et al. Major effects of delayed graft function and cold ischaemia time on renal allograft survival. *Nephrol Dial Transplant*. 2006;21(6):1689–1696.
203. Solez K, Colvin RB, Racusen LC, et al. Banff 07 classification of renal allograft pathology: updates and future directions. *Am J Transplant*. 2008;8(4):753–760.
204. Rush DN, Cockfield SM, Nickerson PW, et al. Factors associated with progression of interstitial fibrosis in renal transplant patients receiving tacrolimus and mycophenolate mofetil. *Transplantation*. 2009;88(7):897–903.
205. Locke JE, Zachary AA, Haas M, et al. The utility of splenectomy as rescue treatment for severe acute antibody mediated rejection. *Am J Transplant*. 2007;7(4):842–846.
206. Lamas S. Cellular mechanisms of vascular injury mediated by calcineurin inhibitors. *Kidney Int*. 2005;68(2):898–907.
207. El-Zoghby ZM, Stegall MD, Lager DJ, et al. Identifying specific causes of kidney allograft loss. *Am J Transplant*. 2009;9(3):527–535.
208. Wiseman AC. Polyomavirus nephropathy: a current perspective and clinical considerations. *Am J Kidney Dis*. 2009;54(1):131–142.
209. Nankivell BJ, Borrows RJ, Fung CL, et al. The natural history of chronic allograft nephropathy. *N Engl J Med*. 2003;349(24):2326–2333.
210. Stegall MD, Park WD, Larson TS, et al. The histology of solitary renal allografts at 1 and 5 years after transplantation. *Am J Transplant*. 2011;11(4):698–707.
211. Kandaswamy R, Humar A, Casingal V, et al. Stable kidney function in the second decade after kidney transplantation while on cyclosporine-based immunosuppression. *Transplantation*. 2007;83(6):722–726.
212. Ojo AO, Held PJ, Port FK, et al. Chronic renal failure after transplantation of a nonrenal organ. *N Engl J Med*. 2003;349(10):931–940.
213. Cosio FG, Gloor JM, Sethi S, Stegall MD. Transplant glomerulopathy. *Am J Transplant*. 2008;8(3):492–496.
214. Magoon S, Zhou E, Pullman J, Greenstein SM, Glicklich DG. Successful transplantation of a donor kidney with diffuse proliferative lupus nephritis and crescents—a case report. *Nephrol Dial Transplant*. 2010;25(12):4109–4113.
215. Myslak M, Amer H, Morales P, et al. Interpreting post-transplant proteinuria in patients with proteinuria pre-transplant. *Am J Transplant*. 2006;6(7):1660–1665.
216. Choy BY, Chan TM, Lai KN. Recurrent glomerulonephritis after kidney transplantation. *Am J Transplant*. 2006;6(11):2535–2542.
217. Opelz G, Zeier M, Laux G, Morath C, Döhler B. No improvement of patient or graft survival in transplant recipients treated with angiotensin-converting enzyme inhibitors or angiotensin II type 1 receptor blockers: a collaborative transplant study report. *J Am Soc Nephrol*. 2006;17(11):3257–3262.
218. Cross NB, Webster AC, Masson P, O'Connell PJ, Craig JC. Antihypertensive treatment for kidney transplant recipients. *Cochrane Database Syst Rev*. 2009(3):CD003598.
219. Fishman JA, Rubin RH. Infection in organ-transplant recipients. *N Engl J Med*. 1998;338(24):1741–1751.
220. Morath C, Mueller M, Goldschmidt H, et al. Malignancy in renal transplantation. *J Am Soc Nephrol*. 2004;15(6):1582–1588.
221. Kliem V, Fricke L, Wollbrink T, et al. Improvement in long-term renal graft survival due to CMV prophylaxis with oral ganciclovir: results of a randomized clinical trial. *Am J Transplant*. 2008;8(5):975–983.
222. Sagedal S, Hartmann A, Nordal KP, et al. Impact of early cytomegalovirus infection and disease on long-term recipient and kidney graft survival. *Kidney Int*. 2004;66(1):329–337.
223. Preiksaitis JK, Brennan DC, Fishman J, Allen U. Canadian society of transplantation consensus workshop on cytomegalovirus management in solid organ transplantation final report. *Am J Transplant*. 2005;5(2):218–227.
224. Richardson WP, Colvin RB, Cheeseman SH, et al. Glomerulopathy associated with cytomegalovirus viremia in renal allografts. *N Engl J Med*. 1981;305(2):57–63.
225. Pouria S, State OI, Wong W, Hendry BM. CMV infection is associated with transplant renal artery stenosis. *QJM*. 1998;91(3):185–189.
226. Humar A, Lebranchu Y, Vincenti F, et al. The efficacy and safety of 200 days valganciclovir cytomegalovirus prophylaxis in high-risk kidney transplant recipients. *Am J Transplant*. 2010;10(5):1228–1237.
227. Kamar N, Rostaing L, Selves J, et al. Natural history of hepatitis C virus-related liver fibrosis after renal transplantation. *Am J Transplant*. 2005;5(7):1704–1712.
228. Sayiner A, Ece T, Duman S, et al. Tuberculosis in renal transplant recipients. *Transplantation*. 1999;68(9):1268–1271.
229. John GT, Thomas PP, Thomas M, et al. A double-blind randomized controlled trial of primary isoniazid prophylaxis in dialysis and transplant patients. *Transplantation*. 1994;57(11):1683–1684.
230. Tolkoff-Rubin NE, Rubin RH. Opportunistic fungal and bacterial infection in the renal transplant recipient. *J Am Soc Nephrol*. 1992;2(12 Suppl):S264–269.
231. Kasiske BL, Snyder JJ, Gilbertson DT, Wang C. Cancer after kidney transplantation in the United States. *Am J Transplant*. 2004;4(6):905–913.
232. Vajdic CM, McDonald SP, McCredie MR, et al. Cancer incidence before and after kidney transplantation. *JAMA*. 2006;296(23):2823–2831.
233. Kiberd BA, Keough-Ryan T, Clase CM. Screening for prostate, breast and colorectal cancer in renal transplant recipients. *Am J Transplant*. 2003;3(5):619–625.
234. Carroll RP, Ramsay HM, Fryer AA, et al. Incidence and prediction of nonmelanoma skin cancer post-renal transplantation: a prospective study in Queensland, Australia. *Am J Kidney Dis*. 2003;41(3):676–683.
235. Shroff R, Rees L. The post-transplant lymphoproliferative disorder—a literature review. *Pediatr Nephrol*. 2004;19(4):369–377.
236. Blaes AH, Peterson BA, Bartlett N, Dunn DL, Morrison VA. Rituximab therapy is effective for posttransplant lymphoproliferative disorders after solid organ transplantation: results of a phase II trial. *Cancer*. 2005;104(8):1661–1667.
237. Stallone G, Schena A, Infante B, et al. Sirolimus for Kaposi's sarcoma in renal-transplant recipients. *N Engl J Med*. 2005;352(13):1317–1323.
238. Kasiske BL, Maclean JR, Snyder JJ. Acute myocardial infarction and kidney transplantation. *J Am Soc Nephrol*. 2006;17(3):900–907.
239. Groth CG, Bäckman L, Morales JM, et al. Sirolimus (rapamycin)-based therapy in human renal transplantation: similar efficacy and different toxicity compared with cyclosporine. Sirolimus European Renal Transplant Study Group. *Transplantation*. 1999;67(7):1036–1042.

240. Holdaas H, Fellström B, Jardine AG, et al. Effect of fluvastatin on cardiac outcomes in renal transplant recipients: a multicentre, randomised, placebo-controlled trial. *Lancet*. 2003;361(9374):2024–2031.
241. Holdaas H, Fellström B, Cole E, et al. Long-term cardiac outcomes in renal transplant recipients receiving fluvastatin: the ALERT extension study. *Am J Transplant*. 2005;5(12):2929–2936.
242. Bruno S, Remuzzi G, Ruggenenti P. Transplant renal artery stenosis. *J Am Soc Nephrol*. 2004;15(1):134–141.
243. Aeberhard JM, Schneider PA, Vallotton MB, Kurtz A, Leski M. Multiple site estimates of erythropoietin and renin in polycythemic kidney transplant patients. *Transplantation*. 1990;50(4):613–616.
244. Julian BA, Laskow DA, Dubovsky J, et al. Rapid loss of vertebral mineral density after renal transplantation. *N Engl J Med*. 1991;325(8):544–550.
245. Rosenbaum RW, Hruska KA, Korkor A, Anderson C, Slatopolsky E. Decreased phosphate reabsorption after renal transplantation: Evidence for a mechanism independent of calcium and parathyroid hormone. *Kidney Int*. 1981;19(4):568–578.
246. Bhan I, Shah A, Holmes J, et al. Post-transplant hypophosphatemia: Tertiary 'Hyper-Phosphatoninism'? *Kidney Int*. 2006;70(8):1486–1494.
247. Nijenhuis T, Hoenderop JG, Bindels RJ. Downregulation of Ca(2+) and Mg(2+) transport proteins in the kidney explains tacrolimus (FK506)-induced hypercalciuria and hypomagnesemia. *J Am Soc Nephrol*. 2004;15(3):549–557.
248. Abbott KC, Kimmel PL, Dharnidharka V, et al. New-onset gout after kidney transplantation: incidence, risk factors and implications. *Transplantation*. 2005;80(10):1383–1391.
249. Johnston O, Rose CL, Webster AC, Gill JS. Sirolimus is associated with new-onset diabetes in kidney transplant recipients. *J Am Soc Nephrol*. 2008;19(7):1411–1418.
250. Cole EH, Johnston O, Rose CL, Gill JS. Impact of acute rejection and new-onset diabetes on long-term transplant graft and patient survival. *Clin J Am Soc Nephrol*. 2008;3(3):814–821.
251. McKay DB, Josephson MA. Pregnancy in recipients of solid organs—effects on mother and child. *N Engl J Med*. 2006;354(12):1281–1293.
252. Le Ray C, Coulomb A, Elefant E, Frydman R, Audibert F. Mycophenolate mofetil in pregnancy after renal transplantation: a case of major fetal malformations. *Obstet Gynecol*. 2004;103(5 Pt 2):1091–1094.
253. Huyghe E, Zairi A, Nohra J, et al. Gonadal impact of target of rapamycin inhibitors (sirolimus and everolimus) in male patients: an overview. *Transpl Int*. 2007;20(4):305–311.

CHAPTER

83 Peritoneal Dialysis

Seth Furgeson • Rajnish Mehrotra • John M. Burkart • Isaac Teitelbaum

Since the first description of continuous ambulatory peritoneal dialysis (CAPD) in 1976, peritoneal dialysis (PD) has become the dominant modality for home dialysis across the globe. Over the last decade, the patterns of utilization rates for PD have changed. Although the proportion of end-stage renal disease (ESRD) patients treated with PD remains low in many Western countries, as well as developing countries in the Middle East and South Asia, the utilization rates are increasing in several Eastern European, South Pacific, and East Asian countries.[1,2] In the United States, the percentage of dialysis patients on PD has decreased over the past decade with a slight increase in 2008; during that year, fewer than 7% of dialysis patients received PD.[3] Lack of adequate patient and physician education regarding PD likely contributes to this pattern of underutilization.[4] Given the absence of a randomized, controlled clinical trial comparing PD and conventional hemodialysis (HD), observational studies comparing incident PD and HD patients provide the best comparisons of the two modalities. Based on these studies, a few key observations can be made. First, patients commencing treatment with PD are younger and have a lower comorbidity burden than those that are treated with HD.[5] Second, there appears to be a modality by time interaction, such that patients commencing PD have a higher probability of survival during the first 2 to 3 years of renal replacement therapy when compared to HD patients; this advantage diminishes over time.[6–8] Third, the relative outcomes of patients treated by HD or PD seem to be modified by their age and diabetic status and the presence or absence of comorbidities. Thus, among individuals with no baseline comorbidity, treatment with PD appears to be associated with a survival advantage among nondiabetic patients (all age groups) and young diabetic patients (age <45 years).[9,10] It remains unclear if these differences in survival reflect a "modality effect" or are due to selection bias undescribed by known comorbidities. Nonetheless, PD treatment is used by thousands of patients around the world and appears poised to remain an important modality for renal replacement therapy. Furthermore, virtually all studies of contemporary cohorts of dialysis patients have demonstrated a similar overall survival from different parts of the world with different levels of PD utilization.[6,9,11,12]

Space precludes us from describing an extensive physiologic basis for PD. We discuss the current major issues of concern for PD in this chapter—the definition of "adequate" therapy and the control or management of therapy-related complications.

PERITONEAL DIALYSIS MODALITIES

PD may be performed manually and/or with the assistance of an automated device, commonly referred to as a "cycler." Similarly, PD therapy may be either continuous or intermittent. In most patients, selection of the PD modality hinges upon which therapy better suits the patient's lifestyle. However, in the absence of residual renal function, it is probably always desirable to use a continuous therapy.

Peritoneal Dialysis Techniques: Continuous Therapies

Continuous Ambulatory Peritoneal Dialysis

Until recently, CAPD was the most commonly used form of PD. Since its original description, there have been few changes in the basic therapy, although there have been many changes in the connection devices or "connectology" used to make the exchange. CAPD is a manual therapy and usually uses less dialysate than automated PD. The usual dialysis prescription for patients on this technique is four exchanges per day using 2.0 to 2.5 L of dialysate. However, in many developing countries, patients are treated using three exchanges with lower fill volumes with similar results. The equivalent results despite a lower dialysate use may, in part, be secondary to smaller body size in these countries.

Continuous-Cycling Peritoneal Dialysis

The utilization of automated peritoneal dialysis (APD), of which continuous-cycling peritoneal dialysis (CCPD) is the most common, is rapidly increasing in many parts of the world, like the United States.[3] Most often, patients undergoing CCPD use an automated cycler to perform exchanges while they sleep with a subsequent "last fill" and single daytime dwell until the following evening; therefore, this is a continuous therapy. Some patients also require a daytime exchange, either to maximize solute clearances or to enhance fluid removal. Although it may be done manually, this exchange is more commonly performed using the cycler as a "docking" station for drain of the last fill instilled in the morning and subsequent instillation of fresh dialysis fluid. APD performed in this fashion is commonly referred to as CCPD with a midday exchange or as "high-dose" CCPD (a misnomer, as the volume of fluid used may well be less than that used by another patient performing "low" dose CCPD).

Peritoneal Dialysis Techniques: Intermittent Therapies

Because intermittent therapies typically use multiple short dwells, they tend to be automated, although they can be done manually. Intermittent PD (IPD) therapies are best suited for patients who are found to be high transporters based on the peritoneal equilibration test (PET). However, they should rarely be used once the patient loses residual renal function. These therapies also may be transiently indicated during peritonitis for some patients experiencing problems with ultrafiltration, or if PD therapy needs to be initiated within 2 weeks of implantation of the PD catheter (early "break-in").

Intermittent Peritoneal Dialysis

By definition, IPD implies that therapy periods alternate with periods when the peritoneum has been drained ("dry abdomen"). As classically performed the patient uses multiple short-dwell exchanges three or four times a week. Techniques include manual IPD, cycler IPD, reverse osmosis machine IPD, intermittent reciprocating dialysis with an extracorporeal reconstituting circuit, and others. In recognition of the importance of small and possibly middle-molecule clearances, IPD is now rarely used.

Nonetheless, classic IPD therapies continue to have their uses. Cycler IPD has been used in areas where technical, social, and economic limitations restrict the use of CAPD. Cycler IPD has been used immediately after abdominal surgery, for elderly patients, patients with refractory heart failure, or for those who are on CAPD and have developed hernias or leaks.[13]

Nightly Intermittent Peritoneal Dialysis

Nightly IPD (NIPD) utilizes a cycler overnight with a subsequent dry day. It is best employed by patients who still have residual renal function regardless of their transport type. Daytime ambulatory peritoneal dialysis (DAPD) is based on the same concept as NIPD, but DAPD is a manual technique, and the patient typically has a "dry time" during the night. The lower the peritoneal membrane transfer rates, the lower the 8-hour NIPD or DAPD clearances, and, in some patients, time spent on NIPD or DAPD has to be prolonged by 10% to 40% to achieve minimal target clearances.[16,17] Like IPD, NIPD can be used for management of patients with heart failure, as transient therapy for postoperative patients, or patients treated with CAPD or CCPD, who have developed hernias or leaks,[18] or for women with rectal or vaginal prolapse.

Tidal Peritoneal Dialysis

Tidal peritoneal dialysis (TPD) is best performed nightly by the use of an automated cycler. It involves the maintenance of an intraperitoneal reservoir of dialysate, which is achieved by incomplete drainage of the fluid at the end of each dwell. Additional amounts of fluid are instilled with each exchange to maintain an optimal intraperitoneal volume. By maintaining an intraperitoneal reservoir of dialysate, it is assumed that tidal dialysis may maintain more continuous contact of dialysate with the peritoneal membrane. Furthermore, the more rapid cycling of dialysis may increase mixing and prevent formation of stagnant intraperitoneal fluid layers. Although preliminary studies suggested that small solute clearances are augmented[14,15] subsequent studies have failed to confirm the ability of TPD to enhance clearances.[16–18] TPD is useful, however, for patients who have pain with either infusion or draining; the reservoir of dialysate minimizes pain during drainage and upon instillation of fresh dialysate.[19] In prescribing tidal peritoneal dialysis, variables to be chosen include reserve volume, tidal outflow volume, tidal replacement volume, flow rates, and frequency of the exchanges. Although TPD may have clinical benefits, the treatment cost will be increased due to the additional dialysate fluid.

DEFINING ADEQUACY OF DIALYSIS USING SMALL SOLUTE CLEARANCES

Minimal Versus Optimal Dialysis

The native kidneys perform excretory and endocrine functions and are pivotal in the maintenance of euvolemia. The loss of these functions in patients with progressive renal failure results in numerous metabolic and vascular abnormalities. In order to return the individual to complete health, some of the goals of optimal renal replacement therapy are summarized in Table 83.1. The concept of "optimal" renal replace-

TABLE 83.1 Goals of End-Stage Renal Disease Replacement Therapy

Improve duration and quality of life
Reverse uremic signs and symptoms
Control acid-base abnormalities
Improve dyslipidemia and cardiovascular risk
Stabilize nutritional status
Remove small and middle sized uremic toxins
Improve abnormalities in mineral and bone metabolism
Minimize patient inconvenience factors
Control blood pressure and maintain euvolemia

TABLE 83.2 **Solute Removal by Dialysis and the Natural Kidney**

Solute Clearance	Natural Kidney	HD Low Flux	HD High Flux	CAPD
Urea (L/wk)	750	130	130	70
Vitamin B_{12} (L/wk)	1,200	30	60	40
Inulin (L/wk)	1,200	10	40	20
B_2-microglobulin (mg/wk)	1,000	0	300	250

HD, hemodialysis; CAPD, continuous ambulatory peritoneal dialysis.
Modified from Keshaviah P. Adequacy of CAPD: a quantitative approach. *Kidney Int Suppl.* 1992;38:S160.

ment therapy, as applied to dialytic therapies, entails that the amount of dialysis delivered is not the rate-limiting step that determines patient outcome. In other words, an "optimal" dialysis prescription eliminates uremia as a potential variable, allows patients to achieve euvolemia, and maximizes quality of life. Given the continuing high risk for morbidity and mortality and poor rehabilitation among the ESRD population, it is clear that the current renal replacement therapies are far from achieving the goal of "optimal" therapy.[20] One of the reasons for this may be that, for a large number of solutes, the dialytic clearances typically replace <10% of the native renal excretory function (Table 83.2).[21] Based on these considerations and the current state of knowledge relating small solute clearances to outcome, it is more reasonable to define clearance goals of dialytic therapy in terms of "minimal acceptable," rather than "optimal," dialysis.

After the widespread introduction of hemodialysis, studies of patients undergoing HD attempted to define a "dose" of hemodialysis sufficient to prevent malnutrition, uremia, and premature death. Based on the initial results and subsequent reanalysis of the National Cooperative Dialysis Study, the concept of urea kinetic modeling was developed to monitor the dose of HD.[22,23] Shortly thereafter, the concept of monitoring the dose of dialysis using urea (and, subsequently, creatinine) kinetic modeling was extended to patients undergoing PD. Thus, over the last two decades, the adequacy of dialysis dose has been based on an assessment of achieved clearances of small solutes.

However, as is clear from Table 83.2, small-solute clearance is substantially lower for PD than HD. Yet, as discussed in the preceding section, the overall outcome is similar between HD and PD patients. It is also clear from Table 83.2 that solute clearances in CAPD exceed those of standard HD for all but the small-molecular-weight solutes. Is the reason that survival rates on CAPD and HD are similar because of comparable "middle-molecule" clearance? Should middle-molecule clearance be measured as the "PD yardstick?" At this time, there are no interventional studies to support such a change in the "PD yardstick." However, it is important to note that strategies that maximize small-solute clearances do not necessarily enhance the clearance of larger-molecular-weight toxins as clearance of the latter is time-dependent (Fig. 83.1).[24]

Small-Solute Clearances and Mortality

Dialysis dose among patients undergoing PD had historically been measured using both urea and creatinine clearances; however, as renal creatinine clearance in ESRD patients is largely a function of creatinine secretion, urea clearance alone is now more commonly used. Because the urea clearance is expressed as a sum of renal and peritoneal clearance, studies evaluating mortality risk and dialysis dose must clearly differentiate between renal and peritoneal Kt/V. Most large, observational studies examining mortality demonstrated that although renal urea clearance is strongly associated with a variety of patient outcomes, peritoneal clearances within the range achieved in clinical practice is substantially less so.[25–35] Furthermore, two randomized, controlled, clinical trials[36,37] have now provided the final confirmatory evidence that increases in peritoneal

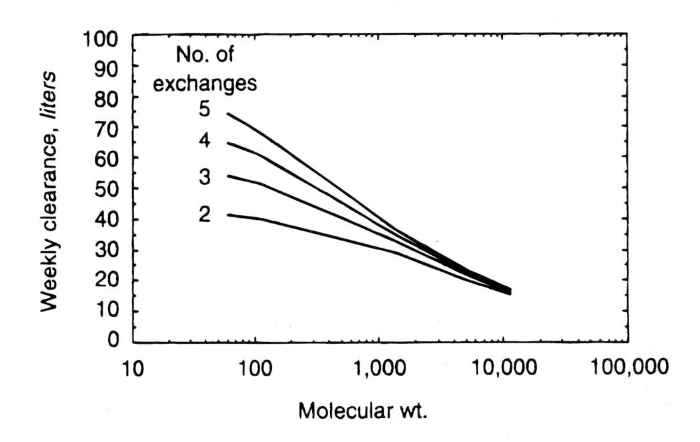

FIGURE 83.1 The influence of the number of exchanges on the weekly solute clearance for solutes with a range of molecular weights derived from a computerized model of peritoneal transport. (From Keshaviah P. Adequacy of CAPD: a quantitative approach. *Kidney Int Suppl.* 1992;38:S160, with permission.)

clearance, within the range achieved in clinical practice, do not result in significant improvement in patient morbidity or mortality (Table 83.3).[52,53] This accumulating body of data should not be taken to mean that peritoneal clearances are biologically irrelevant or that providing peritoneal clearances do not have a survival benefit—an anuric patient would die in the absence of peritoneal clearances. However, these data clearly suggest that within the range of clearances currently achieved in clinical practice, higher peritoneal clearances are unlikely to result in significant improvement in patient survival.

Small-Solute Clearances and Morbidity

ESRD patients suffer considerable morbidity, have impairments in the quality of life, and patients treated with PD continue to have a high rate of transfer off the therapy ("technique failure"). In observational studies, it appears that a low level of small solute clearance is associated with morbid outcome.[28,30,35] Two of the three randomized, controlled trials were unable to demonstrate any beneficial effect of increasing peritoneal clearances on the risk for hospitalization or the number of hospital days or technique survival (Table 83.3).[36,37] In the study by Mak et al., the intervention group had a higher hospitalization rate at the time of entry into the study when compared to the control group. Upon follow-up over 12 months, the hospitalization rate remained unchanged in the intervention group but increased in the control group, such that there were no significant differences in the hospitalization rates between the two groups over the study period.[38]

Furthermore, observational studies have been unable to demonstrate any relationship between small-solute clearances and the quality of life of PD patients.[39,40] These findings have now been confirmed by ADEMEX—a randomized, controlled, clinical trial.[41]

Thus, the existing body of evidence suggests that within the range of clearances currently achieved in clinical practice, higher peritoneal clearances are unlikely to result in significant improvements in hospitalization rate, technique failure, or quality of life of PD patients.

Small-Solute Clearances, Nutritional Status, and Patient Outcome

Due to the high prevalence of protein-energy wasting (PEW) in PD patients and the deleterious long-term consequences of wasting, the impact of small solute clearance on the nutritional status of PD patients has been an actively studied area. As with HD patients, in PD patients there are multiple, imperfect clinical measures of PEW as well as difficult-to-obtain research techniques. Importantly, there is poor correlation amongst the different measurements.[42–44] Low serum albumin and prealbumin levels, poor subjective global assessment (SGA), low fat-free edema-free mass, low dietary protein intake, and diminished hand grip strength are associated with higher morbidity and mortality.[42,43,45–49] Notwithstanding the evidence that the etiology of nutritional decline among ESRD patients is multifactorial (including an important role of inflammation), inadequate dietary intakes are probably important and independent contributors to the high prevalence of PEW among the dialysis population.[50] It follows, then, that if enhancing the dose of dialysis can result in an increase in dietary intakes, the higher dose would have the potential of improving their nutritional status; this, in turn, would be expected to have a salutary effect on patient outcome.

Based on multiple, small studies, there is evidence that increasing dialysis dose can improve nutritional status. Studies that show a relationship between Kt/V_{urea} and nPNA (normalized protein equivalent of nitrogen appearance) are problematic since both equations share common variables.[51,52] However, enhanced solute removal has been associated with improvement in other nutritional parameters: protein intake (as measured by dietary records,[53,54] mid-arm circumference and weight gain,[55] SGA,[53] and albumin[56]). Given data that a factor in uremic serum can induce anorexia in rats, it is plausible that dialytic removal of such a factor would increase appetite.[57] However, notwithstanding the increase in dietary protein intake, recent randomized controlled trials have been unable to demonstrate an improvement in nutritional status with increasing peritoneal clearances (Table 83.3).[37,38]

Minimal Total Solute Clearance Goals

Several organizations around the world have developed clinical practice guidelines to define the target level of small-solute clearances required to optimize the health of patients undergoing PD. As would be expected, these guidelines have evolved with our understanding (as discussed previously), particularly with the availability of the results of two large randomized controlled clinical trials.[37,38] The updated guidelines by organizations in United States, Canada, and Europe are summarized in Table 83.4.[58–62] When compared to guidelines published earlier, the current recommendations differ in several important respects. First, most of the guidelines recommend only one measure of adequacy to define the minimum dose of dialysis (Kt/V_{urea}). Early studies, including the CANUSA study, suggested that patient outcome was more dependent upon total (renal + peritoneal) creatinine clearances rather than total urea clearances.[63] However, the contribution of renal creatinine clearance to total (renal + peritoneal) creatinine clearances is substantially greater than of native renal urea clearances. Because creatinine is secreted and urea is reabsorbed by renal tubules, renal creatinine clearance is always higher than renal urea clearance; on the other hand, peritoneal clearances are dependent on the molecular weight of the solute in question. Thus, creatinine clearance (molecular weight, 113) is always lower than peritoneal urea clearance (molecular weight, 60). Consequently, the expected weekly creatinine clearance is different in a patient who is just starting PD with a residual renal Kt/V_{urea} of 2.0 per week than in an anuric patient with a peritoneal Kt/V_{urea} of 2.0 per week. Thus, although both markers of solute clearance may be predictors of outcome, the target or goal for creatinine clearance may have to change over time as residual renal function decreases and is replaced by peritoneal clearance.

TABLE 83.3 **Summary of Randomized, Controlled Clinical Trials That Have Evaluated the Effect of Increasing Dialytic Clearances on Outcome among Patients Undergoing Peritoneal Dialysis**

				Mean Achieved Clearances[b]				
Author	**Patient Number**	**Follow-up (months)**	**Patient Type[a]**	**Peritoneal Kt/V_{urea}**	**Total Kt/V_{urea}**	**Peritoneal CrCl**	**Total CrCl**	**Key Results**
Mak[38]	66	12	I	1.56 1.92	1.92 2.02	1.67 54.6	54.6 61.9	Higher clearances associated with higher dietary protein intakes. No effect of increased clearances on serum albumin, hospitalization rates, or infectious complications
Paniagua[36,41]	965	22	I + P	1.62 2.13	1.80 2.27	46.1 56.9	54.1 62.9	No effect of increased clearances on patient or technique survival, serum albumin, hospitalizations, infectious complications, or quality of life. More patients in the control group died from congestive heart failure or uremia/hyperkalemia/acidosis.
Lo[37]	320	24	I[c]		1.5–1.7 1.7–.0 > 2.0			No effect of increased clearances on patient survival, nutritional status, or hospitalizations. Higher incidence of anemia and higher Epo requirements in the group with the lowest clearances.

[a]Patient type: *I*, incident; *P*, prevalent; *I* + *P*, incident and prevalent.
[b]For each study, the first line refers to the clearances in the control group and the second line refers to the clearances in the intervention group.
[c]Only those incident patients with renal Kt/V_{urea} <1.0 were eligible to participate.
CrCl, creatinine clearance.

TABLE 83.4 **Targets for Small Solute Clearances Recommended by Various Organizations for Patients Undergoing Chronic Peritoneal Dialysis**

Committee	Nature of Clearances	Kt/V	Creatinine Clearance
United States—NKF-K/DOQI[a]	Renal + peritoneal	1.7	—
European Best Practice Guidelines	Peritoneal	1.7	—
Canadian Society of Nephrology	Renal + peritoneal	1.7[a]	—
International Society of Peritoneal Dialysis	Renal + peritoneal	1.7	—
CARI (Australia)	Renal	>1.6	> 60 L/week (high and high-average transporters) > 50 L/week (low and low-average transporters)

[a]For patients with residual renal function >4 mL/min, a peritoneal Kt/V between 1.0 and 1.7 is recommended.
NKF-K/DOQI, National Kidney Foundation's Kidney Disease Outcome Quality Initiative.

On the other hand, it appears from outcome studies that the Kt/V_{urea} target may not need to change. Furthermore, it is now recognized that the stronger relationship of creatinine clearances to patient outcome was a result of the effect of the confounding effect of residual renal function. There is no evidence that peritoneal creatinine clearances are superior in predicting outcome, when compared to peritoneal urea clearance. In light of these considerations, the various expert groups recommend the use of Kt/V_{urea} alone to determine the dose of dialysis (Table 83.4). Second, the targets for Kt/V_{urea} have been changed, such that Kt/V_{urea} of 1.7 at all times is now considered to be the minimum dose necessary needed for patient well-being. Based on the results of the two recent randomized controlled trials, it is also recognized that some patients may require a higher dose of dialysis to manage uremic symptoms or to achieve euvolemia.[36,37] Third, except in the CARI guidelines, there are no differences in the definition of minimum dose of dialysis based upon the patients' transport type (see below). Fourth, some expert groups (Europe and Australia) have defined the adequacy of dialysis based only on peritoneal clearances, whereas others (Canada and the United States) define it based upon total clearances. Fifth, the targets are the same, irrespective of PD modality (CAPD or APD). Finally, volume control is recognized as an additional dimension to define adequate dialysis (see below).

MONITORING AND ADJUSTING SMALL-SOLUTE CLEARANCES

Determination of Peritoneal Transport

In its function as a dialysis membrane, the peritoneum performs two important processes: diffusion (movement of solute down a concentration gradient) and convection (movement of solute along with water, ultrafiltration [UF]). There is interpatient variation in peritoneal membrane transport characteristics. A variety of methods have been suggested, standardized, and studied to assess the peritoneal membrane function (Table 83.5).[64–68] The most precise method to evaluate diffusive function of the peritoneum is to determine the mass transfer area coefficients (MTAC) of solutes like creatinine.[69] These define transport independent of ultrafiltration (convection-related solute removal) and, consequently, are not influenced by dwell volume or glucose concentration. In order to determine the MTAC, additional laboratory measurements and computer models are necessary, but, once these are obtained, MTAC can be used easily in the clinical setting.[67,69,70]

However, of these various assessments of membrane transport characteristics, the peritoneal equilibration test (PET) is the most widely used.[65] All patients commencing PD therapy should undergo a PET. The first PET should be performed after at least 4 weeks of commencing peritoneal dialysis therapy.[71] Although some centers choose to repeat a PET only if clinically indicated, others perform the test periodically to monitor peritoneal membrane function.

In order to enhance the reproducibility of the test, several steps of the PET are standardized: (1) long (8 to 12 hours) preceding exchange; (2) drain the preceding exchange as completely as possible over 20 minutes; (3) infuse 2 L of 2.5% dextrose dialysate over 10 minutes (time 0); (4) take samples of dialysate of times 0, 120, and 240 minutes; (5) in order to take samples, 200 mL of dialysate is drained into a bag, 10 mL is drawn for testing, and 190 mL is reinfused; (6) a blood sample is taken at 120 minutes; and (7) the dialysate is drained completely at 240 minutes and the drain volume is measured. Dialysate and serum urea, glucose, and creatinine

TABLE 83.5 **Tests to Evaluate Peritoneal Membrane Function**

Test	Parameter Used to Evaluate Solute Removal Function	Parameter Used to Evaluate Fluid Removal Function
Peritoneal equilibration test (4-hour)	D/P creatinine, D/Do glucose	Drain volume
Dialysis adequacy and transport test (24-hour)	D/P creatinine	Drain volume
Standard peritoneal analysis	MTAC creatinine	Drain volume, D/P sodium, and others
Personal dialysis capacity	Area parameter	Ultrafiltration coefficient
Apex	Purification phosphate time	Apex time

are measured. For each dwell time (0, 120, and 240 minutes), dialysate to plasma ratios (D/P) of creatinine and urea are determined, as is the ratio of glucose at the drain time (120 and 240 minutes) to the initial dialysate glucose concentration (D/D_0). These results are plotted against time and compared to known standard curves (Fig. 83.2). Based on the values of D/P creatinine or D/D_0 glucose, patients are classified into one of four categories: low, low average, high average, and high transporters. It should be noted that there is a significant discordance between the categorization of patients' transport type, based upon whether D/P creatinine or D/D_0 glucose is used (Fig. 83.3).[72] Studies suggest that abbreviating the preceding exchange to 2 to 3 hours does not significantly influence the values of D/P creatinine or D/D_0 glucose; thus, patients being treated with APD do not have to change their treatment schedule on the day prior to the PET.[73,74]

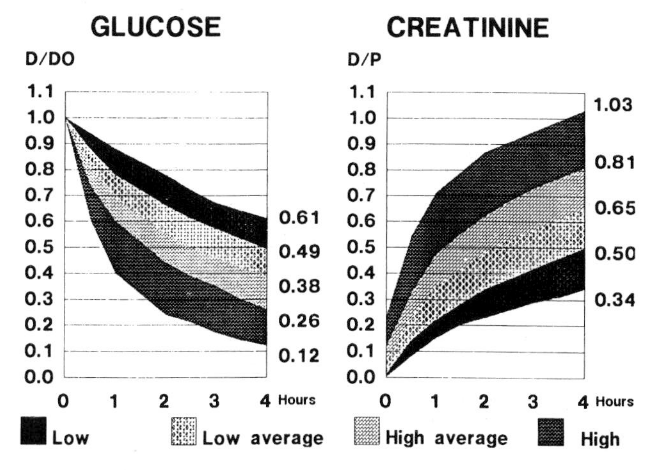

FIGURE 83.2 Dialysate to plasma ratios (D/P) for creatinine and drain time to initial dialysis concentration (D/D_0) ratios for glucose, generated from standard peritoneal equilibration testing. (From Twardowski ZJ. Clinical value of standardized equilibrium tests in CAPD patients. *Blood Purif.* 1989;7:95, with permission.)

As more has become known about ultrafiltration and water transport across the peritoneal membrane, it has been recommended that a 4.25% dextrose PET be used to characterize the ultrafiltration capacity of the peritoneum, including aquaporin-mediated water transport and solute transport.[75] The 4.25% PET has been compared to the 2.5% PET in a cohort of chronic PD patients and no clinically relevant difference in classifying the patients into different transport types was noted, suggesting that the 4.25% PET may be as clinically useful in prescription management as is the 2.5% PET.[76] The 4.25% PET has the added advantage of directly assessing the adequacy of ultrafiltration as well; ultrafiltration is defined as failure of a 4-hour dwell with 4.25% dextrose to yield at least 400 mL of net ultrafiltration.[75]

Clinical Relevance of Characterizing Peritoneal Membrane Function

The PET is used specifically to characterize the patient's peritoneal membrane transport properties. Knowledge of the peritoneal transport allows a physician to choose an appropriate prescription for a patient; this is particularly useful when using computerized, kinetic modeling for prescription management.

In general, rapid transporters of creatinine and urea also tend to be rapid absorbers of dialysate glucose (high D/P creatinine and low D/D_0 glucose). Therefore, although the D/P creatinine ratios for a 4-hour dwell tend to be close to 1, drain volumes tend to be small. Rapid transporters maximize their D/P ratios and intraperitoneal volumes early during the dwell. Once the osmotic gradient dissipates, UF ceases, followed thereafter by net fluid reabsorption. With standard CAPD, these patients may have drain volumes that are actually less than instilled volumes. Short dwell times often are needed to optimize clearance.[77]

On the other hand, in slow transporters, peak UF occurs late during the dwell, and net UF can be obtained even after prolonged dwells because glucose absorption is slow (low

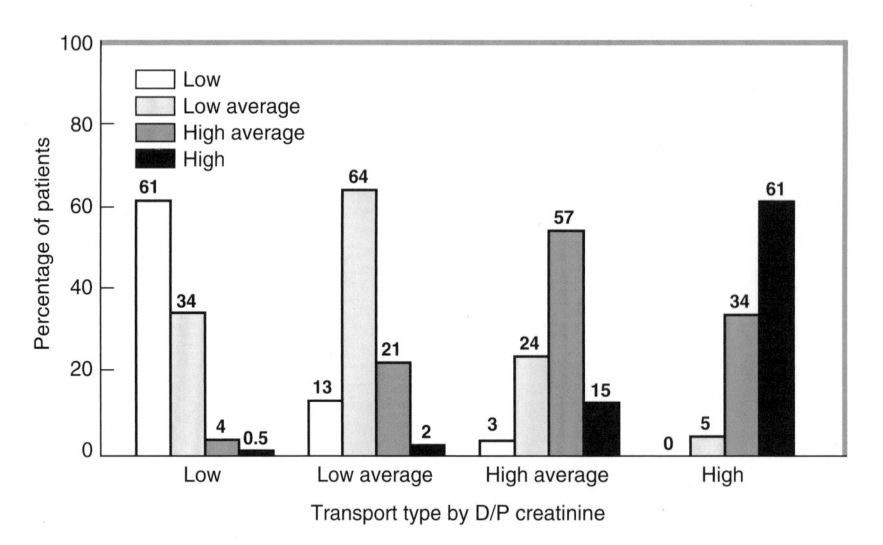

FIGURE 83.3 Discordance between categorization of patients' transport type by D/P creatinine or D/D_0 glucose. Thus, of the patients categorized low transporter by D/P creatinine, 61% of them will be classified as a low transporter by D/D_0 glucose; of the patients classified as low average transporter, 64% will be classified as low average transporter by D/D_0 glucose; of the patients classified as high average transporter, 57% will be classified as high average transporter by D/D_0 glucose; and of the patients classified as high transporter by D/P creatinine, 61% will be classified as high transporter by D/D_0 glucose. (Modified from Mujais S, Vonesh E. Profiling of peritoneal ultrafiltration. *Kidney Int Suppl.* 2002;81:S17, with permission.)

D/P creatinine and high D/D_0 glucose). The D/P ratios for creatinine and urea increase almost linearly during the dwell. For these patients, dwell time is the crucial determinant of overall clearance. They do best with continuous therapies, such as standard CAPD or CCPD. Notwithstanding these considerations, the vast majority of patients have an "average" transport type and they can be successfully treated with either PD modality. Two recent, large studies have demonstrated that there is not a difference in mortality among patients treated with CAPD or APD.[78,79] Furthermore, either PD modality (CAPD or CCPD) can be successfully adapted to even patients at the extreme of transport type (rapid or slow).

The original studies of the PET demonstrated associations between clinical variables and transport status.[65] Diabetes has been commonly linked to high transport status.[80] More recent, larger studies have not demonstrated a firm association with many clinical variables (e.g., diabetes, inflammation, and volume status) and transport status.[81–83] Accordingly, peritoneal membrane function can only be determined by an actual, standardized measurement rather than predicting transport rate from clinical variables. Furthermore, the PET cannot be used as a substitute to measure the dose of dialysis. Although it is possible to estimate daily clearances from PET studies, these estimates can significantly over- or underestimate actual daily clearances.[84]

The PET also provides useful prognostic information for patients treated with CAPD. Brimble et al. performed a meta-analysis of studies examining the consequences of high transport status.[85] Twenty studies representing distinct populations throughout the world were included in the analysis. Increases in D/P Cr were associated with higher mortality risk and treatment failure. Due to rapid dissipation of an osmotic gradient for ultrafiltration, high transporters on CAPD would be expected to more commonly have volume overload. Indeed, within the meta-analysis, the association between high transport and mortality was much diminished in CCPD patients and other data demonstrate that once patients with high transport status transfer to HD, mortality rates equalize.[86] Thus, the present state of knowledge would suggest a careful evaluation and aggressive management of nutritional and volume status and comorbidities among individuals with a higher transport type.

Measurements to Monitor Dialysis Dose

It is recommended that monitoring should include both dialysis dose and nutritional parameters because outcomes correlate with both. In light of emerging data favoring urea clearances over creatinine clearances, however, the consensus of the various expert groups seems to be to use only urea kinetics to monitor the dose of PD (Fig. 83.4). The only major difference appears to be with regard to defining the clearance targets based upon peritoneal or total (renal + peritoneal) Kt/V_{urea}. This is an important consideration since, for a 70-kg man, each 1 mL per minute of renal urea clearance adds approximately 0.25 to the total weekly Kt/V_{urea}.

Collections of dialysate and urine over 24 hours are relatively easy to obtain and can provide most of the clinically relevant data one needs to individualize a patient's prescription and monitor progress. These collections also can be used to calculate PNA, fat-free, edema-free mass (FFEFM), and other variables. The data obtained from 24-hour collections is complementary to that obtained from PET and are routinely used together for developing a patient's dialysis prescription and problem solving.

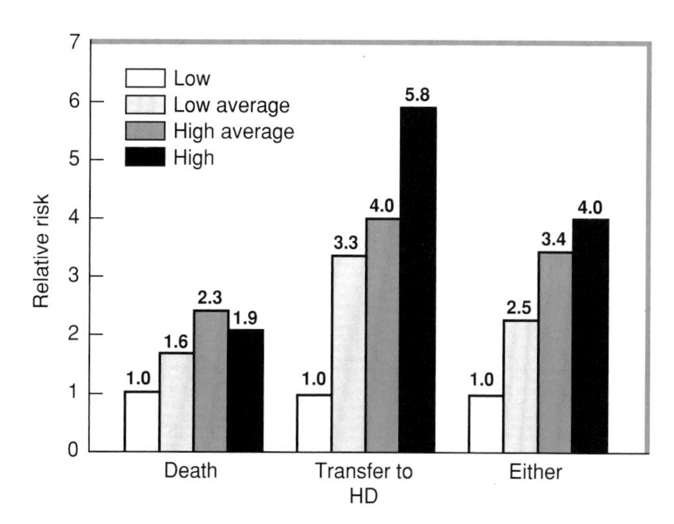

FIGURE 83.4 Relationship between transport type and patient outcome. With increasing permeability of the peritoneum, as defined by the peritoneal equilibration test, there is an increasing risk for death and/or technique failure. (Modified from Churchill DN, Thorpe KE, Nolph KD, et al. Increased peritoneal transport is associated with poor patient and technique survival on continuous ambulatory peritoneal dialysis. *J Am Soc Nephrol.* 1998;9:1285.)

Calculation of Dialysis Dose

To individualize dialysis dose and make comparisons of dose between patients, the solute clearances are typically normalized. If urea kinetics (Kt/V) are used, the sum of the daily dialysate and residual renal urea clearances are then divided by the volume of distribution for urea (V).[29] The urea V can be estimated to be 60% (males) or 55% (females) of the patient's weight in kilograms. More accurate estimations of V can be obtained using standardized nomograms, such as Watson[87] or Hume and Weyers.[88]

Calculation of the urea volume of distribution (V) is complicated by numerous pitfalls.[89] Weight has a different effect on normalization for men or women and, therefore, will affect Kt/V measurements. These differences are most marked when a patient's weight differs significantly from the norm in patients with the same height and frame size. The actual V is different in a patient with the same body weight if the increase in body weight from desirable is owing to overhydration or increase in adipose tissue. The same is true if loss of weight is due to protein energy wasting (PEW) versus amputation.

Calculation of Dietary Protein Intake

Dietary protein intake can be directly measured in metabolic wards, by dietary histories, or food recall records. An advantage of using food records is that they also evaluate total energy intake. Unfortunately, food records are time consuming and difficult to obtain because they require trained dietitians. Therefore, most reports relating dialysis dose to protein intake use estimations, based on urinary and dialysate nitrogen appearances and expressed as the protein equivalent of nitrogen appearance (PNA).[90] The most commonly used formulas to estimate PNA are summarized in Table 83.6.[91–94]

TABLE 83.6 **Commonly Used Formulas for Protein Nitrogen Appearance**

$PNA = 10.76\ (G_{un} + 1.46)$[91]
$PNA = 9.35\ G_{un} + 0.294\ V$ + protein losses[90]
$PNA = 6.25\ (UN_{loss} + 1.81 + 0.031 \times \text{body weight})$[94]
$PNA = 6.25 \times N\ loss$[92]
PNA (g/24 h) = 15.1 + (6.95 × urea nitrogen appearance in g/24 h) + dialysate and urine protein in g/24 h (Bergstrom)[a]
In the absence of direct measurement of urinary and dialysate protein losses, this following less accurate formula may be used: PNA (g/24 hours) = 20.1 + (7.50 × urea nitrogen appearance in g/24 h (Bergstrom)

[a]Bergstrom J, Heimburger O, Lindholm B. Calculation of the protein equivalent of total nitrogen appearance from urea appearance, which formulas should be used? *Perit Dial Int* 1998;18:467. (Modified from Keshaviah P, Nolph K. Protein catabolic rate calculations in CAPD patients. *Trans Am Soc Artif Intern Org.* 1991;37:M400.)

PNA, protein nitrogen appearance; G_{un}, urea nitrogen generation rate; V, volume of urea distribution; UN_{loss}, urea nitrogen loss; N, nitrogen.

The total PNA is then divided by the patient's body weight to determine the "normalized" PNA (nPNA), expressed in grams per kilogram of body weight per day. This term does not take into account differences in frame size and fat-free, edema-free mass (FFEFM). If a patient is markedly obese, the aforementioned calculations give a falsely low nPNA for the patient's actual FFEFM. Conversely, if a patient has PEW and has a less than expected FFEFM, these equations yield a falsely elevated nPNA. Various attempts to avoid this problem have been investigated, but corrections have not been standardized. One modification uses actual measurements of V or data from nomograms that more accurately estimate V. This V is then "normalized" by dividing it by 0.58 kg per L to determine normalized body weight. The PNA is then divided by normalized body weight to get nPNA. An extension of these principles is utilized to determine FFEFM from creatinine kinetics.[95] Finally, there is early evidence that bioimpedance measurements can assist with identifying both the "dry weight" and relative contribution of muscle mass, adipose mass, and fluid.[96]

Adjusting Dialysis Dose and Recognizing Pitfalls in Prescribing Peritoneal Dialysis

The initial PD prescription should be based upon a knowledge of the patient's transport type (determined using a PET), body size, and presence or absence of residual renal function. This can be done by using published algorithms (e.g., K/DOQI guidelines, data from EAPOS) or using computerized kinetic modeling.[97,98] The clearances achieved with the initial prescription should be confirmed with 24-hour collections of urine and dialysate. If the patient is not at goal, the prescription should be adjusted. This adjustment can also be done either empirically or using computerized kinetic modeling programs. There are two general changes that can be made to maximize clearances in an individual patient—either increase the drain volume or increase the D/P ratio in the dialysate effluent. Increasing the instilled volume increases the total drain volume and thus, the convective clearance. By altering dwell time, one can change both the D/P ratio at the end of prescribed dwell and the drain volume. The strategies to maximize the drain volume in patients undergoing PD are summarized in Table 83.7.[4,73,99–104] If a patient does not have a continuously wet abdomen, providing 24-hour dialysis should be the first step to enhance clearances. In a patient with a continuously wet abdomen, increasing the dwell volume should be the first step to enhance clearances. Most patients are able to tolerate the increased fill volumes without any discomfort and, if blinded to the fill volume, many are unable to correctly identify the amount of fluid instilled.[105,106] In order to improve tolerance, the fill volumes may be increased when the patient is lying supine (i.e., for the nighttime exchanges). Furthermore, cycler therapy allows increases in fill volumes in increments of 100 mL and improves tolerance of increasing the volume of instilled dialysate.

Some issues to consider in patients on standard CAPD are: (1) inappropriate dwell times (a rapid transporter would do better with short dwells); (2) failure to increase dialysis dose to compensate for loss of residual renal function; (3) inappropriate instilled volume (patient may only infuse 2 L of a 2.5-L bag); (4) multiple rapid exchanges and one very long dwell (patient may do three exchanges between 9 AM and 5 PM, and a long dwell from 5 PM to 9 AM,

TABLE 83.7 **Strategies to Enhance the Peritoneal Small Solute Clearances**

Continuous Ambulatory Peritoneal Dialysis	Automated Peritoneal Dialysis
Daytime exchanges	Daytime exchanges
Increase dwell volume[100]	Add daytime dwell (if dry day)
Increase ultrafiltration (tonicity of dialysate)	Add midday exchange[101] Increase dwell volume Increase ultrafiltration (tonicity of dialysate or alternative osmotic agents like icodextrin)
Nighttime exchanges	Nighttime exchanges
Increase dwell volume[99,100]	Volume of each dwell[100]
Increase number of exchanges (nighttime exchange device)	Number of nighttime exchanges[104]
Increase ultrafiltration (tonicity of dialysate or alternative osmotic agent like icodextrin)	Number of hours of cycling (8–10 hours)[101] Increase ultrafiltration (tonicity of dialysate)

limiting overall clearances); and (5) inappropriate selection of dialysate glucose for long dwells that may not maximize UF and clearance.

Other problems are specific for those patients on cycler therapy: (1) the drain time may be inappropriately long (more than 20 minutes), (2) inappropriately short dwell times may not maximize clearances, (3) failure to augment total dialysis dose with a daytime dwell ("wet" day versus "dry" day), and (4) inappropriate selection of dialysate glucose may not allow maximization of UF, resulting in less total clearance. One may be able to achieve weekly urea clearance targets, but not creatinine or middle-molecule clearance targets, with short dwell times, as in NIPD. A shortened time with fluid in the peritoneum is accompanied by decreased middle-molecule clearances and this may have an adverse effect on outcomes. It appears reasonable to state that when patients become anuric, they must maximize their "time" (most of day) on dialysis to maintain middle-molecular-weight clearances.

TABLE 83.8 Reported Benefits of Residual Renal Function in Patients Undergoing Peritoneal Dialysis

Reported Benefits
Greater probability of survival[26–29]
Lower morbidity Hospitalizations[108] Peritonitis rates[108] Technique survival
Cardiovascular Lower total body and extracellular water[107] Better control of blood pressure[109] Lower left ventricular mass index[1]
Nutritional status Higher dietary nutrient intakes[53,112] Higher serum albumin[1,27,113] Better nutritional status[2,111,113]
Anemia management Higher hemoglobin[1,113]
Divalent ion metabolism Better control of serum phosphorus[111,113]
Lower levels of circulating putative uremic toxins Low molecular weight like α1-microglobulin, alkaline RNAse[3] "Middle molecules"[115] Advanced glycosylation end-products like carboxymethyllysine[114]
Better quality of life[40,41,116]

RESIDUAL RENAL FUNCTION AND PERITONEAL DIALYSIS

Over the last decade, the centrality of residual renal function (RRF) in maintaining the health and welfare of patients undergoing PD has been established. Multiple studies mentioned previously demonstrated the superiority of renal urea clearance over peritoneal urea clearance. Over the same time period, data has accumulated that patients with significant RRF have a lower morbidity, have a lower severity of numerous complications associated with uremia, and have a better health-related quality of life (Table 83.8).[32,40,41,53,71,107–119] Thus, an understanding of the determinants of and strategies that retard the rate of loss of RRF are critical to the success of PD.

Notwithstanding the beneficial effect of treatment with PD on rate of decline of RRF, residual renal function inexorably declines over time (Table 83.9). Although many comorbidities have been linked to loss of RRF, to date, only one intervention has shown a beneficial effect on RRF. Randomized, controlled trials have shown that treatment with angiotensin-converting enzyme inhibitors (ACEIs, ramipril) or angiotensin-receptor blockers (ARBs, valsartan) significantly slows the rate of decline of RRF.[120,121] Finally, it appears that use of ACEIs and ARBs in patients undergoing PD is safe and does not result in significant elevations in serum potassium.[122] This may be related to the use of PD fluids without any potassium, as currently practiced. An initial, short-term, randomized, cross-over study demonstrated that patients had a higher urine volume when treated with PD solutions with low concentration of glucose degradation products.[123] However, three subsequent clinical trials, with follow-up for up to 12 months, have been unable to substantiate the benefits of these PD solutions on preserving residual renal function.[124–126]

ULTRAFILTRATION

A certain minimal amount of daily UF is necessary to maintain water balance in patients with ESRD. This is achieved by an osmotic pressure gradient between blood and the dialysate using glucose (predominantly) as the effective osmotic agent. During UF, retained solutes are swept along with the bulk solvent flow even in the absence of a concentration difference for diffusion. This contribution to net solute clearance has been termed solvent drag or convection; therefore, overall solute clearance is the sum of that owing to diffusion and convection.

Clinical Physiology

Simultaneous with UF of fluid from the bloodstream into the peritoneal cavity, there also occurs absorption of fluid from the peritoneal cavity, largely across tissue beds and partially via lymphatics.[127] Intraperitoneal volume at any time is determined by the relative magnitudes of transcapillary UF and tissue reabsorption and lymphatic reabsorption. Net

TABLE 83.9 **Summary Results of Some of the Studies That Have Compared the Rate of Decline of Residual Renal Function among Hemodialysis and Peritoneal Dialysis Patients**

Author	Patient no. HD/PD	Study Design	Baseline Measure	Index of Renal Function	% Decline/Month (HD/PD)	PD Decline Rate, % of HD Rate
Rottembourg[4]	25/25	Prospective	Predialysis	C_{cr}	6.0/1.2	80
Cancarini[5]	75/86	Retrospective	Pre- and postdialysis	C_{cr}	5.8/2.9	50
Lysaght[6]	57/48	Retrospective	Pre- and postdialysis	C_{cr}	7.0/2.2	69
Misra[2]	40/103	Retrospective	Postdialysis	Mean	7.0/2.2	69
Lang[7]	30/15	Prospective	Dialysis start	C_{cr}	9.4/5.0	47
Jansen[8]	279/243	Prospective	Predialysis	Mean	10.7/8.1	24
McKane[9] [d]	300/175	Retrospective	Pre- or postdialysis	Urea Cl	Rate of decline similar in HD and PD	

[a]C_{cr}, timed creatinine clearance
[b]*Mean*, mean of timed urea and creatinine clearances.
[c]*Urea Cl*, timed urea clearance.
[d]All HD patients dialyzed with high flux dialyzers and ultrapure water.

UF at the end of any dwell is defined as the difference between drained volume and instilled volume. This definition assumes that the residual intraperitoneal volume is constant, which is often not the case. This variation is insignificant for day-to-day clinical practice.[128,129]

Ultrafiltration rates are highest at the beginning of the dwell. As glucose is absorbed and its concentration is diluted by influx of ultrafiltrate, UF decreases as osmotic equilibrium is approached. Depending on the concentration of instilled glucose, osmotic equilibrium is reached at different times in the dwell cycle. For 2-L solutions containing 1.5% dextrose, osmotic equilibrium and maximal drain volume are reached after about 2 hours of dwell time in patients with average peritoneal membrane transport characteristics. For 4.25% dextrose solutions, peak intraperitoneal volumes are not likely to occur until after 3 or 4 hours.[77] As osmotic equilibrium is approached, intraperitoneal volume and ultimate drain volume decrease owing to isosmotic absorption of fluids. In CAPD patients, this absorption rate ranges from 40 to 60 mL per hour and is attributable both to bulk absorption of fluid across the peritoneal membrane and lymphatic drainage of the peritoneum.[130]

Ultrafiltration Failure

UF failure represents a failure to maintain volume homeostasis. This definition implies that clinically, UF failure can result from either loss of residual renal function, inadequate fluid removal by PD, patient nonadherence to the therapy, or excessive salt and water intake. Furthermore, failure to remove adequate amounts of salt and water by the current PD prescription does not necessarily imply that there must be a pathologic alteration of the peritoneal membrane itself. Other possible causes include catheter malfunction, inadequate selection of tonicity of dextrose or icodextrin, inappropriately long dwell times, fluid sequestration, including, as recently described, retroperitoneal leakage,[131] and failure to match dwell time to peritoneal membrane transport status.[75]

Among CAPD patients, ultrafiltration failure may be defined as clinical evidence of fluid overload despite restriction of fluid intake and the use of three or more hypertonic (4.25% dextrose) exchanges per day.[132] However, other definitions have been used in various publications; therefore, the exact incidence of UF failure is unknown. At one center, UF failure was observed in 6.2% of 227 CAPD patients over 10 years and the risk increased with time on PD.[133] The prevalence was 2.6% after 1 year on PD and 30.9% after 6 years. If one considers a more rigid definition, such as one defined by the ability to generate an UF volume of at least 400 mL after 4 hours of dwell with 4.25% dextrose, the true incidence is rather low. As discussed previously, clinical symptoms consistent with UF failure are not always caused by an actual loss of peritoneal UF capacity. The first steps in the evaluation of a patient with suspected UF failure are to rule out dietary indiscretions, determine urine volume, and establish whether net effluent drain volume and/or peritoneal transport have changed. Apparent loss of UF is potentially reversible if caused by catheter malposition, dialysate leak, or recent peritonitis, but usually is permanent if kinetic studies sug-

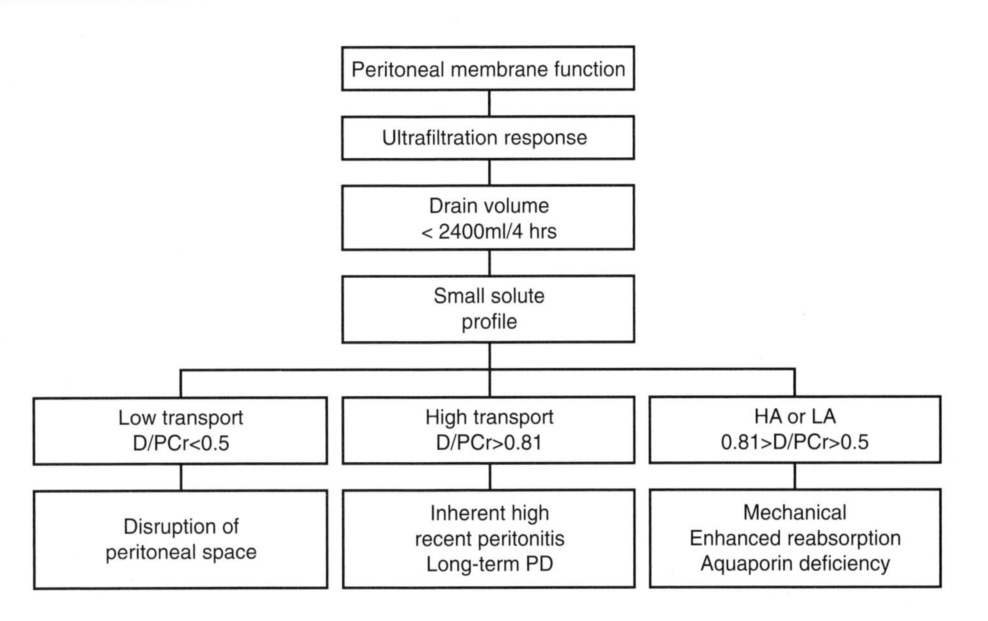

FIGURE 83.5 Algorithm for loss of ultrafiltration in continuous ambulatory peritoneal dialysis (CAPD) patients. *D/P CR,* dialysis:plasma creatinine ratio. (From Mujais S, Nolph K, Gokal R, et al. Evaluation and management of ultrafiltration problems in peritoneal dialysis. International Society for Peritoneal Dialysis Ad Hoc Committee on Ultrafiltration Management in Peritoneal Dialysis. *Perit Dial Int.* 2000;20 Suppl 4:S5–21.)

gest a reduction in UF capacity of the membrane. A rational approach to the patient with suspected UF failure is found in Figure 83.5.

Ultrafiltration Failure and High Solute Transport

Patients with loss of UF and current 4-hour PET ratios of D/D_0 glucose of less than 0.3 and D/P creatinine of greater than 0.81 are characterized as high solute transporters (see Fig. 83.2). These patients tend to have rapid small-molecular-weight solute transport and poor UF owing to high (rapid) glucose absorption and resultant rapid dissipation of the osmotic gradient. These patients are the largest group with true UF failure. Some patients have these transport characteristics at baseline and, if their dwell times are mismatched for their membrane transport characteristics, they often appear to have UF failure as they lose residual renal function and no longer have urine flow to supplement dialysate daily fluid losses. In other patients, the loss of UF is owing to an increase in membrane transport. This increase is caused by either an acquired increase in transport (formerly called type I membrane failure) or membrane changes associated with a recent episode of peritonitis.

Recent Peritonitis

It is a common clinical experience for PD patients to experience fluid retention during peritonitis. Compared to baseline, a PET performed during peritonitis reveals an increase in the D/P ratio for creatinine and a decrease in the D/D_0 ratio for glucose. There is also an increase in dialysate protein losses and a significant decrease in net UF.[134] In order to maintain UF during episodes of peritonitis, patients often need a temporary change in their standard dialysis prescription (shorter dwell times or increased tonicity) to maintain UF. Several studies have indicated that UF during an episode of peritonitis can be maintained with alternative osmotic agents such as icodextrin.[135]

Acquired Increase in Membrane Transport

An acquired increase in peritoneal transport over time on PD (formally called type I membrane failure) can cause chronic UF problems in CAPD. PET confirms high or high average transport rates with resultant rapid glucose absorption, loss of the osmotic gradient, and a decrease in net transcapillary UF. In contrast to the situation seen with peritonitis, where transport changes and protein losses usually are transient, small-solute transport changes and protein losses are more permanent with acquired loss of UF capacity.[136] There also tends to be less of a decline in dialysate sodium owing to the sodium sieving with convective transport. These changes are thought to result from an increase in effective surface area of the peritoneal membrane, supported by biopsy data showing an increase in vascular density in the membranes of long-standing PD patients.[137]

Risk factors for developing membrane changes are not firmly established but the incidence of an increase in membrane transport seems to increase with time on PD, implicating prolonged exposure of the peritoneum to dialysate as a possible cause. Davies et al. retrospectively analyzed glucose exposure in two patient cohorts: those whose transport characteristics were stable over 5 years and those who exhibited an increase in membrane transport over the same length of time. They found that the patients who were destined to exhibit increased transport over time had been exposed to a greater glucose load from the inception of peritoneal dialysis, strongly suggesting a relationship.[138] Similarly, among patients who were followed in the EAPOS study, those on icodextrin were less likely to have ultrafiltration problems than those on glucose.[139] This limited clinical evidence is consistent with a substantially more robust body of laboratory data linking the high glucose degradation products, glucose degradation products, and advanced glycosylation products to the long-term anatomic and functional changes seen in the peritoneal membrane.

Most cases can be managed by shortening dwell times and using icodextrin solution for the long dwell. Because these patients have high (rapid) transport of small solutes, they have adequate urea and creatinine clearances even with short dwell exchanges. Occasionally, resting the peritoneum for at least 4 weeks through temporary transfer to HD has been associated with an improvement.[140]

Patients with apparent ultrafiltration failure due to rapid solute transport should be strongly considered for treatment with icodextrin, a slowly metabolized glucose polymer which acts as a colloid osmotic agent. Clinical studies have shown icodextrin to be a safe and effective alternative to glucose.[141] Although the rate of UF with icodextrin is slower than that with dextrose, the effect of icodextrin persists much longer, making it suitable for ultrafiltration during long dwells of up to 14 to 16 hours. In both CAPD and APD patients, icodextrin has been shown to provide ultrafiltration superior to that with either 2.5% or 4.25% dextrose.[103,142] This is associated with decreases in total body and extracellular fluid water, lower blood pressure, and, possibly, regression of left ventricular hypertrophy (LVH).[143] Although icodextrin is approved for only a single dwell in the United States, it has recently been reported that the use of icodextrin in two daily exchanges in CAPD patients improved volume status and LVH.[144] With the use of a combination of short dwells with dextrose-based solutions and icodextrin for the long dwell, it is usually possible to achieve adequate small-solute clearances and fluid removal in these patients; yet, a minority may require transfer to HD for volume and blood pressure control.

Ultrafiltration Failure and No Change or Average Solute Transport

Loss of UF in patients with no change or average transport characteristics tends to result from catheter malfunction, fluid leaks, excessive lymphatic reabsorption (formerly type III membrane failure), or aquaporin dysfunction. If loss of UF is owing to catheter malfunction or fluid leaks, the patients do not have a functional change in their membrane and usually can be maintained on PD after the problem has been resolved.

Excessive Lymphatic and Tissue Absorption

Excessive lymphatic absorption is a very uncommon cause of membrane failure related to excessive rates of lymphatic and tissue absorption of fluid from the peritoneal cavity.[132] Although these patients may not have a significant change in D/P values when compared to baseline, they do have drain volumes after 4 hours of dwell that are less than baseline values or that which would be expected based on standard therapy. A further diagnostic clue is that these patients tend to have higher dialysate sodium concentration during the dwell than controls (Fig. 83.6).

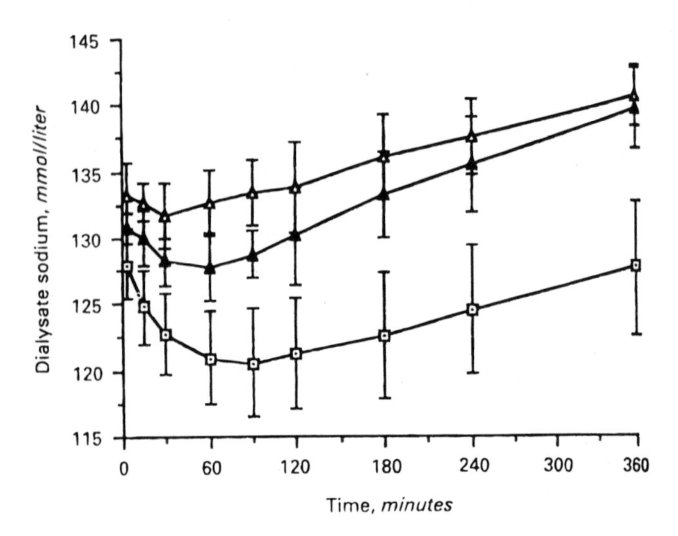

FIGURE 83.6 Dialysate sodium concentrations as a function of time in patients using 4.25% dextrose exchanges over 6-hour dwells. Results are compared in patients with normal ultrafiltration kinetics (*hollow squares*), those with high lymphatic absorption rates (*solid triangles*), and those with high glucose absorption rates (*hollow triangles*). (From Heimburger O, Waniewski J, Werynski A, et al. Peritoneal transport in CAPD patients with permanent loss of ultrafiltration capacity. *Kidney Int.* 1990;38:495, with permission.)

Aquaporin Dysfunction

Aquaporin dysfunction is a very rare condition.[145] Patients with suspected aquaporin dysfunction have damage to, decreased number of, or no water channels (ultra-small pores) that can lead to deficient crystalloid-induced UF.[146] These patients are diagnosed clinically by finding less than 400 mL of UF with a 4.25% PET and lack of sodium sieving early in the dwell. However, one must be careful to exclude patients who are very rapid transporters. Rapid transporters do exhibit sodium sieving, but it occurs so early in the dwell that if looked for after 60 to 90 minutes of dwell time it may be masked. These patients should respond clinically to use of colloid osmotic agents (such as icodextrin), which achieve ultrafiltration through a different mechanism and are not dependent on the water channels for UF.

Ultrafiltration Failure and Low Solute Transport

Patients with UF failure and low (slow) solute transport (D/D_0 glucose of more than 0.5 and a D/P creatinine of less than 0.5) tend to have inadequate small-solute clearances as well. Poor UF occurs despite the maintenance of adequate osmotic gradients. These patients are found to have a loss of functional peritoneum and the differential should include: peritoneal sclerosis (formally called type II membrane failure) or multiple peritoneal adhesions and, at times, patients with high lymphatic absorption rates. These patients often require transfer to HD.

DIALYSATE SOLUTIONS

Over the last three decades, a large number of patients have been successfully treated with conventional peritoneal dialysis solutions (Table 83.10) for long periods of time. However, several concerns have been identified with these solutions. First, the solutions are unphysiologic in that they are hyperosmolar, contain very high concentrations of glucose, and heat-sterilization generates toxic glucose degradation products. A large body of laboratory data and several observational clinical studies suggest that long-term use of conventional solutions results in structural and functional changes in the peritoneal membrane that limits its use as a long-term dialysis membrane. Peritoneal biopsies from patients on long-term peritoneal dialysis demonstrate mesothelial cell denudation, submesothelial fibrosis, neovascularization, and vasculopathy that primarily affects the postcapillary venule. This is associated with an increase in peritoneal solute transport rate and results in ultrafiltration failure in up to 30% of patients after 6 years of the therapy. Second, there are limitations with the use of glucose as an osmotic agent, particularly in the long dwells—these are the overnight dwell in a CAPD patient, and the day dwell in an APD patient. Absorption of glucose across the peritoneal membrane and dilution by the ultrafiltrate results in a progressive decline in glucose concentration, and hence, the ultrafiltration gradient during long dwells. In some patients this can result in net fluid reabsorption during long dwells and make it difficult to achieve euvolemia. Third, systemic glucose absorption can result in unwanted weight gain and is associated with a more atherogenic lipid profile. Fourth, the low pH of the fluid can cause infusion pain, particularly in the presence of peritonitis. Finally, concern has been raised that the unphysiologic peritoneal dialysis solutions can impair neutrophil and phagocyte function and increase the risk for and/or severity of peritonitis.

In order to overcome some of these limitations, several advanced peritoneal dialysis solutions have been introduced and are commercially available in different parts of the world. *Glucose-based, lactate-buffered low glucose-degradation product peritoneal dialysis solution* has been offered as a solution that is potentially more biocompatible. This claim is supported by animal studies and surrogate measures of peritoneal health in humans (higher concentrations of CA-125 and lower concentrations of profibrotic biomarkers). However, there are no data on the long-term effect of these solutions on either the structural or functional characteristics of the peritoneal membrane. Furthermore, the hope for a better preservation of residual renal function with these solutions has not been confirmed in three randomized, controlled trials.[124–126] Although previous studies showed no evidence for reduced episodes of peritonitis with these solutions, the recently published balANZ study reported longer time to the first episode of peritonitis in patients using a neutral pH, low GDP dialysate. Note however, that this study too demonstrated no beneficial effect on residual kidney function.[126a] There is no evidence for lower peritonitis rates with these solutions. Finally, an observational study from Korea demonstrated a lower risk for death in patients treated with low glucose-degradation product solutions.[147] These findings, although provocative, cannot be considered definitive. Thus, there are limited data that support a widespread use of low glucose-degradation product solutions.

Lactate is the most commonly used base but neutrophil function is better preserved with bicarbonate-containing dialysate compared to lactate-containing dialysate although bicarbonate with a high glucose concentration remains cytotoxic.[148] Lactate-containing dialysate with neutral pH is much less inhibitory of superoxide generation by neutrophils compared to standard lactate dialysate and is almost similar to bicarbonate-containing dialysate. Bicarbonate containing dialysate is feasible, in that the bicarbonate and dextrose can be kept in separate compartments and combined prior to infusion.[149] Two-chambered bicarbonate lactate-buffered PD fluid confers better phagocytosis and is associated with lower glucose degradation products compared to standard dialysate.[150] Use of bicarbonate-containing dialysate has been shown to improve peritoneal macrophage function.[151,152] Despite the in vitro data, bicarbonate solutions have not shown protection against peritonitis in patients. In a randomized controlled trial, bicarbonate-based peritoneal dialysis solutions were associated with significant lower severity of infusion pain.[153] Furthermore, a recent observational study from Korea has demonstrated a lower risk for death in patients treated with bicarbonate-based peritoneal dialysis solutions.[147] However, given the non-random assignment of patients to the different PD solutions, these findings cannot be considered definitive.

As mentioned previously, the glucose polymer icodextrin is an alternative to dextrose, particularly in high transporters. Dextrose is rapidly absorbed during a dwell, thus decreasing the osmotic gradient and leading to considerable caloric load. Glucose polymers are isosmolar; UF is obtained through colloid osmosis. Several randomized controlled trials have now demonstrated a higher UF volume, and lower extracellular water in patients treated with

TABLE 83.10 **Dialysate Composition**

Dextrose, measured in g/dL (%) as the hydrous dextrose, available as 1.5%, 2.5%, and 4.25%
Sodium, measured as mEq/L, available at 132
Chloride, measured as mEq/L, available at 102, 96, and 95
Lactate, measured as mEq/L, available at 35 and 40
Calcium, measured as mEq/L, available at 2.5 and 3.5
Magnesium, measured as mEq/L, available at 0.5 and 1.5
Bag volumes, measured in L, available at 0.25, 0.5, 0.75, 1.0, 1.5, 2.0, 2.5, 3.0, 5.0, and 6

icodextrin.[102,103,142,143] This reduction in extracellular volume has been shown to be associated with regression of left ventricular hypertrophy in CAPD patients using icodextrin for the long overnight exchange. Peritonitis results in increased degradation of icodextrin, an increase in dialysate osmolality, and, therefore, increased ultrafiltration, in striking contrast to the changes seen with glucose dialysate in peritonitis.[154] Observational studies demonstrate a better preservation of peritoneal membrane function and lower mortality in patients treated with icodextrin.[139,147] However, none of these findings can be considered conclusive.

Amino acid–containing dialysate has been proposed as an alternative to glucose-containing dialysate. Polymorphonuclear cell function is not impaired by amino acid dialysate in contrast to dextrose-containing dialysate.[155] Amino acid dialysate has similar small- and large-molecular-weight solute transport and UF to equimolar dextrose dialysate.[156] The use of one exchange each day of a 1% amino acid dialysate for 6 months improved nitrogen balance, but did not result in a rise in the serum albumin. Disadvantages of amino acid dialysate include a rise in the blood urea nitrogen level and a fall in the bicarbonate; therefore, close attention must be paid to urea nitrogen clearance to prevent uremia and oral sodium bicarbonate often is necessary during use of amino acid dialysate.[157] Amino acid–containing dialysate is not available in the United States.

CATHETERS

Types of Peritoneal Catheters

The Tenckhoff catheter originally designed by Palmer and modified by Tenckhoff continues to be used in the majority of PD patients.[158–160] A number of variations are available. The straight or curved subcutaneous portion may have one or two cuffs. Double-cuffed catheters are used in the majority of patients. The intra-abdominal portion of the catheter may be straight or coiled. Coiled catheters were designed to decrease outflow problems and infusion pain but appear to have similar complication rates as straight Tenckhoff catheters.[160] Although there are plausible benefits to coiled and double-cuffed catheters, prospective studies comparing different catheter designs have not shown a difference in infections or need for catheter replacement.[161]

To decrease migration of the intra-abdominal portion and exit-site infections, Twardowski and associates[162] designed a catheter with a curved subcutaneous pathway in which both the internal and external exit sites are downward (swan-neck catheters). Prospective comparisons of swan-neck and straight catheters have consisted of small trials. From the trials, it appears that swan-neck catheters have a lower incidence of catheter migration than straight catheters although there is no clear difference in infectious complications or other mechanical complications.[163,164] Given the overall equivalency of outcomes, the choice of a straight or swan-neck catheter often is predicated upon the location of the exit site. An exit site in the upper abdomen that is directly lateral is best achieved with a straight catheter whereas an exit site in the lower abdomen that is pointed downward is best obtained with a swan-neck catheter. A modification of the swan-neck catheter with a presternal exit site had excellent 2-year survival of 95% in the hands of an experienced team.[165] Placement of a 5- to 10-g weight at the tip of the intra-abdominal portion of the catheter has also been shown to decrease catheter migration. Use of this "self-locating" catheter was shown to result in significant decreases in catheter dislocation, peritonitis, tunnel infections, cuff extrusion, leakage, and obstruction with a concomitant improvement in overall catheter survival.[166,167]

Peritoneal Catheter Placement

The location of the exit site should be discussed with the patient prior to catheter placement to avoid the beltline. Preoperative laxatives are indicated for constipation, commonly present in patients because of phosphate binders, and an important cause of catheter malfunction.[168] The patient should void prior to the procedure; if the patient has a neurogenic bladder, then urethral catheterization is performed. Placement can be done either with local anesthesia and sedation or general anesthesia. The patient usually does not require overnight admission. Prophylactic antibiotics (generally a cephalosporin) for catheter placement, given before the skin incision, decrease the risk of catheter-related peritonitis.[169]

Most PD catheters are inserted by a surgeon using a dissection technique. A small paramedian incision is made overlying the rectus sheath down through the muscle to the peritoneum. The catheter is inserted so that the deep cuff is within the rectus muscle and the tip is in the deep pelvis. A purse string of nonresorbable suture (to decrease the risk of subsequent leaks) is placed where the catheter enters the peritoneum. Catheter function is assessed intraoperatively by infusing and draining fluid. The subcutaneous tunnel is formed such that the superficial cuff is 3 cm from the skin surface and is directed downward or pointed laterally. A small exit site wound formed by a tapered tunneling device of the same diameter as the catheter is best for minimizing trauma and decreasing the risk of subsequent exit site infection and catheter-related peritonitis.[170] If needed, the exit site should be closed with Steri-Strips (3M, St. Paul, MN); sutures should be avoided in order to decrease the risk of wound infection with a foreign body.

Placement via a laparoscopy is increasingly commonly used. This technique allows direct intra-abdominal visualization.[171] Adhesions can be avoided and the tip of the catheter placed to allow optimal catheter function. In a randomized comparison of laparoscopic versus conventional dialysis catheter insertion (both done by surgeons) outcomes were not different except that the conventional placement was faster (14 vs. 22 minutes, $P < .0001$).[172] However, a recent report studied the outcomes of over 400 laparoscopically placed catheters in which adjunctive procedures (e.g., rectus sheath tunneling, omentopexy, adhesiolysis, or resection of epiploic appendices) were employed as well. The catheter survival rate was 99% at an average of 21 months follow-up; the revision free survival was 96%.[171] The laparoscope may be particularly useful in patients with previous surgery or when placement by dissection results in a nonfunctioning catheter.

Blind percutaneous catheter placement may be used for placement of a catheter for acute renal failure to be used for a short time. However, for chronic dialysis patients, it does not allow a peritoneal examination nor does it allow surgical repair of intra-abdominal abnormalities, such as herniorrhaphy or omentopexy.[170] Additionally, the risk of bowel perforation makes percutaneous placement a less desirable technique. On the other hand, percutaneous placement under fluoroscopic guidance can be successfully used in a large proportion of uncomplicated cases.[173]

To decrease the risk of peritonitis from the formation of a biofilm, Moncrief and coworkers[174] developed a new insertion technique (Moncrief-Popovich technique). At insertion, the entire external portion of the catheter is buried in abdominal wall subcutaneous tissue. Three to 5 weeks later, the catheter is externalized via a small incision, which becomes the exit site. Burying the external portion of the catheter for up to 2 years does not change technique survival.[174a] Data regarding a possible decrease in infectious rates with this technique are conflicting.[175,176] A recent, large nonrandomized study did show a decrease in infections and leaks and an increase in catheter survival.[177] This technique has been employed for use with presternal as well as abdominal catheters.[178] Of note, however, use of the Moncrief-Popovich technique does appear to allow for earlier patient acceptance of catheter placement, analogous to the early placement of arteriovenous fistulas in patients planning to perform hemodialysis. Furthermore, because of the previous healing period, no "break in" period is required and full dose peritoneal dialysis may be started immediately upon externalization of the catheter.

Children require special consideration. In infants, the exit site is located above the diaper area to prevent contamination. Partial omentectomy is useful to prevent outflow problems. In boys, herniotomy and ligation of patent processus vaginalis at the time of catheter placement decrease the risk of subsequent inguinal hernia and hydrocele.[179]

Perforation of the bladder or bowel or laceration of the spleen is an uncommon occurrence, but adhesions increase the risk. Perforation of a hollow viscus should be considered if the effluent is feculent or when watery diarrhea, polyuria, or watery vaginal discharge occurs with infusion of dialysate. Minor bleeding frequently occurs after catheter insertion, but generally stops quickly and spontaneously.[180] Flushing the catheter with heparinized dialysate (500 U/L) is useful to clear the catheter and prevent blockage by clots.

Postoperative Management and Exit Site Care

If possible, initiation of PD is postponed by about 2 weeks from the time of catheter placement to allow healing and prevent leaks ("break-in"). The break-in period may need to be longer in patients who may have problems with wound healing, patients with a failing kidney transplant, or other conditions for which long-term corticosteroids are prescribed. During the break-in period, the catheter should be flushed several times with 1 L of dialysate or saline until the effluent is clear and then capped until training begins.[160] However, PD can be started within hours of placement of the catheter, if clinically indicated. Under such circumstances, the patient may initiate low-volume supine PD—best achieved with a cycler.[181]

Postoperative sterile dressing changes until healing takes place may help reduce infection risk. The surgical dressing should be left intact for 1 week unless there is bleeding. The exit site should be kept dry until well healed—this may require up to 2 weeks. During this interval, patients should not shower or bathe in tubs—personal hygiene should be performed with sponge baths. Once healed, many centers advise washing the exit site with bactericidal soap and water during routine bathing. Once the exit site is well healed, swimming in chlorinated pools or the ocean is permitted, but swimming in creeks or ponds or the use of hot tubs should be avoided, because this may result in infection.[182]

Mechanical Complications

Early inadequate outflow occurs after 7% of catheter insertions, requiring replacement in one half of these patients.[183,184] Constipation may lead to shifting of the catheter position, drainage failure, but only rarely catheter loss. Ideally, the catheter tip should be in a pelvic gutter, because this location ensures good hydraulic function of the catheter and minimizes risk of omental entrapment.[185] Tip migration to the epigastric or hypochondrial regions is generally associated with dysfunction.[183,184] Poor drainage owing to catheter malposition in the upper quadrants may be corrected by surgical repair (either open or laparoscopically).

There are other causes of catheter dysfunction in addition to catheter malposition. One- or two-way obstruction may result from clots or fibrin within the lumen. Forcibly flushing with heparinized saline may resolve this problem, but fibrinolytic agents may be effective if this fails.[186,187] Omental obstruction may necessitate omentectomy, especially in children.[179,183] Omentopexy or partial omentectomy at catheter placement improves catheter survival; the latter is performed routinely in children.[188]

Peritoneal dialysate leaks, which may occur at several different locations,[189] develop in 5% to 10% of catheters in the immediate postoperative period[183,184] and in 2% to 4%[184] of catheters later in the course of CAPD. Dialysate leaking from the exit site presents as clear fluid that is strongly test strip–positive for glucose. Leaks at the internal cuff may present as abdominal wall edema. These leaks may result from the use of resorbable suture material at the deep cuff, placement in a median rather than paramedian site, early initiation of CAPD, or hernia formation.[190,191] Computed tomography (CT) scan peritoneography (using Omnipaque, 50 mL/L of dialysate) is the best way to evaluate leaks and hernias.[192] A dialysate leak may resolve with PD in the supine position or temporary cessation of PD (using HD).[189] Dialysate leaks from the exit site often are associated with infection; thus prophylactic antibiotics should be given.[193] If a leak occurring more than 1 month after catheter insertion does not resolve within 4 days of reduced dialysate volumes, or if it recurs after full volumes are resumed, surgical correction generally is required.[194]

Diagnosis of Peritoneal Dialysis-Related Infections

A diagnosis of peritonitis is made when a patient has two of the following three: (1) cloudy peritoneal effluent and abdominal pain, (2) white blood cell count ≥100 cells/L with more than 50% polymorphonuclear cells, and (3) positive Gram stain or culture.[195] The patient usually does not have a fever. The effluent white blood cell concentration is a less sensitive indicator of peritonitis if the patient is already on antibiotics or if the patient is on automated PD who has either a dry abdominal cavity or has had fluid for a short period of time at the time of presentation. In these circumstances, the percentage of neutrophils (more than 50%) is more useful than is total white blood cell concentration.

The optimum technique for culture of peritoneal dialysate consists of centrifugation of 50 mL of peritoneal effluent at 3,000 g for 15 minutes followed by resuspension of the sediment in 3 to 5 mL of sterile saline and culture on both solid and liquid media.[195] More commonly, however, 5 to 10 mL of dialysis effluent is injected directly into blood culture bottles. When processed in this fashion the culture is "sterile" in approximately 14% to 20% of episodes that meet the criteria for peritonitis based on cell count.[196] A fastidious microorganism that has not grown in culture probably causes most of these episodes. When subsequently recultured, a microorganism is identified in one third.[197] Also, recent antibiotic exposure can render dialysate "sterile," despite active peritonitis. Mycobacteria always should be considered in peritonitis that is culture negative. Such patients have cloudy effluent, abdominal pain, and fever. Extraperitoneal TB is not necessarily present. Polymorphonuclear cells predominate in the effluent and, thus, do not distinguish *Mycobacterium* peritonitis from bacterial peritonitis. Acid-fast bacillus (AFB) smears of the effluent, even examining three concentrated specimens, are seldom positive; therefore, the diagnosis is generally made on culture, delaying treatment for weeks. Peritoneal tissue cultures are more optimal than culture of peritoneal fluid.

Approximately 6% of patients with culture-positive effluent present with abdominal pain and clear effluent.[198] A delayed effluent cell reaction occurs in two thirds of these patients, but one third never develop an appropriate cellular response to infection. When not experiencing peritonitis, such patients have a lower dialysate cell count (particularly macrophages and CD4 lymphocytes) and a delayed production of interleukin -6 and -8, compared to other patients. Though there are truly noninfectious causes of cloudy dialysate (see later) any patient on PD who presents with abdominal pain should be considered to have peritonitis until proved otherwise.

An exit site infection is defined by the presence of purulent drainage, with or without erythema, at the catheter exit site.[195] Induration and tenderness at the exit site are abnormal and may indicate infection. In the absence of drainage, erythema of the exit site (which is normally flesh colored) does not necessarily indicate the presence of infection; erythema may result from irritation or trauma to the exit site,[199] but is seldom associated with catheter loss unless drainage also is present.[168] Nonpurulent drainage and crusting of the exit site do not necessarily represent infection, nor does a positive culture of a normal-appearing exit site.

An infection of the subcutaneous catheter (or "tunnel infection") is present when there is pain, tenderness, erythema, or induration over the subcutaneous pathway. Tunnel infections most often occur in the presence of an exit site infection.[195] Tunnel infections may be clinically occult. This has been shown by numerous studies using sonography of the subcutaneous tunnel in patients with exit site infections.[200] When peritonitis occurs in conjunction with an exit site infection owing to the same microorganism (particularly *Staphylococcus aureus* or *Pseudomonas aeruginosa*), the presumption should be that there is a tunnel infection.[201]

PD-related infections remain a major problem. Such infections are responsible for the majority of catheter loss and contribute to transfer of the patient to HD.[202,203] Peritonitis is a major cause of hospitalization (Fig. 83.7).[204] Peritonitis occasionally results in death, either directly from sepsis or indirectly from ensuing complications such as cardiovascular disease.[205,206]

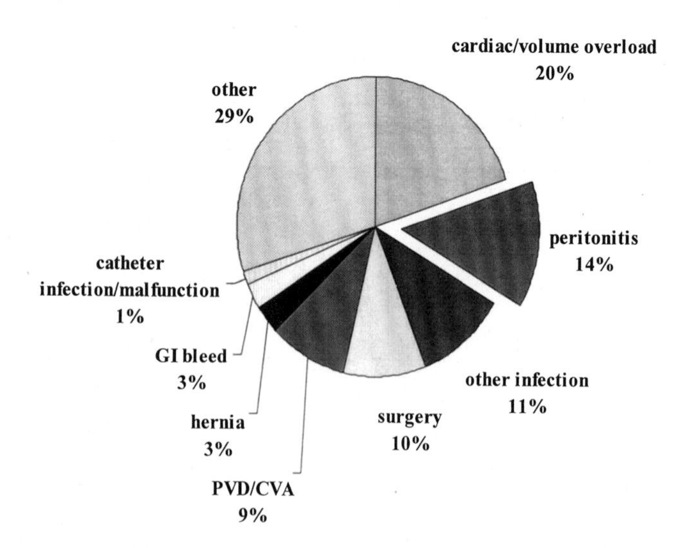

FIGURE 83.7 Causes of 274 hospitalizations for 126 peritoneal dialysis patients, as percentages. (From Fried L, Abidi S, Bernardini J, et al. Hospitalization in peritoneal dialysis patients. *Am J Kidney Dis.* 1999;33:927, with permission.)

Connection Devices

Evolution of connection techniques over time have resulted in a dramatic lowering of peritonitis rates, particularly those owing to organisms such as coagulase-negative *Staphylococcus*. For many years, the standard connection system was a straight line with an empty dialysate bag attached to the patient between dialysis exchanges. The exchange was performed manually. The straight line system has been replaced with safer connection systems, such as the Y-set and double-bag system. With the Y-set, the patient connects the catheter to a Y-set of tubing attached to a full dialysate bag and an empty bag. The patient sequentially flushes dialysate through the line into the drain bag to clear air, then drains the effluent from the peritoneum, infuses the fresh dialysate, and disconnects the Y tubing, either capping the catheter or snapping off the tubing. This strategy is known as "flush before fill" and was initially brought into practice by Buoncristiani.[215] The double-bag system is a further improvement in technology, because both the drain and fill bags are already attached to the Y tubing; therefore, the only possible site of contamination is during the connection the patient makes to the exchange tubing attached to the catheter. Peritonitis rates are significantly lower with the double-bag system compared to the Y-set in high-risk populations; however, there does not appear to be a difference in exit site infections or catheter survival.[216–218] There are lower rates of gram-positive peritonitis with the double-bag as compared to the Y-set, suggesting that this method further reduces the risk of contamination (Fig. 83.8) and, hence, the double-bag system has become the community standard of care in the United States.

The data are conflicting on whether peritonitis rates are lower on the cycler compared to CAPD, although a number of studies suggest that is the case (Fig. 83.9). A recent meta-analysis compared randomized trials of APD versus CAPD. In two out of three trials, peritonitis was significantly less common in APD patients (relative risk 0.75 vs, CAPD).[219] Two out of the three trials were quite small and the meta-analysis was heavily weighted toward the trial by de Fijter et al.[220] In this study, 82 patients were randomized to APD or CAPD. Patients on APD had close to a 50% reduction in peritonitis. However, in an analysis of the USDRS database, patients on CAPD appeared to have a lower peritonitis rate than patients on APD.[221] A small study suggests that NIPD may be associated with lower infection rates, perhaps due to enhanced peritoneal immune function as a consequence of the abdomen being kept dry for a portion of the day.[222] However, most of these studies were undertaken prior to the widespread use of the double-bag system for CAPD; with use of contemporary connectology, the difference in peritonitis rates between CAPD and APD, if any, is small and not clinically significant.

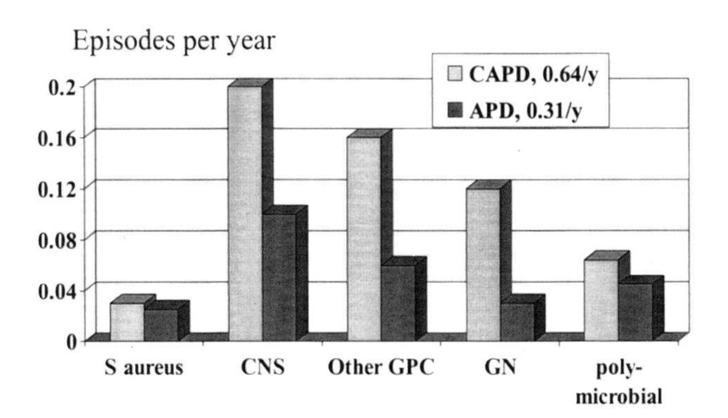

FIGURE 83.9 Episodes of peritonitis per dialysis year at risk in patients on CAPD versus APD. The center uses prophylaxis for *S. aureus* nasal carriers; therefore, *S. aureus* peritonitis rates are very low in both groups. (Modified from Rodriguez-Carmona A, Perez Fontan M, Garcia Falcon T, et al. A comparative analysis on the incidence of peritonitis and exit-site infection in CAPD and automated peritoneal dialysis. *Perit Dial Int.* 1999;19:253, with permission.)

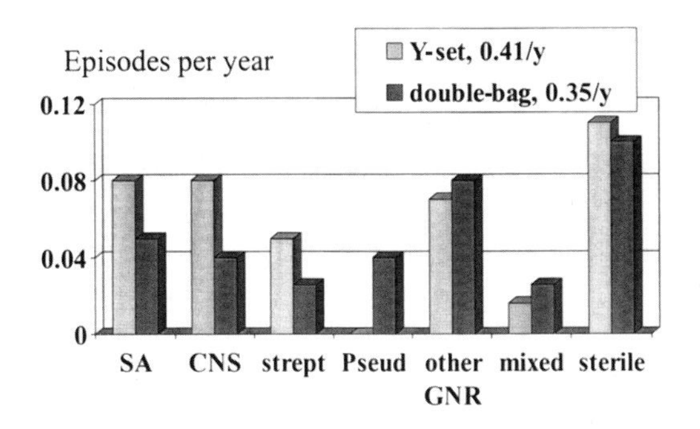

FIGURE 83.8 Episodes of peritonitis per dialysis year at risk in patients randomly assigned to the Y-set or the double-bag system for CAPD. (Modified from Li PK, Szeto CC, Law MC, et al. Comparison of double bag and Y set disconnect systems in continuous ambulatory peritoneal dialysis: a randomized prospective multicenter study. *Am J Kidney Dis.* 1999;33:535.)

Catheter Infections

The International Society for Peritoneal Dialysis has published comprehensive reviews of the approach to infectious complications in the PD patients.[195,223] The reader is referred to those articles for details; the following text is a broad overview.

There is marked variation in reported rates of exit site infections, in part because of differing definitions and because exit and tunnel infections are not always reported separately. Furthermore, much of the infection data precedes recent innovations in connector technology and prophylactic treatment. In a randomized controlled trial of mupirocin versus gentamicin prophylaxis, the rate of exit site infections in the mupirocin group was 0.54, similar to previous studies.[224] The rate of clinically obvious tunnel infection is 0.19 per year[225]; however, when an exit site infection is present, fluid collections along the subcutaneous pathway can be frequently demonstrated by ultrasound examination. Tunnel involvement is common when an exit site infection is concurrent.[200,226]

Microorganisms causing exit site infections are shown in Table 83.11.[227,228] The most common organism causing exit site and tunnel infections is *S. aureus*, which may be difficult

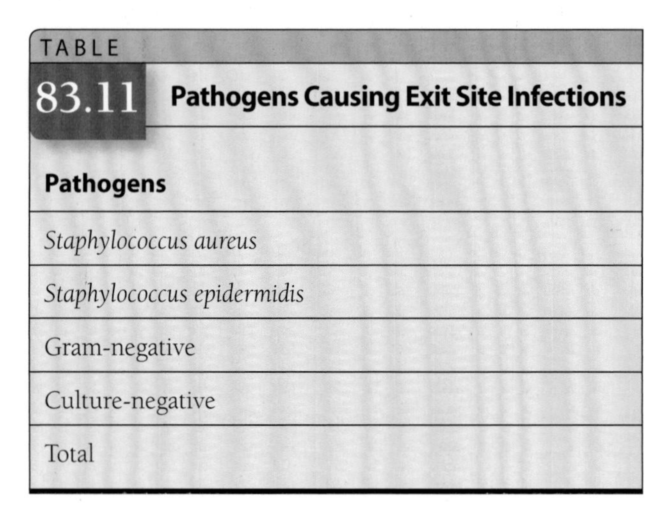

TABLE 83.11 **Pathogens Causing Exit Site Infections**

Pathogens
Staphylococcus aureus
Staphylococcus epidermidis
Gram-negative
Culture-negative
Total

[a]Much lower in programs using *S. aureus* prophylaxis.[H1]
Modified from Flanigan MJ, Hochstetler LA, Langholdt D, et al. Continuous ambulatory peritoneal dialysis catheter infections: diagnosis and management. *Perit Dial Int.* 1994;14:248; Holley JL, Bernardini J, Piraino B. Infecting organisms in continuous ambulatory peritoneal dialysis patients on the Y-set. *Am J Kidney Dis.* 1994;23:569.

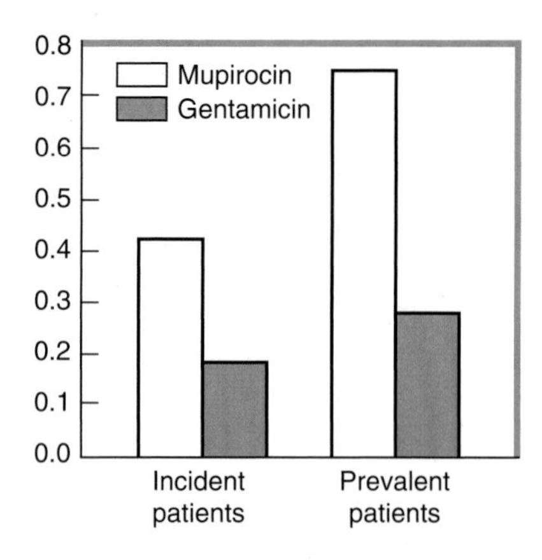

FIGURE 83.10 Rates of exit site infections in incident (on ≤3 months) and prevalent patients (on >3 months). In both groups, those who were using gentamicin exit site cream had significantly lower ($P < .01$) rates than those who were using mupirocin.

to resolve and can lead to peritonitis and catheter loss.[201,203] *P. aeruginosa* is the second most common cause of exit site and tunnel infections and frequently recurs or is refractory to antibiotic therapy and tunnel revision.[229,230] Therefore, early catheter removal is appropriate if the patient does not respond to a course of antibiotics. *Staphylococcus epidermidis* and culture-negative exit site infections are generally nonpurulent, and only infrequently do they cause peritonitis.[231]

The peritonitis rate in patients who have catheter infections is more than twice that of patients who do not.[231] Involvement of the tunnel, especially the inner cuff as demonstrated by ultrasound, predicts subsequent peritonitis.[200] Even in the absence of a clinical tunnel infection and with resolution of exit site infection with therapy, the deep cuff may harbor *S. aureus* or *P. aeruginosa*, resulting in recurrent peritonitis.[232]

A number of studies have demonstrated the efficacy of local antibiotics applied to the exit site to prevent infections. Daily exit site mupirocin is highly effective in reducing *S. aureus* exit site infections.[224,233–235] It must be noted, however, that organisms with low level mupirocin resistance have begun to emerge.[236,237] Although this is not yet a clinical concern, should the organisms acquire high-level resistance (minimum inhibitory concentration [MIC] ≥512 μg per mL), increased infection and/or relapse rates may ensue. Ciprofloxacin otologic solution, 0.5 mL single-dose vial, applied daily as part of routine care, reduced both *S. aureus* and *P. aeruginosa* exit site infections compared to historical controls.[238] However, the use of ciprofloxacin may be prohibitively expensive for many patients. A double-blind study compared the effects of 0.1% gentamicin sulfate versus 2% mupirocin applied to the exit site daily (Fig. 83.10).[224] Use of gentamicin resulted in significantly decreased rates of exit site infections and peritonitis. Gram-negative infections were markedly diminished by the use of gentamicin and there were no infections with *P. aeruginosa*; the frequency of *S. aureus* infections was unchanged. Gentamicin has the added advantage of being far less expensive than is mupirocin. This regimen is likely to become the preferred mode of prophylaxis for catheter-related infections.

Peritonitis

Peritonitis rates appear to be decreasing over the last two decades. In a recent analysis of a large cohort of PD patients (over 40,000), there was a 2% to 3% decline in peritonitis from 2000 to 2003.[239] In an analysis of peritonitis rates in the United States and Canada, Mujais reported peritonitis rates of one per 32.7 months in the United States and one per 27.6 months in Canada.[240] The organisms that most commonly cause peritonitis are listed in Table 83.12.[228,241,242] Szeto et al. have documented that the percentage of *S. epidermidis* peritonitis is significantly decreasing with the use of the disconnect systems and this increases the relative proportion of all peritonitis episodes that are caused by gram-negative organisms.[243] Many other organisms in addition to those listed have been identified in episodes of peritonitis, including those caused by fungi, protozoans, algae, viruses, and mycobacteria.[195] The outcome of peritonitis is highly organism-specific. Etiologies of peritonitis are shown in Figure 83.11.

A number of demographic features are associated with an increased risk for peritonitis. White, nondiabetic patients aged 20 to 59 years have the lowest risk of peritonitis. The reason for the increased risk seen in blacks is not understood.[244,245] Conflicting data exist on whether diabetic patients have an increased risk of peritonitis.[246,247] Age greater than 60 years was a risk factor for peritonitis in some reports, but most studies indicate that elderly patients have similar peritonitis rates as younger patients.[248] Peritonitis rates in children are higher than those of adults.[249] Immunosuppressed patients are also at increased risk, especially for

TABLE 83.12 **Pathogens Causing Peritonitis Using Disconnect Systems**

Pathogens	**Episodes/Year**
Staphylococcus epidermidis	0.1–0.2
Staphylococcus aureus	0.15[a]
Other gram-positive	0.1–0.2
Gram-negative	0.1
Polymicrobial	0.01
Fungi	0.01
Culture-negative	0.01–0.1
Total	0.4–0.6

[a]Approximately one third of this is in programs using *S. aureus* prophylaxis.
Modified from Holey JL, Bernardini J, Piraino B. Infecting organisms in continuous ambulatory peritoneal dialysis patients on the Y-set. *Am J Kidney Dis.* 1994;23:569; Tofte-Jensen P, Klem S, Nielson PK, et al. PD-related infections of standard and different disconnect systems. *Adv Perit Dial.* 1994;10:214; Lupo A, Tarchini R, Carcarini G, et al. Long-term outcome in continuous ambulatory peritoneal dialysis: a 10 year survey by the Italian cooperative peritoneal dialysis study group. *Am J Kidney Dis.* 1994;24:826.

infections owing to *S. aureus* and fungi.[250] Peritonitis risk is also increased after an episode of peritonitis.[251]

Contamination at the time of an exchange, usually but not invariably resulting in coagulase-negative staphylococcal peritonitis, remains a leading cause of peritonitis. *S. epidermidis* peritonitis is not usually caused by a catheter infection or colonization of the skin, nose, or exit site; however, *S. epidermidis* can colonize the peritoneal catheter, producing a slime layer (or biofilm) that can extend from the exit site through the cuff(s) into the peritoneal cavity.[252,253] The rate of bacterial colonization of the catheter is related to the degree of bacterial contamination of the exit site at the time of catheter insertion, but, within 3 weeks of insertion, most catheters are colonized.[254] The relationship of biofilm to peritonitis is unclear. Recurrent or relapsing peritonitis (defined as a second episode owing to the same organism within 4 weeks of stopping antibiotics) is generally caused by *Staphylococcus* and may be related to the presence of biofilm, which shields bacteria from antibiotics.[195] The coagulase-negative staphylococci isolated from patients with peritonitis are more likely to be producers of biofilm than are isolates not associated with peritonitis; however, biofilm formation does not invariably lead to peritonitis.[255,256] The keys to preventing peritonitis caused by coagulase-negative staphylococcal peritonitis are avoidance of connection techniques requiring spiking of bags and extensive training of the patient in aseptic technique. Miller and Findon have demonstrated that proper hand washing and drying prior to performance of an exchange sharply reduces bacterial numbers on the spike connection and in the peritoneal space after touch contamination.[257] Furthermore, patients should be trained how to identify contamination and report to the dialysis unit; prophylactic antibiotics should be administered under appropriate circumstances.[182]

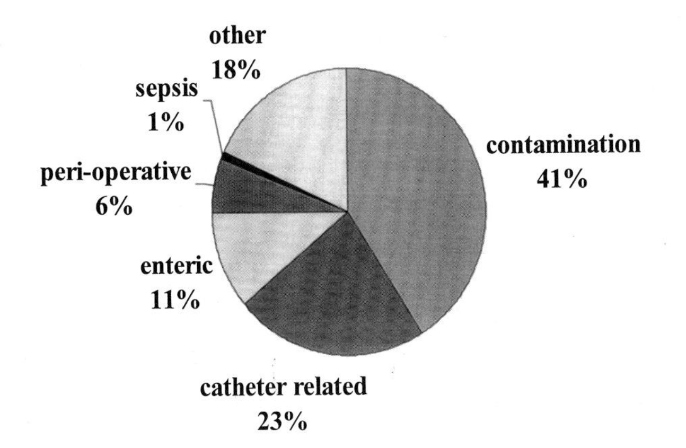

FIGURE 83.11 Etiologies of peritonitis. (Modified from Harwell CM, Newman LN, Cacho CP, et al. Abdominal catastrophe: visceral injury as a cause of peritonitis in patients treated by peritoneal dialysis. *Perit Dial Int.* 1997;17:586, with permission.)

S. aureus carriage and catheter infections are another source of peritonitis. *S. aureus* in the nares, at the exit site, or on the skin is associated with *S. aureus* catheter infection and peritonitis. Prevention of *S. aureus* peritonitis is critical, because the outcome is worse compared to that of other staphylococcal infections. Several antibiotic protocols have been shown to decrease the risk of *S. aureus* infection in PD patients.[216] These predominantly use intranasal mupirocin cream, twice a day for 5 days monthly for carriers, or daily at the exit site. These protocols are uniformly effective in reducing exit site infections but not peritonitis. Exit site mupirocin is also effective in reducing *S. aureus* peritonitis.[233,234] As discussed previously, low-level mupirocin resistance has been reported. Gentamicin is equally efficacious as mupirocin for prophylaxis against *S. aureus* and is superior for the prevention of gram-negative infections.[224]

Gram-negative peritonitis, which is associated with considerable morbidity, is not well understood.[258–260] The bowel may be a source, through translocation of bacteria across the bowel wall or secondary to organ pathology. Constipation and enteritis have both been associated with peritonitis due to enteric organisms.[261,262] Possibly due to the effects on colonic motility, hypokalemia has been associated with an increase in enterobacterial peritonitis as well.[263] Peritonitis can rarely be caused by intra-abdominal pathology and under those circumstances is associated with severe symptoms and commonly results in transfer of the patient to HD or death, especially if surgery is delayed.[260,264] Examples of primary intra-abdominal diseases that can present as PD peritonitis include ischemic bowel, cholecystitis, appendicitis, perforated ulcers, colonic polypectomy, and diverticula (see section on intra-abdominal catastrophes). An elevated amylase level in the dialysate effluent is a clue to the presence of enteric peritonitis.[265]

Procedures, such as colonoscopy, endoscopy with sclerotherapy, dental manipulation, endometrial biopsy, liver biopsy, and laparoscopic cholecystectomy can result in peritonitis; thus, antibiotic prophylaxis is indicated.[266–268] Other unusual causes of peritonitis are vaginal leak of dialysate and the use of intrauterine devices.[269] It is recommended that the abdomen be emptied of fluid prior to procedures involving the abdomen or pelvis.[195]

Fungal peritonitis accounts for 2% to 3% of all peritonitis episodes.[270,271] Abdominal pain may be severe and associated with fever. Patients may be acutely ill and appear to have a surgical abdomen; death may result, particularly if catheter removal is delayed.[272] A recent observational study of Australian patients suggests that mortality from fungal peritonitis may be decreasing. Previous small series described a mortality rate greater than 20%. In the largest series to date (162 patients), mortality rate was 9%.[270] Prior antibiotic therapy and frequent bacterial peritonitis are predisposing causes. Prophylaxis, mainly using nystatin during antibiotic therapy, appears to be most effective in programs with high fungal peritonitis rates (Table 83.13).[273–278] Programs with a low fungal peritonitis rate do not appear to benefit from prophylaxis.

The differential diagnosis for truly sterile cloudy fluid is broad and is best approached by considering whether turbidity is due to cellular or acellular elements.[279] Acellular causes include fibrin and triglycerides; the latter may be due to lymphatic obstruction, superior vena cava syndrome, pancreatitis, or certain dihydropyridine calcium channel blockers. Cellular elements may include polymorphonuclear leukocytes, eosinophils, red blood cells, or malignant cells. Intraperitoneal generic vancomycin and amphotericin may cause chemical peritonitis.[280,281] Icodextrin had been previously reported to cause sterile peritonitis with the number of cases peaking in 2002.[282,283] This was determined to be a consequence of contamination with a bacterial peptidoglycan that was introduced during the manufacturing process.[284] Correction of the manufacturing process has virtually eliminated this problem (incidence now 0.01%).

Treatment of Peritoneal Dialysis-Related Infections

Exit Site Infections

The initial antibiotic for an exit site infection must be active against staphylococci, with subsequent therapy dependent on the specific organism identified. Oral antibiotics are as effective as intraperitoneal antibiotics with the exception of infections with methicillin-resistant *Staphylococcus aureus* (MRSA); these will usually require treatment with vancomycin. Sonography of the tunnel may be useful, although not always necessary, to determine length of therapy (Fig. 83.12).[195] Infections limited to the exit site require an average of 2 weeks of antibiotic therapy, whereas involvement of the superficial tunnel lengthens average therapy to 3 weeks or more. Involvement of the deep cuff requires 2 months or more of antibiotic therapy and may require removal of the catheter to prevent peritonitis.[285] Local care of the exit site is generally intensified and, in mild or equivocal exit site infection when the tunnel is not involved, this may suffice as therapy. If prolonged antibiotic therapy fails to resolve the exit site infection, revision of the tunnel with removal of the external cuff (in two cuffed catheters) may help to prolong the life of the catheter in a select group of patients but there is limited long-term data.[286] An incision is made over the tunnel to expose the cuff, which is carefully shaved

TABLE 83.13 **Fungal Peritonitis without and with Prophylaxis**

Reference	Prophylaxis	Incidence[a]
Zaruba[278]	Nystatin tid	0.20 vs. 0.03
Robitaille[273]	Nystatin or ketoconazole	0.14 vs. 0
Wadhwa[277]	Fluconazole qod	0.08 vs. 0.01
Lo[276]	Nystatin qid	0.02 vs. 0.01
Thodis[275]	Nystatin qid	0.02 vs. 0.02
Williams[274]	Nystatin qid	0.01 vs. 0.01

[a]Antibiotic associated fungal peritonitis, in episodes per year. Rate without prophylaxis given first.

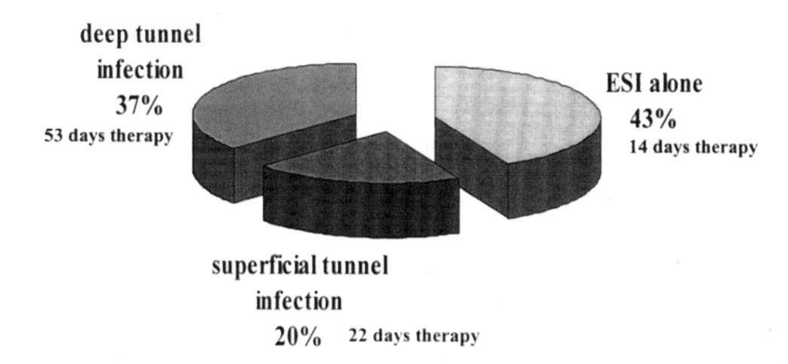

FIGURE 83.12 Extent of *S. aureus* catheter infection ($n = 49$) using sonography with mean days of therapy also shown. (From Vychytil A, Lilaj T, Lorenz M, et al. Ultrasonography of the catheter tunnel in peritoneal dialysis patients: what are the indications? *Am J Kidney Dis.* 1999;33:722, with permission.)

from the catheter. The area of granulation tissue and cellulitis may also be débrided. Cuff shaving and tunnel revision are never effective if catheter-related peritonitis is present.

Pseudomonas exit site infections are particularly prone to recurrence and often lead to peritonitis, which is a devastating complication.[287] Therefore, if the patient has a history of prior exit site infection with *Pseudomonas*, the antibiotic chosen for empiric therapy should be efficacious against that organism (e.g., oral quinolone). Dual therapy is sometimes needed and the duration of therapy may need to be extended to as long as 6 weeks. Recurrent and refractory exit site infections might be best managed with catheter replacement. In such high-risk patients, to prevent recurrence in a new catheter, consideration should be given to using gentamicin or ciprofloxacin otic solution at the exit site, as previously described.

Peritonitis

As discussed previously, not all patients who present with cloudy dialysate will prove to have peritonitis. Nevertheless, to avoid delay in treatment, empiric antibiotic therapy should be started upon presentation with cloudy dialysate.[288,289] Initial therapy should include coverage for both gram-positive and gram-negative organisms.[195] This should be guided by knowledge of both the patient's history and the individual program's pattern of microorganisms responsible for peritonitis and their antibiotic sensitivities.

A first-generation cephalosporin or vancomycin should be used to provide gram-positive coverage. A single daily dose of cefazolin, 15 mg per kg, results in dialysate concentration levels above the MIC over 24 hours for sensitive organisms, allowing once a day dosing (for those without residual renal function).[290] In CCPD patients treated with intermittent dosing with cefazolin, the antibiotic should be administered in a long day exchange (at least 4–6 hours of dwell) immediately preceding the overnight cycling. Alternatively, cefazolin could be administered in every bag for either CAPD or APD patients (500 mg per L loading dose followed by 125 mg per L in each subsequent bag). Antibiotics could be administered with intermittent therapy. Vancomycin is needed in patients with a cephalosporin allergy and could be used in centers with a high incidence of infection with methicillin-resistant organisms. Centers with a high prevalence of methicillin-resistant organisms, however, still may use cefazolin empirically since the relatively high concentration of cefazolin in the dialysate can be effective even in the presence of resistant organisms. Patients on vancomycin generally require dosing at 3- to 5-day intervals—the more frequent dosing is important particularly in patients with significant residual renal function or with frequent cycling at night. The frequency of dosing can be individualized by checking plasma vancomycin levels and levels maintained ≥ 15 μg per mL.

Gram-negative coverage may be provided by a third-generation cephalosporin (e.g., cefepime or ceftazidime) or an aminoglycoside agent (Table 83.14). A single dose of ceftazidime, 15 mg per kg IP, results in serum and dialysate concentrations above the MIC (for susceptible organisms) for more than 24 hours, because the serum elimination half-life is 22 hours.[291] Hence, ceftazidime can be dosed intermittently for both CAPD and APD patients as described above for cefazolin. Alternatively, the drug could be dosed continuously with the antibiotic added to each bag (500 mg per L loading dose followed by 125 mg per L in each subsequent bag). Although a retrospective study suggested long-term aminoglycoside therapy should be avoided when possible to preserve residual renal function a short course of empiric therapy appears to be safe.[292,293] Lui et al. randomized patients with peritonitis to either netilmicin or ceftazidime for 14 days. Both regimens were equally effective and associated with a transient loss of residual function. More importantly, netilmicin did not harm long-term residual renal function.[292,293] Quinolones may be used by centers with documented local sensitivities of gram-negative organisms to this class of drugs. A meta-analysis has confirmed that initial monotherapy with quinolones can be effective.[294] However, the included trials were old and, given the frequent emergence of quinolone resistance, quinolone monotherapy is not recommended.[295]

Subsequent therapy after antibiotic loading depends on the organism isolated. *S. aureus* or *S. epidermidis* may be treated with a first-generation cephalosporin alone, if methicillin-sensitive. Fifty percent or more of *S. epidermidis* causing peritonitis is resistant to cephalosporins.[296,297] These patients should be treated with vancomycin, as should patients with MRSA peritonitis.[298] MRSA peritonitis has a failure rate of 60% when treated with vancomycin alone and, frequently, results not only in catheter loss but also in peritoneal adhesions precluding further PD.[299] Therefore, rifampin should be added to vancomycin therapy. Peritonitis caused by vancomycin intermediate-resistant *S. aureus* has been reported and was successfully treated with rifampin and trimethoprim–sulfamethoxazole.[300]

Streptococcal or enterococcal peritonitis is best treated with ampicillin; an aminoglycoside may be added for synergy in enterococcal infections. Vancomycin-resistant enterococcus (VRE) as a cause of peritonitis in PD patients is still rare but there are many published case reports.[301,302] Colonization had been considered rare although there is data that VRE may be increasing in dialysis units.[303] VRE should be treated with linezolid, quinupristin/dalfopristin, or daptomycin.

Infections due to *S. aureus* or enterococci require 3 weeks of therapy; 2 weeks is generally sufficient for other gram-positive cocci. For any peritonitis, failure to achieve clear dialysis effluent after 5 days of appropriate antibiotic therapy defines refractory peritonitis and is an indication for catheter removal.[195]

The subsequent therapy of gram-negative organisms is dependent on sensitivities. Aminoglycoside therapy should generally be reserved for those infections in which sensitivities dictate the use of these drugs. Once a day dosing of intraperitoneal aminoglycoside, shown to be effective, provides high local levels of the antibiotic, while avoiding systemic toxicity.[304]

P. aeruginosa peritonitis should always be treated with two drugs for a minimum of 3 weeks.[195] Peritonitis caused by *P. aeruginosa* is difficult to treat and can sometimes result in the death of the patient.[230,259,305–307] Aminoglycosides may be used if the isolate is sensitive to the drugs but long courses may result in vestibular toxicity. Ceftazidime, cefepime, piperacillin, or oral quinolones are generally effective. Antibiotic therapy is much more likely to be effective if a catheter infection is not present, although long courses of therapy may be required to prevent relapse. If a *Pseudomonas* catheter infection is present in conjunction with peritonitis, catheter removal is necessary.

Peritonitis owing to *Stenotrophomonas maltophilia* (formerly *Xanthomonas maltophilia*) is difficult to resolve as the organism displays very limited antimicrobial sensitivities. Despite treatment with multiple antibiotics, catheter removal may be necessary.[308,309] Immunosuppression is a risk factor.

Antimicrobial therapy of fungal peritonitis is not generally successful unless the catheter is removed. Amphotericin B has poor diffusion from blood into the peritoneum, whereas intraperitoneal administration results in chemical peritonitis.[281] Flucytosine, ketoconazole, and fluconazole diffuse readily from blood to the peritoneum and are more effective than amphotericin, although catheter removal still is often necessary.[272,310,311] Fluconazole is particularly well tolerated when administered intraperitoneally. Chan and colleagues found a cure rate of 9.5% using fluconazole therapy alone without catheter removal.[312] Fluconazole plus catheter removal cured 67%, whereas 14% required addition of amphotericin. The ISPD recommends prompt catheter removal for fungal peritonitis.

Temporary cessation of PD, which improves peritoneal immune function, has been successfully utilized to assist in resolving peritonitis, in conjunction with antibiotics.[313,314] This approach has been useful in recurrent peritonitis episodes owing to coagulase-negative staphylococcus, but has also been helpful in resolving refractory *S. aureus*.[315,316] It is effective only if catheter infection is absent.

Catheter removal is necessary to resolve the infection in some cases. Peritonitis owing to *S. aureus, P. aeruginosa,* or enteric peritonitis with an intra-abdominal source often requires catheter removal.[195] Catheter-related peritonitis accounts for approximately one third of the catheters removed, although the proportion and rate of catheter removal for isolated peritonitis have decreased with use of improved connection systems.[184,228] Recent data shows that persistence of peritoneal white blood cell (WBC) count ≥1090 cells per mm^3 after 3 days of therapy portends treatment failure and catheter removal should be considered.[317]

Simultaneous catheter removal and replacement are quite successful for recurring peritonitis and tunnel infections.[318,319] This eliminates an interim period on hemodialysis. This approach should be used only when the effluent leukocyte cell count is under 100 per μL. This approach is not recommended for fungal, mycobacterial, or *P. aeruginosa* peritonitis, or when peritonitis is a consequence of intra-abdominal pathology—these episodes require that the patient spend a period of time off PD.

TABLE 83.14 **Antibiotic Doses for Intermittent Therapy for Peritonitis**

Antibiotic	Dose intraperitoneally
Cefazolin or cephalothin	15–20[a] mg/kg once daily
Vancomycin	30 mg/kg once, then 15 mg/kg every 5 d
Ceftazidime	15–20[a] mg/kg once daily
Gentamicin, tobramycin, or netilmicin	0.6 mg/kg once daily

[a]Higher dose for patients with residual renal function.
Modified from Piraino B, Bailie GR, Bernardini J, et al. Peritoneal dialysis related infections recommendations: 2005 update. *Perit Dial Int.* 2005;25:107.

OTHER COMPLICATIONS

Pancreatitis

Pancreatic abnormalities including pancreatitis occur with a higher frequency in uremic patients.[320] The highest incidence of pancreatitis among ESRD patients is in transplant recipients, but within dialysis populations, it is not clear that PD patients have a higher incidence than do HD patients.[321–323] Reports from the mid-1980s suggested a greater incidence in PD due to higher uremic solute concentrations in PD patients or even to the potentially direct toxic effects of dialysate, which bathes a portion of the pancreas. The dialysate dextrose concentration, hypertonicity, hypercalcemia, foreign particulate debris, bacteria, or antibiotics may induce inflammation in the sensitive pancreas.[322,324] That the direct toxicity of dialysate may be causative is supported by the recurrence of pancreatitis after reinstitution of PD after initial resolution.[325] The relevance of those reports from 1980s to the contemporary practice of peritoneal dialysis, however, is unclear and there is no convincing evidence for a higher incidence of pancreatitis in PD than HD today. Hyperlipidemia is both a risk factor for and complication of pancreatitis. The hyperlipidemia seen more frequently in PD patients is low-density lipoprotein hypercholesterolemia, which is not particularly toxic to the pancreas. On the other hand, HD patients are more likely to suffer from hypertriglyceridemia, which is a predisposing factor for pancreatitis when severe enough to be associated with hyperchylomicronemia. The high intake of simple carbohydrates in PD patients may be a factor in inducing hyperlipidemia.

Even though pancreatitis is an infrequent complication of PD, older reports suggested a high mortality rate.[320] The typical clinical presentation for acute pancreatitis in a PD patient is characterized by abdominal pain with normal bowel sounds, nausea, vomiting, absence of fever, hyperamylasemia (more than three times normal), elevated effluent dialysate amylase concentration (more than 100 U per L), and a variable appearance of effluent dialysate, including being clear, hemorrhagic, tea-colored, or even cloudy.[320–322] Amylase levels may be spuriously decreased in patients using icodextrin.

Hyperlipidemia and/or hypercalcemia are frequently present and may be predisposing metabolic abnormalities. Pancreatitis should be strongly considered if appropriately treated "peritonitis" does not resolve because this presentation is quite similar to PD-associated microbial peritonitis. The effluent in pancreatitis is usually sterile, even if hemorrhagic, cloudy, or tea-colored. Burkart and associates have suggested that dialysate effluent amylase concentration is low in bacterial peritonitis, even if slow to resolve, whereas it is more than 100 U per L with pancreatitis or other intra-abdominal pathologies.[265] If a diagnosis of pancreatitis is uncertain, CT is the preferred imaging study. In addition to demonstration of an engorged pancreas, CT may be particularly useful to identify the ominous finding of a pseudocyst.

The principles of management do not differ from those in patients without ESRD. Offending agents should be discontinued and, if that includes dialysate, PD should be halted. However, peritoneal lavage can be helpful in removing inflammatory mediators, especially if the dialysate was not the culprit. There is no evidence to support a recommendation to halt PD in all patients with acute pancreatitis, and discontinuing PD probably does not alter the prognosis.[326] Percutaneous pseudocyst drainage may be preferable to internal (jejunal) drainage and this may preclude continuation of PD. Hyperlipidemia and hypercalcemia should be corrected. The role of lower concentrations of calcium in dialysate is unknown.

Chyloperitoneum

There have been a few scattered case reports of chylous fluid leaking into the peritoneum and draining with effluent dialysate. This topic was recently reviewed.[327] The dialysate is cloudy but, on more careful examination, looks milky, reflecting the lipid rich content of chyle. The most common cause is trauma to intraperitoneal lymph vessels, either catheter-induced or from external trauma. Rocklin and Teitelbaum have recently reported a case of chyloperitoneum due to the superior vena cava syndrome.[328] Certain dihydropyridine calcium channel blockers have also been associated with chyloperitoneum, perhaps due to impaired lymphatic peristalsis.[329] Patients are usually asymptomatic. Treatment initially is conservative, to decrease abdominal lymph production by a low-fat, high-calorie diet supplemented with medium-chain triglycerides. The next step is discontinuation of PD, because the presence of dialysate may retard closure of the leak. If this is unsuccessful, a trial of total parenteral alimentation may be considered. Should these steps fail to resolve the leak, catheter removal is indicated. Lymphangiography may identify the source of the leak should surgery be considered.

Hemoperitoneum

As little as 1 mL of blood in 2 L of dialysate results in readily evident visual hemoperitoneum, and 7 mL results in effluent dialysate that looks like red fruit juice. Fortunately, this is an uncommon occurrence, but, when it does occur, it is often very frightening to the patient.[330] Fortunately, however, hemoperitoneum is almost always benign.[330,331] In Table 83.15 are listed causes of hemoperitoneum in PD patients. Hemoperitoneum occurs in 3.8% to 10% of PD patients and is twice as common in women as in men. When it occurs in women of childbearing age, 64% of the causes are related to ovulation or menses. In one series, this population experienced an almost 90% incidence rate.[332] There does not appear to be a correlation with PD-associated peritonitis, nor does hemoperitoneum adversely impact long-term outcomes on PD.

Menstrual and surgical histories are informative (Table 83.15). If the patient is asymptomatic and the bleeding stops spontaneously, no evaluation is absolutely necessary.

TABLE 83.15 **Causes of Hemoperitoneum in Peritoneal Dialysis Patients**

Causes
Retrograde menstruation
Ovulation
Catheter-induced trauma (omental abrasion, repositioning, constipation)
Bowel disease (ischemic, inflammatory)
Peritonitis
Cysts (ovarian, polycystic kidney, acquired cystic kidney)
Abdominal trauma
Strenuous exercise (including sexual activity)
Systemic bleeding (thrombocytopenia, anticoagulants)
Hypertonic exchanges (hyperemia)
Pancreatitis
Vasculitis (systemic lupus erythematosus)
Sclerosing peritonitis
Adhesions
Granulosa cell tumor
Ectopic pregnancy
Cholecystitis
Colonoscopy
Dissection from adjacent sites (femoral hematoma, spleen, colon)
Previous hepatitis
Enema
Extracorporeal lithotripsy
Splenic infarction

In the absence of active menses, bloody dialysate should be evaluated by effluent cell count and differential, and only if clinically appropriate, Gram stain and culture, and effluent fluid amylase concentration. An abdominal ultrasound may occasionally be informative. Obviously, symptoms referable to the abdomen prompt further evaluation, which ultimately could include a laparotomy. Treatment is directed at the specific cause. However, because patients often are asymptomatic, precluding an extensive evaluation, treatment generally is supportive. Heparin administered intraperitoneally may protect from subsequent catheter occlusion from clots. Three rapid flushes with room-temperature dialysate may induce peritoneal vasoconstriction and stop the bleeding.[333] Dialysate that is significantly cooler than room temperature could precipitate cardiac dysrhythmias. Furthermore, cool dialysate should be avoided where mesenteric perfusion is compromised, because it could exacerbate ischemia of the bowel. This therapy is probably only effective in cases where the bleeding is secondary to a peritoneal membrane bleed. Gynecologic hormone therapy may be indicated in women who demonstrate hemoperitoneum during menses or ovulation.[334]

Defects of the Peritoneal Cavity Boundary

Hernias and Genital and Abdominal Wall Edema

Intra-abdominal pressure rises with increasing intraperitoneal volume, sitting, straining at stool, coughing, and strenuous physical activity. Combined with the extremes of age, debilitation, and poor wound healing from uremia, it is no surprise that hernias are common. A recent study documented a hernia prevalence near 20%.[335] Over 13% of the hernias present are strangulated. Teitelbaum and colleagues reported the largest series of patients with defects of the peritoneal cavity boundary. The overall frequency of hernia in this population of nearly 1900 patients was 6.7%. The most common sites were: inguinal, 25% of total; umbilical, 19%, and ventral, 14.[336] They found hernias to be more common in men than women, although another study demonstrated the converse.[337] Patients with cystic disease as the etiology of ESRD are at higher risk for the development of hernias.[336,338] One-half of the hernias become clinically evident within the first year of PD,[339] but many probably go undetected unless special scintigraphic studies are performed.[340] Most of the scintigraphically diagnosed asymptomatic cases never progress to clinically appreciable disease. Many PD patients have hernias diagnosed prior to initiating PD and herniorrhaphies are performed at the time of catheter insertion. Bargman and colleagues recently documented the outcomes of 50 patients undergoing hernia repair. PD was stopped for 48 hours perioperatively followed by gradual increase in dialysate volume. No hernia recurrences were noted and patients did not require temporary hemodialysis.[341] Other centers have also shown that discontinuation of PD is usually not necessary after hernia surgery.[342,343]

There probably is no benefit from routine screening scintigraphy in adults because clinical manifestations alone dictate the need to repair. Increased intraperitoneal pressure alone is not sufficient to cause hernias—a preexisting anatomic abnormality is often present.[344] In children, some programs routinely perform intraoperative peritoneograms (and herniorrhaphies if positive) at the time of catheter placement. To ensure prompt strength postoperatively, especially for large hernias, supporting prosthetic overlay mesh is inserted at the time of herniorrhaphy.[345] Placement of catheters through the rectus muscle in a paramedian approach probably reduces the incidence of subsequent incisional or catheter site hernias. Postinsertion leakage increases the likelihood of subsequent hernias.

Abdominal wall edema or genital edema is caused by either dialysate leakage through acquired peritoneal defects, such as at the catheter insertion site, traumatic rents such as previous hernias or incisions, or congenital defects that go undetected until PD raises intraperitoneal pressures, opening them (patent processus vaginalis). Thus, the fluid could dissect between tissue layers or through natural pathways. In the study by Teitelbaum and colleagues pericatheter or subcutaneous leaks were present in 3% of the total population.[336] Edema of the scrotum or perineal area is usually owing to a patent processus vaginalis. Scrotal edema may develop in up to 10% of men on CAPD.[346] This can be managed temporarily by supine PD, but surgical correction is generally required, certainly if a hernia is present. Postoperative management may include hemodialysis for 1 week or more.[347] Vaginal leakage of dialysate is rare but serious, because it can lead to recurrent peritonitis, often with fungus. This complication should be suspected in any woman with watery vaginal discharge that is positive for glucose. If the leak is through the fallopian tubes, then tubal ligation is corrective.[348]

The site of a subcutaneous dialysate leak can be located with scintigraphy, ultrasonography, or contrast imaging.[349,350] Surgical closure is recommended, hence the need for precise identification of the leak site. Although watchful waiting is tempting, the collective PD experience suggests that elective operative intervention is the best approach to these complications related to increased abdominal pressure.

Hydrothorax

Fluid migrates from the peritoneal to the pleural space in 0.6% to 5% of patients undergoing PD either via transdiaphragmatic lymphatics or defects in the tendinous portion of the diaphragm.[351] There is an increased incidence in women, patients with polycystic kidney disease or hernias, those prone to peritonitis, and children.[352] Right sided pleural effusions appear to be more common than left.[353] The heart or pericardium probably protects the tendinous portion of the left hemidiaphragm. The hydrothorax can occur abruptly and painfully following exercise or trauma and can be immediately life threatening. A more common presentation is that of gradual progression of orthopnea or dyspnea, usually without pain. One half of the cases present within the first month of PD, and only one fifth present 1 year or more after initiation.[353] Resolution (i.e., being able to continue PD) is more likely in those cases where the presentation is within 1 year of initiating PD.

The simultaneous measurement of the concentrations of albumin, glucose, and lactate dehydrogenase in peritoneal effluent, pleural fluid, and blood may be helpful diagnostically. Peritoneal scintigraphy with radiolabeled albumin is a useful diagnostic maneuver; methylene blue should be avoided because of the pain it causes. Although helpful in localizing the defect, these diagnostic maneuvers probably do not alter management.[351] If the origin of the hydrothorax is dialysate, therapy is indicated regardless of whether there is a distinct leak versus lymphatic transport.

Initial attempts at conservative management should be made by decreasing volumes (decrease fill, decrease UF), performing PD supine, and periods of an empty abdomen. If conservative management fails, video-assisted thoracoscopic surgery is the preferred therapeutic modality. Chemical pleurodesis with tetracycline, blood, N-CWS (*Nocardia rubra* cell wall skeleton), triamcinolone, OK-432, talc, or fibrin adhesive have each been successful; however, these procedures can be very painful and are associated with unpredictable results.[351,353a]

Hyperlipidemia

Compared to HD patients, PD patients demonstrate higher concentrations of total cholesterol, triglycerides, Lp(a), apo A-I, and apo B as well as lower apo A-I: B ratios, and high-density lipoprotein (HDL) cholesterol concentrations.[354] The cause of these abnormalities is multifactorial. Although total caloric intake is equal in PD and HD patients because of absorbed dextrose from peritoneal dialysate, oral caloric intake is actually less in PD patients.[355] This absorbed simple carbohydrate may account for 25% of total caloric intake. Patients who require frequent hypertonic exchanges do so because of increased fluid and/or food intake. Therefore, it is difficult to determine whether hyperlipidemia is secondary to diet or glucose-based dialysate. It should be noted, however, that use of icodextrin has now been shown to improve glucose control, total cholesterol, and LDL levels but not hypertriglyceridemia.[356,357] This supports a role for the caloric load from glucose in the pathogenesis of hyperlipidemia in PD patients. In addition to the above, there is loss into effluent dialysate of oncotic proteins (e.g., albumin) and liporegulatory molecules (e.g., HDL cholesterol, apoproteins).[358,359] This sets the stage for hyperlipidemia and atherosclerosis.

The treatment of hyperlipidemia in PD patients must include an attempt to decrease the use of the most hypertonic exchanges. This should be done in conjunction with dietary restriction of fluids, fats, and simple carbohydrates. Lipid-lowering drugs of several classes have been utilized successfully. The major U.S. experience with fibric acid derivatives is with gemfibrozil, which increases lipoprotein lipase activity, the catabolism of very-low-density lipoproteins (VLDL), and the concentration of HDL_2 and HDL_3.[360] The dose should be reduced by initiation with 300 mg once daily and titrated gradually upward. Gemfibrozil can cause myositis, which may be manifested by increased serum potassium and/or creatine kinase concentrations. Hydroxymethylglutaryl-CoA reductase inhibitors, predominantly used to treat hypercholesterolemia, are safe and effective in PD patients.[361] The recently concluded SHARP study included patients on PD and showed that both simvastatin and ezetimibe are safe in the PD population as well.[362]

Intra-abdominal Pathology in Peritoneal Dialysis Patients

Less than 6% of peritonitis episodes in PD patients are owing to intra-abdominal pathology (IAP) and, although polymicrobial peritonitis may be associated with IAP, most cases are not.[363] Peripheral leukocytosis, an increasing PD cell count on antibiotic therapy, or an expanding pneumoperitoneum are important clues to IAP.[183,363,364] Obvious signs of IAP, such as fecal or biliary material in the dialysate or diarrhea containing dialysate, are not commonly observed. Risk factors for the development of IAP include diverticulosis, constipation and its treatment, and unrepaired hernia.[262] Death from IAP is linked to bowel gangrene; malnutrition; comorbidities such as liver failure, shock, bacteremia, pneumonia, and gastrointestinal or intracerebral hemorrhage; and delayed surgical intervention—therefore, by a broad consensus, early surgical intervention in suspected IAP is strongly recommended.[365,366]

In general, slowly resolving peritonitis warrants close follow-up. Clear dialysate while on antibiotics is not an absolute sign of a benign process. Generalized abdominal peritonitis can mask localized signs and symptoms of IAP. Surgical consultation is urgently needed in the following conditions:

- Localized abdominal pain and tenderness
- Dilated loops of bowel on abdominal radiograph
- Progressive increase in intraperitoneal free air with continued peritonitis
- Hemoperitoneum with measurable dialysate hematocrit

Those perioperative interventions that best allow continuation or quick return to PD postoperatively include:

1. Tight wound closure for prevention of dialysate leakage, possibly using nonresorbable sutures.
2. Drain removal before resuming PD to allow adequate dialysis.
3. Preoperative extensive PD to increase platelet function and allow a few days without PD postoperatively for healing.
4. Elective repair of abdominal wall hernias (see earlier Abdominal Hernias in Continuous Peritoneal Dialysis) both for patient comfort as well as prevention of bowel incarceration.
5. Avoidance of constipation, because impacted stool often accompanies diverticulitis or perforated bowel.
6. Optimization of nutrition to counter the marked protein loss through an inflamed peritoneum.
7. Avoidance of PD with transfer to HD if extensive bowel wall repairs are made. A low threshold for transition to HD is generally a prudent decision.
8. Omentectomy at surgery if the omentum appears threatening to catheter flow function.[367]

ENCAPSULATING PERITONEAL SCLEROSIS

Encapsulating peritoneal sclerosis (EPS) is a potentially devastating complication of peritoneal dialysis. EPS is rare, affecting fewer than 5% of peritoneal dialysis patients and is sometimes diagnosed after renal transplantation.[368,369] Patients with EPS present with anorexia, nausea, vomiting, protein-energy wasting, and intestinal obstruction.[370] A thick-walled membrane "cocoon" is present, entrapping loops of bowel. This gives rise to the classic "sandwich" appearance on abdominal ultrasonography.[371]

The etiology and pathogenesis of EPS are uncertain although time on dialysis is a risk factor.[372] Peritoneal irritants, recurrent peritonitis, long-term use of PD, acetate-containing dialysis, chlorhexidine, beta-blockers, and high transporter status have all been implicated in the pathogenesis.[373] Historically, mortality was severe—as high as 60% within 4 months of diagnosis. However, contemporary data from Australia and New Zealand has demonstrated a considerably lower mortality and suggests that many of the deaths may not be related to EPS.[374]

Treatment consists of corticosteroids, supportive care with parenteral nutrition, and, in extreme cases, surgical enterolysis. ACEI and tamoxifen are considered potential treatments for EPS due to antifibrotic properties but high quality clinical data is lacking.

INTRAPERITONEAL INSULIN

Shortly after the advent of CAPD it was suggested that the intraperitoneal administration of insulin could improve glycemic control.[375] Although easily utilized in CAPD, the use of intraperitoneal insulin in patients performing APD, an increasing segment of the overall PD population, is more complex. Coupled with the trend toward use of longer-acting insulin preparations, this has resulted in a substantial decrease in the utilization of this route for insulin delivery. Furthermore, intraperitoneal insulin has been linked to subcapsular hepatic steatosis.[376]

HYPERTENSION

Volume control and sodium removal by PD are related to numerous factors, including dialysate composition (osmolality created by dextrose and sodium concentrations), peritoneal permeability and UF capacity, splanchnic circulation, and residual renal function.[377] After many months of PD, the antihypertensive effect of PD may be due to other factors as well.[378]At this time, body weight may actually increase, although this could reflect the increased caloric intake from the transperitoneal absorption of dextrose. Because the peritoneal membrane is associated with different transport properties than HD membranes, the more efficient removal of pressor substances by PD is speculated to play a role in this late hypertension control.[378] These pressor compounds could include Na-K–ATPase inhibitors, norepinephrine, and endothelin. However, after a year or more of PD, hypertension is less effectively controlled than after PD initiation.[109] This may be related to the development of peritoneal sclerosis, progressive obesity, dialysis prescription nonadherence, improved appetite and well-being and dietary indiscretion, increased hematocrit, loss of residual renal function, or other as yet unidentified factors.

Recent studies have focused attention on the differences in blood pressure between patients performing CAPD or APD. Some single-center studies have reported that patients performing APD have higher blood pressure and left ventricular mass than do those on CAPD.[379–381] This is likely due to decreased sodium removal and ultrafiltration in APD patients due to the shortened dwell times and high transport, respectively.[379] However, careful attention to APD prescription—limiting the number of cycles to 3 to 5 at night, and avoiding long dwells with glucose-based solutions by leaving the abdomen dry for part of the day, or use of a day exchange, or use of icodextrin—allows for equivalent control of blood pressure and hypervolemia as can be achieved with CAPD.[382,383]

TRANSPLANTATION

Peritoneal dialysis patients may differ from their HD counterparts in several aspects that could influence transplant outcomes. Compared to HD patients, PD patients demonstrate a more normal immune response as characterized by T4:T8 lymphocyte ratios, T cell counts, T cell stimulation, and cell-mediated immunity.[384] However, many observational studies have shown that both the incidence of delayed graft function and long-term transplant outcomes in patients who performed PD prior to transplantation are equivalent—if not superior to—those obtained in patients who performed HD.[385–389] A higher incidence of vascular graft thrombosis after performance of PD has been reported but this remains controversial.[387]

Another difference between PD and HD patients potentially influencing transplantation is that the control of anemia, with or without erythropoietin, is easier with PD.[390] Thus, PD patients are less likely to experience blood transfusions and subsequent enhanced graft tolerance. Furthermore, the decreased transfusion requirement of PD patients makes hepatitis less likely, which is important considering the adverse effects of viral hepatitis on graft survival and the potential need for antiviral therapy prior to transplantation.

When compared to HD patients, PD patients have better blood pressure control and preserved residual renal function, which may affect care in the immediate posttransplant period. Patients receiving intraperitoneal insulin must be converted back to subcutaneous insulin once PD is terminated.

Because of a low frequency of delayed graft function, and because of the location of a pancreatic allograft in adults or the renal allograft in children, it has become common to remove PD catheters at the time of transplantation. If desired, the PD catheter may be kept in place for up to 2 to 3 months after transplantation. In that case, frequent flushing is recommended to maintain catheter patency and to avoid unlubricated or unbuffered bowel contact which, especially in the patient on steroids, may result in abscess formation and potentially even erosion of the catheter through the bowel wall.

A tunnel infection or active peritonitis generally precludes transplantation at that time. A prudent policy is to observe the course of the peritonitis for at least 2 weeks following the discontinuation of antibiotics. If no relapse has occurred, the patient is then reactivated on the recipient list.

There is no difference in the frequency or types of nonperitonitis-related posttransplant infections in recipients previously dialyzed by PD or HD.[391,392] If the PD catheter has been left in place and peritonitis develops, its course is not different from that seen in PD patients who are not receiving immunosuppressive medications. It requires essentially the same treatment with parenteral or intraperitoneal antibiotics, with the exception that allograft function may necessitate larger or more frequent doses. Posttransplant exit site or tunnel infections probably warrant catheter removal, especially if the infection is in proximity to the graft incision.

Posttransplant ascites may develop in PD patients, even with functioning grafts.[393] It is probably related to a hyperemic peritoneum whose mesothelium has been altered by the previous presence of dialysate. It may take weeks, but this does subside spontaneously. The ascites should be drained only when dictated by patient comfort because the protein content is generally high and negative protein balance may ensue.

REFERENCES

1. Wang AY, Wang M, Woo J, et al. A novel association between residual renal function and left ventricular hypertrophy in peritoneal dialysis patients. *Kidney Int.* 2002;62:639–647.

2. Misra M, Nolph KD, Khanna R, et al. Retrospective evaluation of renal kt/V(urea) at the initiation of long-term peritoneal dialysis at the University of Missouri: relationships to longitudinal nutritional status on peritoneal dialysis. *ASAIO J.* 2003;49:91–102.

3. Stompor T, Sulowicz W, Anyszek T, et al. Dialysis adequacy, residual renal function and serum concentrations of selected low molecular weight proteins in patients undergoing continuous ambulatory peritoneal dialysis. *Med Sci Monit*, 2003;9:CR500–504,

4. Rottembourg J, Issad B, Gallego JL, et al. Evolution of residual renal function in patients undergoing maintenance haemodialysis or continuous ambulatory peritoneal dialysis. *Proc Eur Dial Transplant Assoc*, 1983;19:397–403.

5. Cancarini GC, Brunori G, Camerini C, et al. Renal Function Recovery and Maintenance of Residual Diuresis in CAPD and Hemodialysis. *Perit Dial Bull*, 1986;6:77–79.

6. Lysaght MJ, Vonesh EF, Gotch F, et al. The influence of dialysis treatment modality on the decline of remaining renal function. *ASAIO transactions / American Society for Artificial Internal Organs*, 1991;37:598–604.

7. Lang SM, Bergner A, Topfer M, et al. Preservation of residual renal function in dialysis patients: effects of dialysis-technique-related factors. *Peritoneal dialysis international : journal of the International Society for Peritoneal Dialysis*, 2001;21:52–57.

8. Jansen MA, Hart AA, Korevaar JC, et al. Predictors of the rate of decline of residual renal function in incident dialysis patients. *Kidney Int.* 2002;62:1046–1053.

9. McKane W, Chandna SM, Tattersall JE, et al. Identical decline of residual renal function in high-flux biocompatible hemodialysis and CAPD. *Kidney Int.* 2002;61:256–265.

10. Vonesh EF, et al. The differential impact of risk factors on mortality in hemodialysis and peritoneal dialysis. *Kidney Int.* 2004;66(6):2389–2401.

11. Huang CC, Cheng KF, Wu HD. Survival analysis: comparing peritoneal dialysis and hemodialysis in Taiwan. *Perit Dial Int.* 2008;28 Suppl 3:S15–20.

12. Sanabria M, et al. Dialysis outcomes in Colombia (DOC) study: a comparison of patient survival on peritoneal dialysis vs hemodialysis in Colombia. *Kidney Int Suppl.* 2008(108):S165–172.

13. Woywodt A, et al. In-center intermittent peritoneal dialysis: retrospective ten-year single-center experience with thirty consecutive patients. *Perit Dial Int.* 2008;28(5):518–526.

14. Twardowski ZJ, et al. Chronic nightly tidal peritoneal dialysis. *ASAIO Trans.* 1990;36(3):M584–588.

15. Steinhauer HB, et al. Increased dialysis efficiency in tidal peritoneal dialysis compared to intermittent peritoneal dialysis. *Nephron.* 1991;58(4):500–501.

16. Vychytil A, et al. Tidal peritoneal dialysis for home-treated patients: should it be preferred? *Am J Kidney Dis.* 1999;33(2):334–343.

17. Juergensen PH, et al. Tidal peritoneal dialysis: comparison of different tidal regimens and automated peritoneal dialysis. *Kidney Int.* 2000;57(6):2603–2607.

18. Aasarod K, Wideroe TE, Flakne SC. A comparison of solute clearance and ultrafiltration volume in peritoneal dialysis with total or fractional (50%)

intraperitoneal volume exchange with the same dialysate flow rate. *Nephrol Dial Transplant.* 1997;12(10):2128–2132.

19. Juergensen PH, et al. Tidal peritoneal dialysis to achieve comfort in chronic peritoneal dialysis patients. *Adv Perit Dial.* 1999;15:125–126.

20. Morbidity & mortality. *Am J Kid Dis.* 2011;57(1, Supplement 1):e77–e86.

21. Keshaviah P. Adequacy of CAPD: a quantitative approach. *Kidney Int Suppl.* 1992;38:S160–164.

22. Lowrie EG, et al. Effect of the hemodialysis prescription of patient morbidity: report from the National Cooperative Dialysis Study. *N Engl J Med.* 1981;305(20):1176–1181.

23. Gotch FA, Sargent JA. A mechanistic analysis of the National Cooperative Dialysis Study (NCDS). *Kidney Int.* 1985;28(3):526–534.

24. Kim DJ, et al. Dissociation between clearances of small and middle molecules in incremental peritoneal dialysis. *Perit Dial Int.* 2001;21(5):462–466.

25. Jager KJ, et al. Mortality and technique failure in patients starting chronic peritoneal dialysis: results of The Netherlands Cooperative Study on the Adequacy of Dialysis. NECOSAD Study Group. *Kidney Int.* 1999;55(4): 1476–1485.

26. Rocco M, et al. Peritoneal dialysis adequacy and risk of death. *Kidney Int.* 2000;58(1):446–457.

27. Shemin D, et al. Residual renal function in a large cohort of peritoneal dialysis patients: change over time, impact on mortality and nutrition. *Perit Dial Int.* 2000;20(4):439–444.

28. Szeto CC, et al. Importance of dialysis adequacy in mortality and morbidity of chinese CAPD patients. *Kidney Int.* 2000;58(1):400–407.

29. Bargman JM, Thorpe KE, Churchill DN. Relative contribution of residual renal function and peritoneal clearance to adequacy of dialysis: a reanalysis of the CANUSA study. *J Am Soc Nephrol.* 2001;12(10):2158–2162.

30. Szeto CC, et al. Impact of dialysis adequacy on the mortality and morbidity of anuric Chinese patients receiving continuous ambulatory peritoneal dialysis. *J Am Soc Nephrol.* 2001;12(2):355–360.

31. Brown EA, et al. Survival of functionally anuric patients on automated peritoneal dialysis: the European APD Outcome Study. *J Am Soc Nephrol.* 2003;14(11):2948–2957.

32. Szeto CC, et al. Independent effects of renal and peritoneal clearances on the mortality of peritoneal dialysis patients. *Perit Dial Int.* 2004;24(1):58–64.

33. Jansen MA, et al. Predictors of survival in anuric peritoneal dialysis patients. *Kidney Int.* 2005;68(3):1199–1205.

34. Lo WK, et al. Minimal and optimal peritoneal Kt/V targets: results of an anuric peritoneal dialysis patient's survival analysis. *Kidney Int.* 2005;67(5): 2032–2038.

35. Fried L, et al. Association of Kt/V and creatinine clearance with outcomes in anuric peritoneal dialysis patients. *Am J Kidney Dis.* 2008;52(6):1122–1130.

36. Paniagua R, et al. Effects of increased peritoneal clearances on mortality rates in peritoneal dialysis: ADEMEX, a prospective, randomized, controlled trial. *J Am Soc Nephrol.* 2002;13(5):1307–1320.

37. Lo WK, et al. Effect of Kt/V on survival and clinical outcome in CAPD patients in a randomized prospective study. *Kidney Int.* 2003;64(2):649–656.

38. Mak SK, et al. Randomized prospective study of the effect of increased dialytic dose on nutritional and clinical outcome in continuous ambulatory peritoneal dialysis patients. *Am J Kidney Dis.* 2000;36(1):105–114.

39. Moreno F, et al. Quality of life in dialysis patients. A spanish multicentre study. Spanish Cooperative Renal Patients Quality of Life Study Group. *Nephrol Dial Transplant.* 1996;11 Suppl 2:125–129.

40. Merkus MP, et al. Quality of life in patients on chronic dialysis: self-assessment 3 months after the start of treatment. The Necosad Study Group. *Am J Kidney Dis.* 1997;29(4):584–592.

41. Paniagua R, et al. Health-related quality of life predicts outcomes but is not affected by peritoneal clearance: The ADEMEX trial. *Kidney Int.* 2005;67(3):1093–1104.

42. Pollock CA, et al. Total-body nitrogen by neutron activation in maintenance dialysis. *Am J Kidney Dis.* 1990;16(1):38–45.

43. Heimburger O, et al. Hand-grip muscle strength, lean body mass, and plasma proteins as markers of nutritional status in patients with chronic renal failure close to start of dialysis therapy. *Am J Kidney Dis.* 2000;36(6):1213–1225.

44. Jacob V, et al. Nutritional profile of continuous ambulatory peritoneal dialysis patients. *Nephron.* 1995;71(1):16–22.

45. Wang AY, et al. Evaluation of handgrip strength as a nutritional marker and prognostic indicator in peritoneal dialysis patients. *Am J Clin Nutr.* 2005; 81(1):79–86.

46. Sreedhara R, et al. Prealbumin is the best nutritional predictor of survival in hemodialysis and peritoneal dialysis. *Am J Kidney Dis.* 1996;28(6):937–942.

47. Avram MM, et al. Markers for survival in dialysis: a seven-year prospective study. *Am J Kidney Dis.* 1995;26(1):209–219.

48. Blake PG, et al. Serum albumin in patients on continuous ambulatory peritoneal dialysis—predictors and correlations with outcomes. *J Am Soc Nephrol.* 1993;3(8):1501–1507.

49. Chung SH, Lindholm B, Lee HB. Influence of initial nutritional status on continuous ambulatory peritoneal dialysis patient survival. *Perit Dial Int.* 2000;20(1):19–26.

50. Mehrotra R, Kopple JD. Nutritional management of maintenance dialysis patients: why aren't we doing better? *Annu Rev Nutr.* 2001;21:343–379.

51. Harty J, et al. The influence of small solute clearance on dietary protein intake in continuous ambulatory peritoneal dialysis patients: a methodologic analysis based on cross-sectional and prospective studies. *Am J Kidney Dis.* 1996;28(4):553–560.

52. Uehlinger DE. Another look at the relationship between protein intake and dialysis dose. *J Am Soc Nephrol.* 1996;7(1):166–168.

53. Wang AY, et al. Independent effects of residual renal function and dialysis adequacy on actual dietary protein, calorie, and other nutrient intake in patients on continuous ambulatory peritoneal dialysis. *J Am Soc Nephrol.* 2001;12(11):2450–2457.

54. Bergstrom J, et al. Protein and energy intake, nitrogen balance and nitrogen losses in patients treated with continuous ambulatory peritoneal dialysis. *Kidney Int.* 1993;44(5):1048–1057.

55. Davies SJ, et al. Analysis of the effects of increasing delivered dialysis treatment to malnourished peritoneal dialysis patients. *Kidney Int.* 2000;57(4): 1743–1754.

56. Nancy G, Steven F, Robert IL. The effect of improved dialytic efficiency on measures of appetite in peritoneal dialysis patients. *J Renal Nutr.* 1996;6(4): 217–221.

57. Anderstam B, et al. Middle-sized molecule fractions isolated from uremic ultrafiltrate and normal urine inhibit ingestive behavior in the rat. *J Am Soc Nephrol.* 1996;7(11):2453–2460.

58. Peritoneal Dialysis Adequacy Work Group. Clinical practice guidelines for peritoneal dialysis adequacy. *Am J Kidney Dis.* 2006;48 Suppl 1:S98–129.

59. Dombros N, et al. European best practice guidelines for peritoneal dialysis. Adequacy of peritoneal dialysis. *Nephrol Dial Transplant.* 2005;20 Suppl 9:ix24–ix27.

60. Blake PG, et al. Clinical practice guidelines and recommendations on peritoneal dialysis adequacy 2011. *Perit Dial Int.* 2011;31(2):218–239.

61. Lo WK, et al. Guideline on targets for solute and fluid removal in adult patients on chronic peritoneal dialysis. *Perit Dial Int.* 2006;26(5):520–522.

62. Johnson D, et al. The CARI guidelines. Dialysis adequacy (PD) guidelines. *Nephrology (Carlton).* 2005;10 Suppl 4:S81–107.

63. Adequacy of dialysis and nutrition in continuous peritoneal dialysis: association with clinical outcomes. Canada-USA (CANUSA) Peritoneal Dialysis Study Group. *J Am Soc Nephrol.* 1996;7(2):198–207.

64. Van Biesen W, et al. Personal dialysis capacity (PDC(TM)) test: a multicentre clinical study. *Nephrol Dial Transplant.* 2003;18(4):788–796.

65. Twardowski ZJ, et al. Peritoneal equilibration test. *Perit Dial Int.* 1987;7(3): 138–148.

66. Fischbach M, et al. Determination of individual ultrafiltration time (APEX) and purification phosphate time by peritoneal equilibration test: application to individual peritoneal dialysis modality prescription in children. *Perit Dial Int.* 1996;16 Suppl 1:S557–560.

67. Pannekeet MM, et al. The standard peritoneal permeability analysis: a tool for the assessment of peritoneal permeability characteristics in CAPD patients. *Kidney Int.* 1995;48(3):866–875.

68. Rocco MV, Jordan JR, Burkart JM. Determination of peritoneal transport characteristics with 24–hour dialysate collections: dialysis adequacy and transport test. *J Am Soc Nephrol.* 1994;5(6):1333–1338.

69. Krediet RT, et al. Simple assessment of the efficacy of peritoneal transport in continuous ambulatory peritoneal dialysis patients. *Blood Purif.* 1986;4(4): 194–203.

70. Vonesh EF, et al. Kinetic modeling as a prescription aid in peritoneal dialysis. *Blood Purif.* 1991;9(5–6):246–270.

71. Johnson DW, et al. A comparison of peritoneal equilibration tests performed 1 and 4 weeks after PD commencement. *Perit Dial Int.* 2004;24(5):460–465.

72. Mujais S, Vonesh E. Profiling of peritoneal ultrafiltration. *Kidney Int Suppl.* 2002(81):S17–22.

73. Twardowski ZJ, et al. Short peritoneal equilibration test: impact of preceding dwell time. *Adv Perit Dial.* 2003;19:53–58.

74. Figueiredo AE, Conti A, Poli de Figueiredo CE. Influence of the preceding exchange on peritoneal equilibration test results. *Adv Perit Dial.* 2002; 18:75–77.

75. Mujais S, et al. Evaluation and management of ultrafiltration problems in peritoneal dialysis. International Society for Peritoneal Dialysis Ad Hoc

Committee on Ultrafiltration Management in Peritoneal Dialysis. *Perit Dial Int.* 2000;20 Suppl 4:S5–21.
76. Pride ET, et al. Comparison of a 2.5% and a 4.25% dextrose peritoneal equilibration test. *Perit Dial Int.* 2002;22(3):365–370.
77. Twardowski ZJ. Nightly peritoneal dialysis. Why, who, how, and when? *ASAIO Trans.* 1990;36(1):8–16.
78. Mehrotra R, et al. The outcomes of continuous ambulatory and automated peritoneal dialysis are similar. *Kidney Int.* 2009;76(1):97–107.
79. Badve SV, et al. Automated and continuous ambulatory peritoneal dialysis have similar outcomes. *Kidney Int.* 2008;73(4):480–488.
80. Churchill DN, et al. Increased peritoneal membrane transport is associated with decreased patient and technique survival for continuous peritoneal dialysis patients. The Canada-USA (CANUSA) Peritoneal Dialysis Study Group. *J Am Soc Nephrol.* 1998;9(7):1285–1292.
81. Rumpsfeld M, et al. Predictors of baseline peritoneal transport status in Australian and New Zealand peritoneal dialysis patients. *Am J Kidney Dis.* 2004;43(3):492–501.
82. Davenport A, Willicombe MK. Hydration status does not influence peritoneal equilibration test ultrafiltration volumes. *Clin J Am Soc Nephrol.* 2009;4(7):1207–1212.
83. Oh KH, et al. Baseline peritoneal solute transport rate is not associated with markers of systemic inflammation or comorbidity in incident Korean peritoneal dialysis patients. *Nephrol Dial Transplant.* 2008;23(7):2356–2364.
84. Burkart J, Jordan JR, Rocco M. Assessment of dialysis dose by measured clearance versus extrapolated data. *Perit Dial Int.* 1993;13(3):184–188.
85. Brimble KS, et al. Meta-analysis: peritoneal membrane transport, mortality, and technique failure in peritoneal dialysis. *J Am Soc Nephrol.* 2006;17(9): 2591–2598.
86. Wiggins KJ, et al. High membrane transport status on peritoneal dialysis is not associated with reduced survival following transfer to haemodialysis. *Nephrol Dial Transplant.* 2007;22(10):3005–3012.
87. Watson PE, Watson ID, Batt RD. Total body water volumes for adult males and females estimated from simple anthropometric measurements. *Am J Clin Nutr.* 1980;33(1):27–39.
88. Hume R, Weyers E. Relationship between total body water and surface area in normal and obese subjects. *J Clin Pathol.* 1971;24(3):234–238.
89. Tzamaloukas AH, et al. The prescription of peritoneal dialysis. *Semin Dial.* 2008;21(3):250–257.
90. Borah MF, et al. Nitrogen balance during intermittent dialysis therapy of uremia. *Kidney Int.* 1978;14(5):491–500.
91. Randerson DC, Farrell PC. Amino acid and dietary status in long-term CAPD patients. In: Atkins RC, Thomson NM, Farrell PC, eds. *Peritoneal Dialysis.* Edinburgh: Churchill Livingstone; 1981.
92. Kjeldahl J. Neue methode zur bestimmung des stickoffs nin organischen Korpern. *Z Anal Chem.* 1983;22.
93. Keshaviah PR, Nolph KD. Protein catabolic rate calculations in CAPD patients. *ASAIO Trans.* 1991;37(3):M400–402.
94. Teehan BP, Schleifer CR, Sigler MH. A quantitative approach to the CAPD prescription. *Perit Dial Bull.* 1985;5:152–156.
95. Keshaviah PR, et al. Lean body mass estimation by creatinine kinetics. *J Am Soc Nephrol.* 1994;4(7):1475–1485.
96. Kotanko P, Levin NW, Zhu F. Current state of bioimpedance technologies in dialysis. *Nephrol Dial Transplant.* 2008;23(3):808–812.
97. Vonesh EF, Story KO, O'Neill WT. A multinational clinical validation study of PD ADEQUEST 2.0. PD ADEQUEST International Study Group. *Perit Dial Int.* 1999;19(6):556–571.
98. Gotch FA, Lipps BJ. PACK PD: a urea kinetic modeling computer program for peritoneal dialysis. *Perit Dial Int.* 1997;17 Suppl 2:S126–130.
99. Harty J, et al. Impact of increasing dialysis volume on adequacy targets: a prospective study. *J Am Soc Nephrol.* 1997;8(8):1304–1310.
100. Gao H, Lew SQ, Bosch JP. The effects of increasing exchange volume and frequency on peritoneal dialysis adequacy. *Clin Nephrol.* 1998;50(6):375–380.
101. Page DE. Comparing an additional hour of cycler therapy to an additional midday exchange to achieve adequacy targets. *Adv Perit Dial.* 2000;16:102–103.
102. Wolfson M, et al. A randomized controlled trial to evaluate the efficacy and safety of icodextrin in peritoneal dialysis. *Am J Kidney Dis.* 2002;40(5): 1055–1065.
103. Finkelstein F, et al. Superiority of icodextrin compared with 4.25% dextrose for peritoneal ultrafiltration. *J Am Soc Nephrol.* 2005;16(2):546–554.
104. Juergensen PH, et al. Increasing the dialysis volume and frequency in a fixed period of time in CPD patients: the effect on Kpt/V and creatinine clearance. *Perit Dial Int.* 2002;22(6):693–697.
105. Sarkar S, et al. Tolerance of large exchange volumes by peritoneal dialysis patients. *Am J Kidney Dis.* 1999;33(6):1136–1141.
106. Fukatsu A, et al. Clinical benefits and tolerability of increased fill volumes in Japanese peritoneal dialysis patients. *Perit Dial Int.* 2001;21(5):455–461.
107. Konings CJ, et al. Fluid status in CAPD patients is related to peritoneal transport and residual renal function: evidence from a longitudinal study. *Nephrol Dial Transplant.* 2003;18(4):797–803.
108. Szeto CC, et al. Independent effects of residual renal function and dialysis adequacy on nutritional status and patient outcome in continuous ambulatory peritoneal dialysis. *Am J Kidney Dis.* 1999;34(6):1056–1064.
109. Menon MK, et al. Long-term blood pressure control in a cohort of peritoneal dialysis patients and its association with residual renal function. *Nephrol Dial Transplant.* 2001;16(11):2207–2213.
110. Wang AY, et al. Inflammation, residual kidney function, and cardiac hypertrophy are interrelated and combine adversely to enhance mortality and cardiovascular death risk of peritoneal dialysis patients. *J Am Soc Nephrol.* 2004;15(8):2186–2194.
111. Wang AY, et al. Important differentiation of factors that predict outcome in peritoneal dialysis patients with different degrees of residual renal function. *Nephrol Dial Transplant.* 2005;20(2):396–403.
112. Caravaca F, Arrobas M, Dominguez C. Influence of residual renal function on dietary protein and caloric intake in patients on incremental peritoneal dialysis. *Perit Dial Int.* 1999;19(4):350–356.
113. Lopez-Menchero R, et al. Importance of residual renal function in continuous ambulatory peritoneal dialysis: its influence on different parameters of renal replacement treatment. *Nephron.* 1999;83(3):219–225.
114. van de Kerkhof J, et al. Nepsilon-(carboxymethyl)lysine, Nepsilon-(carboxyethyl)lysine and vascular cell adhesion molecule-1 (VCAM-1) in relation to peritoneal glucose prescription and residual renal function; a study in peritoneal dialysis patients. *Nephrol Dial Transplant.* 2004;19(4):910–916.
115. Bammens B, et al. Removal of middle molecules and protein-bound solutes by peritoneal dialysis and relation with uremic symptoms. *Kidney Int.* 2003;64(6):2238–2243.
116. Termorshuizen F, et al. The relative importance of residual renal function compared with peritoneal clearance for patient survival and quality of life: an analysis of the Netherlands Cooperative Study on the Adequacy of Dialysis (NECOSAD)-2. *Am J Kidney Dis.* 2003;41(6):1293–1302.
117. Han SH, et al. Reduced residual renal function is a risk of peritonitis in continuous ambulatory peritoneal dialysis patients. *Nephrol Dial Transplant.* 2007;22(9):2653–2658.
118. Liao CT, et al. Rate of decline of residual renal function is associated with all-cause mortality and technique failure in patients on long-term peritoneal dialysis. *Nephrol Dial Transplant.* 2009;24(9):2909–2914.
119. Fang W, Oreopoulos DG, Bargman JM. Use of ACE inhibitors or angiotensin receptor blockers and survival in patients on peritoneal dialysis. *Nephrol Dial Transplant.* 2008;23(11):3704–3710.
120. Li PK, et al. Effects of an angiotensin-converting enzyme inhibitor on residual renal function in patients receiving peritoneal dialysis. A randomized, controlled study. *Ann Intern Med.* 2003;139(2):105–112.
121. Suzuki H, et al. Effects of an angiotensin II receptor blocker, valsartan, on residual renal function in patients on CAPD. *Am J Kidney Dis.* 2004;43(6):1056–1064.
122. Phakdeekitcharoen B, Leelasa-nguan P. Effects of an ACE inhibitor or angiotensin receptor blocker on potassium in CAPD patients. *Am J Kidney Dis.* 2004;44(4):738–746.
123. Williams JD, et al. The Euro-Balance Trial: the effect of a new biocompatible peritoneal dialysis fluid (balance) on the peritoneal membrane. *Kidney Int.* 2004;66(1):408–418.
124. Szeto CC, et al. Clinical biocompatibility of a neutral peritoneal dialysis solution with minimal glucose-degradation products—a 1-year randomized control trial. *Nephrol Dial Transplant.* 2007;22(2):552–559.
125. Fan SL, et al. Randomized controlled study of biocompatible peritoneal dialysis solutions: effect on residual renal function. *Kidney Int.* 2008;73(2):200–206.
126. Kim S, et al. Benefits of biocompatible PD fluid for preservation of residual renal function in incident CAPD patients: a 1-year study. *Nephrol Dial Transplant.* 2009;24(9):2899–2908.
126a. Johnson DW, Brown FG, Clarke M, et al. Effects of biocompatible versus standard fluid on peritoneal dialysis outcomes. *J Am Soc Nephrol.* 2012;23: 1097–1107.
127. Nolph KD, et al. The kinetics of ultrafiltration during peritoneal dialysis: the role of lymphatics. *Kidney Int.* 1987;32(2):219–226.
128. Struijk DG, et al. Indirect measurement of lymphatic absorption in CAPD patients is not influenced by trapping. *Kidney Int.* 1992;41(6):1668–1675.
129. Imholz AL, et al. Residual volume measurements in CAPD patients with exogenous and endogenous solutes. *Adv Perit Dial.* 1992;8:33–38.
130. Koomen GC, et al. A fast reliable method for the measurement of intraperitoneal dextran 70, used to calculate lymphatic absorption. *Adv Perit Dial.* 1991;7:10–14.

131. Lam MF, et al. Retroperitoneal leakage as a cause of acute ultrafiltration failure: its associated risk factors in peritoneal dialysis. *Perit Dial Int.* 2009;29(5):542–547.
132. Heimburger O, et al. Peritoneal transport in CAPD patients with permanent loss of ultrafiltration capacity. *Kidney Int.* 1990;38(3):495–506.
133. Heimburger O, et al. A quantitative description of solute and fluid transport during peritoneal dialysis. *Kidney Int.* 1992;41(5):1320–1332.
134. Krediet RT, et al. Alterations in the peritoneal transport of water and solutes during peritonitis in continuous ambulatory peritoneal dialysis patients. *Eur J Clin Invest.* 1987;17(1):43–52.
135. Posthuma N, et al. Icodextrin use in CCPD patients during peritonitis: ultrafiltration and serum disaccharide concentrations. *Nephrol Dial Transplant.* 1998;13(9):2341–2344.
136. Krediet RT. The peritoneal membrane in chronic peritoneal dialysis. *Kidney Int.* 1999;55(1):341–356.
137. Williams JD, et al. Morphologic changes in the peritoneal membrane of patients with renal disease. *J Am Soc Nephrol.* 2002;13(2):470–479.
138. Davies SJ, et al. Peritoneal glucose exposure and changes in membrane solute transport with time on peritoneal dialysis. *J Am Soc Nephrol.* 2001;12(5):1046–1051.
139. Davies SJ, et al. Longitudinal membrane function in functionally anuric patients treated with APD: data from EAPOS on the effects of glucose and icodextrin prescription. *Kidney Int.* 2005;67(4):1609–1615.
140. Rodrigues A, et al. Peritoneal rest may successfully recover ultrafiltration in patients who develop peritoneal hyperpermeability with time on continuous ambulatory peritoneal dialysis. *Adv Perit Dial.* 2002;18:78–80.
141. Mistry CD, Gokal R, Peers E. A randomized multicenter clinical trial comparing isosmolar icodextrin with hyperosmolar glucose solutions in CAPD. MIDAS Study Group. Multicenter Investigation of Icodextrin in Ambulatory Peritoneal Dialysis. *Kidney Int.* 1994;46(2):496–503.
142. Davies SJ, et al. Icodextrin improves the fluid status of peritoneal dialysis patients: results of a double-blind randomized controlled trial. *J Am Soc Nephrol.* 2003;14(9):2338–2344.
143. Konings CJ, et al. Effect of icodextrin on volume status, blood pressure and echocardiographic parameters: a randomized study. *Kidney Int.* 2003;63(4):1556–1563.
144. Sav T, et al. Effects of twice-daily icodextrin administration on blood pressure and left ventricular mass in patients on continuous ambulatory peritoneal dialysis. *Perit Dial Int.* 2009;29(4):443–449.
145. Monquil MC, et al. Does impaired transcellular water transport contribute to net ultrafiltration failure during CAPD? *Perit Dial Int.* 1995;15(1):42–48.
146. Goffin E, et al. Expression of aquaporin-1 in a long-term peritoneal dialysis patient with impaired transcellular water transport. *Am J Kidney Dis.* 1999;33(2):383–388.
147. Han SH, et al. Mortality and technique failure in peritoneal dialysis patients using advanced peritoneal dialysis solutions. *Am J Kidney Dis.* 2009;54(4):711–720.
148. Dobos GJ, et al. Bicarbonate-based dialysis solution preserves granulocyte functions. *Perit Dial Int.* 1994;14(4):366–370.
149. Chaudhary K, Khanna R. Biocompatible peritoneal dialysis solutions: do we have one? *Clin J Am Soc Nephrol.* 2010;5(4):723–732.
150. Sundaram S, et al. Effect of two-chambered bicarbonate lactate-buffered peritoneal dialysis fluids on peripheral blood mononuclear cell and polymorphonuclear cell function in vitro. *Am J Kidney Dis.* 1997;30(5):680–689.
151. Mackenzie RK, et al. In vivo exposure to bicarbonate/lactate- and bicarbonate-buffered peritoneal dialysis fluids improves ex vivo peritoneal macrophage function. *Am J Kidney Dis.* 2000;35(1):112–121.
152. Pawlaczyk K, et al. Bicarbonate/lactate dialysis solution improves in vivo function of peritoneal host defense in rats. *Perit Dial Int.* 1999;19 Suppl 2:S370–377.
153. Tranaeus A. A long-term study of a bicarbonate/lactate-based peritoneal dialysis solution—clinical benefits. The Bicarbonate/Lactate Study Group. *Perit Dial Int.* 2000;20(5):516–523.
154. Wang T, et al. Effect of peritonitis on peritoneal transport characteristics: glucose solution versus polyglucose solution. *Kidney Int.* 2000;57(4):1704–1712.
155. Brulez HF, et al. In vitro compatibility of a 1.1% amino acid containing peritoneal dialysis fluid with phagocyte function. *Adv Perit Dial.* 1994;10:241–244.
156. Olszowska A, et al. Peritoneal transport in peritoneal dialysis patients using glucose-based and amino acid-based solutions. *Perit Dial Int.* 2007;27(5):544–553.
157. Tjiong HL, et al. Amino acid-based peritoneal dialysis solutions for malnutrition: new perspectives. *Perit Dial Int.* 2009;29(4):384–393.
158. Palmer RA, et al. Treatment of chronic renal failure by prolonged peritoneal dialysis. *N Engl J Med.* 1966;274(5):248–254.
159. Tenckhoff H, Schechter H. A bacteriologically safe peritoneal access device. *Trans Am Soc Artif Intern Organs.* 1968;14:181–187.
160. Gokal R, et al. Peritoneal catheters and exit-site practices toward optimum peritoneal access: 1998 update. (Official report from the International Society for Peritoneal Dialysis.) *Perit Dial Int.* 1998;18(1):11–33.
161. Strippoli GF, et al. Catheter type, placement and insertion techniques for preventing peritonitis in peritoneal dialysis patients. *Cochrane Database Syst Rev.* 2004(4):CD004680.
162. Twardowski ZJ, et al. The need for a "swan neck" permanently bent, arcuate peritoneal dialysis catheter. *Perit Dial Int.* 1985;5(4):219–223.
163. Lye WC, et al. A prospective randomized comparison of the Swan neck, coiled, and straight Tenckhoff catheters in patients on CAPD. *Perit Dial Int.* 1996;16(Suppl_1):S333–335.
164. Eklund BH, et al. Catheter configuration and outcome in patients on continuous ambulatory peritoneal dialysis: a prospective comparison of two catheters. *Perit Dial Int.* 1994;14(1):70–74.
165. Twardowski ZJ, et al. Six-year experience with Swan neck presternal peritoneal dialysis catheter. *Perit Dial Int.* 1998;18(6):598–602.
166. Bergamin B, et al. Finding the right position: a three-year, single-center experience with the "self-locating" catheter. *Perit Dial Int.* 2010;30(5):519–523.
167. Di Paolo N, Gaggiotti E. The self-locating peritoneal catheter. *Int J Artif Organs.* 2004;27(4):261–264.
168. Flanigan M, Gokal R. Peritoneal catheters and exit-site practices toward optimum peritoneal access: a review of current developments. *Perit Dial Int.* 2005;25(2):132–139.
169. Katyal A, Mahale A, Khanna R. Antibiotic prophylaxis before peritoneal dialysis catheter insertion. *Adv Perit Dial.* 2002;18:112–115.
170. Crabtree JH. Selected best demonstrated practices in peritoneal dialysis access. *Kidney Int Suppl.* 2006(103):S27–37.
171. Crabtree JH, Burchette RJ. Effective use of laparoscopy for long-term peritoneal dialysis access. *Am J Surg.* 2009;198(1):135–141.
172. Wright MJ, et al. Randomized prospective comparison of laparoscopic and open peritoneal dialysis catheter insertion. *Perit Dial Int.* 1999;19(4):372–375.
173. Rosenthal MA, et al. Comparison of outcomes of peritoneal dialysis catheters placed by the fluoroscopically guided percutaneous method versus directly visualized surgical method. *J Vasc Interv Radiol.* 2008;19(8):1202–1207.
174. Moncrief JW, et al. The Moncrief-Popovich catheter. A new peritoneal access technique for patients on peritoneal dialysis. *ASAIO J.* 1993;39(1):62–65.
174a. Elhassan E, McNair B, Quinn M, et al. Prolonged duration of peritoneal dialysis catheter embedment does not lower the catheter success rate. *Perit Dial Int.* 2011;31(5):558–564.
175. Park MS, et al. Effect of prolonged subcutaneous implantation of peritoneal catheter on peritonitis rate during CAPD: a prospective randomized study. *Blood Purif.* 1998;16(3):171–178.
176. Danielsson A, et al. A prospective randomized study of the effect of a subcutaneously "buried" peritoneal dialysis catheter technique versus standard technique on the incidence of peritonitis and exit-site infection. *Perit Dial Int.* 2002;22(2):211–219.
177. Brum S, et al. Moncrief-Popovich technique is an advantageous method of peritoneal dialysis catheter implantation. *Nephrol Dial Transplant.* 2010; 25(9):3070–3075.
178. Kubota M, et al. Implantation of presternal catheter using Moncrief technique: aiming for fewer catheter-related complications. *Perit Dial Int.* 2001;21 Suppl 3:S205–208.
179. Clark KR, et al. Surgical aspects of chronic peritoneal dialysis in the neonate and infant under 1 year of age. *J Pediatr Surg.* 1992;27(6):780–783.
180. Campos RP, Chula DC, Riella MC. Complications of the peritoneal access and their management. *Contrib Nephrol.* 2009;163:183–197.
181. Lye WC, et al. Breaking-in after the insertion of Tenckhoff catheters: a comparison of two techniques. *Adv Perit Dial.* 1993;9:236–239.
182. Bender FH, Bernardini J, Piraino B. Prevention of infectious complications in peritoneal dialysis: best demonstrated practices. *Kidney Int Suppl.* 2006(103):S44–54.
183. Robison RJ, et al. Surgical considerations of continuous ambulatory peritoneal dialysis. *Surgery.* 1984;96(4):723–730.
184. Swartz R, et al. The curled catheter: dependable device for percutaneous peritoneal access. *Perit Dial Int.* 1990;10(3):231–235.
185. Joffe P, Christensen AL, Jensen C. Peritoneal catheter tip location during non-complicated continuous ambulatory peritoneal dialysis. *Perit Dial Int.* 1991;11(3):261–264.
186. Zorzanello MM, Fleming WJ, Prowant BE. Use of tissue plasminogen activator in peritoneal dialysis catheters: a literature review and one center's experience. *Nephrol Nurs J.* 2004;31(5):534–537.
187. Wiegmann TB, et al. Effective use of streptokinase for peritoneal catheter failure. *Am J Kidney Dis.* 1985;6(2):119–123.
188. Nicholson ML, et al. The role of omentectomy in continuous ambulatory peritoneal dialysis. *Perit Dial Int.* 1991;11(4):330–332.
189. Leblanc M, Ouimet D, Pichette V. Dialysate leaks in peritoneal dialysis. *Semin Dial.* 2001;14(1):50–54.

190. Stegmayr B, et al. Absence of leakage by insertion of peritoneal dialysis catheter through the rectus muscle. *Perit Dial Int.* 1990;10(1):53–55.
191. Apostolidis NS, et al. The use of TWH catheters in CAPD patients: fourteen-year experience in technique, survival, and complication rates. *Perit Dial Int.* 1998;18(4):424–428.
192. Litherland J, et al. Computed tomographic peritoneography: CT manifestations in the investigation of leaks and abnormal collections in patients on CAPD. *Nephrol Dial Transplant.* 1994;9(10):1449–1452.
193. Holley JL, Bernardini J, Piraino B. Characteristics and outcome of peritoneal dialysate leaks and associated infections. *Adv Perit Dial.* 1993;9: 240–243.
194. Hirsch DJ, Jindal KK. Late leaks in peritoneal dialysis patients. *Nephrol Dial Transplant.* 1991;6(9):670–671.
195. Piraino B, et al. Peritoneal dialysis-related infections recommendations: 2005 update. *Perit Dial Int.* 2005;25(2):107–131.
196. Sewell DL, et al. Comparison of large volume culture to other methods for isolation of microorganisms from dialysate. *Perit Dial Int.* 1990;10(1):49–52.
197. Alfa MJ, et al. Improved detection of bacterial growth in continuous ambulatory peritoneal dialysis effluent by use of BacT/Alert FAN bottles. *J Clin Microbiol.* 1997;35(4):862–866.
198. Koopmans JG, et al. Impaired initial cell reaction in CAPD-related peritonitis. *Perit Dial Int.* 1996;16 Suppl 1:S362–367.
199. Gonthier D, et al. Erythema: does it indicate infection in a peritoneal catheter exit site? *Adv Perit Dial.* 1992;8:230–233.
200. Plum J, Sudkamp S, Grabensee B. Results of ultrasound-assisted diagnosis of tunnel infections in continuous ambulatory peritoneal dialysis. *Am J Kidney Dis.* 1994;23(1):99–104.
201. Gupta B, Bernardini J, Piraino B. Peritonitis associated with exit site and tunnel infections. *Am J Kidney Dis.* 1996;28(3):415–419.
202. Woodrow G, Turney JH, Brownjohn AM. Technique failure in peritoneal dialysis and its impact on patient survival. *Perit Dial Int.* 1997;17(4):360–364.
203. Piraino B, Bernardini J, Sorkin M. The influence of peritoneal catheter exit-site infections on peritonitis, tunnel infections, and catheter loss in patients on continuous ambulatory peritoneal dialysis. *Am J Kidney Dis.* 1986;8(6):436–440.
204. Fried L, et al. Hospitalization in peritoneal dialysis patients. *Am J Kidney Dis.* 1999;33(5):927–933.
205. Fried LF, et al. Peritonitis influences mortality in peritoneal dialysis patients. *J Am Soc Nephrol.* 1996;7(10):2176–2182.
206. Perez Fontan M, et al. Peritonitis-related mortality in patients undergoing chronic peritoneal dialysis. *Perit Dial Int.* 2005;25(3):274–284.
207. Holmes CJ. Peritoneal host defense mechanisms in peritoneal dialysis. *Kidney Int Suppl.* 1994;48:S58–70.
208. Betjes MG, et al. Analysis of the peritoneal cellular immune system during CAPD shortly before a clinical peritonitis. *Nephrol Dial Transplant.* 1994;9(6): 684–692.
209. Ates K, et al. The longitudinal effect of a single peritonitis episode on peritoneal membrane transport in CAPD patients. *Perit Dial Int.* 2000;20(2):220–226.
210. Lai KN, et al. Changes of cytokine profiles during peritonitis in patients on continuous ambulatory peritoneal dialysis. *Am J Kidney Dis.* 2000;35(4):644–652.
211. Jorres A, et al. Impact of peritoneal dialysis solutions on peritoneal immune defense. *Perit Dial Int.* 1993;13 Suppl 2:S291–294.
212. Posthuma N, et al. Peritoneal defense using icodextrin or glucose for daytime dwell in CCPD patients. *Perit Dial Int.* 1999;19(4):334–342.
213. de Fijter CW, et al. Biocompatibility of a glucose-polymer-containing peritoneal dialysis fluid. *Am J Kidney Dis.* 1993;21(4):411–418.
214. Kim SG, et al. Could solutions low in glucose degradation products preserve residual renal function in incident peritoneal dialysis patients? A 1-year multicenter prospective randomized controlled trial (Balnet Study). *Perit Dial Int.* 2008;28 Suppl 3:S117–122.
215. Buoncristiani U. Continuous ambulatory peritoneal dialysis connection systems. *Perit Dial Int.* 1993;13 Suppl 2:S139–145.
216. Strippoli GF, et al. Catheter-related interventions to prevent peritonitis in peritoneal dialysis: a systematic review of randomized, controlled trials. *J Am Soc Nephrol.* 2004;15(10):2735–2746.
217. Monteon F, et al. Prevention of peritonitis with disconnect systems in CAPD: a randomized controlled trial. The Mexican Nephrology Collaborative Study Group. *Kidney Int.* 1998;54(6):2123–2128.
218. Kiernan L, et al. Comparison of continuous ambulatory peritoneal dialysis-related infections with different "Y-tubing" exchange systems. *J Am Soc Nephrol.* 1995;5(10):1835–1838.
219. Rabindranath KS, et al. Automated vs continuous ambulatory peritoneal dialysis: a systematic review of randomized controlled trials. *Nephrol Dial Transplant.* 2007;22(10):2991–2998.
220. de Fijter CW, et al. Clinical efficacy and morbidity associated with continuous cyclic compared with continuous ambulatory peritoneal dialysis. *Ann Intern Med.* 1994;120(4):264–271.
221. Oo TN, Roberts TL, Collins AJ. A comparison of peritonitis rates from the United States Renal Data System database: CAPD versus continuous cycling peritoneal dialysis patients. *Am J Kidney Dis.* 2005;45(2):372–380.
222. Ramalakshmi S, Bernardini J, Piraino B. Nightly intermittent peritoneal dialysis to initiate peritoneal dialysis. *Adv Perit Dial.* 2003;19:111–114.
223. Li PK, et al. Peritoneal dialysis-related infections recommendations: 2010 update. *Perit Dial Int.* 2010;30(4):393–423.
224. Bernardini J, et al. Randomized, double-blind trial of antibiotic exit site cream for prevention of exit site infection in peritoneal dialysis patients. *J Am Soc Nephrol.* 2005;16(2):539–545.
225. Holley JL, Bernardini J, Piraino B. Risk factors for tunnel infections in continuous peritoneal dialysis. *Am J Kidney Dis.* 1991;18(3):344–348.
226. Holley JL, et al. Ultrasound as a tool in the diagnosis and management of exit-site infections in patients undergoing continuous ambulatory peritoneal dialysis. *Am J Kidney Dis.* 1989;14(3):211–216.
227. Flanigan MJ, et al. Continuous ambulatory peritoneal dialysis catheter infections: diagnosis and management. *Perit Dial Int.* 1994;14(3):248–254.
228. Holley JL, Bernardini J, Piraino B. Infecting organisms in continuous ambulatory peritoneal dialysis patients on the Y-set. *Am J Kidney Dis.* 1994;23(4): 569–573.
229. Kazmi HR, et al. Pseudomonas exit site infections in continuous ambulatory peritoneal dialysis patients. *J Am Soc Nephrol.* 1992;2(10):1498–1501.
230. Bernardini J, Piraino B, Sorkin M. Analysis of continuous ambulatory peritoneal dialysis-related Pseudomonas aeruginosa infections. *Am J Med.* 1987;83(5):829–832.
231. Abraham G, et al. Natural history of exit-site infection (ESI) in patients on continuous ambulatory peritoneal dialysis (CAPD). *Perit Dial Int.* 1988;8(3):211–216.
232. Bayston R, et al. Recurrent infection and catheter loss in patients on continuous ambulatory peritoneal dialysis. *Perit Dial Int.* 1999;19(6):550–555.
233. Thodis E, et al. Decrease in Staphylococcus aureus exit-site infections and peritonitis in CAPD patients by local application of mupirocin ointment at the catheter exit site. *Perit Dial Int.* 1998;18(3):261–270.
234. Bernardini J, et al. A randomized trial of Staphylococcus aureus prophylaxis in peritoneal dialysis patients: mupirocin calcium ointment 2% applied to the exit site versus cyclic oral rifampin. *Am J Kidney Dis.* 1996;27(5):695–700.
235. Tacconelli E, et al. Mupirocin prophylaxis to prevent Staphylococcus aureus infection in patients undergoing dialysis: a meta-analysis. *Clin Infect Dis.* 2003;37(12):1629–1638.
236. Annigeri R, et al. Emergence of mupirocin-resistant Staphylococcus aureus in chronic peritoneal dialysis patients using mupirocin prophylaxis to prevent exit-site infection. *Perit Dial Int.* 2001;21(6):554–559.
237. Perez-Fontan M, et al. Mupirocin resistance after long-term use for Staphylococcus aureus colonization in patients undergoing chronic peritoneal dialysis. *Am J Kidney Dis.* 2002;39(2):337–341.
238. Montenegro J, et al. Exit-site care with ciprofloxacin otologic solution prevents polyurethane catheter infection in peritoneal dialysis patients. *Perit Dial Int.* 2000;20(2):209–214.
239. Mujais S, Story K. Peritoneal dialysis in the US: evaluation of outcomes in contemporary cohorts. *Kidney Int Suppl.* 2006(103):S21–26.
240. Mujais S. Microbiology and outcomes of peritonitis in North America. *Kidney Int Suppl.* 2006;(103):S55–62.
241. Tofte-Jensen P, et al. PD-related infections of standard and different disconnect systems. *Adv Perit Dial.* 1994;10:214–217.
242. Lupo A, et al. Long-term outcome in continuous ambulatory peritoneal dialysis: a 10-year-survey by the Italian Cooperative Peritoneal Dialysis Study Group. *Am J Kidney Dis.* 1994;24(5):826–837.
243. Szeto CC, et al. Change in bacterial aetiology of peritoneal dialysis-related peritonitis over 10 years: experience from a centre in South-East Asia. *Clin Microbiol Infect.* 2005;11(10):837–839.
244. Korbet SM, Vonesh EF, Firanek CA. A retrospective assessment of risk factors for peritonitis among an urban CAPD population. *Perit Dial Int.* 1993;13(2):126–131.
245. Farias MG, et al. Race and the risk of peritonitis: an analysis of factors associated with the initial episode. *Kidney Int.* 1994;46(5):1392–1396.
246. Lye WC, et al. A prospective study of peritoneal dialysis-related infections in CAPD patients with diabetes mellitus. *Adv Perit Dial.* 1993;9:195–197.
247. Viglino G, et al. Ten years experience of CAPD in diabetics: comparison of results with non-diabetics. Italian Cooperative Peritoneal Dialysis Study Group. *Nephrol Dial Transplant.* 1994;9(10):1443–1448.
248. Szeto CC, Kwan BC, Chow KM. Peritonitis risk for older patients on peritoneal dialysis. *Perit Dial Int.* 2008;28(5):457–460.

249. Yinnon AM, et al. Comparison of peritoneal fluid culture results from adults and children undergoing CAPD. *Perit Dial Int.* 1999;19(1):51–55.

250. Andrews PA, et al. Impaired outcome of continuous ambulatory peritoneal dialysis in immunosuppressed patients. *Nephrol Dial Transplant.* 1996;11(6):1104–1108.

251. Port FK, et al. Risk of peritonitis and technique failure by CAPD connection technique: a national study. *Kidney Int.* 1992;42(4):967–974.

252. Read RR, et al. Peritonitis in peritoneal dialysis: bacterial colonization by biofilm spread along the catheter surface. *Kidney Int.* 1989;35(2):614–621.

253. Eisenberg ES, et al. Colonization of skin and development of peritonitis due to coagulase-negative staphylococci in patients undergoing peritoneal dialysis. *J Infect Dis.* 1987;156(3):478–482.

254. Gorman SP, et al. Confocal laser scanning microscopy of peritoneal catheter surfaces. *J Med Microbiol.* 1993;38(6):411–417.

255. Beaman M, et al. Peritonitis caused by slime-producing coagulase negative staphylococci in continuous ambulatory peritoneal dialysis. *Lancet.* 1987;1(8523):42.

256. Swartz R, et al. Biofilm formation on peritoneal catheters does not require the presence of infection. *ASAIO Trans.* 1991;37(4):626–634.

257. Miller TE, Findon G. Touch contamination of connection devices in peritoneal dialysis—a quantitative microbiologic analysis. *Perit Dial Int.* 1997;17(6):560–567.

258. Szeto CC, et al. Enterobacteriaceae peritonitis complicating peritoneal dialysis: a review of 210 consecutive cases. *Kidney Int.* 2006;69(7):1245–1252.

259. Siva B, et al. Pseudomonas peritonitis in Australia: predictors, treatment, and outcomes in 191 cases. *Clin J Am Soc Nephrol.* 2009;4(5):957–964.

260. Troidle L, et al. Differing outcomes of gram-positive and gram-negative peritonitis. *Am J Kidney Dis.* 1998;32(4):623–628.

261. Wood CJ, et al. Campylobacter peritonitis in continuous ambulatory peritoneal dialysis: report of eight cases and a review of the literature. *Am J Kidney Dis.* 1992;19(3):257–263.

262. Singharetnam W, Holley JL. Acute treatment of constipation may lead to transmural migration of bacteria resulting in gram-negative, polymicrobial, or fungal peritonitis. *Perit Dial Int.* 1996;16(4):423–425.

263. Chuang YW, et al. Hypokalaemia: an independent risk factor of Enterobacteriaceae peritonitis in CAPD patients. *Nephrol Dial Transplant.* 2009;24(5):1603–1608.

264. Harwell CM, et al. Abdominal catastrophe: visceral injury as a cause of peritonitis in patients treated by peritoneal dialysis. *Perit Dial Int.* 1997;17(6):586–594.

265. Burkart J, et al. Usefulness of peritoneal fluid amylase levels in the differential diagnosis of peritonitis in peritoneal dialysis patients. *J Am Soc Nephrol.* 1991;1(10):1186–1190.

266. Verger C, Danne O, Vuillemin F. Colonoscopy and continuous ambulatory peritoneal dialysis. *Gastrointest Endosc.* 1987;33(4):334–335.

267. Fried L, Bernardini J, Piraino B. Iatrogenic peritonitis: the need for prophylaxis. *Perit Dial Int.* 2000;20(3):343–345.

268. Troidle L, et al. Continuous peritoneal dialysis-associated peritonitis of nosocomial origin. *Perit Dial Int.* 1996;16(5):505–510.

269. Coward RA, et al. Peritonitis associated with vaginal leakage of dialysis fluid in continuous ambulatory peritoneal dialysis. *Br Med J (Clin Res Ed).* 1982;284(6328):1529.

270. Miles R, et al. Predictors and outcomes of fungal peritonitis in peritoneal dialysis patients. *Kidney Int.* 2009;76(6):622–628.

271. Prasad N, Gupta A. Fungal peritonitis in peritoneal dialysis patients. *Perit Dial Int.* 2005;25(3):207–222.

272. Goldie SJ, et al. Fungal peritonitis in a large chronic peritoneal dialysis population: a report of 55 episodes. *Am J Kidney Dis.* 1996;28(1):86–91.

273. Robitaille P, et al. Successful antifungal prophylaxis in chronic peritoneal dialysis: a pediatric experience. *Perit Dial Int.* 1995;15(1):77–79.

274. Williams PF, Moncrieff N, Marriott J. No benefit in using nystatin prophylaxis against fungal peritonitis in peritoneal dialysis patients. *Perit Dial Int.* 2000;20(3):352–353.

275. Thodis E, et al. Nystatin prophylaxis: its inability to prevent fungal peritonitis in patients on continuous ambulatory peritoneal dialysis. *Perit Dial Int.* 1998;18(6):583–589.

276. Lo WK, et al. A prospective randomized control study of oral nystatin prophylaxis for Candida peritonitis complicating continuous ambulatory peritoneal dialysis. *Am J Kidney Dis.* 1996;28(4):549–552.

277. Wadhwa NK, Suh H, Cabralda T. Antifungal prophylaxis for secondary fungal peritonitis in peritoneal dialysis patients. *Adv Perit Dial.* 1996;12:189–191.

278. Zaruba K, Peters J, Jungbluth H. Successful prophylaxis for fungal peritonitis in patients on continuous ambulatory peritoneal dialysis: six years' experience. *Am J Kidney Dis.* 1991;17(1):43–46.

279. Rocklin MA, Teitelbaum I. Noninfectious causes of cloudy peritoneal dialysate. *Semin Dial.* 2001;14(1):37–40.

280. Wang AY, Li PK, Lai KN. Comparison of intraperitoneal administration of two preparations of vancomycin in causing chemical peritonitis. *Perit Dial Int.* 1996;16(2):172–174.

281. Fabris A, et al. Pharmacokinetics of antifungal agents. *Perit Dial Int.* 1993;13 Suppl 2:S380–382.

282. Gokal R. Icodextrin-associated sterile peritonitis. *Perit Dial Int.* 2002;22(4):445–448.

283. Del Rosso G, et al. A new form of acute adverse reaction to icodextrin in a peritoneal dialysis patient. *Nephrol Dial Transplant.* 2000;15(6):927–928.

284. Martis L, et al. Aseptic peritonitis due to peptidoglycan contamination of pharmacopoeia standard dialysis solution. *Lancet.* 2005;365(9459):588–594.

285. Vychytil A, et al. New criteria for management of catheter infections in peritoneal dialysis patients using ultrasonography. *J Am Soc Nephrol.* 1998;9(2):290–296.

286. Crabtree JH, Burchette RJ. Surgical salvage of peritoneal dialysis catheters from chronic exit-site and tunnel infections. *Am J Surg.* 2005;190(1):4–8.

287. Szabo T, et al. Outcome of Pseudomonas aeruginosa exit-site and tunnel infections: a single center's experience. *Adv Perit Dial.* 1999;15:209–212.

288. Yinnon AM, Jain V, Magnussen CR. Group B Streptococcus (agalactiae) peritonitis and bacteremia associated with CAPD. *Perit Dial Int.* 1993;13(3):241.

289. Officer TP, et al. Group A streptococcal peritonitis associated with continuous ambulatory peritoneal dialysis. *Am J Med.* 1989;87(4):487.

290. Manley HJ, et al. Pharmacokinetics of intermittent intraperitoneal cefazolin in continuous ambulatory peritoneal dialysis patients. *Perit Dial Int.* 1999;19(1):65–70.

291. Grabe DW, et al. Pharmacokinetics of intermittent intraperitoneal ceftazidime. *Am J Kidney Dis.* 1999;33(1):111–117.

292. Shemin D, et al. Effect of aminoglycoside use on residual renal function in peritoneal dialysis patients. *Am J Kidney Dis.* 1999;34(1):14–20.

293. Lui SL, et al. Cefazolin plus netilmicin versus cefazolin plus ceftazidime for treating CAPD peritonitis: effect on residual renal function. *Kidney Int.* 2005;68(5):2375–2380.

294. Wiggins KJ, et al. Treatment of peritoneal dialysis-associated peritonitis: a systematic review of randomized controlled trials. *Am J Kidney Dis.* 2007;50(6):967–988.

295. Fontan MP, et al. Treatment of peritoneal dialysis-related peritonitis with ciprofloxacin monotherapy: clinical outcomes and bacterial susceptibility over two decades. *Perit Dial Int.* 2009;29(3):310–318.

296. Agraharkar M, et al. Use of cefazolin for peritonitis treatment in peritoneal dialysis patients. *Am J Nephrol.* 1999;19(5):555–558.

297. Ng R, et al. Vancomycin-resistant enterococcus infection is a rare complication in patients receiving PD on an outpatient basis. *Perit Dial Int.* 1999;19(3):273–274.

298. Vas S, Bargman J, Oreopoulos D. Treatment in PD patients of peritonitis caused by gram-positive organisms with single daily dose of antibiotics. *Perit Dial Int.* 1997;17(1):91–94.

299. Lye WC, Leong SO, Lee EJ. Methicillin-resistant Staphylococcus aureus nasal carriage and infections in CAPD. *Kidney Int.* 1993;43(6):1357–1362.

300. Smith TL, et al. Emergence of vancomycin resistance in Staphylococcus aureus. Glycopeptide-Intermediate Staphylococcus aureus Working Group. *N Engl J Med.* 1999;340(7):493–501.

301. Huen SC, et al. Successful use of intraperitoneal daptomycin in the treatment of vancomycin-resistant enterococcus peritonitis. *Am J Kidney Dis.* 2009;54(3):538–541.

302. Furgeson SB, Teitelbaum I. New treatment options and protocols for peritoneal dialysis-related peritonitis. *Contrib Nephrol.* 2009;163:169–176.

303. Servais A, et al. Rapid curbing of a vancomycin-resistant Enterococcus faecium outbreak in a nephrology department. *Clin J Am Soc Nephrol.* 2009;4(10):1559–1564.

304. Lye WC, et al. Once-daily intraperitoneal gentamicin is effective therapy for gram-negative CAPD peritonitis. *Perit Dial Int.* 1999;19(4):357–360.

305. Bunke M, Brier ME, Golper TA. Pseudomonas peritonitis in peritoneal dialysis patients: the Network #9 Peritonitis Study. *Am J Kidney Dis.* 1995;25(5):769–774.

306. Tzamaloukas AH, Murata GH, Fox L. Death associated with Pseudomonas peritonitis in malnourished elderly diabetics on CAPD. *Perit Dial Int.* 1993;13(3):241–242.

307. Szeto CC, et al. Clinical course of peritonitis due to Pseudomonas species complicating peritoneal dialysis: a review of 104 cases. *Kidney Int.* 2001;59(6):2309–2315.

308. Szeto CC, et al. Xanthomonas maltophilia peritonitis in uremic patients receiving continuous ambulatory peritoneal dialysis. *Am J Kidney Dis.* 1997;29(1):91–95.

309. Tzanetou K, et al. Stenotrophomonas maltophilia peritonitis in CAPD patients: susceptibility to antibiotics and treatment outcome: a report of five cases. *Perit Dial Int.* 2004;24(4):401–404.

310. Wang AY, et al. Factors predicting outcome of fungal peritonitis in peritoneal dialysis: analysis of a 9–year experience of fungal peritonitis in a single center. *Am J Kidney Dis.* 2000;36(6):1183–1192.
311. Wong PN, et al. Treatment of fungal peritonitis with a combination of intravenous amphotericin B and oral flucytosine, and delayed catheter replacement in continuous ambulatory peritoneal dialysis. *Perit Dial Int.* 2008;28(2):155–162.
312. Chan TM, et al. Treatment of fungal peritonitis complicating continuous ambulatory peritoneal dialysis with oral fluconazole: a series of 21 patients. *Nephrol Dial Transplant.* 1994;9(5):539–542.
313. Glancey GR, Cameron JS, Ogg CS. Peritoneal drainage: an important element in host defence against staphylococcal peritonitis in patients on CAPD. *Nephrol Dial Transplant.* 1992;7(7):627–631.
314. Usberti M, et al. Treatment of acute peritonitis by temporary discontinuation of dialysis and low doses of oral ciprofloxacin in patients on CAPD. *Perit Dial Int.* 1994;14(2):185–186.
315. Cairns HS, et al. Treatment of resistant CAPD peritonitis by temporary discontinuation of peritoneal dialysis. *Clin Nephrol.* 1989;32(1):27–30.
316. Kant KS, et al. Relapsing peritonitis in continuous ambulatory peritoneal dialysis (CAPD): treatment by interruption of CAPD and prolonged antibiotic therapy. *Perit Dial Int.* 1988;8(2):155–157.
317. Chow KM, et al. Predictive value of dialysate cell counts in peritonitis complicating peritoneal dialysis. *Clin J Am Soc Nephrol.* 2006;1(4):768–773.
318. Paterson AD, et al. Removal and replacement of Tenckhoff catheter at a single operation: successful treatment of resistant peritonitis in continuous ambulatory peritoneal dialysis. *Lancet.* 1986;2(8518):1245–1247.
319. Mitra A, Teitelbaum I. Is it safe to simultaneously remove and replace infected peritoneal dialysis catheters? Review of the literature and suggested guidelines. *Adv Perit Dial.* 2003;19:255–259.
320. Rutsky EA, et al. Acute pancreatitis in patients with end-stage renal disease without transplantation. *Arch Intern Med,* 1986;146(9):1741–1745.
321. Gupta A, et al. CAPD and pancreatitis: no connection. *Perit Dial Int.* 1992;12(3):309–316.
322. Caruana RJ, et al. Pancreatitis: an important cause of abdominal symptoms in patients on peritoneal dialysis. *Am J Kidney Dis.* 1986;7(2):135–140.
323. Quraishi ER, et al. Acute pancreatitis in patients on chronic peritoneal dialysis: an increased risk? *Am J Gastroenterol.*2005;100(10):2288–2293.
324. Singh S, Wadhwa N. Peritonitis, pancreatitis, and infected pseudocyst in a continuous ambulatory peritoneal dialysis patient. *Am J Kidney Dis.* 1987;9(1):84–86.
325. Flynn CT, Chandran PKG, Shadur CA. Recurrent pancreatitis in a patient on CAPD. *Perit Dial Int.* 1986;6(2):106.
326. Pannekeet MM, et al. Acute pancreatitis during CAPD in the Netherlands. *Nephrol Dial Transplant.* 1993;8(12):1376–1381.
327. Cheung CK, Khwaja A. Chylous ascites: an unusual complication of peritoneal dialysis. A case report and literature review. *Perit Dial Int.* 2008;28(3):229–231.
328. Rocklin MA, Quinn MJ, Teitelbaum I. Cloudy dialysate as a presenting feature of superior vena cava syndrome. *Nephrol Dial Transplant.* 2000;15(9):1455–1457.
329. Tsao YT, Chen WL. Calcium channel blocker-induced chylous ascites in peritoneal dialysis. *Kidney Int.* 2009;75(8):868.
330. Lew SQ. Hemoperitoneum: bloody peritoneal dialysate in ESRD patients receiving peritoneal dialysis. *Perit Dial Int.* 2007;27(3):226–233.
331. Tse KC, et al. Recurrent hemoperitoneum complicating continuous ambulatory peritoneal dialysis. *Perit Dial Int.* 2002;22(4):488–491.
332. Blumenkrantz MJ, et al. Retrograde menstruation in women undergoing chronic peritoneal dialysis. *Obstet Gynecol.* 1981;57(5):667–670.
333. Goodkin DA, Benning MG. An outpatient maneuver to treat bloody effluent during continuous ambulatory peritoneal dialysis (CAPD). *Perit Dial Int.* 1990;10(3):227–229.
334. Harnett JD, et al. Recurrent hemoperitoneum in women receiving continuous ambulatory peritoneal dialysis. *Ann Intern Med.* 1987;107(3):341–343.
335. Garcia-Urena MA, et al. Prevalence and management of hernias in peritoneal dialysis patients. *Perit Dial Int.* 2006;26(2):198–202.
336. Van Dijk CM, Ledesma SG, Teitelbaum I. Patient characteristics associated with defects of the peritoneal cavity boundary. *Perit Dial Int.* 2005;25(4):367–373.
337. O'Connor JP, et al. Abdominal hernias complicating continuous ambulatory peritoneal dialysis. *Am J Nephrol.* 1986;6(4):271–274.
338. Del Peso G, et al. Risk factors for abdominal wall complications in peritoneal dialysis patients. *Perit Dial Int.* 2003;23(3):249–254.
339. Digenis GE, et al. Abdominal hernias in patients undergoing continuous ambulatory peritoneal dialysis. *Perit Dial Int.* 1982;2(3):115–117.
340. Kopecky RT, et al. Complications of continuous ambulatory peritoneal dialysis: diagnostic value of peritoneal scintigraphy. *Am J Kidney Dis.* 1987;10(2):123–132.
341. Shah H, Chu M, Bargman JM. Perioperative management of periotoneal dialysis patients undergoing hernia surgery without the use of interim hemodialysis. *Perit Dial Int.* 2006;26(6):684–687.
342. Martinez-Mier G, et al. Abdominal wall hernias in end-stage renal disease patients on peritoneal dialysis. *Perit Dial Int.* 2008;28(4):391–396.
343. Crabtree JH. Hernia repair without delay in initiating or continuing peritoneal dialysis. *Perit Dial Int.* 2006;26(2):178–182.
344. Dejardin AS, Robert A, Goffin E. Intraperitoneal pressure in PD patients: relationship to intraperitoneal volume, body size and PD-related complications. *Nephrol Dial Transplant.* 2007;22(5):1437–1444.
345. Imvrios G, et al. Prosthetic mesh repair of multiple recurrent and large abdominal hernias in continuous ambulatory peritoneal dialysis patients. *Perit Dial Int.* 1994;14(4):338–343.
346. Orfei R, Seybold K, Blumberg A. Genital edema in patients undergoing continuous ambulatory peritoneal dialysis (CAPD). *Perit Dial Int.* 1984;4(4):251–252.
347. Schleifer CR, et al. Management of hernias and Tenckhoff catheter complications in CAPD. *Perit Dial Int.* 1984;4(3):146–150.
348. Caporale N, Perez D, Alegre S. Vaginal leak of peritoneal dialysis liquid. *Perit Dial Int.* 1991;11(3):284–285.
349. Schultz SG, Harmon TM, Nachtnebel KL. Computerized tomographic scanning with intraperitoneal contrast enhancement in a CAPD patient with localized edema. *Perit Dial Int.* 1984;4(4):253–254.
350. Johnson BF, et al. A method for demonstrating subclinical inguinal herniae in patients undergoing peritoneal dialysis: the isotope "peritoneoscrotogram." *Nephrol Dial Transplant.* 1987;2(4):254–257.
351. Lew SQ. Hydrothorax: pleural effusion associated with peritoneal dialysis. *Perit Dial Int.* 2010;30(1):13–18.
352. Fletcher S, Turney JH, Brownjohn AM. Increased incidence of hydrothorax complicating peritoneal dialysis in patients with adult polycystic kidney disease. *Nephrol Dial Transplant.* 1994;9(7):832–833.
353. Nomoto Y, et al. Acute hydrothorax in continuous ambulatory peritoneal dialysis—a collaborative study of 161 centers. *Am J Nephrol.* 1989;9(5):363–367.
353a. Mutter D, et al. A recently described laparoscopic technique for the repair of hydrothorax appears promising. *Perit Dial Int.* 2011;31:692–694.
354. Kronenberg F, et al. Prevalence of dyslipidemic risk factors in hemodialysis and CAPD patients. *Kidney Int Suppl.* 2003(84):S113–116.
355. Grodstein GP, et al. Glucose absorption during continuous ambulatory peritoneal dialysis. *Kidney Int.* 1981;19(4):564–567.
356. Paniagua R, et al. Icodextrin improves metabolic and fluid management in high and high-average transport diabetic patients. *Perit Dial Int.* 2009;29(4):422–432.
357. Lin A, et al. Randomized controlled trial of icodextrin versus glucose containing peritoneal dialysis fluid. *Clin J Am Soc Nephrol.* 2009;4(11):1799–1804.
358. Steele J, et al. Lipids, lipoproteins and apolipoproteins A-I and B and apolipoprotein losses in continuous ambulatory peritoneal dialysis. *Atherosclerosis.* 1989;79(1):47–50.
359. Kagan A, et al. Kinetics of peritoneal protein loss during CAPD: I. Different characteristics for low and high molecular weight proteins. *Kidney Int.* 1990;37(3):971–979.
360. Chan MK. Gemfibrozil improves abnormalities of lipid metabolism in patients on continuous ambulatory peritoneal dialysis: the role of postheparin lipases in the metabolism of high-density lipoprotein subfractions. *Metabolism.* 1989;38(10):939–945.
361. Navaneethan SD, et al. HMG CoA reductase inhibitors (statins) for dialysis patients. *Cochrane Database Syst Rev.* 2009;(3):CD004289.
362. Sharp Collaborative Group Study of Heart and Renal Protection (SHARP): randomized trial to assess the effects of lowering low-density lipoprotein cholesterol among 9,438 patients with chronic kidney disease. *Am Heart J.* 2010;160(5):785–794.e10.
363. Tzamaloukas AH, et al. Peritonitis associated with intra-abdominal pathology in continuous ambulatory peritoneal dialysis patients. *Perit Dial Int.* 1993;13(Suppl 2):S335–337.
364. Wakeen MJ, Zimmerman SW, Bidwell D. Viscus perforation in peritoneal dialysis patients: diagnosis and outcome. *Perit Dial Int.* 1994;14(4):371–377.
365. Wellington JL, Rody K. Acute abdominal emergencies in patients on long-term ambulatory peritoneal dialysis. *Can J Surg.* 1993;36(6):522–524.
366. Spence PA, et al. Indications for operation when peritonitis occurs in patients on chronic ambulatory peritoneal dialysis. *Surg Gynecol Obstet.* 1985;161(5):450–452.
367. Fleisher AG, et al. Surgical complications of peritoneal dialysis catheters. *Am J Surg.* 1985;149(6):726–729.
368. Summers AM, et al. Single-center experience of encapsulating peritoneal sclerosis in patients on peritoneal dialysis for end-stage renal failure. *Kidney Int.* 2005;68(5):2381–2388.

369. Fieren MW, et al. Posttransplant encapsulating peritoneal sclerosis: a worrying new trend? *Perit Dial Int.* 2007;27(6):619–624.
370. Chin AI, Yeun JY. Encapsulating peritoneal sclerosis: an unpredictable and devastating complication of peritoneal dialysis. *Am J Kidney Dis.* 2006;47(4):697–712.
371. Campbell S, et al. Sclerosing peritonitis: identification of diagnostic, clinical, and radiological features. *Am J Kidney Dis.* 1994;24(5):819–825.
372. Brown MC, et al. Encapsulating peritoneal sclerosis in the new millennium: a national cohort study. *Clin J Am Soc Nephrol.* 2009;4(7):1222–1229.
373. Kawaguchi Y, et al. Encapsulating peritoneal sclerosis: definition, etiology, diagnosis, and treatment. International Society for Peritoneal Dialysis Ad Hoc Committee on Ultrafiltration Management in Peritoneal Dialysis. *Perit Dial Int.* 2000;20 Suppl 4:S43–55.
374. Johnson DW, et al. Encapsulating peritoneal sclerosis: incidence, predictors, and outcomes. *Kidney Int.* 2010;77(10):904–912.
375. Flynn CT, Nanson JA. Intraperitoneal insulin with CAPD - an artificial pancreas. *Trans Am Soc Artif Intern Organs.* 1979;25:114–117.
376. Torun D, et al. Hepatic subcapsular steatosis as a complication associated with intraperitoneal insulin treatment in diabetic peritoneal dialysis patients. *Perit Dial Int.* 2005;25(6):596–600.
377. De Vecchi AF. Adequacy of fluid/sodium balance and blood pressure control. *Perit Dial Int.* 1994;14 Suppl 3:S110–116.
378. Saldanha LF, Weiler EW, Gonick HC. Effect of continuous ambulatory peritoneal dialysis on blood pressure control. *Am J Kidney Dis.* 1993;21(2):184–188.
379. Wang MC, et al. Blood pressure and left ventricular hypertrophy in patients on different peritoneal dialysis regimens. *Perit Dial Int.* 2001;21(1):36–42.
380. Ortega O, et al. Peritoneal sodium mass removal in continuous ambulatory peritoneal dialysis and automated peritoneal dialysis: influence on blood pressure control. *Am J Nephrol.* 2001;21(3):189–193.
381. Rodriguez-Carmona A, et al. Compared time profiles of ultrafiltration, sodium removal, and renal function in incident CAPD and automated peritoneal dialysis patients. *Am J Kidney Dis.* 2004;44(1):132–145.
382. Boudville NC, et al. Blood pressure, volume, and sodium control in an automated peritoneal dialysis population. *Perit Dial Int.* 2007;27(5):537–543.
383. Davison SN, et al. Comparison of volume overload with cycler-assisted versus continuous ambulatory peritoneal dialysis. *Clin J Am Soc Nephrol.* 2009;4(6):1044–1050.
384. Giacchino F, et al. Improved cell-mediated immunity in CAPD patients as compared to those on hemodialysis. *Perit Dial Int.* 1984;4(4):209–211.
385. Vanholder R, et al. Reduced incidence of acute renal graft failure in patients treated with peritoneal dialysis compared with hemodialysis. *Am J Kidney Dis.* 1999;33(5):934–940.
386. Bleyer AJ, et al. Dialysis modality and delayed graft function after cadaveric renal transplantation. *J Am Soc Nephrol.* 1999;10(1):154–159.
387. Vats AN et al. Pretransplant dialysis status and outcome of renal transplantation in North American children: a NAPRTCS Study. North American Pediatric Renal Transplant Cooperative Study. *Transplantation.* 2000;69(7): 1414–1419.
388. Chalem Y, et al. Access to, and outcome of, renal transplantation according to treatment modality of end-stage renal disease in France. *Kidney Int.* 2005;67(6):2448–2453.
389. Goldfarb-Rumyantzev AS, et al. The role of pretransplantation renal replacement therapy modality in kidney allograft and recipient survival. *Am J Kidney Dis.* 2005;46(3):537–549.
390. Besarab A, Golper TA. Response of continuous peritoneal dialysis patients to subcutaneous recombinant human erythropoietin differs from that of hemodialysis patients. *ASAIO Trans.* 1991;37(3):M395–396.
391. Maiorca R, et al. Kidney transplantation in peritoneal dialysis patients. *Perit Dial Int.* 1994;14 Suppl 3:S162–168.
392. Winchester JF, et al. Transplantation in peritoneal dialysis and hemodialysis. *Kidney Int Suppl.* 1993;40:S101–105.
393. Dutton S. Transient post-transplant ascites in CAPD patients. *Perit Dial Int.* 1983;3(3):164.

CHAPTER

84 Hemodialysis

Scott D. Bieber • Jonathan Himmelfarb

DEFINITION OF DIALYSIS

Dialysis is defined as the bidirectional movement of molecules across a semipermeable membrane. During dialysis, solute (molecules dissolved in a liquid) can be removed and subsequently discarded from the body. If this process takes place across an artificial membrane which is in contact with the blood during extracorporeal circulation it is called hemodialysis. Hemodialysis can be performed in treatment centers which specialize in the delivery of dialysis or, alternatively, it can be performed at home.

The ultimate goal of dialysis is to replace the function of the kidney to alleviate signs and symptoms of uremia and rehabilitate patients with end-stage renal disease (ESRD) so that they may lead productive lives. Thus far, methods of renal replacement outside of kidney transplantation have focused on mechanical methods to purify the blood of toxins, balance fluid and electrolyte levels, and correct acid–base disturbances. The downside to the currently available forms of mechanical renal replacement is they do not address the many other important endocrine and immunologic functions of the kidney. Therefore, despite our many technological advances in the field, dialysis by mechanical means does not completely replace kidney function but rather serves as a substitute.

HISTORY

In 1913 Abel, Rowntree, and Turner at Johns Hopkins University performed the first dialysis on dogs using cellulose trinitrate membranes and hirudin for anticoagulation.[1] The first human hemodialysis was performed by Hass in 1924 in Germany.[2] Hass used the radial carotid artery and portal vein for blood access. In 1943 Kolff developed the rotating drum dialyzer in Holland. Kolff used cellophane membranes (sausage casings) and an immersion bath and reported on the first patient to recover from acute renal failure after treatment. Further work by Kolff would lead to the twin coil dialyzer in 1955.[3] In 1946, Alwall developed a system for applying hydrostatic pressure to achieve ultrafiltration allowing for fluid removal from the circulation during dialysis. In 1960 Kiil developed a flat plate dialyzer that could easily be dismantled and reassembled. The Kiil dialyzer consisted of boards of polypropylene and used more permeable cellulosic cuprophane membranes. Due to low internal resistance, a blood pump was not necessary. Meanwhile, Scribner and Quinton came up with a method to heat Teflon to bend it into a U shape. This allowed a connection between the radial artery and cephalic vein in the forearm that could be used for dialysis access.[4] Prior to this development, dialysis therapy was largely reserved for the treatment of acute renal failure in a few specialized inpatient centers. The Scribner-Quinton shunt was a crucial step that made long-term dialysis for chronic renal failure a reality. Dialysis technology was further refined in 1963 when Babb developed a central proportioning system for the delivery of dialysate to multiple patients. Access to the bloodstream was improved in 1966 when Cimino and Brescia developed the native arteriovenous fistula. More recent times have seen the development of improved technology such as ultrafiltration control, dialysate proportioning systems allowing the use of bicarbonate based dialysate, improved safety mechanisms, more biocompatible dialysis membranes, high flux dialyzers, simplified home dialysis technologies, and even development of wearable artificial kidneys. Advances by researchers and industry coupled with financial support through government subsidized care have led to the expansion of dialysis as we know it today and have solidified chronic hemodialysis as a feasible life-sustaining treatment for thousands of patients who would otherwise be facing terminal ESRD.

EPIDEMIOLOGY

According to the United States Renal Data System (USRDS) atlas of ESRD report,[5] in the year 2008 there were 109,832 new ESRD patients. The rate of ESRD incidence reached 322 per million population for hemodialysis, 20.7 for peritoneal dialysis, and 7.9 for transplant. In the United States, hemodialysis remains the most common form of chronic renal replacement therapy. Hemodialysis as the modality of renal replacement therapy accounted for the bulk of the incident dialysis patients with peritoneal dialysis initiated in only 6,577 patients and renal transplant in only 2,644. Trends over the past few decades have seen increases in percentages of incident hemodialysis patients and decreases or plateauing of the incident patients on peritoneal dialysis. In-center hemodialysis therapies were more frequently utilized with more than 347,000 patients receiving hemodialysis and only 3,826 performing home hemodialysis.

Hemodialysis Outcomes: Morbidity and Mortality

Patients with ESRD are frequently hospitalized for medical complications. Numbers from the USRDS reveal 12.8 hospital days per patient year on hemodialysis (HD), compared with 13.3 hospital days per patient year on peritoneal dialysis (PD) and 5.9 for transplant patients. Over the last few years, hospital admission rates have remained the same for HD (approximately two admissions per year) and declined 9.6% in PD patients. Women appear 16% more likely to be hospitalized than their male counterparts. Common causes for admission to the hospital are cardiovascular complications, infectious complications, and access complications. Admission rates for infection (pneumonia, bacteremia) have risen 19% whereas admission rates for cardiovascular disease have remained similar and admissions for vascular access issues have fallen as more procedures are now performed in the outpatient setting.[5]

ESRD patients have high mortality rates. Adjusted rates for all-cause mortality in dialysis patients are approximately six to eight times higher than in the general population. Five-year probability of survival (1999–2003) among incident ESRD patients was 0.39. This improved 8.4% when compared with 1994–1998. The greatest amount of improvement was seen in the PD population with a 17.6% increase compared with an 8.4% increase in HD patients. There is a large racial disparity in risk for death when comparing Caucasians (21%), African Americans (17%), and other racial groups (14%), with minorities having a clear survival advantage.[5]

MECHANISMS OF SOLUTE REMOVAL

Removal of solute (molecules dissolved in liquid, such as urea) from solvent (the liquid which contains the molecules, such as the bloodstream) is the major function of dialysis. Removal of solute from the body can be accomplished by diffusion, convection, or osmosis.

Diffusion

Diffusion is the movement of particles from areas of higher concentration to areas of lower concentration through random motion. In the example of hemodialytic therapy, diffusion is the driving force that is responsible for the movement of solute dissolved in blood (such as urea) across the membrane of the dialyzer to the area of lower concentration, the dialysate (Fig. 84.1).

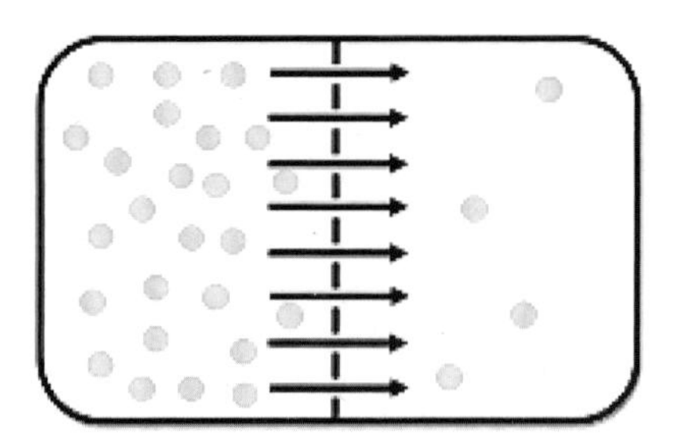

FIGURE 84.1 Diffusion. If two compartments are separated by a semipermeable membrane (*dashed line*) solute tends to move down a concentration gradient from areas of high concentration to areas of lower concentration. For example, in the case of hemodialysis, solute (e.g., urea) dissolved in solvent (blood) passes the semipermeable membrane (dialyzer) to an area of lower solute concentration (dialysate).

Convection

Convection is the movement of molecules within fluids, also known as "solute drag." Convection occurs in hemofiltration when a transmembrane pressure is applied to the blood side of a membrane forcing plasma water through the pores in the membrane. Any solute dissolved in the plasma water smaller than the membrane pore size is subsequently transported (Fig. 84.2). The ability for a particular solute to be removed through convection is dependent on the solute size and the membrane pore size, compared to the diffusive process where removal is also dependent on concentration gradients. The sieving coefficient describes the membrane passage of a particular solute during convection and can be determined by dividing the concentration of the solute in the effluent by the concentration in the blood. For example, urea (small molecule) generally will have a sieving coefficient of 1 which indicates that the

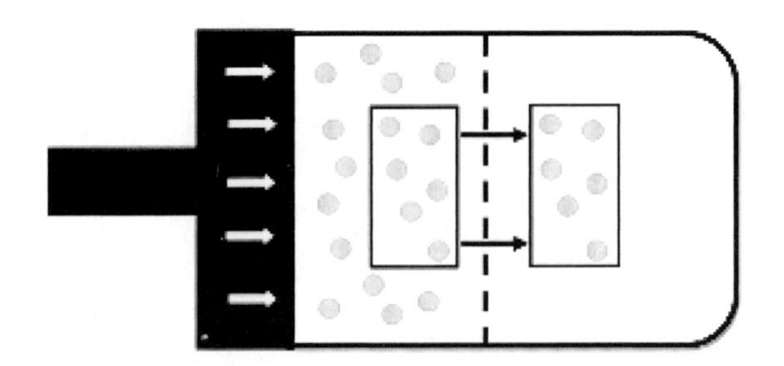

FIGURE 84.2 Convection is the movement of molecules within fluid. In the case of hemofiltration, solute (e.g., urea) is dissolved in plasma water. If a hydrostatic pressure is applied to one side of the semipermeable membrane, water will be forced through the pores of the membrane bringing along the solute which is dissolved in it if the solute particles are smaller than the membrane pore size. This is also known as solute drag.

concentration in the blood is equal to the concentration in the effluent whereas albumin, a molecule which is too large to pass traditionally used membranes, will have a sieving coefficient of 0.

Osmosis

Osmosis is the movement of water molecules across a semipermeable membrane down a water gradient. In other words, osmosis is the movement of water across a semipermeable membrane from an area of low solute concentration to an area of high solute concentration. A clinical example of osmosis is PD where a high dextrose containing fluid is instilled into the peritoneal cavity which creates a osmotic gradient moving water into the peritoneal space.

Ultrafiltration

Ultrafiltration is the movement of fluid across a semipermeable membrane which is caused by a pressure difference. This pressure difference can be a result of osmotic pressure (as is the case with PD) or hydrostatic pressure (as is the case with HD). Ultrafiltration is a form of convective clearance in traditional HD but does not typically account for a significant volume of clearance.

Concept of Clearance in Dialysis

The clearance of a solute is defined as the volume from which the solute is completely removed in a specified period of time and is often expressed in units of milliliters per minute. In HD, the processes of diffusion, convection, and, to a lesser extent, membrane adsorption each contribute to the total clearance of solute. Numerous factors affect the clearance of solute in dialysis including the concentration differences between the blood and dialysate, the rate at which blood is delivered to the dialyzer, and the intrinsic properties of the dialyzer such as surface area, permeability, membrane thickness, pore size, and solute size.

Concentration is the ratio of the amount of solute in a given solvent volume. The clearance of a solute is dependent on the concentration of the solute. It is also important to recognize the relationship between concentration and generation of a solute. Both generation and removal of a solute from the body will affect the concentration and therefore has an effect on clearance. The concept of mass balance and the relationship between concentration, generation, and clearance forms the basis for many of the equations that have been derived to assess the adequacy of dialysis (discussed in more detail below).

DIALYSIS TECHNIQUE

The HD equipment typically consists of a tubing set, dialyzer, and the hemodialysis machine. The tubing set connects the patient's source of blood access to the dialyzer which contains the semipermeable membrane. The entire circuit is connected to the dialysis machine. After negative pressure is applied to the access by a mechanically driven blood pump on the dialysis machine, blood circulates through the arterial limb of the blood tubing and past the dialysis membrane. It is then sent through the venous limb of the tubing and back to the patient via the vascular access (Fig. 84.3).

Blood Access

Ideally HD is performed through a connection between the arterial circulation and the venous system in the form of an arteriovenous fistula (AVF) or an arteriovenous graft (AVG). The AVF is the preferred form of access. The use of the arteriovenous circulation allows intradialytic blood flows that can easily support achieving adequate solute clearance during the dialysis procedure. In the case of the AVF and AVG, needles are placed into the access during each dialysis session. Hemodialysis needles range in size but usually are 17 to 15 gauge with larger needles (15 g) being used in stable accesses with lower risk of bleeding and smaller needles (17 g) used in situations of small diameter access, developing accesses (especially for first cannulation), or higher bleeding risk. Typically two needles are placed in the access, one needle for the inflow to the dialysis machine, and the other needle for the outflow from the dialysis machine. Single needles with a dual lumen are also available but are rarely used due to a higher degree of access recirculation.

The buttonholing technique of dialysis access is sometimes used in patients with an AVF. Through this technique, the AVF is accessed in the same location at the same angle during each dialysis session, preferably by the patients themselves or by the same dialysis caregiver. Over time, the patient develops a scarred tract that eventually allows for the placement of blunt needles down the tract after removal of the scab that serves as a plug. Once established, buttonholes have the advantage of ease of obtaining access, less pain, reduced aneurysm formation, and reduced incidence of hematoma formation.[6] The downside of buttonholes is higher rates of infection, particularly, *Staphylococcus aureus* bacteremia. This increased risk may be mitigated by diligent topical care and the use of agents such as mupirocin.[7]

Catheters placed in the central veins can also be used for dialysis access. Typically these catheters are placed within the internal jugular or femoral vein. The subclavian vein position is associated with greater rates of central stenosis and should be avoided if possible.[8,9] Catheters are less desirable than AVF or AVG due to increased rates of infection,[10] clotting,[11] recirculation,[12] poor blood flows,[13] and higher potential to cause stenosis of the central veins.[14] Catheters that are tunneled and cuffed have lower rates of infectious complications than noncuffed, nontunneled catheters, and, when possible, are preferable in patients

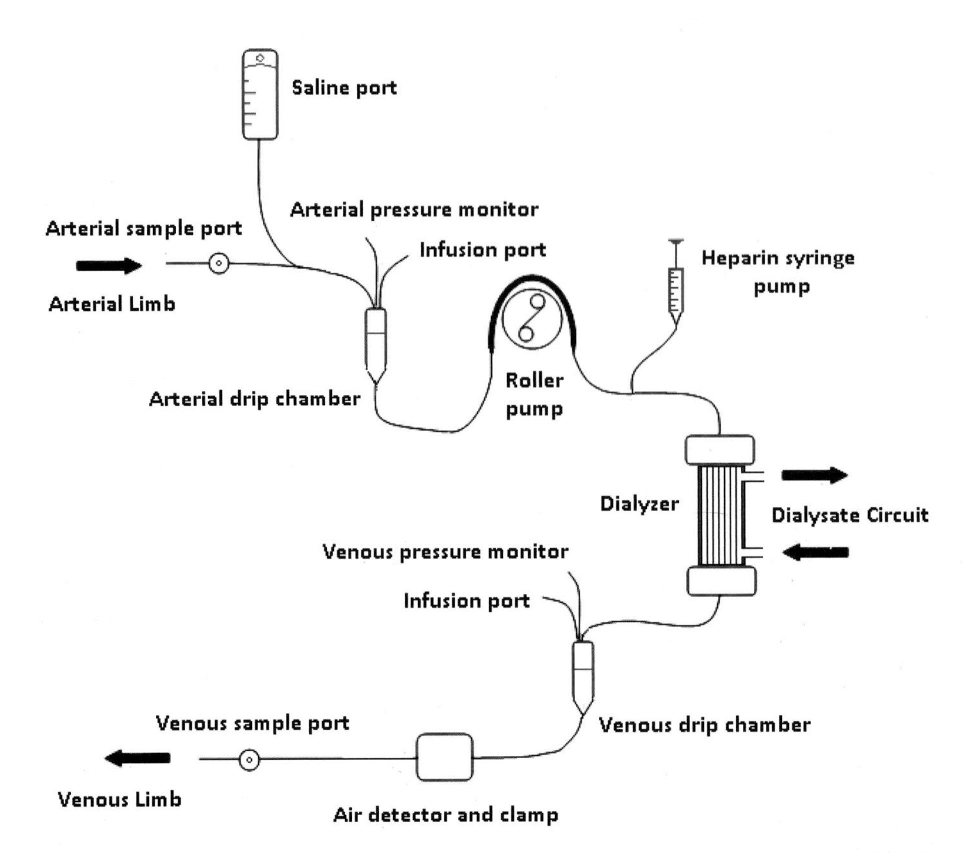

FIGURE 84.3 Drawing of a hemodialysis circuit. Blood flows from the patient access into the arterial limb of the circuit, passes the dialyzer, then is delivered to the venous limb and back to the patient. Note that the location of the arterial drip chamber, which is drawn prepump in this picture, is occasionally postpump in some designs. The location of the infusion ports and sample ports can vary as well.

who have an anticipated need for dialysis that is longer than 2 weeks.[15]

Blood Circuit

The blood circuit is composed of tubing which carries blood from the patient access through the dialyzer and back to the patient. There are two main portions of the dialysis circuit: the arterial and venous limbs. The arterial limb carries blood under negative pressure provided by the blood pump from the access to the dialyzer. It usually includes a drip chamber which serves to remove air from the dialysis circuit. The arterial pressure monitor is frequently located at the top of the arterial drip chamber and blood flows out of the bottom of the drip chamber toward the blood pump. The blood pump is commonly designed in a circular roller fashion that squeezes segments of blood through a portion of arterial tubing as the rollers apply pressure to the line. This configuration leads to an irregular vacillating flow of blood through the circuit. The portion of the arterial limb tubing that comes in contact with the rollers from the pump is reinforced to withstand the extra stress applied by the rollers. The blood pump typically operates at speeds ranging from 150–500 mL per min. There is usually a branching line that connects to an automated heparin syringe pump, typically located after the blood pump.

After the blood passes through the arterial circuit it is delivered to the dialyzer. Post dialyzer the blood enters the venous circuit. Similar to the arterial limb, the venous limb also has a drip chamber and pressure monitor. Furthermore, the venous limb has an air detector and a portion of line which passes through an automated clamp. If air is detected in the venous line, the clamp will be triggered, preventing delivery of air to the patient. This portion of equipment is crucial as an air embolus is a potentially lethal complication. The arterial and venous pressure monitors play an important function in monitoring the progress of dialysis. Arterial pressures are typically negative with pressures ranging from −80 to −200 mm Hg. Venous pressures are usually positive, ranging from 50 to 250 mm Hg. Pressures that fall outside of the acceptable ranges should trigger machine alarms that will stop the blood pump. Tables 84.1 and 84.2 list potential reasons for arterial and venous pressure alarms, respectively.

The ideal tubing set has a smooth inner surface to reduce blood turbulence, is biologically compatible to prevent allergic reactions, and does not narrow or kink. Care should be taken to ensure that the tubing is rinsed completely prior to initiation of dialysis especially in the case of tubing that is sterilized with ethylene oxide. Failure to do so can result in an allergic reaction. For example, if there is a faulty or

TABLE 84.1 Arterial Pressure Alarms

Arterial Pressure (normal −80 to −200)	Potential Problem
0 to −80	Pump speed too low Arterial needle dislodged Saline line open
−200 or more negative	Kink in line or catheter ports Catheter or needle placement suboptimal Clotting of access Vasospasm Infiltration Low patient blood pressure

TABLE 84.2 Venous Pressure Alarms

Venous Pressure (normal 50–250 mm Hg)	Potential Problem
<50	Pump speed too slow Postpump clotting (clotted dialyzer) Dialyzer membrane rupture Kink in line (postpump, prepressure monitor) Venous needle or catheter dislodged
>250	Access stenosis Kink in line or catheter (postpressure monitor) Catheter or needle placement suboptimal Venous drip chamber clotting Clotting of access Access hematoma formation Access vasospasm Bad arm positioning Pump speed too fast

misplaced clamp on a side branch of the circuit, such as the heparin branch, ethylene oxide can backfill into the tubing during rinsing and later is delivered to the patient.

Shear stress applied to blood in dialysis tubing has been associated with hemolysis and should be avoided. Narrowing or kinking of the blood tubing can cause hemolysis.[16] In the past faulty tubing sets were linked to outbreaks of hemolysis in patients on dialysis.[17] High blood flows using small gauge needles,[18] excessively negative arterial pressures, and misalignment of the blood tubing with the blood pump can theoretically cause hemolysis as well.

Dialyzer

The dialyzer is a crucial portion of the hemodialysis apparatus that provides a site for solute transport. Dialyzers are composed of blood and dialysate compartments. These two compartments are separated by a semipermeable membrane and form a closed self-contained system. Although dialysis membranes initially used the parallel plate design, the hollow fiber design is now used almost exclusively (Fig. 84.4). Hollow fiber dialyzers consist of a cylindrical plastic shell. At the opposing ends of the cylinder are headers which provide ports for the blood flow. Blood flows through the header to the potting compound which encases thousands of tiny hollow fibers through which the blood flows. On the side of the cylinder are two ports for the dialysate connections. Blood and dialysate flows are typically run in opposite directions (countercurrent) to improve clearance, but can be run in the same direction if less solute clearance is desired. The hollow fibers are the site of diffusion and convection as each of the hollow fibers contain pores which allow the passage of molecules.

Dialysis membrane biomaterials can be divided into four different types: cellulose, substituted cellulose, mixed cellulose synthetic, and pure synthetic. Cellulose membranes are formed from plant (usually cotton) polysaccharide. They are considered to be less biocompatible and are therefore now used less frequently. Substituted cellulose membranes are formed by removing free hydroxyl groups from cellulose membranes. The removal of these hydroxyl groups attenuates complement activation and therefore is more biocompatible. Cellulosynthetic membranes are cellulose membranes with a synthetic material (tertiary amine structure) added to the surface. Pure synthetic membranes do not contain cellulose materials and are the most commonly used membranes today.

Dialyzer solute clearance characteristics are primarily dependent on surface area and porosity. Dialyzer properties are provided by the manufacturer via dialyzer specification sheets. It is worthy to note that reported clearance data for the dialyzer is based on in vitro testing which tends to overestimate in vivo clearances. It is also important to note that clearance is affected by blood flow, therefore analysis of clearance at varying blood flows is of relevance. In general, the clearance values provided by the manufacturer can give the practitioner an idea of the performance of a particular dialyzer. For example, urea can be used as a marker of small molecule removal, whereas clearance values for B12 provide information about the middle molecule removal. Flux refers to the ability to remove or ultrafilter plasma water. High-flux dialyzers have larger pores capable of removing greater volumes of plasma water. This is denoted by the ultrafiltration coefficient, or K_{uf}, of a dialyzer. Low-flux dialyzers have a K_{uf} of <10 mL/h/mm Hg and high flux dialyzers >20 mL/h/mm Hg. High-flux membranes, by nature of their larger pore sizes, also have higher clearance

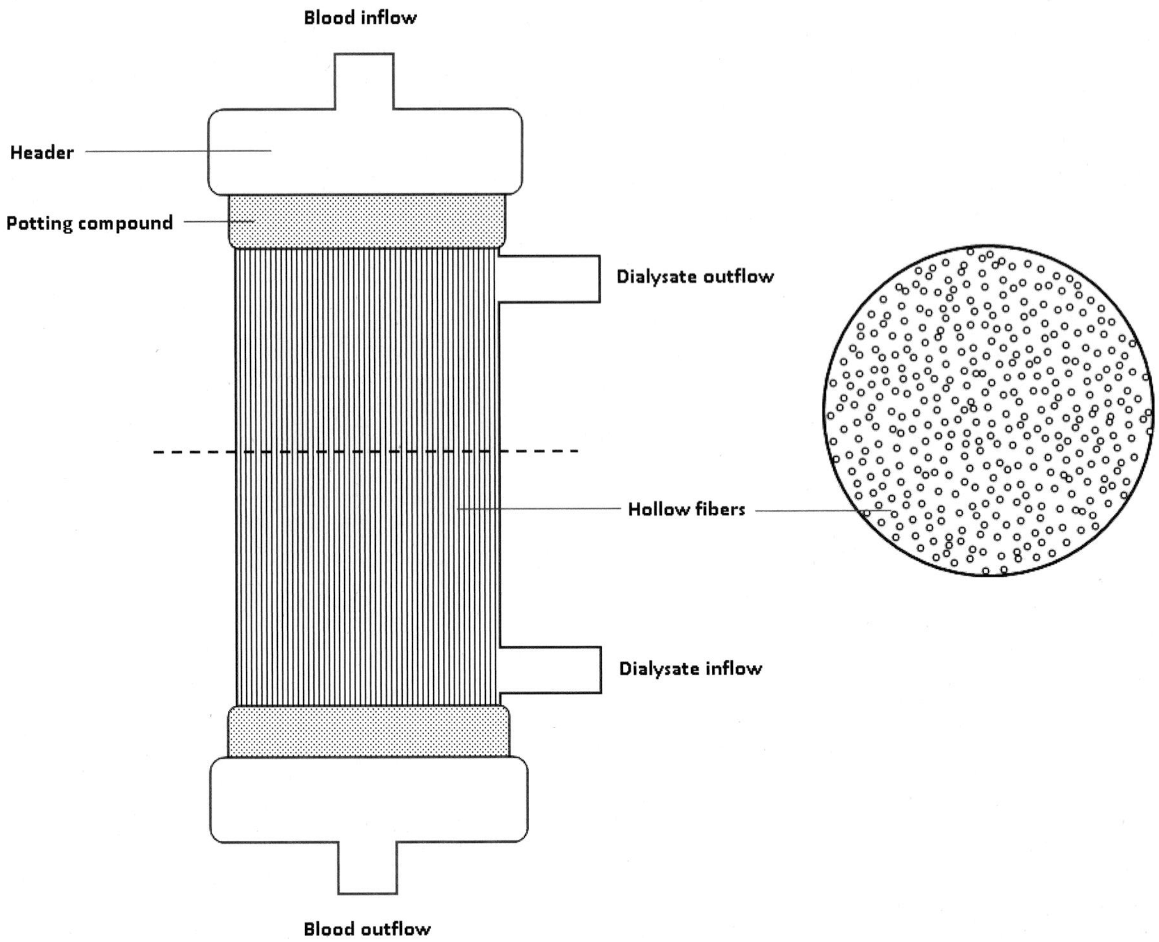

FIGURE 84.4 Hollow fiber dialyzer. In modern times nearly all dialysis setups utilize hollow fiber dialyzers as the membrane site of dialysis. The dialyzer is usually designed as a cylindrical tube which encases hollow fibers. The fibers serve as semipermeable membranes. Blood flows through the cavity of the hollow fiber and dialysate bathes the outside of the fibers. The fibers are held in place by the impermeable potting compound and the dialyzer is capped off by two headers which also serve as the site for the blood hookups. The dashed line above indicates the site of cross-section that is illustrated on the right. Note that blood and dialysate usually run in a countercurrent (opposite) direction to optimize exposure of the blood to fresh dialysate and improve clearance; however, dialysate can also be run in the same direction as the blood if less efficient therapy is required.

of middle molecules with sizes similar to molecules such as vitamin B12 (MW ~1400 Da) and β2-microglobulin (MW ~12000 Da). The efficiency of a dialyzer refers to its ability to remove small molecular solutes such as urea; this is usually denoted by the KoA of urea. The KoA is related to the clearance of a dialyzer (Ko) and the surface area of the dialyzer (A). It should be recognized that the manufacturer-provided clearance values for different dialyzers at different blood flows can be useful to help compare performance, but cannot reliably be used to calculate the dose of dialysis.

The priming volume of the dialyzer and the sterilization method of the dialyzer will also be listed in the dialyzer specifications. The average priming volume ranges from 50 to 150 mL. Sterilization methods of dialyzers include ethylene oxide, gamma beam radiation, and heat/steam sterilization. Sterilization with ethylene oxide has fallen out of favor due to increased rates of allergic reactions. Certain dialyzers can be reprocessed and reused. Reused dialyzers are cleaned with bleach, hydrogen peroxide, or peracetic acid and sterilized with formaldehyde, glutaraldehyde, or heat. Before reuse, the dialyzers have to be tested for residual chemical agents and ability to withstand pressure. Fiber bundle volume is also calculated to ensure the dialyzer has an adequate number of patent hollow fibers to achieve adequate solute clearance. This process can be tedious and labor intensive and can sometimes outweigh the cost of the dialyzer—as a consequence, many dialysis units choose single-use dialyzers.

Dialysate Circuit

The main components of a typical dialysis circuit include the dialysate concentrate, the water input, a proportioning system, and a volumetric control system. The dialysate circuit is usually fitted with monitors including the conductivity monitor, temperature monitor, and a blood leak detector (Fig. 84.5).

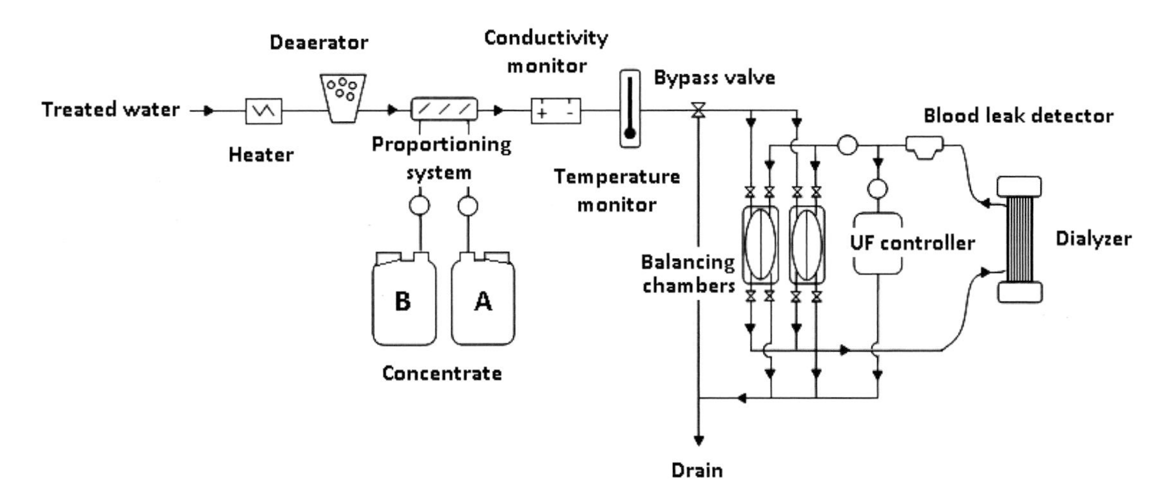

FIGURE 84.5 Drawing of the typical components in a dialysate circuit. Treated water is heated to an appropriate temperature (~35.5°–38°C) and any air bubbles in the water are removed by the deaerator. The water is then mixed with concentrate. In dynamic proportioning systems bicarbonate is usually added followed by the acid concentrate through the proportioning system. The mixed product is then tested by the conductivity monitor and tested to ensure that temperature is appropriate. pH sensors are also sometimes used. If the product is not within acceptable conductivity or temperature range the bypass valve is opened and the dialysate is delivered to the drain preventing delivery to the patient. If the product passes the tests, then it is delivered to the balancing chambers. The balancing chambers are an intricate set of chambers separated by impermeable membranes and inflow and outflow valves. The purpose of the balancing chambers is to balance dialyzer inflow with dialyzer outflow to ensure that the amount of dialysate entering the dialyzer and the amount leaving the dialyzer are equal. The ultrafiltration (UF) controller uses pressure measurements and a separate pump to remove any additional desired volume from the dialyzer effluent. The blood leak detector located on the effluent outflow tract serves to ensure dialyzer membrane integrity.

The job of the proportioning system is to take pretreated pure water and mix it with the bicarbonate and acid concentrates to make final dialysate for delivery to the dialyzer. The common range of components for bicarbonate dialysate are listed in Table 84.3. The level of sodium or bicarbonate in the dialysate can be adjusted by the proportioning system from input provided to the dialysate machine, whereas the concentration of the other electrolytes such as potassium and calcium are relatively fixed and require a change in the concentration in the concentrate. Dialysis machines rely on conductivity to test the dialysate and appropriately proportion the bicarbonate concentrate, acid concentrate, and water prior to delivery to the patient. The flow of electricity through solution is proportional to the amount of ions dissolved in the solution. Pure water is a poor conductor of electricity and salty water conducts electricity more readily. The conductivity monitor ensures that the conductivity of the dialysate, and therefore the overall electrolyte concentrations, are within the appropriate range. If out of range, the dialysate is delivered to the drain via a bypass valve. Machine alarms due to altered conductivity usually represent either inaccurate input of the concentrations of electrolytes in the concentrate, an inappropriately calibrated machine, or problems with the water purification system. These alarms can indicate malfunction of proportioning or contaminated water which can be potentially fatal to the patient if the bypass system is not evoked.

TABLE 84.3 **Typical Dialysate Composition Ranges**

Sodium (mEq/L)	130–145
Potassium (mEq/L)	0–4
Chloride (mEq/L)	98–112
Bicarbonate (mEq/L)	30–40
Magnesium (mEq/L)	0.5–1.5
Calcium (mEq/L)	2.5–3.5
Glucose (mg/dL)	100–200

In most dialysis machines, treated water flows through the dialysate circuit at a constant rate and bicarbonate concentrate is metered into the water at a ratio around 1:20 to 1:30. After mixing of the bicarbonate with the water there is a conductivity check, then the acid concentrate is metered and added to the water in a ratio around 1:33 to 1:45. The product dialysate then undergoes further conductivity testing. It is important to understand that current dialysis technology is not sophisticated enough to measure the exact concentration of electrolytes in the dialysate but rather it relies on conductivity to ensure the correct preparation of dialysate. For example, if a lower bicarbonate concentration is desired in the dialysate then the bicarbonate pump will deliver less of the bicarbonate concentrate to the water stream, therefore, there will be less sodium delivered as well. In order for the machine to prepare dialysate with appropriate conductivity it will need to deliver additional sodium from the acid concentrate, subsequently, other cations in the acid concentrate will also be delivered in a larger proportion as well (e.g., potassium and calcium).

The volumetric control system regulates the amount of plasma water removed (ultrafiltration) during dialysis. It consists of an intricate set of valves coupled with balancing chamber(s), an ultrafiltration pump, pressure monitors, and a computerized ultrafiltration controller. If no ultrafiltration is desired, these components act together to ensure that the amount of fluid entering the dialyzer matches the amount of fluid that leaves the dialyzer. If fluid removal is desired, the amount of fluid in the dialyzer outflow will exceed the dialysate input.

Other safety systems included in the dialysate circuit include the temperature monitor, the blood leak detector, and sometimes a pH detector. Standard dialysate temperature is around 37°C. Lower temperature is associated with shivering and discomfort but may reduce intradialytic hypotension. Higher temperatures (>42°C) can lead to protein denaturation and hemolysis.[19,20] The blood leak detector serves as a method to detect the presence of blood in the dialysate. Given that dialysate water is not sterile, blood should not come in direct contact with the dialysate. If there is a rupture in the dialysis membrane blood will be found in the dialysate effluent. Additionally, high levels of myoglobin or hemoglobin in the dialysate effluent can set off the blood leak detector if a significant amount of pigment is able to pass through the membrane.

Methods of Dialysis

Traditional Intermittent Hemodialysis

In traditional intermittent hemodialysis (IHD) blood flows through a dialyzer at rates from 300 to 500 mL per min against countercurrent flow of dialysate at 500 to 800 mL per min. Typically this is done in 4-hour treatments three to four times weekly. Solute removal in IHD is predominantly from diffusive clearance. Ultrafiltration is usually performed concurrently for volume removal. The resulting convective removal of solute by ultrafiltration is only a small fraction of the overall clearance.

Slow Low Efficiency Dialysis

Slow low efficiency dialysis (SLED) or sustained low efficiency dialysis is an option for patients who are hemodynamically unstable and would not otherwise tolerate traditional intermittent hemodialysis. With SLED, the speed and efficiency of dialysis is decreased and this decreases the rate of osmolar shifts while still providing for solute removal and volume removal if necessary. Blood pump speeds are typically 100 to 200 mL per min and dialysate flows 100 to 300 mL per min. SLED is typically done for longer periods of time or continuously with lower rates of ultrafiltration (0–400 mL per hr), and is primarily used in inpatient hospital settings for the treatment of acute kidney injury (AKI).

Hemofiltration

In hemofiltration (Fig. 84.6) large quantities of plasma water are removed with ultrafiltration by hydrostatic pressure (typically 1–5 L per hr). There is no dialysate, thus, diffusive clearance is nonexistent and resulting solute clearance is primarily convective. Blood pump speeds can vary from slow (100 mL per min) to speeds similar to IHD. The large amount of ultrafiltration performed necessitates use of a replacement fluid; otherwise, plasma volume would be rapidly depleted using this technique. Replacement fluid is added back to the blood circuit either pre- or postfilter (or both). The replacement fluid needs to be sterile or "ultrapure" as it will be delivered directly to the patient. Hemofiltration can be intermittent or slow and continuous. Slow continuous hemofiltration is also known as continuous arteriovenous hemofiltration (CAVH) or continuous venovenous hemofiltration (CVVH). CAVH requires arterial access and has fallen out of favor in recent years. These continuous techniques are primarily used for the treatment of critically ill patients with AKI.

Typically the dose of replacement fluid is set in liters per hour. The ideal dose is controversial but, in general, around 20 to 35 mL/kg/hr is recommended. Care should be taken to account for the difference between the actual delivered dose and the prescribed dose as the two can often be off by 20% due to a variety of technical and logistic problems such as breaks in therapy and clotting issues.[21] There does not seem to be any improvement in outcomes when using higher delivered dosages (>30 mL/kg/hr) for AKI.[21–24] Volume removal in hemofiltration can be achieved by decreasing the amount of replacement fluid given back to the patient in relation to the amount of fluid that is removed.

Hemodiafiltration

Combining diffusive clearance with large amounts of convective clearance (in other words, combining hemofiltration with dialysis) is termed hemodiafiltration. With hemodiafiltration, both use of dialysate and ultrapure replacement fluid administration are necessary. If performed continuously, hemodiafiltration is termed continuous veno-venous hemodiafiltration or CVVHDF (also CVVHD). Hemodiafiltration can be used for the treatment of ESRD and is also frequently used continuously for critically ill patients with AKI.

Pure Ultrafiltration

In patients who require fluid removal without solute clearance, removal of plasma water alone or ultrafiltration can be performed. Fluid removal without simultaneous dialysis has the added benefit of conferring more hemodynamic stability as

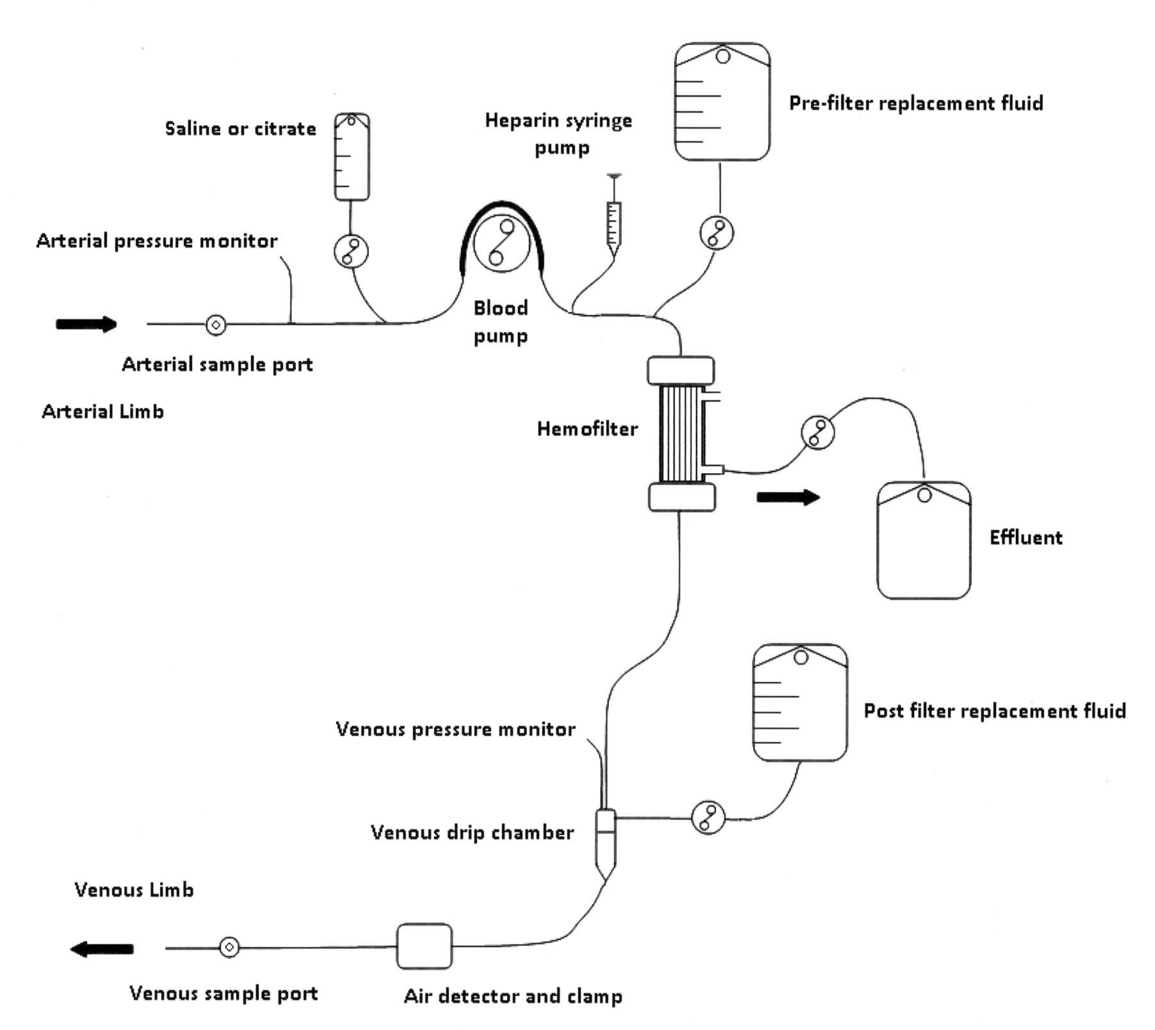

FIGURE 84.6 Drawing of a hemofiltration circuit. Blood enters the arterial limb from the patient dialysis access and flows through a hemofilter where plasma water and solute that is smaller than the hemofilter pore size passes the membrane via convection and is discarded in the effluent bag. Blood then continues to flow through the venous limb and back to the patient. To achieve meaningful clearance of solute, large volumes of plasma water removal are required, thus the need for replacement fluid to prevent excessive volume removal from the patient. Replacement fluid can be delivered prefilter, postfilter, or both pre- and postfilter as illustrated. Anticoagulation options typically include either heparin delivered by a syringe pump or citrate delivered to the arterial limb by a separate pump. Note that the illustration only shows a hemofiltration setup which is similar to setups used for continuous venovenous hemofiltration (CVVH). Many different arrangements are available. If dialysate is hooked up to the filter, the technique can be modified to perform dialysis at the same time as hemofiltration, also known as hemodiafiltration.

osmolar shifts are not taking place in the circulation due to lack of diffusive clearance. For patients who are particularly hemodynamically unstable, slow continuous ultrafiltration (SCUF) is an option. With SCUF blood flows are typically 100–200 mL per min with fluid removal (ultrafiltration rate) ranging from 100–500 mL per hr as tolerated. Small amounts of convective clearance of solute occur with this technique but not at a level that is clinically significant. Pure ultrafiltration or SCUF has also been termed aquaphresis by non-nephrologists.

Water Treatment Systems

To perform hemodialysis, a large amount of pure water is needed. At a dialysate flow rate of 500 to 800 mL per min a standard 4-hour dialysis session will require 120 to 192 L of water. Inpatient and outpatient dialysis units operate using water treatment systems that are able to meet this demand for water (Fig. 84.7). Regular city or well water can contain many contaminants. Some of these contaminants include particulate matter such as sand, clay, and plant matter or metals such as copper, zinc, and lead which can be leeched from pipes during water transport. Water obtained in proximity of agriculture may be contaminated with fertilizers and pesticides. Further, heath authorities of city water systems frequently add agents to water to make it safer or more palpable for consumption. Chlorine and chloramines are added to control microbial contamination, fluorides for dental prophylaxis, and occasionally aluminum sulfate and iron salts are added as flocculating agents to decrease water turbidity.[25] These contaminants and

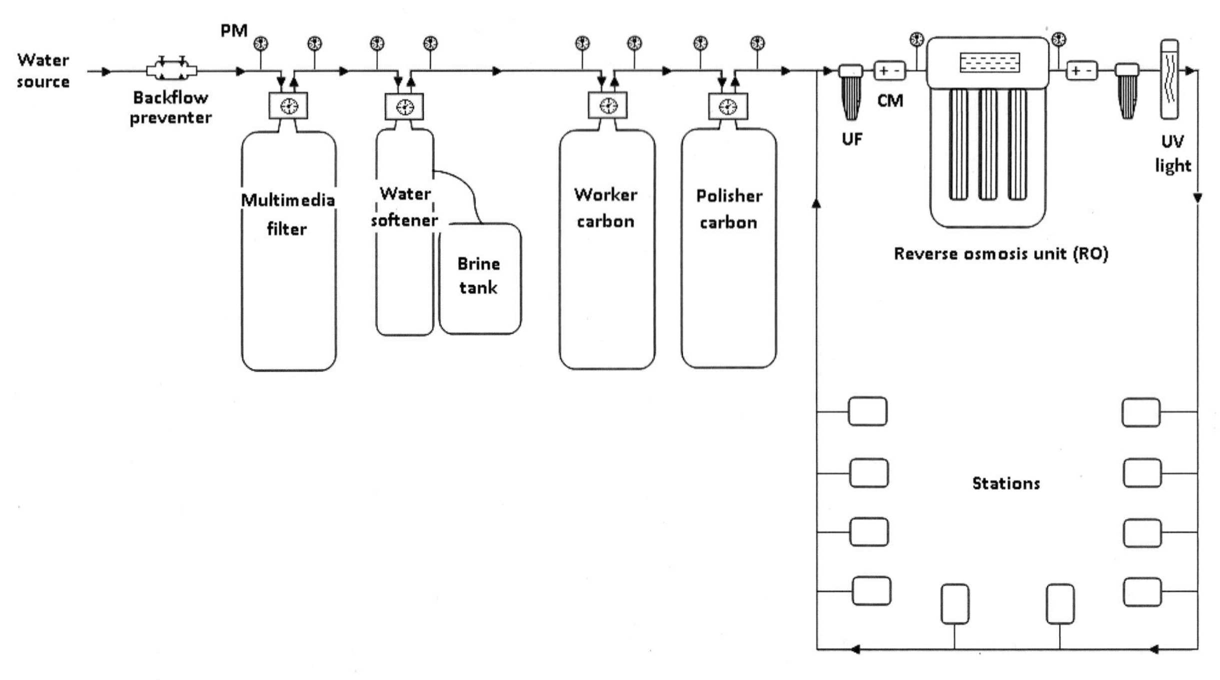

FIGURE 84.7 Simplified drawing of the components of a typical direct feed water treatment system. *Arrows* indicate the direction of flow. City water enters the system and runs through a backflow preventer. Pressure is monitored (PM) at multiple points in the circuit to ensure filtration integrity of the various components. Conductivity monitors (CM) are placed before and after treatment with the reverse osmosis unit. Ultrafilters (UF) and a ultraviolet (UV) light are placed in the loop to prevent microbiologic contamination. Water not used at the dialysis stations in the loop is returned to the circuit pre-RO for reuse. Not drawn but occasionally included in the water treatment system is the storage tank (for indirect feed systems), pressure tank, booster pump, and acid feed system.

additives need to be removed from the water source prior to being used in the production of dialysate.

Treatment guidelines for water purification have been set by the Association for the Advancement of Medical Instrumentation (AAMI) and the European Pharmacopeia. Water treatment systems can vary among institutions and differ based on water supply and local requirements. The water purification circuit generally consists of a back flow preventer, multimedia filter, water softener, activated carbon filters, and a final purification device which can be a de-ionizer or more commonly a reverse osmosis system. The backflow preventer serves to keep water in the circuit from regurgitating into the plumbing circuit of the building. The multimedia filter contains sand and gravel of varying sizes and serves to remove large particulate matter and debris from the water. The water softener contains anion exchange beads which exchange calcium and magnesium in the city water for sodium from the brine tank. Carbon tanks remove chlorine and chloramines from the city water. After passing through these initial steps the water is sent to the final purification unit. Reverse osmosis (RO) is a filtration process by which water is actively forced through a membrane with very small pore sizes that do not allow solute (including sodium) and other organic matter to pass through. De-ionization, an alternative to reverse osmosis, uses an ion exchange process to form water. Supply water percolates around cationic and anionic exchange resins which exchange hydrogen and hydroxide ions for other ions. The H+ and OH− ions then form pure water. De-ionization is effective in removing inorganic ions but has the downside of ineffective removal of organic contaminants and potential bacterial contamination. Water also can be passed through a UV light and ultrafilters to aid in the sterilization process. Once purified, typically, water is sent through a loop which feeds dialysis stations. Depending on the dialysis machine, there may also be a filter at the machine for the dialysate after the water has mixed with the concentrate.[26,27]

Water Quality Issues

Clinical events can manifest when there is a problem with chemical or microbiologic impurities in water. Aluminum, chloramines, and fluoride intoxication have been reported in recent years in hemodialysis units. Aluminum toxicity can lead to progressive central nervous system (CNS) effects, anemia, and low turnover bone disease. High levels can lead to permanent CNS toxicity, dementia, and even death.[27] Blood exposure to chloride and chloramines in the dialysate can lead to symptoms of nausea, vomiting, hypotension, dyspnea, and hemolytic anemia. Patients with hemolysis may present with dark blood in the hemodialysis line. Chloramines are not completely removed by de-ionization or reverse osmosis and require functional activated charcoal columns for removal. Charcoal columns can be exhausted over time and if water flow is too rapid through them, chloramines can pass into the product water. For this reason, purified water for dialysis should be checked every dialysis shift or every 4 hours for chloramines to ensure that this complication is avoided. Fluoride is removed by reverse osmosis and de-ionization. However, if the de-ionizer becomes saturated, large quantities of fluoride can be released into the water as the anion resin preferentially exchanges bound fluoride for anions of higher affinity such as chloride. In the body, fluoride binds to calcium and can disrupt cell membranes leading to hyperkalemia. Toxic effects of fluoride can manifest with pruritus, painful gastrointestinal (GI) symptoms, syncope, tetany, neurologic symptoms, cardiac arrhythmia, and death.[28]

Dialysate water does not have to be sterile because the dialysis membrane does not have pore sizes large enough for transport of microbes. Even so, water-related febrile reactions and related inflammatory problems can occur if the water is excessively contaminated with microorganisms, lipopolysaccharides, or endotoxins. The AAMI recommends that water used for dialysate has less than 200 colony forming units (CFU) per milliliter of water. The European Pharmacopeia guidelines are more strict, recommending less than 100 CFU per mL. Water contaminated with high levels of endotoxins or lipopolysaccharides can cause fevers, chills, and systemic inflammatory response. The acceptable level for endotoxin measured by the LAL test is less than 0.1 EU per mL.[27,29]

The term "ultrapure dialysate" describes fluid that is nearly free of bacteria and endotoxin but should not be confused with sterile fluid which is completely free of pyrogen and bacteria. Ultrapure dialysate has been suggested as beneficial in dialysis patients due to a decreased burden of microbial contamination resulting in less inflammatory response.[30] Ultrapure dialysate water contains bacterial concentrations less than 0.1 CFU per mL if standard techniques are used or less than 0.03 IU per mL if sensitive assays are used.[31] Improving water purification methods have allowed for more interest in online generation of replacement fluid for hemofiltration or hemodiafiltration.[32,33] These techniques usually involve an extra ultrafilter at the dialysis machine to generate ultrapure replacement fluid for infusion into the patient.

Uremic Toxins

Uremic retention compounds are usually classified by molecular weight and degree of protein binding. Many of the known uremic toxins are generated by metabolism of proteins and by modification of amino acids by gut microbes.

Urea, measured by blood urea nitrogen (BUN), is a low molecular weight solute (60 daltons) which is linked to protein metabolism and has been used as a surrogate marker for small, water soluble uremic toxins. Urea itself is not highly toxic and its generation is influenced by many factors such as dietary intake and liver function. In current practice, urea is the predominant marker used to evaluate clearance in dialysis and urea clearance is accordingly associated with dose of dialysis or dialysis adequacy. However, the clinical picture of uremia is complex and involves more than just small molecules.

Middle molecules (500 daltons to 60 kDa) have also been suggested as an important component of the uremic syndrome.[34] This proposal was based, in part, on the observation that peritoneal dialysis patients did quite well with high BUN and creatinine levels and the peritoneal membrane is more permeable to middle size molecules than the dialysis membranes used early on in dialytic therapy.[35] Most middle molecules are peptides. Clearance of middle molecules has improved in recent years with the use of high-flux dialyzers that have larger pore sizes. Clearance of middle molecules can also be improved by lengthening treatment time. Further, convective methods of clearance are gaining in popularity and are more effective than diffusive methods for clearance of middle molecules. The prototype middle molecule is β2–microglobulin (12 kDa). Many of the middle molecules are involved in leukocyte, endothelial cell, smooth muscle cell, and/or thrombocyte function and therefore they likely have an impact on cardiovascular health.[36]

Protein-bound uremic toxins can be of variable size but due to their binding to large molecular weight plasma proteins such as albumin (68 kDa), they are not well cleared with current dialysis technology. Only the smaller, free fraction of these solutes is cleared with diffusion or convection. Phenols, indoles, hippurates, and advanced glycation end products are some examples of uremic toxins that are protein bound.[37] Many uremic toxins, protein bound and otherwise, appear to be generated in the gastrointestinal tract as a result of altered intestinal absorption of nutrients in the uremic state leading to changes in gut flora and microbial metabolism.[38]

Urea as a Marker of Dialysis Adequacy

Single Pool Kt/V (spKt/V)

To quantify the effect dialysis has on the removal of urea over time we can multiply clearance (K, mL/min) by time (t, min) which gives us the expression Kt which is a volume (mL) cleared. To generalize this expression among patients, Kt can be normalized to the volume of distribution of urea or total body water (V, mL) which results in a dimensionless expression of Kt/V.[39] In hemodialysis, this can be thought of as a ratio of the volume cleared of urea to the volume of distribution of urea. In other words, a Kt/V of 1.0 means that a volume of blood equal to the volume of total body water was cleared of urea. The clearance of urea from the blood over time during dialysis follows an exponential pattern. The following equation models the clearance of a substance from the body where that substance decreases in an exponential fashion:

$$Kt/V = \ln(C_{pre} / C_{post})$$

where C_{pre} is predialysis urea and C_{post} is postdialysis urea. This simplified equation provides the basis for urea kinetic modeling. It should be noted that it does not take into account the minimal generation of urea that happens during dialysis, nor does it take into account fluid that is removed with ultrafiltration during dialysis (changing V). It also assumes that the postdialysis urea is equilibrated across all body compartments or a "single pool." This is an erroneous assumption as urea is not distributed equally throughout all body compartments, especially during dialysis with high blood and dialysate flow rates. Other more complex formulas attempt to improve on accuracy and can also be used for the calculation of single pool Kt/V (Table 84.4).[40]

Equilibrated Kt/V (eKt/V)

The concentration of solute removal will be the greatest in the compartments of the body which have the largest amount of blood flow in continuity with the dialysis access—for example, the cardiopulmonary circuit. Other less well perfused areas such as the peripheral capillary beds will equilibrate urea more slowly with the vascular space. The method described above for calculation of Kt/V is the single pool method (spKt/V). This method treats the volume of distribution of urea as if it was a single pool that urea moves in and out of easily. In reality this is not true as solute gradients form between the various body compartments during dialysis and equilibration occurs in a delayed fashion after dialysis is complete. Although access recirculation and the cardiopulmonary circuit are quickly equilibrated, movement from less well perfused areas and cellular compartments continues for up to 60 minutes after dialysis.[41]

Keeping the phenomenon of recirculation in mind, it becomes important to be consistent about the timing of the postdialysis sample. Although measuring the urea concentration 60 minutes after dialysis would allow for equilibration to occur, this expenditure of patient and staff time is not practical in everyday practice. Alternate methods have been developed to estimate the degree of equilibration which are not so time consuming. In one such method ultrafiltration is stopped and the blood pump is slowed to 100 mL per min for 10 seconds, after which a sample is drawn from the arterial port. This maneuver allows for access recirculation to resolve and will yield a measurement that can be used in the calculation of the spKt/V. To account for equilibration of urea between body compartments after dialysis, equations have been developed to estimate the equilibrated Kt/V (eKt/V).[42] These equations (Table 84.5) were developed to serve as estimations extrapolated from urea rebound curves. The lack of significant cardiopulmonary recirculation in patients dialyzing with catheters necessitates the use of a separate formula.

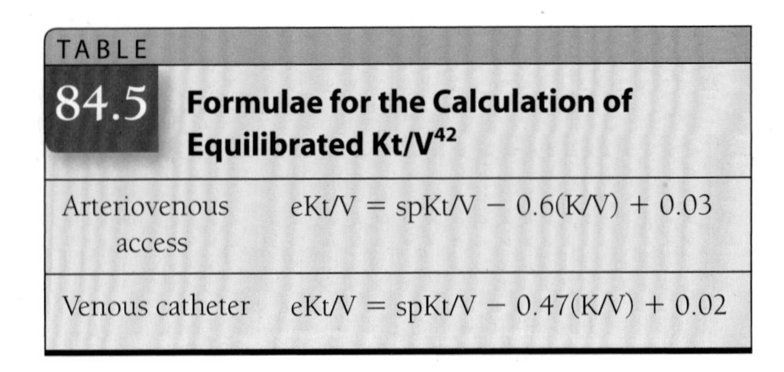

TABLE 84.5 Formulae for the Calculation of Equilibrated Kt/V[42]

Arteriovenous access	$eKt/V = spKt/V - 0.6(K/V) + 0.03$
Venous catheter	$eKt/V = spKt/V - 0.47(K/V) + 0.02$

TABLE 84.4 Formulae for the Calculation of Single Pool Kt/V

$Kt/V = (4 \times URR) - 1.2$
$Kt/V = 1.18 \times -\ln(R)$
$Kt/V = 2.2 - 3.3 \times (R - 0.03 - UF/W)$
$Kt/V = -\ln(R - 0.03) + (4 - 3.5 \times R) \times UF/W$

Accuracy of formulae increases from top to bottom.
URR, pre-post BUN/pre-BUN; UF, volume of fluid removed (L); W, postdialysis weight (kg); R, post/pre-BUN ratio.
From Daugirdas JT. Chronic hemodialysis prescription: a urea kinetic approach. In: Daugirdas JT, Ing TD, eds. *Handbook of dialysis*. 2nd ed. Boston: Little, Brown and Company; 1994:92; with permission.

Standard Kt/V

Measuring the single pool Kt/V (spKt/V) or equilibrated Kt/V (eKt/V) provides data for a single dialysis treatment, and this has limited value for comparing different treatment frequency strategies or for comparing peritoneal dialysis to hemodialysis. In an effort to quantify the dose of dialysis that is delivered continuously, the standard Kt/V (stdKt/V) was developed.[43,44] One can think of the standard Kt/V urea as a continuous clearance over a week of therapy rather than an intermittent clearance, similar to continuous urea clearance provided by residual renal function. The clearance is calculated based on the mean (peak) urea concentrations and the generation rate of urea over a week. It is then normalized to the volume of distribution of urea. This method of quantifying dialysis dose has utility particularly when comparing (or standardizing) patients on continuous therapies such as peritoneal dialysis or those who are receiving more frequent hemodialysis. Equations for calculation of stdKt/V are described in Table 84.6.[44,45]

Urea Reduction Ratio

Compared to formal urea kinetic modeling, the amount of urea removed in a single dialysis treatment can be expressed in a simple way as the fractional reduction of urea. The urea reduction ratio (URR) can then be converted into a percentage of urea reduction for a given dialysis session:

$$\%UR = C_{pre} - C_{post} / C_{pre} * 100$$

Roughly, a %UR of 65 correlates with a single pool Kt/V of 1.2. The URR does not take into account changes

TABLE 84.6 Formulae for the Calculation of Standard Kt/V

Equation 1: Gotch formula[43]

$$stdKt/V = 7*1440[0.184(PCRn - 0.17)]/Co \text{ weekly}$$

PCRn is the normalized protein catabolic rate, Co is the mean peak urea concentration

Equation 2: Leypoldt formula[44]

$$stdKt/V = \frac{10{,}080\,\frac{1 - e^{-eKt/V}}{t}}{\frac{1 - e^{-eKt/V}}{eKt/V} + \frac{10{,}080}{Ft} - 1}$$

eKt/V is the equilibrated Kt/V, t is treatment time in minutes, and F is the frequency of dialysis treatments per week

Equation 3: Adjustment for ultrafiltration and residual renal function[45]

$$stdKt/V = S/(1 - (0.74/F) * UFw/V) + Kru * (0.974/(spKt/V + 1.62) + 0.4) * 10{,}080/V$$

Where t is the treatment time in minutes, S is the result of equation 1, F is the number of sessions per week, UFw is the weekly fluid removal in liters, spKt/V is the single pool Kt/V, Kru is residual renal function, and V is the volume of distribution of urea.

in volume. Larger amounts of fluid removed with dialysis will result in a lower URR. This effect should be realized in patients with large intradialytic weight gains and high ultrafiltration rates.

Protein Catabolic Rate

Measurement of pre- and postdialysis urea concentration also allows the ability to calculate the amount of urea that is generated in the intradialytic period. This in turn can be used as a surrogate measure of protein intake and/or nutritional status. As protein is metabolized by the body, urea is generated. Therefore, measurement of the amount of urea in the body can be viewed as a measurement of net protein breakdown and, in the nutritional steady state, net protein catabolism is equal to dietary protein intake.[46]

There are many equations available for the calculation of normalized protein catabolic rate (Table 84.7). It should be noted that the equations do not take into account the

TABLE 84.7 Formula for the Calculation of Normalized Protein Catabolic Rate[217]

$PCRn = 5.42\ G / V + 0.168$

G is the urea generation rate and V the volume of distribution of urea.

Three times weekly dialysis	
Beginning of week	$C_o / [36.3 + 5.48Kt/V + 53.5/(Kt/V)] + 0.168$
Mid week	$C_o / [25.8 + 1.15Kt/V + 56.4/(Kt/V)] + 0.168$
End of week	$C_o / [16.3 + 4.3Kt/V + 56.6/(Kt/V)] + 0.168$
Twice weekly dialysis	
Beginning of week	$C_o / [48 + 5.14Kt/V + 79/(Kt/V)] + 0.168$
End of week	$C_o / [33 + 3.6Kt/V + 83.2/(Kt/V)] + 0.168$

C_o is the predialysis concentration of urea.

clearance of urea that takes place by native kidneys in persons with residual kidney function. If a significant amount of urea clearance is still present through the native kidneys the PCRn will appear low. Further care should be taken when relating the PCRn to nutrition. Each patient needs to be evaluated for other clinical factors that can affect serum urea levels because the equation assumes that the patient is in a steady state of protein balance. For example, in states of increased protein catabolism, such as acute illness, urea levels will be increased and do not represent increased dietary intake. Taking these potential confounders into account, in general, an nPCR of greater than 1.0 g/kg/day would indicate that the patient has adequate protein intake. Goal PCRn should be in the range of 0.8 g/kg/day to 1.4 g/kg/day.[47]

Pitfalls with Urea-based Measures of Dialysis Adequacy

Urea is used as a surrogate marker of dialysis adequacy but urea itself does not describe the entirety of the uremic milieu. Urea is attractive as a marker of uremic toxicity because levels correlate with protein catabolism and many uremic toxins have been linked to protein metabolism. Urea is also easily measured by blood chemistry. However, urea levels may not correlate with the level of all uremic toxins, particularly in the case of uremic toxins that are not small solutes. Middle molecules and uremic toxins which are protein bound are largely ignored when using urea based methods of measurement of adequacy. Further, putting these inherent properties of urea aside, many other potential inaccuracies exist in the calculation of Kt/V (Table 84.8).

Timing of Initiation of Dialysis

The ideal timing for the initiation of dialysis in the patient with chronic kidney disease (CKD) is dependent on sound clinical judgment which accounts for factors such as age, residual kidney function, rate of progression to ESRD, modality choice, and patient preference. Examples of clear indications for the initiation of dialysis include uremia, uremic pericarditis, and volume excess refractory to diuretic therapy. Over time in the United States, the estimated glomerular filtration rate (eGFR) at which patients are initiated on dialysis continues to increase. In 1996 the mean eGFR at dialysis initiation was between 7 and 8 mL per min whereas in 2008 the mean eGFR was 11 mL per min.[5] It is possible that this increase in eGFR represents changing nephrologist attitudes toward offering dialysis care with a general shift in practice patterns toward offering dialysis earlier. Patients starting dialysis at higher eGFRs may also be sicker than appreciated or sicker than historical patients. Patients starting dialysis with a higher eGFR are generally older, diabetic, and have a higher number of premorbid conditions.[5]

Many recent clinical guidelines and recommendations focus on the estimated GFR as calculated by Cockcroft-Gault or MDRD formulae as a tool to assist with the timing of initiation of dialysis. Use of eGFR is fraught with difficulties because the eGFR does not always correlate well with the actual GFR, particularly at very low levels of renal function as is seen in patients nearing the need for renal replacement therapy. Often patients with malnutrition will have lower creatinine levels reflective of decreased muscle mass and MDRD eGFRs which appear to be higher.

The trend toward starting dialysis earlier based on eGFR is alarming due to lack of clear demonstration of benefit in early start situations. In a prospective registry study comparing the MDRD eGFR and mortality, in a subgroup of patients with measured creatinine clearances, mortality rates were higher in patients with a higher eGFR but this relationship did not hold up when the GFR was calculated by measured creatinine clearance.[48] Furthermore, higher eGFR at initiation of dialysis has been correlated with a greater risk for death. In an evaluation of registry data from Scotland and British Columbia, a progressively increasing hazard ratio of death was seen with increasing eGFR.[49] In a cohort of over 25,000 patients from Canada between 2001 and 2007, increased mortality was seen in the early start group (eGFR >10.5) compared with late start (eGFR <10.5). After adjustment for comorbidities, the increased risk persisted.[50] Retrospective analysis of the USRDS revealed similar associations between increased mortality and early dialysis start when using eGFR >15 mL per min as the definition for early start and <5 mL per min late start, arguing against early start of dialysis based on eGFR alone.[51] Recently, a randomized controlled trial of patients from Australia and New Zealand attempted to define the ideal timing of dialysis based on the eGFR calculated by the Cockcroft-Gault formula (IDEAL study).[52] Patients were randomized to two groups, early start (eGFR 10–14 mL per min) and late start (5–7 mL per min). Enrollment included 828 patients followed between 2000 and 2008. The results showed no difference between early versus late start with regard to death from any cause, cardiovascular complications, infectious complications, or dialysis complications. The conclusion was early start based on eGFR considerations alone does not confer clinical benefit.

The weight of the evidence seems to point away from using eGFR as the sole factor to determine the appropriate timing for initiation of dialysis. Rather, decisions regarding timing of the initiation of dialysis should remain a clinical judgment call made by a physician trained in kidney disease and individualized to meet the patient's needs.

Clinical Trials to Define the Optimal Dialysis Dose

Over the years, clinicians and researchers have attempted to define the optimal dose of dialytic therapy for ESRD patients. Currently, dialysis therapy is delivered in a relatively uniform fashion to nearly all dialysis patients (3 to 4 days a week for 3 to 4 hours). Realization that the appropriate dose of volume and solute removal in dialysis is probably

TABLE 84.8 **Some Potential Pitfalls with Urea-based Methods of Dialysis Adequacy and Their Solutions**

	Problem	Potential Solution
Expected K_{urea}	Clearance data for specific dialyzers relies on information provided by manufacturers measured in artificial situations with urea solutions, not in vivo.	Anticipate that manufacturer listed clearances overestimate in vivo clearances
Sampling error	Clearance calculations can be affected by sampling, if sample is not drawn correctly or there is significant access recirculation results can be overestimated.	Develop consistent quality driven protocols for measurement of pre- and postdialysis urea
Discrepancy between prescribed vs. delivered dose	Loss of fiber bundle volume due to clotting can reduce amount of clearance. This is more of an issue near the end of the dialysis run or in dialyzers that are reused. Lost dialysis time. Staff or patient related factors may create a discrepancy between the prescribed dose of dialysis and the amount of dialysis actually delivered.	Urea kinetic modeling should not be used alone to prescribe a dose of dialysis
Urea rebound	Urea rebound occurs after dialysis. Initially urea is equilibrated in the dialysis access as recirculation is negated, in the following minutes recirculation from the cardiopulmonary circuit resolves and over the following hour urea is redistributed completely from various tissue compartments and cellular spaces. Urea levels drawn immediately after dialysis do not allow enough time for equilibration to occur.	The calculation of equilibrated Kt/V attempts to address this problem
Modeled after traditional intermittent HD	Single pool Kt/V measures the effectiveness of a single dialysis session and is modeled after patients undergoing thrice weekly dialysis for 3–4 hours. The applicability of this method in persons on differing dialysis regimens particularly in cases of more frequent dialysis is unclear.	The calculation of standard Kt/V attempts to address this problem

not the same for every patient led to expanded concepts for adequacy of dialysis by measurement of patient specific factors which could quantify the amount of dialysis delivered.

The National Cooperative Dialysis Study (NCDS) in 1981 was a seminal early study seeking to provide a means for quantitative measurement of the optimal dose for thrice weekly dialysis.[53] Investigators compared time averaged urea clearances (TAC_{urea}) with long or short treatment durations using a factorial randomized study design. Patients were divided into four groups based on their TAC_{urea} and dialysis time (Table 84.9). The TAC_{urea} provides a value for the mean concentration of urea over a dialysis cycle (Fig. 84.8). Investigators found that the patients in groups 2 and 4 with higher TAC_{urea} had more frequent hospitalizations, most commonly due to nausea, anorexia, and other uremic symptoms. As a result, more patients were withdrawn from the high TAC_{urea} groups for medical reasons. With regard to the length of therapy, in the high TAC_{urea} patients (groups 2 and 4), the short duration dialysis group (group 4) was hospitalized more frequently than the long duration dialysis group (group 2). The benefit of longer dialysis was not seen in the two groups with low TAC_{urea} (groups 1 and 3).

The NCDS findings were widely interpreted as suggesting that to prevent morbidity, clearance of urea is more

TABLE 84.9 Four Groups of the National Cooperative Dialysis Study (NCDS)

Group	Td (h)	Predialysis BUN (mg/dL)	TAC_{urea} (mg/dL)	Patients (%)
1 Long Td, low BUN	4.5 to 5.0	60 to 80	50	86
2 Long Td, high BUN	4.5 to 5.0	110 to 130	100	46
3 Short Td, low BUN	2.5 to 3.5	60 to 80	50	69
4 Short Td, high BUN	2.5 to 3.5	110 to 130	100	31

Td, dialysis time; BUN, blood urea nitrogen; TAC_{urea}, time-averaged concentration of BUN.

important than dialysis treatment time. This led to the assumption by many clinicians that dialysis time could be shortened so long as urea clearance remained adequate. Notable caveats of the NCDS study include relatively low urea clearances across all groups, a patient population that was healthier when compared to the dialysis population in more recent times, and the small size of the study which was underpowered to make mortality comparisons.

Following the NCDS study numerous large observational studies, most of them performed in the 1990s, challenged the NCDS findings and suggested that higher Kt/V urea values and higher flux dialysis is associated with better outcomes.[54–61] Subsequently, there was a trend toward lengthening dialysis time and the utilization of high flux membranes.

The Hemodialysis (HEMO) study[62] in 2002 sought to evaluate the effect of dialysis dose and membrane flux on death from any cause. In a schedule of thrice weekly dialysis, investigators used a two by two factorial design to randomize patients to high dose or low dose groups and high flux or low flux groups. They achieved an equilibrated Kt/V (eKt/V) in the low dose group of 1.16 and 1.53 in the high dose group. The low flux and high flux groups had similar mean eKt/V at 1.34. There was no significant improvement in survival seen between standard dose, high dose, low flux, or high flux dialysis groups. The results of the HEMO study were surprisingly negative in contrast to the earlier observational data. Even so, it is notable that on secondary analysis of the HEMO study, high flux dialysis was associated with improved cardiovascular[63] and cerebrovascular outcomes.[64]

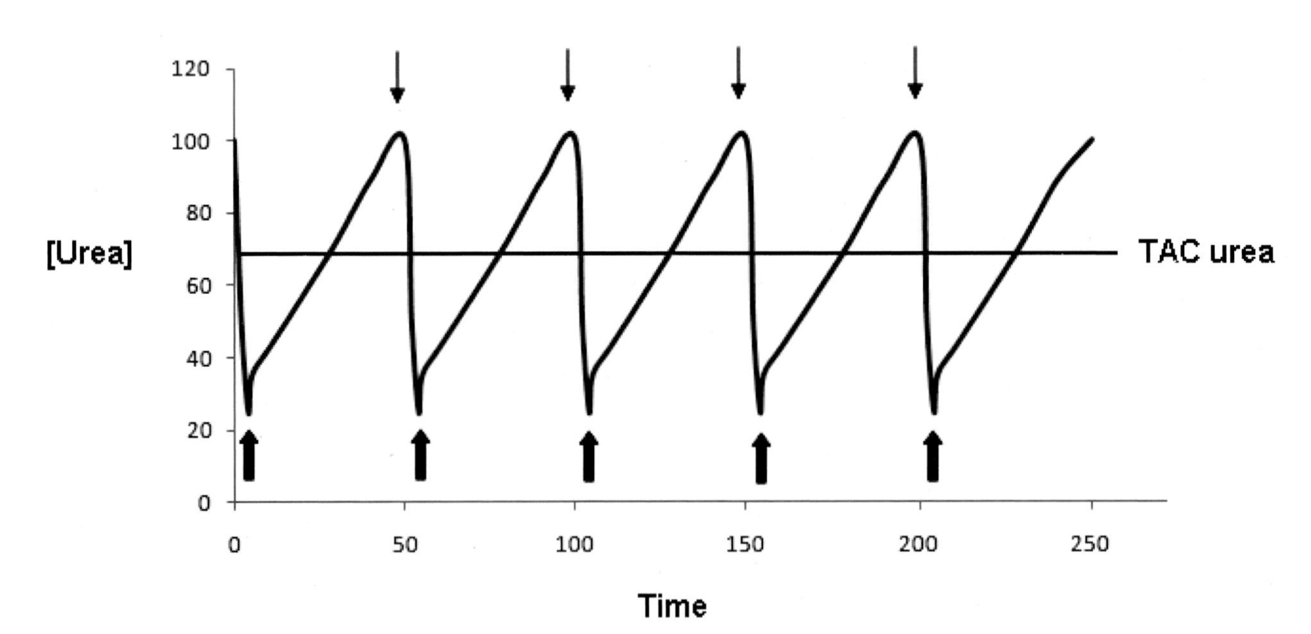

FIGURE 84.8 Time averaged concentration of urea (TAC_{urea}). Graphical representation of the time averaged urea concentration. On the *y* axis is urea concentration (mg/dL), on the *x* axis time (hours). The *thin arrows* indicate the urea concentration predialysis and *thick arrows* postdialysis. The *black line* intersecting the urea curve is the time-averaged urea concentration (approximately 70 mg/dL in this example). Note the brisk upstroke of the urea curve postdialysis which represents equilibration (described previously under equilibrated Kt/V).

The Membrane Permeability Outcome Study Group (MPO study)[65] was also undertaken with a goal of evaluating the effect of membrane permeability on outcomes. Patients were randomized to dialysis with low flux or high flux membranes and stratified according to their serum albumin level (albumin <4 g per dL or albumin >4 g per dL). Both groups were treated with a minimum single pool Kt/V of 1.2. Findings revealed that patients in the low albumin group (<4 g per dL) had significantly higher survival rates when treated with a high flux dialyzer. Further, high flux dialyzers in secondary analysis seemed to improve survival of diabetics regardless of serum albumin. This survival benefit was not seen in patients with higher serum albumin levels or across the group as a whole.

Effect of extended duration of dialysis therapy on patient outcome was not assessed in the aforementioned clinical trials. In 2010 data from the Frequent Hemodialysis Network (FHN) trial[66] was released to help address the issue of the appropriate duration of dialysis. The rationale for the currently used duration of dialysis (three times weekly) is based on limited studies, logistic practicality, cost, and patient acceptance rather than on sound science. The FHN randomized subjects to in-center hemodialysis six times weekly compared with standard thrice weekly dialysis with the hypothesis that more frequent dialysis would improve outcomes. As expected, solute clearance was improved in the frequent dialysis group (weekly standard Kt/V 3.54 vs. 2.49). Results revealed that more frequent dialysis was associated with improvement in left ventricular mass, physical composite health score, hypertension, and phosphorus control. The study was only conducted for 12 months and was underpowered to detect any differences in mortality. There was no difference in the rates of hospitalizations with more frequent dialysis. Results of a trial of extended daily dialysis (nocturnal dialysis) are currently pending and may also contribute to this clinical question.

Anticoagulation

Systemic anticoagulation is usually necessary in hemodialysis patients to prevent clotting of the extracorporeal blood circuit. Due to underlying renal disease, patients with ESRD often have abnormalities of the clotting system. Most classically this is thought of as a bleeding disorder, related to uremic platelet dysfunction. However, it is also worthwhile to note that patients with renal failure frequently have coagulation abnormalities that predispose to clot formation. This may be related to underlying systemic inflammation and endothelial injury which can activate the clotting cascade.[4] The clotting cascade is composed of intrinsic and extrinsic pathways which converge at factor X. Activated factor X (factor Xa) catalyzes the formation of thrombin from prothrombin. Thrombin then converts soluble fibrinogen to fibrin which can be cross-linked to form a clot. The extrinsic pathway is endogenously activated by trauma or injury and endothelial release of tissue factor. The intrinsic pathway, also known as the contact pathway, is activated by artificial surfaces, such as occurs during extracorporeal circulation in hemodialysis.[67] Therefore, the process of dialysis itself can activate the clotting cascade as blood comes in contact with needles, plastic tubing, and dialyzer materials. The movement of blood through the extracorporeal circuit also leads to increased shear stress and turbulent flow, mechanical factors that can activate platelets, and the clotting cascade. Granulocytes and monocytes can adhere to artificial surfaces and subsequently release granules containing tissue factor which can stimulate the coagulation cascade.[26] Risk factors for clotting on hemodialysis include slow blood flow, high hematocrit, and blood transfusion into the extracorporeal circuit. The drip chambers, particularly on the venous limb, are more prone to clotting due to slow blood flow, relative stasis, and air interface which can activate the clotting cascade.

The most widely used agent for anticoagulation during the dialysis procedure is unfractionated heparin (UFH). There is no standard dose for heparin given with dialysis and the prescription should be modified to fit the patient's needs taking into account the risk of bleeding from anticoagulation. As an example, one prescription for low dose heparinization would be a bolus dose of heparin (25–30 U per kg) given at the beginning of dialysis followed by 500–1000 U hourly during the treatment. Heparin can be stopped 30 to 60 minutes before the end of a treatment for the purpose of achieving hemostasis after needles are removed from the dialysis access. For extended or continuous hemodialysis sessions in inpatient settings heparin dosing should be monitored by periodically checking aPTT and titrating to a goal level of anticoagulation (usually between 40 and 60). Heparin has the advantage of being relatively inexpensive, easy to administer and monitor, and there is an available antidote in protamine sulfate. Adverse effects of heparin include osteoporosis, hyperkalemia, hyperlipidemia, and allergic reactions. Heparin related allergic reactions take two main forms: acute allergic reactions (type 1 hypersensitivity reactions) and heparin induced thrombocytopenia (HIT). HIT is estimated to affect 10% of patients who receive heparin though only 17% of patients with HIT experience adverse clinical effects.[68] HIT usually manifests 5 to 10 days after exposure to heparin and presents with a drop in the platelet count and a propensity to form clots ("white clots").

Low molecular weight heparins (LMWH) are also an option for anticoagulation. LMWH has the advantage of more predictable dose effects, ease of subcutaneous administration, and less of the traditional side effects associated with heparin such as HIT. However, LMWH has a long duration of action leading to anticoagulation effects lasting long after dialysis is completed. Furthermore, the effects of anticoagulation are not readily reversible. LMWH is not approved for use with dialysis in the United States but is frequently used in Europe.[26,67]

Occasionally patients cannot receive systemic anticoagulation with heparin while on dialysis due to excessive bleeding risk or allergies. In these cases, often heparin-free dialysis with frequent saline rinses of the circuit (e.g., 200 mL of normal saline every 20 to 30 minutes) is enough to prevent excessive clotting. If this is ineffective, alternative methods of anticoagulation are available but often not utilized in outpatient dialysis units due to technical difficulty and/or excessive cost. Regional forms of anticoagulation involving the dialysis circuit have been developed; the most commonly used is regional citrate anticoagulation. Citrate is infused into the arterial limb of the circuit and acts by chelating free calcium which in turn inhibits the coagulation cascade. Some of the citrate is removed from the circuit as it passes through the dialyzer but diffusion of citrate across the membrane is not complete and some of it is delivered to the patient. Citrate anticoagulation is often very effective at keeping the circuit patent and with proper monitoring can be accomplished safely.[69] Regional citrate anticoagulation is frequently used in inpatient settings when continuous renal replacement therapy is employed but it can also be used for intermittent hemodialysis. Citrate infusion should be monitored closely to ensure that the patient does not develop systemic citrate toxicity. In citrate toxicity, serum total calcium levels will be normal or elevated but ionized calcium levels can be low due to the binding of free ionized calcium to circulating citrate. Patients with liver disease are at particular risk for citrate toxicity over time due to inadequate hepatic citrate metabolism.[70] Citrate toxicity can manifest with all of the symptoms of hypocalcemia such as fatigue, weakness, tetany, cramping, seizures, prolonged QT interval, and arrhythmias. An alternative to administration of citrate in the blood circuit is adding citrate to the dialysate, a method of anticoagulation that is effective, safe, and relatively easy to perform.[71] Other options include direct thrombin inhibitors such as argatroban, heparinoids such as danaparoid, and regional heparin-protamine setups. These options are infrequently used due to cost and difficulty with administration in outpatient settings.

Vascular Access

Establishing reliable, functional, and infection free access to the bloodstream for dialysis has often been described as the Achilles heel of hemodialysis. Recent clinical practice guidelines and clinical initiatives have recognized the importance of appropriate vascular access with goals to increase the numbers of patients with fistulas (the "fistula first" initiative) and decrease the usage of hemodialysis catheters. These guidelines are in part a response to the mortality and morbidity that has been realized in hemodialysis patients with suboptimal access. It is estimated that 20% of hospitalizations in dialysis patients are related to dialysis access problems.[72] Infection is the second leading cause of mortality in dialysis patients and is often related to the dialysis access. Adjusted mortality rates in patients who dialyze through a catheter as opposed to a fistula are 40% to 70% higher,[73] and these rates improve after being switched from a catheter to a fistula or graft.[74] Placement of dialysis access requires close collaboration between nephrologists, primary care physicians, and vascular surgeons to ensure that it happens in a timely fashion. In general, access planning should take into account the level of kidney function, rate of decline, and the time needed for the selected dialysis access to mature.

Fistulas are typically created using a side-to-end anastomosis of the vein to the artery or less frequently a side-to-side anastomosis. Fistulas have the lowest complication rates, the longest patency rates, and require fewer interventions. Maturation time differs among accesses. Fistulas usually take at least 6 to 12 weeks to mature and may take as long as 8 to 9 months. In particular, fistulas tend to take longer to mature in diabetics.[75] Venous mapping through imaging with ultrasonography or venography is recommended to provide surgical planning.[76] In general, for fistula placement, a minimum vein diameter of 2.5 mm is necessary. For grafts the minimum vein diameter is 4 mm. The artery diameter should be at least 2 mm for both fistulas and grafts.[77] Stenosis or thrombosis of proximal portions of the vein that is to be used should be ruled out prior to fistula placement.

If the patient does not have anatomy that is amenable to placement of a native arteriovenous fistula then placement of a graft should be considered. AV grafts are usually composed of synthetic material, most often polytetrafluoroethylene (PTFE). Occasionally deceased donor vein grafts (cryoveins) or bovine carotid arteries are used; however, these have not been found to be superior to synthetic PTFE.[78,79] More recent work using stem cells to create artificial veins has the hope of providing more biocompatible graft materials for use in dialysis access in the future. Grafts often can be used as early as 2 to 3 weeks. Grafts are more prone to infectious complications than native fistulas. If graft material becomes infected the graft needs to be removed and the dialysis access will be lost. Problems with stenoses and thrombosis are also more common with grafts. Stenosis in grafts usually happens at the graft-vein anastomosis.

Catheters should be considered the last resort in patients who need long-term hemodialysis access. Catheters which are used for long-term access are tunneled under the skin and have a cuff whereas temporary catheters usually do not have a cuff or tunnel. The preferred site of insertion is the right internal jugular vein followed by the left internal jugular vein. In patients with difficult access, placement in the femoral veins or translumbar placement into the inferior vena cava can be considered. Subclavian catheters have been associated with higher rates of central stenosis and should be avoided.[8] Catheters should be locked with heparin, citrate, or thrombolytic agents to maintain patency between dialysis sessions.

ACUTE COMPLICATIONS OF DIALYSIS

Intradialytic Hypotension

Hypotension is a common complication of the hemodialysis procedure (Table 84.10) and is estimated to occur in 10% to 50% of treatments.[80] Intradialytic hypotension has been reported to occur more commonly in women, the elderly, diabetics, and patients with autonomic dysfunction.[81] Usually

TABLE 84.10 Acute Complications of Hemodialysis

Complication	Potential Cause
Hypotension	Excessive fluid removal, excessive antihypertensive medication regimen, infection, myocardial infarction, tamponade, anaphylactic reaction
Hypertension	Sodium and water excess, inadequate ultrafiltration
Allergic reactions	Dialyzer, tubing, heparin, iron (especially dextrans), latex or tape reaction
Arrhythmias	Electrolyte imbalance, rapid fluid shifts, dialytic removal of antiarrhythmic medications
Muscle cramping	Rapid ultrafiltration, electrolyte imbalances
Air embolism	Air entry into blood circuit
Dialysis disequilibrium	Osmotic shifts between intracellular and extracellular space leading to cell swelling, cerebral edema. Rapid drop in plasma urea concentration
Dialysate/Water Quality Problems	
Chlorine/chloramines	Hemolysis, usually due to depletion of charcoal columns
Fluoride contamination	Itching, gastrointestinal symptoms, syncope, tetany, neurologic symptoms, arrhythmia; due to exhaustion of de-ionizer, usually not a complication if reverse osmosis is used
Bacterial/endotoxin contamination	Fever, rigors, hypotension; due to contamination of dialysate or water circuit

hypotension is related to aggressive ultrafiltration rates, but intradialytic hypotension can also be a sign of other clinical problems such as underlying infection, myocardial ischemia, or, if severe, an anaphylactic reaction to dialysis components. Excessive removal of volume from the plasma through an ultrafiltration rate that exceeds the plasma refill rate can lead to decreased circulatory volume. If the patient is subsequently not able to increase cardiac output to keep up with the volume lost or move fluid from the interstitium into the plasma compartment quickly enough then hypotension and hemodynamic collapse ensues. In hemodialysis patients there may also be a reduction in the ability of the venous system to appropriately vasoconstrict, possibly due to cardiopulmonary redistribution of blood flow that occurs in patients with arteriovenous accesses.[81] Left ventricular hypertrophy is thought to be a significant factor in intradialytic hypotension. Myocardial hypertrophy can impair ventricular filling by narrowing the ventricular cavity and leading to lower filling volumes. Myocardial hypertrophy and fibrosis can result in a stiff ventricular wall that requires a higher filling pressure to expand. Presence of atrial fibrillation can lead to intradialytic hypotension through decreased ventricular filling due to loss of atrial kick.[82] Autonomic nervous system dysfunction is seen frequently in ESRD, and in patients with intradialytic hypotension, autonomic dysfunction is usually more severe, particularly in diabetic patients.[80]

Treatment of intradialytic hypotension involves measures aimed at restoration of blood volume or vascular tone. If the hypotension is mild and asymptomatic, patients may respond with improvement in blood pressure after simply discontinuing the ultrafiltration for a period of time sufficient enough to allow plasma refill and restoration of blood pressure. In more severe cases of symptomatic hypotension, administration of normal saline is indicated to restore blood volume. Placing the patient in the Trendelenburg position to improve vital cerebral perfusion can also be considered if the patient is symptomatic.

Accurate assessment of dry weight by the clinician is important to prevent iatrogenic excessive ultrafiltration. Key to the avoidance of intradialytic hypotension is patient control of interdialytic weight gains to prevent the need for excessive ultrafiltration rates. This can be accomplished through tight dietary sodium restriction and clinical attention to the amount of sodium delivered through dialysate during the dialysis process. Dialysate sodium levels should be kept low to prevent a net sodium gain during dialysis. Rapid ultrafiltration rates during dialysis (ultrafiltration rate of >10 mL/kg/hr) are associated with higher odds of intradialytic hypotension and a higher risk of mortality.[83]

Intradialytic hypotension can usually be avoided and dry weight goals still met in patients by decreasing the ultrafiltration rate and prolonging dialysis time. This simple yet time and resource intensive maneuver is perhaps the most effective intervention in the prevention of intradialytic hypotension. Cool dialysate has been shown to be an effective method for prevention of hypotension.[84] Alteration of the dialysate chemistry can improve stability as well. Increasing dialysate sodium or sodium modeling has been associated with greater stability but should be avoided to prevent sodium loading and rebound fluid excess. Higher calcium dialysate (3–3.5 mEq per L) may also be helpful but may lead to a positive calcium balance over time. Other methods frequently employed with little definitive data to support their use include colloid infusions such as albumin and medications such as midodrine. Careful adjustment of blood pressure altering medications is necessary when managing intradialytic hypotension.

Intradialytic Hypertension

Changes in blood pressure during dialysis are not always in the hypotensive direction. In approximately 10% to 15% of patients on hemodialysis blood pressure increases during the dialysis run or shortly thereafter. Increased predialysis blood pressure has been shown to have an inverse relationship with mortality in cross-sectional studies.[85] Perhaps this relationship is seen because healthier dialysis patients start out with higher blood pressures. However, this mortality benefit does not seem to hold true when the patient starts out with low or normal blood pressures and the blood pressure elevates with dialysis. In one study of over 400 patients on dialysis there was a twofold increase in the odds of hospitalization or death at 6 months in patients who had a blood pressure that increased with dialysis or failed to decrease by the end of the dialysis run when compared with patients who had a blood pressure decrease with dialysis.[86] Intradialytic hypertension seems more common in patients who are older, lower body weight, lower creatinine, lower albumin, and those on more antihypertensive medications.[87] The mechanism of intradialytic hypertension is unclear but most likely represents a state of salt and volume excess.[88] Other proposed mechanisms include increased sympathetic activity, activation of the renin-angiotensin-aldosterone system, endothelial cell dysfunction, vascular stiffness, erythropoietin stimulating agents, and dialysis related factors such as sodium loading, hypercalcemia, hypokalemia, and removal of antihypertensive medications during dialysis.[87] The majority of cases of hypertension during dialysis reported in the literature respond to increased ultrafiltration or prolonged slow ultrafiltration, suggesting volume excess as the predominant factor.[89]

Allergic Reactions

Allergic or hypersensitivity reactions are fortunately rare in hemodialysis patients but can be clinically devastating if not promptly recognized and treated appropriately. Over the course of hemodialysis technological advances, numerous types of anaphylactic (IgE mediated) and anaphylactoid (non-IgE mediated) reactions have been described. Anaphylactic reactions typically present as an acute event with pruritus, erythema, flushing, urticaria, and angioedema. If the episode is severe patients can develop hypotension, shock, laryngeal edema, and respiratory failure. Generally symptoms happen within minutes of starting dialysis but can manifest 30 to 45 minutes into the dialysis treatment. Ethylene oxide (EtO), an agent used in the sterilization of dialyzers, has been associated with allergic type reactions. This can be seen as a "first use" syndrome of dialyzers sterilized with EtO seen on the first dialysis run and not on subsequent uses of the dialyzer. The majority of dialyzers on the market currently are sterilized with steam or radiation, making this entity less frequent. Formaldehyde can be used in the sterilization and preservation of reuse dialyzers and has also been associated with IgE type anaphylactic reactions as well as delayed hypersensitivity reactions.[90] Dialyzer membranes can also be a source of immune stimulation. Polyacrylonitrile membranes are negatively charged and have been shown to increase bradykinin levels via the contact activation pathway. This reaction can be worsened if the patient is taking angiotensin-converting enzyme (ACE) inhibitors concomitantly due to the prolongation of the biologic half-life of bradykinin and other kinins.[91] Newer "biocompatible" synthetic membranes are generally well tolerated and only rarely precipitate an allergic reaction.[92] Heparin administered to dialysis patients can rarely induce anaphylactoid reactions. Heparin-induced thrombocytopenia (HIT) is a more common immune response to heparin leading to thrombocytopenia and a hypercoagulable state. Iron infusion is common in dialysis patients and known to cause allergic reactions, particularly with the administration of iron dextran. Iron preparations free of dextrans such as iron sucrose and sodium ferric gluconate are well tolerated and only rarely associated with allergic reactions. Patients can form allergies to latex from gloves and contact allergies to tape and adhesive products.

The management of allergic reactions depends on the severity of the reaction. In patients with severe reactions, dialysis should be stopped immediately and the blood in the dialysis circuit should be discarded. Acute management of life threatening situations should include the administration of epinephrine, antihistamines, corticosteroids, and attention to supporting potential airway compromise and hemodynamic collapse.[90]

Arrhythmias

Arrhythmias are a common cause of sudden cardiac death in dialysis patients. In a retrospective review of dialysis patients, ventricular arrhythmias were among the most common causes of cardiac arrest.[93] As one may expect, ventricular arrhythmias are a bad prognostic sign. Approximately one half of the patients survived 24 hours after the arrest, one third survived to discharge from hospital, and only 15%

survived 1 year after the arrest. Another review of a large number of dialysis patients provides insight into the risk factors that are associated with cardiac arrest while on dialysis. Older age, dialysis early in the week (Monday), low (0 or 1 mEq/L) potassium dialysate, diabetes, and use of a catheter for dialysis were all associated with higher risk for cardiac arrest and sudden death.[94]

Arrhythmias during the intradialytic period can be related to electrolyte disturbances. Rapid intradialytic shifts of potassium may play a role in precipitating intradialytic arrhythmias. One group looked at 30 arrhythmia-prone dialysis patients and noted that there was a tendency for ventricular ectopy in patients who dialyzed with a constant potassium level in the dialysate as opposed to a tapering potassium level in the dialysate.[95] Potassium profiling may be useful for patients prone to ventricular arrhythmias.

Atrial fibrillation is often present in dialysis patients. In a retrospective review of 488 Italian dialysis patients, atrial fibrillation was reported in approximately 30%.[96] Atrial fibrillation tended to be more common in older patients, patients with an older dialysis vintage, patients with ischemic heart disease, episodes of pulmonary edema, valvular heart disease, cerebrovascular accidents, increased left atrial diameter, and hyperkalemia. Interestingly, diabetes and hypertension were not associated with higher incidence of atrial fibrillation in this series, in contrast to the association seen in the normal population. In a review of USRDS data a prevalence of 10% was noted. One year mortality was noted to be 39% in the patients with atrial fibrillation compared with 19% in those who did not have the diagnosis.[97] The role of anticoagulation for atrial fibrillation in patients with advanced kidney disease is unclear. Patients with advanced kidney disease have increased incidence of both thromboembolism and bleeding events.[98] Previous studies evaluating the use of warfarin to prevent stroke for atrial fibrillation excluded patients with advanced kidney disease and caution should be used before extrapolating their results to dialysis patients.[99] In a cohort of incident HD patients with atrial fibrillation warfarin use was associated with increased incidence of stroke.[100] The risk–benefit balance should be carefully weighed on an individual basis when treating dialysis patients with warfarin.

Muscle Cramps

Muscle cramps are a common cause of intradialytic discomfort and a frequent patient complaint. Cramping can be a sign that the patient has reached an ideal dry body weight or it can be a sign of ultrafiltration rate that is too rapid. Cramps usually can be remedied by administration of normal saline and by discontinuing the ultrafiltration for a period of time. Hypertonic solutions (saline, dextrose, mannitol) may be useful.[101] Manual techniques such as massage or sequential compression also have a role in the prevention of cramps.[102] Avoidance of cramping during dialysis is of utmost importance. Often, cramping leads to patient dissatisfaction with the dialysis procedure and can cause alienation from dialysis caretakers interfering with the ability to attain adequate dialysis. L-carnitine,[103] vitamin E,[104,105] and quinine sulfate[106] have all been suggested to help treat cramps but clear data to support their routine use is lacking. In the evaluation of persistent muscle cramping with dialysis, other reversible causes of cramping should be investigated and ruled out. These include thyroid disorders, hypomagnesemia, hyponatremia, hypocalcemia, and hypokalemia.

Dialysis Disequilibrium Syndrome

Dialysis disequilibrium syndrome (DDS) is a constellation of acute symptoms that was initially described early on in the history of dialysis in the 1960s.[107] DDS can manifest as a variety of symptoms including headache, nausea, vomiting, dizziness, and, in more severe forms, alteration in mentation, seizures, hypotension, shock, and coma. Symptoms are usually mild, transient, and only rarely have been associated with adverse clinical outcomes such as cerebral demyelination or death. Patients at greater risk for DDS include those with a history of previous CNS lesions, children, and persons with hyponatremia. DDS is caused by the development of cerebral edema in dialysis patients during the end of their dialysis session or shortly after dialysis is complete. The mechanism of DDS is hypothesized to involve urea effect, idiogenic osmoles, and/or changes in pH. Rapid removal of urea from the plasma space during dialysis creates a gradient between the intracellular space (high urea concentration) and the extracellular space (lower concentration) in the brain. If cellular mechanisms to move urea out of the cell have been adaptively suppressed due to chronically high urea concentrations then the movement of urea back into the extracellular space will be delayed allowing water to move up an osmotic gradient into the intracellular space causing cell swelling and cerebral edema. The diagnosis of DDS is largely clinical. DDS usually occurs in patients with chronic uremia when first initiated on dialysis. Rapid intradialytic drop in the plasma BUN concentration can precipitate DDS. Management of DDS is largely supportive and revolves around prevention by starting patients with chronic uremia on slow gentle dialysis initially to bring the urea levels down slowly. In cases where the dialysis needs to be performed more rapidly, consideration can be given to adding urea to the dialysate at a concentration that is 10% less than the serum concentration. Hemofiltration, hemodiafiltration, and PD have not been associated with DDS.[108]

Air Embolism

Air embolism is exceedingly rare but a potentially lethal complication of the hemodialysis procedure. Development of a pump-driven dialysis machine with negative arterial pressures created a higher potential for the introduction of air into the hemodialysis circuit. To remedy this potential problem standard hemodialysis machines come equipped with an air detector on the venous limb. This air detector is associated with a clamping mechanism that will clamp the line if air is detected, preventing delivery to the patient. Due to this technological safeguard, machine-related air embolism in dialysis patients has become exceedingly rare. There are other potential causes of air embolism in dialysis patients that are not machine driven. In a fatal case of flawed technique, air was inadvertently administered to a dialysis patient after saline was pushed into a line full of air.[109] Air embolism can also be a complication of intravenous catheters. In one case of inadvertent laceration of a hemodialysis catheter, a patient presented with air embolism and respiratory compromise.[110] Air embolism can happen after catheter removal, particularly if a well-formed tract is present between the skin and the central vein, as is seen in catheters that have been in place for prolonged periods of time. If the patient has an intracardiac shunt, such as a patent foramen ovale, air can be introduced into the arterial system which can have devastating cerebrovascular effects.[111] To prevent air embolism during catheter removal, it is advisable to place the patient in the Trendelenburg position so that the venous pressure elevates and exceeds the atmospheric pressure thereby preventing a negative pressure which can draw air into the vein. If air embolism is suspected, the patient should be immediately placed in the Trendelenburg and left lateral decubitus position to move the air to the apex of the right ventricle and out of the pulmonary circuit. If a catheter is in place, attempts can be made to aspirate the air from the central line.

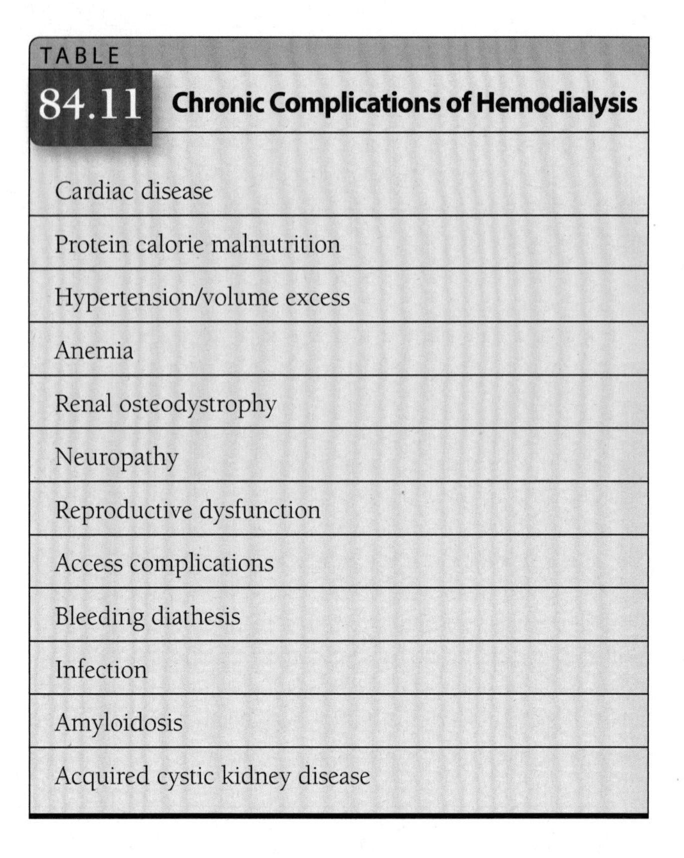

TABLE 84.11 Chronic Complications of Hemodialysis

Chronic Complications of Hemodialysis
Cardiac disease
Protein calorie malnutrition
Hypertension/volume excess
Anemia
Renal osteodystrophy
Neuropathy
Reproductive dysfunction
Access complications
Bleeding diathesis
Infection
Amyloidosis
Acquired cystic kidney disease

CHRONIC COMPLICATIONS OF END-STAGE RENAL DISEASE

The following chronic complications of advanced renal failure (Table 84.11) are described in detail in other chapters of this text: cardiac disease (see Chapter 79), protein calorie malnutrition (see Chapter 85), anemia (see Chapter 76), neuropathy (see Chapter 78), renal osteodystrophy (see Chapter 77), and reproductive dysfunction (see Chapter 80).

Underdialysis

Inadequate delivery of dialysis can be a cause of morbidity in dialysis patients. Underdialysis usually presents subtly with a lack of appetite that can progress to more severe problems such as protein calorie malnutrition. If underdialysis is severe, patients experience the full range of symptoms associated with uremia. Clues to underdialysis lie in the history where patients may complain of pruritus or fatigue in addition to anorexia. Laboratory parameters and urea kinetic modeling may reveal measures of declining solute clearance or even inability to meet monthly adequacy goals. Worsening phosphorus levels or decline in hemoglobin may also be present. Alternatively, if protein calorie malnutrition progresses and is severe enough, patients can have low BUN and phosphorus levels which indicate poor nutrition as opposed to good clearance with dialysis. Underdialysis is most commonly a result of a dysfunctional dialysis access or an inadequate dialysis prescription. Workup of underdialysis should include a close review of the dialysis access for functional problems such as recirculation. In the setting of recirculation, dialysis efficiency is reduced due to blood which is leaving the extracorporeal circuit via the venous limb being taken up by the arterial inflow. In this situation blood which has already been dialyzed is sent through the dialyzer repeatedly leading to a decrease in the overall effectiveness of the therapy systemically. Doppler ultrasonography can be used to evaluate a dysfunctional dialysis access and decide if further intervention is needed to repair or replace it. Recirculation can also be calculated through measurements of arterial, venous, and peripheral blood samples (three-needle method) which can be used to calculate a percent recirculation:

$$\% \text{ Recirculation} = [C_{periph} - C_a / C_{periph} - C_v] * 100$$

Identification of significant recirculation (greater than 15% to 20%) should prompt further investigation of the dialysis access. Recirculation rates tend to be higher when catheters are used for hemodialysis due to the nature of their configuration with the arterial inflow in close proximity of the venous return. Location of the venous catheter tip can also have an effect on catheter recirculation.

After careful evaluation and repair of hemodialysis access problems, treatment of underdialysis involves increasing the dose of dialysis. This most readily can be accomplished by increasing the frequency of dialysis treatments, increasing blood, and/or dialysate flows or by increasing the duration of each dialysis treatment.

Hypertension in End-Stage Renal Disease

The Mechanism of Hypertension in End-Stage Renal Disease *(see also Chapter 41)*

Hypertension is present in 75% to 90% of dialysis patients.[112,113] As a potential risk factor for cardiovascular disease, hypertension has been associated with increased left ventricular mass in dialysis patients.[114,115] Excess sodium and fluid balance is thought to play the predominant role in driving hypertension in ESRD. In particular, large intradialytic weight gains contribute to hypertension in ESRD and may be associated with mortality.[116] In a large cohort study of over 85% of dialysis patients who gained more than 1.5 kg of weight in between dialysis sessions, after controlling for demographics and nutritional factors, higher weight gains were incrementally associated with all-cause and cardiovascular mortality.[117] Endothelial dysfunction, vascular stiffness, activation of the renin–angiotensin–aldosterone system, and increased sympathetic nervous system activity may also contribute.

Ideal Blood Pressure in End-Stage Renal Disease

According to the Joint National Committee on Prevention, Detection, Evaluation, and Treatment of High Blood Pressure (JNC-7) the blood pressure goal for persons with hypertension, diabetes, or renal disease is less than 130/80 mm Hg.[118] These recommendations do not include the ESRD population. In an effort to find the ideal blood pressure for hemodialysis patients, one group studied 5,433 dialysis patients. In the analysis of postdialysis blood pressures they noted a U-shaped curve when graphing relative death rate on the *y*-axis and systolic blood pressure on the *x*-axis. The most favorable postdialysis systolic blood pressures were between 120 and 160 mm Hg. In analysis of the predialysis blood pressures this relationship held true when the blood pressure was low (lower blood pressure was associated with higher mortality). However, higher predialysis systolic hypertension was not associated with higher mortality, forming a J-shaped curve.[85] This relationship between predialysis blood pressures and mortality was confirmed in a study of over 4,000 dialysis patients that were randomly selected[112] and in a subsequent analysis of the HEMO study.[119] Others have argued that blood pressure measurements taken in the ambulatory setting are likely to have a higher prognostic significance than blood pressures that are obtained in center.[120] The relationship between blood pressure and mortality over time may be of importance as well. In a large cohort of nearly 17,000 incident dialysis patients, low systolic blood pressure (<120) was associated with increased mortality in years 1 and 2 after starting dialysis. High blood pressure (>150) was not associated with increased mortality early on but the association was seen in patients who survived over 3 years.[121] Despite these studies, the ideal target for blood pressure in ESRD remains unknown and more study will be needed to define appropriate clinical guidelines.

Treatment Options for Hypertension in End-Stage Renal Disease

Salt restriction and ultrafiltration (preferably through slow, longer dialysis sessions or daily dialysis treatments) are among the most effective options for treatment of hypertension in ESRD. Experience with dialysis patients in Tassin, France, has shown a time-dependent relationship between dialysis and volume control with longer dialysis sessions leading to superior volume control. The benefit of tight volume control has been seen in patients through improved blood pressure values and improved mortality.[122] In a cross-sectional study of ESRD patients from two dialysis centers (~200 patients per center) the differences between a medication intensive therapy versus increased ultrafiltration were evaluated. In one center patients practiced a salt-restricted diet and aggressive ultrafiltration without blood pressure medications. In the other center patients were treated with antihypertensive medications. Blood pressures were similar in both groups but the ultrafiltration group had lower left ventricular mass, lower frequency of left ventricular hypertrophy, and less frequent episodes of intradialytic hypotension.[123] One group performed a randomized controlled trial of 150 hypertensive hemodialysis patients who were randomized to routine dialysis care versus more intensive ultrafiltration to reduce dry weight without increasing duration or frequency of dialysis treatments. Systolic and diastolic blood pressure was reduced in the group with more aggressive ultrafiltration.[89] The downside of aggressive ultrafiltration without increasing the time spent on dialysis is the development of more symptoms associated with rapid fluid removal such as nausea, cramping, dizziness, and intradialytic hypotension. Even so, reduction of dry weight is an effective first step to decreasing blood pressure in dialysis patients.

Therapy with antihypertensive medication is rarely effective without concomitant control of volume status in hemodialysis patients. Often due to financial or time constraints and dietary indiscretion, adequate volume control cannot be achieved in hemodialysis patients through ultrafiltration alone. In such cases, medical therapy may be indicated. First line agents are RAAS blockers, especially in cases with coexisting diabetes and heart disease. RAAS blockers may also be of benefit in preservation of residual renal function. Choosing medical therapies for hypertension in ESRD requires attention to the timing of the dose of medication as well as the clearance of medications with dialysis so as to prevent episodes of intradialytic hypotension. Excessive prescription of antihypertensive agents can lead to the inability to ultrafiltrate and, therefore, inability to achieve adequate volume status.

Vascular Access Complications

Failure of Arteriovenous Fistulae to Mature

The rates of primary fistula failure to mature vary by patient population and center but are estimated to be around 40%.[124] Factors associated with a higher rate of failure to mature include age >65, white race, coronary artery disease, peripheral vascular disease,[125] female gender, and forearm location.[124] Others have found that predialysis vein diameter is the major predictive element in fistula maturity.[126] Fistulae are usually ready for use when they meet the rule of sixes: minimum of 6 mm in diameter, less than 6 mm deep, and blood flows of >600 mL per min. The vessel walls of the fistula should be tough and firm to touch. Reasons for primary failure of fistulae to mature include inadequate anastomosis limiting flow to the fistula, collateral branches off the fistula diverting flow from the main conduit, and thrombosis. Management of fistulae that are failing to mature depends on the clinical scenario but likely will consist of Doppler ultrasonography of the access to evaluate blood flow and identify collateral veins as well as evaluation by a surgeon or nephrologist familiar with the placement of dialysis access.

Access Thrombosis

Access thrombosis can occur at any time in the lifespan of a fistula. Thrombosis is usually due to decreased flow through the fistula which allows blood more time to pool and clot. This can be due to venous outflow stenosis, extrinsic compression to the fistula, or due to arteriovenous anastomotic failure limiting flow to the fistula. Thrombosis occurs more frequently in grafts than native fistulae.[127,128] Patients with thrombosed accesses can present to medical attention following periods of systemic hypotension which precipitated the thrombosis.[129] Access thrombosis can usually be managed by angiography and local mechanical and/or pharmacologic thrombolysis. Percutaneous therapy has been found effective in prolonging survival of fistulae with primary failure due to thrombosis.[130]

Access Stenosis

Vessel intimal and fibromuscular hyperplasia can lead to stenosis of the dialysis access. In the case of PTFE grafts, up to 90% of cases of thrombosis are attributed to venous outflow stenosis developing within 2 to 3 cm of the venous anastomosis of the graft.[131,132] Central venous stenosis is also a common complication of dialysis access with the stenotic lesion developing in the more central venous location in the axillary, subclavian, brachiocephalic, or superior vena cava. Patients who have central vein stenosis can present with facial or neck swelling, extremity swelling, or superficial venous prominence across the chest wall and shoulder. Central venous stenosis is more common in patients with a history of multiple central lines, particularly in the case of central lines placed in the subclavian position or central lines placed on the left side, as well as in patients with pacemakers.[133,134]

Ischemic Injury

Arterial steal is a feared complication of the formation of an arteriovenous access. Particularly in the case of radial artery fistulas, blood can be diverted away from the hand and preferentially circulate through the fistula. Also, a low pressure palmar arch can provide preferential flow for the ulnar artery further diverting blood from the interosseous supply stealing the blood supply to the digits. The end result is ischemic injury to the hand. Symptoms of steal include paresthesias, cool digits, pain, and skin changes. If allowed to persist, steal can result in tissue loss and muscle wasting. Steal syndrome is more common in patients with a history of vascular disease, diabetes, lupus, and hypertension.[135] Steal can occur immediately after the surgical procedure to create the fistula or can present more insidiously over time. Occasionally, a procedure to improve fistula flow such as an angioplasty can exacerbate or unmask symptoms of steal. Treatment of severe steal syndrome usually involves surgical assessment for ligation of the fistula. In certain cases, consideration can be given to performing a distal revascularization and interval ligation (DRIL) procedure which can alleviate the steal while sparing the use of the fistula.[136–139]

Ischemic monomelic neuropathy is a rare form of access steal syndrome where multiple distal neuropathies develop in the limb following placement of the dialysis access. Classically ischemic monomelic neuropathy affects the radial, median, and ulnar nerve distributions (a pan-neuropathy) resulting in loss of motor function, paresthesias, and nerve deficits that are out of proportion to the ischemic findings in other tissues of the hand. As a result, patients can develop functional limitations and a "claw hand." The symptoms usually occur immediately after surgery. Treatment includes efforts at improvement of vascular perfusion and early reversal of the fistula or graft may improve symptoms.[140]

Venous hypertension can also occur in dialysis accesses with chronic thrombosis or stenosis.[141] This typically presents with swelling of the arm or hand distal to the access or distal to the stenotic lesion which can sometimes be in a central location. Digits can also appear cyanotic due to poor venous flow and pooling. Angioplasty of venous stenoses can improve venous hypertension though frequent intervention is often required after a stenosis has been identified in order to maintain the access.[142]

Aneurysms and Pseudoaneurysms

Aneurysms are common late complications of AV fistulas. Most of the time true aneurysms are of little clinical consequence; however, aneurysms can grow to be quite large and should be taken seriously if there are signs of altered integrity that may herald impending rupture. Such signs include skin changes overlying the fistula consistent with thinning, pigment changes, or overt tissue breakdown and scabbing. The presence of a firm aneurysm, pulsatile fistula, or inability of the fistula to collapse upon extremity elevation may point to a venous outflow stenosis or central venous stenosis as the etiology for expansion of an aneurysm. Occasionally, aneurysms can be revised, sparing the function of the fistula.[143] Pseudoaneurysms can be seen with grafts after needle puncture, and if there is an inability to seal off the graft puncture blood can collect under the skin in a hematoma. Rapidly expanding pseudoaneurysms, pain or throbbing, infection, or loss of skin integrity should be taken seriously and require surgical or endovascular repair.[144]

Access Infection

Vascular access infection is common, with infection rates being the highest in catheters, followed by grafts. Infections are rare in the case of the native AVF.[128] Infectious organisms usually are skin flora such as *S. aureus, S. epidermis,* and *Streptococcal* species. Catheters with evidence of a tunnel infection (redness, pus expressed from tunnel, or fluctuance over tunnel) and infected graft material usually need to be removed in order to eradicate the infection.[145] Antibiotic therapy should be tailored to the cultured organism keeping in mind local resistance patterns if culture data is not available. Patients often require prolonged courses of intravenous (IV) antibiotics (6–8 weeks) if endovascular infection is suspected.

Bleeding Diathesis

Under normal conditions, hemostasis is dependent on intricate interplay between the platelet receptor glycoproteins (GPIb, GP IIb/IIIa), von Willebrand factor (vWF), fibrinogen, and the damaged endothelial surface. At areas of injury the subendothelial surface is exposed, vWF binds to the injured surface, platelet glycoprotein GP1b binds vWF, and GP IIb/III3 binds fibrinogen creating a mesh-like network that precipitates further platelet and fibrin aggregation as well as activation of the clotting cascade. Shear stress is required for affinity of the binding of vWF to GPIb.

In uremic states, platelet function is impaired and the normal clotting mechanism is altered. Platelets tend to be hyporesponsive in the setting of bleeding.[146] Typically this results in prolonged bleeding times[147]; however, it should be noted that other defects in platelet and coagulation cascade have been associated with an increased risk of thrombosis in dialysis patients as well.[148] The underlying mechanisms of platelet dysfunction in the uremic environment are unclear. Platelet aggregation may be impaired due to GP IIb/IIIa dysfunction or a uremic toxin that inhibits binding of GP IIb/IIIa to fibrinogen.[149] Abnormalities in the interaction between GPIb and vWF may also play a role. Increased levels of glycocalicin, a cleavage product of GPIb, has been demonstrated in dialysis patients.[150] Other mechanisms involved could include higher levels of prostacyclins and nitric oxide, reduction in platelet ADP levels, abnormal calcium signaling, altered blood rheology, and altered thromboxane-A2 production.[151] It is clear that uremic bleeding is not caused by elevated BUN as evidenced by studies of patients with rare urea disorders in the setting of normal renal function.[152]

Treatment of bleeding diathesis revolves around improvement of the uremic condition. Peritoneal dialysis seems to have a stronger association with clotting abnormalities as opposed to bleeding abnormalities when compared with hemodialysis, possibly due to increased middle molecule clearance, decreased platelet activation via dialysis membranes, and lack of need for anticoagulation with agents such as heparin.[153,154] Correction of anemia is also important as anemia is associated with prolonged bleeding times. In situations of active uremic bleeding, desmopressin (DDAVP) can be administered. DDAVP induces the release of vWF, leading to increased platelet adhesion and has been shown to be effective.[155] Recommended dose is 0.3 μg per kg given IV in 50 mL of NS over 30 minutes. DDAVP will act within 1 hour and the effect lasts up to 8 hours. More than two successive administrations of DDAVP are not likely to be effective due to depletion of vWF stores. Conjugated estrogens, cryoprecipitate, and activated factor VII can also be considered in cases of serious uremic bleeding.[156]

Infectious Complications

The following section is limited to infectious issues pertinent to the dialysis patient but not related to dialysis access.

Tuberculosis

Infection with *Mycobacterium tuberculosis* is more common in dialysis patients than the general population. The increased risk of tuberculosis in dialysis patients is believed to be due to impaired cellular immunity.[157] Risk factors for tuberculosis in dialysis patients in the United States include advanced age, unemployment, Medicaid insurance, reduced body mass index, decreased serum albumin, Asian and Native American race, ischemic heart disease, smoking, illicit drug use, and anemia.[158] Active tuberculosis in dialysis patients often presents with extrapulmonary manifestations which can make the diagnosis difficult.[159] Latent tuberculosis infection (LTBI) is believed to affect anywhere from 20% to 70% of patients.[158] Diagnosis of LTBI can be difficult but is of paramount importance as patients with LTBI on dialysis should be aggressively treated to prevent reactivation of infection and transmission to other patients in the dialysis center. Traditionally, diagnosis of LTBI has relied on the tuberculin skin test; however, this method is less sensitive in dialysis patients owing to high rates of anergy (up to 44%).[160,161] Newer testing strategies with interferon gamma release assays (TSPOT and QuantiFERON-TB) take advantage of two proteins which are specific to *M. tuberculosis* (not found in other forms of mycobacterium, including the BCG vaccine) known as early secretory antigenic target 6 (ESAT-6) and culture filtrate protein 10 (CFP-10). ESAT-6 and CFP-10 are antigenic targets for T cells. When T cells encounter these proteins they release interferon gamma (IFN-γ). Therefore, by measuring T cell secretion of IFN-γ when exposed to ESAT-6 and CFP-10 one can indirectly test for the presence of *M. tuberculosis*. The role of IFN-γ release assays is unclear in the diagnosis of LTBI in dialysis patients; however, they appear to be useful in the setting of previous BCG vaccination,[162] recent exposure,[163] or active infection.[164] Treatment of tuberculosis in hemodialysis patients varies depending upon the activity of disease and location of infection. Care should be taken to dose anti-tuberculin medications after dialysis.[165]

Hepatitis B

Historically, hepatitis B has been a significant pathogen in the hemodialysis population. In 1974, the incidence of newly acquired hepatitis B infection in dialysis patients was 6.2%; this number dropped to 0.06% by 1999 after widespread implementation of guidelines to prevent the spread of hepatitis B in dialysis units.[166] Hepatitis B can cause acute and/or chronic hepatitis and usually has an insidious onset. The hepatitis B virus is transmitted by percutaneous or mucosal transfer of blood or bodily fluids. Hepatitis B is remarkable in that it is stable at room temperature for up to 7 days on artificial surfaces.[167] Due to the potential ability of dialysis staff to transfer virus from one patient to another, guidelines have been developed by the Centers for Disease Control and Prevention (CDC) and endorsed by the Centers for Medicare and Medicaid Services (CMS) as a condition for coverage of a dialysis unit. These guidelines include isolation of dialysis patients with hepatitis B in a separate room, assignment of specific staff to hepatitis B patients alone (preventing simultaneous care for any patients who are hepatitis B susceptible), assignment of dialysis equipment to hepatitis B patients alone without sharing with other patients, assignment of a separate set of supplies, cleaning and disinfection of all equipment before use on another patient, use of gloves and glove changes between patients, and routine cleaning of all environmental surfaces. Dialyzers should not be reused in patients with hepatitis B infection. The guidelines also recommend routine serologic screening for hepatitis B and, in particular, monthly screening for patients who are hepatitis B susceptible.[167] Hepatitis B serologic status should be known for all patients prior to admission to a dialysis unit and testing should be repeated upon transfer to a different dialysis unit.

Hepatitis C

The hepatitis C virus can cause acute and chronic hepatitis. The course of hepatitis C is variable but the disease seems to be milder in dialysis patients. Patients tend to have lower viral loads, lower inflammatory activity, and lower amounts of fibrosis on liver biopsy.[168] Hepatitis C is transmitted through exposure to infected blood. Risk factors for infection include history of blood transfusions, intravenous drug use, and dialysis vintage. The CDC recommends routine screening for hepatitis C with monthly liver enzyme tests and every 6-month checks of hepatitis C antibodies. Liver function tests are of use in screening for hepatitis C because around 90% of hemodialysis patients with hepatitis C will have elevated ALT levels.[166] If unexplained liver enzyme elevations are noted, hepatitis C testing should be pursued with addition of polymerase chain reaction (PCR) for hepatitis C RNA if the enzyme-linked immunosorbent assay (ELISA) for hepatitis C antibody is negative. It has been proposed that hepatitis C infection can be occult in hemodialysis patients manifesting as a negative serum antibody, negative serum PCR for hepatitis C RNA, but detectable hepatitis C virus in mononuclear cells and liver tissue.[169] Occult hepatitis C is a consideration in patients with unexplained persistently elevated ALT levels; however, the clinical significance of occult infection remains unclear. Unlike hepatitis B patients, patients with hepatitis C do not require strict isolation. Rather, they require adherence to routine infection prevention practices applicable to all dialysis patients. Dedicated machines for patients with hepatitis C are not necessary and dialyzers can be reused if processed appropriately.

Patients on hemodialysis can be considered for treatment of hepatitis C, particularly if they are kidney transplant candidates. Typically ESRD patients are treated with dose adjusted standard interferon (IFN): 3 MU three times weekly subcutaneously (SQ) as monotherapy. Length of therapy depends on the genotype and is usually around 48 weeks for genotypes 1 and 4 and 24 weeks for genotypes 2 and 3. Viral load is typically checked at 12 weeks to evaluate the response to therapy.[170] Sustained virologic response to monotherapy in dialysis patients is around 37%,[171] which is higher than rates of persons with normal renal function treated with standard IFN (7% to 16%) and lower than persons treated with dual therapy including ribavirin. Proposed mechanisms for improved efficacy of IFN in dialysis patients include lower viral load, milder histologic disease, lower clearance of IFN, and increased endogenous release of IFN.[172] Pegylated IFN has not been extensively studied in the dialysis population but appears to provide no additional benefit when compared to standard IFN.[170] Ribavirin is usually not used as clearance is impaired in kidney disease and the drug carries an increased risk of hemolytic anemia. Even so, limited case reports have reported on successful use of dual therapy with careful monitoring.[173] Patients on dialysis seem to suffer from higher rates of side effects due to IFN therapy. Dropout rate due to side effects is around 17% for dialysis patients compared with 5% to 9% in patients without kidney disease.[170]

Vaccinations

Clinical practice guidelines recommend annual influenza immunization, hepatitis B immunization, and pneumococcal immunization for all dialysis patients.

Influenza vaccination is recommended on an annual basis. Live attenuated virus should not be used in dialysis patients. Immunization against influenza provides approximately the same rates of seroprotection in dialysis patients as the general population (~80%).[174]

In the general population, 90% to 95% of adults develop protective antibodies to hepatitis B after immunization. The effectiveness of the vaccine in dialysis patients is much lower and patients on dialysis require a higher dose of vaccine or an increased number of administrations. Studies have shown only 64% protection after a standard three dose regimen of hepatitis B vaccination, but this number can be improved to 86% if the vaccine series is increased to four doses. A special hepatitis B vaccine has been developed for dialysis patients which is higher dose (Recombivax HB 40 μg per mL).

Testing for immunogenicity can be performed 1 to 2 months after the last dose of vaccine to ensure patient response (goal hepatitis B surface antibody titer >10 mIU per mL). Booster doses should be administered to patients previously vaccinated if their hepatitis B surface antibody titers fall below 10 mIU per mL.[175] Based on the observation that combined hepatitis A and B immunization improves immunogenicity to hepatitis B in the general population, a randomized controlled clinical trial comparing combined hepatitis A and hepatitis B vaccination with hepatitis B vaccination alone was performed in dialysis patients which showed improvement in seroprotection when hepatitis A was added.[176] Therefore, it is advisable to administer hepatitis A vaccination at the same time or in combination with hepatitis B vaccination.

Pneumococcal vaccination is recommended every 5 years for dialysis patients; however, this interval can be shortened to 3 years if it is felt that the patient is at high risk for a pneumococcal infection.[175] Pneumococcal vaccination in dialysis patients has been associated with lower mortality risk.[177]

Amyloidosis

Dialysis-related amyloidosis is a disease entity seen only in ESRD patients and differs from other forms of systemic amyloidosis. In persons without renal disease, β2-microglobulin is freely filtered by the glomerulus then taken up in the proximal tubule and metabolized.[178] In ESRD clearance of β2-microglobulin is impaired and serum levels rise and accumulation of β2-microglobulin subsequently forms fibrils in tissues. Deposition of amyloid fibrils seems to have a predilection for articular tissues and bone but can deposit in all tissues. Clinically, the afflicted manifest joint pain and stiffness. Chronic arthralgias can progress to a destructive arthropathy. Most commonly the carpal tunnel is involved. The shoulders are another site of frequent involvement. Amyloid can also involve the synovial membranes and tendons of the hand leading to trigger finger or contractures. Amyloid deposits in bone can lead to pathologic fracture of long bones. Vascular deposition of amyloid may play a role in the vascular disease seen in patients with ESRD. Clinically significant visceral involvement is less common but can be found in the GI tract, heart, lung, liver, ovaries, ureter, and subcutaneous tissue.[179] Amyloid has been associated with GI bleeding, bowel infarction, and pseudo-obstruction.[180,181] Amyloidosis of ESRD usually manifests in patients who have been on dialysis for more than 10 years and becomes more common (up to 100%) in patients who have been on dialysis for more than 30 years.[182] The disease appears to be uncommon as the majority of dialysis patients do not live long enough for it to become clinically relevant. Even so, amyloid deposition appears to occur early in the course of ESRD. This observation has been noted on histologic autopsy studies demonstrating presence of amyloid prior to clinically evident disease.[183] Clearance of β2-microglobulin may be better in peritoneal dialysis.[184] Regardless, the histologic prevalence of amyloid in peritoneal dialysis patients did not differ from HD patients in one study of joint samples from continuous ambulatory peritoneal dialysis (CAPD) patients.[185] Newer, commonly used high flux dialyzers are more effective at removing β2-microglobulin from the circulation and probably account for the declining incidence of clinically relevant disease.[186–188] Convective forms of solute removal such as hemofiltration, in combination with dialysis (hemodiafiltration) are also more effective at middle molecule clearance. Management of the dialysis patient with amyloidosis centers around symptomatic treatments and local procedures such as carpal tunnel release. Patients who receive a renal transplantation usually have improvement in symptoms.[189]

Acquired Cystic Kidney Disease

Under circumstances of normal health, even persons without renal disease can acquire cysts in the renal parenchyma as they age. Acquired cystic kidney disease (ACKD) refers to persons with ESRD who develop at least three cysts in a kidney which were not present before the onset of renal failure and which cannot be explained by other inherited renal cystic conditions. Renal cysts are seen in over 80% of patients who have been on dialysis for more than 10 years.[190] Longer time on dialysis is a risk factor for the development of ACKD and this risk is also associated with higher rates of renal cell carcinoma (RCC).[191] The progression of ACKD may exist along a spectrum where cystic lesions evolve from simple to complex and on to form carcinoma.[192] The specific cause of ACKD is unknown but may be related to an increase in proliferation of renal tubular epithelial cells. The observation that cysts can improve after renal transplantation has led some to believe that the underlying mechanism of cyst formation may be related to the uremic environment.[193] Patients with RCC associated with ACKD often have multifocal and bilateral lesions. Clinical features of ACKD are often silent. Rarely patients can present with hematuria, flank pain, or spontaneous retroperitoneal bleeding. ESRD patients rarely die from metastatic RCC. Therefore, screening for disease is controversial and guidelines for screening in ACKD are not universally agreed upon, even in the post-kidney transplantation population.[194]

Neoplasia

It has been proposed that ESRD patients may be at a higher risk for cancer than the general population due to multiple factors. The uremic milieu may contribute to tumor formation. Increased oxidant stress and chronic inflammation seen in dialysis patients can lead to DNA alteration. Depressed immune system function may allow cancerous cells to grow unchecked and allow cancers that are associated with infectious pathogens to proliferate. Further, previous treatment with immunomodulatory medications may predispose to development of cancer (e.g., cyclophosphamide which has been associated with genitourinary cancers or rituximab which has been associated with lymphoproliferative disorders). Early reports and case series did not support the findings of increased rates of cancer in dialysis patients[195,196] but more recent and larger series seem to point toward an association between certain types of cancer and ESRD. In a population-based cohort study an association was seen between patients with ESRD who were receiving renal replacement therapy and higher rates of RCC, liver carcinoma, and lymphomas.[197] In an international collaborative study[198] 831,804 patients who received dialysis from 1980 to 1994 were reviewed. They observed that 25,044 patients were diagnosed with cancer compared with the expected number of 21,185 patients if using normal population incidences. Higher risk was seen in younger patients and decreased with age. Significantly increased cancer risk was confined to specific tissues with cancers of the kidney, bladder, thyroid, tongue, liver, lymphoma, and multiple myeloma being more common. They noted that tumors in these areas are often associated with viral infections (human papilloma virus, Epstein Barr virus, hepatitis C), which suggests a role of impaired immunologic function in tumor pathogenesis. Cancers of the lung, prostate, breast, stomach, and colorectum were not increased compared to the general population. There is also an association between increased risk of kidney and urinary tract cancers in toxic nephropathies such as analgesic nephropathy and Balkan nephropathy. Risk for developing RCC increases with increasing time spent on dialysis whereas risk for developing bladder cancer decreases with time on dialysis.[199]

Consensus screening guidelines for cancer in ESRD do not exist currently. Given that malignancy is not a major cause of mortality in dialysis patients, cancer pathology in ESRD seems to differ from pathology in the general population. Furthermore, the expected longevity of the dialysis population is much less compared with that of the general population. Therefore, applying screening guidelines from the general population to dialysis patients seems inappropriate. The decision to screen ESRD patients for cancer should be customized to the individual dialysis patient taking into account inherent risks, the usefulness of the results obtained with the screening study, and its impact on future management.[200] Over time, as dialysis technology and medical therapy improves, and dialysis patients live longer, further study should guide recommendations for screening which will become more of a clinical necessity to protect the longevity of dialysis patients.

Psychosocial Problems

Psychiatric illnesses seem to be more common in patients with ESRD. When compared with patients with other chronic illnesses, hospitalization with mental disorders was 1.5 to 3 times higher in patients with renal failure. Of all psychosocial problems that dialysis patients suffer from, depression is the most common with estimates of 20% to 30% of dialysis patients afflicted with depression.[201]

Depression in dialysis patients may be driven by feelings of futility, loss of hope, fear, loss of control, loss of employment, financial stress, and altered family relationships. Higher prevalence of comorbid conditions and lower body mass index is associated with depression.[202] Patients on dialysis who have depression have been found to have impaired cognitive function.[203] Elective withdrawal from dialysis has been linked to depression and occurs in 9% to 20% of ESRD patients. Stopping dialysis is a decision seen more often in the elderly, white patients, or women. High disease burden associated with malnutrition, dementia, malignancy, and other chronic disease states is also a risk factor.[204] Withdrawal from dialysis is not considered suicide; however, actual suicide rates are higher in dialysis patients compared with those of the general population. One study showed patients on dialysis were found to have an 84% higher rate of active suicide compared with that of the general population.[205] This was true for all age groups except age 15 to 29 which had lower suicide rates. The increased rate of suicide did not hold true across all races. Whereas whites and Asians had higher suicide rates, African American suicide rates were similar to those of the general population.

Anxiety also appears to be common with 18% seen in the national comorbidity survey[206] and rates up to 27% in other studies.[201,202] Anxiety can adversely affect dialysis patients, particularly when it interferes with their ability to complete a dialysis treatment session.

HOME HEMODIALYSIS

Home hemodialysis has been available since the early days of chronic renal replacement therapy when physicians realized that more patients could be offered hemodialysis if the patient was willing to shoulder some of the burden and cost involved in the administration of their care.[207] Limitations in the availability of in-center dialysis at the time drove many patients to home dialysis. Later, when dialysis therapy began to be financially supported by governments around the world, there was a shift from home to in-center therapies.

The benefits of home hemodialysis may include improved patient independence, flexibility with dialysis schedule, ability to provide more dialysis than what is offered in-center, improved health and quality of life,[208] as well as better survival.[209] Hospitalization rates are lower in home hemodialysis patients when compared to peritoneal dialysis patients.[210] Although these findings may represent a selection bias of healthier patients on home hemodialysis it may also be due to improved well-being and improved dialysis therapy. Home hemodialysis is considered an adequate bridge to transplantation and may even be an adequate substitution for transplant. A cohort study of the USRDS over 12 years showed no difference in survival between patients on home hemodialysis and patients who received a deceased donor transplant.[211] On the other hand, recipients of a living donor transplant tended to do better than home hemodialysis patients.

Home hemodialysis provides flexibility in schedules which can be adjusted to fit the patient. Short daily hemodialysis (SDHD) is usually done 5 to 6 days per week for 2 to 3 hours and nocturnal home hemodialysis (NHHD) is usually done 5 to 6 nights per week for more than 6 hours. Home dialysis can also be done on the more traditional schedule of three times weekly for 4 hours per treatment. NHHD has the added benefit of extended time on dialysis without much intrusion into day-to-day life. Significant barriers exist to implementation of home hemodialysis including the patient's physical capabilities, fear, anxiety, and feelings of being a burden to their family. Remote monitoring, patient counseling, and education can help alleviate some of those fears.[212]

Home hemodialysis is somewhat hindered by access to water purification systems which are expensive to set up and can require extensive plumbing changes. Development of newer compact dialysis technologies using slow dialysate flow and dialysate saturation as well as newer sorbent-based systems should help to work around this problem by providing water-efficient dialysis. Currently used water-efficient dialysis technologies often use sterile dialysate in preformed bags. The anionic base used in the dialysate can be lactate as opposed to bicarbonate. This should be kept in mind in patients with liver disease as metabolism of lactate will be impaired, potentially leading to increased serum lactate concentrations. Other systems utilize streamlined water treatment systems for in-home generation of smaller quantities of dialysate.

Medication changes are common after starting patients on home hemodialysis. Volume control with frequent or daily dialysis is often superior and subsequently there is less need for antihypertensive medications.[213] Phosphorus levels decrease and binder medications often need to be adjusted or discontinued, particularly in patients on NHHD.[214] With more frequent hemodialysis bone marrow responsiveness to erythropoietin therapy improves,[215] although patients on more frequent dialysis may require higher iron and erythropoietin doses to keep up with increased blood loss involved with an increased frequency of dialysis treatment.[216]

REFERENCES

1. Abel JJ, Rowntree LG, Turner BB. On the removal of diffusable substances from the circulating blood by means of dialysis. Transactions of the Association of American Physicians, 1913. *Transfus Sci.* 1990;11(2):164–165.
2. Wizemann V, Benedum J. Nephrology dialysis transplantation 70th anniversary of haemodialysis—the pioneering contribution of Georg Haas (1886–1971). *Nephrol Dial Transplant.* 1994;9(12):1829–1831.
3. Kolff WJ, Berk HT, ter Welle M, van der LA, van Dijk EC, van Noordwijk J. The artificial kidney: a dialyser with a great area. 1944. *J Am Soc Nephrol.* 1997;8(12):1959–1965.
4. Quinton W, Dillard D, Scribner BH. Cannulation of blood vessels for prolonged hemodialysis. *Trans Am Soc Artif Intern Organs.* 1960;6:104–113.
5. Gramaticopolo S, Chronopoulos A, Piccinni P, et al. Extracorporeal CO2 removal—a way to achieve ultraprotective mechanical ventilation and lung support: the missing piece of multiple organ support therapy. *Contrib Nephrol.* 2010;165:174–184.
6. Struthers J, Allan A, Peel RK, Lambie SH. Buttonhole needling of ateriovenous fistulae: a randomized controlled trial. *Asaio J.* 2010;56(4):319–322.
7. Nesrallah GE, Cuerden M, Wong JH, Pierratos A. Staphylococcus aureus bacteremia and buttonhole cannulation: long-term safety and efficacy of mupirocin prophylaxis. *Clin J Am Soc Nephrol.* 2010;5(6):1047–1053.
8. Barrett N, Spencer S, McIvor J, Brown EA. Subclavian stenosis: a major complication of subclavian dialysis catheters. *Nephrol Dial Transplant.* 1988; 3(4):423–425.
9. Fant GF, Dennis VW, Quarles LD. Late vascular complications of the subclavian dialysis catheter. *Am J Kidney Dis.* 1986;7(3):225–228.
10. Hoen B, Paul-Dauphin A, Hestin D, Kessler M. EPIBACDIAL: a multicenter prospective study of risk factors for bacteremia in chronic hemodialysis patients. *J Am Soc Nephrol.* 1998;9(5):869–876.
11. Little MA, O'Riordan A, Lucey B, et al. A prospective study of complications associated with cuffed, tunnelled haemodialysis catheters. *Nephrol Dial Transplant.* 2001;16(11):2194–2200.
12. Twardowski ZJ, Van Stone JC, Jones ME, Klusmeyer ME, Haynie JD. Blood recirculation in intravenous catheters for hemodialysis. *J Am Soc Nephrol.* 1993;3(12):1978–1981.
13. Ash SR. Fluid mechanics and clinical success of central venous catheters for dialysis—answers to simple but persisting problems. *Semin Dial.* 2007; 20(3):237–256.
14. MacRae JM, Ahmed A, Johnson N, Levin A, Kiaii M. Central vein stenosis: a common problem in patients on hemodialysis. *Asaio J.* 2005;51(1):77–81.
15. Weijmer MC, Vervloet MG, ter Wee PM. Compared to tunnelled cuffed haemodialysis catheters, temporary untunnelled catheters are associated with more complications already within 2 weeks of use. *Nephrol Dial Transplant.* 2004;19(3):670–677.
16. Malinauskas RA. Decreased hemodialysis circuit pressures indicating post-pump tubing kinks: a retrospective investigation of hemolysis in five patients. *Hemodial Int.* 2008;12(3):383–393.
17. Duffy R, Tomashek K, Spangenberg M, et al. Multistate outbreak of hemolysis in hemodialysis patients traced to faulty blood tubing sets. *Kidney Int.* 2000;57(4):1668–1674.
18. De Wachter DS, Verdonck PR, Verhoeven RF, Hombrouckx RO. Red cell injury assessed in a numeric model of a peripheral dialysis needle. *Asaio J.* 1996;42(5):M524–529.
19. Misra M. The basics of hemodialysis equipment. *Hemodial Int.* 2005;9(1): 30–36.
20. van der Sande FM, Wystrychowski G, Kooman JP, et al. Control of core temperature and blood pressure stability during hemodialysis. *Clin J Am Soc Nephrol.* 2009;4(1):93–98.
21. Vesconi S, Cruz DN, Fumagalli R, et al. Delivered dose of renal replacement therapy and mortality in critically ill patients with acute kidney injury. *Crit Care.* 2009;13(2):R57.
22. Palevsky PM, Zhang JH, O'Connor TZ, et al. Intensity of renal support in critically ill patients with acute kidney injury. *N Engl J Med.* 2008;359(1):7–20.
23. Tolwani AJ, Campbell RC, Stofan BS, Lai KR, Oster RA, Wille KM. Standard versus high-dose CVVHDF for ICU-related acute renal failure. *J Am Soc Nephrol.* 2008;19(6):1233–1238.
24. Bellomo R, Cass A, Cole L, et al. Intensity of continuous renal-replacement therapy in critically ill patients. *N Engl J Med.* 2009;361(17):1627–1638.
25. Pontoriero G, Pozzoni P, Andrulli S, Locatelli F. The quality of dialysis water. *Nephrol Dial Transplant.* 2003;18 Suppl 7:vii21–25; discussion vii56.
26. Fischer KG. Essentials of anticoagulation in hemodialysis. *Hemodial Int.* 2007;11(2):178–189.
27. Ahmad S. Essentials of water treatment in hemodialysis. *Hemodial Int.* 2005;9(2):127–134.
28. McIvor ME. Acute fluoride toxicity. Pathophysiology and management. *Drug Saf.* 1990;5(2):79–85.
29. Pontoriero G, Pozzoni P, Andrulli S, Locatelli F. [The quality of dialysis water]. *G Ital Nefrol.* 2004;21 Suppl 30:S42–45.
30. Ledebo I. Ultrapure dialysis fluid—how pure is it and do we need it? *Nephrol Dial Transplant.* 2007;22(1):20–23.
31. Ledebo I, Nystrand R. Defining the microbiological quality of dialysis fluid. *Artif Organs.* 1999;23(1):37–43.
32. Vaslaki LR, Berta K, Major L, et al. On-line hemodiafiltration does not induce inflammatory response in end-stage renal disease patients: results from a multicenter cross-over study. *Artif Organs.* 2005;29(5):406–412.
33. Ledebo I. On-line preparation of solutions for dialysis: practical aspects versus safety and regulations. *J Am Soc Nephrol.* 2002;13 Suppl 1:S78–83.
34. Babb AL, Ahmad S, Bergstrom J, Scribner BH. The middle molecule hypothesis in perspective. *Am J Kidney Dis.* 1981;1(1):46–50.
35. Blagg CR. The early history of dialysis for chronic renal failure in the United States: a view from Seattle. *Am J Kidney Dis.* 2007;49(3):482–496.
36. Vanholder R, Van Laecke S, Glorieux G. The middle-molecule hypothesis 30 years after: lost and rediscovered in the universe of uremic toxicity? *J Nephrol.* 2008;21(2):146–160.
37. Jourde-Chiche N, Dou L, Cerini C, Dignat-George F, Vanholder R, Brunet P. Protein-bound toxins—update 2009. *Semin Dial.* 2009;22(4):334–339.
38. Schepers E, Glorieux G, Vanholder R. The gut: the forgotten organ in uremia? *Blood Purif.* 2010;29(2):130–136.
39. Gotch FA, Sargent JA. A mechanistic analysis of the National Cooperative Dialysis Study (NCDS). *Kidney Int.* 1985;28(3):526–534.

40. Daugirdas JT. Second generation logarithmic estimates of single-pool variable volume Kt/V: an analysis of error. *J Am Soc Nephrol.* 1993;4(5):1205–1213.

41. Depner TA. Hemodialysis adequacy: basic essentials and practical points for the nephrologist in training. *Hemodial Int.* 2005;9(3):241–254.

42. Tattersall JE, DeTakats D, Chamney P, Greenwood RN, Farrington K. The post-hemodialysis rebound: predicting and quantifying its effect on Kt/V. *Kidney Int.* 1996;50(6):2094–2102.

43. Gotch FA. The current place of urea kinetic modelling with respect to different dialysis modalities. *Nephrol Dial Transplant.* 1998;13 Suppl 6:10–14.

44. Leypoldt JK. Urea standard Kt/V(urea) for assessing dialysis treatment adequacy. *Hemodial Int.* 2004;8(2):193–197.

45. Daugirdas JT, Depner TA, Greene T, et al. Standard Kt/Vurea: a method of calculation that includes effects of fluid removal and residual kidney clearance. *Kidney Int.* 2010;77(7):637–644.

46. Hakim RM, Depner TA, Parker TF III. Adequacy of hemodialysis. *Am J Kidney Dis.* 1992;20(2):107–123.

47. Shinaberger CS, Kilpatrick RD, Regidor DL, et al. Longitudinal associations between dietary protein intake and survival in hemodialysis patients. *Am J Kidney Dis.* 2006;48(1):37–49.

48. Beddhu S, Samore MH, Roberts MS, et al. Impact of timing of initiation of dialysis on mortality. *J Am Soc Nephrol.* 2003;14(9):2305–2312.

49. Sawhney S, Djurdjev O, Simpson K, Macleod A, Levin A. Survival and dialysis initiation: comparing British Columbia and Scotland registries. *Nephrol Dial Transplant.* 2009;24(10):3186–3192.

50. Clark WF, Na Y, Rosansky SJ, et al. Association between estimated glomerular filtration rate at initiation of dialysis and mortality. *CMAJ.* 2011; 183(1):47–53.

51. Wright S, Klausner D, Baird B, et al. Timing of dialysis initiation and survival in ESRD. *Clin J Am Soc Nephrol.* 2010;5(10):1828–1835.

52. Cooper BA, Branley P, Bulfone L, et al. A randomized, controlled trial of early versus late initiation of dialysis. *N Engl J Med.* 2010;363(7):609–619.

53. Lowrie EG, Laird NM, Parker TF, Sargent JA. Effect of the hemodialysis prescription of patient morbidity: report from the National Cooperative Dialysis Study. *N Engl J Med.* 1981;305(20):1176–1181.

54. Held PJ, Levin NW, Bovbjerg RR, et al. Mortality and duration of hemodialysis treatment. *JAMA.* 1991;265(7):871–875.

55. Hornberger JC, Chernew M, Petersen J, et al. A multivariate analysis of mortality and hospital admissions with high-flux dialysis. *J Am Soc Nephrol.* 1992;3(6):1227–1237.

56. Owen WF Jr, Lew NL, Liu Y, et al. The urea reduction ratio and serum albumin concentration as predictors of mortality in patients undergoing hemodialysis. *N Engl J Med.* 1993;329(14):1001–1006.

57. Port FK, Wolfe RA, Hulbert-Shearon TE, et al. Mortality risk by hemodialyzer reuse practice and dialyzer membrane characteristics: results from the USRDS dialysis morbidity and mortality study. *Am J Kidney Dis.* 2001;37(2): 276–286.

58. Koda Y, Nishi S, Miyazaki S, et al. Switch from conventional to high-flux membrane reduces the risk of carpal tunnel syndrome and mortality of hemodialysis patients. *Kidney Int.* 1997;52(4):1096–1101.

59. Locatelli F, Mastrangelo F, Redaelli B, et al. Effects of different membranes and dialysis technologies on patient treatment tolerance and nutritional parameters. The Italian Cooperative Dialysis Study Group. *Kidney Int.* 1996; 50(4):1293–1302.

60. Collins AJ, Ma JZ, Umen A, Keshaviah P. Urea index and other predictors of hemodialysis patient survival. *Am J Kidney Dis.* 1994;23(2):272–282.

61. Held PJ, Port FK, Wolfe RA, et al. The dose of hemodialysis and patient mortality. *Kidney Int.* 1996;50(2):550–556.

62. Eknoyan G, Beck GJ, Cheung AK, et al. Effect of dialysis dose and membrane flux in maintenance hemodialysis. *N Engl J Med.* 2002;347(25): 2010–2019.

63. Cheung AK, Levin NW, Greene T, et al. Effects of high-flux hemodialysis on clinical outcomes: results of the HEMO study. *J Am Soc Nephrol.* 2003; 14(12):3251–3263.

64. Delmez JA, Yan G, Bailey J, et al. Cerebrovascular disease in maintenance hemodialysis patients: results of the HEMO Study. *Am J Kidney Dis.* 2006;47(1): 131–138.

65. Locatelli F, Martin-Malo A, Hannedouche T, et al. Effect of membrane permeability on survival of hemodialysis patients. *J Am Soc Nephrol.* 2009;20(3):645–654.

66. Chertow GM, Levin NW, Beck GJ, et al. In-center hemodialysis six times per week versus three times per week. *N Engl J Med.* 2010;363(24):2287–2300.

67. Suranyi M, Chow JS. Review: anticoagulation for haemodialysis. *Nephrology (Carlton).* 2010;15(4):386–392.

68. Cronin RE, Reilly RF. Unfractionated heparin for hemodialysis: still the best option. *Semin Dial.* 2010;23(5):510–515.

69. von Brecht JH, Flanigan MJ, Freeman RM, Lim VS. Regional anticoagulation: hemodialysis with hypertonic trisodium citrate. *Am J Kidney Dis.* 1986;8(3): 196–201.

70. Durao MS, Monte JC, Batista MC, et al. The use of regional citrate anticoagulation for continuous venovenous hemodiafiltration in acute kidney injury. *Crit Care Med.* 2008;36(11):3024–3029.

71. Kossmann RJ, Gonzales A, Callan R, Ahmad S. Increased efficiency of hemodialysis with citrate dialysate: a prospective controlled study. *Clin J Am Soc Nephrol.* 2009;4(9):1459–1464.

72. Feldman HI, Kobrin S, Wasserstein A. Hemodialysis vascular access morbidity. *J Am Soc Nephrol.* 1996;7(4):523–535.

73. Clinical practice guidelines for vascular access. *Am J Kidney Dis.* 2006;48 Suppl 1:S176–247.

74. Lacson E Jr, Wang W, Lazarus JM, Hakim RM. Change in vascular access and mortality in maintenance hemodialysis patients. *Am J Kidney Dis.* 2009; 54(5):912–921.

75. Fitzgerald JT, Schanzer A, Chin AI, McVicar JP, Perez RV, Troppmann C. Outcomes of upper arm arteriovenous fistulas for maintenance hemodialysis access. *Arch Surg.* 2004;139(2):201–208.

76. Allon M, Lockhart ME, Lilly RZ, et al. Effect of preoperative sonographic mapping on vascular access outcomes in hemodialysis patients. *Kidney Int.* 2001; 60(5):2013–2020.

77. Maya ID, Allon M. Vascular access: core curriculum 2008. *Am J Kidney Dis.* 2008;51(4):702–708.

78. Madden RL, Lipkowitz GS, Browne BJ, et al. A comparison of cryopreserved vein allografts and prosthetic grafts for hemodialysis access. *Ann Vasc Surg.* 2005;19(5):686–691.

79. Hurt AV, Batello-Cruz M, Skipper BJ, Teaf SR, Sterling WA Jr. Bovine carotid artery heterografts versus polytetrafluoroethylene grafts. A prospective, randomized study. *Am J Surg.* 1983;146(6):844–847.

80. Sato M, Horigome I, Chiba S, et al. Autonomic insufficiency as a factor contributing to dialysis-induced hypotension. *Nephrol Dial Transplant.* 2001; 16(8):1657–1662.

81. Davenport A. Intradialytic complications during hemodialysis. *Hemodial Int.* 2006;10(2):162–167.

82. Sherman RA. Intradialytic hypotension: an overview of recent, unresolved and overlooked issues. *Semin Dial.* 2002;15(3):141–143.

83. Saran R, Bragg-Gresham JL, Levin NW, et al. Longer treatment time and slower ultrafiltration in hemodialysis: associations with reduced mortality in the DOPPS. *Kidney Int.* 2006;69(7):1222–1228.

84. Sherman RA, Rubin MP, Cody RP, et al. Amelioration of hemodialysis-associated hypotension by the use of cool dialysate. *Am J Kidney Dis.* 1985;5(2):124–127.

85. Zager PG, Nikolic J, Brown RH, et al. U curve association of blood pressure and mortality in hemodialysis patients. Medical Directors of Dialysis Clinic, Inc. *Kidney Int.* 1998;54(2):561–569.

86. Inrig JK, Oddone EZ, Hasselblad V, et al. Association of intradialytic blood pressure changes with hospitalization and mortality rates in prevalent ESRD patients. *Kidney Int.* 2007;71(5):454–461.

87. Inrig JK. Intradialytic hypertension: a less-recognized cardiovascular complication of hemodialysis. *Am J Kidney Dis.* 2010;55(3):580–589.

88. Agarwal R, Light RP. Intradialytic hypertension is a marker of volume excess. *Nephrol Dial Transplant.* 2010;25(10):3355–3361.

89. Agarwal R, Alborzi P, Satyan S, et al. Dry-weight reduction in hypertensive hemodialysis patients (DRIP): a randomized, controlled trial. *Hypertension.* 2009;53(3):500–507.

90. Ebo DG, Bosmans JL, Couttenye MM, et al. Haemodialysis-associated anaphylactic and anaphylactoid reactions. *Allergy.* 2006;61(2):211–220.

91. Verresen L, Waer M, Vanrenterghem Y, et al. Angiotensin-converting-enzyme inhibitors and anaphylactoid reactions to high-flux membrane dialysis. *Lancet.* 1990;336(8727):1360–1362.

92. Huang WH, Lee YY, Shih LC. Delayed near-fatal anaphylactic reaction induced by the F10–HPS polysulphone haemodialyser. *Nephrol Dial Transplant.* 2008;23(1):423–424.

93. Davis TR, Young BA, Eisenberg MS, et al. Outcome of cardiac arrests attended by emergency medical services staff at community outpatient dialysis centers. *Kidney Int.* 2008;73(8):933–939.

94. Karnik JA, Young BS, Lew NL, et al. Cardiac arrest and sudden death in dialysis units. *Kidney Int.* 2001;60(1):350–357.

95. Santoro A, Mancini E, London G, et al. Patients with complex arrhythmias during and after haemodialysis suffer from different regimens of potassium removal. *Nephrol Dial Transplant.* 2008;23(4):1415–1421.

96. Genovesi S, Pogliani D, Faini A, et al. Prevalence of atrial fibrillation and associated factors in a population of long-term hemodialysis patients. *Am J Kidney Dis.* 2005;46(5):897–902.

97. Winkelmayer WC, Patrick AR, Liu J, Brookhart MA, Setoguchi S. The increasing prevalence of atrial fibrillation among hemodialysis patients. *J Am Soc Nephrol.* 2011;22(2):349–357.
98. Reinecke H, Brand E, Mesters R, et al. Dilemmas in the management of atrial fibrillation in chronic kidney disease. *J Am Soc Nephrol.* 2009;20(4):705–711.
99. Marinigh R, Lane DA, Lip GY. Severe renal impairment and stroke prevention in atrial fibrillation: implications for thromboprophylaxis and bleeding risk. *J Am Coll Cardiol.* 2011;57(12):1339–1348.
100. Chan KE, Lazarus JM, Thadhani R, Hakim RM. Warfarin use associates with increased risk for stroke in hemodialysis patients with atrial fibrillation. *J Am Soc Nephrol.* 2009;20(10):2223–2233.
101. Canzanello VJ, Hylander-Rossner B, Sands RE, et al. Comparison of 50% dextrose water, 25% mannitol, and 23.5% saline for the treatment of hemodialysis-associated muscle cramps. *ASAIO Trans.* 1991;37(4):649–652.
102. Ahsan M, Gupta M, Omar I, et al. Prevention of hemodialysis-related muscle cramps by intradialytic use of sequential compression devices: a report of four cases. *Hemodial Int.* 2004;8(3):283–286.
103. Lynch KE, Feldman HI, Berlin JA, et al. Effects of L-carnitine on dialysis-related hypotension and muscle cramps: a meta-analysis. *Am J Kidney Dis.* 2008; 52(5):962–971.
104. Khajehdehi P, Mojerlou M, Behzadi S, et al. A randomized, double-blind, placebo-controlled trial of supplementary vitamins E, C and their combination for treatment of haemodialysis cramps. *Nephrol Dial Transplant.* 2001;16(7):1448–1451.
105. El-Hennawy AS, Zaib S. A selected controlled trial of supplementary vitamin E for treatment of muscle cramps in hemodialysis patients. *Am J Ther.* 2010; 17(5):455–459.
106. Kaji DM, Ackad A, Nottage WG, et al. Prevention of muscle cramps in haemodialysis patients by quinine sulphate. *Lancet.* 1976;2(7976):66–67.
107. Kennedy AC, Linton AL, Eaton JC. Urea levels in cerebrospinal fluid after haemodialysis. *Lancet.* 1962;1(7226):410–411.
108. Patel N, Dalal P, Panesar M. Dialysis disequilibrium syndrome: a narrative review. *Semin Dial.* 2008;21(5):493–498.
109. Riddick L, Brogdon BG. Fatal air embolism during renal dialysis. *Am J Forensic Med Pathol.* 2012;33(1):110–112.
110. Tien IY, Drescher MJ. Pulmonary venous air embolism following accidental patient laceration of a hemodialysis catheter. *J Emerg Med.* 1999;17(5):847–850.
111. Yu AS, Levy E. Paradoxical cerebral air embolism from a hemodialysis catheter. *Am J Kidney Dis.* 1997;29(3):453–455.
112. Port FK, Hulbert-Shearon TE, Wolfe RA, et al. Predialysis blood pressure and mortality risk in a national sample of maintenance hemodialysis patients. *Am J Kidney Dis.* 1999;33(3):507–517.
113. Inrig JK. Antihypertensive agents in hemodialysis patients: a current perspective. *Semin Dial.* 2010;23(3):290–297.
114. Foley RN, Parfrey PS, Harnett JD, et al. Impact of hypertension on cardiomyopathy, morbidity and mortality in end-stage renal disease. *Kidney Int.* 1996;49(5):1379–1385.
115. London GM, Pannier B, Guerin AP, et al. Alterations of left ventricular hypertrophy in and survival of patients receiving hemodialysis: follow-up of an interventional study. *J Am Soc Nephrol.* 2001;12(12):2759–2767.
116. Inrig JK, Patel UD, Gillespie BS, et al. Relationship between interdialytic weight gain and blood pressure among prevalent hemodialysis patients. *Am J Kidney Dis.* 2007;50(1):108–118, 118 e101–e104.
117. Kalantar-Zadeh K, Regidor DL, Kovesdy CP, et al. Fluid retention is associated with cardiovascular mortality in patients undergoing long-term hemodialysis. *Circulation.* 2009;119(5):671–679.
118. Chobanian AV, Bakris GL, Black HR, et al. The Seventh Report of the Joint National Committee on Prevention, Detection, Evaluation, and Treatment of High Blood Pressure: the JNC 7 report. *JAMA.* 2003;289(19):2560–2572.
119. Chang TI, Friedman GD, Cheung AK, et al. Systolic blood pressure and mortality in prevalent haemodialysis patients in the HEMO study. *J Hum Hypertens.* 2011;25(2):98–105.
120. Agarwal R. Volume-associated ambulatory blood pressure patterns in hemodialysis patients. *Hypertension.* 2009;54(2):241–247.
121. Stidley CA, Hunt WC, Tentori F, et al. Changing relationship of blood pressure with mortality over time among hemodialysis patients. *J Am Soc Nephrol.* 2006;17(2):513–520.
122. Charra B, Laurent G, Calemard E, et al. Survival in dialysis and blood pressure control. *Contrib Nephrol.* 1994;106:179–185.
123. Kayikcioglu M, Tumuklu M, Ozkahya M, et al. The benefit of salt restriction in the treatment of end-stage renal disease by haemodialysis. *Nephrol Dial Transplant.* 2009;24(3):956–962.
124. Peterson WJ, Barker J, Allon M. Disparities in fistula maturation persist despite preoperative vascular mapping. *Clin J Am Soc Nephrol.* 2008;3(2):437–441.
125. Lok CE, Allon M, Moist L, et al. Risk equation determining unsuccessful cannulation events and failure to maturation in arteriovenous fistulas (REDUCE FTM I). *J Am Soc Nephrol.* 2006;17(11):3204–3212.
126. Lauvao LS, Ihnat DM, Goshima KR, et al. Vein diameter is the major predictor of fistula maturation. *J Vasc Surg.* 2009;49(6):1499–1504.
127. Fitzgerald JT, Schanzer A, McVicar JP, et al. Upper arm arteriovenous fistula versus forearm looped arteriovenous graft for hemodialysis access: a comparative analysis. *Ann Vasc Surg.* 2005;19(6):843–850.
128. Schild AF, Perez E, Gillaspie E, et al. Arteriovenous fistulae vs. arteriovenous grafts: a retrospective review of 1,700 consecutive vascular access cases. *J Vasc Access.* 2008;9(4):231–235.
129. Berger A, Rosenberg N. Hypotension and closure of hemodialysis access shunts. *Am Surg.* 1983;49(10):551–553.
130. Bakken AM, Galaria II, Agerstrand C, et al. Percutaneous therapy to maintain dialysis access successfully prolongs functional duration after primary failure. *Ann Vasc Surg.* 2007;21(4):474–480.
131. Etheredge EE, Haid SD, Maeser MN, et al. Salvage operations for malfunctioning polytetrafluoroethylene hemodialysis access grafts. *Surgery.* 1983;94(3): 464–470.
132. Beathard GA. Percutaneous transvenous angioplasty in the treatment of vascular access stenosis. *Kidney Int.* 1992;42(6):1390–1397.
133. Kundu S. Review of central venous disease in hemodialysis patients. *J Vasc Interv Radiol.* 2010;21(7):963–968.
134. Teruya TH, Abou-Zamzam AM Jr, et al. Symptomatic subclavian vein stenosis and occlusion in hemodialysis patients with transvenous pacemakers. *Ann Vasc Surg.* 2003;17(5):526–529.
135. Morsy AH, Kulbaski M, Chen C, et al. Incidence and characteristics of patients with hand ischemia after a hemodialysis access procedure. *J Surg Res.* 1998;74(1):8–10.
136. Yu SH, Cook PR, Canty TG, et al. Hemodialysis-related steal syndrome: predictive factors and response to treatment with the distal revascularization-interval ligation procedure. *Ann Vasc Surg.* 2008;22(2):210–214.
137. Field M, Blackwell J, Jaipersad A, et al. Distal revascularisation with interval ligation (DRIL): an experience. *Ann R Coll Surg Engl.* 2009;91(5):394–398.
138. Walz P, Ladowski JS, Hines A. Distal revascularization and interval ligation (DRIL) procedure for the treatment of ischemic steal syndrome after arm arteriovenous fistula. *Ann Vasc Surg.* 2007;21(4):468–473.
139. Knox RC, Berman SS, Hughes JD, et al. Distal revascularization-interval ligation: a durable and effective treatment for ischemic steal syndrome after hemodialysis access. *J Vasc Surg.* 2002;36(2):250–255; discussion 256.
140. Wodicka R, Isaacs J. Ischemic monomelic neuropathy. *J Hand Surg Am.* 2010;35(5):842–843.
141. Irvine C, Holt P. Hand venous hypertension complicating arteriovenous fistula construction for haemodialysis. *Clin Exp Dermatol.* 1989;14(4):289–290.
142. Bakken AM, Protack CD, Saad WE, et al. Long-term outcomes of primary angioplasty and primary stenting of central venous stenosis in hemodialysis patients. *J Vasc Surg.* 2007;45(4):776–783.
143. Pasklinsky G, Meisner RJ, Labropoulos N, et al. Management of true aneurysms of hemodialysis access fistulas. *J Vasc Surg.* 2011;53(5):1291–1297.
144. Pandolfe LR, Malamis AP, Pierce K, et al. Treatment of hemodialysis graft pseudoaneurysms with stent grafts: institutional experience and review of the literature. *Semin Intervent Radiol.* 2009;26(2):89–95.
145. Lok CE, Mokrzycki MH. Prevention and management of catheter-related infection in hemodialysis patients. *Kidney Int.* 2011;79(6):587–598.
146. Moal V, Brunet P, Dou L, et al. Impaired expression of glycoproteins on resting and stimulated platelets in uraemic patients. *Nephrol Dial Transplant.* 2003; 18(9):1834–1841.
147. Steiner RW, Coggins C, Carvalho AC. Bleeding time in uremia: a useful test to assess clinical bleeding. *Am J Hematol.* 1979;7(2):107–117.
148. Molino D, De Lucia D, Marotta R, et al. In uremia, plasma levels of anti-protein C and anti-protein S antibodies are associated with thrombosis. *Kidney Int.* 2005;68(3):1223–1229.
149. Gawaz MP, Dobos G, Spath M, et al. Impaired function of platelet membrane glycoprotein IIb-IIIa in end-stage renal disease. *J Am Soc Nephrol.* 1994;5(1):36–46.
150. Himmelfarb J, Nelson S, McMonagle E, et al. Elevated plasma glycocalicin levels and decreased ristocetin-induced platelet agglutination in hemodialysis patients. *Am J Kidney Dis.* 1998;32(1):132–138.
151. Sohal AS, Gangji AS, Crowther MA, et al. Uremic bleeding: pathophysiology and clinical risk factors. *Thromb Res.* 2006;118(3):417–422.
152. Linthorst GE, Avis HJ, Levi M. Uremic thrombocytopathy is not about urea. *J Am Soc Nephrol.* 2010;21(5):753–755.
153. Malyszko J, Malyszko JS, Mysliwiec M. Comparison of hemostatic disturbances between patients on CAPD and patients on hemodialysis. *Perit Dial Int.* 2001;21(2):158–165.

154. Salvati F, Liani M. Role of platelet surface receptor abnormalities in the bleeding and thrombotic diathesis of uremic patients on hemodialysis and peritoneal dialysis. *Int J Artif Organs.* 2001;24(3):131–135.
155. Mannucci PM, Remuzzi G, Pusineri F, et al. Deamino-8–D-arginine vasopressin shortens the bleeding time in uremia. *N Engl J Med.* 1983;308(1): 8–12.
156. Galbusera M, Remuzzi G, Boccardo P. Treatment of bleeding in dialysis patients. *Semin Dial.* 2009;22(3):279–286.
157. Segall L, Covic A. Diagnosis of tuberculosis in dialysis patients: current strategy. *Clin J Am Soc Nephrol.* 2010;5(6):1114–1122.
158. Klote MM, Agodoa LY, Abbott KC. Risk factors for Mycobacterium tuberculosis in US chronic dialysis patients. *Nephrol Dial Transplant.* 2006;21(11): 3287–3292.
159. Abdelrahman M, Sinha AK, Karkar A. Tuberculosis in end-stage renal disease patients on hemodialysis. *Hemodial Int.* 2006;10(4):360–364.
160. Smirnoff M, Patt C, Seckler B, Adler JJ. Tuberculin and anergy skin testing of patients receiving long-term hemodialysis. *Chest.* 1998;113(1):25–27.
161. Shankar MS, Aravindan AN, Sohal PM, et al. The prevalence of tuberculin sensitivity and anergy in chronic renal failure in an endemic area: tuberculin test and the risk of post-transplant tuberculosis. *Nephrol Dial Transplant.* 2005; 20(12):2720–2724.
162. Chung WK, Zheng ZL, Sung JY, et al. Validity of interferon-gamma-release assays for the diagnosis of latent tuberculosis in haemodialysis patients. *Clin Microbiol Infect.* 2010;16(7):960–965.
163. Winthrop KL, Nyendak M, Calvet H, et al. Interferon-gamma release assays for diagnosing mycobacterium tuberculosis infection in renal dialysis patients. *Clin J Am Soc Nephrol.* 2008;3(5):1357–1363.
164. Inoue T, Nakamura T, Katsuma A, et al. The value of QuantiFERON TB-Gold in the diagnosis of tuberculosis among dialysis patients. *Nephrol Dial Transplant.* 2009;24(7):2252–2257.
165. Launay-Vacher V, Izzedine H, Deray G. Pharmacokinetic considerations in the treatment of tuberculosis in patients with renal failure. *Clin Pharmacokinet.* 2005;44(3):221–235.
166. Recommendations for preventing transmission of infections among chronic hemodialysis patients. *MMWR Recomm Rep.* 2001;50(RR-5):1–43.
167. Bond WW, Favero MS, Petersen NJ, et al. Survival of hepatitis B virus after drying and storage for one week. *Lancet.* 1981;1(8219):550–551.
168. Trevizoli JE, de Paula Menezes R, Ribeiro Velasco LF, et al. Hepatitis C is less aggressive in hemodialysis patients than in nonuremic patients. *Clin J Am Soc Nephrol.* 2008;3(5):1385–1390.
169. Barril G, Castillo I, Arenas MD, et al. Occult hepatitis C virus infection among hemodialysis patients. *J Am Soc Nephrol.* 2008;19(12):2288–2292.
170. KDIGO clinical practice guidelines for the prevention, diagnosis, evaluation, and treatment of hepatitis C in chronic kidney disease. *Kidney Int Suppl.* 2008(109):S1–99.
171. Fabrizi F, Martin P, Dixit V, Bunnapradist S, Dulai G. Meta-analysis: Effect of hepatitis C virus infection on mortality in dialysis. *Aliment Pharmacol Ther.* 2004;20(11–12):1271–1277.
172. Badalamenti S, Catania A, Lunghi G, et al. Changes in viremia and circulating interferon-alpha during hemodialysis in hepatitis C virus-positive patients: only coincidental phenomena? *Am J Kidney Dis.* 2003;42(1):143–150.
173. van Leusen R, Adang RP, de Vries RA, et al. Pegylated interferon alfa-2a (40 kD) and ribavirin in haemodialysis patients with chronic hepatitis C. *Nephrol Dial Transplant.* 2008;23(2):721–725.
174. Scharpe J, Peetermans WE, Vanwalleghem J, et al. Immunogenicity of a standard trivalent influenza vaccine in patients on long-term hemodialysis: an open-label trial. *Am J Kidney Dis.* 2009;54(1):77–85.
175. National Center for Immunization and Respiratory Diseases. General recommendations on immunization — recommendations of the Advisory Committee on Immunization Practices (ACIP). *MMWR Recomm Rep.* 2011;60(2):1–64.
176. Tung J, Carlisle E, Smieja M, et al. A randomized clinical trial of immunization with combined hepatitis A and B versus hepatitis B alone for hepatitis B seroprotection in hemodialysis patients. *Am J Kidney Dis.* 2010;56(4): 713–719.
177. Gilbertson DT, Guo H, Arneson TJ, Collins AJ. The association of pneumococcal vaccination with hospitalization and mortality in hemodialysis patients. *Nephrol Dial Transplant.* 2011;26(9):2934–2939.
178. Bernier GM, Conrad ME. Catabolsm of human beta-2–microglobulin by the rat kidney. *Am J Physiol.* 1969;217(5):1359–1362.
179. Dember LM, Jaber BL. Dialysis-related amyloidosis: late finding or hidden epidemic? *Semin Dial.* 2006;19(2):105–109.
180. Mogyorosi A, Schubert ML. Dialysis-related amyloidosis: an important cause of gastrointestinal symptoms in patients with end-stage renal disease. *Gastroenterology.* 1999;116(1):217–220.
181. Dulgheru EC, Balos LL, Baer AN. Gastrointestinal complications of beta2–microglobulin amyloidosis: a case report and review of the literature. *Arthritis Rheum.* 2005;53(1):142–145.
182. Otsubo S, Kimata N, Okutsu I, et al. Characteristics of dialysis-related amyloidosis in patients on haemodialysis therapy for more than 30 years. *Nephrol Dial Transplant.* 2009;24(5):1593–1598.
183. Jadoul M, Garbar C, Noel H, et al. Histological prevalence of beta 2–microglobulin amyloidosis in hemodialysis: a prospective post-mortem study. *Kidney Int.* 1997;51(6):1928–1932.
184. Sethi D, Murphy CM, Brown EA, et al. Clearance of beta-2–microglobulin using continuous ambulatory peritoneal dialysis. *Nephron.* 1989;52(4):352–355.
185. Jadoul M, Garbar C, Vanholder R, et al. Prevalence of histological beta2–microglobulin amyloidosis in CAPD patients compared with hemodialysis patients. *Kidney Int.* 1998;54(3):956–959.
186. Kuchle C, Fricke H, Held E, et al. High-flux hemodialysis postpones clinical manifestation of dialysis-related amyloidosis. *Am J Nephrol.* 1996;16(6): 484–488.
187. Traut M, Haufe CC, Eismann U, et al. Increased binding of beta-2–microglobulin to blood cells in dialysis patients treated with high-flux dialyzers compared with low-flux membranes contributed to reduced beta-2–microglobulin concentrations. Results of a cross-over study. *Blood Purif.* 2007;25(5–6):432–440.
188. Ayli M, Ayli D, Azak A, et al. The effect of high-flux hemodialysis on dialysis-associated amyloidosis. *Ren Fail.* 2005;27(1):31–34.
189. Campistol JM. Dialysis-related amyloidosis after renal transplantation. *Semin Dial.* 2001;14(2):99–102.
190. Matson MA, Cohen EP. Acquired cystic kidney disease: occurrence, prevalence, and renal cancers. *Medicine (Baltimore).* 1990;69(4):217–226.
191. Ishikawa I, Saito Y, Onouchi Z, et al. Development of acquired cystic disease and adenocarcinoma of the kidney in glomerulonephritic chronic hemodialysis patients. *Clin Nephrol.* 1980;14(1):1–6.
192. Hughson MD, Hennigar GR, McManus JF. Atypical cysts, acquired renal cystic disease, and renal cell tumors in end stage dialysis kidneys. *Lab Invest.* 1980; 42(4):475–480.
193. Ishikawa I, Yuri T, Kitada H, Shinoda A. Regression of acquired cystic disease of the kidney after successful renal transplantation. *Am J Nephrol.* 1983; 3(6):310–314.
194. Kasiske BL, Vazquez MA, Harmon WE, et al. Recommendations for the outpatient surveillance of renal transplant recipients. American Society of Transplantation. *J Am Soc Nephrol.* 2000;11 Suppl 15:S1–86.
195. Bush A, Gabriel R. Cancer in uremic patients. *Clin Nephrol.* 1984;22(2): 77–81.
196. Kantor AF, Hoover RN, Kinlen LJ, McMullan MR, Fraumenti JF Jr. Cancer in patients receiving long-term dialysis treatment. *Am J Epidemiol.* 1987; 126(3):370–376.
197. Buccianti G, Ravasi B, Cresseri D, Maisonneuve P, Boyle P, Locatelli F. Cancer in patients on renal replacement therapy in Lombardy, Italy. *Lancet.* 1996;347(8993):59–60.
198. Maisonneuve P, Agodoa L, Gellert R, et al. Cancer in patients on dialysis for end-stage renal disease: an international collaborative study. *Lancet.* 1999; 354(9173):93–99.
199. Stewart JH, Buccianti G, Agodoa L, et al. Cancers of the kidney and urinary tract in patients on dialysis for end-stage renal disease: analysis of data from the United States, Europe, and Australia and New Zealand. *J Am Soc Nephrol.* 2003;14(1):197–207.
200. Holley JL. Screening, diagnosis, and treatment of cancer in long-term dialysis patients. *Clin J Am Soc Nephrol.* 2007;2(3):604–610.
201. Cukor D, Coplan J, Brown C, et al. Depression and anxiety in urban hemodialysis patients. *Clin J Am Soc Nephrol.* 2007;2(3):484–490.
202. Chen CK, Tsai YC, Hsu HJ, et al. Depression and suicide risk in hemodialysis patients with chronic renal failure. *Psychosomatics.* 2010;51(6):528–528. e526.
203. Agganis BT, Weiner DE, Giang LM, et al. Depression and cognitive function in maintenance hemodialysis patients. *Am J Kidney Dis.* 2010;56(4): 704–712.
204. Leggat JE Jr, Bloembergen WE, Levine G, et al. An analysis of risk factors for withdrawal from dialysis before death. *J Am Soc Nephrol.* 1997;8(11): 1755–1763.
205. Kurella M, Kimmel PL, Young BS, et al. Suicide in the United States end-stage renal disease program. *J Am Soc Nephrol.* 2005;16(3):774–781.
206. Kessler RC, Chiu WT, Demler O, et al. Prevalence, severity, and comorbidity of 12–month DSM-IV disorders in the National Comorbidity Survey Replication. *Arch Gen Psychiatry.* 2005;62(6):617–627.
207. Blagg C. Home hemodialysis: a view from Seattle. *Nephrol News Issues.* 1992;6(11):33, 36.

208. Van Eps CL, Jeffries JK, Johnson DW, et al. Quality of life and alternate nightly nocturnal home hemodialysis. *Hemodial Int.* 2010;14(1):29–38.
209. Lockridge RS, Kjellstrand CM. Nightly home hemodialysis: Outcome and factors associated with survival. *Hemodial Int.* 2011;15(2):211–218.
210. Kumar VA, Ledezma ML, Idroos ML, et al. Hospitalization rates in daily home hemodialysis versus peritoneal dialysis patients in the United States. *Am J Kidney Dis.* 2008;52(4):737–744.
211. Pauly RP, Gill JS, Rose CL, et al. Survival among nocturnal home haemodialysis patients compared to kidney transplant recipients. *Nephrol Dial Transplant.* 2009;24(9):2915–2919.
212. Cafazzo JA, Leonard K, Easty AC, Rossos PG, Chan CT. Patient perceptions of remote monitoring for nocturnal home hemodialysis. *Hemodial Int.* 2010;14(4):471–477.
213. McGregor DO, Buttimore AL, Nicholls MG, Lynn KL. Ambulatory blood pressure monitoring in patients receiving long, slow home haemodialysis. *Nephrol Dial Transplant.* 1999;14(11):2676–2679.
214. Kohn OF, Coe FL, Ing TS. Solute kinetics with short-daily home hemodialysis using slow dialysate flow rate. *Hemodial Int.* 2010;14(1):39–46.
215. Chan CT, Liu PP, Arab S, Jamal N, Messner HA. Nocturnal hemodialysis improves erythropoietin responsiveness and growth of hematopoietic stem cells. *J Am Soc Nephrol.* 2009;20(3):665–671.
216. Rao M, Muirhead N, Klarenbach S, Moist L, Lindsay RM. Management of anemia with quotidian hemodialysis. *Am J Kidney Dis.* 2003;42(1 Suppl):18–23.
217. Depner TA, Daugirdas JT. Equations for normalized protein catabolic rate based on two-point modeling of hemodialysis urea kinetics. *J Am Soc Nephrol.* 1996;7(5):780–785.

CHAPTER

85 Dietary Factors in the Treatment of Chronic Kidney Disease

Sreedhar A. Mandayam • William E. Mitch • Joel D. Kopple

INTRODUCTION

Our goal is to provide the reader with an understanding of how chronic kidney disease (CKD) induces metabolic aberrations and how introducing nutritional factors can improve these metabolic problems. Achieving this goal requires knowledge about how the requirements of different nutrients change with the different stages of CKD. For example, diabetes is the most frequent cause of CKD and the incidence of diabetes is growing. In part, this is occurring because of the increasing prevalence of obesity. Clearly, both diabetes and obesity require the manipulation of the diet to improve health and to prevent adverse outcomes. In addition, diabetes and/or obesity is frequently accompanied by high blood pressure and diffuse vascular complications. If the salt intake of these individuals is not controlled, antihypertensive drugs tend to become ineffective.[1,2] There also are the consequences of progressively accumulating waste products leading to uremia (literally, urine in the blood). Because these waste products arise mainly from the metabolism of protein, it is not surprising that symptoms of CKD can be successfully reversed by controlling protein intake.[3–5] Besides ensuring that nutrient requirements are met, the nephrologist must understand how to monitor compliance and how to deal with the progressive loss of kidney function. As will be discussed, there remains uncertainty about the influence of dietary modification on the progression of CKD. Regardless, this is not the sole reason to manipulate the diet of a CKD patient.[6] Other reasons include correcting acidosis, preventing or ameliorating protein-energy wasting (PEW), suppressing uremic bone disease, combating hypertension, and reducing the accumulation of waste products and thereby mitigating uremic syndrome.[7,8] Ignoring these aspects of patient care hastens the need to begin dialysis. But several studies have demonstrated that initiating dialysis earlier (e.g., at glomerular filtration rates [GFR] of about 10 to 12 mL per minute) does not improve the mortality associated with CKD nor does it reduce the complications of CKD.[9–12] This makes it even more important to use dietary modification to prevent the complications of CKD.

Are there specific problems arising in CKD patients attributable to inadequate attention to nutritional principles? Among such problems, there is uremic bone disease. This complication has become more prominent, in part related to a recent and dramatic increase in phosphate additives to processed food.[13] In addition, hyperphosphatemia reduces the effectiveness of angiotensin-converting enzyme (ACE) inhibitors in slowing the loss of kidney function.[14] Likewise, adding sodium chloride to foods, particularly processed foods or fast foods, is a major contributor to increasing difficulties in managing hypertensive patients.[1,15] Another major diet-related problem is the accumulation of waste products when the dietary protein of a CKD patient is unrestricted.[8,16] For example, metabolic acidosis arises from the metabolism of amino acids in protein and acid excretion falls as function is lost.[7] This problem is raised because simply correcting the serum bicarbonate improves protein metabolism, calcium metabolism, and possibly, the progression of CKD.[17–22] Complicating dietary planning are the reports that the average intake of energy, calcium, and a number of vitamins may be inadequate in CKD patients. In short, attention to the diet of patients with CKD is not simply an intellectual exercise; it can produce rapid and sustained benefits as long as the adequacy of the diet is ensured.[6]

The need for and approaches to manipulation of the diet will depend on the degree of renal insufficiency. The most widely used classification of the degree of CKD was developed by the National Kidney Foundation-Kidney Disease Outcomes Quality Initiative (NKF-KDOQI) Committee and includes a level signifying an increase in the risk of progressive loss of kidney function (i.e., individuals with an estimated GFR [eGFR], of <60 mL/min/1.73 m^2). Notably, those with higher eGFR values can still develop complications of CKD.[23] The variables used in the equations that estimate GFR include age, serum creatinine, sex, and race and the interpretation of the eGFR level has several limitations. First, it was derived from individuals in the United States with established kidney disease but without severe PEW or morbid obesity. Second, there is evidence that the equations are inaccurate for other regions of the world, including Asia and Latin America.[24–26] Third, the boundaries for the stages of renal insufficiency are somewhat arbitrary; it seems unlikely there is an absolute threshold identifying all patients who will develop progressive CKD. Fourth, certain activities can acutely reduce GFR (e.g., hypertension therapy with blockers of the renin–angiotensin system [RAS], a very low protein diet). In this case, the stage of CKD can change even though kidney damage has not occurred. Nonetheless, this system can identify patients for whom interventions, including dietary modification, could improve their overall health.

METABOLIC CHANGES IN CHRONIC KIDNEY DISEASE AND TOXINS IN OR DERIVED FROM NUTRIENTS

Although it is possible for one toxin or group of toxins to be responsible for specific signs and symptoms of uremia, the interaction of many toxins more commonly causes the problems of CKD. For example, it was reported that a combination of products of protein metabolism (urea, magnesium, acetoin, 2, 3-butylene-glycol, sulfate, creatinine, T-cresol, and guanidine) impairs oxidative metabolism in slices of the cerebral cortex. When studied at the same concentration but separately, however, none of the potential toxins exerted adverse effects on metabolism.[27] There are a large number of potential uremic toxins: in 2003, the European Uremic Toxin Work Group (EUTOX) identified 90 potential toxins that are accumulated in patients with CKD. Proving they are toxic has been difficult. Bergström [28] noted that the requirement for identifying a uremic toxin should include: (1) its chemical identity; (2) a concentration higher in tissues or plasma from uremic patients compared to levels in normal subjects; (3) a concentration should correlate with specific uremic signs or symptoms that are improved when the substance is removed; and (4) its toxicity in tissues, cells, etc. should be demonstrable at the concentration present in tissue or fluids from uremic patients. Few putative compounds have met these criteria.

Urea

There is some evidence that urea is toxic, but it is difficult to test for toxicity because the short half-life of urea makes it difficult to maintain a high level in blood and tissues. Nephrectomized dogs were treated with peritoneal dialysis and the serum urea nitrogen (SUN) level was raised to ~200 mg per deciliter by adding urea to the dialysate; the dogs developed weakness, anorexia, and decreased attentiveness.[29] Continued therapy led to vomiting, hemorrhagic diarrhea, hypothermia, and death. In humans undergoing maintenance hemodialysis (MHD), a similar strategy was used to increase the urea concentration in the dialysate: at serum urea nitrogen (SUN) levels of 140 to 200 mg per deciliter most patients developed malaise, lethargy, and some evidence of bleeding.[30] Consistent with the idea that urea is toxic at high levels is the recent report that urea can stimulate reactive oxygen species (ROS), leading to insulin resistance.[31] In patients with CKD, insulin resistance could lead to accelerated muscle wasting (see the following).

Urea toxicity could arise following its decomposition to ammonia or cyanate adducts. Cyanate can condense with NH_2-terminal amino groups and amides, altering the tertiary structure of proteins and, hence, interfering with enzyme activity. For example, a variety of lipids are carbamylated to form toxins, including 3-carboxy-4-methyl-5 propyl-2-furaproprionic carboxy-4methyl-5propyl-2furapropionic (CMPF) acid, a major cause of altered drug protein binding in uremia.[32,33] Still, the role of protein carbamylation in uremic toxicity is unsettled.[34] Finally, urea is converted to ammonia and carbon dioxide largely by bacterial ureases, but this does not raise blood ammonia substantially, at least in patients with normal hepatic function.[35] The kidney is another contributor to body ammonium levels but this function is markedly reduced or lost in kidney failure. Thus, hyperammonemia rarely occurs in kidney failure.

LOSS OF NONEXCRETORY KIDNEY FUNCTION AND TOXIC METABOLITES OF PROTEIN

At first glance, many of the manifestations of CKD appear to be due to small, water-soluble toxins that are cleared by hemodialysis or peritoneal dialysis because the removal of urea by dialysis reverses several uremic complications. Besides problems related to urea accumulation, the retention of salt leads to extracellular volume expansion, hypertension, cardiac dilatation, sympathetic nervous system activation, and inflammatory cytokine production. But, the removal of ions or small molecules is only part of the story. First, the loss of metabolic or endocrine functions of the kidney can cause certain complications of CKD. For example, loss of kidney-produced hormones, such as erythropoietin (EPO) or 1,25 hydroxyvitamin D3, can interfere with metabolic functions. Second, the ability to remove larger molecules (so-called middle molecules [0.5 to 3.0 kD] or larger polypeptides including many hormones and cytokines) is progressively diminished as CKD progresses. This interferes with normal cellular metabolism. A more easily understood example is the accumulation of unexcreted acid arising largely from metabolism of sulfur-containing and phosphate-containing proteins and lipids. Acid accumulation causes an increase in the breakdown of protein and essential amino acids. It also causes insulin resistance and abnormalities in endocrine function, including factors affecting bone metabolism.[17,36–39] Fortunately, these problems are largely prevented when metabolic acidosis is corrected.

Other potentially toxic metabolites of dietary protein can affect kidney function indirectly. For example, phenylalanine metabolites can accumulate when dietary protein is unrestricted; the phenylalanine metabolite, phenyl acetic acid, will inhibit the expression of inducible nitric oxide synthase (iNOS) and, hence, may contribute to the development of atherosclerosis.[40]

Guanidino-Containing Compounds

Guanidino compounds are potent organic bases that accumulate in the sera and tissues of uremic patients.[41,42] Their production rises with excess protein intake. However, the production of guanidinosuccinic acid also increases in renal failure independent of protein intake, thus underscoring the metabolic complexities induced by CKD.[43,44] The controversy around the identification of uremic toxins such as guanidine compounds arises in part because of the difficulty measuring the plasma and tissue concentrations of guanidino compounds.[42] In uremic patients, plasma levels may be as high as 8 to 10 mM, but corresponding tissue levels have not been documented. Certain guanidino compounds can have neurotoxic effects: guanidine and methylguanidine are implicated in the development of peripheral neuropathy, and γ-guanidinobutyric acid, taurocyamine, homoarginine, and α-keto-δ-guanidinovaleric acid lower the seizure threshold of experimental animals.[45] The central nervous system excitatory effects of uremic guanidino compounds may reflect an inhibition of depolarization at γ-aminobutyric acid (GABA) receptors, selective activation of N-methyl-D-aspartate (NMDA) receptors by guanidinosuccinic acid, and an intrinsic depolarizing response.[46]

The Arginine Derivative Asymmetric Dimethylarginine

Asymmetric dimethylarginine (ADMA) derived from arginine can inhibit NOS, and its concentration rises in patients with CKD to decrease nitric oxide (NO) and impair vascular responses.[47,48] In experimental animals, ADMA is associated with concentration-dependent pressor and bradycardic responses and vasoconstriction.[49] In CKD patients, a decrease in the actions of NO because of a high ADMA level could aggravate hypertension and, possibly, the progression of renal failure.[50] Despite these intriguing reports, the influence of ADMA on cardiovascular disease is controversial.[48]

Products of Bacterial Metabolism

Uremic toxins can be produced by gut bacteria, and their absorption may be promoted by an increase in the permeability of the gastrointestinal mucosa.[51] The potential of these processes is great because of the huge mass of bacteria (there are more bacterial cells in the colon than in the rest of the human body). Specific uremia-associated problems include bacteria-produced nitrogen-containing waste products and aromatic compounds as well as aliphatic amines (e.g., phenols, indoles, aliphatic amines). With normal kidney function, these compounds do not accumulate because they are rapidly cleared by the kidneys. But, with CKD, some compounds (indoxyl sulfate, hippuric acid, p-cresol, and 3-carboxy-4-methyl-5-propyl-2-furanpropionic acid) initiate toxic reactions in the brain or even contribute to progressive loss of kidney function.

Aromatic Amines

Tryptophan is touted as a major precursor of uremic toxins. It, along with aromatic amines, undergoes deamination and decarboxylation by gut bacteria, yielding metabolites such as indole, indoxyl, skatole, skatoxyl, indican, and indoleacetic acid. Their potential toxicity has been tested by feeding large amounts of the potential toxin and observing changes in organ functions. In the case of indoxyl sulfate, uremic rats were treated with a proprietary resin that absorbs it and other metabolites. The resin not only reduced plasma and urinary levels of indoxyl sulfate, but it also improved metabolism of the kidney and reduced the progression of renal failure.[52] In the United States, a randomized clinical trial of its effectiveness to retard the progression of CKD has shown promise with minimal toxic reactions.[53] This has led to plans for a more extensive trial. Aromatic amines could also exert toxicity by interfering with the binding of drugs to serum proteins yielding abnormal responses at doses used for normal adults. Aromatic amines could also serve as false neurotransmitters.[54] The infusion of phenol or p-cresol into dogs causes a variety of neurologic symptoms, whereas conjugated phenols can inhibit ATPases and ion transport systems to interfere with cellular metabolism.[55] p-Cresol can inactivate β-hydroxylase to interfere with the transformation of dopamine into norepinephrine to develop impaired macrophage function.[56,57]

Aliphatic Amines

Aliphatic amines such as monomethylamine are derived from the metabolism of creatinine. Alternatively, bacterial metabolism of choline or lecithin produces tertiary methylamines that can then be converted to form secondary methylamines.[58] Secondary methylamines accumulate in the blood, the cerebrospinal fluid, and brain tissue, but toxicity has not been demonstrated.

In summary, dietary protein is initially broken down into peptides and amino acids. These compounds in turn can be metabolized by bacteria in the gastrointestinal tract generating compounds that are absorbed. There is evidence that sufficiently high levels of these compounds could impair the function of different organs. However, it has been difficult to assign specific toxic reactions to these compounds because of: (1) difficulties in measuring their concentrations in specific tissues; and/or (2) toxic reactions that could be caused by direct interference with cell functions or through indirect actions that decrease organ function.

Nephrotoxic Compounds Derived from Dietary Protein

In 1905, Folin[59] pointed out that the principal metabolic response to a change in dietary protein intake is a parallel change in urinary urea excretion. This has been confirmed in normal adults and patients with CKD.[60,61] Many of the degradation products of dietary protein are excreted primarily by the kidney. Consequently, products arising from the metabolism of protein will accumulate in patients in direct proportion to the amount of protein eaten and in inverse proportion to the degree of kidney failure. The accumulation of these compounds is in large part responsible for the symptoms and complications of CKD because decreasing dietary protein improves these symptoms.[3–6,62] Therefore, dietary counseling should be directed at reducing the SUN, but only following an assurance that adequate amounts of protein and energy are provided.

Illustrative examples of the principle that excess dietary protein participates in the generation of uremic toxicity are indoxyl sulfate and uric acid. Indoxyl sulfate arises from the metabolism of indoles such as dietary tryptophan.[52] Experimentally, indoxyl sulfate can accelerate kidney damage in models of glomerular sclerosis.[63] As indicated previously, a clinical trial was directed at assessing whether removing indoxyl sulfate by ingested activated charcoal will slow the progression of CKD.[64] Uric acid can contribute to the complications of CKD; a 12-year study of 47,150 previously normal men indicated that diets with high levels of meat or seafood were associated with an increased risk of gout.[65] This is relevant because Johnson and colleagues[30] have described an important association between an increase in uric acid and the development of hypertension. Untreated hypertensive adolescents were found to exhibit a correlation between systolic blood pressure and serum uric acid ($r = 0.8$).[66] In some of these adolescents, their hypertension was largely corrected by administering allopurinol. Notably, in CKD patients, serum uric acid does not rise to the level expected from the degree of lost kidney function because there is extensive metabolism of uric acid, presumably by bacteria in the gastrointestinal tract.[67] The degree to which dietary protein restriction modifies the serum uric acid of CKD patients has not been established, but there is the possibility that allopurinol treatment can help preserve renal function in patients with CKD.

MECHANISMS THAT REGULATE BODY PROTEIN STORES

Robust metabolic mechanisms act to maintain body protein mass following a change in protein intake. These act rapidly and precisely to adjust the rates of amino acid and protein metabolism. Specifically, when dietary protein falls, the major metabolic response is a suppression of the degradation of essential amino acids (EAAs). This response will help to maintain an adequate supply of EAAs for protein synthesis. The ability to decrease EAA degradation, however, is limited, reaching a minimum level when the amount of protein being eaten is at a level that is just adequate for achieving nitrogen balance (i.e., ~0.6 g protein per kilogram of ideal body weight per day). If dietary protein falls further, there also are adaptive responses that suppress protein degradation (protein synthesis may also increase but is less consistently found compared to a decrease in protein degradation). These responses limit the loss of protein stores and are active in normal adults or CKD patients as long as there are no complications such as acidemia or other catabolic illnesses.[68–70] Similar adaptive responses are also active in patients with the nephrotic syndrome.[71]

Protein Metabolism and Protein Stores

All intracellular and extracellular proteins are continually turning over, being degraded to their constituent amino acids and replaced by the synthesis of new proteins. The rapidity of the turnover of individual proteins varies widely, from minutes for some regulatory enzymes or transcription factors, to days or weeks for proteins like actin and myosin in skeletal muscle and months for hemoglobin in red blood cells. The rate of the degradation of proteins must be specific and highly regulated. Otherwise, countless cellular functions as well as the maintenance of protein stores (e.g., in muscle) would be jeopardized. Evidence that these processes are highly regulated includes the following: (1) The daily rates of protein turnover are enormous (3.7 to 4.7 g/kg/day) and therefore, even a small but sustained decrease in the synthesis of proteins or acceleration of protein degradation would result in marked loss of protein stores.[72] (2) Precise changes in the levels of proteins are required for the minute-to-minute regulation of transcriptional events or metabolic pathways. It is surprising, therefore, that the majority of intracellular proteins in all tissues is degraded by a single proteolytic system, the ATP-dependent, ubiquitin-proteasome system (UPS).[72] This specialized system exhibits remarkable specificity by individual proteins for degradation.

The Ubiquitin-Proteasome System

The initial processes of protein degradation by the UPS involve a series of three enzymes that link ubiquitin (Ub) onto proteins.[72,73] The single E1 isoform (Ub-activating enzyme) uses ATP to activate Ub and then transfers Ub to one of 20 to 40 isoforms of the E2 Ub-carrier proteins (Fig. 85.1). These reactions provide some specificity for the degradation of substrate proteins; a specific E2 Ub-carrier conjugates with only some of the more than 1,000 different E3 enzymes. This third enzyme, an E3 Ub-protein ligase, is the key determinant of the specificity of proteolysis; a specific E3 Ub-ligase recognizes a specific protein substrate (or possibly specific classes of proteins) and transfers Ub to a lysine in the protein. This process is repeated until the initial Ub is increased to form a chain of four to five Ubs attached to the substrate protein. This poly-Ub chain is recognized by the 26S proteasome. It also uses ATP to degrade the substrate protein. The proteasome is a very large organelle consisting of >60 proteins that create a 20S, barrel-shaped particle with 19S regulatory particles at either or both of its ends. The 19S regulatory particles not only recognize polyubiquitin chains, but when ATP is present, the 26S proteasome also cleaves the poly-Ub chain from the doomed protein and unfolds the protein's tertiary structure. In the next step, the unfolded substrate protein is translocated through a tunnel-like structure into the 20S particle where it is degraded into peptides. The peptides are released into the cytoplasm and

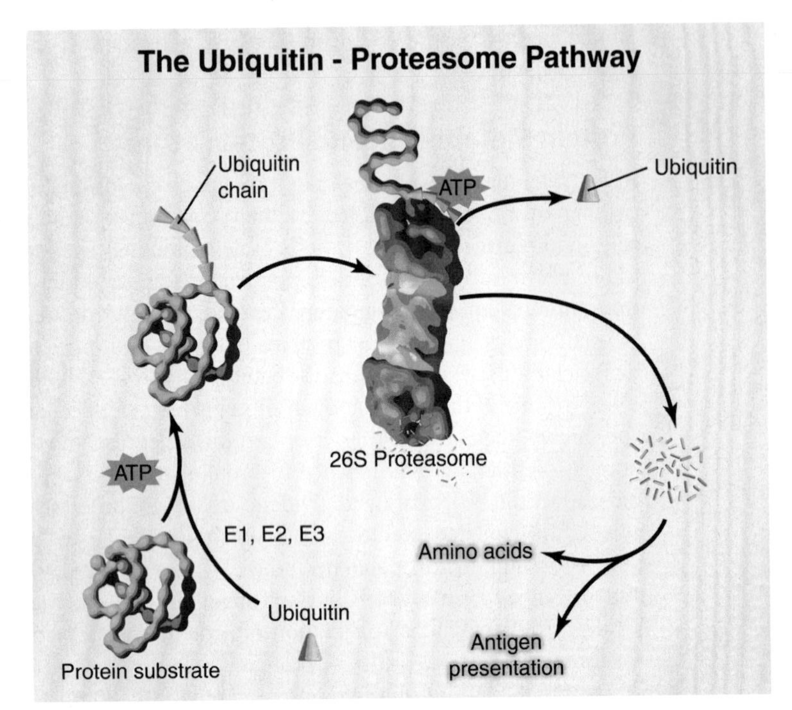

FIGURE 85.1 An illustration of the major components of the ubiquitin–proteasome system. (Lecker SH, Goldberg AL, Mitch WE. Protein degradation by the ubiquitin-proteasome pathway in normal and disease states. *J Am Soc Nephrol.* 2006;17:1807–1819.)

are converted to amino acids by peptidases.[73] The importance of these processes is underscored by the awarding of the 2004 Nobel Prize to Avram Hershko, Aaron Ciechanover, and Irwin Rose for discovering this system (http://nobelprize.org/chemistry/laureates/2004/).

Recent results have uncovered insights into the proteolytic processes that regulate muscle protein breakdown by the UPS and by mechanisms separate from the UPS. For example, in muscle wasting conditions, the expression of two E3 Ub-conjugating enzymes, Atrogin-1 (also known as MAFbx) and MuRF-1, are critical for the breakdown of muscle proteins.[73,74] In models of muscle wasting conditions, the expression of Atrogin-1 and MuRF-1 are increased 8- to 20-fold, serving as a sign that muscle protein breakdown is accelerated.[75,76] The signals that activate these E3 Ub-conjugating enzymes have been extensively studied and at least two transcription factors have been identified as regulators of Atrogin-1/MAFbx and MuRF-1 expression: the Forkhead transcription factors (FoxO) and the inflammatory transcription factor, nuclear factor-kappaB (NF-κB).[73,74]

At least five functions of the UPS have been identified as crucial for maintaining normal cellular functions: (1) It permits cells to adapt rapidly to physiologic changes because the UPS rapidly removes proteins to terminate an enzymatic or regulatory process. (2) The UPS can change gene expression by degrading transcription factors or cofactors/inhibitors that regulate transcription (e.g., the UPS degrades I-κB to activate NF-κB and accelerate inflammatory processes).[73] (3) The UPS eliminates misfolded or damaged proteins (e.g., the mutant transmembrane conductance regulator protein [CFTR] is selectively degraded by the UPS so it does not reach the epithelial cell surface in patients with cystic fibrosis). (4) The UPS presents antigen to the major histocompatibility complex, class I molecules, thereby participating in immunologic responses. (5) The UPS degrades cellular proteins (including muscle proteins), which are used in gluconeogenesis when energy intake is inadequate or in response to catabolic illnesses.

Chronic Kidney Disease Initiates Mechanisms That Cause a Loss of Muscle Protein

Epidemiologic evidence indicates that CKD is associated with a decrease in muscle and fat mass, which in turn is associated with an increased risk of morbidity and mortality.[77] The mechanisms causing protein wasting include CKD-induced acceleration of the degradation of proteins due to defective responses to insulin or insulin growth factor 1 (IGF-1) intracellular signaling. Other stimuli causing protein losses include the accumulation of acid (Table 85.1). In addition, an excess of angiotensin (Ang) II, impaired function of muscle precursor cells (i.e., satellite cells), and/or activation of the muscle protein, myostatin, which is synthesized in muscle and modulates muscle growth, stimulate the loss of protein stores. Although there is evidence that each of these factors controls muscle protein metabolism, it is likely that they often act together to cause a loss of muscle mass.

When is a loss of muscle mass suspected? Besides a loss of body weight, the principal evidence for subnormal protein stores has been hypoalbuminemia. The finding of hypoalbuminemia in CKD patients is generally presumed to be attributable to protein malnutrition.[78,79] However, malnutrition is defined as abnormalities related to an insufficient amount of protein, energy, or other nutrients in the diet or to an imbalance among dietary nutrients.[80] There are at least two reasons that the muscle wasting associated with CKD is not caused

TABLE 85.1 **Evidence That Metabolic Acidosis Induces Protein and Amino Acid Catabolism in Normal Infants and Children as Well as Chronic Kidney Disease Patients**

Subjects Investigated	Measurements of Effectiveness	Outcome of Trial
Infants[226]	Low birth weight, acidotic infants were given $NaHCO_3$ or NaCl	$NaHCO_3$ supplement improved growth
Children[227] with CKD	Children with CKD had protein degradation measured	Protein loss was ~twofold higher when HCO_3 was <16 mM compared to >22.6 mM
Normal adults[228]	Induced acidosis and measured amino acid and protein metabolism	Acidosis increased amino acid and protein degradation
Normal adults[108]	Induced acidosis and measured nitrogen balance and albumin synthesis	Acidosis induced negative nitrogen balance and suppressed albumin synthesis
CKD[229]	Nitrogen balance before and after treatment of acidosis	$NaHCO_3$ improved nitrogen balance
CKD[22]	2 years $NaHCO_3$ therapy vs standard care	Slowed loss of creatinine clearance and improved nutritional status
CKD[17]	Essential amino acid and protein degradation before and after treatment of acidosis	$NaHCO_3$ suppressed amino acid and protein degradation
CKD[230]	Muscle protein degradation and degree of acidosis	Proteolysis was proportional to acidosis and blood cortisol
CKD[231]	Nitrogen balance before and after treatment of acidosis	$NaHCO_3$ reduced urea production and nitrogen balance
CKD[22]	Protein stores after $NaHCO_3$ treatment to slow progression	Serum proteins and weight improved
Hemodialysis[103]	Protein degradation before and after treatment of acidosis	$NaHCO_3$ decreased protein degradation
Hemodialysis[109]	Serum albumin before and after treatment of acidosis	$NaHCO_3$ increased serum albumin
CAPD[104]	Protein degradation before and after treatment of acidosis	$NaHCO_3$ decreased protein degradation
CAPD[106]	Weight and muscle gain before and after treatment of acidosis	Raising dialysis buffer increased weight and muscle mass

CKD, chronic kidney disease; CAPD, continuous ambulatory peritoneal dailysis.

by malnutrition per se: first, if protein malnutrition were the cause of defects in protein stores, then the abnormalities should be corrected by simply altering the diet. This hypothesis has been examined and found to be wanting: Ikizler et al.[81] measured rates of protein synthesis and degradation in fasting hemodialysis patients using labeled amino acid turnover techniques. They studied three protocols and in each instance measured protein metabolism before, during, and at 2 hours after completing dialysis.[82–83]. When dialysis was performed in fasting patients, protein degradation exceeded protein synthesis demonstrating that over days to weeks, these responses would produce a significant loss of body protein stores. In the second protocol, they tested the influence of intravenous parenteral nutrition (IDPN) given during hemodialysis.[82] IDPN did improve both protein synthesis and degradation measured during dialysis, but the increase in protein degradation persisted at 2 hours following the completion of dialysis. In the third protocol, they tested the effects of an oral nutritional supplement versus IDPN. As before, protein balance improved with both supplements but at 2 hours after completing dialysis, protein balance was still negative.[83] Thus, abnormalities in protein metabolism were not eliminated by simply increasing the intake of protein and calories during dialysis. Others report similar conclusions: in a randomized, controlled trial of responses to IDPN, hemodialysis patients were compared to other hemodialysis patients who were not given a dietary supplement. After 2 years, the supplement had not improved mortality, body mass index, laboratory markers of nutritional status, or the rate of hospitalization.[84] Even though the excessive morbidity and mortality occurring in patients with CKD may not be corrected simply by changing the diet or correcting hypoalbuminemia, it is critical to plan the diet of CKD patients in order to ensure that they receive an adequate amount of protein and energy.[78,80] It is also necessary to avoid an excess of dietary protein because the accumulation of waste products will contribute to complications of CKD, especially in the nondialyzed patient with advanced CKD.[8]

What are the signals in CKD that enhance a loss of protein stores? Recent studies in rodent models of CKD have established that the accelerated muscle wasting involves cellular mechanisms that are similar to those causing muscle wasting in other catabolic conditions, such as cancer cachexia, starvation, insulin deficiency/resistance, or sepsis.[72,73] Common to each of these catabolic states is an acceleration of proteolysis via the UPS, which is presumably augmented by higher levels of messenger RNAs (mRNAs) encoding certain components of the UPS.[36] There are also increases or decreases in the expression of about 100 atrophy-related genes called atrogenes. The latter responses indicate that the mRNAs of atrophy-related genes in muscle wasting states are due to changes in gene transcription yielding a common transcriptional program that involves various growth-related genes in atrophying muscle.[85] The strongest evidence for the activation of the UPS in muscles of animals undergoing CKD-induced atrophy from catabolic diseases is that inhibitors of the proteasome block the increase in protein degradation in muscles isolated from rodent models of catabolic diseases.[36,86,87]

In CKD, abnormalities identified as signals that stimulate protein degradation in muscle include the development of metabolic acidosis, defects in insulin/IGF-1 intracellular signaling, or an increase in Ang II levels.[88–90] All three conditions cause muscle atrophy in rodents. Finally, CKD patients frequently have high circulating levels of inflammatory cytokines and this has been shown to cause accelerated muscle protein degradation at least in part by impairing insulin or IGF-1 signaling in muscles.[91,92]

Caspase-3 and Muscle Wasting in Chronic Kidney Disease

Muscle atrophy in catabolic conditions specifically affects contractile proteins, which comprise about two-thirds of the protein in muscle. Notably, the ubiquitin protease system (UPS) readily degrades major components of the myofibril (actin, myosin, troponin, or tropomyosin). But when these same proteins are present in complexes or in intact myofibrils, they are degraded very slowly by the UPS.[93] Therefore, other proteases must initially cleave proteins to break down the complex structure of muscle. The protease functioning in this fashion is caspase-3.[94] Notably, caspase-3 cleaves actomyosin in vitro, and it is stimulated in cultured muscle cells, where myofibrillar proteins are cleaved and subsequently degraded by the UPS. Caspase-3 activation produces a footprint of its activity, a 14kD C-terminal fragment of actin that is found in the insoluble fraction of muscle.[94] For example, accumulation of the 14-kD actin fragment is found in muscles of animals with accelerated protein degradation due to acidosis, diabetes, and Ang II–induced hypertension.[89,94,95] Likewise, the 14-kD actin fragment can be found in muscles of patients with CKD or other causes of muscle wasting. The level of the 14-kD actin fragment in muscle of CKD patients was found to decrease in response to an exercise program directed at increasing the patient's endurance. The level of the fragment was also highly correlated ($r = 0.78$) with the measured rate of protein degradation in muscles of patients undergoing hip replacement for osteoarthritis. Finally, the 14-kD actin fragment that was present in unburned muscle of patients who had a major burn injury to another area of the body was sharply increased.[96] Thus, the level of the 14-kD fragment seems to be closely related to the rate of protein degradation and is present in specific disorders characterized by muscle wasting. Additional testing will be needed to determine if this method could serve as a biomarker of accelerated muscle protein degradation in other conditions causing muscle wasting.

Signals Triggering Muscle Wasting in Chronic Kidney Disease or Other Catabolic States

CKD is associated with several complications that can trigger the UPS to degrade muscle protein, and there is evidence that these complications can function in concert to cause muscle wasting. Metabolic acidosis stimulates muscle protein breakdown by the UPS, but only when there is a concomitant increase in glucocorticoid production and development of insulin resistance.[97,98] Glucocorticoids are also required for the accelerated protein degradation that occurs in models of diabetes, high levels of Ang II, and sepsis.[90,99,100]

Impaired insulin/IGF-1 intracellular signaling is another stimulus for accelerated muscle protein breakdown. The mechanism involves the decreased activation of the phosphatidylinositol 3-kinase(PI3K)/Akt pathway.[89] Specifically, when insulin or IGF-1 signaling is low, PI3K activity falls, reducing the production of phosphadidylinositol-3,4,5 phosphate, the active product of PI3K. This results in decreased phosphorylation and activity of the serine/threonine kinase, Akt, leading to decreased phosphorylation of downstream kinases, gycogen synthase kinase 1 (GSK1) and mTOR/S6kinase, and suppression of protein synthesis.

Decreased PI3K/Akt signaling is a key step that stimulates protein degradation in muscle. Decreased PI3K/Akt signaling induces the expression of caspase-3 and the E3 Ub conjugating enzymes, Atrogin-1 and muscle ring finger protein 1 (MuRF-1), to enhance muscle protein degradation.[89] Expression of these E3 enzymes occurs because there is decreased phosphorylation of the Forkhead family of transcription factors (FoxO1, 3, 4). When these factors are not phosphorylated, they migrate into the nucleus to stimulate the transcription of Atrogin-1 and, potentially, other genes involved in muscle metabolism.[89,101,102] Insulin or IGF-1 blocks this process by stimulating the PI3K/Akt pathway to suppress the expression of Atrogin-1. Together, these results provide evidence that muscle wasting in response to the complications of CKD is due to a common signaling pathway that alters key enzymes modulating protein synthesis and degradation.

Are there methods for correcting the abnormalities in muscle protein metabolism that occur in CKD? In a mouse model of CKD, the mice were paired for SUN and weight and treated with either a humanized antibody or peptibody against myostatin or the diluent.[76] Peptibody treatment increased body and muscle weight while raising muscle protein synthesis and suppressing protein degradation. Interestingly, these beneficial responses were accompanied by an increase in the phosphorylation of Akt and a decrease in the circulating levels of tumor necrosis factor alpha (TNF-α) and interleukin 6 (IL-6). These results suggest that methods could be developed to prevent muscle wasting in CKD patients.

This brief review of changes in muscle protein metabolism caused by progressive CKD emphasizes that activities of caspase-3 and the UPS participate in the turnover of the bulk of proteins in the body. Because the daily turnover of protein is high, even a small but persistent increase in protein breakdown would cause muscle wasting. Specific complications of kidney disease coordinate the activity of proteolytic systems (i.e., caspase-3 and the UPS) to degrade muscle proteins. These responses involve defects in insulin/IGF-1 intracellular signaling pathways and decreased PI3K/Akt signaling, which are initiated by metabolic acidosis or inflammation. In addition, glucocorticoids play a permissive role in stimulating muscle wasting. Understanding these regulatory mechanisms could blunt the muscle wasting that occurs in different catabolic conditions.

Factors Stimulating Loss of Muscle Mass in Chronic Kidney Disease

Abundant clinical evidence indicates that acidemia is an important cause of protein losses (Table 85.1). Reaich et al.[17] found that the rate of protein degradation in acidemic CKD patients is high, but when they were given sodium bicarbonate, protein degradation decreased by 28%. It increased again when the patients developed acidemia in response to eating an equimolar amount of sodium chloride. The stimulatory effect of metabolic acidosis on protein breakdown is also present in hemodialysis or continuous ambulatory peritoneal dialysis (CAPD) patients.[103–105] At least in CAPD patients, increased muscle proteolysis was found to be related to activation of the UPS.[106,107] In normal adults, induction of metabolic acidemia not only increased insulin resistance but also caused negative nitrogen balance and reduced the rate of albumin synthesis.[38,108] Changes in albumin metabolism induced by metabolic acidemia also occur in hemodialysis patients; correcting their serum bicarbonate levels was found to increase serum albumin levels.[109] Despite these reports documenting the catabolic effects of metabolic acidemia, a cross-sectional analysis of dialysis patients suggested there is no relationship between acidemia and hypoalbuminemia, weight loss, etc.[110] There are several problems with this conclusion. First, a cause and effect relationship cannot be evaluated from results of a cross-sectional study.[111] Second, a single serum bicarbonate measurement is not sufficient to define the presence of acidemia, and there are technical problems with measuring serum bicarbonate: a delay in measuring the serum bicarbonate concentration allows for the escape of carbon dioxide, which lowers the bicarbonate artificially.[112] Third, there are many impaired hormonal responses in patients with metabolic acidemia, including the impaired function of growth hormone, the thyroid hormone, and the conversion of vitamin D to its most active form, 1, 25 (OH)2 cholecalciferol.[113–115] All of these could interact and impair the ability of CKD patients to maintain protein stores by indirect mechanisms.

SPECIFIC DIETARY CONSTITUENTS FOR PATIENTS WITH CHRONIC KIDNEY DISEASE

Energy Intake

In patients entering dialysis therapy, anthropometric abnormalities, including suboptimal body weight, could result from an inadequate energy intake.[116–118] Unfortunately, such caloric deficits are difficult to measure; estimates from the resting energy expenditure (REE) may underestimate or overestimate a patient's average activity. Moreover, indirect calorimetry measured during brief periods can yield erroneous conclusions when extrapolated to 24 hours. Estimates of energy intake based on dietary histories or questionnaires can lead to erroneous conclusions.[119,120]

The 1981 Food and Agricultural Organization (FAO)/World Health Organization (WHO)/United Nations (UN) recommended energy requirements based on 11,000 REE determinations made in healthy subjects.[121] But, the regression equations used to derive energy requirements had considerable variability. Extrapolating REE measurements to all activities with this degree of variability suggests caution is required in making decisions based on those types of measurements. Besides these issues, the individual can adapt to different calorie intakes: healthy adults eating an inadequate nutrient intake will decrease their REE value.[122] When normal adults ate diets with barely adequate amounts of EAA, their nitrogen balance improved when energy intake increased.[123] Well-nourished adults achieve energy balance but only by decreasing their activity. With this adaptation, lean body mass can be lost.[118] Nonetheless, virtually all studies of REE by indirect calorimetry as well as studies based on nitrogen balances indicate that both CKD and maintenance dialysis patients have at least normal energy expenditures during resting or with a variety of activities. Patients with advanced kidney failure and those undergoing MHD or CPD usually have decreased daily physical activity. In normal sedentary adults, total daily physical activity is estimated to account for only about 15% to 25% of total daily energy expenditure. Thus, the reduced physical activity of advanced kidney failure or chronic dialysis patients generally does not result in a major reduction in daily energy expenditure in comparison to sedentary normal people without CKD.

Energy Requirements of Chronic Kidney Disease Patients

Unfortunately, there have been few evaluations of the energy requirements of CKD patients or their responses to a reduced-calorie intake. In one landmark study, the energy expenditure of normal subjects, CKD patients, and hemodialysis patients during rest and exercise revealed no differences among the three groups.[124] Notably, when calorie intake was reduced, energy expenditure did not fall, indicating that CKD patients do not develop a special ability to adapt to a low-calorie intake. Thus, an inadequate energy intake when coupled to dietary protein restriction could cause negative nitrogen balance (i.e., a loss of protein stores).[8] Most studies of energy expenditure in CKD and MHD patients support the thesis that energy expenditure is normal, but one group of investigators reported that energy expenditure on both dialysis and nondialysis days was 7% higher in hemodialysis patients compared to normal adults.[124,125] If, indeed, uremia increases energy expenditure, impaired energy use (e.g. insulin resistance) could cause a loss of lean body mass. This is relevant because patients with serum creatinine values >2.4 mg per deciliter or those who are obese or those with metabolic acidosis can develop insulin resistance and impaired energy use.[2,38,126,127] Fortunately, a low protein diet can actually improve insulin resistance.[3,5,128,129] Regarding this conclusion, energy intake in patients with moderate renal insufficiency in the MDRD study was below 30 to 35 kcal/kg/day yet the loss of body mass was infrequent and only a few patients were withdrawn from the trial because of nutritional considerations.[130] On the other hand, the MDRD study used dietary interviews and diaries to estimate energy intake, methods that can give erroneous results, particularly in CKD or MHD patients.[119,120] Regardless, if a patient is losing weight and there is a history of a low energy intake, additional calories are needed. Intake from such a supplement must be monitored closely because it may lead to an increase in body fat rather than larger stores of protein.[131]

The contribution of a low energy intake to nutritional deficiencies in CKD patients is unclear: CKD outpatients who were eating 16 to 20 g per day of protein plus a supplement of EAA had no change in nitrogen balance when their energy intake was varied between 22 and 50 kcal/kg/day.[132] On the other hand, Kopple et. al.[133] fed six CKD patients a constant, minimal protein intake of 0.55 to 0.60 g/kg/day and measured nitrogen balance while calorie intake was varied from 15 to 45 kcal/kg/day. They concluded that the dietary energy requirement for nitrogen equilibrium for CKD patients who are eating low protein diets should be 35 kcal/kg/day in order to maximize dietary protein use. If CKD patients are at or below their ideal body weight, we believe their energy intake should be 35 kcal/kg/day.[134] For overweight patients, energy intake should be restricted to reduce obesity because obesity causes insulin resistance and impairs the use of protein and calories.[2,120, 131]

Protein Requirements

Nitrogen balance (Bn) is a measurable index of changes in body protein stores and serves as the gold standard for assessing dietary protein requirements. A neutral or positive Bn indicates that the body's protein stores are maintained or increased. For healthy adults engaging in moderate physical activity and eating sufficient calories, the World Health Organization (WHO) used Bn values to conclude that the average requirement for protein of mixed biologic value is approximately 0.6 g of protein per kilogram of body weight per day. This average dietary protein requirement plus 2 standard deviations was assigned as the "safe level of intake," or 0.75 g/kg/d; this value should meet the protein requirements of 97.5% or more of healthy adults.[121] There are two caveats: first, not all normal adults will require this amount of dietary protein, but some will need more than 0.75 g/kg/day. Second, for CKD patients, an increase in dietary protein will increase the production of urea and other waste products. If these compounds are not excreted, uremia will develop.[72,135] Adaptive metabolic responses are activated when dietary protein is restricted (see previous). The presumed origin of these metabolic responses is a decrease in plasma insulin leading to the conversion of body protein stores (principally, skeletal muscle) into amino acids, which are converted to glucose in the liver. Insulin is likely to be one of the most potent mediators of these changes in protein turnover because it suppresses protein degradation in normal or diabetic subjects.[136,137] This could explain why diabetic patients (including those with insulin resistance) being treated by hemodialysis are at increased risk of developing an accelerated loss of lean body mass.[138] Because insulin resistance can be present in patients with serum creatinine levels as low as 2.4 mg per deciliter and because metabolic acidosis can cause insulin resistance, insulin-initiated mechanisms could be a key factor regulating whole body protein metabolism.[38,127] In summary, healthy adults successfully adapt to dietary protein restriction by: (1) suppressing the catabolism of EAA and, possibly, NEAA; and (2) suppressing protein degradation while stimulating protein synthesis. A principal mediator of these changes is likely to be insulin.

Protein Requirements for Chronic Kidney Disease Patients

Patients with advanced CKD that is uncomplicated by metabolic acidemia or inflammation, etc. are remarkably efficient at adapting to dietary protein restriction.[68] In response to the limitation of dietary protein from 1.0 to 0.6 g/kg/day, they reduce amino acid oxidation and protein degradation as well as normal adults. The same adaptive responses occur if the diet is restricted to only 0.3 g/kg/day plus a supplement of essential amino acids or their nitrogen-free analogs (ketoacids). These diets are associated with the maintenance of indices of adequate nutrition during more than 1 year of observation.[69,70] Clinically, it must be recognized that compensatory responses will not fully compensate for an inadequate diet and the diet will cause loss of lean mass. Moreover, diabetic patients may not activate adaptive changes to dietary protein restriction as efficiently as do normal adults or CKD patients. Finally, if CKD is complicated by acidemia or inflammatory or chronic illnesses, patients may not be able to activate an adaptive response to dietary restriction.

Protein Requirements for Nephrotic Patients

Patients who are excreting more than 3 to 5 g of protein per day could be at increased risk for protein wasting because their protein intake may not meet minimal requirements. This does not mean that prescribing an excess of protein will improve protein stores. Unfortunately, a high protein diet actually raises the degree of proteinuria in CKD patients.[139,140] This problem is emphasized because patients eating a well-designed low-protein diet can experience a decrease in proteinuria and an increase in serum albumin concentrations compared to patients fed excessive amounts of protein (see the following). The other problem is that feeding a high protein diet increases the likelihood of developing complications of CKD. The other reason to emphasize this problem is the consensus that the degree of proteinuria is closely related to the risk for progressive kidney and cardiovascular diseases.[141] The other factor to consider regarding dietary protein prescriptions for nephrotic patients is that it can activate the same adaptive responses as CKD patients or normal subjects.[71] This ability leads to neutral Bn of nephrotic patients fed 0.8 or 1.6 g/kg/day (plus 1 g of dietary protein for each gram of proteinuria) and 35 kcal/kg/day of energy. There is evidence that even less dietary protein (<0.6 g/kg/day) may not increase the risk of protein wasting in patients with the nephrotic syndrome.[142] In summary, patients with uncomplicated CKD, including those with nephrotic range proteinuria, activate normal compensatory responses to dietary protein restriction by suppressing EAA oxidation and reducing protein degradation. These responses lead to the preservation of lean body mass during long-term dietary therapy. When nephrotic patients excrete ≥10 g of protein per day, there are no clear guidelines for manipulating their dietary protein and calories.

Dietary Sodium and Chloride

Normal adults maintain an extracellular fluid volume that changes by <1 L (1 kg of body weight) and only have minimal changes in blood pressure despite wide variations in daily salt intake. But, if blood pressure rises when sodium chloride intake increases, a patient is labeled salt sensitive and salt balance occurs only slowly. Notably, salt sensitivity can precede established hypertension and it constitutes a cardiovascular risk factor, complicates antihypertensive therapy, contributes to a progressive loss of kidney function in patients with CKD, exacerbates proteinuria, and diminishes the antiproteinuric responses of patients with kidney disease.[143,144] For these reasons, regulating sodium chloride intake is essential for the treatment of patients who have or who are at risk for high blood pressure, for those with kidney disease, and/or for those with cardiovascular risk factors. Treatment with diuretics generally fails in patients who have no dietary guidelines for salt intake because salt intake can cancel the effectiveness of diuretics.[145] Unfortunately, regulating sodium chloride intake is difficult because salt is added to so many foods; it is estimated that, generally, >80% of daily sodium intake is already an integral part of foods.[146,147]

A sodium intake of 2 g per day or 84 mEq per day is widely recommended for patients with hypertension or cardiovascular and kidney diseases. It is important to specify this amount because a no-added-salt diet contains about 4 g of sodium or 168 mEq.[1,148] This level of salt intake exacerbates blood pressure and edema in many CKD patients. Fortunately, a diet of 2 g of sodium per day can be achieved with skilled diet planning.

Salt-sensitive patients with CKD and hypertension can be detected by determining if their blood pressure rises >10% when a low salt diet is switched to a high salt diet. The frequency of salt-sensitive individuals (with the exception of some patients with primary interstitial kidney disease) increases with age, especially when renal function is declining.[147,149,150] Salt restriction is especially important in the treatment of hypertensive CKD patients because antihypertensive agents, with the possible exception of calcium channel blockers, are less effective when sodium intake is unrestricted.[151] Because it is an achievable goal, the ideal sodium intake for hypertensive patients is 2 g per day. A decrease in dietary salt can transiently reduce GFR but this usually reverses within a week. Because most dietary salt is already in foods, especially in prepared or fast foods, it is difficult to predict salt intake. Because ~95% of sodium ingested is excreted by the kidneys, the sodium content of a 24-hour urine sample is the best indicator of sodium intake. With fever, strenuous exercise, or diarrhea, and especially in patients with an ileostomy, there can be significant extrarenal sodium losses. To monitor salt intake, CKD patients should weigh themselves daily and record their weight; if weight is declining, it is most likely due to a loss of extracellular salt and water, and contrariwise, if weight is increasing, it is most likely due to an accumulation of salt and water. In such cases, the diet should be reviewed to determine the source of the unwanted salt. Monitoring body weight is emphasized because sodium excretion fluctuates widely during the day, and a "spot" urine for measurement of the sodium/creatinine ratio does not provide reliable insights into the assessment of dietary salt. Fortunately, even patients accustomed to a high sodium chloride intake experience salt cravings, and they should be reassured that the craving will disappear after a few weeks.[146,152]

In summary, a cornerstone of designing diets for CKD patients is to establish appropriate goals for blood pressure and sodium intake. Home blood pressure recording or ambulatory 24-hour blood pressure recordings are the most reliable in assessing the effectiveness of therapy. Compliance with dietary salt restriction must be monitored by 24-hour urine collections for sodium content. Fortunately, this same collection can be used to determine creatinine clearance and to estimate protein intake from urea excretion (see the following) and the presence of microalbuminuria and other minerals. If sodium excretion is excessive and blood pressure increases, education by the nutritionist and repeated measurements of 24-hour urine sodium collections will make dietary planning easier.

Dietary Potassium

Guidelines from the Institute of Medicine recommend a potassium intake of 4.7 g per day.[153] Fortunately, the ability to excrete this amount of potassium is usually retained until renal insufficiency is very advanced.[154] The ability to eliminate potassium is maintained by increased potassium excretion by both the gut and kidney, making the design of diets to restrict both dietary salt and potassium possible.[154] If hyperkalemia is present, a search is needed to determine if there is acidemia, defects in aldosterone actions, or if treatment has been changed to include nonsteroidal anti-inflammatory drugs (NSAIDs) or blockers of the renin-angiotensin-aldosterone system (RAAS). If these changes are required, dietary potassium must be restricted. The diet is limited to ~1.5 g per day; compliance is monitored from the 24-hour urinary excretion of potassium.

It is fortunate that the ability to excrete potassium is maintained because diets rich in potassium (e.g., fruits and vegetables) reduce the likelihood of developing chronic diseases, such as coronary heart disease and diabetes. Moreover, clinically important reductions in blood pressure have been documented to occur when adults with normal blood pressure or mild hypertension consume a potassium-rich diet. For example, in the DASH (Dietary Approaches to Stop Hypertension) Study,[155] potassium was increased in the diet but a potassium supplement was not supplied. Adults with systolic blood pressures <160 mm Hg and diastolic blood pressure 80 to 95 mm Hg were fed a standard Western diet high in saturated fat and low in fruits and vegetables and calcium. They were then randomly assigned to the same diet, which included a diet rich in fruits and vegetables versus a combined diet rich in fruits, vegetables, and with low-fat dairy products. This last diet had a reduced content of saturated and total fat. For all three groups, sodium intake and body weight were maintained at constant and at similar levels. Systolic and diastolic blood pressures decreased with the fruit and vegetable diet, and a more pronounced reduction in systolic and diastolic pressures occurred with the combination of high fruit and vegetable, and low-fat dairy product diet (−11.4 and −5.5 mm Hg, respectively). The changes in blood pressures were substantially greater in African American participants as compared to Caucasians.[156] This study did not address the effects of these diets in CKD patients but may be applicable because of the adaptations in potassium excretion.

Regarding CKD patients, the National Kidney Foundation's expert panel[157] recommended the restriction of dietary potassium in adults with CKD at stage 4 (estimated GFR <30 mL/min/1.73 m^2). The regulation of the serum potassium concentration at the desired level is complicated because patients with advanced CKD generally have low values of total body potassium, even when the serum potassium is high.[158] More studies are needed to determine the usefulness and dangers of increasing (or limiting) dietary potassium in patients with CKD.

VITAMINS AND TRACE ELEMENTS IN RENAL DISEASE

Micronutrients, vitamins, and trace elements are required for energy production, organ function, and cell growth and protection (e.g., from oxygen free radicals). Consequently, they should be included when planning diets for CKD patients.[159] Besides an insufficient intake, losses of protein-bound elements with proteinuria, decreased intestinal absorption of micronutrients, cellular metabolic changes or circulating inhibitors, and medicines that antagonize some vitamins can cause micronutrient deficiency syndromes. Unfortunately, there is very little information concerning the minimum requirements or the recommended daily allowances (RDA) for these nutrients in CKD patients. For CKD patients, supplements of water-soluble vitamins are routinely prescribed because meat and diary products are routinely restricted in their diets and there can be benefits of a daily supplemental vitamin. The long-term administration of vitamin B6 and folate can improve responses to EPO.[160] Vitamin B1 (thiamine) losses can occur with diuretic therapy or hemodialysis, potentially causing problems when the diet is restricted. However, there are no long-term evaluations detailing the incidence of thiamine deficiency even though some of its cardiovascular and neurologic symptoms can mimic complications of advanced CKD. For MHD patients, the average concentrations of folate, niacin, and vitamins B1, B6, B12, and C in whole blood and erythrocytes are often normal, presumably because the diet protein requirement of 1 g/kg/day is being eaten.[161] However, low or borderline low levels of certain vitamins, particularly vitamins B6 and C, folic acid, and 25-hydroxycholecalciferol and 1,25-dihydroxycholecalciferol, are often reported.[162] The need for some vitamins is increased in kidney failure, so we recommend that a supplement containing the RDA for water-soluble vitamins be prescribed for CKD, hemodialysis, and CAPD patients.

Riboflavin is necessary for normal energy use because it is used to maintain levels of the coenzymes flavin mononucleotide and flavin adenine dinucleotide. Riboflavin is present in meat and dairy products and its deficiency can produce sore throats, stomatitis, or glossitis, which may be mistaken for uremic symptoms. Folic acid is found in fruits and vegetables, but cooking can destroy it, and hence, it could become deficient in patients with restricted diets. Because folic acid is required for adequate EPO treatment and for the synthesis of nucleic acids and for methyl group transfer reactions and because it may decrease homocysteine production, it should be provided as a supplement. Vitamin B6 (pyridoxine) is necessary for many metabolic reactions involving amino acids via transaminase-catalyzed reactions. It is contained in meats, vegetables, and cereals. A deficiency can produce symptoms of a peripheral neuropathy or altered immune function, or host resistance may develop. Because these problems could complicate advanced uremia, a daily pyridoxine HCl supplement providing 5 mg per day for stage 4 and 5 CKD patients and 10 mg per day for MHD and CPD patients is recommended. Vitamin B12 is required for the transfer of methyl groups among metabolic compounds and for the synthesis of nucleic acids. Its major sources are meat and diary products. A deficiency state is unusual because this vitamin is stored in the liver. Also, little vitamin B12 is removed during hemodialysis because its molecular weight is rather high (1,355 Da), and it is largely protein bound in plasma. A daily supplement containing the RDA is recommended even though the likelihood of CKD, MHD, or CPD patients developing a deficiency state is low.[159]

Vitamin C or ascorbic acid protects against antioxidant reactions and is involved in the hydroxylation of proline during collagen formation. It also is contained in meat, dairy products, and most vegetables so a deficiency state is unusual. Unfortunately, dialysis readily removes vitamin C, so a deficiency state can develop in patients eating an inadequate diet. Since high doses of vitamin C are metabolized to oxalate which can precipitate in soft tissues (including the kidney), vitamin C supplements should contain only the RDA amount.

The remaining water soluble vitamins, including biotin, niacin, and pantothenic acid, have been less well studied. Biotin functions as a coenzyme in bicarbonate-dependent carboxylation reactions and is produced by intestinal microorganisms. Consequently, a deficiency state is unusual. Niacin (nicotinic acid) is used as a nicotinamide adenine dinucleotide phosphate coenzyme. It is synthesized from the essential amino acid, tryptophan; a deficiency produces diarrhea, dermatitis, or increased triglycerides. Pantothenic acid is involved in the function of coenzyme A and, hence, in the metabolism of fatty acids, steroid hormones, and cholesterol. Although there is minimal information about the efficacy and consequences of these vitamins in renal disease, a supplement of the RDA of these vitamins appears to be quite safe, and we also recommend supplements, but only at amounts equivalent to the RDA.

In summary, patients eating restricted diets are at risk for developing vitamin-deficiency syndromes. Even MHD and chronic peritoneal dialysis (CPD) patients who are urged to eat generous amounts of protein and energy are at risk for ingesting less than the RDA of vitamins established for normal subjects and the daily requirements at least for vitamin B6 and folate appear to be increased in these patients.[163] We conclude that CKD as well as chronic dialysis patients should have a water-soluble vitamin supplement because it may prevent certain problems from developing and probably does little harm. Because hyperoxaluria and possibly peripheral neuropathy can occur with high doses of vitamin C and pyridoxine, respectively, megavitamin therapy should be avoided.[164]

The requirements for fat-soluble vitamins in patients with CKD have not been established, and there are reasons to suspect that some of these vitamins may even cause complications of CKD. We recommend that fat-soluble vitamins should be given only when there is a well-defined indication. Because many multivitamin preparations contain fat-soluble vitamins, these preparations should be avoided unless there is evidence for a deficiency condition. Notably, plasma vitamin A (retinol) levels are usually increased in CKD patients because the level of retinol-binding protein is high, making it likely that tissue levels are normal or increased.[159] Supplemental vitamin A can contribute to anemia, dry skin, pruritus, bone resorption, and hepatic dysfunction in uremic patients.[165]

The requirements for vitamin E, another fat-soluble vitamin, are not established. Vitamin E has been given in experimental models of CKD, providing some reduction in the degree of renal injury in rats with experimental immunoglobulin A (IgA) nephropathy or glomerulosclerosis following a subtotal nephrectomy or diabetes.[166] Although plasma vitamin E levels are generally reported to be normal in uremic patients, the question of supplementing vitamin E to suppress lipid peroxidation/oxidant stress has not been settled. Vitamin E may reduce the rate of progression of carotid artery stenosis in MHD patients with a history of vascular disease. Other studies have not confirmed a beneficial effect of vitamin E on atherosclerosis in patients with CKD. Another factor to be considered is that vitamin E supplements may be hazardous. The Heart Outcomes Prevention Evaluation (HOPE) Study was carried out in older people who were at a high risk for adverse cardiovascular events; there was no restriction to the presence or absence of CKD. Patients treated with daily vitamin E (400 IU) developed a delayed and significantly increased risk for heart failure and hospitalization for heart failure.[167] The RDA for vitamin E is 15 mg per day, and lower doses of vitamin E could be given to CKD or maintenance dialysis patients. Indeed, some multivitamins contain quantities of vitamin E that are less than the RDA and are provided largely to ensure that the daily vitamin E intake meets the RDA. Although vitamin E might reduce oxidant stress, it is controversial whether routine vitamin E supplements should be given to CKD patients.

The vitamin D analogs, 25-hydroxycholecalciferol and 1,25-dihydroxycholecalciferol, are bound to an alphalike globulin and may be lost in the urine in nephrotic patients.[168] This can lead to decreased ionized and total calcium, and bone disease in some patients and patients with the nephrotic syndrome should have regular surveillance of vitamin D levels. Recommendations for supplemental vitamin D are discussed in Chapter 73.

The need to supplement most trace element supplements for CKD and maintenance dialysis patients is not clear. The controversy arises because of difficulties in determining if body stores are insufficient, adequate, or excessive. A deficiency may not be reversed solely if only more trace elements are supplied.[159] Aluminum has been studied extensively because aluminum-containing antacids have been used to control serum phosphorus and, in the past, dialysates were contaminated with aluminum. Aluminum accumulation can cause bone disease, especially osteomalacia, a progressive dementia, proximal muscle weakness, impaired immune function, and anemia.[169,170] Aluminum retention also can reduce serum iron stores, contributing to resistance to erythropoetin (EPO) therapy.[171] Plasma and leukocyte zinc levels are reportedly decreased and may be associated with endocrine abnormalities such as high plasma prolactin levels.[172] In patients with advanced CKD, the urinary excretion of zinc or fecal zinc may be decreased.[173] Some reports indicate that dysgeusia, poor food intake, and impaired sexual function, which are common problems of uremic patients, may be improved by giving patients zinc supplements.[174] Other studies, however, have not confirmed these results.[175] A zinc supplement has been reported to increase B-lymphocyte counts, granulocyte motility, and taste and sexual dysfunction.[159]

The finding that serum selenium is low in dialysis patients has raised the question of supplementing selenium because selenium participates in the defense against oxidative damage of tissues, which may be increased with kidney failure.[176] The relationship among other trace elements and the occurrence of beneficial or adverse reactions has not been well studied in CKD patients. Hence, with the possible exception of the nephrotic syndrome, we do not recommend routinely giving supplements of trace elements unless there is documentation that trace element intake is low or a deficiency is present. This may be the case for iron, zinc, and selenium. The exception would be patients who are receiving long-term parenteral or enteral nutrition without supplements of trace elements; these individuals should routinely be given trace elements. Finally, the appearance of skin rashes, neurologic abnormalities, or other unexplained problems in maintenance dialysis patients should prompt a search for excessive concentrations of trace elements in the dialysate.

Assessment of Dietary Compliance

The classic report of Folin[59] pointed out that urea excretion is the principal change in urinary nitrogen that occurs when dietary protein changes. This has been repeatedly confirmed and provides a firm foundation for assessing compliance with low-protein diets.[60,61,177] The rate of urea production exceeds the steady-state rate of urea excretion in both normal and uremic subjects because there is an extrarenal clearance of urea. This extrarenal removal of urea is due to its degradation by bacterial ureases present in the gastrointestinal tract.[178–180] In the past, it was believed that urea degradation to ammonia contributes substantially to amino acid synthesis in the liver and, hence, improves the nutritional status of uremic patients.[181] This is incorrect; the ammonia nitrogen is simply used to synthesize urea by reincorporating it into urea.[179,180] Fortunately, the rate of net urea production closely parallels dietary nitrogen[60,177] and net production (i.e., urea appearance [UNA]) is easily calculated because the concentration of urea is equal throughout body water.[154,179] Because water represents ~60% of body weight in nonedematous patients, changes in the urea nitrogen pool can be calculated by multiplying 60% of nonedematous body weight in kilograms by the SUN concentration in grams per liter. The UNA is calculated as the change in the urea nitrogen pool (positive or negative) plus urinary urea nitrogen excretion. If the SUN and weight are stable, urea nitrogen accumulation is zero and UNA equals the excretion rate (Table 85.2).

Nonurea Nitrogen

Unlike urea nitrogen, nonurea nitrogen excretion (i.e., the nitrogen excreted in feces and in urinary uric acid, creatinine, and unmeasured nitrogenous products) does not vary greatly over a large range of dietary protein.[60,61] The nonurea nitrogen excretion averages 0.031 g of nitrogen per kilogram of ideal body weight per day (Fig. 85.2). This average value was derived from patients with ≤ 5 g per day of proteinuria; if proteinuria exceeds 5 g per day, then protein in the diet should be increased by the amount of protein lost in the urine. There is no significant correlation between nonurea nitrogen excretion and dietary protein in patients eating low-protein diet.[61,117] This finding is important because a value of nonurea nitrogen excretion depending on weight provides a method for assessing compliance with protein-restricted diets. We examined results of over 70 nitrogen balance measurements and found no significant correlation between dietary nitrogen and either fecal nitrogen or nonurea nitrogen excretion, at least in CKD patients eating protein-restricted diets.[61] This distinction is important because independence of nonurea nitrogen excretion from dietary protein yields a method of assessing compliance with protein-restricted diets. Compliance is assessed by converting the prescribed protein intake to its nitrogen equivalent by multiplying dietary protein by 0.16 (protein is 16% nitrogen). If nitrogen balance is assumed to be zero, then nitrogen intake equals the sum of UNA (Table 85.2) plus 0.031 g/kg/day of nitrogen.[60] Therefore, the patient is compliant if the intake equals the output. However, when intake is greater or less than nitrogen output, then the assistance of a skilled dietician is needed. The caveat is that this method cannot be used reliably if a patient is receiving total parenteral nutrition or eating completely digestible foods (e.g., astronauts). In summary, total nitrogen

TABLE 85.2 **Estimating Compliance with Dietary Protein Using Urea Turnover**

1. A 70-year-old man with a urea clearance of 10 mL/minute weighs 70 kg. He is taught a diet containing 0.8 g protein/kg/day in order to meet the daily allowance of protein recommended by the World Health Organization. His serum urea nitrogen (SUN) and weight are stable. A 24-hour urine collection contains 6 g of urea nitrogen.

   Because protein is 16% nitrogen, he is eating 9 g of nitrogen daily. His non-urea nitrogen excretion is 70 kg × 0.031 g of nitrogen/kg/day or 2.17 g of nitrogen per day and his total nitrogen excretion is 6 + 2.2 = 8.8 indicating that he is compliant with the prescribed diet.
2. A 60-year-old woman with stage V CKD is admitted to the hospital for plastic surgery. She has been taught a diet that contains 40 g of protein/kg/day (~6.4 g of nitrogen per day because protein is 16% nitrogen). She is excreting 4 g urea nitrogen per day, but on the 2nd day of admission, her SUN rises from 50 to 60 mg/dL.

   Her non-urea nitrogen excretion is estimated as 60 × 0.031 g of nitrogen/kg/day or 1.9 g of nitrogen/day. Thus, her total excretion is 9.5 g of nitrogen/day. (Total nitrogen excretion = 4 g urinary urea nitrogen + 1.9 g non-urea nitrogen + the accumulation of 3.6 g urea nitrogen [36 L as estimated body water × 0.1 g urea nitrogen per liter of body water.]) Her nitrogen excretion substantially exceeds her prescribed intake so a nutrition/dietician consult and a stool sample for blood are obtained.

excretion is calculated from weight, SUN, and urea nitrogen excretion. It is compared to the prescribed protein intake and if the values are different by more than 20%, then reasons for noncompliance or the reasons for a negative nitrogen balance should be investigated.[182] Another equation that takes into account unmeasured losses of nitrogen through respiration, sweat, exfoliated skin, flatus, and sputa is

$$\text{Dietary nitrogen intake in grams per day} = 1.20\ \text{UNA (g/day)} + 1.74.$$

Multiplying the amount of dietary nitrogen intake by 6.25 estimates the protein intake.

Another potential use of the calculated dietary protein is to evaluate a patient's calorie intake. First, the ratio of dietary protein to calories can be estimated from the patient's dietary history. Second, the protein intake calculated from urea nitrogen excretion as just outlined is divided by the

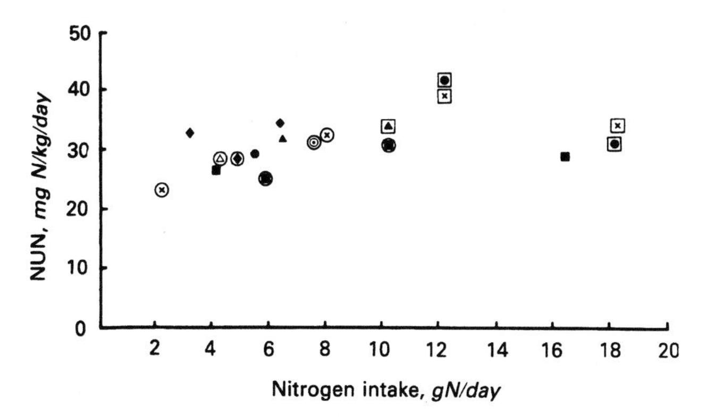

FIGURE 85.2 Calculated values of total nonurea nitrogen (NUN) excretion in normal subjects (*solid symbols*) and patients with chronic renal failure. The average value for patients not being treated by dialysis is 0.031 g of nitrogen per kilogram per day. (From Maroni BJ, Steinman T, Mitch WE. A method for estimating nitrogen intake of patients with chronic renal failure. *Kidney Int.* 1985;27:58.)

calculated protein intake yielding the calorie intake. This type of analysis should be used regularly in patients treated with restricted diets because calorie intake must be sufficient to use protein in the diet efficiently to maintain body protein stores. The importance of using these calculations regularly is highlighted by the report that CKD patients frequently underreport their calorie intake, especially if they are obese.[183]

Other methods of assessing protein intake, including dietary histories, were exhaustively reviewed by Bingham[184]: interview methods are less accurate and, over time, patients learn the appropriate responses to questions about dietary habits. Examples of this problem have been reported by Kloppenburg et al.[120] and Molitch et al.[183] They evaluated food records and anthropometric and oxygen consumption data of dialysis patients and CKD patients. They found that energy intake was grossly underestimated when assessed by diet records. In summary, dietary compliance can and should be calculated from the measured urea nitrogen excretion and the nonurea nitrogen excretion.

DIETARY PROTEIN RESTRICTION AND THE PROGRESSION OF RENAL INSUFFICIENCY

Several conditions related to a loss of kidney function have been identified from studies of experimental kidney damage (Table 85.3). Regarding responses in the patient, beneficial effects of dietary restriction on the progression of CKD were reported in the late 1970s, but the reports were criticized because they relied on changes in the serum creatinine or creatinine clearance to assess progression. There also were difficulties in the study design (including the lack of randomization and retrospective analyses). The Modification of Diet in Renal Disease (MDRD) Study,[185] an intention-to-treat analysis of the largest trial of dietary protein restriction and progression, led

TABLE 85.3 **Experimental Renal Diseases Improved by Dietary Protein Restriction**

Remnant kidney
Nephrotoxic serum nephritis
Doxorubicin nephrosis
DOCA salt hypertension
Spontaneous hypertension with reduced renal mass
Salt-sensitive hypertension with glomerulonephritis
Diabetes mellitus
Spontaneous glomerular sclerosis of aging
Antitubular basement membrane nephritis

DOCA, deoxy-cortisone acetate.

to the conclusion that there was no benefit of protein-restricted diets on progression. There were notable problems with this interpretation but there are other reasons to manipulate the diet of CKD patients, namely to prevent complications of CKD.

Randomized Controlled Trials in Nondiabetic Chronic Kidney Diseases

Clinical trials that satisfy "high quality" requirements[186] include the report of the Northern Italian Cooperative Study Group, which analyzed results from 456 patients categorized according to the National Kidney Foundation (NKF) definition as stage III to IV CKD patients.[187] The patients were examined over at least 2 years following their random assignment to diets containing either 0.6 g of protein per kilogram per day (low-protein diet [LPD]) or 1g/kg/day (control group) plus at least 30 kcal/kg/day. The actual protein intake was determined from the urea nitrogen excretion,[60,61] and unfortunately, varied minimally. The average protein intake was 0.9 g/kg/day for the control group and 0.78 g/kg/day for the LPD group with substantial overlap in the amounts of protein eaten. Thus, the study did not test the hypothesis that eating a low protein diet will slow the loss of kidney function. Because dietary protein differed by 0.12 g/kg/day, it is not surprising that there was only a borderline difference in the primary outcome of renal survival, defined as the start of dialysis or the doubling of serum creatinine between control and LPD groups; slightly fewer patients assigned to the LPD group reached the end point ($P = .059$).

The MDRD study evaluated different levels of protein intake and two levels of blood pressure control in a 2 × 2 design.[185] GFR was measured as the urinary clearance of ^{125}I-iothalamate to determine how rapidly renal function was lost. In Study A (stages III to IV CKD), 585 patients were randomly assigned to a standard diet of >1 g of protein per kilogram per day or a diet containing 0.6 g of protein per kilogram per day and there were targeted mean arterial blood pressures of 105 or 92 mm Hg. In Study B, 255 stage IV CKD were randomly assigned to diets of 0.6 g of protein per kilogram per day or 0.3 g of protein per kilogram per day supplemented with a ketoacid/essential amino acid mixture, very low protein-keto acid (VLP-KA); the same blood pressure goals were sought. Actual protein intakes based on urea nitrogen excretion[60,61] were 1.11 and 0.73 g of protein per kilogram per day, respectively, in Study A and 0.69 and 0.46 g of protein per kilogram per day (plus the supplement in the VLP-KA group), respectively, in Study B. The analysis revealed no statistical difference in the rate of loss of GFR between the two groups in Study A. Results of Study B showed a trend toward a slowing of the loss of GFR for the VLP-KA diet patients ($P < .07$), but the difference was not statistically significant.

There are a number of caveats in the interpretation of this study: (1) In Study A, there was an initial, rapid decrease in GFR in CKD patients assigned to the restricted, 0.6 g/kg/day of protein intake. This response has been ascribed to a physiologic reduction in glomerular hemodynamics.[188] Subsequently, the loss of GFR was slower in CKD patients prescribed the LPD versus those assigned to the control diet (1.11 g of protein per kilogram per day). Thus, if the physiologic response is disregarded because it does not represent kidney damage, the rate of loss of GFR from the end of the initial 4 months until the last measurements yields a significantly lower value in patients assigned to the protein-restricted group. There also was a significant improvement in kidney survival ($P = .009$). (2) ACE inhibitors were prescribed to some patients in both Study A and B, which can influence the rate of loss of kidney function.[141] (3) The trial may have been discontinued prematurely.[182] For example, in the U.S. National Institutes of Health (NIH)-sponsored Diabetes Control and Complications (DCCT) Trial of the risks and benefits of strict blood glucose control, there was no protective effect of the intervention on the progression of kidney disease initially. But, after 4 years of strict glucose control, the development of microalbuminuria or macroalbuminuria was significantly depressed with strict glucose control. (4) Secondary analyses of the MDRD trial, although less robust for assessing efficacy, did identify the slowing of progression in those patients who had a measured decrease in dietary protein.[189,190] A low protein diet reduced the rate of loss of GFR in Study B patients ($P = .011$). There also was a reduction in the frequency of renal death (death or initiation of dialysis; $P = .001$). Specifically, for every 0.2 g/kg/day reduction of dietary protein, there was a 1.15 mL/minute/year reduction in the rate of loss of GFR and a 49% reduction in the frequency of renal deaths. (5) The inclusion of results from these patients with polycystic kidney disease had no benefit of restricting dietary protein or controlling blood pressure. Because polycystic kidney disease patients constituted ~25% of patients enrolled in the MDRD study, including them could have biased the interpretation of the results.[185] Based on an intention-to-treat analysis, restricting dietary protein in the MDRD study did not produce a statistically significant slowing of the rate of loss of GFR.

In an 18-month study, Williams et al.[191] compared three dietary interventions in 95 patients with stage IV to V CKD: (1) 0.6 g of protein per kilogram per day and 800 mg of phosphate intake; (2) 1,000 mg of phosphate per day plus phosphate binders; and (3) unrestricted dietary protein and phosphate. Dietary compliance was estimated from diet records and urea excretion, yielding levels of 0.7, 1.02, and 1.14 g of protein per kilogram per day plus 815, 1,000, and 1,400 mg of phosphorus per day, respectively. Rates of progression were measured by creatinine clearances. There were no differences in the decrease in creatinine clearance over time among the three groups nor were there differences in the numbers of patients who died or began dialysis therapy. Criticisms, however, are that changes in creatinine clearance may not accurately represent changes in GFR. In addition, differences in actual protein intakes were minimal and the number of CKD patients studied was small.

Cianciaruso et al.[192] studied patients with stage IV to V CKD during 18 months of observation following assignment to 0.55 or 0.8 g of protein per kilogram per day. They randomly assigned 212 patients to receive the lower protein intake and 211 CKD patients to receive the higher level of dietary protein. Based on estimates from urea excretion,[60] the protein-restricted group ate 0.72 g compared to 0.92 g of protein per kilogram per day of the high protein diet patients ($P < .05$). The authors found no alteration in body composition or nutritional indices (principally, serum albumin) in either group. Based on an intention-to-treat analysis, 13 patients in the 0.92 g of protein per kilogram per day group versus 9 assigned to the 0.55 g of protein per kilogram per day died or were started on maintenance dialysis during the study.

Munford[193] evaluated if a very low protein intake supplemented with ketoacids might affect the efficiency of EPO therapy in 20 patients who were examined over 2 years. Patients were randomly assigned to 0.49 g/kg/day plus a supplement of ketoacids/amino acids or 0.79 g/kg/day. For the VLPD-KA group, only two had to begin dialysis compared to seven subjects assigned to the higher dietary protein group ($P < .05$). There also was an improvement in EPO responsiveness.

Ihle and colleagues,[194] studied 72 Australian patients with stage IV to V CKD. The patients were randomly assigned to a diet of unlimited protein or 0.4 g of protein per kilogram per day and were observed for 18 months (Fig. 85.3). Based on urea excretion,[60] the dietary protein-restricted group ate 0.69 g of protein per kilogram per day versus 0.8 g of protein per kilogram per day for the control group. The GFR (^{51}Cr-EDTA clearance) progressively declined, but only in patients eating the unlimited diet. The number of patients who had to begin dialysis was also lower in the protein-restricted group ($P < .05$). The authors did note that patients in the protein-restricted group lost weight, but otherwise there were no abnormalities in other anthropometric measures or in serum albumin.[194]

Jungers et al.[195] reported the outcomes of dietary protein manipulation in only 19 stage V CKD patients. Ten patients were randomly assigned to a VLPD-KA regimen, whereas nine were assigned to a conventional low protein diet of 0.6 g of protein per kilogram per day. Unfortunately, the actual amount of dietary protein eaten in the two groups differed by only 0.2 g/kg/day. This factor and the small number of patients limits the interpretation of the results.

Malvy et al.[196] studied 50 stage IV to V CKD patients by randomly assigning them to a VLPD-KA diet or a diet of 0.65 g of protein per kilogram per day. The time until a patient's creatinine clearance decreased below 5 mL/min/1.73 m^2 or until

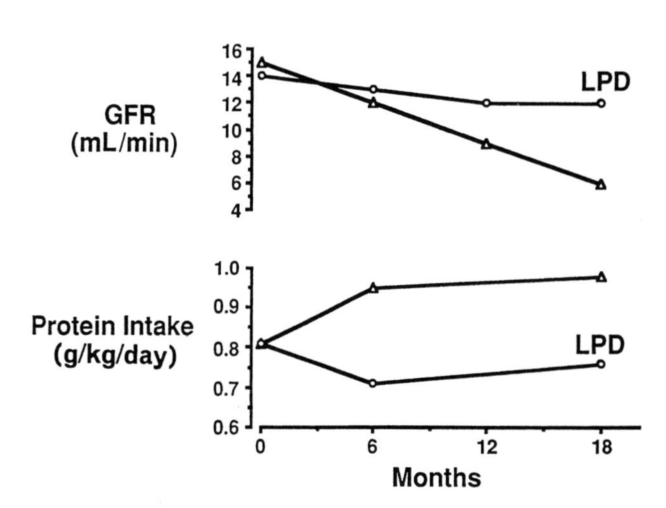

FIGURE 85.3 Changes in glomerular filtration rate (GFR) measured as the plasma clearance of 51 chromium ethylene diaminetetraacetic acid (51Cr-EDTA) in patients prescribed a protein-restricted diet (*open circles*) or an unrestricted diet (*open triangles*). The calculated level of dietary protein based on urea excretion[120] is also shown. The low-protein regimen significantly reduced the decline in GFR. *LPD,* low protein diet. (Figure was drawn from the results of Ihle BU et al.[194] and is reproduced with permission from Mitch WE, Klahr S. *Nutrition and the Kidney.* [2nd ed.]. Boston: Little, Brown, 1993, 254.)

dialysis was required was measured. There was no significant difference in renal survival between the two diets, but the study was underpowered to test the hypothesis adequately. Patients in the VLPD-KA group lost 2.7 kg, including loss of both fat and lean body mass; this was not found in patients prescribed the 0.65 g of protein per kilogram diet. Interpreting these results is difficult because no patients were studied while eating an unrestricted diet. Still, the time for patients to reach a GFR of 15 mL/min/1.73 m^2 or less averaged 9 months for those assigned to the LPD regimen but 21 months for VLPD-KA patients. It was concluded that delaying the need for dialysis can be accomplished by dietary manipulation.

Mircescu et al.[197] assessed the clinical course of 53 stage IV to V CKD patients for 60 weeks. Twenty-six patients were randomly assigned to a diet of 0.6 g of protein per kilogram per day and 27 were assigned to a VLPD-KA diet yielding average protein intakes of 0.59 ± 0.08 g and 0.32 ± 0.07 g of protein per kilogram per day respectively. There were no deaths in either group, but 7 of the 26 patients assigned to the 0.6 g of protein per kilogram per day diet reached end-stage renal disease versus only 1 of the 27 assigned to the VLPD-KA diet ($P = .06$). Other responses to the VLPD-KA diet included a 24% decrease in serum phosphorus ($P < .05$). There were no changes in nutritional status of either group and no significant differences in the loss of GFR from serum creatinine (eGFR), but no conclusion about progression was reached as the number of patients studied was too few to examine this question rigorously (the authors estimated that approximately 100 patients per group would be required to identify significant differences in the number of renal deaths associated with the VLPD-KA diet).

Rosman et al.[198,199] studied the influence of dietary protein restriction in 228 stage III and stage IV to V CKD patients during 2 or 4 years. The control group ate an unrestricted diet, whereas patients assigned to the dietary protein-restricted diets ate different levels of protein: stage III CKD patients were instructed in a diet consisting of 0.6 g of protein per kilogram per day and stage IV to V CKD patients ate a diet of 0.4 g of protein per kilogram per day. After 2 years, the authors found decreased proteinuria and a significant slowing of the progression of kidney failure but only in male patients; patients with polycystic kidney disease had no beneficial responses. After 4 years, there was a survival benefit (i.e., the percentage of patients requiring dialysis) for patients treated by restricting dietary protein (60% versus 30%, $P < .025$).[199] It was concluded that compliance with the diets was fairly good and did not cause signs of malnutrition.

Brunori et al.[200] examined elderly Italian patients with stage V CKD by randomly assigning patients to treatment with a protein-restricted diet or chronic dialysis therapy. Results in the 56 patients treated with the VLPD-KA diet were compared to 56 patients assigned to dialysis. The survival rate was 83.7% and 87.3% in the dialysis and low protein diet, respectively ($P = .6$). Patients assigned to dialysis had a 50% higher degree of hospitalization. Based on an intention-to-treat analysis, the authors found a continuous benefit of the protein-restricted diet over time. The authors concluded that those randomly assigned to the VLPD-KA diet had no difference in life span compared to those treated by hemodialysis. The VLPD group had fewer hospitalizations.

Acidosis and Progression of CKD

Recent results have rekindled interest in a mechanism proposed to explain the loss of kidney function in CKD, namely that acidosis contributes to the loss of function. As noted earlier, the development of metabolic acidosis depends on the amount of protein ingested plus the limited ability to excrete acid and, therefore, dietary factors will influence the degree of acidosis. Nath et al.[201] proposed that acidosis could activate complement, leading to kidney damage. In 2009, CKD outpatients were evaluated and it was concluded that those with serum bicarbonate values ≤ 22 mM had a significantly greater likelihood of progressive loss of eGFR compared to patients with values ≥ 27 mM.[202] Another group reported that the administration of sodium citrate to patients with albuminuria and stage II CKD reduced the production of endothelin and the likelihood of decreasing eGFR.[203] They expanded these studies and performed a randomized clinical trial of administration of sodium bicarbonate to patients with stage II CKD and hypertension.[204] Over a 5-year period, patients treated with sodium bicarbonate had slowing of the loss of eGFR compared to patients treated with equivalent amounts of NaCl. In another randomized clinical trial, deBrito-Ashurst and colleagues[22] demonstrated that the administration of sodium bicarbonate slowed the loss of kidney function and improved nutritional indices (e.g., serum albumin).

Randomized, Controlled Trials in Diabetic Kidney Disease

Clinical trials of the influence of dietary restriction in diabetic, CKD patients generally have been too brief to identify differences in renal deaths compared to patients assigned to unrestricted diets. Consequently, surrogate analyses including a reduction in the degree of microalbuminuria or proteinuria, and/or changes in creatinine clearance or serum creatinine (converted to eGFR using the standard MDRD equation) have been examined to determine the efficacy of protein-restricted diets on the progression of CKD or changes in nutritional factors. In many of the early trials, a confounding factor was the unregulated prescription of ACE inhibitors, which can change the progression. For these reasons, the influence of dietary protein restriction in slowing the progression of diabetic nephropathy is unsettled.

Zeller et al.[205] compared diets containing 1 g of protein per kilogram per day with 0.6 g of protein per kilogram per day in 36 type 1 diabetic CKD patients during an average of 35 months. Changes in creatinine clearance and GFR (iothalamate clearance) were assessed, as were actual protein intakes based on urea excretion. The groups averaged 1.08 g versus 0.72 g of protein per kilogram per day, respectively. The low protein regimen significantly ($P < .02$) reduced the rate of decrease in GFR in patients who initially had eGFR values >45 mL per minute compared to results with the control diet. The nutritional status was not compromised by the low protein diet.

Hansen et al.[206] analyzed results from the longest randomized trial of patients with type 1 diabetes and CKD. The groups were prescribed their usual protein intake or a diet containing 0.6 g of protein per kilogram per day over 4 years. Average protein intakes were 1.02 g/kg/day versus 0.89 g/kg/day, a minimal difference. Not surprisingly, the degree of proteinuria in the two groups was not different. However, the frequency of renal deaths (i.e., progression to end-stage renal disease) was 36% lower in patients consuming the protein-restricted diet. When renal deaths were analyzed, adjusting for cardiovascular disease by the Cox analysis, the benefits of the low protein diet were even more significant ($P = .01$).

Meta-Analyses of Reports of Progression of Chronic Kidney Disease with Low Protein Diets

A meta-analysis provides an alternative approach that is based on analyzing the combined results from all methodologically acceptable clinical trials with the goal of increasing the number of participants available for analyses. The analyses can identify responses in each original study even though that study was sufficiently underpowered to examine the significance of the outcome.[207] Outcomes from large randomized trials are considered to be level one evidence versus evidence from meta-analyses, which are considered to be equal to outcomes derived from small randomized trials. After searching the literature to collect trials, including searches of international databases and often including results from non–English-based journals, a set of rigorous criteria have been established to select or reject reports that are not randomized, controlled trials so that biased results could be minimized.[208] The most frequent outcome in meta-analyses of the influence of dietary protein manipulation is renal death, signified by a patient's death, the need to start dialysis,[209–211] the rate of decline in kidney function,[208] or changes in the degree of proteinuria.[212]

Kasiske et al.[208] studied results from >1,900 patients and found that the protein-restriction reduced the loss of GFR by only 0.53 mL/minute/year ($P < .05$). Although this result can be considered positive in terms of a renal protective effect of the diets, it was concluded that the results were not very important clinically.

Fouque et al.[186] performed a meta-analysis of 10 randomized controlled trials directed at evaluating whether low protein diets slow the loss of kidney function in nondiabetic CKD patients. Renal death was the outcome and the baseline characteristics of the patients in terms of gender and the causes of kidney diseases were equally distributed between the control and the diet-restricted groups. The outcomes of 1,002 patients assigned to dietary protein restriction were compared to the outcomes of 998 patients who had been assigned to higher protein intakes (Fig. 85.4). In the low

Analysis 1.1. Comparison I Low protein versus higher protein diets, Outcome I Renal death.

Review: Low protein diets for chronic kidney disease in nondiabetic adults

Comparison: I Low protein versus higher protein diets

Outcome: I Renal death

Study or subgroup	Low protein n/N	Higher protein n/N	Weight	Risk Ratio M-H, Random, 95% CI
1 0.6 g/kg/d versus higher protein diet				
Locatelli 1991	21/230	32/236	15.7%	0.67 [0.40, 1.13]
MDRD 1994	18/291	27/294	12.9%	0.67 [0.38, 1.20]
Williams 1991	12/33	11/32	9.8%	1.06 [0.55, 2.04]
Subtotal (95% CI)	**554**	**562**	**38.3%**	**0.76 [0.54, 1.05]**
Total events: 51 (Low protein), 70 (Higher protein)				
Heterogeneity: Tau² = 0.0; Chi² = 1.37, df = 2 (P = 0.50); I² = 0.0%				
Test for overall effect: Z = 1.65 (P = 0.099)				
2 0.3–0.6 g/kg/d versus higher/free protein diets				
Cianciaruso 2008	9/212	13/211	6.2%	0.69 [0.30, 1.58]
di Iorio 2003	2/10	7/10	2.5%	0.29 [0.08, 1.05]
Ihle 1989	4/34	13/38	4.1 %	0.34 [0.12, 0.95]
Jungers 1987	5/10	7/9	8.4 %	0.64 [0.32, 1.31]
Malvy 1999	11/25	17/25	15.8%	0.65 [0.39, 1.09]
Mirescu 2007	1/27	7/26	1.0%	0.14 [0.02, 1.04]
Rosman 1989	30/130	34/117	23.7 %	0.79 [0.52, 1.21]
Subtotal (95% CI)	**448**	**436**	**61.7%**	**0.63 [0.48, 0.83]**
Total events: 62 (Low protein), 98 (Higher protein)				
Heterogeneity: Tau² = 0.01; Chi² = 6.27, df = 6 (P = 0.39); I² = 4%				
Test for overall effect: Z = 3.31 (P = 0.00092)				
Total (95% CI)	**1002**	**998**	**100.0%**	**0.68 [0.55, 0.84]**
Total events: 113 (Low protein), 168 (Higher protein)				
Heterogeneity: Tau² = 0.0, Chi² = 8.20, df = 9 (P = 0.51); I² = 0.0%				
Test for overall effect: Z = 3.68 (P = 0.00024)				

0.01 0.1 1 10 100

Less deaths on low | Less deaths on high

FIGURE 85.4 A representation of the results of a meta-analysis of low protein diets in patients with chronic kidney disease. *M-H,* meta-analysis for harm; *MDRD,* modification of diet in renal disease; *CI,* confidence interval. (From Fouque D, Laville M. Low protein diets for chronic renal failure in non-diabetic adults. *Cochrane Database of Systematic Reviews.* Issue 3, Art. No.: CD001892. Copyright Cochrane Collaboration; reproduced with permission.)

protein groups, 113 renal deaths occurred versus 168 patients in the control group, leading to a 0.68 odds ratio for renal death in the low protein group compared to the control group (the 95% confidence interval was 0.55 to 0.84; $P = .0002$). The authors concluded that eating low protein diets can result in a 32% reduction in death or the need to start dialysis therapy when results were compared to eating unlimited amounts of protein.[186]

The number needed to treat (NNT) is a tool for comparing the outcomes of a treatment in different studies, especially when risks of events are quite different between studies.[213] NNT indicates the number of patients that would have to be treated for 1 year to spare one major event (e.g., renal death). The NNT for a low protein diet varied from 2 to 56 for each study.[186] The variation was high because patients had different degrees of renal insufficiency at the start of the trials and the outcomes are confounded because the absolute risk of renal death would be greater in those CKD patients with more impaired kidney function.[195,196] Importantly, this level of NNT is acceptable for analyses of primary and secondary prevention outcomes in part because a low protein diet is far less expensive than dialysis or transplant therapy. In addition, these NNTs compare favorably with examples such as the well-accepted reduction in mortality with statin therapy, in the 4S trial (NNT = 30) or in the WOSCOPS study (NNT = 111).[214]

The discrepancy between the meta-analysis of Kasiske et al.[208] and other investigators may be related to the types of outcomes. Renal death, including the commencement of chronic dialysis therapy, was reported to be significantly and importantly reduced with low protein diets. The finding that renal death was delayed with low protein diets may be due to the slowing of the rate of loss of GFR or to the fact that low protein diets, by generating fewer uremic toxins, may maintain a healthier state for patients with stage 5 CKD. Consequently, physicians may delay the initiation of chronic dialysis therapy until a lower GFR is reached when compared to patients eating less well-controlled diets. It should be emphasized that none of these meta-analyses limited an examination of patients who were highly adherent to their prescribed low protein diets. It is possible that the benefits of low protein diets for these patients would be greater.

Conclusions about a benefit of low protein diets in patients with diabetic nephropathy yield opposing views. Pedrini et al.[210] reported that outcomes based on the combined criteria of microalbuminuria and a decline in renal function improved by 44% ($P < .001$) in patients assigned to low protein diets. More recently, Pan et al.[212] analyzed eight randomized trials with results from 519 patients: 253 in the low protein diet group and 266 in the control group. Changes in GFR or creatinine clearance, HbA1c levels, proteinuria, and serum albumin levels were recorded. No definitive differences in death or dialysis were uncovered with the two diets. Notably, however, the difference in dietary protein was minimal, at 0.36 g/kg/day (1.27 versus 0.91 g of protein per kilogram per day; $P = .04$). Proteinuria did decrease ($P = .003$), and glycosylated hemoglobin improved in seven of eight studies (a mean reduction of 0.31%; $P = .005$). Limitations of this review were the inclusion of results from patients with type I and II diabetes and from patients with early renal disease (e.g., isolated microalbuminuria but no renal insufficiency or only those with macroalbuminuria [>1 g per day]). In addition, four trials lasted only 12 months. Finally, the total number of patients (about 500) might not have been sufficient to detect statistical differences for all measures.

Regardless, this analysis confirms that reducing protein intake in patients with diabetes and CKD improves insulin sensitivity, decreases HbA1c, and reduces proteinuria, two independent factors associated with renal protection.

In summary, the meta-analysis technique indicates that there can be clear benefits for CKD patients eating low protein diets, including a reduced risk of renal death or a substantial delay until dialysis is required. This conclusion stands in sharp contrast to the suggestion by some that dialysis should be started early. Notably, tests of the efficacy of early dialysis have revealed that it does not improve mortality and certainly is more costly.[5,9,10,215] It is controversial whether dietary restriction will slow the loss of kidney function. But, there are other reasons to assess the diets of CKD patients: a well-planned diet can avoid some of the complications of CKD and delay the time until dialysis or transplantation becomes necessary.

Nutritional Impact and Safety of Modified Diets in Chronic Kidney Disease

A critical issue in the evaluation of outcomes with long-term dietary modification is whether a low protein diet is nutritionally sound and safe for patients with CKD. The MDRD Study enrolled 840 patients with different stages of CKD, providing the largest number of patients to address this question.[185] Patients were examined for an average of 2.2 years and a large number of measurements of nutritional status (e.g., body weight and anthropometrics, serum proteins, dietary adherence) were gathered. Based on urea excretion,[60] the average protein intakes of the different groups were significantly different. Kopple et al.[130] concluded there was some decrease in the estimated protein intake of subjects as their renal insufficiency advanced. There also was a decrease in energy intake, but this conclusion is not solid because the reliability of estimating calorie intake from dietary diaries can be problematic.[119,120] Notably, only 2 of the 840 participants had to stop the trial because of concerns about the nutritional status. Assignment to the low protein diet was associated with a small loss of body weight and arm muscle area (an index of muscle mass), but there was a small increase in serum albumin.

In contrast to these rather positive outcomes from the MDRD study, Menon et al.[216] reported that their analysis of results from the U.S. Renal Data System (USRDS) revealed a problem. They gathered data from the USRDS about patients entering dialysis or receiving a transplant and all-cause mortality during the almost 10 years of the study, including the 2.2 years of the actual MDRD study. This led them to conclude that patients assigned to the VLPD-ketoacid diet had an associated increased risk of death. No information was provided about the compliance of the patients during the MDRD study nor were dietary factors examined following the end of the MDRD study. There was no information about other illnesses, dialysis-related factors, or treatments occurring after the end of the MDRD study. It was speculated that there could have been persistent restriction of dietary protein after beginning dialysis, or possibly, an accumulation of an unidentified toxin that somehow influenced the survival. Regarding the former, one group reported that patients trained in low protein diets had a delay of 3 months before their dietary protein was raised after the initiation of dialysis therapy.[217] In contrast, other investigators found no delay in increasing protein intake after dialysis therapy begins.[218] Regarding the possibility that the increased risk of death was related to an accumulation of an unidentified toxin, no such substance was looked for or identified. Importantly, the ketoacid supplements were discontinued at the end of the MDRD study, making it unlikely that nutritional or toxic responses occurring years later were due to ingestion of the ketoacid supplements. Other problems with the Menon et al.[216] analysis have been detailed.[219]

Results compiled by Chauveau and colleagues[5] provide a markedly different outcome. They detailed the long-term survival of 220 stage IV to V CKD patients who had been treated with 0.3 g of protein per kilogram per/day plus a mixture of ketoacids for an average of 33 months (4 to 230 months) before starting dialysis or being transplanted.[5] The authors analyzed the survival of these patients and compared it to a larger cohort of patients who were not treated with a low protein diet but who were treated concurrently by the same investigators. At 1 year after beginning dialysis, the authors concluded that the survival of dialysis patients was 97%, and after 5 years, it was 60%. For the kidney transplant patients, the survival at 5 and 10 years was 97% and 95%, respectively. When compared to the survival of U.S. patients, these results are excellent.[220] On the other hand, results achieved by Chauveau et al.[5] were compared to retrospective control patients who may not have received the same intensity of care as did patients assigned to a more complicated dietary regimen. Because the number of patients treated by Chauveau et al.[5] and those analyzed by Menon et al.[216] are similar, these widely disparate results are unexplained. A notable difference in the reports is that details of treatment and outcomes are provided in the report of Chauveau et al.[5] but not by the Menon et al.[216] publication. The Menon et al.[216] manuscript, however, does compare patients who were randomly assigned to different treatment regimens and who were followed very closely for the first 2 years of a 10-year period. We conclude that low protein diets, including the VLPD-KA regimen, are probably not harmful and do not increase mortality in patients, including in those who progress to a stage requiring dialysis or transplantation.

Conclusions

Patients with CKD can respond to dietary manipulation to reduce the signs and symptoms of uremia. The regimen is nutritionally safe as long as there is no complicating factor such as acidosis, infection, etc. Consequently, dietary manipulation should be included in a treatment program that includes monitoring protein and energy intake in collaboration with a dietician.[60,221] We suggest that such a regimen be implemented for patients with stages III to V CKD, if not earlier. The observation that protein intake may voluntarily decrease as renal insufficiency progresses should not be a signal to raise dietary protein because this will simply increase the degree of uremia (including hyperphosphatemia, metabolic acidosis, aggravate hypertension, etc.) and will not raise serum protein above what a well-designed low protein diet will achieve.[3,222,223] A well-designed protein-restricted diet may increase serum albumin.[6] Regarding benefits on the progression of CKD, a low protein diet could delay the need for dialysis by ameliorating uremic symptoms while maintaining nutritional status. In addition, adherence to a well-designed diet could prove valuable in correcting complications of CKD. For example, the effectiveness of ACE inhibitors in slowing progressive CKD is blunted by increased serum phosphorus, a problem that should be avoided by dietary manipulation.[14] There is strong evidence for the long-term safety of this approach.[224,225] Clearly, successful implementation of dietary therapy requires the motivation of both the patient and the physician. The principal, if not the only disadvantage of such therapy (assuming that it is successful in eliminating uremic symptoms), is the dietary restriction it entails, but it is reasonable to expect that dialysis therapy will be significantly delayed.

Dietary Protein Requirements for Dialysis and Transplant Patients

Maintenance hemodialysis (MHD) patients have increased dietary protein requirements due to losses of amino acids, peptides, and proteins by the dialysis procedure.[232,233] Hemodialysis also stimulates protein catabolism by engendering an inflammatory, catabolic response (Table 85.4).[234] Nitrogen balance results suggest that most maintenance hemodialysis patients require about 1 g of protein per kilogram per day to maintain both protein balance (Bn) and normal total body protein mass.[235] The National Kidney Foundation K/DOQI Clinical Practice Guidelines on Nutrition in Chronic Renal Failure recommend 1.2 g of protein per kilogram of body weight per day.[236] To ensure an adequate intake of essential amino acids, at least half of the dietary protein should be of high biologic value. There are currently no data concerning dietary protein requirements for patients undergoing MHD five or more times per week.

Chronic Peritoneal Dialysis (CPD)

Blumenkrantz and coworkers[237] studied protein and mineral balances in eight clinically stable men who underwent

TABLE 85.4 **Recommended Dietary Nutrient Intake for Patients with Stage III to V Chronic Kidney Disease Not Undergoing Dialysis and for Patients Undergoing Maintenance Hemodialysis or Chronic Peritoneal Dialysis**

	Stage III–V Chronic[a,b,c] Kidney Disease	Maintenance Hemodialysis (MHD)[c]	Continuous Ambulatory Peritoneal Dialysis (CAPD) or Automated Peritoneal Dialysis (APD)
Protein			
Low protein diet	0.60 g/kg/day; protein may be increased up to 0.75 g/kg/ necessary to maintain adequate energy intake or if patient will not accept lower protein diets; 50% of protein is of high biologic value	1.2 g/kg/day; 50% high biologic value protein	1.2–1.3 g/kg/day; 50% high biologic value protein
Energy (kcal/kg/day)	35 kcal/kg/day for individuals <60 years of age and 30–35 kcal/kg/day for patients ≥60 years of age; patients with relative body weight >120% or patients who gain or are afraid of gaining unwanted weight may be prescribed lower energy intakes; energy intake includes energy obtained from diet and, if applicable, from hemodialysate or peritoneal dialysate		
Fat (percent of total energy intake)[d,e]	25–35	25–35	25–35
Polyunsaturated fatty acids [d,e]		Up to 10% of total calories	
Monounsaturated fatty acids [d,e]		Up to 20% of total calories	
Unsaturated fatty acids [d,e]		–<7% of total calories	
Cholesterol [d,e]		–200 mg/day or lower	
Carbohydrate [d,e,f]		50%–65% of total calories	
Total fiber intake (g/day)	20–30	20–30	20–30
Minerals (range of intake)			
Sodium (mg/day)	1,000– 3,000[g]	1,000– 2,000[g]	1,000– 3,000[g]
Potassium (mEq/day)	40–70	40–70	40–70
Phosphorus (mg/kg/day)[h]	10–14	12–17	12–17
Calcium (mg/day)	1,000– 1,500[i]	1,000– 1,500[i]	1,000– 1,500[i]
Magnesium (mg/day)	200–300	200–300	200– 300
Iron (mg/day)	>10– 18[j]	See text	See text
Zinc (mg/day)	15	15	15
Water (mL/day)	Up to 3,000 as tolerated[g]	Usually 750–1,500[g]	Usually 1,000–1,500[g]

Vitamins	Diets to be supplemented with these quantities		
Thiamin (mg/day)	1.5	1.5	1.5
Riboflavin (mg/day)	1.8	1.8	1.8
Pantothenic acid (mg/day)	5	5	5
Niacin (mg/day)	20	20	20
Pyridoxine HCl(mg/day)	5	10	10
Vitamin B12(ng/day)	3	3	3
Vitamin C (mg/day)	60	60	60
Folic acid (mg/day)	1–15[k]	1–15[k]	1–15[k]
Vitamin A	No addition	No addition	No addition
Vitamin D	See text	See text	See text
Vitamin E (IU/day)	15	15	15
Vitamin K	None[l]	None[l]	None[l]

[a]A GFR above 4–5mL/min/1.73 m^2 and less than 30 mL/min/1.73 m^2 (see text for discussion of dietary intake for patients with less severe renal insufficiency).

Note: Patients are to be informed that the ability of low protein diets to reduce progressive chronic renal disease in patients who are receiving angiotensin converting enzyme inhibitors and or angiotensin receptor blockers has not been definitely demonstrated (see text).

[b]The protein intake is increased by 1.0 g/day of high biologic value protein for each gram per day of urinary protein loss.

[c]When recommended intake is expressed per kilogram body weight, this refers to the adjusted edema-to-body weight (see text).

[d]Refers to the percent of total energy intake (diet plus dialysate); if triglyceride levels are very high, the percentage of fat in the diet may be increased to about 40% of total calories; otherwise, 30% or less of total calories is preferable. The recommendations regarding fat, carbohydrate, and fiber intake follow the NCEP TLC (Therapeutic Lifestyle Changes) Diet.[261]

[e]These dietary recommendations are considered less crucial than the others. They are only emphasized if the patient has a specific disorder that may benefit from this modification or is complying well with more important aspects of the dietary treatment (see text).

[f]Should be primarily complex carbohydrates.

[g]Can be higher in CPD patients or in hemodialysis patients or nondialyzed patients with chronic renal failure who have greater urinary losses.

[h]Phosphate binders (e.g., calcium carbonate or acetate, sevelamer HCl or carbonate, lanthanum carbonate or aluminum carbonate, or hydroxide) often are needed to maintain normal serum phosphorus levels.

[i]Dietary intake usually must be supplemented to provide these levels. Higher daily calcium intakes are commonly ingested because of the use of calcium binders of phosphate.

[j]Iron: >10 mg/day for males and nonmenstruating females; >18 mg/day for menstruating females. For individuals receiving erythropoietin, larger iron intakes, usually given intravenously, are usually necessary (see text).

[k]Folic acid, 1 mg/day, is adequate for advanced CKD and maintenance dialysis patients. If hyperhomocysteinemia is present, folic acid, 5 to 15 mg/day, may be more effective at maximizing the reduction in plasma homocysteine concentrations (see text).

[l]Vitamin K supplements may be needed for patients who are not eating and who receive antibiotics.

Note: Patients undergoing hemodialysis more frequently than thrice weekly may have increased tolerance and/or increased requirements for some nutrients.

13 metabolic balance studies of 14 to 33 days' duration in a clinical research center. Patients were fed diets with an average of 0.98 or 1.44 g of protein per kilogram per day (SD) and total energy intake (diet plus dialysate) was 41.3 ± 1.9 or 42.1 ± 1.2 kcal/kg/day with the low and high protein diets, respectively (Fig. 85.5). Bn results adjusted for changes in body urea nitrogen but not for unmeasured losses was +0.35 ± 0.83 g per day with the 1.0 g per kilogram protein diet and +2.94 ± 0.54 g per day with the higher protein intake (P = NS). When nitrogen balances are adjusted by subtracting about 1 g per day for unmeasured losses through skin, respiration, flatus, and blood sampling, Bn was negative with the low protein diet but still positive with the higher protein diet. There was a curvilinear relationship between dietary protein intake and nitrogen balance in the 13 studies.[237] Based on the these reports, we recommend prescribing 1.2 to 1.3 g of protein per kilogram per day to CAPD and automated peritoneal dialysis (APD) patients as recommended by the NKF K/DOQI Clinical Practice Guidelines on Nutrition in CRF for clinically stable CPD patients.[238] As with MHD patients, at least 50% of the dietary protein should be of high biologic value. Protein depleted patients may become anabolic with intakes as high as 1.5 g of protein per kilogram per day. In most CAPD and APD patients, there may be a need to increase the number or volume of dialysate exchanges or at least the volume of dialysate outflow.

Other nitrogen balance studies[239] in MHD or CPD patients have not included either the total nitrogen intake and/or outputs or the duration of these studies was too short to interpret the results rigorously. Patients classified as high peritoneal transporters. by the peritoneal equilibration test tend to lose more protein and amino acids into peritoneal dialysate versus low transporter patients. The high transporters also have, on average, lower serum albumin levels.[240] Dietary protein intakes of 1.2 to 1.3 g per kilogram per day should provide sufficient amounts of protein and amino acids to compensate for the increased peritoneal losses if the synthetic function for serum proteins is normal.

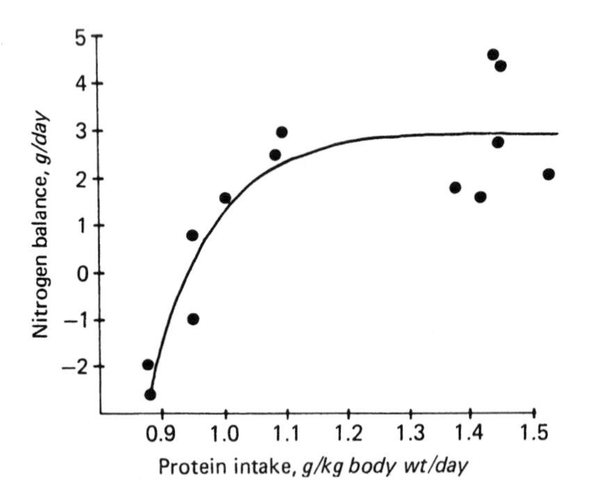

FIGURE 85.5 The relationship between dietary protein intake and nitrogen balance measured in 13 studies in 8 men undergoing CAPD. Each *circle* represents the mean balance data observed in an individual patient fed a constant diet for 14 to 33 days in a clinical research unit. The *curved line* represents the calculated relationship between nitrogen balance and protein intake. (From: Blumenkrantz MJ, Kopple JD, Moran JK, et al. Metabolic balance studies and dietary protein requirements in patients undergoing continuous ambulatory peritoneal dialysis. *Kidney Int.* 1982;21:849, with permission,)

Some nephrologists describe MHD or CPD patients who have dietary protein intakes of about 0.9 to 1.0 g per kilogram per day and do not appear protein depleted and lead physically active, rehabilitated lives. These observations have raised questions as to whether the foregoing recommended dietary protein intake may be excessive for maintenance dialysis (MD) patients. First, the number of MHD or CPD patients who have undergone careful nitrogen balance or other studies of their dietary protein requirements is small, and conclusions concerning their dietary protein needs therefore are imprecise; this is particularly true for MHD. Moreover, some MD patients who appear to be doing well will have evidence for protein depletion. Epidemiologic studies have associated protein depletion, even in mild forms, with increased mortality.[241]

The concept of dietary allowances presupposes that in order to ensure a sufficient nutrient intake for virtually all individuals (i.e., about 97%) in a population, the recommended allowance must be greater than the actual requirement for a large proportion of that population.[242] This reasoning is similar to that used by the WHO and the U.S. National Academy of Sciences when they recommended dietary protein intakes for normal adults. Thus, if the recommended protein allowance is 1.2 to 1.3 g/kg/day, many patients will tolerate lower protein intakes without developing protein depletion. At present, no known method identifies which patients can safely ingest lower levels of protein. To be safe, unless the patient can be shown to maintain a healthy nutritional status, he/she should be prescribed the recommended dietary allowance. Subtle forms of protein losses are particularly difficult to detect and a normal serum albumin concentration for patients may indeed be > 4.0 g/dL to be reassured of desirable clinical outcomes.[243]

Energy

Most studies indicate that energy expenditure measured by indirect calorimetry appears to be normal during resting and sitting or with defined exercise or after ingestion of a standard meal for nondialyzed CKD patients or those treated by MHD or CAPD.[235,244–246] In two studies of nondialyzed CRF or MHD and CPD patients, resting energy expenditure was increased.[247] What is most impressive about the foregoing studies is that there is no report of decreased energy expenditure in CKD, MHD, or CPD patients. Nitrogen Bn measurements indicate that in nondialyzed stage V CKD patients ingesting 0.55 to 0.60 g of protein per kilogram per day the amount of energy intake necessary to ensure neutral or positive nitrogen Bn is approximately 35 kcal/kg/day.[235] In clinically stable MHD patients ingesting 1.13 ± 0.02 (SEM) g of protein per kilogram per day, Bn and anthropometric measurements indicate that close to 38 kcal/kg/day may be necessary to maintain body mass.[246] Virtually every study of stage IV and V CKD patients or MHD and CPD patients indicates that their mean energy intakes are below this level, averaging 24 to 27 kcal/kg/day.[248] Children with chronic renal failure (CRF) also have low energy intakes.[249] Many patients undergoing CPD tend to gain body fat and weight, probably due to the glucose uptake from the dialysate and the subsequent rise in insulin.

The NKF K/DOQI Clinical Practice Guidelines for Nutrition in CRF recommend that the energy intake for stage III CKD patients and for MHD and CPD patients should be 35 kcal/kg/day for individuals $<$60 years of age and 30 to 35 kcal/kg/day for those $>$60 years old (Table 85.4).[238] This intake includes energy derived from the diet plus glucose taken up from dialysate in MHD or CPD patients. The recommended energy intake is somewhat lower for individuals $>$60 years of age because they tend to be more sedentary and have less muscle mass. These recommendations are rather similar to those for normal individuals engaged in light-to-moderate activity as put forth in the RDAs by the Food and Nutrition Board, National Academy of Sciences.[242] Patients with an edema-free body weight greater than 120% of desirable body weight may be treated with lower calorie intakes. Some patients, particularly those with more mild renal insufficiency or younger or middle-aged women, may become obese on this energy intake or may refuse to ingest the recommended calories to avoid obesity and may require a lower energy prescription. It is important to monitor dietary intake and to treat inadequate intakes, even in clinically stable healthy appearing adults with advanced CKD or MHD or CPD patients. To remedy this problem, the dietician can recommend high-calorie foods that are low in protein and sodium and that can be prepared easily.

Lipids

There are several mechanisms that produce abnormal serum lipids and lipoproteins in CKD patients.[250] Stage IV and V CKD patients and patients undergoing MHD and CPD frequently have a high incidence of increased serum triglyceride levels, low-density lipoprotein (LDL), very low LDL (VLDL), and serum lipoprotein (a) (Lp[a]); their serum level of high density lipoprotein (HDL) cholesterol is often low. CPD patients often have higher serum total cholesterol, triglycerides, LDL cholesterol, and apolipoprotein B levels than do MHD patients.[250] Qualitative changes in the apolipoprotein concentrations also occur; among these is an increase in small density LDL (sd LDL).[250,251] Elevated serum triglyceride levels in uremia appear to be caused primarily by the impaired catabolism of triglyceride-rich lipoproteins.[250] Reduced catabolism leads to increased quantities of apoB-containing triglyceride-rich lipoproteins in IDL and VLDL and reduced concentrations of HDL. The key alteration in the apolipoprotein levels appears to be a decreased ratio of apoA-1 to apoC-Ill.[250] Activities of plasma and hepatic lipoprotein lipase and lecithin cholesterol acyltransferase (LCAT) are reduced,[250] and it is often difficult to provide sufficient energy without resorting to a large intake of purified sugars because of other dietary restrictions. CPD, with its attendant glucose load from the dialysate, appears to promote a further increase in serum triglycerides and cholesterol. Patients with the nephrotic syndrome usually have hypertriglyceridemia with an increase in serum total cholesterol and LDL cholesterol. LDLs, intermediate density lipoproteins (IDLs), VLDLs, and LP(a) are increased,[252] and serum HDL tends to be low. Serum phospholipids and apoproteins B, C-II, C-III, and E are increased, whereas apoproteins A-I and A-II are normal. Elevated serum cholesterol is caused by increased hepatic synthesis of lipoproteins and cholesterol and reduction in LDL receptor activity, playing an important role in the clearance of IDLs. These changes are aggravated by urinary albumin losses. Decreased activity of lipoprotein lipase contributes to the elevated serum triglyceride levels. There also is an elevation in plasma cholesterol ester transfer protein (CETP) and decreased catabolism of LDL apolipoprotein, at least by the more typical receptor pathway.

Renal transplant recipients may have high serum total and LDL cholesterol values plus increased LDL and IDL lipoproteins. Increased serum total cholesterol, LDL cholesterol, and triglycerides are more likely to be present in transplant recipients with chronic rejection and to correlate with a decrease in kidney function.[253] Therapy with glucocorticoids, cyclosporine A, sirolimus, tacrolimus, diuretics, or certain antihypertensives plus kidney failure, fasting hyperinsulinemia, and obesity are commonly present in renal transplant recipients and can add to the serum lipid disorders.

Because alterations in lipid metabolism and serum lipids may contribute to the high incidence of atherosclerosis and cardiovascular cerebrovascular and peripheral vascular disease in CKD patients, attention has been directed at reducing serum triglycerides and LDL cholesterol and increasing HDL cholesterol. Treatment strategies to correct abnormal lipid levels and the risk of cardiac and vascular disease should involve three components: nutrient intake, medicines, and exercise. The statins (3-hydroxy-3-methylglutaryl coenzyme A reductase inhibitors) are beneficial in the general population in terms of reducing coronary artery disease at least in certain groups of high risk coronary heart disease patients.[254] Besides the lowering of LDL cholesterol, statins may slightly increase serum HDL cholesterol and may have anti-inflammatory, antithrombotic, and fibrinolytic effects to increase nitric oxide biosynthesis and bioavailability, to decrease synthesis of certain proinflammatory cytokines, to improve impaired endothelial function, and to protect against progressive renal injury in animals.[254] Statins will decrease LDL cholesterol in CKD patients, including patients with the nephrotic syndrome or treated by MHD or following kidney transplantation.[314,315] In the general population, higher doses of statins may be more protective against adverse cardiovascular events.

Unfortunately, in diabetic or nondiabetic MHD patients, statins do not exert benefits from cholesterol lowering[255,256]; adverse cardiovascular events and all-cause mortality were not reduced. On the other hand, statins may reduce adverse cardiovascular events and slow the rate of progression of CKD in patients with mild-to-advanced CKD.[257] We recommend a dietary plan similar to that of the National Cholesterol Education Program (NCEP) Therapeutic Lifestyle Changes (TLC) for all patients with CKD, including MHD and CPD patients, patients with the nephrotic syndrome, and renal transplant recipients, especially if their serum LDL levels are >100 mg per deciliter.[258] Because these patients are at a high risk for cardiovascular, cerebrovascular, and peripheral vascular diseases, we prefer to set a target LDL cholesterol of 70 mg per deciliter. The diet should provide ≤ 25% to 35% of total calories from fat with polyunsaturated fatty acids providing up to 10% of total calories, monounsaturated fatty acids providing up to 20% of total calories, saturated fatty acids providing less than 7% of total calories, and a cholesterol content of 200 mg per day or lower. Carbohydrate intake should be 50% to 60% of total calories and should be derived predominantly from foods rich in complex carbohydrates. Fiber intake should be 20 to 30 g per day.[258] Because this diet may be less palatable, energy intake should be monitored to ensure that it remains adequate (see the subsequent text). Patients should not become obese (i.e., body mass index [BMI] should be <28 kg per square meter). It is recognized that most individuals will not be able to adhere exactly to this diet. But, even an incomplete modification of the diet to lower the serum cholesterol could reduce the risk of adverse vascular events.[259]

Omega-3 fatty acids (e.g., eicosapentaenoic acid and docosahexaenoic acid are found in fish oil) and can lower serum triglycerides and exert variable effects on serum LDL and HDL cholesterol.[260] Fish oil also decreases platelet aggregation and appears to exert anti-inflammatory effects, whereas omega-3 fatty acids may enhance immune function. Low fat diets and lipid-lowering medicines retard the rate of progression of renal failure in animal models,[261] and in humans, some suggest that omega-3 fatty acids may lower the progression of renal failure in renal transplant patients as well as the progression of IgA nephropathy.[262,263]

The fibric acid derivative, fenofibrate, reportedly reduces the progression to albuminuria in type 2 diabetic patients.[264] Fenofibrate may be tried cautiously in patients with high levels of triglycerides because statins or fibric acid derivatives can induce a number of side effects, including myopathy. The combined use of a statin and a fibrate is likely to cause a severe myopathy and both should not be used unless careful and repeated monitoring is available. The reports of patients with CKD being treated with carnitine for hypertriglyceridemia are divided between those that show a lowering of serum triglycerides versus others showing minimal benefit or even a rise in serum triglycerides.[236] Sevelamer HCl acts to bind phosphate in the gastrointestinal tract but also lowers serum LDL cholesterol and increases serum HDL cholesterol. For CPD patients with severe, resistant hypertriglyceridemia, L-carnitine may be given at 500 to 1,000 mg per day. For such patients being treated by MHD, 10- to 20-mg L-carnitine per kilogram thrice weekly could be administered at the end of each dialysis treatment to examine efficacy.

Intensive dietary and lifestyle counseling of diabetic patients may significantly reduce or prevent the magnitude of albuminuria, the rate of progression of CKD, adverse cardiovascular events, and stroke.[265,266] We recommend a TLC NCEP diet for CKD patients or for MHD or kidney transplant recipients. To correct hypertriglyceridemia, we increase dietary lipid intake to <40% of total calories but only when fasting serum triglycerides are very high (i.e., ≥ 500 mg per deciliter). In addition, the dietary carbohydrates should mainly be composed of complex carbohydrates. Occasionally, it may be necessary to add a medicine such as ezetimibe to reduce intestinal cholesterol absorption, a statin or other cholesterol-lowering medicines, plus dietary manipulation to reach acceptable serum LDL cholesterol levels.[267]

Oxidant and Carbonyl Stress, Homocysteine

Antioxidants or antioxidant precursors, such as vitamins E and C or selenium, have been proposed as a method of reducing oxidant stress. Supplemental selenium should be taken with caution as it accumulates because of decreased excretion by the damaged kidney.[268] The body selenium burden is difficult to assess because selenium is protein bound and binding properties are altered in uremia. One glass per day of alcohol (e.g., red wine), statins, and regular exercise reportedly reduce oxidant stress.

Plasma homocysteine is increased in nondialyzed CKD patients and in about 90% of MHD and CPD patients.[269] The mechanism for this increase is unclear but may involve impaired remethylation of homocysteine back to methionine.[270] In the general population, elevated plasma homocysteine is associated with cardiovascular disease through three suggested biochemical mechanisms[271]: homocysteine oxidation generates hydrogen peroxide, it decreases methylation reactions from the accumulation of S-adenosylhomocysteine, and it acylates proteins by homocysteine thiolactone. In MHD, there can be a positive association between an increase in plasma homocysteine and adverse cardiovascular events, but other studies conclude that there is a negative association between these factors. In one large, controlled trial of CKD and MHD patients, large doses of a folic acid, pyridoxine HCl, and vitamin B12 did reduce plasma homocysteine levels but did not improve cardiovascular events or all-cause mortality.[269] To date, the treatment of MHD patients to reduce high plasma homocysteine does not improve their outcome.

Carnitine

Carnitine is a naturally occurring compound that is essential for life because it facilitates the transfer of long chain (>10 carbon) fatty acids into muscle mitochondria.[272] This activity is considered necessary for normal skeletal and cardiac muscle function. Patients undergoing maintenance dialysis, and particularly maintenance hemodialysis, but not patients with advanced CRF, display low serum free carnitine and, in some but not all studies, low skeletal muscle free and total carnitine levels.[236,272] In patients with stage IV or V CKD plus MHD patients, muscle acyl-carnitines (fatty acid-carnitine compounds) are increased, and serum total carnitine (i.e., acylcarnitines plus free carnitine) is normal or elevated.[273] Randomized clinical trials in patients with CKD and MHD or CAPD patients suggest that L-carnitine may provide such clinical benefits as increased physical exercise capacity, increased hematocrit, reduced interdialytic symptoms of skeletal muscle cramps or hypertension, or improvement in overall global sense of well-being or the improvement of various symptoms often found in CKD patients.[236] L-carnitine is also reported to improve nitrogen balance in CAPD patients.[277] The most promising of proposed applications is the treatment of EPO-resistant anemia. Until more definitive studies are available, it seems reasonable to use L-carnitine for MHD or CPD patients who satisfy any of the following conditions: (1) disabling skeletal muscle weakness or cardiomyopathy; (2) muscle cramps or hypotension during hemodialysis treatment; (3) severe malaise; or (4) anemia refractory to EPO therapy. The patient could be given a 3- to 6-month trial of L-carnitine (or 9 months for refractory anemia). The optimal carnitine dose is not defined and a dose of 20 mg per kilogram at the end of each hemodialysis is reasonable.[236]

Magnesium

In CKD or MHD patients, about 40% to 50% of ingested magnesium is absorbed from the intestinal tract.[237,275] Because the absorbed magnesium is excreted primarily by the kidney, hypermagnesemia may occur in kidney failure patients. Magnesium commonly accrues in bone and may play a causal role in renal osteodystrophy.[276] If the patient takes high magnesium substances (e.g., magnesium antacids or laxatives), serum magnesium will increase and the substance should be stopped. A magnesium content of about 1 mEq per liter in the hemodialysate, 0.50 to 0.75 mEq per liter in peritoneal dialysate, plus a dietary magnesium intake of 200 to 300 mg per day will maintain serum magnesium at normal or only slightly elevated levels.[237]

Fiber

Studies in normal adults suggest that a high dietary fiber intake may lower the incidence of constipation, irritable bowel syndrome, diverticulitis, and neoplasia of the colon and, possibly, improve glucose tolerance. In patients with CKD, a high dietary fiber intake may reduce the SUN by enhancing its fecal excretion.[277] Consequently, CKD or MHD patients should have a dietary fiber intake of 20 to 30 g per day.

PRIORITIZING DIETARY GOALS

The number and magnitude of the changes in the dietary intake for stage III to V CKD including MD patients are so great that if they were all presented to the patient at one time, the patient could become demoralized and lose his or her motivation to comply with the diet. We recommend prioritizing goals by emphasizing the importance of controlling the protein, phosphorus, sodium, energy, potassium, and magnesium intake and the need to take calcium and vitamin supplements for stage IV to V CKD patients. Unless the patient has a lipid disorder or other risk factors for adverse cardiovascular events, the adherence to these dietary guidelines are not as strongly emphasized, at least initially. Statins or fibric acid derivatives are usually better tolerated than dietary modifications and their use may enable patients to focus on other pressing aspects of dietary modification. If the patient has complied well with the other elements of dietary therapy but has a lipid disorder that can benefit from dietary therapy or wishes to modify fat, carbohydrate, or fiber intake, then other modifications can be adjusted by encouraging the patient to participate actively in designing the diet.

Adjusted Edema-Free Body Weight

Because the recommended nutrient intakes are often based on body weight, a reference weight should be used in prescribing the diet for individuals with kidney disease. The National Kidney Foundation Clinical Practice Guidelines on Nutrition in CKD published the following statement[236]: "The body weight to be used for assessing or prescribing protein or energy intake is the adjusted edema-free body weight or aBWef. For MHD patients, the weight should be obtained postdialysis, but for PD patients, it should be obtained following drainage of the dialysate." The aBWef is used for CKD and MHD plus CPD patients, who have BWef $<95\%$ or $>115\%$ of the median standard weight of the National Health and Nutrition Examination Survey II (NHANES II) data.[278,279] For patients between these levels, the actual BWef is used. The guideline also notes: "for DEXA measurements of total body fat and fat-free mass, the actual edema-free body weight obtained at the time of the DXA measurement should be used. For anthropometric calculations, the postdialysis (for MHD) or postdrain (for CPD) actual edema-free body weight should be used." The aBWef is calculated as follows[236]:

$$aBWef = BW + [(SBW - BWef) \times 0.25]$$

where BWef is the actual edema-free body weight and SBW is the standard body weight from the NHANES II data.

NUTRITIONAL THERAPY FOR ACUTE KIDNEY INJURY

Patients with acute kidney injury (AKI) have varying degrees of alterations in their metabolic and nutritional status. Patients without catabolism from underlying illnesses are usually not oliguric and the cause of their AKI is typically an isolated event, such as the administration of radiocontrast drugs or aminoglycoside nephrotoxicity. Patients with AKI requiring more complex attention have evidence of increased net protein breakdown (synthesis minus degradation) and disordered fluid, electrolyte, and/or acid–base status. There is often an excess total body water, azotemia, hyperkalemia, hyperphosphatemia, hypocalcemia, hyperuricemia, and a large anion gap metabolic acidosis. Rarely, AKI patients will have net protein degradation that is massive, with net losses as high as 200 to 250 g per day.[280] Patients are more likely to be catabolic when the AKI is associated with shock, sepsis, or rhabdomyolysis. The patients with net protein catabolism may accelerate the increase in plasma concentrations of potassium, phosphorus, nitrogenous metabolites, and non–nitrogen-containing acids. For these reasons, PEW is prevalent in AKI patients and is associated with increased morbidity and mortality.[281]

Results of animal studies indicate that acute uremia causes disorders in amino acid and protein metabolism. The UNA rises rapidly in rats with AKI versus events in control animals. There is increased uptake of several amino acids by livers of acutely uremic rats leading to increased urea synthesis. These animals have enhanced protein degradation and reduced protein synthesis in skeletal muscle.[282,283] Insulin treatment suppresses muscle protein degradation and increases protein synthesis. The insulin responses of the animal with AKI are impaired because of insulin resistance in muscle; this also occurs in patients with AKI.[280] In addition, acidemia contributes to protein catabolism (see previous). These responses can be attributed to AKI alone and when they are complicated with sepsis, hypoxia or trauma catabolism increases substantially. The mechanisms for the catabolic effect responses to AKI include: (1) products of metabolism may be toxic when their concentration rises due to impaired removal by the damaged kidney. (2) Alterations in catabolic hormones in plasma can promote wasting because the infusion of cortisone, epinephrine, and glucagon causes a sustained increase in glucose production, increased protein catabolism, increased energy expenditure, and negative Bn.[284] In addition, hypercatabolic illnesses are often associated with the release of catabolic cytokines or microbial toxins, elevated acute phase reactants, plus increased oxidants and elevated counterregulatory hormone levels (e.g., parathyroid hormone). (3) Acidemia increases the catabolism of amino acids and proteins. (4) There may be increased protease activities in plasma, which degrade proteins, or other changes (e.g., increased myostatin). Other potential causes for PEW in AKI arise because patients are unable to eat adequately due to anorexia or vomiting or impaired gastrointestinal function. Secondly, an underlying medical disorder can stimulate catabolism. Third, there can be losses of nutrients in draining fistulas or with dialysis, and the hemodialysis procedure may stimulate catabolism.

Nutritional Therapy for Acute Kidney Injury

If parenteral nutrition is required for the nutritional support of AKI patients, the nine EAA (including histidine) are used more efficiently for nitrogen or protein conservation compared to mixtures of EAA and nonessential amino acids (NEAA).[280] In addition, the small amount of EAA can decrease the rate of rise of potassium, phosphorus, and magnesium and can decrease the SUN and other potentially toxic products of protein and amino acid metabolism.[285] However, to maintain neutral or near-neutral nitrogen balance or to minimize net protein catabolism, particularly in hypercatabolic AKI patients, parenteral nutrition with larger amounts of EAA and NEAA may be necessary.

Effect of Continuous Venovenous Hemofiltration/Continuous Venovenous Hemodiafiltration on the Nutritional Management of Patients with Acute Kidney Injury

Continuous venovenous hemofiltration (CVVH), CVVHD (CVVH with concurrent hemodialysis), or CVVHDF (continuous venovenous hemodiafiltration) are used for very ill patients with AKI, CKD, or other causes of fluid or nitrogen intolerance (e.g., liver or heart failure). These dialysislike procedures, CVVH/CVVHD/CVVHDF, are performed while requiring only low blood and (for CVVHD) dialysate flow rates; they are usually administered throughout the 24 hours. These procedures offer potential advantages, including: (1) large quantities of water, electrolytes, and metabolites may be removed each day compared to standard 4-hour hemodialysis; (2) the removal of water and electrolytes is slow and, hence, causes less hypotension; (3) it is safe to administer greater amounts of amino acids and other nutrients because of the increased removal of fluid from the patient; (4) the daily clearances of molecules may avoid hemodialysis. These advantages have increased the use of CVVH/CVVHD/CVVHDF but it should be pointed out that these procedures have not improved the mortality or complications for AKI patients when compared to standard hemodialysis therapy. Finally, there is sustained low-efficiency dialysis (SLED) or hemodialysis carried out with low blood and dialysate flow rates similar to the advantages of CVVH/CVVHD/CVVHDF.

Amino acid losses during CWH/CWHD/SLED are influenced by the permeability characteristics of the filter membrane, the ultrafiltration and dialysate flow rates, and the amount of amino acids infused.[286] Approximately 4 to 7 g per day of amino acids are removed with CVVH[286] and this loss represents about 8.9 ± 1.2 (SEM)% and 12.1 ± 2.2% of the daily quantity of amino acids infused into the AKI patient. Amino acid losses with CVVH generally average about 6% to 12% of the daily amino acids infused; this level can be higher when the rate of amino acid infusion rises because the amount removed depends on the plasma concentration. Calcium and magnesium losses during CVVH or CVVHD average 2,800 and 600 mg per day, respectively, and losses of zinc average about 1.20 mg per day.[287] Although the infusion of large quantities of amino acids during CVVH/CVVHD/CVVHDF/SLED will improve the nitrogen Bn, it is not clear that there is a net accrual of protein stores. The infused amino acids might simply increase intracellular and extracellular amino acid levels to produce positive intake but do not improve protein synthesis or suppress protein degradation in AKI patients. Still, results of nonrandomized and randomized prospective clinical trials of AKI patients treated with enteral or parenteral nutrition indicate that Bn is directly related to the intake of protein or amino acids.[288] Regarding actual amounts, about 1.5 g of protein or amino acids per kilogram per day seemed to maintain nitrogen Bn in severely catabolic patients. There also was a greater probability of survival for AKI patients who had an improvement in Bn after adjusting for age, sex, and APACHE II score.[288] This association did not extend to protein or amino acid intake and survival. Possible reasons why intake alone did not improve survival are (1) the degree of protein catabolism was not reduced by increasing amino acid/protein intake; (2) the ability to achieve positive Bn may only identify survivors; and (3) perhaps greater amounts of amino acids would improve survival. Regardless, these results must be interpreted cautiously with regard to the differences in characteristics of the patients, the small number of patients, and the need to include unmeasured nitrogen losses (e.g., respiration/skin losses) in assessing Bn.[289]

Enteral Versus Parenteral Nutrition

Patients with AKI and superimposed illnesses should always be given oral nutrition if feasible. The substitution of liquid formula diets, elemental diets, or tube or enterostomy feeding should be attempted if dietary intake is minimal. For patients requiring feeding by enteric tube or gastrostomy, liquid protein-based or elemental diets can be tried to increase protein and energy intake. It is always prudent to assess what other constituents make up the diet because increasing phosphate intake, etc. can be countereffective. There are reviews of techniques used to achieve enteral feeding and the complications arising when using chemically defined diets and tube feeding.[290] Most of the principles will be applicable to patients with kidney failure. Notably, enteral feeding is extensively used for pediatric patients, particularly infants with CKD.

Patients with AKI requiring enteral nutrition frequently have high residual volumes in the stomach, signifying impaired gastric emptying or nasogastric tube obstruction.[291] Despite these problems, enteral feeding is a safe and effective way to provide nutrition for adults with AKI if attention is given to the rate of delivery and the need to increase intake when there are disruptions due to medical and surgical care.

Peripheral vein parenteral nutrition can be an alternative to total parenteral nutrition (TPN). This is suggested because TPN requires central venous catheters, thus increasing the risks of complications.[291] Like TPN, peripheral parenteral nutrition requires careful monitoring because there are complications. For example, the osmolality of the infusate must be restricted to ≤ 600 mOsmol to prevent thrombophlebitis, and the needles should be changed every 24 to 72 hours to prevent infections. The large quantity of fluid infused in order to provide adequate calories and amino acids represents another problem for patients with limited kidney function. The costs of peripheral parenteral nutrition are similar to those of TPN due to the expenses of administering fluids in order to achieve nutritional requirements. Because the risks of peripheral venous parenteral nutrition are lower, some patients with AKI may be treated with peripheral nutrition as an adjunct to their oral or enteric feeding. For example, a solution containing an 8.5% to 10% amino acid solution plus a 20% lipid emulsion could be used to meet part of the total nutritional requirements in conjunction with the higher osmolality fluids (e.g., carbohydrates) being given by the enteral route.

Why Benefits of Nutritional Therapy Have Not Been Unequivocally Demonstrated

Notwithstanding earlier reports,[285,288] it has not been demonstrated that treatment with amino acids and other nutrients improves either the rate or incidence of recovery of kidney function or the nutritional status. Intuitively, nutritional therapy could benefit patients with AKI and, at least in patients with AKI who have survived for >2 weeks but still have difficulty in meeting nutritional requirements, oral or parenteral nutritional support should improve nutritional status. Why has it been difficult to demonstrate the benefits of nutritional therapy? First, the clinical course of patients with AKI is variable and complex, so large numbers of patients are required for randomized prospective evaluations of nutritional therapy. Second, some of the published comparisons were retrospective or inadequately controlled, leading to unintentional biases. Third, the optimal composition of nutrients in the enteral or parenteral solutions is not defined and the lack of outcome benefits for AKI patients could simply reflect the inadequacy of the nutritional formulations. Fourth, the paucity of randomized, controlled trials with AKI patients have relied on morbidity, mortality, or subsequent quality of life as the key outcome measures. These outcomes may actually reflect the presence of other illnesses, not just the presence of AKI. Fifth, no prospective controlled comparisons have assessed the clinical course of AKI patients with nutritional therapy versus those without nutritional therapy.

Recommended Nutritional Support for Patients with Acute Kidney Injury

The therapeutic approach in Tables 85.4 and 85.5 represents our analysis of published reports and personal experience. Based on the diversity of the clinical status of patients with AKI, the prescription for intakes of nutrients will depend on the patient's nutritional status, estimates of protein catabolic rates, residual GFR, and the indications for initiating intermittent dialysis therapy, SLED, or CVVH/CVVHD/CVVHDF. The malnourished or hypercatabolic patient might receive an excess of nutrients provided during intermittent hemodialysis, SLED, or CVVH/CVVHD/CVVHDF. On the other hand, patients with residual kidney function might also receive excess nutrients because he or she has less of a risk for developing fluid and electrolyte disorders or the accumulation of metabolic waste products. For those with minimal urine flow but who are not very catabolic, water/mineral intake can be limited and calories with small amounts of amino acids—and especially EAA—may be given to decrease the need for dialysis. In general, the fluid intake (including water present in wet foods) should equal the fluid output from urine and other sources (e.g., nasogastric aspirate, fistula drainage) plus about 400 mL per day. This will take into account endogenous water production from metabolism and insensible water losses (e.g., from respiration and skin). If the patient is catabolic and in negative calorie and Bn, fluid intake should be restricted to allow for a loss of 0.2 to 0.5 kg per day. The intake of sodium and other minerals should be restricted to prevent their accumulation as judged by body weight, blood pressure, and the changes in the concentrations of sodium, potassium, phosphorus, etc. Insulin should be used to maintain normal plasma glucose concentrations and because it may improve mortality as was demonstrated in nonuremic patients with catabolic illnesses.[292] Because of the large glucose loads associated with enteral or parenteral feeding, hyperglycemia is common and insulin should be used to keep plasma glucose concentrations at 80 to 100 mg per deciliter.[293] The use of other hormones is less certain. For example, recombinant human growth hormone (rhGH) can improve Bn in patients with acute catabolic stress or with chronic illnesses, but trials of rhGH in critically ill patients indicate that the hormone can increase mortality in severely ill patients.[294]

The following discussion of specific nutrient intakes for patients with AKI can be used with oral, enteral, or intravenous nutrition. Information from TPN is emphasized because it is frequently used for more catabolic patients with AKI and it requires special attention to avoid complications. As noted earlier, the preferred route of feeding is total enteral nutrition (TEN) because it is associated with reduced morbidity.[295] This may reflect better preservation of the mass and physiology of the intestines and elements of host resistance.

Nitrogen Intake

The intake of nitrogen as protein or amino acids should be tailored to the clinical condition and dialysis needs of the patient. The intake is restricted for patients who have low values of urea production (i.e., 4 to 5 g of nitrogen per day but not severe protein malnutrition). These patients are expected to recover kidney function within weeks (Tables 85.4 and 85.5). Because the dialysis procedure causes catabolism (see previous), protein and amino acid intakes are restricted to avoid dialysis or reduce its frequency. For example, EAA with or without arginine may be given at 0.30 to 0.50 g per kilogram aBWef per day. More than 40 g per day of the nine EAAs should not be given in order to avoid serious amino acid imbalances. For patients who can eat, low protein feedings of 0.10 to 0.30 g/kg/day plus 10 to 20 g per day of EAA can be used to avoid rapid accumulation of nitrogenous waste products. Fortunately, these regimens will usually maintain neutral or mildly negative Bn and will reduce the need for dialysis. For patients with residual function (e.g., GFR of 5 to 10 mL per minute) but minimal catabolism, he or she can be treated as a patient with stage III to V CKD. The prescription would be a diet of 0.60 g per kilogram aBWef per day, primarily high biologic value protein or about 0.28 g of protein per kilogram per day supplemented with 6 to 10 g per day of EAA or a mixture of ketoacids and EAA. If the patient requires parenteral nutrition, the prescription is 0.60 g per kilogram aBWef per day of EAA and NEAA intravenously. If there is catabolism and/or a UNA >5 g of nitrogen per day, and the AKI is predicted to last for more than 2 weeks, the prescribed intake should be 1.0 to 1.2 g per kilogram per day for patients undergoing regular hemodialysis 3 times weekly and 1.2 to 1.5 g per kilogram per day for patients requiring standard hemodialysis more than 3 times weekly and approximately 1.5 to 2.5 g per kilogram per day in patients treated by SLED or CVVH/CVVHD/CVVHDF (Table 85.5). It should be noted that the UNA (and hence, the SUN) will invariably rise and this change plus the fluids given to meet these requirements generally increase dialysis needs.

Energy

The energy requirements for patients with AKI are determined by the same factors that affect patients without kidney failure and include weight, age, sex, associated diseases, and physical activity. When energy expenditure rises, it is largely but not entirely due to sepsis or other catabolic illnesses.[247] It is not known whether AKI per se changes energy expenditure. However, AKI treated by CVVH/CVVHD reduces energy expenditure in patients but whether this is hazardous is unknown.[296] Based on the principle that energy intake should rise when nitrogen intake is low, coupled with the need to provide large amounts of protein/amino acids in catabolic patients, the prescription for energy requirements are high and this complicates the provision of TPN and even enteral nutrition. Because patients with AKI provided with higher energy intakes had an improvement in survival, it is important to ensure that their energy requirements are satisfied.[280] A standard method for assessing energy needs is the Harris-Benedict equations that estimate basal energy expenditure (BEE) from age, sex, body weight, and height.

The Harris-Benedict equations are as follows[297]:

For men: $\text{BEE} - 66.5 + (13.8 \times \text{weight [kg]}) + (5.0 \times \text{height [cm]}) - (6.8 \times \text{age [years]})$

For women: $\text{BEE} - 655.1 + (9.6 \times \text{weight [kg]}) + (1.8 \text{ height [cm]}) - (4.7 \times \text{age [years]})$

The calculated BEE is then multiplied by an adjustment factor for the increase in energy expenditure associated with different clinical conditions (Table 85.6). Finally, the BEE is increased by 25% to adjust for individual variability, physical activity, and the potential needs associated with a low nitrogen intake and AKI. For these reasons, the BEE calculated for patients with AKI is

$$\text{Energy requirements} = \text{Estimated BEE} \times \text{Adjustment for illness} \times 1.25$$

TABLE 85.5 **Composition of Solutions for Total Parenteral Nutrition in Patients with Acute Kidney Injury[a]**

			Vitamins	
Essential and nonessential Free crystalline amino acids[b] (4.25–5.0%)	42.5–50	g/L	Vitamin A[f] Vitamin D Vitamin K Vitamin E[g] Niacin	2,000 IU/day see text 7.5 mg/week 10 IU/day 20 mg/day
Essential amino acids (5%)[b]	12.5–25	g/L	Thiamine HC1 (B_1) Riboflavin (B_2)	2 mg/day 2 mg/day
Dextrose (D-glucose)[c]	350	g/L	Pantothenic acid (B_3)	10 mg/day
Lipid emulsion	10% or 20%	in 500 mL	Pyridoxine HC1	10 mg/day
Energy (approximately)	1,140	kcal/L	Ascorbic acid (C) Biotin	60 mg/day 200 mg/day
Electrolytes[d]			Folic acid[g]	1 mg/day
Sodium[e]	40–50	mmol/L	Vitamin B_{12}	3 μg/day
Chloride[e]	25–35	mmol/L		
Potassium	<35	mmol/day		
Acetate	35–40	mmol/day		
Calcium	5	mmol/day		
Phosphorus	8	mmol/day		
Magnesium	4	mmol/day		
Iron	2	mmol/day		
Other trace elements	See text			

[a]The nutrients listed are present in each bottle containing 50 mL of 8.5% to 10% crystalline amino acids or 250 to 500 mL of 5% essential amino acids and 500 mL of 70% D-glucose. The vitamins and trace elements are an exception because they are added to only one bottle per day. For those doses of nutrients that are expressed as concentrations rather than as quantities per day, the dose refers to the quantity present in each liter of dextrose and amino acids, with or without lipids. The patient's fluid status and serum electrolytes and glucose values must be monitored closely. The composition and volume of the infusate may be modified according to the nutritional status of the patient (see text).

[b]For patients who are more catabolic (e.g., UNA >5 g/day), who are undergoing regular dialysis treatments (particularly for 2 or more weeks), or who are very wasted, essential and nonessential amino acids should be infused; about 1.0 to 1.2 g/kg/day for hemodialysis patients and 1.0 to 1.3 g/kg/day for intermittent peritoneal dialysis, CAPD, or APD patients (see text). 1.5 to 2.5 g/kg/day of essential and nonessential amino acids may be given to patients undergoing CVVH/CVVHD/CVVHDF or SLED. For patients who are not very wasted, who are less catabolic, who are not undergoing regular dialysis therapy, and who will not be receiving TPN for more than 2 or 3 weeks, 21 to 40 g per day of the nine essential amino acids may be infused. See text for a discussion of the formulations of amino acids.

[c]70% D-glucose is added as necessary to obtain an energy intake of 30 to 35 kcal/kg/day (see text); lower energy intakes may be used in very obese patients. For the higher levels of energy intake (i.e., 45 kcal/kg/day), additional 70% D-glucose may be added to the solutions. Generally, lipids are infused each day to provide 20%–30% of total calories in order to balance the sources of calories and to prevent essential fatty acid deficiency. For patients who are septic or at high risk for sepsis, about 10%–20% of calories may be given as lipids. The lipids probably should be infused over 12 to 24 hours to reduce the hyperlipidemia that occurs with the intravenous infusion of lipid emulsions and to avoid impairment of the reticuloendothelial system. The lipids may be infused through a separate line or mixed with the amino acid and dextrose solutions and infused soon after mixing (see text). Usually a 20% lipid emulsion (250–500 mL) is used to reduce the water load. The approximate calorie values are dextrose monohydrate, 3.4 kcal/g and amino acids, 3.5 kcal/g.

[d]When adding electrolytes, the amounts intrinsically present in the amino acid solution should be taken into account.

[e]Refers to the final concentrations of electrolytes after any additional 70% dextrose or other solutions have been added.

[f]About 600/xg/day of retinol activity equivalents (RAE) (see text) should be given orally or parenterally and not in the TPN solution because of chemical antagonisms.

[g]May need to be increased with use of lipid emulsions.

APD, automated peritoneal dialysis; CAPD, continuous ambulatory peritoneal dialysis; CVVH, continuous venovenous hemofiltration; CVVHD, continuous venovenous hemofiltration with concurrent dialysis; CVVHDF, continuous venovenous hemodiafiltration; SLED, slow, low-efficiency dialysis; TPN, total parenteral nutrition; UNA, urea nitrogen appearance.

TABLE 85.6 **Adjustment Factors for Estimating Energy Expenditure During Illness**

Type of Stress	Fraction of Normal Basal Energy Expenditure
Malnutrition (chronic, severe)	0.70–1.00
Nondialyzed chronic renal failure	1.00
Maintenance hemodialysis	1.05
Elective surgery	
Early (1–4 days)	1.00
Late (18–21 days)	0.95
Peritonitis	1.15
Soft tissue trauma	1.15
Fractures	1.20–1.25
Infections	
Mild	1.00
Moderate	1.20–1.40
Severe	1.40–1.60
Burns (percent of body surface)	
0%–20%	1.00–1.50
20%–40%	1.50–1.85
40%–100%	1.85–2.05

The basal energy expenditure values during the normal healthy state may be multiplied by these approximate factors to estimate resting energy expenditure during acute or chronic illness.
Adapted from Wilmore DW. *The metabolic management of the critically ill.* New York. Plenum, 1977; and Monteon FJ, Laidlaw SA, Shaib JK, et al. Energy expenditure in patients with chronic renal failure. 1986; *Kidney Int.* 30:741.

The Harris-Benedict equations reportedly overestimate the resting metabolic rate by 10% to 15%,[298] especially in patients with low values of BEE. The WHO equations, compiled from about 11,000 measurements in adults of both genders, all ages, and a wide variety of ethnic groups and body mass indices, are[299]

$$\text{RMR} = 15.4 \times \text{weight (kg)} - 27.0 \times \text{height (m)} + 717$$

Men: 30 to 60: $\text{RMR} = 4.6 \times \text{weight (kg)} + 16.0 \times \text{height (m)} + 901$

Women: 18 to 30: $\text{RMR} = 13.3 \times \text{weight (kg)} + 334.0 \times \text{height (m)} + 35$

30 to 60: $\text{RMR} = 8.7 \times \text{weight (kg)} - 25.0 \times \text{height (m)} + 865$

Where RMR is resting metabolic rate (in kilocalories per day). Indirect calorimetry can be used to estimate energy expenditure and, if multiplied by 1.25 as in the previous equation, the BEE for patients with AKI requiring nutritional support is between 30 and 35 kcal per kilogram aBWef per day. The higher energy intake (i.e., 35 kcal/kg/day) is generally used for patients with higher UNAs who are severely ill and not obese. Using these methods, a rising UNA despite an appropriate amino acid intake could theoretically be corrected by raising energy intake to 35 kcal/kg/day. Larger energy intakes have not been shown to improve patient outcomes and they generate more carbon dioxide from the metabolism of infused carbohydrates and fat, compromising blood gasses if pulmonary function is impaired. A very high-energy intake also can cause obesity and fatty liver. Because AKI patients may not tolerate a large water intake, glucose is usually administered in a 70% solution yielding energy from glucose monohydrate at 3.4 kcal per gram or, for 70% dextrose, about 2.38 kcal per milliliter. Amino acids provide about 3.5 kcal per gram and they can be given simultaneously with carbohydrates (see Table 85.5).

Lipids are commonly given from the onset of TPN, but the optimal amount of fat required is controversial because of the impaired lipid clearance of AKI.[300] Although 25 g per day will prevent essential fatty acid deficiencies, 30% to 40% of calories as lipid emulsions are used to meet energy needs. It has been suggested that lipid emulsions can transiently lower host resistance by inhibiting the function of the reticuloendothelial system.[300] A prudent approach is to infuse lipid emulsions over 12 to 24 hours to minimize high levels of plasma lipids and to interfere with the reticuloendothelial system.[300] Nonseptic patients may be given up to 20% to 30% of calories as lipid emulsions, but those who are septic should not receive intravenous lipids to avoid impaired function of the reticuloendothelial system. Alternatively, the provision of omega-3 fatty acids may enhance immune function and host resistance.[301]

Minerals

Recommendations for mineral intakes are tentative and should be modified according to a patient's clinical status (Table 85.5). If a serum electrolyte concentration rises, the rate of its infusion should be adjusted. But, parenteral nutrition can rapidly lower potassium and phosphorus (and potentially others), related in part to the action of insulin. Alternatively, the low concentration may signal the need for administering a supplement. Note that calcium and magnesium deficiencies may occur during CVVH/CVVHD/CVVHDF treatment.[302] With the exception of iron and possibly zinc, copper, and selenium, supplements of trace elements are probably not needed for AKI patients unless the nutritional support will be extended for 2 to 3 weeks. Low values of plasma selenium can occur with the multiple organ dysfunction syndrome and, in a prospective trial, patients given 535 μg per day of sodium selenite had less morbidity and a reduced need for CVVHD.[303] Nutritional requirements for other trace elements for AKI patients receiving TEN or TPN have not been established.

Vitamins

Requirements for vitamins are not defined for patients with AKI and tentative recommendations for patients receiving parenteral nutrition are listed in Table 85.5. We recommend that AKI patients receive water-soluble vitamins to make up for poor intake and dialysate losses (see previous). During CWH/CVVHD, water-soluble vitamins are lost and require supplements. AKI can also affect the fat-soluble vitamins, A, E, 25-OH vitamin D3, and 1,25-(OH)2 vitamin D,3 and vitamin K. Vitamin D should be used for specified conditions and vitamin A should be given only for demonstrated deficiency because serum vitamin A levels are increased in CKD patients and supplements may cause toxicity. Vitamin E may be beneficial for CKD patients but requirements are poorly established (see Table 85.5). Vitamin K deficiency can occur because of poor appetite and antibiotic treatment of AKI patients (antibiotics suppress vitamin K–producing intestinal bacteria).[304] Vitamin K is given routinely to patients receiving parenteral nutrition (Table 85.5). Regarding water-soluble vitamins, 10 mg per day of pyridoxine hydrochloride and only 60 to 100 mg of ascorbic acid are recommended to avoid toxicity.[305]

Intravenous Nutrition Limited to Hemodialysis

For AKI patients with marginally adequate intakes, supplemental amino acids, glucose, or lipids may be infused during the hemodialysis treatment (i.e., intradialytic parenteral nutrition [IDPN]).[306] This avoids the need to catheterize a central or peripheral vein and reduces the problems of excessive fluid administration. Evidence does not demonstrate a clear benefit of IDPN.[306] IDPN reportedly improves protein synthesis and energy balance during hemodialysis, leading to an increase in serum albumin and BWef, but the studies were not well controlled.[306] Stationary bicycle exercise during hemodialysis in patients receiving IDPN reportedly improves protein balance, but it is not clear if mortality is improved with IDPN.[307,308] Based on these reports, we conclude that IDPN is indicated only for malnourished MHD patients who are unable to eat or tolerate tube feeding. Because most patients requiring IDPN have decreased intakes of energy and nitrogen, we give 40 to 42 g of EAAs and NEAAs and about 200 g of D-glucose (about 150 g of D-glucose if the dialysate contains glucose) and usually 250 mL of a 10% or 20% lipid solution (i.e., 25 to 50 g of fat) throughout the dialysis procedure. The nutrients may be used more efficiently if given continuously rather than as a bolus. Only small amounts of amino acids are lost into hemodialysate during IDPN.[313] Patients with low serum phosphorus levels may need supplements during the IDPN. If the dialysate does not contain glucose, the infusion should be maintained for 20 to 30 minutes after the dialysis to prevent hypoglycemia.

Nutritional Hemodialysis and Nutritional Peritoneal Dialysis

Amino acids and glucose may be added to the dialysate in order to increase their uptake. Lowering the dialysate flow rate may increase the uptake of amino acids and glucose when the nutrients are added to the hemodialysate. Thus, some investigators have reduced the dialysate flow rate to increase the fractional extraction of amino acids and glucose.[310] This reduces the costs of the nutrients but also decreases the efficiency of dialysis. When 46 g of a mixture of 20 amino acids are added to the hemodialysate, the amino acid concentrations are similar to those in the plasma of fasting patients and amino acid losses are reduced.[233] When 139 g of the same amino acid mixture is present, there is a net transfer of about 39 g of amino acids from the dialysate into the patient.

Adding amino acids to the peritoneal dialysate appears to increase Bn, protein synthesis, and the concentrations of several serum proteins.[311] It also allows a reduction in the dialysate glucose concentration. Generally, a mixture of both EAAs and NEAAs are added to a 1.1% dialysate solution. This amount is used for one to two peritoneal dialysate exchanges, and dwell times of 4 to 6 hours are used to ensure an uptake of about 80% of the amino acid content. The calorie load from these solutions is small and it is suggested that the dialysis be undertaken during major meals in order to provide calories and other nutrients with the amino acid load from the dialysate. Still, the patient should be counseled to eat regular food or undertake tube feeding before turning to these more expensive and incomplete nutritional supplements.

DIETARY THERAPY FOR RENAL TRANSPLANTATION

Following a successful kidney transplantation, patients often have an improvement in their appetite, in part due to glucocorticoid therapy. Generally, there is a gain in body weight and fat.[312,313] Other nutritional problems include the development of obesity, insulin resistance and diabetes mellitus,[313] impaired growth in children, protein wasting,[314] altered serum lipid and homocysteine concentrations,[315] and abnormalities in bone, mineral, and vitamin metabolism.[316] These complications are concerning because these patients are at risk for cardiovascular disease. An important cause of these disorders is prednisone because glucocorticoids cause metabolic changes, including enhanced gluconeogenesis, protein degradation, lipolysis, reduced protein synthesis, and increased glucose uptake. They also can increase serum cholesterol, inhibit intestinal calcium absorption, and reduce serum levels of 25-hydroxycholecalciferol and 1,25-dihydroxycholecalciferol.[317] The latter changes participate in negative calcium balance and osteoporosis. In addition, cyclosporine or tacrolimus can cause glucose intolerance. Kidney transplant patients treated with high doses of prednisone have sustained negative Bn[314,318] and this can be aggravated further by proteinuria. A report from a nonrandomized study of kidney transplant patients receiving prednisone at 120 mg per day with tapering to 70 to 90 mg per day over approximately 10 to 14 days had intakes of protein and energy of 1.30 ± 0.06 (SEM) g/kg/day and 33 ± 3 kcal/kg/day.[314] However, their estimated Bn was still negative. This study points out the problems with using glucocorticoids. In another study[318] of 12 nondiabetic kidney transplant recipients with diets of 2 ± 0.03(SD) g protein/kg/day and only 28 ± 2 kcal/kg/day, Bn was more positive and potassium was lower with a more positive sodium balance. Lower doses of prednisone (i.e., 10 mg per day) do not appear to impair body composition or resting energy expenditure.

Kidney transplant patients often have increased serum triglycerides, VLDL triglycerides, and LDL, and total LDL cholesterol concentrations. HDL cholesterol is often low with an increased LDL/HDL cholesterol ratio.[319] Serum triglyceride levels are correlated with the prednisone dose plus obesity and the stage of CKD. These changes are relevant because there is a correlation between increased serum lipids and the risk of cardiovascular disease, graft failure, and fatality in kidney transplant recipients.[320] In most but not all studies, dietary counseling can reduce the energy intake, weight gain, and levels of serum total cholesterol, LDL cholesterol, and triglycerides, without changing the serum HDL cholesterol.[321] A low cholesterol, high fiber diet with a polyunsaturated saturated fatty acid ratio >1.0 was found to lower serum total cholesterol and LDL cholesterol after kidney transplantation.[321] A combination of a similar diet plus regular exercise can improve the plasma lipid pattern.[322] With 3 g per day of omega-3 fatty acids (as in fish oil), given over 3 months, serum triglycerides and VLDL cholesterol were decreased without a change in serum total cholesterol or LDL cholesterol. The effects of diet on the improvement in the serum lipid pattern tend to be modest and we recommend combining dietary therapy with statins as the more effective strategy for reducing serum total and LDL cholesterol.[323]

High plasma homocysteine concentrations could be a risk factor for cardiovascular complications and mortality in kidney transplant patients.[324] The causes of hyperhomocysteinemia include reduced kidney function and, less importantly, a low serum folate level and, possibly, cyclosporine A. There are conflicting reports about cyclosporine A versus tacrolimus and hyperhomocysteinemia.[326] Supplements of folic acid can decrease homocysteine, and it has been suggested that this benefit can be augmented by adding pyridoxine HCl (50 mg per day) and vitamin B12 (0.4 mg per day).[327]

Serum folate levels can be low for prolonged periods after kidney transplantation.[315] This could be linked to the finding that 52% of the patients develop macrocytosis, but even in this case, the patients were treated with azathioprine, which could have increased folate use. After a successful kidney transplant, serum vitamin A may not fall to normal for years.[328] Low plasma and hair zinc and urinary zinc losses have been observed after 1 year in kidney transplant patients.[329] This may be a reflection of more advanced kidney failure. Immunosuppressive medicines may affect the nutritional status of kidney transplant patients because cyclosporine A may increase serum LDL cholesterol and triglycerides, promote potassium retention with hyperkalemia,[320] cause urinary magnesium wasting with hypomagnesemia,[330] and promote early satiety during eating. Tacrolimus and sirolimus also increase serum LDL cholesterol levels.

Recommended Nutrient Intake for Renal Transplant Recipients

The nutritional requirements for kidney transplant patients are not established and our recommendations should be considered tentative. Immediately after kidney transplant surgery, especially if there is catabolism and/or prednisone at ≥30 mg per day, we recommend a diet of 1.3 to 1.5 g of protein per kilogram per day. If treatment with CVVH/CVVHD/CVVHDF or SLED is required, protein intake may be increased to 2.0 g/kg/day. If the daily prednisone dose is <30 mg per day, protein intake should be decreased. Although some reports suggest that low protein diets can retard the progression of kidney failure, it was not determined if the kidney transplant recipients who are receiving angiotensin converting enzyme (ACE) inhibitors or angiotensin receptor blockers (ARBs) had an additional benefit from low protein diets. In general, dietary protein is not restricted when the eGFR is >60 mL per minute unless there is a progressive loss of eGFR. If the patient is receiving >15 mg of prednisone per day, a protein intake of 0.60 to 0.80 g/kg/day is prescribed, but with higher doses of prednisone, the protein intake should be raised to 0.80 to 1.2 g/kg/day. If, however, the patient has an eGFR of 20 to 25 mL per minute or lower progressive less of GFR, then the patient is prescribed 0.6 g of protein per kilogram per day with at least 0.35 g of high biologic protein per kilogram per day. With a GFR of 20 to 25 mL/min or lower, some authorities would prescribe a very low-protein diet supplemented with a ketoacid plus essential amino acid mixture (see previous). Protein intake may be adjusted upward for acute increases in prednisone dosage or for large urinary protein losses as with nephrotic patients.[331]

A diet low in carbohydrates and modestly restricted in calories may reduce glucocorticoid toxicity.[318] However, diets that are moderately restricted in energy intake should be limited to short periods when the prednisone dosage is >40 mg per day in order to minimize the development of protein catabolism. Although a higher protein intake accompanying such diets (e.g., 2 g of protein per kilogram per day) may reduce protein malnutrition, there is the complicated problem of lipid abnormalities developing if lipids are substituted for carbohydrates in an attempt to avoid the Cushingoid complications (glucocorticoid toxicity). Kidney transplant patients should be encouraged to ingest a National Cholesterol Education Program Therapeutic Lifestyle Changes (TLC) diet as described earlier for CKD and MHD patients.[258] Patients also should be encouraged to exercise regularly and to maintain a normal body weight.[278,279] When superimposed catabolic illnesses are present, 30 to 40 kcal per kilogram per day can be prescribed. If dietary therapy does not reduce serum LDL cholesterol to 70 mg per deciliter, statins should be used for patients with cardiovascular disease risk factors.[323]

REFERENCES

1. He FJ, Jenner KH, Macgregor GA. WASH-world action on salt and health. *Kidney Int.* 2010;78:745–753.
2. Wang Y, Chen X, Song Y, Caballero B, Cheskin LJ. Association between obesity and kidney disease: a systematic review and meta-analysis. *Kidney Int.* 2007;73:19–33.
3. Walser M, Mitch WE, Maroni BJ, Kopple JD. Should protein be restricted in predialysis patients? *Kidney Int.* 1999;55:771–777.
4. Beale LS. *Kidney Diseases, Urinary Deposits and Calculous Disorders: Their Nature and Treatment.* 3rd ed. Philadelphia: Lindsay and Blakiston; 1869.
5. Chauveau P, Couzi L, Vendrely B, et al. Long-term outcome on renal replacement therapy in patients who previously received a keto acid-supplemented very-low-protein diet. *Am J Clin Nutr.* 2009;90:969–974.
6. Mitch WE, Remuzzi G. Diets for patients with chronic kidney disease, still worth prescribing. *J Am Soc Nephrol.* 2004;15:234–237.
7. Scialla JJ, Appel LJ, Astor BC, et al. Estimated net endogenous acid production and serum bicarbonate in African Americans with chronic kidney disease. *Clin J Am Soc Nephrol.* 2011;6:1526–1532.
8. Masud T, Mitch WE. Requirements for protein, calories and fat in the predialysis patient. In: Mitch WE, Ikizler TA, eds. *Handbook of Nutrition and the Kidney*. 6th ed. Philadelphia: Lippincott Williams & Wilkins; 2010: 92–108.
9. Traynor JP, Simpson K, Geddes CC, Deighan CJ, Fox JG. Early initiation of dialysis fails to prolong survival in patients with end-stage renal failure. *J Am Soc Nephrol.* 2002;13:2125–2132.
10. Beddhu S, Samore MH, Roberts MS, et al. Impact of timing of initiation of dialysis on mortality. *J Am Soc Nephrol.* 2003;14:2305–2312.
11. Wright S, Klausner D, Baird B, et al. Timing of dialysis initiation and survival in ESRD. *Clin J Am Soc Nephrol.* 2010;5:1828–1835.
12. Cooper BA, Branley P, Bulfone L, et al. A randomized, controlled trial of early versus late initiation of dialysis. *N Engl J Med.* 2010;363:609–619.
13. Sherman RA, Mehta O. Phosphorus and potassium content of enhanced meat and poultry products: implications for patients who receive dialysis. *Clin J Am Soc Nephrol.* 2009;4:1370–1373.
14. Zoccali C, Ruggenenti P, Perna A, et al. Phosphate may promote CKD progression and attenuate renoprotective effect of ACE inhibition. *J Am Soc Nephrol.* 2011;22:1923–1930.
15. Chobanian AV. Shattuck Lecture. The hypertension paradox—more uncontrolled disease despite improved therapy. *N Engl J Med.* 2009;361:878–887.
16. Fouque D, Pelletier S, Mafra D, Chauveau P. Nutrition and chronic kidney disease. *Kidney Int.* 2011;80:348–357.
17. Reaich D, Channon SM, Scrimgeour CM, et al. Correction of acidosis in humans with CRF decreases protein degradation and amino acid oxidation. *Am J Physiol.* 1993;265:E230–E235.
18. Frassetto L, Morris RC Jr, Sebastian A. Potassium bicarbonate reduces urinary nitrogen excretion in postmenopausal women. *J Clin Endocrinol Metab.* 1997;82:254–259.
19. Graham KA, Hoenich NA, Tarbit M, Ward MK, Goodship TH. Correction of acidosis in hemodialysis patients increases the sensitivity of the parathyroid glands to calcium. *J Am Soc Nephrol.* 1997;8:627–631.
20. Green J, Maor G. Effect of metabolic acidosis on the growth hormone/IGF-1 endocrine axis in skeletal growth centers. *Kidney Int.* 2002;57:2258–2267.
21. Sebastian A, Harris ST, Ottaway JH, Todd KM, Morris RC Jr. Improved mineral balance and skeletal metabolism in postmenopausal women treated with potassium bicarbonate. *N Engl J Med.* 1994;330:1776–1781.
22. de Brito-Ashurst I, Varagunam M, Raftery MJ, Yaqoob MM. Bicarbonate supplementation slows progression of CKD and improves nutritional status. *J Am Soc Nephrol.* 2009;20:2075–2084.
23. National Kidney Foundation. K/DOQI clinical practice guidelines for chronic kidney disease: evaluation, classification, and stratification. *Am J Kidney Dis.* 2005;45:S1–S153.
24. Ma YC, Zuo L, Chen JH, et al. Modified glomerular filtration rate estimating equation for Chinese patients with chronic kidney disease. *J Am Soc Nephrol.* 2006;17:2937–2944.
25. Horio M, Imai E, Yasuda Y, Watanabe T, Matsuo S. Modification of the CKD epidemiology collaboration (CKD-EPI) equation for Japanese: accuracy and use for population estimates. *Am J Kidney Dis.* 2010;56:32–38.
26. Soares AA, Eyff TF, Campani RB, et al. Performance of the CKD Epidemiology Collaboration (CKD-EPI) and the Modification of Diet in Renal Disease (MDRD) Study equations in healthy South Brazilians. *Am J Kidney Dis.* 2010;55:1162–1163.
27. Lascelles PT, Taylor WH. The effect upon tissue respiration in vitro of metabolites which accumulate in uraemic coma. *Clin Sci.* 1966;31:403–413.
28. Bergström J. Why are dialysis patients malnourished? *Am J Kidney Dis.*1995;26:229–241.
29. Grollman EF, Grollman A. Toxicity of urea and its role in the pathogensis of uremia. *J Clin Invest.* 1959;38:749.
30. Johnson WJ, Hagge WW, Wagoner RD, Dinapoli RP, Rosevear JW. Effects of urea loading in patients with far-advanced renal failure. *Mayo Clin Proc.* 1972;47:21–29.
31. D'Apolito M, Du X, Zong H, et al. Urea-induced ROS generation causes insulin resistance in mice with chronic renal failure. *J Clin Invest.* 2010;120: 203–213.
32. Bailey JL, Mitch WE. Pathophysiology of uremia. In: Brenner BM, Rector FC, eds. *The Kidney*. 6th ed. New York: W.B. Saunders; 1999: 2146–2157.
33. Depner TA, Gulyassy PF. Plasma protein binding in uremia: extraction and characterization of an inhibitor. *Kidney Int.* 1980;18:86–94.
34. Kraus LM, Jones MR, Kraus AP Jr. Essential carbamoyl-amino acids formed in vivo in patients with end-stage renal disease managed by continuous ambulatory peritoneal dialysis: isolation, identification and quantitation. *J Lab Clin Med.* 1998;131:425–431.
35. Tizianello A, De Ferrari G, Garibotto G, Gurreri G, Robaudo C. Renal metabolism of amino acids and ammonia in subjects with normal renal function and in patients with chronic renal insufficiency. *J Clin Invest.* 1980;65:1162–1173.
36. Bailey JL, Wang X, England BK, et al. The acidosis of chronic renal failure activates muscle proteolysis in rats by augmenting transcription of genes encoding proteins of the ATP-dependent, ubiquitin-proteasome pathway. *J Clin Invest.* 1996;97:1447–1453.
37. Bushinsky DA. The contribution of acidosis to renal osteodystrophy. *Kidney Int.* 1995;47:1816–1832.
38. DeFronzo RA, Beckles AD. Glucose intolerance following chronic metabolic acidosis in man. *Am J Physiol.* 1979;236:E328–E334.
39. Hara Y, May RC, Kelly RA, Mitch WE. Acidosis, not azotemia, stimulates branched-chain amino acid catabolism in uremic rats. *Kidney Int.* 1987;32:808–814.
40. Kalantar-Zadeh K, Horwich TB, Oreopoulos A, et al. Risk factor paradox in wasting diseases. *Curr Opin Clin Nutr Metab Care.* 2007;10:433–442.
41. Ando A, Orita Y, Tsubakihara Y, et al. The effect of low protein diet and surplus of essential amino acids on the serum concentrations and the urinary excretion of methylguanidine and guanidinosuccinic acid in chronic renal failure. *Nephron.* 1979;24:161–169.
42. Marescau B, Deshumkh DR, Kockx M, et al. Guanidino compounds in serum, urine, liver, kidney, and brain of man and some ureotelic animals. *Metabolism.* 1992;41:526–532.
43. Kopple JD, Gordon SI, Wang M, Swenseid ME. Factors affecting serum and urinary guanidinosuccinic acid levels in normal and uremic subjects. *J Lab Clin Med.* 1977;90:303–311.
44. Yokozawa T, Fujitsuka N, Oura H. Studies on the precursor of methylguanidine in rats with renal failure. *Nephron.* 1991;58:90–94.
45. Marescau B, Hiramatsu M, Mori A. α-keto-δ-guanidinovaleric acid-induced electroencephalographic, epileptiform discharges in rabbits. *Neurochem Pathol.* 1983;1:203–211.
46. D'Hooge R, De Deyn PP, Van de Vijver G, et al. Uraemic guanidino compounds inhibit γ-aminobutyric acid-evoked whole cell currents in mouse spinal cord neurons. *Neurosci Lett.* 1999;265:83–86.
47. Anderstam B, Katzaraki K, Bergström J. Serum levels of NG, NG-dimethyl -L-arginine, a potential endogenous nitric oxide inhibitor in dialysis patients. *J Am Soc Nephrol.* 1997;8:1437–1442.
48. Fleck C, Schweitzer F, Karge E, Busch M, Stein G. Serum concentrations of asymmetric (ADMA) and symmetric (SDMA) dimethylarginine in patients with chronic kidney diseases. *Clin Chim Acta.* 2003;336:1–12.
49. Gardiner SM, Kemp PA, Bennett R, Palmer RM, Moncado S. Regional and cardiac haemodynamic effects of NG, NG-dimethyl-L-arginine and their reversibility by vasodilators in conscious rats. *Br J Pharmacol.* 1993;110:1457–1464.
50. Reyes AA, Karl IE, Kissane J, Klahr S. L-Arginine administration prevents glomerular hyperfiltration and decreases proteinuria in diabetic rats. *J Am Soc Nephrol.* 1993;4:1039–1045.
51. Magnusson M, Magnusson KE, Sundqvist T, Denneberg T. Increased intestinal permeability to differently sized polyethylene glycols in uremic rats: effects of low- and high-protein diets. *Nephron.* 1990;56:306–311.
52. Niwa T. Organic acids and the uremic syndrome: protein metabolite hypothesis in the progression of chronic renal failure. *Semin Nephrol.* 1996;16:167–182.

53. Schulman G, Agarwal R, Acharya M, et al. A multicenter, randomized, double-blind, placebo-controlled, dose-ranging study of AST-120 (Kremezin) in patients with moderate to severe CKD. *Am J Kidney Dis.* 2006;47:565–577.

54. Hajjar SM, Fadda GZ, Thanakitcharu P, Smogorzewski M, Massry SG. Reduced activity of Na(+)-K+ ATPase of pancreatic islets in chronic renal failure: role of secondary hyperparathyroidism. *J Am Soc Nephrol.* 1992;2:1355–1359.

55. Wardle EN. Phenols, phenolic acids and sodium-potassium ATPases. *J Mol Med.* 1978;3:319.

56. Goodhart PJ, DeWolf WE Jr, Kruse LI. Mechanism-based inactivation of dopamine beta-hydroxylase by p-cresol and related alkylphenols. *Biochemistry.* 1987;26:2576–2583.

57. Vanholder R, De Smet R, Waterloos MA, et al. Mechanisms of uremic inhibition of phagocytic reactive species production: characterization of the role of p-cresol. *Kidney Int.* 1995;47:510–517.

58. Simenhoff ML, Asatoor AM, Milne MD, Zilva JF. Retention of aliphatic amines in uremia. *Clin Sci.* 1963;25:65–77.

59. Folin O. Laws governing the clinical composition of urine. *Am J Physiol.* 1905;13:67–115.

60. Maroni BJ, Steinman TI, Mitch WE. A method for estimating nitrogen intake of patients with chronic renal failure. *Kidney Int.* 1985;27:58–65.

61. Masud T, Manatunga A, Cotsonis G, Mitch WE. The precision of estimating protein intake of patients with chronic renal failure. *Kidney Int.* 2002;62:1750–1756.

62. Chauveau P, Barthe N, Rigalleau V, et al. Outcome of nutritional status and body composition of uremic patients on a very low protein diet. *Am J Kidney Dis.* 1999;34:500–507.

63. Niwa T, Ise M. Indoxyl sulfate, a circulating uremic toxin, stimulates the progression of glomerular sclerosis. *J Lab Clin Med.* 1994;124:96–104.

64. Niwa T, Tsukushi S, Ise M, et al. Indoxyl sulfate and progression of renal failure: effects of a low-protein diet and oral sorbent on indoxyl sulfate production in uremic rats and undialyzed uremic patients. *Miner Electrolyte Metab.* 1997;23:179–184.

65. Choi HK, Atkinson K, Karlson EW, Willett W, Curhan G. Purine-rich foods, dairy and protein intake, and the risk of gout in men. *N Engl J Med.* 2004;350:1093–1103.

66. Feig DI, Nakagawa T, Karumanchi SA, et al. Hypothesis: uric acid, nephron number, and the pathogenesis of essential hypertension. *Kidney Int.* 2004;66:281–287.

67. Mitch WE. Effects of intestinal flora on nitrogen metabolism in patients with chronic renal failure. *Am J Clin Nutr.* 1978;31:1594–1600.

68. Goodship TH, Mitch WE, Hoerr RA, et al. Adaptation to low-protein diets in renal failure: leucine turnover and nitrogen balance. *J Am Soc Nephrol.* 1990;1:66–75.

69. Masud T, Young VR, Chapman T, Maroni BJ. Adaptive responses to very low protein diets: the first comparison of ketoacids to essential amino acids. *Kidney Int.* 1994;45:1182–1192.

70. Tom K, Young VR, Chapman T, et al. Long-term adaptive responses to dietary protein restriction in chronic renal failure. *Am J Physiol.* 1995;268: E668–E677.

71. Maroni BJ, Staffeld C, Young VR, Manatunga A, Tom K. Mechanisms permitting nephrotic patients to achieve nitrogen equilibrium with a protein-restricted diet. *J Clin Invest.* 1997;99:2479–2487.

72. Mitch WE, Goldberg AL. Mechanisms of muscle wasting: the role of the ubiquitin-proteasome system. *N Engl J Med.* 1996;335:1897–1905.

73. Lecker SH, Goldberg AL, Mitch WE. Protein degradation by the ubiquitin-proteasome pathway in normal and disease states. *J Am Soc Nephrol.* 2006;17:1807–1819.

74. Lecker SH, Mitch WE. Proteolysis by the ubiquitin-proteasome system and kidney disease. *J Am Soc Nephrol.* 2011;22:821–824.

75. Bailey JL, Zheng B, Hu Z, Price SR, Mitch WE. Chronic kidney disease causes defects in signaling through the insulin receptor substrate/phosphatidylinositol 3-kinase/Akt pathway: implications for muscle atroply. *J Am Soc Nephrol.* 2006;17:1388–1394.

76. Zhang L, Rajan V, Lin E, et al. Pharmacological inhibition of myostatin suppresses systemic inflammation and muscle atrophy in mice with chronic kidney disease. *FASEB J.* 2011;25:1653–1663.

77. Huang CX, Tighiouart H, Beddhu S, et al. Both low muscle mass and low fat are associated with higher all-cause mortality in hemodialysis patients. *Kidney Int.* 2010;77:624–629.

78. Stenvinkel P, Heimbürger O, Lindholm B. Wasting, but not malnutrition, predicts cardiovascular mortality in end-stage renal disease. *Nephrol Dial Transplant.* 2004;19:2181–2183.

79. Kaysen GA, Dubin JA, Müller HG, et al. Inflammation and reduced albumin synthesis associated with stable decline in serum albumin in hemodialysis patients. *Kidney Int.* 2004;65:1408–1415.

80. Mitch WE. Malnutrition: a frequent misdiagnosis for hemodialysis patients. *J Clin Invest.* 2002;110:437–439.

81. Ikizler TA, Pupim LB, Brouillette JR, et al. Hemodialysis stimulates muscle and whole body protein loss and alters substrate oxidation. *Am J Physiol Endocrinol Metab.* 2002;282:E107–E116.

82. Pupim LB, Flakoll PJ, Brouillette JR, et al. Intradialytic parenteral nutrition improves protein and energy homeostasis in chronic hemodialysis patients. *J Clin Invest.* 2002;110:483–492.

83. Pupim LB, Majchrzak KM, Flakoll PJ, Ikizler TA. Intradialytic oral nutrition improves protein homeostasis in chronic hemodialysis patients with deranged nutritional status. *J Am Soc Nephrol.* 2006;17:3149–3157.

84. Baumeister W, Walz J, Zühl F, Seemüller E. The proteasome: paradigm of a self-compartmentalizing protease. *Cell.* 1998;92:367–380.

85. Lecker SH, Jagoe RT, Gomes M, et al. Multiple types of skeletal muscle atrophy involve a common program of changes in gene expression. *FASEB J.* 2004;18:39–51.

86. Price SR, Bailey JL, Wang X, et al. Muscle wasting in insulinopenic rats results from activation of the ATP–dependent, ubiquitin-proteasome pathway by a mechanism including gene transcription. *J Clin Invest.* 1996;98:1703–1708.

87. Tawa NE Jr, Odessey R, Goldberg AL. Inhibitors of the proteasome reduce the accelerated proteolysis in atrophying rat skeletal muscles. *J Clin Invest.* 1997;100:197–203.

88. May RC, Kelly RA, Mitch WE. Mechanisms for defects in muscle protein metabolism in rats with chronic uremia. Influence of metabolic acidosis. *J Clin Invest.* 1987;79:1099–1103.

89. Lee SW, Dai G, Hu Z, et al. Regulation of muscle protein degradation: coordinated control of apoptotic and ubiquitin-proteasome systems by phosphatidylinositol 3 kinase. *J Am Soc Nephrol.* 2004;15:1537–1545.

90. Song YH, Li Y, Du J, et al. Muscle-specific expression of IGF-1 blocks angiotensin II-induced skeletal muscle wasting. *J Clin Invest.* 2005;115:451–458.

91. Kimmel PL, Phillips TM, Simmens SJ, et al. Immunologic function and survival in hemodialysis patients. *Kidney Int.* 1998;54:236–244.

92. Zhang L, Du J, Hu Z, et al. IL-6 and serum amyloid A synergy mediates angiotensin II-induced muscle wasting. *J Am Soc Nephrol.* 2009;20:604–612.

93. Solomon V, Goldberg AL. Importance of the ATP-ubiquitin-proteasome pathway in degradation of soluble and myofibrillar proteins in rabbit muscle extracts. *J Biol Chem.* 1996;271:26690–26697.

94. Du J, Wang X, Miereles CL et al. Activation of caspase-3 is an initial step triggering muscle proteolysis in catabolic conditions. *J Clin Invest.* 2004;113: 115–123.

95. Wang X, Hu Z, Hu J, Du J, Mitch WE. Insulin resistance accelerates muscle protein degradation: activation of the ubiquitin-proteasome pathway by defects in muscle cell signaling. *Endocrinology.* 2006;147:4160–4168.

96. Workeneh B, Rondon-Berrios H, Zhang L, et al. Development of a diagnostic method for detecting increased muscle protein degradation in patients with catabolic conditions. *J Am Soc Nephrol.* 2006;17:3233–3239.

97. Hu Z, Wang H, Lee IH, Du J, Mitch WE. Endogenous glucocorticoids and impaired insulin signaling are both required to stimulate muscle wasting under pathophysiological conditions in mice. *J Clin Invest.* 2009;119:7650–7659.

98. May RC, Kelly RA, Mitch WE. Metabolic acidosis stimulates protein degradation in rat muscle by a glucocorticoid-dependent mechanism. *J Clin Invest.* 1986;77:614–621.

99. Mitch WE, Bailey JL, Wang X, et al. Evaluation of signals activating ubiquitin-proteasome proteolysis in a model of muscle wasting. *Am J Physiol.* 1999;276:C1132–C1138.

100. Tiao G, Fagan J, Roegner V, et al. Energy-ubiquitin-dependent muscle proteolysis during sepsis in rats is regulated by glucocorticoids. *J Clin Invest.* 1996;97:339–348.

101. Sandri M, Sandri C, Gilbert A, et al. Foxo transcription factors induce the atrophy-related ubiquitin ligase atrogin-1 and cause skeletal muscle atrophy. *Cell.* 2004;117:399–412.

102. Stitt TN, Drujan D, Clarke BA, et al. The IGF-1/PI3K/Akt pathway prevents expression of muscle atrophy-induced ubiquitin ligases by inhibiting FOXO transcription factors. *Mol Cell.* 2004;14:395–403.

103. Graham KA, Reaich D, Channon SM, Downie S, Goodship TH. Correction of acidosis in hemodialysis decreases whole-body protein degradation. *J Am Soc Nephrol.* 1997;8:632–637.

104. Graham KA, Reaich D, Channon SM, et al. Correction of acidosis in CAPD decreases whole body protein degradation. *Kidney Int.* 1996;49:1396–1400.

105. Szeto CC, Chow KM. Metabolic acidosis and malnutrition in dialysis patients. *Semin Dial.* 2004;17:371–375.

106. Stein A, Moorhouse J, Iles-Smith H, et al. Role of an improvement in acid-base status and nutrition in CAPD patients. *Kidney Int.* 1997;52:1089–1095.

107. Pickering WP, Price SR, Bircher G, et al. Nutrition in CAPD: serum bi-

carbonate and the ubiquitin-proteasome system in muscle. *Kidney Int.* 2002;61: 1286–1292.
108. Ballmer PE, McNurlan MA, Hulter HN, Anderson SE, Garlick PJ, Krapf R. Chronic metabolic acidosis decreases albumin synthesis and induces negative nitrogen balance in humans. *J Clin Invest.* 1995;95:39–45.
109. Movilli E, Zani R, Carli O, et al. Correction of metabolic acidosis increases serum albumin concentration and decreases kinetically evaluated protein intake in hemodialysis patients: a prospective study. *Nephrol Dial Transplant.* 1998;13:1719–1722.
110. Uribarri J, Levin NW, Delmez J, et al. Association of acidosis and nutritional parameters in hemodialysis patients. *Am J Kidney Dis.* 1999;34:493–499.
111. Mitch WE. Getting beyond cross-sectional studies of abnormal nutritional indices in dialysis patients. *Am J Clin Nutr.* 2003;77:760–761.
112. Kirschbaum B. Spurious metabolic acidosis in hemodialysis patients. *Am J Kidney Dis.* 2000;35:1068–1071.
113. Brüngger M, Hulter HN, Krapf R. Effect of chronic metabolic acidosis on the growth hormone/IGF-1 endocrine axis: new cause of growth hormone insensitivity in humans. *Kidney Int.* 1997;51:216–221.
114. Brüngger M, Hulter HN, Krapf R. Effect of chronic metabolic acidosis on thyroid hormone homeostasis in humans. *Am J Physiol.* 1997;272:F648–F653.
115. Krapf R, Vetsch R, Vetsch W, Hulter HN. Chronic metabolic acidosis increases the serum concentration of 1,25-dihydroxyvitamin D in humans by stimulating its production rate. Critical role of acidosis-induced renal hypophosphatemia. *J Clin Invest.* 1992;90:2456–2463.
116. Qureshi AR, Alvestrand A, Danielsson A, et al. Factors predicting malnutrition in hemodialysis patients: a cross-sectional study. *Kidney Int.* 1998;53:773–782.
117. Kopple JD, Gao XL, Qing DP. Dietary protein, urea nitrogen appearance and total nitrogen appearance in chronic renal failure and CAPD patients. *Kidney Int.* 1997;52:486–494.
118. Kopple JD. McCollum Award Lecture, 1996: protein-energy malnutrition in maintenance dialysis patients. *Am J Clin Nutr.* 1997;65:1544–1557.
119. Avesani CM, Kamimura MA, Draibe SA, Cuppari L. Is energy intake underestimated in nondialyzed chronic kidney disease patients? *J Ren Nutr.* 2005;15:159–165.
120. Kloppenburg WD, de Jong PE, Huisman RM. The contradiction of stable body mass despite low reported dietary energy intake in chronic haemodialysis patients. *Nephrol Dial Transplant.* 2002;17:1628–1633.
121. FAO/WHO/UNU. *Energy and Protein Requirements. In Technical Report Series 724.* 1st ed. Geneva: World Health Organization; 1985.
122. Leibel RL, Rosenbaum M, Hirsch J. Changes in energy expenditure resulting from altered body weight. *N Engl J Med.* 1995;332:621–628.
123. Rose WC. The amino acid requirements of adult man. *Nutr Abstr Rev Ser Hum Exp.* 1957;27:631.
124. Monteon FJ, Laidlaw SA, Shaib JK, Kopple JD. Energy expenditure in patients with chronic renal failure. *Kidney Int.* 1986;30:741–747.
125. Ikizler TA, Wingard RL, Sun M, et al. Increased energy expenditure in hemodialysis patients. *J Am Soc Nephrol.* 1996;7:2646–2653.
126. Smith D, DeFronzo RA. Insulin resistance in uremia mediated by postbinding defects. *Kidney Int.* 1982;22:54–62.
127. Kobayashi S, Maesato K, Moriya H, Ohtake T, Ikeda T. Insulin resistance in patients with chronic kidney disease. *Am J Kidney Dis.* 2005;45:275–280.
128. Aparicio M, Gin H, Potaux L, et al. Effect of a ketoacid diet on glucose tolerance and tissue insulin sensitivity. *Kidney Int Suppl.* 1989;27:S231–S235.
129. Rigalleau V, Combe C, Blanchetier V, et al. Low protein diet in uremia: effects on glucose metabolism and energy production rate. *Kidney Int.* 1997;51:1222–1227.
130. Kopple JD, Levey AS, Greene T, et al. Effect of dietary protein restriction on nutritional status in the Modification of Diet in Renal Disease (MDRD) Study. *Kidney Int.* 1997;52:778–791.
131. Cuppari L, Medeiros FAM, Papini HF, et al. Effectiveness of oral energy-protein supplementation in severely malnourished hemodialysis patients. *J Ren Nutr* 1994;4:127–135.
132. Bergstrom J, Furst P, Ahlberg M, Noree LO. The role of dietary and energy intake in chronic renal failure. In: Canzler VH, ed. *Topical Questions in Nutritional Therapy in Nephrology and Gastroenterology*. Stuttgart: Georg Thieme Verlag; 1978:1 –16.
133. Kopple JD, Monteon FJ, Shaib JK. Effect of energy intake on nitrogen metabolism in nondialyzed patients with chronic renal failure. *Kidney Int.* 1986;29:734–742.
134. Kerr GR, Sul Lee E, Lam M-KM, et al. Relationships between dietary and biochemical measures of nutritional status in NHANES I data. *Am J Clin Nutr.* 1982;35:294–308.
135. Shaw JH, Wildbore M, Wolfe RR. Whole body protein kinetics in severely septic patients. The response to glucose infusion and total parenteral nutrition. *Ann Surg.* 1987;205:288–294.
136. Louard RJ, Fryburg DA, Gelfand RA, Barrett EJ. Insulin sensitivity of protein and glucose metabolism in human forearm skeletal muscle. *J Clin Invest.* 1992;90:2348–2354.
137. Nair KS, Ford GC, Halliday D. Effect of intravenous insulin treatment on in vivo whole body leucine kinetics and oxygen consumption in insulin-deprived Type I diabetic patients. *Metabolism.* 1987;36:491–495.
138. Pupim LB, Heimbürger O, Qureshi AR, Ikizler TA, Stenvinkel P. Accelerated lean body mass loss in incident chronic dialysis patients with diabetes mellitus. *Kidney Int.* 2005;68:2368–2374.
139. Kaysen GA, Gambertoglio J, Jimenez I, Jones H, Hutchison FN. Effect of dietary protein intake on albumin homeostasis in nephrotic patients. *Kidney Int.* 1986;29:572–577.
140. Yeun JY, Zakari M, Kaysen GA. Nephrotic syndrome: nutritional consequences and dietary management. In: Mitch WE, Ikizler TA, eds. *Handbook of Nutrition and the Kidney.* 6th ed. Philadelphia: Lippincott Williams & Wilkins; 2010:132–147.
141. Remuzzi G, Bertani T. Pathophysiology of progressive nephropathies. *N Engl J Med.* 1998;339:1448–1456.
142. Walser M, Hill S, Tomalis EA. Treatment of nephrotic adults with a supplemented, very low-protein diet. *Am J Kidney Dis.* 1996;28:354–364.
143. Adrogué HJ, Madias NE. Sodium and potassium in the pathogenesis of hypertension. *N Engl J Med.* 2007;356:1966–1978.
144. Cappuccio FP. Salt and cardiovascular disease. *BMJ.* 2007;334:859–860.
145. Kelly RA, Wilcox CS, Mitch WE, et al. Response of the kidney to furosemide. II. Effect of captopril on sodium balance. *Kidney Int.* 1983;24:233–239.
146. Malik B, Price SR, Mitch WE, Yue Q, Eaton DC. Regulation of epithelial sodium channels by the ubiquitin-proteasome proteolytic pathway. *Am J Physiol Renal Physiol.* 2006;290:F1285–F1294.
147. He FJ, MacGregor GA. Effect of modest salt reduction on blood pressure: a meta-analysis of randomized trials. Implications for public health. *J Hum Hypertens.* 2002;16:761–770.
148. Chobanian AV, Bakris GL, Black HR, et al. Seventh report of the Joint National Committee on Prevention, Detection, Evaluation, and Treatment of High Blood Pressure. *Hypertension.* 2003;42:1206–1252.
149. Ritz E. Lowering salt intake —an important strategy in the management of renal disease. *Nat Clin Pract Nephrol.* 2007;3:360–361.
150. Karppanen H, Mervaala E. Sodium intake and hypertension. *Prog Cardiovasc Dis.* 2006;49:59–75.
151. Esnault VL, Ekhlas A, Delcroix C, Moutel MG, Nguyen JM. Diuretic and enhanced sodium restriction results in improved antiproteinuric response to RAS blocking agents. *J Am Soc Nephrol.* 2005;16:474–481.
152. Kusaba T, Mori Y, Masami O, et al. Sodium restriction improves the gustatory threshold for salty taste in patients with chronic kidney disease. *Kidney Int.* 2009;76:638–643.
153. Panel on Dietary Reference Intakes for Electrolytes and Water. *Dietary Reference Intakes for Water, Potassium, Sodium, Chloride, and Sulfate.*Washington, DC: National Academies Press; 2005:617.
154. Mitch WE, Wilcox CS. Disorders of body fluids, sodium and potassium in chronic renal failure. *Am J Med.* 1982;72:536–550.
155. Appel LJ, Moore TJ, Obarzanek E, et al. A clinical trial of the effects of dietary patterns on blood pressure. DASH Collaborative Research Group. *N Engl J Med.* 1997;336:1117–1124.
156. Svetkey LP, Simons-Morton D, Vollmer WM, et al. Effects of dietary patterns on blood pressure: subgroup analysis of the Dietary Approaches to Stop Hypertension (DASH) randomized clinical trial. *Arch Intern Med.* 1999;159:285–293.
157. Kidney Disease Outcomes Quality Initiative (K/DOQI). K/DOQI clinical practice guidelines on hypertension and antihypertensive agents in chronic kidney disease. *Am J Kidney Dis.* 2004;43:S1–S290.
158. Cotton JR, Woodward T, Carter NW, Knochel JP. Resting skeletal muscle membrane potential as an index of uremic toxicity. *J Clin Invest.* 1979;63: 501–508.
159. Kopple JD. Trace elements and vitamins in renal disease. In: Mitch WE, Klahr S, eds. *Nutrition and the Kidney*. 6th ed. Philadelphia: Lippincott Williams & Wilkins; 2010:163 –176.
160. Mydlík M, Derzsiová K, Zemberová E. Metabolism of vitamin B6 and its requirement in chronic renal failure. *Kidney Int Suppl.* 1997;62:S56–S59.
161. Ramirez G, Chen M, Boyce HW Jr, et al. Longitudinal follow-up of chronic hemodialysis patients without vitamin supplementation. *Kidney Int.* 1986;30:99–106.
162. Bushinsky DA, Nilsson EL. Additive effects of acidosis and parathyroid hormone on mouse osteoblastic and osteoclastic. *Am J Physiol.* 1995;269: C1364–C1370.
163. Rocco MV, Poole D, Poindexter P, Jordan J, Burkhart JM. Intake of vitamins and minerals in stable hemodialysis patients as determined by 9-day food food records. *J Ren Nutr.* 1997;7:17–24.

164. Schaumburg H, Kaplan J, Winderbank A, et al. Sensory neuropathy from pyridoxine abuse. A new megavitamin syndrome. *N Engl J Med.* 1983;309: 445–489.

165. Gleghorn EE, Eisenberg LD, Hack S, Parton P, Merritt RJ. Observations of vitamin A toxicity in three patients with renal failure receiving parenteral alimentation. *Am J Clin Nutr.* 1986;44:107–112.

166. Hahn S, Kuemmerle NB, Chan W, et al. Glomerulosclerosis in the remnant kidney is modulated by dietary alpha-tocopherol. *J Am Soc Nephrol.* 1998;9:2089–2095.

167. Lonn E, Bosch J, Yusuf S, et al. Effects of long-term vitamin E supplementation on cardiovascular events and cancer: a randomized controlled trial. *JAMA.* 2005;293:1338–1347.

168. Levey AS, Greene T, Schluchter MD, et al. Glomerular filtration rate measurements in clinical trials. Modification of Diet in Renal Disease Study Group and the Diabetes Control and Complications Trial Research Group. *J Am Soc Nephrol.* 1993;4:1159–1171.

169. Faugere MC, Malluche HH. Stainable aluminum and not aluminum content reflects bone histology in dialyzed patients. *Kidney Int.* 1986;30:717–722.

170. Tzanno-Martins C, Azevedo LS, Orii N, et al. The role of experimental chronic renal failure and aluminium intoxication in cellular immune response. *Nephrol Dial Transplant.* 1996;11:474–480.

171. Nesse A, Garbossa G, Stripeikis J, et al. Aluminium accumulation in chronic renal failure affects erythropoiesis. *Nephrology.* 1997;3:347–351.

172. Caticha O, Norato DY, Tambascia MA, et al. Total body zinc depletion and its relationship to the development of hyperprolactinemia in chronic renal insufficiency. *J Endocrinol Invest.* 1996;19:441–448.

173. Chen SM, Chen TW, Young TK. Renal excretion of zinc in patients with chronic uremia. *J Formos Med Assoc.* 1990;89:220–224.

174. Mahajan SK, Abbasi AA, Prasad AS, et al. Effect of oral zinc therapy on gonadal function in hemodialysis patients. A double-blind study. *Ann Intern Med.* 1982;97:357–361.

175. Rodger RS, Sheldon WL, Watson MJ, et al. Zinc deficiency and hyperprolactinaemia are not reversible causes of sexual dysfunction in uraemia. *Nephrol Dial Transplant.* 1989;4:888–892.

176. Taccone-Gallucci M, Giardini O, Ausiello C, et al. Vitamin E supplementation in hemodialysis patients: effects on peripheral blood mononuclear cells lipid peroxidation and immune response. *Clin Nephrol.* 1986;25:81–86.

177. Cottini EP, Gallina DL, Dominguez JM. Urea excretion in adult humans with varying degrees of kidney malfunction fed milk, egg or an amino acid mixture: assessment of nitrogen balance. *J Nutr.* 1973;103:11–19.

178. Jones EA, Smallwood RA, Craigie A, Rosenoer VM. The enterohepatic circulation of urea nitrogen. *Clin Sci.* 1969;37:825–836.

179. Mitch WE, Lietman PS, Walser M. Effects of oral neomycin and kanamycin in chronic renal failure: I. Urea metabolism. *Kidney Int.* 1977;11:116–122.

180. Mitch WE, Walser M. Effects of oral neomycin and kanomycin in chronic uremic patients: II. Nitrogen balance. *Kidney Int.* 1977;11:123–127.

181. Giordano C. Use of exogenous and endogenous urea for protein synthesis in normal and uremic subjects. *J Lab Clin Med.* 1963;62:231–246.

182. Franch HA, Mitch WE. Navigating between the Scylla and Charybdis of prescribing dietary protein for chronic kidney diseases. *Ann Rev Nutr.* 2009;29:341–364.

183. Molitch ME, DeFronzo RA, Franz MJ, et al. Nephropathy in diabetes. *Diabetes Care.* 2004;27 Suppl 1:S79–S83.

184. Bingham SA. The dietary assessment of individuals: Methods, accuracy, new techniques and recommendations. *Nutr Abstr Rev.* 1987;57:705–742.

185. Klahr S, Levey AS, Beck GJ, et al. The effects of dietary protein restriction and blood-pressure control on the progression of chronic renal failure. *N Engl J Med.* 1994;330:878–884.

186. Fouque D, Laville M. Low protein diets for chronic renal failure in non-diabetic adults. *Cochrane Database Syst Rev.* 2009;(3):CD001892.

187. Locatelli F, Alberti D, Graziani G, et al. Prospective, randomised, multicentre trial of effect of protein restriction on progression of chronic renal insufficiency. *Lancet.* 1991;337:1299–1304.

188. Hostetter TH. Human renal response to a meat meal. *Am J Physiol.* 1986;250:F613–F618.

189. Levey AS, Greene T, Beck GJ, et al. Dietary protein restriction and the progression of chronic renal disease: what have all the results of the MDRD Study shown? Modification of Diet in Renal Disease Study group. *J Am Soc Nephrol.* 1999;10:2426–2439.

190. Levey AS, Adler S, Caggiula AW, et al. Effects of dietary protein restriction on the progression of advanced renal disease in the Modification of Diet in Renal Disease Study. *Am J Kidney Dis.* 1996;27:652–663.

191. Williams PS, Stevens ME, Fass G, Irons L, Bone JM. Failure of dietary protein and phosphate restriction to retard the rate of progression of chronic renal failure: a prospective, randomized, controlled trial. *Q J Med.* 1991;81:837–855.

192. Cianciaruso B, Pota A, Pisani A, et al. Metabolic effects of two low protein diets in chronic kidney disease stage 4-5—a randomized controlled trial. *Nephrol Dial Transplant.* 2008;23:636–644.

193. Munford RS. Statins and the acute-phase response. *N Engl J Med.* 2001;344:2016–2018.

194. Ihle BU, Becker GJ, Whitworth JA, Charlwood RA, Kincaid-Smith PS. The effect of protein restriction on the progression of renal insufficiency. *N Engl J Med.* 1989;321:1773–1777.

195. Jungers P, Chauveau P, Ployard F, et al. Comparison of ketoacids and low protein diet on advanced chronic renal failure progression. *Kidney Int Suppl.* 1987;22:S67–S71.

196. Malvy D, Maingourd C, Pengloan J, Bagros P, Nivet H. Effects of severe protein restriction with ketoanalogues in advanced renal failure. *J Am Coll Nutr.* 1999;8:481–486.

197. Mircescu G, Gârneaţă L, Stancu SH, Căpuşă C. Effects of a supplemented hypoproteic diet in chronic kidney disease. *J Ren Nutr.* 2007;17:179–188.

198. Rosman JB, ter Wee PM, Meijer S, et al. Prospective randomised trial of early dietary protein restriction in chronic renal failure. *Lancet.* 1984;2: 1291–1295.

199. Rosman JB, Langer K, Brandl M, et al. Protein-restricted diets in chronic renal failure: a four year follow-up shows limited indications. *Kidney Int Suppl.* 1989;27:S96–S102.

200. Brunori G, Viola BF, Parrinello G, et al. Efficacy and safety of a very-low-protein diet when postponing dialysis in the elderly: a prospective randomized multicenter controlled study. *Am J Kidney Dis.* 2007;49:569–580.

201. Nath KA, Hostetter MK, Hostetter TH. Pathophysiology of chronic tubulo-interstitial disease in rats. *J Clin Invest.* 1985;76:667–675.

202. Shah SN, Abramowitz M, Hostetter TH, Melamed ML. Serum bicarbonate levels and the progression of kidney disease: a cohort study. *Am J Kidney Dis.* 2009;54:270–277.

203. Wesson DE, Simoni J, Broglio K, Sheather S. Acid retention accompanies reduced GFR in humans and increases plasma levels of endothelin and aldosterone. *Am J Physiol Renal Physiol.* 2011;300:F830–F837.

204. Mahajan A, Simoni J, Sheather SJ, et al. Daily oral sodium bicarbonate preserves glomerular filtration rate by slowing its decline in early hypertensive nephropathy. *Kidney Int.* 2010;78:303–309.

205. Zeller K, Whittaker E, Sullivan L, Raskin P, Jacobson HR. Effect of restricting dietary protein on the progression of renal failure in patients with insulin-dependent diabetes mellitus. *N Engl J Med.* 1991;324:78–83.

206. Hansen HP, Tauber-Lassen E, Jensen BR, Parving HH. Effect of dietary protein restriction on prognosis in patients with diabetic nephropathy. *Kidney Int.* 2002;62:220–228.

207. Noordzij M, Hooft L, Dekker FW, Zoccali C, Jager KJ. Systematic reviews and meta-analyses: when they are useful and when to be careful. *Kidney Int.* 2009;76:1130–1136.

208. Kasiske BL, Lakatua JDA, Ma JZ, Louis TA. A meta-analysis of the effects of dietary protein restriction on the rate of decline in renal function. *Am J Kidney Dis.* 1998;31:954–961.

209. Fouque D, Laville M, Boissel JP, et al. Controlled low protein diets in chronic renal insufficiency: meta-analysis. *BMJ.* 1992;304:216–220.

210. Pedrini MT, Levey AS, Lau J, Chalmers TC, Wang PH. The effect of dietary protein restriction on the progression of diabetic and nondiabetic renal diseases: a meta-analysis. *Ann Intern Med.* 1996;124:627–632.

211. Fouque D, Wang P, Laville M, Boissel JP. Low protein diets delay end-stage renal disease in non diabetic adults with chronic renal failure. *Nephrol Dial Transpl.* 2000;15:1986–1992.

212. Pan Y, Guo LL, Jin HM. Low-protein diet for diabetic nephropathy: a meta-analysis of randomized controlled trials. *Am J Clin Nutr.* 2008;88:660–666.

213. Altman DG, Andersen PK. Calculating the number needed to treat for trials where the outcome is an event. *BMJ.* 1999;319:1492–1495.

214. Skolbekken JA. Communicating the risk reduction achieved by cholesterol reducing drugs. *BMJ.* 1998;316:1956–1958.

215. Coresh J, Walser M, Hill S. Survival on dialysis among chronic renal failure patients treated with a supplemented low-protein diet before dialysis. *J Am Soc Nephrol.* 1995;6:1379–1385.

216. Menon V, Kopple JD, Wang X, et al. Effect of a very low-protein diet on outcomes: long-term follow-up of the Modification of Diet in Renal Disease (MDRD) Study. *Am J Kidney Dis.* 2008;53:208–217.

217. Pollock CA, Ibels LS, Zhu FY, et al. Protein intake in renal disease. *J Am Soc Nephrol.* 1997;8:777–783.

218. Vendrely B, Chauveau P, Barthe N, et al. Nutrition in hemodialysis patients previously on a supplemented very low protein diet. *Kidney Int.* 2003;63: 1491–1498.

219. Aparicio M, Fouque D, Chauveau P. Effect of a very low-protein diet on long-term outcomes. *Am J Kidney Dis.* 2009;54:183.

220. Division of Kidney UaHDNN. *USRDS 2009 Annual data report: atlas of end-stage renal disease in the United States.* Bethesda: National Institutes of Health; 2003.
221. Rosman JB, Donker-Willenborg MA. Dietary compliance and its assessment in the Groningen trial on protein restriction in chronic renal failure. *Contrib Nephrol.* 1990;81:95–101.
222. Yeh SS, Schuster MW. Geriatric cachexia: the role of cytokines. *Am J Clin Nutr.* 1999;70:183–197.
223. Meireles CL, Price SR, Pererira AM, Carvalhaes JT, Mitch WE. Nutrition and chronic renal failure in rats: what is an optimal dietary protein? *J Am Soc Nephrol.* 1999;10:2367–2373.
224. Walser M, Hill S. Can renal replacement be deferred by a supplemented very-low protein diet? *J Am Soc Nephrol.* 1999;10:110–116.
225. Aparicio M, Chauveau P, De Précigout V, et al. Nutrition and outcome on renal replacement therapy of patients with chronic renal failure treated by a supplemented very low protein diet. *J Am Soc Nephrol.* 2000;11:719–727.
226. Kalhoff H, Diekmann L, Kunz C, Stock GJ, Manz F. Alkali therapy versus sodium chloride supplement in low birthweight infants with incipient late metabolic acidosis. *Acta Paediatr.* 1997;86:96–101.
227. Boirie Y, Broyer M, Gagnadoux MF, Niaudet P, Bresson JL. Alterations of protein metabolism by metabolic acidosis in children with chronic renal failure. *Kidney Int.* 2000;58:236–241.
228. Reaich D, Channon SM, Scrimgeour CM, Goodship TH. Ammonium chloride-induced acidosis increases protein breakdown and amino acid oxidation in humans. *Am J Physiol.* 1992;263:E735–E739.
229. Papadoyannakis NJ, Stefanides CJ, McGeown M. The effect of the correction of metabolic acidosis on nitrogen and protein balance of patients with chronic renal failure. *Am J Clin Nutr.* 1984;40:623–627.
230. Garibotto G, Russo R, Sofia A, et al. Skeletal muscle protein synthesis and degradation in patients with chronic renal failure. *Kidney Int.* 1994;45:1432–1439.
231. Williams B, Hattersley J, Layward E, Walls J. Metabolic acidosis and skeletal muscle adaptation to low protein diets in chronic uremia. *Kidney Int.* 1991;40:779–786.
232. Ikizler TA, Flakoll PJ, Parker RA, et al. Amino acid and albumin losses during hemodialysis. *Kidney Int.* 1994;46:830–837.
233. Chazot C, Shahmir E, Matias B, Laidlaw S, Kopple JD. Dialytic nutrition: provision of amino acids in dialysate during hemodialysis. *Kidney Int.* 1997;52:1663.
234. Lindsay RM, Bergström J. Membrane biocompatibility and nutrition in maintenance haemodialysis patients. *Nephrol Dial Trans.* 1994; 9 Suppl 2:150.
235. Kopple JD, Monteon FJ, Shaib JK. Effect of energy intake on nitrogen metabolism in nondialyzed patients with CRF. *Kidney Int.* 1986;29:734.
236. K/DOQI Nutrition Workgroup. National Kidney Foundation kidney disease outcomes quality initiative. Clinical practice guidelines for nutrition in chronic renal failure. *Am J Kidney Dis.* 2000;35:S42.
237. Blumenkrantz MJ, Kopple JD, Moran JK, Coburn JW. Metabolic balance studies and dietary protein requirements in patients undergoing continuous ambulatory peritoneal dialysis. *Kidney Int.* 1982;21:849.
238. K/DOQI Nutrition Workgroup. National Kidney Foundation kidney disease outcomes quality initiative clinical practice guidelines for nutrition in chronic renal failure. *Am J Kidney Dis.* 2000;35:S1–S140.
239. Borah M, Schoenfeld PY, Gotch FA, et al. Nitrogen balance in intermittent hemodialysis therapy. *Kidney Int.* 1978;14:491.
240. Ahmed KR. Scognamillo B, Kopple JD. Relationship of peritoneal transport kinetics and nutritional status in chronic peritoneal dialysis patients [abstract]. *Perit Dial Int.* 1995;15:S5.
241. Noori N, Kovesdy CP, Dukkipati R, et al. Survival predictability of lean and fat mass in men and women undergoing maintenance hemodialysis. *Am J Clin Nutr.* 2010;92:1060–1070.
242. National Academy of Sciences. *Dietary reference intakes for energy, carbohydrate, fiber, fat, fatty acids, cholesterol, protein, and amino acids.* Washington DC: National Academies Press; 2002.
243. Lowrie EG, Lew NL. Death risk in hemodialysis patients: the predictive value of commonly measured variables and an evaluation of death rate differences between facilities. *Am J Kidney Dis.* 1990;15:458.
244. Monteon FJ, Laidlaw SA, Shaib JK, et al. Energy expenditure in patients with CRF. *Kidney Int.*1986;30:741.
245. Schneeweiss B, Graninger W, Stockenhuber F, et al. Energy metabolism in acute and chronic renal failure. *Am J Clin Nutr.* 1990;52:596–601.
246. Slomowitz LA, Monteon FJ, Grosvenor M, Laidlaw SA, Kopple JD. Effect of energy intake on nutritional status in maintenance hemodialysis patients. *Kidney Int.* 1989;35:704–711.
247. Neyra R, Chen KY, Sun M, et al. Increased resting energy expenditure in patients with end-stage renal disease. *JPEN J Parenter Enteral Nutr.* 2003;7:36–42.
248. Hylander B, Barkeling B, Rössner S. Eating behavior in continuous ambulatory peritoneal dialysis and hemodialysis patients. *Am J Kidney Dis.* 1992;6:592–597.
249. Kalantar-Zadeh K, Kopple JD, Deepak S, Block D, Block G. Food intake characteristics of hemodialysis patients as obtained by food frequency questionnaire. *J Ren Nutr.* 2002;12:17–31.
250. Vaziri N. Altered lipid metabolism and serum lipids in kidney disease and kidney failure. In: Kopple JD, Massry SG, Kalantar-Zadeh K, eds. *Nutritional Management of Renal Disease.* Elsevier; 2012 (in press).
251. Deighan CJ, Caslake MJ, McConnell M, Boulton-Jones JM, Packard CJ. Atherogenic lipoprotein phenotype in end-stage renal failure: origin and extent of small dense low-density lipoprotein formation. *Am J Kidney Dis.* 2000;35:852–862.
252. Joven J, Villabona C, Vilella E, et al. Abnormalities of lipoprotein metabolism in patients with the nephrotic syndrome. *N Eng J Med.* 1990;323:579–584.
253. Diméņy E, Fellström B, Larsson E, Tufveson G, Lithell H. Lipoprotein abnormalities in renal transplant recipients with chronic vascular rejection. *Transplant Proc.* 1992;24:366.
254. K/DOQI Nutrition Workgroup. National Kidney Foundation clinical practice guidelines for managing dyslipidenuas in chronic kidney disease. *Am J Kidney Dis.* 2003;41:S1–S91.
255. Wanner C, Krane V, März W, et al. Atorvastatin in patients with type 2 diabetes mellitus undergoing hemodialysis. *N Engl J Med.* 2005;353:238–248.
256. Fellström BC, Jardine AG, Schmieder RE, et al. Rosuvastatin and cardiovascular events in patients undergoing hemodialysis. *N Engl J Med.* 2009;360:1395–1407.
257. Navaneethan SD, Pansini F, Perkovic V, et al. HMG CoA reductase inhibitors (statins) for people with chronic kidney disease not requiring dialysis. *Cochrane Database Syst Rev.* 2009;(2):CD007784.
258. Expert Panel on Detection, Evaluation, and Treatment of High Blood Cholesterol in Adults. Executive summary of The Third Report of The National Cholesterol Education Program (NCEP) Expert Panel on Detection, Evaluation, and Treatment of High Blood Cholesterol In Adults (Adult Treatment Panel III). *JAMA.* 2001;285:2486.
259. LaRosa JC, Grundy SM, Waters DD, et al. Intensive lipid lowering with atorvastatin in patients with stable coronary disease. *N Engl J Med.* 2005;352:1425–1435.
260. Mozaffarian D, Wu JH. Omega-3 fatty acids and cardiovascular disease: effects on risk factors, molecular pathways, and clinical events. *J Am Coll Cardiol.* 2011;58:2047–2067.
261. Keane WF. O'Donnell MP, Kasiske BL, Schmitz PG. Lipids and the progression of renal disease. *J Am Soc Nephrol.* 1990;1:S69.
262. Homan van der Heide JJ, Bilo HJ, Tegzess AM, Donker AJ. The effects of dietary supplementation with fish oil on renal function in cyclosporine-treated renal transplant recipients. *Transplantation.* 1990;49:523.
263. Donadio JV Jr, Bergstralh EJ, Offord KP, Spencer DC, Holley KE. A controlled trial of fish oil in IgA nephropathy. Mayo Nephrology Collaborative Group. *N Engl J Med.* 1994;331:1194.
264. Ansquer JC, Foucher C, Rattier S, Taskinen MR, Steiner G. Fenofibrate reduces progression to microalbuminuria over 3 years in a placebo-controlled study in type 2 diabetes: results from the Diabetes Atherosclerosis Intervention Study (DAIS). *Am J Kidney Dis.* 2005;45:485.
265. Rachmani R, Slavacheski I, Berla M, Frommer-Shapira R, Ravid M. Treatment of high-risk patients with diabetes: motivation and teaching intervention: a randomized, prospective 8-year follow-up study. *J Am Soc Nephrol.* 2005;16:S22-S26.
266. Tuomilehto J, Lindström J, Eriksson JG, et al. Prevention of type 2 diabetes mellitus by changes in lifestyle among subjects with impaired glucose tolerance. *N Engl J Med.* 2001;344:1343.
267. Pearson TA, Denke MA, McBride PE, et al. A community-based, randomized trial of ezetimibe added to statin therapy to attain NCEP ATP III goals for LDL cholesterol in hypercholesterolemic patients: the ezetimibe add-on to statin for effectiveness (EASE) trial. *Mayo Clin Proc.* 2005;80:587–595.
268. Burk RF, Brown DG, Seely RJ, Scaief CC III. Influence of dietary and injected selenium on whole-body retention, route of excretion, and tissue retention of $^{75}SeO_3^{2-}$ in the rat. *J Nutr.* 1972;102:1049–1056.
269. Jamison RL, Hartigan P, Kaufman JS, et al. Effect of homocysteine lowering on mortality and vascular disease in advanced chronic kidney disease and end-stage renal disease: a randomized controlled trial. *JAMA.* 2007;298:1163–1170.
270. van Guldener C, Kulik W, Berger R, et al. Homocysteine and methionine metabolism in ESRD: a stable isotope study. *Kidney Int.* 1999;56:1064–1071.
271. Perna AF, Ingrosso D, Castaldo P, et al. Homocysteine, a new crucial element in the pathogenesis of uremic cardiovascular complications. *Miner Electrolyte Metab.* 1999;25:95–99.
272. Evans AM, Faull R, Fornasini G, et al. Pharmacokinetics of L-carnitine in patients with end-stage renal disease undergoing long-term hemodialysis. *Clin Pharmacol Ther.* 2000;68:238.

273. Fouque D, Holt S, Guebre-Egziabher F, et al. Relationship between serum carnitine, acylcarnitines, and renal function in patients with chronic renal disease. *J Ren Nutr.* 2006;16:125–131.

274. Kopple JD, Qing DP. Effect of L-Carnitine on nitrogen balance in CAPD patients [abstract]. *J Am Soc Nephrol.* 1999;10:264.

275. Kopple JD, Cobum JW. Metabolic studies of low protein diets in uremia. II. Calcium, phosphorus and magnesium. *Medicine (Baltimore).* 1973;52:597.

276. Wallach S. Effects of magnesium on skeletal metabolism. *Magnes Trace Elem.* 1990;9:1.

277. Rampton DS, Cohen SL, Crammond VD, et al. Treatment of CRF with dietary fiber. *Clin Nephrol.* 1984;21:159–163.

278. Frisancho AR. New standards of weight and body composition by frame size and height for assessment of nutritional status of adults and the elderly. *Am J Clin Nutr.* 1984;40:808–819.

279. Najjar MF, Rowland M. Anthropometric reference data and prevalence of overweight, United States, 1976–1980. *Vital Health Stat 11.* 1987;(238):1–73.

280. Feinstein EI, Blumenkrantz MJ, Healy H, et al. Clinical and metabolic responses to parenteral nutrition in acute renal failure. A controlled double-blind study. *Medicine (Baltimore).* 1981;60:124.

281. Fiaccadori E, Lombardi M, Leonardi S, et al. Prevalence and clinical outcome associated with preexisting malnutrition in acute renal failure: a prospective cohort study. *J Am Soc Nephrol.* 1999;10:581–593.

282. Flugel-Link RM, Salusky IB, Jones MR, et al. Enhanced muscle protein degradation and urea nitrogen appearance (UNA) in rats with acute renal failure. *Am J Physiol.* 1983;244:E615.

283. Clark AS, Mitch WE. Muscle protein turnover and glucose uptake in acutely uremic rats. Effect of insulin and the duration of renal insufficiency. *J Clin Invest.* 1983;72:836.

284. Bessey PQ, Watters JM, Aoki TT, Wilmore DW. Combined hormonal infusion simulates the metabolic response to injury. *Ann Surg.* 1984;200:264.

285. Abel RM, Beck CH Jr, Abbott WM, et al. Improved survival and acute renal failure after treatment with intravenous essential L-amino acids and glucose. *N Eng J Med.* 1973;288:695.

286. Davenport A, Roberts NB. Amino acid losses during continuous high-flux hemofiltration in the critically ill patient. *Crit Care Med.* 1989;17:1010.

287. Klein CJ, Moser-Veillon PB, Schweitzer A, et al. Magnesium, calcium, zinc, and nitrogen loss in trauma patients during continuous renal replacement therapy. *JPEN J Parenter Enteral Nutr.* 2002;26:77.

288. Scheinkestel CD, Kar L, Marshall K, et al. Prospective randomized trial to assess caloric and protein needs of critically ill, anuric, ventilated patients requiring continuous renal replacement therapy. *Nutrition.* 2003;19:909.

289. Kopple JD. Uses and limitations of the balance technique. *JPEN J Parenter Enteral Nutr.* 1987;11:S79.

290. Fiaccadori E, Maggiore U, Giacosa R, et al. Enteral nutrition in patients with acute renal failure. *Kidney Int.* 2004;65:999.

291. Freeman JB, Fairfull-Smith RJ. Physiologic approach to peripheral parenteral nutrition. In: JE Fischer, ed. *Surgical Nutrition.* Boston: Little Brown; 1983:703.

292. Woolfson AM, Heatley RV, Allison SP. Insulin to inhibit protein catabolism after injury. *N Engl J Med.* 1979;300:14.

293. Meyfroidt G, Keenan DM, Wang X, et al. Dynamic characteristics of blood glucose time series during the course of critical illness: effects of intensive insulin therapy and relative association with mortality. *Crit Care Med.* 2010;38: 1021–1029.

294. Takala J, Ruokonen E, Webster NR, et al. Increased mortality associated with growth hormone treatment in critically ill adults. *N Engl J Med.* 1999;341:785.

295. Moore FA, Moore EE, Jones TN, et al. TEN versus TPN following major abdominal trauma—reduced septic morbidity. *J Trauma.* 1989;29:916.

296. Matamis D, Tsagourias M, Koletsos K, et al. Influence of continuous haemofiltration-related hypothermia on haemodynamic variables and gas exchange in septic patients. *Intensive Care Med.* 1994;20:431.

297. Harris JA, Benedict FG. *A Biometric Study of Basal Metabolism in Man. Public No. 279.* Washington, DC: Carnegie Institute; 1919.

298. Garrel DR, Jobin N, de Jonge LH. Should we still use the Harris and Benedict equations? *Nutr. Clin. Pract.* 1996;11:99.

299. World Health Organization. *Energy and Protein Requirements. WHO Tech. Rep. Ser. No. 724.* WHO: Geneva; 1985.

300. Druml W, Laggner A, Widhalm K, et al. Lipid metabolism in acute renal failure. *Kidney Int.* 1983;24:S139.

301. Kinsella JE, Lokesh B, Broughton S, Whelan J. Dietary polyunsaturated fatty acids and eicosanoids: potential effects on the modulation of inflammatory and immune cells: an overview. *Nutrition* 1990;6:24.

302. Klein CJ, Moser-Veillon PB, Schweitzer A, et al. Magnesium, calcium, zinc, and nitrogen loss in trauma patients during continuous renal replacement therapy. *J Parenter Enter Nutr.* 2002;26:77.

303. Berger MM, Shenkin A, Revelly J-P, et al. Copper, selenium, zinc, and thiamine balances during continuous venovenous hemodiafiltration in critically ill patients. *Am J Clin Nutr.* 2004;80:410.

304. Udall JA. Human sources and absorption of vitamin K in relation to anticoagulant stability. *JAMA.* 1965;194:127.

305. Friedman AL, Chesney RW, Gilbert EF, et al. Secondary oxalosis as a complication of parenteral nutrition in acute renal failure. *Am J Nephrol.* 1983;3:248.

306. Dukkipati R, Kalantar-Zadeh K, Kopple JD. Is there a role for intradialytic parenteral nutrition? A review of the evidence. *Am J Kidney Dis.* 2010;55: 352-64.

307. Pupim LB, Flakoll PJ, Levenhagen DK, et al. Exercise augments the acute anabolic effects of intradialytic parenteral nutrition in chronic hemodialysis patients. *Am J Physiol Endocrinol Metab.* 2004;286:E589.

308. Cano NJ, Fouque D, Roth H, et al. Intradialytic parenteral nutrition does not improve survival in malnourished hemodialysis patients: a 2-year multicenter, prospective, randomized study. *J Am Soc Nephrol.* 2007;18:2583.

309. Wolfson M, Jones MR, Kopple JD. Amino acid losses during hemodialysis with infusion of amino acids and glucose. *Kidney Int.* 1982;21:500.

310. Feinstein EI, Collins JF, Blumen Krantz MJ, et al. Nutritional hemodialysis. *Prog Attif Organs.* 1984;1:421.

311. Kopple JD, Bernard D, Messana J, et al. Treatment of malnourished CAPD patients with an amino acid based dialysate. *Kidney Int.* 1995;47:1148.

312. El Haggan W, Vendrely B, Chauveau P, et al. Early evolution of nutritional status and body composition after kidney transplantation. *Am J Kidney Dis.* 2002;40:629.

313. van den Ham EC, Kooman JP, Christiaans MH, et al. Posttransplantation weight gain is predominantly due to an increase in body fat mass. *Transplantation.* 2000;70:241.

314. Cogan MG, Sargent JA, Yarbrough SG, et al. Prevention of prednisone-induced negative nitrogen balance. Effect of dietary modification of urea generation rate in patients on hemodialysis receiving high-dose glucocorticoids. *Ann Intern Med.* 1981;95:158.

315. Zaffari D, Kosekann AF, Santos WC, et al. Effectiveness of diet in hyperlipidemia in renal transplant patients. *Transplant Proc.* 2004;36:889.

316. Renau A, Yoldi B, Farrerons J, et al. Bone mass and mineral metabolism in kidney transplant patients. *Transplant Proc.* 2002;34:407.

317. Jahn TJ, Halstead LR, Baran DT. Effects of short term glucocorticoid administration on intestinal calcium absorption and circulating vitamin D metabolite concentrations in man. *J Clin Endocrinol Metab.* 1981;52:111.

318. Whittier FC, Evans DH, Dutton S, et al. Nutrition in renal transplantation. *Am. J. Kidney Dis.* 1985;6:405.

319. Rajman I, Harper L, McPake D, et al. Low-density lipoprotein subtraction profiles in chronic renal failure. *Nephrol Dial Transplant.* 1998;13:2281.

320. Roodnat JI, Mulder PG, Zietse R, et al. Cholesterol as an independent predictor of outcome after renal transplantation. *Transplantation.* 2000;69:1704.

321. Hines L. Can low-fat/cholesterol nutrition counseling improve food intake habits and hyperlipidemia of renal transplant patients? *J Ren Nutr.* 2000;10:30.

322. Triolo G, Segoloni GP, Tetta C, et al. Effect of combined diet and physical exercise on plasma lipids of renal transplant recipients. *Nephrol Dial Transplant.* 1989;4:237.

323. Foldes K, Maklary E, Vargha P, et al. Effect of diet and fluvastatin treatment on the serum lipid profile of kidney transplant, diabetic recipients: a 1-year follow up. *Transpl Int.* 1998;11:S65.

324. Duclous D, Motte G, Challier B, et al. Serum total homocysteine and cardiovascular disease occurrence in chronic, stable renal transplant recipients: a prospective study. *J Am Soc Nephrol.* 2000;11:134.

325. Ducloux D, Ruedin C, Gibey R, et al. Prevalence, determinants, and clinical significance of hyperhomocyst(e)inaemia in renal-transplant recipients. *Nephrol Dial Transplant.* 1998;13:2890.

326. Fernandez-Miranda C, Gomez P, Diaz-Rubio P, et al. Plasma homocysteine levels in renal transplanted patients on cyclosporine or tacrolimus therapy: effect of treatment with folic acid. *Clin Transplant.* 2000;14:110.

327. Bostom AG, Gohh RY, Beaulieu AJ, et al. Treatment of hyperhomocysteinemia in renal transplant recipients. A randomized, placebo-controlled trial. *Ann Intern Med.* 1997;127:1089.

328. Yatzidis H, Digenis P, Koutsicos D. Hypervitaminosis in CRF after transplantation. *Br Med J.* 1976;2:1075.

329. Mahajan SK, Abraham J, Hessburg T, et al. Zinc metabolism and taste acuity in renal transplant recipients. *Kidney Int.* 1983;24(Suppl. 16):S310.

330. Barton CH, Vaziri ND, Martin DC, et al. Hypomagnesemia and renal magnesium wasting in renal transplant recipients receiving cyclosporine. *Am J Med.* 1987;83:693.

331. Salahudeen AK, Hostetter TH, Raatz SK. et al. Effects of dietary protein in patients with chronic renal transplant rejection. *Kidney Int.* 1992;41:183.

CHAPTER

86 Use of Drugs in Patients with Renal Failure

Ali J. Olyaei • Jessica L. Steffl • William M. Bennett

Chronic kidney disease (CKD) is associated with a great magnitude of morbidity and mortality in the United States. The recent data indicate that approximately 26 million Americans have CKD, including 350,000 patients with end-stage renal disease (ESRD) who require scheduled dialysis several times per week. Despite the advances in the field of dialysis and management of comorbid conditions in these patients, infections, cardiovascular complications, and adverse drug reactions are the most common cause of mortality in patients with CKD.[1,2] A number of studies have documented the role of medication dosing errors in the overall increase in mortality of patients with renal failure.[3–5] Although a number of algorithms and drug dosing recommendations have been proposed over the last two decades, most are not up-to-date, not adequately studied, and have not kept pace with new advances in the field of dialysis.[6] Acute or chronic renal insufficiency alters the pharmacokinetic and pharmacodynamic properties of most commonly used drugs significantly. Kidneys play an important role in the excretion of active drugs and their pharmacologically active metabolites. Drug accumulation and adverse drug reactions can develop rapidly if drug dosages are not adjusted according to reduced renal function in patients with CKD. Most drugs should be adjusted as renal function improves to ensure efficacy and dosage should be reduced if renal function continues to deteriorate. Even in drugs that are mostly metabolized through the liver, patients with renal failure are at greater risk of adverse drug reactions and toxicity.[7] Drug interactions are also a common problem in this population because most patients with renal insufficiency often have serious comorbid conditions requiring pharmacologic intervention.[8–20]

In addition, a large part of the difficulty in prescribing drugs for the rapidly growing numbers of older patients is due to age-related declines in renal function.[3] Finally, renal replacement therapies including hemodialysis are considered the treatment of choice in patients with ESRD. The effects of dialysis on drug elimination and the need for supplemental dosing must also be considered in patients receiving renal replacement therapy.[21–27]

In this chapter, the basic principles of pharmacokinetic modeling and drug dosing in patients with CKD or dialysis are reviewed. The changes in drug pharmacokinetics and pharmacodynamics are highlighted, and practical guidelines for drug dosing in these patients are provided. However, dialysis patients also face the risk of drug–drug and drug–disease interactions, thus, no specific dosing guideline can be given confidently because individual patient factors such as age, gender, nutrition, body fluid volume, and disease states may influence pharmacokinetic and pharmacodynamic parameters significantly. To provide safe and effective pharmacotherapy, the clinician must utilize clinical judgments, knowledge of altered pharmacokinetic properties, and the patient's specific physiologic status to administer drugs safely to a renal patient population. In order to optimize pharmacotherapy and avoid over- and undermedication, these factors should be taken into account and appropriate dosage adjustment should be considered.

PHARMACOKINETIC PRINCIPLES

The term *pharmacokinetics* refers to a mathematical model of the time course of drug concentration in a body compartment. Pharmacokinetic properties of a drug define or predict plasma concentrations and, therefore, drug activity or toxicity at the site of the action. Pharmacokinetics is the study of drug absorption, distribution, metabolism, and elimination. Pharmacokinetics can be thought of as the body's effect on the drug over time. A simplified scheme of drug pharmacokinetics is illustrated in Figure 86.1. The pharmacologic effect of any drug depends on the concentration of the unbound active drug or an active metabolite at the receptor site of action. The blood and tissue levels of a drug are functions of the administered dose, rate of its absorption, concentration, rate of metabolism or biotransformation, and rate of elimination.[9–13]

Drug Absorption

Following extravascular administration, drugs must be transported through a number of physiologic barriers

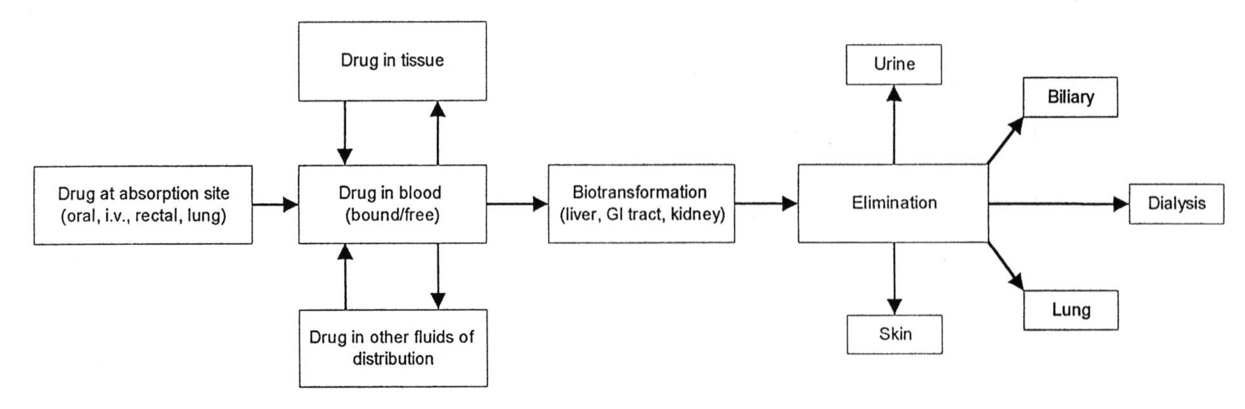

FIGURE 86.1 Pharmacokinetic factors involved in drug distribution.

before reaching the systemic circulation. Drug absorption and bioavailability relate to the amount of drug that reaches the systemic circulation after oral administration. The fraction or percent of administrated drug that reaches systemic circulation is known as bioavailability (F). These parameters are often highly specific for a given compound and vary with the physical and chemical properties of the drug, its formulation, the integrity of the absorptive surface, and the presence of other agents and/or food in the gastrointestinal tract. Absorption rates of most therapeutic agents are slow and unpredictable. Uremia-induced vomiting or sluggish peristalsis secondary to enteropathy may further reduce the onset of action of most agents. In patients with diabetes mellitus, the drug absorption is more variable due to autonomic neuropathy. Both calcium- and aluminum-containing phosphate binders may form insoluble complexes with certain drugs such as antibiotics or ferrous sulfate, thereby impeding absorption. Acidic drugs prefer an acidic environment for optimal absorption whereas weak basic drugs are better absorbed in a more alkalinized small intestine. Use of proton pump inhibitors or phosphate binders presumably reduces the rate of absorption of a number of acidic agents.[14–18] The gastrointestinal tract edema in patients with hypoalbuminemia may also diminish drug absorption.

Propranolol, morphine, and verapamil are examples of drugs that undergo first pass metabolism.[28,29] In first pass metabolism, a significant amount of the absorbed drug molecules are delivered to the liver via the portal vein. A drug is said to undergo significant first pass metabolism when it is metabolized in the liver so extensively upon absorption that only a small percentage of drug concentrations reaches the systemic circulation.[30,31] In addition many drugs may be metabolized via the cytochrome P-450 system in the gastrointestinal tract before reaching the systemic circulation. For example, it is well established that rifampin decreases and erythromycin increases the bioavailability of cyclosporine and calcium channel blockers by induction and inhibition of intestinal and hepatic cytochrome P-450 enzymes, respectively. Finally, patients with renal failure have a higher salivary urea concentration that increases the gastric ammonia levels and increases overall gastric pH. Drugs like iron and ketoconazole whose absorption is dependent on an acidic environment may have reduced bioavailability in renal failure.[29,32]

Volume of Distribution

The volume of distribution (Vd) for a specific drug is derived by dividing the fractional absorption of a dose by the plasma concentration.

$$\text{Volume of distribution (Vd)} = \frac{\text{Amount of drug in body}}{\text{Concentration of drug in plasma or blood (C)}} \quad (86.1)$$

It is important to emphasize that Vd does not signify the total body fluid. Rather, it is an apparent volume needed for equal distribution of drug throughout the body compartment. For example, the plasma volume of a normal 70 kg man is approximately 3 to 3.5 L, whereas the Vd of 0.25 mg of digoxin to obtain a 0.7 ng per dL plasma level is 350 L, which is 10 times greater than the plasma volume. Therefore, Vd does not refer to a specific anatomic compartment per se. Instead, it is the volume of fluid in which the drug would need to be dissolved to give the observed plasma concentration.[33–35] A drug distributes in the body in a characteristic manner based on physiochemical properties of the drug and individual patient variables. Volume of distribution is used mathematically to determine the dose of a drug necessary to achieve a desired plasma concentration. Although the Vd is relatively constant for a given drug, many factors such as obesity, extracellular fluid volume status, age, gender, thyroid function, renal function, and cardiac output influence drug distribution. Volume of distribution echoes the water solubility and protein and tissue-binding characteristics of an individual agent. Drugs with a small Vd (Vd less than ~0.7 L per kg) are usually considered more water soluble. Highly lipid-soluble drugs have a large Vd with little retention of drug in the plasma because the drug tends to stay in the lipophilic tissue compartment. Drugs that are highly tissue bound, such as digoxin, will also have a large Vd. If tissue binding of drugs is decreased by azotemia, a decrease in Vd results. Digoxin is highly bound to cardiac and other tissue Na^+–K^+–ATPase transporters, accounting for its large Vd of 300 to 500 L and very low plasma concentrations. Waste products that accumulate in the azotemic patient serve to displace digoxin from its tissue-binding sites and thus reduce its Vd. Further, such waste products cross-react with the antidigoxin antibody used in drug monitoring assays, producing "therapeutic" digoxin levels in patients not even taking the drug. Insulin and methotrexate similarly have diminished Vd in the uremic state. As a general rule, plasma concentrations of a drug correlate inversely with its Vd.[3,29,36]

Protein Binding

The third important pharmacokinetic concept is protein binding. Only unbound drug or unbound active drug metabolites are able to exert any pharmacologic effects. Disease states that affect total body proteins may significantly alter free drug concentration and increase the risk of drug toxicity. Quantity (binding site) and quality (affinity) of protein binding are substantially altered in patients with renal failure.[37–39] Specifically, uremic toxins may decrease the affinity of albumin for a variety of drugs. Organic acids that accumulate in renal failure compete with acidic drugs for protein binding sites. This results in a larger fraction of acidic compounds existing in the unbound or active state. Conversely, basic drugs bind more readily to nonalbumin serum proteins such as α_1-acid glycoprotein and may demonstrate increased protein binding because this acute phase reactant is often elevated in patients with acute disease states including renal impairment. Malnutrition and proteinuria lower serum protein levels, which may increase the free fraction of a compound as well. Alterations in a drug's protein binding and subsequent effects on drug disposition may be difficult to predict. Drugs that are highly protein bound (>80%) are not removed very effectively during dialysis. In general, drugs that are highly protein bound are largely confined to the vascular space and thus have a Vd of 0.2 L per kg or less. Generally, the Vd for a given agent increases as its protein binding decreases and diminishes as its protein-bound fraction increases.[37–39]

Drug Metabolism or Biotransformation

The total body clearance of a drug is equal to the sum of renal clearance plus nonrenal clearance. Obviously, in patients with renal insufficiency, the contribution of renal clearance to total body clearance will be reduced. Nonrenal clearance, however, may be increased, decreased, or unchanged in such patients. Specifically, hepatic pathways of drug metabolism or biotransformation including acetylation, oxidation, reduction, and hydrolysis may be slowed or accelerated depending on the drug under consideration.[40,41] Sulfisoxazole acetylation, propranolol oxidation, hydrocortisone reduction, and cephalosporin hydrolysis are all slowed in uremic patients. Most drugs undergo biotransformation to more polar but less pharmacologically active compounds that require intact renal function for elimination from the body.[7,42,43] Active or toxic metabolites of parent compounds may accumulate in patients with renal failure. The antiarrhythmic agent procainamide is metabolized to *N*-acetylprocainamide, which is excreted by the kidney. Thus, the antiarrhythmic properties and toxicity of procainamide and its active metabolite are additive, particularly in patients with renal failure. Meperidine, a commonly used narcotic, is biotransformed to normeperidine, which undergoes renal excretion. Although normeperidine has little narcotic effect, it lowers the seizure threshold as it accumulates in uremic patients.[44,45]

Renal Elimination

The most important route of drug elimination is the kidney. Specific processes involved in the renal handling and elimination of drugs include glomerular filtration, tubular secretion and reabsorption, and renal epithelial cell metabolism.[46] All of these functions can be directly or indirectly influenced by renal impairment. Because plasma proteins are too large to pass through a normal glomerulus, only unbound compounds will be freely filtered across this barrier. When proteinuria exists, protein-bound molecules may move into the tubular fluid and be eliminated from the circulation. Changes in renal blood flow may affect both drug reabsorption and secretion. Drugs that are highly protein bound can be eliminated without exerting any pharmacologic effects. For example, binding of furosemide to intraluminal albumin in nephrotic states may contribute to the diuretic resistance characteristic of such conditions. When renal disease reduces nephron numbers, the kidneys' ability to eliminate drugs declines in proportion to the decline in glomerular filtration rate (GFR). As patients progress toward dialysis dependency, drugs usually filtered and excreted begin to accumulate, leading to a high prevalence of adverse reactions unless dosage adjustments are instituted.[47–50]

Drugs that are extensively bound to protein either have a low renal clearance or enter the filtrate by tubular secretion. Tubular handling of a drug is an energy-requiring, active transport process and involves two separate and distinct pathways in the proximal tubule that are used for the secretion and reabsorption of organic acids and bases.[51] These processes are dependent on renal blood flow but not GFR. Accumulation of organic acids in the setting of renal failure competes with acidic drugs for tubular transport and secretion into the urinary space. This, in turn, may lead to drug accumulation and adverse reactions as serum concentrations of agents such as methotrexate, sulfonylureas, penicillins, and cephalosporins rise. Diuretics gain access to their intraluminal sites of action via organic acid secretory pumps. Competition for these secretory pathways by accumulated uremic wastes results in diuretic resistance and necessitates increased diuretic doses to elicit the desired natriuretic effect.

Drug metabolism occurs in the kidney due to a high parenchymal concentration of cytochrome P-450 enzymes. Endogenous vitamin D metabolism and insulin catabolism are examples of processes that decline as renal failure progresses.[35,39–41]

First-order pharmacokinetics describes the manner in which most drugs and their metabolites are eliminated from the body. Specifically, the amount of drug eliminated over time is a fixed proportion of the body stores. The half-life ($t_{1/2}$) of a given agent is most commonly used to express its elimination rate from the body and equals the time required for the drug's plasma concentration to fall by 50%. Half-life can be expressed mathematically as follows:

$$t_{1/2} = \frac{0.693}{Kr + Knr} \qquad (86.2)$$

where *Kr* represents the renal elimination rate constant and *Knr* represents the nonrenal elimination rate constant. As renal elimination declines with renal function, $t_{1/2}$ is prolonged.

DOSAGE ADJUSTMENT FOR THE PATIENT WITH CHRONIC KIDNEY DISEASE

The following outline provides a stepwise approach to prescribing drug therapy for patients with renal failure. Again, it must be emphasized that these steps simply provide a framework for dosage adjustments in patients with renal impairment and must be modified on a case-by-case basis.

Initial Assessment

A history and physical examination constitute the first step in assessing dosimetry in any patient but particularly in those with renal impairment. Kidney injury should be defined as acute or chronic and the cause ascertained if possible. In addition, a history of previous drug intolerance or toxicity should be determined. The patient's current medication list must be reviewed, including both prescription as well as nonprescription and herbal formulations to identify potential drug interactions and nephrotoxins. Calculation of ideal body weight will be based on physical examination findings. For men, the ideal body weight is 50 kg plus 2.3 kg for each 2.54 cm (1 inch) over 152 cm (5 feet). For women, the formula is 45.5 kg plus 2.3 kg per 2.54 cm over 152 cm. An assessment of extracellular fluid volume is also key because significant shifts can affect the Vd of many pharmacologic agents. The presence of hepatic dysfunction may also require additional dosage adjustments.

Calculating Creatinine Clearance

The rate of drug excretion by the kidney is proportional to the GFR. Therefore, it is important to accurately assess renal function and GFR. Serum creatinine alone is an unreliable marker of renal function. Although it overestimates GFR, calculated creatinine clearance (Ccr) more accurately approximates the GFR than serum creatinine and can be estimated conveniently by the Cockcroft and Gault (CG) equation:

$$Ccr = \frac{(140 - \text{age})\ (\text{ideal body weight in kg})}{72 \times \text{serum creatinine in mg/dL}} \qquad (86.3)$$

For women, the calculated value is multiplied by 0.85. The use of this formula implies that the patient is in a steady-state with respect to serum creatinine. There is no accurate method to quantify GFR when renal function is rapidly changing, and as such, it is best to assume a GFR value of less than 10 mL per minute in acute renal failure to avoid drug accumulation and toxicity.[52]

Measured GFR is another method of renal assessment. Inulin is an ideal agent for measuring GFR. Following administration, inulin is filtered by the glomerulus and, in contrast to creatinine, inulin is not secreted, reabsorbed, or metabolized by the kidney. Like other exogenous substances, the inulin test is costly and time consuming and is not available for routine clinical use. Today, isotope tests (51Cr-EDTA, 99Tc-DTPA) have replaced the inulin clearance test for measuring GFR.[53]

Other methods have been suggested to estimate GFR to improve accuracy and reduce estimation errors.[54] However, all newer methods are serum creatinine–based equations and are subject to the same systemic errors as CG method. The Modification of Diet in Renal Disease (MDRD) equation was derived from the 1,628 patients involved in the MDRD study group.[55] In this study, subjects underwent GFR measurement using 125 I-iothalamate, 24–hour creatinine clearance urine collection, and a single measurement of serum creatinine. Multiple variables (i.e., weight, height, sex, ethnicity, diabetes, etc.) were used to determine the most accurate assessment of GFR. Initially, a six-variable equation was determined by the study group. Upon further study, the four-variable equation was found to be as accurate as the six-variable equation. Adding albumin and urea as variables did not improve accuracy or reduces errors.

MDRD6 Equation*

$$GFR = 170 \times [Pcr]^{-0.999} \times [Age]^{-0.176} \times [0.762 \text{ if patient is female}] \times [1.180 \text{ if patient is black}] \times [SUN]^{-0.170} \times [Alb]^{0.318}$$

**Pcr*, serum creatinine concentration; *SUN*, serum urea nitrogen concentration; *Alb*, serum albumin concentration

MDRD4 Equation

$$GFR = 186 \times Scr^{-1.154} \times age^{-0.203} \times 0.742 \text{ [if female]} \times 1.21 \text{ [if black]}$$

The U.S. Food and Drug Administration (FDA) released "Guidance for Industry: Pharmacokinetics in Patients with Impaired Renal Function-Study Design, Data Analysis and Impact on Dosing and Labeling" in 2010, recommending the CG or MDRD4 equations as the method for assessing renal function in pharmacokinetic studies.[56] It is important to emphasize that all different methods of GFR estimation and equations for drug dosing in CKD have small biases when comparing CG to other methods.[57]

Choosing a Loading Dose

Loading doses are intended to achieve a therapeutic steady-state drug level within a short period of time. As such, the loading dose generally is not reduced in the setting of renal failure. Loading doses can be calculated if the Vd and desired peak level are known, as is discussed later. If extracellular volume depletion exists, the Vd may be reduced for certain pharmacologic agents, and slight reductions in the loading dose would be prudent. Specifically, drugs with narrow therapeutic–toxic profiles such as digoxin and ototoxic aminoglycosides should be administered with a 10% to 25% reduction in their loading dose when volume contraction is present in patients with renal failure.

Choosing a Maintenance Dose

Maintenance doses of a drug ensure steady-state blood concentrations and lessen the likelihood of subtherapeutic regimens or overdosage. In the absence of a loading dose, maintenance doses will achieve 90% of their steady-state level in three to four half-lives. One of two methods can be used to adjust maintenance doses for patients with renal insufficiency. The "dosage reduction" method involves reducing the absolute amount of drug administered at each dosing interval proportional to the patient's degree of renal failure. The dosing interval remains unchanged, and more constant drug concentrations are achieved. The "interval extension" method involves lengthening the time period between individual doses of a drug, reflecting the extent of renal insufficiency. This method is particularly useful for drugs with a wide therapeutic range and long half-life.

Monitoring Drug Levels

Blood, serum, and plasma drug concentrations may not be equivalent. As a result, drug levels can only be interpreted if the dosage schedule is known, including the dose administered, timing, and route of administration. A peak level is usually obtained 30 minutes following intravenous administration and 60 to 120 minutes after oral ingestion. It reflects the maximum level achieved after the rapid distribution phase and before significant elimination has occurred. A trough level is obtained just prior to the next dose, reflects total body clearance, and may be a marker of drug toxicity. If the concentration of a drug and its Vd are known, the dose required to achieve a desired therapeutic level can be calculated by the following formula where Vd in L per kilogram is multiplied by ideal body weight (IBW) in kilograms and the desired plasma concentration in milligrams per L (Cp):

$$\text{Dose} = Vd \times IBW \times Cp \quad (86.4)$$

Drug level monitoring is a clinically useful tool when used appropriately. Clinical judgment is paramount because drug failure or toxicity can occur within "therapeutic concentrations." For example, digitalis intoxication can occur in the presence of therapeutic serum levels if hypokalemia or metabolic alkalosis coexists. Phenytoin toxicity is a common problem in patients with renal failure and hypoalbuminemia because of an increase in the unbound or biologically active fraction of phenytoin despite a low total phenytoin plasma concentration. In this setting phenytoin levels should be adjusted for reduced protein binding and the effect of renal failure on phenytoin distributions (Table 86.1).

DIALYSIS AND DRUG DOSING

Patients undergoing renal replacement therapy (dialysis therapy) require special attention in terms of dosage adjustment because dialysis membranes significantly remove many therapeutic agents. An array of modalities including high efficiency, high flux, continuous, and conventional hemodialysis exist and differ from one another based on membrane porosity, surface area, and blood as well as dialysate flow rates. These differences, in turn, affect drug removal. In Table 86.2 are summarized drug properties and dialysis parameters that determine dialytic clearance of pharmacologic agents. In general, in thrice weekly intermittent hemodialysis (IHD), the drug removal is affected by blood and dialysate flow rate, molecular weight (MW) of the drug, fraction of protein binding, and dialyzer surface area. Drugs with MW greater than 500 D and that are highly protein bound (80%), highly tissue bound, and lipophilic are poorly dialyzed by conventional IHD. However, drugs with small MW, low protein binding, small volume of distribution, and of a hydrophilic character are effectively removed by IHD.[58–61]

Drug Properties Affecting Dialytic Clearance

A drug's molecular weight is a major determinant of its dialyzability. Specifically, drugs larger than 500 D are primarily cleared by convection as opposed to diffusion. If too large to pass through a given membrane, the drug will not

TABLE 86.1 **Therapeutic Drug Monitoring**

	Drug Name	Therapeutic Range	When to Draw Sample	When to Check Levels	Time to Reach Steady State	Other Considerations
Antibiotics	Aminoglycosides (conventional dosing) Gentamicin Tobramycin Amikacin	Gentamicin and tobramycin: Peak: 5 to 8 mg/L Trough: <2 mg/L (for moderate to severe non-UTI infections, or CF, peaks should be between 10 to 12) Amikacin Peak: 20 to 30 mg/L Trough: <10 mg/L	Trough: Immediately prior to dose Peak: 30 minutes after a 30 minute infusion or 30 minutes after a 60 minute infusion CF patients: 15 minutes after 30 minute infusion	With third dose for initial therapy or after dose change. For therapy less than 72 hours, levels not necessary. Repeat drug levels if renal function changes.	Steady state is reached in 4 to 5 elimination half-lives; generally by the third dose	Special considerations for renal patients and dialysis: 2 mg/kg then 1 mg/kg, redose if level less than 2 mg/L
	Gentamicin Tobramycin Amikacin	0.5 to 3 mg/L	Obtain random drug level 12 hours after dose	After initial dose. Repeat drug level in 1 week or if renal function changes.	Steady state is not reached in most cases due to insufficient drug accumulation between dosing intervals	24-hour dosing not to be used for patients with burns, CrCl <20, CF, dialysis, endocarditis, neutropenia, pediatrics, pregnancy
	Vancomycin	Peak: 20 to 50 mg/L Trough: 5 to 20 mg/L	Trough: Immediately prior to dose Peak: 60 minutes after a 60-minute infusion	With third dose for initial therapy or after dose change. For therapy less than 72 hours, levels not necessary. Repeat drug levels if renal function changes.	Steady state is reached in 4 to 5 elimination half-lives; generally by the third dose	Special considerations for renal patients—goal trough <15 mg/L

Anticonvulsants	Carbamazepine	4 to 12 μg/mL	Trough: Immediately prior to dosing	2 to 4 days after first dose or change in dose	2 to 5 days	Monitor baseline LFTs, then 2 to 3 months after starting drug
	Phenobarbital	15 to 40 μg/mL	Trough: Immediately prior to next dose	2 weeks after first dose or change in dose. Follow-up level in 1 to 2 months.	14 to 21 days	
	Phenytoin Free phenytoin	10 to 20 μg/mL 1 to 2 μg/mL	Trough: Immediately prior to dosing	5 to 7 days after first dose or change in dose	10 to 14 days	Adjustments necessary for albumin <3.5 g/dL or patients with renal impairment. For acutely ill patients, earlier levels should be considered.
	Valproic acid (includes divalproex sodium)	50 to 100 μg/mL	Trough: Immediately prior to next dose	2 to 4 days after first dose or change in dose.	2 to 4 days	Monitor baseline LFTs, then 2 to 3 months after starting drug

UTI, urinary tract infection; CF, cystic fibrosis; CrCl, creatinine clearance; LFTs, liver function tests.

TABLE 86.2 **Antimicrobal Agents in Renal Failure**

Drugs	Normal Dosage	% of Renal Excretion	Dosage Adjustment in Renal Failure			Comments	HD	CAPD	CVVH
			GFR >50	GFR 10 to 50	GFR <10				
Aminoglycoside Antibiotics						Nephrotoxic, ototoxic Toxicity worse when hyperbilirubinemic Measure serum levels for efficacy and toxicity Peritoneal absorption increases with presence of inflammation Vd increases with edema, obesity, and ascites			
Streptomycin	7.5 mg/kg q12h (1.0 g q24h for TB)	60%	q24h	q24 to 72h	q72 to 96h	For the treatment of TB May be less nephrotoxic than other members of class	1/2 normal dose after dialysis	20 to 40 mg/L/d	Dose for GFR 10 to 50 and measure levels
Kanamycin	7.5 mg/kg q8h	50% to 90%	60% to 90% q12h or 100% q12 to 24h	30% to 70% q12 to 18h or 100% q24 to 48h	20% to 30% q24 to 48h or 100% q48 to 72h	Do not use once-daily dosing in patients with creatinine clearance less than 30 to 40 mL/minutes or in patients with acute renal failure or uncertain level of kidney function	1/2 full dose after dialysis	15 to 20 mg/L/d	Dose for GFR 10 to 50 and measure levels
Gentamicin	1.7 mg/kg q8h	95%	60% to 90% q8 to 12h or 100% q12 to 24h	30% to 70% q12h or 100% q24 to 48h	20% to 30% q24 to 48h or 100% q48 to 72h		1/2 full dose after dialysis	3 to 4 mg/L/d	Dose for GFR 10 to 50 and measure levels

Tobramicin	1.7 mg/kg q8h	95%	60% to 90% q8 to 12h or 100% q12 to 24h	30% to 70% q12h or 100% q24 to 48h	20% to 30% q24 to 48h or 100% q48 to 72h		1/2 full dose after dialysis	3 to 4 mg/L/d	Dose for GFR 10 to 50 and measure levels
Netilmicin	2 mg/kg q8h	95%	50% to 90% q8 to 12h or 100% q12 to 24h	20% to 60% q12h or 100% q24 to 48h	10% to 20% q24 to 48h or 100% q48 to 72	May be less ototoxic than other members of class Peak 6 to 8, trough <2	1/2 full dose after dialysis	3 to 4 mg/L/d	Dose for GFR 10 to 50 and measure levels
Amikacin	7.5 mg/kg q12h	95%	60% to 90% q12h or 100% q12 to 24h	30% to 70% q12 to 18h or 100% q24 to 48h	20% to 30% q24 to 48h or 100% q48 to 72h	Monitor levels Peak 20 to 30, trough <5	1/2 full dose after dialysis	15 to 20 mg/L/d	Dose for GFR 10 to 50 and measure levels
Cephalosporin						Coagulation abnormalities, transitory elevation of BUN, rash, and serum sickness-like syndrome			
Oral Cephalosporin									
Cefaclor	250 to 500 mg tid	70%	100%	100%	50%		250 mg bid after dialysis	250 mg q8 to 12h	N/A
Cefadroxil	500 to 1 g bid	80%	100%	100%	50%		0.5 to 1.0 g after dialysis	0.5 g/d	N/A
Cefixime	200 to 400 mg q12h	85%	100%	100%	50%		300 mg after dialysis	200 mg/d	Not recommended
Ceftibuten	400 mg q24h	70%	100%	100%	50%		300 mg after dialysis	No data: Dose for GFR <10	Dose for GFR 10 to 50

(continued)

TABLE 86.2 **Antimicrobal Agents in Renal Failure *(continued)***

Drugs	Normal Dosage	% of Renal Excretion	Dosage Adjustment in Renal Failure			Comments	HD	CAPD	CVVH
			GFR >50	GFR 10 to 50	GFR <10				
Cefuroxime axetil	250 to 500 mg tid	90%	100%	100%	100%	Malabsorbed in presence of H2 blockers. Absorbed better with food.	Dose after dialysis	Dose for GFR <10	N/A
Cephalexin	250 to 500 mg tid	95%	100%	100%	100%	Rare allergic interstitial nephritis. Absorbed well when given intraperitoneally. May cause bleeding from impaired prothrombin biosynthesis.	Dose after dialysis	Dose for GFR <10	N/A
Cephradine	250 to 500 mg tid	100%	100%	100%	50%		Dose after dialysis	Dose for GFR <10	N/A
IV Cephalosporin									
Cefazolin	1 to 2 g IV q8h	80%	q8h	q12h	q12 to 24h		0.5 to 1.0 g after dialysis	0.5 g q12h	Dose for GFR 10 to 50
Cefepime	1 to 2 g IV q8h	85%	q8 to 12h	q12h	q24h		1 g after dialysis	Dose for GFR <10	Not recommended
Cefmetazole	1 to 2 g IV q8h	85%	q8h	q12h	q24h		Dose after dialysis	Dose for GFR <10	Dose for GFR 10 to 50
Cefoperazone	1 to 2 g IV q12h	20%	No renal adjustment is required			Displaced from protein by bilirubin. Reduce dose by 50% for jaundice. May prolong prothrombin time.	1 g after dialysis	None	None
Cefotaxime	1 to 2 g IV q6 to 8h	60%	q8h	q12h	q12 to 24h		1 g after dialysis	1 g/d	1g q12h

Cefotetan	1 to 2 g IV q12h	75%	q12h	q12 to 24h	q24h		1 g after dialysis	1 g/d	750 mg q12h
Cefoxitin	1 to 2 g IV q6h	80%	q6h	q8 to 12h	q12h	May produce false increase in serum creatinine by interference with assay	1 g after dialysis	1 g/d	Dose for GFR 10 to 50
Ceftazidime	1 to 2 g IV q8h	70%	q8h	q12h	q24h		1 g after dialysis	0.5 g/d	Dose for GFR 10 to 50
Ceftriaxone	1 to 2 g IV q24h	50%	No renal adjustment is required				Dose after dialysis	750 mg q12h	Dose for GFR 10 to 50
Cefuroxime sodium	0.75 to 1.5 g IV q8h	90%	q8h	q8 to 12h	q12 to 24h		Dose after dialysis	Dose for GFR <10	1.0 g q12h
Penicillin						Bleeding abnormalities, hypersensitivity. Seizures.			
Oral Penicillin									
Amoxicillin	500 mg po tid	60%	100%	100%	50% to 75%		Dose after dialysis	250 mg q12h	N/A
Ampicillin	500 mg po q6h	60%	100%	100%	50% to 75%		Dose after dialysis	250 mg q12h	Dose for GFR 10 to 50
Dicloxacillin	250 to 500 mg po q6h	50%	100%	100%	50% to 75%		None	None	N/A
Penicillin V	250 to 500 mg po q6h	70%	100%	100%	50% to 75%		Dose after dialysis	Dose for GFR <10	N/A
IV Penicillin									
Ampicillin	1 to 2 g IV q6h	60%	q6h	q8h	q12h		Dose after dialysis	250 mg q12h	Dose for GFR 10 to 50

(continued)

TABLE 86.2 **Antimicrobal Agents in Renal Failure *(continued)***

Drugs	Normal Dosage	% of Renal Excretion	Dosage Adjustment in Renal Failure			Comments	HD	CAPD	CVVH
			GFR >50	GFR 10 to 50	GFR <10				
Nafcillin	1 to 2 g IV q4h	35%	No renal adjustment is required				None	None	Dose for GFR 10 to 50
Penicillin G	2 to 3 million units IV q4h	70%	q4 to 6h	q6h	q8h		Dose after dialysis	Dose for GFR <10	Dose for GFR 10 to 50
Piperacillin	3 to 4 g IV q4 to 6h		No renal adjustment is required			Sodium, 1.9 mEq/g	Dose after dialysis	Dose for GFR <10	Dose for GFR 10 to 50
Ticarcillin/ clavulanate	3.1 g IV q4 to 6h	85%	1 to 2 g q4h	1 to 2 g q8h	1 to 2 g q12h	Sodium, 5.2 mEq/g	3.0 g after dialysis	Dose for GFR <10	Dose for GFR 10 to 50
Piperacillin/ tazobactam	3.375 g IV q6 to 8h	75% to 90%	q4 to 6h	q6 to 8h	q8h	Sodium, 1.9 mEq/g	Dose after dialysis	Dose for GFR <10	Dose for GFR 10 to 50
Quinolones						Food, dairy products, tube feeding, and $Al(OH)_3$ may decrease the absorption of quinolones.			
Ciprofloxacin	200 to 400 mg IV q24h	60%	q12h	q12 to 24h	q24h	Poorly absorbed with antacids, sucralfate, and phosphate binders. Intravenous dose 1/3 of oral dose. Decreases phenytoin levels.	250 mg q12h (200 mg if IV)	250 mg q8h (200 mg if IV)	200 mg IV q12h

Levofloxacin	500 mg po qd	70%	q12h	250 q12h	250 q12h	L-isomer of ofloxacin: appears to have similar pharmacokinetics and toxicities	Dose for GFR <10	Dose for GFR <10	Dose for GFR 10 to 50
Moxifloxacin	400 mg qd	20%	No renal adjustment is required				No data	No data	No data
Nalidixic acid	1.0 g q6h	High	100%	Avoid	Avoid	Agents in this group are malabsorbed in the presence of magnesium, calcium, aluminum, and iron. Theophylline metabolism is impaired. Higher oral doses may be needed to treat CAPD peritonitis.	Avoid	Avoid	N/A
Norfloxacin	400 mg po q12h	30%	q12h	q12 to 24h	q24h	See above.	Dose for GFR <10	Dose for GFR <10	N/A
Ofloxacin	200 to 400 mg po q12h	70%	q12h	q12 to 24h	q24h	See above.	100 to 200 mg after dialysis	Dose for GFR <10	300 mg/d
Miscellaneous Agents									
Azithromycin	250 to 500 mg po qd	6%	No renal adjustment is required			No drug-drug interaction with CsA/FK	None	None	None
Clarithromycin	500 mg po bid		No renal adjustment is required				None	None	None
Clindamycin	150 to 450 mg po tid	10%	No renal adjustment is required			Increase CsA/FK level	None	None	None
Dirithromycin	500 mg po qd		No renal adjustment is required			Nonenzymatically hydrolyzed to active compound erythomycylamine	None	No data: None	Dose for GFR 10 to 50

(continued)

TABLE 86.2 **Antimicrobal Agents in Renal Failure *(continued)***

Drugs	Normal Dosage	% of Renal Excretion	Dosage Adjustment in Renal Failure			Comments	HD	CAPD	CVVH
			GFR >50	GFR 10 to 50	GFR <10				
Erythromycin	250 to 500 mg po qid	15%	No renal adjustment is required			Increase CsA/FK level, avoid in transplant patients	None	None	None
Ertapenem	1 gm IV q24h		1 gm IV q24h	0.5 gm IV q24h	0.5 gm IV q24h		Dose after dialysis	Dose for GFR <10	Dose for GFR <30
Imipenem/ Cilastatin	250 to 500 mg IV q6h	50%	500 mg q8h	250 to 500 q8 to 12h	250 mg q12h	Seizures in ESRD. Non-renal clearance in acute renal failure is less than in chronic renal failure. Administered with cilastin to prevent nephrotoxicity of renal metabolite.	Dose after dialysis	Dose for GFR <10	Dose for GFR 10 to 50
Meropenem	1 g IV q8h	65%	1 g q8h	0.5 to 1g q12h	0.5 to 1g q24h	Fewer seizures compared to imipenem	Dose after dialysis	Dose for GFR <10	Dose for GFR 10 to 50
Metronidazole	500 mg IV q6h	20%	No renal adjustment is required			Peripheral neuropathy, increase LFTs, disulfiram reaction with alcoholic beverages	Dose after dialysis	Dose for GFR <10	Dose for GFR 10 to 50
Pentamidine	4 mg/kg/ day	5%	q24h	q24h	q48h	Inhalation may cause bronchospasm, IV administration may cause hypotension, hypoglycemia, and nephrotoxicity	None	None	None
Trimethoprim/ sulfamethoxazole	800/160 mg po bid	70%	q12h	q18h	q24h	Increase serum creatinine. Can cause hyperkalemia.	Dose after dialysis	q24h	q18h

Vancomycin	1 g IV q12h	90%	q12h	q24 to 36h	q48 to 72h	Nephrotoxic, ototoxic, may prolong the neuromuscular blockade effect of muscle relaxants Peak 30 to 40. Trough 5 to 10.	500 mg q12 to 24h (high FLX)	1.0 gm q24 to 96h	500 mg q12h
Vancomycin	125 to 250 mg po qid	0%	100%	100%	100%	Oral vancomycin is indicated only for the treatment of *C. diff*.	100%	100%	100%
Antituberculosis Antibiotics									
Rifampin	300 to 600 mg po qd	20%	No renal adjustment is required			Decrease CsA/FK level. Many drug interactions.	None	Dose for GFR <10	Dose for GFR <10
Antifungal Agents									
Amphotericin B	0.5 mg to 1.5 mg/kg/day	<1%	No renal adjustment is required			Nephrotoxic, infusion related reactions, give 250 mL NS before each dose	q24h	q24h	q24 to 36h
Amphotec	4 to 6 mg/kg/day	<1%	No renal adjustment is required						
Abelcet	5 mg/kg/day	<1%	No renal adjustment is required						
AmBisome	3 to 5 mg/kg/day	<1%	No renal adjustment is required						
Azoles and other Antifungals						Increase CsA/FK level			
Fluconazole	200 to 800 mg IV qd/bid	70%	100%	100%	50%		200 mg after dialysis	Dose for GFR <10	Dose for GFR 10 to 50
Flucytosine	37.5 mg/kg	90%	q12h	q16h	q24h	Hepatic dysfunction. Marrow suppression more common in azotemic patients.	Dose after dialysis	0.5 to 1.0 g/d	Dose for GFR 10 to 50

(continued)

TABLE 86.2 **Antimicrobal Agents in Renal Failure *(continued)***

Drugs	Normal Dosage	% of Renal Excretion	Dosage Adjustment in Renal Failure			Comments	HD	CAPD	CVVH
			GFR >50	GFR 10 to 50	GFR <10				
Griseofulvin	125 to 250 mg q6h	1%	100%	100%	100%		None	None	None
Itraconazole	200 mg q12h	35%	100%	100%	50%	Poor oral absorption	100 mg q12 to 24h	100 mg q12 to 24h	100 mg q12 to 24h
Ketoconazole	200 to 400 mg po qd	15%	100%	100%	100%	Hepatotoxic	None	None	None
Miconazole	1,200 to 3,600 mg/day	1%	100%	100%	100%		None	None	None
Posaconazole	200 mg qid	1%	100%	100%	100%				
Terbinafine	250 mg po qd	>1%	100%	100%	100%				
Voriconazole	4–6 mg/kg q12h	1%	100%	100%	100%	Avoid IV formulation in CKD			
Caspofungin	70 mg LD then 50 mg daily	1%	100%	100%	100%				
Micofungin	100–150 mg IV daily	1%	100%	100%	100%				
Anidulafungin	200 mg LD, then 100 mg daily	1%	100%	100%	100%				

Antiviral Agents									
Acyclovir	200 to 800 mg po 5×/day	50%	100%	100%	50%	Poor absorption. Neurotoxicity in ESRD. Intravenous preparation can cause renal failure if injected rapidly.	Dose after dialysis	Dose for GFR <10	3.5 mg/kg/d
Adefovir	10 mg q24h	45%	100%	10 mg q48h	10 mg q72 h	Renal toxicity	10 mg weekly after HD	No data	No data
Amantadine	100 to 200 mg q12h	90%	100%	50%	q96h to 7 days		None	None	Dose for GFR 10 to 50
Cidofovir	5 mg/kg weekly ×2 (induction); 5 mg/kg every 2 weeks	90%	Avoid in CKD	No data: Avoid	No data: Avoid	Dose-limiting nephrotoxicity with proteinuria, glycosuria, renal insufficiency; nephrotoxicity and renal clearance reduced with coadministration of probenecid	No data	No data	Avoid
Delavirdine	400 mg q8h	5%	No data: 100%	No data: 100%	No data: 100%		No data: None	No data	No data: Dose for GFR 10 to 50
Didanosine	200 mg q12h (125 mg if <60 kg)	40% to 69%	q12h	q24h	50% q24h	Pancreatitis	Dose after dialysis	Dose for GFR <10	Dose for GFR <10
Emtricitabine	200 mg q24h	86%	q24h	q48–72h	q 96 h			Dose after dialysis	No data
Entecavir	0.5 mg q24h	62%	q24h	q48–72h	q 96 h			Dose after dialysis	No data
Famciclovir	250 to 500 mg po bid to tid	60%	q8h	q12h	q24h	VZV: 500 mg po tid HSV: 250 po bid. Metabolized to active compound penciclovir.	Dose after dialysis	No data	No data: Dose for GFR 10 to 50

(continued)

TABLE 86.2 **Antimicrobial Agents in Renal Failure *(continued)***

Drugs	Normal Dosage	% of Renal Excretion	Dosage Adjustment in Renal Failure			Comments	HD	CAPD	CVVH
			GFR >50	GFR 10 to 50	GFR <10				
Foscarnet	40 to 80 mg IV q8h	85%	20 to 40 mg q8 to 24 h according to ClCr			Nephrotoxic, neurotoxic, hypocalcemia, hypophosphatemia, hypomagnesemia, and hypokalemia	Dose after dialysis	Dose for GFR <10	Dose for GFR 10 to 50
Ganciclovir IV	5 mg/kg q12h	95%	q12h	q24h	2.5 mg/kg qd	Granulocytopenia and thrombocytopenia	Dose after dialysis	Dose for GFR <10	2.5 mg/kg q24h
Ganciclovir	1,000 mg po tid	95%	1,000 mg tid	1,000 mg bid	1,000 mg qd	Oral ganciclovir should be used ONLY for prevention of CMV infection. Always use IV ganciclovir for the treatment of CMV infection.	No data: Dose after dialysis	No data: Dose for GFR <10	N/A
Indinavir	800 mg q8h	10%	No data: 100%	No data: 100%	No data: 100%	Nephrolithiasis; acute renal failure due to crystalluria, tubulointerstitial nephritis	No data: None	No data: Dose for GFR <10	No data
Lamivudine	150 mg po bid	80%	q12h	q24h	50 mg q24h	For hepatitis B	Dose after dialysis	No data: Dose for GFR <10	Dose for GFR 10 to 50
Maraviroc	300 mg bid	20%	300 mg bid	No data	No data	Drug interaction with CYP III-A	No data	No data	No data
Nelfinavir	750 mg q8h	No data	No data	No data	No data		No data	No data	No data
Nevirapine	200 mg q24h × 14d	<3	No data: 100%	No data: 100%	No data: 100%	May be partially cleared by hemodialysis and peritoneal dialysis	Dose after dialysis	No data: Dose for GFR <10	No data: Dose for GFR 10 to 50

Oseltamivir	75 mg bid	99%	75 bid	75 mg daily	75 mg q48h		Dose after dialysis		
Ribavirin	500 to 600 mg q12h	30%	100%	100%	50%	Hemolytic uremic syndrome	Dose after dialysis	Dose for GFR <10	Dose for GFR 10 to 50
Rifabutin	300 mg q24h	5% to 10%	100%	100%	100%		None	None	No data: Dose for GFR 10 to 50
Rimantadine	100 mg po bid	25%	100%	100%	50%				
Ritonavir	600 mg q12h	3.50%	No data: 100%	No data: 100%	No data: 100%	Many drug interactions	No data: None	No data: Dose for GFR <10	No data: Dose for GFR 10 to 50
Saquinavir	600 mg q8h	<4%	No data: 100%	No data: 100%	No data: 100%		No data: None	No data: Dose for GFR <10	No data: Dose for GFR 10 to 50
Stavudine	30 to 40 mg q12h	35% to 40%	100%	50% q12 to 24h	50% q24h		Dose for GFR <10 after dialysis	No data	No data: Dose for GFR 10 to 50
Telbivudine	600 mg po daily		100%	600 mg q48h	600 mg q96h		Dose for GFR <10 after dialysis	No data	No data: Dose for GFR 10 to 50
Tenofovir	300 mg q24h		100%	300 mg q48–72h	300 mg q96h	Nephrotoxic	Dose for GFR <10 after dialysis	No data	No data: Dose for GFR 10 to 50
Valacyclovir	500 to 1,000 mg q8h	50%	100%	50%	25%	Thrombotic thrombocytopenic purpura/hemolytic uremic syndrome	Dose after dialysis	Dose for GFR <10	No data: Dose for GFR 10 to 50

(continued)

TABLE 86.2 **Antimicrobal Agents in Renal Failure *(continued)***

Drugs	Normal Dosage	% of Renal Excretion	Dosage Adjustment in Renal Failure			Comments	HD	CAPD	CVVH
			GFR >50	GFR 10 to 50	GFR <10				
Valganciclovir	900 mg po daily or bid		100%	50%	25%	Granulocytopenia and thrombocytopenia	Dose after dialysis	Dose for GFR <10	450 mg daily
Vidarabine	15 mg/kg infusion q24h	50%	100%	100%	75%		Infuse after dialysis	Dose for GFR <10	Dose for GFR 10 to 50
Zanamivir	2 puffs bid × 5 days	1%	100%	100%	100%	Bioavailability from inhalation and systemic exposure to drug is low	None	None	No data
Zalcitabine	0.75 mg q8h	75%	100%	q12h	q24h		No data: Dose after dialysis	No data	No data: Dose for GFR 10 to 50
Zidovudine	200 mg q8h, 300 mg q12h	8% to 25%	100%	100%	100 mg q8h	Enormous interpatient variation. Metabolite renally excreted.	Dose for GFR <10	Dose for GFR <10	100 mg q8h

HD, hemodialysis; CAPD, chronic peritoneal dialysis; CVVH, continuous venovenous hemofiltration; GFR, glomerular filtration rate; q, every; TB, tuberculosis; BUN, blood urea nitrogen; tid, three times a day; bid, twice a day; IV, intravenous; po, by mouth; ESRD, end-stage renal disease; *C. diff*, *Clostridium difficile*; CKD, chronic kidney disease; VZV, varicella zoster virus; HSV, herpes simplex virus; ClCr, creatinine clearance; CMV, cytomegalovirus.

be cleared from the circulation. An inverse semilogarithmic relationship exists between molecular weight and dialysis clearance.

Protein binding represents another major determinant of drug dialyzability. Compounds that are highly protein bound have a smaller fraction of unbound drug available for removal by dialysis. Because heparin stimulates lipoprotein lipase, free fatty acid levels may increase during dialysis. Free fatty acid levels may displace sulfonamides, salicylates, and phenytoin from their protein binding sites, resulting in increased free fractions of each drug. In contrast, free fatty acids can increase protein binding of certain cephalosporins. The free fraction of phenytoin is increased by free fatty acids.

As discussed previously, drugs with a large Vd (greater than 2 L per kg) tend to have low concentrations in the intravascular space and are thus not readily dialyzable. The lower the Vd (less than 1 L per kg), the greater the drug's availability to the circulation and, similarly, to the dialyzer.

Larger molecular weight compounds do not equilibrate rapidly between the extracellular and intracellular compartments during dialysis—little change is detected in intracellular concentrations whereas extracellular levels may fall significantly. As such, postdialysis rebound may occur in which pharmacologic agents move down their concentration gradients into the extracellular space. Rebound can be sizable as well as highly unpredictable in its time course, as demonstrated by vancomycin. Ultrafiltration raises the hematocrit, which can influence the dialytic clearance of drugs that partition into red blood cells. Drugs such as ethambutol, procainamide, and acetaminophen partition into red blood cells and demonstrate decreased dialytic clearance due to hemoconcentration following dialysis ultrafiltration.

Thus, parent compounds and their metabolites will be eliminated by dialysis to a greater extent if they possess a low molecular weight, limited Vd, and are water soluble. An increase in drug clearance of 30% or greater by dialytic therapy is considered significant and may warrant supplemental dosing following dialysis.

Dialytic Factors Affecting Drug Clearance

Dialysis membranes, dialysate flow rates, and the dialytic technique used can significantly alter drug clearance (Table 86.3).[62] A wide variety of membranes have been developed including cellulose, cellulose acetate, polysulfone, polyamide, polyacrylonitrile (PAN; AN69), and polymethylmethacrylate (PMMA) in an effort to improve membrane permeability for larger uremic toxins. Similarly, albumin can cross polysulfone membranes to a limited extent.[63] Vancomycin clearance is significantly increased when polysulfone or PAN membranes are used.[59,60] Likewise, cuprammonia rayon membranes allow greater aminoglycoside removal compared to cellulose fibers.[44] Two endogenous compounds that are poorly dialyzed, phosphate and

TABLE 86.3 **Factors Affecting Drug Removal During Dialysis**

Drug Properties	Dialysis System Properties
Renal clearance	Filter properties
Volume of distribution	Blood flow, dialysate flow, and ultrafiltration rates
Water and lipid solubility	
Protein binding	
Drug charge	
Molecular weight	

β_2-microglobulin, undergo enhanced clearance when PAN, PMMA, and polysulfone membranes are used due to the increased surface area of these membranes.[64] The electrical charge of a dialysis membrane as well as the drug may help or hinder clearance. Like charges will repel one another, whereas opposite charges between membrane and drug may lead to drug adsorption to the membrane, ultimately reducing clearance.[65,66]

Drug clearance is achieved primarily by two processes: diffusion and convection. Diffusion of a compound increases as its molecular weight decreases and is negligible when standard membranes are used for substances larger than 1,000 D.[21,67] Diffusion of a drug is enhanced when the concentration gradient between blood and dialysate is maximized by countercurrent flow and increased blood and dialysate flow rates. Flow rates have less impact on the diffusion of middle-sized and large molecules, but the surface area and hydraulic permeability of the membrane assume greater significance. Diffusion can be hindered, however, when high ultrafiltration rates lead to the mixing of dialysate and ultrafiltrate. This results in a decreased concentration gradient between blood and dialysate, reducing diffusive clearance.[68] Convection refers to the movement of solute by way of ultrafiltration, which affects molecules of all sizes but particularly large molecular weight substances, which diffuse poorly. To be removed by dialysis, compounds greater than 1,000 D require ultrafiltration when cellulose membranes are used, whereas those greater than 2,000 D demonstrate limited clearance. Ultrafiltration, and thus convection, can be reduced by protein binding to membrane surfaces during the dialytic procedure, which ultimately diminishes drug removal.[21,22]

Continuous Renal Replacement Therapies and Drug Removal

Critically ill patients may require continuous renal replacement therapies (CRRTs) such as hemofiltration or hemodialysis, and an awareness of drug handling by such procedures is crucial to the patient's outcome. Continuous hemofiltration removes solute by convection. The degree to which a solute can convectively cross a membrane can be quantitated by its sieving coefficient (S), the ratio of solute concentration in the ultrafiltrate to solute concentration in the retentate (returning to the patient's circulation). This can be approximated by the formula:

$$S = UF/A[5] \qquad (86.5)$$

where *UF* is ultrafiltrate and *A* is arterial concentrations of solute, which will remain relatively constant during hemofiltration because blood flow does not affect sieving. Clearance of a solute (drug) is determined by multiplying the ultrafiltration rate by the S for that substance. The sieving coefficient for a given molecule can change, however, when comparing different dialysis membranes and is likely due to drug–membrane binding. Sieving can also be reduced by negatively charged solutes, although exceptions to this exist.[23,25] Because inulin (5,200 D) can readily cross polysulfone hemofiltration membranes, nearly all therapeutic agents would be expected to permeate such membranes given molecular weights less than that of inulin. The drug's degree of protein binding will be the major limiting factor to drug removal during hemofiltration.

In contrast to hemofiltration, drug removal during continuous hemodialysis occurs primarily via diffusion rather than convection. Protein binding again plays a central role whereby unbound drug diffuses more readily than protein-bound drug and molecular weight correlates inversely with diffusion. It should be noted that during continuous hemodialysis with venovenous access and average blood flow rates of 200 mL per minute, a GFR of 20 to 30 mL per minute can be achieved, which may provide greater drug clearance than expected. As previously discussed, when supplemental dosing is indicated, the amount of drug required to achieve a desired blood level can be calculated by multiplying the drug's Vd by the patient's IBW and the difference between the desired drug concentration and the trough concentration.

Lastly, peritoneal dialysis generally provides minimal drug removal, as dialysate flow rates are significantly slower than other forms of dialytic therapy. Drugs that are dialyzable via peritoneal dialysis must be small in size and have a low Vd. Drugs that are highly protein bound, however, may undergo greater clearance with peritoneal dialysis versus hemodialysis given the large protein losses commonly seen with peritoneal therapy.

SPECIFIC CONSIDERATIONS FOR DRUG PRESCRIBING IN RENAL FAILURE

In this section, the effects of renal insufficiency on drug pharmacokinetics and pharmacodynamics are reviewed and dosage adjustment guidelines are provided. It is imperative to reiterate that the following recommendations provide a framework for dosage adjustments that must be applied to individual patients with caution. Continual monitoring and modification of drug therapy are required by concurrent illnesses, clinical response, and side effects present in the individual patient. Drugs are listed in tabular form (Tables 86.3 through 86.13) by generic name in alphabetical order and are grouped into categories based on therapeutic effect. General comments about each group precede the individual dosing table. For reference, the standard dose given to patients with normal renal function is included. Specific dosing guidelines are provided for each drug based on the patient's level of renal function in terms of GFR. It should be remembered that creatinine clearance always overestimates true GFR.

The maintenance dosage regimen may be modified by either extending the interval between doses, decreasing the individual dose while maintaining normal dosing intervals, or a combination of the two methods. As outlined previously, the variable interval method allows a more convenient and less costly dosing schedule but may result in periods of subtherapeutic drug levels. The variable dose method maintains more constant drug levels because the dosing interval remains unchanged but risks greater toxicity because the difference between peak and trough levels is diminished. When the interval extension method (I) is used, the dosing interval length (in hours) is indicated. When the dosage reduction method (D) is used, the percentage of the standard dose normally used is indicated.

The requirement for supplemental dosing after hemodialysis and special dosing considerations for peritoneal dialysis and continuous renal replacement therapies are also included. For many drugs, specific data are not available on dialytic drug clearance, and the likelihood of dialytic removal is based on molecular weight, Vd, and protein binding.

Antimicrobial Agents

Infection is the leading cause of morbidity and mortality in patients with renal failure. Many antibiotics require dosage adjustment in the setting of renal insufficiency due to alterations in pharmacokinetic and pharmacodynamic parameters. An increased incidence of extrarenal toxicity is also observed in patients with renal insufficiency due, in part, to accumulation of drug and/or active metabolites. Specific dosing guidelines for individual antimicrobial agents are provided in Table 86.2. One or more pharmacokinetic parameters may be altered in the patient with renal failure.[69,70] A number of oral antibiotics are now available for the treatment of infections in patients with renal impairments. However, a decreased absorption may occur for some agents such as tetracycline or ciprofloxacin.[71,72] Most antibiotics should be administrated at least 2 to 4 hours after iron and phosphate binder therapy. Although the majority of antibiotics are excreted partially or completely by glomerular filtration, a number of antimicrobials such as trimethoprim–sulfamethoxazole or ciprofloxacin reach the urinary space by tubular secretion. This, in turn, achieves high urinary concentrations of such agents even though the GFR is diminished.[73] This feature is used to therapeutic advantage for treatment of urinary tract infections in patients with renal insufficiency or cyst infections in patients with polycystic kidney disease.

For most drugs, the loading dose will be the same as that used in patients with normal renal function because rapid achievement of therapeutic antibiotic levels are critical for life-threatening infections. Recently, the postantibiotic effect has been observed with a number of antimicrobials including aminoglycosides, newer macrolides, and the penems.[74,75] Clinically, the persistence of antibiotic activity beyond the time point at which blood levels fall below the minimum inhibitory concentration may be used to design extended and more convenient dosing intervals of antimicrobial agents without jeopardizing patient outcomes.

Peritoneal dialysis patients often use the intraperitoneal route of antibiotic administration for treatment of peritonitis. Detailed reviews of this therapeutic modality exist elsewhere, and intraperitoneal antibiotic dosing for peritonitis has been reviewed by Li and colleagues. Patients with renal dysfunction have an increased risk of antimicrobial-induced nephrotoxicity whereby dosage adjustments and close monitoring are required to minimize further renal injury, particularly with aminoglycosides.[55] Less predictably, acute interstitial nephritis often complicates courses of antimicrobial therapy, but no known risk factors or preventive measures exist. Spurious rises in serum creatinine may result when certain cephalosporins interfere with the creatinine assay or trimethoprim blocks tubular secretion of creatinine. Lastly, significant potassium and salt loads may accompany the administration of certain antibiotics, particularly penicillins.

Analgesics and Agents Used by Anesthesiologists

Opioid analgesics remain the primary pain modality for the treatment of pain in patients with renal failure.[76] In Table 86.4 dosage recommendations are summarized for analgesics and agents used by anesthesiologists. Most analgesics are metabolized by the liver and thus require little dosage adjustment, but renal failure tends to increase the sensitivity to the pharmacologic effects of these drugs.[77] Special attention needs to be paid when prescribing meperidine or propoxyphene for patients with reduced renal function. Normeperidine, a meperidine metabolite excreted by the kidneys, has central nervous system excitatory properties that can lower the seizure threshold in patients with renal failure. Similarly, the propoxyphene metabolite has cardiovascular toxicity. Because of these serious adverse effects, both meperidine and propoxyphene should be avoided in patients with renal problems.[76] Acetaminophen should be considered initially for mild or moderate pain. If not effective, opioid analgesics or non-opioid analgesic (tramadol) should be considered. Use of NSAIDs should be avoided or limited in patients with chronic kidney disease. Cycloxygenase-2 inhibitors should be avoided in patients with ischemic heart disease because of its risk of cardiovascular complications.[78–80] Finally, many of the neuromuscular blocking agents are excreted by the kidney and thus may display prolonged action and depolarization in patients with impaired renal function as the effects of the antagonist dissipate.[26,81,82]

Antihypertensive and Cardiovascular Agents

In Table 86.5 dosage recommendations are summarized for antihypertensive and cardiovascular agents. The most common cause of death in the ESRD population is cardiovascular disease. A number of factors contribute to cardiovascular diseases in patients with renal failure. The risk of cardiovascular diseases increases with age, hypertension, hyperlipidemia, smoking, and anemia. Unfortunately, most of the cardiovascular interventional studies have been done in patients with normal renal function and patients with serum creatinine greater than 2 mg per dL have been excluded. It is still strongly recommended to treat these risk factors aggressively. Hypertension complicates the management of most patients with renal insufficiency and impacts adversely on renal disease progression and increases the risk of cardiovascular events.[83]

Patients with renal disease, in particular diabetic patients and patients with the metabolic syndrome, have high serum levels of triglycerides, low-density lipoproteins (LDL), and total cholesterol. All patients with renal insufficiency should have an annual lipid panel and should be managed according to the new ATP III guideline.[84,85]

Endocrine and Metabolic Agents

Dosage recommendations for endocrine and metabolic agents are provided in Tables 86.6, 86.7, and 86.8. Renal failure is associated with peripheral insulin resistance and decreased insulin metabolism by the kidney. In the presence of renal insufficiency, sulfonylureas that are excreted primarily by the kidney should be avoided, as prolonged hypoglycemia may result from the accumulation of such agents. Peritoneal dialysis allows for intraperitoneal insulin therapy, which has been shown to provide better overall control of plasma glucose when compared to standard subcutaneous injection therapy. Hyperlipidemia also complicates renal failure and adds to the increased risk of atherosclerotic complications in this population. Lipid-lowering agents such as bile acids can add to fluid overload and worsen acidosis in patients with renal failure, while other agents, such as lovastatin and clofibrate, have been associated with rhabdomyolysis.[86]

TABLE 86.4 **Analgesic Drug Dosing in Renal Failure**

Analgesics	Normal Dosage	% of Renal Excretion	Dosage Adjustment in Renal Failure			Comments	HD	CAPD	CVVH
			GFR >50	GFR 10 to 50	GFR <10				
Narcotics and Narcotic Antagonists									
Alfentanil	Anesthetic induction 8 to 40 μg/kg	Hepatic	100%	100%	100%	Titrate the dose regimen	N/A	N/A	N/A
Butorphanol	2 mg q3 to 4h	Hepatic	100%	75%	50%		No data	No data	N/A
Codeine	30 to 60 mg q4 to 6h	Hepatic	100%	75%	50%		No data	No data	Dose for GFR 10 to 50
Fentanyl	Anesthetic induction (individualized)	Hepatic	100%	75%	50%	CRRT-titrate	N/A	N/A	N/A
Meperidine	50 to 100 mg q3 to 4h	Hepatic	100%	75%	50%	Normeperidine, an active metabolite, accumulates in ESRD and may cause seizures. Protein binding is reduced in ESRD; 20% to 25% excreted unchanged in acidic urine.	Avoid	Avoid	Avoid
Methadone	2.5 to 5 mg q6 to 8h	Hepatic	100%	100%	50% to 75%		None	None	N/A
Morphine	20 to 25 mg q4h	Hepatic	100%	75%	50%	Increased sensitivity to drug effect in ESRD	None	No data	Dose for GFR 10 to 50

Naloxone	0.4 to 2 mg IV	Hepatic	100%	100%	100%		N/A	N/A	Dose for GFR 10 to 50
Pentazocine	50 mg q4h	Hepatic	100%	75%	75%		None	No data	Dose for GFR 10 to 50
Propoxyphene	65 mg po q6 to 8h	Hepatic	100%	100%	Avoid	Active metabolite norpropoxyphene accumulates in ESRD	Avoid	Avoid	N/A
Sufentanil	Anesthetic induction	Hepatic	100%	100%	100%	CRRT-titrate	N/A	N/A	N/A
Non-Narcotics									
Acetaminophen	650 mg q4h	Hepatic	q4h	q6h	q8h	Overdose may be nephrotoxic Drug is major metabolite of phenacetin	None	None	Dose for GFR 10 to 50
Acetylsalicylic acid	650 mg q4h	Hepatic (renal)	q4h	q4 to 6h	Avoid	Nephrotoxic in high doses. May decrease GFR when renal blood flow is prostaglandin dependent. May add to uremic GI and hematologic symptoms. Protein binding reduced in ESRD.	Dose after dialysis	None	Dose for GFR 10 to 50

GFR, glomerular filtration rate; HD, hemodialysis; CAPD, chronic peritoneal dialysis; CVVH, continuous venovenous hemofiltration; q, every; CRRT, continuous renal replacement therapies; ESRD, end-stage renal disease; IV, intravenous; po, by mouth; GI, gastrointestinal.

TABLE 86.5 **Antihypertensive and Cardiovascular Agent Dosing in Renal Failure**

Antihypertensive and Cardiovascular Agents	Normal Doses		% of Renal Excretion	Dosage Adjustment in Renal Failure			Comments	HD	CAPD	CVVH
	Starting Dose	Maximum Dose		GFR >50	GFR 10 to 50	GFR <10				
ACE Inhibitors							Hyperkalemia, acute renal failure, angioedema, rash, cough, anemia, and liver toxicity			
Benazepril	10 mg qd	80 mg qd	20%	100%	75%	25% to 50%		None	None	Dose for GFR 10 to 50
Captopril	6.25 to 25 mg po tid	100 mg tid	35%	100%	75%	50%	Rare proteinuria, nephrotic syndrome, dysgeusia, granulocytopenia. Increases serum digoxin levels.	25% to 30%	None	Dose for GFR 10 to 50
Enalapril	5 mg qd	20 mg bid	45%	100%	75%	50%	Enalaprilat, the active moiety formed in liver	20% to 25%	None	Dose for GFR 10 to 50
Fosinopril	10 mg po qd	40 mg bid	20%	100%	100%	75%	Fosinoprilat, the active moiety formed in liver. Drug less likely than other ACE inhibitors to accumulate in renal failure.	None	None	Dose for GFR 10 to 50
Lisinopril	2.5 mg qd	20 mg bid	80%	100%	50% to 75%	25% to 50%	Lysine analog of a pharmacologically active enalapril metabolite	20%	None	Dose for GFR 10 to 50

Pentopril		125 mg q24h	80% to 90%	100%	50% to 75%	50%		No data	No data	Dose for GFR 10 to 50
Perindopril		2 mg q24h	<10%	100%	75%	50%	Active metabolite is perindoprilat. The clearance of perindoprilat and its metabolites is almost exclusively renal. Approximately 60% of circulating perindopril is bound to plasma proteins, and only 10% to 20% of perindoprilat is bound.	25% to 50%	No data	Dose for GFR 10 to 50
Quinapril	10 mg qd	20 mg qd	30%	100%	75% to 100%	75%	Active metabolite is quinaprilat. 96% of quinaprilat is excreted renally.	25%	None	Dose for GFR 10 to 50
Ramipril	2.5 mg qd	10 bid	15%	100%	50% to 75%	25% to 50%	Active metabolite is ramiprilat. Data are for ramiprilat.	20%	None	Dose for GFR 10 to 50
Trandolapril	1 to 2 mg qd	4 mg qd	33%	100%	50% to 100%	50%		None	None	Dose for GFR 10 to 50
Angiotensin-II-Receptors Antagonists							Hyperkalemia, angioedema (less common than ACE inhibitors)			
Candesartan	16 mg qd	32 mg qd	33%	100%	100%	50%	Candesartan cilexetil is rapidly and completely bioactivated by ester hydrolysis during absorption from the GI tract to candesartan	None	None	None

(continued)

TABLE 86.5 **Antihypertensive and Cardiovascular Agent Dosing in Renal Failure *(continued)***

Antihypertensive and Cardiovascular Agents	Normal Doses		% of Renal Excretion	Dosage Adjustment in Renal Failure			Comments	HD	CAPD	CVVH
	Starting Dose	Maximum Dose		GFR >50	GFR 10 to 50	GFR <10				
Eprosartan	600 mg qd	400 to 800 mg qd	25%	100%	100%	100%	Eprosartan pharmacokinetics more variable in ESRD. Decreased protein binding in uremia.	None	None	None
Irbesartan	150 mg qd	300 mg qd	20%	100%	100%	100%		None	None	None
Losartan	50 mg qd	100 mg qd	13%	100%	100%	100%		No data	No data	Dose for GFR 10 to 50
Telmisartan	20 to 80 mg qd		<5%	100%	100%	100%		None	None	None
Valsartan	80 mg qd	160 mg bid	7%	100%	100%	100%		None	None	None
Beta Blockers							Decrease HDL, mask symptoms of hypoglycemia, bronchospasm, fatigue, insomnia, depression, and sexual dysfunction			
Acebutolol	400 mg q24h or bid	600 mg q24h or bid	55%	100%	50%	30% to 50%	Active metabolites with long half-life	None	None	Dose for GFR 10 to 50
Atenolol	25 mg qd	100 mg qd	90%	100%	75%	50%	Accumulates in ESRD	25 to 50 mg	None	Dose for GFR 10 to 50

Betaxolol	20 mg q24h	80% to 90%	100%	100%	50%	50%		None	Dose for GFR 10 to 50	Dose for GFR 10 to 50
Bopindolol	1 mg q24h	4 mg q24h	<10%	100%	100%	100%		None	None	Dose for GFR 10 to 50
Carteolol	0.5 mg q24h	10 mg q24h	<50%	100%	50%	25%		No data	None	Dose for GFR 10 to 50
Carvedilol	3.125 mg po tid	25 mg tid	2%	100%	100%	100%	Kinetics are dose dependent. Plasma concentrations of carvedilol have been reported to be increased in patients with renal impairment.	None	None	Dose for GFR 10 to 50
Celiprolol		200 mg q24h	10%	100%	100%	75%		No data	None	Dose for GFR 10 to 50
Dilevalol	200 mg bid	400 mg bid	<5%	100%	100%	100%		None	None	No data
Esmolol (IV only)	50 μg/kg/min	300 μg/kg/min	10%	100%	100%	100%	Active metabolite retained in renal failure	None	None	No data
Labetalol	50 mg po bid	400 mg bid	5%	100%	100%	100%	For IV use: 20 mg slow intravenous injection over a 2-minute period. Additional injections of 40 mg or 80 mg can be given at 10-minute intervals until a total of 300 mg or continuous infusion of 2 mg/minute.	None	None	Dose for GFR 10 to 50

(continued)

TABLE 86.5 **Antihypertensive and Cardiovascular Agent Dosing in Renal Failure *(continued)***

Antihypertensive and Cardiovascular Agents	Normal Doses		% of Renal Excretion	Dosage Adjustment in Renal Failure			Comments	HD	CAPD	CVVH
	Starting Dose	Maximum Dose		GFR >50	GFR 10 to 50	GFR <10				
Metoprolol		50 mg bid	100 mg bid	<5%	100%	100%		None	None	None
Nadolol	80 mg qd	160 mg bid	90%	100%	50%	25%	Start with prolonged interval and titrate	40 mg	None	Dose for GFR 10 to 50
Penbutolol	10 mg q24h	40 mg q24h	<10	100%	100%	100%		None	None	Dose for GFR 10 to 50
Pindolol	10 mg bid	40 mg bid	40%	100%	100%	100%		None	None	Dose for GFR 10 to 50
Propranolol	40 to 160 mg tid	320 mg/day	<5%	100%	100%	100%	Bioavailability may increase in ESRD. Metabolites may cause increased bilirubin by assay interference in ESRD. Hypoglycemia reported in ESRD.	None	None	Dose for GFR 10 to 50

Sotalol	80 bid	160 mg bid	70%	100%	50%	25% to 50%	Extreme caution should be exercised in the use of sotalol in patients with renal failure undergoing hemodialysis. To minimize the risk of induced arrhythmia, patients initiated or re-initiated on sotalol should be placed for a minimum of 3 days (on their maintenance dose) in a facility that can provide cardiac resuscitation and continuous electrocardiographic monitoring.	80 mg	None	Dose for GFR 10 to 50
Timolol	10 mg bid	20 mg bid	15%	100%	100%	100%		None	None	Dose for GFR 10 to 50
Calcium Channel Blockers							Dihydropyridine: headache, ankle edema, gingival hyperplasia and flushing Non-dihydropyridine: bradycardia, constipation, gingival hyperplasia, and AV block			
Amlodipine	2.5 po qd	10 mg qd	10%	100%	100%	100%	May increase digoxin and cyclosporine levels	None	None	Dose for GFR 10 to 50
Bepridil	No data	<1%	No data	No data	No data	Weak vasodilator and antihypertensive		None	No data	No data

(continued)

TABLE 86.5 **Antihypertensive and Cardiovascular Agent Dosing in Renal Failure *(continued)***

Antihypertensive and Cardiovascular Agents	Normal Doses		% of Renal Excretion	Dosage Adjustment in Renal Failure			Comments	HD	CAPD	CVVH
	Starting Dose	Maximum Dose		GFR >50	GFR 10 to 50	GFR <10				
Diltiazem	30 mg tid	90 mg tid	10%	100%	100%	100%	Acute renal dysfunction. May exacerbate hyperkalemia. May increase digoxin and cyclosporine levels.	None	None	Dose for GFR 10 to 50
Felodipine	5 mg po bid	20 mg qd	1%	100%	100%	100%	May increase digoxin levels	None	None	Dose for GFR 10 to 50
Isradipine	5 mg po bid	10 mg bid	<5%	100%	100%	100%	May increase digoxin levels	None	None	Dose for GFR 10 to 50
Nicardipine	20 mg po tid	30 mg po tid	<1%	100%	100%		Uremia inhibits hepatic metabolism. May increase digoxin levels.	None	None	None
Nifedipine XL	30 qd	90 mg bid	10%	100%	100%	100%	Avoid short-acting nifedipine formulation	None	None	None
Nimodipine	30 mg q8h	10%	100%	100%	100%		May lower blood pressure	None	None	Dose for GFR 10 to 50
Nisoldipine	20 mg qd	30 mg bid	10%	100%	100%	100%	May increase digoxin levels	None	None	Dose for GFR 10 to 50

Verapamil	40 mg tid	240 mg/day	10%	100%	100%	100%	Acute renal dysfunction. Active metabolites accumulate particularly with sustained-release forms.	None	None	Dose for GFR 10 to 50
Diuretics							Hypokalemia/hyperkalemia (potassium sparing agents), hyperuricemia, hyperglycemia, hypomagnesemia, increase serum cholesterol			
Acetazolamide	125 mg po tid	500 mg po tid	90%	100%	50%	Avoid	May potentiate acidosis. Ineffective as diuretic in ESRD. May cause neurologic side effects in dialysis patients.	No data	No data	Avoid
Amiloride	5 mg po qd	10 mg po qd	50%	100%	100%	Avoid	Hyperkalemia with GFR <30 mL/minute, especially in diabetics. Hyperchloremic metabolic acidosis.	N/A	N/A	N/A
Bumetanide	1 to 2 mg po qd	2 to 4 mg po qd	35%	100%	100%	100%	Ototoxicity increased in ESRD in combination with aminoglycosides. High doses effective in ESRD. Muscle pain, gynecomastia.	None	None	N/A
Chlorthalidone	25 mg q24h	50%	q24h	q24h	Avoid	Ineffective with low GFR	Not effective on GFR <30 mL/min	N/A	N/A	N/A
Ethacrynic acid	50 mg po qd	100 mg po bid	20%	100%	100%	100%	Ototoxicity increased in ESRD in combination with aminoglycosides	None	None	N/A

(continued)

TABLE 86.5 **Antihypertensive and Cardiovascular Agent Dosing in Renal Failure *(continued)***

Antihypertensive and Cardiovascular Agents	Normal Doses		% of Renal Excretion	Dosage Adjustment in Renal Failure			Comments	HD	CAPD	CVVH
	Starting Dose	Maximum Dose		GFR >50	GFR 10 to 50	GFR <10				
Furosemide	40 to 80 mg po qd	120 mg po tid	70%	100%	100%	100%	Ototoxicity increased in ESRD, especially in combination with aminoglycosides. High doses effective in ESRD.	None	None	N/A
Indapamide	2.5 mg q24h	<5%	100%	100%	Avoid	Ineffective in ESRD.		None	N/A	None
Metolazone	2.5 mg po qd	10 mg po bid	70%	100%	100%		High doses effective in ESRD. Gynecomastia, impotence.	None	None	None
Eplerenone	25 mg daily	200 mg daily	100%	100%	100%					
Spironolactone	100 mg po qd	300 mg po qd	25%	100%	100%	Avoid	Active metabolites with long half-life. Hyperkalemia common when GFR <30, especially in diabetics. Gynecomastia, hyperchloremic acidosis. Increases serum by immunoassay interference.	N/A	N/A	Avoid
Thiazides	25 mg bid	50 mg bid	>95%	100%	100%	Avoid	Usually ineffective with GFR <30 mL/min. Effective at low GFR in combination with loop diuretic. Hyperuricemia.			

Torsemide	5 mg po bid	20 mg qd	25%	100%	100%	100%	High doses effective in ESRD. Ototoxicity.	None	None	N/A
Triamterene	25 mg bid	50 mg bid	5% to 10%	q12h	q12h	Avoid	Hyperkalemia common when GFR <30, especially in diabetics. Active metabolite with long half-life in ESRD. Folic acid antagonist. Urolithiasis. Crystalluria in acid urine. May cause acute renal failure.	Avoid	Avoid	Avoid
Miscellaneous agents										
Amrinone	5 mg/kg/minute daily dose <10 mg/kg	10 mg/kg/minute daily dose <10 mg/kg	10% to 40%	100%	100%	100%	Thrombocytopenia. Nausea, vomiting in ESRD.	No data	No data	Dose for GFR 10 to 50
Clonidine	0.1 po bid/tid	1.2 mg/day	45%	100%	100%	100%	Sexual dysfunction, dizziness, postural hypotension	None	None	Dose for GFR 10 to 50

(continued)

TABLE 86.5 **Antihypertensive and Cardiovascular Agent Dosing in Renal Failure *(continued)***

Antihypertensive and Cardiovascular Agents	Normal Doses		% of Renal Excretion	Dosage Adjustment in Renal Failure			Comments	HD	CAPD	CVVH
	Starting Dose	Maximum Dose		GFR >50	GFR 10 to 50	GFR <10				
Digoxin	0.125 mg qod/qd	0.25 mg po qd	25%	100%	100%	100%	Decrease loading dose by 50% in ESRD. Radioimmunoassay may overestimate serum levels in uremia. Clearance decreased by amiodarone, spironolactone, quinidine, verapamil. Hypokalemia, hypomagnesemia enhance toxicity. Vd and total body clearance decreased in ESRD. Serum level 12 hours after dose is best guide in ESRD. Digoxin immune antibodies can treat severe toxicity in ESRD.	None	None	Dose for GFR 10 to 50
Hydralazine	10 mg po qid	100 mg po qid	25%	100%	100%	100%	Lupus-like reaction	None	None	Dose for GFR 10 to 50
Midodrine	No data	No data	75% to 80%	5 to 10 mg q8h	5 to 10 mg q8h	No data	Increased blood pressure	5 mg q8h	No data	Dose for GFR 10 to 50

Col 1	Col 2	Col 3	Col 4	Col 5	Col 6	Col 7	Col 8	Col 9	Col 10	Col 11
Minoxidil	2.5 mg po bid	10 mg po bid	20%	100%	100%	100%	Pericardial effusion, fluid retention, hypertrichosis, and tachycardia	None	None	Dose for GFR 10 to 50
Nitroprusside	1 μg/kg/min	10 μg/kg/min	<10%	100%	100%	100%	Cyanide toxicity	None	None	Dose for GFR 10 to 50
Amrinone	5 μg/kg/min	10 μg/kg/min	25%	100%	100%	100%	Thrombocytopenia. Nausea, vomiting in ESRD.	No data	No data	Dose for GFR 10 to 50
Dobutamine	2.5 μg/kg/min	15 μg/kg/min	10%	100%	100%	100%		No data	No data	Dose for GFR 10 to 50
Milrinone	0.375 μg/kg/min	0.75 μg/kg/min	100%	100%	100%			No data	No data	Dose for GFR 10 to 50

HD, hemodialysis; CAPD, chronic peritoneal dialysis; CVVH, continuous venovenous hemofiltration; GFR, glomerular filtration rate; ACE; angiotensin-converting enzyme; qd, every day; po, by mouth; tid, three times a day; bid, twice a day; GI, gastrointestinal; ESRD, end-stage renal disease; HDL, high-density lipoprotein; AV, atrioventricular; Vd, volume of distribution; qid, four times a day.

TABLE 86.6 Hypoglycemic Agents Dosing in Renal Failure

	Normal Doses			Dosage Adjustment in Renal Failure						
Hypoglycemic Agents	**Starting Dose**	**Maximum Dose**	**% of Renal Excretion**	**GFR >50**	**GFR 10 to 50**	**GFR <10**	**Comments**	**HD**	**CAPD**	**CVVH**
							Avoid all oral hypoglycemic agents on CRRT			
Acarbose	25 mg tid	100 mg tid	35%	100%	50%	Avoid	Abdominal pain, N/V, and flatulence.	No data	No data	Avoid
Acetohexamide	250 mg q24h	1,500 mg q24h	None	Avoid	Avoid	Avoid	Diuretic effect. May falsely elevate serum creatinine. Active metabolite has $t_{1/2}$ of 5 to 8 hours in healthy subjects and is eliminated by the kidney. Prolonged hypoglycemia in azotemic patients.	No data	None	Avoid
Chlorpropamide	100 mg q24h	500 mg q24h	47%	50%	Avoid	Avoid	Impairs water excretion. Prolonged hypoglycemia in azotemic patients.	No data	None	Avoid
Exenatide	5 μg q12h	10 μg q12h	No data	100%	Use with caution	Avoid				
Glibornuride	12.5 mg q24h	100 mg q14h	No data	No data	No data	No data		No data	No data	Avoid
Gliclazide	80 mg q24h	320 mg q24h	<20%	50% to 100%	Avoid	Avoid		No data	No data	Avoid
Glipizide	5 mg qd	20 mg bid	5%	100%	50%	50%		No data	No data	Avoid

Glyburide	2.5 mg qd	10 mg bid	50%	100%	50%	Avoid		None	None	Avoid
Liraglutide	0.6 mg qd	1.8 mg qd	6%	100%	100%	Avoid	No data on dialysis			
Metformin	500 mg bid	2,550 mg/ day (bid or tid)	95%	100%	Avoid	Avoid	Lactic acidosis	No data	No data	Avoid
Pioglitazone	15 mg qd	45 mg qd	3%	100%	100%	100%	Drug interactions	None	None	NA
Pramlintide	15 μg	60 μg qd	No data	100%	No data	No data				
Repaglinide	0.5 to 1 mg	4 mg tid								
Rosiglitazone	2 mg qd	8 mg qd	3%	100%	100%	100%	Increases LDL	None	None	NA
Sitagliptin	25 mg	100 mg	79%	100%	50%	25%				
Tolazamide	100 mg q24h	250 mg q24h	7%	100%	100%	100%	Diuretic effects	Avoid	Avoid	Avoid
Tolbutamide	1 g q24h	2 g q24h	None	100%	100%	100%	May impair water excretion	None	None	Avoid
Parenteral Agents							Dosage guided by blood glucose levels			
Insulin		Variable	None	100%	75%	50%	Renal metabolism of insulin decreases with azotemia	None	None	Dose for GFR 10 to 50
Lispro insulin		Variable	No data	100%	75%	50%	Avoid all oral hypogly-cemic agents on CRRT	None	None	None

GFR, glomerular filtration rate; HD, hemodialysis; CAPD, chronic peritoneal dialysis; CVVH, continuous venovenous hemofiltration; CRRT, continuous renal replacement therapy; tid, three times a day; N/V, nausea and vomiting; q, every; $t_{1/2}$, half-life; bid, twice a day; LDL, low-density lipoprotein.

TABLE 86.7 **Hyperlipidemic Agents Dosing in Renal Failure**

	Normal Doses			Dosage Adjustment in Renal Failure						
Hypoglycemic Agents	**Starting Dose**	**Maximum Dose**	**% of Renal Excretion**	**GFR >50**	**GFR 10 to 50**	**GFR <10**	**Comments**	**HD**	**CAPD**	**CVVH**
		400 mg SR q24h								
Atorvastatin	10 mg/day	80 mg/day	<2%	100%	100%	100%	Liver dysfunction, myalgia, and rhabdomyolysis with CsA/FK	No data	No data	No data
Bezafibrate		200 mg bid–qid	50%	50% to 100%	25% to 50%	Avoid	No data	No data	No data	
Cholestyramine	4 gm bid	24 gm/day	None	100%	100%	100%		No data	No data	No data
Clofibrate	500 mg bid	1,000 mg bid	40% to 70%	q6 to 12h	q12 to 18h	Avoid		No data	No data	No data
Colestipol	5 gm bid	30 gm/day	None	100%	100%	100%		No data	No data	No data
Fenofibrate	48 mg daily	145 mg daily	30%	100%	100%	50%				
Fluvastatin	20 mg daily	80 mg/day	<1%	100%	100%	100%		No data	No data	No data
Gemfibrozil	600 bid	600 bid	None	100%	100%	100%		No data	No data	No data
Lovastatin	5 mg daily	20 mg/day	None	100%	100%	100%		No data	No data	No data
Nicotinic acid	1 g tid	2 g tid	None	100%	50%	25%		No data	No data	No data
Pravastatin	10 to 40 mg daily	80 mg/day	<10%	100%	100%	100%		No data	No data	No data
Probucol		500 mg bid	<2%	100%	100%	100%		No data	No data	No data
Rosuvastatin	5 mg daily	20 mg daily	<5%	100%	100%	50%				
Simvastatin	5 to 20 mg daily	20 mg/day	13%	100%	100%	100%		No data	No data	No data

GFR, glomerular filtration rate; HD, hemodialysis; CAPD, chronic peritoneal dialysis; CVVH, continuous venovenous hemofiltration; SR, sustained release; bid, twice a day; qid, four times a day; tid, three times a day; q, every.

TABLE 86.8 Antithyroid Dosing in Renal Failure

Antithyroid Drugs	Normal Dosage	% of Renal Excretion	Dosage Adjustment in Renal Failure			HD	CAPD	CVVH
			GFR >50	GFR 10 to 50	GFR <10			
Methimazole	5 to 20 mg tid	7	100%	100%	100%	No data	No data	Dose for GFR 10 to 50
Propylthiouracil	100 mg tid	<10	100%	100%	100%	No data	No data	Dose for GFR 10 to 50

GFR, glomerular filtration rate; HD, hemodialysis; CAPD, chronic peritoneal dialysis; CVVH, continuous venovenous hemofiltration; tid, three times a day.

Gastrointestinal Drugs

Table 86.9 summarizes dosage recommendations for gastrointestinal drugs. Patients with renal insufficiency experience gastrointestinal disorders more often than the general population, particularly peptic ulcer disease. Prior to the development of H_2 blockers, antacid therapy with compounds containing aluminum, calcium, magnesium, or bicarbonate was the mainstay. Excessive intake of calcium carbonate can result in the milk–alkali syndrome, characterized by hypercalcemia, metabolic alkalosis, and renal failure. Aluminum toxicity has been well described with chronic ingestion of aluminum-containing antacids in the setting of renal failure.

Neurologic Agents

Table 86.10 includes the dosage recommendations for neurologic agents. Unfortunately, seizure disorders complicate renal insufficiency and ESRD. Phenytoin is commonly used as an anticonvulsant, but in patients with renal impairment, its Vd increases while its degree of protein binding decreases. As a result, a low total plasma phenytoin level may not reflect subtherapeutic drug levels, as the "free phenytoin" level may be adequate. Following free or unbound phenytoin levels is prudent in patients with markedly reduced renal function.

Rheumatologic Agents

Summarized dosage recommendations for rheumatologic agents are in Table 86.11. Although dosage reductions of nonsteroidal anti-inflammatory drugs (NSAIDs) are generally not required in renal failure, several precautions must be considered. When renal perfusion is reduced as in congestive heart failure or cirrhotic patients, vasodilatory prostaglandins may be key in maintaining renal blood flow. NSAIDs in such settings may cause reversible abrupt declines in renal function due to prostaglandin inhibition. Impaired potassium, sodium, and water excretion have also been attributed to NSAID use.

Patients with gout and renal insufficiency require reductions in allopurinol dosing because accumulation of its metabolite may underlie the complication of exfoliative dermatitis.[87] Similarly, renal failure increases the risk of myopathy and polyneuropathy associated with colchicine use. Use of intravenous (IV) colchicines should be avoided in all patients with renal impairment.[88]

Sedatives, Hypnotics, and Psychiatric Agents

Tables 86.12, 86.13, and 86.14 provide dosage recommendations for sedatives, hypnotics, and psychiatric agents. The majority of drugs in this category are lipid-soluble, highly protein bound, and excreted primarily by hepatic transformation to inactive metabolites, but increased sensitivity to the sedative side effects occurs in patients with renal impairment. Additionally, though dosage reduction generally is not required, increased sensitivity to the side effects of tricyclic antidepressants mandates a cautious approach in their use. Similarly, renal failure may exacerbate extrapyramidal side effects associated with phenothiazine therapy. In contrast, lithium is water-soluble and undergoes renal elimination. Renal syndromes induced by lithium therapy include nephrogenic diabetes insipidus as well as acute and chronic renal failure. Lithium toxicity can be minimized by avoidance of volume depletion and concurrent diuretic therapy. Regular monitoring ensures adequate serum levels and minimizes the risk of toxicity.[89,90]

Miscellaneous Agents

In Tables 86.15 and 86.16 are provided dosage recommendations for a wide variety of miscellaneous agents.

TABLE 86.9 **Gastrointestinal Agents Dosing in Renal Failure**

	Normal Doses			Dosage Adjustment in Renal Failure			
Gastrointestinal Agents	**Starting Dose**	**Maximum Dose**	**% of Renal Excretion**	**GFR >50**	**GFR 10 to 50**	**GFR <10**	**Comments**
Antiulcer agents							
Cimetidine	300 mg po tid	800 mg po bid	60%	100%	75%	25%	Multiple drug-drug interactions; beta blockers, sulfonylurea, theophylline, warfarin, etc.
Famotidine	20 mg po bid	40 mg po bid	70%	100%	75%	25%	Headache, fatigue, thrombocytopenia, alopecia
Lansoprazole	15 mg po qd	30 mg bid	None	100%	100%	100%	Headache, diarrhea
Nizatidine	150 mg po bid	300 mg po bid	20%	100%	75%	25%	Headache, fatigue, thrombocytopenia, alopecia
Omeprazole	20 mg po qd	40 mg po bid	None	100%	100%	100%	Headache, diarrhea
Rabeprazole	20 mg po qd	40 mg po bid	None	100%	100%	100%	Headache, diarrhea
Pantoprazole	40 mg po qd	80 mg po bid	None	100%	100%	100%	Headache, diarrhea
Ranitidine	150 mg po bid	300 mg po bid	80%	100%	75%	25%	Headache, fatigue, thrombocytopenia, alopecia
Metoclopramide	10 mg po tid	30 mg po qid	15%	100%	100%	50% to 75%	Increase cyclosporine/tacrolimus level; neurotoxic
Misoprostol	100 μg po bid	200 μg po qid		100%	100%	100%	Diarrhea, N/V, abortifacient agent
Sucralfate	1 gm po qid	1 gm po qid	None	100%	100%	100%	Constipation, decreases absorption of MMF

GFR, glomerular filtration rate; po, by mouth; tid, three times a day; bid, twice a day; qd, every day; N/V, nausea and vomiting; qid, four times a day; MMF, mycophenolate mofetil.

TABLE 86.10 **Neurologic/Anticonvulsant Dosing in Renal Failure**

	Normal Doses			Dosage Adjustment in Renal Failure						
Anticonvulsants[290]	**Starting Dose**	**Maximum Dose**	**% of Renal Excretion**	**GFR >50**	**GFR 10 to 50**	**GFR <10**	**Comments**	**HD**	**CAPD**	**CVVH**
Carbamazepine	2 to 8 mg/kg/day; adjust for side effect and TDM		2%	100%	100%	100%	Plasma concentration: 4 to 12, double vision, fluid retention, myelosuppression	None	None	None
Clonazepam	0.5 mg tid	2 mg tid	1%	100%	100%	100%	Although no dose reduction is recommended, the drug has not been studied in patients with renal impairment. Recommendations are based on known drug characteristics, not clinical trials data.	None	No data	N/A
Ethosuximide	5 mg/kg/day; adjust for side effect and TDM	20%	100%	100%	100%	Plasma concentration: 40 to 100, headache	None	No data	No data	
Felbamate	400 mg/tid	1,200 mg/tid	90%	100%	50%	25%	Anorexia, vomiting, insomnia, nausea	Dose after dialysis	Dose for GFR <10	Dose for GFR 10 to 50
Gabapentin	150 mg tid	900 mg tid	77%	100%	50%	25%	Fewer CNS side effects compared to other agents	300 mg load, then 200 to 300 after hemodialysis	300 mg qod	Dose for GFR 10 to 50
Lamotrigine	25 to 50 mg/day	150 mg/day	1%	100%	100%	100%	Autoinduction, major drug–drug interaction with valproate	No data	No data	Dose for GFR 10 to 50

(continued)

TABLE 86.10 **Neurologic/Anticonvulsant Dosing in Renal Failure *(continued)***

	Normal Doses			Dosage Adjustment in Renal Failure						
Anticonvulsants[290]	**Starting Dose**	**Maximum Dose**	**% of Renal Excretion**	**GFR >50**	**GFR 10 to 50**	**GFR <10**	**Comments**	**HD**	**CAPD**	**CVVH**
Levetiracetam	500 mg bid	1,500 mg bid	66%	100%	50%	50%		250 to 500 mg after dialysis	Dose for GFR <10	Dose for GFR 10 to 50
Oxcarbazepine	300 mg bid	600 mg bid	1%	100%	100%	100%	Less effect on P450 compared to carbamazepine	No data	No data	No data
Phenobarbital	20 mg/kg/day; adjust for side effect and TDM		1%	100%	100%	100%	Plasma concentration: 15 to 40, insomnia			
Phenytoin	20 mg/kg/day; adjust for side effect and TDM		1%	Adjust for renal failure and low albumin	Plasma concentration: 10 to 20, nystagmus, check free phenytoin level	None	None	None		
Primidone	50 mg	100 mg	1%	100%	100%	100%	Plasma concentration: 5 to 20	1/3 dose	No data	No data
Sodium valproate	7.5 to 15 mg/kg/day; adjust for side effect and TDM		1%	100%	100%	100%	Plasma concentration: 50 to 150, weight gain, hepatitis, check free valproate level	None	None	None

Tiagabine	4 mg qd, increase 4 mg/ day, titrate weekly		2%	100%	100%	100%	Total daily dose may be increased by 4 to 8 mg at weekly intervals until clinical response is achieved or up to 32 mg/day. The total daily dose should be given in divided doses two to four times daily.	None	None	Dose for GFR 10 to 50
Topiramate	50 mg/day	200 mg bid	70%	100%	50%	Avoid		No data	No data	Dose for GFR 10 to 50
Trimethadione	300 mg tid-qid	600 mg tid-qid	None	q8h	q8 to 12h	q12 to 24h	Active metabolites with long half-life in ESRD. Nephrotic syndrome.	No data	No data	Dose for GFR 10 to 50
Vigabatrin	1 g bid	2 g bid	70%	100%	50%	25%	Encephalopathy with drug accumulation	No data	No data	Dose for GFR 10 to 50
Zonisamide	100 mg qd	100 to 300 mg qd-bid	30%	100%	75%	50%	Manufacturer recommends that zonisamide should not be used in patients with renal failure (estimated GFR <50 mL/minute) as there has been insufficient experience concerning drug dosing and toxicity. Zonisamide doses of 100 to 600 mg/day are effective for normal renal function. Dose recommendations for renal impairment based on clearance ratios.	Dose for GFR <10	Dose for GFR <10	Dose for GFR <10 to 50

GFR, glomerular filtration rate; HD, hemodialysis; CAPD, chronic peritoneal dialysis; CVVH, continuous venovenous hemofiltration; TDM, therapeutic drug monitoring; tid, twice a day; CNS, central nervous system; qod, every other day; qd, every day; qid, four times a day; ESRD, end-stage renal disease.

TABLE 86.11 Rheumatologic Dosing in Renal Failure

Arthritis and Gout Agents	Normal Dosage	% of Renal Excretion	Dosage Adjustment in Renal Failure			Comments	HD	CAPD	CVVH
			GFR >50	GFR 10 to 50	GFR <10				
Allopurinol	300 mg q24h	30	75%	50%	25%	Interstitial nephritis. Rare xanthine stones.			
						Renal excretion of active metabolite with $t_{1/2}$ of 25 hours in normal renal function; $t_{1/2}$ one week in patients with ESRD. Exfoliative dermatitis.	½ dose	No data	Dose for GFR 10 to 50
Auranofin	6 mg q24h	50	50%	Avoid	Avoid	Proteinuria and nephritic syndrome	None	None	None
Colchicine	Acute: 2 mg then 0.5 mg q6h	5 to 17	100%	50% to 100%	25%	Avoid prolonged use if GFR <50 mL/minute	None	No data	Dose for GFR 10 to 50
	Chronic: 0.5 to 1.0 mg q24h								
Gold sodium	25 to 50 mg	60 to 90	50%	Avoid	Avoid	Thiomalate proteinuria; nephritic syndrome; membranous nephritis	None	None	Avoid
Penicillamine	250 to 1,000 mg q24h	40	100%	Avoid	Avoid	Nephrotic syndrome	⅓ dose	No data	Dose for GFR 10 to 50
Probenecid	500 mg bid	<2	100%	Avoid	Avoid	Ineffective at decreased GFR	Avoid	No data	Avoid
Pegloticase	8 mg IV q2 week	No data	100%	100%	100%				
Febuxostat	40–80 mg po daily	3%	100%	100%	50%		No data	No data	No data

Nonsteroidal anti-inflammatory drugs						May decrease renal function. Decrease platelet aggregation. Nephrotic syndrome. Interstitial nephritis. Hyperkalemia.			
						Sodium retention			
Diclofenac	25 to 75 mg bid	<1	50% to 100%	25% to 50%	25%		None	None	Dose for GFR 10 to 50
Diflunisal	250 to 500 mg bid	<3	100%	50%	50%		None	None	Dose for GFR 10 to 50
Etodolac	200 mg bid	Negligible	100%	100%	100%		None	None	Dose for GFR 10 to 50
Fenoprofen	300 to 600 mg qid	30	100%	100%	100%		None	None	Dose for GFR 10 to 50
Flurbiprofen	100 mg bid-tid	20	100%	100%	100%		None	None	Dose for GFR 10 to 50
Ibuprofen	800 mg tid	1	100%	100%	100%		None	None	Dose for GFR 10 to 50
Indomethacin	25 to 50 mg tid	30	100%	100%	100%		None	None	Dose for GFR 10 to 50
Ketoprofen	25 to 75 mg tid	<1	100%	100%	100%		None	None	Dose for GFR 10 to 50
Ketorolac	30 to 60 mg load then 15 to 30 mg q6h	30 to 60	100%	50%	25% to 50%	Acute hearing loss in ESRD	None	None	Dose for GFR 10 to 50
Meclofenamic acid	50 to 100 tid-qid	2 to 4	100%	100%	100%		None	None	Dose for GFR 10 to 50
Mefenamic acid	250 mg qid	<6	100%	100%	100%		None	None	Dose for GFR 10 to 50

(continued)

TABLE 86.11 **Rheumatologic Dosing in Renal Failure *(continued)***

Arthritis and Gout Agents	Normal Dosage	% of Renal Excretion	Dosage Adjustment in Renal Failure			Comments	HD	CAPD	CVVH
			GFR >50	GFR 10 to 50	GFR <10				
Nabumetone	1.0 to 2.0 g q24h	<1	100%	50% to 100%	50% to 100%		None	None	Dose for GFR 10 to 50
Naproxen	500 mg bid	<1	100%	100%	100%		None	None	Dose for GFR 10 to 50
Oxaprozin	1,200 mg q24h	<1	100%	100%	100%		None	None	Dose for GFR 10 to 50
Phenylbutazone	100 mg tid-qid	1	100%	100%	100%		None	None	Dose for GFR 10 to 50
Piroxicam	20 mg q24h	10	100%	100%	100%		None	None	Dose for GFR 10 to 50
Sulindac	200 mg bid	7	100%	100%	100%	Active sulfide metabolite in ESRD	None	None	Dose for GFR 10 to 50
Tolmetin	400 mg tid	15	100%	100%	100%		None	None	Dose for GFR 10 to 50

GFR, glomerular filtration rate; HD, hemodialysis; CAPD, chronic peritoneal dialysis; CVVH, continuous venovenous hemofiltration; q, every; $t_{1/2}$, half-life; ESRD, end-stage renal disease; bid, twice a day; IV, intravenous; po, by mouth; qid, four times a day; tid, three times a day.

TABLE 86.12 Sedative Dosing in Renal Failure

Sedatives	Normal Dosage	% of Renal Excretion	Dosage Adjustment in Renal Failure			Comments	HD	CAPD	CVVH
			GFR >50	GFR 10 to 50	GFR <10				
Barbiturates						May cause excessive sedation, increase osteomalacia in ESRD. Charcoal hemoperfusion and hemodialysis more effective than peritoneal dialysis for poisoning.			
Pentobarbital	30 mg q6 to 8h	Hepatic	100%	100%	100%		None	No data	Dose for GFR 10 to 50
Phenobarbital	50 to 100 mg q8 to 12h	Hepatic (renal)	q8 to 12h	q8 to 12h	q12 to 16h	Up to 50% unchanged drug excreted with urine with alkaline diuresis	Dose after dialysis	1/2 normal dose	Dose for GFR 10 to 50
Secobarbital	30 to 50 mg q6 to 8h	Hepatic	100%	100%	100%		None	None	N/A
Thiopental	Anesthesia induction (individualized)	Hepatic	100%	100%	100%		N/A	N/A	N/A
Benzodiazepines						May cause excessive sedation and encephalopathy in ESRD			
Alprazolam	0.25 to 5.0 mg q8h	Hepatic	100%	100%	100%		None	No data	N/A
Clorazepate	15 to 60 mg q24h	Hepatic (renal)	100%	100%	100%		No data	No data	N/A
Chlordiazepoxide	15 to 100 mg q24h	Hepatic	100%	100%	50%		None	No data	Dose for GFR 10 to 50

(continued)

TABLE 86.12 **Sedative Dosing in Renal Failure *(continued)***

Sedatives	Normal Dosage	% of Renal Excretion	Dosage Adjustment in Renal Failure			Comments	HD	CAPD	CVVH
			GFR >50	GFR 10 to 50	GFR <10				
Clonazepam	1.5 mg q24h	Hepatic	100%	100%	100%	Although no dose reduction is recommended, the drug has not been studied in patients with renal impairment. Recommendations are based on known drug characteristics not clinical trials data.	None	No data	N/A
Diazepam	5 to 40 mg q24h	Hepatic	100%	100%	100%	Active metabolites, desmethyldiazepam, and oxazepam may accumulate in renal failure. Dose should be reduced if given longer than a few days. Protein binding decreases in uremia.	None	No data	None
Estazolam	1 mg qhs	Hepatic	100%	100%	100%		No data	No data	N/A
Flurazepam	15 to 30 mg qhs	Hepatic	100%	100%	100%		None	No data	N/A
Lorazepam	1 to 2 mg q8 to 12h	Hepatic	100%	100%	100%		None	No data	Dose for GFR 10 to 50
Midazolam	Individualized	Hepatic	100%	100%	50%		N/A	N/A	N/A
Oxazepam	30 to 120 mg q24h	Hepatic	100%	100%	100%		None	No data	Dose for GFR 10 to 50
Quazepam	15 mg qhs	Hepatic	No data	No data	No data		Unknown	No data	N/A
Temazepam	30 mg qhs	Hepatic	100%	100%	100%		None	None	N/A
Triazolam	0.25 to 0.50 mg qhs	Hepatic	100%	100%	100%	Protein binding correlates with alpha-1 acid glycoprotein concentration	None	None	N/A

Antagonist						May cause excessive sedation and encephalopathy in ESRD			
Flumazenil	0.2 mg IV over 15 sec	Hepatic	100%	100%	100%		None	No data	N/A
Miscellaneous Sedative Agents									
Buspirone	5 mg q8h	Hepatic	100%	100%	100%		None	No data	N/A
Ethchlorvynol	500 mg qhs	Hepatic	100%	Avoid	Avoid	Removed by hemoperfusion. Excessive sedation.	Avoid	Avoid	N/A
Haloperidol	1 to 2 mg q8 to 12h	Hepatic	100%	100%	100%	Hypertension, excessive sedation	None	None	Dose for GFR 10 to 50
Lithium carbonate	0.9 to 1.2 g q24h	Renal	100%	50% to 75%	25% to 50%	Nephrotoxic. Nephrogenic diabetes insipidus. Nephrotic syndrome. Renal tubular acidosis. Interstitial fibrosis. Acute toxicity when serum levels >1.2 mEq/L. Serum levels should be measured periodically 12 hours after dose. $t_{1/2}$ does not reflect extensive tissue accumulation. Plasma levels rebound after dialysis. Toxicity enhanced by volume depletion, NSAIDs, and diuretics.	Dose after dialysis	None	Dose for GFR 10 to 50
Meprobamate	1.2 to 1.6 g q24h	Hepatic (renal)	q6h	q9 to 12h	q12 to 18h	Excessive sedation. Excretion enhanced by forced diuresis.	None	No data	N/A

GFR, glomerular filtration rate; HD, hemodialysis; CAPD, chronic peritoneal dialysis; CVVH, continuous venovenous hemofiltration; ESRD, end-stage renal disease; q, every; qhs, every bedtime; IV, intravenous; $t_{1/2}$, half-life; NSAIDs, nonsteroidal anti-inflammatory drugs.

TABLE 86.13 **Antiparkinson Dosing in Renal Failure**

Antiparkinson Agents	Normal Dosage	% of Renal Excretion	Dosage Adjustment in Renal Failure			Comments	HD	CAPD	CVVH
			GFR >50	GFR 10 to 50	GFR <10				
Carbidopa	1 tab tid to 6 tabs daily	30	100%	100%	100%	Requires careful titration of dose according to clinical response	No data	No data	No data
Levodopa	25 to 500 mg bid to 8 g q24h	None	100%	50% to 100%	50% to 100%	Active and inactive metabolites excreted in urine. Active metabolites with long $t_{1/2}$ in ESRD.	No data	No data	Dose for GFR 10 to 50

GFR, glomerular filtration rate; HD, hemodialysis; CAPD, chronic peritoneal dialysis; CVVH, continuous venovenous hemofiltration; tid, three times a day; bid, twice a day; $t_{1/2}$, half-life; ESRD, end-stage renal disease.

TABLE 86.14 **Antipsychotic Dosing in Renal Failure**

Antipsychotics[334,335]	Normal Dosage	% of Renal Excretion	Dosage Adjustment in Renal Failure			Comments	HD	CAPD	CVVH
			GFR >50	GFR 10 to 50	GFR <10				
Phenothiazines						Orthostatic hypotension, extrapyramidal symptoms, and confusion can occur			
Chlorpromazine	300 to 800 mg q24h	Hepatic	100%	100%	100%		None	None	Dose for GFR 10 to 50
Promethazine	20 to 100 mg q24h	Hepatic	100%	100%	100%	Excessive sedation may occur in ESRD	No data	No data	Dose for GFR 10 to 50
Thioridazine	50 to 100 mg po tid. Increase gradually. Maximum of 800 mg/day.	Hepatic	100%	100%	100%				
Trifluoperazine	1 to 2 mg bid. Increase to no more than 6 mg.	Hepatic	100%	100%	100%				
Perphenazine	8 to 16 mg po bid, tid, or qid. Increase to 64 mg daily	Hepatic	100%	100%	100%				
Thiothixene	2 mg po tid. Increase gradually to 15 mg daily	Hepatic	100%	100%	100%				

(continued)

TABLE 86.14 **Antipsychotic Dosing in Renal Failure *(continued)***

Antipsychotics[334,335]	Normal Dosage	% of Renal Excretion	Dosage Adjustment in Renal Failure			Comments	HD	CAPD	CVVH
			GFR >50	GFR 10 to 50	GFR <10				
Haloperidol	1 to 2 mg q8 to 12h	Hepatic	100%	100%	100%	Hypotension, excessive sedation	None	None	Dose for GFR 10 to 50
Loxapine	12.5 to 50 mg IM q4 to 6h	Hepatic	100%	100%	100%	Do not administer drug IV			
Clozapine	12.5 mg po. 25 to 50 daily to 300 to 450 by end of 2 weeks.	Hepatic	100%	100%	100%				
Maximum: 900 mg daily	Metabolism nearly complete	Hepatic	100%	100%	100%				
Risperidone	1 mg po bid. Increase to 3 mg bid.	Hepatic	100%	100%	100%				
Olanzapine	5 to 10 mg	Hepatic	100%	100%	100%	Potential hypotensive effects			
Quetiapine	25 mg po bid. Increase in increments of 25 to 50 bid or tid. 300 to 400 mg daily by day 4	Hepatic	100%	100%	100%				
Ziprasidone	20 to 100 mg q12h	Hepatic	100%	100%	100%				

GFR, glomerular filtration rate; HD, hemodialysis; CAPD, chronic peritoneal dialysis; CVVH, continuous venovenous hemofiltration; q, every; ESRD, end-stage renal disease; po, by mouth; tid, three times a day; bid, twice a day; qid, four times a day; IM, intramuscular; IV, intravenous.

TABLE 86.15 **Miscellaneous Dosing in Renal Failure**

			Dosage Adjustment in Renal Failure						
Corticosteroids[340]	**Normal Dosage**	**% of Renal Excretion**	**GFR >50**	**GFR 10 to 50**	**GFR <10**	**Comments**	**HD**	**CAPD**	**CVVH**
Betamethasone	0.5 to 9.0 mg q24h	5	100%	100%	100%	May aggravate azotemia, Na^+ retention, glucose intolerance, and hypertension	No data	No data	Dose for GFR 10 to 50
Budesonide	No data	None	100%	100%	100%	Same as above	No data	No data	Dose for GFR 10 to 50
Cortisone	25 to 500 mg q24h	None	100%	100%	100%	Same as above	None	No data	Dose for GFR 10 to 50
Dexamethasone	0.75 to 9.0 mg q24h	8	100%	100%	100%	Same as above	No data	No data	Dose for GFR 10 to 50
Hydrocortisone	20 to 500 mg q24h	None	100%	100%	100%	Same as above	No data	No data	Dose for GFR 10 to 50
Methylprednisolone	4 to 48 mg q24h	<10	100%	100%	100%	Same as above	Yes	No data	Dose for GFR 10 to 50
Prednisolone	5 to 60 mg q24h	34	100%	100%	100%	Same as above	Yes	No data	Dose for GFR 10 to 50
Prednisone	5 to 60 mg q24h	34	100%	100%	100%	Same as above	None	No data	Dose for GFR 10 to 50
Triamcinolone	4 to 48 mg q24h	No data	100%	100%	100%	Same as above	No data	No data	Dose for GFR 10 to 50

GFR, glomerular filtration rate; HD, hemodialysis; CAPD, chronic peritoneal dialysis; CVVH, continuous venovenous hemofiltration; q, every; Na^+, sodium.

TABLE 86.16 Anticoagulant Dosing in Renal Failure

	Normal Doses			Dosage Adjustment in Renal Failure						
Anticoagulants	Starting Dose	Maximum Dose	% of Renal Excretion	GFR >50	GFR 10 to 50	GFR <10	Comments	HD	CAPD	CVVH
Alteplase	60 mg over 1 h then 20 mg/h for 2 h	No data	100%	100%	100%	Tissue-type plasminogen activator [tPa]	No data	No data	Dose for GFR 10 to 50	
Anistreplase	30 U over 2 to 5 minutes	No data	100%	100%	100%		No data	No data	Dose for GFR 10 to 50	
Aspirin	81 mg/day	325 mg/day	10%	100%	100%	100%	GI irritation and bleeding tendency			
Clopidogrel	75 mg/day	75 mg/day	50%	100%	100%	100%				
Dabigatran	150 mg po bid	150 mg po bid	7%	100%	50%	No data				
Dalteparin	2,500 units SQ/ day	5,000 units SQ/ day	Unknown	100%	100%	100%				
Dipyridamole	50 mg tid		No data	100%	100%	100%		No data	No data	N/A
Enoxaparin	20 mg/day	30 mg bid	8%	100%	75% to 50%	50%	1 mg/kg q12h for treatment of DVT. Check anti-factor Xa activity 4 hours after seconnd dose in patients with renal dysfunction. Some evidence of drug accumulation in renal failure.			
Fondaparinux	2.5 mg to 10 mg daily	77%	100%	Avoid	Avoid			No data	No data	No data

Heparin	75 U/kg load then 15 U/ kg/hour	None	100%	100%	100%	Half-life increases with dose		None	None	Dose for GFR 10 to 50
Iloprost	0.5 to 2.0 ng/kg/ min for 5 to 12 h	No data	100%	100%	50%			No data	No data	Dose for GFR 10 to 50
Indobufen	100 mg bid	200 mg bid	<15%	100%	50%	25%		No data	No data	N/A
Streptokinase	25,0000 U load then 10,0000 U/ hour	None	100%	100%	100%			N/A	N/A	Dose for GFR 10 to 50
Sulfinpyrazone	200 mg bid	25% to 50%	100%	100%	Avoid	Acute renal failure. Uricosuric effect at low GFR.		None	None	Dose for GFR 10 to 50
Sulotroban	No data	52% to 62%	50%	30%	10%			No data	No data	No data
Ticlopidine	250 mg bid	250 mg bid	2%	100%	100%	100%	Decrease CsA level and may cause severe neutropenia and thrombocytopenia	No data	No data	Dose for GFR 10 to 50
Tranexamic acid	25 mg/kg tid-qid	90%	50%	25%	10%			No data	No data	No data
Urokinase	4,400 U/kg load then 4,400 U/ kg qh	No data	No data	No data	No data			No data	No data	Dose for GFR 10 to 50
Warfarin	5 mg/day	Adjust per INR	<1%	100%	100%	100%	Monitor INR very closely. Start at 5 mg/day. 1 mg vitamin K IV over 30 minutes or 2.5 to 5 mg po can be used to normal- ize INR.	None	None	None

GFR, glomerular filtration rate; HD, hemodialysis; CAPD, chronic peritoneal dialysis; CVVH, continuous venovenous hemofiltration; GI, gastrointestinal; po, by mouth; bid, twice a day; SQ, subcutaneously; tid, three times a day; q, every; DVT, deep vein thrombosis; CsA, cyclosporin A; INR, international normalized ratio; IV, intravenous.

REFERENCES

1. Manley HJ, Drayer DK, Muther RS. Medication-related problem type and appearance rate in ambulatory hemodialysis patients. *BMC Nephrol.* 2003;4:10.
2. Bedard M, Klein R, Papaioannou A, et al. Renal impairment and medication use among psychogeriatric inpatients. *Can J Clin Pharmacol.* 2003;10(2):78–82.
3. Breton G, Froissart M, Janus N et al. Inappropriate drug use and mortality in community-dwelling elderly with impaired kidney function—the Three-City population-based study. *Nephrol Dial Transplant.* 2011;26(9):2852–2859.
4. Chapin E, Zhan M, Hsu VD, Seliger SL, Walker LD, Fink JC. Adverse safety events in chronic kidney disease: the frequency of "multiple hits." *Clin J Am Soc Nephrol.* 2010;5(1):95–101.
5. Fink JC, Chertow GM. Medication errors in chronic kidney disease: one piece in the patient safety puzzle. *Kidney Int.* 2009;76(11):1123–1125.
6. Mueller BA, Pasko DA, Sowinski KM. Higher renal replacement therapy dose delivery influences on drug therapy. *Artif Organs.* 2003;27(9):808–814.
7. Nolin TD. Altered nonrenal drug clearance in ESRD. *Curr Opin Nephrol Hypertens.* 2008;17(6):555–559.
8. Olyaei AJ, Steffl JL. A quantitative approach to drug dosing in chronic kidney disease. *Blood Purif.* 2011;31(1–3):138–145.
9. Olyaei AJ, Bennett WM. The effect of renal failure on drug handling. In: Webb AJ, Shapiro MJ, Singer M, et al, eds. *Oxford Textbook of Critical Care.* New York: Oxford University Press; 1996.
10. Olyaei AJ, deMattos AM, Bennett WM. Prescribing drugs in renal failure. In: Brenner BM, ed. *Brenner and Rector's The Kidney*, 5th ed. Philadelphia: W.B. Saunders; 1999.
11. Olyaei AJ, deMattos AM, Bennett WM. Drug-drug interactions and most commonly used drugs in transplant recipients. In: Norman DJ, Turks LA, eds. *Primer on Transplantation.* Mt. Laurel, NJ: American Society of Transplantation; 2001.
12. Olyaei AJ, deMattos AM, Bennett WM. Principle of drug usage in dialysis patients. In: Nissenson AR, Fine RN, eds. *Dialysis Therapy*. Philadelphia: Hanley & Belfus Inc. Medical Publishers; 2001.
13. Olyaei AJ, deMattos AM, Bennett WM. Principles of drug dosing and prescribing in renal failure. In: Johnson RJ, Feehally J. *Comprehensive Clinical Nephrology*. St. Louis: Mosby; 2003:1189–1203.
14. Olyaei AJ, deMattos AM, Bennett WM. Drug dosage in renal failure. In: DeBroe ME, Porter GA, Bennett WM, et al, eds. *Clinical Nephrotoxins: Renal Injury from Drugs and Chemicals*, 2nd ed. Dordrecht, The Netherlands: Kluwer; 2003:667–679.
15. Olyaei AJ, deMattos AM, Bennett WM. Drug-drug interactions and most commonly used drugs in renal transplant recipients. In: Weir M. *Medical Management of Kidney Transplantation*. Philadelphia: Lippincott William & Wilkins; 2005:512–532.
16. Olyaei A, deMattos AM, Bennett WM. Drug usage in dialysis patients. In: Nissenson AR, Fine RN, eds. *Clinical Dialysis*. New York: McGraw-Hill; 2005:891–926.
17. Olyaei AJ, Bennett WM. Drug dosing in dialysis and renal failure. In: Feehally J, Johnson RJ, Floege J, eds. *Comprehensive Clinical Nephrology*. St. Louis: Mosby; 2006.
18. Olyaei AJ, Bennett WM. Drug induced renal disease. In: Glassock RJ, ed. *Current Therapy in Nephrology*. St. Louis: Mosby; 2006.
19. Olyaei AJ. Pharmacogenomics. In: Wyne AL, Woo TM, Olyaei AJ, eds. *Pharmacotherapeutics for Nurse Practitioner Prescriber*, 2nd ed. Philadelphia: F.A. Davis Company; 2007.
20. Olyaei AJ. Review of basic principles of pharmacology. In: Wyne AL, Woo TM, Olyaei AJ, eds. *Pharmacotherapeutics for Nurse Practitioner Prescriber*, 2nd ed. Philadelphia: F.A. Davis Company; 2007.
21. Subach RA, Marx MA. Drug dosing in acute renal failure: the role of renal replacement therapy in altering drug pharmacokinetics. *Adv Ren Replace Ther.* 1998;5(2):141–147.
22. Clark WR, Turk JE, Kraus MA, Gao D. Dose determinants in continuous renal replacement therapy. *Artif Organs.* 2003;27(9):815–820.
23. Clark WR, Ronco C. Renal replacement therapy in acute renal failure: solute removal mechanisms and dose quantification. *Kidney Int.* 1998;66:S133–S137.
24. Pea F, Viale P, Pavan F, Furlanut M. Pharmacokinetic considerations for antimicrobial therapy in patients receiving renal replacement therapy. *Clin Pharmacokinet.* 2007;46(12):997–1038.
25. Heintz BH, Matzke GR, Dager WE. Antimicrobial dosing concepts and recommendations for critically ill adult patients receiving continuous renal replacement therapy or intermittent hemodialysis. *Pharmacotherapy.* 2009;29(5):562–577.
26. Bugge JF. Influence of renal replacement therapy on pharmacokinetics in critically ill patients. *Best Pract Res Clin Anaesthesiol.* 2004;18(1):175–187.
27. Clark WR, Ronco C. Renal replacement therapy in acute renal failure: solute removal mechanisms and dose quantification. *Kidney Int.* Suppl 1998; 66:S133–S137.
28. Lam YW, Banerji S, Hatfield C, Talbert RL. Principles of drug administration in renal insufficiency. *Clin Pharmacokinet.* 1997;32(1):30–57.
29. Verbeeck RK, Musuamba FT. Pharmacokinetics and dosage adjustment in patients with renal dysfunction. *Eur J Clin Pharmacol.* 2009;65(8):757–773.
30. Talbert RL. Pharmacokinetics and pharmacodynamics of beta blockers in heart failure. *Heart Fail Rev.* 2004;9(2):131–137.
31. Matzke GR, Frye RF. Drug administration in patients with renal insufficiency. Minimising renal and extrarenal toxicity. *Drug Saf.* 1997;16(3):205–231.
32. Tett SE, Kirkpatrick CM, Gross AS, McLachlan AJ. Principles and clinical application of assessing alterations in renal elimination pathways. *Clin Pharmacokinet.* 2003;42(14):1193–1211.
33. Janku I. Physiological modelling of renal drug clearance. *Eur J Clin Pharmacol.* 1993;44(6):513–519.
34. Westphal JF, Brogard JM. Drug administration in chronic liver disease. *Drug Saf.* 1997;17(1):47–73.
35. Swan SK, Bennett WM. Drug dosing guidelines in patients with renal failure. *West J Med.* 1992;156(6):633–638.
36. Lamy PP. Comparative pharmacokinetic changes and drug therapy in an older population. *J Am Geriatr Soc.* 1982;30(11 Suppl):S11–S19.
37. Muhlberg W, Platt D. Age-dependent changes of the kidneys: pharmacological implications. *Gerontology.* 1999;45(5):243–253.
38. Barre J, Houin G, Brunner F, Bree F, Tillement JP. Disease-induced modifications of drug pharmacokinetics. *Int J Clin Pharmacol. Res.* 1983;3(4):215–226.
39. Nancarrow C, Mather LE. Pharmacokinetics in renal failure. *Anaesth Intensive Care.* 1983;11(4):350–360.
40. Dowling TC, Briglia AE, Fink JC et al. Characterization of hepatic cytochrome p4503A activity in patients with end-stage renal disease. *Clin Pharmacol Ther.* 2003;73(5):427–434.
41. Dreisbach AW, Lertora JJ. The effect of chronic renal failure on drug metabolism and transport. *Expert Opin Drug Metab Toxicol.* 2008;4(8):1065–1074.
42. Naud J, Michaud J, Boisvert C et al. Down-regulation of intestinal drug transporters in chronic renal failure in rats. *J Pharmacol Exp Ther.* 2007;320(3):978–985.
43. Dreisbach AW, Japa S, Gebrekal AB et al. Cytochrome P4502C9 activity in end-stage renal disease. *Clin Pharmacol Ther.* 2003;73(5):475–477.
44. Davies G, Kingswood C, Street M. Pharmacokinetics of opioids in renal dysfunction. *Clin Pharmacokinet.* 1996;31(6):410–422.
45. Yuan R, Venitz J. Effect of chronic renal failure on the disposition of highly hepatically metabolized drugs. *Int J Clin Pharmacol Ther.* 2000;38(5):245–253.
46. Regardh CG. Factors contributing to variability in drug pharmacokinetics. IV. Renal excretion. *J Clin Hosp Pharm.* 1985;10(4):337–349.
47. Falconnier AD, Haefeli WE, Schoenenberger RA, Surber C, Martin-Facklam M. Drug dosage in patients with renal failure optimized by immediate concurrent feedback. *J Gen Intern Med.* 2001;16(6):369–375.
48. Turnheim K. Pitfalls of pharmacokinetic dosage guidelines in renal insufficiency. *Eur J Clin Pharmacol.* 1991;40(1):87–93.
49. Turnheim K. Drug dosage in the elderly. Is it rational? *Drugs Aging.* 1998;13(5):357–379.
50. Levy G. Pharmacokinetics in renal disease. *Am J Med.* 1977;62(4):461–465.
51. van Ginneken CA, Russel FG. Saturable pharmacokinetics in the renal excretion of drugs. *Clin Pharmacokinet.* 1989;16(1):38–54.
52. Cockcroft DW, Gault MH. Prediction of creatinine clearance from serum creatinine. *Nephron.* 1976;16(1):31–41.
53. Coresh J, Stevens LA. Kidney function estimating equations: where do we stand. *Curr Opin Nephrol Hypertens.* 2006;15(3):276–284.
54. Stevens LA, Levey AS. Use of the MDRD study equation to estimate kidney function for drug dosing. *Clin Pharmacol Ther.* 2009;86(5):465–467.
55. Levey AS, Bosch JP, Lewis JB, et al. A more accurate method to estimate glomerular filtration rate from serum creatinine: a new prediction equation. Modification of Diet in Renal Disease Study Group. *Ann Intern Med.* 1999;130(6):461–470.
56. Guidance for Industry Pharmacokinetics in Pregnancy—Study Design, Data Analysis, and Impact on Dosing and Labeling. U.S. Department of Health and Human Services Food and Drug Administration Center for Drug Evaluation and Research (CDER) Clinical Pharmacology October 2010.
57. Michels WM, Grootendorst DC, Verduijn M, et al. Performance of the Cockcroft-Gault, MDRD, and new CKD-EPI formulas in relation to GFR, age, and body size. *Clin J Am Soc Nephrol.* 2010;5(6):1003–1009.

58. Gibson TP. Problems in designing hemodialysis drug studies. *Pharmacotherapy* 1985;5(1):23–29.

59. Nensel U, Rockel A, Hillenbrand T, et al. Dialyzer permeability for low-molecular-weight proteins. Comparison between polysulfone, polyamide and cuprammonium-rayon dialyzers. *Blood Purif.* 1994;12(2):128–134.

60. Touchette MA, Patel RV, Anandan JV, et al. Vancomycin removal by high-flux polysulfone hemodialysis membranes in critically ill patients with end-stage renal disease. *Am J Kidney Dis.* 1995;26(3):469–474.

61. Kerr PG, Lo A, Chin M, Atkins RC. Dialyzer performance in the clinic: comparison of six low-flux membranes. *Artif Organs.* 1999;23(9):817–821.

62. Maduell F, del Pozo C, Garcia H, et al. Change from conventional haemodiafiltration to on-line haemodiafiltration. *Nephrol Dial Transplant.* 1999;14(5): 1202–1207.

63. Agarwal R, Toto RD. Gentamicin clearance during hemodialysis: a comparison of high-efficiency cuprammonium rayon and conventional cellulose ester hemodialyzers. *Am J Kidney Dis.* 1993;22(2):296–299.

64. Teigen MM, Duffull S, Dang L, et al. Dosing of gentamicin in patients with end-stage renal disease receiving hemodialysis. *J Clin Pharmacol.* 2006;46(11):1259–1267.

65. Al-Homrany MA, Irshaid YM, El Sherif AK, et al. Pharmacokinetics of gentamicin in hemodialysis patients: a comparative study between diabetic and non-diabetic patients. *Int Urol Nephrol.* 2009;41(3):663–669.

66. Balant LP, Dayer P, Fabre J. Consequences of renal insufficiency on the hepatic clearance of some drugs. *Int J Clin Pharmacol. Res.* 1983;3(6):459–474.

67. Pea F, Viale P, Pavan F, et al. Pharmacokinetic considerations for antimicrobial therapy in patients receiving renal replacement therapy. *Clin Pharmacokinet.* 2007;46(12):997–1038.

68. Heintz BH, Matzke GR, Dager WE. Antimicrobial dosing concepts and recommendations for critically ill adult patients receiving continuous renal replacement therapy or intermittent hemodialysis. *Pharmacotherapy.* 2009;29(5): 562–577.

69. Choi G, Gomersall CD, Tian Q, et al. Principles of antibacterial dosing in continuous renal replacement therapy. *Crit Care Med.* 2009;37(7):2268–2282.

70. Kuang D, Verbine A, Ronco C. Pharmacokinetics and antimicrobial dosing adjustment in critically ill patients during continuous renal replacement therapy. *Clin Nephrol.* 2007;67(5):267–284.

71. Morabito S, Guzzo I, Solazzo A, et al. Continuous renal replacement therapies: anticoagulation in the critically ill at high risk of bleeding. *J Nephrol.* 2003;16(4):566–571.

72. Turnidge J. Pharmacokinetics and pharmacodynamics of fluoroquinolones. *Drugs.* 1999;58 Suppl 2:29–36.

73. Rodvold KA, Neuhauser M. Pharmacokinetics and pharmacodynamics of fluoroquinolones. *Pharmacotherapy.* 2001;21(10 Pt 2):233S–252S.

74. Roberts JA, Lipman J. Pharmacokinetic issues for antibiotics in the critically ill patient. *Crit Care Med.* 2009;37(3):840–851.

75. Choi G, Gomersall CD, Tian Q, et al. Principles of antibacterial dosing in continuous renal replacement therapy. *Crit Care Med.* 2009;37(7):2268–2282.

76. Kurella M, Bennett WM, Chertow GM. Analgesia in patients with ESRD: a review of available evidence. *Am J Kidney Dis.* 2003;42(2):217–228.

77. Bailie GR, Mason NA, Bragg-Gresham JL, et al. Analgesic prescription patterns among hemodialysis patients in the DOPPS: potential for underprescription. *Kidney Int.* 2004;65(6):2419–2425.

78. Davison SN. Chronic pain in end-stage renal disease. *Adv Chronic Kidney Dis.* 2005;12(3):326–334.

79. Florentinus SR, Heerdink ER, de Boer A, van Dijk L, Leufkens HG. The trade-off between cardiovascular and gastrointestinal effects of rofecoxib. *Pharmacoepidemiol Drug Saf.* 2005;14(7):437–441.

80. Motsko SP, Rascati KL, Busti AJ, et al. Temporal relationship between use of NSAIDs, including selective COX-2 inhibitors, and cardiovascular risk. *Drug Saf.* 2006;29(7):621–632.

81. Scheen AJ. [Withdrawal of rofecoxib (Vioxx): what about cardiovascular safety of COX-2 selective non-steroidal anti-inflammatory drugs?]. *Rev Med Liege.* 2004;59(10):565–569.

82. Pollard BJ. Neuromuscular blocking drugs and renal failure. *Br J Anaesth.* 1992;68(6):545–547.

83. Sica DA. Pharmacologic Issues in treating hypertension in CKD. *Adv Chronic Kidney Dis.* 2011;18(1):42–47.

84. Sica DA. Chlorthalidone - a renaissance in use? *Expert Opin Pharmacother.* 2009;10(13):2037–2039.

85. Sica DA. Fibrate therapy and renal function. *Curr Atheroscler Rep.* 2009; 11(5):338–342.

86. Garcia MJ, Reinoso RF, Sanchez NA, Prous JR. Clinical pharmacokinetics of statins. *Methods Find Exp Clin Pharmacol.* 2003;25(6):457–481.

87. Kobayashi M, Chisaki I, Narumi K, et al. Association between risk of myopathy and cholesterol-lowering effect: a comparison of all statins. *Life Sci.* 2008;82(17–18):969–975.

88. Terkeltaub RA. Colchicine update: 2008. *Semin Arthritis Rheum.* 2009;38(6): 411–419.

89. Costa MG, Chiarandini P, Della RG. Sedation in the critically ill patient. *Transplant Proc.* 2006;38(3):803–804.

90. Darrouj J, Karma L, Arora R. Cardiovascular manifestations of sedatives and analgesics in the critical care unit. *Am J Ther.* 2009;16(4):339–353.

INDEX

Page numbers followed by *f* and *t* indicate figures and tables, respectively.

D

F

G

J

K

L

M

N

O

P

Q

R

S

T